Surgery of Infants and Children

Scientific Principles and Practice

Surgery of Infants and Children

Scientific Principles and Practice

Edited by

Keith T. Oldham, MD
Professor and Chief
Division of Pediatric Surgery
Duke University Medical Center
Durham, North Carolina

Paul M. Colombani, MD
Robert Garrett Professor of Pediatric Surgery
Professor of Surgery, Pediatrics, and Oncology
Chief, Division of Pediatric Surgery
The Johns Hopkins University School of Medicine
Children's Surgeon-in-Charge
The Johns Hopkins Hospital
Baltimore, Maryland

Robert P. Foglia, MD
Associate Professor of Surgery and Pediatrics
Chief, Division of Pediatric Surgery
Washington University School of Medicine
Surgeon-in-Chief
St. Louis Children's Hospital
St. Louis, Missouri

149 Contributors

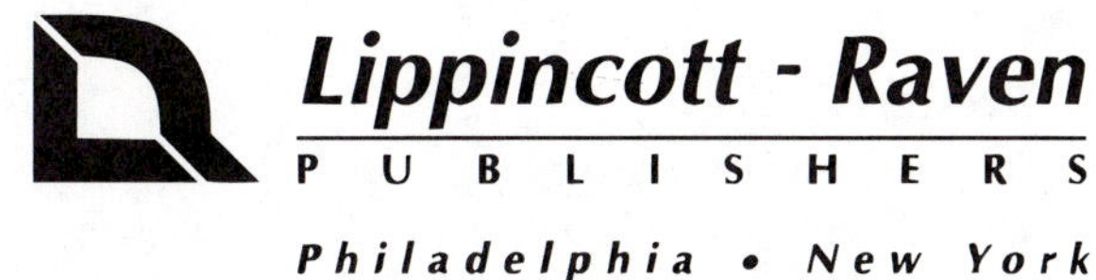

Lippincott - Raven
PUBLISHERS

Philadelphia • New York

Acquisitions Editor: Lisa McAllister
Developmental Editor: Paula Callaghan
Project Editor: Cynthia J. Wells
Production Manager: Caren P. Erlichman
Senior Production Coordinator: Kevin P. Johnson
Design Coordinator: Melissa G. Olson
Indexer: Pilar Wyman
Compositor: Maryland Composition
Printer: Quebecor/Kingsport

Library of Congress Cataloging-in-Publication Data

Surgery of infants and children : scientific principles and practice /
  edited by Keith T. Oldham, Paul M. Colombani, Robert P. Foglia; 149
  contributors.
        p.   cm.
    Includes bibliographical references and index.
    ISBN 0-397-51417-4 (hard cover : alk. paper)
    1. Infants—Surgery.   2. Children—Surgery.   I. Oldham, Keith T.
II. Colombani, Paul M.   III. Foglia, Robert P.
    [DNLM: 1. Surgery, Operative—in infancy & childhood.   WO 925
S9608 1996]
RD137.S83   1996
617.9′8—DC20
DNLM/DLC
For Library of Congress   96-43070
                                                         CIP

9 8 7 6 5 4 3 2 1

We dedicate this endeavor to our wives,
Karen, Nancy, and Linda,
and to our children,
Christian, Brian, Mathew, Stephen, Andrew, Michael, Rob, and Elizabeth.
Without their support neither this nor any professional success would be worthwhile,
and without their sacrifices, none would be possible.

Contributors

E. Stanton Adkins III, MD
Assistant Professor of Surgery and Pediatrics
Thomas Jefferson University School of Medicine
Philadelphia, Pennsylvania
Attending Surgeon
Alfred I. duPont Institute
Wilmington, Delaware

N. Scott Adzick, MD
C. Everett Koop Professor of Pediatric Surgery
University of Pennsylvania School of Medicine
Surgeon-in-Chief
The Children's Hospital of Philadelphia
Philadelphia, Pennsylvania

Walter S. Andrews, MD
Clinical Associate Professor of Surgery
Children's Medical Center
Dallas, Texas

Anna M. August, MD
Assistant Professor of Pediatrics
Washington University School of Medicine
St. Louis Children's Hospital
St. Louis, Missouri

Richard G. Azizkhan, MD
Professor of Surgery and Pediatrics
University of Buffalo
State University of New York
Surgeon-in-Chief
Children's Hospital of Buffalo
Buffalo, New York

Diane S. Bairas, PA-C
Physician Assistant
Department of Pediatric Surgery
Medical College of Georgia
Augusta, Georgia

Françoise Baylis, PhD
Assistant Professor of Philosophy
University of Tennessee
Knoxville, Tennessee

**Spencer W. Beasley, MB, ChB (OTAGO),
  MS (MELB), FRACS**
Senior Lecturer
Department of Paediatrics
University of Melbourne
Consultant Paediatric Surgeon and Head
Postgraduate Education
Royal Children's Hospital
Melbourne, Australia

Jacob Ben-Chaim, MD
Fellow in Pediatric Urology
James Buchanan Brady Urological Institute
Johns Hopkins University School of Medicine
The Johns Hopkins Hospital
Baltimore, Maryland

David A. Bloom, MD
Professor of Surgery
University of Michigan
Chief, Pediatric Urology
Mott Children's Hospital
Ann Arbor, Michigan

Mary L. Brandt, MD
Associate Professor of Surgery and Pediatrics
Department of Surgery
Section of Pediatric Surgery
Baylor College of Medicine
Houston, Texas

Christopher Kane Breuer, MD
Surgical Research Fellow
Harvard Medical School
Boston, Massachusetts

Rebecca H. Buckley, MD
J. Buren Sidbury Professor of Pediatrics
Professor of Immunology
Chief, Division of Allergy and Immunology
Department of Pediatrics
Duke University Medical Center
Durham, North Carolina

Marilyn W. Butler, MD
Associate Professor of Surgery and Pediatrics
Baylor College of Medicine
Houston, Texas

Donna A. Caniano, MD
Associate Professor of Surgery and Pediatrics
Ohio State University College of Medicine
Attending Surgeon
Children's Hospital
Columbus, Ohio

Michael G. Caty, MD
Assistant Professor of Surgery and Pediatrics
The University at Buffalo
State University of New York School of Medicine and Biomedical Sciences
Attending Surgeon
Children's Hospital of Buffalo
Buffalo, New York

Kenneth D. Chavin, MD, PhD
Chief Resident in Surgery
Medical University of South Carolina
Charleston, South Carolina

Walter J. Chwals, MD
Associate Professor of Surgery and Pediatrics
Bowman Gray School of Medicine
Wake Forest University
Winston-Salem, North Carolina

Francisco G. Cigarroa, MD
Assistant Professor in Surgery and Pediatrics
University of Texas Health Science Center
San Antonio, Texas

Robert E. Cilley, MD
Assistant Professor of Surgery and Pediatrics
The Pennsylvania State University College of Medicine
Division of Pediatric Surgery
The Milton S. Hershey Medical Center
Hershey, Pennsylvania

Curt I. Civin, MD
Professor of Oncology and Pediatrics
Johns Hopkins University School of Medicine
The Johns Hopkins Hospital
Baltimore, Maryland

Mark G. Clemens, PhD
Chairman, Biology Department
University of North Carolina at Charlotte
Charlotte, North Carolina

Bernard A. Cohen, MD
Associate Professor of Pediatrics and Dermatology
Johns Hopkins University School of Medicine
Director of Pediatric Dermatology
The Johns Hopkins Hospital Children's Center
Baltimore, Maryland

F. Sessions Cole, MD
Professor of Pediatrics, Cell Biology, and Physiology
Vice Chairman
Department of Pediatrics
Washington University School of Medicine
Director, Division of Newborn Medicine
Regional Medical Director
Pediatrics for the BJC Health System
St. Louis Children's Hospital
St. Louis, Missouri

Paul M. Colombani, MD
Robert Garrett Professor of Pediatric Surgery
Professor of Surgery, Pediatrics, and Oncology
Chief, Division of Pediatric Surgery
The Johns Hopkins University School of Medicine
Children's Surgeon-in-Charge
The Johns Hopkins Hospital
Baltimore, Maryland

Jeffrey G. Dawson, MD
Assistant Professor of Pediatrics
Washington University School of Medicine
St. Louis Children's Hospital
St. Louis, Missouri

Peter W. Dillon, MD
Associate Professor of Surgery and Pediatrics
The Pennsylvania State University College of Medicine
The Pennsylvania State University Children's Hospital
Milton S. Hershey Medical Center
Hershey, Pennsylvania

Steven G. Docimo, MD
Assistant Professor of Pediatric Urology
Johns Hopkins University School of Medicine
Johns Hopkins Bayview Medical Center
Baltimore, Maryland

Maryanne Dokler, MD
Clinical Assistant Professor of Surgery
University of Florida College of Medicine
Nemours Children's Clinic
Pediatric Surgeon
Wolfson Children's Hospital
Jacksonville, Florida

Daniel P. Doody, MD
Assistant Professor of Surgery
Harvard Medical School
Associate Visiting Surgeon
Massachusetts General Hospital
Boston, Massachusetts

David L. Dudgeon, MD
Professor of Surgery and Pediatrics
Case Western Reserve University School of Medicine
Division Chief
Department of Pediatric Surgery
Rainbow Babies and Children's Hospital
Cleveland, Ohio

Barbara A. Duffy, MD, MPH
Instructor
Department of Pediatrics and Oncology
Johns Hopkins Oncology Center
Baltimore, Maryland
Pediatric Consultant
Lutherville, Maryland

Craig DuFresne, MD
Assistant Professor of Plastic Surgery
The Johns Hopkins Hospital
Baltimore, Maryland

Martin R. Eichelberger, MD
Professor of Surgery and Pediatrics
George Washington University School of Medicine
Senior Attending Surgeon
Children's National Medical Center
Washington, DC

R. Alan B. Ezekowitz, MB, ChB, DPhil
Charles Wilder Professor of Pediatrics
Harvard Medical School
Chief of Pediatrics
Massachusetts General Hospital
Boston, Massachusetts

Mary E. Fallat, MD
Associate Professor of Surgery
University of Louisville
Attending Surgeon
Kosair Children's Hospital
Louisville, Kentucky

Robert M. Filler, MD, FRCSC
Professor of Surgery
University of Toronto
Medical Director, External Affairs
Hospital for Sick Children
Toronto, Ontario, Canada

Alan W. Flake, MD
Associate Professor of Surgery and Obstetrics
Wayne State University
Director of Fetal Surgery
Children's Hospital of Michigan
Detroit, Michigan

Robert P. Foglia, MD
Associate Professor of Surgery and Pediatrics
Chief, Division of Pediatric Surgery
Washington University School of Medicine
Surgeon-in-Chief
St. Louis Children's Hospital
St. Louis, Missouri

Judah Folkman, MD
Julia Dyckman Andrus Professor of Pediatric
  Surgery
Professor of Cell Biology
Harvard Medical School
Director, Surgical Research Laboratory
Senior Associate in Surgery
Children's Hospital
Boston, Massachusetts

John W. Foreman, MD
Professor of Pediatrics
Duke University
Chief, Division of Nephrology
Department of Pediatrics
Duke University Medical Center
Durham, North Carolina

Herbert Edgar Fuchs, MD, PhD
Assistant Professor of Neurosurgery
Head of Pediatric Neurosurgical Services
Duke University Medical Center
Durham, North Carolina

Barbara A. Gaines, MD
Resident in Surgery
Vanderbilt University
Nashville, Tennessee

J. William Gaynor, MD
Assistant Professor of Surgery
University of Pennsylvania
Assistant Surgeon
Pediatric Cardiothoracic Surgery
Children's Hospital of Philadelphia
Philadelphia, Pennsylvania

John P. Gearhart, MD
Associate Professor of Urology and Pediatrics
Johns Hopkins University School of Medicine
Director of Pediatric Urology
The Johns Hopkins Hospital and Children's Center
Baltimore, Maryland

David W. Gray, MD
Pediatric Orthopedics
Scottish Rite Children's Medical Center
Atlanta, Georgia

Karen S. Guice, MD
Professor of Surgery
Duke University Medical Center
Durham, North Carolina

Philip C. Guzzetta, Jr., MD
Professor and Chairman, Division of Pediatric
  Surgery
University of Texas Southwestern Medical Center
Chief, Clinical Department of Surgery
Children's Medical Center of Dallas
Dallas, Texas

J. Alex Haller Jr., MD
Professor of Pediatric Surgery, Pediatrics,
  and Emergency Medicine
Johns Hopkins University School of Medicine
Pediatric Surgeon
The Johns Hopkins Hospital
Baltimore, Maryland

Ada Hamosh, MD, MPH
Assistant Professor of Pediatrics
Center for Medical Genetics
Johns Hopkins University School of Medicine
The Johns Hopkins Hospital
Baltimore, Maryland

Michael R. Harrison, MD
Professor of Surgery and Pediatrics
Chief, Division of Pediatric Surgery
Director, Fetal Treatment Center
University of California, San Francisco
San Francisco, California

Robyn M. Hatley, MD
Associate Professor of Surgery and Pediatrics
Medical College of Georgia
Augusta, Georgia

Kurt F. Heiss, MD
Assistant Professor of Surgery
Emory University School of Medicine
Egleston Children's Hospital
Atlanta, Georgia

Ronald B. Hirschl, MD
Associate Professor of Surgery
Section of Pediatric Surgery
University of Michigan
Ann Arbor, Michigan

George W. Holcomb III, MD
Assistant Professor of Pediatric Surgery
Vanderbilt University School of Medicine
Nashville, Tennessee

Charles G. Howell, MD
Professor of Surgery and Pediatrics
Chief, Pediatric Surgery
Medical College of Georgia
Augusta, Georgia

Suzanne T. Ildstad, MD
Professor of Surgery
Department of Surgery
Director of the Institute of Cellular Therapeutics
Allegheny University of Health Sciences
Philadelphia, Pennsylvania

Robert D. Jeffs, MD
Professor
Johns Hopkins University School of Medicine
Director Emeritus, Division of Pediatric Urology
The Johns Hopkins Hospital
Consultant in Pediatric Urology,
Johns Hopkins Bayview Medical Center
Baltimore, Maryland

Kaj Johansen, MD, PhD
Professor of Surgery
University of Washington School of Medicine
Director of Surgical Education
Providence Medical Center
Seattle, Washington

Madelyn Kahana, MD
Associate Professor of Anesthesia and Critical
* Care Medicine*
University of Chicago
Director of Burn Critical Care
Chicago, Illinois

Jessica Kandel, MD
Assistant Professor of Surgery
Division of Pediatric Surgery
Columbia University
College of Physicians and Surgeons
Attending Surgeon
Babies and Children's Hospital
New York, New York

Frederick M. Karrer, MD
Associate Professor of Surgery
University of Colorado School of Medicine
Program Director of Children's Hospital
Denver, Colorado

Aviva L. Katz, MD
Assistant Professor of Surgery and Pediatrics
Jefferson Medical College
Pediatric Surgeon
Thomas Jefferson University Hospital
Philadelphia, Pennsylvania
A.I. duPont Institute
Wilmington, Delaware

Bruce A. Kaufman, MD
Assistant Professor of Neurological Surgery
Washington University School of Medicine
Attending Neurosurgeon
St. Louis Children's Hospital
St. Louis, Missouri

Michael A. Keating, MD
Associate Professor of Pediatric Urology
Indiana University School of Medicine
Attending Urologist
James Whitcomb Riley Hospital for Children
Indianapolis, Indiana

Ilan R. Kirsch, MD
Section Chief
Attending Physician
National Cancer Institute
Bethesda, Maryland

David N. Korones, MD
Assistant Professor of Pediatrics
University of Rochester School of Medicine
Strong Memorial Hospital
Rochester, New York

Ann M. Kosloske, MD, MPH
Professor of Surgery and Pediatrics
The Ohio State University College of Medicine
Attending Surgeon
The Children's Hospital
Columbus, Ohio

Rita A. Kostecke, MD
Resident in Surgery
Brown University
Providence, Rhode Island

Theodore C. Koutlas, MD
Assistant Professor of Surgery
Division of Cardiothoracic Surgery
East Carolina University School of Medicine
Cardiothoracic Surgery Staff
Pitt County Memorial Hospital
Greenville, North Carolina

Deborah W. Kreddich, MD
Associate Dean of Medical Education
Associate Clinical Professor of Pediatrics
Duke University Medical Center
Durham, North Carolina

Thomas M. Krummel, MD
John W. Oswald Professor of Surgery
Chairman, Department of Surgery
Director, Section of Surgical Sciences
Chief, Division of Pediatric Surgery
The Pennsylvania State University College of
* Medicine*
Surgeon-in-Chief
University Hospitals
The Milton S. Hershey Medical Center
Hershey, Pennsylvania

Jacob C. Langer, MD, FRCSC
Associate Professor of Surgery and Pediatrics
Washington University School of Medicine
Attending Pediatric Surgeon
St. Louis Children's Hospital
St. Louis, Missouri

Michael P. LaQuaglia, MD
Associate Professor of Surgery
Cornell University Medical School
Associate Attending Surgeon and Member
Chief, Pediatric Surgical Service
Memorial Sloan-Kettering Cancer Center
New York, New York

Robert W. Letton, MD
Senior Assistant Resident
Department of General Surgery
Bowman Gray School of Medicine
Wake Forest University
Winston-Salem, North Carolina

Terry R. Light, MD
Dr. William M. Scholl Professor and Chairman
Department of Orthopaedic Surgery
Loyola University Chicago
Stritch School of Medicine
Chairman, Orthopaedic Surgery
Foster McGraw Hospital
Maywood, Illinois

Craig W. Lillehei, MD
Assistant Professor of Surgery
Harvard Medical School
Associate in Surgery
The Children's Hospital
Boston, Massachusetts

John R. Lilly, MD†
Professor of Surgery and Pediatrics
The University of Colorado School of Medicine
Chairman of Pediatric Surgery
Children's Hospital
Denver, Colorado

Carson D. Liu, MD
Instructor
Department of Surgery
Division of General Surgery
University of California, Los Angeles, School of
* Medicine*
Los Angeles, California

Lori Luchtman-Jones, MD
Instructor
Department of Pediatrics
Divisions of Hematology/Oncology and Laboratory
* Medicine*
Attending Physician
Director, Hematology Laboratory
St. Louis Children's Hospital
St. Louis, Missouri

Dennis P. Lund, MD
Assistant Professor of Surgery
Harvard Medical School
Associate in Surgery
Children's Hospital
Boston, Massachusetts

† Deceased

David K. Magnuson, MD
Assistant Professor of Surgery and Pediatrics
George Washington University School of Medicine
Attending Surgeon
Children's National Medical Center
Washington, DC

Samuel M. Mahaffey, MD
Assistant Professor
Department of Surgery
Division of Pediatric Surgery
Duke University
Durham, North Carolina

Paul N. Manson, MD
Professor and Chairman of Plastic Surgery
Johns Hopkins Medical Institutions
Attending Surgeon
University of Maryland Shock Trauma Unit
Baltimore, Maryland

Jeffrey L. Marsh, MD
Professor of Plastic and Reconstructive Surgery
Associate Professor of Pediatrics in Surgery
Professor of Radiology in Research
Washington University School of Medicine
Director, Pediatric Plastic Surgery
Director, Craniofacial Deformities Institute
St. Louis Children's Hospital
St. Louis, Missouri

Eugene D. McGahren III, MD
Assistant Professor, Pediatric Surgery
University of Virginia Health Sciences Center
Charlottesville, Virginia

Charles P. McKay, MD
Pediatric Nephrologist
Alfred I. duPont Institute
Children's Hospital
Wilmington, Delaware

Kevin P. McLaughlin, MD
Assistant Professor of Urology
Loma Linda University School of Medicine
Loma Linda, California

Mark J. Mogul, MD
Assistant Professor of Pediatrics
Winship Cancer Center
Emory University School of Medicine
Atlanta, Georgia

Jean Pappas Molleston, MD
Assistant Professor of Pediatrics
Washington University School of Medicine
Division of Gastroenterology and Nutrition
St. Louis Children's Hospital
St. Louis, Missouri

Daniel L. Mollitt, MD
Professor of Surgery
University of Florida College of Medicine
Chief, Division of Pediatric Surgery
University of Florida Health Science Center
Jacksonville, Florida

John B. Mulliken, MD
Associate Professor of Surgery
Harvard Medical School
Senior Associate in Surgery
Children's Hospital
Boston, Massachusetts

Eisuke Nagabuchi, MD
Research Fellow, First Department of Surgery
Hokkaido University School of Medicine
Sapporo, Japan
Research Fellow, Division of Pediatric Surgery
University of Cincinnati College of Medicine
Children's Hospital Medical Center
Cincinnati, Ohio

Kurt D. Newman, MD
Associate Professor of Surgery and Pediatrics
George Washington University School of Medicine
Vice Chairman and Senior Attending Surgeon
Children's National Medical Center
Washington, DC

Keith T. Oldham, MD
Professor and Chief
Division of Pediatric Surgery
Duke University Medical Center
Durham, North Carolina

Charles N. Paidas, MD
Assistant Professor of Surgery, Pediatrics,
  Oncology, Anesthesia, and Critical Care
  Medicine
The Johns Hopkins University School of Medicine
Baltimore, Maryland

Maryland Pao, MD
Assistant Professor, Department of Psychiatry
George Washington University
Director, Pediatric Consultation Liaison
Emergency Psychiatric Services
Children's National Medical Center
Washington, DC
Assistant Professor
Division of Child and Adolescent Psychiatry
Department of Psychiatry
Johns Hopkins University School of Medicine
Baltimore, Maryland

Tae Sung Park, MD
Professor, Neurological Surgery and Pediatrics
Neurosurgeon-in-Chief
St. Louis Children's Hospital
St. Louis, Missouri

Walter Pegoli, Jr., MD
Assistant Professor of Surgery and Pediatrics
Johns Hopkins University School of Medicine
The Johns Hopkins Hospital
Baltimore, Maryland

Alberto Peña, MD
Professor of Surgery
Albert Einstein College of Medicine
Chief, Pediatric Surgery
Schneider Children's Hospital
Long Island Jewish Medical Center
New Hyde Park, New York

David H. Perlmutter, MD
Professor of Pediatrics, Cell Biology, and
  Physiology
Washington University School of Medicine
Director, Division of Gastroenterology and
  Nutrition
St. Louis Children's Hospital
St. Louis, Missouri

Mark D. Plunkett, MD
Visiting Assistant Professor of Surgery
University of California, Los Angeles, School of
  Medicine
Division of Cardiothoracic Surgery
University of California, Los Angeles, Center for
  Health Sciences
Los Angeles, California

Fran L. Porter, PhD
Assistant Professor of Pediatrics and Psychology
Washington University School of Medicine
St. Louis Children's Hospital
St. Louis, Missouri

Prem Puri, MB, MS
Director of Research
Children's Research Centre
Consultant Paediatric Surgeon
Our Lady's Hospital for Sick Children
National Children's Hospital
Crumlin, Dublin, Ireland

Sonja A. Rasmussen, MD
Fellow in Pediatrics
Division of Genetics
University of Florida College of Medicine
Gainesville, Florida

Michael X. Repka, MD
Associate Professor of Ophthalmology and
  Pediatrics
Johns Hopkins University School of Medicine
The Johns Hopkins Hospital
Baltimore, Maryland

Frederick J. Rescorla, MD
Associate Professor
Division of Pediatric Surgery
Indiana University School of Medicine
Attending Pediatric Surgeon
J.W. Riley Hospital for Children
Indianapolis, Indiana

Bradley M. Rodgers, MD
Professor of Surgery and Pediatrics
University of Virginia Health Sciences Center
Chief, Children's Surgery
Children's Medical Center
Charlottesville, Virginia

Joan L. Rosenbaum, MD
Assistant Professor in Pediatrics
Washington University School of Medicine
St. Louis Children's Hospital
St. Louis, Missouri

Thomas A. Rozanski, MD
Chief of Urology
Brooke Army Medical Center
San Antonio, Texas

Frederick C. Ryckman, MD
Associate Professor of Surgery
Division of Pediatric Surgery
University of Cincinnati
Children's Hospital Medical Center
Cincinnati, Ohio

Robert S. Sawin, MD
Associate Professor of Surgery
University of Washington School of Medicine
Chief, General and Thoracic Surgery
Children's Hospital and Medical Center
Seattle, Washington

L.R. Scherer III, MD
Clinical Associate Professor of Pediatric Surgery
Indiana University School of Medicine
Director of Kiwanis-Riley Trauma Life Center
J. W. Riley Hospital for Children
Indianapolis, Indiana

Alan L. Schwartz, MD, PhD
Alumni-Endowed Professor
Chairman, Department of Pediatrics
Professor of Molecular Biology and Pharmacology
Washington University School of Medicine
Pediatrician-in-Chief
St. Louis Children's Hospital
St. Louis, Missouri

Cindy L. Schwartz, MD
Associate Professor of Oncology and Pediatrics
Johns Hopkins University School of Medicine
Associate Director of Clinical Programs in
* Pediatric Oncology*
Johns Hopkins Oncology Center
Baltimore, Maryland

Marshall Z. Schwartz, MD
Professor of Surgery and Pediatrics
George Washington University School of Medicine
Chief of Surgery
Chairman, Department of Pediatric Surgery
Children's National Medical Center
Washington, DC

Curtis A. Sheldon, MD
Associate Professor of Clinical Surgery
Director, Division of Pediatric Urology
University of Cincinnati
Director, Division of Pediatric Urology
Children's Hospital
Cincinnati, Ohio

Robert L. Sheridan, MD
Assistant Professor of Surgery
Harvard Medical School
Assistant Chief of Staff
Shriners Burns Institute
Boston, Massachusetts

Stephen J. Shochat, MD
Professor of Surgery and Pediatrics
University of Tennessee College of Medicine
Chairman and Surgeon-in-Chief
Department of Surgery
St. Jude Children's Research Hospital
Memphis, Tennessee

Nicholas A. Shorter, MD
Associate Professor of Surgery and Pediatrics
Dartmouth Medical School
Director of Pediatric Surgical Services
Children's Hospital at Dartmouth
Lebanon, New Hampshire

Michael A. Skinner, MD
Assistant Professor of Surgery
Division of Pediatric Surgery
Washington University School of Medicine
Attending Pediatric Surgeon
St. Louis Children's Hospital
St. Louis, Missouri

Paul D. Sponseller, MD
Associate Professor and Head of Pediatric
* Orthopaedics*
Johns Hopkins University School of Medicine
The Johns Hopkins Hospital
Baltimore, Maryland

Thomas L. Spray, MD
Professor of Surgery
University of Pennsylvania School of Medicine
Chief, Division of Pediatric Cardiothoracic Surgery
Children's Hospital of Philadelphia
Philadelphia, Pennsylvania

Charles J.H. Stolar, MD
Professor of Surgery and Pediatrics
Columbia University College of Physicians and
* Surgeons*
Attending Surgeon
Babies and Children's Hospital of New York
Columbia-Presbyterian Medical Center
New York, New York

Derya U. Tagge, MD
Assistant Professor of Surgery
Medical University of South Carolina
Assistant Chief of Surgery
Ralph H. Johnson Veterans Affairs Medical Center
Charleston, South Carolina

Edward P. Tagge, MD
Associate Professor of Surgery and Pediatrics
Medical University of South Carolina
Charleston, South Carolina

Ronald G. Tompkins, MD, ScD
Associate Professor of Surgery
Harvard Medical School
Visiting Surgeon
Massachusetts General Hospital
Boston, Massachusetts

Thomas F. Tracy Jr., MS, MD
Professor of Surgery
St. Louis University School of Medicine
Associate Professor of Pediatrics
Cardinal Glennon Children's Hospital and the
* Pediatric Research Institute*
St. Louis University Health Sciences Center
St. Louis, Missouri

William R. Treem, MD
Professor of Pediatrics
Chief, Division of Pediatric Gastroenterology
Duke University Medical Center
Durham, North Carolina

David E. Tunkel, MD
Assistant Professor of Otolaryngology and
* Pediatrics*
Johns Hopkins University School of Medicine
Director of Pediatric Otolaryngology
The Johns Hopkins Hospital
Baltimore, Maryland

Curtis W. Turner, MD
Assistant Professor of Pediatrics
Emory University School of Medicine
Staff Physician
Egleston Children's Hospital
Atlanta, Georgia

Ross M. Ungerleider, MD
Professor of General and Thoracic Surgery
Chief, Pediatric Cardiac Surgery
Duke University Medical School
Durham, North Carolina

Joseph P. Vacanti, MD
Associate Professor of Surgery
Harvard Medical School
Senior Associate in Surgery
Director of Organ Transplantation
Children's Hospital
Boston, Massachusetts

Craig A. Vander Kolk, MD
Associate Professor of Surgery
Johns Hopkins University School of Medicine
Director of Pediatric Plastic Surgery
The Johns Hopkins Hospital
Baltimore, Maryland

Brad W. Warner, MD
Assistant Professor of Pediatric Surgery
University of Cincinnati College of Medicine
Attending Surgeon
Children's Hospital Medical Center
Cincinnati, Ohio

John R. Wesley, MD
Clinical Professor of Surgery
University of California, Davis, Medical School
Section Head, Pediatric Surgery
University of California, Davis, Medical Center
Sacramento, California

Randall C. Wetzel, MB,BS, FCCM
Associate Professor, Departments of
* Anesthesiology, Critical Care Medicine, and*
* Pediatrics*
Johns Hopkins University School of Medicine
Chief, Division of Pediatric Anesthesia
The Johns Hopkins Hospital
Baltimore, Maryland

Karen M. Wickline, MD
Assistant Professor of Pediatrics
Washington University School of Medicine
St. Louis Children's Hospital
St. Louis, Missouri

Delbert R. Wigfall, MD
Assistant Professor of Pediatrics
Director of Pediatric Dialysis
Division of Pediatric Nephrology
Duke University Medical Center
Durham, North Carolina

Andrea L. Winthrop, MD, FRCSC
Assistant Professor of Surgery
Washington University School of Medicine
Medical Director, Pediatric Trauma Service
St. Louis Children's Hospital
St. Louis, Missouri

Peter D. Witt, MD
Assistant Professor of Surgery
Washington University School of Medicine
Plastic and Reconstructive Surgery
St. Louis Children's Hospital
St. Louis, Missouri

Gordon Worley, MD
Associate Clinical Professor of Pediatrics
Duke University Medical Center
Durham, North Carolina

Myron Yaster, MD
Associate Professor, Departments of
* Anesthesiology, Critical Care Medicine, and*
* Pediatrics*
Johns Hopkins University School of Medicine
Director, Pediatric Pain Service
The Johns Hopkins Hospital Children's Center
Baltimore, Maryland

Andrew M. Yeager, MD
Professor of Pediatrics, Anatomy, Cell Biology, and
* Medicine*
Professor, Winship Cancer Center
Director, Division of Pediatric Hematology/
* Oncology and Bone Marrow Transplantation*
Emory University School of Medicine
Chief, Section of Hematology/Oncology and Bone
* Marrow Transplantation*
Egleston Children's Hospital
Atlanta, Georgia

Bevan Yueh, MD
Robert Wood Johnson Clinical Scholar
Instructor
Department of Otolaryngology
Yale School of Medicine
Attending Otolaryngologist
Yale-New Haven Hospital
New Haven, Connecticut

Theodoros Ziambaras, MD
Fellow
Department of Pediatrics
Washington University School of Medicine
St. Louis, Missouri

Moritz M. Ziegler, MD
Professor of Surgery and Pediatrics
The University of Cincinnati College of Medicine
Director, Division of Pediatric Surgery
Surgeon-in-Chief
The Children's Hospital Medical Center
Cincinnati, Ohio

Preface

Modern pediatric surgery evolved over the past several decades in response to the need to treat the unique anatomic anomalies of infants and children. In the course of this evolution, it became clear that the pathologic processes and the physiologic needs of sick children are diverse, complex, and fundamentally different from those of adults. Technologic progress and the consolidation of care in dedicated institutions by fully committed practitioners led to truly remarkable medical and surgical successes. Many such successes occurred after the Second World War, when practitioners began to routinely correct anomalies that had until that time resulted in mortality. Esophageal atresia with tracheoesophageal fistula, Hirschsprung disease, and giant abdominal wall defects are but a few such lesions.

More recently, pediatric surgery, like other surgical disciplines, shifted its focus to areas of residual morbidity and mortality. The critical care of infants and children with respiratory failure, multiorgan dysfunction, trauma, transplanted organs, and other problems became areas of interest and expertise. In the 1980s and '90s, the scope of children's surgery expanded far beyond the traditional realms of anatomy and physiology into areas of molecular and cellular pathophysiology. Current clinical practice and the related scientific investigations would have been inconceivable to our mentors. Fetal diagnosis and intervention are now realities. Contemporary pediatric oncology involves regionalized multidisciplinary care using sophisticated molecular techniques for both diagnosis and therapy. Modern anesthesia and critical care management depend on technologies that did not exist a decade ago. Specific diseases, such as cystic fibrosis, are defined at the genomic and molecular levels, thereby altering medical and surgical therapy forever. Transplantation, immunology, wound healing, nutrition, and many other disciplines have been similarly and rapidly transformed by a torrent of information detailing basic cellular responses. It is apparent that the uniqueness of childhood disease extends to these new frontiers. State-of-the-art clinical practice and future progress require that those who care for children with surgical problems be cognizant of their surgical heritage as well as contemporary scientific progress.

Surgery of Infants and Children: Scientific Principles and Practice is designed to combine a rigorous examination of scientific principles relevant to infants and children with the practice of clinical pediatric surgery. Our intent has been to create a text written by investigators and active, innovative children's surgeons. The result has been a group of contributing authors substantially younger than tradition would suggest for a text of this sort. We believe this has produced a reference work with a unique and contemporary view of pediatric surgery. The first section of the text establishes the scientific foundations for the discussions of clinical problems that follow. Included are chapters that deal with cell structure and function, genetics, the fetus, critical care, respiratory physiology, wound healing, immunology, and other basic disciplines. The remainder of the text is arranged according to organ system, and is designed to provide a succinct yet comprehensive review of clinical problems, emphasizing an analytic rather than empiric approach. Although the line drawings have been rendered with care, we have sought to emphasize surgical principles rather than specific operative techniques.

It is our intent that the text be of value to all students of children's surgery, regardless of scientific background or years in practice. It is our expectation that much of this information will soon be obsolete, as the pace of scientific progress is ever more rapid. Successive generations of surgeons will, no doubt, look back on this as a tentative step in the effort to reconcile these clinical and scientific domains. This view will indicate that pediatric surgeons have continued to contribute to the process of scientific inquiry. It cannot be otherwise. We hope that this effort serves current and future children's surgeons well as they negotiate this course.

Keith T. Oldham, MD
Paul M. Colombani, MD
Robert P. Foglia, MD

Acknowledgments

The production of a textbook of this type involves the considerable time and efforts of many people if it is to be successful. First and foremost, we are indebted to our contributing authors, all of whom devoted many personal hours in the effort to develop succinct and lucid discussions in their areas of expertise.

We have been fortunate to have had the unqualified support of Lippincott-Raven Publishers. In particular, we owe our thanks to Lisa McAllister, Senior Editor for Medical Books, for the impetus to undertake the project. Her colleague, Paula Callaghan, Associate Editor for Medical Books, has sustained us with her good humor and tenacity. Grace Caputo, Associate Managing Editor, has been both tolerant and expert once again.

The unique artistic talents and equanimity of Valorie Loomis, the artist responsible for the line drawings throughout the text, have been essential to the success of the project.

We would be remiss not to acknowledge Lazar J. Greenfield, MD, a friend and mentor whose 1992 textbook of general surgery served as an example of excellence in our pursuit of similar objectives.

Finally, the text would not have come to fruition without the able and tireless skills of Mary Artley, Kim Merritt, and Laura Cornelius, and similar secretarial support from Pat Tighe and Joan Green.

Contents

Section B: Trauma

Section C: Oncology

Section D: Transplantation

Part II: Surgical Practice

Section A: Head and Neck

Section D: Intestine

Section E: Colon

Section F: Liver, Biliary Tract, and Pancreas

Section L: Musculoskeletal System

Section M: Vascular System

Section N: Conjoined Twins

Color Figures appear after Part 1 opening page

Surgery of Infants and Children

Scientific Principles and Practice

Basic Considerations

Color Figures

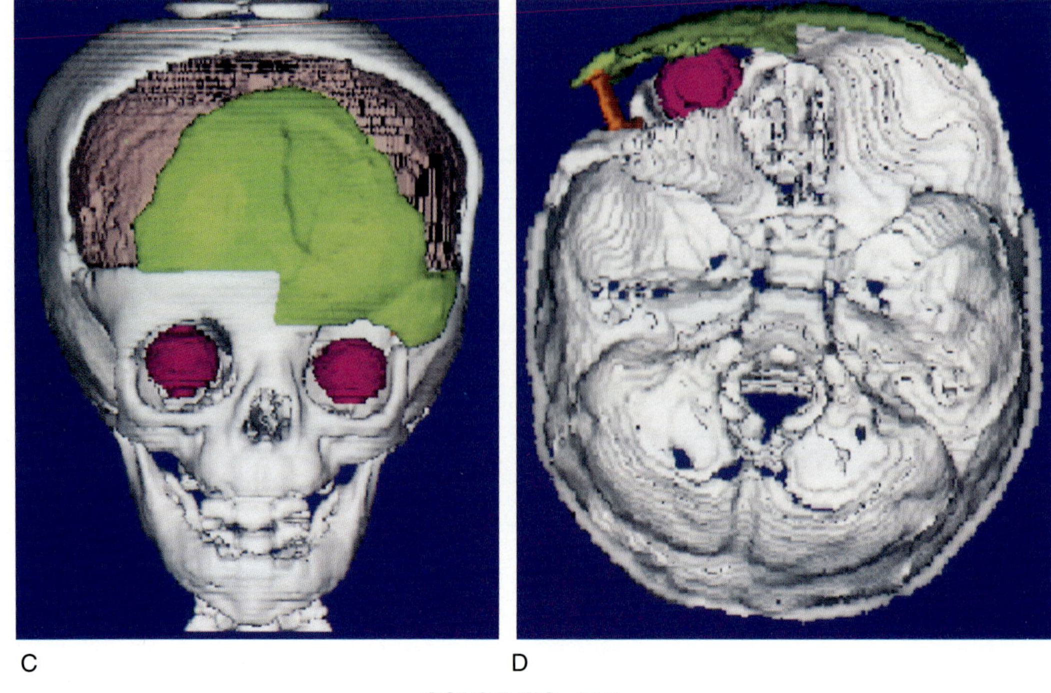

C   D

COLOR FIG. 48-2.

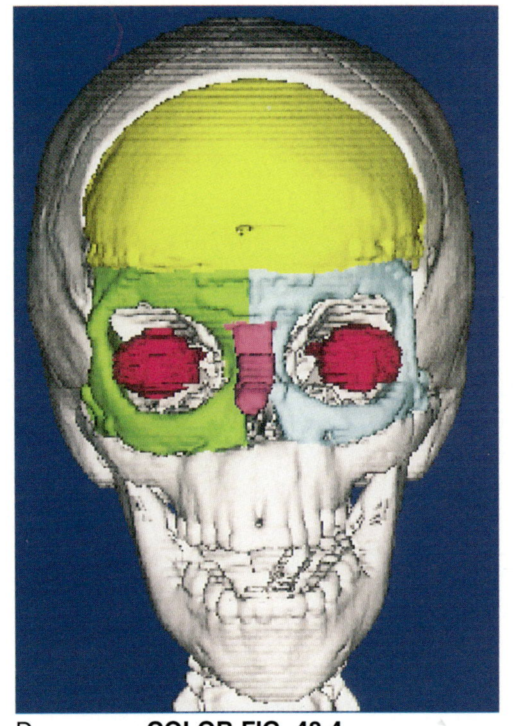

D   **COLOR FIG. 48-4.**

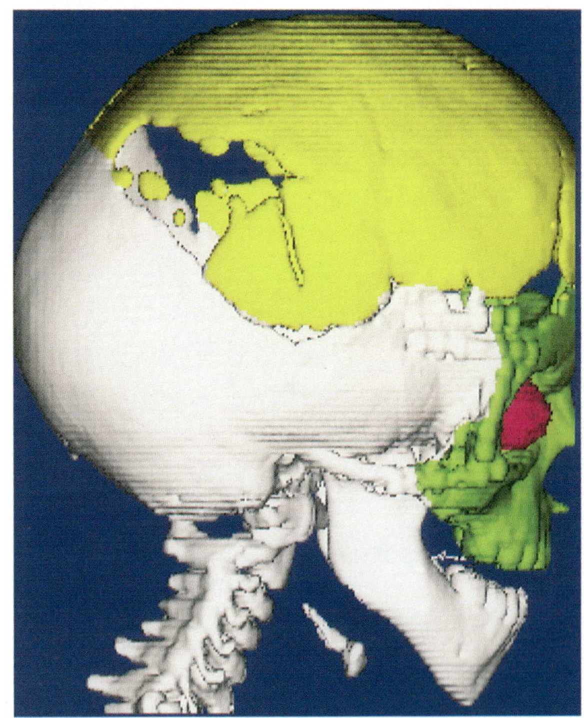

B   **COLOR FIG. 48-6.**

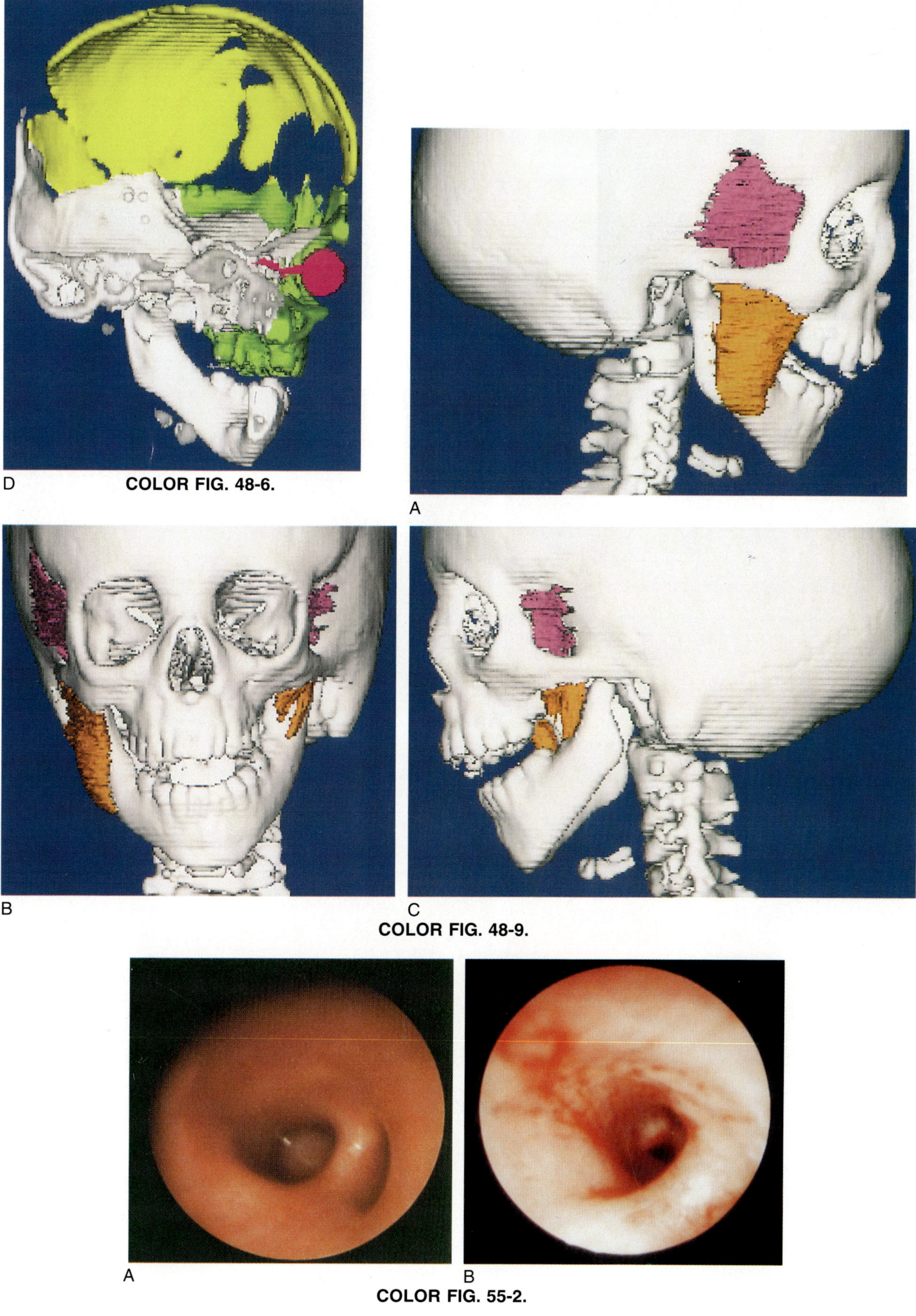

D   **COLOR FIG. 48-6.**

A

B

C   **COLOR FIG. 48-9.**

A

B   **COLOR FIG. 55-2.**

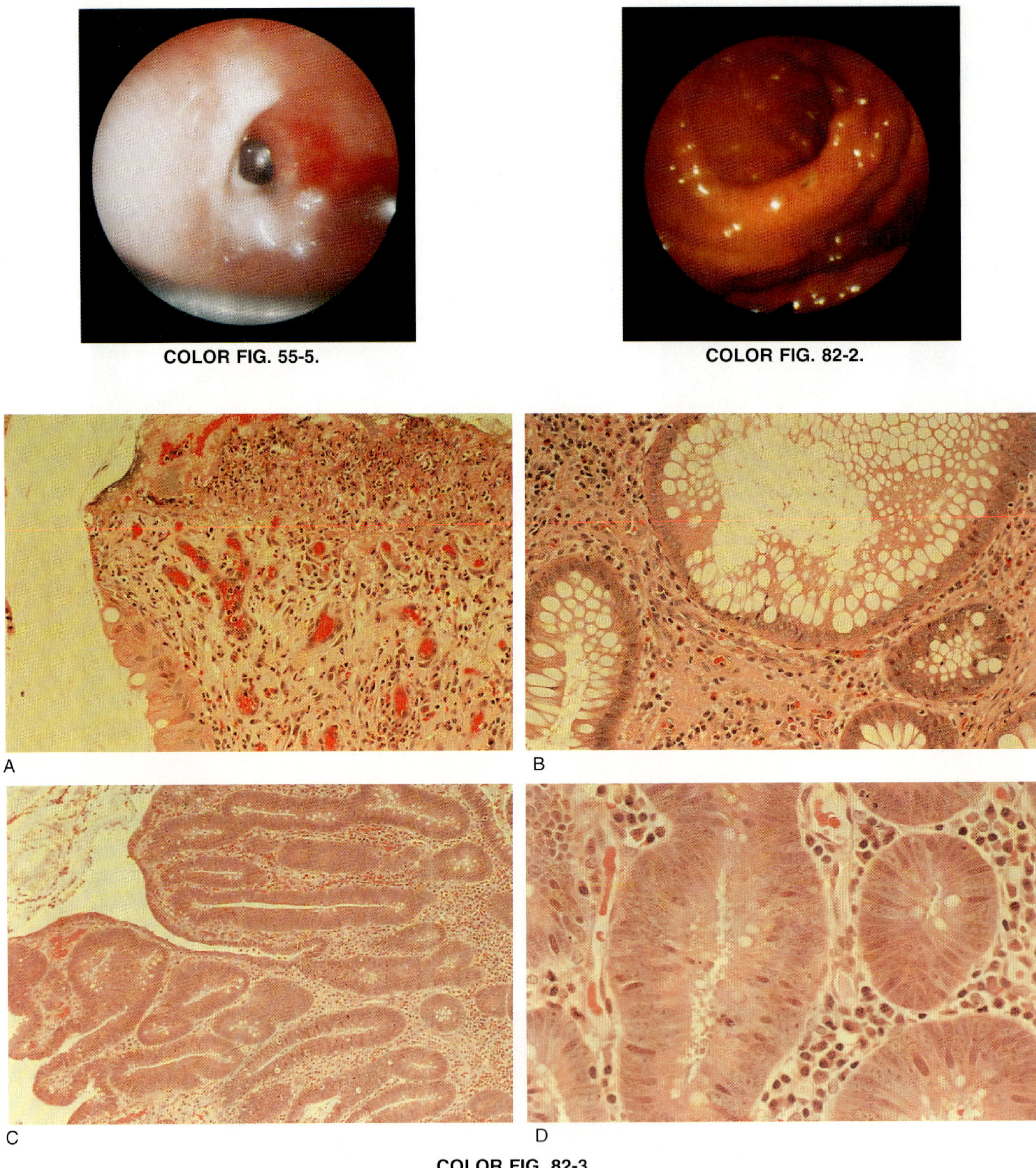

COLOR FIG. 55-5.

COLOR FIG. 82-2.

A

B

C

D

COLOR FIG. 82-3.

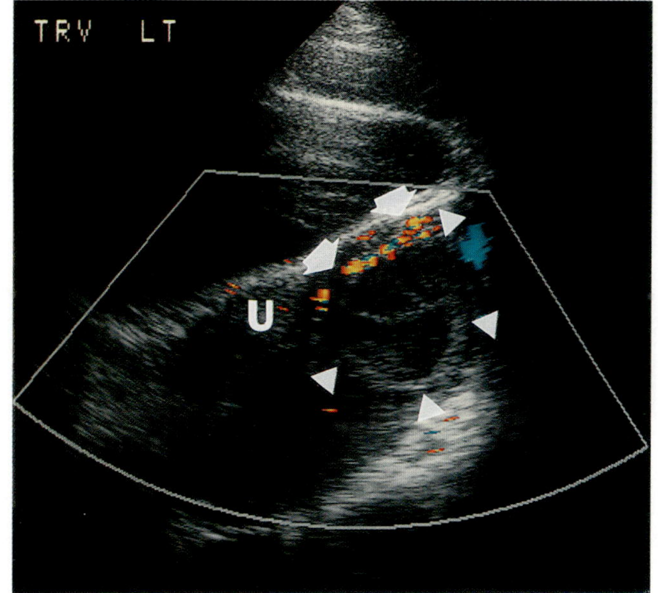

COLOR FIG. 94-4.

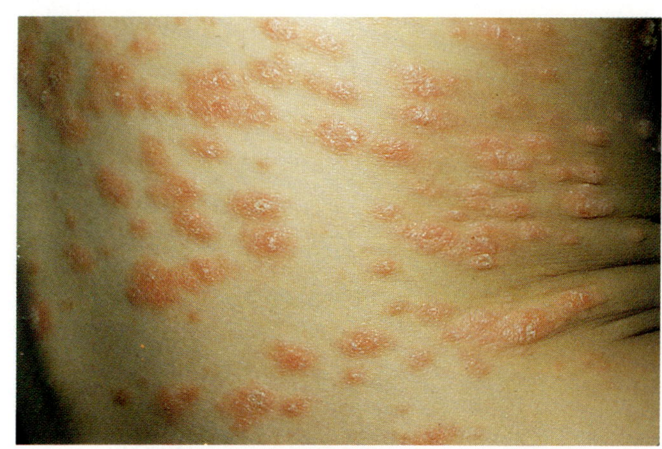

COLOR FIG. 96-2.

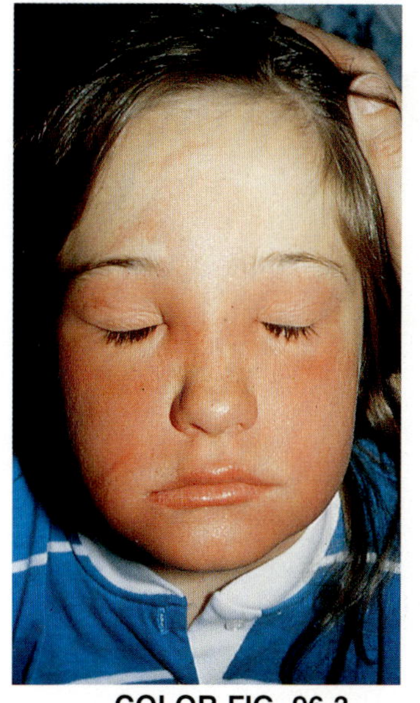

COLOR FIG. 96-3.

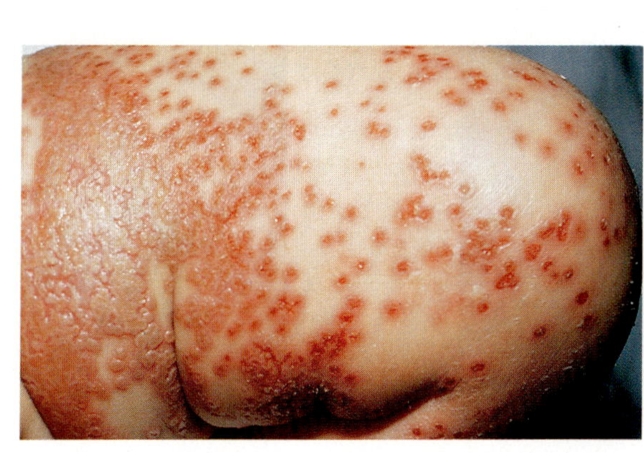

A

B

COLOR FIG. 96-4.

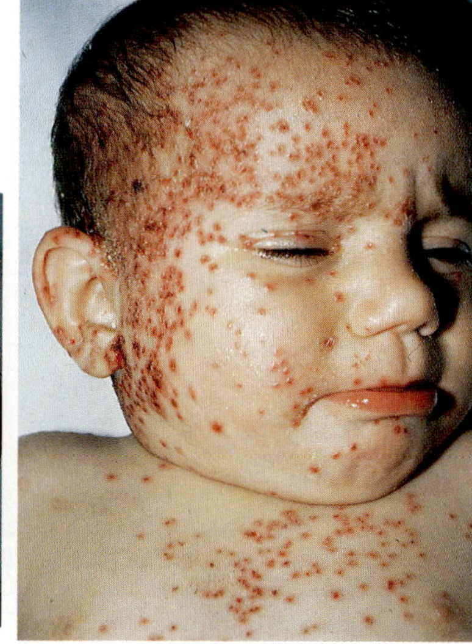

COLOR FIG. 96-5.

COLOR FIG. 96-6.

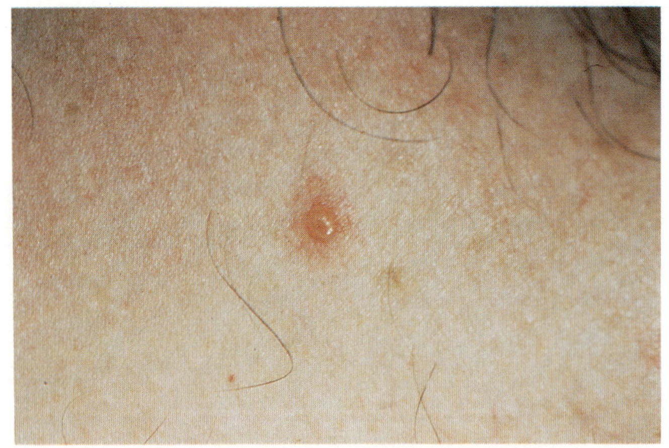

COLOR FIG. 96-7.

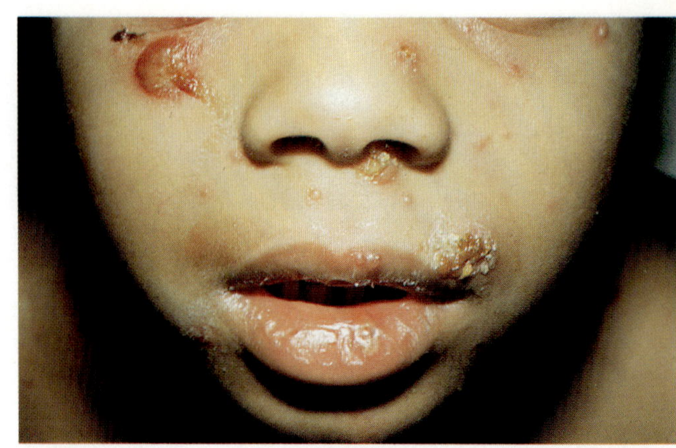

COLOR FIG. 96-8.

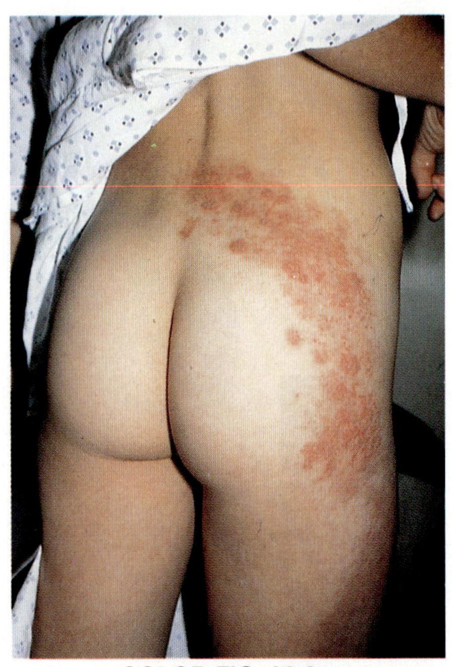

COLOR FIG. 96-9.

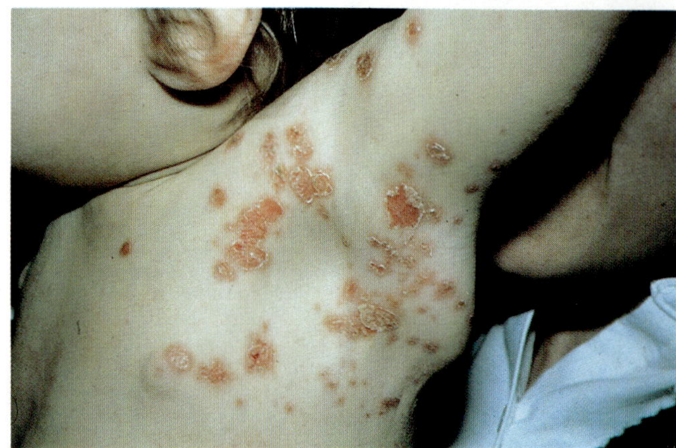

COLOR FIG. 96-10.

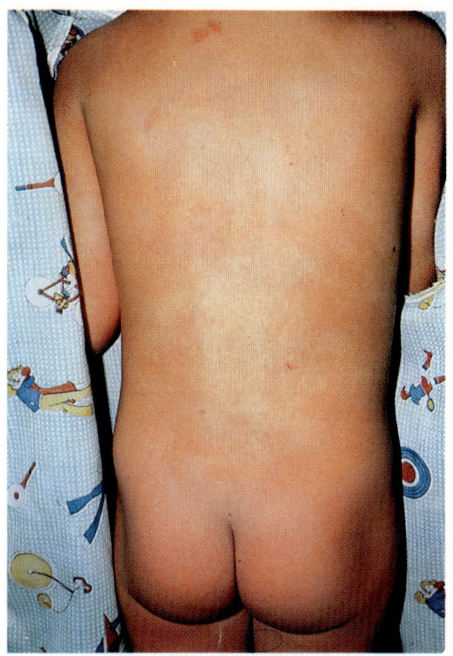

COLOR FIG. 96-11.

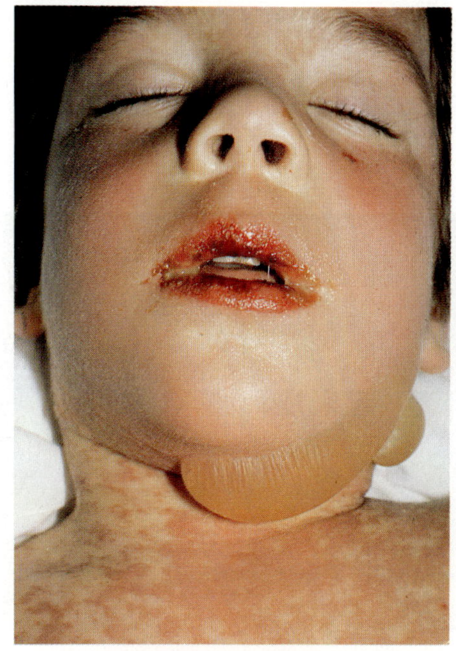

COLOR FIG. 96-12.

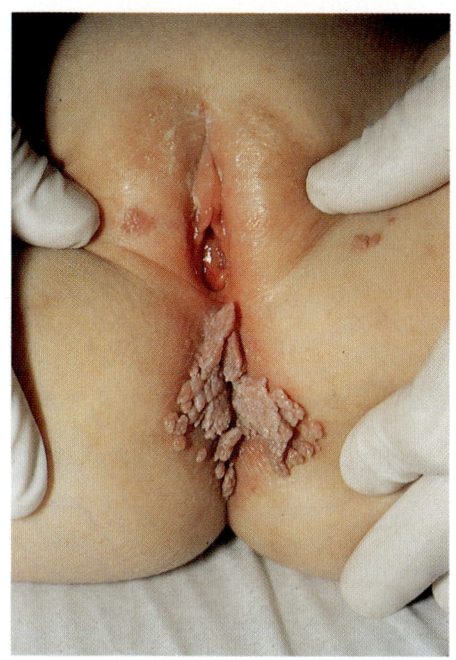

COLOR FIG. 96-13.

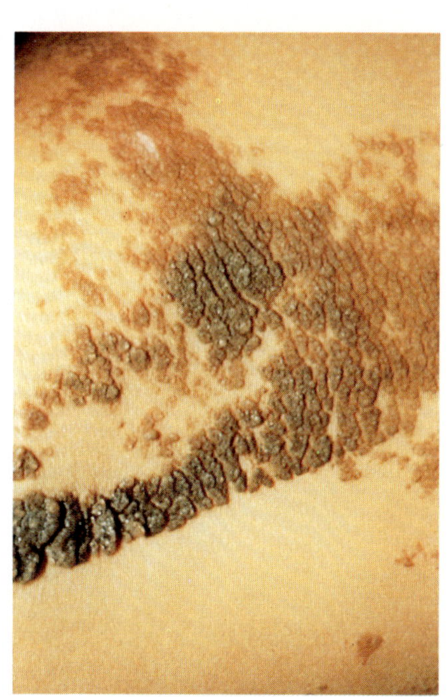

COLOR FIG. 96-14.

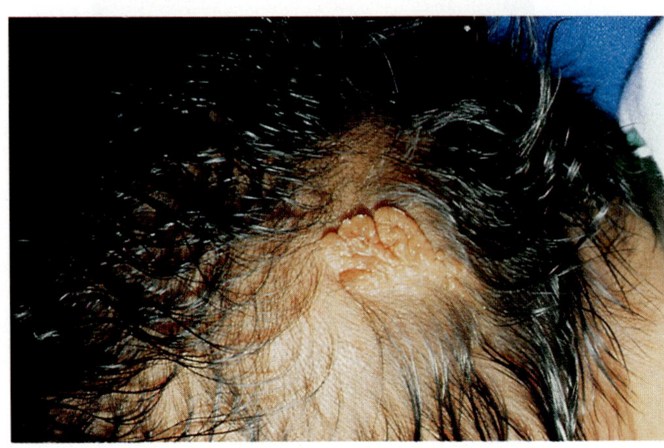

COLOR FIG. 96-15.

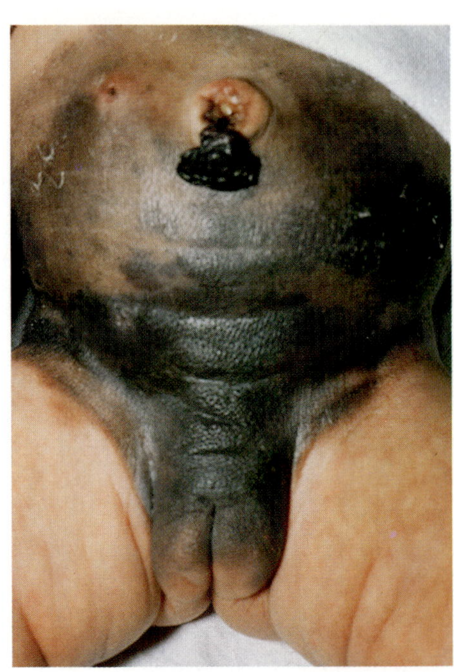

COLOR FIG. 96-16.

SECTION A

Scientific Principles

Surgery of Infants and Children: Scientific Principles and Practice, edited by
Keith T. Oldham, Paul M. Colombani, and Robert P. Foglia.
Lippincott–Raven Publishers, Philadelphia, © 1997.

CHAPTER 1

Cellular and Genetic Fundamentals

Edward P. Tagge, Kenneth D. Chavin, Sonja A. Rasmussen, and Ada Hamosh

1.1 Cell Structure and Function

Edward P. Tagge and Kenneth D. Chavin

All living creatures are made of cells—small, membrane-bounded compartments filled with a concentrated aqueous solution of chemicals. We study cells to learn how they are made from molecules and how they cooperate to make an organism as complex as a human being. More than 250 different types of cells exist in the human body, and these cells have differentiated into a highly integrated and complex system of tissues and organs.

This chapter provides an overview of the major developments in cell biology, a review of the families of small organic molecules that are the building blocks of cells, a discussion of the major components of the eukaryotic cell, and an overview of basic recombinant deoxyribonucleic acid (DNA) technology. This discussion should serve to provide both an introduction for the cell biology neophyte as well as an up-to-date discussion of pertinent cell biology areas for the aficionado. This chapter, however, is not a comprehensive review, but rather attempts to highlight areas of particular interest to the pediatric surgeon.

The modern concept of the cell took shape between 1830 and the early 1900s. The first major step forward was the recognition of the importance of the nucleus by Robert Brown in 1833; previously, emphasis had been placed on the importance of the cell wall. In 1838, T. Schwann and M. Schleiden formalized the postulate that the cell was the underlying unit of structure of all organisms. By 1855, R. Virchow observed that all cells arise from preexisting cells (*omnis cellula e cellula*), directing attention to the cell as the important factor in the transmission of inherited traits. In the 1870s, W. Flemming coined the term *mitosis* to describe the process in which chromatin elongated and then ''split'' lengthwise to be distributed to the two daughter cells at the end of cell division.

To complete the modern version of the cell concept, chromosome structure and function had to be related to the physical appearance. E. van Beneden reported in 1883 that gametes of the roundworm *Ascaris* had one chromosome each, whereas the zygote that formed when egg and sperm fused possessed two chromosomes. In 1905, J.B. Farmer and J.E. Moore coined the term *meiosis,* more fully describing the division events leading to halving of the chromosome number in sexually reproducing species. The 20th century began with the rediscovery of Gregor Mendel's studies of inheritance in garden peas published in 1865, in which he noted that unit factors (genes) governed the development of seven characteristics in pea plants. By 1902, W.S. Sutton and others had provided microscopic evidence in support of gene location within chromosomes, and Sutton formally proposed the Chromosome Theory of Heredity.

Studies of the chemical basis of heredity began in 1871 when Friedrich Miescher announced the discovery of *nuclein*, which he had extracted from white blood cells. In 1889, R. Altmann analyzed nuclein, which he called *nucleic acid,* and identified the specific sugars and nitrogenous bases involved. It was not for 60 years, however, that DNA was accepted as the genetic material. Previously, scientists tenaciously clung to the idea that genes were most likely proteins because proteins were extremely diverse and DNA was a monotonous molecule. In the early 1950s, E. Chargaff provided evidence that DNA was indeed a highly variable molecule; and in 1953, the landmark molecular model of DNA proposed by J. D. Watson and F. H. C. Crick was published. This set the stage for the myriad of discoveries that would usher in the era of recombinant DNA technology. In 1957, Kornberg discovered DNA polymerase, the enzyme used to replicate DNA. Nirenberg, Ochoa, and Khorana elucidated the genetic code in 1966, and Gellert discovered DNA ligase, the enzyme used to join DNA fragments together in 1967. In the early 1970s, Boyer, Cohen, Berg, and colleagues developed DNA cloning techniques, and 1975 saw the development of rapid DNA sequencing methods by Sanger, Maxam, and Gilbert. In the early 1980s, Palmiter and Brinster produced transgenic mice and Kary Mullis developed the polymerase chain reaction (PCR). These and many other molecular techniques allow cell biologists, who previously studied cells using only microscopy, to advance the understanding of the cell structure and function in the past 15 years.

CELLULAR BUILDING BLOCKS

Chemical Components

Carbon, hydrogen, nitrogen, and oxygen make up nearly 99% of a cell's weight. Disregarding the cell's most abundant substance, water, nearly all of the cell's molecules are carbon compounds. Carbon is outstanding among all the elements for its ability to form large molecules, because of its small size and four outer-shell electrons, which can form four strong covalent bonds with other atoms. Most important, it can join to other carbon atoms to form chains and rings, thereby generating large and complex molecules.

Broadly speaking, cells contain just four major families of small organic molecules: simple sugars, fatty acids, amino acids, and nucleotides. These small molecules are carbon compounds with molecular weights in the range 100 to 1000, containing up to 30 carbon atoms. They are usually found free in the cytoplasm, where they form a pool of intermediates from which large polymers, called *macromolecules,* are made. They are also essential intermediates in the chemical reactions that transform energy derived from food into usable forms vital to the cell's existence.

Sugars

Carbohydrates, another name for sugars, are aldehyde or ketone derivatives of polyhydric alcohols, so named because the hydrogen and oxygen are usually in the proportion to form water $(\mathbf{CH_2O})_n$. Glucose, for example, which is a six-carbon sugar, has the formula $C_6H_{12}O_6$ (Fig. 1-1*A*). The triose monosaccharides, glyceraldehyde and dihydroxyacetone, which are three-carbon sugar, are the simplest carbohydrates. Sugars with five- and six-carbon atoms are called *pentoses* and *hexoses,* respectively, with the two most common hexoses being glucose and fructose. The aldehyde or ketone group of these sugars can react with a hydroxyl group of the same molecule, forming a five- or six-membered ring; glucose and fructose are usually ring structures when in physiologic solutions. Monosaccharides have many isomers that differ only in the orientation of their hydroxyl (OH) groups; glucose, galactose, and mannose, for example, are isomers of each other. The hydroxyl groups of a simple monosaccharide can be replaced by other groups; for example, a carboxyl group (COOH) added to glucose produces glucuronic acid, and an amino group (NH_2) added to glucose produces glucosamine. The carbon that carries the aldehyde or the ketone can react with any hydroxyl group on a second sugar molecule to produce a disaccharide by forming a glycosidic bond, such as maltose (glucose α1,4 glucose), lactose (galactose β1,4 glucose), and sucrose (glucose α1,2 fructose). Larger linear and branched molecules can be made from repeating simple sugar units. Short chains are called *oligosaccharides,* and long chains are called *polysaccharides.* Glycogen, for example, is a polysaccharide made entirely of glucose units. In many cases, a sugar sequence is nonrepetitive, and such complex oligosaccharides are usually linked to proteins or lipids.

Fatty Acids

Fatty acids are carboxylic acids with long hydrocarbon tails (see Fig. 1-1*B*). They are water-insoluble biomolecules that have high solubility in organic solvents such as chloroform. These molecules have a variety of biologic roles; they serve as fuel molecules, as highly concentrated energy stores, as components of membranes, and as precursors for steroid hormones.

The systematic name for a fatty acid is derived from the name of its patent hydrocarbon by the substitution of *oic* for the final *e.* For instance, the C18 saturated fatty acid (18:0) is called octadecanoic acid because the parent hydrocarbon is octadecane. A C18 fatty acid with one double bond (18:1) is called octadec*enoic* acid; with two double bonds (18:2), octadeca*dienoic* acid; and with three double bonds (18:3), octadecat*rienoic* acid. Fatty acids with one or more double bonds are said to be *unsaturated.* Fatty acids in biologic systems usually contain an even number of carbon atoms, typically between 14 and 24. The 16- and 18-carbon fatty acids are most common: palmitic acid (C16), stearic acid (C18), and oleic acid (C18:1). The properties of fatty acids and of lipids derived from them are markedly dependent on their chain lengths and on the degree to which they are unsaturated. Unsaturated fatty acids and fatty acids with shorter chain lengths have lower melting points, which enhances the fluidity of fatty acids, an important component of membrane fluidity.

Fatty acids are synthesized in the cytosol by a multienzyme complex called *fatty acid synthetase.* The major product of this enzyme is palmitic acid. Longer fatty acids are formed by elongation reactions catalyzed by two different systems, one in mitochondria and one in the microsomes. Because mammals lack the enzymes to introduce double bonds distal to C9, they cannot synthesize certain fatty acids, such as linoleate (18:2) and linolenate (18:3). Therefore, these are called *essential fatty acids* because they must be supplied in the diet. Fatty acids are frequently complexed, through an ester linkage, to glycerol to form triglycerides, an important fuel molecule for the cell (see Fig. 1-1*B*).

Amino Acids

Amino acids, the building blocks of proteins, contain a carboxylic acid group, an amino group, and a variable side-chain group, all linked to a single carbon atom (see Fig. 1-1*C*). This single α-carbon atom is asymmetric, allowing for two mirror images, D and L. There are 20 major amino acids, all of which are conserved in evolution. All amino acids have a three-letter and one-letter abbreviation, such as glycine (Gly, G), leucine (Leu, L) and lysine (Lys, K). Amino acids are joined together by an amide linkage called a *peptide bond* (see Fig. 1-1*C*). In this bond, the carboxyl group of one amino acid joins with the amino group of another, liberating water. Proteins are long linear polymers of L-amino acids linked by peptide bonds. By convention, protein sequences are written using the one-letter amino acid abbreviations, with the amino terminus toward the left and the carboxyl terminus to the right.

Each amino acid has a different side chain attached to its α-carbon atom. These amino acids can be grouped according to the characteristics of their side chains: acidic, basic, uncharged polar, or nonpolar. Amino acids with uncharged polar side chains are relatively hydrophilic and are usually on the outside of proteins, whereas the side chains on nonpolar amino acids

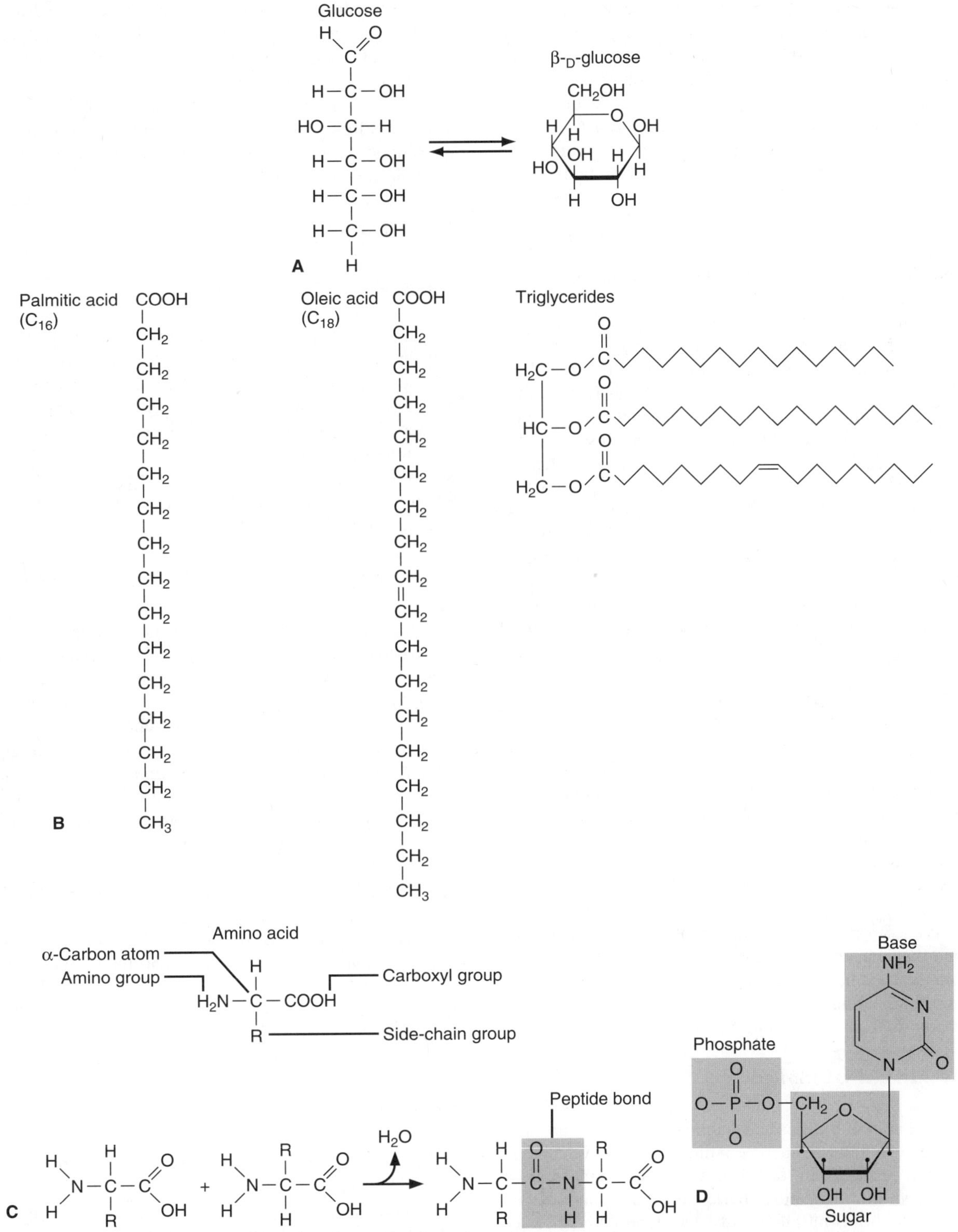

FIG. 1-1. (*A*) The common hexose glucose, with the molecular formula $C_6H_{12}O_6$. In physiologic solutions, glucose forms a ring structure. (*B*) Palmitic acid and oleic acid, two common fatty acids, which are carboxylic acids with long hydrocarbon tails. Fatty acids are stored through an ester linkage to glycerol to form triglycerides. (*C*) The general formula for amino acids, with an amino group (NH_2), carboxyl group (COOH), an α-carbon, and the variable side-chain group (R). Amino acids are commonly joined together by an amide linkage, called a *peptide bond*. (*D*) A nucleotide consists of a nitrogen-containing base, a five-carbon sugar, and one or more phosphate groups.

tend to cluster together on the inside. Amino acids with basic and acidic side chains are very polar and nearly always are found on the outside of protein molecules. One important nonpolar amino acid, cysteine, has a sulfhydryl side chain that allows it to pair with other cysteines through a disulfide bond. The properties of the amino acid side chains, in aggregate, determine the properties of the proteins they constitute and underlie all of the diverse and sophisticated functions of proteins.

Nucleotides

A nucleotide consists of a nitrogenous base, a pentose sugar, and one or more phosphate groups (see Fig. 1-1*D*). There are five different nitrogenous bases, grouped into pyrimidines and purines, all of which are ring compounds that can form hydrogen bonds. The pyrimidines include cytosine (C), thymine (T), and uracil (U), so named because they are derivatives of the six-membered pyrimidine ring. Guanine (G) and adenine (A) are purines, with a second five-membered ring fused to the pyrimidine ring. A, C, G, and T are used in DNA synthesis, while the T is replaced by U in ribonucleic acid (RNA) synthesis. The sugar used in RNA synthesis is β-ribose, while that used in RNA synthesis is β_2-deoxyribose. Each carbon on the sugar is numbered, from 1 to 5. The nitrogenous base is linked to the C1 of the sugar molecule in an *N*-glycosidic bond, while the phosphates are joined to the C5 hydroxyl in an ester linkage. Either one, two, or three phosphates can be added, as in adenosine monophosphate (AMP), adenosine diphosphate (ADP), and adenosine triphosphate (ATP), respectively. The phosphate makes the nucleotide negatively charged. Each nucleotide is named for the unique nitrogenous base that it contains. Nucleotides are joined together, by a phosphodiester linkage between 5′ and 3′ carbon atoms, to form nucleic acids. The linear sequence of nucleotides in a nucleic acid chain is commonly abbreviated by a one-letter code with the 5′ end of the chain written at the left, such as 5′-A-G-T-A-C-C-A-3′.

Nucleotides have a variety of functions. They can act as carriers of chemical energy; in which case ATP, the triphosphate ester of adenine, is the most important. Nucleotide derivatives can also serve as carriers for the transfer of particular chemical groups, and they can combine with other groups to form coenzymes. Finally, a cyclic adenine derivative, cyclic AMP, serves as a universal signaling molecule within cells, controlling the rates of many different intracellular reactions.

ENERGY METABOLISM

Obeying the laws of physics and chemistry, cells convert one form of energy to another to survive. Animal cells derive energy from food in three stages. In stage 1, large polymeric molecules are broken down into their monomeric subunits—polysaccharides into sugars, lipids into their fatty acids and glycerol, and proteins into amino acids. In stage 2, the resultant small molecules enter cells and are further degraded in the cytoplasm. Most of the carbon and hydrogen atoms of sugars are converted into pyruvate, which then enters mitochondria, where it is converted to the acetyl groups of the chemically reactive compound acetyl coenzyme A (acetyl CoA). A limited amount of ATP and NADH is also produced, and these are the only reactions that can yield energy in the absence of oxygen. In stage 3, the acetyl CoA molecules are degraded in mitochondria, yielding

CO_2 and hydrogen atoms. Electrons from the hydrogen atoms are then passed through a complex chain of membrane-bound carriers, eventually reacting with molecular oxygen to form water. Driven by the energy released in these electron-transfer steps, hydrogen ions are transported out of the mitochondria. The resulting electrochemical proton gradient across the inner mitochondrial membrane is harnessed to drive the synthesis of most of the cell's ATP.

Carbohydrates as Fuel

Glycolysis

Glucose is the principal foodstuff of many cells. The first step in the generation of ATP from glucose includes a series of reactions called *glycolysis*. After nine separate reactions, glucose is broken down to pyruvate, with two molecules of ATP produced for every molecule of glucose used. If there is a limited amount of oxygen, the pyruvate is converted to lactate. Much more energy, however, can be extracted aerobically, when the pyruvate molecule is entered into the citric acid cycle and the electron transport chain.

Citric Acid Cycle and Oxidative Phosphorylation

Under aerobic conditions, pyruvate undergoes oxidative decarboxylation to form acetyl CoA. This activated acetyl unit is then completely oxidized to CO_2 in the citric acid cycle, the final common pathway for the oxidation of amino acids, fatty acids, and carbohydrates. The reactions of the citric acid cycle occur inside the mitochondria, in contrast to those of glycolysis, which occur in the cytosol. For every acetyl CoA that enters the citric acid cycle, three NADH molecules, one $FADH_2$ molecule, and one GTP molecule are produced. NADH and $FADH_2$ are energy-rich molecules, containing a pair of electrons that have a high transfer potential. ATP is formed as electrons are transferred from NADH or $FADH_2$ in a process called *oxidative phosphorylation*. Oxidative phosphorylation generates 32 of the 36 ATP molecules that are formed when glucose is completely oxidized. This electron transport is normally tightly coupled to phosphorylation. NADH and $FADH_2$ are oxidized only if ADP is simultaneously phosphorylated to ATP. This coupling, called *respiratory control*, can be disrupted by uncouplers, such as 2,4-dinitrophenol (DNP).

Glycogen Metabolism

Glycogen is a readily mobilized storage form of glucose. It is a branched polymer of glucose residues and has a high molecular weight. The presence of glycogen greatly increases the amount of glucose that is immediately available. An average 70-kg man has an energy content of only 40 kcal available in glucose, while the total body glycogen has an energy content of more than 600 kcal.

Fatty Acids as Fuel

Fatty acids are physiologically important as fuel molecules. They are stored in adipose tissue as triglycerides (neutral fat;

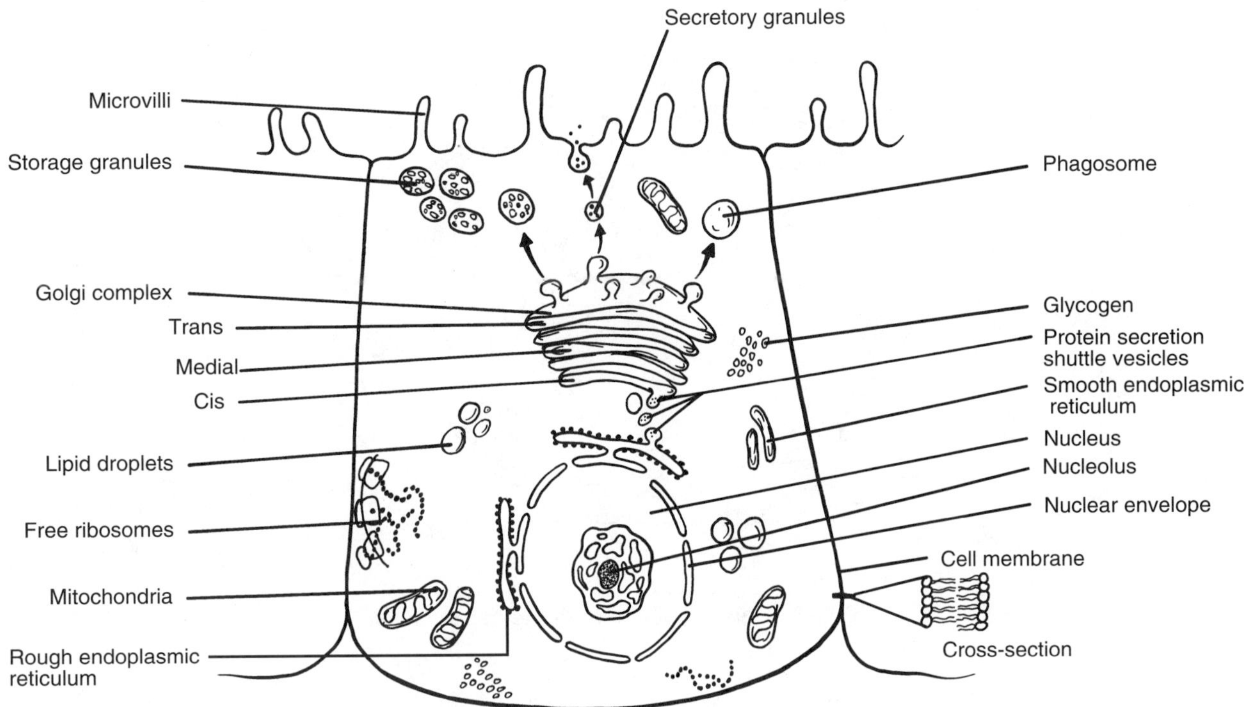

FIG. 1-2. Schematic diagram of a typical epithelial cell, showing the common internal organelles.

see Fig. 1-1*B*), which can be mobilized by the hydrolytic action of lipases. Triglycerides are highly concentrated stores of metabolic energy because they are reduced and anhydrous. The energy yield from the complete oxidation of fatty acids is about 9 kcal/g, in contrast to about 4 kcal/g for carbohydrate and protein. Consider a typical 70-kg man, who normally has fuel reserves of 100,000 kcal in triglycerides, 25,000 kcal in protein (mostly in muscle), 600 kcal in glycogen, and 40 kcal in glucose. Triglycerides constitute about 11 kg of his total body weight, but if this amount of energy were stored in glycogen, his total body weight would be 55 kg greater. The initial event in the use of fat is the hydrolysis of triglycerides by lipases, releasing the individual fatty acids for subsequent β-oxidation. These lipases are regulated by a variety of hormones (epinephrine, norepinephrine, glucagon), stimulating an increase in cyclic AMP. The glycerol formed by lipolysis can also be used for energy by entering the glycolytic pathway.

Fatty acids are activated to acetyl CoAs, transported across the inner mitochondrial membrane by carnitine, and degraded in the mitochondrial matrix by a recurring sequence of four reactions (β-oxidation pathway). The $FADH_2$ and NADH formed in the oxidation steps then transfer their electrons to O_2 through the respiratory chain, whereas the acetyl CoA formed enters the citric acid cycle after condensing with oxaloacetate to form citrate. The complete oxidation of palmitic acid (C16) yields 129 ATP molecules, with an efficiency of energy conservation of about 40%, a value similar to that for the citric acid cycle and oxidative phosphorylation. In some situations, however, such as starvation or diabetes, fat breakdown predominates over carbohydrate degradation (source of oxaloacetate), and acetyl CoA is diverted to give rise to acetoacetate and 3-hydroxybutyrate. Large amounts of acetoacetate, 3-hydroxybutyrate, and acetone (collectively known as *ketone bodies*) then accumulate in the blood because mammals are unable to convert fatty acids into glucose and because there is no pathway for gluconeogenic intermediates from acetyl CoA.

CELLULAR COMPARTMENTS

Unlike a bacterium, which generally consists of a single compartment surrounded by a plasma membrane, a eukaryotic cell is elaborately subdivided into functionally distinct, membrane-bounded compartments (Fig. 1-2). Each compartment, or organelle, contains its own distinct set of enzymes. Complex distribution systems convey specific products from one compartment to another. To understand the eukaryotic cell, it is essential to know what occurs in each of these compartment, how molecules move between them, and how the compartments are created and maintained.

Nucleus

Organization

The nucleus is usually the largest of the cellular organelles, ranging from 3 to 8 μm in diameter. The nucleus is defined by an envelope consisting of two membranes, the inner and outer nuclear membranes (Fig. 1-3). The outer membrane is continuous with the rough endoplasmic reticulum (ER) and is studded with ribosomes. All of the chromosomal DNA is contained within the nucleus and is usually in association with a specialized class of acidic proteins termed *histones*. The nucleus communicates with the cytoplasm by means of openings in the nuclear envelope, termed *nuclear pores*. These ringlike pores are

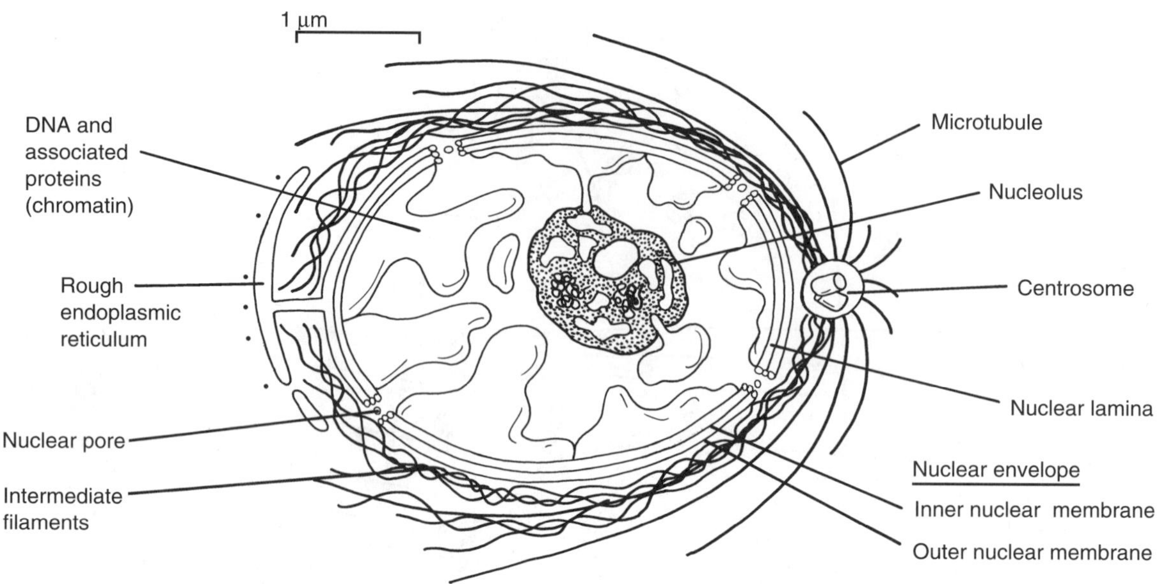

FIG. 1-3. Detailed structure of the cell nucleus.

composed of specialized proteins that function as channels to regulate the movement of material between nucleus and cytoplasm. The nucleus also contains a specialized region, the nucleolus, where ribosomes are assembled.

DNA Structure

DNA is a polymer formed by individual nucleotides, molecules formed by the union of a sugar residue (2-deoxyribose), phosphoric acid, and one of four nitrogenous bases. The four nitrogenous bases found in DNA are adenine (A), guanine (G), cytosine (C), and thymine (T). Each 2-deoxyribose molecule is linked to one of the nitrogenous bases through its 1′ carbon; its 5′ hydroxyl group makes an ester bond with phosphoric acid to form the 2′-deoxynucleoside triphosphates dATP, dGTP, dCTP, and dTTP. Alternating phosphate and sugars residues are the backbone of DNA and are joined in a 3′– 5′ diphosphoester bond. The two phosphate–sugar backbones, running antiparallel to each other, are joined through hydrogen bonds formed between the individual nitrogenous bases. As Watson and Crick initially described, DNA resembles a twisted ladder, with the nitrogenous bases acting as the rungs (Fig. 1-4). Fundamental to the genius of DNA is the fact that these nitrogenous bases have a unique and absolute bonding pattern: adenine with thymine, cytosine with guanine, and vice versa. Thus, if the sequence of bases on one strand is known, the other strand's sequence can be deduced. For instance, if the nitrogenous bases on one strand are 5′-A-C-G-T-T-G-C-A-3′, the other strand must be 3′-T-G-C-A-A-C-G-T-5′.

About 6×10^9 nitrogenous base pairs exist in the DNA of each nucleated human cell. For an appreciation of this complexity, assume that the abbreviation for each nitrogenous base of one strand of DNA was typed into a book, that is, A, T, C, G, and so forth. This book would then have to be 3 million pages long to hold the information contained in a single nucleus. This information is folded into 46 chromosomes, 23 from each parent, reducing the length of relaxed DNA 12,000 fold.

The study of chromosome structure, called *cytogenetics,* can provide useful clinical information. Dividing cells grown in tissue culture are arrested at metaphase (when chromosomes are the most condensed) and stained by a variety of chemicals in a process called *karyotyping.* This staining produces a unique pattern of alternating light and dark bands on each chromosome. Maternal and paternal chromosomes can then be paired and arranged according to their size and banding pattern. A simple nomenclature is then used to describe the chromosome pattern. For instance, p and q represent the short and long arms of a chromosome, respectively. A karyotype is designated by writing sequentially: (1) the total number of chromosomes, (2) the sex chromosomal complement, and (3) any chromosomal abnormality. Chromosomal abnormalities are of two types, numeric and structural. A common numeric abnormality would be 47,XY,+ 21, which describes a male with an extra chromosome 21 (Down syndrome). A common structural abnormality would be 46,XX,del(5p), which depicts a female with the normal number of chromosomes but a deletion of the short arm of chromosome 5 (cri du chat syndrome).

Central Dogma

In 1956, Francis Crick proposed the central dogma hypothesis, which theorized that chromosomal DNA functions as the template for its own replication as well as for the production of RNA and subsequently protein. Other than for rare exceptions, this dogma still remains valid. During DNA replication, the tightly compacted DNA molecule unwinds its complex folding, allowing DNA polymerase enzymes to copy both strands simultaneously, always in a 5′ to 3′ direction. Each strand directs its own replication, based on the previously described nitrogenous base pairing, producing two double helixes identical to the original DNA molecule.

Genes are segments of DNA that directly code for messenger

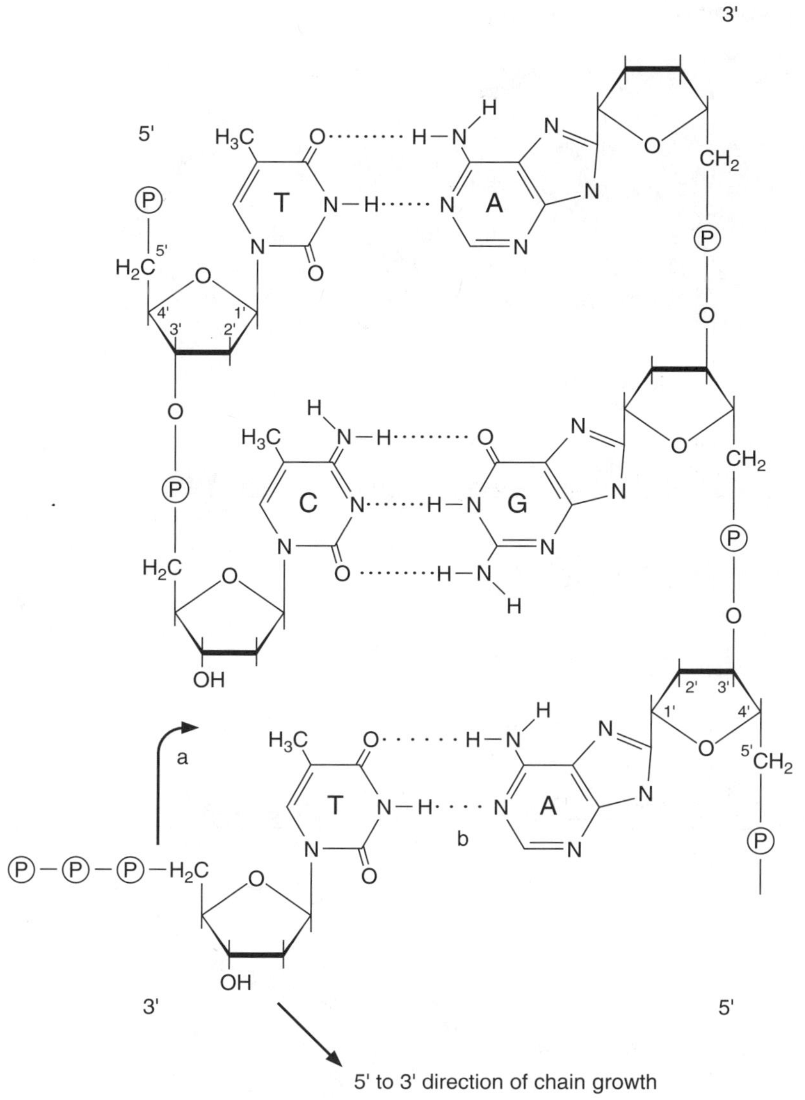

FIG. 1-4. Addition of a 2′-deoxyribonucleoside triphosphate to the 3′ end of a DNA chain is the fundamental step in DNA replication. The addition of the incoming dTTP is determined by the presence of dATP on the opposite strand. The hydrogen bonding between base pairs occurs on the inside of the double helix. Adenine and thymine have two hydrogen bonds, and guanine and cytosine have three hydrogen bonds. The sugar–phosphate backbones on either side run antiparallel to each other.

RNA (mRNA) in a process called *transcription* (Fig. 1-5). Genes make up only a small percentage of the total cellular DNA. There are an estimated 100,000 genes in each human cell, ranging in size from 2000 to 2,000,000 base pairs (average, 5000 base pairs). Genes contain segments, called *exons*, that ultimately directly code for a particular protein, interspersed with segments, called *introns*, that are spliced from the mRNA before protein production. Overall, only 10% of the cell's DNA is ever made into protein. The exact role of the remaining 90%, which includes the large stretches of DNA situated between genes as well as the introns, is largely unknown, although it probably has important regulatory functions.

Cell Cycle

The cell cycle is the sequence of events involved in the growth and division of one cell into two daughter cells. These daughter cells have three possible courses: (1) reentry into a new cell cycle, resulting in two new identical progeny; (2) early cell death; and (3) entry into a permanent or reversible quiescent phase with no increase in cell number. The cell cycle has been classically described by time intervals: DNA synthesis (S phase), cell division or mitosis (M phase), and the gaps of time between these events (G_1 is before DNA synthesis; G_2 is between DNA synthesis and mitosis). G_0 phase has been described for cells not actively proliferating but capable of undergoing cellular division after an appropriate signal.

RNA Synthesis (Transcription)

Ribonucleic acid has a similar structure to DNA, with several important exceptions: (1) RNA is a single-stranded molecule; (2) ribose is the sugar residue used, not 2-deoxyribose, and (3) the nitrogenous base thymine is replaced by uracil (U), although it is still complementary to adenine. There are three major forms of RNA: mRNA, which is the intermediary form between the DNA gene and its protein; ribosomal RNA (rRNA), the predominant form of cellular RNA, which makes up a large portion of ribosomes; and transfer RNA (tRNA), which carries a unique amino acid to the ribosome during protein synthesis.

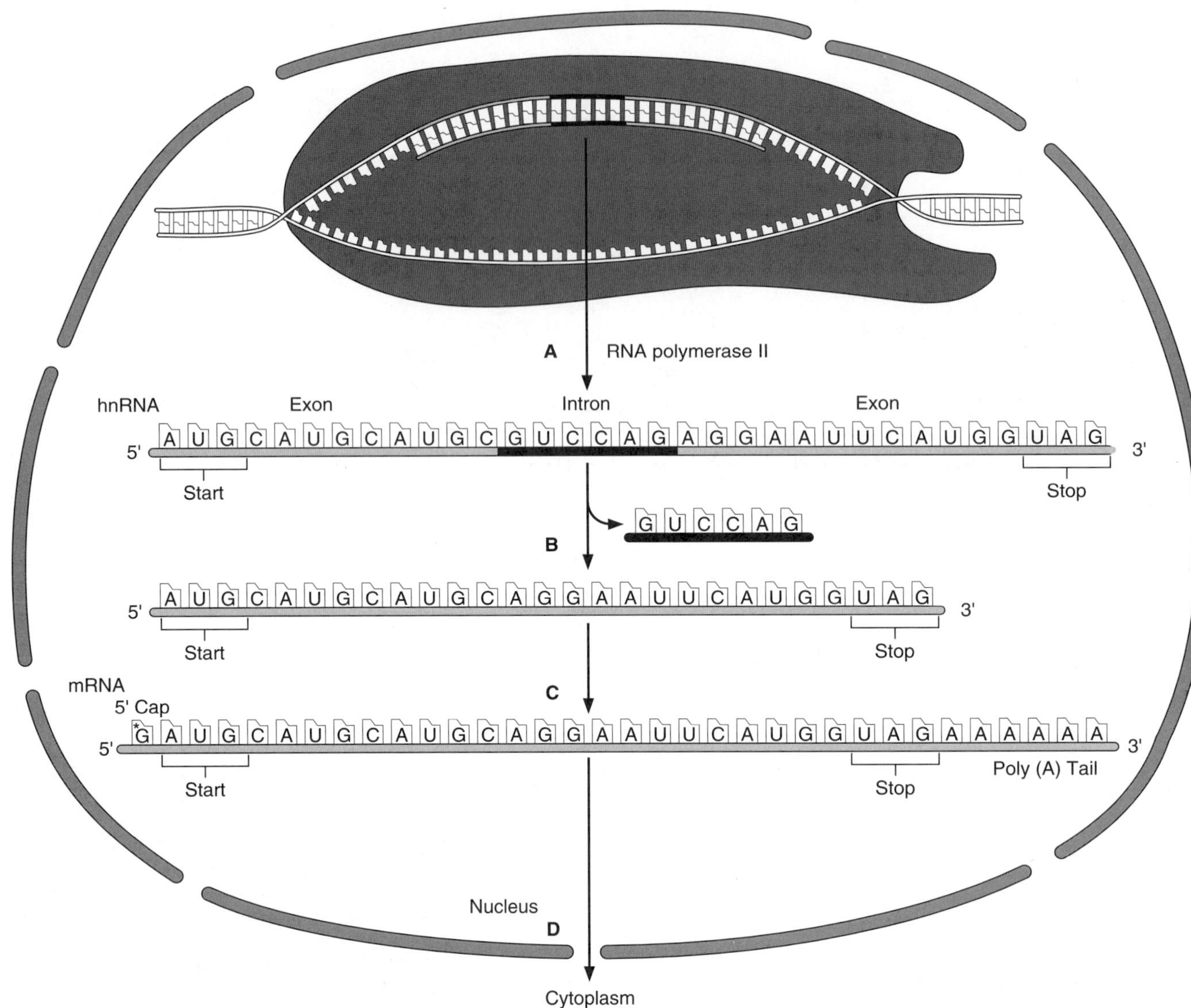

FIG. 1-5. Production of mRNA during transcription. (*A*) A heterogeneous nuclear RNA (hnRNA) molecule is copied directly from one strand of the relaxed DNA molecule by RNA polymerase II, including both the exons (*lightly shaded strand*) and the intron (*darkly shaded strand*). (*B*) The intron is removed, and the exons are joined in a process called *splicing*. (*C*) Multiple adenosine residues (20 to 200) are added to the 3′ end, generating the poly (A) tail, and a "cap" of 7-methylguanosine (*G) is added to the 5′ end. (*D*) The completely processed messenger RNA (mRNA) is transported to the cytoplasm for protein production.

During the process of mRNA synthesis, otherwise known as *transcription,* an RNA polymerase II enzyme binds to a specific site on the DNA and copies one strand (template strand), forming a heterogeneous nuclear RNA (hnRNA) transcript (see Fig. 1-5*A*). This hnRNA initially contains the entire gene sequence, including both exons and introns, but is subsequently processed in two ways: (1) the introns are removed by spliceosomes and the exons joined together (see Fig. 1-5*B*); and (2) multiple (20 to 200) adenine residues are added to the 3′ end (poly [A] tail) and a "cap" of 7-methylguanine is added to the 5′ end (see Fig. 1-5*C*). This final processed mRNA is then transported from the nucleus to the cell's cytoplasm for protein synthesis (see Fig. 1-5*D*).

Cytoplasm

Cytosol

The remainder of the cell, external to the nucleus and contained by the plasma membrane, is termed the *cytoplasm.* The cytoplasm is composed of a nonparticulate "soup," or cytosol, as well as a number of membranous organelles and a filamentous cytoskeleton. The cytosol constitutes more than half the total volume of most cells and is the main site of many of the enzymes involved in protein synthesis and intermediary metabolism. The fibrous cytoskeleton is a collection of filamentous

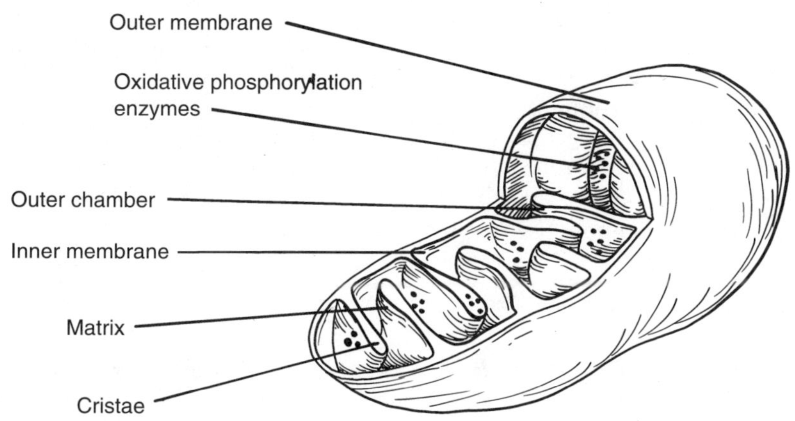

FIG. 1-6. Schematic structure of a typical mitochondrion.

protein structures that allows cells to assume and maintain a variety of shapes, to produce directed movement of organelles within the cell, and to effect movement of the entire cell relative to other cells. These multiple activities depend on three main types of filaments: actin filaments, intermediate filaments, and microtubules. Each type of filament is formed from protein monomers and a variety of accessory proteins that serve to cross-link individual filaments or to attach them to membranes.

About 20% of the cytosol's weight is protein, so it is more appropriate to think of the cytosol as a highly organized gelatinous mass rather than as a simple solution of enzymes. Although small molecules diffuse nearly as quickly in the cytosol as they do in pure water, that is not the case for large particles such as transport vesicles and organelles. To move at useful rates, such particles usually are actively transported by protein ''motors'' that hydrolyze ATP to propel the particles along microtubules or actin filaments.

Mitochondria

Mitochondria are sausage-shaped organelles, 0.2 to 0.5 μm in diameter (Fig. 1-6). Because mitochondria divide by fission and contain their own DNA and ribosomes, they probably originated from symbiotic bacteria during evolution. Mitochondria have a smooth outer membrane and an inner membrane characterized by in-foldings, termed *cristae,* which protrude into a central matrix. The outer membrane contains *porins,* proteins forming large channels that render the membrane permeable to molecules of up to 10 kd. The inner mitochondrial membrane is almost entirely protein, with the lowest lipid content of common biologic membranes. Mitochondria are the major source of energy production in eukaryotic cells. The enzymes involved in electron transport and oxidative phosphorylation exist on small, stalked particles protruding inward from the inner membrane. Oxidative phosphorylation, which occurs at the inner membrane, generates an electrochemical proton gradient, and the downhill movement of H^+ through adenosine triphosphatase (ATPase) molecules provides energy to synthesize ATP. The enzymes involved in the final oxidation of sugars and lipids are also present in the matrix space.

Endoplasmic Reticulum

The ER is a network of interconnected membranes forming closed vesicles, tubules, and saccules. In some cells, the ER has a total membrane surface that is 25 times that of the plasma membrane. It is primarily involved in the synthesis of protein and lipids. The ER is divided into rough ER, which is studded with ribosomes and involved in the synthesis of exportable proteins, and smooth ER, which lacks ribosomes and is involved in the synthesis of fatty acids and lipids. Rough ER is prominent in cells such as pancreatic acinar cells and plasma cells that secrete large amounts of protein, while smooth ER is especially prominent in cells producing lipid derivatives such as the adrenal cortex. Smooth ER also contains enzymes that detoxify endogenous metabolites and foreign molecules such as drugs and pesticides.

The ER plays a central part in cell biosynthesis. The transmembrane proteins and lipids of the ER, Golgi, lysosome, and plasma membrane are synthesized in association with the ER membrane. The ER membrane also makes a major contribution to the mitochondrial membrane by producing most of the lipids for this organelle. In addition, all of the newly synthesized proteins that will reside in the lumen of the ER, Golgi apparatus, or lysosome—as well as those to be secreted to the cell exterior—are initially delivered to the ER lumen. Most of these proteins are glycoproteins, and the covalent addition of sugars to proteins is one of the major biosynthetic functions of the ER (Fig. 1-7). In contrast, few proteins that reside in the cytosol are glycosylated because they are produced on free ribosomes that are not associated with the ER.

Golgi Apparatus

The Golgi apparatus, usually located near the cell nucleus, contains a collection of flattened membrane-bounded cisternae, resembling a stack of plates. Swarms of small vesicles associated with these stacks clustering on the side abutting the ER and along the dilated rims of each cisterna (Fig. 1-8). These vesicles are transport containers that shuttle proteins destined for secretion to and from the Golgi and between the Golgi cisternae. These vesicles are coated by protein complexes, some by clathrin and others by ADP-ribosylation factor in association with *coatomer* (equimolar complex of seven proteins). Proteins exported from the ER enter the first of the Golgi compartments, the cis compartment, then move from the medial compartment to the trans compartment and finally to the *trans-Golgi network* (Fig. 1-9). In the trans-Golgi network, proteins are segregated into different transport vesicles and dispatched to their final

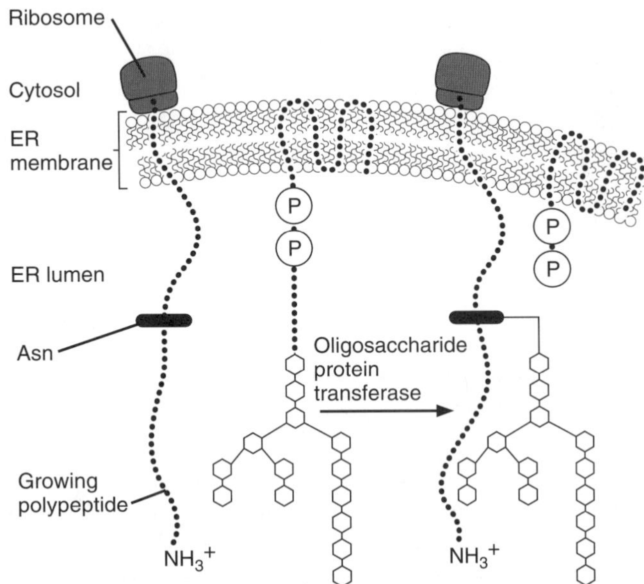

FIG. 1-7. Biosynthesis of an asparagine-linked glycoprotein in the endoplasmic reticulum (ER) lumen. The sugar core is transferred as a preformed unit from a carrier lipid, dolichol phosphate, to the protein as it is being synthesized.

destination. During this transport, secretory proteins are modified in a stepwise fashion. For instance, the removal of mannose residues and the addition of *N*-acetylglucosamine occurs in the medial compartment, while galactose and sialic acid residues are added in the trans compartment. In addition, many polypep-

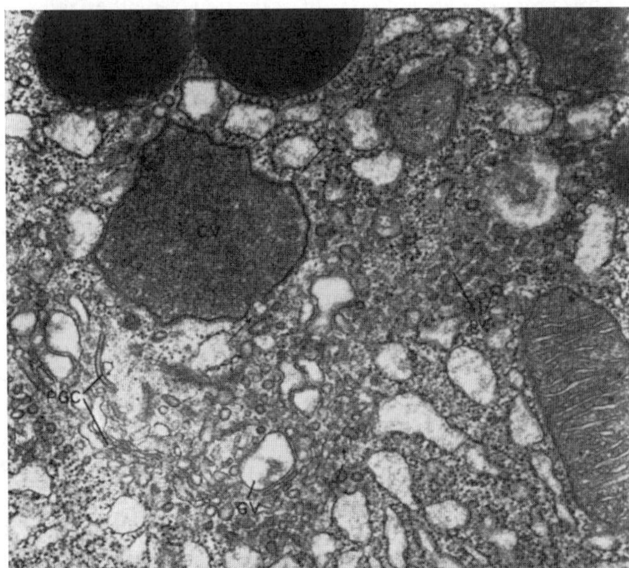

FIG. 1-8. Electron photomicrograph of a portion of a pancreatic acinar cell showing endoplasmic reticulum, Golgi apparatus, and forming secretory granules. An abundance of small transport vesicles shuttle secretory proteins between the various membrane-limited organelles. CV, condensing vacuole; PGC, post-Golgi cisternae; PV, peripheral vesicles; GV, Golgi vacuole; t, transition element of the RER. (Courtesy of J. Jamieson, Yale University, New Haven, CT)

tide hormones that are synthesized as inactive protein precursors are activated in the trans-Golgi network. Finally, the Golgi is the compartment involved in directing secretory proteins into one of three destinations: (1) small vesicles that rapidly move to the periphery of the cell and either release their contents or direct them to the plasma membrane, (2) lysosomes, or (3) secretory granules, where the contents condense and are stored to await a stimulatory signal.

Lysosomes

Lysosomes are membrane-limited organelles containing hydrolytic enzymes that are the principal site for the controlled intracellular digestion of macromolecules. About 40 hydrolytic enzymes are contained in these lysosomes: proteases, nucleases, glycosidases, lipases, phospholipases, phosphatases, and sulfatases. All are acid hydrolases, which work best at an acid pH. The interior of the lysosome is maintained at pH 5.0 by an H⁺-transporting ATPase located in the lysosomal membrane. Lysosomes can obtain the material they degrade by at least three pathways (Fig. 1-10). The best-studied pathway includes digested materials taken up by endocytosis, leading from coated pits to endosomes and eventually the lysosomes. A second pathway involves digestion of obsolete parts of the cell. The third pathway occurs only in cells that are specialized for the phagocytosis of large particles and microorganisms, such as macrophages and neutrophils. These cells can engulf large objects, forming a phagosome, which is converted to a phagolysosome by fusion with a lysosome.

Protein Synthesis (Translation)

To a large extent, cells are made of protein, which constitutes more than half of their dry weight. Proteins determine the shape and structure of the cell and also serve as the main instruments of molecular recognition and catalysis. Although DNA stores the information required to make a cell, it has little direct influence on cellular processes. In computer terminology, the DNA and the mRNA represent the "software"—instructions that a cell receives from its parent. Proteins constitute the "hardware"—the machinery that executes the program stored in the memory.

To initiate protein synthesis, ribosomes, which are a combination of rRNA and proteins, attach to specific ribosomal binding sites on the mRNA. The ribosomes then move along the mRNA strand producing a protein in a process called *translation* (Fig. 1-11). The nitrogenous bases (A, C, G, U) are read in triplet (called *codons*), and each codon directs the addition of a specific amino acid (see Fig. 1-11A). Since there are 64 potential codons (4³), and only 20 amino acids, there is degeneracy in the genetic code (Table 1-1). For instance, there are 6 codons for the amino acid leucine, but only 1 codon for tryptophan. One specific codon, AUG, not only represents methionine but also is the universal *start* codon, where almost all protein synthesis is initiated. Three codons (UAA, UAG, UGA) do not correspond to any amino acid but instead serve as *stop* codons, terminating protein synthesis. Important to note is that all organisms on earth use the same genetic code. This allows an organism as simple as a bacterium to translate a human sequence,

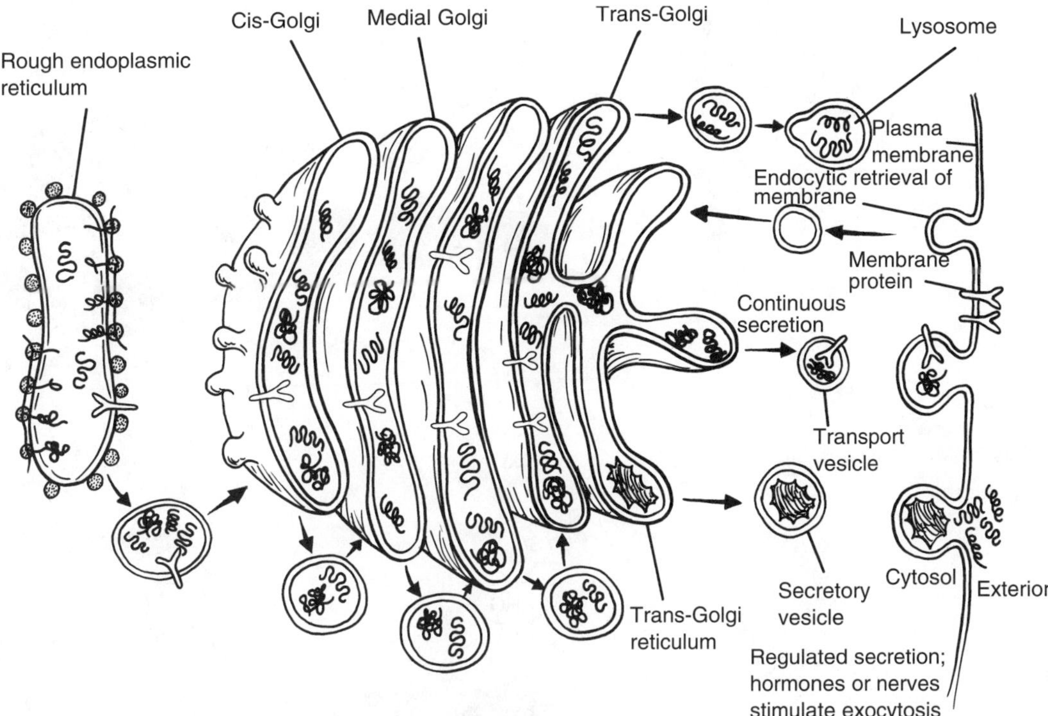

FIG. 1-9. Intracellular transport and sorting of proteins destined for secretion, insertion into the plasma membrane, or targeting to the lysosome. After insertion into the endoplasmic reticulum lumen, movement from one compartment to another is by vesicular transport, which buds off one compartment and fuses with the next. Sorting signals intrinsic to the newly synthesized proteins specify the pathway to be taken.

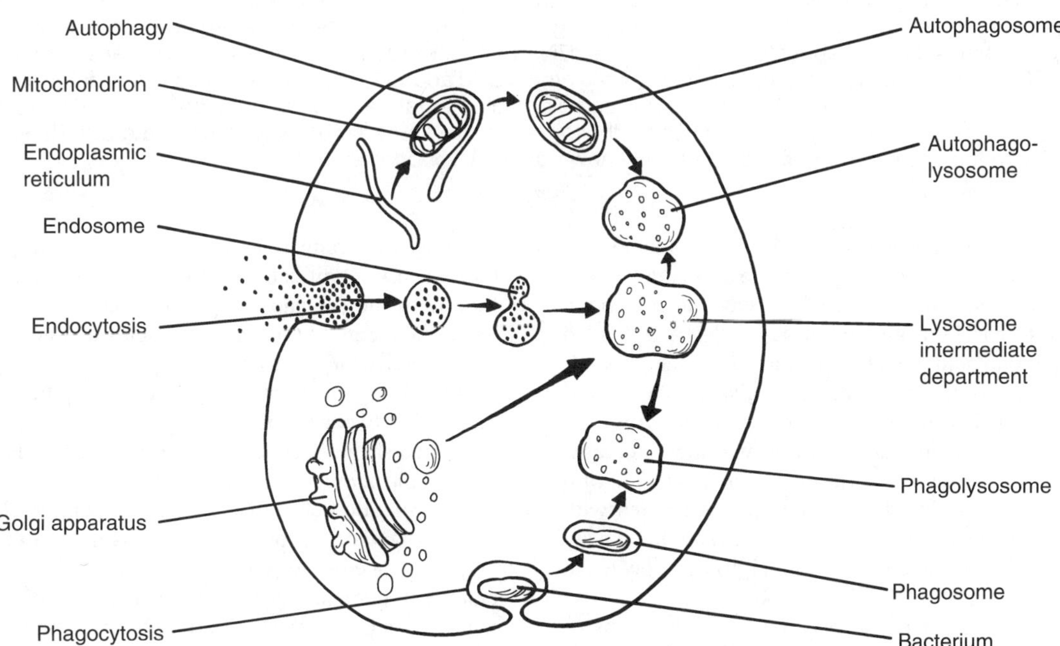

FIG. 1-10. Formation of lysosomes by combination of transport vesicles from the Golgi-containing lysosomal enzymes with material that has been phagocytosed, endocytosed, or internalized by autophagy.

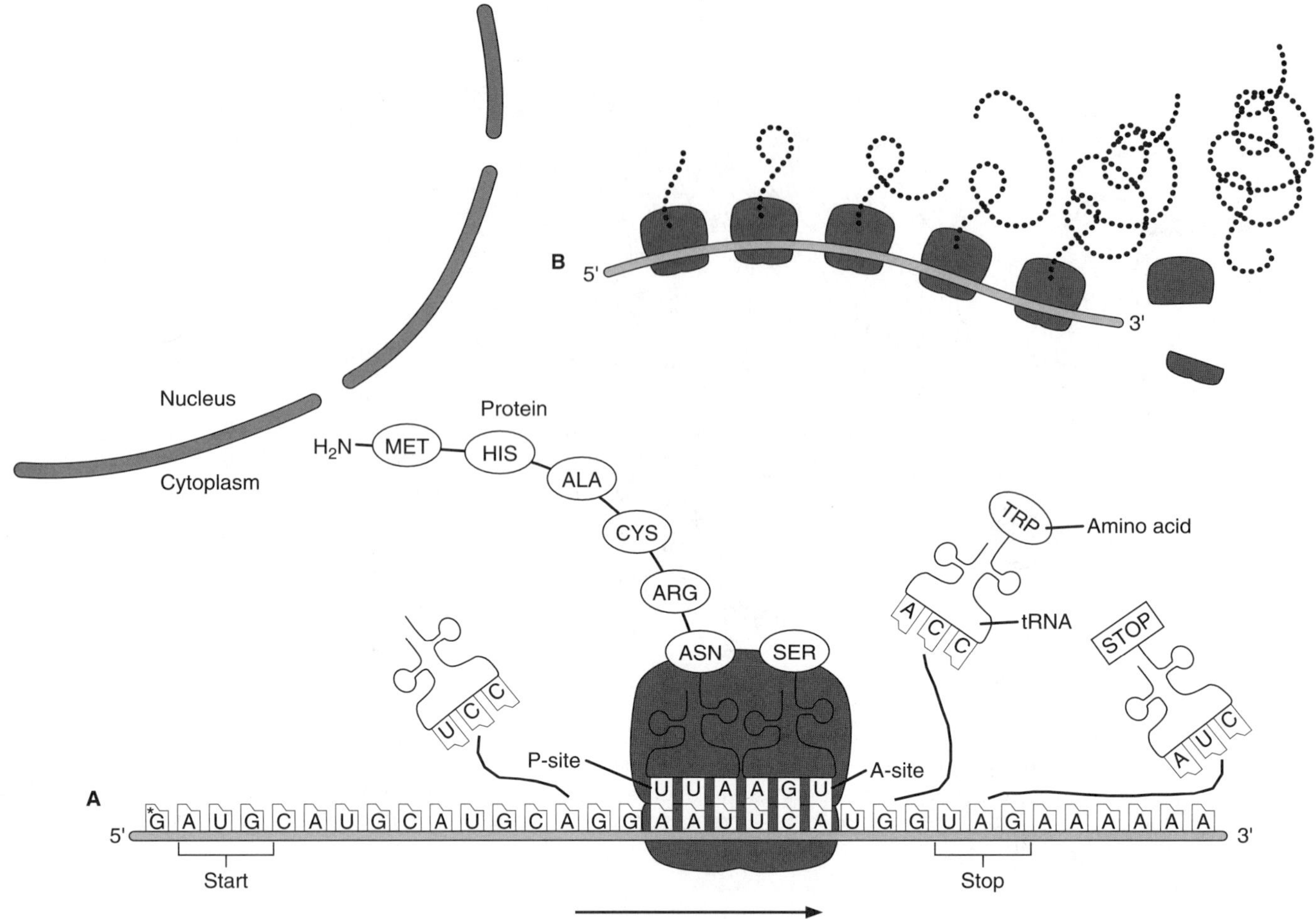

FIG. 1-11. Production of protein during translation. (*A*) As in transcription, mRNA is translated starting from its 5′ end. The growing polypeptide chain is in the P-site. A tRNA molecule loaded with its specific amino acid, serine (SER) in this illustration, brings its amino acid to the A-site on the ribosome, where a new peptide bond is about to be formed. The tRNA that delivered the most recent amino acid, arginine (ARG), can be seen leaving the ribosome. Each amino acid added to the polypeptide chain is determined by base pairing of the codon on the mRNA and a complementary anticodon on each specific tRNA. (*B*) A single mRNA usually has a number of ribosomes at the same time, making separate but identical polypeptide chains; the entire structure is known as a *polyribosome.*

which is one of the fundamental concepts of recombinant DNA technology. Amino acids are brought to the growing protein chain by specific tRNA molecules, which have an *anticodon* complementary to each mRNA codon. Each tRNA is loaded with a specific amino acid, which is then added to the growing peptide chain. This process continues until a stop codon is encountered, at which time the ribosome disassociates from the mRNA. The protein is then either released into the cytoplasm if it has been produced on a free ribosome, or is directed into the ER if it has been produced by a ribosome associated with the rough ER. A number of ribosomes can attach simultaneously to mRNA, producing a number of identical protein species at the same time (see Fig. 1-11*B*).

More than 100 different posttranslational modifications of amino acid side chains have been described. Although the functions of most of these modifications are not known, many must be important for the operation of the cell because they are tightly controlled by specific enzymes. Some of these modifications are permanent; others, such as phosphorylation, are reversible and play important roles in regulating the activity of the proteins. These modifications can occur either in the cytosol or the lumina of the ER and Golgi apparatus.

The sequential order of amino acids making a particular protein is referred to as its *primary structure*. The first three-dimensional folding arrangement is referred to as the *secondary structure*, with two common configurations: the α helix and the β-pleated sheet. Second and third folding levels are commonly termed the *tertiary structure*. The *quaternary* structure is the spatial relation between multiple polypeptide chains.

The shape of a protein molecule is determined by its amino acid sequence because the various amino acid side chains associate with one another and with water. One of the most important factors governing the folding of a protein is the distribution of its polar and nonpolar side chains. The nonpolar hydrophobic side chains in a protein tend to be pushed together into the interior of the molecule, enabling them to avoid contact with the aqueous environment. By contrast, the polar side chains tend to arrange themselves near the outside of the protein molecule,

TABLE 1-1. *The genetic code*

First position (5′ end)	Second position				Third position (3′ end)
	U	C	A	G	
U	Phe	Ser	Tyr	Cys	U
	Phe	Ser	Tyr	Cys	C
	Leu	Ser	Stop	Stop	A
	Leu	Ser	Stop	Trp	G
C	Leu	Pro	His	Arg	U
	Leu	Pro	His	Arg	C
	Leu	Pro	Gln	Arg	A
	Leu	Pro	Gln	Arg	G
A	Ile	Thr	Asn	Ser	U
	Ile	Thr	Asn	Ser	C
	Ile	Thr	Lys	Arg	A
	Met	Thr	Lys	Arg	G
G	Val	Ala	Aap	Gly	U
	Val	Ala	Asp	Gly	C
	Val	Ala	Glu	Gly	A
	Val	Ala	Glu	Gly	G

where they can interact with water and with other polar molecules. Secreted or cell surface proteins often form additional covalent intrachain bonds, such as disulfide bonds, to stabilize their three-dimensional structures.

Protein Function

The human cell synthesizes between 3000 and 6000 different proteins, and the chemical properties of a protein molecule depend almost entirely on its exposed surface residues. When a protein molecule binds to another molecule, the second molecule is commonly referred to as a *ligand.* The region of a protein that associates with a ligand, known as its *binding site,* usually consists of a cavity formed by a specific arrangement of amino acids that are often on widely separated regions of the polypeptide chain. The rest of the protein molecule is necessary to maintain the polypeptide chain in the correct position and to provide additional binding sites for regulatory purposes.

Many proteins have two or more slightly different conformations available to them. By shifting reversibly from one to another, they can alter their functions. Such *allosteric* proteins are essential to the feedback regulation that controls the flux through a metabolic pathway. One form is an active conformation that binds substrate at its active site and catalyzes its conversion to the next substance in the pathway. The other is an inactive conformation that tightly binds the final product of the same pathway at a different place on the protein surface (the regulatory site). Such allosteric proteins are vital for cell signaling because they can reversibly change their shape when ligands bind to their surfaces. The changes produced by one ligand often affect the binding of a second ligand, thereby providing a mechanism for regulating various cell processes.

Intracellular Protein Trafficking

Proteins play a central part in the compartmentalization of a eukaryotic cell. They catalyze the reactions that occur in each organelle and serve as organelle-specific surface markers that direct deliveries of new proteins and lipids to the appropriate organelle. By tracing the protein traffic from one compartment to another, one can begin to make sense of the otherwise bewildering maze of intracellular membranes. The ER, Golgi apparatus, endosomes, and lysosomes all communicate with one another and with the outside of the cell through transport vesicles that bud off from one organelle and fuse with another. Thus, all the spaces enclosed are topologically equivalent to one another and to the cell exterior, and they can be regarded as parts of a single functionally connected complex.

All proteins originate on ribosomes in the cytosol, but the traffic from this point onward diverges into two main branches. The proteins in one branch are released into the cytosol, where most remain, but some are directed to the mitochondria, nucleus, or peroxisomes. The other main branch consists of proteins destined to be secreted from the cell, plus those destined to reside in the ER, Golgi apparatus, plasma membrane, or lysosomes. All of these proteins are transferred through a translocator into the ER as they are being synthesized; (before they assume their normal folding pattern), because of a sorting signal that is generally located at their amino terminus (Fig. 1-12). Once in the ER, proteins destined for secretion are packaged into transport vesicles that pinch off from specialized regions of the ER and fuse specifically with nearby cisternal elements of the Golgi apparatus. After fusion, the constituents of the vesicle membrane become part of the Golgi membrane, while the soluble proteins in the vesicle lumen are delivered to the lumen of a Golgi cisterna. In this way, soluble proteins are selectively carried from one membrane-bounded compartment to another without actually passing across a membrane. By similar cycles of vesicle budding and fusion, proteins are thought to be transported from one Golgi cisterna to another and eventually to the lysosomes, secretory vesicles, or plasma membrane according to their different functions. This intracellular sorting appears to require at least 10 distinct types of transport vesicles, each with a unique set of ''molecular address labels'' on its surface. Thus, the transport vesicles leaving the ER must fuse only with the cis-Golgi compartment, those leaving the cis-Golgi compartment must fuse only with the medial Golgi compartment, and so on. In each step, vesicle budding, vesicle docking, and vesicle fusion are involved, each requiring highly specific recognition events.

The ER and each of the compartments in the Golgi apparatus contain their own unique sets of proteins. These proteins probably are selectively retained in these organelles by a mechanism that depends on ''retention signals'' in the proteins, while the remainder of the flow of materials from ER to the cell surface occurs by default. Transport vesicles designed for immediate fusion with the plasma membrane follow this constitutive secretory pathway. Specialized secretory cells have a second pathway in which soluble proteins and other substances are stored in secretory vesicles for later release—the so-called triggered or regulated secretory pathway. There also exists a third pathway, whereby the acid hydrolases are targeted to the lysosome. Thus, the bulk of the evidence suggests that proteins made in the ER are automatically delivered to the trans-Golgi network and then to the plasma membrane by this constitutive pathway unless they are otherwise diverted or retained by specific sorting signals.

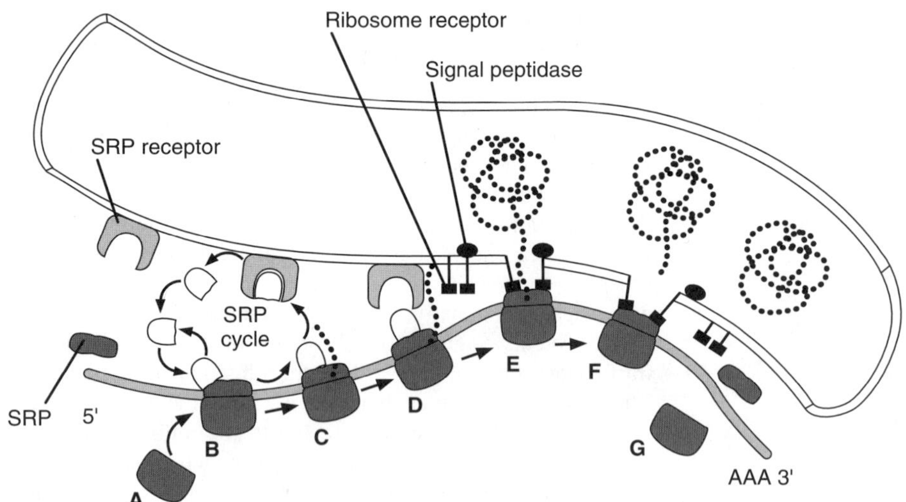

FIG. 1-12. Synthesis and sequestration of secretory protein. Synthesis begins on the left as ribosomal subunits aggregate (*A*) and begin to translate mRNA (*B*). The signal-recognition particle (SRP) binds to the complex and arrests peptide chain elongation (*C*) until SRP binds to a receptor in the endoplasmic reticulum membrane (*D*). The nascent polypeptide is then extruded into the lumen (*E*) with the aid of ribosome receptors, and SRP is released to recycle. The amino-terminal sequence may be cleaved by a signal peptidase (*F*). On chain termination, the ribosome dissociates (*G*), and its subunits can recycle.

Plasma Membrane

The plasma membrane is the essential structure that defines cellular life. Without the presence of the plasma membrane, which acts as a barrier separating the internal aqueous environment from the outside world, life as we know it would not exist. The plasma membrane, however, is more than a simple passive barrier. It is a highly selective filter that maintains a concentration gradient of ions and allows for penetration of nutrients and the excretion of waste. Simply, the plasma membrane is a lipid bilayer with embedded protein and cholesterol molecules (Fig. 1-13). Furthermore, interspersed carbohydrates account for a small but extremely important portion of the plasma membrane.

Membrane Lipids

The three major kinds of membrane lipids are phospholipids, glycolipids, and cholesterol. Phospholipids, which are abundant in all biologic membranes, are derived from the three-carbon alcohol glycerol (are thus called *phosphoglycerides*), or from sphingosine, a more complex alcohol. Two of glycerol's hydroxyl groups are linked to fatty acids, while the third hydroxyl is linked to phosphoric acid, which is further linked to a variety of small polar head groups (alcohols). The fatty acid chains, which can be saturated or unsaturated, usually contain between 14 and 24 carbon atoms. Phosphatidylcholine (lecithin), phosphatidylserine, and phosphatidylethanolamine are the major

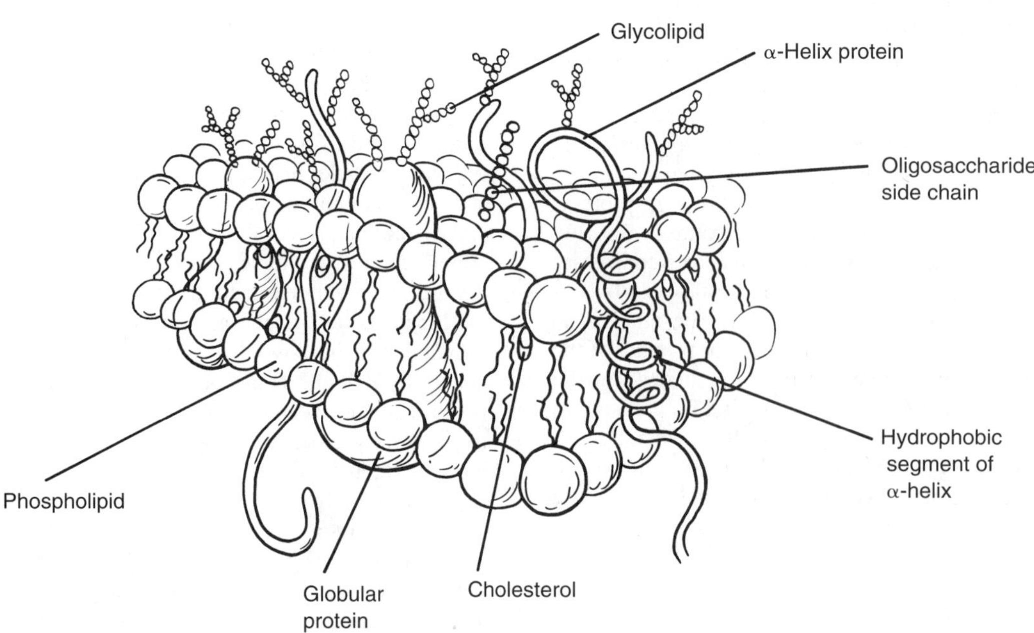

FIG. 1-13. Structure of the cell membrane as a fluid mosaic consisting of a phospholipid bilayer that contains cholesterol and embedded proteins.

phosphoglycerides. Sphingomyelin is the main phospholipid that contains a sphingosine backbone instead of glycerol.

Glycolipids, as their name implies, are sugar-containing lipids. Glycolipids, like sphingomyelin, are derived from sphingosine. Unlike sphingomyelin, however, glycolipids have one or more sugars (rather than phosphoryl choline) linked to sphingosine's primary hydroxyl group. The simplest glycolipid is cerebroside, in which there is only one sugar residue. More complex glycolipids, such as gangliosides, contain a branched chain of as many as seven sugar residues.

Membrane lipids possess a critical common structural theme: they are amphipathic molecules; that is, they contain a hydrophilic polar head and one or two hydrophobic, nonpolar hydrocarbon tails. In an aqueous medium, membrane lipids are arranged as a stable bilayer, with their hydrocarbon tails juxtaposed to form a hydrophobic interior domain, while their hydrophilic polar head groups face the aqueous environment on either side. These sheets serve as a permeability barrier, yet they are fluid. Formation of the lipid bilayer is a self-assembly process, driven by a variety of bonding forces: hydrophobic interactions, van der Waals forces between the hydrocarbon tails, and electrostatic and hydrogen-bonding interactions between the polar head groups and water molecules.

The molecules within the bilayer demonstrate a remarkable degree of lateral and rotational movement, known as *membrane fluidity*. There is a great degree of lateral diffusion, with lipids able to diffuse along the bilayer at about the length of a bacteria per second. An important determinant of membrane fluidity is its cholesterol content, which increases membrane fluidity. Cholesterol also helps stabilize the membrane by partially immobilizing the region of the hydrocarbon chain closest to the polar head group. Finally, cholesterol also helps inhibit temperature-induced phase transition; thus, crystallization of the membrane does not occur with decreasing temperature.

Membrane Proteins and Carbohydrates

Although the lipid bilayer determines the basic structure of biologic membranes, proteins are responsible for most membrane functions, serving as specific receptors, enzymes, transport proteins, and so on. Membrane proteins interact with the lipid bilayer in a variety of ways (see Fig. 1-13). Peripheral proteins are attached superficially by loose bonds and can be removed easily. Transmembrane proteins are amphipathic integral proteins that span the entire membrane in either single or multiple passes, usually as α helices. Other membrane-associated proteins do not span the bilayer but instead are attached to one side of the membrane, either bound by noncovalent interactions with transmembrane proteins, or covalently attached to lipid molecules. In addition, frequently the extracellular domains of integral proteins are bound with oligosaccharide chains. This glycosylation adds considerable diversity to these molecules, and similar proteins can take on unique and specific identities based on the sugar chains that are added.

Membrane Transport of Small Molecules

Due to the effectiveness of the plasma membrane, the transport of materials from the extracellular to the intracellular space

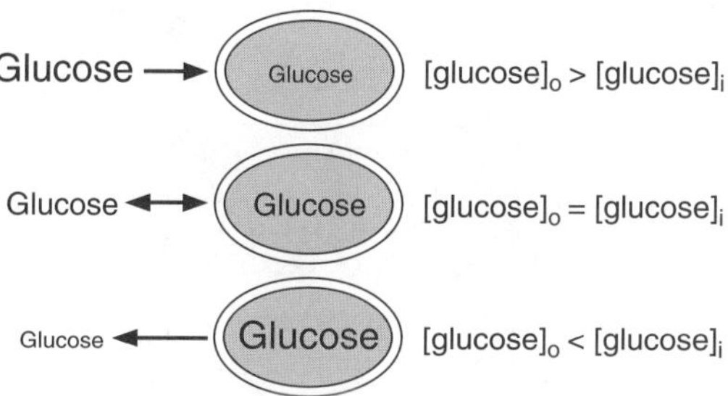

FIG. 1-14. For a substance that moves by a non–energy-dependent transport mechanism, the direction of the net flow is determined by the passive driving force. In this example, the movement of glucose is determined by the orientation of the concentration gradient.

is markedly impeded without the presence of specialized transport mechanisms. The simplest of these mechanisms is simple diffusion, which includes the movement of gases, lipid-soluble materials, and small noncharged particles down a concentration gradient. Some larger molecules use facilitated diffusion, which requires specialized transmembrane proteins that act as channels to the inside of the cell; examples include the transport proteins for glucose and amino acids (Fig. 1-14). Some membrane proteins form ion-specific gates. These channels function in different cells by responding to either a voltage shift or to particular neural transmitters. Finally, some transport proteins are energy dependent and work against specific charge or concentration gradients, consuming ATP (Fig. 1-15).

Membrane Transport of Macromolecules and Particles

Larger molecules are brought into the cell through the process of endocytosis (see Fig. 1-10). The two main types of endocytosis are distinguished on the basis of the size of the endocytic vesicles formed: (1) pinocytosis, which involves the ingestion of fluid and solutes through small vesicles (less than 150 nm) and (2) phagocytosis, which involves the ingestion of microorganisms or cellular debris through large vesicles called *phagosomes* (less than 250 nm). In endocytosis, localized regions of the plasma membrane invaginate, mediated by clathrin-coated pits, and pinch off to form endocytic vesicles, many of which end up fusing with lysosomes.

Receptor-mediated endocytosis is a specialized form of endocytosis that involves cell surface receptors that bind specific extracellular macromolecules (Fig. 1-16). After these molecules are bound, the receptor–ligand complex localizes in specific areas where clathrin-coated pits form and internalize. A variety of viruses, hormones, and other proteins use this pathway to gain entrance to the cell. Once the ingested molecule is digested, the receptor is recycled, returning to the cell surface.

Receptors and Cell Signaling

The communication of a cell with its outside environment involves extracellular signaling molecules, which mediate three kinds of intercellular communication, distinguished by the distance over which they act: (1) in endocrine signaling, hormones are carried in the blood to target cells throughout the body; (2) in paracrine signaling, chemical mediators act only on local cells, and (3) in neurocrine signaling, signaling molecules act across a synapse. Messages may be delivered through ports (channels) that work through ion fluxes, by the acquisition of substances by endocytosis, or through membrane-bound receptors. An ever-increasing number of cell receptors and their specific ligands, involved in cell–cell communication, are being identified. Binding of a ligand to its receptor results in a specific transmembrane signal that is transduced through the receptor's cytoplasmic tail, initiating a cascade of second messengers. These receptor proteins are not only specific, being able to discriminate between various stimuli, but are also able to amplify a particular signal. A variety of receptors and cell signaling molecules exist; this chapter briefly discusses (1) adhesion molecules, (2) cytokines, (3) growth factors, and (4) nitric oxide (Fig. 1-17).

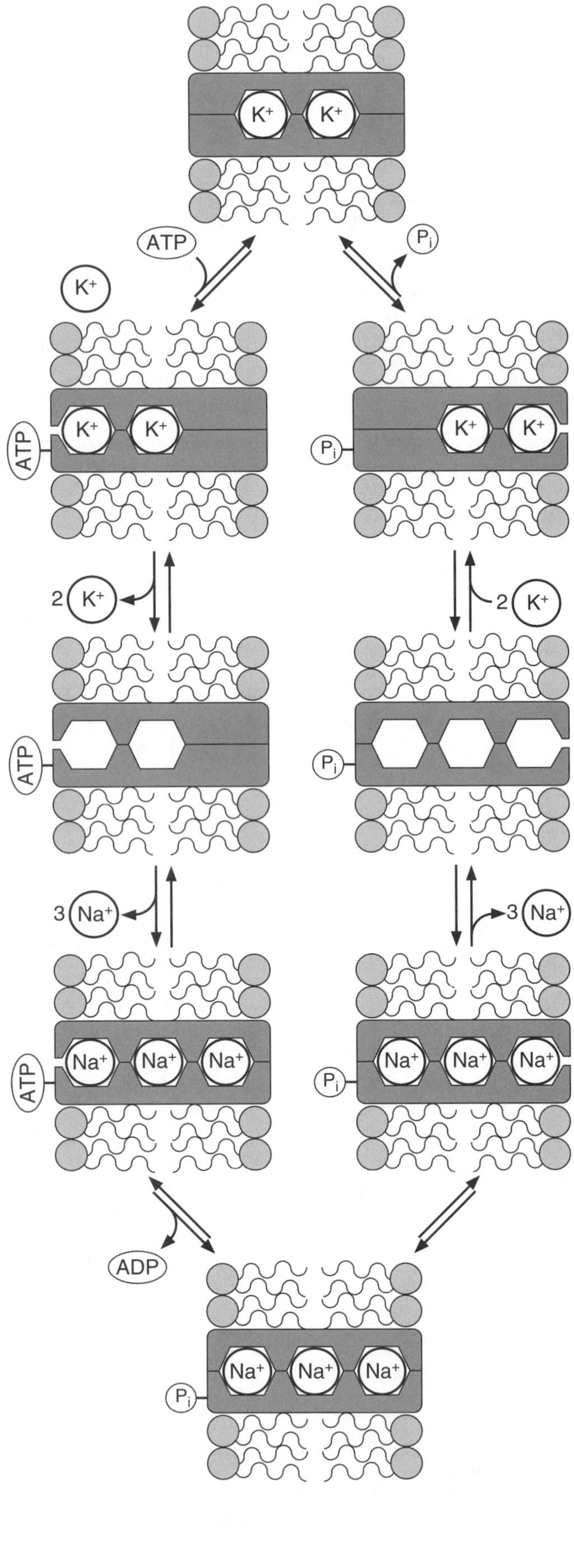

Adhesion Molecules

An integral part of multicellular organisms is a recognition system that allows for cell–cell communication or cell–extracellular matrix communication. This system is critical in embryogenesis, organogenesis, malignant transformation, wound healing, inflammation and sepsis, and transplant immunology. Six families of cell adhesion molecules are known: (1) integrins, (2) selectins, (3) cadherins, (4) the immunoglobulin superfamily, (5) proteoglycans, and (6) mucins. Given the advances in these areas and their importance to the surgical scientist, an overview of the first three categories is presented (see also Chapter 11).

The *integrins* are a supergene family composed of heterodimers that span the cell membrane, binding extracellular proteins while interacting with cytoskeleton elements. They are primarily composed of both an α and β subunit, with the β subunits being the most important. The integrins specifically function in cell–cell or cell–extracellular matrix interactions, and there are two diseases known to be associated with integrin deficiencies: leukocyte adhesion deficiency disease (deficiency of CD18) and Glanzmann thrombasthenia (deficiency in platelet glycoprotein IIb/IIIa).

The seven major integrin subfamilies are identified by their different β subunits. The β_1 subfamily, also know as the *extracellular matrix integrins,* uses six α subunits, called the VLA (*very late after*) antigens, which form a heterodimer with the β_1 subunit. The ligands of the β_1 subfamily include laminin, collagen, fibronectin, and vascular cell adhesion molecule 1 (VCAM-1). An important motif found in the β_1 subunit family is the RGD (arginine, glycine, and aspartic acid) amino acid sequence. The ligands for the β_1 subfamily all recognize this RGD sequence, which thus appears to be critical for the adhesion process.

The β_2 subfamily, also known as the *leukocyte integrins,* includes leukocyte function antigen 1 (LFA-1) and macrophage

FIG. 1-15. The Na$^+$-K$^+$-ATPase pump has a complicated catalytic cycle that involves not only the binding and unbinding of Na$^+$ and K$^+$ but also the binding of ATP, phosphorylation of the protein, and subsequent dephosphorylation, so that one ATP is hydrolyzed per transport cycle.

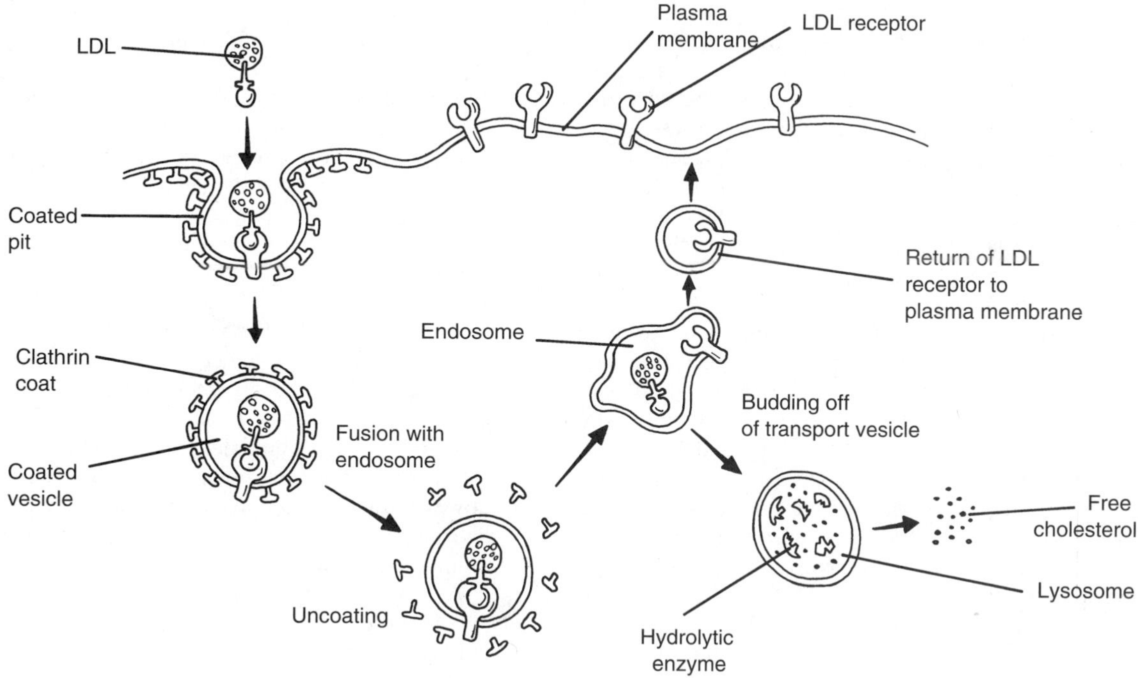

FIG. 1-16. Receptor-mediated endocytosis of low-density lipoprotein (LDL), with resultant degradation of the endocytosed LDL and recycling of the receptor.

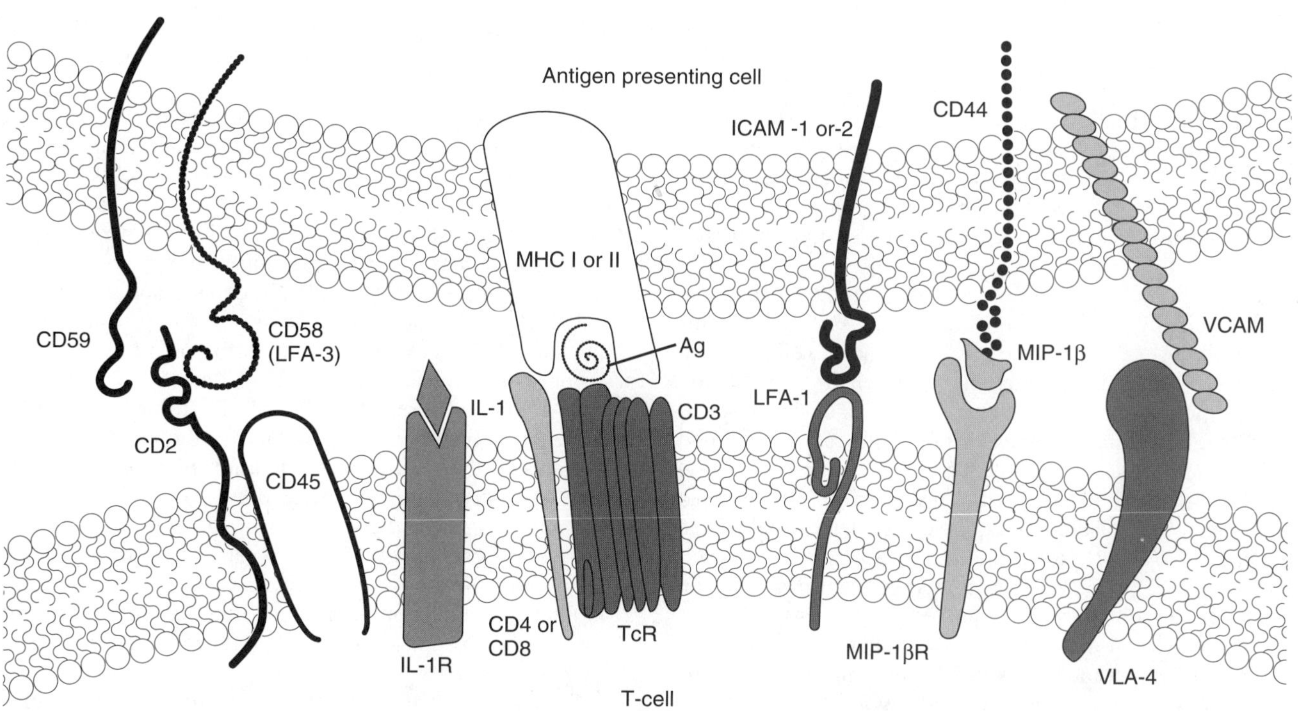

FIG. 1-17. Receptor–ligand interactions. Schematic examples of cell-surface receptors with their cognate ligands. Shown are cytokine–cytokine receptor binding, cell–cell adhesion, selectin–cell-surface receptor adhesion, major histocompatibility complex (MHC)–T-cell receptor (TcR)–CD3 adhesion, and chemokine–chemokine receptor adhesion. LFA, lymphocyte function antigen; ICAM, intracellular adhesion molecule; MIP, macrophage inflammatory protein; VCAM, vascular cell adhesion molecule; VLA, very late antigen.

1 (MAC-1. These leukocyte integrins play a central role in neutrophil and endothelial interactions during inflammation and infection, particularly in the initial steps in diapedesis. MAC-1 and LFA-1 specifically enhance neutrophil and endothelial adhesion after initial stimulation by the chemotactic peptide C5a component of complement, leukotriene B_4, and platelet-activating factor. Interleukin 1 (IL-1) and tumor necrosis factor further amplify this process, resulting in increased endothelial adhesiveness for neutrophils and increased expression of intercellular adhesion molecule 1 (ICAM-1), the only natural ligand of LFA-1. As a result of these steps, neutrophils phagocytose and kill foreign particles. MAC-1 also contributes to natural killer cell activity and has been implicated as mediating adhesive interactions of myeloid cells.

The third major integrin subfamily is the β_3 subfamily, whose major molecules include the platelet glycoprotein IIb/IIIa complex and the vitronectin receptor. Specifically, glycoprotein IIb/IIIa is a calcium-dependent heterodimer that is found on activated platelets and binds fibrinogen, fibronectin, and von Willebrand factor. In addition to being involved in platelet aggregation, glycoprotein IIb/IIIa is expressed on endothelium and may be involved in the spreading of platelets on the subendothelium.

The second important group of adhesion molecules are the *selectins*, also called the LECams (L-lectin, E-epidermal growth factor, C-complement–binding protein), so named because their extracellular domains have regions of homology with the carbohydrate-binding lectins. These molecules appear to mediate adherence of neutrophils, monocytes, and eosinophils during inflammation and thrombosis. E selectin, or endothelial leukocyte adhesion molecule 1 (ELAM-1), is involved in ICAM-1–independent adhesion. ELAM-1 is found on neutrophils and endothelial cells, specifically on the postcapillary venule. L selectin, which is referred to as lymphocyte-homing receptor gp 90^{MEL}, or LECAM-1, is involved in lymphocyte binding to high endothelial venules (HEV) of peripheral lymph nodes, but not to mucosal lymph nodes. P selectin, known as granule membrane protein 140 (GMP-140) and platelet activation dependent granule external membrane protein (PADGEM), is expressed on leukocytes, platelets, and Weibel-Palade bodies of the endothelial cells.

Another group of adhesion molecules are the cadherins, which principally regulate epithelial cell adhesion. Cadherins are a multiple gene family of calcium-dependent cell adhesion molecules with a single-spanning transmembrane structure. Cadherins have two major subfamilies: classic and desmosomal cadherins. The classic cadherins include: (1) E-cadherins, found on adult epithelial cells, (2) N-cadherins, found on adult neural tissue and muscle, and (3) P-cadherins, found on the placenta and epithelial cells. Cadherins require cytoskeletal proteins, like catenin, to bind their cytoplasmic domains. Without this cadherin–catenin complex, cells cannot use the cadherin adhesion system. These molecules are major regulators of such diverse processes as normal morphogenesis and tumor metastasis.

Overall, adhesion molecules have many important biologic roles. The β_1 integrins and cadherins are involved in organogenesis. ICAM-1, E selectins, P selectins, and VCAM-1 are cytokine-responsive during the early stages of inflammation and infection. Wound healing also demonstrates the importance of integrins because platelets bind to exposed matrix through both β_1 and β_2 integrins after injury. Selectins contribute to wound healing by mediating neutrophil migration and thrombosis at the site of injury. Changes in integrin and cadherin expression have been correlated with tumor invasion and metastasis: β_1 expression on squamous cell carcinomas is down-regulated, β_3 expression is up-regulated in melanoma cells, and the RGD peptide has been shown to inhibit melanoma cell migration. Thus, adhesion proteins play critical roles in all aspects of biologic activity, from embryogenesis to malignant transformation.

Cytokines

Cytokines are soluble molecules that instruct cells with appropriate receptors to undergo proliferation, differentiation, or migration. They are an integral part of adhesion molecule expression and cell–cell communication. These molecules are essential for the development of the inflammatory response and thus play an important role in the sepsis syndrome. Frequently, however, there is an imbalance between the beneficial and the detrimental effects of these cytokines in inflammation, autoimmunity, and infection.

At least 60 different cytokines have been identified; these can be grouped into four distinct families: (1) interleukins, (2) colony-stimulating factors, (3) interferons, and (4) chemokines. Clinical applications of cytokines include colony-stimulating factor for patients undergoing chemotherapy, erythropoietin for chronic anemia, the interferons for treatment of certain leukemias and viral infections, and IL-2 for cancer management.

Fifteen *interleukins* have been described, although more are probably yet to be identified. Their exact role in immune responsiveness is poorly understood, owing to the redundancy within the immune system, but these molecules are involved in lymphocyte activation and differentiation. IL-1, IL-2, IL-6, and IL-10 are the most clinically relevant cytokines and are discussed in more detail.

IL-1 is produced by monocytes, macrophages, dendritic cells, natural killer cells, and astrocytes. It induces lymphokine release from T cells, facilitates the growth of fibroblast and synovial cells, stimulates prostaglandin release, and acts as an endogenous pyrogen. It also synergizes with other cytokines during acute infection and shock, resulting in the synthesis of acute-phase proteins, skeletal muscle proteolysis, and the stimulation of the hypothalamic pituitary axis. IL-1 is produced early in the setting of shock and thus is an important cytokine in the systemic inflammatory response syndrome.

IL-2, originally called the T-cell growth factor, is produced by helper T lymphocytes. It induces cytotoxic T lymphocytes and aids in the growth and activation of natural killer cells, B cells, and lymphokine-activated killer cells. Transplantation immunosuppressive therapies attempt to suppress IL-2 production and thus subsequent T-cell expansion. Clinically, IL-2 has been used to treat a variety of cancers, either alone or in combination with lymphokine-activated killer cells or tumor-infiltrating lymphocytes, in an attempt to induce tumor-specific killer lymphocytes.

IL-6 is important not only in the maturation of B cells but also in the acute metabolic response to trauma. It has been found in the circulation after endotoxin injection as well as after elective operations and thermal injury. It is produced by monocytes, fibroblasts, and some tumors. IL-6 induces major histocompatibility class I expression and aids in the production of acute-phase proteins.

IL-10 is produced by helper T cells and acts as a local immunosuppressant. It has been shown to suppress cytokine production, specifically IL-2 and interferon-γ, in helper T cells. Both in vivo and in vitro experiments have demonstrated a decrease in T-cell responsiveness and activation secondary to IL-10. Furthermore, IL-10 has also been shown to regulate the B-cell humoral response.

Colony-stimulating factors stimulate hematopoietic stem cells to mature, differentiate, and expand. The four main colony-stimulating factors are granulocyte colony-stimulating factor, granulocyte-macrophage colony-stimulating factor, macrophage colony-stimulating factor, and erythropoietin. These soluble products, which are primarily produced by T cells, stimulate the bone marrow to increase circulating granulocytes, neutrophils, eosinophils, and macrophages. Clinically, this treatment is frequently used in support of myeloablative chemotherapy regimens and bone marrow transplantation.

The third cytokine family includes the *interferons*. Interferons are a family of glycoproteins normally produced by various mammalian cells in response to viral infections. The three major types are α, β, and γ. These molecules have a variety of dose-dependent immunomodulating effects as well as direct antiproliferative effects that are mediated by binding to cell surface receptors. Interferon-α was the first biologic response modifier approved as an anticancer agent, based on results in hairy cell leukemia. Interferon-γ is a glycoprotein produced almost exclusively by activated T lymphocytes. It appears to have more pronounced immunity-modulating effects on immune cells, including macrophage activation and the increased expression of Fc receptors, which may be important in antibody-mediated cellular cytotoxicity. The interferons have been used as biologic response modifiers in a variety of cancers (eg, hematologic malignancies, melanoma) and viral disease (eg, hepatitis, acquired immunodeficiency syndrome).

Chemokines are a group of cytokines that appear to be both leukocyte chemotactic and activating. These molecules are low-molecular-weight proinflammatory peptides and are divided into two subfamilies: α and β. The α subfamily includes IL-8, melanocyte growth-stimulating activity, and neutrophil-activating peptide 2, all of which affect polymorphonuclear cells but not monocytes. The β subfamily includes monocyte chemotactic and activating factor, macrophage inflammatory protein 1a and 1b, RANTES (*r*egulated on *a*ctivation, *n*ormal *T* *e*xpressed and *s*ecreted), and I-309, which stimulate monocytes, macrophages, T cells, basophils, mast cells, and eosinophils.

Growth Factors

Most cells require growth factors, which are highly potent proteins present in very low concentrations (10^{-9} to 10^{-11} M), to stimulate cell division directly and specifically. Epidermal growth factor, platelet-derived growth factor, transforming growth factor β, IL-2, and the colony-stimulating factors are examples. One new family of growth factors comprises the angiogenic factors. These factors, which are heparin-binding proteins, promote angiogenesis, which is the induction of new blood vessels by a diffusible chemical factor. It appears that the colony-stimulating factors, such as erythropoietin, granulocyte colony-stimulating factor, and granulocyte-macrophage colony-stimulating factor, may also function as angiogenic factors because they work through similar receptors to induce mesoderm and stimulate the formation of blood cells.

This family of heparin-binding growth factors, which initially included only fibroblast growth factor, has now grown to include at least seven members with four known receptors. Additional angiogenesis factors include transforming growth factor β, epidermal growth factor, platelet-derived growth factor, and vascular endothelial growth factors. The principle molecules in the fibroblast growth factor family, the most powerful angiogenic factors, are the acidic and basic fibroblast growth factors. The receptors for these molecules have multiple immunoglobulin-like extracellular domains, a transmembrane domain, and an intracellular tyrosine kinase domain necessary for signal transduction. The tissue distribution of all angiogenesis factors is widespread, including vascular endothelium, vascular smooth muscle, cardiac myocytes, and organs that are heavily vascularized. These molecules have been shown to stimulate most of the individual components of capillary in-growth, including endothelial cell proliferation and release of proteases that digest the basement membrane.

Nitric Oxide

Nitric oxide is a molecule that has an important role in cell–cell interactions and as a second messenger. Nitric oxide is a simple, unstable, potentially toxic gas that is a free radical and is readily diffusible across the cell membrane. Its half-life is between 3 and 50 seconds, and its lability is due to rapid oxidation to nitrates and nitrites. It is synthesized from L-arginine by the enzyme nitric oxide synthetase, which exists in two forms: (1) as a constitutive nitric oxide synthetase, which is calcium dependent, and (2) as an inducible nitric oxide synthetase, which is calcium independent. These enzymes are found in activated macrophages, neutrophils, vascular endothelium, and microglial cells.

Nitric oxide is involved in a wide range of physiologic processes. It controls vascular tone, acts as a neurotransmitter and neuromodulator in the central and peripheral nervous systems, and influences the activity of the immune system. Specifically, nitric oxide is an important determinant of basal vascular tone, myocardial contractility, and platelet–vessel wall interactions. From the perspective of cardiovascular pathophysiology, nitric oxide has been implicated in the pathogenesis of essential hypertension, atherosclerosis, and the hypotension associated with shock states. Nitric oxide also appears to be a selective pulmonary vasodilator and bronchodilator and has been used to treat pulmonary hypertension in infants. High levels of nitric oxide are produced by macrophages in response to endotoxin, interferon, and tumor necrosis factor stimuli as well as tissue damage and graft rejection. Additionally, nitric oxide suppresses leukocyte adhesion and enhances the leukocyte inflammatory response. Thus, nitric oxide, which was once thought to be only a toxic by-product of oxygen free radicals, is in fact a stimulus and an important component of the immune response. Finally, nitric oxide produced by activated lymphocytes can also function in tumor killing, owing to its ability to rupture DNA by nitrosylation as well as by impairing tumor cell mitochondrial enzymes.

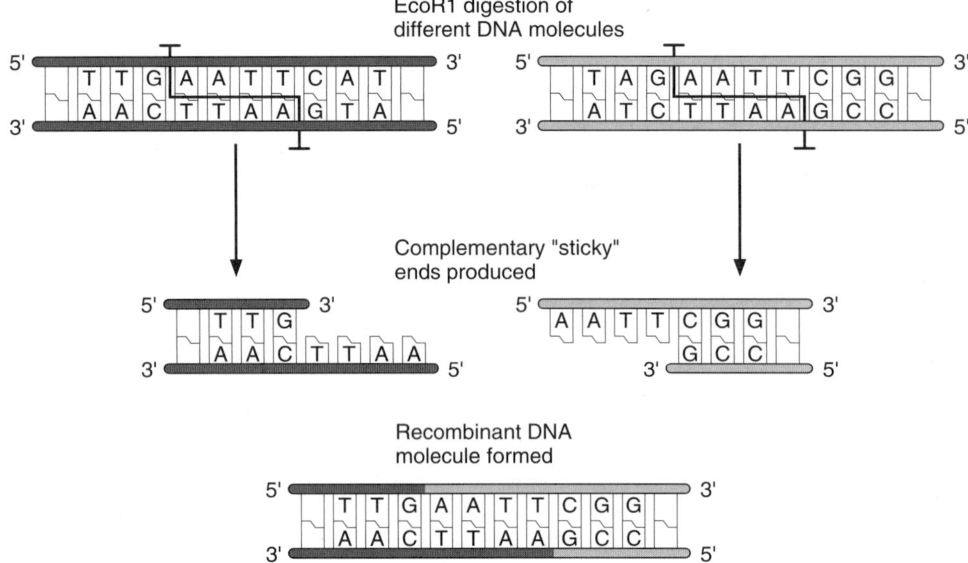

FIG. 1-18. Restriction enzyme digestion and formation of recombinant DNA molecule. Restriction enzymes are bacterial endonucleases that recognize and cleave short stretches of DNA. In this case, the restriction enzyme *Eco*R1, which recognizes the six-nucleotide stretch G-A-A-T-T-C (in the middle of each sequence), is used to cut DNA from two different species, leaving 5′ overhanging ends. Because these ends are complementary, the DNA from the two different species may potentially anneal, forming a recombinant DNA molecule.

RECOMBINANT DNA TECHNOLOGY

The central challenge in modern cell biology is to understand the workings of the cell in molecular detail, particularly examining the structure and function of the cell's DNA. Until the early 1970s, DNA was the most difficult cellular molecule for the biochemist to analyze. Enormously long and chemically monotonous, the nucleotide sequence of DNA could be approached only by indirect means. It is now possible to excise specific regions of DNA in virtually unlimited quantities and to determine the sequence of their nucleotides. By variations of the same techniques, an isolated gene can be altered (engineered) at will and transferred back into cells in culture or into the germ line of animals, where the modified gene becomes incorporated as a permanent functional part of the genome.

Technical breakthroughs have had a dramatic impact on cell biology, by allowing the study of cells and their macromolecules in previously unimagined ways. The most important of these techniques are as follows:

- The specific cleavage of DNA by restriction nucleases
- Nucleic acid hybridization, which makes it possible to find specific sequences of DNA or RNA with great accuracy
- Rapid sequencing of all the nucleotides in a purified DNA fragment
- DNA cloning, whereby a specific DNA fragment is integrated into a self-replicating genetic element (plasmid or virus), allowing the generation of many billions of identical copies in vivo
- PCR, which performs DNA cloning more simply in vitro

Restriction Enzymes

Many of the revolutionary changes that have occurred in the biologic sciences during the past 20 years can be directly attributed to the ability to manipulate DNA. Enzymes that catalyze specific reactions on DNA molecules are one of the major tools used for this genetic manipulation. The discovery of restriction enzymes was probably the breakthrough that ushered in the era of the recombinant DNA technology. Restriction enzymes recognize short nucleotide sequences and cleave double-stranded DNA at specific sites within or adjacent to those sequences (Fig. 1-18). The recognition sequences are generally four to six nucleotides in length and are usually *palindromic* (antiparallel sequences identical). Some restriction enzymes cleave at the axis of symmetry, yielding "blunt" ends. Others make staggered cleavages, yielding overhanging single-stranded 3′ or 5′ ends known as *cohesive* or "sticky" ends. Unrelated DNA molecules, if cut with the same restriction enzyme, can anneal together, forming a recombinant DNA molecule (see Fig. 1-18). This is one of the basic principles used in genetic engineering.

Restriction Fragment Length Polymorphisms

Researchers have been able to locate many human genes using "forward genetics," whereby genes are found through their previously known protein products. Examples include the genes for sickle cell anemia, Tay-Sachs disease, hemophilia, thalassemia, and hypercholesterolemia. Most genetic defects, however, do not yet have an identified defective protein. In the early 1980s, an alternative approach was introduced to permit identification of a gene on the basis of its chromosome location alone, without knowledge of the exact genetic defect. This process was initially termed *reverse genetics* and more recently has been termed *positional cloning*.

Positional cloning has its origin in the work of Thomas Morgan, who mapped the genes of fruit flies. After locating single genes that determined eye color, wing shape, and bristle patterns, Morgan used these genes as markers to help locate the position of other closely linked genes. Constructing such a linkage map in humans initially appeared difficult because almost no genetic markers were known relative to mapped genes. Researchers using restriction enzymes to digest genomic DNA noticed a phenomenon that was to provide the key to gene hunters. When chromosomes of different people were incubated with the same restriction enzyme, the lengths of the resulting DNA fragments often differed. The explanation for this was straightforward: slight individual differences exist in human DNA sequences, and when one of those variations occurs at a restriction enzyme site, the enzyme no longer cuts at that site. This genetic heterogeneity is manifested when these DNA restriction fragments are analyzed by Southern blotting. These variations in restriction fragment lengths are referred to as *restriction fragment length polymorphisms* (RFLPs, dubbed ''riflips''). Because these RFLPs are inherited, they provided the valuable markers required to hunt for elusive genes. Today, many diseases are diagnosed prenatally by RFLP linkage analysis, including hemophilia A and B, Huntington disease, myotonic dystrophy, and Friedreich ataxia.

Hybridization

Gel Electrophoresis

DNA, RNA, and protein samples can be isolated from a variety of tissues (eg, blood, solid tumors, tissue culture cells) based on differential solubility and centrifugation characteristics. These species can than be separated by electrophoresis, a technique that separates ionic solutes by differences in their migration rates in an applied electric field (Fig. 1-19A). Electrophoresis, using either agarose or polyacrylamide gels, also allows purification and subsequent identification of nucleic acid fragments. The technique is simple, rapid, and capable of resolving fragments that cannot be separated adequately by other procedures. Polyacrylamide gels are most effective for separating small fragments of DNA (5 to 500 base pairs), and they can resolve DNA fragments that differ in size by only 1 base pair. Agarose gels have a lower resolving power but a greater range of separation, from 200 base pairs to about 50 kilobase pairs. DNA, which is negatively charged at neutral pH, migrates toward the positively charged anode when an electric field is applied. RNA will also migrate toward the anode after treatment with a denaturing agent such as formaldehyde. Both DNA and RNA migrate through gel matrices at rates that are inversely proportional to the $\log_{10}$ of the number of base pairs. Larger molecules migrate more slowly because of greater frictional drag and because they worm their way through the pores of the gel less efficiently than smaller molecules. Once separated by electrophoresis, nucleic acids within an agarose gel can be detected by staining with the fluorescent dye ethidium bromide (Fig. 1-20). Polyacrylamide gels require more complex detection schema, such as the use of radiolabeled molecules and exposure of the gel to x-ray film (autoradiography).

Detecting specific nucleic acid sequences by hybridization is one of the more fundamental techniques used in molecular biology. Hybridization is based on the fact that single-stranded nucleic acid molecules form a double-stranded molecule when they encounter a complementary strand. This technique is widely used to identify nucleic acid sequences in both DNA (Southern blot) and RNA (Northern blot) samples. This process requires nucleic acid probes, which are short segments of nucleic acids complementary to a particular DNA or RNA molecule. They can be obtained through digestion of naturally purified nucleic acids or created using an automated DNA

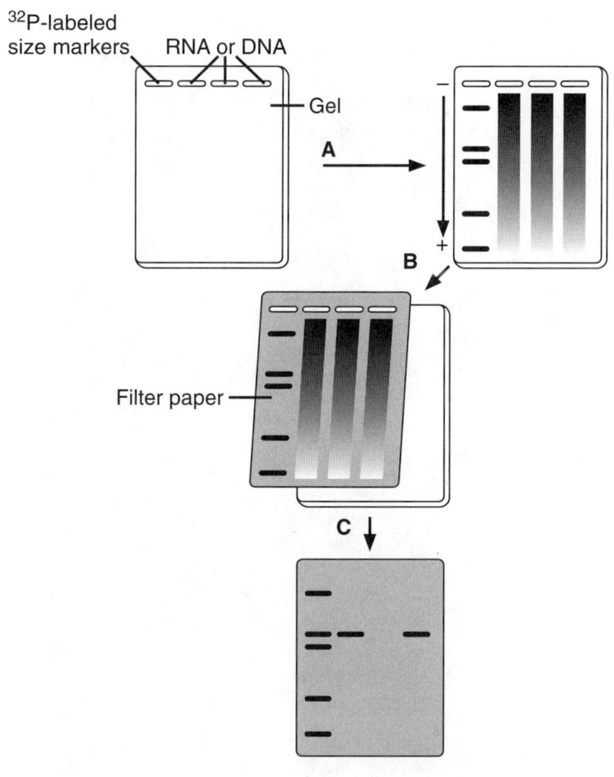

FIG. 1-19. DNA or RNA samples are loaded into a well of agarose gel. (*A*) Nucleic acid samples are separated in an electrical field, based on their size, with the smallest migrating the farthest. (*B*) The samples are transferred from the gel to a filter paper by a variety of methods: capillary action, positive pressure, or vacuum. (*C*) The filter paper is incubated with a radiolabeled probe of the sequence of interest. This filter paper is then used to expose x-ray film, producing the autoradiogram. In this illustration, lanes 2 and 4 have the sequence of interest, but lane 3 does not. Known standard molecular weight markers in lane 1 allow for accurate size determination.

synthesizer. Probes must have a sufficient number of base pairs complementary to the nucleic acid sequence of interest to identify it uniquely, and they must be labeled to determine their presence in a sample. Probes can be labeled a number of ways, with both radionuclides and nonradioactive markers.

Localization of a particular DNA sequence is accomplished by the transfer technique initially described by E.M. Southern. Better known as the Southern blot, genomic DNA is first isolated and then digested by restriction enzymes. These DNA fragments are denatured, separated by gel electrophoresis, and then transferred from the gel to a nitrocellulose or nylon membrane (ie, blotting), maintaining the relative positions of all the DNA fragments (see Fig. 1-19B). The DNA is then permanently attached to the membrane and incubated with a single-stranded radiolabeled nucleic acid probe (hybridization) specific for that DNA sequence. The filter is then washed to remove nonspecific binding of the probe and dried, and autoradiography is performed (see Fig. 1-19C). In a manner analogous to Southern blotting, RNA can be separated by electrophoresis and transferred to a nitrocellulose or nylon membrane. The RNA of inter-

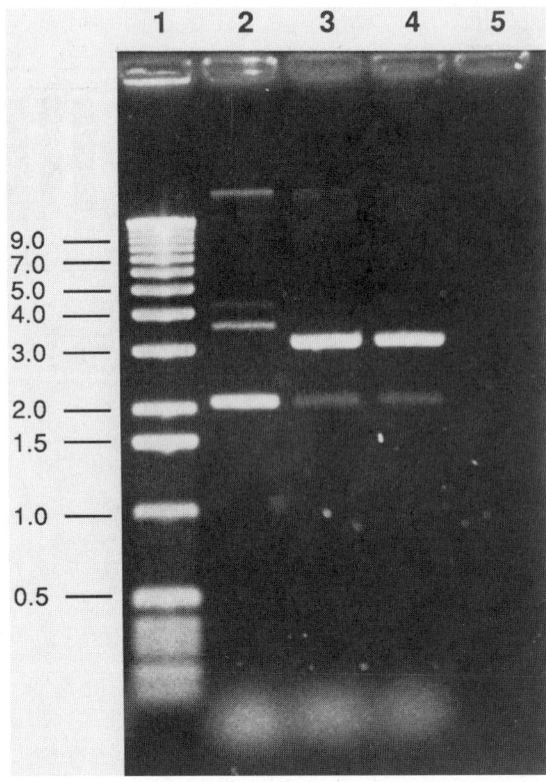

FIG. 1-20. Nucleic acid fragment separation and size determination demonstrated using ethidium bromide–stained agarose gel. A 1% agarose gel is poured, plasmid samples are placed into the wells, and the gel subjected to 50 V. Samples migrate from the wells (*top*) toward the positive node (*bottom*) according to size. The wells contain the following: lane 1, DNA molecular weight standards; lane 2, the circularized plasmid pKS containing the gene from β-actin; lane 3, the plasmid pKS with a small β-actin probe, now linear after digestion by restriction enzyme HindIII; lane 4, the plasmid pKS with a small β-actin probe, now linear after digestion by restriction enzyme KpnI. Nondigested plasmid in lane 2 has several bands, depicting the different forms of the same plasmid depending on how tightly coiled they are. Lanes 3 and 4 have one main band (the linear plasmid pKS–β-actin) and a much lighter band (the highly coiled pKS, which is not fully cut by the restriction enzymes). The smear at the bottom of lanes 2 through 4 represents RNA.

est is then located by autoradiography after incubation with a radiolabeled single-stranded nucleic acid probe.

Protein Detection

In a manner analogous to that for nucleic acids, proteins can also be separated by electrophoresis and detected using a variety of techniques. Proteins are also separated based on molecular weight by the technique of sodium dodecyl sulfate-polyacrylamide gel electrophoresis (SDS-PAGE). SDS coats the proteins, giving them a net negative charge, facilitating their migration in an electrical field. Sample preparation is particularly crucial for accurate separation of proteins based on molecular weight. The proteins must be denatured by exposure to heat in the presence of a denaturing agent such as SDS, and reduced by β-mercaptoethanol or dithiothreitol. This procedure solubilizes and denatures proteins, dissociates polypeptides, and reduces disulfide bonds, making their migration in an electrical field more reproducible of their molecular weight. Their molecular weight is then estimated by comparing their gel mobility to molecular weight standards run at the same time (Fig. 1-21*A*). Detection of the protein species after electrophoresis is usually performed by staining. Coomassie blue (sensitivity, 50 ng) and silver staining (sensitivity, 1 to 5 ng) are the most common nonspecific stains used, while identification of a specific protein, with sensitivities to 10 pg, can be accomplished with the Western blot.

Detection of individual protein species in an immunoblot, or Western blot, is dependent on the specificity of antibody–protein interactions. Either polyclonal (produced by animal immunization) or monoclonal (produced by hybridomas) antibodies must first be raised to the protein of interest. Proteins are separated in an SDS-PAGE gel and electrically transferred to a membrane for immobilization. The membrane is then incubated with the primary antibody, which binds to the protein of interest (Fig. 1-22). After washing off nonspecific binding, the membrane is incubated with a secondary antibody, which recognizes features of the primary antibody. This secondary antibody also carries a reporter enzyme, such as alkaline phosphatase or horseradish peroxidase, which allows detection of the primary antibody–secondary antibody sandwich by catalyzing a chemical reaction. This chemical reaction can produce a visible stained deposit (see Fig. 1-21*B*), or it can generate light using recently developed, highly sensitive chemiluminescence reagents. The resulting light can then directly expose photographic film.

DNA Sequencing

Technique

Knowledge of the exact sequence of nitrogenous bases of a gene is a prerequisite for its further manipulation. During the past several years, investigators have deduced and published the DNA sequence of many genes of personal interest. In an ambitious attempt to sequence the entire human genome, Dr. James Watson organized the Human Genome Project in 1989. This represents a 15-year, $200,000,000 international effort whose main objective is to determine the complete nucleotide sequence of the human genome, localizing all estimated 50,000 to 100,000 genes.

DNA sequencing techniques are based on electrophoretic separation of a heterogeneous population of DNA molecules using high-resolution denaturing polyacrylamide gels. These so-called sequencing gels are capable of resolving up to 500 bases in a single gel. The most common sequencing method employed is the enzymatic dideoxy method originally developed by F. Sanger. This technique imitates DNA replication, employing both a DNA polymerase and all four 2′-deoxynucleoside triphosphates (dNTP corresponds to any one of the four). Sanger's dideoxy sequencing method capitalizes on the ability of the DNA polymerase to also use 2′,3′-dideoxynucleoside triphosphates (ddNTPs), in addition to dNTPs, as substrates (Fig. 1-23). As long as dNTPs are incorporated into the growing

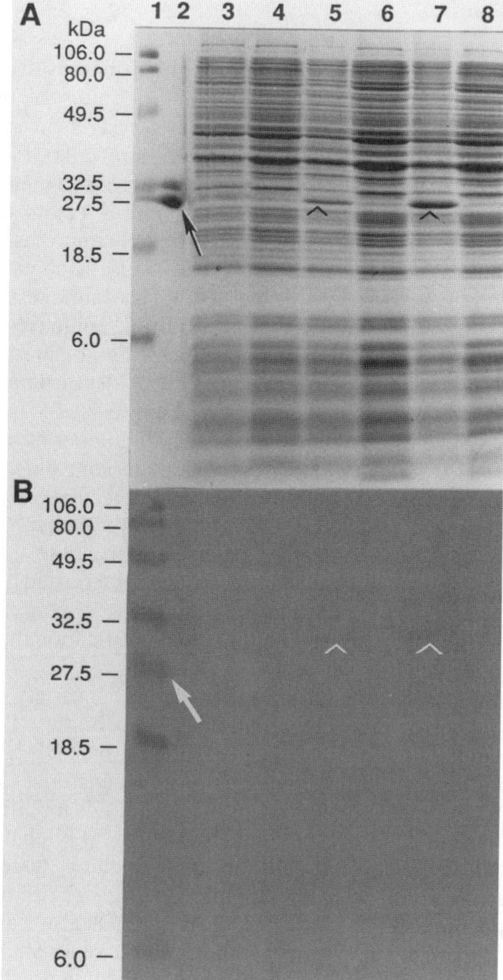

FIG. 1-21. SDS-PAGE protein gel with concomitant Western blot. (*A*) Ricin A chain (RTA), a potent plant hemitoxin, was expressed as an inducible recombinant protein in *Escherichia coli*. Proteins were then extracted from *E coli* lysates, separated SDS-PAGE, and detected by Coomassie brilliant blue staining. Lane 1, protein molecular weight markers; lane 2, control plant RTA (about 30 kd) with two forms due to differential glycosylation (*arrow*); lanes 3 and 4, protein production in *E coli* transformed with the *RTA* gene in both forward (lane 3) and reverse (lane 4) directions, without induction; lanes 5 and 6, protein production in *E coli* transformed with the *RTA* gene in both forward (lane 3) and reverse (lane 4) directions, 3 hours after induction with isopropyl β-D-thiogalactoside (IPTG); lanes 7 and 8, protein production in *E coli* transformed with the *RTA* gene in forward (lane 3) and reverse (lane 4) directions, overnight after induction with IPTG. Arrowheads point to a 30-kd band in lane 5, which increases in intensity in lane 7, representing plant RTA produced by *E coli*. (*B*) Western blot performed on the same SDS-PAGE gel. After electrical transfer of proteins to nitrocellulose paper, the nitrocellulose is incubated with a mouse polyclonal antiricin primary antibody and then a goat antimouse secondary antibody. This secondary antibody also carries the reporter enzyme horseradish peroxidase, which allows detection of the primary antibody–secondary antibody sandwich by catalyzing a chemical reaction and producing a visible stained deposit. Besides the molecular weight markers, the only bands detected are the control plant RTA (*arrow*) and the recombinant RTA (*arrowheads*).

DNA chain, a free 3′ hydroxyl group will be available, which is required for continued polymerization of the new DNA strand. However, ddNTPs lack a 3′ hydroxyl group and thus act as chain terminators when incorporated into the DNA chain. Thus, DNA synthesis in the presence of all four dNTPs (one radioactively labeled) and one ddNTP yields a population of molecules with common 5′ ends but different 3′ ends, depending on the site at which a ddNTP was incorporated. Four separate reactions are performed, each with a different ddNTP. The products of the four reactions are analyzed by electrophoresis through a denaturing polyacrylamide gel, separating the different DNA fragments based on size. After drying the sequencing gel and exposing it to x-ray film, the sequence of the DNA of concern can be read from the autoradiogram.

Computational Sequence Analysis

The number of available gene sequences is doubling about every 22 months. Molecular sequence data has become the "common currency" of biomedical research and often provides exciting and unexpected links between diverse biologic systems. These connections accelerate research progress and may even open up entire new fields of inquiry. For example, the discovery in the early 1980s that the viral oncogene *sis* was 80% identical to human platelet-derived growth factor demonstrated that great advances in understanding the biochemical basis of disease could be made by analyzing sequence data. This process, made possible by the existence of publicly funded electronic data bases, represents one of the essential methods that all molecular biologists must understand.

For the past several years, the National Center for Biotechnology Information has been developing information resources that integrate molecular sequence and structural data with the MEDLINE bibliographic data base. These resources are designed

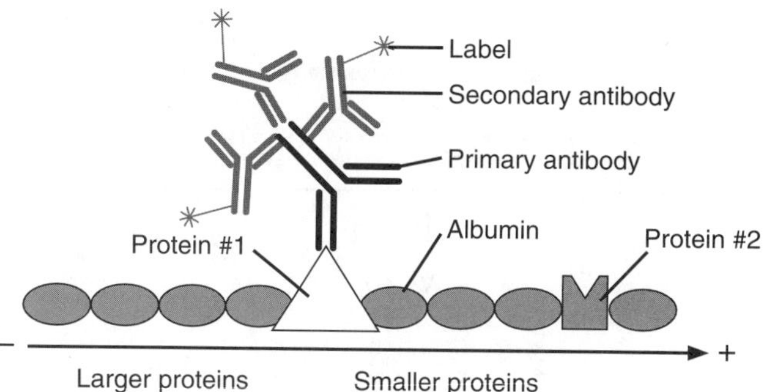

FIG. 1-22. Schematic representation of an immunoblot (Western blot) after the proteins are separated in an electrical field according to size and transferred from a polyacrylamide gel to filter paper. The filter paper is incubated with albumin (to block nonspecific antibody binding) and then with an antibody raised against protein #1 (primary antibody). After gentle washes, the paper is incubated with another antibody (secondary antibody) raised against the immunoglobulins of the species where the primary antibody was made (eg, sheep antirabbit antibody). A label is added to the secondary antibody, which either catalyzes a visible colorimetric reaction, produces chemiluminescence (detected by photography paper), or emits radioactivity (detected by radiograph).

for easy access over national high-speed computer networks or through CD-ROM disks. The BLAST (*basic local alignment search tool*) network service allows one to formulate a data base search locally, transport it thousands of miles over Internet to a remote high-speed computer, and then return the results in a matter of seconds for inspection.

DNA Cloning

Cloning is a method by which an unlimited quantity of a particular DNA segment can be made. Cloning requires the use of a vector, which is a DNA molecule that can propagate in a particular host (bacteria, yeast, or eukaryotic culture cells). Plasmids, which are bacterial self-replicating extrachromosomal DNA molecules, are the most frequently used cloning vectors. In 1981, Stanley Cohen and Herbert Boyer significantly improved the use of plasmids as cloning vectors by including three common features: a replicator, a selectable marker (eg, antibiotic resistance), and a cloning site (a small region with multiple unique restriction enzyme sites). The cloning procedure begins with digestion of a plasmid and foreign DNA of interest with an identical restriction enzyme, chosen to cut in the plasmid's cloning site. When these two DNA species are coincubated, a small number of plasmid-foreign DNA molecules are created through annealing of their complementary ends. These recombinant molecules are then introduced back into bacterial cells in a process called *transformation* and are grown in the presence of the appropriate antibiotic. The plasmids can then be isolated from the bacteria and the DNA insert removed by incubation with the original restriction enzyme. This process permits the in vivo amplification of a DNA fragment.

Plasmids are not the only cloning vectors. A variety of other vectors differ in their DNA insert size capabilities. Plasmids can reliably carry from 0.01 to 10 kilobase pair DNA inserts. Bacteriophages, which are viruses that infect bacteria, can carry 10 to 25 kilobase pair inserts. Cosmids, plasmids modified with bacteriophage genome, can hold from 35 to 50 kilobase pairs, and DNA inserts up to 500 kilobase pairs can be cloned into yeast artificial chromosomes. Some cloning vectors not only can replicate foreign DNA in a host cell but also can direct the production of the foreign protein. These vectors are called *expression vectors,* and a large number of human substances (eg, insulin, tumor necrosis factor, lymphokines, growth factors) are produced in bacteria in this manner.

Transfection

Transfection describes the introduction of foreign DNA into cells of higher eukaryotes. This can be accomplished in a variety of ways. One method uses calcium phosphate, which binds to DNA and increases its uptake. Electroporation involves placing

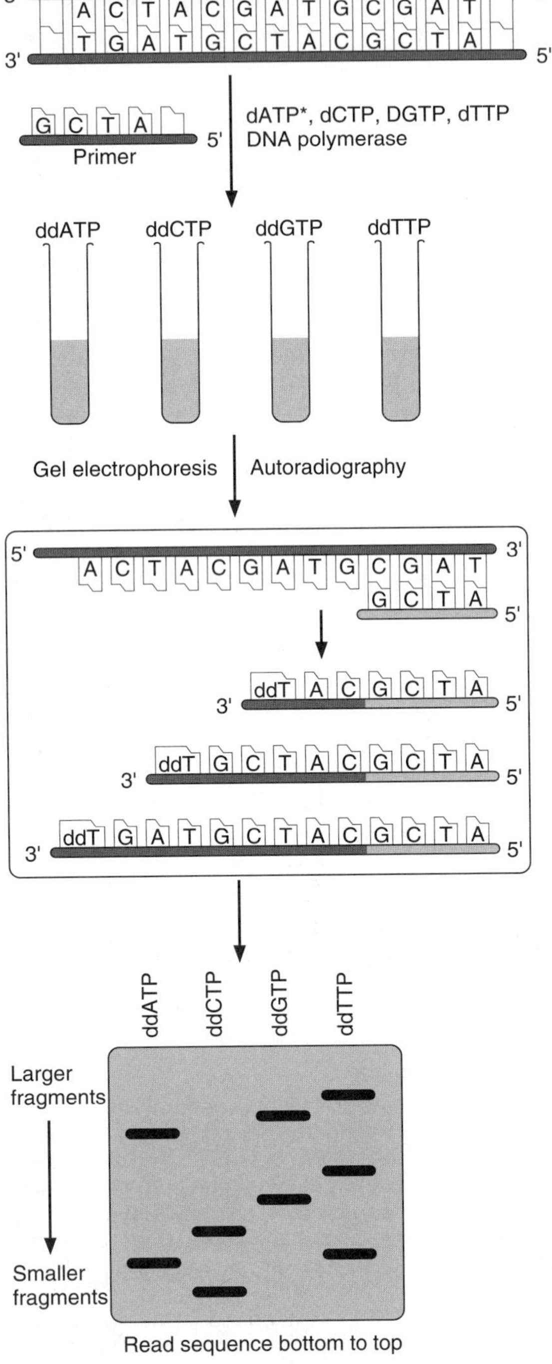

FIG. 1-23. Sanger dideoxy sequencing reaction. This method is based on DNA replication, using DNA polymerase, all four deoxynucleotides (dNTPs) and a small primer in which replication is initiated. In addition, dideoxynucleotides (ddNTPs), which are identical to dNTPs except that they lack a 3′ hydroxyl group, are added to the DNA replication mixture, one per reaction. As long as dNTPs are incorporated into the growing DNA chain, a free 3′ hydroxyl group will be available, which is required for continued DNA polymerization. Because ddNTPs lack a 3′ hydroxyl group, however, they act as chain terminators. Thus, DNA synthesis in the presence of all four dNTPs (one radiolabeled) and one ddNTP yields a population of molecules with common 5′ ends but different 3′ ends (*inset* = one of four sequencing reactions, this one using ddTTP. Three additional reactions would be performed using ddATP, ddCTP and ddGTP). The products of the four reactions are analyzed by electrophoresis, and the sequence of the DNA of interest can be read from an autoradiogram.

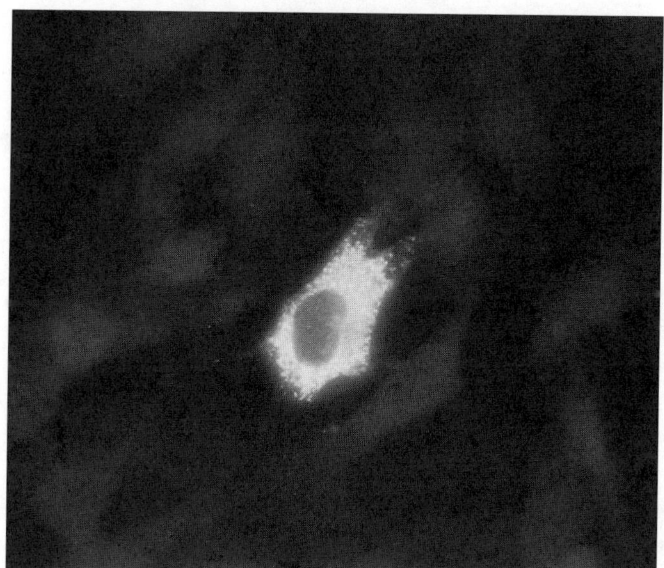

FIG. 1-24. Localization of an antigen expressed by a transfected gene. This image shows the expression of a transfected gene in a large population of cultured cells. The human gene for p55 (disulfide isomerase), a protein antigen expressed in the lumen of the endoplasmic reticulum, was transfected into a population of mouse fibroblasts. The cells were fixed and made permeable. Immunofluorescence was performed that recognizes only the human form of this protein and not the endogenous mouse counterpart. In this field, only one cell has been successfully transfected, and the pattern of the endoplasmic reticulum and nuclear envelope is apparent, whereas neighboring nontransfected cells show no labeling.

cells into an electrical field, which alters their membrane permeability and facilitates the uptake of foreign DNA. Lipofection induces transfection by using lipid vesicles that fuse directly with the cell membrane. Most of these eukaryotic methods are not as efficient as the heat-shock method used to transform bacteria. For example, when cultured mammalian cells are transfected, the percentage of cells in the culture that express the transfected gene and its resulting protein is low, usually less than 5%. Such expressing cells can be detected using sensitive enzyme assays for the entire culture or by immunohistochemical detection of the expressed protein in individual cells (Fig. 1-24). In addition to indicating the percentage of cells transfected, these techniques also provide information about the cellular compartments in which these new proteins are located.

Retroviral strategies have gained popularity. This process uses RNA viruses, which have the ability to inject their nucleic acid directly into a cell. These retroviruses must be genetically engineered by replacing the viral genes necessary for replication with the DNA of interest. Finally, transgenic techniques are the most sophisticated method of introducing foreign DNA into another host. This technique involves direct needle injection of DNA into the male pronucleus of a fertilized oocyte, with subsequent implantation of the manipulated oocyte into a foster mother. Subsequent progeny can then be bred, eventually allowing studies of the functional effects of the DNA inserted into the germline.

Polymerase Chain Reaction

The development of the PCR by Kary B. Mullis and a team of workers at Cetus Corporation is clearly one of the most im-

portant technical advances in molecular biology in the past decade. It is an ingenious new method that has had an effect on molecular biology second only to the description of the DNA molecule.

A major problem in analyzing genes is that they are rare targets in a complex genome. PCR enables one to produce enormous copy numbers (up to 10^9) of a specific DNA sequence without resorting to cloning. Moreover, the ability to propagate DNA from amounts too minute for standard cloning techniques gives the method such extraordinary power and sensitivity that the DNA in fixed pathologic specimens, human hairs, a single sperm cell, or ancient mummies now can be analyzed.

Technique

The PCR is divided into three steps: (1) denaturation of the DNA to single strands by high temperature exposure, (2) annealing of oligonucleotide (15 to 40 base pairs) primers to the DNA single strands on either side of the sequence of interest, and (3) replication of the DNA from the primer–template double-stranded complex by DNA polymerase (Fig. 1-25). These three steps are commonly repeated up to 30 times, generating enormous amplification of the desired DNA sequence.

DNA can be made single stranded by subjecting it to high temperatures (95°C), but most DNA polymerases would be irreversibly denatured at such a high temperature. The discovery of the enzyme *Taq* polymerase, a DNA polymerase isolated from the *Thermus aquaticus* bacterium found in the geysers of Yellowstone National Park, allowed the PCR process to be automated. This polymerase replicates DNA best at temperatures of 75°C but is stable at 95°C, making it ideal for use in PCR.

Although DNA replication requires a single-stranded DNA molecule, initiation of DNA replication must begin at a small double-stranded region. This starting point for DNA replication in the PCR reaction is specified by supplying two oligonucleotide primers (15 to 40 base pairs long), chemically synthesized to be complementary to the flanking regions of the DNA sequence in question. When these primers are added to the DNA specimen, two specific double-stranded areas are created that become the initiation sites for DNA synthesis. Choosing these oligonucleotide primers correctly is important because they must anneal on opposite strands and direct DNA replication toward the opposite primer site. This points out the main drawback of PCR—the sequence of the DNA of interest must be known beforehand (though not in all cases).

The temperature at each PCR step is strictly regulated. Normally, the DNA strands separate at 95°C, anneal with the primers at 55°C, and extend using *Taq* polymerase at 72°C. By rapidly thermoregulating the temperature back to 95°C, the polymerization reaction stops, the double-stranded DNA molecules separate, and the process can be repeated. The development of a low-cost, programmable thermal cycling device has also significantly automated the process.

The importance of extreme care in the performance and interpretation of PCR cannot be overemphasized. Sample contamination is unacceptable because this material may be amplified inadvertently. Negative-control material is extremely valuable in detecting this contamination. To avoid these artifacts, laboratories must implement special procedures, such as the use of

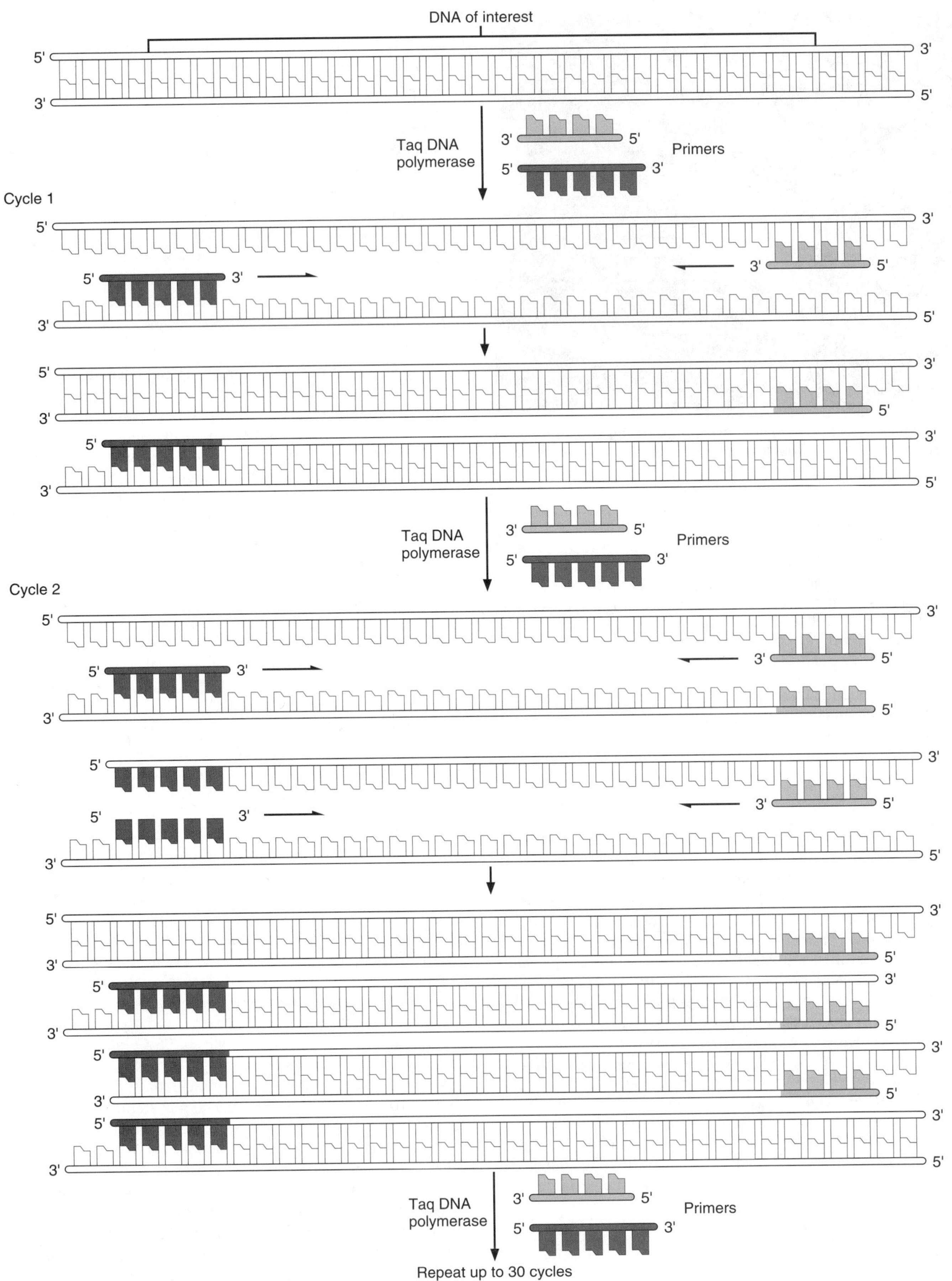

DNA of interest
5'
3'
3'
5'
Taq DNA
polymerase
3' 5'
Primers
5' 3'
Cycle 1
5' 3'
3' 5'
5' 3'
3' 5'
5' 3'
3' 5'
5' 3'
Taq DNA
polymerase
3' 5'
Primers
5' 3'
Cycle 2
5' 3'
5' 3'
3' 5'
5' 3'
5' 3'
3' 5'
5' 3'
3' 5'
5' 3'
5' 3'
3' 5'
5' 3'
3' 5'
Taq DNA
polymerase
3' 5'
Primers
5' 3'
Repeat up to 30 cycles

positive-displacement pipettes and the physical separation of reactions occurring before and after the PCR.

Applications

PCR is most commonly used to determine whether a given sequence of DNA exists in a clinical specimen. There has been significant progress in the rapid diagnosis of infectious disease by PCR, particularly in the detection of the human immunodeficiency virus. PCR also greatly facilitates the prenatal diagnosis of a variety of genetic disorders, including cystic fibrosis, β-thal-

assemia, and hemophilia. PCR plays a major role in cancer research, identifying chromosomal abnormalities, detecting mutations in oncogenes and tumor suppressor genes, and demonstrating the presence of RNA or DNA tumor viruses.

PCR has applications other than in the medical field. It facilitated the construction of phylogenetic trees that confirm the African origin of humans, and DNA from extinct species like the woolly mammoth and the quagga have been subjected to PCR amplification. PCR has also allowed the genetic typing of biologic evidence found at a crime scene by amplifying polymorphic sequences, and it has been applied increasingly in this setting since its first use in 1986 (*Pennsylvania* v *Pestinikis*).

1.2   Principles of Genetics

Sonja A. Rasmussen and Ada Hamosh

Genetic factors contribute significantly to conditions of consequence to pediatric surgeons. Recognition of conditions with a genetic cause is critical to allow for accurate recurrence risk counseling of families. Furthermore, appreciation of these disorders may lead the surgeon to identify other manifestations that could affect the patient's prognosis and surgical management.

Two studies illustrate the contribution of genetic factors to disease in children. The first, performed in the early 1970s, demonstrated the frequency of genetic conditions in hospitalized children.[1] About 25% of patients admitted to a general pediatric hospital had a condition with a significant genetic component. Of these, about 4% had single-gene disorders, 0.6% had chromosomal abnormalities, and 22% had multifactorial or polygenic conditions. With improved control of infectious diseases, it is likely that the contribution of genetic factors to pediatric disease is even higher now than when this study was performed. When evaluated on a population basis, genetic disorders continue to make a significant impact. About 5% of live-born individuals in a population study in British Columbia had a condition with an important genetic component that presented before age 25 years.[2] A similar distribution was observed in this study between single-gene disorders (3.6 in 1000), chromosomal abnormalities (1.8 in 1000), and multifactorial conditions (46.6 in 1000).

DNA AND GENES

DNA, the genetic material, is a double helical structure consisting of four bases (adenine, guanine, cytosine, and thymine) on a sugar and phosphate backbone (see Section 1.1). DNA replication occurs through a semiconservative mechanism; the double

helix separates, and new strands form using the previous strands as templates. During replication, cytosine pairs only with guanine, adenine binds only with thymine. DNA is converted to RNA by transcription, and RNA is converted to a protein by translation. Each set of three bases codes for an amino acid; therefore, the bases comprise a code that determines the entire protein's amino acid sequence. The structure of a gene consists of exons (the portion of the sequence that is translated to protein) and introns (intervening sequences). After DNA is converted to a primary RNA transcript, the intron sequences, as well as sequences at the beginning and end of the genes, must be removed to form the mature messenger RNA. This message is then transferred from the nucleus to the cytoplasm, where translation occurs.

An estimate suggests there are about 60,000 to 70,000 genes in the human genome.[3] These genes are in pairs, with one member of each pair coming from each parent. The term *allele* refers to alternative forms of a gene present at a locus, or location on a chromosome. A person with two of the same alleles at a particular locus is referred to as a *homozygote,* while a person with two different alleles at a locus is called a *heterozygote.* When only one allele is present at a locus (such as in loci on the X chromosome in males), the person is termed *hemizygous.* The alleles present at a particular locus are referred to as *genotype,* and the clinical expression of that genotype in a patient is called *phenotype.*

POLYMORPHISMS AND DISEASE-PRODUCING MUTATIONS

Changes in genetic material are of two types: polymorphisms and disease-producing mutations. Polymorphisms are variations

FIG. 1-25. The polymerase chain reaction (PCR) is divided into three steps: (1) denaturation of the DNA, (2) annealing of oligonucleotide primers to the single-stranded DNA, and (3) replication of the DNA from the primer–template complex by DNA polymerase. The starting point for DNA replication is determined by supplying two oligonucleotide primers that specifically anneal to opposite strands of the DNA, flanking the area of interest. The DNA polymerase used to replicate the DNA must be stable at 95°C (temperature used to denature the DNA). Frequently, more than 30 cycles are performed, generating enormous amounts of the DNA of interest without resorting to cloning.

in the DNA sequence that do not produce disease. These modifications, which occur once in every 500 base pairs, are sometimes helpful for following the inheritance of a nearby gene within a family. Polymorphisms are rare in coding regions of the gene and are more often found in introns or between genes. They can sometimes be detected using restriction endonucleases, which are bacterial enzymes that cut DNA at specific sites. DNA, exposed to a restriction enzyme, is cut at specific sites, resulting in DNA fragments of particular sizes. If a polymorphism occurs at the restriction endonuclease site, the size of the resultant fragments is altered. DNA alterations that change restriction endonuclease sites are called *restriction fragment length polymorphisms* (RFLPs). When near to or within a gene of interest, RFLPs have been used for indirect DNA diagnosis, a topic to be discussed later in this chapter.

Many different types of disease-producing mutations have been identified. A change in a single base pair is referred to as a *point mutation.* This may be either a missense mutation, in which a single amino acid is changed in the protein product, or a nonsense mutation, in which the base pair change results in premature termination of protein translation. The mRNA produced from an allele having undergone a nonsense mutation is often unstable and may result in a significantly reduced amount of protein product.[4,5] Mutations can also alter the initiation codon, and then the initiation of translation does not occur where it should. If a nucleotide changes at or near the intron–exon junction, the splicing mechanism that removes the introns from the coding sequence may be altered. Mutations that change the length of the gene are called *insertions* and *deletions.* If the number of nucleotides added or deleted is not a multiple of three, a frameshift mutation occurs. This means that the reading frame for the DNA sequence following the mutation is incorrect, and therefore all the subsequent codons are altered. This generally results in a premature stop codon, and the effects on the protein level are as with a nonsense mutation, as discussed earlier.

SINGLE-GENE DISORDERS

Single-gene disorders have been documented in McKusick's *Mendelian Inheritance in Man* since the first edition in 1966.[6] Nearly 1500 single-gene conditions were included in the first edition, while in the 11th edition (1994), 6678 conditions are included. Most of these are autosomal dominant (4458), with a lesser number being autosomal recessive (1730) and X-linked (412). Y-linked and mitochondrial conditions were included in this edition for the first time. Because of the rapid advances in this area, this catalog is available as an on-line computerized database. *Mendelian Inheritance in Man* assigns numbers to single-gene conditions, and these are referred to in this chapter as MIM numbers.

Autosomal Dominant Inheritance

In an autosomal (non–sex-linked) dominant condition, an abnormality in one member of the pair is sufficient to cause the condition. Although the strict definition of a dominant condition specifies that the heterozygous person is indistinguishable from the homozygous abnormal person, this is often not the case. Instead, frequently the homozygote is more severely affected than the heterozygote.

Most dominant conditions involve the formation of structural proteins. Two explanations have been proposed for how mutations in one gene of a pair can result in a phenotype; these have been termed *dominant loss of function* and *dominant-negative effect.* Dominant loss of function occurs when the abnormal gene does not produce a protein product; because only one of the pair of genes is working properly, only half of the normal amount of product is formed. The term *dominant-negative effect* has been proposed to describe the situation in which the abnormal gene makes a product that interferes with the normal gene product function (the phenotype is due to an abnormal gene product, not absence of a normal gene product).[7] Evidence suggests that both of these circumstances occur.

Patients with dominant conditions have a 50% risk of passing the condition on to their offspring, and males and females are affected with equal frequency. Patients with autosomal dominant conditions often have other affected family members. Pedigrees in which an autosomal dominant condition is segregating often show a vertical pattern of transmission, with multiple generations affected (Fig. 1-26). Because dominant conditions have a wide variability in expression, a parent might not be identified as having the condition unless he or she is carefully examined for minor manifestations. Rarely, there are no clinical signs in the parent who transmits the mutant gene. This is termed *incomplete penetrance.* In some cases, neither parent is affected, and the child is a sporadic mutation. The frequency of these new mutations increases with increasing parental age.

An example of a common autosomal dominant condition is neurofibromatosis type 1 (NF1; MIM 162200), which occurs in 1 in 3000 people. This condition is characterized by neurofibromas, benign tumors that arise from the peripheral nervous system. Cutaneous neurofibromas are located just underneath the skin and are primarily of cosmetic significance, while plexiform neurofibromas develop from a deeply placed nerve and, because of their size and position, may disrupt growth of other tissues. Other features of NF1, including cafe-au-lait spots (asymptomatic, lightly pigmented macules found on the skin) and Lisch nodules (iris hamartomas that have no effect on vision), are important in establishing the diagnosis. Other features of clinical significance include learning problems or mental retardation, macrocephaly, short stature, scoliosis, hypertension, and increased risk of malignancy.[8] Based on clinical data, about half of the cases of NF1 are believed to be sporadic mutations, which suggests a high mutation rate for the *NF1* gene.

This condition is due to mutations in a gene located on chromosome 17 responsible for encoding a protein called *neurofibromin.* This protein is believed to have a role in keeping *ras* proteins, important in cell proliferation and tumorigenesis, under control.[9] Evidence suggests that the *NF1* gene may be a tumor suppressor gene that, if lost or abnormal, results in tumor development.[10] This could explain the increased risk of malignancy in patients with NF1. This concept of tumor suppressor genes is more fully discussed later in this chapter.

The *NF1* gene is large, spanning about 350,000 bases (or 350 kilobases) of DNA, and contains at least 59 exons.[11] The large size of this gene may be responsible for its high mutation rate. Many different types of mutations have been identified,

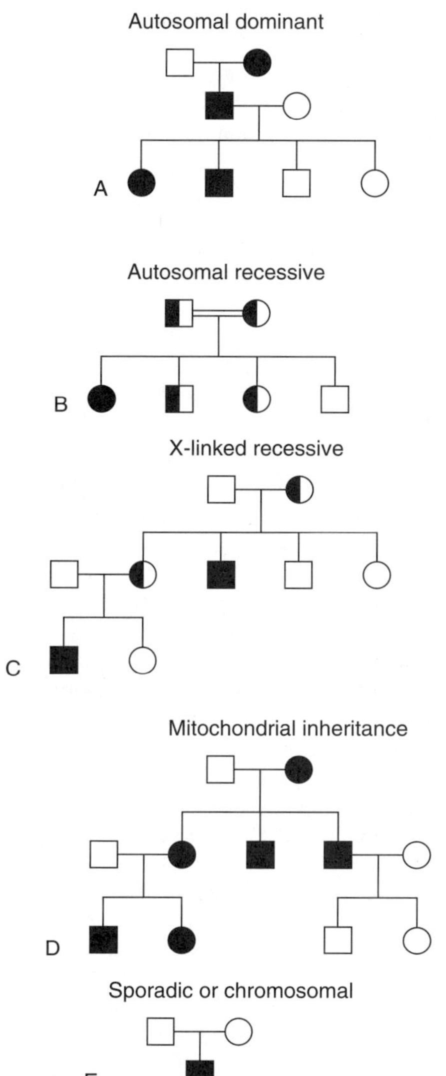

FIG. 1-26. Various modes of traditional and nontraditional inheritance. Squares denote males; circles are females. Shaded symbols are affected; unshaded are unaffected; half-shaded are carriers. The double line in the autosomal recessive figures signifies consanguinity, which increases the risk of recessive disease.

including deletions, insertions, missense mutations, nonsense mutations, and mutations in the introns; and in only a few reported cases has the same mutation been found in unrelated patients. Because of this, the specific mutation responsible for the condition has not yet been identified in many patients.[12] Using polymorphisms within the gene,[13] linkage analysis can be used to follow the gene through an affected family. More detail about linkage analysis follows later in this chapter.

Autosomal Recessive Inheritance

In autosomal recessive conditions, both genes at a locus are abnormal, which results in the absence of normal protein product. Abnormal genes are inherited from both parents, who each have one normal and one abnormal gene (carriers), but who show no clinical evidence of the condition. Many autosomal recessive conditions are due to an absence of an enzyme; carriers often have half the normal amount of enzyme, but this amount is sufficient so they demonstrate no signs or symptoms of the condition. Two carriers of an autosomal recessive condition have a 25% risk of having an affected child with each pregnancy (see Fig. 1-26). It has been estimated that each of us carries 6 to 10 recessive genes. Therefore, these conditions occur more frequently among inbred groups and consanguineous matings because related people are more likely to have inherited the same abnormal recessive gene.

The finding that some autosomal recessive conditions are more frequent in particular ethnic groups has led to population screening for carrier status. Some examples of this strategy include carrier screening of the Ashkenazi Jewish population for Tay-Sachs disease and the African-American population for sickle cell disease.

An example of a condition inherited in an autosomal recessive manner is cystic fibrosis (CF; MIM 219700). This condition, occurring in about 1 in 2500 live births, is characterized by chronic pulmonary disease, pancreatic insufficiency, and elevated sweat chloride concentrations. The condition is due to mutations in the cystic fibrosis transmembrane conductance regulator (CFTR) gene, located on chromosome 7, which codes for a protein that acts as a chloride channel, regulated by cyclic adenosine monophosphate. Therefore, patients with this condition have abnormal chloride conduction across the apical membrane of epithelial cells. The most common mutation in patients with CF (accounting for two thirds of the mutations) results in the deletion of a single amino acid (phenylalanine) from the CFTR protein (termed ΔF508, referring to a deletion of phenylalanine—abbreviated as F—at the codon, or amino acid, numbered 508). Other mutations include missense mutations, frameshift mutations due to addition or deletion of a number of base pairs not a multiple of three, nonsense mutations, and mRNA splicing mutations. ΔF508 and four other mutations account for 85% of CF mutations.[14]

Evaluations of large numbers of CF patients for the CFTR mutation have allowed study of the correlation between the specific mutation (genotype) and the observed clinical manifestations (phenotype). This correlation has demonstrated that certain CFTR mutations are associated with early onset of pancreatic insufficiency, while other mutations have a low frequency of this problem. The occurrence of other common complications and the severity and course of the pulmonary disease, however, do not appear to be predicted by the CF genotype, but are believed to be due to other genetic and environmental factors.[15] These genotype–phenotype correlations are useful for prognostic counseling and may potentially be employed to determine optimal treatment regimens. Determination of genotype has also been shown to be helpful for diagnosis in patients with CF-like lung disease, but in whom sweat chloride values (typically used to make the diagnosis of CF) are normal or borderline.[16]

X-Linked Recessive Inheritance

In the previously discussed autosomal modes of inheritance, males and females are equally likely to be affected, and transmission does not depend on the sex of the parent. This is in contrast to X-linked or sex-linked conditions. X-linked recessive conditions are carried on the X chromosome. When a gene is abnormal on one X chromosome in females, the normal gene on the other X chromosome can compensate for the abnormal one. When a male inherits the abnormal X, however, he is hemizygous because there is no corresponding gene locus on the Y chromosome, and he has the condition. The probability that male offspring of female carriers will be affected is 50%, while female offspring have a 50% chance of being carriers, but are not affected. X-linked inheritance is distinguished from autosomal dominant inheritance by the absence of male-to-male transmission (Fig. 1-26).

Although most females carrying a mutation for an X-linked recessive disorder are asymptomatic, this is not always the case. During embryogenesis in females, one of the X chromosomes undergoes a process known as X-inactivation, or lyonization. This process is random; the maternally and paternally derived X chromosomes have an equal chance of becoming inactivated. The same X, however, remains inactivated in daughter cells of the original cell. If by chance, in a large proportion of cells in the involved organ, the normal X chromosome has been turned off, the woman may show symptoms of the X-linked recessive disorder.

Hemophilia A (classic hemophilia; MIM 306700), the most common of the severe congenital coagulation disorders, is inherited in an X-linked recessive fashion. Patients with this condition have a reduced coagulant activity of antihemophilic globulin or factor VIII in the coagulation cascade, due to either the absence of the protein or formation of an abnormal protein that does not work properly. Reduced factor VIII activity leads to recurrent hemarthrosis, deep muscle hematomas, intracranial bleeds, and hematuria. Patients are also at an increased risk of bleeding after trauma and surgery. The condition occurs in about 1 in 5000 to 10,000 males.[17] In general, the activity of factor VIII in affected males is either absent or severely decreased. Factor VIII activity in carrier females is also reduced, on average, to half of normal. In some carrier females, however, the level of factor VIII activity may be significantly reduced, owing to inactivation of a high proportion of the normal X chromosomes in the cells of the liver. This can sometimes result in a mild bleeding disorder, which may require treatment if the woman undergoes surgery.[18]

Several mutations have been identified in the factor VIII gene. An inversion of exons 1 through 22 has been observed in 45% of patients with severe factor VIII deficiency.[19] Of the remaining mutations, 5% are deletions, and the rest are different single nucleotide substitutions, producing both nonsense and missense mutations.[20] DNA diagnosis must rely on indirect studies in patients with unidentified mutations (discussed later).

DNA Diagnosis

Advances in molecular genetics have led to DNA diagnostic techniques for single-gene conditions. Using these techniques, prenatal diagnosis, presymptomatic diagnosis, and carrier testing are all feasible. These methods are direct or indirect.[21] Direct methods evaluate the DNA for specific mutations. To use a direct method, the gene must have been identified, and an efficient technique for identification of the mutation must be available. Disorders that are ideal for direct DNA analysis are ones in which only one or a few mutations are known. For example, sickle cell disease is due to a single-nucleotide substitution at the sixth codon of the β-globin chain. The mutation changes codon 6 from guanine–adenine–guanine (GAG), which codes for glutamic acid, to guanine–thymine–guanine (GTG), which codes for valine. This single-nucleotide change can be detected using an RFLP. The restriction enzyme cuts the normal DNA sequence, but the mutation changes the cut site so that it is no longer recognized by the enzyme.[22] Diagnosis can then be made by looking at the size of the resulting DNA fragments.

Certain conditions with many different mutations, such as NF1 and hemophilia A, may prove difficult for analysis by direct DNA methods. Indirect methods are based on the fact that loci located near each other on the same chromosome tend to be inherited together. Markers are chosen that are near to or within the gene of interest. These loci, however, can become disassociated through crossing over, an exchange of genetic material that occurs during meiosis. The likelihood of the gene and its marker becoming unlinked is directly related to the distance between them. Therefore, polymorphisms are chosen because of their physical proximity to the gene of interest; the closer the gene and polymorphism are, the more likely they will be inherited together (linked). Indirect methods ideally require study of families with multiple affected members to allow for determination of *phase,* that is, which polymorphism is inherited with the normal or abnormal gene. The phase sometimes cannot be determined, and DNA diagnosis in the particular family is then not possible using that polymorphism (the marker is called *uninformative*). Even when the marker is informative in a family, a crossover event can unlink the gene and its marker. This means that diagnosis is given as a percentage; for example, if crossing over occurs at a frequency of 5%, then presence of the linked marker accurately detects the disease of concern 95% of the time. As more markers are identified, including intragenic markers, the likelihood of an error decreases. Figure 1-27 shows an example of linkage analysis using an intragenic RFLP.

CHROMOSOMAL ABNORMALITIES

Chromosomes, the structures into which the genetic material is packaged, can be examined microscopically. Chromosome analysis is usually performed using lymphocytes, and for this reason, samples for analysis should be obtained from patients before blood transfusions. Other specimens can also be studied, including skin fibroblasts to evaluate for mosaicism (discussed later), bone marrow and other tumor cells to evaluate specific cancers, and chorionic villus cells and amniocytes from amniotic fluid to perform prenatal diagnosis. To make chromosomes visible under the light microscope, the cells to be studied are treated with a chemical that arrests cell division at a point where the chromosomes are spread throughout the cell and can be easily visualized. The samples are then treated with special stains that produce chromosome bands. The specific bands allow the cytogeneticist to identify the 24 chromosomes (22 autosomes, or non-sex chromosomes, and the sex chromosomes, X and Y). The bands also allow detection of missing or extra material. Human chromosome analysis uses a specific nomenclature, which refers to the chromosome number, chro-

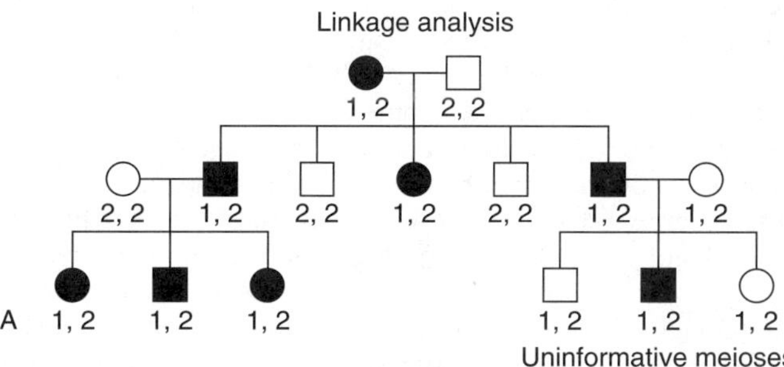

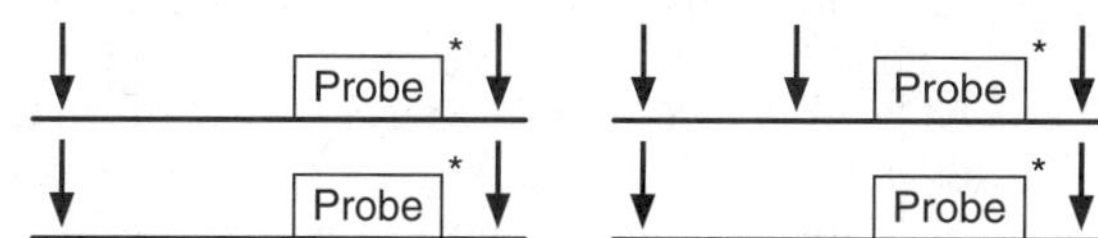

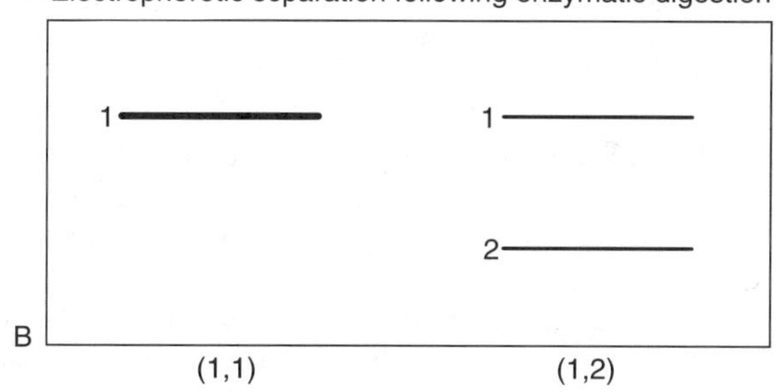

FIG. 1-27. Linkage analysis using restriction fragment-length polymorphism. (*A*) Pedigree demonstrating autosomal dominant inheritance of a phenotype linked to this two-allele locus. In this family, the disease phenotype is linked with the #1 allele, except for the lower right hand corner, where it is impossible to distinguish the affected from unaffected #1 allele. In the latter situation, the marker is said to be *uninformative*. (*B*) Laboratory data that would be seen in this case. A piece of genomic DNA that encompasses the gene of interest is flanked by two endonuclease cut sites and has a variable site within it. When the DNA is digested (cut) by the enzyme, electrophoretically separated, and probed with a labeled piece of complementary DNA, one or two fragments can be seen, depending on whether the person is homozygous or heterozygous at the locus.

mosome arm—p (short) or q (long), and which region and band within that region are involved.[23] For example, 15q13 refers to the long arm of chromosome 15, the third band within the first region.

Chromosomal abnormalities can be divided into two types: abnormality in the chromosome number or in the chromosome structure. The most common abnormalities in chromosome number in live-born infants are Down syndrome (due to an extra dose of genetic information on chromosome 21) and Turner syndrome (due to a single X chromosome).

Abnormalities in chromosome structure that result in missing or extra chromosomal material (deletions and duplications) also have clinical consequences. Translocations in which two chromosomes break and exchange genetic material also occur. These can be unbalanced, in which the total amount of chromosome material is incorrect, or balanced, when the correct amount of material is present, but rearranged. People with balanced translocations are usually phenotypically normal but are at increased risk for offspring with unbalanced chromosome constitutions (these can be either miscarriages, stillbirths, or live-born infants with multiple anomalies). A number of other rearrangements are seen, including ring chromosomes, insertions, inversions, and isochromosomes,[23] but these complex arrangements are beyond the scope of this chapter.

For a duplication or deletion to be detectable by conventional cytogenetic means, it has been estimated that 2 to 3 million base pairs of DNA[24] or 50 to 100 genes[25] must be altered. Advances in the field of cytogenetics have allowed the identification of smaller deletions and duplications through the use of a technique known as *fluorescence in situ hybridization* (FISH).[26] This technique uses probes that can be tagged with fluorescent markers. These probes attach to sites of interest in single-stranded DNA, and the markers can then be visualized under the fluorescence microscope. The presence and copy number of sequences complementary to areas of interest can be determined. For example, when evaluating for a deletion with a FISH probe, two fluorescent markers are normally seen in each cell, one attaching to each member of the chromosome pair. In a patient with a deletion, only one fluorescent marker per cell is observed.

An example of the usefulness of the FISH technique is evident in a set of conditions for which the acronym CATCH 22 (*c*ardiac, *a*bnormal facies, *t*hymic hypoplasia, *c*left palate, and *h*ypocalcemia, associated with a deletion on chromosome *22*) was coined.[27] This term refers to what was previously thought to be two separate conditions, DiGeorge and velocardiofacial (Shprintzen) syndromes (MIM 192430). DiGeorge syndrome is characterized by congenital heart disease, hypocalcemia due to hypoparathyroidism, T-lymphocyte abnormalities due to complete or partial absence of the thymus, and dysmorphic facies,[27] and is often a sporadic event in a family. Typical features of the velocardiofacial syndrome include cleft palate, congenital heart defects, facial characteristics, and learning disabilities, and this condition is inherited as an autosomal dominant trait.[28] These conditions have been shown to be associated with a deletion in chromosome 22q11 in 88% of DiGeorge syndrome and 76% of velocardiofacial syndrome patients.[29] This deletion is often not visible using traditional cytogenetic means but is evident with the use of FISH analysis using chromosome 22–specific probes. The relation of both these conditions to conotruncal heart defects led investigators to evaluate patients with isolated conotruncal defects, and a number of these patients have also been shown to have a deletion in chromosome 22.[30] This group of conditions is now believed to be a spectrum from the most severe (DiGeorge syndrome) to the mildest end (isolated heart defects). FISH analysis allows for identification of patients who fall into this spectrum; in addition, parents of patients with these conditions can be screened for the deletion, and when it is found, genetic counseling regarding a 50% recurrence risk can be provided. In parents with the deletion, prenatal diagnosis can be offered.

MULTIFACTORIAL INHERITANCE

As noted in the introduction, most congenital abnormalities are not due to a single-gene or chromosomal abnormality, but are multifactorial. Multifactorial inheritance refers to conditions in which an interaction between genetic and environmental factors is involved. Most of the congenital malformations (ie, neural tube defects, cleft lip and/or palate, and congenital heart disease), as well as many of the common adult-onset conditions (ie, coronary heart disease, hypertension, and diabetes mellitus), are believed to be due to a combination of genetic and environmental factors. In these conditions, the recurrence risk in families is increased, but there is no obvious pattern when examining pedigrees. In addition, frequently one sex is more often affected than the other in these conditions.

Genetic counseling in multifactorial conditions requires the use of empiric recurrence risk figures (ie, actual observed data from families) because neither the genetic nor environmental factors are well understood. These empiric risks most probably are based on a combination of families with low risk and families with high risk, but the limited knowledge about significant factors do not allow for more accurate risk estimation. Some known important factors should be used to modify the empiric risk for the particular situation, including the severity of the disorder in the patient, the patient's sex, and the presence of other affected family members. These factors function in the following ways[31]:

1. The more severe the condition is in the affected patient, the higher the recurrence risk is for the family.
2. A higher recurrence risk results when more than one family member is affected.

3. If the condition occurs more often in one sex, the risk is higher in relatives of patients of the less frequently affected sex.

Pyloric stenosis, a multifactorial condition occurring in about 1 in 500 births, demonstrates the different recurrence risks based on sex of the affected patient. This condition occurs about five times more frequently in males than females, and the recurrence risk to parents with an affected male is 4%, while the risk to parents of an affected female is 14%.[32]

Advances have identified some of the genetic and environmental factors in the causation of these birth defects. An association has been identified between specific alleles in the transforming growth-factor α (TGF-α) gene and both cleft lip and palate[33] and cleft palate only,[34] suggesting an important role of this gene in craniofacial development. Likewise, an environmental factor of importance in the causation of neural tube defects has been identified. In a study by the British Medical Research Council Vitamin Study Research Group,[35] the recurrence risk of a neural tube defect among folate-supplemented women was 1%, and among women without folate, it was 3.5%. The preventive effect has also been demonstrated in women without a previous occurrence.[36] As geneticists learn more about the causes of these conditions, families can be provided with more accurate recurrence risk information as well as information that can be used in prevention of the defect in future offspring.

APPROACH TO THE EVALUATION OF MALFORMATIONS

When encountering what appears to be an isolated congenital defect, it is essential to evaluate for related syndromes and associations. Many birth defects may be seen as part of a syndrome, and identification of this syndrome can significantly alter prognosis and recurrence risk counseling. Table 1-2 lists some selected syndromes that may be associated with four common congenital malformations. The goal of this table is to demonstrate the wide range of conditions associated with these malformations and is by no means exhaustive; in fact, each malformation is associated with several other syndromes or can be seen in isolation as a multifactorial trait. This table emphasizes the

TABLE 1-2. *Selected syndromes associated with congenital malformations*

Congenital malformation	Associated syndrome	Cause
Cleft lip and/or palate[54]	Trisomy 13	Chromosomal
	Van der Woude syndrome (MIM 119300)	Autosomal dominant
	Meckel syndrome (MIM 249000)	Autosomal recessive; also associated with chromosome 22q deletion
	Velocardiofacial syndrome (MIM 192430)	
Hirschsprung disease[55]	Trisomy 21	Chromosomal
	Waardenburg syndrome (MIM 193500)	Autosomal dominant
	Cartilage-hair hypoplasia (MIM 250250)	Autosomal recessive
Omphalocele[56,57]	Beckwith-Wiedemann syndrome (MIM 130650)	Sporadic, autosomal dominant
	Trisomy 13, trisomy 18 or other chromosomal abnormalities (seen in 35%–58% of cases)	Chromosomal
Hypospadias[58]	Smith-Lemli-Opitz syndrome (MIM 250400)	Autosomal recessive
	Opitz-Frias syndrome (MIM 145410)	Autosomal dominant
	Trisomy 13 or trisomy 18	Chromosomal

importance of evaluating patients with these birth defects not only to provide accurate recurrence risk but also to provide families with information regarding prognosis.

An association is the nonrandom occurrence of birth defects for which no cause is known. Although identification of an association does not provide knowledge about a cause, its consideration assists in identifying other possible defects that may accompany the known defect. For example, when one of the defects included in the VACTERL association (*v*ertebral, *a*nal, *c*ardiac, *t*racheoesophageal fistula, *r*enal, and *l*imb) is observed in a patient, the other parts of the association should be considered.

Another important concept to consider in the evaluation of patients with birth defects is that of the *sequence*. This term refers to the situation when a single problem in prenatal development leads to a cascade of subsequent defects.[37] An example familiar to pediatric surgeons is prune-belly or Eagle-Barrett syndrome. This condition is characterized by abdominal muscle deficiency and excess abdominal skin (giving a wrinkled appearance, or ''prune belly''), undescended testes, and urinary tract anomalies. It has been postulated that this condition is often secondary to a single problem, prenatal urethral obstruction. This obstruction causes bladder distention, which may produce multiple secondary anomalies, including abdominal distention with abdominal muscle deficiency, hydroureter, renal dysplasia (due to the back pressure from the urethral obstruction), cryptorchidism (due to obstruction of testicular descent by the dilated bladder), and malrotation of the colon (due to the enlarged bladder preventing normal gut rotation).[38,39] Although this explanation may not account for all cases of Eagle-Barrett syndrome, analysis of many cases is consistent with this explanation.

NONTRADITIONAL INHERITANCE

Mosaicism

A number of new concepts have been described that have been termed *nontraditional inheritance*,[40] in contrast to the mendelian inheritance patterns described for single-gene conditions. The first of these is *mosaicism*. This term refers to different genotypes (either different chromosome constitution or alleles at a specific locus) in different cells of a single person. Two types of mosaicism are important: somatic and gonadal. Somatic mosaicism refers to a postzygotic event that occurs in a single cell. The daughter cells also have the abnormal genotype, leading to two populations of cells in the person. Although usually the person is less severely affected by the gene mutation than if all cells were affected by the gene change, the actual observed results of this type of change depend on the type of mutation, the gene in which it occurs, the stage in development in which it occurs, and the cell types involved.[41] Probably the most interesting area in which somatic mutations are important is cancer genetics. It appears that a large proportion of cancers are due to a genetic change occurring in a single cell that leads to uncontrolled growth of the daughter cells. This concept is discussed further later.

Another important concept is gonadal mosaicism. This refers to two separate populations of cells with different genotypes in the gonads. This concept can be used to explain how two children with an autosomal dominant condition can be born to normal parents. Using molecular genetic techniques, the occurrence of this phenomenon has been confirmed in multiple genetic conditions. For example, a phenotypically normal father with two offspring with NF1 was shown to have a mutation in the *NF1* gene in about 10% of his spermatozoa. The remainder of his sperm, as well as his lymphocytes, did not demonstrate the mutation.[42]

Imprinting and Uniparental Disomy

Genomic imprinting is a process believed to be set in meiosis, which labels a gene as originating from the father or the mother. This label, which defines the parent of origin, is temporary and is reset in each generation. When the parent-of-origin of a gene affects its expression, the gene is said to be *imprinted.*[43]

A dramatic illustration of genomic imprinting involves two conditions with mental retardation as a major feature, Prader-Willi syndrome and Angelman syndrome. Prader-Willi syndrome is a condition characterized by hypotonia, hypogonadism, failure to thrive in infancy, and later, hyperphagia with resulting obesity. Angelman syndrome is characterized by absent speech, ataxic movements, seizures, and an inappropriate happy affect. About 75% of patients with these conditions have an interstitial deletion of the long arm at chromosome 15q11-13. The parental origin of this deletion differs between these two conditions; when this deletion occurs on the father's chromosome 15, patients have Prader-Willi syndrome, but when it occurs on the mother's chromosome 15, the patients have Angelman syndrome.[44]

In addition, uniparental disomy (UPD) has been recognized in a proportion of these patients without a chromosomal deletion. This phenomenon refers to the inheritance of two copies of a genetic locus or an entire chromosome from only one parent.[45]

Patients with Prader-Willi syndrome due to UPD have inherited both their chromosomes 15 from their mother, while patients with Angelman syndrome due to UPD have inherited both their chromosomes 15 from their father. Therefore, it appears that both maternal and paternal contributions of this region on chromosome 15 are essential for normal development. If the paternal contribution is absent (either through deletion or UPD), then the patient will have Prader-Willi syndrome; in contrast, if the maternal contribution is absent, then the patient will have Angelman syndrome.[44]

At this time, the mechanisms of genomic imprinting are not known, although evidence suggests that DNA methylation and timing of DNA replication are involved. The frequency at which this phenomenon occurs in the human genome is also not known; however, imprinting effects are suspected in several human genes and disorders.[43] It is essential when evaluating pedigrees that this possibility be considered.

Mitochondrial Inheritance

Another form of nontraditional inheritance involves the DNA found in the mitochondria, instead of the nucleus, as previously discussed. The mitochondrial chromosome is circular and contains no introns and little noncoding DNA. Its genetic code is different from that seen in the nucleus. Because the ova, but not the sperm, contain mitochondria, conditions inherited in this manner have a unique pattern of inheritance. Females pass on the condition to their offspring (usually to all, both male and female), but males are unable to pass the condition on, so transmission ends with each son.[40] (see Fig. 1-26.) The mitochondrial genome carries 37 genes; many of these are involved in various steps in oxidative phosphorylation, the process by which mitochondria produce energy in the form of adenosine triphosphate.[7]

PRENATAL DIAGNOSIS

Progress in genetics has made possible prenatal diagnosis of many of the conditions discussed earlier. In the past, most women undergoing prenatal diagnostic techniques were presumed to be at increased risk for offspring with anomalies either because of the mother's age (increased risk of chromosome abnormalities) or because of a previous affected child. Screening programs are now available in which levels of proteins in maternal blood (α-fetoprotein, unconjugated estriol, and human chorionic gonadotropin) are measured and used to identify a proportion of women at increased risk for chromosomal abnormalities, neural tube defects, and some other structural defects.[46] These women are then offered more specific studies for identification of these conditions. In addition, ultrasonography performed for other purposes may identify unsuspected structural birth defects. Chorionic villi sampling and amniocentesis are methods of obtaining samples for biochemical, cytogenetic, or molecular genetic analyses. Chorionic villi sampling, performed between the 9th and 12th weeks of gestation, involves obtaining chorionic cells either through a transcervical or transabdominal technique. Amniocentesis, performed usually at 15 to 16 weeks' gestation, allows transabdominal collection of amniotic fluid to be used for genetic studies.

The options available to couples who have undergone prenatal diagnosis by amniocentesis or chorionic villi sampling are limited; the family may elect to undergo pregnancy termination or to continue an affected pregnancy. This has led workers to study methods of diagnosis before implantation of the embryo, taking advantage of in vitro fertilization techniques. The cells for genetic analysis are obtained either by removal of a cell at an early stage when only a few cells are present (blastomere or blastocyst biopsy) or by examining the polar body formed in meiosis I, and using this to infer the genetic status of the oocyte. Preimplantation diagnostic techniques have been successfully used in a limited number of cases, but technical problems, as well as ethical and societal issues, need to be addressed before these techniques become widely available.[47]

Pediatric surgeons are often involved in the counseling sessions of families in whom a condition amenable to surgical intervention has been prenatally diagnosed. The aim in genetic counseling is to provide the family with adequate information so that an informed course of action appropriate for the family may be chosen by them, a process termed *nondirective counseling*. Some information regarding issues for prenatal counseling by pediatric surgeons is summarized in an article by Wilcox and colleagues.[48]

GENETICS AND CANCER

A relation between genetics and cancer has long been recognized. Several genetic conditions put patients at increased risk

of malignancy. These include chromosome instability syndromes such as ataxia-telangiectasia (MIM 20890), Bloom syndrome (MIM 21090), and xeroderma pigmentosa (MIM 27870); genodermatoses such as neurofibromatosis type 1 (MIM 16220), von Hippel-Lindau syndrome (MIM 19330), and tuberous sclerosis (MIM 19110); immunodeficiency syndromes such as Wiskott-Aldrich syndrome (MIM 30100); and overgrowth conditions such as Beckwith-Wiedemann syndrome (MIM 130650).[49] In addition to these single-gene conditions, chromosomal abnormalities can place patients at increased risk of developing cancer, including patients with Down syndrome (increased risk of leukemia), or deletion in the short arm of chromosome 11 (increased risk of Wilms tumor).

In addition to these genetic conditions with an elevated risk of malignancy, three types of cancer genes have been identified: oncogenes, tumor suppressor genes, and mutator genes. Oncogenes are genes that can cause cells to become malignant when activated. Initially, oncogenes are in an inactivated state, called *protooncogenes*; these are thought to be important in the regulation of normal cells. Activation of the oncogene can occur through a number of mechanisms, including chromosome translocation, retroviral insertion, point mutation, and gene amplification. An example of activation of an oncogene involves the *abl* oncogene, located on chromosome 9, which becomes activated through a translocation to chromosome 22 (called the Philadelphia chromosome). This oncogene activation results in a predisposition to chronic myelogenous leukemia; in fact, the Philadelphia chromosome is seen in 90% of cases of this disease.[50]

Tumor suppressor genes are also important in the etiology of human cancer. These genes serve a growth-constraining role, and their inactivation can lead to uncontrolled growth of tumor cells.[51] In contrast to oncogenes, which tend to be dominant, such that their activity prevails over the normal allele, tumor suppressor genes tend to be recessive. When both alleles at a locus are inactivated, loss of tumor suppressor function occurs, resulting in malignant growth.[52]

A classic example of a tumor suppressor gene involves development of the childhood eye malignancy, retinoblastoma. The inactivation of both copies of the retinoblastoma gene on chromosome 13q14 results in tumor growth. This condition can be sporadic or familial. In the sporadic form, patients must undergo two somatic mutations in the retinoblastoma gene on chromosome 13q14, while in the familial form, the first mutation either can be inherited from the previous generation or can originate from a mutation during gametogenesis, and the second mutation in the retinoblastoma gene is somatic in origin. The familial cases have an earlier age of onset and are more often bilateral than sporadic cases of retinoblastoma. Tumor-suppressor genes have also been shown to be involved in several types of cancers, including Wilms tumor and certain forms of colon cancer, as well as in some of the malignancies associated with multiple endocrine neoplasia types 1 (MIM 131100) and 2 (MIM 171400) and neurofibromatosis types 1 (MIM 162200) and 2 (MIM 10100).[51]

A third type of ''cancer gene'' has been identified, called a *mutator gene*. This gene serves a function in the repair of DNA replication errors, and the accumulation of these errors leads to malignant transformation of cells. This type of gene has been associated with families with hereditary nonpolyposis colon cancer.[53]

Although the field of cancer genetics has made great strides in recent years, much is left to be learned. It is hoped that improved understanding of the genetics of cancer not only will allow for provision of accurate recurrence risks to relatives but also will provide information on the optimal treatment, and some day prevention, of these disorders.

BIBLIOGRAPHY (Chapter 1.1)

Anggard E. Nitric oxide: mediator, murderer, and medicine. Lancet 1994; 343:1199.

Arbeit JM. Molecules, cancer, and the surgeon: a review of molecular biology and its implications for surgical oncology. Ann Surg 1990;212:3.

Aulitzky WE, Schuler M, Peschel C, et al. Interleukins: clinical pharmacology and therapeutic use. Drugs 1994;48:667.

Benton LD, Khan M, Greco RS. Integrins, adhesion molecules and surgical research. Surg Gynecol Obstet 1993;177:311.

Cirelli R, Tyring SK. Major therapeutic used of interferons. Clin Immunother 1995;3:27.

Cowin P. Unraveling the cytoplasmic interactions of the cadherin superfamily. Proc Natl Acad Sci USA 1994;91:10759.

Fidler IJ, Ellis LM. The implications of angiogenesis for the biology and therapy of cancer metastasis. Cell 1994;79:185.

Green ED, Waterson HR. The Human Genome Project: prospects and implications for clinical medicine. JAMA 1991;266:1966.

Hartwell LH, Kastan MB. Cell cycle control and cancer. Science 1994; 266:1821.

Mullis KB. The unusual origin of the polymerase chain reaction. Sci Am 1990;262:56.

Nathan C, Sporn M. Cytokines in context. J Cell Biol 1991;113:981.

Nilsson T, Warren G. Retention and retrieval in the endoplasmic reticulum and the Golgi apparatus. Curr Opin Cell Biol 1994;6:517.

Rio DC. RNA processing. Curr Opin Cell Biol 1992;4:444.

Rothman JE. Mechanisms of intracellular protein transport. Nature 1994; 372:55.

Singer SJ. The structure and insertion of integral proteins in membranes. Annu Rev Cell Biol 1990;6:247.

Thilo L. Endocytosis: aspects of organellar processing. Ann NY Acad Sci 1994;710:209.

Tsokos GC. Lymphocytes, cytokines, inflammation, and immune trafficking. Curr Opin Rheumatol 1994;6:461.

REFERENCES (Chapter 1.2)

1. Hall JG, Powers EK, McIlvaine RT, Ean VH. The frequency and financial burden of genetic disease in a pediatric hospital. Am J Med Genet 1978;1:417.

2. Baird PA, Anderson TW, Newcombe HB, et al. Genetic disorders in children and young adults: a population study. Am J Hum Genet 1988; 42:677.

3. Fields C, Adams MD, White O, et al. How many genes in the human genome? Nat Genet 1994;7:345.

4. McIntosh I, Hamosh A, Dietz HC. Nonsense mutations and diminished mRNA levels. Nat Genet 1993;4:219.

5. Urlaub G, Mitchell PG, Ciudad CJ, Chasin LA.Nonsense mutations in the dihydrofolate reductase gene affect RNA processing. Mol Cell Biol 1989;9:2868.

6. McKusick VA, Francomano CA, Antonarakis SE, Pearson PL. Mendelian inheritance in man: a catalog of human genes and genetic disorders, ed 11. Baltimore, Johns Hopkins University Press, 1994.

7. Herskowitz I. Functional inactivation of genes by dominant negative mutations. Nature 1987;329:219.

8. Wallace MR, Collins FS. Von Recklinghausen neurofibromatosis. Adv Hum Genet 1991;20:267.

9. Viskochil D, White R, Cawthon R. The neurofibromatosis type 1 gene. Annu Rev Neurosci 1993;16:183.

10. Seizinger BR. NF1: a prevalent cause of tumorigenesis in human cancers? Nat Genet 1993;3:97.

11. Colman SD, Wallace MR. Neurofibromatosis type I. Eur J Cancer 1994;13:1974.

12. Heim RA, Silverman LM, Farber RA, et al. Screening for truncated NF1 proteins. Nat Genet 1994;8:218.

13. Jorde LB, Watkins WS, Viskochil D, et al. Linkage disequilibrium in the neurofibromatosis 1 (NF1) region: implications for gene mapping. Am J Hum Genet 1993;53:1038.

14. Beaudet AL. Genetic testing for cystic fibrosis. Pediatr Clin North Am 1992;39:213.

15. Cystic Fibrosis Genotype-Phenotype Consortium. Correlation between genotype and phenotype in patients with cystic fibrosis. N Engl J Med 1993;329:1308.

16. Highsmith WE, Burch LH, Zhou A, et al. A novel mutation in the cystic fibrosis gene in patients with pulmonary disease but normal sweat chloride concentrations. N Engl J Med 1994;331:974.

17. Kazazian HH Jr, Tuddenham EGD, Antonarakis SE. Hemophilia A and parahemophilia: deficiencies of coagulation factors VIII and V. In: Scriver CR, Beaudet Al, Sly WS, et al, eds. The metabolic and molecular bases of inherited disease, vol 1. New York, McGraw-Hill, 1995:3241.

18. Ludlam CA. Congenital disorders of haemostasis. In: Emery AEH, Rimoin DL. Principles and practice of medical genetics. New York, Churchill Livingstone, 1990:1371.

19. Lakich D, Kazazian HH Jr, Antonarakis SE, et al. Inversions disrupting the factor VIII gene are a common cause of severe haemophilia A. Nat Genet 1993;5:236.

20. Antonarakis SE. The molecular genetics of hemophilia A and B in man: factor VIII and factor IX deficiency. Adv Hum Genet 1988;17:27.

21. Antonarakis SE. Diagnosis of genetic disorders at the DNA level. N Engl J Med 1989;320:153.

22. Orkin SH, Little PFR, Kazazian HH Jr, et al. Improved detection of the sickle mutation by DNA analysis: application to prenatal diagnosis. N Engl J Med 1982;307:32.

23. Therman E, Susman M. Human chromosomes: structure, behavior and effects. New York, Springer-Verlag, 1993.

24. Ledbetter DH, Ballabio A. Molecular cytogenetics of contiguous gene syndromes: mechanisms and consequences of gene dosage imbalance. In: Scriver CR, Beaudet AL, Sly WS, et al, eds. The metabolic and molecular bases of inherited disease, vol 1. New York, McGraw-Hill, 1995:811.

25. Aylsworth AS. Genetic counseling for patients with birth defects. Pediatr Clin North Am 1992;39:229.

26. Cohen MM, Rosenblum-Vos LS, Prabhakar G. Human cytogenetics: a current overview. Am J Dis Child 1993;147:1159.

27. Wilson DI, Burn J, Scambler P, Goodship J. DiGeorge syndrome, part of CATCH 22. J Med Genet 1993;30:852.

28. Goldberg R, Motzkin B, Marion R, et al. Velo-cardio-facial syndrome: a review of 120 patients. Am J Med Genet 1993;45:313.

29. Driscoll DA, Salvin J, Sellinger B, et al. Prevalence of 22q11 microdeletions in DiGeorge and velocardiofacial syndromes: implications for genetic counselling and prenatal diagnosis. J Med Genet 1993;30:813.

30. Goldmuntz E, Driscoll D, Budarf ML, et al. Microdeletions of chromosomal region 22q11 in patients with congenital conotruncal cardiac defects. J Med Genet 1993;30:807.

31. Skinner R. Genetic counseling. In: Emery AEH, Rimoin DL, eds. Principles and practice of medical genetics. New York, Churchill Livingstone, 1990:1923.

32. Carter CO. Genetics of common disorders. Br Med J 1969;25:52.

33. Ardinger HH, Buetow KH, Bell GI, et al. Association of genetic variation of the transforming growth factor-alpha gene with cleft lip and palate. Am J Hum Genet 1989;45:348.

34. Shiang R, Lidral AC, Ardinger HH, et al. Association of transforming growth-factor alpha gene polymorphisms with nonsyndromic cleft palate only (CPO). Am J Hum Genet 1993;53:836.

35. MRC Vitamin Study Research Group. Prevention of neural tube defects: results of the Medical Research Council vitamin study. Lancet 1991;338:131.

36. Czeizel AE, Dudas I. Prevention of the first occurrence of neural-tube defects by periconceptional vitamin supplementation. N Engl J Med 1992;327:1832.

37. Jones KL. Smith's recognizable patterns of human malformation. Philadelphia, WB Saunders, 1988.

38. Pagon RA, Smith DW, Shepard TH. Urethral obstruction malformation

complex: a cause of abdominal muscle deficiency and the ''prune belly.'' J Pediatr 1979;94:900.

39. Reinberg Y, Shapiro E, Manivel JC, et al. Prune belly syndrome in females: a triad of abdominal musculature deficiency and anomalies of the urinary and genital systems. J Pediatr 1991;118:395.

40. Austin KD, Hall JG. Nontraditional inheritance. Pediatr Clin North Am 1992;39:335.

41. Hall JG. Somatic mosaicism: observations related to clinical genetics. (Review and hypotheses) Am J Hum Genet 1988;43:355.

42. Lazaro C, Ravella A, Gaona A, et al. Neurofibromatosis type 1 due to germ-line mosaicism in a clinically normal father. N Engl J Med 1994; 331:1403.

43. Hall JG. Genomic imprinting: review and relevance to human diseases. Am J Hum Genet 1990;46:857.

44. Driscoll DJ. Genomic imprinting in humans. In: Friedmann T, ed. Molecular genetic medicine 4. New York, Academic Press, 1994:37.

45. Nicholls RD. Genomic imprinting and uniparental disomy in Angelman and Prader-Willi syndromes: a review. Am J Med Genet 1993;46:16.

46. Wald NJ, Kennard A. Prenatal biochemical screening for Down's syndrome and neural tube defects. Curr Opin Obstet Gynecol 1992;4:302.

47. McGowan KD. Preimplantation prenatal diagnosis. Obstet Gynecol Clin North Am 1993;20:599.

48. Wilcox DT, Karamanoukian HL, Glick PJ. Antenatal diagnosis of pediatric surgical anomalies: counseling the family. Pediatr Clin North Am 1993;40:1273.

49. Schneider KA. Counseling about cancer: strategies for genetic counselors. Dennisport, MA, Graphic Illusions, 1994.

50. Miller DM, Blume S, Borst M, et al. Oncogenes, malignant transformation, and modern medicine. Am J Med Sci 1990;300:59.

51. Weinberg RA. Tumor suppressor genes. Science 1991;254:1138.

52. Goddard AD, Solomon E. Genetic aspects of cancer. Adv Hum Genet 1993;21:321.

53. Fishel R, Lescoe MK, Roa MRS, et al. The human mutator gene homolog MSH2 and its association with hereditary nonpolyposis colon cancer. Cell 1993;75:1027.

54. Lettieri J. Lips and oral cavity. In: Stevenson RE, Hall JG, Goodman RM, eds. Human malformation and related anomalies, vol 2. New York, Oxford University Press, 1993:367.

55. Passarge E, Stevenson RE. Megacolon. In: Stevenson RE, Hall JG, Goodman RM, eds. Human malformation and related anomalies, vol 2. New York, Oxford University Press, 1993:484.

56. Kaplan MS, McGregor SN. Perinatal management of congenital diaphragmatic hernia and anterior abdominal wall defect. Clin Perinatol 1989;16:917.

57. Curry CJR, Honore L, Boyd E. Omphalocele. In: Stevenson RE, Hall JG, Goodman RM, eds. Human malformation and related anomalies, vol 2. New York, Oxford University Press, 1993:879.

58. McGillivray BC. Hypospadias. In: Stevenson RE, Hall JG, Goodman RM, eds. Human malformation and related anomalies, vol 2. New York, Oxford University Press, 1993:554.

Surgery of Infants and Children: Scientific Principles and Practice, edited by Keith T. Oldham, Paul M. Colombani, and Robert P. Foglia. Lippincott–Raven Publishers, Philadelphia, © 1997.

CHAPTER 2

The Fetus

Jacob C. Langer, N. Scott Adzick, and Michael Harrison

2.1   Normal Fetal Development

Jacob C. Langer

Normal organ development in the human embryo and fetus is extremely complex and involves the precise and coordinated timing of cellular signals and responses. The three phases of organ development are morphogenesis, differentiation, and growth. Although embryologists have described the structural changes in great detail, the mechanisms by which these processes occur have only begun to be explored. Normal development depends on a normal genetic code, appropriate response to biochemical signals, and an intrauterine environment that is supportive and nourishing. The causes of most congenital anomalies are unknown, but the embryology has been determined with some degree of accuracy in most cases.

Organs are formed from one of the three embryonic layers that appear about 3 weeks after conception: ectoderm, mesenchyme, and endoderm (Fig. 2-1). Ectoderm gives rise to the epidermis, the nervous system, and several other organs; endoderm forms the epithelium of the respiratory and gastrointestinal tracts; and mesoderm gives rise to striated and smooth muscle, connective tissue, blood vessels, hematopoietic cells, bone, and reproductive and excretory organs.

This chapter does not attempt to give an exhaustive description of human embryology because the standard textbooks are more appropriate for this purpose.[1,2] In addition, the specific embryology of individual systems is covered in detail in many of the following chapters. Instead, this chapter approaches each of the major organ systems encountered by the pediatric surgeon and summarizes both the normal developmental processes and the perturbations that result in common congenital anomalies.

HEAD AND NECK

Organs of the head and neck form as a result of three processes: development and maturation of the branchial apparatus, formation of the facial structures by complex molding and migration of the mesenchyme, and formation of the thyroid gland from midline migration of endodermal elements.[3]

Branchial (Pharyngeal) Apparatus

During the 4th week after conception, neural crest cells migrate into the head and neck region and form four pairs of branchial arches. The grooves between the arches are known as the *branchial clefts.* The inner aspects of the arches are called *pharyngeal pouches,* and the interface between each branchial groove and pharyngeal pouch is known as the *branchial membrane* (Fig. 2-2).

The branchial arches consist of mesenchymal tissue, which goes on to form the cartilage, muscle, and bony structures of the head and neck. Branchial arch mesenchyme also develops into cranial nerves V, VII, IX, and X. The endodermal lining of the pharyngeal pouches gives rise to a number of important organs, including the tympanic membrane and eustachian tube (first pouch), the tonsils (second pouch), the inferior parathyroid glands and thymus (third pouch), and the superior parathyroid glands and thyroid C cells (fourth pouch). The first branchial groove forms the external auditory meatus, and the rest of the grooves ultimately become obliterated. The branchial membranes involute after the 6th week, except for the first branchial membrane, which contributes to the formation of the tympanic membrane.

Disturbances in the development of the branchial apparatus result in various types of branchial cysts, sinuses, and cartilaginous remnants. The location of each anomaly corresponds to the branchial structure involved. Shared origin from the third pharyngeal pouch explains the anomalous location of some inferior parathyroid glands within the thymus, and common origin from the second pharyngeal pouch explains anomalous location of the superior parathyroid glands within the thyroid parenchyma.

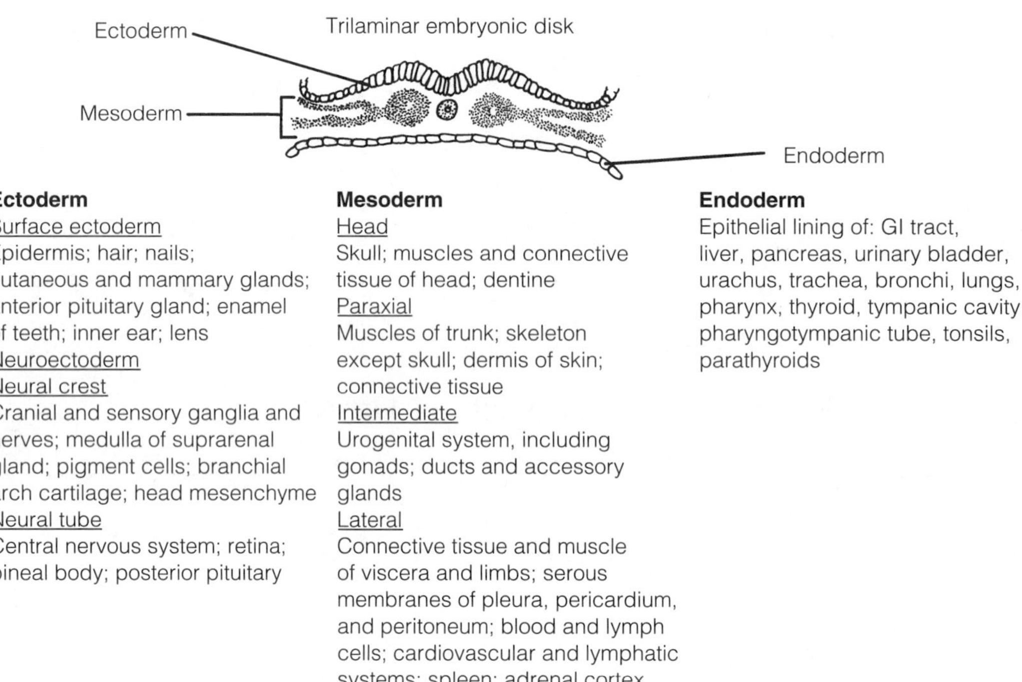

Ectoderm
<u>Surface ectoderm</u>
Epidermis; hair; nails;
cutaneous and mammary glands;
anterior pituitary gland; enamel
of teeth; inner ear; lens
<u>Neuroectoderm</u>
<u>Neural crest</u>
Cranial and sensory ganglia and
nerves; medulla of suprarenal
gland; pigment cells; branchial
arch cartilage; head mesenchyme
<u>Neural tube</u>
Central nervous system; retina;
pineal body; posterior pituitary

Mesoderm
<u>Head</u>
Skull; muscles and connective
tissue of head; dentine
<u>Paraxial</u>
Muscles of trunk; skeleton
except skull; dermis of skin;
connective tissue
<u>Intermediate</u>
Urogenital system, including
gonads; ducts and accessory
glands
<u>Lateral</u>
Connective tissue and muscle
of viscera and limbs; serous
membranes of pleura, pericardium,
and peritoneum; blood and lymph
cells; cardiovascular and lymphatic
systems; spleen; adrenal cortex

Endoderm
Epithelial lining of: GI tract,
liver, pancreas, urinary bladder,
urachus, trachea, bronchi, lungs,
pharynx, thyroid, tympanic cavity,
pharyngotympanic tube, tonsils,
parathyroids

FIG. 2-1. The three germ layers and their derivatives.

Formation of the Face

The orbits, nose, mouth, tongue, and palate form as a result of complex changes in mesenchymal elements between the 4th and 12th weeks after conception. The components of the face begin as prominences around the primitive stomodeum, and changes are induced by the prosencephalic and rhombencephalic organizing centers. The bony and cartilaginous components of the face are derived from neural crest cells originating in the first branchial arches. Facial features, including the nose, orbits, ears, mouth, and palate, are formed through complicated processes of mesenchymal folding, ingrowth, and migration.

Because of the complexity of facial embryology, craniofacial anomalies are relatively common. The most prevalent of these is the spectrum of cleft lip and palate, which is caused by failure of the lateral mesenchymal masses to merge or failure of the lateral mesenchyme to fuse with the medial nasal prominences.

Development of the Thyroid Gland

The thyroid gland begins as a collection of endodermal cells that aggregate in the floor of the primitive pharynx. Between the 4th and 7th weeks after conception, the thyroid migrates

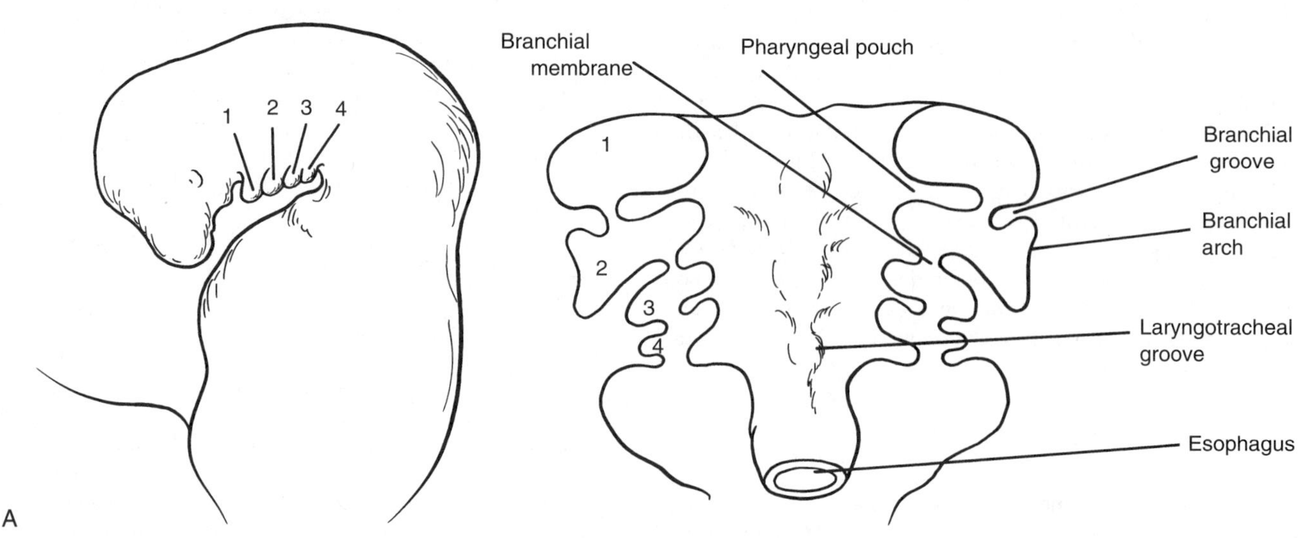

FIG. 2-2. The branchial apparatus.

caudally in the midline toward the trachea. Initially, it remains connected to the base of the tongue at the foramen cecum by the thyroglossal duct, but normally by the 8th week, this structure has disappeared.

Anomalies of thyroid gland development include ectopic thyroid and thyroglossal duct cysts and sinuses. Both of these conditions can occur anywhere along the path of the migrating thyroid from the foramen cecum to the suprasternal notch.

RESPIRATORY SYSTEM AND DIAPHRAGM

Respiratory System

The respiratory system begins during the 4th week after conception as a midline outgrowth from the caudal end of the primitive pharynx, called the *laryngotracheal groove*. This structure then elongates to form the laryngotracheal tube, and the distal end forms a rounded lung bud. Endoderm, lining the laryngotracheal tube, gives rise to the epithelium of the upper airway as well as the pulmonary epithelium, while the cartilage, smooth muscle, and connective tissue of the airways and lung are derived from mesenchymal elements.

By the end of the 5th week, the proximal portion of the laryngotracheal tube has been divided by the tracheoesophageal septum into an anterior tube (the larynx and trachea) and a posterior component (the foregut, or esophagus). A number of anomalies may occur during this process. Incomplete or aberrant formation of the tracheoesophageal septum leads to the various types of esophageal atresia, tracheoesophageal fistula, and laryngeal cleft. In addition, retention cysts may form, resulting in a foregut cyst (eg, esophageal duplication, bronchogenic cyst).

Lung development is usually divided into four stages: pseudoglandular, canalicular, terminal sac, and alveolar.[4] During the pseudoglandular stage (5 to 17 weeks), the lungs and bronchi develop through multiple division of the primitive lung bud. As this process occurs, the expanding lungs grow laterally into the pericardioperitoneal canals, which ultimately form the pleural cavities. During the canalicular stage (16 to 25 weeks), the respiratory bronchioles form, and terminal sacs, or primitive alveoli, begin to appear. In addition, the vascularization of the airways is completed. During the terminal sac period (24 weeks to birth), the alveoli form and develop their capillary and lymphatic networks, and differentiation of the type I and II alveolar pneumocytes occurs. The alveolar period (late fetal period to about 8 years of life) is characterized by an ongoing increase in the number of respiratory bronchioles and alveoli.

Several anomalies occur during lung development (lung bud anomalies). These include congenital lung cyst, cystic adenomatoid malformation, pulmonary sequestration, and pulmonary agenesis. In addition, preterm infants born before maturation of the type II pneumatocytes often suffer from hyaline membrane disease due to surfactant deficiency.

Diaphragm

The diaphragm forms from four structures (Fig. 2-3). The septum transversum is composed of mesoderm, which comes to lie between the pericardium and the abdomen after ventral folding of the embryonic head during the 4th week. This structure eventually forms the central tendon of the diaphragm. The pleuroperitoneal membranes occur on either side of the septum transversum. The dorsal mesentery of the esophagus attaches the developing foregut to the dorsal body wall and ultimately forms the crura of the diaphragm. The fourth component of the diaphragm comes from mesenchyme of the lateral abdominal wall, which grows in to join the other components starting about 12 weeks after conception.

Abnormalities of development can result in diaphragmatic defects, leading to herniation of abdominal viscera into the chest. Diaphragmatic hernias usually occur posterolaterally (foramen of Bochdalek) due to inadequate fusion of the pleuroperitoneal membrane with the other components of the diaphragm. In severe cases, complete diaphragmatic agenesis may be found. Infants with this problem often suffer from pulmonary hypoplasia, likely due to impaired lung growth from compression.

HEART AND GREAT VESSELS

The cardiovascular system is the first to function in the embryo and is mainly formed from mesodermal elements. The heart originates as a single tube into which blood flows from three systems of veins. The vitelline veins come from the yolk sac and disappear by the 10th week. The umbilical veins arise from the chorion and ultimately form a single umbilical vein that provides oxygenated blood from the placenta throughout fetal life. The umbilical vein enters the portal system, but most of the blood bypasses the liver through the ductus venosum and flows directly into the inferior vena cava to the heart. The paired cardinal veins bring blood from the rest of the embryo and form the vena cavae and the azygous system. The arterial system begins as a series of paired arteries associated with the branchial arches, called the *aortic arches*. In addition, a paired dorsal artery forms that quickly fuses to become a single dorsal aorta and runs the entire length of the embryo. Branches to the gut, kidneys, and gonads form as these structures develop.

Morphogenesis of the heart is a complex process during which the heart becomes divided into atria and ventricles, and into right and left. In addition, the heart makes vascular connections with the developing lungs, the vena cavae, and the aorta. The aorta, which begins as a series of paired arches, eventually forms a single arch connecting the left ventricle with the dorsal aorta. To permit most oxygenated blood from the placenta to bypass the lungs, the foramen ovale connects the right and left atrium, and the ductus arteriosus connects the pulmonary artery and the aortic arch.

Anomalies can occur at any point during the complex development of the heart and great vessels. These include inadequate formation of the ventricular or atrial septa, incorrect connection of the aorta and pulmonary artery to the ventricles, incorrect connection of the pulmonary veins or vena cavae to the atria, aberrant aortic arches or branches, persistence of the ductus arteriosus, and narrowing of the aortic arch, or coarctation.

DIGESTIVE TRACT

The intestine begins to form about 4 weeks after conception, incorporating the dorsal yolk sac into a long tube from the primitive mouth (stomodeum) to the anal pit (proctodeum; Fig. 2-4). The epithelial elements of the gut are formed from endo-

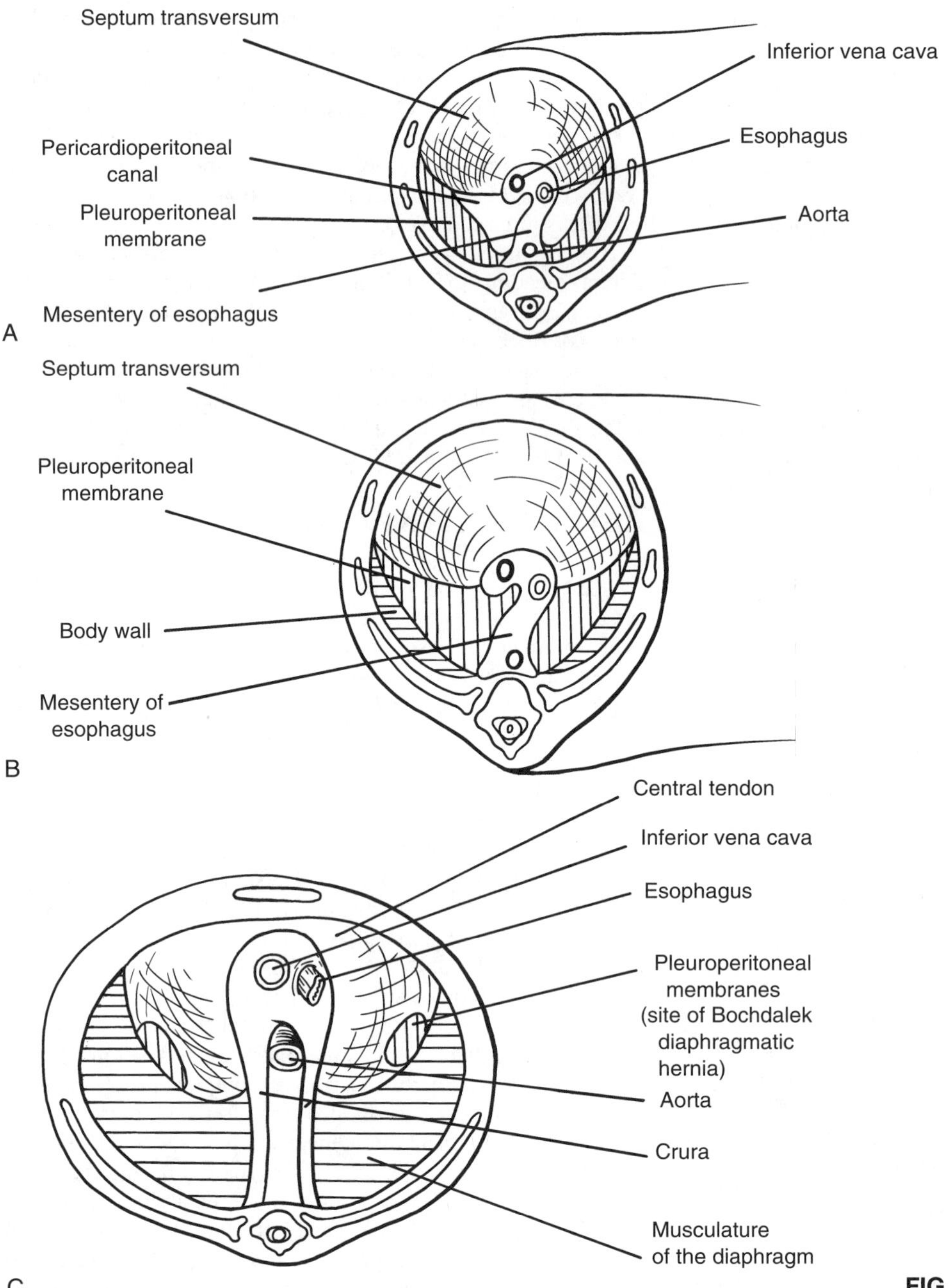

FIG. 2-3. Development of the diaphragm.

derm, and the smooth muscle and connective tissue are formed from surrounding mesoderm. The epithelium of the mouth and anal canal are ectodermal in origin. The enteric nervous system is formed from neural crest cells that migrate into the gut. The digestive system is usually divided into three parts: the foregut, the midgut, and the hindgut.

Foregut

The foregut consists of the pharynx, esophagus, stomach, duodenum, pancreas, liver, and bile ducts. Development of the pharynx and esophagus were described earlier. All the other components of the foregut are supplied by the celiac artery.

The foregut begins as a straight tube. The stomach becomes evident during the 4th week as a small swelling, which rapidly enlarges during the next 2 weeks. The dorsal aspect grows faster than the ventral aspect, creating the greater and lesser curves. As the stomach enlarges, it rotates 90 degrees in a clockwise direction. At the same time, the duodenum (as well as the entire midgut) also grows rapidly and rotates, giving it the characteristic C-loop orientation. During the 5th and 6th weeks, the duodenal epithelium proliferates until the lumen is completely obliterated. Revacuolization due to epithelial degeneration occurs by the end of the 8th week.

The liver begins as a small bud of proliferating endodermal cells from the ventral foregut early in the 4th week after conception. This hepatic diverticulum grows into the septum transver-

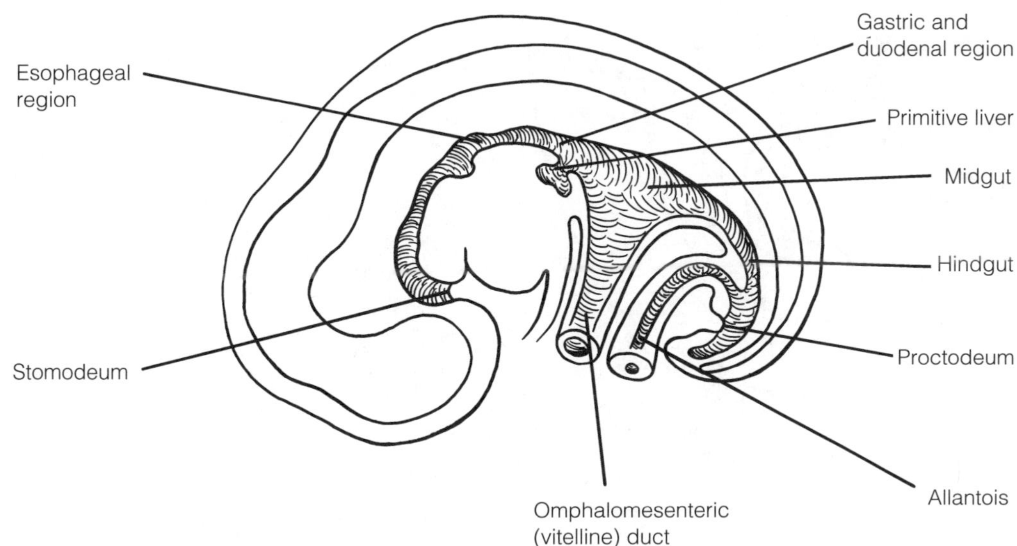

FIG. 2-4. The digestive system 4 weeks after conception.

sum (part of the primitive diaphragm) and between the 5th and 10th weeks fills a large part of the abdominal cavity. The endoderm forms the hepatocytes and the epithelial lining of the biliary tree. The connective tissue, hematopoietic elements, and Kupffer cells are derived from mesenchyme in the septum transversum. The biliary tree, like the duodenum, initially is occluded with proliferating epithelium, but forms a conduit for bile at about the 12th week. Hematopoiesis begins in the liver during the 6th week, but later in fetal life, this responsibility is mostly taken over by the bone marrow. The pancreas develops from two buds of endodermal cells (dorsal and ventral). The ventral bud is carried dorsally with duodenal rotation and eventually fuses with the dorsal bud to form the uncinate process. Both pancreatic exocrine and endocrine cells originate from the endoderm, and the connective tissue arises from the surrounding mesenchyme.

Foregut anomalies are relatively common. Esophageal atresia and tracheoesophageal fistula were mentioned earlier. Failure of recanalization of the duodenum leads to duodenal atresia and stenosis. Annular pancreas and pancreas divisum are caused by incomplete fusion of the ventral and dorsal pancreas. Some cases of biliary atresia may be due to failure of bile duct recanalization, although many are likely acquired in utero and not developmental in origin.

Midgut

The midgut represents those parts of the intestine supplied by the superior mesenteric artery and includes everything from the distal duodenum to the splenic flexure of the colon. Initially, the midgut is connected to the yolk sac by the vitelline or omphalomesenteric duct, which regresses by the 4th week. The midgut then grows rapidly, and during the 6th week begins to herniate into the umbilical cord. Between the 6th and 10th weeks, rotation in a counterclockwise direction around the superior mesenteric artery occurs, and the gut then returns to the abdomen. A further 180 degrees of rotation then occurs in two

planes: around the superior mesenteric artery, and around the umbilicus. Finally, retroperitoneal fixation of the duodenum, ascending colon, and descending colon occurs. Malrotation occurs when rotation is either incomplete or incorrect. Meckel diverticulum is a remnant of the vitelline duct on the intestinal side, but in rare cases, the duct may remain completely intact. Intestinal duplications and atresias likely result from failure or aberrations of recanalization, although some atresias may be the result of an ischemic insult later during gestation. Omphalocele results from failure of the midgut to return to the abdomen in the 10th week.

Hindgut

The hindgut represents the portion of the intestine supplied by the inferior mesenteric artery, including the descending and sigmoid colon, and the organs formed from the cloaca (Fig. 2-5). The cloaca is divided by the urorectal septum into an anterior urogenital sinus and a posterior rectum between the 4th and 7th weeks. At this point, the posterior part of the cloacal membrane becomes the anal membrane, which subsequently ruptures to become the anus.

Abnormal development of the cloaca results in the spectrum of anorectal anomalies, including the various forms of imperforate anus, persistent cloaca, and cloacal exstrophy. Hirschsprung disease usually affects the hindgut and is characterized by absence of enteric ganglion cells. It is controversial whether this is caused by failure of neural crest cell migration or by lack of neural crest cell survival after migration is complete.

GENITOURINARY TRACT

The genitourinary tract is composed of excretory and reproductive components, although the development of these components is closely related.

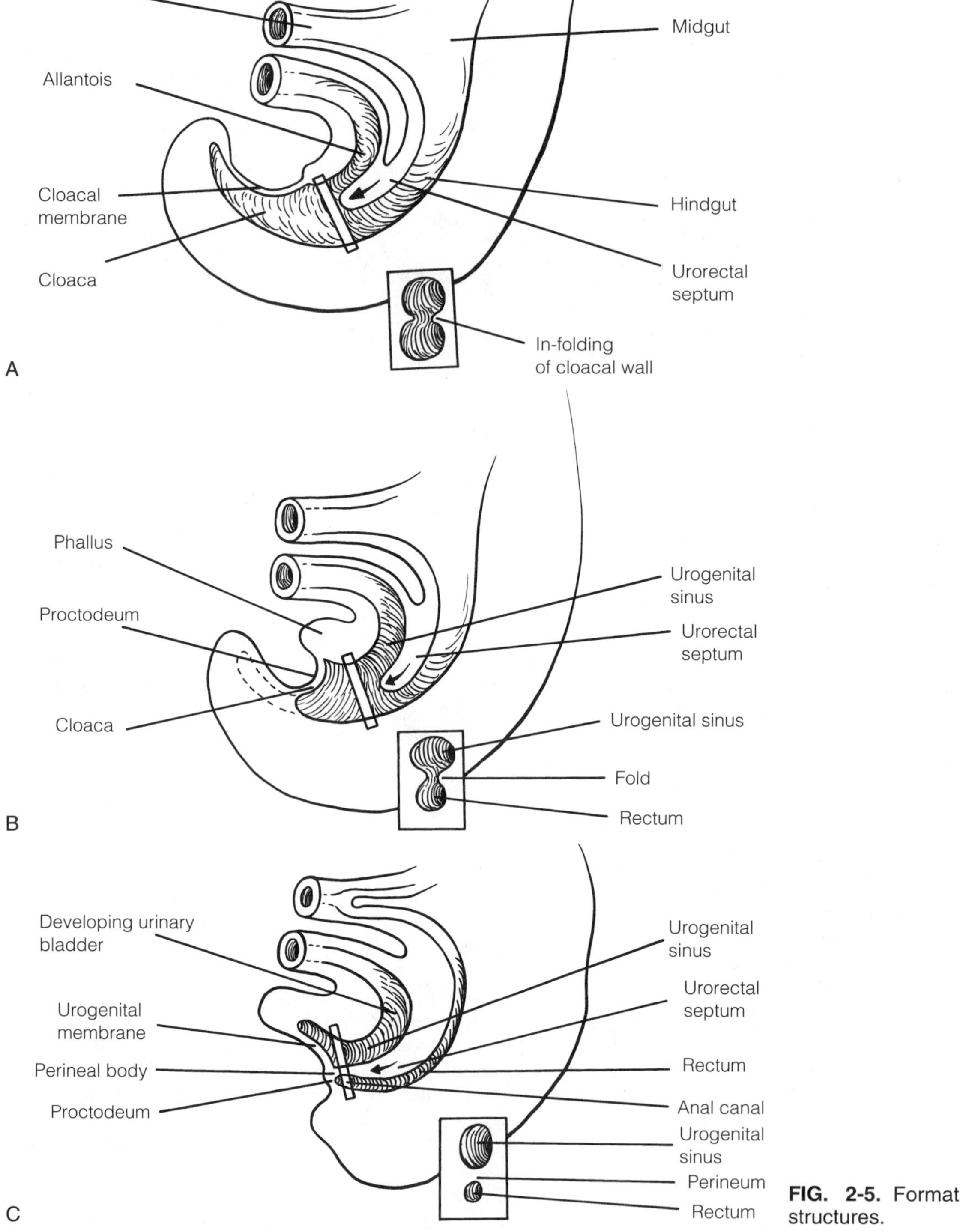

FIG. 2-5. Formation of the cloacal structures.

Urinary System

The kidney forms in three stages. The pronephros appears early in the 4th week after conception and drains into the cloaca through pronephric ducts. The pronephros is then replaced by the mesonephros, which begins to function, and the pronephric ducts become the mesonephric ducts. Finally, the mesonephros is replaced by the metanephros (permanent kidney) toward the end of the first trimester. Urine begins to be produced by the permanent kidneys around the 9th week and through most of fetal life represents the major component of amniotic fluid. The metanephros forms from two sources, both consisting of mesoderm. The metanephric diverticulum (ureteric bud) forms the ureter, renal pelvis, and collecting tubules, and the metanephric mesoderm (metanephrogenic blastema) forms the renal parenchyma.

The bladder and urethra are formed during division of the

cloaca (described earlier), with bladder epithelium arising from endoderm in the urogenital sinus. Early during embryonic life, the bladder is connected to the allantois by the urachus, which subsequently involutes and becomes a fibrous cord.

Anomalies of the kidneys can occur during any of the stages of development and include duplications, dysplastic changes, cysts, and horseshoe kidneys. Persistence of the urachus may result in cysts, sinuses, or fistulae along the anterior abdominal wall.

Reproductive System

The gonads in both males and females are derived from mesothelium in the posterior abdominal wall, which develops medial to the mesonephros during the 5th week. The mesothelium and the surrounding mesenchyme proliferate to form the gonadal ridges. At this point, primordial germ cells from the area of the yolk sac migrate into the area and are incorporated into what are known as the *primary sex cords.* Differentiation into either a testis or ovary then occurs, depending on the presence or absence of a Y chromosome. In males, the testis begins to produce both testosterone and müllerian-inhibiting substance (MIS), which promotes the development of a male phenotype and also leads to normal testicular descent. Absence of a functioning Y chromosome, or inability to respond to testosterone or MIS, results in a female phenotype.

Both male and female embryos have two pairs of ducts: the mesonephric (wolffian) and the paramesonephric (müllerian) ducts. Under the influence of testosterone and MIS, the mesonephric duct becomes the epididymis and vas deferens, and the paramesonephric duct largely disappears. In the absence of testosterone and MIS, the paramesonephric duct contributes to the formation of the uterus and vagina, and the mesonephric duct largely disappears. The external genitalia begin around the 4th week after conception as several collections of mesenchyme, called the *genital tubercle, labioscrotal swellings,* and *urogenital folds.* These form either a male or female phenotype, depending on the presence or absence of a testosterone effect.

A large number of anomalies of the reproductive system occur. These can be caused by faulty morphogenesis (bifid uterus, hypospadias), inability to respond to testosterone (testicular feminization), and abnormally high or low levels of testosterone or MIS (pseudohermaphroditism). In addition, the common problem of cryptorchidism may be related in some cases to defects in hormonal regulation of testicular descent.

CENTRAL NERVOUS SYSTEM

The central nervous system begins during the 3rd week after conception as a small collection of ectoderm called the *neural plate.* Segments of this structure differentiate into the neural crest, which gives rise to most of the peripheral nervous system, enteric nerves, adrenal medulla, melanocytes, and a variety of other cells, and the neural tube, which becomes the central nervous system. The central canal of the neural tube initially communicates with the amniotic fluid, but closes during the 4th week, at about the time a vascular supply to the neural tube is established.

The spinal cord forms from the caudal portion of the neural tube. Three zones of neuroepithelium-derived cells form: the ventricular zone, which forms neurons and macroglial cells; the intermediate zone, which is composed of neuroblasts that go on to develop into neurons; and the marginal zone, which becomes the white matter. As development proceeds, cells from all layers differentiate and form the neurons and supporting cells of the spinal cord. In addition, axons from the developing brain grow into the spinal cord and make connections. The meninges of the spinal cord arise from surrounding mesenchyme, and cerebrospinal fluid (CSF) is formed starting in the 5th week after conception. The development of the spinal cord

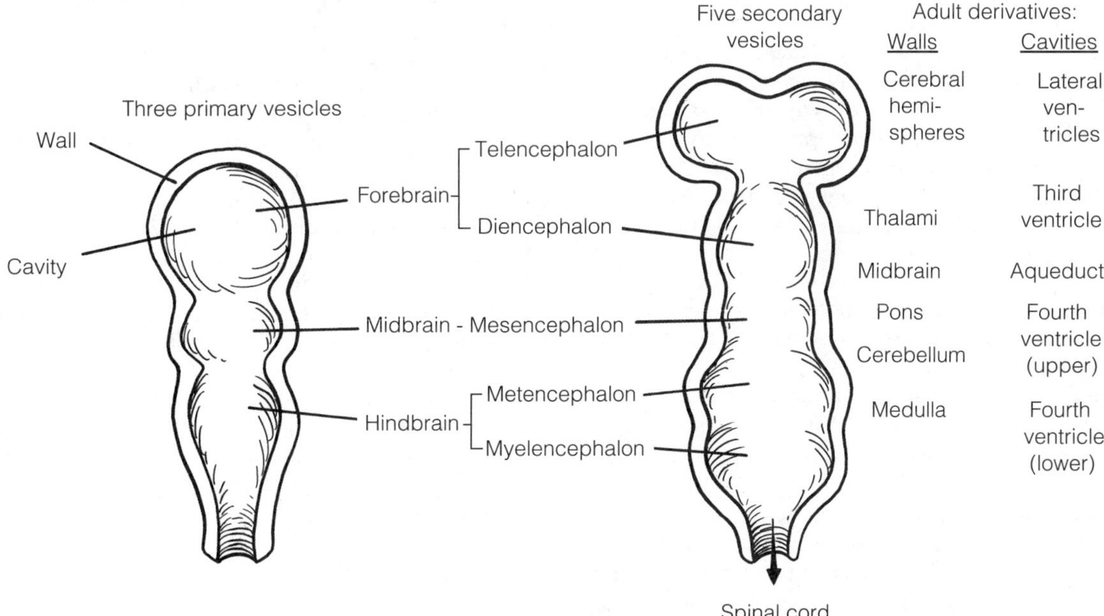

FIG. 2-6. Formation of the brain.

is closely linked to the development of the vertebral column, which originates from the mesenchyme surrounding the primitive notochord. As the neural tube grows, it is surrounded by the developing vertebral bodies.

The brain is formed from the first four somites of the neural tube. During the 4th week after conception, three primary brain vesicles form: the forebrain (prosencephalon), the midbrain (mesencephalon), and the hindbrain (rhombencephalon). During the 5th week, the forebrain again divides into the telencephalon and diencephalon, and the hindbrain divides into the metencephalon and the myelencephalon. Each of these five secondary brain vesicles goes on to form a different part of the mature brain (Fig. 2-6). As with the spinal cord, the meninges are formed from surrounding mesenchyme, and CSF begins to be formed by the choroid plexus in the 5th week.

The most common anomalies of the central nervous system are neural tube defects. These range from spina bifida occulta, which has no neurologic sequelae, to spina bifida with myeloschisis, which is associated with severe neurologic deficit. Similarly, bony defects of the skull can occur either with or without involvement of the underlying brain. Microcephaly or anencephaly occurs as a result of abnormal histogenesis of the brain. Hydrocephalus may result from obstruction to the flow of CSF or from CSF overproduction or underabsorption. Hydrocephalus is often associated with a neural tube defect in the same patient.

2.2　　The Fetus as Patient

N. Scott Adzick and Michael R. Harrison

The diagnosis and treatment of human fetal anatomic abnormalities have evolved rapidly during the past decade because of improved fetal sonographic and sampling techniques and a better understanding of fetal pathophysiology derived from animal models. Fetal therapy is the logical culmination of progress in fetal diagnosis.[5]

The accurate diagnosis of a fetal anomaly permits the physician and parents to decide knowledgeably among various management options for the pregnancy. Although most prenatally diagnosed malformations are best managed by maternal transport, planned delivery near term, and appropriate neonatal therapy, other choices include elective abortion, a change in the timing or mode of delivery, and in utero therapy. A few simple anatomic abnormalities with predictable and life-threatening prenatal pathophysiologic consequences may benefit from surgical correction before birth (Table 2-1).

In the 1960s, direct fetal exposure and catheterization of fetal vessels for exchange transfusion was unsuccessful, and the procedure was abandoned. In the 1970s, increasingly sophisticated sonographic experience led to the accurate diagnosis before birth of many anatomic defects. In the 1980s, the rationale and feasibility of in utero repair for a number of fetal anomalies were explored. The following succession of steps led from the laboratory to the bedside:

1. The pathophysiology of fetal abnormalities was delineated in fetal animal models, and experimental in utero correction was shown to be efficacious.
2. Serial sonographic study of human fetuses with anatomic lesions determined the features that affect clinical outcome and helped craft selection criteria for prenatal intervention.
3. The surgical, anesthetic, and tocolytic techniques for hysterotomy and fetal surgery were developed in nonhuman primates and were finally introduced clinically. In the 1990s, clinical implementation is underway, and critical evaluation of the efficacy, safety, and cost of this new therapeutic approach is anticipated.

PRENATAL DIAGNOSIS

Ultrasonography and Other Imaging Techniques

Ultrasonography, like no other technique of prenatal diagnosis, has permitted the detailed assessment of fetal development and the early recognition of structural defects. The resolution and diagnostic capabilities of ultrasound have increased dramatically during the past decade. Ultrasonography allows accurate prenatal diagnosis without subjecting the mother or fetus to known harmful side effects. In addition, sonographic guidance is routinely employed during other prenatal diagnostic techniques, such as amniocentesis and fetal blood sampling.

The assessment of fetal hemodynamics and cardiac anatomy using echocardiographic techniques deserves special mention. Multiple types of imaging techniques complement each other to provide different types of clinical information. Cross-sectional imaging allows definition of cardiac position and situs. M-mode echocardiography is useful to evaluate ventricular cavity dimension, wall thickness, and valve motion. Pulsed Doppler analysis, especially with the addition of color-coded mapping, is helpful in the analysis of vascular flow patterns, either at the level of the umbilical cord or within the fetal body. In addition to offering a means of evaluating congenital heart defects and arrhythmias, fetal cardiac monitoring has permitted the detailed hemodynamic assessment of the fetus with a noncardiac anomaly.

Other imaging options have emerged for fetal diagnosis. Standard magnetic resonance imaging is difficult to apply to prenatal diagnosis because of fetal movement. A more promising technique is echo planar imaging, which provides a real-time snapshot with the same image quality as magnetic resonance imaging and which may provide a significant improvement in fetal imaging.

Genetic Evaluations

The incidence of abnormal karyotype varies depending on the specific fetal malformation; some examples are: gastroschi-

TABLE 2-1. *Malformations that interfere with development and that may benefit from prenatal surgical relief*

Defect	Effect on development (rationale for treatment)		Treatment
1. Urinary obstruction (urethral valves)	Hydronephrosis	→ Renal failure	Vesicoamniotic shunt
	Lung hypoplasia	→ Pulmonary failure	Video fetoscopic vesicostomy Open vesicostomy
2. Cystic adenomatoid malformation	Lung hypoplasia or hydrops	→ Fetal hydrops and demise	Open pulmonary lobectomy
3. Chylothorax	Lung hypoplasia or hydrops	→ Fetal hydrops and demise	Thoracoamniotic shunt
4. Diaphragmatic hernia	Lung hypoplasia	→ Pumonary failure	Open repair Temporary tracheal occlusion
5. Sacrococcygeal teratoma	High-output failure	→ Fetal hydrops and demise	Resect tumor Video fetoscopic vascular occlusion*
6. Twin–twin transfusion syndrome	Vascular steal through placenta	→ Fetal hydrops and demise	Open fetectomy Video fetoscopic division of placenta
7. Complete heart block	Low-output failure	→ Fetal hydrops and demise	Percutaneous pacemaker Open pacemaker
8. Aqueductal stenosis	Hydrocephalus	→ Brain damage	Ventriculoamniotic shunt Open ventriculoperitoneal shunt*
9. Pulmonary or aortic valve obstruction	Ventricular maldevelopment	→ Heart failure	Percutaneous valvuloplasty Open valvuloplasty*
10. Laryngeal atresia or stenosis	Overdistention by lung fluid	→ Fetal hydrops and demise	Video fetoscopic tracheostomy* Open tracheostomy*

* Not yet attempted in human fetuses.

sis, 1% to 3%; omphalocele, 28% to 52%; and endocardial cushion defect, 70% or more. The combination of two or more anomalies greatly increases the likelihood of aneuploidy. For example, isolated congenital diaphragmatic hernia (CDH) has an 8% to 14% incidence of associated aneuploidy, whereas diaphragmatic hernia and spina bifida are nearly always associated with trisomy 13 or 18. Several alternatives for genetic testing may be available depending on the gestational age of the fetus.

Amniocentesis (14 Weeks to Term)

Since its inception in 1952, second- and third-trimester amniocentesis has been a well-proven gold standard for fetal cell and amniotic fluid sampling for prenatal diagnosis. In addition, late-gestation amniotic fluid sampling, which can be assayed for biochemical markers of pulmonary development, provides guidance for the timing of delivery of the fetus with an anatomic defect. Studies are evaluating the usefulness of amniocentesis before 14 weeks' gestation.

This technique is technically easy and accurate. Amniocentesis requires 10 to 14 days for reliable karyotyping and up to 4 weeks for total turnover time. The principal risk is a low (0.5%) fetal loss rate.

Chorionic Villus Sampling (10 Weeks to Term)

Chorionic villus sampling (CVS) is a *first*-trimester fetal cell sampling procedure that facilitates the prenatal analysis of certain genetic diseases for which specific DNA probes are available. Villi on the implantation side of the gestational sac (chorion frondosum) form the placenta. CVS is performed by biopsy of the placenta using a transcervical or transabdominal approach under ultrasound guidance. Fetal chorionic tissue obtained by CVS is then cultured for specific biochemical or genetic analysis.

Couples at risk for having a fetus with a chromosomal disorder are the largest group to which CVS is applicable. For cytogenetic analysis, an initial chromosomal spread can be obtained within 24 to 48 hours, and final results are completed within 5 to 7 days. Prompt, early diagnosis has obvious advantages for decisions regarding first-trimester abortion.

The major complication of CVS is pregnancy loss (1% to 2%). Concern has also been raised regarding a likely increase in limb abnormalities in fetuses undergoing early CVS (8 to 9 weeks' gestation), so early CVS is generally not recommended unless there are mitigating circumstances. Sources of diagnostic error (1% to 3%) include maternal cell contamination, fetal mosaicism within the chorionic villi, and true false-negative findings for chromosomal abnormalities.

Cordocentesis (18 Weeks to Term)

Cordocentesis, or percutaneous umbilical blood sampling (PUBS), is used for a variety of indications, including prenatal diagnosis of congenital disorders (eg, various hemoglobinopathies, coagulation disorders, and inborn errors of metabolism), detection of prenatal infections (eg, toxoplasmosis and rubella), and rapid karyotyping (2 days versus 10 to 14 days by amniocentesis). The technique requires considerable experience, and the procedure-associated fetal loss rate is 1% to 2%.

A separate and rapidly developing indication for PUBS is fetal intravenous therapy. This application of PUBS is used most often for blood transfusion in fetuses with hemolytic anemia after rhesus alloimmunization. Fetal intravenous therapy also can be used to inject various drugs directly into the fetal circulation, such as agents to treat cardiac arrhythmia.

FETAL SURGICAL MANAGEMENT

Clinical fetal surgical principles are derived from more than 1600 operations in fetal lambs and more than 400 operations in fetal rhesus monkeys performed at our center during the past 15 years. Fetal surgery is a team effort requiring input from the different team members. The operative team consists of two pediatric surgeons, a perinatologist, and a sonographer. The operative steps are performed by the pediatric surgeon with the assistance of the others. Fetal surgery cannot develop and succeed unless a few surgeons are willing to devote considerable time and effort to developing, practicing, and perfecting all aspects of these new procedures: hysterotomy, fetal exposure, and correction; closure of the pregnant uterus; and maternal–fetal perioperative care and control of preterm labor.

Indomethacin and antibiotics are given preoperatively, and halogenated inhalation agents provide anesthesia for both mother and fetus. Perioperative maternal monitoring requires a radial arterial catheter, blood pressure cuff, intravenous and central venous pressure catheters, bladder catheter, electrocardiogram leads, and transcutaneous pulse oximeter.

The uterus is exposed through a low transverse abdominal incision. Fentanyl and pancuronium are injected into the fetus under sterile intraoperative ultrasound guidance to help ablate the fetal stress response. The fetal and placental position are determined sonographically, some amniotic fluid is aspirated through a trocar, the hysterotomy is extended with a specially developed absorbable uterine stapler, and the appropriate fetal part is exposed (Fig. 2-7). For fetal monitoring, a miniaturized pulse oximeter is wrapped around the fetal hand, and an implanted radiotelemetry device reliably measures the fetal electrocardiogram, temperature, and intrauterine pressure both intraoperatively and postoperatively. The fetus and uterus are continually bathed in warm saline. After repair of the defect, the fetus is returned to the uterus, the staples are removed from the uterine edge, a water-tight two-layer uterine closure is performed that is supplemented with fibrin glue to help seal the membranes, and a transparent dressing is placed on the closed laparotomy wound to prevent interference with postoperative sonographic monitoring.

Optimal perioperative management of a fetus and mother requires continuous monitoring of maternal hemodynamics, fetal condition, and uterine contractions in an intensive care setting, usually for 48 hours. Vigilant maternal–fetal monitoring continues on the obstetrics ward for 5 to 7 days postoperatively, followed by outpatient examinations, sonograms, and subcutaneous terbutaline tocolysis given through a portable pump. Cesarean section is performed when either the membranes rupture or labor cannot be controlled, which usually occurs before 36 weeks' gestation.

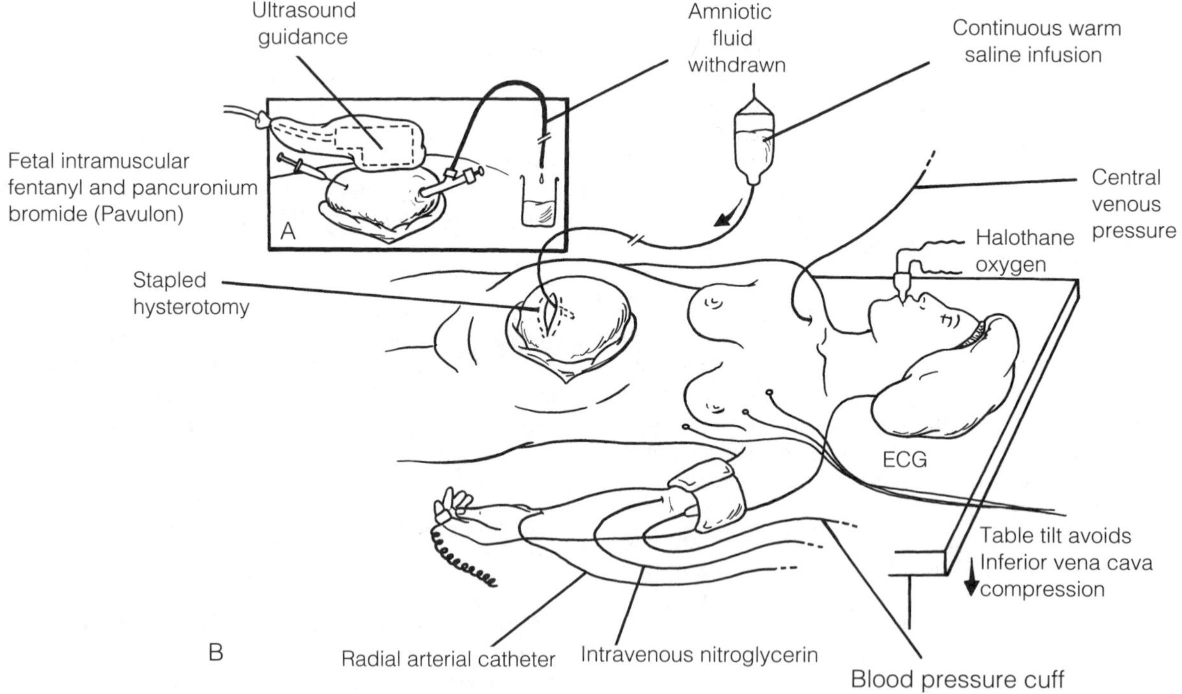

FIG. 2-7. Maternal positioning and monitoring during fetal surgery. (*A*) After laparotomy and uterine exposure, the placenta is localized by ultrasound, fetal blood is withdrawn, and some amniotic fluid is withdrawn to make the uterus softer. (*B*) Maternal positioning includes tilting to avoid compression of the inferior vena cava by the gravid uterus. The hysterotomy is made away from the placenta, and only the pertinent fetal anatomy is exposed. Maternal monitoring includes a radial arterial line and a subclavian central venous catheter. (After Harrison MR, Golbus MS, Filly RA. The unborn patient, ed 2. Philadelphia, WB Saunders, 1990)

Appropriate surveillance and treatment of preterm labor remains the drawback of fetal surgery, and the tocolytic regimen that was successful in the nonhuman primate experiments is fraught with potential clinical difficulties. Indomethacin can cause fetal ductus arteriosus constriction, tricuspid regurgitation, and right-sided heart failure, so serial fetal echocardiographic monitoring is essential. Although deep halogenated anesthesia can provide satisfactory intraoperative uterine relaxation, this regimen can produce fetal and maternal myocardial depression and decrease placental perfusion. Maternal pulmonary edema is a known side effect of magnesium sulfate and β-mimetics used for tocolysis, and fluid restriction to avoid this complication may compromise maternal–placental–fetal circulation and exacerbate preterm labor. Experimental studies suggest that endogenous nitric oxide mediates normal uterine relaxation during pregnancy. Nitric oxide donors have been shown to inhibit hysterotomy-induced uterine contractions in rhesus monkeys,[6] and our own use of the nitric oxide donor nitroglycerin appears effective in the management of uterine contractions during human fetal surgery.

Maternal safety is the cardinal issue. Clearly, the healthy mother accepts some risk to help her unborn child. Although there have been few maternal complications in 47 cases from our center, all patients had uterine contractions after fetal surgery, which accounted for some morbidity from the treatment regimen (one patient developed pulmonary edema from the tocolytic medications). Amniotic fluid leaks developed in five patients: two patients had leaks through the hysterotomy site requiring reoperation and closure, and three other patients had vaginal amniotic fluid leaks that were presumably from fluid dissecting internally from the hysterotomy site to the cervix. There were two infections: one case of pseudomembranous colitis due to parenteral antibiotic therapy that responded promptly to a course of oral vancomycin, and one superficial wound infection. Five patients required blood transfusion.

Because the mid-gestation hysterotomy is invariably in the upper segment of the uterine corpus and thus is comparable to a classic cesarean section, there is potential for uterine disruption during labor. Thus, delivery after the fetal surgery and for all future deliveries should be by cesarean section. Two disruptions occurred in subsequent pregnancies before a cesarean section could be done. Maternal and neonatal outcome were excellent in both cases. Finally, future reproductive potential does not appear to be jeopardized by fetal surgery. Although most fetal operations have taken place in the past 3 years, long-term follow-up from earlier cases revealed that 18 patients have had 19 normal children in subsequent pregnancies.

FETAL THORACIC LESIONS

Prenatal diagnosis provides new insight into the natural history, pathophysiology, and management of fetuses with thoracic lesions such as congenital cystic adenomatoid malformation (CCAM) and pulmonary sequestration. In a series of more than 100 prenatally diagnosed cases, the overall prognosis depended on the size of the lung mass and the secondary physiologic derangement: a large mass causes mediastinal shift, hypoplasia of normal lung tissue, polyhydramnios, and cardiovascular compromise leading to fetal hydrops and death. Hydrops is a harbinger of fetal or neonatal demise and manifests as fetal ascites, pleural and pericardial effusions, and skin and scalp edema. Smaller thoracic lesions can cause respiratory distress in the newborn period, and the smallest masses may be asymptomatic until later in childhood, when infection or pneumothorax may occur.

Prenatal Diagnosis and Natural History

Classically, three types of CCAM (types I to III) have been categorized based primarily on cyst size. We have classified prenatally diagnosed CCAM into two categories based on gross anatomy and ultrasound findings. Macrocystic lesions contain single or multiple cysts that are 5 mm in diameter or larger, appear cystic on prenatal ultrasound, are not frequently associated with hydrops, and have a more favorable prognosis. Microcystic lesions are more solid, appear echogenic on prenatal ultrasound, and are more commonly associated with pulmonary hypoplasia, fetal hydrops, and death. The overall prognosis, however, depends primarily on the *size* of the CCAM rather than on the lesion type.

Pulmonary sequestrations are masses of nonfunctioning lung tissue supplied by an anomalous systemic artery. On prenatal ultrasonography, a pulmonary sequestration appears as a well-defined, echodense, homogeneous mass in the lower chest or even in the abdomen. Detection by color-flow Doppler of a systemic artery from the aorta to the fetal lung lesion is a pathognomonic feature of fetal pulmonary sequestration. The ability to differentiate intralobar and extralobar sequestration before birth is limited unless an extralobar sequestration is highlighted by a pleural effusion or is located in the abdomen. There are no diagnostic hallmarks for the specific prenatal diagnosis of an intralobar sequestration.

Because polyhydramnios is a common obstetric indication for ultrasonography, a prenatal diagnostic marker exists for many large fetal lung tumors. Polyhydramnios is likely due to esophageal compression by the thoracic mass, with consequent interference with fetal swallowing of amniotic fluid. Support for this concept comes from the absence of fluid in the fetal stomach in some of these cases, and the alleviation of polyhydramnios (and the return of visible gastric fluid) after effective fetal treatment. Although there is some association of both polyhydramnios and hydrops with fetal CCAM, our experience indicates that either can occur independently of the other.

Differences in survival rate of patients with CCAM previously were ascribed to the histologic type of the lesion, but our experience is that an unfavorable outcome is associated most closely with fetal hydrops. The hydrops is secondary to vena caval obstruction and cardiac compression from huge tumors causing an extreme mediastinal shift. Like CCAMs, fetal extralobar pulmonary sequestrations can also cause fetal hydrops, and the mechanism is usually a tension hydrothorax from fluid or lymph secretion from the sequestration into the pleural space.

Although sonographic prenatal diagnosis is becoming increasingly sophisticated, diagnostic errors are possible. Diaphragmatic hernia can be distinguished either by careful sonographic assessment or by amniography with or without computed tomography. Other possibilities in the ultrasonographic differential diagnosis of fetal thoracic masses include bronchogenic and enteric cysts, mediastinal cystic teratoma, and bronchial atresia or stenosis.

Fetal Chylothorax

Congenital pleural effusions are often due to fetal chylothorax (FCT) and can be diagnosed as early as 16 weeks' gestation. Small effusions may be harmless, but large effusions may result in pulmonary compression, pulmonary hypoplasia, and hydrops.

We have reported on a series of 32 cases.[7] The overall mortality rate was 53%. Polyhydramnios was present in 22 cases and was not associated with a higher mortality rate. Early diagnosis (less than 32 weeks' gestation) and hydrops were associated with a higher mortality rate. Pleural fluid was available in 12 patients, all of which had more than 80% lymphocytes on cell count, which confirmed the diagnosis of FCT.

Small effusions diagnosed late in gestation often have a satisfactory outcome without prenatal treatment, and some resolve spontaneously. In these cases, serial ultrasound examinations should be performed, with appropriate postnatal follow-up. For large effusions causing hydrops, in utero decompression may offer the only hope for survival. Although success with repeated thoracenteses in utero has been reported, we have used a percutaneously placed thoracoamniotic shunt successfully in several cases to decompress the FCT after a single aspiration failed to drain the fetal chest permanently. Rodeck and colleagues[8] reported the successful placement of a thoracoamniotic shunt in eight fetuses with massive FCT. Six of these infants survived, five without respiratory difficulty postnatally. Lung reexpansion was seen in all of the survivors, but not in the two who died.

Disappearing Fetal Lung Lesions

Although a large pulmonary lesion diagnosed in utero might appear to be an ominous finding, the natural history of prenatally diagnosed pulmonary lesions is variable. Some large fetal lung lesions can decrease in size and even disappear before birth. We have reported nine cases of prenatally diagnosed large pulmonary lesions (three CCAMs and six sequestrations) associated with contralateral mediastinal shift that dramatically decreased in size during the course of the pregnancy.[9] None of these fetuses had signs of hydrops. Thus, the natural history of fetal pulmonary lesions is dynamic and variable. Initial impressions concerning the prognosis of large pulmonary lesions should be tempered with the understanding that they can occasionally shrink in size or even disappear.

The exact mechanism by which these lesions shrink is unclear. The masses that shrank in our series were all echodense lesions. The echogenic appearance on ultrasonography is due to the large number of tissue–fluid interfaces. As the lung lesions decreased in size, they also became less echogenic, implying that they were losing tissue–fluid interfaces. CCAMs and sequestrations usually do not communicate directly with the tracheobronchial tree, although abnormal channels to the airway and the gastrointestinal tract can occur. Perhaps the lesions shrink owing to decompression of fetal lung fluid through these abnormal channels. Another possible explanation is that the pulmonary lesions outgrow their vascular supply and involute. It is unlikely that the lesions actually stayed the same size but appeared to shrink relative to the growing fetus because some of these lesions disappeared completely on prenatal ultrasonography.

Experimental Studies: Rationale for Fetal Surgery

Experimental studies have elucidated the pathophysiologic consequences of fetal intrathoracic masses and have demonstrated that fetal pulmonary resection is straightforward. Simulation of the thoracic mass effect with an intrathoracic balloon in the third-trimester fetal lamb resulted in pulmonary hypoplasia and death at term due to respiratory insufficiency,[10] whereas lambs that underwent simulated resection of the mass by balloon deflation in the middle of the third trimester had sufficient lung growth to permit survival at birth.[11] In addition, intrauterine pneumonectomy in fetal lambs is technically feasible at early and mid-gestation and can induce compensatory growth of the remaining lung by term.[12]

To study the cause of hydrops associated with huge fetal lung masses, we created a fetal sheep model in which a surgically implanted intrathoracic tissue expander was gradually inflated over several days while monitoring fetal arterial, venous, intrathoracic, and intraamniotic pressures and while monitoring for sonographic indications of hydrops.[13] Balloon inflation resulted in hydrops as a result of cardiac venous obstruction and increasing central venous pressure. Simulation of prenatal resection of the fetal thoracic mass by deflating the expander resulted in complete resolution of the hydrops and return of pressures to normal. This model may be used to further evaluate the pathophysiologic and sonographic features of large fetal chest masses.

Fetal Surgery Experience

Fetuses with life-threatening CCAM were selected for prenatal treatment according to predetermined guidelines, including the gestational age of the fetus, the size of the intrathoracic lesion, maternal health, and the development of fetal hydrops. The finding that fetuses with large tumors and hydrops are at high risk for fetal or neonatal demise led to several therapeutic maneuvers. Fetal thoracentesis alone was ineffective because of rapid reaccumulation of cyst fluid. Thoracoamniotic shunting was attempted in five cases that had at least one predominant cyst, but shunting provided reliable long-term decompression only in two cases. Fetal thoracoamniotic shunts can be used to decompress the tension hydrothorax that can be associated with extralobar pulmonary sequestration. Multicystic or predominantly solid CCAM lesions do not lend themselves to catheter decompression and require resection.

Fetal surgical resection of the massively enlarged pulmonary lobe (fetal lobectomy) was performed between 21 and 27 weeks' gestation in eight cases, with five survivors[14] (Table 2-2). In the first case, resection was too late because preoperative labor and maternal preeclampsia could not be reversed, leading to premature delivery of a nonviable infant. In cases two, three, four, five, and eight, CCAM resection led to resolution of the hydrops, impressive in utero lung growth, and normal postnatal development with follow-up of 6 to 40 months (Fig. 2-8). After resection, fetal hydrops resolved in 1 to 2 weeks, and the mediastinum returned to the midline within 3 weeks. Right middle and lower lobe resection in the sixth fetus at 21 weeks' gestation was successful, but subsequent inexplicable fetal demise highlights the need for better postoperative fetal monitoring and treatment. Case seven was unsuccessful because of uncontrolled intraoperative uterine contractions leading to fetal death. This series demonstrates that in highly selected

TABLE 2-2. *Congenital cystic adenomatoid malformation resections*

Case no.	Fetal hydrops	Surgery (gestational wk)	Prenatal course	Follow-up (gestational wk)	Outcome	Lesion location
1	Yes	27	Preterm labor and mirror syndrome	28	Died from lung hypoplasia at 40 h	RML
2	Yes	23	Hydrops resolved 1 wk after surgery	30	Ventilated for 2 d; left pneumothorax; alive and well at 4 y	LLL
3	Yes	26	Failed shunt at 25 wk; hydrops resolved 2 wk after surgery	34	Ventilated for 6 d; alive and well at 2½ y	LLL
4	Yes	26	Hydrops resolved 1 wk after surgery	33	Ventilated for 2 d; alive and well at 2½ y	LLL
5	Yes	24	Postoperative indocin-induced ductus arteriosus constriction; preterm labor and delivery 2 wk after surgery	26	Ventilated for 4 wk; right pneumothorax; PDA ligation; alive and well at 2 y	RML
6	Yes	21	Fetal demise 8 h after surgery; autopsy showed no known cause of death	21	—	RML, RLL
7	Yes	25	Intraoperative fetal demise secondary to uterine contractions	—	—	RUL
8	Yes	24	Minimal uterine activity on nitroglycerin; hydrops resolved 1 wk after surgery	30	Ventilated for 10 d; alive and well at 1 y	RML, RLL

RML, right middle lobe; LLL, left lower lobe; RLL, right lower lobe; RUL, right upper lobe; PDA, patent ductus arteriosus.

cases, fetal CCAM resection is reasonably safe, is technically feasible, reverses hydrops, and allows sufficient lung growth to permit survival.

The first case showed that the maternal hyperdynamic state referred to as the *mirror syndrome* cannot be reversed solely by treatment of the underlying fetal condition. This preeclamptic state is associated with molar pregnancies and fetal conditions that cause placentomegaly (also seen in severe cases of fetal sacrococcygeal teratoma [SCT] and fetal neuroblastoma) and that may be caused by a factor released by poorly perfused

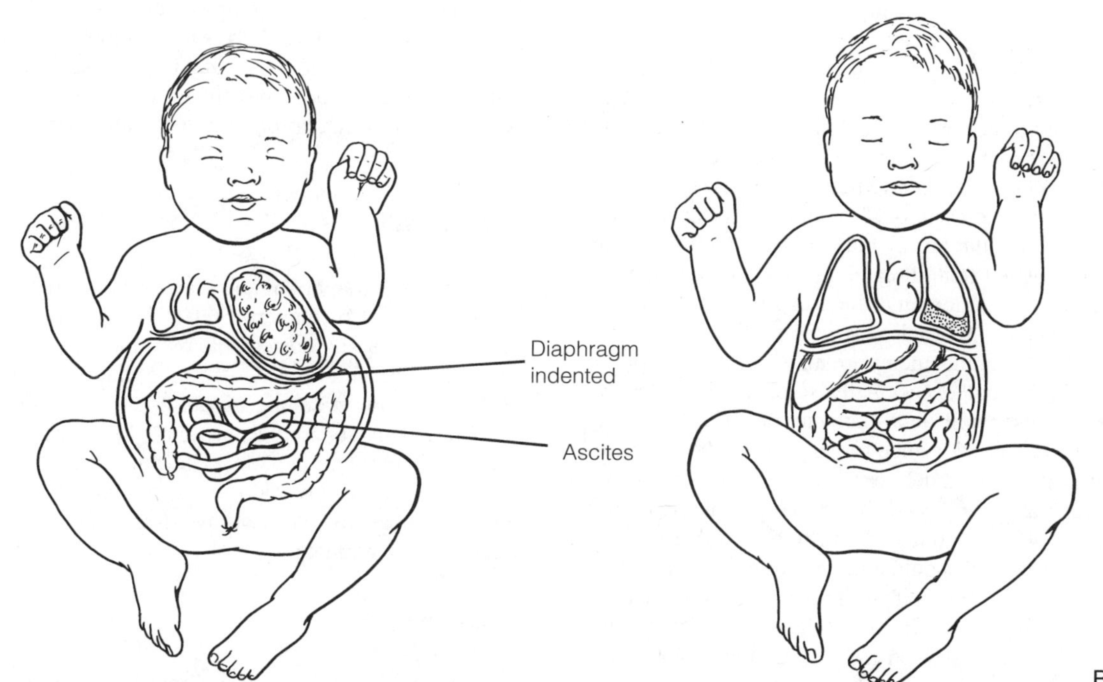

FIG. 2-8. Fetal anatomy preoperatively (*A*) and 6 weeks after fetal surgery (*B*).

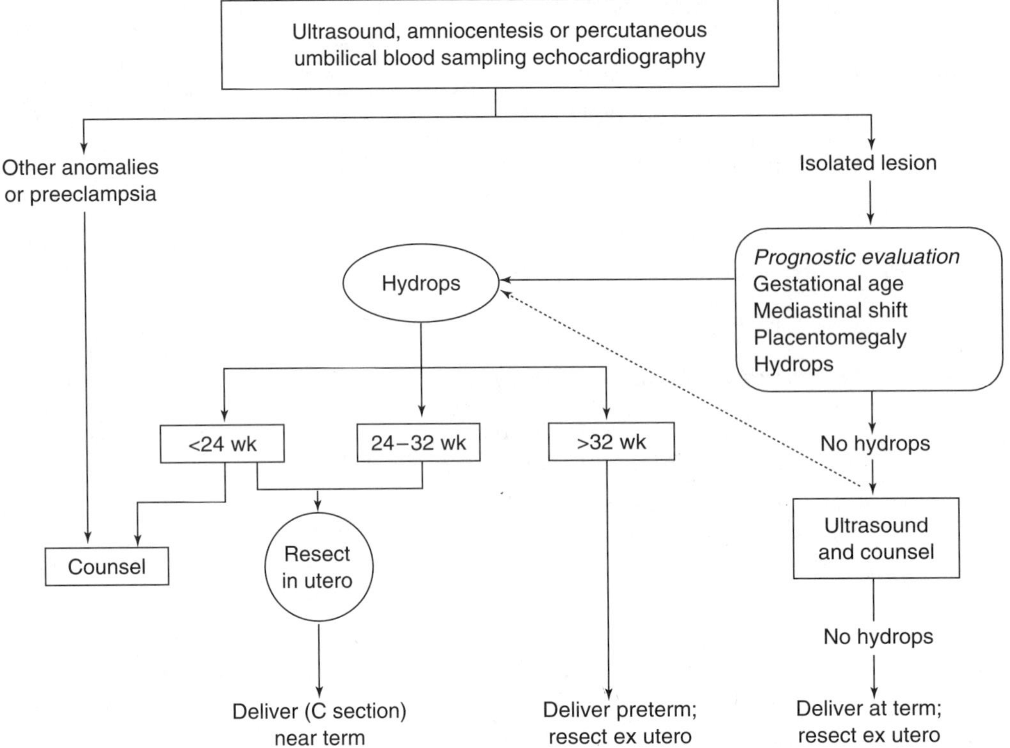

FIG. 2-9. Management algorithm for the fetus with a cystic adenomatoid malformation. (Adzick NS, Harrison MR, Flake AW, et al. Fetal surgery for cystic adenomatoid malformation of the lung. J Pediatr Surg 1993;28:806)

placental tissue that leads to endothelial cell injury. Until the pathophysiology of the maternal mirror syndrome is understood, earlier intervention before the onset of placentomegaly and the related maternal preeclamptic state may be the only approach to salvage these fetuses.

A proposed algorithm for management of the fetus with a thoracic mass is shown in Figure 2-9. Initial evaluation begins with an ultrasound to confirm the diagnosis, amniocentesis or PUBS to exclude chromosomal anomalies, and a fetal echocardiogram to detect congenital heart disease. If an associated life-threatening anomaly is present or if the mother is sick with the mirror syndrome, then the family may choose to terminate the pregnancy. For isolated fetal thoracic masses, the fetus undergoes a prognostic evaluation, and there is a wide spectrum of severity. If fetus is not hydropic, then the mother is followed by serial ultrasound. Arrangements are made for the best possible care after birth, and occasionally some of these lesions shrink in size. Fetuses with fetal thoracic masses who do not have hydrops have a good chance for survival in the setting of maternal transport, planned delivery, and immediate resuscitation and surgery at a facility with extracorporeal membrane oxygenation (ECMO) capability. At birth, babies that have an antenatal shrinking lesion should undergo surgery if the pulmonary mass is symptomatic or if the lesion is large enough to be seen on chest radiograph. In the absence of symptoms and radiologic anomalies, as seen in the rare disappearing lesion, expectant management is reasonable.

If the fetus is hydropic at presentation or if hydrops develops during serial follow-up, then management depends on the gestational age. For those fetuses greater than 32 to 34 weeks' gestation, early delivery should be considered so that the lesion can be resected ex utero. For those fetuses less than 32 weeks' gestation, there is a new therapeutic option, which is to treat the lesion before birth. With prenatal identification of fetal thoracic tumors comes the potential for in utero intervention in severe cases to prevent fatal progression of pulmonary hypoplasia and hydrops.

CONGENITAL DIAPHRAGMATIC HERNIA

Congenital diaphragmatic hernia is a frustrating clinical problem (see also chapter 54). CDH is an anatomically simple defect that is easily correctable by removing the herniated viscera from the chest and closing the diaphragm. Many infants with CDH, however, die of pulmonary insufficiency despite optimal postnatal care because their lungs are too hypoplastic to support extrauterine life. The pulmonary hypoplasia seen with CDH has been well documented clinically and experimentally; it appears to be caused by compression of the developing fetal lung by herniated bowel.

Fetal Lamb Model

To study the pulmonary hypoplasia that accompanies CDH and the possibility of reversing these changing by correcting the CDH in utero, a model was developed in which a conical, silicone-rubber balloon was progressively inflated in the left hemithorax of fetal lambs during the last trimester to simulate compression of the growing fetal lung by abdominal viscera.[10] Lambs with inflated intrathoracic balloons deteriorated rapidly and died of respiratory insufficiency despite maximal resuscitation and ventilatory support. Deflation of the balloon midway through the third trimester (simulated correction) allowed sufficient lung growth to alleviate respiratory insufficiency and to ensure survival in all of five lambs delivered by cesarean section.[11] Simulated correction produced a significant increase in lung weight, air capacity, compliance, and area of the pulmonary vascular bed.

Although the balloon model established the efficacy of in utero repair, it could not be used to study the feasibility of correction or to develop the surgical techniques necessary for actual successful fetal surgical repair. For this purpose, actual fetal diaphragmatic hernias had to be created and then repaired. We created diaphragmatic hernias in fetal lambs by making a hole in the left diaphragm and demonstrated that herniated viscera produced pulmonary hypoplasia comparable to that produced by the balloon. We then tried to repair the CDH surgically at a second operation.[15]

The first attempts at repair were unsuccessful because increased intraabdominal pressure secondary to replacement of the viscera into the abdomen resulted in severely compromised umbilical venous blood flow. It became clear that the abdominal cavity would need to be enlarged to prevent increased intraabdominal pressure after CDH repair. Incorporating a piece of Silastic into the abdominal wall proved to be a satisfactory solution, allowing the abdominal contents to be accommodated without increased pressure. When these techniques were used to repair fetal CDH, the lambs survived at term, and at sacrifice, the lungs were well expanded, histologically mature, and much larger than those of uncorrected animals. Subsequent pulmonary morphometric studies have shown that an early gestational CDH lamb model simulates the morphologic features that correlate with fatal outcome for human neonates with CDH and persistent fetal circulation, and that fetal surgical repair ameliorates these vascular changes and permits compensatory lung growth and development.[16]

Prenatal Diagnosis and Natural History

The prenatal diagnosis of CDH by sonogram has made it possible to define the natural history of this lesion and elucidate the important pathophysiologic features. Experienced sonographers can make the prenatal diagnosis of CDH accurately, and current techniques can detect lethal nonpulmonary anomalies and prevent diagnostic errors. Serial sonographic studies have demonstrated that fetal CDH is a dynamic process and that there is a broad range of severity; nonsurvivors have larger diaphragmatic defects and a greater volume of viscera displaced into the chest at an earlier stage of development. Fetuses diagnosed late in gestation, often after a previously normal-appearing ultrasound examination, may have herniated only late in gestation and may not have significant lung compression from a dilated stomach or liver in the chest.

Polyhydramnios is both a common prenatal marker for CDH and a predictor for mortality. The association of polyhydram-

nios with poor prognosis may be explained by obstruction of the esophagus or duodenum (Fig. 2-10). For example, herniation of the stomach into the chest can kink the duodenum and produce gastric outlet obstruction, which has been documented at autopsy. Gastric outlet obstruction produces both polyhydramnios and gastric dilation with significant intrathoracic volume displacement and compression of the lungs. Thus, the severity of pulmonary hypoplasia may be directly linked to polyhydramnios by partial gastric outlet obstruction.

A wide discrepancy can be found in the outcomes reported for infants with CDH. Survey data derived from neonatal centers underestimate the incidence and mortality of CDH because the more severely affected infants often die before the anomaly is recognized. Minimum incidence figures derived from various sources range from 1 in 2400 to 1 in 5000 live births; the true incidence, including stillborn fetuses, is probably about 1 in 2200 births. Tertiary neonatal referral centers report that up to 80% of neonates with CDH can be saved, whereas reliable data on more than 200 fetuses with this condition show that less than 25% can be saved despite optimal, planned tertiary care that includes ECMO.[17,18] This discrepancy between the visible mortality reported from children's centers that treat only those infants who survive gestation, birth, resuscitation, transport, and often major surgery, and the true mortality based on all prenatally diagnosed cases has been called the *hidden mortality* of CDH. The magnitude of the hidden mortality for CDH is not known and cannot be accurately determined from a birth defects monitoring program because many cases in stillborn infants go unrecognized unless there is an autopsy.

On the other hand, reports from prenatal diagnostic specialists that CDH mortality rates exceed 75% are overly pessimistic. Fifteen to 40% of these fetuses have other life-threatening chromosomal and anatomic anomalies, which often preclude treatment or survival. Clearly, the estimated mortality for the re-

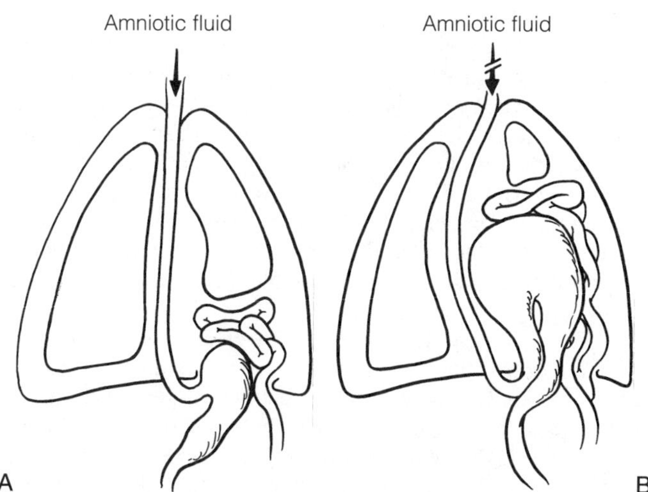

FIG. 2-10. The pathophysiologic link between polyhydramnios and mortality is related to herniation of the fetal stomach into the chest. A dilated stomach with partial outlet obstruction results in interference with fetal swallowing of amniotic fluid with resultant polyhydramnios as well as severe lung compression and hypoplasia.

maining potentially salvageable fetuses with isolated CDH is lower than the overall mortality for all fetuses with CDH.

It would seem that antenatal diagnosis of CDH would result in immediate postnatal repair and survival. Our initial reported experience with fetal CDH, however, was disappointing: no survivors in seven fetuses prospectively diagnosed before birth. This led to a multicenter survey that documented the natural history and clinical outcome of fetal CDH in 94 cases.[17] This study demonstrated that the prenatal sonographic diagnosis is accurate, the mortality rate is high (80%), and polyhydramnios is a prenatal predictor of poor clinical outcome. A subsequent study of 38 prenatally diagnosed cases from Boston Children's Hospital permitted a detailed assessment of prognostic factors and evaluation of the impact of ECMO on outcome.[18] This study found that survival was poor despite optimal postnatal therapy that included ECMO, and that both polyhydramnios and an early gestational diagnosis were associated with a dismal outcome.

A Prospective Study

Because retrospective estimates of mortality for CDH vary widely and are flawed by a hidden mortality of unknown magnitude, we performed a prospective study to settle the question of outcome for potentially salvageable fetuses with isolated CDH diagnosed before 25 weeks' gestation.[19] Eighty-three such fetuses were identified that were referred to our Fetal Treatment Center from 1989 to 1993. These fetuses had well-documented diaphragmatic hernias diagnosed before 25 weeks' gestation without associated chromosomal or anatomic abnormalities. Outcome was determined after planned delivery at tertiary neonatal centers with ECMO availability.

These patients were candidates for in utero repair, but the families chose conventional management with delivery at a neonatal center. Fifty-eight percent (48 of 83) died despite optimal postnatal care. Of the 48 fetuses who did not survive, 7 died in utero, an unexpectedly high rate of fetal demise. Of these 7, 4 fetuses died spontaneously near term, one after attempted version, and two others after chorioamnionitis developed after PUBS. Four neonates died after premature delivery (29 to 32 weeks' gestation), attributable to massive polyhydramnios secondary to fetal CDH. Sixteen neonates had severe respiratory distress at birth and could not be resuscitated sufficiently to receive ECMO. Twenty newborns died despite successful resuscitation and urgent ECMO support lasting from 2 to 30 days. Twenty-two of the 35 survivors received ECMO, and 9 of these have severe chronic illness attributable to the intensive management.

This prospective study revealed three reasons why retrospective studies from tertiary centers often underestimate the hidden mortality of CDH. First, patients reported from tertiary centers are selected. For example, 3 newborns in this series were delivered at an ECMO center that has reported an 80% survival for diaphragmatic hernia. Two died immediately after birth, and the third died after ECMO treatment; only the last patient would be reported as an ECMO failure. Second, 7 fetuses suffered intrauterine demise, and 4 others were delivered prematurely at 29 to 32 weeks' gestation because of severe polyhydramnios. Most of these would not be counted as deaths due to CDH unless an autopsy was performed. Third, 16 neonates died immediately after birth before ECMO could be started; some of these may have gone unrecognized, and none would be reported in the mortality figures of an ECMO registry.

Experience With Treatment Before Birth

The pulmonary hypoplasia that limits survival is an underdevelopment of both the pulmonary parenchyma and vascular bed and appears to be reversible both experimentally and clinically. Many weeks or even months are required for treatment, however. ECMO is limited to 1 to 2 weeks, and while useful for marginal babies, it clearly cannot salvage severely affected babies. Long-term support or replacement of lung function after birth requires either an artificial placenta or neonatal lung transplantation. Repair before birth with continued support on the placental ECMO while the fetal lung grows and recovers would be ideal. Repair in utero with continued gestation, however, has proved to be a formidable challenge. Initial attempts to repair six fetuses with diaphragmatic hernia showed that although the repair was feasible, there were significant technical difficulties, particularly from herniated liver.[20]

From 1989 to 1991, fetal repair was attempted in 14 fetuses with severe isolated left CDH diagnosed before 25 weeks' gestation.[21] Five fetuses died intraoperatively from technical problems related to reduction of incarcerated liver and uterine contractions. Nine patients were successfully repaired. Four patients survived, two were delivered prematurely and died, and three died in utero within 48 hours of repair. This series demonstrated that issues of patient selection and many intraoperative technical problems have been overcome. The factors limiting successful outcome are now postoperative physiologic management of the maternal–fetal unit and effective tocolysis to control preterm labor.

Many fetuses with left diaphragmatic hernias have some liver herniated into the chest. This comes as a surprise because pediatric surgeons seldom see liver in a CDH patient after birth. This is because newborns who make it to surgery often already have the liver reduced from the chest by positive-pressure ventilation. Reduction of the liver after birth either by the respirator or by the surgeon causes little problem because there is no blood flow through the umbilical vein. Reduction of the liver before birth is devastating because it compromises the umbilical circulation (Fig. 2-11). Herniated liver accounted for most failures. Disturbance of the umbilical circulation during or after liver reduction was implicated in all five intraoperative deaths and in the three early postoperative deaths.

The problem of accurate preoperative assessment of the extent of liver herniation has finally yielded to careful evaluation of the umbilical vein and ductus venosus by color-flow Doppler. Fetuses with the vessels above the level of the diaphragm cannot be repaired completely by current techniques and can be excluded. In these cases, the entire liver is torqued into the chest and cannot be reduced without compromising umbilical flow. This is also true for right-sided diaphragmatic hernias because reduction of the torqued liver kinks not only the sinus venosus but also the inferior vena cava.

The toughest lesson was that the subcostal incision that works so well after birth provides inadequate exposure to deal with the severe defects encountered in those fetuses. The solution is a carefully planned two-step approach employing both a thora-

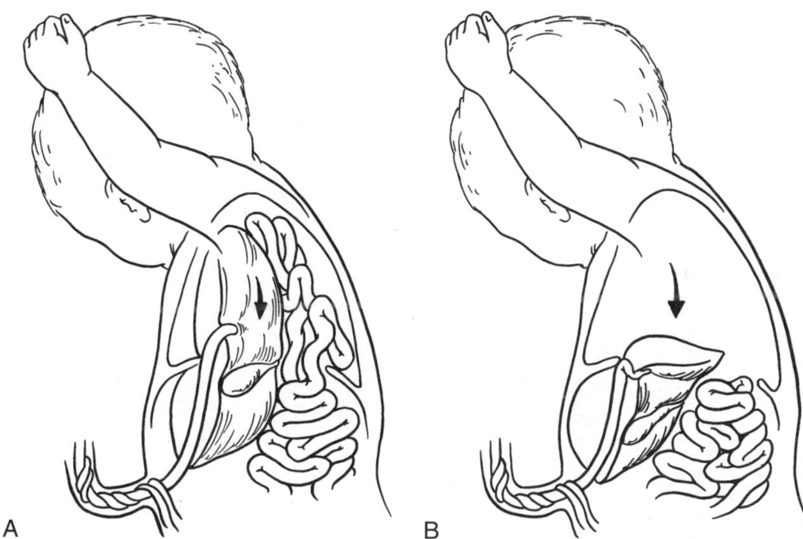

FIG. 2-11. Attempts to reduce the herniated fetal liver cause fetal deterioration and demise; autopsy and angiogram studies have documented kinking of the umbilical vein with compromise of venous return. (After Harrison MR, Adzick NS, Longaker MT, et al. Successful repair in utero of a fetal diaphragmatic hernia after removal of herniated viscera from the left thorax. N Engl J Med 1990;322:1582)

cotomy and a subcostal incision. This method allows reduction of viscera using a push–pull technique and reconstruction of the diaphragm with a prosthetic patch.

Plug the Lung Until it Grows: A Potential Method to Treat Congenital Diaphragmatic Hernia in Utero

Even with these advances, complete repair of CDH in utero remains challenging. We have long sought another approach to improve fetal lung growth that does not require the extensive manipulation necessary for total repair. The simple expedient of creating an abdominal wall defect and leaving the viscera externalized has proved unsatisfactory: decompression of the chest is inadequate, and damage to the viscera can be significant.[20] A potential therapeutic strategy for treatment of CDH in utero is to block the normal outflow of fetal lung fluid through the trachea. The fetal lungs normally produce fluid under positive pressure, which flows through the airway into the amniotic fluid. A positive-pressure differential (relative to the amniotic fluid) within the fetal lungs is necessary for normal fetal lung development. Impeding the egress of fetal lung fluid by tracheal occlusion in fetal lambs with surgically created CDH can markedly enlarge the hypoplastic lungs, push the viscera back into the abdomen, and dramatically improve lung function.[22] This PLUG (*p*lug *l*ung *u*ntil it *g*rows) procedure is being applied clinically[23] and may be used to treat other causes of pulmonary hypoplasia in the fetus or neonate.

Amniotic Fluid Phospholipid Analysis

Is the CDH fetus surfactant deficient? Clinically, amniocentesis-derived lecithin/sphingomyelin (L/S) ratio and phosphatidylglycerol (PG) data are used to assess fetal lung maturity. We performed amniotic fluid phospholipid analyses in 18 consecutive fetuses with prenatally diagnosed CDH at 33 to 38 weeks' gestation to determine fetal lung maturity, plan optimal timing for delivery, and delineate indications for prenatal glucocorticoid or postnatal surfactant therapy.[24] The L/S ratio was measured by thin-layer chromatography, and the presence of PG was determined by slide agglutination or thin-layer chromatography. Compared with published control values from uncomplicated pregnancies, there was no difference in the L/S ratio or PG in the CDH fetus. Based on amniotic fluid phospholipid data, the human CDH fetus is not surfactant deficient, so empiric antenatal glucocorticoid treatment or postnatal surfactant replacement therapy are not warranted.

Algorithm for Prenatal Management

Figure 2-12 shows a proposed algorithm for management. Once a diaphragmatic hernia is diagnosed by ultrasound, the patient should be referred for chromosomal analysis by amniocentesis or PUBS, screening for other anatomic abnormalities by an experienced obstetric sonographer, and evaluation for cardiac abnormalities by fetal echocardiography. When associated serious anomalies are discovered, the family may choose to terminate the pregnancy.

Sonographic studies have shown that there is a wide spectrum of CDH severity. Some mildly affected fetuses are detected later in gestation, develop polyhydramnios later or not at all, and have a smaller volume of viscera in the chest. These fetuses should be followed by sonogram and delivered at an appropriate tertiary perinatal center after the lungs are mature. Unfortunately, most fetuses with CDH are on the severe end of the spectrum and do not survive, even with optimal conventional prenatal and postnatal management. In general, these fetuses are detected earlier, develop polyhydramnios earlier, and have a larger volume of viscera in the chest (dilated stomach, impressive mediastinal shift, little lung visible in either thorax).

Now that careful preoperative evaluation of the umbilical vein and ductus venosus with color-flow doppler ultrasonography can detect fetal liver herniation, fetuses with vessels above the level of the diaphragm can be excluded from complete in utero repair. For fetuses with liver herniation, the therapeutic strategy for treatment of CDH in utero by blocking the normal outflow of fetal lung fluid through the trachea (PLUG) is being applied clinically and appears promising.[23] In the future, prena-

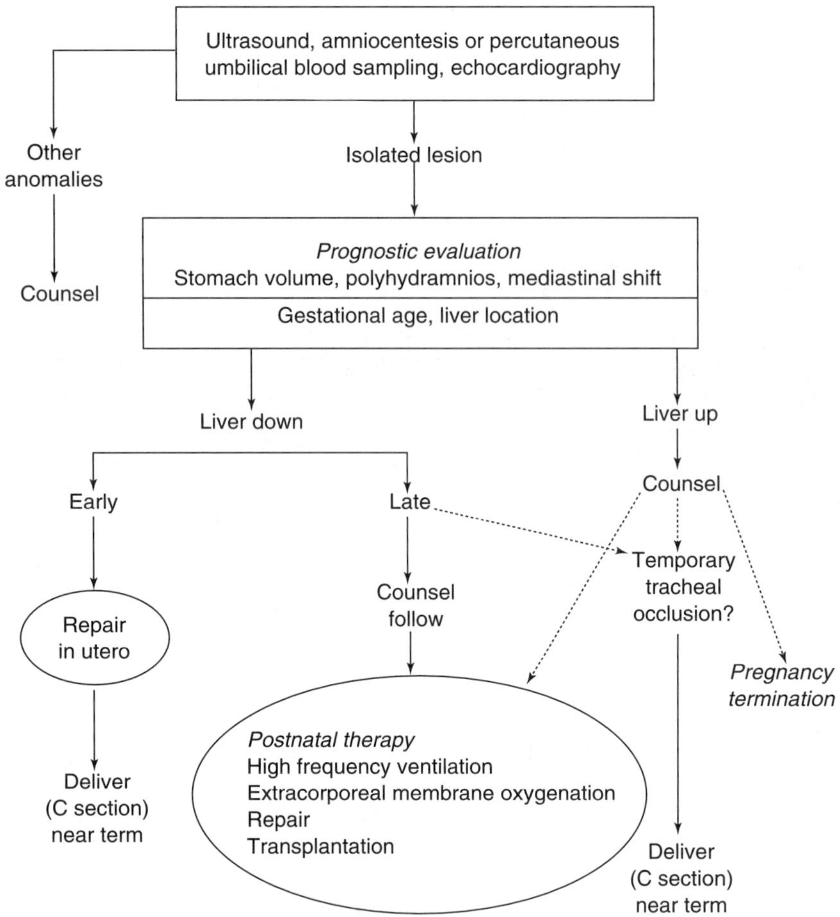

FIG. 2-12. Algorithm for management of the fetus with congenital diaphragmatic hernia.

tal tracheal occlusion with less invasive video fetoscopic techniques may simplify the surgical approach to diaphragmatic hernia.

Some severely affected CDH fetuses without liver herniation may be saved by treatment in utero. A clinical trial funded by the National Institutes of Health is underway to compare the efficacy, safety, and cost-effectiveness of repair before birth to conventional postnatal care. If the results from a series of fetal surgery patients treated in the first year of the study appear to justify a prospective randomized trial, randomization to one of the two treatment groups will occur as soon as patient suitability for fetal surgical treatment is confirmed and maternal consent to enter the trial is obtained.

URINARY TRACT OBSTRUCTION

Unrelieved urinary tract obstruction interferes with fetal development. The severity of damage at birth depends on the type, degree, and duration of the obstruction. Although infants born with partial bilateral obstruction may have only mild hydronephrosis that is reversible with decompression after birth, male fetuses with high-grade urethral obstruction secondary to urethral valves develop renal dysplasia. In addition, oligohydramnios secondary to decreased fetal urine output produces fatal pulmonary hypoplasia.

Animal studies have demonstrated that these devastating renal and pulmonary consequences can be alleviated by urinary tract decompression before birth.[25] Sonographic study of hundreds of human fetuses with urinary tract obstruction has helped trace the natural history of this fetal condition, and selection criteria for in utero treatment have been developed. The sonographic detection of renal cortical cysts or increased renal echogenicity is predictive of renal dysplasia. High levels of sodium, chloride, calcium, and β_2-microglobulin in fetal urine obtained by a percutaneous fetal bladder aspiration correlate with poor fetal renal function.[26]

A proposed algorithm for management of fetal obstructive uropathy is shown in Figure 2-13. Most fetuses with obstructive uropathy do not require intervention. If bilateral hydronephrosis is an isolated condition and the amniotic fluid volume is adequate, the mother should be followed by serial ultrasound, and the fetus should be evaluated and treated postnatally. If moderate to severe oligohydramnios develops, then the fetus should undergo a complete prognostic evaluation to determine the potential for normal renal and pulmonary function at birth. For the fetus with predicted renal dysplasia, aggressive obstetric care or in utero decompression is not indicated. For the fetus with predicted preserved renal function, early delivery for postnatal decompression is indicated if the lungs are mature. If the lungs are immature, in utero decompression is recommended using either a double-pigtail catheter shunt placed percutaneously under sonographic guidance or creation of a vesicostomy using open fetal surgical techniques.[26] Survival after catheter

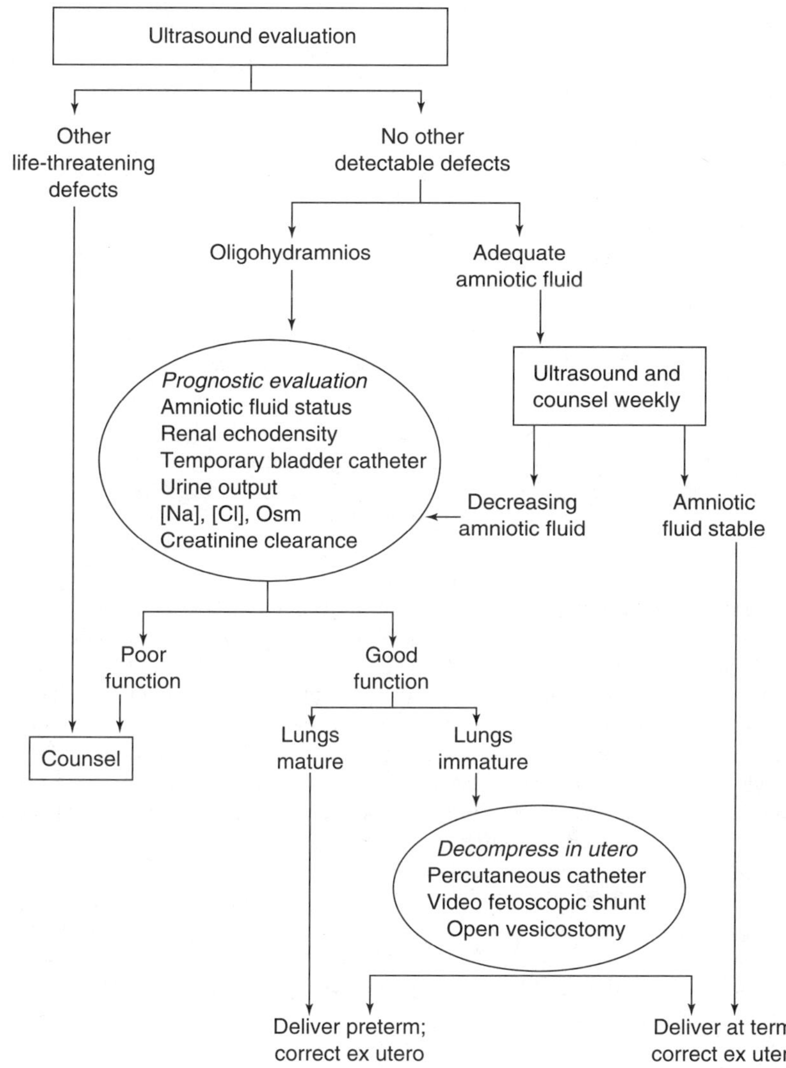

FIG. 2-13. Algorithm for management of the fetus with obstructive uropathy. (Estes JM, Harrison MR. Fetal obstructive uropathy. Semin Pediatr Surg 1993;2:932)

placement is about 70% in appropriately selected male fetuses with posterior urethral valves. A newly developed fetoscopic technique for placement of an expandable mesh stent may solve some of the technical problems encountered with double-pigtail catheters (ie, occlusion, dislodgement, abdominal wall disruption) and avoid the potential morbidity of open surgery.[27]

Important lessons have been gleaned from more than a decade of clinical experience. Patient selection is accurate enough to avoid intervention in cases that do not need it. In utero decompression with restoration of amniotic fluid can prevent the development of fatal oligohydramnios-induced pulmonary hypoplasia. It is still unclear if fetal treatment can arrest or reverse renal dysplastic changes initiated before birth that may compromise renal function as demand increases during postnatal growth.

FETAL THERAPY FOR OTHER ANATOMIC LESIONS

A number of surgical lesions (conditions 5 through 10 in Table 2-1) may be treated prenatally once their pathophysiology is deciphered and new methods of fetal treatment are developed.

Sacrococcygeal Teratoma

Sacrococcygeal teratoma is the most common neonatal tumor. Most SCTs are diagnosed in newborns when the malignant potential is low and the prognosis is good. Prenatal sonographic diagnosis, however, has identified fetuses with large teratomas and associated hydrops who die. A review our experience confirmed the high mortality of fetal SCT, with 22 of 42 patients dying either in utero or at birth.[28] When placentomegaly or hydrops occurred, 15 of 15 fetuses died precipitously. An additional prognostic indicator was that when a maternal indication for sonography such as polyhydramnios was present, 22 of 32 fetuses died, whereas 9 of 10 fetuses detected by routine screening ultrasound survived. Although diagnosis before 30 weeks' gestation was associated with poor outcome, the incidental finding of SCT was favorable at any gestational age.

SCT frequently causes fetal death but not by the malignant degeneration mechanism usually responsible for death in children. Instead, death appears to result from a variety of mechanisms that are secondary effects of the SCT. These can be divided into complications related either to the tumor mass or the tumor physiology (Fig. 2-14).

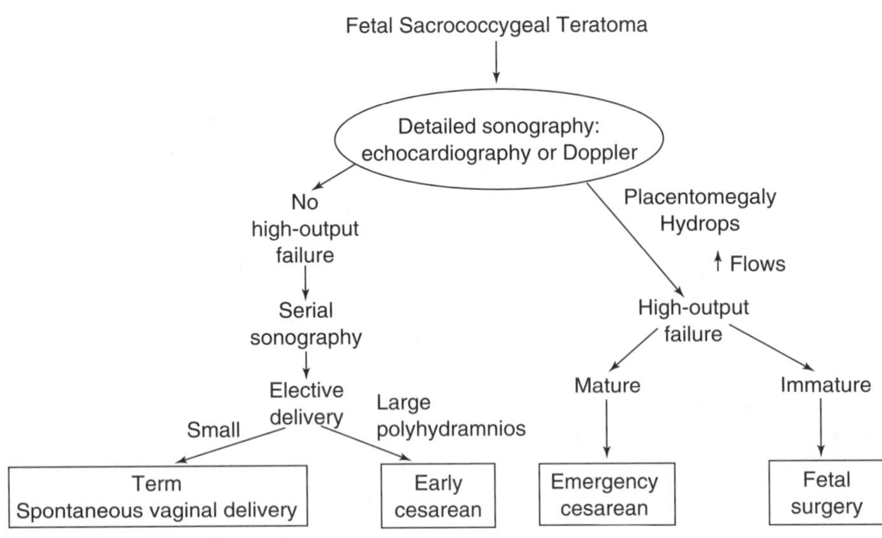

FIG. 2-14. Pathophysiology of fetal sacrococcygeal teratoma, which can cause fetal morbidity or mortality by a variety of mechanisms.

Mass effects include dystocia secondary to tumor bulk and premature delivery. Dystocia can result in traumatic tumor rupture and hemorrhage during vaginal or cesarean delivery. The unexpected presence of a large SCT is a classic cause of arrested delivery. Probably the greatest contribution of prenatal diagnosis of SCT is prevention of dystocia by elective or emergent cesarean delivery. Tumor mass effect with or without polyhydramnios can also result in preterm delivery induced by uterine distention. Massive polyhydramnios is a frequent finding with large fetal SCT, but the underlying pathophysiology of polyhydramnios is unclear in this circumstance.

Evidence supporting high-output failure due to vascular steal is convincing. Doppler ultrasound of these tumors can demonstrate a large arteriovenous fistula, with markedly increased distal aortic blood flow and shunting of blood away from the placenta and to the tumor. The fetal demise presumably occurs because of high-output cardiac failure associated with the vascular steal of the tumor. This tumor pathophysiologic process leads to fetal hydrops and placentomegaly. The development of placentomegaly and hydrops is also associated with the potentially devastating maternal complication of the mirror syndrome.

The uniformly fatal outcome of immature fetuses who develop placentomegaly and hydrops suggests that in utero tumor resection might reverse hydrops and prevent fetal demise. Our limited experience with two clinical cases indicates that fetal teratoma excision leads to resolution of hydrops, but resection must be done before initiation of placentomegaly and the associated mirror syndrome.[28] Less invasive sonographically guided or video fetoscopic techniques may soon be used to occlude the tumor vessels selectively and to interrupt the vascular steal.

Twin–Twin Transfusion

Abnormalities of twin pregnancies that may require in utero treatment occur when abnormal placental chorionic vessels connect the circulations of the twins, leading to an imbalance of blood flow. This parabiosis can put both twins in jeopardy because of marked changes in amniotic fluid volume, growth retardation, and hydrops. Both twin–twin transfusion syndrome

and heart failure of the normal "pump" twin in an acardiac twin pregnancy are associated with high perinatal mortality secondary to premature birth or in utero death, especially when these conditions occur in previable pregnancies when delivery is not an option. Therapy has focused on interrupting the abnormal placental vascular circulation by severing the abnormal placental vessels. For twin–twin transfusion syndrome, these vessels have been divided using a fetoscopically directed laser. For the acardiac twin pregnancy, the normal twin has been salvaged by occluding the umbilical circulation of the abnormal twin, by removing the abnormal fetus through a hysterotomy at 26 weeks' gestation or less (four of five normal twins survived at our center), or by umbilical cord ligation under video fetoscopic guidance.[29,30] Future studies will determine the most effective approach.

Cardiac Conditions

Fetal aortic valvular stenosis often causes irreversible left ventricular damage, and percutaneous balloon catheter dilation of the stenotic fetal aortic valve has been performed.[31] Fetal complete heart block in the setting of maternal collagen vascular disease can lead to cardiac failure, hydrops, and fetal demise. After establishing the efficacy of pacing for heart block in fetal lambs, a pacemaker was successfully placed in a 22-week hydropic fetus, but the heart was already irreversibly damaged by more than 6 weeks of heart failure, so earlier intervention may be required.

Hydrocephalus

Progressive ventriculomegaly due to obstruction of the aqueduct of Sylvius can compress and injure the developing brain. A large multicenter experience with in utero drainage procedures for fetal hydrocephalus has not clearly improved outcome, and a moratorium for fetal treatment of this condition has been observed because of inadequacies in diagnosis, ineffective fetal shunting techniques, and improper selection criteria.[32] If these shortcomings can be overcome, then some hydrocephalic fetuses may benefit from ventricular decompression before birth.

Laryngeal Obstruction

Fetuses with laryngeal atresia develop large lungs distended with fetal lung fluid that can lead to cardiac compression and hydrops. These fetuses may be salvaged in utero by decompressing the obstructed trachea (fetal tracheostomy). If hydrops is not present, then planned near-term cesarean delivery permits airway access by tracheostomy while the fetus remains connected to the placenta.[33]

Fetal Neuroblastoma

We have experience with five fetal neuroblastomas detected by routine prenatal sonography.[34] All were adrenal tumors diagnosed between 26 and 39 weeks' gestation. The adrenal glands are the site of most neuroblastomas, and the fetal adrenals can be reliably imaged before 26 weeks' gestation. The sonographic image of fetal adrenal neuroblastoma is variable and ranges from cystic to solid to hyperechoic to mixed foci of calcification. All five tumors were completely resected postnatally, and the patients have remained disease free for 1 to 10 years after resection without adjuvant therapy.

A literature review collated 16 other cases of fetal neuroblastoma detected by sonography between 29 and 38 weeks' gestation. These cases included 1 cervical, 1 thoracic, and 14 adrenal tumors. Thirteen neonates had Evans stage I or II tumors, and three had more advanced disease. Eleven mothers did not have hypertension or preeclampsia during pregnancy, and the neonates all had stage I or II disease. Four mothers had hypertension or preeclampsia. Three of these neonates had stage IV or IVS disease with liver metastases, and all three had fetal hydrops.

Review of the congenital neuroblastoma literature documented 71 cases diagnosed soon after birth, and several of these cases had unusual features that could have been detected by prenatal ultrasound. Four of the tumors were so large that dystocia resulted and fetal dismemberment was required for delivery. Eight of the tumors metastasized to the placenta, and one metastasized to the umbilical cord with fetal demise.

Thus, neuroblastoma can metastasize in utero. Severely affected fetuses with metastatic disease tend to be hydropic and the pregnancy complicated by maternal hypertension or other signs of preeclampsia. The cause of hydrops in neuroblastoma is not understood, but there are several possibilities. Tumor production of catecholamines with consequent fetal hypertension, constriction of the ductus arteriosus, or heart failure could lead to hydrops. Liver invasion from metastases could cause fetal hydrops by occluding the inferior vena cava or by compromising fetal liver function with resultant hypoproteinemia. Placentomegaly associated with hydrops may result in the maternal mirror syndrome.

The prenatal diagnosis of neuroblastoma may confer the advantages of diagnosis at an early stage as well as offering the potential for early therapy and improved survival. Because of the inverse relation between patient age and survival, early diagnosis and treatment may be critical to improve outcome. A proposed algorithm for the prenatal management of neuroblastoma is shown in Figure 2-15.

PRENATAL FINDINGS IN NEWBORN GASTROINTESTINAL CONDITIONS

Fetal Gastrointestinal and Biliary Obstruction

Many causes of fetal gastrointestinal obstruction have been identified, including congenital atresia, stenosis, webs, other mechanical causes (midgut volvulus, internal hernias), intraluminal obstruction (meconium ileus), and disturbed motility (Hirschsprung disease). The fetal gastrointestinal tract is characterized by rapid growth in a unique environment, so it is not surprising that obstruction has a number of important consequences. Amniotic fluid is swallowed and absorbed by the fetus. Evidence suggests that amniotic fluid plays an important role in fetal nutrition and gastrointestinal tract development. Proximal obstruction interferes with normal amniotic fluid dynamics, resulting in polyhydramnios and mild growth retardation. Distal obstruction may or may not result in polyhydramnios, depending on how much intestinal surface is available to absorb swallowed amniotic fluid. Swallowing starts at 16 to 17 weeks' gestation in humans, which explains why polyhydramnios develops only after mid-gestation with fetal gastrointestinal obstruction.

Proximal obstructing lesions include those of the esophagus and duodenum. In some cases of esophageal atresia, the sonographic findings include a dilated proximal esophageal pouch and polyhydramnios associated with lack of fluid in the stomach. Fetuses with esophageal atresia and an associated distal tracheoesophageal fistula, however, frequently do not develop polyhydramnios, presumably because amniotic fluid enters the gastrointestinal tract through the fistula. Duodenal atresia has a characteristic double-bubble appearance on prenatal ultrasound, resulting from the dilation of the fluid-filled stomach and proximal duodenum.

The sonographic features that most accurately diagnose distal obstructive lesions, such as jejunoileal atresia and meconium ileus, are dilated bowel loops with increased peristalsis. Echogenic meconium may be apparent in dilated small bowel in cases of meconium ileus, and cystic fibrosis is the frequent underlying problem. If prenatal intestinal perforation occurs, there is a spectrum of prenatal sonographic findings for the consequent meconium peritonitis, including peritoneal calcifications, fetal ascites, bowel dilation, and polyhydramnios.

Causes of colonic obstruction, such as Hirschsprung disease and anorectal atresia, are rarely diagnosed in utero. The explanation for this fact is unclear but may be related to the relative lack of peristalsis in the fetal colon or to an as yet unrecognized ability of the fetal colon to absorb fluid secreted by the proximal small bowel.

The incidence of associated chromosomal and structural anomalies in infants with gastrointestinal tract obstruction appears to be lower than in other prenatally diagnosed surgical conditions, such as omphalocele and CDH. However, there are well-known associations between duodenal atresia and trisomy 21 and between esophageal atresia and other trisomies. Consequently, both fetal karyotyping and careful sonographic assessment are indicated when a diagnosis of proximal obstruction is

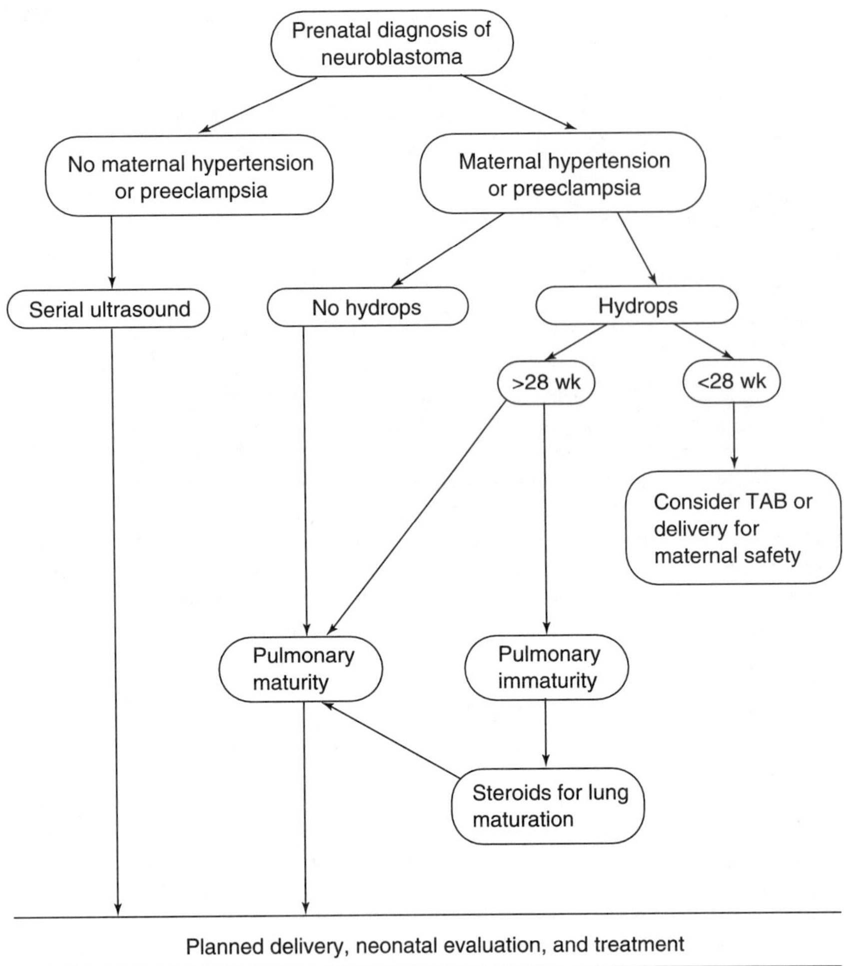

FIG. 2-15. Algorithm for management of the fetus with neuroblastoma. TAB, therapeutic abortion. (After Jennings RW, LaQuaglia MP, Leong K, et al. Fetal neuroblastoma: prenatal diagnosis and natural history. J Pediatr Surg 1993;28:1168)

made. When distal obstruction is evident, karyotyping is not necessary, unless other abnormalities are detected sonographically. A family history of cystic fibrosis should be sought in all cases of distal obstruction. A number of techniques have been developed to diagnose cystic fibrosis prenatally.

In addition to leading to early detection of associated lethal anomalies and appropriate genetic counseling, prenatal diagnosis of gastrointestinal tract obstruction permits planned delivery with prompt resuscitation, fluid administration, operative intervention under controlled circumstances, and improved neonatal outcome.[35]

Choledochal cyst has been diagnosed by antenatal ultrasound as early as 15 weeks' gestation and should be distinguished from ovarian or mesenteric cysts, intestinal duplication cysts, and cystic neuroblastomas. Biliary atresia cannot be accurately diagnosed by prenatal ultrasound. Choledochal cyst is partly due to prenatal distal biliary obstruction, the anatomic basis of which is an abnormal pancreaticobiliary ductal union. Although the specific cause of biliary atresia is unknown, evidence is accumulating that this disease is a dynamic process that also begins weeks before birth. Biliary atresia has been diagnosed and treated surgically in the first week of life.[36] Analysis of fetal gastrointestinal enzymes in amniotic fluid provides insight into the temporal onset of biliary atresia. Gamma-glutamyl transpeptidase (GGTP) is an enzyme synthesized in the liver and excreted in the bile. High levels of GGTP are present in the amniotic fluid between weeks 14 and 24 of gestation, owing to fetal defecation. This time period corresponds to the opening of the anal membrane at 14 weeks followed by the functional innervation and closure of the anal sphincter at 21 to 24 weeks. Muller and colleagues analyzed amniocentesis fluid in 10,000 cases.[37] In this study, only three fetuses had very low levels of GGTP (first percentile) at 18 to 20 weeks' gestation. All three of these patients were found to have biliary atresia after birth. Mid-gestational biliary obstruction in these fetuses indicates that an in utero process led to the biliary atresia. Of interest, fetuses with gastrointestinal obstruction (eg, duodenal atresia) have markedly elevated amniotic fluid GGTP levels owing to prenatal bilious vomiting. Amniotic fluid GGTP enzyme analysis may aid in the prenatal diagnosis of biliary atresia or other gastrointestinal anomalies and permit earlier postnatal intervention with improved survival.

Fetal Abdominal Wall Defects

Abdominal wall defects, including gastroschisis, omphalocele, and various degrees of exstrophy (bladder and cloacal), can be diagnosed and differentiated prenatally by sonography during the second trimester. The diagnosis of omphalocele should not be made until after 12 weeks' gestation, when the abdominal viscera normally return to the abdominal cavity. Although gastroschisis and omphalocele are both congenital defects of the abdominal wall, certain features on sonography distinguish between them. In omphalocele, a membranous sac covers the herniated viscera; in gastroschisis, the viscera float in the amniotic fluid. The cord insertion can be seen arising from the apex of the sac in omphalocele; whereas in gastroschisis, the cord arises to the side of the defect, and the bowel herniates through a right paramedian abdominal wall defect. Another important difference that affects prognosis is the presence of major malformations and chromosomal anomalies. They are common with omphalocele (particularly those without liver in the sac) and rare with gastroschisis. Prenatal counseling for fetuses without associated life-threatening anomalies should reflect a good prognosis.

The variable appearance and functional capacity of neonatal bowel in gastroschisis is well recognized. In some newborns with gastroschisis, the eviscerated intestines are covered with a thick inflammatory peel and may not function properly for weeks to months, necessitating parenteral nutrition. In others, the intestines have a smooth pink serosal surface, and enteral nutrition is tolerated shortly after the abdominal wall closure is completed. Both amniotic fluid exposure and gradual constriction of the bowel at the abdominal wall defect have been implicated. We have developed a reproducible model of gastroschisis in the fetal lamb that closely approximates the human condition grossly and histologically.[38] The findings with this model suggest that the fibrous peel is formed as a reaction to amniotic fluid exposure and that bowel dilation and thickening are caused by gradual constriction at the level of the abdominal wall defect, with resultant chronic venous and lymphatic obstruction late in gestation. The defect in bowel motility appears to be caused by both amniotic fluid and bowel constriction, and these effects are both independent and additive.

Theoretically, preterm delivery of the fetus with gastroschisis and evidence of bowel dilation and thickening on ultrasound could prevent ongoing damage and improve outcome. Langer and associates[39] studied a group of fetuses with gastroschisis and reported a significantly longer time to oral feeding and increased need for bowel resection in infants with maximal bowel diameter (MBD) of 18 mm or greater on prenatal sonography.

To determine whether prenatal sonographic features of the bowel can accurately predict postnatal outcome in fetuses with gastroschisis, we retrospectively reviewed the sonograms of 24 gastroschisis fetuses for fetal bowel features, including bowel dilation and bowel wall thickening.[40] MBD correlated with the length of time to full oral feeding. MBD also correlated with the need for postnatal bowel resection, but 11 mm was the cutoff for this group, not 18 mm. Furthermore, MBD was not a highly reproducible measurement between two sonographers. Despite this experience, we made the same MBD measurement in less than 30% of the fetuses. Our measurements differed by 2 mm or greater in over 65% of the cases, with more than 20% showing a 5 mm or greater discrepancy. Distinguishing between small bowel and colon is also difficult on ultrasound. Finally, an overall subjective assessment of the fetal bowel condition was an even poorer predictor of postnatal bowel complications than the measurement of MBD. In light of these findings, basing clinical decisions on a single cutoff measurement for MBD

or a subjective assessment of fetal bowel condition may be impractical and misleading. Therefore, sonography cannot accurately predict impending bowel damage and should not be used to make a decision to deliver a fetus before term.

Appropriate timing and mode of delivery of the fetus with an abdominal wall defect remain controversial. There is no compelling evidence to support routine cesarean section for most abdominal wall defects. Cesarean section is reserved for giant omphaloceles and for mothers who require it for obstetric indications.

UNANTICIPATED RESULTS: LESSONS FROM FETAL BIOLOGY

Investigative studies that were initially focused on prenatal diagnosis and treatment have led to other potential benefits that extend beyond the nascent field of fetal surgery. The natural history and pathophysiologic consequences of a growing list of fetal anatomic abnormalities have been clarified for perinatologists, neonatologists, and pediatric surgical specialists. A uterine stapling device containing absorbable staples that was developed to open quickly and bloodlessly the gravid uterus during fetal surgery has been applied to routine cesarean sections. Continuous transmission of intrauterine pressure and fetal electrocardiogram by a fetal radiotelemeter may prove useful in the management of high-risk pregnancies threatened with preterm labor. Nitric oxide donors may provide a promising new approach to the broader problem of preterm labor.

Fetal endoscopic surgery may permit fetal surgery through small puncture sites in the uterus, thereby obviating the potential morbidity of a large hysterotomy. Video fetoscopic techniques have been developed in fetal lambs and monkeys for in utero bladder and pleural fluid decompression, temporary tracheal occlusion for pulmonary hypoplasia, umbilical cord ligation for acardiac twin pregnancies, and cleft lip and palate repair.[27,41] Using video fetoscopic visualization, extraamniotic catheterization of chorionic vessels for chronic fetal vascular access may provide a portal for fetal blood sampling, transfusion, hematopoietic stem cell transplantation, and gene therapy.[42]

The fetus has taught us some important lessons about fetal biology. By serendipity, we learned that the fetus heals surgical incisions without scar. This observation has fostered a multidisciplinary approach to unravel the biology of scarless fetal wound healing. This unique repair process is not dependent on the sterile, aqueous intrauterine environment. The differences between fetal and adult skin healing reflect processes intrinsic to fetal tissue, such as an extracellular wound matrix rich in hyaluronic acid and a markedly reduced inflammatory infiltrate and cytokine profile.[43] By mimicking the scarless fetal wound healing "blueprint," therapeutic strategies have emerged to ameliorate scar in children and adults.[44]

Fetal immune tolerance permits stable, long-term chimerism after in utero transplantation of normal fetal hematopoietic stem cells without graft-versus-host disease or the need for immunosuppression.[45] This tactic to avoid transplant rejection may allow a wide variety of prenatally diagnosed inherited diseases, such as thalassemia and Hurler disease, to be cured by fetal hematopoietic stem cell transplantation. Furthermore, fetuses diagnosed with impending organ failure may undergo the prenatal infusion of allogeneic or xenogeneic hematopoietic stem cells to render them tolerant for donor-specific organ transplantation after birth.

REFERENCES

1. Moore KL, Persaud TVN. The developing human: clinically oriented embryology, ed 5. Philadelphia, WB Saunders, 1993.
2. England MA. A color atlas of life before birth: normal fetal development. Chicago, Year Book Medical Publishers, 1990.
3. Sperber GH. Craniofacial embryology, ed 4. London, Butterworths, 1989.
4. Liggins GC. Growth of the fetal lung. J Dev Physiol 1984;6:237.
5. Harrison MR, Golbus MS, Filly RA. The unborn patient, ed 2. Philadelphia, WB Saunders, 1990.
6. Jennings RW, MacGillivray TE, Harrison MR. Nitric oxide inhibits preterm labor in the rhesus monkey. J Maternal Fetal Med 1993;2:170.
7. Longaker MT, Laberge JM, Dansereau J, et al. Primary fetal hydrothorax: natural history and management. J Pediatr Surg 1989;24:573.
8. Rodeck CH, Fisk NM, Fraser DI, et al. Long-term in utero drainage of fetal hydrothorax. N Engl J Med 1988;319:1135.
9. MacGillivray TE, Harrison MR, Adzick NS. Disappearing fetal lung lesions. J Pediatr Surg 1993;1321.
10. Harrison MR, Jester JA, Ross NA. Correction of congenital diaphragmatic hernia in utero. I. The model: intrathoracic balloon produces fatal pulmonary hypoplasia. Surgery 1980;88:174.
11. Harrison MR, Bressack MA, Churg AM, et al. Correction of congenital diaphragmatic hernia in utero. II. Simulated correction permits fetal lung growth with survival at birth. Surgery 1980;88:260.
12. Adzick NS, Harrison MR, Hu LM, et al. Compensatory growth after pneumonectomy in fetal lambs: a morphologic study. Surg Forum 1985;37:309.
13. Rice HE, Estes JM, Hedrick MH, et al. Congenital cystic adenomatoid malformation: a sheep model of fetal hydrops. J Pediatr Surg 1994;29:692.
14. Adzick NS, Harrison MR, Flake AW, et al. Fetal surgery for cystic adenomatoid malformation of the lung. J Pediatr Surg 1993;28:806.
15. Harrison MR, Ross NA, deLorimier AA. Correction of congenital diaphragmatic hernia in utero. III. Development of a successful surgical technique using abdominoplasty to avoid compromise of umbilical blood flow. J Pediatr Surg 1981;16:934.
16. Adzick NS, Outwater KM, Harrison MR, et al. Correction of congenital diaphragmatic hernia in utero. IV. An early gestational model for pulmonary vascular morphometric analysis. J Pediatr Surg 1985;20:673.
17. Adzick NS, Harrison MR, Glick PL, et al. Diaphragmatic hernia in the fetus: prenatal diagnosis and outcome in 94 cases. J Pediatr Surg 1985;20:357.
18. Adzick NS, Vacanti JP, Lillehei CW, et al. Fetal diaphragmatic hernia: ultrasound diagnosis and clinical outcome in 38 cases from a single medical center. J Pediatr Surg 1989;24:654.
19. Harrison MR, Adzick NS, Estes JM, Howell LJ. A prospective study of the outcome for fetuses with diaphragmatic hernia. JAMA 1994;271:382.
20. Harrison MR, Adzick NS, Longaker MT, et al. Successful repair in utero of a fetal diaphragmatic hernia after removal of herniated viscera from the left thorax. N Engl J Med 1990;322:1582.
21. Harrison MR, Adzick NS, Flake AW, et al. Correction of congenital diaphragmatic hernia in utero. VI. Hard-earned lessons. J Pediatr Surg 1993;28:1411.
22. Hedrick MH, Estes JM, Sullivan KM, et al. Plug the lung until it grows (PLUG): a new method to treat congenital diaphragmatic hernia in utero. J Pediatr Surg 1994;29:612.
23. Harrison MR, Adzick NS, Flake AW, et al. Treatment of fetal diaphragmatic hernia by temporary tracheal occlusion. J Pediatric Surg 1996 (in press).
24. Sullivan KM, Hawgood S, Flake AW, et al. Amniotic fluid phopholipid analysis in the congenital diaphragmatic hernia fetus. J Pediatr Surg 1994;29:1020.
25. Adzick NS, Harrison MR, Flake AW, et al. Fetal urinary tract obstruction: experimental pathophysiology. Semin Perinatol 1985;9:79.
26. Estes JM, Harrison MR. Fetal obstructive uropathy. Semin Pediatr Surg 1993;2:932.
27. Estes JM, Macgillivray TE, Hedrick MH, et al. Fetoscopic surgery for the treatment of congenital anomalies. J Pediatr Surg 1992;27:950.
28. Flake AW. Fetal sacrococcygeal teratoma. Semin Pediatr Surg 1993;2:113.
29. Fries MH, Goldberg JD, Golbus MS. Treatment of acardiac-acephalus twin gestations by hysterotomy and selective delivery. Obstet Gynecol 1992;79:601.
30. Quintero RA, Reich H, Puder KS, et al. Umbilical-cord ligation of an acardiac twin by fetoscopy at 19 weeks gestation. N Engl J Med 1994;330:469.
31. Maxwell D, Allan L, Tynan MJ. Balloon dilatation of the aortic valve in the fetus: a report of two cases. Br Heart J 1991;65:256.
32. Manning FA, Harrison MR, Rodeck CH, et al. Catheter shunts for fetal hydronephrosis and hydrocephalus. (Special report) N Engl J Med 1986;315:336.
33. Martinez-Ferro M, Hedrick MH, Flake AW, et al. Prenatal diagnosis of congenital high airway obstruction (CHAOS): potential for perinatal intervention. J Pediatr Surg 1994;29:271.
34. Jennings RW, LaQuaglia MP, Leong K, et al. Fetal neuroblastoma: prenatal diagnosis and natural history. J Pediatr Surg 1993;28:1168.
35. Langer JC, Adzick NS, Filly RA, et al. Gastrointestinal tract obstruction in the fetus. Arch Surg 1989;124:1183.
36. MacGillivray TE, Adzick NS. Biliary atresia begins before birth. Pediatr Surg Int 1994;9:116.
37. Muller F, Oury C, Dumez Y, et al. Microvillar enzyme assays in amniotic fluid and fetal tissues at different stages of development. Prenat Diagn 1988;8:189.
38. Langer JC, Longaker MT, Crombleholme TM, et al. Etiology of bowel damage in gastroschisis. I. Effects of amniotic fluid exposure and bowel constriction in a fetal lamb model. J Pediatr Surg 1989;24:992.
39. Langer JC, Khanna J, Caco C, et al. Prenatal diagnosis of gastroschisis: development of objective sonographic criteria for predicting outcome. Obstet Gynecol 1993;81:53.
40. Babcook CJ, Hedrick MH, Goldstein RB, et al. Gastroschisis: can sonography of the fetal bowel accurately predict postnatal outcome? J Ultrasound Med 1994;13:701.
41. Estes JM, Whitby DJ, Lorenz HP, et al. Endoscopic creation and repair of fetal cleft lip. Plast Reconstr Surg 1992;90:743.
42. Hedrick MH, Jennings RW, MacGillivray TE, et al. Chronic fetal vascular access. Lancet 1993;342:1086.
43. Adzick NS, Longaker MT, eds. Fetal wound healing. New York, Elsevier Scientific, 1992.
44. Adzick NS, Lorenz HP. Cells, matrix, growth factors, and the surgeon: the biology of scarless fetal wound repair. Ann Surg 1994;220:10.
45. Flake AW, Harrison MR, Adzick NS, et al. Transplantation of fetal hematopoietic stem cells in utero: the creation of hematopoietic chimeras. Science 1986;233:776.

Surgery of Infants and Children: Scientific Principles and Practice, edited by
Keith T. Oldham, Paul M. Colombani, and Robert P. Foglia.
Lippincott–Raven Publishers, Philadelphia, © 1997.

CHAPTER 3

The Neonate

Jeffrey G. Dawson, Anna M. August, Joan L. Rosenbaum, Fran L. Porter,
Karen M. Wickline, and F. Sessions Cole

3.1   Complications of Premature Infants

Jeffrey G. Dawson, Anna M. August, F. Sessions Cole

EPIDEMIOLOGY OF PRETERM DELIVERY

Despite continuing technologic advances in the care of premature infants that have lowered the infant mortality rate in the
United States from 26 in 1000 live births (1960) to 8.9 in 1000
(1991), the rate of preterm delivery of premature infants (less
than 37 weeks of gestation or less than 2500 g birthweight),
which is the largest contributor to infant mortality, has not
changed significantly. The United States ranks between 20th
and 30th among countries around the world in infant mortality
and premature delivery rates.[1]

Epidemiologic investigations have identified important population-based risk factors for premature delivery:

- African American race
- Poverty
- Low maternal educational attainment
- Substance abuse (tobacco, cocaine, alcohol) during pregnancy
- No or inadequate prenatal care (prenatal care initiated after the
  first trimester and fewer than five visits through 37 completed
  weeks of gestation)
- Previous adverse pregnancy outcome (preterm delivery, more
  than two spontaneous abortions, stillbirth, or neonatal death)

One of the more prominent findings is the two-fold greater
risk of African-American women for delivery of low-
birthweight infants (13.3% in 1992) than for white women
(5.8%) and for most Hispanic women (7.1%).[2] The mechanisms
by which ethnic background impacts on pregnancy outcome
are poorly understood. Tools for understanding the interactions
between environmental and socioeconomic factors and genetic
predisposition to preterm delivery are being developed.[3]

CLINICAL CAUSES OF PREMATURE DELIVERY

Maternal, fetal, placental, and environmental factors may act
individually or together to cause premature delivery (Table
3-1). Individualized risk assessment is important in planning for
optimal outcomes for both mother and infant. This assessment
should ideally be completed before conception, and prenatal
care should be initiated within 4 weeks of the first missed menstrual period. Ongoing risk assessment during pregnancy permits matching of biologic risk of mother and fetus with appropriate availability of skilled personnel, technology, and
facilities.

Uterine anomalies can be congenital (eg, uterus didelphys or
abnormal cervix after in utero diethylstilbestrol exposure) or
acquired (eg, increased risk of premature delivery after cervical
conization procedures). Both placenta previa and chronic placental abruption are associated with increased risk of preterm
labor. Many women with recurrent second- and third-trimester
losses have immunologic diseases (eg, systemic lupus erythematosus or antiphospholipid antibody syndrome) that disrupt
immunologic adaptation necessary for maternal tolerance to paternal antigens on fetal and placental cells. Increased uterine
volume and myometrial stretching in multiple-gestation pregnancies and in pregnancies characterized by polyhydramnios
suggest a potential mechanism to account for the 40% to 50%
rate of preterm delivery associated with these conditions.

Nutritional deficiencies and substance abuse provide important opportunities for preventive interventions. Several studies
have implicated potentially reversible iron-deficiency anemia
and calcium deficiency as causes of preterm delivery. Tobacco
is the most significant and preventable cause of low-birthweight
infants in the United States. Cessation of smoking among all

TABLE 3-1. *Preconceptual and prenatal risk assessment*

MATERNAL FACTORS
Uterine or cervical anomalies
Previous adverse pregnancy outcome*
Nutritional deficiencies
Family history in first-degree relatives of fetal or neonatal
  deaths or diseases
Maternal medical conditions

FETAL FACTORS
Multiple gestations
Fetal growth abnormalities
Amniotic fluid volume abnormalities

PLACENTAL FACTORS
Placenta previa
Placental abruption
Abnormalities of umbilical cord

ENVIRONMENTAL FACTORS
Maternal infections
Substance use during pregnancy†
Exposure to toxic substances‡

  * Preterm delivery, more than two spontaneous abortions,
stillbirth, or neonatal death
  † Tobacco, cocaine, or alcohol
  ‡ For example, exposure to ionizing radiation or known teratogens

reproductive-age women in the United States would result in about a 25% reduction in the low-birthweight rate.

Prevention of infectious processes may also significantly reduce the frequency of preterm delivery.[4] The pathway between infection and preterm labor or preterm rupture may involve both weakening of amniotic membranes by bacterial products and decidual inflammation elicited by bacterial invasion. Prostaglandins, potent participants in the normal process of labor, are found in high concentrations in amniotic fluid of women with histologic chorioamnionitis. Cytokines, including interleukin-1, interleukin-6, and tumor necrosis factor, are also found in high concentrations in the amniotic fluid of pregnancies with proven chorioamnionitis. They may act by stimulating prostaglandin production. The frequency of preterm delivery among patients with early chorioamnionitis and elevated cytokine concentrations in amniotic fluid has been reduced by maternal antibiotic treatment.

DIAGNOSIS OF PREMATURITY

The diagnosis of prematurity can be based on antenatal estimation of duration of gestation or on physical characteristics of the infant noted postnatally.[5] Use of the last menstrual date alone has been shown to overestimate the prevalence of prematurity when compared with antenatal ultrasound assessment of gestational stage. Antenatal ultrasound estimate of gestational dating is based on empirically observed rates of change in specific fetal measurements, including crown–rump length, femur length, abdominal circumference, and head circumference. Because fetal growth rates can be influenced by a variety of factors at different stages of pregnancy, estimates of gestational age are difficult when fetuses have birth defects that alter these measurements. For example, congenital diaphragmatic hernia reduces abdominal circumference. Estimating gestational age in a fetus with this defect solely with abdominal circumference would consistently underestimate fetal maturity. The most accurate estimates use multiple fetal measurements, are obtained during the first half of pregnancy, and are accurate within 4 days. Estimates based on third-trimester fetal ultrasound measurements have potential errors of 1.5 to 4 weeks.

Use of neuromuscular maturity, anthropometric measurements, and physical findings of the newborn infant permit postnatal estimation of gestational age.[6] The Ballard examination (Fig. 3-1) and modified Dubowitz examination provide the most reliable postnatal estimates of gestational age.

FETAL CIRCULATION AND PATIENT DUCTUS ARTERIOSUS

In the fetus, 69% of combined ventricular output is oxygenated blood that travels from the placenta to the fetal right atrium through the umbilical vein, ductus venosus, and inferior vena cava (Fig. 3-2). A portion of oxygen-rich blood that enters the right atrium from the inferior vena cava (27% of combined ventricular output) is shunted preferentially across the atrial septum through the foramen ovale to the left atrium. This richly oxygenated blood is pumped into the ascending aorta by the left ventricle and is thus more available to the coronary arteries and subclavian and carotid arteries than to the systemic circulation. The remaining portion of blood from the inferior vena cava mixes with blood from the superior vena cava and from the coronary sinus return and is pumped into the pulmonary artery by the right ventricle. Because only about 7% of fetal right ventricular output goes to the lungs, owing to supersystemic pulmonary vascular resistance during fetal life, the right ventricle performs about twice as much work as the left ventricle during fetal life. About 90% of right ventricular output flows to the systemic circulation through the ductus arteriosus. The two umbilical arteries that originate from iliac arteries just inferior to the aortic bifurcation carry blood from the systemic circulation back to the placenta. Fetal oxygen tension is usually 25 to 30 mmHg.

The ductus arteriosus shunts blood flow from the pulmonary artery into the aorta. Within hours to days after delivery in normal, full-term infants, as pulmonary vascular resistance falls and arterial oxygenation increases, the ductus arteriosus closes by constriction of vascular smooth muscle in its wall, which shortens and narrows its lumen.[7] Intimal cushions protrude into the lumen and also contribute to functional closure. After several weeks, fibrous proliferation and hemorrhage with necrosis occur in the intima, and a fibrous ligamentum arteriosus remains. Failure of the ductus arteriosus to close after postnatal reduction in pulmonary vascular resistance results in left-to-right shunting from aorta to pulmonary artery, pulmonary hyperperfusion, high-output congestive heart failure, and a diastolic steal syndrome, which reduces perfusion to the splanchnic and renal vascular beds. Failure of closure with persistently supersystemic postnatal pulmonary vascular resistance results in

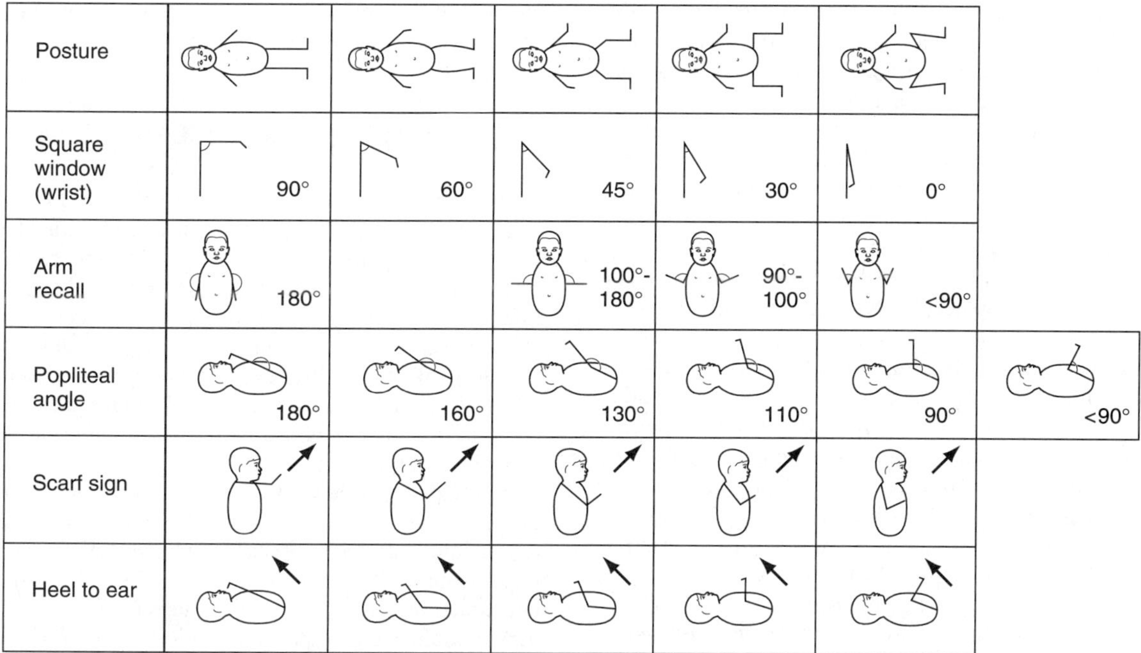

FIG. 3-1. The Ballard examination provides the most reliable postnatal estimates of gestational age based on neuromuscular maturity, anthropometric measurements, and physical findings.

right-to-left shunting from pulmonary artery to aorta and systemic hypoxia proportional to the magnitude of the pulmonic–aortic pressure gradient.

Regulation of ductal closure requires complex interactions among vascular smooth muscle of the ductus arteriosus, physiologic changes in hemodynamic relations between the systemic and pulmonary vascular beds, arterial oxygen tension, vasoactive factors, and neurohumoral substances.[7] Prostaglandin E_2 (PGE_2) is the most potent dilator of the ductus arteriosus and is synthesized locally by ductal tissue. PGE_2 serum concentrations are higher in preterm infants than full-term infants and may contribute significantly to the increased incidence of hemodynamically significant patency of the ductus arteriosus in preterm infants. Increased arterial oxygen tension constricts the

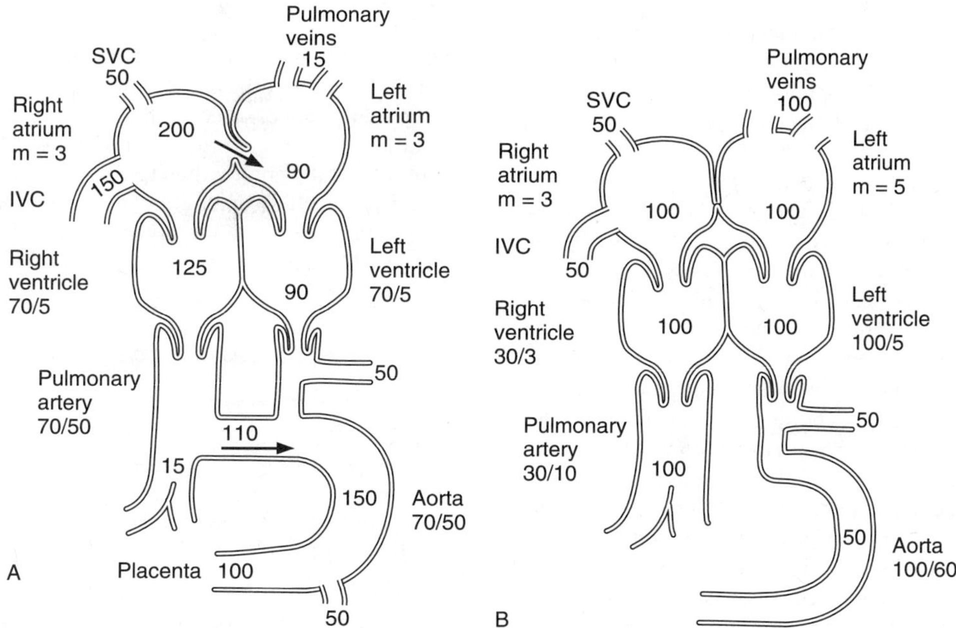

FIG. 3-2. (A) Fetal circulation is in parallel. (B) Mature circulation is in series, and the amount of blood carried by the two ventricles is about the same as before birth. IVC, inferior vena cava; SVC, superior vena cava.

ductal lumen. The mechanism of this effect has not been established. Reduction in PGE_2 production associated with increased arterial oxygen tension may contribute significantly to ductal closure during normal fetal–neonatal transition.

In the full-term newborn infant, functional closure occurs within 24 to 48 hours, with anatomic closure by 2 months of age. Persistent postnatal hypoxia due to supersystemic pulmonary artery pressure and resultant right-to-left shunting may contribute to maintenance of ductal patency in full-term infants. Increased pulmonary vascular resistance is observed in full-term infants with chronic uteroplacental dysfunction, in infants with abnormal extension of pulmonary vascular smooth muscle to distal pulmonary arterial vessels, and in infants with anatomic reduction in pulmonary vascular cross-sectional surface area due to interruption in early gestation of pulmonary vascular development (eg, by congenital diaphragmatic hernia). The diagnosis of supersystemic pulmonary arterial pressure can be established by echocardiographic visualization of right-to-left ductal flow throughout the cardiac cycle and transductal arterial saturation gradient of more than 10%. In contrast to the premature infant in whom treatment has focused on ductal closure, treatment to reduce pulmonary vascular resistance in full-term infants by mechanical ventilation, pharmacologic pulmonary vasodilation, or extracorporeal membrane oxygenation has been successful in different clinical situations.[8]

In the preterm infant, functional closure is often delayed. Clinical evidence of a hemodynamically significant patent ductus arteriosus includes a systolic or continuous murmur that can be detected under the left clavicle as well as along the left sternal border, bounding pulses with widened (more than 20 mmHg) pulse pressure, hyperdynamic precordium, tachypnea, tachycardia, hepatomegaly, and worsening respiratory failure characterized by hypercarbia and worsening pulmonary compliance. About 30% of patients with symptomatic patent ductus arteriosus have cardiomegaly and pulmonary plethora on chest radiograph. Echocardiographic findings include evidence by color-flow Doppler assessment of ductal patency, quantification of the magnitude of the left-to-right shunt, determination of the direction of the shunt throughout the cardiac cycle, and enlargement of the left atrial diameter when compared with aortic diameter.

Management of premature infants with patent ductus arteriosus must be individualized. For infants with hemodynamically significant patent ductus arteriosus, pharmacologic interruption with indomethacin, which irreversibly inhibits cyclooxygenase activity and reduces synthesis of PGE_2, should be considered. Symptoms of patent ductus arteriosus respond to treatment with indomethacin in about 70% of infants.[9] Symptoms recur in about 30% of these infants, owing to reopening of the ductus arteriosus. These infants require additional treatment with indomethacin or surgical ligation. Success of indomethacin is increased if used in infants younger than 21 days. Because of side effects of indomethacin therapy, which include inhibition of platelet function, reduction of splanchnic blood flow, and reduction of renal blood flow, treatment of infants with asymptomatic patent ductus arteriosus remains controversial.[10,11]

Surgical interruption of the ductus arteriosus is a safe alternative to indomethacin treatment in infants unresponsive to indomethacin or in those whose clinical situation contraindicates its use. The operative mortality rate at centers where experienced surgical teams are available is less than 1%. The morbidity of the procedure is also low.[12]

HYALINE MEMBRANE DISEASE

Hyaline membrane disease (HMD) has a characteristic pathologic appearance, biochemical cause, and clinical phenotype, and contributes significantly to morbidity and mortality among premature infants.[13] The pathologic appearance of premature infant lungs affected by this disease includes eosinophilic, proteinaceous material that fills alveolar spaces and forms characteristic hyaline membranes. The primary biochemical abnormality in HMD is deficiency of the pulmonary surfactant, a complex mixture of phospholipid and protein produced in alveoli by the type II pneumocyte, a pulmonary epithelial cell. The pulmonary surfactant lowers surface tension at the air–liquid interface in alveoli and thereby reduces atelectasis at end expiration. Deficiency of surfactant production or function can result from multiple mechanisms (Table 3-2). Reduced surfactant function leads to increased atelectasis, worsening pulmonary compliance, and progressive respiratory failure characterized by hypercarbia, hypoxemia due to ventilation–perfusion mismatch, and acidosis due to hypercarbia and inadequate tissue oxygenation. Clinical signs of surfactant deficiency occur within the first 12 hours of life and include tachypnea, grunting, nasal flaring, and chest retractions. Early descriptions of the natural history of HMD indicated that infants who survive usually exhibit worsening pulmonary function for the first 3 to 4 days of life. As pulmonary surfactant production increases, functional pulmonary abnormalities resolve. Long-term follow-up of survivors of HMD suggests persistent abnormalities in pulmonary function testing, increased susceptibility to reactive airways disease and pulmonary infections, and development of bronchopulmonary dysplasia (BPD) in the most severely affected infants.[14]

The diagnosis of HMD is based on clinical, biochemical, and radiographic characteristics. In addition to the clinical symptoms noted earlier, the chest radiograph shows a homogeneous, ground-glass appearance with visible air bronchograms. Biochemical evidence of surfactant deficiency may be available from antenatal amniotic fluid testing of pulmonary phospholipid maturity. A lecithin/sphingomyelin ratio of less than 2, absence of detectable phosphatidylglycerol, or lack of stabilization of bubbles at an air–liquid interface (the shake test) each suggest

TABLE 3-2. *Causes of deficiency of surfactant production or function*

REDUCED SURFACTANT PRODUCTION
Inadequate population of type II pneumocytes
Lack of hormonal signals for surfactant production
Immaturity of type II pneumocyte synthesis or secretion of surfactant proteins or phospholipids

REDUCED SURFACTANT FUNCTION
Inhibition of surfactant function by plasma proteins, plasma cholesterol, bacterial products
Pulmonary hemorrhage
Meconium aspiration

surfactant deficiency. These tests can also be performed on gastric aspirate fluid obtained within 60 minutes of delivery or on tracheal aspirate fluid. Results of any of these tests that indicate surfactant sufficiency exclude HMD. Frequently, the clinical presentation of HMD is indistinguishable from pulmonary or systemic bacterial infection. This clinical ambiguity requires careful evaluation for infection in all infants treated for HMD and initiation of systemic antibiotic coverage until clinical, biochemical, and microbiologic testing excludes bacterial infection.

Treatment of HMD begins with a high index of clinical suspicion. Because pulmonary function in untreated infants with HMD deteriorates during the first 3 to 4 days of life, prompt initiation of oxygen therapy and mechanical ventilation to reduce atelectasis and improve gas exchange are often indicated. The classic ventilatory strategy for infants with HMD includes positive end-expiratory pressure to maintain alveolar patency at end expiration, maintenance of adequate minute ventilation with pressure-cycled ventilators, and administration of adequate inspired oxygen to maintain oxygen delivery to tissues.[15] Alternative ventilatory strategies, including jet ventilation or high-frequency oscillatory ventilation, have been useful in clinical situations characterized by onset of pulmonary interstitial emphysema or multiple pneumothoraces within the first 24 hours of life.[16] Because of the rapid changes in pulmonary compliance and surfactant production that can occur during the first week of life, rigorous attention to gas exchange and ventilatory strategy must be provided to ensure that potential pulmonary sequelae of HMD caused by barotrauma and oxygen toxicity are minimized. In addition, cardiopulmonary complications frequently encountered in premature infants, including bacterial infection, patent ductus arteriosus, and pneumothorax, must be promptly evaluated and treated.

After extensive clinical evaluation during the 1980s, surfactant replacement therapy was approved for use in the United States in 1990.[17] Pharmacologic preparations with surfactant activity (synthetic phospholipid mixtures or extracts of bovine lung with both phospholipid and protein) can be administered to affected infants directly into the tracheobronchial tree through the endotracheal tube. These preparations spread rapidly to distal alveoli, reduce surface tension, and improve pulmonary compliance. Use of these preparations has been shown to reduce the frequency of pneumothorax among infants with HMD and reduce mortality of HMD. Surfactant replacement may be administered to symptomatic infants within the first 12 to 24 hours of life or may be given to high-risk infants prophylactically in the delivery room.[17] Infants who respond to the first dose of surfactant by improved pulmonary compliance and reduced need for oxygen administration may require up to four doses during the first 48 hours of life. Lack of response to surfactant replacement among symptomatic infants has been associated with increased risk of death from HMD.[18]

Other therapies for premature infants with HMD include administration of steroid preparations to improve pulmonary compliance by interrupting inflammation. Duration of dependence on mechanical ventilation and oxygen administration is reduced by steroid administration within the first 2 to 4 weeks of life.[19] Catabolic nutritional effects of glucocorticoids, enhanced susceptibility to infection, and improvement in long-term neurodevelopmental outcome have not been fully evaluated. Other therapies, such as diuretic treatment, supplementation with vitamins

A and E, prophylactic pharmacologic closure of the patent ductus arteriosus with indomethacin, and fluid restriction have shown inconsistent results.

Although mortality from HMD has significantly decreased since introduction of oxygen administration, mechanical ventilation, and surfactant replacement therapy, prevention of prematurity through improved access to prenatal care and use of antenatal glucocorticoids to accelerate pulmonary surfactant maturation represent the two most effective strategies to improve outcomes of premature infants. Antenatal glucocorticoids given over 48 hours before unpreventable preterm birth reduce significantly the frequency and severity of HMD in singleton gestations.[20,21] This clinical benefit cannot be duplicated by postnatal administration to the newborn infant, probably because of the role of the placenta in metabolizing prenatally administered glucocorticoids to steroid derivatives that are active on fetal lung.

Although HMD is uncommon in full-term infants, delay in maturation of surfactant production or inhibition of surfactant function can occur. Genetic, developmental, anatomic, and infectious mechanisms may be responsible for abnormal surfactant function. An inherited deficiency in one of the surfactant-associated proteins, surfactant protein B, has been shown to cause lethal respiratory failure within the first 6 months of life in full-term infants.[22] These infants present with clinical, radiologic, and biochemical characteristics typical of premature infants with HMD, do not respond to surfactant replacement, antenatal or postnatal steroids, ventilatory support, or extracorporeal membrane oxygenation. The only two survivors of this genetic deficiency have undergone successful lung transplantation. In addition to genetic causes, full-term infants with group B streptococcal infections or with total anomalous pulmonary venous drainage with obstruction may present with similar clinical phenotypes. Prompt consideration of the multiple causes of surfactant deficiency among full-term infants will lead to rapid and appropriate diagnosis and treatment.

BRONCHOPULMONARY DYSPLASIA

BPD, or chronic lung disease, in infants is the most common pulmonary sequela of prematurity or mechanical ventilation in full-term infants. It is defined by the need for supplemental oxygen or an abnormal chest radiograph at 28 days of age. The term was originally used to describe the radiologic and pathologic changes observed in premature infants who did not recover within 4 weeks from HMD.[23] BPD is now used to describe chronic lung disease that results from any condition in the neonatal period. Despite the diverse diseases that lead to the development of BPD, infants with BPD share clinical and pathologic characteristics.

The incidence of BPD among premature infants is inversely proportional to gestational age and birthweight. Up to 70% of infants with birthweights less than 1000 g develop BPD. With the increased use of antenatal steroids, surfactant replacement, improved methods of ventilation, and increased attention to nutritional needs of the sick infant, the birthweight-specific incidence of BPD is decreasing. Continued improved survival of sick infants, however, has increased the size of the population at risk for developing this disease.

Many factors play a role in the development of BPD (Table

TABLE 3-3. *Risk factors for development of bronchopulmonary dysplasia*

ANTENATAL FACTORS: REDUCED LUNG GROWTH
Oligohydramnios
Reduced fetal breathing due to neurologic or neuromuscular
    diseases
Reduced fetal urine output
Congenital diaphragmatic hernia

NEONATAL FACTORS
Pulmonary infection
Patent ductus arteriosus
Compromised nutrition
Chronic aspiration
Barotrauma
Oxygen toxicity
Surfactant deficiency
Structural tracheobronchial immaturity

3-3). The most significant factors are the degree of pulmonary structural and functional immaturity at birth and the degree and length of ventilatory and oxygen support. Pathologically, there is progression from alveolar and interstitial edema, atelectasis, and necrosis of bronchial mucosa to alternating areas of atelectasis and emphysema, metaplasia of airway mucosa, and fibrosis. The chest radiograph progresses to show areas of atelectasis and cystic changes with overexpansion. Clinically, these infants show signs of respiratory distress with tachypnea, retractions, wheezing, and need for supplemental oxygen. Pulmonary function testing may show increased resistance as a result of airway injury, bronchospasm, or interstitial edema. Lung compliance may also be decreased. Hypoxemia may result from ventilation–perfusion mismatch and from loss of surface area for gas exchange. Pulmonary hypertension and cor pulmonale may develop as a result of chronic hypoxemia.[24]

Treatment of BPD must begin with strategies to prevent prematurity and other conditions that lead to development of this disease. Improved access to prenatal care, prolongation of pregnancy, and antenatal glucocorticoid administration to accelerate fetal lung maturation will reduce the frequency of BPD by reducing the population of infants at risk for development of the disease.[25]

Postnatal prevention and treatment of BPD require early identification of at-risk infants and strategies to minimize the inflammatory effects of barotrauma and oxygen toxicity. Both the reduction of ventilatory requirements and the use of surfactant replacement therapy decrease the severity of BPD. Early attention to nutritional support is critical to optimize lung growth and recovery in infants with BPD. They frequently exhibit growth failure due to high-energy expenditure and require high caloric density formulas. Other therapies early in the disease, including vitamin A supplementation, antioxidant administration, fluid restriction, and diuresis, have not shown consistent benefit.[26]

Although the heterogeneity of BPD makes extrapolation from clinical trials to individual patients difficult, there are several pharmacologic interventions that should be considered for infants with BPD. The maintenance of adequate oxygen delivery to tissues by administration of low-flow oxygen ($\frac{1}{32}$ to $\frac{3}{4}$ L/min) by nasal cannula is critical to optimize outcome of these infants. More severely affected infants may require supplemental oxygen for months after discontinuation of other pharmacologic agents. Because interstitial and peribronchiolar pulmonary edema play a role in BPD, diuretics have been useful in improving lung mechanics. Furosemide, 1 mg/kg twice daily, intravenously or orally, reduces edema and pulmonary vascular resistance while increasing surfactant secretion. Electrolyte and mineral imbalances that occur with chronic furosemide administration must be carefully monitored and corrected. Treatment of clinical and histologic evidence of airway reactivity with bronchodilators (eg, β-adrenergic agonists, anticholinergics, and methylxanthines) have all been used successfully. The use of long-term corticosteroids (eg, dexamethasone, 1 mg/kg/d, tapering over 7 to 42 days) in the treatment of BPD to reduce airway reactivity and pulmonary inflammation remains controversial. Available data show short-term improvement in lung mechanics, but longer-term benefit has not been established.[19] When chronic administration is instituted, use of steroid preparations that minimize mineralocorticoid effects (eg, oral prednisone) should be considered.[27]

The contribution of gastroesophageal reflux to worsening BPD must be individually assessed. Although gastroesophageal reflux is a relatively common problem during infancy, chronic aspiration can exacerbate bronchospasm associated with BPD and with pulmonary sequelae of congenital diaphragmatic hernia and surgically repaired tracheoesophageal anomalies.[28] Chronic aspiration can be further exacerbated by oral bronchodilators like theophylline. An initial approach to evaluation of these problems includes documentation of the effects of chronic aspiration on growth, pulmonary radiographic appearance, and respiratory compromise. Further evaluation can include an upper gastrointestinal series, 24-hour pH probe monitoring, and radionuclide gastric emptying study. Initial therapeutic efforts should be medical: thickening of feedings, maintenance of upright position after feedings, and reduction in use of theophylline for bronchodilation. If gastroesophageal reflux is contributing to worsening lung disease and medical therapy is unsuccessful, infants with reduced pulmonary reserve due to BPD, neurologic compromise, and clinical, biochemical, and radiologic evidence of chronic aspiration may benefit from fundoplication.[29,30] The risk of recurrence of symptoms or a mechanical problem with the fundoplication in this high-risk group of infants must be carefully evaluated.[31,32]

As infants with BPD grow, pulmonary symptoms (bronchospasm, chronic cough, shortness of breath) generally improve, and reliance on daily medications (low-flow oxygen, diuretics, bronchodilators) is reduced. Long-term sequelae of BPD detected by pulmonary function testing, somatic growth, and neurodevelopmental progress, however, are seen in more than half of survivors. Follow-up of infants 20 years after premature birth (birthweights of more than 1000 g) indicated that 76% of survivors showed abnormalities in pulmonary function.[14] In addition, among survivors, growth (height and weight) was reduced, neurologic sequelae were more frequent, and educational outcomes were significantly worse. Because of the heterogeneity of mechanisms that lead to BPD, treatment of infants with BPD requires individualization of therapies, consistent interactions between physician and family, and attention to support and education of parents.

INTRACRANIAL HEMORRHAGE

The most common form of brain injury in preterm infants is intraventricular–periventricular hemorrhage (IV/PVH).[33] Risk of intracranial hemorrhage is directly associated with degree of prematurity. Severe brain injury with immediate (hemodynamic instability, seizures, rapid increase in anterior fontanelle pressure, anemia) and long-term (deafness, blindness, seizures, cerebral palsy) consequences is observed in 6% to 7% of very-low-birthweight (less than 1500 g) infants who survive intracranial hemorrhage. Prematurity, however, is not the sole determinant of prognosis; several studies have documented a decrease in the incidence of IV/PVH during the past decade without a change in infants at risk from extreme prematurity. Estimates suggest that 16% to 25% of very-low-birthweight infants sustain some degree of IV/PVH, while 6% to 7% of this same population sustain severe IV/PVH.[37,38]

Two mechanisms account for the susceptibility of preterm infants to IV/PVH. First, these hemorrhages arise in the germinal matrix, an area just ventrolateral to the lateral ventricles, with a rich vascular system that appears to be relatively fragile. The normal involution of this structure during the third trimester by about 34 weeks of gestation partially explains the decreasing risk of significant hemorrhage that accompanies increasing gestational age. Second, in contrast to rigorous autoregulation in adults, regulation of cerebral blood flow in premature infants is pressure passive. This dysfunctional autoregulation leads to greater pressure variations in the fragile vascular system of preterm infants. Both arterial and venous blood pressure can contribute to the pathogenesis of hemorrhage, particularly in instances of increased intrathoracic pressure associated with pneumothorax. Rapid changes in serum osmolality have also been implicated in the development of IV/PVH. These observations have led to more judicious use of rapid volume expansion in premature infants, slower administration of intravenous medications with high osmolality (eg, sodium bicarbonate), and avoidance of rapid intravenous administration of solutions with glucose concentrations greater than 10%.

In light of the heterogeneous pathogenesis of IV/PVH, attempts at prevention have taken several routes. Prenatally, the most important interventions are prolongation of the healthy pregnant state and delivery at a site where optimal neonatal resuscitation efforts are available. Administration of antenatal steroids to accelerate fetal phospholipid pulmonary maturation has also been noted to reduce the postnatal risk of IV/PVH. Postnatally, the accessibility of rapid resuscitation and stabilization, as well as avoidance of rapid changes in intrathoracic and intravascular pressure, are important in preventing IV/PVH. Pharmacologic interventions aimed at stabilization of blood flow velocity (eg, muscle relaxation) and prevention or correction of coagulation disturbances have also been attempted with varying degrees of success.

The prognosis after IV/PVH depends on initial severity and on the development of posthemorrhagic hydrocephalus. Severity of injury is described by the extent of bleeding assessed by cranial ultrasound examination (Table 3-4). When hemorrhage is limited to the area of the germinal matrix alone (grade I), no adverse immediate or long-term outcomes have been observed in careful clinical studies. More extensive hemorrhage into the lateral ventricles (grade II), from which the blood eventually

TABLE 3-4. *Grading of severity of intraventricular–paraventricular hemorrhage by ultrasound scanning*

Grade I	Germinal matrix hemorrhage without intraventricular hemorrhage
Grade II	Intraventricular hemorrhage
Grade III	Intraventricular hemorrhage with ventricular dilation
Grade IV	Hemorrhagic intracerebral involvement or other parenchymal lesion

(Adapted from Volpe JJ, Neurology of the newborn, ed 2. Philadelphia, WB Saunders, 1987:331)

is cleared, is associated with major neurologic sequelae (eg, blindness, deafness, cerebral palsy, seizure disorder) in 10% to 15% of infants. Some infants with intraventricular hemorrhage develop varying degrees of ventricular enlargement (grade III), presumably secondary to reactive arachnoiditis as blood degradation products collect at the arachnoid granulations and impair cerebrospinal fluid reuptake. Rapid (within days), severe ventricular enlargement is associated with adverse outcome in about 40% of infants. Additionally, large intraventricular hemorrhages may be accompanied by hemorrhagic infarctions in the surrounding periventricular white matter (grade IV). In contrast to the isolated germinal matrix hemorrhage or the intraventricular hemorrhage without significant ventriculomegaly, both extensive hydrocephalus and significant periventricular injury are associated with a more than 90% risk of major, long-term neurodevelopmental sequelae. About half of infants with ventriculomegaly associated with intraventricular hemorrhage require some treatment for relief of hydrocephalus. These interventions include serial lumbar punctures for 7 to 14 days, an external ventriculostomy, or a ventriculoperitoneal shunt.

BACTERIAL SEPSIS

Despite improvement in morbidity and mortality from neonatal bacterial sepsis during the past 30 years, the incidence of sepsis during the first week of life has been unchanged and about five-fold greater among premature infants (5 in 1000 preterm infants) than full-term infants (about 1 in 1000 term newborns). In addition, 25% to 33% of premature infants who require longer than 2 weeks of hospitalization during the neonatal period develop at least one episode of systemic bacterial infection. The systemic pathogen most commonly recovered after the first week of life is coagulase-negative staphylococcus.

The high rate of invasive disease among premature infants is caused by humoral, cellular, and environmental factors[34] (Table 3-5). Transplacental transport of maternal immunoglobulin G (IgG) provides the full-term infant with concentrations of IgG equal to or greater than maternal concentrations. This transport process increases significantly after 20 weeks of gestation; about two-thirds of the IgG acquired by the fetus during pregnancy is transported during the last third of gestation. Lack of transplacentally acquired IgG in the extremely premature infant results in quantitative and qualitative humoral susceptibility to bacterial infection. In addition, concentrations of the principal nonspecific humoral effector response proteins of the classic and alternative pathways of complement activation are

TABLE 3-5. *Immunologic susceptibility of preterm infants to bacterial infections*

HUMORAL FACTORS
Specific humoral immunity: quantitative and qualitative reduction in serum immunoglobulin G concentrations
Nonspecific humoral immunity: reduced concentrations of complement proteins

CELLULAR FACTORS
Reduced antibody synthesis due to altered T and B lymphocyte interactions
Reduced phagocyte function

ENVIRONMENTAL FACTORS
Prolonged clinical need for arterial and venous access
Antibiotic-resistant organisms
Reduced skin integrity
Suboptimal nutritional status

(Cole FS. Immunology. In: Taeusch HW, Ballard RA, Avery ME, eds. Schaffer and Avery's diseases of the newborn, ed.6. Philadelphia, Harcourt Brace Jovanovich, 1991:305.)

also significantly lower than in adults and do not reach adult levels until 3 to 6 months of age.

Immunologic cellular defense is impaired by the premature infant's reduced ability to respond to antigenic stimulation, owing to altered T lymphocyte–B lymphocyte cooperation in antigen recognition and antibody synthesis. In addition, functional deficiencies in neonatal phagocytes, including impaired migration, aggregation, and adherence, reduce the clearance of invading microorganisms from sites of inflammation.

Environmental factors frequently encountered among premature infants with prolonged need for neonatal intensive care also increase the risk for systemic bacterial infection. The need for prolonged use of arterial or central venous catheters, even when they are fastidiously maintained, provides potential sites for nosocomial bacterial invasion. Poor skin integrity and catabolic nutritional status may also contribute to enhanced susceptibility to systemic infection.

Although the morbidity and mortality of systemic bacterial infection in premature infants are significant, the initial clinical symptoms of sepsis may be subtle and nonspecific until infection is significantly advanced.[35] Early detection and treatment prompted by consideration of sepsis as a possible cause whenever clinically significant deterioration occurs are critical in optimizing outcome. Clinical presentation of sepsis may range from mild feeding intolerance or an increase in frequency of apnea, both frequently seen in premature infants in response to noninfectious stimuli, to rapidly evolving hypotension and shock. Laboratory investigations may assist in the diagnosis; metabolic acidosis and hypoxemia, leukopenia, neutropenia, or thrombocytopenia may be important indicators of evolving infection. Antibiotic coverage is frequently indicated before results of appropriate systemic cultures, usually of blood, urine, and possibly cerebrospinal fluid, are available. Choice of antibiotics varies with the specific clinical situation, but use of a penicillin and an aminoglycoside has been effective in many different clinical settings.

The organisms most commonly seen in septic infants in the first week of life include group B β-hemolytic streptococcus (about 33%), *Escherichia coli* and other gram-negative enteric organisms (about 33%), and a group of less common organisms, including *Listeria monocytogenes* and nontypable *Haemophilus influenzae*. Initial antibiotic choices to cover these organisms are usually ampicillin and an aminoglycoside. After the first week of life, coagulase-negative staphylococci are the most commonly encountered organisms. Fungal pathogens may also contribute significantly to serious infections after the first week of life. The most commonly encountered fungi are species of *Candida* and *Malassezia*, opportunistic organisms that require additional antifungal coverage (usually amphotericin B) for successful eradication. Because of the pronounced changes in glomerular filtration rate, hepatic blood flow, volume of drug distribution, and hemodynamic stability that occur during the first weeks of life in premature infants and during episodes of systemic infection, careful monitoring of antibiotic pharmacokinetics is critical to avoid toxicity or subtherapeutic concentrations of antibiotics. The dosing of these agents must also be carefully monitored.

3.2　Common Problems of Full-Term Infants

Joan L. Rosenbaum

RESPIRATORY DISORDERS

Transient Tachypnea of the Newborn

Transient tachypnea of the newborn (TTN) is a benign, self-limiting cause of respiratory distress in full-term infants. About 70% of term infants with respiratory distress carry this diagnosis.[36] This disease process results from delayed clearance of lung fluid by the lymphatic system.[39] Conditions that cause

elevation of central venous pressure may also present as transient tachypnea.

The clinical characteristics of TTN include "comfortable" tachypnea within 12 to 24 hours of birth, mild hypoxemia secondary to ventilation–perfusion mismatch, prominent perihilar streaking, and fluid in the interlobar fissures on chest radiograph.[40] Because of the benign course of the disease, treatment is usually supportive. Rarely, symptoms are more severe; grunting, retracting, and cyanosis suggest other respiratory diseases, such as surfactant deficiency or pneumonia.[36] Because of the similarity between symptoms of TTN and those of more serious diseases of the neonatal period (eg, sepsis, congenital heart disease), inclusion in the evaluation of tests to exclude other diseases must be considered. TTN should be considered a diagnosis of exclusion.

Meconium Aspiration

Meconium is a substance that accumulates in the fetal intestine during gestation. Mainly composed of water, it lacks the intestinal bacteria necessary to convert primary bile acids to secondary bile acids. The protein, lipid, and sterol contents of meconium mimic those found in amniotic fluid.[41,42]

Meconium staining of amniotic fluid is a common phenomenon that occurs in 8% to 20% of all deliveries.[43] The presence of meconium in amniotic fluid has historically been associated with fetal acidosis and hypoxia, although its exact relation to fetal distress remains unclear.[44]

Intrauterine hypoxia may initiate fetal gasping respirations and passage of meconium in utero. Meconium causes chemical inflammation and airway obstruction. Air trapping in the distal airways may result in hyperexpansion of alveoli or atelectasis. This leads to uneven ventilation and intrapulmonary shunting. Hypoxemia and acidosis may follow. Air leaks may occur in an many as half of infants with meconium aspiration syndrome. Vasoactive substances present in meconium may act directly on the pulmonary vasculature, causing vasoconstriction and pulmonary hypertension, or they may indirectly contribute to pulmonary hypertension by inducing platelet aggregation and release of thromboxane.[45]

The diagnosis of meconium aspiration syndrome should be suspected in the clinical setting of meconium-stained amniotic fluid and fetal distress. The infant may be past due or show clinical signs of placental insufficiency. Respiratory distress is common with cyanosis, grunting, flaring, and retractions. The diagnosis can be confirmed by suctioning meconium from the trachea or chest radiograph, which has the typical appearance of irregular pulmonary densities creating a snowstorm appearance.[43,45]

Management strategies focus first on prevention. Amnioinfusion has been used to correct oligohydramnios and variable decelerations secondary to cord compression. Improved outcome variables include 1-minute Apgar test and cord pH, less meconium below the cords, and lower incidence of operative deliveries.[46,47]

It has been shown that suctioning the nasopharynx immediately after delivery of the head removes 90% of meconium from the airway.[48] After delivery and before spontaneous respirations are established, the vocal cords should be visualized and suctioned through an endotracheal tube when thick or particulate meconium-stained amniotic fluid is present.[49–51]

Treatment for established disease is symptomatic. Attention to adequate oxygenation and ventilation is imperative. Coexisting metabolic acidosis may require correction. Mechanical ventilation is helpful for pulmonary toilet and treatment of pulmonary hypertension. For infants who do not respond to conventional therapy, administration of nitric oxide or extracorporeal membrane oxygenation may be helpful.[52–54]

Pneumothorax

Pneumothorax is a frequent cause of respiratory distress in the neonatal period. The term refers to the accumulation of air from a ruptured alveolus in the mediastinum or pleural cavity. The overall incidence of spontaneous pneumothorax is high (about 1%),[55] probably because of the high transpleural pressure (up to 80 cm H_2O) frequently generated by the infant with onset of respiration.[56] The presence of pulmonary pathology, such as hyaline membrane disease or meconium aspiration, may increase the incidence of pneumothorax because of uneven aeration. Other diseases that require high-pressure ventilation, such as pulmonary hypoplasia or congenital diaphragmatic hernia, also have a high incidence of corresponding pneumothorax.

The diagnosis of pneumothorax should be suspected in any infant who experiences a rapid deterioration in clinical condition. Tachypnea, grunting, retracting, and cyanosis are common findings. Breath sounds may be absent or decreased on the affected side. The point of maximal cardiac impulse may be shifted, and signs of hypotension may be present. Transillumination, a simple bedside test, may be helpful in diagnosing pneumothorax. Asymmetry of chest wall illumination when a fiberoptic light is placed on the infant's chest wall permits identification of the affected side and drainage of the accumulated gas in emergent situations before confirmation by chest radiograph. Chest radiograph showing localization of extrapulmonary air remains the gold standard for diagnosis.

The management of pneumothorax should be dictated by the clinical condition of the infant. When there is no underlying lung disease, the pneumothorax is small, and the infant is not receiving positive-pressure ventilation, close observation may be sufficient. Reabsorption of intrapleural air has also been shown to increase by allowing infants to breathe 100% oxygen for 6 to 24 hours.[55] When underlying lung pathology is present or mechanical ventilation is required, however, percutaneous needle drainage followed by thoracostomy tube insertion should be considered. Long-term drainage is accomplished by thoracostomy tube (10F to 12F). Great care should be taken to avoid iatrogenic lung puncture, rib fracture, or damage to the nipple.[57]

Pneumonia and Sepsis

Congenital pneumonia is a frequent cause of neonatal respiratory distress and has been observed in 5% of all live births.[58] Most of these infections becomes symptomatic in the first 3 days of life. Invading microorganisms are commonly acquired by the fetus by the transplacental route from the maternal circulation or by the ascending route from the maternal genitourinary tract.

Common bacterial pathogens include group B streptococcus (about 33%), *Escherichia coli* and other gram-negative enteric organisms, and, less frequently, *Listeria monocytogenes*, *Enterococcus* sp, nontypable *Haemophilus influenzae*, *Pseudomonas* sp, and *Staphylococcus aureus*. Viruses, including herpes, varicella, enterovirus, and adenovirus, account for about 1% to 10% of neonatal infections.[59]

The clinical presentation of pneumonia can vary. Frequently, there is a history of fetal tachycardia without maternal fever, fetal blood loss, or maternal chronotropic agents. Delay in initiation of the first breath at the time of delivery can occur, followed by respiratory distress. Signs and symptoms also can nonspecific (eg, apnea). Diagnosis begins with a high index of suspicion and is confirmed by a thorough clinical examination to help exclude other causes of respiratory distress (eg, congenital heart disease), laboratory evaluation (eg, complete blood count with differential and platelet count, blood culture, urine latex agglutination for group B streptococcal antigen, blood gases), and chest radiograph. Although the indications for evaluation of cerebrospinal fluid must be individualized, meningitis should be suspected in the setting of multiple maternal risk factors, maternal pretreatment with antibiotics, or an infant with symptoms referable to the central nervous system (eg, seizures, lethargy). Antibiotic therapy should be strongly considered at the time of evaluation. Treatment should provide broad-spectrum coverage, including a penicillin and an aminoglycoside, until a specific organism is identified.[59]

In addition to antibiotics, pulmonary, hemodynamic, and metabolic supportive measures may be required. Mechanical ventilation may be required for persistent apnea, hypoxemia and respiratory acidosis, pulmonary hypertension, or pulmonary toilet. When septicemia is present, the infant should have close cardiorespiratory monitoring with frequent blood gas analysis and correction of metabolic acidosis. Hypotension or decreased perfusion may require vigorous fluid resuscitation, use of inotropic agents, or both. Metabolic abnormalities, such as hypocalcemia, hyponatremia, and glucose imbalance, should be monitored. The presence of disseminated intravascular coagulation may necessitate transfusion of blood products.

The duration of antibiotic therapy is usually 7 to 14 days, depending on clinical presentation, culture results, and organ system involvement. When meningitis is present, 21 days of antibiotic therapy is indicated. Although immunotherapies, such as human immunoglobulin replacement, neutrophil transfusion, and steroid administration, have been investigated, consistent benefit from these interventions has not been shown in clinical studies.[60–63] Selective intrapartum chemoprophylaxis with antibiotics to decrease the incidence of invasive neonatal disease caused by group B streptococcus has been effective.[64] Prevention of congenital pneumonia and neonatal sepsis, however, requires development of strategies to enhance transplacentally acquired immunologic defenses (eg, maternal vaccination) or neonatal immunologic responsiveness (eg, cytokine administration).

HYPOXIC–ISCHEMIC INJURY

Hypoxic–ischemic cerebral injury is the most frequently recognized cause of neurologic morbidity in the term infant. The developing fetus can experience decreased oxygen transfer as a result of multiple mechanisms. These include alterations in maternal cardiopulmonary function, decrease in oxygen transport by maternal blood (eg, severe maternal anemia, smoking), or decrease in placental blood flow due to maternal disease (eg, diabetes mellitus or hypertension). Oxygen delivery is also decreased when placental–fetal blood flow is reduced (eg, placental abruption, umbilical cord occlusion).

The fetal impact of a change in oxygen delivery is determined by the acuity and duration of the alteration and fetal responses to the change. The fetus can adapt to reduced oxygen delivery by increasing oxygen extraction while maintaining oxygen consumption. When oxygen delivery is decreased by about half, metabolic acidosis ensues. If chronic reduction in oxygen delivery occurs, oxygen consumption is reduced by decreased fetal movement and growth before brain injury occurs.

The biochemistry of brain injury after hypoxia is multifactorial. One of the most important phenomena is the disruption of energy metabolism, with depletion of high-energy phosphate reserves and accumulation of reducing substances (NADH, FADH). These changes lead to cessation of oxidative phosphorylation and to increase of glycolysis with a net reduction in adenosine triphosphate formation. Adenosine triphosphate–dependent processes cease functioning, with accumulation of intercellular water, mitochondrial dysfunction, and uncoupling of oxidative phosphorylation. Decreased reuptake of glutamate after hypoxia leads to cell death secondary to ion shifts and osmotic lysis.[65]

Although several neuropathologic patterns, including selective neuronal necrosis, status marmoratus, parasagittal brain injury, periventricular leukomalacia, and focal ischemic necrosis, have been observed in hypoxic–ischemic encephalopathy, the neuron is the primary site of injury. Selective neuronal necrosis may coexist with any one of these patterns and is characterized by increased eosinophilia of the cytoplasm, loss of endoplasmic reticulum, and fragmentation of the nucleus, followed by cell necrosis and the appearance of microglia and astrocytes. Cavity formation can occur. Parasagittal brain injury is the most common lesion seen in full-term infants. It is characterized by bilateral necrosis of the cortex and immediately adjacent white matter in the parietal occipital regions of the cerebral cortex in an area known as the *watershed area. Periventricular leukomalacia* refers to necrosis of white matter adjacent to the angles of the lateral ventricles. It is the most common ischemic injury in preterm infants.[66]

Risk factors for hypoxic–ischemic injury include a history of fetal distress, placental insufficiency, abnormalities in fetal heart rate tracing, and acute blood loss. Evidence of multiple organ system dysfunction due to abnormalities of oxygen delivery or perfusion is often present, including acute tubular necrosis and myocardial dysfunction.[67]

The immediate clinical neurologic syndrome after hypoxic–ischemic insult has been staged, based on level of consciousness, as mild, moderate, or severe.[68] Infants with mild encephalopathy are usually alert and have subtle abnormalities of tone and behavior, including irritability and feeding difficulty. Those with severe encephalopathy are comatose, are flaccid, and frequently have seizures that are refractory to treatment.

Clinical investigators have examined multiple variables in an attempt to predict outcome. Obstetric factors, cord pH, Apgar scores, presence of seizures, and brain imaging were examined and found to have limited usefulness in predicting outcome. The best predictor of outcome is the severity of the neonatal encephalopathy. In general, those with mild encephalopathy survive without sequelae, while those with severe encephalopathy either die or survive with major neurologic morbidity.[69]

3.3 Assessment and Management of Pain in the Newborn Infant

Fran L. Porter

PHYSIOLOGIC MEASURES OF RESPONSE TO PAIN

Pain assessment and pain management are important challenges for those who care for newborn infants. Although it is now acknowledged that pain, or nociperception, can be perceived by the most premature infant, no alternatives to verbal report or pain behaviors used by adults have been standardized for use in newborn infants.[70] Physiologic measures that quantify pain in the newborn infant have suggested both pharmacologic and nonpharmacologic techniques for managing pain in infants. These promising new developments are reviewed in this section.

The Context of Pain

The normal newborn infant (eg, heel sticks or unanesthetized circumcision) and the ill newborn infant (eg, insertion of vascular catheters or thoracostomy tubes, lumbar punctures, and surgical procedures) are regularly subjected to procedures and to environmental stimuli that older children and adults would consider to be painful.[71] The potential impact of pain on outcomes of newborn infants raises concerns about the iatrogenic hazards of medical care for newborn infants. Both animal and human studies have suggested that these effects of neonatal pain may be permanent.[70–74]

Physiologic Indices of Pain in Healthy Infants

A variety of physiologic parameters have been examined experimentally to assess pain in infants. These include measures of cardiac and respiratory activity, blood pressure, blood gas levels, neurochemical and neurohormonal concentrations, and palmar sweating. These parameters have been selected for study because they have been found to accompany verbally reported pain in adults. The underlying assumption is that these parameters can be used to index pain in those who are not able to report pain or exhibit behaviors indicative of pain.

Cardiovascular and cardiorespiratory measures have been recognized as sensitive and clinically relevant because of the physiologic link between the regulation of these measures (eg, the baroreceptor reflex) and systems (eg, the endogenous opioid system) that modulate the perception of pain.[70,75] In healthy full-term infants, for example, heart rate is significantly greater during heel stick and circumcision than during preparatory handling and restraint.[76] In healthy premature infants, more invasive procedures (eg, heel stick versus circumcision) elicit greater elevations in heart rate and blood pressure, although the magnitude of these responses is less than that seen in full-term infants. Differences have also been observed for behavioral (eg, facial expression, behavioral state changes) parameters, suggesting that standardizing pain indices among developmentally diverse patients is difficult.

Physiologic Indices of Pain in Acutely Ill Infants

A broad range of hormonal, neurochemical, metabolic, cardiorespiratory, and cardiovascular changes have been documented among newborn infants born prematurely or with acute illnesses or conditions that require surgical intervention. During operating room procedures performed with minimal anesthesia, significant increases in catecholamines, growth hormone, glucagon, and corticosteroids have been reported.[77] These changes result in the breakdown of carbohydrate and fat stores, which can facilitate tissue repair but can also precipitate severe metabolic, cardiovascular, hematologic, and infectious complications, even leading to organ failure. Controlled clinical trials have demonstrated that these responses can be attenuated with more potent anesthetics.[78] It has also been shown that endogenous opioids are released in the fetus and newborn in response to noxious stimuli but are 10,000 times less potent than those known to mask pain in adults.[77] Thus, although the system that transmits pain appears to be functional in the newborn, the pain modulation system may not be functionally mature until long after birth. Newborn infants may experience pain even more exquisitely than older infants and children.

Premature, sick newborn infants display considerably more cardiorespiratory and cardiovascular variability, even during undisturbed periods, than full-term infants. Also, the pattern of their responses differs from that of healthy infants. In acutely ill newborn infants, heart rate and blood pressure increased significantly during preparation for lumbar puncture but returned toward baseline during the procedure. The only cardiorespiratory measure that continued to change during the procedure was transcutaneous P_{O_2}.[76] This change may have been due to prolonged positioning or pain. These findings underscore the difficulty in relying on a single physiologic parameter as a pain index.

Pain Scoring Systems for Infants

Several different scoring systems for infant pain have been developed. These range from subjective questionnaires that prompt care providers to consider neonatal pain treatment to more objective questionnaires that scale the magnitude of physiologic, motor, behavioral, and acoustic responses of infants to interventions.[79] The disadvantage of these scoring systems is that they are not appropriate for a broad clinical or developmental sample of infants whose responses may be altered by immaturity or pharmacologic agents. Another type of scoring system targeted for neonatal surgical patients details the amount of blood loss, visceral trauma, and severity of surgery as a means of standardizing the interventions for comparisons of therapeutic effectiveness.[80] The advantage of this scoring system is that it allows comparison of hormonal and metabolic responses of infants with the degree of surgical stress. It is not appropriate, however, for the many bedside procedures performed in the neonatal intensive care environment.

A Physiologic Stress and Pain Index for Newborn Infants

A promising physiologic measure of response to stressful or painful stimuli is the amplitude of respiratory sinus arrhythmia. Because the degree of heart rate change due to respiratory activity is determined by vagal efferent input to the sinoatrial node of the heart, a measure of that vagal input is believed to provide an index of neural response to stimulation. The amplitude of respiratory sinus arrhythmia has been operationalized by Porges'[81,82] cardiac vagal tone measure. In healthy full-term infants during unanesthetized circumcision, vagal tone decreased with increasingly invasive stimuli.[83,84] More provocative is the finding that individual differences in vagal tone in healthy newborn infants before circumcision predict the magnitude of heart rate responses to circumcision.[84] Similar findings that vagal tone before heel stick procedures in healthy newborns predicts heart rate, and neurochemical responses to heel stick have since been reported.[85] These relations have been extended to acutely ill infants who exhibited a significant decrease in vagal tone in response to handling and positioning for lumbar punctures. In addition, their baseline measures of vagal tone predicted the magnitude of their heart rate response to handling.[86]

PHARMACOLOGIC MANAGEMENT OF PAIN IN THE NEWBORN INFANT

Pain management in newborn infants has traditionally been neglected for the following reasons: (1) the putative physiologic inability among newborn infants to perceive pain, owing to lack of complete myelination at birth—although in adults, pain is primarily transmitted by unmyelinated or thinly myelinated fibers; (2) the inability of newborn infants to report or remember early pain; and (3) the fear of inducing cardiorespiratory instability or addiction by inappropriate levels of anesthesia. Although these reasons have been discarded in light of more recent data, the complexity of providing adequate pain relief in the neonatal period remains high. For example, because neonatal pharmacokinetics differ markedly from those used in older infants and children, anesthetics that are safe and effective in the latter population may not be appropriate for neonates or have not yet been evaluated. Delivery of pain relief may also be a function of the provider's gender, age, experience, and profession (physician versus nurse), which influence perception of need for pain relief in infants.[87] A brief review of some of the more effective and safe medications that have been used in newborn infants is presented next.

Opioid anesthetics are the most effective agents for pain relief in adults, children, and newborn infants, although age-related risks have been identified. Studies of young rat pups demonstrated that 2-day-old animals required higher doses of morphine to achieve anesthesia but were more sensitive to the respiratory depressant effects than 14-day-old animals.[88] Of the opioids, *fentanyl* is the primary anesthetic agent used in acutely ill newborns. It has a rapid onset of action (less than 1 minute), has a brief duration of action (30 to 45 minutes), and offers greater hemodynamic stability than morphine. Fentanyl effectively reduces cardiovascular, cardiorespiratory, neurochemical, and endocrine responses to noxious interventions.[88] One of its most serious side effects, chest wall rigidity, can be attenuated with muscle relaxants. *Sufentanil*, a fentanyl derivative that is 5 to 10 times more potent than fentanyl, offers cardiovascular stability similar to that of fentanyl but with greater attenuation of the hormonal and metabolic responses to pain. *Alfentanil* is 3 to 10 times less potent than fentanyl and has an even shorter duration of action, making it an option for brief, mild to moderately noxious procedures.

Sedatives such as *benzodiazepines* do not have pain relieving effects but can reduce the dose of opioid required for sedation when used in combination with opioids. These combinations are particularly effective in mechanically ventilated infants or in nonventilated infants with chronic lung disease to reduce agitation. For infants who require extracorporeal membrane oxygenation, benzodiazepines are also frequently used to achieve sedation, in combination with fentanyl, after cannulation.

Nonsteroidal antiinflammatory agents, commonly used in older patients, are rarely used to relieve pain in newborn infants because they are delivered only orally or rectally.

Local anesthetics block conduction of pain impulses and are delivered to the immediate area of the nerves to be blocked. They are particularly useful for procedure-related pain and for infants who may not be able to tolerate opioids. Traditionally, procedure-related pain has been denied or ignored by clinicians or, alternatively, "controlled" by the use of physical restraint. This strategy has led to both acute and chronic adverse effects associated with medical procedures for newborn infants.[88] Fortunately, local anesthetics have been shown to eliminate much of this pain with few potential side effects at recommended clinical dosages. For example, dorsal penile nerve block with lidocaine effectively and safely blocks pain responses to circumcision.[89] In many medical communities, however, physicians remain reluctant to use it. For acutely and critically ill infants, few studies have been conducted to evaluate the effectiveness and safety of local anesthesia.[90] In a controlled clinical trial of lidocaine for lumbar punctures, no significant differences in response to lumbar punctures were observed between lidocaine-treated and untreated acutely ill infants. This finding was less likely a failure of anesthesia than a failure of the lumbar puncture to elicit the anticipated pain reaction.[76] Developmentally and clinically diverse populations of newborn infants may require different pain relief strategies than older, healthier populations of children and adults.

NONPHARMACOLOGIC MANAGEMENT OF PAIN IN THE NEWBORN INFANT

Unless severe or prolonged pain is anticipated, nonpharmacologic methods of reducing pain should be considered before delivering drugs. This nonpharmacologic strategy provides an adjunct to effective pharmacologic pain management.

Nonpharmacologic methods to minimize pain include the following strategies:

- To reduce the agitation of infants before performing painful procedures by protecting the infant from excessive light, noise, and handling procedures characteristic of hospital nurseries and by providing boundaries for the infant (eg, by swaddling)
- To reduce the overall toll of pain on the patient by temporally grouping required invasive procedures
- To provide patients with comfort aids, such as a sucrose-dipped pacifier, hand-to-mouth sucking, or holding during painful procedures
- To use distraction or counterirritation to reduce the effects of pain

It is known that immobilization in animals blunts pain reactions; studies are underway to investigate whether the restraint required by lumbar punctures is responsible for the attenuated response of acutely ill newborns to lumbar punctures.

3.4   Outcome Studies

Karen M. Wickline

PRIMARY DETERMINANTS OF INFANT OUTCOME

The infant mortality rate (annual deaths among infants younger than 1 year per 1000 livebirths) has declined during the past 20 years. The four leading causes of infant death are congenital anomalies, sudden infant death syndrome, disorders related to short gestation and unspecified low birthweight, and respiratory distress syndrome.[91] The lowest mortality rates occur among infants with birthweights between 3000 and 3500 g. Low-birthweight infants (2500 g or less) constitute about 7% of all infants at birth. Low birthweight, however, is a major determinant of neonatal mortality due to respiratory distress.[92] Much of the decline in infant mortality during the past 20 years has resulted from a decrease in neonatal mortality. Survival of high-risk newborn infants has improved as a result of advances in the understanding of neonatal physiology and in perinatal care and technologic improvements. Survival of the smallest infants has shown the most dramatic improvement: 20 years ago, less than 10% of infants with birthweights of less than 1000 g survived; the current survival rate of infants with birthweights less than 750 g is about 50%, and for infants with birthweights of 751 to 1000 g, the survival rate is about 72%.[93]

Despite improved outcomes for infants with birthweights of more than 1000 g, the overall morbidity rate among infants who require intensive care has remained constant owing to the morbidity associated with improved survival of the extremely low-birthweight infant (less than 1000 g). Infants with birthweights of less than 1500 g are at increased risk for a number of health problems, including cerebral palsy, seizure disorders, growth disturbances, chronic lung disease, deafness, and blindness. The rate of handicap is inversely correlated with gestational age. About 70% to 80% of extremely low-birthweight infants who survive are free of major neurodevelopmental handicaps.[93]

Considerable heterogeneity in outcome has been reported in the literature, partly due to differing definitions of disability, developmental delay, neurologic impairment, and handicap. Risk for poor outcome may be due to biologic or environmental risk factors. Primary determinants of neurodevelopmental outcome include birthweight, gestational age, intracranial pathology, socioeconomic status, and maternal level of education. In general, the lower the birthweight and gestational age, the higher the incidence of developmental delay and neurosensory deficits. The incidence of major developmental disability ranges from 5% to 10% for infants with birthweights below 1500 g and up to 20% for infants with birthweights below 1000 g. About 30% to 40% of all infants born before 32 weeks of gestation develop intraventricular–periventricular hemorrhage, posing additional risk for disability and handicap.[94] During the past 10 years, however, the incidence of intraventricular hemorrhage has decreased.[38,95]

Social class plays a role in cognitive scores at 3 years of age; children from lower social classes show a decline in mental scores with time, and those in higher social classes show improvement with time.[96] Studies have shown that socioeconomic status, level of parental education, and the home environment all influence cognitive development.[97,98] In infants without intracranial hemorrhage or parenting risk factors, severe chronic lung disease is not related to neurologic or cognitive outcome.[99] The outcome for infants with bronchopulmonary dysplasia is no different from that for the premature population in general.

OPHTHALMOLOGIC OUTCOME

Preterm infants are at risk for retinopathy of prematurity (ROP), a vasoproliferative disorder of the developing retina. In most infants, ROP is a benign, self-limiting disease. In about

10% of affected infants, however, untreated ROP progresses to retinal detachment and blindness. Rigorous attention to regular ophthalmologic surveillance of the at-risk population is critical in preventing significant vision loss.

The cause of this problem is not well understood, but ROP it is thought to be a reaction to injury of the immature retinal capillary bed from the time of birth.[100] Postnatal events, such as prolonged hyperoxia, sepsis, asphyxia, and shock, may be contributing factors by altered oxygen delivery or decreased blood flow to the retina.

ROP incidence and severity increase as birthweight and gestational age decrease.[101] Increasing survival of more extremely low-birthweight infants has been associated with a rising incidence of ROP.[102] Incidence of any ROP is 80% for those infants with birthweights of less than 1000 g or who were delivered before 28 weeks of gestation. The natural course of stage I and II ROP is regression. Stage III with ''plus'' disease, involving five contiguous or eight cumulative 30-degree sectors in zone 1 or 2, is considered ''threshold'' disease if left untreated; about half of these patients progress to retinal detachment. Effective treatment is available with cryotherapy or laser photocoagulation, which can reduce the risk of retinal detachment.[103,104] These children should be followed for sequelae of regressed ROP, which include myopia, strabismus, and amblyopia.

American Academy of Pediatrics guidelines recommend ophthalmologic examinations for all infants born before 35 weeks of gestational or with birthweights of less than 1800 g who received supplemental oxygen.[105] Examinations should be done before discharge or at 5 to 7 weeks after birth when the infant is at least 32 weeks postconception age. The need for subsequent examinations is determined by the ophthalmologist.

AUDIOLOGIC OUTCOME

The ill infant, term or preterm, is at risk for damage to the auditory system. Etiologic factors include congenital infections, shock, hypoxia, hyperbilirubinemia, and the use of ototoxic drugs. Between 2% and 12% of survivors of neonatal intensive care develop moderate to profound hearing loss.[106] Preterm infants with birthweights of less than 1500 g are at highest risk, with 9% to 17% affected.[107] Early detection of hearing impairment is critical for optimizing speech and language development. The risk factors that identify neonates (28 days old or younger) who are at risk for sensorineural hearing impairment include the following[110]:

- Family history of congenital or delayed-onset childhood sensorineural hearing impairment
- Congenital infection known or suspected to be associated with sensorineural hearing impairment, such as toxoplasmosis, syphilis, rubella, cytomegalovirus, and herpes
- Craniofacial anomalies, including morphologic abnormalities of the pinna and ear canal, absent philtrum, and low hairline
- Birthweight less than 1500 g (about 3.3 lb)
- Hyperbilirubinemia that exceeds indication for exchange transfusion
- Ototoxic medications used for more than 5 days, including but not limited to the aminoglycosides (eg, gentamicin, tobramycin, kanamycin, streptomycin), and loop diuretics used in combination with aminoglycosides

- Bacterial meningitis
- Severe depression at birth, which includes infants with Apgar scores of 0 to 3 at 5 minutes or those who fail to initiate spontaneous respiration by 10 minutes or those with hypotonia persisting to 2 hours of age
- Prolonged mechanical ventilation for 10 days or longer (eg, persistent pulmonary hypertension)
- Stigmata or other findings associated with a syndrome known to include sensorineural hearing loss (eg, Waardenburg or Usher syndrome)
- Need for extracorporeal membrane oxygenation

The NIH Consensus Panel on the Early Identification of Hearing Impairment in Infants and Young Children has concluded that all infants should be screened for hearing impairment because current criteria fail to identify 50% to 70% of the children born with hearing impairment.[109] The screening procedure recommended by the panel is a quick, inexpensive, accurate test of hearing sensitivity that measures otoacoustic emissions. Universal screening of all infants is not yet in place. In those high-risk infants who fulfill at least one of the risk criteria, an auditory brain-stem response should be performed before discharge from the nursery or when the infant is at least 35 weeks postconception age, but no later than 3 months of age.[108] It is a sensitive method of screening newborn infants with sensorineural hearing loss. If the auditory brain-stem response screen is abnormal or equivocal, the infant should be referred for otologic, audiologic, and neurodevelopmental follow-up.

EDUCATIONAL OUTCOME

The determinants of educational outcome for high-risk, low-birthweight infants are still being defined. Those born with a birthweight of less than 750 g are at highest risk for poor school performance and behavioral problems.[110] Other predictors of educational outcome may include race, low socioeconomic status, sensory impairment, or physical impairment.[111]

Follow-up extending beyond infancy into school age has revealed that normal developmental progress in infancy does not predict continued normal development in extremely low-birthweight (less than 1000 g) infants.[112] Emerging developmental sequelae are being recognized, such as behavior problems, poor visual–motor integration, deficits in spatial relations, and language disorders. At age 5 years, about half of extremely low-birthweight children may be at mild to high risk for future learning disabilities.[113] On the other hand, just as motor deficits may improve with time, cognitive outcome may also improve over the years. Intellectual assessment at age 5.5 years may actually show improvement from that at age 2 years.[114]

As the duration of follow-up increases, outcomes for extremely low-birthweight infants should be better understood. Some of these children may eventually overcome their academic difficulties.

ENHANCING OUTCOME

Enhancement of neurodevelopmental outcome should begin before discharge from the neonatal intensive care unit. The convalescing neonate may benefit from occupational therapy, physical therapy, and speech therapy on a regular basis. Other aspects of developmental care include decreasing environmental stressors, such as bright lights, noise, and temperature fluctuations. Calming techniques, such as positioning or providing a pacifier, have been shown to decrease stress and pain. Developmental care may prove to be cost-effective by decreasing the infant's length of hospital stay.[73]

Many level III nurseries have a high-risk infant follow-up program designed to assess growth and neurodevelopment longitudinally. Through these programs, the infant may be referred for multidisciplinary evaluation and early intervention services. Federal Law 99-457 requires state programs to provide intervention services to high-risk infants. Prompt initiation of postdischarge intervention programs may improve ultimate outcome.[115,116]

REFERENCES

1. Miller CA. Maternal and infant care: comparisons between western Europe and the United States. Int J Health Sci 1993;23:655.
2. Ventura SJ, Martin JA, Taffel SM, et al. Advance report of final natality statistics, 1992: monthly vital statistics report. 1994;43:5.
3. Kempe A, Wise PH, Barkan SE, et al. Clinical determinants of the racial disparity in very low birth weight. N Engl J Med 1992;327:969.
4. Gibbs RS, Romero R, Hillier SL, et al. A review of premature birth and subclinical infection. Am J Obstet Gynecol 1992;166:1515.
5. Alexander GR, deGunes F, Hulsey TC, et al. Validity of postnatal assessments of gestational age: a comparison of the method of Ballard et al. and early ultrasonography. Am J Obstet Gynecol 1992;166:891.
6. Ballard JL, Khoury JC, Wedig K, et al. New Ballard score, expanded to include extremely premature infants. J Pediatr 1991;119:417.
7. Clyman RI. Present status of patent ductus arteriosus. Int J Technol Assess Health Care 1991;1:70.
8. Roberts JD, Shaul PW. Advances in the treatment of persistent pulmonary hypertension of the newborn. Pediatr Clin North Am 1993;40:983.
9. Gersony WM, Peckham GJ, Ellison RC, et al. Effects of indomethacin in premature infants with patent ductus arteriosus: result of a national collaborative study. J Pediatr 1983;102:895.
10. Mahoney L, Carnero V, Brett C, et al. Prophylactic indomethacin therapy for patent ductus arteriosus in very low birth weight infants. N Engl J Med 1982;306:506.
11. Mahoney L, Caldwell RL, Girod DA, et al. Indomethacin therapy on the first day of life in infants with very low birth weight. J Pediatr 1985;106:801.
12. Edmunds LH. Operation or indomethacin for the premature ductus. Ann Thorac Surg 1978;26:586.
13. Thurlbeck WM. Prematurity and the developing lung. Clin Perinatol 1992;19:497.
14. Northway WH, Moss RB, Carlisle KB, et al. Late pulmonary sequelae of bronchopulmonary dysplasia. N Engl J Med 1990;323:1834.
15. Stark AR, Frantz ID. Respiratory distress syndrome. Clin Perinatol 1986;33:533.
16. Clark R. High frequency ventilation. J Pediatr 1994;124:661.
17. Jobe AH. Pulmonary surfactant therapy. N Engl J Med 1993;328:861.
18. Hamvas A, Devine T, Cole FS. Surfactant therapy failure identifies infants at risk for pulmonary mortality. Am J Dis Child 1993;147:665.
19. Cummings JJ, D'Eugenio DB, Gross SJ. A controlled trial of dexamethasone in preterm infants at high risk for bronchopulmonary dysplasia. N Engl J Med 1989;320:1505.
20. Doyle LW, Kitchen WH, Ford GW, et al. Effects of antenatal steroid therapy on mortality and morbidity in very low birth weight infants. J Pediatr 1986;108:287.
21. Collaborative Group on Antenatal Steroid Therapy. Effect of antenatal dexamethasone administration on the prevention of respiratory distress syndrome. Am J Obstet Gynecol 1981;141:276.
22. Hamvas A, Nogee LM, deMello DE, et al. Pathophysiology and treatment of surfactant protein-B deficiency. Biol Neonate 1995;67(Suppl 1):18.
23. Northway WH, Rosan RC, Porter DY. Pulmonary disease following respiratory therapy of hayline membrane disease: bronchopulmonary dysplasia. N Engl J Med 1967;276:357.
24. Goodman G, Sperling DR, Hicks DA, et al. Pulmonary hypertension in infants with BPD. J Pediatr 1988;112:67.
25. VanMarter LJ, Leviton A, Kuban KCK, et al. Maternal glucocorticoid therapy and reduced risk of bronchopulmonary dysplasia. Pediatr Pulmonol 1990;86:331.
26. Frank L. Antioxidants, nutrition and bronchopulmonary dysplasia. Clin Perinatol 1992;19:541.
27. Rush MG, Hazinski TA. Current therapy for bronchopulmonary dysplasia. Clin Perinatol 1992;19:563.
28. Glassman M, George D, Grill B. Gastroesophageal reflux in children: clinical manifestations, diagnosis, and therapy. Gastroenterol Clin North Am 1995;24:71.
29. Bliss D, Hirschl R, Oldham K, et al. Efficacy of anterior gastric fundoplication in the treatment of gastroesophageal reflux in infants and children. J Pediatr Surg 1994;29:1071.
30. Martinez DA, Ginn-Pease ME, Caniano DA. Sequelae of antireflux surgery in profoundly disabled children. J Pediatr Surg 1992;27:267.
31. Gluffre RM, Rubin S, Mitchell I. Antireflux surgery in infants with bronchopulmonary dysplasia. Am J Dis Child 1987;141:648.
32. Smith CD, Othersen HB, Gogan NJ, Walker JD. Nissen fundoplication in children with profound neurologic disability: high risks and unmet goals. Ann Surg 1992;215:654.
33. Volpe JJ. Neurology of the newborn, ed 2. Philadelphia, WB Saunders, 1987:311.
34. Cole FS. Immunology. In: Taeusch HW, Ballard RA, Avery ME, eds. Schaffer and Avery's diseases of the newborn, ed 6. Philadelphia, Harcourt Brace Jovanovich, 1991:305.
35. Gerdes J. Clinicopatholgic approach to the diagnosis of neonatal sepsis in clinics. Perinatology 1991;18:361.
36. Taeusch HW, Ballard RA, Avery ME, eds. Schaffer and Avery's diseases of the newborn, ed 6. Philadelphia, Harcourt Brace Jovanovich, 1991:504.
37. Hanigan WC, Morgan AM, Anderson RJ, et al. Incidence and neurodevelopmental outcome of periventricular hemorrhage and hydrocephalus in a regional population of very low birth weight infants. Neurosurgery 1971;29:701.
38. Philip AGS, Allan WC, Tito AM, et al. Intraventricular hemorrhage in preterm infants: declining incidence in the 1980s. Pediatrics 1989;84:797.
39. Avery ME, Gatewood OB, Brumley G. Transient tachypnea of newborn: possible delayed resorption of fluid at birth. Am J Dis Child 1986;111:380.
40. Kuhn JP, Fletcher BD, deLemos RA. Roentgen findings in transient tachypnea of the newborn. Radiology 1969;92:751.
41. Lackkainen TJ, Lentonen PJ, Hess AE. Fetal sulfate and nonsulfate bile acids in intrahepatic cholestasis of pregnancy. J Lab Clin Med 1978;92:185.
42. Miettinen TA, Laa Kkainen TJ. Gas liquid chromatographic and mass spectrometric studies on sterols in vernix caseosa, amniotic fluid and meconium. Acta Chem Scand 1968;22:2603.
43. Avery GB, ed. Neonatology, pathophysiology, and management of the newborn, ed 3. Philadelphia, JB Lippincott, 1987:438.
44. Abramovic A, Brandes JM, Fuchs K, et al. Meconium during delivery: a sign of compensated fetal distress. Am J Obstet Gynecol 1974;118:251.
45. Co E, Vidyasagar D. Meconium aspiration syndrome. Compr Ther 1990;16:34.
46. Wenstrom KD, Parsons MT. The prevention of meconium aspiration in labor using amnioinfusion. Obstet Gynecol 1989;73:647.
47. Sadovsky Y, Amon E, Bade ME, et al. Prophylactic amnioinfusion during labor complicated by meconium: a preliminary report. Obstet Gynecol 1989;161:613.
48. Carson BS, Losey RW, Bowes WA, et al. Combined obstetric and pediatric approach to prevent meconium aspiration syndrome. Am J Obstet Gynecol 1976;126:712.
49. Benny PS, Malani S, Hoby MS, et al. Meconium aspiration: role of obstetric factors and suction. Aust N Z J Obstet Gynecol 1987;27:36.

50. Cunningham AS, Lawson EE, Martin RJ, et al. Tracheal suction and meconium: a proposed standard of care. J Pediatr 1990;116:153.

51. Hageman JR, Conley M, Francis K, et al. Delivery room management of meconium staining of the amniotic fluid and the development of meconium aspiration syndrome. J Perinatol 1988;8:127.

52. Barlett RH, Roloff DW, Cornell RG, et al. Extracorporeal circulation in neonatal respiratory failure: a prospective randomized study. Pediatrics 1985;76:479.

53. Short BL, Miller MK, Anderson KD. Extracorporeal membrane oxygenation in management of respiratory failure of the newborn. Clin Perinatol 1987;14:737.

54. Kinsella JP, Neish SR, Ivy DD, et al. Clinical responses to prolonged treatment of persistent pulmonary hypertension of the newborn with low doses of inhaled nitric oxide. J Pediatr 1993;123:103.

55. Chernick V, Avery, ME. Spontaneous alveolar rupture at birth. Pediatrics 1963;32:816.

56. Nelson NM. The onset of respiration. In: Avery G, ed. Neonatology: pathophysiology and management in the newborn, ed 3. Philadelphia, JB Lippincott, 1987:178.

57. Allen RW, Jung AL, Lester PD. Effectiveness of chest tube evacuation of pneumothorax in neonates. J Pediatr 1981;99:629.

58. Taeusch HW, Ballard RA, Avery ME, eds. Schaffer and Avery's diseases of the newborn, ed 6. Philadelphia, Harcourt Brace Jovanovich, 1991:527.

59. Remington JS, Klein JO, eds. Infectious diseases of the fetus and newborn. Philadelphia, WB Saunders, 1990:17.

60. Christensen RD, Rothstein G, Anstall HB, et al. Granulocyte transfusion in neonates with bacterial infection, neutropenia, and depletion of bone marrow neutrophils. Pediatrics 1982;70:1.

61. Christensen KK, Christensen P. Intravenous gammaglobulin in the treatment of neonatal sepsis with special reference to group B streptococci and pharmacokinetics. Pediatr Infect Dis 1986;5(3 Suppl):3189.

62. Kliegman RM, Clapp DW. Rational principles for immunoglobulin prophylaxis and therapy of neonatal infection. Clin Perinatol 1991; 18:303.

63. Magny JF, Bremard-Oury C, Brault D, et al. Intravenous immunoglobulin therapy for prevention of infection in high risk premature infants: report of a multicenter, double blind study. Pediatrics 1991;88:437.

64. Boyer KM, Gotoff SP. Prevention of early onset group B streptococcal disease with selection intrapartum chemoprophylaxis. N Engl J Med 1986;314:1665.

65. Rothman S. Synaptic release of excitatory amino acid neurotransmitter mediates anoxic neuronal death. J Neurosci 1984;4:1884.

66. Volpe J. Neurology of the newborn, ed 2. Philadelphia, WB Saunder, 1987:209.

67. Carter BS, Hauerkamp AD, Merenstein GB, The definition of acute perinatal asphyxia. Clin Perinatol 1993;20:287.

68. Volpe J. Neurology of the newborn, ed 2. Philadelphia, WB Saunder, 1987:236.

69. Robertson C, Finer N. Term infants with hypoxic-ischemic encephalopathy: outcome at 3–5 years. Dev Med Child Neurol 1985;27:473.

70. Fitzgerald M, Anand KJS. Developmental neuroanatomy and neurophysiology of pain. In: NL Schechter, CB Berde and M Yaster (eds). Pain in infants, children and adolescents. Baltimore, Williams & Wilkins, 1993:11.

71. Franck LS, Gregory GA. Clinical evaluation and treatment of infant pain in the neonatal intensive care unit. In: NL Schechter, CB Berde and M Yaster (eds). Pain in infants, children and adolescents. Baltimore, Williams & Wilkins, 1993:519.

72. Porter F. Pain assessment in children: infants. In: NL Schechter, CB Berde and M Yaster (eds). Pain in infants, children and adolescents. Baltimore, Williams & Wilkins, 1993:87.

73. Als H, Lawhon G, Brown E, et al. Individualized behavioral and environmental care for the very low birth weight preterm infant at high risk for bronchopulmonary dysplasia: neonatal intensive care unit and developmental outcome. Pediatrics 1986;78:1123.

74. Volpe JJ, ed. Neurology of the newborn, ed 3. Philadelphia, WB Saunders, 1995:410.

75. Randich A, Maixner W. Interactions between cardiovascular and pain regulatory systems. Neurosci Biobehav Rev 1984;8:343.

76. Porter FL, Miller JP, Cole FS, et al. A controlled clinical trial of local anesthesia for lumbar punctures in newborn infants. Pediatrics 1991; 88:663.

77. Anand KJS, Hickey PR. Pain and its effects in the human neonate and fetus. N Engl J Med 1987;317:1321.

78. Anand KJS, Sippell WG, Aynsley-Green A. Randomized trial of fentanyl anaesthesia in preterm babies undergoing surgery: effects on the stress response. Lancet 1987;1:62.

79. Weatherstone KB, Rasmuessen LB, Erinberg A, et al. Safety and efficacy of a topical anesthetic for neonatal circumcision. Pediatrics 1993;92:710.

80. Anand KJS, Aynsley-Green A. Measuring the severity of surgical stress in newborn infants. J Pediatr Surg 1988;23:297.

81. Porges SW. Method and apparatus for evaluating rhythmic oscillations in aperiodic physiological response systems. Patent Number 1985;4: 510,944.

82. Porges SW. Respiratory sinus arrhythmia: physiological basis, quantitative methods, and clinical implications. In: Grossman P, Janssen K, Vait D, eds. Cardiorespiratory and somatic psychophysiology. New York, Plenum, 1986:101.

83. Porter FL, Miller RH, Marshall RE. Neonatal pain cries: effect of circumcision on acoustic features and perceived urgency. Child Dev 1986;57:790.

84. Porter FL, Porges SW, Marshall RE. Newborn pain cries and vagal tone: parallel changes in response to circumcision. Child Dev 1988; 59:495.

85. Gunnar MR, Porter FL, Wolf CM, et al. Neonatal stress reactivity: predictions to later emotional temperament. Child Dev 1995;66.

86. Porter FL, Miller JP. Vagal response to handling in acutely ill newborn infants. Unpublished data.

87. Porter FL, Wolf C, Gold J, et al. Doctors and nurses: what are you thinking (about infant pain?). Accepted for presentation at the Society for Research in Child Development, Indianapolis, March 1995.

88. Yaster M, Maxwell LG. Opioid agonists and antagonists. In: Schechter NL, Berde CB, Yaster M, eds. Pain in infants, children and adolescents. Baltimore, Williams & Wilkins, 1993:145.

89. Stang HJ, Gunnar MR, Snellman L, et al. Local anesthesia for neonatal circumcision: effects on distress and cortisol response. JAMA 1988; 259:1507.

90. Martin TW, Sanders EG. Anesthesia for procedures in the neonatal intensive care unit. Prob Anesth 1992;6:475.

91. National Center for Health Statistics. Advance report of final mortality statistics, 1991. Monthly vital statistics report. Hyattsville, MD, Public Health Service, 1993;2S:52.

92. McCormick MC. The contribution of low birth weight to infant mortality and childhood morbidity. N Engl J Med 1985;312:82.

93. Bregman J, Kimberlin LVS. Developmental outcome in extremely premature infants: impact of surfactant. Pediatr Clin North Am 1993; 40:937.

94. van de Bor M, Ens-Dokkum M, Schreuder AM, et al. Outcome of periventricular-intraventricular hemorrhage at five years of age. Dev Med Child Neurol 1993;35:33.

95. Järvenpää AL, Vlrtanen M, Pohjavouri M. The outcome of extremely low birth weight infants. Ann Med 1991;23:699.

96. Ross G, Lipper EG, Auld PAM. Consistency and change in the development of premature infants weighing les than 1,501 grams at birth. Pediatrics 1985;76:885.

97. Resnick MB, Stralka K, Carter RL, et al. Effects of birth weight and sociodemographic variables on mental development of neonatal intensive care unit survivors. Am J Obstet Gynecol 1990;162:374.

98. Weisglas-Kuperus N, Baetrs W, Smrkovsky M, et al. Effects of biological and social factros on the cognitive development of very low birth weight children. Pediatr 1993;92:658.

99. Leonard CH, Clyman RI, Piecuch RE, et al. Effects of medical and social risk factors on outcome of prematurity and very low birth weight. J Pediatr 1990;116:620.

100. Phelps DL. Retinopathy of prematurity. Pediatr Clin North Am 1993; 116:620.

101. Palmer EA, Flynn JT, Hardy RJ, et al. Incidence and early course of retinopathy of prematurity. Ophthalmology 1991;98:1628.

102. Valentine PH, Jackson JC, Kalina RE, et al. Increased survival of low birth weight infants: impact on the incidence of retinopathy of prematurity. Pediatrics 1989;84:442.

103. Cryotherapy for Retinopathy of Prematurity Cooperative Group. Multicenter trial of cryotherapy for retinopathy of prematurity. Arch Ophthalmol 1988;106:471.

104. McNamara JA, Tasman W, Brown GC, et al. Laser photocoagulation for stage 3 + retinopathy of prematurity. Ophthalmology 1991;98: 576.

105. Guidelines for perinatal care, ed 3. Elk Grove Village, IL, and Washington, DC, American Academy of Pediatrics and American College of Obstetricians and Gynecologists, 1992:110.
106. Sanders R, Durieux-Smith A, Hyde M, et al. Incidence of hearing loss in high risk and intensive care nursery infants. J Otolaryngol 1985;14:28.
107. Bergman I, Hirsch RP, Fria TJ, et al. Cause of hearing loss in the high risk premature infant. J Pediatr 1985;106:95.
108. Joint Committee on Infant Hearing. 1990 position statement. ASHA 1991;33:3.
109. Early identification of hearing impairment in infants and young children. NIH Consensus Statement, 1993.
110. Hack M, Taylor G, Klein N, et al. School-age outcomes in children with birth weights under 750 g. N Engl J Med 1994;331:753.
111. Ramey CT, Stedman DJ, Borders-Patterson A, et al. Predicting school failure from information at birth. Am J Ment Defic 1978;82:525.
112. Collin MF, Halsey CL, Anderson CL. Emerging developmental sequelae in the ''normal'' extremely low birth weight infant. Pediatr 1991;88:115.
113. Saigal S, Szatmari P, Rosenbaum P, et al. Intellectual and functional status at school entry of children who weighed 1000 grams or less at birth: a regional perspective of births in the 1980s. J Pediatr 1990;116:409.
114. Kitchen WH, Ford GW, Rickards AL, et al. Children of birth weight <1000 g: changing outcome between ages 2 and 5 years. J Pediatr 1987;110:283.
115. The Infant Health and Development Program. Enhancing the outcomes of low-birth-weight, premature infants: a multisite, randomized trial. JAMA 1990;263:3035.
116. McCormick MC, Brooks-Gunn J, Workman-Daniels K, et al. The health and developmental status of very low-birth-weight children at school age. JAMA 1992;267:2204.

Surgery of Infants and Children: Scientific Principles and Practice, edited by
Keith T. Oldham, Paul M. Colombani, and Robert P. Foglia.
Lippincott–Raven Publishers, Philadelphia, © 1997.

CHAPTER 4

Homeostasis

4.1   Fluid and Electrolyte Management

Robert W. Letton and Walter J. Chwals

Managing fluids and electrolytes in critically ill children requires dynamic monitoring and frequent adjustment. Subtle differences in the perioperative management of these patients can be amplified more so than in adults. The pediatric surgeon should understand the evolving physiologic parameters and fluid compartment values particular to infants and children as well as the physiologic mechanisms involved in controlling this balance.

Fluid and electrolyte balance should be viewed from three perspectives: the total amount of water and solute in the body, the distribution of water and solute in the various body compartments, and the osmolar concentration of each in these various compartments. Increasing numbers of premature infants with more complex anatomic and physiologic pathology are being treated earlier in gestation. Technologic advances allow more accurate methods of monitoring these patients than past calculations based on outdated standard formulas and tables.

This chapter reviews the standard physiology involved in fluid and electrolyte balance and applies this information to the fluid management of pediatric surgery patients. In addition, newer techniques and areas of debate are discussed as they relate to infants and children.

BODY COMPOSITION AND HOMEOSTASIS

Body Fluid Compartments

The most abundant component of the human body is water. Total body water (TBW) can be divided into extracellular fluid (ECF) and intracellular fluid (ICF) compartments. The major components of the ECF compartment are an intravascular component (plasma volume) and an interstitial component. The interstitial component contains most of the ECF and is found in the space between the cells. It is composed of the fluid phase of connective tissues and the lymphatic fluid. A third component of the ECF compartment is the transcellular fluid, which consists of cerebrospinal, pleural, peritoneal, and synovial fluid as well as fluids compartmentalized in the various glands of the body. It is often the sequestration of fluids in one or more

of these volumes during pathologic states that results in what is commonly termed the *third-space* fluid.

The principal cation of the ECF compartment is sodium; the principal anions are chloride and bicarbonate. In the ICF compartment, potassium is the principal cation, while phosphates and nondiffusible proteins are the principal anions. The ICF compartment consists of the fluid found inside the cells of the body. It is separated from the ECF compartment by the cell membrane. ICF volume is estimated as the difference between TBW and ECF volumes. Because cell membranes are freely permeable to water, the osmolality values of the ICF and ECF are always equal. These membranes are not freely permeable to cations and anions, however. Therefore, any acute changes in concentration on either side of the membrane can result in fluid shifts until an equilibrium of 280 to 295 mOsm/L is reached. This concept is essential to understanding many of the disorders of abnormal fluid and electrolyte metabolism.

Developmental Changes in Composition

During the course of gestation, there is a decrease in the percentage of body weight represented by TBW and a relative decrease in the ECF/ICF compartment ratio. Isotopic measurements have demonstrated that the TBW compartment represents about 80% to 90% of total body weight in fetuses, 70% to 80% in normal neonates, and 60% in adults.[1,2] At 20 weeks' gestation, TBW accounts for 85% of total weight, three fourths of which is in the ECF (60% of body weight), and one fourth of which is in the ICF (25% of body weight). At term, the TBW compartment is equal to roughly 80% of the total body weight, with near equal distribution between the ECF and ICF compartments (45% and 35% of body weight, respectively). These changes are represented in Figure 4-1. Because fetuses and newborn infants have relatively larger ECF compartments than ICF compartments, they have more sodium and chloride per kilogram of body weight than adults. By 18 months of age, fluid and electrolyte distribution reaches adult proportions, with the TBW compartment representing 60% of total body weight, two-thirds of which is now intracellular (40% body weight), and one third of which is extracellular (20% body weight).[2] The

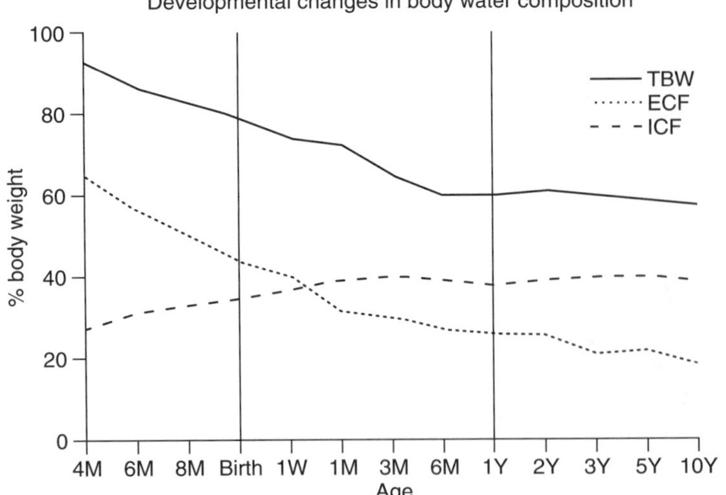

FIG. 4-1. Changes in the proportion of body weight involved in each of the body water compartments during maturation of the fetus into an adult. TBW, total body water; ECF, extracellular fluid; ICF, intracellular fluid (Modified from Friis-Hansen B. Changes in body water compartments during growth. Acta Pediatr 1957; 46[Suppl 110]:1)

plasma compartment in newborn infants represents about 8% of total weight and decreases to the adult volume of 6% of total weight by 12 to 18 months of age.

The Premature or Small-for-Gestational-Age Infant

Preterm infants are born with relatively high percentages of TBW and ECF compared with term infants. The process of eliminating this excess water and solute, which would normally occur over weeks to months in utero, is accelerated and occurs within a matter of days to weeks postnatally. Infants with earlier gestational age require a greater amount of postnatal time to achieve the equivalent fluid compartment ratios of term infants. Both premature and term infants require an initial period of physiologic diuresis and weight loss to remove excess TBW and solute. Replacing fluid lost during this physiologic diuresis can lead to volume excess, especially in premature infants. Even in the face of excess fluid administration, however, preterm infants can regulate renal water and sodium excretion to complete this elimination process (up to 140 mL/kg/d).[3]

Studies show that excess intravenous fluids in premature infants may alter the clinical outcome by increasing the incidence of patent ductus arteriosus, left ventricular failure and congestive heart failure, respiratory distress syndrome, bronchopulmonary dysplasia, and necrotizing enterocolitis. In infants who weigh less than 1500 g, the period of diuresis-associated weight loss extends through the first 2 weeks of life and primarily involves volume decrease within the ECF compartment (plasma volume constant). During the second week of life, TBW, as determined by deuterium oxide dilution, increases while the volumes of the ECF and plasma compartments remain stable. This positive fluid balance reflects changes in interstitial volume because TBW and plasma volume have not changed.[4]

Controversy persists in the management of fluids in premature infants. Preterm infants may tolerate fluid restriction better than fluid excess, owing to changes that appear to affect primarily the interstitial fluid space. The tendency is toward more conservative fluid management.

The total body content of the major extracellular electrolytes (especially sodium and chloride) decreases in proportion to the changes in the ECF/ICF compartment ratio during the first week of life. Increased urinary sodium excretion results in a negative sodium balance and may be the physiologic mechanism involved in initiating postnatal diuresis. Increasing the sodium content of intravenous fluids does not reduce this fluid contraction, but instead results in increased sodium excretion.[5] In addition, infants of older gestational age, but with intrauterine growth retardation, have compartmental water volumes similar to those of less mature infants of the same birthweight.[6] They also undergo a mandatory physiologic diuresis, and replacement of this volume should not be calculated into their fluid requirements.

Fluid and Sodium Regulation During Gestational and Postnatal Maturation

The manner in which the fetus detects changes in the ECF volume and regulates urinary sodium excretion is dependent on developmental maturation. Most of the mechanisms that sense volume changes exist in the plasma compartment. A very sensitive, low-pressure cardiopulmonary reflex exists during the first week of life. This mechanism leads to increased sodium excretion during periods of hypervolemia, and its sensitivity diminishes with postnatal development.[7] This reflex may act by triggering a surge in atrial natriuretic peptide in response to increased left atrial stretch as pulmonary vascular resistance decreases.[8] High-pressure receptors in the carotid sinus and aorta that regulate renal sympathetic nerve activity undergo a similar decline in sensitivity with increasing postnatal age.[9,10] The immature juxtaglomerular apparatus responds to decreased perfusion by releasing renin; as the infant matures, the trigger pressure increases.[11,12]

The immature kidney has an elevated fractional excretion of sodium (FE_{Na}). This can be seen in the differences between preterm and term neonatal kidneys and between term neonatal kidneys and those of older children.[13] Functional glomerulotubular imbalance, in which the number and activity of the glomeruli is greater than that of the distal tubules, may be partly responsible for this elevated FE_{Na}.[14,15] As the kidney matures, the ratio of glomeruli to distal tubules decreases, leading to a decrease in FE_{Na}. Sympathetic nervous input to the kidney, which would normally decrease sodium excretion, is attenuated in the immediate postnatal period.[16] Despite the increased excretion of sodium, the immature kidney has a lower capacity to excrete a sodium load, owing to a decrease in tubular Na^+-K^+-ATPase activity and functional immaturity of the tubular basolateral cell membranes.[17,18] Dopamine infusion increases glomerular filtration rate and sodium excretion to a similar degree in adults and neonates.[19] Some developmental differences may be present, however, because there is an increased adenylate cyclase response and an attenuated Na^+-K^+-ATPase inhibition in the neonatal kidney as compared with the adult kidney.[20,21] The renin–angiotensin system is active and well developed in the neonate; however, the immature kidney is less responsive to exogenous aldosterone, most likely owing to decreased Na^+-K^+-ATPase activity.[22,23]

The difficulty involved in managing postnatal fluids, especially in premature neonates, relates to the balance between the physiologic need for diuresis and the functional immaturity of the kidney, which primarily regulates this process. Premature infants have a decreased glomerular filtration rate and concentrating capacity. In contrast to the volume-loaded preterm infant kidney, which can adequately clear free water, the inefficient concentrating capability of the immature kidney necessitates adequate volume replacement during periods of dehydration, and a delicate balance must be maintained.

Insensible Water Loss

Water expenditure in neonates and infants can be divided into insensible water loss, excretion of renal solute, water loss in stool, and water and electrolytes lost during normal homeostasis. Insensible losses are free water losses that occur through the skin and respiratory tract. The rate of loss through the respiratory tract is dependent on tidal volume, respiratory rate, temperature, and the humidity of inspired and expired air. In term and near-term infants (more than 32 weeks' gestation), respiratory losses can account for up to one third of insensible losses. Although infants have greater insensible losses at earlier gestational ages, respiratory losses in this population are proportionally less, owing to increased loss through the skin.

In all infants, regardless of age, transepithelial water loss (TEWL) makes up most insensible losses. The degree of TEWL varies inversely with body weight and age. Younger infants have a higher ratio of body surface area to body weight. Environmental factors also play a significant role. Using radiant warmers and phototherapy can increase temperature and decrease humidity, exacerbating evaporative losses. Extremely low-birthweight infants have poorly developed insulating white fat layer and skin that is not yet keratinized, allowing for increased cutaneous loss of free water. In infants, TEWL can be reduced significantly during transport by use of an impermeable plastic cover. Fever can increase insensible losses by about 7 mL/kg/d for each degree above 37.2°C (99°F).[24] In very-low-birthweight infants, TEWL can exceed the volume of fluid excreted by the kidneys, but transcutaneous losses decrease steadily as postnatal age increases. Free water should be used to replace insensible losses. Complications of fluid loss include hyperosmolality, which can lead to an increased risk of intracerebral hemorrhage.

TABLE 4-1. *Transepithelial water loss (mL/kg/24 h) as a function of birthweight*

Postnatal age (wk)	Birth weight (g)		
	751–1000	1001–1250	1251–1500
1	65	55	40
2	60	50	30
3	45	35	30
4	45	35	30

(Modified from Bell EF, Oh W. Fluid and electrolyte balance in very low birth weight infants. Clin Perinatol 1979;6:139)

Tables are available to aid in estimating TEWL in neonatal patients. These either use weight or postnatal and gestational age to compare the amount of TEWL in the respective groups. The simplest of these tables estimates TEWL at 30 to 60 mL/kg/d for neonates who weigh less than 1500 g, and 15 to 35 mL/kg/d in neonates who weigh more than 1500 g.[25] Further refinement of this weight-based scale is presented in Table 4-1and accounts for postnatal age as well as gestational weight. Values for TEWL that account for both postnatal age and gestational age are presented in Table 4-2. As computers become more available in the intensive care setting, the use of specific and detailed mathematic formulas may allow more precise fluid delivery in neonates.[26]

Body Fat

The body fat compartment is generated during the last 2 months of gestation and reaches about 10% of total body weight at term. Most body fat is contained in white adipose tissue, which serves as an insulating blanket against energy loss and for the storage of caloric energy. A second type of fat is stored as brown adipose tissue (BAT), which can comprise up to 10% of total body fat at term. Infants with intrauterine growth retardation have markedly reduced total body fat, exhibited by decreased skin fold thickness and ponderal index, defined as birthweight in grams times 100, divided by body length in centimeters.[27] Ponderal index and skin fold thickness correlate with lean body mass as calculated by dual photon absorptiometry in

TABLE 4-2. *Transepithelial water loss (mL/kg/24 h ± SD) in newborns as a function of gestational age*

Postnatal age (d)	Gestational age (wk)			
	25–27	28–30	31–36	37–41
<1	129 ± 39	42 ± 13	12 ± 5	7 ± 2
1	110 ± 27	39 ± 11	11 ± 5	6 ± 1
3	71 ± 9	32 ± 9	12 ± 4	6 ± 1
5	51 ± 7	27 ± 7	12 ± 4	6 ± 1
7	43 ± 9	24 ± 7	12 ± 4	6 ± 1
14	32 ± 10	18 ± 6	9 ± 3	6 ± 1
21	28 ± 10	15 ± 6	8 ± 2	6 ± 0
28	24 ± 11	15 ± 6	7 ± 1	7 ± 1

(Modified from Hammarlund K, Sedin G, Stromberg B. Transepidermal water loss in newborn infants. VIII. Relation to gestational age and post-natal age in appropriate and small for gestational age infants. Acta Pediatr Scand 1983;72:721)

premature and neonatal infants. As gestational age increases in both small-for-gestational-age and appropriate-for-gestational-age infants, there is a significant decrease in percentage of lean body mass relative to total body weight, indicating increased adipose tissue stores.[27]

Nonshivering Thermogenesis

Infants undergo a tremendous temperature shock at birth, coming from a protected thermoneutral environment into the cool surroundings of the external world. To survive, evolution has provided a means by which infants can generate heat and maintain their temperature. Two mechanisms exist by which an infant can generate heat. These are shivering thermogenesis, in which muscle contraction generates heat, and nonshivering thermogenesis, which is due to the presence of BAT.

No parallel organ to BAT exists in cold-blooded animals. There are species-specific differences in the development of BAT.[8] Alitricial newborns are born as members of a litter and must huddle to keep warm. Their recruitment of BAT is a slow process that starts at birth and reaches a maximum days later. Immature newborns, including marsupials, are not able to respond at birth to changes in environmental temperature and are technically poikilothermic. Precocial newborns are born singly or in small litters and have well-recruited BAT stores that atrophy postnatally. The physiologic development of the human infant is similar to that of precocial newborn animals at birth, but BAT stores are not as extensive and must mature similar to that in alitricial newborns.

BAT can generate large amounts of heat and can convert thyroxine to triiodothyronine (T_3). Biochemically, it is identical to white fat, except for the presence of thermogenin, an uncoupling protein that allows BAT to generate heat.[8] Electron transport in the mitochondrion becomes uncoupled from adenosine triphosphate (ATP) synthesis by this unique mitochondrial protein.[28] A proton translocator dissipates the proton gradient in the mitochondrion and allows a high rate of mitochondrial respiration. In infants, BAT comprises 1% to 2% of birthweight and is concentrated in the axillary and perirenal areas, but no particular advantage has been suggested for these locations.[29] During periods of cooling, there is a rapid redistribution of cardiac output, resulting in increased blood flow to the BAT.[30] Excess energy used to generate heat can rapidly lead to a depletion of energy stores needed for homeostasis, and BAT is strongly dependent on an adequate supply of lipids. Even routine nursing procedures performed on the premature infant while in an incubator can lead to a temperature drop as great as 2° to 3°C, requiring up to 2 hours to restore thermoneutrality.[31]

At birth, human infants are completely dependent on nonshivering thermogenesis for maintaining body temperature. The onset of nonshivering thermogenesis is delayed by a placental factor that is thought to inhibit thermogenin. As this factor disappears during the first few days of neonatal life, there is a gradual increase in BAT thermogenin activity.[32] The thermoregulatory control center is located in the posterior hypothalamus. The initiation of nonshivering thermogenesis is related to both an increase in T_3[33] and stimulation of the sympathetic nervous system by the posterior hypothalamus, causing the release of norepinephrine in the BAT.[8] As the BAT is slowly replaced by white adipose tissue, the infant becomes dependent on shivering thermogenesis.

Very premature infants carry out nonshivering thermogenesis poorly, owing to inadequate BAT stores (which develop during the last 3 months of gestation). Full-term infants can keep their body temperature at a level much higher than that of the environment, while premature infants tend to be more poikilothermic. The rate of lipid depletion in BAT and the loss of nonshivering thermogenesis capability are accelerated in malnourished and sick infants. There also appears to be an important link between T_3 and nonshivering thermogenesis: low levels of T_3 can lead to hypothermia and even death, an effect that is more pronounced in the premature infant.[34] The successful metabolic adaptation of the neonate is linked to BAT function in conjunction with maintenance of T_3 levels.

Respiratory drive also may be related to BAT function. While BAT is being replaced with white adipose tissue, the metabolic and respiratory rates of the infant decrease.[35] The exposure of infants with increased BAT stores to warm ambient conditions can cause irregular respiration and even apnea.[36] The depletion and conversion of BAT to white adipose tissue is significantly delayed in sudden infant death syndrome victims. Impaired BAT function resulting from exposure to warm ambient temperature in conjunction with a high degree of thermal insulation may explain why these conditions are related to sudden infant death syndrome.[37]

ELECTROLYTE COMPOSITION: HOMEOSTATIC AND PATHOPHYSIOLOGIC

Sodium

Sodium is the principal cation of the ECF compartment, and therefore sodium balance plays a major role in the maintenance of the ECF volume. As primary changes occur in the volume of the ECF, feedback mechanisms, primarily in the kidney, act to keep the total amount of sodium in the ECF compartment constant. For example, with a loss of ECF volume and its sodium content, the feedback loop would attempt to preserve sodium through renal mechanisms. The total amount of sodium present in the whole body, not just the serum concentration of sodium, determines the ECF volume.

Changes in the ECF volume can be accompanied by a decrease, an increase, or no change in the sodium concentration. The total amount of sodium in the body is about 60 mEq/kg; 6.5 mEq/kg is present in the plasma compartment, 17 mEq/kg in the interstitial compartment, 1.5 mEq/kg in the ICF compartment, and 25 mEq/kg in bone. The remainder can be found in dense connective tissue and cartilage. The sodium content of the fetus is much higher, about 85 to 90 mEq/kg, owing to the proportionally increased ECF compartment as compared with that in adults.

Absorption of sodium primarily occurs in the jejunum, catalyzed by a mucosal Na^+-K^+-ATPase. Sodium is excreted in the urine, sweat, and feces. The concentration in sweat ranges from 5 to 40 mEq/L, with increased amounts in infants with cystic fibrosis. In the absence of diarrhea, losses in stool are minimal. Viral gastroenteritis, however, which induces diarrhea and vomiting, can commonly cause hyponatremia. The kidney is primarily responsible for the regulation of sodium, and, under normal conditions, changes in glomerular filtration rate do not affect sodium homeostasis. Two thirds of the filtered sodium is reabsorbed in the proximal convoluted tubule and the ascending limb of the loop of Henle. The fine modulation of sodium homeostasis occurs in the distal convoluted tubule and collecting ducts. The end result of activation of the renin–angiotensin system is increased levels of aldosterone, which result in increased sodium reabsorption in the distal convoluted tubule in exchange for potassium or hydrogen.

Sodium is actively pumped out of the cell by Na^+-K^+-ATPases to maintain the intracellular concentration at about 10 mEq/L, as opposed to 140 mEq/L in the ECF. About 80% of serum osmolality depends on the sodium concentration, but it also depends on urea nitrogen and glucose concentrations and can be estimated with the following formula:

$$2[Na^+] \; + \; \text{blood urea nitrogen}/2.8 \; + \; \text{glucose}/18$$

Intracellular sodium content is relatively constant, with changes in total body sodium reflecting changes in the extracellular sodium.

Hyponatremia

Hyponatremia is defined as a serum concentration of sodium less than 135 mEq/L. Symptoms usually do not become apparent until the level drops to below 120 mEq/L. These symptoms are usually associated with the manifestation of some concurrent disease state and may occur with hypovolemia, euvolemia, or hypervolemia. Although central nervous system effects are usually the most apparent, cardiovascular and musculoskeletal effects can also become clinically significant.

Serum osmolality is dependent on serum sodium concentration, and a decrease in serum sodium causes an alteration in the osmotic gradient, which can lead to fluid shifts. Water can cross the blood–brain barrier into the central nervous system. Symptoms arise due to cerebral overhydration and include apathy, nausea, vomiting, headache, seizures, and coma. The rate and magnitude of the shift determines the degree of symptoms. Acute hyponatremia, which occurs over a period of 24 hours or less, is associated with the most rapid onset of symptoms. Chronic changes that occur over several days are better tolerated and lead to less significant changes, such as weakness, ataxia, and hemiparesis.

Rapid movement of water into the brain initiates protective mechanisms in the central nervous system, so that swelling is less than would be predicted owing to osmotic shifts alone. An increase in the hydrostatic pressure of the cerebral interstitial fluid accelerates water clearance into the cerebrospinal fluid and is then returned to the systemic circulation through the arachnoid villi. This fluid shift also removes sodium and potassium, which, in turn, acts to decrease the osmotic gradient. As hyponatremia continues, intracellular amino acids and potassium are lost in conjunction with reduced cellular swelling. Because of these changes, the brain is particularly susceptible to dehydration during the fluid and electrolyte correction phase. Rapid correction of the low plasma sodium increases the plasma osmolality in advance of correction in the cerebral intracellular compartment, and a net shift of fluid out of the brain can occur, leading to further damage. Therapeutic correction of hypona-

tremia should occur over 24 to 48 hours to avoid secondary injury from this mechanism.

The cardiovascular response to hyponatremia depends primarily on the overall fluid status of the patient. In a volume-depleted child, hyponatremia leads to a further decrease in intravascular volume as fluid shifts to the intracellular compartment. Release of antidiuretic hormone (ADH) in the hypovolemic state exacerbates this hyponatremia by increasing water reabsorption in the renal tubules. It also acts as a potent vasoconstrictor to increase peripheral vascular resistance and redistribute blood flow.

The renal response to hyponatremia is to produce dilute urine, but this can be complicated by release of ADH. Urine sodium concentration may provide clues to the underlying condition causing the hyponatremia. Urine sodium concentrations less than 10 mEq/L indicate that renal sodium handling is intact and that effective blood volume is decreased. A sodium concentration greater than 20 mEq/L indicates intrinsic renal tubular damage or a natriuretic response to a state of hypervolemia.

The causes of hyponatremia are many and depend on the volume status of the patient. It must first be determined if hyponatremia is actually present. Pseudohyponatremia can develop in states of hyperlipidemia and hyperproteinemia due to a decreased percentage of plasma water in the sample. Because these molecules are large and do not contribute to the osmolality, the plasma remains isotonic, and laboratory measurements often are artificially lowered. On the other hand, factitious hyponatremia due to hyperglycemia or presence of mannitol is associated with a true hyponatremia and is due to redistribution of water from the intracellular to extracellular space. This occurs in the face of an abnormally high serum osmolality. As the underlying condition is corrected, the sodium concentration returns to normal.

Hypovolemic hyponatremia occurs with losses of sodium in relative excess to water and is associated with total body sodium depletion and ECF volume contraction. The most common cause is secondary to increased gastrointestinal losses from vomiting, diarrhea, or fistula output. Increased losses through perspiration can occur, especially in infants with cystic fibrosis and adrenal insufficiency. Intake of hypotonic solutions then leads to a hyponatremic hypovolemic ECF volume. The hyponatremia is maintained by the kidney's inability to excrete sufficient free water. Diuretics can lead to a hypovolemic hyponatremia by means of the excessive renal loss of sodium. Adrenal insufficiency should be suspected when hypovolemic hyponatremia exists in conjunction with hyperkalemia and renal sodium wasting (urinary sodium greater than 20 mEq/L) despite normal renal function. Intrinsic renal disease can lead to an impaired ability to conserve sodium, resulting in hyponatremia.

''Euvolemic'' hyponatremia is rarely euvolemic and usually exists in a state of increased ECF volume, often associated with a normal amount of total body sodium. The syndrome of inappropriate secretion of ADH (SIADH) is the most common cause in children. It is diagnosed by exclusion and is found in certain malignancies, pulmonary diseases, and disorders of the central nervous system. SIADH is a problem of water retention, not decreased sodium. Attempts to correct this condition with the administration of saline solutions usually causes an increase in renal sodium excretion with little change in serum sodium. Postoperatively, increased levels of ADH, coupled with the infusion of hypotonic fluids, can place the infant at risk of iatrogenic hyponatremia. Acute water intoxication is rare but can occur in infants owing to their inability to excrete a water load effectively.

Patients with hypervolemic hyponatremia present with peripheral and pulmonary edema. Despite the low serum concentration of sodium, they usually have elevated total body sodium and body water. This condition can occur in infants with congestive heart failure, cirrhosis of the liver, nephrotic syndrome, and renal failure. The hyponatremia is a result of a decreased effective blood volume, which leads to an increased release of ADH and results in water retention. A decreased glomerular filtration rate leads to increased water reabsorption, and, with active sodium reabsorption, urine sodium is usually less than 20 mEq/L. In surgical patients, hypervolemic hyponatremia can be seen in patients who have received generous amounts of crystalloid and who have had concomitant stimulation of aldosterone and ADH. This results in a disproportionate amount of retained water.

Any patient with significant symptoms of hyponatremia and a serum sodium concentration of less than 120 mEq/L should receive hypertonic saline to increase the sodium concentration rapidly (over 4 hours) to 125 mEq/L. An estimate of sodium necessary for adequate correction can be obtained with the following formula:

$$\text{mEq Na required} = (\text{desired [Na]}^- \text{actual [Na]}) \times 0.6 \times \text{kg}$$

Further correction toward normal should then occur more slowly during the next 24 to 48 hours. Subsequent therapy is based on the patient's volume status. Hypovolemic patients should receive isotonic saline or isooncotic colloid solutions. Euvolemic patients with SIADH require fluid restriction. If symptoms persist with little change in serum sodium, furosemide followed by hypertonic saline may be effective.[38] In chronic SIADH, lithium and demeclocycline can inhibit the renal response to ADH. Hypervolemic patients require both salt and water restriction. In instances of renal failure, diuretics and dialysis also help correct the hyponatremia.

Hypernatremia

Hypernatremia is defined as a serum sodium concentration of greater than 145 mEq/L. Symptoms become severe at levels above 160 mEq/L. This condition usually represents a deficiency of water relative to total body sodium and is most often a disorder of water balance as opposed to sodium balance. Total body sodium content may be high, normal, or low in relation to TBW content, depending on the cause of the hypernatremia. ADH secretion is increased and stimulation of thirst occurs in response to increased tonicity of the ECF. Cellular dehydration occurs as water is shifted from the intracellular to extracellular compartment.

The most common cause of hypernatremia in children is the loss of hypotonic fluid without adequate water intake. This results in a TBW volume that is decreased to a greater extent than total body sodium content. Although diarrhea most often leads to isonatremic or hyponatremic dehydration, when it is additionally associated with decreased fluid intake or prolonged vomiting, hypernatremic dehydration can occur. Excess sodium intake is unusual but can occur iatrogenically if infants are fed an inappropriately concentrated formula. It can also result from overzealous sodium bicarbonate administration during resuscitation. Newborns are at particular risk owing to their decreased ability to excrete a sodium load. The loss of pure water that occurs in diabetes insipidus is characterized by decreased secretion of ADH (primary) or end-organ unresponsiveness (secondary). Excessive sweating or increased insensible losses, especially in premature infants, result in increased free water loss.

Hypernatremic dehydration is associated with extremely dry mucous membranes and doughlike skin. Periods of lethargy and irritability, increased muscle tone, seizures, and coma can occur. Hypernatremia resulting in central nervous system cellular dehydration can lead to permanent damage. Intracerebral hemorrhage results from the tearing of cerebral vessels caused by the shrinkage of brain matter associated with ICF losses. Acute changes are more likely to lead to symptoms than are chronic changes. In response to persistent hypernatremia, the accumulation of intracellular amino acids, particularly taurine, occurs in an attempt to increase the osmotic gradient for the intracellular return of water.[39]

Hypernatremic dehydration should first be treated using isotonic crystalloid solutions to promote volume expansion. When urine output has been reestablished, hypotonic solutions should be used to correct the hypernatremia over 48 hours. Rapid rehydration leads to cell swelling and cerebral edema and increases the likelihood of permanent neurologic deficit. Hypocalcemia is commonly associated with hypernatremia and may also require correction. In cases of central diabetes insipidus, the administration of vasopressin can be used cautiously as an adjunct to volume expansion to help correct the hypernatremia.

Potassium

The most important function of the potassium ion is the role it plays in regulating the electrical activity of biologic systems. Disorders of potassium homeostasis occur frequently in hospitalized children and can lead to signs and symptoms ranging from muscle weakness to cardiac arrhythmias. Potassium is the principal intracellular cation, remaining primarily unbound and osmotically active. Although it is not freely diffusible through the cytoplasmic membrane, it is more easily diffusible than sodium or calcium.

Cytoplasm is composed of salts that are dissociated into their free ionic form. Although inorganic ions, such as sodium, potassium, and calcium, can diffuse through the cell membrane, larger organic anions within the cytoplasm cannot freely diffuse. In addition, a membrane bound Na^+-K^+-ATPase actively pumps sodium out of and potassium into the cell at a ratio of about $3:2$. In electrically excitable cells, nondiffusible anions and Na^+-K^+-ATPase act to form a resting membrane potential of -90 mV relative to the outside of the cell. The cell membrane has a low permeability with respect to sodium and a high permeability with respect to potassium. Therefore, the resting potential is dependent on the concentration of potassium in the ECF. Low plasma potassium concentrations result in a shift of potassium out of the cell and make the membrane hyperpolarized, owing to increased negativity within the cell. High plasma potassium concentrations have the opposite effect, shifting potassium into the cell and causing a relative depolarization.

The cell generates an action potential when the membrane

rapidly depolarizes owing to the influx of sodium. The point at which the cell completely depolarizes and generates an action potential is known as the *threshold potential*. Although extracellular potassium affects the resting membrane potential, it has no effect on the threshold potential. The difference between the resting potential and the threshold potential determines the ability of the cell to depolarize. Increasing extracellular potassium results in a net depolarization of the cell, moving the membrane potential closer to its threshold potential and making the cell more excitable. Hypokalemia hyperpolarizes the cell, making it less likely to generate an action potential. Clinically, hypokalemia is associated with muscle weakness and ileus. Symptoms develop more rapidly in conditions associated with acute potassium changes. When the loss of potassium occurs slowly, both the intracellular and extracellular potassium are changed in a proportional fashion, maintaining the membrane potential.

The extracellular potassium is controlled by both renal and extrarenal mechanisms. The proximal convoluted tubule reabsorbs about 65% of the potassium filtered by the glomerulus. The ascending limb of the loop of Henle reabsorbs another 30%. The distal convoluted tubule and the collecting ducts are primarily responsible for the secretion of potassium into the urine, a process dependent on electrical and chemical gradients. With a high urinary flow rate, a maximal potassium gradient between the tubule cells and the urine is maintained, thereby promoting secretion of potassium. In addition to the stimulated reabsorption of sodium, aldosterone also generates an electrical gradient and increases the rate of potassium of secretion. The rate of potassium secretion is always less than the rate of sodium reabsorption because hydrogen can also be exchanged for sodium in the kidney.

The absorption of potassium is relatively complete in the upper gastrointestinal tract, with some exchange for sodium in the distal colon. Insulin and β-catecholamines can promote the hepatic and muscle uptake of potassium. The release of insulin from the pancreas can be stimulated by increased potassium concentrations.[40] α-Adrenergic agents impair the extrarenal disposal of potassium and can result in elevated serum potassium levels.[41] Acid–base balance can affect intracellular shifts of potassium, with metabolic acidosis resulting in movement of potassium out of the cell. Potassium loss also occurs in the feces and sweat but is not significant, except in cases of secretory diarrhea.

Hypokalemia

Hypokalemia is frequently associated with the use of diuretics without appropriate potassium replacement. The diuretic promotes potassium secretion by increasing both urine flow and the delivery of sodium to the distal nephron. In addition, the diuretic-induced depletion of sodium triggers the release of aldosterone, which further aggravates the hypokalemia.

Renal potassium losses are seen under conditions in which proximal and distal tubular transport are affected. Diseases associated with proximal renal tubular acidosis (RTA) cause profound sodium and potassium wasting. Drugs that cause interstitial nephritis with high urine output lead to increased potassium losses. Glucocorticoids increase potassium losses by increasing the urinary flow rate.

In addition to renal loss, extrarenal potassium losses also occur, and the urine concentration of potassium can be helpful in distinguishing between the two. A urine concentration of potassium that is less than 15 mEq/L indicates renal conservation of potassium, suggesting loss from an extrarenal source. Increased gastrointestinal losses through vomiting and diarrhea lead to a dehydrated, contracted physiologic state that can be associated with significant potassium losses. In the adolescent population, bulimic patients, who try to control their weight by inducing emesis and abusing laxatives, can have significant hypokalemia.[42] Increased levels of hormones, such as insulin and catecholamines, cause a significant shift of potassium into the cells, leading to a loss of extracellular potassium, even though total body potassium remains constant.

Depending on the extent of hypokalemia, the time interval over which the condition develops can result in a varied clinical presentation. Signs and symptoms are more often encountered with acute losses than with chronic losses and are usually related to hyperpolarization of excitable membranes. Both skeletal and smooth muscle can be affected, leading to generalized weakness and ileus. Arrhythmias can occur and are especially prominent if the patient is taking digitalis. Electrocardiographic changes include decreased T waves and the presence of a U wave.

Treatment of mild hypokalemia in symptomless patients may not be necessary, except in patients receiving digitalis preparations (to whom supplements should be given). In severe depletion, potassium replacement should be given parenterally. Up to 1mEq K^+/kg/h can be given to correct significant hypokalemia. Concentrations of 40 mEq/L can be tolerated in peripheral veins, but if higher concentrations are needed, central access with continuous heart monitoring is required. Because potassium is located intracellularly, it is difficult to calculate the exact deficit; therefore, frequent monitoring of the plasma potassium level should be performed as repletion is continued. Generally, a 1 mEq/L decrease in serum potassium (due to actual decrease in total body potassium) represents a loss of about 5% to 10% of body potassium. In patients with significant hypochloremic alkalosis, potassium is difficult to replace until the chloride is corrected. This is also true for patients who have significant hypomagnesemia.

Hyperkalemia

Hyperkalemia is most often present in patients who have impaired renal excretion. Children with congenital urologic abnormalities, such as reflux nephropathy and prune belly syndrome associated with bilateral hydronephrosis, have an associated dysfunction of the tubular epithelium. If this involves the epithelium responsible for potassium secretion, an associated hyperkalemic, hyperchloremic metabolic acidosis can ensue. This type of RTA is resistant to aldosterone administration because the hormone-responsive epithelial cells are damaged, and the resultant non–anion gap metabolic acidosis aggravates the hyperkalemia by shifting potassium out of the cell and into the ECF.

Adrenal insufficiency causes hyperkalemia due to impaired secretion of potassium in the kidney and colon (secondary to decreased mineralocorticoid production). Insulin-dependent diabetes mellitus limits the ability of muscle and liver to take up potassium. Severe crush injuries associated with trauma or the lysis of tumor cells associated with chemotherapy can lead to acute life-threatening hyperkalemia. Excess hydrogen ion, which neutralizes intracellular anions, decreases the membrane electrical gradient, allowing potassium to follow its chemical gradient out of the cell into the ECF. This form of hyperkalemia is not associated with an increase in total body potassium, just a shift from one compartment to another.

Potassium loss in the urine is affected by potassium-sparing diuretics such as spironolactone. Angiotensin-converting enzyme inhibitors limit the release of aldosterone and β-blockers, inhibiting the catecholamine-induced shift of potassium into cells. This may not have a significant effect in patients with normal renal function but can become significant in those with mild to moderate renal impairment. The membrane-depolarizing action of succinylcholine can lead to a transient hyperkalemia, especially in patients with spinal cord injuries and significant burns. Hyperkalemia can be caused by the use of sodium substitutes that contain potassium in patients on a limited sodium diet, and by the administration of antibiotics in the form of potassium salts. Spurious hyperkalemia can be seen with hemolysis of the sample, such as with the heel sticks performed in newborns. Thrombocytosis (with platelet aggregation in the sample) elevates potassium. This can be avoided by drawing a venous sample in a heparinized container.

Hyperkalemia causes clinical sequelae by depolarizing electrically excitable cells. Early electrocardiograms show peaked T waves that progress to a lengthening of the P-R interval and a widening of the QRS complex. If hyperkalemia persists, the child is at risk for life-threatening arrhythmias, including asystole. When the QRS complex is widened or asystole is present, immediate infusion of intravenous calcium increases the threshold potential, allowing cells to repolarize and once again generate action potentials. The hyperkalemia should be treated with an infusion of insulin and glucose, which shifts potassium into the intracellular compartment. If a metabolic acidosis also exists, the administration of bicarbonate shifts potassium into the intracellular compartment. These maneuvers transiently lower the extracellular potassium concentration for a few hours, allowing time to reduce total body potassium more definitively. Loop diuretics are effective at removing potassium in patients with adequate renal function. In patients without adequate renal function and with severe hyperkalemia, the administration of sodium polystyrene sulfonate (Kayexalate), a cation-exchange resin, into the gastrointestinal tract bonds potassium and removes it from the system. Kayexalate is usually administered with sorbitol to enhance its removal from the gastrointestinal tract and avoid obstruction caused by concretion formation. Cation-exchange resin therapy requires hours for adequate effect; poor retention and significant ileus limit its use. In the event that these measures are unsuccessful, hemodialysis or peritoneal dialysis is effective at correcting the hyperkalemia as well as the associated metabolic acidosis.

Calcium

About 99% of the body's total calcium is found in bone. The total body calcium content in infants is proportionately less than in adults owing to decreased mineralization. In healthy people, the nonosseous extracellular pool of calcium remains stable despite constant exchange with the mineralized compartment.

The body's pool of extracellular calcium is divided into three different compartments. Free ionized calcium (45% to 50% of total) is the physiologically active form of calcium and is available for transmembrane participation in events such as neural transmission and muscle contraction. Calcium complexed with sulfate and phosphate (10% to 15% of total) is present (and can be measured) but is not readily available for electrical events. A third calcium fraction is protein bound (40% of total).

The gastrointestinal tract, kidney, and bone are the primary regulators of the body's total calcium. Calcium is absorbed in the small intestine under the influence of parathyroid hormone (PTH) and $1,25(OH)_2D_3$, the active form of vitamin D_3. Hypocalcemia results in an increase in PTH secretion, which increases the 1α-hydroxylase enzyme activity in the kidney, inducing the formation of $1,25(OH)_2D_3$. PTH also increases calcium levels by stimulation of bone reabsorption, while calcitonin decreases serum calcium by encouraging deposition, rather than absorption, in the bone. Calcium is filtered in the glomerulus, and 99% is reabsorbed in the renal tubules under the influence of PTH and $1,25(OH)_2D_3$. Reabsorption in the proximal convoluted tubule and loop of Henle (85%) follows sodium reabsorption, while that in the distal tubule and collecting duct (15%) is independent of sodium transport. The urinary excretion of calcium may be increased by diuretics, growth hormone, thyroid hormone, and glucagon. Increased absorption occurs in sarcoidosis, leukemia, and multiple myeloma, all conditions known to increase levels of $1,25(OH)_2D_3$. Increased gastric motility, decreased small bowel length, and states of protein depletion may result in decreased absorption.

The total calcium reflects the sum of the ionized, complexed, and protein-bound pools. The ionized form of calcium is most important physiologically. There is a great potential for movement of calcium between the various extracellular pools. These shifts can change the ionized component without causing a reliable or accurate change in the measured total calcium. Hyperproteinemia and alkalosis increase the proportion of protein-bound calcium at the expense of ionized calcium. The addition of complexing agents such as citrate, as occurs with exchange transfusions, result in an increase in the complexed pool at the cost of free calcium. Albumin levels drop with stress-induced catabolism (especially sepsis) and can result in hypoalbuminemia with a subsequent decrease in protein-bound calcium. Other mechanisms, however, act simultaneously to reduce the free pool of calcium, and the end effect on ionized calcium is often unpredictable. Hyperparathyroidism increases the total calcium pool in addition to the ionized pool, but in hypoalbuminic states, the total calcium may not reflect this increase in ionized calcium. Additional factors that can contribute to a poor correlation between free and total calcium include pH effects on protein binding, variation in binding kinetics between patients, unusual serum proteins, calcium complexers, and free fatty acids.

Nomograms that estimate ionized calcium values on the basis of albumin and total calcium levels are frequently inaccurate. Pediatric patients exhibit an abundance of complicating conditions that can affect the ionized calcium pool. The complexed, non–protein-bound calcium pool is not incorporated into many nomograms, which may account for some of the variability observed.

Hypocalcemia

Hypocalcemia is relatively common in neonates. An exaggerated primary parathyroid response may persist into adulthood, but with a relatively benign course.[43] The immunologic compromise associated with DiGeorge syndrome results in a hypoparathyroid hypocalcemia that requires aggressive management. Neonatal hypocalcemia can be seen in infants of mothers with maternal diabetes[44] and may be related to hypomagnesemia.[45] In this condition, a postprandial fall in ionized calcium fails to elicit an appropriate parathyroid response.[46,47] States of maternal hypocalcemia, hypercalcemia, hypomagnesemia, and hypermagnesemia predispose the neonate to calcium abnormalities.

Calcium concentrations in healthy term and preterm infants decrease during the first 24 to 36 hours postnatally. By 6 days, levels rise to greater than those present at birth.[48] Severe hypocalcemia can occur when the early physiologic fall occurs in an infant with decreased parathyroid response. Very-low-birthweight infants have extremely low ionized calcium during the early postnatal period. Vitamin D metabolites may be of some benefit,[49] but intravenous calcium remains the conventional treatment despite uncertain optimal regimens.[50] Hypomagnesemia is a known, correctable cause of resistant hypocalcemia, and adequate magnesium repletion should be provided to hypocalcemic infants. Late-onset hypocalcemia can occur with increased phosphorous intake. Maternal hyperparathyroidism may suppress the fetal glands in utero and lead to late-onset hypocalcemia. Hypocalcemia in critically ill children is relatively common. The inverse relation between blood pH and ionized calcium seen with hyperventilation and other conditions of acid–base pathology in critically ill adults may also occur in neonates.

Hypocalcemia results in seriously diminished cardiac function. Rate, rhythm, contractility, and afterload are all dependent on the maintenance of ionized calcium within a physiologic range. The range at which ionized calcium remains physiologic is also dependent on other variables, such as adrenergic activity, preload, and oxygen delivery. Left ventricular contractility increases with calcium administration in hypocalcemic states. When given to a normocalcemic person, however, blood pressure elevations are more likely to occur, owing to increased peripheral resistance.[51] Calcium boluses can be dangerous, resulting in acute cardiac decompensation in patients who are hypokalemic or receiving digitalis. Calcium therapy only benefits patients with cardiac arrest associated with hyperkalemia or due to hypoglycemia-induced arrhythmias.[52,53] When calcium therapy is required, calcium chloride or calcium gluconate should be administered slowly, preferably by continuous infusion into high-flow veins.

Decreases in both total and ionized calcium have been observed in septic shock models,[54,55] are associated with alterations in cardiac contractility and peripheral resistance, and may be related to defects in vitamin D metabolism and parathyroid dysfunction. In hypocalcemic patients in septic shock, calcium administration results in increased cardiac output.[56]

Intraoperative changes in ionized calcium can occur, and patients at risk should have calcium levels corrected preoperatively. Ventilatory changes in pH, the need for large intraoperative transfusion (with associated chelation of calcium), the use of anesthetic agents, and initiation of cardiopulmonary bypass can all result in hypocalcemia. States of acute and chronic renal failure, the use of parenteral lipid solutions, changes in serum free fatty acid concentrations, and calcium-lipid complexes resulting from pancreatitis with an associated parathyroid dysfunction can lead to hypocalcemia.

Hypercalcemia

Many disease states in neonates can result in hypercalcemia. The clinical expression of familial hypercalcemic hypocalciuria is variable and is related to a neonatal state of hyperparathyroidism that requires initial aggressive resuscitation and may potentially necessitate parathyroidectomy.[57] Patients receiving hyperalimentation or vitamin supplements can develop hypercalcemia secondary to hypervitaminosis A or to hypophosphatemia. Hyperthyroid patients, during periods of immobilization, are subject to hypercalcemia, and hypothyroidism can cause hypercalcemia secondary to associated calcitonin insufficiency. Solid tumors, which can cause hypercalcemia secondary to paraneoplastic syndromes, are not as common in infants and children as in adults, but tumors with metastases to bone and multiple myeloma may cause hypercalcemia in children. Hypercalcemia can predispose patients to pancreatitis due to increased pancreatic duct permeability.

Chloride

Chloride is the major anion of the ECF, and its intake and output parallel that of sodium. It follows electrochemical gradients created largely by movement of sodium by passive diffusion. Active transport occurs in the ascending limb of the loop of Henle. Adjustments are made in the levels of bicarbonate; chloride often shifts in a reciprocal fashion. Chloride must be given in addition to potassium to correct hypokalemia, and chloride administration is necessary to correct most forms of metabolic alkalosis. Administration of potassium and sodium chloride results in excretion of bicarbonate into the urine and correction of the alkalosis. Renal correction of metabolic alkalosis results in reabsorption of chloride in excess of sodium and potassium. In distal RTA, increased reabsorption of chloride occurs in the proximal tubule of the kidney.

The measurement of chloride is necessary for calculation of the anion gap. The concentration of sodium is greater than the sum of chloride and bicarbonate, resulting in an anion gap of 8 to 16 mEq/L under normal conditions. This is due to the presence of unmeasured anions that exceed the concentration of unmeasured cations.

Magnesium

Magnesium plays a major role in intracellular enzymatic activity and is the fourth most abundant cation in the body. It is a crucial cofactor in glycolysis and also in the stimulation of ATPase. Sixty percent of the body's total magnesium is bound in bone, with only one third of this freely exchangeable. The remaining magnesium is intracellular, most in muscle and liver, and is bound to proteins, RNA, and ATP. Extracellular magnesium is maintained at a low level within a narrow physiologic range and is freely interchangeable with the bone pool. Absorption of magnesium occurs in the upper gastrointestinal tract and is enhanced by vitamin D, parathyroid hormone, and increased sodium absorption. It remains incomplete, however, with only one third being absorbed.

Renal reabsorption maintains the balance of magnesium, with only 5% of the filtered load appearing in the urine. Absorption occurs in the proximal tubule and in the ascending limb of the loop of Henle. Resorption parallels that of sodium and calcium, with competition between magnesium and calcium for transport. This resorption is stimulated by volume contraction, calcitonin, and PTH. Increased excretion occurs with ECF volume expansion, diuretics, glucagon, and calcium loading. During periods of magnesium deficiency, the release of PTH is stimulated, causing increased magnesium resorption in the kidney and also release of calcium and magnesium from the bone pool.

The serum concentration of magnesium may remain normal despite severe magnesium depletion. Symptoms are related primarily to increased neuromuscular irritability and arrhythmias and do not correlate well with serum levels because these do not accurately represent total body content. Hypomagnesemia often coexists with hypocalcemia because the release of PTH is dependent on adequate magnesium levels. Because the kidney can filter large magnesium loads, hypermagnesemia is often related to decreased renal function. In patients with renal insufficiency, magnesium-containing laxatives, antacids, and intravenous fluids should be avoided. Hypermagnesemia may also be seen in infants born to preeclamptic mothers who received magnesium prenatally. In this situation, elevated magnesium levels tend to return to normal spontaneously within 3 days. Hypermagnesemia is characterized by hypotonia, hyporeflexia, respiratory depression, and even coma. These can be rapidly reversed with intravenous calcium administration.

FLUID RESUSCITATION

Maintenance Fluids and Electrolytes

Maintenance intravenous fluids and electrolytes are the amounts of fluids and solutes required for basal needs and to replace the usual daily losses from the respiratory, integumentary, gastrointestinal, and genitourinary systems. The amounts required can be estimated by measuring the metabolic energy expenditure or by employing formulas based on body weight or body surface area. Fluid and electrolyte maintenance are related to the metabolic rate because increased metabolism results in increased endogenous water production from the oxidation of endogenous substrates. The oxidation of 1 g of carbohydrate, fat, and protein generates 0.56 g, 0.41 g, and 1.07 g, respectively, of water.[58] In addition, increased urinary solute excretion is associated with concomitant urinary water loss. Predicted energy expenditure is only an estimate of basal metabolism; therefore, adjustments must be made for level of activity and other variables, such as fever or hypermetabolic states, that increase the fluid requirement.

Maintenance fluid volume replacement can be estimated by the use of a number of standard formulas. The most common

TABLE 4-3. *Estimation of maintenance fluid requirements*

Body weight	Fluid
First 10 kg	100 (ml/kg/d)
Second 10 kg	50 (ml/kg/d)
Each additional kg	20 (ml/kg/d)

of these is expressed in Table 4-3. The infant liver, especially in the premature baby, is low in glycogen reserves, and replacement with $D_{10}\frac{1}{4}$ normal saline is recommended to provide some carbohydrate caloric supplement. In older infants, $D_5\frac{1}{2}$ normal saline is an appropriate choice for maintenance. Both neonates and older infants should have about 2 mEq/kg/d of potassium added to their maintenance fluids to replace daily potassium losses. These maintenance fluid estimates should be reduced in the first 2 to 5 days of life, owing to the neonate's physiologic need for diuresis. This principle is countered by the increase in TEWL in the very premature neonate. Although there is some controversy, a general guideline would be to deliver 70 to 80 mL/kg/d for term and neoterm newborns. With size and earlier gestational age, increases in maintenance fluid needs are appropriate in the first several days of life. After this period of physiologic diuresis, the neonate can tolerate the same maintenance volume per kilogram as an older infant.[3,4]

The loss of water and electrolytes in stool is usually negligible unless diarrhea is present. The presence of significant emesis or daily nasogastric tube losses should be accounted for in calculating replacement fluids. Daily fistula losses and other surgical drainage also need to be calculated into maintenance requirements. These losses should be accurately measured and replaced on a volume-to-volume basis with appropriate fluids. Table 4-4 provides the electrolyte composition of the commonly encountered gastrointestinal fluids. The electrolyte composition of the commonly used parenteral fluids is provided in Table 4-5. Gastric losses from above the pylorus contain sodium, chloride, potassium, and hydrogen ion. The hydrogen ion concentration $[H^+]$ is 100 mEq/L at a pH of 1.0, 10 mEq/L at a pH of 2.0, and so on, in a logarithmic fashion. Because an infant's gastric pH is usually 3.0 to 4.0, gastric electrolyte losses can be replaced readily with half-normal to normal saline containing 10 to 20 mEq of potassium chloride per liter. Intestinal losses distal to the pylorus are ultrafiltrates of plasma and are readily replaced with a balanced salt solution such as lactated Ringers. Urinary loss of sodium is about 2 to 3 mEq/kg/d, with a loss of potassium of 1 to 2 mEq/kg/d. Usual daily maintenance replacement should include 3 to 4 mEq of sodium and 2 mEq of

TABLE 4-4. *Electrolyte composition of gastrointestinal fluids*

Fluid	Na⁺ (mEq/L)	K⁺ (mEq/L)	Cl⁻ (mEq/L)	HCO₃⁻ (mEq/L)
Saliva	10	26	10	30
Stomach	60	10	130	—
Duodenum	140	5	80	—
Bile	145	5	100	35
Pancreas	140	5	75	115
Ileum	140	5	104	30
Colon	60	30	40	—

TABLE 4-5. *Electrolyte composition of parenteral fluids*

Fluid	Na$^+$ (mEq/L)	K$^+$ (mEq/L)	Ca^{2+} (mEq/L)	Cl$^-$ (mEq/L)	HCO$_3^-$ (mEq/L)	Glucose (g/dL)
Lactated Ringer	130	4	3	109	28	0
Normal saline (0.9% NaCl)	154	0	0	154	0	0
D$_{10}$ ½ normal saline	77	0	0	77	0	10
D$_{10}$ ¼ normal saline	38.5	0	0	38.5	0	10
3% Saline	513	0	0	513	0	0

potassium per kilogram in the form of the chloride salts. Unusually large daily electrolyte losses, such as those encountered with a high small bowel fistula, can be accurately calculated by measuring the content of electrolytes in an aliquot of the drainage and multiplying these values by the 24-hour volume output of the fistula.

Crystalloid Versus Colloid as Resuscitation Fluid

The choice of fluid for resuscitating patients from shock has remained a controversial issue in the scientific literature. In animal hemorrhagic shock models, both colloid and isotonic crystalloid solutions can restore hemodynamics to appropriate levels without significant pulmonary edema. Hemorrhagic shock alone does not constitute a major threat for developing noncardiogenic pulmonary edema.[59] A metaanalysis of studies examining colloid versus crystalloid resuscitation of hemorrhagic shock reported a higher mortality due to pulmonary complications in those subjects treated with colloids.[60] It was thought that if acute lung injury exists, then colloid extravasates and exacerbates lung injury.[61] Patients with burns and sepsis are at increased risk for endothelial injury, which results in a colloid leak with increased interstitial oncotic pressure and resultant pulmonary edema.[62]

The volume of colloid required to reexpand plasma volume can often be only one fourth of the volume of crystalloid.[64] Isotonic fluids, such as lactated Ringers, have the same osmolarity as body fluids; therefore, no osmotic drive exists for water to either enter or leave the intracellular space. Isotonic fluid distribution within the extracellular space is the same as the distribution of water: 25% intravascular and 75% interstitial. Therefore, effective fluid resuscitation of the vascular space with isotonic crystalloid solutions requires the administration of four times the vascular deficit. Despite the increased volume of crystalloid needed for resuscitation, crystalloid is much less expensive than colloid and is the resuscitation fluid of choice.

The most common complications of crystalloid infusion are related to inadequate volume resuscitation resulting in inadequate perfusion, progressive shock and acute renal failure. For a number of trauma patients, crystalloid alone is inadequate, and colloid in the form of blood products is often necessary. Some investigators have suggested that, compared with colloid, crystalloid infusion may cause increased tissue edema, and overzealous administration can worsen this syndrome. Tissue edema decreases the tissue oxygen tension, contributes to ongoing metabolic acidosis, and negatively impacts wound healing.[65]

Advantages of colloid transfusion are predicated on no evidence of a capillary leak and a circumstance in which significant hypoalbuminemia exists. At albumin levels below 2 g/dL, infusion of albumin can raise oncotic pressure significantly and cause flux of water into the plasma space. The infusion of either 5% or 25% albumin can cause an increase in preload, improved cardiac output and renal plasma flow, and subsequent diuresis.

Endogenous albumin persists in the body for 18 to 20 days, but the intravascular half-life of exogenous albumin is only 2 to 24 hours.[66] Other colloids available for resuscitation include the hydroxyethylated amylopectins and dextran. Hydroxyethylated amylopectin (Hespan) has a wide range of molecular weights, with an intravascular life of up to 24 hours. Metabolites can last in the body for up to 60 days. Hespan has a specific effect on the coagulation cascade by lowering the serum concentration of factor VIII:C. This effect is not of clinical significance at volumes of less than 20 mL/kg/d.[67] Hespan interferes with typing and crossmatching, but the effect can be reversed by washing the cells with normal saline. Dextran can cause a significant anaphylactic reaction owing to dextran-reactive antibodies and interferes with the crossmatching of blood, an effect that cannot be reversed by washing the cells. In addition, dextran is known to alter hemostasis by interfering with factor VIII activity, but it may be useful at low doses for prevention of embolism.

ACID–BASE PHYSIOLOGY

Basic Physiology

The pH of ECF is regulated to remain between 7.35 and 7.45. Many disease states encountered in the pediatric surgical population result in acid–base disorders. These are classified as either metabolic or respiratory. Metabolic acidosis or alkalosis occurs when the concentration of plasma bicarbonate deviates from normal. Respiratory acidosis or alkalosis occurs when arterial carbon dioxide tension is altered. Metabolic disorders result in an attempted compensation by the respiratory system, while respiratory disorders result in metabolic compensation. Simple acid–base disorders consist of one primary defect and its resultant compensation. Mixed acid–base disorders occur from a combination of primary events. When mixed disorders occur to drive the pH in the same direction, the infant is in jeopardy of serious or life-threatening complications, and suitable therapy should be instituted quickly.

The normal range for extracellular hydrogen ion concentration is 35 to 45 mEq/L, corresponding to a pH of 7.35 to 7.45. Normal metabolism generates volatile acids (carbonic acid [H_2CO_3] is the most abundant acid produced) and fixed acids (such as lactic acid and the ketoacids). H_2CO_3 is readily converted to carbon dioxide (CO_2) and water (H_2O) and excreted by ventilation. Fixed acids are first buffered by extracellular

HCO_3^-, and then the kidneys excrete the H^+ as ammonium and regenerate the HCO_3^-. Severe acidosis (pH < 7.2) depresses myocardial function, lowers the arrhythmia threshold, decreases systemic vascular resistance leading to hypotension, and predisposes the infant to pulmonary edema. Severe alkalosis (pH > 7.55) leads to tissue hypoxia, muscle irritability, a decreased seizure and arrhythmia threshold, and mental obtundation.

The first line of defense to maintain normal pH is the extracellular buffering system, consisting primarily of HCO_3^- and serum proteins. An intracellular buffering system composed of proteins, hemoglobin, and phosphates exists but takes hours to become effective. The extracellular buffering system can be assessed clinically by measuring blood gas pH and P_{CO_2} and the serum HCO_3^- (total CO_2 content). The relation between HCO_3^- and H_2CO_3 to pH is expressed in the Henderson-Hasselbalch equation:

$$pH = pK + \log([HCO_3^-]/[H_2CO_3])$$

where: the pK of water is 6.1, dependent on the concentration ratio of P_{CO_2} to HCO_3, and not on their absolute values.

An increase in P_{CO_2} or decrease in HCO_3^- leads to acidosis, while a decrease in P_{CO_2} or increase in HCO_3^- leads to alkalosis. When both values are changed proportionally, the pH remains constant.

Correction to a normal pH occurs when the primary defect is corrected. Partial compensation by the kidneys and lung can only approximate the normal pH. Overcompensation is not physiologically possible, and mixed disorders should be considered if that condition appears to exist. Respiratory compensation begins immediately but does not reach steady state for 12 to 24 hours. Acute metabolic compensation, which occurs within 24 hours, is due to recruitment of intracellular buffer systems. Chronic metabolic compensation occurs in the kidney and reaches steady state in 1 to 2 days but often requires 3 to 5 days for completion.

Using the basic guidelines of blood gas interpretation (Table 4-6), one can determine whether a primary or mixed defect is present. For an acute change in P_{CO_2} of 10 mmHg, there is an associated change in the pH of 0.08 units. If the patient's P_{CO_2} is subtracted from the normal value of 40, the pH can be predicted according to the preceding rule. If the predicted pH is equal to the measured pH, the changes are purely respiratory in origin. Any difference that exists between predicted and measured pH is due to an associated metabolic alkalosis or acidosis.

Metabolic Acidosis

Metabolic acidosis occurs when a primary decrease in HCO_3^- concentration results in a pH of less than 7.35. HCO_3^-

TABLE 4-6. *Clinical guidelines for blood gas interpretation related to acid-base status*

1. An acute increase in P_{CO_2} of 10 mmHg is associated with a decrease in pH of 0.08 units.
2. An acute increase in base of 10 mEq/L is associated with an increase in pH of 0.15 units.
3. Total bicarbonate deficit equals base deficit (mEq/L) times patient's weight (kg) times 0.3.

concentration can be decreased by dilution of the ECF with HCO_3^--free solutions, by the loss of HCO_3^- in body fluids, or by the addition of free acids that are buffered by the extracellular HCO_3^-. Respiratory compensation occurs in the form of deep rapid respirations to decrease P_{CO_2}. The anion gap, which is the difference in unmeasured anions and cations, can be useful in determining the cause of a metabolic acidosis. It can be estimated by the formula:

$$\text{Anion gap} = [Na^+] - ([Cl^-] + [HCO_3^-])$$

A normal anion gap (range, 8 to 16 mEq/L) suggests that the loss of HCO_3^- has occurred through the kidneys or gastrointestinal tract, or that rapid HCO_3^- dilution has occurred. A normal anion gap acidosis usually occurs with a proportionally increased concentration of serum Cl^-. In conditions causing an increased anion gap, acids have been added to the system, either by increased production of endogenous acids or by the addition of exogenous acids. An increase in sodium or total protein, or a decrease in potassium, magnesium, or calcium, can also lead to an elevated anion gap.

Normal Anion Gap Metabolic Acidosis

The most common cause of normal anion gap metabolic acidosis in children is diarrhea. Under these conditions, the stool contains a large amount of HCO_3^- and K^+ and a small amount of Cl^- compared with plasma. The combination of hypokalemia and metabolic acidosis stimulates renal ammonium excretion to raise the urine pH above 5.5. The presence of a hyperchloremic metabolic acidosis in the face of a urine pH greater than 6.0 is also consistent with RTA. The two can be distinguished by measuring urinary ammonium excretion, which is high in patients with diarrhea but low in patients with RTA.

Other gastrointestinal (small bowel, biliary, and pancreatic) fluids are also high in HCO_3^- and low in Cl^-, and their external drainage by tube or fistula can result in a normal anion gap acidosis. Ureteral diversion to the small bowel or colon results in the exchange of mucosal HCO_3^- for the Cl^- present in the urine. Hyperchloremic, hypokalemic metabolic acidosis can then develop in conduits that are too long or that are stenotic and allow prolonged contact between urine and mucosa. Bladder augmentation with intestine in children with myelodysplasia, posterior urethral valves, and other lower urinary tract disorders is associated with similar metabolic problems.

Exogenous chloride-containing compounds, such as $CaCl_2$ and $MgCl_2$, allow ready absorption of Cl^-. The Ca^{2+} and Mg^{2+} react with HCO_3^- in the lumen, become insoluble, and are excreted in stool. Cholestyramine, the anion exchange resin used to treat hypercholesterolemia, exchanges Cl^- for HCO_3^-, which is then excreted in the stool. Treatment with cholestyramine can lead to a net increase in Cl^- combined with loss of HCO_3^-, and non–anion gap acidosis can result.

RTA is a condition in which a hyperchloremic metabolic acidosis exists in the face of elevated urine pH, and reduced excretion of ammonium occurs in the face of a normal or minimally reduced glomerular filtration rate. In type I RTA (distal RTA), the distal nephron has an idiopathic inefficient ability to secrete H^+, and the urinary pH is greater than 6.0 in both mild and severe acidosis. Other problems include HCO_3^- wasting, especially during rapid growth phases. Severe acidosis can develop when oral HCO_3^- supplements cannot be tolerated. After 6 years of age, supplements can usually be decreased. Untreated children have hypokalemia and hypercalciuria, with or without nephrocalcinosis.

Type II RTA (proximal RTA) is characterized by increased loss of HCO_3^- in the urine, and the urinary pH is greater than 6.0 during mild, but not severe, acidosis. Proximal RTA is associated with carbonic anhydrase inhibition or deficiency. During periods of severe acidosis, urine pH drops below 5.5, and ammonium excretion is normal. Hypokalemia is invariably a component of type II RTA, and patients usually require high doses of alkali and potassium to correct this condition. The other clinically significant RTA is type IV. This condition is characterized by hyperkalemia, with the ability to decrease urinary pH during periods of severe acidosis. A resistance to aldosterone in the distal renal tubule is common to the various disorders in type IV RTA. A state of pseudohypoaldosteronism is responsible for the most common subgroup of patients. Despite increased renin and aldosterone activity, these patients have hyponatremia and are usually volume depleted, losing sodium chloride in the urine. This form of RTA is usually familial, is treated with increased dietary sodium chloride, and can resolve in early childhood.

A less common subset of type IV RTA is characterized by mineralocorticoid resistance and severe hypertension, but the plasma levels of renin and aldosterone are reduced. These patients retain sodium chloride and potassium and are in a state of volume overload. Sodium chloride restriction, in addition to diuretic administration, effectively corrects the acidosis and hyperkalemia. Primary aldosterone deficiency, which occurs in congenital adrenal hyperplasia, can result in a clinical condition that is similar to type IV RTA but that can be successfully treated with mineralocorticoid replacement.

Increased Anion Gap Metabolic Acidosis

Increased anion gap metabolic acidosis is usually a normochloremic acidosis and is most often due to overproduction of endogenous acids, ingestion of acids, or decreased clearance, such as occurs in renal failure. In diabetic ketoacidosis, insulin deficiency leads to underuse of the ketoacids β-hydroxybutyric and acetoacetic acid. Insulin treatment causes use of the remaining ketoacids and increases net acid excretion by the kidneys, generating HCO_3^-. Despite an initial hyperkalemia secondary to the metabolic acidosis, saline administration with potassium and magnesium supplementation is necessary for restoration of organ function and can also prevent rebound hypokalemia with resultant metabolic alkalosis. Ketoacidosis is also a feature of many inborn errors of metabolism and glycogen storage diseases.

Tissue hypoxia secondary to shock or sepsis, as well as some inborn errors of carbohydrate or pyruvate metabolism, can lead to lactic acidosis. The morbidity of lactic acidosis is not so much related to the degree of acidosis as to the inability to correct the underlying cause. Correcting the lactic acidosis without attention to the underlying shock or metabolic derangements does not improve survival.

Anion gap acidosis secondary to ingestion of toxic materials is especially common in children. Overdose involving aspirin initially causes respiratory center stimulation and respiratory alkalosis. To buffer the salicylic acid later in the metabolic course, there is a depletion of extracellular HCO_3^-, a ketoacidosis, and a lactic acidosis. Nausea and vomiting, induced by the overdose or resulting from treatment, also complicate this clinical condition, often leading to mixed metabolic acidosis and alkalosis. Acidosis is more likely to develop with chronic, rather than acute, ingestion.[68]

Methanol and ethylene glycol are metabolized in the liver by alcohol and aldehyde dehydrogenases to form formic acid and glycolic acid, respectively. Their accumulation can lead to an anion gap in excess of 30 mEq/L and an increased osmolality gap greater than 10 mOsm/L (measured serum osmolality minus calculated serum osmolality). An osmolality gap greater than 10 mOsm/L should warrant an investigation for the presence of unmeasured osmotic particles like methanol, ethanol, and ethylene glycol. Methanol ingestion is more common in adult alcoholics. Ethylene glycol is found in antifreeze and cleaning solutions, and as little as 15 mL in a 2-year-old may be lethal.[69] Its by-product, glycolic acid, can be converted to oxalate with subsequent crystal deposition in the kidney, brain, heart, and lung, leading to organ failure and death. Gastric lavage and ethanol infusion, which competitively inhibit the metabolism of methanol and ethylene glycol, should be instituted in conjunction with immediate hemodialysis for severe ingestion.

Acute and chronic renal failure commonly lead to an increased anion gap metabolic acidosis. Hydrogen ion generated by normal metabolism cannot be excreted as renal failure progresses and renal ammonium production decreases, and HCO_3^- is consumed. In children with congenital renal anomalies (see earlier), a non–anionic gap acidosis may develop secondary to HCO_3^- wasting from renal tubular damage.

Metabolic Alkalosis

A net loss of H^+, gain of HCO_3^-, or loss of fluid containing more Cl^- than HCO_3^- leads to metabolic alkalosis. The kidneys must be unable to excrete HCO_3^- adequately for the alkalosis to persist. A common cause of metabolic alkalosis in children is severe vomiting with a net loss of H^+. The loss of HCl by vomiting or by nasogastric tube suction results in a rise in plasma HCO_3^- concentration. Dehydration secondary to this loss of fluid results in volume contraction and promotes the renal absorption of sodium at the cost of H^+ and K^+, maintaining the alkalosis and causing a paradoxic aciduria. Histamine-2–receptor antagonists can reduce the volume of gastric fluid and the amount of H^+ generated and minimize the associated alkalosis.

Diuretics and mineralocorticoids lead to excessive loss of H^+ by the kidney. Diuretics can also increase the loss of Na^+ and Cl^-, which leads to extracellular volume contraction, stimulation of the renin–angiotensin system, and increased reabsorption of Na^+ at a cost of H^+ and K^+, thus generating a hypokalemic metabolic alkalosis. A hypokalemic metabolic alkalosis in the face of volume expansion occurs in patients with excess endogenous mineralocorticoid production who have normal sodium chloride intake. In addition, posthypercapneic metabolic alkalosis can occur after rapid correction of chronic respiratory acidosis.

To maintain metabolic alkalosis, factors preventing excretion of HCO_3^- by the kidney must be present. These include decreased glomerular filtration rate (due to decreased delivery of HCO_3^-) and volume contraction (which stimulates the renin–angiotensin system). Potassium depletion (which stimulates proximal reabsorption of HCO_3^-), distal excretion of H^+, and renal ammoniagenesis also all maintain metabolic alkalosis.

Measurement of urinary chloride concentration is a useful test to determine the cause of metabolic alkalosis. Urine Cl^- concentration less than 10 mEq/L indicates increased Cl^- reabsorption, such as occurs in severe vomiting, nasogastric aspiration, and severe Cl^--wasting diarrhea. This is a saline-responsive metabolic alkalosis, and these patients require saline volume expansion to correct the disorder. If the urinary Cl^- is greater than 20 mEq/L, the alkalosis is saline resistant and requires treatment of the underlying disorder, especially if profound hypokalemia if present.

Respiratory Disorders

Respiratory acidosis occurs as a result of decreased alveolar ventilation, which results from an increase in P_{CO_2} and a resultant decrease in pH. Causes include acute airway obstruction, bronchospasm, pneumonia, and chronic obstructive lung diseases such as cystic fibrosis. Other causes can include sedation and overproduction of CO_2 due to large parenteral carbohydratic loads. The increase in P_{CO_2} is initially buffered by intracellular systems, with a significant renal contribution occurring after 12 to 24 hours. Renal reabsorption of HCO_3^- rarely results in a serum concentration greater than 32 mEq/L in acute conditions. With chronic respiratory acidosis, however, HCO_3^- concentrations can be as high as 40 to 45 mEq/L. Appropriate management consists of treating the underlying pulmonary condition, decreasing sedation, or adjusting the carbohydratic intake.

Respiratory alkalosis results from a primary decrease in P_{CO_2}. It is usually caused by hyperventilation from anxiety, fever, high altitude, sepsis, central nervous system disorders, and mechanical ventilation. The initial change in pH is buffer-compensated by the intracellular mechanisms mentioned previously. Later, renal compensation occurs, usually within the first 24 to 48 hours. With chronic adaptation, the renal compensation can actually return the pH to normal, as is the case in high-altitude populations.

4.2   Nutrition

Walter J. Chwals

The importance of appropriate nutrient support during the growth and development of the healthy child has been a major concern for practitioners since the inception of pediatrics as a specialty. Just as our knowledge has increased about the physiologic changes that occur as the fetus matures, so too has the care of the preterm neonate improved. Attention has focused on the metabolic changes in response to injury that occur in children, especially infants, in contrast to those of adults. This consideration is particularly crucial in children who require surgery, not only owing to the acute injury of the operation itself, but also, more importantly, because of the frequency of severe primary illness that necessitates the surgical intervention.

A growing understanding of the basic pathophysiologic alterations that accompany acute injury states has led to a heightened awareness of the importance of specialized nutrition in the critical care setting. A reduction in mortality and morbidity following injury has evolved from advances in knowledge about the metabolism and nutritional needs of acutely ill patients. Implicit in this evolution is a more comprehensive understanding of the mechanisms underlying the response of the human body to acute metabolic stress.

The principles of nutritional support during critical illness are more in keeping with a general concept of metabolic resuscitation than with maintenance of standard nutritional parameters. The nutritional requirements to meet metabolic demands during injury states are more extensive and different from basal nutritional needs. Although many putatively beneficial effects of therapeutic modifications have been described, the most convincing are those that result in improved clinical outcome.

This chapter is designed to address not only the nutritional needs of the healthy child but also the specialized requirements due to prematurity, the importance of route of nutrient administration, and the dangers of overfeeding and how to avoid them.

Although much of the data included have been generated through the study of animal and adult human subjects, they provide an important foundation for ongoing investigations of the injury response in children.

NUTRITIONAL REQUIREMENTS AND DELIVERY IN THE HEALTHY CHILD

Nutritional needs can be divided into the general categories of energy, protein, nonprotein, and noncaloric substrate delivery. Amounts differ in children as compared with adults, primarily because of increased requirements for growth and activity in children. This is especially true during early infancy when visceral organ growth is rapid and extensive relative to muscle and fat growth[70]

Energy Requirements

Energy can be partitioned into maintenance metabolic needs (basal metabolic rate, activity, and heat loss to the environment) and growth needs. Energy requirements are age-related and are three to four times higher for infants than for adults (Table

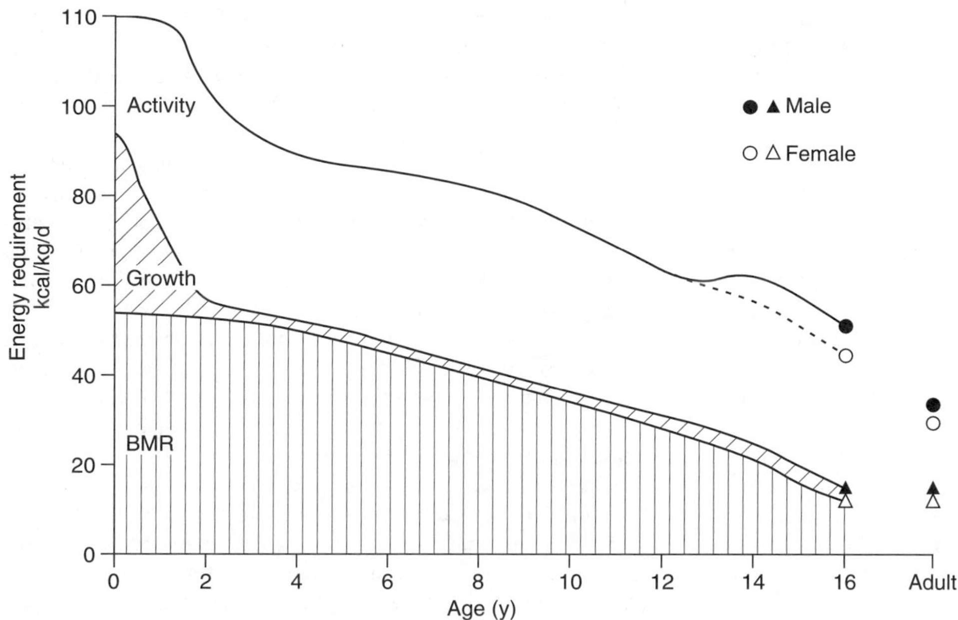

FIG. 4-2. Change in energy requirement per kilogram of body weight during growth. (Holliday MA. Body composition and energy needs during growth. In: Falkner F, Tanner JM, eds. Human growth: a comprehensive treatise, ed 2. Postnatal neurobiology, vol 2. New York, Plenum, 1986:102)

4-7). In premature infants, daily needs may increase to 150 kcal/kg/d.[71] Normal healthy infants use about 35% to 40% of their daily caloric intake for growth (energy cost of tissue synthesis and energy stored in new tissue) during the first 6 months of life. At 2 years of age, only about 2% to 5% of energy intake is used for this purpose[70] (Fig. 4-2). The basal metabolic rate is about 50 to 55 kcal/kg/d in infancy and gradually declines to about 20 to 25 kcal/kg/d during adolescence.

Protein Requirements

Protein requirements correlate with the basal metabolic rate (as assessed by resting energy expenditure) and decrease with age.[72] Protein caloric delivery is therefore relatively constant and should constitute about 7% to 10% of total caloric intake. In hospitalized patients, this requires 2.5 to 3 g/kg/d in infants younger than 2 years of age, 1.5 to 2 g/kg/d for children 2 to 10 years of age, and 1 to 1.5 g/kg/d thereafter.

TABLE 4-7. *Age-adjusted energy requirements**

Age (yr)	Energy delivery§	
	(kcal/kg/d)	(kcal/d)
0–1	120–90	500–1000
1–7	90–75	1000–1500
7–12	75–60	1500–2000
12–18	60–30	2000
>18	30–25	2000–1300

* (After Wretlind A *Nutr Metabol* 1972;14 (suppl):1.)
§ Values on left in each column indicate requirements at lowest age of the interval (eg, 120 kcal/kg/d or 500 kcal/d at 0 yr).

Nonprotein Requirements

Most infant formulas provide a relatively balanced delivery of nonprotein calories, in the ranges of 45% of total caloric intake each for carbohydrate and fat. In the postnatal period, infant metabolism is characterized by a greater dependence on lipid substrate for energy needs.[73] There is substantial evidence that premature infants, because of impaired fat absorption by immature gut, may benefit from increased concentrations of medium-chain triglycerides (MCTs) in enteral formulas.[74] Carbohydrates remain important as a source of energy and are optimally provided in the form of starches, such as those found in cereals, vegetables, and flour. Simple sugars, such as sucrose, should be limited and are generally overused in the American diet.

Noncaloric Requirements

Infants require increased supplements of calcium, phosphorus, folate, and iron. Vitamin C and D requirements are reported to be greater for infants than for older children.[75] In critically ill infants, increased supplements of vitamins E and C may be beneficial in reducing oxidative stress by facilitating removal of superoxide radicals. Recommendations for pediatric multivitamin delivery are 2 mL/d (maximum, 5 mL/d).[76] Infants have higher trace element requirements, especially zinc.[77] This is particularly true when there are excessive gastrointestinal losses due to diarrhea, ostomies, or fistula output. Copper and manganese requirements increase in association with jejunal losses. Administration of these trace elements, however, should be reduced in patients with severe liver dysfunction. Selenium, chromium, and molybdenum delivery should be reduced in infants with renal failure.

Special Considerations in Low-Birthweight Infants

The principal goal of protein-calorie nutritional support in low-birthweight (LBW) infants is to generate postnatal growth rates that match intrauterine growth. Preterm infants are developmentally immature and have low energy stores in the form of hepatic glycogen content and subcutaneous adipose tissue. Caloric reserves in the 1000-g infant are about 100 kcal/kg/d, in contrast to those of the term baby, which measure 1500 to 1800 kcal/kg/d. Total caloric requirements for LBW infants are 130 to 150 kcal/kg/d, depending on gestational age, versus 110 to 120 kcal/kg/d in the term neonate.[78]

Because of accelerated organ growth rates, protein requirements are 3 to 4 g/kg/d in otherwise healthy LBW infants to achieve the desired weight gain of 15 g/kg/d.[79] Cysteine, proline, taurine, and histidine are viewed as conditionally essential amino acids in these infants, owing to decreased endogenous synthesis rates stemming from immature development of enzyme systems.[80,81]

Physiologic jaundice is increased and prolonged in LBW infants as a result of an inability to conjugate bilirubin. Because fatty acids compete with bilirubin for albumin-bonding sites, parenteral lipid administration should be reduced to decrease the risk of kernicterus. As a guideline, lipid delivery is reduced to 1 g/kg/d if albumin is less than 2.5 g/dL, associated with serum bilirubin concentrations of greater than 12 mg/dL during the first 2 postnatal weeks. Moreover, increased carnitine administration may be useful to improve fatty acid use (improved transmitochondrial membrane transport) in these infants.[71]

Requirements for elemental calcium (5 to 7.5 mEq/kg/d) and phosphate (1 to 2 mEq/kg/d) in LBW infants are generally impossible to achieve, either enterally or parenterally, because they precipitate out of solution at these concentrations, owing to the lower pH of infant amino acid formulas. The use of calcium glycerophosphate or monobasic phosphate, however, allows for greater quantities of calcium and phosphate delivery. Increased magnesium administration is also required, especially with hepatic dysfunction due to diseases such as neonatal hepatis or biliary atresia.

Vitamin requirements for LBW infants are controversial. There is growing concern that these needs, particularly of the lipid-soluble vitamins, may be overestimated, although conclusive data are lacking.

Trace elements are essential for growth and development, and requirements are increased in LBW infants.[76]

NUTRITIONAL ASSESSMENT

Accurate nutritional and metabolic assessment is particularly difficult in the neonatal and pediatric intensive care settings. The metabolic events that accompany acute injury states are incompletely understood and frequently cause changes that render standard techniques based on assumptions derived from nonstressed subjects invalid.

Anthropometry

The standard for assessing the adequacy of nutritional delivery in the healthy nonstressed child is growth. Growth may be assessed by body weight norms for age and sex[78] and have been revised for premature infants. Body length, head circumference, and body weight are commonly used in infants, as is height in older children. Malnutrition in nonstressed children more

accurately can be determined by weight-for-height and height-for-age evaluation.[82] Acute and chronic malnutrition can approach 15% to 50%, respectively, in hospitalized children.

Anthropometric techniques of body composition analysis are based on measurements of skin fold thickness and limb circumference. These methods rely on the assumption that single or multiple measurements, taken at various anatomic sites, accurately reflect the fat mass and lean body mass of the entire subject, a controversial premise. There are several important problems involved with anthropometric techniques in critically in patients, particularly in neonates. A wide variability in body compartment composition exists, and infant body composition changes rapidly as a function of differential growth and development.[70] The rate of these changes may be significantly different in premature infants, or in children with growth retardation. Even healthy infants and children have a broad range of normal growth for any given age and sex. It is difficult to assess body composition using these techniques in children, and impossible to evaluate growth unless previous sequential data have been gathered over a longer term. The main problem in the intensive care setting, however, is that patients tend to increase weight, because of third-space fluid gains, during acute metabolic stress at the very time when catabolism of endogenous protein, fat, and carbohydrate stores is taking place. This phenomenon can lead to spurious results using the standard anthropometric techniques.

ROUTE OF DELIVERY

Enteral Delivery

A large body of literature now exists to establish the substantial advantages of enteral, as compared with parenteral, nutritional delivery. The advantages include better maintenance of the structural and functional integrity of the gastrointestinal tract, decreased risk of bacterial translocation, greater ease and safety of administration, more physiologic and efficient use of nutrient substrates, decreased risk of hepatobiliary complications, improved outcome, and improved cost-effectiveness.[86]

Breastfeeding remains the optimal method for nutritional support of the healthy neonate. In addition to fostering bonding between mother and child, breast milk provides optimal nutrient content to support growth and provides immunoactive substrates. Breast milk can be fortified with commercially available protein and calcium supplements. Supplemental iron and vitamin D are suggested if breast milk is continued after 4 months. Primarily because of inadequate calcium deposition, fortified breast milk is recommended for premature infants.

Infant enteral formulas generally mimic breast milk in caloric density but provide more protein, calcium, phosphorus, and iron. Products designed for premature infants contain even higher concentrations of these constituents, and many include a substantial portion of fat substrate as MCT. Formulas designed to meet the specific protein-calorie and noncaloric nutrient requirements of LBW infants are available in 24 and 27 kcal/oz concentrations. To facilitate carbohydrate absorption in the immature gut, up to half is provided in the form of lactose, and the rest as maltodextrins. Whey protein is used to reduce curd formation and promote gastric emptying. Most formulas are within an isoosmolar range. Gastric emptying is inversely proportional to caloric density and osmolarity, so concentrated preparations must be used with caution because they can predispose to aspiration. In premature infants, the initial use of a carefully placed, soft gastric or transpyloric feeding tube for continuous drip feedings may be beneficial until gastric function improves and swallow coordination matures. In older children who have prolonged tube-feeding needs, placement of a gastrostomy tube may be performed. When gastric or nasogastric tube feeding is initiated or increased, residual gastric volumes should be checked.

Although enteral feeding is generally safer than parenteral feeding, complications can occur due to improper use, poor gastric emptying, tube migration, bacterial contamination of the formula, underlying illness, or medications.[87] The most frequent serious complication is the pulmonary aspiration of formula. This risk can be reduced by elevating the upper torso to a 30-degree angle or by keeping the child in a prone position and by advancing the tube to a transpyloric position, preferably beyond the ligament of Treitz.

Inadequate absorption can result in poor growth or diarrhea. Measuring the biochemical products of malabsorption are better than measuring the volume of diarrhea to evaluated feeding intolerance.[88] Carbohydrate malabsorption can be documented by a fecal pH of less than 5.5 and the presence of greater than 0.25 g/dL of reducing substances in the stool. Fat malabsorption is assessed by measuring the fat content of a 72-hour stool collection. After 6 months of age, healthy infants should absorb 90% of ingested fat.

Parenteral Delivery

Parenteral nutrition is necessary in patients who are unable to tolerate adequate enteral nutritional delivery for an extended time period (usually 5 days or more), owing to prolonged gastrointestinal dysfunction. The clinical feasibility of total parenteral nutrition (TPN) led to the successful nutrition of babies with gastroschisis and short bowel syndrome. In addition, parenteral nutrition is frequently used to supplement protein-calorie needs in critically ill patients who can tolerate only limited enteral nutritional delivery. Because highly concentrated (greater then 12.5 g/dL) carbohydrate solutions quickly induce thrombophlebitis in peripheral veins, TPN must be administered through a central venous catheter. The catheter tip is usually advanced to the junction of the superior vena cava with the right atrium to facilitate rapid dilution of the infused hyperosmolar solution with blood in a large, high-flow chamber. The development of small-caliber, soft, polyurethane catheters has reduced complications associated with erosion of the catheter tip through the vessel wall. The addition of heparin (1 U/mL) to solution may reduce the risk of central vein thrombosis.

Peripheral-vein parenteral nutrition (PPN) may be useful for periods of 1 to 2 weeks, either as the sole source of nutritional support or to supplement enteral nutrient delivery.[89] To reduce the risk of thrombophlebitis, solution osmolality should not exceed 600 mOsm/L, and dextrose concentrations should not exceed 12.5 g/dL. The addition of lipid emulsions, either in combination with protein and carbohydrate (three-in-one compounded solutions), or piggybacked into polyurethane catheters with protein-carbohydrate solutions, can decrease the irritative effects of hypertonic carbohydrate infusion. This enables the safe nutrient delivery of up to 85 kcal/kg/d (about 850 mOsm). PPN avoids the complication of central vein thrombosis as well as the tech-

nical and mechanical complications (pneumothorax, catheter tip-induced central vein, and right atrial erosion or perforation) associated with the placement of central catheters. The short-term use of femoral venous catheters has been shown to be a safe alternative for PPN delivery, associated, in one study, with a low catheter sepsis rate (2%).[90]

In infants requiring long-term TPN, cyclic delivery has been shown to be safe and effective.[91] The cyclic administration of carbohydrate mimics, to some extent, the intermittent nature of oral feeding. When TPN is cycled off, serum glucose and insulin concentrations fall, lipid oxidation increases, and lipid storage decreases. All these factors have putative benefit in reducing liver dysfunction, a complication frequently observed in infants receiving long-term TPN.

The complications associated with parenteral feeding, some of which were discussed earlier, may be categorized as mechanical or technical (catheter, pump, and placement related); metabolic (fluid, electrolyte, and organ function related); nutritional (related to excessive or inadequate nutrient delivery); and infectious. In one study, the overall infection rate associated with TPN administration was 5%, with considerable variability based on site of placement and lumen number.[92] The risk of many of these complications is substantially reduced if a complete nutritional support team, including well-trained physicians, nurses, dietitians, and pharmacists, takes part in nutritional delivery.

Drawbacks of Total Parenteral Nutrition

A substantial number of randomized, prospective trials have compared TPN to enteral nutritional delivery in acutely stressed high-risk patients (including children). Metaanalysis of eight of these trials (involving high-risk surgical patients) shows a significant reduction in septic complications (18% versus 35%) in the enterally fed patient group.[93] A study of burn patients demonstrated significantly increased mortality (63% versus 26%) in the group randomized to receive TPN supplementation of enteral calories versus enteral calories alone.[94] A study of adult trauma patients has shown that the enteral group infection rate is significantly lower than that of the parenteral group, as determined by fewer cases of pneumonia and intraabdominal abscesses.[95]

These data support the preferential use of enteral nutritional delivery to the degree clinically feasible.

METABOLIC ASSESSMENT

Acute Metabolic Stress: Overview

Among the early features of injury response (eg, trauma, sepsis, acute inflammatory conditions) is the release of cytokines followed rapidly by important alterations in the hormonal environment: increased counterregulatory hormone levels associated with insulin and growth hormone (GH) resistance (Fig. 4-3). A sequence of metabolic events is initiated that includes the catabolism of endogenous stores of protein, carbohydrate, and fat to provide essential substrate and energy to fuel the ongoing response process. Amino acids from catabolized proteins flow to the liver where they provide substrate for synthesis of acute phase proteins and glucose (gluconeogenesis). The acute metabolic stress response represents a hypermetabolic,[96] hypercatabolic state[97] that results in the loss of endogenous tissue and can lead to poor clinical outcome in the absence of appropriate exogenous support.[98] As the acute response resolves, adaptive anabolic metabolism ensues to restore catabolic losses.[99] In children, this phase is characterized by the resumption of somatic growth. The goal of metabolic and nutritional resuscitation in the critically ill child is to promote the earlier and more complete evolution to growth recovery.

Cytokines

Over the past several years, intense interest has focused on a group of peptides that are secreted by a number of cells, including macrophages, monocytes, lymphocytes, and vascular smooth muscle, in response to a variety of metabolic stress stimuli. These peptides, called cytokines, appear to have important regulatory functions in mediating the metabolic and immune responses to injury. Several prominent cytokines are tumor necrosis factor (TNF), interleukin-1 (IL-1), interleukin-2 (IL-2), interleukin-6 (IL-6), and interferon-γ (IFN-γ). Though these peptides are secreted in small amounts and have relatively short serum half-lives, they appear, individually or synergistically, to mediate a cascade of events with widespread metabolic and immunologic effects. Cytokines have been shown to play an important role in the host response mechanism to a variety of inflammatory, neoplastic, and acute injury states. Specific cytokine characteristics and interactions, as they pertain to inflammation and cellular metabolism, are described in Chapter 11. While these effects are important stress factors, one of the most significant consequences of cytokine release, in terms of the acute metabolic stress response, related to the potent cytokine stimulus of counter-regulation hormone release.

Hormonal Alterations and the Catabolic Response

Insulin is a potent anabolic hormone, responsible for glycogen synthesis and the storage of carbohydrate, lipogenesis and the storage of fat, and new protein synthesis. Insulin and insulin-like growth factor 1 (IGF-1) are essential hormones for somatic growth in infants and children. Acute metabolic stress in characterized by substantial increases in serum concentrations of catecholamines, glucagon, and cortisol, referred to as *counterregulatory hormones* because they counteract, or oppose, the anabolic effects of insulin. Glucagon induces glycolysis and gluconeogenesis. These effects counteract the synthetic effects of insulin. Increased glycolysis, which results in increased serum lactate and alanine levels, thus providing the substrate necessary for the endogenous regeneration of glucose (Cori cycle and alanine cycle), is a major contributor to altered carbohydrate metabolism during acute metabolic stress.[100]

Cortisol induces muscle proteolysis and promotes gluconeogenesis. The major amino acid sources for gluconeogenesis are alanine[101] and glutamine[102] from skeletal muscle and gut. Hepatic uptake of these amino acids is accelerated during acute metabolic stress. Like glucagon, cortisol also causes insulin resistance. Although insulin levels may be elevated during acute metabolic stress, the anabolic effects of insulin are inhibited.

Catecholamines cause hyperglycemia by promoting hepatic glycogenolysis; by causing conversion of skeletal muscle glycogen to lactate, which is then transported to the liver for conversion to glucose (Cori cycle); and by suppression of the pancreatic secretion of insulin. Catecholamines also induce lipolysis, which results in the mobilization of free fatty acids. Finally, catecholamines, in addition to glucagon and cortisol, induce hypermetabolism, which results in an increase in the basal metabolic rate.

Visceral Protein Status

The liver normally synthesizes a number of proteins that constitute labile pools within the serum compartment (Fig. 4-4). Among others, they include albumin, transferrin, prealbumin, and retinol-binding protein. These proteins, sometimes referred to as *reserve proteins*, constitute labile protein stores. They

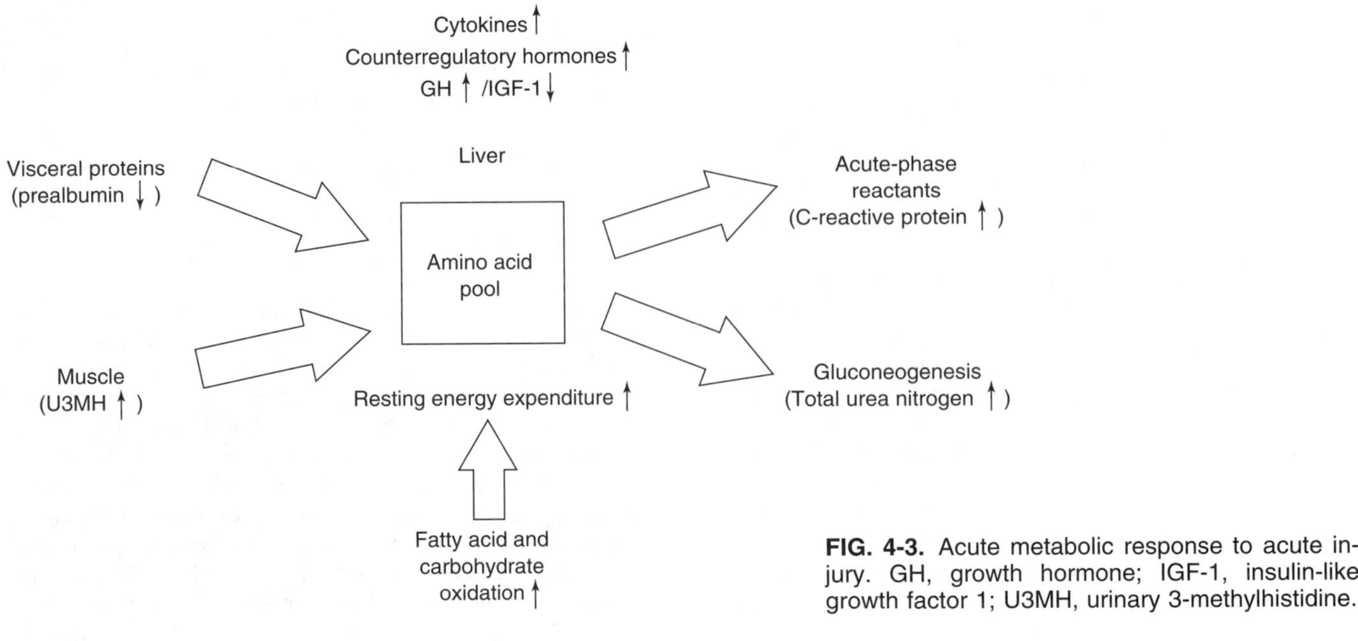

FIG. 4-3. Acute metabolic response to acute injury. GH, growth hormone; IGF-1, insulin-like growth factor 1; U3MH, urinary 3-methylhistidine.

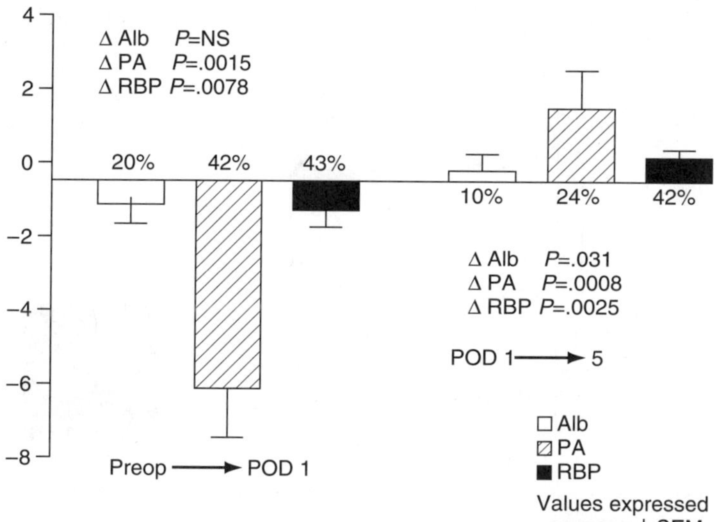

FIG. 4-4. Mean percentage change (Δ) of visceral proteins during acute metabolic stress. Statistical analysis used the paired t-test. Alb, serum albumin (g/dL); PA, serum prealbumin (mg/dL); RBP, serum retinol-binding protein (mg/dL); Preop, within 24 hours before surgery; POD, postoperative day.

account for early nitrogen losses resulting from the catabolism induced by injury or starvation[91] (Fig. 4-5). As compared with albumin (half-life, 20 days), both prealbumin (half-life, 2 days) and retinol-binding protein (half-life, 10 hours) have shorter serum half-lives and constitute smaller protein pools. Visceral proteins with shorter half-lives correlate better than albumin with other variables of malnutrition in response to surgical trauma. Prealbumin concentrations appear to be more signifi-cantly depressed than serum albumin during visceral protein catabolism (Figs. 4-6 through 4-8).

Total Urinary Nitrogen

Protein and fat catabolism during acute metabolic stress re-sults in increased urinary nitrogen losses. Protein catabolism

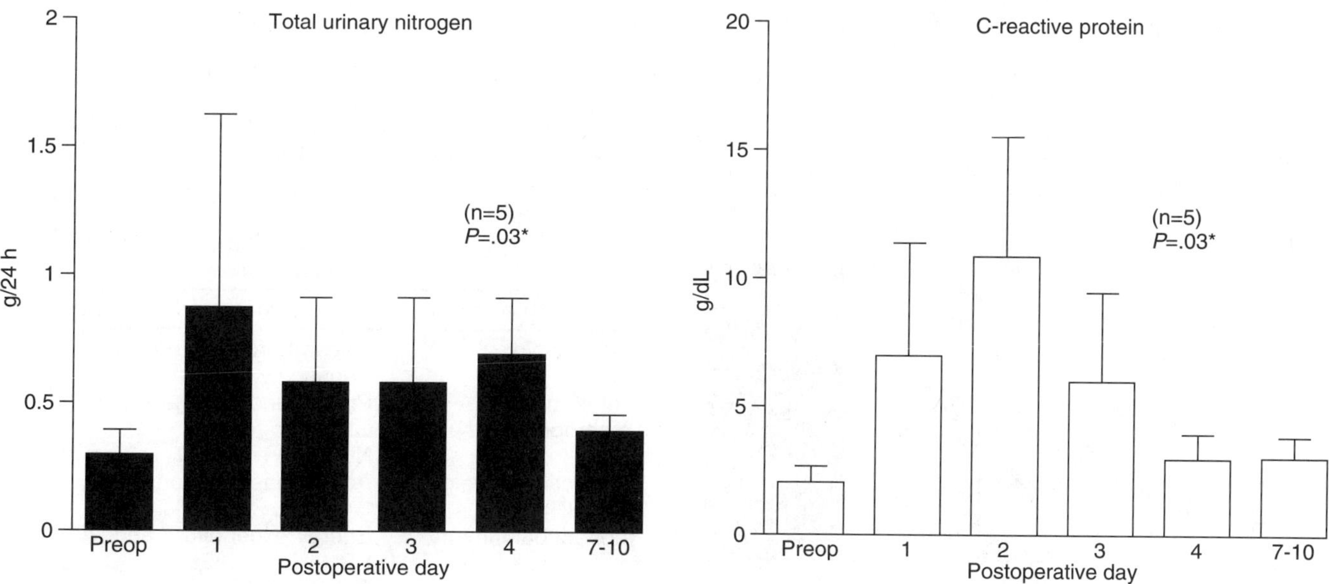

FIG. 4-5. Infant metabolic response to surgical stress. Preoperative values obtained within 24 hours before surgery.

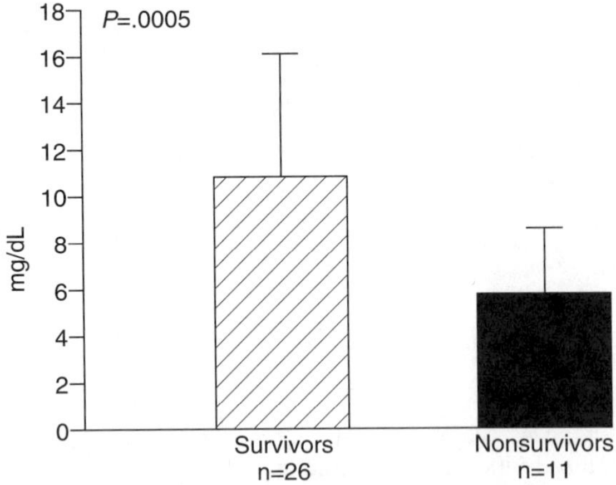

FIG. 4-6. Preoperative serum prealbumin concentrations obtained within 24 hours before surgery. n, Number of patient data points obtained during this time interval.

increases the size of the hepatic free amino acid pool. The liver deaminates a substantial portion of these amino acids to synthesize glucose (gluconeogenesis), resulting in increased nitrogen, which is then excreted in the urine as urea[103] or ammonia. Fat catabolism (lipolysis) yields increased free fatty acids, which when oxidized, cause ketone body formation. These ketoacids are buffered by ammonia and excreted in the urine.[104] Because urea nitrogen losses correlate poorly with ammonia nitrogen losses in the urine during injury states, it is preferable, in assessing catabolism, to measure 24-hour total urinary nitrogen (TUN).[105] Serial urinary nitrogen measurements reflect the degree and duration of catabolism resulting from various categories of injury and correlate grossly with hypermetabolism (increased stress-related energy expenditure).[97] This technique can be used to monitor the acute metabolic stress response and may also be valuable in determining injury severity.[106] There is often a small (0.2 to 0.5 g N_2), but significant, increase in TUN during

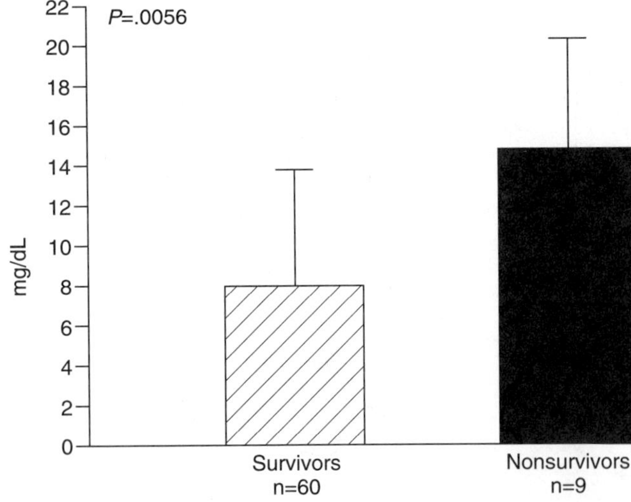

FIG. 4-7. Peak postoperative serum C-reactive protein concentrations obtained within 48 hours after surgery. n, Number of patient data points obtained during this time interval.

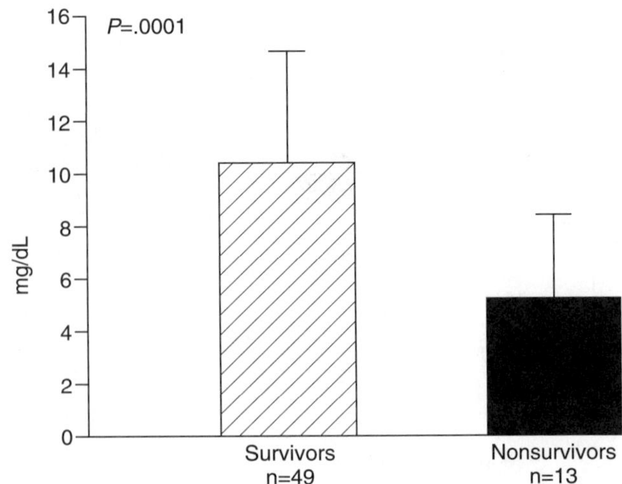

FIG. 4-8. Late postoperative serum prealbumin concentrations obtained on postoperative days 4 through 7 (average values). These prealbumin concentrations in surviving infants represent a substantial increase from postoperative day 1 levels. This was not observed in the nonsurvivors, thus indicating ongoing acute metabolic stress in the nonsurvivor group. n, Number of patient data points obtained during this time interval.

the first 2 to 4 days after major surgery in infants. These values return to normal levels by postoperative days 7 through 10 (see Fig. 4-5) and may also reflect nutritional repletion as the acute stress response resolves.[107]

Precise 24-hour urinary output measurements are required. Bladder catheterization is often unnecessary because carefully applied urine collection bags can be adequate. Diapers must be weighed so that leakage volume can be accurately tabulated if it occurs. If 24-hour nitrogen intake (N_1) is calculated (24-hour protein intake (g) divided by 6.25), then daily nitrogen balance (NB) can be calculated for infants as follows:

$$NB = N_I - [TUN + 75 \text{ mg/kg } N_2]$$

This equation assumes about 50 to 60 mg/kg N_2 daily fecal losses[108] and 15 mg/kg daily cutaneous N_2 losses (Table 4-8).

TABLE 4-8. *Guidelines for infant metabolic monitoring during acute stress*

Parameter	Stress characteristics evaluated*
Prealbumin	Visceral protein catabolism Hepatic synthesis
Total urinary nitrogen (TUN)	Protein and fat catabolism Gluconeogensis $NB = N_1 - [TUN + 75 \text{ mg/kg } N_2]$
C-reactive protein (CRP)	Acute phase response
Indirect calorimetry	Energy expenditure and RQ $EB = E_1 - MEE$ $RQ = V_{CO_2}/V_{O_2}$

* NB, nitrogen balance; N_1, 24-hour nitrogen intake; EB, energy balance; E_1, energy intake; MEE, measured energy intake; RQ, respiratory quotient

Appropriate modifications can be easily made with minimal or absent fecal excretion. Negative nitrogen balance is generally observed during acute metabolic stress, whereas positive nitrogen balance is associated with growth (anabolism).

Acute-Phase Response

A key feature of the acute metabolic stress response is an increase in the hepatic synthesis of certain specialized proteins. These acute-phase proteins appear in response to a variety of stimuli, such as tissue injury, inflammation, bacterial infection, antigen–antibody interactions, and endotoxin challenge.[109] As the synthesis of acute-phase proteins in increased, the synthesis of visceral proteins is retarded. These proteins carry out a number of important immunologic and repair functions during the acute stress period[109] (see Chap. 5). C-reactive protein (CRP) is an acute-phase protein that, among its several known biologic functions, is capable of activating the complement pathway in the absence of immunoglobulin. In the presence of activated complement, it can also induce monocyte phagocytosis of bacteria, enhancing natural killer (NK) cell activity. After injury, there is a latent period of 6 to 16 hours followed by increased serum levels that generally peak at 26 to 48 hours. Since serum half life is 4 to 6 hours, decreases in the hepatic synthesis of CRP (as the acute metabolic stress response resolves) are promptly reflected in decreased serum levels of this acute phase protein. In children, CRP increases after a variety of metabolic stress stimuli.[110,111] In infants, this same effect has been noted in response to bacterial causes,[112,113] although the response may be decreased in neonates owing to hepatic functional immaturity.[114] The perioperative acute-phase response in healthy infants is characterized by significant increases in serum CRP concentrations on postoperative day 1 (relative to preoperative values), which return toward normal values by postoperative day 4. These changes in serum acute-phase protein levels appear to coincide with urinary nitrogen excretion, demonstrating two important aspects of altered protein metabolism during acute metabolic stress (see Fig. 4-5).

Indirect Calorimetry

Energy expenditure is a measurable feature of metabolism based on the amount of heat released. This is the principle of direct calorimetry,[115] in which energy release is quantified by the amount of heat required to raise the temperature of 1 mL of water by 1°C from 15 to 16°C (1 calorie). Because this methodology involves confining the subject in a closed calorimeter for extended time periods, it is impractical for clinical use. In contrast, indirect calorimetry can be carried out at the patient's bedside. It involves the measurement of the differences in O_2 and CO_2 concentrations between a known volume (minute ventilation) of inspired and expired gas. In this way, oxygen consumption ($\dot{V}O_2$) and carbon dioxide production ($\dot{V}CO_2$) can be calculated. These calculations[116] are based on known and constant relations between $\dot{V}O_2$, $\dot{V}CO_2$, and heat produced (energy expenditure) for many metabolic processes. Such processes include, among others, the oxidation of various carbohydrates, fats, and proteins, and also lipogenesis.[117] The respiratory quo-

TABLE 4-9. *Guidelines for infant nutritional support during acute stress*

POST-INJURY NUTRITION (ENTERAL OR PARENTERAL)
Protein 2.5 g/kg/d
Fat 1–3 g/kg/d
Carbohydrate 10–20 g/kg/d
INCREASE NUTRITION INTAKE (ENTERAL ROUTE PREFERRED)
Respiratory quotient (<1.05 or decreased × 48 h)

tient (RQ), which may be expressed as $\dot{V}CO_2/\dot{V}O_2$ (Table 4-9), is also specific and constant for each of these processes; for instance, for the total oxidation of carbohydrate (RQ = 1) or fat (RQ = 0.7). For lipogenesis (the synthesis of fat from carbohydrate), RQ equals 2.75.[118]

The value of indirect calorimetry in the intensive care setting lies in the fact that estimations of energy expenditure based on other clinical criteria are notoriously inaccurate.[119] Actual measured energy expenditure (MEE) is frequently much less than predicted values based on clinical grounds.[120,121] Although average MEE values in large patient series tend to differentiate various degrees of injury,[97] individual subjects can respond to similar injury states with widely diverse MEE values.[122] An improved understanding of the metabolic stress response in infants may eventually provide other indices that adequately predict energy expenditure, but for now, the only available accurate clinical means of determining daily energy expenditure in the critical care setting is to measure it.

Energy expenditure measurements correlate well with weight gain after nutritional repletion of malnourished children.[123] In the critical care setting, indirect calorimetry may be useful in accurately determining caloric needs during acute metabolic stress to avoid overfeeding and promote optimal growth recovery (see Nutritional Repletion During Metabolic Stress and Growth Recovery).

Metabolic cart technology, employing pneumotachometers that precisely measure small tidal volumes, is available and has been validated in infant populations.[123–125] These carts are easily used in the intensive care setting and can measure energy expenditure in mechanically ventilated, as well as nonventilated, infants. Accurate MEE can be obtained in mechanically ventilated infants with noncuffed endotracheal tubes if no audible air leak is present.[126] Adequate MEE usually requires 20 to 30 minutes and correlates well with 24-hour MEE values in both acutely stressed adult and infant populations.[127,128]

Assessment of Injury Severity

Recent studies have suggested that metabolic response parameters may be useful in predicting mortality in the pediatric intensive care setting.[86,87] Metabolic monitoring has been used to stratify injury response based energy expenditure[39,88] and urinary nitrogen excretion.[39] A metabolic stress scoring system has been devised using modified nitrogen balance calculations.[58] Both CRP[71,87,89] and prealbumin[87,90] have reported value in injury stratification and outcome. Serum TNF concentrations have been found to correlate with mortality in critically ill adult and pediatric patients following infection.[91–93]

Serial monitoring of the metabolic response of the infant surgical population to acute injury (Figure 4-3) should include treatment of daily energy expenditure (MEE), serum protein indices (CRP and prealbumin), and total urinary nitrogen (TUN) throughout the perioperative period (preoperatively and on post-operative days [POD] 1-5, 7, and 10) (Table 4-8). In addition, when infants are evaluated perioperatively with respect to post-operative mortality (within 30 days of surgery), significant differences in serum prealbumin and peak CRP levels between survivors and non-survivors exist. (87). These findings support the potential predictive value of such metabolic indices for serial perioperative evaluation in acute stressed surgical infants (Figures 4-6 and 4-7). The strongest potential predictor appears to be day five prealbumin levels (Figure 4-8). Failure of the liver to resume visceral protein synthesis by this time (indicating continued acute metabolic stress) is associated with the most significant increase in infant mortality seen in out critical care population.

In additon to establishing injury severity, the early detection of postoperative complicating resulting in inflammation can be facilitated by serial monitoring of the acute metabolic stress response. Studies of surgical infants have demonstrated significant increases of both serum CRP and IL-6(95) concentrations in the detection of perioperative sepsis.

METABOLIC CONSEQUENCES OF OVERFEEDING

Overfeeding involves the delivery of calories or substrate in excess of the amounts required to meet metabolic needs. These requirements may vary substantially with altered metabolic states as determined by subject age, state of health, and nutritional status. During acute metabolic stress states, the nature of the injury insult can cause a varied metabolic response, as is the case with sepsis in contrast to traumatic injury.[129] In addition, there may be considerable intersubject response variability to the same type of injury.

From a clinical standpoint, the harmful effects of overfeeding may result in respiratory compromise, hepatic dysfunction, and an increased risk of dying. Subjects at particular risk are those with severe injury and those at the extremes of age (ie, infants, especially preterm infants, and the elderly).

Effects on Respiration

Carbohydrate overfeeding, either with or without excessive caloric delivery, can have a significant negative impact on respiration. Lipogenesis is an energy-requiring process characterized by an increase in $\dot{V}CO_2$ relative to $\dot{V}O_2$. The RQ for pure lipogenesis is 2.75.[118] Lipogenesis represents the only metabolic process with an RQ consequence of greater than 1. Because other metabolic processes with RQs of 1 or less also occur simultaneously in vivo (ie, lipid oxidation, RQ = 0.7; carbohydrate oxidation, RQ = 1; and protein oxidation, RQ = 0.8), and the measured RQ represents the net effect of all of these processes, RQ values in excess of 1 represent high lipogenic activity and are usually associated with overfeeding. In infants, increased CO_2 production, resulting from excess carbohydrate administration, can cause an increase in respiratory rate, necessary to re-

move excess CO_2.[130] Excess protein delivery has been shown to exacerbate this effect in adults by increasing respiratory sensitivity to CO_2.[131] Substituting lipid for some of the carbohydrate administered, usually 25% to 35%, is effective (in both infant and adult studies) in reducing CO_2 production and lipogenesis, thus resulting in decreased RQ.[130,132–135]

In acute injury states, particularly with severe metabolic stress, hypermetabolism (increased MEE) resulting from increased $\dot{V}O_2$ accompanies the increases in $\dot{V}CO_2$ due to over-feeding. Overfeeding in these stressed patients can result in increased respiratory requirements caused by increased CO_2 production,[136–138] even though these changes may not be accurately reflected in total RQ.[139] Maximum glucose oxidation rates exist for metabolically stressed, as well as nonstressed, subjects. Glucose administered in excess of maximum oxidation rates undergoes fat biosynthesis (lipogenesis), resulting in substantial increases in CO_2 production.[137] The importance of avoiding excessive nutritional delivery is confirmed by studies that demonstrate that overfeeding can result in ventilatory dependency in patients with decreased pulmonary reserve.[131,140,141] This ventilatory dependency is due to the inability of patients with limited pulmonary function to eliminate adequately increased CO_2 produced when excessive total caloric and, particularly, carbohydrate intake is metabolized. Preterm infants are especially vulnerable to the respiratory effects of overfeeding, owing to their immature pulmonary development and limited respiratory reserve.

Effect on Hepatic Morphology and Function

A number of metabolic alterations are the result of total caloric overfeeding and carbohydrate overfeeding. In healthy subjects and clinically stable patients, excessive glucose intake induces increased insulin levels, resulting in decreased fatty acid oxidation, reduced ketogenesis, increased glucose oxidation, and increased lipogenesis. In addition, the insulin/glucagon ratio increases in the portal vein, associated with increased hepatic deposition of fat (steatosis) and increased serum levels of hepatic enzymes, indicating hepatic cellular injury.[142] In one study of stable adult patients overfed (average, 177% of predicted energy expenditure) with glucose-based TPN, liver biopsy results showed fatty infiltration and incipient intrahepatic cholestasis within 5 days of the initiation of intravenous nutrition.[143] After 21 days, biopsy results showed bile duct proliferation, canalicular bile plugs, centrilobular cholestasis with the bile pigment in hepatocytes, and periportal inflammation. Liver function tests were elevated in 83% of the subjects by a mean of 14 days, and the number of abnormal liver function tests increased in proportion to the increased amount of carbohydrate calories infused. These changes are typical of a number of similar studies involving overfed subjects.[137,142,144,145] Similar alterations have been documented in several studies involving clinically stable infants receiving glucose-based TPN; however, the onset of these changes is more rapid, particularly in preterm neonates. This phenomenon may be due to hepatic functional immaturity.[146]

Acute metabolic stress increases lipolysis and free fatty acid oxidation relative to glucose oxidation, owing to counterregulatory hormone-induced insulin resistance. These endocrine effects reduce the efficiency with which exogenous carbohydrate is metabolized. With excessive carbohydrate delivery, serum insulin, glucose, glucose oxidation, and fatty acid oxidation increase, and lipogenesis remains high.[129] These metabolic events further predispose the liver to hepatic cellular injury resulting in hepatic dysfunction. Furthermore, glucose oxidation is dependent on pyruvate dehydrogenase for entry of pyruvate into the tricarboxylic acid cycle. During acute injury due to sepsis, increased serum concentrations of lactate and alanine suggest that pyruvate dehydrogenase activity may be inhibited as part of the metabolic stress response.[147] Excess glucose administration increases the hepatic work demand to metabolize increased amounts of these substrate intermediates.[129]

Lipid overfeeding with long-chain triglyceride (LCT) formulations can inhibit the ability of the reticuloendothelial system of the liver to clear bacteria during acute injury states.[148] Decreased hepatic clearance is associated with increased bacterial sequestration in the lung, resulting in increased pulmonary neutrophil activation and the release of inflammatory mediators. LCT contains high concentrations of linoleic acid, an arachidonic acid precursor, which increases substrate availability for prostaglandin synthesis. Replacing LCT with MCT, which is absorbed directly into the blood from the gut and does not pass through the liver, restores liver reticuloendothelial system function and reduces lung bacterial sequestration.

Stress metabolism cannot be reversed by overfeeding during critical illness, further increasing the negative impact of stress by increasing the hypermetabolic demands associated with it and by augmenting the hepatic work load.[138] Finally, hepatic compromise due to overfeeding during nonstress periods may decrease hepatic metabolic function in response to subsequent acute injury, especially sepsis. Cecal ligation and puncture in rats previously overfed enterally for 6 days resulted in marked decreases in hepatic (and whole-body) protein synthesis relative to the normal intake group.[149] Hepatomegaly was 67% greater in the overfed group, but liver protein per gram of tissue was significantly less relative to normally fed animals. It is particularly noteworthy that hepatic dysfunction and pathomorphology due to carbohydrate-based TPN nutritional delivery not only are observed earlier in infants than adults, but also, among this infant population, evolve most rapidly in patients who are severely stressed, especially those who are septic.[144]

Effect on Survival

It is logical to assume that the damaging aspects of overfeeding during acute metabolic stress would have a negative impact on survival, but proof of this hypothesis remains elusive in many human studies, owing to the different nature of various injury stimuli and the diverse responses they induce in individual patients. Also, the limitations in the design of experimental human protocols preclude the more definitive methods of evaluation available in more rigidly controlled animal studies.

As previously discussed, the increased metabolic demands imposed by overfeeding result in increased glucose production, glucose and lipid oxidation, CO_2 production associated with lipogenesis, insulin/glucagon ratio, and lactate and alanine cycling. Although whole-body protein synthesis rates increase in some stressed populations, protein breakdown is not substantially decreased in response to overfeeding.[150] These alterations result in increased respiratory work demand to remove excess CO_2 and increased hepatic work demand to metabolize the excess substrates created. Excessive substrate caloric administration augments energy requirements to process the increased substrate load, resulting in further hypermetabolism due to diet-induced thermogenesis. Overfeeding has been documented to increase hypermetabolism (MEE) by 34% in acutely stressed adult subjects after the initiation of excess protein-caloric delivery.[138]

The effects of caloric overfeeding with high carbohydrate delivery were evaluated in postoperative adults retrospectively grouped based on RQ higher than 0.95 (high-caloric) versus RQ of less than 0.95 (low-caloric) values.[151] The high-caloric group received 150% MEE, and the low-caloric group received 100% MEE. Glucose calories were 77% of the total caloric intake in the high-caloric group (yielding an average RQ of 1.12), as compared with glucose calories of 60.6% (yielding an RQ of 0.73) in the low-caloric group. Mortality was significantly greater in the overfed group than in the group delivered calories equal to MEE (40% versus 28%; $P < .05$).

In a prospective study of septic guinea pigs grouped by caloric intake (100, 125, 150, or 175 kcal/kg/d), there was a significant increase in mortality and decrease in survival time in the animals fed 150 and 175 kcal/kg/d (the mortality rate was 100% in both groups).[152] On the other hand, 175 kcal/kg/d was optimal for guinea pigs subjected to thermal injury.[153] This underscores the differing nutritional requirements based on the nature of the injury insult and the metabolic stress response that it induces. As discussed previously, data on septic stress suggest that pyruvate dehydrogenase activity is inhibited as part of the metabolic stress response.[147] In contrast, data generated in burned children show that pyruvate dehydrogenase activity is not decreased but rather is amplified during this type of acute injury.[100] In sepsis, glucose infusion results in increased levels of lactate and alanine; whereas in thermal stress, increased glucose oxidation occurs, and less lactate and alanine are generated. This may help to explain why the increased nutritional delivery appropriate for burn injury might constitute overfeeding during sepsis in the same animal model.

Another consideration involves the impact of prestress overfeeding on the subsequent metabolic stress response. When acute bacterial peritonitis was induced in rats after 6 days of enteral overfeeding (175% of normal intake), the mortality rate increased to 53%, in contrast to the 14% mortality rate observed in normal-intake animals. These changes were associated with decreased hepatic and whole-body protein synthesis, which may reflect a reduced metabolic capability to meet the demands of acute injury in the overfed group.

NUTRITIONAL REPLETION DURING METABOLIC STRESS AND GROWTH RECOVERY

The acute metabolic stress response represents a predominantly catabolic state. Endogenous tissue stores of protein, carbohydrate, and fat are invariably decreased during this period, and growth is impeded (Fig. 4-9). Cytokine-induced decreases in IGF-1[154] likely play an important role in stress-related growth retardation. About 30% to 35% of predicted energy requirements for healthy infants are needed for growth[70] (see Fig. 4-2). In addition, because of the reductions in activity and the insensible losses typically observed in sedated infants in a ther-

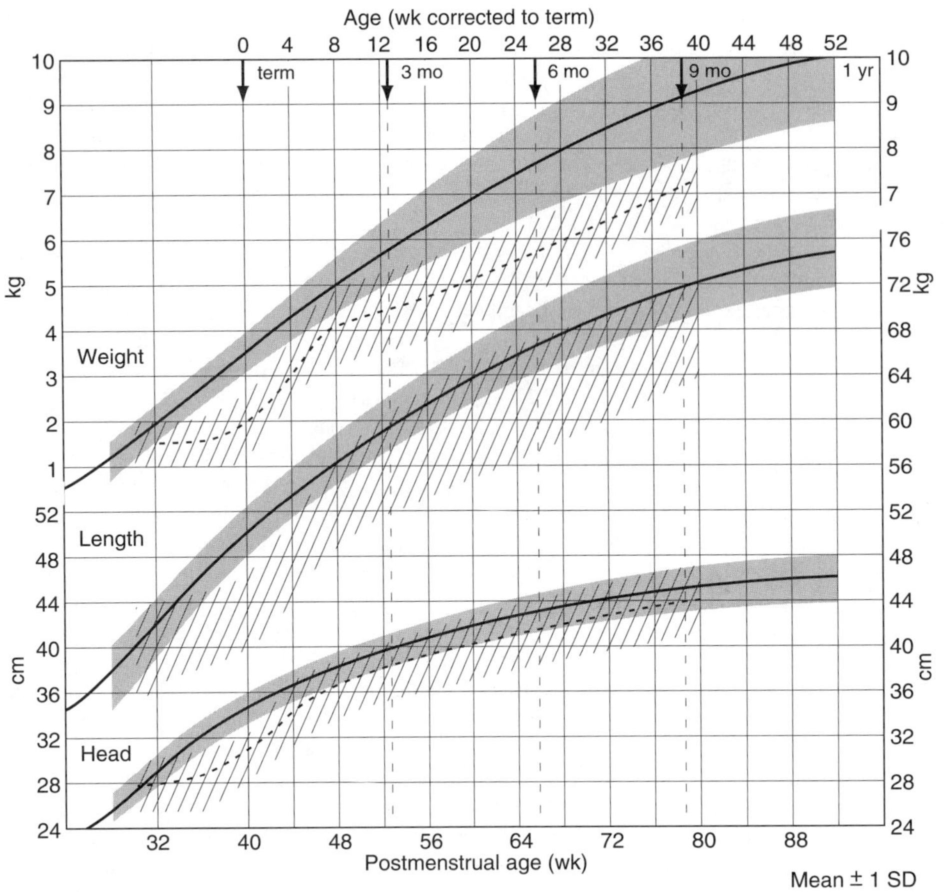

FIG. 4-9. Longitudinal growth (*diagonal shading*) of sick preterm infants (28 to 32 weeks' gestation), superimposed on the Babson curve for postnatal growth in healthy infants. Note the growth cessation during acute illness. (Maisels MJ, Marks KH. J Pediatr 1981;88:663)

moneutral intensive care environment, caloric requirements during acute metabolic stress are reduced to amounts necessary to meet basal metabolic needs alone. Therefore, if caloric repletion based on the predicted requirements for healthy infants is administered during the acute phase of metabolic stress in critically ill infants, when the energy required for growth is negligible, substantial overfeeding is likely.[124]

Infant energy expenditure after uncomplicated surgical procedures does not increase substantially over measured baseline values[155,156] unless preoperative stress is severe.[157] This finding has been demonstrated in an acutely stressed population of surgical infants.[157] In addition, substantial interpatient variability was found to exist independent of preoperative clinical status, further suggesting that the serial measurements of acute changes in metabolic parameters, such as energy expenditure, are more accurate than diagnostic category in assessing injury response.

As discussed previously, because RQ equals $\dot{V}_{CO_2}/\dot{V}_{O_2}$, and because overfeeding causes increased lipogenesis (and thus increased $\dot{V}_{CO_2}$ relative to $\dot{V}_{O_2}$[118]), excessive caloric intake (especially excessive carbohydrate intake[130,132–134]) generally results in RQ greater than 1.

Infants frequently have RQ values above 1 after nutritional support has been initiated in the immediate postoperative period. This finding suggests overfeeding due to lipogenesis during acute metabolic stress. At constant substrate and caloric delivery rates, the RQ usually falls below 1 in conjunction with resolution of the injury response (as confirmed by serum and urine metabolic stress parameters), usually within 5 days of surgery. This effect likely occurs, at least in part, because of increased energy needs resulting from the resumption of anabolic metabolism (growth).[157]

Somatic growth is characterized by a positive energy balance (EB), which, for healthy infants, is usually greater than 45 to 50 kcal/kg/d.[108] In addition, positive EB is associated with recovery of hepatic visceral protein synthesis after surgery in infants.[158] A gross calculation of EB can be made as follows:

$$EB = E_1 - MEE$$

where E_1 represents energy intake.

To reduce the likelihood of overfeeding-induced lipogenesis, we recommend limiting caloric intake to about 65 kcal/kg/d (about half of predicted requirements for healthy neonates) in infants immediately after surgery. The authors compared EB with RQ and CRP values obtained simultaneously and found that the EB was near zero when associated with high CRP values and an RQ greater than 1 on postoperative day 1 (Fig. 4-10*A*). This RQ value suggests some overfeeding even at reduced energy intake rates. By postoperative day 4, the CRP values decreased to near normal, and RQ decreased to 1, indicating resolution of acute metabolic stress. EB values increased despite constant energy and substrate intake (see Fig. 4-10*B*). These findings demonstrate that some calories were now being used for the resumption of anabolic metabolism. At this point, caloric administration was progressively increased. By postoperative day 9, positive EB values had risen to levels consistent with

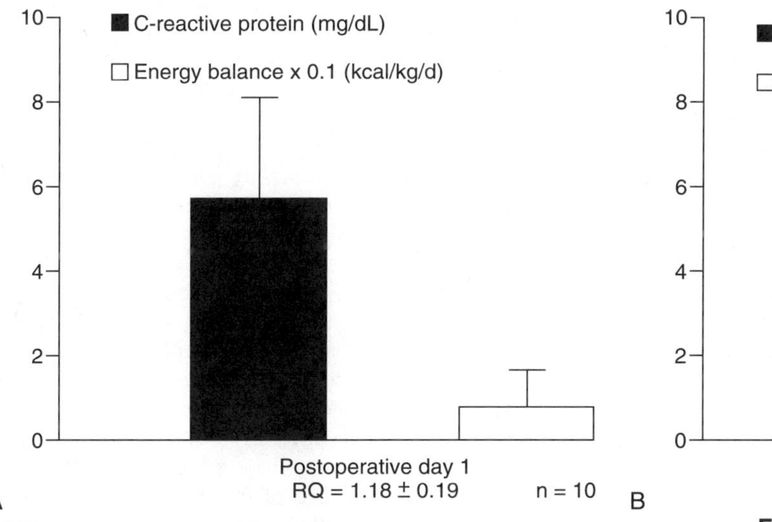

Resumption of anabolic metabolism

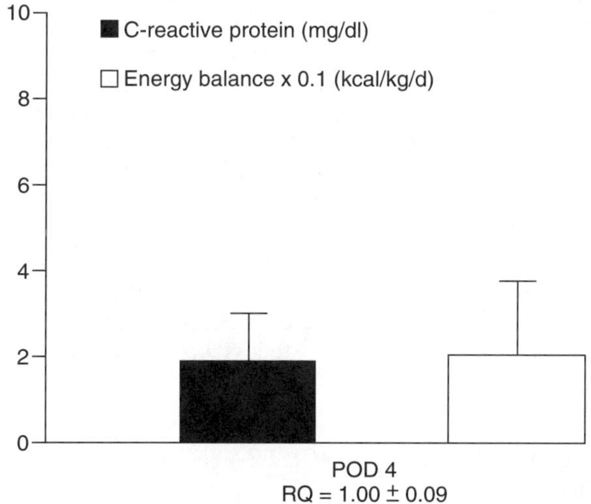

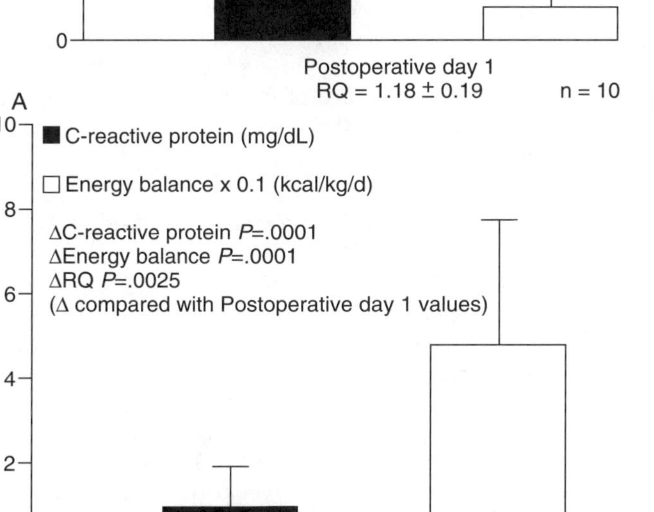

FIG. 4-10. (*A*) Initial postoperative catabolism. Despite predictably low energy balance associated with basal energy delivery, the respiratory quotient (RQ) is more than 1.0 during acute metabolic stress. C-reactive protein concentrations are high, suggesting substantial lipogenesis at a caloric intake that is moderately in excess of energy expenditure on postoperative day 1. (*B*) Resumption of anabolic metabolism. A two-fold increase in energy balance at constant basal energy intake is associated with decreasing RQ and return of C-reactive protein concentrations toward normal. This suggests increasing use of caloric intake for anabolic metabolism as acute stress response resolves. (*C*) Normal growth recovery after acute injury. After an increase in energy delivery to normal, nonstress caloric intake and energy balance reach values appropriate for adequate growth. This is associated with an RQ of less than 1.0 and low C-reactive protein concentrations. Changes (*Δ*) in C-reactive protein concentrations, energy balance, and RQ values on postoperative day 9 are statistically significant relative to postoperative day 1 values.

normal growth, and these were associated with a RQ of less than 1 and normal, nonstressed CRP levels[159] (see Fig. 4-10*C*). A follow-up study to assess substrate use at a reduced caloric delivery rate of 65 kcal/kg/d in acutely stressed surgical neonates demonstrated that significant lipogenesis occurs during the early postoperative period in this patient population.[160] This study further shows a significant correlation between carbohydrate intake and $\dot{V}CO_2$. These data suggest that caloric requirements during acute metabolic stress are likely equal to actual MEE values, and that caloric administration in excess of MEE values results in overfeeding.

To avoid overfeeding infants during the acute metabolic stress period, the authors provide adequate protein supplements while limiting calorie repletion to MEE values. Nutritional delivery during this period consists of protein (2.5 g/kg/d), fat (1 to 3 g/kg/d), and carbohydrate (10 g/kg/d), administered at rates necessary to meet maintenance daily fluid requirements (see Table 4-9). This provides from 50 to 75 kcal/kg/d, depending

on the MEE-established requirement. Initially, peripheral vein parenteral delivery may constitute most of the caloric intake budget; however, in nearly all cases, 2 mL/h enterally (using a soft, transpyloric feeding tube) can be provided. This small amount of enteral nutrient delivery has been shown to protect gut hormone homeostasis in TPN-fed infants.[161] It is likely, therefore, that minimal enteral feeding can decrease TPN-associated gut atrophy, and it may also be useful in decreasing TPN-induced liver complications.[162] Initial postoperative enteral nutrient delivery is provided at continuous rate (not a bolus) from elemental formulations containing short-chain polypeptides as the major portion of protein substrate. As the acute phase of metabolic stress resolves, the adaptive (anabolic) phase ensues and results in resumption of somatic growth. Recovery is characterized by decreasing levels of CRP and TUN, increasing serum levels of prealbumin, and stress resolution trends based on indirect calorimetric measurements. Recovery can be established by the serial postinjury monitoring of these parameters.[157,160] When serial measurements of these metabolic parameters demonstrate resolution of the acute stress phase, nutritional supplements are increased, preferably using the enteral route. To avoid premature increments in caloric delivery, daily indirect calorimetric measurements are carried out to assess the RQ. When RQ decreases on two consecutive postoperative days, or when RQ is less than 1.05, the authors advance caloric intake above MEE values (see Table 4-9). This method provides a potentially useful guide to advance caloric delivery and optimize growth recovery without overfeeding infants during the acute phase of the metabolic response to injury. If calorimetric measurement capabilities are not possible, predicted *basal* metabolic rates should be used to estimate caloric delivery until serum CRP concentrations are less than or equal to 2 mg/dL.[160]

GUT INTEGRITY AND ACUTE METABOLIC STRESS

The gut plays a supportive role in acute injury states. The metabolic, immunologic, and infectious pathophysiologic states of this important organ system are key factors in determining the metabolic stress response.

Because the intestines contain bacteria and endotoxin, maintenance of gut barrier function is essential. The gut barrier includes the intestinal mucosa and submucosa, the lymphatic system of the mesentery, the reticuloendothelial system, and other immunocompetent cells within the splanchnic bed. A substantial number of investigations have shown that physical or functional disruption of this barrier can result in the translocation of gut-derived bacteria and endotoxin. Translocation can lead to systemic bacteremia or endotoxemia, culminating in increased morbidity and mortality.[163] Three basic mechanisms for translocation are (1) intestinal bacterial overgrowth, especially with gram-negative organisms, (2) impairment of host immune defenses, and (3) physical disruption of the gut mucosal barrier.[164,165] Groups at high risk for translocation include immunocompromised and malnourished patients, burn and trauma victims, critically ill patients with multisystem organ failure,[163,166] and newborn infants.[167,168] Studies suggest that clinical outcome depends on the balance between injury severity and the adequacy of host defense mechanisms. For instance, translocation is more extensive as injury severity increases.[169] Excessive translocation can lead to impaired systemic immunity[170] and overwhelm reticuloendothelial system clearance capacity, resulting in injury to postsplanchnic organ systems.[171] In contrast, low levels of translocation may cause salutary immune system activation, resulting in protection against infectious challenge.[172] Neonatal gut mucosal barrier function may be altered owing to immaturity, especially in preterm infants. Newborn piglet gut allows increased transmucosal bacterial passage compared with the gut of older, weaning piglets.[167,168]

REINFORCING MUCOSAL BARRIER INTEGRITY

Enteral Versus Parenteral Delivery

Enteral nutritional delivery is critical in preventing bacterial translocation.[173] Parenteral nutrition (without glutamine supple-mentation) is associated with mucosal atrophy. In contrast, enteral formulations stimulate trophic gut hormone secretion and nourish the mucosa. Enterally fed, stressed humans have fewer postoperative septic-related complications when compared with those fed parenterally.[95,174] In guinea pigs, early versus late enteral feeding has been shown to reduce the hypermetabolic response to burn injury and promote gut mucosal growth.[175] This effect on energy expenditure is possibly due to decreased translocation resulting in a decreased metabolic stress response. In rats, immediate postoperative enteral feeding is associated with improved wound strength and less weight loss when compared with late feeding.[176] In addition, enteral feeding, even in small amounts, appears to protect the liver against TPN-related complications.[162] A prospective study of severely injured adult trauma patients has demonstrated increased constitutive and decreased acute-phase protein levels after enteral versus parenteral nutrient delivery, suggesting early resolution of the acute metabolic stress response if the gut is supported.[177] In all of these studies, better maintenance of intestinal barrier function with early, enteral nutrition is the most probable reason for improved outcome.

Short-Chain Polypeptides Versus Free Amino Acids

Considerable debate has focused on whether short-chain polypeptide (two- to five-carbon length) diets are absorbed better than formulations consisting primarily of free amino acids by intestinal mucosa. In unstressed animals, polypeptide versus amino acid diets are associated with decreased translocation, improved bowel growth, improved trophic gut hormone secretion, and improved somatic growth and IGF-1 production. Polypeptide diets also improve early somatic growth recovery and survival,[178–180] compared with amino acid diets in metabolically stressed animals. Finally, these diets have been shown to be superior to amino acid diets in decreasing diarrhea, improving visceral protein synthesis, and decreasing hospital stay in trauma patients.[181]

Glutamine

Glutamine is the most abundant amino acid in plasma and skeletal muscle, but serum levels fall precipitously after acute metabolic stress, primarily owing to increased uptake and metabolism by the gut.[182] Glutamine is a major energy source for intestinal mucosa and may stimulate increased protein synthesis in enterocytes during acute injury states such as sepsis.[183] It is also deaminated by the gut to form alanine, which then flows through the splanchnic circulation to the liver. During acute stress, this gut-to-liver pathway provides a major contribution to the hepatic amino acid pool.[184] Provision of standard parenteral nutrition is associated with atrophy of the intestinal mucosa.[185] In contrast, glutamine-enriched parenteral nutrition has been shown to increase gut mucosal weight and DNA content, stimulate villous growth, and improve gut glutamine use.[186] Moreover, glutamine-supplemented TPN decreases bacterial translocation, compared with standard TPN.[187] Parenteral glutamine supplementation may have an additional beneficial role in protecting the liver against TPN-induced hepatic steatosis.[186,188] The safety of parenteral glutamine administration has been demonstrated in humans.[189]

During acute metabolic stress, gut glutamine uptake is enhanced. Improved survival has been achieved with glutamine-enriched TPN in septic rats.[183,190] This effect may be due to enhancement of the immunologic, rather than the physical, gut barrier function. In addition to its role as a primary fuel source for enterocytes and colonocytes, glutamine is an important fuel source for lymphocytes and macrophages. Although it is considered nonessential in health, glutamine appears to become essential during acute metabolic states, when uptake by the intestinal mucosa and by immunologically active cells exceeds its synthesis and release from skeletal muscle. Glutamine has been shown to decrease the incidence of infection and improve nitrogen balance in neutropenic adults after bone marrow transplantation.[189]

Glutamine has been used safely in infants[191] and appears to be a valuable parenteral adjunct to gut nutrition when enteral delivery is contraindicated.

Peptide Growth Factors

Peptide growth factors are naturally occurring proteins that induce cell proliferation. The removal of these growth factors from cell culture causes cessation of proliferation, even in the presence of adequate nutrient substrate. Investigations designed to establish the role of peptide growth factors in gastrointestinal growth and function have focused primarily on epidermal growth factor (EGF), transforming growth factor α (TGF-α), and IGF-1.

Both EGF and TGF-α are synthesized by gut mucosa and are known to stimulate proliferation of intestinal mucosa.[192] The administration of EGF in malnourished rat models has resulted in increased mucosal weight, villus height, and crypt cell production.[193] These effects are enhanced by the addition of glutamine,[193] perhaps owing to increased (EGF-induced) glutamine transport by intestinal mucosa.[194] Mucosal EGF levels increase after gastrointestinal ulceration. The administration of EGF[195] and the induction of increased endogenous EGF production (using GH—releasing factor)[196] have both been associated with improved ulcer healing.

The role of peptide growth factors present in mammalian milk may be especially important in infant gut maturation. In newborn rat models, EGF has a pronounced trophic effect on intestinal mucosa[197] and has also been found to promote hepatic growth.[198] The importance of IGF-1 in neonatal gastrointestinal growth and development has also been intimated using a porcine model.[199] Intestinal growth, macromolecular transport, and functional maturation in this model were all quantitatively related to variations in IGF-1 protein content and receptor numbers. Furthermore, it is possible that enteral nutrition provided when the fetus swallows amniotic fluid containing a variety of growth factors, including EGF and IGF-1, supports gut maturation and growth during gestation.

MODIFICATIONS OF NUTRITIONAL SUPPORT DURING INJURY STATES

Hormonal Supplementation

Although the timely provision of nutrient substrates can promote recovery from acute metabolic stress states, it is also clear that aggressive nutritional repletion alone may be insufficient to overcome the catabolic effects caused by more severe injury stimuli, especially in patients with low endogenous substrate reserves.[200,201] This consequence may be at least partially due to compromised hepatic (and skeletal muscle) use of available protein substrates, and investigations have focused on the adjunctive use of GH during acute metabolic stress to promote anabolic metabolism and blunt endogenous substrate catabolism.[202–204] The anabolic effects of GH, especially as they affect protein metabolism, are mediated primarily by IGF-1.[205] It has been demonstrated that, with moderate stress, GH administration can optimize use of adjuvant nutritional support and counteract protein catabolic effects of the injury response by increasing protein synthesis and by inducing IGF-1 synthesis and release. Consequently, protein breakdown decreases, and nitrogen retention improves. As a result, body cell mass is preserved and even restored, wound healing is promoted, immunologic function is enhanced, and hospital stay is shortened.[202–204,206–208]

With increased injury severity (particularly sepsis), the GH-induced IGF-1 response is blunted, and exogenous GH is relatively ineffective in promoting anabolic metabolism,[209,210] although increased serum IGF-1 levels have been demonstrated in some clinically septic patients receiving longer dosage schedules of GH175. To circumvent this type of stress-related GH resistance, the exogenous use of IGF-1 during severe metabolic stress states has been proposed.[211] It has been well documented that serum levels of IGF-1 drop rapidly after acute metabolic stress insult,[212] and that this decrease is reflective of the degree of injury. Furthermore, the stress-related fall in IGF-1 levels occurs despite a concomitant increase in serum GH concentrations, reinforcing the concept that GH resistance exists relative to IGF-1 during the acute metabolic stress period. Data on the regulation of IGF-1 metabolism during acute injury states are becoming available. In an endotoxin-induced rat metabolic stress model, decreased serum IGF-1 after acute injury is associated with an insulin-independent increase in serum levels of IGF-1–binding protein 1,[213] a mediator known to inhibit IGF-1 activity. Furthermore, evaluation of organ-specific IGF-1 levels using this model has demonstrated decreased hepatic levels, suggesting decreased hepatic synthesis of IGF-1 during acute metabolic stress states. Although its effects in the acute stress setting have yet to be adequately evaluated, IGF-1 administration has been found to promote improved postoperative nitrogen balance, bowel trophic effects, and total body weight gain in rats undergoing an 80% small bowel resection.[214] Improved nitrogen retention may be due, in part, to increased amino acid delivery to the liver. Short-term administration of IGF-1 (1.5 μg/kg/min for 180 minutes) increased hepatic amino acid uptake in a canine acute injury model.[215] In healthy adult humans, IGF-1 can attenuate nitrogen losses caused by hypocaloric feeding while conserving cellular amino acid stores.[216] In contrast to insulin, IGF-1 does not appear to suppress lipolysis in nonstress states.[217] In a prospective, randomized trial,[218] adults with acute head injuries who were administered 0.24 mg/kg/d of IGF-1 for 7 to 14 days demonstrated improved immunologic function over those who were administered placebo.

Adjunctive hormonal therapy of this nature may be of particular benefit in acutely stressed infants. Acute illness in infants is associated with growth retardation that is generally followed by a period of accelerated ``catch-up'' growth when the injury response resolves.[219,220] Catch-up growth after acute metabolic stress, however, may be inadequate to achieve normal anthropometric standards, resulting in associated mental retardation and neuromotor functional handicaps.[221,222] Shortening the interval of catabolic response to injury and promoting earlier recovery of anabolic metabolism through the use of adjunctive hormonal therapy possibly could facilitate complete growth recovery and perhaps avoid the long-term consequences of growth retardation. This represents an important area of future clinical investigation.

Branched-Chain Amino Acids

The predominant metabolic effects during acute stress result in catabolism and reduced total body protein synthesis. The demands placed on the liver are extensive during this period, and hepatic protein synthesis actually increases. Amino acids mobilized from visceral protein pools, muscle, and gut are taken up by the liver and used for synthesis of acute-phase proteins and glucose (gluconeogenesis). The eventual failure of the liver to respond to these demands, owing to the magnitude or duration of the stress insult, is associated with increased mortality. Although 40% to 100% of most amino acids are metabolized as they pass through the liver, branched-chain amino acids (BCAAs—leucine, isoleucine, and valine) are thought to undergo minimal hepatic degradation and are therefore available to support muscle. Solutions enriched with these amino acids reduce skeletal muscle proteolysis, increase protein synthesis, and decrease the release of aromatic amino acids from muscle.[223] BCAAs, particularly leucine, are also associated with increased hepatic acute-phase protein synthesis and decreased urea production. In septic rats, enriched BCAA solutions have resulted in significant muscle-sparing effects and improved nitrogen balance.[224] Clinical studies in metabolically stressed humans have shown similar effects.[224,225] Because BCAAs lower aromatic amino acid production and decrease ureagenesis, solutions enriched with BCAAs may be of benefit in treating hepatic encephalopathy.[226,227] Most studies suggest BCAA enrichment should approach 45% to 50% for optimal effect.

Modified Lipid Substrates

Medium-chain triglyceride preparations contain saturated fatty acids with 6- to 12-carbon chain lengths. They are directly absorbed into the circulatory system from the gut and do not require bile for absorption. They are rapidly cleared from the bloodstream, exhibit rapid mitochondrial uptake, and do not require carnitine for metabolism. In contrast to LCT,[228] MCT preparations do not appear to impair reticuloendothelial system clearance of bacteria.[148,229] They are incorporated in several enteral formulations and can improve fat absorption from dysfunctional bowel. Studies also have demonstrated potentially beneficial effects of short-chain fatty acids (butyrate) in promoting intestinal growth delivered both enterally[230] and parenterally.[231]

NUTRITIONAL IMMUNOMODULATION

Data have suggested that several dietary components can exert a variety of effects on the immune system. Because in-creased metabolic stress severity is associated with substantially increased immunocompromise, the potential ability to enhance immunologic function by dietary alterations offers the possibility of improving clinical outcome after injury. Research interest has focused on three major substrate subgroups: $\omega 3$ fatty acids, nucleotides, and arginine.

$\omega 3$ Polyunsaturated Fatty Acids

In addition to providing important substrate for energy, essential fatty acids, fat-soluble vitamins, and cell membranes, lipid metabolism may also modulate immune function through arachidonic acid synthetic pathways.[232] Increased intake of linoleic acid (ω_6 polyunsaturated fatty acid), an important precursor of arachidonic acid, has been shown to inhibit immune function by impeding neutrophil chemotaxis, phagocytosis, and bacteriocidal activity; reducing macrophage phagocytosis; and reducing lymphocyte proliferation. The metabolism of linoleic acid by the cyclooxygenase pathway yields monoenoic and dienoic prostaglandins (such as prostaglandin E_2) known to have widespread macrophage and lymphocyte immunosuppressant effects at the high serum concentrations (more than 10^{-8} M) associated with severe metabolic stress conditions such as sepsis and burn trauma.[233]

In contrast, diets high in $\omega 3$ polyunsaturated fatty acids (such as fish oil) result in comparatively less arachidonic acid production and yield the less potent trienoic prostaglandins. As a result, prostaglandin E_2 production is decreased, and immunosuppression is reduced. Diets rich in $\omega 3$ versus $\omega 6$ polyunsaturated fatty acids have been shown to improve immunologic function in burned animals[234] and have been associated with improved survival in acutely stressed humans[235] and animals,[236] although this effect may be model dependent.[237]

Nucleotides

In vitro investigations have suggested that the metabolism of stimulated lymphocytes is nucleotide dependent.[238] Enhanced immunologic function has been demonstrated in animal studies by showing increased allograft rejection, greater resistance to bacterial challenge,[239] and improved delayed hypersensitivity[240] associated with nucleotide-supplemented versus nucleotide-free diets. Immunosuppression resulting from the absence of dietary nucleotides appears to be due primarily to increased helper T-cell suppression and decreased interleukin-2 production. These findings appear to be uracil dependent.[240]

Arginine

The immune effects of in vitro arginine are to enhance lymphocyte activation (improve mitogenesis and increase synthesis of nucleic acids and protein).[241] Arginine administration increases T-cell immunity and is associated with increased thymic mass and cellularity. It has been suggested that arginine becomes an essential amino acid during acute metabolic stress states, owing to insufficient endogenous production to meet increased demands. Animal studies demonstrate improved survival with arginine-supplemented diets after burn injuries and peritonitis,[242,243] presumably by improving T-lymphocyte–dependent immunocompetence. This concept is supported by investigations in postoperative human subjects showing that the mitogenic response of circulating lymphocytes is increased as a result of arginine supplementation.[241,244] Arginine-enriched diets are associated with improved wound healing[245] and may inhibit the growth and development of malignant tumors, owing to enhanced immune function.[241] Arginine is a precursor for nitric oxide synthesis. Arginine-induced augmentation of macrophage and natural killer cell activity may be due, in part, to enhanced nitric oxide production. Furthermore, arginine induces increased pituitary GH secretion and may be necessary for optimal growth in healthy infants.[241]

REFERENCES

1. Moore FD. Determination of total body water and solids with isotopes. Science 1946;104:157.
2. Friis-Hansen B. Body water compartments in children: changes during growth and related changes in body composition. Pediatr 1961;28:169.
3. Lorenz JM, Kleinman LI, Kotgol UR. Water balance in very low birth weight infants: relationship to water and sodium intake and effect on outcome. J Pediatr 1982;101:423.
4. Bauer K, Bovermann G, Rothmaither A, et al. Body composition, nutrition, and fluid balance during the first two weeks of life in preterm neonates weighing less than 1500 grams. J Pediatr 1991;118:615.
5. Bidiwala KS, Lorenz JM, Kleinman LI. Renal function correlates of postnatal diuresis in preterm infants. Pediatrics 1988;82:50.
6. Peterson S, Gotfredsen A, Knudsen FU. Lean body mass in small for gestational age and appropriate for gestational age infants. J Pediatr 1988;113:886.
7. Smith FG, Klinkefus JM, Robillard JE. Effects of volume expansion on renal sympathetic nerve activity and cardiovascular and renal function in lambs. Am J Physiol 1992;262:R651.
8. Tulassay T, Seri I, Rascher W. Atrial natriuretic peptide and extracellular volume control after birth. Acta Pediatr Scand 1987;76:444.
9. Smith FG, Klinkefus JM, Robillard JE. Baroreceptor mediated changes in sympathetic activity during development. (Abstract) Pediatr Res 1989;25:245A.
10. Tomomatsu E, Nishi K. Comparison of carotid sinus baroreceptor sensitivity in newborn and adult rabbits. Am J Physiol 1982;243:H546.
11. Anderson DF, Parks CM, Faber JJ. Arterial pressure after chronic reductions in suprarenal aortic flow in fetal lambs. Am J Physiol 1987;253:H838.
12. Binder ND, Anderson DF. Resetting of the relationship between renal perfusion pressure and plasma renin activity at birth. (Abstract) Pediatr Res 1991;29:37A.
13. Engleke SC, Shah BV, Vasan V. Sodium balance in very low birth-weight infants. J Physiol 1978;93:837.
14. Merlet-Benichou C, deRouffignac C. Renal clearance studies in fetal and young guinea pigs: effect of salt loading. Am J Physiol 1977;232:F178.
15. Rodriguez-Soriano J, Vallo A, Oliveros R. Renal handling of sodium in premature and full-term neonates: a study using clearance methods during water diuresis. Pediatr Res 1983;17:1013.
16. Rozycki JH, Baumgart S. Atrial natriuretic factor and postnatal diuresis in respiratory distress syndrome. Arch Dis Child 1991;66:43.
17. Fukuda Y, Bertorello A, Aperia A. Ontogeny of the regulation of Na/K-ATPase activity on the renal proximal convoluted tubule cell. Pediatr Res 1991;30:131.
18. Linshaw MA, Welling LW. Basolateral membrane properties in proximal convoluted tubules of the newborn rabbit. Am J Physiol 1983;244:F172.
19. Tulassay T, Seri I, Machay T. Effects of dopamine on renal functions in premature neonates with respiratory distress syndrome. Int J Pediatr Nephrol 1983;4:19.
20. Bertorello A, Aperia A. Short term regulation of Na/K-ATPase activity by dopamine. Am J Hypertens 1990;3(Suppl):51.
21. Kinoshita S, Jose PA, Felder RA. Ontogeny of the dopamine (DA1) receptor in rat renal proximal convoluted tubule (PCT). (Abstract) Pediatr Res 1989;25:68A.
22. Aperia A, Larsson L, Zetterstrom R. Hormonal induction of Na-K-ATPase in developing proximal convoluted tubule cells. Am J Physiol 1981;241:F356.
23. Stephenson G, Hammet M, Hadaway G. Ontogeny of mineralocorticoid receptors and urinary electrolyte response in the rat. Am J Physiol 1984;247:F665.
24. Mirkin G. Insensible weight loss in infants with fever. Pediatrics 1962;30:279.
25. Roy RN, Sinclair JC. Hydration of the low birth-weight infant. Clin Perinatol 1975;2:393.
26. Ultman JS. Computational model for insensible water loss from the newborn. Pediatrics 1987;79:760.
27. Forbes GB. Methods for determining composition of the human body. Pediatrics 1962;29:477.
28. Cannon B, Nedergaard J. The biochemistry of an inefficient tissue: brown adipose tissue. Essays Biochem 1985;20:110.
29. Alexander G, Bell AW. Quantity and calculated oxygen consumption during summit metabolism of brown adipose tissue in newborn lambs. Biol Neonate 1975;26:214.
30. Stern L. Physiology of the newborn infant. II. Thermoregulation. Prog Pediatr Surg 1978;12:23.
31. Nedergaard J, Cannon B. Brown adipose tissue: development and function. In: Polin RA, Fox WW, eds. Fetal and neonatal physiology. Philadelphia, WB Saunders, 1992:314.
32. Power GG. Biology of temperature: the mammalian fetus. J Dev Physiol 1989;12:295.
33. Polk DH. Thyroid hormones effects on neonatal thermogenesis. Semin Perinatol 1988;12:151.
34. Cabello G. Endocrine reactivity (T3, T4 and cortisol) during cold exposure in pre-term and full-term lambs. Biol Neonate 1983;44:224.
35. Andrews DC, Symonds ME, Johnson P. Thermoregulation and the control of breathing during N-REM sleep in the lamb. J Dev Physiol 1991;16:27.
36. Andrews DC, Symonds ME, Johnson P. The interaction of the upper airway and thermometabolism on respiratory rhythm during N-REM sleep in the developing lamb. J Dev Physiol 1991;16:37.
37. Fleming PJ, Gilbert R, Azaz Y, et al. Interaction between bedding and sleeping position in the sudden infant death syndrome. Br Med J 1990;301:85.
38. Goldberg M. Hyponatremia. Med Clin North Am 1981;65:251.
39. Stevenson JG. Fluid administration in the association of patent ductus arteriosus complicating respiratory distress syndrome. J Pediatr 1977;90:257.
40. DeFronzo RA, Bia M. Extrarenal potassium homeostasis. In: Seldin DW, Giebisch GH, eds. The kidney: physiology and pathophysiology. New York, Raven Press, 1985:1179.
41. Williams ME, Rosa RM, Silva P. Impairment of extrarenal potassium disposal by an adrenergic stimulation. N Engl J Med 1984;311:145.
42. Fleming BJ, Genuth SM, Gould AB. Laxative induced hypokalemia, sodium depletion, and hyperreninemia. Ann Intern Med 1975;83:60.
43. Lillquist K, Illum N, Jacobsen BB. Primary hyperparathyroidism in infancy associated with familial hypocalciuric hypercalcemia. Acta Pediatr Scand 1983;72:625.
44. Tsang RC, Kleinman LI, Sutherland JM. Hypocalcemia in infants of diabetic mothers: studies on calcium, phosphorus, and magnesium metabolism and parathyroid hormone responsiveness. J Pediatr 1972;30:284.
45. Mimouni F, Tsang RC, Hertzberg VS. Polycythemia, hypomagnesemia, and hypocalcemia in infants of diabetic mothers. Am J Dis Child 1986;140:798.
46. Venkataraman PS, Blick KE. Lowered serum Ca, blood ionized Ca, and unresponsive serum parathyroid hormone with oral glucose ingestion in infants of diabetic mothers. J Pediatr Gastroenterol Nutr 1987;6:931.
47. Venkataraman PS, Blick KE, Rao R. Decline in serum calcium, magnesium, and phosphorous values with oral glucose in normal neonates: studies of serum parathyroid hormone and calcitonin. J Pediatr 1985;70:543.
48. Wandrup J, Kroner J, Pryds O. Age-related reference values for ionized calcium in the first week of life in premature and full-term neonates. Scand J Clin Lab Invest 1988;48:255.

49. Fleischman AR, Rosen JF, Nathenson G. 25-Hydroxycholecalciferol for early neonatal hypocalcemia. Am J Dis Child 1978;132:973.

50. Brown DR, Salsburey DJ. Short-term biochemical effects of parenteral calcium treatment of early-onset neonatal hypocalcemia. J Pediatr 1982;100:777.

51. Scheidegger VD. The analysis of ionized calcium in the intensive-care ward. Fortschr Med 1985;103:39.

52. Hughes WG, Ruedy JR. Should calcium be used in cardiac arrest? Am J Med 1986;81:285.

53. Paraskos JA. Cardiovascular pharmacology. III. Atropine, calcium, calcium blockers, and b-blockers. Circulation 1986;74(Suppl 4):IV87.

54. Cardenas-Rivero N, Chernow B, Stoiko MA. Hypocalcemia in critically ill children. J Pediatr 1989;114:946.

55. Sanchez GJ, Vankataraman PS, Pryor RW. Hypercalcitoninemia and hypocalcemia in acutely ill children: studies in serum calcium, blood ionized calcium, and calcium regulating hormones. J Pediatr 1989;114:953.

56. Furhman BP. Hypocalcemia and critical illness in children. (Editorial) J Pediatr 1989;114:990.

57. Cooper L, Wertheimer J, Levey R. Severe primary hyperparathyroidism in a neonate with two hypercalcemic parents: management with parathyroidectomy and heterotopic autotransplantation. Pediatrics 1986;78:263.

58. Bursztein S, Elwyn DH, Askanazi J, et al. The theoretical framework. In: anonymous energy metabolism, indirect calorimetry, and nutrition. Baltimore, Williams & Wilkins, 1989:27.

59. Garvey JW, Hagstrom JWC, Veith FJ. Pathologic pulmonary changes in hemorrhagic shock. Ann Surg 1975;181:870.

60. Moss GS, Rice CL, Sehgal LR. Management of traumatic and hemorrhagic shock. Anesth Rev 1990;17:25.

61. Holcroft JW, Trunkey DD. Pulmonary extravasation of albumin during and after hemorrhagic shock in baboons. J Surg Res 1975;18:91.

62. Zikria BA, King TC, Stanford J. A biophysical approach to capillary permeability. Surg 1989;105:625.

63. Mackersie RC, Durelle J. Differential clearance of colloid and crystalloid solutions from the lung. J Trauma 1993;35:448.

64. Dawidson I, Ottosson J, Reisch J. Infusion volumes of Ringer's lactate and 3% albumin solution as they relate to survival after resuscitation of a lethal intestinal ischemic shock. Circ Shock 1986;18:277.

65. Heughan C, Niinikoski J, Hunt TK. Effect of excessive infusion of saline solution on tissue oxygen transport. Surg Gynecol Obstet 1972;135:257.

66. Velanovich V. Crystalloid versus colloid fluid resuscitation: a meta-analysis of mortality. Surgery 1989;105:65.

67. Kapiotis S, Quehenberger P, Eichler HG, et al. Effect of hydroxyethyl starch on the activity of blood coagulation and fibrinolysis in healthy volunteers: comparison with albumin. Crit Care Med 1994;22:606.

68. Gaudreault P, Temple AR, Lovejoy FH. The relative severity of acute versus chronic salicylate poisoning in children: a clinical comparison. Pediatrics 1982;70:566.

69. Kaehny WD, Gabow PA. Pathogenesis and management of metabolic acidosis and alkalosis. In: Schrier RW, ed. Renal and electrolyte disorders, ed 3. Boston, Little, Brown, 1986:141.

70. Holliday MA. Body composition and energy needs during growth. In: Falkner F, Tanner JM, eds. Human growth: a comprehensive treatise, ed 2. New York, Plenum, 1986.

71. Reichman BL, Chessex P, Putet G. Partition of energy metabolism and energy cost of growth in the very low-birth weight infant. Pediatrics 1982;69:446.

72. Young VR, Stefee WP, Pencharz PB, et al. Total human body protein synthesis in relation to protein requirements at various ages. Nature 1975;253:192.

73. Carlson SE, Barness LA. Macronutrient requirements for growth. In: Walker WA, Watkins JB, eds. Nutrition in pediatrics. Boston, Little, Brown, 1985.

74. Dupont C, Rocchiccioli F, Bougneres PF. Urinary excretion of dicarboxylic acids in term newborns fed with 5% medium-chain triglycerides-enriched formula. J Pediatr Gastroenterol Nutr 1987;6:313.

75. Schwarz KB. Vitamins. In: Walker WA, Watkins JB, eds. Nutrition in pediatrics. Boston, Little, Brown, 1985.

76. Greene HL, Hambidge KM, Schanler R, et al. Guidelines for the use of vitamins, trace elements, calcium, magnesium, and phosphorus in infants and children receiving total parenteral nutrition: report of Subcommittee on Pediatric Parenteral Nutrient Requirements from the Committee on Clinical Practice Issues of the American Society of Clinical Nutrition. Am J Clin Nutr 1988;48:1324.

77. Hambidge KM. Trace elements in human nutrition, In: Walker WA, Watkins JB, eds. Nutrition in pediatrics. Boston: Little, Brown, 1985.

78. Hamill PVV, Drizd TA, Johnson CL. Physical growth: National Center for Health Statistics percentiles. Am J Clin Nutr 1993;32:607.

79. Zlotkin SH, Bryan MH, Anderson GH. Intravenous nitrogen and energy intakes required to duplicate in utero nitrogen accretion in prematurely born human infants. J Pediatr 1981;99:115.

80. Laidlaw SA, Kopple JD. Newer concepts of the indispensable amino acids. Am J Clin Nutr 1987;46:593.

81. Miller RG, Jahoor F, Jaksic T. Decreased cysteine and proline synthesis in parenterally fed, premature infants. J Pediatr Surg 1995;30:953.

82. Waterlow JR. Classification and definition of protein-calorie malnutrition. Br Med J 1972;3:566.

83. Nyboer J, Bogna S, Nimo LF. The electrical impedance plethysmograph: an electrical volume recorder. NRC Report 149. Washington, DC, National Academy Press, 1943.

84. Schoeller DA, Van Santen E, Peterson DW, et al. Total body water measurement in humans with ^{18}O and ^{2}H labeled water. Am J Clin Nutr 1984;33:2686.

85. Mayfield RS, Uauy R, Waidelich D. Body composition of low-birth-weight infants determined by using bioelectrical resistance and reactance. Am J Clin Nutr 1991;54:296.

86. Chellis MJ, Price MB, Dean JM. Cost effectiveness of early enteral feeding in critically ill children. Crit Care Med 1994;22:A156.

87. Brown RO, Carlson SD, Cowan GSM, et al. Enteral nutritional support management in a university teaching hospital: team versus non-team. JPEN 1987;11:52.

88. Roberts P, Meredith JW, Black K, et al. Diarrhea does not alter impaired small bowel absorption following trauma. JPEN 1993;17:348.

89. Payne-James JJ, Khawaja HT. First choice for total parenteral nutrition: the peripheral route. JPEN 1993;17:468.

90. Friedman B, Kanter G, Titus D. Femoral venous catheters: a safe alternative for delivering parenteral alimentation. Nutr Clin Pract 1994;9:65.

91. Collier S, Crouch J, Hendricks K, et al. Use of cyclic parenteral nutrition in infants less than 6 months of age. Nutr Clin Pract 1994;9:65.

92. Kemp L, Burge J, Choban P, et al. The effect of catheter type and site on infection rates in total parenteral nutrition patients. JPEN 1994;18:71.

93. Moore FA, Feliciano DV, Andrassy RJ, et al. Early enteral feeding, compared with parenteral, reduces postoperative septic complications. Ann Surg 1992;216:172.

94. Herndon DN, Barrow RE, Stein M, et al. Increased mortality with intravenous supplemental feeding in severely burned patients. J Burn Care Rehabil 1989;10:309.

95. Kudsk KA, Groce MA, Favian TC, et al. Enteral *versus* parenteral feeding. Ann Surg 1992;215:503.

96. Frankenfield DC, Wiles CE, Bagley S, et al. Relationships between resting and total energy expenditure in injured and septic patients. Crit Care Med 1994;22:1796.

97. Long Cl, Schaffel N, Geiger JW, et al. Metabolic response to injury and illness: estimation of energy and protein needs from indirect calorimetry and nitrogen balance. JPEN 1979;3:452.

98. Cerra RB. Hypermetabolism, organ failure, and metabolic support. Surgery 1987;101:1.

99. Moore FD. Bodily changes in surgical convalescence. I. The normal sequence: observations and interpretations. Ann Surg 1953;137:28.

100. Wolfe RR, Jahoor F, Herndon DN, et al. Isotopic evaluation of the metabolism of pyruvate and related substrates in normal adult volunteers and severely burned children: effect of dichloroacetate and glucose infusion. Surgery 1991;110:54.

101. Consoli A, Nurjhan N, Reilly JJ, et al. Contribution of liver and skeletal muscle to alanine and lactate metabolism in humans. Am J Physiol 1990;259:E677.

102. Smith RJ, Wilmore DW. Glutamine nutritional and requirements. JPEN 1990;14(Suppl):94S.

103. Pacitti AJ, Austgen TR, Souba WW. Adaptive regulation of alanine transport in hepatic plasma membrane vesicles from the endotoxin-treated rat. J Surg Res 1991;51:46.

104. Felig P, Marliss EB, Cahill GF, Jr. Metabolic response to human growth hormone during prolonged starvation. J Clin Invest 1971;50:411.

105. Loder PB, Kee AJ, Horsburgh R, et al. Validity of urinary urea nitrogen as a measure of total urinary nitrogen in adult patients requiring parenteral nutrition. Crit Care Med 1989;17:309.

106. Bistrian BR. A simple technique to estimate severity of stress. Surg Gynecol Obstet 1979;148:675.

107. Helms RA, Mowatt-Larssen CA, Boehm KA, et al. Urinary nitrogen constituents in the postsurgical preterm neonate receiving parenteral nutrition. JPEN 1993;17:68.

108. Catzeflis C, Schutz Y, Micheli JL, et al. Whole body protein synthesis and energy expenditure in very low birth weight infants. Pediatr Res 1985;19:679.

109. Pepys MD, Baltz ML. Acute phase proteins with special reference to C-reactive protein and related proteins (Pentaxins) and serum amyloid A protein. Adv Immunol 1983;34:14.

110. Daniels JC, Larson DL, Abston S, et al. Serum protein profiles in thermal burns. J Trauma 1974;14:153.

111. Peltola H, Ahlqvist J, Rapola J, et al. C-reactive protein compared with white blood cell count and erythrocyte sedimentation rate in the diagnosis of acute appendicitis in children. Acta Chir Scand 1986; 152:55.

112. Sabel KG, Wadsworth C. C-reactive protein (CRP) in early diagnosis of neonatal septicemia. Acta Paediatr Scand 1979;68:825.

113. Pourcyrous M, Bada HS, Korones SB, et al. Significance of serial C-reactive protein responses in neonatal infection and other disorders. Pediatrics 1993;92:431.

114. Baker RD, Long S. Acute phase proteins in neonatal rabbits: diminished C-reactive protein response. J Pediatr Gastroenterol Nutr 1990; 11:534.

115. Wilmore DW. The metabolic management of the critically ill. New York, Plenum Press, 1977.

116. Weir JB. New methods for calculating metabolic rate with special reference to protein metabolism. J Physiol 1949;109:1.

117. Burstzein S, Elwyn DH, Askanazi J, et al. Energy metabolism, indirect calorimetry, and nutrition. Baltimore, Williams & Wilkins, 1989:55.

118. McGilvery RW. Biochemistry: a functional approach ed 2. Philadelphia, WB Saunders, 1979:532.

119. Cortes V, Nelson LD. Errors in estimating energy expenditure in critically ill surgical patients. Arch Surg 1989;124:287.

120. Baker JP, Detsky AS, Stewart S. Randomized trial of total parenteral nutrition in critically ill patients: metabolic effects of varying glucose-lipid ratios as an energy source. Gastroenterology 1984;87:53.

121. Fredrix EW, Soeters PB, Von Meyenfeldt MF, et al. Resting energy expenditure in cancer patients before and after gastrointestinal surgery. JPEN 1991;15:604.

122. Swinamer DL, Phang PT, Jones RL, et al. Twenty-four hour energy expenditure in critically-ill patients. Crit Care Med 1987;15:637.

123. Salas JS, Dozio E, Goulet OJ, et al. Energy expenditure and substrate utilization in the course of renutrition of malnourished children. JPEN 1991;15:288.

124. Chwals WJ, Lally KP, Woolley MM, et al. Measured energy expenditure in critically ill infants and young children. J Surg Res 1988;44:467.

125. Alverson D, Isken V, Cohen R. Effect of booster transfusions on oxygen utilization in infants with bronchopulmonary dysplasia. J Pediatr 1988;113:722.

126. Chwals WJ, Lally KP, Woolley MM. Indirect calorimetry in mechanically-ventilated infants and children: measurement accuracy with absence of audible airleak. Crit Care Med 1992;20:768.

127. Powell K, Albernaz L, Skipper E, et al. Does measurement of 20 minute energy expenditure represent the 24 hours energy expenditure in the critically ill? JPEN 1991;15:37S.

128. Pierro A, Carnielle V, Filler RM, et al. Partition of energy metabolism in the surgical newborn. J Pediatr Surg 1991;26:581.

129. Burstzein S, Elwyn DH, Askanazi J. Energy metabolism and indirect calorimetry in critically-ill and injured patients. Acute Care 1988; 14–15:91.

130. Piedboeuf B, Chessex P, Hazan J, et al. Total parenteral nutritional in the newborn infant: energy substrates and respiratory gas exchange. J Pediatr 1991;118:97.

131. Askanazi J, Weissman C, Lasala P, et al. Effects of increasing protein intake on ventilatory drive. Anesthesiology 1984;60:106.

132. Bresson JL, Bader B, Rocchiccioli F, et al. Protein-metabolism kinetics and energy-substrate utilization in infants fed parenteral solutions with different glucose-fat ratios. Am J Clin Nutr 1991;54:370.

133. Van Aerde JEE, Sauer PJJ, Pencharz PB, et al. Effect of replacing glucose with lipid on the energy metabolism of newborn infants. Clin Sci 1989;76:581.

134. Salas-Salvado J, Molina J, Figueras J, et al. Effect of the quality of infused energy on substrate utilization in the newborn receiving total parenteral nutrition. Pediatr Res 1993;33:112.

135. Delafosse B, Bouffard Y, Viale JP, et al. Respiratory changes induced by parenteral nutrition in postoperative patients undergoing inspiratory pressure support ventilation. Anesthesiology 1987;66:393.

136. Elwyn DH, Kinney JM, Jeevanandam M, et al. Influence of increasing carbohydrate intake on glucose kinetics in injured patients. Ann Surg 1979;190:117.

137. Burke JF, Wolfe RR, Mullany CJ. Glucose requirements following burn injury. Ann Surg 1979;190:274.

138. Askanazi J, Carpentier YA, Elwyn DH, et al. Influence of total parenteral nutrition on fuel utilization in injury and sepsis. Ann Surg 1980; 191:40.

139. Askanazi J, Rosenbaum S, Hyman R. Respiratory changes induced by the large glucose loads of total parenteral nutrition. JAMA 1980; 243:1444.

140. van den Berg B, Stam H. Metabolic and respiratory effects of enteral nutrition in patients during mechanical ventilation. Intensive Care Med 1088;14:206.

141. Askanazi J, Nordenstrom J, Rosenbaum SH, et al. Nutrition for the patients with respiratory failure: glucose versus fat. Anesthesiology 1990;54:373.

142. Nussbaum MS, Fischer JE. Pathogenesis of hepatic steatosis during total parenteral nutrition. In: Nyhus LM, ed. Surgery annual. Norwalk, CT, Appleton & Lange, 1991:1-11.

143. Lowry SF, Brennan MF. Abnormal liver function during parenteral nutrition: relation to infusion excess. J Surg Res 1979;26:300.

144. Payne-James JJ, Silk DB. Heptobiliary dysfunction associated with total parenteral nutrition. Dig Dis 1992;9:106.

145. Freund HR. Abnormalities of liver function and hepatic damage associated with total parenteral nutrition. Nutrition 1991;7:1.

146. Das JB, Cosentino CM, Levy MF, et al. Early hepatobiliary dysfunction during total parenteral nutrition: an experimental study. J Pediatr Surg 1993;28:14.

147. Vary TC, Siegel JH, Nakatani T, et al. Effects of sepsis on activity of pyruvate dehydrogenase complex in skeletal muscle and liver. Am J Physiol 1986;250:E634.

148. Sobrado J, Moldawer LL, Pomposelli JJ, et al. Lipid emulsions and reticuloendothelial system function in healthy and burned guinea pigs. Am J Clin Nutr 1985;42:855.

149. Yamazaki K, Maiz A, Moldawer LL, et al. Complications associated with the overfeeding of infected animals. J Surg Res 1986;40:152.

150. Koea JB, Shaw JHF. Total parenteral nutrition in surgical illness: how much? how good? Nutrition 1992;8:275.

151. Vo NM, Waycaster M, Acuff RV, et al. Effects of postoperative carbohydrate overfeeding. Am Surg 1987;53:632.

152. Alexander JW, Gonce SJ, Miskell PW, et al. A new model for studying nutrition in peritonitis. Ann Surg 1989;209:334.

153. Dominioni L, Trocki O, Fang CH, et al. Enteral feeding in burn hypermetabolism: nutritional and metabolic effects of different levels of calorie and protein intake. JPEN 1985;9:269.

154. Lazarus DD, Lowry SF, Moldawer LL. Cytokines acutely decrease circulating insulin-like growth factor-1 (IGF-1) and IGF binding protein-3 (IGFBP-3). Surg Forum 1992;43:92.

155. Shanbhogue RL, Lloyd DA. Absence of hypermetabolism after operation in the newborn infant. JPEN 1992;16:333.

156. Gebara BM, Gelmini M, Sarnaik A. Oxygen consumption, energy expenditure, and substrate utilization after cardiac surgery in children. Crit Care Med 1992;20:1550.

157. Chwals WJ, Letton RW, Jamie A, et al. Stratification of injury severity using energy expenditure response in surgical infants. J Pediatr Surg 1995;30:1161.

158. Chwals WJ, Fernandez ME, Charles BJ, et al. Serum visceral protein levels reflect protein-calorie repletion in neonates recovering from major surgery. J Pediatr Surg 1992;27:317.

159. Chwals WJ, Fernandez ME, Charles BJ. Adjustment of nutritional repletion using bedside indirect calorimetry in infants recovering from surgical stress. Crit Care Med 1992;20:S11.

160. Letton RW, Chwals WJ, Jamie A, et al. Early postoperative alterations

in infant energy utilization increases the risk of overfeeding. J Pediatr Surg 1995;30:988.

161. Lucas A, Bloom SR, Aynsley-Green A. Gut hormones and minimal enteral feeding. Acta Paediatr Scand 1986;75:719.

162. Zamir O, Nussbaum MS, Bhadra S, et al. Effect of enteral feeding on hepatic steatosis induced by total parenteral nutrition. JPEN 1994;18:20.

163. Border JR, Hassett J, LaDuca J, et al. The gut origin of septic states in blunt multiple trauma (ISS = 40) in the ICU. Ann Surg 1987;206:427.

164. Deitch EA, Berg RD, Specian R. Endotoxin promotes the translocation of bacteria from the gut. Arch Surg 1987;122:185.

165. Deitch EA, Bridges W, Baker J, et al. Hemorrhagic shock-induced bacterial translocation is reduced by xanthine oxidase inhibition or inactivation. Surgery 1988;104:191.

166. Deitch EA, Ma WA, Ma L, et al. Protein malnutrition predisposes to inflammatory-induced gut origin septic states. Ann Surg 1990;211:560.

167. Smith SD, Cardona M, Wishnev S, et al. Unique characteristics of the neonatal intestinal mucosal barrier. J Pediatr Surg 1992;27:333.

168. Go LL, Ford HR, Watkins SC, et al. Quantitative and morphologic analysis of bacterial translocation in neonates. Arch Surg 1994;129:1184.

169. Mainous MR, Tso P, Berg RD, et al. Studies of the route, magnitude, and time course of bacterial translocation in a model of systemic inflammation. Arch Surg 1991;126:33.

170. Deitch EA, Xu D, Qi L, et al. Bacterial translocation from the gut impairs systemic immunity. Ann Surg 1991;109:269.

171. Caty MG, Guice KS, Oldham KT, et al. Evidence for tumor necrosis factor-induced pulmonary microvascular injury after intestinal ischemia-reperfusion injury. Ann Surg 1990;212:694.

172. Alexander JW. Nutrition and translocation. JPEN 1990;14(Suppl):170S.

173. Alverdy JC, Aoys E, Moss GS. Total parenteral nutrition promotes bacterial translocation from the gut. Surgery 1988;104:185.

174. Moore FA, Feliciano DV, Andrassy RJ, et al. Early enteral feeding, compared with parenteral, reduces postoperative septic complications. The results of a meta-analysis. Ann Surg 1992;216:172.

175. Mochizuki H, Trocki O, Dominioni L, et al. Mechanism of prevention of postburn hypermetabolism and catabolism by early enteral feeding. Ann Surg 1984;200:297.

176. Bortenschlager L, Zaloga G, Black KW, et al. Immediate post-operative enteral feeding decreases weight loss and improves wound healing following abdominal surgery in rats. Crit Care Med 1992;20:115.

177. Kudsk KA, Minard G, Wojtysiak SL, et al. Visceral protein response to enteral versus parenteral nutrition and sepsis in patients with trauma. Surgery 1994;116:516.

178. McAnena OH, Harvey lP, Bonau RA, et al. Alteration of methotrexate toxicity in rats by manipulation of dietary components. Gastroenterology 1987;92:354.

179. Trocki O, Mochizuki H, Dominioni L, et al. Intact protein versus free amino acids in the nutritional support of thermally injured animals. JPEN 1986;10:139.

180. Zaloga GP, Knowles R, Ward K, et al. Total parenteral nutrition (TPN) increases mortality following hemorrhage. Crit Care Med 1991;19:54.

181. Meredith JW, Dietsheim JA, Zaloga GP. Visceral protein levels in trauma patients are greater with peptide diet than intact protein diet. J Trauma 1990;30:825.

182. Souba WW, Smith RJ, Wilmore DW. Glutamine metabolism by the intestinal tract. JPEN 1985;9:608.

183. Yoshida S, Leskiw JM, Schluter MD, et al. Effect of total parenteral nutrition, systemic sepsis, and glutamine on gut mucosa in rats. Am J Physiol 1992;263:E368.

184. Souba WW, Herskowitz K, Austgen RT, et al. Glutamine nutrition: theoretical considerations and therapeutic impact. JPEN 1990;14(Suppl):237S.

185. O'Dwyer ST, Smith RJ, Hwang TL, et al. Maintenance of small bowel mucosa with glutamine enriched parenteral nutrition. JPEN 1989;13:579.

186. Grant J. Use of L-glutamine in total parenteral nutrition. J Surg Res 1988;44:506.

187. Burke D, Alverdy JC, Aoys E, et al. Glutamine supplemented TPN improves gut immune function. Arch Surg 1989;124:1396.

188. Li S, Nussbaum MS, McFadden DW, et al. Addition of L-glutamine to total parenteral nutrition and its effects on portal insulin and glucagon and the development of hepatic steatosis in rats. J Surg Res 1990;49:421.

189. Ziegler TR, Young LS, Benfell K, et al. Clinical and metabolic efficacy of glutamine-supplemented parenteral nutrition after bone marrow transplantation: a randomized, double-blind-controlled study. Ann Intern Med 1992;116:821.

190. Inoue Y, Grant JP, Snyder PJ. Effect of glutamine-supplemented intravenous nutrition on survival after Escherichia coli-induced peritonitis. JPEN 1993;17(Suppl):41.

191. Crouch J, Wilmore D. The use of glutamine-supplemented parenteral nutrition (PN) in very-low birth weight infants. JPEN 1991;15(Suppl):25S.

192. Thompson JS, Sharp JG, Saxena SK, et al. Stimulation of neomucosal growth by systemic urogastrone. J Surg Res 1987;42:402.

193. Jacobs DL, Evans DA, Mealy K, et al. Combined effects of glutamine and epidermal growth factor on the rat intestine. Surgery 1988;104:358.

194. Salloum RM, Schultz GS, Souba WW. Regulation of small intestinal glutamine transport by epidermal growth factor. Surgery 1993;113:552.

195. Olsen PS, Poulsen SS, Therkelsen K, et al. Oral administration of synthetic human urogastrone promotes healing of chronic duodenal ulcers in rats. Gastroenterology 1986;90:911.

196. Konturek SJ, Brzozowski T, Dembiniski A, et al. Interaction of growth hormone-releasing factor and somatostatin on ulcer healing and mucosal growth in rate: role of gastrin and epidermal-growth factor. Digestion 1988;41:121.

197. Berseth CL. Enhancement of intestinal growth in neonatal rats by epidermal growth factor in milk. Am J Physiol 1987;253:G662.

198. Berseth CL, Go VL. Enhancement of neonatal somatic and hepatic growth by orally-administered epidermal growth factor in rats. J Pediatr Gastroenterol Nutr 1988;7:889.

199. Schober DA, Simmen FA, Hadsell DL, et al. Perinatal expression of type I IGF receptors in porcine small intestine. Endocrinology 1990;126:1125.

200. Shaw JH, Wildbore M, Wolfe RR. Whole-body protein kinetics in severely septic patients. Ann Surg 1987;205:288.

201. Streat SJ, Beddoe AH, Hill GL. Aggressive nutritional support does not prevent protein loss despite fat gain in septic intensive care patients. J Trauma 1987;27:262.

202. Jiang ZM, He GZ, Zhang SY, et al. Low-dose growth hormone and hypocaloric nutrition attenuate the protein-catabolic response after major operation. Ann Surg 1989;210:513.

203. Ziegler TR, Young LS, Manson JM, et al. Metabolic effects of recombinant human growth hormone in patients receiving parenteral nutrition. Ann Surg 1988;208:6.

204. Voerman HJ, Strack van Schijndel JM, Groeneveld ABJ, et al. Effects of recombinant human growth hormone in patients with severe sepsis. Ann Surg 1992;216:648.

205. Zapf J, Froesch ER. Insulin-like growth factors/somatomedins: structures, secretion, biological actions and physiological role. Horm Res 1986;24:121.

206. Gore DC, Honeycutt D, Jahoor F, et al. Effect of exogenous growth hormone on whole-body and isolated-limb protein kinetics in burned patients. Arch Surg 1991;126:38.

207. Zaizen Y, Ford EG, Costin G, et al. The effect of perioperative exogenous growth hormone and wound bursting strength in normal and malnourished rats. J Pediatr Surg 1990;25:70.

208. Gatzen C, Scheltinga MR, Kimbrough TD, et al. Growth hormone attenuates the abnormal distribution of body water in critically ill surgical patients. Surgery 1992;112:181.

209. Dahn MS, Lange MP, Jacobs LA. Insulin-like growth factor 1 production is inhibited in human sepsis. Arch Surg 1988;123:1409.

210. Gottardis M, Benzer A, Koller W, et al. Improvement of septic syndrome after administration of recombinant human growth hormone (rhGH)? J Trauma 1991;31:81.

211. Chwals WJ, Bistrian BR. Role of exogenous growth hormone and insulin-like growth factor-I in malnutrition and acute metabolic stress: a hypothesis. Crit Care Med 1991;19:1317.

212. Ross RJM, Miell JP, Holly JMP, et al. Levels of GH binding activity, IGFBP-1, insulin, blood glucose, and cortisol in intensive care patients. Clin Endocrinol 1991;35:361.

213. Fan J, Molina PE, Gelato MC, et al. Differential tissue regulation of insulin-like growth-factor-I content and binding proteins after endotoxin. Endocrinology 1994;134:1685.

214. Lemmey AB, Martin AA, Read LC, et al. IGF-I and the truncated analogue des-(1-3)IGF-I enhance growth in rats after gut resection. Am J Physiol 1991;260:E213.

215. Roth E, Valentini L, Holzenbein T, et al. Acute effects of insulin-like growth factor I on inter-organ amino acid flux in protein-catabolic dogs. Biochem 1993;296:765.

216. Thompson WA, Coyle SM, Lazarus D, et al. The metabolic effects of a continuous infusion of insulin-like growth factor (IGF-1) in parenterally fed men. Surg Forum 1991;42:23.

217. Elahi D, McAloon-Dyke M, Fukagawa NK, et al. Effects of recombinant human IGF-I on glucose and leucine kinetics in men. Am J Physiol 1993;265:E831.

218. Kudsk KA, Mowatt-Larssen C, Bukar J, et al. Effect of recombinant human insulin-like growth factor-I and early total parenteral nutrition on immune depression following severe head injury. Arch Surg 1994;129:66.

219. Marks KH, Maisels MJ, Moore E, et al. Head growth in sick premature infants: a longitudinal study. J Pediatr 1979;94:282.

220. Prader A, Tanner JM, Moore E, et al. Catch-up growth following illness or starvation. J Pediatr 1963;62:646.

221. Gross SJ, Oehler JM, Eckerman CL. Normative early head growth in very-low-birth-weight infants. J Pediatr 1983;103:946.

222. Hack M, Gordan D, Merkatz I, et al. The prognostic significance of postnatal growth in very low birth weight infants. Pediatr Res 1980;14:434.

223. Fischer JE. Branched-chain-enriched amino acid solutions in patients with liver failure: an early example of nutritional pharmacology. JPEN 1990;14(Suppl):249S.

224. Brennan MF, Cerra F, Daly JM, et al. Report of a research workshop: branched chain amino-acids in stress and injury. JPEN 1986;10:446.

225. Desai SP, Bistrian BR, Polombo JR, et al. Branched chain amino acid administration in surgical patients. Arch Surg 1987;127:760.

226. Abel RM, Beck CH Jr, Abbott WM, et al. Improved survival from acute renal failure after treatment with intravenous essential L-amino acids and glucose. N Engl J Med 1973;288:695.

227. Cerra RB, Cheung NK, Fischer JE, et al. Disease-specific amino acid infusion (FO 80) in hepatic encephalopathy: a prospective, randomized, double-blind, controlled trial. JPEN 1985;9:288.

228. Katz S, Plaisier BR, Folkening WJ, et al. Intralipid adversely affects reticuloendothelial-bacterial clearance. J Pediatr Surg 1991;26(8):921.

229. Hamawy KJ, Moldawer LL, Georgieff M, et al. Effect of lipid emulsions on the reticuloendothelial system function in the injured animal. JPEN 1985;9:559.

230. Kripke SA, Fox AD, Berman JM, et al. Stimulation of intestinal growth with intracolonic infusion of short-chain fatty acids. JPEN 1989;3:109.

231. Koruda MJ, Rolandelli RH, Zimmaro DM, et al. Parenteral nutrition supplemented with short-chain fatty acids: effect on the small bowel mucosa in normal rats. Am J Clin Nutr 1989;51:685.

232. Kinsella JE, Lokesh B, Broughton S, et al. Dietary polyunsaturated fatty acids and eicosanoids: potential effects on the modulation of inflammatory and immune cells: an overview. Nutrition 1990;6:25.

233. Kinsella JE, Lokesh B. Dietary lipids, eicosanoids, and the immune system. Crit Care Med 1990;18(Suppl):S94.

234. Alexander JW, Saito H, Trocki O, et al. The importance of lipid type in the diet after burn injury. Ann Surg 1986;204:1.

235. Alexander JW, Gottschlich MD. Nutritional immunomodulation in burn patients. Crit Care Med 1990;18(Suppl):S149.

236. Peck MD, Ogel CK, Alexander JW. Composition of fat in enteral diets can influence outcome in experimental peritonitis. Ann Surg 1991;214:74.

237. Clouva-Molyvdas P, Peck MD, Alexander JW. Short-term dietary lipid manipulation does not affect survival in two models of murine sepsis. JPEN 1992;16:343.

238. Rudolph FB, Kulkarni AD, Fanslow WC, et al. Role of RNA as a dietary source of pyrimidines and purines in immune function. Nutrition 1990;6:45.

239. Kulkarni AD, Fanslow WC, Rudolph FB, et al. Modulation of delayed hypersensitivity in mice by dietary nucleotide restriction. Transplantation 1988;44:847.

240. Kulkarni AD, Fanslow WC, Rudolph FB, et al. Effect of dietary nucleotides on response to bacterial infections. JPEN 1986;10:169.

241. Barbul A. Arginine and immune function. Nutrition 1990;6:53.

242. Madden HP, Breslin RJ, Wasserkrug HL, et al. Stimulation of T cell immunity enhances survival in peritonitis. J Surg Res 1988;44:658.

243. Saito H, Trocki O, Wang S, et al. Metabolic and immune effects of dietary arginine supplementation after burn. Arch Surg 1987;122:784.

244. Daly JM, Reynolds JV, Thom A, et al. Immune and metabolic effects of arginine in the surgical patient. Ann Surg 1988;208:512.

245. Nirgiotis JG, Hennessee PJ, Andrassy RJ. The effects of an arginine-free enteral diet on wound healing and immune function in the postsurgical rat. J Pediatr Surg 1991;26:936.

Surgery of Infants and Children: Scientific Principles and Practice, edited by Keith T. Oldham, Paul M. Colombani, and Robert P. Foglia. Lippincott–Raven Publishers, Philadelphia, © 1997.

CHAPTER 5

Metabolism

Mark G. Clemens and Charles N. Paidas

The metabolic response to injury, disease, or surgical stress is complex and multifactorial. These stresses encompass humoral, inflammatory, and ischemic components, all of which influence metabolic response. Moreover, these components are not independent of one another. On the other hand, the nature of the metabolic response depends on the relative magnitude of these influences and the order in which they occur. In this context, the diverse components of the response to injury and their physiologic sequelae have been described under the heading of a broadly defined syndrome: the systemic inflammatory response syndrome (SIRS). This syndrome describes a set of characteristic manifestations of the response to stresses of diverse causes. Although this makes it of limited value in designing broad-based therapies, it constitutes a useful starting place for discussion of the basic mechanisms by which diverse pathologies can produce metabolic alterations with recognizable similarities. Therefore, the purpose of this chapter is to present a summary of cellular metabolism relevant to the response seen in SIRS. This is not intended to be a comprehensive presentation of basic metabolic biochemistry, but rather a review of the fundamental pathways, presented in a context of what is relevant to an understanding of the metabolic response to surgical stress. This chapter includes a summary of the basic metabolic pathways, followed by a review of the current thinking concerning how regulation of these pathways is altered in response to surgical stress. By necessity of available space and the diverse causes of the systemic inflammatory response syndrome, this discussion is directed at identifying unifying themes rather than a detailed comparison of response to individual stressors. In particular, these responses are presented in terms of acute versus chronic and compensatory versus decompensatory responses.

ENERGY PRODUCTION

A major goal of cellular metabolism is the provision of energy in the form of high-energy phosphates for the maintenance of endergonic cellular processes. The magnitude of the task of energy production and the energetically precarious position in which the cell exists typically are not fully appreciated. For example, isolated perfused rat livers have been reported to have a basal oxygen consumption of about 2 mL/min/g of liver tis-

sue.[1] This level of metabolism is required to maintain cellular homeostasis by providing energy to ion pumps and by supporting essential biosynthetic pathways. In response to metabolic stimulation with lactic acid (to stimulate gluconeogenesis), this increases by 50% to 3 mL/min/g of tissue, and it increases again to 5 mL/min/g with hormonal stimulation. When these figures are expressed in terms of the amount of adenosine triphosphate (ATP) consumed that would be replenished by oxidative phosphorylation, these levels of oxygen consumption range from 5.4 to 13.4 μmol ATP/min/g. How does this compare with the ATP content of the typical liver cell? Under normal conditions, liver tissue contains about 3.5 μmol ATP per gram of tissue. Thus, even under basal conditions, ATP consumption in 1 minute exceeds the cell's total stores. Clearly, the uninterrupted generation of ATP is vital to the continuation of normal function in these cells. Although the exact ATP contents and rates of energy consumption vary among different tissues, the consumption/production ratio is similar in most tissues.

Generation of high-energy phosphates is accomplished by transferring the energy released through the conversion of large (in a thermodynamic sense, ordered) molecules into smaller (less ordered) molecules. In most mammalian cells, the bulk of ATP production is performed aerobically through oxidative phosphorylation. This process occurs in the mitochondria and is the end stage of a series of steps to conserve the energy of catabolism in the form of reducing equivalents (see later). Generally, for different classes of substrates, these step are as follows: (1) preparation for entry into the Krebs cycle, (2) generation of reduced pyridine nucleotides in the Krebs cycle, and (3) electron transport and oxidative phosphorylation. Step 1 differs substantially for different substrates, while steps 2 and 3 are the same for all substrates, with only minor variations. Therefore, the common final steps are presented first, and the preparation steps are presented in the context of the mechanisms by which the precursors converge on the Krebs cycle.

The Krebs Cycle

Oxidative metabolism of carbohydrates, fats, and amino acids requires entry into the Krebs cycle. In this pathway, the energy released by increasing the disorder of the substrates is conserved by transferring it in the form of electrons to nicotinamide adenine dinucleotide (NAD) or its phosphorylated form (NADP). The resulting reduced forms, NAD or NADPH, then serve as the source of reducing equivalents to drive electron transport and the resulting ATP production in the mitochondria as well as to drive various dehydrogenase, oxidase, and reductase reactions. Some examples of these reactions that are particularly relevant to surgical stress are lactic dehydrogenase, which catalyzes the interconversion between lactic and pyruvic acid; NADPH oxidase, which transfers an electron from NADPH to oxygen to produce superoxide in phagocytic cells; and glutathione reductase, which catalyzes the regeneration of reduced glutathione, which is consumed in detoxifying H_2O_2 through the glutathione peroxidase reaction. As such, it is important to consider pathways that generate reduced NAD or NADP not only in the context of ATP synthesis but also in supplying reducing power for many other cellular processes.

A substrate can enter the Krebs cycle by one of two mechanisms: generation of acetyl coenzyme A (acetyl-CoA), or generation of specific intermediates in the cycle (see Preparation for Entry Into the Krebs Cycle for details). The cyclic nature of the Krebs cycle implies that the intermediates are not consumed but rather recycled. This is true for carbon added to the cycle by acetyl-CoA. On the other hand, the intermediates in the cycle are not physically constrained. In fact, competition for substrates among pathways is extremely important in the overall regulation of metabolism. Examples can be found in the reciprocal regulation of gluconeogenesis and ureagenesis, both of which use some Krebs cycle intermediates, as well as in the impact of accelerated gluconeogenesis on ketogenesis through the depletion the Krebs cycle intermediate oxaloacetate. These mechanisms are discussed in more detail in the sections regarding the specific pathways. The implication is that substrates can enter or exit in mid-cycle, generating reducing equivalents in the process.

Conceptually, the Krebs cycle accepts two carbons from acetyl-CoA to form citric acid from oxaloacetate. In a series of enzymatic reactions, two carbons are lost as CO_2 (although not the same carbons as were donated by the acetyl-CoA), 3 mol of NAD are reduced to NADH, 1 mol of flavin adenine dinucleotide (FAD) is reduced to $FADH_2$, and 1 mol of guanosine diphosphate (GDP) is phosphorylated to guanosine triphosphate (GTP). The product, oxaloacetate, can then combine with another acetyl-CoA and begin the cycle again. Thus, with the exception of the 1 mol of GTP formed, which can form ATP by the reaction GTP + adenosine diphosphate (ADP) → GDP + ATP, all of the energy conservation resulting directly from complete oxidation of the two-carbon units of acetyl-CoA is through the transfer of reducing equivalents to NAD or FAD. As already discussed, these reduced intermediates have significant inherent utility in driving vital cellular processes. Nevertheless, for most energy-requiring reactions, it is necessary that the energy be provided as ATP. Conversion of the energy contained in NADPH and $FADH_2$ occurs in the mitochondria through electron transport and oxidative phosphorylation.

ELECTRON TRANSPORT AND OXIDATIVE PHOSPHORYLATION

The final common energy currency of the cell is ATP. Contrary to popular belief, the terminal phosphate of ATP is not the highest energy bond in the cell, nor is it inherently chemically unstable. To the contrary, the moderately high–energy bond has sufficient inherent energy to drive reactions, but the energy bond also is low enough to allow it to be synthesized (within the constraints that the theoretic energy released by breaking a bond is equal to that required to synthesize the bond). In reality, the inefficiency of energy transfer results in a greater energy requirement for synthesis than can be effectively recovered in an energy-using reaction. Thus, with the moderately high energy of the terminal phosphate bond of ATP, sufficient energy is contained to fuel cellular processes, but the bond can still be rapidly regenerated. The chemical stability of the molecule allows it to be degraded selectively by specific enzymatic reactions rather than by spontaneously hydrolyzing. As a result, the energy released is coupled to useful cell work. In addition, the specific effect of phosphorylation on protein conformation and function provides a mechanism by which the energy contained in the high-energy bond can be effectively used to perform cellular work as well as to effect cellular signaling. This ATP-dependent signaling can result from generation of cyclic adenosine monophosphate (AMP) from ATP or the allosteric regulation of specific proteins by kinase-dependent protein phosphorylation.

Oxidative phosphorylation takes place in the mitochondria and is absolutely dependent on structural and functional properties of the mitochondria as well as on the availability substrates and oxygen. Conceptually, there are three major components of oxidative phosphorylation: (1) the electron transport chain, (2) establishment of a chemiosmotic potential, and (3) conservation of the energy contained in this potential by synthesizing ATP.

The inner mitochondrial membrane differs from the other membrane systems of eukaryotic cells in its extremely high protein content. A large portion of these proteins are components of the electron transport chain. The electron transport chain comprises a series of enzyme complexes made up of iron-containing proteins called *cytochromes*. This cytochrome chain accepts a pair of electrons from NADPH or $FADH_2$ and transfers them down the chain, with O_2 as the ultimate electron acceptor. The net reaction of $NADH + H^+ + \frac{1}{2} O_2 \rightarrow H_2O + NAD$ is highly exergonic, with a standard free-energy change of 220 kJ/mol. At three sites in the chain, this energy is used to pump a proton from the inner matrix to the space between the inner and outer mitochondrial membranes. The result is the establishment of a pH (H^+) and a charge gradient, both of which strongly favor the movement of the protons into the mitochondrial matrix. These gradients result in a chemiosmotic potential equivalent to a membrane potential of about -300 mV.

How is this potential converted into ATP? Also in the inner mitochondrial membrane is an H^+-ATPase (the F_1 ATPase), which is oriented so that it pumps H^+ out of the matrix, using the hydrolysis of ATP to ADP as the source of energy. In energized mitochondria, however, the energy of H^+ electrochemical gradient sufficiently exceeds the energy of hydrolysis of ATP, so that the reaction runs in reverse. H^+ enters the mitochondrion through the F_1 ATPase, and ADP is phosphorylated to yield ATP. The ATP formed inside the mitochondrial matrix must then be transported into the cytoplasm using a carrier (the adenine nucleotide translocase) that transports it in exchange for ATP. The tight coupling of H^+ influx to ATP synthesis is absolutely dependent on the extremely low permeability of the inner mitochondrial membrane to H^+ at sites other than the F_1 ATPase. Damage to the inner membrane can result in increased permeability to protons and *uncoupling* of the mitochondria. This means that oxygen consumption proceeds, usually at elevated rates, but ATP is not synthesized. This process, which results from the futile cycling of protons, can be of biologic utility, such as in thermogenesis in brown fat. When associated with cell injury, however, uncoupling results in a hypercatabolic state in which ATP production is depressed.

Another potentially serious consequence of uncoupling is accelerated generation of reactive oxygen intermediates. Even under normal conditions, transfer of electrons to O_2 is imperfect. In addition to the generation of water, some single (unpaired) electrons are transferred, resulting in the generation of superoxide. When the rate of electron transport is elevated, and in particular when there has been damage to the inner membrane, the rate of superoxide production is increased. This may be of significant biologic importance in cell signaling as well as in the genesis of injury because mitochondria-derived oxidants have been proposed to be a significant activator of the transcription factor Nuclear factor Kappa B (NFKB) in response to metabolic overload.

Uncoupling alone is rarely seen in injured cells. To the contrary, a decreased efficiency of ATP production is typically observed in conjunction with decreased total rates of oxygen consumption. This *inhibition* of oxidative phosphorylation in injured cells can result from damage to the electron transport chain, so that the electrons cannot be transferred to oxygen. It can also result from inhibition of the adenine nucleotide translocase, so that synthesized ATP accumulates in the mitochondrial matrix and causes product inhibition of ATP production. A significant contributor to inhibition of the adenine nucleotide translocase under pathologic conditions is the accumulation of free fatty acids as a result of phospholipase activation.[2]

PREPARATION FOR ENTRY INTO THE KREBS CYCLE

Carbohydrates

Carbohydrates are available to tissues in the form of circulating (plasma) glucose and intracellular stores of glycogen. Both sources are of substantial importance, but their relative importance varies depending on the tissue. Neural tissue, blood cells, and tissue macrophages are particularly dependent on plasma glucose. Hypoglycemic coma has long been recognized as a result of inadequate supply of circulating glucose to the central nervous system. It more recently has been shown that a substantial portion of the increase in total body glucose use during stress responses, such as after endotoxemia, results from increased metabolism by phagocytic cells such as tissue macrophages and infiltrating neutrophils. Normally, supply of plasma glucose is primarily from the liver by glycogenolysis and gluconeogenesis and, to a lesser extent, from the kidney by gluconeogenesis. Induction of stress rapidly depletes liver glycogen, thus increasing the dependence on gluconeogenesis. Control of gluconeogenesis is discussed in more detail later.

Once glucose enters a cell, it is immediately phosphorylated by the enzyme hexokinase (or glucokinase in the liver) to form glucose-6-phosphate. This step serves several purposes: (1)

phosphorylation of glucose adds negative charges, thus making it impermeant through the plasma membrane; (2) this step helps maintain the intracellular levels of glucose low, so that uptake can continue; and (3) the phosphate attached in the hexokinase reaction eventually is transferred to ADP to generate ATP. In addition, glucose-6-phosphate constitutes the branch point between glycolysis and the pentose shunt (see later). This step and a subsequent step (catalyzed by phosphofructokinase, PFK) use ATP to prime the pathway. Additional phosphates that eventually are used for ATP synthesis are derived from inorganic phosphates. As a result, the net ATP generation is 2 mol of ATP per 1 mol of glucose. Ultimately, the six carbons of the 1 molecule of glucose that entered glycolysis yield 2 molecules of the three-carbon pyruvic acid. Depending on the redox state of the cell, pyruvate can either enter the Krebs cycle or be converted to lactic acid.

A unique feature of glycolysis is that it allows energy in the form of ATP to be produced in the absence of oxygen. Although the energy yield is low compared with oxidative metabolism, the ATP produced in glycolysis is essential for homeostasis during hypoxia in all cells; and in some cells (eg, blood cells and central nervous system neurons), it is essential at all times. Therefore, regulation of glycolysis is closely tied to cellular ATP content. The two major regulatory enzymes in glycolysis—PFK and pyruvate kinase—are allosterically regulated by the cellular levels of ATP and ADP such that they are activated by low levels of ATP and high levels of ADP. This manner of regulation results in acceleration of glycolysis when oxidative ATP production is inhibited by hypoxia. This relation was first observed by Louis Pasteur in yeast, which eliminates the pyruvate generated during glycolysis by alcoholic fermentation. In mammals, pyruvate is converted into lactic acid. This reaction, catalyzed by lactic dehydrogenase, is facilitated during hypoxia by the accumulation of NADH in the absence of oxygen, thus shifting the equilibrium toward the conversion of pyruvate to lactate, with subsequent release of lactate into the blood (pyruvate + NADH $\rightarrow$ lactate + NAD).

Under aerobic conditions, on the other hand, the redox potential favors the equilibrium to be shifted toward conversion of lactate to pyruvate or at least inhibition of the conversion of pyruvate to lactate. In most cells, the alternative pathway for pyruvate is to enter the Krebs cycle by conversion to acetyl-CoA by the pyruvate dehydrogenase (PDH) complex. In liver and kidney, pyruvate can also be reconverted to glucose by gluconeogenesis (see later). PDH is an enzyme complex located in the mitochondria that catalyzes the oxidative decarboxylation of pyruvate (three carbons) to acetyl-CoA (two carbons in the acetyl group), with the release of CO_2 and the reduction of NAD to NADH. PDH is made up of three separate enzymes requiring five different coenzymes. It is also the primary site of regulation of entry of pyruvate into the Krebs cycle. Because of this regulatory role, activity of PDH is a major determinant of cellular rate of oxidative glucose consumption. During the hypometabolic phase of stresses resembling SIRS, PDH has been shown to be down-regulated. The contribution of this down-regulation to decreased glucose turnover during hypometabolic states is discussed later.

The total energy yield for glucose that is completely oxidized in the Krebs cycle is considerably higher than that for glycolysis alone. As described earlier, the net ATP yield from glycolysis is 2 mol of ATP per 1 mol of glucose. In addition, 2 mol of NAD are reduced to NADH. In the presence of oxygen, these reducing equivalents can be transferred into the mitochondrion to yield another 6 mol of ATP. Conversion of each of the 2 mol of pyruvate formed during glycolysis to acetyl-CoA yields another 1 mol of NADH with another 3 mol of NADH, 1 mol of $FADH_2$, and one substrate-level phosphorylation of GDP to GTP. The net result is 2 mol of ATP, 2 mol of GTP, 10 mol of NADH, and 2 mol of $FADH_2$, or an ATP equivalent of 38 mol of ATP per 1 mol of glucose. With the exception of the 2 mol of ATP that are produced in glycolysis, all of the ATP production is dependent on the continued availability of oxygen.

Alternative Pathway: The Pentose Shunt

An alternative metabolic route for glucose-6-phosphate is entry into the pentose shunt. This is catalyzed by glucose-6-phosphate dehydrogenase, which shunts the glucose-6-phosphate to 6-phosphoglucono-δ-lactone instead of to fructose-6-phosphate for glycolysis. This pathway results in the conversion of glucose-6-phosphate to ribose-5-phosphate and CO_2. In the process, NADP is reduced to NADPH. The ribose-5-phosphate can then serve as a precursor for nucleotide synthesis or be recycled to glucose-6-phosphate. This recycling pathway uses a complex interconversion among three-, four-, five-, six-, and seven-carbon sugars but does not require oxidation of NADPH. As a result, the recycling of glucose-6-phosphate through the pentose shunt serves as the major source of cellular NADPH for use in specific redox reactions. The most notable of these are fatty acid synthesis; NADPH oxidase, which generates superoxide anion in phagocytic cells; glutathione reductase, which regenerates reduced glutathione after it has been oxidized in detoxifying glutathione peroxidase; and all isoforms of nitric oxide synthase.

Gluconeogenesis

Because of the extreme importance of maintaining relatively constant plasma glucose levels, a mechanism for synthesizing glucose from other substrates when dietary sources are unavailable is essential. This is accomplished by gluconeogenesis, which occurs primarily in the liver with additional contribution by the kidney. In mammals, de novo synthesis of glucose can be accomplished using a variety of substrates as precursors. The most important of these are pyruvate, lactate, and specific glucogenic amino acids. Fatty acids and ketone bodies cannot serve as precursors for gluconeogenesis. In general, gluconeogenesis can be considered as glycolysis in reverse. There are, however, some important distinctions. First, three of the steps in glycolysis are energetically irreversible under physiologic conditions. This necessitates the existence of bypass steps to circumvent these obstacles. Second, gluconeogenesis is costly in terms of energy consumed to convert the three-carbon precursor pyruvate into the more ordered six-carbon glucose. In contrast to glycolysis, which provides a net yield of 2 mol of ATP per 1 mol of glucose catabolized, gluconeogenesis consumes 6 mol of ATP (4 mol of ATP and 2 mol of GTP) for each 1 mol of glucose synthesized. It is thus obvious that gluconeogenesis is not useful for supplying glucose as a fuel to the hepatocyte that engages in gluconeogenesis. It is, however, essential for interorgan metabolic regulation by the liver. This role is well illustrated by the Cori cycle. Essentially, the Cori cycle provides a mechanism by which peripheral tissues relying on anaerobic glycolysis consume glucose and release lactic acid into the blood. The lactate is then taken up by the liver, where glucose is resynthesized by gluconeogenesis. Even though this process requires a net input of energy in the liver, it provides a mechanism by which other tissues can maintain metabolic integrity even with compromised oxygen supply, as might occur with redistribution of cardiac output during SIRS.

The three steps of gluconeogenesis that require alternate enzymatic pathways are the conversion of pyruvate to phosphoenolpyruvate, fructose-1,6-bisphosphate to fructose-6-phosphate, and glucose-6-phosphate to glucose. Of these, the conversion of pyruvate to phosphoenolpyruvate is the most pertinent. This is a multistep, multicompartment reaction in which pyruvate is first converted into oxaloacetate by pyruvate carboxylase and then to phosphoenolpyruvate by phosphoenolpyruvate carboxykinase (PEPCK). This series requires both cytoplasmic and mitochondrial steps and is strongly influenced by the redox potential of the cell. In addition, the maximal rate of gluconeogenesis is regulated by the relative abundance of PEPCK. This enzyme is transcriptionally regulated and shows large fluctuations in abundance in response to nutritional state (ie, it is induced by starvation). Most significantly, PEPCK levels are suppressed in SIRS-related animal models as a result of the hepatocytes becoming refractory to stimuli (eg, glucagon) that normally induce the PEPCK gene.

Lipids

The major sites of lipid storage in the body are as triacylglycerols in adipose tissue and in circulating lipoproteins and chylomicrons. Mobilization of fatty acids from these sources is discussed later (see Metabolic Regulation). Free fatty acids released from adipose tissue are transported in the blood bound to protein, especially serum albumin. Because of their hydrophobic nature, free fatty acids readily enter cells in peripheral tissue. Once intracellular, the fatty acids can be reesterified to form either triacylglycerol or phospholipids, or they can be catabolized by β-oxidation. For β-oxidation to occur, the fatty acids must first enter the mitochondria by a process that involves attachment of the fatty acid to acetyl-CoA to form cytoplasmic acyl-CoA; transfer of the fatty acid to carnitine to form acyl-carnitine, which is transported into the mitochondrion; and finally, transfer of the fatty acid back to intramitochondrial acetyl-CoA to form acyl-CoA once again. The transport from the acyl-carnitine carrier is the rate-limiting step in the entrance into β-oxidation; however, as discussed later, the entry of the acetyl-CoA that is produced during β-oxidation into the Krebs cycle can constitute another important regulatory step in the complete oxidation of fatty acids versus the generation of ketones. Regulation of the rate of transport of the acyl-carnitine also contributes to the regulation of fatty acid synthesis under anabolic conditions. The first intermediate formed in the conversion of glucose to fatty acid is malonyl CoA. Malonyl CoA is an inhibitor of the acyl-carnitine transferase and thus inhibits the entry of fatty acids into the catabolic pathway during periods of fat synthesis when glucose abundance exceeds the needs of energy metabolism and glycogen synthesis.

Conceptually, β-oxidation can be considered to be a series of passages through a pathway that removes the CoA with the two adjoining carbons (α and β) to form acetyl-CoA and adds another CoA to the remnant fatty acid to form an acyl-CoA that is shorter by two carbons. This process continues until the final two-carbon remnant forms acetyl-CoA. Thus, 1 mol of a 16-carbon fatty acid, such as palmitate, yields 8 mol of acetyl-CoA that can enter the Krebs cycle. In the process of oxidizing the fatty acid to release acetyl-CoA, each cycle through β-oxidation reduces 1 mol of FAD to FADH$_2$ and 1 mol of NAD to NADH. As described earlier, these reducing equivalents can then donate their electrons to the mitochondrial electron transport chain to provide the energy for synthesis of 2 (FADH$_2$) or 3 (NADH) mol of ATP. In addition, each mole of acetyl-CoA can then generate another 3 mol of NADH, 1 mol of FADH$_2$, and one substrate-level phosphorylation (GTP), which can be converted to ATP. Two concepts can be derived from these calculations. First, complete oxidation of a fatty acid is potentially a rich source of energy. Oxidation of 1 mol of palmitate can yield 131 mol of ATP. Second, with the exception of the 1 mol of GTP per acetyl-CoA (16 mol of GTP per palmitate), all ATP production has a direct requirement for O_2 as an electron acceptor. Even the generation of GTP proximately requires O_2 to maintain the Krebs cycle operational. Thus, energy generation from fatty acids absolutely requires a continues supply of oxygen.

Ketogenesis

Entry of acetyl-CoA produced by β-oxidation into the Krebs cycle is regulated primarily by the availability of oxaloacetate for the formation of citric acid. As discussed earlier, the intermediates of the Krebs cycle are not fixed in a cyclic conformation, nor are their levels constant. These intermediates are shared by multiple pathways. As such, the intramitochondrial levels of these intermediates may fluctuate substantially, depending on the metabolic state of the cell. In addition to being vital to the Krebs cycle, oxaloacetate is a component of the gluconeogenic pathway. As a result, when hepatic gluconeogenesis is stimulated, such as during fasting (or in uncontrolled diabetes), mitochondrial oxaloacetate is depleted, resulting in inhibition of entry of acetyl-CoA into the Krebs cycle. In such cases, the acetyl-CoA formed in β-oxidation takes an alternate pathway to form ketone bodies. In two successive steps, three acetyl-CoA molecules are condensed to form acetoacetyl-CoA and then β-hydroxy-β-methylglutatryl-CoA. One molecule of acetyl-CoA is then released, leaving acetoacetate. Acetoacetate can be further metabolized to acetone plus CO_2. Excretion of acetone by the lungs gives the characteristic ketone breath. Acetoacetate also is readily reduced using NADH as the cofactor for reducing equivalents to form β-hydroxy butyrate. This reaction is readily reversible, and the equilibrium between acetoacetate and β-hydroxy butyrate is determined by the ratio of NAD to NADH, such that β-OH butyrate/acetoacetate $\propto$ NADH/NAD.

The ketone bodies are freely released from the liver and can be transported through the blood to other tissues, such as heart, muscle, and brain, that can use them as fuel for oxidative metabolism. In addition, the relative levels (ratio) of acetoacetate and β-hydroxy butyrate in arterial blood have been found to correlate with their levels in the liver. Because these ketone bodies are in equilibrium with the NAD/NADH ratio in the liver where they are formed, it has been proposed that the ratio of the arterial ketone bodies (typically abbreviated AKBR) can be used to estimate the redox potential of the liver.[3] This technique has been used both experimentally[3–5] and clinically[6] to estimate hepatic redox potential as an indicator of hepatic ischemia. Although it is well documented that hypoxia (ie, shortage of the ultimate electron acceptor in the mitochondrial electron transport chain) results in an accumulation of NADH and a depletion of NAD, many other factors can contribute to this balance, making the reliability of the arterial ketone body ratio of questionable value as a quantitative tool in determining level of hepatic oxygenation. Nevertheless, a number of both laboratory and clinical studies have shown good predictive value for this parameter with respect to outcome in a critical care setting.

Proteins and Amino Acids

Unlike carbohydrates and fats, there is no pure storage form for amino acids. On the other hand, the potential pool of amino acids that can be mobilized from proteins in all cells of the body is extensive. Similar to the manner in which dietary protein is made available for metabolism by the proteolytic action of specific proteases in the small intestine, cellular protein can also be degraded, resulting in the release of small peptides and, ultimately, individual amino acids. Turnover of cellular protein is constantly occurring under normal conditions and is an essential mechanism for cellular homeostasis. Not only is proteolysis necessary for the removal of damaged tissues or cellular components, but it is also important for the regulation of the level of activity of key enzymes that, because of their very short half lives and absence of significant allosteric regulation, can have their cellular activity regulated by rate of new protein synthesis. The longevity of the protein in the cell is determined by its susceptibility to proteolytic degradation.

Once a protein is reduced to its individual amino acids, these amino acids can be used as building blocks to synthesize new protein, or they can be further catabolized to provide energy. Unlike the catabolic pathways for the carbohydrates and fats, which are relatively few in number, the diverse structure of the amino acids requires many different pathways for catabolism. Despite this extreme diversity in the early steps of catabolism, eventually all of the amino acids feed into the Krebs cycle. A detailed presentation of the pathways that individual amino acids take in preparation for entry into the Krebs cycle is beyond the scope of this text; however, the amino acids can be grouped according to the sites at which they enter the Krebs cycle. This is of primary importance because of the differentiation between amino acids that can serve as precursors for gluconeogenesis as an alternative to immediate oxidation and those that give rise to ketones.

Irrespective of the amino acid, the first step in catabolism is to remove the amino group. This is accomplished by transamination reactions in which the amino group is transferred to an α-keto acid to form alanine, glutamate, or aspartate. Although this may appear to be futile cycling, these amino acids can then transfer the amino group as ammonia into the urea cycle in the liver. In humans, the urea cycle is the primary mechanism for excretion of nitrogen. In this process, called the *alanine cycle*, amino acids to be catabolized transfer their amino group to

α-ketoglutarate to form glutamate. Glutamate then transfers its amino group to pyruvate to form alanine and regenerate α-ketoglutarate. The advantage of this two-step process is that it preserves cellular α-ketoglutarate, while pyruvate is constantly supplied as the end product of glycolysis. The alanine is then released from the cell and is taken up by the liver. In the liver, the amino is transferred back to α-ketoglutarate to form glutamate and pyruvate. Finally, the amino group is transferred into the urea cycle, and the pyruvate becomes a substrate for gluconeogenesis. The glucose returns to the skeletal muscle cell to provide substrate for glycolysis and completes the cycle. In this manner, the nitrogen removed during catabolism of amino acids in all peripheral tissues is transported to the liver, which is the site of the only significant activity of the urea cycle.

The urea cycle receives 2 mol of ammonia (1 mol from either glutamate or glutamine and 1 mol from aspartate) and one carbon from HCO_3 to form urea, which is then released from the liver and is excreted in the urine. To accomplish this synthesis, the hepatocyte uses substrates from both the mitochondria and cytoplasm and expends energy in the form of 3 mol of ATP, which are converted to 2 mol of ADP and 1 mol of AMP. As described earlier with respect to the intermediates of the Krebs cycle, the intermediates of the urea cycle are shared with other pathways. The most notable of these pathways are the Krebs cycle, gluconeogenesis, and nitric oxide synthase, although the possibility that separate intracellular substrate pools might exist has been suggested. These overlaps in intermediates can result in competition between pathways because of a relative shortage of key intermediates. This competition has been shown to limit the rate of gluconeogenesis from amino acids in animal models with peritonitis because entry of the amino acid–derived nitrogen is accelerated.[7,8]

Once an amino acid transfers its amino group, it undergoes a catabolic pathway that is unique for each amino acid; nevertheless, the end products are more limited. Essentially, the amino acids are funneled into acetyl-CoA, pyruvate, or one of the intermediates of the Krebs cycle.

METABOLIC REGULATION

Many interrelated factors regulate flux through the metabolic pathways described earlier. In general terms, these can be grouped into the following categories: substrate levels, allosteric regulators, hormonal regulators, and changes in the levels of regulatory enzymes. Alternatively, regulation can be considered in terms of the time scale of regulation. The effects of substrate levels and allosteric regulators are exerted over a course of seconds to minutes. Some of the effects of hormonal regulation are also expressed in this short time frame. On the other hand, regulation can also occur by means of a more fundamental remodeling of the responsiveness of the cells by changing the levels of key proteins in the cell. These proteins may be enzymes, signaling factors (eg, adenylate cyclase or G proteins, channels, transcription factors), or even structural components. Because these responses require the transcription, translation, and posttranslational processing of new proteins, the time course of expression is longer than 30 minutes. Moreover, these changes may lead to chronic remodeling of the responsiveness of the cell. As such, the discussion of regulation presented here is considered in terms of acute and chronic mechanisms that alter the metabolic response and responsiveness of the cell. These two cannot really be separated because in vivo response consists of acute regulation superimposed on a variable underlying level of responsiveness determined by chronic regulation.

For purposes of this discussion, acute response is considered to comprise the moment-to-moment regulation of rates of the various metabolic pathways. This section first summarizes the mechanisms responsible for acute regulation of metabolism under normal conditions and then addresses the changes that occur as a result of conditions related to SIRS. These changes are divided into two sections covering substrate and allosteric regulators and hormonal control. In both sections, the presentation is an overview with emphasis on mechanisms relevant to surgical stress.

Conceptually, substrate and allosteric control can be differentiated in that substrate level regulation depends on mass action (substrate/product ratio), while allosteric regulation allows rates of enzymatic processes to be regulated somewhat independent of actual substrate but tied to another important signal related to the pathway. An example of this is regulation of PFK by cellular levels of ATP. Since ATP is a substrate for PFK, one would predict based on substrate effects that elevated levels of ATP would increase the rate of the reaction. To the contrary, ATP binds to PFK at a regulatory site and decreases the affinity of the enzyme for its substrate fructose-6-phosphate. As a result, the activity of PFK is *inhibited* by ATP. Because PFK is the major rate-limiting step in glycolysis, this allosteric regulatory mechanism allows the rate of the entire pathway to be regulated by the levels of its ultimate end product. This is the basis of the Pasteur effect.

The most common incidence of unstressed regulation of metabolism by changes in substrate levels is in the fluctuations that occur as a result of nutritional intake. The mechanisms for the transition between storage and mobilization of energy as a function of transition from the fed to fasted state provide an overall paradigm for metabolic regulation. These mechanisms also serve as a useful backdrop for the discussion of alterations with the development of stress conditions and thus are presented in some detail.

In general terms, the transition from the fed to fasted state is one of a change from substrate storage to substrate production. In the fed state, free substrate levels (glucose, amino acids, and lipids) are relatively high as a result of intestinal absorption. As illustrated in Figure 5-1, the substrate levels of the postprandial state drive the pathways for synthesis of storage forms such as glycogen and triacyl glycerol. At the same time, high insulin levels relative to glucagon result in favoring the storage pathways and inhibiting the liberation of substrates from storage forms as well as de novo synthesis of glucose. In addition, in tissues such as skeletal muscle, in which glucose uptake is highly insulin dependent, high insulin levels result in enhanced uptake of glucose and flux through glycolysis. As a result, mitochondrial acetyl-CoA derived from pyruvate is plentiful, as is oxaloacetate. The result is a rise in levels of citrate, the precursor to cytoplasmic acetyl-CoA. This tends to drive fatty acid synthesis. Simultaneously, the generation of malonyl CoA, the first intermediate in fatty acid synthesis, inhibits transport of acyl-carnitine into the mitochondria. The end result is inhibition of fatty acid degradation. Finally, the abundance of glucose to feed into the pentose shunt provides the NADPH that is a necessary cofactor for fatty acid synthesis. The overall effect is an increase

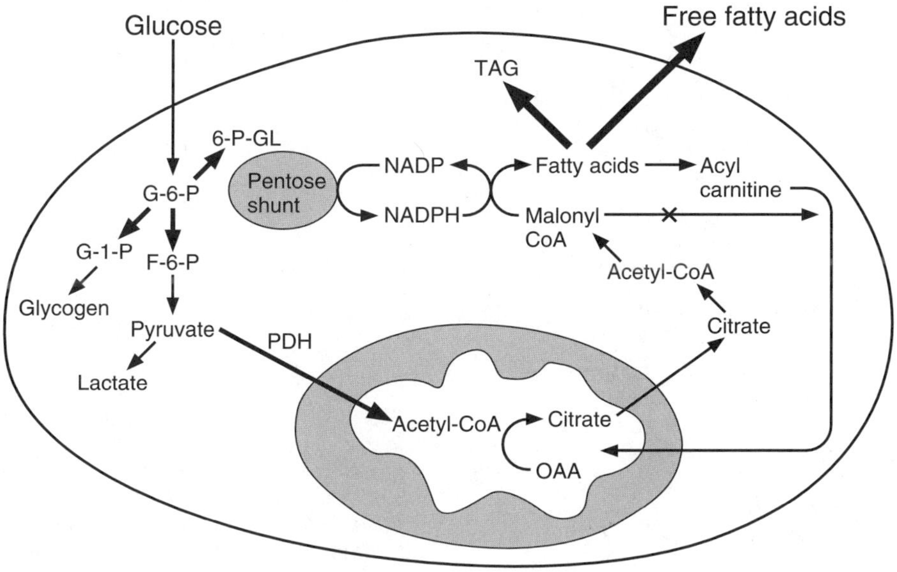

FIG. 5-1. Substrate interactions during the fed state. The diagram is representative of the response in most cell types. Triacylglycerol synthesis takes place largely in adipocytes. G-6-P, glucose-6-phosphate; G-1-P, glucose-1-phosphate; 6-P-GL, 6-phosphogluconolactone; TAG, triacylglycerol; PDH, pyruvate dehydrogenase; F-6-P, fructose-6-phosphate.

in the net synthesis of fatty acids. On an interorgan level, the increase in fatty acid synthesis in the liver is accompanied by inhibition of lipolysis and stimulation of lipogenesis in adipose tissue.

Amino acids also contribute to substrate storage (not depicted in Fig. 5-1). The amino acids that do not contribute directly to protein synthesis are catabolized and serve as substrate for fatty acid synthesis.

In the fasted state, substrate flow is reversed. Plasma glucose levels are decreased, and the availability of other substrates from dietary sources is eliminated. The response is to release substrates from storage depots. The first recourse for maintenance of plasma glucose is to liberate glucose from glycogen while at the same time shifting the fuel for oxidative metabolism from glucose to fatty acid and ketone bodies. De novo synthesis of glucose by means of gluconeogenesis is also increased. This shift is partly dependent on substrate availability but is strongly dependent on the shift in insulin/glucagon ratios. The high glucagon (and catecholamine) levels directly stimulate glycolysis, gluconeogenesis, and lipolysis. This effect is manifested in minutes as a result of alterations in the rates of substrate flux catalyzed by existing levels of enzymes. During prolonged starvation, glycogen stores become depleted, and gluconeogenesis remains the sole source for replenishing plasma glucose levels to provide the needs of glucose-dependent tissues such as the central nervous system and blood cells. In keeping with the increased demands for gluconeogenesis, chronic remodeling of the hepatocyte gluconeogenic capacity occurs through transcriptional induction of key enzymes in the gluconeogenic pathway. The most extensively studied of these is PEPCK. This enzyme, which is essential for bypassing the irreversible conversion of phosphoenolpyruvate to pyruvate, can constitute a rate-limiting step in gluconeogenesis. Induction of this enzyme is glucagon dependent, but unlike the acute stimulation of glycogenolysis and gluconeogenesis that occurs in minutes early in starvation, enzyme induction has a lag time of at least 1 hour. This mechanism is also of particular interest because it has been identified as a negatively regulated stress protein (see later).

Induction of gluconeogenesis has implications for the handling of fatty acids that provide a substantially higher portion of the substrate for oxidative metabolism during prolonged fasting. As shown in Figure 5-2, oxaloacetate is an important precursor to glucose in gluconeogenesis. With accelerated gluconeogenesis, oxaloacetate is depleted. Because acetyl-CoA entry into the Krebs cycle occurs in combination with oxaloacetate, the acetyl-CoA is unable to enter and is shunted into the formation of acetoacetate and acetate, giving rise to ketosis.

EFFECT OF INFLAMMATORY STRESS ON THE METABOLIC RESPONSE

In many ways, the effect of inflammatory stress can be considered to be a set of specific disturbances of the response to prolonged fasting. Essentially, all of the hormonal regulators of the response to fasting are present, but the response of the organism is modified by the superimposition of the effects of inflammatory mediators such as the cytokines. These alterations are exerted both acutely (eg, through elevated catecholamines) and chronically through remodeling of the underlying responsiveness. In addition to changes related to energy production or storage, the induction of significant oxidative stress during an inflammatory response imposes additional burdens on the metabolic machinery to support pathways that protect against oxidative damage.[9] Finally, there is evidence that oxidative stress directly influences the expression of specific programs of stress-related proteins and peptides by activation of key transcription factors such as NFKB.[2] These responses are discussed in the context of their relevance to the metabolic response.

As described earlier, the most notable component of the change in metabolic response in the transition from fed to fasting is the making available of substrates from storage sites and the maintenance of plasma glucose by glycogenolysis and gluconeogenesis. Surgical stress, with its attendant inflammatory (cytokine) response, can profoundly alter both the use and availability of substrates.

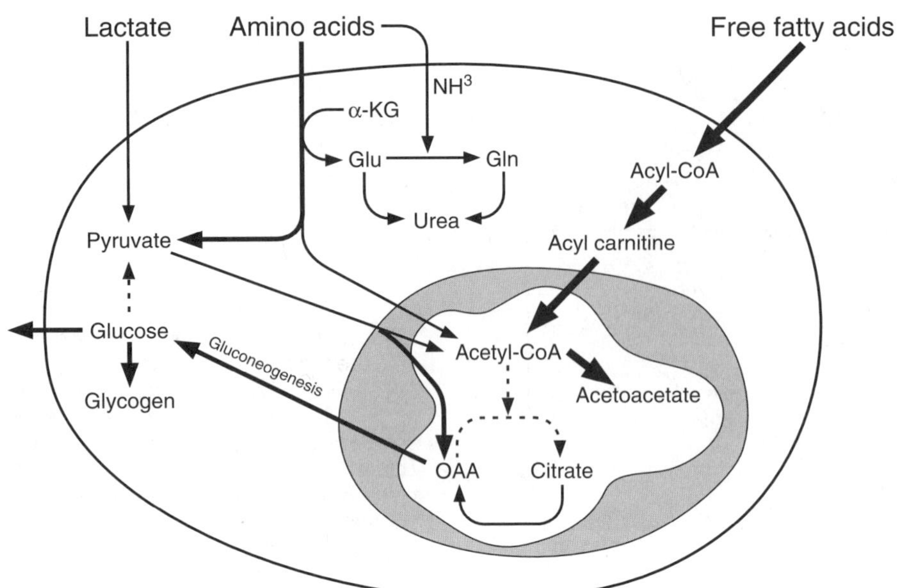

FIG. 5-2. Substrate interactions in the fasted state. These reactions take place primarily in hepatocytes to provide a constant source of plasma glucose. α-KG, α-ketoglutarate; Glu, glutamate; Gln, glutamine; OAA, oxaloacetate.

Carbohydrates

In general, SIRS without the development of hypodynamic shock results in a substantial increase in glucose use as well as in absolute rates of gluconeogenesis.[10] Although this response has classically been considered in terms of increased glucose use by tissue parenchymal cells, it is now realized that the response is more complex. In simplistic terms, the gross increase in glucose turnover can be considered to be the result of two factors. First, an increase in rates of glycolytic flux in parenchymal cells[11,12] results in lactic acid as an end product. Second, there is a dramatic increase in glucose use by activated inflammatory cells, such as macrophages and neutrophils, and most likely also by vascular endothelial cells.[13]

The increase in glucose consumption resulting in lactate release has long been considered to be evidence of tissue hypoxia despite the fact that increased glucose turnover is often observed in the presence of elevated cardiac output. The association of increased lactate production with narrowing of arteriovenous oxygen contents has led to the alternative suggestion that fundamental cellular changes occur, resulting in an impairment of the cell's ability to use oxygen. It is likely that both mechanism contribute. Studies of microvascular perfusion of tissues during systemic inflammatory states indicate that the development of microvascular heterogeneity contributes to the appearance of microregional ischemia despite adequate or even luxurious whole organ perfusion.[14–16] This appears to suggest that narrowed arteriovenous oxygen gradients are the result of flow–demand mismatch and that lactate release is from the ischemic tissue. On the other hand, the elusive mechanism for a putative defect in the ability of cells to consume oxygen has begun to be elucidated. This mechanism is related to the induction of the inducible form of nitric oxide synthase during inflammatory states. This enzyme is responsible for the profuse and poorly regulated production of nitric oxide in response to inflammation. Nitric oxide, or more likely, the product of its reaction with superoxide, peroxynitrite, has been shown to impair the mitochondrial respiratory chain directly[17] and to inhibit the

Krebs cycle enzyme aconitase,[18] which catalyzes the conversion of citrate to isocitrate. The end results are decreased substrate flux through the Krebs cycle and an impaired ability to convert any reducing equivalents (NADH) formed by other pathways into energy conserved as ATP. The implications for alterations in substrate balance are the same as those for hypoxia. Indeed, this mechanism has been suggested for the altered ketone body ratio seen in hyperdynamic SIRS. The net effect is an increase in the dependence on anaerobic glycolysis, with increased lactate production and recycling by gluconeogenesis in the Cori cycle (see earlier).

The mechanisms controlling glucose use in cells other than the parenchymal cells of the tissues (eg, blood cells, macrophages, endothelial cells) are substantially different. For sake of this discussion, cells are grouped into two classes: (1) phagocytes, which are oxidant generators, and (2) targets of oxidative stress. In both cases, a significant portion of excess glucose consumption supports generation of NADPH by means of flux through the pentose shunt.

In the case of phagocytic cells, inflammatory activation results in stimulation of oxidative burst. In these cells, the primary source of oxidants is generation by the membrane-associated NADPH oxidase system. This enzyme complex uses NADPH as a cofactor to donate an electron to oxygen to form the superoxide anion. Ideally, generation of superoxide is restricted to secretion into a phagosome that contains an invading microorganism. The result is bacterial killing. In the process, NADPH is used and must be regenerated through the pentose shunt.[19] In this case, oxygen consumption, which is dramatically increased, is not primarily related to mitochondrial respiration but rather to superoxide generation using NADPH as the electron donor.

In addition to its importance for providing unpaired electrons for superoxide generation, NADPH is an essential component of antioxidant defense mechanisms.[20] This role is mediated by the contribution of NADPH to the regeneration of reduced glutathione by the enzyme glutathione reductase.[9] Glutathione is a tripeptide with an exposed sulfhydryl group on a cysteine.

Reduced glutathione can serve as an important antioxidant defense by virtue of its reaction with hydrogen peroxide catalyzed by glutathione peroxidase. In this reaction, 2 mol of glutathione combine with hydrogen peroxide to form an oxidized glutathione complex, in which the 2 mol of glutathione are linked by a disulfide bond and water. Although this reaction is effective in detoxifying hydrogen peroxide, the energy cost of the system would be prohibitive if it were necessary to synthesize reduced glutathione de novo to replace that which is consumed as a substrate for glutathione peroxidase. The reduced form can be regenerated, however, through the action of glutathione reductase, using NADPH as the source of reducing equivalents. This requires increased flux through the pentose shunt.[21] Note that all three enzymes involved in this antioxidant defense mechanism (glutathione peroxidase, glutathione reductase, and glucose-6-phosphate dehydrogenase, which controls entry of glucose-6-phosphate into the pentose shunt) are transcriptionally induced in response to oxidative stress.

To supply the increased needs of glucose consumption in the face of glycogen depletion with a prolonged inflammatory response, gluconeogenesis must be stimulated. Indeed, absolute rates of gluconeogenesis in vivo are accelerated during the hyperdynamic shock.[10,22,23] This is largely due to the increase in substrate availability and to a hormonal milieu that favors gluconeogenesis.[12,24] As such, with the ready availability of intravenous glucose solutions, a primary importance of gluconeogenesis in a patient in the intensive care unit is likely to be removal of gluconeogenic substrates such as lactate and amino acids. Even though the absolute rates of gluconeogenesis are accelerated, substantial evidence suggests that the liver's maximal capacity for glucose production is impaired even in the relatively early stages of infection and transiently as a result of relatively mild surgical stress.[1,25] Progressive impairment of gluconeogenesis eventually leads to the intractable hypoglycemia that typically accompanies hypodynamic septic shock.[26]

Proteins

Although accelerated proteolysis with wasting of lean body mass is typical of prolonged starvation, it is suppressed by feeding. In contrast, a prolonged stress response results in extensive proteolysis that is not readily suppressible by dietary supplement. This profound, intractable proteolytic response, which results in severe negative nitrogen balance, has been referred to as *septic autocannibalism*.[27] This response appears to be largely dependent on elevation of cytokines, especially interleukin-1.[28–31] This response makes available elevated levels of free amino acids, which can serve as substrates for gluconeogenesis or, particularly in the case of glutamine and branched-chain amino acids, can serve directly as fuel for energy production in specific tissues.

Lipids

During unstressed fasting, lipids become an extremely important source of energy production. The energy yield from oxidative metabolism is substantially greater than the yield from metabolism of either glucose or amino acids. On the other hand, energy production from fat absolutely requires oxidative metabolism. As discussed earlier, there is evidence that effective tissue perfusion is impaired in stress conditions even when cardiac output is normal or even elevated. In such situations, relatively ischemic tissues are not capable of effectively using fat for fuel.

In addition to the potential problems of hypoxic tissue using fat, the balance between storage and mobilization of fat from storage forms is impaired during surgical stress. Mobilization is impaired in two ways. First, there is substantial experimental evidence to suggest that hormonal activation of adipocyte lipase is impaired by inflammatory stress.[32] Although the exact mechanism of this response has not been completely elucidated, it is most likely the result of remodeling of signal transduction pathways.[32] Whatever the mechanism, the result is a blunted response to hormonal activation of liberation of free fatty acids from triacyl glycerol in adipose tissue.

Second, at the same time that liberation of fatty acids from adipose tissue is suppressed, mobilization from circulating lipoproteins through the action of lipoprotein lipase is also suppressed. This suppression of lipoprotein lipase is a well-recognized action of tumor necrosis factor.[33] The end result is an overall impairment of mobilization of fatty acids from storage forms and thus limited availability for metabolism. This limitation in fat availability leads to increased dependence on other substrates, such as amino acids, for energy production.

REFERENCES

1. Clemens MG, Chaudry IH, McDermott PH, et al. Regulation of glucose production from lactate in experimental sepsis. Am J Physiol 1983; 244:R794.
2. Pahl HL, Baeuerle PA. Oxygen and the control of gene expression. Bioessays 1994;16:497.
3. Tanaka J, Ozawa K, Tobe T. Significance of blood ketone body ratio as an indicator of hepatic cellular energy status in jaundiced rabbits. Gastroenterology 1979;76:691.
4. Yamamoto M, Tanaka J, Ozawa K, et al. Significance of acetoacetate/B-hydroxybutyrate ratio in arterial blood as an indicator of the severity of hemorrhagic shock. J Surg Res 1980;28:124.
5. Hirai F, Aoyama H, Ohtoshi M, et al. Significance of mitochondrial enhancement in hepatic energy-metabolism in relation to alterations in hemodynamics in septic pigs with severe peritonitis. Eur Surg Res 1984;16:148.
6. Ozawa K, Kamlyama Y, Kimura K, et al. Contribution of the arterial blood ketone body ratio to elevate plasma amino acids in hepatic encephalopathy of surgical patients. Am J Surg 1983;146:299.
7. Ohtake Y, Clemens MG. Interrelationship between hepatic ureagenesis and gluconeogenesis in early sepsis. Am J Physiol 1991;260:E453.
8. Paidas CN, Clemens MG. Hormone effects on hepatic substrate preference in sepsis. Shock 1994;2:94.
9. Yu BP. Cellular defenses against damage from reactive oxygen species. Physiol Rev 1996;74:139.
10. Long CL, Kinney JM, Geiger JW. Nonsuppressability of gluconeogenesis by glucose in septic patients. Metabolism 1976;25:193.
11. Lang CH, Bagby GJ, Bornside GH, et al. Sustained hypermetabolic sepsis in rats: characterization of the model. J Surg Res 1983;35:201.
12. Lang C, Bagby GJ, Spitzer JJ. Carbohydrate dynamics in the hypermetabolic septic rat. Metabolism 1984;33:959.
13. Meszaros K, Bojta J, Bautista AP, et al. Glucose utilization by Kupffer cells, endothelial cells, and granulocytes in endotoxemic rat liver. Am J Physiol 1991;260:G7.
14. Bauer M, Zhang JX, Bauer I, et al. Endothelin-1 induced alterations of hepatic microcirculation: sinusoidal and extrasinusoidal sites of action. Am J Physiol 1994;267:G143.
15. Clemens MG, Bauer M, Gingalewski C, et al. Heterogeneity of hepatocellular response: role of intercellular communication. In: Faist E, Schildberg F, Baue A, eds. Host defense dysfunction in trauma, shock and sepsis, ed 2. Berlin, Springer Verlag, 1994.

16. Clemens MG, Bauer M, Gingalewski C, et al. Hepatic intercellular communication in shock and inflammation. Shock 1994;2:1.
17. Radi R, Rodriquez M, Castro L, et al. Inhibition of mitochondrial electron transport by peroxynitrite. Arch Biochem Biophys 1994;308:89.
18. Hausladen A, Fridovich I. Superoxide and peroxynitrite inactivate aconitases but nitric oxide does not. J Biol Chem 1996;269:29405.
19. Spolarics Z, Bautista AP, Spitzer JJ. Primed pentose cycle activity supports production and elimination of superoxide anion in Kupffer cells from rats treated with endotoxin in vivo. Biochim Biophys Acta 1993;1179:134.
20. Spolarics Z, Spitzer JJ. Augmented glucose use and pentose shunt activity in hepatic endothelial cells after in vivo endotoxemia. Hepatology 1996;17:615.
21. Spolarics Z, Novarro L. Endotoxin stimulates the expression of glucose-6-phosphate dehydrogenase in Kupffer and hepatic endothelial cells. J Leukocyte Biol 1994;56:453.
22. Gump FE, Long CL, Geiger JW, et al. The significance of altered gluconeogenesis in surgical catabolism. J Trauma 1975;15:704.
23. Gump FE, Long C, Killian P, et al. Studies of glucose intolerance in septic injured Patients. J Trauma 1974;14:378.
24. Lang CH, Bagby GJ, Spitzer JJ. Glucose kinetics and body temperature after lethal and nonlethal doses of endotoxin. Am J Physiol 1985;248:R471.
25. Clemens MG, Chaudry IH, Daigneau N, et al. Insulin resistance and depressed gluconeogenic capability during early hyperglycemic sepsis. J Trauma 1984;24:701.
26. Filkins JP, Cornell RP. Depression of hepatic gluconeogenesis and the hypoglycemia of endotoxin shock. Am J Physiol 1974;227:778.
27. Cerra FB, Siegel JH, Coleman B, et al. Septic autocannibalism: a failure of exogenous nutritional support. Ann Surg 1980;192:570.
28. Clowes GHA Jr, George BC, Villee CA Jr, et al. Muscle proteolysis induced by a circulating peptide in patients with sepsis or trauma. N Engl J Med 1983;308:545.
29. Jeevanandam M, Horowitz GD, Lowry SF, et al. Cancer cachexia and protein metabolism. Lancet 1984;1(8392):1423.
30. Yang RD, Moldawer LL, Sakamoto A, et al. Leukoycte endogenous mediator alters protein dynamics in rats. Metabolism 1983;32:654.
31. Hasselgren PO, Pederson P, Sax HC, et al. Current concepts of protein turnover and amino acid transport in liver and skeletal muscle during sepsis. Arch Surg 1988;123:992.
32. Nelson KM, Spitzer JA. Alteration of adipocyte calcium homeostasis by Escherichia coli endotoxin. Am J Physiol 1985;248:R331.
33. Price SR, Olivecrona T, Pekala PH. Regulation of lipoprotein lipase synthesis by recombinant tumor necrosis factor: the primary regulatory role of the hormone 3T3-L1 adipocytes. Arch Biochem Biophys 1986;251:738.

Surgery of Infants and Children: Scientific Principles and Practice, edited by Keith T. Oldham, Paul M. Colombani, and Robert P. Foglia. Lippincott–Raven Publishers, Philadelphia, © 1997.

CHAPTER 6

Renal Physiology and Pathophysiology

John Foreman, Delbert Wigfall, and Charles McKay

RENAL PHYSIOLOGY

Renal Blood Flow and Glomerular Filtration

The major role of the kidney is to maintain body water and electrolyte homeostasis. This homeostasis is dependent on the formation of an ultrafiltrate of the plasma and the subsequent reabsorption of the bulk of the water and solute by a complex series of interactions along the nephron. These interactions have led to the segmentation of the nephron on both a functional and a histologic basis (Fig. 6-1).

The first step in water and solute homeostasis by the kidney is the production of the glomerular filtrate from the renal plasma.[1] The glomerular filtration rate (GFR) is dependent on renal plasma flow, which in turn is dependent on blood pressure and circulating volume. The kidneys receive about 20% to 30% of the cardiac output, and this is maintained over a wide range of blood pressures through changes in renal vascular resistance. Numerous hormones play a role in this autoregulation, including the vasodilators (prostaglandins E and I_2, dopamine, and endothelin-derived relaxing factor [nitric oxide]) and the vasoconstrictors (angiotensin II, thromboxane, adrenergic stimulation, and endothelin). Congestive heart failure and volume contraction severely limit the kidney's ability to maintain autoregulation in the face of changes in blood pressure.

In neonates, renal blood flow, adjusted for body surface area, doubles during the first 2 weeks of postnatal life and continues to rise until it reaches adult values by the age of 2 years.[2,3] This results from both an increase in cardiac output and a fall in renal vascular resistance. Paralleling these changes in renal blood flow, the GFR, adjusted for body surface area, also doubles over the first 2 weeks of postnatal life and continues to rise until it reaches adult values by the age of 1 to 2 years. The initial GFR and the rate of rise correlate directly with gestational age at birth, such that the GFR of an infant of 28 weeks' gestation is half that of a full-term infant.

At the level of the glomerular capillary, the GFR is dependent on the balance of the hydrostatic pressure forcing fluid through the capillary wall into Bowman's, space, the oncotic pressure from plasma proteins retarding this flow, the capillary surface area available for filtration, and the permeability of the capillary wall.[1] The net hydrostatic pressure is dependent on the intraglomerular capillary pressure and the pressure in Bowman's space. Autoregulation maintains intraglomerular capillary pressure over a wide range of systemic blood pressures, although this is blunted by volume contraction. The pressure in Bowman's space rarely plays a role in determining the GFR, except during some forms of acute renal failure (ARF) with tubular blockage by cellular debris and acute urinary tract obstruction. Changes in plasma oncotic pressure also have little influence on the GFR because these changes are counteracted by changes in the surface area available for filtration.

The whole-kidney GFR is the sum of the GFR of each nephron, of which humans have about 1 million in each kidney. The formation of these nephrons is complete by 36 weeks of gestational age. Individual nephrons can alter their GFR in response to several stimuli, including protein loading and nephron loss. In healthy individuals, the GFR can increase by 50% after a large protein meal. Renal donors can increase the GFR in their remaining kidney such that the average donor has a GFR that is 70% of the preoperative value. Children with congenital absence of a kidney have a more marked increase in the size and GFR of the remaining kidney after birth, such that their GFR is comparable to that of their peers with two kidneys. However, clinically apparent changes in the GFR are not seen with renal disease until 70% of the nephrons are damaged because the unaffected nephrons increase their individual GFR.

The GFR is measured by determining the clearance of a solute that is freely filtered, not protein bound, and not secreted or reabsorbed by the tubule. The "gold standard" for GFR measurements has been inulin, but handling and measuring inulin levels is laborious and difficult, limiting the use of inulin clearance measurements to research studies. Creatinine clearance measurements traditionally have been used to approximate the GFR because there is no need for an intravenous infusion and creatinine can be measured in any hospital laboratory. However, creatinine is secreted into the urine, so creatinine clearance levels are about 20% higher than inulin clearance levels. This percent "error" increases as the GFR falls. Creatinine clearance measurements also necessitate accurate urine collection, which is not easily done in young children and adds another source of potential error. The variation in repeated serum creatinine measurements, especially when done by the Jaffé method, is

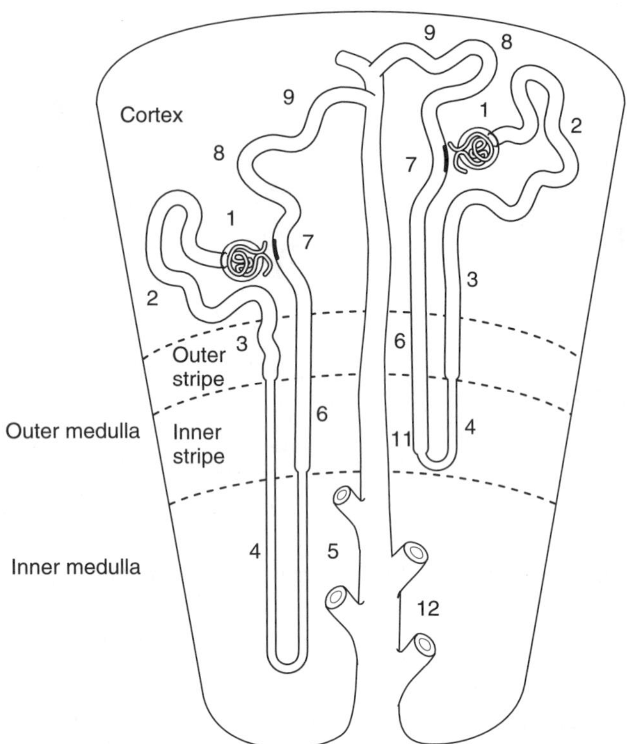

FIG. 6-1. Structure of the nephron. Long- and short-loop nephrons are shown with the following segments: (1) glomerulus, (2) proximal convoluted tubule, (3) proximal straight tubule, (4) descending thin limb, (5) ascending thin limb, (6) ascending thick limb, (7) macula densa, (8) distal convoluted tubule, (9) connecting tubule, (10) cortical collecting duct, (11) outer medullary collecting duct, and (12) inner medullary collecting duct. (After Kriz W, Bankir L. A standard nomenclature for structures of the kidney. The Renal Commission of the International Union of Physiological Sciences (IUPS). Am J Physiol 1988;254:F1.)

0.2 mg/dL, which adds another significant source of error to this approach. This is especially true for young children, whose serum creatinine levels are less than 0.6 mg/dL. An estimate of creatinine clearance can be made from the serum creatinine level and the height, according to the following formula:[4,5]

$$\text{creatinine clearance (mL/min/1.73 m}^2) = \frac{\text{height (cm)} \times \text{k}}{\text{serum creatinine}}$$

where: k = 0.55 for children and 0.45 for infants

Although simple to perform, this formula gives only an approximation of the GFR.

Radionuclides, such as diethylenetriamine pentaacetic acid (DTPA), can be used to measure the GFR accurately and easily. DTPA is freely filtered by the glomerulus and not reabsorbed or secreted by the renal tubule, making it an ideal substance for GFR measurements. One method is to inject a single dose of the radionuclide and plot the fall in radioactivity with timed blood samples. The decline in radioactivity is proportional to the GFR. These GFR measurements also can be combined with renal imaging studies. The GFR in each kidney can be estimated by determining the radioactivity in each kidney over time. Although this method obviates the need for blood-drawing, it is not as accurate as the first method. The disadvantage of these studies is the necessary, albeit small, exposure to radioactivity. In place of a radionuclide, the disappearance of a single injection of radiocontrast material also has been used to measure the GFR, although this requires special instrumentation. The GFR also can be estimated from the constant infusion of a suitable material, such as inulin or iothalamate. If the plasma level is stable, then the GFR is equal to the infusion rate. Such methodology requires an accurate infusion pump and significant amounts of time to achieve a stable plasma level, although part of the infusion can be done at home with a portable pump.

Sodium Handling

One of the major roles of the kidney is to regulate total body sodium balance and maintain a normal extracellular and circulating volume.[6] The kidneys of a normal adult filter 25,000 mEq of sodium a day, yet excrete less than 1% through extremely efficient reabsorption mechanisms along the nephron. The driving force for most of this sodium reabsorption is the enzyme Na^+-K^+-adenosine triphosphatase (Na^+-K^+-ATPase) located on the basolateral membrane. This enzyme exchanges three intracellular sodium ions for two extracellular potassium ions using the energy from the hydrolysis of adenosine triphosphate (ATP). This exchange maintains a low (less than 20 mEq/L) intracellular sodium concentration and a negative intracellular-to-extracellular charge. These two forces provide energy to drive sodium ions from the lumen of the tubule into the tubular cell through numerous membrane transporters and channels. These sodium ions then are extruded from the cell, mainly by Na^+-K^+-ATPase, and move from the renal interstitial space into the peritubular capillary. Movement from the interstitial space into the capillary is dependent on the difference between the tissue and the capillary hydrostatic pressures and the capillary oncotic pressure, especially in the proximal tubule.

The proximal tubule reabsorbs 50% to 70% of the filtered sodium. Sodium enters the proximal tubule cell by the luminal membrane through two general types of transporters (Fig. 6-2). One of these cotransports organic solutes and phosphate, and the other exchanges intracellular hydrogen ion for sodium. Sodium exits the cell mainly through the Na^+-K^+-ATPase. The descending limb of the loop of Henle does not play a role in sodium balance, whereas the ascending limb, especially the thick portion, reabsorbs about 25% of the filtered sodium. The luminal entry step in this segment is by cotransport with one potassium and two chloride ions (Na^+-K^+-$2Cl^-$ pump; Fig. 6-3). The distal nephron accounts for 10% of overall sodium reabsorption by cotransport with chloride in the distal tubule and through sodium channels in the collecting duct (Fig. 6-4).

The kidney must be able to adapt to marked changes in sodium intake and defend against changes in extracellular volume. Several factors play a role in these adaptations. First, these changes must be recognized, and it is clear that alterations in both circulating volume and total extracellular volume are "sensed" by the body, although the exact location of all these sensors has not been determined. There is good evidence for sensors in the cardiac atria, carotid sinus, and kidney. There also may be intracranial sensors. Once changes in extracellular volume are recognized, several factors are set in motion to adjust urinary sodium excretion.

One of these factors is a change in the GFR. Increasing di-

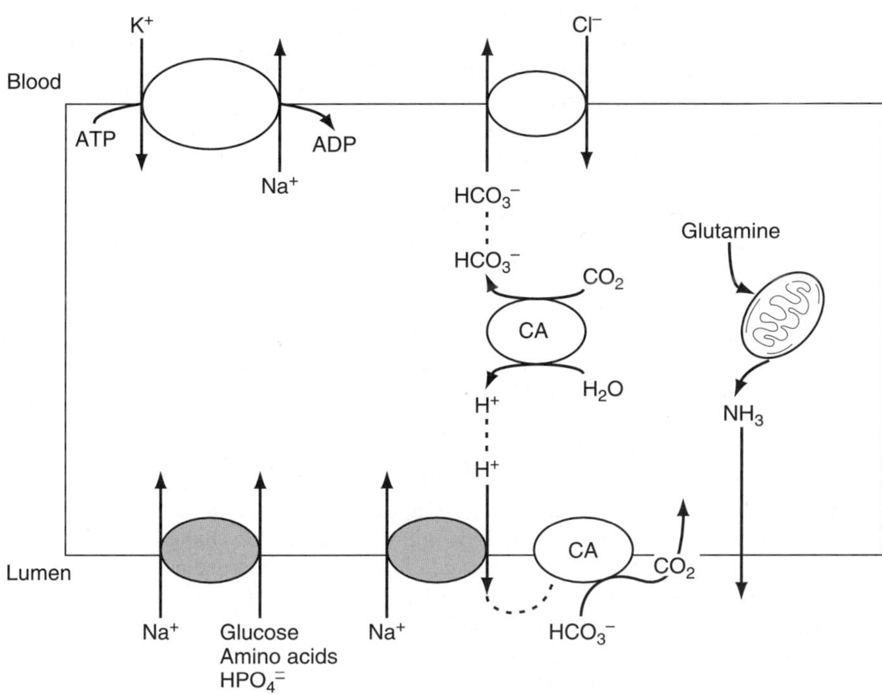

FIG. 6-2. Proximal tubule cell. Sodium enters the cell through cotransport with an organic solute such as glucose or an amino acid, or through exchange with H^+. Sodium exits the cell mainly through the Na^+-K^+-ATPase pump. H^+, formed from CO_2 and H_2O by cytosolic carbonic anhydrase (CA), is exchanged for luminal Na^+ and combines with luminal HCO_3^- to form H_2CO_3. This is rapidly decomposed to CO_2 and H_2O by luminal CA. The newly formed CO_2 enters the cell, where CA combines it with H_2O to form H_2CO_3, which decomposes to H^+ and HCO_3^-. The HCO_3^- exits the cell in exchange for Cl^-. The net result is the reclamation of the filtered HCO_3^-. The proximal tubule cell also generates NH_3 from amino acids, principally glutamine, that is later "trapped" in the cortical collecting duct as NH_4^+. ATP, adenosine triphosphate; ADP, adenosine diphosphate.

etary sodium intake or intravenous volume expansion increases the GFR, just as volume contraction decreases it. Volume contraction lowers the GFR by increasing renin release, both directly from the kidney and through the renal nerves. This in turn increases the angiotensin II level, which reduces the capillary surface area available for filtration and renal plasma flow. These changes are antagonized by prostaglandins released by the kidney. This reduction in the GFR decreases the filtered sodium load. Volume loading has the opposite effect. However, these changes in filtered load are blunted by changes in proximal

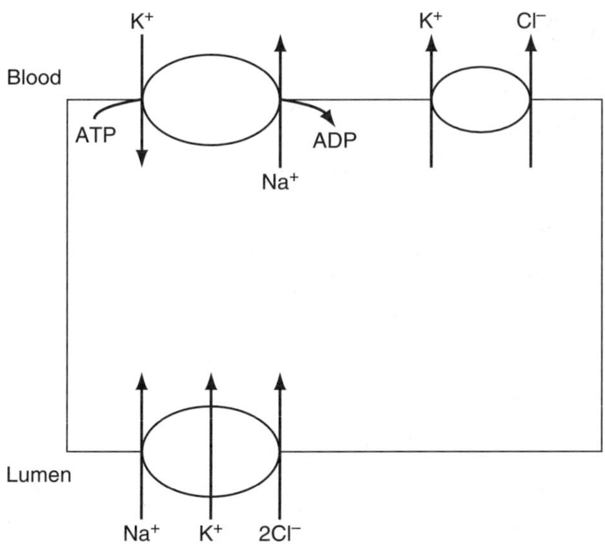

FIG. 6-3. Ascending limb of the loop of Henle. Sodium, potassium, and chloride are reabsorbed from the lumen through the Na^+-K^+-$2Cl^-$ pump. Sodium is pumped out of the cell by Na^+-K^+-ATPase. Potassium and chloride exit the cell through a cotransport pathway. ATP, adenosine triphosphate; ADP, adenosine diphosphate.

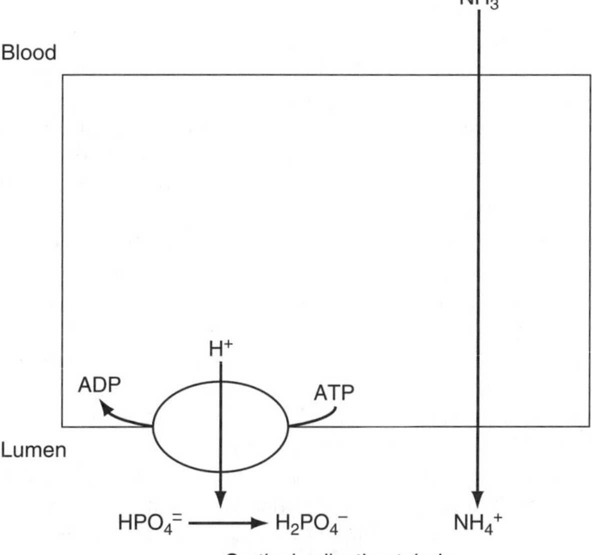

FIG. 6-4. Cortical collecting tubule. H^+ is pumped into the lumen through the H^+-ATPase pump. H^+ then can combine with $HPO_4^=$ (titratable acid) or NH_3, leading to net acid secretion. ADP, adenosine diphosphate; ATP, adenosine triphosphate.

tubule sodium reabsorption. This has been termed *glomerulotubular balance.*

Proximal tubule sodium reabsorption is regulated mainly by changes in peritubular capillary hydrostatic and oncotic pressure. Volume depletion leads to an increase in angiotensin II levels that constricts the glomerular arterioles, especially the efferent arteriole. This decreases renal perfusion pressure, renal plasma flow, and the GFR. Renal plasma flow is reduced more than the GFR, increasing the fraction of plasma filtered and the protein concentration of the plasma entering the peritubular capillaries. This increases the capillary oncotic pressure. This increase in capillary oncotic pressure and the decrease in capillary hydrostatic pressure promotes the movement of the reabsorbed sodium and water from the interstitial space into the capillary and increases luminal sodium reabsorption. Volume loading has the opposite effect.

In addition to the GFR and physical factors influencing proximal tubule reabsorption, two other factors, the renin–angiotensin–aldosterone system and atrial natriuretic peptide (ANP), play significant roles in regulating sodium excretion. Angiotensin II levels influence the GFR and proximal tubule capillary pressures. Angiotensin II also stimulates the release of aldosterone from the adrenal cortex, and this increases sodium uptake by the cortical collecting duct. ANP is released from the cardiac atria in response to changes in pressure and stretching. ANP increases the GFR by dilating the afferent glomerular arteriole and possibly increasing the capillary surface area available for filtration. ANP also inhibits sodium reabsorption in the inner medullary collecting duct.

The maximal increase in the GFR on changing from a low-sodium diet (10 mmol/d) to a high-sodium diet (600 mmol/d) would be from 100 to 150 mL/min, which would increase the filtered load of sodium by 10,000 mmol/d. However, glomerulotubular balance would limit the increase in excreted sodium to 60 mmol/d. Decreased renin production from the sodium loading, which in turn would limit angiotensin and aldosterone production, would increase sodium excretion by two-fold. Changes in peritubular physical factors would only increase sodium excretion by two-fold. Increased release of ANP, as a consequence of volume expansion from the high-sodium diet, would increase sodium excretion by 10-fold. Sodium balance is maintained by a combination of these four factors.

A precise understanding of the regulation of sodium balance in neonates is not clear. Neonates are born with expansion of the extracellular volume. This excess water and solute are excreted during the first week of life. Newborns also have higher circulating levels of renin, angiotensin II, aldosterone, and ANP compared with adults.[7] ANP may play a role in this physiologic neonatal diuresis and natriuresis as these levels decrease to normal levels with the diuresis. Maintenance of a high sodium intake will prevent this fall. However, in spite of these higher hormonal levels, neonates are less able to excrete a sodium load or to conserve sodium when compared with older children. This is especially true in premature infants. As a result, neonates are less able to respond to marked changes in dietary sodium intake or to defend against diarrheal losses.

Water Regulation

Serum osmolality is tightly regulated through changes in arginine vasopressin (AVP) release and the appreciation of thirst.[8]

AVP, also called *antidiuretic hormone,* is a nonapeptide synthesized in the neurons of the paraventricular and supraoptic regions of the anterior hypothalamus, and transported down their axons into the posterior pituitary, where it is stored and released. Separate cells, osmoreceptors, in the anterior hypothalamus are able to sense changes in plasma osmolality and signal the release of AVP and the sensation of thirst. Plasma osmolality below 280 mOsm/kg (the osmotic threshold) completely or nearly completely inhibits AVP secretion, allowing maximal free water excretion by the kidney. As the plasma osmolality rises above 280 mOsm/kg, AVP secretion rises nearly linearly, leading to an increasingly concentrated urine. As the plasma osmolality reaches 295 mOsm/kg, thirst is sensed. However, these changes in plasma osmolality affect AVP secretion only if they are caused by solutes with limited cellular permeability, such as sodium. Increased plasma osmolality from high levels of urea has little effect on AVP secretion.

AVP also is released in response to a fall in circulating volume or hypotension, although detectable changes in AVP secretion are not observed until the blood volume is reduced by 10% to 15%.[9] The rise of plasma AVP in response to circulating volume changes is exponential and can markedly exceed levels observed as a consequence of osmolality changes. Other stimuli also have been purported to release AVP. Nausea, even in the absence of vomiting, can markedly increase AVP release.[10] Less clear are the roles of stress and opiates. Early studies indicated that stress and noxious stimuli could release AVP. More recent studies do not support this concept when controlled for other factors, such as hypotension and nausea. Opiates in subemetic and hypotensive doses actually inhibit AVP release.

AVP decreases free water excretion by the kidney by increasing the water permeability of the collecting duct. Water movement out of the collecting duct is dependent on the establishment of a hypertonic interstitium in the medulla. This occurs through the unique arrangement of water and sodium transport in the loop of Henle. Isosmotic fluid enters the descending limb of the loop. This segment is permeant to water but not sodium, whereas the ascending limb is impermeant to water but actively pumps sodium into the interstitium. The active transport of sodium into the medullary interstitium increases its tonicity and abstracts water from the descending limb, concentrating the luminal sodium in this segment. Sodium then moves passively along its concentration gradient out of the ascending thin limb, adding to the medullary tonicity. This arrangement causes fluid entering the distal tubule to be hypotonic relative to the plasma. This hypotonic fluid then proceeds down the collecting duct, which is impermeant to water in the absence of AVP. With the binding of AVP to the basolateral membrane of the collecting duct, intracellular cyclic adenosine monophosphate is formed that results in an increase in luminal membrane permeability to water. Water then moves from the lumen through the cell and into the hypertonic interstitium, where it is removed by the vasa recta. This countercurrent mechanism elaborates both a hypotonic and a hypertonic urine. Hypokalemia, hypercalcemia, prostaglandins, lithium, and demeclocycline interfere with urinary concentrating ability.

The ability of neonates to conserve or excrete water is limited compared with older infants.[11] Full-term neonates can produce urine with an osmolality of 50 mOsm/kg, whereas premature infants can lower the osmolality to only 70 mOsm/kg. Despite these relatively low urine osmolalities, the excretion of a water load is prolonged, presumably because of the low GFR. Maximal urine-concentrating ability also is reduced, but reaches adult levels by 4 to 6 months of age. This can be hastened with protein loading, suggesting that some of the decreased concentrating ability is related to the low solute content of infant formula.

Potassium Regulation

In general, the kidney excretes about 10% to 15% of the filtered load of potassium, but under certain conditions, it can excrete more than the filtered load. The proximal tubule reabsorbs about 50% of the filtered potassium load through passive diffusion. Potassium is secreted into the descending limb of the loop of Henle from the medullary interstitium, which has a higher concentration. The ascending limb of the loop of Henle actively reabsorbs potassium from the lumen through the Na^+-K^+-$2Cl^-$ pump. This pump, which can be inhibited by loop diuretics, reduces the potassium content of the tubular fluid entering the distal tubule to 10% of the filtered load. The regulation of potassium excretion occurs in the cortical collecting duct. The principal cell of this nephron segment actively secretes potassium into the lumen, and this secretion is regulated by the intracellular potassium concentration and aldosterone. A potassium-rich diet raises the serum potassium level and enhances basolateral membrane Na^+-K^+-ATPase activity and principal cell uptake of potassium. This raises the intracellular concentration of potassium and promotes potassium movement into the lumen. Such a diet also stimulates aldosterone secretion, which stimulates Na^+-K^+-ATPase activity and increases the number of open channels in the luminal membrane for potassium to exit into the lumen. With decreased potassium intake, aldosterone secretion is inhibited and principal cells decrease or stop secreting potassium. Another, but much less numerous, cell type in the cortical collecting duct, the intercalated cell, continues to reabsorb potassium, leading to net potassium reabsorption. The medullary collecting duct passively reabsorbs a small amount of potassium, and this is the source of the potassium that is secreted into the descending limb of the loop of Henle.

Newborns are much less efficient at excreting potassium loads compared with adults.[12] The normal range of serum potassium concentrations is higher in newborns. This appears to be related, at least in part, to a decrease in secretion by the principal cell of the cortical collecting duct. Principal cells from newborn animals have fewer organelles, mitochondria, and plasma membrane surface area. Na^+-K^+-ATPase activity is decreased in newborns, although intracellular potassium concentrations are comparable to those of adults. This indicates that the decreased potassium secretion is related to a decrease in potassium permeability of the luminal membrane or a less favorable gradient for potassium movement into the lumen. The decreased potassium secretion is not related to decreased aldosterone secretion, because these levels are higher in newborns. The tubular response to aldosterone, however, is blunted. This appears to be related to a postreceptor phenomenon, because the receptor density is comparable to that of adults.

Renal Acid–Base Regulation

The kidney plays a major role in the day-to-day regulation of acid–base balance and the response to the stress of illness.

The initial role of the kidney is the reclamation of the 4000 mEq/d of bicarbonate that is filtered by the glomeruli. Eighty to 90% of this occurs in the proximal tubule, with the remaining bicarbonate absorbed in the collecting duct, such that the final urine is virtually free of bicarbonate under usual physiologic circumstances. Bicarbonate ion is reabsorbed through a series of steps involving the secretion of hydrogen ion (Fig. 6-5). In the proximal tubule, H^+ is exchanged for a luminal Na^+. This H^+ combines with filtered HCO_3^- to form H_2CO_3. This is rapidly converted into H_2O and CO_2 by carbonic anhydrase on the luminal membrane. The CO_2 easily traverses the luminal membrane and enters the cell, where it is recombined with H_2O to form H_2CO_3 by intracellular carbonic anhydrase. Carbonic acid rapidly decomposes into H^+ and HCO_3^-. The bicarbonate is exchanged for Cl^- across the basolateral membrane. The net effect is the movement of HCO_3^- from the lumen to the blood. A similar sequence of events occurs in the intercalated cells of the collecting duct, except that they lack carbonic anhydrase on the luminal surface. Therefore, the intraluminal breakdown of carbonic acid into CO_2 and H_2O is much slower and occurs to some extent in the lower urinary tract.

The next role of the kidney in acid–base balance is the formation of "new" bicarbonate to replace that lost in the neutralization of acid generated by the normal combustion of food, especially protein, and the formation of bone. New bicarbonate is generated within the cell from the decomposition of H_2CO_3 from H_2O and CO_2 by carbonic anhydrase, after which it enters the peritubular blood (see Fig. 6-5). The H^+ also generated from the decomposition of this H_2CO_3 is pumped into the lumen of the collecting duct, where it combines with urinary buffers, chiefly HPO_4^{2-} and NH_3.

Most of the H^+ secreted in the proximal tubule is used in the reclamation of filtered HCO_3^- and does not result in the addition of new HCO_3^- to the body. However, the intercalated cells in the collecting duct actively pump H^+ into the lumen, where it combines with HPO_4^{2-} and other urinary buffers, forming "titratable" acid. With acidosis, the secretion of H^+ increases, lowering the urine pH to about 4.4, which converts all the filtered HPO_4^{2-} to $H_2PO_4^-$, increasing the amount of acid excreted.

The other means of eliminating H^+ is the formation of NH_4^+. Ammonia is generated in the proximal tubule cell from the catabolism of amino acids, mainly glutamine, and is rapidly converted to NH_4^+ because the intracellular pH is much lower than the pK_b of ammonia (see Fig. 6-5). Ammonium ion is transported into the lumen in exchange for Na^+ and excreted. With acidosis, the generation of NH_4^+ can be increased many-fold and is the principal way of responding to a prolonged acidosis. Hypokalemia also stimulates glutamine catabolism and ammonia generation, whereas hyperkalemia has the opposite effect.

Infants, especially newborns, maintain slightly lower values of pH (7.37) and plasma bicarbonate (22 mEq/L) when compared with older children and adults (pH, 7.39; HCO_3^-, 24 to 28).[13] They can maintain acid–base homeostasis, but are limited in the ability to respond to an acid load. This is especially true for premature infants.

This lower plasma HCO_3^- in infants appears to be the result of a lower "threshold" or the plasma concentration at which HCO_3^- no longer is completely reabsorbed by the kidney. The explanation for this is unclear, but may relate to decreased activ-

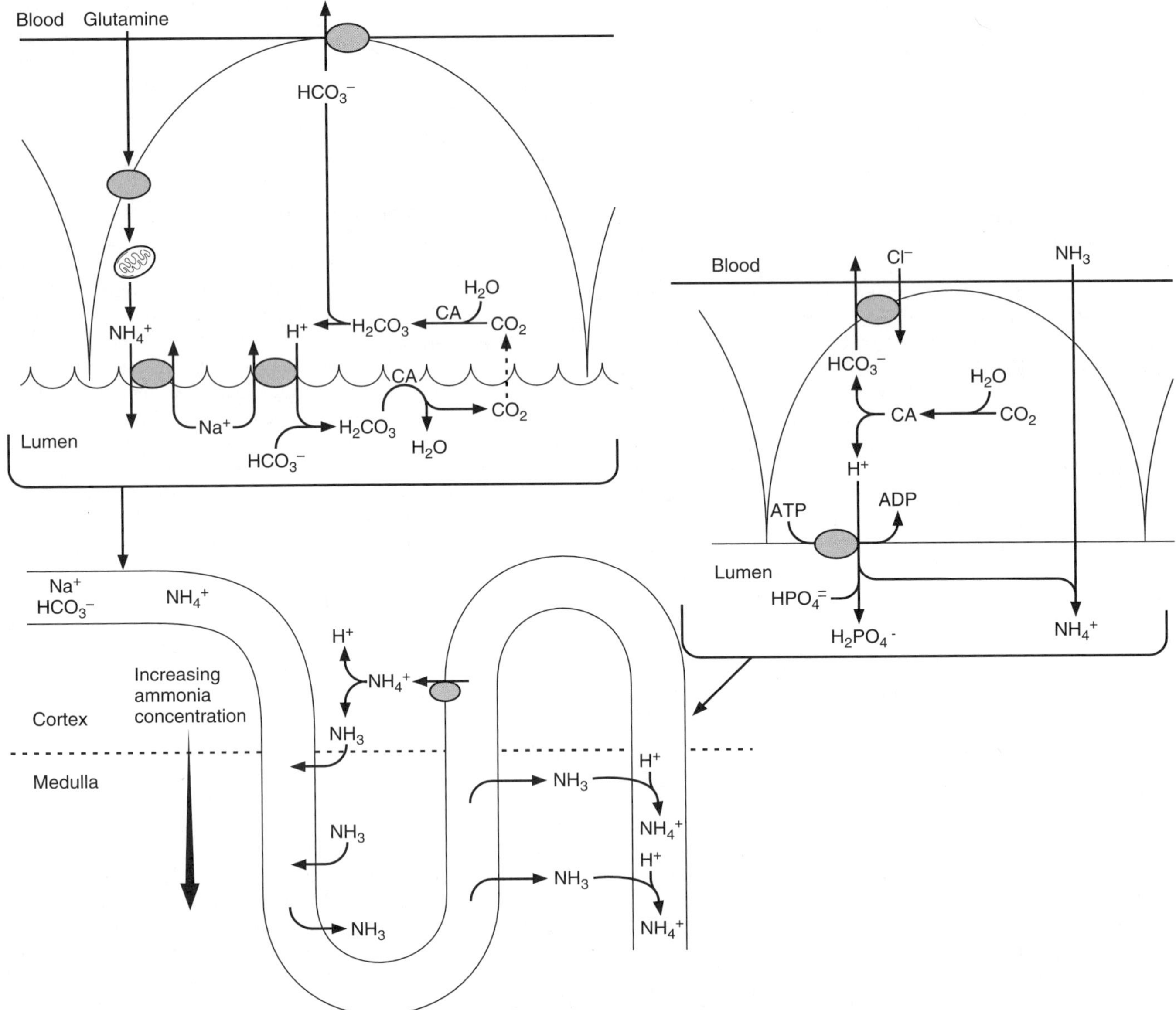

FIG. 6-5. Acid–base physiology. Na^+ and HCO_3^- are filtered by the glomerulus. The Na^+ is reabsorbed by the proximal tubule in exchange for NH_4^+ or H^+. NH_4^+ is formed from the catabolism of amino acids, principally glutamine. Intracellular carbonic anhydrase (CA) combines CO_2 and H_2O to form H_2CO_3. This splits into H^+, which is exchanged for luminal Na^+, and HCO_3^-, which is transported out of the cell and into the blood. Luminal H^+ combines with filtered HCO_3^- to form H_2CO_3. This is converted to H_2O and CO_2 by CA on the luminal membrane. CO_2 diffuses back into the proximal tubule cell, where it can be recycled for more H^+. The net effect is the reclamation of filtered HCO_3^-. Ammonia is recycled and concentrated in the medulla by active transport out of the ascending limb of the loop of Henle and the countercurrent concentrating mechanism. In the collecting duct, intercalated cells actively pump the H^+ formed by intracellular CA into the lumen. There, the H^+ combines with filtered $HPO_4^=$ or NH_3 that has passively diffused from the medulla into the lumen. HCO_3^- is exchanged for Cl^-. This results in the net excretion of H^+. ATP, adenosine triphosphate; ADP, adenosine diphosphate.

ity of carbonic anhydrase or greater heterogeneity between superficial and deep cortical tubules for bicarbonate reabsorption related to differences in maturation. In contrast, the maximal rate for bicarbonate reabsorption is comparable to that of adults.

Infants in the first month of life respond less well to an acid load than do older infants and adults. This is true in terms of both an increase in urine ammonia and titratable acid. High-protein feeding can result in acidosis in the first weeks of life. Possible explanations are that the kidneys are excreting acid at nearly maximal rates on a normal diet, so the ability to increase acid excretion further is limited, that their urine contains less phosphate buffer because breast milk and formula contain limited amounts, and that there are fewer precursors for ammoniagenesis because of a lower protein intake.

The limited ability to respond to an acid load is magnified in premature infants. Premature infants in the first 3 postnatal weeks do not consistently lower their urine pH below 6 with acid loading and have excretion rates for titratable acid, ammonia, and net acid that are half those of full-term infants.[14] Ammonia excretion does not approach that of full-term infants until the second postnatal month.

Renal Calcium Excretion

About 60% of the plasma calcium is filtered by the glomeruli, of which 98% to 99% is reabsorbed. Sixty to 70% of this reabsorption occurs passively in the proximal tubule. Another 20% is reabsorbed in the thick ascending limb of the loop of Henle, although the exact mechanism is unclear. This reabsorption can be inhibited by loop diuretics.

The major site of regulation of calcium excretion is the distal tubule, where up to 10% of the filtered load is actively reabsorbed. Parathyroid hormone, vitamin D, thiazide diuretics, and estrogen increase distal calcium reabsorption, whereas acidosis decreases it. Saline loading and glucocorticoids also increase calcium excretion by undefined mechanisms. The cortical collecting duct actively reabsorbs a small fraction of the filtered load, less than 5%.

Urinary calcium excretion appears to decrease with age. The median of 131 24-hour urinary calcium samples from 21 healthy full-term infants between 8 and 179 days of age was 5 mg/kg, whereas the 95th percentile was 11 mg/kg.[15] This is similar to the 95th percentile of 8.9 mg/kg for healthy premature infants.[16] Older children and adults excrete less than 4 mg/kg/d.[17] The urine calcium:creatinine ratio (mg:mg) also fell with maturation. The 95th percentile for infants younger than 7 months of age was 0.86. For infants 7 to 18 months of age, it was 0.60, and for children 19 months to 3 years of age, it was 0.42. The upper limit of the normal urine calcium:creatinine ratio in older children and adults is 0.20 to 0.25.

Renal Phosphate Handling

The kidney plays a major role in regulating the plasma concentration of phosphate. About 5% to 10% of the plasma phosphate is bound to protein, and therefore, only 90% is available for filtration by the glomerulus. Of the filtered phosphate, 99% is reabsorbed by newborns, 90% to 95% by children, and 80% by adults, corresponding to growth rates.[18] The renal tubule normally operates at nearly maximal capacity for phosphate reabsorption, especially in infants and children. Increases in dietary phosphate intake lead to increases in phosphate excretion, maintaining plasma levels without necessarily leading to changes in tubular transport. On the other hand, reductions in phosphate intake signal the renal tubule to increase tubular transport independently of factors known to influence phosphate transport, such as parathyroid hormone.

Virtually all phosphate reabsorption occurs in the proximal tubule through a sodium cotransport system on the luminal membrane. A small amount is reabsorbed in the more distal nephron. Several factors increase phosphate excretion by inhibiting proximal phosphate reabsorption, including parathyroid hormone (the most potent factor on phosphate reabsorption),

acidosis, and glucagon. Vitamin D, growth hormone, and insulin increase phosphate reabsorption. The higher growth hormone levels found in infants and children may explain, in part, their higher phosphate reabsorption rates and, consequently, their higher plasma phosphate levels.

Renal Magnesium Handling

About 80% of the plasma magnesium is ultrafilterable and 97% is reabsorbed by the kidney. About 20% to 30% is reabsorbed in the proximal tubule by passive mechanisms. Another 50% to 60% is reabsorbed in the thick ascending limb of the loop of Henle, probably driven by the positive luminal charge relative to the interstitial fluid from the Na^+-K^+-$2Cl^-$ pump. The distal tubule and collecting duct account for another 2% to 5%. No specific hormone has been shown to regulate magnesium excretion, but parathyroid hormone, glucagon, AVP, and calcitonin enhance magnesium reabsorption. Mannitol, furosemide, ethacrynic acid, and, to some extent, thiazides increase magnesium excretion. Aminoglycosides, cisplatin, and cyclosporine can cause markedly increased magnesium excretion.

RENAL RESPONSE IN STRESS STATES

To maintain the internal milieu, the kidney must respond to many perturbations to the steady state. These conditions activate renal and extrarenal compensatory mechanisms that attempt to restore homeostasis. In an attempt to maintain the vital body functions, these mechanisms may result in trade-offs. For example, in response to cardiac failure, the kidney retains sodium and water that may result in edema and its attendant problems.

Hypovolemia

The volume of the extracellular fluid compartment is regulated by control of the content of its osmotically active solute, which is mainly sodium.[19] Changes in the sodium content result in parallel changes in the plasma volume, which is monitored by sensors of central blood volume and blood pressure. It is the "effective blood volume" that is detected, and this volume may not always correlate with the actual extracellular fluid volume (Fig. 6-6). This is commonly the case in edema-forming states. In response to hypovolemia, the atrial stretch receptors decrease their rate of firing, which lessens their inhibitory feedback on the cardioinhibitory and vasomotor centers in the brain. As a result, sympathetic nerve activity increases, resulting in vasoconstriction and elevated heart rate.[20] Renal sympathetic nerve activity stimulates proximal renal tubular sodium reabsorption and renin secretion. In addition, renin secretion also is activated by intrarenal baroreceptors. Renin activates angiotensin II formation, which is a major effector hormone responding to hypovolemia. Angiotensin II directly stimulates renal tubular sodium reabsorption, vasoconstricts arterioles, and stimulates aldosterone secretion from the adrenal glomerulosa. Aldosterone also is secreted in response to adrenocorticotropic hormone, the secretion of which also is stimulated by hypovolemia. Angiotensin II also has central nervous system effects

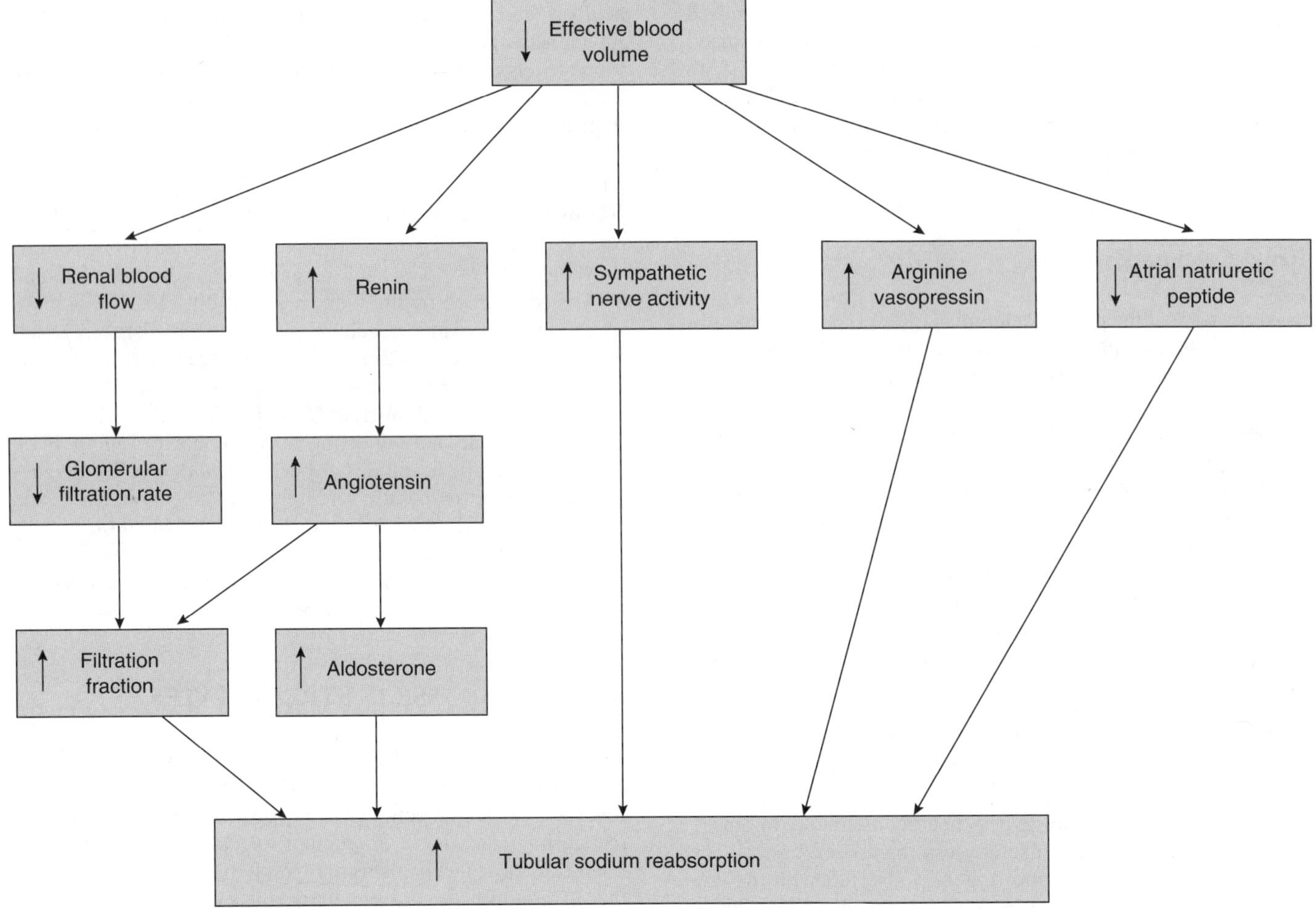

FIG. 6-6. Activation of renal sodium reabsorption occurs with a decrease in effective blood volume. In response to the activation of a variety of hormonal and nonhormonal factors, the kidney reacts to a decrease in the effective blood volume by increasing renal tubular sodium reabsorption. Vascular responses involve changes in the renal blood flow, glomerular filtration rate, and filtration fraction. Hormonal mediators include arginine vasopressin and the atrial natriuretic peptide.

of stimulating AVP and adrenocorticotropic hormone release, thirst, sodium appetite, and sympathetic activity.

Hyporolemia stimulates nonosmotic secretion of AVP.[9] In addition to the enhancement of water reabsorption in the collecting duct, AVP also stimulates sodium reabsorption in the thick ascending limb of the loop of Henle and, in combination with aldosterone, stimulates sodium reabsorption in the collecting tubule. Finally, AVP displays vasoconstrictor properties that support blood pressure and contribute to sodium conservation.

In addition to their neural effects, atrial stretch receptors control the secretion of ANP. In response to volume depletion, ANP secretion is decreased and its multiple effects promoting sodium excretion are diminished. Also as a result of decreased ANP secretion, there is lessened venous dilation, resulting in increased central venous pressure, increased renin and aldosterone secretion, and increased sodium reabsorption in the medullary collecting duct, where ANP normally inhibits reabsorption. Renal tubular sodium excretion also is diminished as result of decreased ANP activation of the GFR and medullary blood flow.

These are some of the major effector mechanisms by which the body protects the integrity of the vascular volume in response to decreased effective plasma volume. There are potential side effects of these effector mechanisms. The antidiuretic effects of AVP secreted in response to a nonosmotic stimulus contribute to the hyponatremia that is present in many of the conditions associated with decreased effective plasma volume. Potassium wasting and hypokalemia may result from the action of aldosterone on the collecting tubule. The protection of the effective blood volume stimulates sodium reabsorption, which may result in peripheral edema that may become severe. Teleologically, these responses are less of a threat than that of vascular collapse.

Hypernatremia and Hyponatremia

The osmolality of the body fluids is maintained by regulation of the quantity of total body water. Water freely and rapidly crosses virtually all plasma membranes, equalizing the osmolalities of intracellular and extracellular fluids. Total osmolality is composed of both effective and ineffective osmoles.[21] Substances such as urea that freely cross cell membranes do not cause transmembrane shifts of water and are ineffective osmoles. In contrast, substances such as sodium or glucose that cause shifts in water between the intracellular and extracellular compartments are effective osmoles. The control of water balance determines the osmolality of the body fluids.

Total body water is controlled by the osmoregulatory center in the brain, which regulates water excretion by control of AVP secretion and water intake by control of thirst.[22] Receptors in the hypothalamus in the vicinity of the supraoptic nucleus sense changes in effective osmolarity. These osmoreceptors are stimulated by changes in plasma osmolarity greater than 280 mOsm/kg, with maximal stimulation of AVP occurring when the plasma osmolarity reaches 295 mOsm/kg. It is at this point that thirst also is stimulated. A rise in the plasma osmolarity to 285 mOsm/kg results in a rise in the circulating AVP level from 1 to 2 pg/mL, which doubles the urine osmolarity and decreases the urine volume by half. A further increase in plasma osmolarity to 295 mOsm/kg, raises circulating AVP levels to more than 5 pg/mL and maximally concentrates the urine. The response of AVP secretion to an osmotic stimulus is enhanced dramatically in the presence of hypovolemia.

In the presence of hyponatremia and a plasma osmolarity of less than 280 mOsm/kg, circulating AVP would be expected to be less than 1 pg/mL and the urine maximally dilute. Yet more than 90% of patients with hyponatremia have elevated concentrations of AVP for the level of plasma osmolarity, resulting in a urine that is less than maximally dilute. The cause of this usually is nonosmotic stimulation of AVP secretion as result of a low effective blood volume. The presence of a low effective blood volume in this setting is indicated by a urine sodium level of less than 10 mEq/L. AVP also activates the secretion of ANP, which increases urinary sodium loss, actively contributing to the hyponatremia. Therefore, hyponatremia usually does not result solely from dilution by excess total body water, but also involves urinary sodium losses.

Hyperkalemia

The body responds to surfeits and deficits of potassium through both renal and extrarenal mechanisms.[23] With 98% of the total body potassium being located in the intracellular water, the distribution of potassium across the plasma membrane plays an important role in the serum concentration of potassium. Even small shifts of potassium between the intracellular and extracellular compartments can profoundly change the plasma potassium concentration. The transcellular potassium gradient is maintained largely by the activity of the plasma membrane Na^+-K^+-ATPase. Factors influencing the transcellular distribution of potassium include insulin, catecholamines, and pH.

In response to an intravenous load of potassium (0.5 mEq/kg) delivered over 1 hour, the kidneys normally excrete 40% of this load by the end of the infusion, and by 3 hours, the entire load is excreted into the urine and the serum potassium returns to baseline. In contrast, only 50% of an oral load is excreted over the first 3 to 6 hours after ingestion. The renal mechanisms for handling a potassium load include increased secretion by the principal cells and aldosterone-mediated secretion by the renal tubule. Finally, hyperkalemia inhibits sodium and water reabsorption in the proximal tubule, which increases potassium excretion by increasing the flow rate in the distal nephron.

An oral load of 0.5 mEq/kg would be expected to increase serum potassium by a clinically significant 2.5 mEq if the load was distributed only in the extracellular fluid. With an apparent volume of distribution of 70% to 80% of body weight, such a potassium load results in a rise in serum potassium of 0.6 mEq/L. This results from a large buffering capacity for potassium by the intracellular space. This aptitude decreases as the cellular capacity is approached, resulting in significant and potentially dangerous increases in serum potassium. The intracellular stores similarly act as a reservoir during potassium depletion, minimizing the fall in serum potassium. The largest pool of intracellular potassium is in skeletal muscle, which is responsible for most of the ability of the body to respond to changes in potassium content.

Important regulators of extrarenal potassium metabolism include insulin, β-catecholamines, aldosterone, and hydrogen ion concetration. Insulin responds to increases in serum potassium of 1.0 to 1.5 mEq/L with a two- to three-fold increase in peripheral levels. Insulin, independent of its effects on glucose metabolism, enhances potassium uptake into skeletal muscle and the liver by stimulating Na^+-K^+-ATPase. Activation of β_2-catecholamine receptors on skeletal muscle cells and hepatocytes also enhances potassium uptake by a cyclic adenosine monophosphate–mediated activation of Na^+-K^+-ATPase. β-Adrenergic stimulation of potassium uptake into cells plays a role in the protection from hyperkalemia after eating and after vigorous exercise. In addition to its renal effects, aldosterone also participates in extrarenal potassium metabolism. Aldosterone is increased in response to elevations in serum potassium and stimulates cellular uptake of potassium into muscle and potassium secretion into saliva, sweat, and the intestine. Finally, an increased hydrogen ion concentration (acidosis) from most causes increases potassium movement out of the cell, and a low concentration (alkalosis) has the opposite effect.

Acidosis and Alkalosis

The kidney is the primary organ for the control of the acid–base status of the body.[24] This is achieved by the processes of bicarbonate reabsorption plus acid and ammonium excretion to generate new bicarbonate. The source of this new bicarbonate has long been thought to be from the H_2CO_3 that it uses for H^+ secretion in the distal nephron, but Halperin and colleagues have stressed that the source of the bicarbonate actually is the metabolism of the 2-oxoglutarate that is formed in the proximal tubule when NH_4^+ is produced from glutamine.[25] In addition to normal endogenous acid production, many stress states (eg, the trauma of burns or surgery, fever, starvation, exercise) and certain drugs (eg, corticosteroids) can increase endogenous acid production by increasing catabolism. With its ability to quadruple NH_4^+ excretion to 670 mEq/d, the kidney is largely responsible for maintaining normal acid–base status in the presence of these conditions as well.

In response to metabolic acidosis, there is an increase in acid excretion by the kidneys that begins within 1 to 2 days of the onset and continues until its resolution. Decreased serum pH is a potent stimulus for increased acid excretion, but acid excretion also increases in response to enhnaced endogenous acid production without notable changes in pH or serum bicarbonate. Acidosis associated with the administration of chloride typically is more severe than that associated with an organic anion. This is because chloride administration initially augments sodium excretion. This is followed by decreased sodium delivery to the collecting tubule, which then limits distal H^+ secretion. In contrast, organic anions, which are poorly reabsorbed by the renal tubule, result in persistent sodium delivery to the collecting tubule.

The major adaptive mechanism to increase renal acid excretion is enhanced NH_4^+ formation. Increased excretion of H^+ as NH_4^+ in response to systemic acidosis requires increased synthesis in the proximal tubule followed by increased excretion into the urine. The initial response to acute metabolic acidosis that results in enhanced formation of NH_3 is activation of the pH-sensitive enzyme, 2-oxoglutarate dehydrogenase. Greater adaptation occurs with chronic metabolic acidosis as the basolateral uptake of glutamine into the proximal renal tubular cells is stimulated.

Ammonia production in the proximal tubule does not ensure that enhanced excretion of NH_4^+ and de novo production of bicarbonate will occur. Ammonia formed in the proximal renal tubule can enter the renal tubule, where it eventually is trapped in the urine, or it can enter the bloodstream, where it is metabolized into urea in the liver in a process that negates the de novo formation of bicarbonate. Therefore, the processes that lead to the trapping and excretion of NH_4^+ in the urine play an essential role in the formation of de novo bicarbonate. Normally, only one third of the NH_4^+ that is formed in the proximal tubule is excreted in the urine. In response to metabolic acidosis, there is increased secretion of NH_4^+ into the luminal fluid by an undefined mechanism. After reabsorption in the loop of Henle, the transfer of NH_4^+ across the collecting duct into the urine also is enhanced with metabolic acidosis.

In response to chronic respiratory acidosis, the kidney increases NH_4^+ excretion through a process that includes activation of H^+ secretion by the collecting tubule. The stimulus for this adaptation is Pa_{CO_2} rather than pH. If hypercapnia is sustained, a steady state is reached during which increased bicarbonate delivery offsets increased ammonia excretion, resulting in a fall of net acid excretion and return of the serum pH close to normal. The opposite process occurs in respiratory alkalosis. Acutely, bicarbonate is excreted into the urine until the serum bicarbonate falls. This is followed by a chronic adaptation in which collecting duct H^+ secretion is diminished, but is appropriate for the reduced delivery of bicarbonate, resulting again in a steady state.

Metabolic alkalosis can result in varied renal responses depending on other influences on the kidney.[26] With the administration of a large alkali load, the kidneys in the absence of significant metabolic alkalosis can excrete up to 24 mEq/kg/d of HCO_3^-. Early studies showing the presence of a threshold above which HCO_3^- is excreted into the urine suggest that there is a point near the normal serum HCO_3^- level that the proximal renal tubular reabsorption of HCO_3^- is saturated. More recent studies suggest that the capacity of the proximal renal tubule to reabsorb HCO_3^- in vitro is much greater, but there is adaptation in the H^+ secretion in the proximal renal tubule in response to alkalosis. The collecting duct responds to alkalosis by increasing the excretion of HCO_3^-, and that of citrate, which is metabolically equivalent to HCO_3^- excretion.

Certain clinical conditions causing metabolic alkalosis, such as gastrointestinal loss of acid or diuretic abuse, also are associated with volume, chloride, and potassium depletion. In these states, the kidney responds inappropriately in relation to the pH and acts to maintain the alkalosis. In response to volume contraction, there is a decreased filtered load of HCO_3^- as a result of a decreased GFR, decreased backleak of HCO_3^- into the proximal renal tubular lumen, and enhanced H^+ secretion in the proximal tubule, which augments HCO_3^- reabsorption. In addition, the hypochloremia results in increased H^+ secretion by the medullary collecting duct. If the volume depletion is severe enough to activate the renin–angiotensin–aldosterone axis, there may be enhanced distal tubular exchange of K^+ for Na^+, resulting in potassium depletion. Potassium depletion can work to maintain the alkalotic state by increasing proximal renal tubular H^+ secretion, enhancing NH_4^+ synthesis and increasing H^+ secretion by the collecting duct. These processes are responsible for the so-called paradoxic aciduria of metabolic alkalosis. The relative importance of the volume, potassium, and chloride depletion are controversial, but the repletion of each of these deficits results in renal correction of the alkalosis.

RENAL ACTIONS OF DIURETICS

Diuretics are a group of chemically diverse agents that increase the renal excretion of salt and water.[27] Their use in surgical patients usually is to treat extracellular volume overload associated with renal, cardiac, or hepatic disease. In contrast to the excretion of 1% of the filtered load of sodium, diuretics can acutely increase sodium excretion 25-fold. These agents can be divided into groups according to the segment of the renal tubule they affect (Table 6-1). The mechanism of action, relative effectiveness, and other actions can be understood through knowledge of the normal renal physiology of each of these segments. A more complete review of the pharmacology and action of diuretics in children is provided elsewhere.[28]

Proximal Tubule Diuretics

Mannitol and acetazolamide act primarily to increase salt and water excretion by their action on the proximal renal tubule. Mannitol is an inert substance that is freely filtered, but subsequently neither reabsorbed nor metabolized. Hence, mannitol acts as an osmotically active agent in the renal tubule and decreases salt and water reabsorption. Acetazolamide is a carbonic anhydrase inhibitor that blocks the reabsorption of bicarbonate in the proximal renal tubule. This non-reabsorbed bicarbonate directly inhibits sodium and water reabsorption in the proximal nephron and acts as a non-reabsorbable anion in the distal nephron. Acetazolamide is most effective in the presence of metabolic alkalosis. Because of the renal loss of bicarbonate, prolonged use of acetazolamide can result in metabolic acidosis, which lessens its effectiveness. Despite the fact that most of the salt and water is reabsorbed in the proximal tubule, neither of these agents result in the excretion of more than 5% of salt and water because of enhanced reabsorption in the more distal segments of the nephron.

TABLE 6-1. *Site of action of diuretics*

Tubular segment	Percent of filtered sodium reabsorbed	Diuretics active at segment
Proximal tubule	50–60%	Mannitol, acetazolamide
Thick ascending limb-loop of Henle	35–40%	Furosemide, bumetanide, ethacrynic acid
Distal tubule	8%	Thiazides, chlorthalidone, metolazone
Cortical collecting tubule	2%	Amiloride, spironolactone, triamterene

Loop Diuretics

Agents acting at the thick ascending loop of Henle are the most powerful group of diuretics. The major members of this group are furosemide and bumetanide, which inhibit the Na^+-K^+-$2Cl^-$ cotransporter, and ethacrynic acid, whose mechanism of action is not known. The site of action of these agents, and of the other diuretics discussed later in this chapter, with the exception of spironolactone, is at the luminal side of the tubule. Therefore, to be active, these drugs must be filtered or secreted into the lumen of the renal tubule. Secretion into the tubule is by the organic anion transporter in the case of the loop diuretics and thiazides, and by the organic cation transporter in the case of amiloride and triamterene. In the presence of renal insufficiency or with inhibition of the anion transporter by probenecid, there is decreased diuretic effectiveness as a result of insufficient delivery to the active site. Because 35% to 40% of filtered sodium is reabsorbed in the loop of Henle, loop diuretics can result in the excretion of up to 25% of the filtered sodium and water. By inhibiting the Na^+-K^+-$2Cl^-$ cotransporter, loop diuretics directly inhibit the reabsorption of potassium and chloride, and indirectly inhibit the reabsorption of calcium and magnesium by blocking formation of the lumen-positive potential that drives divalent cation reabsorption. Clinically significant losses and depletion of these ions can occur with prolonged use of loop diuretics.

Distal Tubule Diuretics

The distal tubule diuretics include the thiazides and the longer-acting chlorthalidone, and metolazone, which is structurally unrelated but probably acts at the same site. These drugs block sodium reabsorption by competing for the chloride site of the NaCl cotransporter. Through this mechanism, the distal tubule diuretics can result in the excretion of 5% to 10% of the filtered load of sodium. These agents can be used in combination with loop diuretics for increased effectiveness. In contrast to the calciuretic effect of loop diuretics, the distal tubule diuretics decrease calcium excretion, a property used in the treatment of hypercalciuria. Similar to loop diuretics, significant potassium depletion can occur with long-term use.

Potassium-Sparing Diuretics

Spironolactone, amiloride, and triamterene are the major drugs referred to as potassium-sparing diuretics. These agents inhibit sodium reabsorption by the principal cells in the renal collecting tubule, but by different mechanisms. Spironolactone is a progesterone analogue that inhibits aldosterone-induced activation of sodium reabsorption by competing for its intracellular receptor. Amiloride and triamterene probably act by binding to and inhibiting the luminal sodium channel. Spironolactone reaches its site of action from the basilar (blood) side of the cell, whereas amiloride and triamterene are active only at the luminal side. Because the lumen-negative potential is necessary for potassium secretion, inhibition of sodium reabsorption by the collecting tubule inhibits potassium excretion. This characteristic can result in significant hyperkalemia, but is potentially beneficial when used to counteract the potassium and magnesium wasting induced by the administration of loop and distal tubule diuretics.

Resistance to Diuretics

Whereas the initial response to diuretic administration is significant excretion of sodium and water, prolonged administration characteristically results in a diminution of the diuretic response.[29] In a patient with significant edema in whom it is desirable to remove large amounts of fluid, the development of this relative resistance to the action of diuretics is a problem. Diuretics in general are only effective at the luminal surface, so the degree of diuresis is largely equal to the amount of diuretic excreted. Therefore, administering an intravenous dose of diuretics to overcome defects in absorption, or increasing the dose to compensate for decreased renal tubular delivery (as may be present in renal or cardiac disease) usually results in significant improvements in effectiveness.

There usually is a diminution of the effectiveness of diuretic therapy with continued administration. Reasons for the subsequent development of resistance include systemic factors such as volume depletion and decreased renal perfusion, and activation of systemic compensatory mechanisms such as angiotensin II, aldosterone, and norepinephrine, which are secreted in an attempt by the body to restore actual or apparent intravascular volume depletion. There is rebound sodium reabsorption after even a single dose of a short-acting loop diuretic that diminishes the effectiveness of the therapy. Constant infusion of loop diuretics potentially minimizes this effect and avoids this rebound phenomenon. Intrarenal mechanisms that interfere with the effectiveness of long-term diuretic therapy include hypertrophy of the distal renal and collecting tubules resulting in enhanced sodium reabsorption by these segments. The combination of distal tubule diuretics or potassium-sparing diuretics with loop diuretics counteracts the enhanced reabsorption at these sites and potentiates the diuretic effect. Whereas metolazone has been suggested to be particularly effective in this circumstance, especially in the presence of renal insufficiency, thiazides may be equally effective when used at equivalent doses.

Other practical factors that may limit diuretic effectiveness in controlling edema include noncompliance, uncontrolled sodium and water intake, and postural effects resulting in pooling of fluid in the lower extremities. In addition, appropriate adjustment must be made when switching from intravenous to oral dosing. For example, an oral dose twice the intravenous dose is needed for an equivalent effectiveness with furosemide, whereas the intravenous and oral doses of bumetanide are equivalent because of virtually complete gastrointestinal absorption of the orally administered form.

Complications of Diuretic Therapy

Diuretics cause complications as a result of their action on the renal tubule and through other, unrelated mechanisms. Diuretics in proportion to their potency cause several fluid and electrolyte abnormalities. As a result of their ability to increase sodium and water flow through the renal tubule, diuretics cause salt and water depletion. In its most extreme uncompensated form, volume depletion can result in prerenal azotemia, hypotension, and syncope. All diuretics except the potassium-sparing agents promote potassium loss and hypokalemia. This is the result of increased delivery of sodium and volume to the distal tubule stimulating potassium secretion. Through related mechanisms, magnesium loss and hypomagnesemia also can result. Potassium-sparing diuretics have the opposite effect by their actions on the collecting tubule. Metabolic alkalosis is another complication of diuretic use that results from potassium and volume depletion with its associated activation of aldosterone secretion. Acetazolamide, by inhibiting carbonic anhydrase, may cause metabolic acidosis, as can spironolactone by inhibiting aldosterone-stimulated hydrogen secretion. In part because of their effects on intravascular volume, diuretics stimulate uric acid reabsorption and may cause hyperuricemia.

Hyponatremia is another common complication of diuretic therapy. Hyponatremia is not caused by simple sodium wasting in the kidney. In response to volume depletion, there is nonosmotic stimulation of antidiuretic hormone (AVP), which results in water reabsorption in the renal collecting duct. Loop diuretics prevent the formation of a dilute urine in the diluting segment of the renal tubule, which inhibits the ability of the kidney to excrete a hypotonic urine. Other nonrenal mechanisms contributing to hyponatremia include an intracellular shift of sodium in response to potassium depletion.

ACUTE RENAL INSUFFICIENCY

Acute renal insufficiency or failure (ARF) can be defined as an abrupt deterioration in the kidney's ability to clear nitrogenous wastes, such as urea and creatinine. Concomitantly, there is a loss of ability to handle appropriately other solute excretion, as well as salt and water balance, resulting in intravascular and extravascular volume derangements. These factors all interact, resulting in the clinical picture of hypertension, hyperkalemia, and uremia that often ensues in patients with ARF.

The term *acute renal failure* often is incorrectly used interchangeably with *acute tubular necrosis.* Acute tubular necrosis usually refers to a rapid deterioration in renal function occurring minutes to days after an ischemic or nephrotoxic event. Although acute tubular necrosis is an important cause of ARF, it is not the sole cause, and the terms are not synonymous. Nonetheless, acute tubular necrosis, as an entity, may occur in many of the immediately reversible causes of ARF, such as dehydration or urinary tract obstruction, if they go unrecognized.

Etiology and Pathophysiology

To understand the treatment of ARF, it is important to understand its causes and pathophysiology. The causes of ARF are varied, but overall can be classified as follows:

Prerenal—implies poor renal perfusion
Renal—implies intrinsic renal disease or damage
Postrenal—implies an obstruction to urine excretion

The various causes of ARF are summarized in Table 6-2.

Prerenal insults are a common cause of ARF, accounting for up to 70% of all cases. Prerenal failure usually results from extracellular fluid loss, such as that which accompanies burns, hemorrhage, or postobstructive diuresis. It also can be seen in the setting of cardiac failure or sepsis. The common feature of these conditions is a marked reduction in cardiac output, and as a result, diminished renal perfusion. In response to the reduction in flow, there is a compensatory increase in afferent tone, with a reduction in glomerular filtration and an increase in salt and water retention. The net effect of these events is a drastic reduction in urine volume, often resulting in oliguria or anuria. If the underlying problem is recognized and treated aggressively, progressive renal insufficiency may be averted.

Patients who concomitantly receive nonsteroidal antiinflammatory drugs or angiotensin-converting enzyme inhibitors are more prone to the development of frank renal failure because of the intrinsic hemodynamic effects of these drugs. Patients who chronically have poor renal perfusion as a result of hypovolemia or hypotension often have renal perfusion that is supported by endogenously produced prostaglandin vasodilative compounds. Inhibition of these agents by treatment with nonsteroidal antiinflammatory drugs results in increased afferent tone, decreased glomerular perfusion, and decreased glomerular filtration. This effect is aggravated by the effects of increased circulating vasoconstrictors (eg, norepinephrine, angiotensin II), which are likely to be present because of the lack of adequate perfusion.[30]

In addition, in hypovolemic patients or patients with renal artery stenosis, renal perfusion is supported by increased vascular tone induced by angiotensin II. The use of angiotensin-converting enzyme inhibitors can result in a dramatic decline in renal function by reducing systemic pressure, and hence perfusion, and also by inducing renal arteriolar efferent relaxation, decreasing transglomerular pressure.[31] The net effect of these changes is to reduce glomerular filtration. Early recognition of drug-induced reduction of renal perfusion and prompt cessation of the offending agent usually results in restoration of function.

ARF resulting from parenchymal disease or injury accounts for 20% to 30% of cases of abrupt renal insufficiency. Prolonged prerenal azotemia may result in overt renal injury. Similarly, intrarenal obstruction to blood flow (thrombi) or vasculitis may be a cause of renal failure. In addition, drugs (eg, aminoglycosides, amphotericin B) or other nephrotoxins (including ra-

TABLE 6-2. *Etiology of acute renal failure*

Prerenal	Renal	Postrenal

a) Hypovolemia
  1. Volume loss
  2. Gastrointestinal, renal losses
  3. Sequestration (burns,
    postoperative)
b) Hypotension
  1. Shock
  2. Vasodilators
c) Decreased effective blood flow
  1. Low cardiac output
  2. Cirrhosis
  3. Nephrotic syndrome
d) Renal hypoperfusion
  1. Use of ACE inhibitors
  2. Nonsteroidal and
    antiinflammatory drugs
  3. Hepatorenal syndrome
e) Vascular occlusion
  1. Thromboembolic phenomenon
  2. Aortic dissection
  3. Renal vein thrombosis
    (dehydration, hypercoagulable
    state, neoplasm)
	a) Acute glomerulonephritis
	  1. Postinfectious
	  2. Membranoproliferative
	    glomerulonephritis
	  3. Rapidly progressive
	    glomerulonephritis
	  4. Glomerulonephritis secondary to
	    systemic disease (eg, HUS,
	    DIC, SLE)
	b) Acute interstitial nephritis
	  1. Drug-induced hypersensitivity
	    (penicillin)
	  2. Infections
	c) Tubular disease
	  1. ATN (ischemic, nephrotoxic)
	  2. Intratubular obstruction (uric
	    acid, oxalate)
	d) Cortical necrosis
	  1. Gram-negative sepsis
	  2. Hemorrhage
	  3. Shock
	e) Acute renal failure
	  1. Toxins
	  2. Organic solvents
	  3. Heavy metals
	  4. Insecticides
	  5. Other
	    • Hemoglobin
	    • Myoglobin
	f) Chronic renal failure
	  1. Chronic interstitial nephritis
	  2. Chronic glomerulonephritis
	  3. Chronic glomerulosclerosis
	  4. Nephrocalcinosis
	  5. Obstructive uropathy
	  6. Hypertension
		a) Obstruction
		  1. Intrinsic (papillary necrosis
		    secondary to diabetes, sickle
		    cell disease, or analgesic
		    nephropathy)
		  2. Intrarenal abnormalities, ureteral
		    obstruction, obstruction of the
		    bladder or urethra
		  3. Extrinsic (tumor compression,
		    lymphadenopathy)

ACE, angiotensin-converting enzyme; HUS, hemolytic-uremic syndrome; DIC, disseminated intravascular coagulation; SLE, systemic lupus erythematosus; ATN, acute tubular necrosis.

diocontrast agents) may induce ARF through tubular injury, or cause interstitial injury as a result of allergic reactions (as can be seen with penicillins).

The remaining causes of ARF are the result of obstruction to urine flow. These conditions, as a group, account for less than 10% of all cases of ARF, and may occur within the collecting system of the kidney (intrarenal) or in the ureter or urethra (extrarenal). Intrarenal obstruction may be seen clinically in the setting of tumor lysis syndrome with deposition of uric acid crystals, with direct tubular toxicity as seen from acyclovir, or with multiple myeloma in which proteinaceous debris may result in tubular obstruction. The extrarenal collecting system may become obstructed by stones, lymph nodes (external compression), or tumor. As in all other instances, recognition and appropriate intervention to relieve an obstruction may prevent catastrophic declines in renal function.

The pathophysiology of ARF is an area of active investigative interest. The initial events that characterize ARF are thought to evolve in response to profound vasoconstriction. The initial hypothesis for the evolution of ARF was that an insult in the renal tubular epithelium resulted in the release of vasoactive compounds that increased cortical vascular resistance, decreasing renal blood flow and perpetuating injury to the tubule (Fig. 6-7). The same compounds then could cause the constriction of afferent and efferent arterioles within the glomerulus, resulting in diminished urine output or oliguria. Several compounds have been implicated as having a pathogenic role in ARF, including angiotensin, prostaglandins, adenosine, and endothelin. Although all these agents do exert profound vasoconstrictive influences peripherally and within the kidney, their specific roles in the pathogenesis of ARF are not clear.[32] Vasoconstriction is a well-defined factor in initiating ARF, but vasodilatation alone does not ameliorate ARF. In addition, the infusion of potent vasodilators, such as dopamine or prostaglandins, does not result in ongoing improvement in the GFR.[33] Although hemodynamic factors are important in initiating ARF, these alterations themselves do not explain the evolution of this condition.

Factors resulting from direct injury to nephronal elements also contribute to the manifestations of ARF (Fig. 6-8). Injury of the tubular epithelium results in sloughing of the brush border, swelling, mitochondrial condensation, and disruption of cell morphology. These changes, occurring within minutes of an ischemic event, are believed to contribute to the observed reduction in the GFR, and to decrease physically filtration by obstructing tubular lumina.[32] In addition, ultrastructural changes in the epithelium also contribute to a backleak phenomenon. As has been demonstrated experimentally and in patients with acute tubular necrosis, the loss of tubular integrity results in the backleak of tubular fluid. This backleak has been demonstrated by a decrease in the clearance of inulin and graded dextrans.[32,34,35] If waste products are filtered, but then returned to the circulation through backleak, the measured renal clearance of these compounds is diminished.

There also are individual cellular derangements, such as a decline in cellular ATP levels,[36] and direct cell membrane injury by reactive oxygen molecules.[37] In addition, changes in the metabolism of membrane phospholipids may contribute to membrane instability and result in cell death.[32] The decline of ATP levels observed within the cells may adversely affect ATP-dependent calcium pumps, resulting in an accumulation of intracellular calcium. High intracellular calcium levels have been associated with cell death, although a direct pathophysiologic explanation is lacking.[38,39]

In general, therapeutic interventions for ARF are supportive, so it is critical that appropriate diagnostic studies be used early in these patients. Early diagnosis and appropriate intervention offer the best chance of improved survival.

Diagnostic Procedures

The laboratory assessment of patients with ARF includes simple measurements of urea, creatinine, and electrolytes. Using this information, in addition to detecting overt distur-

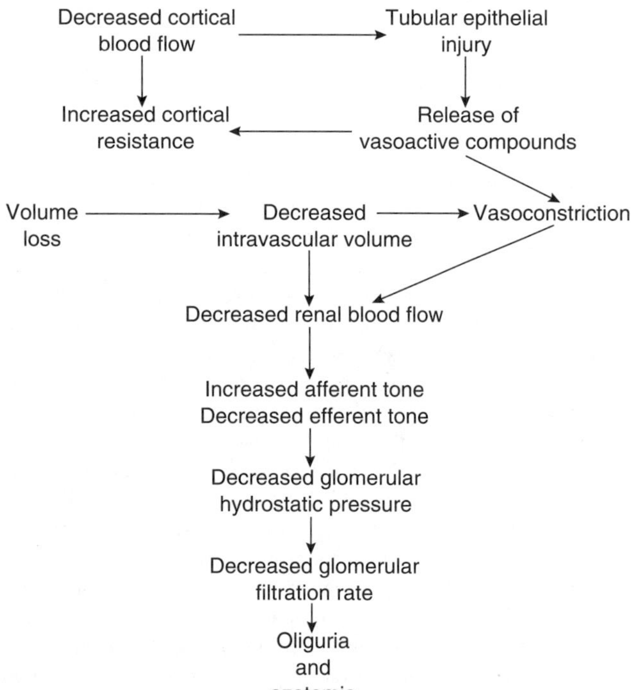

FIG. 6-7. Hemodynamic factors in the pathogenesis of acute renal failure.

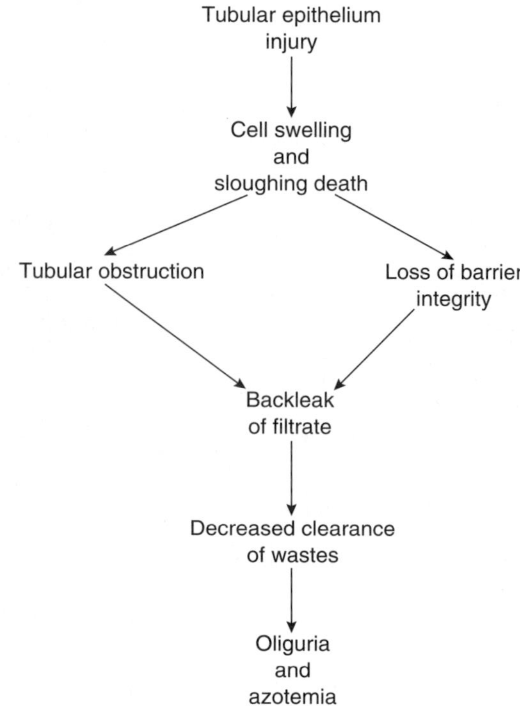

FIG. 6-8. Influences of specific injury to the nephron in the pathogenesis of acute renal failure.

bances in electrolytes, the level of urea can be compared with that of creatinine. In cases of prerenal azotemia, the ratio of blood urea nitrogen to creatinine usually is greater than 20. In cases of renal parenchymal dysfunction, this ratio usually is 10. It is important to perform a urinalysis with an examination of the urinary sediment. It is common in cases of ARF to observe both hematuria and proteinuria. In cases of overt glomerulonephritis, there may be additional findings of cellular casts. In simple dehydration, there often are findings of granular casts. In cases of glomerulonephritis complicated by nephrotic syndrome, there often are oval fat bodies on microscopic examination.

One commonly used and useful test of renal function is the fractional excretion of sodium (FE_{Na}). To calculate the FE_{Na}, the urine sodium, urine creatinine, serum sodium, and serum creatinine must be measured. The FE_{Na} is calculated using the following equation:

$$FE_{Na} = \frac{U_{Na} \times P_{Cr}}{P_{Na} \times U_{Cr}} \times 100\%$$

The normal FE_{Na} is less than 1% for adults and children, and less than 2.5% for infants. The FE_{Na} usually is elevated in cases of frank renal insufficiency resulting from renal parenchymal insult. In cases of prerenal azotemia, the FE_{Na} usually is normal.

The radiologic assessment of patients with ARF may include ultrasound and nuclear renography (renal scanning). A well-performed ultrasound can define asymmetry in size and changes in parenchymal density, and can indicate obstruction. The last would be evidenced by dilatation within the collecting system. In patients in whom obstruction is demonstrated by ultrasound, a bladder catheterization and voiding cystourethrogram may be indicated. The voiding cystourethrogram evaluates for lower tract obstruction and vesicoureteral reflux. Renal blood flow and renal function can be assessed by nuclear renography. The one limitation of this study is that the quality of images obtained in patients who have a creatinine clearance of less than 30 mL/min/m^2 may be inadequate for assessment.

Therapeutic Interventions

Therapeutic interventions in patients with ARF usually are aimed at improving renal function or urine flow. A variety of pharmacologic interventions have been incorporated into the care of patients with ARF in hopes of improving function. These include volume expansion, diuretics, and vasoactive agents such as dopamine. Correction of existing hypovolemia is necessary to provide adequate cardiac output and organ perfusion. Appropriate fluids include isotonic solutions such as normal saline, Plasmanate, or blood products (if indicated), infused in volumes of 20 mL/kg over 30 to 60 minutes. The volume resuscitation can be repeated if necessary, especially if there is ongoing volume loss. Patients with oliguria secondary to hypovolemia usually respond within 4 to 6 hours with urine output.

If the patient is hypervolemic, the initial management includes fluid restriction and diuretics in an attempt to return the patient to euvolemia. A trial of intravenous mannitol, 0.5 g/kg over 5 minutes, or furosemide, 1 to 5 mg/kg, may be attempted in a patient with oliguria for less than 48 hours who has not responded to adequate hydration. This may be especially beneficial in a patient with ARF resulting from tubular obstruction (myoglobinuria, hyperuricuria, or hemoglobinuria). There are theoretic reasons why mannitol, furosemide, or other loop diuretics might ameliorate ARF. Mannitol is purported to improve ARF because it may help flush tubular obstructions (casts) and reestablish urine flow. In addition, in animal models, mannitol has been demonstrated to decrease hypoxic cell swelling. The administration of mannitol results in an expansion of the plasma volume, with the benefit of reducing the hematocrit, and therefore serving to prevent erythrocyte aggregation after ischemia.[40]

Furosemide binds to the luminal membrane in the thick ascending loop of Henle, inhibiting the Na$^+$-K$^+$-2Cl$^-$ cotransporter and thereby inhibiting chloride transport, with a resultant natriuresis. In so doing, the Na$^+$-K$^+$-ATPase activity at the basolateral membrane decreases, and the cell enters a resting state with decreased need to expend energy or consume oxygen. This response to diuretics theoretically could protect the cell of the loop of Henle from hypoxic injury by decreasing oxygen consumption and preserving ATP.[41] Loop diuretics also may flush out tubular casts, much like mannitol.

Neither mannitol nor loop diuretics can predictably convert an oliguric patient with ARF to a polyuric patient. There are numerous reports of individual patients with improved output and recovery from ARF who were treated with mannitol or furosemide, but no controlled studies are available. Neither agent is capable of reducing the need for more aggressive support (including dialysis), and neither agent improves the morbidity or mortality of patients with ARF. If a patient proves refractory to diuretic therapy, it is appropriate to discontinue the agent until urine output returns. Continued use of diuretics in an anuric or oliguric patient, especially if circulating volume has not been adequately replaced, may aggravate preexisting prerenal azotemia and worsen renal insufficiency. It is probable that, even during the recovery phase of ARF, the patient will remain poorly responsive to diuretics.

The role of dopamine in the prevention and management of ARF has been a controversial subject. Those who support and encourage the use of dopamine argue that the agent acts as a predominant or selective renal vasodilator, increasing renal blood flow, GFR, urinary solute, and water clearance. Dopamine stimulates α-adrenergic receptors on systemic arterial resistance vasculature, resulting in vasoconstriction; cardiac β_1-adrenergic receptors, resulting in increased cardiac contractility, heart rate, and cardiac index; and β_2-adrenergic receptors on systemic arterial resistance vasculature, resulting in vasodilation. In addition, dopamine stimulates DA$_1$ and DA$_2$ receptors. DA$_1$ receptors mediate increases in renal blood flow and decreases in tubular resorption of sodium and water, whereas DA$_2$ receptors regulate neurotransmitter release. The threshold for DA$_1$ effects is 0.5 μg/g/min, with a 100% maximal effect reached by 3 μg/kg/min. The threshold for α, β_1, and β_2 effects is 3 μg/kg/min, with a 100% maximal effect reached by 20 μg/kg/min. The beneficial effects of dopamine can be used selectively in ARF by carefully titrating the dose of the agent.[33,42]

Three separate groups have shown that patients who remain oliguric in spite of volume expansion, mannitol, and loop diuretics may begin to have urine output if they are given low-dose dopamine. In euvolemic critically ill patients who were oliguric, urine flow was improved by dopamine infusion, and diminished when dopamine was discontinued.[40,43] However, the improvement in renal function in all these patients may be the result of more favorable changes in systemic hemodynamic parameters (eg, cardiac index, oxygen uptake, oxygen delivery). There have been no controlled studies in humans that demonstrate isolated beneficial effects of dopamine on the kidney in the setting of ARF.

If medical management fails to halt a progressive decline in renal function, or if a patient becomes refractory to medical management, renal replacement therapy (dialysis) is indicated. The concept of dialysis is an old one, first described in 1854. Dialysis first was performed successfully in an animal in 1912; however, hemodialysis as a treatment modality for humans was not widely available until the 1960s. There are three variations of renal replacement available to the practicing nephrologist for the support of critically ill children or adults: hemodialysis, peritoneal dialysis, and hemofiltration. Although the modalities differ technically, they all are based on the same principles (Fig. 6-9). The aim of all renal replacement therapies is to promote the removal of nitrogenous wastes (urea), excess fluid, and excess solute (especially potassium). This is achieved by exposing blood to a salt solution (dialysate), with the two separated by a semipermeable membrane. The movement of solute is encouraged by both diffusion (with solute moving across the membrane in response to a concentration gradient) and ultrafiltration (osmotic or hydrostatic pressures). The rate of removal of water and solute waste is dependent on membrane characteristics (pore size and selectivity), diffusion, and ultrafiltration.[44]

These characteristics can be altered selectively to enhance the clearance of a particular waste or volume. The actual permeability characteristics and surface areas are known for specific membranes used in hemodialysis and hemofiltration. The peritoneum serves as the dialysis membrane in peritoneal dialysis and remains physically unalterable, but it can be influenced

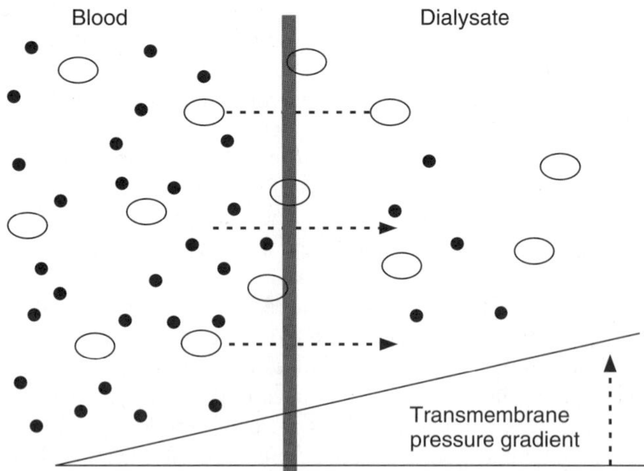

FIG. 6-9. Principles of dialysis. Solute (*closed circles*) moves from the blood to the dialysate (*dashed arrows*) in response to a concentration gradient (diffusion). There is an obligate passive movement of water (*open circles*) to attempt to maintain appropriate osmolarity. This flux of solute and water (ultrafiltration) may be enhanced by increased osmotic pressure (ie, glucose in peritoneal dialysis fluid) or by increased hydrostatic pressure (created mechanically as transmembrane pressure in hemodialysis).

functionally by alterations in the rate of diffusion or in ultrafiltration. The rate of diffusion can be altered by the addition of solute to the dialysate. For example, if it is desirable to maintain the serum potassium concentration, potassium can be added to the dialysate, blunting the concentration gradient, and as a result, slowing passive diffusion. Ultrafiltration also can be influenced by increases in transmembrane pressure, as a mechanical force (in conventional hemodialysis) or an increased osmotic force (in peritoneal dialysis). In all forms of renal replacement therapy, the therapeutic prescription is individualized for the patient.[45]

Hemodialysis

The indications for dialysis are hypervolemia, hyperkalemia, uremia, and, because of the inherent clearance capabilities of the modality, some instances of drug overdose or ingestion. In the last situation, in which renal function may remain relatively normal, the use of dialysis may result in rapid clearance of toxins, improving survival. There are relative contraindications to hemodialysis, including marked vascular instability or hypotension and advanced liver disease with hepatorenal syndrome. The decision to embark on a protracted course of dialysis must be made cautiously in any patient with advanced multisystem disease in whom the therapy is not likely to alter the prognosis.

Adequate vascular access is essential to successful treatment. The most common technique for achieving access in children is the insertion of a double-lumen catheter into the subclavian or femoral vein. Infrequently, a single-lumen catheter is used for access and return of blood. In patients with chronic renal failure managed by hemodialysis, access may be achieved by permanent placement of a vascular catheter into the superior vena cava, or by the creation of a permanent arteriovenous fistula, using native vessels or interpositioning a synthetic conduit between the artery and vein. Seemingly simple vascular access procedures often are fraught with complications, including hematoma formation and obstruction to flow from edema, bleeding, or thrombosis.

Hemodialysis often requires systemic anticoagulation as a practical matter, and when heparin is used, its clinical effectiveness is monitored by the activated clotting time. It is possible to perform dialysis without the use of an anticoagulant, especially if the patient has a bleeding diathesis, liver disease, or is at risk for bleeding complications (after surgery). In situations where anticoagulants are not used, clotting is discouraged by the use of rapid blood flow rates and frequent rinsing of the blood flow circuit with saline. There is an active interest in the use of regional anticoagulation to prevent the bleeding complications of systemic therapies, but these techniques have not gained widespread use in children or adults.

In addition to the risk of bleeding, hemodialysis is associated with several other complications. The most common side effect is hypotension, which can be related to aggressive volume removal (a target dry weight that is too low), sepsis, or the cytokine and autokine release that results from the passage of blood cells over the hemodialysis membrane surface. Muscle cramps also occur frequently, often as the result of conditions predisposing to hypotension, but also as a result of electrolyte imbalance (especially sodium and calcium). Headache, nausea, and vomiting also are encountered commonly and may result from a described disequilibrium syndrome.

The disequilibrium syndrome is related to rapid removal of solute from the bloodstream (especially urea), with lack of equilibration between the blood and tissues. This is especially true in the brain, where lack of equilibration may result in relative hyperosmolarity within the cell, leading to an influx of water and cell swelling. The swelling of brain tissue is manifested by headache, but may progress to obtundation, seizures, or coma. The disequilibrium syndrome often is seen in the acute setting in new patients who undergo aggressive dialysis, and usually can be avoided by stepwise increases in the dialysis treatment. It also is helpful to treat patients with intravenous mannitol, not as a diuretic, but as an agent that remains in the circulation as an osmotically active particle.

In patients who are unable to tolerate the rapid hemodynamic changes intrinsic to hemodialysis, alternative therapeutic renal replacement modalities are peritoneal dialysis or hemofiltration. The volume changes associated with these modalities are more gentle; however, their clearance capabilities may not always approach that of conventional hemodialysis.

Peritoneal Dialysis

Peritoneal dialysis is a technique developed in the 1970s as a widespread renal replacement modality. It has gained popularity because it is relatively effective, and inexpensive. Peritoneal dialysis involves the direct instillation of dialysate fluid into the peritoneum, with removal of waste products by active and passive diffusion and removal of water by ultrafiltration. Because the peritoneum serves as the dialysis membrane and is porous, there also is passage of some proteins. The resistance of the peritoneal membrane to the passage of proteins and solute is increased by sclerosis and decreased by inflammation (peritonitis).

Peritoneal dialysis necessitates access, which can be achieved by the insertion of an indwelling catheter. By convention, the acute catheter is left in place for a maximum of 72 hours because of the probability of infection if it is left any longer. If dialysis is required for more than 3 days, the catheter is replaced or a permanent catheter is inserted surgically. Several types of permanent catheters are available. They vary in shape (eg, curled, straight) and have a single cuff (placed at the peritoneum) or a double cuff (one placed at the peritoneum and the other near the exit site). The cuffs anchor the catheter through the ingrowth of fibrous tissue.

Peritoneal dialysis may be performed manually, instilling and draining dialysate from the abdomen at prescribed intervals. This method is known as continuous ambulatory peritoneal dialysis. In continuous cycler-assisted peritoneal dialysis, the patient is physically connected to the cycler by extension tubes to the peritoneal catheter, and is dialyzed at predetermined intervals. By varying the interval between exchanges, the dextrose concentration of the dialysate, and the volume of the exchange, the clearance of solute and ultrafiltration of water can be influenced selectively.

The principal complications of this form of dialysis include infection and mechanical problems related to the catheter and circuit. Mechanical problems include poor inflow or outflow from the catheter, often related to physical obstruction from omentum or bowel. The catheter may leak at its point of insertion, or at the exit site. Given the physical presence of dialysate dwelling in the abdomen, hernias may develop or become manifest that require surgical repair before the use of large dialysis volumes. Infectious complications include local infection at the exit site, more extensive involvement of the subcutaneous tunnel, and peritonitis. Peritonitis always is treated as a medical emergency, and depending on the offending organism, may require removal of the peritoneal catheter.

Overall, peritoneal dialysis is believed to be better tolerated hemodynamically, and allows for more steady-state homeostasis than does hemodialysis. However, given the porosity of the peritoneum, with its potential for protein loss and its vulnerability to injury and infection, peritoneal dialysis may not be the modality of choice for a given patient. It may be possible to achieve comparable hemodynamic stability using more controlled hemodialysis, and such is the case with hemofiltration.

Hemofiltration and Hemodiafiltration

Hemofiltration first was described by Kramer[45a] in 1977, and is an extracorporeal method of removing excess fluid and solutes by continuous arteriovenous hemofiltration. Since that time, the modality has been applied widely to the treatment of both adults and children. It has been used successfully to control hypervolemia and clear metabolic wastes. Since its inception, continuous arteriovenous hemofiltration has been intended to be a bedside modality that works through the generation of a plasma water ultrafiltrate across a highly permeable membrane. The rate at which the ultrafiltrate forms (Qf) is directly dependent on the permeability of the membrane (K, the coefficient of membrane permeability) and the blood flow rate through the circuit. The blood flow rate ultimately is dependent on arterio-

venous blood pressure differences, which in addition are responsible for the generation of a transmembrane pressure gradient (TMP). The relation is described by the following equation:

$$Qf = K \times TMP$$

Since its initial description, continuous arteriovenous hemofiltration has been modified by the addition of dialysis to allow for more effective solute clearance (continuous arteriovenous hemodiafiltration).

More recently, with the inclusion of an external blood pump, patients have successfully undergone hemofiltration using only a venous access (continuous venovenous hemofiltration). In continuous arteriovenous hemofiltration, continuous arteriovenous hemodiafiltration, continuous venovenous hemofiltration, and continuous venovenous hemodiafiltration, the ultrafiltrate is replaced by a fluid of appropriate electrolyte content, occasionally with the addition of parenteral nutrition. When necessary, using arteriovenous or venovenous access, patients can undergo slow volume removal, or ultrafiltration, without volume replacement. The choice of modality, the rate of volume removal, and the choice of and volume of fluid replacement are tailored to the individual patient.

The indications for hemofiltration are analogous to those of peritoneal dialysis or hemodialysis and include acute renal insufficiency, hypervolemia refractory to medical management, and electrolyte and acid–base disturbances accompanying these conditions. This treatment modality causes less hemodynamic instability than standard hemodialysis and is used in the clinical setting of renal failure in patients with shock, sepsis, burns, or hepatic failure.

The rate of volume removal can be defined as the ultrafiltration rate and other volume output minus the replacement fluid. Actual solute and waste clearance is a function of blood flow through the circuit and resultant ultrafiltrate formation, and the degree of protein binding. The propensity for a solute to be cleared also is influenced by its molecular size relative to the membrane's pore size. The rate of ultrafiltrate formation can be augmented by increasing negative pressure across the membrane by lowering the collection vessel below the level of the ultrafiltration circuit and filter. For each centimeter below the level of the circuit, 0.74 mmHg of negative pressure is generated.

Like all renal replacement therapies, this treatment modality has inherent risks. The use of systemic anticoagulation places patients at risk for hemorrhage, and debilitated patients have a significant risk of intracerebral or intraventricular hemorrhage. Patients may remain uremic as a result of the filter's inadequate clearance capabilities. Alternatively, volume depletion, caused by high ultrafiltrate formation, and secondary hypotension may complicate the care of critically ill patients.

CHRONIC RENAL INSUFFICIENCY AND FAILURE

Electrolyte Abnormalities

The loss of functioning renal mass results in a compensatory increase in filtration by the remaining renal tissue.[46,47] After a unilateral nephrectomy, there is a demonstrable increase in the GFR and evidence of contralateral renal hypertrophy within the first 48 hours. By 2 to 4 weeks, the GFR has returned to 80% of normal and there is no clinical evidence of renal dysfunction. With the loss of 50% to 75% of the renal mass, there is an increase in the residual function to 50% to 80% of normal and often little evidence for clinical renal insufficiency. When the residual renal function falls to 30% to 50% of normal, the term *chronic renal insufficiency* applies. At this point, acute illness and other stress states may result in acidosis, hyperkalemia, and dehydration. It is only when the residual function falls to less than 30% of normal that the term *chronic renal failure* is used. At this point, electrolyte abnormalities begin to appear and, more importantly, there is limited ability of the kidney to adjust to variations in fluid and electrolyte homeostasis (Table 6-3). The term *uremia* refers to the symptoms of anorexia, nausea, lethargy, and somnolence that develop as a result of chronic renal failure. Uremia ultimately results in death unless dialysis therapy or renal transplantation is performed. The performance of dialysis or renal transplantation is referred to as end-stage renal disease care.

The adaptive response of the kidney to the loss of functioning renal tissue is remarkable. The excretion of sodium, potassium, and water is maintained until the GFR is only 10% to 20% of normal. The factors responsible for these adaptive phenomena vary. For example, sodium is regulated independently from phosphorus, and involves both intrinsic renal and extrarenal elements. In response to these adaptive mechanisms, there may be "trade-offs," such as hypertension associated with enhancement of sodium excretion by the natriuretic hormone and secondary hyperparathyroidism associated with control of calcium and phosphorus metabolism.

One of the most important consequences of these adaptive processes is the limitation in the ability of the kidney to maintain homeostasis in response to stress or further injury. Whereas patients with normal renal function can respond to extremes in water intake of 1 to 12 L/m^2/d, patients with renal failure may tolerate an intake of only 2 to 3 L/m^2/d without the development of hyponatremia or hypernatremia (Fig. 6-10). This is because each functioning nephron is required to increase the fraction of filtered solute and water it excretes to maintain balance. At a normal GFR, 1% of the filtered sodium is excreted; with a reduction to a GFR of 10% of normal, 10% of the filtered sodium must be excreted to maintain sodium balance. This is referred to as the *magnification phenomenon*. The damaged kid-

ney is able to respond to changes in the intake of a substance, but it may take days rather than hours to adapt.

Despite losses of up to 90% of renal function, sodium homeostasis usually is well maintained in chronic renal failure. In the presence of large decreases in the GFR, the kidney maintains a normal serum sodium by increasing the FE_{Na} from less than 1% up to 25% to 30%, largely through decreases in distal tubular reabsorption. Some of the hormonal factors involved in this adaptation include aldosterone, atrial natriuretic factor, and a poorly characterized natriuretic hormone that inhibits Na$^+$-K$^+$-ATPase. With chronic renal failure, the ability of the kidney to handle a wide range of sodium intake, from 1 to 250 mEq/m^2/d, is lost. Instead, the kidney may be able to handle an intake of only 100 to 150 mEq/m^2/d. It may be possible to decrease this obligatory excretion of sodium to 5 to 20 mEq/m^2/d, but only after weeks of decreasing the sodium intake slowly. Certain children with renal disease, especially those with obstructive uropathy or tubulointerstitial disease, may be unable to adjust to a decreased sodium intake and display a "salt-losing" nephropathy. These patients are prone to dehydration with salt restriction and may need salt supplementation for normal growth. In others, a regular diet may lead to sodium retention, volume overload, and hypertension. Sodium intake must be individualized to fit the limitations of each patient.

Water balance also is affected by chronic renal failure. There is an obligatory total osmolar excretion that limits the ability of the kidney to excrete free water. In addition, the concentrating ability of the kidney is affected, limiting its ability to make a maximally concentrated or dilute urine. These limitations may result in both water retention and hyponatremia or dehydration if water is administered in amounts exceeding the kidney's capabilities. These limitations must be considered in the treatment of children with chronic renal failure in such clinical situations as the time before surgery when free access to water is restricted.

In the presence of chronic renal failure, normal serum potassium levels usually are maintained until the GFR is less than 10% of normal. Potassium excretion in normal and uremic states is maintained by potassium secretion in the distal nephron.[48] In response to an increase in potassium intake or loss of renal mass, there is an increase in Na$^+$-K$^+$-ATPase in the remaining collecting tubules that seems to be partly responsible for augmented excretion of potassium per nephron. Excretion of potassium at a rate six-fold greater than normal and 1.5 times the filtered potassium load can be demonstrated in renal tubules from uremic animals. Partial adaptation can occur in the absence

TABLE 6-3. *Common complications of chronic renal failure in children*

Condition	Pathophysiology	Treatment
Anemia	Inadequate erythropoietin production	Recombinant erythropoietin
	Iron, folate deficiency	Iron, folate
	Hemolysis	
	Inhibitors of erythropoiesis	
Bleeding	Inhibitors of platelet function	Adequate dialysis DDAVP
Renal osteodystrophy	Decreased excretion of phosphate	Calcium carbonate
	Decreased production of 1,25 (OH)$_2$ vitamin D	1,25 (OH)$_2$ vitamin D
Hypertension	Salt and water retention	Control of dry weight
	Increased renin, angiotensin II	Angiotensin-converting enzyme inhibitors
Acidosis	Decreased ammonia excretion	Sodium bicarbonate or sodium citrate

DDAVP, 1-deamino-8-D-arginine vasopressin.

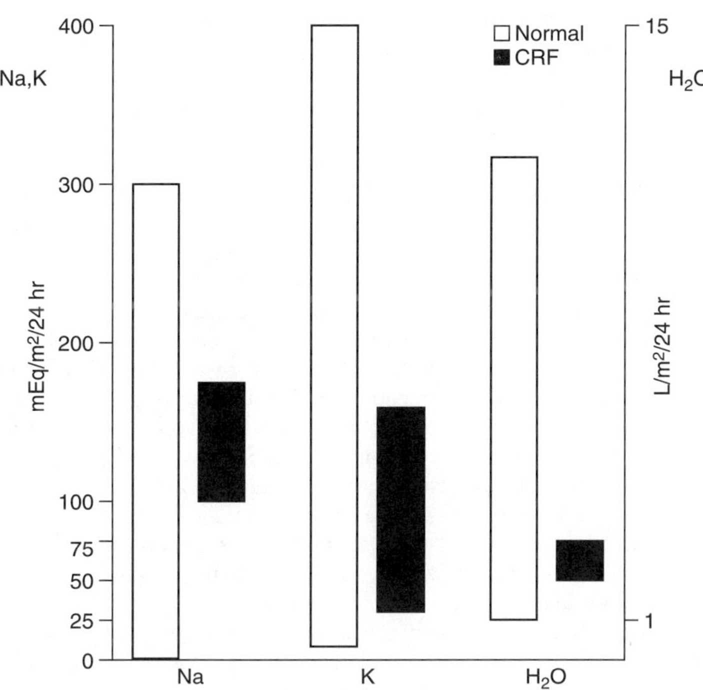

FIG. 6-10. Handling of salt and water in chronic renal failure (CRF). The kidneys in CRF do not tolerate maximal or minimal intakes of sodium, water, and potassium. This results in relatively narrow ranges of intake to maintain homeostasis.

of aldosterone, but aldosterone plays an important role in the maintenance of normal potassium homeostasis. This is demonstrated by the presence of hyperkalemia in patients with hyporeninemic hypoaldosteronism or in those treated with the aldosterone antagonist spironolactone.

The colon normally is responsible for the excretion of less than 13% of dietary potassium. In the presence of chronic renal failure, this can be increased to 50% by the activation of colonic Na^+-K^+-ATPase. Aldosterone plays a role in this augmentation of colonic Na^+-K^+-ATPase. An additional mechanism that plays an essential role in the adaptation to an acute potassium load is the redistribution of potassium from the extracellular to the intracellular compartment, which is dependent on insulin, β-adrenergic catecholamines, aldosterone, and pH. Despite the presence of total body potassium depletion in uremia, there is impaired uptake of potassium into the cells. This contributes to the intolerance of an acute potassium load in uremia despite the ability to excrete a potassium load.

Hyperkalemia is a major problem in chronic renal failure. In contrast, significant hypokalemia is unusual in the absence of potassium restriction, alkalosis, or diuretic therapy. Hyperkalemia can result from an extrinsic potassium load, but it also can be caused by fasting or acidosis, in which case the source of the potassium is the intracellular compartment. This can be a particular problem when a patient is fasted before surgery, and can be ameliorated by an infusion of glucose and insulin. Drugs that can cause hyperkalemia in renal failure include spironolactone, β-adrenergic blockers, and angiotensin-converting enzyme inhibitors. When clinically significant hyperkalemia develops in a patient with chronic renal failure, it is treated best initially by stabilizing the myocardium with calcium gluconate and redistributing the potassium into the intracellular compartment with insulin and glucose. More definitive correction of hyperkalemia is accomplished by removing potassium from the body using dialysis or Kayexalate. Nebulized albuterol at eight

times the normal asthma dose also has been found to be effective in stimulating potassium redistribution, whereas $NaHCO_3$ administration has not.

Metabolic acidosis commonly is present with chronic renal failure.[49] The metabolic acidosis is associated with a normal anion gap in moderate renal insufficiency, but with severe renal insufficiency, there is retention of phosphate, sulfate, and organic acids, resulting in an elevated anion gap. The primary cause of metabolic acidosis in chronic renal failure is inability of the remaining proximal renal tubule to increase ammonium formation to keep pace with the loss of renal mass. The kidney becomes unable to generate the 1 to 3 mEq/kg/d of new bicarbonate that is necessary to compensate for that lost to buffer endogenous acid production. Previous studies have suggested a major role for decreased reabsorption of bicarbonate by the proximal renal tubule in chronic renal failure. Although this may occur in the presence of volume overload, severe secondary hyperparathyroidism, and disorders such as Fanconi's syndrome, it is not a major mechanism causing acidosis in chronic renal failure. Except for severe phosphate depletion, decreased excretion of phosphate as a titratable acid normally does not contribute to metabolic acidosis.

One of the earliest manifestations of chronic renal failure is secondary hyperparathyroidism.[50] Secondary hyperparathyroidism resulting from inadequate formation of 1,25-$(OH)_2$ vitamin D develops in moderate renal insufficiency in the presence of normal serum concentrations of calcium and phosphorus. With more severe renal insufficiency, overt hypocalcemia and hyperphosphatemia often develop. Hypocalcemia results from decreased calcium absorption from the gastrointestinal tract as a result of true deficiency of 1,25-$(OH)_2$ vitamin D. In addition, diminished release of calcium from bone occurs as a result of resistance to the action of parathyroid hormone, and calcium and phosphate are deposited in soft tissues as a consequence of hyperphosphatemia.

The kidney plays a key role in the maintenance of normal phosphate homeostasis by regulating its excretion. In the presence of a normal GFR, the kidney excretes 5% to 15% of the filtered load of phosphate, whereas in chronic renal failure, the kidney can increase the fractional excretion of phosphate to 60% to 80%. Through this adaptation, the kidneys in chronic renal failure are able to maintain phosphate balance, but at a higher serum phosphate level. However, they have no reserve with which to increase phosphate excretion in response to a phosphate load. A large phosphate load, such as can occur with the administration of a phosphate-containing enema, can lead to life-threatening hyperphosphatemia and hypocalcemia in chronic renal failure.

Hematologic Problems

One of the most common manifestations of chronic renal failure is anemia. The anemia of chronic renal failure results from impaired erythropoiesis, hemolysis, and bleeding. Of these, impaired erythropoiesis is most important and usually is the result of a deficiency of erythropoietin production. Erythropoietin is synthesized and secreted by peritubular cells in the renal cortex in response to decreased tissue oxygenation. It acts on receptors on the erythroid burst-forming units and erythroid colony-forming units, and leads to erythropoiesis. With loss of renal mass, erythropoietin secretion does not respond adequately to hypoxia, and anemia results. With the advent of recombinant human erythropoietin therapy, patients with chronic renal failure now are treated routinely with erythropoietin.[51] Current recommendations are to treat patients with chronic renal failure in whom the hematocrit is less than 30%, starting at a dosage of about 50 to 150 units/kg intravenously three times a week. When a target hematocrit of 36% is reached, a maintenance dosage of about 75 units/kg is instituted. Subcutaneous administration of erythropoietin has been found to be more effective on a per-unit basis, can be given only once a week, and obviates the need for intravenous injections. Dosages of greater than 150 units/kg increase the hematocrit faster than lesser dosages, but both therapies take 4 to 8 weeks to reach target hematocrit values of 33% to 36%. The most common cause for failure of erythropoietin to be effective is concurrent iron deficiency. Current recommendations are to maintain serum ferritin levels above 250 ng/mL and transferrin saturation above 25%. Other causes for failure of erythropoietin to increase or maintain the hematocrit are occult infections, hemolysis, aluminum overload, severe hyperparathyroidism, or occult bleeding. Complications of erythropoietin therapy include worsening of hypertension and a possible increased incidence of thrombosis of polytetrafluoroethylene vascular grafts.

The other major hematologic problem in chronic renal failure is bleeding. This is a classic and lethal complication in patients with terminal uremia and results from platelet dysfunction in the presence of a normal coagulation profile and normal platelet counts. The best indicator of platelet dysfunction in patients with chronic renal failure is prolonged bleeding time. The platelet dysfunction is the result of poorly described abnormalities attributed to the uremic environment, and platelet transfusions are ineffective. Dialysis improves the platelet dysfunction, as does improvement in the hematocrit with transfusion or erythropoietin therapy. The vasopressin analogue, 1-deamino-8-D-argi-nine vasopressin, has been shown to be effective in improving the bleeding time in patients with uremia when it is administered at an intravenous dosage of 0.3 μg/kg, and it has been used effectively before surgery.

Hypertension and Cardiovascular Complications

Hypertension is one of the most common complications of chronic renal failure and contributes significantly to the morbidity and mortality of these patients. The cause is multifactorial and includes volume overload and hormonal abnormalities, such as increased secretion of renin, that result from the underlying renal disorder. In patients receiving dialysis, volume overload is the result of inadequate removal of volume by the process of ultrafiltration during dialysis. The goal of ultrafiltration is to remove sufficient salt and water to achieve the ''dry weight'' that is appropriate for each patient. The dry weight is that weight at which the patient has no signs of volume overload, but below which the patient has hypotension. The initial response to volume overload is to increase the cardiac output. Later, the cardiac output returns to normal, but the peripheral resistance becomes elevated because of peripheral vasoconstriction, resulting in hypertension. These patients may have no other signs of volume overload, such as edema, but with a reduction in total body salt and water content, the blood pressure can be controlled with little or no antihypertensive medication.

In other patients, intrinsic renal abnormalities play a primary role in hypertension. In these patients, bilateral nephrectomy may be necessary to control the hypertension, although it usually can be controlled with oral antihypertensive agents. Of the mechanisms that cause hypertension in these patients, increased renin secretion is the best understood. Renin activates the formation of angiotensin I, which, when converted to angiotensin II, is a powerful vasoconstrictor. Patients with renin-dependent hypertension respond poorly to control of blood pressure by salt and water removal alone, but respond well to angiotensin-converting enzyme inhibitors such as captopril.

Cardiovascular disease is the most common cause of death in patients receiving long-term dialysis, including children.[52] Patients with chronic renal failure can have abnormalities of the pericardium, myocardium, cardiac valves, and coronary arteries. Most important is the increased incidence of premature death caused by coronary artery disease that is occurring in adults, who are surviving longer with improved end-stage renal disease care. Lipid abnormalities, hypertension, and other abnormalities associated with chronic renal failure contribute to ischemic heart disease in older adults. Another cardiac manifestation, pericarditis, has long been recognized as a complication of uremia. Whereas it once was considered a sign of the terminal phase of uremia, it now is present in 15% of patients receiving dialysis and can be symptomatic or clinically silent. In nondialyzed uremic patients with pericarditis, intensive dialysis often results in its resolution within about 2 weeks. In certain patients, surgical procedures such as pericardiocentesis, pericardial drainage with a catheter or through a pericardial window, and even pericardiectomy are required.

Left ventricular failure also is a common complication of chronic renal failure. In older patients, coronary artery disease may lead to myocardial dysfunction, severely limiting cardiac output. Volume overload and hypertension, which increase preload and afterload, respectively, are important causes of heart failure. With proper fluid management and antihypertensive medication, these abnormalities can be controlled. Anemia is another contributing factor that can be controlled with the use of erythropoietin therapy. Finally, an array of metabolic abnormalities associated with chronic renal failure, such as secondary hyperparathyroidism, electrolyte and acid–base imbalances, and the accumulation of nonspecific uremic toxins, all contribute to abnormal myocardial function.

Anesthesia in Patients With Renal Failure

Patients with chronic renal failure frequently require surgery, but have several problems that complicate the required anesthesia.[53] These problems stem mainly from fluid and electrolyte abnormalities, complications of chronic renal failure such as hypertension, and differences in the pharmacokinetics of anesthetic agents in chronic renal failure. In patients with some renal function, AVP secretion and activation of renin secretion during anesthesia may result in clinically significant water and sodium overload. Hypertension and hypotension pose major problems during anesthesia. In patients with poorly controlled hypertension before surgery, severe rises in blood pressure can occur, especially during light anesthesia. This usually can be controlled by a variety of antihypertensive agents. On the other end of the spectrum, patients receiving dialysis who are volume depleted before surgery are prone to the development of hypotension during anesthesia because of inadequate intravascular volume. Hypotension probably is handled best by the administration of colloid or packed red blood cells, especially if the patients are anemic.

In chronic renal failure, increased tissue water, muscle wasting, increased cardiac output, decreased renal clearance, and abnormal protein binding of drugs can alter the metabolism of anesthetic agents. Volatile anesthetics are taken up more rapidly, but actually take longer to reach the alveolar anesthetic concentration to achieve the required brain anesthetic tension. Fluoride-containing agents such as enflurane may create unacceptable problems with fluoride toxicity in renal failure, whereas halothane usually is well tolerated and is preferred. Opiates, tranquilizers, and barbiturates can be used safely, but may be associated with more rapid awakening in patients with chronic renal failure. Muscle relaxants should be used with caution in patients with renal failure, especially if there is significant muscle atrophy. Despite concerns expressed in the literature, succinylcholine can be used safely in the absence of hyperkalemia. Decamethonium and the nondepolarizing muscle relaxants gallamine and metocurine are relatively contraindicated because of significantly prolonged half-lives with chronic renal failure. Curare and pancuronium can be used, but are not ideal.

The choice of anesthesia is an important consideration in patients with renal failure. The use of regional anesthesia, such as upper extremity blocks when achieving vascular access or epidural or spinal anesthesia when appropriate for other procedures, avoids many of the complications of general anesthesia. Careful evaluation of each patient's condition, age, and required procedure facilitates the correct anesthetic choice.

REFERENCES

1. Maddox DA, Brenner BM. Glomerular ultrafitration. In: Brenner BM, Rector FC Jr, eds. The kidney, ed 4. Philadelphia, WB Saunders, 1991: 205.
2. Fawer C-L, Torrado A, Guignard J-P. Maturation of renal function in full-term and premature neonates. Helv Paediat Acta 1979;34:11.
3. Aperia A, Borberger O, Elinder G, et al. Postnatal development of renal function in pre-term and full-term infants. Acta Paediatr Scand 1981; 70:183.
4. Schwartz GJ, Haycock GB, Edelmann CM Jr, Spitzer A. A simple estimate of glomerular filtration rate in chidren derived from body length and plasma creatinine. Pediatrics 1976;58:259.
5. Schwartz GJ, Feld LG, Langford DJ. A simple estimate of glomerular filtration rate in full-term infants during the first year of life. J Pediatr 1984;104:849.
6. Sonnberg H. Renal regulation of salt balance: a primer for non-purists. Pediatr Nephrol 1990;4:354.
7. Tulassay T, Seri I, Rascher W. Atrial natriuretic peptide and extracellular volume contraction after birth. Acta Paediatr Scand 1987;76:444.
8. Robertson GL. Physiology of ADH secretion. Kidney Int 1988; 32(Suppl 21):20.
9. Baylis PH. Osmoregulation and control of vasopressin secretion in healthy humans. Am J Physiol 1987;253:R671.
10. Rowe JW, Shelton RL, Helderman JH. Influence of the emetic reflex on vasopressin release in man. Kidney Int 1979;16:729.
11. Svenningsen NW, Aronson AS. Postnatal development of renal concentrating capacity as estimated by the DDAVP-test in normal and asphyxiated neonates. Biol Neonate 1974;25:23.
12. Tudvad F, McNamara H, Barnett HL. Renal response of premature infants to administration of bicarbonate and potassium. Pediatrics 1954; 13:4.
13. Edelmann CM Jr, Rodriguez-Soriano J, Boichis H, et al. Renal bicarbonate reabsortion and hydrogen ion excretion in normal infants. J Clin Invest 1967;46:1309.
14. Svenningsen NW, Lindquist B. Postnatal development of renal hydrogen ion excretion capacity in relationship to age and protein intake. Acta Paediatr Scand 1974;63:721.
15. Sargent JD, Stukel TA, Kresel J, Klein RZ. Normal values for random urinary calcium to creatinine ratios in infancy. J Pediatr 1993;123:393.
16. Rowe JC, Goetz CA, Carey DE, Horak E. Achievement of *in utero* retention of calcium and phosphorus accompanied by high calcium excretion in very low birth weight infants fed a fortified formula. J Pediatr 1987;110:581.
17. Ghazali S, Barrett TM. Urinary excretion of calcium and magnesium in children. Arch Dis Child 1974;49:97.
18. Brodehl J, Gellissen K, Kaas WP, et al. The postnatal development of tubular phosphate reabsorption. Kidney Int 1978;13:526.
19. Gonzalez-Campoy J, Knox FG. Integrated responses of the kidney to alterations in extracellular fluid volume. In: Seldin DW, Giebisch G, eds. The kidney: physiology and pathophysiology, ed 2. New York, Raven Press, 1992:2041.
20. Dzau VJ. Renal and circulatory mechanisms in congestive heart failure. Kidney Int 1987;31:1402.
21. Sterns RH, Ocdol H, Schrier RW, Narins RG. Hyponatremia: pathophysiology, diagnosis, and therapy. In: Narins RG, ed. Clinical disorders of fluid and electrolyte metabolism, ed 5. New York, McGraw-Hill, 1994:583.
22. Robertson GL. The use of vasopressin assays in physiology and pathophysiology. Semin Nephrol 1994;14:368.
23. Brown RS. Extrarenal potassium homeostasis. Kidney Int 1986;30:116.
24. Gennari FJ, Maddox DA. Renal regulation of acid-base homeostasis, integrated response. In: Seldin DW, Giebisch G, eds. The kidney: physiology and pathophysiology, ed 2. New York, Raven Press, 1992:2695.
25. Halperin ML, Kamel KS, Ethier JH, et al. Biochemistry and physiology of ammonium excretion. In: Seldin DW, Giebisch G, eds. The kidney: physiology and pathophysiology, ed 2. New York, Raven Press, 1992: 2645.
26. Alpern RJ, Emmett M, Seldin DW. Metabolic alkalosis. In: Seldin DW, Giebisch G, eds. The kidney: physiology and pathophysiology, ed 2. New York, Raven Press, 1992:2733.
27. Rose BD. Diuretics. Kidney Int 1991;39:336.
28. Wells TG. The pharmacology and therapeutics of diuretics in the pediatric patient. Pediatr Clin North Am 1990;37:463.

29. Brater DC. Resistance to diuretics: mechanisms and clinical applications. Advances in Nephrology 1993;22:349.
30. Kirschenbaum MA, Anderson DA. Nephropathies of nonsteroidal anti-inflammatory agents. In: Massry SG, Glassock RJ, eds. Textbook of nephrology. Baltimore, Williams & Wilkins, 1989:823.
31. Hricik DE, Dunn MJ. Angiotensin-converting enzyme inhibitor induced renal failure: causes, consequences, and diagnostic uses. J Am Soc Nephrol 1990;1:845.
32. Seigel NJ, Gaudio KM, Van Why SK, et al. Acute renal failure: pathophysiological mechanisms. In: Holliday MA, Barratt TM, Avner ED, eds. Pediatric nephrology, ed 2. Baltimore, Williams & Wilkins, 1994: 1176.
33. DiBona GF. Hemodynamic support: volume management and pharmacological cardiovascular support. Semin Nephrol 1994;14:33.
34. Myers BD, Hilberman M, Spencer RJ, Jamison RL. Glomerular and tubular function in non-oliguric acute renal failure. Am J Med 1982; 72:642.
35. Myers BD, Chui F, Hilberman M, Michaels AS. Transtubular leakage of glomerular filtrate in human acute renal failure. Am J Physiol 1979; 237:F319.
36. Avison MJ, van Waard A, Stromski ME, et al. Metabolic alterations in the kidney during ischemic acute renal failure. Semin Nephrol 1989; 9:98.
37. Andreoli SP. Reactive oxygen molecules, oxidant injury and renal disease. Pediatr Nephrol 1991;5:733.
38. Berridge MJ. The biology and medicine of calcium signalling. Mol Cell Endocrinol 1994;98:119.
39. Fischereder M, Trick W, Nath KA. Therapeutic strategies in the prevention of acute renal failure. Semin Nephrol 1994;14:41.
40. Shilliday I, Allison MEM. Diuretics in acute renal failure. Ren Fail 1994;16:3.
41. Shanley PF, Johnson GC. Adenine nucleotides, transport activity and hypoxic necrosis in the thick ascending limb of Henle. Kidney Int 1989; 36:823.
42. Szerlip HM. Renal-dose dopamine: fact and fiction. Ann Intern Med 1991;115:153.
43. Flancbaum L, Choban P, Dasta J. Quantitative effect of low-dose dopamine (DA) on urine output (UO) in oliguric SICU patients (pts). Crit Care Med 1992;20:S21.
44. Jameson MD, Wiegmann TB. Principles, uses, and complications of hemodialysis. Med Clin North Am 1990;74:945.
45. Mehta R. Therapeutic alternatives to renal replacement for critically ill patients in acute renal failure. Semin Nephrol 1994;14:64.
45a. Kramer P, Wigger W, Rieger J, Matthaei D, Scheler F. Arteriovenous hemofiltration: a new and simple method for the treatment of overhydrated patients resistant to diuretics. Klin Wochenschr 1977;55:1121.
46. Fine LG, Kurtz I, Woolf AS, et al. Pathophysiology and nephron adaptation in chronic renal failure. In: Schrier RW, Gotschalk CW, eds. Diseases of the kidney, ed 5. Boston, Little, Brown, 1993:2703.
47. Fildes RD, Jose PA. Disturbances in salt and water balance. In: Edelmann CM, ed. Pediatric kidney disease, ed 2. Boston, Little, Brown, 1992:609.
48. Allon M. Treatment and prevention of hyperkalemia in end-stage renal disease. Kidney Int 1993;43:1197.
49. Warnock DG. Uremic acidosis. Kidney Int 1988;34:278.
50. Feinfeld DA, Sherwood LM. Parathyroid hormone and $1,25(OH)_2D_3$ in chronic renal failure. Kidney Int 1988;33:1049.
51. Eschbach JW. Erythropoietin: the promise and the facts. Kidney Int 1994;45(Suppl 44):S70.
52. Harnett JD, Parthey PS. Cardiac disease in uremia. Semin Nephrol 1994;14:245.
53. Gronert GA. Anesthetic considerations. In: Eknoyan G, Knochel JP, eds. The systemic consequences of renal failure. Orlando, Grune & Stratton, 1984:519.

Surgery of Infants and Children: Scientific Principles and Practice, edited by
Keith T. Oldham, Paul M. Colombani, and Robert P. Foglia.
Lippincott–Raven Publishers, Philadelphia, © 1997.

CHAPTER 7

Cardiopulmonary Critical Care and Shock

Ronald B. Hirschl and Kurt Heiss

Support of oxygen delivery is essential to the care of the critically ill. Whether through interventions designed to correct deviations in cardiac output, oxygenation, or hemoglobin content, the overall therapeutic goal is to maintain perfusion and oxygen delivery to the tissues. Lactic acidosis, impairment of organ function, and eventual death of the organism are the sequelae of inadequate oxygen delivery. This chapter discusses the hemodynamic evaluation and management of critically ill patients, with particular emphasis on the assessment and maintenance of optimal oxygen delivery (Do_2) and oxygen consumption ($\dot{V}o_2$) relations.

OXYGEN KINETICS

Oxygen Consumption

Oxygen based metabolism is necessary to maintain cell life. The cellular milieu typically requires an oxygen tension of about 1 to 4 mmHg to sustain baseline $\dot{V}o_2$ levels.[1] Intravascular venous oxygen tensions of at least 20 mmHg are required to maintain an appropriate oxygen gradient to achieve these minimal levels of intracellular oxygen tension.[2] Oxygen is necessary to provide reduction of cytochromes A and A3 to allow oxidative phosphorylation to occur (Fig. 7-1).[3] Hypoxemia results in a decrease in the availability of oxygen to mitochondria. The consequence is inhibition of Kreb cycle activity with reduction in adenosine triphosphate (ATP) production. With a decrease in perfusion, metabolism of other substrates such as glucose by the glycolytic pathway is necessary to maintain cellular metabolic processes. As ATP stores diminish, cellular synthetic and transport functions become impaired and eventually stop. With continued hypoxia, mitochondrial and endoplasmic reticulum swelling is observed, and lysosomal rupture and intracellular proteolysis follow.

The oxygen consumption of the organism is the sum of the metabolic needs of all of the individual cells. In adults, $\dot{V}o_2$ is typically 3 mL/kg/min (120 mL/m^2/min) under basal conditions.[4] It can range as high as 8 mL/kg/min, depending on the size of the patient. The $\dot{V}o_2$ levels are greater in smaller patients, in whom the surface area/body mass ratio is high. The basal metabolic rate is regulated by the hypothalamus with control by thyroid hormone and catecholamine availability. The $\dot{V}o_2$ levels decrease in the settings of hypothermia, hypothyroidism, and paralysis. In contrast, muscular activity, hyperthermia, hyperthyroidism, catecholamine production or administration, and cytokine expression all increase $\dot{V}o_2$. Examination of total body oxygen consumption, however, fails to reflect the variation found in individual organs. Especially high $\dot{V}o_2$ levels are observed in the heart (30 to 80 mL/kg/min), the liver (25 to 50 mL/kg/min), and the alimentary tract (25 mL/kg/min). Oxygen consumption can vary even within an individual organ; for example, an increase in heart rate or afterload can result in up to a three-fold increase in $\dot{V}o_2$ in the heart.[5] A similar increase may be observed in the gastrointestinal tract after consumption of food, the musculoskeletal system with exercise, and the musculoskeletal system with labored breathing (Table 7-1).

Precise measurement of oxygen consumption in the intensive care unit is often difficult. Three methods are in reasonably frequent use: (1) closed-circuit rebreathing volumetric analysis; (2) mixed expired gas analysis; and (3) calculations based on the Fick equation.[6] Closed-circuit breathing volumetric spirometry is the gold standard because it directly measures the actual volume of oxygen; the circuit contains a spirometer and a carbon dioxide scrubber[7,8] (Fig. 7-2). Any leak in the system has a large effect on the volumetric measurement and, therefore, introduces substantial error into oxygen consumption assessment. This technique is most easy applied, therefore, to mechanically ventilated patients with endotracheal tubes because concerns regarding nose and mouth closure during analysis are obviated.

The second method of measuring oxygen consumption is by inspired and expired gas analysis[9,10] (Fig. 7-3). Precise measurement of the oxygen concentration in both the inspired (F_{IO_2}) and expired (F_{EO_2}) gas is performed. The difference is multiplied by the minute volume ventilation to yield $\dot{V}o_2$. Three potentially imprecise measurements are required: F_{IO_2}, F_{EO_2}, and minute volume ventilation. This technique is most suitable for the patient breathing air because the inspired gas oxygen concentration may be assumed rather than measured. Unfortunately, most critically ill patients require an increase in inspired gas and large minute volumes for effective ventilation, both of which increase the potential for error associated with oxygen consumption assessment by mixed expiratory gas analysis.

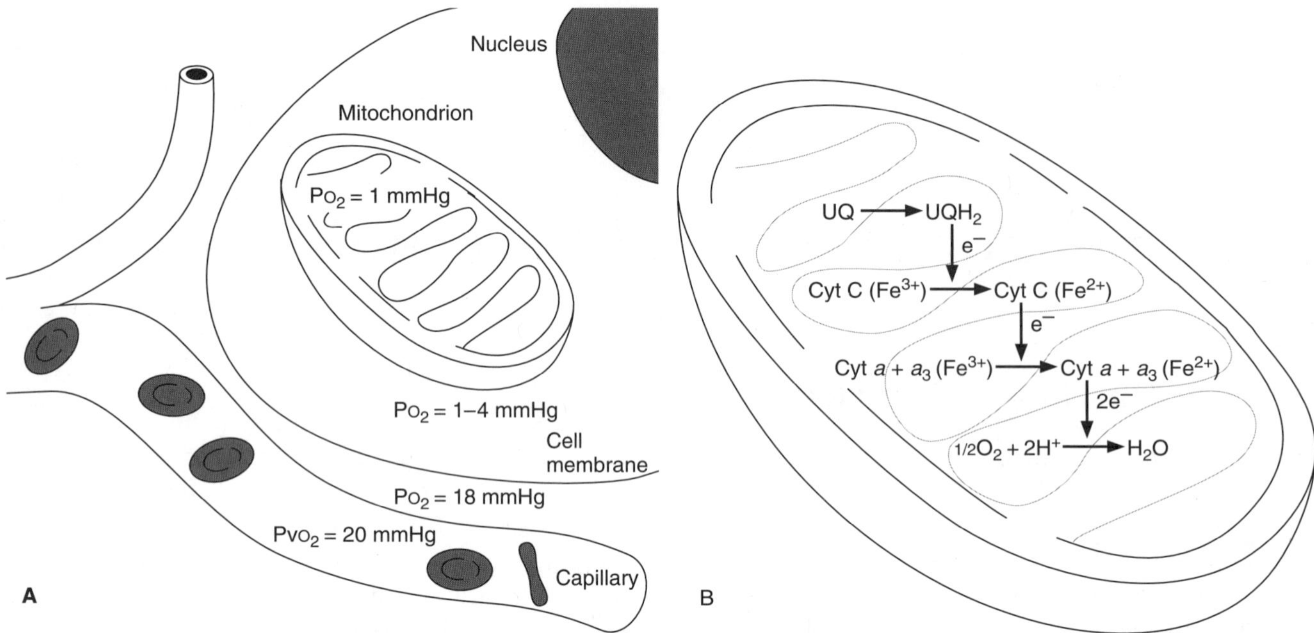

FIG. 7-1. The metabolic functions of the mitochondria are dependent on an uninterrupted supply of oxygen. (*A*) Estimated critical levels of venous capillary (Pvo₂) tissue and of cell membrane and mitochondrial Po₂ are shown. (*B*) The process of cytochrome-dependent reduction required for oxidative phosphorylation is illustrated.

The third technique for oxygen consumption measurement applies Fick's axiom, which states that the $\dot{V}_{O_2}$ is exactly equal to the amount of oxygen taken up in the pulmonary capillaries from the airway.[11] This may be expressed by the equation:

$$\dot{V}_{O_2} = Q \times (Ca_{O_2} - Cv_{O_2})$$

where Q = cardiac output,
$\quad$ Ca$_{O_2}$ = oxygen content of arterial blood, and
$\quad$ Cv$_{O_2}$ = oxygen content of venous blood

Because mixed venous blood must be analyzed, this technique is only applicable to the patient with a pulmonary artery catheter in place. Because of the error introduced by both cardiac output measurements and blood gas analysis, this technique is the least accurate and should only be used to provide a rough estimate of oxygen consumption or in situations in which the two previously discussed techniques cannot be used.

Oxygen consumption measurements must be converted from atmospheric temperature–pressure–saturated (ATPS) to standard temperature–pressure–dry (STPD) units. The conversion adjusts the $\dot{V}_{O_2}$ measurement by 15% to 20%.

Oxygen Delivery

Three clinical factors are manipulated in an attempt to improve oxygen delivery: cardiac output, hemoglobin concentration, and arterial blood oxygen saturation (Sao₂). Although we tend to address each individually, it is the product of the three that allows one to achieve sufficient oxygen delivery. The following calculation reveals the relation of these three factors to one another and to the D_{O_2}[12] (Fig. 7-4):

$$D_{O_2} = Q \times [(1.36 \times \text{serum hemoglobin concentration} \times Sa_{O_2}) + (0.003 \times Pa_{O_2})]$$

Note that the contribution of the partial pressure of arterial oxygen (Pao₂) to oxygen delivery is minimal and, therefore, may be disregarded in many circumstances. Each gram of hemoglobin combines with up to 1.36 mL of oxygen. If the hemoglobin concentration of the blood is normal (15 g/dL) and the hemoglobin is 100% saturated, the amount of oxygen bound to hemoglobin is 20.4 mL/dL. In addition, about 0.3 mL of oxygen is physically dissolved in each deciliter of plasma, which makes

TABLE 7-1. *Factors contributing to alterations in oxygen consumption*

INCREASE IN OXYGEN CONSUMPTION
Sepsis
Burns
Agitation
Seizures
Exercise, muscle activity, respiratory distress
Fever
Increased catecholamine production
Catecholamine administration
Hypocarbia

DECREASE IN OXYGEN CONSUMPTION
Paralysis
Hypothermia
Sedation
β-blockade
Mechanical ventilation
Hypercarbia

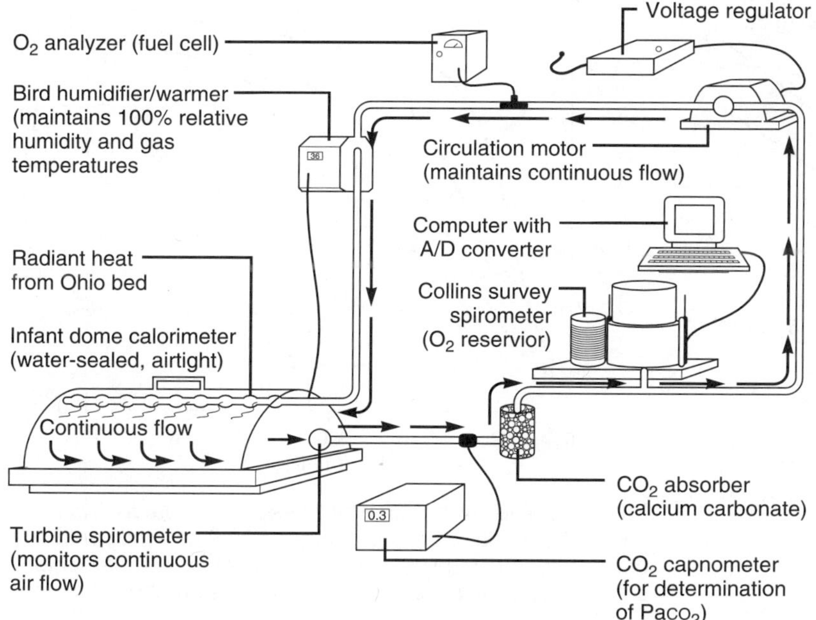

FIG. 7-2. Depiction of a device used for volumetric determination of oxygen consumption in infants. The infant is placed inside the water-sealed chamber, and oxygen consumption is determined by volume loss from the spirometer.

the oxygen content of normal arterial blood equal to about 20.7 mL/dL. Similar calculations reveal that normal venous blood oxygen content is about 15 mL/dL. Typically, Do$_2$ is 12 to 15 mL/kg/min or 500 to 600 mL/kg/min, which is four to five times greater than the associated oxygen consumption[4] (Fig. 7-5). Note that the product of the cardiac output and arterial oxygen content must be multiplied by a factor of 10 dL/L because cardiac output is measured in liters per minute, but arterial oxygen content is measured in milliliters per deciliter. Oxygen kinetic measurements are normalized to either body surface area (mL/m^2/min) or weight (mL/kg/min).

Oxygen content is the most important measure of oxygen in blood, although partial pressure of oxygen (Po$_2$) and oxyhemoglobin saturation are more commonly assessed in the intensive care unit (Fig. 7-6). The partial pressure of oxygen is measured in a blood gas machine using a silver wire anode and platinum cathode. These are encased in glass, surrounded by silver chloride electrolyte and covered with a polyethylene membrane that is permeable to oxygen.[13] When oxygen-containing gases or fluids are exposed to the membrane, current flow is generated

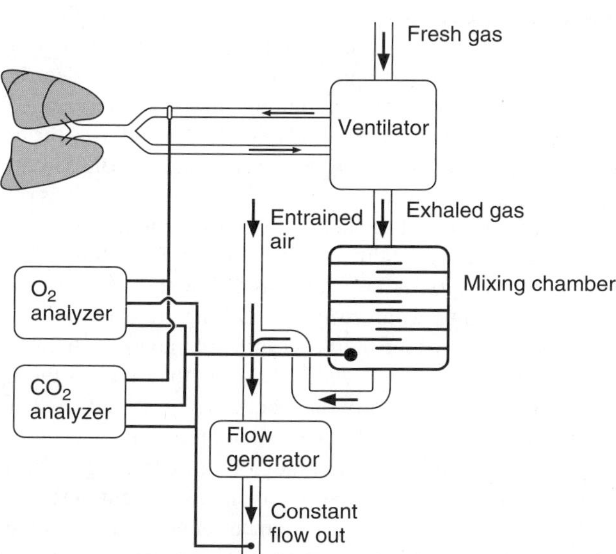

FIG. 7-3. Determination of oxygen consumption by expired gas analysis. Both inspired and expired gas are assessed by the O$_2$ and CO$_2$ analyzers.

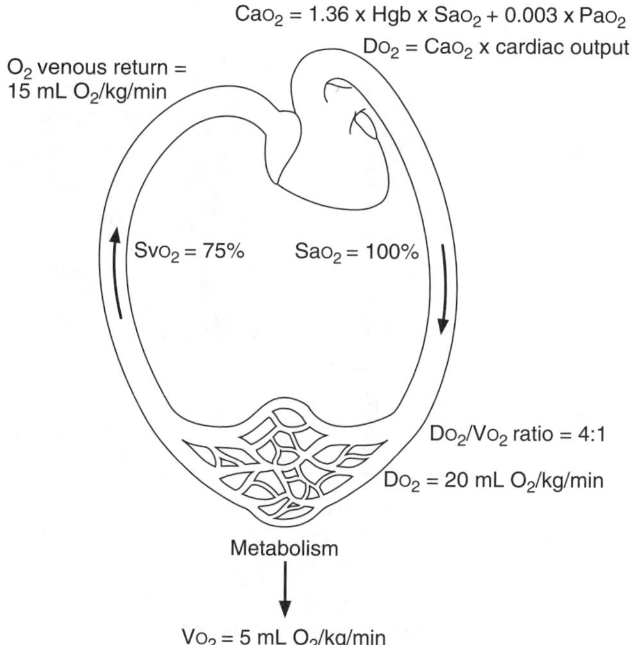

FIG. 7-4. This schematic illustration of oxygen kinetics demonstrates the relation of oxygen consumption (V̇o$_2$), oxygen delivery (Do$_2$), and the mixed venous oxygen saturation (Svo$_2$).

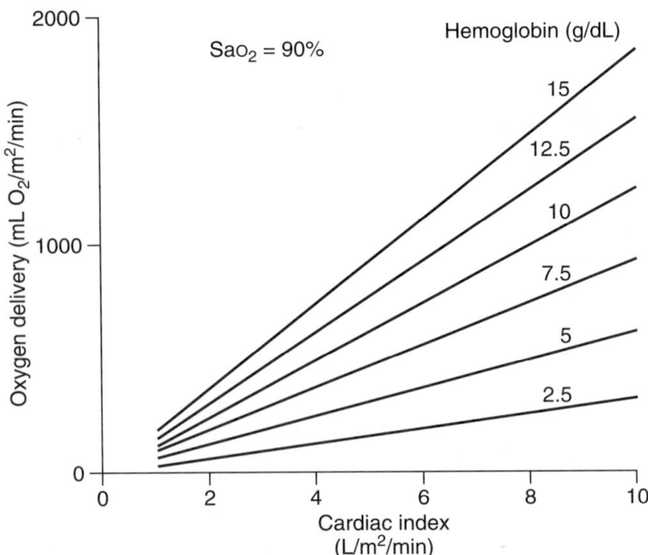

FIG. 7-5. Oxygen delivery can be calculated if hemoglobin concentration and cardiac output data are available.

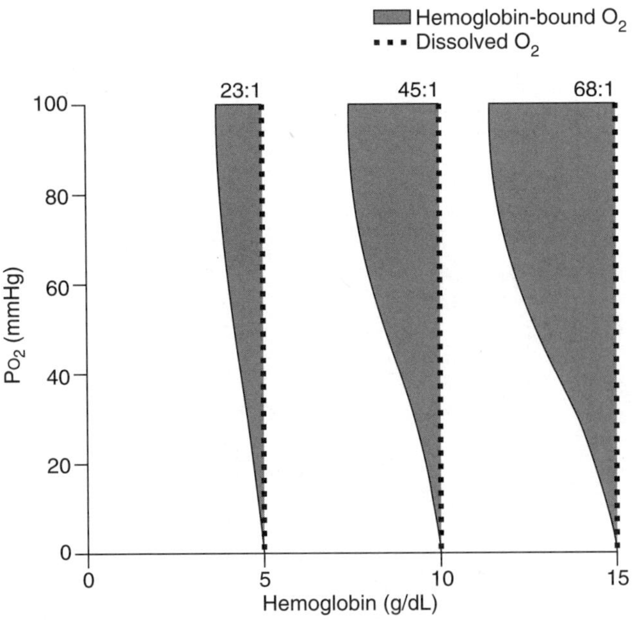

FIG. 7-6. Oxygen content in the dissolved and hemoglobin-bound phases of blood is shown at hemoglobin concentrations of 5, 10, and 15 g/dL as a function of Po$_2$. Note the predominant effect of hemoglobin concentration on blood oxygen content. The numbers above each oxygen content diagram indicate the ratio of hemoglobin-bound to dissolved oxygen at an O$_2$ tension of 100 mmHg.

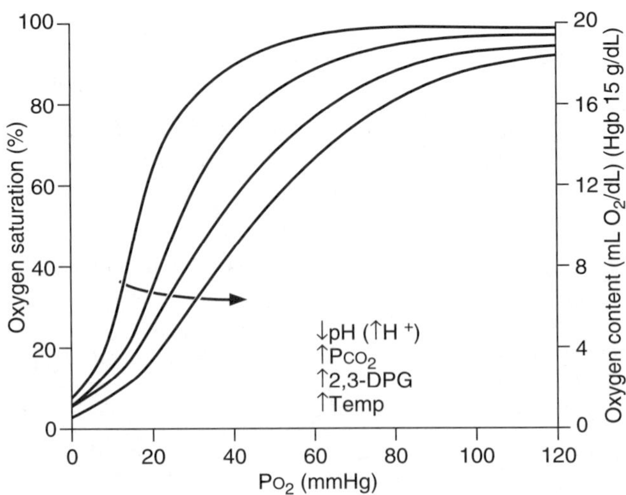

FIG. 7-7. The oxyhemoglobin dissociation curve. The relation of the partial pressure of oxygen to the hemoglobin oxygen saturation or the oxygen content of blood at a hemoglobin concentration of 15 g/dL is affected by a number of factors.

within the electrode, and this is used to determine oxygen concentration.

The amount of oxygen carried in plasma is minimal at one atmosphere pressure, although supersaturated oxygen solutions capable of carrying up to 16 times as much oxygen are being investigated.[14] The most efficient way to increase oxygen content in a patient is to increase the oxygen-carrying capacity of the blood by increasing red blood cell mass. Normal hemoglobin contains two α and two β chains, with four associated iron heme groups. Oxygen forms a reversible covalent bond with the ferrous ion within the heme molecule. Arterial hemoglobin saturation is a function of the Pao$_2$ and the affinity of oxygen for hemoglobin. This is described by the oxyhemoglobin dissociation curve[15] (Fig. 7-7). At the normal physiologic arterial Pao$_2$ of 100 mmHg, arterial oxygen saturation is 100%, while at a normal venous Po$_2$ of 40 mmHg, the mixed venous oxygen saturation (Svo$_2$) is 75%. The normal Po$_2$ that achieves a hemoglobin saturation of 50% (P$_{50}$) is 27 mmHg. Hemoglobin–oxygen affinity may be altered by a number of factors: increases in H$^+$ ion (decreased pH), Paco$_2$, temperature, and erythrocyte 2,3-diphosphogycerate (2,3-DPG) concentration all induce a shift of the oxyhemoglobin dissociation curve to the right, which means that the hemoglobin oxygen saturation is decreased if free Pao$_2$ remains constant.[15] In contrast, decreases in these variables increase hemoglobin affinity for oxygen. This may increase oxygen content and delivery, but reduces the efficiency of oxygen off-loading at the tissue level. Based on the measured Pao$_2$, temperature, and pH, blood gas machines often provide an estimate of the hemoglobin saturation. These calculated values often contain substantial error. Therefore, the hemoglobin saturation is best measured directly with a spectrophotometer known as an *oximeter*. During standard oximetry, a small sample of whole blood is aspirated into a cuvette, where the hemoglobin is hemolyzed.[16] Light is then passed through the cuvette, and the absorption spectrum is assessed at each of four wavelengths, allowing determination of the concentration of oxyhemoglobin, reduced hemoglobin, methemoglobin, and carboxyhemoglobin. Simultaneously, measurement of reflected light intensity also allows measurement of hemoglobin content. When total hemoglobin content, hemoglobin oxygen saturation, Po$_2$ of oxygen dissolved in plasma, and cardiac output are known, oxygen content and oxygen delivery can both be calculated.

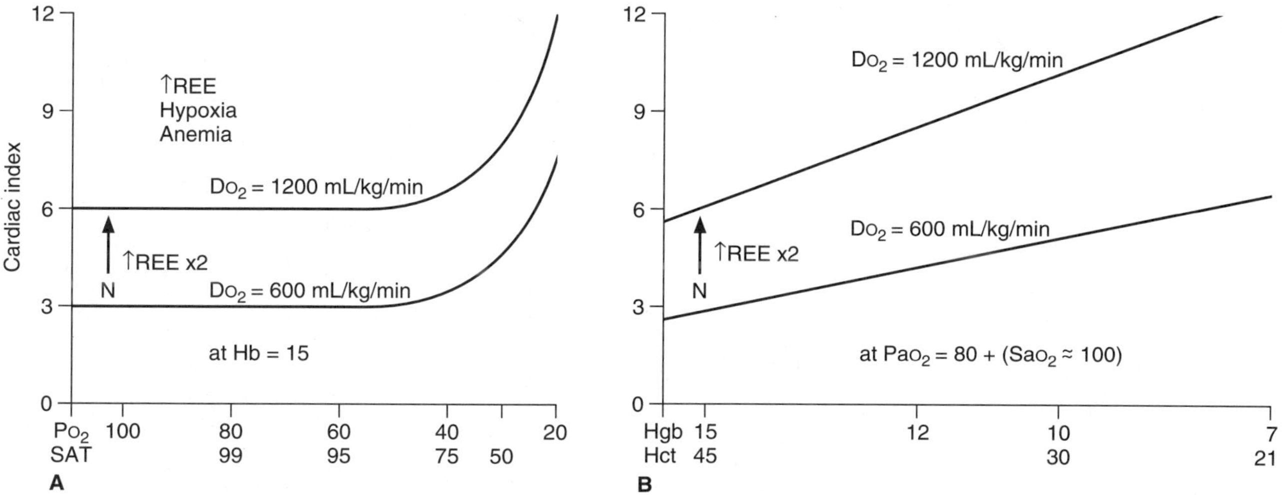

FIG. 7-8. The alterations in cardiac response required to maintain a stable oxygen delivery/consumption ratio are shown. Illustrated physiologic responses in cardiac index to a reduction in arterial oxygen saturation (*A*), a reduction in hemoglobin concentration and a two-fold increase in oxygen consumption (*A* and *B*). REE, resting energy expenditure; SAT, hemoglobin saturation; Hgb, hemoglobin content in grams/dL; Hct, hematocrit %.

Autoregulation of Oxygen Delivery

Acute changes in oxygen delivery are the result of alterations in cardiac output (or cardiac index; Fig. 7-8). The stimulus for an increase in cardiac output in response to reduced oxygen delivery is unclear, although there is evidence that cells similar to those of the carotid body may reside at the bifurcation of the main pulmonary artery (glomus pulmonale) and regulate cardiac output in response to changes in venous oxygen or carbon dioxide levels.[17] The cardiac output response to reductions in Pao$_2$ or hemoglobin content results in an increase only to the level necessary to reestablish normal oxygen delivery. If the cardiac output response is inadequate to normalize Do$_2$ on a chronic basis, red-cell mass can be increased through erythropoietin production. When cardiac output does not respond adequately to normalize Do$_2$, total body oxygen extraction may increase from a normal of 25% up to a maximum of 50% to 60%. Further reductions in Do$_2$ are met with pathologic reductions in oxygen consumption (see later).

Oxygen Consumption and Delivery Relations in Normal Metabolic States

The relation of oxygen consumption and oxygen delivery in normal humans follows a biphasic distribution. Specifically, a given rate of oxygen consumption is constant and independent of oxygen delivery as long as an excess of oxygen is delivered. This area of the $\dot{V}o_2$ and Do$_2$ relation is characterized by a stable $\dot{V}o_2$ plateau at which the $\dot{V}o_2$ is supply independent (Fig. 7-9). As oxygen delivery falls, however, a critical level is attained at which the rate of oxygen consumption becomes dependent on delivery. $\dot{V}o_2$ then becomes supply dependent. It is below this critical point of oxygen delivery (Do$_2$ crit) that onset of metabolic acidosis with increasing lactate production occurs. This Do$_2$ crit has been estimated in adult patients undergoing cardiac operations to be 8.2 mL/kg/min or 330 mL/m^2/min.[18]

The Do$_2$ crit appears to be the same whether the reduction in Do$_2$ is secondary to a decrease in hemoglobin, Sao$_2$, or cardiac output.[19]

Oxygen Consumption and Delivery Relations in Altered Metabolic States

Animal studies have documented that the $\dot{V}o_2$ plateau is lower in hypometabolic states, such as hypothermia, and is associated with a lower Do$_2$ crit.[20] In contrast, hypermetabolic, exercising dogs have a higher plateau $\dot{V}o_2$ and a higher Do$_2$ crit.

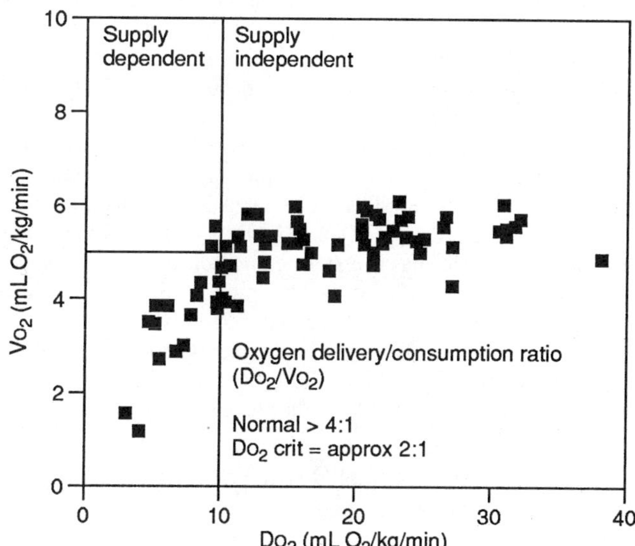

FIG. 7-9. The oxygen consumption ($\dot{V}o_2$)/oxygen delivery (Do$_2$) ratio in normal canines. Oxygen delivery is decreased by a reduction in cardiac output. The supply-dependent and supply independent oxygen consumption states are demonstrated. The critical Do$_2$/$\dot{V}o_2$ ratio (Do$_2$/$\dot{V}o_2$ crit) is about 2.

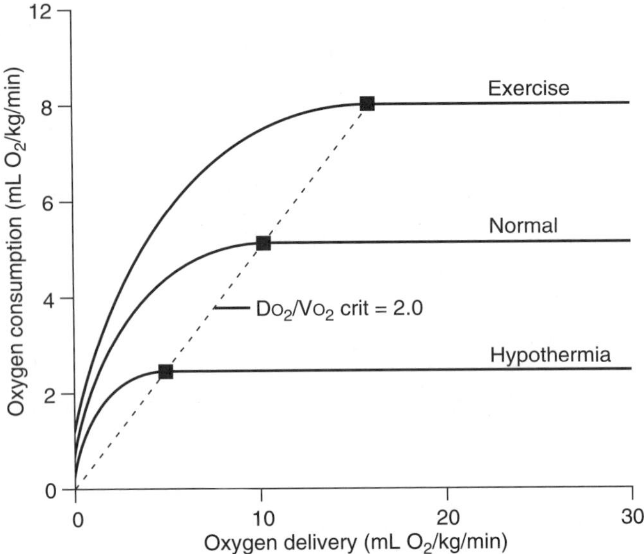

FIG. 7-10. Theoretic depiction of the oxygen consumption ($\dot{V}O_2$) and delivery (DO_2) relation in hypometabolic (hypothermic), normal, and hypermetabolic (exercise) states. Critical DO_2 (DO_2 crit) is greater (further to the right) with increasing levels of $\dot{V}O_2$. The critical $DO_2/\dot{V}O_2$ ratio ($DO_2/\dot{V}O_2$ crit), however, remains the same.

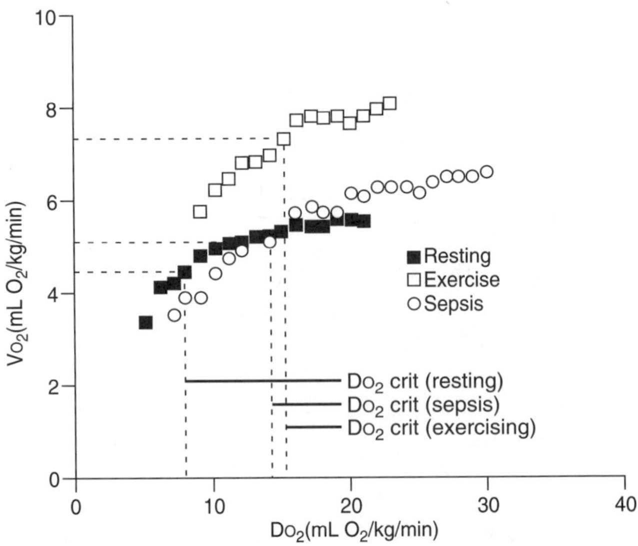

FIG. 7-11. The oxygen consumption ($\dot{V}O_2$) and oxygen delivery (DO_2) relation in resting, septic, and exercising canines is shown. The critical DO_2 (DO_2 crit) is greater (further to the right) in the exercising, hypermetabolic animals than in the normal animals. The critical $DO_2/\dot{V}O_2$ ratio ($DO_2/\dot{V}O_2$ crit), however, is about the same in both groups (about 2). The level of oxygen delivery at which oxygen consumption begins to decrease (DO_2 crit) and the oxygen delivery/consumption ratio at that point ($DO_2/\dot{V}O_2$ crit) in septic animals are greater than expected, perhaps reflecting fundamental alterations in the $DO_2/\dot{V}O_2$ ratio in the septic state.

(P. Bongiorno and colleagues, unpublished data, Department of Surgery, University of Michigan, 1994; Fig. 7-10). The ratio of the DO_2 crit to the plateau $\dot{V}O_2$ is a constant factor that determines the shift from supply-dependent to supply-independent oxygen consumption. Some have suggested that this relation follows a Michaelis-Mentin equation.[21] As DO_2 decreases and $\dot{V}O_2$ remains stable, the ratio of oxygen delivery to oxygen consumption falls until the critical $DO_2/\dot{V}O_2$ ratio is reached. At this point, supply-dependent oxygen consumption begins. This $DO_2/\dot{V}O_2$ crit marks the onset of supply-dependent oxygen consumption at all levels of metabolism. Most studies suggest that the $DO_2/\dot{V}O_2$ crit in the laboratory setting is about 2, while clinical studies suggest that humans have a critical $DO_2/\dot{V}O_2$ ratio of about 3.[18,20,22–25]

Controversy exists about whether these $DO_2/\dot{V}O_2$ ratios are similar in patients with the acute respiratory distress syndrome and sepsis.[26–28] Some studies suggest that $\dot{V}O_2$ is uniformly and continuously dependent on DO_2 regardless of the delivery rate in such patients. This has been termed *pathologic supply dependency*. Other studies dispute such findings. Further data are required to resolve this controversy, but it is likely that the critical $DO_2/\dot{V}O_2$ ratio is higher is patients with sepsis or acute respiratory distress syndrome, and this would result in $\dot{V}O_2$ remaining supply dependent at higher levels of DO_2 (Fig. 7-11).

Relation of Mixed Venous Oxygen Saturation to Oxygen Kinetics

The hemoglobin saturation by oxygen in mixed venous blood obtained from the pulmonary artery is referred to as the SvO_2. This directly reflects the $DO_2/\dot{V}O_2$ ratio. As oxygen delivery increases or oxygen consumption decreases, more oxygen remains in the venous blood. The result is an increase in SvO_2.

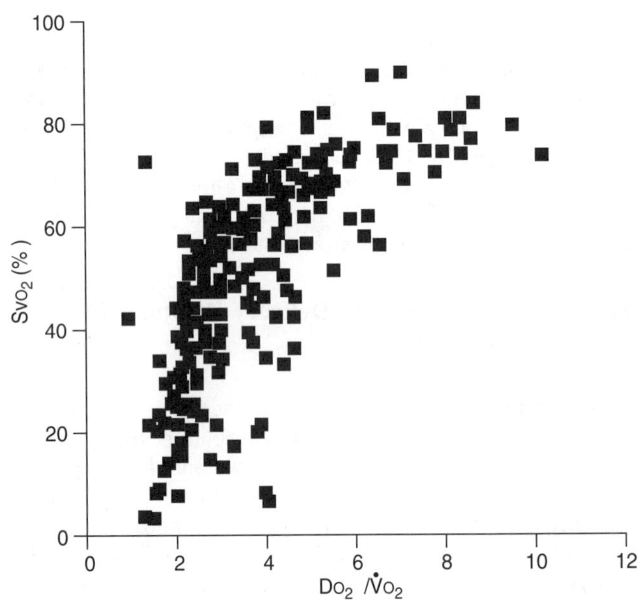

FIG. 7-12. The relation of the mixed venous oxygen saturation (SvO_2) and the ratio of oxygen delivery to oxygen consumption ($DO_2/\dot{V}O_2$) in normal (eumetabolic), hypermetabolic (septic), and hypermetabolic (exercising) canines is shown.

In contrast, if delivery decreases or consumption increases, relatively more oxygen is extracted from the blood, and therefore, less oxygen remains in the venous blood. A decrease in Svo_2 is the result. The Svo_2 serves as an excellent monitor of oxygen kinetics because it specifically assesses the adequacy of oxygen delivery in relation to oxygen consumption[29] (Fig. 7-12). Clinical studies suggest that the critical Svo_2 is in the 35% to 50% range, which correlates with a critical $Do_2/\dot{V}o_2$ ratio of about 2.[30,31] Simply put, at this point, half of the oxygen available is consumed. Technologic advances have allowed development of a fiberoptic, continuous Svo_2 monitor that accurately reflects the measured pulmonary artery Svo_2. Continuous Svo_2 monitoring provides early identification of cardiopulmonary instability, rapid assessment of the response to therapy, and cost savings in critically ill patients because of a diminished need for other data such as sequential blood gas monitoring.[29,32] The accuracy of Svo_2 monitoring may be diminished under certain circumstances in which arteriovenous shunting occurs, such as in some patients with cirrhosis or sepsis. Importantly, this means that in situations in which vasoregulation is altered, the Svo_2 may be normal even though the oxygen delivery at the tissue level is inadequate.

HEMODYNAMIC MONITORING IN THE INTENSIVE CARE UNIT

Noninvasive Monitoring

Noninvasive cardiopulmonary monitoring is an important aspect in the care of all critically ill patients. It is especially important in critically ill newborns and infants because invasive monitoring may be more difficult and is at times less reliable. The physical examination is an integral part of the assessment of cardiopulmonary status. For instance, warmth and color of extremities and capillary refill allow assessment of perfusion. Pink extremities and central color should make one suspicious of the validity of a low pulse oximeter value. Intravascular volume status can be evaluated by (1) assessment of oral and ocular mucous membranes and axillary moistness, (2) urinary output measurement in the patient without renal insufficiency, (3) warmth of peripheral extremities, and (4) the fullness of the anterior fontanelle in newborns and infants. Information gained from the physical examination should be integrated with data gained by invasive and noninvasive monitoring to assess the cardiopulmonary status. Although monitors are an essential part of modern critical care, they are designed to supplement rather than replace clinical judgment (Table 7-2).

TABLE 7-2. *Noninvasive clinical parameters indicative of inadequate perfusion*

Weak, rapid pulse
Hypotension
Extremities cool, mottled, with capillary refill >2 s
Urine output <0.5–1 mL/kg
Mental status inappropriate, lethargic
Anterior fontanelle flat
Sclera, mucous membranes, axillae dry
Orthostatic hypotension (blood pressure decrease ≥20 mmHg or heart rate increase ≥20 beats/min with head of bed up)
Internal jugular veins flat

Electrocardiographic Monitoring

Electrocardiographic (ECG) monitoring is among the most basic of noninvasive monitoring procedures and should be used routinely in all critically ill patients. In addition to accurate heart rate assessment, ECG monitoring provides evidence of dysrhythmias, metabolic abnormalities, and myocardial ischemia.[33] Most intensive care unit ECG systems use adhesive chest leads onto which clip adapters are placed. These leads are typically located on the right upper chest, the left upper chest, and the left lower chest in the anteroaxillary line, potentially providing data from leads I, II, and V_1, although lead II is the most commonly used for monitoring.

ECG monitoring systems are subject to failure. Movement of the patient, incomplete electrode contact, or separation of the electrode from the patient can result in artifacts that simulate arrhythmias, including ventricular tachycardia and asystole. For this reason, the 12-lead ECG is a much more specific and complete means of evaluation and should be used when monitoring raises suspicion for cardiac abnormalities in the critically ill patient. The various ECG intervals and segments can be evaluated, as can trends throughout all leads of the heart. Most dysrhythmias can be classified into those that are too fast, too slow, or disorganized or absent and those that are atrial or ventricular. Any arrhythmia that results in cardiovascular instability should be managed with synchronized cardioversion or defibrillation at a dose of 0.5 to 4 J/kg.[34]

Atrial tachyarrhythmias include both sinus tachycardias and supraventricular tachycardias. The former require identification and treatment of the underlying cause (fever, agitation, hypovolemia, pain). The latter can generally be treated in a more elective fashion with adenosine in infants and children or verapamil in children older than 1 year. Ventricular tachycardia is more hazardous and should be managed promptly with intravenous bolus lidocaine, 1 mg/kg, followed by a 20 to 50 μg/kg/min infusion.[34] Tachyarrhythmias occur secondary to spontaneous or accelerated firing of particular regions of the conducting system. This may be due to stimulation by catecholamines, digitalis, hypoxemia, electrical irritability, or other causes. For all of these arrhythmias, the patient should be evaluated for evidence of hypoxia, acidosis, electrolyte imbalance, or specific medication toxicity (Fig. 7-13).

Bradyarrhythmias are often secondary to inadequate ventilation and oxygenation. Less often, slow rhythms are secondary to vagal stimulation, sinus node abnormalities, heart block, hypercalcemia, or hypermagnesemia. Administration of intravenous atropine, 0.02 mg/kg, isoproterenol, 0.1 to 1 μg/kg/min, and epinephrine, 0.01 mg/kg of 1:10,000 IV bolus or an infusion of 0.1 to 1 μg/kg/min, may increase heart rate, conduction velocity, and contractility.[34]

Temperature Monitoring

Critically ill children are at substantial risk for hypothermia if body temperature is not monitored and appropriate warming techniques used. In neonates, skin temperature probes reflect core body temperature accurately, while in infants and children beyond the neonatal period, rectal probes are effective for continuous temperature monitoring. In neonates and young infants, these temperature probes may be used to servoregulate over-

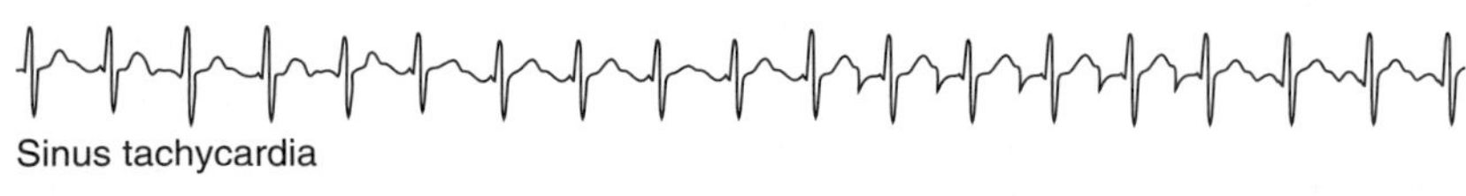

Sinus tachycardia

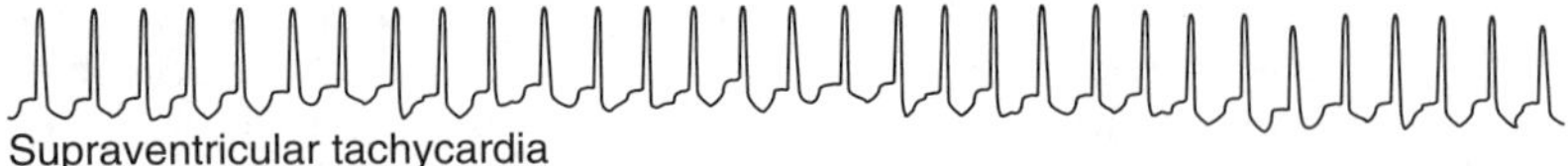

Supraventricular tachycardia

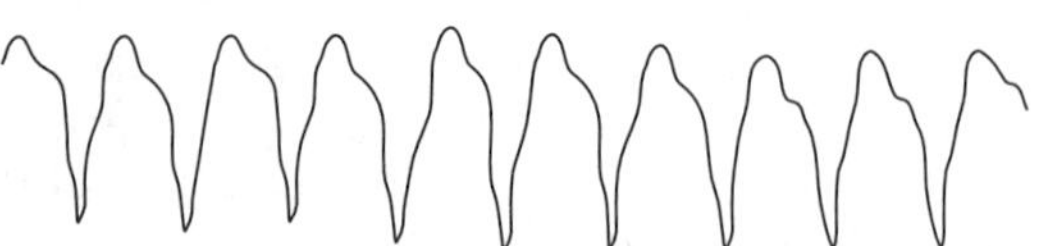

Ventricular tachycardia

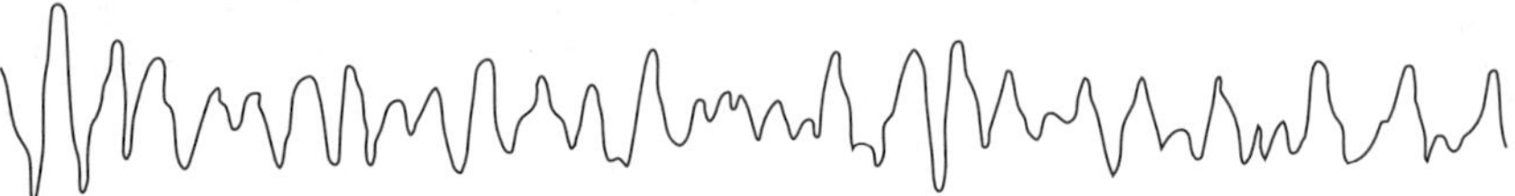

Course ventricular fibrillation

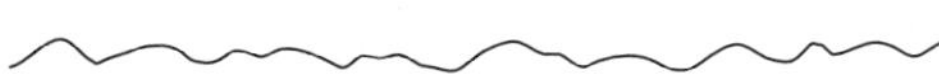

Fine ventricular fibrillation

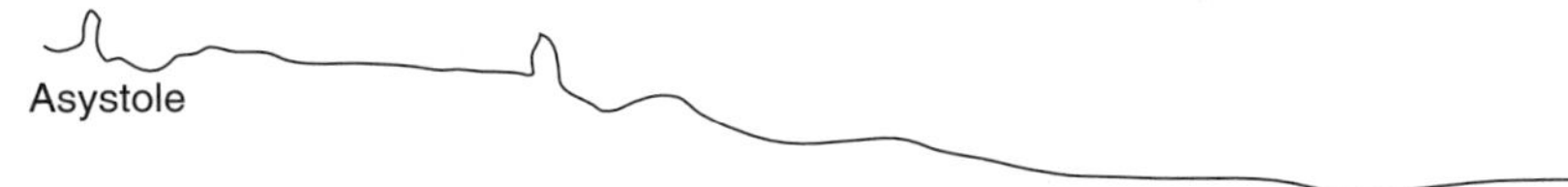

Asystole

FIG. 7-13. Electrocardiographic tracing demonstrating several common arrhythmias, from top to bottom: regular rhythm and P, QRS, and T sequences of sinus tachycardia at 180 beats/min; rapid, regular rhythm of supraventricular tachycardia at 320 beats/min; wide QRS complex of ventricular tachycardia; disorganized depolarizations of both coarse and fine ventricular fibrillation; and flat line of asystole.

bed warmers to maintain stable body temperature. Additional ways of warming, such as under-body and over-body warming blankets, warming of the ventilating gas, warming of administered fluids and blood products, and warming of ambient temperature, should all be considered in children at risk for hypothermia.[35]

Sphygmomanometry

Blood pressure determination using sphygmomanometry should be done in all patients even when more invasive means of blood pressure monitoring are in use. In children, it is critical that the cuff be of appropriate size. The bladder in the cuff should be placed over an appropriate artery. The width of the bladder should be 40% of the extremity circumference at the midpoint of the limb, and the length should be twice the recommended width.[36,37] The cuff is inflated to a level well above the expected systolic blood pressure and then deflated rapidly as the approximate systolic blood pressure is identified by either an aneroid or mercury manometer. The cuff should then be reinflated to a point just above this level with subsequent slow deflation as the systolic pressure is identified at the point at which the first of the five phases of Korotkoff sounds are audible.[37] The diastolic pressure is noted as the point at which those sounds disappear or are abruptly muffled (phase IV or V). The blood pressure may be difficult to obtain by this technique in the settings of hypotension, elevated peripheral vascular resistance, and poor perfusion. In such situations, a Doppler probe may be used to ascertain systolic blood pressure by identifying return of pulsatile arterial flow distal to a deflating proximal extremity blood pressure cuff. Automatic blood pressure devices are frequently used in the intensive care unit.[38] These devices can be programmed to measure blood pressure accurately and automatically at various intervals.[39,40] The inflated cuff determines blood pressure and simultaneously identifies the presence of minute alterations in cuff pressure that are associated with the appearance and disappearance of the Korotkoff sounds.[41] These automated devices determine the systolic pressure on first identification of changes in cuff pressure, mean blood pressure at the point of maximum amplitude of such changes, and diastolic blood pressure on disappearance or the abrupt decrease in the amplitude of the cuff pressure changes. Automated devices that can measure blood pressure using a forefinger cuff have been developed[42] (Fig. 7-14).

Pulse Oximetry

The pulse oximeter is one of the most important advances in noninvasive cardiopulmonary monitoring in critically ill children (Fig. 7-15). Information about oxygenation, heart rate, and perfusion is provided.[43–45] Pulse oximeters emit light at two wave lengths, usually 660 nm (red) and 940 nm (near infrared), and this is transmitted through tissue to a photodetector.[46] The intensity of the transmitted light remains constant except for alterations in absorbency due to the pulsatile nature of arterial flow. The pulsatile waveform change of light absorbency allows determination of the pulse rate. In addition, because light is differentially absorbed by reduced hemoglobin and oxyhemo-

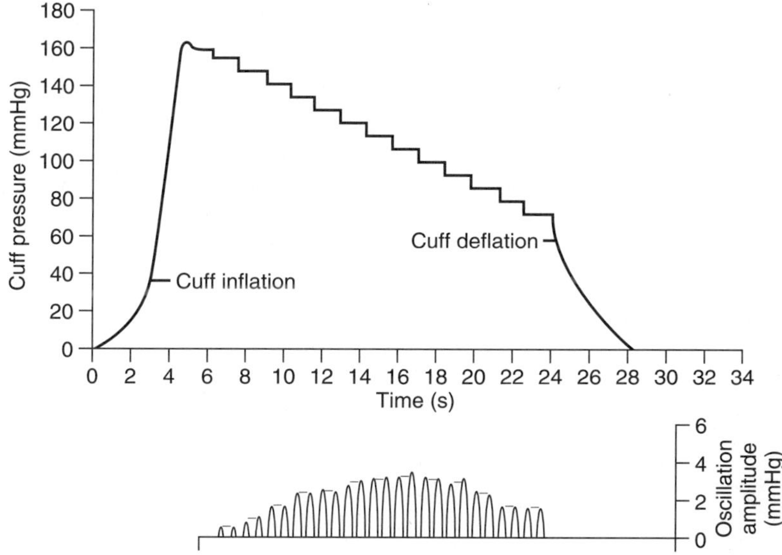

FIG. 7-14. The relation between Korotkoff sounds and blood pressure during automatic measurement. The amplitude of sound oscillation increases and then decreases with cuff deflation, allowing identification of systolic pressure at first detection, mean pressure at maximum amplitude, and diastolic pressure at disappearance of the sound oscillation.

globin, variable absorbency at the two wavelengths allows estimation of hemoglobin saturation. In the setting of poor peripheral perfusion, patient motion, or methemoglobinemia, the default saturation reading of the pulse oximetry device is 85%.[46] This is often seen in states of low cardiac output, hypothermia, and increased vascular resistance. Therefore, if hemoglobin saturation abruptly decreases to 85%, the patient and device should be assessed for pulse oximeter artifact by noting whether a valid heart rate is displayed by the pulse oximeter. Other sources of error in pulse oximeter analysis include the presence of venous blood pulsation (arteriovenous fistula), the presence of nail polish or similar materials on the skin, ambient room light affecting the photodetector, and high levels of carbon monoxide when the oximeter cannot differentiate carboxyhemoglobin from oxyhemoglobin and therefore overestimates the true hemoglobin

oxygen saturation.[47] The accuracy of the pulse oximeter–derived oxygen saturation may be limited at levels less than 70% to 80%.[48] Intravascular administration of methylene blue or fluorescein induces a falsely low reading because of absorption of light at the particular wavelengths used.

The absorbency levels of fetal hemoglobin are similar to those of hemoglobin A at the two wavelengths used in the pulse oximeter. Therefore, the presence of hemoglobin F does not have a significant effect on the hemoglobin saturation measurements.[46,49] The pulse oximeter probe is usually placed on the fingers or toes. If the probes fail to function appropriately at those sites, more central locations, such as the ears, lips, and nose, can be used. Pulse oximeters can also be placed on extremities with questionable arterial perfusion to provide continuous localized monitoring when necessary.

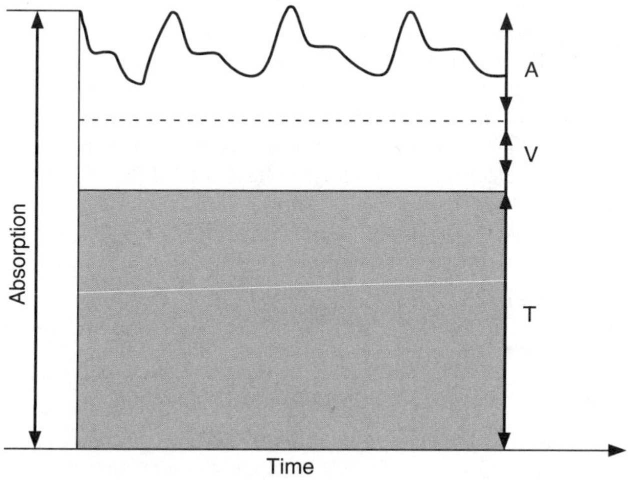

Carbon Dioxide Monitoring

End-tidal carbon dioxide (etCO₂) monitors assess the absorption of infrared light as it passes through expired gas (Fig. 7-16). Two techniques are used: sidestream monitoring, in which a sample of expired gas is continuously aspirated and

FIG. 7-15. The absorption of light for assessment of hemoglobin saturation by a pulse oximeter. Light is absorbed by tissue (T), venous blood (V), and arterial blood (A). The variation in light absorption results from alterations in arterial blood volume with each pulsation.

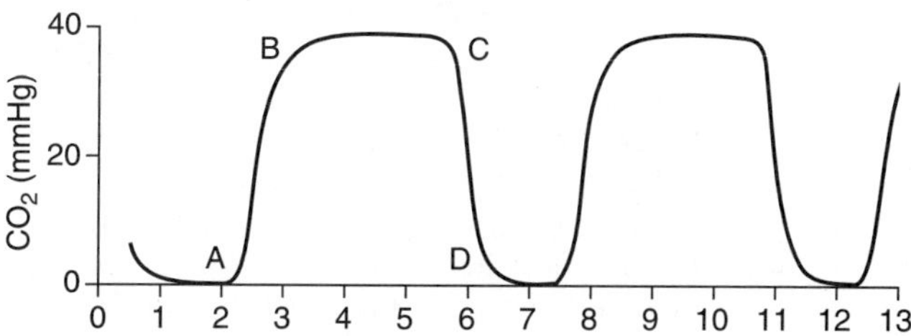

FIG. 7-16. Waveform generated by a CO_2 analyzer during tidal breathing. The partial pressure of CO_2 is 0 mmHg at the beginning of expiration (A) because of the dead space in the conducting airways. The B-to-C interval represents the alveolar P_{CO_2}, and the end-tidal P_{CO_2} is at point C. The P_{CO_2} then decreases during inspiration (D) before the cycle is repeated.

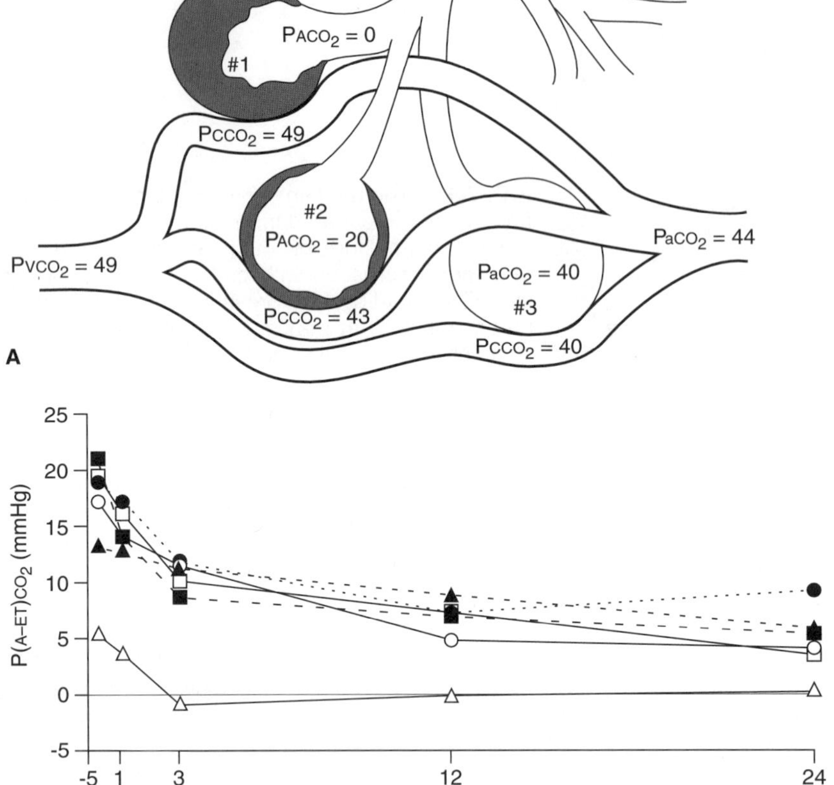

FIG. 7-17. The alveolar P_{CO_2} (P_{ACO_2}) and, therefore, the end-tidal P_{CO_2} (ET_{CO_2}) are lower than the arterial P_{CO_2} (P_{aCO_2}) in the setting of ventilation–perfusion mismatch. (*A*) In alveoli 1 and 2, gas exchange is compromised, and therefore, the P_{ACO_2} is less than the P_{aCO_2}. This contributes to an increase in the P_{aCO_2}–ET_{CO_2} gradient. (*B*) The P_{aCO_2}–ET_{CO_2} gradient diminishes after lung transplantation as ventilation–perfusion matching improves transplantation occured at time 0 h on the horizontal axis.

assessed; or mainstream monitoring, which evaluates gas as it is exhaled.[50] A disadvantage of the sidestream technique is that tidal volume and minute ventilation measurements may be inaccurate. A disadvantage of the mainstream method is that it requires additional dead space in the ventilating circuit. The techniques are equivalent with regard to accuracy.

Airway P_{CO_2} monitoring is helpful to document effective ventilation of the airway after endotracheal tube placement and to evaluate trends in P_{aCO_2} during ventilator manipulation.[51] In healthy patients without respiratory insufficiency, the maximal value assessed over a few minutes provides a relatively good approximation of the true P_{aCO_2}. Unfortunately, ventilation–perfusion mismatch in the setting of respiratory insufficiency often results in a decrease in $etCO_2$ relative to P_{aCO_2}.[52,53] In these patients, the difference between the $etCO_2$ and P_{aCO_2} may be variable and significant, and therefore, it is useful only for trend analysis. The arterial P_{CO_2}–$etCO_2$ gradient and the arterial P_{CO_2}/$etCO_2$ ratio, however, reflect the degree of ventilation–perfusion mismatch and are useful to monitor therapy[54] (Fig. 7-17).

Transcutaneous Blood Gas Monitoring

Transcutaneous P_{O_2} (tcP_{O_2}) and P_{CO_2} (tcP_{CO_2}) electrodes assess the diffusion rates of oxygen and carbon dioxide through the skin. The tcP_{O_2} electrode consists of a gold and platinum wire surrounded by a silver anode that donates electrons when molecular oxygen is reduced to OH^-.[50] The rate of electron flow is proportional to the rate of diffusion of oxygen at the electrode surface. In similar fashion, the tcP_{CO_2} electrode functions to assess changes in pH when CO_2 combines with water to form $HCO_2^- \rightarrow H$ and HCO_3^-. The two electrodes can be combined into a single instrument, and this is commonly done.

The P_{O_2} at the skin is substantially lower (about 53 mmHg) than arterial P_{O_2}. To counteract this diffusion-induced reduction in P_{O_2}, the electrode and skin are heated to 44°C, which increases capillary P_{O_2} by about 45 mmHg, causing the measured tcP_{O_2} and P_{aO_2} to be about equal[55] (Fig. 7-18). However, if the hemoglobin–oxygen dissociation curve is shifted, the standardized heating procedure produces inaccurate estimations of P_{aO_2}. In addition, both the tcP_{O_2} and tcP_{CO_2} are unreliable in patients in shock with low cardiac output and poor perfusion.[46] The tcP_{O_2}, however, does appear to accurately reflect the P_{aO_2} in children and young adults, especially at P_{aO_2} levels of less than 60 mmHg.[56,57] Because production of CO_2 by the skin is enhanced during heating, the tcP_{CO_2} measurement may be 20 to 30 mmHg higher than the P_{aCO_2}.[55,58] However, both the tcP_{O_2} and tcP_{CO_2} monitors under most conditions can at least provide relevant information on trends in arterial P_{O_2} and P_{CO_2} when transcutaneous values are inaccurate.[59] Transcutaneous blood gas assessment is dependent on the location in which the elec-

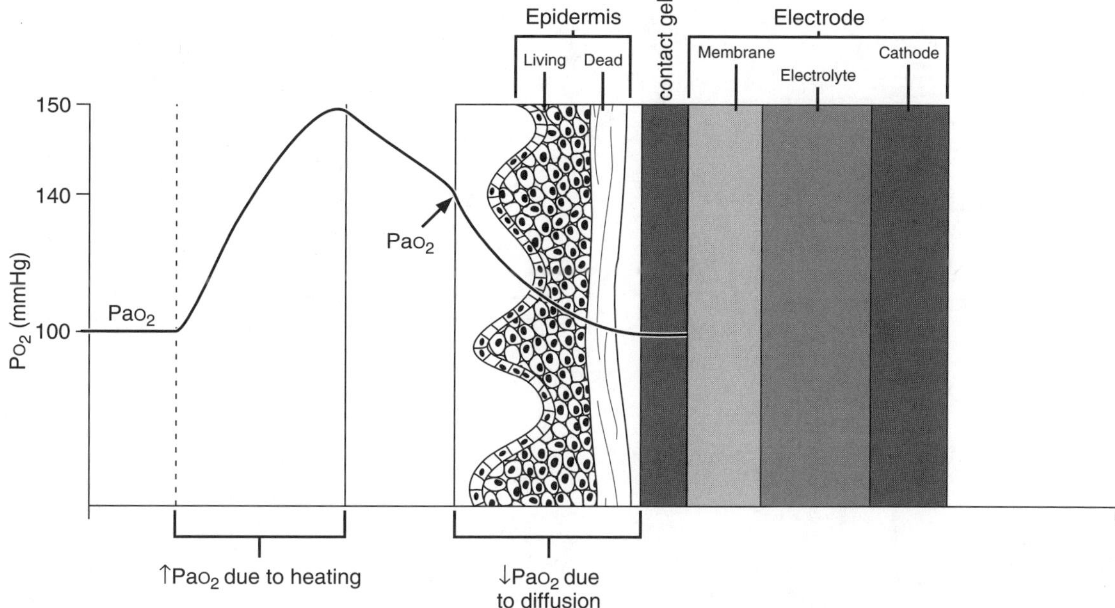

FIG. 7-18. Diffusion of oxygen during transcutaneous O_2 monitoring. The capillary Po_2 is increased by heating, which shifts the hemoglobin–oxygen dissociation curve to the right. The oxygen tension decreases about the same amount during diffusion to the skin surface, resulting in a capillary Po_2 that approximates the Pao_2.

trode is placed. The trunk is preferred because central perfusion is less often compromised there than in the periphery. Areas with thick skin or hair should be avoided. Because of the risk of burns, the position of the heated electrode should be changed every 6 hours.

Measurement of Cardiac Output

Noninvasive estimations of cardiac output include thoracic electrical bioimpedance measurement, suprasternal Doppler ultrasound assessment, and transesophageal or transtracheal Doppler ultrasound evaluation. Transthoracic electrical bioimpedance requires placement of electrodes on the neck and lower chest[60,61] (Fig. 7-19). Low-amplitude current is passed between pairs of electrodes. The measured change in thoracic resistance is a function of the pulsatile change in the fluid volume of the thoracic cavity with each cardiac cycle. An equation based on the patient's height, weight, sex, and deviation from ideal body weight can be used to convert measured changes in impedance to cardiac output. Although problems of reliability tempered interest in the past, technical advances have substantially improved reproducibility and accuracy of cardiac output estimation.[62–64] The validity of this technique in children has been demonstrated, and it may offer one practical means of measuring cardiac output in neonates.[65]

Continuous Doppler ultrasound can be used to assess the velocity of blood flow within the aorta through probes placed at the suprasternal notch, esophagus, or trachea[66–69] (Fig. 7-20). The cross-sectional area of the aorta is determined either by ultrasound measurement or through a nomogram based on age, sex, height, and weight.[70] Once velocity of blood flow and aortic cross-sectional area are known, cardiac output can be calculated. Although studies regarding accuracy and reliability of Doppler-determined cardiac output vary, validity is improved when direct measurement of the aortic diameter is used instead of a nomogram and when transesophageal or transtracheal ultrasound is used.[70] The Doppler technique cannot be used in patients with anatomic abnormalities that disturb aortic blood flow, such as aortic stenosis or insufficiency.[71] Also, this technique is highly dependent on the ultrasound operator. Experience using cardiac output measurements with this technique is limited, but encouraging, in children and neonates.[72–75]

Invasive Monitoring

Systemic Arterial Catheters

Indications for arterial access include the need for continuous monitoring of blood pressure or the need for frequent arterial blood gas samples. Blood pressure monitoring is frequently required in patients with hemodynamic instability, sepsis, vasoactive drug therapy, mechanical ventilation, and other critical care needs. Although noninvasive monitoring has partially replaced the need for frequent blood gas assessment, the requirement for more than two or three blood gas samples per day is an indication for intraarterial access.

The most common arterial access site used in nonneonates is the radial artery (70%), followed by the posterior tibial and femoral arteries.[76] Peripheral arteries are best used because of the low complication rate should thrombosis occur.[77] The femoral artery, however, is frequently cannulated in children with few complications.[78] The superficial temporal artery is easily identified and cannulated in neonates, but concern regarding retrograde flow of air or debris into the carotid artery circulation

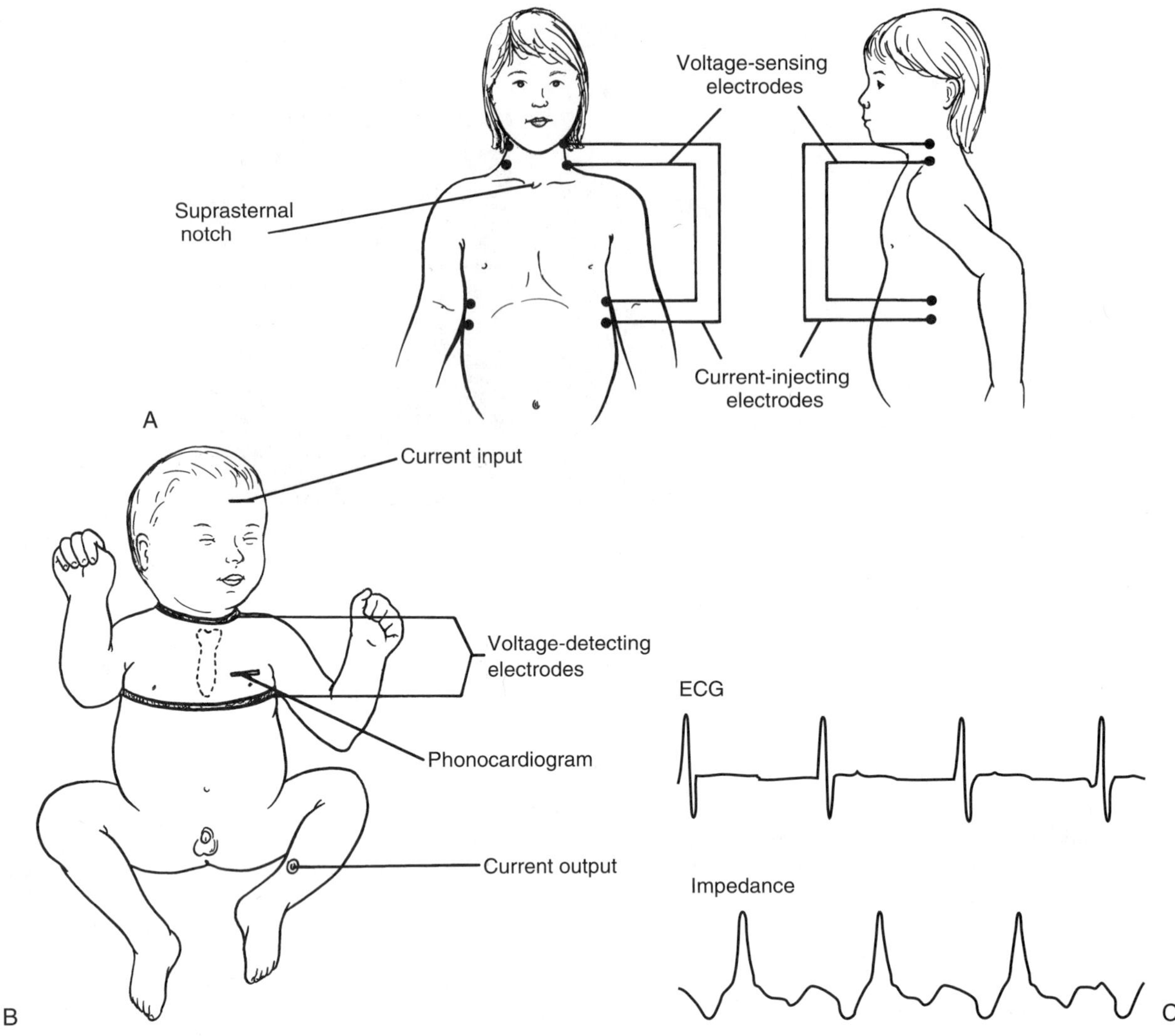

FIG. 7-19. Chest lead placement for thoracic impedance cardiac output assessment in older children (*A*) and neonates (*B*). (*C*) The relation of impedance (hence cardiac output) to the cardiac cycle.

makes this site less then optimum. If used, extreme care must be taken during flushing of the catheter.

Cannulation in children can be performed using either percutaneous or open methods. Percutaneous insertion is attempted in most circumstances[79] (Fig. 7-21). Typical catheters for arterial cannulation in neonates and small children are 24-gauge or 22-gauge polyethylene cannulas. Two methods of cannulation are commonly used: the direct cannulation method and the transfixion technique.[80] For radial artery cannulation, the authors prefer the transfixion technique, in which the catheter and needle are advanced through the artery to the head of the radius as the pulse is palpated. A flash of blood from the needle is observed on withdrawal of the catheter, at which point the needle and catheter are advanced once again. The needle is then removed, the catheter is withdrawn until blood return is visualized, and the catheter is advanced down the lumen of the artery. The catheter is sutured in place and secured. A flexible guide wire can be used to guide the catheter into the artery when difficulties are encountered. An arterial cutdown to the radial or dorsalis pedis arteries may be necessary in neonates and infants (Fig. 7-22). It is rare that artery ligation is required.

The umbilical artery provides an excellent site for arterial access in neonates who are younger than 10 days of age. Umbilical artery catheters are placed in up to 30% of neonates admitted to the neonatal intensive care unit.[81] An incision on the inferior aspect of the umbilicus about 1 to 2 cm above skin level should allow identification of one of the two ventrally located umbilical arteries (Fig. 7-23). If the artery cannot be located or cannulated in the umbilical stump, another option is to perform an infraumbilical curvilinear incision with identification of the umbilical artery posterior to the linea alba and anterior to the peritoneum. The catheter is advanced gently because resistance is often met at a point about 5 to 6 cm from the umbilicus as the catheter passes from the umbilical artery into the iliac artery. Final catheter position should be either above the mesenteric vessels (T-6 to T-11) or below the renal vessels (L-4).[82] The data from Figure 7-24 may be used to estimate the insertion length of the umbilical artery catheter (Fig. 7-24).[83] Otherwise, one can advance the catheter either a length equivalent to the distance between the umbilicus and the shoulder plus the weight of the patient in kilograms plus the length of the umbilical stump, which will place the catheter in the T-6 to T-11 region, or twice

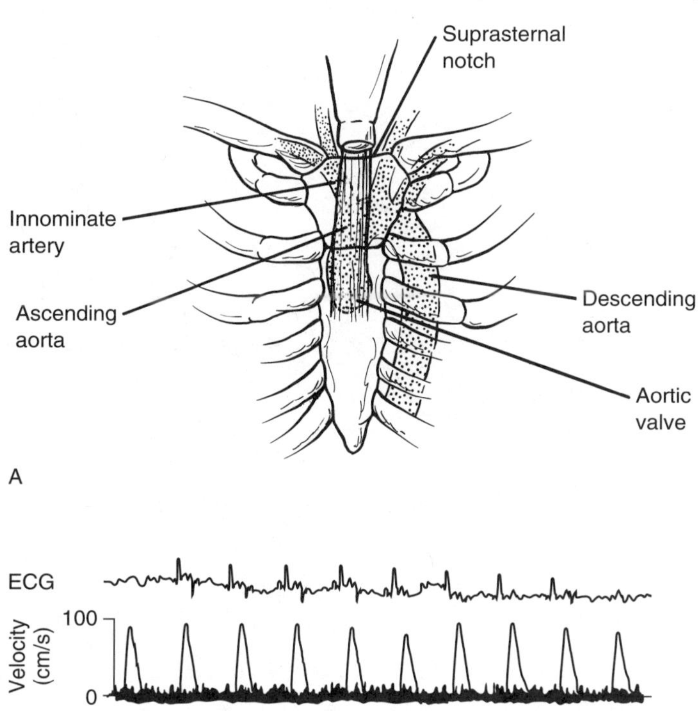

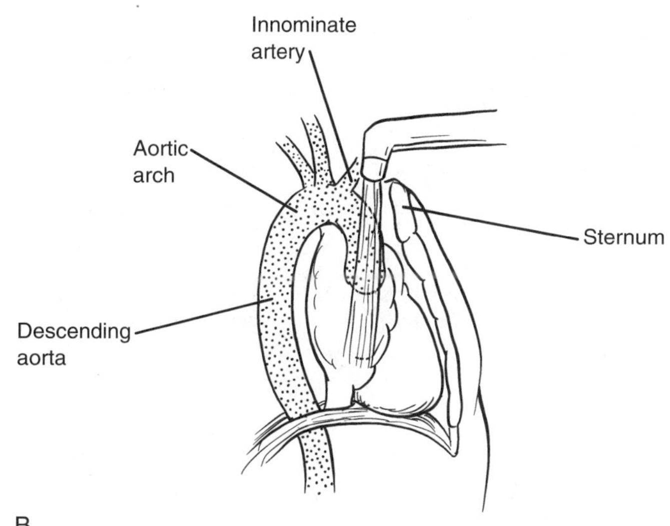

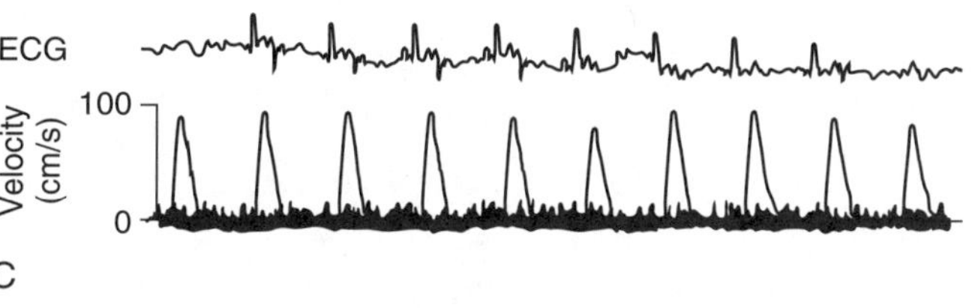

FIG. 7-20. (*A* and *B*) Technique of Doppler ultrasound imaging of the aorta. (*C*) Measurement of blood flow velocity and its correlation to the cardiac cycle. This information along with aortic cross-sectional area, allows calculation of cardiac output.

the distance between the symphysis pubis and the umbilicus plus the length of the umbilical stump, which will place the tip in the L-4 vertebral region.

After placement, the arterial catheter is connected to a transducer using short, noncompliant, clear tubing, and the system is flushed through an intervening stopcock so that the entire line is free of debris and air. Continuous-flow systems flush the catheter with heparinized saline or dextrose water and minimize the incidence of catheter failure.[80] Particularly in small neonates, it is important that the continuous-flow device *not* be used to flush the catheter by bolus because large volumes of fluid may be introduced. Studies have demonstrated that material can appear in the neonate's carotid artery circulation after injection of only 0.3 to 0.75 mL into the radial artery.[84]

A number of techniques can be used to obtain blood gas samples for analysis. Care should be taken to minimize waste of aspirated blood, especially from small neonates. In older patients, systems that provide on-line information with regard to Pao_2, $Paco_2$, and pH have been developed. Their reliability remains a problem, however, and frequent calibration of the devices is required.

Systolic and diastolic blood pressure measures using indwelling arterial cannulas may be inaccurate for a variety of reasons.[85] These include air or clot in the system, inappropriate tubing, and inadequate calibration of monitors. Systolic and diastolic arterial pressures obtained from peripheral arterial catheters are often greater and less, respectively, than those measured in the aorta. The mean arterial pressure, however, is the same. The mean arterial pressure is estimated by adding one third of the pulse pressure to the diastolic blood pressure. Because diastolic and systolic pressures are related more to the compliance and resistance of the monitoring circuit, and because systolic and diastolic pressures in the radial artery are different than those measured in the aorta, the mean arterial pressure is most reliable (Fig. 7-25).

Complications of arterial catheter placement are surprisingly few. Distal embolization or ischemia is rare if the catheter is managed appropriately and prospective evaluation for collateral flow is done. If this does occur, the catheter should be removed and anticoagulation with heparin considered. Tissue loss is rare. Thrombosis of the vessel occurs frequently in the radial artery in small newborns and infants after prolonged catheterization. Most obstructed arteries, however, recanalize after catheter removal. Acute vascular injury to the femoral artery can lead to chronic ischemia and limb length discrepancies. If the pulse is lost in the lower extremity after femoral arterial catheter placement, the catheter should be removed.[80] If the limb is acutely threatened, surgical exploration must be undertaken in most circumstances.[86] In neonates and infants, however, femoral artery exploration is technically difficult and often unrewarding. In these instances, heparin anticoagulation or thrombolytic therapy with streptokinase or urokinase may result in improved limb perfusion.

Thrombotic complications of umbilical artery catheters are frequent. Some Doppler studies have shown that up to 30% of infants develop thrombus within the aorta after umbilical artery cannulation.[87,88] The incidence of clinically significant aortic thrombus formation is 3% to 6%.[89] The likelihood of adverse thromboembolic events appears to be greater in these patients with low (L-4 or lower) abdominal umbilical artery catheters, although the incidence of intracranial hemorrhage is lower when the catheter is in the low position.[82] Aortoiliac thrombosis often can be managed with supportive care alone. Systemic heparinization, fibrinolytic therapy, and surgical thrombectomy are reserved for specific problems, such as limb-threatening ischemia, renal failure, visceral compromise, and systemic acidosis (Table 7-3).[90–93] Sepsis occurs in less than 1% of patients with radial artery catheters and in 2% to 5% of patients with umbilical artery catheters.[79,94]

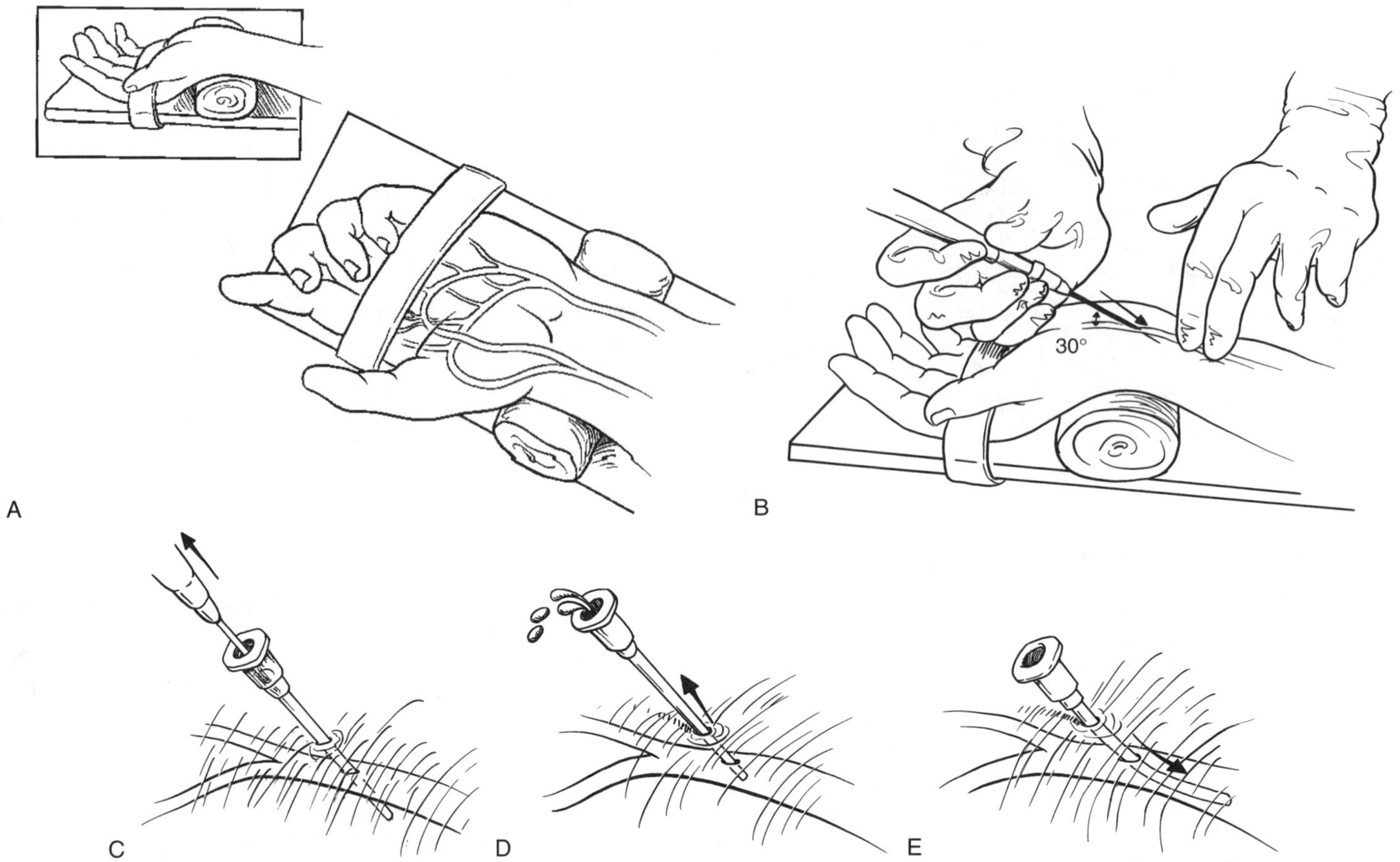

FIG. 7-21. Percutaneous insertion of a catheter into the radial artery. (*A*) The hand is taped securely to an arm board with a roll placed under the wrist. (*B*) The radial pulse is palpated, and the needle and catheter are guided at about a 30-degree angle through the artery. As the needle and catheter are withdrawn and pass into the artery, blood may be observed to flow into the hub. The needle and catheter are then advanced a second time; the needle is removed (*C*), and the catheter is withdrawn until blood return is observed (*D*) and then advanced into the lumen of the artery (*E*).

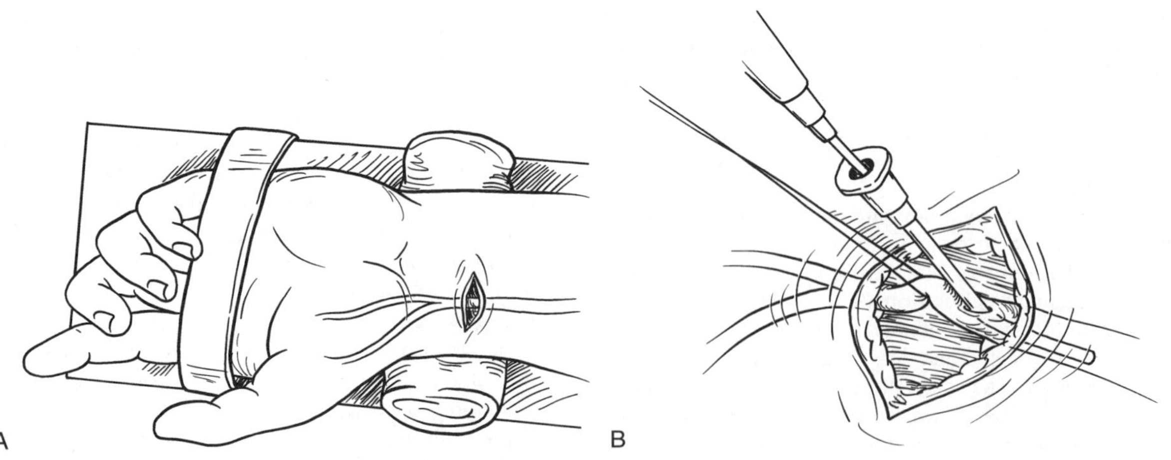

FIG. 7-22. Insertion of a catheter into the radial artery by the cutdown technique. (*A*) A 1-cm incision is made over the area of the radial artery just proximal to the wrist. (*B*) The artery is identified on the head of the radius and retracted distally with a suture as a needle and catheter are advanced into the lumen of the artery. Ligation of the artery is usually not necessary.

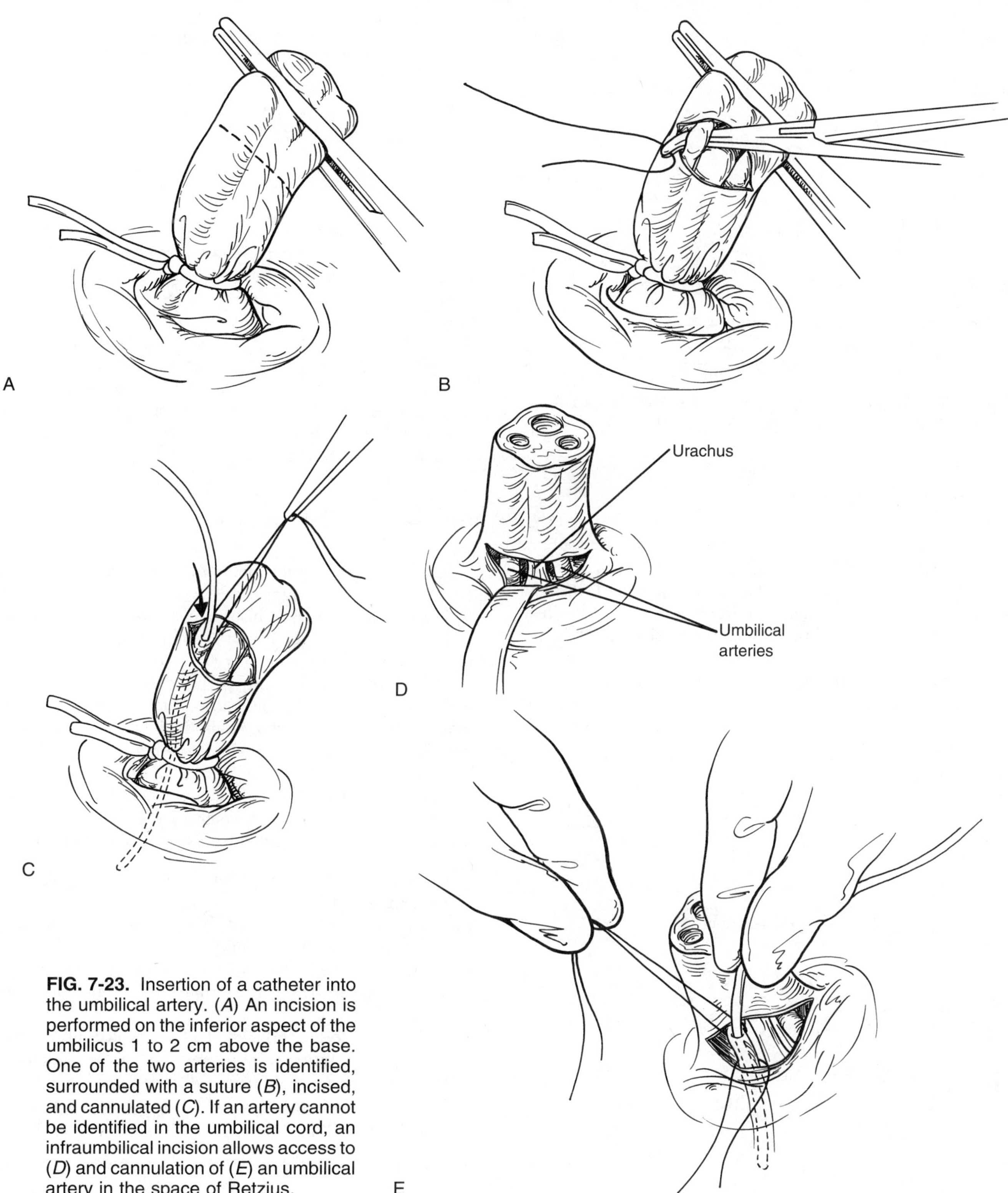

FIG. 7-23. Insertion of a catheter into the umbilical artery. (*A*) An incision is performed on the inferior aspect of the umbilicus 1 to 2 cm above the base. One of the two arteries is identified, surrounded with a suture (*B*), incised, and cannulated (*C*). If an artery cannot be identified in the umbilical cord, an infraumbilical incision allows access to (*D*) and cannulation of (*E*) an umbilical artery in the space of Retzius.

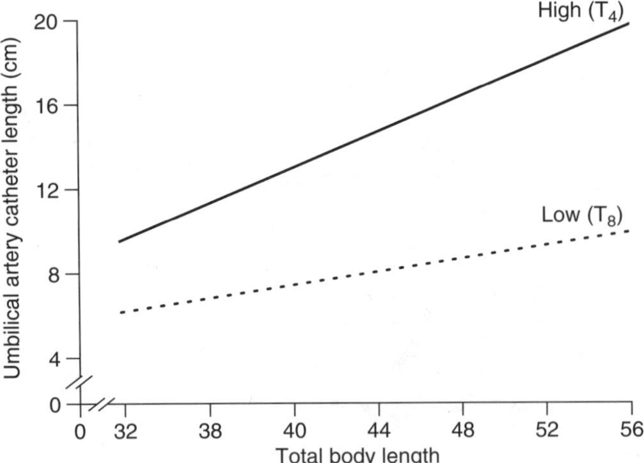

FIG. 7-24. Umbilical artery catheter insertion length as a function of patient total body length.

Central Venous Catheters

Central venous catheters are most commonly placed for purposes of administration of parental nutrition, antibiotics, or chemotherapeutic agents. In addition, measurement of central venous pressure (right atrial pressure) serves as an excellent monitor of intravascular volume status, especially in children. Indeed, in children, central venous pressure is as reliable as pulmonary artery or pulmonary capillary wedge pressure assessment for patients with normal cardiac function in the absence of high positive and end-expiratory pressures during mechanical ventilation.

The technical aspects of central venous catheter insertion and

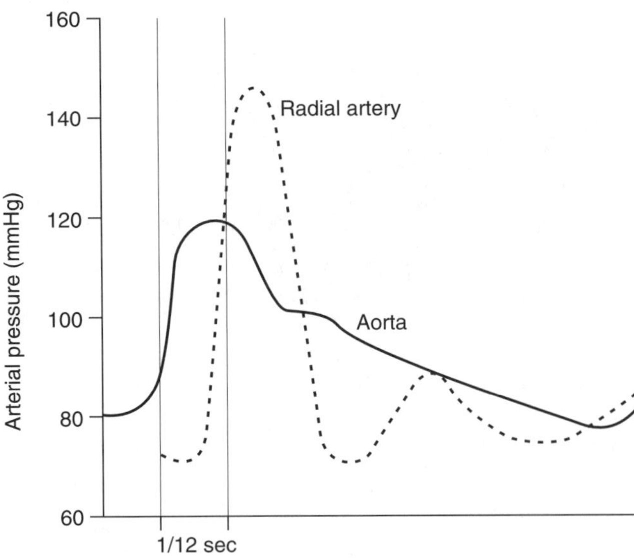

FIG. 7-25. A comparison of aortic and radial arterial waveforms. The systolic and diastolic pressures are higher and lower, respectively, the more distal the point of blood pressure measurement.

TABLE 7-3. *Complications of arterial catheter placement*

Thrombosis
Intimal flap formation
Distal ischemia or necrosis
Arterial embolus
Sepsis
Bleeding

care are detailed in Chapter 103. Assessment of central venous pressure should be performed at end-expiration because it is least affected by the patient's ventilatory status at this point. Pressure measurement should be performed using a transducer with a short, noncompliant tubing connector placed between the catheter and transducer. The transducer should be placed at the level of the right atrium when all hemodynamic measurements are performed. Variation in central venous pressure with the cardiac cycle should be documented. Normal right atrial pressure is 5 to 10 mmHg.

Pulmonary Arterial Catheters

In most children, assessment of cardiopulmonary status can be performed using noninvasive means or a right atrial catheter. Patients with pulmonary insufficiency, renal dysfunction, or cardiac failure, however, often benefit from the additional information provided by a pulmonary arterial catheter. Patients who remain hypotensive or poorly perfused despite apparently adequate volume resuscitation, those who require perioperative monitoring, and those who require inotropic therapy may also benefit from pulmonary artery monitoring.

Two sizes of pulmonary arterial catheters can be used in children: 5F and 7F. The 5F catheter is usually appropriate for patients up to 25 to 30 kg in weight. The catheters have five or six ports, each of which provides a specific function, including:

- An inflation port for injection of air into an inflatable balloon at the catheter tip
- A thermistor probe near the tip for estimation of cardiac output by thermodilution techniques
- A fiberoptic bundle, which emits a light signal and also provides computer input for determination of pulmonary artery Svo_2
- A port distal to the inflatable balloon, which allows assessment of pulmonary arterial pressures when the balloon is deflated, and left atrial pressures when inflated
- One or two additional proximal infusion or pressure monitoring ports usually placed in the right ventricle or right atrium

Pulmonary arterial catheters are most often placed using a subclavian or internal jugular vein approach. In children younger than 2 years, the femoral venous approach may ease placement because of the difficulty in achieving the appropriate curvature of the catheter through the right atrium, right ventricle, and into the pulmonary artery from the superior vena cava. Catheter placement is usually accomplished by on-line monitoring of the distal port pressures as the catheter traverses the right heart into the pulmonary artery[95] (Fig. 7-26). Occasionally, placement requires use of fluoroscopy to guide catheter inser-

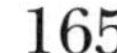

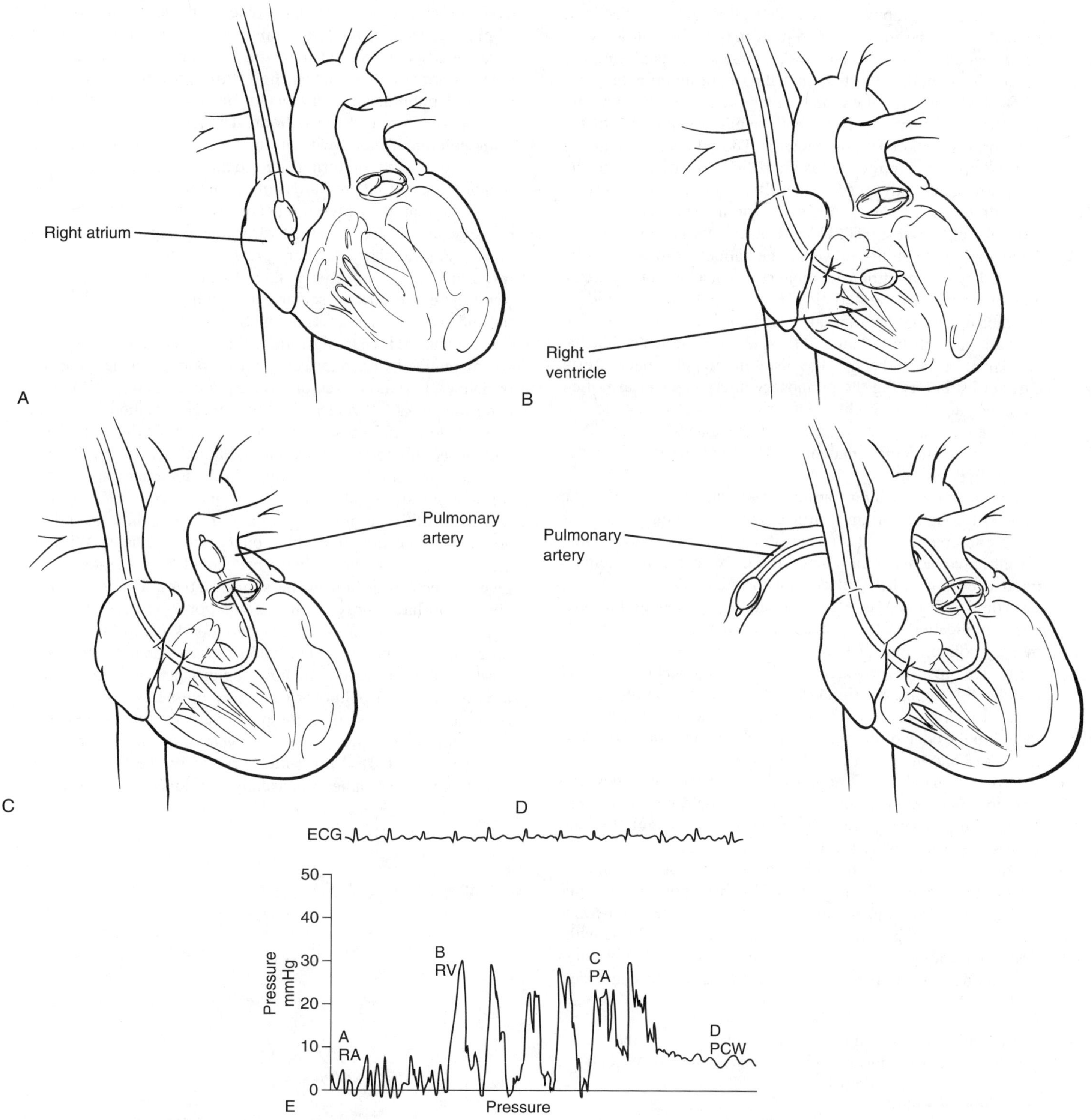

FIG. 7-26. Pulmonary artery catheter placement. Vascular pressure waveforms are used to monitor passage of the catheter through the (*A*) right atrium (RA), (*B*) right ventricle (RV), and (*C*) pulmonary artery (PA), and (*D*) into the wedged position in the pulmonary artery (pulmonary capillary wedge, PCW). (*E*) The pressure waveforms during transit of the distal aspect of the catheter through the RA, RV, PA, and into PCW position is demonstrated.

tion. Echocardiography (ECG) localization of the catheter at the bedside in the intensive care unit may be helpful as well. Once venous access is established, an introducer is placed; the balloon is inflated and tested; and all monitoring infusion ports are flushed. The pressure monitoring system is zeroed, and the tip of the catheter is shaken gently while ascertaining that a waveform is recorded on the monitor. The catheter is advanced past the tip of the introducer as the balloon is inflated, and the catheter is gently advanced further. Right atrial, right ventricular, pulmonary arterial, and, finally, pulmonary wedge waveforms should be observed. Correct placement is confirmed by documenting the ability to wedge the balloon at the end of the 1.5 mL-balloon inflation with rapid return of a pulmonary artery pressure waveform on deflation. Chest radiographs should be obtained to confirm appropriate placement. The ability to wedge the balloon with less than 1 mL of air may indicate that the placement of the catheter is too distal in the pulmonary artery. Difficulties in passing the pulmonary artery catheter are often secondary to coiling in the right atrium or ventricle, or to impingement on one of the ventricular trabeculae. Catheter placement may be difficult in patients with right ventricular dysfunction or hypertrophy.

Ventricular arrhythmias are common during passage of the catheter through the right ventricle, but rarely require pharmacologic intervention.[95] Lidocaine should be administered only if ventricular tachycardia is induced. The balloon should remain inflated during catheter placement to reduce the incidence of arrhythmias. Rupture of the pulmonary artery is a rare but serious complication of this procedure. Hemoptysis or cardiopulmonary collapse may be observed after inflation of the balloon for wedge pressure measurement. These complications are best avoided by keeping the tip of the catheter in the central pulmonary circulation less than 3 to 5 cm from the midline or 2 cm lateral to the edge of the spine on the chest radiograph. In addition, the balloon should be inflated with the minimal volume necessary to achieve a wedge tracing, and the frequency and duration of wedge pressure assessment should be limited. Patients with pulmonary artery hypertension and coagulation disorders are at highest risk for this complication.

Distal migration, with permanent wedging of the catheter, may result in pulmonary infarction. The distal port of the catheter should be continuously monitored for evidence of a permanent wedge tracing. If this occurs, the catheter should be withdrawn until appropriate pulmonary artery and wedge tracings are obtained. A number of other rare complications can occur. These include:

- perforation of the ventricle during catheter placement
- valvular damage during withdrawal with an inflated balloon
- right bundle-branch block
- pulmonary embolus
- knotting of the catheter in the right ventricle

Measurement of Pulmonary Artery Pressure

As noted, the right atrial pressure in children usually represents the intravascular volume status accurately and, therefore, is a useful indicator of left ventricular preload. Patients with sepsis, complex positive-pressure ventilation needs, pulmonary hypertension, pulmonary embolus, pulmonary fibrosis, cardiac

dysfunction, and other similar problems, however, may benefit from assessment of the left atrial pressure as an approximation of left ventricular end-diastolic volume. This is critical management information (see later). Left atrial pressure is measured by distal pulmonary artery occlusion during inflation of the pulmonary artery catheter balloon. The measurement creates a static column of blood without intervening valves between the catheter pressure monitoring site and the left atrium. Determination of the left atrial pressure is important for two reasons. First, pulmonary capillary pressure is approximated by the left atrial pressure, and this reflects the hydrostatic forces in alveolar capillaries. A pulmonary capillary pressure greater than 25 mmHg in normal lungs and greater then 18 mmHg in injured lungs (with increased microvascular permeability) results in interstitial and alveolar edema formation. Second, left ventricular function is enhanced when diastolic filling pressures (and volumes) are maintained in a relatively narrow normal range (Starling principle). Left atrial pressure usually correlates well with these determinants of left ventricular function. Hence, there is clinical value to left atrial pressure monitoring in critically ill patients and those with abnormal myocardial function (Fig. 7-27). Factors that potentially can invalidate this approach include the following: states of altered cardiac compliance (sepsis, restrictive pericarditis, cardiomyopathy), mitral valve disease, and inappropriate position of the pulmonary artery catheter. With regard to the latter, the catheter tip should be posterior to the level of the left atrium in the supine patient. This is because alveolar inflation pressure in the anterior (non-dependent) regions of the lungs may exceed pulmonary capillary pressure during positive-pressure ventilation, thus invalidating the catheter-derived information. In lung regions posterior to the left atrium, the mean pulmonary vascular pressures exceed those of the alveoli. Therefore, this pulmonary vasculature remains patent throughout the respiratory cycle, allowing accurate assessment of left atrial pressure. Fortunately, the flow-directed pulmonary artery catheter is usually positioned at or below the

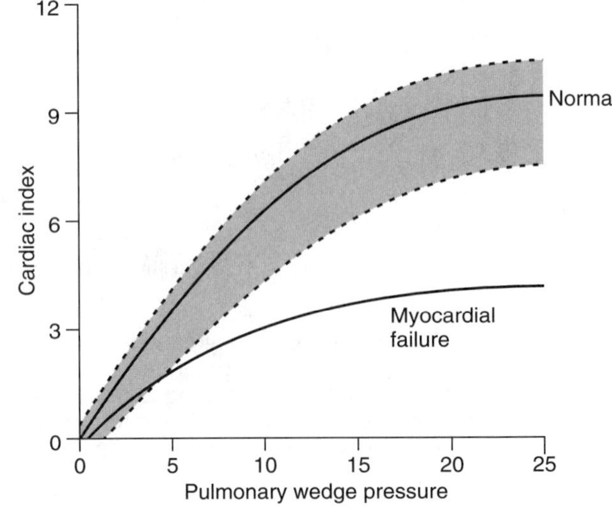

FIG. 7-27. Starling curve demonstrating an increase in cardiac index related to an increase in pulmonary wedge pressure in normal patients and in those with myocardial failure.

left atrium because a predominance of blood flow is distributed to the dependent regions of the lungs.

Application of positive end-expiratory pressure (PEEP) may result in overestimation of left atrial pressure because the intrathoracic pressure is transmitted from the left atrium to the monitoring catheter. This effect is observed in compliant normal lungs and less so in injured, noncompliant lungs. In the latter circumstance, the measured pulmonary artery occlusion pressure exceeds left atrial pressure by about 1 mmHg for every 5 cm H_2O increase in applied PEEP.[96] Generally, pulmonary wedge pressures are measured and reported without correction for the PEEP level because this effect is relatively minor and because trends, rather than absolute values, are most important. No effort is made to obtain the catheter measurements without PEEP because most of these patients are highly sensitive to interruptions of PEEP.

By convention, pulmonary capillary wedge pressure is assessed at end-expiration because the effects of ventilation on intrathoracic pressures may be significant: intrathoracic pressure is closest to atmospheric pressure at end-expiration.

Measurement of Cardiac Output

Two invasive methods of cardiac output estimation are in common clinical use: the temperature dilution technique and the Fick method. Both are based on the concept of Fick that the rate of indicator dilution in the circulation is directly related to cardiac output.[11] Fick used oxygen as the indicator. For the temperature dilution technique, a bolus of iced or room-temperature saline is injected rapidly as the indicator into the central venous circulation. This can be injected into any central venous port and does not have to be administered through a pulmonary catheter proximal port. The indicator mixes with blood in the right ventricle and is then assessed by a thermistor at the tip of the pulmonary artery catheter. Once the initial blood temperature, the volume of injectate, the injectate temperature, and the change in blood temperature as a function of time are known, cardiac output can be determined.[97] If the cardiac output is high, then the decrease in blood temperature will be small and sustained only for a short period. In contrast, if the cardiac output is low, the decrease in blood temperature will be relatively greater and result in a longer period of temperature reduction (Fig. 7-28).

In practice, cardiac output measurements are performed in triplicate, and irregular curves or curves that deviate by more than 10% are discarded. The individual measurements are averaged, and the result has an approximate accuracy of ±10%. It is important to inject the bolus rapidly and at a consistent point in the respirator cycle. The colder the indicator solution, the greater the amplitude of the change. Although iced fluids tend to warm during passage through conduit tubing, they generally increase accuracy when compared with room-temperature saline injections.[98] In general, 5- or 10-mL injectate volumes are used, except in small children, in whom 1-mL injections are preferred.

Measurement of oxygen consumption and mixed venous and arterial oxygen content allows determination of cardiac output using the Fick equation[11]:

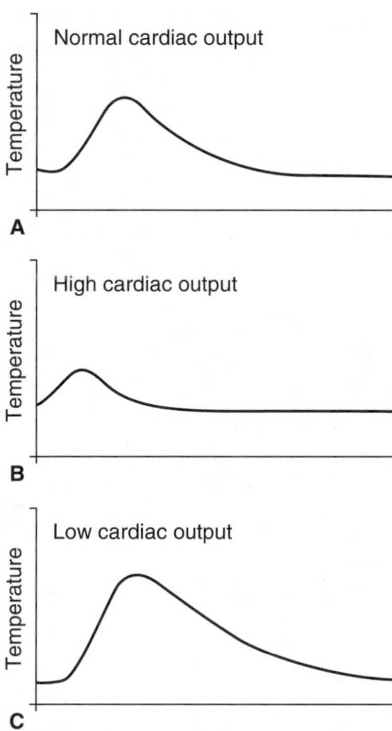

FIG. 7-28. Thermodilution cardiac output determination during periods of normal, high, and low cardiac output. The magnitude and duration of the changes in temperature are inversely proportional to the cardiac output.

$$\text{Cardiac output (L/m}^2\text{/min)}$$
$$= \text{(Arterial oxygen saturation [mL/m}^2\text{/min]}$$
$$- \text{Mixed venous oxygen saturation [L/dL])}$$
$$\times \text{ Hemoglobin (g/dL)} \times 1.36 \, \dot{V}_{O_2} \times 10$$

$$\text{Cardiac Index (L/m}^2\text{/min)}$$
$$= \frac{V_{O_2} \, (\text{mLo}_2\text{/m}^2\text{/min}) \times 10 \, \text{L/dL}}{\begin{array}{l}\text{(Arterial oxygen saturation}\\ - \text{ Venous oxygen saturation)}\\ \times \text{ Hgb (gm/dL)}\\ \times 1.36 \, (\text{mLo}_2\text{/gm})\end{array}}$$
$$= \frac{V_{O_2} \, (\text{mLo}_2\text{/m}^2\text{/min}) \times 10 \, \text{L/dL}}{(\text{SaO}_2 - \text{SvO}_2) \times \text{Hgb (gm/dL)} \times 1.36 \, (\text{mLo}_2\text{/gm})}$$

Because this calculation requires knowledge of the mixed venous blood oxygen saturation, a pulmonary artery catheter must be placed. Because of the inherent error present in each of the variables, the Fick cardiac output has an error of about ±5%.[96] In general, the Fick-calculated cardiac output exceeds the thermodilution cardiac output by about 5% to 10%. A number of studies have demonstrated the clinical feasibility of on-line Fick calculation of cardiac output using data obtained from continuous oxygen consumption monitoring, arterial pulse oximetry, and mixed venous oximetry[99,100] (Fig. 7-29).

Mixed Venous Oximetry Monitoring

Many pulmonary arterial catheters contain fiberoptic bundles that provide continuous mixed venous oximetry data. Emitted

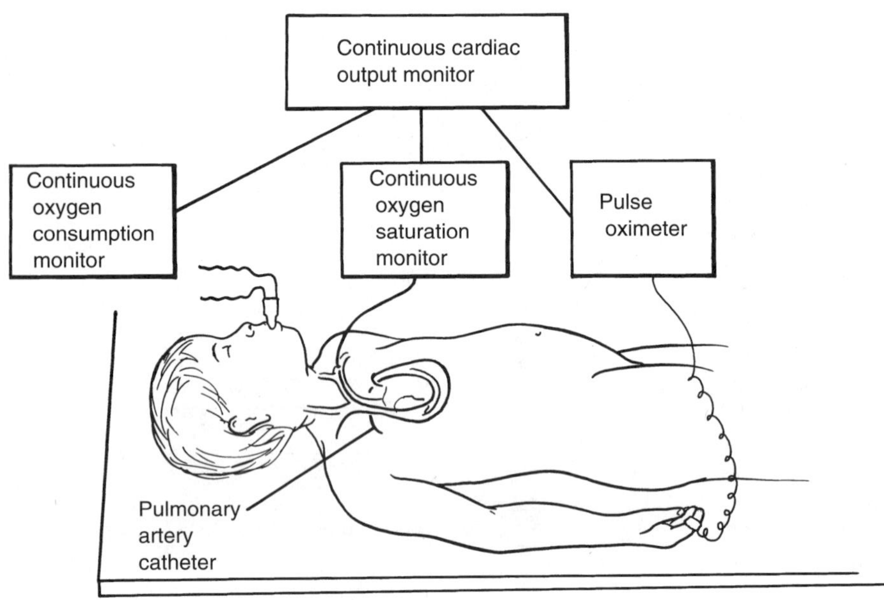

FIG. 7-29. Continuous Fick cardiac output monitoring is illustrated schematically.

light is reflected from circulating blood cells and transmitted through the receiving fiberoptic bundle to an analyzer, where accurate determination of hemoglobin oxygen saturation is done. Calibration is done by withdrawing a sample of pulmonary arterial blood and assessing oxygen saturation with an oximeter. Mixed venous oximetry provides a means for continuously assessing the adequacy of oxygen delivery.[101] A decrease in Svo_2 to less than 65% or a change of more than 5% to 10% at any time should be investigated by assessing cardiac output, arterial oxygen saturation, and the hemoglobin level, as detailed earlier.

Gastric Tonometry

Global estimates of oxygenation may underestimate the presence of occult visceral ischemia and abnormalities of tissue oxygen extraction. Septic shock, for example, appears to disrupt the cellular ability to use oxygen, despite adequate microvascular oxygenation. Tissue pH has been presented as a potentially more effective means to assess adequacy of oxygenation. Gastric tonometry is a technique in which changes in gastric mucosal blood flow are used to reflect mucosal tissue acidosis from ischemia.[102] For this, a nasogastric tube with a saline-filled balloon is placed in the stomach and allowed to equilibrate. Simultaneous measurements of the saline Pco_2 and arterial bicarbonate are performed. The presence of tissue acidosis is determined using the Henderson-Hasselbach equation. This provides an indirect measure of tissue oxygenation in the stomach and is correlated to oxygenation in the splanchnic vascular bed. Use of type II histamine blockers improves the reliability of this assessment by reducing the amount of CO_2 produced by mixture of gastric acid and pancreatic bicarbonate. The clinical application of this technique has been limited and remains controversial. Insufficient data are available for a meaningful analysis with specific regard to infants and children.

SHOCK

Shock is a clinical state in which the cardiopulmonary system fails to deliver oxygen adequately to the tissues. In addition, the removal of metabolic wastes and carbon dioxide from the peripheral tissues is inadequate. Shock is often accompanied by hypotension. The shock state in children and adults often is associated with a reduction in cardiac performance. Because of the small size of pediatric patients, direct monitoring of cardiac function can be difficult using traditional invasive measures. With the inherent size limitations, the physical examination and other noninvasive forms of monitoring, such as echocardiography, become increasingly important. Because of these challenges, an understanding of the response of cardiac function to shock is essential.

Cardiac Function

Preload refers to the diastolic filling pressure of the ventricles. It is determined by the intravascular volume of the patient and by the flow characteristics of the patient's circulatory system. Preload determines whether the ventricles fills appropriately, hence whether the cardiac output is optimal. The preload volume is difficult to assess directly, so measurements of central venous and left atrial pressure are commonly used alternatives in clinical practice. With abnormal ventricular wall compliance, or in the presence of certain forms of congenital heart disease, right atrial pressure may not represent preload accurately. In children, cardiovascular dysfunction is often due to hypovolemic shock. The treatment of shock begins with the establishment of adequate preload before the use of inotropic agents. If evidence of inadequate cardiac output exists, attempts should be made to increase right atrial pressures to 10 to 15 mmHg, a range that generally provides adequate cardiac filling.

Significant lung disease accompanying shock often requires

the addition of PEEP and an increase in mean airway pressure to maintain oxygenation. In a patient with healthy lungs, increasing PEEP or mean airway pressure can significantly increase intrathoracic pressure, impair right heart filling (preload), and thus decrease cardiac output. Although patients with significant lung disease have a more permissive response to high airway pressures because of reductions in pulmonary compliance, application of PEEP and high ventilator pressures may compromise patients who are hypotensive or hypoperfused. Volume administration may resolve the cardiovascular sequelae of applied PEEP.[103] Measurements of oxygen delivery at various levels of PEEP are required, however, to optimize oxygen delivery in this scenario.

Afterload refers to the resistance against which the ventricle must work to eject blood. It is dependent on the systemic vascular resistance and the myocardial wall tension. Systemic vascular resistance is calculated by dividing the difference of the mean arterial and central venous pressure by the cardiac output. Myocardial contractility is indirectly related to afterload. Increased afterload causes a decrease in myocardial contractility, and vice versa. Decreasing afterload by vasodilator therapy may be beneficial when cardiac output is inadequate despite adequate intravascular blood volume.

The inotropic state of the heart reflects the ability of the cardiac muscle to shorten and eject blood. The left ventricular ejection fraction is a common measurement of contractility. Poor contractility can occur in the presence of acidemia, hypoxemia, sepsis, and congenital heart disease. Poor cardiac function that persists after optimization of preload, afterload, and correction of hypoxemia and acidosis necessitates use of inotropic agents, such as dopamine, dobutamine, amrinone, epinephrine, and others.

Increasing the heart rate is the most common and effective way of increasing cardiac output and oxygen delivery. The infant is uniquely dependent on this mechanism because the ability to regulate blood volume and myocardial contractility is more limited. Extremes in cardiac rate induce their own form of pathophysiology. Pathologic tachycardia can prevent adequate time for complete atrial filling and impairs cardiac output. In contrast, bradycardia is often a reflection of a prearrest state. If not corrected, a low heart rate can progress to asystole. The appearance of bradycardia in a child should prompt immediate and aggressive resuscitative measures.

Vascular Resistance

Systemic vascular resistance is a calculated number used to represent the resistance the heart must overcome to provide effective blood flow to the tissues. In the presence of shock, vasoconstriction can be profound and the systemic vascular resistance high. In the acute phase of shock, vasoconstriction allows the child to maintain blood pressure, but the result is decreased flow to the extremities and to visceral organs such as the kidney and gut. In the extreme shock state, a child shunts blood away from the periphery to maintain perfusion centrally. In this circumstance, peripheral vasoconstriction may lead to a blood pressure that cannot be measured. The physical examination is notable for central pallor, poor capillary refill in the extremities, decreased urinary output, and altered mentation. In children, overt hypotension is a late and ominous event during

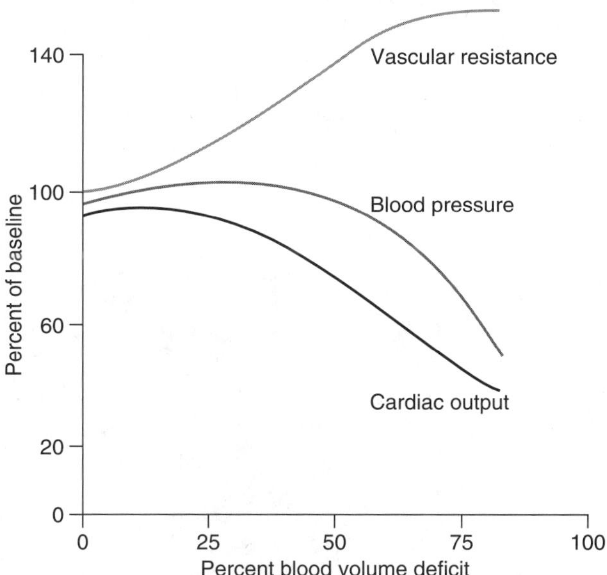

FIG. 7-30. Blood pressure, heart rate, cardiac output, and systemic vascular resistance are shown in relation to progressive hypovolemia in children. Blood pressure is initially compromised after 30% volume depletion and only after all other hemodynamic reserve is exhausted.

shock (Fig. 7-30).[104] It requires emergency intervention for reversal.

The pulmonary circulation also has the capacity to vasoconstrict and dilate in response to many influences. Similar to the systemic circulation, a numeric estimate can be calculated for the resistance of the pulmonary circulation to right heart blood flow. This is termed *pulmonary vascular resistance*. Hypoxia, endogenous inflammation, and airway obstruction can cause significant pulmonary vasoconstriction, which may result in the shunting of pulmonary blood flow and further hypoxia. In newborns, the potential for vasoconstriction can be extremely important. The transitional circulation of newborns is sensitive to hypoxia, acidosis, and hypercarbia. Pulmonary vasoconstriction and shunting exacerbate respiratory insufficiency and can result in persistent fetal circulation with additional right to left cardiac shunts through the patent foramen ovale and ductus arteriosus. The resulting hypoxia can induce further vasoconstriction and exacerbate shunting. The cycle is potentially lethal. In addition, pulmonary hypertension exposes the right heart to significant afterload. Suprasystemic pressures in the pulmonary artery can cause the volume-dependent right ventricle to fail in the face of an afterload that it is not able to overcome (Fig. 7-31).

In acute conditions of hypovolemic shock, the systemic vascular resistance increases to maintain perfusion pressure. Restoration of intravascular volume results in normal vasomotor tone in the peripheral circulation. Crystalloid volume infusions are effective, but saline remains in the intravascular space for a limited time. In conditions such as sepsis, in which microvascular permeability is increased, this may be only a matter of minutes. In contrast, blood and colloid solutions remain in the intravascular compartment longer and may help further by creating an osmotic gradient away from the extravascular space. Prolonged periods of increased vascular resistance can result in a

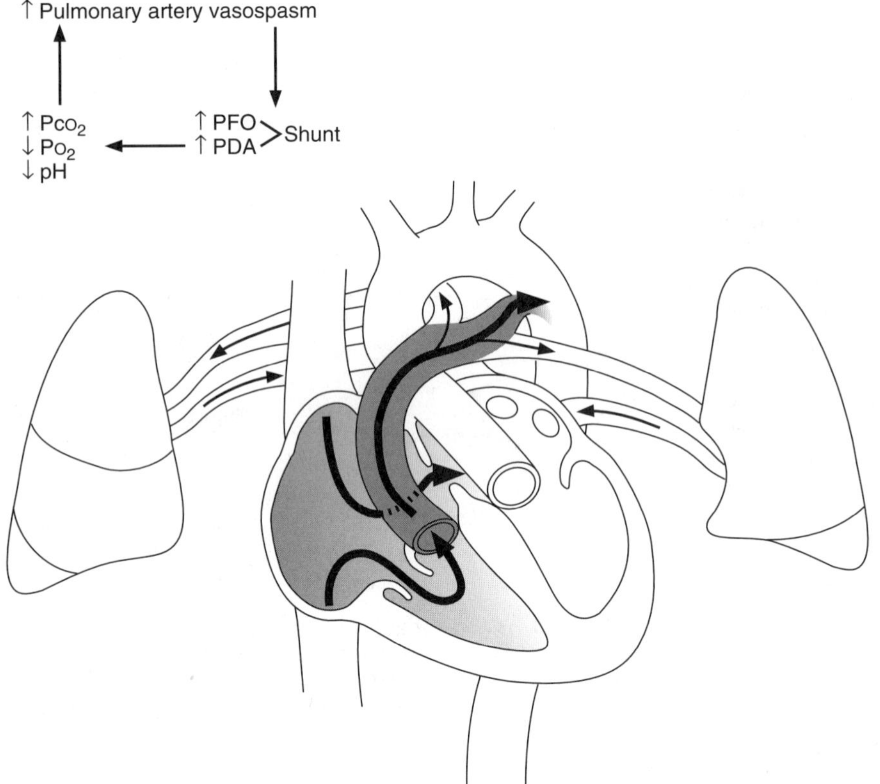

FIG. 7-31. The pathophysiology of persistent fetal circulation. Venous blood returning to the right heart preferentially flows (shunts) through the patent foramen ovale (PFO) or the patent ductus arteriosus (PDA) in the setting of severe pulmonary hypertension. This results in hypoxia, hypercarbia, and acidosis, which induce further increases in pulmonary hypertension and worsen the shunt. A vicious cycle of pulmonary hypertension and deteriorating gas exchange develops and can lead to the demise of the patient if not interrupted.

state of relative hypovolemia, such as with a pheochromocytoma. Volume resuscitation in conjunction with α-adrenergic antagonist administration returns the patient to a normal volume state preoperatively. In contrast, loss of sympathetic tone in patients with sepsis, spinal cord injuries, anaphylaxis, and adrenocortical insufficiency results in decreased systemic vascular resistance and shock. These patients are noted to be warm and well perfused, but hypotensive. The hypotension may not respond to volume resuscitation alone. α-Adrenergic agonists are often necessary to attain acceptable blood pressure levels in these patients. Normal adrenocortical function is required to support vascular tone. Patients with acute adrenal insufficiency have vascular collapse, requiring administration of hydrocortisone to restore normal vascular tone and perfusion.

Compensatory Responses to Shock

Many compensatory mechanisms are invoked by the shock state. These include the sympathetic nervous system response, release of vasoactive agents and hormones, release of endorphins, and activation of coagulation and endogenous inflammatory systems.[105] Hypovolemic shock produces a classic response from the sympathetic nervous system. Adrenergic neurotransmitters constrict large-capacitance venous blood vessels, displacing blood into the central circulation. Increased cardiac filling pressures result, cardiac output increases, and oxygen delivery to essential tissues is enhanced. The heart responds by increasing both contractility and heart rate, thus additionally increasing cardiac output and oxygen delivery. Vasoactive hormones, such as vasopressin and angiotensin II, are released into the circulation and selectively increase vascular resistance. This helps maintain oxygen delivery to critical organs. In addition, renal arterial vasoconstriction occurs and protects intravascular volume by decreasing urine output. Vasoconstriction has a number of physiologic benefits. Blood flow is diverted from skeletal muscle, visceral organs, skin, and fat. In addition, vasoconstriction may increase the velocity of microvascular blood flow in specific vascular beds, resulting in increased blood flow and oxygen delivery to ischemic tissues.

Vasoconstriction also decreases the amount of plasma–interstitial fluid exchange that occurs in countercurrent circulation systems such as in the kidney, gut, and other sites. In the normal state, large dilated arteries are adjacent to similarly dilated venules in the mucosal layer of the gut. The amount of oxygen and carbon dioxide exchanged by diffusion between these adjacent vessels is significant. With vasoconstriction, this countercurrent exchange is substantially decreased, resulting in increased oxygen content of the arterial blood as it returns to the microcirculation. In addition, the inability of waste products, such as carbon dioxide, to back-diffuse into the arterial system may have important effects on the pH of the microcirculation. Vasoconstriction by the large arterioles decreases capillary hydrostatic pressure and allows for the flux of interstitial fluid into the vascular space, thereby increasing intravascular fluid volume (Fig. 7-32). Hormones, such as epinephrine, cortisone, and glucagon, are also released in response to shock. Collectively, these hormones increase extracellular glucose concentrations and osmolarity in both the vascular and interstitial compartments. The net movement of fluid from the intracellular to the intravascular space is of fundamental importance in shock and hypovolemia.

In aggregate, these compensatory mechanisms are effective,

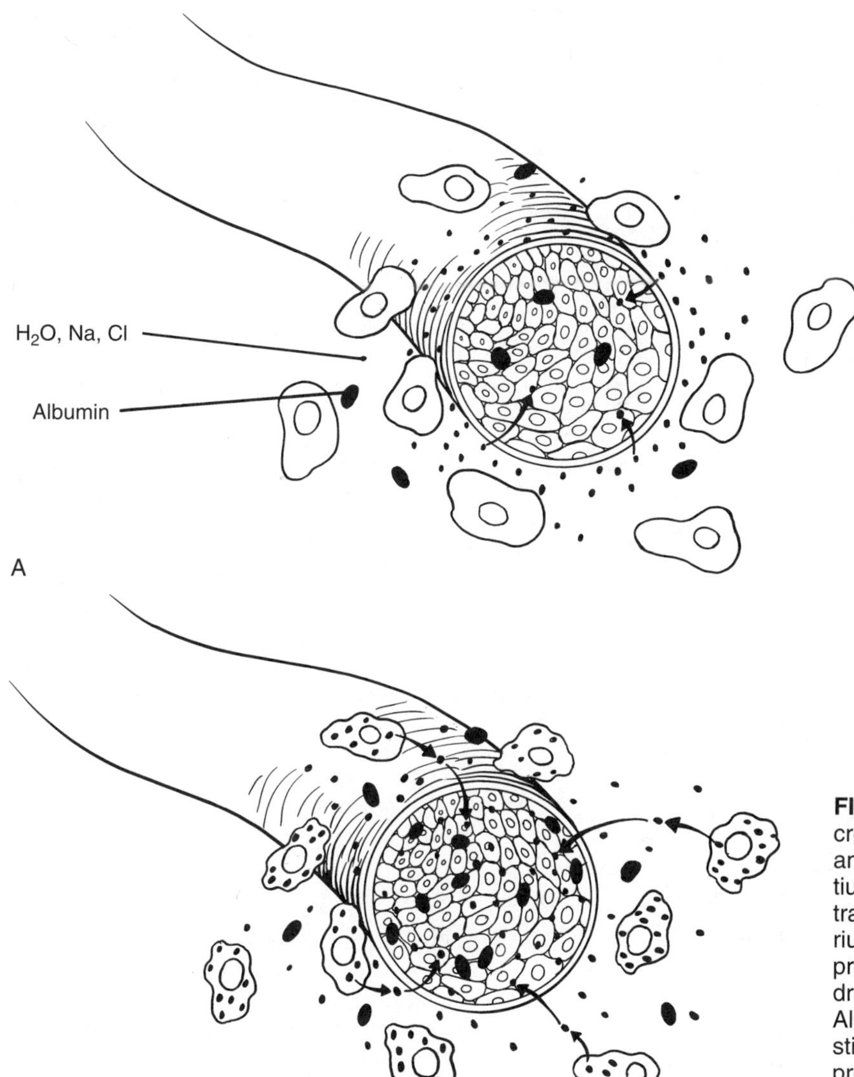

FIG. 7-32. (*A*) Hypovolemic shock results in decreased microvascular pressure, allowing a limited amount of protein-free fluid to flow from the interstitium into the vascular space. As albumin concentration in the interstitum increases, a new equilibrium is reached between oncotic and hydrostatic pressures. (*B*) Increased extracellular glucose draws water out of the cells into the interstitium. Albumin-rich lymph flows from the engorged interstitium into the vascular space, increasing oncotic pressure and encouraging movement of water and electrolytes into the vascular space.

but their ability to respond to shock is limited. Adults can generate a net movement of 1 to 2 L of interstitial and intracellular fluid into the vascular space, and children are proportionately limited. Although these compensatory mechanisms are essential in the face of major injury, they serve principally to keep a patient alive until the underlying problem can be corrected.

Many of these compensatory mechanisms have potentially adverse cardiovascular effects as well. With prolonged or severe shock, arterioles lose the ability to constrict, while postcapillary sphincters retain this capacity. The result is capillary pooling of blood. This allows extravasation of fluid from the vascular space, exacerbating the underlying problem and resulting in local edema formation. Particularly in the lung, this leads to physiologically dangerous organ dysfunction. Endorphin release is a consequence of shock and leads to a sense of well-being, increased strength, and pain tolerance, allowing the injured person to fight or flee. Endorphins dilate the vascular system, however, and thus counteract other compensatory mechanisms.

The shock state stimulates macrophages to release tumor necrosis factor, which activates inflammatory and coagulation cascades. Activated neutrophils release proteases and highly reactive oxygen radicals, causing vascular endothelial damage. Loss of vascular endothelial integrity results in increased microvascular permeability and the sequestration of large quantities of fluid into the surrounding tissues (Fig. 7-33). Experimental efforts to block these cytokine mediators in septic or hypovolemic shock have decreased mortality rates. Large randomized studies using cytokine antagonists in patients with septic or hemorrhagic shock, however, have not resulted in consistent clinical benefit.

Shock and Myocardial Function

Both systemic and pulmonary hypertension can result in obstructive forms of shock. Obstructive shock results from the inability of the myocardium to generate an adequate cardiac output with normal filling pressures and contractility. In pulmonary hypertension, the pulmonary vascular bed presents an abnormal afterload to the right ventricle, preventing effective emptying. This may be a primary problem, as with persistent

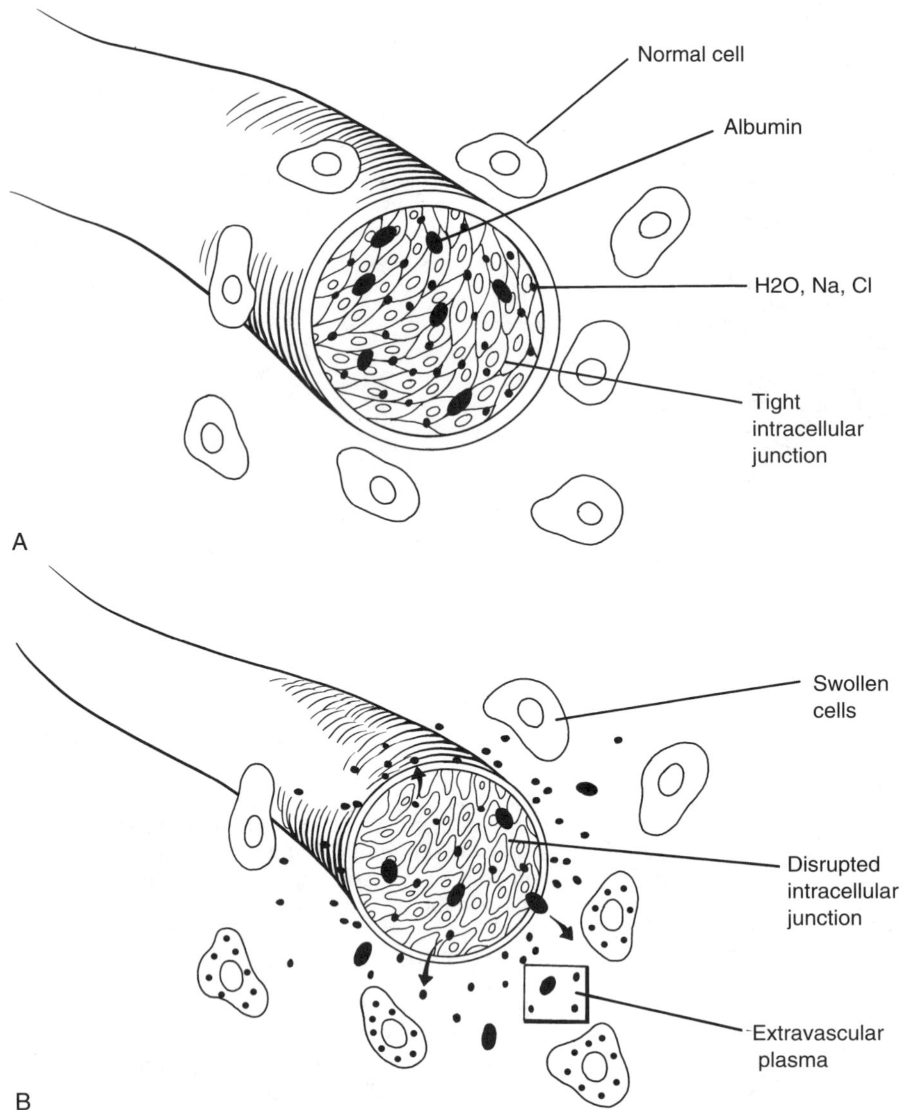

FIG. 7-33. (*A*) Release of inflammatory mediators causes endothelial cell injury disrupting tight intracellular junctions and allowing plasma to extravasate into the interstitium. (*B*) Cellular swelling occurs in end-stage shock, further worsening hypovolemia.

fetal circulation, or a secondary problem, as in a patient with a pulmonary embolus. Other situations that can result in right ventricular decompensation include application of excessive positive-pressure ventilation, tension pneumothorax, and congenital heart disease, such as pulmonary stenosis. The left ventricle is more tolerant of afterload elevations because it has evolved to supply the systemic circulation; however, it can still fail with extreme or chronic systemic hypertension.

Most shock states in children are associated with changes in peripheral blood pressure late in their course. Because of compensatory vasoconstriction in childhood, adequate blood pressures are maintained until the intravascular volume or cardiac output drops to 30% or 40% below normal levels.[104] Thereafter, hypotension and cardiovascular collapse can be precipitous.

Hypotensive shock states can be associated with either increased or decreased cardiac output. Low cardiac output is most often due to hypovolemia from either hemorrhage or dehydration. This is characterized by low cardiac filling pressures. Normal or increased right atrial pressures are found in states of primary myocardial dysfunction, such as myocarditis or cardio-

myopathy. Valvular heart disease may result in output failure with an increase in cardiac filling pressures.

As outlined earlier, diminished cardiac output may also result specifically from right ventricular failure. Common causes of this problem in the newborn period include congenital heart disease, such as pulmonary stenosis, various forms of neonatal respiratory failure, and primary pulmonary hypertension. The thin right ventricle responds effectively to volume distention but is less capable of compensating for high afterload. The impaired cardiac output is compounded by right to left shunting and inadequate pulmonary perfusion.

Shock also can result from cardiac tamponade or tension pneumothorax. The acute filling of the pericardial space with fluid or blood results in substantial increases in filling pressures required to maintain cardiac output. Although this can be reasonably compensated in the chronic state, an acute increase in pericardial fluid rapidly exceeds right heart filling pressures and dramatically decreases cardiac output and oxygen delivery. Similarly, the mediastinal shift that occurs with tension pneumothorax can induce obstruction of the superior and inferior vena cavae, resulting in diminished venous return to the right heart. In addition, collapse of the ipsilateral lung and compression of the contralateral lung result in hypoxia and further impairment of oxygen delivery.

Systemic hypotension with adequate cardiac output is referred to as *distributive shock*. It is associated with conditions such as sepsis, anaphylaxis, endocrine failure, and neurogenic shock. Sepsis results in the release of vasodilating mediators that decrease systemic vascular tone. The decrease in systemic vascular resistance may be sufficient to cause hypotension. In most patients, the myocardium responds by increasing cardiac output. Although oxygen delivery may increase, blood flow may be inappropriately distributed, hence the term. The cellular extraction of oxygen is impaired owing to sepsis-induced cellular dysfunction. Myocardial function may be compromised in early sepsis. There is evidence of transient functional cardiomyopathy with a decreased left ventricular ejection fraction. Some have suggested the existence of a specific myocardial depressant substance that impairs myocardial contractility. This has been a controversial point for many years, and it remains so today. Many circulatory mediators are released during sepsis, some of which may lead to myocyte dysfunction. Because intravascular volume resuscitation does not account for the underlying problem in these patients, the use of vasoactive agents, such as dopamine, norepinephrine, and dobutamine, is frequently required.

Anaphylaxis is characterized by the loss of systemic vascular tone due to an allergic response to exogenous antigen. This results in a profound decrease in systemic vascular resistance, which is usually associated with an increase in cardiac output. Neurogenic shock occurs when spinal cord injury results in generalized sympathectomy. The decreased vascular resistance is also associated with an increase in cardiac output. The patient appears warm and well perfused and is not tachycardic despite hypotension. The initial treatment of anaphylaxis includes administration of intravenous diphenhydramine, 1 to 2 mg/kg, or epinephrine, 0.01 mL/kg of 1 : 1000 solution (maximum, 0.5 mL), or both, by subcutaneous or intramuscular injection.[106] Blood pressure support in the setting of anaphylactic or neurogenic shock may require adrenergic agents.

Finally, normal adrenal function is necessary to maintain adequate systemic vascular resistance. It appears that glucocorticoids potentiate catecholamine effects, supporting normal peripheral vascular resistance. Cortisol also appears necessary to maintain normal synaptic transmission, particularly in multisynaptic regions. Adrenal insufficiency is characterized by a low systemic vascular resistance and inadequate circulating levels of glucocorticoids. In the setting of hypotension due to adrenocortical insufficiency, hydrocortisone should be administered with adrenergic drugs, such as dopamine, epinephrine, or norepinephrine, as needed to support blood pressure and perfusion.

Ischemia–Reperfusion Injury

One result of resuscitation after shock is reperfusion injury. In the presence of preexisting ischemia, reperfusion causes generation of highly reactive oxygen metabolites, including hydroxyl ion, hydrogen peroxide, hypochlorous acid, and superoxide anion.[107] The oxygen radicals are created by the reintroduction of oxygen into ischemic tissue in the presence of the enzyme xanthine dehydrogenase. Neutrophil-derived, NADPH-oxidase-

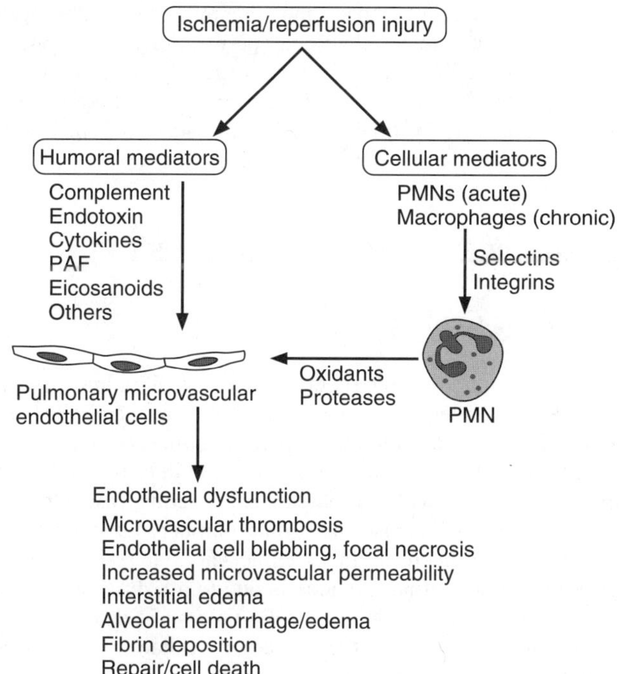

FIG. 7-34. Ischemia–reperfusion injury activates both and cellular mediators of acute inflammation. These mediators target pulmonary and other vascular endothelial cell beds. PMN, polymorphonuclear leukocytes; PAF, platelet-activating factor.

generated oxidants contribute significantly as well. Oxygen radicals are cytotoxic because of their ability to peroxidize lipid cell membranes and disrupt protein metabolism. In addition, oxygen radicals activate complement, generating C5a, a potent chemoattractant that effectively recruits neutrophils to the site of reperfusion injury. When activated, neutrophils roll along activated vascular endothelium, eventually adhering to adhesion molecules expressed on both the neutrophil and the endothelial cell (see Chap. 11). This allows transmigration of the leukocytes into the adjacent tissues with release of neutrophil proteases and further oxidative injury. Reperfusion injury also generates vasoactive metabolites and cytokines, which act locally and systemically. Platelet-activation factor, prostaglandin I_2, and thromboxane are involved with prostaglandin production and can worsen local tissue ischemia by reducing regional blood flow. It has become evident that tumor necrosis factor and several interleukins (ILs), such as IL-2, IL-6, and IL-8, are involved in the systemic inflammatory injury during reperfusion (Fig. 7-34).

The role of nitric oxide in reperfusion injury is being intensely studied.[108] It appears that nitric oxide acts both locally and regionally through several mechanisms. Endotoxin has been shown to stimulate macrophages, resulting in the L-arginine–dependent production of nitric oxide. Nitric oxide synthase inhibitors have been shown to inhibit experimental inflammation, while L-arginine enhances injury in similar models. This may be the result of oxidative injury from nitric oxide, which is itself a highly reactive oxidative species. Local vasodilation mediated by nitric oxide appears to be important as well.

The outcome of these various events is injury to the vascular endothelium. The nonspecific immune response focuses oxygen radicals, proteases, cytokines, and other mediators on the vascular endothelium. Increased vascular permeability and interstitial edema result. This leads to multiple organ dysfunction, which, for purposes of a critical care discussion, is most notable in the lung. Physiologic dysfunction follows rapidly, and the clinical problem becomes one of paramount importance.

CARDIOPULMONARY MANAGEMENT

Optimizing Cardiac Output

The principal physiologic tasks of the cardiopulmonary system are the delivery of oxygen and removal of metabolic waste and carbon dioxide from the peripheral tissues. Shock is a failure of the system. Shock is characterized either by a reduction in cardiac output with an increase in systemic vascular resistance, or by an increase in cardiac output with hypotension secondary to a decrease in systemic vascular resistance. Decreased cardiac output in shock is due to a reduction in either heart rate or stroke volume. Stroke volume is determined by myocardial contractility, the degree of cardiac filling, and afterload status. Therefore, shock must result from one or more of the following: a decrease in systemic vascular resistance, a lower heart rate, diminished myocardial contractility, inadequate preload volume, or an increase in afterload resistance (Fig. 7-35).

Shock in most neonatal and pediatric patients is secondary to low cardiac output from hypovolemia, inadequate preload, and poor cardiac filling. A cardinal manifestation of shock is a reduction in blood pressure. The lower limit of normal systolic blood pressure in children can be approximated by the formula: $80 + (2 \times \text{age in years})$.[109] Minimum monitoring in the setting of impaired perfusion would include serial blood pressure measurement, determination of the pulse and respiratory rate, and continuous ECG monitoring. Important physical findings indicating poor perfusion or hypovolemia include poor skin turgor, cool extremities with pale color, dry mucous membranes, and capillary refill of more than 2 seconds. Collapsed peripheral veins, a rapid and weak pulse, rapid and shallow breaths, and reduced glomerular filtration rate and renal blood flow as mani-

fested by oliguria are more serious indicators of hypoperfusion. Restlessness, anxiety, agitation, unresponsiveness, or other change in the level of consciousness suggest greatly impaired oxygen delivery. Extremity temperature can be useful as an indicator of perfusion status. Resuscitation results in the improvement of these physical signs as perfusion improves (Fig. 7-36).

Volume resuscitation for shock should be initiated with the intravenous administration of 10 mL/kg boluses of crystalloid solutions or 5% albumin. Each should be administered in a 15- to 20-minute period, followed by reassessment of blood pressure, clinical perfusion, and urine output. It is not unusual for a hypovolemic, hypoperfused patient to require 40 to 60 mL/kg of crystalloid before resuscitation is adequate. The hematocrit should be followed closely to avoid significant dilution of the hemoglobin concentration, which results in reduction of the oxygen-carrying capacity. In neonates, the general approach is to maintain the hemoglobin concentration at more than 13 g/dL; in older infants and children, a hemoglobin concentration of 10 to 12 g/dL is adequate if normal cardiac output and arterial oxygen saturation can be achieved. Patients with inadequate oxygen saturation or low cardiac output are maintained at a hemoglobin concentration of more than 13 g/dL to optimize oxygen delivery.

Patients with additional organ system failure, such as pulmonary, renal, or cardiac insufficiency, often require invasive monitoring to establish that adequate volume resuscitation has been achieved. A central venous pressure of more than 10 mmHg is usually associated with sufficient volume repletion. Continuing shock despite volume administration should lead to concern for ongoing blood loss or other causes of hypotension, such as cardiac tamponade, tension pneumothorax, adrenocortical insufficiency, sepsis, neurogenic shock, or anaphylaxis. Arrhythmias that contribute to the hypoperfused state should be treated. Persistence of hypoperfusion is an indication for pulmonary arterial catheter placement for pulmonary artery and left atrial pressure measurement and determination of mixed venous blood oxygen saturation and cardiac output assessment. This information is critical in establishing the contributions of cardiac output and vascular tone to the shock state and directs subsequent pharmacologic intervention. In patients too small for pulmonary artery pressure monitoring, or in whom the cause of cardiac insufficiency remains unclear, echocardiography is a safe and noninvasive method of evaluating cardiac function. Echocardiography allows near quantitative evaluation of cardiac output, ventricular filling, ventricular size, and myocardial contractility. In addition, the presence of congenital heart disease, intracardiac shunting, and pericardial effusion, as well as more refined indicators of cardiac function, such as the change in pressure over time and ventricular wall function, can be assessed.

Patients with hypotension and reduced systemic vascular resistance are best managed initially with a continuous intravenous infusion of dopamine. Dopamine is an endogenous catecholamine that results in enhancement of renal and splanchnic blood flow at doses between 1 and 5 μg/kg/min.[110] β-adrenergic receptor effects become apparent between 5 and 10 μg/kg/min, and α-adrenergic receptor–induced vasoconstriction develops at doses between 10 and 20 μg/kg/min. Therefore, dopamine provides enhancement of myocardial contractility at lower doses, but splanchnic and peripheral vasoconstriction at higher

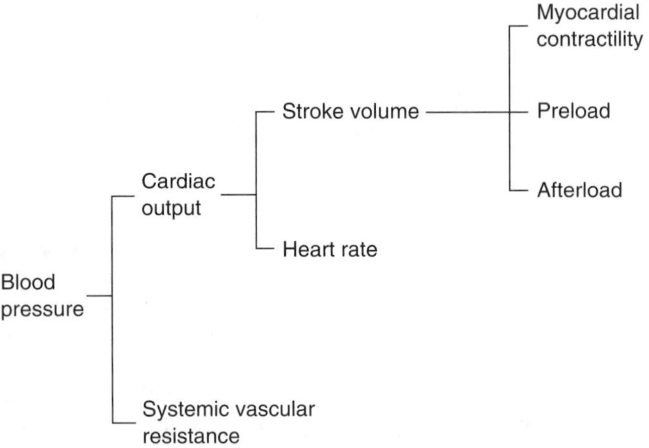

FIG. 7-35. Factors affecting blood pressure.

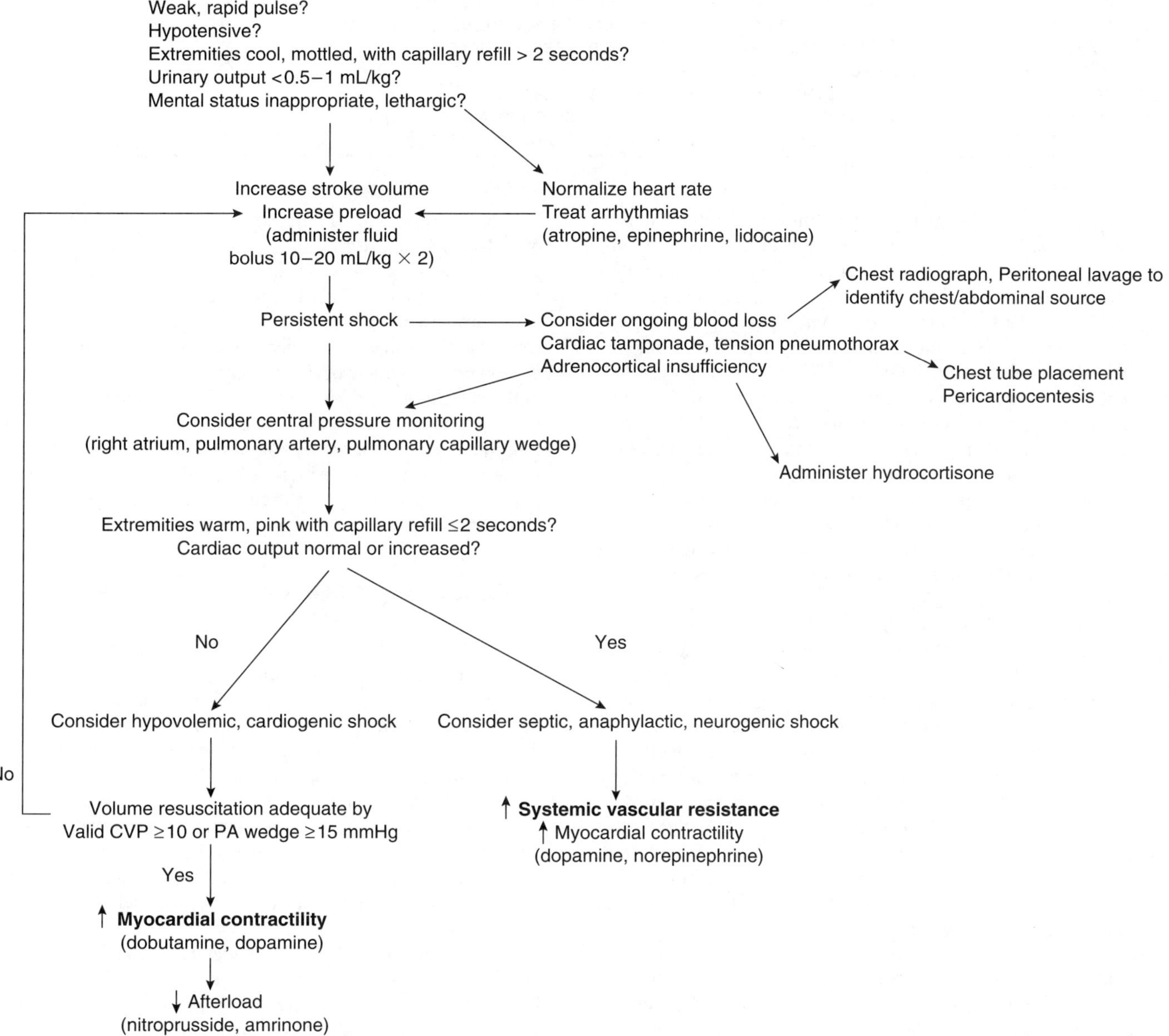

FIG. 7-36. Algorithm for managing the patient in shock. CVP, central venous pressure; PA, pulmonary artery.

infusion rates. Complications of dopamine administration are relatively few and include the induction of arrhythmias, peripheral ischemia at high infusion rates, and skin loss after extravasation. Total body oxygen consumption and carbon dioxide production increase 15% to 30% with the use of dopamine, epinephrine, and norepinephrine in normal adults. Most patients benefit from monitoring of the mixed venous blood oxygen saturation during periods of pressor support. Careful assessment and specific titration of pressors ensure that the benefits of an increase in oxygen delivery outweigh the costs in increased oxygen consumption (Table 7-4).

At times, dopamine infusion may be inadequate to produce the desired hemodynamic response. For example, patients in septic shock may benefit from the infusion of norepinephrine to induce vasoconstriction and increase blood pressure. Doses in the range of 0.05 to 1 μg/kg/min are typical.[111] Potential complications of norepinephrine administration are similar to those of dopamine, but more common.

For patients in cardiogenic shock (low cardiac output and high systemic vascular resistance), intravascular volume resuscitation is directed by right or left atrial pressure monitoring (see earlier). In addition, cardiac function is best promoted by administration of the synthetic, selective β-adrenergic agent dobutamine.[110] Myocardial contractility, stroke volume, and car-

TABLE 7-4. *Agents commonly administered in the setting of cardiac insufficiency*

Drug	Dose	Effect
Dopamine	2–20 μg/kg/min	Renal and splanchnic vasodilation at low dose; inotrope; vasoconstrictor
Dobutamine	2–20 μg/kg/min	Predominant inotrope
Epinephrine	0.1–1 μg/kg/min	Inotrope; vasoconstrictor
Nitroprusside	0.2–10 μg/kg/min	Vasodilator
Amrinone	5–10 μg/kg/min	Inotrope; vasodilator
Isoproterenol	0.1–1 μg/kg/min	Inotrope; chronotrope
Norepinephrine	0.05–1 μg/kg/min	Inotrope, vasoconstrictor

diac output typically increase, and pulmonary capillary wedge pressure falls. Infusions are titrated from initial doses of 2 to 5 μg/kg/min until the desired effect is achieved or a maximum of 20 μg/kg/min is reached. Minimal alteration in heart rate or systemic vascular resistance is noted with dobutamine, although myocardial oxygen consumption is usually increased. Epinephrine at doses of 0.1 to 1 μg/kg/min may be used to provide potent α- and β-adrenergic effects in patients who are unresponsive to either dopamine or dobutamine infusions.[34] Patients with cardiogenic shock and elevated systemic vascular resistance may benefit from simultaneous administration of a systemic vasodilator. The purpose is to reduce cardiac afterload resistance, decrease myocardial stroke work, and increase stroke volume. In addition, venous and arterial vasodilation can lead to reductions in right and left atrial pressures, which may be of benefit if myocardial dysfunction is associated with pulmonary edema. The overall result is improvement in both gas exchange and cardiac output.[111] Systemic vasodilators, such as sodium nitroprusside (initial dose, 0.2 to 0.5 μg/kg/min; maximum, 10 μg/kg/min) and phentolamine (1 to 20 μg/kg/min) can be used in conjunction with pressors to enhance myocardial function and cardiac output.[111] Amrinone is a useful agent as well. It is a phosphodiesterase inhibitor that enhances cardiac contractility while inducing systemic arterial vasodilation.[112] Amrinone may provide an optimal combination of these effects in patients with cardiogenic shock. Importantly, the pressor-induced increase in oxygen consumption is not observed during the administration of amrinone. The loading dose of amrinone is 0.75 mg/kg over 5 to 10 minutes, followed by a continuous infusion of 5 to 10 μg/kg/min.

Lactic acidosis is often observed in the setting of shock as ATP production shifts to the glycolytic pathway. Because of the untoward effect of metabolic acidosis on myocardial function and the pH dependence of inotropes, a normal pH is a necessity in patients with cardiac dysfunction. A plasma pH of less than 7.2 should be corrected by hyperventilation if the $Paco_2$ is greater than 40 mmHg or, if otherwise necessary, correction is by the administration of intravenous sodium bicarbonate, initially 1 mEq/kg. The distinction between respiratory and metabolic acidosis is best determined by assessing the level of $Paco_2$ and noting that an acute change in $Paco_2$ of 10 mmHg is associated with an increase or decrease in pH of 0.08 units.[34] At the same time, a base deficit of 10 mEq/L results in a change in pH of 0.15 units. By applying these estimates to the observed pH and $Paco_2$, one can determine whether acidosis is secondary to a respiratory or metabolic disorder. The total bicarbonate deficit can be estimated by the following equation[113]:

$$\text{Total } HCO_3 \text{ deficit (mEq)} = \text{Base deficit (mEq/L)}$$
$$\times \text{ Weight (Kg)} \times 0.3$$

To correct this, half of this dose can be given intravenously over 1 to 2 hours, followed by administration of the remainder over the ensuing 24 to 48 hours. Administration of sodium bicarbonate in the setting of hypoventilation can result in hypercarbia from the related increase in the production of CO_2. Therefore, in patients in whom hypercarbia is of concern, trishydroxymethylaminomethane (THAM) may serve as an effective buffer in the setting of metabolic acidosis. A 3.6% solution of THAM is administered at a dose of 6 to 8 mL/kg over 20 minutes. The total dose of THAM over 24 hours should not exceed 40 mL/kg. Adverse effects may include hypoglycemia, hyperkalemia, hypervolemia, and hypernatremia. For this reason, THAM should be used with caution in patients with renal insufficiency.

Optimizing Arterial Oxygen Saturation (Sao_2)

Support of the Sao_2, often through application of supplemental oxygen or positive-pressure ventilation, is critical to the maintenance of oxygen delivery in the critically ill child. Application of PEEP and positive-pressure ventilation are limited by the effects on cardiac output and the incidence of barotrauma.[114] Aside from pneumothorax and pulmonary interstitial emphysema, application of peak inspiratory pressures greater than 30 to 40 cm H_2O place a patient at high risk for ventilator-induced acute lung injury.[115,116] In neonates, particularly preterm neonates, this injury threshold is much lower. When exceeded for prolonged periods, pulmonary fibrosis and end-stage lung disease can follow.

Assessment of the best PEEP identifies that level of PEEP at which oxygen delivery and Svo_2 are optimal.[117] This should be estimated in any patient requiring an Fio_2 in excess of 60%. The Fio_2 should be adjusted to maintain the Sao_2 greater than 85%. Additional interventions, such as high-frequency oscillation, prone positioning, inverse ratio ventilation, nitric oxide administration, liquid ventilation with perfluorocarbon, and surfactant administration, may all enhance Sao_2. These are considered in Chapter 8.

Optimizing Hemoglobin Concentration

One of the most efficient ways to enhance oxygen delivery is to increase the oxygen-carrying capacity of the blood. Blood viscosity is increased, however, during isovolemic blood transfusion, and this may result in a reduction in cardiac output. Therefore, the benefits are potentially limited. Blood substitutes, such as stroma-free hemoglobin and perfluorocarbon solutions, may enhance oxygen-carrying capacity. Indeed, some perfluorocarbon blood substitutes have the potential to unload up to nine times more oxygen at the tissue level than can an equivalent volume of blood.[118]

Optimizing Oxygen Consumption

Oxygen consumption is elevated in patients with sepsis, burns, agitation, seizures, hyperthermia, hyperthyroidism, increased catecholamine production, and a variety of other problems. A number of strategies reduce oxygen consumption. In the intensive care unit, appropriate sedation, adequate analgesia, mechanical ventilation, and correction of the underlying problem are frequent necessities. Paralysis can enhance the effectiveness of mechanical ventilation while simultaneously reducing oxygen consumption.[119,120] Occasionally, indirect hypothermia may be appropriate because it is associated with reductions of 7% in $\dot{V}o_2$ for each 1°C decrease in core temperature.[121]

Optimizing Mixed Venous Blood Oxygen Saturation

The Svo_2 is an excellent monitor of oxygen kinetics because it specifically assesses the adequacy of oxygen delivery in relation to oxygen consumption. As detailed earlier, a fiberoptic, continuous Svo_2 monitor as part of pulmonary artery catheterization may enhance the ability to optimize oxygen consumption and delivery relations. For instance, the best PEEP is determined by continuous monitoring of the Svo_2 as the PEEP is sequentially increased over a short period. The point at which the Svo_2 is maximum indicates the PEEP where oxygen delivery is optimal. Likewise, the result of various interventions designed to increase cardiac output can be assessed by the effect on the Svo_2. For example, a patient who responds to inotropic agent administration with an increase in oxygen consumption without a simultaneous increase in cardiac output has diminished oxygen delivery and an associated reduction in Svo_2. Therefore, continuous monitoring of the Svo_2 can be of critical clinical value (Fig. 7-37).

Extracorporeal Life Support

Extracorporeal life support (ECLS) can be used to provide both cardiac and respiratory support. It involves the use of extra-

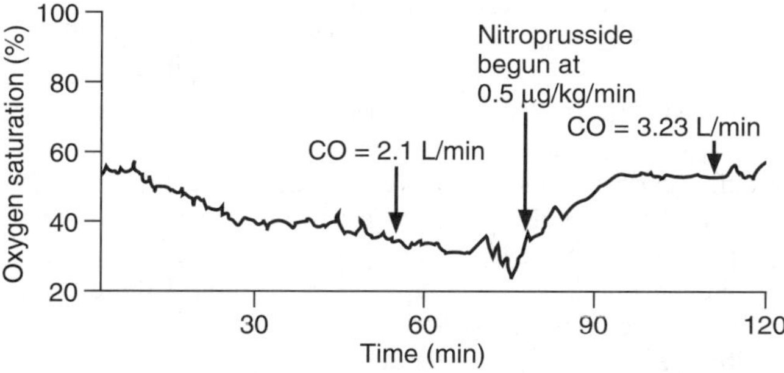

FIG. 7-37. Alterations in mixed venous blood oxygen saturation are shown as sodium nitroprusside is administered to reduce left ventricular afterload in the setting of cardiac insufficiency.

thoracic vascular cannulation and a modified heart–lung machine to allow prolonged extracorporeal support.[122] The indications for ECLS include acute, reversible respiratory or cardiac failure unresponsive to optimal ventilator and pharmacologic management. The ECLS device may be thought of as an oxygen delivery device that can be used to enhance and, in some situations, provide total oxygen delivery in patients who are in shock due to application of high ventilator pressures or hypoxemia as well as in patients in cardiogenic shock. ECLS may also be useful in the setting of septic shock; administration of vasoactive agents may increase vascular tone, while adequate perfusion and oxygenation are provided by the ECLS device. This subject is discussed in Chapter 8.

CARDIAC ARREST

Cardiopulmonary Resuscitation

Cardiopulmonary arrest is the consequence of a variety of clinical problems. Situations in which cardiac rhythms are disorganized (ventricular fibrillation) or absent (asystole) are among these. Every physician must be schooled in the principles of cardiopulmonary resuscitation. The response to an unplanned cardiac arrest begins with institution of the ABCs (*a*irway, *b*reathing, *c*irculation) of cardiopulmonary resuscitation. The first priority is the airway. Unresponsiveness and breathlessness should be established by inspection. The jaw thrust or head tilt and chin lift maneuvers should be performed to open the airway. As soon as possible, the airway is cleared, and endotracheal intubation is performed. Breathing is instituted as soon as an airway is established. Mouth-to-mouth respirations or preferably bag-mask ventilation should be performed. Circulation is next evaluated. If carotid or brachial artery pulses are absent,

TABLE 7-5. *Medications used during management of cardiac arrest*

Drug	Dose and Instruction
Atropine	IV/IM/ET IO/IN (0.02 mg/kg; min 0.1 mg, max 0.5 mg infant/child & 1 mg adult; may repeat × 1)
Sodium bicarbonate	IV (1 mEq/Kg), give slowly based on blood gas analysis
Epinephrine	1st dose: 0.01 mg/kg (0.1 mL/kg of 1:10,000) IV/IO/ET 0.1 mg/kg (0.1 mg/kg of 1:1000) ET Subsequent doses: 0.1 mg/kg (0.1 mL/kg of 1:1000) q 3–5 min IV/IO/ET
Lidocaine	1 mg/kg IV/ET/IM slowly, repeat q 5 min PRN; then begin intravenous infusion
Bretylium	Initial dose: IV 5 mg/kg Subsequent doses 10 mg/kg

IV, intravenous; IM, intramuscular; ET, endotracheal tube instillation; IO, intraosseus IN = Intranasal.

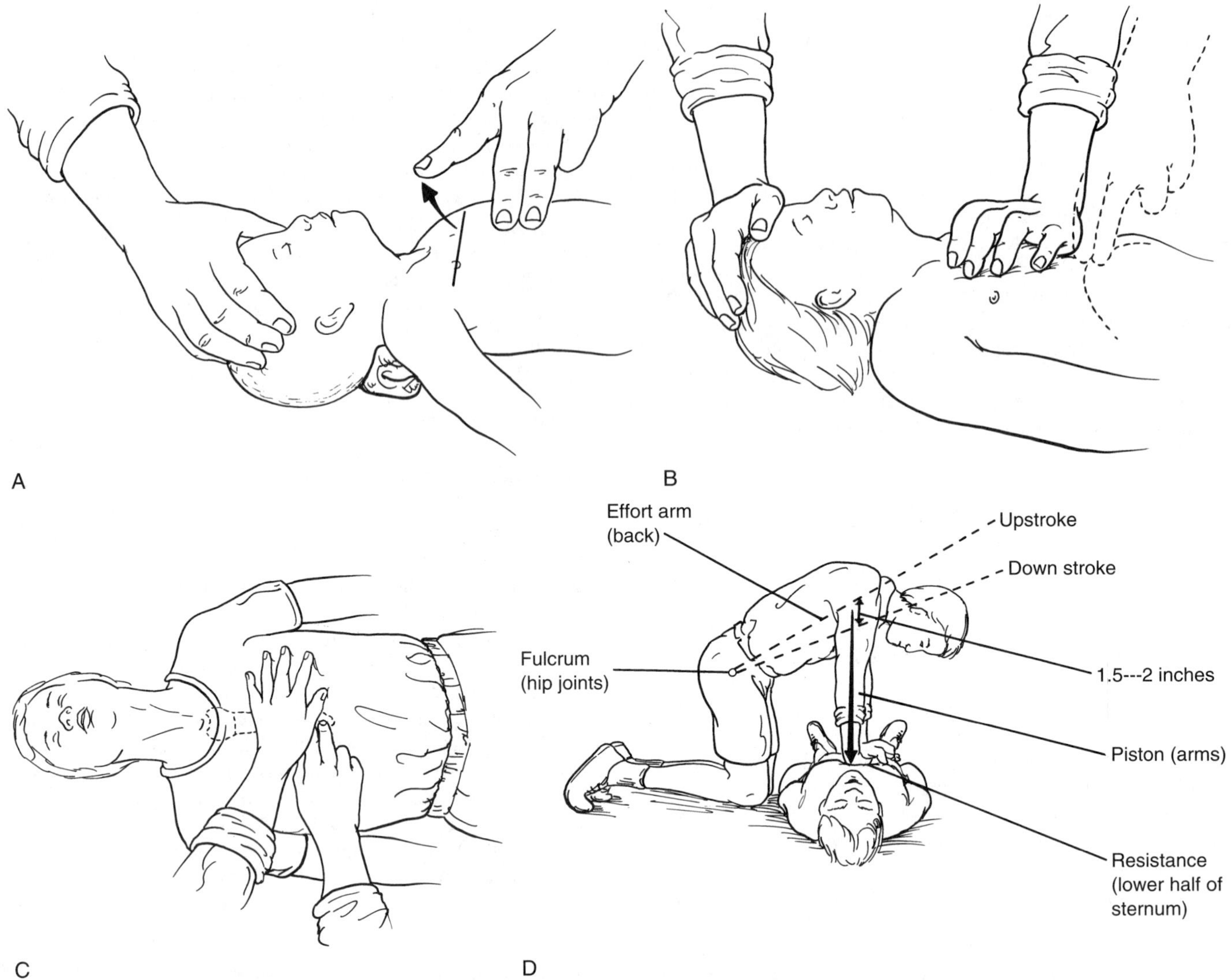

FIG. 7-38. The proper application of chest compressions during cardiopulmonary resuscitation in a neonate (*A*), child (*B*), and child older than 8 years of age (*C*). The proper technique of cardiopulmonary resuscitation is demonstrated. (*D*)

external cardiac massage is instituted by chest compressions. In infants, the sternum is compressed to a depth of 1 to 2.5 cm at a rate of 100 times per minute using 2 or 3 fingers placed over the lower sternum just inferior to the intermammary line.[34] In children older than 1 year of age, the sternum is compressed 2.5 to 4 cm at a rate of 80 to 100 times per minute using the heel of one hand placed over the lower aspect of the sternum. In children older than 8 years of age, adult methods using the heel of one hand on top of the second to compress the lower half of the sternum 4 to 5 cm at a rate of 80 to 100 times per minute should be applied (Fig. 7-38). The compression/ventilation ratio should be maintained at 5:1. If intravenous access is not available, resuscitation medications, such as atropine, epinephrine, and lidocaine, may be administered through the endotracheal tube. When doing so, medications should be diluted in 1 to 2 mL of normal saline and injected into the endotracheal tube, followed by application of positive-pressure ventilation. All cardiac arrest medications, except for bicarbon-

ate, may be administered through the endotracheal tube. During cardiac arrest, intravenous fluids should be administered to correct hypovolemia; positive-pressure ventilation and oxygen should be provided to correct hypoxemia; and sodium bicarbonate should be administered in an initial dose of 1 mEq/kg, as directed by blood gas analysis, to correct metabolic acidosis.[34] Other medications of use in cardiac arrest include atropine to accelerate the cardiac rate; epinephrine to increase systemic vascular resistance and blood pressure and to increase myocardial contractility and automaticity; and lidocaine or bretylium for the child with ventricular tachycardia or ventricular fibrillation. Suggested doses and frequency of dosing of these drugs during cardiac arrest are demonstrated in Table 7-5. If ventricular fibrillation is present, external defibrillation should be performed with an initial setting of 2 J/kg.[34] If unsuccessful, these should be repeated immediately with 4 J/kg. It is critical that the underlying cause of the cardiac arrest be identified: hypoventilation, hypoxia, hypokalemia, hyperkalemia, and hypovo-

Asystole

Check 2 leads
Intubate/IV access
EPI 0.1 mL/kg of 1:10,000 IV
▽
Atropine 0.02 mg/kg IV
(min 0.1 mg; max 1 mg)
▽
EPI 0.1 mL/kg of 1:1000 IV
q 3–5 min
▽
Consider EPI drip

Consider hypoxia, ↑K+, ↓K+,
acidosis, overdose, hypothermia

V FIB/Pulseless VT

Asynch shock 2 J/kg
▽
Asynch shock 4 J/kg × 2
▽
CPR
Intubate/IV access
EPI per asystole protocol
q 3–5 min
Asynch shock 4 J/kg
▽
Lidocaine 1 mg/kg IV
Asynch shock 4 J/kg
▽
Bretylium 5 mg/kg IV
Asynch shock 4 J/kg
▽
Bretylium 10 mg/kg IV
Asynch shock 4 J/kg
▽
Repeat Lido or Bret,
then shock again 4 J/kg

(Repeat EPI every 3–5 min)

Pulseless Electrical
Activity (PEA/EMD)

CPR
Intubate/IV access
EPI 0.1 mL/kg of 1:10,000 IV
▽
EPI 0.1 mL/kg of 1:1000 IV
q 3–5 min

Consider EPI drip

Assess for:
1. Hypovolemia
2. Tamponade
3. Tension PTX
4. Hypothermia
5. Hypoxia/acidosis

V TACH

Unstable:
IV access (defibrillate immediately if
critically unstable)
Otherwise, consider sedation
Cardiovert (synch) 1 J/kg
▽
Cardiovert (synch) 2 J/kg
▽
Cardiovert (synch) 4 J/kg × 2
▽
If recurs add lidocaine
and cardiovert

Stable:
Lidocaine 1 mg/kg IV
▽
Lidocaine drip
Sedate
▽
Cardiovert (synch)
0.5–2 J/kg
▽
Bretylium 5 mg/kg IV
▽
Bretylium 10 mg/kg IV
▽
Overdrive pacing

Symptomatic Bradycardia
(poor perfusion, hypotension, resp distress)

Airway/IV access
▽
EPI 0.1 mL/kg of 1:10,000 IV
▽
Atropine 0.02 mg/kg IV
repeat × 1 q 5 min
▽
EPI 0.1 mL/kg of 1:10,000 IV
repeat q 3–5 min
▽
Consider EPI drip

SVT

Unstable:
Cardiovert (synch)
0.5–1 J/kg
▽
Cardiovert (synch)
2 J/kg
▽
Cardiovert (synch)
4 J/kg

Stable:
1. Vagal maneuvers
2. Adenosine
3. Dig/β-blocker
4. Verapamil *(avoid if <1 yr)*

> ▽ = *Assess pt, continue if no*
> *response*

FIG. 7-39. Cardiac arrest algorithms. Protocols are demonstrated for patients in asystole; pulseless electrical activity (PEA) or electromechanical dissociation (EMD); bradycardia; ventricular fibrillation (V FIB); pulseless ventricular tachycardia (VT); stable ventricular tachycardia (V TACH) or V TACH with hemodynamic compromise; and supraventricular tachycardia (SVT). PTX, pneumothorax; synch, synchronous; asynch, asynchronous; EPI, epinephrine; DIG, digoxin; Lido, lidocaine; Bret, bretylium.

lemia are among the most frequent causes of cardiac arrest in children. Electromechanical dissociation, indicated by the presence of organized electrical activity on ECG with ineffective myocardial contractions, is relatively commonly observed during cardiac arrest. Possible causes include tension pneumothorax, cardiac tamponade, hypovolemia, and hypocalcemia.

Algorithms for the management of specific cardiac rhythm disturbances during cardiopulmonary resuscitation are shown in Figure 7-39.

Intraosseous Needle Placement

Peripheral intravenous or central venous access should be obtained as rapidly as possible during cardiac arrest. In infants and children younger than 2 years of age, intravenous line placement can be especially difficult. Alternative access includes intraosseous needle placement about two finger breadths below the tibial tuberosity on the flat anteromedial portion of the tibia

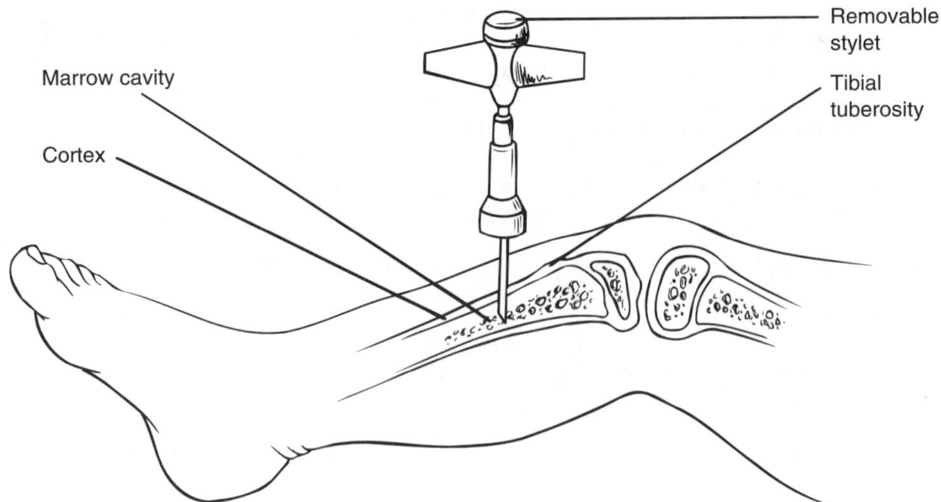

FIG. 7-40. Intraosseous needle placement.

(Fig. 7-40). The needle is angled away from the growth plate as a screwing motion is used to pass the needle through the cortex of the bone.[123] Entry into the marrow cavity is palpable as the needle moves from the hard cortical bone into the softer marrow. Bone marrow may then be aspirated and the drugs infused. Studies have documented that drugs infused into the marrow appear in the right atrium within 1 minute of administration. In addition, marrow aspiration samples can be evaluated for blood gas and electrolyte data and sent for typing and cross-matching for blood transfusion. Complications of intraosseous cannulation are rare but include development of osteomyelitis and compartment syndrome if drugs and fluid are inadvertently infused into the muscle compartment.

REFERENCES

1. Forster RD. Diffusion as a limiting factor in oxygen transport in cells. New York, Hafner Publishing, 1966:16.
2. Jones D. Intracellular diffusion gradients of O_2 and ATP. Am J Phys 1986;250:C663.
3. Lehninger AL, Nelson DL, Cox MM. Principles of biochemistry with an extended discussion of oxygen-binding proteins, ed 2. New York, Worth Publishers, 1993.
4. Bartlett RH. Use of the mechanical ventilator, vol 1. New York, Scientific American, 1993.
5. Sidi A, Davis RF. Cardiovascular physiology: essential concerns, ed 2. Philadelphia: JB Lippincott, 1992.
6. Branson RD. The measurement of energy expenditure: Instrumentation, practical considerations, and clinical application. Respir Care 1990;35:640.
7. Bartlett RH, Dechert RE, Mault JR, et al. Measurement of metabolism in multiple organ failure. Surgery 1982;92:772.
8. Dechert RE, Wesley JR, Schafer LE, et al. A water-sealed indirect calorimeter for measurement of oxygen consumption (VO_2), carbon dioxide production (VCO_2), and energy expenditure in infants. JPEN 1988;12:256.
9. Rasanen J. Continuous breathing circuit flow and tracheal tube cuff leak: sources of error during pediatric indirect calorimetry. Crit Care Med 1992;20:1335.
10. Westenskow DR, Cutler CA, Wallace WD. Instrumentation for monitoring gas exchange and metabolic rate in critically ill patients. Crit Care Med 1984;12:183.
11. Fick A. On the measurement of the blood quantity in the ventricles of the heart. Proceedings of the physiological-medical society of Wurzburg 1870.
12. Hirschl RB. Oxygen delivery in the pediatric surgical patient. Curr Opin Pediatr 1994;6:341.
13. Clark L Jr, Clark EW. A personalized history of the Clark oxygen electrode. Int Anesthesiol Clin 1987;25:1.
14. Spears J, Brereton G. Potential intravascular oxygenation with oxygen clathrate hydrate. Circulation 1992;86(Suppl I):I97.
15. Davenport HW. The ABC of acid-base chemistry, ed 6. Chicago, University of Chicago Press, 1974.
16. Langston PG, Jarvis DA, Lewis G, et al. The determination of absorption coefficients for measurement of carboxy-hemoglobin, oxy-hemoglobin, reduced hemoglobin, and met-hemoglobin in sheep using the IL482 CO-Oximeter. J Anal Toxicol 1993;17:278.
17. Dolezel S, Kovalcik V, Kriska M. Monoamines in the glomus pulmonale. Experientia 1968;24:442.
18. Shibutani K, Komatsu T, Kubal K, et al. Critical level of oxygen delivery in anesthetized man. Crit Care Med 1983;11:640.
19. Cilley RE, Scharenberg AM, Bongiorno PF, et al. Low oxygen delivery produced by anemia, hypoxia, and low cardiac output. J Surg Res 1991;51:425.
20. Gutierrez G, Warley AR, Dantzker DR. Oxygen delivery and utilization in hypothermic dogs. J Appl Physiol 1986;60:751.
21. Mault JR, Heinle JS, Ungerleider RM, et al. Michaelis-Menten (MM) kinetics predict and define the oxygen delivery (DO_2)–oxygen consumption (VO_2) relationship. Crit Care Med 1992;20:S14.
22. Cain SM. Supply dependency of oxygen uptake in ARDS: myth or reality? (Review) Am J Med Sci 1984;288:119.
23. Lugo G, Arizpe D, Doninguez G, et al. Relationship between oxygen consumption and oxygen delivery during anesthesia in high-risk surgical patients. Crit Care Med 1993;21:64.
24. Mohsenifar Z, Goldbach P, Tashkin DP, et al.. Relationship between O_2 delivery and O_2 consumption in the adult respiratory distress syndrome. Chest 1983;84:267.
25. Komatsu T, Shibutani K, Okamoto K, et al. Critical level of oxygen delivery after cardiopulmonary bypass. Crit Care Med 1987;15:194.
26. Danek S, Lynch JP, Weg JG, et al. The dependence of oxygen uptake on oxygen delivery in the adult respiratory distress syndrome. Am Rev Respir Dis 1980;122:387.
27. Clark C, Edwards JD, Nightingale P, et al. Persistence of supply dependency of oxygen uptake at high levels of delivery in adult respiratory distress syndrome. Crit Care Med 1991;19:497.
28. Weg JG. Oxygen transport in adult respiratory distress syndrome and other acute circulatory problems: relationship of oxygen delivery and oxygen consumption. Crit Care Med 1991;19:650.
29. White KM. Completing the hemodynamic picture: SvO_2. Heart Lung 1985;14:272.
30. Wever KT, Janicki JS, Maskin CS. Pathophysiology of cardiac failure. Am J Cardiol 1985;56:3B.
31. Kasnitz P, Druger GL, Yorra F, et al. Mixed venous oxygen tension and hyperlactatemia: survival in severe cardiopulmonary disease. JAMA 1976;236:570.

32. Orlando R. Continuous mixed venous oximetry in critically ill surgical patients: ''high-tech'' cost-effectiveness. Arch Surg 1986;121:470.

33. Gravenstein N, Good ML. Noninvasive assessment of cardiopulmonary function, ed 2. Philadelphia, JB Lippincott, 1992.

34. Chameides L. Textbook of pediatric advanced live support. Dallas, American Heart Association, 1994.

35. Smith RM. Temperature monitoring and regulation. Pediatr Clin North Am 1969;16:643.

36. Kirkendall WM, Keinbeib M, Freis ED, et al. Recommendations for human blood pressure determination by sphygmomanometers. AHA Committee Report 1980:1146A.

37. Perloff D, Grim C, Flack J, et al. Human blood pressure determination by sphygmomanometry. Circulation 1993;88:2460.

38. Ramsey MI. Blood pressure monitoring: automated oscillometric devices. J Clin Monit 1991;7:56.

39. Ling J, Ohara Y, Orime Y, et al. Clinical evaluation of the oscillometric blood pressure monitor in adults and children based on the 1992 AAMI SP-10 standards. J Clin Monit 1995;111:123.

40. Bald M, Kubel S, Rascher W. Validity and reliability of 24hr blood pressure monitoring in children and adolescents using a portable, oscillometric device. J Hum Hypertens 1994;8:363.

41. Gunderson LP, Cusson RM. Instrumentation in neonatal research: arterial blood pressure monitoring. Neonat Netw 1994;13:51.

42. Lyew MA, Jamieson JW. Blood pressure measurement using oscillometric finger cuffs in children and young adults: a comparison with arm cuffs during general anaesthesia. Anaesthesia 1994;49:895.

43. Talke P, Nichols R Jr, Traber DL. Does measurement of systolic blood pressure with a pulse oximeter correlate with conventional methods? J Clin Monit 1990;6:5.

44. Johnson N, Johnson VA, Bannister J, et al. Measurement of fetal peripheral perfusion with a pulse oximeter. Lancet 1989;1:898.

45. Poets CF, Seidenberg J, Wilken M, et al. Accuracy of measurements of Kontrol 7840, Nellcor N200 and Radiometer OX13 pulse oximeters in infants and young children. Klin Pediatr 1993;205:107.

46. Poets CF, Southall DP. Noninvasive monitoring of oxygenation in infants and children: practical considerations and areas of concern. Pediatr 1994;93:737.

47. Bowes W3, Corke BC, Hulka J. Pulse oximetry: a review of the theory, accuracy, and clinical applications. Obstet Gynecol 1989;74:541.

48. Fanconi S. Pulse oximetry for hypoxemia: a warning to users and manufacturers. Intensive Care Med 1989;15:540.

49. Dziedzic K, Vidyasagar D. Pulse oximetry in neonatal intensive care. Clin Perinatol 1989;16:177.

50. Harris K. Noninvasive monitoring of gas exchange. Respiratory Care 1987;32:544.

51. Curley MA, Thompson JE. End-tidal CO_2 monitoring in critically ill infants and children. Pediatr Nurs 1990;16:397.

52. Swedlow DB. Respiratory gas monitoring. Int Anesthesiol Clin 1992; 30:1.

53. Shimada Y, Yoshiya I, Tanaka K, et al. Evaluation of the progress and prognosis of adult respiratory distress syndrome: simple respiratory physiologic measurement. Chest 1979;76:180.

54. Jellinek H, Hiesmayr M, Simon P, et al. Arterial to end-tidal CO_2 tension difference after bilateral lung transplantation. Crit Care Med 1993;21:1035.

55. Severinghaus JW. Transcutaneous blood gas analysis. Respir Care 1982;27:152.

56. Wimberley PD, Frederiksen PS, Witt-Hansen J, et al. Evaluation of a transcutaneous oxygen and carbon dioxide monitor in a neonatal intensive care department. Acta Paediatr Scand 1985;74:352.

57. Yahav J, Mindorff C, Levison H. The validity of the transcutaneous oxygen tension method in children with cardiorespiratory problems. Am Rev Respir Dis 1981;124:586.

58. Hand IL, Shepard EK, Krauss AN, et al. Discrepancies between transcutaneous and end-tidal carbon dioxide monitoring in the critically ill neonate with respiratory distress syndrome. Crit Care Med 1989; 17:556.

59. Tremper KK, Shoemaker WC, Shippy CR, et al. Transcutaneous PcO_2 monitoring on adult patients in the ICU and the operating room. Crit Care Med 1981;9:752.

60. Preiser JC, Daper A, Parquier JN, et al. Transthoracic electrical bioimpedance versus thermodilution technique for cardiac output measurement during mechanical ventilation. Intensive Care Med 1989; 15:221.

61. Wong DH, Tremper KK, Stemmer EA, et al. Noninvasive cardiac output: simultaneous comparison of two different methods with thermodilution. Anesthesiology 1990;72:784.

62. Thomas AN, Ryan J, Doran BR, Pollard BJ. Biomedance versus thermodilution cardiac output measurement: the Bomed NCCOM3 after coronary bypass surgery. Intensive Care Med 1991;17:383.

63. Castor G, Klocke RK, Stoll M, et al. Simultaneous measurement of cardiac output by thermodilution, thoracic electrical bioimpedance and Doppler ultrasound. Br J Anaesth 1994;72:133.

64. Shoemaker WC, Wo CC, Bishop MH, et al. Multicenter trial of a new thoracic electrical bioimpedance device for cardiac output estimation. Crit Care Med 1994;22:1907.

65. Sexson WR, Gotshall RW, Miles DS. Cardiothoracic variables measured by bioelectrical impedance in preterm and term neonates. Crit Care Med 1991;19:1054.

66. Kobayashi I, Kawana S, Watanabe H, et al. Cardiac output measurement with transtracheal Doppler in children. Masui 1993;42:166.

67. Nishimura RA, Callahan MJ, Schaff HV, et al. Noninvasive measurement of cardiac output by continuous-wave Doppler echocardiography: initial experience and review of the literature. Mayo Clin Proc 1984;59:484.

68. Gorcsan JE, Diana P, Ball BA, et al. Intraoperative determination of cardiac output by transesophageal continuous wave Doppler. Am Heart J 1992;123:171.

69. Abrams JH, Weber RE, Holmen KD. Continuous cardiac output determination using transtracheal Doppler: initial results in humans. Anesthesiology 1989;71:1.

70. Cerny JC, Ketslakh M, Poulos CL, et al. Evaluation of the Velcom-100 pulse Doppler cardiac output computer. Chest 1991;100:143.

71. Huntsman LL, Stewart DK, Barnes SR, et al. Noninvasive Doppler determination of cardiac output in man: clinical validation. Circulation 1983;67:593.

72. Mellander M, Sabel KG, Caidahl K, et al. Doppler determination of cardiac output in infants and children: comparison with simultaneous thermodilution. Pediatr Cardiol 1987;8:241.

73. Wippermann CF, Schranz D, Huth R, et al. Determination of cardiac output by an angle and diameter independent dual beam Doppler technique in critically ill infants. Br Heart J 1992;67:180.

74. Hudson I, Houston A, Aitchison T, et al. Reproducibility of measurements of cardiac output in newborn infants by Doppler ultrasound. Arch Dis Child 1990;65:15.

75. Koide M, Imai Y, Hoshino S, et al. Measurement of cardiac output by Doppler echocardiography: clinical validation in pediatric patients after open heart surgery. Kyobu Geka 1993;46:210.

76. Sellden H, Nilsson K, Larsson LE, et al. Radial arterial catheters in children and neonates: a prospective study. Crit Care Med 1987;15: 1106.

77. Randel SN, Tsang BH, Wung JT, et al. Experience with percutaneous indwelling peripheral arterial catheterization in neonates. Am J Dis Child 1987;141:848.

78. Sheridan RL, Weber JM, Tompkins RG. Femoral arterial catheterization in pediatric burn patients. Burns 1994;20:451.

79. Furfaro S, Gauthier M, Lacroix J, et al. Arterial catheter-related infections in children: a 1-year cohort analysis. Am J Dis Child 1991;145: 1037.

80. Cilley RE. Arterial access in infants and children. Semin Pediatr Surg 1992;1:174.

81. Fletcher MA, Brown DR, Landers S, et al. Umbilical arterial catheter use: report of an audit conducted by the Study Group for Complications of Perinatal Care. Am J Perinatol 1994;11:94.

82. Schick JB, Beck AK, DeSilva HN. Umbilical artery catheter position and intraventricular hemorrhage. J Perinatol 1989;9:382.

83. Klaus MH, Fanaroff AA. Care of the high-risk neonate, ed 4. Philadelphia, WB Saunders, 1993.

84. Edmonds JF, Barker GA, Conn AW. Current concepts in cardiovascular monitoring in children. Crit Care Med 1980;8:548.

85. Abrams JH, Cerra F, Holcroft JW. Cardiopulmonary monitoring, vol 1. New York, Scientific American, 1989.

86. Waller DA, Sivanathan UM, Diament RH, et al. Iatrogenic vascular injury following arterial cannulation: the importance of early surgery. Cardiovasc Surg 1993;1:251.

87. Seibert JJ, Taylor BJ, Williamson SL, et al. Sonographic detection of neonatal umbilical-artery thrombosis: clinical correlation. AJR 1987; 148:965.

88. Horgan MJ, Bartoletti A, Polansky S, et al. Effect of heparin infusates in umbilical arterial catheters on frequency of thrombotic complications. J Pediatr 1987;111:774.

89. Berger C, Durand C, Francoise M, et al. Ultrasonographic survey of the effect of umbilical arterial catheterization in newborn infants. Arch Pediatr 1994;1:998.

90. Colburn MD, Gelabert HA, Quinones-Baldrich W. Neonatal aortic thrombosis. Surgery 1992;111:21.

91. Martin J Jr, Moran JF, Cook LS, et al. Neonatal aortic thrombosis complicating umbilical artery catheterization: successful treatment with retroperitoneal aortic thrombectomy. Surg 1989;105:793.

92. Richardson R, Applebaum H, Touran T, et al. Effective thrombolytic therapy of aortic thrombosis in the small premature infant. J Pediatr Surg 1988;23:1198.

93. Krueger TC, Neblett WW, O'Neill JA, et al. Management of aortic thrombosis secondary to umbilical artery catheters in neonates. J Pediatr Surg 1985;20:328.

94. Landers S, Moise AA, Fraley JK, et al. Factors associated with umbilical catheter-related sepsis in neonates. Am J Dis Child 1991;145:675.

95. Urbach DR, Rippe JM. Pulmonary artery catheter placement and care, ed 1. Intensive Care Med 1985;43–57.

96. Bartlett RH. Critical care physiology. Boston, Little, Brown, 1995.

97. Weisel RD, Berger RL, Hechtman HB. Measurement of cardiac output by thermodilution. N Engl J Med 1975;292:682.

98. Renner LE, Morton MJ, Sakuma GY. Indicator amount, temperature, and intrinsic cardiac output affect thermodilution cardiac output accuracy and reproducibility. Crit Care Med 1993;21:586.

99. Carpenter JP, Nair S, Staw I. Cardiac output determination: thermodilution versus a new computerized fick method. Crit Care Med 1985;13:576.

100. Davies GG, Jebson PJR, Glasgow BM, et al. Continuous Fick cardiac output compared to thermodilution cardiac output. Crit Care Med 1986;14:881.

101. Nelson L. Continuous venous oximetry in surgical patients. Ann Surg 1986;203:329.

102. Fiddian-Green RG, Haglund U, Guiterrez G, et al. Goals for resuscitation of shock. Crit Care Med 1993;21:525.

103. Shapiro B, Cane R, Harrison R. Positive end-expiratory pressure therapy in adults with special reference to acute lung injury: a review of the literature and suggested clinical correlations. Crit Care Med 1984;12:127.

104. Schwaitzberg SD, Bergman KS, Harris BH. A pediatric trauma model of continuous hemorrhage. J Pediatr Surg 1988;23:605.

105. Holcroft JW, Robinson MK. Shock in the care of the surgical patient, vol 1. New York, Scientific American, 1992.

106. Greene MG. The Harriet Lane handbook, ed 12. St Louis, Mosby-Year Book, 1991.

107. Turnage RH, Guice KS, Oldham KT. Pulmonary microvascular injury after intestinal reperfusion. New Horizons 1994;2:463.

108. Valance P, Moncada S. Role of endogenous NO in septic shock. New Horizons 1993;1:77.

109. Advanced trauma life support program for physicians, ed 5. Chicago, First Impression, 1993.

110. Silverberg RA, Weil MH. The pharmacologic approach to the critically ill patient. London, Williams & Wilkins, 1983.

111. Perkin RM, Levin DL. Shock. In: Essentials of pediatric intensive care. St Louis, Quality Medical Publishing, 1990.

112. Rice CL. Pharmacologic support of the failing heart, vol 1. New York, Scientific American Surgery, 1989.

113. Pestana C. Fluids and electrolytes in the surgical patient, ed 2. Baltimore, Williams & Wilkins, 1981.

114. Trang TT, Tibballs J, Mercier JC, et al. Optimization of oxygen transport in mechanically ventilated newborns using oximetry and pulsed Doppler-derived cardiac output. Crit Care Med 1988;16:1094.

115. Marini JJ. Pressure-targeted, lung-protective ventilatory support in acute lung injury. Chest 1994;105(Suppl 3):109S.

116. Parker JC, Hernandez LA, Peevy KJ. Mechanisms of ventilator-induced lung injury. Crit Care Med 1993;21:131.

117. Suter PM, Fairley HB, Isenberg MD. Optimum end-expiratory airway pressure in patients with acute pulmonary failure. N Engl J Med 1975;292:284.

118. Weers JG. A physicochemical evaluation of perfluorochemicals for oxygen transport applications. J Fluorine Chem 1993;64:73.

119. Palmisano BW, Fisher DM, Willis M, et al. The effect of paralysis on oxygen consumption in normoxic children after cardiac surgery. Anesthesiology 1984;61:518.

120. Coggeshall JW, Marini JJ, Newman JH. Improved oxygenation after muscle relaxation in adult respiratory distress syndrome. Arch Intern Med 1985;145:1718.

121. Ganong WF. Energy balance, metabolism, and nutrition. In: Review of medical physiology, ed 9. Los Altos, CA, Lange Medical Publications, 1979.

122. Bartlett RH. Current problems in surgery, vol 27. St Louis, Mosby-Year Book, 1990.

123. Fiser DH. Intraosseous Infusion. N Engl J Med 1990;322:1579.

Surgery of Infants and Children: Scientific Principles and Practice, edited by
Keith T. Oldham, Paul M. Colombani, and Robert P. Foglia.
Lippincott–Raven Publishers, Philadelphia, © 1997.

CHAPTER 8

Respiratory Physiology and Extracorporeal Life Support

Robert E. Cilley

Every day, pediatric surgeons care for patients with lung pathology. For infants and children with developmental abnormalities of the lung, we respond as surgeons by removing the abnormal part. Newborns with congenital diaphragmatic hernias undergo mechanical correction of their defects, but the cure for the abnormal lung function and development that characterize this disease remains elusive. In other infants, lung injuries result from the activation of an inflammatory response that may protect them from infection under some circumstances, but can cause lung injury when it is prolonged and unchecked. Some children sustain direct mechanical injury to the lung as a result of externally applied forces. The very cure that often is applied to treat respiratory insufficiency, mechanical ventilation, may be the ultimate culprit that results in the progression of lung injury, and prevents lung recovery. Even in the so-called routine practice of pediatric surgery, respiratory function is altered by the incisions that are made and the anesthetic techniques that are relied on. All surgeons should have a thorough understanding of the lung in health and disease, and a working knowledge of the methods of treating respiratory insufficiency.

PULMONARY ANATOMY, PHYSIOLOGY, AND PATHOPHYSIOLOGY

Developmental Anatomy of the Lung

Although all lung disease is not explained by embryology gone awry, an appreciation of the lung in health and disease is based on an understanding of its normal development. The normal function of the lung is dependent on the coordinated development of the airway conducting system in conjunction with a specialized vasculature within an active interstitial matrix.

The uniform nomenclature that is used to describe the developmental stages of human lung growth derives from the meeting of the International Congress of Anatomists in Leningrad in 1970. Lung development has been divided into the embryonic, pseudoglandular, canalicular, and terminal sac periods based on the histologic appearance. The terminal sac period blends imperceptibly into the alveolar period.[1,2]

Embryonic Period

The embryonic period of lung development begins with the appearance of the median pharyngeal groove on the 22nd day after ovulation. At this time, the embryo is about 4 mm long and has seven somites. The median pharyngeal groove is an outpouching on the ventral surface of the primitive foregut. The lung bud probably develops solely from this ventral outpouching, and the separation between the esophagus and trachea (the future larynx) remains stationary throughout development. It is unlikely that lateral indentation of the foregut tube to form an anterior tracheal tube and a posterior esophageal tube actually occurs, although this mechanism has been invoked to explain developmental abnormalities of the esophagus and trachea. Shortly after the lung bud appears, it elongates, descending into the mesenchymal tissue of the thorax, and immediately divides into left and right components, which grow dorsally around the esophagus. Already, the left bronchus has a more horizontal orientation than the right, and the lobar divisions of the lower respiratory tract are identifiable (5th and 6th embryonic weeks). During the 7th week of development, splanchnopleural mesoderm is organizing to form bronchial smooth muscle and cartilage. Segmental and first-generation subsegmental bronchi develop at this stage in a variable fashion, explaining the many variations of bronchial anatomy seen in the mature lung. The truncus arteriosus also separates into the aorta and pulmonary artery at this time, and the pulmonary capillary plexus develops, ensheathing the bronchial tree. The pulmonary capillary plexus becomes confluent with the sixth aortic arch (pulmonary artery) and the pulmonary veins. Distinct lobar architecture is now visible. It also is during this 8th week of gestation that the pleuroperitoneal canals close.

Pseudoglandular Period

The pseudoglandular period of lung development extends from the 8th to the 16th week of development. The future airways develop in an asymmetric, dichotomous fashion and are lined by columnar epithelium that contains glycogen. In histologic sections of the lung at this stage, the future airways appear as multiple round structures that resemble glands, hence the name, pseudoglandular. During this period, the number of airway generations increases from about 4 to as many as 27 in some parts of the lung. Essentially all axial branching of the bronchial tree has taken place by the end of this phase of development such that the entire conducting airway system to the level of the terminal bronchiole has developed. In the pulmonary interstitium, the developing vasculature follows the development of the airways. Cartilage, smooth muscle, and the pulmonary capillary plexus continue to develop in the loose mesenchymal tissue into which the future airways are proliferating. Cellular differentiation of the epithelial lining cells is first seen during the pseudoglandular stage. The epithelial cells take on a more pseudostratified appearance and the first ciliated cells appear. Mucous glands appear in the trachea, and a few goblet cells can be seen. Neuroepithelial cells also are found at this time.

Canalicular Period

The next stage of lung development is defined by the appearance of the acinus or respiratory unit of the lung, and its invasion by the developing capillaries. The acinus consists of a terminal bronchiole, 2 to 4 respiratory bronchioles, and a cluster of several generations of budding epithelium that ultimately become the saccules. The cells of the peripheral airway are now distinctly cuboidal, in contrast to the more columnar bronchiolar epithelium. The "canalization" of the acinus, or insertion of capillary processes among these budding respiratory epithelial cells, gives its name to this stage of lung development. The canalicular period spans the 4th to the 6th month (16th to 26th week) of development. The critical process of capillary invasion of the acinus is a relatively long process. Capillary invasion begins first at the points of division of the branching epithelial buds that ultimately become the saccules (see later). Capillary invasion progresses to include the entire acinus. Capillaries are plentiful by the 22nd week of gestation and the interstitium is gradually thinning, making gas exchange at least theoretically possible. The respiratory bronchiole is the last portion of the acinus to be vascularized. In addition, during the later part of this period of lung development, the epithelial cells of the acinus begin to differentiate, and thinned-out septal cells (type I pneumocytes) can be distinguished from the larger alveolar cells (type II pneumocytes). The appearance of lamellar bodies in the type II cells heralds the production of pulmonary surfactant.

Terminal Sac Period

After canalization or vascularization of the acinus is complete by the 26th week, the growth of the lung is characterized by proliferation and progressive thinning of the cells of the terminal lung buds into clusters consisting of several generations of saccules lined by "capillarized" epithelium. The connective tissue septa that separate the saccules continue to become progressively thinner during this stage of development. This stage of development is called the terminal sac period, or saccular

TABLE 8-1. *Lung development*

EMBRYONIC PERIOD (3 TO 8 WEEKS)
Epithelial lung bud penetrates mesenchyme of the thorax
Pulmonary capillary plexus develops
Pleuroperitoneal canal closes

PSEUDOGLANDULAR PERIOD (8 TO 16 WEEKS)
Airway conducting system develops to the level of the terminal bronchiole
Developing vasculature follows the airways
Cellular differentiation of the epithelium occurs

CANALICULAR PERIOD (16 TO 26 WEEKS)
Capillary processes invade the acinus
Interstitum of the acinus thins
Gas exchange is possible by the end of this period

SACCULAR PERIOD (26 WEEKS AND BEYOND)
Terminal lung bud progressively thins
Epithelium is capillarized
Type II pneumocytes produce surfactant
Blends imperceptibly into the alveolar phase

phase. The saccules are relatively smooth-walled cylindrical structures. The saccules then are subdivided by the ingrowth of ridges that protrude into the saccule, drawing the surrounding capillaries in with them. Opinions differ on when the developing saccule should be termed an alveolus. True alveoli may be seen as early as 32 weeks of gestation and are present in all fetuses by 36 weeks of gestation. The terminal sac phase of growth results in an enormous increase in the potential surface available for gas exchange. There are more than 20 million of these saccules at the time of birth. The type II pneumocyte has matured and is capable of producing surfactant properly, completing the functional maturity of the lung by 32 to 36 weeks of gestation. These events are summarized in Table 8-1.

"Alveolarization" of the lung begins late in gestation and continues for the first 8 years of life, and perhaps even beyond. The acini, or respiratory units of the lung (defined as the airspaces associated with a terminal bronchiole), are about 1 mm long at birth, growing to 1.75 mm at 2 months, 2.1 mm at 6 months, 4 mm at 7 years, and 7.5 mm in adulthood, when they number about 50,000. The total number of alveoli increases to about 300 million by 8 years of age. After this, alveoli increase in size, but only minimally in number. Alveolar surface area increases from 6.5 m^2 at 3 months, to 32 m^2 at 8 years, to 75 m^2 in adulthood. The Lambert ducts (bronchoalveolar ducts), first seen during childhood, are outgrowths from terminal bronchioles that penetrate adjacent alveoli. These ducts, along with interalveolar pores of Kohn, provide collateral ventilation, speed up the diffusion of gases, and permit ventilation of respiratory units with obstructed bronchioles.

Formation of the Pulmonary Vasculature

The adult lung has a double arterial supply and, to some degree, a double venous drainage. The pulmonary artery supplies blood for respiratory gas exchange, whereas the bronchi themselves and the walls of large blood vessels are supplied by systemic arteries. Bronchial veins account for a small amount of systemic venous drainage into the azygous system, but the pulmonary veins capture the pulmonary blood flow and much of the systemic arterial flow.[3]

Two morphogenetic processes contribute to the development of the vasculature of the lung.[4] *Vasculogenesis* refers to the differentiation of endothelial cell precursors from the lung mesenchyme that coalesce to form vascular channels (arteries, veins, or lymphatics). These cells contribute to the differentiation of the surrounding mesenchyme such that smooth muscle cells form around or are attracted to the coalescing blood vessels. *Angiogenesis* refers to new blood vessels that are formed by sprouting from preexisting primitive vascular channels. The development of these vessels is synchronized to the development of the airways, implying that the regulation of their development is interdependent. These vessels that are intrinsic to the developing lung later join the developing pulmonary arteries that are derived from the sixth aortic arch. The sixth and last of the paired aortic arches that connect the dorsal and ventral aortas is seen during the fifth week of human embryonic development. (The first and second arches have already disappeared. The third arch forms the carotid system and the fourth arch becomes the aorta. The fifth arch is rudimentary.) The left sixth arch becomes the pulmonary artery. These developments have been completed such that right ventricular blood enters the lungs by the eighth week of development. The pulmonary veins develop a little later than the pulmonary artery. Venous drainage begins as a single primitive pulmonary vein that grows out of the atrium toward the lung buds. After connection is made with the developing intrapulmonary venous system, the first branches of the pulmonary vein are resorbed into the atrium, giving rise typically to four pulmonary veins. During this early period of vascular development of the lung, there are additional segmental arteries from the supraceliac aorta that supply lung tissue. In addition, before the lung is linked to the heart by the pulmonary veins, there are venous vessels that drain into the systemic venous system. These vessels normally regress, and their persistence can be seen in pathologies such as lung sequestrations and systemic pulmonary venous return.

Molecular Embryology of Lung Development

The destinies of individual cell lineages that form specific organs have been described in simple organisms. Some of the genes that control these cell lineages also have been described. It is possible that homologous or similar human genes may determine the lung cell–specific lineages that arise from the floor of the hypopharynx in early human lung development. Someday, it may be possible to determine the master gene switches that initiate genetic cascades controlling cellular development.

Adhesive glycoproteins, collagen, proteoglycans, and other components of the extracellular matrix play key roles in the mesenchymal-epithelial interactions that are responsible for organogenesis. Branching of the developing conducting airway system is wholly dependent on these interactions such that epithelial cells will not undergo branching when separated from lung mesenchyme. It is probable that peptide growth factors elaborated by mesenchymal cells control epithelial proliferation, and that the extracellular matrix controls the patterns of branching and growth. Fibronectin, an adhesive glycoprotein

that forms high-molecular-weight polymers that interact with embryonic cells during migration, differentiation, and organogenesis, probably is a key part of the extracellular matrix in lung morphogenesis. The commitment to cell lines such as type II alveolar cells occurs early in development and also is dependent on epithelial-mesenchymal interactions. Transforming growth factors-β_1, $-\beta_2$, and $-\beta_3$ (polypeptide dimers of about 25,000 M_r) are involved in cell differentiation, proliferation, chemotaxis, and formation of the extracellular matrix in embryonic tissues. Transforming growth factor-β messenger RNA localization and mapping of the protein itself show a widespread distribution in developing lung. Epidermal growth factor also has a particularly important role in airway branching morphogenesis during lung development. Autocrine and paracrine interactions between mesenchymal and epithelial cells probably control the proliferation of cells and the commitment to cell lines. Extracellular matrix proteases and their inhibitors play an important role in determining the patterns and shape of the developing lung. All the events of development are coordinated in a time- and position-specific manner.[5,6]

Respiratory Physiology

The most important and unique contribution of the lung to the maintenance of homeostasis is as the organ of gas exchange with the environment. Although the nonkeratinized skin of premature infants theoretically is capable of some gas exchange, and the highly vascularized intestines may transfer some gases across their large epithelial surfaces, for practical purposes, all respiratory gas exchange occurs across the alveolar-capillary barriers of the pulmonary acinus. Under basal conditions, as little as 2 to 3 mL/kg/min of oxygen need be transferred from the environment to the circulation, whereas under conditions of maximal exercise, as much as 60 mL/kg/min may be required. With this enormous reserve, the respiratory transfer of gases rarely limits the uptake and use of oxygen or the removal of carbon dioxide by the body. Under conditions of respiratory failure, gas exchange may be limited in such a way that normal levels of oxygen and carbon dioxide are not maintained. Transfer of oxygen across the alveolar-capillary barrier for delivery to the tissues or removal of carbon dioxide from the blood then may be inadequate.

Muscular Activity of Normal Respiration

The coordinated activity of skeletal muscle is required both to maintain the patency of the upper airway and to provide energy for the movement of air into and out of the lungs. Normal aerodigestive function requires that the laryngeal inlet be open during respiration and protected during the initial phase of swallowing. The muscles of ventilation include all the truncal muscles that can contribute to changing the intrapleural pressure or altering the volume of the thorax. The function of some muscles is directed primarily at ventilation (diaphragm, intercostals); other muscles are normally a part of ventilation but have other important functions (abdominal wall muscles); and still other muscles normally provide little assistance with ventilation, except perhaps to stabilize the movement of the thorax, and are called into play under pathologic conditions (accessory muscles of respiration).

The diaphragm is dome-shaped and has a longer vertically oriented component than usually is depicted in anatomic diagrams, a fact that is well known to surgeons who perform tube thoracostomy placement or operations in the upper retroperitoneum. The zone of diaphragmatic apposition refers to this long, vertically oriented portion of the diaphragm that lies in direct contact with the inner surface of the thorax. The zone of apposition is disproportionately short in infants compared with adults. Diaphragmatic contraction primarily pulls the diaphragm downward, increasing the intrathoracic volume. The vertical orientation of the zone of apposition provides maximal mechanical advantage during inspiration. Lowering of the intrapleural pressure that occurs with contraction and vertical descent of the diaphragm during inspiration tends to collapse the portion of the rib cage that overlies the lungs. This phenomenon is especially apparent in infants, with their compliant chest walls, and may limit the effectiveness of diaphragmatic function during respiratory failure.

The muscles of the chest wall change the anteroposterior and transverse diameter of the chest by elevating and depressing the ribs, increasing or decreasing the intrathoracic volume. The muscles of inspiration rotate the ribs about their costovertebral articulation such that the sternal end of the rib moves up and the middle of the rib moves upward and outward. (These movements have been called the *pump-handle* and *bucket-handle* motion of the ribs.) The ribs are much more horizontally oriented in infants than in older children, so active rib movement contributes less to ventilation. The muscles of inspiration include the levator costae, external intercostals, parasternal intercostals, scalenes, and sternocleidomastoids. The muscles of expiration rotate the ribs downward and inward, and include the subcostals, internal intercostals, transversus thoracis, rectus abdominis, oblique and transverse abdominal muscles, and quadratus lumborum. Muscles of the shoulder girdle also can be recruited for respiration.

Pulmonary Mechanics and Respiratory Gas Flow and Distribution

Respiratory gas exchange is dependent on the flow of gases from the environment to the alveolus, where gas exchange takes place. Gas flow is possible only when there is a pressure gradient between the airway and the alveolus. During spontaneous respiration, that pressure gradient is the result of negative intrapleural pressure that results from the muscular activity of the chest wall and the diaphragm. The energy requirements for the movement and distribution of respiratory gases normally constitute less than 3% of the total body energy expenditure. Under conditions of respiratory failure, this energy expenditure can increase many times that amount and may not be sustainable. Respiratory work, the work of breathing, is a form of pressure-volume work. Pressure is required to move a tidal volume of fresh gas into and out of the thorax. The work of spontaneous breathing can be summarized for one breath as:

$$W = (P_i + P_e)V$$

where: W = work of breathing

P_i = pressure required to move fresh gas into the thorax

P_e = pressure required to move a tidal volume (V) of fresh gas out of the thorax

During spontaneous breathing and mechanical ventilation, the expiratory component of the work of breathing usually is zero, because exhalation is largely passive as a result of the elastic properties of the lungs and chest wall. It may be significant in obstructive airway disease when active muscular activity is used to aid exhalation. The work of breathing is increased when higher pressures are needed to generate a given tidal volume, minute ventilation increases by an increase in the tidal volume, or minute ventilation increases by higher respiratory rates.

Work, by definition, is the application of force over a distance. The force applied by the respiratory muscles is exerted to overcome two major forces: the total respiratory compliance (contributed by the lung parenchyma, the chest wall, and the abdomen) and the resistance to ventilatory gas flow in the large and small airways. Compliance is defined as the lung volume change that results from a given change in pressure, and it reflects the elastic properties of the entire ventilatory apparatus:

$$C = \Delta V/\Delta P$$

The pressure that must be generated to move a given tidal volume increases as compliance decreases. Almost any acute parenchymal lung process, such as pneumonia, systemic inflammatory response syndrome, or hydrostatic pulmonary edema, results in a decrease in lung parenchymal compliance. A decrease in compliance probably is the first and most sensitive indicator of lung injury.[7] Similarly, abdominal distention, ascites, bony abnormalities of the thorax (eg, severe kyphoscoliosis), pleural effusions, and generalized edema also may contribute to decreased total respiratory compliance.

In addition to the pressure needed to overcome the compliance of the respiratory apparatus, pressure also is needed to overcome the resistance to flow within the airways. Resistance is defined by the pressure gradient required to produce a given flow within a conducting system:

$$R = \Delta P/flow$$

Resistance is the net result of factors that tend to retard the flow of gas through the airways and is determined by the physical properties of the respiratory gases (density and viscosity), the length and diameter of the conduit through which they must travel, and the velocity of gas flow. As airway resistance increases, more pressure is required to maintain respiratory gas flow. Airway diameter is the most critical determinant of resistance, and any condition that narrows the airway will have a large effect on resistance. Even under ideal circumstances of laminar flow of respiratory gases within the airways, resistance changes inversely with the fourth power of the diameter of the airway. Therefore, small changes in the airway diameter can have large effects on resistance and on the pressure (ie, work) required to move tidal volumes. Turbulent flow, which always is present in large airways, accentuates the effect of airway diameter on resistance. Similarly, disease states that result in airway narrowing (bronchospasm) markedly affect the resistive work of breathing. The contribution of the peripheral airways to total airway resistance is proportionally greater in infants and small children than in adults. As a result, they are more susceptible to respiratory failure in diseases that affect the small airways, such as bronchiolitis. In addition, when airway resistance increases, the compliant chest walls of infants may limit their ability to generate adequate pressure to maintain gas flow.

To describe the mechanics of respiration, the lung can be thought of as a compliant reservoir that empties and fills according to first-order kinetics. The time course of volume change in a compliant reservoir that obeys first-order kinetics is defined by the compliance of the reservoir and the resistance to flow into or out of the reservoir according to the natural logarithmic function:

$$V_+ = V_0 e^{\pm (1/RC)\tau}$$

where: V_+ = volume at a given time
V_0 = initial volume
R = resistance
C = compliance
e = sign of the exponent, which is positive during filling and negative during emptying
τ = time constant

The time constant of such a compliant reservoir is defined as the product of its compliance and resistance. It is a measurement of the time required to equilibrate lung volume and airway pressure after a rapid change in airway pressure, such as occurs at the beginning of inspiration and at the beginning of expiration. According to the equation, one time constant in emptying is the time required to reduce the volume of the lungs to e^{-1} of their original volume (ie, to 63% of their original volume). Three time constants are required to equilibrate 95% of a tidal volume and five time constants are required to equilibrate 99% of a tidal volume. Normally, the time constant of the lung is short in comparison with inspiratory and expiratory times, and only becomes important in disease states.

Diseases that decrease compliance, such as respiratory distress syndrome (RDS), result in a shortening of the time constant. The time required to equilibrate the volume of the lung is shortened; inflation and deflation are completed in a shorter time than in normal lungs and higher respiratory rates may be tolerated than in normal lungs. Likewise, patients with high expiratory resistance, such as occurs in children with reactive airway disease and in infants with bronchiolitis, have a long time constant and rapid respiratory rates may not allow sufficient time for expiration. This phenomenon results in elevation of the lung volume at end expiration (elevated functional residual capacity [FRC]) and may manifest itself as air trapping, carbon dioxide retention, impaired venous return to the heart, and reduced cardiac output.

In an ideal elastic reservoir, the pressure-volume relation is the same whether the reservoir is expanding or contracting. In the lung, the time constant (ie, the resistance and compliance) that characterizes inflation (inhalation) differs from the time constant of deflation (exhalation). This physical property of the lungs is responsible for the phenomenon of hysteresis. At a given distending pressure, the lung volume is different depending on whether the lung is being inflated from FRC or deflated from maximum volume. Further, the human lung is not an ideal compliant reservoir and does not obey first-order kinetics perfectly. In both health and disease, the lung behaves like a reservoir with multiple compartments in parallel, each of which has a different time constant. The behavior of the lung as a whole is a summation of the multiple compartments.

When the lung is inflated with positive pressure from FRC, collapsed alveoli or atelectatic areas require the application of relatively high pressures to open.[8,9] Initial compliance is low,

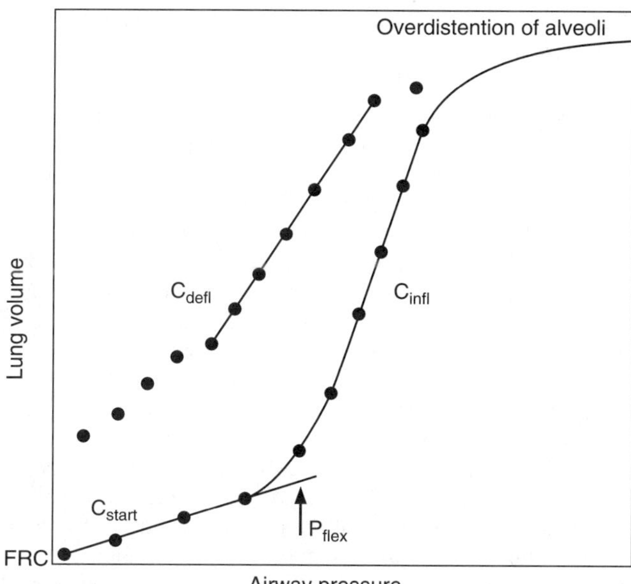

FIG. 8-1. Static pressure-volume curve. C_{start} reflects the poor distensibility of the lung at low volumes. High pressures are needed to open airways that are closed. P_{flex} is the point at which recruitable alveoli are open. C_{infl} is the compliance of the respiratory system when all recruitable airspaces are open. Compliance decreases dramatically when the lung is overdistended. In injured lungs, overdistention may occur at relatively small total volumes. C_{defl} differs from the inflation limb because of hysteresis. FRC, functional residual capacity.

corresponding to the initially flat portion of the compliance curve seen in Figure 8-1, and is referred to as starting compliance (Cstart). The portion of the lung that expands in this fashion is referred to as *recruitable* and represents areas that may be maintained open under the influence of positive end-expiratory pressure (PEEP) when mechanical ventilation is required. The normal lung has few areas of atelectasis and, therefore, little in the way of recruitable volume. However, when subjected to positive-pressure ventilation, even normal lungs develop atelectasis if they are allowed to equilibrate to atmospheric pressure at end-expiration, such as occurs when endotracheal intubation is used without PEEP. Diseased lungs may have significant amounts of recruitable volume. The next portion of the compliance curve is steep, representing the distention of normal alveoli, which requires only small changes in pressure to effect relatively large increases in volume. This is where normal respiration takes place. When all recruitable alveoli have been fully distended, large pressures are required to effect a small change in volume. The compliance curve again becomes flat above this second inflection point. In normal lungs, this is the total lung capacity. Even diseased lungs in patients with ''diffuse'' lung injury, such as adult RDS, have small portions that retain near-normal compliance characteristics. This is the portion of the lung that is preferentially ventilated and also the portion that is most vulnerable to injury from high-pressure mechanical ventilation. When high pressures are used in conjunction with mechanical ventilation, the more normal portion of the lung is most likely to be overdistended and injured.

Pulmonary Blood Flow and Pulmonary Vascular Resistance

During intrauterine life, only about 10% of the right ventricular output actually circulates through the pulmonary vasculature. Most of the blood flow is directed to the systemic circulation at the level of the ductus arteriosus and foramen ovale. In spite of this lack of blood flow, the pulmonary vasculature develops with the potential to receive all the cardiac output almost immediately after birth, when the transition to pulmonary gas exchange must occur abruptly. This is a truly remarkable developmental phenomenon in which form anticipates function.

The pulmonary vasculature is highly compliant and can accept large changes in blood flow with minimal changes in pressure. Pulmonary blood flow is highly dependent on gravity. The effect of gravity is to create a hydrostatic gradient that favors blood flow to the dependent regions of the lung.[10] The zones of the lung describe the relations among pulmonary arterial pressure, alveolar pressure, and pulmonary venous pressure. In the upper areas of the lung (zone 1), alveolar pressure theoretically exceeds arterial pressure, and there is no flow. It is unlikely that this occurs in healthy lungs, but it may be important during mechanical ventilation that exposes the alveoli to extremely high pressures. In zone 2, the gradient between arterial pressure and alveolar pressure determines pulmonary blood flow; both are greater than pulmonary venous pressure. Most of the lung operates under zone 3 conditions in healthy individuals. Here, flow is determined by the pulmonary arteriovenous pressure gradient; both pressures exceed alveolar pressure.

The pulmonary circulation must change profoundly during the transition from intrauterine to extrauterine life. Pulmonary blood flow increases with the first expansion of the lungs that occurs with the first breath. Pulmonary vascular resistance falls dramatically and the ductus arteriosus closes over the course of several days. Less blood also is shunted at the atrial level and the infant achieves true parallel circulation between the pulmonary and systemic circulations. "Fetal" circulation persists (persistent pulmonary hypertension of the newborn) when pulmonary vascular resistance remains elevated and blood is shunted at the atrial and ductal levels, resulting in admixture of venous blood to the systemic circulation and hypoxia. Because hypoxia is one of the most potent stimuli of pulmonary vasoconstriction, a deteriorating cycle may begin. Acidosis and hypercarbia that accompany the hypoxia also may contribute to the pulmonary vasospasm. Excessive muscularization of the pulmonary arteries that is characteristic of the lungs in congenital diaphragmatic hernia contributes to pulmonary hypertension.

Gas Exchange: The Functions of Oxygenation and Ventilation

Under normal conditions, oxygenation and ventilation occur simultaneously and harmoniously. Apnea results in both hypoxia and hypercarbia, whereas restoration of breathing reestablishes gas exchange. This phenomenon is so much a part of everyday experience that it is intuitive to think of oxygenation and ventilation together. However, oxygenation and ventilation are separable functions of the lung, and under pathologic conditions, may even interfere with each other.[11]

Oxygen and carbon dioxide are transferred across the alveolar-capillary membrane by passive processes of diffusion. Gas transfer is proportional to the difference between the partial pressures of the gas in the alveolus and the pulmonary capillary blood, and is similar for oxygen and carbon dioxide. Only about one third of the 0.75 seconds that the blood spends in the pulmonary capillary are necessary for equilibration; diffusing capacity must be reduced significantly to result in abnormal pulmonary gas exchange. Abnormal thickening of the alveolar-capillary membrane, reduced transit time in the capillary, and alveolar hypoxia may contribute to inadequate gas exchange as a result of a diffusion abnormality. Increases in the fraction of inspired oxygen (FIO_2) overcome hypoxemia resulting from diffusion abnormalities.

Carotid body and central nervous system chemoreceptors continuously monitor the arterial partial pressure of carbon dioxide ($PaCO_2$) and adjust alveolar ventilation to maintain a value within a narrow range, regardless of the amount of metabolic carbon dioxide produced. Hyperventilation is defined as excessive alveolar ventilation for the level of carbon dioxide production. Hypoventilation results when alveolar ventilation is inadequate to remove metabolically produced carbon dioxide and hypercarbia results. An increase in dead-space ventilation (reducing alveolar ventilation for the same minute ventilation) or lack of normal coupling between the $PaCO_2$ and minute ventilation by the respiratory centers of the brain (eg, central nervous system depression, brain stem injury, neuromuscular disease, musculoskeletal disease of the chest, upper airway obstruction) may result in hypoventilation. Any elevation of the alveolar partial pressure of carbon dioxide (PCO_2) obligatorily causes a fall in the alveolar partial pressure of oxygen (PO_2), as defined by the alveolar gas equation (simplified form):

$$P_{alveolar}O_2 = P_{inspired}O_2 - \left(\frac{P_{alveolar}CO_2}{\text{respiratory quotient}}\right)$$

The relation between ventilation and perfusion (VA/Q) determines to a large degree the adequacy of pulmonary gas exchange. The relation may vary from areas of the lung with no ventilation and some blood flow ($VA/Q = 0$, true shunt) to areas with ventilation and no perfusion ($VA/Q = $ infinity, dead space). Normally, the mean VA/Q is 1, varying from 0.6 to 3. The most common VA/Q abnormality is a reduction. The respiratory center responds by increasing minute ventilation, which is preferentially distributed to already ventilated areas, resulting in a fall in their postcapillary $PaCO_2$ and a rise in their postcapillary PO_2. This does not effect a rise in the arterial partial pressure of oxygen (PaO_2) because the arterial oxygen content (CaO_2) of the postcapillary blood is changed little by a rise in the PO_2 as most of the oxygen is carried by the already saturated hemoglobin. However, the $PaCO_2$ is normalized, because carbon dioxide content is proportional to the PCO_2. If the VA/Q abnormality becomes too great, minute ventilation cannot compensate and $PaCO_2$ will rise. If the rise in the $PaCO_2$ is gradual, it may be well tolerated and part of the compensation for respiratory failure because it increases the efficiency of the compromised respiratory system (the higher the alveolar PCO_2, the more CO_2 eliminated at a given minute ventilation). Marked elevations in $PaCO_2$ can be tolerated if they occur gradually and are compensated for. If the rise in the $PaCO_2$ is acute and results in central nervous system depression and acidosis, alveolar ventilation must be assisted. The hypoxemia of V_A/Q abnormalities responds to supplemental oxygen administration, becoming more resistant as the abnormality worsens.

The admixture of venous blood with blood returning from ventilated alveolar-capillary units results in a shunt. The normal "physiologic" shunt is about 1% to 3% of the cardiac output and is a result of the return of the bronchial circulation to the left side of the heart and to the intracardiac veins (thebesian veins) that return to the left ventricle. High pressure in the pulmonary arterial circulation predisposes to shunting. Blood that passes through the capillaries of collapsed alveoli (atelectasis) or those filled with inflammatory exudate or edema fluid results in a shunt. Pulmonary arteriovenous malformations and cyanotic congenital heart disease also result in shunts. The hypoxemia associated with shunted blood is resistant to increases in the F_{IO_2}. Even breathing 100% oxygen makes only a small change in the Pa_{O_2} in the presence of a true shunt.

Under normal circumstances, a fall in the mixed venous P_{O_2} such as that which occurs during exercise or other states of increased oxygen consumption (V_{O_2}) does not result in hypoxia. Ventilation normally is able to increase far greater than cardiac output. In lung disease, gas exchange may not be able to improve during exercise or stress to maintain oxygenation of the blood (ie, V_A/Q falls) and hypoxia results.

Pulmonary Surfactant

It first was recognized in the 1950s that lungs contain substances that lower surface tension, and that these substances, called pulmonary surfactant, are deficient in the lungs of infants with respiratory distress related to prematurity. Pulmonary surfactant, by reducing surface tension at the air-liquid interface of the alveolar lining, stabilizes the alveoli at low lung volumes and prevents alveolar collapse at end-expiration. RDS of the newborn is characterized by surfactant deficiency and alveolar collapse (atelectasis). It occurs primarily in premature infants, but others, such as infants of diabetic mothers, also are at risk. RDS is the leading cause of perinatal mortality and morbidity in developed countries. Its high prevalence, treatment, and prevention have enormous economic and social implications.

All mammalian species display augmented surfactant production after about 85% of gestation is complete. Pulmonary surfactant is produced in the type II alveolar lining cells that comprise 10% to 15% of the cell population of the lung. The surfactant-producing type II cells are distinguished ultrastructurally by the presence of lamellar bodies, which are the intracellular storage form of surfactant. Lamellar bodies are secreted into the alveolar space by the process of exocytosis. Conformational changes then occur in the lamellar body substances that facilitate the spreading of surfactant over the alveolar surface.

Pulmonary surfactant has a lipid component and a protein component. The lipid component is primarily composed of glycerophospholipids, of which dipalmitoylphosphatidylcholine is the most abundant compound and the major surface-active component. Surfactant contains several proteins that assist in its distribution over the alveolar surface and contribute to its surface-active properties. Surfactant replacement therapy has changed dramatically the treatment of RDS (see later).

The major protein component of pulmonary surfactant is a 28- to 36,000-molecular-weight glycoprotein (surfactant protein-A, SP-A) that is highly conserved across mammalian species and is composed of two major domains, one with collagen-like properties and one with lectin-like carbohydrate-binding properties. SP-A has the ability to bind lipids and carbohydrates, and to bind to specific cell surface receptors. SP-A, along with other surfactant proteins (SP-B, SP-C, SP-D), promotes the rapid formation of surfactant surface films that coat the alveolus and reduce surface tension. SP-A also is important in the binding and recycling of surfactant material by the type II cells through the process of endocytosis that involves specific receptors for SP-A.

The synthesis of the glycerophospholipid component of pulmonary surfactant is subject to multifactorial control, and many substances, including glucocorticoids, prolactin, thyroid hormones, estrogens, androgens, insulin, and catecholamines acting through cyclic adenosine monophosphate, are important in its control.[12] The genes encoding SP-A, SP-B, and SP-C are regulated independently during fetal lung development. SP-A gene expression is undetectable in the human lung before 20 weeks of gestation. Differentiated type II cells that contain a few lamellar bodies are observed by 22 weeks, and active surfactant secretion begins to occur after 30 weeks of gestation. The expression of SP-B and SP-C is detectable much earlier in development than that of SP-A. Cyclic adenosine monophosphate and glucocorticoids play an important role in the regulation of SP-A gene expression.

Term infants of diabetic mothers have an increased incidence of RDS. Fetal hyperinsulinemia in response to maternal hyperglycemia may play a role in the abnormal development of surfactant-producing capability. It also has been observed that fetal "stress" associated with maternal hypertension and uteroplacental insufficiency results in accelerated lung maturation. Such infants usually are small and yet have a decreased incidence of RDS. It may be that elevated levels of glucocorticoids and other stress hormones, such as catecholamines, enhance lung maturation and accelerate SP-A expression, phospholipid synthesis, and surfactant secretion. Antenatal glucocorticoid treatment results in enhanced maturation of the lung and is used therapeutically to promote lung maturation when preterm delivery is anticipated.

Non–Gas Exchange Functions of the Lung

The lung is more than simply a gas-exchanging organ. It is composed of living cells and accounts for 1% to 3% of the body's V_{O_2}. The lung is ideally suited as a metabolic organ because the entire cardiac output must contact the pulmonary vascular endothelium. Substances metabolized or altered by the pulmonary vascular endothelium include angiotensin I, bradykinin, prostaglandins, serotonin, and norepinephrine.[13]

The lung also serves as a filter, removing particulate debris, thrombi, and bacteria from the circulation. The lung is a major determinant of right ventricular afterload and left ventricular preload. It provides buoyancy in aquatic environments.

Respiratory Pathophysiology

An extensive list of causes of respiratory failure in infants and children is given in Table 8-2. A comprehensive discussion

TABLE 8-2. *Causes of respiratory failure in infants and children*

EXTRATHORACIC AIRWAY OBSTRUCTION
Choanal atresia
Laryngomalacia
Pierre Robin syndrome
Tracheomalacia
Vocal cord paralysis
Epiglottitis
Hemangioma, lymphangioma
Subglottic stenosis (congenital, acquired)
Subglottic swelling (infection, trauma)
Foreign body
Cervicofacial trauma

INTRATHORACIC AIRWAY OBSTRUCTION
Vascular ring
Tracheal stenosis or malacia
Bronchial stenosis or malacia
Reactive airway disease
Mucous plugging
Bronchiolitis
Pulmonary interstitial emphysema
Bronchial adenoma (carcinoid)
Inflammatory pseudotumor
Bronchiogenic carcinoma
Other rare benign and malignant intrabronchial tumors
Hodgkins disease/non-Hodgkins lymphoma
Other mediastinal tumors
Cystic fibrosis

PARENCHYMAL LUNG DISEASE
Pneumonia (bacterial, viral)
Meconium aspiration
Contusion
Surfactant deficiency (respiratory distress syndrome)
Pulmonary edema (cardiogenic, permeability, oncotic)
Oxygen toxicity
Bronchopulmonary dysplasia
Pulmonary hypoplasia

ABNORMAL PULMONARY PERFUSION
Congenital heart disease
Persistent fetal circulation
Pulmonary hypertension
Pulmonary embolus

OTHER
Shock/hypoperfusion
Systemic inflammatory response syndrome/sepsis
Central nervous system depression
   Trauma
   Drugs (narcotics, muscle relaxants)
   Seizures
   Encephalopathy
   Apnea
   Intracranial hemorrhage
Neuromuscular disorders
   Spinal cord injury and disease
   Myopathies
   Thoracic deformities
   Phrenic nerve injuries
Pleural effusion
Diaphragmatic hernia
Congenital lobar overinflation
Congenital cystic adenomatoid malformation
Pulmonary sequestration
Abdominal distention

of each of these diseases is beyond the scope of this chapter. Several pathologic processes and diseases are discussed because of their particular relevance to pediatric surgeons.

Abnormalities of Lung Development

Normal human lung development has been reviewed earlier. Developmental abnormalities can occur in relation to any of the components of the lung. These are summarized here and discussed in detail elsewhere in the text. Abnormal development of the large airways may result in atresia or agenesis of the trachea or bronchi, which may result in respiratory failure at birth. In pulmonary sequestration, lung tissue develops separate from the tracheobronchial tree and in association with an abnormal blood supply from the systemic circulation. Bronchogenic cysts contain respiratory epithelium lining a fibromuscular wall that may contain cartilage and muscle. They may communicate with a bronchus or be entirely separate. Cystic adenomatoid malformations are characterized by disorganized parenchymal lung growth that includes a marked increase in tissue at the terminal bronchiolar level, lined by abnormal ciliated columnar epithelium, surrounded by an interstitium with disorganized elastic tissue and smooth muscle, and without mature alveoli. Vascular abnormalities such as arteriovenous malformations are treated with surgery or embolization. Disordered lymphatic development (pulmonary lymphangiectasia) may result in chylothorax and respiratory failure.

Lung Hypoplasia

A variety of newborn anomalies of great interest to pediatric surgeons are associated with lung hypoplasia. The study of hypoplastic lung development may hold the key to therapeutic strategies that may be helpful in treating many different diseases. Hypoplastic lung development, in which the lung is inadequately developed relative to the gestational age, usually is found in association with other fetal anomalies, but can occur in isolation. There is a spectrum of hypoplastic lung development ranging from severe forms that are incompatible with survival to mild forms in which the diagnosis is only suspected. Hypoplastic lung development is distinguished from the respiratory insufficiency of prematurity, because the latter represents normal lung development interrupted by the premature institution of pulmonary gas exchange; however, the parallels are obvious and therapies may be similar.

The pathologic criteria for establishing the diagnosis of pulmonary hypoplasia include a lung-to-body weight ratio more than one standard deviation below normal (normal, 0.018 ± 0.003) and a low morphometric radial alveolar count (number of alveoli encountered on a straight line drawn between a bronchiole and the periphery of the acinus; low-normal, 4.1). These measurements are not clinically helpful. Prenatal estimations of pulmonary hypoplasia have been made using ultrasound to measure the fetal chest circumference-to-abdominal circumference ratio, with good correlation to postnatal pathologic findings.[14] The modulation of fetal ductus arteriosus flow by fetal breathing movements also has been proposed as a clinically useful predictor of pulmonary hypoplasia.[15]

Pulmonary hypoplasia occurs in association with many other

TABLE 8-3. *Conditions associated with pulmonary hypoplasia*

SPACE-OCCUPYING LESIONS OF THE CHEST
Diaphragmatic hernia
Eventration of the diaphragm
Extralobar lung sequestration (nonfunctioning lung tissue)
Massive bilateral pleural effusions
Chylothorax
Hydrothorax
Cystic adenomatoid pulmonary malformation
Paratracheal hemangioma
Nonimmune hydrops fetalis
Bronchogenic cyst
Thoracic neuroblastoma

CARDIAC LESIONS
Hypoplastic left heart
Ebstein anomaly
Hypoplastic right heart
Pulmonic stenosis

RENAL ANOMALIES
Bilateral renal agenesis
Infantile polycystic kidney disease
Multicystic dysplastic kidneys
Bilateral congenital hydronephrosis
Bladder outlet obstruction

ABDOMINAL WALL DEFECTS
Omphalocele
Gastroschisis
Prune-belly syndrome

OLIGOHYDRAMNIOS
Prolonged preterm rupture of membranes
Extraamniotic pregnancy
Abdominal pregnancy

SKELETAL MALFORMATIONS
Osteogenesis imperfecta
Thanatophoric dwarfism
Asphyxiating thoracic dystrophy
Other types of short limb dwarfism
Short rib polydactyly syndrome
Congenital scoliosis
Arthrogryposis multiplex
Chondrodysplasia

NEUROMUSCULAR PATHOLOGIES
Amyoplasia of the diaphragm
Agenesis of the phrenic nerve

CENTRAL NERVOUS SYSTEM
Anencephaly
Arnold-Chiari malformation

PRIMARY PULMONARY HYPOPLASIA

Modified from Sherer DM, Davis JM, Woods JR. Pulmonary hypoplasia: a review. Obstet Gynecol Surv 1990;45:792.

conditions[16] (Table 8-3). Prolonged compression of the fetal thorax has been postulated to explain pulmonary hypoplasia in oligohydramnios associated with renal agenesis (Potter syndrome), urinary obstruction, and cases of prolonged amniotic fluid leak. Intrathoracic compression caused by fluid or a mass effect similarly could explain pulmonary hypoplasia associated with a space-occupying lesion of the chest. Absent or reduced fetal breathing movements also have been associated with pulmonary hypoplasia. Agenesis of the phrenic nerve and agenesis of the muscle within the diaphragm illustrate this most clearly. It also is possible that amniotic fluid contains growth factors that are necessary for normal lung development.

Experimental models have duplicated some of these clinical observations, including the surgical creation of diaphragmatic hernia in fetal lambs and the teratogenic creation of diaphragm defects with nitrofen.[17] Fetal lamb tracheostomy resulting in unrestricted egress of fetal lung fluid causes pulmonary hypoplasia, whereas fetal pharyngostomy does not, implying that distending pressure in the developing fetal airways is of critical importance to normal lung development.[18,19] Further evidence of the importance of "back-pressure" in the developing airways comes from the observation that tracheal ligation may reverse the hypoplastic development of experimentally created diaphragmatic hernia.[20] Fraser syndrome (simultaneous occurrence of renal agenesis and laryngeal atresia), a fatal anomaly, results in non-hypoplastic, more normal lung development.[21]

Treatment strategies designed to prevent pulmonary hypoplasia include in utero shunting of intrathoracic fluid, intra-amniotic fluid instillation to counteract the effects of oligohydramnios, fetal surgery to remove space-occupying lesions of the thorax, fetal diaphragmatic hernia repair, temporary tracheal ligation to promote lung growth, and fetal urinary tract diversion. The therapeutic implications of manipulating the "airway pressure" of the fetus and the newborn as a method of promoting lung development are only beginning to be understood.

Respiratory Failure of Prematurity

The respiratory failure associated with premature birth is an enormous health problem, accounting for most admissions to neonatal intensive care units (ICUs) in developed countries. The primary pathology is surfactant deficiency resulting in elevated alveolar surface tension, alveolar collapse, atelectasis, and respiratory insufficiency. The use of mechanical ventilation to support gas exchange may result in further lung injury. The greatest therapeutic advance in the care of RDS of prematurity has been the use of exogenous surfactant. Its use has resulted in a measurable decrease in premature infant mortality.[22,23] Premature infants treated for respiratory failure with supplemental oxygen, endotracheal intubation, and mechanical ventilation are at risk for the development of bronchopulmonary dysplasia. Bronchopulmonary dysplasia is defined clinically as oxygen dependence that is present for more than 28 days after the use of mechanical ventilation, along with persistent abnormalities on the chest radiograph. Pathologic findings include epithelial necrosis, squamous metaplasia, organization of hyaline membranes in the airways, and fibroblast proliferation in the lung interstitium. The beginnings of these changes may be seen as soon as a few days after birth. The relative contribution of oxygen, airway pressure, and intubation to the pathogenesis are unknown. In its worse form, chronic lung disease results in pulmonary hypertension, cor pulmonale, and death. This severe form is relatively uncommon; however, less severe forms that result in chronic oxygen dependence or the need for prolonged mechanical ventilation with ultimate recovery are common.

The best therapy for bronchopulmonary dysplasia is prevention, through reduction in premature birth and avoidance of excessive oxygen exposure, along with strategies of mechanical ventilation that use low airway pressures. Once bronchopulmonary dysplasia is established, these infants require an approach to care that is somewhat different than the acute-care phase of the respiratory failure of prematurity. Weaning strategies from mechanical ventilation include such concepts as "weaning schedules," in which ventilator changes are made according to a predesigned plan. Continuous monitoring using pulse oximetry, along with the ability of the bedside caregiver (nurse or parent) to make immediate changes in the F_{IO_2} in response to changes in oxygen saturation, prevents prolonged periods of hypoxia and hyperoxia. Nutritional support with both parenteral and enteral nutrition to ensure progressive accrual of lean body mass is of paramount importance. Pharmacologic therapy with antibiotics and bronchodilators is used as needed. Infant stimulation is an essential part of therapy for these infants, who are at increased risk for developmental delay. The use of systemic corticosteroids may result in improvement in lung function and facilitate weaning from mechanical ventilation.[24] The role of tracheostomy remains uncertain. Any infant who will require mechanical ventilation for more than 1 month should be considered for tracheostomy.

Acute Lung Injury

The lung, in injury and disease, assumes a role of critical importance perhaps more than any other organ. The lung may be developmentally abnormal (eg, hypoplastic) or simply too immature to carry out the function of gas exchange (eg, respiratory failure of prematurity). The lung may lack normal defense mechanisms as a result of genetic abnormalities such as cystic fibrosis or immune deficiencies. The lung may be primarily injured as a result of infection, aspiration of acidic gastric contents, or externally applied forces (eg, blunt injury from trauma). The lung also may function abnormally as a result of pathologic conditions that initially target other organ systems, and then generate a systemic inflammatory response that results in lung injury (eg, burns, pancreatitis, tissue necrosis, abscesses, circulating endotoxin or bacteria, ischemia-reperfusion injury). Any disease process may derange the body's homeostatic mechanisms sufficiently to result in respiratory failure. When respiratory failure progresses to the point that gas exchange cannot be maintained, mechanical ventilation and supplemental oxygen are the mainstays of therapy. These treatments themselves may be injurious to the lung, and are responsible for ventilator-induced lung injury and oxygen toxicity.

Although there are many types of lung injury, the lung seems to have a limited repertoire of response to injury.[25] The general pattern of lung injury is as follows: endothelial permeability increases, fluid and protein accumulate in the interstitium of the lung, and increased epithelial permeability results in alveolar flooding. At any point in this continuum, if injury is reversed, the lung may recover, or gas exchange may become impaired sufficiently to preclude survival. Under some circumstances, ongoing inflammation leads to fibrosis, resulting in chronic lung disease or late death. Many endogenous mediators and the cells that produce them have been implicated in acute lung injury. The host defense mechanisms that are protective against some injuries can be "overexpressed" and result in a strong generalized reaction that may cause widespread organ injury.

Acute Lung Injury at the Cellular Level

Neutrophils are the most important cell in the development of acute lung injury. Normally, there is a large pool of neutrophils in the vascular space of the lung. This population of neutrophils increases dramatically under the influence of chemoattractants that are elaborated by endothelial cells, monocytes, and other neutrophils in the injured lung. Neutrophils in the intravascular space contact the endothelial lining cells during their traverse through the pulmonary circulation. The phenomena of neutrophil adherence and migration are regulated largely by the complementary action of the neutrophil cell surface adhesion molecule receptors and the vascular endothelial adhesion molecules. Some of these adhesion molecules are expressed constitutively and others are upregulated in response to cytokines (particularly interleukin-1 and tumor necrosis factor) and proinflammatory stimuli (see Chap. 11). Neutrophils are larger than pulmonary capillaries and must deform to pass through them. Because neutrophils are less deformable when activated, their contact with the pulmonary capillary endothelial cells is enhanced. In acute lung injury, the adherent neutrophils and those recruited into the interstitium of the lung are a major source of oxygen radicals (molecular oxygen, superoxide, hydroxyl) and proteases (elastase, collagenase, gelatinase) that result in tissue injury (see later). Neutrophils that leave the vascular space to enter the interstitium then may enter the alveolus. Endothelial cell damage is not necessary for this migration to occur.

The importance of neutrophils in the pathogenesis of acute lung injury is supported by several lines of evidence. Neutrophils and their products are present in increased numbers in the bronchoalveolar lavage fluid of patients with acute lung injury. Pathologic specimens show increased numbers of sequestered neutrophils in acute lung injury. Neutrophil depletion attenuates experimental mediator-induced lung injury, as does functional manipulation of neutrophils, such as inhibition of cyclooxygenase with ibuprofen. Although adult RDS may occur in neutropenic patients, lung function may worsen when neutropenia resolves.

Pulmonary vascular endothelium also is actively involved in acute lung injury. The cell surface adhesion molecules are upregulated in lung injury and affect neutrophil adherence. The contact between neutrophils and endothelial cells is increased and prolonged, providing a microenvironment protected from circulating antioxidants and antiproteases and favoring endothelial cell injury. With damage to the integrity of the endothelial cell-endothelial cell barrier, permeability increases and interstitial edema results. Impairment of the normal metabolism of serotonin, norepinephrine, prostaglandins, bradykinin, and angiotensin I by the endothelial cells probably occurs in lung injury. In addition, endothelial cells produce chemoattractants that augment and perpetuate injury.

The macrophage/monocyte cell line also is important in acute lung injury. Resident macrophages respond to inflammatory mediators and become activated. Activated macrophages produce the same toxic products as neutrophils, including oxygen radicals and proteases. Lung macrophages also release tumor necrosis factor and interleukin-1. The population of interstitial macrophages increases in the first several days after an inflammatory response is initiated. This may be the most important event in the perpetuation of the inflammatory response that results in ongoing lung injury even after the systemic factors that initiated the response have been controlled. The long life of lung macrophages, measured in days, compared with neutrophils, which may only survive for hours, also contributes to the perpetuation of the inflammatory response. Macrophages also play an important role as bactericidal cells and phagocytic cells in injured lungs. Macrophages participate in the regulation of fibroblast function and probably play a role in the fibrosis that can result when lung injury is perpetuated.

Platelets have a less certain role in acute lung injury, and may be involved secondarily; however, sequestered platelets commonly are found in acute lung injury. Platelet release of serotonin, proteases, and prostaglandins may contribute to lung injury.

Biochemical Mediators of Lung Injury

The cellular components that characterize acute lung injury elaborate products that perpetuate and alter the injury. When neutrophils and macrophages are activated by the complement cascade or other injury, cytokines, phospholipid metabolites, and oxygen radicals are produced. These products influence the activity and function of the cells around them and participate in the activation of enzymatic cascades related to inflammation. The array of compounds and their effects is dizzying and indicates the complexity of the inflammatory response in the lung (see Chap. 11).

Among them, cytokines and products of arachidonic acid metabolism are especially important. Interleukin-1, interleukin-2, interleukin-6, tumor necrosis factor, and interferon-γ probably are the most important cytokines. The activity of phospholipases is increased in activated inflammatory cells, which in turn increases the cleavage of arachidonic acid from membrane phospholipids. The action of cyclooxygenase on arachidonic acid results in the production of prostaglandins, thromboxanes, and prostacyclin. Thromboxane is a potent agonist for platelet aggregation and smooth muscle contraction, and is implicated in the pulmonary hypertension and bronchoconstriction associated with sepsis and acute lung injury. Prostacyclin functions in an opposing fashion, by inhibiting platelet aggregation and causing vasodilation, and may be in part responsible for the systemic vasodilation associated with the systemic inflammatory response. Other prostaglandins are primarily vasodilators. During lung injury, these compounds and others may have exaggerated local and systemic effects. The key events of acute lung injury are summarized in Figure 8-2.

Overdistention Lung Injury and Pressure-Volume Lung Injury

The role of mechanical ventilation in lung injury is difficult to determine precisely. In clinical practice, it has long been recognized that patients can be sustained almost indefinitely using mechanical ventilation. Patients with normal lungs may undergo both positive-pressure and negative-pressure ventila-

tion without deleterious effects. Likewise, long-term animal experiments failed to show pathologic lung changes that can be attributed to mechanical ventilation itself when normal ventilating pressures and volumes were used. In acute respiratory failure, however, mechanical ventilation is being applied to already injured lungs, and abnormally high pressures and tidal volumes may be necessary to achieve adequate gas exchange. Under these circumstances, although necessary as a life-sustaining measure to maintain pulmonary gas exchange, the use of mechanical ventilation may be responsible for lung injury. Several lines of evidence, both clinical and experimental, implicate the use of mechanical ventilation as both a culprit and a cure for respiratory failure.[26]

The multi-institutional, randomized, prospective trial of extracorporeal membrane oxygenation (ECMO) for adult respiratory failure sponsored by the National Institutes of Health concluded that ECMO was not more effective in the treatment of severe respiratory failure than conventional mechanical ventilation.[27] A more appropriate conclusion would have been that when life is sustained using ECMO and irreversible lung injury already has taken place, survival is not improved. ECMO was applied more appropriately to neonates, for whom the methods of mechanical ventilation available at the time were failing. In this population, respiratory failure that was rapidly fatal using conventional means was treated with extracorporeal support and "lung rest." The rapidity with which respiratory failure progressed to become life-threatening may be the feature that allowed lung rest to result in recovery, before the effects of high pressures and high oxygen concentrations became irreversible. During ECMO, the mechanical ventilator was turned down to pressures that presumably were not injurious. The concept that lung rest could result in the complete reversal of fatal respiratory failure of short duration emphasized that mechanical ventilation itself may be injurious to the lung. In neonates with severe respiratory failure, simply eliminating mechanical ventilation can result in the rapid return of respiratory function within a few days.

When the use of routine mechanical ventilation was still in its infancy, Greenfield and colleagues demonstrated that pulmonary edema developed in dogs that were subjected to high-volume mechanical ventilation using a pressure of 30 cm H_2O for several hours.[28] This was the first study that demonstrated that mechanical ventilation could alter lung function and cause lung injury. The morphologic characteristics of the lung injury associated with the application of high pressure to normal lungs in rats included injury that progressed from perivascular edema, to interstitial edema with detachment of endothelial cells from their basement membrane, to type I cell damage, denuding of the epithelial side of the basement membrane, alveolar edema, and the formation of hyaline membranes consisting of cellular debris and protein.[29] The question of whether pressure or volume of distention was the primary culprit responsible for this kind of lung injury then was addressed. Using microvascular permeability changes to assess lung injury, positive-pressure ventilation and negative-pressure ventilation (using a small "iron lung") to equivalent degrees of lung overdistention (40 to 45 mL/kg) resulted in identical lung injuries.[30] The investigators further showed that thoracoabdominal strapping ablated the injury associated with high-pressure ventilation. Others have demonstrated in similar experiments that when lung overexpansion is prevented (using a body cast), high airway pressures are

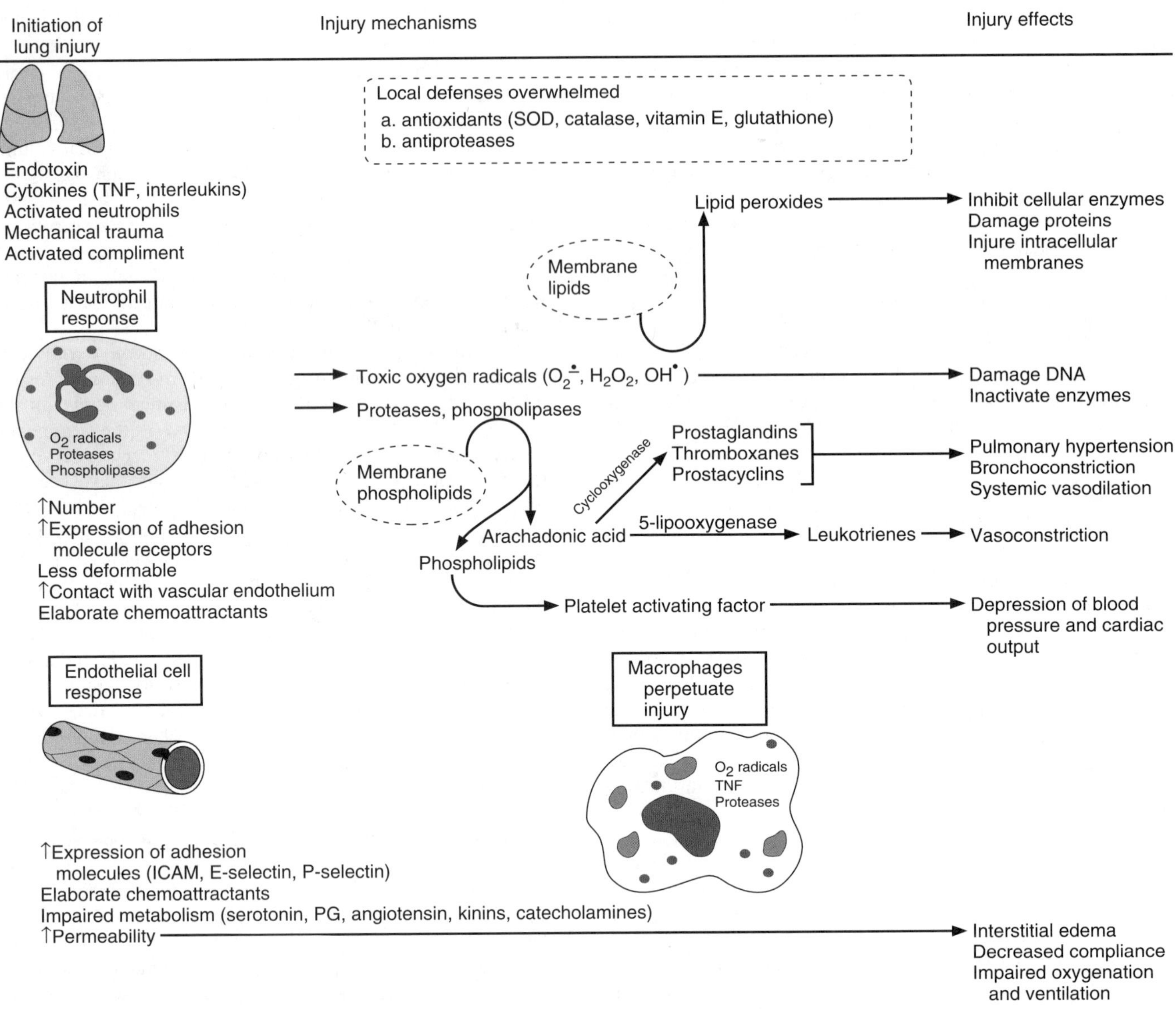

FIG. 8-2. Summary of the events of acute lung injury. (See text for details.) TNF, tumor necrosis factor; SOD, superoxide dismutase; ICAM, Intercellular adhesion molecule.

tolerated without lung injury, and that when low pressures are applied to the lung and there is no restriction to its expansion (ex vivo), severe alterations in microvascular permeability result.[31] Dreyfuss and Saumon also demonstrated that the most important determinant of overdistention lung injury is the absolute lung volume at end-inspiration, with similar injuries produced by high-FRC/low–tidal volume ventilation and low-FRC/high–tidal volume ventilation.[32] Large swings in tidal volume with zero end-expiratory pressure are not tolerated as well and PEEP tends to preserve gas exchange and reduce edema to some extent. It may be that PEEP decreases the shear stress associated with the repetitive opening and closing of the terminal airways. Overdistention can cause injury beyond the lung itself, and Kolobow and colleagues demonstrated that prolonged mechanical ventilation with excessive tidal volumes resulted in a syndrome of multiple organ failure.[33]

It is clear from these experiments that the most significant determinant of lung injury in normal lungs exposed to excessive pressures and volumes is the absolute level of lung volume achieved at end-inspiration. The mechanism by which this injury takes place is not clear. However, striking ultrastructural similarities have been shown between the endothelial and epithelial lesions that result from elevated *capillary* transmural pressure and the lesions of lung *airway* overdistention. This phenomenon, associated with elevation of the pulmonary capillary transmural pressure to levels greater than 40 mmHg, has been called capillary stress failure. The pressure required to produce capillary stress failure is reduced by increased lung volume.[34] It may be that lung overdistention results in capillary stress failure, and that elevated vascular pressures act in synergy with airway overdistention to produce lung injury. This may be of particular importance in neonatal respiratory failure, where pulmonary hypertension plays such a prominent role and mechanical ventilation may result in lung overdistention.

Lung overdistention experiments have been conducted largely on normal animals and in initially healthy lungs. The combined effects of lung overdistention and oleic acid injury, inactivation of pulmonary surfactant, or hydrochloric acid injury result in more severe injury than does overdistention or chemical injury alone. This raises the possibility that lung overdistention may be even more harmful to diseased lungs than to healthy lungs.

Work by Gattinoni and associates using computed tomography in adults with RDS has demonstrated that the lung in RDS has three components[35]:

- Healthy tissue that has a fairly normal appearance on computed tomographic scanning, has essentially normal compliance, and may be overexpanded under the influence of excessive airway pressures and excessive PEEP
- Recruitable lung that may be expanded under the influence of variable levels of PEEP
- Injured tissue that does not respond to increases in airway pressure

Under conditions of severe lung injury, mechanical ventilation may result in overdistention of the most normal portion of the lung and cause further injury.

Recognition of the phenomenon of overdistention lung injury and the possible deleterious effects of mechanical ventilation using high pressures and volumes has resulted in a change in the way that mechanical ventilation is practiced today in comparison with methods used just 10 years ago. The concept of minimal-excursion ventilation is a direct result of this understanding.

Local tissue alkalosis also may play a role in lung injury associated with mechanical ventilation. When a large intrapulmonary shunt is present in respiratory failure, the P_{CO_2} in the ventilated alveoli and their associated capillaries must be far less than 40 mmHg to achieve a "normal" Pa_{CO_2} of 40 mmHg. The more normal areas of the lung with appropriate matching of ventilation and perfusion must be "hyperventilated" to achieve a normal Pa_{CO_2} after mixing with blood of a higher P_{CO_2} that has traversed perfused but unventilated portions of the lung. In theory, the P_{CO_2} in the ventilated areas of the lung could be low enough to result in tissue-damaging alkalosis.[36] It is unknown whether this mechanism is clinically important.

Deleterious Effects of Oxygen

One of the primary functions of the lung is to permit the transfer of molecular oxygen from the respiratory gas mixture to the blood. Supplemental oxygen often is added to the respiratory gas mixture to treat respiratory failure that results in arterial hypoxemia and tissue hypoxia. Oxygen is a drug, however, and its pharmacologic properties must be recognized. Oxygen administration also may cause direct cellular injury as a result of the increased production of oxygen free radical–containing species that overwhelm the natural protective mechanisms that normally scavenge these highly reactive molecules.

In patients with chronic hypoxia and hypercarbia, ventilatory drive may be unusually dependent on hypoxia. The administration of supplemental oxygen with "normalization" of arterial oxygen levels actually may depress ventilation and worsen respiratory failure during spontaneous breathing. This phenomenon is seen clinically in older patients with chronic obstructive pulmonary disease, in children with chronic lung disease such as advanced cystic fibrosis, and in infants with bronchopulmonary dysplasia. Oxygen administration may depress erythropoiesis, but this is unlikely to be of clinical significance. One pharmacologic use of oxygen is as a pulmonary vasodilator. It is important in the treatment of pulmonary hypertension for this reason. In addition, absorption atelectasis can occur when poorly ventilated areas of the lung contain only oxygen and no inert gases. As oxygen is slowly absorbed, these areas of the lung tend to become atelectatic. Apart from the lung, chronic oxygen exposure in neonates can result in retinopathy (retrolental fibroplasia, retinopathy of prematurity). Hyperbaric exposure to oxygen causes central nervous system injury manifested as seizures and paralysis.

The direct lung injuries associated with oxygen exposure include tracheobronchitis, acute alveolar-capillary injury, and chronic lung injury. A variety of physiologic changes have been described with continuous hyperoxia.[37] Early in exposure, mucociliary clearance is decreased. Macrophage phagocytic function is depressed. Vital capacity and compliance fall, and adult volunteers uniformly report chest pain after only a few hours of breathing at an F_{IO_2} (Fraction of inspired oxygen) of 1. Surfactant production decreases and lung water increases. Vital capacity and diffusing capacity do not return to normal for 2 weeks after only 3 days of breathing at an F_{IO_2} of 1. Primates survive for about a week under such exposure. Pathologic changes associated with hyperoxic exposure are seen after a latent period of 24 to 72 hours that varies among species and among individuals. This latent period is followed by a period of acute injury and inflammation, then by a destructive phase. Endothelial cells show injury first, and many endothelial cells undergo destruction. This is followed by type I epithelial cell damage and an increase in the number of type II pneumocytes. Interstitial edema develops, followed by alveolar edema. Many neutrophils and monocytes infiltrate the interstitial space coincident with the beginning of cellular injury. The initiation of injury probably results as follows: Hyperoxia increases the substrate for reactions that normally produce toxic oxygen species. The protective mechanisms that scavenge these toxic products are overwhelmed and the cycle of tissue injury begins. Resident neutrophils and monocytes become activated and release cytokines that result in the recruitment of more leukocytes to the lung, which in turn become activated and perpetuate the injury.

The highest "safe" concentration of inspired oxygen that can be tolerated indefinitely is unknown. F_{IO_2} concentrations of less than 0.6 result in minimal morphologic changes in rodents. F_{IO_2} concentrations of less than 0.5 seem to be tolerated indefinitely by both children and adults. In premature infants, minimal elevations in the F_{IO_2} may be associated with retinopathy.

Barotrauma

The subtle morphologic and physiologic changes that can result from overdistention of the lung have been referred to as a form of barotrauma; however, other descriptive names, such as volutrauma, overdistention lung injury, and pressure-volume lung injury, better describe these injuries. The term *barotrauma* is best used to refer to the appearance of extra-alveolar gas as a result of the gross mechanical disruption of the airways. The clinical manifestations of barotrauma include pneumothorax, tension pneumothorax, pneumomediastinum, tension pneumomediastinum, pneumopericardium, pulmonary interstitial emphysema, pneumoperitoneum, pneumoretroperitoneum, subcutaneous emphysema, pneumatocele, bronchopleural fistula, and intravascular air embolism.

When high pressures and corresponding high volumes are created in the lungs, large pressure gradients may be present between the bronchovascular sheaths and adjacent alveoli. Alveoli may rupture into the interstitial tissues of the bronchovascular sheath and allow gas to be introduced. Both high airway pressures and underlying lung disease are necessary to cause barotrauma, as evidenced by the fact that adults with normal lungs can sustain seemingly enormous increases in airway pressure without developing extra-alveolar air. Coughing, sneezing, Valsalva maneuver, weight lifting, and playing wind instruments result in airway pressures that may exceed 200 cm H_2O.

Barotrauma should be regarded as a sign of lung injury associated with the use of mechanical ventilation. Therapy for barotrauma should be directed at the primary disease and consideration given to changing the method of mechanical ventilation. Life-threatening effects of barotrauma may need to be treated immediately. Any pneumothorax that occurs while a patient is on positive-pressure ventilation must be considered a potential tension pneumothorax and should be decompressed by tube thoracostomy. Tube drainage (best performed under ultrasound guidance) of pneumopericardium may be necessary. Ventilator strategies that reduce PEEP, tidal volume, and inspiratory pressure should be used. Permissive hypercapnia may be helpful. Neonates with pulmonary interstitial emphysema may benefit from high-frequency oscillatory ventilation (HFOV). Pneumoperitoneum always presents a diagnostic dilemma for the surgeon because critically ill patients are at risk for stress ulcers and intestinal ischemia that may result in visceral perforation. Excluding a surgical cause of pneumoperitoneum may be difficult. Contrast studies may be of some benefit, along with serial examinations, in making a decision about the need for laparotomy or laparoscopy.

TREATMENT OF RESPIRATORY INSUFFICIENCY: ASSISTING THE FAILING LUNG

The treatment of respiratory failure must be designed to permit healing of the injured lung while preserving the remaining uninjured lung. The goals of treatment include improving the inadequate pulmonary gas exchange that results in hypoxemia and acute respiratory acidosis, relieving respiratory distress by decreasing the work of breathing, and altering lung mechanics to improve lung compliance and treat atelectasis.[38]

General Measures

Position of the Patient

In the mathematic description of the mechanical properties of the lung given earlier, the lung is assumed to be homogeneous. However, the lung is inhomogeneous in both health and disease. Position and gravity play an important role in determining the inflation, distribution of ventilation, and distribution of perfusion of both healthy and sick lungs.

In normal, supine individuals, regional lung inflation decreases exponentially from ventral to dorsal, with the most inflated alveoli near the ventral surface and the most compressed alveoli in the dependent, dorsal regions. In the prone position, regional lung inflation changes; the dorsal portions of the lung are the most inflated and the dependent (ventral) lung is the most compressed. Regional inflation is more homogeneous in the prone than in the supine position. Lung weight and hydrostatic pressure probably play the major role in determining the distribution of lung inflation.

In adults with acute respiratory failure, lung weight may be two or three times that of normal lungs. This lung edema is distributed relatively uniformly throughout the lung tissue and does not accumulate preferentially in dependent regions of the lung.[39] Total lung gas volume is markedly decreased, whereas total lung dimensions are unchanged (ie, interstitial fluid replaces gas volume and FRC is decreased). The rate of decrease in lung inflation along the vertical axis is greater in acute respiratory failure than in normal lungs. In acute respiratory failure, the most dependent regions of the lung also are subject to high hydrostatic pressures from the weight of the homogeneously distributed edema fluid (10 to 15 cm H_2O in adults). As in the normal lung, the prone position usually results in greater inflation in the dorsal regions and less inflation in the ventral regions of the lung.

In supine, spontaneously breathing individuals, ventilation is distributed primarily to the dependent portions of the lung. These portions of the lung have a greater capacity to expand because they are relatively more compressed at end-expiration. The action of the diaphragm also results in a greater ventilation of the dependent lung. In mechanically ventilated patients, ventilation is preferentially distributed to the nondependent portion of the lung because the dependent regions are more likely to be totally collapsed. In addition, the diaphragm is passive and its upper (ventral) portion faces less intraabdominal pressure.

In the normal lung, blood flow is distributed largely by gravity. In the diseased lung, factors such as vasoconstriction, vessel obliteration, the effect of microemboli, and extrinsic vessel compression play a role in the distribution of blood flow.

Prone positioning can make a dramatic change in the respiratory function of adults with RDS.[39] There are no comparable studies in children. In supine patients, ventilation goes primarily to the anterior portions of the lung, whereas perfusion goes primarily to the posterior aspects of the lung, creating the ventilation-perfusion mismatch that results in hypoxemia. It seems prudent to use frequent position changes in patients with respiratory failure. Dependent, compressed portions of the lung may be expanded. Pooling of respiratory secretions also may be prevented. Ventilation-perfusion mismatch may be minimized. Because prone positioning is not practiced routinely in children and adults, and has obvious dangers, side-to-side position changes should be carried out. Diligent nursing is required to ensure that patients actually are turned fully lateral during these position changes. It is difficult to break the habit of routine supine positioning in the ICU. It is noteworthy that nurses who handle newborns with respiratory failure are aware of the position that ''the baby likes.'' With the instantaneous feedback afforded by continuous pulse oximetry, these fragile infants are positioned empirically in such a way that their oxygenation is optimized.

Heat and Humidification

Any therapeutic gas delivery system should match the normal heat and humidity at the point of entry into the respiratory system. Gas delivered to the nose should have a temperature of 22°C and a relative humidity of 50%, whereas gas delivered to the trachea should be 34°C and have a relative humidity of 100%. During spontaneous respiration, inspired gases are heated and become saturated with water, reaching 100% humidity and 37°C just below the carina. The airway above this point adds heat and humidity to the inspired gas and extracts heat and humidity from the expired gas, acting as a heat and moisture exchanger. When the upper airway is bypassed during endotracheal intubation, excessive heat and moisture are lost if the ventilating gases are not humidified. Heat loss results largely from the heat of vaporization when the inspiratory gases are humidified by the lungs. Air has a relatively low specific heat and the warming of the gases themselves accounts for relatively little heat loss. The trachea and upper bronchi are most affected by inadequate humidification of the respiratory gases, with resultant moisture loss. With inadequate humidification, ciliary action is decreased and ultimately lost, mucous glands are damaged, and the mucosa becomes ulcerated. Compliance and surfactant activity decreases; atelectasis and hypoxia may result. Heating and humidifying the respiratory gases is not an effective method of rewarming a hypothermic patient, but it is important in preventing further heat loss.

Technical issues related to the delivery of warmed, humidified gases to mechanically ventilated infants can be complex. When ventilator tubing passes through the room at an ambient temperature of 23°C and subsequently into an incubator at 36°C, or is exposed to radiant warmers, the performance of the heating and humidifying devices can be unpredictable and result in inadequate humidification and heating.

Suctioning and Postural Drainage

Gravity can be used to advantage to help clear airway secretions. Specific positions allow dependent drainage of the lobar bronchi. Adjuncts such as vibration and percussion (manual or by mechanical devices) also may help mobilize secretions.

Suctioning is important in the care of intubated patients because cough mechanisms are disrupted by mechanical airways. Suctioning the airways of nonintubated patients is a lost art. Eliciting a deep cough to clear airway secretions and forcing a vital capacity breath may be facilitated by intratracheal suctioning. Suctioning as it usually is practiced involves the placement of a catheter in the hypopharynx. True intratracheal suctioning can be accomplished in much the same way as nasotracheal intubation in spontaneously breathing patients. A catheter with a curved tip is passed through the nose and positioned in the hypopharynx. The catheter is manipulated until respirations are audible through it and then is advanced rapidly with inspiration. Proper entry into the trachea is obvious. The use of fiberoptic bronchoscopy as an adjunct to suctioning is controversial. Bronchoscopy does allow directed suctioning to be performed, but it is doubtful that it is more helpful than properly performed catheter suctioning in intubated or nonintubated patients.

Prevention of Atelectasis, Incentive Spirometry, and Positive-Pressure Ventilation

Sustained inspiration is the most effective method of both preventing and treating atelectasis.[40] During normal respiration, deep, sustained breaths are taken several times each hour in the form of a sigh or yawn. This normal mechanism may not be present in perioperative or critically ill patients and must be encouraged or substituted for. Coughing does little to promote full lung inflation, whereas a sustained inspiratory effort is effective in fully expanding the lungs. Nonintubated children who can cooperate benefit from incentive spirometry. Proper use of an incentive spirometer requires a sustained, gentle inspiratory effort. The object is not to create the greatest negative inspiratory pressure, but to create sustained inspiratory effort. ''Blowing'' maneuvers such as blowing bubbles are less effective in lung expansion, but may be performed more easily by younger children. Children who are too young to participate in voluntary maneuvers may benefit from the lung expansion that results from crying. Although pain should be controlled adequately, oversedation that results in continual somnolence and shallow breathing must be avoided. Intermittent positive-pressure breathing is not used frequently, but in selected settings may be beneficial in promoting full lung expansion. Failure of positive-pressure breathing results more from improper technique than from any other cause. Properly fitting mouthpieces, good coaching, and frequent treatment are needed to achieve good results.

Intubated patients benefit from intermittent lung expansion to full lung capacity. Routine ''bagging and suctioning'' as a part of the respiratory care of all intubated patients provides acceptable lung expansion. Intermittent large tidal volume ''sigh'' breaths provided by the mechanical ventilator do not really recapitulate the normal mechanisms of full lung inflation and carry a risk of lung injury in diseased lungs. A more physiologic approach to atelectasis treatment and prevention is provided by a sustained breath at 35 to 40 cm H_2O that is held for 5 seconds or longer and repeated three times. This pattern should be repeated each hour.

Pharmacologic Agents

Antibiotics

When respiratory insufficiency is caused by bacterial infections involving the lung itself (pneumonia), or when bacterial infections involving other organs results in respiratory failure (eg, necrotizing enterocolitis), antibiotic therapy is used. Appropriate cultures are obtained, including blood, sputum, urine, and cerebrospinal fluid, as indicated by the disease presentation and the age of the child, and broad-spectrum antibiotic coverage is begun. Antibiotic therapy then is tailored to specific organisms based on culture results.

Patients who are intubated and receiving mechanical ventilation for any reason are at great risk for acquired bacterial pneumonia; however, prophylactic antibiotics are not indicated when mechanical ventilation is instituted. Gram-negative organisms and *Staphylococcus* species are the most common infectious agents in intubated patients. The diagnosis of pneumonia and the decision to institute antibiotic therapy in intubated patients can be difficult to make. Decisions to institute or change antimicrobial therapy should be based on multiple clinical variables, including worsening gas exchange, end-organ signs of sepsis, changes in the chest radiograph, changes in the quantity or quality of respiratory secretions, and the results of respiratory tract cultures.

Microscopic examination and culture of respiratory secretions may be helpful in making treatment decisions, but their limitations must be recognized. Semiquantitative grading of neutrophils and bacteria in tracheal aspirates is imprecise; however, abundant neutrophils and intracellular organisms are associated with pneumonia. The results of tracheal aspirate cultures may be difficult to interpret because they are likely to include many oropharyngeal and upper airway organisms that may not be the pathogenic agent. Significant bacterial pneumonia is improbable in the absence of cultured organisms, but organisms frequently are cultured even when pneumonia is not present.

The use of fiberoptic bronchoscopy to perform directed bronchoalveolar lavage, in association with quantitative culture techniques, may allow specimens to be obtained that more reliably indicate pathogens. Another bronchoscopic technique uses the protected specimen brush to obtain samples closer to the site of actual lung infection that more meaningfully reflect the infectious organisms. In this technique, a protected brush contained within a catheter is inserted through a fiberoptic bronchoscope. Bronchoalveolar lavage and the protected specimen brush have been used widely in adults and their relative merits are still controversial; however, they seem to be able to provide fairly reliable lower respiratory tract specimens for microscopic examination and quantitative culture. The efficacy and safety of these techniques have not been reported in children.

Diuretics and Fluid Management

In diffuse lung injury, the increase in interstitial fluid results primarily from increased capillary permeability, although hydrostatic forces still may be a contributing factor. Reduction of intravascular volume using diuretics may improve lung function. The goal of diuretic therapy is to reduce hydrostatic pressure in the lungs while maintaining intravascular volume such that other organs are well perfused. Central hemodynamic monitoring using right atrial pressure or pulmonary artery occlusion pressures may be necessary to guide the use of diuretics. Fluid restriction and diuresis are used to produce the lowest possible central venous or pulmonary artery pressures that do not result in a fall in cardiac output or end-organ perfusion. In the absence of invasive cardiac monitoring, the empiric use of diuretics is not likely to be harmful if end-organ perfusion is monitored carefully. A difficult clinical condition to interpret is that of total body fluid overload with intravascular depletion, a situation that is encountered frequently in patients with systemic inflammatory response syndrome who require an intraabdominal operation. In this situation, visibly edematous patients may require intravascular fluid administration to maintain intravascular vol-

ume in the perioperative period. If the inflammatory response is reversed, diuresis most often begins spontaneously and may be augmented by diuretics. Another condition encountered by pediatric surgeons is stable infants in the neonatal unit with chronic lung disease from prematurity who must undergo surgical procedures. The operative fluid administration associated with major intraabdominal procedures (eg, colon resection for stricture) or even with seemingly minor procedures (eg, inguinal hernia repair) may result in deterioration of lung function and benefit from the use of diuretics in the early postoperative period.

Bronchodilators

Many drugs have bronchodilator properties and have been used therapeutically for this effect. Side effects and toxicity have limited the usefulness of many agents, including epinephrine and isoproterenol. Inhaled albuterol, a selective β_2-agonist, is the most widely used agent in the United States and combines a potent bronchodilator effect with good selectivity and low toxicity (tremor and tachycardia). Methylxanthines are used less often.

Corticosteroids

Because the inflammatory process contributes to the lung damage associated with acute lung injury, the use of antiinflammatory therapies might reduce lung injury. Adult studies have shown no benefit from the use of high-dose corticosteroids administered early in the course of adult RDS. However, corticosteroids may be beneficial when administered during the fibroproliferative phase of lung injury in adult RDS, which typically occurs 5 to 10 days after the onset of disease.[41] There are no studies that support this practice in children; however, corticosteroids are often used in pediatric respiratory failure that is unresponsive to supportive care.

Corticosteroids also have been used therapeutically in neonatal respiratory failure. The use of dexamethasone in mechanically ventilated infants with bronchopulmonary dysplasia has been shown to decrease the duration of mechanical ventilation.[24,42] Dexamethasone also is used empirically to treat worsening respiratory failure in neonates and may even be beneficial when given during the first week of life to premature infants with RDS.[43] Beneficial effects must be weighed against the known harmful effects, such as hyperglycemia, hypertension, pituitary and adrenal depression, and gastrointestinal side effects.

Pulmonary Vasodilators

Newborn respiratory failure associated with pulmonary hypertension and hypoxic right-to-left shunting at the ductal level should improve if pulmonary vascular resistance falls. The pulmonary vasculature of newborns may be sensitive to oxygen, carbon dioxide, and pH. Hypoxia, hypercarbia, and acidosis raise pulmonary artery pressure, increasing the right-to-left shunting. Oxygen and hyperventilation may be used therapeutically to reduce pulmonary artery pressure. Nitroprusside, nitroglycerin, tolazoline, calcium-channel blockers, and other vaso-dilators have been used as pulmonary vasodilators, with limited success. The common failing of these agents is that each also is a systemic vasodilator. When administered into the systemic circulation, or even when delivered directly into the pulmonary artery, they usually result in reduced systemic vascular resistance and pulmonary vascular resistance. Hypoxic right-to-left shunting is not reduced, and the resulting systemic hypotension may lead to inadequate perfusion.

Nitric Oxide

Before the last decade, nitric oxide was considered biologically important only as an environmental pollutant. In 1987, nitric oxide was shown to be the endothelium-derived relaxing factor that was necessary to cause the relaxation of vascular smooth muscle.[44] It is now known to have many important functions, both as a signaling agent and as a cytotoxic molecule. Nitric oxide is a colorless gas. Although lipophilic, it has good solubility in water and a relatively long aqueous half-life of about 3 seconds. Nitric oxide is produced biologically from the action of the nitric oxide synthases on the guanidino-nitrogen group of L-arginine. These enzymes exist in three isoforms found in endothelial cells, brain, and macrophages. Many of the biologic actions of nitric oxide, including the relaxation of vascular smooth muscle, are mediated by guanylyl cyclase and cyclic guanosine monophosphate (cGMP). Nitric oxide is a small molecule that diffuses easily to adjacent cells and enters the cytosol. Within the cell, it binds to the iron of the heme component of guanylate cyclase, moving iron out of the plane of the porphyrin ring, activating the enzyme, and increasing the levels of intracellular cGMP. The rise in intracellular cGMP inhibits the release of calcium from the sarcoplasmic reticulum and prevents calcium entry into cells, reducing intracellular calcium concentration and causing relaxation of vascular and non-vascular smooth muscle.[45] Nitric oxide also has cGMP-independent functions, including the activation of cyclooxygenase, inhibition of cytochrome P-450, alteration of protein synthesis, modulation of gene transcription and translation, and free-radical cytotoxicity.

Nitric oxide is found in atmospheric air at concentrations up to 9 ppm and in cigarette smoke at concentrations up to 1000 ppm. Inhaled nitric oxide is administered therapeutically at concentrations up to 80 to 100 ppm. It rapidly penetrates cell membranes and theoretically is able to cause relaxation of airway and vascular smooth muscle cells of the lung. Nitric oxide that enters the bloodstream is metabolized rapidly to form nitrate (NO_3^-, associated with the conversion of hemoglobin to methemoglobin) and nitrite (NO_2^-). Clinical and laboratory data have shown that nitric oxide does cause a dose-dependent reduction in pulmonary artery pressure that often is associated with a rise in the systemic Pao_2. Unlike with other pulmonary vasodilators, no change in systemic vascular resistance is seen.

The ability to administer nitric oxide as an inhaled gas that might selectively encounter the pulmonary vasculature led to predictions that this agent would be the ''magic bullet'' that would treat pulmonary hypertension associated with respiratory failure. Inhaled nitric oxide has been used to treat persistent pulmonary hypertension of the newborn, pulmonary hypertension associated with congenital heart disease, idiopathic pulmo-nary hypertension, adult RDS, chronic obstructive airway disease, and pneumonia.[46] Newborn pulmonary artery hypertension in association with right-to-left shunting at the ductal level is physiologically well suited to treatment with nitric oxide. However, results have been inconsistent, and the use of nitric oxide has not eliminated the need for extracorporeal life support (ECLS) in all centers that offer both these modalities. In the experience of this author, nitric oxide has been responsible for dramatic improvement in some infants who otherwise would have met the criteria for the institution of ECLS, but has resulted in only transient improved oxygenation in others. The best use for inhaled nitric oxide in the treatment of respiratory failure remains to be determined and awaits validation by randomized, prospective studies.

Therapy Directed Against Mediators of Acute Lung Injury

Therapy directed at specific targets in the inflammatory process associated with acute lung injury might be expected to modify lung injury. However, no agent has been shown to influence greatly the progression or recovery of acute lung injury. Antioxidants such as acetylcysteine, superoxide dismutase, and catalase might be protective against the injuries of oxygen free radicals.[47] Ketoconazole inhibits the synthesis of thromboxane and leukotrienes.[48] Pentoxifylline inhibits the activation and chemotaxis of polymorphonuclear neutrophils.[49] Antibodies to tumor necrosis factor, endotoxin, and interleukin-1 have not been shown to alter the outcome of respiratory failure associated with sepsis. All studies have been performed in adults with RDS.

It is unlikely that a simple pharmacologic ''cure'' for inflammatory lung injury will be forthcoming. The multiple pathways that lead to lung injury and the precise timing of the intervention required to alter the injury make clinical effectiveness nearly impossible to achieve.

Mechanical Ventilation

History

In ancient times, it was recognized that the lungs could be inflated artificially with the use of a reed in the trachea. During the Middle Ages, artificial ventilation using an intratracheal reed and a bellows to provide tidal volume prolonged the beating of the heart during vivisection. In response to the number of drowning victims in The Netherlands and England in the 17th century, there was great popular interest in the idea of artificial respiration as a form of resuscitation. Techniques were developed that included intratracheal tube placement and bellows ventilation. Complications associated with overzealous bellows ventilation and lack of effectiveness in the treatment of drowning victims caused these techniques to fall into disfavor in Western medical practice for more than 100 years. Positive-pressure ventilation was relegated primarily to animal physiology experiments during this time. Ingenious devices for both positive- and negative-pressure ventilation are of historical interest. Positive-pressure ventilation found greater use in the early 20th century in the operating room, where it allowed better airway protection during procedures performed in and about the mouth. Positive-pressure ventilation also expanded the ability of surgeons to operate within the thorax. The modern era of positive-pressure ventilation for use outside the operating room was ushered in by the polio epidemics of the mid-20th century. Respiratory muscle paralysis from poliomyelitis at that time was treated by negative-pressure ventilation using an iron lung. Although effective, these apparatuses were cumbersome and were not available in large numbers throughout the world. The polio epidemic that struck Copenhagen in 1952 resulted in the first successful widespread use of positive-pressure ventilation (initially supplied by manual effort). This experience provided impetus for the development of practical mechanical ventilators. The act of grouping together patients who required mechanical ventilation and its attendant intensive nursing care provided the framework for the subsequent development of ICUs. Product development over the ensuing 50 years has centered on improving the reliability and safety of mechanical ventilators, altering ventilatory pressure and flow to achieve the best respiratory gas exchange with the least possibility of injuring the lung, and creating communication between the mechanical ventilator and the spontaneously breathing patient to allow the most physiologically beneficial interaction possible.[50]

Objectives and Indications

Endotracheal intubation and mechanical ventilation should be considered when pulmonary gas exchange is inadequate, as evidenced by inadequate alveolar ventilation or arterial oxygenation, or when the work of breathing is excessive and cannot be maintained. Mature clinical judgment is required to make the decision to intubate the trachea and initiate mechanical ventilation. Both the severity and the rapidity of progression of the respiratory failure should be taken into account in making the decision, in addition to the possibility of a response to other treatments. Objective measurements provide only guidelines for this decision-making process. Equal degrees of hypoxemia may respond to supplemental oxygen and diuretic therapy in some patients, but require mechanical ventilation in others. Normal arterial blood gases may be maintained in some patients with excessive work of breathing in whom mechanical ventilation should be initiated, yet some infants can tolerate extraordinary tachypnea for long periods without difficulty. Clinical objectives of mechanical ventilation include maintaining arterial oxygenation, controlling alveolar ventilation, and relieving respiratory distress.[51]

Maintenance of Arterial Oxygenation

With the other techniques available to improve arterial oxygenation, such as supplemental oxygen and continuous positive airway pressure (CPAP), this often is not the sole reason for initiating mechanical ventilation. If the arterial oxygen saturation (Sao_2) cannot be maintained greater than 90%, corresponding to a Pao_2 of about 60 mmHg, mechanical ventilation may be needed. There is no evidence that increasing the Sao_2 to levels much higher than 90% is advantageous. Lower values may be tolerated during mechanical ventilation if tissue oxygen delivery is adequate. Because the primary goal of increasing arterial oxygen levels is to improve tissue oxygenation, the other components of tissue oxygen delivery, including hemoglobin level and cardiac output, also must be considered in therapy. Higher levels of arterial oxygen may be used therapeutically in infants with pulmonary hypertension. In these circumstances, oxygen is being used for its pharmacologic properties as a pulmonary vasodilator. The toxic effects of high levels of inspired oxygen and the association of excessive oxygen use with retinopathy of prematurity always must be kept in mind. Infants with cyanotic congenital heart disease may have adequate tissue oxygen delivery in the face of severe hypoxemia as a result of the admixture of unoxygenated venous blood in the systemic circulation.

Control of Alveolar Ventilation

Alveolar hypoventilation with acute respiratory acidosis marked by a rising $Paco_2$ (above 50 to 60 mmHg) and a falling pH (below 7.20 to 7.25) requires intubation and mechanical ventilation. Once mechanical ventilation has been initiated, there is no mandatory physiologic target $Paco_2$ that must be achieved, and as long as the pH is kept above 7.20 to 7.25, hypercarbia may be part of a therapeutic strategy to limit the possibility of injury from mechanical ventilation. Deliberate hyperventilation also may be used as a therapeutic strategy (eg, hypocarbia to reduce intracranial pressure, induced alkalosis to treat pulmonary vasospasm in infants with pulmonary hypertension).

Relief of Respiratory Distress

When the work of breathing is increased by elevated airway resistance or reduced lung compliance, intubation and mechanical ventilation may be necessary. Elevated airway resistance may be at the level of the proximal airways, such as in subglottic stenosis or airway edema. In this case, mechanical bypass of the obstruction by tracheostomy or endotracheal intubation is the primary treatment. Elevated airway resistance also may be in the distal airways, as in reactive airway disease and bronchiolitis. Reduced compliance is the hallmark of RDS associated with surfactant deficiency. Mechanical ventilation may be necessary to maintain FRC and prevent atelectasis.

Other

Endotracheal intubation and mechanical ventilation may be necessary to manage excessive respiratory secretions and provide a means of suctioning. Occasionally, therapeutic bronchoscopy is indicated if multiple episodes of directed suctioning are necessary to maintain the patency of a particularly affected lung region. Mechanical ventilation permits the sedation and neuromuscular blockade that may be necessary for operative anesthesia or procedures in the ICU. Flail chest associated with chest wall instability may be stabilized by mechanical ventilation. When systemic oxygen delivery and utilization are compromised by low cardiac output, anemia, or sepsis, and hemodynamic compromise is present (ie, shock), mechanical ventilation should be instituted. Any of the causes of respiratory failure listed in Table 8-2 may require an artificial airway and mechanical ventilation.

Intubation and Artificial Airways

Definitive tracheal intubation can be accomplished by the orotracheal route, by the nasotracheal route, or with a tracheostomy. Orotracheal intubation is most readily performed. It should be preceded by preoxygenation using a bag-mask device, and the cervical spine must be protected using in-line axial stabilization whenever cervical spine injury is a possibility. Paralysis with a neuromuscular blocking agent such as vecuronium (high dose, 0.3 mg/kg) and a narcotic and amnestic combination (fentanyl 1 to 5 mg/kg and diazepam 0.1 mg/kg) ideally should be given. Awake intubation can be performed in newborns and infants. Orotracheal tubes can become dislodged relatively easily, and excursions of a centimeter or two can result in extubation or bronchial intubation in small infants. Tube size should permit a small air leak at high airway pressures. Cuffed tubes usually are not used in infants. Airway injury causing subglottic stenosis may result from excessive tube movement and snug fitting. Children with teeth may be able to occlude the endotracheal tube by biting. Nasotracheal intubation is advocated by some to reduce the risk of accidental extubation and tube biting, and to improve oral hygiene. This technique requires greater skill to manipulate the endotracheal tube into the larynx by the nasal route (by blind passage in spontaneously breathing patients or using a forceps for assistance). Nasal septal necrosis, an increased incidence of sinusitis, and inadequate tube size are potential disadvantages.

Tracheostomy should be considered when prolonged mechanical ventilation is probable. Rigid guidelines are inappropriate. If mechanical ventilation will be required for more than 2 to 3 weeks in older children, tracheostomy is warranted. Infant tracheostomy carries a higher risk of short-term problems related to airway occlusion and long-term problems related to tracheal injury. Infants may remain translaryngeally intubated for periods exceeding 1 month. Complications related to tracheostomy include obstruction caused by granulation tissue, tracheomalacia, stenosis at the cannulation site, and erosion into surrounding structures such as the innominate artery or esophagus (these are extremely uncommon in children). The method of tracheostomy is presented in Chapter 55.

Conventional Modes of Mechanical Ventilation

Infants and children with respiratory failure are cared for in several hospital settings. Newborns are treated in neonatal ICUs in cooperation with neonatologists, whereas older children are cared for in pediatric ICUs in cooperation with pediatric intensivists. In some hospitals, separate pediatric surgical ICUs exist. Many children are treated in "adult" ICUs. Each ICU develops its own strategy for mechanical ventilation based on such factors as the equipment used (ie, the brand of ventilator in that hospital) and the philosophy of ventilation of the physicians who prescribe its use. A bewildering array of equipment options is available, each with different "knobs and dials" and formidable user's manuals. Depending on the hospital setting, surgeons

may be responsible for all aspects of critical care in the ICU, or they may share responsibilities with medical intensivists. However, in any ICU setting in which surgical patients are treated, it is of utmost importance that surgeons be knowledgeable about the use of mechanical ventilators. Surgeons must critically appraise the use of mechanical ventilation in their patients.

All modern mechanical ventilators use electronic timing devices or microprocessors to control valves and flow regulators that modify the delivery of pressurized inspiratory gases to expand the lungs. The mode of ventilation is determined by the manner in which the pressure, flow, and volume of inspiratory gases are controlled, and by the use of sensors and monitors that allow the ventilator to respond to the patient's spontaneous respiratory efforts. Although there is no firm physiologic rationale for it, mechanical ventilators have evolved along two different lines: ventilators that generate flow by rapidly pressurizing the ventilator circuit (pressure-controlled or pressure-limited ventilation) and ventilators that control the flow of inspiratory gas to deliver a predetermined tidal volume (volume-controlled ventilation). Most infant ventilators have been pressure controllers that operate in a continuous-flow, time-cycled, pressure-limited mode. Most ventilators used for older children and adults have been flow-volume controllers. The current generation of standard infant, pediatric, and adult ventilators are capable of working as both pressure and volume ventilators. In addition to the pressure and volume mode, the response of the ventilator to the patient can be determined by selecting various modes of ventilation. Properties of the commonly available modes of mechanical ventilation are given in Table 8-4.

Volume-Controlled Versus Pressure-Controlled Ventilation

Idealized airway pressure, alveolar pressure, lung volume, and gas flow for volume-controlled and pressure-controlled ventilation are illustrated in Figure 8-3. During volume-controlled ventilation, modern ventilators function as flow controllers, delivering a constant flow of inspiratory gases. There is an initial instantaneous rise in the airway pressure that is caused by the airway resistance to flow. The pressure to overcome airway resistance is maintained throughout inspiration because flow is constant. Airway pressure and alveolar pressure then rise gradually as the lung expands. Lung volume corresponds to alveolar pressure according to the compliance of the lung. By design of the ventilator, flow is constant. (Inspection of control consoles on modern ventilators reveals that "sinusoidal," "ascending ramp," and "descending ramp" flow may be chosen instead of truly constant flow. These modes of ventilation should be viewed as variations of constant flow or volume ventilation. Their advantages are largely theoretic.) During pressure-controlled ventilation, the ventilator initiates a breath by instantaneously elevating the pressure within the ventilator circuit to the preset maximum inspiratory pressure. Alveolar pressure lags behind airway pressure on the basis of airway resistance to flow. Lung volume again corresponds to alveolar pressure according to the compliance of the lung. Flow is initially high, but falls rapidly (exponentially) as alveolar pressure approaches the pressure applied by the ventilator, finally ceasing (flow = 0) when there is no driving pressure between the

TABLE 8-4. *Modes of mechanical ventilation*

INTERMITTENT MANDATORY VENTILATION (IMV)

The ventilator is time cycled and delivers a breath without regard for the patient's spontaneous respiratory effort. May be volume controlled or pressure controlled. Ventilators in effect are working in this mode when patients are not breathing spontaneously, as is the the case with pharmacologic paralysis, heavy sedation, or neurologic injury.

Disadvantages: Spontaneous respiration is unlikely to be synchronous with the ventilator (because it is entirely dependent on the patient to create the synchrony). Therefore, the likelihood of patient agitation and increased work of breathing is high (ie, "fighting the ventilator"). There is a greater need for sedation and paralysis.

Careful use of this mode by experienced practitioners has been effective in the treatment of newborn respiratory failure.

ASSIST-CONTROL (A/C)

In this mode, the ventilator is intended to support every patient-initiated breath by delivering a full machine breath. A back-up control ventilatory rate is set, but the patient may breathe at any rate above this. A/C ventilation is secure because a back-up rate is set, and has the possibility of synchronizing the breathing rhythm of the patient and the ventilator. A/C mode almost always has been used with volume-controlled ventilation, but newer ventilators may have pressure-limited or pressure-targeted A/C modes in which pressure level, inspiratory time, and rate are set.

Disadvantages: Excessive patient work may be required if the ventilator cannot sense the patient's inspiratory effort. This is the primary problem encountered with infants and small children. Although A/C mode provides synchrony between the initiation of a patient breath and a machine breath, there is not necessarily synchrony between machine and patient inspiratory mechanics. Inadequate inspiratory flow may not meet patient demands, and inspiratory time (breath termination) may not coincide with that of the patient. Tachypnea and agitation result in excessive machine breaths, increased minute ventilation, and respiratory alkalosis, and may require significant sedation to control. There is potential for worsening of air-trapping in patients with obstructive lung disease.

SYNCHRONIZED INTERMITTENT MANDATORY VENTILATION (SIMV)

SIMV is used as a ventilating and weaning mode. It is the most commonly used ventilating mode for children and adults. It provides a preset number of mandatory ventilator breaths while allowing the patient to breathe spontaneously. Machine breaths are given if the patient fails to breathe spontaneously. In this mode, the ventilator awaits a patient-initiated breath for a given period; if none is sensed, the ventilator provides a breath. The ventilator does not deliver a mandatory breath while it is sensing a spontaneous breath. Spontaneous breaths are supported by fresh gas flow after the ventilator senses them, not by elevated pressure within the ventilator circuit. This means that spontaneous patient breaths, in addition to being sensed by the ventilator, must overcome the resistance of the endotracheal tube and the ventilator circuit. As with A/C mode, SIMV traditionally has been used with volume-controlled ventilation; however, newer ventilators also may offer a pressure-targeted form of SIMV. SIMV mode may be used in ventilator weaning as the level of support is reduced gradually from total to minimal.

Disadvantages: The significant work of breathing associated with SIMV mode make it unsatisfactory for use as a weaning mode for infants. There is no convincing evidence that SIMV weaning is superior to T-piece trials in weaning from mechanical ventilation.

PRESSURE-SUPPORT VENTILATION (PSV)

In the PSV mode, the patient has significant control over the delivery of the machine breath. The patient controls both breath initiation and breath termination. When the ventilator senses a patient breath, the pressure rises rapidly to a preset positive pressure that is maintained throughout the inspiration. The patient can regulate his or her own inspiratory time and tidal volume. In some ventilators, the inital pressure waveform is adjustable. Breath termination occurs when the ventilator senses deceleration of the inspiratory flow (ie, the breath is flow cycled, made possible by the incorporation of sensitive pneumotachographs into the ventilator circuit). PSV allows the patient and the ventilator to work in synchrony. PSV allows for a wide variation in the level of support provided by the ventilator. When set at high pressure levels, it can provide near total support, whereas lower levels can be used simply to compensate for the resistance of the endotracheal tube and the ventilator circuit. It has versatility as a weaning mode.

PSV may be used in combination with SIMV to decrease the work of breathing associated with spontaneous breaths.

Disadvantages: Tidal volume is not controlled in PSV and, therefore, minute ventilation is not assured. Unstable patients in whom apnea is a risk should have a back-up SIMV rate to ensure that minute ventilation is maintained. Some patients poorly tolerate the inspiratory flow patterns generated with PSV and, as with all modes of assisted ventilation, the smallest children may not be able to trigger the ventilator adequately without excessive work of breathing.

---

airways and the alveolus. During each form of mechanical ventilation, expiration is passive, driven by the elastic recoil of the lungs and chest wall.

This idealized representation does not reflect perfectly the behavior of the lungs during mechanical ventilation, because the lungs are heterogeneous and different portions have different compliance and resistance properties. In addition, in real lungs, compliance and resistance are not constant throughout the inspiration and expiration cycle, and rapid respiratory rates may not allow complete equilibration between the alveolus and the proximal airways.

Neonatal and Infant Ventilation

Time-cycled, pressure-limited infant ventilators are conceptually simple. Continuous flow is provided past the endotracheal tube adapter at rates of about 4 to 10 L/min. An adjustable fixed

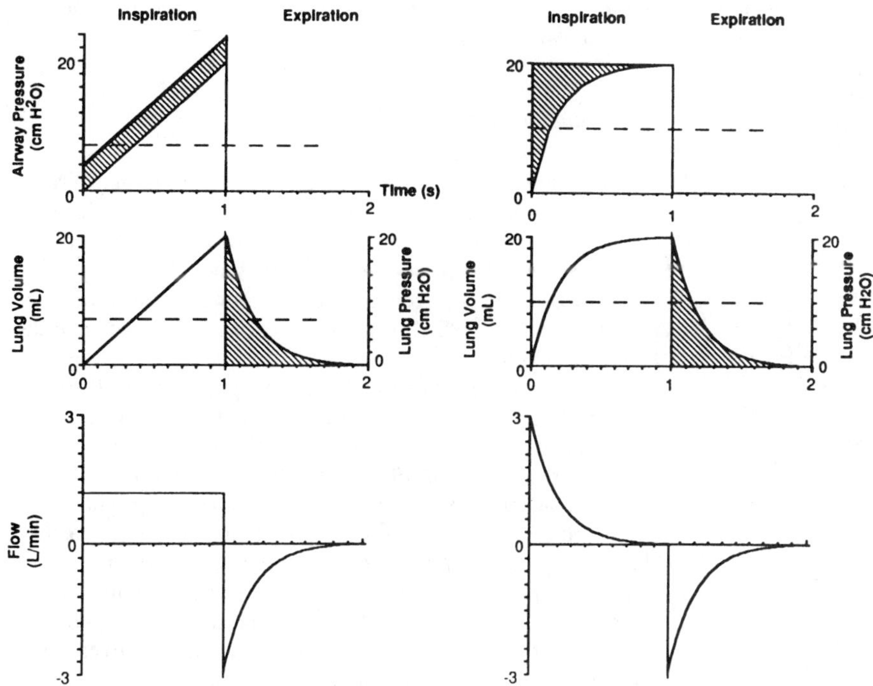

FIG. 8-3. Idealized pressure, volume, and flow during mechanical ventilation. A 20-mL tidal volume is delivered during a 1-second inspiratory time. (*Left*) Constant-inspiration flow ventilation (volume-controlled ventilation). During volume ventilation at constant flow, the initial rise in airway pressure is needed to overcome airway resistance. Thereafter, airway pressure, lung volume, and lung pressure are defined by the compliance of the lung. (*Right*) Constant inspiratory pressure ventilation (pressure-controlled ventilation). During pressure ventilation, lung volume, lung pressure, and flow are exponential functions of time. Airway peak inspiratory pressure is higher and mean airway pressure lower in volume ventilation compared with pressure ventilation. In the lungs, however, peak pressure is the same. [Shaded areas represent the pressure required to overcome flow resistance. Unshaded areas represent the pressure required to overcome elastic properties of the lung.] (Chatburn RRT. Respiratory Care 1991;36:569)

resistance is included in the expiratory limb of the ventilator to control PEEP. An occlusion valve also is present in the expiratory limb of the circuit that is controlled by a timing device. The duration of closure of the valve determines the inspiratory time, and the time between closures or the duration of expiration determines the respiratory rate. The degree of closure of the occlusion valve and the gas flow rate determine the pressure that is applied to the airways. In its most basic form, this type of ventilator is working in an intermittent mandatory ventilation (IMV) mode. The infant's spontaneous breathing efforts do not alter the operation of the ventilator. Using this mode of ventilation, tidal volume can be increased by increasing the gas flow in the ventilator circuit, lengthening the inspiratory time, or increasing the occlusion of the inspiratory valve (increase in peak inspiratory pressure). Infant ventilators of this variety are compact, relatively inexpensive, and easy to use. When properly used, they can provide adequate mechanical ventilatory support for most infants; however, certain limitations must be recognized. The actual tidal volume delivered to the infant is unknown and is affected by leaks around the noncuffed endotracheal tube. In most pressure-limited infant ventilators, tidal volume is not assured and is dependent on compliance. When compliance is zero (eg, the endotracheal tube is mechanically occluded), most infant ventilators of this variety continue to function in spite of the fact that the infant is not being ventilated. Likewise, when compliance rapidly improves (eg, after the therapeutic administration of surfactant), tidal volume can increase dramatically, and lung injury such as pneumothorax can occur. Close attention is required to prevent inadequate or excessive ventilation.

Infant ventilators with more advanced capabilities are being marketed. Technology to monitor tidal volume is available and reasonably accurate. Pressure, flow, and timing changes can be made in a more rational manner by observing the effect on tidal volume. Infant ventilators also are available that allow synchronization with the patient's ventilatory effort. During normal spontaneous respiration, the sequence of events for any breath is as follows: brain stem signal, phrenic nerve action potential, diaphragm contraction, thoracic pressure changes, and air movement. Synchronization based on pressure changes in the ventilator circuit already is beginning too late and is delayed even more by functions of the ventilator that take time, such as the triggering of pressure sensors or demand valves and the function of flow regulators. Adult ventilators usually have used pressure sensors in the ventilator circuit to determine when a spontaneous breath is initiated to "trigger" the ventilator to deliver a breath or to time the machine breaths to coincide properly with the patient's breathing. Pressure sensors have lacked the sensitivity to respond to the small pressure changes created by infant breathing. The delay inherent in this method of interaction between patient and machine is accentuated by the rapid rates at which infants breathe. When ventilator breaths must be initiated by the infant, the work of breathing may be markedly increased. Better synchronization for infant ventilators is theoretically possible by monitoring abdominal wall or chest motion, or intrathoracic pressure changes (monitored by esophageal pressure). Ventilators with sensitive inspiratory flow or pressure monitors are available that provide synchronized IMV for infants.[52,53] It is uncertain whether this mode of ventilation will result in more rapid ventilator weaning or a lower incidence of complications such as pneumothorax and intracranial hemorrhage. Infant ventilators also are available that function in a volume mode.

Ventilator settings are chosen according to the nature of the respiratory failure. In infants with relatively normal lungs, the respiratory rate is set to approximate normal breathing rates for infants of 20 to 40 breaths per minute. PEEP is used at low levels (2 to 4 cm H_2O, physiologic PEEP) to prevent the atelectasis that results when FRC is established at atmospheric pressure, such as occurs when an endotracheal tube is in place.

Inspiratory pressures are set at 12 to 20 cm H_2O, which results in "normal" lung expansion of 4 to 6 mL/kg depending on the size of the patient and the compliance of the lungs and chest wall. Inspiratory times of 0.5 to 1 second are used. Less compliant lungs may require shorter inspiratory times at higher pressures and rates to achieve adequate oxygenation and ventilation.

Pediatric Mechanical Ventilation

Volume ventilation has been used for children primarily because of product availability. The descendants of the first practical mechanical ventilators that delivered tidal volumes on the basis of a rotating crank and piston were applicable to children. Modern pediatric and adult ventilators use a combination of hardware (gas source, transducers, and flow controllers) and electronics (microprocessors) to control the flow of gas precisely and generate a variety of inspiratory waveforms. Adding somewhat to the confusion over the choice of ventilator modes, most modern ventilators used for children also are capable of working in a pressure-controlled mode.

In children with normal lungs who require mechanical ventilation, it is doubtful that the mode of ventilation is important. Typically, volume ventilation is used. Rates that approximate normal breathing are chosen, ranging from 10 to 20 breaths per minute. PEEP is chosen at low levels to prevent atelectasis (2 to 4 cm H_2O). Tidal volumes are chosen to deliver 5 to 6 mL/kg. The use of tidal volumes of 10 to 15 mL/kg is unlikely to offer any advantage over the smaller volumes that more nearly approach normal tidal volumes. However, tidal volumes up to 15 mL/kg are not harmful to normal lungs. Atelectasis is prevented by the use of PEEP and the use of sustained inspiratory pressures during respiratory care and suctioning. If the patient is breathing spontaneously, most ventilators have the ability to provide "pressure support" to overcome the work of breathing associated with the resistance of the endotracheal tube. Pressure-support breathing provides high inspiratory flows at low pressures in response to patient breaths. Because it is triggered by pressure or flow changes sensed by transducers in the ventilator circuit, it always is delayed in time from the true initiation of the patient's respiratory effort. In many patients, 2 to 5 cm H_2O of pressure support can overcome the work of breathing associated with the endotracheal tube and permit better patient-machine interaction.

In children with more severe respiratory failure and poor lung compliance, oxygenation may be inadequate using volume ventilation modes that result in high inspiratory pressures. If oxygenation cannot be supported with elevation of PEEP to 8 to 10 cm H_2O, and peak airway pressures are markedly elevated (above 35 to 40 cm H_2O), pressure-controlled ventilation should be tried. It is important to measure tidal volumes during pressure-controlled ventilation. Frequency is adjusted to maintain the Pa_{CO_2} at the highest acceptable level, and PEEP is adjusted to permit reduction of the F_{IO_2} below 0.60 if possible.

Children with reactive airway disease (bronchial asthma or bronchiolitis) may have a long time constant of ventilation and require especially long expiratory times to return to an appropriate FRC. Rapid respiratory rates result in gas-trapping, inadvertent PEEP, carbon dioxide retention, impaired venous return, and low cardiac output. This is one common form of pediatric respiratory failure that benefits from ventilation with relatively large tidal volumes at slow rates.

PEEP and Intrinsic PEEP

The application of PEEP to mechanical ventilation is a powerful mechanism to improve oxygenation and maintain arterial oxygenation on the upper portion of the oxyhemoglobin dissociation curve (oxygen delivery is increased). The use of PEEP also increases intrathoracic pressure, limiting venous return and right heart filling, which decreases cardiac output (oxygen delivery is decreased). The ultimate effect of PEEP on oxygen delivery is determined by the balance between improved arterial oxygenation and decreased cardiac output. Small amounts of PEEP usually are used, even when no lung injury is present, in an effort to maintain FRC and prevent atelectasis. (FRC decreases considerably when changing from the upright to the supine position, primarily as a result of changes in the position of the diaphragm and the redistribution of circulating blood volume to the thorax from the extremities.) The application of PEEP to injured lungs increases FRC through the distention of already ventilated alveoli and the recruitment of nonventilated terminal airspaces. PEEP may prevent airway collapse, reducing shear forces produced by the opening of coapted terminal airways. By recruiting lung volume and preventing airway collapse, PEEP improves oxygenation. PEEP is increased to allow the F_{IO_2} to be reduced to safe levels (less than 0.6). Elevation of PEEP to levels greater than 10 to 12 cm H_2O usually is not helpful. In injured lungs, the initial portion of the pressure-volume compliance curve is flat (ie, compliance is low), corresponding to the "recruitable" lung volume (alveoli that can be expanded). At a certain pressure, there is an inflection point above which the compliance curve is steep, corresponding to the inflation of the more normal portions of the lung (see Fig. 8-1). This inflection point represents a rational physiologic minimum PEEP. PEEP does not actually decrease overall lung edema, but may result in a redistribution of fluid from the alveoli to the interstitial space. By augmenting mean airway pressure, it may avoid the use of large tidal volumes and counteract the hydrostatic forces that tend to collapse the dependent portions of the lung in diffuse lung injury. The effect on preload probably is the primary reason for the reduction in cardiac output with PEEP; however, right ventricular afterload also is increased from the elevation of pulmonary vascular resistance associated with PEEP. Cardiac output can be augmented by volume loading and the use of inotropes, although hypervolemia should be avoided. The elevated intrathoracic pressure associated with the use of PEEP also may impede venous return from the head, elevate intracranial pressure, and reduce cerebral blood flow. There is some evidence that PEEP augments the transcapillary migration of leukocytes in the lung as a result of compression of the pulmonary capillaries by the distended alveoli.[54]

The difference between alveolar pressure and proximal airway pressure at end-expiration is referred to as auto-PEEP (the terms *intrinsic PEEP, air trapping,* and *dynamic hyperinflation* also are used to refer to this phenomenon). Alveolar pressure remains higher than external PEEP throughout expiration, and consequently, expiratory flow continues until the onset of the next inspiration. Dynamic hyperinflation occurs most commonly in the setting of severe obstruction to airflow. Under such circumstances, expiratory resistance may be several times that of inspiratory resistance, and the expiratory time constant is correspondingly long. It has effects similar to those of extrinsic PEEP and may cause the tidal volume to cycle near total lung capacity (ie, when compliance is reduced and the risk of overdistention lung injury is greater). It also may reduce cardiac output.

Continuous Positive Airway Pressure

The application of continuous pressure throughout the respiratory cycle increases FRC, improves and stabilizes oxygenation, and may assist in maintaining the patency of the upper airway by its splinting action on the hypopharynx. CPAP can be delivered through an endotracheal tube, a hypopharyngeal tube, nasal prongs, or a head box. In older children and adults, a mask can be used. CPAP is used to treat the apnea of prematurity and mild RDS that does not require endotracheal intubation. It also is useful as a mode of weaning from mechanical ventilation. In addition, patients with sleep apnea may benefit from CPAP. Pressures in the range of 2 to 6 cm H_2O are used.

Newer Modes of Mechanical Ventilation

Conventional mechanical ventilation depends on the bulk flow of ventilating gases to deliver tidal volumes to the distal lung, where gas exchange takes place. In diseased lungs, these strategies may not provide adequate oxygenation or clearance of carbon dioxide. High airway pressures may result in alveolar overdistention and lung injury. When conventional ventilators are used at progressively higher rates, inadequate expiratory times result in gas trapping, with its deleterious consequences. By using noncompliant tubing and a ventilator with hardware capable of delivering small tidal volumes rapidly, along with the appropriate choice of inspiratory time, conventional ventilation can be performed at rates up to about 150 breaths per minute. Beyond this rate, ventilators that rely on unusual physical properties of the movement of gases through conducting systems must be used. These devices use rates typically between 5 and 15 Hz (300 to 900 breaths per minute). By using ventilator frequencies that are much higher than usual, along with small tidal volumes, adequate oxygenation and ventilation can be provided in a less injurious manner. High-frequency ventilation may help to prevent the wide swings in lung volume (in which collapsed alveoli are recruited with each tidal volume) and alveolar overdistention that have been implicated in ventilator-induced lung injury.[55]

The two forms of high-frequency ventilation that have been used extensively in children, high-frequency jet ventilation (HFJV) and HFOV, deliver small tidal volumes. The tidal volumes produced by these ventilatory modes are smaller than the conventionally understood dead space of the lung. Intuitively, this seems impossible, and it does violate the fundamental requirement of bulk flow conventional mechanical ventilation that alveolar ventilation is the product of the frequency and the difference between tidal volume and dead-space volume ($V_A = f[V_T - V_D]$). Mechanisms in addition to conventionally understood bulk flow of gases must be invoked.[56,57] These mechanisms are similar for HFJV and HFOV, but have been mathematically modeled most satisfactorily for HFOV. The feasibility of these modes depends on the behavior of gases in conducting systems of narrow diameter subjected to rapid pressure changes. A combination of several mechanisms may be responsible for the transport of gas to provide ventilation at these rapid rates:

1. Bulk convectional flow is responsible for part of the movement of gas into the large airways and subsequently into proximally located alveolar units.
2. *Taylor dispersion* is a complex physical phenomenon that describes the movement of gases when high-velocity flow alternates between laminar flow and turbulent flow, resulting in net gas transport.
3. *Pendelluft* refers to the mixing of gases among lung units with different impedance characteristics (ie, different time constants). It may be responsible for considerable movement of gases at the distal airway level.
4. The vibratory action of the heart itself may improve the mixing of gases in the distal airways.
5. Gas mixing in the terminal airspaces probably is governed by molecular diffusion during high-frequency ventilation, just as it is during conventional ventilation.
6. Asymmetric velocity profiles are conceptually the easiest mechanism to account for the flow of gases during high-frequency ventilation.

If the gas flow profile is parabolic during the inspiratory phase of the ventilatory cycle and square during the expiratory phase, there can be a net forward flow of gas in the center of the airway and a coaxially oriented flow around the periphery in the opposite direction (Fig. 8-4). Rather than flowing in and out of the conducting system, as is the case in conventional tidal volume ventilation, the moving gas distributes itself within the conducting system such that flow away from the driving pressure source (ie, toward the peripheral airways) is found in the center of the conducting system, whereas return flow (from the peripheral airways) swirls around the periphery of the conducting system. Oxygenation is understood more easily during the use of high-frequency techniques. Simply maintaining the alveolar units open in the presence of oxygen-containing gas mixtures results in adequate oxygenation under most circumstances. Totally collapsed or fluid-filled alveoli (V/Q ratio = 0) still result in hypoxia, but the mean airway pressure in the ventilator circuit functions as "constant PEEP," maximizing oxygenation.

During high-frequency ventilation, oxygenation is largely dependent on mean airway pressure (mean alveolar pressure), as it is during conventional ventilation. Alveolar ventilation is a function of frequency (f) and tidal volume (V_T):

$$\text{alveolar ventilation} = k(f \times V_T n)$$

where: k = small proportionality constant
n approaches 2 as nonbulk flow mechanisms of gas transport become more important

Because k is small, the ventilator output ($f \times V_T$) must be large compared with conventional ventilation.

HFJV uses a high-pressure source to deliver gas through a small-bore cannula incorporated into the infant's endotracheal tube. The Bunell Life Pulse (Salt Lake City, UT) is the most

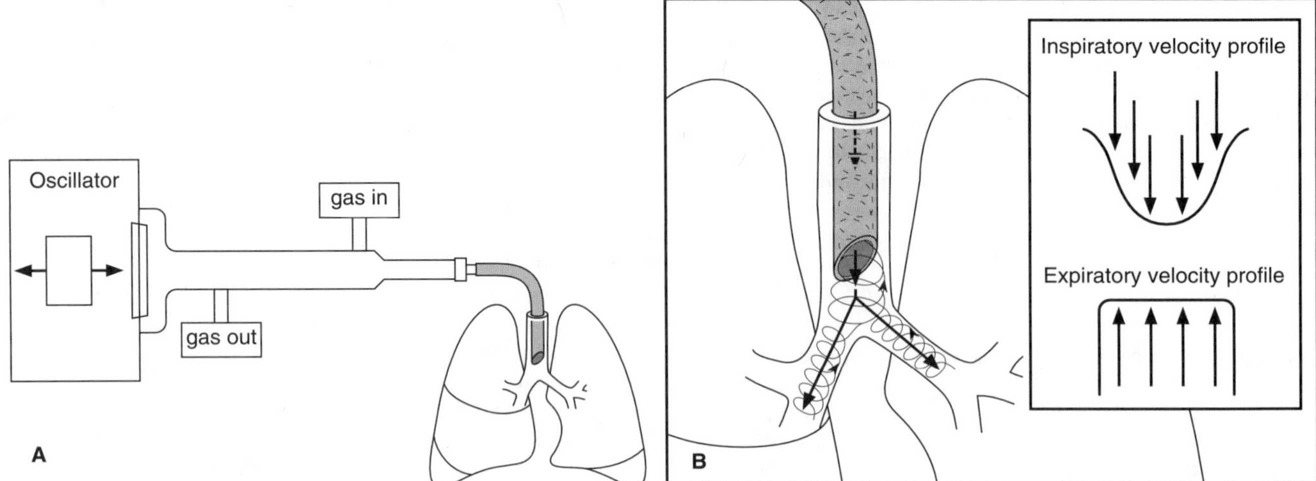

FIG. 8-4. (*A*) High-frequency ventilation schematic: oscillatory movement applied to gas flowing within the ventilator circuit. (*B*) Asymmetric inspiratory and expiratory velocity profiles result in net gas movement in different parts of the conducting system, with inspiratory flow located more centrally and expiratory flow oriented coaxially. Other mechanisms also account for gas transport during high-frequency ventilation (see text).

widely used infant jet ventilator. Using frequencies of 150 to 600 breaths per minute, jet "drive" pressure, inspiratory time, and PEEP are used to control oxygenation and ventilation. Exhalation is passive. Predicting the response to changes in ventilator settings can be difficult during HFJV because tidal volume cannot be measured accurately. Equivalent gas exchange is achieved at lower peak and mean airway pressures. Clinical parameters are used to guide ventilator changes. HFJV results in more rapid resolution of interstitial emphysema and decreases the output from bronchopleural fistulas. Ventilation may be efficient and respiratory alkalosis can occur. Air trapping may limit the application of HFJV and humidification is difficult. Controlled trials have not indicated a clear-cut advantage of HFJV in treating newborn RDS compared with conventional ventilation. It is used primarily as a salvage therapy for patients in whom conventional ventilation fails.

The SensorMedics 3100 (Yorba Linda, CA) is available for infant and pediatric oscillatory ventilation. HFOV delivers small tidal volumes at high rates using the to-and-fro motion of a rapidly cycling piston pump or an acoustic speaker as an energy source. Unlike other forms of mechanical ventilation, it provides active exhalation by the ventilator. Pressure oscillations are superimposed on an adjustable airway pressure that is controlled by altering the gas flow into the circuit (bias flow) and the outflow resistance of the ventilator circuit. Oscillator frequency is controlled between 200 and 1000 breaths per minute (3 to 18 Hz). Piston displacement, which generates the ventilator pressure amplitude and percent inspiratory time, are under user control. As with HFJV, tidal volume is difficult to control and depends on many factors. Clinical parameters must be used to guide ventilator changes.

In an initial randomized, prospective study of HFOV, this technique showed no advantage over conventional ventilation in the treatment of newborn RDS and was associated with increased intraventricular hemorrhage, dampening the enthusiasm of many practitioners.[58] Subsequent studies using the SensorMedics device have suggested greater safety and improved outcome.[59] Other reports have demonstrated the usefulness of HFOV in pediatric patients.[60,61]

Other modes of mechanical ventilation, such as inverse ratio ventilation and airway pressure release ventilation, have not found wide application in infants and children.

Permissive Hypercapnia

Physicians customarily measure and respond to blood gas tensions in monitoring mechanical ventilation. Because the Pa_{CO_2} and Pa_{O_2} always appear adjacent to each other on laboratory reports and bedside flow charts, and because the clinically relevant values are in similar ranges (eg, 40 to 80 mmHg), they tend to be thought of similarly. However, hypoxia and hypercarbia do not represent equal threats to patients. The human body stores little oxygen in the blood or lungs. In the absence of breathing, if no supplemental oxygen is administered, stores are depleted in minutes, metabolic acidosis develops as anaerobic metabolism begins, and hypoxic tissue injury occurs. Intolerant organs such as the brain and heart suffer irreversible damage promptly; other organs, such as muscle and skin, may tolerate hours of hypoxia. In contrast, when hypercarbia is not accompanied by hypoxia, it often is well tolerated. Blood pH is inversely proportional to the blood CO_2 content, and not to the Pa_{CO_2}. It is true that the Pa_{CO_2} and the CO_2 content are linearly related over much of the physiologic range of changes in the Pa_{CO_2}, and pH falls as the Pa_{CO_2} rises, up to a Pa_{CO_2} of about 80 mmHg. However, as the Pa_{CO_2} continues to rise beyond this level, the CO_2 content does not rise linearly and pH is less affected. In spontaneously breathing patients, progressive hypercarbia results in narcosis, further respiratory depression, and, ultimately, hypoxia, with all its serious consequences. In patients undergoing mechanical ventilation, hypercarbia is well tolerated, especially if it is allowed to progress gradually. Normal renal compensation for acidosis results in bicarbonate retention and the development of a compensatory metabolic alkalosis. A Pa_{CO_2} of greater than 100 mmHg is well tolerated in otherwise healthy individuals who are maintained apneic but normoxic by the intratracheal insufflation of oxygen during bronchoscopy.

As recently as 10 years ago, the standard practice of mechanical ventilation used "target" blood gas determinations to guide the choice of ventilator settings in all patients. A normal Pa_{CO_2} is 40 mmHg, and mechanical ventilation was used to create similar levels of Pa_{CO_2}. This tactic works well in situations in which the lung is not severely injured. In conditions of severe lung impairment, such as adult RDS or respiratory failure of prematurity, the cost of maintaining normocarbia in terms of further damage to the lungs may be extremely high. In such pathologic states, in which ventilation is directed primarily at the most normal remaining lung, the regional hyperventilation required to achieve arterial normocarbia may be injurious. High volumes of inflation with alveolar overdistention and local tissue alkalosis are implicated in this process. Potential deleterious effects of hypercapnia include headache, somnolence, coma, increased cerebral blood flow, increased intracranial pressure, pulmonary hypertension, systemic hypertension, electrolyte abnormalities, and excessive acidosis with myocardial dysfunction.

With proper patient selection, permissive hypercapnia can be applied safely to the treatment of respiratory failure. Its use may lessen the injury of mechanical ventilation superimposed on the already injured lungs of patients with respiratory failure. Guidelines have been published for the use of mechanical ventilation in adults with RDS.[51] These include maintaining the Sa_{O_2} above 90%, reducing the tidal volume to maintain inspiratory plateau pressures of less than 35 cm H_2O if possible, and, if no contraindication exists, allowing the gradual rise of the Pa_{CO_2} that accompanies the lowering of the tidal volume. There are no consensus statements regarding the use of permissive hypercapnia in the treatment of neonates and children with diffuse lung injury. Many neonatologists have become more accepting of hypercapnia in premature infants with lung immaturity and RDS, but practices vary widely among the neonatologists, intensivists, and surgeons who direct mechanical ventilation.

Supplemental Carbon Dioxide Ventilation

In some circumstances, hypocarbia may be specifically harmful and some degree of hypercarbia beneficial. Infants with cyanotic congenital heart disease who undergo construction of a systemic-to-pulmonary artery shunt may be exquisitely sensitive to changes in pulmonary vascular resistance. Hypocarbia may cause pulmonary vascular resistance to fall and result in excessive pulmonary blood flow, "flooding" of the lungs, and inadequate systemic perfusion. However, oxygenation may suffer and atelectasis result if small tidal volumes and slow ventilator rates are chosen. The addition of dead space to prevent hypocarbia is difficult to control precisely. Supplemental carbon dioxide, added to the ventilator gas supply, allows these infants to be ventilated with volumes that maintain lung inflation and prevent atelectasis while the Pa_{CO_2} is controlled precisely.[62]

Liquid Ventilation

Pulmonary surfactant deficiency and abnormal surfactant function are implicated in the pathogenesis of infant and adult respiratory failure and result in decreased lung compliance and atelectasis. Liquid ventilation, using perfluorocarbons, replaces the gas phase of the lung with liquid and delivers liquid tidal volumes. Gas exchange is accomplished by circulating the perfluorocarbons through a membrane lung, where oxygen is added and carbon dioxide removed. The high solubility of oxygen and carbon dioxide in perfluorocarbons allows adequate gas exchange to take place at the (fluid-filled) alveolar-capillary membrane. The biologic inertness of perfluorocarbons prevents damage to the lungs. Elimination of the air–fluid interface in the terminal airway and alveolus greatly reduces surface tension and improves lung compliance. Specialized equipment is necessary to provide liquid ventilation. In addition, the work of breathing is high because of the high resistance associated with liquid viscosity, making spontaneous breathing impossible. Perfluorocarbon liquid ventilation has been shown to improve lung mechanics and gas exchange in animal studies and in a few premature human infants.[63] A modification of liquid ventilation using intratracheally administered perfluorocarbons combined with conventional mechanical ventilation (ie, liquid FRC and gas tidal volumes) has been shown to improve lung mechanics and gas exchange.[64,65] This technique is referred to as perfluorocarbon-associated gas exchange or partial liquid ventilation. This technique is especially intriguing because it requires no special apparatus to implement. It is uncertain what role liquid ventilation and partial liquid ventilation will play in the treatment of respiratory failure.

Discontinuation of Mechanical Ventilation

The need to institute mechanical ventilation often is obvious, whereas the determination that mechanical ventilation can be withdrawn safely may be far less straightforward. The term *weaning* usually is used to describe the gradual reduction of mechanical support and the assumption by the patient of the work of breathing. Support may be withdrawn abruptly when mechanical ventilation is used temporarily in situations such as general anesthesia as soon as the effects of the anesthetics resolve. What physicians refer to as weaning actually may be the discovery that the patient has the capacity to support gas exchange adequately without the assistance of the ventilator. Often, the gradual withdrawal of mechanical support coincides with the reduced work of breathing that results from improved compliance of the recovering lung. In some instances, such as chronic respiratory insufficiency and prolonged ventilator support, weaning may be a form of gradual reconditioning of the respiratory muscles to accept the demands of spontaneous breathing. Discontinuation of mechanical ventilation should not be attempted until shock has been reversed, heart failure has been controlled, compliance is nearly normal, and any precipitant cause of respiratory failure has been treated or eliminated.

Certain aspects of mechanical ventilation may make it particularly difficult to determine when a patient is able to be liberated from the ventilator. The small endotracheal tubes used for infants and children have high resistance to airflow, making it excessively difficult for them to breathe spontaneously. The

TABLE 8-5. *Predictive indices of successful weaning from mechanical ventilation*

$Pa_{O_2} \geq 60$ mmHg with $F_IO_2 \leq 0.35$
Pa_{O_2}/F_IO_2 ratio >200
Alveolar-arterial oxygen gradient <350 mmHg
Maximum inspiratory pressure (negative inspiratory force) in excess of 30 mmHg
Minute ventilation <10 L/min (adults)
Maximum voluntary ventilation (MVV) more than twice the resting minute ventilation
Vital capacity 10–15 mL/kg
Rapid shallow breathing index (frequency/tidal volume (liters) <100 predicts successful weaning)
"Weaning index" is an integrative index that incorporates a measure of ventilatory endurance and an index of gas exchange
CROP index incorporates compliance, rate, oxygenation, and pressure measurements.

Modified from Tobin MJ, Alex CG. Discontinuation of mechanical ventilation. In: Tobin MJ, ed. Principles and practice of mechanical ventilation. New York; McGraw-Hill, 1994:1177.

decision to remove an endotracheal tube is by definition empiric, representing a best guess that it will be tolerated by the patient.

Several predictive indices have been proposed to assist in discontinuance of mechanical ventilation. These indices have been used primarily in adults and are only somewhat helpful in children. They offer limited help in the weaning of infants from the ventilator. The number of indices and the continual appearance of new ones is evidence that none is able to predict accurately when a given patient can be liberated safely from mechanical ventilation. The indices are summarized in Table 8-5.[66] These predictive indices do not evaluate the patient's upper airway function, which is of critical importance in sustaining spontaneous respiration.

Several techniques of discontinuing mechanical ventilatory support commonly are used, including spontaneous respiration through the endotracheal tube ("T-tube trials" with or without CPAP), IMV weaning, and pressure-support ventilation.[67] The response of the patient to T-tube breathing for as little as 30 minutes or as long as several hours has been used to assist in the decision to extubate. T-tube breathing is tolerated poorly by infants and may be supplemented by CPAP. The high resistance of the endotracheal tube and ventilator circuit limit the applicability of this method to infants and smaller children. In IMV weaning, the ventilator rate is decreased progressively and the patient is required to provide more of the work of breathing. When low rates are achieved, the decision is made to extubate. The work of breathing associated with spontaneous respiration through a small, high-resistance endotracheal tube and IMV ventilatory support may be excessive. In general, the smaller the patient, the higher the rate at which IMV weaning is stopped and extubation attempted. The use of pressure-support ventilation as a weaning mode alone, or in conjunction with IMV, allows the work of breathing to be shared between the patient and the ventilator. Pressure-support ventilation assists the patient's spontaneous ventilation and may be adjusted to low levels intended to overcome the resistance of the endotracheal tube and the ventilator circuit. Even with the aid of predictive indices

and weaning techniques, the decision to discontinue mechanical ventilation and extubate the patient remains empiric. Experienced clinical judgment and observation of the patient's response to changes in the level of mechanical ventilator support are necessary to predict the ability of a given patient to tolerate extubation. Each extubation is an experiment based on the hypothesis that the patient is capable of supporting spontaneous ventilation.

Factors that affect the success of weaning include the degree of residual lung disease present, the degree of immaturity in premature infants, and the neurologic status of the patient. Adequate nutritional support is an essential component of successful ventilator weaning. In theory, overfeeding can result in excessive carbon dioxide production through lipogenesis, increasing ventilation requirements. In a patient with no ventilatory reserve, this may hinder weaning from mechanical ventilation. In practice, nutritional support that results in the gradual accrual of lean body mass (slow weight gain in a fluid-stable patient) does not hinder ventilator weaning. After mechanical ventilation has been discontinued, CPAP may help support oxygenation and maintain a patent airway in infants. Dexamethasone may decrease airway edema after extubation, whereas caffeine and theophylline are respiratory stimulants that may enhance respiratory drive.

Paralysis and Sedation

The use of neuromuscular blocking agents varies greatly among ICUs. They are used most often in conjunction with analgesics, sedatives, and amnestics in the ICU setting to facilitate mechanical ventilation and reduce the risk of accidental extubation. They also are used in the ICU to facilitate endotracheal intubation, to prevent motion in patients undergoing procedures and those with indwelling devices or tenuous surgical repairs, to reduce intracranial pressure, to prevent combativeness and agitation that cannot be controlled with analgesics and sedatives, to assist in the treatment of muscular rigidity (eg, tetanus), and to limit V_{O_2} in patients with hemodynamic instability (especially important when there is a risk of shivering with its attendant dramatic elevation in metabolic rate).[68,69]

Although there is an ever-growing array of non-depolarizing neuromuscular blocking agents available, pancuronium and vecuronium remain the most commonly used agents in ICUs. Typically, pancuronium is administered as intermittent bolus therapy because of its long duration of action (up to several hours), whereas vecuronium often is given by constant infusion. These agents bind to the postsynaptic nicotinic cholinergic receptors on the motor end plate at the neuromuscular junction and inhibit the binding of acetylcholine, producing neuromuscular blockade. Neuromuscular blockade monitoring, although used in only a few ICUs, is the safest method to determine the level of blockade and prevent excessive drug administration. Using the "train-of-four" technique (four twitches with supramaximal stimulus at a 0.5-second interval), bolus therapy with neuromuscular blocking agents should not be administered until at least a single twitch returns. Continuous therapy should be titrated to retain one or two twitches. Administering bolus therapy at the return of spontaneous movement is a common practice. Neuromuscular blocking agents typically undergo some degree of hepatic metabolism and require some degree of renal elimination, and must be used cautiously in patients with hepatic and renal insufficiency. In addition, there are active 3-hydroxy metabolites of both pancuronium and vecuronium that may accumulate with prolonged administration. In addition to a prolonged duration of action based on excessive dosing, poor elimination, and the accumulation of active metabolites, a second, more serious pattern of neuromuscular dysfunction has been recognized with the prolonged use of neuromuscular blocking agents. An acute generalized myopathy has been reported in several adult patients that appears to be related to the concurrent use of these agents and corticosteroids. Great caution should be exercised when neuromuscular blocking agents are used in the presence of renal failure or concurrently with steroids.[70]

Opioid and benzodiazepine combinations frequently are used to provide analgesia and sedation during mechanical ventilation. Opioids are excellent analgesics and also have sedative, respiratory depressant, and antitussive effects that facilitate mechanical ventilation. The respiratory depressant effects may hinder weaning from mechanical ventilation, whereas hypotension is the primary adverse hemodynamic response. Morphine and fentanyl are the most commonly used opioids in the ICU. Benzodiazepines provide sedation and amnesia, but also may add to the confusion and disorientation associated with ICU care. Diazepam is administered appropriately as intermittent therapy, titrated to effect, because of its long half-life. Midazolam frequently is used as a continuous infusion. The safety of long-term continuous infusion of fentanyl and midazolam, and their effects on development are unknown.

Monitoring of Patients on Mechanical Ventilation

In addition to physical assessment and cardiorespiratory monitoring, patients who undergo mechanical ventilation require monitoring of oxygenation and ventilation. Traditionally, arterial blood gas measurement consisting of three measured values (Po_2, Pco_2, and pH) and various calculated values (HCO_3^-, base excess) has been used to guide the changes made in ventilator settings during mechanical ventilation. The availability of noninvasive monitoring devices has allowed mechanical ventilation to be performed safely with far less need for arterial blood gas determination. The end-tidal carbon dioxide level reflects the alveolar Pco_2 and correlates closely with the $Paco_2$ under most circumstances. Peripheral pulse oximetry provides reliable and accurate information about Sao_2. It does not allow hyperoxia to be assessed. The instantaneous information it provides about the most critical component of survival, adequacy of oxygenation, has made it indispensable as a monitoring method in critical care, in anesthesia, and during transport of sick patients. Transcutaneous electrodes measure the cutaneous Po_2 and Pco_2, which correlate with arterial values over the ranges usually encountered clinically.

Although not often required in the treatment of children with respiratory failure, invasive cardiac monitoring may be necessary to optimize cardiac output in mechanically ventilated children. Pulmonary artery catheters with the capacity to measure mixed venous oxygen saturation (Svo_2) provide the most important physiologic information about the relation between tissue oxygen supply and oxygen utilization. Right atrial oxygen saturation correlates well with pulmonary artery saturation and may provide useful information in patients with central venous cath-

eters without the need to pass a pulmonary artery catheter (see Chap. 7).

Phrenic Nerve Stimulation and Other Ventilatory Assist Devices

Electrical stimulation of the phrenic nerve can be used to provide ventilatory support to patients who otherwise are dependent on long-term mechanical ventilator support.[71] Infants and children who may benefit from diaphragmatic pacing include those with high spinal cord injuries, central hypoventilation syndromes (including sleep apnea and Ondine's curse), spinal muscle atrophy, and idiopathic diaphragmatic paralysis. Electrodes are placed on the phrenic nerve through a cervical incision in older children and through a thoracotomy in infants and small children. These electrodes are attached to a radio receiver implanted under the skin on the anterior chest wall. A radio frequency transmitter sends signals and power through an external antenna placed over the receiver. Bursts of electrical pulses applied to the phrenic nerve result in contraction of the diaphragm and inhalation. The only commercially available device is from Avery Laboratories in Glen Cove, New York. It has been shown that diaphragmatic pacing can be performed safely for more than 20 years, that many patients who undergo diaphragmatic pacing no longer require tracheostomy, and that there may be a cost savings related to decreased needs for intensive care. More than 200 children have undergone implantation of these devices.

Negative-pressure ventilators, negative-pressure assist devices, and nonintubated positive-pressure breathing using custom mouthpieces may be helpful in patients with neuromuscular diseases.[72,73] Expiratory assist devices (to generate artificial cough and enhance clearance of secretions) also are available. Glossopharyngeal breathing (gulping, frog-breathing) represents a method of generating tidal volume (6 to 10 gulps of 60 to 100 mL each) that does not use the conventional muscles of respiration.

Philosophy of Mechanical Ventilation

The clinical practice of mechanical ventilation varies from those who stress complete control of the patient's ventilatory function through the liberal use of sedatives and paralysis (often using paralysis as a sedative) to those who seek to intervene as little as possible in the spontaneous respiration of the patient and merely support that effort as necessary.[74] There may be specific times and circumstances when each of these techniques is needed, but this author's personal bias is for an approach that recognizes that mechanical ventilation can cause great harm as well as good and should be used with a sense of trepidation. There are clear trends among those who practice critical care indicating a greater recognition of the harmful effects of mechanical ventilation, as evidenced by the abundance of published articles that discuss the injury of pressure and overdistention on healthy and diseased lungs. In addition, when there is a lack of "cooperation" between the patient and the ventilator, the machine should be implicated first and altered (by changing the settings, mode, or type of ventilator). The decision to force the patient to cooperate (paralysis) should be made thoughtfully.

EXTRACORPOREAL LIFE SUPPORT FOR THE MANAGEMENT OF RESPIRATORY FAILURE

The short-term application of extracorporeal circulation using a mechanical pump and an artificial means of gas exchange ushered in the modern era of cardiac surgery. The development of membrane oxygenators using a gas-permeable surface to avoid direct contact between blood and gas phases opened the door to long-term ECLS. Two important developments have occurred over the past 25 years: the technology of ECLS has been refined to the point that injured lungs can be supported for several days or, if necessary, several weeks in newborns, children, and adults; and patient populations with potentially reversible respiratory failure have been identified for whom ECLS can be used with reasonable hope of lung recovery.[75,76] Because prolonged extracorporeal circulation may involve all lung functions and may not use membrane oxygenators, the term *extracorporeal life support* (ECLS) is preferred over *extracorporeal membrane oxygenation* (ECMO) to describe prolonged extracorporeal circulation without thoracotomy.

Abbreviated History of ECLS

The earliest devices to substitute for the function of the heart and lungs, heart–lung machines, exposed blood directly to gas mixtures to provide oxygenation and carbon dioxide removal. Extracorporeal circulation was provided by the insertion of a cannula directly into the heart or great vessels. Extracorporeal circulation for cardiac surgery using these devices was limited to several hours' duration. A time-dependent response occurred that resulted in thrombocytopenia, hemolysis, coagulopathy, generalized edema, and multiorgan failure. The first attempts to separate the blood phase from the gas phase (similar to what occurs in the native lung) used semipermeable membranes, such as cellophane or polyethylene. Silicone rubber membranes (dimethylpolysiloxane) with much greater permeability to oxygen and carbon dioxide allowed practical membrane oxygenators to be built in the 1960s. In the absence of direct gas exposure to blood, extracorporeal circulation could be carried out for weeks without hemolysis, significant capillary leak, or organ deterioration. In addition, the use of partial heparinization was important in the development of ECLS. Heparin anticoagulation sufficient to produce an infinite clotting time had been used since the development of the first heart–lung machines. Much lower doses of heparin could be used safely for long-term ECLS. Heparin administration then could be regulated to prevent thrombosis in the extracorporeal circuit with a prolonged but measurable clotting time, reducing bleeding complications.

A method to support the failing lungs had such far-reaching implications that enormous interest was generated in developing these techniques. In 1975, the National Institutes of Health ECMO study, a multicenter, prospective, randomized study of ECMO in life-threatening respiratory failure in adults, was begun. The study was terminated at 92 patients (less than one-third the projected study size) when the survival rates of the ECMO and control groups both were less than 10%.[27] Death frequently was the result of technical complications, and autopsies uniformly revealed extensive pulmonary fibrosis (ie, an irreversible injury). As a result of the study findings, ECMO

therapy for adults essentially ceased in the United States. The application of ECMO to patients who already had irreversible pulmonary fibrosis did not work.

Bartlett and colleagues foresaw the application of the technique to a select population of patients with life-threatening respiratory failure that was reversible.[77] Neonates with respiratory failure characterized by pulmonary hypertension with right-to-left hypoxic shunting were amenable to ECLS treatment. The nature of respiratory failure in neonates was such that there was a rapid progression to death before irreversible lung injury occurred (ie, before mechanical ventilation had been used for an extended period, with its resultant injury). The technique of neonatal ECLS involved the extrathoracic cannulation of the right internal jugular vein and right common carotid artery for partial venoarterial cardiopulmonary bypass. Partial heparinization using a whole blood activated clotting time was used to prevent circuit thrombosis and minimize hemorrhagic complications. The most physiologically significant concept to come from this experience was that of *lung rest.* It became apparent that even profoundly injured lungs could recover if they were allowed to heal without the application of high-pressure mechanical ventilation and high concentrations of oxygen.

More recently, venovenous extracorporeal support using a single cannula placed in the internal jugular vein has been used to provide extracorporeal support with excellent results in newborns.[78] With the success of ECLS in newborns, ECLS is being applied to both pediatric and adult patients for respiratory support at some centers. The ECLS techniques also have been used for prolonged cardiac support on a more limited basis in patients of all ages. Key events in the history of ECLS are presented in Table 8-6.[79]

Physiology

Hemodynamics and Characteristics of Different Methods

During venoarterial ECLS, venous blood is drained from the central circulation, pumped through an artificial lung, and returned to a central artery (Fig. 8-5*A*). Blood bypasses the pulmonary circulation. Both cardiac and pulmonary function can be supported with venoarterial bypass. The total aortic blood flow reflects a combination of the pump flow and the native cardiac output. The Cao_2 and Po_2 in systemic arteries result from the relative contribution of oxygen delivery from these two sources. During venoarterial bypass, essentially nonpulsatile flow is delivered by the extracorporeal circuit into the aorta or its branches. The resulting pulse contour of the arterial pressure wave is dampened. However, it is unusual for the arterial pressure trace to be flat, because 10% to 50% of the total aortic flow is contributed by the native cardiac output.

During venovenous ECLS, venous blood is circulated through the artificial lung and returned to the venous circulation. A separate vein, most often the common femoral vein, has been used for returning oxygenated blood to the body. A single-lumen catheter system that alternates venous drainage with the reinfusion of oxygenated blood also has been used. A single catheter with two lumens that allows continuous drainage and reinfusion has been developed for newborn ECLS, and now is used routinely (see Fig. 8-5*B*). During venovenous bypass,

TABLE 8-6. *Key events in the history of Extracoporeal Life Support for respiratory failure*

Date	Event
1965–1975	Unsuccessful attempts to support infants with both bubble and membrane oxygenators
1972	First successful treatment of adult respiratory distress syndrome with ECMO using partial venoarterial bypass for 3 days by Hill
1975	First neonatal ECMO survivor at University of California-Irvine, by Bartlett and colleagues
1975	Copenhagen meeting of ECMO investigators hosted by Zapol and Qvist
1975–1979	National Institutes of Health ECMO study of adults with respiratory failure shows 10% survival rate in treatment and control groups
1979	First neonatal ECMO seminar leading to the development of ECMO research teams in Richmond, Pittsburgh, and Detroit
1980	Neonatal ECMO project moves from California to University of Michigan in Ann Arbor
1982	Forty-five newborn cases with 23 survivors reported by Bartlett and colleagues
1985, 1989	Randomized, prospective studies of ECMO for neonatal respiratory failure show superiority to conventional therapy
1986	Gattinoni reports 49% survival rate using extracorporeal carbon dioxide removal in the adult respiratory distress syndrome; others report similar results
1988	Treatment of select adult patients resumes in United States
1988	ECMO registry report: 795 cases at 18 centers with greater than 80% survival rate
1989	Extracorporeal Life Support Organization (ELSO) study group formed
1995	Overall survival rate of 81% in nearly 10,000 newborns

Cilley RE, Bartlett RH. Extracorporeal life support for respiratory failure. In: Gravlee GP, Davis RF, Utley JR, eds. Cardiopulmonary bypass: principles and practice. Baltimore, Williams & Wilkens, 1993:655.
ECMO, extracorporeal membrane oxygenation.

oxygenated venous blood is returned to the venous circulation and mixed with systemic venous blood, raising its oxygen content. Some of this oxygenated venous blood returns to the extracorporeal circuit through recirculation, whereas most enters the right ventricle and traverses the pulmonary vasculature, or is shunted, to the left heart and finally to the systemic arterial circulation. Venovenous ECLS is limited by the amount of systemic venous return that can be "captured" by the extracorporeal circuit. If insufficient systemic venous return is removed by the venous cannula, adequate support may not be achieved. Venovenous ECLS depends solely on the cardiac output to provide flow, and is most useful in pure respiratory failure or in respiratory failure that is accompanied by cardiac failure that is solely attributable to hypoxia or to the excessive intrathoracic pressures generated by mechanical ventilation.

Arteriovenous bypass has not found practical clinical application. The concept of an artificial placenta is appealing, and has been investigated in lambs.[80]

Tissue Oxygen Delivery During Extracorporeal Support

Vo_2 reflects the aerobic metabolic activity of tissues. Newborns use 5 to 8 mL/kg/min of oxygen, children use 4 to 6 mL/kg/min, and adults use 3 to 5 mL/kg/min. Vo_2 is decreased by hypothermia, sedation, and complete paralysis. Vo_2 is increased by exercise, shivering, catecholamines, hyperthermia, and infection. Under normal steady-state conditions, the amount of oxygen taken up across the lungs into the pulmonary blood is equal to the amount of oxygen consumed by the tissues (the Fick principle). Vo_2, under most circumstances, is independent of oxygen delivery. Normally, oxygen delivery exceeds Vo_2 by a factor of about 4 : 1. If arterial blood is nearly saturated, this corresponds to an Svo_2 of about 75%. When oxygen delivery is reduced significantly in mammalian species, Vo_2 becomes supply-limited and falls, resulting in acidosis, hypotension, and a rise in blood lactate (ie, shock). The ratio of oxygen delivery to Vo_2 is more important than the absolute quantities of the individual components of oxygen delivery, namely hemoglobin, Sao_2, and cardiac output.[81] ECLS most often is applied to treat low oxygen delivery in the face of arterial hypoxia (hypoxic shock). Systemic oxygen delivery during ECLS is a combination of oxygen delivery from the extracorporeal circuit and oxygen delivery across the native lung. This is understood most easily when applied to the situation of venoarterial ECLS. Here, total oxygen delivery is expressed as follows:

$$Do_2 = \text{(extracorporeal circuit flow)(membrane lung } Cao_2) \\ + \text{(native cardiac output)(left ventricle } Cao_2)$$

A rise in the systemic arterial Po_2 at constant extracorporeal flow may reflect different physiologic conditions. Improving lung function results in greater oxygen saturation of left ventricular blood, correspondingly improving the Po_2 in systemic arterial blood. However, decreased contribution from the native circulation likewise results in a rising Po_2 because a greater proportion of the systemic arterial blood is being contributed by the extracorporeal circuit. A rising Pao_2 in the face of a deteriorating patient on ECLS might be seen under conditions of pneumothorax, hemothorax, or pericardial tamponade.

The best monitor of the adequacy of tissue oxygenation is the Svo_2. Continuous venous oxygen monitoring is performed routinely during ECLS. During ECLS, oxygen delivery is controlled primarily by the extracorporeal flow rate. Extracorporeal flow is set at the minimum amount that results in a normal Svo_2. Pump flow is increased to treat a falling Pao_2 and Svo_2. Pump flow may be decreased as the Pao_2 rises when the Svo_2 is normal, usually indicating lung recovery. Air-oxygen sweep gas mixtures can be used to reduce the Po_2 of the perfusate if significant arterial hyperoxia is present. In venovenous bypass, the Pao_2 is identical to the mixed right atrial Po_2, assuming there is no contribution from native lung gas exchange. Because of the return to the right ventricle of unsaturated blood not captured by the venous drainage catheter, right atrial saturation rarely can be raised to greater than 80% to 90%. The resulting Pao_2 in arterial blood may be as low as 40 mmHg. The patient will be relatively hypoxic and even cyanotic, but if the cardiac output is normal and the hemoglobin adequate, oxygen delivery is adequate and recovery can occur. Under these circumstances,

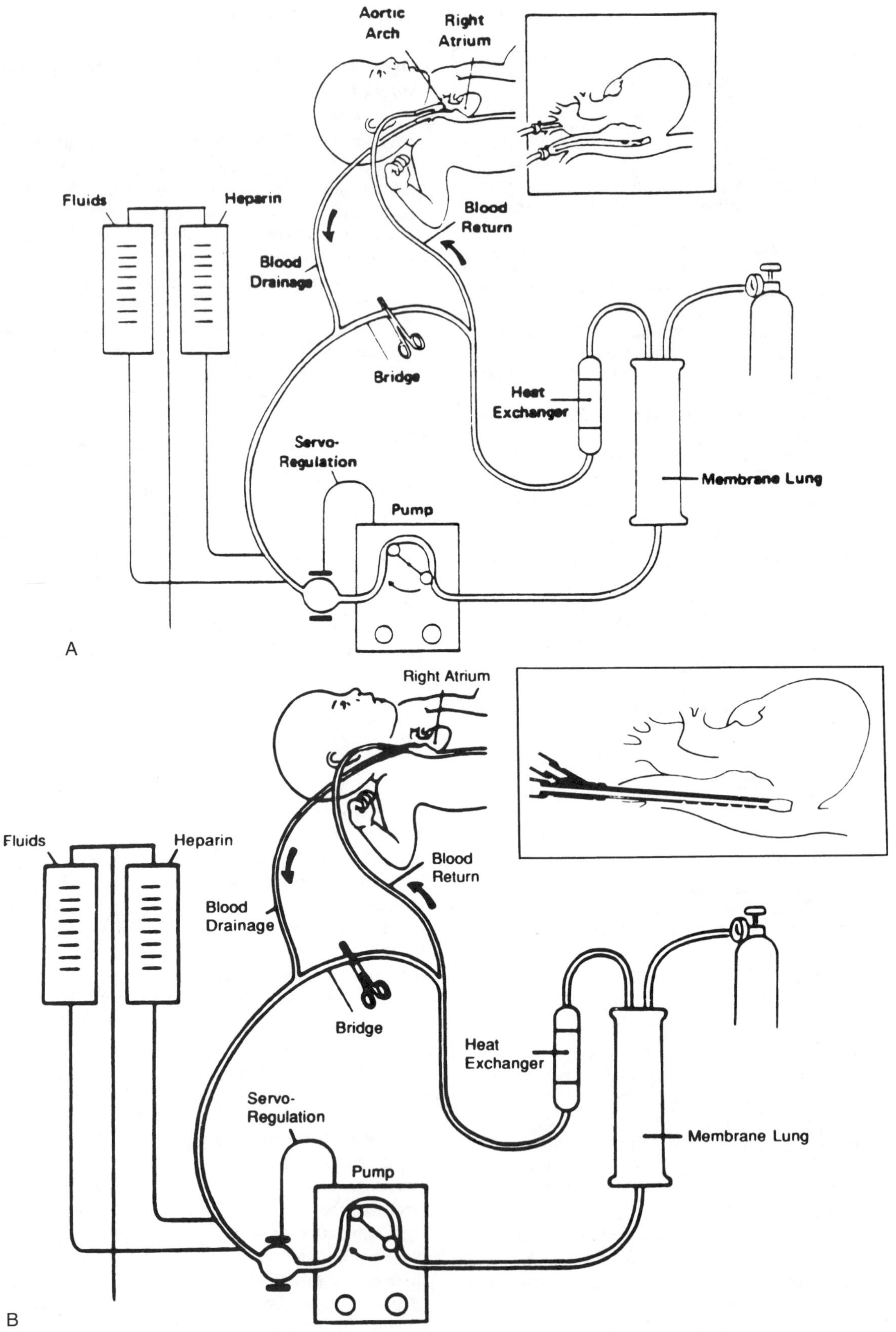

FIG. 8-5. Two modes of extracorporeal circulation. (*A*) Venoarterial access. (*B*) Venovenous access. (*A* from Bartlett RH, Andrews AF, Toomasian JM, Haiduc NJ, Gassainiga AB. Extracorporeal membrane oxygenation for newborn respiratory failure: 45 cases. Surgery 1982;92:426. *B* from Anderson HL, Otsu T, Chapman RA, Bartlett RH. Venovenous extracorporeal life support in neonates using a double lumen catheter. ASAIO Trans 1989;35:650)

recovery is heralded by an increase in the arterial Po_2 as the native lung contributes oxygen to the pulmonary blood flow.

An interesting physiologic property of lung function has been recognized with the application of ECLS. Even the most severely injured lungs (as might be found in severe adult RDS) can support oxygenation if they are not required to provide any ventilatory function. This is the rationale behind extracorporeal carbon dioxide removal and so-called apneic oxygenation as developed by Gattinoni and associates.[82] The lungs are inflated to a moderate pressure (15 to 20 cm H_2O) and oxygen is supplied to meet metabolic oxygen demand, while carbon dioxide is removed by low-flow partial venovenous bypass.

Carbon Dioxide Removal During Extracorporeal Support

During extracorporeal circulation, the major determinants of carbon dioxide removal are the surface area of the artificial lung and the flow rate and composition of the sweep gas. Under most circumstances, carbon dioxide removal is more efficient than oxygen transfer. Because an extracorporeal circuit is designed to meet Vo_2 needs, it may be capable of removing excessive amounts of carbon dioxide. Excessive levels of hypocarbia are prevented by adding carbon dioxide to the ventilating gas for the artificial lung, allowing the $Paco_2$ to be set at any desired level.

Control of Coagulation

Whenever blood contacts any foreign surface, the enzymatic cascades are initiated that result in the production of fibrin, complement, kinins, and plasmin. Blood in the extracorporeal circuit may be exposed to Silastic, polyvinylchloride, polyurethane, polycarbonate, and stainless steel. Activation of the coagulation cascade, if not modified, will result in thrombosis of the extracorporeal circuit. Systemic heparinization customarily is used to prevent thrombosis, maintaining a minimum level of anticoagulation. A loading dose of heparin, 40 to 150 U/kg, is followed by a continuous heparin infusion, 20 to 70 U/kg/h. Heparin effect is monitored by whole blood activated clotting time. Although thrombocytopenia and procoagulant depletion also prevent circuit thrombosis, they are associated with hemorrhagic complications. Thrombocytopenia must be prevented by platelet transfusions as necessary to maintain platelet counts greater than 50,000/μL, and preferably greater than 100,000/μL. Heparin effect alone is used to maintain anticoagulation, whereas fibrinogen levels and prothrombin time should be kept near normal and fibrin degradation products should not appear in excess. The administration of fresh frozen plasma or cryoprecipitate may be necessary to achieve this. The accepted practice for prolonged extracorporeal circulation is to maintain the whole blood activated clotting time at about 200 seconds (1.5 to 2 times the normal clotting time of 120 seconds). Heparin is excreted in the urine and bound to platelets. Therefore, heparin administration must be increased during periods of diuresis and platelet transfusion.

Effects on Blood Components, Fluids, and Electrolytes

Potential sources of red blood cell damage during long-term ECLS include mechanical injury from the pumping device and negative pressure surges within the circuit. The roller pump is adjusted to near occlusion and Servo-regulation is used to interrupt the pump if there is inadequate venous return to minimize these risks. There is negligible red blood cell loss attributable to the use of modern membrane lungs over prolonged periods. The surface of the extracorporeal circuit becomes "pacified" because of the dense protein monolayer that forms on the membrane lung and other circuit surfaces in the first few minutes of blood contact. Plasma free hemoglobin levels usually are less than 40 mg/dL, and the urine is clear during ECLS.

Platelets adhere to the prosthetic surface within minutes of exposure. They tend to adhere most to areas where fibrin has been deposited, attracting other platelets and causing platelet aggregates to form. These "clumps" of platelets, which also include some leukocytes (and red blood cells in more stagnant areas of the circuit), are released into the circulating blood and infused into the patient. They subsequently "disaggregate" and eventually are removed by the reticuloendothelial system. Platelets are consumed continuously during ECLS. If consumption is balanced by increased production, platelet counts stabilize in the range of 30,000 to 60,000. In newborns and children, platelet production does not match destruction, and platelet transfusion almost always is required.

The effects of prolonged ECLS on leukocytes are less well known. Total leukocyte counts during ECLS range from 5000 to 15,000/μL under most circumstances. The differential leukocyte count is nearly normal during ECLS. Leukocyte function is adequate, because bacterial infections usually resolve with antibiotic treatment.

Increased capillary permeability resulting from complement activation occurs to some degree when ECLS is initiated. There often is an initial weight gain and visible edema. Whether this is a result of extracorporeal circulation itself or a reperfusion injury is unknown. Edema usually resolves within 1 or 2 days, and diuresis results in a return to the baseline weight.[83] Hemofiltration may be necessary if renal function is abnormal or edema is significant. Although it rarely is a problem, significant amounts of free water are lost from the membrane lung. Cool, dry sweep gas exits the membrane lung warmed and saturated with water vapor. An infant can lose more than 150 mL/d of free water in this fashion.

Serum ionized calcium may fall to dangerous levels when extracorporeal circulation is started, and may result in cardiac dysfunction if not treated.[84] This is most important when venovenous ECLS is initiated, and can result in significant hypotension from low cardiac output. It is unclear whether this is caused by the citrate present in banked blood or a dilutional phenomenon. There are no other electrolyte abnormalities that are peculiar to ECLS. Electrolytes are monitored as they would be in any critically ill patient, and requirements are administered intravenously.

Effects on Other Organ Systems

Parenteral nutrition customarily is used during ECLS. However, there is no evidence that gastrointestinal function is impaired specifically by ECLS. Gastric aspirates typically test positive for occult blood, and small amounts of formula or antacids may be given to reduce the risk of bleeding from gastritis. Patients receiving ECLS continue to have bowel movements.

Renal function usually is normal during ECLS. Both loop diuretics and osmotic agents can be used to treat fluid overload or edema. Preexisting renal failure can be treated by dialysis using a hemofilter placed within the circuit.

The function of the central nervous system appears to be unaffected by prolonged ECLS. Infants may be awake, alert, and even playful, and adults may be communicative during ECLS. The effect of microembolization from the extracorporeal circuit, although potentially dangerous, seems to be of less practical importance. Organ function remains nearly normal for many weeks, and tissue infarcts are not found at autopsy.

Native Lung During Extracorporeal Life Support

During venoarterial bypass, a significant portion of the pulmonary blood flow is diverted through the extracorporeal circuit. There appear to be no major deleterious effects of reduced pulmonary blood flow, unless normal ventilation is maintained. With normal ventilation of the native lungs during venoarterial extracorporeal circulation, pulmonary capillary pH can be as high as 8.0. Hemolysis and pulmonary hemorrhage can result, even without marked systemic hypocarbia.[85,86] When ECLS is initiated, ventilator settings are decreased rapidly to prevent further damage from overdistention, and to prevent local tissue alkalosis. There is no standard approach to management of the native lung during ECLS. It may not be important whether a low respiratory rate and normal inspiratory pressure are chosen, or whether the patient is placed on CPAP. A few sustained inflations above the alveolar opening pressure are provided periodically to prevent total lung collapse.

During venovenous bypass, right ventricular output is normal and probably higher than before the institution of ECLS, because cardiac output increases after severe hypoxemia is corrected. This may have the salutary effect of exposing the pulmonary vasculature to blood with a relatively high P_{O_2}, which may be beneficial in the treatment of pulmonary hypertension.

Severely injured lungs can recover if placed ''at rest'' using ECLS. The period necessary for recovery spans several days to several weeks. The presence of extensive fibrosis precludes recovery. If ECLS is initiated before fibrosis occurs or is irreversibly initiated, recovery can be expected unless technical complications ensue. The radiographic appearance of a typical newborn with meconium aspiration before, during, and after ECLS is shown in Figure 8-6.

Technical Aspects of Extracorporeal Life Support

Equipment

Basic ECLS circuits, used in their most common application, neonatal venoarterial and neonatal venovenous ECLS, are depicted in Figure 8-5. Venous blood, from a centrally placed catheter, drains by gravity through a collapsible ''bladder'' and then to a roller pump. Servo-regulation prevents negative pressure application to the venous side of the circuit by interrupting

pump flow if venous return is inadequate. Blood is pumped through the artificial lung and subsequently through a heat exchanger, and then is returned to the patient. Components of the circuit are affixed to a mobile cart. The oxygenated blood is returned to the patient through a major artery during venoarterial bypass, or to a major vein during venovenous bypass. Standard priming techniques include carbon dioxide flushing of the circuit, vacuum application to the membrane lung gas phase, and crystalloid priming. The circuit then is coated with albumin, followed by blood priming. Circuit electrolytes and gas partial pressures are measured and adjusted in preparation for the initiation of ECLS. The ECLS circuits are made of the same components used in operative cardiopulmonary bypass. As long as the patient's blood volume is adequate, the venous drainage catheter limits extracorporeal flow. Appropriately sized venous catheters, tubing, and reinfusion catheters must be chosen to allow adequate blood flow to support a given patient.

During ECLS, gas transfer occurs across the artificial lung. The silicone rubber used in commercially available membrane lungs has excellent gas transfer capabilities. Oxygen diffusion through the thin film of venous blood within the artificial lung is the limiting factor that determines the membrane lung's oxygenating capacity. Carbon dioxide transfer is much more efficient than oxygen transfer.

An ideal membrane lung would have low thrombogenicity, high oxygen transfer per unit surface area, a relatively large gas space to minimize water condensation within the membrane lung, low blood path resistance, and small priming volume. It also should be relatively inexpensive and easy to prime. The most widely used membrane lung for ECLS is the SciMed-Kolobow lung (Avecor Cardiovascular, Plymouth, MN), consisting of a long, spirally wound envelope of silicone rubber. Gas circulates within the envelope and blood passes lengthwise between the windings of the spiral. This device requires high perfusion pressures to overcome its high resistance; however, excellent gas exchange and low priming volume are achieved.

Hollow-fiber oxygenators also have been used for ECLS. Microporous capillaries, around which the blood flows, conduct the sweep gas. These devices have low resistance and low priming volumes, but their use for this clinical application has been limited by a tendency to leak plasma into the gas phase after 24 to 48 hours.

Direct drive roller pumps are used by most ECLS centers. These pumps can generate extreme negative pressures when venous return is inadequate. They also can generate large positive pressures when outflow is occluded, sufficient to cause circuit rupture. Roller occlusion can contribute to red blood cell damage and hemolysis. Tubing fatigue of the raceway segment can result in catastrophic raceway rupture. In spite of these potential problems, with proper Servo-regulation (see later), these pumps are relatively safe and reliable, and cause minimal blood damage. Other pumping mechanisms include centrifugal pumps and passive filling pumps.

A collapsible bladder or pressure monitor is used in the venous return line to regulate pump flow. It is critical that the pumping mechanism not apply high negative pressure to the venous filling line. Small amounts of negative pressure can cause significant hemolysis and air entrainment within the circuit. Right atrial and superior vena cava damage may occur if they are sucked into the catheter. Premembrane and postmem-

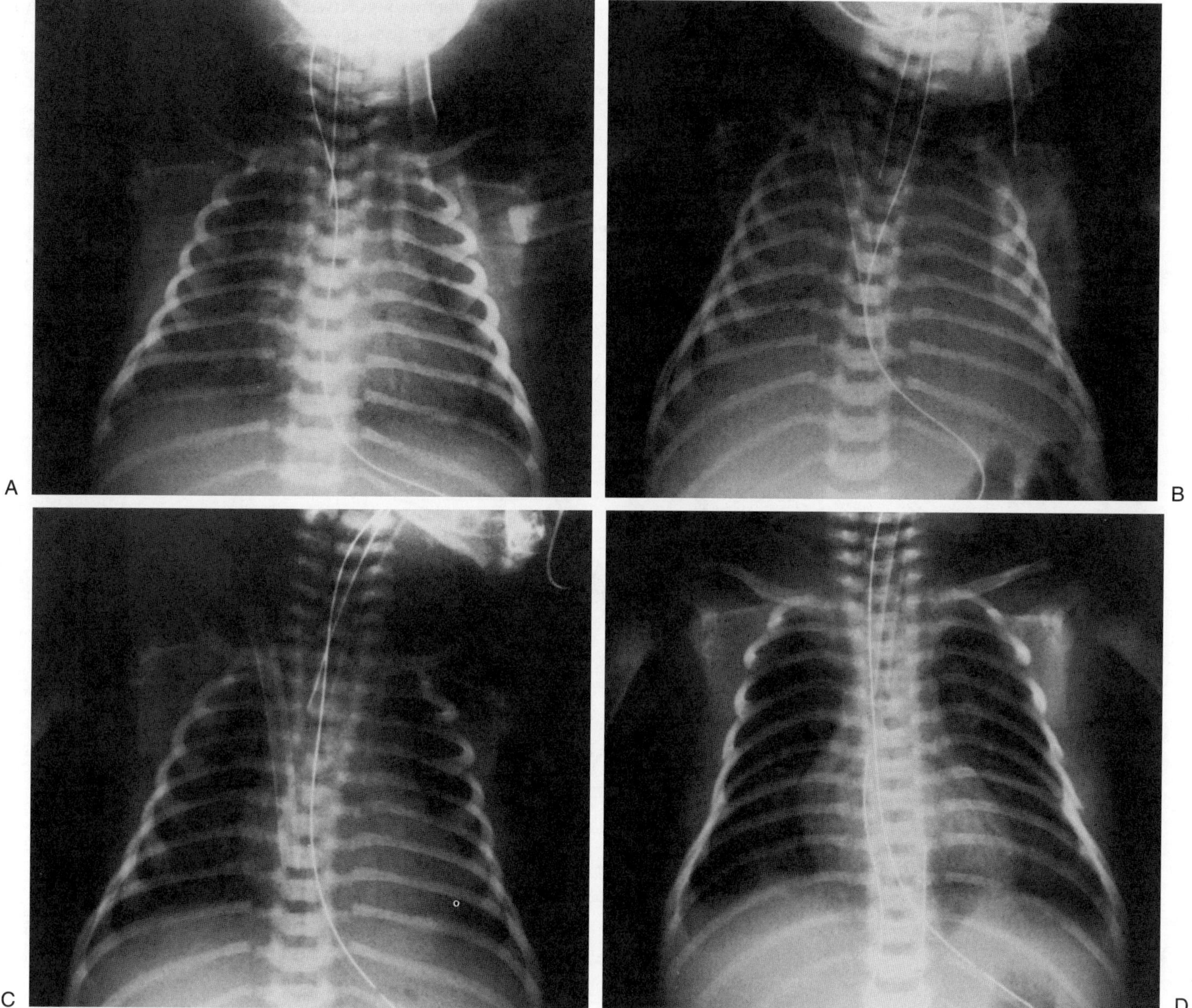

FIG. 8-6. Radiographic appearance of a newborn with meconium aspiration syndrome. (*A*) Appearance before the institution of extracorporeal life support (ECLS) of a patient on maximal ventilator settings (PaO$_2$ of 35). (*B*) The second day on ECLS, the ventilator settings are reduced for lung rest and a double-lumen venovenous cannula is placed in the right atrium. There is a typical "whiteout" appearance of the lungs. (*C*) Lung recovery after 4 days of ECLS with the ventilator still at low settings. (*D*) The patient as maintained on low ventilator settings after decannulation from ECLS. (Cilley RE, Bartlett RH. Extracorporeal life support for respiratory failure. In: Gravlee GP, Davis RF, Utley JR, eds. Cardiopulmonary bypass: principles and practice. Baltimore, Williams & Wilkins, 1993:644)

brane pressure monitors and continuous venous oxygen saturation monitoring should be included within the circuit. Continuous monitoring of the oxygen and carbon dioxide concentrations of the membrane lung sweep gases adds another measure of safety to the conduct of ECLS.

A hemofilter can be incorporated within the extracorporeal circuit.[87] In fluid-overloaded patients who are unresponsive to diuretics but still require significant volumes of parenteral fluids, a hemofilter can provide slow, continuous ultrafiltration.

The volume of extracellular fluid to be removed is regulated by simply controlling the ultrafiltrate flow from the hemofilter. Continuous arteriovenous hemofiltration provides some clearance of uremic toxins by replacing the continuous output of the hemofilter with a plasma-like electrolyte solution. When catabolic acute renal failure and uremia requiring high solute clearance are present, continuous arterial venous hemofiltration with dialysis can be used. In this technique, the hemofilter ultrafiltrate compartment is perfused with a dialysis solution.

Vascular Access

Cervical cannulation is the site of choice for most ECLS applications. The largest cannula that can be inserted in the internal jugular vein will permit adequate venous drainage for ECLS. Although ligation of the common carotid artery is unappealing, infants and children (and adults) have collateral circulation such that the risk of acute stroke is minimal. With an experience of several thousand common carotid artery ligations, there have been minimal neurologic sequelae that can be attributed to the ligation of these vessels. Other venous and arterial access sites also can be used. In general, the largest cannula that will fit into the internal jugular vein and common carotid artery will provide adequate flow for almost every patient. Cannulation is performed as an operative procedure in the ICU where ECLS is to be performed. Anesthesia consists of locally infiltrated lidocaine (Xylocaine), an intravenous narcotic, and a neuromuscular blocker. Complete operating room staffing is optimal, including a nurse or technician and a circulating nurse. Electrocautery and headlights are brought to the ICU. Cannulation occurs concurrently with circuit preparation and priming.

The cannulation technique involves minimal handling of the vessels, especially the vein, to prevent spasm (Fig. 8-7). In neonates, intimal stay sutures are placed to prevent dissection

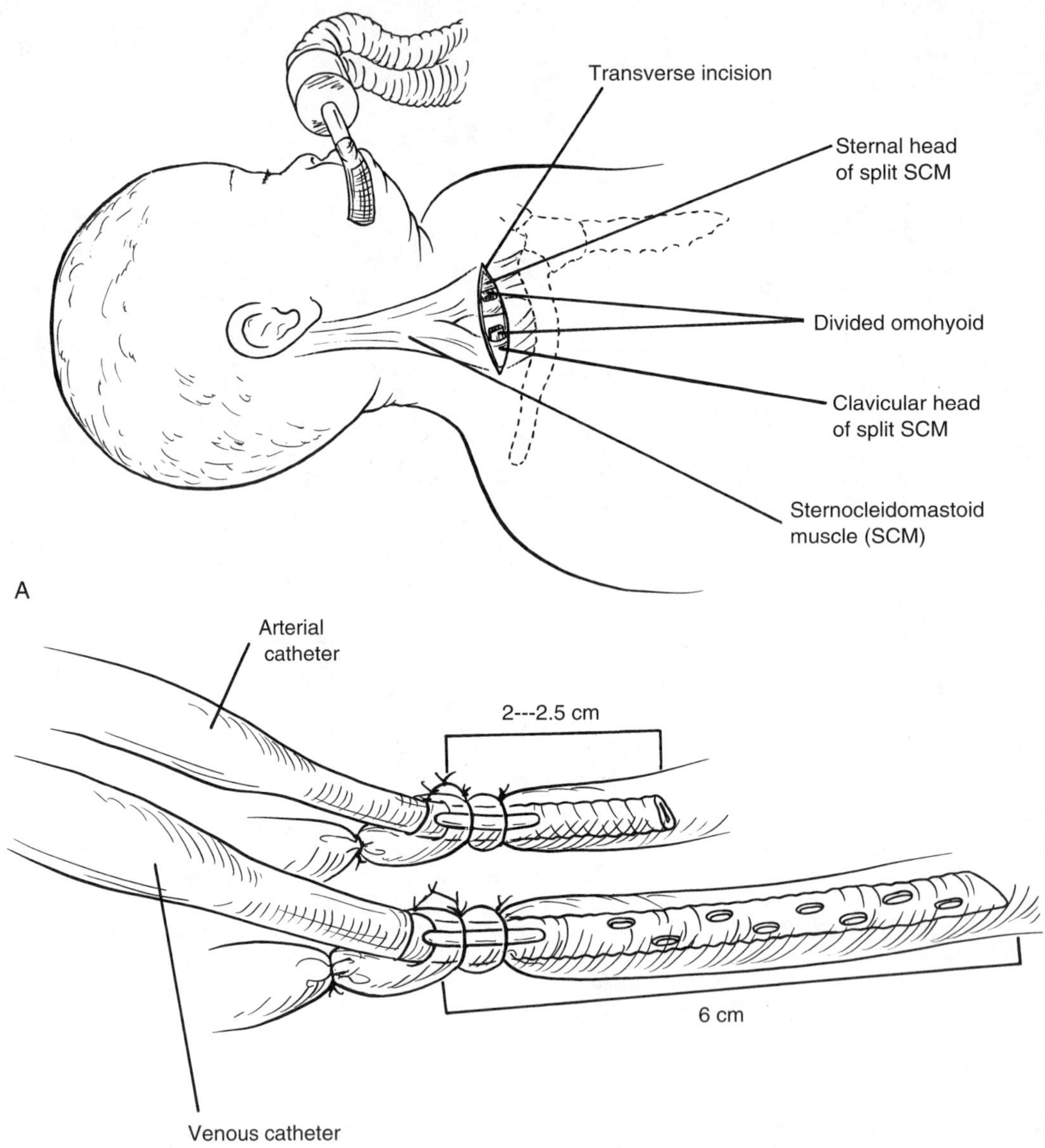

FIG. 8-7. Technique of vascular access for neonatal extracorporeal life support. (*A*) A transverse or vertical incision is made over the lower sternocleidomastoid muscle (SCM). The sternal and clavicular heads of the muscle are split. The omohyoid is divided. (*B*) A 6F, 8F, or 10F arterial catheter is inserted 2 to 2.5 cm. A 10F, 12F, or 14F venous catheter is inserted 5.5 to 6.5 cm. Stay sutures (not shown) are placed through the arterial wall to prevent intimal dissection during catheter insertion. Two ligatures around the vessel are tied over the vessel loop "boot" to allow safe suture removal at decannulation. A marking suture is tied to the vascular cannula to aid in accurate insertion length.

of the delicate arterial intima on introduction of the catheter. The artery is mobilized even when venovenous bypass is anticipated in case a rapid conversion to venoarterial bypass is required. Electrocautery is used liberally to minimize bleeding. The catheter is secured within the vessels using sutures tied over a short segment of silicone rubber tape (vessel loop). When the catheter is removed, the sutures can be cut against the silicone rubber tape, preventing damage to the native vessels. Repair of the carotid artery and jugular vein is possible after ECLS.[88,89] Greater experience is needed to define the long-term benefit of vessel reconstruction, and whether it can be performed without complication.

Patient Care

Infants and children on ECLS require one-on-one nursing, in addition to a perfusionist or technical specialist to regulate the extracorporeal circuit.

The feared complication of intracranial hemorrhage (occurring in 14% of neonatal ECLS patients) may be heralded by obvious neurologic deterioration and seizures or an unexplained increase in platelet consumption, or it may be clinically silent. In neonates, cranial ultrasound is useful for assessing intracranial hemorrhage, and is performed frequently throughout their time on ECLS.

Parenteral nutrition is used to meet nutritional requirements. Routine electrolytes, including sodium, chloride, bicarbonate, phosphorus, and magnesium, are monitored daily, or more frequently if changes are occurring. More frequent monitoring may be required during periods of high-volume hemofiltration. Glucose, urea nitrogen, creatinine, albumin, hepatic transaminases, and bilirubin also are measured daily. Hematologic values, including leukocyte count, fibrinogen, fibrin degradation products, and serum hemoglobin, also are checked. Potassium, calcium, hematocrit, and platelets require more frequent monitoring and correction. Patient and oxygenator blood gas tensions are checked periodically. In the past, many patient blood gas determinations were made; now, with a greater reliance on continuous venous oximetry and pulse oximetry, these can be checked a few times throughout the day.

Excessive bleeding occurs from minor wounds as a result of partial heparinization. No intramuscular injections are given. No percutaneous arterial or venous samples are obtained. New intravenous catheters are not started. Capillary blood gases, requiring heel or digital puncture, are not performed. Urethral catheters are neither inserted nor removed, if possible. Endotracheal tubes can be changed with extreme care. Tracheal suctioning should be performed gently with soft catheters.

Sedation and analgesia are provided as necessary. Patients are given broad-spectrum parenteral antibiotics throughout ECLS. Specific infections mandate specific antibiotic treatment. It is surprisingly uncommon to have a patient deteriorate during ECLS from an infection. Topical antifungal agents are used liberally.

Critically ill patients and their families always require emotional support and sensitivity. ECLS adds another factor to the emotional turmoil that families experience. Most centers provide information booklets to help families understand this treatment. Patients who were sick enough to die, and may have been dying when ECLS was initiated, often become ''well'' and may

appear almost normal. If treatment proceeds with resolution of the disease and recovery, the results are gratifying to all. If, however, the lungs fail to recover, life support must be terminated or allowed to continue until a fatal complication results. This kind of outcome can be emotionally devastating to all involved. Support from nursing personnel, social workers, and the clergy is helpful.

Surgical Procedures and Management of Bleeding

Minor surgical procedures may be required during ECLS, and should not be taken lightly. Bleeding complications have occurred after seemingly trivial procedures. Arterial cutdown may be needed if appropriate access can not be obtained before the initiation of ECLS, or if the access is lost. Tube thoracostomy may be required to drain hemothorax or pneumothorax. Cannulation sites may bleed, requiring reexploration. Skin incisions can be made with the cutting mode of an electrocautery instrument. Muscles should be cauterized, and not torn (this is especially important during chest tube insertions). Fibrin glue (cryoprecipitate, calcium, and thrombin solution) applied to wounds decreases bleeding complications.

Major operative procedures can be performed during ECLS. Although bleeding may be a significant problem, liberal use of cautery, application of fibrin glue, and a low threshold for reexploration permit nearly any procedure to be performed.

When bleeding occurs during ECLS, several strategies can be used. Laboratory evaluation may reveal correctable forms of coagulopathy. The prothrombin time should be normal; if not, it should be corrected with fresh frozen plasma. Low fibrinogen levels (less than 100 mg/dL) are corrected with cryoprecipitate. Platelet counts should be elevated to greater than 150,000 by platelet transfusion. Activated clotting times are allowed to fall to 160 to 180 seconds. High circuit flow rates should be maintained during times when activated clotting times are low. Activated clotting times can be lowered further to the range of 120 to 140 seconds and heparin can be discontinued for several hours if bleeding persists. When activated clotting times are this low, a back-up, saline-primed circuit should be immediately available in the ICU. If these measures fail to stop the bleeding, operative therapy is indicated. A rule of thumb is to explore the appropriate body cavity or wound for bleeding that exceeds one half a blood volume in 24 hours. ϵ-Aminocaproic acid (Amicar) infusion during ECLS has resulted in a decreased incidence of intracranial hemorrhage and less bleeding after surgical procedures.[90]

Weaning and Discontinuation

The return of pulmonary gas exchange heralds lung recovery in patients treated with ECLS.[91] This usually is seen as an increase in the venous oxygen saturation and arterial P_{O_2}, or as a decrease in the arterial P_{CO_2} without a change in the ventilator settings or the level of ECLS. Lung compliance improves and chest radiographs clear. Serial compliance measurements may provide an easy means of gauging lung recovery.[92] Extracorporeal flow is decreased progressively, allowing more pulmonary blood flow. When low levels of support have been achieved (about 25% of the initial flow), patients should be ''trialed off''

TABLE 8-7. *Summary of patient management during extracorporeal life support (ECLS)*

Patient identified as meeting criteria for ECLS; no contraindications present

Cannulation of vessels in the intensive care unit; preparation of ECLS circuit

ECLS initiated

ECLS management:

    Extracorporeal circuit flow adjusted using arterial oxygen tension and mixed venous oxygen saturation to provide adequate oxygen delivery

    Sweep gas flow and composition adjusted to normalize arterial carbon dioxide tension

    Ventilator placed at rest settings

    Systemic blood pressure regulated by volume administration and inotropes as necessary

    Hemoglobin maintained at 14–15 g/dL by transfusion and ultrafiltration if necessary

    Platelet count maintained at greater than 100,000/μL

    Activated clotting time maintained at 200 seconds by continuous heparin infusion

    Central nervous system function, nutrition, and renal function monitored and supported

Native lung recovery occurs (chest radiograph improved, lung compliance improved, rising Pao_2, lower ECLS flow, appearance of CO_2 in endotracheal tube)

"Trial-off" at moderate or low ventilator settings

Decannulation, ventilator weaning and extubation

---

with moderate ventilator support, and if stable, decannulated. The weaning procedure often is more of a discovery that patients have improved sufficiently that ECLS no longer is required. In patients who are unable to be taken off ECLS at low ventilator settings, sequential trials off ECLS at moderately high ventilator settings are performed once or twice daily. Continued improvement with serial trials indicates that ECLS should be continued. Failure to improve after several trials off may indicate residual, static lung disease and ECLS should be discontinued, in the anticipation that prolonged mechanical ventilation will be required. During prolonged trials off bypass, anticoagulation of both the patient and the circuit must be maintained.

The decision to discontinue ECLS is made in a similar fashion during venovenous bypass. In this situation, a trial off ECLS can be accomplished much more simply. Capping the oxygenator gas inlet port allows the circuit oxygen to be consumed and equilibrate the entire extracorporeal circuit with the patient's mixed venous blood. Extracorporeal flow and anticoagulation need not be changed; there is no concern about circuit, catheter, or patient thrombosis. Hemodynamics remain constant, without the abrupt changes in pulmonary blood flow and aortic pressure that are associated with initiating and stopping venoarterial bypass. Patient management during ECLS is summarized in Table 8-7.

Logistics and Cost

Providing ECLS requires a significant investment of personnel, time, and financial support. The best examples of how to establish ECLS centers come from the neonatal ECMO experience. Guidelines for neonatal ECMO have been proposed, and provide some insight into the support structure that is required to perform safe ECLS.[93] ECLS should be based at a tertiary care center with an appropriately staffed ICU for support. Each center needs a medical director. An ECLS coordinator usually is required to supervise staff training, equipment maintenance, and data recording. Most centers have found that a specially trained perfusionist, nurse, or respiratory therapist is necessary to manage the extracorporeal circuit. The primary responsibility of this technical specialist is to regulate blood flow, control membrane lung function, and adjust anticoagulation. Perhaps most importantly, this individual also must diagnose and treat patient and circuit emergencies (circuit disruption, membrane lung failure, power loss, and thrombosis). Under most circumstances, each patient also has a one-on-one ICU nurse in addition to the ECLS technical specialist. A follow-up team of neonatologists, neurologists, or developmental specialists is needed. Dedicated ICU space is needed, with on-site back-up equipment for all ECLS components. Operating capability within the ICU is required. ECLS centers need a well-defined program for staff training and certification. This requires didactic teaching, laboratory training with live animals, and bedside training. The ECLS system is a team undertaking that requires institutional support, personal commitment from the leadership, and continuous updating and training.

In 1996, most institutions should count on start-up costs in excess of $100,000. This includes the salary and benefits of a full-time clinical coordinator ($40,000 to $70,000) and primary and back-up equipment ($25,000 $\times$ 2). In addition, laboratory animal training exercises must be conducted and disposable items purchased. ECLS adds about $2000 per day to the cost of caring for a newborn in a neonatal ICU using a mechanical ventilator. There is evidence that this cost is offset by a shorter neonatal ICU stay and, ultimately, less significant residual lung disease.[94]

Clinical Applications

Neonatal Respiratory Failure

Neonatal respiratory failure can be severe, progressive, and rapidly fatal, characteristics that make it ideally suited for a treatment such as ECLS. Its severity and potential for mortality justify the use of extraordinary life-saving means. The rapidity with which neonatal respiratory failure can progress ensures that "sick lungs" will not be irreversibly injured by the application of mechanical ventilation by the time ECLS is used. Most causes of neonatal respiratory failure result in pulmonary artery hypertension. Hypoxia, hypercarbia, and acidosis cause pulmonary vasoconstriction that results in right-to-left shunting at the atrial, ductal, and intrapulmonary levels. Shunting worsens the hypoxia, which in turn increases pulmonary vascular resistance, creating a vicious cycle. ECLS and lung rest provide one method of breaking this cycle. As many as 5% of neonates do not respond to conventional treatment such as paralysis, induced respiratory alkalosis, vasodilators, and nitric oxide, and may benefit from ECLS.

Candidates for neonatal ECMO include infants with persistent pulmonary hypertension of the newborn and meconium aspiration syndrome. A few of these babies do not respond to conventional therapy. Infants with congenital diaphragmatic hernia continue to have a high mortality rate and may benefit from ECLS. Early use of ECLS should be considered in these patients given the increased vulnerability of the congenitally hypoplastic lung to mechanical ventilation. Severe pulmonary hypoplasia may preclude recovery. Infants with sepsis and severe respiratory failure who do not respond to conventional therapy may benefit from ECLS. In these infants, the underlying lung injury often is more severe and the systemic inflammatory response generated by sepsis results in more profound multiple organ dysfunction. The mortality rate is higher in these infants and the duration of ECLS is prolonged. Newborn RDS occurs in some infants greater than 35 weeks of gestation who may benefit from ECLS.

Initially, ECLS/ECMO was offered as a salvage therapy to patients who were believed to be moribund and unlikely to survive. More objective criteria have evolved over the ensuing years. The two most widely used objective measures are the alveolar-arterial oxygen gradient and the oxygenation index. The normal alveolar-arterial oxygen gradient is about 50 mmHg. A gradient above 610 mmHg for 8 hours defines a mortality risk of about 80%. An oxygenation index ([mean airway pressure in cm H_2O][Fio_2] $\times$ 100/[postductal Pao_2 in mmHg]) consistently greater than 25 defines a mortality risk of about 50%, whereas an oxygenation index greater than 40 defines a mortality risk of about 80%.[95,96] Each center performing neonatal ECLS should corroborate the applicability of objective criteria to its own neonatal population.

A cranial ultrasound should be obtained to rule out intracranial hemorrhage before instituting ECLS. In addition, an echocardiogram should be obtained to rule out significant structural heart disease. Total anomalous pulmonary venous return can present with apparent respiratory failure meeting ''ECLS criteria.''

Contraindications to neonatal ECLS include profound neurologic impairment, congenial anomalies incompatible with prolonged or meaningful survival, and irreversible lung disease already present (eg, bronchopulmonary dysplasia). Mechanical ventilation of more than 7 days' duration is a relative contraindication, whereas mechanical ventilation for more than 10 days is considered an absolute contraindication.

The high risk of intracranial hemorrhage in the early newborn experience (about 30%) was associated with a gestational age of less than 35 weeks.[97] It also has been observed that when intracranial hemorrhage is present, it may expand rapidly under the condition of partial heparinization. A grade III or IV intracranial hemorrhage is a contraindication to ECLS. Patients with grade I or questionable grade II intracranial hemorrhage can be considered for treatment using lower heparin doses, higher platelet counts, and aminocaproic acid. A gestational age of less than 35 weeks constitutes a relative contraindication to ECLS in the newborn. Premature newborns (32 weeks of gestation or less) have been treated on an individualized basis using higher platelet counts, lower activated clotting times, and a cephalad jugular venous drainage catheter, with encouraging results.[98]

The major complications of neonatal ECLS include bleeding associated with heparin anticoagulation, mechanical failure of circuit components, and long-term neurologic and pulmonary sequelae. Bleeding complications (primarily intracranial hemorrhage and bleeding from an operative site) occur in 30% of patients. The incidence of intracranial hemorrhage and technical

TABLE 8-8. *Neonatal Extracorporeal Life Support cases and survival by diagnosis*

Primary diagnosis	Total	Number of survivors	Percent surviving
Meconium aspiration syndrome	3607	3374	94
Respiratory distress syndrome	1093	914	84
Congenital diaphragmatic hernia	1960	1143	58
Pneumonia/sepsis	1528	1163	76
Air leak syndrome	44	32	73
Persistent pulmonary hypertension of the newborn	1313	1097	84
Other	366	285	78
Totals	9911	8008	81

ELSO registry. Ann Arbor, MI, Extracorporeal Life Support Organization, 1995.

complications has fallen as experience has progressed. Jugular and carotid ligation is surprisingly well tolerated. Symptoms of right hemispheric dysfunction have been minimal.

A survival advantage using ECLS in newborn respiratory failure has been shown in two randomized, prospective studies.[99,100] These patients represent a population with a high mortality rate (about 80%). There is no control group with which they can be compared for follow-up. About one fourth of the newborns with severe respiratory failure who are treated by mechanical ventilation alone, without extracorporeal support, have developmental or neurologic impairment.[101,102] Follow-up data from experienced neonatal ECLS centers demonstrate that most patients (75%) are normal or nearly normal.[103,104] There are more than 70 centers using ECLS for the treatment of newborn respiratory failure in North America. With nearly 10,000 newborn cases reported, the overall survival rate is 81%[105] (Table 8-8). More than 1000 patients a year were treated from 1988 to 1993, whereas in 1994 the number decreased to 816 neonates. It is uncertain whether the use of ECLS will continue at its current level.

It is remarkable that extracorporeal support results in the routine recovery of infants who are moribund with respiratory failure. There can be nothing therapeutic about anticoagulation and extracorporeal circulation. Lung recovery results from ''resting'' the lung from high pressure and high oxygen concentration, and sustaining the life of the infant through a few days. This phenomenon suggests that there is something about the customary ventilator and pharmacologic management of this group of term infants that contributes to pulmonary dysfunction.

Pediatric Respiratory Failure

The favorable experience with neonatal ECLS has renewed interest in the application of ECLS to older children. About 15 centers offer ECLS for respiratory failure in children, with a reported survival rate of 50%.[106] As applied to children, ECLS is indicated in acute, potentially lethal respiratory failure that does not respond to conventional therapy when the underlying condition is reversible. ECLS is used as salvage therapy, when survival otherwise would not be expected. Further studies are needed to define its place in the treatment of respiratory failure outside the newborn period.

It is difficult to identify potentially reversible respiratory failure in infants and children. Unlike neonates, older children are more likely to have irreversible disease from interstitial inflammation leading to pulmonary fibrosis. It is perhaps unfortunate that these patients can be treated with high-pressure mechanical ventilation successfully for so long. Acceptable arterial blood gases may be generated at the expense of ongoing lung injury from the application of high-pressure mechanical ventilation. The rapid progression to lethality and earlier application of ECLS in newborns protect their lungs from the injuries that may result from many days of mechanical ventilation.

Future Directions

The future of ECLS as a therapy for respiratory failure is uncertain. When properly applied, this technology can be life-saving. Safer ECLS may find earlier application and more widespread use in the treatment of moderate respiratory failure. Percutaneously placed venous catheters used for venovenous ECLS and a nonthrombogenic circuit that does not require systemic heparinization potentially could be used with relatively low risk. Alternatively, ECLS may be supplanted by safer, less injurious mechanical ventilation. Improved drug therapies to relax pulmonary arterioles are needed to break reliably the cycle of pulmonary artery hypertension. Nitric oxide has some potential to reduce the need for ECLS. Agents to control the deleterious effects of the inflammatory response in the lung also are needed.

REFERENCES

1. Boyden EA. Development and growth of the airways. In: Hodson WA, ed. Development of the lung. New York, Marcel Dekker, 1977: 3.
2. Thurlbeck WM. Prematurity and the developing lung. Clin Perinatol 1992;19:497.
3. Hislop A, Ried LM. Formation of the pulmonary vasculature. In: Hodson WA, ed. Development of the lung. New York, Marcel Dekker, 1977:37.
4. Morin FC, Stenmark KR. Persistent pulmonary hypertension of the newborn. Am J Respir Crit Care Med 1995;151:2010.
5. Warburton D, Lee M, Berberich MA, Bernfield M. Molecular embryology and the study of lung development. Am J Respir Cell Mol Biol 1993;9:5.
6. DiFiore JW, Wilson JM. Lung development. Semin Pediatr Surg 1994;3:221.
7. Byrne K, Cooper KR, Carey PD, et al. Pulmonary compliance: early assessment of evolving lung injury after onset of sepsis. J Appl Physiol 1990;69:2290.
8. Gattinoni L, Pesenti A, Avalli L, et al. Pressure-volume curve of total respiratory system in acute respiratory failure. Am Rev Respir Dis 1987;136:730.
9. Shapiro MB, Bartlett RH. Pulmonary compliance and mechanical ventilation. Arch Surg 1992;127:485.
10. West JB, Dollery CT, Naimark A. Distribution of bloodflow in isolated lung: relation to vascular and alveolar pressures. J Appl Physiol 1964;19:713.
11. Dantzker DR. Pulmonary gas exchange. In: Scharf SM, ed. Cardiopulmonary physiology in critical care. New York, Marcel Dekker, 1992: 291.
12. Mendelson CR, Boggaram V. Hormonal and developmental regulation of pulmonary surfactant synthesis in fetal lung. Baillieres Clin Endocrinol Metab 1990;4:351.
13. Pitt BR, Lister G. Interpretation of metabolic function of the lungs. Clin Chest Med 1989;10:1.
14. Ohlsson A, Fong K, Rose T, et al. Prenatal ultrasonic prediction of autopsy-proven pulmonary hypoplasia. Am J Perinatol 1992;9:334.
15. Van Eyck J, Van der Mooren K, Wladimiroff JW. Ductus arteriosus flow velocity modulation by fetal breathing movements as a measure of fetal lung development. Am J Obstet Gynecol 1990;163:558.
16. Sherer DM, Davis JM, Woods JR. Pulmonary hypoplasia: a review. Obstet Gynecol Surv 1990;45:792.
17. DiFiore JW, Wilson JM. Lung liquid, fetal lung growth and congenital diaphragmatic hernia. Pediatric Surgery International 1995;10:2.
18. Fewell JD, Hislop AA, Kitterman JA, Johnson P. Effect of tracheostomy on lung development in fetal lambs. J Appl Physiol 1983;55:1103.
19. Fisk NM, Parkes MJ, Moore PJ, et al. Mimicking low amniotic pressure by chronic pharyngeal drainage does not impair lung development in fetal sheep. Am J Obstet Gynecol 1992;166:991.
20. Hedrick MH, Estes JM, Sullivan KM, et al. Plug the lung until it grows (PLUG): a new method to treat congenital diaphragmatic hernia in utero. J Pediatr Surg 1994;29:612.
21. Wigglesworth JS, Desai R, Hislop AA. Fetal lung growth in congenital laryngeal atresia. Pediatr Pathol 1987;7:515.
22. Morley CJ. Surfactant treatment for premature babies: a review of clinical trials. Arch Dis Child 1991;66:445.
23. Berry DD. Neonatology in the 1990's: surfactant replacement therapy becomes reality. Clin Pediatr (Phila) 1991;30:167.
24. Collaborative Dexamethasone Trial Group. Dexamethasone therapy in neonatal chronic lung disease: an international placebo-controlled trial. Pediatrics 1991;88:421.
25. Demling RH. Adult respiratory distress syndrome: current concepts. New Horiz 1993;1:388.
26. Cilley RE, Wang JY, Coran AG. Lung injury produced by moderate lung overinflation in rats. J Pediatr Surg 1993;28:488.
27. Zapol WM, Snider MT, Hill JD, et al. Extracorporeal membrane oxygenation in severe acute respiratory failure. JAMA 1979;242:2193.
28. Greenfield LJ, Ebert PA, Benson DW. The effect of positive pressure ventilation on surface tension properties of lung extracts. Anesthesiology 1964;25:312.
29. Dreyfuss D, Basset G, Solar P, Saumon G. Intermittent positive pressure hyperventilation with high inflation pressures produces pulmonary microvascular injury in rats. Am Rev Respir Dis 1985;132:880.
30. Dreyfuss D, Soler P, Basset G, Saumon G. High inflation pulmonary edema. Am Rev Respir Dis 1988;137:1159.
31. Hernandez LA, Peevy KJ, Moise AA, Parker JC. Chest wall restriction limits high airway pressure-induced lung injury in young rabbits. J Appl Physiol 1989;66:2364.
32. Dreyfuss D, Saumon G. Role of tidal volume, FRC, and end-inspiratory volume in the development of pulmonary edema following mechanical ventilation. Am Rev Respir Dis 1993;148:1194.
33. Kolobow T, Moretti MP, Fumagalli R, et al. Severe impairment in lung function induced by high peak airway pressure during mechanical ventilation. Am Rev Respir Dis 1987;135:312.
34. Fu Z, Costello ML, Tsukimoto K, et al. High lung volume increases stress failure in pulmonary capillaries. J Appl Physiol 1992;73:123.
35. Gattinoni L, D'Andrea L, Pelosi P, et al. Regional effects and mechanism of positive end-expiratory distress syndrome. JAMA 1993;269:2122.
36. Mascheroni D, Kolobow T, Fumagalli R, et al. Acute respiratory failure following pharmacologically induced hyperventilation: an experimental animal study. Intensive Care Med 1988;15:8.
37. Jenkinson SG. Oxygen toxicity. New Horiz 1993;1:504.
38. Tobin MJ. Mechanical ventilation. N Engl J Med 1994;330:1056.
39. Gattinoni L, Pelosi P, Valenza F, Mascheroni D. Patient positioning in acute respiratory failure. In: Tobin MJ, ed. Principles and practice of mechanical ventilation. New York, McGraw-Hill, 1994:1067.
40. Bartlett RH, Brennen MC, Gazzaniga AB, Hanson EL. Studies on the pathogenesis and prevention of postoperative pulmonary complications. Surg Gynecol Obstet 1973;137:925.
41. Kollef MH, Schuster DP. The acute respiratory distress syndrome. N Engl J Med 1995;332:27.
42. Ng PC. The effectiveness and side effects of dexamethasone in preterm infants with bronchopulmonary dysplasia. Arch Dis Child 1993;68:330.
43. Sanders RJ, Cox C, Phelps DL, Sinkin RA. Two doses of early intrave-

nous dexamethasone for the prevention of bronchopulmonary dysplasia in babies with respiratory distress syndrome. Pediatr Res 1994; 36:122.

44. Palmer RMJ, Ferrige AG, Moncada SA. Nitric oxide release accounts for the biological activity of endothelium derived relaxing factor. Nature 1987;327:524.

45. Szabo C. Alterations in nitric oxide production in various forms of circulatory shock. New Horiz 1995;3:2.

46. Cioffi WG, Ogura H. Inhaled nitric oxide in acute lung disease. New Horiz 1995;3:73.

47. Suter PM, Domenighetti G, Schaller MD, et al. N-acetylcysteine enhances recovery from acute lung injury in man: a randomized, double-blind, placebo-controlled clinical study. Chest 1994;105:190.

48. Yu M, Tomasa G. A double-blind, prospective, randomized trial of ketoconazole, a thromboxane synthetase inhibitor, in the prophylaxis of the adult respiratory distress syndrome. Crit Care Med 1993;21:1635.

49. Montravers P, Fagon JY, Gilbert C, et al. Pilot study of cardiopulmonary risk from pentoxifylline in adult respiratory distress syndrome. Chest 1993;103:1017.

50. Colice GL. Historical perspective on the development of mechanical ventilation. In: Tobin MJ, ed. Principles and practice of mechanical ventilation. New York, McGraw-Hill, 1994:1.

51. Slutsky AS. Mechanical ventilation. Chest 1993;104:1833.

52. Donn SM, Nicks JJ, Becker MA. Flow-synchronized ventilation of preterm infants with respiratory distress syndrome. J Perinatol 1994; 14:90.

53. Servant GM, Nicks JJ, Donn SM, et al. Feasibility of applying flow-synchronized ventilation to very low birth-weight infants. Respiratory Care 1992;37:249.

54. Loick HM, Wendt M, Rotker J, Theissen JL. Ventilation with positive end-expiratory airway pressure causes leukocyte retention in human lung. J Appl Physiol 1993;75:301.

55. Gerstmann DR, deLemos RA, Clark RH. High-frequency ventilation: issues of strategy. Clin Perinatol 1991;18:563.

56. Froese AB, Bryan AC. State of the art: high frequency ventilation. Am Rev Respir Dis 1987;135:1363.

57. Chang HK. Mechanisms of gas transport during ventilation by high frequency oscillation. J Appl Physiol 1984;56:553.

58. Rigatto H, Davi M, Frantz ID, et al (the HIFI Study Group). High-frequency oscillatory ventilation compared with conventional mechanical ventilation in the treatment of respiratory failure in preterm infants. N Engl J Med 1989;320:88.

59. Clark RH, Gerstmann DR, Null DM, deLemos RA. Prospective randomized comparison of high-frequency oscillatory and conventional ventilation in respiratory distress syndrome. Pediatrics 1992;89:5.

60. Arnold JH, Truog RD, Thompson JE, Fackler JC. High-frequency oscillatory ventilation in pediatric respiratory failure. Crit Care Med 1993;21:272.

61. Arnold JH, Hanson JH, Toro-Figuero LO, et al. Prospective randomized comparison of high-frequency oscillatory ventilation and conventional mechanical ventilation in pediatric respiratory failure. Crit Care Med 1994;22:1530.

62. Jobes DR, Nicolson SC, Steven JM, et al. Carbon dioxide prevents pulmonary overcirculation in hypoplastic left heart syndrome. Ann Thorac Surg 1992;54:150.

63. Greenspan JS, Wolfson MR, Rubenstein SD, et al. Liquid ventilation of human preterm neonates. J Pediatr 1990;117:106.

64. Tutuncu AS, Faithfull NS, Lachmann B. Intratracheal perfluorocarbon administration combined with mechanical ventilation in experimental respiratory distress syndrome: dose-dependent improvement of gas exchange. Crit Care Med 1993;21:962.

65. Leach CL, Fuhrman BP, Morin FC. Perfluorocarbon-associated gas exchange (partial liquid ventilation) in respiratory distress syndrome: a prospective, randomized, controlled study. Crit Care Med 1993;21:1270.

66. Tobin MJ, Alex CG. Discontinuation of mechanical ventilation. In: Tobin MJ, ed. Principles and practice of mechanical ventilation. New York, McGraw-Hill, 1994:1177.

67. Esteban A, Frutos F, Tobin MJ, et al. A comparison of four methods of weaning patients from mechanical ventilation. N Engl J Med 1995; 332:345.

68. Isenstein DA, Venner DS, Duggan J. Neuromuscular blockade in the intensive care unit. Chest 1992;102:1258.

69. Coursin DB. Neuromuscular blockade: should patients be relaxed in the ICU? Chest 1992;102:988.

70. Hansen-Flaschen J, Cowen J, Raps EC. Neuromuscular blockade in the intensive care unit: more than we bargained for. Am Rev Respir Dis 1993;147:234.

71. Dobelle WH, D'Angelo MS, Goetz BF. 200 Cases with a new breathing pacemaker dispel myths about diaphragm pacing. ASAIO J 1994; 40:244.

72. Bach JR. Update and perspectives on noninvasive respiratory muscle aids. Part 1: The inspiratory aids. Chest 1994;105:1230.

73. Bach JR. Update and perspective on noninvasive respiratory muscle aids. Part 2: The expiratory aids. Chest 1994;105:1538.

74. James LS, Wung JT. Neonatal problems treated with ECMO: pathology, prevention, alternative therapies. In: Wright LL, ed. Report of the Workshop on Diffusion of ECMO Technology. US Department of Health and Human Services, Rockville, MD, 1993:43.

75. Bartlett RH. Extracorporeal life support for cardiopulmonary failure. Curr Probl Surg 1990;27:621.

76. Bartlett RH, Gazzaniga AB. Extracorporeal circulation for cardiopulmonary failure. Curr Probl Surg 1978;15:1.

77. Bartlett RH, Gazzaniga AB, Jefferies R, et al. Extracorporeal membrane oxygenation (ECMO) cardiopulmonary support in infancy. ASAIO Trans 1976;22:80.

78. Anderson HL, Otsu T, Chapman RA, Bartlett RH. Venovenous extracorporeal life support in neonates using a double lumen catheter. ASAIO Trans 1989;35:650.

79. Cilley RE, Bartlett RH. Extracorporeal life support for respiratory failure. In: Gravlee GP, Davis RF, Utley JR, eds. Cardiopulmonary bypass: principles and practice. Baltimore, Williams & Wilkins, 1993: 655.

80. Schmidt S, Dudenhausen JW, Langner K, et al. A new perfusion circuit for the newborn with lung immaturity: extracorporeal CO_2 removal via an umbilical arterio-venous shunt during apneic O_2 diffusion. Artif Organs 1984;8:478.

81. Cilley RE, Scharenberg AM, Bongiorno PF, et al. Low oxygen delivery produced by anemia, hypoxia, and low cardiac output. J Surg Res 1991;51:425.

82. Gattinoni L, Presenti A, Mascheroni D, et al. Low-frequency positive-pressure ventilation with extracorporeal CO_2 removal in severe acute respiratory failure. JAMA 1986;256:881.

83. Anderson HL III, Coran AG, Drongowski RA, et al. Extracellular fluid and total body water changes in neonates undergoing extracorporeal membrane oxygenation (ECMO). J Pediatr Surg 1992;27:1003.

84. Meliones JN, Moler FW, Custer JR, et al. Hemodynamic instability after the initiation of extracorporeal membrane oxygenation: role of ionized calcium. Crit Care Med 1991;19:1247.

85. Foster AH, Kolobow T. A potential hazard of ventilation during early separation from total cardiopulmonary bypass. (Letter) J Thorac Cardiovasc Surg 1987;93:150.

86. Kolobow T, Spragg RH, Pierce JE. Massive pulmonary infarction during total cardiopulmonary bypass in unanesthetized spontaneously breathing lambs. Int J Artif Organs 1981;4:76.

87. Heiss KF, Pettit B, Hirschl RB, et al. Renal insufficiency and volume overload in neonatal ECMO managed by continuous ultrafiltration. ASAIO Trans 1987;33:557.

88. Spector ML, Wiznitzer M, Walsh-Sukys MC, Stork EK. Carotid reconstruction in the neonate following ECMO. J Pediatr Surg 1991; 26:357.

89. Moulton SL, Lynch FP, Cornish JD, et al. Carotid artery reconstruction following neonatal extracorporeal membrane oxygenation. J Pediatr Surg 1991;26:794.

90. Wilson JM, Bower LK, Fackler JC, et al. Aminocaproic acid decreases the incidence of intracranial hemorrhage and other hemorrhagic complications of ECMO. J Pediatr Surg 1993;28:536.

91. Cilley RE, Wesley JR, Zwischenberger JB, et al. Pulmonary recovery predicted by measurement of pulmonary and membrane lung gas exchange during extracorporeal membrane oxygenation. Surg Forum 1985;36:294.

92. Garg M, Lew CD, Ramos AD, et al. Serial measurement of pulmonary mechanics assists in weaning from extracorporeal membrane oxygenation in neonates with respiratory failure. Chest 1991;100:770.

93. American Academy of Pediatrics Committee on Fetus and Newborn. Recommendations on extracorporeal membrane oxygenation. Pediatrics 1990;85:618.

94. Schumacher R, Roloff DW, Chapman CA, et al. Extracorporeal membrane oxygenation in term newborns: a prospective cost-benefit analysis. ASAIO J 1993;39:873.

95. Shanley CJ, Hirschel RB, Schumacker RE, et al. Extracorporeal life support for neonatal respiratory failure: a twenty year experience. Ann Surg 1994;220:269.

96. Bartlett RH, Gazzaniga AB, Toomasian J, et al. Extracorporeal membrane oxygenation (ECMO) in neonatal respiratory failure: 100 cases. Ann Surg 1986;204:236.

97. Cilley RE, Zwischenberger JB, Andrews AF, et al. Intracranial hemorrhage during extracorporeal membrane oxygenation in neonates. Pediatrics 1986;78:699.

98. Bui KC, La Clair P, Vanderkerhove J, Bartlett RH. ECMO in premature infants: review of factors associated with mortality. ASAIO Trans 1991;37:54.

99. Bartlett RH, Andrews AF, Toomasian JM, et al. Extracorporeal circulation in neonatal respiratory failure: a prospective randomized study. Pediatrics 1985;76:479.

100. O'Rourke PP, Crone R, Vacanti J, et al. Extracorporeal membrane oxygenation and conventional medical therapy in neonates with persistent pulmonary hypertension of the newborn: a prospective randomized study. Pediatrics 1989;84:957.

101. Cohen RS, Stevenson DK, Malachowkski N, et al. Late morbidity among survivors of respiratory failure treated with tolazoline. J Pediatr 1980;97:644.

102. Brett C, Dekl M, Leonard CH, et al. Developmental follow-up of hyperventilated neonates: preliminary observations. Pediatrics 1981;68:588.

103. Hofkosh D, Thompson AE, Nozza RJ, et al. Ten years of extracorporeal membrane oxygenation: neurodevelopmental outcome. Pediatrics 1991;87:459.

104. Schumacher RE, Palmer TW, Roloff DW, et al. Follow-up on infants treated with extracorporeal membrane oxygenation for newborn respiratory failure. Pediatrics 1991;87:451.

105. Extracorporeal life support organization registry. Ann Arbor, MI, University of Michigan Press, 1995.

106. Moler FW, Custer JR, Bartlett RH, et al. Extracorporeal life support for severe pediatric respiratory failure: an updated experience 1991-1993. J Pediatr 1994;124:875.

Surgery of Infants and Children: Scientific Principles and Practice, edited by Keith T. Oldham, Paul M. Colombani, and Robert P. Foglia. Lippincott–Raven Publishers, Philadelphia, © 1997.

CHAPTER 9

Wound Healing

Thomas M. Krummel

Critical to the survival of every higher organism is the ability to repair wounded tissue rapidly and efficiently. The processes by which hemostasis is attained, invasion by microorganisms repelled, and function restored are key determinants of survival after injury. Should any of these steps prove inadequate or, at the other extreme, too exuberant, the potential for significant morbidity or even mortality is high. For this reason, the clinical aspects of wound healing have long been of interest to the surgeon. The past decade has seen renewed interest in understanding the mechanisms of tissue repair, particularly with regard to the possible manipulation of wounded tissue to improve healing and prevent adverse consequences of the repair process where it is deficient (dehiscence) or excessive (keloids, strictures, fibrosis).

This renewed interest in wound repair stems from two areas. The discovery and characterization of a family of peptide growth factors, now known to orchestrate the events of repair, has served to reenergize wound healing research on both the basic science and commercial fronts. But even more exciting have been first reports of the attempted in utero repair of specific fetal anomalies. A new appreciation of the fact that the mammalian fetus appears to heal without scar formation has arisen from this experience. Wound repair in mid-gestation mammals may have as at least as much in common with the regenerative capabilities of axolotls as with the fibrotic response of adult mammals (Fig. 9-1). What has arisen during the past decade is a large body of research directed toward discerning the differences between the mechanisms of fetal and of adult tissue repair. Driving this research is the hope of one day turning these differences to clinical advantage, using the unique properties of fetal wound healing to ameliorate the undesirable consequences of inadequate or overexuberant adult tissue repair.

Before considering fetal wound healing, the characteristics of the adult response to wounding must be understood. It has long been taught that adult wound healing consists of three phases: inflammation, proliferation, and remodeling (Fig. 9-2). This teaching, although somewhat simplistic, serves as an acceptable framework from which to consider tissue repair in more detail. Although these three phases overlap, each appears at a clearly definable time after wounding, has a distinct complement of events occurring within it, and is becoming relatively well characterized in terms of its cellular and biochemical mediators (Fig. 9-3).

INFLAMMATION

The inflammatory phase after injury can perhaps best be thought of as a delivery period. During this phase, the wound is secured by the host's hemostatic mechanisms, devitalized tissues are débrided, and the milieu is conditioned for the enormous mobilization of cellular and noncellular elements into the repair site. The successful completion of this phase is vital to the subsequent repair process; the regulation of this period is equally important, however, because an uncontrolled inflammatory response can soon spread beyond the boundaries of a local reaction and engulf the affected organism in a life-threatening systemic response.

Hemostasis

The disruption of tissue results in the exposure of circulating blood elements to subendothelial collagen. The subsequent aggregation of platelets, vasoconstriction, and activation of the coagulation cascade achieve hemostasis through the formation of a fibrin-based hemostatic plug (Fig. 9-4). The platelets trapped within this network release stored mediators—including chemoattractants (platelet-activating factor, platelet-derived growth factor [PDGF]), growth factors (transforming growth factor β [TGF-β], fibroblast-derived growth factor), and vasoactive substances (prostaglandin E_2, serotonin—that initiate and amplify the inflammatory response. In addition, similar mediators stored within the wounded tissues are released into the wound environment, further amplifying and maintaining the inflammatory response.[1]

Chemotaxis and Adhesion

Drawn by the release of chemoattractants from aggregating platelets and wounded tissue, numerous inflammatory cells infiltrate the wound site, with the type of infiltrating cell following a predictable time course. Early in the inflammatory period, polymorphonuclear leukocytes are the predominant infiltrating cells, leaving the microvasculature and migrating through the endothelial pores of wounded tissue. They function primarily as

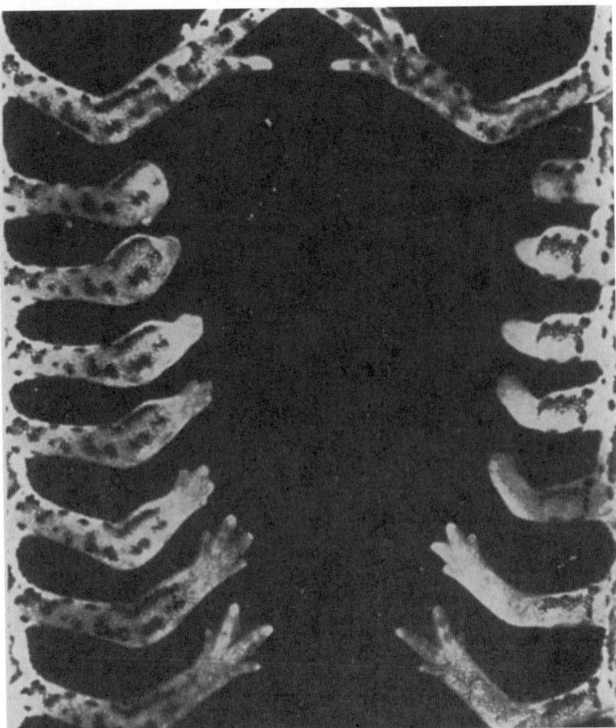

FIG. 9-1. Sequence photographs showing limb regeneration in an axolotl.

a first line of defense, working to phagocytize microorganisms invading through the breached integument, in addition to removing devitalized tissue. Later in this stage, macrophages and lymphocytes migrate to the wound site, where through complex signals they perpetuate and amplify the repair cascade. The ultimate goal of these actions is recruitment of the fibroblast, necessary for the deposition of collagen and restoration of tensile strength in the wounded tissue (Fig. 9-5).

PROLIFERATION

Fibroblasts, migrating in response to chemoattractants such as TGF-β, populate the wound site in increasing numbers throughout the first two phases of wound healing. Initial activities center around the deposition of extracellular matrix (ECM), the proteoglycan-rich framework around which the reparative architecture is constructed. Later in the repair process, the fibroblast is responsible for the deposition of new collagen. Along with this accumulation of collagen-producing cells, two other events highlight this phase (Fig. 9-6).

Neovascularization

Essential to the maintenance of the repair process and the resulting newly synthesized tissue is a delivery mechanism for nutrients. Early on, diffusion and cellular migration supply the wound site; however, new vasculature must develop to maintain the delivery of cells active in repair, provide them with adequate nourishment, and remove the by-products of metabolism. This process of neovascularization begins as an outgrowth of fine capillaries from the existing bed in adjacent unwounded tissue. In time, a larger system develops, although the newly deposited scar tissue never achieves the same degree of vascularization as the original tissue.

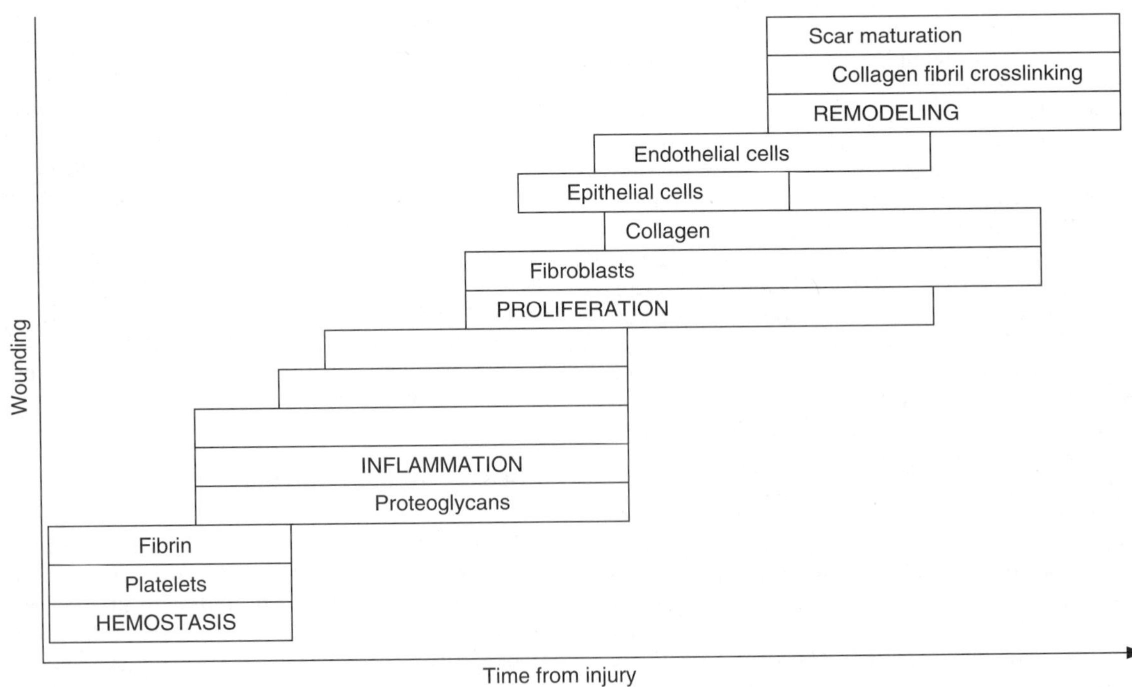

FIG. 9-2. Timeline of the events of wound healing.

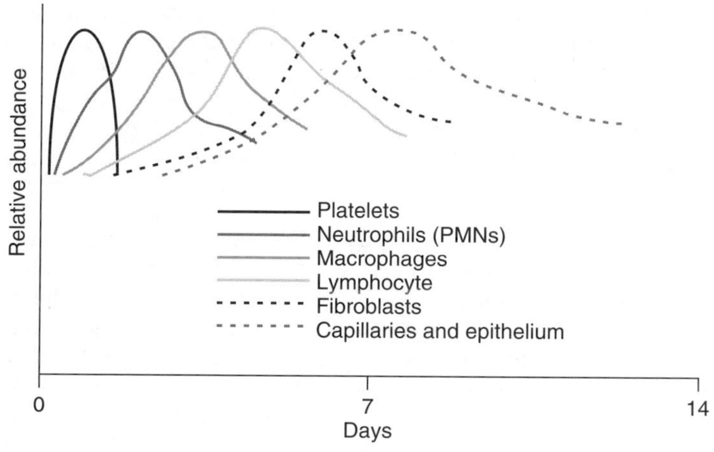

FIG. 9-3. Time course of cellular infiltration of the wound site.

Epithelialization

Although the neutrophil provides the initial defense against invasion through the wounded integument, surface closure of the defect must be achieved. By a relatively early point in the repair process, basal epithelial cells from the wound edges have migrated under the fibrin eschar to close the wound. This process provides wound closure, not wound strength, and is helped enormously in the clinical setting by proper coapting of the wound edges at the conclusion of an operation. The relatively early occurrence of this process suggests an important role, in addition to barrier reconstitution. Some researchers have suggested cell-to-cell communication, but these mechanisms are poorly understood.

REMODELING

Collagen Turnover

New collagen exists in a dynamic state after its synthesis. The degrading action of collagenases, opposed by further collagen deposition by residing fibroblasts, results in a wound that sustains a marked remodeling for months to years (Fig. 9-7). In this phase, the overlap of the separate phases can be seen. Deprived of nutrients and substrates to support continued collagen synthesis, the wound site breaks down over time, as seen historically in scurvy-stricken naval recruits. At the opposite end of the repair spectrum, the failure to control synthesis at this stage accounts for many of the cosmetic and functional deficits seen by the practicing clinician.

Contraction

Through the action of specialized cells possessing contractile elements, the wound site undergoes a centripetally directed contraction, reducing the scar's size and visibility. Such action, however, can be detrimental in wounds located over joints. The process of wound contraction in this situation can result in a contracture, rendering the joint nonfunctional (Fig. 9-8).

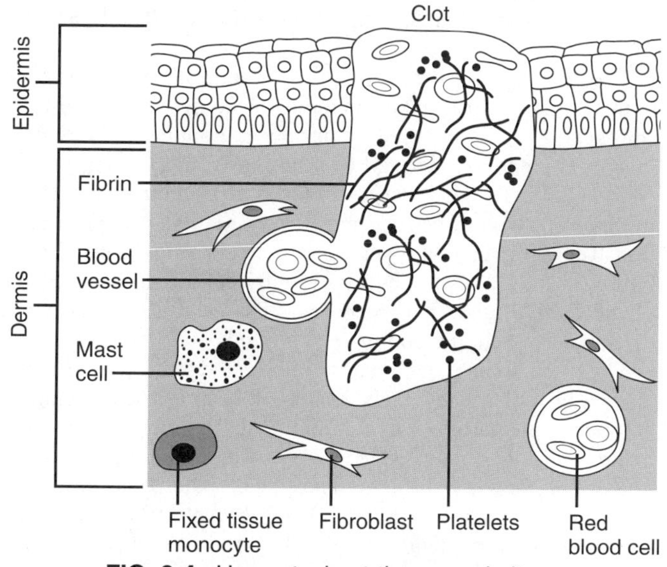

FIG. 9-4. Hemostasis at the wound site.

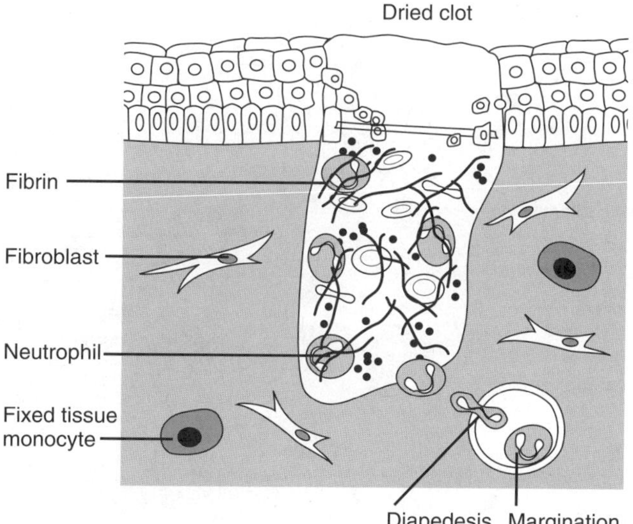

FIG. 9-5. Inflammatory phase of wound healing.

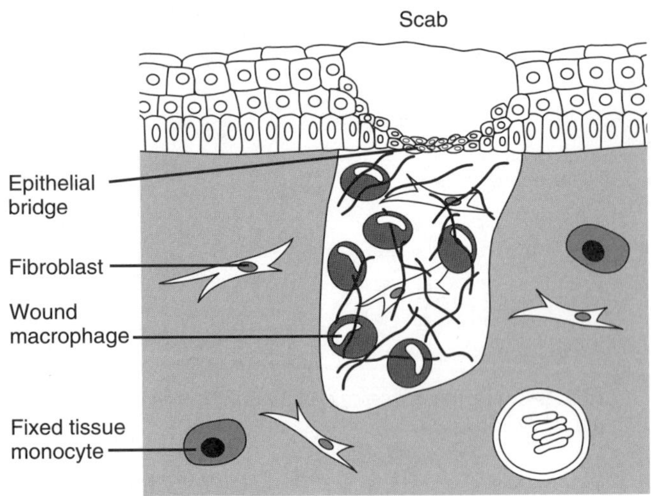

FIG. 9-6. Fibroplasia at the wound site. Fibroblasts infiltrate the wound site in response to signaling from wound macrophages.

GROWTH FACTORS

Perhaps the predominant advance in wound healing research during the past decade was the discovery of the role that the cytokines play in mediating tissue repair. Although much remains to be learned about the spectrum of events mediated by these compounds, they have become a prime investigative target, not only of the basic scientist but also of the clinician seeking methods to manipulate the wound environment.

The cytokines involved in wound healing all share characteristics of the hormones, particularly in the way in which they are secreted and then affect cells remote from the site of synthesis. This similarity has led to the concept of the ''wound hormone''; as for the conventional hormones of the endocrine system, these compounds can be broadly classified based on the cells targeted for their actions[2] (Fig. 9-9):

Endocrine substances act on a cell distant from the site of production. This target cell is reached through the systemic circulation.

Paracrine factors act on cells adjacent to the cell of production. The range of the factor's action is limited by diffusion.

Autocrine cytokines are secreted by the producer cell and act on the membrane of the producing cell.

Intracrine factors remain inside the cell of production, exerting their effects without leaving the confines of the cell membrane.

Of the cytokines implicated in wound healing, TGF-β has generated the greatest interest, for its roles in both tissue repair and development. Released at the wound site by degranulating platelets, this 34-kd peptide is chemotactic to both the monocyte and fibroblast lines. TGF-β appears to have as its most basic repair function the promotion of fibrosis, stimulating fibroblasts to migrate, proliferate, and deposit collagen, while at the same time inhibiting collagenase production.[3] Wound implants treated with TGF-β show markedly increased collagen deposition[4]; in contrast, neutralizing antibodies directed against TGF-β reduce collagen deposition in adult wounds.[5]

PDGF is released from platelets aggregated at the wound site and is one of the earliest factors present. This factor is important to the cellular inflammatory response, providing a potent chemotactic signal to macrophages and, to a lesser extent, fibroblasts. PDGF also plays a role in the production of collagenases and as such may provide a balance to the actions of TGF-β.[6] Epidermal growth factor is closely related to TGF-α. This peptide is a known mitogen for fibroblasts as well as epidermal cells. It has been shown to accelerate the healing of experimental wounds in mammals and can accelerate reepithelialization in both adult and fetal wounds. Additional cytokines that contribute to wound healing are summarized in Table 9-1.

EXTRACELLULAR MATRIX

The ECM may prove to be the critical factor in determining the type of repair that occurs in wounded tissue. This complex framework of glycoproteins, glycosaminoglycans, and proteoglycans—all relatively complex macromolecules composed of varying proportions of modified peptide and carbohydrate moieties—provides the environment within which cell migration, cytodifferentiation, and secretion occur (Fig. 9-10 and Table 9-2).

The fibrin plug forms the initial wound matrix. In addition to providing hemostasis, fibrin rapidly becomes associated with fibronectin. Both delivered by platelet α granules and circulating plasma and synthesized by fibroblasts, macrophages, and endothelial cells, fibrinectin, a 440-kd glycoprotein, functions in the promotion of cellular motility, migration, and proliferation. Tenascin, another glycoprotein seen in only limited distribution in the ECM of adults, is rapidly deposited in the ECM of the fetal wound. This compound has been associated with the rapid epithelialization of fetal wounds.[7]

The provisional wound matrix of both the fetus and the adult is rapidly replaced by a glycosaminoglycan-rich environment composed primarily of hyaluronic acid. Hyaluronic acid is a macromolecule composed primarily of repeating disaccharide units of *N*-acetylglucosamine and glucuronate. It accumulates in polyvinyl alcohol sponge implants at levels 10 times higher than in surrounding fetal skin.[8] Produced by fibroblasts, hyaluronic acid exists in the ECM in a strongly hydrated state, occupy-

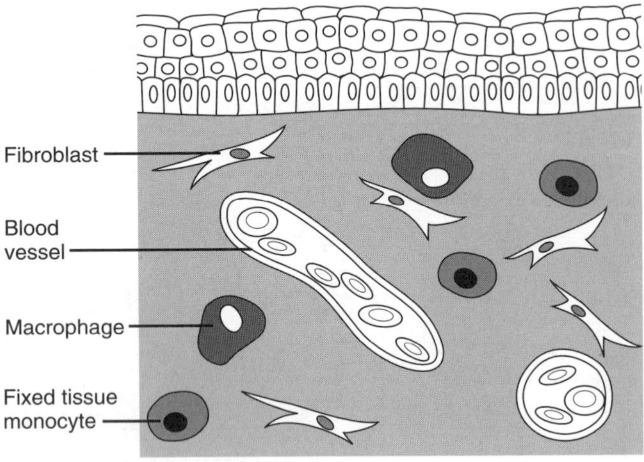

FIG. 9-7. Remodeling phase at the wound site.

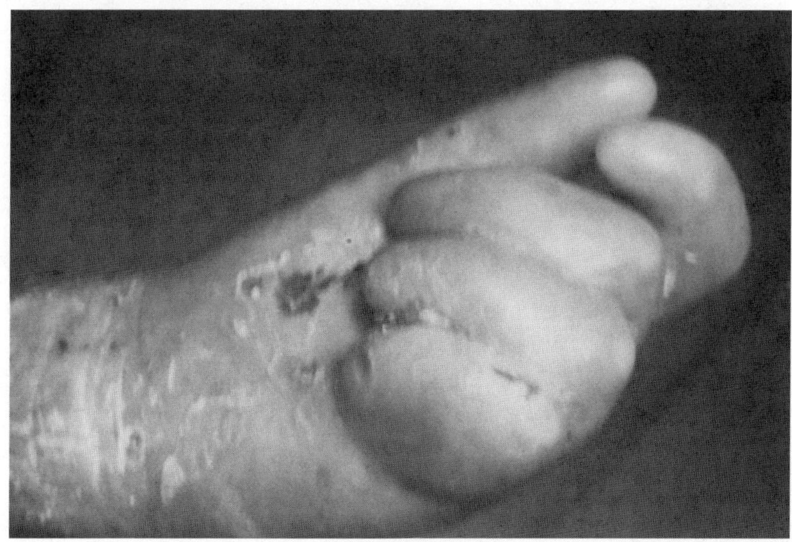

FIG. 9-8. Patient's hand rendered nonfunctional by scar contraction. (Courtesy of Randall Hauck, MD, Hershey Medical Center, Hershey, PA)

ing a relatively large volume. This characteristic results in a matrix that is highly permissive to cell migration, and it provides a framework for the highly organized reticular pattern of collagen deposition seen in fetal wounds (Fig. 9-11 and Table 9-3).

Unique to fetal fluids, including serum, amniotic fluid, and wound fluid, is a glycoprotein that stimulates the production of hyaluronic acid. This compound, known as hyaluronic acid–sti-mulating factor, appears unique to the fetal environment. The elaboration of this compound by fetal tissues may account for the persistence of hyaluronic acid in the fetal wound matrix, resulting in the highly ordered deposition of collagen.[9] This is in contrast to the adult wound, in which the hyaluronic acid–based matrix rapidly gives way to an environment populated by highly sulfated glycosaminoglycans, which are themselves replaced by a dense collagen scar.

COLLAGEN

Ultimately, all wound extracellular matrices contain collagen as their primary component. The biology and chemistry of this ubiquitous compound have been well characterized. At least 16 types of collagen have been described; characteristics of the first six are listed in Table 9-4.

The collagens have as their common structure a triple helical conformation composed of similar but nonidentical polypeptides. A high frequency of the tripeptide sequence glycine–proline–x is demonstrated, with x being hydroxyproline in about 10% of the sequences. The heavy glycine content is essential to the helical structure that predominates in the collagens. Glycine, the smallest amino acid, with a side chain composed of a single hydrogen atom, provides a chemical swivel around which the repeated coiling can occur (Fig. 9-12).

The types of collagen in tissues have been closely correlated with the function of these tissues. Type I collagen, for example, imparts a rigid structure to tissues and is therefore the predominant collagen found in bone. Type III collagen is found in elastic structures, constituting as much as 70% of the total collagen content in large arteries. Skin exhibits properties of both strength and elasticity, and its collagen makeup is about 80% type I and 20% type III. Of the remaining collagens, type II is the predominant collagen in cartilage, whereas type IV is found primarily as a component of basement membranes.

Collagen is assembled in a complex series of steps that require numerous cofactors for proper synthesis. Before collagen is secreted from the cell, hydroxylation of numerous proline and lysine residues occurs. Oxygen, ferrous iron, α-ketogluta-

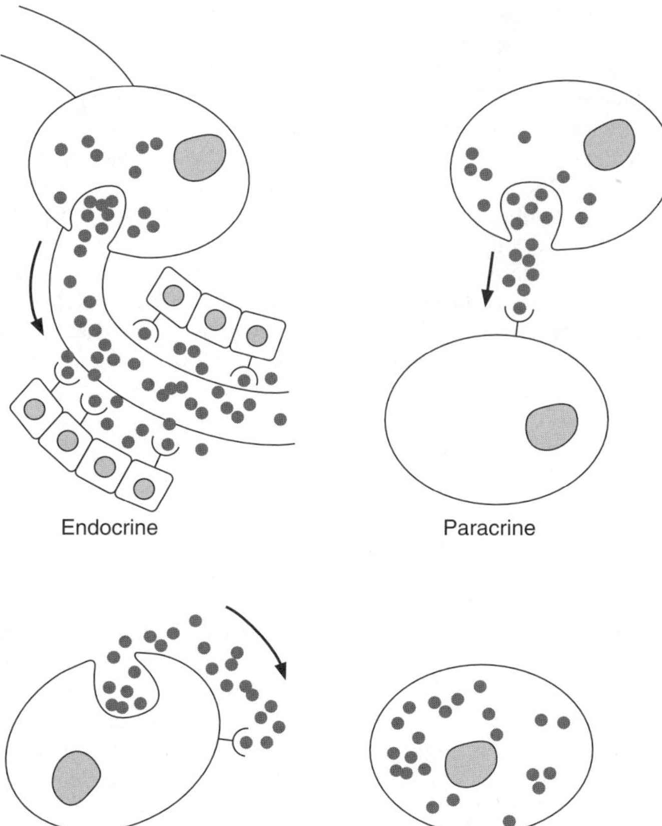

FIG. 9-9. Cell signaling by the cytokines.

TABLE 9-1. *Cytokines implicated in tissue repair*

Factor	Abbreviation	Source	Functions regulated
Platelet-derived growth factor	PDGF	Platelets and macrophages	Fibroblast proliferation, chemotaxis, and collagenase production
Transforming growth factor β	TGF-β	Platelets, polymorphonuclear neutrophil leukocytes, T lymphocytes, and macrophages	Fibroblast proliferation, chemotaxis, collagen metabolism, and action of other growth factors
Transforming growth factor α	TGF-α	Activated macrophages and many tissues	Similar to epidermal growth factor functions
Interleukin-1	IL-1	Macrophages	Fibroblast proliferation
Tumor necrosis factor	TNF	Macrophages, mast cells, and T lymphocytes	Fibroblast proliferation
Fibroblast growth factor	FGF	Brain, pituitary, macrophages, and many other tissues and cells	Fibroblast proliferation, stimulates collagen deposition and angiogenesis
Epidermal growth factor	EGF	Saliva, urine, milk, and plasma	Stimulates epithelial cell proliferation and granulation tissue formation
Insulin-like growth factor	IGF	Liver, plasma, and fibroblasts	Stimulates synthesis of sulfated proteoglycans, collagen, and cell proliferation
Human growth factor	HGF	Pituitary and thus plasma	Anabolism

(Cohen IK, Diegelmann FR. Wound healing. In: Greenfield LJ, Mulholland MW, Oldham KT, et al, eds. Surgery: scientific principles and practice. Philadelphia, JB Lippincott, 1992:89)

rate, and ascorbate are cofactors critical to the proper function of the hydroxylases catalyzing these events. Additionally, manganese is required for the subsequent glycosylation of hydroxylysine residues. Deficiencies of any of these cofactors (eg, hypoxia, vitamin C or manganese deficiency) can result in impaired wound healing secondary to the rapid breakdown of unstable collagen structures in the ECM.

Collagen is secreted into the ECM in its triple helical form but as procollagen, with a number of peptides remaining at both the carboxy and amino terminals. These extension peptides are rapidly cleaved from procollagen, resulting in a functional collagen molecule. At this point, lysyl oxidase catalyzes the stabilizing formation of stable intermolecular and intramolecular cross-links. This results in a longitudinal alignment of the collagen molecules into fibrils, yielding a characteristic overlap pattern with a periodicity of 68-nm when viewed by electron microscopy. These cross-links are critical to normal collagen synthesis, as seen by the deficient collagens that result when pharmacologic agents such as β-amino propionitrile or D-penicillamine are administered. β-Amino propionitrile impairs collagen synthesis directly through its inhibition of lysyl oxidase, and D-penicillamine impairs collagen synthesis by binding to collagen at the sites of cross-link formation, thereby inhibiting their development.[10,11]

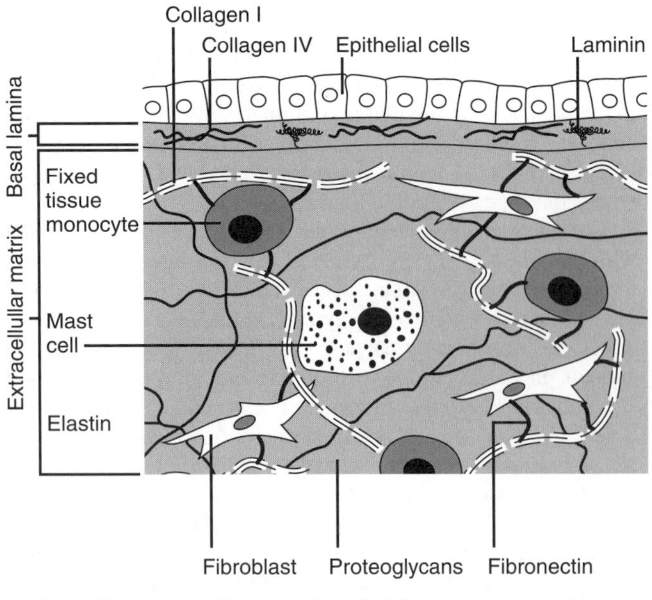

With regard to matrix formation, type I collagen forms the predominant collagen in the adult wound. The fetus is unique, however, in that a relatively greater amount of type III collagen is deposited. The deposition of this type of collagen favors organization into the fine reticular pattern characteristic of scarless repair, as opposed to the dense, poorly ordered fibers seen in adult scars.

FETAL REPAIR

Surgeons have long had an empirical sense that very young patients enjoy an advantage in tissue repair, with a more rapid return to function and a superior cosmetic result after many surgical procedures. In addition, the concept of fetal tissue repair as an entity distinct from adult repair was discussed in the first half of this century with the observation that embryonic extracts applied topically to wounds promote healing. In 1970, Somasundaram and Prathap[12] described scarless repair in fetal rabbits; in 1971, Burrington[13] demonstrated the scarless healing of linear incisions in fetal lambs. In 1979, these observations were extended to humans when Rowlatt[14] reported on the heal-

FIG. 9-10. Extracellular matrix. GAG, glycosaminoglycan.

TABLE 9-2. *Extracellular matrix components*

Component	Structure	Function
Collagen	Triple helical glycoprotein molecules rich in proline, hydroxyproline, and glycine	Strength, support, and structure for all tissues and organs
Elastin	Stretchable hydrophobic protein interacting with glycosylated microfibrils	Allows tissues and structures to expand and contract
Fibronectin	Specialized adhesive glycoprotein	Mediates cell–matrix adhesion
Laminin	Large, complex, adhesive glycoprotein	Binds cells to type IV collagen and heparan sulfate
Proteoglycans	Heterogeneous, long glycosaminoglycan chains covalently linked to a core protein	Moisture stores, shock absorption, sequestration of cytokines
Hyaluronic acid	Very large, specialized, nonsulfated glycosaminoglycan	Provides a fluid environment for cell movement and differentiation, and binds to cytokines

ing of limb amputations, probably caused by amniotic constriction bands, in a stillborn fetus of 20 weeks' gestation. Subsequently, Hallock[15] described in utero cleft lip repair first in A/J mice and then in rhesus monkeys, making a strong case for someday being able to turn the unique repair capabilities of the fetus to clinical advantage.

These seminal observations have stimulated a large body of research in the past decade devoted to understanding the mechanisms of fetal tissue repair. A number of key differences in tissue repair between mid-gestation fetuses and adults have emerged:

1. In fetuses, little inflammatory response appears after wounding.
2. Hyaluronic acid plays a prominent role in constituting the ECM of the healing wound.
3. Collagen deposition is markedly reduced in fetuses, and the collagen deposited is far more ordered.
4. Secondary to this ordered collagen deposition, a marked remodeling phase is not seen in fetuses.
5. T lymphocytes, which ultimately constitute most of the

invading cells in the adult wound, are relatively fewer in fetuses.

Repair in Specific Fetal Tissues

Despite the discovery of the unique properties of repair exhibited by fetuses, nearly all of the research has focused on the dermis. Relatively little is known about repair in other fetal organs. Summarized here are observations about the responses of nonintegumentary fetal organs to wounding.

Skeletal Muscle

The first reports of experience with fetal surgery suggest that fetal muscle heals with a tendency to greater scar formation than does the dermis. Anecdotal reports of previous in utero surgical patients who later underwent operation for postnatal

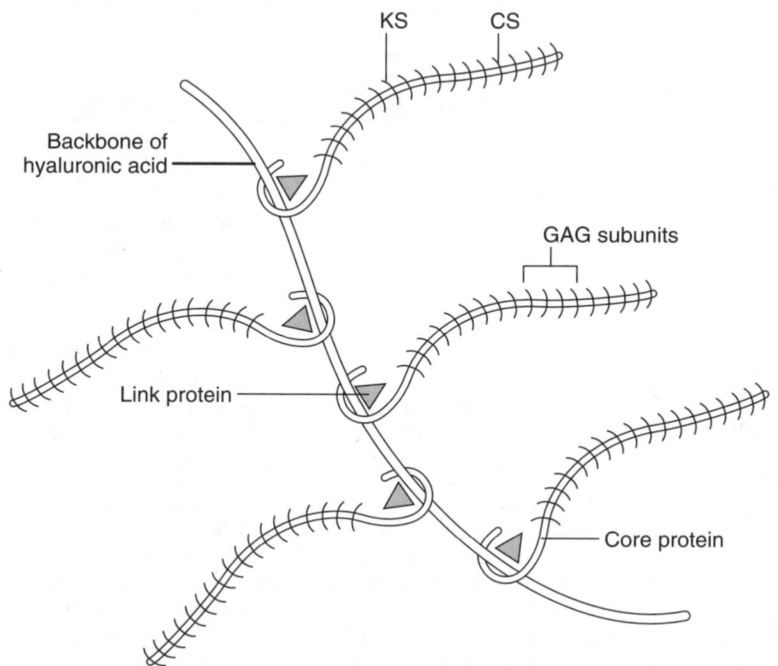

FIG. 9-11. Structure of a representative proteoglycan demonstrating bottle-brush architecture.

TABLE 9-3. *Glycosaminoglycans and their tissue distributions*

| Glycosaminoglycan | Molecular weight | Repeating disaccharide (A-B) | | Linked to protein | Tissue distribution |
		Monosaccharide A	Monosaccharide B		
Hyaluronic acid	4000 to 8×10^8	D-Glucuronic acid	N-acetyl-d-glucosamine	−	Most connective tissues, skin, cartilage, and synovial fluid
Chondroitin sulfate	5000–50,000	D-Glucuronic acid	N-acetyl-d-galactosamine	+	Cartilage, bone, and skin
Dermatan nitrate	15,000–40,000	D-Glucuronic acid or L-iduronic acid	N-acetyl-d-galactosamine	+	Skin and blood vessels
Heparan sulfate	5000–12,000	D-Glucuronic acid or L-iduronic acid	N-acetyl-d-glucosamine	+	Lungs, arteries, and cell surfaces
Heparin	6000–25,000	D-Glucuronic acid or L-iduronic acid	N-acetyl-d-glucosamine	+	Skin, lungs, liver, and mast cells
Keratan sulfate	4000–19,000	D-Galactose	N-acetyl-d-glucosamine	+	Cartilage and intervertebral disk

(Cohen IK, Diegelmann FR. Wound healing. In: Greenfield LJ, Mulholland MW, Oldham KT, et al, eds. Surgery: scientific principles and practice. Philadelphia, JB Lippincott, 1992:97)

conditions record scar formation in the diaphragm in conjunction with densely adherent intestine and stomach. Burd and colleagues[16] confirmed this observation in fetal lambs, demonstrating that diaphragmatic incisions heal with scar formation whether or not they are exposed to amniotic fluid. In contrast, the wounded musculature in full-thickness lip wounds heals without scar formation.

Myocardium

Fetal myocardial healing has been studied in the organ culture system. Using these methods, fetal murine myocardium has been shown to heal without scar formation in mid-gestation, with a transition to an adult-like healing pattern by late gestation.[17]

Lung

The murine fetal lung has also been investigated in organ culture. The lung appears to retain scarless healing capabilities late into gestation, with a transition to definite adult-type healing seen only in the neonatal period.[18]

Tendon

Tendon healing has been investigated in the fetal lamb model. Reconstitution of collagen fibers along the long axis of the fetal tendon was seen 2 weeks after wounding, along with restoration of a smooth, gliding surface. This is in contrast to healing of the adult tendon, which had a much slower restoration of collagen fiber orientation, without a resulting smooth, gliding surface.[19]

Bone

Fracture healing has been investigated in fetal rabbits. Femur fractures produced in utero were observed to undergo a much smaller inflammatory reaction and less prominent hematoma formation than fractures produced in neonates. Proliferative activity in the fetal periosteum and endosteum was more intense and began earlier after wounding. Finally, fetal callus was more abundant and showed a more rapid differentiation into cartilaginous bone precursors than did similarly wounded neonatal controls.[20]

Investigative Methods

Stimulated by observations such as these, a number of investigative methodologies have been developed for the study of

TABLE 9-4. *Molecular structure of collagen types I through VI*

Type	Molecular configuration*	Distribution
I	$[\alpha 1(I)]_2 \alpha 2(I)$	All connective tissues except cartilage and basement membranes
II	$[\alpha 1(II)]_3$	Cartilages and vitreous humor
III	$[\alpha 1(III)]_3$	Distensible connective tissues (eg, fetal skin, blood vessels, and uterus)
IV	$[\alpha 1(IV)]_2 \alpha 2(IV)$	Basement membranes
V	$[\alpha 1(V)]_2 \alpha 2(V)$	Essentially all tissues
VI	$[\alpha 1(VI), \alpha 2(VI), \alpha 3(VI)]$	Essentially all tissues

* α Chains are composed of about 1000 amino acids and are rich in glycine, proline, and hydroxyproline. Most collagens contain three α chains interacting in a helical structure.
(Cohen IK, Diegelmann FR. Wound healing. In: Greenfield LJ, Mulholland MW, Oldham KT, et al, eds. Surgery: scientific principles and practice. Philadelphia, JB Lippincott, 1992:93)

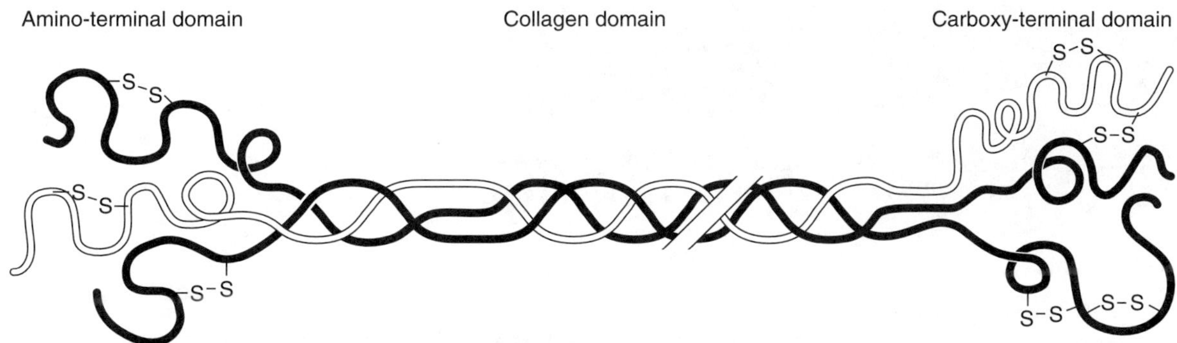

FIG. 9-12. Structure of the type I procollagen molecule

fetal wound healing. A few of the techniques and models devised for the study of wound healing are discussed next.

Cell Culture

Standardized methods for the maintenance of cell lines have been used for the culture of cells implicated in the repair process, particularly the fibroblast. These techniques have proved invaluable for studying cellular characteristics, but they have as a limitation the complete absence of anything resembling the architecture of the native environment. Despite this limitation, cell culture techniques have been useful in determining the effects of many putative mediators of the repair process.

Collagen Lattices

Bell and colleagues[21] popularized the culture of fibroblasts in strictly defined conditions within a circular collagen framework. These collagen lattices can be reduced in size by the fibroblasts cultured within them; what has resulted is an extremely powerful tool for the study of wound contraction (Fig. 9-13). This well-defined system can be manipulated with a high degree of specificity, allowing the investigation of the factors influencing wound contraction.

Implants

Several types of subcutaneous implants have been developed for the study of the wound environment. These implants include those used for the collection of wound fluid, such as the Hunt-Schilling chamber, as well as those designed to accept the deposition of wound matrix, that is, the polyvinyl alcohol sponge (Fig. 9-14). Although some have argued that the infiltration of these structures represents more of a foreign body reaction than tissue repair, the infiltration of these structures is viewed by other investigators as a reasonable approximation of the granulation process.[22]

Organ Culture

Techniques for the culture of whole organs from small fetal mammals have allowed the study of the response to wounding

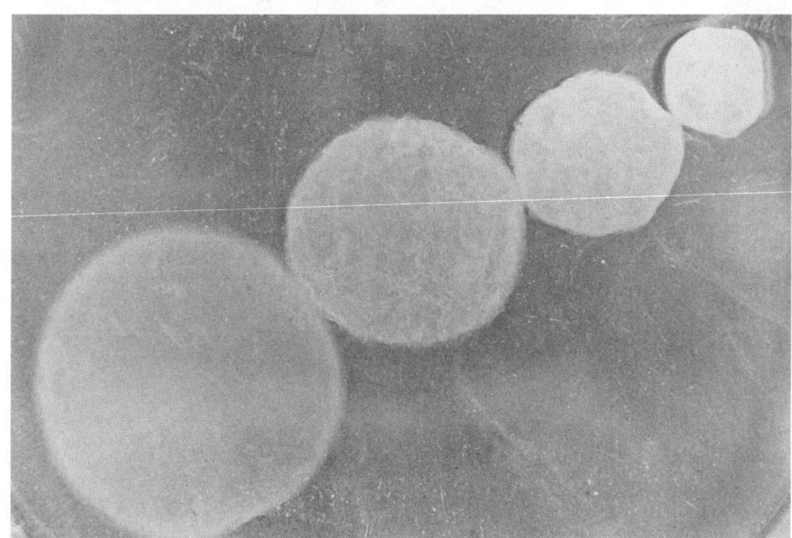

FIG. 9-13. Fibroblast-populated collagen lattices in varying degrees of contraction. (Courtesy of H. Paul Ehrlich, PhD, Hershey Medical Center, Hershey, PA)

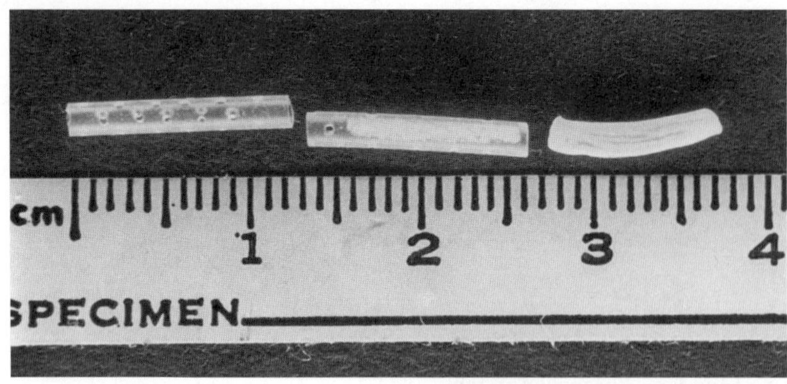

FIG. 9-14. Polyvinyl alcohol sponge implants, shown with fenestrated Silastic encasements.

in fetal tissues in an environment that retains its native architecture. In addition to their preservation of architecture, wounded tissue explants exist in an unperfused state, such that the observed repair occurs without a contribution from the usual circulating mediators of the host. Finally, the culture of these tissues in chemically defined media, without the aid of serum, provides an environment that can be precisely manipulated with respect to the presence or absence of soluble growth factors. Using this technique for the culture of the developing murine forelimb, Bleacher and associates[23] demonstrated the ability of the midgestation fetal integument to undergo scarless repair in the absence of circulating factors. The technique has been applied to demonstrate the ability of certain nonintegumentary organs to repair mechanical wounds in a similar fashion.

Fetal Skin Transplantation

Using athymic mice, murine fetal skin can be engrafted onto nude mice in both external and subcutaneous sites. The model is attractive in that it allows comparison of fetal skin in conditions approximating the protected intrauterine environment with conditions of external exposure. Furthermore, it provides an immu-

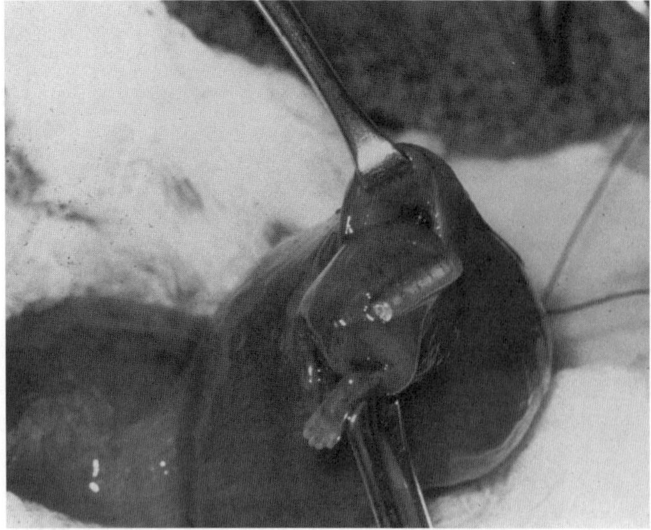

FIG. 9-15. Fetal rabbit undergoing in utero operation for the placement of a polyvinyl alcohol sponge implant.

nologically nonthreatening environment for the study of repair.[24]

Fetal Manipulation

Techniques for the manipulation of mammalian fetuses in utero have been described for numerous species, particularly the fetal rabbit (Fig. 9-15). Although somewhat more labor and resource intensive, thereby limiting the sample size that can be achieved, these models provide the best means of studying repair in the native fetal wound environment.

WOUND MANAGEMENT

Wound management has been of central interest to surgeons for thousands of years. Historically, the management of wounds has existed on a pendulum, swinging from minimalist care to heavy-handed intervention. In ancient times, knowledge of tissue débridement, gentle cleansing, and reapproximation were observed to yield superior wound healing. Through the Middle Ages, with the discovery and use of gunpowder in the warfare of Western civilizations, the trend was toward a more aggressive management of wounds, with attempts at harsh cleansing and débridement by the application of substances such as scalding water or burning oil. It was not until the mid-16th century that Ambroise Paré rediscovered the concept of the minimalist approach to wound care, an approach necessitated by supply shortages at the Battle of Villaine.[25] The investigations and clinical practices of the leading clinicians of succeeding generations confirmed that the best approach to the wound is by enabling of the body to perform repair in as natural a state as possible. The removal of contaminants, the débridement of devitalized tissue, and ultimately the tension-free coapting of wound edges have been shown to provide the body with the greatest chances of successful tissue repair.

Types of Repair

Primary

The most commonly encountered wound repair is that initiated virtually every day at the conclusion of most operations.

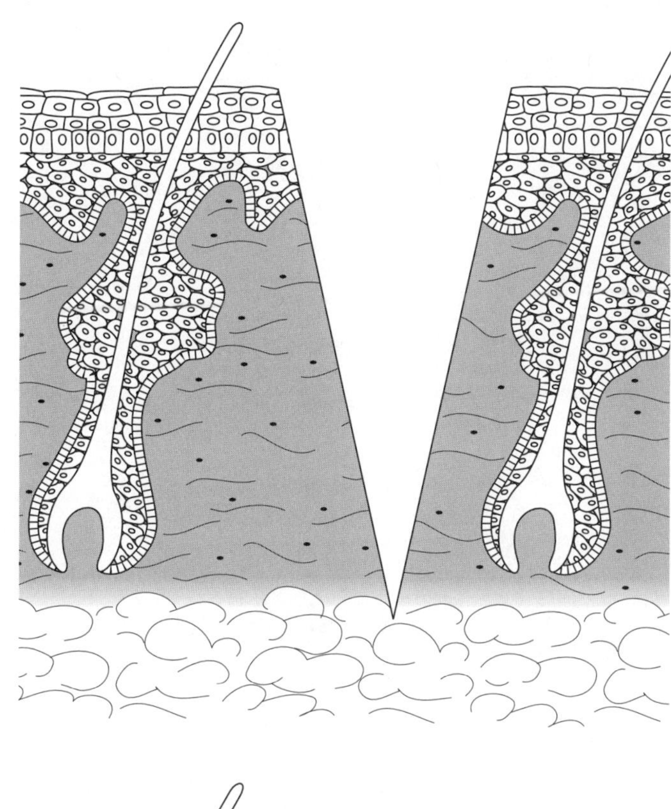

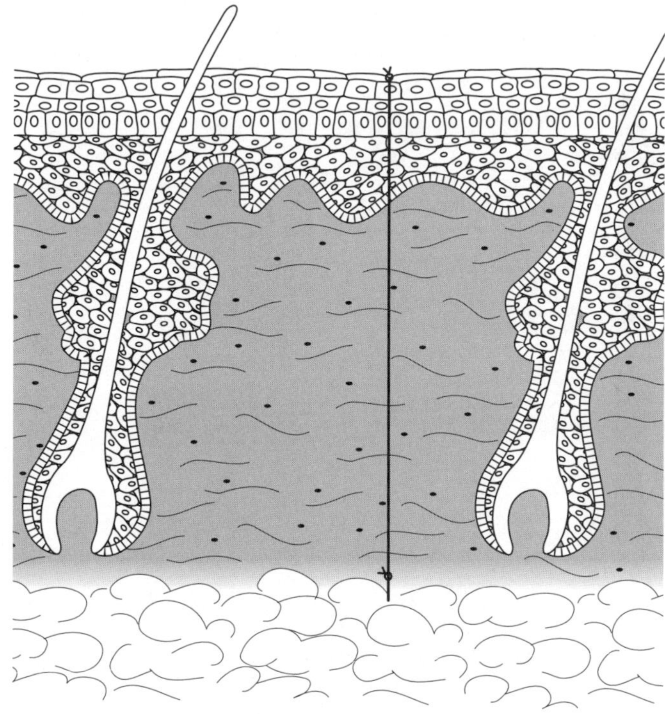

FIG. 9-16. Schematic depiction of primary healing.

Wounded tissue edges are approximated using staples, sutures, or adhesive strips within a few hours of creation of the wound. Issues of contamination usually are not a factor, but if they are, they are dealt with by aggressive irrigation and débridement of the wound before closure. After this type of closure, repair is accomplished through collagen synthesis and epithelialization (Fig. 9-16).

Secondary

After completion of a contaminated case such as one involving perforated colon, or delayed presentation of a wounded patient, the skin and subcutaneous tissues are generally packed open with moist gauze. Serial wet-to-dry dressing changes in the postoperative period provide an ongoing mechanical débridement, allowing the formation of highly vascular granula-

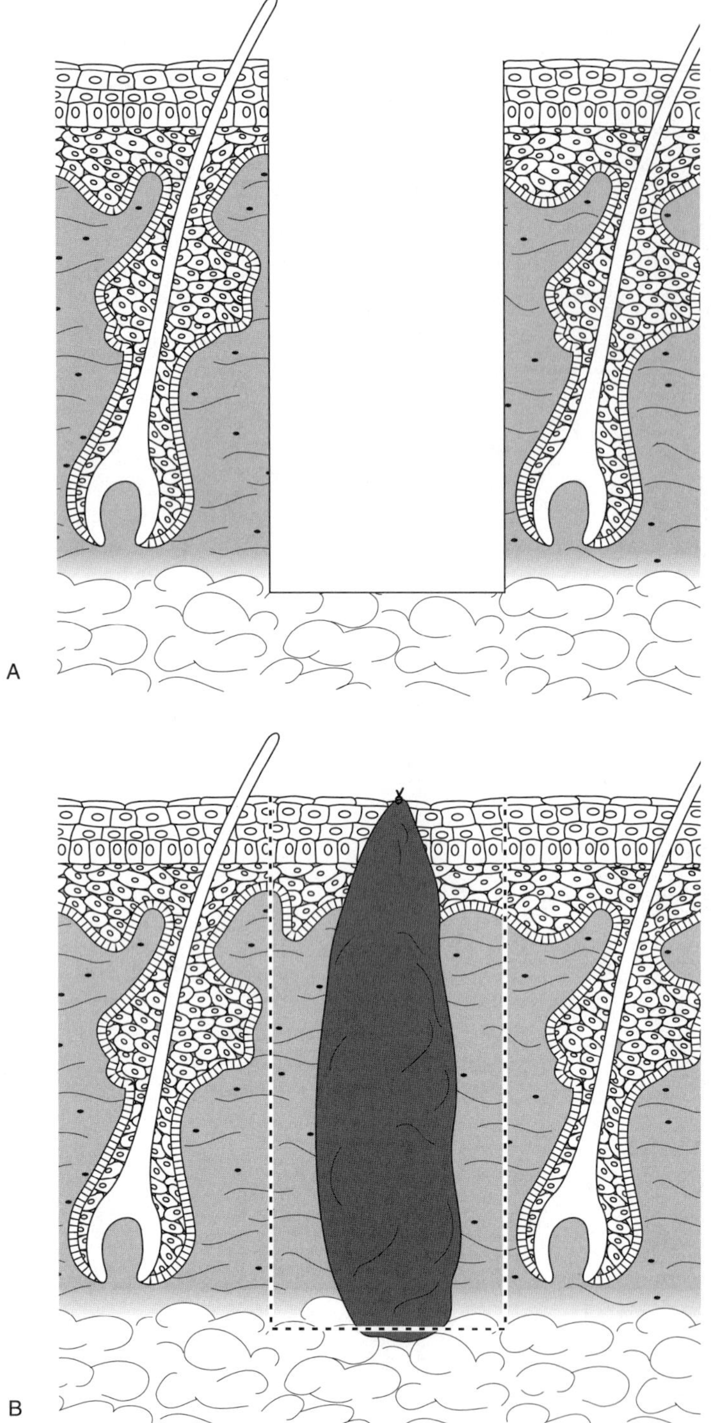

FIG. 9-17. Schematic depiction of wound healing by secondary intention.

tion tissue. Over time, centripetally directed contraction reduces the area of the wound, and epithelialization completes the visible repair process (Fig. 9-17).

Delayed Primary

In an attempt to derive the benefits of both systems, a slightly or questionably contaminated wound is often packed open for 3 to 5 days after operation. At the end of this period, tissue edges are approximated as in a primary closure (Fig. 9-18). In theory, this method provides a period of débridement and allows for the enrichment of the wound edges by ingrowth of new vessels. Closure is achieved before the onset of the bulk of new collagen synthesis. Many of these wounds must be reopened because of infection, leading some clinicians to advocate quantitative wound cultures, with a bacteria count of less than 105 per gram of tissue being a prerequisite for closure.

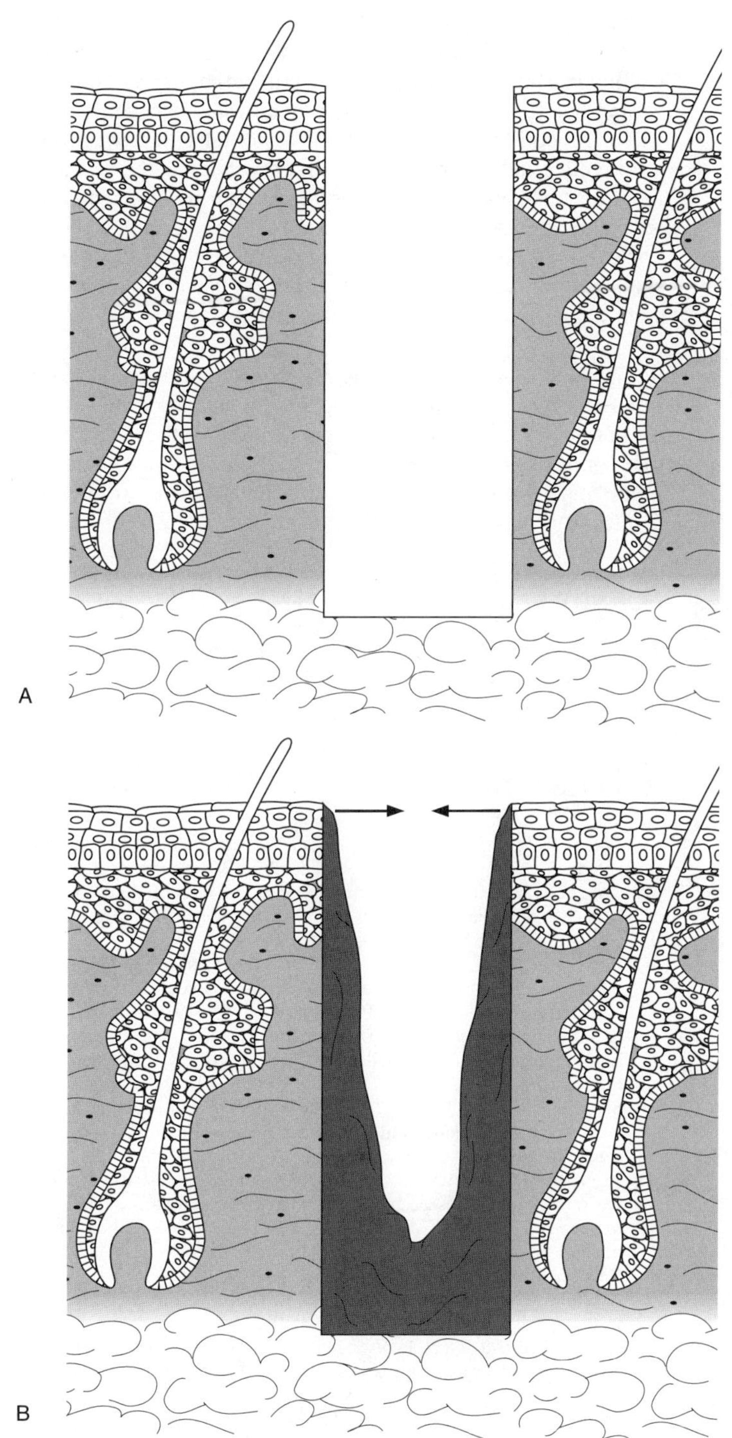

FIG. 9-18. Schematic depiction of delayed primary healing.

Pediatric Wounds

Wounds in children are generally treated according to the principles of adult wound care. Several physiologic and psychologic considerations, however, affect clinical decision making in this group of patients. Generally speaking, children have less subcutaneous adipose tissue, resulting in a decreased potential for contaminated dead space. This difference, in addition to a circulatory system far less impaired by systemic illnesses such as diabetes and atherosclerosis, allows for the closure of numerous wounds that would be considered appropriate only for healing by secondary intention in adults. Wounds such as the incision created for removal of a ruptured appendix. or even the defect remaining after a colostomy takedown, are considered candidates for primary closure or at least a loose dermal approximation.

In choosing closure materials and methods, two major factors should be kept in mind. First, the outcome should be as cosmetically appealing as possible. Second, suture removal can be as traumatic to young children as the actual wound repair. To this end, absorbable sutures are highly desirable for skin closure. Furthermore, sutures placed in a subcuticular fashion are cosmetically more acceptable and avoid the ''railroad track'' scar that can result from full-thickness dermal sutures.

Excessive Scarring

Despite the best efforts of surgeons, some patients experience collagen deposition out of the range of normal even for a prominent scar. The two classes of excessive scars encountered in clinical practice are known as hypertrophic scars and keloids. Although both have in common the deposition of a collagen scar beyond that seen in normal repair, these two entities exhibit distinct clinical properties.

A *hypertrophic scar* is distinguished by its restriction to the boundaries of the original wound. These lesions have a tendency to regress over time and infrequently cause functional impairment. As such, their removal is rarely indicated.

In contrast, a *keloid* usually extends beyond the borders of the original wound (Fig. 9-19). Keloids can cause functional impairment of joint mobility secondary to encroachment into these regions. They can contain mast cells and can become intensely pruritic as the result of histamine release. As a rule, keloids do not regress over time and frequently recur after removal. For these reasons, their removal is indicated only for functional impairment or severe cosmetic deficit. A modest amount of success has been achieved in reducing keloid size by the intralesional injection of steroids such as triamcinolone; however, an even more important aspect of therapy is the counseling of afflicted patients to avoid wound-creating practices, such as ear piercing.

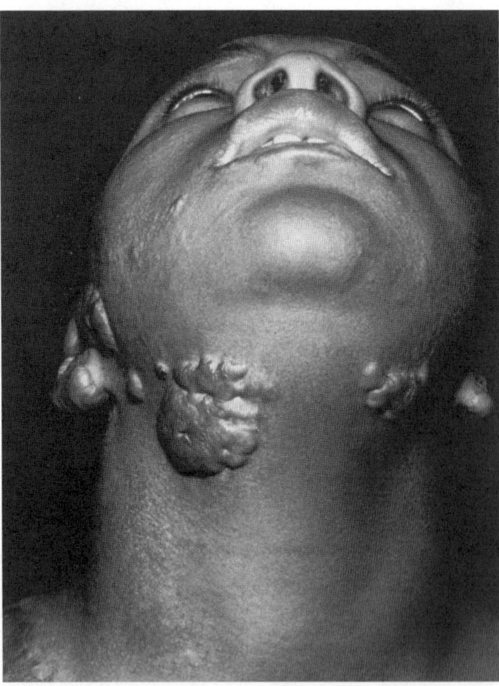

FIG. 9-19. Patient afflicted with severe keloid formation at sites of previous wounding. (Courtesy of H. Paul Ehrlich, PhD, Hershey Medical Center, Hershey, PA)

The topic of burns receives a thorough treatment elsewhere in this text (see Chap. 29). The results of the natural pattern of healing in a burn wound often place it in the category of problem wound healing. This is most often manifested as a contracture, when the contractile properties of a wound extending over a joint render the joint nonfunctional. Prevention is the best treatment for this condition, with early skin grafting and aggressive rehabilitation used to maintain joint mobility. Established contractures can be alleviated by surgical release accompanied by skin grafting, but some functional deficit usually remains, despite aggressive postoperative physical therapy.

The field of wound care has undergone a substantial evolution for several centuries. Advances in molecular biology promise not only a more complete understanding of the mechanisms that control tissue repair but also the ability to control and manipulate the wound environment to decrease the morbidity that results from adverse wound healing.

ACKNOWLEDGMENT

The author gratefully acknowledges the major contributions of Christopher J. Blewett, MD, Surgical Research Fellow, in the preparation of this chapter.

REFERENCES

1. Cohen IK, Diegelmann RF, Lindblad WJ, eds. Wound healing: biochemical and clinical aspects. Philadelphia, WB Saunders, 1992.
2. Cohen IK, Diegelmann RF. Wound healing. In: Greenfield LJ, Mulholland MW, Oldham, KT, et al, eds. Surgery: scientific principles and practice. Philadelphia, JB Lippincott, 1993:86.
3. Roberts A, Sporn M, Assoian R, et al. Transforming growth type β: rapid induction of fibrosis and angiogenesis in vivo and stimulation of collagen formation in vitro. Proc Natl Acad Sci 1986;83:4167.
4. Krummel TM, Nelson JM, Diegelmann RF, et al. Fetal response to injury and its modulation with transforming growth factor beta. Surg Forum 1987;38:622.
5. Shah M, Foreman DM, Ferguson MW. Control of scarring in adult wounds by neutralising antibody to transforming growth factor β. Lancet 1992;339:213.
6. Aggarwal BB, Gutterman JU, eds. Human cytokines: handbook for basic and clinical research. Boston, Blackwell Scientific, 1992.
7. Whitby DJ, Longaker MT, Harrison MR, et al. Rapid epithelialisation of fetal wounds is associated with the early deposition of tenascin. J Cell Sci 1991;99:583.
8. Krummel TM, Nelson J, Diegelmann R, et al. Fetal response to injury in the rabbit. J Pediatr Surg 1987;22:601.
9. Longaker M, Adzick N, Jackson L, et al. Studies in fetal wound healing. VII. Fetal wound healing may be modulated by hyaluronic acid stimulating activity in amniotic fluid. J Pediatr Surg 1990;25:430.
10. Flinsenmayer TF. Collagen. In: Hay ED, ed. Cell biology of extracellular matrix, ed 2. New York, Plenum, 1991:7.
11. Fleischmayer R, Olsen BR, Kulin K, eds. Biology, chemistry, and pathology of collagen. New York, New York Academy of Sciences, 1985.
12. Somasundaram K, Prathap K. Intra-uterine healing of skin wounds in rabbits foetuses. J Pathol 1970;100:81.
13. Burrington JD. Wound healing in the fetal lamb. J Pediatr Surg 1971; 6:523.
14. Rowlatt U. Intrauterine wound healing in a 20 week human fetus. Arch A Pathol Anat Histol 1979;381:353.
15. Hallock GG. In utero repair in A/J mice. Plast Reconstr Surg 1985; 75:785.
16. Burd DAR, Longaker MT, Adzick NS, et al. Foetal wound healing in a large animal model: the deposition of collagen is confirmed. Br J Plast Surg 1990;43:571.
17. Blewett CJ, Cilley RE, Ehrlich HP, et al. Regenerative healing of inci-

sional wounds in murine fetal lungs maintained in organ culture. J Pediatr Surg (in press).

18. Blewett CJ, Cilley RE, Blackburn JH, et al. Regenerative healing of incisional wounds in midgestation murine hearts. Abstracts from 23rd Annual Meeting, Association for Academic Surgery, Albuquerque, 1994.

19. Al-Qattan MM, Posnick JC, Kant YL, et al. Fetal tendon healing: development of an experimental model. Plast Reconstr Surg 1993;92:1155.

20. Ris PM, Wray JB. A histological study of fracture healing within the uterus of the rabbit. Clin Orthop 1972;87:318.

21. Bell E, Ivarsson B, Merrill C. Production of a tissue-like structure by contraction of collagen lattices by human fibroblasts of different proliferative potential in vitro. Proc Natl Acad Sci USA 1979;76:1274.

22. Adzick NS. Fetal animal and wound implant models. In: Adzick NS, Longaker MT, eds. Fetal wound healing. New York, Elsevier, 1992.

23. Bleacher JC, Adolph VR, Dillon PW, et al. Isolated fetal mouse limbs: gestational effects on tissue repair in an unperfused system. J Pediatr Surg 1993;28:1312.

24. Lorenz HP, Longaker MT, Perchocka LA, et al. Scarless wound repair: a human fetal skin model. Development 1992;114:253.

25. Madden JW, Arem AJ. Wound healing: biological and clinical factors. In: Sabiston DC, ed. Textbook of surgery, ed 14. Philadelphia, WB Saunders, 1991:164.

Fetal Wound Healing Reviews

Adzick NS, Lorenz HP. Cells, matrix, growth factors, and the surgeon: the biology of scarless fetal repair. Ann Surg 1994;220:10.

Bleacher JC, Adolph VR, Dillon PW, et al. Fetal tissue repair and wound healing. Dermatol Clin 1993;11:677.

Dostal GH, Gamelli RL. Fetal wound healing. Surg Gynecol Obstet 1993;176:299.

Longaker MT, Adzick NS. The biology of fetal wound healing: a review. Plast Reconstr Surg 1991;87:788.

Surgery of Infants and Children: Scientific Principles and Practice, edited by Keith T. Oldham, Paul M. Colombani, and Robert P. Foglia. Lippincott–Raven Publishers, Philadelphia, © 1997.

CHAPTER 10

Infection

Francisco Cigarroa and Walter Pegoli, Jr.

Humans exist in equilibrium with an ecosystem that contains innumerable microbes, most of which have a symbiotic relationship with us. Evolutionary pressure has allowed this coexistence to persist by the development of several defenses against microbial invasion, including physical, chemical, and immunologic barriers. A fault in any of these barriers can lead to bacterial proliferation and subsequent infection, the severity of which depends on the virulence of the organism and the competence of the host.

NONIMMUNE HOST DEFENSES

The human skin is the largest organ in the body and provides an effective barrier against infection. It is constantly desquamating, resulting in a continual change of surface flora. Intact, the skin is a harsh environment for many nonresident organisms. Resident flora vary dependent on location, but *Corynebacterium* and *Propionibacterium* species predominate.[1] These bacteria and the stratum corneum provide a low pH, which make the skin surface inhospitable to nonresident flora. The skin surface is coated by lipids, which are known to possess antibacterial properties that suppress *Staphylococcus epidermidis* and *aureus.*[2]

Mucous membranes within the airways and gastrointestinal tract contain resident flora that inhibit the growth of pathogenic organisms. Antibiotics can alter airway flora, resulting in tracheitis and bronchopneumonia. In the pharynx and tracheobronchial tree, organisms are engulfed by mucus and propelled outward by ciliary movement. Damage to cilia by noxious agents can impair this protective mechanism, resulting in pneumonia. Cough suppression owing to pain from surgical procedures or oversedation results in decreased clearance of pathogens. Tears, saliva, and secretions of the nasopharynx contain lysozyme, which damages bacterial cell walls.

In the gastrointestinal tract, the low gastric pH is bacteriostatic. Antacids can alter gastric pH and lead to the proliferation of yeast and other pathogens. Peristalsis is an important means of clearing bacteria from the gut. Intestinal stasis promotes proliferation of pathogenic bacteria and mucosal damage. Mucosal injury leads to increased gut permeability with resultant bacterial translocation and subsequent systemic sepsis. Resident intestinal flora are also intrinsically protective because they occupy sites that could otherwise house pathogenic species. Administration of antibiotics can alter this flora, allowing proliferation of organisms such as *Clostridium difficile,* resulting in pseudomembranous colitis.

EFFECTOR MECHANISMS OF THE IMMUNE SYSTEM

The immune system is the human's fortress against pathogens. A deficiency in any of its effector mechanisms inevitably results in infection. An understanding of humoral and cell-mediated immunodefenses is essential to treat infections in children successfully.

Macrophages

The macrophage is a ubiquitous cell found in many parts of the body. This cell is involved in host defense, inflammation, and reactions against invading microbes. The precursor of this cell develops from pluripotential stem cells in the bone marrow and is under the influence of colony-stimulating factors.[3–4] Colony-stimulating factors are produced by a variety of cells, and their concentration increases during infection. These factors promote the growth and prolong the survival of macrophages.

Macrophages exhibit characteristics that vary with location and differentially express class II major histocompatibility (MHC) proteins.[5] These cells have receptors that are sensitive to their environment, and they have been shown to be motile in response to chemotactic factors. Receptors to the Fc fragment of immunoglobulin G (IgG) and to complement allow uptake of antibodies and complement-coated proteins.[6–8] CR1 and CR3 are complement proteins that influence phagocytosis of particles and also promote cellular cytotoxicity. Macrophages can endocytose microorganisms opsonized by antibodies and complement. Endocytosis of foreign material results in formation of superoxide and hydroxyl radicals that have antimicrobicidal and cytocidal activity.[9–10]

Macrophages play a dominant role in eliciting inflammatory responses. They secrete prostaglandins, thromboxane, leukotriens, and complement when activated by lymphokines and bacterial products. Macrophages are initiators of the acute-phase response, releasing interleukin-1 (IL-1) and IL-6 and tumor necrosis factor (TNF). Circulating lymphokines elicit fever, leukocytosis, and increases in insulin, haptoglobin, C-reactive protein, and C3.

Macrophages are intimately involved in the regulation of immune responses. These cells express class II MHC, process and present antigen to lymphocytes, and release lymphokines. IL-1 stimulates B-cell proliferation and T-cell responsiveness.[11] TNF promotes natural killer cells to release interferons, which have an antiviral effect.[12] Interferon-γ increases expression of a class II MHC protein important in cell-mediated immune responsiveness.

Interferons

Interferons are virally induced host proteins that possess antiviral activities and immunoregulatory properties.[13,14] The three types of interferons are: α, secreted by virus infected leukocytes; β, synthesized by fibroblasts; and γ, produced by stimulated lymphocytes.[14]

The antiviral properties of interferon are the result of the production of $2',5'$-oligosynthetase and a protein kinase that result in viral RNA degradation and inhibition of viral protein synthesis. Interferon-α and interferon-β increase the antigen-presenting accessory cell functions of macrophages.[15] Macrophages exposed to interferons increase synthesis of lysosomal hydrolases, esterases, and proteases, promoting the destruction of pathogens. Activated cells produce IL-1 and TNF.[16] Interferon increases Fc receptor expression in macrophages, which results in increased phagocytosis of opsonized proteins and increased capacity to lyse antibody-coated bacteria.[17] Interferon-γ is a potent enhancer of the antigen-presenting functions of macrophages.

Defense against virus-infected cells by natural killer cells is enhanced by interferon.[18] Exposure increases natural killer cell function by promoting expression of adhesion molecules and synthesis of cytolytic proteins. Studies have shown an increased susceptibility to viral infections in mice treated with antibodies to interferon.[19] Patients who are interferon deficient or produce inhibitors of interferon are at increased risk of acquiring hepatitis B and C and herpesvirus infections.

Complement

Complement is a complex system of serum proteins involved in opsonization, cell lysis, and inflammation. This system has been divided into the classic and alternate complement pathways.[20] The classic pathway is activated by antigen–antibody complexes; the alternate pathway can be activated directly by endotoxin, polysaccharides, and foreign proteins. The alternate pathway is a first-line defense against antigen.

The classic pathway is activated by the C1 QRS complex after binding IgG or IgM that has linked antigen. The alternate pathway is initiated when alternate factors D and B are activated. This can occur through direct contact with foreign proteins or by IgG4 binding to antigen. C4b2a or C3bBb complexes are C3 convertases that amplify conversion of C3, which in turn drives the complement cascade. Each pathway functions similarly after activation of C3 (Fig. 10-1).

Activation of the complement system produces a number of reactive proteins.[21] C3b is an opsonin that binds to surface receptors on neutrophils and macrophages. This results in phagocytosis and bacterial death if IgM or IgG is bound to the bacterial cell wall. Activation of C8 and C9 by C5–C6–C7 complex leads to penetration of the bacterial wall and osmotic lysis of the pathogen. C5a is a chemoattractant to leukocytes and macrophages, leading to additional humoral and cellular defenses to areas of inflammation. C3a, C4a, and C5a are potent activators of basophils and mast cells, which release histamine, an agent known to increase vascular permeability.

Interleukins

The interleukins are cytokines that have immunomodulatory activities important to the host response to pathogens and foreign proteins. They function to prime the humoral and cell-mediated immune systems. The main sources of IL-1 are monocytes and macrophages.[22] IL-1 has a stimulatory effect on B cells, increases IL-2 receptor synthesis in activated T cells, and stimulates production of other lymphokines.[23] IL-1 is responsible for initiating the synthesis and release of prostaglandins and thromboxanes.

IL-2 stimulates cytolytic T cells and enhances natural killer cell activity through interferon-γ synthesis.[24,25] IL-2 binding to T cells with appropriate receptors causes T cells to proliferate. TNF production is enhanced by the presence of IL-2.[26] IL-2 produces the fever and hypotension associated with endotoxemia.

IL-3 stimulates proliferation of basophils and mast cells, both active participants in the inflammatory response. IL-3 has been shown to induce pluripotent stem cell proliferation.[27]

IL-4 results in the proliferation of activated B lymphocytes as well as increased synthesis of immunoglobulin.[28,29] It induces expression of class II MHC genes on the surfaces of lymphocytes important in immunomodulation,[30] and it triggers cytolytic T-cell development.

IL-5 enhances IgA production and stimulates proliferation of eosinophils, which are thought to be important in the defense against parasites.

Cytokines constantly regulate the immune system and are responsible for many of the clinical events exhibited in sepsis. They provide a proper microenvironment for optimal function of the immune system in the body's battle against invading pathogens.

Humoral and Cell-Mediated Defenses

A fundamental division in the immune system is apparent. Humoral immune responses are mediated by B lymphocytes, and cell-mediated immune responses by T lymphocytes. Both arms of the immune system are intricately involved in the host defense against microorganisms. Antigen, which may be protein specific to an invading microbe, is presented to helper T cells by either macrophages or dendritic cells.

Activated helper T cells produce a number of lymphokines, such as IL-4, necessary for the growth and differentiation of B

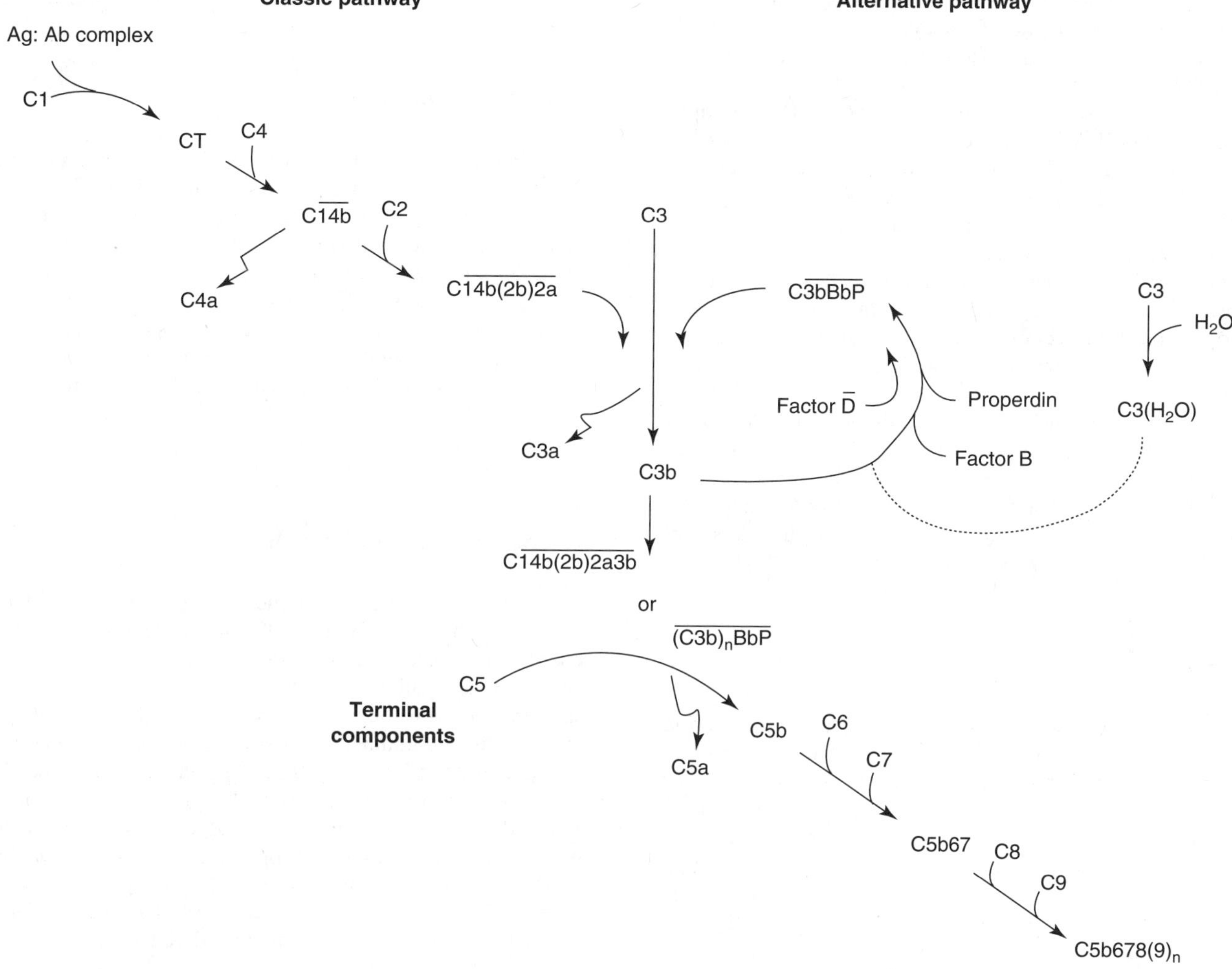

FIG. 10-1. Schematic diagram of complement activation. Regulatory proteins, side reactions, and inactive fragments have been omitted for clarity. Enzymatically active species are designated by overbars. (After Frank MM, Fries LF. Complement. In: Paul WE, ed. Fundamental immunology, ed 2. New York, Raven Press, 1989:679)

cells into antibody-producing cells. Interferon-γ, which induces class II MHC molecules, and IL-2, which is necessary for growth and differentiation of T cells, are also produced by activated helper T cells. In the presence of specific lymphokines, T cells can differentiate into suppressor cells, which downregulate the immune response. B cells differ from T cells in that activation can occur in the absence of T cells by direct interaction with antigen through their surface immune globulin receptors.

IMMUNODEFICIENCIES

The immune system is adversely affected by prematurity, malnutrition, infection, and trauma. An infant's immune system requires a period of maturation to achieve full immunocompetence. Efficient T-cell and B-cell responses require previous exposure to an antigen. The fetus is at a disadvantage in this respect because of its protection from the external environment. Additionally, fetal B cells are not fully programmed to synthe-

size the complete spectrum of immunoglobulins. Passive immunity to the fetus is provided by maternal transfer of IgG during the third trimester.[31] The level of IgG in premature infants is proportional to gestation age. Postnatally, IgG levels decline during the first 4 months. Prematurity, therefore, results in a hypogammaglobulinemic state in the fetus and in the first few months of life. These infants manifest suboptimal protection against gram-negative organisms and exhibit deficiencies in opsonization, increasing the risk of infections from streptococcus B, *Escherichia coli,* and *Serratia* sp.[32] Complement components are decreased in the newborn period but rise rapidly postnatally. Low levels of complement adversely affect opsonization.

The fetus begins to produce IgM at 10 weeks' gestation but at birth only has 10% the normal adult level.[33] The infant's humoral response to an antigen is an elevation of IgM, but it may be inadequate to protect effectively against severe infections. IgA is not detected until near term and does not achieve normal levels until puberty.[34] Diseases whose defenses depend primarily on secretory IgA, such as respiratory syncytial virus, remain prevalent throughout infancy.

Trauma affects various aspects of the immune system. Total neutrophil counts rise, but chemotaxis and phagocytosis are decreased. There is a decrease in the number of T-cell lymphocytes. IL-1 and IL-2 levels decrease, adversely affecting lymphocyte differentiation.[35,36] Cutaneous anergy can occur in the setting of a significant traumatic injury.

Malnutrition, secondary to chronic disease or poverty, is detrimental to the immune response. Patients with marasmus and kwashiorkor have depressed cell-mediated immune responses.[37] Malnourished children suffer increased viral, fungal, and opportunistic infections, such as cytomegalovirus (CMV), disseminated herpes zoster virus, and *Pneumocystis carinii* infection. Delayed cutaneous hypersensitivity reactions, chemotaxis, and phagocytosis are also diminished. The humoral immune system is largely spared in malnutrition, but total immunoglobulin levels are below normal.[38]

A number of congenital and acquired disorders that affect the immune system have been described. Those disorders pertinent to the pediatric surgeon are reviewed in the following sections.

Asplenia

Asplenia often occurs in association with complex cardiac defects, but it can occur as an isolated deficit. The peripheral blood smear demonstrates increased Howell-Jolly bodies. Affected infants have a decreased ability to opsonize encapsulated organisms. These children have a 2% chance of dying from sepsis, compared with a rate of 0.7% in children with intact spleens.[39] An asplenic child should receive penicillin prophylaxis to decrease the risk of developing pneumococcal sepsis.

Common Variable Agammaglobulinemia

Common variable agammaglobulinemia is likely a hereditary disease, but the mode of transmission is not known. The primary deficit is a low level of immunoglobulin. T-cell abnormalities can be present, resulting in increased susceptibility to viral, fungal, and opportunistic infections. Therapy involves intravenous immunoglobulin replacement (IVIG).

X-Linked Agammaglobulinemia

In X-linked agammaglobulinemia, plasma cells, germinal centers, and follicle formation are all absent from lymphoid tissue. The immunologic defect involves an arrest of B-lymphocyte differentiation.[40] T lymphocytes are spared. Children develop recurrent infections with pneumococci, streptococci, and *Haemophilus influenzae,* but not until maternal IgG is depleted. Treatment is with IVIG replacement.

Immunoglobulin A Deficiency

In immunoglobulin A deficiency, secretory and serum IgA are deficient. The predominant infection involves encapsulated bacteria. Administration of IVIG does not significantly elevate IgA levels,[41] and treatment involves organism-specific antibiotics.

DiGeorge Syndrome

DiGeorge syndrome is a cell-mediated deficiency associated with thymic hypoplasia and hypoparathyroidism. There is an arrest in development of the third and fourth pharyngeal pouches during the 6th week of gestation.[42] The cellular immune deficits are the result of thymic hypoplasia. There is a wide clinical spectrum. The defect can involve only cell-mediated factors or can involve the humoral system. These patients are susceptible to viral and fungal infections. Therapy for the immune dysfunction has involved intramuscular or intraperitoneal implantation of a 14- to 16-week fetal thymus.[43] Bone marrow transplantation has also been attempted with some success.[44]

Severe Combined Immunodeficiency Disease

Children with severe combined immunodeficiency disease manifest both T- and B-cell deficiencies. This is an inherited disorder that occurs in an X-linked and autosomal recessive pattern. Half of patients with the autosomal recessive form have deficient adenosine deaminase levels.[45] The thymus is dysplastic. Lymphocyte numbers are deficient, and available cells are unresponsive to stimulation. These patients are anergic and are subject to recurrent infections with opportunistic organisms. Affected children die within the first 2 years of life without therapy. Bactrim is used for prophylaxis against *Pneumocystis* sp. Bone marrow transplantation is the therapy of choice for these patients.[46] Gene replacement therapy has been performed in patients with adenosine deaminase deficiency.

Chédiak-Higashi Syndrome

Patients with Chédiak-Higashi syndrome have abnormal cytotoxic granules within phagocytic cells. Bacterial killing is impaired because phagocytes are unable to degranulate. Neutropenia is common, and chemotaxis is abnormal. Specific therapy with antibiotics is required. Bone marrow transplantation has had variable results.[47]

Human Immunodeficiency Virus and the Acquired Immunodeficiency Syndrome

The human immunodeficiency virus (HIV) is a retrovirus that selectively infects CD4 cells. CD4 cells are circulating lymphocytes that are responsible for modulating the immune response. HIV is an RNA retrovirus that penetrates the CD4 cell. Reverse transcriptase, an intracellular enzyme, then produces complementary DNA. Double-stranded DNA is incorporated into the genome of the CD4 cell. Loss of CD4 cells results in a deficiency in cell-mediated immunity.

Viral transmission is usually followed in 1 to 6 weeks by an acute febrile condition that resembles infectious mononucleosis. These symptoms are associated with a high-grade viremia and usually resolve spontaneously. It is during this time that

TABLE 10-1. *Diagnosis of HIV infection in children*

Diagnosis: HIV infected
A child <18 months of age who is known to be HIV seropositive or born to an HIV-infected mother and has positive results on two separate determinations (excluding cord blood) from one or more of the following HIV detection tests:
HIV culture
HIV polymerase chain reaction
HIV antigen (p24)

or

meets criteria for AIDS diagnosis based on the 1987 AIDS surveillance case definition
A child ≥18 months of age born to an HIV-infected mother or any child infected by blood, blood products, or other known modes of transmission (eg, sexual contact) who
is HIV-antibody positive by repeatedly reactive enzyme immunoassay (EIA) and confirmatory test (eg, Western blot or immunofluorescence assay [IFA])

or

meets any of the criteria listed above
Diagnosis: Perinatally Exposed (Prefix E)
A child who does not meet the criteria above who
is HIV seropositive by EIA and confirmatory test (eg, Western blot or IFA) and
is <18 months of age at the time of test

or

has unknown antibody status, but was born to a mother known to be infected with HIV

(Data from the Centers for Disease Control.)

antibodies form. Seroconversion generally takes place in about 6 to 12 weeks.

The usual CD4 count in healthy, uninfected people is 600 to 1400 cells/mm^3. The average patient infected with HIV has a decline of 60 to 100 CD4 cells/mm^3/y. It is thought that the critical level is 100 to 200 cells/mm^3. As host immunity wanes, opportunistic infections begin to occur. By definition, acquired immunodeficiency syndrome (AIDS) can be diagnosed in any person with a CD4 count of less than 200/mm^3, regardless of symptoms (data from the Centers for Disease Control).

Vertical (perinatal) transmission continues to be the most common mode of HIV infection in infants and children. The standard test for detection of HIV is a screening enzyme-linked immunosorbent assay (ELISA) followed by a Western blot. These serologic tests are remarkably accurate. Using standard criteria for a positive test, false-positive results in one study

were found in only 135,000 tests (0.0007%).[48] Nevertheless, repeat testing is advocated. False-negative results can occur in the window period (usually 6 to 12 weeks) between the time that the infection is acquired and the time of seroconversion. The recommendation is to repeat the test in 2 or 3 months to exclude the possibility that a person is in the process of seroconversion (Tables 10-1 and 10-2).

A number of AIDS indicator diseases are present among children. The most common of these continue to be opportunistic infections with *P carinii* (pneumonia) and *Candida albicans* (esophagitis). Once the diagnosis of AIDS is made, the median life expectancy can range from 13 months to 3 years.[49] With therapy, life expectancy can be prolonged, and the progression of disease can be slowed. Therapy for HIV infection is targeted at inhibition of viral replication and prevention of opportunistic diseases when they occur.

Antiretroviral therapy is based on inhibition of HIV reverse transcription with nucleoside analogue drugs. The most common of this category of agents is zidovudine (AZT). Zidovudine is the first line of antiviral therapy. It has been proved effective in preventing transmission of HIV from mother to infant. In one study, treatment of women with zidovudine in the second and third trimesters of pregnancy and of infants during the first 6 weeks of life decreased the rate of transmission from 25% to 8%.[50] Recently pharmacologic agents used in combination have been shown to offer substantial promise of long-term efficacy. The combination therapies appear to combat the problem of drug resistance. The three categories of agents include nucleoside and nonnucleoside reverse transcriptase inhibitors and protease inhibitors. Prospective studies to define optimal regimens are now beginning.

PHARMACOKINETICS

The effectiveness of an antibiotic is dependent on its absorption and its concentration at the site of infection. The concentration of the antibiotic at the involved site must be within the minimal inhibitory concentration for an offending organism and should remain sufficiently high for an adequate period of time to achieve the desired result.

Pharmacokinetics involves the absorption, distribution, biotransformation, and excretion of a drug. The rate of absorption affects the duration and intensity of action. It is dependent on the route of administration, the solubility and concentration of the drug, and local tissue factors.

After absorption, antibiotics distribute into extracellular and

TABLE 10-2. *Pediatric HIV classification*

	Clinical categories			
Immunologic category	N: No signs or symptoms	A: Mild signs or symptoms	B:* Moderate signs or symptoms	C:* Severe signs or symptoms
1. No evidence of suppression	N1	A1	B1	C1
2. Evidence of moderate suppression	N2	A2	B2	C2
3. Severe suppression	N3	A3	B3	C3

Note: Children whose HIV infection is not confirmed are classified by using the above grid with a letter E (for perinatally exposed) placed before the appropriate classification code (eg, EN2).
* Both category C and lymphoid interstitial pneumonitis in category B are reportable to state and local health departments as acquired immunodeficiency syndrome.
(Data from the Centers for Disease Control.)

intracellular compartments. The initial phase of distribution reflects cardiac output and regional blood flow. Highly perfused organs, such as the heart, kidney, liver, and brain, are exposed to more drug during its first pass. Delivery of the drug to muscle, fat, and skin is slower, with a resultant delay in equilibration at these sites. Membrane permeability also plays a factor in a drug's ability to penetrate tissues. Binding of drug to a protein can limit tissue concentration because only unbound drug is in equilibrium across membranes.

Important to the initial metabolism of a drug is its passage across the cell membrane. Drug transfer across cell membranes, a dynamic phospholipid bilayer, may involve passive transfer, facilitated diffusion, or active transport. In passive transfer, the drug is transported along a concentration gradient through aqueous pores in the membrane or by dissolving in the membrane. The degree of drug transfer is dependent on the concentration gradient across the membrane and the lipid/water partition coefficient of the drug. The greater the partition coefficient, the more efficient the diffusion. After a steady state is obtained, the concentration of the free drug is the same on both sides of the membrane. Drugs that have ionic charges develop a steady state dependent on pH and the electrochemical gradient across the membrane.

Facilitated diffusion involves a carrier-mediated transport process that is not energy dependent and cannot occur across concentration or electrochemical gradients. This process becomes important when passive diffusion is inadequate for a physiologic action. In contrast to passive and facilitated diffusion, active transport is an energy-dependent process that can move against concentration and electrochemical gradients. This mechanism is selective, is susceptible to competitive inhibition, and can be saturated.

Many antibiotics are lipid-soluble, weak organic acids, or bases that are not readily eliminated from the body. To aid in excretion, they must be transformed into polar compounds. Biotransformation often results in deactivation of the parent compound and enhances drug elimination through excretion. The hepatic microsomal enzyme systems are responsible for the biotransformation of most drugs. The kidney is the most important organ for elimination of drugs and their metabolites through glomerular filtration, active tubular secretion, and passive tubular readsorption.

A consideration of pharmacokinetics in the clinical setting allows intelligent decisions concerning not only the choice of antibiotic but also the dose, method, and interval of administration. Knowledge of the volume of distribution of a drug allows an accurate assessment of the concentration at a specific site. For example, first-generation cephalosporins have a low concentration in cerebrospinal fluid but are highly concentrated in the bile. On the other hand, chloramphenicol readily crosses the blood–brain barrier. The methods of biotransformation and excretion of a drug are also clinically important because toxic levels can occur in hepatic and renal disease. Moreover, many agents can affect enzyme systems involved in biotransformation, resulting in either subtherapeutic or toxic levels of a drug.

ANTIBIOTICS

Louis Pasteur established the principles of infection by attributing the infectious process to bacteria. In 1865, Joseph Lister introduced antisepsis by using carbolic acid, which was known to kill bacteria. Sir Alexander Fleming discovered penicillin in 1928, and sulfa drugs were introduced in the mid-1930s. The era of antimicrobial therapy began in 1941 when penicillin was administered as an antibiotic and produced in large quantities for patients.

Since the introduction of sulfas, many antibiotics have been developed with different spectra of activities and modes of action (Tables 10-3 through 10-5). The vast array of antibiotics can sometimes make it difficult to choose the appropriate drug. The patient's clinical status and site of infection can help in selecting the proper therapeutic agent. The use of antibiotics can involve prophylactic, empiric, or directed therapy.

The aim of prophylactic therapy is to decrease bacterial counts to minimize the risk of infection. The efficacy of prophylaxis has been well documented. In 1960, Burke[51] demonstrated that prophylactic antibiotics suppress staphylococcal infections at the surgical wound if administered appropriately. The critical interval begins at the time of the surgical incision and ends within 3 hours. Antibiotics had no effect on infection if the antibiotics were given 3 hours after bacteria entered the tissues. Polk and Lopez-Majoy[52] conducted a double-blind, prospective, randomized trial on the effect of cephaloridine or a placebo given preoperatively and 5 and 11 hours postoperatively to patients undergoing emergency operations. The infection rate fell from 30% in the control group to 7% in the treated group. In their conclusion, the authors advised that antibiotics should be started 2 hours before incision and continued for no more than 48 hours after surgery. Antibiotics have been shown to decrease the incidence of wound infection after a number of surgical procedures. Whatever benefit that may exist, however, must be weighed against the following risks: toxic and allergic reactions, development of resistant bacteria, and superinfection. Prophylaxis should be considered only for operations that have high infection risks or when infection could be associated with catastrophic consequences. Pediatric literature on this topic is wanting; therefore, such information has been extrapolated from adult studies (Table 10-6).

Prophylactic therapy is important for the prevention of bacterial endocarditis in patients with prosthetic cardiac valves, congenital cardiac defects, and valvular disease. Penicillin treatment is recommended if a procedure is done involving the oral cavity or respiratory tract. If a gastrointestinal or genitourinary procedure is performed, ampicillin and gentamicin are recommended.

In transplant recipients, prophylaxis against *Pneumocystis* sp, *Candida* sp, herpesvirus, and CMV is recommended. Bactrim is used to decrease the risk of *Pneumocystis* sp infection during the first year after transplantation. While patients are on high immunosuppressive regimens, nystatin mouth rinse or clotrimazole (Mycelex) troches is prescribed to reduce oral and esophageal candidiasis. Acylovir is used to reduce the incidence of herpesvirus and CMV infection during the first 3 months after solid organ transplantation.

Empiric therapy is used when infection is suspected but not proved. The selection of antibiotics depends on the presumed site of infection and the clinical status of the patient. This mode of therapy is begun without the benefit of culture data; therefore, a broad spectrum of activity is often required. Empiric therapy requires consideration of the risks and benefits to the patient. Antibiotics may have adverse effects, can interact with other drugs, and increase patient expenses. During treatment, there must be a search for the infectious agent and a defined limit to the length of therapy if no organism is identified. An example of the complexities involved in empiric therapy is a transplant recipient who presents with fever and a right upper lobe infiltrate on chest radiograph. Evaluation of this patient should include bronchoscopy, bronchoalveolar lavage, and transbronchial biopsies. After these are performed and blood cultures obtained, broad-spectrum antibiotics should be initiated, which often include vancomycin and cefotaxime for bacterial causes of pneumonia. Bactrim is administered because of the risk of *P carinii* being the cause of the pneumonia. Erythromycin is also prescribed because *Legionella* sp may be the causative organism. Erythromycin may result in elevated levels of either cyclosporine or tacrolimus. Finally, ganciclovir is begun to protect against CMV pneumonia. These agents are quickly tapered as information returns from the bronchoscopic and peripheral blood cultures.

Antibiotic-directed therapy is based on the identification of the responsible organism and sensitivities obtained from culture data. An organism is considered susceptible if the concentration of antimicrobial agent necessary to inhibit growth is lower than that usually attainable in body fluids, such as blood, cerebrospinal fluid, or urine. Based on the organism, the physician must also consider whether single- or double-agent therapy is required. In certain situations, such as the treatment of *Pseudomonas* sp infections, administration of multiple agents is essential to the achievement of optimal therapy.

Antibiotics vary in their final modes of action. They are classified into two broad groups. *Bactericidal agents* cause death of the bacteria, while *bacteriostatic antibiotics* inhibit or retard their growth (Table 10-7). The following sections describe the mechanisms of action and spectra of the most commonly used antibiotics.

Antibacterial Agents

Penicillins

Penicillins possess a 6-aminopenicillanic acid nucleus in which the β-lactam ring is essential for antibacterial activity. The bactericidal activity of penicillins results from binding to receptors and blocking the synthesis of bacterial cell wall mucopeptide.[53] In actively growing bacteria, interference with biosynthesis of the peptidoglycan structure increases osmotic fragility, resulting in cell lysis. Resistant organisms produce β-lactamases that hydrolyze the β-lactam ring of penicillin. Semisynthetic penicillins have been constructed by adding side chains to the aminopenicillanic acid nucleus, making them resistant to the β-lactamases.[54] The natural penicillins are penicillin, benzathine penicillin G, procaine penicillin G, and penicillin V. Penicillins are the drug of choice for infections produced by pneumococci, streptococci, non–β-lactamase–producing staphylococci, meningococci, gonococci, clostridia, actinomycetes, treponemas, and most anaerobes, excluding *Bacteroides fragilis*. Penicillinase-resistant penicillins are indicated for staphylococcal infections that produce β-lactamases. These agents include methicillin, oxacillin, nafcillin, cloxacillin, and dicloxacillin.

Aminopenicillins are ampicillin and amoxicillin. These are active against many strains of *E coli, Proteus mirabilis, Salmonella* sp, *Shigella* sp, *Listeria* sp, and *H influenzae*. They are bacteriostatic to *Streptococcus faecalis* but bactericidal when an aminoglycoside is added. All strains of *Pseudomonas* sp are resistant. Aminopenicillins are sensitive to β-lactamases.

Carboxypenicillins include carbenicillin and ticarcillin. Carbenicillin has an antibacterial range similar to ampicillin with the added benefit of activity against certain strains of *Pseudomonas aeruginosa, Proteus* sp, and *Enterobacter* sp. The spectrum of activity of ticarcillin is similar to that of carbenicillin, but it is more active against *P aeruginosa*.

The ureidopenicillins include mezlocillin, azlocillin, and piperacillin. They are semisynthetic penicillins derived from the ampicillin molecule with an acyl derivative of urea. This group has activity against streptococci, enterococci, *Enterobacter* sp, *Pseudomonas* sp, and many anaerobes. The ureidopenicillins are susceptible to β-lactamases. Their advantage is that they achieve high concentrations in bile and have increased activity against *P aeruginosa* and *Klebsiella* sp.

Clavulanate, sulbactam, and tazobactam are β-lactam inhibitors that can augment the effect of β-lactam agents. Clavulanate has been combined with amoxicillin, ticarcillin, and piperacillin.[55]

The main adverse side effect of all penicillins is hypersensitivity, which can occur in 2% of treated patients. Anaphylaxis occurs in 0.02% of patients receiving penicillin. The reaction is the result of antibodies formed against penicilloate and its metabolites.

Cephalosporins

Cephalothin was the first cephalosporin to be introduced as an antibiotic. This drug is derived from *Cephalosporium acremonium*. The cephalosporin structure consists of a dehydrothiazine ring fused to a β-lactam ring. This group of antibiotics inhibit bacterial cell wall synthesis. Side chains have been substituted at the number 3 carbon position of the six-membered ring and at the acyl side chain of the cephalosporin nucleus. Substitutions at the acyl chain lead to differences in antibacterial activity and β-lactamase stability.

Three variables determine the antimicrobial spectrum of cephalosporins: (1) the ability of the drug to penetrate the outer cell wall of the bacterium, (2) the ability to inhibit penicillin-binding protein enzymes (transpeptidases and carboxypeptidases) that are involved in cell wall synthesis, and (3) the ability to resist β-lactamase activity.

Cephalosporins are divided into four generations based on increasing gram-negative activity (Table 10-8). First-generation cephalosporins are effective against most aerobic gram-positive cocci. This group demonstrates activity against *E coli, Klebsiella pneumoniae,* and *P mirabilis*. Resistance to these gram-negative organisms may reach 30%. First-generation cephalosporins include cephalothin, cefazolin, cephapirin, cephalexin, cephradine, and cefadroxil.

Second-generation cephalosporins possess the same spectrum of activity as the first generation and also have a wider spectrum of activity toward gram-negative organisms. They are effective against *H influenzae,* indole-positive *Proteus* sp, and some *Neisseria* and *Enterobacter* species. The minimal inhibitory concentration required to kill staphylococci is variable.

TABLE 10-3. *Penicillins, imipenem, aztreonam,*

Organisms	Penicillin G	Penicillin V	Pen'ase Res. Penicillins					Aminopenicillins			
			Methi-cillin	Naf-cillin	Oxa-cillin	Cloxa-cillin	Dicloxa-cillin	Ampi-cillin	Amoxi-cillin	Amox/Clav	Amp/Sulb
GRAM-POSITIVE											
Strep, Group A,B,C,G	+	+	+	+	+	+	+	+	+	+	+
Strep. pneumoniae	+	+	+	+	+	+	+	+	+	+	+
Strep. viridans	+	+	+	+	+	+	+	+	+	+	+
Strep. faecalis	0	0	0	0	0	0	0	+	+	+	+
Strep. faecium	0	0	0	0	0	0	0	+	+		
Staph. aureus (MSSA)	0	0	+	+	+	+	+	0	0	+	+
Staph. aureus (MRSA)	0	0	0	0	0	0	0	0	0	0	0
Staph. epidermidis	0	0	±	±	±	±	±	±	±	+	+
C jeikeium	0	0	0	0	0	0	0	0	0	0	0
L monocytogenes	+	0	0	0	0	0	0	+	+	+	+
GRAM-NEGATIVE											
N gonorrhoeae	0	0	0	0	0	0	0	0	0	+	+
N meningitidis	+	0						+	+	+	+
M catarrhalis†	0	0	0	0	0	0	0	0	0	+	+
H influenzae	0	0	0	0	0	0	0	±	±	+	+
E coli	+	0	0	0	0	0	0	±	±	+	+
Klebsiella sp	0	0	0	0	0	0	0	±	±	+	+
Enterobacter sp	0	0	0	0	0	0	0	0	0	+	+
Serratia sp	0	0	0	0	0	0	0	0	0	0	0
Salmonella sp	±	0	0	0	0	0	0	+	+	+	+
Shigella sp	0	0	0	0	0	0	0	+	±	+	+
Proteus mirabilis	+	±	0	0	0	0	0	+	+	+	+
Proteus vulgaris	0	0	0	0	0	0	0	0	0	+	+
Providencia sp	0	0	0	0	0	0	0	0	0	+	+
Morganella sp	0	0	0	0	0	0	0	0	0	0	+
Citrobacter sp‡	0	0	0	0	0	0	0	0	0	0	0
Aeromonas sp	0	0	0	0	0	0	0	0	0	+	+
Acinetobacter sp	0	0	0	0	0	0	0	0	0	0	±
P aeruginosa	0	0	0	0	0	0	0	0	0	0	0
P cepacia	0	0	0	0	0	0	0	0	0	0	0
X maltophilia	0	0	0	0	0	0	0	0	0	0	0
Y enterocolitica	0	0	0	0	0	0	0	0	0	±	±
Legionella sp	0	0	0	0	0	0	0	0	0	0	0
P multocida	+	+	0	0	0	0	0	+	+	+	+
H ducreyi								0	0	+	+
MISC.											
Chlamydia sp	0	0	0	0	0	0	0	0	0	0	0
M pneumoniae	0	0	0	0	0	0	0	0	0	0	0
ANAEROBES											
Actinomyces	+	0	0	0	0	0	0	+	+	+	+
Bacteroides fragilis	0	0	0	0	0	0	0	0	0	+	+
P melaninogenica†	+	0	0	0	0	0	0	+	+	+	+
Clostridium difficile	+										+
Clostridium (not difficile)	+	0						+	+	+	+
Peptostreptococcus sp	+	+	+	+	+	+	+	+	+	+	+

* This table includes data based on both clinical trials and in vitro susceptibility tests; the clinical significance of the latter is often uncertain without clinical trials. Antimicrobials such as rufloxacin have high tissue penetration, hence in vivo activity may exceed in vitro activity.

† *Moraxella catarrhalis* renamed *Branhamella catarrhalis*; *B melaninogenicus* renamed *Prevotella melaninogenica*.

‡ *C freundii:* most strains resistant to cephalothin. *C diversus:* most strains resistant to ampicillin, carbenicillin.

+, sensitive; ±, variable; 0, resistant; blank, data not available; *Ticar/Clav,* ticarcillin clavulanate; *Amp/Sulb,* ampicillin sulbactam; *Amox/Clav,* amoxicillin clavulanate; *MSSA,* methicillin-sensitive *Staph. aureus*; *MRSA,* methicillin-resistant *Staph. aureus*; *Pip/Tazo,* piperacillin tazobactam.

(Sanford JP, ed. The Sanford guide to antimicrobial therapy. Antimicrobial Therapy Inc., Dallas, 1994)

metronidazole, fluoroquinolones

Antipseudomonal penicillins								Fluoroquinolones				
Ticar-cillin	Ticar/Clav	Pip/Tazo	Mezlo-cillin	Pipera-cillin	Imipenem	Aztreonam	Metroni-dazole	Cipro-floxacin	Oflox-acin	Lomeflox-acin	Peflox-acin	Ruflox-acin
+	+	+	+	+	+	0	0	±	±	0	0	±
+	+	+	+	+	+	0	0	±	±	0	0	±
+	+	+	+	+	+	0	0	0	0			
0	0	+	+	+	+	0	0	+	+		0	0
0	0	±		±	±	0	0	0	0		0	
0	+	+	0	0	+	0	0	+	+		+	+
0	0	0	0	0	0	0	0	0	0		0	
±	±	+	0	0	+	0	0	+	+		+	+
0	0		0	0	0	0	0	0	0			
+	+		+	+	+	0	0	+				
+	+	+	+	+	+	+	0	+	+		+	+
+	+	+	+	+	+	+	0	+	+		+	+
0	+	+	0	±	+	+	0	+	+		+	+
±	+	+	±	±	+	+	0	+	+		+	+
±	+	+	+	+	+	+	0	+	+		+	+
0	+	+	+	+	+	+	0	+	+		+	±
+	+	+	+	+	+	+	0	+	+		+	±
+	+	+	+	0	+	+	0	+	+		+	+
+	+		+	+	+	+	0	+	+		+	+
+			+	+	+	+	0	+	+		+	+
+	+	+	+	+	+	+	0	+	+		+	+
+	+	+	+	+	+	+	0	+	+		+	+
+	+	+	+	+	+	+	0	+	+		+	+
+	+	+	+	+	+	+	0	+	+		+	
+	+	+	+	+	+	+	0	+	+			+
0	0	+	0	0	+	0	0	+	±			+
+	+	+	+	+	+	+	0	+	±			
0					+	0	0	0	0			
	+	0	±	+	0	0	0	+	+			
±	+		+	+	+	+	0	+	+		+	
0	0		0	0	0	0	0	+	+			0
+	+		+	+	+	+	0	+	+		+	
0	0	0	0	0	0	0	0	+	+	+	+	+
0	0	0	0	0	0	0	0	+	+		0	
				+	+	0	0	0	±			
±	+	+	+	+	+	0	+	0	+	0	0	0
+	+	+	+	+	+	0	+	0	0	0		
				+	+	0	+					
+	+	+	+	+	+	0	+	±	±	0		+
+	+	+	+	+	+	0	+	±	±	0		

TABLE 10-4.

Organisms	Generation		2nd generation					
	Cefazolin	Cephalothin	Cefamandole	Cefmetazole	Cefonicid	Cefotetan	Cefoxitin	Cefuroxime
GRAM-POSITIVE								
Strep, Group A,B,C,G	+	+	+	+	+	+	+	+
Strep. pneumoniae	+	+	+	+	+	+	+	+
Strep. viridans	+	+	+	+	+	+	+	+
Strep. faecalis	0	0	0	0	0	0	0	0
Staph. aureus (MSSA)	+	+	+	+	+	+	+	+
Staph. aureus (MRSA)	0	0	0	0	0	0	0	0
Staph. epidermidis	±	±	±	±	±	±	±	±
C jeikeium	+		0	0	0	0	0	0
L monocytogenes	0	0	0	0	0	0	0	0
	0	0						
GRAM-NEGATIVE								
N gonorrhoeae	+	+	+	+	+	+	+	+
N meningitidis	0	0	+	+	+	+	+	+
M catarrhalis†	+	+	+	+	+	+	+	+
H influenzae	+	+	+	+	+	+	+	+
E coli	+	+	+	+	+	+	+	+
Klebsiella sp	+	+	+	+	+	+	+	+
Enterobacter sp	0	0	0	0	+	±	0	±
Serratia sp	0	0	0	0	0	+	0	0
Salmonella sp		+	0	+		+		+
Shigella sp		+	0	+		+		+
Proteus mirabilis	+	+	+	+	+	+	+	+
Proteus vulgaris	0	0	±	+	+	+	+	0
Providencia sp	0	0	+	+	+	+	+	+
Morganella sp	0	0	+	+	+	+	+	±
Citrobacter sp		0	±	±	+	±		±
Aeromonas sp	0	0	±	+	+	+	±	+
Acinetobacter sp	0	0	0	0	0	0	0	0
P aeruginosa	0	0	0	0	0	0	0	0
P cepacia	0	0	0	0	0	0	0	0
X maltophilia	0	0	0	0	0	0	0	0
Y enterocolitica	0	0				+	±	+
Legionella sp	0	0	0	0	0	0	0	0
P multocida				+				
M ducreyi		+					+	
ANEROBES								
Actinomyces		+						
Bacteroides fragilis	0	0	0	+	0	±	+	0
P melaninogenica†			+	+		+	+	+
Clostridium difficile						+	0	
Clostridium (not difficile)			+	+	+	+	+	+
Peptostreptococcus sp			+	+	+	+	+	+

* This table includes data based on both clinical trials and in vitro susceptibility tests; the clinical significance of the latter is often uncertain without clinical trials.

† *Moraxella catarrhalis* renamed *Branhamella catarrhalis*; *B melaninogenicus* renamed *Prevotella melaninogenica.*

+, sensitive; ±, variable, 0, resistant; blank, data not available; *MSSA,* methicillin-sensitive *Staph. aureus; MRSA,* methicillin-resistant *Staph. aureus.*

(Sanford JP, ed. The Sanford guide to antimicrobial therapy. Antimicrobial Therapy, Inc., Dallas, 1994)

Cefoxitin and cefmetazole have significant activity against anaerobes, including *B fragilis.* Second-generation cephalosporins include cefamandole, cefaclor, cefuroxime, cefonicid, ceforanide, loracarbef, cefprozil, cefoxitin, cefotetan, and cefmetazole.

Third-generation cephalosporins have the broadest activity against gram-negative organisms but the least activity against gram-positive cocci. They are active against enteric gram-negative bacilli, *Serratia* sp, *Citrobacter* sp, *H influenzae,* and *Neisseria gonorrhoeae* and are moderately active against *Pseudomonas* sp.

Adverse effects of cephalosporins include hypersensitivity reactions, hypoprothrombinemia, and alcohol intolerance.

Aminoglycosides

Aminoglycosides are composed of two or more amino sugars bound by glycosidic linkage to a central hexose nucleus. This group of antibiotics binds irreversibly to the 30S bacterial ribosome and interferes with protein synthesis. Cell penetration is a requirement for activity and is an energy-dependent process.

*Cephalosporins**

3rd generation						Oral agents									
Cefotaxime	Ceftizoxime	Ceftriaxone	Cefoperazone	Ceftazidime	Cefepime	Cefadroxil	Cephalexin	Cefaclor	Cefprozil	Cefurox. axetil	Loracarbef	Cefixime	Ceftibuten	Celetamet-Piv.	Cefpodoxime-Prox.
+	+	+	+	+	+	+	+	+	+	+	+	+	+	+	+
+	+	+	+	+	+	+	+	+	+	+	+	+	±	+	+
+	+	+	+	+	+	+	+	+	0	+	+	+		±	+
0	0	0	+	0	0	0	0	0	0	0	0	0		0	
+	+	+	+	+	+	+	+	+	+	+	+	0	0	0	+
0	0	0	0	0	0	0	0	0	0	0	0	0	0	0	
±	±	±	±	±	±	±	±	±	±	±	±	0			±
0	0	0	0	0		0	0	0	0	0	0	0			
0	0	0	0	0	0	0	0	0	0	0	0	0			
+	+	+	+	+	+		0	+	+	+	+	+		+	+
+	+	+	+	+	+		0	+	+	+	+	+			
+	+	+	+	+	+	+	+	+	+	+	+	+	+	+	+
+	+	+	+	+	+		+	+	+	+	+	+	+	+	+
+	+	+	+	+	+	+	+	+	+	+	+	+	+	+	0
+	+	+	+	+	+	+	+	+	+	+		+	+		0
+	+	+	+	+	+	0	0	0	0	±		0		0	0
+	+	+	+	+	+	0	0	0	0	0		±	±	0	0
+	+	+	+	+	+		0	+	+	+		+	+	+	
+	+	+	+	+	+		0	+	+	+		+	+	+	
+	+	+	+	+	+	+	+	+	+	+	+	+	+	+	+
+	+	+	+	+	+	0	0	0	0	0		+		+	±
+	+	+	+	+	+	0	0	0	0	+		+		+	
+	+	+	+	+	+	0	0	0	0	±		0		0	0
+	+	+	+	+	+	0	±	0	±	±		+		±	+
+	+	+	+	+	+					+		+		+	
+	+	+	0	+	±	0	0	0	0	0		0		0	
±	+	±	+	+	+	0	0	0	0	0		0		±	0
+	+	+	+	+	±	0	0	0	0	0		0		+	+
0	0	0	±	±	0	0	0	0	0	0		0			
+	+	+	+	+	+							+		+	+
0	0	0	0	0		0	0	0	0	0	0	0			0
	+	+	+									+			
+	+	+		+								+		+	
±	±	+	0	±	0		0	0	0			0	0	0	0
+	+	+	+	+	0			+	+	+		+		+	
0	0		0		0							0			
+	+	+	+	+			+	+	+	+		0			
+	+	+	+	+	+		+	+	+	+		+			

Aminoglycoside uptake is facilitated by the presence of inhibitors of cell wall synthesis such as a β-lactam antibiotic.[56] This group of antibiotics exhibit bactericidal activity by disrupting calcium homeostasis.

Aminoglycosides are active primarily against aerobic and facultative gram-negative bacilli. Resistance is related to ineffective cell transport, inability to bind ribosomal receptor, or enzymatic degradation of the drug. Aminoglycosides can also be inactivated by β-lactam antibiotics in high concentrations. This is due to formation of a covalent bond between the carboxyl group of a broken β-lactam ring and an amino group of the aminoglycoside.

Available aminoglycosides include streptomycin, kanamycin, neomycin, gentamicin, tobramycin, amikacin, netilmicin, and sisomicin. Streptomycin is effective against *Mycobacterium tuberculosis, Francisella tularensis, Yersinia pestis,* and *Brucella* sp. Amikacin has the broadest activity against gram-negative organisms, owing to its relative resistance to enzymatic degradation. Adverse effects of aminoglycosides are primarily nephrotoxicity and ototoxicity.

Tetracyclines

Tetracyclines inhibit protein synthesis and are bacteriostatic. These agents require active transport into the cell. Inside the cell, tetracyclines inhibit synthesis of protein by binding to the 30S ribosome and preventing aminoacyl transfer RNA from gaining access to the messenger RNA–ribosome complex.

Tetracyclines are broad-spectrum antibiotics, active against

TABLE 10-5. *Aminoglycosides, macrolides, glycopeptides,*

Organisms	Aminoglycosides					Chloram-phenicol	Clinda-mycin	Macrolides		
	Kana-mycin	Genta-micin	Tobra-mycin	Ami-kacin	Netil-micin			Erythro-mycin	Azithro-mycin	Clarithro-mycin
GRAM-POSITIVE										
Strep, Group A,B,C,G	0	0	0	0	0	+	+	+	+	+
Strep. pneumoniae	0	0	0	0	0	+	+	+	+	+
Strep. faecalis	S	S	S	S	S	0	0	0	0	
Strep. faecium	S	S	0	0	0	0	0	0		
Staph. aureus (MSSA)	+	+	+	+	+	±	+	±	+	+
Staph. aureus (MRSA)	0	0	0	0	0	0	0	0	0	0
Staph. epidermidis	±	±	±	±	±		+	+	0	
C jeikeium	0	0	0	0	0	0	0	0	0	0
GRAM-NEGATIVE										
N gonorrhoeae	±	0	0	0	0	+	0	+	+	+
M catarrhalis†		+				+		+	+	+
H influenzae	+	+	+	+	+	+	0	±	+	+
Aeromonas sp						+				
E coli	+	+	+	+	+	+	0	0	0	0
Klebsiella sp	+	+	+	+	+	±	0	0	0	0
Enterobacter sp	0	+	+	+	+	0	0	0	0	0
Serratia marcescens	+	+	+	+	+	0	0	0	0	0
Proteus vulgaris	+	+	+	+	+	±	0	0	0	0
Acinetobacter sp	0	0	+	0			0	0	0	0
P aeruginosa	0	+	+	+	+	0	0	0	0	0
P cepacia	0	0	0	0	0	+	0	0	0	0
X maltophilia	0	0	0	0	0	+	0	0	0	0
F tularensis		+				+				
Brucella sp		+				+	0			
Legionella sp								+	+	+
H ducreyi	+					+	+	+	+	
V vulnificus		0	0	0	+					
MISCELLANEOUS										
Chlamydia trachomatis	0	0	0	0	0	+		+	+	+
M pneumoniae	0	0	0	0	0	+	0	+	+	+
Rickettsia sp	0	0	0	0	0	+		±		
Mycobacterium avium				+					+	+
ANAEROBES										
Actinomyces sp	0	0	0	0	0	+	+		+	+
Bacteroides fragilis	0	0	0	0	0	+	+		0	0
P melaninogenica†	0	0	0	0	0	+	+		+	+
Clostridium difficile	0	0	0	0	0	±				
Clostridium (not difficile)‡						+		±	+	+

* This table includes data based on both clinical trials and in vitro susceptibility tests; the clinical significance of the latter is often uncertain without clinical trials. Antimicrobials such as azithromycin have high tissue penetration and some, such as clarithromycin, are metabolized to more active compounds, hence in vitro activity may exceed in vivo activity.

† *Morazella catarrhalis* renamed *Branhamella catarrhalis; B melaninogenicus* renamed *Prevotella melaninogenica.*

‡ Vancomycin, metronidazole active against *C difficile.*

+, sensitive; ±, variable; 0, resistant; S, synergistic with penicillins (ampicillin); blank, data not available; *TMP/SMX,* trimethoprim-sulfamethoxazole; *MSSA,* methicillin-sensitive *Staph. aureus; MRSA,* methicillin-resistant *Staph. aureus.*

(Sanford JP, ed. The Sanford guide to antimicrobial therapy. Antimicrobial Therapy, Inc., Dallas, 1994)

many gram-positive and gram-negative organisms, *Treponema* sp, and *Mycobacterium marinum.* These drugs have been shown to inhibit the growth of *Actinomycetes, Rickettsiae, Mycoplasma, Chlamydia,* and *Brucella* sp and *Vibrio cholerae.*

Resistance to the tetracyclines is mediated by plasmids. They impart resistance by coding for proteins that interfere with active transport of the drug into the bacteria. A microorganism resistant to one tetracycline is resistant to the others.

Adverse effects of tetracyclines include inhibition of bone growth and yellow discoloration of teeth if given during the early stages of calcification. Liver damage has been noted at higher concentrations. Gastrointestinal disturbances are com-

mon secondary to alterations of the enteric flora. Staphylococcal enterocolitis and pseudomembranous colitis have occurred in patients treated with tetracyclines. Azotemia can occur in patients with renal insufficiency. Minocycline can result in vestibular toxicity.

Erythromycin

Erythromycin is a macrolide that inhibits protein synthesis by binding to the 50S ribosomal subunit of susceptible microbes. Erythromycin is active against many gram-positive organisms

and urinary tract agents

Doxycycline	Minocycline	Glycopeptides		Fusidic acid	Trimethoprim	TMP/ SMX	Urinary tract agents			Rifampin	Metronidazole
		Vancomycin	Teicoplanin				Nitrofurantoin	Norfloxacin	Enoxacin		
±	+	+	+	±	+	+	+	0	0	+	0
+	+	+	+	±	±	+	+	0	±	+	0
0	0	+	+	+	+	+	±	0	0	±	0
0	0	±	±		0	0	0	0	0	0	0
±	+	+	+	+	±	+	+	±	+	+	0
0	0	+	+	+	0	0	0	0	0	0	0
		+	±	+	+			±	+	+	0
0	0	+	+	+	0	0	0	0	0	0	0
±	±	±		+	0	±	+	+	+	+	0
+	+					+		+	+	+	0
+	+				±	±	+	+	+	+	0
+						+					
±	±	0	0	0	+	+	+	+	+	0	0
0	0	0	0	0	+	+	±	+	+	0	0
0	0	0	0	0	±	±	±	+	+	0	0
0	0	0	0	0	0	±		0	+	0	0
0	0	0	0	0	0	0	0	+	+	0	0
0	±	0	0	0	0	0	0	0	±	0	0
0	0	0	0	0	+	+	0	+	+	0	0
0	0	0	0	0	+	+	0	0	0	0	0
+	+	0	0	0	0	+	0	0	0		0
+	+	0	0		+	+				+	0
				±	+	+				+	0
0	0	0		0		±		+			0
+				0							
+	+				0	0		0	0	+	0
+	+				0						0
+	+	0	0		0						0
											0
+	+	+									
±	±	0		+	0			0	0		+
+	+	0		+				0	0		+
		+								0	+
+	+	+	+	+							+

TABLE 10-6. *Prophylactic antibodies: therapeutic suggestions*

Procedure	Antibiotic	Duration
Gastroduodenal	Cefazolin, 100 mg/kg/d q6°*	24 h
Biliary tract	Cefazolin, 100 mg/kg/d q6	24 h
Appendectomy	Cefoxitin, 100 mg/kg/d q6	24 h
Colorectal	Oral: neomycin; erythromycin base	Oral, 24 h before operation
	IV: Cefoxitin or ampicillin and gentamacin (<1 y old)	15–24 h after operation
Head and neck	Cefazolin or clindamycin	48 h
Noncardiac thoracic	Cefazolin	48 h
Colorectal	Oral: Neomycin (100 mg/kg divided among 3 doses; erythromycin base, 50 mg/kg divided among 3 doses	Preoperative
	IV: Cefoxitin, 100 mg/kg/d q6; or ampicillin, 100 mg/kg/d q6; and gentamicin, 3 mg/kg/d q8	25 h

* Intravenous prophylactic antibiotics should be administered up to 2 h *before* incision.
(Fallat M. Personal communication.)

TABLE 10-7. *Antibiotics: Classification by mode of therapy*

BACTERICIDAL

Aminoglycosides
Aztreonam
Bacitracin
Cephalosporins
Imipenem
Vancomycin
Penicillins
Polymyxins
Quinolones

BACTERIOSTATIC

Sulfonamides
Clindamycin
Trimethoprim
Chloramphenicol
Erythromycin
Tetracyclines

and is the agent of choice for *Mycoplasma* and *Legionella* sp. The drug may be used to treat gonorrhea and syphilis in patients unable to tolerate penicillin or tetracycline. It is active against actinomycosis. Bacterial resistance is common with long-term therapy. The major adverse effect is gastrointestinal disturbance.

Lincosamides

The lincosamides include lincomycin and clindamycin. Lincomycin is now rarely used because it is less active in vitro and has no advantage over clindamycin. Clindamycin binds to the 50S subunit of bacterial ribosomes and suppresses the protein synthesis. Clindamycin, erythromycin, and chloramphenicol act at the same site and may therefore compete against each other.

Clindamycin is used in the treatment of anaerobic infections. It is active against many gram-positive organisms. Plasmid-mediated resistance to clindamycin can occur with prolonged therapy. Adverse effects include diarrhea, pseudomembranous colitis, and rarely neutropenia.

TABLE 10-8. *Features of cephalosporins*

First generation (P Ceph 1)—cephalothin, cefazolin, cefazolin, cephapirin, cephradine, cefazaflur (investigational): Most active against gram-positive cocci. Enterococci are resistant. Limited activity against aerobic gram-negative bacilli: *E coli, K pneumoniae, P mirabilis.*

Second generation—cefamandole, cefoxitin, cefuroxime, cefmetazole, cefonicid, ceforanide, cefotetan

    Cefuroxime subgroup (P Ceph 2): About equal to first-generation cephalosporins against gram-positive cocci. More active against *E coli, K pneumoniae, P mirabilis.* Also active against *H influenzae;* some *Enterobacter, Serratia, Anaerobes, Neisseria* sp. NOT active against *Pseudomonas* sp.

    Cephamycin subgroup (P Ceph 2): Less active than 1st generation vs Gram + aerobes and Gram + anaerobes. Are most active against bacteroides spp.

Third generation

    Modest antipseudomonal activity (P Ceph 3)—cefotaxime, moxalactam, ceftizoxime, ceftriaxone: Less active than first generation against gram-positive cocci. Most active against *E coli, Klebsiella* sp, *Proteus* sp. Inconsistent against *Serratia, Enterobacter, Acinetobacter* and *Pseudomonas* sp. Only modest activity against anaerobes.

    Enhanced antipseudomonal activity (P Ceph 3 AP)—cefoperazone, ceftazidime, cefsulodin (investigational): Least active against aerobic gram-positive cocci. Similar to P Ceph 3 against aerobic gram-negative bacilli. Most active against *P aeruginosa.*

Fourth generation (P Ceph 4)—cefepime, cefpirome: activity against gram positive cocci more than P Ceph 3. increased activity over P Ceph 3 against *Enterobacteriaceae* sp. and *P aeruginosa.*

| | | Comparative in vitro activity | | | | |
| | First generation | Second generation | | Third generation | | Fourth generation |
Organism		Cefuroxime	Cefoxitin	P Ceph 3	P Ceph 3 AP	
Staphylococci	+ + +	+ +	+ +	+ + +	+ +	+ + +
Streptococci	+ + +	+ +	+ +	+ + +	+ +	+ + +
Enterococci	—	—	—	+	—	+
E coli, Klebsiella sp, *Proteus mirabilis*	+ +	+ + +	+ + +	+ + +	+ + +	+ + +
Enterobacter cloacae, Serratia marcescens	—	+ +	+	+ +	+ +	+ + +
Haemophilus influenzae	+ +	+ + +	+ +	+ + +	+ + +	+ + +
P aeruginosa	—	—	—	+	+ +	+ +
B fragilis	—	+ +	+ + +	+ +	—	—

—, <50% strains susceptible; +, 50%–80%; + +, 81%–95%; + + +, >95%; *P Ceph 3,* cefotaxime, ceftriaxone; *P Ceph 3 AP,* ceftazidime.

(Adapted from Sader HS, Jones RN, *Antimicrobic Newsletter* 1992; 8:75)

Chloramphenicol

Chloramphenicol is a broad-spectrum antibiotic. It is bacteriostatic and acts by inhibiting protein synthesis by binding to the 50S ribosomal subunit. It prevents the amino acid–containing end of aminoacyl-tRNA from binding to the ribosome. Resistance occurs as a result of production of an acetyltransferase, which inactivates the drug.

Chloramphenicol is active against *Salmonella typhi* and is effective in the treatment of bacterial meningitis caused by susceptible organisms. In patients who cannot tolerate tetracyclines, chloramphenicol can be used to treat rikettsia diseases, psittacosis, or lymphogranuloma venereum.

Chloramphenicol should not be the first-choice antibiotic because of its potential toxicity. Bone marrow suppression is a known complication and is a dose-related phenomenon. Bone marrow suppression occurs when the drug concentration exceeds 25 μg/mL. Idiosyncratic bone marrow suppression is rare and occurs in 1 in 40,000 courses of therapy. Premature infants treated with chloramphenicol can develop circulatory collapse known as *gray syndrome.*

Vancomycin

Vancomycin is derived from *Nocardia orientalis.* It is a bactericidal drug that acts by inhibiting the biosynthesis of peptidoglycan. Vancomycin is primarily effective against gram-positive organisms. It is the agent of choice for methicillin-resistant *Staphylococcus aureus* and is also active against *S faecalis, Actinomyces* sp, and *C difficile.* A notable adverse effect of vancomycin is circulatory collapse (red man syndrome) if administered too rapidly. The incidence of nephrotoxicity is low if blood levels are closely monitored.

Carbapenems

Imipenem-cilastin falls into the carbapenem category of penicillin analogue antibiotics. Carbapenems possess a nucleus containing a β-lactam ring and a thiazolidine ring. Imipenem exhibits a broad spectrum of activity against aerobes and anaerobes such as *B fragilis, Actinomyces* sp, *C difficile,* and peptostreptococcus. It is not active against methicillin-resistant *S aureus, Xanthomonas maltophilia,* or *Legionella, Mycoplasma,* or *Chlamydia* sp.

Monobactams

Aztreonam is a monocyclic β-lactam antibiotic that lacks the thiazolidine ring found in penicillins. This drug is active against gram-negative organisms only. It is not active against *Acinetobacter* sp, *X maltophilia,* or *Legionella* sp.

Quinolones

The quinolones include ciprofloxacin, norfloxacin, enoxacin, pefloxacin, and ofloxacin. These drugs are active against *S faecalis* and *Staphylococcus, Listeria, Chlamydia,* and *Mycoplasma* sp. They are not very effective against anaerobic infections. Cross-resistance to all quinolones is observed.

Trimethoprim-Sulfamethoxazole

The antimicrobial activity of this drug results from its action on the synthesis of tetrahydrofolic acid. Sulfonamide inhibits the incorporation of paraaminobenzoic acid into folic acid, and trimethoprim prevents the reduction of dihydrofolate to tetrahydrofolate. The interaction between trimethoprim and sulfamethoxazole is synergistic. The antibacterial spectrum includes *Streptococcus pneumoniae, C diphtheriae, Neisseria meningitidis, S aureus* and *S epidermidis, S faecalis, E coli, P aeruginosa,* and *Enterobacter, Salmonella, Shigella, Serratia, Klebsiella, Nocardia,* and *Legionella* sp.

Metronidazole

Metronidazole possesses a selective activity against anaerobic and microaerophilic microorganisms. The nitro group of metronidazole is reduced by electron transport proteins with low redox potentials. It acts as an electron sink and deprives the cell of required reducing equivalents. It is believed that the reduced form of the drug produces the biochemical lesions that lead to death of the pathogen. Metronidazole is effective against *B fragilis, Prevotella melaninogenica, C difficile,* and *Trichomonas* and *Giardia* sp.

Antifungal Agents

Amphotericin

Amphotericin is an antifungal agent derived from *Streptomyces nodosus.* It is a polyene antibiotic. The antifungal activity of the drug is dependent on its binding to a sterol moiety present in the membrane of fungi. It has a high binding affinity to ergosterol. Sterol binding results in the formation of pores, weakening the fungal membrane. Adverse effects of this drug include anaphylaxis, thrombocytopenia, fever, anemia, and renal toxicity.

Fluconazole

Fluconazole (Diflucan) is a synthetic biz-triazole antifungal agent with activity against *Cryptococcus neoformans* and *Candida* sp. It inhibits fungal cytochrome P-450 sterol C-14 α-demethylation, leading to accumulation of 14 α-methyl sterols in fungi. It is useful in the treatment of oropharyngeal and esophageal candidiasis.

Nystatin

Nystatin is derived from *Streptomyces noursei.* Its antifungal activity is dependent on binding to a sterol moiety, primarily ergosterol. Binding creates pores or channels that increase the permeability of the membrane, resulting in cell death. It is effective against *Candida, Cryptococcus, Histoplasmosis, Blastomyces, Trichophyton, Epidermophyton,* and *Microsporum* sp. Absorption of this drug from the gastrointestinal tract is negligible. Nystatin is used primarily to treat candidal infections of skin, mucous membranes, and intestinal tract.

Flucytosine

Flucytosine is converted in fungal cells to fluorouracil by cytosine deaminase. Fluorouracil is metabolized to 5-fluoro-deoxyuridylic acid, which inhibits thymidylate synthetase. Flucytosine is used in combination with amphotericin B for the treatment of cryptococcal meningitis.

Antiviral Agents

Acyclovir

Acyclovir is a synthetic nucleoside analogue with antiviral properties against herpesvirus. It interferes with DNA polymerase of herpesvirus, inhibiting viral replication. It is effective in the treatment of herpes simplex virus types 1 and 2 encephalitis and cutaneous infections. Acyclovir is also active against varicella zoster virus. Adverse reactions include nephrotoxicity, gastrointestinal disturbances, and bone marrow suppression.

Ganciclovir

Ganciclovir is an acyclic nucleoside related to acyclovir but with greater activity toward CMV. It inhibits replication of CMV by interfering with cellular DNA. Adverse reactions include bone marrow suppression, mild nephrotoxicity, and elevation of hepatic enzymes.

Foscarnet

Foscarnet is a pyrophosphate derivative that results in inhibition of herpesvirus DNA polymerases and retrovirus reverse transcriptases. It is used in the treatment of acyclovir-resistant herpes infection and in AIDS patients with CMV retinitis.

Testing of Susceptibility

The microbiology laboratory is essential to the proper selection of antibiotics. It provides the ability to isolate and identify the invading microbe and to determine antibiotic sensitivities.

A simple Gram stain can identify gram-positive and gram-negative organisms, fungi, and inflammatory cells. This stain provides important information regarding the morphology of a microbe, identifying it as a rod or a cocci. A diagnosis of an infection secondary to *N gonorrhoeae* can be made from the Gram stain, allowing the proper selection of an antibiotic for therapy. An acid-fast stain can make the diagnosis of tuberculosis. Phase-contrast microscopy is helpful in making the diagnosis of syphilis by demonstrating the presence of spirochetes. An India ink stain reveals *Cryptococcus* sp in cerebrospinal fluid, providing a diagnosis of cryptococcal meningitis. Fluorescent antibody stains are helpful in detecting *Legionella sp, F tularensis,* and *Y pestis.*

Many organisms are fastidious and difficult to isolate. It is important for the clinician to have good communication with the microbiology laboratory so that proper handling of a specimen occurs and appropriate culture media are selected to provide the best growth environment. Anaerobic organisms quickly die on exposure to oxygen. An anaerobic environment is important for isolation of both facultative and obligate anaerobes. Isolation of a virus also requires appropriate specimen collection and inoculation into animals or onto appropriate cell lines. The identity of isolated viruses can be confirmed by using specific antisera that inhibit viral growth.

Isolation and growth of an organism allows in vitro susceptibility testing to antimicrobial agents. Susceptibility testing should be done when the isolated organism is likely to be resistant to several antibiotics, such as occurs in *Pseudomonas, Enterobacter,* or *Staphylococcus* sp or enterococci. Organisms are screened for β-lactamase production.

Antimicrobial susceptibility is determined by agar dilution or disk diffusion. An organism is considered susceptible if the concentration of an antibiotic necessary to inhibit its growth is lower than that attained in body fluids such as blood, cerebrospinal fluid, or urine. The agar technique provides quantitative results that are expressed as the minimal concentration of antibiotic that inhibits the growth of the isolated organism. An organism is sensitive to an antibiotic when the minimal inhibitory concentration equals one eighth of the achievable peak blood level of the drug. The disk diffusion method provides a qualitative measure of susceptibility. Commercially available paper disks containing specific amounts of antibiotics are placed on agar plates that contain a standard inoculum of bacteria. A zone of growth inhibition occurs around each active antibiotic. The size of the zone of inhibition determines the susceptibility of the organism. The organism is identified as susceptible, intermediate, or resistant to the tested antibiotic.

IMMUNE MODULATION

Modulation of the immune system is not a new concept. In 1798, Jenner published his work on vaccination for the prevention of smallpox. Since this publication, vaccination has resulted in the control of pertussis, tetanus, diphtheria, polio, and hepatitis B. Passive immunization has been used in recent years for treatment against hepatitis B, CMV, and herpesvirus.

A better understanding of the effector mechanisms of the immune system has led to a focus on developing biologic modifiers of the immune response. Monoclonal antibodies have been developed to inactivate endotoxin for treatment of gram-negative sepsis. Antibodies directed against TNF are also being developed. Recombinant technology has allowed large-scale synthesis of granulocyte-stimulating factor, interleukins, and interferons, making them available for therapy. These agents can be used to prime both humoral and cell-mediated immune events, allowing some control over their response to pathogens.

INFECTION

Nosocomial Infection

Hospital-acquired infections are a major problem in newborn infants. One to 2% of fetuses are infected in utero, and as many as 10% of infants are infected before 2 months of age.[57]

The fetus and neonate are immunocompromised compared with the older child or adult. The skin and mucous membranes of newborns are more permeable to exogenous antigen. There is poor development of the stratum corneum before 26 weeks' gestation. After 2 weeks of age, regardless of gestational age, the skin matures, and the stratum corneum develops. This immature barrier to infection is a common source of bacterial entry into the newborn, specifically the premature newborn.

Many factors affect the infection risk of the developing fetus. The mother's immunity and exposure to infection are of prime concern. Transplacental spread of maternal infection (eg, rubella, syphilis, toxoplasmosis, CMV, varicella, tuberculosis, or bacterial infection) can cause significant fetal disease.

The microorganisms colonizing the maternal birth canal are those that the baby will become exposed to with rupture of membranes and during descent through the birth canal. Normal flora include group B streptococcus, herpesvirus B, and herpes simplex virus.

Nosocomial infections in neonatal intensive care populations can be problematic. Hemming and colleagues,[58] in a study of 904 infants, showed a 15.3% overall infection rate; 14% of these infections were bacteremias, 29.3% pneumonias, 8.1% postoperative wound infections, and 4.5% urinary tract infections. Nosocomial infection rates were significantly greater in infants with birthweights of less than 1500 g.

Neonatal Sepsis

A child who presents with sepsis needs to be treated empirically with broad-spectrum antibiotics until the offending organism is identified and culture data obtained. In directing therapy for the child, a differential diagnosis of the pathogen is required. For example, susceptibility to infection is different for the neonate than for an adolescent, owing to differences in the maturity of the immune system.

The symptoms and signs of sepsis in the newborn are nonspecific. Infants may present with apnea, ileus, lethargy, seizures, jaundice, hypoglycemia, fever, hypothermia, or poor feeding. A normal white count or leukopenia is not uncommon secondary to limited bone marrow reserves. Sepsis must be considered in an infant with any of those symptoms. Blood, cerebrospinal fluid, and urine should be cultured.

Neonatal sepsis has been classified into that which occurs during and after the first week of life. Early neonatal sepsis is associated with prematurity and maternal risk factors, such as a prolonged rupture of membranes and chorioamnionitis. The common offending organisms during this time period are group B streptococcus and *E coli*. Less common are *S epidermidis* and *Listeria monocytogenes*. Herpes simplex virus must be considered if the mother has a history of herpes simplex infection. Ampicillin and gentamicin are suggested for the treatment of early neonatal sepsis, and acyclovir should also be added if there is a history of maternal herpes simplex virus. Early neonatal sepsis carries a mortality rate as high as 50%.

After the first week of life, infections are usually secondary to organisms that have colonized the mother. These infections have a significantly better outcome than early neonatal sepsis. Most infants have meningitis. Infants who have an extended hospitalization begin developing nosocomial infections with *S aureus*, gram-negative organisms, and *Candida* sp. After the first month of life, the spectrum of infections changes, with streptococcal pneumonia, *N meningitidis*, and *H influenzae* type II becoming common pathogens.

Soft Tissue Infections

Cellulitis

Cellulitis is an infection that involves the skin and subcutaneous tissues. The clinical presentation involves a tender area surrounded by edema and erythema. Common organisms involved in this type of infection are *Streptococcus* sp, *Staphylococcus* sp, and *H influenzae*. Streptococcus often causes a rapidly advancing cellulitis secondary to secretion of hyaluronidase. Certain strains of staphylococcus can cause an exfoliative dermatitis. Surgical débridement is rarely necessary, and treatment with an antibiotic with activity toward gram-positive organisms often suffices.

Necrotizing Fasciitis

Necrotizing fasciitis is a life-threatening condition. The patient is toxic and manifests extensive fascial necrosis. Edema extends beyond the area of erythema, and the involved area can have paresthesias. The offending pathogen is often β-hemolytic streptococcus and staphylococcus. Patients who acquire this entity are often immunosuppressed or in a low-flow state. Treatment must be emergent and requires wide surgical débridement of the overlying skin and necrotic fascia. Delay leads to patient demise. High-dose antibiotic therapy active against streptococci, penicillinase-producing staphylococci, gram-negative organisms, and anaerobes is indicated. These patients often require multiple débridement procedures with eventual skin grafting for wound closure.

REFERENCES

1. Marples MJ. The normal flora of the human skin. Br J Dermatol 1969; 81(Suppl 1):2.
2. Larson, EL, McGinley, KJ, Foglia, AR, et al. Composition and antimicrobic resistance of skin flora in hospitalized and healthy adults. J Clin Microbiol 1986;23:604.
3. Nicola NA, Metcalf D. Specificity of action of colony stimulating factors in the differentiation of granulocytes and macrophages. In: Biochemistry of macrophages. Ciba Foundation Symposium. London, Pitman, 1986;118:7.
4. Stanley ER. Action of the colony stimulating factor CSF-1. In: Biochemistry of macrophages. Ciba Foundation Symposium. London, Pitman, 1986;118:29.
5. Unanue ER. Antigen presenting function of the macrophage. Annu Rev Immunol 1984;3:973.
6. Unkeless JC, Scigliano E, Friedman V. Structure and function of human and murine receptors for IgG. Annu Rev Immunol 1988;6:25.
7. Fearon DT, Wong WW. Complement ligand–receptor interactions that mediate biological responses. Annu Rev Immunol 1983;1:243.
8. Schreiber RD. The chemistry and biology of complement receptors. Springer Semin Immunopathol 1984;7:221.
9. Babior BM. Oxygen dependent microbial killing by phagocytes. N Engl J Med 1978;298:659.
10. Badwey JA, Karnovsky ML. Active oxygen species and the functions of phagocytic leukocytes. Annu Rev Biochem 1980;49:695.
11. Hofman MK, Gilbert KM, Hirst JA, et al. An essential role for IL-1

and a dual function for IL-2 in the immune response of murine B lymphocytes to sheep erythrocytes. J Mol Cell Immunol 1987;3:29.

12. Kohase M, Henriksin-de Stefano D, May LT, et al. Induction of B-2-interferon by TNF: a homeostatic mechanism in the control of cell proliferation. Cell 1986;45:659.

13. Isaacs A, Lindemann J. Virus interference. I. The interferon. Proc Natl Acad Sci 1957;147:258.

14. Friedman RM. Interferons. In: Oppenheim JJ, Shevach EM, eds. Textbook of immunophysiology. New York, Oxford Press, 1988.

15. Chen B, Najor F. Macrophage activation by interferon alpha and beta is associated with a loss of proliferative capacity. Cell Immunol 1987;106:343.

16. Rhodes J, Ivanyi J, Cozens P. Antigen presentation by human monocytes: effects of modifying MHC class II antigen expression and IL-1 production by using recombinant interferons and corticosteroids. Eur J Immunol 1986;16:370.

17. Vogel SN, Finfloom DS, English KE, et al. Interferon induced enhancement of macrophage Fc receptor expression: B-interferon treatment of C3H/HeJ macrophages results in increased numbers and density of Fc receptors. J Immunol 1982;130:1210.

18. Ortaldo JR, Herberman RB. Augmentation of natural killer activity in immunobiology of natural killer cells, vol 2. Boca Raton, FL, CRC Press, 1986:145.

19. Pfau CJ, Gresser I, Hunt KP. Lethal role of interferon in lymphocytic choriomeningitis virus induced encephalitis. J Genet Virol 1983;64:1827.

20. Frank MM, Fries L. Complement. In: Paul WE, ed. Fundamental immunology. New York, Raven Press, 1989:679.

21. Law SKA, Reid KBM. Complement. Oxford, UK, IRL Press, 1988.

22. Duran SK, Schmidt JA, Oppenheim JJ. Interleukin 1: an immunologic perspective. Annu Rev Immunol 1986;3:263.

23. Mannel DN, Mizel SB, Diamanstein T, et al. Induction of IL-2 responsiveness in thymocytes by synergistic action of interleukin 1 and interleukin 2. J Immunol 1985;134:3108.

24. Smith KA. T cell growth factor. Immunol Rev 1980;51:337.

25. Kuribayashi K, Gillis S, Kern DE, et al. Murine NK cell cultures: effects of interleukin 2 and interferon on cell growth and cytotoxic reactivity. J Immunol 1981;126:2321.

26. Aggarwall BB, Moffat B, Harkins RN. Human lymphotoxin: production by a lymphoblastoid cell line, purification, and initial characterization. J Biol Chem 1984;259:686.

27. Lopez AF, To LB, Jany J, et al. Stimulation of proliferation, differentiation, and function of human cells by primate interleukin 3. Proc Natl Acad Sci USA 1987;84:2761.

28. Howard M, Farrar J, Hilfiker M, et al. Identification of a T cell derived B cell growth factor distinct from interleukin 2. J Exp Med 1982;155:914.

29. Coffman R, Carty J. A T cell activity that enhances polyclonal IgE production and its inhibition by interferon gamma. J Immunol 1986;136:949.

30. Smith CA, Rennick DM. Characterization of a murine lymphokine distinct from interleukin 2 and interleukin 3 possessing a T cell growth factor activity and a mast cell growth factor activity that synergizes with interleukin 3. Proc Natl Acad Sci USA 1986;83:1857.

31. Kohler PF, Farr RS. Elevation of cord over maternal IgG immunoglobulin: evidence for an active placental IgG transport. Nature 1966;210:1070.

32. Dossett JH, Williams RC Jr, Quie PG. Studies on interaction of bacteria serum factors and polymorphonuclear leukocytes in mothers and newborns. Pediatrics 1969;44:49.

33. Cates KL, Rowe JC, Ballow M. The premature infant as a compromised host. In: Current problems in pediatrics. Chicago, Year Book Medical Publishers, 1983:1.

34. Allansmith M, McClennan BH, Butterworth M, et al. The development of immunoglobulin levels in man. J Pediatr 1968;72:276.

35. McRitchie DI, Girotti MJ, Rotstein OD, et al. Impaired antibody production in blunt trauma: possible role for T cell dysfunction. Arch Surg 1990;125:91.

36. Ertel W, Faist E, Nestle C, et al. Kinetics of IL-2 and IL-6 synthesis following major mechanical trauma. J Surg Res 1990;48:622.

37. Schlesinger L, Stekel A. Impaired cellular immunity in marasmic infants. Am J Clin Nutr 1974;27:615.

38. Cunningham-Rundles S. Nutritional factors in immune response. In: White PL, Selvey N, eds. Malnutrition: determinants and consequences. New York, Alan R Liss, 1984:233.

39. McCool RE, Catalona WJ. Current management of iatrogenic splenic injuries in children. J Urol 1981;125:549.

40. Mensenk EJ, Thompson A, Schot JD, et al. Genetic heterogeneity in X-linked agammaglobulinemia complicates carrier detection and prenatal diagnosis. Clin Genet 1987;31:91.

41. McFarlin DE, Strober W, Wochner RD, et al. Immunoglobulin A production in ataxia telangiectasia. Science 1965;150:1175.

42. Harrington H. Absence of the thymus gland. Lond Med Gaz 1829;3:314.

43. August CS, Levay RH, Berkel AI, et al. Establishment of immunological competence in a child with congenital thymic aplasia by a graft of fetal thymus. Lancet 1970;1:1980.

44. Goldsobel AB, Haas A, Stiehm ER. Bone marrow transplantation in DiGeorge syndrome. J Pediatr 1987;111:40.

45. Giblett ER, Anderson JE, Cohen F, et al. Adenosine deaminase deficiency in two patients with severely impaired cellular immunity. Lancet 1972;2:1067.

46. Levy RH, Klemperer MR, Gelfand EW, et al. Bone marrow transplantation in severe combined immunodeficiency. Lancet 1971;2:571.

47. Good RA. Bone marrow transplantation symposium: bone marrow transplantation for immunodeficiency diseases. Am J Med Sci 1987;294:68.

48. Chaisson RE, Bartlett JG. What the surgeon needs to know about AIDS. In: Cameron JL, ed. Current surgical therapy. St Louis, CV Mosby, 1995:955.

49. Cooper A. Human immunodeficiency virus and acquired immunodeficiency syndrome: recent developments and their implications for pediatric surgeons. Semin Pediatr Surg 1995;4:252.

50. Connor EM, Sperling RS, Gelker R, et al. Reduction of maternal infant transmission of human immunodeficiency virus type 1 with zidovudine treatment. N Engl J Med 1994;331:1173.

51. Burke JF. The effective period of preventive antibiotic action in experimental incisions and dermal lesions. Surgery 1961;50:161.

52. Polk HC, Lopez-Majoy JF. Post-operative wound infection: a prospective study of determinant factors and prevention. Surgery 1969;66:97.

53. Tomasz A. From penicillin binding proteins to the lysis and death of bacteria: a 1979 view. Rev Infect Dis 1979;1:434.

54. Gubert DN, Sanford JP. Methicillin: critical appraisal after a decade of experience. Med Clin North Am 1970;54:1113.

55. Meylan PR, Calandra T, Casey PA, et al. Clinical experience with Timentin in severe hospital infections. J Antimicrob Chemother 1986;17(Suppl C):127.

56. Moellering RC Jr, Weinbert AN. Studies on antibiotics synergism against enterococci. II. Effect of various antibiotics on the uptake of 14-carbon labeled streptomycin by enterococci. J Clin Invest 1971;50:2580.

57. Plotkin SA, Starr SE. Symposium on perinatal infections. Clin Perinatol 1981;8:617.

58. Hemming VQ, Overall JC, Britt MR. Nosocomial infections in a newborn intensive care unit: results of forty-one months of surveillance. N Engl J Med 1976;294:1310.

Surgery of Infants and Children: Scientific Principles and Practice, edited by
Keith T. Oldham, Paul M. Colombani, and Robert P. Foglia.
Lippincott–Raven Publishers, Philadelphia, © 1997.

CHAPTER 11

Inflammation

Karen S. Guice and Keith T. Oldham

Darwinian selection has given all animals endogenous defenses that prevent their consumption by microbes. Host defense can be likened to a military engagement; foreign microbes invade while the immune system defends with an arsenal of lymphocytes, neutrophils, macrophages, antibodies, complement proteins, oxidants, cytokines, and other weapons. Acute inflammation includes the collateral tissue injury resulting from this conflict. Using this analogy, the battlefields are the host tissues; therefore, triumph of the immune system is ultimately a prerequisite for survival of the species. It is not surprising that a complex and highly efficient immune system has evolved.

In conjunction with anatomic barriers, the immune system normally maintains a constant level of activity to prevent entry of organisms from the external environment. In addition, it routinely aids in the removal of tumor cells, senescent cells, and devitalized host tissues. Clinical evidence of inflammation results when injury or infection exceeds this norm. Foreign antigen is recognized as nonself by the immune system through specific T-cell receptors and immunoglobulins. Nonspecific recognition of foreign antigen also occurs and may be mediated directly by phagocytic cells or by alternative pathway activation of the complement system. These are all highly conserved and tightly regulated processes, because inflammation would destroy the host if allowed to proceed without control. The distinction between an efficient defense and pathologic injury of host tissues can be extremely narrow. Exuberant or misdirected inflammatory responses have important roles in many contemporary pediatric surgical disease processes.

The potential for endogenous inflammatory injury was recognized during the First World War when it was observed that serum sickness resulted from antigen-antibody–mediated tissue injury in the host. Subsequently, the fundamental importance of acute inflammation and its role in diverse diseases such as atherosclerosis, arthritis, adult respiratory distress syndrome, multiorgan failure syndrome, bronchopulmonary dysplasia, trauma, thermal injury, acute pancreatitis, ischemia-reperfusion injury, sepsis, transplant rejection, and wound healing were demonstrated. As antibiotics and immunizations have reduced human dependence on host defenses against microbes, other stimuli that generate a systemic inflammatory response have become increasingly important. For example,

adult respiratory distress syndrome was recognized in the late 1960s during the treatment of victims of modern warfare who would have died in previous eras. It is recognized now that this is a syndrome of acute respiratory failure resulting from a systemic inflammatory response to trauma, but not necessarily infection. The inflammatory response generates leukocyte-mediated injury to the pulmonary microvasculature, resulting in interstitial edema, alveolar flooding, impaired gas exchange, and respiratory failure. The mortality rate remains 50% or more in most reports and is essentially unchanged since its original description. Specific therapy has not been forthcoming despite a substantial mechanistic understanding of the processes involved.

This chapter is designed to provide an overview of the immune system, with particular attention to nonspecific immunity, acute inflammation, and tissue injury. Other relevant aspects of the immune system, including transplantation, tumor immunology, specific infections, and autoimmune disease, are detailed elsewhere in the text. In particular, many of the basic aspects of the specific immune response and immunodeficiencies are reviewed in Chapter 12.

INDIVIDUAL COMPONENTS OF THE IMMUNE SYSTEM

Redness (rubor), edema (tumor), heat (calor), and pain (dolor) were recognized as cardinal manifestations of inflammation more than 2000 years ago. It is recognized now that vasodilation with enhanced local blood flow is the cause of redness and heat; increased microvascular permeability leads to edema. Extravasation of plasma proteins and leukocyte recruitment to the injury site generate pain.

In the early 20th century, Ehrlich and Metchnikoff were awarded Nobel prizes for recognizing the two basic components of this immune response, humoral (antibody-mediated) and cellular elements. For years thereafter, incremental progress was made toward understanding these relations. In the last decade, modern molecular and cell biology techniques have yielded an enormous amount of data detailing the specific components and regulatory mechanisms. The current task is to translate this

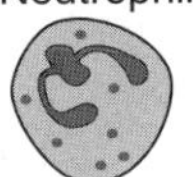
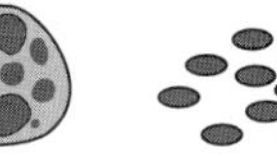
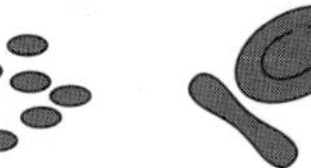
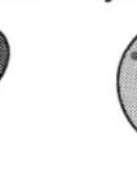
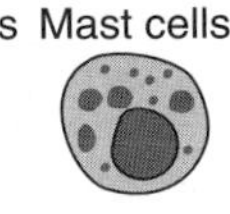

FIG. 11-1. The several components of the lymphorecticular system are illustrated. The bone marrow, an essential but dispersed element, is not shown in this diagram. SALT, skin-associated lymphoid tissue; GALT, gut-associated lymphoid tissue; BALT, bronchus-associated lymphoid tissue. (See also Figures 11-11 through 11-13.)

information into an understanding of relevant human disease and to develop applicable therapies.

The immune system has several fundamental characteristics. These include the ability to differentiate self and nonself antigens using antibodies (immunoglobulins) and T-cell receptors, a high degree of specificity in discriminating among antigens, and the ability to discriminate among many antigens. The immune response is derived from the lymphoreticular system, which has both circulating and fixed elements (Fig. 11-1). Fixed elements are localized in specialized organs with the primary function of supply and support (ie, the bone marrow, spleen, liver, lymph nodes, and thymus), and in specialized cells that contribute to the response within organs (ie, the skin, gastrointestinal, respiratory, and urogenital tracts). In the circulation, both formed elements (cells and platelets) and soluble (humoral) factors participate. Cellular participants include lymphocytes, granulocytes, monocytes, macrophages, erythrocytes, and mast cells. Platelets usually are considered here also. Humoral factors include complement, cytokines, kinins, eicosanoids, and various other soluble molecules. These and other molecular species participate through autocrine, paracrine, and humoral mechanisms.

Circulating cellular elements (Fig. 11-2) are derived from common progenitor cells that originate in the embryonic yolk sac. During the 6th week of human gestation, the fetal liver is populated with yolk sac–derived stem cells and becomes a site for hematopoietic activity. By the 12th week of gestation, the spleen begins to produce blood cells, and at 20 weeks of gestation, the thymus, lymph nodes, and bone marrow are all active sites of hematopoiesis. It is at this time that the two major lymphocyte subsets, T cells and B cells, first become differentiated. At term, only the bone marrow normally remains as a source for the production of new blood cells.

Cellular Elements

T Lymphocytes

Bone marrow–derived precursors become differentiated into T lymphocytes in the thymus. In this peripheral site, the T cell acquires a specific receptor for antigen binding and also the associated proteins that constitute the entire T-cell receptor complex (CD3). Additional subsets of membrane receptors (clusters of differentiation or CD antigens) also are acquired by T cells in the thymus. Most notable are the CD8 cytotoxic/suppressor antigens and the CD4 helper/inducer antigens, which functionally differentiate T-cell subsets. After maturation, T cells enter into the circulation.[1] The process is illustrated schematically in Figure 11-3, and additional details are provided in Chapter 12.

B Lymphocytes

B lymphocytes are categorized on the basis of membrane-bound antigen-specific immunoglobulins. Mature B lymphocytes differentiate into plasma cells programmed to synthesize and release into the circulation the specific immunoglobulin present on the cell surface. Memory and the ability to manufacture highly specific antibodies in large quantities are unique features of these cells. As a population, B cells possess a large repertoire of immunoglobulin responses, although each B cell is specific in its product. Their extraordinary potential for clonal expansion is a fundamental aspect of the immune response and acquired immunity.[1] These issues are summarized schematically in Figure 11-3 and detailed in Chapter 12.

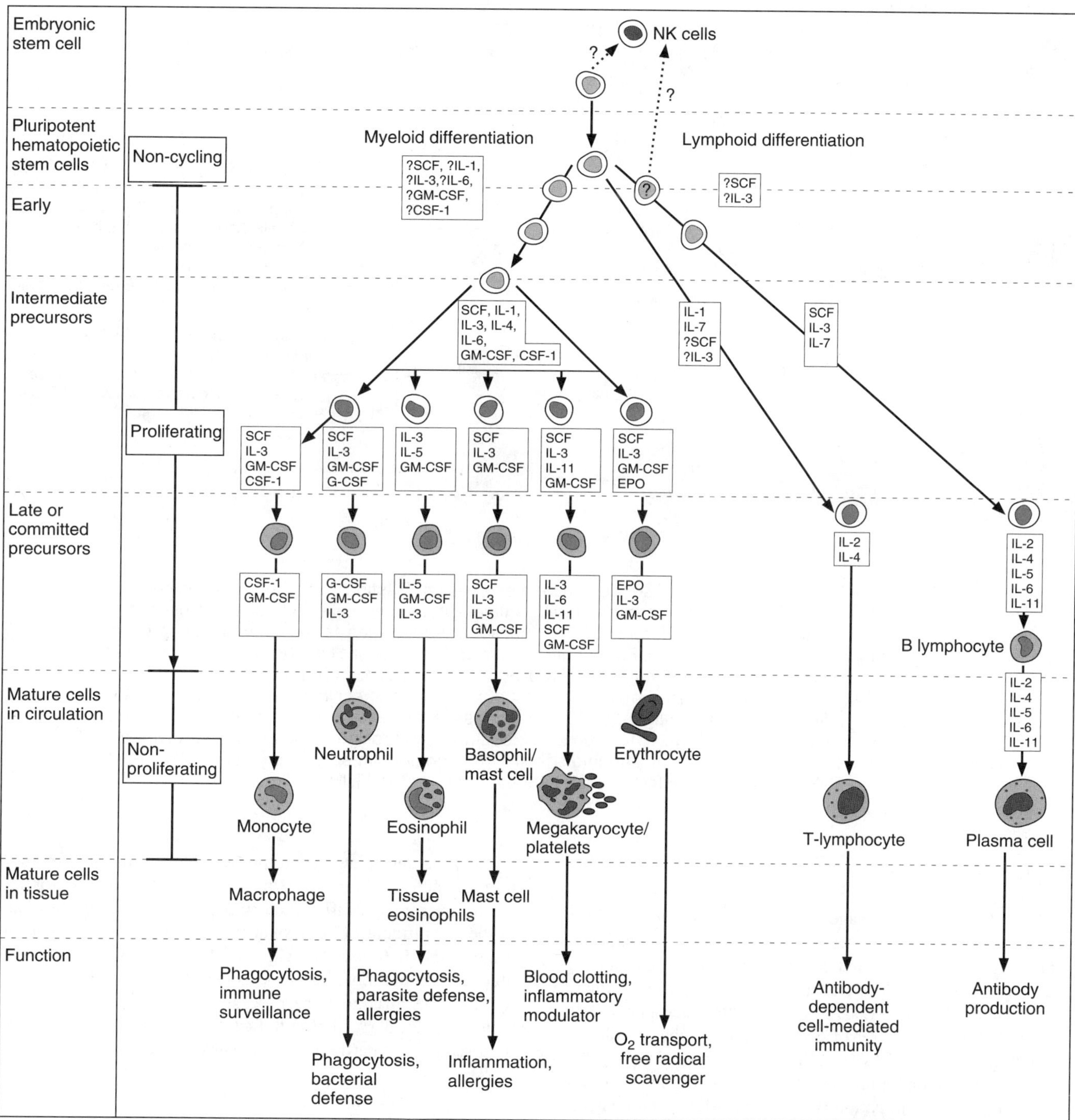

FIG. 11-2. Hematopoietic cells are derived from embryonic stem cells, which differentiate into pluripotential lymphoid and myeloid precursors within the bone marrow. The lymphoid lineage yields B lymphocytes, which undergo further differentiation into plasma cells. This occurs within peripheral lymphoid tissues. Likewise, T lymphocytes undergo differentiation into subclasses, a process in which the thymus plays an important role. Natural killer (NK) cell differentiation also occurs from this lineage, but the process is poorly understood. Granulocytes, mast cells, erythrocytes, and megakaryocytes are derived from this stem cell population. Circulating monocytes become macrophages when they exit the circulation and enter the tissues. SCF, stem cell factor; GM-CSF, granulocyte-macrophage colony-stimulating factor; CSF-1, colony-stimulating factor-1; G-CSF, granulocyte colony-stimulating factor; EPO, erythropoietin; IL, interleukin.

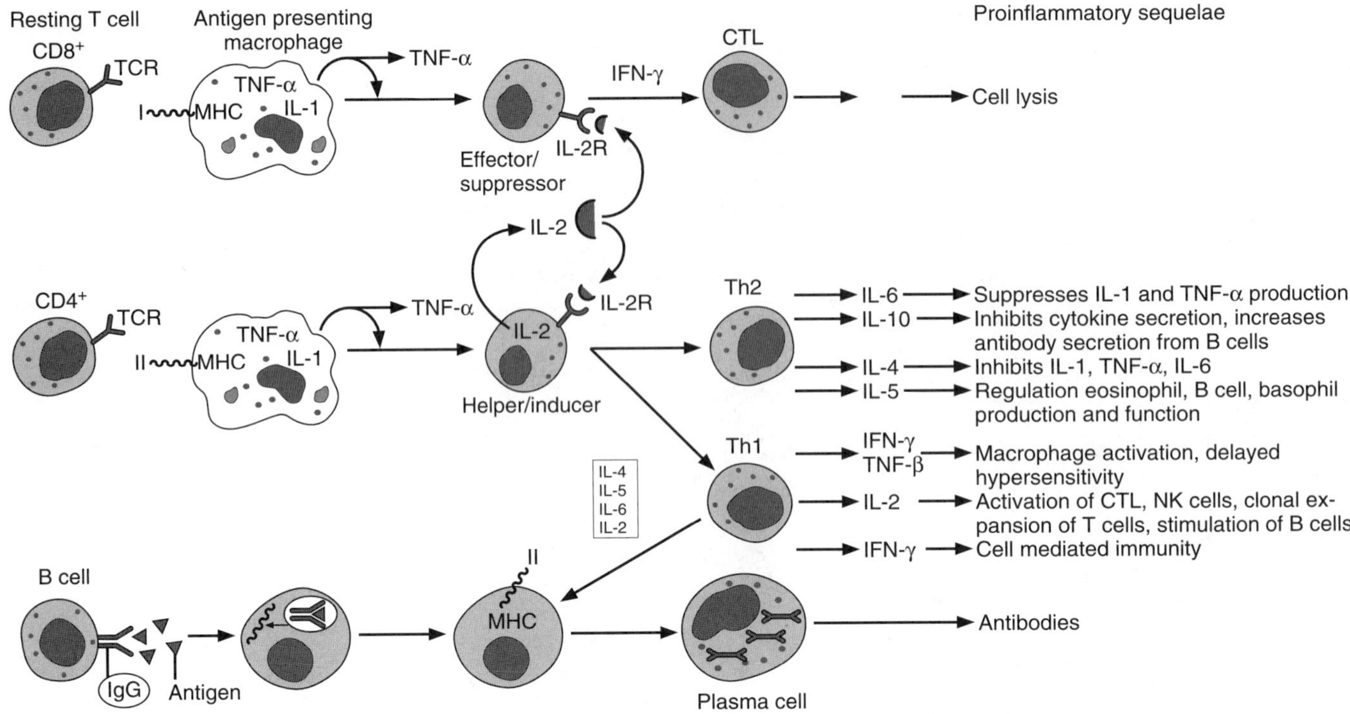

FIG. 11-3. T cells are classified by cell surface antigen expression. Resting T cells are grouped conventionally into CD4+ or CD8+ cells. On contact with antigen-presenting cells (and in the presence of interleukin-2 [IL-2], these T cells differentiate into functional subclasses termed effector/suppressor (CD8+) or helper/inducer (CD4+) cells. Further differentiation into cytotoxic lymphocytes (CTLs) occurs in the case of CD8+ cells or into T helper 1 (Th1) or T helper 2 (Th2) cells in the case of CD4+ cells. B lymphocytes are characterized by membrane-bound antigen-specific immunoglobulins. IgG is illustrated here. After binding with antigen, the B cell processes the antigen into a complex with class II major histocompatibility complex (MHC) molecules. Modulated by cytokines produced by TH1 lymphocytes, activated B lymphocytes differentiate into specific immunoglobulin-secreting plasma cells. TCR, T-cell receptor; TNF, tumor necrosis factor; IFN, interferon; NK, natural killer.

Monocytes/Macrophages

Monocytes and macrophages are essential effector cells for host defense and wound healing. Monocytes are produced within the bone marrow and enter the peripheral circulation under the regulation of several growth factors and cytokines, notably interleukin (IL)-1, IL-3, granulocyte-macrophage colony-stimulating factor (GM-CSF), and macrophage colony-stimulating factor (M-CSF).[2,3] They are characterized by the presence of immunoglobulin receptors and by both class I and class II major histocompatibility complex (MHC) antigens on the cell surface. Their cytoplasm contains lysosomal granules that aid in the digestion of engulfed bacteria. Monocytes adhere to and traverse the microvascular endothelium to reach specific peripheral tissues. This tissue homing may be part of the terminal differentiation process whereby circulating monocytes become antigen-presenting cells and tissue macrophages capable of phagocytosis. Organ-specific differentiated macrophages include the Kupffer cells within the liver, microglial cells in the central nervous system, and Langerhans cells in the skin.

In response to foreign protein such as bacteria and viruses, the monocyte/macrophage secretes IL-1, tumor necrosis factor-α (TNF-α), IL-6, and IL-12.[4–6] These cytokines activate a variety of cells and induce acute-phase protein synthesis. In addition, the activated monocyte/macrophage secretes chemokines (IL-8, macrophage inflammatory peptides 1 and 2). These aid in the recruitment of additional inflammatory cells. Finally, it secretes IL-10, transforming growth factor-β (TGF-β), and soluble IL-1 receptor, which serve as feedback inhibitors to downregulate the inflammatory process. The macrophage also secretes platelet-derived growth factor, which, with TGF-β, is an important early participant in the wound repair process (Fig. 11-4).

Neutrophils

Neutrophils are derived from pluripotential stem cells, and more than 90% of the mature population resides within the bone marrow. Their maturation and proliferation are under the control of several cytokines and growth factors,[7,8] and this is detailed in Chapter 12 and in Figure 11-2. Their release from the bone marrow into the circulation is a complex and incompletely understood process.

Neutrophils are the primary cells responsible for phagocytosis in acute inflammation. As such, they are of fundamental

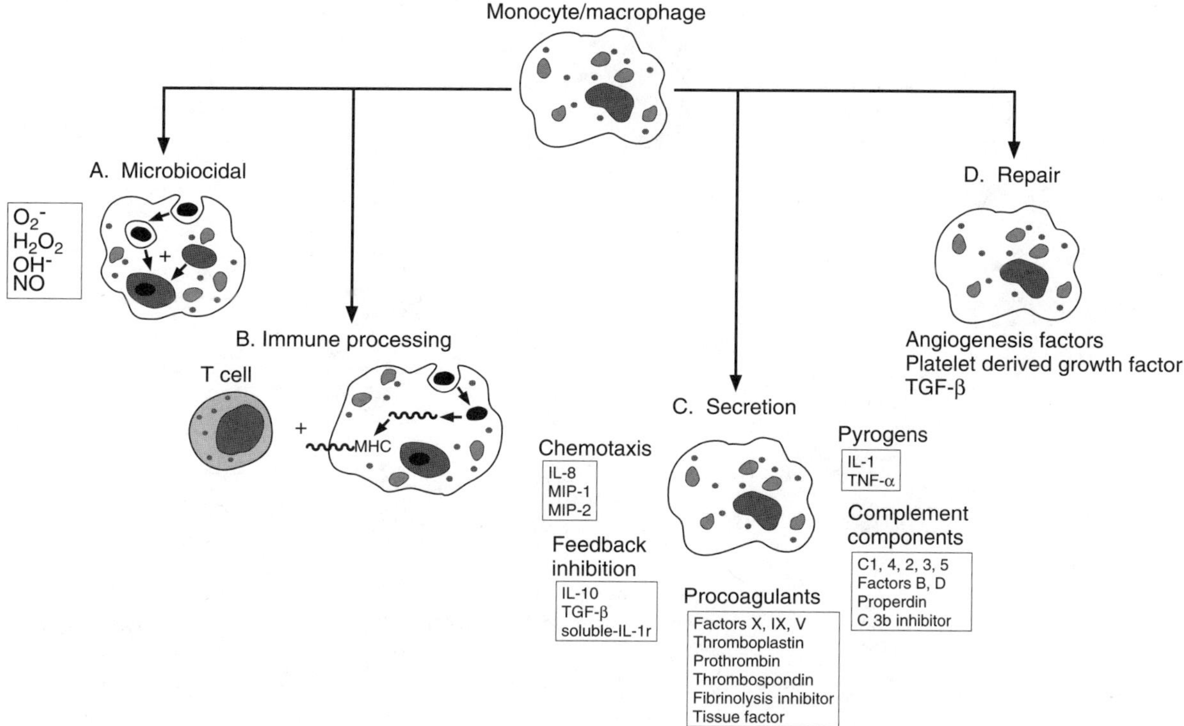

FIG. 11-4. Monocytes are migratory phagocytes that become macrophages after they leave the circulation and enter into tissues. Macrophages have several major functions: (*A*) They ingest and kill pathogens using a variety of microbicidal compounds. (*B*) They serve as antigen-presenting cells. (*C*) They secrete a wide variety of cytokines, complement components, and chemotactic substances. (*D*) They play a central role in wound repair and chronic inflammation. MHC, major histocompatibility complex; IL, interleukin; MIP, macrophage inflammatory peptide; TGF, transforming growth factor; TNF, tumor necrosis factor.

importance in inflammatory tissue injury. They are equipped with a variety of surface ligands and receptors that are conduits for the regulatory signals that govern activation, chemotaxis, endothelial adherence, phagocytosis, and cell killing (Fig. 11-5 and Table 11-1).[7–16] Complement, immunoglobulins, endotoxin, growth factors, chemoattractants, and adhesion molecules are among the mediators of neutrophil function.

Neutrophils contain a variety of secretory products that react with pathogens and host tissues; proteinases and cationic proteins are among the most important of these. These products are stored in specific cytoplasmic granules that do not take up hematoxylin or eosin stains, hence the neutrophil designation. When the neutrophil is activated, the granules fuse with phagolysosomes or become exported to the cell surface. Dependent on this, granule contents are targeted to intracellular or extracellular locations and destruction of the pathogen follows (see Fig. 11-5*A*). Table 11-2 provides a partial inventory of neutrophil granule contents.[17–19]

In addition, a key functional aspect of neutrophil activation is the generation of reactive oxygen products at the cell membrane (see Fig. 11-5*B*). These products include the superoxide anion (O_2^-), hydrogen peroxide (H_2O_2), hypochlorite (HOCl), and the hydroxyl radical (OH·). All are nascent, highly reactive free radicals. In addition, neutrophils produce chloramines, oxidants with relatively long biologic half-lives. Oxidants account for many relevant biochemical interactions[20] (see Fig. 11-5*C*). Among these are protein oxidation, DNA strand breakage, and

membrane lipid peroxidation, all of which contribute to the death of an invading pathogen or a targeted host cell. Oxidant injury by free radicals is a major mechanism for neutrophil-mediated cell killing. Significant synergy has been demonstrated for neutrophil-derived oxidants and proteinases.[19] Oxidant- and proteinase-mediated killing expose host cells to potential injury.[21,22] Their regulation in general is precise, and a variety of endogenous antiproteinases and antioxidants have evolved. These are highly conserved phylogenetically. Among the most important of these regulatory enzymes are α_1-antiproteinase, α_2-macroglobulin, superoxide dismutase, and catalase.

Basophils/Eosinophils

Basophils and eosinophils are granulocytes derived from a common hematopoietic stem cell. IL-3 is the principal cytokine responsible for basophil growth and differentiation. Although early workers believed that basophils were circulating mast cells because of their histamine content, recent evidence suggests that basophils and eosinophils are functionally similar.

Basophils constitute less than 1% of the circulating leukocyte population. They usually remain in the circulation; however, they may be found in the skin or airway after local antigen stimulation. Patients with active allergies or asthma have increased numbers of circulating basophils. Basophils have cell surface receptors for IgE; IgG; complement (C3aR, C5aR, CR1,

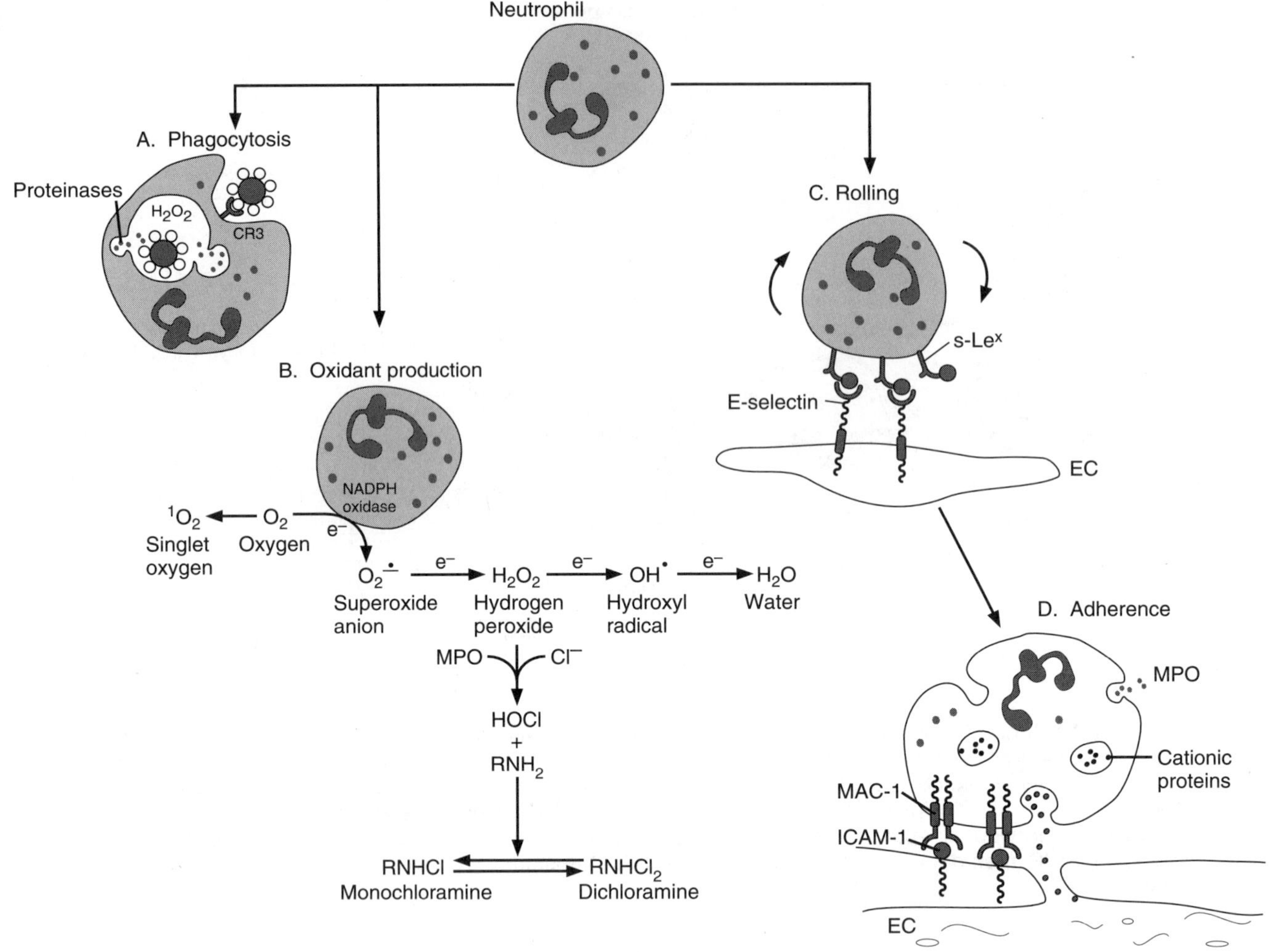

FIG. 11-5. The neutrophil is a primary effector cell in the acute inflammatory process. Like the monocyte, it is a mobile phagocytic cell. Its primary function is to isolate, ingest, and kill pathogens (phagocytosis; *A*). To accomplish their mission, polymorphonuclear neutrophils secrete a wide variety of proteinases and other proinflammatory peptides. (*B*) In addition, cytotoxic oxidants are generated by a membrane-bound NADPH oxidase system. (*C* and *D*) Neutrophils function through directed adherence to vascular endothelium that creates a microenvironment protected from circulating antiproteinases and antioxidants (see text). MPO, myeloperoxidase; EC, endothelial cell; ICAM, intercellular adhesion molecule, MAC, membrane attack complex.

CR3 p150,95); cytokines (IL-2, IL-8, monocyte chemoattractant protein, IL-3, IL-4, IL-5, GM-CSF, interferon (IFN)-γ, TNF-α); platelet-activating factor (PAF); and histamine.[23] Histamine and proteoglycans reside within basophils as preformed mediators that are promptly released on cell stimulation. In addition, basophils have an important capacity to synthesize and release leukotriene C_4.

Eosinophil differentiation within the bone marrow is regulated principally by GM-CSF, IL-3, and IL-5. Once released from the bone marrow, eosinophils circulate briefly (13 to 18 hours) before transvascular migration into peripheral tissues. Eosinophils usually are found in tissues exposed to the external environment, such as the skin, respiratory, gastrointestinal, and genitourinary tracts. Eosinophils have many receptors on their cell surfaces, including those for IgG (Fc), C1q, C3b/C4b (CR1), C3bi (CR3), C5a, IgE, IL-3, IL-5, and GM-CSF. In addition, MHC class II proteins and CD4 are expressed on the eosinophil cell surface. The presence of the CD4⁺ receptor suggests that eosinophils can respond to lymphocyte chemoattractants and also act to present antigen to T cells. Similar to other granulocytes, eosinophils possess a variety of proinflammatory proteins within cytoplasmic granules. Granule constituents include lysophospholipase, collagenase, and peroxidase. Eosinophils also produce a wide range of cytokines, including GM-CSF, IL-1, IL-3, IL-5, IL-6, and IL-8. In addition, eosinophils produce PAF, leukotriene C_4, and leukotriene D_4, all potent mediators of inflammation. Eosinophil activation may be induced by GM-CSF, IL-3, IL-5, TNF-α, IFN-γ, IFN-α, and PAF.[24,25]

Mast Cells

Mast cells are derived from CD34⁺ pluripotent progenitor cells within the bone marrow, and their growth and maturation

TABLE 11-1. *Some of the important polymorphonuclear neutrophil receptors and ligands*

Receptor	Ligand	Function
COMPLEMENT		
Complement receptor-1 (CR1)	C3	↑ Immune complex binding
Complement receptor-3 (CR3)	C3bi	↑ Phagocytosis, adherence
Complement C5a receptor (C5aR)	C5a	↑ Adherence, chemotaxis, degranulation, oxygen radical release
IMMUNOGLOBULINS		
FcγRII, FcγRIIIB	IgG	↑ Phagocytosis, migration, degranulation
FcαR	IgA	? Migration, synergy with CSFs
Mac-2/ϵ-binding protein (S-lectin)	IgE	↑ Respiratory burst
BACTERIAL PEPTIDES AND ENDOTOXIN		
Formyl Peptide Receptor (FPR)	F-met-leu-phe (FMLP)	↑ Chemotaxis, and respiratory burst
CD14	Lipopolysaccharide (LPS, endotoxin)	
COLONY-STIMULATING FACTORS (CSF)		
Granulocyte colony-stimulating factor receptor (G-CSFR)	G-CSF	PMN priming, ↑ phagocytosis
Granulocyte-macrophage colony-stimulating factor receptor (GM-CSFR)	GM-CSF	↑ Phagocytosis, ↑ superoxide production, ↑ margination, ↑ adhesion
CHEMOATTRACTANTS		
Neutrophil-activating peptide receptor (NAP-1/IL-8 R)	NAP-1/IL-8, NAP-2, gro/MGSA	↑ Chemotaxis
Leukotriene B$_4$ receptor (LTB$_4$R)	LTB$_4$	
Platelet-Activating Factor Receptor (PAFR)	PAF	Chemotaxis, PMN activation
ADHESION MOLECULES		
β_2-Integrins		
CD11a/CD18	ICAM-1, -2, -3	↑ Adherence to endothelium
CD11b/CD18	ICAM-1	↑ Adherence to endothelium
CD11c/CD18	ICAM-1	↑ PMN-endothelium binding
L-selectin	Heparin-like ligand on endothelial cells	↑ Leukocyte rolling
OTHERS		
Tumor necrosis factor-α receptor (TNF-αR)	TNF-α	Potentiates activation by other factors
Atrial natriuretic peptide receptor (ANP R)	ANP	
A$_2$R	Adenosine	

IL-8, interleukin-8; PMN, polymorphonuclear neutrophil.

are regulated by several soluble factors. Mast cells usually are considered as two distinct populations dependent on location: connective tissue mast cells are found in the skin and peritoneal cavity, and mucosal mast cells reside within the lamina propria of hollow viscera. Both reach functional maturity in the peripheral tissues, but they differ in the types of surface proteoglycans present and the types of proteinases found in their cytoplasmic granules. When activated, mast cells release preformed mediators from intracellular granules and also synthesize eicosanoids (notably prostaglandin D$_2$, leukotriene B$_4$, and leukotriene C$_4$) and PAF. These responses contribute to increases in microvascular permeability, peripheral vasodilation, platelet aggregation, and leukocyte adherence. Pulmonary vasoconstriction, bronchoconstriction, and alveolar edema formation are important effects of mast cell degranulation in the lung. Mast cell products include histamine, proteoglycans, serine proteinases, and carboxypeptidase A. A wide range of cytokines, including TNF-α, IL-1, IL-2, IL-3, IL-4, IL-5, IL-6, GM-CSF, IFN-γ, and macrophage inflammatory proteins 1α and 1β, also are

elaborated by mast cells. Tissue mast cells release serotonin when activated, and this promotes the infiltration of other leukocytes.[26]

Unlike neutrophils, mast cells are capable of new protein synthesis and persist in the local microenvironment after degranulation. It is probable that they contribute to chronic inflammation in this way. In addition, mast cells synthesize collagen, laminin, and heparan sulfate proteoglycans, all of which are essential structural components of basement membrane. These observations suggest that mast cells have an important role in wound healing and tissue repair. The initial signal for fibroblast migration into a wound may be mast cell collagen synthesis and secretion.

Platelets

Platelets are anucleated, membrane-bound circulating elements with an essential role in hemostasis and coagulation, and

TABLE 11-2. *Partial inventory of neutrophil granule constituents**

Constituent	Function
AZUROPHIL GRANULES	
Lysozyme	Targets bacterial cell wall peptidoglycan
Myeloperoxidase	Catalyzes conversion of hydrogen peroxide and hydrogen chloride to hypochlorous acid, molecular chlorine, and chloramines
Bacterial permeability–increasing protein/CAP57	Targets gram-negative bacteria
Defensins (human neutrophil proteins [HNP] 1–4)	Target gram-positive and gram-negative bacteria and some fungi and viruses, weak monocyte chemoattractants
Azurocidin/CAP37	Interferes with bacterial membranes, monocyte chemoattractant
Acid phosphatase	Hydrolysis of phosphate monoesters
β-Glucosaminidase	Acid hydrolase
α-Mannosidase	Acid hydrolase
α-Fucosidase	Cleaves oligosaccharides
Cathepsin G	Targets gram-negative bacteria
Cathepsin D	Acid hydrolase
Elastase	Serine protease
Phospholipase A	Cleaves membrane phospholipids
Deoxyribonuclease	Hydrolysis of polymerized DNA
5′-Nucleotidase	Hydrolysis of nucleotides
Collagenase	Degrades collagen
β-Glycerophosphatase	Acid hydrolase
β-Glucuronidase	Acid hydrolase
SPECIFIC GRANULES	
Lactoferrin	Binds free iron (required for bacterial viability)
Cytochrome B-558	Critical to respiratory burst
Procollagenase	Degrades collagen
Mac-1/C3bi receptor	Mediates binding to endothelial cells and matrix proteins; binds complement component C3bi
Formyl peptide receptor	Binds to portions of bacterial cell wall
B_{12} binding protein	Binds to vitamin B_{12}
Histaminase	Oxidative deamination of histamine

* Data from references 17 through 19.

in the inflammatory response. They are derived from bone marrow polynuclear megakaryocytes and have a half-life of 8 to 10 days in the circulation. Like granulocytes, platelets store a variety of proteins in granules, and these are used to regulate critical events such as leukocyte adherence, complement activation, microvascular tone and permeability, eicosanoid production, and chemotactic and growth factor production[27] (Table 11-3).

Erythrocytes

Although erythrocytes usually are not considered primary participants in the inflammatory response, they do provide an important source of antioxidant enzymes and quenching of nitric oxide (NO). These features may prove beneficial at sites of wounding by limiting oxidant- and NO-mediated injury.

Soluble Components of Inflammation

Immunoglobulins

Immunoglobulins are synthesized by cells of B-lymphocyte lineage in five forms: IgG, IgA, IgM, IgD, and IgE. Each is composed of two identical light and two identical heavy polypeptide chains. There are two isotypes for light chains, κ and λ, and five for heavy chains, α, δ, Σ, γ, and μ. Antibodies are described by their heavy chain because it is that portion that mediates antibody function. This structure is illustrated in Figure 11-6. Immunoglobulin structure and function is summarized briefly here, and the ontogeny is considered in Chapter 12.[28]

The amino-terminal Fab portion of the immunoglobulin molecule is a complex three-dimensional structure with hypervariable regions that form specific antigen-binding sites. Most antibody effector function is mediated through the constant Fc (carboxy terminus) region. The formation of antigen-antibody complexes results in complement activation or immunoglobulin binding to Fc receptors, which are found on monocytes, macrophages, neutrophils, and natural killer cells. When complement binds to the antigen-antibody complex, phagocytosis is enhanced in a process referred to as opsonization.

Membrane-bound IgM on the B cell frequently is the point of initial antigen contact. Antigen binding initiates clonal B-cell expansion, and more antibody is formed. Therefore, primary antibody responses typically induce IgM synthesis. Secondary antigen exposure usually results in a rapid IgG response, yielding antibodies of greater affinity and in greater quantity than the primary IgM response. Individual plasma cells produce a specific IgG antibody in response to antigen stimulation. IgG binding neutralizes carriers of antigen recognized as foreign.

TABLE 11-3. *Platelet granule contents and function*

Granule constituent	Function
Fibronectin	↑ Fibrin formation
Fibrinogen	↑ Platelet aggregation, fibrin precursor
Thrombospondin	↑ Platelet aggregation, ↑ monocyte adherence
von Willebrand factor	↑ Platelet adherence
Plasminogen	Precursor of plasmin
α_2-Plasmin inhibitor	Inhibits fibrinolysis
Platelet-derived growth factor	↑ Chemotaxis
Platelet factor 4	↑ Chemotaxis, histamine release, ↑ angiogenesis
Transforming growth factor α and β	↑ Chemotaxis
Basic fibroblast growth factor	↑ Chemotaxis for fibroblasts and endothelial cells, ↑ angiogenesis
GMP-140 (*P*latelet *a*ctivation *d*ependent, *g*ranule-external *m*embrane protein, PADGEM)	↑ Leukocyte adherence
LAMP-1 (*l*ysosomal-*a*ssociated *m*embrane *p*rotein)	↑ Cell-to-cell adhesion
Factors D and H	Complement regulation
Decay-accelerating factor	Complement regulation
Serotonin	Vasodilation or vasoconstriction depending on specific vascular receptors, ↑ collagen synthesis, ↑ fibroblast proliferation
Adenosine diphosphate	↑ Platelet activation and aggregation
Calcium	↑ Platelet activation and aggregation

It also enhances phagocytosis by opsonization, and activates complement by the classic pathway. About 85% of antibody in serum is of the IgG class.

IgA is found predominantly in saliva, tears, bile, and respiratory and enteric secretions. Although IgA can bind to foreign antigen, it lacks an Fc moiety and is incapable of activating complement. A primary function of secretory IgA appears to be binding at enteric and respiratory epithelial surfaces to prevent adherence of potentially pathogenic organisms. Whereas IgA synthesis is demonstrable in the small intestine and lung by the 26th week of gestation, most IgA synthesis occurs after birth.[29]

IgD and IgE have relatively low serum levels when compared with the other major circulating immunoglobulins. IgD is coexpressed with IgM on the surface of B lymphocytes and appears to aid in antigen recognition and subsequent lymphocyte activation. In humans, IgE normally is present in low concentrations. It is an important component of the acute allergic response. After antigen binding, the Fc portion of the IgE molecule binds to mast cells and basophils, triggering histamine and serine proteinase release, and prostaglandin and cytokine (TNF-α, IL-1, IL-3, and IL-4) synthesis. IgE has an important role in the host response to certain parasites.

Complement

Recognition of foreign antigen by antibody normally is the first step in the process of eliminating a pathogen. Although the repertoire of existing antibodies is extensive in a mature and immunocompetent individual, the naive or immature host requires a mechanism to recognize and remove newly presented novel antigen. The phylogenetically primitive complement system offers this essential function. This system is composed of about 25 plasma proteins, several membrane-bound glycoproteins, and their regulatory enzymes. It is presented in detail in Chapter 12 and in several published reviews.[30-32] It is summarized briefly

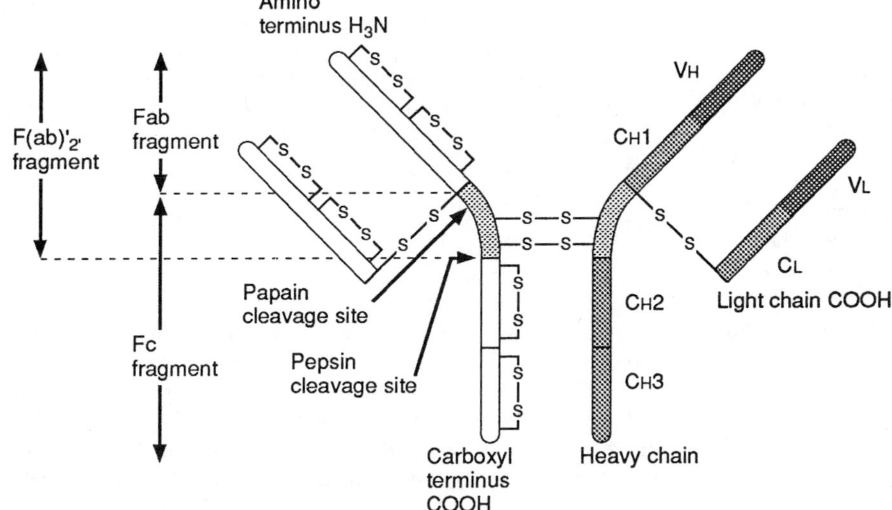

FIG. 11-6. The basic structure of the immunoglobulins consists of a constant (C) region (or Fc fragment) and a variable (N) region (or Fab fragment). Antigen binds to the Fab portion and antibody effector function is mediated by the Fc portion.

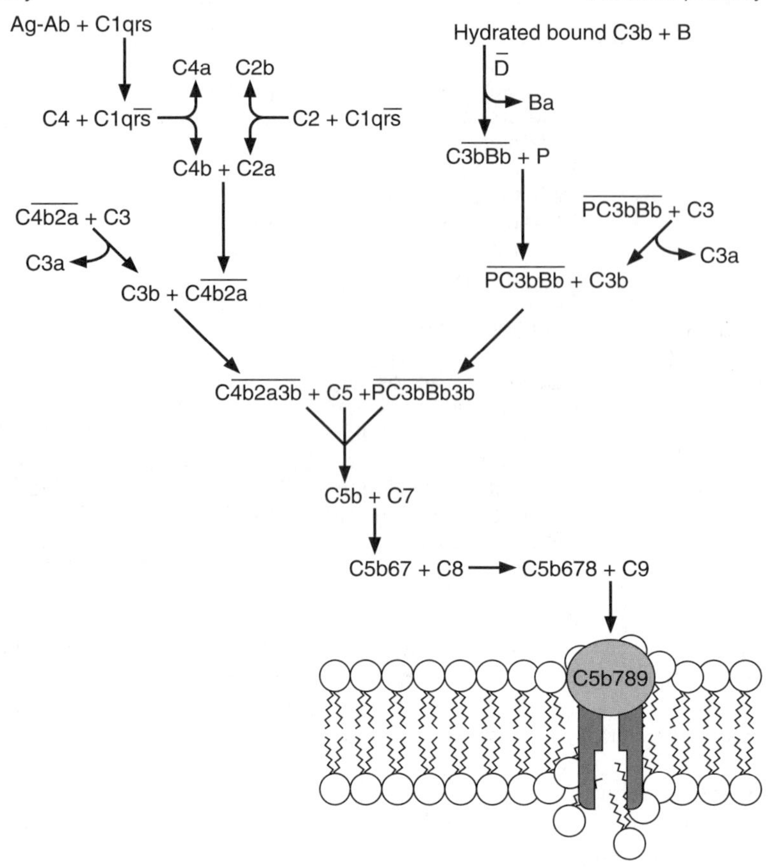

FIG. 11-7. Classic and alternate complement pathways. Ag-Ab, antigen-antibody.

in Figure 11-7 and is discussed here in the context of its physiologic role rather than its biochemistry. The protein products that result from complement activation interact to opsonize, or in some cases, directly kill pathogens. In addition, certain complement products modulate important aspects of the immune system, such as local blood flow and leukocyte trafficking. Complement activation is initiated by the classic pathway, through antigen-antibody complex formation, or by the alternative pathway after exposure to a variety of noxious stimuli, such as endotoxin, chemical toxins, or mechanical tissue injury. This latter pathway is of particular surgical interest because surgical injuries such as acute pancreatitis, burns, and other forms of trauma act by this conduit. Both pathways are illustrated in Figure 11-7.

Although it is apparent that the complement system lacks specificity, it is a critical contributor to host defense that is capable of both amplification of inflammation and tissue injury (Fig. 11-8). It is intuitive that it must be regulated strictly to avoid injury to host tissues. Under normal circumstances, this is done with a variety of plasma inhibitors and feedback mechanisms by C1 inhibitor, CR1, CR2, C4-binding protein, decay-accelerating factor, and membrane cofactor protein. When these controls fail or activation is excessive, host injury results in important clinical problems, such as posttraumatic acute lung injury, the multiorgan failure syndrome, and transplant rejection.

Cytokines

Cytokines are a group of polypeptides and glycoproteins ranging in molecular weight from 8 to 30 kD. Lymphokines, monokines, ILs, TNF, IFNs, colony-stimulating factors, and a variety of other growth factors are among these. The cytokines usually are short-lived, essential mediators of immunity and inflammation that are induced in response to cellular activation rather than synthesized constitutively. Typically, they function through autocrine or paracrine rather than hormonal mechanisms, although their plasma levels are measured and often reported. Correlation of plasma cytokine levels with tissue events may be difficult, and this represents a fundamental concern with much of the available clinical data. Cytokines function principally as intercellular signals using high-affinity cell surface receptors to regulate cell growth, differentiation, and phenotypic behavior. A complete review is beyond the scope of this text, but many contemporary discussions are available.[33–45] Some of the key functions related to acute inflammation are illustrated in Figure 11-9 and summarized in Table 11-4 and later in this text.

Tumor Necrosis Factor-α

Tumor necrosis factor-α is a proximal and central mediator of acute inflammation. Convincing data show that TNF-α is a moiety through which the effects of endotoxin are transmitted.[46–48] Injection of endotoxin or recombinant TNF-α produces host responses that are indistinguishable: fever, chills, nausea, headache, and, in higher doses, shock. Pretreatment with blocking antibody to TNF-α protects against this response when endotoxin is injected. More recent data suggest that TNF-

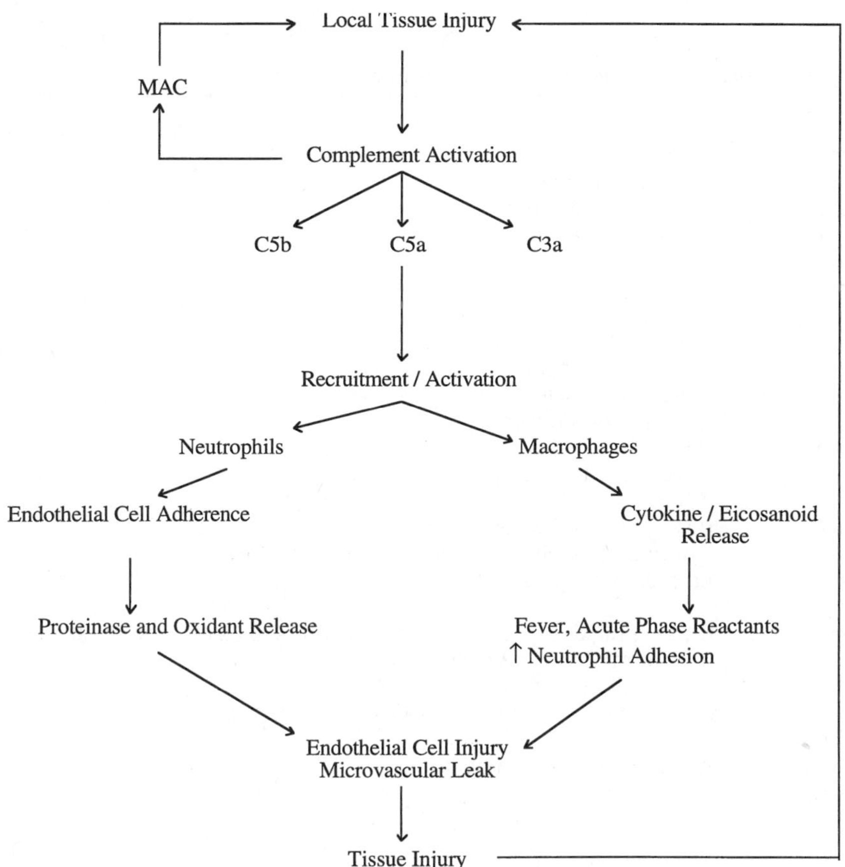

FIG. 11-8. Complement activation is a proximal and early event in the sequence of acute inflammation. Unregulated complement activation may lead to systemic or local injury of host tissues. (MAC, membrane attack complex)

α itself acts through a cytokine network of low-molecular-weight chemokines with a cysteine motif (C-X-C family).[49]

TNF-α is produced principally by monocytes, macrophages, and cells derived from this lineage, such as Kupffer cells. It is induced in large quantities by endotoxin, C5a, and IL-1. Endothelial cells, mast cells, and natural killer cells also produce TNF-α under certain conditions.

Receptors for TNF-α are found on most cell types. Type I receptors are expressed on cells of epithelial origin, whereas type II receptors appear on cells of myeloid origin. Some cell lines express both TNF receptors.[50] Site-specific responses are initiated by ligand-receptor binding. For example, TNF-α binding to endothelial cell receptors results in an increase in vascular permeability and enhances neutrophil-endothelial cell adhesion and transvascular migration. In hepatocytes, TNF-α increases anaerobic glycolysis; in skeletal muscle, proteolysis is stimulated; and in fat, lipolysis results. The catabolic response to this peptide in patients with tumors led to its discovery and initial name, cachectin.

TNF-α activates neutrophils, induces IL-1 gene expression,

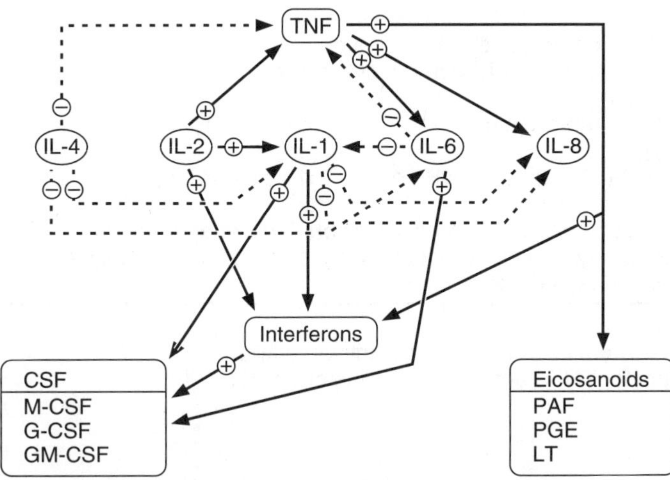

FIG. 11-9. Overview of some key cytokine interactions with the immune system as they relate to acute inflammation. Tumor necrosis factor-α (TNF) is produced primarily by cells of myeloid origin. TNF induces the synthesis of IL-6, IL-8, interferons, and eicosanoids. It in turn is upregulated by IL-2 and downregulated by IL-6 and IL-4. IL-1 increases the expression of IL-6, IL-8, colony-stimulating factors (CSFs) and the interferons. IL-1 production is increased by IL-2 and diminished by IL-6 and IL-4. This complex set of interactions apparently has evolved to provide tight, local regulatory control of the inflammatory process (see text). PAF, platelet-activating factor; PGE, E series prostaglandins; LT, leukotrienes; IL, interleukin; M-CSF, macrophage colony-stimulating factor; G-CSF, granulocyte colony-stimulating factor; GM-CSF, granulocyte-macrophage colony-stimulating factor.

TABLE 11-4. *Inventory of key interleukin (IL) functions relevant to acute inflammation**

Interleukin	Origin	Effector cells	Functions

IL-1	Monocytes
	Macrophages
	Endothelial cells
	Keratinocytes
	Neutrophils
	B lymphocytes
		Macrophages
		Fibroblasts
		Synovial cells
		Endothelial cells
		Hepatocytes
		Osteoclasts
			↑ Synthesis of:
			  C-reactive protein
			  Complement proteins
			↑ Serum concentrations of:
			  ACTH
			  Cortisone
			  Insulin
			↓ Blood pressure
			↓ Systemic vascular resistance
			↑ Fibroblast proliferation
			↑ Collagen production

IL-2	T lymphocytes	B lymphocytes T lymphocytes NK lymphocytes	Proliferation of B cells ↑ Antibody synthesis ↑ IFN-γ Proliferation of T cells Proliferation of NK cells, differentiation to LAK cells
IL-3	T lymphocytes	Eosinophils Mast cells	Hematopoietic growth factor
IL-4	T lymphocytes Mast cells	B lymphocytes Endothelial cells Mast cells Macrophages	↑ Class II MHC expression, proliferation of B cells, ↑ IgE synthesis, proliferation of Th2 cells, CTLs ↑ Increased expression of VCAM-1 Inhibits TNF-α, IL-1, PGE$_2$, NO synthesis, and IFN-γ effects
IL-6	Monocytes Macrophages Fibroblasts T lymphocytes Keratinocytes Endothelial cells	Plasma cells T lymphocytes	↑ Acute-phase protein synthesis
IL-8	Monocytes Macrophages Neutrophils Fibroblasts Endothelial cells Synovial cells Keratinocytes Epithelial cells Melanocytes T lymphocytes Hepatocytes Mesangial cells Chondrocytes	Neutrophils Basophils	↑ Adhesion molecules ↑ Chemoattraction
IL-9	T lymphocytes	Megakaryocytes	Growth factor
IL-10	T lymphocytes B lymphocytes Macrophages	T lymphocytes B lymphocytes	↓ Cytokine secretion ↑ Proliferation and antibody secretion

IL-11	PU34 cells
	  (primate
	  stromal cell
	  line)
		B lymphocytes
		Megakaryocytes
			↑ Clonal expansion of B lymphocytes
			↓ Adipogenesis
			↑ Acute-phase proteins

IL-12	Phagocytic cells B cells	NK and T cells	↑ IFN-γ, ↑ cytotoxicity of NK cells, ↑ Th1 cell activity
IL-13	Th2 cells	Monocytes and macrophages	Regulates surface antigen expression, inhibits antibody-dependent cytotoxicity and NO production, ↓ proinflammatory cytokine and chemokine synthesis

* See text for additional review. Data from references 33 through 45.

NK, natural killer; ACTH, adrenocorticotropic hormone; IFN, interferon; LAK, lymphokine-activated killer; MHC, major histocompatibility complex; CTL, cytotoxic T lymphocyte; TNF, tumor necrosis factor; PGE$_2$, prostaglandin E$_2$; NO, nitric oxide.

and enhances MHC class I antigen expression. It increases the production of prostaglandin E_2 and collagenase from fibroblasts. All these individual responses contribute to its role as a primary proinflammatory mediator.

Interleukins

The ILs and their individual roles in the inflammatory process are summarized in Table 11-4. Several features also are presented briefly here. IL-1 and TNF-α are similar and synergistic in their functional properties, although the structure and receptors for each are distinct. IL-1α and IL-1β are recognized by the same receptor and elicit similar biologic responses. They are considered jointly here. Like TNF-α, IL-1 has effects on many different cell types, including macrophages, fibroblasts, synovial cells, endothelial cells, hepatocytes, and osteoclasts. Also like TNF-α, IL-1 exists preformed and bound within cellular membranes. The hepatocyte response to IL-1 is to synthesize acute-phase proteins such as C-reactive protein, complement, clotting factors, serum amyloid A, and metalloproteins. In addition, IL-1 depresses hepatocyte cytochrome P-450 activity, thereby impairing drug metabolism. Endothelial cells respond to IL-1 by expressing β_2 integrins and other cell surface molecules that regulate leukocyte adherence. IL-1 also activates basophils and eosinophils.[51]

IL-1 has several other endocrine and physiologic effects, including the ability to increase plasma levels of adrenocorticotropic hormone, cortisone, and insulin while decreasing blood pressure and systemic vascular resistance. As a growth factor, IL-1 appears to sensitize bone marrow progenitor cells to the effects of other colony-stimulating factors, and it induces fibroblast proliferation and collagen production. Among other important IL-1 effects are the stimulation of TNF-α, IL-2, IL-6, and IL-8 production. It causes the proliferation of CD4$^+$ T cells and B cells, and it is pyrogenic.

IL-1 receptors exist on most cells and appear to be of two types. Type I receptors initially were described on the surface of T lymphocytes and fibroblasts, whereas type II receptors are on macrophages and B lymphocytes. Data suggest that glucocorticoid-stimulated monocytes express both types I and II.[52] The presence of structurally distinct receptors implies separate signal transduction pathways and provides a mechanism by which IL-1 can induce such protean biologic responses.

Interleukin-2. IL-2 is essential for T-cell and B-cell proliferation and for the activation of natural killer and certain T-cell subsets. IL-2 binding to its receptor initiates T-cell proliferation and leads to clonal expansion specific for the antigen of activation.[40] IL-2–mediated responses are an important aspect of immune surveillance and provide the tumoricidal host response to tumor antigens. IL-2 administration in humans has been shown to produce lymphokine-activated killer cells with cytotoxic potentials. This is an area of immunotherapy that is under investigation.[53] At least 10 clinical trials of IL-2 gene therapy for cancer have been approved.[54]

IL-2 induces IL-1, IFN-γ, TNF-α, and TNF-β synthesis, but inhibits both granulocyte-macrophage colony formation and erythropoiesis in the bone marrow. Cyclosporin A and corticosteroids inhibit IL-2 production, probably a critical aspect of their therapeutic actions.

Interleukin-4. IL-4 is produced by Th2 lymphocytes and mast cells. B lymphocytes respond to IL-4 by increasing class II MHC expression, increasing IgG (isotype 1) and IgE synthesis, and decreasing the secretion of IgG isotypes 2 and 3. IL-4 increases antigen presentation and the tumoricidal activity of macrophages. It inhibits IL-1 and TNF-α expression and regulates the induction of endothelial cell adhesion molecules, ELAM-1 and ICAM-1.[55] Other relevant actions include inhibition of macrophage superoxide production,[56] diminished production of macrophage chemotactic factors,[57] and inhibition of IL-6 secretion by monocytes.[58] Collectively, these actions provide important regulatory restraint on certain aspects of the inflammatory process.

Interleukin-6. The effects of IL-6 in general are similar to those of IL-1 and TNF-α. IL-6 supports terminal differentiation of plasma cells, provides for T-lymphocyte activation and induction of IL-2 receptors, activates cytotoxic T cells, and exhibits synergy with IL-2. It also induces acute-phase protein production in the liver and produces a febrile response when injected into experimental animals. IL-6 is a growth factor in the bone marrow. IL-6 production is stimulated by IL-1, TNF-α, platelet-derived growth factor, and endotoxin. IL-6 suppresses IL-1 and TNF-α production and may serve as a critical feedback inhibitor in the process of acute inflammation.[34,36]

Interleukin-8. IL-8 is a member of the C-X-C chemokine network through which TNF-α exerts its biologic effects.[49] Therefore, it is predictable that the actions of TNF-α and IL-8 are similar. These include neutrophil chemoattraction and activation, T-cell and basophil chemoattraction, and upregulation of macrophage/monocyte adhesion molecules. Its production is stimulated by IL-1, TNF-α, and endotoxin.

Interferons

IFNs α, β, and γ are the protein products of a multigene family with important regulatory functions in acute inflammation. Most cells possess receptors for all the IFN types.

IFN-α is produced by stimulated mononuclear cells, and a primary function is the regulation of the host response to viruses and other intracellular parasites. IFN-α is cytostatic for tumor cells. It induces fever, stimulates B-lymphocyte proliferation and differentiation, inhibits T-lymphocyte proliferation, and enhances the cytotoxicity of macrophages, neutrophils, natural killer cells, and T lymphocytes.[59]

IFN-β is produced by fibroblasts and epithelial cells after stimulation by IL-1, IL-2, and TNF-α. It shares many of the regulatory properties of IFN-α, but does not stimulate B lymphocytes or inhibit T-cell proliferation.

IFN-γ is produced by both CD4$^+$ and CD8$^+$ T lymphocytes. It shares many properties of IFN-α and IFN-β, and is a particularly potent mitogen. It inhibits B-cell proliferation, stimulates lymphokine-activated killer cells, induces macrophage tumoricidal activity, aids macrophage antigen presentation, and enhances oxidant generation by phagocytic cells. Like IFN-α, IFN-γ has important antiviral properties. Other effects include the regulation of antigen presentation to lymphocytes and upregulation of IL-1, M-CSF, and granulocyte colony-stimulating factor (G-CSF) expression.

Lymphotoxin

Formerly named TNF-β, lymphotoxin is a peptide secreted by activated T lymphocytes and some B cells, often in conjunction with IFN-γ. It activates neutrophils and vascular endothelial cells in vitro. Although the amino acid sequence is only 28% homologous to TNF-α in humans, it competes for binding to the same receptors. Therefore, functional responses can resemble those of TNF-α. It is of limited biologic relevance because of the relatively low levels found in vivo.

Growth Factors

Several growth factors have been characterized with regard to structure and function.[60] Some have been developed commercially and incorporated into clinical practice. More will surely follow. Their relevance to acute inflammation is varied and not necessarily clear. A brief summary follows (see Tables 11-4 and 11-5).

These factors are grouped functionally into one of three categories. The first is composed of those that regulate cell proliferation by inducing pluripotential stem cells and progenitor cells to form colonies (IL-3, GM-CSF). The second consists of those glycoproteins that act preferentially on early progenitor cells to stimulate cell differentiation (IL-1, IL-4, IL-6). In general, these act synergistically with other factors. The last category is made up of those that regulate the terminal differentiation of progenitor cell lineages into mature effector cells. For example, G-CSF induces the differentiation of mature granulocytes. These are reviewed briefly later.

Erythropoietin

Erythropoietin is produced in the kidneys (90%) and the liver (10%). It was the earliest growth factor characterized, and recombinant erythropoietin is now in routine clinical use for the stimulation of erythroid cells, although there is evidence to suggest that it also stimulates granulocyte, macrophage, and megakaryocyte cell lines.[60] Erythropoietin acts in concert with other growth factors, such as GM-CSF and IL-3. Its role in inflammation is limited, although erythrocytes are an important source of antioxidant enzymes.

Macrophage Colony-Stimulating Factor

As the name suggests, M-CSF acts principally to enhance the proliferation and differentiation of macrophage stem cells. It also appears to be synergistic with other growth factors, such as GM-CSF. M-CSF also induces mature monocytes to produce G-CSF, IFNs, TNF-α, IL-1, prostaglandins, plasminogen-activating factor, ferritin, and superoxide dismutase.

Granulocyte-Macrophage Colony-Stimulating Factor

The differentiation of granulocyte, macrophage, and eosinophil cell lines is directed by GM-CSF. Like M-CSF, it also influences the phenotypic behavior of mature cells. In particular, it enhances phagocytic activity and superoxide production in neutrophils. It inhibits neutrophil migration while enhancing margination and adhesion to endothelial cells. GM-CSF also enhances antibody-dependent cell-mediated cytotoxicity.

Granulocyte Colony-Stimulating Factor

It appears that G-CSF has important effects on the differentiation and maturation of bone marrow neutrophil-progenitor stem cells and differentiated neutrophils. These functional effects on mature granulocytes include priming neutrophils for oxidant generation and antibody-dependent cell-mediated phagocytosis. G-CSF also induces terminal differentiation of some tumor cell lines.

Transforming Growth Factor-α

Secreted by macrophages and some tumor cells, TGF-α is structurally similar to epidermal growth factor and exerts its effect on cells through binding to the epidermal growth factor receptor. TGF-α is mitogenic for fibroblasts, endothelial cells, and epithelial cells. It may be responsible for chronic inflammation and pulmonary fibrosis if produced in excessive amounts.[61]

Transforming Growth Factor-β

Activated T cells and monocytes secrete TGF-β. TGF-β inhibits T-cell proliferation and the maturation of cytotoxic T lympho-

TABLE 11-5. *Partial summary of growth factors*

Name	Origin	Function
Erythropoietin (EPO)	Kidneys Liver	Stimulates erythroid cells
Macrophage colony-stimulating factor (M-CSF)	T lymphocytes	Stimulates proliferation and differentiation of macrophage stem cells
Granulocyte-Macrophage colony-stimulating factor (GM-CSF)	Bone marrow T lymphocytes Endothelial cells Fibroblasts Macrophages	Directs differentiation of stem cells Increases neutrophil phagocytic activity, superoxide production, and margination and adhesion
Granulocyte colony-stimulating factor (G-CSF)	Bone marrow Macrophages Endothelial cells Fibroblasts	Directs differentiation of stem cells Primes neutrophils for oxidant generation and antibody-mediated phagocytosis

TABLE 11-6. *Physiologic effects of eicosanoids on inflammation*

PROSTAGLANDINS
Vasodilation
Bronchodilation
Inhibition of platelet aggregation

LEUKOTRIENES
Bronchoconstriction
Vasoconstriction
Increased vascular permeability
Chemotaxis

THROMBOXANES
Vasoconstriction
Increased platelet aggregation

LIPOXINS
Increased polymorphonuclear neutrophil oxidant generation
No chemoattractant properties

cytes. It also appears to promote angiogenesis (see Chap. 32). Of significance, TGF-β appears to downregulate the production and activity of several potent proinflammatory mediators.

Eicosanoids

Eicosanoids are 20-carbon fatty acid derivatives that include the prostaglandins, leukotrienes, thromboxanes, and lipoxins, all of which have important roles in inflammation. All eicosanoids result from biochemical modification of arachidonic acid, which is derived from membrane phospholipids by phospholipase enzymes. None are stored in cellular or extracellular depots; instead, they are rapidly synthesized, secreted, and cleared. Their half-lives in plasma are short, so their biologic effects are local, through paracrine and autocrine mechanisms. Stimuli are variable, but specific depending on the tissue of origin. Stimuli include trauma, thermal injury, sepsis, ischemia-reperfusion injury, and many other relevant clinical events. Virtually all cells are capable of eicosanoid production, and all appear to be carefully regulated in this regard.

The biologic effects of eicosanoids are complex. Some of the relevant effects are summarized briefly in Table 11-6. Most mediate particular aspects of the inflammatory response. Prostaglandins, especially E_2 and I_2, relax smooth muscle, leading to vasodilation and bronchodilation. Leukotrienes usually have an opposite effect on smooth muscle, and also have profound effects on phagocyte migration and activation. Leukotriene B_4 is one of the most potent endogenous chemoattractants known.

The biosynthetic pathways involved in the eicosanoid process are summarized in Figure 11-10. As illustrated, cyclooxygenase is the rate-limiting enzyme for the synthesis of the prostaglandins and thromboxanes. The 5-lipoxygenase enzyme serves a similar purpose for leukotriene synthesis. Many aspirin-related and other nonsteroidal antiinflammatory drugs act by inhibiting cyclooxygenase activity, reversibly or irreversibly. Likewise, specific lipoxygenase inhibitors have been developed for antiinflammatory use. Glucocorticoids exert antiinflammatory effects

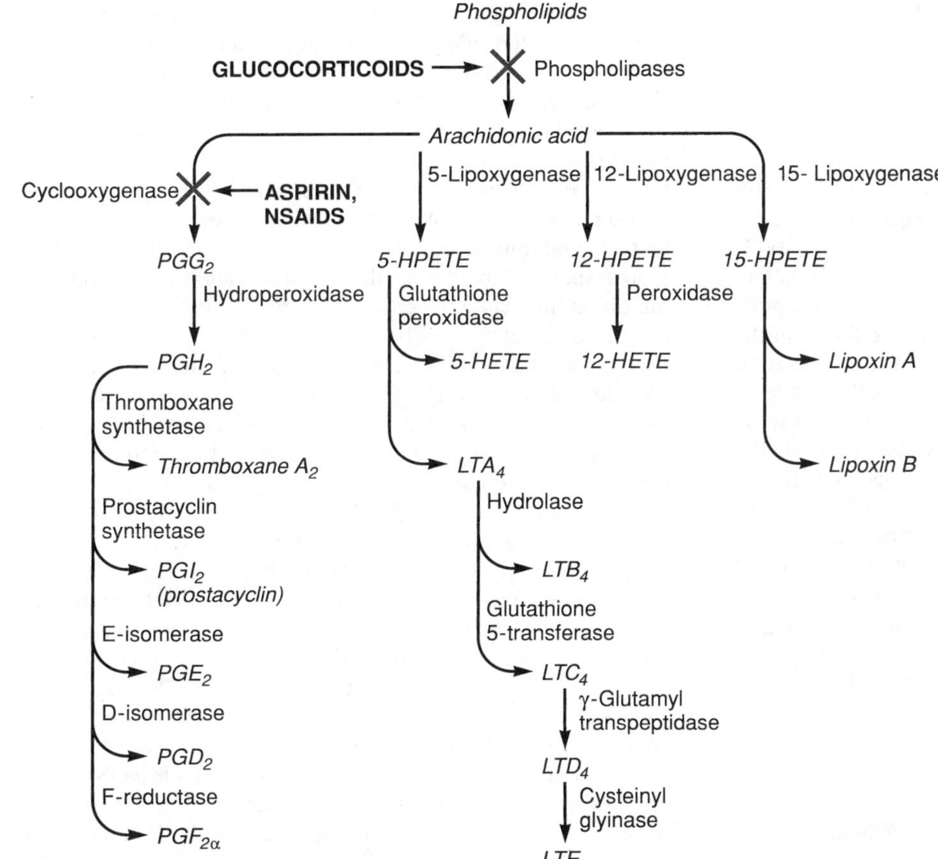

FIG. 11-10. Pathways of eicosanoid production. Inflammatory mediators are derived from arachidonic acid. Sites of inhibition by inflammatory drugs are shown. NSAID, nonsteroidal antiinflammatory drug (Omann GM, Hinshaw DB. Inflammation. In: Greenfield L, Mulholland MW, Oldham K, et al, eds. Surgery: scientific principles and practice. Philadelphia, JB Lippincott, 1993:132)

in part by inhibiting phospholipase-dependent arachidonic acid synthesis; as a result, both lipoxygenase and cyclooxygenase products are blocked by corticosteroid therapy.

Platelet-Activating Factor

The term *platelet-activating factor* actually refers to a heterogenous family of ether phosphocholines derived from membrane phospholipids through a process initiated and controlled by phospholipase A_2 with calcium. Because ether phosphocholines often contain arachidonic acid, PAF and eicosanoid generation are jointly regulated by phospholipase A_2. The effect of PAF on the inflammatory process is similar to that of certain of the eicosanoids, such as leukotrienes (B_4, C_4, D_4) and prostaglandins (E_2, I_2, D_2). PAF synthesis is upregulated rapidly in response to specific stimuli because it is not stored. Leukocytes and endothelial cells are particularly relevant PAF sources. As the name suggests, a prominent effect of PAF is platelet aggregation and granule release; however, some of the most important biologic actions occur independent of platelets. Among these are the regulation of leukocyte chemotaxis and adhesion, neutrophil activation, and smooth muscle tone. PAF given to experimental animals induces systemic hypotension, bronchoconstriction, and multiorgan microvascular injury, with particular effect on the intestine, kidneys, and lungs. The effect is dose-dependent, but shock and death may result.[62]

PAF production is induced by trauma, ischemia-reperfusion, sepsis, and many other similar events. PAF acts through widely distributed, specific cell surface receptors. A notable pharmacologic antiinflammatory strategy now in commercial development involves the use of PAF receptor antagonists. In experimental animals with inflammatory tissue injury, PAF receptor antagonists appear to be of significant benefit; however, human clinical trials are incomplete.[63,64]

Histamine

The primary source of histamine is the mast cell.[26] Stimuli for histamine release include antigen-IgE complexes, C3a, C5a, substance P, vasoactive intestinal peptide, somatostatin, IL-1, IL-3, IL-8, and GM-CSF. After release, histamine diffuses into surrounding tissues, where it interacts with histamine receptors of three types (H_1, H_2, and H_3). H_1 receptors are found in the brain, retina, adrenal medulla, liver, endothelial cells, cerebral microvasculature, and lymphocytes, and on smooth muscle of the airways, intestine, genitourinary tract, and vascular system. H_1 receptor activation results in smooth muscle and endothelial cell contraction. In addition, prostacyclin, PAF, factor VIII, and NO are released by endothelial cells in response to H_1 receptor activation. H_2 receptors are found in brain, gastric mucosa, adipocytes, and vascular smooth muscle, and on basophils and neutrophils. H_2 receptors mediate increases in gastric acid secretion and downregulate several lymphocyte functions. An H_3 receptor has been isolated from brain tissue and also may be present in some peripheral tissues. The functional significance is unknown.

Kinins/Coagulation

When blood vessels are disrupted and the coagulation cascade is initiated, activated Hageman factor promotes the conversion of prekallikrein to kallikrein. Kallikrein cleaves kininogen, forming bradykinin, a small but potent vasoactive peptide that is responsible for some of the increased vascular permeability and vasodilation that occur with the acute phase of the inflammatory response. Bradykinin also activates phospholipase A_2, contributing to the formation of arachidonic acid metabolites.[65]

Nitric Oxide

It has become evident that products of the L-arginine–NO pathways are unique and crucial for many essential biologic functions. Among these are neurotransmission, regulation of vasomotor tone, mediation of the coagulation system, and contributions to specific and nonspecific immunity.[66]

Stuehr observed in 1985 that activated murine macrophages generated large quantities of nitrite and nitrate in response to endotoxin exposure.[67] It subsequently was shown that this process involved the formation of the NO gas, that it was dependent on L-arginine, and that it could be inhibited by selected L-arginine analogues.[68] Products of the L-arginine–NO pathways were shown to be responsible for the cytotoxic effects of macrophages on tumor cells and various bacteria.[69] It is these properties that initially suggested the involvement of NO in inflammation. Evidence suggests an in vivo role for NO in inflammatory tissue injury. For example, in rats with acute inflammation, adjuvant arthritis, and immune complex–induced endothelial cell injury in the lung and skin, treatment with NO synthase inhibitors reduces the degree of inflammation, whereas, in each instance, the injury is enhanced by L-arginine.[66] Myocardial ischemia-reperfusion injury also is reduced by inhibition of NO synthase, although the mechanisms are less clear because of relevant NO-dependent regulation of regional blood flow.

NO is involved in the inflammatory process in at least three fundamental ways. The first results from smooth muscle relaxation, vasodilation, and a primary role in the regulation of local blood flow. The second has to do with the cytotoxic effects of phagocyte- and endothelium-generated NO. The third is related to NO regulation of leukocyte adhesion. In particular, it appears that NO inhibits neutrophil–endothelial cell adherence.[70] In vivo responses involve all these considerations. NO synthase inhibition limits NO-dependent vasodilation but abrogates NO-dependent cytotoxicity. Because of these several roles, there may be substantial risk in manipulation of the NO system in complex clinical settings. For example, NO inhibition in sepsis prevents systemic hypotension, but severe vasoconstriction with irreversible end-organ damage results.[66] Impaired bacterial clearance also remains an undesirable possibility. A thorough understanding and carefully designed therapies are necessary if the L-arginine–NO endothelial cell pathway is to be manipulated successfully to treat human disease.

Calcium-calmodulin–dependent constitutive isoforms of NO synthase (cNOS) from brain and endothelial cells have been purified, cloned, and sequenced.[71,72] These are referred to as neuronal and endothelial constitutive NOS (ncNOS and ecNOS, [or NOS1 and NOS3] respectively). Relatively low levels of spontaneous NO production result from cNOS expression, and this is readily available for cell signaling. Inducible NOS (iNOS or NOS_2) from macrophages[73] and hepatocytes[74] has been similarly characterized. This enzyme appears to be highly conserved across species. In general, the inducible form of the enzyme requires several hours for new protein synthesis, but the quantitative NO response is much greater than for cNOS and is not calcium dependent. Both constitutive and inducible NOS isoforms require cofactors such as the reduced form of nicotinamide adenine dinucleotide phosphate, flavin adenine dinucleotide, flavin mononucleotide, and, most importantly, tetrahydrobiopterin (BH₄).[75] Although it is clear that BH₄ is synthesized by some cells, it is not known whether regulation of this synthetic process is a relevant physiologic control mechanism for NO production. Glucocorticoids inhibit NOS induction but do not affect activity of the NOS enzyme itself. Experimental regulation of NO generation can be achieved by a variety of approaches, including the use of competitive inhibitors that are L-arginine analogues, the manipulation of substrate (L-arginine) or cofactor availability, and exposure to endotoxins and cytokines (particularly TNF-α, IFN-γ, and IL-1).[66]

Barriers to the External Environment

Protective mechanisms against invading organisms include a variety of mechanical and functional barriers in the skin and other epithelial surfaces exposed to the external environment.

Skin

The skin is composed of a thin external layer, the epidermis, and a somewhat more complex supporting structure, the dermis. The two are separated by a basement membrane. The epidermis is composed largely of keratinocytes. Its principal product, keratin, is a mechanical barrier to toxins and microorganisms from the external environment. Specific cellular elements within the epidermis and the dermis participate in local and systemic immune responses and together form the skin-associated lymphoid tissue[76–78] (Fig. 11-11).

Keratinocytes have important metabolic and immunologic functions. For example, they release IL-1α, IL-1β, TNF-α, and IL-6 when injured, and these in turn induce the production of other cytokines, chemokines, and vascular adhesion molecules. This contributes to amplification of inflammation by sequestered leukocytes at the injury site. Other relevant keratinocyte responses include the induction of GM-CSF, IL-8, monocyte chemotactic peptide-1, and IL-6 synthesis.

Langerhans cells are found in the epidermis. They are derived from hematopoietic precursors in the bone marrow and possess several unique surface antigens, including Fc IgG receptors type II, Fc IgE receptors type I, C3bi receptors, and MHC class II antigens.[76] Their primary function appears to be antigen presentation to memory and effector T cells. They are essential for the induction of cutaneous delayed hypersensitivity responses and epidermal allosensitization. When the keratin stratum corneum is penetrated, Langerhans cells phagocytose particulate debris and migrate through the basement membrane to dermal lymphatic channels and thereafter to regional lymph nodes. Within the lymph nodes, these cells adopt the phenotype of a lymphoid dendritic cell and, as such, present the transported antigen to naive or primed T cells to induce mitogenesis and differentiation.

The dermis is populated by substantial numbers of mast cells and fibroblasts. Mast cell–derived vasoactive amines such as

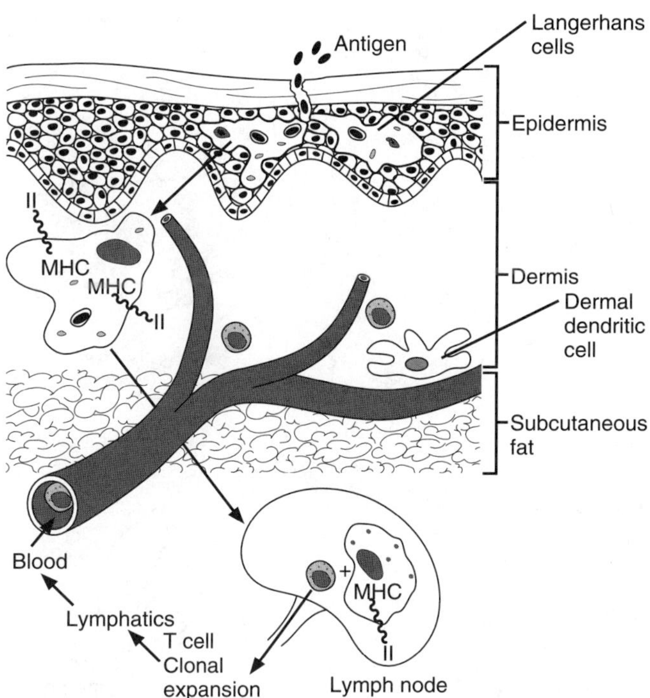

FIG. 11-11. Skin-associated lymphoid tissue (SALT). The skin is composed of the epidermis and the dermis. Within the epidermis, Langerhans cells serve as the primary phagocytes. Functionally, these are the macrophages of the skin. These cells ingest and process pathogens or foreign material. Activated Langerhans cells migrate to nearby lymph nodes, where antigen major histocompatibility complex (MHC) II is presented to T cells, which then undergo differentiation and clonal expansion. After leaving the lymph nodes, the T cells may enter the lymphatic system and return to the site through the circulation, or they may enter the skin directly. In addition, dermal dendritic cells usually are located in the perivascular areas of the skin and have functional characteristics similar to those of Langerhans cells.

histamine enhance vascular permeability, edema formation, and P-selectin expression. In addition, they produce cytokines with relevant effects, including IL-4 and TNF-α. Fibroblasts synthesize cytokines such as GM-CSF, G-CSF, and selected chemokines after stimulation by IL-1 or TNF-α. In addition, fibroblasts present antigen to T lymphocytes under certain conditions. Fibroblasts are more relevant to the processes of chronic inflammation and collagen formation.

Gastrointestinal Epithelium

The mucosal lining of the gastrointestinal tract absorbs essential nutrients and also provides an effective barrier to the foreign antigen that is always present. The barrier function is derived from many contributions, including nonimmune defenses such as gastric hydrochloric acid, pancreatic proteinases, active peristalsis, the mucous layer, the enteric microflora, and the intrinsic capacity for rapid regeneration of epithelium. These are beyond the scope of this discussion.

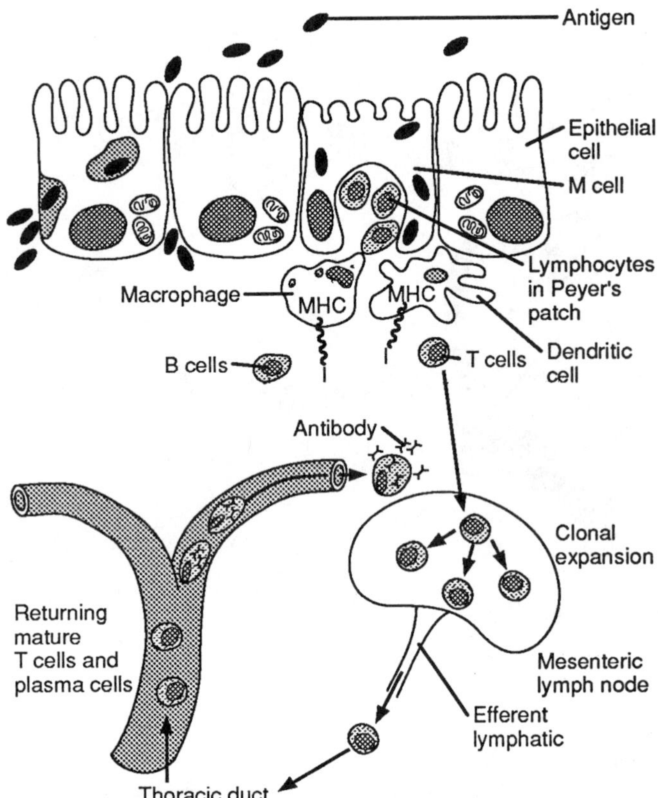

FIG. 11-12. Gut-associated lymphoid tissue (GALT). GALT is composed of specialized cells within the epithelium of the gastrointestinal tract. One key element is the M cell population, which is adjacent to the lymphocytes in underlying Peyer's patches. M cells transport antigen to macrophages or dendritic cells, which process and present the antigen to the lymphocytes. Subsequent lymphocyte clonal expansion occurs in the neighboring lymph nodes, and these differentiated lymphocytes then enter the lymphatic system and return or "home" through the circulation. MHC, major histocompatibility complex.

The enteric immune system is comprised of gut-associated lymphoid tissue.[79] It has both localized and distributed components (Fig. 11-12). Aggregated lymphoid follicles (Peyer's patches), isolated follicles, and mesenteric lymph nodes are the localized structures. Peyer's patches contain primarily B lymphocytes, although some T cells are present. Antigen-presenting cells within Peyer's patches include dendritic cells, macrophages, and specialized adjacent epithelial cells known as M cells. The diffuse components of the gut-associated lymphoid tissue system consist primarily of effector T lymphocytes and immunoglobulin-producing plasma cells distributed throughout the lamina propria and epithelium.

The human fetus develops lymphoid follicles and differentiated T cells between 11 and 20 weeks of gestation. However, the T-cell population is limited and follicular development is incomplete until postpartum enteric antigen exposure occurs. Mature IgA expression in enteric fluids is not complete until after the neonatal period. Although breast milk is a source of enteric IgG for infants, its principal effect on intestinal immune function appears to be derived from epidermal growth factor, which enhances functional maturation of the gastrointestinal epithelium.

Penetration and absorption of antigen is greatest when enteric barrier function is altered or damaged. Antigens initiate a mucosal immune response by passing between or through epithelial cells, or by activating the epithelial M cells overlying Peyer's patches. Regardless of the pathway, luminal enteric antigen then is presented to B or T cells, which clonally expand and migrate to mesenteric lymph nodes. Further maturation and expansion occur within the lymph node, followed by lymphocyte entry into the circulation through the thoracic duct. Because of the unique homing capability of enteric immune cells, these challenged and now mature T cells and B cell–derived plasma cells return to the gastrointestinal tract site as effector cells. Completion of this cycle with generation of antigen-specific IgA takes about 1 week after initial exposure in immunocompetent individuals.

Respiratory Epithelium

Like the gastrointestinal system, the respiratory tract is continually exposed to foreign antigen; therefore, it has developed an immune system similar to that of the gut. It is referred to as the bronchus-associated lymphoid tissue[80–82] (Fig. 11-13). Also like the gut, the lung has nonimmune defense mechanisms, such as the mucous layer, that trap microbes for clearance by mucociliary activity. This mechanism removes more than 80% of inhaled particles as they are swept into saliva, swallowed, and subsequently cleared by the gastrointestinal tract

Submucosal lymphoid follicles, analogous to the gastrointestinal Peyer's patches, are found in the upper respiratory tract. These follicles are composed predominantly of B cells, although T cells are located in the periphery. The overlying epithelium contains unique cells that are functionally similar to the enteric M cell. Continuous antigen sampling is facilitated by the lack of ciliated cells or goblet cells in these regions. Antigen is transported into the lymphoid follicle and presented to dendritic macrophages. Clonal expansion occurs as in the gut, and is followed by migration of lymphocytes to lymphatic channels, entry into the circulation, maturation, and, eventually, homing for return as effector cells to the site of origin.

Extracellular Matrix

The extracellular matrix (ECM) is composed of collagens, proteoglycans, and noncollagenous structural glycoproteins derived principally from fibroblasts. Although its fundamental role as a supporting framework for organs and specialized tissues is evident, ECM constituents also have important regulatory and supportive roles in acute inflammation.[83,84] The term *fibroblast* refers to the ubiquitous cells that provide much of the ECM. Phenotypic and morphologic heterogeneity is characteristic of fibroblasts. The most important subtypes are fibrocytes and myofibroblasts. Fibrocytes are matrix- and protein-synthesizing cells that appear in wounds about 6 to 12 days after injury. Myofibroblasts are contractile cells that appear between 3 and 30 days after injury. All fibroblasts are mesodermally derived and appear early in fetal development. Organogenesis depends on fibroblast regulation and overall

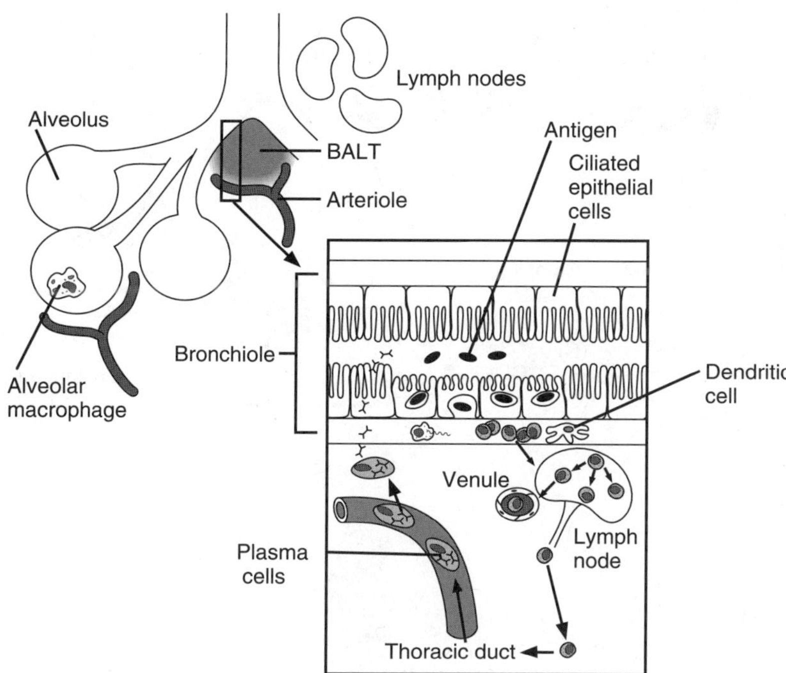

FIG. 11-13. Bronchus-associated lymphoid tissue (BALT). Like the skin and gastrointestinal tract, the respiratory system has a well-developed antigen-processing system. The BALT system is most developed at branching points of the tracheobronchial tree. Nonciliated epithelial cells are adjacent to collections of lymphocytes in a manner analogous to the intestinal M cell and Peyer's patches. The process of antigen presentation also appears similar (see Figures 11-11 and 11-12).

organization of the skeleton and muscle groups in addition to the individual visceral organs. In adults, fibroblasts have primary roles as effectors of wound healing. They produce enzymes capable of both protein degradation and synthesis. Through carefully regulated mechanisms that are not fully understood, they direct ECM remodeling. Fibroblasts elaborate many cytokines and growth factors, such as GM-CSF and G-CSF, in response to stimulation by IL-1 and TNF-α.

The major secretory proteins of cytokine-stimulated fibroblasts are collagens, the most abundant proteins in the human body. At least 14 different types of collagen are known, and these provide the structural matrix for all organs. They are grouped into fibrillar, fibril-associated, and nonfibrillar collagens. Fibrillar collagens have high tensile strength and substantial rigidity, and are found in supportive connective tissues of organs such as skin, bone, tendons, and ligaments. Nonfibrillar collagens form the basement membranes and provide the cytoskeleton for individual cells. Fibril-associated collagens are primarily those that provide molecular cross-links to fibrillar collagens. Collagen is degraded and remodeled by a variety of collagenases derived from neutrophils, mast cells, and fibroblasts themselves.

Elastin is an important fibroblast product that is found in specialized ligaments, lung fibrocartilage, and the media of large blood vessels. Tissues that possess elastic properties owe these properties to the elastin protein.

Proteoglycans, composed of sulfated polysaccharide chains linked to a protein core, first were identified in the ECM. Extracellular or matrix proteoglycans are responsible for providing mechanical support and regulating collagen synthesis, cell migration, and the binding of other matrix molecules. These are synthesized by many cell types and are found within the cell and on its surface. Proteoglycans regulate cell motility, adhesion, proliferation, differentiation, and morphogenesis.

Structural glycoproteins include fibronectin, tenascin, and vitronectin. Fibronectin is synthesized by a variety of cells, and its specific structure is dependent on the cell of origin. It is involved in interactions with the extracellular environment. Specifically, fibronectin serves as a fibroblast chemoattractant that supports anchorage and growth within the ECM. Fibronectin also promotes cellular differentiation among certain inflammatory cells. Tenascin is synthesized by fibroblasts, glial cells, and mesenchymal cells. It is found in rapidly growing and differentiating tissues, including neoplasms. Although its role is not clear, it may regulate cell-to-cell adhesion and serve as a signal for other responses. Vitronectin is synthesized by fibroblasts and hepatocytes, and is found in plasma, urine, platelets, amniotic fluid, and connective tissue. It affects cell differentiation, proliferation, and migration. A portion of the vitronectin molecule has been found to bind the complement components C7, C8, and C9, and to inhibit membrane attack complex–mediated cell lysis.

When cells adhere to matrix proteins, the cytoskeleton may be reorganized, resulting in conformational changes and functional alterations in cell surface receptor affinity. This is one mechanism by which the individual constituents of the ECM may influence the phenotypic behavior of various cells. ECM composition is known to influence cytokine and growth factor synthesis by fibroblasts and other cells. Degraded matrix proteins in a wound also serve a regulatory role for inflammatory cells and fibroblasts.

ACUTE INFLAMMATION

Acute inflammation results from the orderly recruitment of mature effector cells and their products to a site of injury or microbial invasion. Inflammation begins with the release of preformed chemical mediators at the site where foreign antigen first is recognized. These mediators begin to isolate the area of

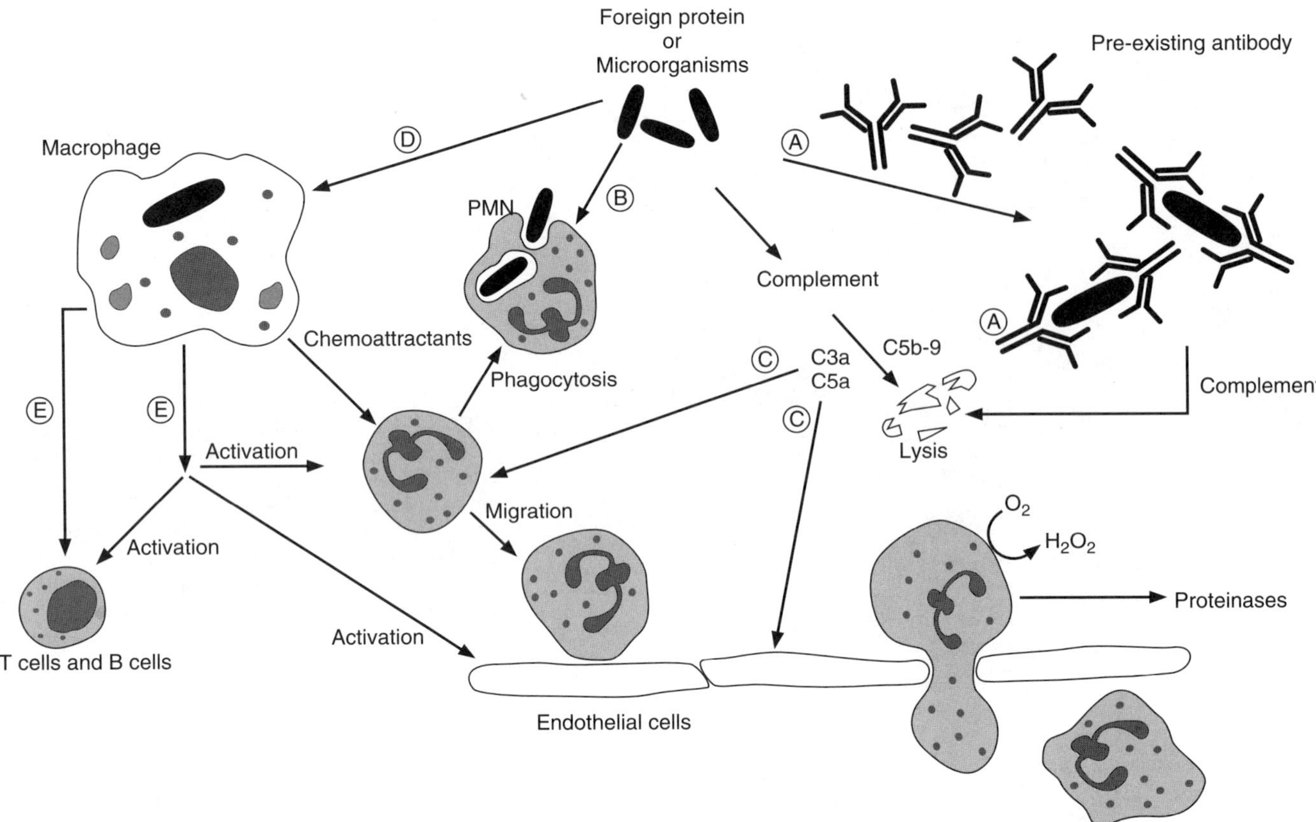

FIG. 11-14. Acute inflammation. When foreign proteins or microorganisms penetrate physical barriers to reach host tissues, several possible mechanisms are available for their removal. (*A*) The foreign antigen can come into contact with preexisting antibody, which then coats the surface. This is followed by complement binding and lysis. Alternatively, complement is capable of direct lysis in some circumstances. (*B*) Phagocytic cells such as neutrophils can ingest the foreign material and, using a variety of oxidants and proteinases, destroy it. Macrophages have similar capabilities. (*C*) Complement products activate and recruit leukocytes to the area of injury. In addition, complement products activate adjacent endothelium, promoting neutrophil adherence and transvascular migration. Secreted products from activated neutrophils contribute to the destruction and removal of invading microorganisms. Macrophages process foreign protein (*D*) and present this antigen to T and B cells (*E*), leading to specific antibody production and to the proliferation of cytoxic T cells.

injury and stimulate the local vascular endothelium, and then recruit inflammatory cells directly or through secondary signals. After initial localization, an increase in regional blood flow results and allows the influx of activated neutrophils. Adhesion of these and other inflammatory effector cells to the endothelium occurs. Transendothelial migration of these phagocytic cells into the extravascular tissues follows. Finally, the inflammatory cells and their regulatory systems target and destroy the foreign antigen. This is illustrated schematically in Figure 11-14. In some circumstances, chronic inflammation follows the acute process. Certain aspects of this latter process are presented here, but it is discussed in more detail in Chapter 9.

Injury Isolation

When a wound is created, injured blood vessels respond immediately with vasoconstriction and coagulation of blood. Serving the needs of hemostasis and injury isolation. The process begins with prothrombinase complex formation with activated factor X (Xa), activated factor V (Va), ionized calcium, and factor II (prothrombin). This complex catalyzes the formation of thrombin from prothrombin and yields a firm clot through fibrin polymerization. In addition to the obvious hemostatic effect, the clot entraps microorganisms or cellular debris. Platelet and collagen interaction also liberates serotonin and thromboxane, both of which contribute to the initial local vasoconstriction. Vasoconstriction and clot formation is followed by the release of histamine and chemotactic factors from platelets. This allows leukocytes to be recruited and then access the wound through newly opened collateral blood vessels. Bradykinin and kallikrein also are products of the coagulation cascade. Bradykinin contributes to vasodilation, whereas kallikrein is a chemotactic and activating factor for neutrophils.

Arachidonic acid metabolites are produced by mechanical injury. Of these, thromboxane A_2 is an important stimulus for platelet aggregation and vasoconstriction, prostaglandins produce vasodilation and increase microvascular permeability, and leukotrienes have important chemotactic properties. Whether

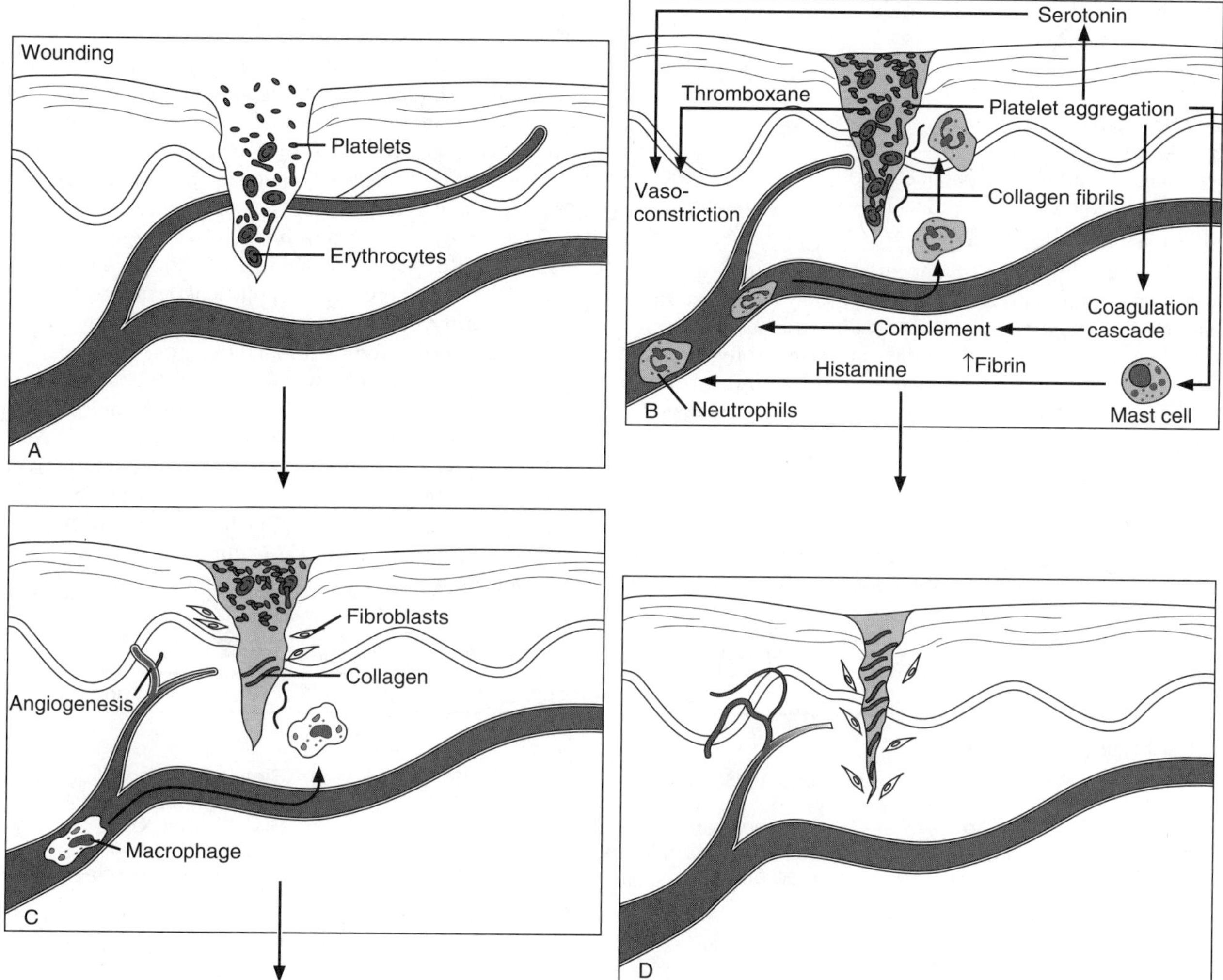

FIG. 11-15. (*A*) The acute inflammatory response can be divided into several distinct phases after wounding. (*B*) First is the vascular response and platelet activation phase. Vasoconstriction is mediated by activated platelets, which produce serotonin and thromboxane. After hemostasis, histamine-mediated vasodilation and complement activation occurs. These, in turn, lead to the activation of endothelium, and this allows various circulating cells to reach the site. Neutrophils are sequestered in the area, microvascular permeability increases, and edema formation results. Foreign material is phagocytosed. (*C*) By the third or forth day after injury, macrophages appear in the wound site. In addition, fibroblasts appear and collagen deposition begins. Angiogenesis follows. (*D*) Finally, the wound becomes relatively acellular and enters a final phase, that of collagen remodeling.

the stimulus is microbial invasion or mechanical tissue injury, the immediate host response is rapid deployment of these chemical mediators to isolate the site (Fig. 11-15).

Complement activation also is an early response to tissue injury. Complement proteins are readily available and bind rapidly to foreign protein, such as that found in viral or other membranes. Complement prevents the attachment of foreign protein to host cell receptors and contributes to the phagocytosis of foreign cells by opsonization or direct lysis. In addition, activation of the complement system generates peptide products such as the anaphylactins (C3a, C4a, C5a), which regulate secondary events, including local vasodilation, microvascular permeability, and leukocyte chemoattraction and activation.

Leukocyte Recruitment and Activation

Successful host defense requires the recruitment of leukocytes from elsewhere in the body and localization at the site of inflammation. This normally involves the release of chemoattractants into the circulation, whereupon leukocytes move from the bone marrow and other locations to the site of injury. This process involves chemotaxis, which is defined as the unidirectional migration of cells along a chemical gradient. Endogenous chemotactic factors include kallikrein, plasminogen-activating factor, fibrinopeptides, collagen fragments, complement products, bacterial peptides, and various lymphokines. A partial inventory of these important chemoattractants includes the following:

- Complement products, especially C5a
- Leukotrienes, especially B_4
- PAF
- IL-8
- Neutrophil-activating peptide-2
- Growth-related cytokine-α
- Macrophage inflammatory peptide-1α
- Macrophage inflammatory peptide-1β
- Formyl peptide (F-met-leu-phe)

In tissue, acute injury brings an influx of neutrophils that occurs within minutes and lasts for hours or days. Chronic inflammation is characterized by monocyte/macrophage infiltration, which occurs over a period of days and remains for weeks or months. Chemotactic factors often serve the additional role of activating effector cells to release cytoplasmic granules or generate oxidants.

Adherence and Migration

Regardless of cell type, leukocytes travel in the circulation to the site of inflammation and then enter tissues through an elegantly orchestrated series of interactions with the endothelium.

This discussion emphasizes neutrophil adherence because this is the fundamental event in acute inflammation; however, the principles involved also relate to other leukocytes. Leukocyte adherence is regulated by four classes of adhesion molecules: selectins, integrins, members of the immunoglobulin gene superfamily, and CD44. The key molecules are inventoried in Table 11-7,[85–92] and their function with regard to neutrophil adherence is depicted schematically in Figure 11-16.

Selectins are expressed by both leukocytes and endothelial cells. These glycoproteins bind carbohydrates on the cell surface and are responsible for the initial interaction that leads to leukocyte rolling on endothelium, a process that allows the leukocyte to sample the intravascular microenvironments and select a point of ''firm'' or ''static'' attachment. L-selectin (LAM-1 or LECAM-1) is constitutively expressed on the neutrophil cell surface and establishes relatively weak adherence between the leukocyte and endothelium, initiating this leukocyte rolling process. After leukocyte activation, L-selectin is shed from the cell surface and firm adhesion occurs through CD11/CD18 binding, as

TABLE 11-7. *Inventory of key leukocyte adhesion molecules**

Name	Site of expression	Ligands
SELECTIN FAMILY		
L-selectin (LAM-1, LECAM-1)	All leukocytes	Sialylated, fucosylated, sulfated glycoproteins
E-selectin (ELAM-1, LECAM-2)	Postcapillary venule endothelial cells	Sialyl Lewis X
P-selectin (PADGEM, GMP-140, LECAM-3)	Platelet alpha granules, endothelial cell Weibel-Palade bodies	Sialyl Lewis X–related
IMMUNOGLOBULIN SUPERGENE FAMILY		
ICAM-1	Endothelial cells	CD11a/CD18, CD11b/CD18,CD11c/CD18
ICAM-2	Endothelial cells	CD11a/CD18
ICAM-3	Endothelial cells	CD11a/CD18
VCAM-1	Leukocytes	VLA-4
INTEGRIN FAMILY		
B1 (VERY LATE ACTIVATION)		
VLA-1 (very late activation-1)	Activated T and B lymphocytes, monocytes	Collagen, laminin
VLA-2	T lymphocytes, monocytes, CTL, LAK	Collagen, laminin
VLA-3	CTL, LAK, monocytes	Collagen, laminin, fibronectin
VLA-4	Lymphocytes, monocytes, thymocytes	Fibronectin, VCAM-1
VLA-5	Monocytes	Fibronectin
VLA-6	T lymphocytes, monocytes	Laminin
B2 (LEUKOCYTE CELL ADHESION MOLECULES)		
CD11a/CD18 (LFA-1)	T and B lymphocytes, monocytes, macrophages, granulocytes, NK lymphocytes	ICAM-1, ICAM-2, ICAM-3
CD11b/CD18 (MAC-1, MO-1, CR3)	Monocytes, macrophages, granulocytes, NK lymphocytes	ICAM-1, C3bi, fibronectin
CD11c/CD18 p150/95	Monocytes, macrophages, NK lymphocytes	C3bi
B3 (CYTOADHESINS)		
Platelet glycoprotein IIb/IIIa	Platelets	Fibrinogen
Vitronectin receptor	Endothelial and epithelial cells	Vitronectin, fibrinogen, thrombospondin, von Willebrand factor
CD44 (LYMPHOCYTE HOMING MOLECULE)		
CD44	Lymphocytes, fibroblasts, smooth muscle, epithelium	Hyaluronic acid

* Data from references 85 through 92.
CTL, cytotoxic T lymphocyte; LAK, lymphokine-activated killer cell; NK, natural killer cell.

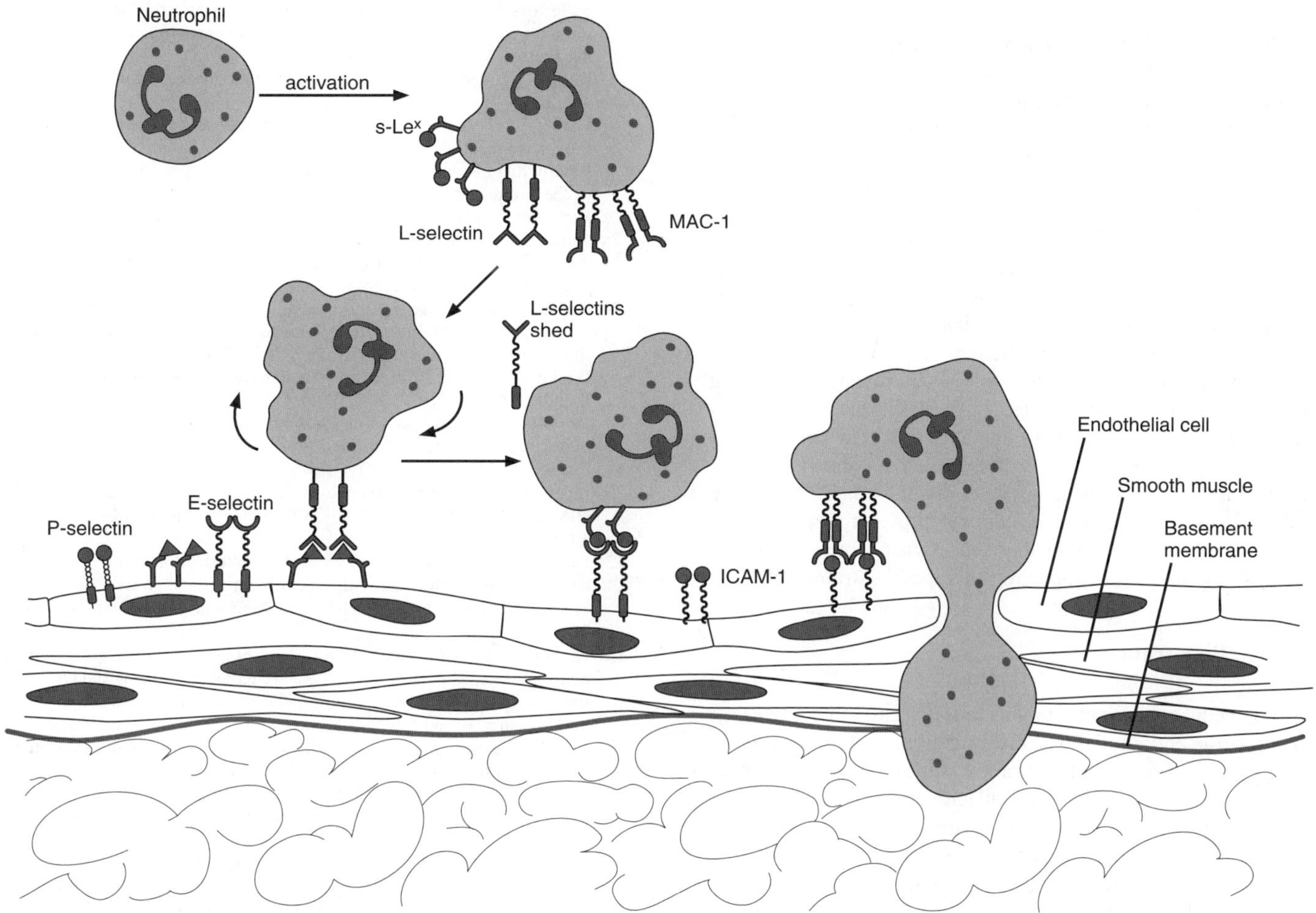

FIG. 11-16. Neutrophils and endothelial cells are activated by a variety of inflammatory mediators. Upregulation of ligands and receptors occurs on both cell surfaces. Neutrophils express L-selectin, which binds to a receptor on the activated endothelial cell. This initiates the "rolling" of neutrophils along the endothelium. L-selectin is shed once the neutrophil undergoes "static" binding by the integrins membrane adhesion complex-1 (MAC-1) and intercellular adhesion molecule-1 (ICAM-1; see text). P-selectin is expressed on the endothelium within seconds or minutes of endothelial cell activation. This also contributes to the process of leukocyte rolling, and perhaps also to transvascular migration. E-selectin appears later in the course of endothelial cell activation, and has a complementary role. Collectively, the selectins initiate leukocyte adherence to endothelium. It appears that selectin-mediated rolling allows the neutrophil to sample the endothelial microenvironment and select a specific site (presumably one of injury) for firm adherence and entry into the tissues where destruction of microbes or foreign antigen can occur. The later stages of the process are regulated largely by the integrins. Together, these mechanisms allow precise targeting by the neutrophil to reach the site of necessity.

detailed later. L-selectin is involved with both neutrophil and monocyte targeting of to injured tissues.[86,93]

P-selectin is expressed by platelets and endothelial cells. It is preformed and stored in alpha granules and Weibel-Palade bodies, respectively. It is mobilized to the cell surface within seconds of stimulation when activation occurs by thrombin, histamine, complement products, oxidants, or leukotrienes. The corresponding ligand on leukocytes is not known, although evidence suggests that P-selectin recognizes sialyl-Lewis X and CD15 on neutrophils. P-selectin also contributes to the neutrophil rolling process.

E-selectin (ELAM-1) is expressed only on postcapillary venule endothelium after cytokine or endotoxin stimulation. Because E-selectin expression requires new protein synthesis, there is a delay in its appearance. Evidence suggests that L-selectin and E-selectin are functionally similar, but that their roles are temporally distinct, with L-selectin mediating the immediate response and E-selectin being involved hours later.

The integrins are heterodimers composed of one β and one α subunit. They are classified by the β chain ($\beta 1$ through $\beta 8$). Integrins of the $\beta 2$ chain are responsible for static neutrophil binding to endothelium. These commonly are denoted as CD11a/CD18, CD11b/CD18, and CD11c/CD18. CD11a/CD18, or lymphocyte function-associated antigen (LFA-1), is expressed on all lymphocytes and is particularly important in T-lymphocyte adhesion. CD11b/CD18 (MAC-1, Mo 1, CR3) is expressed on neutrophils, monocytes, and natural killer cells. CD11c/CD18 is expressed on monocytes, some T cells, and neutrophils. Integrin expression is upregulated by exposure to TNF-α, GM-CSF, leukotriene B$_4$, some bacterial peptides, C5a, and other stimuli.

Endothelial cell ligands for these leukocyte integrins are members of the immunoglobulin gene superfamily and include the intercellular adhesion molecules (ICAM-1 and ICAM-2). ICAM-1 is constitutively expressed on endothelial cells and is upregulated by TNF-α, IL-1, endotoxin, and IFN-γ. ICAM-1 is a ligand for CD11a/CD18 and CD11b/CD18. ICAM-2 also is expressed constitutively and binds to CD11a/CD18. Platelet-endothelial cell adhesion molecule-1 (CD31) is found at endothelial cell junctions and may facilitate the transendothelial migration of adherent neutrophils.

The mechanisms by which leukocytes reach a specific site of injury have been elucidated in the last decade. The ability to manipulate this aspect of the inflammatory response is a potentially powerful tool. Because much of the tissue injury attributable to acute inflammation results from the discharge of oxidants, proteinase, and cationic proteins from activated, adherent neutrophils and other leukocytes, timely attenuation of this response is an appealing therapeutic strategy.

Tissue Penetrance

To reach extravascular targets, intravascular leukocytes must traverse the endothelial basement membrane. This is composed of type IV collagen and laminin, whereas the subjacent matrix is composed of types I and II collagen and other tissue-specific components. Nonactivated leukocytes demonstrate little adherence to ECM proteins. However, after stimulation, phagocytic cells show substantial activity, with polarization and an increase in both random and directed migration.[84] The precise mechanisms that allow penetration of the ECM are not known. It does appear that specific adhesion receptors for matrix proteins are involved, and also that leukocyte-derived proteolytic enzymes are used to degrade the matrix proteins. This appears to be particularly true for neutrophil transmigration from the vasculature.

Lymphocytes have receptors for many of the known ECM proteins, but it is unlikely that all serve locomotor functions. Some data suggest that lymphocytes migrate by wrapping cytoplasmic projections around individual matrix proteins independent of specific adhesion receptors.[84]

SUMMARY

The cellular and humoral elements that comprise the acute inflammatory response are detailed above. Whether the response is initiated by invading microorganisms, by accidental injury, or by a planned operative procedure, these elements are fundamental in the pathogenesis of the clinical problems discussed subsequently.

REFERENCES

1. Goust J. Lymphocyte ontogeny and membrane markers. Immunol Ser 1993;58:161.
2. Demetri G. Hematopoietic growth factors. In: Ozols REA, ed. Current problems in cancer. St Louis, Mosby-Year Book, 1992;179.
3. Sallerfors B. Endogenous production and peripheral blood levels of granulocyte-macrophage (GM-) and granulocyte (G-) colony-stimulating factors. Leuk Lymphoma 1994;13:235.
4. Rees R. Cytokines as biological response modifiers. J Clin Pathol 1992;45:93.
5. Lowry S. Cytokine mediators of immunity and inflammation. Arch Surg 1993;128:1235.
6. Belardelli F. Role of interferons and other cytokines in the regulation of the immune response. APMIS 1995;103:161.
7. Rapoport A, Abboud C, DiPersio J. Granulocyte-macrophage colony-stimulating factor (GM-CSF) and granulocyte colony-stimulating factor (G-CSF): receptor biology, signal transduction, and neutrophil activation. Blood Rev 1992;6:43.
8. Loike J, Silverstein R, Wright S, et al. The role of protected extracellular compartments in interactions between leukocytes, and platelets, and fibrin/fibrinogen matrices. Ann NY Acad Sci 1992;667:163.
9. Walker B, Ward P. Priming and signal transduction in neutrophils. Biol Signals 1992;1:237.
10. Ferrante A. Activation of neutrophils by interleukins-1 and -2 and tumor necrosis factors. Immunol Ser 1992;57:417.
11. Capsoni F, Minonozio F, Colombo G, et al. Membrane expression and function of complement receptors CR1 and CR3 on neutrophils from HIV-infected subects: modulation by rTNF-α and RGM-CSF. Scand J Immunol 1992;36:541.
12. Dent G, Ukena D, Chanez P, et al. Characterization of PAF receptors on human neutrophils using the specific antagonist, WEB 2086: correlation between receptor binding and function. FEBS Lett 1989;244:365.
13. Kishimoto T, Warnock R, Jutila M, et al. Antibodies against human neutrophil LECAM-1 (LAM-1/Leu-8/DREG-56 antigen) and endothelial cell ELAM-1 inhibit a common CD18-independent adhesion pathway in vitro. Blood 1991;78:805.
14. Lo SK, Detmers PA, Levin SM, Wright SD, Transient adhesion of neutrophils to endothelium. J Exp Med 1989;169:1779.
15. Vaporciyan A, Ward P. Enhanced generation of O2 − by human neutrophils via a complement iC3b/Mac-1 interaction. Biol Signals 1993;2:126.
16. Worthen GS, Avdi N, Vukajlovich S, Tobias PS. Neutrophil adherence induced by lipopolysaccharide in vitro. J Clin Invest 1992;90:2526.
17. Borregaard N, Kjeldsen L, Lollike K, Sengelov H. Granules and secretory vesicles of the human neutrophil. Clin Exp Immunol 1995;101(Suppl 1):6.
18. Bainton D. Neutrophilic leukocyte granules: from structure to function. Adv Exp Med Biol 1993;336:17.
19. Baird BR, Cheroncis JC, Sanglhaus RA, et al. O2 metabolites and neutrophil elastase synergistically cause edematous injury in isolated rat lungs. J Appl Physiol 1986;61:2224.
20. Ward P. Mechanisms of endothelial cell killing by H2O2 or products of activated neutrophils. Am J Med 1991;91:86S.
21. Varani J, Ward P. Mechanisms of neutrophil-dependent and neutrophil-independent endothelial cell injury. Biol Signals 1994;3:14.
22. Anderson B, Brown J, Harken A. Mechanisms of neutrophil-mediated tissue injury. J Surg Res 1991;51:170.
23. Bochner B. Basophils. In: Frank M, Austen KF, Claman HN, et al, eds. Samter's immunologic Diseases. New York, Little, Brown, 1995:259.
24. Weller P. Eosinophils: structure and functions. Curr Opin Immunol 1994;6:85.
25. Abu-Ghazaleh R, Kita H, Gleich G. Eosinophil activation and function in health and disease. Immunol Ser 1992;57:137.
26. McNeil H, Austen K. Biology of the mast cell. In: Frank M, Austen KF, Claman HN, et al, eds. Samter's immunologic diseases. New York, Little, Brown, 1995:185.
27. Weksler B. Platelets. In: Gallin J, Goldstein I, Snyderman R, eds. Inflammation: basic principles and clinical correlates. New York, Raven Press, 1992:727.
28. Carroll W, Korsmeyer S. Immunoglobulins. In: Frank M, et al, eds. Samter's immunologic diseases. New York, Little, Brown, 1995:33.
29. Moro I, Saito I, Asano M, et al. Ontogeny of the secretory Ig system in humans. Advances in Experimental Medicine and Biology 1991;310:51–57.
30. Frank M. Complement system. In: Frank M, Austen KF, Claman HN, et al, eds. Samter's imunologic diseases. Boston, Little, Brown, 1995:331.

31. Morgan B, Walport M. Complement deficiency and disease. Immunol Today 1991;12:301.

32. deBoer J, Wolbink G, Thijs L, et al. Interplay of complement and cytokines in the pathogenesis of septic shock. Immunopharmacology 1992;24:135.

33. Kruskal B, Ezekowitz A. Cytokines in the treatment of primary immunodeficiency. Biotherapy 1994;7:249.

34. Akira S, Taga T, Kaishimoto T. Interleukin-6 in biology and medicine. Adv Immunol 1993;54:1.

35. Sehgal P, Wand L, Rayanade R, et al. Interleukin-6-type cytokines. Ann NY Acad Sci 1995;762:1.

36. Molloy R, Mannick J, Rodrick M. Cytokines, sepsis and immunomodulation. Br J Surg 1993;80:289.

37. Lotz M. Interleukin-6. Cancer Invest 1993;11:732.

38. Marchant A, Bruyns C, Vandenabeeele P, et al. The protective role of interleukin-10 in endotoxin shock. Prog Clin Biol Res 1994;388:417.

39. Neben S, Turner K. The biology of interleukin 11. Stem Cells (Dayt) 1993;11(Suppl 2):156.

40. Gaulton G, Williamson P. Interleukin-2 and the interleukin-2 receptor complex. Chem Immunol 1994;59:91.

41. Zurawski G, de Vries J. Interleukin 13 elicits a subset of the activities of its close relative interleukin 4. Stem Cells (Dayt) 1994;12:169.

42. Trinchieri G. Interleukin-12: a proinflammatory cytokine with immunoregulatory functions that bridge innate resistance and antigen-specific adaptive immunity. Annu Rev Immunol 1995;13:251.

43. Quesniaux VFJ, Mayer P, Liehl E, et al. Review of a novel hematopoietic cytokine, interleukin-11. Int Rev Exp Pathol 1993;34A:205.

44. Costello R, Imbert J, Olive D. Interleukin-7: a major T-lymphocyte cytokine. Eur Cytokine Netw 1993;4:253.

45. Guy G, Bee N, Peng C. Lymphokine signal transduction. Progress in Growth Factor Research 1990;2:45.

46. van der Poll T, Lowry S. Tumor necrosis factor in sepsis: mediator of multiple organ failure or essential part of host defense? Shock 1995;31:1.

47. Strieter R, Kunkel S, Bone R. Role of tumor necrosis factor-alpha in disease states and inflammation. Crit Care Med 1993;21(Suppl 10):S447.

48. Tracey K, Cerami A. Tumor necrosis factor: an updated review of its biology. Crit Care Med 1993;21(Suppl 10):S415.

49. Colletti L, Kunkel S, Walz A, et al. Chemokine expression during hepatic ischemia/reperfusion-induced lung injury in the rat: the role of epithelial neutrophil activating protein. J Clin Invest 1995;95:134.

50. Leotscher H, Schlaeger E, Lahm H-W, et al. Purification and partial amino acid sequence analysis of two distinct tumor necrosis factor receptors from HL60 cells. J Biol Chem 1990;265:20131.

51. Warren J. Interleukins and tumor necrosis factor in inflammation. Crit Rev Clin Lab Sci 1990;28:37.

52. Spriggs M, Lioubin P, Slack J. Induction of an interleukin-1 receptor (IL-1R) on monocytic cells: evidence that the receptor is not encoded by a T-cell type IL-1R mRNA. J Biol Chem 1990;265:22499.

53. Grimm E, Mazumber A, Ahang H, Rosenberg S. Lymphokine activated killer cell phenomenon: lysis of natural killer-resistant fresh solid tumour cells by interleukin-2-activated autologous human peripheral blood lymphocytes. J Exp Med 1982;155:1823.

54. Anderson W. End-of-year-potpourri-1994. Hum Gene Ther 1994;5:1431.

55. Thornhill M, Haskard D. IL-4 regulates endothelial cell activation by IL-1, tumor necrosis factor, or IFN-gamma. J Immunol 1990;145:865.

56. Abramson S, Gallin J. IL-4 inhibits superoxide production by human mononuclear phagocytes. J Immunol 1990;144:625.

57. Standiford T, Strieter R, Chensue S, et al. IL-4 inhibits expression of IL-8 from stimulated human monocytes. J Immunol 1990;145:1435.

58. Cheung D, Hart P, Vitti G, et al. Contrasting effects of interferon-gamma and interleukin-4 on the interleukin-6 activity of stimulated human monocytes. Immunology 1990;71:70.

59. Schreiber R, Chaplin D. Cytokines, inflammation, and innate immunity. In: Frank M, Austen KF, Claman HN, et al, eds. Samter's immunologic diseases. New York, Little, Brown, 1995:279.

60. Robinson B, Quesenberry P. Hematopoietic growth factors: overview and clinical applications, part II. Am J Med Sci 1990;300:237.

61. Perkett E. Role of growth factors in lung repair and diseases. Curr Opin Pediatr 1995;7:242.

62. Chao W, Olson M. Platelet-activating factor: receptors and signal transduction. Biochem J 1993;292:617.

63. Nguyen P, Petitfrere E, Potron G. Mechanisms of the platelet aggregation induced by activated neutrophils and inhibitory effect of specific PAF receptor antagonists. Thromb Res 1995;78:33.

64. Koike H, Imanishi N, Natsume Y, Morooka S. Effects of platelet activating factor receptor antagonists on intracellular platelet activating factor function in neutrophils. Eur J Pharmacol 1994;269:299.

65. Wakefield T. Hemostasis. In: Greenfield L, Mulholland M, Oldham K, et al., eds. Surgery: scientific principles and practice. Philadelphia, JB Lippincott, 1993:102.

66. Moncada S, Higgs A. The L-arginine-nitric oxide pathway. N Engl J Med 1993;329:2002.

67. Stuehr D, Marletta M. Mammalian nitrate biosynthesis: mouse macrophages produce nitrite and nitrate in response to Escherichia coli lipopolysaccharide. Proc Natl Acad Sci USA 1985;82:7738.

68. Marletta M, Yoon P, Iyengar R, Leaf C, Wishnok JS. Macrophage oxidation of L-arginine to nitrite and nitrate: nitric oxide is an intermediate. Biochemistry 1988;27(24):8706.

69. Feldman P, Griffith O, Stuehr D. The surprising life of nitric oxide. Chemical and Engineering News 1993;71(51):26.

70. Zimmerman G, Prescott S, McIntyre T. Endothelial cell interactions with granulocytes: tethering and signaling molecules. Immunol Today 1992;13:93.

71. Yui Y, Hattori R, Kosuga K, et al. Purification of nitric oxide synthase from rat macrophages. J Biol Chem 1991;266:12544.

72. Bredt D, Hwand P, Glatt C, Lowenstein C, Reed R, Snyder S. Cloned and expressed nitric oxide synthase structurally resembles cytochrome P-450 reductase. Nature 1991;351:714.

73. Stuehr DJ, Cho HJ, Kwon NS, et al. Purification and characterization of the cytokine-induced macrophage nitric oxide synthase: an FAD- and FMN-containing flavoprotein. Proc Natl Acad Sci USA 1991;88:7773.

74. Billiar T, Curran R, Stuehr D, et al. Inducible cytosolic enzyme activity for the production of nitrogen oxides from L-arginine in hepatocytes. Biochem Biophys Res Commun 1990;168:1034.

75. Tayeh MA, Marletta MA. Macrophage oxidation of L-arginine to nitric oxide, nitrite and nitrate. J Biol Chem 1989;264:19654.

76. Stingl G. The skin: initiation and target site of immune responses. Recent results in cancer research. 1993;128:45.

77. Bos JD, Kapsenberg ML. The skin immune system: progress in cutaneous biology. Immunol Today 1993;14:75.

78. Salmon JK, Armstrong CA, Ansel JC. The skin as an immune organ. West J Med 1994;160:146.

79. Shanahan F. The intestinal immune system. In: Johnson LR, Alpen DH, Christensen J, et al, eds. Physiology of the gastrointestinal tract. New York, Raven Press, 1994:643.

80. Sminia T, Brugge-Gamelkoorn G, Jeurissen S. Structure and function of bronchus-associated lymphoid tissue (BALT). Crit Rev Immunol 1989;9:119.

81. Holt P. Regulation of antigen-presenting cell function(s) in lung and airway tissues. Eur Respir J 1993;6:120.

82. Bienenstock J. Mucosal immunological protection mechanisms in the airways. European Journal of Respiratory Diseases 1986;69(Suppl 147):62.

83. Cohen I, Diegelmann R. Wound healing. In: Greenfield L, Mulholland M, Oldham K, et al, eds. Surgery: scientific principles and practice. Philadelphia, JB Lippincott, 1993:86.

84. Ratner S. Lymphocyte migration through extracellular matrix. Invasion Metastasis 1992;12:83.

85. Kishimoto TK, Anderson DC. The role of integrins in inflammation. In: Gallin J, Goldstein I, Snyderman R, eds. Inflammation: basic principles and clinical correlates. New York, Raven Press, 1992:353.

86. Lasky LA, Rosen SD. The selectins: carbohydrate-binding adhesion molecules of the immune system. In: Gallin J, Goldstein I, Snyderman R, eds. Inflammation: basic principles and clinical correlates. New York, Raven Press, 1992:407.

87. Killam I. Lymphocyte homing to sites of inflammation. Curr Opin Immunol 1992;4:287.

88. Pitzalis C. Adhesion and migration of inflammatory cells. Clin Exp Rheumatol 1993;11(Suppl 8):S71.

89. Albelda SM. Endothelial and epithelial cell adhesion molecules. Am J Respir Cell Mol Biol 1991;4:195.

90. Korthuis RJ, Anderson DC, Granger DN. Role of neutrophil-endothelial cell adhesion in inflammatory disorders. J Crit Care 1994;9:47.

91. Patel K, Lorant E, Jones D, et al. Juxtacrine interactions of endothelial cells with leukocytes: tethering and signaling molecules. Behring Inst Mitt 1993;92:144.

92. Albelda S, Smith C, Ward P. Adhesion molecules and inflammatory injury. FASEB J 1994;8:504.

93. Bevilacqua MP, Nelson RM. Selectins. J Clin Invest 1993;91:379.

Surgery of Infants and Children: Scientific Principles and Practice, edited by Keith T. Oldham, Paul M. Colombani, and Robert P. Foglia. Lippincott–Raven Publishers, Philadelphia, © 1997.

CHAPTER 12

Immunology and Immunodeficiencies

Rebecca H. Buckley

CELLULAR AND HUMORAL BASES OF THE IMMUNE RESPONSE

Cells of the Immune System

The immune system consists of lymphoid and phagocytic cells, their secreted products, and the complement proteins. Lymphocytes that have the ability to differentiate into antibody-forming cells are referred to as *B cells* because of their origin in the bone marrow. *T cells* are so named because they develop in the thymus. Although T cells do not produce antibodies, they play a central role in all specific immune responses by producing soluble factors (cytokines) that influence the function of many types of cells.[1] They and the other cells of the immune system also bear adhesion molecules on their surfaces that facilitate cell–cell interaction, a necessary component of immune responses.[2] Adhesion molecules are also crucial for the trafficking of immune cells to lymphoid organs and tissues and to sites of inflammation. In contrast to T and B lymphocytes, which have antigen-specific recognition capabilities, natural killer (NK) cells mediate non–antigen-specific cytotoxicity; they originate from both the bone marrow and the thymus. NK cells are thought to assist in protection against viral infections, in tumor surveillance, and in immunoregulation. The immune system thus has a crucial role in all host defense. Its ability to recognize foreign antigens also accounts for its ability to reject organ and tissue grafts and to produce allergic reactions. In addition, the immune system serves to protect against autoimmune diseases and malignancy.

Development of Cells and Organs of the Immune System

Stem cells appear in the yolk sac and fetal liver by 5 weeks' gestation; they later reside in the bone marrow, where they remain throughout life. Lymphoid and phagocytic cells arise from these stem cells. Lymphoid stem cells differentiate into T, B, or NK cells, depending on the organs or tissues to which

they migrate (Fig. 12-1). The initial migration and development, as well as the continued differentiation of lymphoid cells throughout life, occur through the interaction of the previously mentioned lymphocytic and tissue cell-surface adhesion molecules (Table 12-1) and under the influence of cytokines (Table 12-2) secreted by the involved cells.[1,2] Primary lymphoid organ (thymus, bone marrow) development begins during the middle of the first trimester of gestation and proceeds rapidly; secondary lymphoid organ (spleen, lymph nodes, tonsils, Peyer patches, lamina propria) development soon follows. This process is almost complete by the end of the first trimester of gestation.[3]

Clusters of Differentiation Classification of Human Leukocyte Differentiation Antigens

The World Health Organization has developed an official classification of well-characterized surface molecules present on immune cells.[2] Each molecule is given a number that is preceded by the letters *CD*, which stand for clusters of differentiation (see Table 12-1). This terminology is used throughout this chapter in referring to the cells of the immune system and other cells with which they interact.

Development and Function

T Cells

The primitive thymic rudiment is formed from the ectoderm of the third branchial cleft and endoderm of the third branchial pouch at 4 weeks' gestation. Blood-borne T-cell precursors (pro-T cells) from the fetal liver bear surface proteins CD7 and CD34 and begin to colonize the perithymic mesenchyme at 8 weeks' gestation; they are found intrathymically soon thereafter (see Fig. 12-1). Some early thymocytes also coexpress CD4, a protein present on the surfaces of mature T-helper cells, and CD8, a protein found on both mature cytotoxic T cells and NK cells. In addition, some cells bear single T-cell receptor (TCR) chains (β, δ, or γ), but none bear complete TCRs. The mature TCR is a heterodimer of two chains, either α and β or γ and

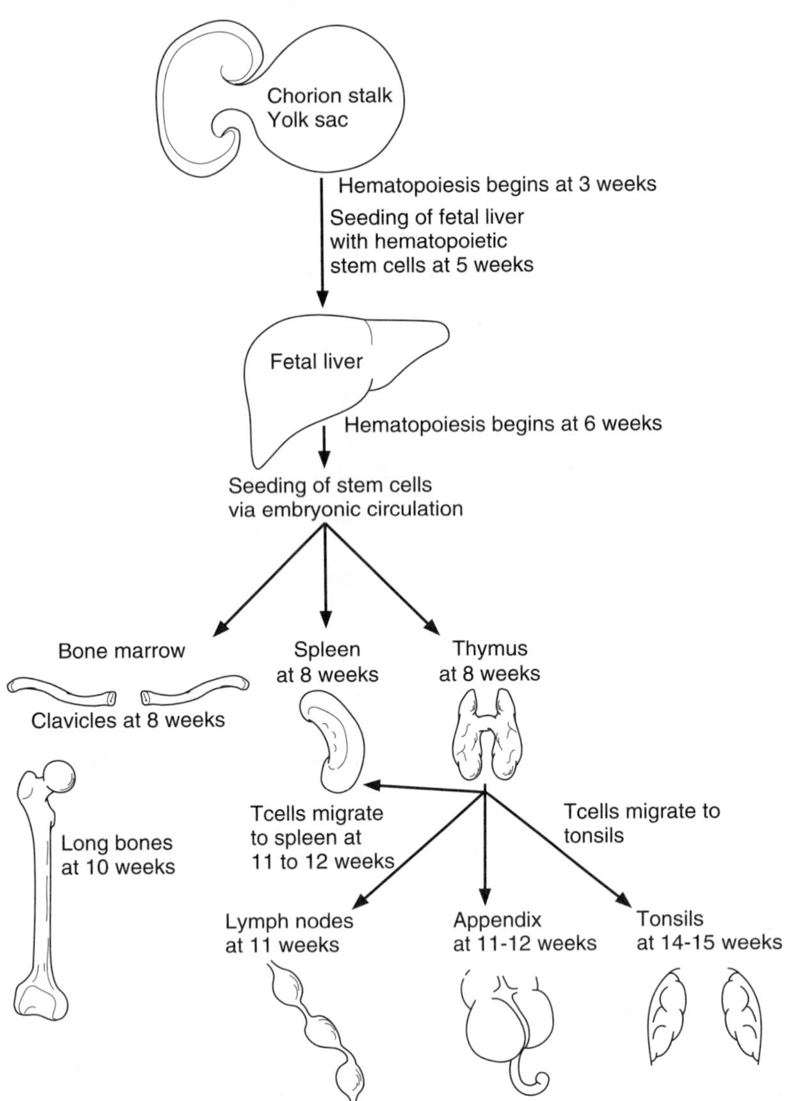

FIG. 12-1. Migration patterns of hematopoietic stem cells and mature lymphocytes during human fetal development. (After Haynes BF, Denning SM. Lymphopoiesis. In: Stamatoyannopoulis G, Nienhuis A, Majerus P, et al, eds. Molecular basis of blood diseases, ed 2. Philadelphia, WB Saunders, 1994:429)

δ; it is coexpressed on the cell surface with CD3, a complex of five polypeptide chains (γ, δ, ϵ, ζ, η) at about 10 weeks' gestation. TCR gene rearrangement occurs by a process in which noncontiguous blocks of DNA are spliced together. These segments, known as V (variable), D (diversity), and J (joining) regions, each have a number of variants, and they randomly combine to produce a large number of distinct TCRs. It is this enormous diversity that enables the immune system to recognize millions of different antigens. Rearrangement of TCR genes signifies commitment of pro-T cells to T-lineage development, that is, to become pre-T cells. TCR$\alpha\beta+$ cells gradually increase in number during embryonic life and represent more than 95% of thymocytes postnatally.[3]

Cortical thymocytes are among the most rapidly dividing cells in the body, with a mean generation time of 6 to 8 hours; they increase in number by 100,000-fold within 2 weeks after stem cells enter the thymus. Owing to processes referred to as *positive selection* and *negative selection,* 97% of all cortical thymocytes die in situ. Positive selection occurs through the interaction of immature thymocytes (which express low levels of TCR) with major histocompatibility complex (MHC) anti-

gens present on cortical thymic epithelial cells. In this manner, thymocytes with TCRs capable of interacting with foreign antigens presented on self MHC molecules are selected and activated to develop to maturity. Mature thymocytes that survive positive selection are either CD4+ and restricted to self class II HLA molecules or CD8+ and restricted to self class I HLA molecules when they interact with foreign antigens presented by these MHC molecules. Negative selection is mediated through interaction of the remaining thymocytes, which now have much higher levels of TCR expression, with HLA class I or II antigens present on bone marrow–derived thymic macrophages and dendritic cells. This results in programmed cell death (apoptosis) of the autoreactive thymocytes. The surviving cells are singly positive for either CD4 or CD8 and migrate to the medulla. T-cell functions are acquired with the development of single-positive thymocytes, but they are not fully developed until the cells emigrate from the thymus.[3]

T cells begin to leave the thymic medulla through the bloodstream at 11 to 12 weeks of embryonic life and are distributed throughout the body, with heaviest concentrations in the paracortical areas of lymph nodes, the periarteriolar areas of the

TABLE 12-1. *Clusters of Differentiation (CD) classification of some lymphocyte surface molecules*

CD number	Other names	Tissue and lineage	Function
CD1	T6	Cortical thymocytes: Langerhans cells	Antigen presentation to TCR$\gamma\delta$ cells
CD2	SRBC receptor	T and NK cells	Binds LFA-3 (CD58); alternative pathway of T-cell activation
CD3	T3, Leu 4	T cells	TCR-associated; transduces signals from TCR
CD4	T4, Leu3a	Helper T-cell subset	Receptor for HLA class II antigens; associated with p56 *lck* tyrosine kinase
CD7	3A1, Leu 9	T and NK cells and their precursors	Comitogenic for T lymphocytes
CD8	T8, Leu2a	Cytotoxic T-cell subset; also on 30% of NK cells	Receptor for HLA class I antigens; associated with p56 *lck* tyrosine kinase
CD11a	LFA-1a α chain	T, B, and NK cells	With CD18 ligand for ICAMS 1, 2, and 3
CD11b,c	MAC-1, CR3; CR4	NK cells	With CD18, receptors for C3bi
CD16	FCγRIII	NK cells	FcR for IgG
CD19	B4	B cells	Regulates B-cell activation
CD20	B1	B cells	Mediates B-cell activation
CD21	B2	B cells	C3d and EBV receptor; CR2
CD34	My10	Precursor cells	?
CD40	—	B cells	Signals Ig class-switching
CD45	Leukocyte common antigen, T200	All leukocytes	Tyrosine phosphatase that regulates lymphocyte activation; CD45R0 isoform on memory T cells, Cd45RA isoform on naive T cells
CD54	ICAM-1	Endothelial cells, many activated cells	Binds CD18/CD11a
CD56	N-CAM; NKH-1	NK cells	Mediates NK homotypic adhesion

TCR, T-cell receptor; ICAM, intracellular adhesion molecule; NK, natural killer; EBV, Epstein-Barr virus.

spleen, and the thoracic duct lymph. They are found in rudimentary tonsils by 14 to 15 weeks' gestation. The homing of lymphocytes to peripheral lymphoid organs is directed by the interaction of a lymphocyte adhesion molecule, L-selectin, with carbohydrate moieties on specialized lymphoid organ vasculature called *high endothelial venules.*[2] By 12 weeks' gestation, T cells are able to proliferate in response to phytohemagglutinin and to allogeneic cells; antigen-binding T cells have been found by 20 weeks' gestation. Hassall corpuscles (swirls of terminally differentiated medullary epithelial cells) appear in the thymic medulla by 16 to 18 weeks of embryonic life.

T cells are present in higher numbers in cord blood than in that of children and adults, but most bear the CD45RA (naive) isoform. This dominance of CD45RA + over CDRO + (memory) T cells persists during the first 2 to 3 years of life, after which time there is gradual equalization of the numbers of cells bearing these two isoforms. Helper T (T$_H$) cells are further subdivided according to the cytokines they produce when activated. T$_H$1 cells produce interleukin-2 (IL-2) and interferon-γ (IFN-γ), thereby promoting cytotoxic T-cell or delayed hypersensitivity types of responses, whereas T$_H$2 cells produce IL-4, IL-5, IL-6, and IL-13, which promote B-cell responses and allergic sensitization (see Table 12-2). Newborn T cells have the capacity to respond normally to the T-cell mitogen, PHA, and to allogeneic cells. The absence of these responses by cord blood lymphocytes provides evidence of profound primary T-cell dysfunction. The normal newborn infant also has the ability to reject foreign cells and the capacity to develop other antigen-specific T-cell responses. Because T-cell function may be lacking in infants with unrecognized severe congenital T-cell defects, many hospitals now irradiate all blood products given to

young infants to avoid graft-versus-host disease (GVHD) from transfused lymphocytes.[4]

Two of the main functions of T cells are (1) to provide cytotoxic activity against facultative intracellular pathogens (mycobacteria, fungi) and virally infected cells or tumor cells, and (2) to provide cytokines (see Table 12-2) to help B cells make antibody. For the T cell to carry out these functions, it first must bind to the target cell or to the antigen-presenting cell (APC), respectively. For high-affinity binding of T cells to target cells or APCs, several molecules on T cells in addition to TCRs bind to molecules on their respective target cells (Fig. 12-2). CD8 molecules on cytotoxic T cells bind to MHC class I molecules on target cells. CD4 molecules on helper T cells bind to MHC class II molecules on APCs. Lymphocyte function antigen 1 (LFA-1) molecules on T cells bind to intracellular adhesion molecule 1 (ICAM-1 or CD54) on APCs. CD2 molecules on T cells bind to LFA-3 or CD58 on APCs. With the adhesion of cytotoxic T cells to their targets, they are stimulated to kill the target; and with the adhesion of helper T cells to APCs, they are stimulated to produce cytokines, which stimulate B cells and other cells. Many other adhesion pairs participate in these important cell–cell interactions.

B Cells

B-cell development begins in the fetal liver before 7 weeks' gestation and slightly later in the bone marrow.[3] Antigen-independent stages of B-cell development have been defined according to immunoglobulin gene rearrangement patterns and the surface proteins the cells bear. The *pro-B cell* is the first descen-

TABLE 12-2. *Functional classification of cytokines**

CYTOKINES INVOLVED IN NATURAL IMMUNE RESPONSES
Type I interferons—IFN-α and IFN-β—inhibit viral replication, inhibit cell proliferation, activate NK cells, up-regulate class I MHC molecule expression
TNF-α—mediates host response to gram-negative bacteria and other infectious agents
IL-1α and β—mediate host inflammatory response to infectious agents
IL-1Ra—is a natural antagonist of IL-1, blocks signal delivered by IL-1
IL-6—mediates and regulates inflammatory responses
Chemokines (IL-8, monocyte chemotactic protein 1, RANTES, and others)—mediate leukocyte chemotaxis and activation

LYMPHOCYTE REGULATORY CYTOKINES
IMMUNOSTIMULATORY OR GROWTH PROMOTING
IL-1—costimulates activation of T cells
IL-2—growth factor for T, B, NK cells; activates effector cells
IL-4—T-cell and B-cell growth factor; stimulates IgE production; up-regulates class I and II MHC molecule and FcRϵII expression on macrophages; expansion of T_H2 subset
IL-5—B-cell growth and activation
IL-6—growth factor for B cells
IL-7—stromal cell factor; growth factor for precursor B and T cells
IL-10—growth and differentiation factor for B cells
IL-9—growth factor for T cells
IL-12—expansion of T_H1 subset; activates effector cells
IL-13—growth and differentiating factor for B cells; stimulates IgE production; up-regulates class I and II MHC molecule and FcRϵII expression on macrophages
TNF-β—stimulates effector cell function
IFN-γ—activates macrophages, NK cells; up-regulates class I and II MHC molecule expression; inhibits IL-4– or IL-13–induced IgE production

IMMUNOSUPPRESSIVE
IL-1Ra—regulates IL-1 activities
TGF-β—antagonizes lymphocyte responses
IL-10—inhibits activities of T_H1 cells

HEMATOPOIESIS-REGULATING CYTOKINES
Granulocyte-macrophage, granulocyte, and macrophage colon-stimulating factors
Erythropoietin—differentiation of erythroid precursors
IL-3, SCF, *c-kit* receptor—regulate stem cell development
IL-4—mast cell development
IL-5—eosinophil differentiation and proliferation
IL-6—differentiation of B cells
IL-7—differentiation of B and T cells

PROINFLAMMATORY CYTOKINES
IL-1, TNF-α, IL-6—participate in the acute-phase response and synergize to mediate inflammation, shock, and death

ANTIINFLAMMATORY CYTOKINES
IL-4—reduces endotoxin-induced TNF and Il-1 production
IL-6—inhibits TNF production
IL-10—suppresses lymphocyte functions and down-regulates production of proinflammatory cytokines
IL-13—down-regulates functions of macrophages, suppresses production of proinflammatory cytokines
TGF-β—has immunosuppressive effects, inhibits IL-1 and TNF gene expression
IL-1Ra—competes with the binding of IL-1 to its cell-surface receptors and blocks IL-1R
TNFsR—soluble TNF receptors, by binding TNF, block interaction of TNF with the target cell

* This is not an exhaustive list.
(Modified from Whiteside TL. Cytokine measurements and interpretation of cytokine assays in human disease. *J Clin Immunol* 1994;14:329)
SCF, stem cell factor; TNF, tumor necrosis factor; NK, natural killer; IL, interleukin; MHC, major histocompatibility complex; IgE, immunoglobulin E; IFN, interferon; T_H, helper T cells.

dent of stem cells committed to the B lineage and is identified by the presence of both CD34 and CD10 on its surface. The next stage is the *pre-pre-B cell*, during which immunoglobulin genes are rearranged, but there are no cytoplasmic or surface μ heavy chains of immunoglobulin M (IgM). The *pre-B cell* is next; these cells are distinguished by the expression of cyto-

plasmic μ heavy chains but no surface IgM because as yet no immunoglobulin light chains are produced. Next is the *immature B cell*, during which surface IgM is expressed (because light chain genes have now been rearranged) but not surface IgD. The last stage of antigen-independent B-cell development is the *mature* or *virgin B cell*, which coexpresses both surface

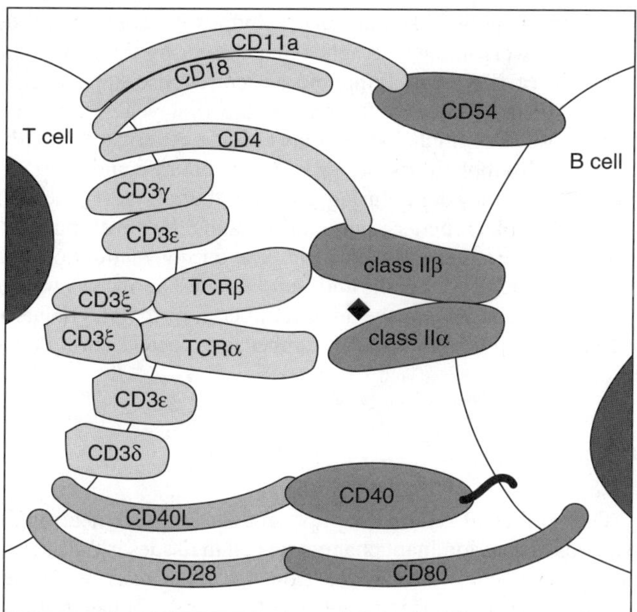

FIG. 12-2. Cell surface molecules and their respective ligands important in T-cell–B-cell interactions.

IgM and surface IgD. *Pre-B cells* can be found in fetal liver at 7 weeks' gestation, surface IgM + and surface IgG + B cells at between 7 and 11 weeks' gestation, and surface IgD + and surface IgA + B cells by 12 to 13 weeks' gestation. By 14 weeks of embryonic life, the percentage of circulating lymphocytes bearing surface IgM and surface IgD is the same as in cord blood and slightly higher than in the blood of adults.[3,4]

Antigen-dependent stages of B-cell development occur after the mature or virgin B cell is stimulated by antigen; the outcome is the differentiation of the cell and its progeny into surface immunoglobulin-positive memory B cells and plasma cells, which synthesize and secrete antibodies. There are five immunoglobulin classes or isotypes (defined by unique heavy chain antigens present on each): IgM, IgG, IgA, IgD, and IgE. IgG and IgM are the only isotypes that fix complement; they are the most important immunoglobulins in the internal body fluids for protection against infectious agents. IgM is confined primarily to the intravascular compartment because of its large size, whereas IgG is present in all internal body fluids. IgA is the major protective immunoglobulin of external secretions, that is, those of the gastrointestinal, respiratory, and urogenital tracts, but it is also present in the circulation. IgE, present in both internal and external body fluids, plays a major role in host defense against parasites. Because of high-affinity IgE receptors on basophils and mast cells, however, IgE is the principal if not sole mediator of allergic reactions of the immediate type. The function of IgD is still unknown. Immunoglobulin subclasses include four subclasses of IgG (IgG1, IgG2, IgG3, and IgG4) and two subclasses of IgA (IgA1 and IgA2). These subclasses each have different biologic roles; for example, antipolysaccharide antibody activity is found predominantly in the IgG2 subclass. Secreted IgM and IgE have been found in aborted fetuses as young as 10 weeks, and IgG as early as 11 to 12 weeks. Despite the capacity of fetal B lymphocytes to differentiate into immunoglobulin-synthesizing and immuno-

globulin-secreting cells, plasma cells are not usually found in lymphoid tissues of the fetus until about 20 weeks' gestation because of the sterile environment of the uterus. Peyer patches have been found in significant numbers by the fifth intrauterine month, and plasma cells have been seen in the lamina propria by 25 weeks' gestation. Before birth, there may be primary follicles in lymph nodes, but secondary follicles are usually not present.

The fetus begins to receive significant quantities of maternal IgG transplacentally at about 12 weeks' gestation, and the quantity increases rapidly until birth, when cord serum contains a concentration of IgG comparable to or greater than that of maternal serum. IgG is the only class to cross the placenta to any significant degree, and all four subclasses do this, but IgG2 does so least well. A small amount of IgM (10% of adult levels) and a few nanograms of IgA, IgD, and IgE are normally found in cord serum; because none of these proteins cross the placenta, they are of fetal origin.

Newborn infants are overly susceptible to infections with gram-negative organisms because they have not received IgM antibodies (ie, heat-stable opsonins) to these organisms from their mothers. Maternally transmitted IgG antibodies serve adequately as heat-stable opsonins for most gram-positive bacteria, and IgG antibodies to viruses afford adequate protection against those agents. There is a relative deficiency of the IgG2 subclass, however, and antibodies to capsular polysaccharide antigens may be deficient. Because premature infants have received less maternal IgG by the time of birth than full-term infants, their serum opsonic activity is low for all types of organisms.

B lymphocytes are present in cord blood in considerably higher numbers than in the blood of children and adults. Cord blood B cells, however, do not synthesize the range of immunoglobulin isotypes made by B cells from older children and adults when stimulated with either pokeweed mitogen or anti-CD40 plus IL-4 or IL-10, producing primarily IgM and at a much reduced quantity.[5]

The infant begins to synthesize antibodies of the IgM class at an increased rate soon after birth in response to antigens in the new environment. Premature infants appear to be as capable of doing this as full-term infants. About 6 days after birth, the serum concentration of IgM rises sharply. This rise continues until adult levels are achieved by about 1 year of age. IgA is usually not detectable in cord serum unless there has been an intrauterine infection. Serum IgA is normally first detected at around the 13th day of postnatal life; the level steadily increases during early childhood until adult levels are achieved between 6 and 7 years of age. Cord serum contains an IgG concentration comparable to or greater than that of maternal serum. Maternal IgG gradually disappears during the first 6 to 8 months of life, while the rate of infant IgG synthesis increases (IgG1 and IgG3 faster than IgG2 and IgG4 during the first year) until adult concentrations of total IgG are reached and maintained by 7 to 8 years of age. The total immunoglobulin level in the infant usually reaches a low point at about 4 or 5 months of age. The rate of development of IgE has generally been found to follow that of IgA. After adult concentrations of each of the three major immunoglobulins are reached, these levels remain remarkably constant for a given normal person. The ability to produce specific antibodies to protein antigens is present at the time of birth. Normal infants, however, usually cannot produce antibodies to polysaccharide antigens until after age 2 years unless the polysaccharide is conjugated to a protein carrier, as in the HIB vaccine.

In the primary antibody response, native antigen is carried to a lymph node draining the site of entry, taken up by specialized cells called follicle-stimulating cells (FSCs), and expressed on their surfaces. Virgin B cells bearing surface immunoglobulin specific for that antigen then bind to the antigen; if the affinity of the B-cell surface immunoglobulin for the antigen present on the FSCs is high, and if other signals are provided by activated helper T cells, the B cell develops into an antibody-producing plasma cell. If the affinity is not high enough, or if T-cell signals are not received, the B cell dies by apoptosis. The signals provided by activated helper T cells include those from cytokines they secrete (IL-4, IL-5, IL-6, IL-10, and IL-13)[1]; see Table 12-2) and the signal from a surface T-cell molecule, gp39, which binds to CD40 on the B-cell surface[5] (see Fig. 12-2) Cross-linking of CD40 on B cells or by allowing CD40 to interact with gp39 in the presence of certain cytokines causes the B cells to undergo proliferation and to initiate immunoglobulin synthesis. In the primary immune response, usually only IgM antibody is made, and most of it is of relatively low affinity. Some B cells become memory B cells during the primary immune response. These cells have switched their immunoglobulin genes so that IgG, IgA, or IgE antibodies of higher affinity are formed on a secondary exposure to the same antigen. The secondary immune response occurs when these memory B cells again encounter that antigen. Plasma cells form, just as in the primary response; however, many more cells are rapidly generated, and IgG, IgA, and IgE antibodies of increased affinity are produced. The exact pattern of isotype response to antigen varies, depending on the type of antigen and the cytokines present in the microenvironment.

Natural Killer Cells

Natural killer lymphocytes are derived from bone marrow stem cells and are defined by their functional capacity to mediate non–antigen-specific cytotoxicity. NK cell activity has been found in human fetal liver cells by 8 to 11 weeks' gestation. Unlike T and B cells, NK cells do not rearrange antigen-receptor genes during their development. All NK cells express CD56, and most also bear CD16 (Fcγ receptor III [FcγRIII]) on their cell surfaces. Because NK cells share surface antigens with T and myeloid cells, the lineage relation of NK cells is still unclear. NK cells have been found in the thymus, but most experimental studies suggest that thymic processing is not necessary for NK cell development. After release from bone marrow, NK cells enter the circulation or migrate to the spleen; there are few NK cells in lymph nodes. The percentage of NK cells in cord blood is usually lower than in the blood of children and adults (constituting 10% of lymphocytes), but the absolute number of NK cells is about the same, owing to a higher lymphocyte count. The capacity of cord blood NK cells to mediate target lysis in either NK cell assays or antibody-dependent cell-mediated cytotoxity assays is roughly two thirds that of adults.[3]

Lymphoid Organs

At the time of birth, lymphoid organs are proportionally small but microscopically well-developed; they mature rapidly during the postnatal period. The neonate's thymus is about two thirds its mature weight, and it reaches that weight by the end of the first year of life. Most lymphoid structures also appear to be mature histologically by the end of the first year. Peripheral blood absolute lymphocyte counts reach a peak by 9 months of age. All lymphoid tissues continue to enlarge and even exceed adult dimensions during the prepubertal years, then all except the spleen undergo involution coincident with puberty. The spleen gradually increases in size during maturation and does not reach full weight until adulthood. The mean number of Peyer patches is half the adult number at birth and gradually increases until the adult mean number is exceeded during adolescent years.[3]

Phagocytic Cells

The principal circulating phagocyte is the neutrophil, whereas the predominant phagocytic cell in tissues is the macrophage. Monocytes are derived from the bone marrow; subsequently, they can differentiate into tissue macrophages. Bone marrow neutrophil maturation is influenced by several factors secreted by stromal cells, monocytes, and T lymphocytes.[6] These cytokines include IL-7, IL-3, granulocyte colony-stimulating factor and granulocyte-monocyte colony-stimulating factor.[1] Mature neutrophils migrate from the bone marrow into the circulation. To carry out their roles, phagocytes must be produced in adequate numbers and mobilized at the appropriate time. To perform their functions, neutrophils must marginate from the intravascular compartment, be deformable enough to undergo diapedesis, migrate along a chemotactic gradient to the site of inflammation, phagocytose, and have adequate lysosomal constituents and oxidative metabolism to kill microorganisms. A defect in any of these characteristics can lead to increased susceptibility to infection. Many functions are dependent on the presence of adhesion molecules on the phagocytic cell surface that facilitate attachment to other cells or that bind complement and immunoglobulin.[6]

Neutrophil adhesion molecules include members of the integrin and selectin families of cell-surface molecules.[7] Integrins are a family of heterodimers, each composed of one α and one β chain. Multiple α chains can pair with each β chain. The two main subfamilies are the β_1 and β_2 families. The LFA-1 heterodimer (CD11a plus CD18) is one member of the β_2-integrin family. LFA-1 binds to ICAM-1 (CD54) on the surfaces of activated endothelial and other cells. Selectins have only one polypeptide chain; these chains contain short consensus repeats found in many complement regulatory proteins. An example found on neutrophils is leukocyte-selectin (L-selectin, or CD62L); it binds to a variety of sialomucins present on activated endothelium. Near a site of infection, endothelium expresses both sialomucins and ICAM-1. The selectin–sialomucin interaction makes the neutrophil start to roll along the endothelium instead of flowing in the bloodstream. Once the neutrophil has been slowed enough to roll, it can then be bound more avidly to ICAM-1 on the endothelium through the integrin LFA-1. The selectin molecules are shed from the neutrophil, and the neutrophil then migrates across the endothelium to the site of the infection.

The ability of neutrophils and monocytes to adhere to antibody and complement in immune complexes or coated on microorganisms is also mediated by cell membrane receptors specific for these proteins. Complement receptors include complement receptor type 1, CR1 (CD35); CR2 (CD21); and CR3 (CD18/CD11b). The structure of CR1 is similar to that of other complement-regulatory proteins, containing many short consensus repeats. It is present on T and B lymphocytes and red blood cells, and it binds C3b. CR2 (CD21) is the Epstein-Barr virus (EBV) receptor; it also binds C3d, and it is part of an activation complex on B cells. CR3 is another member of the β_2-integrin family; it is present on neutrophils. FcγR binds the Fc portion of IgG.

The ability of a neutrophil to migrate requires both a normal actin–myosin system and normal assembly and disassembly of microtubules. Several factors can activate neutrophils and induce their chemotaxis, including the synthetic peptide f-methionine-leucine-phenylalanine, which is structurally related to chemotactically active products of bacteria, and the complement-derived proteins C3a and C5a.[6] Within minutes of encountering such a stimulus, the neutrophil changes from a round cell with a smooth membrane to an elongated cell with undulating pseudopods and cytoplasmic granules oriented toward the chemoattractant. These morphologic changes are accompanied by ion fluxes, changes in membrane potential, microtubule assembly, increased glycolysis, and production of oxygen radicals. Binding of the stimulant or attractant to receptors on the cell surface triggers a series of biochemical events that ultimately lead to synthesis of proteins.

Phagocytosis is the process by which cells ingest particles encountered in their microenvironment so as to contain or destroy them. It is facilitated by a variety of substances known as *opsonins*. The most important opsonins are heat-stable IgG antibodies and the heat-labile complement components C3 and C5.[8] Particles, such as bacteria, are coated with these substances; interaction with phagocytic cell membrane receptors for the opsonins (IgG and C3b) initiates ingestion of the particles. They then enter a phagocytic vacuole that ultimately fuses with specific and azurophilic granules. Destruction of microorganisms requires generation of reactive oxygen molecules through a phagocytic cell respiratory burst. These oxygen radicals interact with myeloperoxidase and a halide ion to generate hypochlorite (HClO), which is extremely toxic to organisms. Azurophilic granules contain lytic enzymes, including acid hydrolase, lysozyme, and myeloperoxidase. Specific granules contain lysozyme and lactoferrin. Movement and fusion of granules is dependent on the microtubular system. The combination of these aerobic and anaerobic neutrophil bactericidal systems effects destruction of the bacterium.

Complement Proteins

The complement system consists of more than 20 native serum proteins, 12 of which act sequentially to amplify the effects of antibody-mediated immunity, cell-mediated immunity, and phagocytosis and to generate elements of the inflammatory response[8] (Fig. 12-3). This system is one of the major

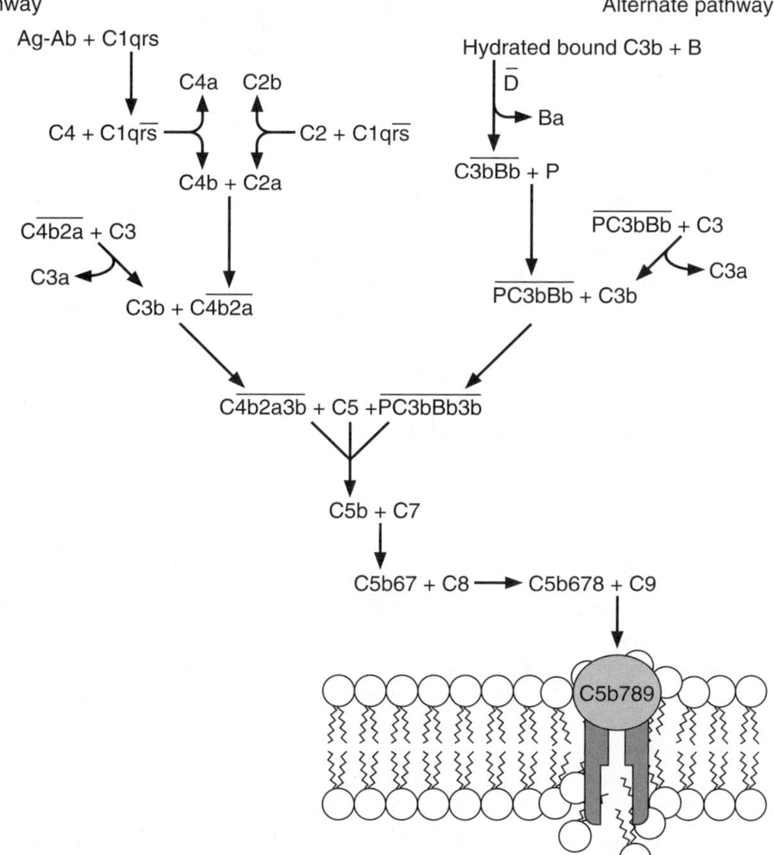

FIG. 12-3. Classic and alternative pathways of complement activation, showing the central role of C3. Cleavage fragments are indicated by letters after the component numbers.

effector arms in host defense. It can effect a primitive non–antigen-specific defense against invading microorganisms, but it can also be triggered by antibody to provide antigen-specific host defense. The molecular weights of the 12 serum proteins that act sequentially in the complement cascade vary from 24,000 to 400,000 kd. Their serum concentrations vary from about 150 mg/dL (C3) to nanogram amounts. The gene encoding properdin is on the short arm of the X chromosome, but the genes encoding all of the other complement proteins are on autosomal chromosomes.[8]

Three major known functions of the complement system are to: (1) cause lysis of organisms and cells, (2) promote opsonization of particles by coating them with peptides recognized by specific receptors on phagocytic cells, and (3) generate inflammatory peptides, which cause smooth muscle dilatation, immigration of inflammatory cells (chemotaxis), and histamine release. Two major pathways of complement activation are known. The more primitive pathway, termed the *alternative pathway* because of its discovery after the original pathway, is important as a first line of defense against invasion. This pathway functions in the absence of antibody, but it can also function more rapidly in the presence of antibody. The proteins that make up the alternative pathway include factors B, D, and properdin as well as C3 and the later components of the complement cascade (see Fig. 12-3). Known activators of the alternative pathway include complex polysaccharides, lipopolysaccharides (such as bacterial endotoxins), immune complexes containing IgA and IgG4, cell-surface constituents of certain intact fungi, erythrocyte membranes, and lymphoid cells. The *classic pathway,* so termed because it was the first pathway to be discovered, is activated by IgM and by IgG1, IgG2, and IgG3 antibodies. This pathway proceeds through the interaction of a series of complement proteins (C1, C4, and C2) to activate C3 and later proteins in the complement cascade. The third component of complement is the substrate for the C3-cleaving enzyme of the classic pathway, that is C4b2a, which is a complex of fragments of the fourth and second complement components, respectively. The C3-cleaving enzyme of the alternative complement pathway contains fragments of factor B (Bb) and C3b (C3bBb). Properdin can stabilize C3bBb by binding to the complex. The C3bBb enzyme activates positive feedback that amplifies the entire complement pathway. Factor D and magnesium ion are necessary for the generation of Bb from factor B, whereas properdin protects Bb from breakdown by serum factors. Thus, both the classic and alternative complement pathways consist of a series of glycoproteins that, when activated, form a C3-cleaving enzyme, termed C3 *convertase,* that cleaves C3 (see Fig. 12-3). The cleavage of C3 generates C5 convertase, which then activates the terminal complement sequence. Interactions between C5b, C6, C7, C8, and C9 produce a channel in the membrane of the bacterium, virus, or red cell, leading to membrane lysis. Receptors for C3b exist on many cells, including polymorphonuclear cells and macrophages, and the specific adherence of C3b to both a bacterium and a phagocyte enhances phagocytosis. Three complement factors (C3a, C4a, and C5a) affect smooth muscle contraction and are termed *anaphylatoxins.* C5a and C567 have chemotactic activity. Binding of C4 to a viral surface may act to neutralize viruses independent of other immune mechanisms.[8]

As with antibody-mediated and cell-mediated immunity, not all complement-mediated reactions are beneficial. When activated under inappropriate circumstances, complement can cause autoimmune disease by mediating tissue damage. The anaphylatoxins can produce nonspecific systemic reactions resembling specific IgE-mediated allergic reactions. The adherence of complement (in addition to antibody) to certain cells can result in their lysis, as in Coombs-positive hemolytic anemia. Circulating antigen–antibody complement complexes can deposit in the kidney and initiate immune complex disease.[8]

Complement does not cross the placenta. Its production begins in the first trimester of gestation, along with all other components of the immune system. At birth, however, full-term infants have only about half of the adult serum concentrations of Clq, C4, C2, C3, and C7. Function of the classic complement pathway, as assessed by total hemolytic complement activity in sera, is subnormal in about half of term infants. Both component concentration and biologic activity of the alternative complement pathway are more frequently abnormal in newborn sera than are those of the classic pathway.[8]

PRIMARY IMMUNODEFICIENCY DISEASES

Primary, or genetically determined, immunodeficiencies are more common in children than in adults, but they are still rare in both age groups. They can involve any of the components of the immune system. More than 50 immunodeficiency syndromes have been described in the past 40 years.[9] Little was known, however, of the primary biologic errors underlying most of these conditions until recently. Several of the primary immunodeficiency diseases involving T, B, and NK cells have been mapped to specific chromosomal locations, and the molecular bases have been identified for a significant number of them[10] (Table 12-3). Most are recessive traits, some of which are caused by mutations in genes on the X chromosome, and others by mutations on autosomal chromosomes.[9]

B-Cell Defects

Defects affecting antibody-forming cells occur more often than those affecting any other component of the immune system (Table 12-4). Selective absence of IgA is the most common, with a reported incidence ranging from 1 in 333 to 1 in 16,000 people in different races. By contrast, it has been estimated that agammaglobulinemia occurs with a frequency of only 1 in 50,000 people.

X-Linked (Bruton) Agammaglobulinemia

Most boys afflicted with X-linked agammaglobulinemia (XLA) are well during the first 6 to 9 months of life owing to protection by maternally transmitted IgG antibodies.[9] Thereafter, they frequently develop infections with high-grade extracellular pyogenic organisms, such as pneumococci, streptococci, and *Haemophilus* sp, unless given antibiotics or immunoglobulin therapy. Mycoplasma infections are also frequent. Chronic fungal infections are not usually present, and *Pneumocystis carinii* pneumonia does not usually occur unless there is an associated neutropenia. Viral infections are self-limiting, except for hepatitis viruses and enteroviruses. The lat-

TABLE 12-3. *Chromosomal map locations for faulty genes in primary immunodeficiency diseases*

Chromosome	Disease
1q25	Chronic granulomatous disease (gp67[phox])*
2	MHC class II antigen deficiency (RFX5)*
2p11	κ-chain deficiency*
2q12	CD8 lymphocytopenia (ZAP70)*
6p21.3	MHC class I antigen deficiency (*TAP2*)*
6p21.3	? Common variable immunodeficiency and selective IgA deficiency
7q11.23	Chronic granulomatous disease (gp47[phox])*
11	CD3 γ-chain deficiency*
11q22.3	Ataxia-telangiectasia (PI-3-like kinase)*
14q13.1	Purine nucleoside phosphorylase deficiency*
14q32.3	Immunoglobulin heavy-chain deletion*
15	MHC class II antigen deficiency (CIITA)*
16q24	Chronic granulomatous disease (gp22[phox])*
19p13.3	Janus kinase 3 (JAK3) deficiency
20q13-ter	Adenosine deaminase deficiency*
21q22.3	Leukocyte adhesion deficiency (CD18)*
22q11.2	DiGeorge syndrome*
Xp21.1	Chronic granulomatous disease (gp91[phox])*
Xp11.22-11.23	Wiskott-Aldrich syndrome (proline-rich protein, WASP)*
Xq13	Severe combined immunodeficiency (γ-chain of IL-2R, IL-2Rγ)*
Xq22	X-linked agammaglobulinemia (Bruton tyrosine kinase)*
Xq24-26	X-linked lymphoproliferative syndrome
Xq26	Immunodeficiency with hyper-IgM (CD40 ligand—gp39)*

* Gene cloned and sequenced, gene product known.
MHC, major histocompatibility complex; IgA, immunoglobulin A; IgM, immunoglobulin M; WASP, Wiskott-Aldrich syndrome protein.

ter susceptibility suggests a primary role for secretory IgA antibody in host defense against hepatitis and enteroviruses because normal T-cell function has been present in all XLA patients with persistent enterovirus infections reported thus far.

The diagnosis of XLA is confirmed when serum concentrations of IgG, IgA, IgM, and IgE are very low and there is a family history of similarly affected lateral maternal male relatives.[10] Tests for antibodies to blood group substances and to diphtheria, tetanus, *Haemophilus influenzae*, or pneumococcal vaccine antigens are useful in distinguishing this disorder from transient hypogammaglobulinemia of infancy. Hypoplasia of adenoids, tonsils, and peripheral lymph nodes is the rule; germinal centers are not found, and plasma cells are rare. Pre-B cells are present in the bone marrow, but blood B lymphocytes are usually absent. The abnormal gene in XLA was mapped to q22 on the long arm of the X chromosome and found to encode a B-cell protein-tyrosine kinase, now named *Bruton tyrosine kinase* (BTK) in honor of the discoverer of this condition.[11] BTK is a member of the Src-related nonreceptor tyrosine kinase family, which includes Lck, Fyn, and Lyn; this molecular family is involved in signal transduction in many hematopoietic cells. BTK is expressed at high levels in all B-lineage cells, including pre-B cells; it has not been detected in any cells of T lineage, but has been found in myeloid cells. BTK has been hypothesized to have a role in B-cell differentiation at all stages. Thus far,

all males with known XLA (by family history) have had low or undetectable BTK mRNA and kinase activity. Carriers can be detected by the finding of nonrandom X-chromosome inactivation in B cells.[11]

The fact that BTK is also expressed in cells of myeloid lineage is of interest because boys with XLA often have neutropenia at the height of an acute infection. In most XLA patients, the percentage of T cells is increased owing to the missing B cells, ratios of T-cell subsets are normal, and T-cell function is intact. The thymus has appeared morphologically normal in all autopsies. A condition that resembles XLA phenotypically and functionally has also been reported in girls—that is, there is an absence of circulating B cells. The molecular basis for that autosomal recessive defect will soon be reported. XLA has also been observed in association with growth hormone deficiency in nine cases.

Common Variable Immunodeficiency

Common variable immunodeficiency (CVID), also known as acquired hypogammaglobulinemia, can appear clinically similar in many respects to XLA. The kinds of infections experienced and bacterial etiologic agents involved are generally the same for the two defects. In CVID, however, there is an almost equal sex distribution, generally a later age of onset, somewhat less severe infections, a tendency for autoantibody formation, and normal-sized or enlarged tonsils and lymph nodes. Splenomegaly is present in about 25% of affected patients. CVID has also been associated with a spruelike syndrome, with or without nodular follicular lymphoid hyperplasia of the intestine; thymoma; alopecia areata; hemolytic anemia; gastric atrophy; achlorhydria; and pernicious anemia. Lymphoid interstitial pneumonia, pseudolymphoma, amyloidosis, and noncaseating granulomas of the lungs, spleen, skin, and liver have also been seen. There is a 438-fold increase in lymphomas in women affected in the fifth and sixth decades of life.[12]

The serum immunoglobulin and antibody deficiencies in CVID can be as profound as in XLA. Despite normal numbers of circulating immunoglobulin-bearing B lymphocytes and the presence of lymphoid cortical follicles, blood B lymphocytes from CVID patients do not differentiate normally into immunoglobulin-producing cells when stimulated with pokeweed mitogen in vitro, even when cocultured with normal T cells. Recent studies have shown, however, that CVID B cells can be stimulated to both isotype-switch and to synthesize and secrete immunoglobulin when stimulated with anti-CD40 plus IL-4 or IL-10. T cells and T-cell subsets are usually present in normal percentages, although T-cell function has been depressed in some patients.[12] Rarely, CVID has been reported to resolve transiently or permanently when these patients were infected with human immunodeficiency virus (HIV).

CVID occurs in first-degree relatives of patients with selective IgA deficiency, and some patients with IgA deficiency later become panhypogammaglobulinemic. Therefore, it is possible that these diseases have a common genetic basis. The high incidence of abnormal immunoglobulin concentrations, autoantibodies, autoimmune disease, and malignancy in families of both types of patients also suggest a shared hereditary influence. This concept is supported by the finding of a high incidence of C4A gene deletions and C2 rare gene alleles in the class III MHC region in patients with either IgA deficiency or CVID,

TABLE 12-4. *Characteristics of some genetic defects in the immune system*

Disorder	Functional deficiencies	Molecular defect
X-linked agammaglobulinemia	Antibody	Mutations in Bruton tyrosine kinase
Common variable immunodeficiency ("acquired" hypogammaglobulinemia)	Antibody	Unknown, ? in MHC Class III region
Selective IgA deficiency	IgA antibody	Unknown, ? in MHC Class III region
Immunodeficiency with elevated IgM	IgG and IgA antibodies	Mutations in CD40 ligand on activated T cells
Transient hypogammaglobulinemia of infancy	None; immunoglobulins low, but antibodies present	Unknown
Antibody deficiency with near-normal immunoglobulins	Antibody	Unknown; ? related to common variable immunodeficiency
X-linked lymphoproliferative disease	Anti-EBV nuclear antigen antibody	B cell; ? also T cell
DiGeorge syndrome	T cellular; some antibody	Mutations in gene at Xp21.1
Nezelof syndrome (including with PNP deficiency)	T cellular; some antibody	Unknown; PNP deficiency
Severe combined immunodeficiency syndromes (autosomal recessive; ADA deficiency; X-linked recessive; reticular dysgenesis)	Antibody and T cellular; phagocytic in reticular dysgenesis	Mutations in genes for ADA or JAK3 in some autosomal, in gene for IL-2Rγ in X-linked; unknown defects
Wiskott-Aldrich syndrome	Antibody and T cellular; platelets	Mutations in gene for proline-rich protein, WASP
CD3 deficiency	T cellular	Mutations in gene for CD3γ
CD8 lymphocytopenia	T cellular	Mutations in ZAP70
Hyperimmunoglobulinemia E syndrome	Specific immune responses; excessive IgE	Unknown
Ataxia-telangiectasia	Antibody; T cellular	Gene for PI-3–like kinase at 11q22.3
Leukocyte adhesion deficiency 1	Cytotoxic lymphocytes; phagocytic cell adhesion	Mutations in CD18
Leukocyte adhesion deficiency 2	Phagocytic cell adhesion	Unknown; Sialyl Lewis X not expressed

Ig, immunoglobulin; IL, interleukin; PNP, purine nucleoside phosphoylase; ADA, adenosine deaminase; EBV, Epstein-Barr virus; WASP, Wiskott-Aldrich syndrome protein; JAK3, janus kinase 3.

suggesting that the susceptibility genes are in this region on chromosome 6[13] (see Tables 12-3 and 12-4). These studies have also shown that a small number of HLA haplotypes are shared by patients affected with CVID and IgA deficiency, with at least one of two particular haplotypes being present in 77% of those affected. Environmental factors, particularly drugs such as phenytoin, D-penicillamine, gold, and sulfasalazine, have been suspected to trigger disease expression in patients with the permissive genetic background.

Selective Immunoglobulin A Deficiency

Absence or near absence of IgA is the most common primary immunodeficiency, with a frequency of 1 in 333 being reported among some putatively healthy US blood donors. This condition, however, is also commonly associated with ill health. As would be expected, infections occur predominantly in the respiratory, gastrointestinal, and urogenital tracts. Bacterial agents responsible are essentially the same as in other types of antibody deficiency syndromes. There is no clear evidence that patients with this disorder have an undue susceptibility to viral agents. Serum concentrations of other immunoglobulins are usually normal in patients with selective IgA deficiency, although IgG2 and other IgG subclass deficiencies have been reported, and IgM (usually elevated) may be monomeric.

As is the case for CVID, the basic defect leading to IgA deficiency is unknown (see Tables 12-3 and 12-4). Phenotypically normal blood B cells are present in both conditions. IgA deficiency has been known to remit spontaneously or after discontinuation of phenytoin (Dilantin) therapy. On the other hand, IgA deficiency has also been noted to evolve into CVID. Similar to patients with CVID, IgA-deficient patients have an increased incidence of malignancy.

Serum antibodies to IgA have been reported in as many as 44% of patients with selective IgA deficiency. These can lead to severe or fatal anaphylactic reactions after intravenous administration of blood products (including immunoglobulin preparations) containing IgA; IgE antibodies to IgA have been implicated as the cause.[14] For this reason, only five-times-washed normal donor erythrocytes or blood products from other IgA-absent people should be administered to these patients.

Other B-Cell Defects

Unlike patients with XLA or CVID, patients with *transient hypogammaglobulinemia of infancy* can usually synthesize antibodies to diphtheria and tetanus toxoids by 6 to 11 months of age, well before their immunoglobulin concentrations become normal.[15] Other patients have been reported to have *IgG subclass deficiencies* despite normal or elevated total serum IgG concentrations. Most with absent or very low concentrations of IgG2 have been patients with IgA deficiency. In others, continued follow-up revealed an evolving pattern of immunodeficiency (into CVID), suggesting that the presence of IgG subclass deficiency may be a marker for more general immune dysfunction. In this group of patients, it is important to ascertain the patient's capacity to make specific antibodies to protein and polysaccharide antigens before embarking on immunoglobulin therapy. Completely symptomless patients have been described who totally lack IgG1, IgG2, IgG4, or IgA1, owing to gene deletions. Conversely, profound deficiencies of antipolysaccharide antibodies have been noted in other patients, even in the presence of normal concentrations of IgG2.

X-linked lymphoproliferative disease (XLP), also referred to as *Duncan disease,* is a recessive trait characterized by an inadequate immune response to infection with EBV. The defective gene in XLP has been localized to chromosome Xq25-26. Affected patients are apparently healthy until they experience infectious mononucleosis; the mean age of presentation is younger than 5 years. The most common outcome is severe, fatal mononucleosis, primarily due to extensive liver necrosis caused by cytotoxic T cells that recognize EBV-infected autologous B cells. Most patients who survive the primary infection develop global cellular immune defects involving T, B, and NK cells, lymphomas, or hypogammaglobulinemia.

T-Cell Defects

In general, patients with defects in T-cell function have infections or other clinical problems that are of a more severe nature than those with antibody deficiency disorders (see Table 12-4).

Thymic Hypoplasia (DiGeorge Syndrome)

DiGeorge syndrome results from developmental abnormalities in the third and fourth pharyngeal pouches during early embryogenesis, leading to hypoplasia or aplasia of the thymus and parathyroid glands.[9] Other structures forming at the same age are also frequently affected, resulting in anomalies of the great vessels (right-sided aortic arch), esophageal atresia, bifid uvula, congenital heart disease (atrial and ventricular septal defects), a short philtrum of the upper lip, hypertelorism, an antimongoloid slant to the eyes, mandibular hypoplasia, and low-set, often notched ears. The syndrome is often first suggested by the presence of hypocalcemic seizures during the neonatal period.

Since the original description of the DiGeorge syndrome, it has become apparent that a variable degree of hypoplasia of the thymus and parathyroid glands is more frequent than total aplasia in this condition. Patients with variable hypoplasia are referred to as having *partial* DiGeorge syndrome; they may have little trouble with infections and grow normally. On the other hand, those with *complete* DiGeorge syndrome resemble patients with severe combined immunodeficiency (SCID) syndrome in their susceptibility to infections with low-grade or opportunistic pathogens (eg, fungi, viruses, and *P carinii*) and to GVHD from nonirradiated blood transfusions.

Serum immunoglobulins are usually near normal for the patient's age, but IgA can be diminished and IgE elevated. Lymphocyte counts are usually only moderately low for age. CD3-positive T cells are uniformly decreased in number, the degree of decrease corresponding to the degree of thymic hypoplasia; as a result, the percentage of B cells is increased. The CD4/CD8 ratio is usually normal. Lymphocyte proliferative responses to PHA and other T-cell mitogens, like intradermal delayed hypersensitivity responses, are absent, reduced, or normal, depending on the degrees of thymic deficiency. Thymic tissue, when found, does contain Hassall corpuscles and a normal density of thymocytes; corticomedullary distinction is present. Cortical follicles are usually present in lymph nodes, but paracortical areas and thymus-dependent regions of the spleen show variable degrees of T-cell depletion. Microdeletions of specific DNA sequences from chromosome 22q11.2 (the DiGeorge chromosomal region) have been shown in most patients.[16] A disrupted candidate gene has been identified in this region.[17]

X-Linked Immunodeficiency With Elevated Immunoglobulin M

Clinically, X-linked immunodeficiency with elevated IgM is characterized by very low serum concentrations of IgG and IgA but usually a markedly elevated concentration of polyclonal IgM. Like patients with XLA, affected boys become symptomatic during the first or second year of life, with recurrent pyogenic infections, including otitis media, sinusitis, pneumonia, and tonsillitis. In contrast to patients with XLA, however, the frequent presence of lymphoid hyperplasia often leads away from a diagnosis of immunodeficiency. Thymic-dependent lymphoid tissues and T-cell functions are usually described as normal, but some affected patients have been shown to have decreased T-cell function.

High titers of specific antibodies to blood group substances and to salmonella O antigen have been found in some patients, but no protective antibodies have been noted in most. There is an increased frequency of autoantibody-mediated disorders, particularly Coombs-positive hemolytic anemia and immune thrombocytopenia. Patients also often have transient, persistent, or cyclic neutropenia, not always on an autoimmune basis. Patients with elevated IgM usually have normal numbers of circulating B cells. B lymphocytes from boys with the X-linked form of this defect were shown several years ago to be capable of synthesizing not only IgM but also IgA and IgG when cocultured with a switch T-cell line, suggesting that the defect lay in T-lineage cells rather than in B-lineage cells. Until recently, this condition was classified as a B-cell defect. One form of this disorder, however, has been shown to be caused by mutations in a gene at chromosome Xq26 encoding a T-cell surface protein on activated CD4+ T_H cells, called gp39 (or CD40L), the ligand for CD40 on B cells.[10,11] Such mutations result in an inability of the T_H cell to signal B cells to undergo isotype switching, accounting for the production of only IgM. The T-cell defect is also considered a possible explanation for the occurrence of *P carinii* pneumonia and extensive verruca vulgaris lesions in some boys with this condition. Not all males with elevated IgM levels, however, have a mutation in the CD40L. In addition, there are females with this disorder, indicating that this phenotype has more than one genetic cause.[10]

Other T-Cell Defects

Defective expression of the TCR–CD3 complex was first found in two brothers in a Spanish family. One presented with severe infections and died at 31 months of age from autoimmune hemolytic anemia and viral pneumonia. The defect in this family was shown to be due to mutations in the CD3γ chain. The first type of defective cytokine production to be described was a selective inability to produce IL-2; two examples of this have been reported. Both patients presented in infancy with severe recurrent infections. The IL-2 gene was present in both, but no IL-2 message or protein was produced. Other T-cell cytokines were produced normally. A second type of cytokine deficiency was characterized by defective transcription of several lymphokine genes, including IL-2, IL-3, IL-4, and IL-5. The latter problem was attributed to abnormal binding of nuclear factor of activated T cells to response elements in IL-2 and IL-4 enhancers.[10]

Patients with *CD8 lymphocytopenia* present during infancy with severe, recurrent, often fatal infections. They have normal or elevated numbers of blood B cells and low to elevated serum immunoglobulin concentrations. Their blood lymphocytes exhibit normal expression of the T-cell surface antigens CD3 and CD4, but there is a near-total absence of CD8 + cells, and the CD4 + lymphocytes fail to respond to mitogens or to allogeneic cells in vitro or to generate cytotoxic T lymphocytes. By contrast, NK activity is normal. The thymus of one patient exhibited normal architecture; there were normal numbers of CD4 and CD8 double-positive thymocytes but an absence of CD8 single-positive thymocytes. This condition has been shown to be due to mutations in the gene on chromosome 2q12 encoding ZAP70, a non–Src family protein tyrosine kinase important in T-cell signaling.[18] Patients with other forms of *T-cell activation defects* have phenotypically normal T cells that fail to proliferate or produce cytokines in response to stimulation with mitogens, antigens, or other signals delivered to the T-cell antigen receptor. Most of these conditions remain to be characterized at a molecular level.

Defects Affecting Both T and B Cells

Severe Combined Immunodeficiency

The SCID syndrome is characterized by absence of T-cell and B-cell function from birth and great genetic diversity[19] (see Tables 12-3 and 12-4). SCID infants present within the first few months of life with frequent episodes of diarrhea, pneumonia, otitis, sepsis, and cutaneous infections. Growth may appear normal initially, but severe wasting begins soon after infections and diarrhea start. Persistent infections with opportunistic organisms, such as *Candida albicans*, *P carinii*, cytomegalovirus, EBV, parainfluenzae 3 virus, respiratory syncytial virus, adenovirus, varicella, and *bacille Calmette-Guérin* lead to death. These infants also lack the ability to reject foreign tissue and are, therefore, at risk for chronic GVHD from maternal immunocompetent T cells that cross the placenta or fatal GVHD from T lymphocytes in nonirradiated blood products or allogeneic bone marrow. Death usually occurs before the second birthday.

Profound lymphopenia, delayed cutaneous anergy, and an absence of lymphocyte proliferative responses to mitogens, antigens, and allogeneic cells in vitro characterize infants with SCID. They have very low (or absent) concentrations of serum immunoglobulins, and no antibody formation occurs after immunization. Monoclonal antibody analyses of SCID lymphocytes have demonstrated marked heterogeneity but characteristic phenotypic patterns among the different genetic types of SCID. Despite the uniformly profound lack of T or B cell function, patients with X-linked and januse kinase 3 (JAK3) deficient autosomal recessive SCID have elevated percentages of B cells. Monoclonal antibody studies have generally shown extremely low percentages of T cells and subsets in all types of SCID. All or most of the circulating lymphocytes in some infants with autosomal recessive SCID are large granular lymphocytes with NK cell phenotype and function, whereas NK cells and function are very low in X-linked and januse kinase 3 (JAK3) deficient autosomal recessive SCID patients, and all lymphocyte subsets are very low in adenosine deaminase (ADA)-deficient SCID. Patients with the SCID syndrome uniformly have very small thymuses (less than 1 g), which usually fail to descend from the neck, contain few thymocytes, and lack corticomedullary distinction and Hassall corpuscles. In contrast to the situation in the thymuses of patients with acquired immunodeficiency syndrome, in which there is marked epithelial atrophy, thymic epithelium appears histologically normal in all forms of SCID. Peripheral lymph nodes are either not found or are depleted of lymphocytes in all areas in SCID patients; tonsils, adenoids, and Peyer patches are absent or extremely underdeveloped. The fact that T-cell–depleted haploidentical bone marrow stem cells can correct these defects indicates that the thymuses in patients with SCID syndrome have normal capacities to differentiate stem cells into T cells.[20]

The first type to be described was *autosomal recessive SCID*, reported initially by Swiss workers in 1958. Patients with autosomal recessive SCID not due to ADA or JAK3 deficiency usually appear similar to those with the X-linked and JAK3-deficient forms, except that they generally have lower percentages of B cells and higher percentages of NK cells. The molecular bases of other autosomal recessive forms of SCID are unknown, but one is likely due to a defective recombinase mechanism, similar to abnormalities seen in SCID mice. *ADA deficiency*, due to a variety of mutations in the ADA gene (on chromosome 20q.13-ter), has been observed in about 15% of patients with SCID.[21] Excessive accumulations of adenosine, 2′-deoxyadenosine, and 2′-O-methyladenosine lead directly or indirectly to lymphocyte toxicity, which causes the immunodeficiency. ADA-deficient SCID infants usually have more profound lymphopenia than any other type, with severe reductions in T, B, and NK cells. Despite the low number of NK cells, however, they usually have normal NK function, in contrast to their profound T-cell deficiency. ADA-deficient SCID is also distinguished by multiple skeletal abnormalities of chondroosseous dysplasia at the costochondral junctions, at the apophyses of the iliac bones, and in the vertebral bodies.

X-linked SCID is probably the most common form of SCID in the United States. Blood B cells are usually higher in number in this defect than in any other form of SCID except JAK3 defiency; nevertheless, B-cell function is extremely abnormal. In addition, NK cell number and function are very low. The abnormal gene responsible for X-linked SCID was mapped by restriction fragment-length polymorphism analysis to chromosome Xq13 and identified as the gene encoding the γ chain of the IL-2 (T-cell growth factor) receptor (IL-2Rγ).[11] IL-2 plays a key role in intracellular signaling in T cells and, consequently, in the development, function, and regulation of the immune system. IL-2Rγ has also been shown to be a component of receptors for several other cytokines that regulate the function and development of the immune system, including IL-4, IL-7, IL-9, IL-15 and several others.[10] Carriers can be detected by demonstration of nonrandom X-chromosome inactivation in their T lymphocytes.[11] Recently an autosomal recessive form of SCID phenotypically similar to X-linked SCID was shown to be due to mutations in the gene on chromosome 19 encoding JAK3, the primary signal transducer for γc.

Reticular dysgenesis was first described in 1959 in identical twin male infants who exhibited a total lack of both lymphocytes and granulocytes in their peripheral blood and bone marrow. Infants with this defect die in early infancy from overwhelming infections.

Combined Immunodeficiency

Infants with combined immunodeficiency present slightly later than infants with SCID but also can have recurrent or chronic pulmonary infections, failure to thrive, oral or cutaneous candidiasis, chronic diarrhea, recurrent skin infections, gram-negative sepsis, urinary tract infections, and severe varicella.[9] Concentrations of all classes of serum immunoglobulins may be normal or elevated, but selective IgA deficiency and marked elevations of IgE and IgD have also been seen. Plasma cells are usually abundant in the lamina propria and lymph nodes. These patients may have neutropenia and eosinophilia.

T-cell function is markedly depressed in all patients with combined immunodeficiency, as evidenced by delayed cutaneous anergy to ubiquitous antigens, lymphopenia, and extremely low (but not absent) lymphocyte proliferative responses to mitogens, antigens, and allogeneic cells in vitro. Because of the presence of normal or elevated immunoglobulins and low but not absent T-cell function, this condition is the one primary immunodeficiency most likely to be confused with the acquired immunodeficiency syndrome in children. Paracortical areas of peripheral lymph nodes are depleted of T cells, as is the spleen. The thymuses are small and have a paucity of thymocytes and usually no Hassall corpuscles. Both males and females are affected, consistent with autosomal recessive inheritance.

Purine nucleoside phosphorylase (PNP) deficiency, resulting from mutations in the PNP gene on chromosome 14q13.1, has caused combined immunodeficiency in more than three dozen patients.[22] Unlike in patients with ADA deficiency, serum and urinary uric acid are markedly deficient, and no characteristic physical or skeletal abnormalities have been noted. All but a few of these children have died from generalized vaccinia, varicella, lymphosarcoma, or GVHD mediated by allogeneic T cells in nonirradiated blood or bone marrow. Neurologic abnormalities ranging from spasticity to mental retardation were noted in two thirds of these patients. Autoimmune diseases were seen in one third of the patients, the most common of which was autoimmune hemolytic anemia. Lymphopenia is profound, due primarily to a marked deficiency of T cells and T-cell subsets; T-cell function is decreased to varying degrees. Cells with NK phenotype and function are increased in number. Prenatal diagnosis is possible.

Immunodeficiency With Thrombocytopenia and Eczema (Wiskott-Aldrich Syndrome)

The Wiskott-Aldrich syndrome is characterized by atopic dermatitis, thrombocytopenic purpura, and undue susceptibility to infection.[9] There are normal-appearing megakaryocytes but small, defective platelets. Initially, infections (eg, otitis media, pneumonia, meningitis, sepsis) are caused by pneumococci and other bacteria with polysaccharide capsules. Later, infections with agents such as *P carinii* and the herpesviruses also develop. Survival beyond the teenage years is rare; infections or bleeding can cause death, but there is also a 12% incidence of fatal malignancy in this condition.

Wiskott-Aldrich patients have a severely impaired humoral immune response to polysaccharide antigens. Titers of antibodies to protein antigens also fall with time, and anamnestic responses are often poor or absent. There is an accelerated rate of synthesis and hypercatabolism of immunoglobulins, resulting in variable serum immunoglobulin concentrations. The usual pattern is low serum IgM, elevated IgA and IgE, and normal or slightly low IgG concentrations. Surprisingly, IgG2 subclass concentrations are normal. There are moderately reduced percentages of CD3, CD4, and CD8+ T cells, lymphocyte responses to mitogens are moderately depressed, and cutaneous anergy is a frequent finding. The abnormal gene is on the short arm of the X chromosome near the centromere; it was isolated and found to encode a 501−amino acid, proline-rich cytoplasmic protein (WASP), shown to be an effector for CDC242Hs, a member of the Rho family of GTP important in actin polymerization.[23] Nonrandom X-chromosome inactivation has been found in several hematopoietic cell lineages in female carriers of this defect.[11]

Ataxia-Telangiectasia

The most prominent clinical features of ataxia-telangiectasia are progressive cerebellar ataxia, oculocutaneous telangiectasia, chronic sinopulmonary disease, a high incidence of malignancy, and variable humoral and cellular immunodeficiency.[9] The cerebellar ataxia typically becomes evident soon after the child begins to walk, and the neurologic abnormalities progress until the child is confined to a wheelchair, usually by the age of 10 to 12 years. Telangiectasias develop in patients between 3 and 6 years of age, depending on the amount of sun exposure. Recurrent bacterial infections occur in most of these patients. Common viral infections do not result in untoward sequelae, but varicella can be fatal.

Selective IgA deficiency occurs in from 50% to 80% of these patients; hypercatabolism of IgA is also known to occur. IgD and IgE concentrations are usually low, and the IgM produced may be of the low-molecular-weight variety. Total IgG may be decreased, or IgG2 may be selectively absent. Specific antibody titers may be decreased or normal. In vitro tests of lymphocyte function have generally shown moderately depressed proliferative responses to T-cell and B-cell mitogens. CD3 and CD4+ T cells are reduced in number, while CD8+ cells are normal or increased. The thymus has a decreased number of thymocytes, is hypoplastic, exhibits poor organization, and is lacking in Hassall corpuscles.[9]

This defect is inherited in an autosomal recessive pattern. The mutated gene (ATM) responsible for this defect was mapped by restriction fragment-length polymorphism analysis to the long arm of chromosome 11 (11q22-23)[24,25] and has been cloned.[26] The gene product is similar to phosphotidyl inositol-3′ kinases involved in mitogenic signal transduction, meiotic recombination, and cell cycle control. Cultured cells from patients and from heterozygotes demonstrate increased sensitivity to ionizing radiation, defective DNA repair, and frequent chromosomal abnormalities. In more than half of cases, chromosomal breakage involves genes that code for the TCR and immunoglobulin heavy chains, possibly accounting for the combined T-cell and B-cell abnormalities seen. Malignancies are most often of the lymphoreticular type, but adenocarcinomas have also been seen, and there is an increased incidence of malignancy in unaffected relatives.[9]

Hyperimmunoglobulinemia E Syndrome

The hyperimmunoglobulinemia E syndrome is characterized by recurrent severe staphylococcal abscesses and markedly elevated levels of serum IgE.[27] This relatively rare primary immunodeficiency was first reported in 1972; many other examples have since been reported. Staphylococcal abscesses involving the skin, lungs, joints, and other sites develop first during infancy; persistent pneumatoceles develop as a result of recurrent staphylococcal pneumonias. There is a pruritic dermatitis that is not typical atopic eczema; it does not always persist; respiratory allergic symptoms are usually absent.

These patients have a pronounced blood and sputum eosinophilia. Serum IgE concentrations are usually exceptionally high; serum IgD concentrations may also be elevated. In vitro studies suggest a high level of endogenous IL-4 production. IgG, IgA, and IgM concentrations are usually normal, but there are often abnormally low anamnestic antibody responses and poor antibody- and cell-mediated responses to neoantigens. Blood CD2, CD3, CD4, and CD8 + lymphocytes are present in normal number. Most patients have normal T-lymphocyte proliferative responses to mitogens but low or absent responses to soluble antigens or to allogeneic cells from family members. Blood, sputum, and histologic sections of lymph nodes, spleen, and lung cysts show striking eosinophilia. Hassall corpuscles and thymic architecture are normal. The primary cause of this disorder is unknown.[27]

Phagocytosis and bacterial killing are normal in all patients. Total hemolytic complement activity is also normal. Variable chemotactic defects have been reported in some patients, but most do not have such abnormalities; hence, defective chemotaxis cannot be the basic problem. Both men and women have been affected, as have members of succeeding generations, suggesting an autosomal dominant form of inheritance with incomplete penetrance. Treatment for this condition is lifelong administration of therapeutic doses of a penicillinase-resistant penicillin, with the addition of other antibiotics or antifungal agents as required for specific infections. Surgery should be undertaken to remove superinfected pneumatoceles or large cysts persisting beyond 6 months.[28]

Defective Expression of Major Histocompatibility Complex Antigens

The two main forms of defective expression of MHC antigens are class I MHC antigen deficiency (bare lymphocyte syndrome) and class II MHC antigen deficiency.[29] Isolated deficiency of MHC class I antigens is rare, and the deficiency is much milder than in SCID, resulting in a later age of presentation. There is a deficiency of CD8 + but not of CD4 + T cells. Two siblings from a Moroccan family presented with relatively late-onset, recurrent, severe bacterial pulmonary infections and were found to have a nonsense mutation in one of two genes within the MHC locus on chromosome 6 that encode the antigenic peptide transporter protein known as TAP.[30] The genes are designated TAP1 and TAP2; the affected siblings had a nonsense mutation in TAP2. Both had a deficiency of CD8 + cells and lacked MHC class I antigens on their lymphocytes. TAP functions to transport antigenic peptides from the cytoplasm across the Golgi apparatus membrane to join the α chain of MHC class I antigens and β_2-microglobulin, which are then assembled into an MHC class I complex that can move to the cell surface. If the assembly of the complex cannot be completed because there is no antigenic peptide, the MHC class I complex is destroyed in the cytoplasm.

MHC class II deficiency is also an autosomal recessive syndrome, but the defects identified do not segregate with the MHC genes, which are encoded on chromosome 6 (6p21.3).[29] Many affected are of North African descent. Immunologic studies reveal a deficiency of CD4 + T cells but normal or elevated numbers of CD8 + T cells. The MHC class II antigens, HLA-DP, HLA-DQ, and HLA-DR, are undetectable on blood B cells and monocytes, even though B cells are present in normal number. MHC antigen–deficient B cells fail to stimulate allogeneic cells in MLC and present antigen poorly. Lymphocyte proliferation studies show normal responses to mitogens but no response to antigens. The thymus and other lymphoid organs are severely hypoplastic. MHC class II antigen deficiency is genetically heterogeneous; three different complementation groups have been reported. Two different molecular defects have been defined thus far; both cause impairment in the coordinate expression of MHC class II molecules on the surfaces of B cells and macrophages. In one, there is a mutation in the gene on chromosome 2 that encodes a protein called RFX5, a promoter protein that binds to the MHC class II gene promoter region X box.[31] In the other, there is a mutation in the gene on chromosome 15 that encodes a novel MHC class II transactivator, called *CIITA*, that coordinates the binding of proteins to the MHC class II gene promoter region.[32] The associated defects of both B-cell and T-cell immunity and of HLA expression emphasize the important biologic role for HLA determinants in effective immune cell cooperation.

Other Defects Affecting Both T and B Cells

Cartilage hair hypoplasia is a form of short-limbed dwarfism characterized by undue susceptibility to infection.[9] Severe and often fatal varicella infections and vaccine-associated poliomyelitis have been observed. Disease severity varies; in one series, 11 of 77 patients died before 20 years of age, but two were still alive at 76 years of age. Affected patients have short and pudgy hands; redundant skin; hyperextensible joints of hands and feet; and fine, sparse light hair and eyebrows. Radiographically, the bones show scalloping and sclerotic or cystic changes in the metaphyses. There are decreased numbers of T cells and defective T-cell proliferation in vitro due to an intrinsic defect related to the G_1 phase, resulting in a longer cell cycle for individual cells. NK cells are increased in number and function in these patients. This condition appears to be inherited in an autosomal recessive pattern, with variable penetrance.

Omenn syndrome is characterized by combined immunodeficiency with hypereosinophilia and elevated serum IgE. It is a fatal, autosomal recessively inherited condition with profound infection susceptibility. T-cell infiltration of skin, gut, liver, and spleen leads to an exfoliative erythroderma, lymphadenopathy, hepatosplenomegaly, and intractable diarrhea. Affected infants have a persistent leukocytosis, with low IgG, IgA, and IgM, and impaired T-cell function due to restricted heterogeneity of the host T-cell repertoire.[9] A T_H2-like cell dominance has been reported.[10]

Phagocytic Cell Disorders

Phagocytic cell disorders are most commonly due to an insufficient number of phagocytic cells, as in aplastic anemia. In some conditions, however, the number of cells is normal, but the function is impaired for a variety of reasons.[6] These disorders are characterized by recurrent infections and by impaired wound healing, both problems of substantial surgical importance.

Congenital Neutropenias

Some of the congenital forms of neutropenia are severe—such as Kostmann syndrome, in which neutrophil counts are less than $100/\mu L$—but there are other less severe forms. Neutropenia can also be associated with pancreatic insufficiency (Shwachman syndrome) and several primary immunodeficiency disorders, including XLA, hyper IgM, and reticular dysgenesis. Cyclic neutropenia is an autosomal dominant disorder that usually presents in infancy and occurs as an isolated abnormality. The molecular cause is not known for any of the neutropenias, but the association of some of them with other immunologic disorders suggests the possibility of abnormal cytokine production. Others are thought to be due to myeloid maturation arrests.[6]

Leukocyte Adhesion Defects

Leukocyte adhesion defect type 1 (LAD-1) is a syndrome characterized clinically by delayed separation of the umbilical cord, persistent leukocytosis, and recurrent necrotic infections of the skin, mucous membranes, and gastrointestinal tract.[7] Despite the elevated number of circulating polymorphonuclear cells, few leukocytes are found in the local lesions. The defect in these patients is due to mutations in the gene encoding CD18, a 95,000-kd member of the β_2-integrin family of cell-surface proteins. CD18 serves as the common β chain of three different $\alpha\beta$-heterodimer adhesion molecules: leukocyte function antigen 1 (LFA-1), complement receptor type 3 (CR3), and complement receptor type 4 (CR4). LFA-1 is found on nearly all immune cells and mediates lymphocyte adhesion. Thus, natural killer cell activity and T-cell–mediated cytotoxicity are absent in LAD-1 because adhesion molecules are critical for effector-to-target cell binding. LFA-1 also participates in the mobilization of leukocytes to infected or inflamed tissues by causing

their firm binding to endothelial cells. A ligand for all of these molecules is ICAM-1, which is widely distributed on lymphocytes, macrophages, and activated endothelial cells. CR3 is found on monocytes, granulocytes, macrophages, and NK cells; CR4 is found on monocytes and neutrophils. In addition to binding ICAM-1, CR3 also binds the C3bi fragment of complement to promote phagocytosis and respiratory burst activity. The ability of LAD-1 phagocytic cells to kill intracellular microorganisms is normal, but because the cells cannot be mobilized to the sites of infection and complement-mediated phagocytosis is impaired, the result is a lack of phagocytic cell function. Patients with less than 0.5% normal amounts of CD11/18 usually die of overwhelming microbial infections within the first few years of life, whereas those with with 3% to 10% have a much better prognosis for survival. These patients, however, are plagued by recurrent ulcers of the mucous membranes, severe periodontal disease, and recurrent skin infections.[7]

LAD-2 was described in two unrelated Israeli children who were products of consanguinous parents.[10] Both presented with severe mental retardation, short stature, and distinctive facies. They had recurrent severe bacterial infections, including pneumonia, peridontal disease, otitis media, and cellulitis, despite a marked leukocytosis. Expression of CD18 was normal, as was NK function. The patients were found to have the Bombay (hh) blood phenotype and were secretor-negative and Lewis-negative. Both lacked Sialyl-Lewis X (CD15) on their neutrophils; Sialyl-Lewis X is the ligand for E-selectin on endothelial cells. Production of the red-cell H antigen and secretor status require the presence of a distinct α1,2-fucosyl transferase, and production of Sialyl-Lewis X requires an α1,3-fucosyltransferase, so LAD-2 is thought to be due to a general defect (as yet undefined) in fucose metabolism.[10]

Chronic Granulomatous Disease

Chronic granulomatous disease (CGD) is a syndrome characterized by defective intracellular killing of bacterial and fungal organisms despite normal chemotaxis and phagocytosis; the defects are due to an inability of the phagocytic cell to mount a respiratory burst.[6] Patients have an increased incidence of infections with catalase-positive organisms, such as *Staphylococcus aureus, Escherichia coli, Serratia marcescens, Salmonella* sp, *Candida albicans*, and *Aspergillus* sp, but not with catalase-negative organisms, such as *Streptococcus pneumoniae*, which provide the oxygen radicals needed for phagocytic cell killing.[33] Most patients develop cutaneous, lymphoid, or visceral abscesses that respond poorly to antibiotics; these lesions often require surgical drainage. As a result of ineffective destruction of phagocytized organisms and compensatory responses by lymphoid cells, granulomatous lesions are also formed, especially in the liver, gastrointestinal, and urinary tracts. Osteomyelitis caused by bacteria (particularly *Serratia marcescens*) or fungi (especially *Aspergillus* sp) is a frequent complication.[33]

Different molecular defects in the electron transport chain have been identified in four different types of CGD. About 65% of patients have an X-linked (X-CGD) defect, and the remainder have autosomal recessive (AR-CGD) inheritance.[6] X-CGD is due to mutations at Xp21.1 in the gene encoding the heavy chain of cytochrome b-245, a glycoprotein of 91 kd (gp91[phox]). In about 5% of patients with CGD, there are mutations in the gene on chromosome 16q24 that encodes the light chain of cytochrome b-245, a 22-kd glycoprotein (p22[phox]). Other autosomal recessive forms of CGD are due either to mutations in the gene at chromosome 7q11.23 encoding a 47-kd cytosolic factor (gp47[phox]) essential for oxygen generation (25% of all patients) or in the gene at chromosome 1q25 encoding a 67-kd cytosolic factor (gp67[phox]), also essential for oxygen generation (5% of all patients).[6]

The diagnosis of CGD is made by demonstrating an inability of neutrophils from the patient to undergo a respiratory burst after phagocytosis or to kill bacteria, such as *S. aureus* or gram-negative bacteria.

Aggressive treatment with antibiotics, especially trimethaprim-sulfamethoxazole, antistaphylococcal penicillins, and aminoglycosides, has reduced the frequency and severity of bacterial infections in these patients.[33] Fungal infections, especially those due to aspergillus, currently account for most deaths. Amphotericin B, with or without alternate-day normal granulocyte transfusions, is the initial treatment of choice. Once aspergillus infections are brought under control with the latter therapy, chronic therapy with itraconazole appears to be effective in preventing recurrences.

Disorders of the Complement System

Deficiencies in almost all of the complement proteins have been discovered.[34] The extraordinary rarity of these defects attests to the importance of complement proteins in host defense. By contrast, heterozygosity for complement protein deficiencies is relatively common in the population. Such heterozygotes fortunately do not have a higher incidence of infections or autoimmune disease than is found in the general population.

Complement deficiencies can be classified generally into those involving proteins of the alternative pathway, those involving proteins of the classic pathway, or those involving late components of complement.[34] Clinically, patients with either classic pathway or late-component deficiencies tend to do relatively well, except when stressed by septicemia or any infection with a high-grade pathogen. Patients deficient in components of the alternative pathway tend to have frequent and severe infections early in life because this pathway serves as a major host defense mechanism against first infections.[35] These patients develop antibodies to specific infectious agents. Thus, complement-deficient adults are often less susceptible than very young infants with even normal complement levels who have not yet made such antibodies.

A high incidence of autoimmune disease is also seen in patients with inherited complement deficiencies, possibly due to defects in removing normally generated immune complexes from the circulation. This however, is not a clearly defined function for complement proteins. These complexes may then localize in the kidneys and other tissues, causing inflammatory reactions.

Early-Component Deficiencies

C1q, C1r, C1s, C2, and C4 deficiencies are inherited in an autosomal recessive pattern. About 1 person in 10,000 has no detectable serum C2, making this defect the most common inherited complement deficiency state.[34] Each of the classic pathway component deficiencies can result in increased susceptibility to infections with encapsulated bacteria, but this susceptibility is less than in alternative pathway deficiencies. Some patients with C2 deficiency have had recurrent septicemia, meningitis, or osteomyelitis; however, clinically normal people with C2 deficiency have also been described.[35]

Each of the classic pathway component deficiencies may also result in a syndrome similar to discoid lupus or systemic lupus erythematosus (SLE). In patients with SLE-like syndrome, disease begins at an early age, with marked photosensitivity and a low but clinically significant incidence of renal disease. Patients with C2 or C4 deficiency have an increased incidence of Henoch-Schönlein purpura as well as glomerulonephritis. In addition, dermatomyositis, vasculitis, cold urticaria, inflammatory bowel disease, Hodgkin disease, and CVID have each been reported in these patients.[34]

Alternative-Pathway Deficiencies

Alternative-pathway defects often predispose to recurrent infections due to encapsulated pyogenic organisms, manifesting as pneumonia, otitis media, or sinusitis.[35] One example is C3 deficiency, a rare syndrome due to either hypercatabolism or hyposynthesis of C3. Patients with C3 hypercatabolism have increased serum levels of C3 inactivator. C3 deficiency is often associated with repeated infections with both low-grade and high-grade pathogens.

Late-Component Deficiencies

Hereditary deficiency of the terminal complement components (C5, C6, C7, C8) may be present in healthy people or may be associated with an increased incidence of infection or autoimmune disease. Deficiencies of these late complement components lead to a high incidence of disseminated neisserial infections, such as recurrent meningococcal meningitis or gonococcal arthritis. Mere opsonization of neisserial organisms appears to be inadequate for their elimination because C3—the principal opsonin generated by complement—is normal in these patients; lysis is required for the destruction of these organisms. Although some patients with C5 deficiency are clinically healthy, some have been reported to have SLE and associated Raynaud phenomena, arthritis, diffuse membranoproliferative glomerulonephritis, recurrent pneumococcal pneumonia, or disseminated gonococcal infection. C7 and C8 deficiencies may also be associated with autoimmune diseases such as SLE and rheumatoid arthritis.[34]

A diagnosis of hereditary complement protein deficiency should be considered in any child with recurrent infections with high-grade encapsulated organisms, with or without the presence of an autoimmune disease. The diagnosis of deficient terminal complement components should be suspected in any patient with recurrent neisserial infections. The total hemolytic complement assay (CH50) is the most useful screening procedure because the CH50 is profoundly low in most of these defects. Many of the individual complement components can be quantified only in research laboratories.[34]

TREATMENT OF IMMUNODEFICIENCIES

B-Cell Defects

Judicious use of antibiotics and regular administration of antibodies have been shown to be effective for this group of disorders.[36] The most common form of replacement therapy is intravenous immune serum globulin (IVIG). Broad antibody deficiency should be carefully documented before IVIG therapy is initiated. The rationale for the use of these preparations is to provide missing antibodies, not to raise the serum IgG concentration. Seven IVIG preparations have been approved by the Food and Drug Administration and are available in the United States; nearly three dozen more are under investigation or marketed abroad. HIV is inactivated by the ethanol used in preparation of immune serum globulin for intramuscular (ISG) and intravenous immune globulin (IVIG); such preparations have also been modified by the addition of a detergent to ensure that they are free of hepatitis viruses. All commercial lots are produced from plasma pooled from 3000 to 6000 donors and, therefore, contain a broad spectrum of antibodies. Each pool must contain adequate levels of antibody to antigens in various vaccines. There is no standardization based on titers of antibodies to clinically relevant organisms, such as *S pneumoniae* or *H influenzae*.[36]

In general, the preparations available in the United States have similar efficacy and safety. There has been no documented transmission of HIV infection by any of them. Before the detergent-modified preparations became available, however hepatitis C was transmitted by a few such preparations in late 1993. Experience suggests that 400 mg/kg/mo of IVIG permits achievement of trough IgG levels close to the normal range. Systemic reactions to IVIG can occur but only rarely true anaphylactic reactions. Anaphylactic reactions caused by IgE antibodies (in the patient) to IgA (in the IVIG preparation) may, however, occur in patients with CVID who lack serum IgA or in those with selective IgA deficiency.[14] All newly diagnosed patients with CVID should be screened for anti-IgA antibodies through the American Red Cross before undergoing IVIG therapy. If such antibodies are detected, IVIG therapy may still be possible by use of the one available IVIG preparation containing almost no IgA (Gammagard, Baxter-Hyland); carefully screened lots of Gammagard can be used safely in patients who have antibodies to IgA.[36]

Complement Deficiencies

Antibiotics are used to treat acute infections in patients with complement deficiencies and, in some patients, for prophylaxis against future infections.[34] Complement components cannot yet be replaced; even if this were possible, it is likely that antibodies would be produced to the missing protein. All of the complement proteins and regulator genes have been sequenced, and many have been cloned. Gene therapy is, therefore, a potential future form of therapy for patients with inborn errors of the complement system.[37]

Bone Marrow Transplantation

The treatment of choice for patients with fatal T-cell or combined T-cell and B-cell defects is transplantation of normal bone marrow stem cells.[20] In addition to the usual problem of potential rejection of the graft by immune cells of the recipient, allogeneic marrow transplantation is complicated by specific problems not usually encountered in solid organ transplantation. Immunosuppressive agents commonly used to ensure the acceptance of solid organ grafts have deleterious effects on the very cells one is trying to engraft in patients with genetically determined immunodeficiency. Therefore, immunosuppressive and myeloablative agents must be given *before* infusion of the marrow to avoid injury to the donor cells. Except in infants with SCID or complete DiGeorge syndrome who have absent T-cell function and are therefore unable to reject allografts, all other immunodeficient recipients have to be preconditioned with chemotherapeutic agents to prevent graft rejection. The most important problem unique to bone marrow transplantation is that donor T cells in the transplanted marrow can also "reject" the recipient, causing GVHD. Earlier efforts to circumvent the lack of a match by fractionating HLA-nonidentical bone marrow on albumin density gradients or by using transplants of fetal liver or thymus were thwarted either by the recipient developing lethal GVHD from residual donor T cells or by failure of immune reconstitution from fetal tissue transplants. These initial attempts taught us that, unlike the situation in solid organ transplantation, HLA identity (at least for class II) between donor and recipient was required for successful unfractionated bone marrow transplantation. Because of these unique problems, bone marrow transplantation had until recently required strict HLA-D locus compatibility. Nevertheless, even in HLA-identical marrow transplantation, GVHD occurs, and it is severe or fatal in a significant proportion of recipients who require pretransplantation conditioning with chemotherapeutic agents.

HLA was discovered in 1968. From 1968 to 1977, however, only 14 (or 29%) of 48 infants with SCID worldwide were long-term survivors of successful HLA class II compatible bone marrow transplantations. Fortunately, the results of bone marrow transplantation have improved considerably during the past decade, owing to earlier diagnosis before untreatable opportunistic infections develop, the availability of better antimicrobials to treat infections, and the development of techniques to deplete all postthymic T cells from donor marrow. The latter techniques employ either incubation with monoclonal antibodies to T cells plus complement or soybean lectin incubation, followed by sheep erythrocyte rosette–depletion. Both methods enrich the final cell suspension for stem cells, but the degree of T-cell depletion is almost a log greater with the latter technique. T-cell depletion has permitted the safe and successful use of haploidentical (half-matched) bone marrow cells for the correction of SCID and other fatal immunodeficiency syndromes without fatal GVHD. After T-cell–depleted normal marrow is transplanted into a SCID infant, it takes 90 to 120 days for T cells to appear in the circulation, whether the stem cells are HLA-identical or haploidentical (half-matched) to the infant. This is in contrast to the results with unfractionated HLA-identical marrow, in which immune function can be seen as early as 2 to 3 weeks after transplantation, owing to adoptive transfer of donor mature T and B cells. The long-term results, however, are similar (Fig. 12-4).

I recently conducted a worldwide survey of physicians performing bone marrow transplantations in immunodeficiency patients and found that 195 of 243 patients (80%) with primary immunodeficiency who received HLA-identical transplanted

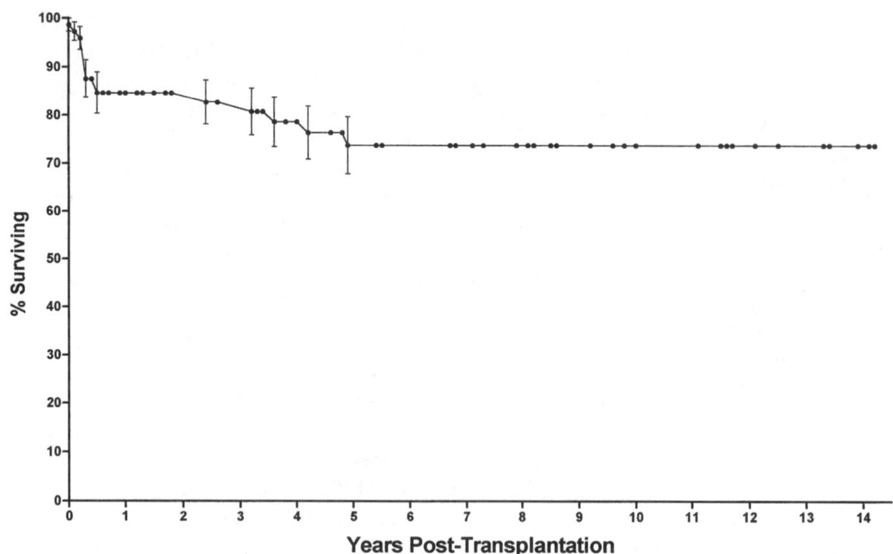

FIG. 12-4. Kaplan-Meier survival curve for 74 infants with severe combined immunodeficiency syndrome (SCIDS) who received bone marrow transplants from 12 HLA-identical or 62 haploidentical donors. To date sixty-eight patients survived for 1 month to 14 years after transplantation.

marrow during the past 26 years survived. In addition, the results of T-cell–depleted haploidentical (half-matched) marrow transplantations in patients with primary immunodeficiency are most encouraging: 535 of these transplantations were performed during the past 12 years, and 291 (or 54%) survived. Most of the 535 recipients would have died had not the new T-cell depletion techniques been developed. In addition to SCID, the immune deficiency in the complete DiGeorge syndrome can also be corrected by unfractionated HLA-identical bone marrow without prior immunosuppression. The latter is effective because of adoptive transfer of mature T cells present in the donor marrow; these infants do not have a thymus to ''educate'' the donor stem cells.

Patients with less severe forms of cellular immunodeficiency (eg, Nezelof syndrome, ataxia-telangiectasia, Wiskott-Aldrich syndrome, cytokine deficiency, MHC antigen deficiency) reject even HLA-identical marrow grafts unless they are cytoreduced with immunosuppressive agents before transplantation. Bone marrow transplantation has corrected the immune defects in three patients with PNP deficiency, and gene therapy is a possibility for the future. Several patients with Wiskott-Aldrich syndrome, LAD, and other forms of partial cellular immunodeficiency have also been treated successfully with (usually HLA-identical) bone marrow transplants after immunosuppression. Several children with LAD-1 have been cured by transplantation of allogeneic bone marrow from a haploidentical parent (using T-cell–depleted marrow). The gene for CD18 has been cloned and successfully transfected into LAD-1 lymphoblasts in vitro, with resultant surface expression of CD18. Thus, it may be possible to correct this defect in the future by inserting a normal CD18 gene into LAD-1 stem cells. Bone marrow transplantation has not been successful in reconstituting phagocytic cell function in CGD patients, primarily because full cytoreduction is necessary to gain graft acceptance by CGD patients, and many have chronic indolent bacterial or fungal infections that could not be controlled if such chemotherapy were to be given. As with the many other immunologic defects for which the molecular bases are being discovered, once the technical problems preventing adequate gene insertion therapy into hematopoietic stem cells are overcome, patients with CGD will be ideal candidates for this type of therapy.[37] Until somatic cell gene therapy is more fully developed, however, bone marrow transplantation remains the most important and effective therapy for inborn errors of the immune system.

Other Therapies

Enzyme replacement therapy with polyethylene glycol-modified bovine ADA (PEG-ADA) administered subcutaneously once weekly has resulted in both clinical and immunologic improvement in about 30 ADA-deficient patients.[10] Bone marrow transplantation remains the treatment of choice, however, so PEG-ADA therapy should be withheld if this is planned because it confers graft-rejection capability. Attempts to correct the immunologic and enzymatic deficiencies of PNP-deficient patients by enzyme or other metabolic replacement therapy have not been successful. Cytokine-deficient patients have been treated with recombinant IL-2 with some clinical improvement. In addition, a double-blind placebo-controlled study of the efficacy and safety of subcutaneous injections of IFN-γ reported a significant reduction in the number of infections requiring hospitalization in CGD patients who received IFN-γ subcutaneously three times a week, as compared with the number of infections in placebo-treated CGD patients.[6] There was no improvement, however, in phagocytic cell oxidative or microbicidal functions.

Surgical Procedures

Surgical procedures are often needed in the management of patients with primary immunodeficiency diseases, particularly in the diagnosis of obscure infections and in the maintenance of nutrition during critical and prolonged illnesses.

Diagnostic and Management Procedures

Some types of defects characteristically require certain types of surgical procedures more often than others. For example, patients with phagocytic cell defects and those with the hyperimmunoglobulinemia E syndrome frequently require incision and drainage of abscesses, including those involving subcutaneous tissues, lymph nodes, liver, lung, and other sites. Patients with a CGD often require bone biopsies of apparent osteomyelitic lesions. Patients with primary immunodeficiency diseases who develop pneumonia frequently have unusual or opportunistic etiologic agents that require bronchoscopy or open lung biopsy for identification of the pathogen, chest tubes to resolve empyema or pneumothoraces, resection of bronchiectatic lobes or entire lungs, and at times performance of tracheostomies for prolonged ventilator support. Infants with T-cell deficiencies of any type are also likely to require placement of central lines to provide total parenteral nutrition, fluid, electrolyte, and antibiotic delivery and access for frequent laboratory testing. This is true, in particular, for those who are undergoing bone marrow transplantations. Many infants with SCID, DiGeorge syndrome, and other lethal primary immunodeficiencies also have significant gastroesophageal reflux and require Nisson fundoplications to prevent aspiration, and gastric tube placement for nutritional support. As already noted, infants with DiGeorge syndrome usually have significant cardiac anomalies, and many require correction early in life. The use of irradiated blood products is absolutely essential during any surgical procedure on infants or children when there is any possibility of T-cell deficiency. By contrast, nonirradiated blood should be used during any surgical procedure for patients with phagocytic cell functional defects (eg, CGD, LAD) who do not have T-cell defects so that the function of the transfused normal phagocytic cells is not impaired.

Thymic Transplantations

Infants with complete DiGeorge syndrome who do not have an HLA-identical donor cannot benefit from T-cell–depleted haploidentical normal stem cell transplantations because they do not have a thymus gland in which such stem cells can develop into mature and functional T cells. In contrast to SCID infants, DiGeorge patients do have normal stem cells. Therefore, it has seemed logical for many years that thymic transplantation might benefit such infants, and the first attempt at this was made in 1968, with reportedly good success. Because the T cells that emerged were usually of host origin, however, it was difficult to prove that the T-cell function that developed after these transplantations was truly due to "education" of the host's stem cells in the transplanted thymus. Because the partial form of this syndrome is far more common, the alternate possibility is that there was gradual development of T-cell function in the tiny residual host thymic tissue. In a review of all published cases of DiGeorge syndrome patients who had received thymic tissue transplantations before 1987, Goldsobel and coworkers[38] reported that there were few survivors and that there was no objective evidence that the survivors' T-cell function was due to the thymic tissue implants. Moreover, most had received thymic tissue obtained from aborted fetuses, and the others received frozen fetal thymuses provided by the Marsden Tissue

Bank in England. Therefore, the viability of the tissues is unknown. Later, slices of mature thymic tissue that had been cultured for a period of time in vitro such that most donor thymocytes had died were implanted at various sites in a number of patients with DiGeorge syndrome and other T-cell deficiencies, with varying degrees of success. However, few, if any, patients survived long term. Recent improvements in this approach include (1) attempts to match at least one HLA class II antigen (and one or more class I antigens if possible) of the thymus donor with that of the recipient, (2) attempts to follow the status of the thymic graft carefully with frequent biopsies, and (3) attempts to use molecular techniques to establish the origin and repertoire of the T cells that emerge later in the recipient. Early results with this new approach appear promising.

REFERENCES

1. Whiteside TL. Cytokine measurements and interpretation of cytokine assays in human disease. J Clin Immunol 1994;14:327.
2. Schlossman SF, Boumsell L, Gilks W, et al. Leucocyte typing. V. White cell differentiation antigens. Oxford, UK, Oxford University Press, 1994 (in press).
3. Haynes BF, Denning SM. Lymphopoiesis. In: Stamatoyannopoulis G, Nienhuis AW, Majarus P, et al, eds. Molecular basis of blood diseases, ed 2. Philadelphia, WB Saunders, 1994:425.
4. Hannet I, Erkeller-Yuksel F, Lydyard P, et al. Developmental and maturational changes in human blood lymphocyte subpopulations. Immunol Today 1992;13:215.
5. Noelle RJ, Roy M, Shepherd DM, et al. A 39-kDa protein on activated helper T cells binds CD40 and transduces the signal for cognate activation of B cells. Proc Natl Acad Sci USA 1992;89:6550.
6. Dinauer MC. Leukocyte function and nonmalignant leukocyte disorders. Curr Opin Pediatr 1993;5:80.
7. Kishimoto TK, Springer TA. Human leukocyte adhesion deficiency: molecular basis for a defective immune response to infections of the skin. Curr Prob Dermatol 1989;18:106.
8. Frank MM. The complement system. In: Frank MM, Austen KF, Claman HN, et al, eds. Samter's immunologic diseases, ed 5. Boston, Little, Brown, 1994:331.
9. WHO Scientific Group. Primary immunodeficiency diseases: report of a WHO scientific group. Clin Exp Immunol 1995;99:1.
10. Buckley RH. Breakthroughs in the understanding and therapy of primary immunodeficiency. Pediatr Clin North Am 1994;41:665.
11. Puck JM. Molecular and genetic basis of X-linked immunodeficiency disorders. J Clin Immunol 1994;14:81.
12. Cunningham-Rundles C. Clinical and immunologic analyses of 103 patients with common variable immunodeficiency. J Clin Immunol 1988;9:22.
13. Schaffer FM, Palermos J, Zhu ZB, et al. Individuals with IgA deficiency and common variable immunodeficiency share complex polymorphisms of major histocompatibility complex class III genes. Proc Nat Acad Sci 1989;86:8015.
14. Burks AW, Sampson HA, Buckley RH. Anaphylactic reactions after gamma globulin administration in patients with hypogammaglobulinemia. N Engl J Med 1986;314:560.
15. Tiller TL, Buckley RH. Transient hypogammaglobulinemia of infancy: review of the literature, clinical and immunologic features of 11 new cases, and long-term follow-up. J Pediatr 1978;92:347.
16. Driscoll DA, Budarf ML, Emanuel BS. A genetic etiology for DiGeorge syndrome: consistent deletions and microdeletions of 22q11. Am J Hum Genet 1992;50:924.
17. Budarf ML, Collins J, Gong W, et al. Cloning a balanced translocation associated with DiGeorge syndrome and identification of a disrupted candidate gene. Nature Genet 1995;10:269.
18. Elder ME, Lin D, Clever J, et al. Human severe combined immunodeficiency due to a defect in ZAP-70, a T cell tyrosine kinase. Science 1994;264:1596.
19. Fischer A. Severe combined immunodeficiencies. Immunodef Rev 1992;3:83.

20. Buckley RH, Schiff SE, Schiff RI, et al. Haploidentical bone marrow stem cell transplantation in human severe combined immunodeficiency. Semin Hematol 1993;30:92.
21. Hirschhorn R. Adenosine deaminase deficiency. Immunodef Rev 1990; 2:175.
22. Markert ML. Purine nucleoside phosphorylase deficiency. Immunodef Rev 1991;3:45.
23. Derry JMJ, Ochs HD, Francke U. Isolation of a novel gene mutated in Wiskott-Aldrich syndrome. Cell 1994;78:635.
24. Gatti RA, Boder E, Vinters HV, et al. Ataxia-telangiectasia: an interdisciplinary approach to pathogenesis. Medicine 1991;70:99.
25. Swift M. Genetic aspects of ataxia telangiectasia. Immunodef Rev 1990;2:67.
26. Savitsky K, Bar-Shira A, Gilad S, et al. A single ataxia telangiectasia gene with a product similar to PI-3 kinase. Science 1995;268:1749.
27. Buckley RH, Sampson HA. The hyperimmunoglobulinemia E syndrome. In: Franklin EC, ed. Clinical immunology update. New York, Elsevier North-Holland, 1981:147.
28. Merten DF, Buckley RH, Pratt PC, et al. The hyperimmunoglobulinemia E syndrome: radiographic observations. Radiology 1979;132:71.
29. Klein C, Lisowska-Grospierre B, LeDeist F, et al. Major histocompatibility complex class II deficiency: clinical manifestations, immunologic features, and outcome. J Pediatr 1993;123:921.
30. de la Salle H, Hanau D, Fricker D. Homozygous human TAP peptide transporter mutation in HLA class I deficiency. Science 1994;265:237.
31. Reith W, Barras E, Satola S. Cloning of the major histocompatibility complex class II promoter binding protein affected in a hereditary defect in class II gene regulation. Proc Nat Acad Sci 1989;86:4200.
32. Steimle V, Siegrist CA, Mottet A, et al. Regulation of MHC class II expression by interferon-γ mediated by the transactivator gene CIITA. Science 1994;265:106.
33. Mouy R, Fischer A, Vilmer E, et al. Incidence, severity, and prevention of infections in chronic granulomatous disease. J Pediatr 1989;114:555.
34. Frank MM. Complement in disease: inherited and acquired complement deficiencies. In: Frank MM, Austen KF, Claman HN, et al, ed. Samter's immunologic diseases, ed 5. Boston, Little, Brown, 1994:489.
35. Figueroa JE, Densen P. Infectious diseases associated with complement deficiencies. Clin Microbiol Rev 1991;4:359.
36. Buckley RH, Schiff RI. The use of intravenous immunoglobulin in immunodeficiency diseases. N Engl J Med 1991;325:110.
37. Blaese RM, Culver KW. Gene therapy for primary immunodeficiency disease. Immunodef Rev 1992;3:329.
38. Goldsobel AB, Haas A, Stiehm ER. Bone marrow transplantation in DiGeorge syndrome. J Pediatr 1987;111:40.

Surgery of Infants and Children: Scientific Principles and Practice, edited by Keith T. Oldham, Paul M. Colombani, and Robert P. Foglia.
Lippincott–Raven Publishers, Philadelphia, © 1997.

CHAPTER 13

Rheumatic Diseases

Deborah W. Kredich

The rheumatic diseases of childhood present a wide variety of intriguing problems to the surgeon.[1] The most common of these diseases is juvenile rheumatoid arthritis (JRA). JRA involves chronic arthritis in children for whom there is no other obvious cause for arthritis. By definition, the arthritis must be present for at least 6 weeks to be classified as JRA. The etiology is unknown. The three definite forms of the disease have different presentations, manifestations, and complications. Some believe they represent three different diseases, but others suggest that differing stimuli in differing hosts produce variable manifestations of the same disease (Table 13-1).

SYSTEMIC JUVENILE RHEUMATOID ARTHRITIS

The systemic onset form of JRA is accompanied by at least 2 weeks of fever, with temperatures spiking to more than 39.5°C (103°F), usually with rash and prominent systemic features such as malaise, hepatosplenomegaly, myalgia, lymphadenopathy, and arthralgia.[2-4] Systemic onset JRA is the least common form (10% of all JRA patients), but these patients usually are referred to tertiary care medical centers because of the impressive nature of the debility and the difficulty in making a diagnosis. Frequently, these children fail to develop clear-cut arthritis for weeks to months after the onset of the fever. They generally are evaluated carefully for malignancy or hidden infection before the diagnosis of probable JRA is determined by exclusion. Nearly all of these children have a skin rash—a maculopapular, salmon-colored eruption most prominent on the trunk and proximal extremities. Laboratory features of this form of disease are nonspecific. These children generally have anemia, which can be profound and is the anemia of chronic disease. They usually have an impressive leukocytosis with a shift to the left, high sedimentation rates, and other parameters of systemic inflammation, but serologic testing is generally negative for rheumatoid factors or antinuclear antibody (ANA) titers. There are no specific diagnostic laboratory tests at this time.

About a fourth of these children have intermittent episodes of febrile illness for many years; there can be prolonged periods of excellent health between. Others progress to a polyarticular form of disease, lose the hectic fevers and severe systemic illness, but persist with chronic debilitating arthritis.

Surgical complications of systemic onset JRA may relate to the fact that many of these children have prominent serositis. Consequently, pericarditis can ensue; this is rarely of such a magnitude to produce tamponade but can be associated with acute chest pain. Constrictive pericarditis is rare. Pericardiocentesis may be required for diagnosis. Persistent pericardial effusion, not responsive to therapy, may require a pericardial window.

In like manner, the pleura is often involved in the inflammatory process. The pleural effusions in these children can be either symptomatic or asymptomatic. Occasionally, the pleural effusion is an early manifestation of this disease and requires thoracentesis for diagnosis. Recurrent massive pleural effusions are not common with systemic onset JRA.

Rarely, abdominal serositis occurs; if it is the initial feature of the JRA, it presents as an acute abdominal crisis with peritoneal pain, ascites, fever, and leukocytosis. Because of the leukocytosis, the shift to immature granulocytes, and the acute abdominal pain, these children may undergo abdominal exploration for suspected appendiceal perforation or other acute surgical emergency. Generally, the serositis in patients with systemic onset JRA is a helpful clinical finding but not a cause for surgical intervention.

Treatment of systemic onset JRA requires high doses of nonsteroidal antiinflammatory drugs (NSAIDs). Periodically, corticosteroids are added, and then the potential for peptic ulcer disease is great. Even in the absence of systemic steroids, acute gastritis and peptic ulcers are possible sequelae in treated JRA patients. Many of these children are very young, and anorexia and weight loss rather than pain are the dominant symptoms.

POLYARTICULAR JUVENILE RHEUMATOID ARTHRITIS

In chronic polyarticular JRA, five or more joints are involved in the first 6 months of disease. Most children with polyarticular JRA have symmetric small and large joint involvement, so that more than 20 joints are involved. Many of these children exhibit low-grade signs of systemic illness, with moderate fever, mild hepatosplenomegaly and lymphadenopathy, and an anemia of chronic disease. Most do not have leukocytosis. Children with

TABLE 13-1. *Clinical features of juvenile rheumatoid arthritis*

Subtype	Pauciarticular	Polyarticular	Systemic
Presentation	Healthy child with 4 or fewer joints involved	Often chronically ill child, 5 or more joints involved	Very ill child with temperature >103°F for 2 weeks with or without joint findings
Proportion of total JRA	50%	40%	10%
Other physical findings	None	± Hepatosplenomegaly ± Lymphadenopathy	Prominent rash Hepatomegaly Splenomegaly Lymphadenopathy
Laboratory findings	+ ANA 40% − RF ± Elevated ESR	+ ANA 25% + RF 20% ± Thrombocytosis Anemia Elevated ESR	− ANA − RF Anemia Leukocytosis Thrombocytosis Elevated ESR
Complications	Chronic uveitis Leg-length discrepancy Contractures	Growth failure Pericarditis Pleuritis Ulcer Contractures Localized growth disturbances	Growth failure Pericarditis Pleuritis Abdominal serositis Myocarditis Ulcer Contractures

ANA, antinuclear antibodies; RF, rheumatoid factor; ESR, erythrocyte sedimentation rate.

polyarticular JRA are further subdivided into those who are negative and those who are positive for rheumatoid factor. A minority of patients with JRA have positive rheumatoid factors; most of these are older children and teenagers with polyarticular disease. Children who are seropositive for rheumatoid factor are much more likely to have erosive articular disease that is refractory to NSAIDs. Seropositive children have erosive disease within the first year of active arthritis.

As with systemic onset disease, initial treatment for this form of JRA is with NSAIDs. If there is erosive articular disease or if the disease is not controlled satisfactorily, second-line agents, such as parenteral gold, sulfasalazine, or low-dose methotrexate, are used.

Potential surgical complications of polyarticular JRA, in addition to those described with systemic onset disease, include contractures of and around joints. A child with painful arthritis tends to keep the involved joint in a position of comfort (flexion). Contractures can develop rapidly, and if they are left unattended as the child grows, irreversible abnormalities of soft tissue development can result. Soft tissue releases around joints are occasionally necessary. Iliotibial band tightness is a common concern that causes the pediatric rheumatologist to refer a child for surgical release.

Cervical spine involvement is predictable with polyarticular JRA and is occasionally seen in children with systemic disease as well. Fusion of apophyseal joints, especially at C-2 and C-3, and of the posterior spinal elements occurs early in some children. Early loss of the ability to extend the neck beyond a neutral position occurs. Atlantoaxial subluxation can follow, and it is important that the anesthesiologist and surgeon are aware of this risk. If a child has any cervical spine involvement, particularly fusion of the cervical spine, access to the airway is potentially limited, and nasal endotracheal intubation is generally preferable. Cervical hyperextension, fracture of fused vertebrae, and cord compression are the potentially catastrophic sequelae of manipulation of a child's neck when JRA is present.

Epiphyseal growth is markedly altered in many patients with JRA. For instance, overgrowth of the distal ulnar epiphysis results in radial deviation of the hand in many children with polyarticular JRA. For unknown reasons, there is often overgrowth at the lateral femoral and proximal tibial epiphyses as well, producing severe genu valgum. These conditions may require surgical correction.

PAUCIARTICULAR JUVENILE RHEUMATOID ARTHRITIS

Pauciarticular JRA is the most common form of the disease, and it accounts for half of all children with chronic arthritis. Pauciarticular arthritis is most common in young girls, with a peak incidence at about 2 years of age. Children with this form of disease are generally well otherwise and are often referred first to an orthopedic surgeon because the swollen joint is assumed to have been injured. These children rarely have a skin rash and virtually never have systemic manifestations of disease such as fever or lymphadenopathy. In fact, a significant number of these children do not even have pain with their arthritis and are not referred until a contracture becomes obvious or someone finally notices a markedly enlarged joint.

All laboratory parameters are normal in the child with pauciarticular JRA, with the exception of the ANA titer. Many of these children have positive ANA results, and this correlates with the increased incidence of chronic uveitis. The chronic uveitis of JRA is typically asymptomatic until scarring has occurred. Blindness can result, and careful ophthalmologic follow-up is mandated. Every child with JRA should be screened with a slit lamp examination by an ophthalmologist semiannually; the child with pauciarticular JRA and a positive ANA should be screened every 3 months for possible uveitis. Treatment of this complication is generally with topical corticosteroids and mydriatics. The consequences of failure to make diagnosis and treat this disease are potentially devastating.

Second-line agents are rarely necessary for children with pauciarticular JRA. Response to NSAIDs is generally good, if not dramatic.

For reasons that are unknown, most children develop quiescence of pauciarticular JRA in a matter of years, some having only one episode of active synovitis and others having two or three, which may be separated by several years of normal joint function. Most, however, have no active disease by adulthood.

The major complication of pauciarticular JRA other than uveitis is that of limb overgrowth. The knee is the most common joint involved in pauciarticular JRA. If knee involvement is asymmetric, ipsilateral growth can exceed that of the asymptomatic extremity. This can produce leg-length inequality and, if severe, a pelvic tilt. Historically, stapling procedures were done for children with leg-length inequalities to slow the growth of the involved leg; this has generally been abandoned. The current approach involves the temporary use of shoe lifts because it has become apparent that compensatory growth occurs in the shorter limb as the acute synovitis resolves. For those children in whom this is not adequate, osteotomies and long-bone lengthening procedures are well accepted.

SYSTEMIC LUPUS ERYTHEMATOSUS

Systemic lupus erythematosus (SLE) is an autoimmune disease with protean manifestations.[5] Virtually every organ system can be involved. The disease is much more common in females than males and does not differ significantly in children and adults. The hallmark of the disease is the production of autoantibodies, some of which have a clear-cut etiologic relation to the disease process. In particular, autoantibodies to native DNA appear to be responsible for the microvascular injury characteristic of glomerulonephritis. A number of these are described that may be simply markers for the disease without attendant organ damage. For example, antithyroid antibodies may be detectable in the circulation in a clinically euthyroid patient. A diagnosis of SLE is assigned by convention when 4 of the 11 American College of Rheumatology criteria are met. These are detailed in Table 13-2.[5]

SLE is a chronic disease characterized by exacerbations and remissions. Ultraviolet light exposure is a stimulus known to produce flares of disease in a number of sun-sensitive patients. Endocrine changes, particularly termination of pregnancy, are associated with changes in disease activity. Treatment of SLE depends on the clinical manifestations. Arthritis is generally well controlled with NSAIDs. Hydroxychloroquine is an effective medication, when coupled with sun avoidance and use of sunscreens, in the treatment of lupus skin disease. If lupus involvement of the central nervous system is associated with seizures, anticonvulsant medications are necessary in addition to high-dose systemic steroids. If nephritis is severe, high-dose corticosteroids plus cyclophosphamide therapy may be necessary.

As with JRA, polyserositis presents many of the potential surgical complications in patients with SLE. Pericarditis in SLE is more likely to progress to tamponade than is pericarditis in JRA. Pleuritis is frequent and often recurrent. Abdominal serositis is occasionally a problem, but patients with SLE also

TABLE 13-2. *Clinical diagnostic criteria for systemic lupus erythematosus**

PHYSICAL SIGNS
Butterfly rash (malar)
Discoid lupus
Photosensitivity
Oral or nasopharyngeal ulcers
Nonerosive arthritis (two or more joints with effusion and tenderness)
Pleuritis or pericarditis
Seizures or psychosis in absence of metabolic toxins or drugs

LABORATORY DATA
RENAL DISEASE
Proteinuria (>500 mg/24 h) *or*
Cellular casts (red blood cells, granular, tubular)
HEMATOLOGIC DISEASE
Hemolytic anemia with reticulocytosis *or*
Leukopenia (<4000 on two occasions) *or*
Lymphophenia (<1500 on two occasions) *or*
Thrombocytopenia (<100,000)
SEROLOGIC DATA
Positive anti-dsDNA antibody *or*
Positive anti-Sm *or*
Positive lupus erythematosus prep *or*
False-positive VDRL for more than 6 mo
Positive antinuclear antibody in absence of drugs
known to induce lupus

* 1982 revised criteria for diagnosis of systemic lupus erythematosus. A patient must have 4 of the 11 criteria to establish the diagnosis. These criteria can be present simultaneously or at different times during the patient's illness.

have an increased incidence of acute pancreatitis. This is particularly true when treatment includes systemic corticosteroids, so an acute abdomen cannot be presumed to be from abdominal serositis. Additionally, the SLE patient is immunosuppressed by the disease as well as by the therapy, and is therefore particularly prone to a variety of local and systemic infections. Renal involvement is universal in SLE patients, although its severity and its clinical relevance vary. Renal biopsies are routinely performed in patients with SLE because not all patients with diffuse SLE nephritis have abnormal urinary sediments, and accuracy of diagnosis directs subsequent therapy. Occasionally, lupus nephritis progresses to end-stage renal disease, requiring hemodialysis and the host of related surgical issues. Fortunately, this occurs far less frequently with systemic therapy with steroids and cytotoxic agents.

Some patients with SLE have a constellation of findings referred to as the *anti–cardiolipin antibody syndrome*. These patients often have false-positive VDRL serology and possess an anti–phospholipid antibody that makes them particularly prone to deep venous thrombosis and its complications, such as pulmonary embolus. This syndrome also accounts in part for the increased risks in pregnant women with SLE, in whom thrombosis has resulted in placental infarction.

NEONATAL LUPUS SYNDROME

The neonatal lupus syndrome results when there is transplacental passage of the Ro antibody from mother to infant. The mother may have clinical diseases such as SLE, Sjögren syndrome, or rheumatoid arthritis, but more often she does not have symptoms. The infant syndrome is characterized by a light-sensitive skin eruption, thrombocytopenia, and hepatosplenomegaly, which is transient. In other infants, congenital heart block develops, usually after the 16th week of gestation. Pathologic sections of hearts of infants who succumb to this syndrome show total obliteration of the cardiac conducting system by fibrosis. Children born with congenital heart block do not show resolution; if present, congenital heart block is a permanent condition.

In the absence of structural cardiac anomalies, congenital heart block occurs in about 1 in 20,000 live births.[6] Virtually all of these infants have antibody-associated heart block. Some of these infants' mothers who do not have symptoms go on to develop a connective tissue disease in subsequent years.

When heart block is apparent in utero, the infant is observed closely with sequential ultrasonography and is delivered promptly if hydrops fetalis develops. Some of these children develop cardiac failure soon after birth, and most require pacemaker placement in the neonatal period. Others do not develop clinical evidence of heart failure until their activity level as toddlers outstrips their cardiac reserve.

DERMATOMYOSITIS

Dermatomyositis of childhood results from a systemic inflammatory process that targets the microvasculature of the skin, striated muscle, and gastrointestinal tract.[7] The natural history of the disease involves a period of activity for about 2 years and then long-term quiescence. Most children appropriately treated completely recover from dermatomyositis without sequelae. Attempts have been made to link common viral pathogens with the onset of childhood dermatomyositis, but the data do not support a single infectious cause.

Childhood dermatomyositis is more frequent in girls than boys and generally presents between 7 and 12 years of age. The history is one of insidious but progressive muscle weakness, beginning in proximal limb muscles but progressing to involve all skeletal muscles. Most affected children have the classic skin rash, which consists of purplish discoloration of the upper eyelid (heliotrope), often with erythema and edema of the upper and lower lids. There may be a malar flush and erythema of the lateral neck and the sun-exposed area of the chest. There is a nonspecific papular erythema of the knees and elbows and a characteristic erythema over the metacarpophalangeal and proximal phalangeal and proximal interphalangeal joints, with plaque-like formations called Gottron papules. Muscle weakness with this characteristic rash warrants a search for enzymatic evidence of muscle destruction (elevated creatinine kinase, aldolase, aspartate aminotransferase, alanine aminotransferase, and lactic dehydrogenase isoenzyme plasma levels). Electromyography and muscle biopsy show characteristic vasculitis and dropout of peripheral muscle fibers.

Except for evidence of elevation of muscle enzymes, the laboratory evaluation of patients with childhood dermatomyositis can be totally normal. Not all children have elevated sedimentation rates, and a small number have an elevated ANA titer. The specificity of the disease can be striking. For example, only one of the muscle enzymes may be elevated in a given child, and this is the enzyme that is most likely to be elevated with subsequent flares. A number of children with dermatomyositis have normal serum creatinine kinase levels throughout their illness.

Treatment of the disease is with corticosteroids, and resolution is usually prompt. Treatment is best continued for the natural course of the disease, which is about 2 years. If diagnosed and treated in this manner, most children have normal strength and function once the disease has resolved.

Ten to 15% of children with dermatomyositis have cutaneous vasculitis associated with the disease. Actually, the rash is a vasculitic rash, and there are times when telangiectasias and dilated vessels are apparent in the nail beds or in the heliotrope rash of the upper lids. When cutaneous vasculitis occurs, it can be associated with significant scarring. Some suggest that cutaneous vasculitis portends a worse outcome of the disease.

A more serious complication of dermatomyositis is gastrointestinal vasculitis, which can result in frank perforation of a viscus or in massive gastrointestinal bleeding. Although both of these conditions are amenable to surgical intervention, further complications can develop. The bleeding is occasionally massive, and exsanguination is a risk. Occasionally, multiple bleeding sites make the achievement of hemostasis difficult. It is essential to localize bleeding sites preoperatively using endoscopy, angiography, or nuclear scintigraphy. Most of these children have been on and will continue to need high-dose corticosteroid therapy, so wound healing is severely compromised. Although any gastrointestinal site can be involved, the colon is a particularly difficult surgical problem because of the severity of the illness and the attendant risks of sepsis. The mortality rate in this setting is high, but the incidence is low.

SCLERODERMA

Scleroderma is rare in childhood.[8] The term literally means ''hard skin.'' When it occurs in children, two forms of disease are appreciated. The first is limited scleroderma; the second is systemic disease or progressive systemic sclerosis (PSS). The cause of neither form is understood. A variety of chemical toxins, however, are known to induce scleroderma-like disease, including polyvinyl chloride, bleomycin, and pentazocine. Ingestion of contaminated cooking oil in Spain in 1981 affected 20,000 people and produced scleroderma-like symptoms in many victims. Other causes are also known; for example, chronic graft-versus-host disease may be accompanied by similar skin changes and visceral disease.

Limited scleroderma can take the form of hardened patches of dermis on the trunk (in which case it is termed *morphea*) or linear areas of sclerosis on limbs (called *linear scleroderma*). Linear scleroderma can also involve the scalp and face; when this occurs, deeper structures can also be involved. Some children with linear scleroderma of the scalp have seizures because of underlying brain involvement. When limbs are involved, there can be tightening of the skin and appendages as well as muscle and bone. The affected limbs can have severe growth retardation and contracture formation. Limited scleroderma is not associated with major organ system disease beyond the skin and musculoskeletal system.

Early in the course of limited scleroderma, there is an inflammatory phase characterized by edema and purplish discoloration of the edges of the involved skin. This quickly progresses to an atrophic phase, in which depression of the area and often hypopigmentation or hyperpigmentation, loss of secondary skin appendages, and tactile hardening can be seen. Localized scleroderma may progress rapidly or may involve only a small area and never progress. The course is capricious, and the physician's ability to predict outcome is limited. Surgery is occasionally needed with limited scleroderma when the involved limb is markedly different in size from the noninvolved limb or when joint release is necessary. Amputation is occasionally necessary to improve function.

PSS, or generalized scleroderma, is a far more serious entity and also has no known cause. Some patients with PSS have associated autoantibodies, including the scleroderma 70 antibody, but the importance of these antibodies to pathogenesis remains unclear.

The usual course of scleroderma is one of progression for several years. Many patients experience softening of the skin and cessation of the progression of the systemic manifestations after an average of 3 years. Raynaud phenomenon is often associated with scleroderma and, when severe, can result in gangrene or loss of integrity of the peripheral digits. Many patients with scleroderma experience sclerodactyly or loss of tuft of the terminal phalanx with associated loss of subcutaneous finger pad pulp. PSS can involve the intestines at any site, resulting in a stiff, immobile intestinal tract in which peristalsis diminishes and digestion and absorption are compromised. Esophageal involvement is relatively common, and small bowel pseudoobstruction is well described. In general, the best management is medical and supportive, with surgery reserved for specific mechanical complications. Involvement of renal vessels in the sclerotic process can lead to severe hypertension; if this is not treated aggressively, renal failure can ensue. Some patients have severe lung involvement with both restrictive disease and decreased diffusion capabilities. Occasionally, pulmonary hypertension is a presenting feature without associated lung disease; this complication has a dire prognosis.

The various surgical problems associated with scleroderma are obvious from this list of potential complications. If the esophagus is involved and there has been significant reflux, strictures are common, and dilation may be necessary, sometimes on a frequent basis. Likewise, fundoplication may be required, although this is a problem in a patient with proximal dysmotility. Gut immobility involving the small intestine can lead to inanition and the necessity for total parenteral nutrition. Since scleroderma is a disease without effective treatment, this presents a clear ethical dilemma.

Raynaud phenomenon can be a severe problem and can lead to gangrene or amputation. It may be amenable to medical therapy with calcium-channel blockers or nitroglycerin paste, or to behavioral therapy in the form of biofeedback. Children with pulmonary hypertension have been considered candidates for heart lung transplantation. The use of oral D-penicillamine in patients with some aspects of scleroderma may be efficacious, but no clear-cut data support this approach. D-Penicillamine is particularly used in the treatment of patients with diffuse lung disease in an effort to diminish pulmonary fibrosis and pulmonary hypertension.

VASCULITIS

Henoch-Schönlein Purpura

Henoch-Schönlein purpura (HSP) is a common childhood vasculitis[9] that is generally recognized and treated by the prac-

ticing pediatrician without referral to a major medical center. HSP is diagnosed in an otherwise healthy child who develops palpable purpura, confined mainly to the buttocks and lower extremities, and whose hematologic parameters are normal. In particular, thrombocytopenia is not characteristic. The children are typically 3 to 8 years of age, and the disease has a slight male predominance. Although linkage to streptococcal or other infection has been made, there are no conclusive data about cause.

Leukocytoclastic vasculitis of the skin, synovium, gastrointestinal tract, and kidney are seen pathologically. Associated arthritis can occur that is extremely painful but that never progresses to chronic arthritis. Purpura can involve the intestinal tract, producing severe abdominal pain. The kidneys also can be involved, with hematuria and occasionally hypertension. Renal involvement in childhood HSP rarely progresses to chronic renal insufficiency, in contrast to HSP in the adult, which has a much higher incidence of associated chronic nephropathy. The usual course of HSP is one in which there is predictable and complete remission of disease activity after about 6 to 8 weeks. In some children, HSP resolves in 2 to 3 weeks, with new crops of lesions developing later. There is no need for therapy of the primary process.

Two thirds of children with HSP have abdominal pain, and thus it is common for surgeons to become involved in their care. Gastrointestinal hemorrhage occasionally occurs and can be life-threatening. Intestinal infarction can occur as well. An area of gut purpura can form the lead point for small bowel intussusception, requiring surgical intervention. Children with HSP who have severe bowel pain often are treated empirically with systemic corticosteroids. No convincing data show that this shortens the course of the disease, although relief of symptoms can be obtained.

Kawasaki Disease

Kawasaki disease (mucocutaneous lymph node syndrome) appears to be a new entity, first described in 1978 in Japan.[10] Since that time, more than 20,000 children with Kawasaki disease have been registered in Japan, although it occurs in the rest of the world as well. For reasons that are unknown, it is more prevalent in children of Japanese extraction.

No definite cause of Kawasaki disease has been recognized, although the most recent work has focused on superantigens as possible etiologic factors. It occurs almost exclusively in very young children. The usual age of onset is 2 years or younger, and it is unusual to see Kawasaki disease in children older than 5 years. A diagnosis is made if five of the following six criteria are present and there is no other disease to explain the symptoms:

- High fever (*must* be present 5 days), plus four of five:
  Conjunctival injection
  Changes in oral mucosa or lips
  Rash, polymorphous
  Extremity changes (edema of the dorsum, of hands and feet, or intense erythema of the palms and soles)
  Lymph node enlargement greater than 1.5 cm, usually cervical

There are many other clinical features of Kawasaki disease related to the systemic vasculitis. Most notable are pneumonia, arthritis, myocarditis, abdominal pain, diarrhea, and hepatocellular dysfunction. Hydrops of the gallbladder is a finding in a number of children and is particularly impressive on ultrasound of the abdomen; it generally resolves spontaneously and requires no therapy. In the untreated child, fever persists for 10 to 14 days, and 15% to 20% of these children to develop coronary artery aneurysms. Intravenous γ-globulin treatment has been shown to be exceedingly effective, reducing the incidence of coronary artery aneurysms to 2% to 3% if administered within the first 10 days of illness. Children who have the worst prognosis are boys younger than 1 year of age. Extreme irritability is a hallmark of the acute phase of Kawasaki disease. Many of these children are admitted to hospitals because of their irritability and refusal to take fluids.

If the lymphadenopathy of Kawasaki disease is deep in the cervical chain, it can cause a mass effect, displacing the tonsillar area in a manner to suggest a retropharyngeal abscess. The lymph nodes of Kawasaki disease do not suppurate and therefore do not need to be drained. The importance of making the appropriate diagnosis is obvious.

Arterial aneurysm formation is the most feared of the sequelae of Kawasaki disease. Usually, these aneurysms occur in the coronary arteries, but children have developed aneurysms in other sites, such as the axillary arteries or visceral vessels. Obviously, rupture of these aneurysms is a potentially life-threatening event and requires preventive surgical intervention if possible.

Aneurysms also are sites for potential thrombosis with distal embolization. In the convalescent phase of Kawasaki disease, the child experiences extreme thrombocytosis that, coupled with this propensity, can lead to life-threatening complications. Myocardial infarction secondary to coronary artery thrombosis is devastating. Rarely, ventricular aneurysms are seen. Coronary artery bypass surgery and heart transplantations have been attempted.

Occasionally, 2 to 3 weeks into the illness, gangrene of digits occurs. Some children require amputation for this unusual complication.

REFERENCES

1. Cassidy JT, Petty RE. Textbook of pediatric rheumatology. New York, Churchill Livingstone, 1990.
2. Kredich DW. Chronic arthritis in childhood. Med Clin North Am 1986; 70:305.
3. Kredich DW, Patrone NA. Pediatric spondyloarthropathies. Clin Orthop 1990;259:18.
4. Lang BA, Shore A. A review of current concepts on the pathogenesis of juvenile rheumatoid arthritis. J Rheumatol 1990;21(Suppl):1.
5. Lang BA, Silverman ED. A clinical overview of systemic lupus erythematosus in childhood. Pediatr Rev 1994;14:194.
6. Waltuck J, Buyon JP. Autoantibody associated congenital heart block: outcome in mother and children. Ann Intern Med 1994;120:544.
7. Pachman LM. Juvenile dermatomyositis: a clinical overview. Pediatr Rev 1990;12:117.
8. Singsen BH. Scleroderma in childhood. Pediatr Clin North Am 1986; 33:1119.
9. Lanzkowsky S, Lanzkowsky L, Lanzkowsky P. Henoch-Schöenlein purpura. Pediatr Review 1992;13:130.
10. Melish M, Hicks RV. Kawasaki syndrome: clinical features, pathophysiology, etiology and therapy. J Rheumatol 1990;24(Suppl):2.

Surgery of Infants and Children: Scientific Principles and Practice, edited by
Keith T. Oldham, Paul M. Colombani, and Robert P. Foglia.
Lippincott–Raven Publishers, Philadelphia, © 1997.

CHAPTER 14

Blood

Lori Luchtman-Jones and Alan L. Schwartz

NORMAL HEMATOPOIESIS

Hematopoiesis in the human embryo and fetus can be divided
into three overlapping phases: mesoblastic, hepatic, and myeloid.[1] The earliest blood cells produced belong to the erythroid
series, and areas of erythropoiesis have been detected at day
14 of gestation within the blood islands of the yolk sac. By
day 35, erythropoiesis is initiated in the liver. Granulopoiesis
and thrombocytopoiesis occur subsequently. From 3 to 6
months' gestation, the liver plays the major role in hematopoiesis, although hematopoiesis occurs in the spleen, thymus, and
lymph nodes as well. In month 4 to 5 of fetal development,
hematopoiesis begins in the bone marrow, signaling the onset
of the myeloid phase. Monocyte and lymphocyte production
also begins at this time. By the final 3 months of normal
gestation, the bone marrow has become the major site of
hematopoiesis. After birth and through early childhood, most
of the bone marrow space is occupied by red (hematopoieti-
cally active) marrow. As the child ages, much of the marrow
space slowly fills with fat, unless a pathologic process intervenes and results in alteration of the normal pattern of hematopoiesis. In some diseases, usually associated with anemia,
extramedullary hematopoiesis occurs in liver, spleen, lymph
nodes, adrenals, and even kidneys.

Fetal erythrocytes differ markedly from those produced in
infancy and adulthood (Fig. 14-1). Differences in mean corpuscular volume, membrane properties, hemoglobin content, metabolic profile, and life-span have all been well described. Hemoglobin production shifts from embryonic forms (Gower 1,
Gower 2, Portland) to fetal forms ($\alpha_2\gamma_2$) to the adult hemoglobins ($\alpha_2\beta_2$, $\alpha_2\sigma_2$) during gestation. In the newborn infant, 70%
to 90% of the hemoglobin is of fetal type. Fetal hemoglobin is
gradually replaced by adult hemoglobin during the next few
months, and it is only after this time period that hemoglobinopathies involving abnormalities of the β chain of hemoglobin are
detectable. Hemoglobinopathies characterized by abnormalities
of the α or γ chain result in abnormalities of the red blood cells
present at birth. The life-span of the red blood cell increases
from 50 to 60 days in the fetus to 120 days in the adult.

Because of the lower oxygen saturation of fetal blood, coupled with the relatively poor oxygen release to the tissues by
fetal hemoglobin, the reticulocyte count, hemoglobin, and hematocrit are elevated in the immediate newborn period relative
to later in infancy. Because the normal ranges for hemoglobin,
hematocrit, mean corpuscular volume, and reticulocyte count
vary depending on the age of the patient, it is important to
consult a standardized chart of age-appropriate values (Table
14-1). The leukocyte count and differential change markedly
from birth to infancy to childhood and on to adulthood. Platelet
counts are relatively stable from the birth of a full-term infant
to adulthood.

ANEMIA

The usual definition of anemia is the presence of a hemoglobin or hematocrit value that is more than two standard
deviations below the mean for age and sex. Because the
primary function of the red blood cell is to transport oxygen
from the pulmonary bed to other tissues for release, anemia
may result in decreased oxygen-carrying capacity, compromising tissue oxygenation. Tissue oxygenation is a complex
concept involving not only the concentration of hemoglobin
or the percentage of hematocrit but also the oxygen affinity
of the hemoglobin within the patient's red cells and the
cardiorespiratory status of the patient. The only absolute indications for rapid correction of anemia by red cell transfusion
are to restore tissue oxygenation and to expand blood volume
after acute loss. Unfortunately, little information exists about
the level of hematocrit or hemoglobin necessary for adequate
delivery of oxygen to the tissues. Observations on the changes
in the coronary sinus oxygen saturation in dogs with varying
degrees of acutely induced anemia[2] and the surgical experience among Jamaican patients with sickle cell disease[3] suggest
that otherwise healthy young adults can tolerate short-term
anemia with a hematocrit value between 20% and 25% (hemoglobin level exceeding 7 g/dL) without adverse outcome. In
many pediatric centers, the sicker patients, particularly those
with cardiorespiratory dysfunction, undergo transfusion to
maintain the hemoglobin and hematocrit values close to normal in an attempt to maximize tissue oxygenation.

In the broadest sense, anemia is caused by a defect in red
cell production, by accelerated loss or destruction of red cells,

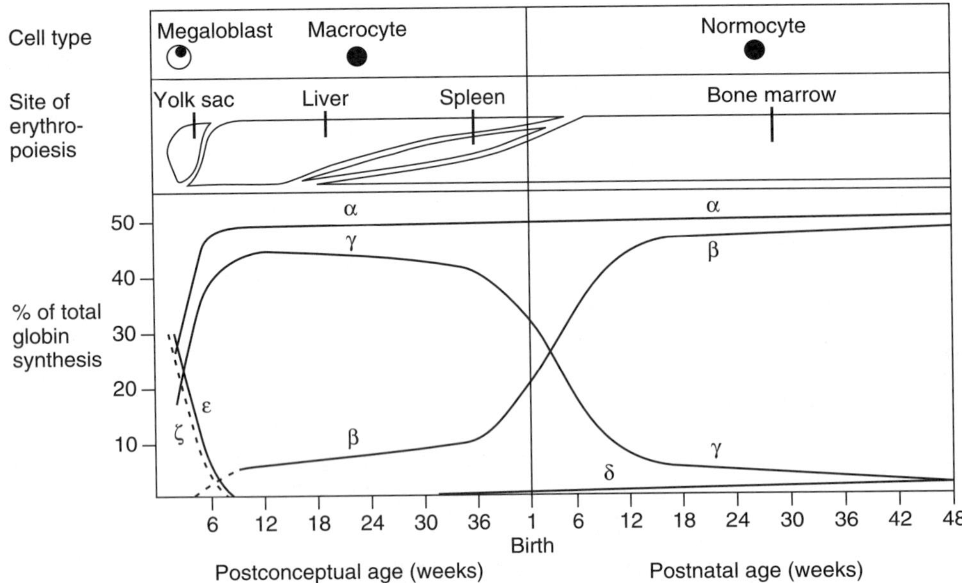

FIG. 14-1. Alterations in the production site, hemoglobin composition, and morphology of red blood cells during the prenatal and early postnatal periods. (After Weatherall DJ, Clegg JB. The thalassemia syndromes, ed 3. Cambridge, Blackwell Scientific, 1981:64)

or by both mechanisms, which is often the case. Defects can be congenital or acquired and can be intrinsic (eg, abnormal hemoglobin) or extrinsic (eg, immune-mediated hemolysis) to the red blood cell. Anemias can also be differentiated morphologically by considering the indices and morphologic appearance of the red cells. Using the latter method, the anemia is classified as microcytic, normocytic, or macrocytic, based on the mean corpuscular volume of the red blood cells (Table 14-2). Hypochromicity, abnormal red cell shapes, polychromasia, and cellular inclusions such as stippling or Howell-Jolly bodies also can provide valuable clues to the cause of the anemia.

The workup for anemia begins with a careful patient history, which includes diet, details of prior anemia or transfusions, pica, evidence for blood loss, and family history of anemia, transfusions, gallbladder disease, or splenectomy. Prescription and over-the-counter drugs, patent medicine ingestion, and exposure to lead or other toxins should be evaluated. The physical examination should focus on identifying dysmorphic or skeletal abnormalities as well as documenting appropriate growth, development, and general health. The adequacy of the cardiovascular system should be assessed. The presence of hepatosplenomegaly or jaundice should be documented. Testing of stool specimens for occult blood should be done. Laboratory tests include a complete blood count with red cell indices, a reticulocyte count, and evaluation of the blood smear. The results of this preliminary workup dictate the need for further laboratory testing, such as hemoglobin electrophoresis, serum ferritin and iron levels, Coombs testing, serum haptoglobin level, free erythrocyte protoporphyrin level, lead level, quantitative or qualitative testing for glucose-6-phosphate dehydrogenase deficiency, osmotic fragility testing, or bone marrow aspirate or biopsy.

TABLE 14-1. *Age-specific values for complete blood count*

Age	Hemoglobin (mean %)	Hematocrit (mean %)	Mean corpuscular volume	Reticulocytes (%)	WBC/ μL $\times$ 1000 (mean)	Neutrophils (%)	Lymphocytes (%)	Monocytes (%)	Eosinophils (%)	Platelets $10^3/\mu$L (mean)
26–30 wk gestation	13.4	41.5	118.2	—	4.4	—	—	—	—	254
28 wk	14.5	45.0	120.0	5–10	—	—	—	—	—	275
32 wk	15.0	47.0	118.0	3–10	—	—	—	—	—	290
Term (cord)	16.5	51.0	108.0	3–7	18.1	—	—	—	—	290
1–3 d	18.5	56.0	108.0	1.8–4.6	18.9	—	—	—	—	192
2 wk	16.6	53.0	105.0	—	11.4	—	—	—	—	252
1 mo	13.9	44.0	101.0	0.1–1.7	10.8	—	—	—	—	
2 mo	11.2	35.0	95.0	—	—	—	—	—	—	
6 mo	12.6	36.0	76.0	0.7–2.3	11.9	32	61	5	3	
6 mo–2 y	12.0	36.0	78.0	—	10.6	31	61	5	3	150–350
2–6 y	12.5	37.0	81.0	0.5–1.0	8.5	42	50	5	3	150–350
6–12 y	13.5	40.0	86.0	0.5–1.0	8.1	53	39	4	2	150–350
12–18 y										
Male	14.5	43	88	0.5–1.0	7.8	57	35	4	3	150–350
Female	14.0	41	90	0.5–1.0	7.8	57	35	4	3	150–350

(Adapted from Johnson KB, ed. The Harriet Lane handbook, ed 13. St Louis, Mosby, 1993:231)

TABLE 14-2. *Morphologic approach to diagnosis of anemia**

MICROCYTIC
Iron deficiency
Thalassemia
  α
  β
Lead poisoning
Chronic disease
Severe protein deficiency

MACROCYTIC
Reticulocytosis
Hepatic disease
Hypothyroidism
Trisomy 21
Megaloblastic
  Folate deficiency
  Vitamin B_{12} deficiency
  Orotic aciduria

NORMOCYTIC
LOW RETICULOCYTE COUNT
Normal WBC count and platelets
  Red cell aplasia
    Congenital
    Acquired
  Infection
  Drugs
Low WBC count and platelets
  Bone marrow infiltration
  Aplastic anemia
Normal or low WBC count and platelets
  Renal disease
  Infection
  Drugs
  Splenomegaly
HIGH RETICULOCYTE COUNT
Abnormal RBC morphology
Spherocytes
  Hereditary spherocytosis (check Coombs test for
    immune hemolysis)
Elliptocytes, stomatocytes, other membrane, defects
Target cells or sickle cells (send hemoglobin
  electrophoresis)
Red cell fragments
  Hemolytic–uremic syndrome
  Disseminated intravascular coagulation
  Microangiopathic disease
Normal morphology
  Blood loss
  Enzyme deficiencies
  Unstable hemoglobin

---

* The initial distinction is based on red cell size. Subsequent decisions take into consideration the reticulocyte count, clinical history, other laboratory testing, and additional morphologic abnormalities of the red blood cells.
(Adapted from Nathan DG. The differential diagnosis of anemia. In: Nathan DG, Oski FA, eds. Hematology of infancy and childhood, ed 4. Philadelphia, WB Saunders, 1993:352)

Iron-Deficiency Anemia

Although the incidence of iron-deficiency anemia in the United States has decreased, it remains the leading cause of anemia in infancy and childhood. Factors associated with the decline in the incidence of iron-deficiency anemia include the increasing number of infants receiving breast milk, the extensive use of iron-supplemented infant formulas and baby cereals during the first year of life, and the avoidance of the introduction of cow milk in the infant's diet until 9 to 12 months of age.[4]

The amount of iron stored in the body of the newborn infant is proportional to body weight and, for the full-term infant, should be sufficient for the first 4 to 6 months of life. Preterm infants, however, weigh less at birth, have a much more rapid rate of postnatal growth, and often develop iron deficiency within the first 3 months of life unless their diets are supplemented with iron. Infants who experience accelerated iron losses secondary to blood loss from repeated laboratory testing, trauma, surgery, or anatomic abnormalities also become iron deficient if supplementation is not instituted early.

The American Academy of Pediatrics suggests that full-term infants receive at least 1 mg/kg of iron daily from age 4 months to 3 years. Premature or low-birthweight infants should be supplemented with 2 mg/kg/d from 2 months of age, and very-low-birthweight infants (those weighing less than 1000 g at birth) should receive 4 mg/kg/d from the age of 2 months. The higher rates of iron supplementation should be continued through the first year of life. Children 4 to 10 years of age require 10 mg/d; the recommended supplementation for adolescents is 18 mg/d. Ideally, the iron requirement should be met by dietary intake, but in instances of high requirements or low dietary intake of iron, additional supplementation may be needed.[4]

Although both breast milk and cow milk contain iron, the bioavailability of the iron in breast milk is superior. Healthy term infants who are breastfed should not require iron supplementation until about 6 months of age. Those who are formula-fed should be given an iron-supplemented formula (12 mg/L). Infant cereal fortified with iron should be one of the earliest solid foods introduced. Because the protein in cow milk can cause occult gastrointestinal bleeding in neonates, and because of the poor bioavailability of iron in cow milk, it is recommended that infants not be given cow milk until after 1 year of age.

Infancy is a period of rapid growth during which most of the diet is composed of foods that are relatively poor sources of iron. Adolescence is another period of rapid growth during which poor dietary intake can result in iron-deficiency anemia. Iron-deficiency anemia can occur at any time when rapid growth outstrips the ability of diet and body stores to supply iron requirements. Evaluation of dietary iron intake is part of the diagnostic workup of anemia. After infancy, however, the possibility of iron-deficiency anemia secondary to blood loss becomes increasingly likely. Malabsorption of iron should also be considered in a patient with the appropriate medical history.

Early in iron deficiency, the bone marrow stores are depleted, and the red cell distribution width increases. Subsequently, the iron transport levels fall, resulting in lower serum iron, ferritin, and transferrin levels. Finally, erythrocyte production is affected. A hypochromic, microcytic anemia becomes apparent, accompanied by elevated free erythrocyte protoporphyrin levels. Although severe iron deficiency is not difficult to diagnose, it can be a problem distinguishing milder deficiency distinguish from other causes of microcytic anemia, especially in patients with chronic illness. Occasionally, the results of the screening tests are inconclusive, and in these cases, a therapeutic trial of iron can be undertaken. Ferrous sulfate in a dose of 3 mg/kg/d can be given for 1 month.[4] If the hemoglobin rises by at least 1 g/dL in 1 month (in the absence of ongoing blood loss), the diagnosis of iron deficiency is made, and the iron supplementation should be continued until 1 or 2 months after the hemoglobin and hematocrit are in the normal range.

Hemolytic Anemias

Accelerated destruction of red blood cells is the end point of a host of causes of anemia. Extrinsic influences on the red blood cell include immune or autoimmune hemolysis and destruction of red cells by the vasculature or the reticuloendothelial system. A variety of intrinsic abnormalities can affect the life-span of the red blood cell, including enzymatic defects, disorders of the red cell membrane, and certain hemoglobinopathies.

A classic example of hemolytic anemia secondary to red cell membrane disorders is hereditary spherocytosis.[5] Defects in membrane proteins spectrin, protein 4.2, ankyrin, and protein 3 have been described, any of which reduce the stability and deformability of the red cell cytoskeleton. Although it was originally described as an autosomal dominantly inherited disorder, 25% of cases are thought to be autosomal recessive in inheritance, or rarely, dominantly inherited with reduced penetrance. Most patients are identified in childhood, although diagnosis in infancy or adulthood is not uncommon. The presenting features, in order of frequency, are: spherocytic anemia, jaundice, splenomegaly, and positive family history. The clinical course can be extremely variable. Most patients do not have symptoms except for splenomegaly and mild hemolysis. Complications of the disease include aplastic crisis, hemolytic crisis, and gallbladder disease. Patients with gallbladder disease and those with substantial anemia are candidates for splenectomy. If possible, splenectomy is deferred until after 6 years of age because the risk of postsplenectomy sepsis, while elevated in all patients, is especially high in infants and young children. Candidates for splenectomy should receive pneumococcal and *Haemophilus influenzae* vaccines. Prophylactic antibiotic therapy, usually with penicillin, is recommended for young patients who undergo splenectomy; but this therapy is complicated and controversial in adolescents and adults.

Sickle Cell Anemia

Sickle cell disease is a common medical problem in the United States, where the incidence in the black population is about 8%. Normal adult hemoglobin is composed of two pairs of globin subunits, each consisting of an α chain and a β chain. Sickle cell trait (hemoglobin AS) is diagnosed when one normal β-globin gene (hemoglobin A) and one abnormal β-globin gene coding for hemoglobin S (hemoglobin S) are inherited. Sickle cell anemia (hemoglobin SS) occurs with the inheritance of two abnormal β-globin genes. There are a number of other sickle hemoglobinopathies in which one gene coding for hemoglobin S is inherited along with a second abnormal β-globin gene coding for another hemoglobin, such as hemoglobin C or β-thalassemia. The clinical courses of disease in these patients may be indistinguishable from, or milder than, the course of hemoglobin SS disease. Heterozygotes for hemoglobin S (hemoglobin AS) are thought to be clinically unaffected, except for an increased incidence of hematuria and occasional reports of sudden death related to high altitude and extreme exercise. The absence of α-globin genes (α-thalassemia) inherited along with hemoglobin SS disease also occurs, although whether the clinical course of sickle cell disease is altered in these patients is unclear.

The first description of sickle cell anemia appeared in 1910, and its associations with hemolytic anemia and vasoocclusive crises were subsequently made. It is now understood that the presence of hemoglobin SS results in numerous direct and indirect effects in the red cell. The abnormal hemoglobin polymerizes readily under conditions of low pH, high ionic strength, or hypoxemia and adheres to the cell membrane, resulting in the characteristic sickled shape of affected red cells. Even cells that are not sickled in shape demonstrate rigidity and adherence and have a host of alterations in cell structure and function.

The clinical hallmark of the disease is hemolytic anemia with reticulocytosis and the appearance of irreversibly sickled cells on the peripheral blood smear. Tremendous clinical variability exists within the population of patients with hemoglobin SS disease, but most affected patients suffer from vasoocclusive crises and require hospitalization one or more times in their lives for hydration and pain management. Chronic vasculopathy and tissue ischemia result in dysfunction of many organs, including the heart, kidneys, lungs, skin, and central nervous system. After early childhood, irreversible organ damage is the most frequent cause of death in these patients. Because of splenic dysfunction from early childhood onward, bacterial infections have historically been a major cause of mortality and morbidity in young children with sickle cell disease. With the advent of penicillin prophylaxis in the 1980s,[6] as well as immunization against *Streptococcus pneumoniae* and *H influenzae*, newborn screening, and improvements in supportive care, the death rate from infection has decreased. Infection continues to be a major threat to survival, especially in patients younger than 6 years of age (Table 14-3). Acute abdominal pain is a common

TABLE 14-3. *Cause of death by age in patients with sickle hemoglobinopathies**

	Age at time of death		
Cause	<3 y (%)	3–10 y (%)	10–20 y (%)
Infection	60.7	26.7	23.3
Cerebrovascular accident	3.6	6.7	23.3
Other	10.7	26.7	33.3
Unknown	25.0	40.0	20.0

* Patients entered into a cooperative study on sickle cell disease when less than 20 years of age.

(Adapted from Leikin SL, Gallagher MS, Kinney TR, et al. Mortality in children and adolescents with sickle cell disease. Pediatrics 1989;84:500)

occurrence in the schoolage or older patient and poses difficult diagnostic dilemmas. Pain may be due to mesenteric sickling, vertebral infarction, sequestration crisis, hepatitis, or acute cholecystitis in addition to the usual causes. Priapism is a distressing, often recurrent problem that causes sexual dysfunction in almost half of affected patients.

Because of the high incidence of morbidity and mortality related to organ dysfunction, and because of the often severe anemia associated with this disease, transfusion therapy has been a cornerstone of treatment for decades. Initially, attempts were made to improve tissue oxygenation by increasing the hematocrit value. Subsequently, it became obvious that transfusion also diluted the concentration of hemoglobin SS–containing cells and diminished the production of additional abnormal cells by reducing erythropoietin levels. As clinical and laboratory evidence accumulates, it is recognized that the decision to transfuse red cells to improve oxygen delivery is a complicated undertaking. Oxygen delivery to the tissues is dependent on multiple variables, including the oxygen affinity of the hemoglobin, vascular perfusion, blood volume, hemoglobin and hematocrit, and viscosity. Because of the many intrinsic abnormalities in cells containing hemoglobin SS, these cells have increased viscosity that is aggravated by, but not confined to, the deoxygenated state. The adverse effects of hematocrit on viscosity can be seen even with a sickle hematocrit value (proportional to percentage of hemoglobin SS–containing cells multiplied by total hematocrit) of 20% to 25%. Increasing the hematocrit by simple transfusion can worsen oxygen delivery to the tissues by raising blood viscosity. Alternatively, oxygen delivery can be improved by exchanging normal (hemoglobin A) cells for sickle cells while maintaining a stable hematocrit. Recommendations for optimal values for hematocrit and percentage of hemoglobin SS–containing cells vary depending on the clinical situation; however, data from controlled, randomized studies are lacking. In general, red cell levels below the patient's baseline level in the setting of acute illness can be treated by simple transfusion. Ideally, transfusions should be given slowly, in small aliquots, with diuretic administration as needed. If rapid correction is needed in the setting of borderline cardiac function or volume status, or if management or prevention of venoocclusive events is desired, red cell exchange transfusion is recommended.[7]

Although perioperative morbidity and mortality rates in sickle cell disease are improving, the potential for serious complications remains. Ongoing prospective trials are evaluating

preoperative transfusion to increase the hemoglobin level to 10 g/dL and reduce the hemoglobin SS–containing cells to either 60% or 30% of the red cell count. Standard practice is to offer chronic or exchange transfusion to raise the hemoglobin to 10 g/dL with or without reducing hemoglobin SS levels to 30% for major surgical or ophthalmologic procedures.

Whether a particular patient with sickle cell disease requires transfusion depends on age and the clinical severity of disease. Other risk factors have not been clearly identified, but most affected patients undergo transfusion at least once. It is recommended that all patients with sickle hemoglobinopathies receive the hepatitis B immunization series. These patients have the usual risks of blood transfusion as well as problems with hyperviscosity and iron overload. Alloimmunization rates in patients with sickle cell disease are higher than those in the general population, approaching 20% in most series (Table 14-4). The likelihood of antibody formation depends in part on the frequency of exposure to a foreign antigen, the antigenicity of the antigen, and the immunologic responsiveness of the recipient. Using donations from a racially discordant donor pool enhances the risk of foreign antigen exposure. Historically, the major antigens are Rhesus (Rh), Kell (K), Duffy (Fy), and Kidd (Jk). Many of the antibodies fall to undetectable levels in the blood over time, so an anamnestic response to further antigen exposure is a serious problem in these patients. Strategies to prevent and manage alloimmunization include attempting to match the donor–recipient pool more closely, routine extended red cell phenotyping of recipients, and phenotyping of donor units for the additional problematic antigens. Antigen-negative blood is cryopreserved and stored through the American Red Cross Rare Donor Registry.[7]

QUANTITATIVE AND QUALITATIVE PLATELET ABNORMALITIES

Platelets participate in the first phase of hemostasis, during which a platelet plug forms at the site of blood vessel injury. Platelets limit blood loss at the site of endothelial disruption within injured blood vessels and provide a framework to facilitate fibrin clot formation by the members of the plasma phase of coagulation. Platelets circulate as smooth disks; but on exposure to various agonists released in response to vascular injury, they become activated, aggregate, and adhere to the site of disrupted endothelium. During platelet activation, arachidonic acid

TABLE 14-4. *Alloimmunization frequency in sickle cell anemia compared with other chronic anemias*

Diagnosis	Number of patients	Number of patients given transfusions	Average number of transfusions	Number of patients with alloantibodies
Sickle cell anemia				
Total	158	107		32 (30%)
Children (1–17 y)	85	42		10 (24%)
Adults (18–41 y)	73	65		22 (34%)
No alloantibodies	75	—	13 (1–45)	
Alloantibodies	32	—	23 (3–46)	
Chronic anemia (age 1–18 y)	19	19	131 (3–600)	1 (5%)

(Adapted from Vichinsky EP, Earles A, Johnson RA, et al. Alloimmunization in sickle cell anemia and transfusion of racially unmatched blood. N Engl J Med 1990;322:1617)

and its metabolites trigger release of platelet granules into the extracellular environment. More platelets are then recruited and activated, resulting in platelet aggregation and rapid formation of a platelet plug.

A number of platelet membrane glycoproteins participate in primary hemostasis by serving as receptors for adhesive polymeric proteins.[8] Identification of many of these glycoproteins and elucidation of their functions have been achieved by examination of platelets from patients with qualitative, congenital defects of platelet function. Von Willebrand factor binds the platelet glycoprotein Ib–glycoprotein IX complex and subendothelial matrix protein, resulting in platelet adhesion to the vessel wall. As platelets become activated and recruit additional platelets, neutrophils, and monocytes to the area, the plug is formed by linking platelets and fibrinogen through the glycoprotein IIb/IIIa receptors. Von Willebrand factor can also participate in the cross-linking of platelets.

Normal circulating platelet counts for all ages are between 150,000 and 400,000. Usually, this constitutes two thirds of the total body platelets. The other one third of platelets are located in the spleen. The amount of the platelet pool sequestered within the spleen, however, increases in proportion to the size of the spleen. The average platelet life-span is 7 to 10 days, although survival of transfused platelets in the thrombocytopenic recipient is decreased in proportion to the severity of the thrombocytopenia.

In contrast to the deep muscle hematomas and hemarthrosis associated with defects in the fluid phase of coagulation, qualitative and quantitative platelet abnormalities typically produce epistaxis, petechiae, purpura, ecchymoses, gastrointestinal bleeding, excessive bleeding from superficial cuts and abrasions, and menorrhagia.

Initial evaluation of a patient with an abnormal platelet count must include a review of the peripheral blood smear to confirm that the manual platelet count agrees with the automated count. Some of the congenital qualitative platelet abnormalities are also characterized by alterations in the size or appearance of the platelets, and abnormally sized platelets may be missed by an automated counter. Pseudothrombocytopenia can result from aggregation of the platelets in the syringe or blood tube. These platelet clumps are often best seen at the periphery of the blood smear. Finally, some causes of both thrombocytopenia and thrombocytosis are associated with abnormalities of the other blood cell components. Once a determination is made that the thrombocytopenia is not artifactual, examination of the patient for splenomegaly indicates whether the quantitative abnormality is likely due to splenic sequestration. If the spleen is enlarged, a greater percentage of the total platelet mass is stored there. In general, splenic sequestration results in mild thrombocytopenia. Platelet counts of less than 50,000 should be investigated for other causes.

Quantitative defects of platelets are due to either decreased production or increased destruction. The most common cause of thrombolytic thrombocytopenia is immune mediated. When antibodies are directed against either an autoantigen or an alloantigen on the platelet membrane or against an antigen adsorbed onto the membrane, accelerated clearance of the cells by the reticuloendothelial system results. Circulating immune complexes can also be deposited on the platelet surface Fc receptor. In idiopathic (immune) thrombocytopenia (ITP), an otherwise well child develops bruising and petechiae with isolated thrombocytopenia. For most young children, the disease is self-limiting (generally within 6 months), and therapeutic intervention is necessary only to prevent serious bleeding. Reports of intracranial bleeding in patients with platelet counts lower than 10,000 have justified consideration of treatment for these patients, especially if extensive mucosal bleeding or retinal petechiae exist. If therapy is undertaken, the most common frontline agents are corticosteroids, 1 to 2 mg/kg/d of methylprednisolone or the equivalent for 2 to 3 weeks with subsequent taper, and intravenous immunoglobulin, 2 g/kg total dose, given over 2 to 5 days. Patients who respond initially and subsequently relapse can be successfully retreated with these same agents. If ITP persists beyond 6 months, splenectomy is strongly considered in patients who are older than 6 years of age and whose thrombocytopenia results in significant risk of problematic bleeding. Because of the risk of postsplenectomy sepsis from encapsulated organisms, vaccinations against *S pneumoniae* and *H influenzae* should be given before surgery. Intensive family education and postsplenectomy penicillin prophylaxis are also advised. In the event of a life-threatening hemorrhage, a multimodality therapeutic approach that includes intravenous immunoglobulin, steroids, and emergency splenectomy is often used. Most patients (65% to 88%) with chronic ITP respond to splenectomy. Often, there is an immediate rise in the platelet count to more than 1,000,000 in the postoperative period, with subsequent equilibration at a lower level. If the patient relapses after an initial good response to splenectomy, the possibility of an accessory spleen should be considered. Other therapies for refractory, chronic ITP use chemotherapeutic agents or other immunomodulatory agents with variable records of success and toxicity.

Alloimmunization as the cause of thrombocytopenia can occur in the neonatal period when a mother who is negative for the platelet antigen Pl^{A1} (HPA-1) produces immunoglobulin G antibodies against a the platelets of her Pl^{A1}-positive fetus. The resultant thrombocytopenia is often severe, albeit transient, with serious morbidity and mortality rates of about 15%. Posttransfusion purpura is a rare syndrome that occurs most commonly in multiparous women; it also occurs in nulliparous women and in men. All affected patients are Pl^{A1} negative and received blood transfusions about 10 days before diagnosis. The thrombocytopenia is severe, and significant bleeding episodes occur commonly.

Drugs can cause thrombocytopenia by suppression of bone marrow production or by immune-mediated mechanisms, such as drug–antidrug immune complex deposition, by exposure of platelet neoantigens by the drug, or by induction of autoantibodies. These idiosyncratic, immune-mediated reactions are commonly associated with heparin, quinidine, penicillin, digoxin, and anticonvulsants.

Nonimmune thrombolytic thrombocytopenia may be due to an increase in platelet activation, as seen in thrombotic thrombocytopenia and hemolytic–uremic syndrome. In these syndromes, platelets clump within the microvasculature and damage the circulating erythrocytes. Another common cause of thrombocytopenia, disseminated intravascular coagulation, is a result of activation of plasma coagulation factors and subsequent intravascular thrombosis and fibrinolysis with increased platelet consumption. Thrombocytopenia can also be associated with the polycythemia of cyanotic congenital heart disease and may be improved by phlebotomy. In neonates, asphyxia, respiratory distress, or meconium aspiration may be associated with low platelet counts. Infants with unexplained thrombocytopenia should be evaluated for the presence of a giant hemangioma causing a reduction in platelet survival, the Kasabach-Merritt syndrome. This generally remits in the first few years of life as the lesions regress.

Quantitative defects of platelets may be due to decreased megakaryocytopoiesis from bone marrow infiltration with malignancy, storage diseases, granulomas, fibrosis, or histiocytoses. Congenital amegakaryocytic thrombocytopenia can be idiopathic, inherited, or due to a congenital viral infection. Thrombocytopenia with absent radii is characterized by megakaryocytopenia, autosomal recessive inheritance, and skeletal abnormalities of the radii or other parts of the upper extremities. Other platelet abnormalities with quantitative and qualitative components include Wiskott-Aldrich syndrome, May-Hegglin anomaly, and Bernard-Soulier syndrome.

BLOOD TRANSFUSION

The practice of blood transfusion originated in the 1650s as therapy for a diverse collection of psychiatric and systemic illnesses. In those days, transfusion was a surgical procedure in which blood was directly transferred from donor to recipient, and outcomes ranged from apparent cure of disease to sudden death of the transfusion recipient. Several critical discoveries in the 20th century enabled transfusion of blood components to become a cornerstone of supportive and therapeutic care in children. In 1901, Landsteiner described the ABO blood groups and ushered in the study of immunohematology. Storage of blood for up to 10 days became possible after the discovery of the anticoagulant sodium citrate in 1920. The use of disposable plastic collection systems for blood, which began in the 1950s, eliminated many sources of contamination that had resulted in febrile transfusion reactions and even death in transfusion recipients.

The field of transfusion medicine has expanded enormously in the past two decades, and a variety of blood-component products and a number of different collection and manipulation strategies are now offered.[9] Unfortunately, those same problems with stability, compatibility, and delivery of an uninfected blood product, which first surfaced in the 1600s, raise concerns about transfusion therapy today. An understanding of the indications and strategies for proper administration of blood products remains critical.

The anucleate red blood cells use glucose by means of anaerobic metabolism to generate adenosine triphosphate (ATP) and to maintain the function of the membrane's Na^+-K^+-ATPase pump. Immediately on removal of the red cell from the donor, a number of changes in the function and deformability of the membrane begin to occur. Progressive losses of ATP and 2,3-diphosphoglycerate (2,3-DPG), as well as other biochemical alterations, have been observed, leading to cellular swelling, decreased posttransfusion survival, and impaired delivery of oxygen to the tissues in the banked red blood cell. Although the cause of these alterations is not well understood, incubation with nutrient substances formulated to maintain ATP levels in the cells results in restoration of normal red cell morphology and improved posttransfusion viability. For this reason, most red cells are stored in a nutrient solution, such as Adsol or Nutricel, which results in a 42-day shelf life. An adenine-supplemented anticoagulant solution that yields a 35-day shelf life is also available. Standard practice is to add 450 mL of donor blood to 63 mL of a citrate-phosphate-dextrose solution and then add the nutrient solution after a holding period of up to 8 hours at room temperature. This results in a decrease of 2,3-DPG levels of about 25%. The determination of the appropriate duration of storage depends on the posttransfusion viability of the cells. On the last day of storage, 24 hours after transfusion, the red cells must demonstrate a mean survival of 75% and result in less than 1% hemolysis.[9]

Table 14-5 lists the composition of whole blood and packed red blood cells after various additions and periods of storage. Red cell products also can be manipulated in various ways to remove the non–red cell components. Most of the available blood products are discussed next.

Whole blood units are less available and have limited indications for use in children. The advantages of transfusing fresh whole blood (less than 48 hours in storage) over red blood cells alone can be seen in situations in which the effects of massive transfusions, resulting in depletion of coagulation factors and platelets, cannot be easily counteracted by the additional infusions of fresh frozen plasma, cryoprecipitate, and stored platelets. Fresh whole blood that has been stored for less than 48 hours has higher levels of stable coagulation factors and 2,3-DPG and lower levels of potassium and ammonia than blood stored for longer periods. Although infrequently used, fresh whole blood can be considered in neonatal exchange transfusion and in the rare situation in which massive use is anticipated in neonatal cardiac surgery.

Packed red blood cells are used for most red cell replacement therapy. If the cells are prepared and stored in the anticoagulant solution, the average hematocrit value of the product is 80%. Further dilution of the cells by addition of a nutrient solution drops the average hematocrit value to 50% to 60%.

Leukocyte depletion of red blood cells was initiated because most febrile, nonhemolytic transfusion reactions are caused by recipient human leukocyte antigen (HLA) sensitization. The importance of transmission of white cell–associated infections, including cytomegalovirus (CMV), and the benefit of leukodepletion in preventing HLA sensitization in potential allograft recipients have been recognized. The most efficient and commonly used method of white-cell removal uses the third-generation leukocyte filters, either at the bedside or in the blood bank. These filters remove 99.9% (three logs) of the white cells from a unit of red cells or platelets.

Irradiation of blood products is intended to impair the proliferative capacity of the lymphocytes without affecting the function of other cellular components to prevent transfusion-associated graft-versus-host disease (TAGVHD) in recipients with congenital or acquired immunodeficiency.

TAGVHD occurs when transfused lymphocytes are allowed to proliferate in a susceptible host and initiate a cellular immune response. It typically occurs within 6 to 10 days after transfusion but can occur as long as 2 months after. Patients considered to be at high risk of TAGVHD who should receive irradiated blood products include the following:

- Fetuses receiving intrauterine or periumbilical simple exchange transfusions
- Neonates weighing less than 1 kg

TABLE 14-5. *Composition of available red cell products*

Product	Viable cells 24 h posttransfusion (%)	Plasma pH at 37°C	ATP (% of initial value)	2,3-DPG (% of initial value)	Plasma (%)	Polymorpho-nuclear leukocytes (%)	Lymphocytes (%)	Coagulation factors (%)	Platelets
Whole blood									
<48 h					100	100	100	Decreased factors V and VIII	<1
<4 h					100	100	100	100	>90
Whole blood in CPD									
0 d	100	7.2	100	100					
7 d	98	7.0	97	99					
21 d	85	6.9	86	31					
Whole blood nutrient solution									
0 d	96	7.0	100	75					
7 d	96	6.9	96	51					
35 d	80	6.8	89	3					
42 d	75	6.5	82	0					
Packed cells					20–50	100	100	10	<1
Leukofiltered cells					5	0.15	0.05	10	<1
Washed packed cells					<1	10	10	<1	<1
Frozen deglycerolized cells					<1	<5	<5	<1	<1

ATP, adenosine triphosphate; CPD, citrate-phosphate-dextrose; 2,3-DPG, 2,3-diphosphoglycerate.
(Data from Technical manual of the American Association of Blood Banks. Fayetteville, IN, Roberts Press, 1990)

- Patients with congenital or acquired immunodeficiencies
- Patients receiving immunosuppressive therapies
- Patients undergoing solid organ transplantation of organs containing lymphoid tissue
- Bone marrow transplant candidates and recipients
- Patients receiving donor cells from a first-degree relative or from any other HLA partially identical, HLA homozygous donor

Immunologically, normal recipients who are heterozygous for HLA proteins do not reject lymphocytes from a donor homozygous for one of the recipient's haplotypes. For this reason, blood products from first-degree relatives should be irradiated before transfusion. Survival of irradiated red blood cells and platelets is essentially unchanged.

Washed red blood cells have been processed with three to four washes of normal saline and a final resuspension in normal saline to remove most traces of plasma and plasma proteins. The major indications for use of this product are in patients with multiple, refractory urticarial or anaphylactic transfusion reactions and in patients with immunoglobulin A deficiency.

Before the advent of leukocyte depletion through filters, frozen, deglycerolized red blood cells were often used when leukocyte removal was indicated. Because the freezing and thawing of the red cells involves extensive washing with solutions of varying osmolarities, 92% to 95% of the white cells and 90% of the plasma are incidentally removed. The major indication at present is in the transfusion of patients with preexisting red cell antibodies requiring extensive antigen matching. The more rare types of red blood cells are frozen for long-term storage.

Special Situations

The fetus is adapted to the lower intrauterine oxygen tension by maintenance of a higher hematocrit and by the presence of fetal hemoglobin. Neonates are born with a predominance of fetal hemoglobin and a hematocrit value that, although it varies by the type of delivery and the gestational age, is higher than the normal range in childhood or adulthood. Infants with cardiorespiratory dysfunction may benefit not only from correction of anemia but also from the addition of hemoglobin A–containing cells with normal deformability, in contrast to the poorly deformable fetal red blood cells. Compatibility testing for neonates must include ABO and Rh typing of the mother as well as the newborn, antibody screening, and tests to detect maternal immune anti-A and anti-B antibodies. Because the neonatal immune system is fairly unresponsive to antigenic stimulation by red blood cells, if the initial antibody screen is negative, repeated cross-matching and antibody screening are not necessary in the first 4 months of life. If antibody is found in the initial maternal or neonatal screening, compatibility testing and screening must be done before each transfusion. Because of the small circulating blood volume of neonates, an ill newborn may lose 10% to 15% of blood volume each day from laboratory testing. The ideal hematocrit for an ill infant is not known, but the general guideline is that patients with cardiorespiratory compromise or severe illness should have their hematocrit maintained closer to the normal value for age (target range for hematocrit of 30% to 40%). The role of transfusion therapy for premature and small-for-gestational-age infants in the recovery phase of their care is less clearly understood, and studies evaluating the relation between weight gain and hemoglobin concentration have produced conflicting results. If transfusion is necessary, the small volume of blood required, the frequency of anticipated transfusions, and the desire to limit the number of donor units to which each infant is exposed have inspired the practice of splitting donor blood units into smaller aliquots for use as needed. In addition, because the ill neonate is more susceptible to hypothermia and hypocalcemia, the blood should be prewarmed and low in citrate.

Newborns with severe jaundice or severe isoimmune hemolytic anemia may require exchange transfusion. In this case, the cells should be group compatible with mother and infant, and the plasma should be group compatible or type AB. The red cells should be less than 5 days old.

Immunocompromised Hosts

Neonates with a birthweight of less than 1 kg and others who are considered to be immunocompromised and therefore at risk for developing TAGVHD should receive irradiated cellular blood products as discussed earlier. Because of the serious risk of introducing CMV or other white cell–associated infections in these patients, the products should also be leukodepleted. Many centers also reserve CMV-negative products for those patients who have no evidence of prior infection with CMV.

Massive Transfusion

Massive blood transfusion is usually considered to occur when more than one blood volume is administered within 6 hours. Children, especially those with liver or renal dysfunction, are susceptible to citrate toxicity and require monitoring for hypocalcemia. The awake child may complain of abdominal pain; otherwise, hypotension can be an early sign of hypocalcemia. Replacement therapy can use either calcium gluconate or calcium chloride. As the citrate in the blood unit is metabolized to bicarbonate, the massively transfused patient becomes alkalotic. Potassium is driven into the cells, and the patient may become hypokalemic. If a child receives replacement therapy with packed red blood cells in fresh frozen plasma and crystalloids, a dilutional coagulopathy may result, requiring replacement with platelets, additional fresh frozen plasma, and cryoprecipitate.

Sickle Cell Disease

Donor red blood cells should be screen negative for sickle cell disease, and units less than 5 days old are preferred because of their higher levels of 2,3-DPG. Because most donor blood is racially discordant with the recipient, alloimmunization with minor blood group antigens and difficulty in cross-matching recipients are major problems.[7] Strategies to encourage donations by family members or a more antigenically concordant group and extended phenotyping of donor and recipient red cells are being undertaken to minimize this problem. Indications for transfusion are discussed in the section on sickle cell anemia.

Autologous Donation

In patients scheduled for elective surgery who are thought likely to require blood transfusion, autologous donation has become popular. Generally accepted criteria include a donor hematocrit value of 30% and weight of 60 lb or more.

Platelet Transfusion

As recognition of the infectious risks of blood transfusions increased in the late 1980s, transfusions of red cells, fresh frozen plasma, and purified clotting factors decreased. Only the incidence of platelet transfusions has continued to rise, in part owing to the increasing number of transplantation programs and more toxic chemotherapeutic regimens. Platelets can be prepared from a single unit of whole blood. This random donor product yields 5 to 7 $\times$ 10^{10} platelets in 50 to 70 mL, and transfusion of one such unit per 10 kg of patient weight is predicted to increase the platelet count by 40,000 to 50,000/μL. Apheresis is the second method of preparation, and the demand for this single donor platelet product is increasing sharply. These units contain 3 to 4 $\times$ 10^{11} platelets in 200 to 300 mL of plasma. Transfusion of one such unit per square meter of patient body surface area should cause an increase in the platelet count of 40,000/μL.

Either platelet product can be filtered, washed, and irradiated as needed. The indications for these procedures were described for red cells. The survival of the transfused platelets is usually somewhat less than the estimated platelet lifespan of 7 to 10 days. In patients who are febrile, severely thrombocytopenic, or actively consuming or sequestering platelets, the platelet survival time may be dramatically shortened. Efficacy of transfusion can be documented by determining platelet counts just before, 1 hour after, and 24 hours after infusion of platelets. If the platelet count is less than expected 1 hour after transfusion, immune-mediated destruction of the platelets, involving either an autoantibody, an HLA-specific antibody, or platelet-specific antigens might have occurred. If the platelet count drops rapidly between the 1- and 24-hour postinfusion counts, non–immune-mediated destruction from fever, sepsis, splenic sequestration, and other mechanisms is suspected. Patients who are refractory to platelet transfusions at 1 hour after the infusion may benefit from leukocyte-poor products. Some patients show improvements with ABO- and HLA class I–matched platelets. Irradiated products from family members also may be better tolerated.

Although apheresis platelet products markedly reduce the exposures to foreign HLA and other antigens as well as the infectious risks of transfusion, the risks as outlined for red cell transfusions still exist. The decision to transfuse platelets must include consideration of the clinical situation, the platelet count, and the expected function of the platelets. In patients who lack platelet dysfunction, serious spontaneous bleeding does not generally occur when the platelet count is greater than 10,000. Major surgical procedures have been safely undertaken with platelet counts of greater than 50,000. In the face of platelet dysfunction, either acquired or congenital, or when other coagulation disorders are coexistent, higher platelet counts, clotting factor correction, and reversal of anticoagulation agents may be needed.

A patient who was previously pregnant or who has undergone an earlier transfusion may develop signs and symptoms of posttransfusion purpura 7 to 10 days after the transfusion of platelets or red cells. This occurs usually, but not exclusively, in the 2% of the population who test negative for the platelet antigen Pl^{A1}. The immune-mediated destruction is nonspecific, so transfused and recipient platelets are affected. Treatment with intravenous γ-globulin or plasmapheresis is recommended. Subsequent platelet transfusions, if necessary, should be Pl^{A1} negative, washed, and leukocyte depleted. Washed red cells are also recommended for these patients.

Transfusion Reactions

The most commonly reported transfusion reaction is the urticarial reaction. This can occur even in previously untransfused patients, and the exact cause is unknown. Allergic reaction to a soluble antigen or protein is commonly suggested. If a localized reaction occurs, the transfusion should be interrupted and an antihistamine administered. Patients who experience repeated urticarial reactions to blood product transfusion should be pretreated with antihistamines with or without corticosteroids. Those who continue to exhibit symptoms should receive washed cells or frozen, deglycerolized red cells.

The next most common type of transfusion reaction is the febrile, nonhemolytic reaction characterized by chills, diaphoresis, or fever during a blood product transfusion. These reactions occur in patients previously sensitized either by pregnancy or prior transfusion and are due to a reaction against plasma or leukocyte protein alloantigens in the blood product. Treatment includes the use of antipyretics, corticosteroids, and narcotics. Future cellular transfusion products should be leukodepleted.

The most severe transfusion reactions are due to antigenic incompatibility. The hemolytic transfusion reaction is generally due to ABO incompatibility, and this is most commonly due to clerical errors. The antigen–antibody interaction activates complement and results in intravascular hemolysis. Symptoms include abdominal and lower back pain, fever, chills, tachycardia, hypotension, shock, and renal failure. Anemia with spherocytosis, hemoglobinemia, hemoglobinuria, low haptoglobin levels, disseminated intravascular coagulation, and a positive direct Coombs test are seen. Treatment includes immediate cessation of the transfusion, collection of specimens to document the cause of the reaction, and supportive care with fluids, mannitol, blood pressure control, and corticosteroids as needed to maintain circulation and assist in maintaining urine output.

Delayed transfusion reactions commonly occur 3 to 10 days after a transfusion and are generally due to an anamnestic response to a minor blood group antigen. Although usually milder in nature than those caused by ABO incompatibility, the symptoms and signs are similar. The diagnosis is made in a recently transfused patient with anemia or bilirubinemia and is confirmed by a positive direct Coombs test and identification of a new red cell antibody in the patient.

Infectious Risks

A number of bacterial, viral, and parasitic diseases have reportedly been transmitted through blood transfusion, and infection remains the most common cause of morbidity and mortality resulting from transfusion therapy. The risks of infection transmission have been minimized by the use of increasingly sensitive assays for detection of infected donors and by the elimina-

tion from the donor pool of paid donors and certain groups of people considered at high risk for having certain viral infections. The incidence of transfusion-associated hepatitis B infection in the United States is estimated to be 1 in 10,000. For this reason, the administration of the hepatitis B vaccine series is advised for any patient who requires chronic transfusion therapy. An antibody against the major cause of non-A, non-B hepatitis, hepatitis C virus, is also included in the routine testing of blood products. The incidence of anti–hepatitis C antibody is about 0.6% in the United States donor population. CMV is a common viral infection, carried in and transmitted by lymphocytes, that usually causes a mild mononucleosis-type illness in the immunocompetent host. If the infection is transmitted to a patient with congenital or acquired immunodeficiency, a lethal illness can result. Neonates and others at risk of infection should receive leukocyte-depleted or CMV-negative blood products. Most attention concerning infection transmission by blood products has focused on human immunodeficiency virus type I. This lethal retroviral infection is propagated in helper or inducer T lymphocytes and induces an immunodeficiency state. Death occurs as a result of opportunistic infection or malignancy. A serologic test for human immunodeficiency virus antibodies has been used to screen donor blood units in the United States since 1985, and in conjunction with donor history screening, this has greatly reduced the incidence of transfusion-associated infection. None of the preventative strategies are completely effective at eliminating infected donor units. Thus, the physician is responsible for understanding the many risks of blood transfusion and using transfusion therapy judiciously.

Transfusion of Plasma and Plasma Derivatives

The study of coagulation and hemostasis has exploded with new discoveries in the past few decades. The coagulation and hemostatic proteins coexist in an elegantly balanced system, and deficiency of one of the components can result in excessive bleeding or thrombosis. As the roles for the individual factors have been described, identification of deficiency states and replacement of missing factors has become possible. Early attempts at replacement therapy focused on hemophilia A (factor VIII deficiency), and the history of the treatment of this disease clearly demonstrates the progression of technologic advances toward products that are relatively infection free, safe, effective, convenient, and affordable.

Many patients with acquired factor deficiencies benefit most from correction of their underlying disorder. The approach to treatment of disseminated intravascular coagulation is a classic example of this principle. The patient with laboratory abnormalities but no serious bleeding or thrombosis should be treated supportively while rapid correction of the underlying illness is attempted. If the disease is severe, a common practice is to maintain the platelet count at about 50,000 with platelet transfusions and to transfuse with fresh frozen plasma as needed to restore many circulating hemostatic and antithrombotic proteins and to maintain the plasma fibrinogen level at 100 mg/dL or greater. Cryoprecipitate and heparin are also used in some cases. Vitamin K deficiency states can result in low levels of factors II, VII, IX, and X, as well as of proteins C and S, and administration of the vitamin can result in correction of the abnormalities within hours or days. For many factor-deficiency states, meticulous attention to local control of bleeding is a cornerstone of treatment. Alteration of the fibrinolytic pathway through the use of agents such as aminocaproic acid (Amicar) is useful in selected situations, such as minor dental surgery in a patient with mild hemophilia. Finally, infusion of the synthetic vasopressin analogue, 1-desamino-(8-D-arginine)-vasopressin in patients with mild to moderate hemophilia A and in those with certain types of von Willebrand disease may release endogenous stores of these deficient components and alleviate the need for transfusion.

The most important aspects of factor-replacement therapy are the correct identification of the underlying abnormality and the clear understanding of when and to what degree correction of the abnormality is needed. Factor replacement is usually reserved for the patient who is actively bleeding or who is reasonably expected to do so as a result of surgery or other hemostatic challenge. In each situation, the physician must estimate the minimum hemostatic level needed, calculate the dose of product needed to raise the plasma level of factor to the desired level, and anticipate repeated dosing of the product, if necessary, based on the half-life of the factor infused and the clinical situation, to maintain the minimum hemostatic level for the necessary period.[10]

Reasonably safe, pure replacement products are available for factors VIII and IX. A factor XI replacement product is undergoing clinical trials. Fresh frozen plasma at 10 to 20 mL/kg is generally used for replacement of factors II, VII, X, XIII, and fibrinogen. Higher plasma levels of factors II, VII, IX, and X are achievable with prothrombin complex concentrates, but these products are associated with increased risks of infectious and thrombotic side effects. Factor V deficiency is treated with fresh frozen plasma, preferably less than 1 month old. Factor XI deficiency is usually treated with fresh frozen plasma as well, although cryoprecipitate and a prothrombin complex concentrate, Konyne 80 (Cutter/Miles, Berkeley, CA), may be used when higher levels are required. Cryoprecipitate has also been used for replacement therapy in factor XIII deficiency, hypofibrinogenemia, and dysfibrinogenemia.

Treatment principles for anticoagulant protein deficiencies also center on treatment of patients with symptoms, correction of underlying disease, and local control measures. A recombinant antithrombin III product is available. Fresh frozen plasma can be used to replace antithrombin III or protein C deficiency.

HEMOSTASIS

Tissue injury triggers a series of host reactions designed to maintain the integrity of the blood vessel while repair efforts are undertaken. Within seconds of tissue disruption, the normally quiescent participants in hemostasis become activated. Platelets form the first line of defense. The platelet plug not only prevents blood loss from the injured vessel but also, along with other activated cell membranes, provides a scaffolding on which the fibrin clot can form. After exposure to agonists such as thrombin and collagen, platelets become activated and undergo a multitude of morphologic and biochemical changes, resulting in degranulation, adherence to the injured vessel surface, binding to neutrophils and monocytes, and aggregation into a platelet plug. Second, a fibrin clot must form, but only at the site of injury. Disruption of the blood vessel exposes tissue factor, which is

constitutively expressed on the subendothelium, to the circulating plasma components of hemostasis. These proteins circulate in their inactive forms, awaiting activation by critical proteolytic cleavage events. Platelet membrane phospholipids provide a surface on which complexes of coagulation factors and calcium can efficiently interact and generate a fibrin clot. Finally, the clot must be lysed at the completion of the repair process.

Early theories about hemostasis stated that coagulation was initiated by the exposure of plasma to injured tissues.[11] The critical substance was identified as tissue thromboplastin (factor III), later renamed *tissue factor*. With the development of the prothrombin time (PT) assay, in which a large amount of tissue factor is added to induce clotting, it was observed that hemophiliac plasma clotted normally. This observation, coupled with the severe clinical picture of patients with factor VIII or IX deficiency, suggested that a coagulation pathway existed that was independent of tissue factor and that was probably more important. In 1964, the coagulation cascade or waterfall hypothesis was introduced[12,13] (Fig. 14-2). According to this theory, coagulation could be initiated either through the intrinsic pathway, so named because all of the components existed within the plasma, or by the extrinsic pathway, which required the participation of tissue factor from the subendothelium. Both pathways would activate factor X for use in the common pathway. In the common pathway, factor Xa, in combination with cofactor Va, calcium, and phospholipids, would proteolytically activate prothrombin to thrombin. Thrombin would cleave fibrinogen, and a fibrin clot would result. The extrinsic and intrinsic pathways could be tested separately by the PT and partial thromboplastin time (PTT) assays, respectively.

Although the PT and PTT assays have proved invaluable for identifying factor deficiencies, it soon became clear that the

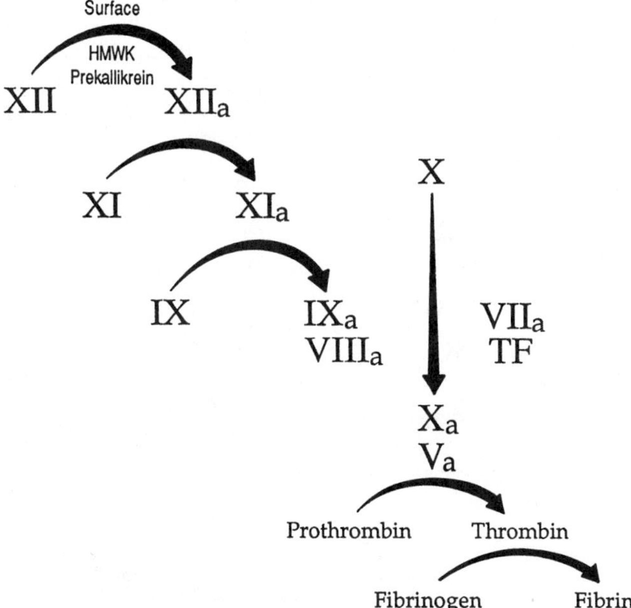

FIG. 14-2. The cascade, or waterfall, hypothesis of blood coagulation. In this scheme, coagulation is initiated by the extrinsic or intrinsic pathways, both of which lead to thrombin-mediated fibrin clot formation through a common pathway involving factor Xa, factor Va, calcium, and phospholipids.

cascade or waterfall hypothesis did not adequately explain a number of clinical and experimental observations. A physiologic activator of the intrinsic pathway's contact activation system has yet to be identified, and patients with deficiency of the contact activation factors (factor XII, high-molecular-weight kininogen, prekallikrein) do not have bleeding problems. Although patients with severe deficiencies of intrinsic pathway members factor VIII or IX have severe clinical bleeding, patients with severe factor XI deficiency have a different course. These patients do not spontaneously bleed, but they do exhibit hemorrhagic tendencies after surgery, especially if the involved tissues have a high fibrinolytic rate. Furthermore, patients with severe factor VII deficiency also have bleeding problems. The factor VIIa/tissue factor complex activates both factors X and IX,[14] suggesting a more central role for factor VII. In contrast to the PT assay results, if small amounts of tissue factor are added to induce clot formation, factors VIII and IX are necessary for optimal clot formation.[15] Resurgent interest in the serine protease inhibitor, tissue factor pathway inhibitor (TFPI), and reports by two groups in 1991 that thrombin could activate factor XI[16,17] and that autoactivation of factor XI was also possible,[18] suggest an alternative mechanism for in vivo coagulation.

In 1991, a revised hypothesis of blood coagulation was proposed[17] (Fig. 14-3). According to this theory, clotting is initiated by the exposure of subendothelial tissue factor to circulating factor VII. The factor VIIa/tissue factor complex (the extrinsic "tenase" complex) proteolytically activates some factor Xa and factor IXa. The factor IXa, in combination with cofactor VIIa, calcium, and phospholipids (the intrinsic tenase complex), participates in additional factor Xa production. Part of the factor Xa continues in the activation process to produce thrombin and fibrin, and the remainder of the factor Xa complexes with TFPI, becomes inactivated, and, in a factor Xa–dependent manner, produces feedback inhibition of the factor VIIa/tissue factor complex. In this system, initial clot formation requires cofactor VIIIa and factor IXa as well as factor VIIa. If additional factor Xa is needed to consolidate clot formation, thrombin can activate factor XI, and factor XIa proteolytically cleaves factor IX to factor IXa. Additional factor XIa may be generated by autoactivation. In cases of ongoing fibrinolysis or hemostatic stress, factor XI deficiency results in clinical bleeding. Importantly, according to this scheme, deficiency of the contact activation factors does not impair blood clotting. Intriguing therapeutic potentials exist for TFPI in the treatment of excessive thrombosis due to ongoing activation of the coagulation system (such as in disseminated intravascular coagulation) and for anti-TFPI antibodies in the treatment of bleeding hemophiliacs.

The fibrin monomers produced by thrombin-mediated cleavage spontaneously polymerize into strands. Factor XIII is a transglutaminase that covalently cross-links the fibrin strands into a stable clot. Cross-linking is not measured by the PT, activated partial thromboplastin time (aPTT), or bleeding time. The clinical symptoms of factor XIII deficiency include umbilical cord bleeding, breakdown and dehiscence of wounds, and posttraumatic bleeding. If deficiency of this factor is suspected, a factor XIII assay should be performed.

Many endogenous mechanisms exist for the regulation of coagulation so that a competent localized blood clot forms, yet systemic thrombosis is avoided.[19] Effective clot localization depends on cellular interactions as well as inhibitory proteins. One important defense against unbridled thrombus formation is that the components of hemostasis exist in an inactive state. Vascular injury triggers platelet activation, and these platelets then marginate against the vessel wall in the injured area and localize other participants in the coagulation and repair processes to the area. Platelets activated by thrombin or other substances express factor VIIIa binding sites, release platelet factor V, and also release microparticles with receptors for factors VIIIa and Va. Endothelial cells are nonthrombogenic in their unactivated state. The initial source of tissue factor is in the subendothelium of the damaged area of blood vessel, but endothelial cells and monocytes exposed to thrombin or other substances can be induced to express tissue factor, further consolidating localized clot formation. Endothelial cells are also a source of heparan sulfate and thrombomodulin.

Thrombin generated by the early stages of coagulation can activate additional factors XI, VIII, and V in the vicinity of the injury, in addition to cleaving fibrinogen. Thrombin is an active member of localized clot formation, but it can also complex with thrombomodulin and activate protein C, two components

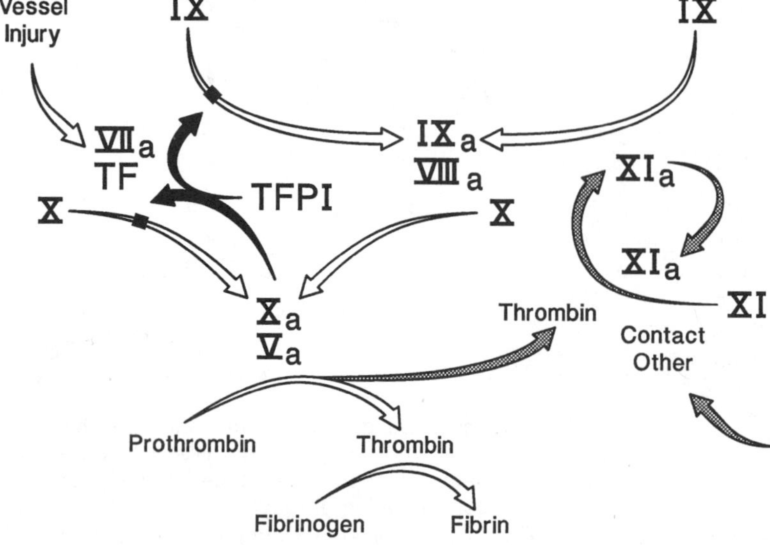

FIG. 14-3. A revised hypothesis of blood coagulation in which coagulation is initiated by factor VIIa and tissue factor–mediated activation of factors X and IX, sustained through the participation of factors VIIIa and IXa, and consolidated by factor XIa. Tissue factor pathway inhibitor inhibits factor Xa and, in a factor Xa–dependent fashion, feeds back and inhibits the factor VIIa and tissue factor complex.

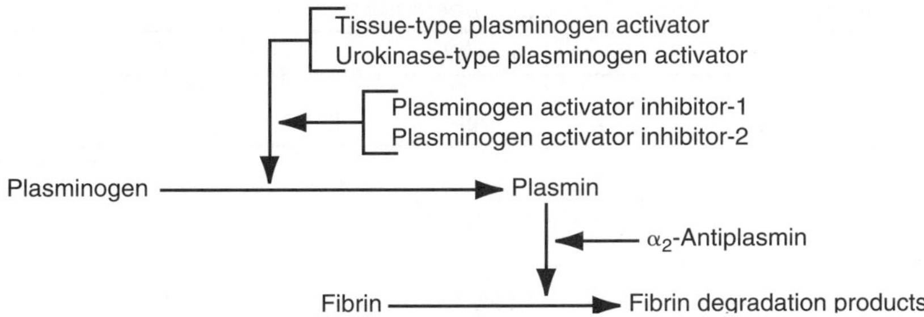

FIG. 14-4. Plasminogen activation cascade. The proenzyme plasminogen is activated to the enzyme plasmin by tissue-type plasminogen activator or urokinase-type plasminogen activator. These latter two enzymes can be inactivated after reaction with PAI-1 or PAI-2. Plasmin is capable of degrading fibrin clots to low-molecular-weight fibrin degradation products. Plasmin can be inactivated by α_2-antiplasmin.

that limit clot formation. Protein C, with its cofactor protein S, proteolytically inactivates cofactors Va and VIIIa. Circulating antithrombin III serves to inactivate proteases that drift from the clot site. Its most important substrate is thrombin, but it also inactivates factors XIa, Xa, IXa, and plasmin. Its action is greatly accelerated by heparan sulfate, which is present on endothelial cells. The anticoagulant effect of heparin is probably largely mediated by enhancement of the inactivation of thrombin and factor Xa by antithrombin III. Another serine protease inhibitor, heparin cofactor II, also performs heparin-enhanced thrombin inactivation.

FIBRINOLYSIS

Tissue-type plasminogen activator (tPA) and urokinase-type plasminogen activator (uPA) and their inhibitors modulate the physiologic regulation of fibrinolysis. The inactive proenzyme, plasminogen, is converted by plasminogen activators to plasmin, a proteolytic enzyme that degrades the fibrin network associated with blood clots. Inhibition of the fibrinolytic system can occur at the level of plasminogen activators by plasminogen-activator inhibitors types 1 and 2 (PAI-1 and PAI-2), or at the level of plasmin, mainly by α_2-antiplasmin (Fig. 14-4). The bioactivity of tPA is largely localized to the vasculature, owing to its affinity for fibrin, which facilitates its physiologic activity on clot lysis. uPA, on the other hand, predominantly functions within the extravascular compartments. Plasminogen activation within tissues contributes to a variety of cell–cell and cell–extracellular matrix interactions,[20] including trophoblast implantation, postlactational mammary gland involution, wound healing, spermatogenesis, and prostate involution. The regulation of fibrinolysis in physiologic and pathophysiologic states within the clinical setting has received increasing attention as thrombolytic therapy has become an effective means of pharmacologic clot dissolution, especially for occluded coronary arteries associated with acute myocardial infarction[21] (see Thrombolytic Therapy).

The physiologic importance of the fibrinolytic system is demonstrated by the association between abnormal fibrinolysis and a tendency toward bleeding or thrombosis. Impairment of fibrinolysis represents the most commonly observed hemostatic abnormality associated with thrombosis. It can result from defective synthesis or release of tPA from the vessel wall, deficiency or defect in the plasminogen molecule, or increased levels of plasminogen-activator inhibitors or inhibitors of plasmin (eg, α_2-antiplasmin). For example, many families have been described with severe bleeding as a result of homozygous α_2-antiplasmin deficiency. Heterozygotes (50% decreased activity)

display mild clinical bleeding. On the other hand, congenital plasminogen deficiency presents as severe thrombotic disease early in life.

Clinically, the relative imbalance between normal coagulation (as discussed earlier) and fibrinolysis results in either bleeding or thrombosis. Venous thrombosis can involve any vein in the body, although it most commonly occurs in the lower limbs. Deep calf venous thrombosis is generally less serious than proximal vessel disease. Numerous situations predispose to venous thrombosis. Venous thrombosis and its major complication, pulmonary embolism, are major pathophysiologic states that are discussed elsewhere. Arterial thrombosis, on the other hand, almost always occurs in association with atherosclerosis. As such, arterial thrombosis, while common in adults (eg, myocardial infarction, cerebrovascular disease or stroke, peripheral arterial disease), is rare in children unless there is acute injury to the artery.

Evaluation of children for thrombotic disease should include consideration of abnormalities in both coagulation and fibrinolytic systems. A defect in coagulation cofactor V that renders it resistant to cleavage inactivation by activated protein C is emerging as a common risk factor in venous thrombosis. As discussed earlier, antithrombin III, protein C, protein S, and heparin cofactor II deficiencies should be considered. In addition, dysfibrinogenemias and plasminogen deficiency or dysplasminogenemias can be involved.

EVALUATION OF INHERITED AND ACQUIRED DEFECTS IN THE HEMOSTATIC SYSTEM

Although laboratory testing can provide important etiologic information in the bleeding patient, a thorough medical history and physical examination are essential. The patient history should focus on identifying any chronic or acute organ dysfunction; details of previous episodes of excessive bleeding, bruising, or petechiae; medications; menstrual history; and response to dental extractions or circumcision. The possibility of vitamin K deficiency should be explored. Any family history of a bleeding tendency should also be recorded. Physical examination should document the extent of the bleeding, bruising, or petechiae. A search for evidence of acute or chronic disease should be undertaken. The results of these components of the evaluation dictate whether general testing for organ dysfunction, infection, or collagen vascular disorders is needed. They should also predict whether platelet dysfunction or factor deficiency or inhibition is more likely. The usual workup of a bleeding patient includes a complete blood count, PT, aPTT, fibrinogen level, and fragment D dimer assay. Levels of coagulation factors vary

TABLE 14-6. *Coagulation data for adults, children, and neonates*

	Screening test		Coagulation factors (%)								
	aPTT (s)	PT (s)	I (mg/dL)	II	V	VII + X	VIII	IX	XI	XII	XIII
Adult or child	44	13	315 ± 60	100	100	100	100	100	100	100	100
Fetus: 10–15 wk	—	—	120	—	81	18	—	—	—	—	—
Preterm infant: 27–31 wk	—	23	—	270 ± 140	30 ± 10	72 ± 25	32 ± 15	70 ± 30	27 ± 10	—	100
Preterm infant: 32–36 wk	70	17 (12–21)	226 ± 70	35 ± 12	91 ± 23	39 ± 14	98 ± 40	—	—	30	100
Term infant	55 ± 10	10 (13–20)	246 ± 55	45 ± 15	98 ± 40	56 ± 16	105 ± 35	28 ± 8	30	51	100

aPTT, activated partial thromboplastin time; PT, prothrombin time.
(Adapted from Hathaway WE. Semin Hematol 1975;12:175)

in the newborn, so factor assay results and PT and aPTT values should be compared to age-adjusted normal values (Table 14-6). A bleeding time may also be useful, although it is abnormally prolonged in most patients with platelet counts of less than 100,000 and is abnormal in all patients with platelet counts of less than 50,000. If the PT or aPTT is abnormal, further tests may be required, such as thrombin time, 50:50 mix of patient plasma with control plasma in the PT and aPTT tests, von Willebrand disease panel, and individual factor assays. Other laboratory evaluations include platelet function studies and factor XIII assay.

PREOPERATIVE COAGULATION TESTING

Preoperative patients must be questioned about their general health as well as about personal or family history of excessive bleeding. If a detailed medical history fails to uncover bleeding problems, many authorities recommend no further testing. If there is a history of excessive bleeding, PT, aPTT, fibrinogen level, platelet count, and bleeding time are recommended. Further testing can include factor XIII levels, qualitative and quantitative fibrinogen assays, α_2-antiplasmin levels, and von Willebrand panel (Table 14-7).

For surgical procedures associated with a risk of operative or postoperative bleeding, the screening tests should include a platelet count, PT, aPTT, fibrinogen level, and fragment D dimer assay. It is important to recognize that patients with autoimmune disorders or malignancy can develop clotting factor inhibitors that can cause serious postoperative bleeding. These patients should also have a preoperative laboratory evaluation.

ANTIPLATELET AGENTS

Platelets serve a critical role in maintaining the integrity of the vascular system. Under normal conditions, vascular injury triggers formation of a platelet plug at the site of injury. Occasionally, the aggregation of platelets occurs at other locations, resulting in thrombosis and tissue ischemia. Many attempts have been made to develop pharmacologic agents that interrupt the pathologic thrombotic process without affecting the normal hemostatic function of platelets. Only the most widely used class of agents, the cyclooxygenase inhibitors, is discussed here.

Arachidonic acid, a normal component of membrane phospholipids, is converted to prostaglandin H_2 by the enzyme cyclooxygenase. Prostaglandin H_2 is then converted by platelet thromboxane synthase to thromboxane A_2 and by prostacyclin synthase in the blood vessel wall to prostacyclin. Thromboxane is a potent vasoconstrictor and proaggregatory agent; prostacyclin has the opposite effects. Aspirin and the other nonsteroidal antiinflammatory agents, such as indomethacin and ibuprofen, inhibit cyclooxygenase for the 7- to 10-day life-span of the platelet in the circulation. This is presumed to be the cause of the prolongation of the template bleeding time observed in patients treated with nonsteroidal antiinflammatory agents. Endothelial and smooth muscle cells in the lining of the blood vessels, however, are capable of synthesizing new enzyme, so that prostacyclin synthesis could be recovered with time. The lack of selectivity with respect to inhibition of thromboxane A_2 versus prostacyclin biosynthesis has triggered interest in agents that could potentially inhibit specifically thromboxane A_2 synthesis. Aspirin has also been shown to acetylate the lysine groups of fibrinogen, yielding a molecule that aggregates platelets poorly and is more susceptible to plasmin-mediated fibrinolysis.

ANTICOAGULANT THERAPY

Pathologic functioning of the coagulation system can result in arterial or venous thrombosis and associated significant morbidity and mortality. Attempts to develop pharmacologic agents that successfully restore the physiologic balance to the coagulation system have been legion. Heparin and warfarin are the two most commonly prescribed agents.

Heparin therapy for anticoagulation traditionally uses unfractionated heparin, which is a mixture of linear heteropolysac-

TABLE 14-7. *Laboratory data in common bleeding disorders*

Disorder	Bleeding time	Partial thromboplastin time	Prothrombin time	Thrombin time	Corrected by normal plasma mix	Other tests
Hemophilia A	N	A	N	N	Y	Factor VIII level
Hemophilia B	N	A	N	N	Y	Factor IX level
Von Willebrand disease	A	N/A	N	N	Y	Ristocetin cofactor, factor VIIIc, vWF, ristocetin-induced cofactor activity
Afibrinogenemia	A	A	A	A	Y	—
Dysfibrinogenemia	N	N/A	A	A	Y	Reptilase time
Factor II deficiency	N	A	A	N	Y	—
Factor V deficiency	N	A	A	N	Y	Factor V level
Factor VII deficiency	N	N	A	N		Factor VII level
Factor X deficiency	N	A	A	N	Y	Factor X level
Factor XI deficiency	N	A	N	N	Y	Factor XI level
Factor XII deficiency	N	A	N	N	Y	Factor XII level
Factor XIII deficiency	N	N	N	N	Y	Factor XIII level

N, normal; A, abnormal; N/A, either normal or abnormal; Y, yes; vWF, von Willebrand factor.
(Adapted from Bithell TC. Hereditary coagulation disorders. In: Lee GR, Bithell TC, Foerster J, et al, eds. Wintrobe's clinical hematology, ed 9. Philadelphia, Lea & Febiger, 1993:1430)

charide molecules with monomer lengths ranging from 10 to greater than 100. Several low-molecular-weight heparin preparations, consisting of molecules between 15 and 20 monomers in length, are being studied for their potential superior clinical performance and safety. The anticoagulant effect is thought to be mediated by conformational changes in antithrombin III resulting from heparin binding. Antithrombin III inhibition of several plasma proteases, including factor Xa and thrombin, is markedly accelerated in the presence of heparin and is dependent on the presence of a specific pentamer sequence within the heparin molecule. Only about 30% of unfractionated heparin molecules contain the necessary sequence, and thus the entire anticoagulant activity is possessed by this 30%. Enhanced thrombin inhibition by antithrombin III also requires that the heparin molecule be at least 18 monosaccharides in length, although heparin molecules of any length enhance factor Xa inhibition. The results of clinical studies indicate that low-molecular-weight heparin is as effective as unfractionated heparin in preventing thrombosis while causing an equal number or fewer bleeding complications. These results can be explained by attributing the anticoagulation effect to accelerated inhibition of factor Xa and assuming that enhanced antithrombin activity by the predominantly longer monosaccharides in unfractionated heparin may result in bleeding complications. Results of clinical trials in the United States and in Europe require further evaluation to determine whether use of the more costly low-molecular-weight heparin preparations is warranted.

At the site of thrombus formation, the activity of heparin is not well understood. Thrombin, once bound to fibrin in a clot, is highly resistant to antithrombin III–induced inactivation. Activated platelets secrete large amounts of platelet factor 4, which binds strongly to heparin and prevents its interaction with antithrombin III. A second plasma inhibitor of thrombin, heparin cofactor II, also accelerates thrombin inhibition in the presence of heparin, but the physiologic significance of this inhibitor during heparin therapy is unknown.

Therapeutic uses for heparin include treatment of thrombosis, prophylaxis against the occurrence of thrombosis in patients known to be at high risk, and as an adjunct to fibrinolytic ther-

apy. The unfractionated drug can be administered intravenously as an intermittent bolus or continuous infusion or subcutaneously. High-, medium-, and low-dose regimens have be used. An initial loading dose of 75 U/kg followed by a continuous infusion of 10 to 25 U/kg can be used for initial, rapid anticoagulation. Long-term anticoagulation with an agent such as sodium warfarin (Coumadin) can be initiated 2 or 3 days later. The most commonly used method for monitoring the heparin effect is the aPTT. For treatment of active thrombosis, a prolongation of the aPTT to 1.5 to 2.5 times the control value is considered adequate therapy. The effect of heparin can be immediately reversed by the infusion of protamine sulfate at a dose of 1 mg per 100 units of heparin estimated to be in the circulation.

HEPARIN-INDUCED THROMBOCYTOPENIA

Heparin-induced thrombocytopenia (HIT) is a clinical syndrome characterized by a drop in the platelet count, usually below 100,000/μL, after administration of heparin. Typically, onset occurs 6 to 12 days after initiation of therapy, although patients who were previously exposed to heparin may experience thrombocytopenia within hours of repeated administration. Intravenous administration of bovine lung heparin is associated with an incidence of about 9%, although the subcutaneous route of administration or the use of porcine mucosal heparin results in a much lower incidence. It is thought that HIT is an immune-mediated phenomenon because serum IgG from affected patients causes aggregation of donor platelets and serotonin release in the presence of unfractionated heparin. There have been cases of HIT reported with the use of low-molecular-weight heparin, as well.

Although laboratory tests for HIT exist, their limited sensitivity and specificity dictate that HIT be a diagnosis of exclusion. The most widely used test measures donor platelet aggregation in the presence of unfractionated heparin and patient serum. The more sensitive tests detect serotonin release from the donor platelets rather than platelet aggregation. Unfortunately, no laboratory test or clinical features can predict distinguish patients who will follow the typical clinical course (ie, no major sequelae and resolution of thrombocytopenia after discontinuation of heparin therapy) from those who will develop the rare but dreaded white clot syndrome. In this syndrome, platelets aggregate to form arterial thrombi, which can cause limb ischemia, myocardial infarction, or central nervous system infarction.

For patients whose heparin anticoagulation can be discontinued, no other therapy is necessary. If anticoagulation is medically necessary, alternative anticoagulant agents that are not derived from unfractionated heparin should be considered. Case reports have documented successful results with a change to porcine mucosal heparin in patients with HIT. Clinical trials of specific inhibitors of thrombin as second-line therapy are also underway.

WARFARIN

Although several oral anticoagulant preparations are available, warfarin is by far the most commonly used. All of the oral anticoagulants interfere with the vitamin K–dependent, postribosomal, γ-carboxyglutamation of procoagulant factors II, VII, IX, and X, and anticoagulant proteins C and S. γ-Carboxylation of the glutamic acid residues of these proteins allows calcium binding and subsequent conformational changes that promote efficient activation of the coagulation system through coagulation factor complex formations on cell membrane surfaces. The effect of the oral anticoagulants is not apparent until about 4 days after the onset of therapy because only newly synthesized factors are affected. Traditionally, the PT has been used to estimate efficacy of anticoagulation, but variations in the ability of various thromboplastin reagents used to initiate blood clotting in the PT assay have yielded inconsistent results. Many laboratories report their results as the international normalized ratio, which requires that the thromboplastin reagents be standardized against a World Health Organization reference preparation.

The most common complication of warfarin therapy is bleeding, but warfarin-induced skin necrosis and teratogenicity associated with maternal use during the first trimester are also known to occur. Many prescription and over-the-counter drugs interact with or alter the action of warfarin.

Reversal of warfarin's effect is achieved by administration of vitamin K. Correction of the PT occurs during the next 24 hours or more as new procoagulant proteins are synthesized.

THROMBOLYTIC THERAPY

Thrombolytic therapy has become standard treatment for acute myocardial infarction and consists of the pharmacologic dissolution of the blood clot through the intravenous administration of plasminogen activators, which activate the fibrinolytic system. As discussed earlier, the fibrinolytic system consists of an inactive proenzyme, plasminogen, which, by the action of plasminogen activators, is converted to plasmin, a proteolytic enzyme that degrades the fibrin network associated with blood clots. Inhibition of the fibrinolytic system can occur at the level of plasminogen activators, mainly by plasminogen activator inhibitor type 1, or at the level of plasmin, mainly by α_2-antiplasmin (see Fig. 14-4). Controlled clinical trials in adult patients with acute myocardial infarction have demonstrated that a number of thrombolytic agents can recanalize occluded coronary arteries and thus reduce infarct size, preserve ventricular function, and reduce mortality rates.[21]

The agents in use include streptokinase (a protein produced by β-hemolytic streptococci), uPA, and tPA. Each of these agents and their newer modified forms (eg, the so-called second-generation tPAs and uPAs) all have the potential to cause a systemic lytic state, in which an increased risk of bleeding results from conversion of plasminogen to plasmin in the circulation. Most commonly as an adjunct to thrombolytic therapy, heparin is administered to minimize reocclusion. Numerous large clinical trials have compared the efficacy and side effects of various thrombolytic therapies in adults with acute myocardial infarction. No one regimen is clearly superior in terms of treatment outcome, side effects, and cost. No trials have involved children.

Thrombolytic therapy for venous thrombosis generally involves heparin or warfarin therapy, although several clinical trials in adults suggest a role for thrombolytics (streptokinase, urokinase, etc.). Potential and real complications of serious bleeding must be weighed against potential efficacy of clot dissolution. Heparin or warfarin therapy is generally prolonged and adjusted to maintain slightly prolonged coagulation parameters (eg, aPTT 1.5 times control). Again, no pediatric clinical trials are available.

REFERENCES

1. Sieff CA, Nathan DG. The anatomy and physiology of hematopoiesis. In: Nathan DG, Oski FA, eds. Hematology of infancy and childhood, ed 4. Philadelphia, WB Saunders, 1993:156.
2. Case RB, Berglund E. Ventricular function. VII. Changes in coronary resistance and ventricular function resulting from acutely induced anemia and the effect thereon of coronary stenosis. Am J Med 1955;10:397.
3. Homi J, Reynolds J. General anaesthesia in sickle cell disease. BMJ 1979;1:1599.
4. Oski FA. Iron deficiency anemia in infancy and childhood. N Engl J Med 1993;329:190.
5. Benz EJ Jr. The erythrocyte membrane and cytoskeleton: structure, function, and disorders. In: Nathan DG, Oski FA, eds. The molecular basis of blood diseases, ed 2. Philadelphia, WB Saunders, 1994:257.
6. Gaston MH, Verter JI, Woods G, et al. Prophylaxis with oral penicillin in children with sickle cell anemia. N Engl J Med 1986;314:1593.
7. Wayne AS, Kevy SV, Nathan DG. Transfusion management of sickle cell disease. Blood 1993;81:1109.
8. Beardsley DS. Platelet abnormalities in infancy and childhood. In: Nathan DG, Oski FA, eds. Hematology of infancy and childhood, ed 4. Philadelphia, WB Saunders, 1993:1561.
9. Westphal RG, ed. Handbook of transfusion medicine. Fayetteville, IN, Roberts Press, 1990.
10. Bithell TC. Hereditary coagulation disorders. In: Lee RG, Bithell TC, Foerster J, et al, eds. Wintrobe's clinical hematology, ed 9. Philadelphia, Lea & Febiger, 1993:1422.
11. Bauer KA, Broze GJ Jr, Kasper CK, et al. Coagulation/hemostasis. Hem 1993: the education program of the American Society of Hematology, 1993:83.
12. Davie EW, Ratnoff OD. Waterfall sequence for intrinsic blood clotting. Science 1964;145:1310.
13. MacFarlane RG. An enzyme cascade in the blood clotting mechanism, and its function as a biochemical amplifier. Nature 1964;202:498.
14. Osterud B, Rapaport S. Activation of factor IX by the reaction product of tissue factor and factor VII: additional pathway for initiating blood coagulation. Proc Natl Acad Sci USA 1977;74:5260.
15. Biggs R, MacFarlane RG. The reaction of hemophiliac plasma to thromboplastin. J Clin Invest 1951;4:445.

16. Naito K, Fujikawa K. Activation of human blood coagulation factor XI independent of factor XII: factor XI is activated by thrombin and factor XIa in the presence of negatively charged surfaces. J Biol Chem 1991;912:909.
17. Gailani D, Broze GJ Jr. Factor XI activation in a revised model of blood coagulation. Science 1991;912:909.
18. Gailani D, Broze GJ Jr. Factor XII-independent activation of factor XI in plasma: effects of sulfatides on tissue factor-induced coagulation. Blood 1993;82:813.
19. Broze GJ Jr, Tollefsen DM. Regulation of blood coagulation by protease inhibitors. In: Stamatoyannopoulos G, Nienhuis AW, Majerus PW, et al, eds. The molecular basis of blood diseases, ed 2. Philadelphia, WB Saunders, 1994:629.
20. Collen D, Lijnen HR. Fibrinolysis and the control of hemostasis. In: The molecular basis of blood diseases, ed 2. Philadelphia, WB Saunders, 1992:725.
21. Anderson HV, Willerson JT. Thrombolysis in acute myocardial infarction. N Engl J Med 1993;329:703.

Surgery of Infants and Children: Scientific Principles and Practice, edited by Keith T. Oldham, Paul M. Colombani, and Robert P. Foglia. Lippincott–Raven Publishers, Philadelphia, © 1997.

CHAPTER 15

Pediatric Anesthesia

Myron Yaster and Randall Wetzel

It has been conservatively estimated that 10% to 15% of all surgery performed in the United States involves children. In many pediatric surgical procedures, the perioperative anesthetic plan depends more on the child's age and the site and nature of the surgery than on the underlying disease or the technical details of the surgical procedure. In other cases, the underlying medical condition, associated anomalies, pathophysiology, and surgical procedure dictate the anesthetic plan. Technologic advances permit more sophisticated diagnoses and have vastly expanded the range of treatment options and operations available to surgeons. Additionally, technologic, physiologic, and pharmacologic advances in anesthesiology allow the pediatric surgeon to contemplate longer, more extensive, and more innovative operations on younger and more critically ill patients than ever before. Almost all surgical procedures present recurring anesthetic concerns, including preoperative anxiety and fear, positioning, airway management, blood loss and fluid replacement, conservation of body temperature, and postoperative pain management. This chapter presents an overview of these issues.

GOALS OF ANESTHESIA

The goals of anesthesia are to provide physiologic stability while achieving conditions in which successful surgical treatment is possible (Table 15-1).

Analgesia

It was long believed that newborns neither responded to nor remembered painful events because of immaturity of the developing nervous system. In the extreme, this concept resulted in newborn infants undergoing major surgery with little or no anesthesia. We now know that this underlying premise is untrue. All of the neural pathways required to perceive and respond to pain are present and functioning by the 24th week of gestation. Indeed, the failure to provide adequate analgesia and anesthesia results in increased morbidity and mortality. The need to provide adequate analgesia has been extended beyond the operating room and has led to improved analgesic care for children in all areas of medicine.[1–3]

Amnesia and Altered Consciousness

A crucial goal of anesthesia is to prevent patients from retaining their ability to encode, store, and recall information presented to them immediately before and during anesthesia. This involves blocking explicit and implicit memory and producing retrograde and anterograde amnesia. *Retrograde amnesia* refers to the inability to recollect events and information learned before the administration of a drug. *Anterograde amnesia* refers to the inability to recollect events and information learned after the administration of a drug. *Explicit memory* entails conscious recollection of events. *Implicit memory* is expressed independently of conscious awareness, by changes in task performance that are attributable to past events. Virtually all potent anesthetic agents block explicit memory, but implicit memory may be preserved. This underscores the need for careful attention to what is said and what a patient may hear during surgery.

The need to ensure an absence of awareness and amnesia is clear. Memory of perioperative events (unrelieved pain, paralysis without loss of consciousness) and conversations in the operating room may have tremendous impact on subsequent development and behavior in children. Furthermore, the fear that a child may be awake and suffering during surgery is a powerful emotional issue for parents. Providing and ensuring amnesia and analgesia are crucial to the anesthetic care of children and their families.

Akinesia

The necessity to ensure the intraoperative absence of movement is obvious. To ensure immobility, most anesthesiologists routinely use muscle relaxants as part of their anesthetic plan. Muscle relaxants, however, have no analgesic or amnestic properties. Paralyzing a child without providing sedation and analgesia is an unacceptable practice, whether in the operating room or intensive care unit.

Homeostasis

Provision of intraoperative physiologic support for the child is a major anesthetic goal. Attention to cardiorespiratory, renal,

TABLE 15-1. *Goals of anesthesia*

Analgesia
Altered consciousness (hypnosis)
Amnesia
Akinesia (the absence of movement)
Homeostasis

hepatic, and endocrine function in the perioperative period provides an opportunity to improve the patient's condition, not merely to provide intraoperative support.

DEVELOPMENTAL IMPLICATIONS

The most characteristic and significant feature of childhood is development. Every organ system undergoes distinct development that is relevant to the anesthetic management of that child. The mind set required is not that of understanding adult anesthesia and adapting it to children, but rather of approaching children as they grow from fetuses to adults. A specific, developmentally appropriate anesthetic plan must be designed for each child.

Growth is not simply a process of proportional enlargement. Body composition, including fluid content, the relation of head and body size, and cardiorespiratory physiology, change disproportionately during development. Body composition is especially important because it determines relevant pharmacologic responses. In the fetus, 90% of total body weight is water; at term, 75% is water; and by 1 year of age, 60% is water, as in adults. In addition, intracellular fluid increases from about 20% of body weight in the premature infant, to 30% in the term neonate, to 40% in the adult. Likewise, extracellular fluid falls as a proportion of body weight from 60% in the premature infant, to 45% at term, to 20% in the adult. The proportion of body weight that is muscle in premature infants is less than 20%, increasing to 50% by adulthood. Fat also increases with age. Regional blood flow is age related. It is not surprising that the uptake and distribution of inhalation anesthetics is different between adults and children.[4]

Respiratory System

Several important differences in the adult and pediatric airway are illustrated in Figure 15-1. Infants usually are described as having anterior, cephalad larynx compared to the adult. The infant airway forms an inverse cone (Fig. 15-2), with the narrowest segment at the cricoid cartilage. This remains true until puberty. To minimize the risk of subglottic edema, cuffed endotracheal tubes are avoided in children younger than 8 to 10 years of age. Airway maturation begins to occur after 2 years of age, and the adult configuration is achieved sometime near puberty. Anatomic differences in the airway have a major impact on intubation techniques in children. For example, a straight laryngoscope blade (eg, Miller blade) can lift the infant epiglottis away from the larynx, whereas the curved laryngoscope blade (eg, McIntosh blade) used in older children and adults may not.

Airway caliber undergoes continuous developmental change, from the nares to the small conducting airways. The significance of airway edema is greater in younger children. An increase in mucosal thickness increases resistance to a greater extent in children because proportional thickening diminishes the airway caliber to a greater extent. Airway resistance decreases about 15 times from infancy to adulthood, with the most dramatic change occurring near the age of 8 years. This decrease in resistance with increasing age is largely due to an increase in diameter of the small airways.[5] Infants are obligate nose-breathers, therefore, nasal obstruction, from an ordinary technique such as nasogastric tube

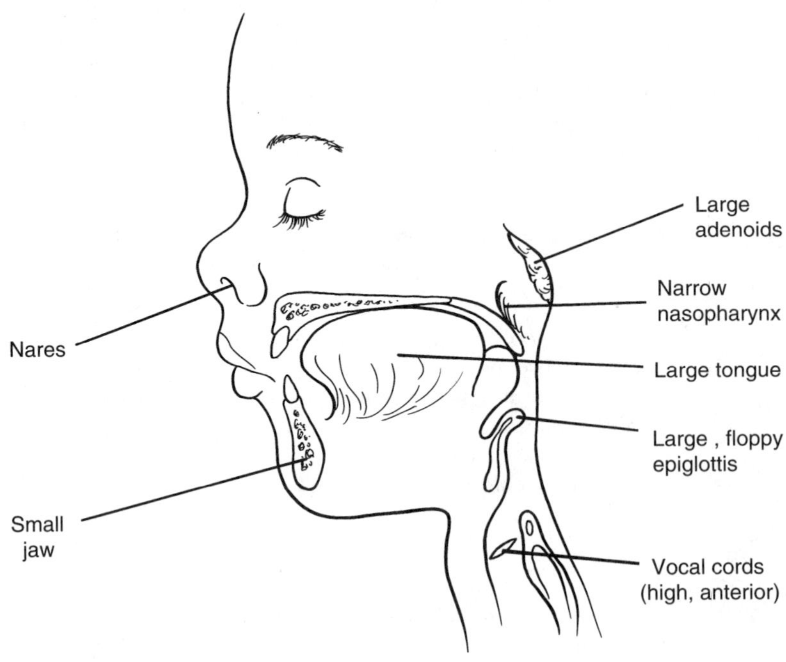

FIG. 15-1. This profile illustrates the major differences between the adult and infant airways. In children, the upper airway is limited by the nares and the narrow nasopharynx, which is additionally diminished by large adenoids. The oropharynx is reduced by the large tongue. Further narrowing results from the small jaw and the relatively large and floppy, omega-shaped epiglottis. The vocal cords are more cephalad and anterior than in adults. Visualization of the vocal cords can be more difficult in children.

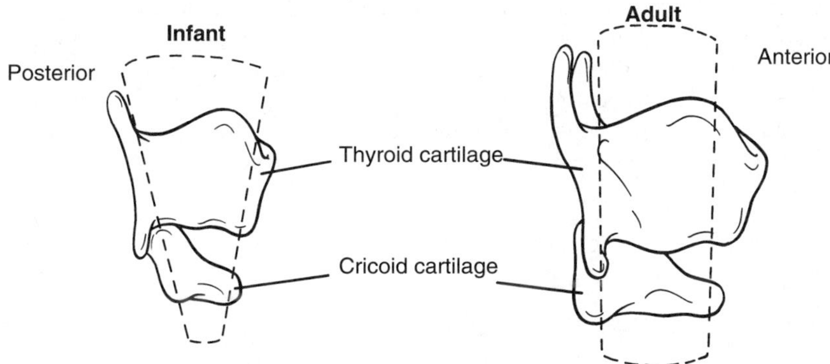

FIG. 15-2. The larynx of a child (*left*) is funnel shaped in comparison with the cylindric shape of an adult larynx (*right*). The narrowest point is at the cricoid ring. (After Cote CJ, Todres DI. The pediatric airway. In: Cote CJ, Ryan JF, Todres DI, et al. A practice of anesthesia for infants and children. Philadelphia, WB Saunders, 1993:61)

drainage, can cause significant respiratory embarrassment, especially in premature infants.[6]

Respiratory mechanics change dramatically from birth to adulthood (Fig 15-3; see Chap. 8). The respiratory system undergoes significant neuromuscular development. Central respiratory control, muscle fiber makeup, and neural innervation of the chest wall show distinct developmental changes.[7] The neonate demonstrates apnea with hypoxia,[8] rather than tachypnea, as would occur in the adult. Clearly, the impact of hypoxia in the presence of this immature response can be catastrophic in the newborn. This infantile pattern of respiratory control determines the risk of postanesthetic apnea in neonates.[9] Both infants and adults demonstrate depression of the normal CO_2 response by potent inhalational anesthetic agents and opioids.[10]

The distribution of diaphragm muscle type does not reach the adult pattern until about 2 years of age. The infantile distribution predisposes the infant to fatigue. Reflex responses and spindle innervation of the thoracic cage also undergo developmental changes. In part, this reflects the change in compliance of the thoracic wall. The Herring-Brauer response is accentuated in preterm infants, compared with full-term infants. These characteristics have a significant impact on cyclic respiration.[11]

In children, normal tidal volume approximates the closing volume. In small infants, airway closure may occur even during tidal respiration. Induction of anesthesia is associated with decreased elastic recoil and airway tone; therefore, a lung volume decrease is expected, possibly with tidal volume falling below the closing volume. In part, this accounts for the rapid onset of hypoxemia in apneic infants on the induction of anesthesia. In addition, infants have higher rates of oxygen consumption than adults. In newborn infants, oxygen consumption is about 7 mL/kg/min, about twice that of adults. This decreases with age. A number of important developmental differences between infants and adults in respiratory physiology are summarized in Table 15-2.

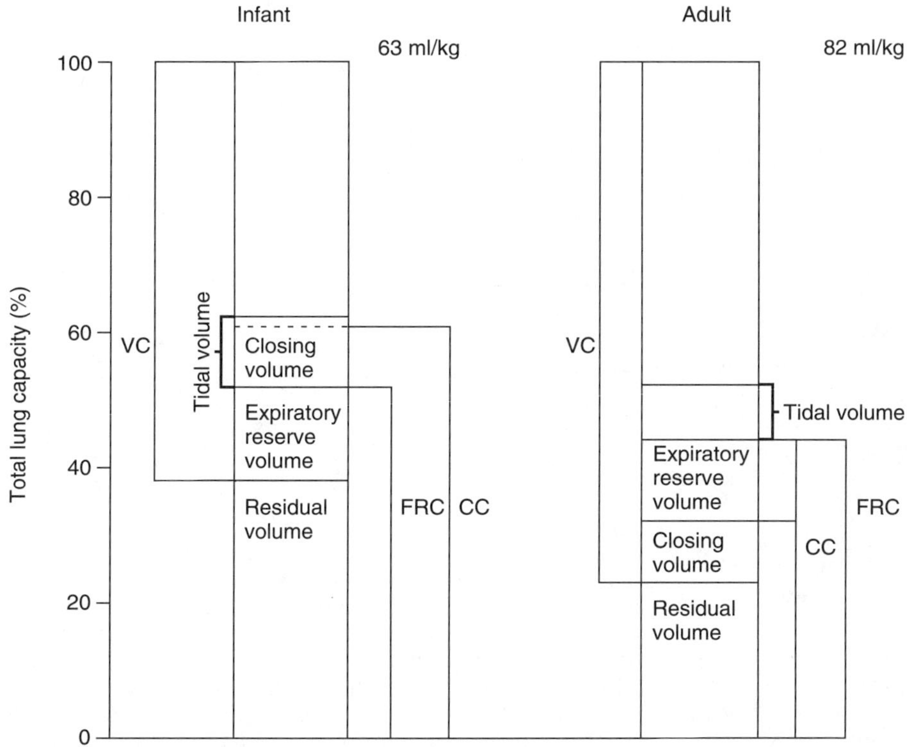

FIG. 15-3. Graphs representing the proportional lung volumes in infants (*left*) and adults (*right*). Note the important relation of functional residual capacity (FRC) to closing volume, and how this changes with age. CC, closing capacity; VC, vital capacity. (After Smith CA, Nelson NM. The physiology of the newborn infant. Springfield, IL, Charles C Thomas, 1976)

TABLE 15-2. *Normal respiratory mechanics*

Parameters	Infants	Adults
Respiratory frequency (breaths/min)	30–40	12–16
Inspiratory time (s)	0.4–0.5	1.2–1.4
Inspiratory/expiratory ratio	1:1.5–1:2	1:2–1:3
Inspiratory flow (L/min)	2–3	24
Tidal volume		
mL	18–24	500
mL/kg	6–8	6–8
Functional residual capacity (FRC)		
mL	100	2200
mL/kg	30	34
Vital capacity		
mL	120	3500
mL/kg	33–40	52
Total lung capacity		
mL	200	6000
mL/kg	63	86
Total respiratory compliance		
mL/cm H_2O	2.6–4.9	100
mL/cm H_2O/mL FRC	0.04–0.06	0.04–0.07
Lung compliance		
mL/cm H_2O	4.8–6.2	170–200
mL/cm H_2O/mL FRC	0.04–0.07	0.04–0.07
Specific airway conductance (mL/cm H_2O/mL FRC)	0.24	0.28
Respiratory insensible water loss (mL/24 h)	45–55	300

(Adapted from Martin LD, Rafferty JF, Walker LK, et al. In: Rogers MC, ed. Textbook of pediatric intensive care. Baltimore, Williams & Wilkins, 1992:147)

Cardiovascular System

The cardiovascular system also undergoes striking developmental changes, particularly in the perinatal period. This is discussed in detail in Chapter 7. Contributors to pulmonary hypertension, such as infection, acidosis, hypoxia, hypercarbia, hypothermia, and aspiration, can lead to a serious decrease in cardiac output and hence hypoxemia and hypotension.

Myocardial performance is age related.[12] Although myocardial ischemia only rarely plays a role in the anesthetic management of children, these factors and the varying responses to pharmacologic agents can lead to rapid and occasionally catastrophic hemodynamic decompensation in children undergoing anesthesia. Cardiac function parameters and their relation to age are illustrated in Figure 15-4.

In newborns and infants, heart rate is the predominant determinant of cardiac output.[13] The infant heart is able to sustain higher heart rates than the adult heart while maintaining preload, contractility, and myocardial oxygenation. Bradycardia can drastically and seriously decrease the cardiac output in infants and children. Increasing cardiac output by increasing heart rate should be considered an early response to intraoperative reduction in cardiac output as manifested by hypotension. Bradycardia results from the predisposition to parasympathetic hyperto-

nia common in young children and can be induced by painful stimuli or hypoxia. Laryngoscopy, intubation, eye surgery, airway manipulation, abdominal traction, and herniorrhaphy are frequently associated with marked increases in vagal tone and profound bradycardia. Under these circumstances, the cardiac output can significantly decrease. Anesthetic suppression of

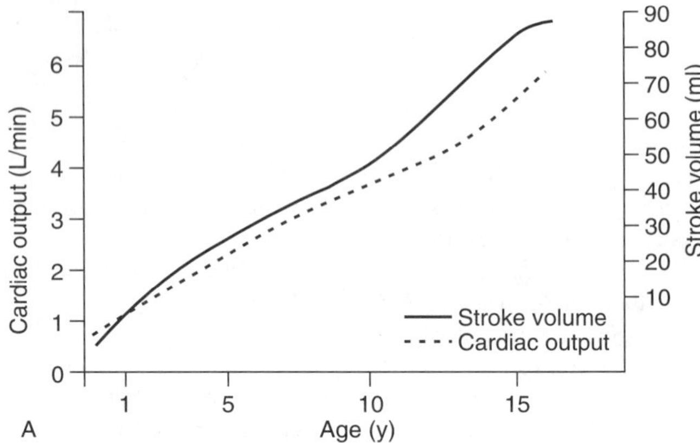

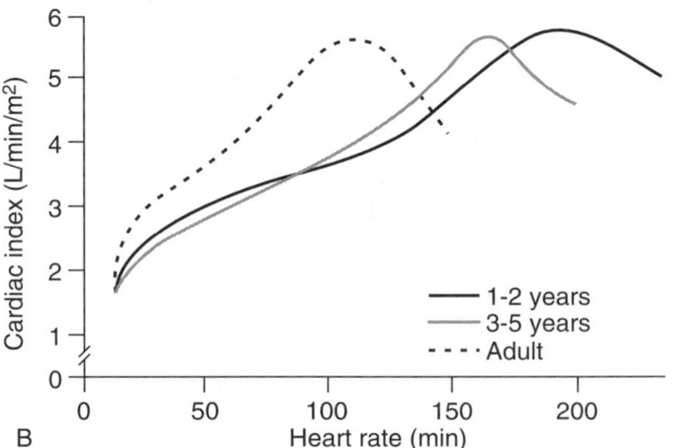

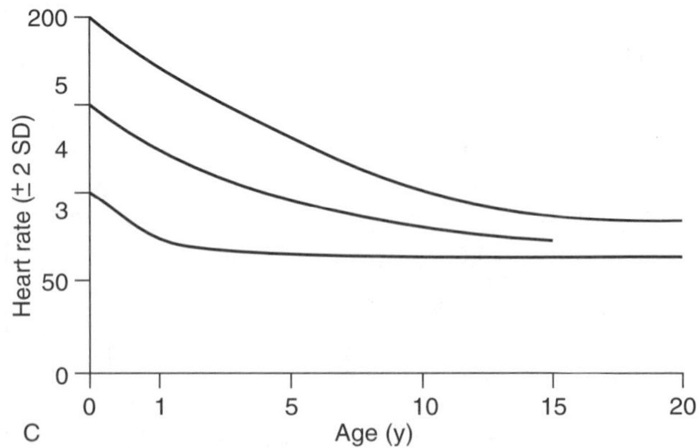

FIG. 15-4. Hemodynamic relations to age. (*A*) Cardiac output and stroke volume as functions of age. (*B*) Relation between heart rate and cardiac output at different stages of development. (*C*) Normal heart rates as a function of age. (After Wetzel RC, Rogers MC. Pediatric hemodynamic monitoring. In: Shoemaker WC, Thompson WL, eds. Critical care: state of the art. Fullerton, CA, Society of Critical Care Medicine, 1983)

atrial conduction can lead to nodal escape arrhythmias, and the result can be hemodynamically significant. This can be readily treated with atropine and is the reason many anesthesiologists include atropine as part of any inhalational anesthetic plan in infants and small children.

The immature myocardium is relatively insensitive to volume loading because it has both lower contractility and compliance than the adult heart. Optimal cardiac output is achieved at lower filling pressures than for adults.[14] Normal adult contractility and compliance are generally achieved by 1 to 2 years of age. The other determinant of cardiac output, afterload, also changes with age. At birth, systemic resistance greatly increases with removal of the placenta, while afterload in the pulmonary circuit decreases dramatically. Right and left ventricular mass and wall thickness are relatively equal in the newborn. During the first year or so of life, the left ventricle becomes markedly dominant. Congenital heart defects also affect all of the determinants of cardiac output: heart rate, contractility, preload and afterload. Thus, the careful evaluation of all of these aspects of cardiac function is necessary in assessing children with congenital heart disease.

Hemoglobin content and oxygen affinity also vary with age.[15] In the term infant, the normal hemoglobin concentration falls in the first year of life, reaching a nadir at about 2 to 3 months. This is referred to as the *physiologic anemia of infancy*.[15] Although the hematocrit at this age can be below 30%, a hemoglobin concentration of more than 10 g/dL is rare. In the preterm infant, however, the hemoglobin concentration may fall normally to between 6 to 8 g/dL within the first 6 to 8 weeks of life.[16] Although this is common, it should not be considered physiologic, and correction may be necessary perioperatively.

In newborns, circulating blood volume is greater on the basis of body weight than in adults. The intravascular blood volume for a newborn is generally 80 to 90 mL/kg. The following formula is useful for estimating how much blood a child can lose before the hematocrit is unacceptably low:

$$ABL = EBV \times \frac{Hct_1 - Hct_2}{mean\ Hct}$$

where ABL is allowable blood loss,
      EBV is estimated blood volume,
      Hct_1 is initial hematocrit,
      Hct_2 is allowable hematocrit, and
      mean Hct is simple arithmetic mean of Hct_1 and Hct_2

Thus, in a 12-kg, 1-year-old child with an initial hematocrit of 37% in whom a final hematocrit of 25% is acceptable, the allowable blood loss would be:

$$ABL = \left[12\ kg \times \frac{80\ ml}{kg} \right] \times \frac{0.37 - 0.25}{0.5(0.25 + 0.37)} = 247\ mL$$

A comparison of the estimate of expected intraoperative loss to the estimate of allowable loss should be made before surgery, and preoperative therapy should be designed, if possible, to decrease the need for blood transfusion. Iron and nutritional supplements may be beneficial, and consideration of recombinant erythropoietin therapy is worthwhile for major elective surgeries.

Renal Function

Renal function also changes substantially with age[17] (see Chap. 6). The glomerular filtration rate per 1.7 m^2 increases from less than 40 mL/min at birth, to 100 mL/min at 1 year, to 130 mL/min in adulthood. The neonatal kidney cannot retain sodium efficiently, and thus there is a tendency toward hyponatremia in premature and full-term neonates. The ability of the infant kidney to concentrate urine is limited, and maximal osmolarity may be only 700 mOsm/kg.[18] Thus, a water load can lead to excess sodium loss in infants. In addition, neonates are less able to preserve intravascular volume if they are water deprived. Complete maturation of renal function usually occurs by about 2 years of age. These concerns require compulsive fluid management in neonates as well as attention to sodium and potassium balance.

Gastrointestinal System

Gastroenterologic development has an impact on a child's response to anesthesia. The reflex coordination of swallowing and lower esophageal sphincter function is not mature until 6 months of age, so gastroesophageal reflux is common in this age group.[19] The need for low residual gastric volumes as determined by NPO policies must be balanced against the risk of hypoglycemia in fasting children.[19] This is especially so in premature, small for gestational age, and nutritionally deprived infants. Children with fever, sepsis, respiratory disease, and other conditions are also at increased risk for reflux and aspiration. For these reasons, a suitable period of preoperative fasting and preoperative intravenous supplementation with dextrose-containing solutions are required, especially in small, ill children.

Thermoregulation

Perhaps no area is more greatly emphasized by pediatric anesthesiologists than the need to maintain normal body temperature perioperatively. During anesthesia, environmental challenges to temperature integrity must be minimized. Cold stress in neonates can lead to increased oxygen consumption, hypoxia, acidosis, respiratory distress, depletion of glycogen stores, hypoglycemia, pulmonary vasoconstriction, shock, and even disseminated intravascular coagulation. In addition, variable drug metabolism, emergence from anesthesia, prolongation of the effects of neuromuscular blocking agents, and other pharmacologic effects emphasize the need for thermoregulatory control intraoperatively in children.[20]

Conductive heat losses can be eliminated by minimizing the contact of children with cold surfaces. Warming pads or heating blankets can eliminate heat loss to the cold operating room table. In addition, warming of the operating room greatly reduces heat loss. Convective heat losses can be further reduced by the use of an incubator as well as by draping and warming blankets. Radiation heat losses must also be minimized. Heat is radiated to objects of lower temperature. Warming objects in the patient's environment decreases radiant losses. This is the principle that underlies radiant neonatal warmers. Transportation of neonates to the operating room in double-walled isolettes is optimal, but the use of radiant warmers where convective loss is minimized is also acceptable. Finally, evaporative loss is the single most important method of heat loss. Evaporative losses are minimized by wrapping a child in plastic wrap or bags.

The use of warmed solutions for skin preparation and irrigation is important. Heated, humidified air for ventilation also contributes greatly to thermoregulatory control in children.

In newborns and small neonates, the operating room should be maintained at 80°F; for infants to 6 months of age, it should be 78°F; and for children 6 months to 2 years of age, it should be 76°F. The humidity should be at least 80%. Warming of all intravascular fluids, including rapidly transfused blood, is also necessary. Covering a child, particularly with plastic (wrap or bag) is the single most important method of minimizing heat loss.

GENERAL PRINCIPLES OF PEDIATRIC PHARMACOLOGY

The pharmacokinetic principles that govern the distribution and metabolism of anesthetic agents in adults are not necessarily applicable to children. Assumptions about converting adult doses to children's doses on a per kilogram, surface area, or age basis have at times proved incorrect. Perhaps no other area demonstrates more clearly that children are not small adults. Volumes of distribution, elimination half-lives, clearance rates, drug sensitivity, side effects, target effects, and organ and protein binding all undergo significant changes with age.

Hepatic maturation is an important illustration as it relates to the development of specific enzyme systems and to alterations in hepatic blood flow. Functional hepatic immaturity is reflected also by a lowered concentration of serum albumin in neonates. This leads to decreased protein binding of many pharmacologic agents (more free or unbound drug), which alters their pharmacodynamics and their pharmacodynamics and thus their pharmacologic effect. Hepatic function is generally mature within the first few months of life.

Drug Administration

Anesthetic agents can be delivered orally, rectally, transnasally, percutaneously, conjunctivally, intramuscularly, intravenously, and by inhalation. Sedatives and induction agents absorbed transrectally are useful in children. Methohexital, midazolam, thiopental, and ketamine are all noteworthy in this regard. Analgesic agents (eg, acetaminophen) can also be administered by this route, allowing mild analgesia without the need for oral administration in the perioperative period. This route is acceptable to most children under 3 to 5 years of age.

Intranasal and transconjunctival administration of benzodiazepines, ketamine, and opioids have all been reported.[21,22] Formulation, solubility characteristics, concentrations, and the desired end-points all affect the rapidity of sedation, its duration, and its depth, and thus define suitability as an agent to induce anesthesia. Novel formulations, such as oral transmucosal fentanyl citrate, have been investigated in recent years but have yet to find a place in routine clinical practice.[23]

Intramuscular drug administration is unpopular in pediatric anesthesia owing to the associated pain. Induction agents, neuromuscular blocking agents, and analgesic agents, however, may all be administered intramuscularly when the need exists. Intramuscular ketamine, 3 to 7 mg/kg, generally achieves anesthetic induction within 5 to 7 minutes.

Drug Distribution

Free, non-bound, water-soluble drug in the circulation is required for an agent to cross the endothelium and other cell membranes, where the effect is achieved, as well as for plasma clearance. Major protein binding is to albumin and α_1-acid glycoprotein. The concentration of the latter and therefore its contribution to protein binding appears to be greater in children than in adults. Infants have very low concentrations of α_1-acid glycoprotein, and they therefore may have a larger, unbound circulating concentration of certain drugs.[24] Curare, metocurine, propranolol, lidocaine, bupivacaine, digoxin, barbiturates, and opioids all demonstrate a significant protein binding. Because the protein-bound fraction acts as a reservoir for a drug, substances (such as bilirubin) that displace drugs from binding sites affect pharmacologic responses. The blood–brain barrier is immature at birth. Because many anesthetic drugs are lipid soluble, more rapid uptake of these agents occurs in neonates than in adults. In addition, blood flow to the brain is much higher in the neonate, and receptor affinities and density vary with age.

The termination of a drug's effect depends on its distribution, metabolism, and excretion. The enzyme systems responsible for drug metabolism undergo distinct developmental differences, especially the cytochrome P-450 system in the liver.[25] Developmental differences in renal function may also affect the clearance and termination of drug effects.

EFFECTS OF ANESTHESIA AND SURGERY

Anesthetic agents are broadly separated into two categories: inhalational agents, of which the most commonly used are halothane and isoflurane; and intravenous agents, the most common of which are benzodiazepines, opioids, and barbiturates. In addition, muscle relaxants are an integral part of most general anesthetic plans. Regional analgesia provides profound sensory analgesia by inducing blockade of nerve transmission, while not altering mentation or obtunding airway reflexes. It has limited use in neonates and, when used, is frequently combined with sedation or general anesthesia.

Cardiovascular Effects of Anesthesia

All anesthetic agents in use are cardiovascular depressants; their mechanisms are summarized in Table 15-3.[26,27] The cardiovascular depressant effects of anesthesia mandate optimal cardiovascular monitoring and support in the perioperative period. The neonate's intravascular volume status should be optimally adjusted to support perfusion, urine output, and metabolic demands. Inotropic support should be considered. The requirements for both intravascular volume and inotropic support increase with general anesthesia. Correction of acid–base imbalance before surgery is required. Although it may be optimal to have the neonate fluid restricted from a respiratory view-

TABLE 15-3. *Causes of cardiovascular depression with inhalational anesthetics*

Rapid uptake of inhalational agents
  1. High minute ventilation in comparison to functional residual capacity; rapid increase in alveolar concentration
  2. Rapid distribution to periphery and central nervous system
Decreased sympathetic tone
Bradycardia
Decreased myocardial contractility
Vasodilation
  1. Decreased venous return
  2. Decreased systemic vascular resistance
Inhibition of baroreceptor responses

TABLE 15-4. *Metabolic responses to surgical stress*

Apnea
Increased oxygen demand
Increased catecholamine release
Hyperglycemia
Glycosuria
Catabolism
Temperature instability

point, the effects of anesthetizing a hypovolemic child can include catastrophic hypotension and cardiac arrest. Anesthetic agents also decrease cardiovascular reserve. The lingering effects of anesthesia in the postoperative period enhance cardiovascular vulnerability in premature infants, and thus postoperative cardiovascular monitoring is required.

Anesthetic Effects on the Respiratory System

All anesthetic agents are respiratory depressants by means of their effects on CNS regulation of ventilation.[9,28–30] There is a primary loss of lung volume and a decrease in functional residual capacity as well. The loss of lung volume on induction of general anesthesia may approach 30%. Because the induction of anesthesia may decrease functional residual capacity below closing volume in an infant, intrapulmonary shunting increases, and the anesthetized neonate has a higher oxygen requirement. The changes in lung volume also decrease compliance.[30,31] The percentage of dead-space tidal ventilation may be as high as 50% to 80% during surgery. During anesthesia, this necessitates an increase in both the tidal volume and frequency (and thus airway pressure) of ventilation. In addition, surgical trauma to the thorax or the abdomen with chest wall instability or increased abdominal pressure grossly affects respiratory mechanics and leads to a marked increase in the need for ventilatory support.

Inhalational anesthetics are airway irritants. They increase secretions and induce coughing.[31,32] The effects in a child with bronchopulmonary dysplasia and hyperactive airways may be significant. In high doses, inhalational anesthetics are bronchorelaxants. The use of potent inhalational anesthetics, particularly halothane is one therapeutic modality useful in resistant asthma. At low doses used for induction and recovery from inhalational anesthesia, however, airway reflexes are generally increased. Inhalational anesthesia also underlies the well-recognized perioperative phenomenon of laryngospasm. Laryngospasm is an acute, vice-like closure of the glottis that leads to total airway obstruction. Finally, in newborn infants, the incidence of apnea is increased in the postanesthetic period regardless of anesthetic technique.

Oxygen Transport

The induction of general anesthesia in the perioperative period has a significant negative effect on oxygen transport. This mandates a logical approach to ensure oxygenation and ventilation in the perioperative period. It is occasionally better to take additional time to ensure stable cardiorespiratory function before subjecting the neonate to surgery, than to rush to the operating room. This approach has changed the management strategy of children with congenital diaphragmatic hernia and other neonatal surgical emergencies, such as omphalocele and tracheoesophageal fistula.

Temperature Regulation

Anesthetic agents decrease the neonate's ability to respond to thermal stress. This is because these agents cause cutaneous vasodilation and also blunt the normal shivering response. Inhalational anesthetics directly interfere with nonshivering thermogenesis.[33] It has become clear that brown fat metabolism is inhibited by inhalational anesthetic agents, and the intrinsic thermoregulatory pathways are blunted as well.[34]

The Stress Response to Surgery

Whereas in the past it was believed that minimizing the administration of anesthetic agents optimized outcomes from surgery, it has become clear that inadequate anesthesia does not blunt deleterious perioperative stress responses. Ansley-Green and Anand clearly demonstrated that adequate intraoperative analgesia greatly blunts the deleterious autonomic, catecholamine, and metabolic responses to surgery[1–3,35] (Table 15-4). This realization has led to new strategies for perioperative and other pain management.

The beneficial effects of intravenous opioid and inhalational halothane anesthesia have been demonstrated (Table 15-5). Perioperative complications are significantly decreased in

TABLE 15-5. *Intraoperative stress responses*

Stress response	Effect of adequate anesthesia
24-h increase in plasma epinephrine levels	Episodes decreased or reversed
Increased glucagon, pyruvate, lactate release	Abolished
Hyperglycemia	Reduced to one-third shorter duration
Hypercortisolemia	Blunted
Increased plasma 3-methylhistadine level	Abolished

TABLE 15-6. *Comparative perioperative complications in anesthetized premature infants*

Complication	Control (n = 8)	Fentanyl (n = 8)
Frequent bradycardia	4	1
Hypotension, poor circulation	4	0
Glycosuria	1	0
Acidosis	2	0
Increased ventilatory requirements	4	1
Intraventricular hemorrhage	2	0
TOTALS	17	2

(Anand KJS, Sippell WG, Aynsley-Green A. Randomized trial of fentanyl anesthesia in preterm babies undergoing surgery: effects on the stress response. Lancet 1987;1:243)

young patients who receive halothane or opioid.[35,36] Table 15-6 compares the incidence of complications in eight premature infants who received fentanyl and eight premature infants who received nitrous oxide and oxygen. Results show that perioperative complications are decreased by adequate analgesia.[35] Thus, it appears that anesthetic amelioration of hormonal and metabolic responses to surgical stress is important to ensure neonatal perioperative stability.[37,38]

INHALATIONAL ANESTHETICS

Inhalational anesthetics are liquids at room temperature that are vaporized to provide accurately controlled concentrations in the inspiratory gases of children receiving anesthesia. The introduction of halothane made safe inhalational anesthesia possible for infants. Nevertheless, the negative effects of inhalational anesthesia on the cardiorespiratory status of premature and full-term neonates are significant. Therefore, intravenous anesthetic agents are often used in these circumstances. In the past, this has included barbiturates (thiopental, pentobarbital) and ketamine; more recently, synthetic opioids, such as fentanyl, have been used.

Halothane

Halothane remains the cornerstone of pediatric inhalational anesthesia. Like all anesthetics, it is an airway irritant and a mild sialagogue. Its use is associated with laryngospasm. Although this does not differ qualitatively from the older inhalational anesthetics (enflurane and isoflurane) or the newer anesthetics (sevoflurane and desflurane), it is clearly the least irritating. Halothane has a blood/gas partition coefficient of 2.4, which yields a slower rate of increase in alveolar concentration than isoflurane (1.4) or enflurane (1.8). Theoretically, the lower solubility coefficients correlate with a more rapid rise in alveolar concentration, resulting in a more rapid agent for inhalational anesthesia in children, but this is not demonstrable in practice.

When compared with ether and chloroform for rapidity and smoothness of induction, airway irritability, and sialagogic effect, halothane is a vastly better agent. Its potency and rapidity of induction may cause cardiorespiratory depression. As anesthesiologists became more familiar with this drug, however, they realized that halothane's advantages far outweigh these concerns.

The concerns with halothane are several. Like other inhalational anesthetics, it is a direct myocardial depressant.[26] This occurs in all age groups and has significant implications in neonates and in children with congenital heart disease. Children with impaired myocardial contractility may become significantly hypotensive before they are adequately anesthetized, and alternative means occasionally must be used. In children with low cardiac output, alveolar concentrations rise more rapidly and are difficult to reverse. Cardiac depression may occur readily. Baroreceptor reflexes are depressed by inhalational anesthetics, and this is more significant in younger animals.[39] This has significant effect on heart rate, contractility, and vascular resistance. Halothane is a direct peripheral vasodilator, although to a lesser degree than other agents, and this also contributes to hypotension.

A further concern about inhalational anesthetics is that they sensitize the myocardium to circulating catecholamines, whether endogenous and exogenous. This effect is aggravated by acidosis, especially respiratory acidosis.[40] This may be the mechanism for the frequency of ventricular extrasystole and bigeminy in children breathing spontaneously who are anesthetized with halothane. The most common causes of arrhythmias during inhalational anesthesia are inadequate depth of anesthesia (with endogenous catecholamines release) and inadequate ventilation with hypercarbia. Thus, the first line therapy for ventricular ectopy in anesthetized children is hyperventilation. This clears CO_2, thus correcting respiratory acidosis, and increases the depth of anesthesia. The administration of exogenous catecholamines during head and neck, neurosurgical, and orthopedic procedures to decrease blood loss is common under halothane anesthesia.[41] Most evidence indicates that up to 10 μg/kg can be given safely subcutaneously or injected extravascularly in children with minimal risk of cardiac dysrhythmias.[42]

A notable concern with halothane anesthesia is the risk of hepatitis.[43] The incidence of halothane-associated hepatitis is not clear, but it is very low. Halothane and its metabolites impair hepatic function, especially with hypoxia or ischemia. A few deaths of children have been reported that appear to be related to halothane hepatitis.[44] A few episodes of hepatitis may be attributable to halothane anesthesia after repeated exposure.[43,45,46] If halothane hepatitis were a significant clinical risk, one would have expected dozens of deaths and perhaps hundreds of cases of hepatitis for an agent so widely used. The safety record of halothane after thousands, and perhaps millions, of uses worldwide is better than for most drugs. The results of the National Halothane Study, published in 1966, remain pertinent:[46] a complete absence of halothane hepatitis in infants and prepubertal children. Although the anesthesiologist needs to be aware of this issue, its impact on the selection of anesthetic agent is minimal. There may be some wisdom in using other inhalational anesthetic agents in children with liver impairment, or in limiting the repeated use of halothane in a child to no more than four or five times in 6 months, if only to avoid confusion.

Enflurane

Enflurane, introduced in 1972, has little application in pediatric anesthesia. Enflurane is a pungent, irritating anesthetic and not suitable for inhalational induction. In addition, it lowers the seizure threshold, especially in hypocarbic patients, and this has made it less useful in pediatric anesthesia.[47] It appears to have no advantages over halothane, and its use has therefore remained minimal in pediatric anesthesia.

Isoflurane

The introduction of isoflurane in 1981 offered the theoretic advantage of more rapid induction. This agent, however, has proved too irritating, causing respiratory pauses, coughing, choking, and occasional laryngospasm, resulting in slower inductions in children.[48] It has not become an agent of choice for inhalational induction in children. Its characteristics after intravenous induction and airway intubation are generally similar to halothane.

Isoflurane is less of a myocardial depressant than halothane but is a more potent peripheral vasodilator than other commonly used inhalational anesthetics.[49,50] In general, cardiac function appears better maintained with isoflurane than with halothane. Although blood pressure may be similarly decreased, as with isoflurane, heart rate and myocardial contractility are better maintained and therefore support cardiac output better. This suggests a slight advantage in children with congenital heart disease. One area in which isoflurane may have particular advantage is for children with elevated intracranial pressure or primary CNS lesions because it appears to better preserve cerebral blood flow than halothane.[51]

Nitrous Oxide

Nitrous oxide (N_2O) is a clear, colorless, odorless, nonirritating gas that is frequently used to provide analgesia and to augment the other potent general anesthetic agents. It cannot be used in high enough concentrations to provide surgical anesthesia, but it is used to potentiate virtually every pediatric anesthetic agent. Nitrous oxide has moderate cardiovascular effects, including mild myocardial depression. A major problem is that it may increase pulmonary artery pressure in adults. This has caused some concern in infants at risk for pulmonary hypertension. Nitrous oxide must be used in concentrations of less than 70%. These features limit its use in patients with pulmonary hypertension and in those who require higher inspired oxygen tensions. Nitrous oxide is also more soluble than nitrogen and therefore transfers from blood to air-filled spaces rapidly. This can lead to bowel distention and expansion of a pneumothorax. Nitrous oxide is contraindicated when gas expansion may be deleterious to the child's health. It is rapidly exhaled at the end of surgery and facilitates rapid awakening, leaving little postanesthetic effect.

INTRAVENOUS ANESTHESIA

Sodium thiopental is an ultrashort-acting barbiturate that has been routinely used to induce anesthesia for 50 years. This agent is both a negative inotrope and a peripheral vasodilator. With its ability to blunt autonomic output, hypotension is an inevitable consequence of its use. This effect is profound in volume-depleted patients. Although thiopental can be used safely to induce unconsciousness and general anesthesia, it is a poor analgesic agent. It is relatively contraindicated in children who are hemodynamically unstable or of an uncertain intravascular volume status. It can be used to induce anesthesia in healthy, hemodynamically stable neonates.

Ketamine can be used to induce anesthesia and provide adequate operative analgesia. Ketamine releases endogenous catecholamines and thus tends to increase heart rate and support myocardial function. This, however, has limitations. In children who have attained maximal sympathetic support, ketamine may not further augment hemodynamic support. In addition, ketamine is intrinsically a negative inotrope and may decrease cardiac output. It is particularly useful in children with congenital heart disease and in patients with asthma. Although intravenous ketamine is probably the safest agent with which to induce anesthesia in a hemodynamically compromised or volume-compromised patient, it may still cause hypotension. Ketamine is a relatively long-acting intravenous agent, and the effects of analgesia and respiratory obtundation may last for several hours, especially in higher doses. In neonates, excretion is delayed, and the effect may be prolonged. Ketamine has a minimal effect on respiratory drive, and spontaneous ventilation is better maintained with ketamine than with opioids.

Opioids

Morphine is a time-honored analgesic agent for use in critically ill children, although its prolonged respiratory effects and hemodynamic effects limit its use both in the intensive care unit and in the operating room. Fentanyl is a synthetic opioid agent with a wider margin of safety and more hemodynamic stability. It is the most widely used intravenous anesthetic agent to provide anesthesia for premature neonates. In 1981, Robinson and Gregory[52] demonstrated that it was possible to provide safe and effective analgesia with fentanyl in infants weighing less than 1500 g. Fentanyl, in combination with nitrous oxide, has also been demonstrated to blunt the stress response to surgery.[1,2] Subsequent studies have shown that neonates tolerate doses up to 50 to 60 μg/kg, if necessary, without adverse hemodynamic effects. Although these high doses can be tolerated, the median effective dose of fentanyl is 10 to 12.5 μg/kg to provide adequate analgesia for up to 75 minutes of surgery.[53] Another means of administering fentanyl is to give a 2 μg/kg bolus, followed by 2 to 3 μg/kg/h as a continuous intravenous infusion. This method has been extended to provide analgesia in the postoperative period. Fentanyl also attenuates pulmonary hypertensive crisis and is therefore useful for children with pulmonary hypertension.

Fentanyl has a rapid onset of action when given intravenously. It is mainly metabolized in the liver, thus its clearance is highly variable in neonates, making it necessary to individualize the dose. By several months of age, the clearance of fentanyl is greater in infants than in adults. When liver blood flow is compromised, fentanyl levels may remain high for some time. The phenomenon of rapid tolerance to fentanyl has been described in children receiving extracorporeal membrane oxygenation.[54] Although fentanyl is a potent analgesic, its ability to blunt awareness is questionable. For this reason, benzodiazepines are frequently added as anxiolytic agents and sedatives when using intravenous fentanyl.

All opioids are potent respiratory depressants. Opioids penetrate the neonatal CNS much more rapidly than in adults and achieve two to four times the concentration.[55] The opioid μ-receptors in neonates are exquisitely sensitive, and respiratory depression readily occurs. Thus, the therapeutic window for opioids is more narrow in premature infants than in older children. This, in addition to the fact that postoperative premature infants are at risk for apnea, makes it prudent to provide careful respiratory monitoring and consider mechanical ventilatory support after surgery. Because the clearance of fentanyl in neonates is variable, weaning of ventilation should be titrated to the infant's needs. As noted, this variability occurs more in patients with poor hepatic clearance, increased abdominal pressure, and low blood flow states.

Fentanyl is the cornerstone of modern intraoperative anesthetic management of critically ill neonates. Familiarity with its use in the operating room has led to its use in other neonatal settings. Its apparent ability to blunt clinical deterioration in response to pain has made it useful for providing analgesia outside the operating room in critically ill children, such as those with diaphragmatic hernia or pulmonary hypertension.

With all opioids, tolerance, withdrawal, dependence, and addiction can occur. The relevance of the term *addiction* to neonates is questionable. Because addiction generally requires a drug-seeking behavior, the term is best avoided in this setting. Neonates do develop physiologic tolerance, requiring increasing doses of opioid anesthetics. They also demonstrate dependence by manifesting withdrawal phenomena. *Dependence,* defined as the physiologic state created by administration of exogenous opiates, does occur in premature infants who have received opioids for several days. The effects of neonatal withdrawal are well described, especially in maternally addicted infants. They include cardiorespiratory instability, temperature instability, agitation, fearfulness, crying and fretting, increased muscle tone, sweating, poor feeding, vomiting, and diarrhea. Whenever these symptoms appear, a review of the record of analgesia and opioids is indicated. Symptoms can be treated with gradual withdrawal of opioids.

PREOPERATIVE EVALUATION

The preoperative evaluation is an important aspect of pediatric anesthesia and is summarized briefly in this chapter. The reader is referred elsewhere for more detailed discussion.[56,57]

Laboratory Investigations

The American Society of Anesthesiologists, the American College of Surgeons, and the American Academy of Pediatrics do make specific recommendations for preoperative testing in children. Specific laboratory testing indicated by the chart review, history, and examination of the child is fairly straightforward. Routine testing for healthy children has remained controversial. In the past, guidelines developed for adults were applied to children. These included a complete blood count, urinalysis, electrolytes, and chest radiograph. Recent studies have revealed that unless a history or physical examination suggests otherwise, routine preoperative laboratory testing is unnecessary.[56,58]

Hematology

If major blood loss is not anticipated, routine hematologic testing (complete blood count, hematocrit, platelet counts, coagulation profiles) is unnecessary. When done, it is important to recognize the developmental differences in levels of hematocrit. For years, ''normal'' hematocrits were required for elective surgery. The lower limit of normal, usually defined as a hematocrit of greater than 30% or a hemoglobin concentration of greater than 10 g/dL in nearly all age groups, was the previous requirement. With recent concerns about blood-borne pathogens, this dogma has become less attractive.[59] Generally, elective surgery should await attaining this level, short of transfusion. Iron and nutritional support are indicated. In the emergent situation, transfusion therapy is directed by patient need, such as anticipated blood loss and cardiorespiratory status. Transfusion should not rely on some arbitrary definition of normal hemoglobin levels.

Screening for Sickle Cell Disease

The recommendations of American Academy of Pediatrics for the screening for sickle cell disease require that a sickle preparation or other screening test be performed in all black children.[56] It is not reasonable, however, to insist on the results of a sickle cell preparation in all such children requiring anesthesia and surgery. Clearly, anesthetizing a child with sickle cell disease who is anemic, with 95% sickle hemoglobin, poses a major threat to that child. The likelihood, however, that a child older than 2 years with a normal hemoglobin has sickle cell disease is extremely low. For children with sickle cell disease who require elective surgery, preoperative management is directed at reducing the sickle hemoglobin level to less than 40%. Chronic transfusion, exchange transfusion, and acute blood transfusion have all been reported to be useful. Management is directed at minimizing the risk of sickling. This includes avoiding hypoxia, dehydration, hyperthermia, hypothermia, and tourniquet use.

Drug Levels

In children receiving therapeutic drugs, it is frequently worthwhile to know whether a therapeutic level has been achieved. Two major groups of children in whom this is of concern are those with epilepsy and asthma. Obtaining routine blood levels of theophylline and anticonvulsants to ensure compliance with therapy and adequate levels for the perioperative management appears to be a wise precaution. It is reassuring to determine that the child is receiving appropriate therapy, in which case the surgery can proceed. Preoperative assessment for elective surgery should be done in a timely enough fashion to allow specific investigations before surgery. Consultation with other services and other procedures, such as computed tomographic scans, electrocardiograms, and echocardiograms, should be timed so that the results are available before the induction of anesthesia. Deciding that such information is important preoperatively, but acting before it is adequately obtained, sets the stage for medical or legal misadventure.

TABLE 15-7. *Endocarditis prophylaxis*

INDICATIONS
Congenital or acquired valvular heart disease
Surgically constructed shunts (eg, Waterston, Blalock-Taussig, Potts)
Subaortic stenosis
Mitral valve prolapse
Rheumatic heart disease
Prosthetic valves

PROCEDURES
All genitourinary or gastrointestinal surgery
All dental procedures
Incision and drainage procedures
Adenoidectomy or tonsillectomy
Airway surgery or bronchoscopy

Prophylaxis not necessary for patients with secundum atrial septal defect or patent ductus arteriosus repaired
   more than 6 months earlier

REGIMENS
DENTAL AND RESPIRATORY

Amoxicillin (PO)	1 h before surgery	50 mg/kg (max, 3g)
	6 h after initial dose	25 mg/kg (max, 1.5 g)
or		
Penicillin G (IV)	30–60 min before surgery	50,000 U/kg
	6 h after initial dose	
For maximal protection:		
Ampicillin (IV) and Gentamicin (IV)	30 min before surgery	50 mg/kg
	Repeat 8 h after initial dose	2 mg/kg
For penicillin-allergy:		
Erythromycin (PO)	1 h before surgery	20 mg/kg (max, 1 g)
or		
Vancomycin (IV)	6 h after initial dose	10 mg/kg (max, 1500 mg)
	1 h before surgery	20 mg/kg (max, 1 g)

GASTROINTESTINAL OR GENITOURINARY PROCEDURE
Routine:

Ampicillin (IV) and Gentamicin (IV)	30 min before surgery	50 mg/kg
	Repeat 8 h after initial dose	2 mg/kg
Minor or repetitive in low-risk children:		
Amoxicillin (PO)	1 h before surgery	50 mg/kg (max, 3 g)
	6 h after initial dose	25 mg/kg (max, 1.5 g)
For penicillin allergy:		
Vancomycin (IV)	1 h before surgery (repeat once)	20 mg/kg (max, 1 g)
Gentamicin (IV)	8–12 h after first dose	2 mg/kg

Endocarditis Prophylaxis

An important preoperative concern is whether a child is at risk for the development of bacterial endocarditis. The approach to this issue is outlined in Table 15-7.

PREOPERATIVE PREPARATION

The goals of the preoperative evaluation are not only to guide intraoperative management but also to guide preoperative optimization of the child's condition. Every effort should be made to optimize the cardiorespiratory status, ensuring an adequately perfused, well-oxygenated and ventilated neonate before sur-

gery. In addition, the child's temperature and thermal environment should be ideal. Nutrition should be maintained if possible and electrolyte abnormalities corrected. These requirements mandate the full support of modern neonatal intensive care.

Preoperative Fasting

Pulmonary aspiration of gastric contents is a serious complication of general anesthesia. The aspiration of gastric contents causes an acute, potentially life-threatening inflammatory pneumonitis. Acid aspiration is impossible with an empty stomach. These facts provide the rationale for preoperative fasting.[60] Factors that increase the risk of aspiration pneumonitis include gastric outlet obstruction, delayed gastric emptying, hiatal her-

TABLE 15-8. *Preoperative fasting guidelines*

Healthy infants for elective surgery
    NPO for solids 8 h before surgery
    NPO for clear liquids (may or may not include breast milk)
       4 h before surgery
Intubated infants with nasogastric feeding
    NPO for solids 8 h before surgery
    NPO for clear liquids (may or may not include breast milk)
       4 h before surgery
Critically ill infants or infants with surgical abdomen
    NPO for at least 8 h, if possible.

nia, gastroesophageal dysmotility, solids or particulate matter, and acid pH (less than 2.5). During the induction of anesthesia, any increase in intraabdominal pressure can cause acid reflux. If the airway reflexes (cough, gag, and vocal cord apposition) are lost, aspiration can occur.

To prevent or minimize the risk of aspiration, anesthesiologists have traditionally ordered a preoperative fast (NPO after midnight) for all liquids and solids. We now realize that small infants and children with their unique glucose and fluid requirements are not benefited by prolonged fasts before surgery. Significant hypovolemia with intraoperative hypotension and hypoglycemia can result. Concerns have also been raised about hypoglycemia occurring in older children after prolonged fast.[61,62] There is little evidence in normal children that prolonged fasting (more than 6 to 8 hours) is required to obtain minimal gastric volumes. Clearly, fasting for solid foods and large meals is appropriate for 8 hours before surgery because gastric volumes can be increased up to 6 hours after a solid meal. This is not so with clear liquids. Ad lib clear liquids until 2 hours before surgery are actually associated with lower gastric volumes at higher pH than for starved patients.[63] Investigators from the Children's Hospital of Philadelphia conclusively demonstrated the safety of ad lib clear liquids 2 hours before surgery.[60] In this study, no patient aspirated despite liberal preoperative drinking guidelines.

Gastric emptying is facilitated by clear, sweet liquids. These can probably be given safely until 2 hours before anesthesia. There has been no change in the recommendation that solid foods not be given for 8 hours before surgery (Table 15-8). A question arises concerning breast milk. Authorities differ on whether breast milk enhances or decreases gastric motility and emptying, and some consider breast milk (not formula) a clear liquid, while others do not. Some allow breast milk to be given up to 4 hours before surgery.[60] This depends on the protocol of the individual institution. Clear liquids (eg, sugar water, Pedialyte) can be given to healthy infants until 2 hours before surgery (Table 15-9).

TABLE 15-9. *Clear liquids*

Pedialyte
Apple juice
Ice popsicles
Plain gelatin
Carbonated drinks
5% Glucose water
Clear broth
(NOT orange juice)

Premedication

Because most children are anxious before the induction of anesthesia, premedication is commonly administered to ease the separation from parents and to smooth the induction of anesthesia. Various drugs and routes of administration are used. Midazolam, a water-soluble, rapidly acting benzodiazepine, is the most commonly used premedicant. It can be administered orally, nasally, rectally, intravenously, or intramuscularly. Other, less commonly used premedicants include oral transmucosal fentanyl, rectal methohexital, nasal sufentanil, and intramuscular cocktails of pentobarbital, meperidine, and atropine.

Parental Presence in the Operating Room

Although it is common to allow parents to accompany children until the time they lose consciousness for most pediatric anesthetics, this requires discretion. For critically ill neonates, when transport to the operating room may be accompanied by rapid changes in the child's condition, the presence of parents can be a problem. Because the induction of anesthesia in neonates, especially those who are critically ill, requires great vigilance and rapid responses, parental presence in the operating room or during induction is probably unwise. The family should certainly be allowed to see, talk to, and touch the infant as much as possible in the preoperative period. They must be reassured that the same care will continue when they are not with their child.[63]

Endotracheal Intubation

In the past 30 years, great advances have been made in our understanding of what is required of pediatric endotracheal tubes. The composition and design of endotracheal tubes have become largely uniform. Several factors are recognized as important in the selection of endotracheal tubes.[64] Most endotracheal tubes are made of polyvinylchloride, although Silastic endotracheal tubes are also becoming popular. All of these have been implant tested to ensure low irritability to the tracheal mucosa. The tube should be of uniform external diameter throughout. Ideally, it should be possible to tell the size and design of the endotracheal tube when it is in place. Tubes with markings of length from the distal end so that depth of insertion can be determined are also recommended. The only major drawback of polyvinylchloride tubes is that they are flammable and thus not indicated for use in laser surgery unless they are suitably wrapped with reflective tape.[65]

The selection of endotracheal tube size and internal diameter relies on multiple factors. From an airway management point of view, a large endotracheal tube that allows access for suctioning airway secretions is optimum. In addition, because resistance is directly proportional to the fourth power of the radius, a larger tube is desirable to facilitate ventilation at low airway pressures. A key consideration, however, is the potential for tracheal injury. An endotracheal tube may readily pass the vocal cords but still impinge on the narrowest part of the child's airway—the subglottic area at the cricoid ring. Tracheal injury occurs most frequently at this site. Mucosal injury occurs with any endotracheal tube, generally within minutes of placement. Ischemia appears to be an aggravating factor, and if lateral pressure from the endotracheal tube excludes capillary flow in the submucosal area, serious injury can be expected. Thus, ensuring the presence of an adequate air leak around the endotracheal tube is a crucial factor in endotracheal tube maintenance.[65–67] The air leak test around an endotracheal tube is performed by slowly increasing airway pressure while noting the airway pressure at which audible air begins to leak around the endotracheal tube through the glottis. The safe range is considered to be between 10 and 30 cm H_2O. A higher leak pressure must be accepted in patients with decreased lung compliance. If the tube is required for a prolonged period (hours), then replacing a tube with no leak at 30 cm H_2O is probably indicated because the trauma of reintubation is probably less than that of ischemia to the subglottic region.

Other factors also play a role in the development of tracheal injury and subglottic stenosis. These include the presence of infection, hemodynamic instability, patient movement, seizure activity, the piston movement of the tube caused by the ventilator, and the difficulty and frequency of reintubation.[68,69] Balancing the potential risks and the potential benefits requires individualized judgment of endotracheal tube size for each child.

The variability in the anatomy of children means that formulas and tabulated recommendations for endotracheal tube size only serve as guidelines. Two practical guidelines for determining the appropriate endotracheal tube are recommended. This first compares the external endotracheal tube diameter to the width of the fifth finger at the distal interphalangeal joint. The other compares the diameter of the tube to the nares. Neither of these have been rigorously evaluated, but both are commonly used. We prefer the formula (16 + age in years) ÷ 4. This formula is correct to ½ mm tube size. The primary need is to ensure that the endotracheal tube is appropriate for the individual child. It should pass easily into the trachea with an acceptable air leak. Whenever a child is intubated, the appropriate-sized suction catheters should be available (Table 15-10).

PREMEDICATION AND INDUCTION

The goal of anesthetic induction is to move the child from the awake to the anesthetized state in a manner that is calm and stress free for child, parent, surgeon, and if possible, anesthesiologist. Variation in technique for the induction of childhood anesthesia is much greater than for adults. This arises from the special physiologic and psychologic needs of children and their families. The range of techniques makes it possible to modify the induction method to the needs of the child, rather than forcing the child into a preconceived induction plan. The goals of anesthetic management are similar in adults and children (ie, amnesia, analgesia, good operating conditions for the surgeon, and patient safety). In addition, the child's emotional needs must be addressed.

Premedication

The issue of premedication must be reviewed before discussing anesthetic induction. The traditional goals of administration of preoperative medication include: (1) decreasing airway secretions; (2) blockade of detrimental autonomic (vagal) reflexes; (3) provision of sedation or anxiolysis; (4) facilitation of the smooth induction of general anesthesia; (5) supplementation of general anesthetic technique; (6) provision of preoperative analgesia to patients with pain; and (7) diminution of volume and acidity of gastric contents.

The negative aspects of premedication (ie, intramuscular injection, respiratory depression, possible airway obstruction), the fact that modern, less pungent volatile anesthetic agents eliminate the need for an antisialagogue in most patients, and the effectiveness of psychologic preparation and parental support have led to a decline in the use of classic premedication. In addition, the increase in outpatient surgery demands the elimination of the use of premedications that outlast the surgical procedure, prolong somnolence, and therefore delay discharge. Despite the decreasing use of premedication, there remain children for whom premedication is beneficial, although seldom by the intramuscular route.

Preoperative treatment with an antisialagogue was essential in the era of ether. Modern inhalational agents are much less irritating to the airway, and therefore drying of secretions is necessary only in patients who have excessive airway secretions or require antisialagogues for other reasons, such as airway endoscopy or laser surgery.[70] In most cases, atropine, 0.02 mg/kg, minimum dose 0.15 mg, is given intravenously after induction to prevent bradycardia, but it is an effective antisialagogue. If the specific drying effect is desired preoperatively, oral atropine, 0.05 mg/kg 1 hour before surgery, is effective. Atropine in the same dosage may be added to rectally administered drugs.

When psychologic preparation fails to achieve a calm, cooperative child, sedative premedication may be desirable. This is most common in adolescents, children who have had extensive hospitalizations with multiple prior procedures, and children in pain. Many oral premedication cocktails are as safe and effective as intramuscularly administered premedications and, when properly administered, do not delay discharge after outpatient surgery.[71,72]

Sedative premedication is unnecessary in healthy infants younger than 8 months of age because they have no anxiety because they do not perceive what is to occur. Infants less than 6 months of age are more prone to airway obstruction and respiratory depression after sedation. Sedative premedication should be avoided in children with CNS disease (abnormal central ven-

---

TABLE 15-10. *Sizes of endotracheal tubes and suction catheters suggested for infants and children*

| | Endotracheal tube | | |
| | | | |
Age	Internal diameter (mm)	Length (mm)*	Suction catheter (French)
Premature	2.5–3	9	6
0–6 mo	3–3.5	10–11	6
6–12 mo	3.5–4	12	8
1–2 y	4	13	8
2–4 y	4.5	14	8
4–6 y	5	15	10
6–8 y	5.5	16	10
8–10 y	6–6.5 optional cuff	17	10–12
10–12 yr	7.5–8 optional cuff	18	12
>12 y	7.5–8 cuffed	19–22	12

* Teeth to mid-trachea.

tilatory control mechanisms, hyperventilation, increased intracranial pressure) or airway abnormalities. There is still a role for opioid premedication in children older than 1 year of age who are in pain and in children with congenital heart disease who are at risk for undesirable hemodynamic responses to pain and anxiety. In contrast to the preceding caution about CNS disease, children with intact intracranial aneurysms or vascular malformations without increased intracranial pressure benefit from preoperative opioid premedication to smooth anesthetic induction and avoid hypertension.

Premedication is most often administered to older children and adolescents. In adolescents, the effects of a usual adult oral dose of diazepam, 0.15 mg/kg, are variable, with some patients becoming calm and others remaining totally unaffected. More consistent sedation has been seen when large doses (0.3 mg/kg) are administered, but postoperative sedation can be prolonged, especially when the surgery is relatively brief. Droperidol is an effective oral premedication in children at a dose of 0.03 mg/kg. Droperidol is an antiemetic with effects that persist into the postoperative period. The incidence of CNS side effects (eg, dysphoria, restlessness, extrapyramidal reactions) has diminished its use in adults, but these side effects are rare in children.

Newer techniques of sedation have been developed in which relatively fast-acting drugs are administered by innovative routes before anesthetic induction while the patient is close to the operating room (preinduction sedation). They include intranasal and oral (lollipop) administration of opioids (fentanyl, sufentanil),[73,74] which reduces perioperative analgesic requirements but also can be associated with chest wall rigidity and delayed waking at higher doses. Oral, rectal, and nasally administered midazolam is safe and rapidly renders children calm and happy. It is not associated with airway obstruction or hyperventilation.[75–77] Mask induction is smooth and pleasant for both child and parent.

Induction Techniques

No one anesthetic induction technique is best for all children. The ideals are to minimize unpleasant experiences and morbidity while ensuring the safety of the patient and expediting the achievement of good operating conditions. Risks include airway obstruction, vomiting and aspiration, hypotension, arrhythmias, and death. Psychologic preparation, premedication, and parental presence can contribute to a safe induction of anesthesia because calm, cooperative children have less stormy inductions.

The major categories of anesthetic induction are intravenous, inhalational, and rectal. Although intramuscular induction is possible, it is used rarely because it is less safe, owing to the absence of venous access, and it is frightening and painful to the patient. Intravenous induction of anesthesia is fast, reliable, and safe in the healthy, normovolemic child. The reason intravenous induction is less commonly used than other methods is that most children are terrified of needles. It is important to give children older than 5 years some choice in the manner in which they will go to sleep, and many will not choose a ''shot'' even if it is guaranteed to be painless. Risks of intravenous induction include extravascular infiltration of anesthetic agents (which, in the case of thiopental, can lead to tissue loss). Another major risk of intravenous induction occurs in patients with unrecognized abnormalities in airway anatomy who may be difficult to ventilate once asleep.

Thiopental and methohexital are similar in onset, but methohexital has a shorter duration of action. Methohexital should be avoided in children with a history of seizures because it may be epileptogenic. Thiopental, although it causes histamine release, does not precipitate bronchospasm. Because it lacks analgesic properties, however, endotracheal intubation after a relatively small dose of thiopental (4 mg/kg) may cause bronchospasm owing to light anesthesia. Therefore, asthmatic patients who are induced with thiopental should receive a sufficient induction dose (5 to 7 mg/kg) to attain an adequate depth of anesthesia for intubation. Intravenous lidocaine, 1 to 1.5 mg/kg, should also be administered to blunt airway reflexes. Alternatively, increased depth of anesthesia can be achieved with increasing concentrations of inhalation agent, using either spontaneous, assisted, or controlled ventilation.

Because of its catecholamine-stimulating properties, ketamine may be chosen for intravenous induction in children who are hypovolemic or hemodynamically unstable. In addition, it is frequently used in children with cyanotic congenital heart disease in whom decreased systemic vascular resistance, as caused by thiopental, is undesirable. Ketamine is also used in children with asthma for its bronchodilating properties.[78] Asthmatic children in whom a rapid sequence induction is indicated may be most safely induced with ketamine because it provides rapid attainment of profound analgesia and bronchodilation.[79] When ketamine is administered by any route, it should be preceded or accompanied by the administration of atropine or glycopyrrolate to attenuate the increase in airway secretions that occurs. The addition of a benzodiazepine is recommended to lessen the dysphoric emergence that can occur with ketamine.

The newest intravenous induction agent is propofol.[80,81] Its use is associated with pain on administration. This may be attenuated by adding 2% lidocaine to the drug immediately before administration (1:10 dilution, final concentration of lidocaine 2 mg/mL). Slow injection and the use of larger (eg, antecubital) veins is also associated with decreased pain. In children, propofol causes the smooth onset of loss of consciousness. Hypotension can occur after rapid bolus injection. The use of propofol is associated with excellent amnesia but little analgesia. Propofol is rapidly distributed after bolus administration, and its elimination half-life is short. These pharmacokinetic characteristics lead to a rapid decline in serum concentration after administration by bolus or infusion and are associated with rapid emergence.

Inhalational Induction

Inhalational induction of anesthesia is well tolerated and accepted by healthy infants 1 to 6 months of age and by well-prepared children older than 4 years of age. An inhalational technique has the advantage of being painless. Children for urgent surgery, with full stomachs, or who are unable to tolerate inhalational induction requires intravenous an induction.

The major complication that occurs during inhalational induction is airway obstruction. As the patient becomes progressively anesthetized, airway tone is lost. The tongue and pharyngeal muscles, large tonsils, and floppy epiglottis may all obstruct the airway. The other major cause of airway obstruction is laryngospasm. Airway irritability is enhanced during inhalation induction in stage II. Sudden, absolute glottic closure can occur. Positive airway pressure up to 10 to 20 cm H_2O may help and should be maintained. If the laryngospasm does not respond within seconds or the oxygen saturation is falling, succinylcholine should be given and the airway intubated. Attempts to intubate without paralysis are dangerous, harmful, and usually futile. Patients with upper respiratory infections and increased secretions are at greater risk for laryngospasm. In these circumstances, elective operations should be postponed.

During induction, until the airway is secure, any sudden or painful stimulus, such as reducing the patient's hernia, may precipitate laryngospasm. For this reason, the patient is not examined or manipulated until the anesthesiologist has secured the airway or achieved adequate anesthetic depth.

Intramuscular Induction

Intramuscular induction may be chosen for children who are uncooperative or unresponsive to psychologic preparation (eg, mental retardation); who lose control during attempted inhalational induction; who become agitated rather than sedated after premedication; or who require rapid sequence induction but have no venous access.

The most commonly used drug for intramuscular induction is ketamine, 8 to 10 mg/kg, 10% solution. It should be combined with atropine, 0.02 mg/kg, to reduce secretions and may be administered in the same syringe with succinylcholine, 4 mg/kg, for rapid sequence induction. A smaller dose of ketamine, 2 to 3 mg/kg, may be used to calm children who are uncooperative for subsequent mask induction or intravenous catheter placement. When the larger dose of ketamine is used for the induction of anesthesia, prolonged emergence with the necessity for maintaining postoperative intubation may occur after short surgical procedures. On the other hand, for short procedures, adequate analgesia may be achieved by ketamine alone. In addition to atropine, a small dose of midazolam, 0.05 to 0.1 mg/kg, should be administered intravenously to ameliorate any emergence delirium caused by the ketamine. This emergence delirium occurs more commonly in older children. Complications of intramuscular induction include pain at the injection site, sterile abscess formation, and unpredictable uptake of drug from tissue, especially in the presence of decreased peripheral perfusion.

Rectal Induction

Children between the age of separation fears (about 8 months) and the age of reason (5 to 6 years) are poor candidates for mask induction. These children, if healthy, are ideal candidates for rectal induction of anesthesia. The use of the rectal route is usually well accepted because it avoids both mask and needle, and the child may fall asleep peacefully in the parent's arms in the induction area, with no memory of struggle in the operating room. After the drug is administered, the child must be continuously observed by the anesthesiologist for signs of airway obstruction, coughing, and apnea until the child is asleep and ready to be taken into the operating room. On transfer to the operating table, primary attention should be devoted to the maintenance of a patent airway and deepening the level of anesthesia by mask while an assistant or nurse attends to monitor placement.

Thiopental, methohexital, and ketamine have all been used for rectal induction. Rectal administration of anesthetic agents is associated with a 10% to 15% incidence of defecation, which usually does not interfere with the onset of sleep. Drugs are administered by syringe through a 14F suction catheter that has been cut to 10 cm in length and lubricated. A volume of air is instilled from the syringe to flush all the agent from the catheter into the rectum, and the parent holds the buttocks together for 2 minutes to encourage retention of the medication.

MUSCLE RELAXANTS

Much has been learned about the developmental aspects of the neuromuscular function.[82] There are differences in the density and sensitivity of the postsynaptic acetylcholine receptor, in the rate of neuromuscular transmission, and in muscle fiber types. Because all inhalational anesthetics potentiate neuromuscular blockade, it is not surprising that at equal anesthetic concentrations, the extent of neuromuscular blockade is age dependent. Most studies indicate that neonates have increased sensitivity to nondepolarizing neuromuscular blocking agents, but that they require the same dose when indexed to body surface area, owing to their larger volume of distribution.[83,84]

Long-acting, nondepolarizing neuromuscular agents have been the cornerstone of neonatal anesthesia, providing immobility, ideal intubating conditions, controlled ventilation, and optimal surgical conditions. These agents also reduce the required concentrations of inhalational anesthetics, improving the safety of neonatal anesthesia. Until recently, combining nitrous oxide, oxygen, and muscle relaxation was the standard approach for neonatal anesthesia. This allowed cardiorespiratory stability and good surgical conditions. It did not provide sufficient analgesia. This technique is supplemented with small amounts of potent inhalational agents to provide adequate analgesia, hemodynamic stability, and amnesia in older children and infants. Alternatively, supplementation of the paralysis, nitrous oxide, and oxygen technique with opioids such as fentanyl has become a standard alternative and provides remarkable hemodynamic stability.[1–3]

The most widely used long-acting neuromuscular blocking agent in pediatric anesthesia practice is pancuronium bromide. The major reasons are the vagolytic effect of pancuronium and its release of catecholamines.[85] This generally leads to an increased heart rate in small infants and children and thus is beneficial, as previously outlined. Intubation doses of 0.1 to 0.15 mg/kg have a duration of effect of from 50 to 70 minutes. This is variable.[82] Neonates who have been receiving pancuronium for a period of time appear to have some degree of tachyphylaxis and may require dosage as frequently as every 30 minutes.[86] This variability necessitates neuromuscular blockade monitoring when using this potent agent. Pancuronium is an ideal neuromuscular blocking agent for prolonged paralysis. After many weeks, an effect on neuromuscular function, similar to disease atrophy, may be seen, and slow weaning from mechanical ventilation may be required.[87]

Vecuronium is a steroidal neuromuscular relaxing agent, similar to pancuronium, that has few cardiac effects.[81,88] There appears to be no change in heart rate or blood pressure with vecuronium administration. This decreases its usefulness in neonatal anesthesia; but in older children, it is an established and useful neuromuscular blocking agent. Vecuronium has a shorter duration of action than pancuronium in children.[89] In infants, the duration of blockade and recovery time are prolonged when compared with children and adults. The duration of vecuronium effect from time of injection to 90% recovery is 73 minutes in infants, 35 minutes in children, and 53 minutes in adults. The use of vecuronium for short surgical procedures in children older than 2 years has become increasingly popular.[90]

Atracurium is a shorter-acting muscle relaxant with a slower onset of paralysis than the other nondepolarizing agents.[91] Neonates are particularly sensitive to atracurium.[92] The ED50 dose of atracurium is lowest in neonates and higher in children and adolescents. An ED95 dose of atracurium lasts between 25 and 35 minutes, making it useful for short surgical procedures in older children. The ED95 dose of atracurium varies from 0.3 mg/kg in neonates to 0.5 mg/kg in older children.[93] Histamine release also occurs, although this has not been reported to be a problem in infants and neonates. Because of a novel method of elimination that does not rely on renal excretion, atracurium may be preferentially used in patients with renal impairment.[91] It is possible that decreased renal clearance of other nondepolarizing muscle relaxants, such as vecuronium, pancuronium, and curare, in immature neonates accounts for their longer duration of action. Atracurium requires a much reduced dose in neonates.[91]

Mivacurium is a new agent with a short duration of activity. After an ED95 dose in adults, recovery begins to occur within 10 minutes. Recovery after infusion in children occurs within 5 minutes.[92] This and other short-acting nondepolarizing muscle relaxants may well supplant the use of succinylcholine in pediatric anesthesia. Two major drawbacks of nondepolarizing muscle relaxants are their relatively slow onset of action and their prolonged effect, making their use for rapid-sequence intubation less than optimum.[93]

Succinylcholine

Succinylcholine is the only depolarizing muscle relaxant in clinical use.[94] In children younger than 1 year, 2 mg/kg is the recommended dose. Others have suggested the use of even higher doses in neonates. This is almost certainly due to an increased volume of distribution, despite the relatively low pseudocholinesterase activity in infants. Complete, reliable muscle relaxation occurs within 90 seconds. Recovery starts to occur within 5 to 7 minutes and is complete within 10 to 15 minutes. In general, succinylcholine has a shorter duration of action in children than in adults. Succinylcholine may also be administered intramuscularly in doses of 4 to 5 mg/kg. Reliable muscle relaxation occurs within 4 to 7 minutes. When the dose is given intramuscularly, the effect is prolonged, and 20 to 30 minutes should be allowed before complete recovery is expected. In an emergency situation in which intravenous access is not available, succinylcholine can be administered intraosseously quite effectively and also into a muscle with high blood flow, such as the tongue. In infants and small children, the onset of muscle relaxation with intramuscular administration

probably is not rapid enough to maintain apneic oxygenation. In full stomach situations, rapid sequence intubation, cricoid pressure, and gentle manual ventilation may be required to avoid serious hypoxemia.

Succinylcholine has a myriad of potential side effects in children. Increased sensitivity to the vagal effects of succinylcholine, with profound bradycardia and asystole, occasionally occurs in children and is a major concern.[94,95] Atropine is recommended even before the first administration of succinylcholine. A second dose of succinylcholine is virtually always associated with a decreased heart rate and is likely to result in profound bradycardia and hypotension. Succinylcholine should never be used without atropine immediately available, and a second dose should never be given without prior administration of atropine. Intravenous atropine is required to abrogate these vagal effects. Intramuscular premedication with atropine is less efficacious. Atropine is not as critical when the drug is given intramuscularly.

Multiple complications can arise from the use of succinylcholine. Rhabdomyolysis, myoglobinuria, myoglobinemia, renal injury, hyperkalemia, masseter spasm, and pulmonary edema all have been reported with the use of this agent in children.[96,97] Malignant hypothermia is a significant concern in pediatric anesthesia, possibly seen more frequently in children owing to the routine use of inhalational anesthetics with succinylcholine.[98] The incidence of life-threatening hyperkalemia precludes its use in burned[99] or traumatized[100] children and in those with neuromuscular disease,[101] although not apparently cerebral palsy. These complications have decreased the routine use of succinylcholine in children.[102]

Reversal of Neuromuscular Blockade

The use of prolonged nondepolarizing neuromuscular blockade in children necessitates familiarity with the principles of antagonism of neuromuscular blockade. Virtually every child who is expected to maintain spontaneous ventilation independently and has received neuromuscular blockade should have the blockade reversed at the end of the procedure. This is especially true in infants and small children, in whom the duration of neuromuscular blockade is variable and prolonged. Reversal of blockade in children who are hypothermic (temperature less than 35.5°C) can quite difficult.[103] There are only two neuromuscular blockade reversing agents from which to choose: neostigmine and edrophonium. Neostigmine has the advantage of being a familiar agent whose use is time honored, whereas edrophonium appears to have a more rapid onset of action and thus allows a more prompt reversal of neuromuscular blockade.

The time for 50% reversal of neuromuscular blockade from a continuous curare infusion differs between adults and children.[104] In infants and children, 15 μg/kg of neostigmine is effective to produce 50% antagonism, whereas in adults, 23 μg/kg is required. The time to 70% antagonism of the blockade is 5 to 8 minutes regardless of age. It appears that the duration of antagonism is equally long in all age groups. Both of these agents have a significant vagomimetic effect, and in all cases, this should be antagonized by the co-administration of atropine. It is recommended that atropine administration precede the neuromuscular relaxant. For neostigmine, a larger dose of atropine is required (15 to 30 μg/kg). For edrophonium, 10 to 20 μg/ kg is the appropriate dose. In no case should less than 0.15 mg

TABLE 15-11. *Infant and child maintenance fluid requirements*

Weight	Water per hour	Water per day
≤10 kg	4 mL/kg	100 mL/kg
10–20 kg	40 mL + 2 mL/kg > 10 kg	1000 mL + 50 mL/ kg > 10 kg
> 20 kg	60 mL + 1 mL/kg > 20 kg	1500 mL + 25 mL/ kg > 20 kg

be given for any child because of paradoxical bradycardia, which can occur if the dose is too low.[103]

Fluid Management

Generally, half of routine fluid requirements for the NPO fasting period are replaced in the first 1 to 2 hours of surgery, while continuing to give maintenance fluid and replace ongoing losses (Table 15-11). Calculating the deficits, the maintenance needs, and the losses frequently gives a greater volume of fluid than is necessary to maintain adequate heart rate and blood pressure in children. Any sign of hemodynamic instability, decreased urine output, tachycardia, borderline hypotension, or decreased perfusion should be treated initially with volume to be certain of restoration of all calculated needs before introducing other therapies or attributing tachycardia and hemodynamic instability to other causes. Thus, deficit plus maintenance plus replacement of estimated losses is indicated intraoperatively. Blood can be replaced by crystalloid solution (generally Ringers lactate or normal saline) on a 3 : 1 basis. When the hematocrit is unacceptably low, blood transfusion is indicated on a milliliter-for-milliliter basis. Every attempt should be made to quantitate blood loss by the use of pediatric suction bottles, weighing sponges, and accurate estimation of blood losses in the operative field. In small children, blood removed for diagnostic purposes may make a significant contribution to blood loss; this should be limited and replaced when necessary.

Third-space losses must also be estimated and are generally related to the type and duration of surgery. Immobility and trauma alter the microvascular integrity. Plasma leaks into the interstitium. Even during minor surgery, this third-space loss can be 1 to 3 mL/kg/h. When more extensive surgery is undertaken, greater losses can be expected. Thoracotomy can be associated with 3 to 5 mL/kg/h third-space losses, and laparotomy may require 5 to 7 mL/kg/h replacement. Large tissue exposure, infection, large areas of tissue trauma, and handling of the bowel may increase third-space losses beyond 7 to 10 mL/kg/h. These third-space losses can exceed those for maintenance fluid. Although third-space fluid losses result in postoperative edema, especially in dependent tissues, this is not the result of aggressive fluid therapy; rather, the microvascular dysfunction is an indication for aggressive fluid therapy.

Regional Anesthesia

Because of the deleterious effects of inhalational and intravenous anesthetics, there has been a resurgence of interest in neonatal regional anesthesia. Regional anesthesia causes loss of pain perception during consciousness. Regional anesthesia can be achieved by spinal anesthesia or epidural anesthesia, and in some cases by local anesthetic infiltration. Regional anesthesia blunts all pain responses and also blunts the response to surgical stress. Infants appear to tolerate spinal or caudal epidural anesthesia up to the mid-thoracic level without respiratory complications, bradycardia, or hypotension; however, caution should always be exercised in anesthetizing a hemodynamically unstable infant, even with regional anesthesia. The contraindications to regional anesthesia are time (urgency), potential for hemodynamic instability, extensive surgery for which regional anesthesia will not provide adequate anesthesia, and the presence or potential development of a coagulopathy, owing to the risk of spinal and epidural hematomas. Thus, hemodynamically unstable, septic, ill neonates who require surgery for necrotizing enterocolitis or thoracic procedures are not candidates. Regional anesthesia is most common in premature infants who require inguinal herniorrhaphy. These children can safely receive a spinal anesthetic or caudal epidural anesthetic for this surgery.[105,106]

Epidural anesthesia is induced by inserting a catheter in the epidural space. In neonates, this is best achieved through a caudal approach. The caudal space can be approached through the sacral hiatus, at the sacrococcygeal junction at the base of the spine. A catheter can be advanced to provide continuous epidural anesthesia, even as high as the thoracic level. Epidural analgesia can effectively be provided for critically ill and premature neonates.[107,108] An additional advantage is that a catheter may be left in situ for postoperative pain management. This technique has been used for hundreds of high-risk infants. In addition to using isolated epidural analgesia, epidural analgesia supplementation of general anesthetics is widely practiced. This diminishes the amount of inhalational or opioid anesthetic given to a child while still blunting the stress responses. This also makes it possible to provide postoperative analgesia without the need for opioids or other depressant drugs during recovery of the neonate. Familiarity with the use of continuous, anesthetic infusion and with the use and potential for epidural opioids is necessary to ensure this form of pain management for the neonate postoperatively.

Spinal analgesia has been used for more than 100 years in critically ill neonates, but it became less popular with the advent of safer general anesthetics. The use of spinal anesthesia for critically ill neonates requiring herniorrhaphy has become popular.[109,110] This has led to a resurgence in the interest in spinal anesthesia. Spinal anesthesia can generally provide proper operative conditions for up to 90 minutes.

The indications for regional anesthesia are surgery below the level of the umbilicus, short duration (less than 2 hours), an elective operation, no gastrointestinal disease, and no threat of reflux and vomiting.

NEONATAL RECOVERY FROM ANESTHESIA

Recovery from anesthesia for premature infants occurs in the neonatal intensive care unit. Attention to the airway is paramount. Overall care and extubation for the neonate are usually best done in this environment. In addition to the physiologic disturbance consequent to the primary disease of the infant, postoperative complications include delayed awakening, residual neuromuscular paralysis, temperature instability, hemodynamic instability, depressed airway reflexes, depressed respiratory control, nausea and vomiting, and surgical pain. Recognition of the deleterious effects of general anesthesia guides monitoring in the postoperative period.

Probably the most significant cause of delayed awakening from anesthesia in neonates is hypothermia. This delays the metabolism of intravenous anesthetic agents and the excretion of inhaled anesthetic agents, and potentiates their negative physiologic consequences. Neuromuscular blockade is also aggravated by hypothermia. Therefore, precise thermal regulation is required in the postoperative period. Prolonged neuromuscular paralysis or weakness after anesthesia raises the possibility of pseudocholinesterase deficiency or delayed metabolism of nondepolarizing muscle relaxants. Because the use of succinylcholine has become increasingly rare in pediatric anesthesia, the former is unlikely to be seen. Excretion of neuromuscular blocking agents in neonates, however, can be prolonged. Prolonged postoperative ventilatory requirements indicate the need for reversal of neuromuscular paralysis and reassessment of the child's muscle function.

Postanesthetic Apnea

The respiratory depressant effects of anesthetic agents have been described. In addition, the neonatal response to stress includes apnea. Preterm and former preterm infants have a propensity for apnea, periodic breathing, and bradycardia. The postoperative incidence of life-threatening apnea and bradycardia in neonates and former preterm infants is significant.[111] In one study,[112] 12% of all preterm infants developed significant apnea in the first 12 hours after operation. Other reports indicate a similar or even greater risk.[113] Kurth and colleagues[10] reported a 37% incidence of significant prolonged postoperative apnea in former preterm infants with postconceptual ages between 32 and 55 weeks. Former preterm infants younger than 60 weeks' postconceptual age required postoperative apnea monitoring for at least 12 hours. Studies since then have demonstrated that monitoring and the provision of mechanical ventilation can decrease the risk of postoperative apnea, that postoperative apnea occurs in infants younger than 55 weeks' postconceptual age whether the anesthetic was inhalational or regional, and that the administration of caffeine can decrease this incidence. Anemia also increases the perioperative likelihood of apnea in preterm infants.[114]

In the authors' institution, infants younger than 44 weeks' postconceptual age and premature and former premature infants younger than 52 weeks' postconceptual age are considered at increased risk of perioperative apnea.[114] These infants, where therapy for apnea can be expeditiously provided, receive cardiorespiratory monitoring for 12 to 24 hours after surgery. These infants are not routinely treated with caffeine because this does not eliminate the risk. It is advisable, whenever possible, to delay surgery beyond these dates. If surgery cannot be deferred, then outpatient surgery is clearly not advisable, and monitoring is provided postoperatively.

Some recommend caffeine, 10 mg/kg intravenously, after surgery.[114] Treatment of anemia with iron supplementation and erythropoietin should be considered.

Anesthesia Mortality and Morbidity

Adverse events during anesthesia and occasional perioperative mortalities were common in the past. In a recent study of overall anesthetic practice, the risk of complications in infants was about 4.3 in 1000. This is eight times greater than in older children.[115] Death occurs in up to 1 in 600 anesthetized neonates; obviously this is related to the complexity of the patient's underlying medical condition.[116]

PEDIATRIC PAIN MANAGEMENT

Even when their pain is obvious, children frequently receive inadequate analgesic treatment.[117–119] Unfortunately, physicians often fail to prescribe potent analgesics or to give adequate doses. Their concern is that children may be harmed by the use of these drugs. This is not surprising because physicians are trained that opiates cause respiratory depression, cardiovascular collapse, depressed levels of consciousness, vomiting, and, with repeated use, addiction. The therapeutic use of these drugs is discussed rarely. It is now clear that children have significant physiologic and psychologic responses to pain and that physicians must be attentive to this need.

Pain Neurophysiology

Pain management is best understood or designed in terms of afferent pain pathways and descending pain modulation. Pain can be relieved in the following ways:

- By reducing the sensory input from damaged tissue (by prostaglandin inhibitors or local anesthetics administration)
- By modulating the transmission of the nociceptive input through the CNS (by transcutaneous electrical nerve stimulation, pharmacologic opioid administration, or administration of local anesthetics)
- By altering the patient's emotional responses to such actual or perceived sensory input (by antidepressants, hypnotics, or amnestics)

Effective pain treatment requires accurate measurement of pain.

Pain Assessment

Because pain is a subjective experience, the child's perspective of pain is an indispensable facet of pediatric pain management and an essential consideration in the study of childhood pain. Pain assessment and management are interdependent. The goal of pain assessment is to provide accurate data about the location and intensity of pain as well as about the effectiveness of measures used to alleviate or abolish it.[120]

Validated, reliable instruments measure and assess pain in children older than 3 years.[121] These instruments are self-report measures and make use of pictures or word descriptors to describe pain. Pain intensity or severity can be measured in children as young as 3 years of age by using picture scales[120,121] (Fig. 15-5).

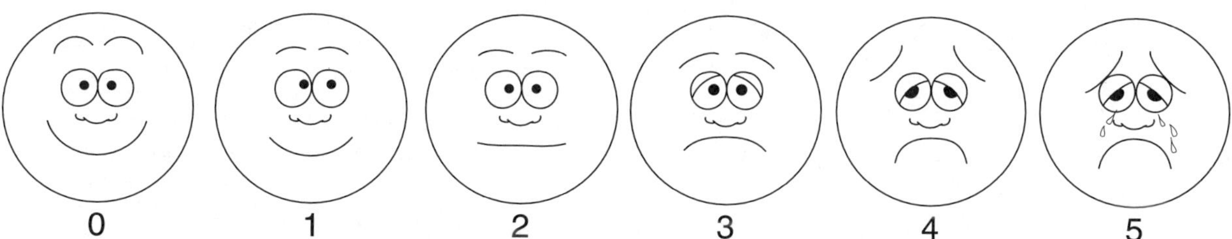

Faces pain rating scale

FIG. 15-5. Visual analogue scales used in pain assessment in children. The higher the score, the greater the child's pain. (After Wong DL, Baker CM. Pain in children: comparison of assessment scales. Pediatr Nurs 1988;14:9)

Pain Management

Nonopioid Analgesics

Mild analgesics, of which acetaminophen (Tylenol), salicylate (aspirin), and ibuprofen (Motrin) are the classic examples, constitute a heterogeneous group of nonsteroidal antiinflammatory drugs (NSAIDs) and nonopioid analgesics. They provide pain relief primarily by blocking peripheral prostaglandin production. These analgesic agents are administered orally or, on occasion, rectally. They are particularly useful for inflammatory, bone, or rheumatic pain. New parenterally administered NSAIDS, such as ketorolac, are available when the oral or rectal routes of administration are not possible. Unfortunately, regardless of dose, the nonopioid analgesics reach a ceiling effect, above which pain cannot be relieved by these drugs alone (Table 15-12). Because of this, these weaker analgesics are often administered in combination with more potent opioids.

Aspirin, one of the oldest and most effective nonopioid analgesics, has been largely abandoned in pediatric practice because of its possible role in Reye syndrome, its effects on platelet function, and its gastric irritant properties. Despite these problems, a new salicylate product, choline-magnesium trisalicylate is increasingly used in pediatric pain management, particularly in the management of postoperative pain and in children with cancer. Choline-magnesium trisalicylate is a unique aspirin-like compound that does not bind to platelets and therefore has no effect on platelet function. It is a convenient drug to give to children because it is available in both a liquid and tablet form and is administered only twice a day (see Table 15-12). The association of salicylates with Reye syndrome will limit its use, even though the risk of developing this syndrome postoperatively is extremely low.

The most commonly used nonopioid analgesic for children remains acetaminophen. Unlike aspirin and the NSAIDs, acetaminophen has minimal, if any, antiinflammatory activity. In usual doses (ie, 10 to 15 mg/kg orally or rectally; the first rectal dose can be as high as 40 mg/kg), acetaminophen has few serious side effects, is an antipyretic, and like all enterally administered NSAIDs, takes about 40 to 60 minutes to provide effective analgesia.

Opioids

The discovery of endorphins and opioid receptors has necessitated a reclassification of opiates into agonists, antagonists,

TABLE 15-12. *Dosage guidelines for commonly used nonsteroidal antiinflammatory drugs*

Generic name	Brand name	Dose (mg/kg) and frequency	Maximum adult daily dose (mg)	Comments
Salicylates (aspirin)	Many brand names, eg, Bayer, Bufferin, Anacin, Alka-Seltzer	10–15 q 4 h	4000	Inhibits platelet aggregation, GI irritability, Reye syndrome
Acetaminophen	Many brand names, eg, Tylenol, Panadol, Tempra	10–15, q 4 h	4000	Lacks antiinflammatory activity
Ibuprofen	Many brand names, eg, Motrin, Advil, Medipren	8–12 q 6–8 h	2400	Available as an oral suspension
Naproxyn	Naprosyn	5–10, q 12 h	1000	Available as an oral suspension
Indomethacin	Indocin	0.3–1, q 6 h	150	Commonly used in NICU to close patent ductus arteriosus
Ketorolac	Toradol	IV or IM: load 0.5; Maintenance: 0.2–0.5, q 6 h	120	May be given orally; adult IM dosing: load 30 mg, followed by 15–30 mg q 6 h
Choline magnesium trisalicylate	Trilisate	8–10, q 8–12 h	3000	Does not bind to platelets, see salicylate

TABLE 15-13. *Commonly used μ-agonist opiates*

Agonist	Equipotent IV dose (mg/kg)	Duration (h)	PO absorption (%)	Comments
Morphine	0.1	3–4	20–40	Seizures in newborns, also in all patients at high doses; histamine release, vasodilation; avoid in asthmatic patients and in patients with circulatory compromise; MS Contin, 8–12 h duration
Meperidine	1.0	3–4	40–60	Catastrophic interactions with monoamine oxidase inhibitors; tachycardia; negative inotrope; metabolite produces seizures; not recommended for routine analgesic therapy; low dose (0.25 mg/kg) stops shivering
Methadone	0.1	6–24	70–100	Can be given IV even though the package insert says SQ or IM
Fentanyl	0.001	0.5–1		Bradycardia; minimal hemodynamic alterations; chest wall rigidity (>5 μg/kg rapid IV bolus); prescribe naloxone, succinylcholine, or pancuronium; oral transmucosal preparation, 10 μg/kg
Codeine	1.2	3–4	40–70	PO only; prescribe with acetaminophen
Oxycodone (Tylox)	0.1	3–4	60–80	PO only; usually prescribed with acetaminophen

and mixed agonist–antagonists based on receptor-binding properties. Morphine and related opiates are agonists. Drugs that block the effects of opiates, such as naloxone, are antagonists. Opioids interact with specific receptors. These are widely distributed throughout the CNS. Although there are as many as eight different opioid receptors, four are of major importance to pain management. These are the μ, δ, κ, and σ receptors. The μ receptor and δ receptor are related to analgesia, respiratory depression, euphoria, and physical dependence. The respiratory depression and analgesia produced by opiates involve different receptor subtypes. These receptors change in number in an age-related fashion and can be blocked by naloxone.[122,123] The newborn is particularly sensitive to the respiratory depressant effects of the opioids by what may be an age-related receptor phenomenon.[124] Obviously, this has important clinical implications for the use of narcotics in newborn infants (see below).

Despite the confusion of terminology and the plethora of available drugs, at equipotent analgesic doses, all commonly used opioids produce similar degrees of respiratory depression, sedation, euphoria, nausea, biliary tract spasm, and constipation. Mixed agonist–antagonist drugs, such as pentazocine (Talwin), nalbuphine (Nubain), and butorphanol (Stadol), produce significantly less respiratory depression and biliary spasm than pure agonist drugs such as morphine. They are significantly less potent analgesics than the pure agonists and reach a ceiling above which no further analgesia can be achieved. Furthermore, they can cause reversal of previously induced narcotic analgesia and should never be used in patients chronically using (or addicted to) opioids. Although many opioids are available for clinical use, the drugs listed in Table 15-13 are the most commonly used.

Opioids are usually administered at fixed time intervals despite enormous variability in patient response. It is not uncommon to provide doses that are too small and at intervals that are too long for individual patient needs (Fig. 15-6). Rational use of opioids requires a flexible, patient-oriented approach to allow for variability in individual pain experience and tolerance as well as both the beneficial and adverse effects of the particular drug being used.

Morphine

Morphine is the standard for analgesia against which all other opioids are compared. When small doses (0.1 mg/kg intrave-

nously or intramuscularly) are administered to patients in pain, analgesia occurs rapidly without loss of consciousness. The relief of tension, anxiety, and pain usually results in drowsiness and sleep as well. Mental clouding, drowsiness, lethargy, sleep, and inability to concentrate can occur after morphine administration even in the absence of pain. Less advantageous CNS effects of morphine include nausea and vomiting, miosis, and at high doses, seizures. Seizures are a particular problem in newborns because they can occur at commonly prescribed doses. The nausea and vomiting with morphine is due to stimulation of the chemoreceptor trigger zone in the brain stem.

Morphine and all other opioids at equipotent doses depress respiration, principally by reducing the sensitivity of the brainstem respiratory centers to arterial CO_2 content.[29] Infants younger than 1 to 2 months of age are particularly sensitive. This is of such great concern that the use of any narcotic in children younger than 2 months of age must be limited to a monitored environment.

Although morphine produces peripheral vasodilation and venous pooling, it has minimal hemodynamic effect in normal, euvolemic, supine patients. The vasodilation associated with morphine is primarily due to histamine release. Significant hypotension can occur when sedatives such as diazepam are concurrently administered. Otherwise, morphine produces virtually no cardiovascular effects when used alone. It causes significant hypotension in hypovolemic patients, and its use in trauma is therefore limited.

Opiates inhibit intestinal smooth muscle function. This decrease in peristalsis and increase in sphincter tone explains the historic use of narcotics in the treatment of diarrhea as well as the side effect of constipation when treating chronic pain. Morphine potentiates biliary colic by causing spasm of the sphincter of Oddi and should be used with caution in patients with, or at risk for, cholelithiasis (eg, sickle cell disease). Finally, to minimize the complications associated with intravenous opioid administration, the dose should be titrated at the bedside until the desired level of analgesia is achieved.

Morphine and most μ-agonists (meperidine, methadone, fentanyl) are biotransformed in the liver before excretion. Many of these reactions are catalyzed in the liver by microsomal mixed-function oxidases that require the cytochrome P-450 system, NADPH, and oxygen. Morphine is primarily metabolized by

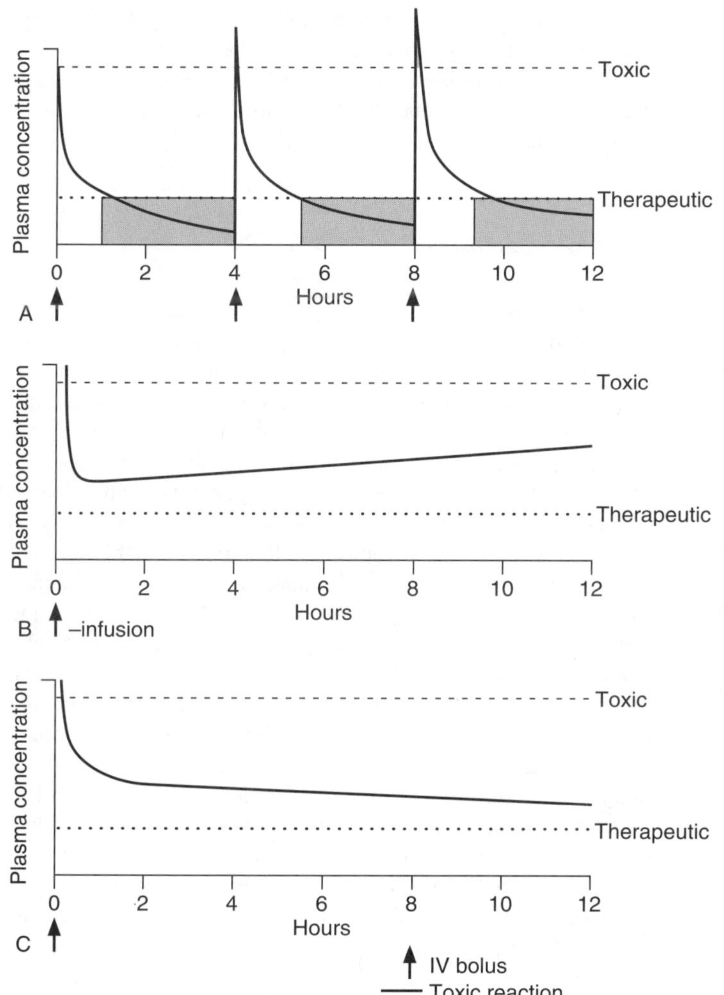

FIG. 15-6. Simulated blood concentration–dose relations for opioids by different administration regimens. (*A*) IV bolus administration of morphine sulfate (elimination half-life, 4 hours) every 4 hours. (*B*) IV bolus administration of morphine sulfate followed by continuous IV infusion. (*C*) IV bolus infusion of methadone (elimination half-life, 19 hours). There is an absence of pain periods in *B* and *C*. Arrows indicate time of IV bolus administration. (After Yaster M, Maxwell LG. Opioid agonists and antagonists. In: Schechter NL, Berde CB, Yaster M. Pain in infants, children, and adolescents. Baltimore, Williams & Wilkins, 1993:145)

glucuronidation into two forms—an inactive form (morphine-3-glucuronide) and an active form (morphine-6-glucuronide). Both glucuronides are excreted by the kidney. In children with renal failure, morphine-6-glucuronide can accumulate and cause toxic side effects, including respiratory depression. This is important not only when prescribing morphine but also when administering other opioids, such as methadone and codeine, that are metabolized into morphine.

Finally, only about 30% of orally administered morphine reaches the systemic circulation. In the past, this led many to believe that morphine was ineffective when administered orally. This is not true. When converting a patient's intravenous morphine requirements to oral maintenance, one needs to multiply the intravenous dose by three to four. Oral morphine is available as a liquid (20 mg/mL), tablet, and sustained release preparation (MS Contin; Table 15-13). MS Contin can not be crushed and given via a feeding tube.

Fentanyl

Because of its rapid onset and brief duration of action, fentanyl has become a favored analgesic for short procedures, such as bone marrow aspirations, fracture reductions, suturing lacera-tions, endoscopy, and dental procedures. Fentanyl is about 100 times more potent than morphine; that is, the equal analgesic dose is 0.001 mg/kg (see Table 15-13), and it is devoid of hypnotic or sedative activity. Fentanyl blocks nociceptive stimuli without hemodynamic instability. It is the drug of choice for trauma, cardiac, or intensive care patients. In addition to its ability to block the systemic and pulmonary hemodynamic responses to pain, fentanyl also prevents the biochemical and endocrine stress (catabolic) response to painful stimuli that can be detrimental in critically ill patients. Fentanyl has the serious side effect of chest wall rigidity after rapid infusions of 0.005 mg/kg or greater. This may make ventilation difficult or impossible. Chest wall rigidity can be treated with either muscle relaxants, such as succinylcholine or pancuronium, or the opioid antagonist, naloxone.

Fentanyl is a highly lipophilic drug and rapidly penetrates all membranes, including the oral mucosa and skin. This feature has made transmucosal and transdermal preparations of this drug possible. Fentanyl is rapidly eliminated from plasma as a result of its extensive uptake by body tissues. Repeated doses of fentanyl for maintenance of analgesic effects lead to tissue accumulation with ventilatory depressant effects. Large doses (0.05 to 0.10 mg/kg, as used in anesthesia) can be expected to induce long-lasting effects because plasma fentanyl levels do not fall below the threshold for spontaneous ventilation during the distribution phases.

Meperidine

Meperidine (Demerol) is a synthetic narcotic that is most commonly used in children as either a premedicant for anesthesia, as sedation, or as treatment for postoperative pain. It is a potent analgesic with pharmacokinetic properties similar to morphine, producing analgesia, sedation, euphoria, dysphoria, miosis, and respiratory depression. At equal analgesic doses (1 mg/kg; see Table 15-13), there is little quantitative difference between meperidine and morphine in producing these effects. Its effects on respiration and on gastrointestinal motility are similar to all of the other μ-agonist opioid analgesics. Thus, it is a potent respiratory depressant and antitussive. Some studies suggest that meperidine exerts less of an effect on the biliary tract, including the common bile duct, than morphine. Other studies dispute this.

Meperidine's principal metabolite, normeperidine, may produce tremors, muscle twitching, hyperactive reflexes, and convulsions. Because of the accumulation of this metabolite, the prolonged use of meperidine is discouraged. The authors have abandoned the routine use of meperidine in their pain management practice. On the other hand, they prescribe meperidine for shivering. When administered at low doses (0.25 to 0.5 mg/kg) intravenously, meperidine has the unique property of stopping shivering regardless of its cause.

Meperidine is commonly administered intramuscularly for moderate to severe pain or as part of a sedative cocktail (meperidine, promethazine, and chlorpromazine) in a dose of 1 to 2 mg/kg. The authors, however, do not recommend intramuscular administration of analgesics in children, nor the use of this cocktail.

Codeine and Oxycodone

Codeine and oxycodone (the opioid in Tylox and Percocet) are frequently used for pain control in both children and adults. Although effective when administered either orally or parenterally, they are most commonly administered orally, usually in combination with acetaminophen. In equipotent doses (see Table 15-13), codeine and oxycodone approach the analgesic and respiratory depressant effects of morphine and other narcotics on the CNS. Codeine commonly causes nausea, and many patients state this as an allergy. Nausea and vomiting are less common with oxycodone. Both drugs delay gastric emptying and can increase biliary tract pressure. Finally, codeine, like all μ-agonist opioids, has potent antitussive properties and is commonly prescribed for this effect.

Codeine and oxycodone have a bioavailability of about 60% after oral ingestion. The analgesic effects occur as early as 20 minutes after ingestion and reach a maximum at 60 to 120 minutes. The plasma elimination half-life is 2.5 to 3 hours. Codeine undergoes nearly complete metabolism in the liver before its final excretion in urine. About 10% of codeine is metabolized into morphine, and it is this fraction that is responsible for codeine's analgesic effect. Interestingly, about 10% of the population cannot metabolize codeine into morphine.

Codeine and oxycodone are available in liquid, tablet, and capsule form. Typically, codeine is prescribed in a dose of 0.5 to 1 mg/kg, and oxycodone is prescribed in a dose of 0.05 to 0.1 mg/kg. Both may be concurrently administered with acetaminophen, 10 mg/kg.

Opioid Antagonists

Naloxone is a pure opioid antagonist with no agonist activity. It antagonizes the effects of pure agonists, such as morphine, as well as the mixed agonist–antagonist drugs, such as butorphanol. It is the most commonly used opioid antagonist in clinical practice. Naloxone not only reverses sedation, respiratory depression, and gastrointestinal effects of the opioid agonists but also reverses the analgesia. The antagonism of narcotic agonist effects must be done with great caution, particularly in children receiving prolonged opioid therapy who exhibit opioid dependence or extreme pain because it may be accompanied by overt withdrawal symptoms. Occasionally a life-threatening (overshoot) phenomenon occurs in these patients, with the development of tachypnea, tachycardia, hypertension, nausea and vomiting, and sudden death. In healthy young adults, this phenomenon may be accompanied by the onset of pulmonary edema. Mechanical ventilation is recommended as a safer treatment for narcotic-induced respiratory depression in dependent patients or in patients in severe pain. Obviously, the magnitude of the withdrawal syndrome is dependent on the dose of naloxone administered as well as on the degree of the patient's physical dependence and needs. On the other hand, when naloxone is administered to patients who have not received opioids, it produces minimal to no effects and has no inherent properties that induce physical dependence or tolerance. After intravenous administration, it reverses opioid effects virtually instantaneously. It has a plasma half-life of elimination of only 60 minutes and a duration of action that is shorter than the agonists it is used to antagonize. Therefore, when naloxone is used to reverse narcotic-induced respiratory depression, patients must be monitored for return of the depression based on the half-life of the opiate agonist. This may require repeat intravenous doses, intramuscular (depot) injection, or a continuous intravenous infusion.

Naloxone is supplied as a parenteral solution (1 mg/mL, 0.4 mg/mL, or 0.02 mg/mL). The usual initial dose in children (and adults) is 0.01 to 0.10 mg/kg given intravenously. If an intravenous route is not available, naloxone may be administered intramuscularly or subcutaneously. Doses as low as 0.001 to 0.002 mg/kg may be effective at reversing opioid-induced respiratory depression (or other unwanted side effects, such as pruritus or biliary spasm) without reversing analgesia. If the initial dose of naloxone does not result in the desired degree of clinical improvement, subsequent doses of 0.02, 0.04, 0.08, and 0.1 mg/kg may be administered in a step-wise manner. The highest dose, 0.1 mg/kg, is used to treat cardiopulmonary arrest. When used to antagonize neonatal respiratory depression (from narcotics administered to the mother in labor), the usual initial dose is the same dose as used in older children (0.01 mg/kg of the 0.02 mg/mL solution).

Patient-Controlled Analgesia

Because of the enormous individual variations in pain perception and opioid metabolism, the administration of fixed doses at specific time intervals makes little sense. Based on the pharmacokinetics of the opioids, it should be clear that intravenous boluses of morphine or meperidine may need to be given at intervals of 1 to 2 hours to avoid marked fluctuations in plasma drug levels (see Fig. 15-6). Continuous intravenous infusions can provide steady analgesic levels but are not a panacea because the perception and intensity of pain is not constant. The most common method of opioid administration in adults and children is intramuscular injection. It is well known that children will suffer in silence and underreport their level of pain, rather than ask for another painful stimulus. Thus, we avoid intramuscular injections in children. To give children some measure of control over their pain therapy, demand analgesia or patient-controlled analgesia (PCA) devices have been developed. These are microprocessor driven pumps with a button that the patient presses to self-administer a small dose of opioid.

PCA devices administer small amounts of an analgesic whenever the child feels a need for more pain relief. The opioid, usually morphine, is administered either intravenously or subcutaneously. The dosage of opioid, number of boluses per hour, and time interval between boluses (the lock-out period) are programmed into the equipment by the pain service physician to allow maximum patient flexibility and sense of control with minimal risk of overdosage (Table 15-14). Generally, because patients know they can obtain relief immediately, many prefer dosing regimens that result in mild to moderate pain in exchange for fewer side effects, such as nausea or pruritus. Typically, morphine is prescribed initially, 20 μg/kg per bolus, at a rate of five boluses per hour, with a 6- to 8-minute lock-out interval between each bolus (see Table 15-14). Variations include larger boluses (30 to 50 μg/kg), shorter time intervals (5 minutes), and so forth. Hydromorphone has fewer side effects than morphine and is often used when pruritus and nausea complicate morphine PCA therapy. The PCA pump memory stores the number of boluses the patient has received as well as how many attempts the patient has made. This allows the physician to evaluate how well the patient understands the use of the pump and provides information to program the pump more efficiently. Many PCA units allow low continuous infusions (morphine, 20 to 30 μg/kg/h) in addition to self-administered boluses. This is sometimes called *PCA-plus*. A continuous background infusion is particularly useful at night and often provides more restful sleep by preventing the patient from awakening in pain. It also increases the potential for overdosage. Although the literature on pain does not support the use of continuous background infusions, it has been the authors' experience that continuous infusions are often necessary when treating children.

PCA requires that the patient have enough intelligence, manual dexterity, and strength to operate the pump. Thus, it was initially limited to adolescents and teenagers, but the lower age limit continues to fall. In fact, any child who is able to play computer games can operate a PCA pump (5 to 6 years of age). Furthermore, nurses and parents can initiate PCA boluses and use this technology in children even younger than 1 year. Difficulties with PCA include its increased costs, patient age limitations, and the bureaucratic (physician, nursing, and pharmacy) obstacles (protocols, education, storage arrangements) that must be overcome before its implementation. Contraindications include inability to push the bolus button (weakness, arm restraints), inability to understand how to use the machine, and desire not to assume responsibility for his or her own care.

Intrathecal and Epidural Opioid Analgesia

The presence of high concentrations of opioid receptors in the spinal cord makes it possible to achieve analgesia with small doses of opioids administered either in the subarachnoid or epidural spaces. Bypassing the blood and the blood–brain barrier, small doses of agonist are effective because they reach the receptor directly.[125] Using these routes, cerebrospinal fluid (CSF) opioid levels are several thousand times greater than those achieved by the parenteral route (see below). These high levels produce profound and prolonged analgesia.

Epidurally administered agonists cross the dura into the CSF at a rate dependent on their lipid solubility. Once in the CSF, opioids must pass from the water phase to the lipid phase of the underlying neuraxis to reach the receptor. Hydrophilic agents, such as morphine, have a greater latency and duration of action than more lipid-soluble agents, such as fentanyl. On the other hand, the lipid-soluble agonists produce more segmental analgesia with less rostral spread than the less lipid-soluble agonists.

When administered by the caudal route, epidural morphine provides effective postoperative analgesia after abdominal, thoracic, and cardiac surgery. Krane and associates[126] reported that 0.03 mg/kg of caudal–epidural morphine is as effective as 0.1 mg/kg for postoperative analgesia, although the higher dose provides a significantly longer duration of analgesia (13.3 $\pm$ 4.7 versus 10 $\pm$ 3.3 hours, respectively). Side effects were the same in both groups, although one patient who was adminis-

TABLE 15-14. *Intravenous patient-controlled analgesia (PCA) treatment guidelines*

Drug (concentration, mg/mL)	Basal rate range (mg/kg/h)	Bolus rate range (mg/kg)	Lock-out interval range (min)	Number of boluses per hour range
Morphine (1.0)	0.01–0.03	0.01–0.03	5–10	2–6
Fentanyl	0.0005 (0.5 μg)	0.0005–0.001	5–10	1–6
0.01 in children <20 kg		(0.5–1.0 μg)		
0.05 in childre >20 kg				
Hydromorphone	0.003–0.005	0.003–0.005	5–10	2–6
0.2 in children <50 kg	(3.0–5.0 μg)	(3.0–5.0 μg)		
0.5–1.0 in children >50 kg				

tered the 0.1 mg/kg dose developed late respiratory depression. These investigators suggest starting with the lower dose when using this technique. Whether lower doses are effective is not known.

Neuraxis spinal opiates produce analgesia without altering autonomic or neuromuscular function. Additionally, both light touch and proprioception are preserved. Thus, unlike local anesthetics, spinal opioids allow ambulation without orthostatic hypotension. Common side effects include facial or segmental pruritus, urinary retention, nausea, vomiting, and respiratory depression. These effects occur more frequently when opioids are administered intrathecally as opposed to epidurally. Except for urinary retention, reversal of adverse side effects, with maintenance of adequate analgesia, can be achieved through the use of a low-dose, intravenous (0.001 to 0.002 mg/kg) naloxone infusion. Pruritus and nausea can also be treated with intravenous or oral diphenhydramine, 0.5 to 1 mg/kg, or hydroxyzine (Vistaril, Atarax). Urinary retention is unusual in these children because most have bladder catheters as part of their postoperative management regimen.

Although rare, respiratory depression is a significant risk with intrathecal and epidural opioids. Attia and associates[127] demonstrated that the ventilatory response to CO_2 was depressed for as long as 22 hours after the administration of 0.05 mg/kg of morphine epidurally. After intrathecal morphine administration, 0.02 mg/kg, in children between 3 months and 15 years of age, Nichols and colleagues[128] reported significant depression of the ventilatory response to hypercarbia for up to 18 hours. The greatest respiratory depression correlated with the highest CSF morphine levels (2863 ± 542 ng/mL), and this occurred 6 hours after administration. This depression persisted despite decreased CSF morphine levels 12 hours (641 ± 219 ng/mL) to 18 hours (223 ± 152 ng/mL) later. This confirms the clinical impression that respiratory depression usually occurs within the first 6 hours after the administration of epidural or intrathecal morphine and may persist as long as 18 hours afterward.

Respiratory depression most commonly occurs when intravenous and intramuscular narcotics are concurrently administered. The risk of respiratory depression is minimized when smaller doses of supplemental narcotics are used. Shorter-acting, more lipid-soluble agents (fentanyl, sufentanil) are an alternative. Because of their shorter action, fentanyl and sufentanil are increasingly being administered by continuous epidural infusion, either alone or in combination with dilute bupivacaine, 1/16% (0.0625 mg/mL), or lidocaine, 3 to 5 mg/mL, solutions. Typically, the epidural solution contains 1 to 5 μg/mL of fentanyl and is administered at rates ranging between 0.5 and 1 μg/kg/h. This provides effective analgesia for postoperative acute and chronic medical pain. Higher doses usually result in pruritus.

Regardless of the opioid and route of administration, a regular system of monitoring for respiratory depression is necessary. Clinical signs that predict impending respiratory depression include somnolence, small pupils, and small tidal volumes (shallow respirations). Oxyhemoglobin saturation monitoring (pulse oximetry) is standard, particularly during the first 24 hours of this therapy.

Pharmacology and Pharmacokinetics of Local Anesthetics

Local anesthetics are tertiary amines of two types[129]: either esters (eg, tetracaine [Pontocaine], procaine [Novocain], chlo-

TABLE 15-15. *Comparative pharmacology of local anesthetics*

Classification	Relative potency	Onset	Duration after infiltration (min)
ESTERS			
Procaine	1	Slow	45–60
Chloroprocaine	4	Rapid	30–45
Tetracaine	16	Slow	60–180
AMIDES			
Lidocaine	1	Rapid	60–120
Mepivacaine	1–2	Slow	90–180
Bupivacaine	4–8	Slow	240–480
Etidocaine	4–8	Slow	240–480
Prilocaine	1	Slow	60–120

roprocaine [Nesacaine], cocaine) or amides (lidocaine [Xylocaine], prilocaine, bupivacaine [Marcaine, Sensorcaine]; Table 15-15). They are all weak bases that block nerve conduction by a primary effect on the sodium channel. To reach the sodium channel, the local anesthetic must cross the nerve membrane; it is only the nonionized (base) form of drug that can do this. The amount available to cross the nerve membrane depends on the pKa of the drug and the pH of the local extracellular fluid. Thus, the lower the pKa of the drug, the more nonionized drug is available to cross the nerve cell membrane at physiologic pH. For example, 28% of lidocaine exists in the base form at pH 7.4, compared with only 2.5% for chloroprocaine because the pKa of these drugs is 7.9 and 9, respectively. Acidosis and hypercapnia, by significantly affecting tissue drug uptake, also increase the toxicity of local anesthetics. In rats, both hypercarbia and acidosis lower the convulsive threshold of local anesthetics and elevate total plasma and tissue concentrations of drug.

The standard of local anesthetic potency is Cm, or the minimum concentration of local anesthetic necessary to block impulse conduction along a given nerve fiber. A variety of factors affect Cm, including fiber size and degree of myelination, pH, local calcium concentration, and the rate at which a nerve is stimulated. Relatively unmyelinated fibers, such as the A-delta and C fibers, carry nociceptive information and have a lower Cm than heavily myelinated fibers that control muscle contraction. Because of the lower Cm, less local anesthetic is necessary to block the transmission of pain than to produce muscle paralysis. Concentrated local anesthetic solutions (eg, 2% versus 1% lidocaine) increase the quality of sensory blockade only minimally. On the other hand, a concentrated local anesthetic increases the incidence of local motor blockade and also the risk of systemic toxicity. Because the process of myelinization is not completed until about 18 months of age, Cm may be reduced in younger children. Newborns and infants may develop complete analgesia and motor blockade when even dilute concentrations of local anesthetics are used.

Other factors influence the quality and duration of a nerve block. These include the addition of a vasoconstrictor to the anesthetic mixture, the use of a combination of local anesthetics, and the site of drug administration. Vasoconstrictors, particularly epinephrine, are frequently added to local anes-

TABLE 15-16. *Suggested maximal doses of local anesthetics (mg/kg)**

Drug (concentration)†	Caudal, lumbar, or epidural	Peripheral	Subcutaneous
ESTERS			
Chloroprocaine (1.0% infiltration; 2%–3% epidural)	8–10	8–10	8–10
Procaine	NR	8–10	8–10
AMIDES			
Lidocaine 0.5%–2.0%; 0.5%–1.0% infiltration; 1%–2% peripheral, epidural, subcutaneous; 5% spinal	5–7	5–7	5–7
Bupivacaine 0.0625%–0.5%; 0.125%–0.25%	2–3	2–3	2–3
Prilocaine 0.5%–1% infiltration; 1%–1.5% peripheral; 2%–3% epidural	5–7‡	5–7‡	5–7‡

* These are suggested safe upper limits; direct intraarterial or intravenous injection of even a fraction of these doses may result in systemic toxicity or death. The higher dose is recommended only with the concomitant use of epinephrine 1:200,000. Epinephrine should never be added to a local anesthetic solution administered in area of an end artery (eg, digital or penile nerve block). The minimal effective dose in children <10 kg is 1.5–2 mg.

† Concentrations are in mg/mL; for example, a 1% solution contains 10 mg/mL.

‡ Total adult dose should not exceed 600 mg. Drug should be used with caution in neonates.

NR, not recommended.

thetic solutions. Epinephrine decreases the rate of vascular reabsorption of local anesthetic from the site of administration and thereby lengthens the duration of sensory blockade. Epinephrine also improves the intensity of anesthesia achieved and increases the effectiveness of dilute concentrations of local anesthetics. Because of the risk of vasoconstriction, epinephrine should never be injected into areas supplied by end arteries, such as the penis or digits, because tissue ischemia or necrosis can result. Epinephrine is most commonly added to local anesthetic solutions in concentrations of 0.005 mg/mL (1:200,000).

Toxicity

The systemic effects of local anesthetics are determined by the total dose of drug administered and by the rapidity of absorption into the blood. This belies the idea of accepted maximal doses of these drugs because even small fractions of these dosages produce toxic systemic effects if injected intraarterially, intravenously, or into any highly vascular location (see Table 15-15). In general, peak absorption of local anesthetic is dependent on the site of the block. The approximate order of absorption from highest to lowest is as follows:

• Intercostal or intratracheal
• Caudal or epidural
• Brachial plexus
• Distal peripheral
• Subcutaneous

Peak local anesthetic blood levels are also directly related to the total dosage of drug administered. The most dilute concentration of a local anesthetic should be used. At recommended clinical dosages (Table 15-16), plasma levels usually remain well below recognized toxic concentrations. A continuum of toxic effects exists and is dependent on the rate of

rise and the total plasma concentration achieved after drug administration. Mild side effects (tinnitus, light-headedness, visual and auditory disturbances, restlessness, muscular twitching) occur at low plasma concentrations, and severe side effects (seizures, arrhythmias, coma, cardiovascular collapse, respiratory arrest) occur as plasma levels increase. Thus, emergency airway and resuscitative equipment must be available for immediate use before the administration of any local anesthetic agent. Finally, bupivacaine as a cause of arrhythmias and cardiovascular collapse is particularly worrisome because it is relatively refractory to treatment. The ventricular arrhythmias caused by bupivacaine that precede the cardiovascular collapse may be effectively treated with intravenous phenytoin or bretylium.[130]

Drug allergy is uncommon with amide local anesthetics but does occur with the ester family of drugs. Usually, a previous history of allergies to local anesthetics or to suntan lotions that contain paraaminobenzoic acid can be obtained.

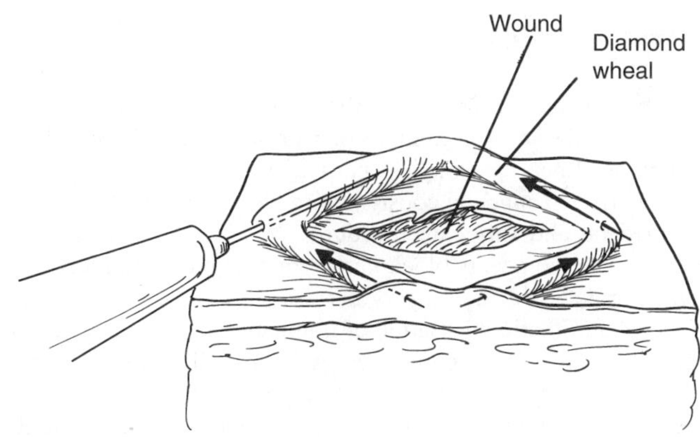

FIG. 15-7. Technique of infiltration of local anesthetic. (After Yaster M, Greenberg RS, Tobin JR. Pain control and sedation. In: Nichols DG, Yaster M, Lappe DG, eds. The golden hour, ed 2. St Louis, Mosby–Year Book, 1996:325)

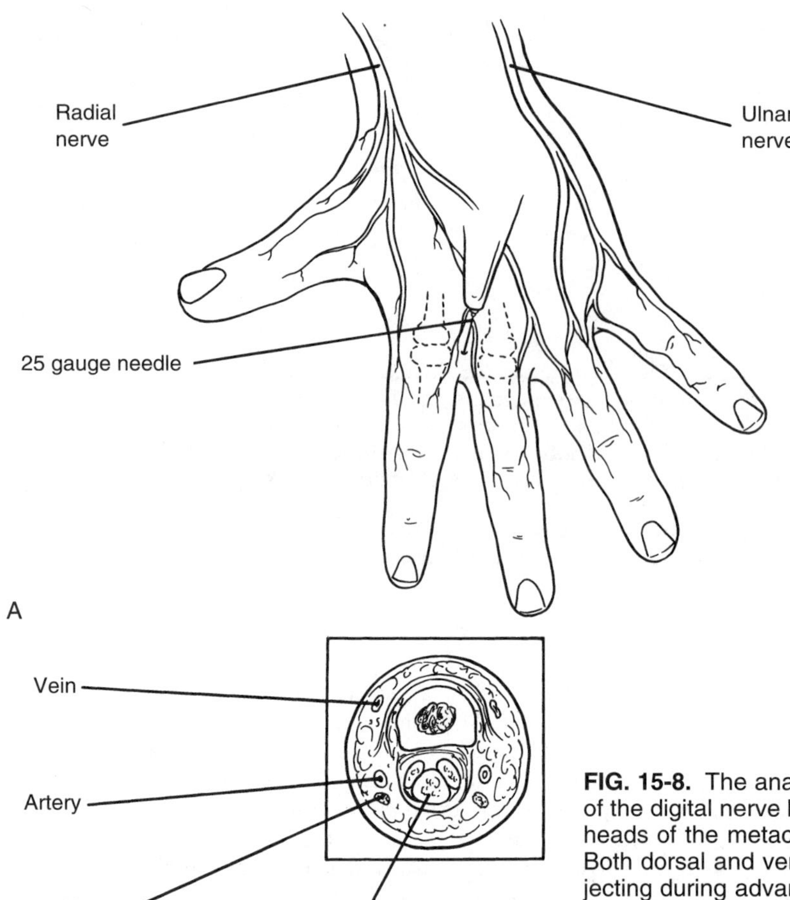

FIG. 15-8. The anatomy of the digital nerves of the hand and technique of the digital nerve block. (*A*) A 25-gauge needle is inserted between the heads of the metacarpals on either side of the digit to be anesthetized. Both dorsal and ventral nerve branches are blocked by continuously injecting during advancement of the needle from the dorsal surface to the palm at this proximal point. (*B*) In the distal digit, the ventral (proper) digital nerve continues, but the dorsal branch arborizes. The anatomic relation of the digital nerves and arteries is shown in this distal cross section.

Local anesthetic allergy is rare and is often mistakenly attributed to adverse experiences occurring during dental anesthesia.

Regional Anesthetic Techniques

Subcutaneous Injection

Subcutaneous infiltration of the skin with a local anesthetic solution is the most commonly performed regional anesthetic technique. Local anesthetics, particularly lidocaine, are commonly injected subcutaneously before the performance of painful medical and surgical procedures. When used in this way, local anesthetic agents block nerve conduction at the most terminal branches of the sensory nerves.

Local anesthetic infiltration of traumatic lacerations requires special mention. Commonly, the wound is dirty and requires extensive scrubbing and irrigation. Administration of the local anesthetic before the cleansing may introduce dirt and bacteria into the surrounding tissue. Injecting the local anesthetic through intact skin adjacent to the wound before the wound is cleaned is recommended[131] (Fig. 15-7). Alternatively, blocking the peripheral nerve that supplies the injured area more proximally results in use of smaller amounts of local anesthetic and fewer injections.

Because local anesthetics are manufactured at a pH of 4 to 5 and are administered by injection, they are painful. This pain can be minimized by using buffered anesthetic solutions and small needles. Buffering a local anesthetic solution, such as lidocaine or bupivacaine, with sodium bicarbonate (9 mL of lidocaine combined with 1 mL of bicarbonate, a 10:1 solution; or 29 mL of bupivacaine with 1 mL bicarbonate) may make the injection painless and shorten the onset of analgesia.[129] Local anesthetics are not manufactured with buffer because the buffering affects the shelf life of the drug.

EMLA Cream

EMLA (eutectic mixture of local anesthetics) cream, a topical emulsion composed of prilocaine and lidocaine, produces complete anesthesia of intact skin after application. For best effect, EMLA cream must be applied and covered with an occlusive dressing for 60 to 90 minutes before a procedure is performed. This limits its use in the emergency room or office unless the site is prepared well in advance of anticipated use. Furthermore, if the procedure is a venipuncture, multiple sites must be prepared in case the initial attempt is unsuccessful.

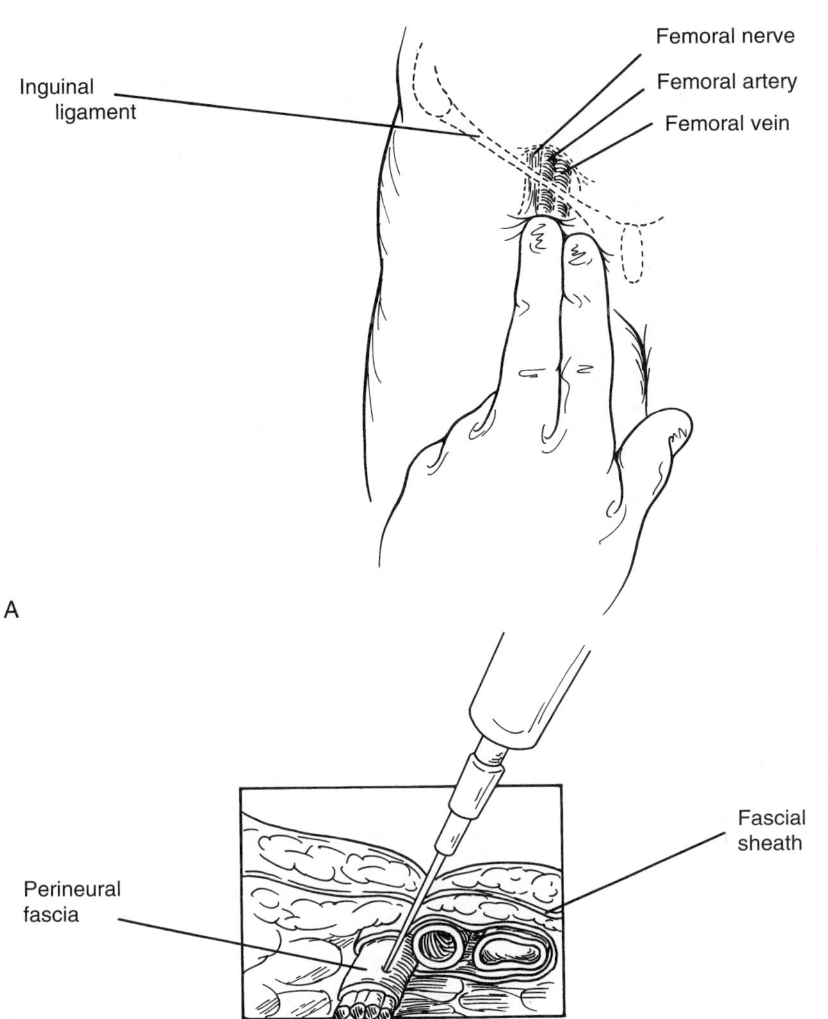

FIG. 15-9. Femoral nerve block. After a skin wheal is placed, the physician's nonoperative hand compresses the femoral artery and nerve against the underlying tissue and bone immediately below the inguinal ligament. A 22- or 25-gauge needle is then inserted perpendicularly, about 0.5 to 1 cm lateral to the pulsation of the femoral artery into the perineural fascia of the femoral nerve. The needle is inserted to a depth clearly deeper than the artery. After a negative aspiration for blood, 5 to 10 mL of local anesthetic is injected, deep and lateral to the artery. The maximal dose of 0.25% bupivacaine is 1 mL/kg. (After Yaster M, Greenberg RS, Tobin JR. Pain control and sedation. In: Nichols DG, Yaster M, Lappe DG, eds. The golden hour, ed 2. St Louis, Mosby–Year Book, 1996:325)

EMLA cream has been compared with injected lidocaine in an effort to reduce the pain associated with venipuncture.[77] Both an observer and a physician performing the procedure judged pain relief to be virtually complete in both groups. The children involved were not so sanguine and were equally dissatisfied with both methods. Despite the fact that two observers thought that the child was pain free, the child's cooperation with venipuncture did not improve. Therefore, it is not clear whether the delay involved in the use of EMLA is justified. On the other hand, EMLA may be more effective in children accustomed to frequent medical procedures or for procedures in which the child cannot see the needle, such as lumbar puncture or bone marrow aspiration.

Peripheral Nerve Blocks

Emergency airway and resuscitative equipment, as well as those trained in using it, must be available for use before the performance of a peripheral nerve block. Additionally, if a patient is to be sedated during the placement of a nerve block, one member of the health care team must be responsible for the patient's overall well being.[132] This person is responsible for monitoring vital signs, assessing the adequacy of the airway, and alerting other members of the health care team if a problem occurs.

Digital Nerve Blocks

The digital nerve block provides excellent anesthesia for surgery performed on either the fingers or toes. It is particularly useful for incision and drainage of an abscess (paronychia). The alternative, local anesthetic infiltration, may fail because the acidic pH of infected tissue may not allow the active (nonionized, base) form of the local anesthetic to reach the nerve membrane.

Digital nerve block is performed in a similar fashion for both the fingers and toes. Each digit is supplied by two pairs of nerves (palmar and dorsal) that travel on either side of that digit. One half to one mL of epinephrine-free local anesthetic is injected between the metacarpal or metatarsal heads on either side of the digit, as shown in Figure 15-8.[131] The 25-gauge needle is kept perpendicular to the plane of the hand or foot and advanced from the dorsal to the palmar surface. Local anesthetic is injected continuously. Complications are few. Obviously, the digital nerve block should never be performed when there is any question of the digit's blood supply. Even when

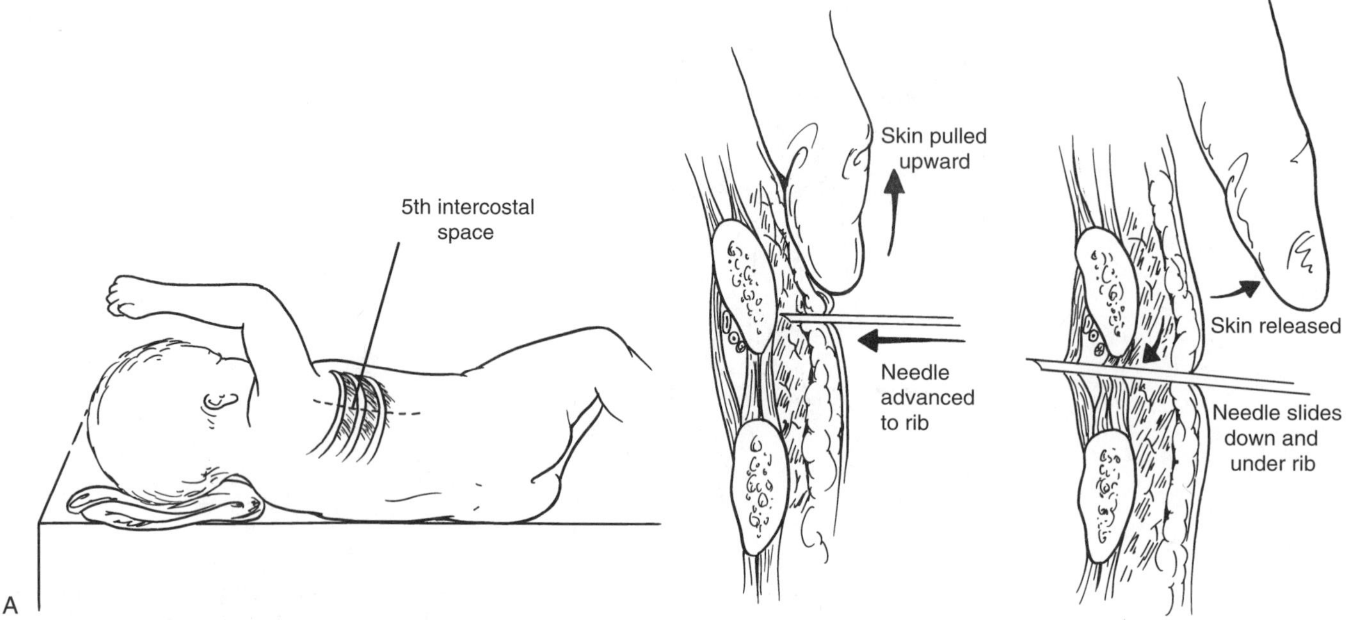

FIG. 15-10. Intercostal nerve block. (After Yaster M, Greenberg RS, Tobin JR. Pain control and sedation. In: Nichols DG, Yaster M, Lappe DG, eds. The golden hour, ed 2. St Louis, Mosby–Year Book, 1996:325)

epinephrine is not used, the most serious complication of this block is caused by the use of too large a volume of local anesthetic. A large volume within a closed fascial space may result in vascular compression (compartment syndrome).

Femoral Nerve Block

The femoral nerve block (L2, L3, L4) is a rapid, reliable, and effective technique for relieving the pain of a femoral shaft fracture. When using bupivacaine without epinephrine in a femoral nerve block, fracture patients are provided with adequate anesthesia for the application of traction as well as for the necessary manipulations that occur during radiologic examinations. The duration of analgesia is 3 to 6 hours, and peak plasma levels of bupivacaine average less than 1 μg/mL. This is depicted in Figure 15-9.

Intercostal Nerve Block

The intercostal nerve block is a safe and versatile block that can provide complete sensory analgesia of the chest and abdominal walls, and it is remarkably easy to perform. It is particularly useful before chest tube insertion and for patients with broken ribs. When used for rib fractures, the analgesia produced is nothing short of remarkable. Patients can sit up, take deep breaths, cough, and ambulate almost as soon as the needle is removed. This technique is greatly underused because of misconceptions about the risk of pneumothorax and the time and effort required to perform these blocks. The intercostal nerve block is illustrated in Figure 15-10), and the technique is similar to that described for a femoral nerve block. This block provides 4 to 10 hours of pain relief. Continuous analgesia with indwelling intercostal catheters is also possible. Finally, for blocking more than one rib, the maximum bupivacaine dosage that can be used is 2.5 mg/kg.

REFERENCES

1. Anand KJ. Neonatal stress responses to anesthesia and surgery. Clin Perinatol 1990;17:207.
2. Anand KJ, Hickey PR. Pain and its effects in the human neonate and fetus. N Engl J Med 1987;317:1321.
3. Schechter NL, Berde CB, Yaster M, eds. Pain in infants, children, and adolescents: an overview. In: Pain in Infants, children and adolescents. Baltimore, Williams & Wilkins, 1993:3.
4. Wetzel RC, Maxwell LG. Anesthesia for children. In: Rogers MC, Tinker JH, Covino BG, et al, eds. Principles and practice of anesthesiology, vol 2. St Louis, Mosby Year Book, 1993:2157.
5. Hogg JC, Williams J, Richardson B, et al. Age as a factor in the distribution of lower airway conductance and in the pathologic anatomy of obstructive lung disease. N Engl J Med 1970;282:1283.
6. Miller MJ, Carlo WA, Strohl KP, et al. Effect of maturation on oral breathing in sleeping premature infants. J Pediatr 1986;109:515.
7. Keens TG, Bryan AC, Levinson H, et al. Developmental pattern of muscle fiber types in human ventilatory muscles. J Appl Physiol 1978;44:909.
8. Rigatto H, Brady JP. Periodic breathing and apnea in the preterm infant: evidence for hypoventilation possibly due to central depression. Pediatrics 1972;50:202.
9. Knill RL, Gelb AW. Ventilatory responses to hypoxia and hypercarbia during halothane sedational anesthesia in man. Anesthesiology 1978;49:244.
10. Kurth CD, Spitzer AR, Broennie AM, et al. Postoperative apnea in preterm infants. Anesthesiology 1987;66:483.
11. Hertzka RE, Gauntlett IS, Fisher DM, et al. Fentanyl-induced ventilatory depression: effects of age. Anesthesiology 1989;70:213.
12. Friedman WF. The intrinsic physiologic properties of the developing heart. In: Friedman WF, Lesch M, Sonnenblick EH, eds. Neonatal heart disease. New York, Grune & Stratton, 1973.
13. Rudolph AM, Heyman MA. Cardiac output in the fetal lamb: the effects of spontaneous and induced changes of heart rate on right and left ventricular output. Am J Obstet Gynecol 1976;124:183.

14. Romero TE, Friedman WF. Limited left ventricular response to volume overload in the neonatal period: a comparative study with the adult animal. Pediatr Res 1979;13:910.

15. Buchanan GR. Hematopoietic diseases. In: Oski FA, DeAngelis CD, Feigin RD, et al, eds. Principles and practice of pediatrics. Philadelphia, JB Lippincott, 1990.

16. Stockman JA III. Anemia of prematurity: current concepts in the issue of when to transfuse. Pediatr Clin North Am 1986;33:111.

17. Chantler C. The kidney. In: Godfrey S, Baum JD, eds. Clinical paediatric physiology. Oxford, Blackwell Scientific, 1979.

18. Arant BS Jr. Renal and genitourinary disease. In: Oski FA, DeAngelis CD, Feigin RD, et al, eds. Principles and practice of pediatrics. Philadelphia, JB Lippincott, 1990.

19. Belknap WM. Developmental disorders of gastrointestinal function. In: Oski FA, DeAngelis CD, Feigin RD, et al, eds. Principles and practice of pediatrics. Philadelphia, JB Lippincott, 1990.

20. Stern L. The newborn infant and his thermal environment. Curr Prob Pediatr 1970;1:3.

21. Aldrete JA, Roman-deJesus JC, Russell LJ, et al. Intranasal ketamine as induction adjunct in children: preliminary report. Anesthesiology 1987;67:A514.

22. Walbergh EJ, Willis RJ, Eckhert J. Plasma concentrations of midazolam in children following intranasal administration. Anesthesiology 1991;74:233.

23. Asburn MA, et al. Oral transmucosal fentanyl citrate in paediatric outpatients. Can J Anaesth 1990;37:857.

24. Wood M, Wood AJJ. Changes in plasma drug binding and A-1-glycoprotein in mother and newborn infant. Clin Pharmacol Ther 1981;29:522.

25. Sereni F. Principals of developmental pharmacology. Am Rev Pharmacol 1968;8:453.

26. Barash PG, Glanz S, Katz JD, et al. Ventricular function in children during halothane anesthesia: an echocardiographic evaluation. Anesthesiology 1978;49:79.

27. Gregory GA. The baroresponses of preterm infants during halothane anaesthesia. Can Anaesth Soc J 1982;29:195.

28. Shulman D, Bar-Yishay E, Beardsmore C, et al. Determinants of end expiration volume in young children during ketamine or halothane anesthesia. Anesthesiology 1987;66:636.

29. Way WL, Costley EC, Way EL. Respiratory sensitivity of the newborn infant to meperidine and morphine. Clin Pharmacol Ther 1965;6:454.

30. Kupferberg JH, Way EL. Pharmacologic basis for the increased sensitivity of the newborn rat to morphine. J Pharmacol Exp Ther 1963;141:105.

31. Motoyama EK. Respiratory physiology in infants and children. In: Moyoyama EK, Davis PJ, eds. Smith's anesthesia for infants and children, ed 5. St Louis, CV Mosby, 1990:11.

32. Pounder DR, Blackstock D, Steward DJ. Tracheal extubation in children: halothane versus isoflurane, anesthetized versus awake. Anesthesiology 1991;74:653.

33. Dicker A, Ohlson KBE, Johnson L, et al. Halothane selectively inhibits nonshivering thermogenesis: possible implications for thermoregulation during anesthesia of infants. Anesthesiology 1995;82:491.

34. Ohlson KBE, Mohell N, Cannon B, et al. Thermogenesis in brown adipocytes is inhibited by volatile anesthetic agents: a factor contributing to hypothermia in infants? Anesthesiology 1994;81:176.

35. Anand KJS, Sippell WG, Aynsley-Green A. Randomized trial of fentanyl anaesthesia in preterm babies undergoing surgery: effects on the stress response. Lancet 1987;1:243.

36. Anand KJS, Sippell WG, Schofield NM, et al. Does halothane anaesthesia decrease the metabolic and endocrine stress responses of newborn infants undergoing operation? Br Med J 1988;296:668.

37. Anand KJS, Hansen DD, Hickey PR. Hormonal-metabolic stress responses in neonates undergoing cardiac surgery. Anesthesiology 1990;73:661.

38. Hickey PR, Hansen DD, Wessell DL, et al. Blunting of stress responses in pulmonary circulation of infants by fentanyl. Anesth Analg 1985;64:1132.

39. Duke PC, Fownes D, Wade JG. Halothane depresses baroreflex control of heart rate in man. Anesthesiology 1977;46:184.

40. Katz RL, Matteo RS, Papper EM. The injection of epinephrine during general anesthesia. 2. Halothane. Anesthesiology 1962;23:597.

41. Ueda W, Hirakawa M, Mae O. Appraisal of epinephrine administration to patients under halothane anesthesia for closure of cleft palate. Anesthesiology 1983;58:574.

42. Karl HW, Swedlow DB, Lee KW, et al. Epinephrine-halothane interactions in children. Anesthesiology 1983;58:142.

43. Garvin JP, Warner EJ. Halothane and children: the first quarter century. Anesth Analg 1984;63:838.

44. Smith RM. Pediatric anesthesia in perspective. Anesth Analg 1978;59:186.

45. Kenna JG, Neuberger J, Mieli-Vergani G, et al. Halothane hepatitis in children. Br Med J 1987;294:1209.

46. Summary of the National Halothane Study. JAMA 1966;197:775.

47. Rosen I, Soderbug M. Electroencephalographic activity in children under enflurane anesthesia. Acta Anaesthesiol Scand 1975;19:361.

48. Phillips AJ, Brimacombe JR, Simpson DL. Anaesthetic induction with isoflurane or halothane: oxygen saturation during induction with isoflurane or halothane in unpremedicated children. Anaesthesia 1988;43:927.

49. Stevens WC, Cromwell TH, Halsey MJ, et al. The cardiovascular effects of a new inhalation anesthetic, forane, in human volunteers at constant arterial carbon dioxide tension. Anesthesiology 1971;35:8.

50. Wolf WJ, Neal MB, Peterson MD. The hemodynamic and cardiovascular effects of isoflurane and halothane anesthesia in children. Anesthesiology 1986;64:328.

51. Michenfelder JD, Sundt TM, Fode N, et al. Isoflurane when compared to enflurane and halothane decreases the frequency of cerebral ischemia during carotid endarterectomy. Anesthesiology 1987;67:336.

52. Robinson S, Gregory GA. Fentanyl-air-oxygen anesthesia for patent ductus arteriosus in preterm infants. Anesth Analg 1981;60:331.

53. Yaster M. The dose response of fentanyl in neonatal anesthesia. Anesthesiology 1987;66:433.

54. O'Rourke PP, Crone RK, Vacanti JP, et al. Extracorporeal membrane oxygenation and conventional medical therapy in neonates with persistent pulmonary hypertension of the newborn: a prospective randomized study. Pediatrics 1989;84:957.

55. Pasternak GW, Zhang AZ, Tecott L. Developmental differences between high and low affinity opiate binding sites: their relationship to analgesia and respiratory depression. Life Sci 1980;27:1185.

56. Maxwell LG, Deshpande JK, Wetzel RC. Preoperative evaluation of children. Pediatr Clin North Am 1994;41:93.

57. Korsch BM. The child and the operating room. Anesthesiology 1975;43:251.

58. Pasternak LR. Preoperative evaluation of the ambulatory surgery patient. Anesth Rep 1990;3:8.

59. NIH and FDA Perioperative Red Blood Cell Transfusion Consensus Conference, Bethesda, MD, April, 1988.

60. Schreiner MS. Preoperative and postoperative fasting in children. Pediatr Clin North Am 1994;41:111.

61. Jensen BH, Werberg M, Adersen M. Preoperative starvation and blood glucose concentration in children undergoing inpatient and outpatient anesthesia. Br J Anaesth 1982;54:1071.

62. Wellborn LG, McGill WA, Hannallah RS, et al. Perioperative blood glucose concentrations in pediatric outpatients. Anesthesiology 1986;65:543.

63. Meakin G, Dingwall AE, Addison GM. Effects of fasting and oral premedication on the pH and volume of gastric aspirate in children. Br J Anaesth 1987;59:678.

64. Chodoff P, Helrich M. Factors affecting pediatric endotracheal tube size: a statistical analysis. Anesthesiology 1967;28:779.

65. Berry FA, Yemen TA. Pediatric airway in health and disease. Pediatr Clin North Am 1994;41:153.

66. Black AE, Hatch DJ, Nauth-Misir N. Complications of nasotracheal intubation in neonates, infants and children: a review of 4 years' experience in a children's hospital. Br J Anaesth 1990;65:461.

67. Finholt DA, Audenaert SM, Stirt JA, et al. Endotracheal tube leak pressure and tracheal lumen size in swine. Anesth Analg 1986;65:667.

68. Hawkins DB. Pathogenesis of subglottic stenosis from endotracheal intubation. Ann Otol Rhinol Laryngol 1987;96:116.

69. Orlowski JP, Willis NG, Amin NP, et al. Complications of airway intrusion in 100 consecutive cases in a pediatric ICU. Crit Care Med 1980;8:324.

70. Falick YS, Smiler BG. Is anticholinergic premedication necessary? Anesthesiology 1975;43:472.

71. Brzustowicz RM, Nelson DA, Betts EK, et al. Efficacy of oral pre-

medication for pediatric outpatient surgery. Anesthesiology 1984;60: 475.

72. Nicolson SC, Betts EK, Jobes DR, et al. Comparison of oral and intramuscular preanesthetic medication for pediatric inpatient surgery. Anesthesiology 1989;71:8.

73. Feld LH, Champeau MW, Van Steennis CA, et al. Preanesthetic medication in children: a comparison of oral transmucosal fentanyl citrate versus placebo. Anesthesiology 1989;71:374.

74. Henderson JM, Brodsky DA, Fisher DM, et al. Pre-induction of anesthesia in pediatric patients with nasally administered sufentanil. Anesthesiology 1988;68:671.

75. Spear RM, Yaster M, Berkowitz ID, et al. Preinduction of anesthesia in children with rectally administered midazolam. Anesthesiology 1991;74:670.

76. Saarnivaara L, Lindgren L, Klemola UM. Comparison of chloral hydrate and midazolam by mouth as premedicants in children undergoing otolaryngological surgery. Br J Anaesth 1988;61:390.

77. Wilton NC, Leigh J, Rosen DR, et al. Preanesthetic sedation of preschool children, using intranasal midazolam. Anesthesiology 1988; 69:972.

78. Tobias JD, Martin LD, Wetzel RC. Ketamine by continuous infusion for sedation in the pediatric intensive care unit. Crit Care Med 1990; 18:819.

79. Waxman K, Shoemaker WC, Lipmann M. Cardiovascular effects of anesthetic induction with ketamine. Anesth Analg 1980;59:355.

80. Borgeat A, Popovic V, Meier D, et al. Comparison of propofol and thiopental/halothane for short-duration ENT surgical procedures in children. Anesth Analg 1990;71:511.

81. Hannallah RS, Baker SB, Case W, et al. Propofol: effective dose and induction characteristics in unpremedicated children. Anesthesiology 1991;74:217.

82. Gronert BJ, Brandom BW. Neuromuscular blocking drugs in infants and children. Pediatr Clin North Am 1994;41:73.

83. Fisher DM, O'Keefe C, Stanski DR, et al. Pharmacokinetics and pharmacodynamics of d-tubocurarine in infants, children and adults. Anesthesiology 1982;55:203.

84. Fisher DM, Miller RD. Neuromuscular effects of vecuronium (ORG NC45) in infants and children during N_2O, halothane anesthesia. Anesthesiology 1983;58:519.

85. Cabal LA, Siassi B, Artal R, et al. Cardiovascular and catecholamine changes after administration of pancuronium in distressed neonates. Pediatrics 1985;75:284.

86. Goudsouzian NG, Crone RD, Todres ID. Recovery from pancuronium blockade in the neonatal intensive care unit. Br J Anaesth 1981;53: 1303.

87. Rutledge ML, Hawkins EP, Langston C. Skeletal muscle growth failure induced in premature newborn infants by prolonged pancuronium treatment. 1986;109:883.

88. O'Connor JP, Ramsay JG, Wynands JE, et al. The incidence of myocardial ischemia during anesthesia for coronary artery bypass surgery in patients receiving pancuronium or vecuronium. Anesthesiology 1989;70:230.

89. Meistelman C, Loose JP, Saint-Maurice C, et al. Clinical pharmacology of vecuronium in children. Br J Anaesth 1986;58:996.

90. Meistelman C, Agoston S, Kersten UW, et al. Pharmacokinetics and pharmacodynamics of vecuronium and pancuronium in anesthetized children. Anesth Analg 1986;65:1319.

91. Fisher DM, Canfell PC, Fahey MR, et al. Elimination of atracurium in humans: contribution of Hofmann elimination and ester hydrolysis versus organ-based elimination. Anesthesiology 1986;65:6.

92. Sarner JB, Brandom BW, Woelfel SK, et al. Clinical pharmacology of mivacurium chloride (BW B1090U) in children during nitrous oxide–halothane and nitrous oxide–narcotic anesthesia. Anesth Analg 1989;68:116.

93. Montgomery CJ, Steward DJ. A comparative evaluation of intubating doses of atracurium, d-tubocurarine, pancuronium and vecuronium in children. Can J Anaesth 1988;35:36.

94. Durant NN, Katz RL. Suxamethonium. Br J Anaesth 1982;54:195.

95. McLeskey CH, McLeod DS, Hough TL, et al. Prolonged asystole after succinylcholine administration. Anesthesiology 1978;49:208.

96. Cook DR, Westman HR, Rosenfeld L, et al. Pulmonary edema in infants: possible association with intramuscular succinylcholine. Anesth Analg 19;81;60:220.

97. Ryan JF, Kagen LJ, Hyman AI. Myoglobinuria after a single dose of succinylcholine. N Engl J Med 1971;285:824.

98. Foster CA. Muscle pain that follows administration of suxamethonium. Br Med J 1960;2:24.

99. Schaner PJ, Brown RL, Kirsey RD, et al. Succinylcholine induced hyperkalemia in burned patients. Anesth Analg 1969;48:76;4.

100. Frankville DD, Drummond JC. Hyperkalemia after succinylcholine administration in a patient with closed head injury without paresis. Anesthesiology 1987;67:264.

101. Azar I. The response of patients with neuromuscular disorders to muscle relaxants: a review. Anesthesiology 1984;61:173.

102. Delphin E, Jackson D, Rothstein P. Use of succinylcholine during elective pediatric anesthesia should be reevaluated. Anesth Analg 1987;66:1190.

103. Nugent SK, Laruvuso R, Rogers MC. Pharmacology and use of muscle relaxants in infants and children. J Pediatr 1979;94:481.

104. Smith SM. The use of curare in infants and children. Anesthesiology 1947;8:176.

105. Harper RG, Garcia A, Sia C. Inguinal hernia: a common problem of premature infants weighing 1000 grams or less at birth. Pediatrics 1975; 56:112.

106. Dohi S, Naito H, Takahashi T. Age related changes in blood pressure and duration of motor block in spinal anesthesia. Anesthesiology 1979;50:319.

107. Payen D, Ecoffey C, Carli P, et al. Pulsed Doppler ascending aortic, carotid, brachial, and femoral artery blood flows during caudal anesthesia in infants. Anesthesiology 1987;67:681.

108. Spear RM, Deshpande JK, Maxwell LG. Caudal anesthesia in the awake, high-risk infant. Anesthesiology 1988;69:407.

109. Abajian JC, Mellish RWP, Browne AF, et al. Spinal anesthesia for surgery in the high-risk infant. Anesth Analg 1984;63:359.

110. Steinbrook RA, Concepcion M. Respiratory effects of spinal anesthesia: resting ventilation and single-breath CO_2 response. Anesth Analg 1991;72:182.

111. Malviya S, Swartz J, Lerman J. Are all preterm infants younger than 60 weeks postconceptual age at risk for postanesthetic apnea? Anesthesiology 1993;78:1076.

112. Steward DJ. Preterm infants are more prone to complications following minor surgery than are term infants. Anesthesiology 1982; 56:304.

113. Liu LMO, Cote CJ, Goudsouzian NG, et al. Life-threatening apnea in infants recovering from anesthesia. Anesthesiology 1983; 59:506.

114. Welborn LG, Greenspun JC. Anesthesia and apnea: perioperative considerations in the former preterm infant. Pediatr Clin North Am 1994; 41:181.

115. Tiret L, Nivoche Y, Hatton F, et al. Complications related to anaesthesia in infants and children: a prospective survey of 40,240 anesthetics. Br J Anaesth 1988;61:263.

116. Holzman RS. Morbidity and mortality in pediatric anesthesia. Pediatr Clin North Am 1994;41:239.

117. Schechter NL. The undertreatment of pain in children: an overview. Pediatr Clin North Am 1989;36:781.

118. Schechter N, Berde C, Yaster M. Pain in infants, children, and adolescents. Baltimore, Williams & Wilkins, 1993.

119. Schechter NL, Allen DA, Hanson K. Status of pediatric pain control: a comparison of hospital analgesic usage in children and adults. Pediatrics 1986;77:11.

120. Wong DL, Baker CM. Pain in children: comparison of assessment scales. Pediatr Nurs 1988;14:9.

121. Beyer JE, Wells N. The assessment of pain in children. Pediatr Clin North Am 1989;36:837.

122. Yaster M, Deshpande JK. Management of pediatric pain with opioid analgesics. J Pediatr 1988;113:421.

123. Yaster M, Maxwell LG. Opioid agonists and antagonists. In: Schechter NL, Berde CB, Yaster M, eds. Pain in infants, children, and adolescents. Baltimore, Williams & Wilkins, 1993:145.

124. Zhang AZ, Pasternak GW. Ontogeny of opioid pharmacology and receptors: high and low affinity site differences. Eur J Pharmacol 1981;73:29.

125. Cousins MJ, Mather LE. Intrathecal and epidural administration of opioids. Anesthesiology 1984;61:276.

126. Krane EJ, Tyler DC, Jacobson LE. The dose response of caudal morphine in children. Anesthesiology 1989;71:48.

127. Attia J, Ecoffey C, Sandouk P, et al. Epidural morphine in children: pharmacokinetics and CO_2 sensitivity. Anesthesiology 1986;65:590.
128. Nichols DG, Yaster M, Lynn AM, et al. Disposition and respiratory effects of intrathecal morphine in children. Anesthesiology 1993;79:733.
129. Yaster M, Tobin JR, Maxwell LG. Local anesthetics. In: Schechter NL, Berde CB, Yaster M, et al. Pain in infants, children, and adolescents. Baltimore, Williams & Wilkins, 1993:179.
130. Maxwell LG, Martin LD, Yaster M. Bupivacaine-induced cardiac toxicity in neonates: successful treatment with intravenous phenytoin. Anesthesiology 1994;80:682.
131. Yaster M, Greenberg RS, Tobin JR. Pain control and sedation. In: Nichols DG, Yaster M, Lappe DG, et al, eds. The golden hour, ed 2. St Louis, Mosby Year Book, 1996:325.
132. American Academy of Pediatrics Committee on Drugs. Guidelines for monitoring and management of pediatric patients during and after sedation for diagnostic and therapeutic procedures. Pediatrics 1992;89:1110.

Surgery of Infants and Children: Scientific Principles and Practice, edited by Keith T. Oldham, Paul M. Colombani, and Robert P. Foglia. Lippincott–Raven Publishers, Philadelphia, © 1997.

CHAPTER 16

Surgical Problems of Children With Physical Disabilities

Gordon Worley and Keith T. Oldham

Inclusion of a chapter about children with physical disabilities (cerebral palsy, spina bifida, spinal cord injury, and Down syndrome) in a textbook of pediatric surgery is recognition of the unusual nature of the surgical problems of these patients. It also demonstrates the cooperative relationship between developmental pediatricians and pediatric surgeons that is needed to manage these children's medical problems successfully. Children with disabilities have benefited from this relationship in the following ways:

1. By jointly managing problems, surgeons and developmental pediatricians have improved and simplified the care provided to children by parents, improved quality of life, and increased longevity.
2. The long-standing relationships between parents and developmental pediatricians and between developmental pediatricians and pediatric surgeons have meant that decisions about surgical interventions have been made in an atmosphere of trust and thoughtfulness.
3. The benefits and potential problems to patients of specific surgical interventions have been well understood by all concerned (parents, developmental pediatricians, and surgeons), which has been useful in helping families when adverse outcomes occur (and when surgery for children with physical disabilities has more risk than for normal children).
4. Good communication between developmental pediatricians and surgeons has resulted in appropriate selection of surgical candidates and expeditious evaluations of problems preoperatively, reducing lengths of hospitalization for surgery.

This chapter discusses surgical contributions to the management of four of the most common developmental disabilities: cerebral palsy, spina bifida, spinal cord injury, and Down syndrome. Although the term *developmental pediatrician* is used to describe the kind of pediatrician managing the medical problems of children with physical disabilities, such care is also provided by committed pediatric neurologists, pediatric physiatrists, and some interested general pediatricians.

The importance of surgical solutions to some of the problems of children with physical disabilities is amply illustrated in Table 16-1. In one developmental pediatrician's practice (GW), 55 patients had new problems diagnosed that required surgery during 1 year. Pediatric surgeons received the most referrals, but patients were also referred to pediatric neurosurgeons, pediatric orthopedic surgeons, pediatric urologic surgeons, and others. In return, the developmental pediatrician was referred patients for chronic medical care by surgeons. This cooperative relationship works well because it respectfully recognizes both that pediatric surgeons can do the most benefit for children by spending their time addressing surgical problems rather than by case management and that developmental pediatricians have a commitment to provide chronic care for their patients, managing medical problems successfully and independently.

In summary, the establishment of cooperative relationships between pediatric surgeons and developmental pediatricians improves patient care, encourages referral of patients for needed surgery, and provides developmental pediatricians patients to treat who need chronic care. All benefit.

In this chapter, the ethical foundations underlying the care of children with physical disabilities are reviewed. Ethics are discussed in more detail elsewhere. For each of the disabilities mentioned earlier (cerebral palsy, spina bifida, Down syndrome, and spinal cord injury), background information is provided to enable pediatric surgeons to place necessary surgery in the context of children's conditions and lives; specific surgical contributions to the care of children with each disability are reviewed, with an emphasis on the unusual aspects of the differential diagnosis of surgical conditions; and special considerations of which surgeons should be aware are mentioned.

ETHICAL CONSIDERATIONS

Ethical theory and medical ethics are presented in detail in Chapter 18. The purpose of this section is to review aspects that require emphasis for the treatment of children with physical disabilities.

The principles on which decision making are based for children with disabilities are the same as for normal children: auton-

TABLE 16-1. *Patient referrals for surgery by one developmental pediatrician, January 1, 1994, to December 31, 1994*

Procedure	Patients referred
PEDIATRIC SURGERY	**27**
Gastrostomy and fundoplication	10
Gastrostomy alone	7
Fundoplication alone	1
Central line placement or removal	4
Miscellaneous	5
PEDIATRIC OPHTHALMOLOGY	**11**
Strabismus	
PEDIATRIC NEUROSURGERY	**8**
Rhizotomy	3
Central nervous system tumors (new diagnoses)	2
Subdural hematoma	1
Tethered cord	1
Hydrocephalus	1
PEDIATRIC ORTHOPEDICS	**4**
MISCELLANEOUS	**5**
TOTAL	**55**

omy, beneficence, justice, nonmaleficence, veracity, and fidelity.[1] Parents and legal guardians are recognized legally as substitute decision makers for neurologically impaired children.

It is important for developmental pediatricians and pediatric surgeons to discuss openly and forthrightly their approaches toward the treatment of severely cognitively impaired children. Agreement on principles is essential to provide best care. When conflicts arise, helpful mediation by a single member of a hospital's Ethics Committee can be useful, without being cumbersome and time-consuming. If true conflicts exist over specific cases, then formal consideration by the hospital Ethics Committee can help with resolution,[2] although this is rarely required.

Advance Directives

In contrast to the situation for normal children, in which it is assumed that there is no limitation to the intensity of care that will be provided in an emergency,[1] for children who are profoundly retarded, are hopelessly ill, or have a progressive degenerative neurologic disease, it is important to determine in advance if parents want care limited. If parents request DO NOT RESUSCITATE (DNR) status for their child, it is useful to have them sign a DNR statement in the medical record, both for clarity and for protection of physicians. In discussing limitations of care, a distinction should be made between initiation of life support and prolonged life support; in our experience, many parents want the technique of resuscitation applied in the event their child is found dying but not dead, but want life support terminated if subsequently their child's condition is found to be hopeless.

A distinction also should be drawn between DNR status and COMFORT MEASURES ONLY status. This two-tiered approach to limitation of care recognizes that vigorous therapeutic interventions may be appropriate to prolong life, even if the prognosis

is bleak.[3] DNR orders limit care only in circumstances that would otherwise be at the end of a patient's life. The goal of treatment is still to prolong life. For patients with COMFORT MEASURES ONLY status, it is recognized that the patient's condition is hopeless (terminal), and the goal of treatment is no longer to prolong life but instead only to prevent suffering. Patients who have COMFORT MEASURES ONLY status also must have DNR status. Therefore, many patients who are profoundly retarded have DNR status but, despite this, receive surgery to prolong life because their parents want medical intervention up to the point of resuscitation.

Exceptions to DNR Orders

DNR orders do not apply to cardiopulmonary arrest resulting from an iatrogenic cause. Therefore, for examples, if a patient has an anaphylactic reaction to a medication, or if a patient aspirates gastric contents after a fundoplication and arrests, then resuscitation is necessary, even if the patient has DNR status.

Parents of a child with DNR status who is undergoing surgery should be informed that during the perioperative period, the DNR status may not apply because most causes of cardiopulmonary arrest occurring in this setting are iatrogenic.[1]

Changing Attitudes of Pediatricians and Surgeons Toward Life-Saving Therapy for Newborns

During the past 20 years, physicians' attitudes toward providing comprehensive medical and surgical care for children with disabilities have changed. A survey of members of the Massachusetts chapter of the American Academy of Pediatrics (which includes pediatric surgeons) was done in 1974–1975 and again in 1984–1985 to determine attitudes toward life-saving therapy for newborns with poor prognoses.[4] The most useful of the three case scenarios presented to assess physician attitudes involved an infant with Down syndrome and duodenal atresia. In 1974–1975, only a minority of physicians (46%) would have recommended surgery to parents for duodenal atresia, but in 1984–1985, most (73%) would. This change was attributed by physicians to their experiences with similar situations in the interval, rather than to the Baby Doe federal regulations of 1982. In 1984–1985, 68% indicated that they would even seek a court order on behalf of the newborn to countermand parents' lack of consent for surgery, if necessary. This survey reflects the fact that aggressive management for potentially life-threatening problems in severely disabled but medically stable patients has become the standard of care, in keeping with the recognition of the rights of disabled people.

CEREBRAL PALSY AND PROFOUND RETARDATION

Background

For purposes of discussion, cerebral palsy and severe and profound retardation without motor involvement are linked because they share many of the same surgical problems. The focus of this discussion is on children with cerebral palsy because they are preponderantly the larger group needing surgery.

A consensus definition of *cerebral palsy* is that it is "an umbrella term covering a group of nonprogressive, but often changing, motor impairment syndromes secondary to lesions or anomalies of the brain arising in the early stages of its development."[5] Most cases of cerebral palsy and retardation are caused by abnormal brain development in the first trimester. Among 189 children with cerebral palsy, Nelson and Ellenberg[6] found that only 40 (21%) had evidence suggestive of perinatal asphyxia; of these 40, 17 had no major congenital malformation or other intrinsic defect of a congenital basis, suggesting that only for these 17 (9%) was hypoxia the cause of cerebral palsy. Therefore, 80% of cases of cerebral palsy are due to dysmorphogenesis of the brain in utero alone, 11% to the combination of dysmorphogenesis and of asphyxia, and only 9% to asphyxia alone. Because it is not known how to prevent brain dysmorphogenesis, it is not surprising that the birth incidence of cerebral palsy, 1.5 to 2.5 per 1000 live births, has increased only slightly in the last 40 years, despite the increased rate of cerebral palsy per 1000 live births in the smallest surviving premature infants.[7]

Cerebral palsy is classified according to the pattern of motor involvement of extremities (hemiplegia, one side; diplegia, lower extremities involved, upper extremities only mildly so; quadriplegia, all extremities involved) and by the type of neurologic dysfunction (spastic, hypotonic, dystonic, athetotic, or a combination).[7] Associated neurologic problems include seizure disorder, strabismus, visual field defects, sensorineural hearing loss, retardation, learning disabilities, and emotional problems. Half of all children with cerebral palsy have normal intelligence, however, and some (especially among those with athetotic cerebral palsy) have superior intelligence.

The life expectancy of people with mental retardation is shorter than that of the general population. Those with the mildest of disabilities can have a nearly normal life span. The most severely involved patients (who are also those who most frequently need surgery) have a much shorter than normal life expectancy. Eyman and colleagues[8] studied a large number of retarded people to determine survival probabilities, separating patients into subgroups based on four characteristics: defective cognitive function, limitations on mobility, incontinence, and inability to eat without assistance. Life table analyses of four subgroups of patients, based on these four characteristics, were presented. In the subgroup with the worst prognosis (those who had profound or severe retardation, were completely immobile, were not toilet trained, and required tube feeding), 42% of infants had died by their first birthdays and 79% by their fifth birthdays. It is against this bleak prognosis that the efficacy of surgery for potentially life-threatening problems needs to be viewed.

Surgical Considerations

Children with cerebral palsy often have problems for which surgery is the only effective, long-term treatment. In this section, the following issues are addressed:

- The three most common presenting problems in patients with cerebral palsy that may eventually require surgical treatment (failure to thrive, upper airway obstruction, and pneumonia), emphasizing differential diagnostic considerations and an approach to medical evaluation and treatment before surgery
- Evaluation of children for enteral feedings
- Indications for gastrostomy tube placement
- Gastroesophageal reflux in children with cerebral palsy
- Complications of gastrostomy and fundoplication in neurologically abnormal children
- Results of gastrostomy and fundoplication in neurologically abnormal children
- Long-term outcomes after gastrostomy and fundoplication in neurologically abnormal children
- Issues for collaborative research

In children with cerebral palsy and malnutrition, recurrent vomiting, pneumonia and lower airway problems, and upper airway disease are all caused most frequently by a combination of neurologic abnormalities: oral motor dysfunction, gastroesophageal reflux, and esophageal and gastric dysmotility. Oral motor dysfunction can result in the inability to consume food at an adequate rate, resulting in malnutrition, and also in the inability to protect the airway from aspiration.

Gastroesophageal reflux causes esophagitis, which can result in pain, food refusal, anemia, and esophageal stricture. When gastric contents are refluxed into the pharynx, aspiration can occur, which can result in upper airway obstruction, asthma, chronic bronchitis, pneumonia, and even death of apnea resulting from laryngospasm.

Some retarded children, as a self-stimulating behavior (rumination), chew gastric contents refluxed into the pharynx. In infants and toddlers, the pain of postprandial reflux causes movement of the neck and torso, resembling torsion dystonia, which enhances esophageal motility to clear the esophagus of acid (Sandifer syndrome).

Failure to Thrive (Malnutrition)

A multidisciplinary assessment of the malnourished child with cerebral palsy by a "feeding team" composed of a developmental pediatrician, a speech therapist, and an occupational therapist is useful in determining the cause of malnutrition and in developing appropriate therapy because unnecessary surgery may be avoided. The general definition of *malnutrition* for children with cerebral palsy is the same as for normal children: weight beneath what is expected for height. It is common in children with cerebral palsy. Of 154 children with cerebral palsy who were surveyed in a clinic, 30% were undernourished as assessed by body weight or triceps skin fold thickness.[9] Younger children were more frequently malnourished than older ones, perhaps because some malnourished young children die.

As a general rule, even for well-nourished children with cerebral palsy, the more severe the motor involvement, the smaller the child.[10] Undernourishment can play a major role in poor growth, however, as evidenced by improvement in weight/height ratios after gastrostomy.[11] Validated growth charts for well-nourished children with spastic quadriparesis, the group for which such charts would be most useful, are not available. The adequacy of nutritional status, therefore, should be assessed by the physician who is experienced in examining subcutaneous fat on the face, ribs, abdomen, and buttocks.

The most common causes of malnutrition in children with cerebral palsy are oral motor dysfunction, recurrent vomiting, and behavior-based food refusal. The evaluation begins with an assessment of the effectiveness and safety of swallowing. The severity of swallowing dysfunction can be roughly determined by the time it takes parents to feed the child. Children who require more than 45 minutes a meal and who are fed more than four meals a day are rarely adequately nourished. Calorie counts determined by a food diary usually confirm this.[12] A history of coughing or choking during mealtimes, especially when drinking liquids, is suggestive of aspiration.[13]

In children with cerebral palsy, the usual neurologic findings associated with dysphagia are hypotonic lips, poor lingual function (resulting in inability to remove food from a spoon), delayed swallow reflex, and poor pharyngeal peristalsis. These neurologic abnormalities result in slow oral transit time, which causes slow feeding and thereby inadequate nutrition; poor bolus formation with food escaping into the pharynx before triggering the swallowing reflex and laryngeal closure; and slow pharyngeal transit with pharyngeal residue.[14] A gag reflex that is both difficult to elicit and has little palatal movement is associated with dysphagia and aspiration. Likewise, an extremely active gag reflex with repeated retching is also associated with disordered swallowing. Coughing during the clinical assessment, especially when drinking liquids, suggests aspiration.

Videofluoroscopic investigation is helpful in both defining problems more precisely and in developing therapeutic approaches to increasing oral caloric consumption safely. Under fluoroscopic observation, children are fed four textures of food (thin liquids, thickened liquids, pureed foods, and chopped foods), all mixed with barium. The phases of swallowing are observed and abnormalities noted. Optimal positioning for safe swallowing, success at increasing consumption by different techniques of feeding, and whether the temperature of food affects swallowing ability (cold food is usually swallowed better) are all determined. Using this information, a feeding program for parents to follow at home is devised.

Incorporation of parents in the processes of assessment and of developing a feeding program is essential. What may work in a hospital setting may not at home, so parental advice should be sought in formulating plans. Further, if parents participate in developing a feeding program, and it fails to result in weight gain over a predetermined period of time, then they are much more likely to accept the need for gastrostomy and enteral feedings. After parents are taught effective feeding techniques, children are followed as outpatients.

Of the first 100 patients with cerebral palsy evaluated by this approach for failure to thrive at Duke University Medical Center, 45 eventually needed enteral feedings (33 had gastrostomy and fundoplication, 10 a gastrostomy alone, and 2 a feeding jejunostomy), but 55 gained weight adequately at home on the feeding program, at least during the short term. It is, therefore, essential that children with cerebral palsy and malnutrition be evaluated by a feeding team before surgery for enteral feedings, to avoid unnecessary surgery.

Children with cerebral palsy who have severe reflux esophagitis can learn to associate swallowing with pain, and thereby acquire behavior-based food refusal. Treatment with a potent histamine-2 (H_2) blocker and a prokinetic agent, such as cisapride, can be helpful in relieving symptoms in some children. After treatment with medication or surgery, a behavior modification program may be necessary to teach children to overcome their aversion to eating.

Pulmonary Problems

The fundamental cause of the pulmonary problems of children with cerebral palsy is inadequate protection of the airway due to glossopharyngeal dysfunction. Dysphagia in children with cerebral palsy is common. In one series, it was found in 27% of 56 children and was associated with slowness of oral intake, poor trunk control, inability to feed independently, coughing with meals, choking, and history of pneumonia.[15] Hypoxemia during feedings is a useful indicator of clinically significant aspiration.[16] In children with severe dysphagia, aspiration of saliva can cause chronic bronchitis.

Dysphagia in children with severe cerebral palsy is usually associated with gastroesophageal reflux.[17] The pulmonary symptoms caused by gastroesophageal reflux are the same in children with cerebral palsy as in the general population (chronic asthma, bronchitis, bronchiectasis, aspiration pneumonia, atelectasis, hemoptysis, apnea, and hoarseness).[18] Aspiration can be documented by videofluoroscopic swallowing study.[19]

Upper Airway Obstruction

Upper airway obstruction in children with cerebral palsy can be acute or chronic. It can be continuous or present only while asleep. Minor degrees of upper airway obstruction may be manifest only when asleep. The common causes of upper airway obstruction in children with cerebral palsy include the following:

- Hypertrophy of tonsils and adenoids
- Hypotonia of the palate
- Subglottic edema from acute or chronic aspiration
- Laryngotracheomalacia from chronic aspiration of gastric acid
- Subglottic stenosis from prolonged neonatal intubation
- Nocturnal epilepsy
- Vocal cord paralysis

All patients with upper airway obstruction should be evaluated for gastroesophageal reflux because aspiration of gastric contents can cause both subglottic edema, resulting in stridor, and laryngotracheomalacia.[20] Reflux also causes chronic adenoidal inflammation and hypertrophy, which can be seen on a lateral neck radiograph. An extended (24-hour) pH probe study (while the patient is not taking an H_2 blocker) is an essential part of the evaluation. This can be done as part of a polysomnographic study to determine whether reflux is associated with hypoxemia or with arousal from sleep. If the patient has a seizure disorder, an electroencephalogram can be part of the sleep study to determine whether interictal epileptiform discharges are associated with sleep arousal.[21] Laryngoscopy to assess for inflammation and vocal cord paralysis can be useful, if ambiguity about the role of reflux in causing upper airway obstruction exists. If adenoidal hypertrophy is the cause of upper airway obstruction, adenoidectomy is necessary even if the hypertrophy is caused by reflux. Medical treatment of adenoidal hypertrophy is usually ineffective.

Reflux in older children with cerebral palsy that is severe enough to cause upper airway obstruction must also be treated surgically, in our experience. If palatal hypotonia is thought to be the only cause of upper airway obstruction in a child with cerebral palsy, and if the upper airway obstruction is severe, then an uvulopalatopharyngeoplasty should be considered. Success was described in 10 children with cerebral palsy and palatal hypotonia who had significant relief of upper airway obstruction from the procedure and did not require tracheostomy. No significant complications were reported.[22]

Tracheostomy is discussed in Chapter 55. Every effort should be made to address the underlying cause of the upper airway obstruction, to be able to avoid tracheostomy. Although the mortality rate for children with tracheostomy has improved with the advent of home nursing care,[23] the cost of care for a child with a tracheostomy at home is formidable. In one experience, 74% of children with tracheostomies had home nursing care for an average of 11 hours a day.[23] Conservatively estimating reimbursement for nursing care at $25 an hour, the cost to provide home care for a child with a tracheostomy can be over $100,000 per year.

Enteral Feedings

The principal indications for enteral feedings are inability to consume sufficient calories by mouth for growth, inability of parents to continue to nourish children who eat very slowly, repeated hospitalizations due to dehydration during episodes of gastroenteritis in children who cannot drink enough during illnesses, and aspiration of oral feedings. Long-term nasogastric tube feedings are not safe and are uncomfortable. Gastrostomy is the most common procedure done for enteral feedings, although other surgical options are available (see Chap. 4).

Evaluation of Children for Surgery for Enteral Feedings

It is the practice of most pediatric surgeons to evaluate children with cerebral palsy who are candidates for enteral feedings for gastroesophageal reflux because reflux is so common in this patient population. The evaluation for reflux is discussed at length in Chapter 62. Although the evaluation and the management of reflux are controversial and recommendations somewhat arbitrary, it is routine in many institutions to obtain the following studies before gastrostomy surgery: a modified swallow with esophagogram and gastric follow-through to assess for aspiration, esophageal stricture, hiatal hernia, and malrotation; an extended pH probe study to detect gastroesophageal reflux; and a liquid-phase radioisotope gastric emptying study to determine whether gastric emptying is delayed.[24]

Delayed gastric emptying is associated with gastroesophageal reflux in neurologically impaired children. Fonkalsrud and associates[24] reported that 75% of neurologically impaired children who required a fundoplication had delayed gastric emptying (defined as greater than 50% gastric retention of isotope at 90 minutes), compared with 25% of neurologically normal children.

It has been established that medical management of gastro-

esophageal reflux in children with cerebral palsy is of little or no long-term value[25–27]; neither vomiting nor aspiration of refluxed gastric contents is prevented. Even cisapride, a relatively new gastrointestinal prokinetic agent that is more effective than metoclopramide, has been shown not to work well in treating reflux in children with cerebral palsy.[27] H_2 blockers, such as ranitidine, alkalinize gastric acid, but alkaline gastroesophageal reflux still occurs and can result in esophagitis.[28] Therefore, if it is concluded that gastroesophageal reflux requires long-term treatment in children with cerebral palsy, then the treatment should be surgical (fundoplication).

The indications for an antireflux procedure in children with cerebral palsy generally relate to either malnutrition or pulmonary problems. These include recurrent vomiting, causing failure to thrive; persistent reflux esophagitis, causing hematemesis, stricture, pain, or food refusal due to pain when swallowing; and aspiration of gastric contents.

A protective antireflux operation has been recommended with feeding gastrostomy in mentally retarded children, even if no reflux is demonstrated by extended pH probe study preoperatively because a few of these children develop reflux-related symptoms subsequent to gastrostomy.[29–33] Table 16-2 presents a compilation of the five case series addressing this issue. Of the 126 mentally retarded children with no reflux preoperatively who had a gastrostomy alone, 33 (25%) eventually required a fundoplication for symptoms. A larger number developed reflux detected by pH probe study and might have subsequently needed surgery. Two children (2%) died from complications of reflux before a fundoplication was done. The controversy about this issue is compounded by the diagnostic limitations of even the extended pH probe study (eg, it cannot detect alkaline reflux). Most surgeons elect not to perform an antireflux procedure if the patient has no symptoms of reflux, has a normal extended pH probe study, and has normal gastric emptying because the difference in operative morbidity between gastrostomy and gastrostomy with fundoplication is substantial.

If gastric emptying is delayed, a pyloroplasty or a pyloroant-

TABLE 16-2. *Outcome of mentally impaired patients with no gastroesophageal reflux who underwent gastrostomy without fundoplication*

Series	Patients	Patients who eventually had fundoplication	Patients who died from reflux symptoms before fundoplication
Jolley et al, 1985[29]	9	3 (33%)	1 (1%)
Mollitt et al, 1985[30]	16	4 (25%)	0
Langer et al, 1988[31]	50	17 (34%)	1 (1%)
Grunow et al, 1989[32]	10	3 (30%)	0
Wheatley et al, 1991[33]	43	6 (14%)	0
TOTAL	126	33 (25%)	2 (2%)

eroplasty is warranted with the fundoplication because delayed gastric emptying after fundoplication can cause disruption of the fundoplication.

Complications of Gastrostomy and Fundoplication

Table 16-3 presents the frequency of major complications after Nissen fundoplication in retarded children from 15 case series published from 1981 to 1992, modified from Spitz and colleagues.[34] The complication rate averaged 36%. Failures of Nissen fundoplication occur predominantly in children with neurologic impairment. Of 36 fundoplication failures reported by Wheatley and associates,[35] 31 occurred in neurologically impaired children. Factors that predispose to fundoplication failure and other complications in this group of patients include esophageal dysmotility, increased intraabdominal pressure from spasticity, kyphoscoliosis, chronic constipation, seizure activity, and athetosis. Other factors shared by normal children, but more common in children with cerebral palsy, include vomiting, retching, aerophagia, and chronic respiratory disease causing coughing.[35,36]

Table 16-4 presents the early and late postoperative complications in approximate order of frequency of occurrence, compiled from the referenced case series. Several deserve specific comment. Retching can be caused by either delayed or too-rapid gastric emptying.[37–39] A radionuclide gastric emptying study can be helpful in diagnosis. Delayed gastric emptying is often a transient postoperative problem. Continuous infusion of formula and treatment with cisapride can improve feeding tolerance until gastric volume increases. Some children with normal gastric emptying preoperatively have delayed gastric emptying after gastrostomy and fundoplication and require subsequently pyloroplasty. Children with rapid gastric emptying after a fundoplication (with or without a pyloroplasty) can have the dumping syndrome. These children have retching associated with diarrhea and symptoms of hypoglycemia (pallor, sweating, and tachycardia). Symptoms often can be controlled satisfactorily using a lactose-free diet and either continuous infusion of formula or small, frequent feedings.[38]

A gastrostomy tube that has migrated into the duodenum can cause duodenal obstruction and gastric distention, increasing intragastric pressure and resulting in disruption of the fundopli-

TABLE 16-3. *Major complications of antireflux procedures in retarded children in 15 published series, 1981 to 1992*

Total patients	1297
Average per series	86
Complication rate	
Range	10%–59%
Average	36%
Intestinal obstruction	
Range	2%–76%
Average	16%
Wrap hernia or dysfunction	
Range	2%–15%
Average	7%

(Modified from Spitz L, Roth K, Kiely EM, et al. Operation for gastroesophageal reflux associated with severe mental retardation. Arch Dis Child 1933;68:347)

TABLE 16-4. *Early and late complications after gastrostomy and fundoplication in neurologically impaired children**

EARLY COMPLICATIONS
Atelectasis and pneumonia
Wound infection or dehiscence
Esophageal narrowing (tight wrap)
Small bowel obstruction
Esophageal perforation
Gastric perforation
Pancreatitis
Splenic injury
Obstructive jaundice
Vagal nerve dysfunction

LATE COMPLICATIONS
Gastrostomy leakage
Aerophagia (gas bloat)
Delayed gastric emptying (retching)
Rapid gastric emptying (dumping syndrome with retching)
Malpositioned gastrostomy tube, causing vomiting
Fundoplication disruption
   Slipped fundoplication
   Paraesophageal hernia
Small bowel obstruction
Esophageal stricture

* Complications are listed in approximate frequency of occurrence and were compiled from 19 case series.[26,27,29,30,34–38,40–49]

cation. This is an important and common event in these children. Parents should be instructed on techniques to keep the tube from migrating and detecting when it has. A "button" feeding device for a gastrostomy eliminates this complication and can be placed as soon as the gastrostomy tract matures.

Small bowel obstruction, caused by adhesions, is a significant early and late complication, usually presenting with abdominal distention[40] (see Table 16-4). Because these patients have limited ability to vomit, intestinal distention and bowel necrosis can progress rapidly in this circumstance. Sensitivity to this risk and a low threshold for early operative intervention are necessary when a small bowel obstruction is suspected in a patient with a fundoplication.

Hypophosphatemia is an infrequently reported but serious complication of nutritional rehabilitation. In a series of 45 malnourished patients, phosphate concentrations were measured in only 9, of whom 5 had hypophosphatemia.[50] Profound hypophosphatemia causes hemolytic anemia, rhabdomyolysis, glucose intolerance, and reversible obtundation and cardiomyopathy. Parenteral phosphate administration is the treatment for phosphate concentrations of less than 1 mg/dL and for patients with symptoms. Enteral sodium phosphate can be used in other circumstances.

Outcome

The surgical options for managing gastroesophageal reflux are discussed at length in Chapter 62. The discussion in this chapter of outcome after Nissen fundoplication is confined to results in neurologically abnormal children. Experience with the anterior fundoplication is increasing, but the number of neurologically abnormal children in published series who have had this operation is still too small for comment about its long-term success. Generally, the circumferential (Nissen) fundoplication is considered when results of surgery for gastroesophageal reflux are reported.

In general, in published series, outcomes after gastrostomy with and without fundoplication have been combined, resulting in difficulty in determining the contribution of each operation to quality of life and survival. Therefore, gastrostomy with and without fundoplication are discussed together in this section.

It has been shown that quality of life generally improves after gastrostomy for malnourished children with cerebral palsy who also have a history of pneumonia[13,25,26,35,41,44,46,47,49] and frequency of hospitalizations diminishes.[44] A weight gain averaging 3 kg in the first 3 months after gastrostomy has been reported. In the four series in which it is possible to determine the percentage of patients with a good surgical outcome (good weight gain, improved respiratory condition, decreased rehospitalizations for pneumonia, and no complications), 75% of patients did well.[35,46,47,49] Parental satisfaction has been reported to be as high as 91%.[13]

The life expectancy of the typical gastrostomy candidate with cerebral palsy is only 4 to 8 additional years of life.[8] Only McGrath and colleagues[49] have presented survival data after gastrostomy in a Kaplan-Meier plot. The 4-year survival rate of their patients after gastrostomy was 67%. Assuming that most patients who had surgery would have had the 50% 4-year survival rate of Eyman's[8] worst-prognosis group, gastrostomy and fundoplication probably resulted in an improvement in longevity of about 33%.

Blane and associates[48] reported follow-up of 46 children 5 to 9 years after Nissen fundoplication for reflux. Eleven (11) had died. Assuming again that these children would have fallen into the worst-prognosis group, this mortality rate is about half what might have been expected.

In conclusion, it is likely, but unproven, that gastrostomy and fundoplication (if reflux is present) improves the life-span of children with cerebral palsy.

Directions for Future Clinical Research

Each year, many retarded children at many institutions have gastrostomies with or without antireflux procedures. Yet, there has been no concerted effort to study prospectively the unresolved issues presented in Table 16-5. Of major interest is whether gastrostomy (with or without fundoplication) improves longevity. To determine this, retarded children requiring surgery should be classified into the prognostic subgroups of Eyman and associates[8] (see earlier), and the survival probabilities of the prognostic subgroups of retarded children who have had surgery should be compared with the survival probabilities of all retarded children in the prognostic subgroups (only some of whom have had gastrostomy with or without fundoplication).

Other Surgical Problems

Severe Gastric Distention (Superior Mesenteric Artery Syndrome)

Recurrent emesis in children with severe cerebral palsy can be caused not only by gastroesophageal reflux but also by rumi-

TABLE 16-5. *Unresolved issues in the management of failure to thrive and aspiration from reflux in neurologically impaired children*

How effective are oral feeding programs for malnourished children with cerebral palsy?
If gastric emptying is delayed, does pyloroplasty reduce the frequency of complications after antireflux procedures?
Does a risk or cost/benefit analysis demonstrate that fundoplication is necessary with gastrostomy, even if no reflux is demonstrated preoperatively?
What is the effect of gastrostomy and an antireflux procedure on survival, compared with the natural history (classifying patients as by Eyman and colleagues[8])?
How do the following antireflux procedures compare in terms of quality of life and longevity in neurologically impaired children who need a gastrostomy?
Nissen fundoplication
Nissen fundoplication by laparoscopy
Other fundoplication techniques
Feeding jejunostomy
Gastrostomy with gastroduodenal tube insertion

nation, fecal impaction, and sigmoid volvulus.[51] In addition to the these causes, recurrent vomiting is associated with severe gastric distention in malnourished children with cerebral palsy.[52] This syndrome, first named *superior mesenteric artery syndrome,*[53] occurs after surgical treatment of scoliosis, after marked weight loss, or after a rapid gain in height without a gain in weight.[53,54] Barium contrast studies reveal a dilated stomach and proximal duodenum with obstruction in the third portion of the duodenum. This obstruction has been attributed to increased angulation of the superior mesenteric artery over the duodenum at this point, but it may also be due to loss of fat stores resulting in the duodenum draping over the spine without support.[52] Gastric rupture can result.[52] Nutritional rehabilitation usually results in resolution of symptoms. The duodenal obstruction should be bypassed for feeding by a nasoduodenal or gastroduodenal tube, advanced beyond the point of obstruction. Continuous gastric suction may be necessary during the refeeding process. The patient should be in the left lateral decubitus position during continuous fusion feedings to promote gastric emptying.[52] Gastrostomy feedings may be necessary after resolution of gastric distention to prevent recurrence. Other surgical intervention is not usually indicated, although parenteral nutrition may also be helpful.

Cryptorchidism

Spasticity of the cremasteric muscle results in an increased prevalence of cryptorchidism in boys with cerebral palsy. The frequency of cryptorchidism in this group increases with age.[55] No data are available about the rate of testicular malignancies in children with cerebral palsy who have undescended testes.

SPINA BIFIDA

Background

Spina bifida (meningomyelocele) is a result of failure of the neural tube to form properly during the first month of gestation.

In consequence, the vertebral bodies are splayed open, and the spinal cord is malformed. The defect can occur at any vertebral level from thoracic to sacral. Neurologic and morphologic consequences depend on the pattern of innervation beneath the level of lesion. Outcome can be improved by delivery by cesarean section after fetal lung maturity (about 36 weeks' gestation) but before a trial of labor. Surgical closure of the spinal lesion is usually undertaken in the first or second day of life to minimize the risk of bacterial infection of the spinal cord because meconium is sterile at birth. Ninety percent of patients have hydrocephalus that requires placement of a ventriculoperitoneal shunt. The Chiari type II malformation of the brain stem (see Chap. 98) is invariably present but causes symptoms in only one third of patients. Prognosis for ambulation depends on the level of lesion. Most patients with lesions beneath lumbar levels 3 and 4, who have intact quadriceps function, are ambulatory, at least during childhood. Perception of acute pain beneath the level of lesion may be diminished or even completely absent.[56]

Folic acid taken by women before conception and through the first trimester can reduce the birth prevalence of spina bifida. For women who have had a child with spina bifida, 4 mg/d of folic acid for 3 months before conception and through the first trimester is recommended to reduce the risk of subsequent pregnancies from about 5% to 1%. For all other women of childbearing age in the general population, 400 μg/d has been shown to be effective. The birth incidence of spina bifida is decreasing worldwide and is now about 5 per 10,000 population in the United States.

Children with spina bifida are best followed in a multidisciplinary clinic staffed by a pediatric neurosurgeon, a pediatric orthopedic surgeon, a pediatric urologist, and a developmental pediatrician. With good care, 70% of children have normal intelligence and most are ambulatory, continent of urine, and continent of stool.[57]

Surgical Considerations

Only problems with treatments that fall within the domain of pediatric surgeons are discussed in this section. Neurosurgical, orthopedic, and urologic management are not addressed here.

Apnea and Upper Airway Obstruction

Brain-stem dysfunction from the Chiari type II malformation (Arnold-Chiari) results in potentially life-threatening problems in early infancy. Infants with spina bifida are born without brain-stem dysfunction, but about one third develop symptoms by 6 months of age. These problems include central apnea, obstructive apnea, dysphagia resulting in aspiration, stridor from paralysis of the recurrent laryngeal nerve resulting in vocal cord abductor paralysis, and gastroesophageal reflux. Neurosurgical decompression of the brain stem is controversial.[58] For patients with obstructive apnea, a tracheostomy can be lifesaving.[59] Some children outgrow the need for a tracheostomy.[59]

Esophagitis

Although gastroesophageal reflux is present in infancy in many children with spina bifida and causes mild symptoms, esophagitis and hematemesis are predominantly problems of older children and adolescents. There are three probable causes of gastroesophageal reflux in patients with spina bifida: abnormal innervation of the lower esophagus from the brain stem[60,61]; anticholinergic effects of oxybutynin (given for the neurogenic bladders), which relaxes the gastroesophageal junction; and increased intraabdominal pressure related to posture and immobility. If hematemesis or other severe symptoms recur after medical management with omeprazole and cisapride, a fundoplication should be considered.

Acute Abdominal Signs and Symptoms

An approximate incidence of the development of acute abdominal signs or symptoms in patients with spina bifida is 1 per 300 patients per year, based on our experience at Duke University Medical Center. Underlying conditions associated with spina bifida cause more problems in aggregate than do unrelated causes of an acute abdomen. These underlying conditions are hydrocephalus with a ventriculoperitoneal shunt, neurogenic bowel, neurogenic bladder, and chronic antibiotic administration, predisposing to *clostridium difficile* enterocolitis.

The ventriculoperitoneal shunt causes acute abdominal signs and symptoms in one of three ways. Shunt infection is the most common cause. If a patient has a shunt infection, acute peritonitis resulting from drainage of infected cerebrospinal fluid into the peritoneum can result. (Conversely, ventriculitis can result from ascending infection from primary peritonitis.) A shunt infection caused by bacteria of low pathogenicity can result in a loculated cerebrospinal fluid pseudocyst in the peritoneum; *Staphylococcus epidermidis* is most common. About 40% of pseudocysts are infected by bacteria. Likewise, ascites can result from a shunt infection caused by bacteria of low pathogenicity. The ascites can be a transudate with few polymorphonuclear leukocytes. The second shunt-related complication involves hollow visceral perforation. The ventriculoperitoneal shunt has been reported to perforate or erode nearly any contiguous structure. Intestine, bladder, and vagina are perforated most commonly, but stomach, gallbladder, and liver perforations have also been reported. The third group of complications relate to mechanical effects of the catheter or the cerebrospinal fluid. Voluvulus of the bowel around shunt tubing, a knot of shunt tubing around bowel, and persistent patency of the processus vaginalis from either shunt tubing or from cerebrospinal fluid, predisposing to inguinal hernia, can all cause acute abdominal signs and symptoms.

The neurogenic bladder can cause acute abdominal signs and symptoms in several ways as well. The first way is by predisposing to pyelonephritis, which can cause ileus. The second is by way of bladder perforation during clean intermittent catheterization. Finally, erosion of the bladder wall by chronic infection (candida and pseudomonal organisms combined) has resulted in bladder perforation.

The neurogenic bowel in children with spinal bifida can predispose to an acute abdomen in two ways. The first way is by predisposing to urinary tract infection. Chronic constipation with rectal distention may prevent complete drainage of urine from the bladder by intermittent catheterization, and thereby can predispose to urinary tract infection. The second way is by causing chronic constipation, which results in fecal impaction and even colonic obstruction.[62] We have encountered two cases of toxic megacolon resulting from obstruction; one resulted in perforation of the transverse colon. Finally, chronic prophylactic antibiotic administration can cause *C difficile* enteritis resulting in diffuse abdominal pain.

Several historical features are helpful in making the correct diagnosis in these patients. Vague lower abdominal pain and frank blood in the urine suggest bladder perforation. A recent history of failure of compliance with the bowel regimen is a clue that the acute abdomen may be the result of constipation or an associated cause. Recent urinary tract infection symptoms (primarily wetness between catheterizations) often occur before the development of acute symptoms of pyelonephritis. Fever, headache, stiff neck, or a change in alertness suggest a ventriculoperitoneal shunt infection. A history of diarrhea suggests either *C. difficile* infection or overflow from chronic constipation.

The physical examination is often not as helpful in making the diagnosis of acute abdomen in children with spina bifida as it is in normal children. Because patients with a thoracic-level meningomyelocele often have an insensate or partially insensate abdomen, the severity of pain cannot be used as a guide to the severity of the underlying condition, and the location of the pain is not as helpful as usual in determining cause. Diffuse peritonitis, originating in the lower abdomen may be perceived only as epigastric pain in patients with a thoracic level lesion of T-7 or higher.

As is the case with acute abdomen in spinal cord injury, fever and tachycardia suggest peritonitis, but the absence of fever does not preclude peritonitis. Patients with spina bifida have been reported to have autonomic dysreflexia, so patients with a high-level (thoracic) lesion may have bradycardia and hypertension caused by peritonitis.

Signs of shunt obstruction or infection should be elicited (eg, a change in sensorium, stiff neck, erythema or tenderness along the shunt tubing, signs of peritonitis, ascites, abdominal mass [pseudocyst]). The absence of ileus does not preclude peritonitis, as is the case also in the acute abdomen of spinal cord injury. Rebound is unreliable because of abnormal motor innervation.

Because the sigmoid colon is commonly elongated in children with spina bifida, the absence of stool in the rectum does not necessarily eliminate an obstructive impaction from consideration. Stool should be tested for blood by the guaiac test. We have seen a patient with a neurenteric cyst present with fecal blood loss and severe anemia from hemorrhage related to an ulcer in ectopic gastric mucosa within the cyst. It should be remembered that adolescent girls with spina bifida are teenagers first. Ectopic pregnancies and sexually transmitted disease occur in this population, just as in normal teenagers. A pelvic examination is therefore necessary.

The laboratory evaluation should, of course, be directed by the history and physical examination. The laboratory evaluation should be similar to that for an acute abdomen in a normal child.

In our experience, abdominal computed tomography is preferred over abdominal ultrasound for establishing a diagnosis. Often, constipation (common in people with spina bifida) limits an ultrasound examination. Free fluid in the peritoneum can be cerebrospinal fluid or urine from a bladder perforation. Bladder perforation should be ruled out in all cases of an acute abdomen in people with spina bifida. Nonionic contrast material should

be used, since ionic contrast material has been reported to cause chemical ventriculitis, by ascending either through the shunt itself or along the shunt tract.

If a pseudocyst or ascites is found, the yield of culturing a bacteria of low pathogenicity can be improved by filtering a volume of cerebrospinal fluid through a sterile filter apparatus and then culturing the filter paper.

Finally, there are often concerns in the evaluation of an acute abdomen in people with spina bifida. Chronic low-grade bladder infection (resulting in pyuria) and constipation are present in many patients with spina bifida, and neither should be assumed to be the cause of serious signs or symptoms until other more serious possibilities have been eliminated. Persistence and careful observation are necessary to make a diagnosis. Despite careful evaluation, diagnostic laparotomy or laparoscopy is sometimes the only means by which the diagnosis can ultimately be made.

The causes of abdominal signs and symptoms encountered in children with spinal bifida at Duke University Medical Center are presented in Table 16-6. Cause reported by others are listed at the bottom of the table.

Fat Embolus Syndrome

The fat embolus syndrome has been reported following femur fracture in adolescents with thoracic level spina bifida.[64,65] Pulmonary difficulties can often precede the diagnosis of femur fracture because the legs are insensate. Abdominal ileus also occurs in the syndrome. It is possible, that the bone marrow of children with spinal bifida is more fatty at a younger age than normal.

Latex Allergy Resulting in Intraoperative Anaphylaxis

For reasons that are unclear, 20% to 40% of patients with spina bifida are allergic to latex.[66] A relation exists between the number of surgical procedures and the incidence of latex allergy, suggesting that intraoperative latex exposure sensitizes

TABLE 16-6. *Causes of abdominal signs or symptoms in children with spina bifida requiring hospitalization*

Infected ventriculoperitoneal shunt
   Peritonitis
   Pseudocyst
Fecal impaction
Urosepsis
Passage of renal stone (renal colic)
Ruptured bladder
Pseudomembranous enterocolitis
Appendicitis
Fractured femur
Infected orthopaedic spinal instrumentation

Causes previously reported by others
   Cerebrospinal fluid
   Ruptured vesicocecoplasty anastomosis[63]
   Perforation of stomach, gallbladder, intestine, bladder, and vagina by ventriculoperitoneal shunt tubing
   Volvulus around the shunt tubing
   Abdominal ascites

patients. Some patients who have never had surgery, however, are also allergic to latex, possibly as a consequence of latex catheters or gloves. It is also conceivable that there is some predilection toward the development of latex allergy that is intrinsic to patients with spina bifida.

Intraoperative anaphylaxis from latex allergy is common in patients with spina bifida. During a 13-month period at one hospital, for instance, it occurred in 10 patients.[66] Most hospitals with large spina bifida clinics have had at least one case of intraoperative anaphylaxis from latex allergy. Many institutions have instituted hospital-wide latex avoidance for all patients with spina bifida, whether or not they have had a previous reaction to latex. This practice should prevent latex sensitization as well as ensure that no allergic child has an anaphylactic reaction while in the hospital. Latex exposure resulting in anaphylaxis is common enough and well enough described in this population to be a potential medicolegal risk. For patients with known latex allergy, premedication before surgery with antihistamines and methylprednisolone should be considered.[67]

Cryptorchidism

Patients with spinal lesions at level L-2 or above have cryptorchidism more frequently than those with lower-level spinal lesions.[68]

Neurogenic Bowel

About 80% of patients with spina bifida can achieve continence of stool (ie, no more than two episodes of fecal incontinence per month).[62] Patients with intact bulbocavernosal and anocutaneous reflexes are more likely to achieve continence on a simple, consistently timed, reflex-triggered bowel management program. Beginning the program when the child is younger than 6 years of age results in a greater success rate. Bisacodyl enemas can also be used every other day beginning at 5 or 6 years of age to establish a bowel habit. Large-volume saline enemas, 20 mL/kg up to 1 L once a day administered by a nonlatex delivery system, are effective in two thirds of patients with flaccid anal sphincters.[68] Saline is made by adding table salt to tap water in the ratio of 1 measuring teaspoon to 500 mL. Only 1% of patients (2 of 300) have needed a colostomy for incontinence in our institution, and both patients required them for the management of decubitus ulcers.

PEDIATRIC SPINAL CORD INJURY

Background

Pediatric spinal cord injury is defined as trauma to the spinal cord resulting in sensory or motor neurologic abnormalities.[68] Fortunately, it is rare in childhood. An epidemiologic study of acute spinal cord injuries in children in 18 northern California counties during 1970 and 1971 revealed that about 9% of spinal cord injuries occur in children 15 years old and younger.[69] Half of these children do not survive to discharge from the hospital. Therefore, of surviving spinal cord injury victims, about 5% are children.[69] Extrapolating from the data from northern Cali-

fornia, there are about 750 new pediatric spinal cord injury patients in the United States each year.

The external causes of trauma resulting in spinal cord injury in children, in decreasing order of frequency in a total of 58 cases, are: pedestrian car accidents (29%), passenger in an automobile accident (21%), athletic injuries (17%), autobike accidents (12%), falls (7%), firearm injuries (7%), motorcycle accidents (3%), and birth trauma (3%).[69]

Spinal cord injury without radiologic abnormality is more common in children than in adults.[70] Persistent neck pain after trauma associated with any neurologic abnormality should be assessed not only by neck flexion and extension films but also by computed tomography and magnetic resonance imaging of the cervical spine. The ''burning hand syndrome,'' extremity numbness or tingling, or ''sparking'' pain in extremities, all warrant magnetic resonance imaging of the spine because damage to spinothalamic tracts causes these symptoms.[71,72] Ligamentous laxity, spinal cervical stenosis, acquired herniation of intervertebral disks, and degenerative changes all lead to cord concussion in children.[72] Detection of these abnormalities in patients with minimal symptoms can prevent paralysis.

Treatment with high-dose methylprednisolone within 8 hours of spinal cord injury results in significant improvement in motor function when compared with placebo.[73] It is given at a bolus dose of 30 mg/kg within 8 hours of injury and at a maintenance dose of 5.4 mg/kg/h for 23 hours. The difference in motor function between the treated group and the placebo group was still evident at 1 year and is probably permanent.

About 5% of patients hospitalized with traumatic spinal cord injury die during acute hospitalization or during rehabilitation. The cumulative 12-year survival rates for those injured between ages 1 and 24 years are 93.5% for complete paraplegia and 87.1% for complete quadriplegia; these rates are much better than for those injured at age 50 years or older.[74] For patients with no motor function beneath the zone of spinal cord injury and no perianal sensation 72 hours after the injury, the prognosis is bleak. Few make a functional recovery. For patients with incomplete lesions, however, improvement can continue for up to 1 year. Other neurologic abnormalities resulting from spinal cord injury include neurogenic bowel and bladder, insensate skin, and insensate abdomen.

Autonomic Dysreflexia

Autonomic dysreflexia, also called *autonomic hyperreflexia* or the *mass reflex*, is a syndrome that commonly affects patients with spinal cord injuries at or above vertebral level T-6. It occurs in 48% to 90% of quadriplegic and high-level paraplegic patients. A noxious stimulus beneath the level of the spinal cord lesion causes, by an uninhibited reflex, a massive release of epinephrine and norepinephrine from the adrenal gland, resulting in severe hypertension. The ordinary cortical inhibition of this reflex is absent because of the spinal cord injury. The carotid sinus and aortic body, sensing the hypertension, cause bradycardia and reflex vasodilation above the level of the cord lesion, induced by the vagal nerve. In consequence, patients have the combination of severe hypertension, a slow pulse rate, a pounding headache, flushing above and pallor beneath the level of spinal cord injury, and sweating above the level of injury. Adult patients with a cardiovascular disease who have autonomic dysreflexia can die from stroke or myocardial infarction. Because this problem is most common in patients with a complete lesion who are quadriparetic, patients are unaware of the provoking cause of the autonomic dysreflexia. Painful stimuli that can provoke the reflex include urinary retention, fecal impaction, skin pinched in clothing or zippers, toes flexed in shoes not put on carefully, skin irritation from sitting on a sharp object or on an uneven seating surface, and more serious causes, such as fractures, abdominal emergencies, urinary tract infections, and decubitus ulcers. Treatment is first and foremost to eliminate the cause of the pain. A decrease in blood pressure is prompt when this is done. The head of the bed should be elevated, tight clothing removed, the bladder catheterized, and stool disimpacted from the rectum. If symptoms persist, a 10-mg capsule of nifedipine (adult dose) should be broken open and the contents squeezed under the tongue. Further emergency treatment includes nitroprusside and other agents.[75]

Surgery in patients with high spinal cord lesions often provokes autonomic dysreflexia. Anesthesiologists should be informed of this potential complication and be ready to treat it so surgery can proceed.

Deep Vein Thrombosis

Deep vein thrombosis is relatively rare in pediatric spinal cord injury patients, compared with adults, but should be considered in patients older than 12 years of age with fever of unknown cause after surgical procedures. Likewise, acute respiratory distress in adolescents with spinal cord injury rarely can be due to pulmonary embolism.

Acute Abdomen

The acute abdomen in spinal cord injury patients is a diagnostic challenge for both physicians and surgeons. Detection is difficult in patients who have an insensate or partially insensate abdomen. The presence of the neurogenic bowel and bladder expand the differential diagnosis. Yet abdominal problems are reasonably common among spinal cord injury patients. Gore and associates[76] reported that gastrointestinal complications were encountered in 63 (11%) of 567 consecutive adult spinal cord injury patients.

Surgical Considerations

At our institution, five pediatric spinal cord injury patients have developed an acute abdomen. The causes were urosepsis, fecal impaction, and appendicitis in one patient each, and acute pancreatitis in two patients. Acute abdominal problems have not previously been reported in pediatric patients with spinal cord injury, to our knowledge.

The causes of acute abdominal signs and symptoms in children are probably similar to those in adults, but underdiagnosed. Therefore, a compilation of diagnoses from the five largest case series in adult patients with spinal cord injuries and acute abdo-

TABLE 16-7. *Causes of severe abdominal signs and symptoms in spinal cord–injured adults**

Cause	Number
Fecal impaction	50
Ileus	26
Appendicitis	26
Peptic ulcer disease	
Without perforation	23
With perforation	11
Upper GI bleeding (unknown source)	18
Pancreatitis	18
Cholecystitis or cholelithiasis	13
Ruptured viscus	11
Volvulus	7
Ruptured bladder	5
Gastric dilation	3
Superior mesenteric artery syndrome	3
Cancer	2
Ruptured spleen	1
Retroperitoneal hemorrhage	1
Unknown	1
TOTAL	100

* Compiled from five case series.[76–80]

mens is presented in Table 16-7, as a guide to the problem in children.[76–80] Within the first 2 weeks after injury in adults, acute abdominal emergencies are most commonly caused by peptic ulcer disease (with or without perforation), pancreatitis, and upper gastrointestinal bleeding from an unknown cause.[78] The use of glucocorticoids and presence of a high-level spinal lesion are risk factors for gastrointestinal bleeding and pancreatitis.[78]

Within the first 4 weeks after injury, intraabdominal pathology is seen in about 5% of cases. Patients with complete cord lesions above level T-5 are most at risk.

Occasionally, the hypercalcemia seen in patients with spinal cord injury can present with an ileus and abdominal pain.

The symptoms of an acute abdomen are often vague in spinal cord injury patients. Anorexia, nausea, and salivation are early signs of increased vagal tone caused by abdominal problems. Most patients (75%) have vague abdominal or flank pain, even those with high-level lesions. Shoulder pain is an ominous sign that reflects peritonitis, which is most commonly caused by a perforated ulcer, ruptured viscus, ruptured bladder, or appendicitis.

Tachycardia is present in most spinal cord injury patients with acute abdomens. A substantial percentage (about 15% in cumulative series) of patients, however, have autonomic dysreflexia provoked by abdominal pain and, therefore, hypertension and bradycardia. Fever suggests peritonitis or urosepsis. Half of patients have tenderness to palpation, but only one fourth each have ileus or guarding.[80] Diagnosis is delayed in about one third of adult patients for 2 days to 1 month. It is more difficult to diagnose an acute abdomen in a patient with a high-level lesion than in a patient with a low-level lesion. Diagnosis is even more different in pediatric patients.

The laboratory evaluation is dictated by the signs and symptoms. Although abdominal ultrasound and computed tomography can be helpful, laparotomy or laparoscopy is often necessary because appropriate preoperative evaluation can confirm the diagnosis in 77% of cases.[80] The surgeon should not be reluctant to operate when in doubt of diagnosis because these patients do well postoperatively.[77]

DOWN SYNDROME

Background

Down syndrome results from triplicated chromosome 21. It is one of the most common developmental disabilities. There are more than 300,000 people with Down syndrome in the United States, and the syndrome occurs in 1 in 670 live births.[81] More than 10,000 children are born each year in the United States with the condition. The birth incidence of Down syndrome increases with increasing maternal age.[82] Full trisomy 21 explains 94% of cases, with translocation and mosaicism causing the rest.

The features that allow ready identification in the newborn period have been outlined succinctly.[83] Mental deficiency is almost universal. Forty percent of patients have a cardiac anomaly. The most common of these, in decreasing order of frequency, are: atrioventricularis communis, ventricular septal defect, patent ductus arteriosus, atrial septal defects, and aberrant subclavian arteries. Thyroid disorders, leukemia, and Alzheimer disease are also more common in Down syndrome patients than in the general population.[83]

Surgical Considerations

It is for the management of congenital anomalies of the gastrointestinal tract that the pediatric surgeon is most needed for children with Down syndrome.

In a compilation of five series that included 3338 patients with Down syndrome,[84–88] 164 (4.9%) had a gastrointestinal congenital anomaly that required surgery. These anomalies are listed in Table 16-8.

Duodenal stenosis or atresia is the most common gastrointestinal anomaly that occurs in Down syndrome patients. It presents in the newborn period with vomiting, abdominal distention, and the classic double-bubble sign on abdominal radiograph.[88] A duodenoduodenostomy is performed if possible

TABLE 16-8. *Gastrointestinal anomalies in children with Down syndrome**

Anomaly	Occurrence
Duodenal stenosis or atresia	72 (45%)
Imperforate anus	31 (19%)
Annular pancreas	17 (10%)
Hirschsprung disease	17 (10%)
Pyloric stenosis	8 (5%)
Hypoplasia of small bowel	5 (3%)
Bile duct atresia	5 (3%)
Malrotation	5 (3%)
Hiatal hernia	2 (1%)
Meckel diverticulum	2 (1%)
TOTAL	164 (100%)

* Compiled from five case series.[88–92]

(see Chap. 68). The mortality rate is high because of the associated conditions of cardiac malformation, immune compromise, and gastroesophageal reflux. In four series,[88–92] the mortality rate averaged 38% (range, 13% to 56%), despite early recognition of duodenal obstruction and management by skilled surgeons.

The usual anorectal malformation associated with Down syndrome is a low-lying rectal pouch without a urinary fistula. It can often be adequately treated by a perineal anoplasty.[93] Others have found a more even distribution of high and low imperforate anus anomalies.[88]

Quinn and colleagues[94] reported their experience with Hirschsprung disease in children with Down syndrome. Of the 17 children with the two conditions (of 135 patients with Hirschsprung disease), 9 presented in the neonatal period, with intestinal obstruction (5 cases), enterocolitis (2 cases), or perforation of the colon (2 cases). Eight presented after the neonatal period with constipation. The rectosigmoid colon was by far the most common site of transition (12 of 17), as it is typically. After definitive surgery, long-term bowel function was poor, with only 1 of 14 patients being continent. There were two deaths, one from enterocolitis and the other from congenital cardiac disease.

Esophageal dysmotility is common in children with Down syndrome, perhaps as part of a widespread disorder of gastrointestinal motility.[95] Medical treatment alone is usually ineffective in managing severe gastroesophageal reflux in children with Down syndrome. The indications for an antireflux procedure or gastrostomy are the same as those for children with retardation and cerebral palsy. Esophageal strictures have been reported in children with Down syndrome and have been associated with mortality.[88] Diaphragmatic hernia has also been associated with Down syndrome.[96]

Obstructive Sleep Apnea

Obstructive sleep apnea is common in children with Down syndrome.[97] Its causes are hypotonia of the pharynx, hypotonia of the tongue with obstruction of the upper airway by it, and enlarged tonsils and adenoids.[97] Polysomnography can document hypoxia associated with obstructive apnea episodes. In children with Down syndrome, surgical relief of the obstruction by an adenoidectomy or uvuloveloplasty can result in improvement in cognitive function. Careful preoperative evaluation is necessary to determine how much adenoid tissue to remove. Failure to anticipate this can lead to hypernasality due to velopalatine incompetence.[98]

Operative Considerations

Atlantoaxial subluxation is associated with Down syndrome. Hyperextension of the neck for endotracheal intubation has resulted in acute paralysis due to spinal cord injury.[99] Cervical spinal cord injury can occur without evidence of subluxation on lateral spine films. Therefore, it is prudent for the anesthesiologist to treat all children with Down syndrome as if they had cervical spine instability, taking this into consideration in positioning and in techniques of intubation.

The hepatitis B infection carrier state is common among non-institutionalized children and adults with Down syndrome.[100] Up to 20% of those with Down syndrome test positive for hepatitis B surface antigen, have no overt clinical signs of liver disease, and have normal transaminase levels. Therefore, all children with Down syndrome undergoing surgery should be isolated by enteric precautions or should be tested for hepatitis B surface antigenemia.[100]

REFERENCES

1. Freeman JM, McDonnell K. Ethical theory and medical ethics. In: Tough decisions. New York, Oxford University Press, 1987:144.
2. Lo B. Behind closed doors: promise and pitfalls of ethics committees. N Engl J Med 1987;317:46.
3. Jonsson MV, McNamce M, Campion EW. The "do not resuscitate" order: a profile of its changing use. Arch Intern Med 1988;148:2373.
4. Todres ID, Guillemin J, Grodin MA, et al. Life-saving therapy for newborns: a questionnaire survey in the state of Massachusetts. Pediatrics 1988;81:643.
5. Mutch L, Alberman E, Hagberg B, et al. Cerebral palsy epidemiology: where are we now and where are we going? Dev Med Child Neurol 1992;34:547.
6. Nelson KB, Ellenberg JH. Antecedents of cerebral palsy. N Engl J Med 1986;315:81.
7. Kuban KCK, Leviton A. Cerebral palsy. N Engl J Med 1994;330:188.
8. Eyman RR, Grossman HJ, Chaney RH, et al. The life expectancy of profoundly handicapped people with mental retardation. N Engl J Med 1990;323:504.
9. Stallings YA, Charney EB, Davies JC, et al. Nutrition-related growth failure of children with quadriplegic cerebral palsy. Dev Med Child Neurol 1993;35:126.
10. Spender QW, Cronk CE, Charney EB, et al. Assessment of linear growth of children with cerebral palsy: use of alternate measures to height or length. Dev Med Child Neurol 1989;31:206.
11. Shapiro BK, Green P, Krick J, et al. Growth of severely impaired children: neurological versus nutritional factors. Dev Med Child Neurol 1986;28:729.
12. Gisel EG, Patrick J. Identification of children with cerebral palsy unable to maintain a normal nutritional state. Lancet 1988;1:283.
13. Splaingard ML, Hutchins B, Sulton LD, et al. Aspiration in rehabilitation patients: videofluoroscopy vs. bedside clinical assessment. Arch Phys Med Rehabil 1989;69:637.
14. Jones PM. Feeding disorders in children with multiple handicaps. Dev Med Child Neurol 1989;31:398.
15. Waterman ET, Koltai PJ, Downey JC, et al. Swallowing disorders in a population of children with cerebral palsy. Int J Pediatr Otolaryngol 1992;24:63.
16. Rodgers BT, Arvedson J, Msall M, et al. Hypoxemia during oral feeding of children with severe cerebral palsy. Dev Med Child Neurol 1993;35:3.
17. Reyes AL, Cash AJ, Green SH, et al. Gastroesophageal reflux in children with cerebral palsy. Child Care Health Dev 1993;19:109.
18. Barish CF, Wu WC, Castell DO. Respiratory complications of gastroesophageal reflux. Arch Intern Med 1985;145:1882.
19. Griggs CA, Jones PM, Lee RE. Videofluoroscopic investigation of feeding disorders of children with multiple handicap. Dev Med Child Neurol 1989;31:303.
20. Neilson DH, Heldt GP, Tooley WH. Stridor and esophageal reflux in infants. Pediatrics 1990;85:1034.
21. Kotagal S, Gibbons VP, Stith JA. Sleep abnormalities in patients with severe cerebral palsy. Dev Med Child Neurol 1994;36:304.
22. Seid AB, Martin PJ, Pransky SM, et al. Surgical therapy of obstruction sleep apnea in children with severe mental insufficiency. Laryngoscope 1990;100:507.
23. Duncan BW, Howell LJ, de Lorimier AA, et al. Tracheostomy with home emphasis on home care. J Pediatr Surg 1992;27:432.
24. Fonkalsrud EW, Ellis DG, Show A, et al. A combined hospital experience with fundoplication and gastric emptying procedure for gastroesophageal reflux in children. J Am Coll Surg 1995;180:449.
25. Wilkinson JP, Dudgeon DL, Sondheimer JM. A comparison of medical and surgical treatment of gastroesophageal reflux in severely retarded children. J Pediatr 1981;99:202.
26. Vane DW, Harmel RP, King DR, et al. The effectiveness of Nissen fundoplication in neurologically impaired children with gastroesophageal reflux. Surgery 1985;98:662.
27. Brueton MJ, Clarke GS, Sandhu RV. The effects of cisapride on gastroesophageal reflux in children with and without neurologic disorders. Dev Med Child Neurol 1990;32:629.
28. Malthaner RA, Newman KD, Parry R, et al. Alkaline gastroesophageal reflux in infants and children. J Pediatr Surg 1991;26:980.
29. Jolley SG, Smith EI, Tunell WP. Protective antireflux operation with feeding gastrostomy: experience with children. Ann Surg 1985;201:736.
30. Mollitt DL, Golladay S, Seibert JJ. Symptomatic gastroesophageal reflux following gastrostomy in neurologically impaired patients. Pediatrics 1985;75:1124.
31. Langer JC, Wesson DE, Ein SH, et al. Feeding gastrostomy in neurologically impaired children: is an antireflux procedure necessary? J Pediatr Gastroenterol Nutr 1988;7:837.
32. Grunow JE, Al-Hafidh AS, Tunell WP. Gastroesophageal reflux following percutaneous endoscopic gastrostomy in children. J Pediatr Surg 1989;24:42.
33. Wheatley MJ, Wesley JR, Tkach DM, et al. Long term follow-up of brain damaged children requiring feeding gastrostomy: should an antireflux procedure always be performed?. J Pediatr Surg 1991;26:301.
34. Spitz L, Roth K, Kiely EM, et al. Operation for gastroesophageal reflux associated with severe mental retardation. Arch Dis Child 1933;68:347.
35. Wheatley MJ, Coran AG, Wesley JR, et al. Redo fundoplication in infants and children with recurrent gastroesophageal reflux. J Pediatr Surg 1991;26:758.
36. Caniano DA, Binn-Pease ME, King D. The failed antireflux procedure: analysis of risk factors and morbidity. J Pediatr Surg 1990;25:1022.
37. Jolley SG, Tunell WP, Leonard JD, et al. Gastric emptying in children with gastroesophageal reflux. II. The relationship to retching symptoms following antireflux surgery. J Pediatr Surg 1987;22:927.
38. Maddern GJ, Jamieson GG, Chatterton BE, et al. Is there an association between failed antireflux procedures and delayed gastric emptying? Ann Surg 1986;202:162.
39. Meyer S, Deckelbaum RJ, Lux E. Infant dumping syndrome after gastroesophageal reflux surgery. J Pediatr 1981;99:235.
40. Jolley SG, Tunell WP, Hoelzer DJ, et al. Postoperative small bowel obstruction in infants and children: a problem following Nissen fundoplication. J Pediatr Surg 1986;21:407.
41. Fonkalsrud EW, Ament ME, Berquist W. Surgical management of the gastroesophageal reflux syndrome in childhood. Surgery 1985;97:42.
42. Stringel G, Delgado M, Guertin L, et al. Gastrostomy and Nissen fundoplication in neurologically impaired children. J Pediatr Surg 1989;24:1044.
43. Turnage RH, Oldham KT, Coran AG, et al. Late results of fundoplication of gastroesophageal reflux in infants and children. Surgery 1989;105:457.
44. Bui H, Dang CV, Chaney RH, et al. Does gastrostomy and fundoplication prevent aspiration pneumonia in mentally retarded persons? Am J Ment Retard 1989;94:16.
45. Smith CP, Biemann Othersen H, Gogan HJ, et al. Nissen fundoplication in children with profound disability, high risks and unmet goals. Ann Surg 1992;215:654.
46. Martinez DA, Ginn-Pease, Caniano DA. Sequelae of antireflux surgery in profoundly disabled children. J Pediatr Surg 1992;17:267.
47. Pearl RH, Robie DR, Ein SH, et al. Complications of gastroesophageal antireflux surgery in neurologically impaired versus neurologically normal children. J Pediatr Surg 1990;25:1169.
48. Blane CE, Turnage RH, Oldham KT, et al. Long-term radiographic follow-up of the Nissen fundoplication in children. Pediatr Radiol 1989;19:523.
49. McGrath SJ, Splaingard ML, Alba HM, et al. Survival and functional outcome of children with severe cerebral palsy following gastrostomy. Arch Phys Med Rehabil 1992;73:133.
50. Mezoff AG, Gremese DA, Farrell MK. Hypophosphatemia in the nutritional recovery syndrome. Am J Dis Child 1989;143:1111.

51. Roy A, Simon GB. Intestinal obstruction as a cause of death in developmentally disabled patients. J Ment Defic Res 1987;31:193.

52. Del Beccaro MA, McLaughlin JF, Polage DL. Severe gastric distention in patients with cerebral palsy. Dev Med Child Neurol 1991;33:912.

53. Wayne ER, Burrington JD. Duodenal obstruction by the superior mesenteric artery in children. Surgery 1972;72:762.

54. Hines JR, Gore RM, Ballantyne GH. Superior mesenteric artery syndrome: diagnostic and therapeutic approaches. Am J Surg 1984;148:630.

55. Smith JA, Hutson JM, Beasley SW, et al. The relationship between cerebral palsy and cryptorchidism. J Pediatr Surg 1989;24:1305.

56. Liptak GS, Bloss JW, Briskin H, et al. The management of the child with spinal dysraphism. J Child Neurol 1988;3:3.

57. McLone DG, Dias L, Kaplan WE, et al. Concepts in the management of spina bifida. Concepts Pediatr Neurosurg 1985;5:97.

58. Worley G, Schuster JM, Oakes WJ. Survival at five years of a cohort of newborns with myelomeningocele. Dev Med Child Neurol (in press).

59. Oren J, Kelly DH, Todres ID. Respiratory complications in patients with myelodysplasia and Arnold-Chiari malformation. Am J Dis Child 1986;140:221.

60. Park TS, Hoffman HJ, Hendrick EB, et al. Experience with surgical decompression of the Arnold-Chiari malformation in young infants with myelomeningocele. Neurosurgery 1983;13:147.

61. Pollack IF, Pang D, Kocoshis S, et al. Neurogenic dysphagia resulting from Chiari malformations. Neurosurgery 1992;30:709.

62. King JC, Currie DM, Wright E. Bowel training in spina bifida:. importance of education, patient compliance, age, and anal reflexes. Arch Phys Med Rehabil 1994;75:243.

63. Rushton HG, Woodard JR, Parrott TS, et al. Delayed bladder rupture after augmentation enterocystoplasty. J Urol 1988;140:344.

64. Kenny NW, Parkinson RW. Simultaneous bilateral hip fractures presenting as an acute abdomen. Br J Accident Surg 1993;24:681.

65. Limbard TJ, Ruderman RJ. Fat embolism in children. Clin Orthop Rel Res 1978;135:267.

66. Kelly KJ, Perarson ML, Krurup VP, et al. A cluster of anaphylactic reactions in children with spina bifida during general anesthesia: epidemiologic features, risk factors, and latex hypersensitivity. J Allergy Clin Immunol 1994;94:53.

67. Kwittken PL, Becker J, Oyefara B, et al. Latex hypersensitivity reactions despite prophylaxis. Allergy Proc 1992;13:123.

68. Kewalramai LS. Spinal cord trauma in children. Spine 1980;5:11.

69. Kewalramai LS, Kraus JF, Sterling HM. Acute spinal cord injuries in a pediatric population: epidemiologic and clinical features. Paraplegia 1980;18:206.

70. Chesire DJE. The paediatric syndrome of traumatic myelopathy without demonstrable vertebral injury. Paraplegia 1977–1978;15:74.

71. Wilberger JE, Abla A, Maroon JC. Burning hands syndrome revisited. Neurosurgery 1986;19:1038.

72. Rathbone D, Johnson G, Letts M. Spinal cord concussion in pediatric athletes. J Pediatr Orthop 1992;12:616.

73. Bracken MB, Shepard MJ, Collins WF, et al. A randomized, controlled trial of methylprednisolone or naloxone in the treatment of acute spinal cord injury. N Engl J Med 1990;322:1405.

74. DeVivo MJ. Life expectancy and causes of death for persons with spinal cord injuries. In: Apple DF, Hudson LM, eds. Spinal cord injury: the model. Proceedings of the National Consensus Conference on Catastrophic Illness and Injury. December 1989. Atlanta, Shepherd Center for Treatment of Spinal Injuries, 1990:61.

75. Braddom RL, Rocco JF. Autonomic dysreflexia: a survey of current treatment. Am J Phys Med Rehabil 1991;70:234.

76. Gore RM, Mintzer RA, Calenoff L. Gastrointestinal complications of spinal cord injury. Spine 1981;6:538.

77. Charney KJ, Juler GL, Coman AE. General surgical problems in patients with spinal cord injuries. Arch Surg 1975;110:1083.

78. Berlly MH, Wilmot CB. Acute abdominal emergencies during the first four weeks after spinal cord injury. Arch Phys Med Rehabil 1984;65:687.

79. Juler GL, Eltorai IM. The acutely affected abdomen in spinal cord injury patients. Paraplegia 1985;23:118.

80. Neumayer LA, Ball DA, Mohr JD, et al. The acutely affected abdomen in paraplegic spinal cord injury patients. Ann Surg 1990;212:561.

81. Stoll C, Alembik Y, Dott B, et al. Epidemiology of Down syndrome in 118,265 consecutive births. Am J Med Genet 1990;7(Suppl):79.

82. Hook EB, Fabia JJ. Frequency of Down syndrome in live births by single-year maternal age interval: results of a Massachusetts study. Teratology 1978;17:223.

83. Smith DW, Jones KL. Recognizable patterns of human malformation. Philadelphia, WB Saunders, 1982.

84. Carter CO. A life table for mongols with the causes of death. J Ment Defic Res 1958;2:64.

85. Rowe RD, Uchida IA. Cardiac malformation in mongolism. Am J Med 1961;31:726.

86. Fabia J, Drolette M. Malformations and leukemia in children with Down syndrome. Pediatrics 1970;45:60.

87. Knox GE, Tein-Bensel RW. Gastrointestinal malformations in Down syndrome. Winn Med 1972;55:542.

88. Buchin PJ, Levy JS, Schullinger JH. Down syndrome and the gastrointestinal tract. J Clin Gastroenterol 1986;8:111.

89. Fonkalsrud EW, DeLorimier AA, Hays DM. Congenital atresia and stenosis of the duodenum: a review compiled from the members of the surgical section of the American Academy of Pediatrics. Pediatrics 1969;43:79.

90. Wesley JR, Mahour GH. Congenital intrinsic duodenal obstruction: a twenty-five year review. Surgery 1977;83:716.

91. Harberg FJ, Pokorny WJ, Hahn H. Congenital duodenal obstruction: a review of 65 cases. Am J Surg 1979;138:825.

92. Puri P, O'Donnell B. Outlook for surgery for congenital intrinsic duodenal obstruction in Down syndrome. Lancet 1981;2:802.

93. Black CT, Sherman JO. The association of low imperforate anus and Down syndrome. J Pediatr Surgery 1989;24:92.

94. Quinn FM, Surana R, Puri P. The influence on trisomy-21 on outcome in children with Hirschsprung's disease. J Pediatr Surg 1994;29:781.

95. Hellemeier C, Buchin PJ, Graboski J. Esophageal dysfunctions in Down syndrome. J Pediatr Gastroenterol Nutr 1982;1:101.

96. Elawad ME. Diaphragmatic hernia in Down syndrome. Ann Trop Paediatr 1989;9:43.

97. Marcus CL, Keens TG, Bautista DB, et al. Obstructive sleep apnea in children with Down syndrome. Pediatrics 1991;88:132.

98. Cavaugh RT, Kahane JC, Kordan B. Risks and benefits of adenotonsillectomy for children with Down syndrome. Am J Ment Defic 1986;91:22.

99. Williams JP, Sommerville GM, Miner ME, et al. Atlantoaxial subluxation and trisomy-21: another perioperative complication. Anesthesiology 1987;67:253.

100. Renner F, Andrle M, Horak W, et al. Hepatitis A and B in noninstitionalized mentally retarded patients. Hepatogastroenterology 1985;32:175.

Surgery of Infants and Children: Scientific Principles and Practice, edited by Keith T. Oldham, Paul M. Colombani, and Robert P. Foglia. Lippincott–Raven Publishers, Philadelphia, © 1997.

CHAPTER 17

Neuropsychiatric Development

Maryland Pao

Children are active, continually evolving, complex organisms who develop in concert with their environments. As they grow and adapt psychosocially, they are subject to many pressures. Physical illness during childhood can place additional stress on children and their families. Medical and surgical specialists working with children should be familiar with child development and the factors influencing psychosocial adaptation, including the following: the child's intelligence, temperament, and social competence; the child's developmental capacity and maturational stage; the child's previous experiences, such as with other illnesses; the nature and severity of the child's illness; the required treatment modalities; and family and community factors. It is important to elicit and document information about these factors whenever possible. Some illness experiences, although unpleasant, can actually be strengthening. Anticipation of potential areas of stress can enhance resilience and result in better treatment outcomes for the child with a severe illness requiring surgery or hospitalization.

This chapter gives a brief overview of normal child development and the impact of chronic illness on development. Children's responses to hospitalization are described, and strategies for coping in the hospital are discussed. Psychiatric aspects of transplantation also are discussed.

NORMAL DEVELOPMENTAL MILESTONES

Norms based on healthy children with intact nervous systems have been established for age, physical growth, and adaptive, cognitive, and social capacities and can be found in most pediatric textbooks. A summary of the highlights of physical, psychologic, and social development and theory can be found in Table 17-1. These norms are not absolute and are meant to be used as a guide. Gestational age assessment criteria are shown in Figure 17-1.

HOW CHILDREN UNDERSTAND ILLNESS

Children's theories about illness and germs generally parallel the acquisition of causal understanding as outlined by Piaget and others.[1] These researchers demonstrated that cognitive development progresses though a systematic and predictable sequence. The *sensorimotor stage* (birth through age 24 months) is characterized by a nonsymbolic understanding of the environment acquired through the senses and motor reflexes. Children learn through the effects of the environment and how it is modified by a caregiver. For example, when children perceive cold, they cry, and the caregiver wraps them in a warm blanket. The hallmark of the *preoperational stage* (age 2 to 7 years) is the development of object permanence and mental representations of objects even when they are removed. It is important to children that even in separation from the caregiver, they can picture the person in their mind and derive comfort from this image. The use of symbols coincides with the rapid expansion of vocabulary. Children normally have difficulty seeing another person's point of view. They generally perceive one aspect of a situation at a time, using immediate temporal and spatial clues. The *concrete operational stage* (age 7 to 11 years) is characterized by the child's ability to classify, serialize, and understand conservation and reversibility. The child is capable of direct observation and understanding cause and effect. The child can see more than one dimension of an object or situation. Finally, the *formal operational stage* (age 11 years to adulthood) is considered the culmination of cognitive development with the ability to reason in abstract terms and to make deductions. Children can more completely differentiate between self, events, and objects in the world and are therefore able to see multiple possibilities in a situation.

Obviously, a child's cognitive stage strongly influences his or her ability to understand an illness and its causes, treatments, and prognosis. Studies have shown that clinicians frequently overestimate the abilities of young children to understand medical explanations and underestimate the cognitive abilities of older children (age 9 years and older). It is important to communicate directly with the patient about the imminent procedure and the medical process. Studies have also shown that physicians communicate almost exclusively with parents, leaving children as passive recipients, which adds to their sense of helplessness.

An assessment of the family's reasoning capacity using the model given earlier also is often useful when communicating important information to parents.

Young children frequently believe that illness is some form

TABLE 17-1. *Physical, psychologic, and social development in children*

Period/age	Physical growth	Gross and fine motor	Language/cognitive	Affect/social	Theory	Stresses
INFANCY						
≤6 mo	Doubles birthweight Eruption of deciduous central incisors	Sits Grasps, transfers toys	Startles to loud/sudden sounds Responds to own name Babbles	Recognizes warning, angry, friendly voices Displays curiosity Reaches in anticipation of being picked up	Attachment/bonding (Bowlby) Oral stage (Freud) Basic trust (Erickson) Sensorimotor stage (Piaget)	Separation from caregivers Difficulty transferring care
12 mo	Triples birthweight Anterior fontanelle of head closes	Walks with help Dislikes any restraint Finger feeds/feeds self Uses index finger to point Neat pincer grasp	First words in addition to mama, dada Understands and uses gestures	Expresses many feelings May recognize feelings in others Stranger anxiety (9 mo) Enjoys active games: peek-a-boo, chasing		Developmental regressions
TODDLERHOOD						
18 mo	Eruption of deciduous first molars	Walks fast, runs stiffly Tries to climb out of crib Shows hand preference Builds tower of 3–4 cubes Scribbles spontaneously Imitates a writing stroke	Follows one-step command Points to own body parts Speaks about 10 words, 2 together Understands simple questions "No" is chief word	Difficulty tolerating frustration Short attention span Temper tantrums with fatigue, anger, or frustration No concept of sharing Pretends Carries special toy or doll	Anal stage (Freud) Autonomy vs shame/doubt (Erikson)	Tendency to tantrum Noncompliance with medical regimens
24 mo	Increase in lymphoid tissue	Runs well, kicks ball Up and down stairs alone without alternating feet Builds tower of 6–7 cubes Right- or left-handed Imitates vertical and circular strokes	Speaks about 50+ words Associates names with most familiar objects Limited understanding of time; language focuses on here and now May reverse pronouns	Has strong positive or negative reactions, "negativistic" Intense sense of self-importance Likes to order others around Anticipates routine events Can help put away toys Parallel play		Coping mechanisms unstable Tendency to regress

Age	Physical	Motor/Adaptive	Language/Cognitive	Social	Developmental theory	Reactions/Concerns
EARLY CHILDHOOD						
3 y	Deciduous teeth calcified Doubles birth height	Hops on one foot Rides a tricycle Can undress self Anal sphincter muscles in control Builds tower of 9–10 cubes Imitates three-cube bridge Copies a circle	Understands about 500 words Can give first and last name Uses three- to four-word sentences Can match four colors Can remember three directions at a time	Frequent mood swings Understands taking turns Enjoys helping others Gender identity: knows own sex, body parts Beginning to play with others	Initiative/imagination versus guilt (Erikson) Preoperational thought (Piaget)	Phobias Susceptible to fears of bodily mutilation Imminent justice, magical thinking Cognitive distortions
4–6 y	Brain, spinal cord, nerves almost adult size Eruption of permanent first molars and central incisors	Walks downstairs one step per tread Skips (5 y), rides two-wheel bike (6 y) Ties shoe laces (6 y) Complete sphincter control Copies cross (4 y), square (4½ y), triangle (5 y), name (6 y)	Speech becomes intelligible, fluent, gramatically correct Understands cause and effect Understands joke, sense of time Can give name and address	Developing guilt Coping with anger, fears of the dark, heights, dogs, death Sensitive to blame and praise Has preferred playmates Play groups along sex lines Curious about birth, marriage, death	Phallic stage (Freud) Industry versus inferiority (Erikson) Concrete operational thought (Piaget) Latency stage (Freud)	Relapse of bedwetting Interference with school learning, social development, motor development
SCHOOL AGE						
7–9 y	Slowest skeletal growth Frontal sinuses develop Cranial sutures harden	Copies diamond (7 y) Copies cross (8 y) Copies cylinder (9 y)	Categorizes, seriates Conserves quantity, weight, and numbers Names days of week (7 y) Repeats five digits forward (8 y)	Competes with partners Ritualistic play Hobbies	Moral development	Decreased mastery, poor self-esteem
10–12 y	Budding of nipples in girls	Copies 3D square (11 y)	Able to rhyme, knows seasons (9 y) Can define brave, nonsense		Identify versus role diffusion (Erikson)	
ADOLESCENCE						
13–15 y	Increased vascularity of penis and scrotum in boys Pubic hair develops Growth spurt (girls before boys) Menses onset		Can define nitrogen, microscope Can divide 72 by 4 without pencil and paper (12 y) Can repeat 6 digits forward	Adjusting to changing body Loosens ties to family Cliques Girls: importance of relationships Boys: sense of masculinity from physical and sexual prowess	Identity versus role diffusion (Erikson) Formal operational stage (Piaget)	Noncompliance Concerns about appearance and medication side effects, surgical scars Wanting to be normal Denial, sense of
15+ y	Growth of testes and penis Facial hair Voice changes in boys			Understands death Able to conceptualize future	Genital stage (Freud)	Denial, sense of invincibility is threatened

Neuromuscular maturity

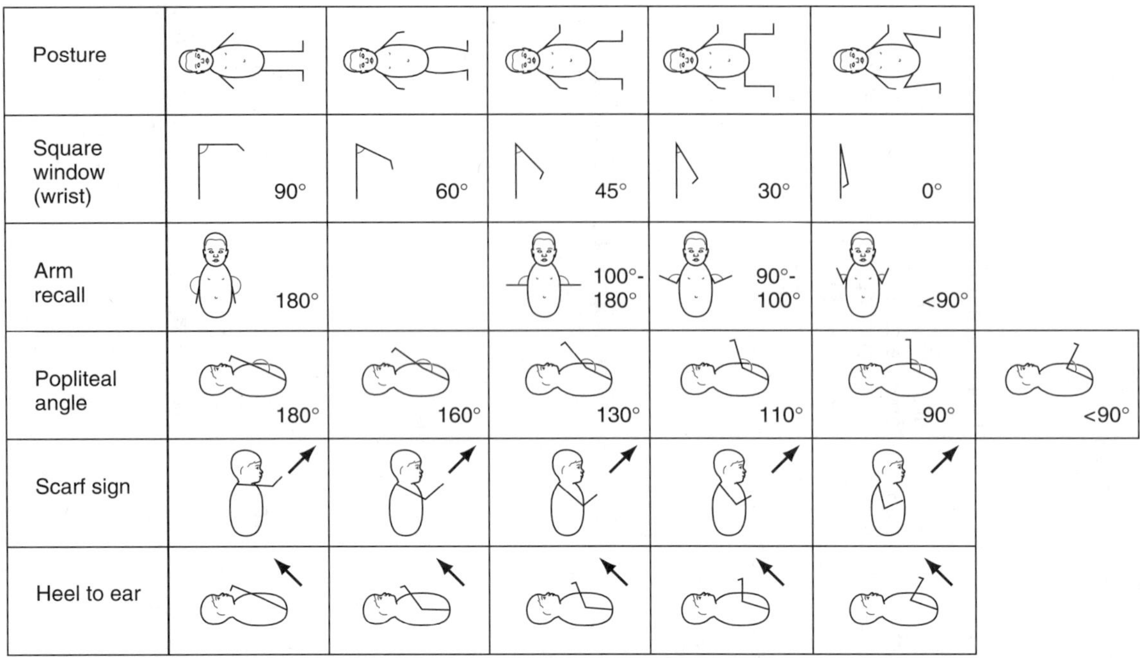

FIG. 17-1. Gestational age assessment based on neuromuscular maturity. The six morphologic and six neurologic criteria, in aggregate, yield an estimation of gestational age. (After Balard J, Novac KK, Driver M, et al. A simplified score of assessment of fetal maturation of newly born infants. J Pediatr 1979;95:769)

of punishment. The concept of *imminent justice* is defined as "the belief that a form of natural justice can emanate from inanimate objects."[1] Children often believe that a bad action or thought can be punished; this can lead to feelings of personal guilt and shame about an illness. Children may not talk about their illnesses because of *magical thinking*—the egocentric be-lief that they can make it go away by not talking about it. In addi-tion, children often initially perceive medical interventions as punishment. Direct inquiry into a child's views and understand-ing is the best way to identify the child's level of comprehension and to appreciate the child's unique misconceptions and con-cerns. It is important to use simple and clear language when talk-

TABLE 17-2. *Psychosocial issues facing parents*

Preoperative	Perioperative	Long-term postoperative
INITIAL HOSPITAL EXPERIENCE	FIRST 24 H	RETURN HOME
Loss of control	Anxiety	Adaptation of new parenting role
Denial of medical reality	Numbness and shock	Fear of rejection or death
Building trust in staff		Readjustment in family structure
	FIRST 2 WK	
WAITING AT HOME	Exhilaration about new beginning	LONG-TERM ISSUES
Concrete tasks	Cease-fire period	Continued public involvement in
Financial burdens	Realignment in parent–child interaction	transplantation issues
Public involvement	Emotional integration of organ	Uncertainties about the future
Guilt		
Death of donor	REMAINDER OF HOSPITALIZATION	
Competition for limited organs	Rollercoaster period	
Burden of informed consent	Fear of rejection or infection	
Anger	Lack of control/powerlessness	
Loss of control	Continued guilt or fear of death	
Feeling forgotten or abandoned	Isolation or marital stress	
Depression		
Endless wait	PREPARATION FOR DISCHARGE	
Child's deteriorating condition	Realization of hospital dependency	
	Building confidence	

(Gold LM, Kirkpatric BS, Fricker FJ, et al. Psychosocial issues in pediatric organ transplantation: the parents' perspective. Pediatrics 1986;77:738)

ing with children and to point out connections between treatment and symptom reduction (eg, elixir for pain relief).

GENERAL REACTIONS TO ILLNESS AND HOSPITALIZATION

Normal children have a number of predictable psychologic and behavioral stress responses to illness and hospitalization. These include regression, which is seen among patients of all ages. In a young child, regression can manifest as a return to the bottle when already weaned or as a setback in new skills, such as walking, talking, or toileting. The child may be more clingy, negative, or restless. The adolescent may become irritable and dependent and be preoccupied, although not always openly, with fear of disfigurement and mutilation of the body. Other commonly described reactions are depression and mood swings; feelings of helplessness, anxiety, denial, and guilt; difficulty sleeping; and acts of aggression and defiance. The patient with a premorbid history of psychopathology may experience aggravation of their psychiatric symptoms. Concerned parents may react with fear, anxiety, guilt, or anger.

Adaptive responses of children and their families to stress depend on many interacting factors, including the following: a history of previous illness and the developmental stage during which it occurred; constitutional endowments, such as the child's temperament; the nature and severity of the illness; parental and other environmental supports; and other psychosocial stressors.

Acute stress can affect endocrine regulation by increasing cortisol secretion, catecholamines, growth hormone, and prolactin and by decreasing testosterone levels. Immune function can also be affected by acute or chronic stress. Studies have shown improved outcomes in adults with breast cancer, melanoma, and acquired immunodeficiency syndrome when stress reduction techniques are introduced to the surgical and medical treatment regimen. No clinical studies on this issue, however, have been reported for children.

Risk factors for developing psychologic disturbances during or after hospitalization include the following: poor parent–child relationship; infancy age group; premorbid psychopathology; the nature and severity of the illness; the amount and kind of preparation necessary for hospitalization; a psychiatric disorder in either parent; parental cognitive understanding of the illness, including unrealistic expectations; and parental feelings of helplessness and pessimism.[2]

PSYCHIATRIC CONSIDERATIONS

Recurrent hospitalizations, particularly before a child is 5 years old, increase the risk for psychiatric symptoms when compared with nonhospitalized controls. About 13% of chronically ill children have emotional problems. A single stressor is not usually enough to cause a significant disorder. Generally, psychiatric disorders arise from experiencing multiple stressors. In the hospital or during or after surgery, children often develop acute stress reactions that manifest as a greater intensity of the symptoms described earlier. These can last hours to days and usually resolve with support.[2]

If a child's response to a known stressor (other than physical illness) is in the form of emotional or behavioral symptoms that last more than 3 months, such as multiple physical complaints, anxious or depressed mood, or aggressive outbursts, the child may be diagnosed with an adjustment disorder in the absence of specific criteria for other syndromes. The symptoms at this juncture generally cause significant impairment in social, occu-

TABLE 17-3. *Possible central nervous system side effects of immunosuppressants and antiinfectious agents*

Agent	Potential neuropsychiatric side effects
IMMUNOSUPPRESSANTS	
Cyclosporine	Tremor, anxiety, delirium, ataxia, seizures, visual hallucinations, disorientation
	Less common: cerebral blindness, paresthesias, dysarthria, paresis
Corticosteroids	Depression, delirium, mania
Azathioprine	None
OKT3	Tremor, aseptic meningitis, seizures, delirium, encephalopathy (?)
FK-506	Headache, anxiety, tremor, restlessness, insomnia, paresthesias, vivid dreams, nightmares, delirium (especially with plasma levels >3 ng/mL)
ANTIINFECTIOUS AGENTS	
Antivirals	
Acyclovir	Tremor, confusion, lethargy, major depression with psychotic features, seizures, agitation, confusion, abnormal electroencephalogram patterns
Dehydroxyphenylglycol	Headache, confusion, seizures, and hallucinations
α-Interferon	Irritability, depression, anxiety, delirium
Antibiotics	
Ciprofloxacin	Restlessness, dizziness, tremor, headache, insomnia, hallucinations, delirium
Cephalosporins	Disorientation, restlessness, anxiety, hallucinations
Sulfonamides	Depression, ataxia, visual and auditory hallucinations
Antifungals	
Amphotericin B	Restlessness, confusion, delirium
Metronidazole	Depression, hallucinations, agitation

(Adapted from Trzepacz PT, DiMartini A, Tringali P. Psychopharmacologic issues in organ transplantation. I. Pharmacokinetics in organ failure and psychiatric aspects of immunosuppressants and anti-infectious agents. Psychosomatics 1993;34:199).

pational, or academic functioning. It has been estimated that between 5% and 15% of children have adjustment disorders. The symptoms should not last longer than 6 months. If they do, another disorder should be considered, even if the adverse circumstance is enduring and it will take longer to reach an effective adaptation. The prognosis for adjustment disorders is much better than for other psychiatric disorders, such as major depression.

If the stress is due to physical illness, psychologic factors may be affecting the child's medical condition. Few outcome data are available for this group. Psychiatric referral is appropriate to help identify stressors, to clarify the role of accompanying developmental changes (which often present with psychologic symptoms, such as in adolescence), and to provide additional support and counseling as needed.

Other symptoms commonly seen by the psychiatric consultation team on surgical services include delirium that is prolonged or exacerbated by serial operations requiring general anesthesia in a short period of time, depression, somatoform disorders, reactions to major pediatric treatment techniques, and family decompensation. In these cases, it is appropriate to seek psychi-atric consultation for additional monitoring, pharmacologic intervention, or counseling.

STRATEGIES FOR FACILITATING COPING IN THE HOSPITAL

Preparing the child and the family for hospitalization and surgical procedures is the most useful and effective tactic to reduce miscommunication and enhance cooperation. If the hospitalization is elective, this can include touring the hospital in advance and explaining in detail the nature and purpose of the procedure and expected related events using age-appropriate language and content. It is helpful and reassuring to describe the feelings and experiences of other children with similar problems. In the acute emergency setting, a member of the team should be assigned to educate and listen to the children and families. Frequent repetition of explanations may be more necessary in the acute setting, when hearing the initial diagnosis sometimes precludes hearing the rest of the discussion.

Additional efforts should be made to discuss the inevitability

---

TABLE 17-4. *Interventions to assist transplant recipients*

INFANCY AND EARLY CHILDHOOD

Minimize separations and number of hospitalizations, allow parents to be present for procedures if tolerable

Encourage transitional objects; continuity of nursing care if possible

Help parents maintain a caregiving role, regain confidence in parenting abilities, and foster normal relationship patterns

Help parents tolerate regression while still encouraging the development of autonomy and self-regulating abilities

Work with parents on helping them distinguish between physical symptoms and signs and emotional distress and to understand their child's experience of illness

Adequate analgesia and cognitive–behavioral techniques during procedures (distraction, storytelling)

Preparation for procedures, including transplantation itself, through play, to foster a sense of active participation and control, turning passive into active; continue to allow working through after surgery and procedures through play; involvement of child life department

Minimize intramuscular injections

Honest explanations in a developmentally informed manner

Be concrete: prehospitalization visits; allow child to touch and hold instruments; use analogies to describe what will happen based on the child's prior experiences; more direct interventions (heating pads, rubbing forehead)

Foster a sense of control: into which arm to have intravenous line put, which test first if there is a choice

LATENCY AGE

Try to maintain continuity with school, peers: visits from teachers, having homework brought to hospital; phone calls, letters

Use the child's growing cognitive abilities to help adjust to transplantation through the use of drawings, reading material, video-tape; reassurance, correction of cognitive distortions; increased use of anatomic and physiologic explanations

Participant modeling and contact with other transplant recipients

Group therapy may be helpful

Denial and suppression are important ego defenses: supportive maneuvers rather than confrontation may be more helpful

ADOLESCENCE

Teach to manage own medication and facilitate development of autonomy

Openness and acceptance of illness and associated feelings may predict better adjustment; role of psychotherapy: denial or suppression may lead to noncompliance

Contact with peers who are also transplant recipients as well as friends from home

Help with issues of who to tell about the transplant, and reintegration into the social milieu

Help find ways to use diet and exercise to control weight gain

Concrete suggestions about how to deal with hirsutism (bleaching, shaving)

Be direct about noncompliance as a major comorbid phenomenon from the beginning, and actively confront if late rejection is in evidence

Help with defining identity and the realization that there are differences between a transplant recipient and his or her peers, although many aspects of adolescent life are similar

Physiologic explanations of illness

(Slater JA. Psychiatric aspects of organ transplantation in children and adolescents. Child Adolesc Psychiatry Clin North Am 1994;3:557).

of some parent separation from the child during the hospitalization, to elicit any fears and anxieties of the child and family so they can be directly addressed, and to reduce potential isolation and disorientation by allowing familiar objects at the bedside or by bringing a clock or a calendar. Identifying anticipated problems in coping allows earlier intervention by nursing, child life, social work, or psychiatry staff. Identifying and adequately managing pain in children are crucial in the treatment of anxiety. The implementation of techniques, such as guided imagery, biofeedback, play therapy, psychotherapy, group therapy, and hypnosis, can enhance a patient's usual coping mechanisms. Community resources, such as religious leaders and specialized camps (eg, diabetes camp), should not be overlooked as additional nonmedical supports for the patient and family.

Over time, parents are encouraged to accept the reality of diagnosis, treatment, and prognosis for their chronically ill child. They should be told that a reasonable degree of regressed and dependent behavior can be expected from the child, but they should also be strongly supported in their efforts to set appropriate and flexible limits and to enforce the necessary restrictions. Parents need encouragement to promote, whenever possible, self-care, regular school attendance, and reasonable physical activities with peers.

Patients and parents emphasize in personal communications that a major contribution by the medical and surgical staff and treatment teams to improved coping is the maintenance of a positive attitude and hope.

PSYCHIATRIC ASPECTS OF ORGAN TRANSPLANTATION

As organ transplantation becomes a more accepted method of treatment for a growing number of disorders, a number of ethical, legal, and psychologic issues surrounding this complex process have been identified and reviewed.[3,4] Children frequently present in the neonatal or infancy period and may never have known what it is like to be completely healthy. Parents face the monumental tasks of accepting a difficult life-threatening diagnosis and treatment program, not to mention the anxiety of determining a donor or waiting for an organ.

The transplantation experience is generally considered in three major stages: the preoperative stage, the perioperative stage, and the long-term postoperative stage. The broad range of psychosocial issues in these stages is outlined in Table 17-2. Preoperative psychiatric and psychosocial evaluation centers around a comprehensive history to identify risk factors for mal-

adaptive coping mechanisms and to identify strengths to promote during the process. Frequently, psychiatric consultation is sought for living donors as well. After transplantation, organic mental changes are not uncommon. Table 17-3 provides a summary of central nervous system side effects of medications frequently used in transplantation patients. Substantial readjustment for the patient and the family ensues after transplantation. Interventions to assist transplant recipients are listed in Table 17-4.

The psychiatric aspects of transplantation are myriad, begin long before the actual operation, and extend far beyond the operating room. This is an area in which thoughtful integration of the consultation and liaison psychiatric teams can play an important role in assessment, treatment, and compliance, helping to promote improved long-term outcomes for the patients and their families.

REFERENCES

1. Schoenfeld DJ. The child's cognitive understanding of illness. In: Lewis M, ed. Child and adolescent psychiatry: a comprehensive textbook. Baltimore, Williams & Wilkins, 1991:949.
2. Lewis M. Introduction to hospital child and adolescent psychiatry consultation-liaison in pediatrics. In: Lewis M, ed. Child and adolescent psychiatry: a comprehensive textbook. Baltimore, Williams & Wilkins, 1991:941.
3. Slater JA. Psychiatric aspects of organ transplantation in children and adolescents. Child Adolesc Psychiatric Clin North Am 1994;3:557.
4. Stuber ML. Psychiatric aspects of organ transplantation in children. Psychosomatics 1993;34:379.

RECOMMENDED READINGS

Caplan F, Caplan T. The second twelve months of life. New York, Bantam Books, 1990.
Caplan F, Caplan T. The early childhood years: the two to six year old. New York, Bantam Books, 1984.
Harris JC. The biopsychosocial approach to pediatrics. In: Oski FA, DeAngelis CD, Feigin RD, et al, eds. Principles and practice of pediatrics. Philadelphia, JB Lippincott, 1990:636.
Lewandowski LA, Baranoski MV. Psychological aspects of acute trauma: intervening with children and families in the inpatient setting. Child Adolesc Psychiatric Clin North Am 1994;3:513.
Parmalee AH. The child's physical health and the development of relationships. In: Sameroff AJ, Emde RN, eds. Relationship disturbances in early childhood: a developmental approach. New York, Basic Books, 1989:145.
Trzepacz PT, DiMartini A, Tringali R. Psychopharmacologic issues in organ transplantation. I. Pharmacokinetics in organ failure and psychiatric aspects of immunosuppressants and anti-infectious agents. Psychosomatics 1993;34:199.

Surgery of Infants and Children: Scientific Principles and Practice, edited by Keith T. Oldham, Paul M. Colombani, and Robert P. Foglia. Lippincott–Raven Publishers, Philadelphia, © 1997.

CHAPTER 18

Medical Ethics and the Pediatric Surgeon

Françoise Baylis and Donna A. Caniano

Advances in pediatric surgery since the mid-1960s have presented pediatric surgeons, neonatologists, and pediatricians with difficult moral problems. Particularly troubling are those clinical situations that involve decisions about the denial or withdrawal of life-saving or life-sustaining treatment for newborns, infants, and children. These decision-making situations have been further complicated by questions concerning the appropriate use of limited health care resources.

In this chapter, a number of moral issues that frequently confront pediatric surgeons are briefly summarized. Each case report is followed by a commentary that focuses on one or more of the central issues raised in the case. But first, a few introductory remarks on medical ethics in general, and ethical decision-making in particular, are appropriate.

WHAT IS ETHICS?

Ethics is a branch of philosophy concerned with questions of right and wrong. It outlines the principles, standards, and rules of conduct that should govern our behavior and guide us in resolving our everyday moral problems. Consider, for example, the maxim *primum non nocere*—"above all, do no harm"—or the principle of beneficence that entreats physicians "to do or promote good." It is from such standards and principles that we derive the physician's commitment to sustain life and relieve suffering.

This social commitment is expressed in professional codes of both ethics and law. The overlap between law and ethics is not surprising given that, in many respects, the law institutionalizes what might be termed a *minimum ethic*—the law articulates a minimum set of legal rules of conduct so that we may live together in relative harmony. The relation between law and ethics, however, is more complicated and controversial than one might first suppose. In addition to areas of overlap, there are important areas of difference, not the least important of which is that the law may be unethical.

WHAT IS A MORAL PROBLEM?

Much of medical ethics focuses on the moral dilemma—a type of moral problem that arises when two (or more) conflict-

ing principles support mutually inconsistent actions. A classic example of a moral dilemma in health care is the conflict that arises between the principles of autonomy and beneficence when the patient makes a choice that does not coincide with the physician's assessment of what is in the patient's best interests. In such instances, the physician can act either in accordance with the patient's expressed wishes or on the basis of the physician's personal estimate of what is in the patient's best interests.

Two other types of moral problems that frequently arise in the health care setting are problems of moral uncertainty and moral distress.[1] Moral uncertainty arises in situations in which the nature of the moral problem is unclear. For example, one might experience some uneasiness at the fact that research subjects have quicker access to specific health care interventions, without being certain which specific moral principles and values are in conflict. As well, there is the problem of moral distress. In this case, one is confident that one understands the nature of the presenting moral problem and knows which principles and values are involved; however, one cannot pursue the chosen course of action or inaction (and "do the right thing") because of institutional constraints, lack of decision-making authority, and so forth. These three types of moral problems are illustrated in the case reports described later.

HOW TO RESOLVE A MORAL PROBLEM

Moral problems can be addressed from a personal or group perspective. That is, efforts at resolving a moral problem can focus on a personal assessment of the rightness or wrongness of a particular course of action or inaction, or the concern can be with group decision-making. Because there is good reason to promote effective shared decision making between physicians and patients,[2] and because contemporary health care is now—in theory, if not always in practice—a team endeavor, the focus here is on decision making in a group context.

A number of steps are necessary to "bring about a concert of moral interests within a team"[3]:

1. The team must develop a common moral language for discussion of moral issues.

2. Team members must have cognitive and practical training in how to articulate rationally their feelings about issues.
3. Value clarification exercises are needed.
4. The team must have common experiences on which to base workable moral policies.
5. The team must develop a moral decision-making method for all to use.

The last of these points merits further commentary. To promote the effective resolution of difficult moral problems, it is imperative that health care teams develop and follow guidelines for moral decision making. For illustrative purposes, a set of guidelines and maxims for decision-making are provided[4]:

GUIDELINES FOR DECISION-MAKING

1. Identify the decision makers. In the case of children, this may be the patient (if the child is an emancipated or mature minor), the parent, or the legal guardian. Hereinafter, parents are referred to as the decision makers because this reflects common practice. It is understood, however, that all claims regarding parents as decision makers apply equally to emancipated or mature minors and to legal guardians.
   Is the patient competent?
   Has the incompetent patient previously expressed feelings or preferences?
   Who is the legal guardian?
2. Gather all medical data.
   What is the illness and its prognosis?
   Is observation, consultation, or testing necessary for further clarification?
3. Define the available treatment options.
   What options are available?
   With each option, what is the likelihood of cure or amelioration?
   What are the risks of an adverse effect?
4. Determine the professionally accepted treatment options.
   To a reasonable medical certainty, does each option offer the possibility of cure, amelioration of illness, or diminution of pain and suffering?
5. Solicit value data from all involved parties.
   Who are the involved parties?
   What is their degree of closeness to the patient?
   Who holds conflicting feelings or values?
   Has the basis for the conflict been clarified?
6. Achieve a consensus resolution.
   Have all parties articulated their viewpoint?
   Is acceptance of the chosen option voluntary?
   Might correction of factual deficiencies resolve the dispute?
   Would a mediator (eg, ethics consultant) or ethics committee be helpful?
   Support all parties despite the outcome.

MAXIMS FOR DECISION-MAKING

1. Good ethics begins with good facts.
2. Rational people of good will may hold views that are opposite and irreconcilable.
3. The best decision is one reached by a consensus of all concerned parties.
4. Legal guardianship resides with parents, but the medical team establishes the minimal level of care.
5. Decisions should not be made in haste.
6. In severe illness, there are rarely happy solutions.
7. In severe illness, all decisions are painful.

In pediatrics and pediatric surgery, difficult moral problems confront physicians and parents when there is severe illness and limited treatment options. The mere passage of time does not make these problems go away, nor does it necessarily make them any easier to deal with. An agreed-on methodology for addressing these problems, however, can do much to promote effective communication between physicians and parents and among members of the health care team. In turn, this makes possible the resolution of controversial moral problems.

CASE 1

Michael, a 4-hour-old 2.3 kg infant, was transferred from a community hospital 50 miles away. The pregnancy had been uncomplicated and considered routine. At birth, the infant experienced immediate respiratory distress and required intubation and ventilatory support. Multiple congenital anomalies were noted (Fig. 18-1). Michael had an enlarged head, cyanosis with a systolic murmur, a large lumbosacral neural tube defect with absence of the skin over the lower half of the back, a low omphalocele, a cloacal exstrophy, two hemibladders with penile remnants, and bilateral club feet. Ultrasound examination of the head, heart, and kidneys showed moderate ventriculomegaly, tetralogy of Fallot, and a single left kidney.

Michael's father, visibly upset and crying, arrived at the hospital with the maternal grandparents. He explained to the nurses that he and his wife were schoolteachers and that they had two other children, girls aged 3 and 5 years. An hour-long conference was held with the pediatric surgeon, who reviewed each of the infant's anomalies, the plan of management, including gender reassignment, and the expected prognosis for each of the anomalies. The father, somewhat overwhelmed by all of the information, asked several questions: What kind of life will our baby have? Are these defects so severe that our baby would be better off not living? Could we decide not to proceed with all of these operations? Would we be doing too much in trying to save this baby?

Commentary

Typically, parents are authorized to consent to or refuse medical treatment on behalf of their children (provided their children are neither emancipated nor mature minors). This authority is conferred on parents in the belief that they are best suited to make decisions that will promote their children's well-being—parents usually care deeply for their children and understand their children's needs. It is also widely recognized that parents bear ultimate responsibility for their children's care and therefore should be actively involved in making health care decisions. It is also held that because parents are responsible for shaping their children's values and beliefs, it is reasonable for them to make health care choices based on the values they would normally teach their children.[5,6]

Parental authority, however, is not absolute. To quote the President's Commission for the Study of Ethical Problems in

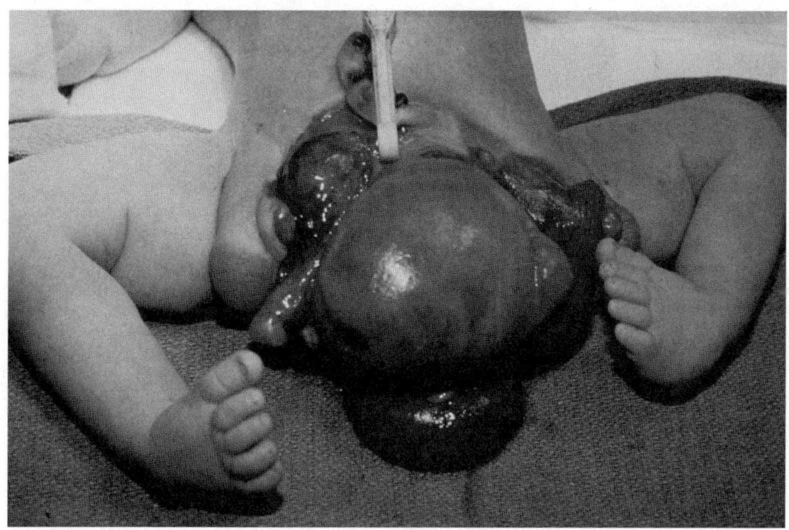

FIG. 18-1. Infant with multiple congenital anomalies.

Medicine and Biomedical and Behavioral Research, "there is a presumption, strong *but rebuttable*, that parents are the appropriate decisionmakers for their infants" (italics added).[7] Specifically, when parents fail to act in the best interests of their children, the state can intervene and exercise its parens patria power to override parental choice and to promote the child's best interests.

But what does it mean to act in a child's best interests?[8,9] In this case, is early surgical intervention followed by repeated surgical interventions (to treat the various congenital anomalies and any sequela from previous surgery) in Michael's best interests? Or, could one reasonably argue that the anticipated benefits of the multiple surgeries are extremely limited, that aggressive treatment likely will result in a life of extreme suffering, and as such that surgery is not in the infant's best interests? To be sure, the prognosis is poor—even if the surgeries are successful, there is a high probability that Michael's life will be one of dependence, chronic physical and mental disability, and multiple life-long hospitalizations. Then again, the final outcome cannot be predicted with certainty, which necessarily complicates the decision making. As John Lantos and Arthur Kohrman write:

> The central ethical principle which guides decision making in pediatrics is that decisions should reflect the best interest of the child. This ethical principle can be applied straightforwardly only in situations in which the facts are clear and well-defined. In conditions of uncertainty, it is difficult to interpret or act on this ethical principle.[10]

What is in Michael's best interests? In the abstract, *best interests* might reasonably be understood as shorthand for: "On balance, given the nature of the anticipated benefits and harms and their likelihood of occurrence, it is believed that the benefits outweigh the harms." On this understanding, a course of action with a low probability of minor harm and a high probability of significant benefit would be in the best interests of the patient. Alternatively, a course of action with a high probability of significant harm and a low probability of minor benefit would *not* be in the best interests of the patient. But, "in the face of inescapable perplexity, ambiguity, ignorance, uncertainty, and conflict,"[11] who determines, and on what basis, which actions

and which outcomes are beneficial or harmful? Is the determining value sanctity of life, quality of life, relief of suffering, parental autonomy, family stability and well-being, or respect for religious and cultural beliefs? Many of these values are clearly incompatible—hence the potential for conflict among the concerned parties (eg, physicians, other members of the health care team, and parents) in determining what is in a child's best interests.

In addition to concerns about the child's best interests, there may be concerns about the family's best interests.[12] Whereas some argue that family interests are irrelevant and that an ethically sound decision requires a narrow focus on the child,[13] others insist that family interests should not be ignored, especially when the proposed treatment will provide little or no benefit for the child but will impose serious burdens on the family.[14] In Michael's case, there are both the short- and long-term emotional, physical, and financial consequences for the family of proceeding with aggressive treatment. For some, these consequences are not incidental to any discussion concerning the ethically appropriate course of action.

This debate aside, suppose that the family and the physician agree not to proceed with surgery (based on the child's best interests, the family's best interests, or some other interests). A further moral question then arises: How should Michael be managed? For example, should fluids be withheld? Should Michael be extubated? These and similar questions cannot be answered in the abstract because input from all involved parties is required (as per the guidelines for decision-making cited earlier). An overriding consideration, however, is that neither the infant nor the family be abandoned. To state the obvious, in *specific* cases, it may be appropriate to withhold or withdraw aggressive treatment, but it is never appropriate to withhold or withdraw care and compassion. On this view, if a decision were made to forgo treatment (ie, the multiple surgeries), Michael would still need to be provided with warmth, sustenance (ie, enteric feeding and hydration), *adequate* pain control (ie, medication in doses not intended to hasten death or to have a persistently sleeping child), and physical contact; and his family may require emotional support.

Contrary to the view of many physicians, this approach is

not prohibited by the so-called Baby Doe regulations—the 1984 amendments to the Child Abuse Prevention and Treatment Act[15] and the regulations issued by the Department of Health and Human Services.[16] Specifically, the Child Abuse Amendments of 1984, introduced in response to the Baby Doe experience,[17,18] stipulate that to qualify for federal child abuse and neglect funds, the state must have programs or procedures for responding to reports of medical neglect, including the withholding of medically indicated treatment from a disabled infant with a life-threatening condition. Medically indicated treatment is defined as "treatment (including appropriate nutrition, hydration, and medication) that, in the treating physician's reasonable medical judgment, will be most likely to be effective in ameliorating or correcting all such [life-threatening] conditions."[19]

According to the Act,[19] treatment other than appropriate nutrition, hydration, and medication may be withheld only in those cases in which:

1. The infant is chronically and irreversibly comatose.
2. The provision of such treatment would merely prolong dying or not be effective in ameliorating all of the infant's life-threatening conditions, or otherwise be futile in terms of the survival of the infant.
3. The provision of such treatment would be virtually futile in terms of the survival of the infant, and the treatment itself under such circumstances would be inhumane.

To be clear, the Act does *not*,[17]

> . . . create federally mandated standards of medical care for newborns, nor does it set standards to which the parents of newborns must comply when deciding about treatment for their child . . . . Legally, because the application of the Baby Doe law is linked to the funding of states by the federal government, the only entity that can violate the Baby Doe law is a state that has accepted a child abuse prevention grant.

It follows that the Baby Doe regulations do not impose on physicians and parents a duty to treat aggressively all impaired newborns.

CASE 2

Kelly, an 8-year-old, is admitted to the hospital for evaluation of fever, generalized bone pain, and an abdominal mass. She is diagnosed with stage IV neuroblastoma with metastases to the cranium, long bones, liver, and bone marrow. The abdominal tumor involves the entire upper retroperitoneum encasing the celiac and proximal aorta. Biopsy of the tumor confirms the pathology to be Shimada, unfavorable histology, with an n-myc amplification greater than 25. The pediatric surgeon and the oncologist meet with Kelly's parents to discuss proceeding with aggressive treatment and including Kelly in a national children's cancer study. The plan of management would include multiagent chemotherapy, radiation therapy, eventual resection of the abdominal tumor, and bone marrow transplantation.

Kelly's parents ask about the survival of other children with advanced neuroblastoma. They are told that almost no children with a disease as involved as their daughter's have been long-term survivors. The parents then wonder out loud if it is right to subject their daughter to the ordeal of prolonged aggressive treatment if she is going to die anyway. They ask about alternative measures, such as comfort care, hospice, and pain medication. Next, they request time to consult with their priest and other family members.

Commentary

A first question to consider is whether it is appropriate for the pediatric surgeon and the oncologist to recommend aggressive intervention when the chance of survival is extremely poor. More generally, when should physicians accept the limits of medicine and recommend palliative care? To quote Hippocrates,[20] "the functions of medicine are three-fold: to relieve pain, to reduce the violence of disease and to refrain from trying to cure those whom disease has conquered, acknowledging that in such cases medicine is powerless."

From another perspective, one might ask whose interests are served by enrolling Kelly in the national children's cancer study—Kelly's? her parent's? society's? With the previous case, the discussion focused on the patient's and the family's best interests. This case extends the discussion to consider the interests of others because the knowledge that may be gained from the clinical trial potentially could benefit future patients with similar disease. Should physicians encourage parents to consider potential benefits to others in decisions regarding their children's health care? In this case, the issue is complicated because care and research are inextricably linked.

As noted previously, parents are expected to consent to medically indicated treatments (ie, established therapies deemed to be in their children's best interests.) There is, however, no presumed parental obligation to consent to research (eg, experimental interventions that could result in harm). Rather, consent to research involving children is generally at the parents' discretion, provided the research is scientifically and ethically valid.

Federal regulations governing research involving children[21] (based on the recommendations of the National Commission for the Protection of Human Subjects of Biomedical and Behavioral Research[22]) permit research in three broad categories: (1) research not involving greater than minimal risk, (2) research presenting the prospect of direct benefit to the individual subjects, and (3) research involving greater than minimal risk and no prospect of direct benefit to individual subjects, but likely to yield generalizable knowledge about the subject's disorder or condition. In the regulations,[23] " 'minimal risk' means that the risks of harm anticipated in the proposed research are not greater, considering probability and magnitude, than those ordinarily encountered in daily life or during the performance of routine physical or psychological examinations or tests."

Case 2 falls within the second category of acceptable research involving children. For such research to proceed, the Institutional Review Board must find that[21]:

• The risk is justified by the anticipated benefit to the subjects
• The relation of the anticipated benefit to the risk is at least as favorable to the subjects as that presented by available alternative approaches
• Adequate provisions are made for soliciting the assent of the children and permission of their parents or guardians . . . when, in the judgment of the Institutional Review Board, the children are capable of providing assent

The risk of harm in this case includes morbidity from the interventions as well as pain and emotional suffering—all of which could significantly detract from Kelly's future quality of life. For some, this potential harm compares favorably with the risk of harm that Kelly "ordinarily encounters in daily life," given that she is afflicted with a lethal condition for which there "is no available treatment alternative other than aggressive multimodality interventions." Also, the potential for direct benefit to the subject—namely, the prolongation of life—arguably justifies the risk of harm. Longer life might allow Kelly to achieve personal goals (eg, Special Wish) and to access future, possibly more effective, treatments. Kelly's parents could choose to begin the aggressive treatment and to enroll their daughter in the national cancer trial, provided that Kelly were involved in the relevant decision making to the extent that she was capable, taking into consideration her age, maturity, and psychological state.

Whereas in the past, practice has been to shelter dying children from the truth, it is now more widely accepted that children should be told the truth and included in relevant discussions regarding their care. Children cannot provide a morally or legally valid consent to or refusal of treatment or research, but they can meaningfully participate in decisions concerning their care by way of assent or dissent. This viewpoint has most recently been endorsed by the American Academy of Pediatrics. The *Guidelines on Forgoing Life-Sustaining Medical Treatment* explicitly state that: "[C]hildren should have the opportunity to participate in decisions about LSMT [Life-Sustaining Medical Treatment] to whatever extent their abilities allow."[23] On this view, Kelly and her parents, in consultation with their physician, are best suited to decide whether to proceed with the aggressive treatment and the cancer trial.

CASE 3

Timothy is a 16-year-old resident of a chronic care facility. He has profound developmental disabilities, including blindness, spastic cerebral palsy, seizures, and kyphoscoliosis. He is completely bedridden and has minimal responses to external stimuli. Recently, Timothy developed recurrent pneumonia and was diagnosed with aspiration secondary to gastroesophageal reflux. With the consent of his legal guardian, he was admitted to hospital for an antireflux procedure, and his case was presented on rounds by the attending pediatric surgeon.

After a discussion of the pathophysiology of gastroesophageal reflux, a colleague asked the attending physician why this patient was admitted for the antireflux procedure. In his view, the intervention was futile, given the patient's very limited quality of life.

Commentary

The claim that a certain treatment is futile is very powerful. Why? Because there is no moral imperative to do that which is not possible. From this, it follows that there is no moral obligation to provide futile medical treatment. But notice, this claim presumes that the term *futile* corresponds with that which is not possible, as when life-saving or life-supporting treatment is "physiologically futile"—that is, when there is *no* probability of medical benefit. For example, mechanical ventilation is physiologically futile if it will not maintain adequate ventilation and oxygenation. Similarly, cardiopulmonary resuscitation (CPR) is physiologically futile if it will not maintain adequate cardiac output and respiration (eg, when there is a cardiac rupture or a severe outflow obstruction).

In contemporary health care, however, this is not the understanding of futility that most health professionals have when they label a particular intervention futile. More often, the term futile is used when there is a *very small* probability that the proposed intervention will achieve its goal. The problem with this understanding of futility is that often there is disagreement within the health care team or between physicians and patients (or parents) about the goals of the intervention and the minimal acceptable probability of success. For example, with CPR, is the goal to survive resuscitation (ie, to restore pulse and blood pressure)? Is the goal short-term survival in hospital (conscious and not dependent on intensive medical care)? Or, is the goal survival until hospital discharge? Second, is a 0.05%, 0.1%, 2%, or 5% chance of success sufficient for CPR (or some other life-saving intervention) not to be considered futile?

A third understanding of futility is perhaps even more controversial. It is believed by some that although a proposed intervention may achieve its medical goal, it may nevertheless be undesirable from a medical standpoint because its probable effectiveness is low *and* the patient's quality of life (either before or after the life-saving or life-supporting treatment) is unacceptable. This understanding of futility is the one relied on by the physician who questioned the decision to admit Timothy for the antireflux procedure. Timothy is in a near-vegetative state, his quality of life is very poor, and in the view of at least some physicians, a major surgical intervention *may not be appropriate.*

Notice here the intentional shift on our part, as authors, away from the language of futility, to the language of appropriate care. This marks an attempt to sidestep the definition debate about futility, and to focus instead on what care is appropriate in a given case, the objective being not to impose on patients treatment that is disproportionately burdensome.

As regards the case of Timothy, the overriding concern should be whether the proposed antireflux procedure imposes more burdens than benefits. In focusing on this question, physicians and other members of the health care team are in a better position to ascertain whether aggressive intervention, conservative management, or palliative care (relieving symptoms, easing pain, maximizing comfort and dignity) is most appropriate. The next step is to initiate a discussion with his legal guardian[24]:

> Where a doctor considers a life-prolonging treatment not to be physiologically futile, but nonetheless "futile" in another sense of the word because of the low probability of success or because of the low quality of life that would remain, then decisions about the withholding or withdrawal of such treatments should be made in the context of full and open discussion of the nature and extent of the "futility" of the treatment with the patient or the patient's representative.

In more general terms, if we are not talking about what is or is not possible, but about what is or is not worth doing, then we must take into consideration the value of all parties involved in the decision-making. As John Lantos and colleagues write[25]:

By suggesting that futility determinations cannot be based on reasonable medical judgement alone, but must include an explicit consideration of patient [or parent/legal guardian] values, we challenge many ethical, legal, and policy presumptions about futility claims and question the appropriateness of unilateral decisions to forego therapy . . . the framework for these determinations should be one of shared decision-making.

CASE 4

Kara is a 3-week-old, 720-g, 26-week–gestation infant who required aggressive resuscitation at delivery and continued respiratory support. At 2 weeks of age, she developed rapidly progressive necrotizing enterocolitis with pneumoperitoneum. At operation, the bowel was necrotic from the proximal ileum to the sigmoid colon. The bowel was resected and end stomas were created.

Kara has since had a complicated postoperative course with ongoing sepsis, worsening of lung disease necessitating escalation of ventilatory support, and a grade III to IV intraventricular hemorrhage. Her renal function is deteriorating with minimal urine output and rising serum blood urea nitrogen and creatinine levels. From the outset, Kara's mother has been insistent that everything possible be done for her daughter, while the father has questioned the prognosis for Kara and stated that he would not want her to be handicapped. As Kara's condition worsens, the pediatric surgeon and neonatologist decide that further aggressive treatment is not beneficial. They approach the parents about Kara's declining status and request that the parents agree to a do-not-resuscitate (DNR) order. Kara's mother becomes upset and refuses to agree, while her father says that no further treatment should be done.

Commentary

It is widely assumed that parents speak in one voice when making health care decisions for their children. In practice, however, it is not uncommon for spouses to disagree with each other regarding what constitutes their child's best interests. Although physicians may be legally entitled to act on the expressed wishes of one parent, there are compelling moral and psychological reasons for considering the views of both parents and trying to have them make a joint decision.

To this end, when there is conflict between parents concerning the care and treatment of their child, it is imperative that physicians engage in repeated dialogue with the parents and other members of the health care team to ensure that all treatment decisions are made in an effective and timely manner. At the discretion of the concerned parties, these discussions may be held with both parents present or with one parent at a time.

If this attempt at facilitation is unsuccessful, the next step is to involve one or more people with social, ethical, or spiritual expertise. In turn, if this initiative fails, some recommend recourse to a multidisciplinary institutional ethics committee. For example[26]:

> The American Academy of Pediatrics believes that hospital-based ''infant bioethics committees,'' consisting of both physicians and non-physicians, can provide consultation and review, ensuring sensitive treatment decisions made in a rea-

soned, informed, and caring manner. Infant bioethics committees can . . . offer consultation to providers and families facing a range of ethical problems or questions about medical treatment of infants.

It is only appropriate to consult an institutional ethics committee, however, if the committee is skilled in case review. Some ethics committees are new and lack experience in case analysis; other committees are designed primarily to address the educational and policy-making needs of the institution. Case review by these committees may be little more helpful than review by the courts, which is usually a last resort. This being said, experience suggests that the key to a successful resolution of parental conflict is time and continued dialogue with concerned parties in a supportive and caring environment. In this context, it is not uncommon for a resolution of the conflict to emerge as one of the parents shifts viewpoint, perhaps having developed a better understanding of the medical situation through witnessing the child's deterioration.

CASE 5

Joseph, a 16-year-old with Duchenne muscular dystrophy, has a tracheostomy and is ventilatory dependent. He has recently been admitted for a left lower lobe pneumonia and a pleural effusion. Despite aggressive antibiotics and chest tube drainage, he has developed an empyema with continued high fever and a worsening clinical status. Although Joseph and his parents have previously agreed to a DNR order with their primary physician, they want to proceed with operative management of the empyema. The anesthesiologist is concerned about the DNR order during the intraoperative period.

Commentary

All hospitals seeking accreditation from the Joint Commission on Accreditation of Healthcare Organizations must have a DNR policy.[27] Surprisingly few of these policies, however, include specific guidelines regarding DNR orders in the operating room.[28] This leaves unanswered a critical question: How should pediatric surgeons and anesthesiologists proceed when parents consent to palliative surgery for their children, but also want to forgo resuscitation in the event of cardiac arrest? Typically, pediatric surgeons and anesthesiologists are not involved in the original DNR decision, nor are they consulted about how to implement it during surgery.

Many pediatric surgeons and anesthesiologists maintain that DNR orders should be suspended during the intraoperative period, given the distinctive nature of cardiac arrest and resuscitation during surgery. A cardiac arrest in the intraoperative period usually can be reversed with little or no adverse effects, thereby allowing the patient to achieve his or her surgical objective (eg, palliation). By comparison, a cardiac arrest in the intensive care unit or on the general medical ward that results from the patient's underlying disease has a higher likelihood of resulting in severe brain damage, irreversible coma, or significant morbidity. Moreover, in these settings, resuscitation clearly thwarts the patient's or parents' objective not to prolong the dying process.

Another unique feature of cardiac arrest and resuscitation in the intraoperative period, from the surgeon's and anesthesiologist's perspective, concerns personal responsibility for a reversible arrest precipitated by a surgical or anesthetic complication. As Charles Bosk writes[29]:

> The specific nature of surgical treatment links the action of the physician and the response of the patient more intimately than in other areas of medicine. In many branches of internal medicine the physician's interventions are relatively nonspecific. This fact allows internists to attribute failure to the inevitable pathophysiology of the disease process rather than to the nature of the treatment itself . . . . When the patient of an internist dies, the natural question his colleagues ask is, ''What happened?'' When the patient of a surgeon dies, his colleagues ask, ''What did you do?'' By the nature of his craft and his beliefs about it, the surgeon is more accountable than other physicians and he also has much more to account for. Of course, this is not to say that every time a surgical patient dies the surgeon is at fault, only that it is much harder for him to claim that he had no hand in it than it is for other colleagues.

For these and other reasons, some DNR policies require the automatic suspension of DNR orders in the operating room.[30] In hospitals in which such policies (or practices) are in effect, ethics demands (at the very least) that patients, their parents, or both be informed of the policy (practice) so that they can weigh the anticipated benefits of palliation against the potential harms of unwanted resuscitation when deciding about whether to consent to surgery.

Other hospitals do not require the automatic suspension of DNR orders before surgery. This practice is consistent with the view that ''[a]dmission to the operating room should not be ruled out solely because there is a DNR order.''[31] Advocates of this viewpoint propose, as an alternative, a ''required reconsideration'' of the DNR status; the objective is to encourage shared decision making. In dialogue with the patient, the parents, or both the physician explains the distinctive nature of cardiac arrest and resuscitation in the intraoperative period, the increased likelihood of successful resuscitation in the operating room, and the commitment to withdraw ineffective life support (such as ventilator and vasopressors) when recovery is unlikely. It is expected that this conversation will lead to a temporary suspension of the DNR order.

This flexible approach promotes shared decision making involving the patient, the parents, the surgeon, and the anesthesiologist. It helps to ensure that all parties are clear about the unique aspects of cardiac dysfunction or arrest during anesthesia and the relative ease with which such cardiac events can be reversed. At one major children's hospital where this flexible approach is practiced, most patients and parents agree to suspend the DNR order during the intraoperative period, in light of the anticipated benefits of the operation.[32]

If a DNR order is to be suspended during the intraoperative period, decisions about the timing of its reinstatement must be addressed before the surgical procedure is undertaken. Questions to consider include: At what point should ventilatory assistance be withdrawn after the operation? If there is a postoperative infection, should antibiotics be prescribed? The resolution of such issues depends, in part, on the patient's clinical status, but ultimately rests on the patient's and family's desires, beliefs, and values.

Disagreement arising from differences in values and beliefs requires a sound methodology for conflict resolution. Moral problems in pediatric surgery can be approached through shared decision-making.

> Consensus does not meant that everyone thinks that the decision made is necessarily the best one possible, or even that they are sure it will work. What it does mean is that in coming to that decision, no one felt that her position on the matter was misunderstood or that it wasn't given proper hearing.[33]

Shared decision-making is the key to effective resolution of difficult moral problems, particularly as the health and well-being of the next generation is at stake.

REFERENCES

1. Jameton A. Nursing practice: the ethical issues. Englewood-Cliff, NJ, Prentice-Hall, 1984:6.
2. Brock DW. The ideal of shared decision making between physicians and patients. Kennedy Institute of Ethics Journal 1991;1:28.
3. Thomasma D. Moral education in interdisciplinary teams. Surg Tech 1982;2:17.
4. Radetsky M. Decisions to limit, diminish, or withdraw therapy. In: Nussbaum E, ed. Pediatric intensive care, ed 2. Mount Kisco, NY, Futura, 1989:143, 156.
5. Baylis F. When a child objects to medical treatment: the case of Philip. Ethics in medical practice 1993;3:1.
6. Brock DW. Children's competence for health care decision making. In: Kopelman LM, Moskop JC, eds. Children and health care: moral and social issues. Boston, Kluwer Academic Publishers, 1989:181.
7. President's Commission for the Study of Ethical Problems in Medicine and Biomedical and Behavioral Research. Deciding to forego life-sustaining treatment: ethical, medical and legal issues in treatment decisions. Washington, DC, US Government Printing Office, 1983:212.
8. Brody H. In the best interests of . . . . Hastings Center Report 1988; 18:37.
9. Bartholome WG. In the best interest of . . . . Hastings Center Report 1988;18:39.
10. Lantos JD, Kohrman AF. Ethical aspects of pediatric home care. Pediatrics 1992;89:922.
11. Bartholome WG. In the best interest of . . . . Hastings Center Report 1988;18::40.
12. Hardwig J. What about the family? Hastings Center Report 1990;20: 5.
13. Weir R. Selective nontreatment of handicapped newborns: moral dilemmas in neonatal medicine. New York, Oxford University Press, 1984.
14. Strong C. The neonatologist's duty to patients and parents. Hastings Center Report 1984;14:10.
15. US Child Abuse Prevention and Treatment Amendments of 1984, Public Law 98–457.
16. US Department of Health and Human Services. Child abuse and neglect prevention and treatment program. 50 Fed Reg 14878, 1985.
17. Nelson LJ. Perinatology/neonatology and the law: looking beyond Baby Doe. In: Oski FA, Stockman JA, eds. Year book of pediatrics. Chicago, Year Book Medical Publ, 1988:5.
18. Strain JE. The American Academy of Pediatrics comments on the ''Baby Doe II'' regulations. N Engl J Med 1983;309:443.
19. US Department of Health and Human Services. Child abuse and neglect prevention and treatment program. 50 Fed Reg 14878, 1985.
20. Jones WHS, translator. Hippocratic corpus: the art. Quoted in: Jonsen AR. Imitations of futility. Am J Med 1994;96:107.
21. Additional protections for children involved as subjects in research. 45 CFR 46; 48 Fed Reg 9818, 1983.
22. National Commission for the Protection of Human Subjects of Biomedical and Behavioral Research. Research involving children: report and recommendations. DHEW Publ no (OS) 77-0004, Washington DC, 1977.
23. American Academy of Pediatrics. Guidelines on forgoing life-sustaining medical treatment. Pediatrics 1994;93:532.
24. The Appleton international conference: developing guidelines for deci-

sions to forgo life-prolonging medical treatment. J Med Ethics 1992; 18(Suppl):6.

25. Lantos JD, Singer PA, Walker RM, et al. The illusion of futility in clinical practice. Am J Med 1989;87:83.

26. Infant Bioethics Task Force and Consultants. American Academy of Pediatrics guidelines for infant bioethics committees. Pediatrics 1984; 74:306.

27. Joint Commission on Accreditation of Healthcare Organizations. Accreditation manual for hospitals. Chicago, Joint Commission of Accreditation of Healthcare Organizations; 1991:77.

28. Personal communications with Monagle JF, Thomasma DC. Medical ethics: policies, protocols, guidelines and programs. Gaithersburg, MD, Aspen Publishers, 1993.

29. Bosk CL. Forgive and remember: managing medical failure Chicago, University of Chicago Press, 1979:29.

30. Truog RD. Do-not-resuscitate orders during anaesthesia and surgery. Anaesthesiology 1991;74;606.

31. Cohen CB, Cohen PJ. Do-not-resuscitate orders in the operating room. N Engl J Med 1991;325:1880.

32. Couper C. DNR in the OR. (Letter) JAMA 1992;267:1465.

33. Women's encampment for a future of peace and justice: Seneca Army Depot. New York: 42.

SECTION **B**

Trauma

Surgery of Infants and Children: Scientific Principles and Practice, edited by
Keith T. Oldham, Paul M. Colombani, and Robert P. Foglia.
Lippincott–Raven Publishers, Philadelphia, © 1997.

CHAPTER 19

Approach to the Pediatric Trauma Patient

David K. Magnuson and Martin R. Eichelberger

BASIC CONSIDERATIONS

Scope of the Problem

Trauma disrupts more young lives and exacts a higher socioeconomic price than any other pediatric health-related issue in the
industrialized world. More children between 1 and 14 years of
age die each year of injuries than from all other diseases combined (Fig. 19-1). This is a sobering fact when one considers
the level of public attention and concern over other diseases,
such as cancer and the acquired immunodeficiency syndrome.
Perhaps this is because childhood injuries, both accidental and
intentional, and their prevention are more inextricably linked
to intransigent social behavior than are most other disease processes.

Consider that more than 20,000 children and adolescents die
of their injuries each year, and that about 50,000 suffer permanent disability, most of which is neurologic.[1] The societal cost,
in terms of both direct medical expenses for care and rehabilitation and lost opportunities for socioeconomic contribution, is
staggering. Except for prevention, the component of trauma
management that offers the greatest chance of limiting or mitigating this carnage is rapid and effective resuscitation.

This chapter discusses some of the biochemical and physiologic derangements that are caused by both injury and resuscitation, reviews salient features of resuscitation techniques with
emphasis on the child, and describes some areas of controversy
and investigation. Its goal is to create a framework of biologic
principles and clinical observations within which basic trauma
management can be applied to the injured child.

Definition of Resuscitation and Impact on Outcome

Resuscitation of the injured child essentially includes all the
judgments and actions necessary to reverse and control the sudden alterations in physiologic homeostasis that occur as the
result of mechanical trauma. It begins with the recognition of
serious injury and progresses through basic first aid, advanced
prehospital care rendered by paramedics, aggressive and invasive maneuvers performed in the emergency department, and
definitive stabilization in the operating room and intensive care
unit. Resuscitation is not complete until injuries have been definitively treated and the child displays physiologic stability
without continued intervention. This chapter focuses, however,
on a narrower definition of resuscitation—the acute restoration,
maintenance, and monitoring of physiologic function immediately after injury.

Differences between children and adults with respect to patterns of injury, physiologic presentation, and management are
well recognized. These differences, however, are blurred both
by the continuum of ages treated by pediatric surgeons and by
trends of increasing injury severity as children and adolescents
become victims of societal violence. Nevertheless, important
distinctions do exist, and those who treat pediatric trauma must
recognize and understand these nuances so that the resuscitation
process addresses the special needs of the injured child.

The principle of a trimodal pattern of trauma-related mortality and morbidity in adults must be modified for children. In
the trimodal model, early deaths that occur within minutes of
the traumatic event invariably result from extreme physiologic
derangement that exceeds the body's ability to compensate. Prevention through social awareness and behavior modification is
the only avenue likely to reduce this mortality. A second mortality peak occurs several hours after the insult. Although initial
physiologic compensation may have been sufficient to achieve
some temporary accommodation, progressive dysfunction and
exhausted reserves bring about a critical impairment of oxygen
delivery and the patient's eventual demise. This group has been
impacted most effectively and positively by advances in the
aggressive and systematized delivery of emergency medical services.

A third mortality peak occurs days to weeks after the initial
injury and represents the end result of processes that begin
within hours after injury, and that persist and progress despite
successful early intervention. Accepted paradigms attribute
these deaths to uncontrolled systemic autoinflammation leading
to *multiple organ failure syndrome,* also referred to as *systemic
inflammatory response syndrome*. This generalized, unregulated inflammatory response can be initiated by ischemia–reperfusion injury, infection, and products of tissue destruction,
and can generate a widespread cascade of cytokine and cellular
responses.[2] This late peak in trauma-related mortality is infrequently observed in younger children. As physicians involved

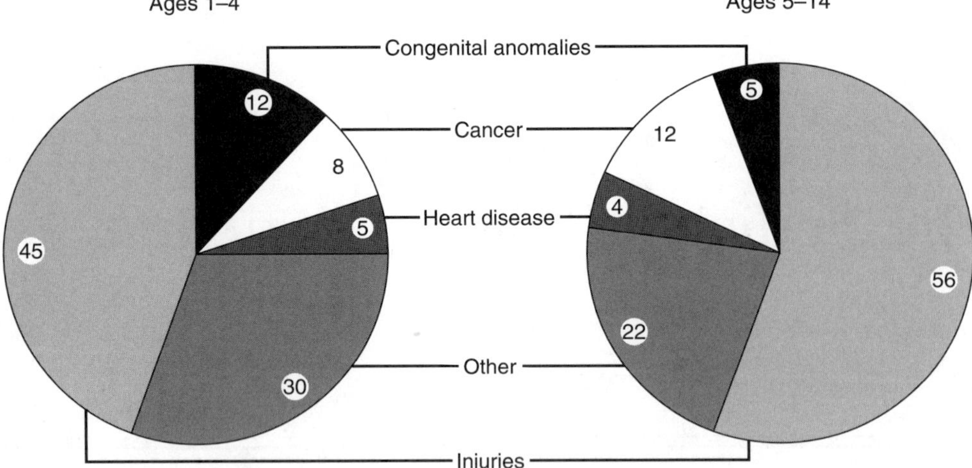

FIG. 19-1. Percentage of childhood deaths by cause.

with pediatric trauma are confronted with the accelerating incidence of severe nonaccidental trauma in young patients, an increased experience with multiple organ failure syndrome can be anticipated.

PATHOPHYSIOLOGY OF INJURY AND RESUSCITATION

Most of the serious morbidity and mortality that occur in the early posttraumatic period are caused by impaired oxygen delivery to vital organs due to global circulatory insufficiency (shock) and reduced oxygen content in circulating blood. Hypoxemia results from many causes, including airway obstruction, ventilatory failure, and compromised cardiac output from hemorrhage and impaired venous return. The immediate consequences of hypoxemia and hypoperfusion after mechanical trauma are progressive cellular ischemia leading to dysfunction and cell death. Although effective resuscitation can limit and ultimately reverse cellular ischemia, biochemical changes have already occurred that instigate an ongoing pathologic cascade of neuroendocrine messengers, inflammatory mediators, cytokines, and activated cells. Furthermore, reperfusion of ischemic tissues generates a deleterious autoinflammatory and cytotoxic process, referred to as *ischemia–reperfusion injury.*

Oxygen Delivery, Ischemia, and Reperfusion

Oxygen delivery to metabolically active cells is determined by two parameters—cardiac output and blood oxygen content—which are in turn dependent on variables that are altered by both injury and therapeutic intervention. Cardiac output is the product of stroke volume and heart rate:

$$\text{cardiac output} = \text{stroke volume} \times \text{heart rate}$$

Heart rate depends on the chronotropic effects of circulating catecholamines that exist in increased concentrations immediately after trauma. Stroke volume reflects myocardial performance and is dependent on three determinants: preload, contractility, and afterload.

Preload depends on venous return and is manifest physiologically as left ventricular end-diastolic volume (LVEDV), which is estimated with variable precision by pulmonary artery wedge pressure or central venous (right atrial) pressure. As LVEDV increases, so does stroke volume (Starling's law). This relation is consistent for any contractile state; the increase in stroke volume does not reflect a change in contractility, but rather a positive shift along the Starling curve for that given contractile state.

The *contractile state,* experimentally defined as the rate of force generation during contraction, determines the position and shape of the Starling curve. An increase in contractility shifts the whole curve to the left, so that a given LVEDV generates a larger stroke volume (Fig. 19-2). Contractility is determined by the level of catecholamine stimulation and the availability of oxygen.

Afterload describes the systemic vascular resistance (SVR) to

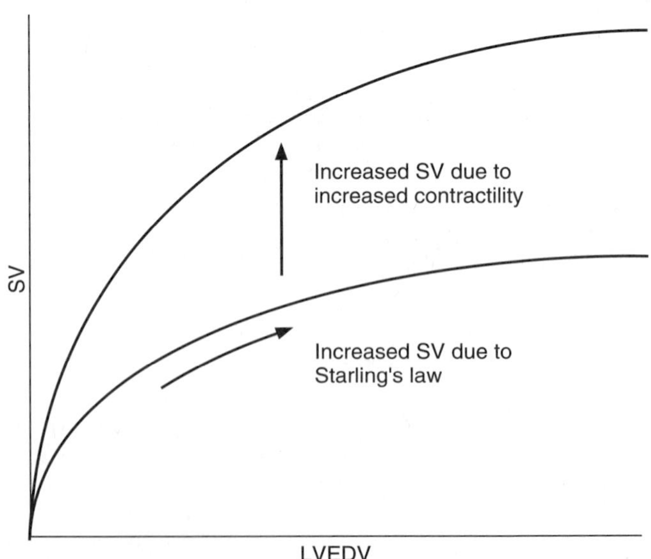

FIG. 19-2. Cardiac response to increased preload (LVEDV) and contractility.

left ventricular outflow and is determined largely by vasomotor constriction within arteriolar resistance vessels. SVR is compensatorily increased in hemorrhagic shock and reduced in septic and neurogenic shock. Sepsis is also characterized by a pathologic redistribution of flow through precapillary shunts, circumventing metabolically active tissue.

The other main determinant of oxygen delivery, blood oxygen content, is determined by the concentration of hemoglobin and its oxygen saturation. Dissolved oxygen represents a trivial amount and is generally ignored in most clinical situations. This may change with the development of synthetic perfluorocarbon resuscitation solutions that dissolve large quantities of oxygen. Oxygen saturation of hemoglobin is dependent on P_{O_2} and the affinity of hemoglobin for oxygen, which is altered by acidosis, temperature, and P_{CO_2}.

Compromised oxygen delivery in the injured child occurs by many mechanisms, including reduced P_{O_2} from hypoventilation or parenchymal lung injury, reduced hemoglobin due to hemorrhage, reduced myocardial contractility and hemoglobin affinity due to acidosis, and preload reduction from hypovolemia, tension hemopneumothorax, and cardiac tamponade. Virtually every resuscitative intervention is directed at manipulating these variables. In most cases, inadequate oxygen delivery is produced primarily by circulatory insufficiency, a condition loosely referred to as shock.

Shock is classically defined as a circulatory state in which perfusion is inadequate to meet the global demands of metabolically active cells. The causes of shock include bleeding (hemorrhagic or hypovolemic shock), myocardial dysfunction or tamponade (cardiogenic shock), and vasomotor instability secondary to endotoxemia (septic shock) or spinal injury (neurogenic shock). Although hemorrhage is the most common cause of shock in the injured child, other causes require prompt recognition for specific treatment. Cardiogenic shock with tension pneumothorax is due to both elevated intrathoracic pressure and mediastinal displacement with mechanical distortion of the large veins that return blood to the right atrium. Pleural decompression dramatically improves both problems. Cardiogenic shock from myocardial contusion, although rare in children, may require invasive hemodynamic monitoring and inotropic support. Cardiac tamponade limits stroke volume by preventing normal cardiac filling in diastole. This can sometimes be temporized by volume infusion to increase central venous pressure and overcome the decreased effective compliance, but often requires pericardiocentesis or thoracotomy. Neurogenic shock, characterized by hypotension, bradycardia, and hypothermia secondary to acute interruption of sympathetic outflow, responds initially to volume expansion but may also require vasopressor therapy.

As oxygen delivery falls, oxygen extraction increases. About 25% of available oxygen is used under normal conditions. The extraction process is limited by a declining P_{O_2} gradient between capillary blood and intracellular mitochondria, resulting in a maximal extraction ratio of 50% to 70%. Therefore, a significant fraction of the oxygen content is not available under any circumstances. As oxygen delivery falls below the level at which maximal extraction occurs, cell function shifts to less efficient anaerobic metabolism, which generates lactic acid.

As these processes are evolving, cell membrane dysfunction due to failure of the Na^+-K^+-ATPase pump occurs, altering membrane permeability and allowing entry of sodium and water. The result is massive cell swelling and contraction of the interstitial fluid compartment. With further ischemia, oxidative phosphorylation is uncoupled, leading to failure of cellular respiration and depletion of ATP. These events are followed rapidly by swelling of the endoplasmic reticulum, the appearance of blebs on the surface membrane, and changes in microfilament and microtubule function. Irreversible cell injury is indicated by mitochondrial swelling, protein denaturation, nucleic acid condensation, and disruption of membrane structure.

Even if ischemia is reversed by restoration of oxygen delivery, the process of reperfusion can cause direct cellular injury. This paradox, referred to as ischemia–reperfusion injury, is explained by the fact that enzymatic pathways are induced in ischemic cells, which convert molecular oxygen to a variety of toxic oxygen metabolites. In the normal recycling of nucleic acids, purines are sequentially degraded to hypoxanthine, xanthine, and uric acid by xanthine dehydrogenase, which uses NAD^+ as the electron acceptor during oxidation. During cellular ischemia, xanthine dehydrogenase is converted to xanthine oxidase, which performs the same degradation but requires oxygen as the electron acceptor. During ischemia, large quantities of hypoxanthine accumulate from the breakdown of ATP to adenosine, and during reperfusion, these are converted to xanthine and uric acid. This reaction occurs in the presence of available oxygen and generates multiple toxic oxygen metabolites, including superoxide radical ($^\bullet O_2^-$), hydrogen peroxide (H_2O_2), and highly reactive hydroxyl radicals (Fig. 19-3).

Toxic oxygen metabolites produce cellular damage in a variety of ways: they oxidize nucleic acids and cause DNA nicking; they cause membrane lipid peroxidation, which alters membrane fluidity and results in leakage; and they cross-link and degrade proteins, rendering them nonfunctional. These metabolites also initiate proinflammatory and chemotactic signals that recruit activated neutrophils (PMNs) to the reperfused tissue.[3] Microvascular endothelial and intestinal epithelial cells contain particularly high concentrations of xanthine oxidase. Diffuse injury to these barriers by reactive oxygen metabolites can have profound consequences for cellular integrity. Studies have documented an association between experimental ischemia–reperfusion injury of the intestine and diffuse lung injury that is mediated by cytokines and PMNs and has histologic and clinical similarities to adult respiratory distress syndrome (ARDS).[4] The premise that such processes are clinically important is supported by investigations that documented protection against ischemia–reperfusion injury by pretreatment with a variety of free-radical scavengers and inhibitors, such as allopurinol, superoxide dismutase, and catalase.

Neuroendocrine Responses

At the time of injury, a number of noxious stimuli are detected by the peripheral nervous system and integrated by the central nervous system (CNS). The CNS responds by elaborating humoral substances that counteract acute alterations in physiology and protect the organism against further injury. Neuroendocrine mediators generally have systemic effects on intravascular volume, cardiovascular performance, and metabolism.

Some of the stimuli that evoke an acute neuroendocrine adaptive response include pain, hypotension, hypovolemia, hypo-

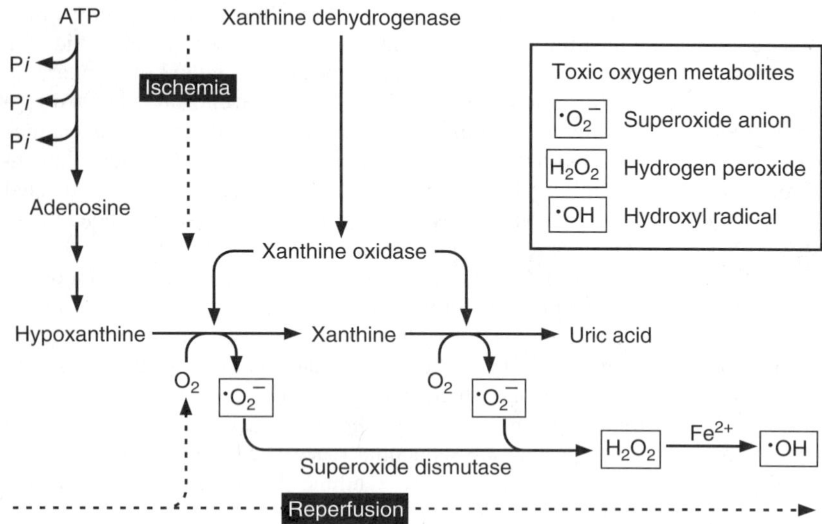

FIG. 19-3. Generation of toxic oxygen metabolites in ischemia–reperfusion injury.

xemia, and extremes of temperature. Pain elicits the production of a variety of endocrine substances, including adrenocorticotropic hormone (ACTH), antidiuretic hormone (ADH), and endorphins. Pain also stimulates sympathetic-mediated secretion of catecholamines from the adrenal medulla and renin from the kidney. Emotional states associated with trauma (eg, fear and anger) potentiate the effects of pain on neuroendocrine outflow.

Hypovolemia and hypotension produced by hemorrhage are also potent stimuli of the neuroendocrine axis. Low-pressure stretch receptors in the heart and high-pressure baroreceptors in the aorta, carotid sinus, and renal arteries monitor intravascular pressure, volume, and their rates of change. When negative changes occur, secretion of ACTH, ADH, growth hormone, endorphins, catecholamines, and renin is increased. Circulating catecholamines result from sympathetic stimulation of the adrenal medulla, a process that requires both baroreceptor and stretch-receptor stimulation of the CNS centers. Renin is elaborated by the renal juxtaglomerular apparatus (JGA) in response to adrenergic signals, and also through intrinsic properties of the JGA that allow it to function as a local intrarenal stretch receptor.

Chemoreceptors in the carotid bifurcation and aortic arch respond to alterations in Po₂, Pco₂, and pH. These highly specialized neuroreceptors transduce alterations in oxygen, carbon dioxide, and hydrogen ion concentrations into autonomic afferent activity, which brings about an increase in ventilatory rate. A reduction in core temperature directly augments the secretion of ACTH, ADH, growth hormone, and thyroid-stimulating hormone. Hypothermia also stimulates sympathetic outflow to produce increased levels of circulating epinephrine, which redistributes blood flow to central core organs.

The hormonal environment that results from neuroendocrine activation in the setting of acute mechanical trauma induces a physiologic state characterized by changes in metabolism, fluid balance, cardiac performance, and vascular tone (Fig. 19-4). This state involves the interrelated functions of a wide variety of molecules and their target organs. The result is a highly redundant and complex system of functional adaptations evolved to promote survival in the acute posttraumatic period, but which can have disadvantageous effects when prolonged

for long periods after the injury. Some of the principal neuroendocrine mediators are discussed in the following sections (Table 19-1).

Cortisol

Cortisol production by the adrenal cortex is regulated by ACTH. Cortisol binds to cytoplasmic receptors, which migrate into the nucleus and bind to specific DNA regulatory regions (glucocorticoid regulatory elements) that increase the transcription of a specific set of genes. The effects of cortisol increase available substrates for energy production in the posttraumatic period. In peripheral tissues such as skeletal muscle, cortisol inhibits insulin-dependent glucose uptake and metabolism. It also promotes catabolism of skeletal muscle proteins with the release of free amino acids into the circulation. In adipocytes, it increases lipolysis and inhibits lipogenesis. These actions tend to increase blood levels of glucose, fatty acids, glycerol, and amino acids. In the liver, these substrates are taken up and enter various biosynthetic pathways; gluconeogenesis and glycogen deposition are increased, and acute-phase protein synthesis is stimulated. Brain, myocardium, and erythrocytes are insensitive to the glucose-inhibitory effects of cortisol, allowing these critical tissues to use glucose as an energy substrate during stress.

Aldosterone

Stimulation of aldosterone synthesis and secretion by the adrenal cortex is governed by three factors: ACTH, angiotensin II, and potassium; during acute stress states, ACTH-mediated processes predominate. The effects of aldosterone on target cells are mediated through cytoplasmic receptor mechanisms similar to cortisol. The principal target cells for aldosterone are in the distal convoluted tubule and proximal collecting duct of the renal nephron, where aldosterone enhances Na^+-K^+-ATPase–dependent sodium and water resorption.

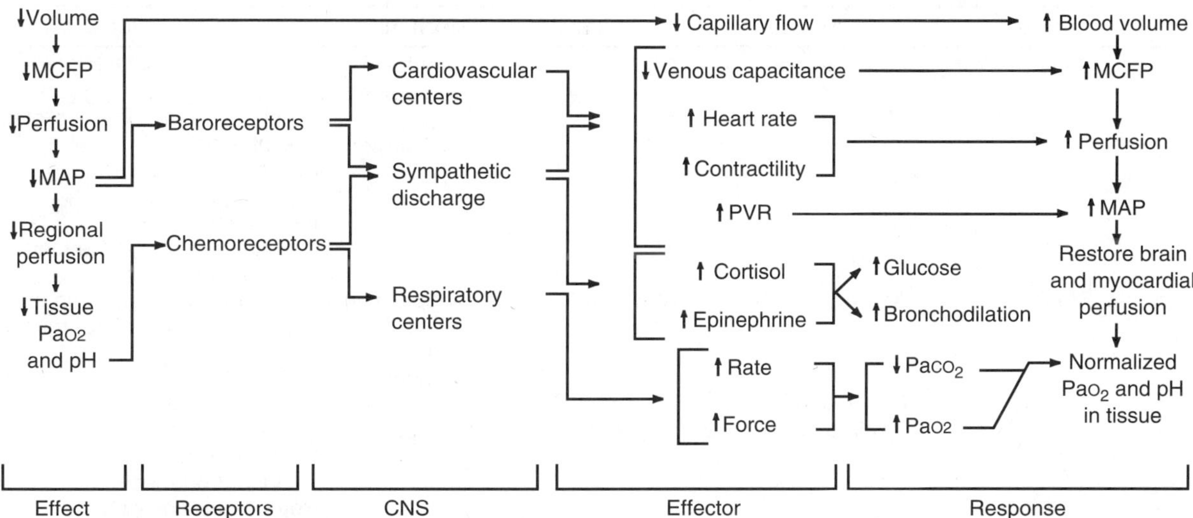

FIG. 19-4. Physiologic response to hemorrhage. MCFP, mean circulating filling pressure; MAP, mean arterial pressure; PVR, pulmonary vascular resistance.

Renin and Angiotensin II

The synthesis and secretion of renin occurs in the renal JGA, a highly specialized cellular network that bridges the afferent and efferent arterioles. The JGA responds to diminished chloride presentation, decreased intravascular pressure, and increased adrenergic outflow. In the circulation, renin catalyzes the conversion of hepatic angiotensinogen to the decapeptide angiotensin I, which is hydrolyzed by angiotensin-converting enzyme in pulmonary microvascular endothelial cells to the octapeptide angiotensin II. Angiotensin II is one of the most potent and rapid direct vasoconstrictors identified. It is also an important inducer of aldosterone production. Other important effects of angiotensin II in the traumatized patient include an increase in the inotropic and chronotropic states of the myocardium, potentiation of adrenal epinephrine secretion, stimulation of vasopressin (ADH) release, and up-regulation of hepatic glycogenolysis and gluconeogenesis.

Catecholamines

This class of mediators includes the neurotransmitters dopamine and norepinephrine and the amine hormone epinephrine. Catecholamines bind to ubiquitous cell-surface adrenergic receptors (α_1, α_2, β_1, and β_2) and have differing effects determined by their relative affinities for the various receptor subclasses. α_1-Receptors mediate arterial and venous vasoconstriction, hepatic glycogenolysis and gluconeogenesis, and pancreatic islet cell inhibition. α_2-Receptor stimulation results in platelet aggregation and mediates presynaptic feedback mechanisms. β_1-Receptors are found in the myocardium; they govern the positive inotropic and chronotropic effects of catecholamines and increase atrioventricular conduction velocities. Other important β_1-mediated effects are lipolysis and ketogenesis in adipose and hepatic tissue. β_2-Receptors are found on smooth muscles cells of the arterial and bronchial trees, and they mediate relaxation and dilation. They also exert a stimulatory effect on pancreatic glucagon secretion, exert an inhibitory effect on peripheral insulin-dependent glucose use, and augment glycogenolysis in muscle.

The three physiologically relevant catecholamines—epinephrine, norepinephrine, and dopamine—have receptor-specific effects that appear to be dose dependent. Epinephrine tends to exert β-mediated effects at lower doses, while α-mediated effects prevail at higher concentrations. Norepinephrine appears to exert primarily α-mediated effects through the entire concentration range, although some β-mediated activity is present. Because of these differences, epinephrine tends to increase myocardial contractility and heart rate and cause peripheral vasodilation, resulting in increased cardiac output, mean systemic pressure, and systolic pressure and decreased diastolic pressure. Norepinephrine, on the other hand, augments systolic, mean, and diastolic arterial pressures, but can result in an unchanged or even lowered cardiac output due to increased afterload. Both agents cause an increase in myocardial oxygen consumption and predispose to dysrhythmia. Dopamine stimulates dopaminergic receptors in the renal and mesenteric vasculature at low doses, but causes β- and α-receptor stimulation at intermediate and high concentrations, respectively. The effects of increased sympathetic and adrenomedullary outflow after injury, therefore, include enhancement of cardiac output, elevation of blood pressure, mobilization of fatty acids, and maintenance of the hyperglycemia required by certain glucose-dependent tissues.

Vasopressin

Vasopressin (ADH) is synthesized in the hypothalamus and released from the posterior pituitary in response to increased serum osmolarity, hypotension, and hypovolemia. Vasopressin release is potentiated by trauma, pain, and hypoxemia and is inhibited by alcohol. The actions of vasopressin are multiple. Serum osmolarity and volume are restored by increases in the permeability of renal collecting ducts to free water resorption. Blood pressure is augmented by systemic arteriolar vasoconstriction, particularly in the splanchnic bed. This mechanism

TABLE 19-1. *Neuroendocrine mediators*

Agent	Structure	Source	Stimuli	Mechanism	Effects
Cortisol	Steroid	Adrenal cortex	ACTH	Cytoplasmic receptor DNA binding	↑ Proteolysis, lipolysis, gluconeogenesis, glycogenolysis, hepatic acute-phase protein synthesis Potentiates catecholamines and glucagon Insulin antagonism Inhibits phospholipase cleavage of arachidonic acid
Aldosterone	Steroid	Adrenal cortex	ACTH, K^+ Angiotensin II	Cytoplasmic receptor DNA binding	↑ Na and H_2O resorption in renal tubule and intestinal mucosa
Angiotensin II	Peptide	Pulmonary microvasculature	↓ Glomerular filtration rate	Membrane receptor	↑ Cardiac contractility and rate, vasoconstriction ↑ Aldosterone, ADH, gluconeogenesis Potentiates epinephrine
Epinephrine	Catecholamine	Adrenal medulla	Sympathetic outflow	Membrane receptor	↑ Cardiac contractility and rate, cardiac output, mean arterial pressure, atrioventricular conduction Vasodilation, bronchodilation ↑ Lipolysis, ketogenesis, insulin antagonism
Norepinephrine	Catecholamine	Sympathetic neurons	Sympathetic outflow	Membrane receptor	↑ Cardiac contractility and rate, mean arterial pressure, arrhythmias ± Cardiac output Vasoconstriction, bronchoconstriction
Dopamine	Catecholamine	Sympathetic neurons	Sympathetic outflow	Membrane receptor	Low dose: ↑ renal and splanchnic blood flow Medium dose: β-adrenergic effects High dose: α-adrenergic effects
Vasopressin	Polypeptide	Posterior pituitary	↑ Osmolality, ↓ blood pressure, ↓ volume	Membrane receptor	↑ Renal H_2O resorption Vasoconstriction ↑ Gluconeogenesis, glycogenolysis
Glucagon	Polypeptide	Pancreatic α cells	Hypoglycemia Adrenergic stimulation	Membrane receptor	↑ Gluconeogenesis, glycogenolysis, ketogenesis
Insulin	Polypeptide	Pancreatic β cells	Hyperglycemia, ↑ amino acids, ↑ fatty acids	Membrane receptor	Glucose and amino acid uptake, glycogen synthesis ↓ Gluconeogenesis, glycogenolysis, proteolysis, lipolysis
β-Endorphin	Polypeptide	Central nervous system	Fear, pain, shock	Opiate receptor	↓ Pain, anxiety, catecholamine activity ↑ Cardiac contractility, vasodilation

(Eichelberger MR. Pediatric trauma. St Louis, Mosby–Year Book, 1993:63)

may contribute to the development of nonocclusive mesenteric ischemia observed in low-flow states during shock. Other effects of vasopressin include enhancement of hepatic glycogenolysis and gluconeogenesis.

Glucagon and Insulin

The balance between these two counterregulatory hormones contributes significantly to the overall metabolic milieu in the postinjury state. The cumulative effects of their actions determine the flow and use of energy substrates. Glucagon and insulin are both under the control of substrate concentrations and the autonomic nervous system, and changes in one hormone are usually countered by reciprocal changes in the other. Their effects are generally not significant during the acute posttraumatic phase except for a shift toward glucagon-mediated metabolism, in which a state of hyperglycemia and increased substrate availability exists. The enhanced availability of substrate to glucose-obligate tissues (brain, renal medulla, red blood cells [RBCs], leukocytes) during the first several hours after an injury is an important consequence of this hormonal milieu (Fig. 19-5).

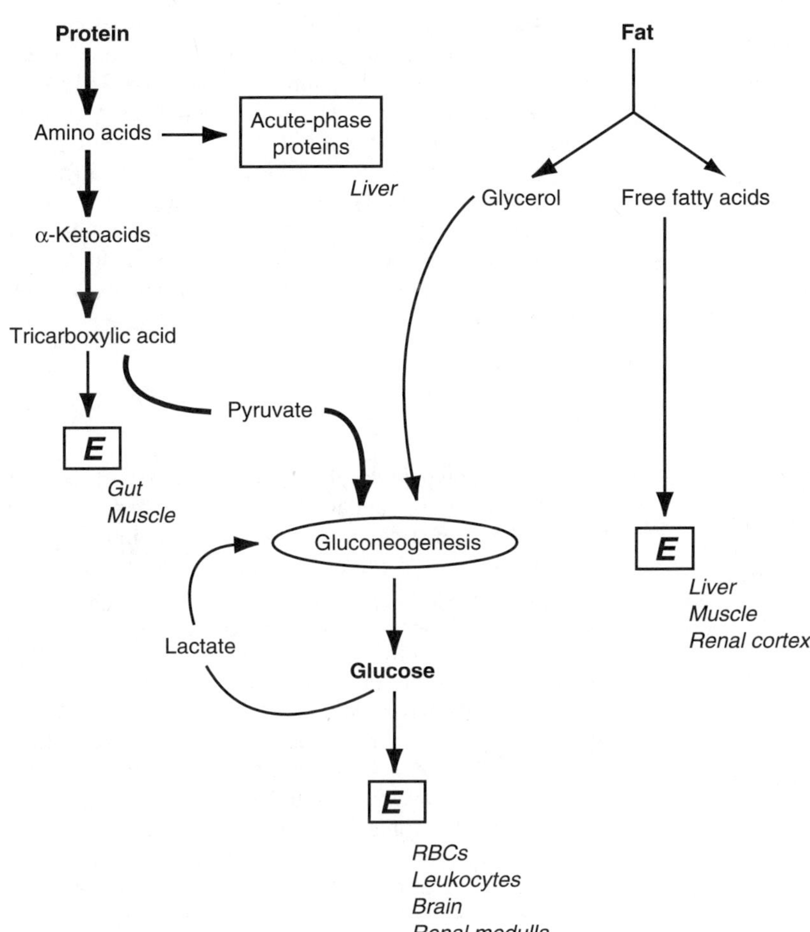

FIG. 19-5. Metabolic profile of acute trauma.

Endorphins

This family of endogenous neuropeptides comprises a large number of substances that share a common pentapeptide sequence at their amino terminus. Although they appear to act mainly within the CNS as neurotransmitters or modulators, certain peptides such as β-endorphin have been observed in elevated concentrations in circulating blood during hemorrhagic shock. The effects of endorphins on the physiologic response to injury are varied. They occupy opiate receptors on neural tissue and blunt the perception of noxious stimuli, thus producing a sense of well-being and hypothetically allowing the patient to function despite the pain associated with trauma. Endorphins also elicit a number of physiologic changes that are counterproductive in the posttraumatic state; these include a depression of myocardial contractility, inhibition of sympathetic activity, and peripheral vasodilation.

Inflammatory Mediator Responses

A significant portion of the acute and chronic pathophysiologic response to injury results from the large number of immunoinflammatory mediators generated by ischemic tissue and bacterial contamination of the wound. Causes of bacterial inoculation include bowel perforation, open soft tissue wounds or fractures, and pulmonary aspiration. Several noncytokine humoral mediators—complement, eicosanoids, and platelet-activating factor (PAF)—appear to be important in the early stages of the injury response.

Complement

The complement system consists of several enzymes that play prominent roles in localized and systemic inflammatory responses. After activation by a variety of stimuli, including bacterial lipopolysaccharides (LPS) and antigen-complexed immunoglobulin G or M, the enzymatic cascade ultimately creates a transmembrane pore complex that inserts into microbial cell membranes and causes osmotic lysis. Peptide fragments generated by the enzymatic hydrolysis of complement precursors also have important biologic functions, causing histamine-mediated increases in microvascular permeability (C3a, C5a), opsinization of microorganisms (C3b), and the recruitment and activation of inflammatory cells such as PMNs (C5a).

Eicosanoids

Eicosanoids have protean effects on the modulation of host responses to shock and sepsis that are mediated through autocrine, paracrine, and endocrine mechanisms.[5] Arachidonic acid, a ubiquitous 20-carbon polyunsaturated fatty acid found in the lipid bilayer of cell-surface membranes, is cleaved from membrane phospholipids by phospholipases in response to cell-specific stimuli. This initial step is inhibited by glucocorticoids, accounting for the antiinflammatory properties of steroid hormones. Arachidonic acid is degraded by one of two membrane-associated enzymes: cyclooxygenase or lipoxygenase. Products of the cyclooxygenase pathway include the prostaglandins (eg, PGE_2, prostacyclin (PGI_2), and thromboxane (TxA_2). This pathway is inhibited by nonsteroidal antiinflammatory drugs, such as indomethacin, ibuprofen, and aspirin. The lipoxygenase pathway results in the production of leukotrienes.

TxA_2 is produced primarily by platelets and macrophages, and elevated plasma levels occur during posttraumatic shock and endotoxemia. TxA_2 causes platelet aggregation, contraction of pulmonary and systemic vascular smooth muscle, and bronchial smooth muscle contraction. Some of the principal biologic consequences of TxA_2 activity are therefore vasoconstriction, stasis, and microvascular thrombosis. These properties contribute to the development of early pulmonary hypertension commonly observed after shock and endotoxemia.

PGI_2 inhibits platelet aggregation and causes relaxation of bronchial, pulmonary vascular and systemic vascular smooth muscle. PGI_2 is one of the principal eicosanoids produced by endothelial cells in response to hemorrhagic shock, and it serves a homeostatic function by counteracting the effects of TxA_2 within intact vascular beds where thrombosis would be inappropriate. Although PGI_2 has no direct effects on microvascular permeability, its vasodilatory properties augment fluid efflux in vascular beds where barrier function has already been compromised by other inflammatory mediators.

PGE_2 release is observed in the renal medulla, gastric submucosa, and endothelium during hemorrhagic shock and after experimental splanchnic ischemia–reperfusion injury. In addition to causing bronchial and microvascular dilation and nonvascular smooth muscle contraction, as well as inhibiting platelet aggregation, PGE_2 also modulates lymphocyte and macrophage function, renal tubular sodium absorption, and neurotransmission. It is a primary regulator of renal and gastric microperfusion and therefore has protective and functional effects on both organs.

Leukotrienes are produced from arachidonic acid by the action of lipoxygenase. Previously known as *slow-reacting substances of anaphylaxis,* they are potent bronchoconstrictors and vasoconstrictors. Some dilate microvessels, increase capillary permeability, and stimulate mucous production. Others augment PMN function through enhanced chemoattraction, adherence, diapedesis, lysosomal enzyme release, and toxic oxygen radical generation.

Platelet-Activating Factor

Platelet activating factor is derived from the phosphoglyceride backbone of arachidonic acid in PMNs, macrophages, platelets, and endothelial cells in response to a wide variety of inflammatory stimuli. One principal effect of PAF is systemic hypotension. It is postulated that leukocyte-derived PAF causes profound pulmonary vasoconstriction, bronchoconstriction, and capillary leak. This results in acute elevations in pulmonary vascular resistance, followed by right ventricular decompensation, left ventricular preload reduction, and systemic hypotension. Hypoxemia secondary to pulmonary interstitial and alveolar edema also ensues. PAF has also been implicated in acute bowel mucosal injury. When infused into the mesenteric circulation, PAF appears to act synergistically with both LPS and tumor necrosis factor to produce necrotic lesions in intestinal mucosa, a potential implication for posttraumatic intestinal barrier dysfunction and bacterial translocation. A similar role for PAF in the causation of hepatic and myocardial dysfunction after shock has been postulated.

Cytokine-Mediated Responses

Cytokines are polypeptides that are synthesized and secreted from a wide variety of stimulated immunocompetent cells and function in the regulation of immune and inflammatory responses[6] (Table 19-2). Unlike the classic stress hormones, it is likely that most cytokines exert physiologic effects both as paracrine agents in local environments and as systemic mediators within the general circulation. Localized and appropriately directed cytokine activity in response to microbial invasion or local trauma clearly has beneficial effects for the host. When the inflammatory response becomes generalized and unfocused, however, pathologic events mediated by disseminated cytokines ensue that can have profoundly deleterious consequences. This occurs through a complex process of cytokine networking in which a cascade of inflammatory mediators is generated, resulting in diffuse activation of multiple molecular and cellular cytotoxic mechanisms. Acute elevations of cytokines are commonly observed after exposure to LPS and other microbial products. Evidence is accumulating that certain cytokines may be present in increased concentrations acutely after mechanical trauma and hypotension.

Tumor Necrosis Factor

Tumor necrosis factor (TNF) is a 17-kd polypeptide produced primarily by cells of the macrophage line (eg, circulating monocytes, alveolar and peritoneal macrophages, Kupffer cells), lymphocytes, and endothelial cells in response to bacterial endotoxins, exotoxins, and other microbial products. The effects of TNF on immune and inflammatory function, metabolic activity, and hemodynamic parameters are widespread. TNF infusions mimic closely the known effects of acute endotoxemia: hypotension, tachycardia, fever, acidosis, disseminated intravascular coagulation, and increased capillary permeability. These effects are manifested by diffuse organ damage involving the kidneys, adrenals, lungs, and gut. Because the lethal effects of LPS infusions in animals can be blocked experimentally by passive immunization or by pretreatment with monoclonal antibodies to TNF, this agent is thought to be a central mediator in the pathophysiology of septic shock. Other effects of TNF include PMN and monocyte–macrophage activation, increased lymphokine production, enhanced adherence of PMNs to endothelial cells, increased endothelial procoagulant activity, and increased hepatic acute-phase protein synthesis accompanied by peripheral proteolysis and lipolysis.

TABLE 19-2. *Cytokine mediators*

Cytokine	Structure	Sources	Stimuli	Effects
TNF-α	17-kd polypeptide	Monocytes–macrophages, lymphocytes, endothelium	LPS, exotoxins, fungi, viruses	Hypotension, shock; PMN release, activation, adherence; macrophage proliferation, activation; endothelial activation, leak; ↑ lymphokine production; ↑ acute-phase protein synthesis, proteolysis, lipolysis
IL-1β	17-kd polypeptide (soluble)	Monocytes–macrophages, lymphocytes, PMNs, endothelium	LPS, TNF	PMN release, adherence; macrophage release, activation; endothelial activation; T-cell proliferation, activation, lymphokine production; ↑ acute-phase protein synthesis, proteolysis, lipolysis; fever
IL-2	15-kd polypeptide	T lymphocytes	IL-1	T-cell proliferation, activation, lymphokine production; hypotension, capillary leak
IL-6	Phosphoglycoproteins	Monocytes–macrophages, endothelium	LPS	T-cell proliferation and cytotoxicity; ↑ B-cell antibody production; ↑ acute-phase protein synthesis
IL-8	Polypeptide	Monocytes–macrophages	LPS	PMN chemotaxis, activation
IFN-γ	Glycoprotein	T lymphocytes	Bacteria, viruses, IL-2	Macrophage activation; antigen presentation; ↑ B-cell antibody production; PMN activation

LPS, lipopolysaccharides; PMNs, polymorphonuclear neutrophils.
(Eichelberger MR. Pediatric trauma. St Louis, Mosby–Year Book, 1993)

Interleukins

Interleukin-1α (IL-1α; membrane-associated) and IL-1β (soluble) interact with the same specific cell-surface receptors on target cells. IL-1 is synthesized primarily by macrophages in response to LPS, but also by PMNs, lymphocytes, and endothelial cells in response to other stimuli. IL-1 increases circulating numbers of PMNs and monocytes and also activates macrophages. It is a potent stimulus for T-lymphocyte proliferation, activation, and lymphokine production. IL-1 causes increased hepatic acute-phase protein synthesis at the expense of peripheral proteolysis. IL-1 is also the original endogenous pyrogen, responsible for resetting the hypothalamic thermoregulatory center and producing the febrile response to infection and trauma. IL-1 has important effects on vascular endothelium, including up-regulation of surface procoagulant activity, stimulation of PAF and IL-1 release, and expression of cell-surface adhesion molecules. The role played by IL-1 in the acute hemodynamic response to trauma is unclear, but it is an important mediator of both beneficial and deleterious inflammatory events during the posttraumatic period.

Several other interleukins may also participate to a lesser extent in the posttraumatic state. IL-2 is elaborated by T cells in response to IL-1 and serves an amplification feedback function by activating T cells, promoting T-cell proliferation, and further stimulating lymphokine production. Although exogenous administration of IL-2 causes profound hypotension and capillary leak, its role in the posttraumatic state is undefined. IL-6 comprises a family of related phosphoglycoproteins produced by macrophages and endothelial cells in response to other cytokines and LPS. This cytokine family stimulates both B and T lymphocytes and enhances antibody production and cytotoxic potential. Like IL-1 and TNF, IL-6 also augments hepatic acute-

phase protein synthesis. Elevated levels of these peptides are found circulating in response to trauma, endotoxemia, and thermal injury. IL-8 is a newly described product of LPS-stimulated macrophages that acts as a potent chemoattractant and activator of PMNs. Its role in the posttraumatic state is still undefined, but it has been detected in bronchoalveolar lavage fluid from patients with ARDS, suggesting a possible role in posttraumatic lung injury.

Interferons

In addition to its antiviral and lymphocyte-stimulatory properties, interferon-γ (IFN-γ) has been shown to be a potent stimulator of macrophage–monocyte cytotoxicity by enhancement of respiratory burst activity. It also enhances antigen presentation by up-regulating membrane HLA-DR expression. The observations that these events are both inhibited by PGE_2 and that IFN-γ levels are reduced in the posttraumatic period suggest that PGE_2-inhibition of IFN-γ may be one mechanism by which immunosuppression associated with severe injury is brought about. The efficacy of enhancing immune function and preventing infectious complications in multiple-injury trauma patients by administering exogenous IFN-γ is under investigation. Preliminary results suggest that administration of exogenous recombinant IFN-γ may reduce infection-related deaths after trauma.[7]

RESUSCITATION PRINCIPLES

Prehospital Care

The major focus of this chapter is the systematized approach to posttraumatic stabilization and management that evolves from the first moment when an injured child presents in the emergency department. The resuscitation process begins, however, when the child is first encountered in the field by emergency transport personnel. The fate of any given child can turn on the decisions and interventions that transpire during these first crucial moments.

In general, children fare worse than adults in the out-of-hospital phase of resuscitation. The injury-adjusted death rate for children is twice that of adults.[8] Similarly, the survival rate for out-of-hospital cardiac arrest in children is only half that of adults. Although part of this discrepancy results from the different causes of cardiac arrest in children and adults, an equal part is probably due to unfamiliarity and inadequate training with children. Indeed, the failure rate for resuscitation interventions in the field is about twice as high in children as adults. Many series report failure rates for prehospital endotracheal intubation of injured children that approach 50%.[9] Unfamiliarity with pediatric skills is understandable because although trauma is the most common indication for pediatric ambulance runs, such runs account for less than 10% of total paramedic patient volume in most metropolitan areas.

The most important objectives for emergency personnel in the field are as follows:

- Recognition and treatment of immediately life-threatening problems
- Assessment of the mechanism of trauma and extent of injuries
- Physiologic stabilization for transport
- Gathering of pertinent medical data, if available
- Triage to the appropriate-level pediatric trauma facility

Add to these the additional challenges of comforting a terrified and hurt child, as well as a distraught parent, and the paramedic's task becomes formidable. For these reasons, and because opportunities to resuscitate children in the field are infrequent, field personnel function best by adopting strict protocols to treat the injured child. The priorities and techniques associated with pediatric field resuscitation are similar to those described later for emergency department care.

Primary Survey and Treatment of Life-Threatening Injuries

When the injured child encounters medical personnel, whether in the field or in the emergency room, events transpire in rapid sequence that are dictated by a systematic protocol to recognize and treat acute injuries. This approach is designed to standardize diagnostic and treatment decisions so that individual variations in patterns of injury do not distract caregivers from recognizing and treating apparently subtle injuries that can have a profound impact on morbidity and mortality. This systematic framework comprises a primary survey, a resuscitation phase, and a definitive secondary survey (Fig. 19-6). The primary survey is the initial process of identifying and temporizing injuries that are potentially life-threatening. It is characterized by its reliance on simple observations to assess physiologic derangement and immediate intervention to prevent death. The components of this approach include attention to *a*irway, *b*reathing, *c*irculation, *d*isability, and *e*xposure: the ABC's of resuscitation.

Airway and Cervical Spine Control

The primacy of airway control is perhaps the least controversial of all priorities in trauma management. Lethal hypoxemia occurs in minutes if the airway is inadequate. Airway compromise can be caused by many things in the injured child: altered sensorium; foreign bodies, blood, and secretions in the oral cavity; maxillofacial trauma with injury to supporting structures; and direct laryngotracheal trauma. Assessment of the airway includes inspection of the oral cavity; manual removal of debris, loose teeth, and soft tissue fragments; and aspiration of blood and secretions with mechanical suction. If a child is neurologically intact, phonates normally, and is ventilating without stridor or distress, invasive airway management can be withheld. Airway patency can be improved in the spontaneously breathing child by use of the jaw-thrust or chin-lift maneuvers.

An airway that is unsecured because of coma, combativeness, shock, or direct airway trauma requires endotracheal intubation. Nasopharyngeal and oropharyngeal airways can improve airway management during bag-mask ventilation but are temporizing measures until definitive control is established. In most cases, orotracheal intubation with in-line cervical spine stabilization is the preferred approach to airway control. Although nasotracheal intubation is recommended in nonapneic adults with potential cervical spine injury, this approach is unnecessary and poorly tolerated in children. Because unbalanced axial traction can further disrupt injured cervical ligaments in children, the neck should be manually stabilized in a neutral position, not pulled, during intubation.[10]

Several unique aspects of pediatric airway anatomy affect management technique. The child's larynx is anatomically higher and more anterior than the adult's, necessitating an upward angulation of the laryngoscope to place the endotracheal tube properly. Removing the anterior half of the rigid cervical collar allows access to the neck for gentle cricoid pressure. The pediatric epiglottis is shorter, less flexible, and tilted posteriorly over the glottic inlet. Because of this, direct control of the epiglottis with a straight Miller blade is usually necessary for proper visualization of the vocal cords. The cords themselves are more fragile and easily damaged. The narrowest point in the pediatric airway is the subglottic trachea at the cricoid ring, as opposed to the glottis in adults. Therefore, passage of the endotracheal tube through the cords does not guarantee safe advancement into the trachea or avoidance of subglottic injury. The pediatric airway is shorter than the adult's, and endobronchial intubation is a common mistake in unfamiliar hands.

The selection of an appropriate endotracheal tube is an important nuance of pediatric resuscitation that rarely requires much consideration in adults. Internal diameter sizes can range from 3.0 to 3.5 mm in newborns to 4.5 mm at 1 to 2 years of age. After 2 years of age, internal diameter can be estimated by the following formula:

$$\text{internal diameter} = \frac{\text{age}}{4} + 4$$

Approximating the diameter of the patient's little finger is also useful. Because of the narrower subglottic trachea, uncuffed tubes should be routinely used in children 8 years of age or younger.

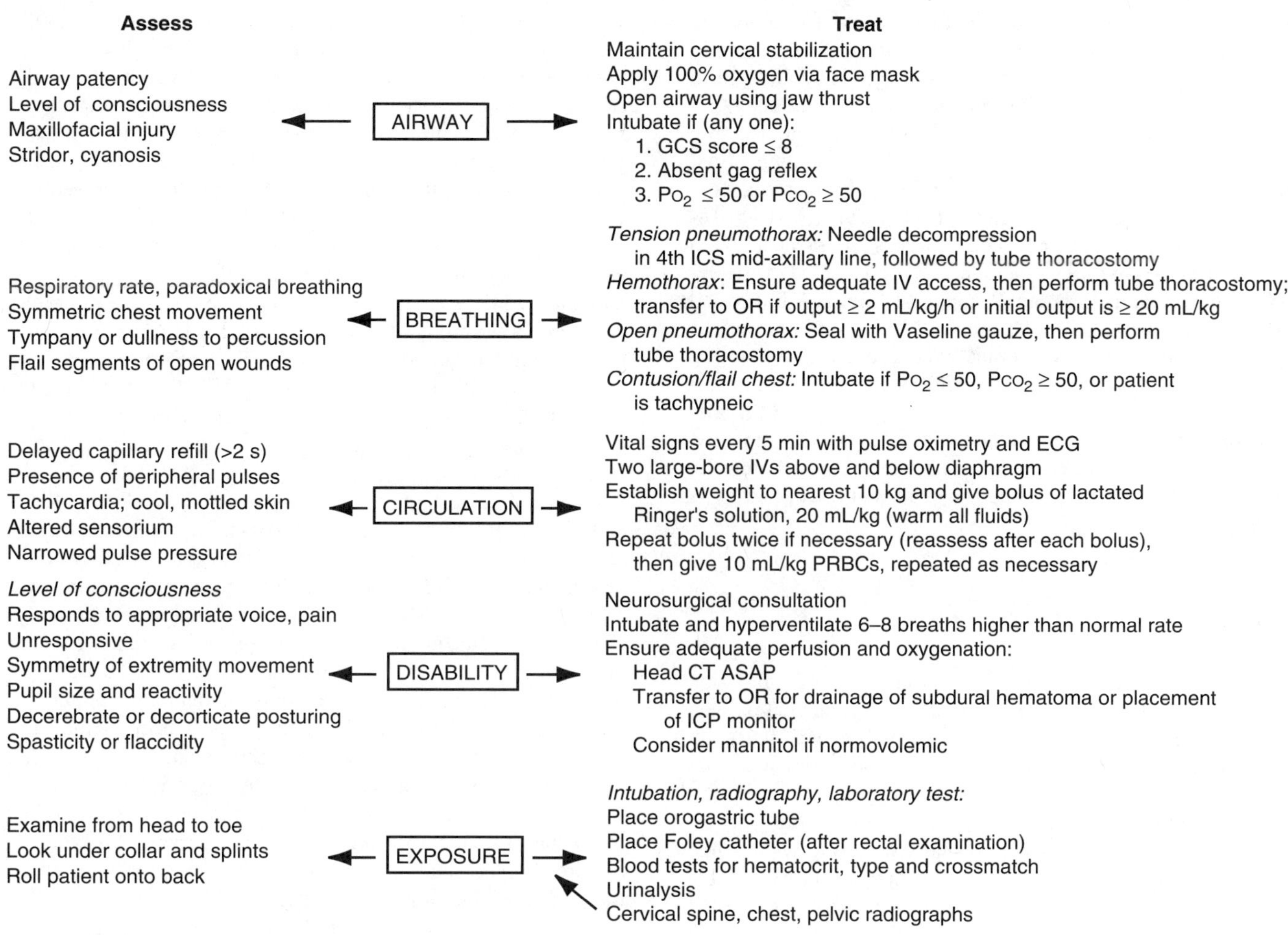

FIG. 19-6. Primary survey with resuscitation guidelines. GCS, Glasgow Coma Scale; ICS, intercostal space; OR, operating room; ICP, intracranial pressure monitoring.

The technique of intubation depends on the urgency of establishing an airway. In the hypotensive, hypoxemic, comatose child, orotracheal intubation is accomplished without delay as an integral part of the resuscitation. In a more elective situation, however, more attention is given to adequate preoxygenation and premedication. An adequate oxygen saturation (ie, more than 95%), as measured by pulse oximetry, is attempted by bag-mask ventilation with 100% oxygen. Thoracic trauma can preclude normal gas exchange and make attainment of an adequate oxygen saturation impossible before intubation. Although not commonly measured, inducing hypocarbia by hyperventilation is advantageous in preventing carbon dioxide accumulation during attempted intubation—a condition that can exacerbate intracranial hypertension.

Premedication with intravenous sedatives and muscle relaxants is also helpful in preventing exacerbations of intracranial hypertension. Appropriate sedatives include short-acting barbiturates (thiopental or thiamylal, 2 to 4 mg/kg) or benzodiazepines (midazolam, 0.02 mg/kg, or diazepam, 0.1 mg/kg). Muscle relaxation is achieved with short-acting nondepolarizing agents (vecuronium, 0.1 mg/kg) or shorter-acting depolarizing agents (succinylcholine, 1 to 2 mg/kg). The presence of burns and devitalized tissue precludes the use of succinylcholine be-cause of the risk of hyperkalemia. All sedatives have myocardial depressant effects and should be avoided in the presence of hypotension. In children younger than 10 years of age, in whom vagally mediated bradycardia is a risk during tracheal manipulation, premedication with atropine, 0.02 mg/kg, or glycopyrrolate, 0.01 mg/kg, may be helpful.

In the rare circumstance when tracheal intubation is not possible (because of maxillofacial trauma, laryngotracheal trauma, or unusual airway anatomy), provision of a surgical airway is mandatory. For larger adolescents, the preferred approach is surgical cricothyrotomy. The cricothyroid membrane is a readily identifiable subcutaneous structure, lying immediately subjacent to the thyroid cartilage. This membrane is easily exposed through a transverse skin incision and can be incised horizontally to accommodate a small, uncuffed endotracheal tube. Because the membrane is in a superficial location, fewer complications related to inadvertent venous injury occur than with emergency tracheostomy. Tracheostomy, a rare procedure in injured children, is more difficult to perform in the emergency setting because of the trachea's deeper location and the possibility of vascular injury or thyroidal laceration. Conversion of a cricothyrotomy to a formal tracheostomy within 48 hours is prudent in most instances to avoid subglottic stenosis. A laryngeal mask airway may provide another means of establishing emergency airway control for ventilation of the comatose child who cannot otherwise be intubated, although its application in the injured child has not yet been adequately evaluated.

In smaller children, the cricoid cartilage is a delicate structure easily injured by cricothyrotomy. To avoid this complication, children younger than 10 years of age should undergo needle cricothyrotomy and jet insufflation of the trachea. A 16- to 18-gauge intravenous catheter is used to access the tracheal lumen through the cricothyroid membrane, and is connected to a 100% oxygen source at a flow rate of about 12 L/min. A bifurcated connector is interposed in the tubing, leaving one limb of the connector open to air. By alternately covering and uncovering this side limb, oxygen is insufflated into the trachea under pressure. By providing an inspiration/expiration ratio of 1:3, adequate oxygenation can be maintained indefinitely. This method is limited by carbon dioxide accumulation to about 20 minutes, after which endotracheal intubation or formal tracheostomy is necessary.

Breathing

Once a secure airway is confirmed, adequacy of ventilation is evaluated and ventilatory support with supplemental oxygen provided. Compromised ventilation in the trauma victim usually results from one of two general causes: head injury with loss of spontaneous ventilatory drive, or thoracic injury causing interference with mechanical bellows function and lung expansion. Recognition of the former is usually straightforward, while recognition of the latter requires a deliberate survey of the thorax. Impaired bellows function can result from any of the following: filling of the pleural space with air or fluid, causing collapse and displacement of the lung; reduction in pulmonary compliance; loss of chest wall integrity; or loss of diaphragmatic function. The potential seriousness of these injuries is underscored by the fact that mortality rates for thoracic trauma in children approach 25%.[11]

The pleural space may be occupied by air (pneumothorax), blood (hemothorax), and rarely lymph (chylothorax) or viscera (ruptured diaphragm). The resulting compression of pulmonary parenchyma causes an impairment of gas exchange sufficient to produce respiratory distress. In the case of traumatic rupture of the diaphragm, loss of muscular integrity also has a direct effect on bellows function. If the contents of the pleural space are under increased pressure or tension, the mediastinum is displaced to the opposite side, causing compression of the contralateral lung. The distortion of mediastinal vascular structures, along with the elevated intrathoracic pressure, can result in a critical reduction of venous return to the right atrium. Because the pediatric mediastinum is extremely mobile, these hemodynamic complications occur at lower pressures and with greater frequency in children than in adults.

Loss of chest wall integrity presents in two ways. Flail chest, a rare occurrence in children, occurs when multiple tandem rib fractures create an isolated segment of the thoracic cage that is disarticulated from the remainder, resulting in paradoxical movement and impairment of the patient's ability to increase intrathoracic volume during inspiration. This problem is most pronounced during spontaneous negative-pressure breathing and does not apply during assisted positive-pressure breathing. The more clinically relevant problem in flail chest is the underlying pulmonary contusion that invariably results from the transfer of energy. Regions of parenchymal hemorrhage and edema impair ventilation–perfusion matching, and the decreased pulmonary compliance can dramatically increase the work of breathing; these effects can precipitate sudden ventilatory failure. A second manifestation of chest wall injury is the open pneumothorax, a rare injury in civilian blunt trauma. The cross-sectional area of these wounds offers less resistance to air flow than does the tracheobronchial tree. This causes preferential air flow through the wound during inspiration, resulting in hypoventilation and lung collapse. This injury can produce tension pneumothorax if the exit of air from the wound is prevented by loose tissue acting like a flap–valve mechanism. The pathophysiology of this injury is also limited to negative-pressure breathing and is mitigated by assisted ventilation.

Recognition of ventilatory compromise is usually not difficult, especially with a high index of suspicion. The sound of air movement at the mouth and nares is assessed, as are the rate, depth, and effort of respirations. On inspection, asymmetric excursion of the chest wall suggests a ventilatory abnormality. Percussion elicits dullness or hyperresonance, depending on the presence of fluid or air in the pleural space. Breath sounds are reduced in all cases. In the case of tension hemopneumothorax, mediastinal shift may be detected by tracheal deviation, displacement of the point of maximal impulse, and distended neck veins caused by mediastinal venous hypertension.

Mechanical ventilatory failure is life-threatening and requires immediate treatment during the primary survey. All children require supplemental oxygen by nasal cannula, mask, or endotracheal tube. Endotracheal intubation and assisted ventilation are sufficient to treat hypoventilation due to head injury, pain from rib fractures, flail chest, and pulmonary contusion. Simple hemopneumothorax may be well tolerated with supplemental oxygen until tube thoracostomy can be performed after the primary survey. In cases of massive hemopneumothorax, thoracostomy is required immediately, often combined with tracheal intubation and intravenous access for rapid fluid infusion. If tension is present, the hemodynamic derangements can be mitigated by equalizing intrathoracic and atmospheric pressures with a needle in the second intercostal space at the mid-clavicular line, allowing time for definitive thoracostomy. An open chest wound requires placement of a semiocclusive dressing that allows egress of air followed by thoracostomy.

After establishment of a patent airway and proper ventilation, delivery of supplemental oxygen is essential. If the child is breathing spontaneously, a nasal cannula delivering 5 to 12 L/min of oxygen is adequate. If a higher inspired F_{IO_2} is desired, a Venti mask or rebreather mask with 100% entrained oxygen is necessary. When endotracheal intubation has been performed, 100% oxygen should be administered. Initially, volume-cycled ventilation should be employed, delivering tidal volumes of 12 to 15 mL/kg at a rate or 12 to 20 cycles/min. Minute ventilation should be increased to induce respiratory alkalosis in children with traumatic brain injury.

Application of positive end-expiratory pressure (PEEP) should not exceed 3 to 5 cm H_2O. PEEP can have deleterious effects on the hypovolemic child with a pulmonary contusion. Increasing intrathoracic pressure with PEEP reduces the gradient that drives venous return to the heart, thereby reducing preload and cardiac output. In addition, the use of high levels of PEEP with focal lung injury is hazardous because increased pressure is transmitted to the normal, more compliant alveoli. This increases capillary resistance and impairs flow through the uninjured gas-exchange units, which worsens ventilation–perfusion mismatch and exacerbates hypoxemia. There is no evidence that the prophylactic use of PEEP is efficacious in preventing or reducing the severity of posttraumatic ARDS.

Tube thoracostomy is accomplished during this phase of resuscitation for symptomatic hemopneumothorax. A chest tube of adequate caliber to evacuate blood and air is inserted into the pleural cavity. The narrow intercostal space of a small child usually limits the size of the tube to 18F to 20F, but a general dictum is to use the largest-caliber tube that can be safely placed. The tube should be placed in the mid-axillary line at about the nipple level (fourth or fifth intercostal space) to avoid intraabdominal placement through an elevated diaphragm. The tube should be directed posteroapically to evacuate both blood and air. The tube is immediately connected to a closed-suction drainage device under water-seal drainage and aspirated at -15 to -20 cm H_2O suction.

The need for surgical control of intrathoracic bleeding is uncommon but can be predicted by the rate of continued bleeding after the pleural space is initially evacuated. Most parenchymal bleeding is low pressure and stops with lung expansion and apposition of the visceral and parietal pleura. Persistent drainage of 1 to 2 mL/kg/h is an indication for thoracotomy and suggests persistent bleeding from a hilar vessel, an intercostal artery, or a mediastinal structure.

Circulation

The third priority in the sequence of the primary survey is the rapid assessment of circulatory adequacy. Healthy children possess a remarkable cardiovascular reserve that allows them to compensate for the early effects of hemorrhage and that delays hemodynamic signs of hypovolemia until relatively late in their physiologic decline. When cardiovascular decompensation does occur in children, it is frequently marked by progressive bradycardia. A high index of suspicion based on the mechanism of injury and careful scrutiny of physiologic parameters and clinical signs must be applied at all times to avoid the precipitous decompensation that inevitably accompanies unrecognized injuries.

A reliable sign of adequate perfusion pressure is a normal mental status. The child who has been in a bicycle accident and arrives in the emergency department conversing with the paramedics is most likely not in shock. Conversely, the comatose child may have an altered level of consciousness due to either traumatic brain injury or shock. A more precise estimate of cardiac output is obtained by observing peripheral signs of perfusion: the rate, strength, and character of peripheral and central pulses (radial, femoral, and carotid); skin color; temperature gradients over the extremities and trunk; and capillary refill in the nail beds and digits. Because children rarely have preexisting atherosclerotic vascular disease, these parameters are sensitive and immediate barometers of cardiac output.

When evidence for circulatory insufficiency exists, it is imperative to determine the cause of shock so that immediate steps to correct cardiovascular dysfunction can be taken. Differentiation between the various types of shock is usually possible. In hemorrhagic and cardiogenic shock, evidence of compromised peripheral perfusion is present. Level of consciousness is depressed; pulses are weak and thready, with a noticeable discrepancy between peripheral and central pulses; heart rate is rapid until bradycardia supervenes in the later stages; the skin is cool, pale, and diaphoretic; and capillary refill takes longer than 2 seconds. In children, intense peripheral vasoconstriction in response to decreasing cardiac output maintains systemic blood pressure in a normal range until blood loss approaches 40% of total blood volume (Fig. 19-7). The severity of hemorrhagic shock can be estimated by these parameters and categorized according to approximate blood volume loss (Table 19-3). An estimate of blood loss helps guide resuscitation volumes, the choice of crystalloid or blood products, and the likelihood of surgical intervention. In cardiogenic shock of all varieties, central venous pressure is elevated and neck veins are distended; these signs may be equivocal with concurrent hemorrhage. In tension hemopneumothorax, mediastinal shift causes tracheal deviation and displacement of the heart tones; in tamponade, the trachea is midline and heart tones are muffled. Septic and neurogenic shock both involve a loss of systemic vasomotor tone, resulting in bounding pulses and warm, flushed skin. Pre-

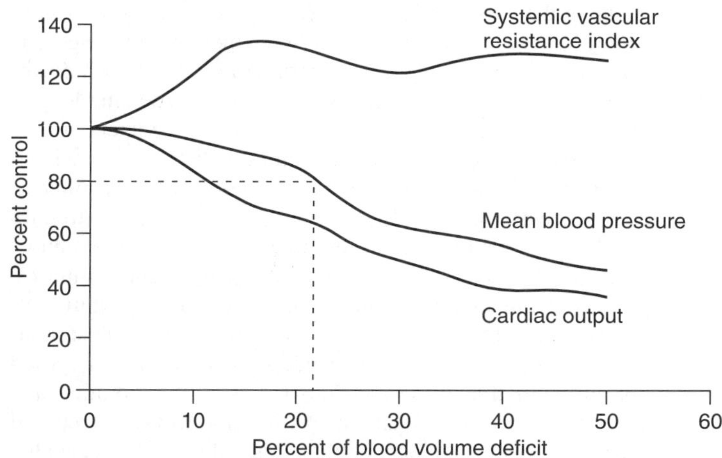

FIG. 19-7. Hemodynamic responses to increasing hemorrhage.

TABLE 19-3. *Clinical signs of hemorrhage in pediatric patients*

	Early: <25% blood volume loss	Prehypotensive: 25% blood volume loss	Hypotensive: 40% blood volume loss
Cardiac	Increased heart rate; weak, thready pulse	Increased heart rate, thready pulse, positive tilt test	Frank hypotension, tachycardia to bradycardia
CNS	Normal, anxious, irritable, combative	Confused, lethargic, dulled response to pain	Comatose
Skin	Cool, clammy	Cyanotic, decreased capillary refill, cold extremities	Pale, cold

(Eichelberger MR. Pediatric trauma. St Louis, Mosby–Year Book, 1993:182)

capillary shunting due to endotoxemia accounts for the perfusion deficit in the septic child.

Disability

A rapid neurologic evaluation is included in the primary survey to identify serious injuries that may have immediate consequences for airway management and that may require early therapeutic measures to prevent secondary brain injury. A thorough assessment is deferred until the secondary survey, but a rapid method for describing gross cerebral function is the AVPU pneumonic: *a*lert, *v*oice responsive, *p*ain responsive, or *u*nresponsive. An assessment of pupillary responsiveness and symmetry is also performed at this time. Transtentorial herniation secondary to an expanding intracranial hematoma causes ipsilateral pupillary dilation and loss of light reflex. Direct trauma to the eye is an equally common cause of unilateral anisocoria. Characterization of extremity posturing as decorticate or decerebrate indicates the loss of cortical or global brain function, respectively.

In the comatose child with a unilateral fixed and dilated pupil, or in the child who develops one during resuscitation, immediate measures to reduce intracranial pressure (ICP) are imperative. These include intubation and hyperventilation to induce respiratory alkalosis and hypocarbia, both of which cause cerebral vasoconstriction and decrease cerebral blood flow. This lowers brain volume and ICP and therefore increases cerebral perfusion pressure (CPP). The reverse Trendelenburg position, in which the head is slightly elevated by 30 degrees, can also reduce intracranial hypertension but should not be employed in the patient with compromised cardiac output of any cause. The cerebral injury caused by global hypoperfusion is just as devastating as that caused by direct head trauma.

Exposure

The final phase of the primary survey is complete exposure of the patient. Although this principle is straightforward and generally unchallenged, a few points can be made in reference to the special needs of children. A conscious child does not understand the need for such action, so exposure must be done delicately and tempered by need in every child. The skillful examiner can often perform a thorough primary survey on a stable child with a normal sensorium without removing all items of clothing. Children are particularly apprehensive about exposing an injury that had previously been covered. Attention to the

special sensitivities of the child in this regard frequently results in a more efficient resuscitation.

A critical concern relating to exposure is the inevitable heat loss that results in the emergency department environment. Because the small child's surface area/mass ratio is larger than the older patient, radiated heat loss is greater, and intrinsic mechanisms for heat production are less effective. Hypothermia significantly impacts important physiologic parameters, such as cognitive function, cardiac activity, and coagulation, so maintenance of a core temperature above 35° to 36°C is important. Resuscitation fluids should be run through warming circuits, and inhaled gases warmed and humidified. The use of warm blankets and heat lamps is also helpful. Radiant warmers of the type used in the intensive care nursery are also helpful in the emergency room evaluation of the injured infant.

Resuscitation Phase

After life-threatening injuries have been identified and managed in the primary survey, the resuscitation phase is entered in which hemodynamic stability is restored and more objective physiologic information is obtained to assess the severity of the original injury and to monitor the child's response to therapy. The cornerstone of resuscitation is continual reappraisal of the patient's response to every therapeutic intervention. Deterioration at any point should be addressed by returning to the basic priorities of the primary survey.

Vascular Access

One of the most challenging aspects of resuscitation is establishing intravenous access in the hypovolemic child. Because resistance to flow is inversely proportional to the fourth power of the conduit radius and directly proportional to conduit length, multiple short, large-gauge peripheral venous catheters are the preferred access option. Two functioning catheters are best in all cases of significant mechanical trauma; more may be required in the hypotensive or unstable patient. At least one upper extremity catheter is preferable, given the potential for extravasation of resuscitation fluids from occult intraabdominal venous injuries.

If percutaneous placement is not successful after initial attempts, surgical cutdown for venous exposure is the most reliable technique. The greater saphenous veins are easily exposed through short transverse incisions 0.5 to 1 cm proximal and anterior to the medial malleoli. An incision in the antecubital fossa may yield three accessible veins—the basilic, cephalic, and median antecubital. The exposed vein can be suspended over a silk ligature, and the largest appropriate intravenous catheter introduced into the vessel lumen under direct vision. The vein need not be ligated or transected (Fig. 19-8).

Central venous catheterization is reserved for the unusual circumstance when measurement of central venous pressure is desirable, such as with suspected cardiac contusion or tamponade. Large-diameter introducer sheaths, such as those used for pulmonary artery catheterization, can be useful for volume resuscitation in larger children. The internal jugular veins are not accessible during resuscitation, so options are limited to the femoral and subclavian veins. The femoral route is preferred

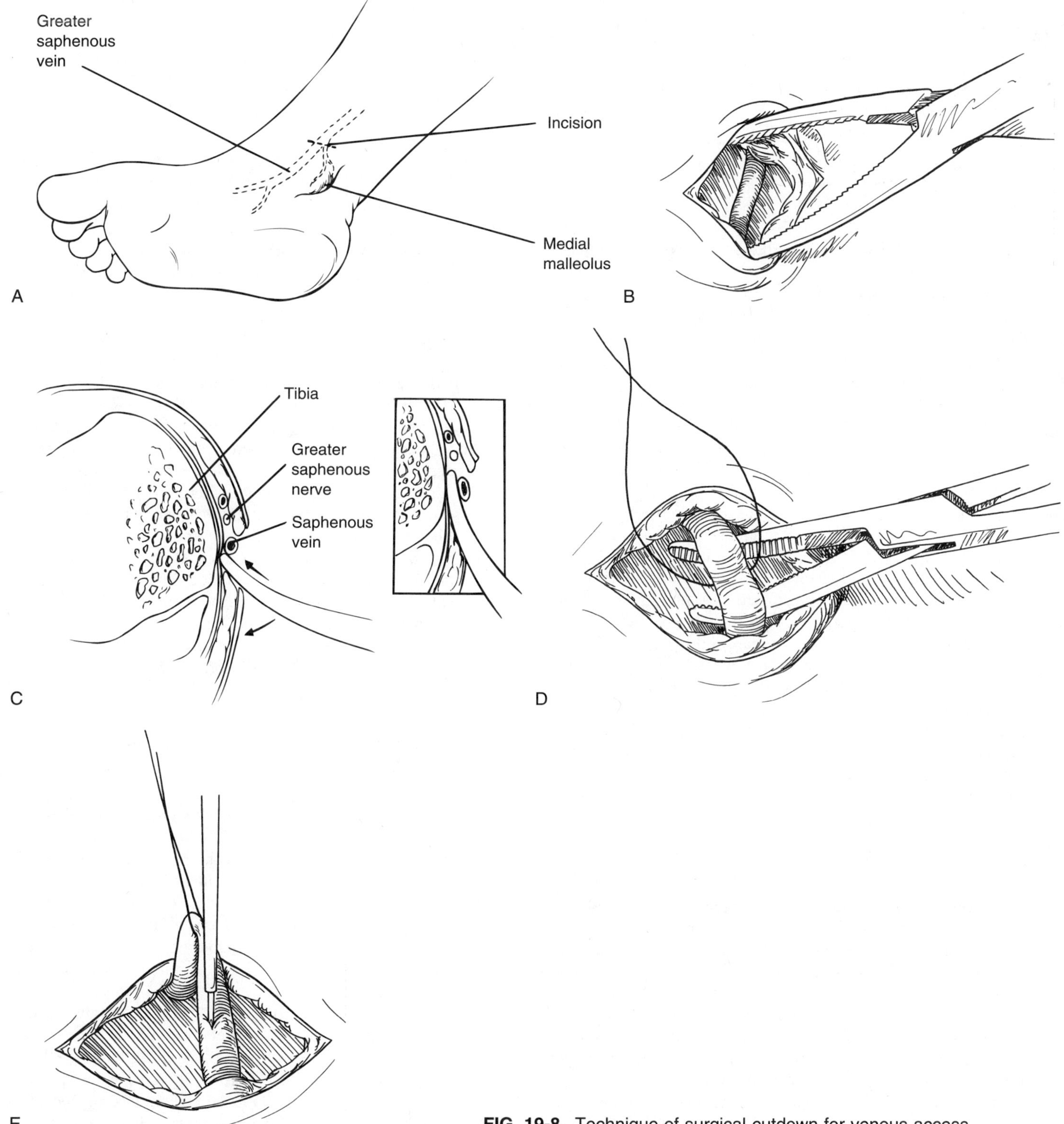

FIG. 19-8. Technique of surgical cutdown for venous access.

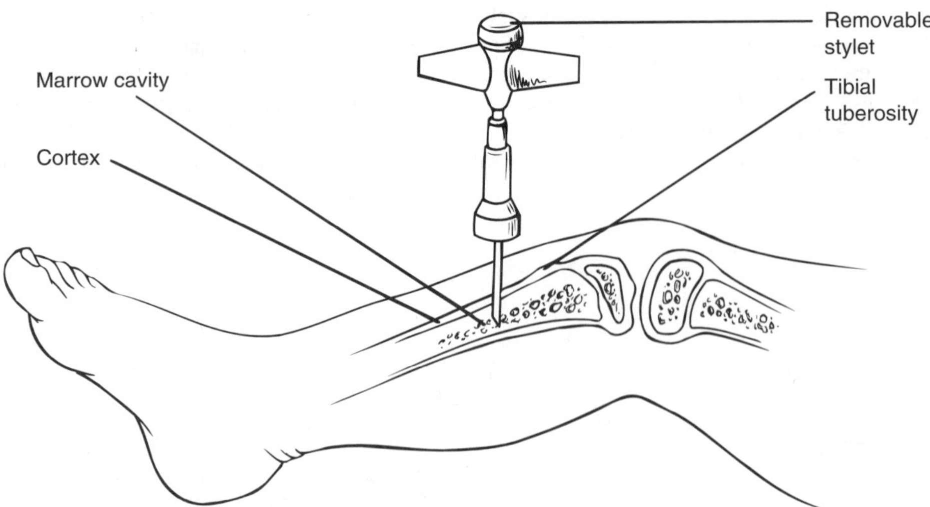

FIG. 19-9. Technique of intrasseous cannulation.

because of the inherent complications of the subclavian technique.

In children for whom intravenous access cannot be obtained, intraosseous cannulation is a simple, reliable, and safe route for administration of fluids, blood products, and resuscitative drugs. The technique is applicable primarily to children 5 years of age and younger because the well-perfused "red" marrow of early childhood is replaced by "yellow" marrow at about this time. Recent reports of successful intraosseous access in adult resuscitation, however, support the application of this technique in older children for whom intravenous access cannot be established.

The preferred site for intraosseous insertion is on the flat anteromedial surface of the tibia, about 2 to 3 cm below the tibial tuberosity (Fig. 19-9). The needle is angled 60 degrees from horizontal and pointed toward the foot. The cortex is penetrated and the marrow cavity detected by aspirating blood and particulate material. Alternative sites include the midline distal femur, 3 cm above the condyles in small children (pointed cephalad), and the distal tibia above the medial malleolus or the proximal humerus in the adolescent. Any 14- to 16-gauge needle can be used, but a bone marrow aspiration needle with a trocar is preferable. Reported complications include osteomyelitis, cellulitis, fracture, growth plate injury, fat embolism, and compartment syndrome. In practice, however, the complication rate is low.

Fluid Resuscitation

As soon as vascular access is established, fluid resuscitation with measured boluses is begun and the physiologic response to each bolus assessed. Generally, isotonic crystalloid solutions, such as lactated Ringer solution, are given in 20 mL/kg increments. If evidence of hypovolemia persists after 40 mL/kg (two boluses) have been given, transfusion of ABO-matched packed RBCs is initiated in boluses of 10 mL/kg. Packed RBCs have the desirable qualities of raising colloid oncotic pressure and effecting a more rapid and sustained intravascular expansion than crystalloid as well as providing hemoglobin to increase oxygen-carrying capacity. All fluids (crystalloid, colloid, and blood) should be warmed during infusion. This can be accomplished by microwave heating of crystalloid solutions and running all other solutions through a standard warming device or countercurrent heat-exchange system.

It is critical to reassess the child's response to resuscitation continually to characterize the nature and extent of the injuries as well as to avoid the complications of excessive fluid resuscitation. As perfusion is restored, the rate of fluid infusion is gradually reduced to avoid unnecessary fluid administration. Although peripheral edema is of little consequence, and pulmonary edema rarely occurs in otherwise normal lungs regardless of the infused volume, considerable morbidity can result from fluid sequestration in areas of pulmonary and cerebral contusion. If hemodynamic stabilization does not ensue with aggressive crystalloid and blood resuscitation, the various causes of continued instability must be considered. These include ongoing occult hemorrhage from an intraabdominal or pelvic source; cardiac dysfunction due to tamponade, contusion, or tension hemopneumothorax; devastating cerebrospinal injury, such as atlantooccipital dissociation; and profound hypothermia.

Decompressive Tubes, Electrocardiogram, and Laboratory Studies

In children, acute gastric dilation can cause both respiratory compromise and vagally mediated bradycardia. Gastric decompression to evacuate the stomach and reduce the risk of vomiting and aspiration is important in all injured children. In older children with stable midface and no evidence of cerebrospinal fluid (CSF) rhinorrhea, an adequate tube can usually be placed through the nose. In small children, or in anyone with severe maxillofacial trauma, the gastric tube is best inserted through the mouth.

A urinary catheter is also placed at this time. A digital rectal examination should precede catheter insertion in the injured boy to detect mobility of the prostate—an indicator of urethral transection. Urinary catheter insertion should be deferred in instances of prostatic mobility, meatal bleeding, scrotal ecchymosis, and unstable anterior pelvic fractures. In these circumstances, a retrograde urethrogram can identify or exclude urethral injury before manipulation of the urethra.

An electrocardiogram is essential to monitor cardiac rhythm. Primary rhythm disturbances in the trauma setting are rare. Secondary abnormalities are occasionally seen and include: sinus bradycardia due to advanced shock; electromechanical dissociation from hypovolemia, tension pneumothorax, or pericardial tamponade; and ventricular fibrillation due to hypothermia or acidosis. Ventricular ectopy, low voltages, and signs of ischemia can accompany myocardial contusion. Beyond evaluating the actual rhythm, diffusely low voltages may be the first indication of hemopericardium. Treatment of these secondary rhythm disturbances places priority on correction of inciting causes. Virtually all resuscitation medications can be given by the intraosseous route, and intratracheal administration is effective for lidocaine, atropine, naloxone, and epinephrine.

After vascular access, blood for laboratory analysis is obtained. The only imperative studies are hematocrit, type and crossmatch, potassium, glucose, and arterial blood gas analysis. A platelet count and serum amylase can be helpful. Blood alcohol levels and toxicology screens are discretionary. There has been a resurgence of interest in the use of serum lactate levels as indicators of anaerobic metabolism due to inadequate perfusion. This test appears to correlate closely with metabolic acidosis induced by hemorrhage in animals, and a prospective, randomized multiinstitution study evaluating its clinical usefulness is ongoing.

Routine Radiologic Evaluation

Films essential to the resuscitation process include a lateral cervical spine film, supine anteroposterior chest radiograph, and pelvis film. Because of their impact on treatment, these films are frequently obtained during the resuscitation phase in severely injured children and are used to guide the management of injuries. Although the eventual radiographic work-up of the cervical spine can include anteroposterior, open-mouth odontoid, flexion–extension, oblique, and computed tomography (CT) studies, most radiographically detectable injuries are discernible on an adequate lateral study.

Evaluation of the lateral cervical spine film involves examining the anterior and posterior borders of the vertebral bodies to detect displacement, which may indicate injury to the anterior or posterior spinal ligaments. Distinct bony abnormalities and subtle soft tissue abnormalities are also sought. Most cervical spine injuries in young children are located in the upper levels because of the rotational forces generated by the large head. In older children and adolescents, injuries are concentrated in the middle and lower levels. It is important to obtain a lateral view of the entire cervical spine, including the C-7 to T-1 junction; if this is not possible with simple traction on the arms during exposure, a transaxillary ''swimmer's'' view is helpful.

Interpretation of cervical spine films in the acutely injured child is difficult because of the wide spectrum of normal variations in the pediatric cervical spine. Variations include ligamentous laxity leading to hypermobility, soft tissue widening in the prevertebral space, absence of normal cervical lordosis, and the presence of growth plates that often resemble fractures. Pseudosubluxation at C-2 to C-3 and C-3 to C-4 is common. This abnormality should not exceed 4 mm and should resolve with gentle extension. The thickness of the prevertebral soft tissue plane should not exceed two thirds of the C-2 vertebral body width in the quiet child. Crying and agitation can increase this tissue plane unpredictably. In any child who is refractory to hemodynamic resuscitation and who lacks evidence of ongoing hemorrhage or other causes of shock, the cervical spine film should be scrutinized for atlantooccipital dislocation. Devastating and irreparable injury to the brain stem and upper spinal cord are common with this injury.

Many injuries detectable on the chest radiograph can have profound and immediate consequences for resuscitation management. The following injuries require prompt intervention or further evaluation: hemopneumothorax (with or without tension), pericardial effusion (tamponade), mediastinal emphysema (suggesting tracheobronchial or esophageal injury), mediastinal widening (suggesting aortic injury), diaphragmatic rupture, rib fractures and pulmonary contusion, and diffuse lung injury indicative of aspiration, drowning, or inhalation injury. The position of tubes and catheters must be checked, and the thoracic spine can frequently be evaluated for gross deformities. Mediastinal widening usually indicates hematoma formation from injury to small mediastinal veins, and suggest deceleration forces sufficient to cause aortic disruption at the ligamentum arteriosum. Other indicators of mediastinal hematoma include pleural capping, tracheal deviation, and effacement of the aorticopulmonary window. If any of these signs is present and the mechanism of injury is consistent with an aortic tear, further investigation is warranted. If spinal injury can be excluded in the alert child, an upright posteroanterior chest radiograph confirms the impression of a wide mediastinum. Aortography is diagnostic.

The pelvis film is evaluated for the presence and severity of pelvic fractures as well as the degree of comminution and displacement of the anterior fragments. A severely comminuted pelvic fracture in a boy suggests the need for a retrograde urethrogram and cystogram. Identification of a massive pelvic injury also explains ongoing hemorrhage and may prompt angiography or external fixation to control bleeding. Hip dislocations and lumbar spine fractures are also identifiable.

Secondary Survey and Directed Radiology

Vital Signs

After the primary survey, quantitative measures of blood pressure, heart rate, and respiratory rate are made. Because pediatric resuscitation relies heavily on weight-indexed doses of fluids and drugs, an estimate of weight based on age or length is also mandatory. One method assumes a roughly linear relation between age and weight during the preadolescent years, beginning with a weight of 10 kg at 1 year of age, and increasing by 5-kg increments every 2 years through 11 years of age. Weight then increases by 10 kg every 2 years after 11 years of age. Alternatively, one may use the following formula:

$$\text{weight (kg)} = (\text{age} \times 2) + 10$$

The upper limits of normal heart rates decline in children from about 160 beats/min at birth to 140 beats/min during the preschool stage, and 120 beats/min in preadolescent patients. Blood pressure, on the other hand, rises steadily with increasing age (Table 19-4). A useful formula for estimating the lower

TABLE 19-4. *Age-related vital signs in children*

	Heart rate (beats/min)	Minimum systolic blood pressure (mmHg)	Respiratory rate (breaths/min)
Infant	100–160	60	30–40
Preschooler	80–140	70	20–30
Adolescent	60–110	90	16–20

(Eichelberger MR. Pediatric trauma. St Louis, Mosby–Year Book, 1993)

limit of normal systolic blood pressure in children older than 2 years of age is as follows:

$$SBP_{min} = 7 + (age \times 2)$$

where: SBP_{min} = minimum acceptable systolic blood pressure

In adolescence, hemodynamic parameters correspond roughly to adult values. A narrowed pulse pressure with a normal systolic and elevated diastolic pressure can indicate marked peripheral vasoconstriction in response to acute hypovolemia. Blood pressures should be obtained in both upper extremities if mediastinal injury is suspected.

Head and Neck

Inspection of the head should include palpation for lacerations, fractures, and cephalohematomas. A small child can lose significant blood volume from a head wound and may present in shock from an isolated scalp laceration. Direct pressure is usually adequate to provide hemostasis. Palpable skull fractures in the alert child should put the examiner on guard for the possible development of an epidural hematoma. The examination should continue by evaluating the ears for hemotympanum, blood in the mastoid air cells (Battle sign), or periorbital ecchymoses without contusion (''raccoon eyes'')—all of which suggest basilar skull fracture. A thorough examination of the eyes and orbits is performed. The midface and mandible are evaluated for fracture and mobility. CSF rhinorrhea and midface instability are contraindications for nasal placement of a gastric decompression tube during the resuscitation phase. The oral cavity is examined again for loose teeth, bony fractures, foreign objects, and soft tissue injuries.

The neck must be examined in neutral position, with the anterior half of the rigid cervical collar temporarily removed, focusing attention on bony vertebral pain or palpable deformities. In the awake child who has no radiographic evidence of spinal injury, the neck may be carefully manipulated to rule out instability. Assessment of carotid pulses and lateral neck hematomas and bruits is undertaken. The central neck is examined for tracheal position, laryngotracheal integrity, and subcutaneous emphysema. When the examination is complete, the anterior half of the rigid cervical collar is reapplied until radiographic and clinical examination of the neck is concluded.

Chest

The chest is examined again for wounds, point tenderness, and instability by applying gentle compressive pressure along the rib cage. Inspection of chest wall excursion in the spontaneously breathing child can reveal paradoxical movement associated with a flail segment and retractions due to injuries that decrease compliance and increase the work of breathing. Because the thoracic cage is extremely compliant in childhood, significant pulmonary contusions can exist in the absence of rib fractures. The sternum is also examined because sternal fractures imply an impact of considerable force and alert the examiner to the possibility of cardiac contusion and aortic injury. Auscultation of both hemithoraces is performed to confirm intact ventilation or to identify a hemopneumothorax. Auscultation also evaluates the regularity of cardiac rhythm, displacement of the point of maximal impulse due to mediastinal shift, and distant or muffled sounds, which suggest hemopericardium.

The diagnosis of cardiac tamponade can be difficult in the emergency department. Cardiac tamponade is occasionally associated with the Beck triad—hypotension, venous distention, and muffled heart tones. A more reliable indicator is pulsus paradoxus (a decline in systolic blood pressure of more than 10 mmHg during inspiration). If a central venous catheter has been placed, or if the neck veins are easily visualized, a drop in venous pressure with inspiration (Kussmaul sign) can also suggest pericardial tamponade. Urgent echocardiography in the emergency department establishes the diagnosis in the stable child. Subxyphoid pericardiocentesis in the unstable child provides temporary hemodynamic improvement and allows for timely surgical exploration.

Traumatic asphyxia is a syndrome that occurs predominantly in children and produces dramatic clinical effects. The mechanism of injury requires extreme compressive pressure imparted to the thorax in a child with a closed glottis or other tracheobronchial obstruction. Because air is trapped within the lung and airways, the force causes rapid displacement of blood from the atrium and major veins of the mediastinum. The pressure is transmitted principally to the upper body and head because the absence of valves in the large veins allows for a free retrograde flow of blood from the right atrium through the superior vena cava. These factors produce retinal hemorrhages. If the pressure is applied long enough, as in a sustained crush injury, the upper body displays diffuse cyanosis, petechiae, and edema. Pulmonary contusion is common, as are liver injuries. Brain dysfunction is also common and is caused by either hypoxemia or hypoperfusion due to reduced CPP. Despite the dramatic presentation, children who survive to reach the hospital have a good prognosis.

Abdomen

A careful abdominal examination is crucial to the proper evaluation of the injured child. A soft, flat, nontender abdomen in an alert child rules out significant intraabdominal trauma with reasonable certainty, but positive findings on examination may not discriminate between trivial injuries and those requiring surgery. Distention can be caused by acute gastric dilation from air swallowing or bag-mask ventilation, hemoperitoneum, or retroperitoneal or pelvic hematoma. Findings of focal tenderness or diffuse peritonitis in the alert child can be important and may dictate surgical exploration without further evaluation. Flank ecchymoses may suggest retroperitoneal or splenic hemorrhage, or a later manifestation of a pancreatic injury.

Attention to the presence of lap-belt contusions across the lower abdominal wall is important. These injuries are common in restrained vehicle passengers, especially those who are too small to allow the lap belt to restrain the pelvic girdle correctly. The presence of a lap belt contusion is associated with an increased incidence of intraabdominal injury—especially hollow viscus perforation. The likelihood of an injury necessitating surgery is even higher when a lap belt contusion and spinal fracture coexist.[12]

CT is the standard technique for assessment of intraabdominal and retroperitoneal injuries. Indications for radiographic evaluation of the abdomen in the stable child include inability to obtain a reliable examination in a child when the mechanism of injury suggests the possibility of visceral injury, equivocal findings in the alert child, unexplained blood loss, gross hematuria, and the coexistence of a lap-belt contusion and lumbar spine fracture. CT can reliably identify solid organ and most hollow viscus injuries in the peritoneal cavity and retroperitoneum.

Although diagnostic peritoneal lavage (DPL) is less useful than CT in the evaluation of abdominal trauma in the stable child, DPL still has an occasional role in identifying intraabdominal hemorrhage as the cause of hemodynamic instability in a comatose, unstable patient with an equivocal abdominal examination. The technique obviates a lengthy radiologic procedure and expedites surgical exploration. Although the Seldinger technique has proved useful in adults, open catheter placement is safer in the small child. Aspiration of the catheter detects gross hemoperitoneum. Warm lactated Ringer solution or normal saline is instilled at a volume of 15 mL/kg, and effluent is evaluated for blood and enteric contents. Historical correlations in adults between lavage findings of 100,000 RBCs/μL and the coexistence of injuries requiring surgery do not apply to children.

Penetrating injuries are unhappily more common in children now than in the past. Although virtually all gunshot wounds to the abdomen are still best evaluated in the operating room, stab wounds to the front, back, and flank are increasingly evaluated by nonoperative means. Anterior wounds that penetrate the muscular fascia can be evaluated by DPL, avoiding formal exploration if the lavage effluent contains less than 1,000 RBCs/μL. In the past, flank and back wounds were thought to be absolute indications for abdominal exploration, but CT imaging with enteral contrast has proved to be a sensitive technique to rule out visceral injury. The child who sustains a penetrating abdominal injury should receive a parenteral second-generation cephalosporin (eg, cefoxitin, 30 mg/kg) as prophylaxis against intraabdominal infection.

Pelvis and Genitourinary Tract

The pelvis is evaluated for instability by applying both compressive and downward pressure on the iliac crests. Infraumbilical distention and ecchymoses can also indicate preperitoneal extension of a pelvic hematoma. Hemodynamic instability in a patient with an unstable pelvic fracture and no other explanation for ongoing hemorrhage is an indication for urgent management to obtain hemostasis. Application of a pneumatic antishock garment is helpful in temporary controlling pelvic hemorrhage until definitive therapy is provided. This is the only situation in which a pneumatic antishock garment is useful in children.

Evidence suggests that pelvic fractures can be graded according to geometric criteria and that increasing severity correlates with both blood transfusion requirements and need for specific therapeutic intervention.[13] Radiographic evidence of simultaneous anterior and posterior fractures, especially if bilateral, predicts an increased need for blood transfusion and invasive therapy. Definitive therapy usually involves angiographic embolization of disrupted pelvic vessels or surgical placement of an external-fixation frame.

Children occasionally sustain perineal injuries from bicycles, straddle toys, jungle-gyms, and sexual abuse. Careful examination of the external genitalia for lacerations and hematomas is crucial. Because pelvic fracture fragments can cause injury to internal pelvic organs, an examination of the vaginal introitus and vestibule for blood and a digital rectal examination are both done at this time if not previously. Proctoscopic examination of the rectal vault with the child under anesthesia is sometimes necessary to identify lacerations from penetrating injuries that require fecal diversion.

Extremities

Examination of the extremities focuses on identifying and classifying injuries to bones, joints, and soft tissues. Special attention to identifying open fractures, bony instability that can cause secondary injury, and evidence of combined neurovascular trauma is important. Certain injuries, such as posterior knee dislocations and midshaft humerus fractures, are associated with a high incidence of injuries to adjacent neurovascular bundles. Such bony deformities must be reduced and immobilized and neurovascular status reassessed to determine the need for urgent operative repair. Routine angiography of high-risk injuries is gradually being replaced by selective angiography based on discrepancies in Doppler pressures between injured and uninjured extremities.[14] With comminuted fractures and vascular injuries, measurement of compartment pressures may be appropriate. Children who sustain open fractures should receive prophylaxis against osteomyelitis and nonunion with a parenteral first-generation cephalosporin (eg, cefazolin, 25 mg/kg).

Back

The back should be examined in the log-roll position. Palpation of the entire thoracic, lumbar, and sacral spine should be performed to identify point tenderness and anatomic deformity. Penetrating injuries not identified on the anterior body may become apparent at this time. The presence of a lap-belt injury is associated with an increased incidence of lumbosacral spine fracture or dislocation.

Neurologic Examination

A thorough neurologic examination completes the secondary survey, unless severe head injury is obvious and detailed assessment is necessary sooner to prioritize management. The three general components of the examination are evaluation of cortical function, which includes calculating a Glasgow coma scale (GCS) score; assessment of cranial nerve and brain-stem reflex

TABLE 19-5. *Glasgow Coma Scale*

Activity	Best response	Score
Eye opening	Spontaneous	4
	To verbal stimuli	3
	To pain	2
	None	1
Verbal	Oriented	5
	Confused	4
	Inappropriate words	3
	Nonspecific sounds	2
	None	1
Motor	Follows commands	6
	Localizes pain	5
	Withdraws to pain	4
	Flexion to pain	3
	Extension to pain	2
	None	1

function; and thorough evaluation of extremity function and posturing. This phase of the trauma resuscitation is crucial because of the extreme morbidity associated with neurologic injury.

The GCS grades level of consciousness by evaluating the eye, voice, and motor responses to verbal or tactile (noxious) stimuli (Table 19-5). Any persistent posttraumatic depression of cortical function is significant and requires CT evaluation, but GCS scores of 8 or below indicate a poor prognosis. These patients require urgent CT evaluation and early intervention to manage intracranial hypertension, such as intubation and hyperventilation, to prevent permanent secondary brain injury.

Cranial nerve and brain-stem testing during the secondary survey reveal clues pertaining to severe intracranial injury. The most useful tests are pupillary responses, extraocular movements, corneal reflexes, cold caloric vestibular reflexes, and the gag reflex. Asymmetry of the pupillary responses with anisocoria suggests transtentorial herniation. Absence of the other cranial nerve reflexes can indicate global, devastating brain injury, usually combined with secondary ischemic injury.

In addition to a careful examination of the neck and vertebral column, functional signs of spinal cord or nerve root injury must be sought. Reflexes, strength, and sensation are evaluated in all extremities. The presence of a normal cervical spine radiograph is reassuring but cannot by itself exclude spinal injury. A syndrome of spinal cord injury without radiographic abnormality occurs in younger children and is best evaluated by magnetic resonance imaging. These injuries are due to sudden traction, rotation, or compression of the cord without bony vertebral injury. They can present as complete spinal interruptions, or can initially cause transient motor and sensory abnormalities before progressing to complete lesions. The administration of corticosteroids to reduce cord edema in acute spinal injury (less than 12 hours old) is recommended.[15] Methylprednisolone is given intravenously as a 30 mg/kg bolus, followed by a continuous infusion of 5.4 mg/kg/h for the next 23 hours.

SPECIFIC ISSUES AND CONTROVERSIES

Crystalloid, Colloid, and Hypertonic Resuscitation

Considerable controversy continues to exist about the optimal approach to fluid resuscitation in hemorrhagic shock. As in other facets of trauma management, most experience and investigation have focused on adults. With few exceptions, these findings can be carefully applied to injured children of all ages. The debate can be reduced to three primary questions:

1. What are the relative advantages and risks of crystalloids versus colloids?
2. Is there a role for hypertonic resuscitation in hemorrhagic shock?
3. Should hemodynamic resuscitation be delayed in certain circumstances?

Colloids Versus Crystalloids

During the past two decades, the merits of resuscitation fluids with enhanced capabilities of expanding intravascular volume have been intensively studied.[16] Isotonic crystalloid (salt) solutions rapidly redistribute throughout the extracellular compartment after intravascular administration. Because the intravascular space accounts for only 25% of the total extracellular fluid compartment, expansion of the intravascular space by a given volume requires infusion of roughly four times that volume of isotonic fluid. The isotonic crystalloids used most commonly in resuscitation are lactated Ringer solution and normal saline.

In contrast, isotonic colloidal resuscitation fluids, in which the osmotically active particles are proteins or carbohydrates of sufficient size to prevent diffusion through the capillary membrane, remain in the intravascular compartment longer. A commonly used colloid is human albumin in concentrations of 5% or 25% diluted in normal saline. Because these solutions are expensive and carry the theoretical risk of disease transmission, synthetic colloids have become popular. The most common synthetic colloids are hydroxyethyl starch (Hetastarch) and the dextrans (Dextran 40 and 70). Hetastarch is a mixture of complex carbohydrates similar to glycogen, with an average molecular weight of 69 kd, and is available in a 6% solution in normal saline with an osmolarity of 310 mOsm/L. Dextran 70 is mixture of glucose polymers derived from the bacterial modification of sucrose, with an average molecular weight of 70 kd, and is also available as an isotonic 6% solution in normal saline. Both synthetic colloids have intravascular half-lives of about 24 hours, in contrast to the 2 to 6 hours for salt solutions.

Proponents of colloid resuscitation argue that colloids result in a more rapid and prolonged intravascular expansion with smaller infused volumes. The colloid is less likely to diffuse through capillary membranes, so less tissue edema is produced than is by crystalloids that freely redistribute 75% of their volume into the interstitium. Because the lung is a common organ involved in posttraumatic organ dysfunction, any protective effect that colloids might have on pulmonary function would be considered advantageous.

Advocates of crystalloid resuscitation point out that experience confirms effective intravascular repletion can be easily accomplished with lactated Ringer solution or normal saline, albeit requiring greater volumes. Crystalloid redistribution reconstitutes the interstitial fluid compartment, which is known to be contracted through shock-induced cell membrane dysfunction, resulting in translocation of sodium and water from the interstitium into the intracellular compartment. The attendant peripheral edema is mobilized after several days and usually causes no further problems. No convincing evidence has shown an increased incidence of lung edema or pulmonary dysfunction after crystalloid resuscitation of trauma victims, perhaps because rapid redistribution prevents left atrial and pulmonary venous pressures from rising abruptly and generating the hydrostatic forces necessary to promote pulmonary edema. Furthermore, in both pulmonary contusion and posttraumatic ARDS, the injured capillary endothelium no longer presents a barrier to the diffusion of even large colloid molecules. A metaanalysis comparing the use of crystalloids and colloids in the resuscitation of adult trauma victims concluded that crystalloid resuscitation conferred a 12% survival advantage over colloid resuscitation.[17] Interestingly, colloids appeared to have a slight advantage (8%) in the resuscitation of nontrauma patients. Finally, crystalloids are inexpensive and are not associated with the potential risks of colloids, which include hypersensitivity, coagulopathy, and platelet dysfunction.

Hypertonic Resuscitation

From a theoretic standpoint, hypertonic fluids are attractive alternatives to the standard isotonic fluids employed for the resuscitation of trauma victims. The underlying principle is simple: hypertonic solutions administered intravascularly promote the osmotic transfer of free water from the intracellular space, which is enlarged because of the effects of shock on cell membrane function, into the extracellular space, where it is distributed between the intravascular and interstitial compartments at a volume ratio of 1:3. The extracellular expansion is driven by exogenous osmotic particles in the resuscitation fluid but is accomplished by endogenous water transfer. Although the end result is the same as with isotonic resuscitation—namely, the expansion of the interstitial and intravascular compartments—it can be effected with a much smaller volume of infused fluid, hence the term *small-volume resuscitation*.

A prompt vascular expansion has been observed in animal studies, but, like isotonic crystalloid infusions, the effect is transient. For this reason, most contemporary studies of hypertonic resuscitation in animals and humans have combined hypertonic saline with an isotonic dextran mixture, which prolongs the vascular expansion effect. The fluid used most commonly is 7.5% NaCl in 6% Dextran 70 (hypertonic saline–dextran [HSD]), which generates an osmolarity of about 2500 mOsm/L.

Animal studies of HSD resuscitation have confirmed a rapid vascular expansion with small infused volumes.[18] Although experimental studies have suggested that the vascular compartment is expanded by only 12% to 25% of the infused volume for crystalloids, and by roughly 100% for isotonic colloids, the expansion observed after HSD resuscitation is about three times the infused volume. Virtually all studies measuring physiologic parameters during experimental or clinical resuscitation with HSD have confirmed more rapid improvements in blood pressure, cardiac output, and peripheral perfusion. Hypothetical advantages of HSD, in addition to rapid intravascular expansion, include vagally mediated venoconstriction, direct enhancement of myocardial contractility, and improved microcirculatory perfusion due to rheologic effects on blood and osmotic shrinkage of injured capillary endothelium. A major multiinstitutional pilot study comparing HSD with isotonic resuscitation in adult trauma victims failed to show a significant difference in overall mortality rates, but it did document improved survival in the subgroup that required surgery.[19] The complications associated with HSD have been limited largely to transient hypernatremia. In both experimental and clinical uses, serum sodium concentrations have been elevated during HSD infusion, but adverse neurologic consequences (eg, seizures and central pontine myelinolysis) have not been observed. Complications of dextran infusion have not been reported. The ability to effect hemodynamic resuscitation in the field with very small fluid volumes is particularly attractive in severely injured children, especially those with interosseous access in whom infusion rates are significantly constrained. Recommendations for HSD in children should wait until its risks and benefits have been evaluated in this special group.

Postponed Fluid Resuscitation

Although anathema to many practitioners of trauma resuscitation, the question has been thoughtfully raised of whether prehospital resuscitation is either beneficial or necessary. The debate actually involves two separate issues. First, how much time, if any, should be allocated to establishing intravenous access in the field? This is particularly critical for pediatric trauma victims, in whom establishing intravenous access can be difficult even in the best circumstances. Second, provided intravenous access can be established, is not fluid administration in the face of uncontrolled internal hemorrhage counterproductive? If internal bleeding cannot be controlled, is it not more rational to permit a certain degree of hypotension to limit further blood loss?

The first question has been adequately addressed. Most studies have shown a distinct advantage to advanced life support transport, including intravenous access, as opposed to basic life support transport for equally injured patients. Nevertheless, most would agree that prolonged attempts to start an intravenous line in the field on an injured child are counterproductive if they delay transport. This is particularly true when the anticipated transport time is short. Furthermore, studies have confirmed that attempts to establish intravenous access in adults during transport are as successful as before transport. Hence, if access cannot be obtained rapidly during stabilization, transport should be initiated and venous access attempted en route.

The second question is less easily resolved. Proponents of delayed resuscitation observe that most animal models of hemorrhage and resuscitation involve controlled blood loss that is curtailed before resuscitation. When models of uncontrolled hemorrhage have been used, resuscitated animals bled more and had a higher mortality rate than did unresuscitated animals.[20] In a follow-up study, animals resuscitated with HSD had a survival rate intermediate between the unresuscitated and isotonic resuscitated animals.[21] Similar findings were reported in a clinical study comparing immediate versus delayed fluid resuscitation in hypotensive victims of penetrating torso trauma.[22] In this study, duration of hospitalization, complication rate, and mortality rate were all reduced in the group that did not receive intravenous fluid resuscitation before admission to the emergency department. The rationale for this approach remains to be established both for children and for blunt trauma victims.

Cerebral Resuscitation

Traumatic brain injury is a common manifestation of pediatric trauma and causes a disproportionate amount of mortality and morbidity. It is estimated that over 100,000 children are admitted to hospitals with significant traumatic brain injury each year in the United States.[23] Of all children who die of their injuries, about 70% are judged to have died primarily of brain injury. In general, the outcome for children older than 3 years of age is better than for adults with comparable injuries and presenting GCS scores.[24,25] Children younger than 3 years of age, however, do not enjoy this same advantage. Nonfatal injuries of both the brain and spine constitute an even greater cause of permanent disability in children.

Traumatic brain injury can be defined as either primary or secondary. *Primary brain injury* is the structural derangement of cerebral architecture that occurs at the instant of energy transfer. It includes cranial fractures, cerebral lacerations and contusions, vascular disruptions leading to intracranial hematomas, and microscopic injury to neuronal axons and myelin sheaths, referred to as *diffuse axonal injury*. Children suffer from focal intracranial lesions, such as subdural hematoma and intraparenchymal hemorrhage and contusion, less frequently than adults. Children, however, have a higher incidence of epidural hematomas, perhaps because the thinner, less rigid skull is more apt to fracture and lacerate meningeal arteries. Although children develop fewer intracranial hematomas than adults, they have an increased propensity for diffuse axonal injury. This lesion is histologically characterized by disruption of ascending and descending axonal tracts, particularly in the corpus callosum and internal capsule, and is caused by shear forces generated by rapid angular and rotational acceleration. The proportionately larger size of the cranium in children, along with a less muscular and more flexible ligamentous cervical spine, may account for the increased incidence of diffuse axonal injury in children.

Secondary brain injury occurs as a result of decreased cerebral perfusion after the traumatic event. The deleterious effects of secondary brain injury are additive to those of the primary injury and are the only aspects of traumatic brain injury that can be reversed or mitigated by therapeutic intervention. Secondary traumatic brain injury is caused primarily by increased ICP and can be understood in terms of the following equation relating ICP, CPP, and mean arterial pressure (MAP):

$$CPP = MAP - ICP$$

Because the cranium is noncompliant, expansion of an extracerebral hematoma or an increase in parenchymal volume secondary to hemorrhage and edema must be offset by a decrease in either CSF or blood volume. As this volume buffer is exhausted, further progression of cerebral edema or intracranial hematoma volume generates exponential increases in ICP, which can be measured by a number of methods. When ICP exceeds venous outflow pressure, it acts as a Starling resistor and determines the pressure gradient for cerebral blood flow as defined in the preceding equation.

Normal CPP values range between 50 and 70 mmHg in adults but are not established in infants and children. Although CPP may still be marginally adequate for substrate and oxygen delivery at levels of 25 to 30 mmHg, a sustained CPP of less than 50 mmHg is considered dangerous. This corresponds roughly to an ICP of 20 mmHg or greater. In the normal brain, perfusion is maintained relatively constant over a wide range of CPP levels by alterations in locoregional cerebrovascular tone, a process referred to as *cerebral autoregulation*. Because autoregulation is impaired in traumatic brain injury, nutrient blood flow to the injured brain may be abnormally dependent on a normal CPP, and inappropriate vasodilation may lead to increases in cerebral blood volume and ICP. Malignant intracranial hypertension, thought to be due to markedly impaired autoregulation, is more common in children than adults. When CPP falls below some critical threshold, because of either increased ICP or decreased MAP, cerebral ischemia occurs.

Efforts to reduce secondary brain injury focus not only on normalization of MAP but also on reduction and control of ICP. A number of avenues are available to accomplish this. The most expeditious method is intubation and controlled hyperventilation, reducing P_{CO_2} to 26 to 30 mmHg to induce a respiratory alkalosis. Hypocarbia and alkalosis promote cerebral vasoconstriction, limiting cerebral blood volume and lowering ICP. The effect is rapid but can be limited in duration by reequilibration of CSF pH balance. The maximal duration of the effect is unknown but may range from several hours to several days. Hyperventilation should not be rapidly withdrawn because rebound elevations in ICP are common.

Recommendations to raise the head 30 degrees have been made, but the efficacy of this maneuver is unclear, given that venous pressure does not determine CPP when it is exceeded by ICP. A head-up position can, however, have a detrimental effect on MAP and thereby reduce CPP. Another traditional intervention to lower ICP acutely during resuscitation is to induce an osmotic diuresis. Mannitol, 0.25 to 1 g/kg, often coupled with a loop diuretic like furosemide, stimulates the osmotic translocation of intracellular and interstitial fluid into the vascular compartment, from which it is excreted by the kidneys. This strategy is effective acutely but is hazardous in the face of concurrent hypovolemia from hemorrhage. Its use is also limited by hyperosmolarity and should not be administered when serum osmolarity exceeds 320 mOsm/L.

A development in brain resuscitation is the use of hypertonic crystalloids, such as 7.5% NaCl. Hypertonic saline rapidly expands the intravascular compartment by inducing an osmotic transfer of fluid out of the intracellular compartment, but it does not cause an inappropriate osmotic diuresis. This osmotic transfer reduces cerebral edema and ICP. Any increase in urine output is largely due to increased renal perfusion. Initial studies in animals have found hypertonic saline as efficacious as mannitol in reducing ICP caused by space-occupying lesions,[26] and experience in clinical settings is accumulating.

Generalized tonic clonic seizures are common after traumatic brain injury, occurring more frequently as the severity of brain injury increases. A child who experiences a single seizure immediately after the event, but is neurologically normal thereafter, probably does not require treatment. The severely brain-injured child who has a documented seizure during resuscitation requires prompt intervention, however, because seizure activity exacerbates intracranial hypertension. Immediate seizure control with a benzodiazepine (eg, diazepam, 0.1 mg/kg), followed by maintenance therapy with phenytoin or phenobarbitol, is indicated. Whether the comatose child who has not demonstrated seizure activity requires anticonvulsant prophylaxis during the resuscitation process is a controversial issue.

Emergency Department Thoracotomy

The clinical futility of emergency department thoracotomy in adult victims of blunt trauma, as well as the high cost and perceived risks of exposure to communicable diseases, has led to a much more limited role for emergency thoracotomy in adults now than in the past.[27–30] Guidelines limit emergency thoracotomy in adults to cases of penetrating chest trauma and to selected cases of blunt or extrathoracic penetrating trauma in which the victim exhibits signs of life before cardiac arrest and has a nonidioventricular rhythm, either initially or after successful cardioversion. Emergency thoracotomy is still commonly attempted in prepubertal children regardless of injury mechanism. This posture is predicated on the belief that children are more resistant to the effects of ischemia and are therefore more likely to respond to desperate resuscitative efforts despite ominous objective signs such as idioventricular cardiac rhythm.

Although anecdotal experience may support limited optimism, this impression is not borne out by objective data. A retrospective study of emergency department thoracotomy in pediatric patients confirmed the futility of this approach in moribund victims of blunt trauma.[31] The authors concluded that indications for emergency department thoracotomy in children should be identical to those for adults: penetrating chest trauma with recent signs of life in the field or emergency department and a cardiac rhythm. A review of injured children receiving cardiopulmonary resuscitation in the field found no survivors in any group when cardiopulmonary resuscitation was required after arrival at the receiving hospital.[32] Unfortunately, there were no victims of penetrating trauma in this study. Based on the available data, then, it seems prudent to restrict emergency department thoracotomy in children to those with penetrating injury, signs of life at some point during evaluation, and electrical cardiac activity.

Emergency thoracotomy in children is performed through a fourth intercostal space anterolateral thoracotomy on the side of the injury. Exsanguinating pulmonary vascular hemorrhage and bronchial disruptions are treated by hilar cross-clamping. The pericardium is opened to decompress potential tamponade, and specific cardiac injuries are addressed. Open cardiac massage is initiated and combined with intracardiac injection of resuscitative drugs, such as epinephrine, atropine, and sodium bicarbonate. If the heart is empty, the descending thoracic aorta is occluded to redirect perfusion to the brain and myocardium. Coronary air embolism is treated by cross-clamping the aortic root and forcibly compressing the heart, driving the trapped air bubbles through the coronary microvasculature. If an explanation for traumatic arrest is not found in the opened chest, the contralateral hemithorax can be entered by manually puncturing the mediastinal pleura anterior to the heart. If a large return of air or blood under pressure is obtained, the thoracotomy can be extended across the sternum into the contralateral fourth interspace and pulmonary hilar control gained. If sustainable cardiac activity can be salvaged, the child is taken to the operating room for definitive management.

Hypothermia

Children have special needs related to thermal control. Their large surface area/mass ratio accounts for a greater rate of heat loss. Because many children are injured in outdoor activities as pedestrians or bicycle riders, by falls, and by drownings, environmental exposure and long stabilization and transport times commonly result in varying degrees of hypothermia when the child arrives at the hospital.

The regulation of core body temperature depends on manipulating the two determinants of temperature, that is, heat production and heat loss. Heat production is a direct result of metabolic rate and oxygen consumption, both of which may be elevated in the posttrauma setting. The increase in metabolic rate is a consequence of increased energy requirements, not an attempt to raise core temperature primarily. Shivering, which begins as core temperature falls to about 32° to 33°C, is a reflex response to hypothermia designed to increase oxygen consumption and generate heat. When oxygen delivery falls below an anaerobic threshold during shock, regardless of cause, oxygen consumption and metabolic rate also fall (supply-dependent oxygen consumption). Therefore, the hypoperfused child is ill equipped to generate heat and maintain core temperature.

Heat loss occurs through evaporation, radiation, conduction, and convection and can be significantly increased in the emergency department setting. Prolonged exposure, contact with clothing and sheets soaked with cold fluid and blood, ventilation with unwarmed gases, uncontrolled hemorrhage, and the administration of unwarmed fluids in large volumes all cause accelerated heat loss and can result in the deleterious effects of hypothermia. Toddlers and young children who are rapidly growing have increased surface area/volume ratios, less insulating fat, and less muscle mass for shivering, and therefore are more susceptible to heat loss. Infants may have lower surface area/volume ratios but also have far less muscle mass and reduced abilities to generate heat, and therefore are also at high risk for hypothermia in the resuscitation environment.

The consequences of hypothermia are significant. The myocardium is particularly sensitive to temperature changes, and hypothermia is accompanied by increased ventricular irritability to potassium and calcium concentrations. Premature ventricular contractions are seen at about 30° to 32°C, with a threshold for ventricular fibrillation at about 28° to 30°C. Cold also shifts the oxyhemoglobin dissociation curve to the left, increasing the affinity of hemoglobin for oxygen and impairing peripheral oxygen unloading. Other effects of hypothermia include CNS depression, respiratory depression, coagulopathy, and loss of peripheral vasomotor tone. All of these effects can initiate or exacerbate metabolic acidosis, hemodynamic instability, and organ dysfunction. Because of the profound effects of hypothermia on cardiovascular function, resuscitation measures need to be continued until rewarming is accomplished, before the response to resuscitation, and therefore prognosis, can be evaluated.

Rapid rewarming is desirable under most circumstances but is often frustrating and difficult to accomplish. Warming all infused fluids and ventilator gases, removing wet clothes and drying the child's skin, providing warm blankets and head covers, and using radiant heaters can all be helpful in small children. Beyond this, lavage of body cavities with warm isotonic fluid is probably the technique that best lends itself to the emergency room setting. Gastric and bladder lavage through catheters is commonly practiced but is not very effective. Continuous lavage of the peritoneal cavity and thorax through peritoneal dialysis catheters and chest tubes is occasionally successful in rewarming a hypothermic patient. The use of cardiopulmonary bypass or extracorporeal membrane oxygenation is theoretically appealing but is limited by practical obstacles in the emergency setting.

New techniques of rapid rewarming that rely on extracorporeal warming of the patient's blood by a countercurrent heat exchanger, similar to those found in bypass circuits but driven by the patient's blood pressure rather than a pump mechanism, have been successful in adults.[33] The application of this technology to small children has been limited by the high resistances imparted by small-diameter cannulas. Further work in this area is required before such methods are a viable option for children.

Coagulopathy

Dysfunctional coagulation related to trauma occurs in the early postinjury period in several scenarios: extreme hypothermia, massive transfusion, and severe brain injury. Hypothermia, discussed earlier, causes excessive bleeding simply by retarding the enzymatic processes that cause coagulation. *Massive transfusion,* defined as the acute administration of blood products equal to or greater than one blood volume (65 to 80 mL/kg), causes coagulopathy by several mechanisms, one of which is iatrogenic hypothermia. Another mechanism is explained by the fact that packed RBCs are stored in anticoagulants containing ethylenediaminetetraacetic acid or citrate (citrate-phosphate-dextrose), both of which chelate calcium and inhibit the calcium-dependent steps of the coagulation cascade. Acute hypocalcemia is therefore another consequence of massive transfusion.

The most common mechanism by which massive transfusion causes coagulopathy, however, is dilutional thrombocytopenia. Coagulopathy due to dilution of clotting factors is much less common because a much greater functional reserve of factors exists. As continued hemorrhage depletes circulating platelets and blood is replaced with RBCs, a progressive reduction in the platelet count ensues. This does not occur as quickly as predicted by washout models; hence, platelet mobilization from the bone marrow and spleen is postulated. In chronic disease, platelet levels of 20,000 to 30,000/μL are usually adequate to prevent bleeding. In the acute trauma setting, however, an acute decrease to 50,000/μL can produce oozing and surgical bleeding.[34] Such drastic reductions in platelet levels require a massive transfusion of at least two blood volumes. During massive transfusion, platelet counts should be regularly checked. Levels below 100,000/μL signify impending coagulopathy, and levels of 50,000/μL or less mandate platelet transfusion. Administration of ABO-matched platelets at an initial dose of 0.1 U/kg raises the platelet level by about 40,000/μL. Prophylactic platelet administration during massive transfusion has not proved efficacious.[35]

Severe head injury is also associated with a coagulopathic state unrelated to platelet dilution. Presumably, large concentrations of procoagulant tissue thromboplastins are released from cerebral lacerations. These thromboplastins initiate disseminated intravascular coagulation, resulting in a consumptive coagulopathy in which clotting factors and fibrinogen are depleted as well as platelets. Coagulopathy after head injury is a grim prognostic sign. Treatment requires administration of matched fresh frozen plasma at a dose of 15 to 30 mL/kg. Cryoprecipitate contains large amounts of fibrinogen, factor VIII, factor XIII, and von Willebrand factor, and can be given at a dose of 0.1 U/kg in addition to fresh frozen plasma. Administration of fresh frozen plasma, cryoprecipitate, or both may also be required in the setting of preexisting coagulopathies such as hemophilia, von Willebrand disease, and advanced liver disease.

REFERENCES

1. Moront ML, Williams JA, Eichelberger MR, et al. The injured child: an approach to care. Pediatr Clin North Am 1994;41:1201.
2. Magnuson DK, Maier RV. Pathophysiology of injury. In: Eichelberger MR, ed. Pediatric trauma: prevention, acute care, rehabilitation. St Louis, Mosby–Year Book, 1993:59.
3. Reilly PM, Schiller HJ, Bulkley GB. Reactive oxygen metabolites in shock. In: Wilmore DW, Brennan MF, Harken AH, et al, eds. Care of the surgical patient. New York, Scientific American, 1991:4;8.
4. Caty MG, Guice KS, Oldham KT, et al. Evidence for tumor necrosis factor-induced pulmonary microvascular injury after intestinal ischemia–reperfusion injury. Ann Surg 1990;212:694.
5. Jaffe BM, LaRosa CA, Kimura K. Prostaglandins and surgical diseases. Curr Prob Surg 1988;25:715.
6. Fong Y, Moldawer LL, Shires GT, et al. The biological characteristics of cytokines and their implications in surgical injury. Surg Gynecol Obstet 1990;170:363.
7. Dries DJ, Jurkovich GJ, Maier RV, et al. Effect of interferon gamma on infection-related death in patients with severe injuries: a randomized, double-blind, placebo-controlled trial. Arch Surg 1994;129:1031.
8. Ramenofsky ML, Luterman A, Quindlen E, et al. Maximum survival in pediatric trauma: the ideal system. J Trauma 1984;24:818.
9. Losek JD, Bonadio WA, Walsh-Kelly C, et al. Prehospital pediatric endotracheal intubation performance review. Pediatr Emerg Care 1989; 5:1.
10. Bivins HG, Ford S, Bezmalinovic Z, et al. The effect of axial traction during orotracheal intubation of the trauma victim with an unstable cervical spine. Ann Emerg Med 1988;17:25.
11. Peclet MH, Newman KD, Eichelberger MR, et al. Thoracic trauma in children: an indicator of increased mortality. J Pediatr Surg 1990;25:961.
12. Sivit CJ, Taylor GA, Newman KD, et al. Safety-belt injuries in children with lap-belt ecchymosis: CT findings in 61 patients. AJR 1991;157:111.
13. McIntyre RC, Bensard DD, Moore EE, et al. Pelvic fracture geometry predicts risk of life-threatening hemorrhage in children. J Trauma 1993;35:423.
14. Lynch K, Johansen K. Can Doppler pressure measurement replace "exclusion" arteriography in the diagnosis of occult extremity arterial trauma? Ann Surg 1991;214:737
15. Bracken MB, Shepard MJ, Collins WF, et al. A randomized, controlled trial of methylprednisolone or naloxone in the treatment of acute spinal-cord injury: results of the Second National Acute Spinal Cord Injury Study. N Engl J Med 1990;322:1405.
16. Gould SA, Sehgal LR, Sehgal HL, et al. Hypovolemic shock. Crit Care Clin 1993;9:239.
17. Velanovich V. Crystalloid versus colloid fluid resuscitation: a meta-analysis of mortality. Surgery 1989;105:65.
18. Dubick MA, Wade CE. A review of the efficacy and safety of 7.5% NaCl/6% dextran 70 in experimental animals and in humans. J Trauma 1994;36:323.
19. Mattox KL, Maningas PA, Moore EE, et al. Prehospital hypertonic saline/dextran infusion for post-traumatic hypotension: the U.S.A. Multicenter Trial. Ann Surg 1991;213:482.
20. Bickell WH, Bruttig SP, Millnamow GA, et al. The detrimental effects of intravenous crystalloid after aortotomy in swine. Surgery 1991;110:529.

21. Bickell WH, Bruttig SP, Millnamow GA, et al. The use of hypertonic saline/dextran versus lactated Ringer's solution as a resuscitation fluid following uncontrolled aortic hemorrhage in anesthetized swine. Ann Emerg Med 1992;21:1077.

22. Bickell WH, Wall MJ Jr, Pepe PE, et.al. Immediate versus delayed fluid resuscitation for hypotensive patients with penetrating torso injuries. N Engl J Med 1994;331:1105.

23. Shapiro K. US government central nervous system trauma status report. Bethesda, NIH, 1985:243.

24. Berger MS, Pitts LH, Lovely M, et al. Outcome from severe head injury in children and adolescents. J Neurosurg 1985;62:194.

25. Becker DP, Miller JD, Ward JD, et al. The outcome from severe head injury with early diagnosis and intensive management. J Neurosurg 1977;47:491.

26. Freshman SP, Battistella FD, Matteucci M, et al. Hypertonic saline (7.5%) versus mannitol: a comparison for treatment of acute head injuries. J Trauma 1993;35:344.

27. Esposito TJ, Jurkovich GJ, Rice CL, et al. Reappraisal of emergency room thoracotomy in a changing environment. J Trauma 1991;31:881.

28. Lorenz HP, Steinmetz B, Lieberman J, et al. Emergency thoracotomy: survival correlates with physiologic status. J Trauma 1992;32:780.

29. Boyd M, Vanek VW, Bourguet CC. Emergency room resuscitative thoracotomy: when is it indicated? J Trauma 1992;33:714.

30. Mazzorana V, Smith RS, Morabito DJ, et al. Limited utility of emergency department thoracotomy. Am Surg 1994;60:516.

31. Sheikh AA, Culbertson CB. Emergency department thoracotomy in children: rationale for selective application. J Trauma 1993;34:323.

32. Moront M, Gotschall CS, Eichelberger MR, et al. Predictors of survival and death for injured children receiving pre-hospital cardiopulmonary resuscitation. Surg Forum 1994;45:87.

33. Gentilello LM, Cobean RA, Offner PJ, et al. Continuous arteriovenous rewarming: rapid reversal of hypothermia in critically ill patients. J Trauma 1992;32:316.

34. Cote CJ, Liu LM, Szyfelbein SK, et al. Changes in serial platelet counts following massive blood transfusion in pediatric patients. Anesthesiology 1985;62:197.

35. Reed RL, Ciavarella D, Heimbach DM, et al. Prophylactic platelet administration during massive transfusion: a prospective, randomized, double-blind clinical study. Ann Surg 1986;203:40.

Surgery of Infants and Children: Scientific Principles and Practice, edited by Keith T. Oldham, Paul M. Colombani, and Robert P. Foglia. Lippincott–Raven Publishers, Philadelphia, © 1997.

CHAPTER **20**

Head Injury and Intracranial Pressure

Bruce A. Kaufman and Tae Sung Park

EPIDEMIOLOGY

Head trauma is a significant cause of death and disability among children. The yearly incidence of head injury in the United States has been estimated at 200 per 100,000 of the pediatric population.[1] Nearly 10% of these patients die from their head injuries; and up to three fourths of all pediatric trauma deaths are due to cranial injuries.

The morbidity in those who survive varies greatly. Minor injuries can be associated with reversible deficits, whereas more serious injuries often result in lifelong disability. The magnitude of morbidity in children with head injuries clearly overshadows the mortality and represents the greatest expense to the patients' families and society.

The mechanisms of injury in children are distinct from those in adults and often relate to the individual child's age and developmental stage.[2] Infants suffer disproportionately from falls, such as accidentally being dropped from a table or a person's arms. As children become more mobile, recreational activities and vehicle-related accidents predominate. Older children are more often victims in higher-speed accidents that involve bicycles or motor vehicles. Overall, motor vehicles are the leading cause of accidental head injuries in children that result in death.

Popular changes in the care of children can also affect the type and degree of injury. One example is the use of infant walkers, which has led to a dramatic increase in the number of severe head injuries in this age group. These infants, barely able to crawl on their own, are rendered capable of moving independently and quickly, allowing them to fall down stairs or reach dangerous objects before the supervising adult can recognize and intervene.

Criminal assault is the most common cause of head injury in children younger than 2 years old.[3] Abuse and neglect account for the higher mortality rate documented in infants compared with older children. Since a history of a fall is usually given, abuse is likely to be an underreported cause of head injury.

The mortality rate in children with head injuries is significantly less than that in adults. This mortality rate decreases just after infancy (when the incidence of abuse and neglect declines) and then rises slowly until early adolescence.[4] The rate then rises quickly because of the larger number of patients involved in high-speed motor vehicle accidents.

Better survival rates from head trauma in children than in adults do not necessarily mean better outcomes. Children have a neuronal plasticity related to the degree of myelination and the establishment of neuronal interconnections. This plasticity may allow a given focal injury to produce a less severe deficit than the same focal injury in a mature brain. This same lack of maturity, however, can also make the infant more susceptible to a diffuse injury, resulting in far greater cognitive deficits than in adults.[5]

PATHOPHYSIOLOGY

Normal Anatomy and Physiology

A number of anatomic differences between children and adults can affect their responses to head trauma. The head of a young infant or child is a large mass relative to the whole body (15% of an infant's mass compared with 3% of an adult's). The accelerations and decelerations encountered in pediatric trauma, therefore, result in a greater momentum of force applied to the brain. The neck musculature is underdeveloped and poorly controlled and offers no significant diminution of these forces.

The skull of the infant is thin, soft, and pliable, becoming progressively thicker and more brittle in the first few years of life. The fontanelles and sutures begin to close in the first year and are effectively closed within 3 years. These changes affect the types of injury received from blunt trauma.

The character of the intracranial contents in children also varies significantly from that in adults. The cerebrospinal fluid (CSF) spaces, both intraventricular and subarachnoid, are present in children, but the relative volumes are much smaller than in adults. The infant's brain tissue has a greater water content. Myelination occurs during months 6 through 24, and most of the synaptic and dendritic arborization also occurs during the first few years. These factors directly affect the consistency of the brain tissue—the infant's brain is soft and easily disrupted.

Intracranial pressure (ICP) is derived from the inherent pressure of the components within the cranial and spinal compartments—the brain, blood vessels, and CSF spaces. Any increase in volume of one component decreases the volume of another

417

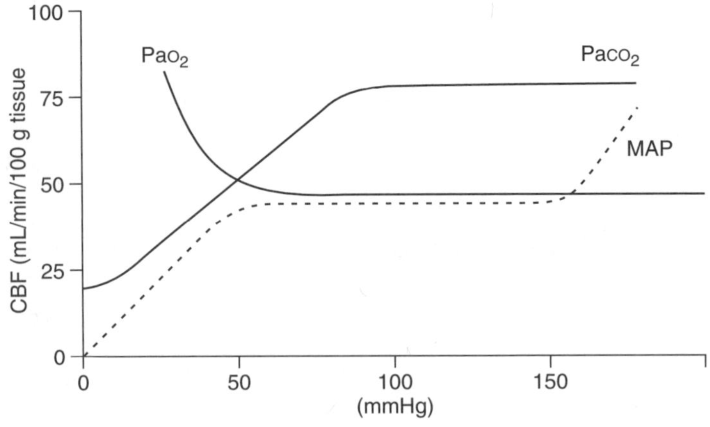

FIG. 20-1. Autoregulation graph showing little variation of cerebral blood flow (CBF) in response to changes over the wide range of normal mean arterial pressure (MAP) or partial pressure of arterial oxygen (Pao$_2$). A rather direct change in CBF occurs in response to changes in the partial pressure of CO$_2$ (Paco$_2$) until high levels are achieved.

and raises the ICP, if compensatory changes are not possible. Brain or intracranial blood volume changes are initially modulated by displacement of CSF from the intracranial space to the intraspinal space. The ICP shows normal variations with both respiration and cardiac pulsation. Marked but transient increases in ICP with activity are normal, particularly with straining and coughing, which increase the venous blood pressure and distend the veins in the spinal and intracranial spaces.

Autoregulation closely regulates cerebral blood flow through a tight coupling of cerebral metabolism with regional blood flow (Fig. 20-1). Mean arterial blood pressure has little effect on blood flow over the normal ranges of pressure. Arterial hypoxia does not usually affect cerebral blood flow until the Pao$_2$ drops below 50 mm Hg. A 1 mm Hg change in the Paco$_2$ can cause a rapid drop in the blood flow of 1.5 to 2 mL/100 g of brain, which can be regional. During the early years of infancy, there are ongoing changes in the degree of normal autoregulation and thus variations in the abnormal responses.

The brain depends on constant blood flow so that oxygen and glucose can maintain the brain's metabolic state; the brain has no significant anaerobic metabolic capability or energy reserves. If blood flow is insufficient, ischemia and disruption of function result. If the ischemia is severe or prolonged, irreversible injury (infarction) results. *Cerebral perfusion pressure* (CPP) is defined as the difference between mean arterial pressure and ICP and is a useful estimation of overall blood flow. The lower limit of normal CPP in adults is 40 to 50 mm Hg. Infants have a much lower normal systemic blood pressure and thus a low CPP. The minimal normal CPP for infants and children is not well defined.[6]

Pathophysiology

As an aid to diagnosis and treatment, it is useful to classify head injuries as *primary* or *secondary*. Primary injuries are those inflicted immediately by the trauma, such as skull fractures, subarachnoid hemorrhage, cerebral contusions or lacerations, intracranial or intracerebral hematomas, and axonal injuries. Ischemia, hypoxia, hypotension, hydrocephalus, seizures, infection, or increased ICP subsequent to the trauma can cause secondary injuries to brain tissue. Secondary injuries are potentially preventable and thus are the focus of most treatment plans.

Compared with adults, children have relatively few subdural or epidural hematomas. Children with epidural hematomas usually present in better neurologic condition than adults and rarely

present in coma after a lucid interval. Children are more likely to have low-pressure venous bleeding from overlying skull fractures than to have dural arterial lacerations causing epidural hematomas. Young children, however, may be at greater risk of dural lacerations, shear, and parenchymal injury with subsequent edema because of a greater transmission of force through the thin bone of the skull and the open cranial sutures. Unique to the young infant whose intracranial volume is relatively large compared to body size, a large intracranial hemorrhage can actually drop the hematocrit or hemoglobin.

Diffuse axonal injury is a primary injury that results from shear stresses on the brain imparted by acceleration–deceleration forces, particularly when combined with angular or rotatory motion. The typical sites of this injury include the internal capsule, corpus callosum, cerebellar peduncle, and brain stem. Even minimal shearing injury in these regions can result in severe neurologic deficits. Shearing is more common in infants and small children than in older children because of the greater rotational forces from the larger momentum of force. Microscopically, the spectrum of injury can vary from a functional disturbance of the neuron that is quickly reversible to a complete disruption of the axons that is an irreversible injury with permanent loss of function.[7] Disruption of the myelin sheath around the axons can result in severe loss of function that is only potentially reversible.

Secondary injuries are frequently due to increased ICP. Increased ICP results from the expansion of one or several components of the intracranial space: cerebral blood volume (both venous and arterial), brain tissue volume, hematomas (intracerebral, subdural, epidural), and CSF spaces. Increased ICP can result in direct compression and injury of brain structures, such as herniation under the falx cerebri or through the tentorium cerebelli (Fig. 20-2). Indirect injury from increased ICP can occur through decreased cerebral blood flow (as a result of decreased CPP), with resulting focal or diffuse secondary ischemic injury. Increased ICP is more common in severely injured patients.

The normal CSF spaces can be displaced in response to the expansion of other components, acting as a buffer for increasing ICP. CSF spaces that are trapped or obstructed, as can happen with subarachnoid or intraventricular hemorrhage, act as additional masses and increase ICP. Children tend to have less CSF buffering capacity despite an open fontanelle or sutures, probably related to a smaller spinal CSF volume. This puts them at risk for more sudden decompensation from smaller changes in ICP.[8]

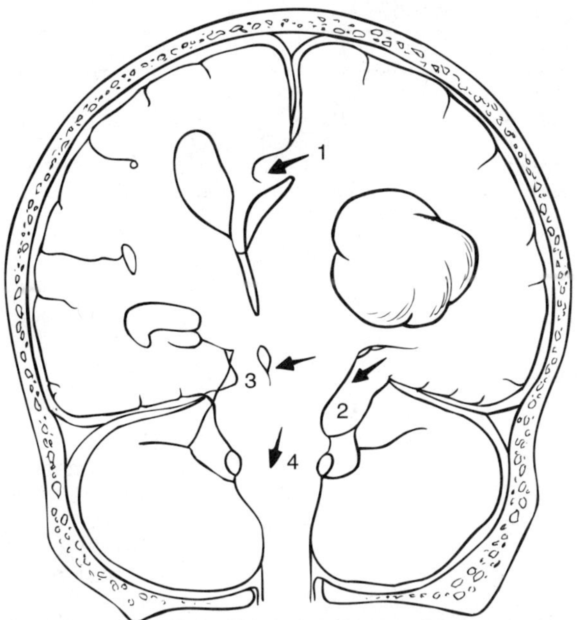

FIG. 20-2. Schematic depiction of herniation types. The intracranial cavity is functionally divided by relatively rigid meningeal membranes—the falx cerebri and the tentorium cerebelli. An intracranial mass lesion, whether a hematoma or region of cerebral edema, can cause herniation around these structures and injure brain remote from the mass lesion. Subfalcian herniation (1) can trap the anterior cerebral artery against the falx and result in an extensive infarction of medial frontal and parietal lobe tissue. A supratentorial mass can cause the uncus to herniate through the tentorial incisura (2) or compress the brain stem against the opposite side of the tentorium (3). Both of these can result in third-nerve palsies and possible compression of the posterior cerebral artery. Generalized increased supratentorial pressure can result in rostral to caudal distribution of force (4) and the classic symptoms of cerebral herniation with a gradually decreasing level of consciousness, followed by signs of midbrain dysfunction and ultimately brain-stem dysfunction and death.

ICP can also rise as a result of interstitial edema of the brain tissue. A focal area of edema can be particularly deleterious if it impinges directly on the brain stem or obstructs the CSF flow. If an area of brain loses autoregulation, vasodilation unrelated to hypercarbia or metabolic demands (hyperemia) can cause a significant increase in tissue volume and thus in ICP.[8] Some children with relatively minor head injuries can suffer from global hyperemia with rapid deterioration and death.[9] Isolated diffuse axonal injuries are less likely to result in increases in ICP, probably because of global decreased metabolic activity and intact autoregulation.

EVALUATION AND DIAGNOSIS

The clinical history in the child with a head injury should include determination of the mechanism of injury and of whether any changes in the patient's clinical examination have occurred since the injury. A high-speed, high-force mechanism of injury raises a greater level of concern for a significant injury regardless of the clinical appearance. A decline in the child's level of function, even if subtle, may be the only clue to an underlying significant injury.

During the physical examination, emphasis should be placed on the trend of serial examinations as well as the presence of *any* focal neurologic findings, including lethargy and irritability. The patient with a deteriorating neurologic examination requires more urgent and aggressive treatment than the patient who is initially comatose and then improves. Systemic hypotension or hypoxia should be promptly corrected because of the brain's dependence on blood flow for normal metabolism. An artificially decreased neurologic examination may be the result of these states and can quickly reverse with their correction.

The typical signs of increased ICP are frequently absent or incomplete in children, even those with significantly elevated ICP levels. Pupillary changes can develop long after significant ICP changes have occurred because third-nerve palsies are the result of nerve compression by displaced cerebral tissue. Papilledema requires days to develop and does not present in acute trauma. The Cushing response to increased ICP (bradycardia with systemic hypertension) is not as predictable in children and may be a preterminal event.

The Glasgow Coma Scale (GCS) is the standard tool for assessing and reporting the neurologic status of a trauma victim. It is based on the patient's best response in three categories: motor activity, verbal response, and eye opening. The GCS score has been validated as an easily applied measure that accurately portrays the severity of the injury and allows for a temporal comparison of the patient's condition. It has been modified for pediatric patients, allowing its use with the nonverbal infant or child[10] (Table 20-1). The usual definitions of severity used in the literature are defined in the GCS as follows: *severe* is a GCS score of 8 or lower; *moderate*, 9 to 12; and *mild*, 13 to 15. Based on evaluations of outcome, it is clear that all mild head injuries, as defined by a GCS score of 13 or higher, are not the same. Patients with a score of 13 or 14 can have significant intracranial injury or morbidity on recovery.

Radiologic evaluation has routinely used plain skull radiographs. Although inexpensive, they define only skull fractures. Only depressed or open fractures are clinically important in themselves, and they are usually well defined by clinical examination combined with computed tomography (CT). The presence of a skull fracture, however, is associated with an increased risk of intracranial injury.[11,12] The absence of a skull fracture, however, does not reliably exclude a significant intracranial injury. Harwood-Nash and colleagues[13] found that 8% of children without skull fractures had brain injuries—subdural hematomas or epidural hematomas. Hahn and McLone[14] reported epidural hematomas in 3% and subdural hematomas in 1.5% of children with head injuries but without skull fractures.

CT is the procedure of choice for evaluating head trauma.[15] CT allows for the prompt identification and treatment of those injuries that are potentially reversible, such as intracranial hemorrhagic masses and depressed fractures. Now nearly ubiquitous at hospitals, the newest scanners are fast, with slice acquisition times of several seconds, which negate most patient motion. Cerebral contusions and shifting of the brain structures can be seen directly, and increased ICP can be inferred from obliteration of normal CSF spaces (Fig. 20-3). When the images are adjusted to evaluate bone density, depressed fractures and most clinically important linear skull fractures are identified.

Radiographic evaluation using CT is indicated for patients who present with GCS scores of 13 or below; immediate scan-

TABLE 20-1. *Glasgow Coma Score modified for children**

Score	>5 y	2–5 y	0–23 mo
VERBAL RESPONSE			
5	Oriented, converses	Appropriate words and phrases	Babbles, coos appropriately
4	Confused	Inappropriate words	Cries, but consolable
3	Inappropriate words	Persistent crying and screaming	Persistent crying and screaming
2	Incomprehensible words	Grunts and moans to pain	Grunts and moans to pain
1	None	None	None
EYE OPENING		>1 Year old	<1 Year old
4		Spontaneous	Spontaneous
3		To verbal command	To shout
2		To pain	To pain
1		None	None
MOTOR RESPONSE			
6		Obeys commands	Spontaneous
5		Localizes pain	Localizes pain
4		Withdraws to pain	Withdraws to pain
3		Flexion to pain (decorticate posturing)	Flexion to pain
2		Extension to pain (decerebrate posturing)	Extension to pain
1		None	None

* The Glasgow Coma Scale score is the sum of best scores in eye-opening, verbal response, and motor response categories.

(Adapted from Simon JE. Accidental injury and emergency medical services for children. In: Behrman RE, ed. Nelson textbook of pediatrics. Philadelphia, WB Saunders, 1992:216)

ning is necessary for severely injured patients (GCS score up to 8). Plain radiographs have no acute diagnostic role in these patients unless indicated for surgical planning. Debate is ongoing regarding the proper radiographic evaluation of minor head injury (ie, GCS score of 15). Significant abnormalities have been detected by CT in 10% of patients with GCS scores of 15, often with no other findings except a history of loss of consciousness or amnesia.[16–18]

The authors recommend CT scanning for any child with a head injury who has any neurologic deficit or a GCS score of 14 or lower. CT scanning regardless of the GCS is warranted when factors such as a high-force mechanism of injury, changes in the level of consciousness, or planned interventions with a loss of the clinical examination are present. The threshold for scanning is also reduced for children younger than 2 years of age because of their thin, deformable skulls.

Magnetic resonance imaging has little utility in the acute management of head injury when determination of surgically treatable lesions is necessary. It is relatively insensitive to acute hemorrhage, and the image quality is easily degraded by even minimal motion. Magnetic resonance imaging does have a role in the evaluation of spinal injury and the subacute care of some patients with head injuries patients. It is extremely sensitive in detecting diffuse and deep shear injuries of the brain and brain stem, allowing a more accurate assessment of the extent of injury and the prognosis for recovery.[15]

MANAGEMENT

Minor Head Injury

No schema has been universally accepted for the evaluation and treatment of children with minor head injuries. The goal

FIG. 20-3. CT scans from different pediatric patients illustrating cerebral injuries. (*A*) Normal. The scan at this axial level clearly shows open cerebrospinal fluid (CSF) cisterns (*arrowheads*). The ventricles are midline and normal in size for a child. Occasionally, subarachnoid space can be seen peripherally and in the sylvian fissures (*arrows*). (*B*) Epidural—the epidural hematoma is seen as a hyperdense lenticular mass in the left frontal region. Bone windows showed an overlying skull fracture. The ventricles are normal and midline, and the cisterns are open. (*C*) Diffuse edema. No subarachnoid or ventricular CSF spaces are seen; the cisterns are completely obliterated by the diffuse edema. There is a slight increased density along the tentorium cerebelli (posterior portion of the brain) that suggests subarachnoid blood. A small amount of subarachnoid blood can render the CSF isodense with the brain and simulate the appearance of diffuse edema. (*D*) Contusion. There is extensive hemorrhagic contusion of the inferior right frontal lobe. This is a typical location for contusion, because the brain is bruised on impact with the rough surface of the orbital roof. Contusion of the temporal lobes can be difficult to see because of beam-hardening artifact from the surrounding skull. They are also particularly dangerous: enlargement and swelling can place pressure directly on the midbrain (*arrowhead*).

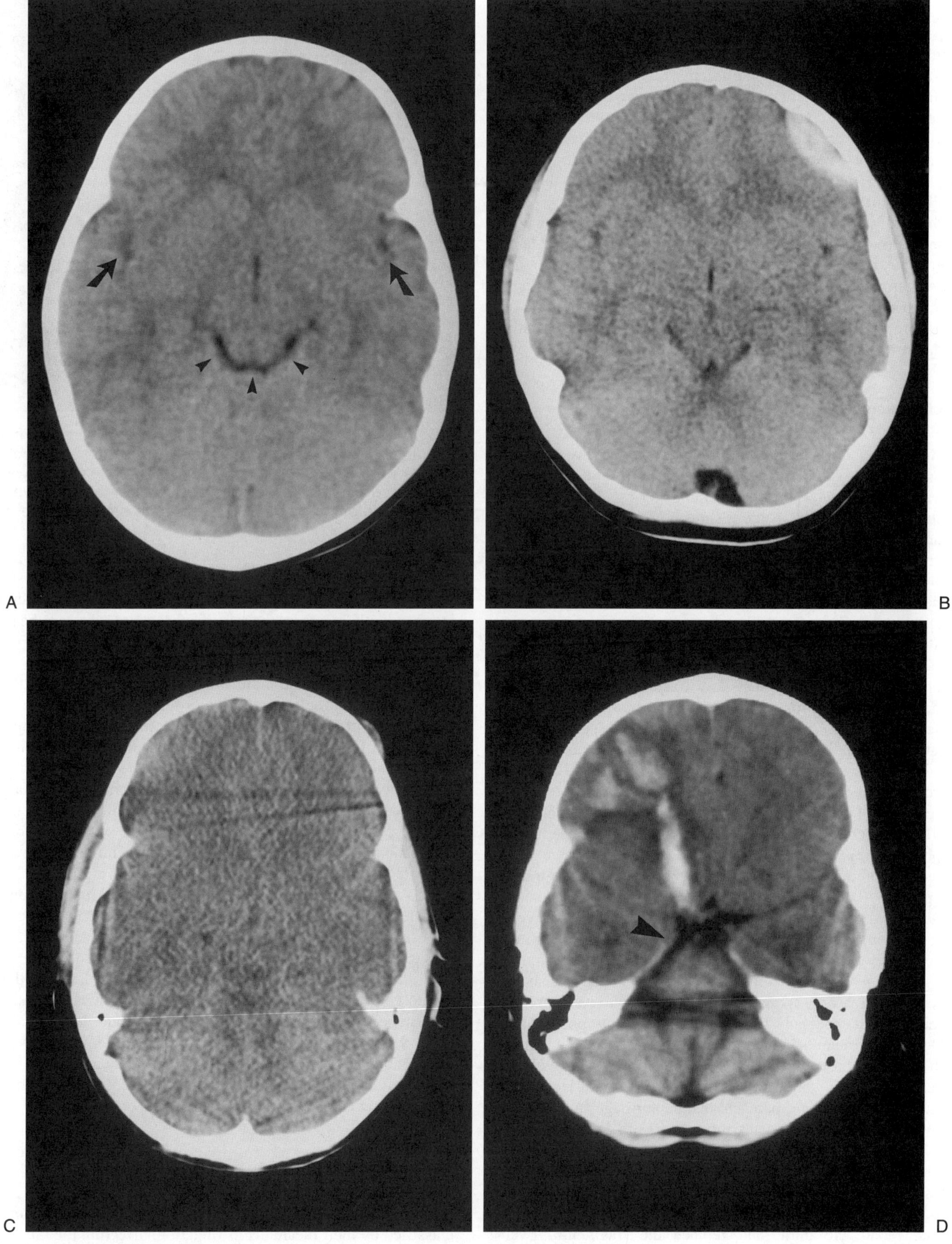

is to identify all significant injuries while minimizing resource use and costs. Any child with a neurologic deficit, known or suspected skull fracture, or documented loss of consciousness should undergo a CT scan. Patients older than 1 year of age who have normal CT scans are usually discharged home with supervision. Any patient younger than 1 year old who has a decreased level of consciousness or a skull fracture usually is admitted for observation regardless of the CT findings. These patients can become dehydrated quickly from vomiting, and they may continue to deteriorate at home without signs that the family can observe.

Physicians have always been concerned that a patient will be sent home with an undetected but significant injury and later deteriorate, the so-called talk-and-die patient. In previously reported cases, however, the patient had manifested some neurologic deficit or had a GCS score of less than 15 at the time of initial presentation. Rarely did these patients have a surgically treatable lesion.[14,19,20]

Skull Fractures

The treatment of isolated skull fractures is relatively straightforward. Linear skull fractures, particularly in infants, are not necessarily associated with intracranial injury. Patients with fractures that cross dural venous sinuses are at risk for delayed epidural hematomas and are admitted for observation. Patients older than 1 year with normal examinations are admitted only for open or depressed fractures; other patients can be discharged home with supervision.

Children who have linear skull fractures in the first few years of life are at risk of developing a ''growing'' fracture of childhood or leptomeningeal cyst and must be followed. This late complication is due to a linear skull fracture that lacerates the dura, allowing pulsation of the underlying brain or arachnoid to act on the inner edges. This pulsation, combined with the constant pressure of a growing brain, remodels the bone, causing significant resorption and enlargement of the fracture. When detected, the repair involves a craniotomy to expose, patch, and close the dural defect; the dural defect is always larger than the overlying fracture. The cranial defect is usually closed with a split-thickness calvarial graft. There is almost always some underlying brain injury, and the significance of this brain injury has probably been underestimated[21] (Fig. 20-4).

Depressed skull fractures can require acute surgical intervention. In neonates, the Ping-Pong ball type of fracture, with no discontinuity of the bone and no underlying parenchymal injury, is most frequent. If elevation of the fracture is needed, usually for cosmetic reasons, a small burr hole is used to pass a probe in the epidural space and lever the fragments into position.

Depressed fractures in the older child are often due to a blow with a sharp object and are more likely to be open, with an underlying dural or brain injury. Evidence of dural laceration includes intracranial air, parenchymal hemorrhage, and depression of the fracture fragments more than 3 to 5 mm or more than half the thickness of the skull. Fractures without evidence of dural laceration can be followed nonoperatively. Other depressed fractures and all open fractures require operative exposure to débride the wound and brain, carefully remove the fragments, repair the dura, and replace the fragments. Even fragments that have been soiled can be cleaned and safely re-

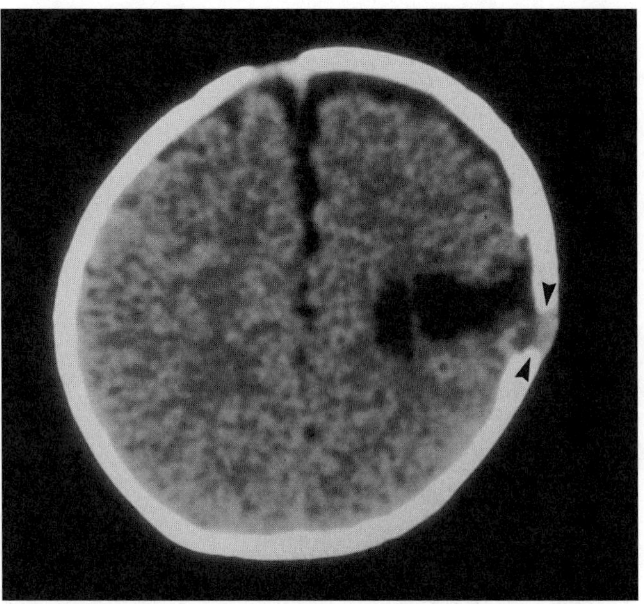

FIG. 20-4. CT scan of growing skull fracture. The skull fracture and underlying parenchymal injury (hypodense infarcted tissue) are easily seen. Growing skull fractures are always associated with a dural defect, usually larger than the overlying bony defect, which must be closed to effect treatment.

turned to the repair after wound débridment and dural closure. There is no clinical evidence that the depression of a fracture independently increases the risk of subsequent seizures; the risk of seizures is related to the underlying parenchymal injury.

Basilar skull fractures in children are most frequently seen in the petrous temporal bone and along the frontal fossa floor into the cribriform plate and orbital roof. Most of the morbidity associated with these fractures results from cranial nerve injury. The frontal fractures must be assessed for impingement on the optic canal, nerve, and orbital muscles. The petrous fractures can involve the middle ear or the petrous portion of the facial nerve, with impairment of hearing and facial motor function. Further evaluation of these fractures is done with thin-section CT scanning, and with electromyography and audiometry when indicated.

CSF leakage can result from these fractures, manifesting as otorrhea or rhinorrhea. The CSF leak usually resolves spontaneously within 7 days, and leaks associated with facial fractures may cease with fixation of the fractures. Although there is a risk of infection (meningitis) with continued CSF leakage, there are no good indications for prophylactic antibiotics. Such therapy can select out a resistant organism or cloud the evaluation of fever or infection in these often multiple-injury patients. Leaks that persist for more than 7 days may require further radiologic investigation to determine the site of leakage and to plan the operative repair.

Severe Head Injury

The various treatments for severe intracranial injury can be classified by their mechanisms of action, affecting the intracranial volume, cerebral blood flow, or cerebral metabolism:

INTRACRANIAL VOLUME
- Mass lesion evacuation
- CSF drainage or ventriculostomy
- Osmotic diuretic use
- Resection of brain

CEREBRAL BLOOD FLOW
- Decrease in jugular vein obstruction
- Elevation of head
- Decrease in positive end-expiratory pressure and ventilation pressure
- Hyperventilation

CEREBRAL METABOLISM
- Anticonvulsant use
- Hypothermia
- Barbiturate-induced coma

A progressive escalation of treatment intensity can be followed, aimed at reducing the ICP and limiting any secondary injury (Fig. 20-5). Although elevated ICP can begin immediately after the trauma, it usually manifests in the first few days and peaks within a week. In some cases, treatment for increased ICP needs to be continued for several weeks. Unfortunately, the ICP is not always controllable, and the patient may die regardless of the treatment.

The child with a severe head injury should be treated like any other major trauma victim, with immediate attention to establishing an unobstructed and protected airway, maintaining ventilation, and supporting adequate circulation. Any patient who is unconscious, unable to maintain an open airway, or

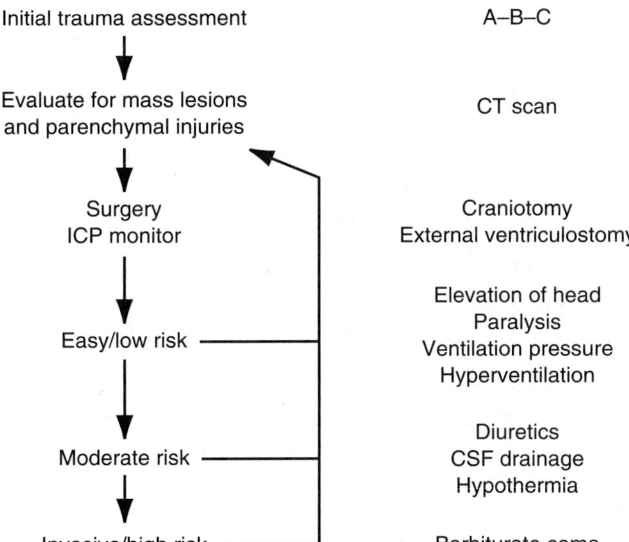

FIG. 20-5. Flow chart for the treatment of a patient with a severe head injury. The management of increased intracranial pressure from head injury can be considered a series of treatment escalations. Surgical lesions are promptly diagnosed and treated, then treatment progresses from easily undertaken and low-risk interventions through more invasive treatments with significant potential morbidity. Whenever a range of treatment becomes ineffective or the intracranial pressure changes unexpectedly, repeated imaging is necessary to rule out the interim development of a surgical lesion.

agitated yet needs additional diagnostic or therapeutic interventions should promptly undergo endotracheal intubation. If possible, a pharmacologic technique using preoxygenation, a nondepolarizing muscle relaxant, and a rapid-acting anesthetic is employed to minimize any increase in the ICP as a result of the stimulation of intubation.

Although it is usually routine to obtain cervical spine radiographs to look for spinal trauma, establishing an airway should not be delayed to take these films. Children are much less likely than adults to have a cervical fracture detectable on lateral spine plain radiographs, and more than half the children with spinal cord injuries do not have a radiographic abnormality.

Also, the levels and types of spinal injury vary with age. Younger children tend to have C-1 through C-3 injuries, often with some component of distraction. Cervical spine alignment should be maintained on a backboard with in-line traction or a Philadelphia collar until evaluation can be carried out. Occasionally, cervical collars applied to small infants and children do not fit well, do not truly immobilize the neck, and can aggravate the injury. Children older than 8 years have a pattern of lower cervical injuries and can be treated similarly to adults.

Fluid resuscitation should use isotonic intravenous fluids. Although colloid has theoretic advantages over crystalloid with respect to ICP, crystalloid is readily available and should be used. Hypotonic solutions should be avoided. Animal experiments suggest that hypotonic fluids contribute free water and aggravate brain edema. Brain-injured patients also have some degree of inappropriate secretion of antidiuretic hormone and can easily become severely hyponatremic if given hypotonic solutions. Dehydration has no role in head injury. It does not limit the development of cerebral edema and can result in decreased end-organ perfusion, causing cerebral ischemia and renal dysfunction.

Lesions and masses that require surgical treatment should be identified as quickly as possible using a CT scan, and then any indicated surgery is undertaken promptly. Burr holes placed while in the emergency room are rarely if ever indicated in children. Most cases of sudden deterioration in children are due to diffuse swelling, and acute extracerebral hematomas have a jelly-like consistency. Neither is effectively treated through a small burr hole. If necessary, a craniotomy can be performed simultaneously with thoracic and abdominal procedures. Separate surgical teams are needed to expeditiously handle the simultaneous operations.

Surgically treated lesions include hematomas (epidural, subdural, intracerebral), skull fractures (open, depressed, those with in-driven bone fragments), and obstructive hydrocephalus. Hydrocephalus can be treated simply by placement of a draining catheter (ventriculostomy). The ventriculostomy can also be used to drain CSF as a therapeutic maneuver for increased ICP. Some small hematomas do not need surgery. With large hematomas, there is usually high ICP and the risk of sudden hypotension when the clot is evacuated. The high ICP stimulates increased peripheral vascular resistance to maintain blood pressure and thus CPP. To obtain a relative hypovolemic state, osmotic diuretic treatment has frequently been given before clot removal. With removal of the clot, however, the ICP can drop, the peripheral resistance drops, and hypotension can result.

Children are more likely to have cerebral contusions than intracranial hematomas (Fig. 20-6). Contused brain tissue is not usually resected because it can recover function, but it may be

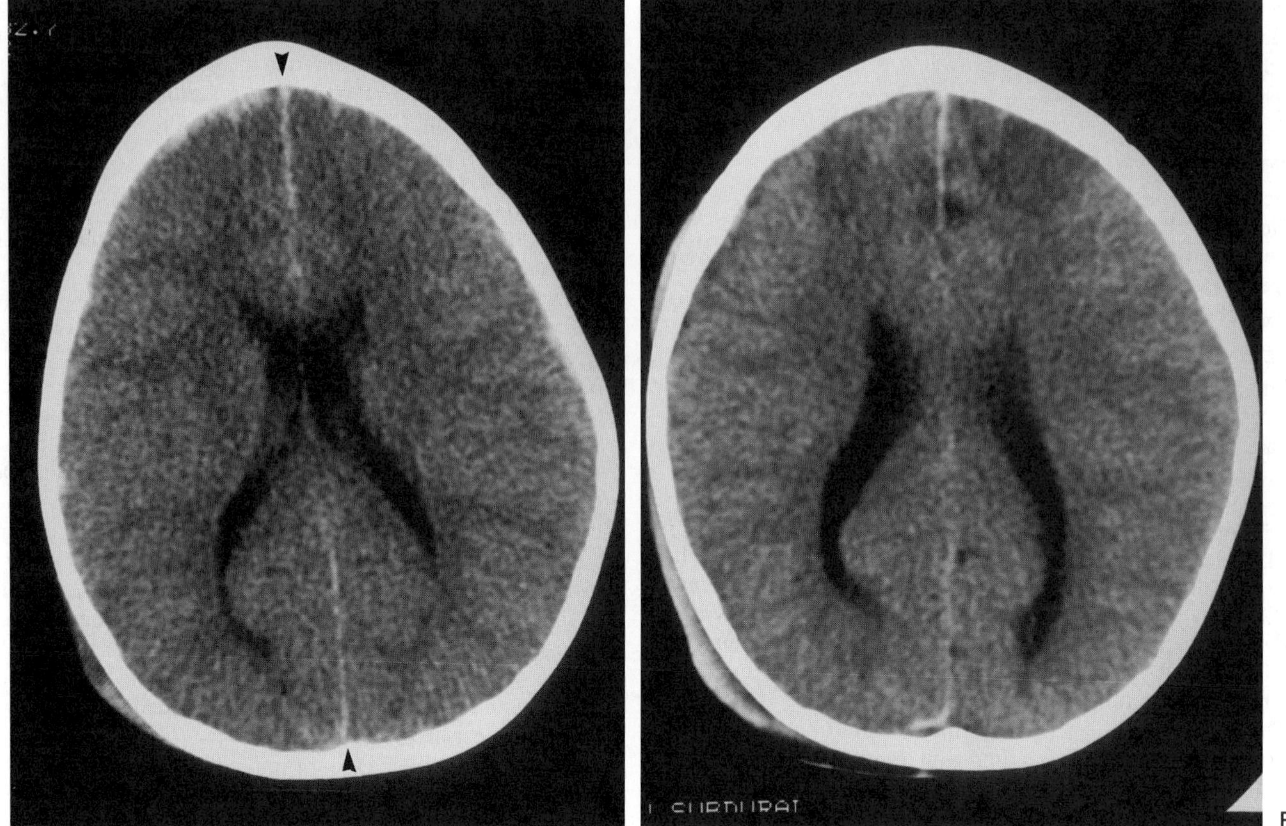

FIG. 20-6. Progressive contusion. (*A*) CT scan from admission shows definite subarachnoid blood along the falx (*arrowheads*) and loss of the differentiation between gray and white matter in the frontal lobes, suggesting contusion. (*B*) Two days later, CT scan shows the bifrontal contusions, which are clearly demarcated by the edema that has developed.

resected to decompress life-threatening increased ICP unresponsive to other treatment. Temporal lobe contusions are particularly serious; developing edema can cause direct compression of the cerebral peduncles, with coma developing rapidly rather than the gradually declining level of consciousness typically associated with more rostral masses. Cerebral contusions that swell with edema may not be seen on the initial CT unless there is some hemorrhagic component.

After any necessary immediate surgical therapy, attention is directed to monitoring and attempting to maintain normal ICP. ICP monitoring is indicated in all patients with GCS scores lower than 9, in those with GCS scores lower than 13 and decreasing levels of consciousness, and sometimes in those who have lesions on CT that are at increased risk of swelling (ie, severe contusions). Patients who are at risk for swelling and are under anesthesia, or who may be kept intubated and paralyzed for other injuries, also require monitoring. Millimeter-sized cable and fiberoptic catheters have been developed that can be quickly placed through a small hole in the skull into the subarachnoid space, cerebral tissue, or cerebral ventricles and can maintain accurate ICP measurements for many days. These monitors can be inserted while in the emergency room or in the intensive care unit. The ICP monitor can also be placed through a ventriculostomy, allowing both monitoring of pressure and treatment through CSF drainage.

The initial medical treatment of increased ICP uses relatively simple maneuvers. Cerebral blood volume can be reduced by minimizing venous outflow obstructions. There should be no compression of the jugular veins in the neck (ie, do not tie the endotracheal tube in place; carefully position cervical collars), the head of the bed is elevated, and ventilator end-expiratory pressures are kept to the minimum required.

Cerebral blood flow is reduced through hyperventilation and induced hypocarbia, keeping the initial $Paco_2$ between 30 and 35 mm Hg, and reducing it to 20 to 25 mm Hg if needed. Unlike adults, children do not lose vasoreactivity after prolonged hypocarbia. Also, this treatment exploits the normal autoregulation of the cerebral vasculature, and areas of injury may have altered autoregulation and not respond. There has been concern that severe hypoventilation may result in regional ischemia, induced by severe vasoconstriction in areas with intact autoregulation or from blood flow steal by areas without vasoreactivity.[22] The $Paco_2$ should be lowered only as needed, and attempts should be made to raise the $Paco_2$ slowly when possible, to prevent these side effects. Hyperventilation, however, remains one of the best treatments for increased ICP.

Neuromuscular blockade is necessary to hyperventilate these patients effectively. Muscular actions such as coughing, gagging, and fighting the ventilator increase intrathoracic and intra-abdominal pressure, decrease venous return, and increase ICP. Adequate sedation and analgesia should be maintained to avoid responses to noxious stimuli that would increase ICP. Use of short-acting narcotics allows for quick reversal and interval assessment of the patient's neurologic condition. The response to endotracheal suctioning, which is noxious and increases the ICP severely, can be blunted by pretreatment with intravenous lidocaine, 1 mg/kg, immediately before suctioning.

Hyperpyrexia increases cerebral metabolism, and thus blood flow and ICP, by as much as 10% for every 1°C above normal. Fever should therefore be treated aggressively with cooling blankets and antipyretics. Moderate systemic hypothermia, with temperatures approaching 34°C, has been used to some benefit in patients with severe head injuries. Coagulation studies, which may already be abnormal in patients with severe head injuries, are not obviously affected by moderate hypothermia.[23] Severe hypothermia also lowers the ICP but is avoided because of the associated morbidity of decreased cardiac output, arrhythmia, hypotension, renal dysfunction, and possible increased risk of infection from depressed leukocyte function.

Seizure activity also increases cerebral metabolism and blood flow and should be aggressively treated. Seizures occur in one third of patients with severe head injuries, usually manifesting within the first few days. Prophylactic loading of a parenterally administered anticonvulsant (phenobarbital or phenytoin) is undertaken on admission. Any subsequent seizure activity is promptly treated with short-acting benzodiazepines and reassessment of the longer-acting anticonvulsant levels. Occult seizure activity should be considered in the paralyzed or sedated patient with unexplained changes in vital signs, respiration, or ICP. If the seizures are difficult to control, or if the patient is paralyzed, an electroencephalogram (EEG) may be required to confirm the diagnosis and assist in treatment.

More aggressive therapy uses CSF drainage to reduce ICP. The compliance of the brain, defined as change in volume/change in pressure ratio, decreases as the ICP increases, and very small changes in the intracranial volume result in large changes in the ICP. Removal of as little as 1 mL of CSF can dramatically reduce the ICP. If not already in place, consideration should be given to placing a ventriculostomy for drainage. The risks of ventriculostomy placement include intraparenchymal hemorrhage and a slowly increasing risk of infection. Extremely small ventricles may not be easily cannulated.

Osmotic diuretics, such as mannitol, are effective at transiently reducing the ICP. The exact mechanism of action for mannitol is highly debated. Mannitol was initially thought to reduce ICP by creating an osmotic gradient between brain tissue and the cerebral vasculature, causing the flow of free water into the vessels and reducing the brain bulk. Other studies suggest an effect on blood viscosity and volume.[24] Regardless, it does cause a transient decrease in ICP, lasting up to several hours. Mannitol should be given as an intravenous bolus, in doses of 0.25 to 1 g/kg, until the measured serum osmolality approaches 300 to 310 mOsm/L. Osmolality above 320 mOsm/L can cause renal dysfunction and rebound cerebral edema and is avoided.

Barbiturate-induced coma is an even more aggressive therapy that reduces the cerebral metabolic rate and thus blood flow and ICP. It has no proven prophylactic role in head injury and is usually undertaken when ICP remains refractory to other treatments. Because of the often severe hypotension and cardiac depression that accompany barbiturate use, invasive cardiopulmonary monitoring (Swan-Ganz catheterization) and the availability of pressure support are needed. A short-acting barbiturate, such as pentobarbital, is administered until burst suppression is noted and maintained on EEG monitoring, usually achieved when the serum concentration of pentobarbital approaches 20 mg/L. A loading dose is infused over 2 hours, followed by a constant infusion of 1 mg/kg/h, while actively monitoring the blood pressure, ICP, and EEG and adjusting the dose as necessary.

Maintenance of cerebral metabolism is one goal during the treatment of increased ICP. A number of techniques have been developed in an attempt to monitor metabolism, several using the direct correlation with cerebral oxygen requirements. Insertion of a monitoring catheter into the jugular bulb allows direct measurement of the blood return from the brain; the jugular bulb receives nearly all its blood flow from intracranial sources. Determining the degree of jugular bulb oxygenation allows calculation of the extraction of oxygen by the brain, the $AVDo_2$. Older catheters required simultaneous sampling of the jugular bulb and arterial blood for blood gas determinations, but newer catheters use fiberoptic spectrophotometric sensors to measure hemoglobin states directly. This technique is limited by the size of the catheters to larger children, and it is not sensitive to regional metabolic changes.

A spectrophotometric device can also be inserted through a burr hole to measure directly from the surface of the brain. This technique is limited by its invasiveness and by the focal region of measurement. Percutaneous near-infrared spectroscopy can measure regional intracerebral hemoglobin states and cerebral oxygen saturation. It is noninvasive and allows continuous monitoring, but its utility and limitations have yet to be defined.

Single photon emission computed tomographic and positron emission tomographic scanning have been suggested as alternatives that would directly measure cerebral metabolism and allow discrimination of regional differences. They require injection of isotopes and scanners that are usually not near the intensive care unit, and positron emission tomographic scanning also requires expensive equipment and dedicated personnel. In addition, they scans lack the ability to monitor the metabolic state continuously and therefore are of limited value while aggressive therapy is actively changing.

The goals of treatment are to maintain the ICP in the normal range and to limit secondary injury. Therapy intensity and invasiveness are escalated to maintain the lower ICP and adequate CPP. As the therapy becomes more aggressive, however, the side effects can become more significant, including hypotension and electrolyte and acid–base imbalances. Any significant change in the ability to control the ICP requires promptly reevaluating the patient, ensuring adequate ventilation (blood gases, chest radiograph, ventilator check), repeating a CT scan to assess for the interval development of surgical lesions (hematomas, hydrocephalus), and assessing for any other unexpected events (electrolytes, osmolality, temperature, seizure) that require changes in treatment.

Experimental Therapies

All of the therapies discussed earlier are directed at preventing secondary insults to brain tissue. A number of biochemical reactions have been recognized that result in cell death and the extension of injury to adjacent cells. Excitatory amino acids, such as glutamate, can have toxic effects on cells and are released with brain injury. The generation of oxygen-derived free radicals and their role in cytotoxic injury has also received increasing attention. One process, lipid peroxidation, is increasingly thought to play a significant role in traumatic central nervous system tissue injury. Lipid peroxidation is a chain reaction of oxidative degradation of the unsaturated fatty acids composing the cellular membrane, allowing calcium influx. Calcium activates phospholipases, further degrading the cellular membrane and producing free fatty acids. The free fatty acids are converted to inflammatory prostaglandins, thromboxanes, and additional free radicals that continue the cycle.

A number of medications are being developed that attempt to interrupt these various reactions. Direct glutamate antagonists, calcium-channel blockers, and inhibitors of lipid peroxidation are being examined for their role in reducing the secondary injuries of brain. Although aminosteroids, such as lazaroids, are being investigated for effects on brain injury, there are no beneficial effects of using corticosteroids in head trauma.

SEQUELAE

In children, seizures due to head trauma occur in up to 10% of all head injuries; 35% occur in patients with severe head injuries and 5% in patients with minor head injuries.[25] Nearly all posttraumatic seizures occur within the first 24 hours of injury. Patients with seizures that occur after 24 hours are more likely to have a later seizure or seizure disorder. The presenting factors highly associated with seizures include a severe head injury (GCS score of 3 to 8), the presence of diffuse cerebral edema, or an acute subdural hematoma. Patients with open depressed skull fractures are at a slightly increased risk of seizures, and those with abnormalities on CT are twice as likely to have a seizure as those without CT findings.

The evaluation of outcome in closed head injury cannot be limited to measurements of mortality. The mortality rate for patients sustaining minor head injuries is extremely low, and even in those who sustain severe head injuries, it approaches only 25%. Even severely injured patients can have good outcomes, but the definition of good outcome is important to consider when comparing studies. Survivors at either end of the spectrum of injury can have morbidity that is severely debilitating, particularly when it involves memory impairment. Most children who survive a moderate to severe injury have some combination of neuropsychologic disturbances, including inattention, hyperactivity, irritability, aggressiveness, and inappropriate behavior. These can also be seen to varying degrees in patients with only minor head injuries.

It has been difficult to identify factors at presentation that can accurately predict outcome, particularly the more subtle disturbances of function mentioned earlier.[26,27] Absent oculovestibular reflexes portend a dismal outcome, with nearly 100% mortality, but merely altered reflexes are not useful in prognostication. A GCS score of 8 or lower on arrival is highly associated with death or serious disability, but patients whose GCS score is higher than 8 still have a significant chance of serious morbidity. There is even a greater degree of variation when outcome is correlated with duration of coma. A patient in coma for less than 6 hours rarely has a gross neurologic deficit or severe neuropsychologic disability, and some patients survive extended comas and recover to functional independence.

CHILD ABUSE AND THE SHAKEN BABY SYNDROME

The clinician involved in the evaluation and treatment of children with closed head injuries must be thoroughly versed in the symptoms and signs of child abuse. A changing history or a history incompatible with the observed injuries may be the initial clue to the abuse. One third of abused children have head injuries, and as many as two thirds have skull fractures.[28] These children may present only with irritability or may have signs of severe brain injury.

The whiplash shaken infant syndrome recognizes the association of significant brain injury with retinal hemorrhages.[28] The shaken child is subjected to acceleration–deceleration and rotational forces that can result in white-matter shear lesions, interhemispheric subdural hematomas, and retinal hemorrhages.[28] Retinal hemorrhages have not been observed in children suffering mild to moderate accidental trauma, and they are extremely rare even with severe trauma.[23,29] Retinal hemorrhages should always raise the suspicion of abuse, and in the child with less than severe trauma, they are diagnostic of a shaking injury.

The outcome in this group of patients is much worse than for accidental trauma in the same age group, and the mortality is higher when the child is unconscious at presentation. The injuries from abuse tend to be more severe and diffuse, with

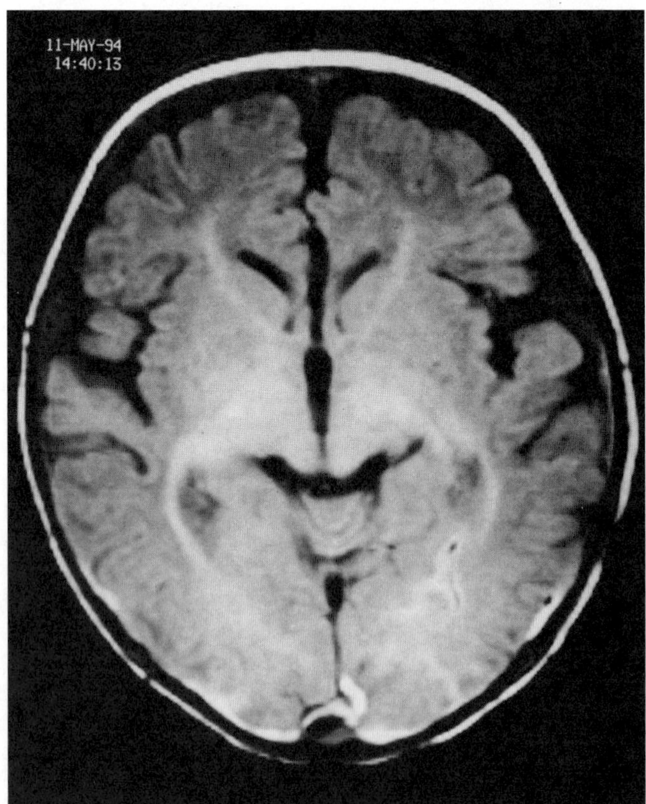

FIG. 20-7. MR image of shaken baby. The brain is atrophied, with chronic subdural hematomas visible bilaterally (two different signal intensities in area outside brain). There were areas of signal change within the brain on T2-weighted images, suggesting deep shear injuries.

nearly half of patients ultimately showing severe cognitive or neurologic deficits (Fig. 20-7). These injuries can be aggravated by hypoxia, hypercarbia, and increased ICP if the child with a depressed level of consciousness is neglected immediately after the assault, often out of guilt or in an attempt to deflect blame.

It is imperative that caregivers maintain a high level of concern in suspecting abuse and promptly evaluate and report their suspicions to the appropriate authorities. When abuse is suspected, evaluation should include careful examination of the patient's entire unclothed body to look for external signs of trauma. A skeletal survey should be performed to look for acute and old fractures; a "babygram" is not adequate because of the lack of detail and variations in exposure that may not detect small epiphyseal fractures. Both retinas must be visualized to rule out hemorrhage. A head CT should be obtained to look for signs of old trauma, such as chronic subdural hematomas, or fresh intracranial hemorrhage. A social service evaluation should be undertaken in an attempt to define any concerns that can affect the determination of nonaccidental trauma.

REFERENCES

1. Goldstein FC, Levin HS. Epidemiology of pediatric closed head injury: incidence, clinical characteristics and risk factors. J Learn Disabil 1987; 20:518.
2. Kraus JF, Black MA, Hessol N, et al. The incidence of acute brain injury and serious impairment in a defined population. Am J Epidemiol 1984;119:186.
3. McClelland CQ, Rekate H, Kaufman B, et al. Cerebral injury in child abuse: a changing profile. Child's Brain 1980;7:225.
4. Luersson TG, Klauber MR, Marshall LF. Outcome from head injury related to patient's age: a longitudinal prospective study of adult and pediatric head injury. J Neurosurg 1988;68:409.
5. Kriel RL, Krach LE, Panser LA. Closed head injury: comparison of children younger and older than 6 years of age. Pediatr Neurol 1989; 5:296.
6. Shapiro K, Smith LP. Special considerations for the pediatric age group. In: Cooper PR, ed. Head injury, ed 3. Baltimore, Williams & Wilkins, 1993:427.
7. Gennarelli TA, Thibault LF, Adams TH, et al . Diffuse axonal injury and traumatic coma in the primate. Ann Neurol 1982;12:564.
8. Bruce DA, Raphaely RC, Goldberg AI, et al. Pathophysiology, treatment, and outcome following severe head injury in children. Childs Brain 1979;5:174.
9. Bruce DA, Alavi A, Bilaniuk L, et al. Diffuse cerebral swelling following head injuries in children: the syndrome of "malignant brain edema." J Neurosurg 1981;54:170.
10. Simon JE. Accidental injury and emergency medical services for children. In: Behrman RE, ed. Nelson's textbook of pediatrics. Philadelphia, WB Saunders, 1992:216.
11. Bonadio WA, Smith DS, Hillman S. Clinical indicators of intracranial lesion on computed tomographic scan in children with parietal skull fracture. Am J Dis Child 1989;143:194.
12. Dacey RG, Alves WM, Rimel RW, et al. Neurosurgical complications after apparently minor head injury: assessment of risk in a series of 610 patients. J Neurosurg 1986;65:203.
13. Harwood-Nash DC, Hendrick EB, Hudson AR. The significance of skull fractures in children. Pediatr Radiol 1971;101:151.
14. Hahn YS, McLone DG. Risk factors in the outcome of children with minor head injury. Pediatr Neurosurg 1993;19:135.
15. Orrison WW, Gentry LR, Stimac GK, et al. Blinded comparison of cranial CT and MR in closed head injury evaluation. AJNR 1994;15:351.
16. Stein SC, Ross SE. The value of computed tomographic scans in patients with low-risk head injuries. Neurosurgery 1990;26:638.
17. Jeret JS, Mandell M, Anziska B, et al. Clinical predictors of abnormality disclosed by computed tomography after mild head trauma. Neurosurgery 1993;32:916.
18. Dietrich AM, Bowman MJ, Ginn-Pease ME, et al. Pediatric head injuries: can clinical factors reliably predict an abnormality on computed tomography? Ann Emerg Med 1993;22:1535.
19. Humphreys RP, Hendrick EB, Hoffman HJ. The head-injured child who "talks and dies": a report of 4 cases. Child's Nerv Syst 1990;6:139.
20. Snoek JW, Minderhoud JM, Wilmink JT. Delayed deterioration following mild head injury in children. Brain 1984;107:15.
21. Tandon PN, Banerji AK, Bhatia R, et al. Cranio-cerebral erosion (growing fracture of the skull in children). II. Clinical and radiological observations. Acta Neurochir (Wein) 1987;88:1.
22. Muizelaar JP, Marmarou A, Ward JD, et al. Adverse effects of prolonged hyperventilation in patients with severe head injury: a randomized clinical trial. J Neurosurg 1991;75:731.
23. Resnick DK, Marion D, Darby J. The effect of moderate therapeutic hypothermia on the development of coagulopathy in severely head-injured patients. (Abstract) AANS Annu Mtg 1994;447.
24. Pilmer SL, Duhaime AC, Raphaely RC. Intracranial pressure control. In: Eichelberger MR, ed. Pediatric trauma: prevention, acute care, rehabilitation. St Louis, Mosby–Year Book, 1993:200.
25. Hahn YS, Fuchs S, Flannery AM, et al. Factors influencing posttraumatic seizures in children. Neurosurgery 1988;22:864.
26. Ghajar J, Hariri RJ. Management of pediatric head injury. Pediatr Clin North Am 1992;39:1093.
27. Hahn YS, Chyung C, Barthel MJ, et al. Head injuries in children under 36 months of age: demography and outcome. Childs Nerv Syst 1988; 4:34.
28. Caffey J. The whiplash shaken infant syndrome: manual shaking by the extremities with whiplash-induced intracranial and intraocular bleedings, linked with residual permanent brain damage and mental retardation. Pediatrics 1974;54:396.
29. Buys YM, Levin AV, Enzenauer RW, et al. Retinal findings after head trauma in infants and young children. Ophthalmology 1992;99:1718.

Surgery of Infants and Children: Scientific Principles and Practice, edited by
Keith T. Oldham, Paul M. Colombani, and Robert P. Foglia.
Lippincott–Raven Publishers, Philadelphia, © 1997.

CHAPTER 21

Facial Trauma

Paul N. Manson, Craig A. Vander Kolk, and Craig DuFresne

Facial fractures are uncommon in children younger than 5 years of age.[1,2] They begin to resemble those of adults in pattern, frequency, mechanism, and treatment at puberty.[3] Children are exposed to a different spectrum of injury mechanisms and forces.[4–6] In general, smaller traumatic forces are involved than are seen in adults.

The basic principles of management of facial trauma in children differ from those in adults in the potential influence of injury and treatment on growth and development; the different patterns of facial skeletal injuries in children; the anatomic, physiologic, and psychological factors related to the various periods of childhood; the presence of tooth buds; and the marked potential for restitutional remodeling in children.[7–13] Special considerations relate to difficulties with obtaining an adequate history, performing a thorough physical examination, and enlisting cooperation, and with the developing nature of physical structures and the rapidity of healing.[13–17]

Posttraumatic facial deformities in children may result from injuries to bone or soft tissue structures, uncorrected displacement of structures, or arrested development. Although most children grow and develop normally after injury,[18] developmental malformations in adolescents and adults occasionally are the result of early trauma.[19–21] Therefore, the parents of injured children must be informed that asymmetric or incomplete development or growth may occur, especially if an injury involves the nasomaxillary complex[22] or the mandibular condyles at an early age.[23,24]

POSTNATAL GROWTH OF THE FACE

The early growth of the face is rapid.[18] The face reaches 40% of adult size at 3 months of age, 70% at 2 years of age, and 80% at 5.5 years of age. The proportions of the face change dramatically during growth.[15,16] At birth, the skull demonstrates a relatively large cranium and a smaller facial component. The ratio of the skull to the face is 8:1 at birth, 4:1 at 5 years of age, and 2:1 in adulthood. These changes are attributed to growth of the facial complex and modification of facial proportions.[15] Facial proportions also differ with regard to sex and genetic heritage. In infants, the frontal lobes are large and the forehead is high and protrusive. Children's heads are proportionately

much larger than those of adults. This heavier head mass may explain in part the high frequency of head injuries, especially involving the frontal bone. The frontal skull forms a prominent portion of the protuberant area of the face, making it susceptible to trauma.[15]

Half the postnatal increase in brain volume occurs during the first year of life, and the brain attains 75% of its adult size by 2 years of age. Compared with adults, the brain case seems disproportionately large, even in children 7 to 8 years of age. Growth of the brain case and face progresses through rapid and slow periods rather than as a steady progression.

The facial skeleton contains cavities for the eyes, nose, and mouth. In the infant facial skeleton, the nasal cavity is small, the perinasal sinuses are almost absent, and the mouth is small. The lower jaw often is diminutive. The nose and sinuses essentially are a single structure in infants, but the sinuses then increase in size, starting with the ethmoid and maxillary sinuses, which begin to develop from the nasal cavity during the latter part of pregnancy. The growth of the maxillary sinuses parallels that of the face. The maxillary sinuses are narrow in newborns and do not reach the level of the orbit. The floor of the maxillary sinuses does not reach the level of the floor of the piriform aperture until at least 7 years of age. It extends below the level of the floor of the nose only after the eruption of the permanent dentition and the increased development of the alveolar process of the maxilla. The maxillary sinuses are not fully developed until 16 years of age; as the sinuses develop, they permit growth of the orbit and fractures of the orbital floor.

The frontal sinus develops as an evagination from the nasal cavity and the ethmoid during the latter portion of pregnancy and cannot be distinguished from the ethmoid sinuses until after 5 years of age. The frontal sinuses usually are asymmetric; vary greatly in size, shape, and septation; grow slowly; and reach adult size only in late puberty.

The frontal cranium, in contrast, has a major growth increase within the first 2 years of life. The first 6 months of life are characterized by a period of rapid growth. A period of slower growth follows from 6 months to 4 years of age. An increase in the vertical dimension of the face results from the development and eruption of the dentition and the growth of the sinuses.[18] Rapid growth in the face occurs between 4 and 7 years of age; a slower period of growth extends from 9 to 15 years of age. A final period of rapid growth occurs from 15 to 19 years of age. The facial bones continue to grow until 21 years of age (Fig. 21-1).

Most facial growth is complete before puberty. The orbits attain adult size by 7 years of age. By 6 years of age, the palate and maxilla are two thirds of adult size. In contrast, the nasal bones exhibit major growth during adolescence. The increase in facial height is greater in the middle third of the face than in the lower third. The increase in the anterior and posterior dimensions of the face is greater in the mandible than in the maxilla. The face often widens more in the mandibular area than in the maxillary region. From a surgical standpoint, growth of the nose may be considered relatively complete by 16 years of age (Fig. 21-1).

The mandible develops by condensation and proliferation from the first pharyngeal arch. It grows by development of the teeth and alveolar processes, and by growth of the bone. Further projection of the mandible is a consequence of growth in the ramus and condylar regions. The mandible is constantly undergoing remodeling, resorption, and deposition, with resultant changes in form and growth.[25–28]

Growth in the condylar region is a result of endochondral ossification. The condyle is capped by a narrow zone of fibrovascular tissue that contains connective tissue cells and cartilage cells. The inner layer of this zone is chondrogenic, and gives rise to hyaline cartilage cells that form the cartilaginous zone. Condylar cartilage differs from long-bone cartilage by virtue of the fibrous tissue cover. Trauma, particularly before the age of 5 years, may damage the fibrous tissue cover and result in hypoplasia of the mandible. Early trauma to the area of the condyle can result in overgrowth, undergrowth, or no disturbance in subsequent growth of the mandible.

Facial growth is controlled by a ''functional matrix''[29–32] composed of the nonskeletal elements of the face, including spaces, muscles, soft tissue, and surrounding ligaments. The relation between trauma and the growth and development of the face remains unclear, although the septum has long been considered to be an important growth force in the midface,[22,32,33] as has the condyle in the mandible.[19–21,34,35] Damage to the septum and nasoethmoidal area during childhood can contribute to hypoplasia of the midface.[32,36–40]

CLINICAL EXAMINATION

Clinical examination of a facial injury often reveals the pathology with surprising accuracy. The clinical examination of a child often is difficult. The patient frequently is unable or unwilling to provide a history. The parents may not be present or may not volunteer detailed information of use to the examining physician. The history should indicate the mechanism of injury and can provide clues to other areas that might have been injured.

Children frequently are uncooperative and easily become frightened and apprehensive. Their fears and anxiety may be heightened by the presence of parents, who often unwittingly add to the confusion. The participation of parents is an individual choice of the examining physician and depends on the particular circumstances. The assessment of the patient demands individual consideration, patience, psychiatric education, and gentle but firm determination. Children should always be dealt with truthfully. Sedation may be considered *if* head injury observation is not indicated. In some cases, general anesthesia is required in children for examination and treatment of injuries that might be accomplished without such measures in adults.

Associated injuries in children are common.[41,42] Skull fractures,[35,43–46] brain injuries,[14,47–50] and cervical spine injuries are common in patients with facial injuries. They should be suspected as ''geographic injuries'' to the head and neck region. The subtle symptoms and signs of head injury can be masked by the emotional response to the accident, and the initial symptoms of cerebral compression often are anxiety and a subtle confusion.

An orderly clinical examination should be initiated and progress through the face using the techniques of observation, palpation, and functional evaluation.

Lacerations, contusions, and bruises are soft tissue injuries that identify specific areas of concern. A fracture or damage to deep soft tissue elements (eg, nerves) may be present (Fig. 21-2). Palpation of all bony surfaces begins in the skull and forehead, and includes the rims of the orbits, the nose, and the zygomatic arches. The dentition should be assessed for tenderness or instability, fractured teeth, or mucosal lacerations. Signs such as tenderness, bone irregularity, step or level discrepancies in the alignment of teeth, crepitus, lacerations, or bleeding may be present. These provide clues to the presence of fractures. The surfaces of the mandible and maxilla are palpated both outside and inside the mouth. Intraoral lacerations, hematomas, and fractured, loose, or missing teeth provide clues to the presence of alveolar, mandibular, or maxillary fractures.[1,51–58] Lateral pressure on the mandibular and maxillary dental arches determines instability or pain.

RADIOLOGIC EVALUATION

Radiographic evaluation of fractures in children is difficult and often requires sedation.[59] Children's bones are cancellous

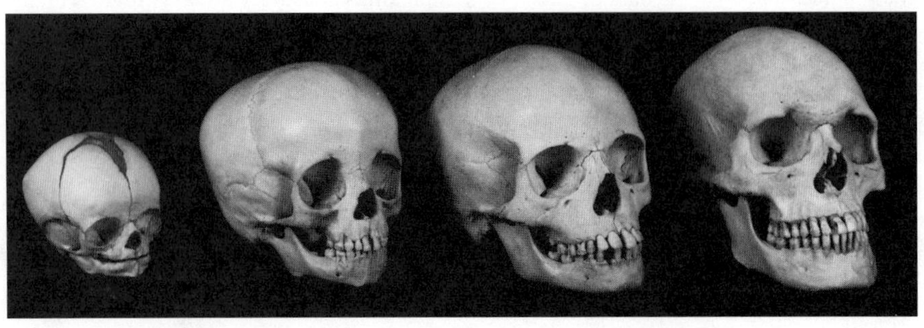

FIG. 21-1. The relative dimensions of the various portions of the face are seen in these skulls, which range in age from infancy to adulthood.

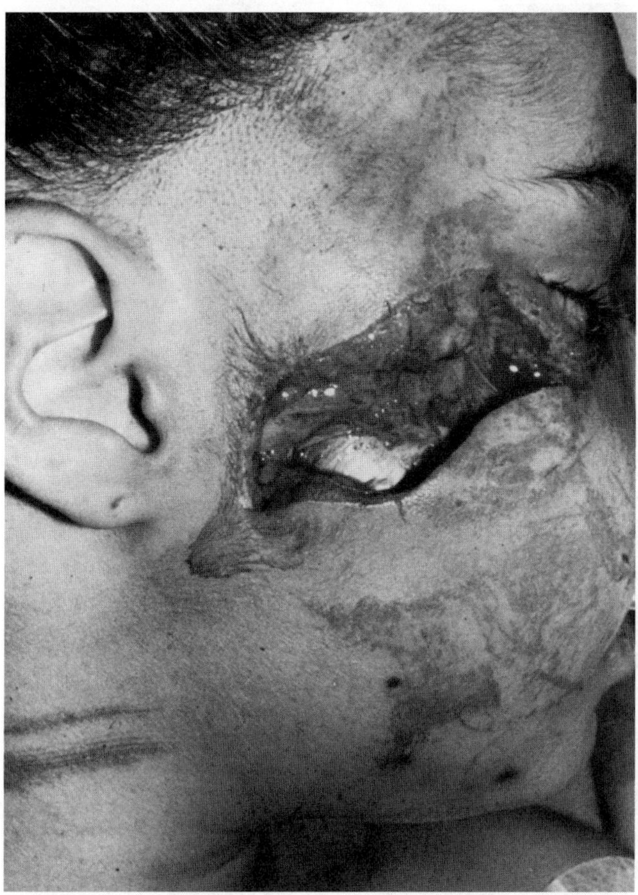

FIG. 21-2. Lacerations, contusions, or bruises can be a symptom of deeper injury. Damage to deep soft tissue elements such as nerves or ducts may be present. This patient had orbital fractures and a zygomatic fracture.

and fractures are more difficult to observe on plain radiographs.[59] Movement blurs the radiographs, further increasing the difficulty of interpretation. Plain films largely have been replaced by computed tomographic (CT) scans (Fig. 21-3). The one exception is the Panorex examination of the mandible (Fig. 21-4), which requires patient cooperation and often is unobtainable. In some cases, undisplaced fractures are difficult to delineate on CT scans or plain films, and these usually are the fractures that produce minimal symptoms. Suspected fractures may be treated without absolute radiographic confirmation.

Imaging studies such as CT scans may require sedation. Care must be exercised in sedating patients with suspected brain injury. Early bone healing in children does not permit delay in diagnosis because treatment must be instituted. The clinician is challenged to achieve a rapid, accurate assessment and to provide alignment and fixation of facial bones to minimize functional disturbances and maximize future growth potential and development.

AIRWAY MANAGEMENT IN CHILDREN

The pharynx and trachea in children are small and easily obstructed by blood, secretions, mucus, fractured teeth, or for-

eign objects[60–63] (Fig. 21-5). When the mandible is fractured bilaterally, it may fall backward, producing pharyngeal obstruction (Fig. 21-6). Forward traction on the mandible in these situations or use of the prone position can improve respiration. Usually, respiratory obstruction can be managed by orotracheal or nasotracheal intubation; tracheostomy in children should be avoided if possible because it involves special considerations.[60,61,64]

The endotracheal tubes used in children frequently are not "cuffed," so a throat pack should be used to protect the respiratory tree from aspiration. The small size of the trachea makes obstruction a genuine concern after intubation. Specific attention to the humidification of inspired air, use of tracheal suction, and administration of mucolytic agents is required in the management of tracheostomies. Some surgeons believe that half of all children undergoing tracheostomies have related complications, most of which occur in patients younger than 5 years of age. Such complications include pneumothorax, emphysema, bleeding, infection, tracheal erosion or stenosis, occlusion of the cannula, displacement of the tube, and difficulty in decannulation. The prolonged use of an endotracheal tube allows the development of tracheal stenosis. Stenosis is minimized by attention to hygiene and positioning, and possibly by the use of stents and corticosteroids in appropriate patients. Radiographic studies of the airway can be used to identify patients with constriction of the tracheal lumen. Patients with identified tracheal narrowing are treated by endoscopic removal of granulation tissue, administration of corticosteroids, and placement of an endotracheal stent.

BLEEDING IN CHILDREN

Hemorrhage accompanies most facial fractures and usually presents through the nose and mouth. Hemorrhage tends to be most severe in fractures of the maxilla. It also can be profuse when the basal skull is fractured, lacerating the major dural veins or carotid artery. The blood volume in children is small and circulatory compromise can occur rapidly. Profuse nasopharyngeal bleeding usually responds to anteroposterior nasal packing (Fig. 21-7). If it does not, manual reduction of the maxilla with maxillomandibular fixation usually rapidly improves nasopharyngeal bleeding from LeFort fractures. Sometimes, a soft compressive bandage wrapped around the face is helpful. Rarely, angiography is indicated and selective embolization or, even more rarely, ligation of the superficial temporal and external carotid artery on the affected side is necessary.

INCIDENCE OF FRACTURES IN CHILDREN

Children are protected from fractures by environmental and anatomic factors. As they grow, their environment changes and so do the types of injuries and patterns of fractures. In general, the incidence of fractures is lower in children than adults because of the large cancellous structural ratio, which renders the bones relatively supple. The more solid structure of the maxilla in children, with the absent sinuses and the presence of developing dentition, changes the usual pattern of LeFort fractures.

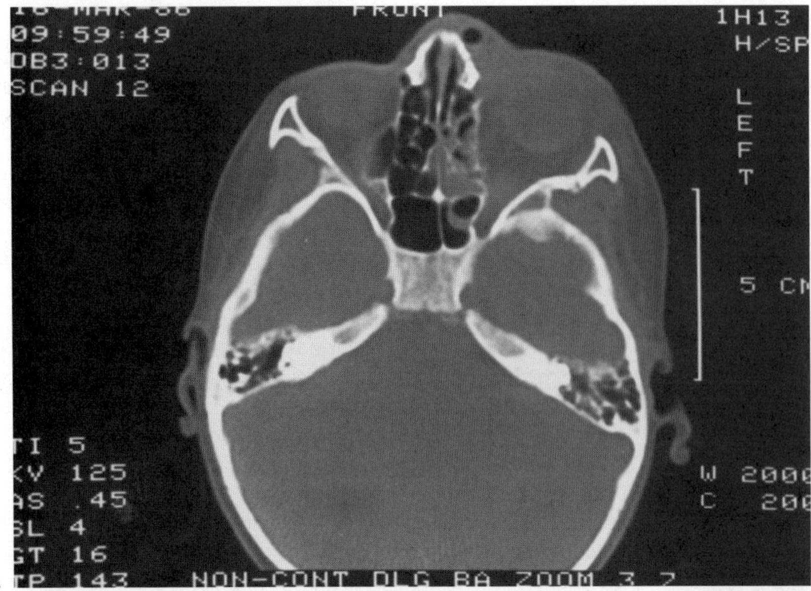

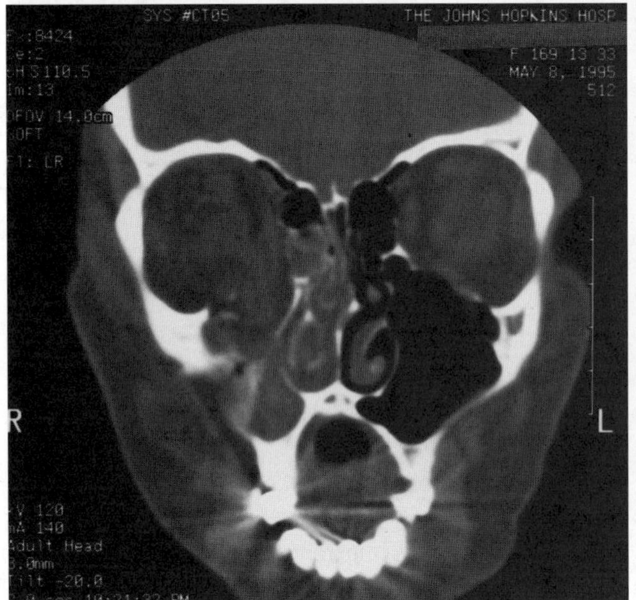

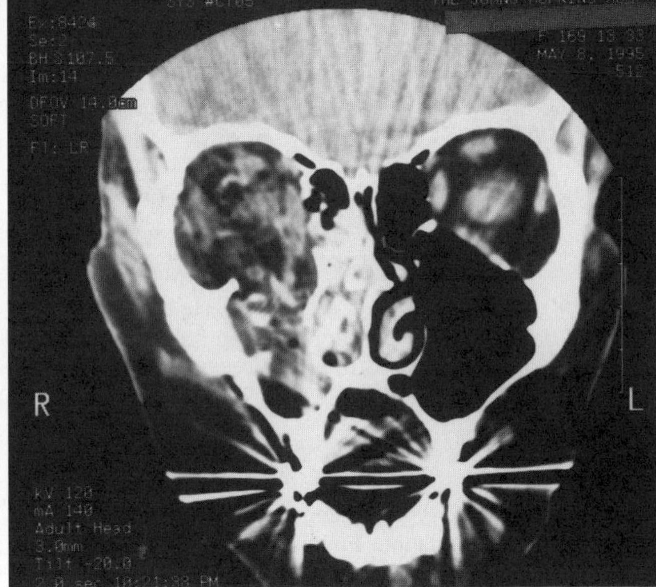

FIG. 21-3. CT scans should include both axial (*A*) and coronal sections, and bone (*B*) and soft tissue (*C*) windows.

Once the sinuses develop, the pattern resembles that of adults. Young children are subject to falls in which the forces involved are much smaller than those sustained in the bicycle or automobile accidents that older children experience. The prominent forehead in young children is the area usually injured in a fall. Incomplete or ''greenstick'' fractures are relatively common in children because of the cancellous structure of the bone and its elasticity. The protruding frontal skull in young children serves to protect the face, which is smaller and relatively recessed (Fig. 21-8). In addition, the soft tissues in children are proportionately thick and padded by layers of fat, which also protect the bones from injury. Frontal skull and supraorbital fractures are common in young children, whereas fractures in the middle and lower facial areas are more common in older children. Because patterns of exposure to environmental factors change during childhood, it is appropriate to consider an age-grouped analysis of injury patterns.

PRENATAL AND BIRTH INJURIES

Skull Fracture and Hematoma

Intrauterine compression can cause some prenatal facial deformities. Birth injuries also can result in facial fractures.[65,66] Prolonged labor, difficult passage through the birth canal, and the use of obstetric forceps are known to induce certain injuries (eg, nasal fractures, facial nerve or brachial plexus traction injuries).[67] Most injuries from obstetric forceps create hematomas over the skull; recovery usually occurs without residual problems, but patients must be observed for the development of a chronic cavity or the need for evacuation or aspiration. Infant skulls are pliable and their segmental arrangement, flexibility, resiliency, and softness contribute to a great tolerance to deformity and fracture. Skull fractures

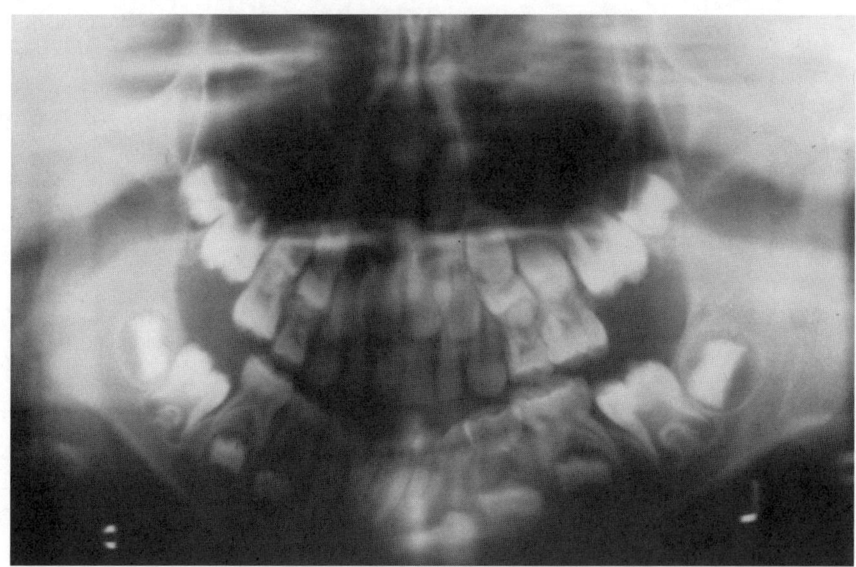

FIG. 21-4. The Panorex examination allows visualization of the entire mandible. This examination usually requires that the patient be cooperative and able to sit upright safely.

may be seen after forcible delivery or other birth injuries. Skull fractures may be suspected on the basis of a hematoma. A shallow grove may be present after resolution of the hematoma. An elliptic or round depression sometimes occurs posterior to the coronal suture. These injuries are "growing skull fractures" (Fig. 21-9) and should be diagnosed by serial radiographs.[68,69] Children with skull fractures should be followed up with plain radiographs 1 year later, at which time growing skull fractures can be recognized easily as radiolucent areas. The components necessary to create a growing skull fracture include a skull fracture that is treated by closed reduction and a dural laceration (which permits cerebral tissue to press on the bone edges, promoting resorption). Repair of the dura usually is all that is necessary, because the bone often regenerates spontaneously in young patients.

Nasal Fracture

Because of its prominent position, the nose also is frequently subjected to birth trauma[65,66] and forceps compression. Facial nerve palsy caused by forceps manipulation usually recovers spontaneously. Other reported injuries include intraorbital hemorrhage, temporomandibular joint ankylosis, and fractures of the mandible. In general, these fractures involve separation at the symphysis and often heal spontaneously without treatment.[57,70] Residual deformity is unusual. Injury to the sternomastoid muscle may result in spasm, contracture, or torticollis, which usually is treated by manipulation and exercise.

During the first year of life, it is estimated that half of all infants fall from a high place, such as a bed, crib, or infant dressing table. The injuries caused by such falls usually consist

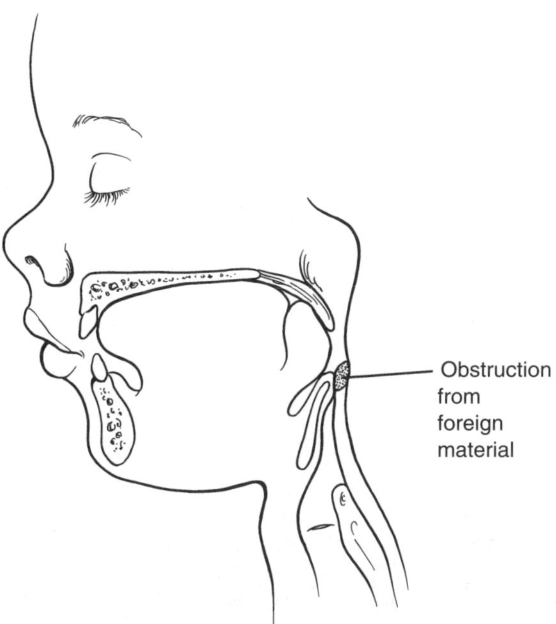

FIG. 21-5. Respiratory obstruction can occur from blood, secretions, mucus, fractured teeth, or foreign objects.

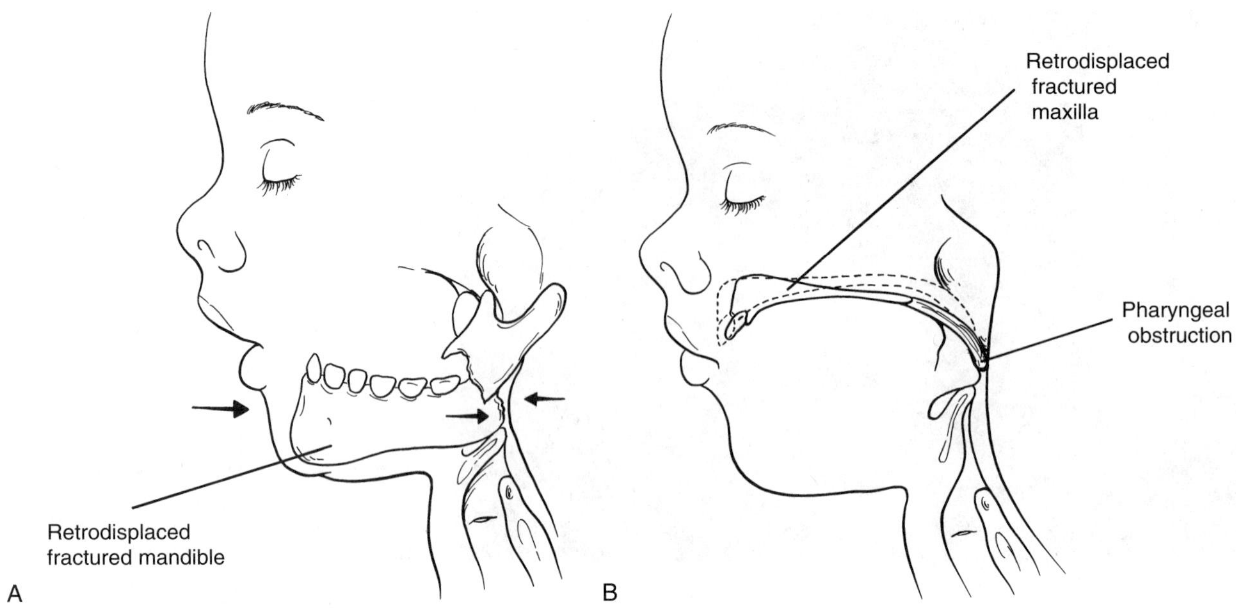

FIG. 21-6. The mandible (*A*) or maxilla (*B*), if fractured and displaced posteriorly, can produce pharyngeal obstruction.

of bruising and hematomas. Undisplaced fractures occur less commonly, and displaced fractures requiring reduction are rare. CT scans usually are required to assess the significance of these fractures.

Among infants who are learning to walk, falls are frequent. Accidents with toys, animal bites, and trauma resulting from inquisitive exploration are common. Occasionally, the battered baby syndrome[71–76] is seen, which includes lacerations (partic-

ularly of the middle section of the upper lip), contusions, facial and skull fractures, and cervical spine and cerebral injuries. Burns also are common in this age group.

After 5 years of age, the incidence of athletic injuries, injuries from airborne objects, and vehicular trauma increases.[9,10,14,77] The "guest passenger injury" refers to the phenomenon of an unrestrained young child becoming a missile during a motor vehicle accident.[10,12]

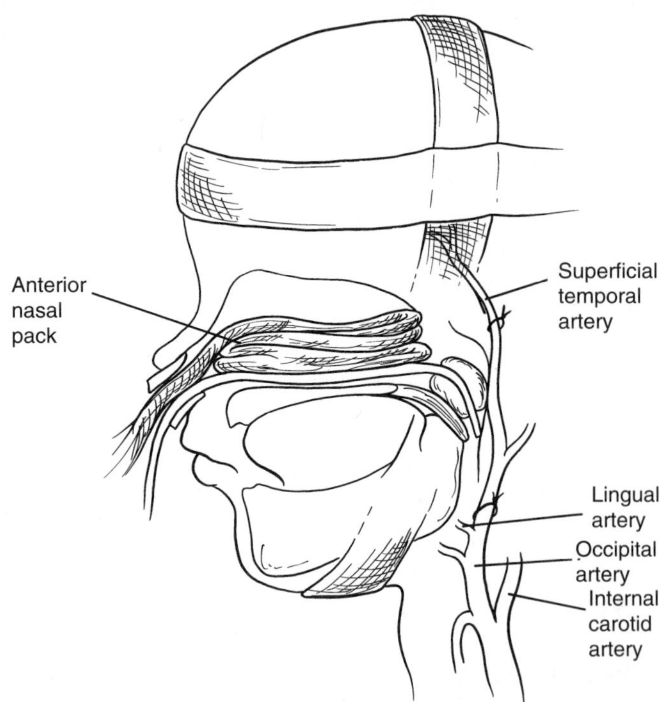

FIG. 21-7. Profuse nasopharyngeal bleeding usually responds to anteroposterior nasal packing (1 and 2). Rarely, a compression dressing (3), intermaxillary fixation (5), or ligation of the superficial temporal and external carotid artery (4) is required.

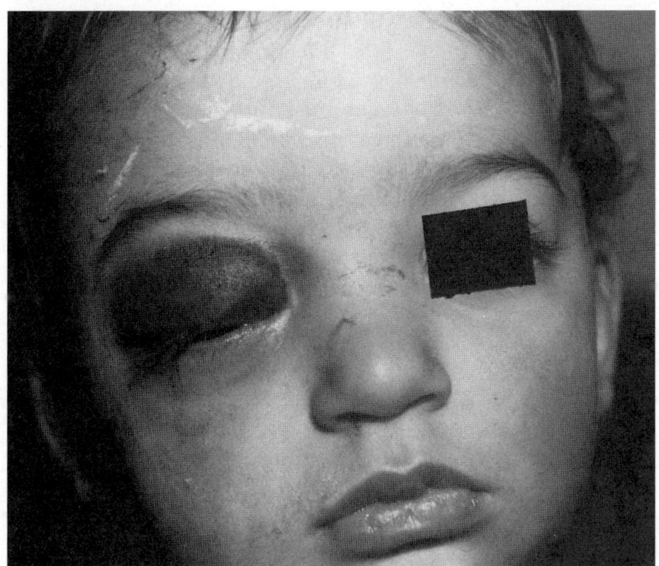

FIG. 21-8. In the young child, the frontal area is large and protruding in comparison with the rest of the face; therefore, frontal and supraorbital fractures are common. The physical sign of a supraorbital fracture is a "spectacle hematoma," which extends within the eyelid to the insertion of the orbital septum. An upper eyelid spectacle hematoma is a reliable sign of an anterior fossa fracture.

SYMPTOMS OF FACIAL INJURIES

The symptoms of facial injuries in children include bruises, hematoma, lacerations, swelling, pain, numbness or deficient function in the distribution of a cranial nerve, and visual disturbances (decreased visual acuity, double vision, or inability to open an eyelid). Bleeding from the nose can occur with any fracture of the midface, orbit, nose, or base of the skull. It is a nonspecific but important symptom. Oral bleeding usually arises from lacerations of the tooth-bearing alveolar surfaces, which suggest fracture of the mandible or maxilla. In the case of fracture of the jaws, malocclusion, difficulty chewing, painful excursion of the jaw, bruising, and ecchymosis indicate a bony injury. When bruising is present around the orbit, exophthalmos or protrusion of the globe may be present. In the later injury period, certain orbital fractures create an enlargement of the orbital cavity, which can contribute to recession of the globe (enophthalmos). The presence of a cerebrospinal fluid (CSF) leak indicates a communication of the frontobasilar region of the skull with the nose, orbit, or ear. Usually, dural tears present with CSF rhinorrhea. The cranial base is partially cartilaginous in children. Leakage from the middle cranial fossa usually is manifested by otorrhea. Blood coming from the ear canal can be from a basal skull fracture, a fracture of the condyle of the mandible, or simply a laceration of the ear canal. The presence of subcutaneous emphysema may be seen in the midface and periorbital area when air from the sinuses enters the tissue from fractures of the midface.[78,79]

INCIDENCE OF FACIAL FRACTURES

Fractures are seen infrequently in children, even in large medical centers. The total fracture experience of surgeons caring for children usually is more limited than in adult trauma. Children initially live in a protected environment and are under close parental supervision. Accidents are uncommon. In the mandible, the tooth-to-bone ratio is high and the bone is elastic because of its cancellous nature. The small size of the perinasal sinuses does not weaken the bone of the maxilla in children. In addition, large cartilaginous growth centers and the small volume ratio of the jaws as compared with the cranium protect facial bones from injury. Fractures are uncommon before 5 years of age. They increase in frequency between 5 and 10 years of age, at which time the frequency pattern and distribution begin to resemble those of adults. With the development of the permanent dentition, the sinuses, behavior patterns, and activities begin to parallel those of adults.

The incidence of fractures varies among reported series. In the United States, nasal and maxillary alveolar fractures, the two most common midfacial injuries, usually are treated on an outpatient basis and have escaped in-hospital record keeping for years. The apparently low incidence of midfacial fractures in children may reflect the limited number who are admitted to the hospital.

In general, the proportion of facial injuries seen in children accounts for no more than 5% of the total number of facial injuries observed in all age groups. In a study of facial injuries performed at Johns Hopkins,[15] fewer than 5% of about 300 pediatric trauma admissions each year involved facial fractures. Sixty percent of the patients in this series had significant head injuries. The facial bones are protected by the smaller size of the face in relation to the head and by the resilient soft tissue bone structure in children.

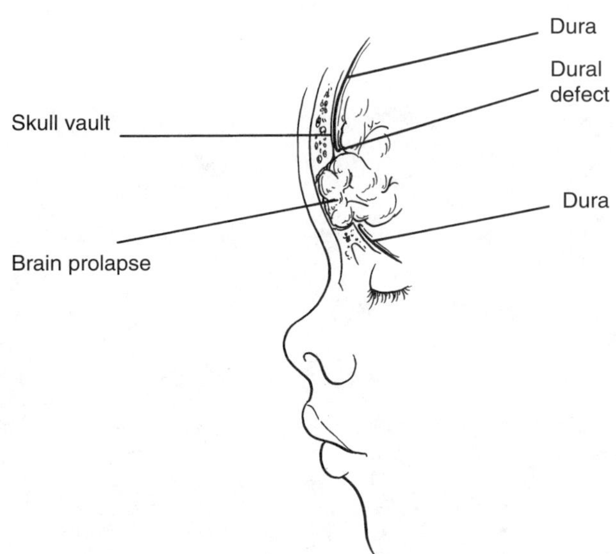

FIG. 21-9. The mechanism of a growing skull fracture includes a skull fracture with an unrepaired dural tear. The pressure from the expanding brain causes the bone edges to resorb. Treatment is by closure of the dura. Reossification of the bone occurs spontaneously in young individuals.

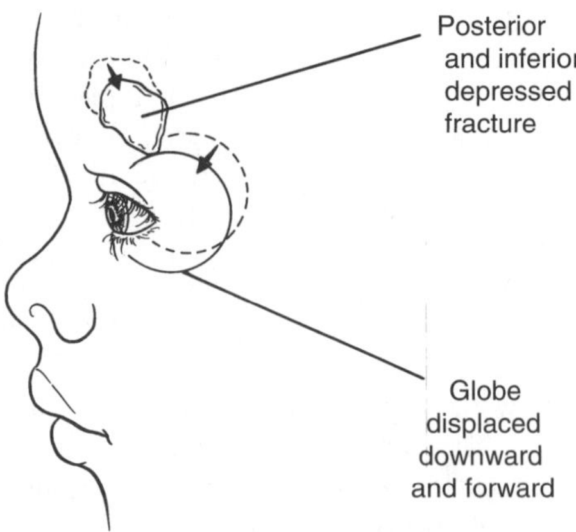

FIG. 21-10. Supraorbital fractures usually are displaced posteriorly and inferiorly. As a result, they displace the globe downward and outward, causing proptosis.

REGIONAL ANALYSIS OF FRACTURES

Fractures of the Frontal and Supraorbital Regions

Fractures of the frontal and supraorbital regions represent a large proportion of the injuries seen in children younger than 5 years of age (Fig. 21-10). Frequently, these fractures are linear, traverse the roof of the orbit and the frontal bone, and create considerable periocular swelling and proptosis. If a significant hematoma exists in the roof of the orbit, the ocular globe usually is displaced inferiorly and anteriorly.[80] If significant displacement or a pulsatile globe is present, the dura may have been torn and the fracture fragments require repositioning. Dural repair and orbital roof reconstruction are indicated.[49] The predominant symptoms of these fractures involve the orbital structures and the symptoms of intracranial injury. The frontal lobe injury may be ''silent,'' with confusion, difficulty in thinking, and the mild symptoms of a head injury.[47–50,81] If a fracture both penetrates the dura and communicates with the nasal cavity, CSF rhinorrhea will occur.[9,82–84] Fractures that traverse the base of the skull[46,85,86] may contuse the optic nerve and result in loss of visual acuity. In addition, some compromise of pituitary gland function may occur from fractures that traverse the base of the skull and penetrate the pituitary fossa.

Radiographic evaluation of the fractured area and displacement is accomplished with an axial and coronal CT scan (Fig. 21-11). The displacement observed determines the necessity for operative treatment. The phenomenon of growing skull fracture should be considered. The symptoms of fracture in the frontal bone consist of a bruise, hematoma, or lacerations. In the orbit, a periorbital and subconjunctival ecchymosis is produced in the upper lid with an anterior cranial fossa fracture; the characteristic ''spectacle hematoma'' occurs, which is a hematoma in the eyelid confined by the distribution of the orbital septum.

Treatment

The surgical treatment of fractures of the frontal region is a combined undertaking involving both neurosurgeons and plastic surgeons (Fig. 21-12). Broad exposure of both orbital

rims and the frontal skull is obtained through a coronal incision. Localized incisions do not provide the access or flexibility that treatment sometimes requires. The treatment consists of subperiosteal exposure of the bone fragments and dissection of all the involved fractured area. Usually, cranial fracture fragments are removed and orbital roof fracture fragments are repositioned.[86] Any necrotic brain tissue is débrided and the dura is repaired using a dural patch of temporoparietal fascia or fascia lata, if required. The fracture fragments often can be cleaned and reassembled on a backtable while neurosurgery to repair the dural and cerebral injury is performed. The reassembled fracture fragments then can be positioned into the bone defect and rapidly secured with marginal rigid fixation (Fig. 21-13). Usually, the microsystem or plates from the 1.2-mm systems are appropriate for these injuries. The fragments of the roof of the orbit must be repositioned accurately to prevent abnormal globe position. It is unclear whether orbital defects of the roof can routinely lead to an encephalocele or a pulsating globe.[49] Those who advocate orbital roof bone repair believe that it prevents these sequelae and provides more predictable eye position.

Fractures of the Nasal Skeleton and Nasal Ethmoid Region

In early childhood, the nasal skeleton is cartilaginous in its distal two thirds.[38,39] This makes the diagnosis of a nasal fracture more difficult because radiographs do not define cartilaginous injury. For small children, general anesthesia may be required for intranasal examination, adequate skeletal examination, and treatment. The midline nasal suture is not ossified in children and may open and allow overriding of nasal bones on the maxilla. Such fractures require lateral compression for reduction and fixation. In significant posteriorly displaced vasal fractures, the arch of the nasal bones may collapse, including the septum.[38,39] The nose may shorten and develop a dorsal

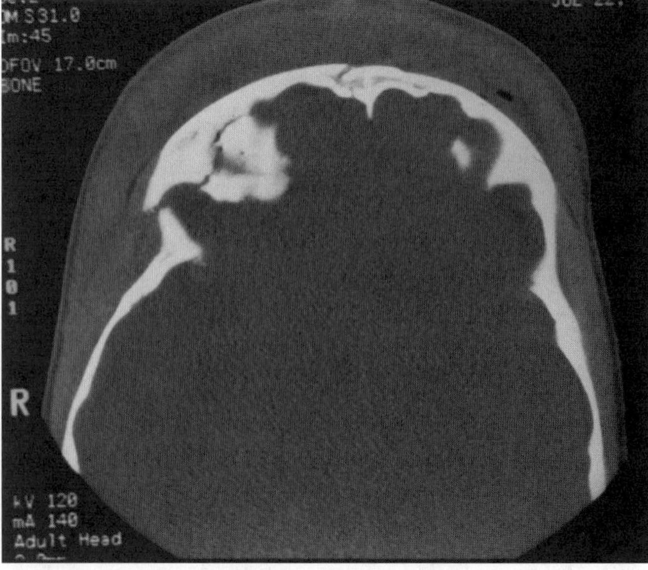

FIG. 21-11. Radiograph of a supraorbital fracture.

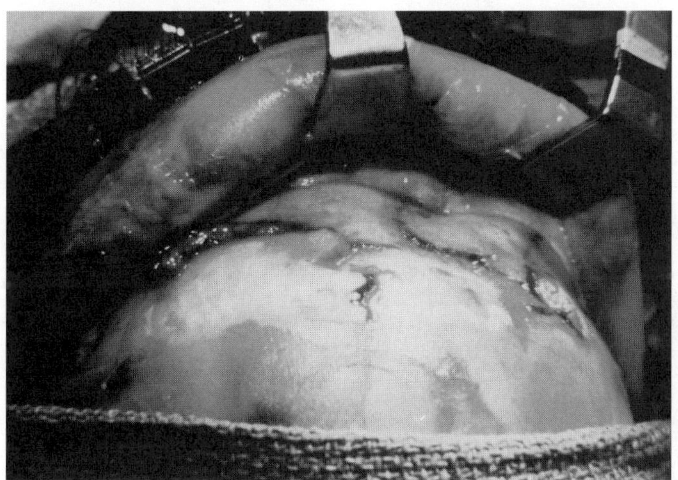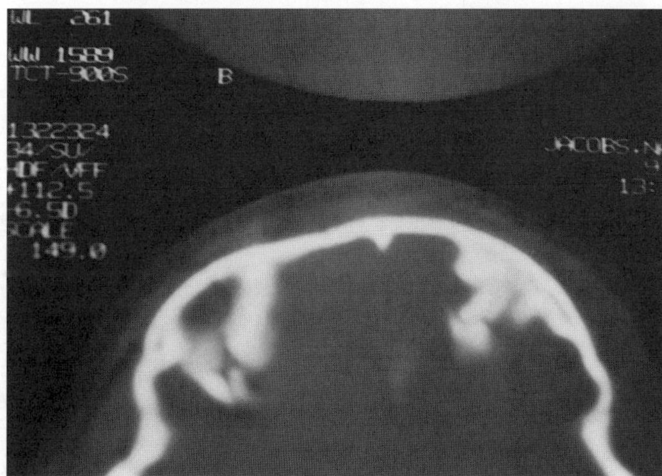

FIG. 21-12. Operative correction (*A*) and CT (*B*) of a supraorbital fracture.

''saddle'' or sinking and an upturned vasal tip. The septum may be seen to be overlapping on intranasal examination (Fig. 21-14).

Fracture-dislocation of the septum uniformly accompanies significant nasal fractures. Small hematomas of the septum are common; large hematomas creating nasal obstruction are uncommon, but should be evacuated. A light compressive packing should be applied within the nose, or an intranasal splint should be used. Hematoma of the septum, although rare, is a potentially serious complication in children because of the implications of pressure necrosis of the septum with subsequent effects on nasal growth.[32,87]

All bone fractures heal rapidly in children,[17] and this healing may prevent adequate reduction after 5 to 7 days. A greenstick fracture of the nasal bones occasionally is seen in children; reduction requires completion of the fracture with lateral osteotomy. A dorsal depression is a common sequela to nasal injury. It is postulated that the nasal septum is one of the major driving forces for forward growth of the maxilla. Therefore, injury to the septum can have potential late sequela in terms of growth and midfacial development.

Nasal bone fractures can be diagnosed radiographically by plain films or CT scans. Plain films sometimes are not diagnostic. In questionable cases, CT scans are advisable. These also may exclude injury to adjacent structures, such as the nasoethmoidal region and the orbit.

The treatment of closed nasal fractures is by internal manipulation of the displaced bone and splinting (see Fig. 21-14). Undisplaced fractures do not require treatment. Open fractures are amenable to open repair. In open injuries, the cartilages often are separated from the nasal septum and can be stabilized by direct suture approximation. When the nasal bones are fractured and the laceration exposes the bone injury, a direct approximation may be accomplished with microplate-and-screw fixation.

Orbital Fractures

Orbital fractures usually are considered to be fractures of the internal portion of the orbit.[88–90] The orbit consists of a rim, an internal middle section, and a posterior section. The posterior section is strong.

The orbital rim is divided into three section. The superior orbital rim and frontal sinus are the upper rim section (Fig. 21-15). The lateral and inferior portions of the orbital rim are the zygoma. Medially in the rim is the nasoethmoidal area.[79] With regard to the internal orbit, the middle third of the orbit can be divided into

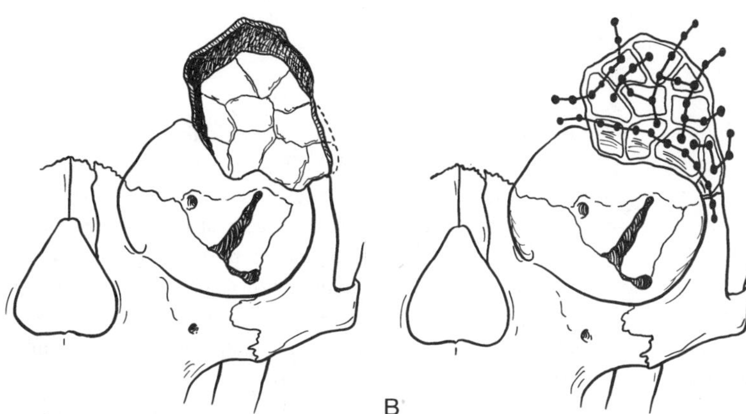

FIG. 21-13. Schematic diagram of marginal rigid fixation of a frontal bone fracture.

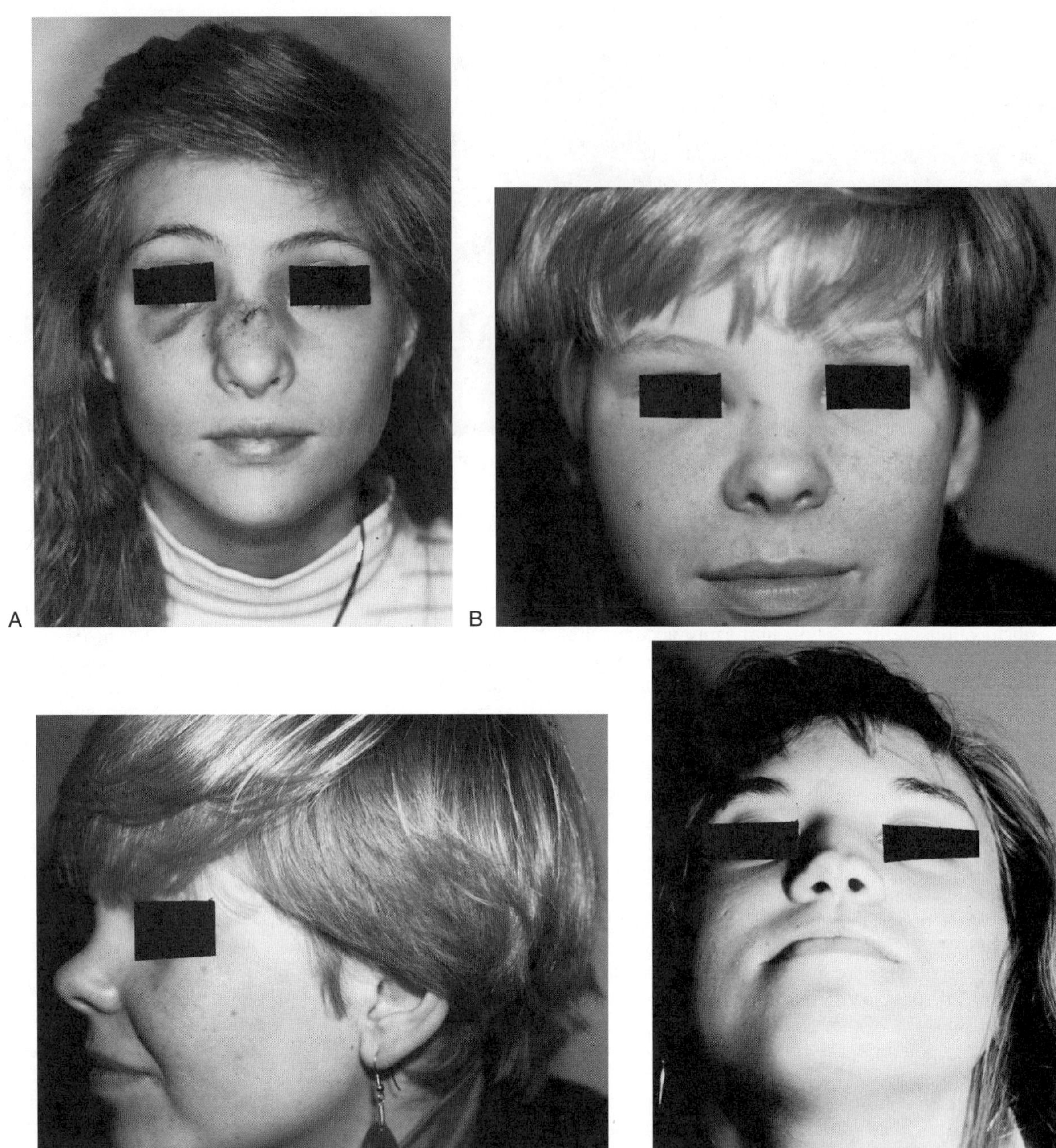

FIG. 21-14. The displacement from a nasal fracture can be lateral (*A*) or posterior (*B* and *C*). External splint fixation sometimes is needed. (*D* and *E*) This latter child sustained a hematoma at the site of the nasal tip at 2 years of age. Unilateral contraction of the nose was observed at that time. Displacement and irregularity and lack of development of the cartilages are present now. *(continued)*

four sections: the roof, the medial wall, the lateral wall, and the orbital floor.

Orbital Floor Fractures

Orbital floor fractures in children are uncommon until the maxillary sinuses begin to pneumatize the midface and orbital floor, weakening the bone.[88,89,91,92] This creates the potential for fractures of the orbital floor. Orbital floor fractures produce symptoms of orbital enlargement and double vision when looking superiorly or inferiorly.[93] The eye sinks medially, posteriorly, and inferiorly. The patient has numbness in the infraorbital nerve distribution. The double vision occurs through the mechanism of impingement of the musculofibrous system of the orbit (Fig. 21-16). Impingement of the orbital fat in an inferior blow-out fracture can restrict the action of an extraocular muscle through the interconnection of the orbital fat and the extraocular muscle. In young children, orbital fractures often are small and linear, and occasionally incarcerate the inferior

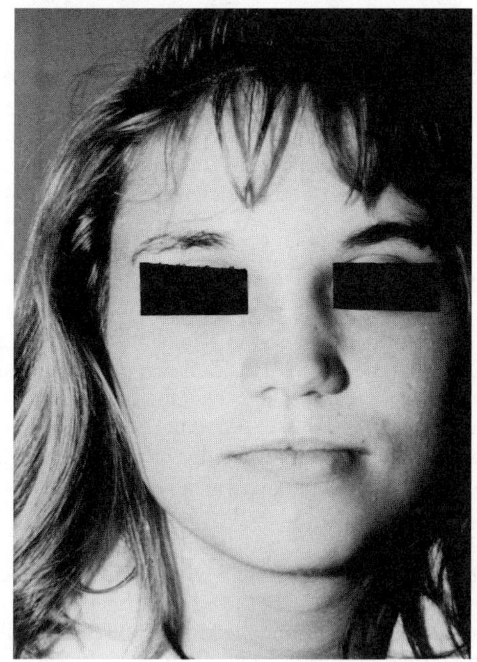

FIG. 21-14. *(continued)*

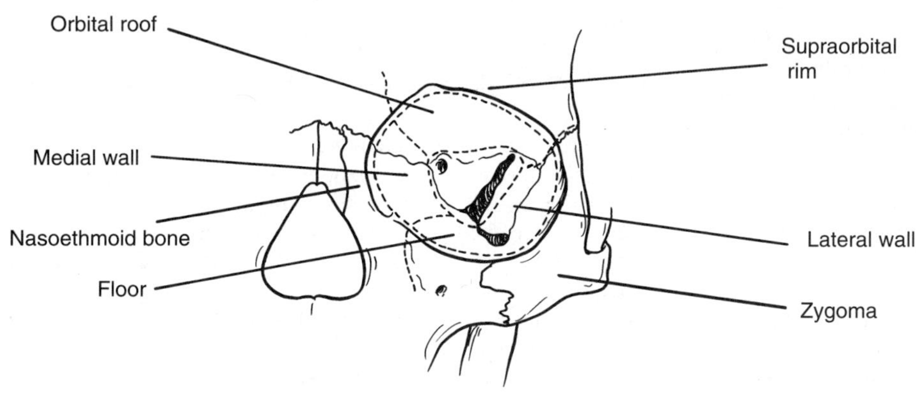

FIG. 21-15. The three sections of the orbital rim are the supraorbital section superiorly, the nasoethmoid section medially, and the zygoma laterally and inferiorly. The orbit can be divided into three sections from anterior to posterior: the rim, the middle third of the orbit, and the posterior third of the orbit. The middle section is divided into the roof, the medial wall, the lateral wall, and the floor.

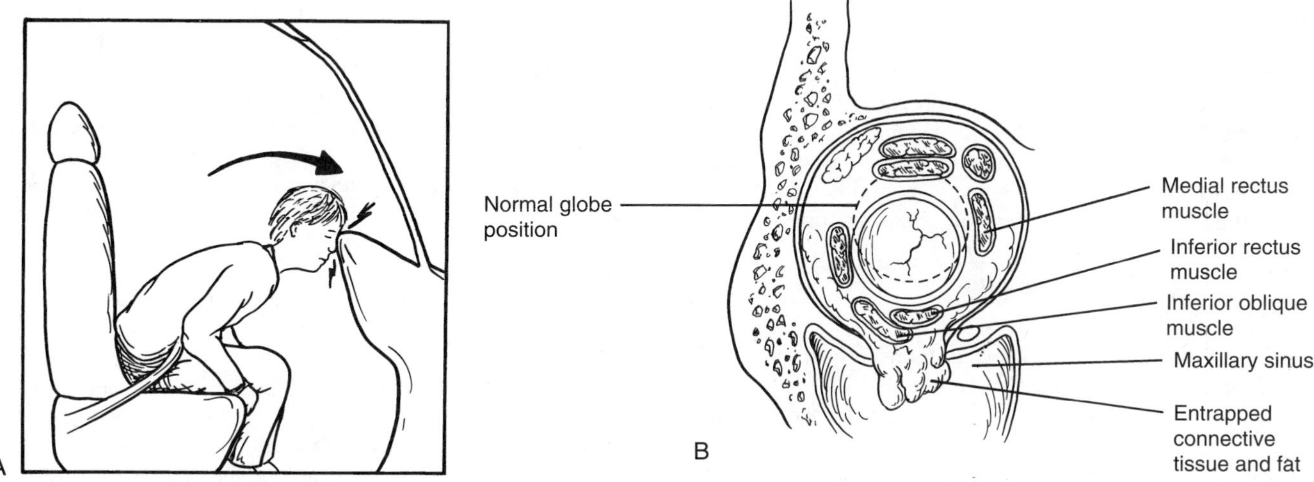

FIG. 21-16. A system of ligaments connects all orbital soft tissue. Therefore, entrapped fat, through its ligamentous attachments, can limit the excursion of the muscular system. (*A*) Blunt injury forces soft tissue into the fracture site. (*B*) Entrapped soft tissue limits extraocular excursion.

rectus muscle directly.[90] These fractures tend to interfere with the blood supply to the inferior rectus muscle, and immediate decompression is indicated. Acutely, these patients have pain, a small fracture, and absolute inability to look upward. A CT scan usually is diagnostic of muscle entrapment, which requires immediate release. Confirmation of the diagnosis of a significant fracture of the orbital floor rests on information provided by axial and coronal CT scans with bone and soft tissue windows.

Medial Blow-Out Fractures

The treatment of medial blow-out fractures requires operative consideration if the area of the defect is sufficient to produce enophthalmos.[88,89,92] After a medial blow-out fracture, the eye is displaced medially, posteriorly, and inferiorly. Muscle entrapment rarely occurs with medial blow-out fractures, but muscle contusion is common and results in diplopia.

The symptoms of medial blow-out fractures include periorbital ecchymosis and a subconjunctival hematoma and epistaxis. With inferior orbital fractures, numbness is present in the infraorbital nerve distribution, which includes the ipsilateral lip, ipsilateral nose, and anterior maxillary teeth. Fractures in the medial portion of the orbit usually are approached with a coronal incision or a local incision at the bridge of the nose. Fractures of the inferior and medial portion of the orbit are approached with a lower eyelid incision and may require bone grafting or the use of alloplastic material to span the defect. Bone sources may include the rib, the iliac crest, and, in older children, the calvarium.

Fractures of the Nasoethmoidal Region

Fractures of the nasoethmoidal region are encountered less frequently in children than in adults.[92,94] In younger children, they often consist of linear fractures that divide the nasoethmoidal region into two half-sections. In these fractures, the pieces are large and easily reassembled. Fractures of the nasoethmoidal region produce a communication between the nose and the cranial base. CSF rhinorrhea and pneumocephalus may be present. The fractures may extend into the region of the frontal sinus.[95] Nasoethmoidal fractures are accompanied by flattening of the nasal bridge, foreshortening of the nose, crepitus, epistaxis, and telecanthus or increased intercanthal distance.[94] Occasionally, nasoethmoidal fractures are dislocated medially and impacted to produce an increased length of palpebral fissure. Nasoethmoidal fractures are diagnosed by CT scan. They require open reduction with plate-and-screw fixation and bone grafting.

Fractures of the Frontal Sinus

Fractures of the frontal sinus occur more frequently in children older than 10 years of age.[95] The frontal sinus is not large enough to permit sinus involvement of significance until puberty.

The significance of sinus involvement relates to two problems[78,96]: sinus obstruction and posterior wall sinus fractures that damage the dura, producing CSF leak and brain injury.

Any posterior wall sinus fracture that is displaced more than the thickness of the posterior wall should be considered for operative exploration. Frontal sinus fractures that result in opacification of the sinus must be presumed to have compromised sinus function (duct obstruction). Sinus fractures that show simultaneous displaced fractures of the anterior and posterior walls should be managed by operative exploration. Most fractures of both walls are sufficiently complicated that sinus function cannot be preserved, and the sinus must be considered for "obliteration" or "cranialization." In the "obliterative" technique, the sinus mucosa is removed and the sinus area is bone grafted so that the previously present sinus becomes a portion of the cranial bone. The sinus is effectively eliminated. "Cranialization" involves removal of the mucosa and posterior sinus wall so that the sinus becomes a portion of the intracranial cavity, with the brain and meninges coming forward to occupy the space. Displaced fractures of the anterior wall alone that do not affect duct function can be managed by anterior wall reconstruction without eliminating the sinus.

Nondisplaced fractures of the anterior wall alone can be managed with observation. If there is a question about sinus function, serial CT scans should be performed at intervals of 1 month to document that the sinus clears. Sinuses that initially are opacified (filled with fluid) opaque need to be serially evacuated in this manner to make sure that they clear and adequate sinus function is ensured. An obstructed sinus results in abscess formation.

Fractures of the Zygoma

Fractures of the zygoma are rare in young children, but their incidence in older children begins to approach that of the adult population as one of the most common injuries.[1-4] The incidence of pure pediatric zygomatic fractures is about 5%, and the incidence of zygomatic fractures with significant orbital fractures is about 15%.[77] Some investigators have shown that the incidence of zygomatic fractures necessitating operative intervention is 0.3%. As in adults, treatment involves repositioning of the zygoma. Plate-and-screw fixation of some type usually is used at the zygomaticofrontal suture and the inferior orbital rim. Zygomatic fractures should be treated within 5 to 7 days because of early healing. Healed zygomatic fractures may not be amenable to correction by refracture of the bone if it is believed that refracture might damage the tooth roots.[78]

Zygomatic fractures vary widely in their severity. Fractures with medial displacement of the arch can be managed with anterior approaches (lower lid and intraoral approaches alone). Fractures that display lateral displacement of the malar eminence require a coronal incision. Zygomatic fractures contuse the infraorbital nerve and produce hypesthesia of the upper lip, nose, and medial cheek, and may produce the same symptoms as orbital fractures. Initially, periorbital and subconjunctival hematomas are present and are characteristic of orbital fractures. The lateral canthus may be displaced inferiorly, resulting in an antimongoloid slant to the palpebral fissure. The malar eminence may be depressed once the swelling has abated. Posterior displacement of the fracture may impinge the body of the zygoma against the coronoid process, and medial displacement of the zygomatic arch may impinge the arch against the coronoid process, which both result in trismus. This may produce a minor malocclusion or the subjective sense of malocclusion in patients affected by swelling.

Malalignment in zygomatic fractures occurs when the diagnosis is missed or the reduction is faulty. Most authors report about a 10% incidence of malalignment in zygomatic fracture reduction. Poor results are more common with conservative (closed) reduction, so open reduction procedures are favored. Many zygomatic fractures are so minimally displaced that they do not benefit from any reduction maneuver at all, and open reduction can be reserved for patients with significant fractures. Zygomatic fractures in children are observed commonly after automobile accidents and after sports-related injuries such as a baseball blow to the cheek. On plain radiographs, separation at the frontozygomatic suture is one of the major indications for operative intervention. In addition, separation of the inferior orbital rim with downward displacement of the floor requires treatment.

On physical examination, palpation of the inferior orbital rim may demonstrate a palpable step-off of the displaced fractures. Tenderness usually is present over the fracture sites and a hematoma may be observed in the upper buccal sulcus. Zygomatic and orbital fractures are accompanied by unilateral epistaxis, which occurs from bleeding within the fractured maxillary sinus exiting through the nose. Isolated fractures of the zygomatic arch occasionally occur; they produce (after resolution of the swelling) a slight depression in the lateral cheek. Their main functional symptom is interference with movement of the mandible by impingement on the coronoid process.

Standard plain radiographs assess displacement in zygomatic fractures. A CT scan with axial and coronal cuts of the orbit is preferred to plain films for the evaluation of all zygomatic fractures. In clinical practice, plain films can be omitted if a CT scan is obtained. Plain films in children may be difficult to interpret, and fracture lines and the soft tissue contents of the orbit may be difficult to identify.

Indications for open reduction of zygomatic fractures are deformity, enophthalmos, and positional abnormalities of the zygoma that are visible on physical examination. In addition, any interference with the mandible requires zygomatic repositioning. Most zygomatic fractures can be stabilized with plate fixation. If the lateral canthus is detached in the reduction, it should be replaced, reattaching it toward the zygomaticofrontal suture. The orbital floor defect is explored routinely as part of the operative treatment of a zygomatic fracture. Depending on the integrity of the floor, a bone graft or artificial material may be used to cover the bone defect. Linear orbital fractures usually are reduced, with alignment of the rest of the zygoma. The orbital dissection must progress until all normal edges of the orbital defect are located precisely so that the exact contour of the orbit can be re-created by the reconstructive material.

Fractures of the Alveolus of the Maxilla

Fractures of the maxillary alveolus are frequent injuries in children. The teeth usually survive if they are replaced and supported for several weeks by an arch bar or orthodontic bonded brackets.[97] The teeth in children have the potential to regain their blood supply and survive because the root structure is incompletely developed.[1,51–56] In some cases, teeth can be replanted successfully and subsequently treated with root canal therapy. To have the best chance of success, they should be replanted within half an hour. If the teeth are removed, the rough edges of the alveolar process should be débrided and the mucosa sutured closed.[98,99] Any bone fragments that are attached to soft tissue usually are preserved.

Fractured crowns of teeth without exposed pulp should be protected by dental methods because restoration with capping usually is successful. Exposed dental pulp requires tooth capping and partial pulpectomy. Such treatment is most successful in young teeth, in which the apexes are still open. Fractures involving the root structures of the teeth or those occurring near the crowns of the teeth ultimately may cause tooth loss that requires extraction. The teeth can be stabilized and treated expectantly in anticipation of possible early root canal treatment. Damage to permanent tooth buds may result from injury. This can produce deformed teeth, false eruption, or irregular arrangement of teeth within the dental arch.

Traditionally, dental injuries are categorized according to whether they involve the deciduous teeth or the permanent dentition.[90,99–101] Deciduous tooth injuries occur between 1 and 3 years of age, when children are learning how to walk. The relative softness of the bone in this age group occasionally allows displacement of teeth up into the bone of the alveolus, which can produce intrusion. Partial dislocation toward the tongue or cheek, or total tooth avulsion can be managed by tooth replacement in the proper position. If a tooth has been out of its socket for less than 1 hour, it usually is a satisfactory candidate for replacement. Intruded teeth can be managed expectantly; they frequently erupt again in the subsequent weeks and may erupt fully in 4 to 6 months. Children younger than 2.5 years of age have incomplete root formation, and intruded teeth may regain normal vitality after another eruption. In older children, there may be calcific degeneration and pulp necrosis after re-eruption of intruded teeth.

Root fractures, particularly those involved in the coronal portion of the tooth, require extraction. Surgical removal of the apical portion of the fractured root is necessary in some cases to prevent interference with the eruption of permanent teeth and infection.

Mandibular Fractures

Mandibular fractures are some of the most common injuries in young children.[57,70,102] The condyle is particularly subject to fracture, and "greenstick" (incomplete) fractures are common before the eruption of the permanent or secondary dentition, when developing tooth follicles occupy most of the body of the mandible.[23,71,103,104] To prevent injury to tooth buds, this anatomic characteristic must be considered when using rigid fixation. In the period of mixed dentition, the absence of teeth and the shape of the crowns of the deciduous teeth may make it difficult to use the teeth as abutments for intermaxillary fixation. Skeletal wires should be used to support the arch bars in these circumstances. The treatment of mandibular fractures in infants and in children in whom the teeth are only partially erupted may involve taking an impression of the mandible under anesthesia and fabricating an acrylic splint. In children older than 9 years of age, the procedure is similar to routine intermaxillary fixation in adults. In children with mixed dentition, the proper occlusion may be more difficult to determine. A minor degree of malocclusion is not a disaster in a child because adaptive adjustment occurs with eruption of the secondary dentition. The

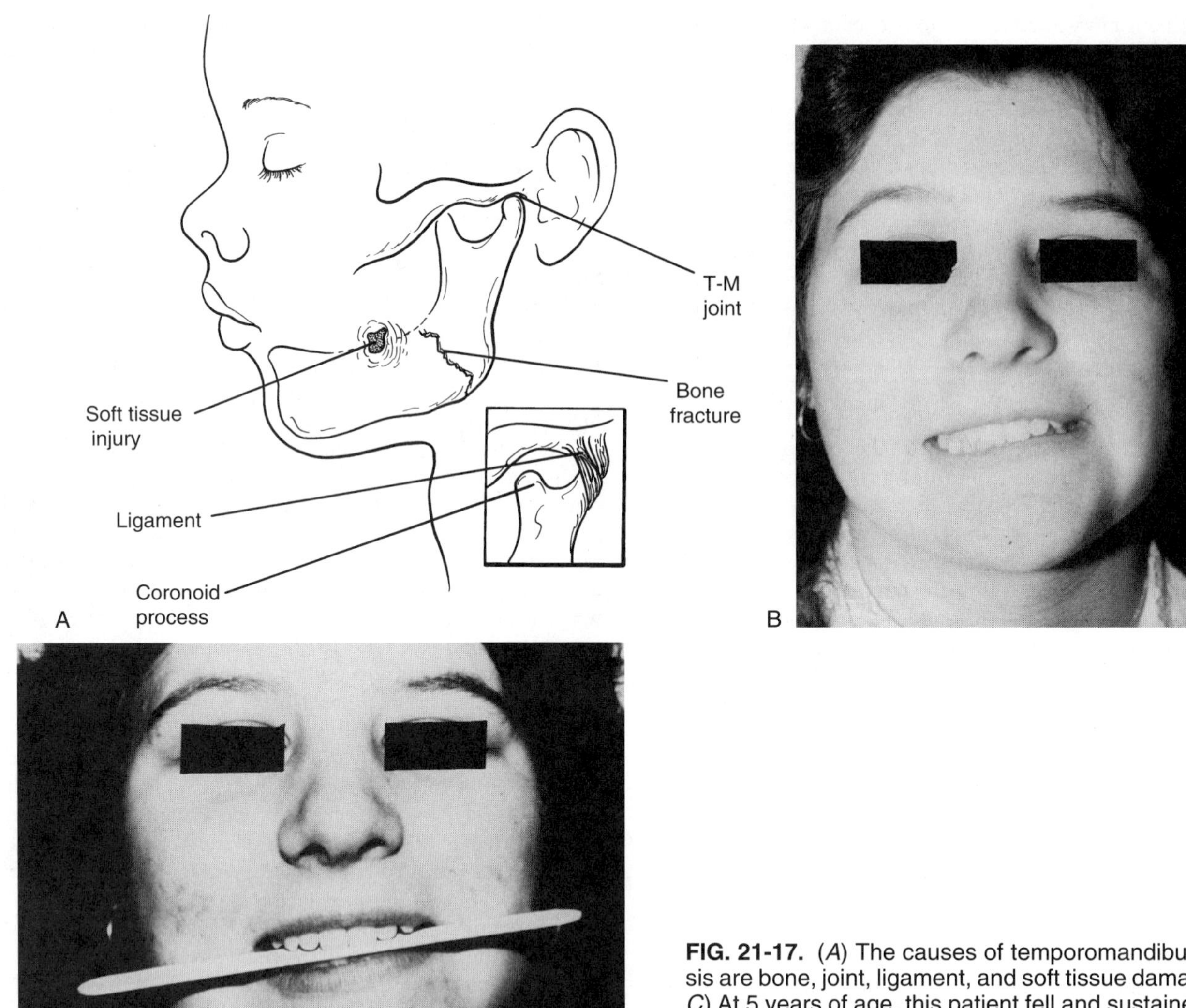

FIG. 21-17. (*A*) The causes of temporomandibular ankylosis are bone, joint, ligament, and soft tissue damage. (*B* and *C*) At 5 years of age, this patient fell and sustained a unilateral subcondylar fracture, resulting in a unilateral occlusal cant and facial asymmetry. In her 20s, she is seen for this surgical correction.

early dentition has a significant ability to adapt, a characteristic that is not present in adults.

Injuries to the articular surfaces of the bone and the temporomandibular joint[105] should be suspected in any child who has sustained a blow to the chin. Radiographic studies may demonstrate fractures of one or both mandibular condyle areas without displacement. If the child is able to bring the occlusion into a normal relation, the injury can be observed without immobilization. Any condylar injury should be viewed with concern because of the possibility of late growth disturbance.[25–28] Injuries to the articular surface of the joint rarely may result in hemarthrosis with fibrosis and subsequent ankylosis.[106]

In young children, the neck of the condyle is a blunt, stubby, thick structure. With growth, it transforms into the long, slender condylar neck of adults. The condyle in young children is more easily crushed than fractured. In the more mature condylar neck area, the fractures often are of the greenstick type and usually are not accompanied by significant disturbances of the temporomandibular joint. Fortunately, fractures in the condylar area

in children are not followed routinely by ankylosis or growth disturbance.[19–21,34,57]

Temporomandibular ankylosis occasionally follows an injury to the condyle.[106,107] Often, less apparent injuries are found on clinical and radiographic examinations performed months after the initial trauma to evaluate a limitation in motion of the mandible with partial ankylosis (Fig. 21-17).

Fractures of the Maxilla (LeFort Maxillary Fractures)

The maxilla fractures in patterns.[108–110] The patterns described for adult maxillary fractures include the LeFort I fracture, a horizontal fracture through the lower aspect of the piriform aperture separating the lower maxilla from the upper maxilla (Fig. 21-18). The LeFort II fracture is a pyramidal fracture that involves the distal nose or the frontal bone at the nasofrontal suture. The LeFort II fracture involves segments of both orbital rims medially and laterally, and the nasofrontal junction.

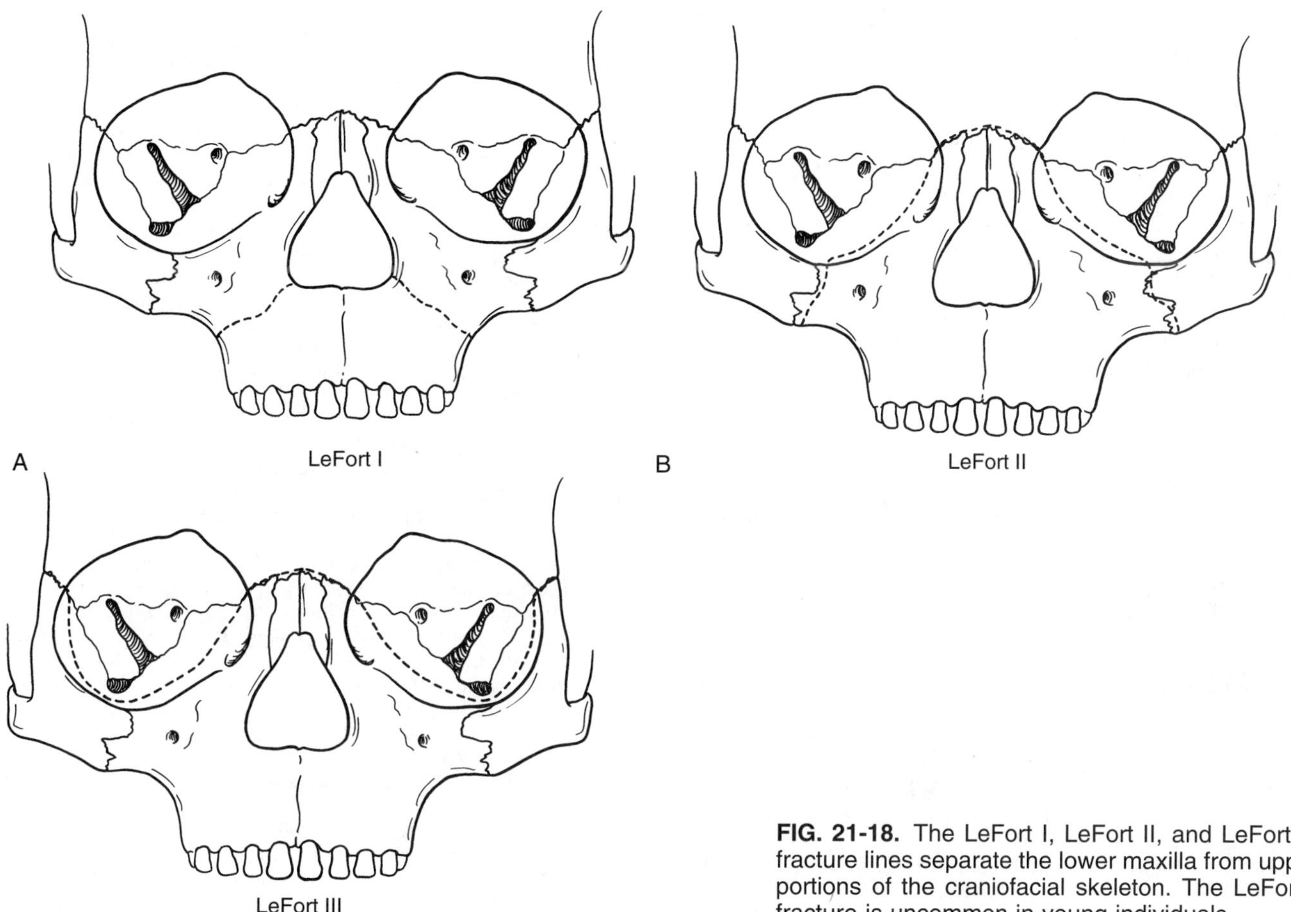

A — LeFort I

B — LeFort II

C — LeFort III

FIG. 21-18. The LeFort I, LeFort II, and LeFort III fracture lines separate the lower maxilla from upper portions of the craniofacial skeleton. The LeFort I fracture is uncommon in young individuals.

LeFort I fractures are observed infrequently in young children because of the absence of the maxillary sinuses and the presence of the developing dentition. The LeFort fracture lines usually occur above these structures. The LeFort II fracture is the most commonly seen fracture in children. A split palate is not unusual because of the incomplete fusion of the midpalatal suture in this age group.[111] Malunion is prevented best by early or immediate exploration and open reduction. The split palate can be plated in the roof of the mouth, the piriform aperture, or both. Treatment should not be delayed until after the edema resolves because solid healing in malunion occurs early in the pediatric population. Placement of the maxillary teeth in occlusion with the mandible is an essential treatment that prepares the position of the maxilla for open reduction.[108,109] The LeFort III fracture, or craniofacial dysjunction, separates the facial bones from the cranial skeleton through the orbits. These fracture lines extend across the zygomatic region from the zygomaticofrontal suture across the lateral orbit and orbital floor to enter the nasal ethmoid area. The nose is separated from the frontal bone or is comminuted, producing nasal-ethmoidal-orbital fractures. LeFort III fractures rarely are a single fragment, but are comminuted, involving zygomatic fractures and a LeFort II fracture. The LeFort II segment carries the maxillary dentition.

In significant midface fractures, bilateral symptoms of a midface injury are observed, such as periorbital and subconjunctival hematomas, bleeding from both nostrils, and considerable swelling. If primary treatment is not rendered for several days, the midface usually is perceived to be elongated and retruded.

The maxilla often drops downward and backward, especially posteriorly, and has a premature contact with the mandible that causes an anterior open bite or failure of the anterior teeth to occlude. Profuse nasopharyngeal bleeding occasionally accompanies a LeFort fracture and may require anteroposterior nasal packing. The facial swelling in these patients is massive. CSF leaks can accompany high LeFort (II or III) fractures. Pneumocephalus may be present if the fracture extends to the cranial base, producing a communication with the nose that allows air to penetrate the meninges.

The radiographic evaluation of a LeFort fracture consists of plain films, but these are of limited value. A CT scan is recommended in all patients for a precise evaluation of the orbital, nasoethmoidal, and maxillary areas. Particular attention should be paid to the orbit with narrow CT cuts through this anatomic region, and axial and coronal sections with bone and soft tissue windows are recommended.

The problems with fixation and treatment in the maxilla are similar to those described in the mandible in children, in that the fixation appliances and arch bars may be difficult to attach to young dentition. Plate-and-screw fixation should be used as appropriate for older children, but the tooth buds must be avoided. Midfacial fractures may lead to midfacial retrusion as a result of an injury to the growth center of the maxilla and the nasal septum. The driving force for lower maxillary growth and nasal growth is believed to be present in the nasal septum. Severe injuries, especially those with incomplete reduction and immobilization, predispose to these complications. In addition, complications of elongation or reduction of facial height, flattening of the face, and malocclusion are seen in the pediatric age group. Malunion is best prevented by early exploration and open reduction and satisfactory fixation. Mobilization of maxillary fracture malunions in children is difficult after 1 week, and reduction should be completed before that time.

Because the palatal suture is a midline suture that does not complete ossification until the end of the second decade of life, hemipalatal fractures are relatively common in young children.[111] Their occurrence is suggested by a labial and mucosal laceration. The fracture is documented on physical examination by eliciting lateral movement of the maxillary dentition, and is corroborated by CT scans. The diagnosis of a LeFort fracture usually is confirmed by maxillary mobility. In rare instances, the maxilla is impacted (or incompletely fractured), in which case mobility may *not* be present, but malocclusion is observed. The malocclusion may be minor and difficult to confirm when the maxilla is only slightly displaced.

Treatment of LeFort fractures consists of open reduction and, possibly, intermaxillary fixation.

REFERENCES

1. Bales CR, Randall P, Lehr HB. Fractures of the facial bones in children. J Trauma 1972;12:56.
2. Berger MS, Pitts LH, Cowely M, Edwards MSB, Bartkowski HM. Outcome from severe head injury in children and adolescents. J Neurosurg 1985;62:194.
3. Dufresne C, Manson PN. Pediatric facial trauma. In: McCarthy JG, ed. Plastic surgery vol 2. Philadelphia, WB Saunders, 1990:1142.
4. Freihofer HP Jr. Results of osteotomies of the facial skeleton in adolescence. Journal of Maxillo-Facial Surgery 1977;5:267.
5. Gilbert GG. Growth of the nose and the postrhinoplastic problem in youth. Arch Otolaryngol 1958;68:673.
6. Hall RK. Facial trauma in children. Aust NZ J Surg 1974;19:336.
7. Rasmussen PS. Acute traumatic liquorrhea. Acta Neurol Scand 1965;41:551.
8. Reilly, Lee H. Unpublished research.
9. Roberts R, Shopfnex CE. Plain skull roentgenograms in children with head trauma. AJR Am J Roentgenol 1972;114:230.
10. Rowe NL. Fractures of the jaws in children. Journal of Oral Surgery 1969;27:4987.
11. Sanders B. Pediatric oral and maxillofacial surgery. St Louis, CV Mosby, 1979;42.
12. Sarnat BG, Gans BJ. Growth of bones: methods of assessing and clinical importance. Plast Reconstr Surg 1952;9:140.
13. Scott JH. Further studies on the growth of the human face. Proceeding of the Royal Society of Medicine 1959;52:263.
14. Kaplan SL, Mark HI. Bilateral fractures of the mandibular condyles and fracture of the symphysis menti in an 18-month-old child: two year preliminary report with a plea for conservative treatment. Oral Surgery 1962;15:136.
15. Manson PN, Shack RB, Leonard LG, Su CT, Hoopes JE. Sagittal fractures of the maxilla and palate. Plast Reconstr Surg 1983;72:484.
16. Proffitt WR, Vig KW, Turvey TA. Early fractures of the mandibular condyles: frequently an unsuspected cause of growth disturbances. Am J Orthod 1980;78:1.
17. Riefkohl R, Georgiade NL. Facial fractures in children. In: Serafin D, Georgiade NL, eds. Pediatric plastic surgery. St Louis, CV Mosby, 1984.
18. Fearon B, Edmonds B, Bird R. Orbito-facial complications in children. Laryngoscope 1979;89:947.
19. Carrington KW, Taren JA, Kahn EA. Primary repair of compound skull fractures in children. Surg Gynecol Obstet 1960;110:203.
20. Cohen RA, Kaufman RA, Myers PA, Towbin RB. Cranial computed tomography in the abused child with head injury. American Journal of Radiology 1986;146:97.
21. Jones KM, Bauer BS, Pensler JM. Treatment of mandibular fractures in children. Ann Plast Surg 1989;23:280.
22. Berkowitz R, Ludwid S, Johnson R. Dental trauma in children and adolescents. Clin Pediatr (Phila) 1980;19:166.
23. Putterman AM, Stevens T, Vrist MJ. Non-surgical management of fractures of the orbital floor. Am J Ophthalmol 1974;77:232.
24. Walker RV. Traumatic mandibular condylar fracture dislocations: effect of growth in the Macaca Rhesus monkey. Am J Surg 1960;100:850.
25. Ortiz-Monasterio F, Olmedo A. Corrective rhinoplasty before puberty: a long-term follow-up. Plast Reconstr Surg 1981;68:381.
26. Schettler D, Rehrmann A. Long-term results of functional treatment of condylar fractures with the long bridle according to A Rehrmann. Journal Maxillofacial Surgery 1975;3:14.
27. Schultz RC. Pediatric facial fractures. In: Kernahan DA, Thompson HG, Bauer BS, eds. Symposium on pediatric plastic surgery. St Louis, CV Mosby, 1982.
28. Sekhar LN, Scarff TB. Pseudogrowth of skull fractures in childhood. Neurosurgery 1980;6:285.
29. Moss ML. The primacy of functional matrices in orofacial growth. Dental Practitioner 1968;19:65.
30. Moss ML, Salentijn L. The capsular matrix. Am J Orthod 1969;56:474.
31. Muller D. Long-term results after rhinoplasty of nose trauma in childhood. Laryngology, Rhinology and Otolaryngology 1983;62:116.
32. Mulliken JB, Kaban LB, Evans CA, Strand D, Murray JE. Facial skeletal changes following hyperteorbitism correction. Plast Reconstr Surg 1986;77:7.
33. Panagopoulos AP. Management of fractures of the jaws in children. Journal of the International College of Surgeons 1957;28:806.
34. Lehman JA Jr, Saddawi ND. Fractures of the mandible in children. J Trauma 1976;16:773.
35. Gillingham FJ. Neurosurgical experiences in northern Italy. Br J Surg 1947;1:81.
36. Oliver P, Richardson JR, Clubb RW, Flake CG. Tracheostomy in children. N Engl J Med 1962;267:632.
37. Otherson HB. Intubation injuries of the trachea in children. Ann Surg 1979;189:601.
38. Steinhauser EW. The treatment of ankylosis in children. Int J Oral Surg 1973;2:129.
39. Tate RJ. Facial injuries associated with the battered child syndrome. Br J Oral Surg 1981;9:41.
40. Waite DE. Pediatric fractures of the jaw and facial bones. Pediatrics 1973;51:551.
41. Korneeff L. Current concepts on the management of orbital blow-out fracture. Ann Plast Surg 1982;9:185.
42. Messinger A, Radkowski MA, Greenwald MJ, Pensler JM. Orbital roof fractures in the pediatric population. Plast Reconstr Surg 1989;84:213.
43. Bergland O, Borchgrevink H. The role of the nasal septum in midfacial growth in man elucidated by the maxillary development in certain types of facial clefts: a preliminary report. Scand J Plast Reconstr Surg 1974;8:42.
44. Bruce DA, Alovi A, Bilaniuk L, Dolinskas E, Obrist W, Uzzeu B. Diffuse cerebral swelling following head injuries in children: the syndrome of malignant brain edema. J Neurosurg 1981;54:170.
45. Caffey J. Multiple fractures in the long bones of infants suffering from chronic subdural hematoma. AJR Am J Roentgenol 1946;56:163.
46. Coccaro PJ. Restitution of mandibular form after condylar injury in infancy: a 7-year study of a child. Am J Orthod 1969;55:32.
47. Hall RK. Injuries of the face and jaws in children. Int J Surg 1972;19:336.
48. Huang CS, Ross RB. Surgical advancement of the retrognathic mandible in growing children. Am J Orthod 1983;82:89.
49. Miller JD, Becker DP, Ward JD. Significance of intracranial hypertension in severe head injury. J Neurosurg 1977;47:503.
50. Thomson HG, Farmer AW, Lindsay WK. Condylar neck fractures of the mandible in children. Plast Reconstr Surg 1964;34:452.
51. Andreasen JO. Luxation of permanent teeth due to trauma. Scandinavian Journal of Dental Research 1970;78:273.
52. Andreasen JO. Etiology and athogenesis of traumatic dental injuries: a clinical study of 1,298 cases. Scandinavian Journal of Dental Research 1970;78:329.

53. Andreasen JO. Prognosis of permanent teeth involved in jaw fractures. Scandinavian Journal of Dental Research 1970;78:343.

54. Andreasen JO. Treatment of fractures and avulsed teeth. Journal of Dentistry in Childhood 1971;38:29.

55. Andreasen JO, Ravn JJ. The effect of traumatic injuries to primary teeth on their permanent successors. II. A clinical and radiographic follow-up study of 213 teeth. Scandinavian Journal of Dental Research 1971;79:284.

56. Andreasen JO, Sundstrom B, Ravn JJ. The effect of traumatic injuries to primary teeth on their permanent successors. I. A clinical and histologic study of 117 injuries to permanent teeth. Scandinavian Journal of Dental Research 1971;79:284.

57. Grote W. Traumatische liquorfisteln in kinds and jurgdendalter. Zeitschrift Kinderchirurgie Greoziegeb 1966;3:11.

58. Rowe NL. Injuries to teeth and jaws. In: Mustarde JC, ed. Plastic surgery in infancy and childhood. Edinburgh, Churchill Livingstone, 1979.

59. Rowe NL. Fractures of the facial skeleton in children. Journal of Oral Surgery 1968;26:505.

60. Brook F, Itghak, Friedman EM. Intracranial complications of sinusitis in children. Annals of Otolaryngology 1982;91:41.

61. Enlow DH. Handbook of facial growth, ed 2. Philadelphia, WB Saunders, 1982.

62. O'Ryan F, Epker BN. Deliberate surgical control of mandibular growth. Oral Surgery 1982;53:2.

63. Ousterhout DK, Vargervik K. Maxillary hypoplasia secondary to midfacial trauma in childhood. Plast Reconstr Surg 1987;80:491.

64. Harwood DC. Fractures of the petrous and tympanic parts of the temporal bone in children: a tomographic study of 35 cases. Radiology 1970;110:598.

65. Jennes M. Corrective nasal surgery in children. Arch Otolaryngol 1964;79:145.

66. Stucer FJ Jr, Bryarly C, Shockley W. Management of nasal trauma in children. Arch Otolaryngol 1984;110:190.

67. Mayer T, Matlak M, Johnson D, Walker M. The modified injury severity scale in pediatric multiple trauma patients. J Pediatr Surg 1980;15:719.

68. Graham GG, Peltier RJ. Management of mandibular fractures in children. Journal of Oral Surgery 1960;18:416.

69. Silverman FN. The roentgen manifestations of unrecognized skeletal trauma in infants. AJR Am J Roentgenol 1953;69:413.

70. Posnick J. Pediatric facial fractures. In: Yaremchuk M, Gruss J, Manson PN, eds. Rigid fixation of the facial skeleton. Butterworths, 1990.

71. Caffey J. The whiplash shaken infant syndrome: manual shaking by the extremities with whiplash-induced intracranial and intraocular bleeding, linked with residual permanent brain damage and mental retardation. Pediatrics 1974;54:396.

72. Caldicott WJH, Nortte JB, Simpson DA. Traumatic cerebrospinal fluid fistulae in children. J Neurosurg 1973;38:1.

73. Converse JC. Orbital blow-out fractures: a 10 year survey. Plast Reconstr Surg 1967;39:20.

74. Stacher FJ, Bryarly RC, Shockley WW. Management of nasal trauma in children. Arch Otolaryngol 1984;11:190.

75. Tai RY, Zee CE, Apthop JS, Dixon GH. Computer tomography in child abuse head trauma. Computerized Tomography 1980;4:277.

76. Teasdale G, Jennett B. Assessment of coma and impaired consciousness. Lancet 1974;2:81.

77. MacLennan WD. Fractures of the mandible in children under the age of six years. Br J Plast Surg 1956;9:125.

78. Fortunato M, Fielding AF, Guernsey LH. Facial bone fractures in children. Oral Surg Oral Med Oral Pathol 1982;53:225.

79. Manson PN. Treatment of pan facial fractures. Journal of Craniofacial Trauma 1995;1:43.

80. Kravitz H, Dreissen G, Gomberg R, Korach A. Accidental falls from elevated surfaces in infants from birth to one year of age. Pediatrics 1969;44:869.

81. Henreick EB, Harwood DC, Hudson AR. Head injuries in children: a survey of 4465 consecutive cases at the Hospital for Sick Children. Clin Neurosurg 1964;11:46.

82. Campbell RL, Moore RF. Fractures of the condyle in a 3-month-old infant. Oral Surgery 1975;40:4547.

83. Gruszkiewicz J, Doron Y, Peyser E. Recovery from severe craniocerebral injury and brain stem lesions in childhood. Surg Neurol 1973;1:197.

84. Reil B, Kranx S. Traumatology of the maxillofacial region in childhood. Journal of Maxillo-Facial Surgery 1976;4:197.

85. Hendrick EB. The use of hypothermia in severe brain stem lesions in childhood. Arch Surg 1959;79:362.

86. McCoy FJ, Chandler RA, Crow ML. Facial fractures in children. Plast Reconstr Surg 1966;37:209.

87. Gilhuus-Moe O, ed. Fractures of the mandibular condyle in the growth period. Stockholm, Scandinavian University Book, 1969.

88. Manson PN, Grivas R, Rosenbaum A, Vannier M, Zinreich J, Iliff N. Studies on enophthalmos. II: The measurement of orbital injuries and their treatment by quantitative computed tomography. Plast Reconstr Surg 1986;77:203.

89. Manson PN, Iliff N. Management of blow out fracture of the orbital floor: early repair of selected injuries. Surv Ophthalmol 1991;35:280.

90. Moffett B. The morphogenesis of the temporomandibular joint. Am J Orthod 1966;52:401.

91. Boyne PJ. Osseous repair and mandibular growth after subcondylar fractures. Journal of Oral Surgery 1967;25:300.

92. Converse JC. Facial injuries in children. In: Mustarde JC, ed. Plastic surgery in infancy and childhood. Edinburgh, Churchill Livingstone, 1979.

93. Rakower W, Protzell A, Rosencrans M. Treatment of displaced condylar fractures in children: report of cases. Journal of Oral Surgery 1961;19:517.

94. May M, Fria TJ, Blumenthal F, Curtin H. Facial paralysis in children: differential diagnosis. Otolaryngol Head Neck Surg 1981;89:841.

95. Williams AF. Children killed in falls from motor vehicles. Pediatrics 1981;68:576.

96. Bruce DA, Schut L, Bruno LA, Wood JH, Sutton LN. Outcome following severe head injuries in children. J Neurosurg 1978;48:679.

97. Lyerly JG. The treatment of depressed fractures of the skull with special reference to the cranial defect. Am Surg 1957;23:1115.

98. Bernstein L. Maxillofacial injuries in children. Otolaryngol Clin North Am 1969;2:397.

99. Georgiade NG, Pickrell KL. Treatment of maxillofacial injuries in children. Journal of the International College of Surgeons 1967;27:640.

100. MacLennan WD, Simpson W. Treatment of fractured mandibular condylar process in children. Br J Plast Surg 1967;18:423.

101. Rowe NL, Williams JCI. Children's fractures. In: Maxillofacial injuries. New York, Churchill Livingstone, 1985:538.

102. MacLennan WD. Injuries involving the teeth and jaws in young children. Arch Dis Child 1957;32:492.

103. Bridges CP, Ryan RF, Longenecker CG, Vincent RW. Tracheostomy in children: a twenty year study at Charity Hospital in New Orleans. Plast Reconstr Surg 1966;37:117.

104. Ramba J. Fractures of the facial bones in children. Int J Oral Surg 1985;14:472.

105. Moos K, El-Attar A. Mandible and dental injuries. In: Mustarde JC, Jackson IT, eds. Plastic surgery in infancy and childhood, ed 3. New York, Churchill Livingstone, 1988:345.

106. Stolsted P, Schonsted-Madsen V. Traumatology of the newborn's nose. Rhinolaryngology 1979;17:77.

107. Kissoon N, Dreyer J, Walia M. Pediatric trauma: differences in pathophysiology, injury patterns and treatment compared with adult trauma. Can Med Assoc J 1990;142:27.

108. Manson PN. Skull and midface injuries. In: Mustarde JC, Jackson IT, eds. Plastic surgery in infancy and childhood, ed 3. New York, Churchill Livingstone, 1986.

109. Manson P, Clifford C, Su CT, Iliff NT, Morgan R. Mechanisms of global support and post-traumatic enophthalmos inframuscular cone orbital fat. Plast Reconstr Surg 1986;77:193.

110. Morgan WC. Pediatric mandibular fractures. Oral Surgery 1975;40:320.

111. Manson PN, Crawley WA, Yaremchuk M, Rochman GM, Hoopes JE, French JH. Midface fractures: advantages of immediate extended open reduction and bone grafting. Plast Reconstr Surg 1985;76:1.

Surgery of Infants and Children: Scientific Principles and Practice, edited by
Keith T. Oldham, Paul M. Colombani, and Robert P. Foglia.
Lippincott–Raven Publishers, Philadelphia, © 1997.

CHAPTER 22

Neck Trauma

Mary L. Brandt and Marilyn W. Butler

Cervical trauma is a relatively uncommon but potentially lethal injury in childhood, with the rates of mortality for civilian penetrating trauma to the neck reported as approximately 2% to 6%.[1,2] These injuries require rapid evaluation and treatment to avoid the significant morbidity and mortality that can occur. It is important to understand the anatomy, how to evaluate and stabilize the child, and how to treat definitively individual injuries of the neck in children.

The recorded history of neck trauma begins in 1552, when Ambroise Paré stopped hemorrhage from the neck of a soldier wounded in a duel by ligating the common carotid and internal jugular vein. By the time of the Civil War, mortality had decreased to 15%, and by World War II mortality was approximately 7% for penetrating neck wounds.[1,2] Controversy concerning exploration versus noninvasive evaluation began during World War II with the proposal for early exploration of cervical hematomas.[1,2] By 1956, a report in the adult literature showed a 35% mortality in late exploration of penetrating neck wounds versus a 6% mortality in early exploration. In part because of this report, mandatory cervical exploration for penetrating wounds became the gold standard of therapy.[1–3] The rate of negative explorations resulting from this policy rose to as high as 75%.[4,5]

ANATOMY OF THE NECK IN CHILDHOOD

The neck is an area of highly complex and compact anatomy. Organs from the cardiovascular, respiratory, digestive, endocrine, and central nervous system are present and are prone to injury from both blunt and penetrating trauma. The relationship between these structures are the same in children as in adults, but there are important anatomic differences that contribute to the morbidity and mortality of trauma to the head and neck. Children, because of a proportionately larger head, are more likely to suffer trauma to the head than adults. The neck is proportionately somewhat shorter in children, making the arrangement of the structures in the neck even more compact. The bones of the head and neck are less dense in childhood, and the ligaments are more elastic. In penetrating trauma, there is a greater risk of injury to the central nervous system, eyes, and vessels of the head because of the lower density of the bones in the face and skull.[6] With blunt trauma, the elastic

ligaments of the neck may allow subluxation of the vertebrae, with spinal cord injury. This may occur without evidence of injury on cervical spine radiographs, a syndrome referred to as SCIWORA (spinal cord injury without radiologic abnormality).[7,8] Because of these anatomic differences, children improperly restrained with adult lap–shoulder seat belts may suffer extensive damage to the cervical spine.[9]

Trauma to the neck can be described by anatomic zones. The neck is divided into anterior and posterior sections that are marked by the transverse processes of the cervical vertebrae. Posterior to the transverse cervical processes are the supporting muscles of the neck. The anterior neck zones are divided into the anterior triangle and posterior triangle, or, more physiologically, can be considered in zones (Fig. 22-1). Zone I, at the base of the neck, extends from the clavicle to the cricoid cartilage. Zone II, or the middle of the neck, extends from the cricoid cartilage to the angle of the mandible. Zone III, in the upper neck, extends from the angle of the mandible to the base of the skull.

The structures of the neck are enclosed within both a deep and a superficial fascia. Although these fascial layers can serve to contain bleeding from injured vessels, they can lead to increased pressure within the neck compartments and cause airway compromise. Vascular and lymphatic structures at risk from injury include the carotid, vertebral, and subclavian arteries, subclavian and jugular veins, and the thoracic duct. Other structures at risk include the trachea, larynx, pharynx, and the thyroid gland. The parathyroid glands are at risk but are in fact rarely injured. In addition to the cervical spine located within the vertebral column, the numerous cranial and peripheral nerves, including the vagus, phrenic, recurrent laryngeal, hypoglossal, spinal accessory, and the brachial plexus, can be injured. Because of the complexity of the neck, those who assess and treat these injured children should have a thorough knowledge of the anatomy of the neck.

MECHANISMS OF INJURY

Most pediatric trauma is caused by a blunt mechanism of injury. Children involved in motor vehicle accidents may be subjected to rapid deceleration forces that can cause shearing

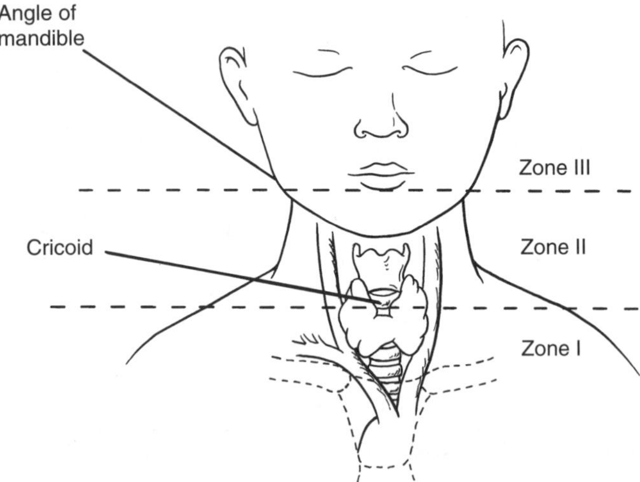

FIG. 22-1. The anterior neck can be divided into zones I, II, and III.

or compression injuries in the neck. Falls can result in cervical spine injury and injury to other neck structures. Roller skating or riding a bicycle into a suspended line can cause a "clothesline injury," resulting in sudden hyperextension of the neck or in direct blunt trauma to the larynx and anterior zone II of the neck. This hyperextension commonly causes a sprain or a strain of the neck or cervical fracture dislocation. With extensive hyperextension, weakness at the hypopharyngeal junction can cause perforation, and the pharynx and larynx can be sheared by extended vertebral bodies during deceleration.[10] Child abuse, or intentional injury, most commonly in the form of strangulation or choke injuries to the neck, may result in direct injury to the larynx. Injury to the carotid artery may occur after direct trauma, or by stretching of the artery during hyperextension of the neck.[11,12] Blunt trauma to the internal carotid artery in the tonsillar fossa may occur after a fall with an object in the child's mouth, the so-called "pencil point injury."[13,14] If neurologic symptoms occur, it is usually within 24 hours of injury.[13] Some children may present with delayed thrombosis of the carotid artery or jugular vein secondary to infection.[15]

Penetrating trauma of the neck ranges from superficial to impalement with a variety of objects. In stab wounds or impalements, the tract usually travels in a straight line. The potential for serious injury can often be deduced by determining the site of entry and direction of the impalement. On the other hand, gunshot wounds have unpredictable pathways because the bullet may travel in fascial planes or ricochet off bony objects. The pathway for a cervical gunshot wound may include the chest, shoulders, and head in addition to cervical structures.

EVALUATION OF THE CHILD WITH CERVICAL INJURY

History

History should be obtained by witnesses at the scene and by whoever transported the child to the hospital. The mechanism of injury should be detailed because these vectors of force can be useful in determining which potential injuries may have occurred. The child should be asked if there is pain in the neck, difficulty breathing, or pain or difficulty swallowing. If there is delay of several hours from the time of injury to the time the patient is seen in the emergency department, the lack of problems during the several hours since the injury should not lessen the concern regarding a potential injury.

Physical Examination

The neck is examined carefully for ecchymoses, swelling, and tenderness. If penetrating trauma has occurred, the wound should *not* be explored by probing. If there is an underlying vascular injury, clot can be disrupted with subsequent hemorrhage. Small penetrating wounds can be locally anesthetized and the wound extended to retract the edges and determine whether the injury has penetrated the platysma. If the platysma is intact, it is safe to close the wound without invasive tests or exploration. If a hematoma or active bleeding is present, it is a reliable indicator of significant injury, and surgical exploration is indicated. However, the absence of a hematoma does not eliminate this possibility. Bleeding may be contained in the superficial or deep fascia, with subtle or absent findings on physical examination. The neck should be examined for presence of pulses and bruits.

The neck is palpated gently for localized tenderness and subcutaneous emphysema. The presence of subcutaneous emphysema in neck trauma suggests injury to the trachea, larynx, or esophagus, but may also be caused by a pneumothorax that has tracked along fascial planes from the mediastinum to the neck. The subcutaneous emphysema resolves spontaneously when the underlying cause is eliminated.

The child is assessed for respiratory compromise, stridor, or other adventitious airway sounds. The patient is asked to speak, if possible, to detect any change in phonation. Hoarseness can be caused by direct laryngeal injury or, less commonly, laryngeal nerve injury. Respiratory distress can be life threatening and, in the presence of neck injury, represents a surgical emergency. In cases of extreme compromise, emergency tracheostomy in the emergency room may be indicated. When possible, the patient should be taken emergently to the operating room where the neck can be explored, hematomas evacuated, and control of the airway established.

Hemoptysis is suggestive of injury to the airway. Although hematemesis may be indicative of injury to the upper gastrointestinal tract, it is more commonly the result of nasopharyngeal bleeding and swallowed blood. A nasogastric tube should be placed in the operating room rather than in the emergency room in patients with likely cervical injury because placement may dislodge a clot or lead to coughing and retching, which in turn may dislodge the clot.[1]

A neurologic examination should be performed. Localized findings of hemiplegia or hemiparesis may be indicative of either intracranial hemorrhage or trauma or carotid or vertebral injury with ischemia. Brachial plexus injury is suggested by a motor or sensory deficit in the arms. Drooping of the corner of the mouth, deviation of the tongue, or Horner syndrome suggest injury as well. Symptoms due to the carotid artery injury include presence of a hematoma, Horner syndrome, transient ischemic attacks, amaurosis fugax, and limb paresis in an otherwise alert patient.[1]

Initial Stabilization

As in all trauma, the primary survey should be done during the initial stabilization of a patient with a cervical injury. Active bleeding should be controlled with pressure until the patient can be taken emergently to the operating room. The evaluation and treatment of airway compromise is particularly important in patients with cervical trauma. Immediate airway compromise can occur from direct laryngeal or tracheal injury. Gradual compromise can occur from an expanding hematoma between tight fascial planes. Indications for intubation in these patients include acute respiratory distress, airway compromise from blood or secretions, extensive subcutaneous emphysema with compression of the airway, tracheal shift, severe alteration in mental status, or need for hyperventilation with intracranial injury.[16] Protective intubation may be indicated in patients with significant penetrating neck trauma because progressive swelling or hemorrhage may result in loss of the airway. All patients with cervical injuries should be assumed to have cervical spine injury, especially patients who have suffered blunt trauma. Nasotracheal intubation in children is often technically difficult and is seldom preferred. Because of the anatomy of the pediatric oropharynx, in-line immobilization is used and orotracheal intubation is performed without hyperextension of the neck.[17] In clear cases of major injury or disruption of the larynx or trachea, no attempt at intubation should be made because further injury may occur. The preferred emergency airway until a definitive surgical airway can be obtained is percutaneous needle cricothyroidotomy with oxygen insufflation. This technique provides adequate oxygenation but leads to respiratory acidosis and therefore is useful only for the 15 to 30 minutes necessary to reach the operating room for definitive repair.[18,19] When possible, a tracheostomy should be performed in the operating room rather than the emergency room. In the prepubertal child, cricothyroidotomy is associated with a significant incidence of vocal cord injury and, for that reason, a tracheostomy is preferred. The tracheotomy should be longitudinal or vertical rather than transverse, because tracheal stenosis may occur in the smaller-diameter trachea of the child.[20]

The initial radiographic studies in all patients with cervical trauma include chest and cervical films. The entrance site of any missile or open wound from impalement should be marked with a radiopaque marker before obtaining these films. On chest radiography, the position of the trachea should be assessed as well as the presence of an associated pneumothorax or hemothorax. Other findings on chest radiographs that suggest injury to the great vessels include a widened mediastinum, presence of an apical cap, and deviation of a nasogastric tube.[21] Lateral and anteroposterior cervical radiographs are obtained to evaluate the cervical spine, the position of tracheal and esophageal air columns, and to look for extraluminal air. In blunt trauma, a computed tomography (CT) scan is obtained to evaluate the larynx and to look for signs of esophageal and airway injury.[22]

MANAGEMENT OF CERVICAL INJURIES

The management of trauma to the neck depends on the zone of injury and the mechanism of injury. Zones I and III are surgically difficult to access and are treated by selective management, based on the diagnostic evaluation. In zone II, virtually all injuries are accessible to surgical exploration. Blunt cervical injuries without indications for immediate surgical exploration should be evaluated by plain radiographs to rule out cervical spine injury and CT scan to rule out laryngeal injury. Initial carotid Doppler examination should be obtained. If indicated, a repeat examination to rule out delayed carotid thrombosis is carried out subsequently. In patients for whom there is a high level of suspicion of carotid injury, an arteriogram should be obtained.

Excluding those patients with obvious indications for surgical exploration (Table 22-1), there is considerable controversy surrounding the assessment and management of patients with penetrating cervical trauma in zone II.[23] Some believe that mandatory exploration guarantees that injuries will not be missed, and, therefore, that the potential morbidity and mortality of these injuries is decreased or eliminated. On the other end of the spectrum are those who argue that most patients with neck trauma can be observed, with selective exploration for those in whom signs of true injury develop. In the middle are those who advocate evaluation by endoscopy and angiography, with surgery reserved for patients who have evidence of injury based on this evaluation. Almost all of the literature considering mandatory versus selective exploration of these injuries is based on either prospective or retrospective studies in adults. In children, the decision of whether to operate is further complicated by the size of the child and the issues concerning complications of angiography and endoscopy in small children.

Pros and Cons of Mandatory Exploration

Mandatory exploration virtually ensures that injuries are identified and repaired, avoiding the complications of a missed injury or delayed repair. Major injuries may be asymptomatic and can be found at the time of exploration, despite a negative physical examination and diagnostic studies.[5] Mandatory exploration does not prolong the hospital stay, results in minimal complications, and the total cost is actually less than the cost of

TABLE 22-1. *Absolute indications for exploration in cervical trauma*

Expanding or pulsatile hematoma
Uncontrolled or ongoing bleeding
Obvious open airway
History of extensive blood loss
Shock
Pulse deficit or bruit
Paralysis of the diaphragm
Neurologic deficits
Hemoptysis
Subcutaneous emphysema
Hoarseness
Hematemesis
Dysphagia

the prolonged hospitalization and special examinations required with selective evaluation and observation.[2] In addition, there may be a high morbidity associated with delayed therapy of some injuries.

The argument against mandatory exploration is the high negative exploration rate, which can be up to 76%.[5] In a review of 26 series with a total of 4369 patients with neck trauma, 10 series had mandatory exploration in all patients with zone II injuries and had a negative exploration rate of 46%. In the 16 series with selective exploration, the negative exploration rate was 30%.[2]

Pros and Cons of Selective Exploration

An alternative approach to patients with neck trauma is to evaluate the structures of the neck using angiography and endoscopy to select patients at higher risk for injury for surgical exploration. The primary advantage of selective management in adults is a lower negative exploration rate, without an increase in complications.[2,24,25] Most series report very few patients admitted for observation who subsequently required operation.[2] In addition, it has been shown that if missed injuries are diagnosed and treated within 24 hours, there is no added morbidity or mortality.[26]

The disadvantages of the selective approach are the risk of overlooking an injury, the potential morbidity associated with invasive (arteriography, endoscopy) procedures, and the need for general anesthesia in younger patients (Table 22-2). In addition to having smaller vessels, the vasculature of children is more prone to vasospasm, increasing the risk of thrombosis.[27–29] The reported rate of injury or thrombosis requiring medical or surgical treatment after cardiac catheterization varies from 4% to 45%.[28–31] The rates of thrombosis after cardiac catheterization have been decreased by the use of systemic heparinization.[28] Heparinization is contraindicated in most pediatric trauma patients, and, therefore, the rate of thrombosis in these patients would be expected to be higher. Thrombectomy is not always successful, and in severe cases, arterial occlusion may result in gangrene.[28,31] Chronic complications include muscle atrophy, weakness, loss of nerve function, and delayed

TABLE 22-2. *Risk of diagnostic procedures in children with selective management of cervical trauma*

Angiography
  General anesthesia
  Hematoma
  False aneurysm
  Ischemic limb with delayed limb growth
  Thrombus/embolus
  Contrast nephropathy
  Contrast reaction
Bronchoscopy
  General anesthesia
  Perforation
  Pneumothorax
Esophagoscopy
  General anesthesia
  Perforation

limb growth.[28,31,32] Although no prospective or extensive studies of duplex scanning in the neck for injuries have been performed, this may prove to be a useful adjunct in the pediatric population in particular for evaluating the carotid arteries.[33]

The contrast esophagogram, although frequently used, is usually not accurate enough to exclude reliably an esophageal injury. In 118 adult patients examined with endoscopy and barium swallow before surgical exploration, barium swallow was shown to be 80% sensitive in one view and 89% sensitive with two views. Rigid esophagoscopy was 89% sensitive in this series. The flexible endoscope was shown to be only 50% sensitive in defining esophageal injury, and is not recommended in this setting. The combination of contrast esophagogram with endoscopy, if the esophagogram is equivocal, led to diagnosis of injury in all patients in this series.[34]

Observation Alone

Because of the high risk associated with missing a cervical injury, a number of authors believe that observation alone is not advised for adults.[23,35,36] Others contend that with a careful physical examination, and a low threshold for surgical exploration in the presence of physical findings, observation can be safe.[23,37–39] Hall and colleagues[23] reported that 56% of children with penetrating zone II injuries had negative physical examinations on arrival to the hospital. These children were all observed, and none had subsequent problems.

Proposed Management of Cervical Trauma in Children

In children, the risks of angiography and endoscopy increases with decreasing size and age. These risks are weighed against the low morbidity of surgical exploration. Most algorithms proposed for the management of cervical trauma in adults cannot be uniformly applied to the pediatric population. Algorithms for the management of pediatric cervical injury should be based on the zone of injury, the probability of injury, and the size of the child. In general, patients with a low risk of injury can be observed. (Small patients with a high risk of injury should undergo exploration. In older children (20-30 kg) with a high risk of injury, selective management may be indicated. This size distinction varies by institution and should be based on the experience of the angiographers, endoscopists, and surgeons.[8]

OPERATIVE MANAGEMENT OF SPECIFIC INJURIES

Preoperative Preparation

All patients undergoing exploration of the neck should be resuscitated, given antibiotics to cover the flora associated with esophageal or tracheal injuries (ie, gram-positive, gram-negative, and anaerobic flora), and blood crossmatched.

Exploration of Cervical Injuries

The preparation should include shoulders, chest, abdomen, and groins in addition to the neck. Betadine paint alone can be used because scrubbing may dislodge a clot.[1] The head is extended and turned to the contralateral side. Two surgical approaches can be used, depending on the location of the injury. The incision can be placed along the anterior border of the sternocleidomastoid muscle, which is then retracted posterolaterally. If the injury is bilateral, the same incision can be made bilaterally, joined across the sternal notch, and this anterior flap raised if the injury crosses the midline. Alternatively, a transverse collar-type incision affords excellent exposure.[1]

Approach to Zone I Injuries

Zone I injuries to the neck have a high mortality rate primarily because of injury to the great vessels and the difficult surgical approaches required to control hemorrhage in this setting.[40] If patients are hemodynamically stable, arteriography should be performed to delineate the extent and location of all injured vessels. Documented injuries to the aorta or innominate artery are best approached by median sternotomy. Proximal left subclavian injuries can be approached by a left anterior thoracotomy in the fourth intercostal space. Proximal carotid injuries can be approached by the same cervical incision with resection of the head of the clavicle if necessary to obtain more proximal control. However, a median sternotomy may be necessary, and it is prudent to have a sternal saw available. Proximal right subclavian injuries are best approached by median sternotomy with a clavicular extension.

Approach to Zone III Injuries

The most life-threatening and difficult injury to manage in zone III is trauma to the distal carotid. Direct repair should be performed when possible, although exposure of the artery is difficult. Additional exposure of distal carotid injuries at the base of the skull can be obtained by anterior subluxation of the jaw, vertical division of the ramus of the mandible with elevation of the posterior segment of the mandible, detachment of the sternocleidomastoid from the mastoid process, and division of the digastric muscle.[41,42] Another approach to this difficult injury is to place a Fogarty balloon catheter into the distal stump to occlude the artery. The Fogarty catheter is then brought out of the wound and sutured securely into position. Several days or even weeks after exploration, the balloon can be slowly deflated and the catheter removed if no bleeding is noted.[1] (In patients with very distal injury, embolization at the time of arteriography may be the management of choice.[40])

Carotid Artery Injury

Carotid artery injuries should be repaired when technically possible. Ligation of the internal carotid artery results in substantial neurologic deficit in many patients[43] while common carotid ligation can be done with relative impunity. The only exception to primary repair is the patient with a neurologic deficit after injury. In patients with significant neurologic deficits, repair of the artery can lead to death from intercerebral

hemorrhage caused by reperfusion.[44] In patients with a severe neurologic deficit, angiography is performed before exploration. If the artery is patent, repair can be performed. If the distal segment is occluded, the artery is ligated to avoid a postperfusion hemorrhagic infarct.[45,46] If repair of the artery is not technically feasible, or in patients with a documented neurologic deficit and no antegrade flow in the carotid, the vessel can be ligated. Results of neurologic examination in patients in shock may be more abnormal than would otherwise be expected. In one study, 12 of 13 patients with an equivocal neurologic examination improved with repair in this setting.[47]

Most patients with documented intimal injury after blunt trauma should undergo resection of the area and repair of the carotid.[41] In patients with minor injury or injury too diffuse to allow easy repair, observation may be indicated.[41] Heparin, or antiplatelet drugs such as aspirin, have been used empirically by some surgeons in this setting.[11]

The approach to a carotid artery injury is to obtain proximal and distal control, including the common internal and external carotid vessels proximal and distal to the area of injury. The injured segment of artery is excised, including sections with intimal tears. In distal injuries, it may not be possible to mobilize the artery sufficiently to allow placement of vascular clamps. In this case, a Fogarty catheter can be placed in the lumen of the distal artery and inflated, occluding the lumen and achieving vascular control.[41]

External carotid artery injuries can be managed by ligation. Internal carotid injuries should be repaired, when technically possible. If the artery can be mobilized to allow primary anastomosis, this is performed with interrupted 6-0 or 7-0 Prolene suture. In small children, the use of the operating microscope and 8-0 or 9-0 suture may be indicated. The external carotid can be ligated distally and transposed to serve as a graft to replace a segment of internal carotid if necessary. When technically possible, this may be the procedure of choice in children to minimize aneurysm formation in a saphenous vein graft. In some cases, however, a graft must be used, and in these cases, saphenous vein is the conduit of choice. In larger children, such as teenagers, polytetrafluoroethylene graft is a reasonable choice.[40]

Anticoagulation is not routinely used for carotid artery injuries.[41] Shunts are rarely needed unless diminution of backflow is noted.[41] If there is an associated injury to the trachea or esophagus, muscle such as the sternocleidomastoid should be placed between the esophagus or trachea and the carotid artery.[48] Drains placed for injury to the esophagus should be directed away from the artery and should be removed as rapidly as possible in the postoperative period.[41]

Vertebral artery injuries are rare, comprising less than 1% of all vascular injuries of the neck.[49] This is an injury usually caused by penetrating trauma, although it can be occasionally caused by blunt trauma with spinal fracture, chiropractic manipulation, prolonged extension of the neck, and exercise.[50,51] It only rarely results in ischemic neurologic injury. There are reports of death from uncontrolled hemorrhage, and the development of arteriovenous fistula.[2] Physical examination is negative in approximately 75% of patients with vertebral artery injury diagnosed by angiography.[50] Injury to the vertebral artery can be approached by surgery, by embolization, or with observation. Operative therapy consists of proximal and distal ligation if there is a normal contralateral vertebral artery. If the injured artery provides the sole occipital blood supply to the brain, repair is recommended if possible. The access to this artery is difficult. The proximal artery can be approached at the takeoff of the subclavian. In distal injuries, an anterior approach at the C1–C2 interspace is recommended to ligate the vessel.[1,42,49] Between C2 and C6, the artery travels within the bony canal of the spinal vertebrae. Access at this level is obtained by removing the costal face of the cervical transverse process.[1,42] Embolization may be effective especially in the setting of arteriovenous fistula.[49,50] Given the low mortality and morbidity and the infrequency of diagnosis before angiography, many authors recommend nonoperative therapy if the patient is not actively bleeding.[52]

Venous Injury

Venous injuries are the most common vascular injuries in the neck. Smaller veins can be ligated. Both the subclavian and internal jugular veins should be repaired when possible with lateral venorrhaphy, patch venoplasty, or resection with anastomosis.[41] If extensive debridement is required, ligation is appropriate. Interposition grafts are not advocated. The exception to this would be injury to both internal jugular veins. In this setting, one jugular can be sacrificed to serve as an interposition graft for the contralateral jugular vein.[41] Air embolism is a potential intraoperative hazard in the presence of a large venous injury, and placement of the patient in a mild reverse Trendelenburg position decreases the risk of air embolus.[41]

Thoracic Duct

The thoracic duct traverses the base of the left neck just posterior and lateral to the head of the clavicle before returning into the subclavian vein, brachiocephalic vein, or internal jugular vein.[1] Injury to the thoracic duct in the neck may be difficult to diagnose at the time of exploration. It is recognized more commonly after exploration by persistent drainage from the neck or chylothorax. This injury is treated by exploration and ligation of the thoracic duct.

Larynx

Laryngeal trauma is best diagnosed and defined by CT scan and flexible fiberoptic laryngoscopy.[48,53,54] In patients with small lacerations or hematomas without a detectable fracture, conservative management with observation, voice rest, humidified air, and elevation of the head is appropriate.[53,54] In patients with more severe injury, airway control, before the onset of edema, is of critical importance. This can most often be accomplished with careful intubation with a small tube, performed by one experienced with intubation in children.[53,54] In patients with extensive injury, or if there is any difficulty with attempted intubation, a tracheostomy should be performed. Repair of the laryngeal injury can then be accomplished. In patients with unstable fractures or tears, stenting of the injured larynx may be required as well.[53,54]

Trachea

Injury to the cervical trachea may be obvious on physical examination, or more subtle, requiring bronchoscopy for diagnosis. It is critically important to recognize these injuries early because there is substantial morbidity and mortality associated with a delay in diagnosis.[55] Tracheal trauma may be either penetrating or blunt in nature. The first step is control of the airway. Endotracheal intubation is preferred, when it can be safely accomplished without further injury to the trachea. When the injury is massive, or intubation is otherwise not safe, a tracheostomy should be performed. The trachea is repaired primarily, usually with a single layer of absorbable suture. Mobilization of the trachea can be accomplished both proximally and distally to allow tension-free anastomosis of most injuries.[56] On occasion, large defects in the trachea may require a fascial flap or synthetic patch.[55] Protective tracheostomy should be considered for all major injuries of the cervical trachea, especially in the setting of a bilateral injury, because of the expected postoperative edema. The tracheostomy should always be placed at least one ring below the injury. A tracheostomy is not needed for simple injuries amenable to primary repair. In cases of combined tracheoesophageal injuries, a strap muscle or sternocleidomastoid muscle vascularized flap should be placed between the two sutured structures and the area drained away from the carotid artery.[56,57]

Pharynx and Esophagus

As with tracheal injury, injury to the pharynx and esophagus can occur with penetrating or blunt trauma.[10,38] Early identification of these injuries is critical because life-threatening sepsis may develop in patients with a delay in diagnosis.[38,58] The mortality rate ranges from 23% to 100% in missed injuries.[59] Mortality increases as the delay in diagnosis and treatment increases. Reports cite a 9% mortality if the injury was recognized in less than 12 hours versus 40% in over 12 hours, and 92% of patients dying if the injury was untreated for 48 hours.[34,60] Although diagnosis may be made by esophagography, injuries can be missed by this technique.[58] If the index of suspicion is high enough, patients should undergo esophagoscopy and, if necessary, exploration. In isolated perforations of the pharynx and esophagus, nonoperative management may be indicated in selected patients. Nonoperative management can be undertaken only in patients with small perforations with no extravasation into the mediastinum or the neck. If the contained perforation easily drains back into the esophagus on esophagography, these patients can be managed with total parenteral nutrition or a nasogastric feeding tube with intravenous antibiotics.[61,62] Most perforations, however, require surgical exploration, closure, and suction drainage, and are best protected with adjacent tissue or a vascularized muscular flap.[6,57,61,63] At the time of exploration, small esophageal perforations may be difficult to identify. Identification may be aided by injecting air, saline, or methylene blue through a nasogastric tube that is pulled proximally into the pharynx.[59] Simple drainage for small to moderate injuries can be considered.[59,62] These drains should be directed anteriorly or through the contralateral neck to avoid the carotid artery. In patients who have massive injury or delayed diagnosis, primary repair or drainage usually is not possible. In massive injuries in which treatment was delayed, a cutaneous esophagostomy with gastrostomy and jejunostomy for feeding may be necessary.[59] Esophageal injuries are notoriously difficult to heal, and an anastomotic leak is a frequent complication with a fistula to skin or trachea. Only 50% of these fistulas are symptomatic; therefore, patients should have postoperative esophagograms 1 week after repair and before feeding.[64] Other complications include mediastinal abscess, mediastinitis, wound infection, and localized infection, all of which can even lead to carotid artery blowout.[57]

Other Injuries in the Neck

Thyroid injury is uncommon in cervical trauma. The surgical treatment is suture repair when recognized. On rare occasions, for extensive injury, a lobectomy may be indicated.

When nerve injuries are identified during surgical exploration, the treatment is debridement and microvascular primary repair if possible. If the nerve is unable to be repaired or the patient is not stable enough to tolerate this, the nerve end should be tagged for future identification and repair.

REFERENCES

1. Thal ER. Injury to the neck. In: Moore EE, Mattox KL, Feliciano DV, eds. Trauma, ed 2. East Norwalk, CT: Appleton & Lange, 1991:305.
2. Asensio JA, Valenziano CP, Falcone RE, et al. Management of penetrating neck injuries. Surg Clin North Am 1991;71:267.
3. Fogelman MJ, Stewart RD. Penetrating wounds of the neck. Am J Surg 1956;91:581.
4. Menawat SS, Dennis JW, Laneve LM, et al. Are arteriograms necessary in penetrating zone II neck injuries? J Vasc Surg 1992;16:397.
5. Meyer JP, Barrett JA, Schuler JJ, et al. Mandatory vs selective exploration for penetrating neck trauma. Arch Surg 1987;122:592.
6. Martin WS, Gussack GS. Pediatric penetrating head and neck trauma. Laryngoscope 1990;100:1288.
7. Pang D, Pollack I. Spinal cord injury without radiographic abnormality in children: the SCIWORA syndrome. J Trauma 1989;29:654.
8. Pollack IF, Pang D, Sclabassi R. Recurrent spinal cord injury without radiographic abnormalities in children. J Neurosurg 1988;69:177.
9. Hoy GA, Cole WG. The paediatric cervical seat belt syndrome. Br J Surg 1993;24:297.
10. Beal SL, Pottmeyer EW, Spisso JM. Esophageal perforation following external blunt trauma. J Trauma 1988;28:1425.
11. Martin RF, Eldrup-Jorgensen J, Clark DE, et al. Blunt trauma to the carotid arteries. J Vasc Surg 1991;14:789.
12. Davis JW, Holbrook TL, Hoyt DB, et al. Blunt carotid artery dissection: incidence, associated injuries, screening and treatment. J Trauma 1991;30:1514.
13. Hellmann JR, Shott SR, Gootee MJ. Impalement injuries of the palate in children: review of 131 cases. Int J Pediatr Otorhinolaryngol 1993;26:157.
14. Pearl PL. Childhood stroke following intraoral trauma. J Pediatr 1987;110:574.
15. Singer JI. Management strategy for penetrating oropharyngeal injury. Pediatr Emerg Care 1989;5:250.
16. Eggen JT, Jorden RC. Airway management, penetrating neck trauma. J Emerg Med 1993;11:381.
17. Nakayama DK, Venkataraman SG, Orr RA, et al. Emergency airway management in pediatric trauma. Trauma Quarterly 1992;8:22.
18. Cote CJ, Eavey RD, Todres ID, et al. Cricothyroid membrane puncture: oxygenation and ventilation in a dog model using an intravenous catheter. Crit Care Med 1988;16:615.
19. Nakayama DK, Gardner MJ, Rowe MI. Emergency endotracheal intubation in pediatric trauma. Ann Surg 1990;211:218.
20. Handler SD. Trauma to the larynx and upper trachea. Int Anesthesiol Clin 1988;26:39.
21. Mattox KL. Injury to the thoracic great vessels. In: Moore EE, Mattox KL, Feliciano DV, eds. Trauma, ed 2. East Norwalk, CT: Appleton & Lange, 1991:393.
22. Ben-Ami T, Rozenman J, Yahav J, et al. Computed tomography in children with esophageal and airway trauma. J Pediatr Surg 1988;23:919.
23. Hall JR, Reyes HM, Meller JL. Penetrating zone-III neck injuries in children. J Trauma 1991;31:1614.
24. Golueke PJ, Goldstein AS, Sclafani SJA, et al. Routine vs selective exploration of penetrating neck injuries: a randomized prospective study. J Trauma 1984;24:1010.
25. Velmahos GC, Souter I, Degiannis E, et al. Selective surgical management in penetrating neck injuries. Can J Surg 1994;37:487.
26. Shepherd RL, Raffensperger JG, Goldstein R. Pediatric esophageal perforation. J Thorac Cardiovasc Surg 1977;74:261.
27. Richardson JD, Fallat M, Nagaraj HS, et al. Arterial injuries in children. Arch Surg 1981;116:685.
28. Wessel DL, Keane JF, Fellows KE, et al. Fibrinolytic therapy for femoral arterial thrombosis after cardiac catheterization in infants and children. Am J Cardiol 1986;58:347.
29. Burrows PE, Benson LN, Williams WG, et al. Iliofemoral arterial complications of balloon angioplasty for systemic obstructions in infants and children. Circulation 1990;82:1697.
30. Shaker IJ, White JJ, Signer RD, et al. Special problems of vascular injuries in children. J Trauma 1976;16:863.
31. White JJ, Talbert JL, Haller JA. Peripheral arterial injuries in infants and children. Ann Surg 1968;167:757.
32. Bloom JD, Mozersky DJ, Buckley CJ, et al. Defective limb growth as a complication of catheterization of the femoral artery. Surg Gynecol Obstet 1974;138:524.
33. Bynoe RP, Miles WS, Bell RM, et al. Noninvasive diagnosis of vascular trauma by duplex ultrasonography. J Vasc Surg 1991;14:346.
34. Weigelt JA, Thal ER, Snyder WH, et al. Diagnosis of penetrating cervical esophageal injuries. Am J Surg 1987;154:619.
35. Narrod JA, Moore EE. Initial management of penetrating neck wounds: a selective approach. J Emerg Med 1984;2:17.
36. Elerding SC, Manart FD, Moore EE. A reappraisal of penetrating neck injury management. J Trauma 1980;20:695.
37. Atteberry LR, Dennis JW, Menawat SS, et al. Physical examination alone is safe and accurate for evaluation of vascular injuries in penetrating zone II neck trauma. J Am Coll Surg 1994;179:657.
38. Sheely CH, Mattox KL, Reul GJ, et al. Current concepts in the management of penetrating neck trauma. J Trauma 1975;15:895.
39. Jurkovich GJ, Zingarelli W, Wallace J, et al. Penetrating neck trauma: diagnostic studies in the asymptomatic patient. J Trauma 1985;25:819.
40. Rao P, Ivatury RR, Sharma P, et al. Cervical vascular injuries: a trauma center experience. Surgery 1993;114:527.
41. Perry MO. Injuries of the carotid and vertebral arteries. In: Bongard FS, Wilson SE, Perry MO, eds. Vascular injuries in surgical practice. East Norwalk, CT: Appleton & Lange, 1991:95.
42. Smith LL, Catalano RD. Exposure of vascular injuries. In: Bongard FS, Wilson SE, Perry MO, eds. Vascular injuries in surgical practice. East Norwalk, CT: Appleton & Lange, 1991:11.
43. Hughes CW. Arterial repair during Korean War. Ann Surg 1958;147:555.
44. Bradley EL. Management of penetrating carotid injuries: an alternative approach. J Trauma 1973;13:248.
45. Thal ER, Snyder WH, Hayes RJ, et al. Management of carotid artery injuries. Surgery 1974;76:955.
46. Liekweg WG, Greenfield LJ. Management of penetrating carotid arterial injury. Ann Surg 1978;188:587.
47. Richardson JD. Management of carotid artery trauma. Surgery 1988;104:673.
48. Minard G, Kudsk KA, Croce MA, et al. Laryngotracheal trauma. Am Surg 1992;58:181.
49. Meier DE, Brink BE, Fry WJ. Vertebral artery trauma: acute recognition and treatment. Arch Surg 1981;116:236.
50. Golueke P, Sclafani S, Phillips T, et al. Vertebral artery injury: diagnosis and management. J Trauma 1987;27:856.
51. Ko GD, Berbrayer D. Childhood stroke after minor neck trauma: case report. Arch Phys Med Rehabil 1990;71:923.
52. Reid JDS, Weigelt JA. Forty-three cases of vertebral artery trauma. J Trauma 1988;28:1007.

53. Schaefer SD. The acute management of external laryngeal trauma: a 27-year experience. Arch Otolaryngol Head Neck Surg 1992;118:598.
54. Bent JP, Silver JR, Porubsky ES. Acute laryngeal trauma: a review of 77 patients. Otolaryngol Head Neck Surg 1993;109:441.
55. Sheely CH, Mattox KL, Beall AC. Management of acute cervical tracheal trauma. Am J Surg 1974;128:805.
56. Sulek M, Miller RH, Mattox KL. The management of gunshot and stab injuries of the trachea. Archives of Otolaryngology 1983;109:56.
57. Feliciano DV, Bitondo CG, Mattox KL, et al. Combined tracheoesophageal injuries. Am J Surg 1985;150:710.
58. Spenler CW, Benfield JR. Esophageal disruption from blunt and penetrating external trauma. Arch Surg 1976;111:663.
59. Defore WW, Mattox KL, Hansen HA, et al. Surgical management of penetrating injuries of the esophagus. Am J Surg 1977;134:734.
60. Blichert-Toft M. Spontaneous oesophageal rupture. Scand J Thorac Cardiovasc Surg 1971;5:111.
61. Hagan WE. Pharyngoesophageal perforations after blunt trauma to the neck. Otolaryngol Head Neck Surg 1983;91:620.
62. White RK, Morris DM. Diagnosis and management of esophageal perforations. Am Surg 1992;58:112.
63. Flynn AE, Verrier ED, Way LW, et al. Esophageal perforation. Arch Surg 1989;124:1211.
64. Winter RP, Weigelt JA. Cervical esophageal trauma: incidence and cause of esophageal fistulas. Arch Surg 1990;125:849.

Surgery of Infants and Children: Scientific Principles and Practice, edited by
Keith T. Oldham, Paul M. Colombani, and Robert P. Foglia.
Lippincott–Raven Publishers, Philadelphia, © 1997.

CHAPTER **23**

Thoracic Trauma

L. R. Scherer III

EPIDEMIOLOGY

Thoracic injuries are the result of blunt trauma in 75% to
80% of all pediatric trauma admissions. In the urban setting,
most trauma services experience a greater incidence of penetrating trauma. There are several characteristics to the injury patterns in children that are different from those in adults. Although
thoracic injuries are present in less than 10% of injured children,
one quarter of fatal injuries include chest trauma. The mechanisms of injury in children are well recognized, and include
pedestrian–motor vehicular, passenger–motor vehicular, falls,
and penetrating. The largest group of children injured consists
of those with pedestrian injuries (37%), and the second largest
is those involved in passenger–motor vehicle crashes (31%).[1]

In children with isolated thoracic trauma, the mortality rate
is 5%. If the children suffer an abdominal injury in addition to
their thoracic injury, the mortality rate increases to 20%, or if a
head injury concomitantly occurs, the mortality rate approaches
35%. Most of these deaths are caused by the head injury.

In comparing the patterns of injury between adults and children, more adult deaths are delayed and result from pneumonia,
adult respiratory distress syndrome, systemic inflammatory response syndrome, and multisystem organ failure; whereas most
deaths in children occur in the acute phase of injury. Although
rib fractures in adults with blunt trauma to the chest occur in
70% of patients, the incidence is only 30% in children. Conversely, pulmonary contusions in children occur in as much as
50%, versus 30% of adults. Flail chest and aortic tear (rupture)
rarely occur in children. Pneumothorax is common in both
groups, but the incidence of tension is much higher in children.
The pathophysiologic considerations of these injuries are discussed later in this chapter.

ANATOMY AND PHYSIOLOGY OF THE THORAX

The physical factors that create injury are related to the mass
(the victim and the colliding object), the velocity (the victim
and colliding object), the rate of change in the velocity, and
the area or volume of body tissues involved in the transfer of
kinetic energy. The body's response to these physical forces
depends on biomechanical features of human tissue, including
tensile strength, compliance, elasticity, and compressive
strength.

In children, the airway may have less than one half the cross-
sectional diameter of the adult airway. Whereas 1 to 2 mm of
edema in the adult may cause less than 50% narrowing of the
airway, in the child, this may result in greater than 75% narrowing and clinical airway obstruction. The internal diameter of
the trachea in a small child is often less than 6 mm, and therefore
1 to 2 mm of edema within the tracheal lumen may create a
significantly obstructed airway. This is even more problematic
in the smaller airways of each lung. The length of the trachea
in young children is as short as 5 cm in an infant and 10 cm
in the school-age child.

There are certain anatomic and physiologic characteristics to
the thorax that are important to the biomechanics of injury. The
chest wall is very compliant because of the elastic nature of its
tissues. The thoracic cage is mainly cartilage, with minimal
skeletal ossification. The pectoralis, intercostal, shoulder girdle,
and paraspinal musculatures are often not fully developed. This
creates a compliant chest wall that results in minimal damage
to the thoracic cage and the transmission of kinetic energy to
the parenchyma.

In children, there is no prominent point of fixation of the
middle mediastinum to the posterior mediastinum. Therefore,
the heart, thoracic great vessels, and vena cava may freely shift
within the chest cavity. A pneumothorax with a tension component can shift the middle mediastinum significantly to impede
venous return, decrease cardiac output, and lead to shock.

The cardiopulmonary physiology of the child provides significant buffer to the potential devastating consequences of trauma.
The injured child often does not suffer from the comorbidity
of underlying cardiac, renal, or hepatic illnesses. This often
masks the hemodynamic effects of hypovolemia, hypoxia, and
hypercarbia until late into the physiologic decline. The cardiac
output of a child is maintained by a relatively fixed stroke volume, and increases in cardiac output are determined by increases in heart rate. In the hypovolemic child, the cardiac output is similarly maintained by increases in heart rate and
vasoconstriction. Tachycardia is the earliest sign of hypovolemia. Other signs include capillary refill of less than 2 seconds,

thready pulses, and cool extremities. Because the child can maintain hemodynamic stability with blood loss up to 30%, and late and complete decompensation occurs with a blood loss in excess of 40%, the clinician must be aware of the subtle hemodynamic changes of hypovolemia.

PATHOPHYSIOLOGY OF THORACIC INJURIES

Blunt forces are the most common etiology in serious injury to the thorax in children. Ninety percent of injuries result from blunt forces in young children, whereas penetrating trauma is involved in 15% to 20% of injuries in adolescents. The underlying pathophysiology of the injuries is often based on the mechanism of injury. As described earlier, blunt forces may effect direct tissue damage by compression, crush, or shear forces, or by rotational or accelerating–decelerating forces.[1,2]

The upper airway is particularly susceptible to direct forces to the trachea. The larynx is well protected by the mandible, and therefore rarely injured. Injuries to the upper airway may present with airway obstruction, subcutaneous emphysema, or both. The airway obstruction may be caused by tracheal deviation, crush disruption, or mucosal edema. The deviation is most often the result of an associated vascular or intrathoracic injury causing a mass effect or shifting of the mediastinum. A direct blow to the trachea causing varying degrees of disruption results in rapid airway compromise due to mucosal edema and marked subcutaneous emphysema from the positive intraairway pressure during expiration.

Because of its cartilaginous makeup and thin muscular, the chest wall is very compliant in children. Therefore, kinetic energy is not absorbed by the thoracic cage as in the ossified ribs of the adult, and is transmitted to the pulmonary parenchyma and mediastinum. There can be severe pulmonary contusions in the absence of rib fractures, and unexplained hypoxemia without clinical or radiologic evidence of major chest wall injury. Likewise, in the acute setting in the emergency department, almost all chest radiographs are obtained in a supine position. Free fluid may be difficult to see in this position. The parenchymal hemorrhage and edema causing the hypoxemia result from loss of alveolar capillary integrity with immediate intrapulmonary shunting. The presence of a rib fracture increases the risk of life-threatening thoracic injury. The biomechanics of a rib fracture depend on the direct or indirect nature of transmission of the kinetic energy. Direct blows to the chest result in the inward displacement of the rib and a fracture on the inner surface of the rib. The more global forces of a crush injury bow the ribs outward either laterally or posteriorly, resulting in a fracture on the outer surface. Likewise, the direct forces from squeezing may result in a series of inner fractures. Because of the significant kinetic energy necessary to cause rib fractures, the resultant head and thoracic injuries are critical and the risk of death is much higher. In one study, rib fractures were present in 25% of trauma-related deaths, and 42% of children with rib fractures died. The two most frequent mechanisms of injury were child abuse and motor vehicle crash.[1]

In the adult, if several rib fractures are noted, the examiner has a high index of suspicion for a lung parenchymal injury such as a pulmonary contusion. The same high index of suspicion would hold for an aortic injury if there were a first rib fracture. Unfortunately, if no fractures are seen because of the relative compliance of the child's chest, the examiner may not be as attuned to the possibility of an intrathoracic injury.

Biomechanically, traumatic hemothorax or pneumothorax from blunt forces to the chest can result from two different mechanisms. Although infrequent in children, pulmonary parenchyma penetration from a fractured rib is well recognized as a cause of hemothorax and pneumothorax. In children, pneumothorax occurs more commonly when external compression produces a sudden, marked increase in the internal pressure within the lung, resulting in rupture of distal bronchioles and leakage of air from the visceral pleura.[3] When a child inspires and closes the glottis, trapping air within the lung, pneumothorax results.

Another injury related to the mobility of the mediastinum is a tear of the tracheobronchial tree. Partial or complete disruption is caused either by shear forces that occur at relatively fixed points, such as the carina or segmental branches, or by severe crush injuries resulting in high intrabronchial pressures with a closed glottis.[3] Another mechanism involves the crush or impact that decreases the anteroposterior diameter of the chest, displacing and distracting the lung laterally from the main tracheobronchial structures.

Injury to the heart or great vessels requires traumatic events at high velocity. The typical mechanism of injury from blunt trauma involves rapid acceleration or deceleration in a motor vehicle crash as a passenger or pedestrian, or a fall from a great height. Because of the highly mobile mediastinum, aortic tearing or rupture is rare in children, particularly in those younger than 10 years of age.[4] The tear results from the relatively fixed portion of the aorta at the ligamentum arteriosum shearing from the more mobile proximal aorta. Survival (less than 25% from the scene) depends on the rupture being contained within the posterior mediastinum. Equally rare, cardiac rupture or papillary muscle tears are caused by rapid changes in speed or severe crush injury.[5] Cardiac rupture most commonly involves the inferior or superior vena cava and the right atrium in deceleration injuries, and the right atrium when compressed during diastole. Papillary muscle disruption is thought to occur by the same mechanism. There is evidence that valvular insufficiency may be either acute or delayed after a traumatic injury.[1]

IDENTIFICATION AND INITIAL MANAGEMENT OF INJURIES IN THE AGONAL PATIENT

Agonal patients must have some sign of life (spontaneous respiration, response to stimuli, cardiac activity, or palpable pulse) during the prehospital resuscitation if there is to be any hope of salvaging them. In this situation, the physician or surgeon must continue to follow the essentials of the primary survey (see Chap. 19) before identifying injuries. The approach to chest injuries in the agonal patient depends on the mechanism of injury. Penetrating injuries to the chest carry a better chance of survival than blunt ones, but only with signs of life. The next step after the primary survey in the agonal patient with penetrating injuries is a resuscitative left anterolateral thoracotomy, even with right-sided injuries.[2] The importance of this procedure lies in the immediate resuscitation of the heart, resolution of a tension pneumothor or pericardial tamponade, and allows for open cardiac massage, and cross-clamping of the descending aorta. Left hilar injuries, parenchymal hemorrhage, and air leaks can be controlled by clamping across the hilum of the lung. Cardiac wounds can be controlled by the surgeon's finger. Injuries involving the right chest can also be controlled after the resuscitative thoracotomy by extending the anterior thoracotomy across the sternum into the right chest. Once the child has been resuscitated and hemorrhage controlled, definitive repair can occur in the superior environment of the operating room. Children suffering blunt injuries who present to the emergency department without signs of life have most often undergone primary respiratory and secondary cardiac failure. Despite heroic efforts at emergent resuscitative thoracotomy, the survival rate is nil after this anoxic injury. Therefore, in blunt injury, the resuscitative thoracotomy is effective only in children who present to the emergency department with signs of life.[1,2,4,5] Other resuscitative maneuvers during thoracotomy are no different after a penetrating injury other than the assessment and treatment of extrathoracic exsanguinating hemorrhage after control of the descending thoracic aorta.

IDENTIFICATION AND INITIAL MANAGEMENT OF INJURIES IN THE UNSTABLE PATIENT

The unstable patient is categorized as having positive vital signs, but an abnormal ventilatory pattern, poor skin perfusion, tachycardia, hypotension, altered sensorium, or decreased urinary output. This patient requires immediate stabilization of the airway and immediate venous access. In evaluating the patient for life-threatening thoracic injury, the surgeon must determine if the derangement results from ventilatory or cardiac failure. Injuries leading to ventilatory instability include tracheal injury, disruption of the tracheobronchial tree, open pneumothorax, and flail chest. These injuries are recognized by subcutaneous emphysema, tracheal deviation, chest wall crepitus, and unilateral or bilateral impairment of ventilation. Flail chest often presents with paradoxic chest wall motion with inspiration. Correction of ventilatory instability begins with establishment of a secure airway and positive pressure ventilation. In the presence of a tracheal injury, an emergency surgical airway may be necessary if endotracheal intubation is unsuccessful. Disruption of a major bronchial segment presents initially with inadequate ventilation, often requiring endotracheal intubation and positive-pressure ventilation. A simple pneumothorax is now converted into a tension pneumothorax.[3] Immediate decompression of the affected thorax is required by catheter in the second intercostal space in the midclavicular line. This is followed by tube thoracostomy along the anterior axillary line at the fourth to sixth intercostal space. With a significant bronchial injury, there is a persistent air leak from a tube thoracostomy, and a collapsed segment or lobe appears on chest radiography.

Cardiac or pulmonary failure, or both, is seen in tension pneumothorax, hemothorax, and pericardial tamponade. The pathophysiology of each of these injuries is diminished venous return leading to inadequate end-diastolic volume. Clinically, this is apparent with hypotension, distended neck veins, and absent breath sounds (hemothorax–pneumothorax) or diminished heart tones and paradoxic pulses (pericardial tamponade).[2,5]

The clinical features of hemothorax–pneumothorax include decreased breath sounds, tracheal deviation and hyperresonance (pneumothorax) or dullness (hemothorax) to percussion.[1,4] Emergent care of these injuries requires placement of a large-diameter anterolateral tube thoracostomy for decompression. In children, the size of the chest tube should equal the size of the child's thumb. If the patient remains hemodynamically unstable with distended neck veins (elevated central venous pressure) after placement of tube thoracostomy, the surgeon or emergency physician must suspect pericardial tamponade. If the patient is unstable, this condition requires needle pericardiocentesis. To evacuate the pericardial sac, a needle is inserted in the left xyphocostal angle and directed posteriorly at a 45-degree angle toward the ipsilateral scapula. When the needle enters the pericardial space, there will be return of nonclotting blood and there should be hemodynamic improvement in the child. This can occur with a return of as little as 5 mL of blood in infants. This procedure only temporizes an unstable situation, and the patient still requires pericardial exploration.

Unstable Pediatric Patient With Tracheobronchial Injury

Instability of the airway in this situation manifests signs and symptoms of persistent bleeding into the airway, tension pneumothorax, or massive air leak causing hypoxia or hypercarbia, requiring emergent control of the tracheobronchial tree.[3] This can be done immediately by directing the endotracheal tube into the right or left main stem bronchus. Operative control of the distal airway is the next step. The patient is initially positioned supine and the neck, torso, and upper thighs are prepared and draped freely. An anterolateral thoracotomy on the suspected side of injury should provide exposure and control of injured parenchyma by manual compression. If this is unsuccessful, the inferior pulmonary ligament can be divided and a vascular clamp placed across the hilum. After control is obtained, the tracheobronchial injury should be definitively repaired (see Treatment of Specific Injuries).

Unstable Pediatric Patient With Uncontrolled Hemorrhage Into the Thoracic Cavity

Unstable patients with a blood-filled chest cavity on radiography may require an emergent thoracotomy. The criteria for uncontrolled or persistent bleeding remain variable, but for children a conservative recommendation includes initial recovery of greater than 15 mL/kg of blood out of the chest tube, greater than 2 to 3 mL/kg/hour collected for 3 consecutive hours, or inability to evacuate the hemothorax after placement of a chest tube.[1,2] The approach to uncontrolled hemorrhage also depends on the mechanism of injury. Persistent bleeding because of blunt injury is likely from an intercostal artery, and less frequently because of a hilar vascular injury. Because of the low pressure of the pulmonary vasculature, bleeding from the pulmonary parenchyma rarely causes hemorrhage requiring operative intervention.

Penetrating injuries to the thorax with uncontrolled bleeding also require a systematic approach, depending on the site of injury.[2] The indications for exploration of the chest are similar to those in blunt injuries; in addition, injuries that cross the mediastinum should also be explored. Injuries involving blood in the right thorax may require a right anterolateral thoracotomy, and if the injury is below the nipple, exploration of the abdomen should precede thoracotomy. A potential cervicomediastinal vascular injury involving blood in the right chest requires exposure through a median sternotomy. The incision may be extended into the right neck for exposure of the subclavian and carotid arteries. Injuries involving the left chest may be approached through an anterior left thoracotomy, and, if necessary, the left neck and thoracic outlet can be approached by the addition of the trapdoor incision. Each of these approaches allows for exposure and control of the origin of the great vessels, and, by dividing the pulmonary ligament, the pulmonary hilum can be controlled with a vascular clamp.

IDENTIFICATION AND INITIAL MANAGEMENT OF INJURIES IN THE STABLE PATIENT

The patient with stable vital signs (pulse rate, urine output, blood pressure, ventilation, and oxygenation) usually can undergo a more thorough evaluation of potential thoracic injuries before decisions about definitive treatment are undertaken. During the initial assessment, the surgeon should evaluate the patient as if they were potentially unstable, and perform maneuvers to ensure an airway, ventilation, and oxygenation, control external bleeding, and provide intravenous access. Anteroposterior chest and lateral cervical spine radiographs should be obtained if the patient has any symptoms or signs of injury to the head, neck, or torso. The remainder of the work-up depends on the mechanism of injury and the structures of the chest that may be at risk for injury.

The evaluation of penetrating injury requires a diagnostic approach to identify injuries in proximity to the penetrating wounds.[2] Assessment of these injuries begins with estimation of the path of the wounding agent and whether there is an exit wound. The surgeon may be able to determine the path of the missile by locating the bullet by plain radiography or fluoroscopy. Bullets normally travel in a straight line, but the apparent trajectory noted by examining the patient may be quite different. Also, the path of the missile may have been altered by varying tissue density or bone deflection. Stab wounds to the base of the neck that penetrate the platysma must be considered as deep and potentially injurious to the great vessels, esophagus, or trachea. A stab wound with a hemothorax–pneumothorax is by definition a deep wound, and the surgeon must be aware that a parasternal wound may puncture the heart without entering the pleural cavity. An entrance wound below the nipple line offers the potential for an injury below the diaphragm.

The presence of a penetrating wound to the base of the neck or upper parasternal area with a history of pulsatile, bright red bleeding, expanding hematoma, a bruit, blood in the pleural cavity or a widened mediastinum, a pulse deficit, lateralizing neurologic deficit, or unequal blood pressures between any extremities suggests a high risk of vascular injury and therefore sudden exsanguination. The patient should be taken immediately to the operating room, where operative exposure provides

the diagnosis. For injuries involving the parasternal area and the base of the right neck to the medial aspect of the left neck, a median sternotomy provides excellent exposure of the proximal great vessels, except the left subclavian artery. Injuries to the base of the left neck are best approached thorough a left anterolateral thoracotomy. Stable patients with wounds at risk for great vessel injury but without the aforementioned signs should undergo immediate arteriography; an exploratory thoracotomy can be prevented with a negative study. In patients with parasternal penetrating wounds, injuries to structures within the pericardium often present with unstable vital signs. The stable patient may have distended neck veins, muffled heart tones, or paradoxic blood pressure. Further evaluation may include continuous intraarterial and central venous pressure monitoring, echocardiography, or pericardiocentesis.

Penetrating injury to the tracheobronchial tree is unusual and is evident when present[3]; the child has subcutaneous emphysema or an air leak. The presence of a persistent air leak suggests a major airway injury, and rigid or flexible tracheobronchoscopy should be performed. Penetrating wounds to the esophagus are most commonly iatrogenic but still occur in the conventional trauma setting as well. These often presenting with dysphagia, hematemesis, widened mediastinum, pleural effusion, or signs of systemic inflammation. If the patient is going to the operating room for other procedures, rigid or flexible esophagoscopy can be performed. Otherwise, a water-soluble contrast esophagogram should be performed. If negative, this should be followed by a barium contrast study. Endoscopy and radiography are equally sensitive, and in the high-risk patient the studies are additive.

The evaluation of blunt injuries of the thorax in a stable patient requires an approach similar to that in penetrating injuries, but the range of injuries is much greater.[1,3–5] In children younger than 10 years of age, a transected thoracic aorta is extremely rare and is most often seen in pedestrian–automobile crashes or side impact automobile crashes. Clinical signs include a widened mediastinum on anteroposterior chest radiography, blood in the left pleural space, apical capping, fractures of the upper ribs, loss of the aortic knob, right deviation of the nasogastric tube or trachea, and depression of the left main bronchus. The optimal imaging study is thoracic aortography. Other modalities for screening and, with experience, diagnosis, include transesophageal echocardiography, magnetic resonance imaging, and spiral computed tomographic angiography. Blunt injuries to the structures within the pericardium are rare and usually fatal because they often involve avulsion of the atrium from the vena cava. In children who survive the transport to the emergency department, the clinical presentation and diagnostic work-up for pericardial tamponade is similar to that for penetrating injuries. Tracheobronchial disruption is common in children exposed to high-velocity blunt forces to the chest. The clinical features of extrapleural air and persistent air leak are similar to those seen in penetrating trauma.

IATROGENIC THORACIC INJURIES

Hospital-acquired thoracic injuries also occur in neonates and children. In large part, these injuries are related to the increasingly small patients who are treated and the various mechanical devices and technology available in their treatment. Parenchymal lung injury can be caused by aggressive chest tube placement, especially with the use of a trocar. This can be seen in particular in the neonate or child in whom a loculated pneumothorax is present and a portion of the lung is tethered to the parietal pleura. If the lung does not drop away from the chest wall when the parietal pleura is opened, as the chest tube is placed it can tear the lung adherent to the chest wall. Mechanical ventilation with high pressure can cause barotrauma with resultant pneumothorax or pulmonary interstitial emphysema. The technique of endotracheal suctioning can lead to a bronchial tear and pneumothorax. If the suction catheter is passed too far distal beyond the carina, a perforation may result. The typical clinical scenario is an intubated neonate who was otherwise well, was suctioned, had blood noted on the tracheal suction catheter, and then had a drop in arterial oxygen saturation. Finally, esophageal perforation occurs in approximately 1% of patients after esophageal dilation or endoscopy and biopsy.

TREATMENT OF SPECIFIC INJURIES

Intrapericardial Injuries

Blunt or penetrating injuries to the heart or intrapericardial vessels are rare in children, but when these injuries do occur they are hemodynamically unstable. Usually, the approach to cardiac injuries begins with a left anterolateral thoracotomy, which can be extended into a transsternal anterolateral thoracotomy or a posterolateral thoracotomy depending on the location of the injuries.[1,2,5] Penetrating cardiac injuries are best repaired by direct suturing using a horizontal mattress stitch and Teflon pledgets for ventricular wounds. Before repair, the wounds can be controlled by the surgeon's finger, Foley catheter, or a partial occlusion (Satinsky) clamp. Intrapericardial great vessel injury is more difficult to repair. Often, control of the inferior and superior venae cavae just before they enter the right atrium provides a clear enough field to visualize and repair the laceration or rupture. Unfortunately, only 25% of these patients survive, if they reach the hospital with signs of life. After surgery, penetrating injuries to the heart require echocardiographic evaluation of potential intracardiac injuries.

In blunt trauma, myocardial contusion is more common, and it should be suspected in any patient suffering blunt thoracic trauma in whom a dysrhythmia develops in the emergency department. Mechanical dysfunction is confirmed by echocardiography and serum enzyme profiles similar to myocardial infarction patients may be seen. Most of these injuries are of no hemodynamic consequence, and only patients with dysrhythmias require prolonged continuous monitoring. Fluid resuscitation should be continued because the child is often in a hyperdynamic state due to associated injuries, and cardiac output responds appropriately with the administration of fluids.

Pleural Injuries

Because of the significantly elastic and compliant nature of the chest wall, the visceral pleura is more often involved in the injuries causing pneumothoraces or hemothoraces. A tension pneumothorax creates hemodynamic instability because of shifting of the mediastinum and decreased venous return. This is a true emergency that requires immediate decompression, followed by a tube thoracostomy. The open pneumothorax of a sucking chest wound in the spontaneously breathing child can cause severe respiratory compromise. This is particularly true if the wound is larger than the cross-sectional area of the trachea, as the wound provides a low resistance conduit that then bypasses tracheal ventilation. Treatment requires the reestablishment of the integrity of the chest wall with an occlusive dressing and tube thoracostomy.

The presence of blood in the thoracic cavity in children may be innocuous or fatal depending on the source.[1-3] Major vascular or hilar injuries are often fatal. The more common pulmonary laceration is easily treated with complete evacuation of blood and reexpansion of the lung with effective tamponade of the low-pressure pulmonary vasculature. Because rib fractures are uncommon in children, intercostal or internal mammary artery laceration causing hemorrhage is uncommon. Initial hemorrhage of more than 15 mL/kg of blood out of the chest tube or continued hemorrhage of more than 2 mL/kg/hour for 3 consecutive hours requires thoracotomy to control hemorrhage of either the chest wall, pulmonary parenchyma, or hilum. Operative control of pulmonary lacerations often requires only suture or staple ligation, whereas major injuries with hemorrhage may require lobectomy or pneumonectomy.

Tracheobronchial Disruption

The clinical presentation of this injury includes the signs and symptoms of tension pneumothorax and significant subcutaneous emphysema.[1,3] There is a continued air leak after tube thoracostomy. With a significant tracheobronchial disruption, there may be lobar or whole lung atelectasis because of inability to ventilate through the disrupted bronchus. Rigid or flexible bronchoscopy is diagnostic, but often underestimates the damage. The injury most often involves the membranous portion of the trachea or bronchus just beyond the carina or the lobar branches. With a tracheobronchial injury and continued air leak and atelectasis, prompt operative repair yields the best results.

If ventilation is compromised because of a massive air leak, control of the leak can be obtained through a double-lumen tube in older children or selective intubation of the uninvolved lung. A median sternotomy should be used if the injury is to the anterior or lateral trachea; a right posterolateral thoracotomy should be used for injuries to the right lateral or posterior trachea or right lung bronchi; and a left posterolateral thoracotomy should be used for left lung bronchial injuries. Lacerations or disruptions to the trachea or major bronchi can be repaired primarily with absorbable suture. The repair is best secured by buttressing with a vascularized segment of a pleural flap. Major injuries to the pulmonary parenchyma most often are treated by suture approximation or as a last-resort, resection of damaged parenchyma. Long-term follow-up is required for patients successfully repaired because of the risk of stenosis in this type of injury.

Pulmonary Contusion

Pulmonary contusion is the most frequent thoracic injury seen in children, and it is often evident as a localized infiltrate on chest radiography or on computed tomography scans during evaluation of blunt abdominal trauma.[1,2] Mild contusions require little more than observation, pain control, pulmonary toilet, and early mobilization.

Because the intraparenchymal hemorrhage, edema, and alveolar fluid result in intrapulmonary shunts and a decrease in pulmonary compliance, more severe contusions may require more aggressive pulmonary support, including mechanical ventilation and positive end-expiratory pressure. The associated injuries in these patients require the same degree of cardiovascular resuscitation to maintain the euvolemic state as in those without contusion. Hypovolemia places the patient at risk for multiorgan system failure including the lung potentiated by hypoperfusion. Severe injuries may require further monitoring support with a pulmonary artery catheter to monitor fluid management, cardiac output, and inotropic support. If severe injury results in marked impairment in oxygenation or ventilation, therapy may have to advance to simultaneous independent lung ventilation for unilateral pulmonary contusion, or extracorporeal life support. Prophylactic antibiotics are not indicated for these injuries, but secondary pneumonitis is a significant risk; therefore the surgeon must be aware of this complication and vigilance is necessary.

Flail Chest

This is an infrequent but severe injury in children.[1] Associated injuries may include hemothorax–pneumothorax and pulmonary contusion. If there is instability of the chest wall, positive-pressure ventilation is required for pulmonary support and stabilization of the chest wall. In general, therapy is directed to the underlying lung injury rather than the chest wall. The use of regional and systemic analgesia can provide benefit to those patients with a stable chest wall but ineffective ventilation because of pain and splinting.

Traumatic Asphyxia

Subconjunctival hemorrhage, cyanosis, head and thoracic petechiae, and pulmonary and central nervous system dysfunction comprise the essential features of traumatic asphyxia. The pathophysiology represents central venous hypertension secondary to crush or restrictive forces on the thoracic cavity with closure of the glottis or tracheal obstruction; the clinical circumstance is most often seen in children whose chest is run over by a car or truck. This results in the development of venous hypertension transmitted from the right atrium into the valveless superior vena cava and the head and neck. The apparent vascular cutaneous signs are noted in other tissues, including the brain, but do not affect outcome.

The clinical sequelae of this injury depend on the severity of hypoxemia. Mortality is rare and is seen only in children with severe injury and, most often, immediate death. Children may require early ventilatory support, and the surgeon should be aware of associated injuries (blunt hepatic and pulmonary contusion), but most survive. The outlook for return of normal cognitive function in the pediatric population is excellent.

Transection of the Thoracic Aorta and Injury to the Great Vessels

This is a rare lesion in children and is due to a rapid deceleration.[1,4] Often this injury causes immediate exsangvination. If the aorta remains intact, these patients are often relatively hemodynamically stable when seen in the emergency department, but often have other associated injuries. The clinical features and the work-up of these patients have been discussed earlier (see Identification and Initial Management of Injuries in the Stable Patient).

After documentation of aortic transection by aortography, this injury must be repaired promptly. Life-threatening abdominal injuries must be ruled out or repaired before approaching the contained transected aorta. The repair of the transected descending aorta is through a posterolateral thoracotomy, and there is still controversy regarding the use of partial bypass to prevent the risk of paraplegia from spinal cord ischemia. The transection may be repaired primarily if there is little tissue loss, but circumferential defects often require significant dissection of collateral vessels, and the repair is under tension. The use of synthetic bypass enables a superior repair in these instances.

Blunt or penetrating injuries to other great vessels within the chest are uncommon except in the urban environment. The identification, work-up, and emergent care of these injuries were discussed previously. Many of these injuries can be repaired primarily; with extensive tissue loss, autologous bypass graft reconstruction may be necessary.

Esophageal Perforation

The diagnosis of an esophageal injury is made before surgery by esophagography or esophagoscopy, or in the operating room during exploration for other injuries. The contained mediastinal injury without systemic signs may be treated with a nasogastric tube, suspension of oral feedings, and broad-spectrum antibiotics. Injuries that present with hydrothorax–pneumothorax, leakage into the pleural cavity, mediastinitis (systemic signs of inflammation), or subcutaneous emphysema require definitive operative repair.

Upper and mid-esophageal injuries are approached through a right posterolateral thoracotomy, and lower esophageal wounds require a left posterolateral thoracotomy. Primary repair is performed, but requires viable tissue with debridement of all devitalized tissue. Many surgeons buttress the repair with a vascularized flap of pleura or intercostal muscle. The area is widely drained with mediastinal and pleural drains. A gastrostomy tube is used to decompress the stomach and prevent gastroesophageal reflux. Total parenteral nutrition is a useful adjunct in those patients who should be NPO for at least 1 week. Rarely in children is it necessary to divert these wounds proximally with a cervical esophagostomy. In selected high risk cases, use of total esophageal isolation be necessary.

REFERENCES

1. Rielly JP, Brandt ML, Mattox KL, et al. Thoracic trauma in children. J Trauma 1992;34:329.
2. Peterson RJ, Tiwary AD, Kissoon N, et al. Pediatric penetrating thoracic trauma: a five-year experience. Pediatr Emerg Care 1994;10:129.
3. Hancock BJ, Wiseman NE. Tracheobronchial injuries in children. J Pediatr Surg 1991;26:1316.
4. Eddy AC, Rusch VW, Flinger CL, et al. The epidemiology of traumatic rupture of the thoracic aorta in children: a 13-year review. J Trauma 1990;30:989.
5. Langer JC, Winthrop AL, Wesson DE, et al. Diagnosis and incidence of cardiac injury in children with blunt thoracic trauma. J Pediatr Surg 1989;24:1091.
6. Bromberg BI, Mazziotti MV, Canter CE, et al. Recognition and management of nonpenetrating cardiac trauma in children. J Pediatrics 1996; 128:536–541.

Surgery of Infants and Children: Scientific Principles and Practice, edited by Keith T. Oldham, Paul M. Colombani, and Robert P. Foglia. Lippincott–Raven Publishers, Philadelphia, © 1997.

CHAPTER 24

Abdominal Trauma

Robert P. Foglia and Andrea L. Winthrop

Approximately half of all deaths in children are trauma related. Isolated abdominal trauma is present in approximately 5% of all children admitted to the hospital after injury. Abdominal injuries account for 10% to 15% of all trauma-related deaths in children. In a prospective study of over 25,000 children admitted to pediatric trauma centers, abdominal injuries accounted for 8% of admissions.[1] Approximately half of all deaths in children are trauma related. The specific mechanism and type of injury and the unique physiologic responses of the child are integral to the successful evaluation and treatment of this patient. In decreasing frequency, abdominal injuries are caused by motor vehicle accidents, falls, recreational and sports-related injuries, and assault and child abuse. In the area of motor vehicle accidents, the child is a pedestrian in 80% of the accidents, and a passenger in the remaining 20%. Specific injury patterns are seen that depend on the activity at the time of injury. Since the early 1970s, an increasing body of information regarding injury response to specific organ injuries has led to changes in management. This has resulted in the greater use of nonoperative treatments for many abdominal injuries. Since the mid-1980s, urban violence has made gunshot and stabbing wounds more common than they had been previously. The management of these children closely follows the algorithm used in the management of adults with penetrating trauma. In principle, violation of the peritoneal cavity due to a gunshot wound or stabbing in a child warrants laparotomy. Notwithstanding the aforementioned societal changes, 90% of abdominal injuries in children are blunt in nature.

ANATOMY

The trauma evaluation can be aided by dividing the abdomen into four zones, the intrathoracic abdomen, the true abdomen, the pelvic abdomen, and the retroperitoneum (Fig. 24-1). Although the true abdomen can be relatively easily assessed, the other three areas are more difficult to evaluate on physical examination. There are several anatomic considerations that make the infant and child different from the adult patient. The bony thorax is much more compliant in children. Because of this, force directed to the inferior thorax can be more directly transmitted to the underlying abdominal viscera. In addition, in in-

fants and toddlers, the bladder is not protected by the bony pelvis and is more a "true abdominal" organ.

The intrathoracic abdomen contains the diaphragm, liver, spleen, and stomach. Because the diaphragm can rise to the level of the fourth thoracic vertebra, any penetrating injury below the nipple line should be considered potentially to cause an abdominal injury. The true abdomen contains portions of the small and large intestine and the bladder, when distended. Physical examination is often more straightforward with an injury to these organs, especially if perforation or peritonitis is present. The pelvic abdomen is defined by those structures within the bony pelvis. This includes part of the small intestine, the distal sigmoid colon, rectum, bladder, urethra, and in women the ovaries, fallopian tubes, and uterus. These structures are in part intraperitoneal and part extraperitoneal. Trauma in this area can be the result either of penetrating or blunt causes. Because of containment in the pelvis, diagnosis may be difficult. A high index of suspicion and the use of appropriate imaging studies are helpful. The retroperitoneal area contains the great vessels, kidneys, ureters, pancreas, and the second and third portions of the duodenum. Because of containment in the retroperitoneum, injury in this area may not manifest itself with the typical signs of peritonitis. Likewise, a peritoneal lavage may be of little use. In a similar manner, if the retroperitoneal duodenum is perforated, pneumoperitoneum may not be seen on plain radiographs or computed tomography (CT) scan. Findings may be more subtle, and the appearance of small bubbles or froth in the area of the retroperitoneal duodenum may be the only suggestion of a perforation. Because of the proximity of a number of retroperitoneal structures, there may be concomitant injury to several organs.

BIOMECHANICS OF INJURY

Kinetic energy in blunt trauma is transmitted either in the form of a direct compressive force or a shearing force caused by rapid deceleration. Examples of the former include direct trauma in a motor vehicle accident to the flank or lower chest wall causing a liver or splenic injury. This can often be a burst or stellate injury. Another example would be a pancreatic or duodenal injury caused by a bicycle handle bar "spearing" the

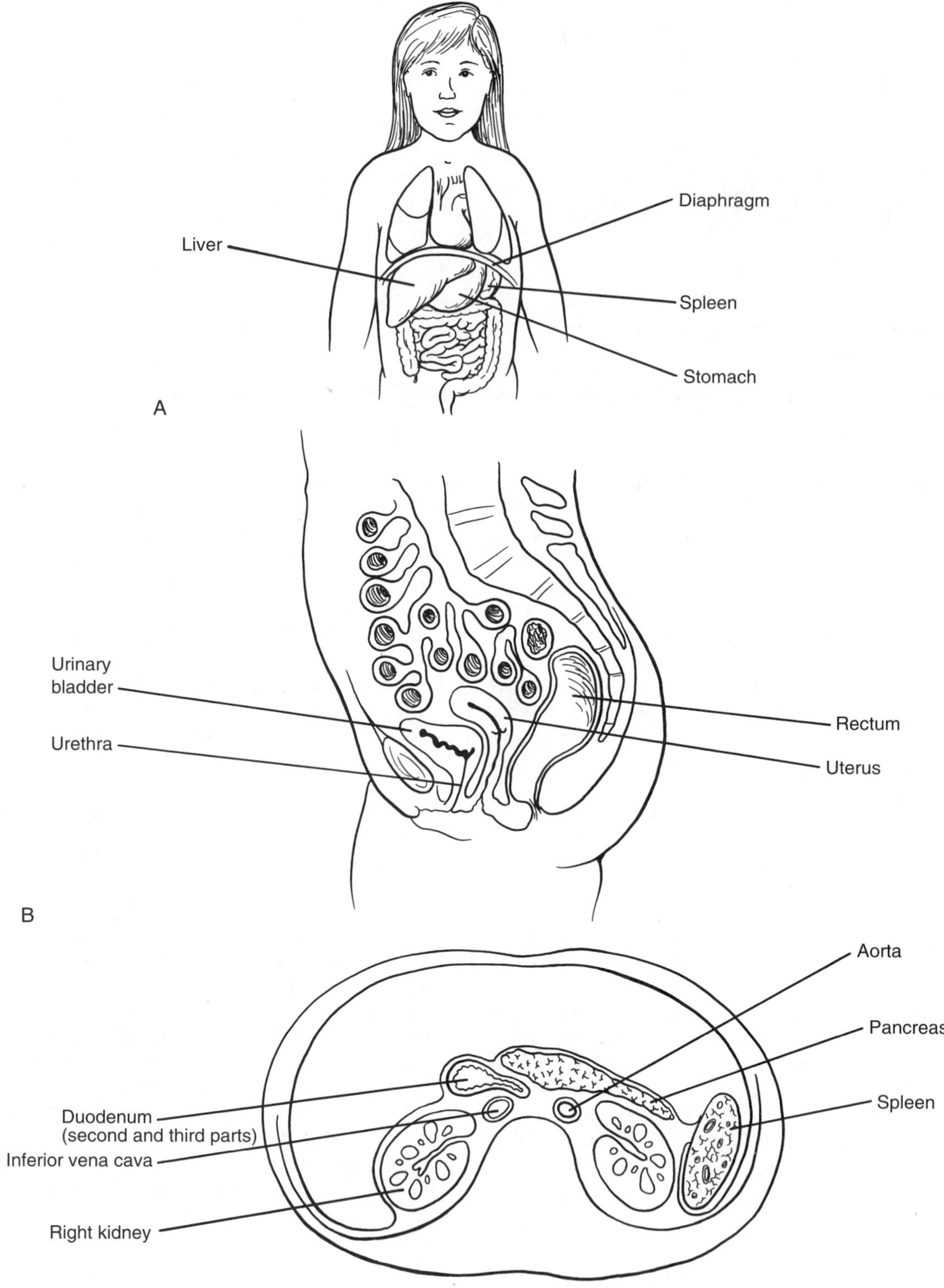

FIG. 24-1. Separation of the abdomen into three of the four anatomic zones—thoracic abdomen (*A*); pelvic abdomen (*B*); and retroperitoneal zone (*C*); —and a listing of the organs present in each zone. Small intestine, prostate (in males), and ureter are not illustrated.

mid-epigastrium. Solid organs are more likely to be injured by direct compressive forces than a hollow viscus. The rapid deceleration injury is seen with a fall from a height or with a seat belt-type injury. The inertia of the abdominal organ causes it to continue along a given vector while the bony skeleton has stopped forward movement. An injury to a hollow viscus such as the small intestine results from these types of biomechanical forces. In a seat belt injury, there is often a vertebral fracture and trauma to one or more organs. The mechanism of injury consists of a sudden deceleration with the child held in place by the seat belt, which acts as a fulcrum.[2] On impact, there is the combination of both a shearing force injury plus compression between the seat belt and spine. There can also be a sudden increase in intraluminal pressure, which can cause rupture of a hollow viscus. In a study of children restrained in a car at the time of accident, 45% sustained abdominal wall bruising due to the seat belt. Blunt visceral injuries affected multiple organs, including liver, spleen, bowel, and kidney.[3] The risk of multiple organ injury in blunt trauma is much higher than in the victim of a penetrating injury. With multiple organ systems involved, there can be a synergistic effect with dysfunction in one organ affecting other organ systems. This increases the potential for multiorgan system failure and death.

DIAGNOSIS AND MANAGEMENT

Prehospital treatment focuses on the identification of any life-threatening problems, assessing the obvious injuries, stabilizing the patient, obtaining intravenous (IV) access, obtaining a history of injury, and carrying out rapid transport to the hospital. With regard to the abdomen, direct pressure with a dressing should be applied to any obvious source of bleeding. If eviscerated bowel is present, no attempt should be made to reduce it back into the peritoneal cavity. It should be covered with a moist dressing. Any foreign object penetrating the chest or abdomen should be left in place.

Hospital Evaluation

On arrival, the basic principles of a primary survey are initiated. Efforts are directed at assessing vital physiologic parameters—airway, breathing, and circulation. Initial resuscitative maneuvers are focused on securing a patent airway and adequate ventilation and restoring a satisfactory circulating blood volume. In the unstable patient with abdominal injuries, diagnosis and resuscitation often occur concurrently (Fig. 24-2). Large-bore IV access is obtained at two sites. Generally, central venous access is not a necessity. At least one IV access should be in an upper extremity or the neck so that drainage is into the superior vena cava. In the patient with an abdominal injury, the potential for a retrohepatic caval injury exists. The surgeon must ensure the ability of infused fluids and blood products to reach the heart. Coincident with the initial assessment and beginning secondary survey, someone should attempt to obtain a history regarding the events of the injury. Pertinent information includes if there was a motor vehicle accident, and the patient was a pedestrian, was he or she thrown by the vehicle after being struck? If the patient was a passenger in a motor vehicle accident, was he or she ejected from the car? Was there penetration of the interior of the vehicle, how fast was the vehicle traveling, and was there a loss of consciousness? Was the child unrestrained? If there was a gunshot wound or stab wound, what type of weapon caused the injury (high- versus low-velocity bullet, length of the knife)? The likelihood of preexisting medical problems is low in children, but an attempt should be made to ascertain whether there is any pertinent medical history, including imunization status.

Physical Examination

The goals of the abdominal examination are to identify whether there is an abdominal injury, and if so, whether it requires operative treatment. The two major types of injury that require laparotomy are uncontrolled hemorrhage and a perforated viscus. The presentation of either may be confusing in the child who has sustained a blunt injury. The child may maintain blood pressure despite significant blood loss, and peritonitis may be confused with tenderness due to a muscle wall hematoma or rib or pelvic fracture.

In the victim of blunt trauma, a rapid assessment of the patient who is in shock should first identify if there is any external source of bleeding. If there is none, the trachea and chest are examined. A tension pneumothorax can decrease venous return to the point of causing hypotension. Significant blood loss in the chest could also account for shock. If there is no evidence to support an external source of bleeding (major laceration) or a chest (tension pneumothorax, hemothorax) or cardiac injury, then the abdomen is the most likely source of the problem. If the abdomen is markedly distended, pneumoperitoneum or hemorrhage is possible. Percussion of the abdomen with resultant tympany can identify the former. Massive distention of the abdomen with air can diminish venous return, leading to shock. Abdominal radiographs can confirm the clinical diagnosis. In the emergency circumstance, a needle paracentesis can be life saving. When the abdomen is distended and is dull to percussion, and there is no evidence of cardiogenic or spinal shock, the abdomen is likely the source of hemorrhage. The bleeding may be in the peritoneal cavity itself, or retroperitoneal or pelvis. Differentiation is important because the pelvic injury is often better treated nonsurgically by radiographic means. Likewise, if there is no ongoing bleeding, a retroperitoneal hematoma will tamponade itself and can be well managed nonoperatively. In contrast, if there is ongoing intraperitoneal bleeding, operative intervention more often is required. Significant hemoperitoneum may lead to ecchymosis in the flank or periumbilical region.

If a pelvic fracture occurs significant blood loss is common. On physical examination, there can be blood at the urethral meatus; the pelvis may be asymmetric, and on palpation may be tender and unstable. Blood at the urethral meatus raises suspicion of a urethral injury, and a retrograde urethrogram is obtained. If there is hemodynamic evidence of continued bleeding, and if the pelvis is fractured, two goals should be pursued, the stabilization of the pelvic fracture and control of blood loss. Pediatric antishock trousers are used in selected cases for this purpose; they can immobilize the fractured components of the pelvis, and often this controls bleeding. When these trousers are used, each leg segment should be inflated first, and then the abdominal portion. Conversely, when deflating the unit, the abdomen is completely deflated first. If there is greater than a 5- to 10-mm Hg blood pressure drop while the unit is being deflated, no further deflation occurs until the blood pressure has been stabilized with volume infusion. The use of pediatric antishock trousers may allow a period of stabilization in the emergency unit until definitive treatment can be instituted. Continued bleeding from a pelvic fracture requires embolization, fracture stabilization, or operative control.

Besides abdominal distention, other signs of abdominal trauma include transverse ecchymoses across the abdominal

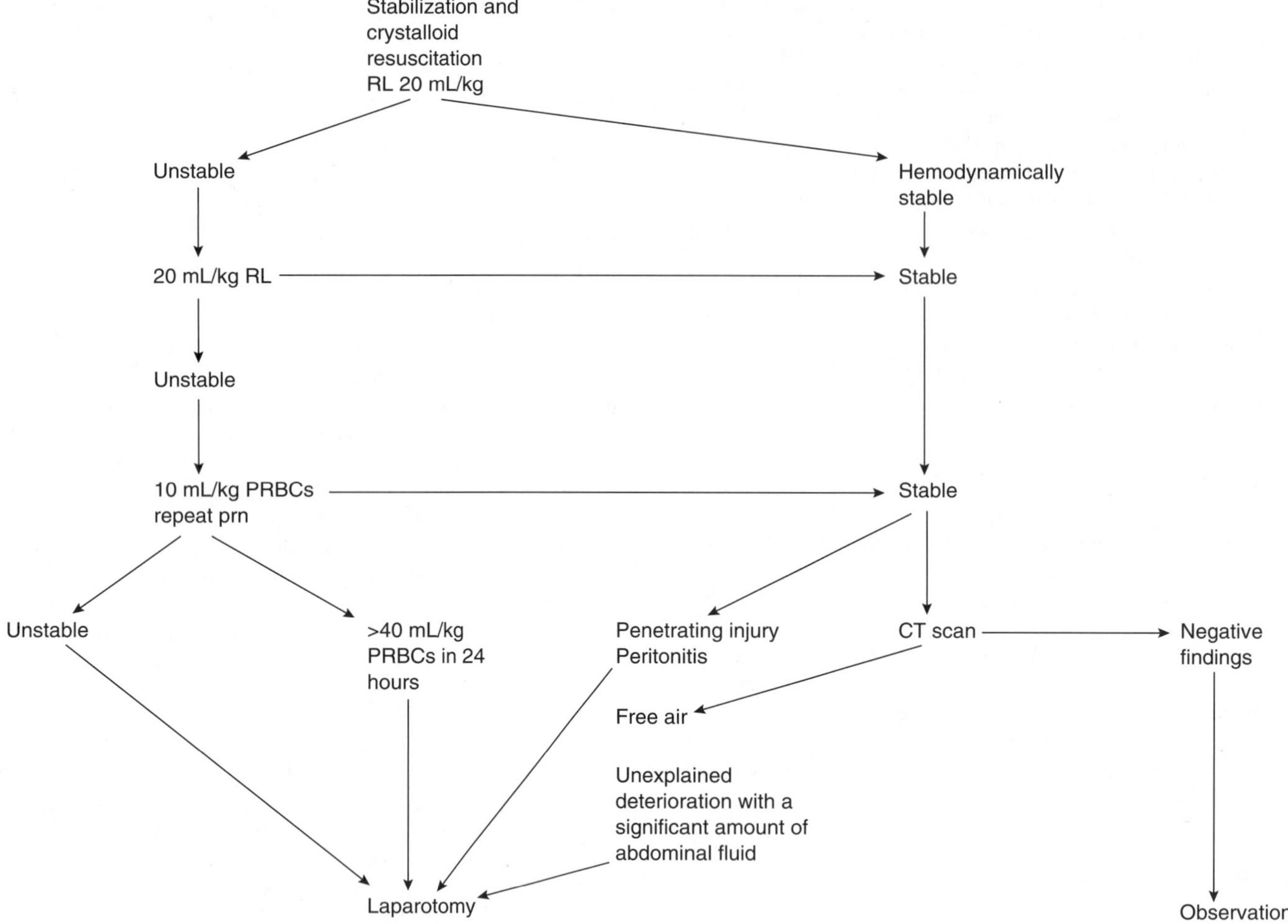

FIG. 24-2. Algorithm for treatment of a patient with abdominal trauma. The patient is initially stabilized and resuscitated with crystalloid consisting of lactated Ringer (RL) solution. The decision tree is based on the patient's hemodynamic status. If the patient is unstable after administration of two 20 mL/kg RL bolus infusions, blood transfusion is performed. If the patient remains unstable after transfusion, laparotomy is indicated. If the child is initially stable or becomes stable after fluid resuscitation, diagnostic imaging studies are undertaken. PRBC, packed red blood cells.

wall in a restrained passenger in a motor vehicle accident, the "seat belt sign." The patient in the emergency unit should be log rolled and examined to ascertain that no back or flank injury is missed. Any sign of penetrating injury should be marked. In the cooperative child, a soft, nontender, nondistended abdomen is a strong negative finding for any significant abdominal trauma. However, the examination of the uncooperative patient may be much more difficult and the abdominal examination may be unreliable. The anxious or frightened child often is crying, which can lead to aerophagia and a marked degree of gastric dilatation. This can cause abdominal distention and also puts the child at increased risk for emesis and aspiration of gastric contents into the tracheobronchial tree. Decompression of the stomach with a nasogastric tube should be routinely carried out in any patient when significant abdominal trauma is suspected. The tube should be placed by a nasal route unless there is a nasal or midface fracture. In those circumstances, an oral route is used to obviate the potential for creating or contributing to the injury.

Laboratory Data

In patients with significant abdominal trauma, an array of blood tests referred to as a "trauma panel" is obtained. This typically includes the following:

- Complete blood count
- Electrolytes
- Blood urea nitrogen and creatinine
- Amylase
- Liver function panel, including serum transaminases
- Coagulation screen
- Type and crossmatch
- Urinalysis

The most significant tests obtained in the patient with suspected abdominal trauma are the hematocrit, serum transaminases, and urinalysis. Serum electrolytes, blood urea nitrogen, creatinine, glucose, white blood cell count, and platelet count are routinely obtained, although they function primarily as baseline values. It is not unusual to see a hematocrit drop because of the liberal use of crystalloid during the resuscitative phase. More important is the correlation of a falling hematocrit with ongoing volume needs in the patient with a suspected abdominal injury. The presence of hematuria should be evaluated in any patient with abdominal trauma.

Threshold values of serum glutamic oxaloacetic transaminase (SGOT) greater than 200 IU and serum glutamic pyruvic transaminase (SGPT) greater than 100 IU provide a useful screen for hepatic trauma.[2] The incidence of hepatic trauma with transaminase levels less than these values is almost nil, whereas there is approximately a 60% likelihood of liver trauma when the serum levels exceed the threshold values. Serum amylase elevation may indicate pancreatic or intestinal injury, although facial trauma can produce hyperamylasemia because of salivary gland injury. Correlation of the amylase elevation with the abdominal examination or persistent elevation strongly suggest a pancreatic injury.

Diagnostic Imaging Studies

All patients with potential abdominal trauma should have an abdominal obstructive series and chest film. If there is evidence for significant abdominal injury, a CT scan of the abdomen should be done urgently, and this is done instead of the abdominal series. Other imaging studies that can give information regarding abdominal injury include an intravenous pyelogram, retrograde urethrogram, abdominal ultrasound examination, radionuclide scan, and arteriography. The plain films can show a pneumoperitoneum, inferior rib or vertebral fractures, loss of psoas shadow, retroperitoneal air, gastric dilatation, air fluid levels, or a marked displacement of viscera by intraperitoneal fluid. Free air is much better seen in either an upright (not usually taken in the trauma setting) or a left lateral decubital film. The chest film can give information regarding abdominal injuries. Examples include a sympathetic pleural effusion with an upper quadrant injury, and rib fractures in association with liver or spleen injuries. The abdominal film can show a pelvic fracture (Fig. 24-3). Pelvic fractures, much like fractures of the orbit, are usually in multiple locations.

CT Scan

The CT scan is the single most useful diagnostic imaging test for blunt abdominal trauma.[4] It is noninvasive and permits detailed evaluation of the inferior chest, abdomen, pelvis, and retroperitoneum. The study is usually carried out with double contrast, both IV and enteral contrast. It gives excellent information regarding the presence of free fluid, solid organ injury, and the viability of organs as noted by perfusion. It also is an excellent way to identify active hemorrhage by means of acute extravasation of contrast material. In addition, a diagnosis of organ hypoperfusion can be made on the basis of the scan.[5] Some think that the CT scan is not as specific for injuries to a hollow viscus; in fact, free air on CT scan may be noted in only one of three children with bowel perforation.[6] The indications for CT scan include the following:

- High-energy mechanism with significant potential for intraabdominal or multisystem injury
- Head injury with altered mental status
- Planned general anesthesia for other injuries (in which case a catastrophic event in the abdomen could go unrecognized)
- Gross hematuria
- Elevated transaminase levels (SGOT above 200 IU and SGPT above 100 IU)
- Evidence suggestive of injury to the liver, spleen, or kidneys
- Equivocal physical examination

Diagnostic Peritoneal Lavage

Diagnostic peritoneal lavage (DPL) is an excellent method to identify if bleeding is present in the peritoneal cavity, and has a sensitivity of greater than 95%. In addition, it is an excellent test to detect a perforated viscus. In the past, the finding of a positive ''tap'' or lavage would mandate laparotomy in a child. However, the liver and spleen account for 75% to 80% of visceral injuries due to blunt trauma and are the source of bleeding in most of these cases. Nonoperative management protocols for these injuries are successful in over 80% to 90% of

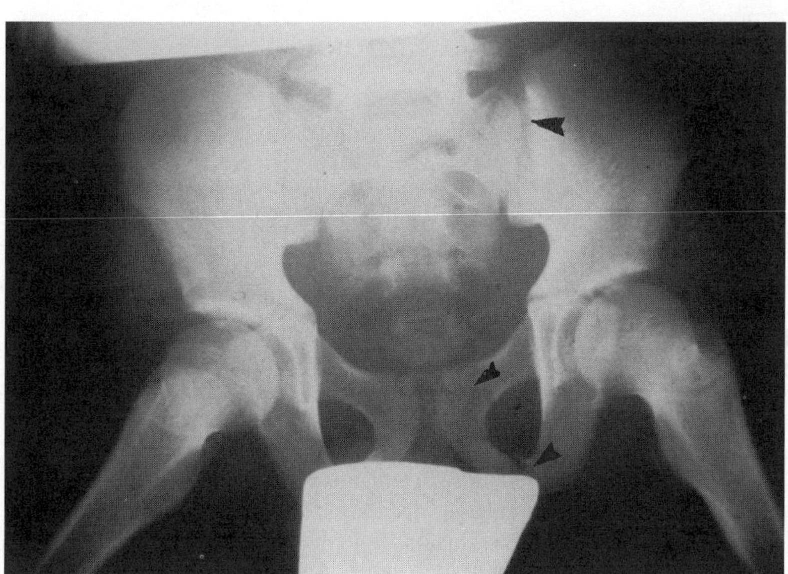

FIG. 24-3. Radiograph demonstrating multiple pelvic fractures (*arrows*) in a child. This injury carries a high risk for significant pelvic bleeding and urethral injury.

cases. Because of these findings, the utility of DPL in pediatric patients has declined. The CT scan can give information regarding a specific organ injury as well as identify the presence of fluid in the peritoneal cavity. DPL does have an advantage in the ability to identify a perforated viscus in some circumstances. The disadvantages for DPL include the lack of specificity when bleeding is identified, the change in abdominal examination after the DPL, and false-positive results. False-positive results can occur in patients with pelvic fractures because of blood dissecting along the anterior inferior abdominal wall. Also, when using a closed technique to place the lavage catheter, there may be placement off the midline, which can cause muscle wall bleeding. DPL is useful in selected cases in which the abdominal physical examination is equivocal regarding peritonitis, and if there is a question as to the character of free intraperitoneal fluid. In patients who require emergency operation for other injuries, DPL is a quick way to rule out major abdominal injury. With the advent of spiral CT scanning, similar information can be obtained in a much shorter period of time than was possible previously. In the true emergency situation, DPL maintains an important role in detecting the presence of hemorrhage or a perforated viscus.

DPL is performed with both the stomach and bladder drained with catheters. An infraumbilical open approach is recommended, with infiltration of the skin and subcutaneous tissue with a local anesthetic. The linea alba is opened under direct vision and a pediatric peritoneal dialysis catheter inserted and directed toward the left lower quadrant. A positive study consists of either 5 mL or more of gross blood return with catheter placement, or a positive lavage. The lavage consists of 15 mL/kg of lactated Ringer solution instilled into the peritoneal cavity and drained by gravity. Positive findings include greater than 100,000 red blood cells/mm^3, greater than 500 white blood cells/mm^3, and the presence of bile, bacteria, or amylase. The incision in the linea alba should be closed to prevent leakage of any fluid and to prevent development of a hernia.

Treatment

An algorithm describing the management of the child with abdominal trauma is outlined in Figure 24-2. Initial attempts at stabilization occur in the field and in the emergency unit. Fluid resuscitation is begun with crystalloid at 20 mL/kg, and concomitant examination is performed. If there is evidence of a penetrating injury that enters the peritoneal cavity, or if peritonitis is diagnosed, laparotomy is indicated. If the patient remains unstable after the initial 20 mL/kg of crystalloid fluid, another 20-mL/kg bolus is given. If the patient becomes hemodynamically stable, a diagnostic work-up is begun to delineate any abdominal trauma. If, after a total of 40 mL/kg of crystalloid, the patient continues to be unstable, packed red blood cell transfusion (10 mL/kg) is started. Indications for laparotomy include ongoing hemodynamic instability, despite blood transfusion and greater than 40 mL/kg packed red cell transfusion over 24 hours. If the patient is stable, serial examinations and appropriate diagnostic imaging studies are obtained. If the child remains stable and the imaging studies do not show injury requiring operative intervention, the patient is transferred to the intensive care unit (ICU) or ward for observation. If the CT scan shows free air, active hemorrhage, or a significant amount of intraabdominal fluid associated with unexplained patient deterioration, then laparotomy is indicated.

Indications for laparotomy based on clinical examination and CT scan include peritonitis, ongoing bleeding, or clinical deterioration with abdominal distention. Appropriate IV access must be ensured, rapid attempts made to correct obvious blood chemistry abnormalities, and broad-spectrum antibiotic coverage begun. Operative findings and culture results should dictate postoperative coverage.

The procedure is started with a generous midline incision. If necessary, this can be extended to give good exposure to the entire abdomen, or extended into a median sternotomy for control of the supradiaphragmatic aorta and vena cava. On entering the peritoneal cavity, blood and fluid is evacuated. If there is a significant amount of blood present and if there is brisk, active bleeding, hemodynamic parameters may decline as the tamponade effect of the closed abdomen is lost. Conversely, ventilation may improve as pressure on the diaphragm is lessened. The anesthesiologist should be ready rapidly to infuse volume to the patient. A warmer should be used to heat the infused fluids. It may be necessary to pack the abdomen to control bleeding until hemodynamic parameters are stabilized. A sequential examination of each quadrant of the abdomen is then carried out. Obvious sources of bleeding are controlled. The gastrointestinal tract from the gastroesophageal junction to the peritoneal reflection is carefully examined. Any perforation of the alimentary tract should be closed temporarily to prevent further contamination; after assessment of the entire peritoneal cavity, decisions can be made either to suture or resect the perforations. If significant bleeding is ongoing, proximal control of the aorta is obtained at the diaphragmatic hiatus. Careful examination of the retroperitoneum is carried out. If a hematoma is present, and not expanding, it is left alone and not opened. If it is expanding, control must be obtained. Subsequently, a systematic examination in each portion of the abdomen—thoracic, true, pelvic, and retroperitoneal—is performed and injuries assessed and treated. During the procedure, every effort is made to continue vigorous resuscitation and correct hypovolemia, hypothermia, and any concomitant coagulopathy.

SPECIFIC ORGAN INJURIES

Diaphragm

Injury to the diaphragm is most commonly diagnosed by significant elevation of the diaphragm or the presence of abdominal viscera in the pleural space. Chest radiography can have a false-negative rate of up to 50%; thus, a number of diaphragmatic injuries are not identified before laparotomy. Therefore, careful examination of the diaphragm is required at laparotomy. Eighty to 90% of these injuries are on the left side. The injury is treated by reducing any viscera out of the chest, assessing that there has been no ischemic damage to the viscera, and then closing the defect. This can usually be done with interrupted sutures. In selected situations, the diaphragmatic defect needs to be enlarged to allow for examination of the pleural space. A radial incision in the hemidiaphragm should be used to minimize the risk of injury to diaphragmatic innervation.

Liver and Spleen Injuries

Bleeding from these organs constitutes over 80% of abdominal visceral bleeding. Strategies for nonoperative management are similar if injury to either or both organs is identified by CT scan. If the child is hemodynamically stable and there is no other reason for laparotomy, they are admitted to the ICU and kept NPO; gastric decompression is continued and IV hydration carried out. Vital signs are monitored, serial physical examinations are performed, and repeat hematocrit determinations are obtained. If evidence of peritonitis develops, exploration is performed. If hemodynamic parameters deteriorate (increased heart rate, decreased blood pressure), further IV fluids are given. Blood transfusion is given if the hematocrit drops significantly. Before the infection-related risks of transfusion had been appreciated, packed red blood cells were transfused more liberally; now, a stable hemoglobin of 7 g/dL is considered acceptable. If the patient become recurrently unstable, nonoperative management ceases and laparotomy is performed.

If the patient remains stable and if the abdominal upper quadrant tenderness resolves, they are transferred out of the ICU after approximately 1 to 2 days and are maintained on bed rest. By days 4 to 5, they are allowed out of bed and are discharged home at approximately the seventh day after injury if there is no other problem necessitating hospitalization. It is unusual to require transferring the patient back to the ICU, and rare for a patient to have a delayed hepatic or splenic hemorrhage that requires laparotomy more than 2 days after the injury. The length of time before the child can resume strenuous physical activity is controversial. In a study of 50 splenic injuries followed by abdominal CT scan at 6 weeks after injury, over 75% of small to moderate (grade I and II) splenic injuries were fully healed. In contrast, less than 10% of grade III through V injuries were fully healed 6 weeks after injury.[7] Patients are advised that they can gradually increase their physical activity after discharge, but should avoid contact sports for 3 months. Ultrasound or abdominal CT scan can be used to follow these injuries if needed. This management strategy has resulted in successful nonoperative management of CT-documented hepatic or splenic injuries in over 90% of cases.[8]

Spleen

The diagnosis of a splenic injury is suspected based on a history of blunt left-sided abdominal or flank trauma by such mechanisms as either a motor vehicle accident as a pedestrian or a fall. Physical examination may elicit left upper quadrant tenderness or identify left shoulder pain, which is referred discomfort due to diaphragmatic irritation from blood. Radiographs may show a left inferior rib fracture. This is seen in only 10% of children with splenic injuries, a smaller percentage than in adults with splenic injuries. Abdominal films may also show a medial position of the gastric air bubble because of splenic enlargement or free blood. In addition, a left pleural fusion is occasionally seen. The CT scan is the imaging study of choice (Fig. 24-4).

''Injuries of the spleen demand excision of gland. No evil effects follow its removal while the danger of hemorrhage is effectively stopped,'' claimed E. T. Kocher in 1911. This tenet of management was held to be fundamental until the 1970s. As early as 1952, it was observed that patients who had undergone splenectomy had a higher risk of death from bacterial sepsis.[9] A number of subsequent studies confirmed this initial observation and showed that although the risk for postsplenectomy sepsis is small, approximately 1.5%, the mortality risk with this sepsis is approximately 50%.[10] It also appears that this risk of fatal infection is highest in young children and gradually declines. However, the adolescent is still at high risk for the development of overwhelming postsplenectomy infection (OPSI). The mechanism of this postsplenectomy sepsis results from the child's inability to clear encapsulated bacterium, most commonly *Streptococcus pneumoniae* and *Haemophilus influenzae*. Alterations in bacterial opsonization and alterations in neutrophil function also play a significant role.

Pediatric surgeons began a course of nonoperative management in the 1970s. This strategy of management was initiated because of the combination of the ability to identify specific splenic injuries by means of radionuclide scans and the advent of the CT scan, and the observation that at operation, splenic bleeding often had stopped spontaneously. This, coupled with the risk of OPSI, made the nonoperative treatment of a splenic injury attractive.

The management principles for nonoperative treatment of splenic injuries have been outlined previously. This strategy can lead to a successful conclusion in approximately 90% of patients. Previous studies with nonoperative management showed that up to 50% of patients required blood transfusion, and that transfusion requirements were up to 20 mL/kg. Increased awareness of transfusion risks has led to management strategies in children with splenic injuries in which blood transfusion is required in less than 20% of cases.[11]

The operative management of the patient with a splenic injury falls into two categories. In the first, the patient requires emergency laparotomy because of unstable vital signs or peritonitis. If there is a major uncontrolled hemorrhage, a life-threatening situation, and a splenic injury is identified, major efforts to repair the spleen are inappropriate. In this case, control of the splenic hilum and splenectomy are indicated. The second scenario is one in which the patient is stable and a splenic injury is identified. Here, splenorrhaphy should be attempted. Part of the reason for successful treatment of splenic injuries lies in the spleen's blood supply. The splenic artery branches into four to five vessels just before entering the spleen itself. The vessels follow a radial course from this point. Most splenic injuries are transverse in nature and thus do not cross a large number of splenic vessels (Fig. 24-5), which allows for spontaneous cessation of bleeding in a large number of cases. In those children who require operation, suture closure of the bleeding area often can be accomplished. The spleen with a subcapsular hematoma and with bleeding and disruption of a portion of the capsule may be difficult to suture. The use of topical hemostatic agents is helpful in this circumstance. In the case of a fragmented spleen, partial splenectomy can be performed if necessary. There is controversy regarding the minimum amount of splenic tissue required to allow normal immune function and prevent OPSI; the implantation of splenic fragments in the omentum does not prevent OPSI.[12] It is thought that at least 25% of the spleen is required. Patients who have undergone splenectomy

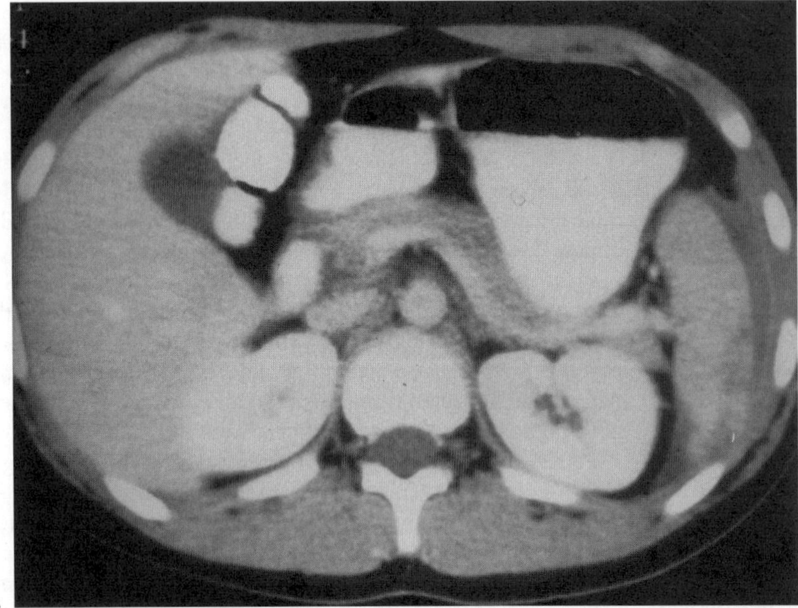

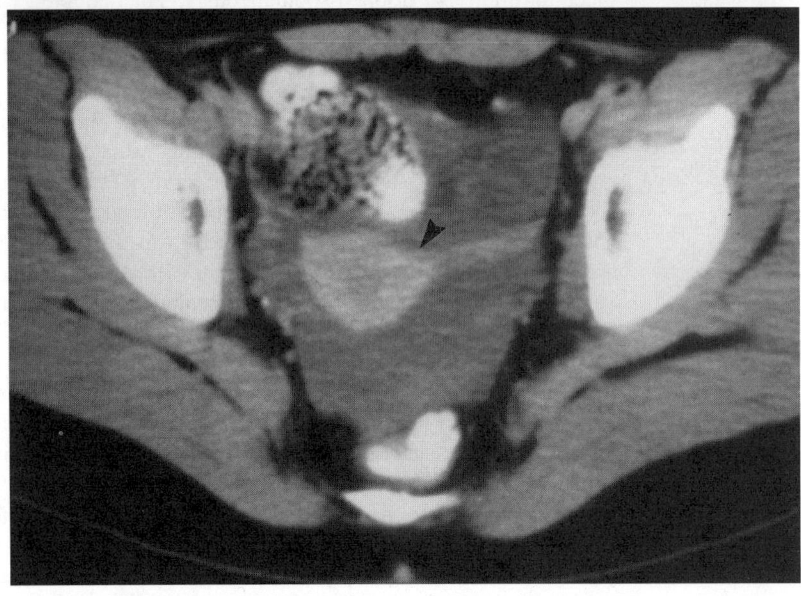

FIG. 24-4. CT scan of a 14-year-old with a splenic injury with free intraperitoneal fluid (*A*), and with extension of the fluid into the pelvis surrounding the uterus (*B; arrow*).

should be immunized with polyvalent pneumococcal and *H influenzae* vaccine. It is imperative that the caregiver be aware of the risk of OPSI in the child. Fever or other signs of illness should be evaluated promptly. In children, prophylactic treatment with penicillin is also useful to decrease the risk of infection, although there is controversy over how long this should continue.

The experience in children who require operation because of splenic bleeding is that splenorraphy is successful in approximately half of the cases. This results in an overall splenic preservation rate of approximately 95% in children with documented splenic injuries. Although a significant number of children often have a concomitant intraabdominal injury, selective nonoperative management is not associated with an increased risk of morbidity from missed associated injuries.[13] There is no question that in children, attempts to salvage the spleen should be made unless there is a life-threatening concurrent problem. The information regarding management in adults less clear.

Liver

The liver is the largest organ in abdomen, and it is increasingly recognized that it is injured almost as frequently as the spleen. Major liver injuries are second only to central nervous system injuries as a cause of death in the pediatric trauma patient. Evaluation and management of a liver injury is much the same as for the spleen. In the hemodynamically stable patient, CT scan of the abdomen is the imaging study of choice (Fig. 24-6).[11] Because of the liver's large size, there is often injury to an adjacent organ. Nonoperative management of liver injuries can be carried out following the guidelines previously noted, and should result in a successful outcome in most patients.

If operation is required, control of hemorrhage is the fundamental goal. Many hepatic injuries that have not spontaneously stopped bleeding can be controlled with a suture ligation. If a large raw liver surface exists because of a stellate or avulsion injury, the use of topical hemostatic agents and suture ligation

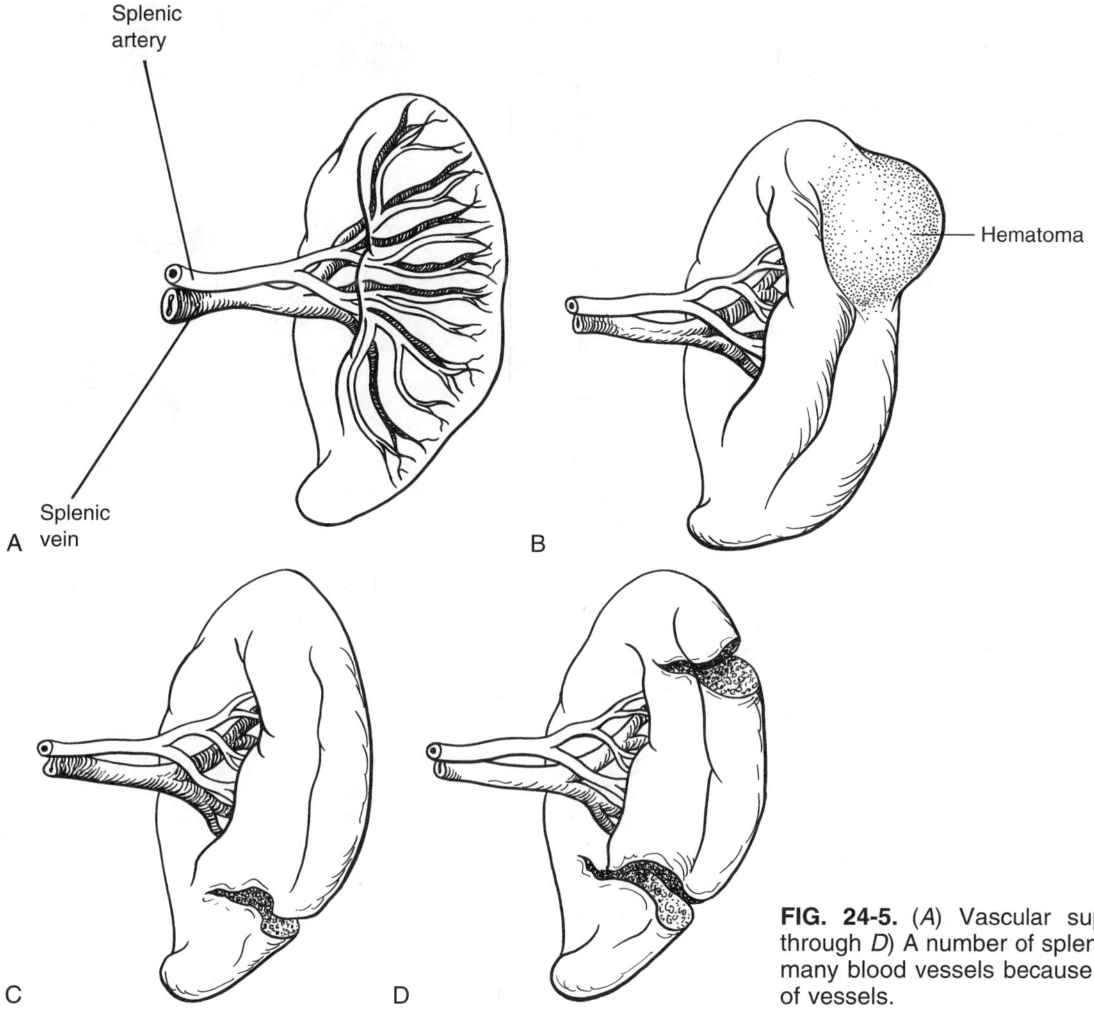

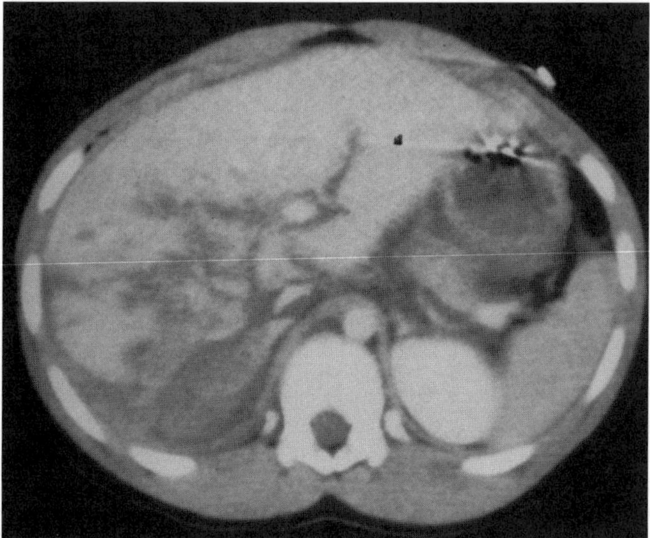

FIG. 24-5. (*A*) Vascular supply to the spleen. (*B* through *D*) A number of splenic injuries do not disrupt many blood vessels because of the radial distribution of vessels.

of vessels is effective. If significant bleeding persists, control at the portal triad by a Pringle maneuver may allow temporary control of the bleeding so that the sources of hemorrhage can be identified and controlled more precisely. Adequate exposure is facilitated by mobilizing the hepatic flexure of the colon and the duodenum. Specific control of bleeding sites is important, and can be problematic when there is a laceration deep into the liver parenchyma. If left untreated, bleeding can persist and lead to hemobilia. Careful dissection and control of bleeding vessels avoids this problem. Areas of necrotic, devitalized tissue are debrided. Resection of small avulsed segments of liver can be carried out as needed. It is unusual to require liver lobectomy; major hepatic resections with lobectomy are associated with high mortality. Appropriate mobilization of the liver by division of the triangular ligaments may be necessary. If there is evidence of a major retrohepatic caval injury, the midline wound can be extended into a median sternotomy. Placement of an atriocaval shunt to bypass the caval injury can be life saving. However, such injuries carry a low likelihood of survival in children.

Pancreas

An injury to the pancreas can occur with any trauma to the upper abdomen and is more often associated with blunt trauma

FIG. 24-6. CT scan of a 7-year-old with multiple liver fractures and a lack of perfusion to the right kidney.

(eg, bicycle handlebar, fall, fist with child abuse). Because of its location, there is often an associated injury to the duodenum or the left kidney. The diagnosis is made on the basis of the mechanism of injury, laboratory data (amylase, lipase), and imaging studies. Both the ultrasound and the CT scan are helpful to identify edema, hematoma, or disruption (Fig. 24-7). Most pancreatic injuries are well treated nonoperatively. The decision to operate depends on the mechanism of injury and the physical findings. A pancreatic injury due to penetrating trauma requires laparotomy, as does a blunt pancreatic injury with associated peritonitis. The findings with a pancreatic injury are often more subtle than those with injuries to other organs, in part because of the pancreas' retroperitoneal position. The CT scan is helpful in identifying pancreatic anatomy and fluid accumulation in the retroperitoneum. The patient with evidence of a blunt injury who is hemodynamically stable and does not have peritonitis can be managed nonoperatively with IV hydration and bowel rest. Serial physical examinations and biochemical determinations for evidence of pancreatic injury are carried out. Indications for operative management in these patients include persistent and worsening pain, fever, and persistent hyperamylasemia.

Complications after pancreatic injuries include pseudocyst formation and the development of a pancreatic fistula. Pseudocysts are associated with the identification of a mass in approximately two thirds of children, and almost all patients have persistent hyperamylasemia. Pancreatic pseudocysts commonly present with a partial obstruction, either gastric or small intestinal, or as an intraabdominal abscess. CT scan can well document the pseudocyst and its relation to adjacent organs (Fig. 24-8). If an abscess is identified, it is drained externally. Percutaneous techniques under ultrasonic or fluoroscopic guidance are effective and have less morbidity than laparotomy and external drainage. If the pancreatic pseudocyst has been present for several weeks and has not decreased in size, internal drainage is the treatment of choice.[14] Internal drainage is performed into the adjacent portion of the gastrointestinal tract, and most commonly involves a cystogastrostomy. If this is not technically

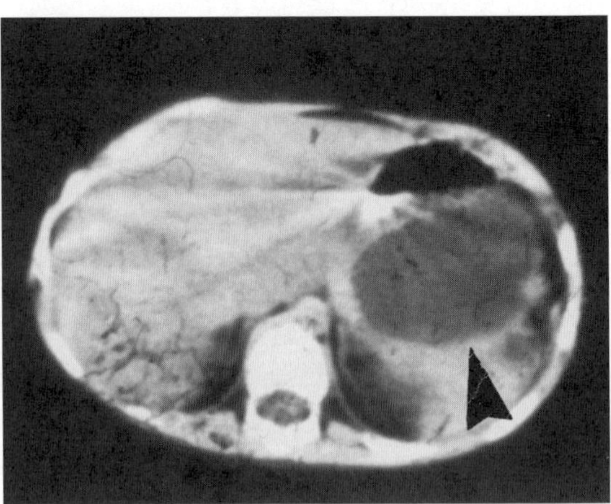

FIG. 24-8. CT scan demonstrating a pancreatic pseudocyst (*arrow*) in a retrogastric position.

feasible, a Roux-en-Y drainage to the jejunum is carried out. Pancreatic fistulas are distinctly unusual in children. Most respond to nonoperative treatment with bowel rest, total parenteral nutrition, and the use of somatostatin analogues. In selected cases, an internal drainage procedure is required. The patient with persistent epigastric pain after a pancreatic injury may have either a fistula or a pancreatic ductal disruption. Endoscopic retrograde cholangiopancreatography can demonstrate ductal anatomy and delineate any area of poor drainage.

Gastrointestinal Injuries

Injuries to the gastrointestinal hollow viscus structures are far less common than hepatic or splenic injuries. The small intestine is the most commonly injured organ. Injuries can be caused by either blunt trauma (compressive force), rapid deceleration (shear force), or a combination of both. Injuries to the stomach are relatively infrequent, but must be suspected in any trauma patient. The diagnosis can be relatively easily made by injecting air through a nasogastric tube, or by obtaining a radiograph after instilling a small amount of contrast into the stomach. At laparotomy, the stomach should be completely examined by opening the lesser sac to examine the posterior surface, as well as examining the anterior surface. Small bowel injuries can occur anywhere, but have a higher frequency at several locations. The duodenum can be subjected to compressive force against the vertebral spine; the classic seat belt injury caused by rapid deceleration can result in such a duodenal injury. This type of injury can also be seen in a patient who has had a transverse fracture through a lumbar vertebra. The mechanism in both cases is rapid deceleration. The resultant duodenal hematoma is in a subserosal location and can cause complete obstruction. Over 85% of duodenal hematomas resolve spontaneously over 1 to 3 weeks time (Fig. 24-9).[15] Treatment consists of gastric decompression and, if a protracted course is expected, total parenteral nutrition. If operation is required for a duodenal hematoma, or if one is encountered during laparotomy, the hematoma can be evacuated. An incision through the serosa evacuates the clot. The submucosa is usually intact, and the overlying serosa and muscularis can be approxi-

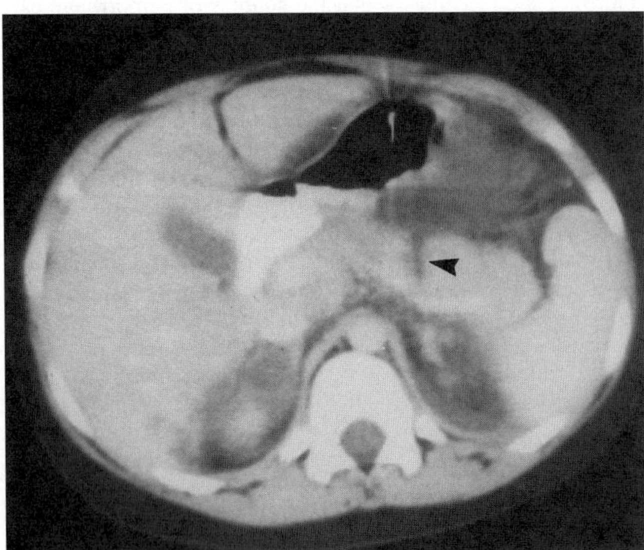

FIG. 24-7. CT scan showing pancreatic edema, parenchymal disruption (*arrow*), free peritoneal fluid, and medial displacement of the stomach.

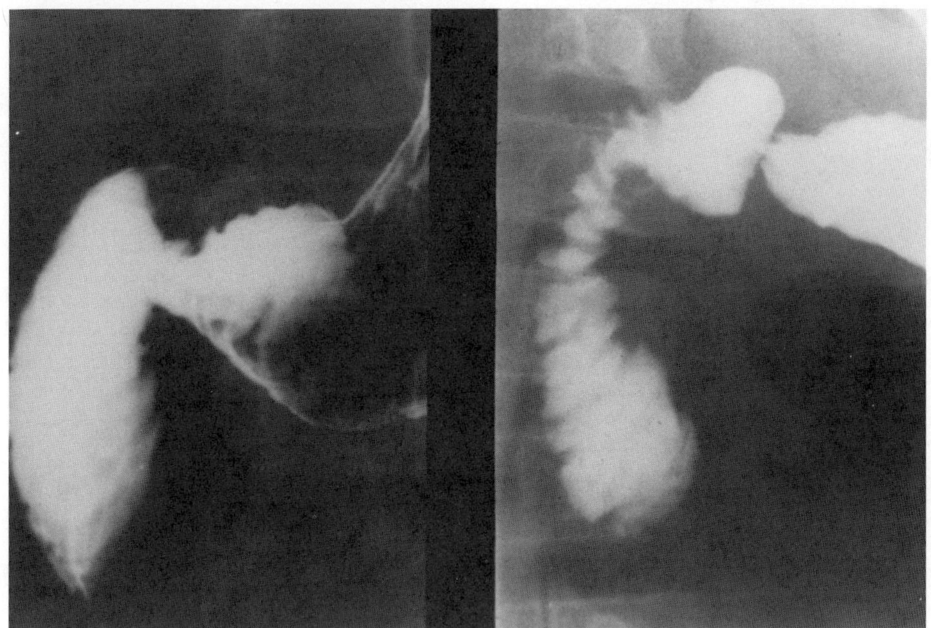

FIG. 24-9. Upper gastrointestinal study demonstrating a complete cut-off of contrast in the duodenum caused by an intramural duodenal hematoma.

mated. Subsequent duodenal leakage is unusual. Another type of intestinal injury results from a sudden increase in intraluminal pressure in a fluid-filled loop of bowel that is trapped between two fixed points of a high-riding lap belt restraint. This can lead to a hematoma or perforation. A duodenal perforation in its retroperitoneal course usually does not manifest itself with free air; rather, there may be only a small amount of air in the retroperitoneum. The CT scan can show this air and can also show any extravasation of contrast material. Exploration and repair with drainage of the duodenum is required in this circumstance.

The small bowel can be injured at points where it is well anchored by the mesentery, such as at the ligament of Treitz and the ileocecal valve. Here, the bowel is tethered, and rapid deceleration causes the bowel to continue to move forward inertially while the peritoneum holds it. This type of injury to the proximal jejunum or terminal ileum should be suspected. A third type of deceleration injury is seen in patients in whom the small bowel is literally torn from its mesentery (Fig. 24-10). Diagnosis of such an injury can be particularly problematic; there is no leakage of contrast material on an initial CT scan. These injuries can go on to perforation several days later because of further ischemia and frank necrosis, or they can heal with stricture formation. The clinician should maintain a strong index of suspicion with regard to this type of injury. A missed diagnosis is particularly likely when no intraabdominal injury had been diagnosed previously and the patient's abdominal pain was ascribed to ''soft tissue'' abdominal wall trauma. If abdominal pain persists for more than several days, intraabdominal injury should be considered, and a repeat CT scan of the abdomen may be diagnostic. Treatment consists of segmental resection and anastomosis.

Genitourinary Injury

Injuries of the kidneys, ureters, bladder, and urethra comprise approximately 10% of all abdominal injuries and are more often associated with blunt trauma. The incidence of trauma-related injuries increases in patients with genitourinary (GU) congenital anomalies. Not infrequently, an anomaly of the GU tract is identified during the work-up for hematuria after a traumatic injury. The kidneys, because of their size and position, are the most commonly injured GU structure. With blunt trauma, a compressive injury can cause significant damage to the renal parenchyma, the collecting system, or the vascular supply. Other areas of injury in the GU tract include the ureters, commonly at the ureteropelvic junction, and at the ureterovesicular junction, especially in patients with pelvic fractures. Injuries also can occur to the bladder and the urethra, associated with pelvic fractures. Hematuria is found in 90% of children with a GU injury. Gross hematuria requires diagnostic evaluation because of the likelihood of a significant underlying injury. In the adult experience, gross hematuria or microscopic hematuria with a period of hypotension correlate with significant renal injuries, and these findings require radiographic evaluation while microscopic hematuria alone may not indicate a significant injury. In children, the presence of hematuria alone, either gross or microscopic, is associated with significant GU injury.[16–18] Either no hematuria or microscopic hematuria may be found in up to 30% of patients with significant renal trauma. It appears that significant bladder and urethral injuries more commonly have gross hematuria.[14] The presence of either a flank mass or hematuria should lead to evaluation with a CT scan with IV contrast (Fig. 24-11). The scan shows the position of the kidneys, perfusion, evidence of parenchymal damage, extravasation, obstruction, ureteral position, dilation if present, and the status of the bladder. If there is significant concern regarding a bladder or urethral injury, a cystourethrogram is a more specific and sensitive diagnostic imaging study.

Over 90% of renal injuries are managed without surgery. The major indications for operation are vascular disruption and the loss of a significant amount of renal tissue. If bleeding is controlled, there may be a better salvage of renal tissue. Contro-

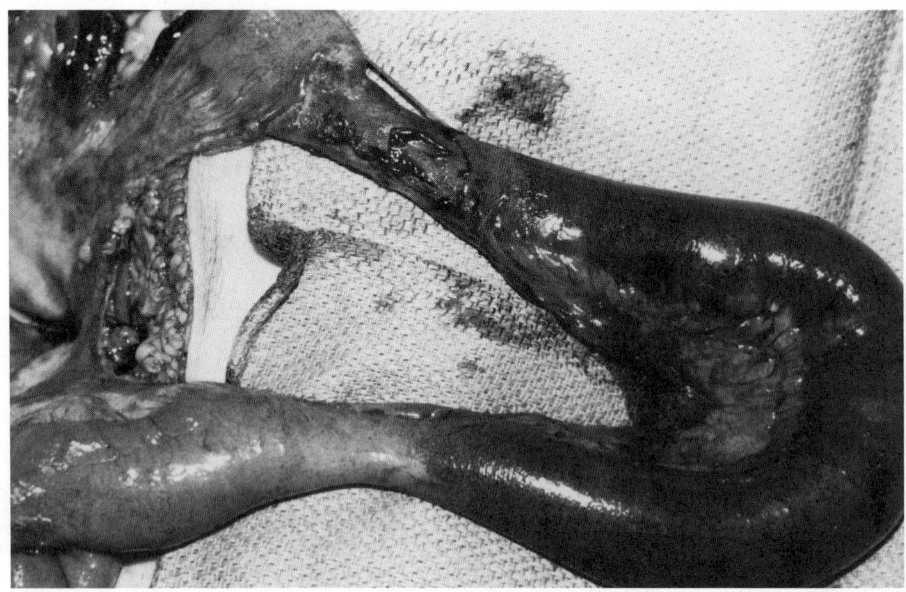

FIG. 24-10. Avulsion of the small bowel from its mesentery in a 14-year-old patient who suffered a rapid deceleration injury in a motor vehicle accident.

versy exists regarding the need for arteriography. This test defines the renal vascular anatomy, identifies vascular anomalies, and gives precise information regarding renal perfusion. Some believe that although it is helpful in some cases, the amount of time required to obtain an arteriogram at some centers is too long. Rather, if the diagnosis of renal artery occlusion was made on the basis of a CT scan with nonvisualization, prompt operative intervention would allow for more prompt repair and a potentially increased renal salvage rate.[19] If a significant extravasation is identified on the CT scan, this should be followed closely. Most are managed nonoperatively. If it continues to increase in size, percutaneous drainage can be performed. Appropriate catheter position can be achieved with placement under ultrasonic or fluoroscopic guidance. Ultrasound is also an effective way to follow serially a urinoma or hematoma. Longitudinal follow-up of children who have incurred renal

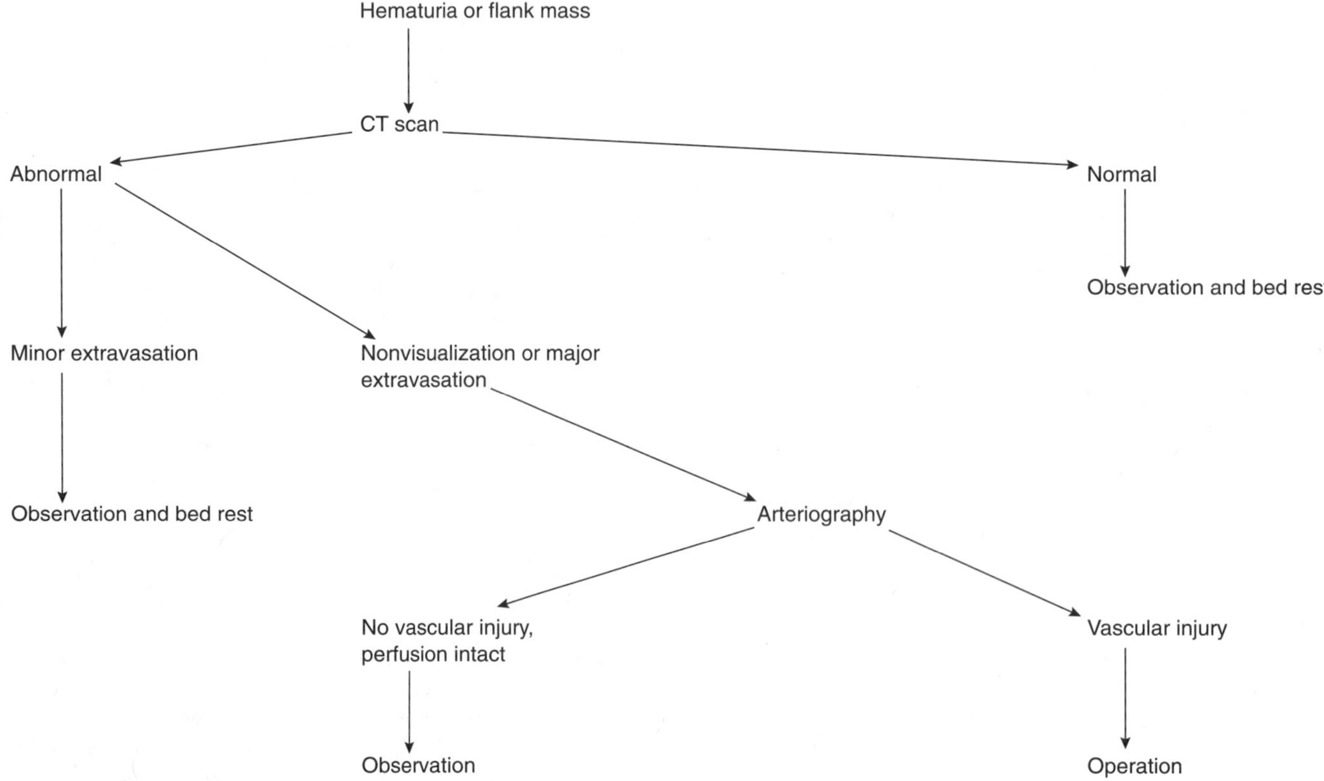

FIG. 24-11. Algorithm for management of blunt renal trauma.

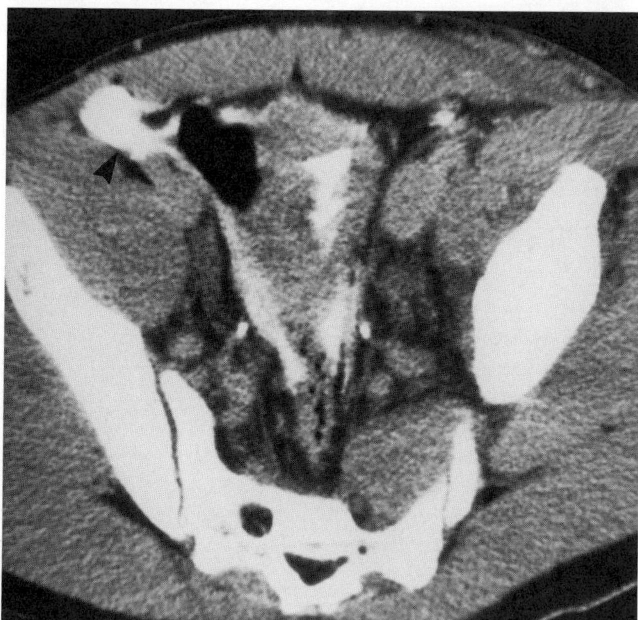

FIG. 24-12. CT scan demonstrating an intraperitoneal bladder rupture. The arrow shows extravasated contrast material.

trauma is important. Up to 20% of children in one study had evidence of renal scarring at follow-up at a mean of 5 years after injury.[20] Patients who have suffered significant renal injuries are at risk for the development of hypertension, and they should be screened for this.

Bladder injuries are commonly identified because of concerns raised by an associate pelvic fracture, and almost always have the finding of gross hematuria. Bladder rupture is sustained more frequently in children with a full bladder, and can occur either into the peritoneal cavity or extraperitoneally. Diagnosis can be made with CT scan if delayed films are taken with the bladder adequately distended, however in the trauma setting, a retrograde cystogram is often faster and more reliable. Either the CT scan or the cystogram can show whether the rupture is into the peritoneal cavity (Fig. 24-12). Free peritoneal rupture requires operative intervention and repair. Extraperitoneal rupture can be managed either with operation or catheter drainage.

A variety of urethral injuries occur because of blunt trauma. These include straddle-type injuries, such as with a bicycle seat, and injuries in association with pelvic fractures. The diagnosis should be suspected in a child who has blood at the urethral meatus. If this is found, Foley catheter passage is contraindicated because of the likelihood of making a false passage. In-

stead, a retrograde urethrogram should be performed with the catheter just within the urethra. If a urethral injury has been sustained, proximal drainage with a suprapubic tube should be carried out. In most cases, delayed repair of the urethra is the treatment of choice.

REFERENCES

1. Cooper A, Barlow B, DiScala C, et al. Mortality and truncal injury: the pediatric perspective. J Pediatr Surg 1994;29:33.
2. Oldham KT, Guice KS, Ryckman F, et al. Blunt liver injury in childhood: evolution of therapy and current perspective. Surgery 1986;100:542.
3. Tso EL, Beaver BI, Haller JA. Abdominal injuries in restrained passengers. J Pediatr Surg 1993;28:915.
4. Taylor GA, Sivit CJ. Computed tomography imaging of abdominal trauma. Semina Pediatr Surg 1992;1:253.
5. Taylor GA, Kaufman RA, Sivit CJ. Active hemorrhage in children after thoracoabdominal trauma: clinical and CT features. AJR Am J Roentgenol 1994;162:401.
6. Bulas DI, Taylor GA, Eichelberger MR. The value of CT in detecting bowel perforation in children after abdominal trauma. AJR Am J Roentgenol 1987;153:561.
7. Pranikoff T, Hirschl RB, Schlesinger AE, et al. Resolution of splenic injury after nonoperative management. J Pediatr Surg 1994;29:1366.
8. Haller JA, Papa P, Drugas G, et al. Nonoperative management of solid organ injuries in children: is it safe? Ann Surg 1994;219:625.
9. King II, Shumacher HB. Splenic studies: Susceptibility to infection after splenectomy performed in infancy. Ann Surg 1952;136:239.
10. Singer DB. Postsplenectomy sepsis. In: Rosenberg HS, Bolande RP, eds. Perspectives in pediatric pathology, vol I. Chicago, Yearbook Medical Publishers, 1973:285.
11. Bond SJ, Eichelberger MR, Gotschall CS. Nonoperative management of blunt hepatic and splenic injury in children. Ann Surg 1996;223:286.
12. Moore GE, Stevens RE, Moore EE, et al. Failure of splenic implants to protect against fatal postsplenectomy infection. Am J Surg 1983;146:413.
13. Morse MA, Garcia VF. Selective nonoperative management of pediatric blunt splenic trauma: risk for missed associated injuries. J Pediatr Surg 1994;29:23.
14. Cooney DR, Grosfeld JL. Operative management of pancreatic pseudocysts in infants and children. Ann Surg 1975;182:590.
15. Holgersen LO, Bishop HC. Nonoperative treatment of duodenal hematomata in childhood. J Pediatr Surg 1977;12:11.
16. Stein JP, Kaji DM, Eastham J, et al. Blunt renal trauma in the pediatric population: indications for radiographic evaluation. Urology 1994;44:406.
17. Levy JB, Baskin LS, Ewalt DH, et al. Nonoperative management of blunt pediatric major renal trauma. Urology 1993;42:418.
18. McAleer IM, Kaplan GW, Scherz HC, et al. Genitourinary trauma in the pediatric patient. Urology 1993;42:563.
19. Smith SD, Gardner MJ, Rowe MI. Renal artery occlusion in pediatric blunt abdominal trauma: decreasing the delay from injury to treatment. J Trauma 1993;35:861.
20. Surana R, Khan A, Fitzgerald RJ. Scarring following renal trauma in children. Br J Urol 1995;75:664.

Surgery of Infants and Children: Scientific Principles and Practice, edited by
Keith T. Oldham, Paul M. Colombani, and Robert P. Foglia.
Lippincott–Raven Publishers, Philadelphia, © 1997.

CHAPTER 25

Orthopedic Principles for Trauma

David W. Gray and Paul D. Sponseller

Skeletal injuries account for about 10% to 15% of all pediatric trauma.[1] In 30% to 50% of patients with multiple traumatic injuries, an extremity injury is present. Residual morbidity after the accident is often due to orthopedic and neurologic injuries.[2,3] To minimize these sequelae, the basic orthopedic principles of treatment should be understood.

SKELETAL DEVELOPMENT

The skeleton develops by both membranous and endochondral ossification. Endochondral bone formation is the primary developmental process of the axial and appendicular skeleton. This developmental mechanism allows the orderly transformation of a cartilage precursor to mature bone and simultaneously creates longitudinal growth. The long bones have several distinct anatomic regions. The *diaphysis* is the shaft area. The *metaphysis* is the region that widens or expands toward the bone end. The *physis,* or growth plate, is present in the immature skeleton. The *epiphysis* is the end of the long bone. The epiphysis and the physis constitute the area of the endochondral growth mechanism (Fig. 25-1). Initially, the epiphysis is made of cartilage; however, as maturation proceeds, a secondary ossification center develops within it. As maturity progresses, the epiphysis changes from cartilage to bone.

The periosteum is the outer connective tissue envelope of the bone. This layer is better developed in children than adults. It provides for bone growth by apposition (ie, expanding the circumference of the shaft by sequential deposition of bone). Periosteal bone deposition also plays an important role in fracture healing.

PATHOPHYSIOLOGY AND BIOMECHANICS OF FRACTURES

The immature skeleton is biologically and mechanically different from the adult skeleton. As bone matures, it undergoes changes in apparent porosity, collagen fiber composition, and mineral content. The elasticity of bone in children allows incomplete fractures and plastic deformation to occur, such as buckle and greenstick fractures. Immature bone can also absorb more energy before breaking.[4]

The angulation of a child's bone after fracture can often be corrected; this is termed *remodeling.* In the immature skeleton, contouring or reshaping occurs simultaneously with bone growth. Because of this prolific biologic activity, most childhood fractures can be treated without surgical intervention. Fractures that occur in the metaphyseal region of the bone in young children are the most conducive to remodeling. Conversely, patients near skeletal maturity can expect little nonsurgical correction of bone alignment. Although these angular deviations can improve, rotational malalignment after a fracture does not effectively correct itself. Therefore, close attention to the rotational alignment of the fracture fragments is mandatory in patients of all ages.

PATIENT EVALUATION

Clinical Examination

The Advanced Trauma Life Support guidelines are well known and provide excellent treatment for polytrauma patients. From the orthopedic standpoint, the areas of concern are the spine, the pelvis, and the extremities. Much can be learned from simple palpation of the skeletal system. Assessment is made of the ability of the patient to voluntarily move the arms and legs, with evaluation of muscle and tendon continuity and neurologic integrity. The neurovascular examination of an injured extremity should be carefully documented. Rectal tone should be documented in any patient with a suspected spinal column injury. Specifics of spinal column evaluation are discussed with spinal cord injuries later in this chapter.

Radiography

Radiography in the polytrauma patient initially includes cervical spine, chest, and pelvis radiographs, although some investigators believe think that a cervical spine radiograph is unnecessary in some adult patients.[5] If there is any question regarding the mental status of the patient, or if the child is not old enough to communicate effectively and localize symptoms, cervical spine radiography should be performed. The cross-table lateral

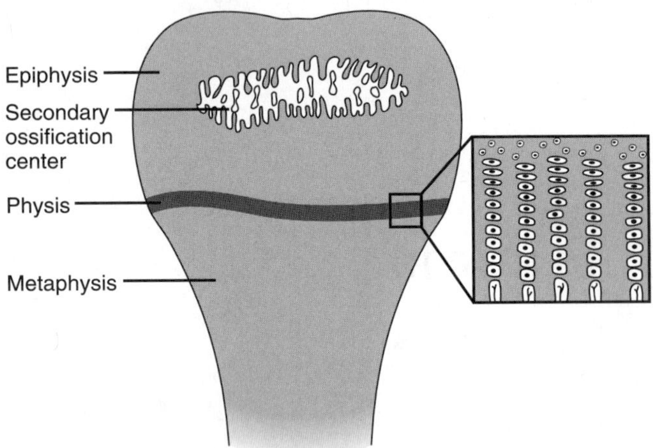

FIG. 25-1. Cartilage cells in the physis hypertrophy and calcify, making the matrix on which ossification occurs. This produces longitudinal growth.

radiograph of the cervical spine can be a useful screen, but it has been shown to have a false-negative rate as high as 26% in adults.[6] The upper cervical spine, especially at the C-1 and C-2 junction, can be difficult to evaluate on lateral radiograph.

Radiography of the extremities should be undertaken in the presence of obvious deformity, pain on palpation, swelling, or concern about retained foreign debris. If a long bone is found to have a fracture, the radiographs should include the entire long bone, not just the area of injury. Multilevel injury to a single long bone does occur. If tenderness or signs of trauma along the spinal column are seen, spine radiographs should be included in the evaluation. In seat belt injuries, radiographs of the thoracolumbar spine should be taken because of the association with flexion–distraction injuries of the spine (see Thoracic and Lumbar Spine Fractures).

GENERAL FRACTURE CARE

The basic tenet of fracture care is to provide immobilization of the bone so that soft tissue and bony healing can occur, allowing full return of function. This can be accomplished by a number of means. Splints are an effective way to immobilize an extremity if there is concern about applying a rigid circular dressing (ie, a cast) in the face of soft tissue swelling. Casting has been the time-honored method of treatment, but it requires skill to achieve both comfort and bony alignment.

More invasive means of fracture care have evolved. Not every fracture can be adequately aligned or maintained in a satisfactory position within a cast. Traction can be an effective tool but is seldom used as definitive treatment. Percutaneous pin fixation in conjunction with a cast has proved useful in pediatric fractures, especially elbow injuries. External fixation is becoming more widespread in its applications for children. In the past, external fixation was used mainly in open fractures. It is now being used for some closed pediatric fractures as well. Internal fixation using screws, plates, and intramedullary rods has given the orthopedist even more options.

GROWTH PLATE INJURY

About 15% of children's fractures involve the physis.[3] Inherent to the physis is a zone of hypertrophic cartilage cells that constitutes a weak area. It is through this zone that a fracture can occur and propagate. An injury to the epiphysis and physis is an injury to the area of endochondral bone formation and can produce long-term sequelae. Complete growth arrest (premature closure of the growth plate) leads to a discrepancy in the length of an arm or a leg. A partial growth arrest can lead to a discrepancy in length and can also create an angular deformity.

A classification system that is commonly used in North America for growth plate fractures is the Salter-Harris system.[7] Modifications of this classification are abundant, but the following constitutes the basic system (Fig. 25-2):

Type I: The epiphysis separates from the metaphysis, with low likelihood of later growth disturbance.
Type II: The epiphysis separates with a metaphyseal fracture fragment—the most common type of physeal fracture.
Type III: Intraarticular type of fracture through the epiphysis and the physis
Type IV: Intraarticular fracture that involves epiphysis, physis, and metaphysis. These typically require anatomic reduction of the fracture to guard against growth disturbance.
Type V: Crush injury to the physis. Because there is often no displacement, these can be difficult to diagnose at the time of injury.

With intraarticular fractures, there is greater need for anatomic alignment. This is necessary both to restore joint congruity and to realign the growth plate. Treatment consists of accurately reducing these fragments by manipulation with or without percutaneous fixation. If this is unsuccessful, open reduction with internal fixation is indicated.

OPEN FRACTURES

Open fractures typically result from a greater magnitude of energy than closed fractures. This increased amount of force not only breaks the bone but also drives the bone fragments through the overlying muscle and skin. Open fractures have more associated soft tissue damage. The initial treatment consists of irrigation and débridement of the wound. This decreases the bacterial count in the wound. Necrotic tissue and particulate debris are removed. Bone stabilization at this time is provided to promote soft tissue recovery. In fact, for fracture healing to occur, a healthy soft tissue envelope must first be present. Again, a classification system has been proposed and is widely used for open fractures.

The Gustilo and Anderson system is as follows:

Type I (grade I): There is an open fracture in a clean wound less than 1 cm in length.
Type II (grade II): There is an open fracture with a laceration more than 1 cm long.
Type III (grade III): There is an open fracture with extensive soft tissue injury. Typically, the wounds are greater than 10 cm in length, and often require flap coverage. Open, severely comminuted fractures, as well as farm and barnyard injuries,

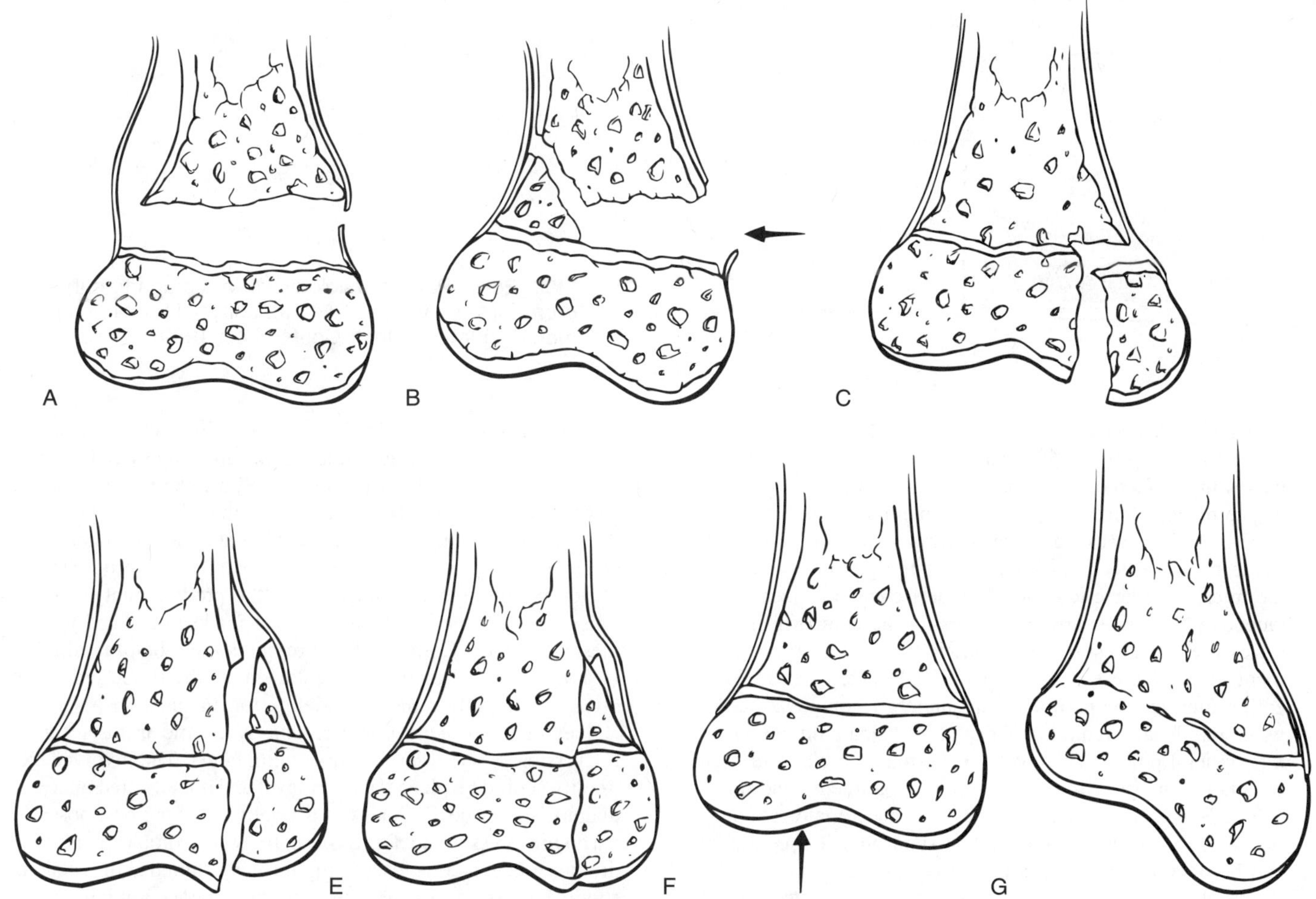

FIG. 25-2. The Salter-Harris classification system for fractures. (*A*) Type I. (*B*) Type II. (*C*) Type III. (*D*) Type IV. (*E*) Type IV fracture with malunion of the fragments, demonstrating the importance of anatomic alignment. (*F* and *G*) Type V fracture showing the initial injury (*arrow in F*) and subsequent growth disturbance (*G*).

are considered grade III injuries regardless of wound size. Traumatic amputations are also grade III injuries.[8]

The basic principles for treatment are débridement and irrigation (about 6 L), antibiotic therapy, fracture stability, and soft tissue closure. Follow-up irrigation and débridement should be done every 24 to 48 hours until the wound is clean and free of necrotic debris. Wound closure can be accomplished using delayed primary closure, skin grafting, or soft tissue flaps.

Antibiotic coverage consists of a first-generation cephalosporin for type I and II injuries. In a type III injury, an aminoglycoside is usually added. Farm injuries are grade III injuries because of the contamination with barnyard and soil organisms, especially clostridia. In these cases, penicillin is added to the cephalosporin and aminoglycoside antibiotic regime.

The duration of antibiotic treatment depends on wound severity, amount of contamination, patient's immune status, and number of surgical débridements needed to achieve a clean wound. In most clinical scenarios, antibiotic coverage continues for 48 hours after each débridement and after the final wound closure. Because patients with type III injuries often return for two or three débridements, antibiotic treatment often lasts for 1 week to 10 days.

The goal of wound treatment is to provide soft tissue coverage for the bone without infection. Not until a stable soft tissue environment is present can bone healing occur. Even with aggressive treatment, infection rates for type III injuries remain as high as 10%. Chronic osteomyelitis resulting from an open fracture can have a significant impact on quality of life.

COMPARTMENT SYNDROME

A compartment syndrome occurs when the tissue pressure in a closed fascial space reaches a critical level, reducing perfusion and creating tissue ischemia. If tissue pressure is not reduced, permanent loss of function ensues. Compartment syndromes are most frequently seen in the leg but can occur in the arm, hand, foot, thigh, shoulder, and buttocks, so that any closed fascial space can be potentially involved. Compartment syndromes are seen with fractures (including open fractures), crush injuries, burns, hemorrhage into a closed space, and after revascularization of ischemic limbs.

Signs and symptoms of a compartment syndrome include pain out of proportion to the clinical setting (the earliest symptom), pain on passive stretch of the involved compartment's

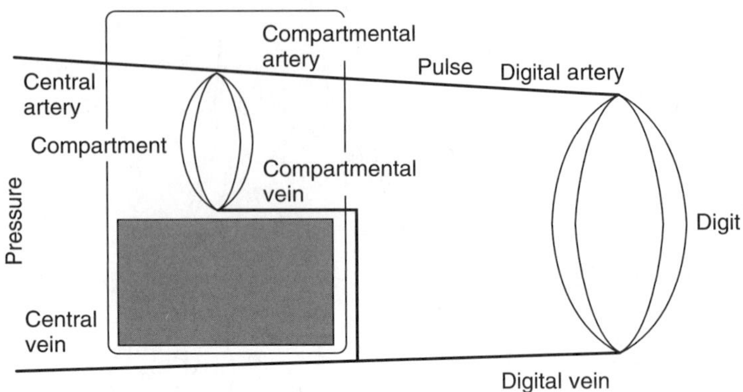

FIG. 25-3. Pathophysiology of a compartment syndrome. (After Matsen FA. Pathophysiology of compartment syndromes. Instr Course Lect 1989)

muscles, a tense muscle compartment on palpation, and hypoesthesia (a late finding). A patient can have normal intact distal pulses in the face of a compartment syndrome.

The pathophysiology of a compartment syndrome should be understood. Perfusion to the cells is impeded as the surrounding tissue pressure becomes greater than the pressure gradient in the microvascular circulation. Tissue ischemia ensues. Simultaneously the major arteries traversing the compartment have a pressure gradient sufficient to allow flow through the compartment, thereby preserving the peripheral pulse (Fig. 25-3). An entire muscle compartment can undergo complete necrosis while the distal circulation is deemed adequate on the basis of a peripheral pulse.[9] Therefore, the peripheral pulse and digital circulation are poor indicators of a compartment syndrome.

Tissue pressure monitoring has become a major adjunct in the early diagnosis of compartment syndrome. Tissue pressure can be obtained by using a needle or catheter connected by a fluid column to a pressure transducer or manometer (Fig. 25-4). Normal resting muscle compartment pressures are 0 to 5 mmHg. There is disagreement about what absolute pressure constitutes a compartment syndrome; however, the threshold for considering decompression in an acute compartment syndrome is about 30 mmHg. The patient's hemodynamic status should also be considered. If the compartment pressure is within 10 to 30 mmHg of the diastolic blood pressure, there should be concern whether perfusion is adequate at the tissue level.[9,10]

Diagnosis is made by clinical examination and compartment pressures. In the awake patient, both pain and pain on passive stretch of the involved muscles are the predominant features. This is the time the diagnosis should be made, not when hypoesthesia develops. Compartment pressures are a helpful adjunct. In a patient with an altered mental status, the tissue pressures often are the only reliable guideline for diagnosis.

Treatment of acute compartment syndrome is fasciotomy. Irreversible tissue injury occurs within hours. The involved extremity should be placed at heart level and not elevated once the diagnosis is made. This allows the delivery of the best possible perfusion pressure to the tissues. In acute compartment syndrome, subcutaneous fasciotomy through limited skin incisions should be avoided because the skin acts as a noncompliant envelope.[11] In lower leg fibulectomy in children, fasciotomy may cause subsequent ankle deformity. The two-incision technique of fasciotomy in the lower leg is preferred.[12]

FRACTURE CARE IN THE POLYTRAUMA PATIENT

In adult polytrauma patients, early orthopedic intervention has been shown to decrease morbidity and mortality.[13] Traditionally, closed fracture treatment in children has been common. It is becoming clear, however, that early operative stabilization of fractures is of benefit in children as well.[2] Problems resulting from immobilization in bed, such as pneumonia, and prolonged hospital stays are refocusing the discussion about operative fracture intervention for some of these children.[14]

HEAD INJURY

Head injuries in children pose a few special problems in fracture care. Increased muscle tone and agitation can make controlling long bone fracture alignment difficult. Casting in patients is not without risk because of the potential for skin ulceration under the cast. Because many of these children regain the ability to walk, long bone malunions can be a source of morbidity and should be avoided. These issues have led to the

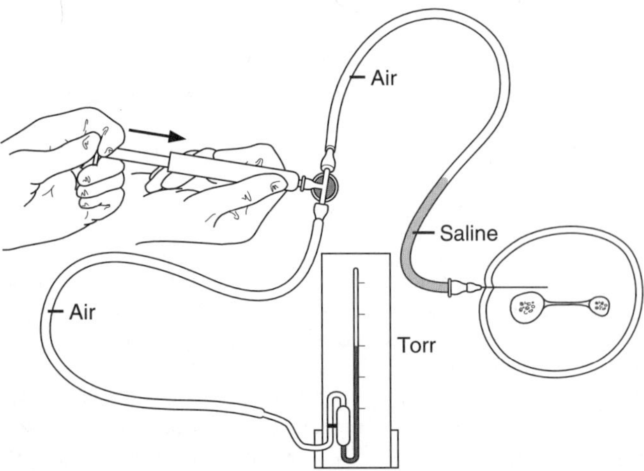

FIG. 25-4. A needle, IV tubing, three-way stopcock, syringe, and mercury manometer can be used to measure compartmental pressure. When the saline–air meniscus in the tubing moves, the pressure on the manometer is recorded. Digital pressure transducers are also available. (After Rang M. Children's fractures, ed 2. Philadelphia, JB Lippincott, 1983)

use of internal or external fixation in patients with injuries resulting in muscle spasticity.[15]

Care should be taken in the acute phase of head injury management to prevent joint and muscle contractures.[16] Contractures can have a detrimental effect on the patient's rehabilitation. Both range-of-motion therapy and splinting are necessary to avoid deformity. The muscular spasticity can be strong enough to break splints and to cause skin ulcerations, so diligence is necessary.

VASCULAR INJURY

Vascular injury associated with a closed fracture is uncommon in children; however, it can occur with essentially any fracture.[11] At the moment of fracture, the bone ends become widely displaced, stretching the accompanying soft tissues, including the neurovascular bundle. This can create intimal injury or direct laceration and can lead to entrapment of the vessels between the fracture fragments.

Several fractures can cause vascular insult. These include the supracondylar humerus fracture with brachial artery injury, fractures around the knee with distal superficial femoral or popliteal vessel injury, and open fractures in general. Associated clavicle and first rib fractures and sternoclavicular separations can injure the innominate and subclavian vessels.

CERVICAL SPINE

Neck injuries in children are usually the result of significant trauma. They differ from adult neck injuries in the following ways:

1. They occur less frequently in children.
2. A child's head is large in proportion to the rest of the body in infancy and early childhood. This, in combination with lack of muscular head control, leads to unique patterns of injury. Most children's cervical spine injuries occur in the upper three vertebrae. In the mature skeleton, the injuries are more common in the lower cervical spine.
3. Ligamentous laxity, the presence of growth plates, and large amounts of unossified cartilage also contribute to the unique features of pediatric spine injuries.[17,18]

Most cervical spine injuries in young children are due to birth trauma, motor vehicle accidents (as passengers), or shaken baby syndrome. Children struck as pedestrians infrequently sustain cervical fractures. In older children, sports, falls from heights, and gunshot wounds are significant causes.

Growth and Development

Some stages of growth simulate traumatic abnormalities. The first cervical vertebra or atlas develops from three ossification centers: one anteriorly in the midline, which may not appear until late in the first year, and one on each side posterolaterally to complete the ring. The ring may not fuse posteriorly for several years.

The axis or second cervical vertebra contains four centers. Its unique feature is the peglike odontoid process (also called the dens), which embryologically is derived from part of the body of C-1 but in reality is not connected to it. It serves to stabilize C-1 and C-2 during rotation, flexion, and extension. There is a physis at the bottom of the odontoid at the junction with the body of C-1.[19] This usually fuses by 6 years of age. This physis can be mistaken for a fracture. There is also a small ossicle at the tip of the odontoid, the ossiculum terminale, which fuses by 12 years of age.

The odontoid is stabilized against the ring of C-1 by the transverse ligament. The normal space between C-1 and the dens in children is up to 4 mm in flexion (Fig. 25-5). The space inside of the ring of C-1 can be conceptualized in thirds: one third of the diameter is occupied by the spinal cord, one third is occupied by the odontoid, and one third is free space.

The vertebral bodies in childhood are not as rectangular as in adulthood. This may give the appearance of a compression

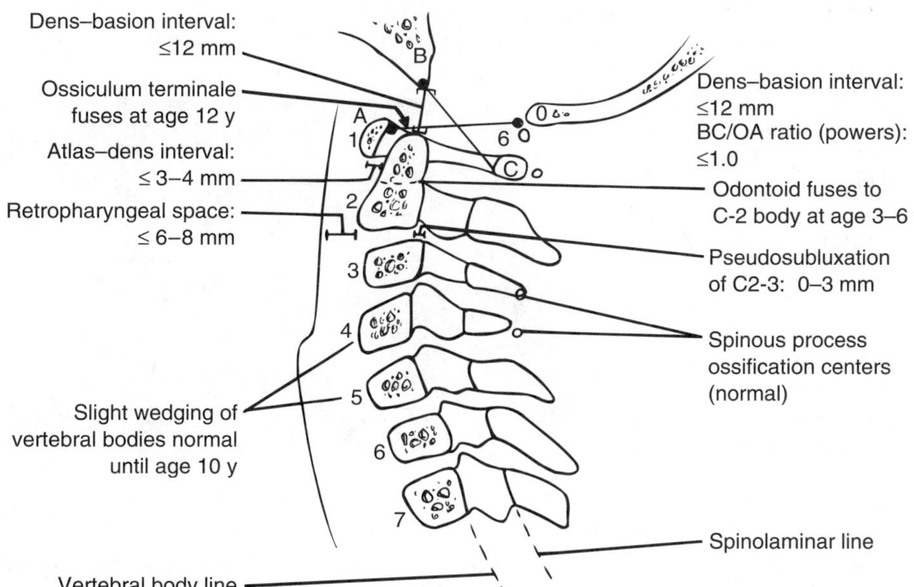

FIG. 25-5. Normal values on the pediatric lateral cervical radiograph.

injury but is simply due to the lack of complete ossification of the rectangular cartilaginous mold.

Physical Examination and Immediate Care

In the trauma setting, a spine injury should always be presumed to be present until proven otherwise. The neck should be palpated for tenderness or swelling. Motor function can be assessed by looking for movement at each major joint, and sensation should be tested at each limb segment. Head injuries or facial lacerations should increase the level of suspicion of cervical spine injuries.[20] Neck guarding, stiffness, or holding the head still with the hands can all be signs of an injury to the spine in an awake patient. Pulmonary arrest or the presence of clonus without decerebrate rigidity also may be a sign of spine trauma. The unconscious patient should be kept immobilized until radiographs show no signs of injury. This should include a backboard for the entire spine and sandbags and tape for the head. Hard cervical collars are often available, but they permit some degree of motion and are best supplemented with sandbags and tape. Foam cervical collars have no value and give a false sense of immobilization.

The head in a young child is relatively large, so placing it flat on a backboard forces the neck into relative flexion.[21] It is therefore recommended that adult backboards be modified by either a cut-out for the head or an extra mattress beneath the trunk. This applies in children 8 years of age and younger.

If a child is injured with an athletic helmet on, it should be left on during transport. This avoids the additional movement of removing it. The face mask should be removed to allow for airway control.

If intubation is needed, it should be done carefully. Avoid flexing and extending the neck. Theoretically, nasotracheal intubation can be done with less movement than orotracheal, but the orotracheal route is easier to carry out.

Radiography

Cervical radiography may not be indicated in a trauma patient who is conscious and able to verify absence of neck pain. The indications for radiography are the presence of neck pain, trauma to the head or face, or an unconscious patient. The lateral film is by far the most important. Anteroposterior and open mouth views may add additional information. Oblique views rarely add additional information owing to the rarity of subaxial subluxations in young children and the availability of better imaging modalities.

The film should be scrutinized for all seven cervical vertebrae (see Fig. 25-5). The alignment of the posterior vertebral bodies and the spinal laminae should form a smooth curve with no step-offs. The retropharyngeal space (in front of the cervical spine) should be less than 7 mm at C-2, and the retrotracheal space less than 14 mm at C-6. These figures may be increased somewhat by inspiration, but if greatly increased, may signal bleeding from an injury. The occipitoatlantal interval should also be scrutinized. A gap of over 10 mm between the basion and the dens or a Powers ratio of greater than 1 may signal disruption at his level. (*Powers ratio* is the distance from the front of the foramen magnum to the posterior cortex of C-1, divided by the distance between the posterior border of the foramen magnum to the anterior cortex of C-1.) Even when one spinal injury is seen, the rest of the spine should be carefully examined because multiple fractures occur in over 15% of all spinal injuries.

Children also may have spinal cord injury without radiographic abnormality (SCIWORA).[22] SCIWORA may be related to the elasticity of the spinal column when subjected to distraction forces. The spine tolerates four times as much stretch as does the spinal cord before failure (tearing) occurs. Other theories about the cause of SCIWORA include cord ischemia, cord compression by a hematoma, and compression by an epiphyseal cartilage end-plate fracture that is not seen on plain radiographs. These injuries account for 5% to 10% of all spinal cord injuries in children. An end-plate disruption can leave the spinal column unstable, so patients with SCIWORA should be immobilized until further workup is completed.

Immobilization

Many different devices are available for immobilization of the cervical spine, and they provide trade-offs in degree of immobilization and patient tolerance. A soft *cervical* (foam) *collar* allows almost full neck rotation and limits flexion and extension minimally. Therefore, it should not be used for unstable injuries. Its main role is for comfort in stable injuries. A *Philadelphia collar* fits around the mandible and over the upper thoracic spine. It is much more effective in controlling the upper cervical spine, but it does not control the lower cervical spine well.

Control of the lower cervical spine is better done with a *SOMI brace* (*s*terno*o*ccipito*m*andibular *i*mmobilizer), which extends over the upper thorax. The greatest rigidity is provided by the *halo vest* (Fig. 25-6) or the *Minerva* cast. The halo anchors to the skull with four to six pins. Its advantages are adjustability and freedom of jaw movement. The Minerva cast is used in younger children, with softer cranial bones, when the adjustability of the halo is not mandatory. The cast is more difficult to apply and provides less access for skin and wound care.

Care of the Patient With Spinal Cord Injury

About one third of cervical spine injuries include cord injury. It is impossible to judge the extent of the neurologic lesion until

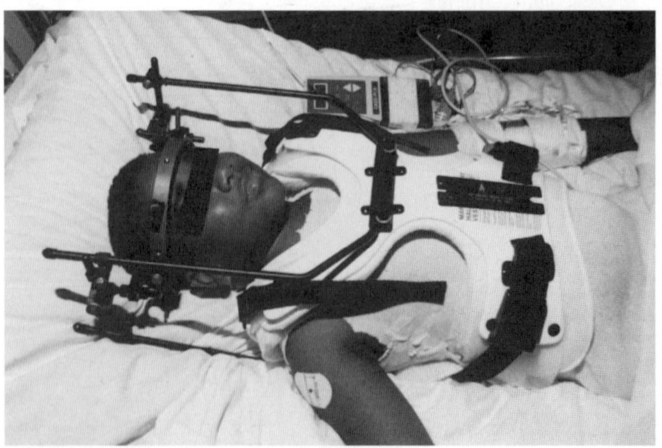

FIG. 25-6. Halo vest used to immobilize unstable cervical spine injury in a child. It is adjustable in multiple planes.

the end of spinal shock, as shown by the return of bulbocaverno-sus reflex. It is important to maintain systemic blood pressure to ensure cord perfusion. This may at times require special effort because neurogenic shock may mandate the use of extra volume or vasopressors. Intubation can also cause hypotension owing to vagal stimulation.

The use of steroids in acute spinal cord injuries is controversial. There is some evidence that high doses may protect the cord if given within 6 hours of injury. The usual dose is methylprednisolone, 30 mg/kg bolus, followed by 5.4 mg/kg/h for an additional 23 hours.[23]

Late effects of spinal cord injury include deformity, contractures, pressure sores, and autonomic dysreflexia. Spinal column deformity develops in nearly all children who sustain a cervical or thoracic paraplegia before the age of 10 years.[24]

Kyphosis can occur if there has been a laminectomy. Contractures can be minimized by paying attention to range of motion from the early stages of the injury. Prompt referral to an experienced rehabilitation facility is essential.

Specific Injuries

Occipitoatlantal Dislocation

The rare injury of occipitoatlantal dislocation poses the risk of complete pentaplegia. It is seen more commonly in hospitals because survival past the accident scene is occurring more frequently with modern emergency care. This injury is more common in children than adults because of the combination of a large head and relative laxity. Radiographic findings are a dens to basion distance of more than 1 cm or a Power ratio of greater than 1. When an occiput C-1 dislocation is seen, traction should be minimal to avoid stretching the cord. If the neurologic lesion is complete, functional recovery is unlikely; however, some patients have no neurologic injury.

Regardless of neurologic function, most physicians treat these injuries with posterior fusion. There have been a few reports of successful stabilization by a period of halo immobilization and no fusion, but the risk of occipitoatlantal instability is greater with this method.

Atlas (C-1) Fracture

This fracture, also known as a Jefferson fracture, is due to direct axial loading, with the occipital condyles splitting the ring of C-1. It is best evaluated by computed tomography (CT) because C-1 is largely a transversely oriented structure. Minimally displaced fractures can be immobilized in a Philadelphia collar. If significant spread of the lateral masses over 4 to 7 mm is seen on the anteroposterior radiograph, traction can be used to help reduce the fragments.

Traumatic Disruption of the Transverse Atlantal Ligament

Disruption of the transverse atlantal ligament is rare in children. If it occurs, it may allow increased translation in flexion and extension between C-1 and C-2 without obvious fracture. CT may reveal evidence of a bony avulsion, with a small fragment of C-1 attached to the avulsed transverse ligament. For acute transverse ligament disruptions, posterior fusion is recommended.

Other causes of C-1 to C-2 instability that are typically chronic in nature include juvenile rheumatoid arthritis, Down syndrome, and many of the skeletal dysplasias. In chronic cases, if there is more than 5 mm of C-1 to C-2 translation, restriction from contact sports is advised. If there is greater than 10 mm of chronic subluxation or any neurologic change, posterior fusion is advised.

Atlantoaxial Rotatory Subluxation

Atlantoaxial rotatory subluxation can be traumatic or atraumatic. In atraumatic cases, it usually follows a pharyngitis that causes ligamentous laxity, allowing one side of C-1 to slip forward and down on C-2. Plain films are notoriously difficult to interpret for this injury because there is no true anteroposterior plane for the radiograph. CT scans are helpful in making this diagnosis (Fig. 25-7). For the CT scan, the patient should be positioned in the scanner with the head appearing centered and

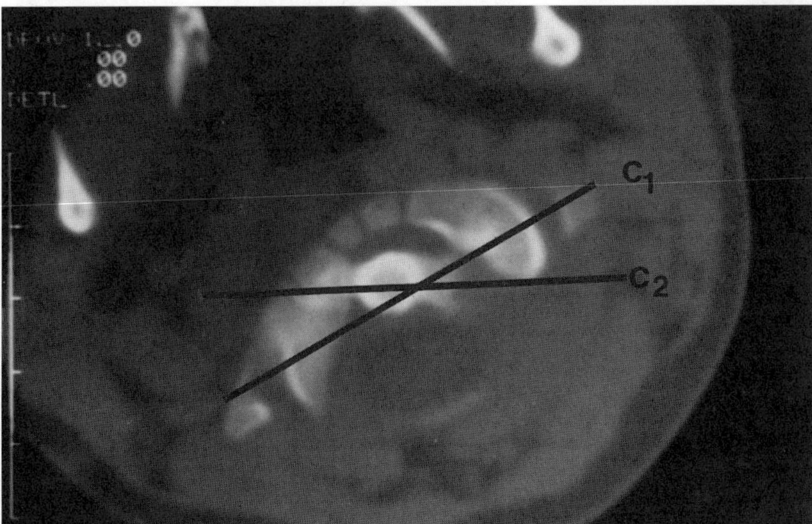

FIG. 25-7. Appearance of C-1-C-2 rotatory subluxation on CT.

neutrally rotated so that any malalignment of C-1 or C-2 can be judged as abnormal. In addition, if desired, CT images with voluntary right and left head rotation can be done.

The clinical appearance is that of torticollis. The head is rotated in one direction and laterally flexed in the other direction—a typical "cock robin" appearance. Treatment depends on the duration of symptoms.[25] If less than 1 week, a soft cervical collar, combined with rest and stretching exercises, may allow the subluxation to reduce spontaneously. If this is not successful, or if symptoms have persisted for more than 4 weeks, halter (soft) traction in bed should be tried. If reduction is still not possible, halo traction may be needed. If the subluxation does not reduce, a fusion in situ at C-1 to C-2 usually results in the clinical appearance of normal head alignment, even if the C-1 to C-2 rotation is not perfectly reduced.

Odontoid Fractures

Odontoid fractures usually occur at the level of the dens physis (Fig. 25-8). They have an excellent healing rate in children. They should be treated with rigid immobilization in a Minerva cast or halo. The halo can also be used for manipulation or traction if the fracture alignment is not adequate. Six to eight weeks of immobilization are needed, followed by an additional month in a protective orthosis.

Os Odontoideum

Os odontoideum is a large ossicle at the level of the dens that is not joined to the body of C-2. It allows instability of C-

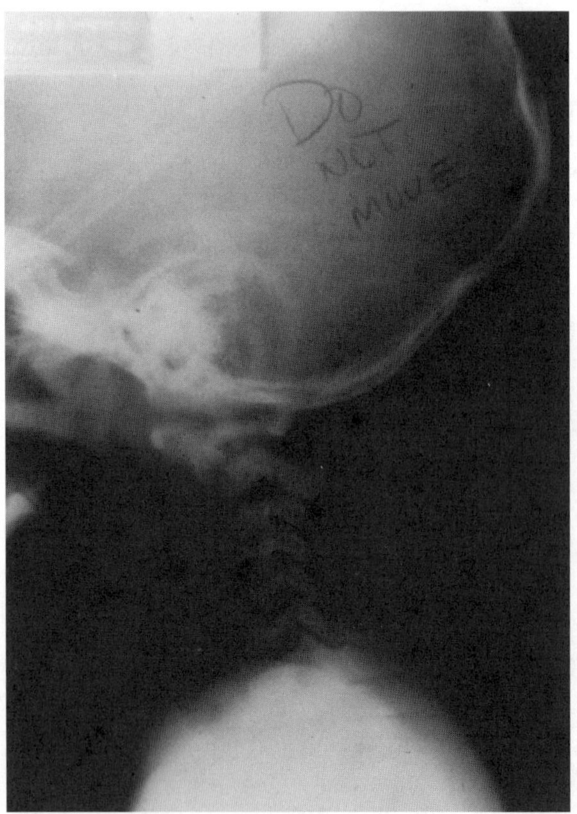

FIG. 25-8. Odontoid fracture before reduction.

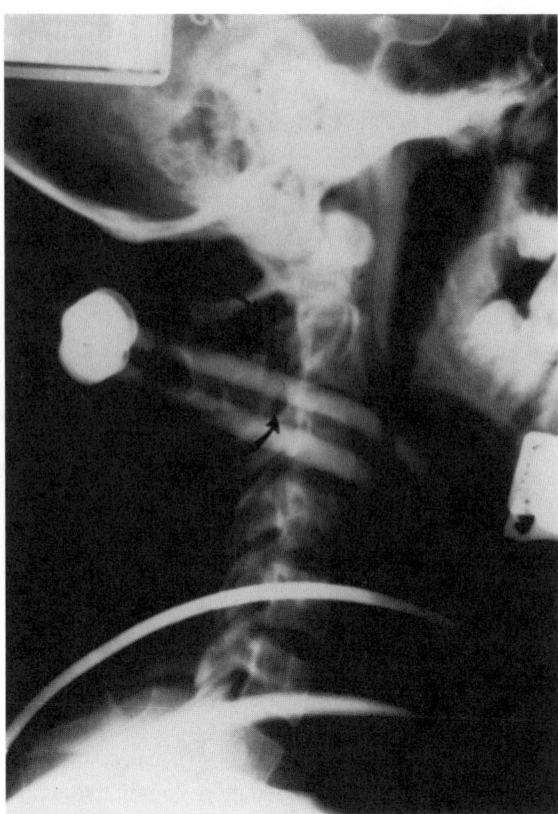

FIG. 25-9. Hangman's fracture or spondylolysis of C-2 is a hyperextension injury with fracture.

1 on C-2. This was previously considered to be a congenital anomaly, but Fielding[26] reported on a series of patients with previously normal odontoids on radiographs who presented much later with os odontoideum. Therefore, it is now thought to be an unrecognized fracture that develops into chronic non-union. Treatment guidelines are the same as for chronic transverse ligament avulsion.

Pedicle Fracture of C-2 (Hangman's Fracture)

Hangman's fracture is due to forced hyperextension—hence the name (Fig. 25-9). Usually, it is minimally displaced.[27] Most cases are stable because of an intact C-2 to C-3 disk anteriorly that maintains stability. These fractures can be treated with a Philadelphia collar or a Minerva cast. If a disk disruption occurs, evidenced by widening of the disk space or an avulsion fracture on the vertebral body margin, instability may be present. In this case, the alignment of the bony elements should be carefully checked, and the patient should be immobilized in a halo, with consideration given to fusion.

Pseudosubluxation of C-2 on C-3

Up to 3 mm of apparent subluxation may be normal in children. This is the level of greatest intervertebral translation, owing to the relatively horizontal facets. To differentiate physiologic subluxation from pathologic subluxation, the Swischuk line is drawn between the laminae of C-1 and C-3. If the lamina of C-2 falls more than 2 mm anterior to this line, the subluxation is not physiologic. Pathologic subluxation is rare, however.

Subaxial Injuries (Below C-2)

Lower cervical injuries occur mainly after 8 years of age, when childhood injury patterns begin to resemble those of adults.[20] Vertebral body fractures usually can be treated by immobilization. Subluxation and dislocation should have a trial of reduction by traction, followed by open reduction if needed. In the case of complete dislocation, a magnetic resonance (MR) imaging scan should be obtained to rule out an associated disk herniation before any attempt is made to achieve reduction with traction. This disk herniation could produce acute cord compression once the dislocation is reduced, creating neurologic injury. If a disk herniation is present, it is removed first in this situation.

THORACIC AND LUMBAR SPINE

Developmental Anatomy and Biomechanics

The thoracic and lumbar spinal vertebrae are developmentally less variable than the cervical spine.[1] Each vertebra develops from three main ossification centers: one in the center of the vertebral body and one on each side, posterolaterally, forming the neural arch. All of these growth regions are fused by 4 to 6 years of age. Further longitudinal growth of the vertebral bodies is provided by the vertebral end plate. The conus medullaris is at the level of L-1.

Biomechanically, orthopedic surgeons conceptualize the thoracic and lumbar spine as being made of three columns. The middle column is the key. This is the posterior one third of the vertebral body and its associated ligaments. The anterior and posterior columns are on either side of the middle column.

Several biomechanical features are unique in a child's spine. First, the ligaments between the vertebrae are stronger in tension than the bone or the growth plates. This means that fractures often occur in tension through either the growth plate (physis) or the bone.[28] Second, the bone is stronger in compression loading than adult bone, so burst and compression fractures are not as common in children. If they happen, the amount of bony collapse is usually not as great as that seen in adults. Multiple fractures in different areas are also common in children.

Biologically, children have an advantage over adults in that they undergo more rapid healing and have lower nonunion rates. They also have a greater ability to reconstitute vertebral height if there is a compression fracture because of further skeletal growth. Typically, childhood spinal injuries start to assume the characteristics of adult injuries after 12 years of age.

Physical Examination

The patient with back pain or a loss of responsiveness after severe trauma should be kept on a backboard until complete evaluation is possible. If turning is necessary, it should be done as a unit. This "logrolling" is done by moving the pelvis, shoulders, and neck at the same time, keeping them in the same relative alignment.

Physical examination should include scrutiny for telltale skin bruising from lap belts as well as abdominal tenderness. Palpation for tenderness should be done posteriorly to localize the level of injury, both in the midline and in the paraspinous muscles. The neurologic examination of the extremities should include motor, sensory, and reflex testing. A rectal examination should be done by some member of the team and documented. Neurologic status may change, so the neurologic examination should be repeated at least daily and any time there is a significant event such as a transfer.

Radiography

Plain radiographs provide at least 90% of the necessary information, especially the alignment and displacement. A CT scan is not necessary in many childhood spinal fractures. CT is necessary, however, to discover bony fragments impinging on the spinal canal. CT studies can be reconstructed in the coronal and sagittal planes, but there is usually a significant "step" artifact, unless the original cuts are requested in small increments, such as 2 mm. Plain tomograms may be preferable if the primary goal is to obtain detailed information about the sagittal plane.

MR imaging provides excellent visualization of soft tissue problems, such as herniated nucleus pulposus, hematoma in the canal or cord, or posttraumatic cyst. Therefore, MR imaging should be done on almost every child with a neurologic deficit. It is unable, however, to provide the fine bony architectural detail seen with plain radiography or CT scans. In general, the imaging studies should be ordered after consultation with the orthopedic surgeon or neurosurgeon who is helping to manage the patient.

One of the goals of the evaluation is to understand the mechanism of injury. This helps the treating physician to determine the stability of the spinal column as well as understand the mechanism of neurologic injury. Different forces applied to the spine generate different injuries. Common force vectors are flexion, flexion–distraction, and axial loading.

Specific Injuries

Compression (Flexion) Fractures

In compression fractures, the anterior portion of the vertebra is compressed, with preservation of the structures around the spinal canal (the middle column is intact). This type of fracture results from flexion around an axis within the vertebral body, that is, a forward "crunch." The importance of this axis becomes clear when compared with seat belt injuries, discussed on the following page. Usually, the compression of the vertebra is less than 20%, which is of little long-term significance. Clinically, because the middle column (the bone anterior to the cord) is intact, neurologic injury is rare. More than one vertebra may be fractured in the same area owing to the elasticity of the spine, and this possibility should be explored on the radiographs. Plain films are generally satisfactory for evaluating this injury.

If the amount of compression is less than 20%, the patient usually is comfortable within a few days and can be mobilized as symptoms permit without any external immobilization. If the compression is greater than this, or if multiple vertebrae are involved, a cast or brace may be needed.

Burst Fractures

Burst fractures differ from compression fractures in that they involve the middle column of the vertebra. There is a risk of neurologic injury from bone impinging on the spinal canal. The amount of vertebral collapse is greater than in a compression fracture. On plain radiographs, if the middle column is severely fractured, there may be widening of the space between the pedicles on the anteroposterior view and a decrease in posterior cortical height on the lateral film.

If the patient has no neurologic compromise, and the deformity is not excessive (less than 20 degrees angulation), the treatment may be nonoperative, with early mobilization in a cast or brace.[29] If there is a neurologic deficit or an unacceptable deformity, decompression and reduction with internal fixation are recommended. This may be done through an anterior or a posterior approach, depending on the surgeon's preference. In most cases of incomplete neurologic deficit, at least some improvement occurs with time.

Flexion–Distraction (Seat Belt) Fractures

Patients subjected to a sudden deceleration while in seat belts without shoulder harnesses are vulnerable to this unique pattern of spinal fracture. Although the body undergoes forcible flex-

ion, the axis of flexion is outside the body; it is the seat belt around which the body is stretched. Therefore, the spine is actually *distracted*. The injury involves all three columns of the spine. The fracture line can travel through the bone or through the growth plate, or the disruption can occur through the ligaments (dislocation).[30,31] The spinal cord can be stretched. In extreme cases, there can be dural rupture. The pressure from the seat belt often produces a characteristic ecchymosis on the anterior abdomen (Fig. 25-10A) and can produce internal visceral damage such as renal contusion or intestinal disruption.

Children appear more prone to this injury than adults because they often will not or cannot wear shoulder harnesses. These harnesses often rest across the face or neck of a small child, and the smaller iliac crest of the child does not provide much purchase for the seat belt. The problem is made worse by the fact that the seat may be too wide for the smaller legs to rest on comfortably, thereby encouraging children to slouch on the seat. A booster seat may help the child be more safely restrained by increasing the child's effective height (for the shoulder harness) and allowing the knees to flex and the seat belt to anchor the pelvis better.

A seat belt–type visceral injury should lead to a search for spinal fractures, and vice versa, because these associated injuries are sometimes missed (see Fig. 25-10B). Treatment of the fracture usually involves reduction by hyperextension of the patient. Rolling the patient supine on top of a padded bolster may accomplish this. If the fracture reduces and the injury is through the bony elements only, it can be treated with a hyperextension cast. Patients in hyperextension and body casts should be watched for superior mesenteric artery syndrome. If the in-

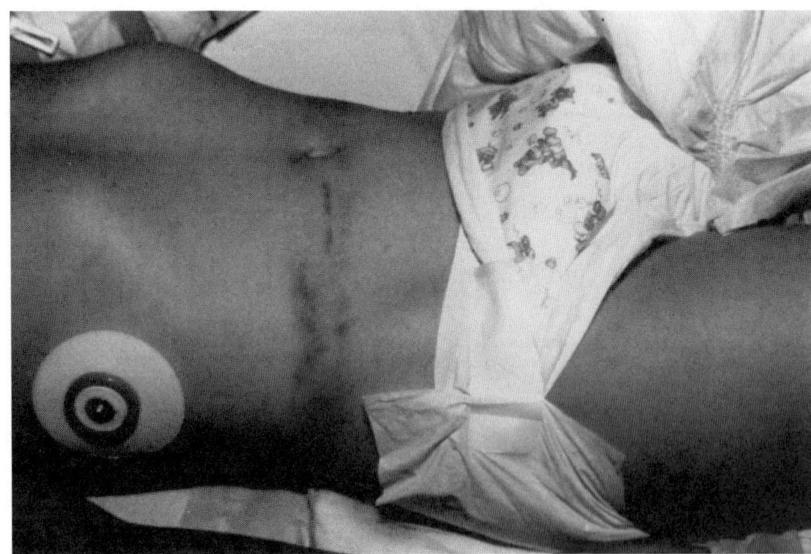

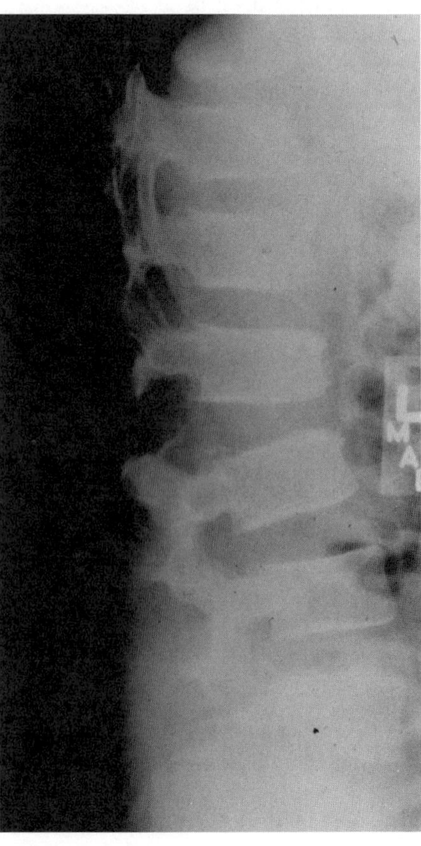

FIG. 25-10. (*A*) Seat belt injury without shoulder harness produces a classic tread-like abdominal ecchymoses. (*B*) Radiograph of a flexion–distraction spine injury.

jury is primarily a dislocation, healing probably will not be adequate to provide spinal stability, and fusion may be needed.

Flexion–Rotation Injury

Flexion–rotation injury occurs rarely in children. This injury has a high incidence of neurologic damage. Closed reduction is often not possible. Otherwise, principles follow those outlined for seat belt injuries.

Spinal Cord Injury Without Radiographic Abnormality

In SCIWORAs, the bony elements can be stable or unstable. Therefore, it is advisable to immobilize the patient until MR imaging can shed some light on the pathology.

Spondylolysis

Spondylolysis is a fracture of the pars interarticularis. It is most common at L-5. Usually, this is an unrecognized developmental injury that occurs in early childhood. Later, trauma may cause the spondylolysis to become recognized as an incidental finding, or it may become symptomatic. Oblique radiographs focused on the affected vertebra usually show the pars defect; at times, a CT scan is needed. If the fracture has sclerotic edges, it is old and can be treated symptomatically with rest followed by gradual mobilization and exercises. In rare cases, however, spondylolysis is caused by the new trauma. These patients should be treated with a cast or brace for 6 to 8 weeks to try to achieve fracture healing.

If there is question about the age of the fracture, a bone scan may resolve the issue. It should only show increased activity if the fracture is recent.

''Minor Injuries'' of the Spinous Process or Transverse Process

Injuries that do not involve the axial load-bearing elements of the spine are stable. They may, however, signal injury to more important structures, such as the pelvis or viscera. In addition, there may be significant muscle spasm because these processes serve as muscle attachment sites. No specific treatment is required other than analgesics.

Pelvic Fractures

Pelvic fractures are typically high-impact injuries. A large amount of force must be applied to create a fracture of the pelvic ring. Contrary to the adult scenario, a child's pelvis is more elastic and thus can have a single break in the pelvic ring (the adult must have at least two fractures in the ring for displacement to occur).

Physical examination often shows tenderness to palpation around the pelvis. Destot sign—a hematoma at the inguinal ligament or in the scrotum—may be present. Radiography should include an anteroposterior view of the pelvis. If a fracture

is seen or suspected, additional views allow formulation of a treatment plan. These include inlet and outlet views of the pelvis, or alternatively, CT. Care should be taken in transporting these patients during initial evaluation because there is always the possibility of significant intrapelvic hemorrhage.

Because the pelvic fracture indicates significant trauma, associated injuries are usually present.[32] Head injuries are common. The same force that creates the fracture can also cause injuries to the genitourinary system, the intraabdominal viscera, and peripheral nerves. Life-threatening hemorrhage can occur from arterial injury or tearing of the plexus of veins within the pelvis.

Evaluation of the skeletal injury of the pelvis centers around the concept of stability. If the fracture fragments are going to maintain their relative alignment, and if there is no ongoing soft tissue injury from the motion of the fracture fragments, the injury is considered stable. The forces that create the injury can be directed either in the anteroposterior direction, from the lateral side, or as vertical shear (directed in a cephalad to caudad vector).[33] These force vectors can be deduced in part from the radiographs. Depending on the pattern of injury, associated ligamentous injury around the pelvis can be predicted, and an assessment of stability can be made (Fig. 25-11A). The unstable fractures are of concern because of possible continued soft tissue injury and hemorrhage caused by the movement of the bony fragments.

Most childhood pelvic fractures are stable, requiring only minimal intervention, such as bed rest. Long-term sequelae in these cases are unusual. If there is bony instability, external fixation to stabilize the bone fragments can be applied rapidly (see Fig. 25-11B). This decreases the motion of the disrupted pelvis, limits ongoing soft tissue injury, and helps control hemorrhage.

LOWER EXTREMITY

Hip Fractures

Hip fractures in children carry the potential for significant lifelong morbidity. Operative intervention is often prudent. Avascular necrosis, nonunion, malunion, and growth disturbances with subsequent deformity are all known complications after these fractures. Depending on the level of the fracture along the femoral neck, the rate of avascular necrosis ranges from 14% at the intertrochanteric level to nearly 100% at the physeal level.[1] These sequelae have pronounced lifelong consequences.

Unlike in adults, children's hip fractures are usually related to severe trauma. On examination, there is pain and often shortening and external rotation of the lower extremity. Fractures of the femoral neck are typically managed by pin fixation to control alignment.

Femoral Shaft Fractures

Femur fractures occur in a wide variety of circumstances. They can be related to severe trauma, such as an auto–pedestrian or motor vehicle accident, and they can occur at home or on the playground. These fractures have excellent healing

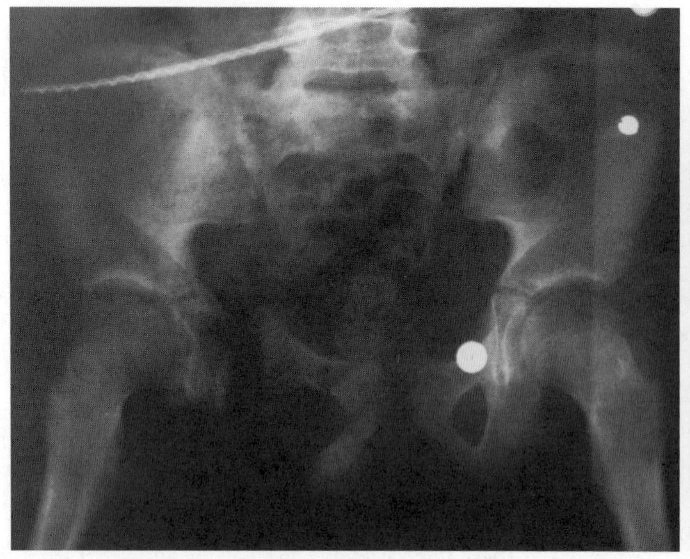
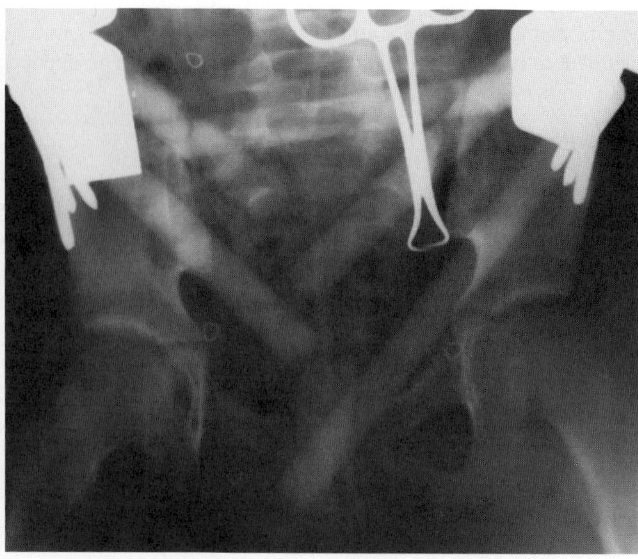

FIG. 25-11. (*A*) Pelvic fracture resulting from an anteroposterior-directed force. There is wide displacement of the fractures through the superior and inferior pubic rami on the right side of the patient. The right hemipelvis has been "hinged" open (similar to opening a book). (*B*) An external fixator has been applied, and the right hemipelvis is closed.

potential, and fracture union occurs even with wide displacement of the fracture ends.

Diagnosis is usually obvious on physical examination, with shortening and external rotation of the involved extremity. The traction splints in which patients are transported by ambulance personnel should be removed as soon as possible to avoid skin complications from the traction straps.

Once removed from the traction splint, simple splinting with plaster, or skin traction applied using adhesive tapes on a thin layer of cast padding, provides satisfactory control of the leg during the trauma evaluation.

Traction and casting provide good results in most patients. Children between the ages of 2 and 10 years often demonstrate overgrowth of the extremity after a femur fracture. Thus, the physician can accept 1 to 2 cm of shortening of the fracture fragments in a cast. In fact, slight overlap of the fracture fragments is preferable in this age group. Overgrowth is much less predictable in children older than 10 years of age, and the amount of fracture fragment shortening should be minimized in these patients.

Using these concepts, early spica (body) casting has gained favor. Children with isolated femur fractures can have casts applied and be discharged from the hospital within 1 or 2 days, instead of spending several weeks in traction before casting. When using this method of treatment, close radiographic follow-up is necessary. If excessive shortening (more than 2 to 2.5 cm in the 2- to 10-year age group) occurs, the treatment modality should be modified to regain length. This includes using traction, a combination of percutaneous pins and a cast, external fixation, or internal fixation.

The treatment regimen for children is evolving. Prolonged inpatient traction is becoming less acceptable for both economic and social reasons. Children older than 10 years of age do not reliably demonstrate overgrowth. Patients with closed head injuries, bilateral femur fractures, multiple visceral injuries, and open fractures are not as easily managed by casting or traction

modalities. In these groups, other treatment options are being used. These include intramedullary rod fixation, external fixation, and internal fixation with compression plates. The treatment regimens employed are becoming more individualized based on the age of the patient, the family situation, and the concomitant injuries (Fig. 25-12).

Fractures of the Supracondylar Femur and Distal Femoral Physis

Fractures of the supracondylar femur and distal femoral physis are notable for their sequelae. They are difficult to hold well aligned with a cast alone and often require pin fixation or internal fixation. About 65% of the growth of the leg occurs around the knee, with the distal femur contributing about 35% of the entire length of the leg. Leg length discrepancies and angular deformities occur in about one third of these patients when the area of the growth plate is involved.[34] Although reports of vascular injury with these fractures are rare, vascular injury can occur because of the close relation with the popliteal vessels and the displacement of the bone.

Fractures of the Proximal Tibial Physis

Fractures of the proximal tibial physis are uncommon injuries; however, vascular compromise is a distinct possibility after these fractures, and patients should be carefully observed. The popliteal artery is at risk. Both complete laceration and occlusion of the popliteal artery have been reported, resulting in amputation.[35]

Tibial Fractures

Tibial shaft fractures can result from twisting forces or from a direct blow. These fractures can present with minimal defor-

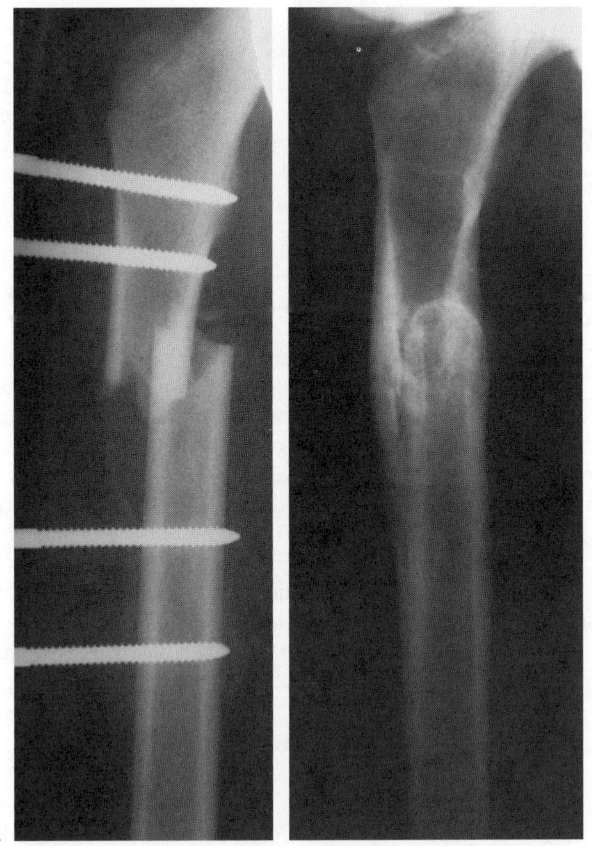

FIG. 25-12. (*A*) Femur fracture treated with an external fixator. The fracture ends were overlapped in this patient, anticipating overgrowth. (*B*) The fracture as remodeled.

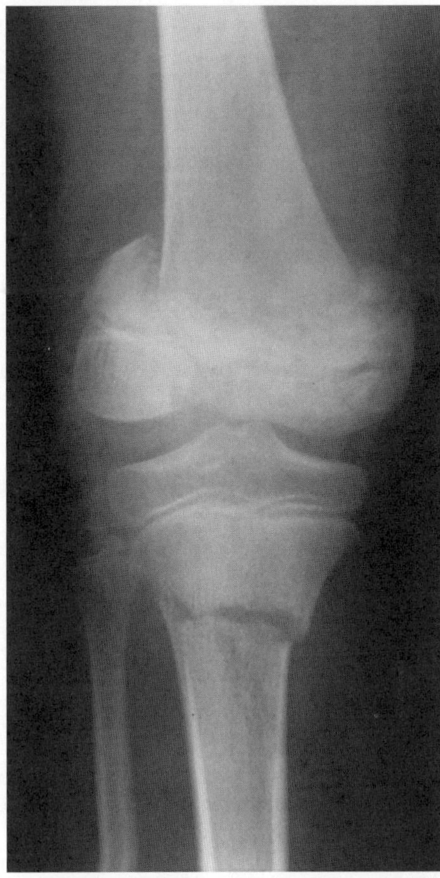

FIG. 25-13. Comminuted Salter-Harris type IV fracture of the distal femur with a proximal tibia fracture. The distal femur requires open reduction and internal fixation. Operative stabilization of the tibia with internal or external fixation simplifies postoperative fracture care and helps permit range-of-motion exercises earlier.

mity and little displacement, so that on clinical examination, only pain and localized swelling are noticeable. They also can have wide displacement and obvious deformity. It is important to evaluate the neurovascular status and to be wary for signs of a compartment syndrome.

Fractures of the tibia can often be managed by closed manipulation and cast immobilization. Like femur fractures, other considerations, such as head injury, open fractures, concomitant injuries, and inability to maintain adequate alignment, can alter treatment plans. The wide array of fixation options includes external fixation and intramedullary rod placement.

Floating Knee

''Floating knee'' occurs with ipsilateral fractures of the femur and tibia, and are typically seen after significant trauma, such as an auto–pedestrian accident. It is difficult to control the alignment of both fractures in a cast at the same time. Stabilization of at least one of these fractures using surgical means simplifies management and improves results[36] (Fig. 25-13).

Fractures of the Distal Tibial and Fibular Physis

The problems associated with fractures of the distal tibial and fibular physis are related to growth disturbance, angular deformity, and articular surface incongruity. For the inju-

rieswith greater than 2 mm of articular surface displacement, surgical reduction and fixation are recommended.

UPPER EXTREMITY

Clavicular Shaft Fractures

The clavicular shaft fracture is one of the most common fractures in children. These fractures usually can be treated using either a sling or a figure-of-eight dressing that wraps around the shoulders, holding them retracted. During healing and afterward, the fracture callus creates a bump that is noticeable to the patient and the family. It is helpful to counsel the family ahead of time regarding this cosmetic appearance.

Neurovascular compromise has been reported but is rare. The combination of a clavicle fracture and a first rib fracture should alert the physician to the possibility of vascular injury.

Sternoclavicular Injuries

Fractures and dislocations involving the medial end of the clavicle at the sternum are unusual. When posterior displacement occurs, compression of mediastinal structures is possible.

The patient typically presents holding the involved upper extremity to keep it still. There is pain to palpation over the area of injury. The swelling in the area of injury can mask the position of the medial clavicle and its relation to the sternum. Plain radiographs do not reveal this area well, and a 40-degree cephalad projection of the radiographic beam can be of help.[1] CT visualizes this well.

If posterior displacement is present with impingement on the mediastinum, as evidenced by diminished upper extremity pulses, venous engorgement, or difficulty with breathing, prompt closed reduction is desired. This is most easily done under general anesthesia with extension of the shoulder girdle using a bolster between the scapulae. A towel clip can then be used to pull the medial clavicle forward.[25] Vascular surgery consultation is a wise precaution.

Proximal Humerus and Humeral Shaft Fractures

Proximal humerus and humeral shaft fractures in children usually are treated with simple immobilization. A sling and swath are often all that is needed. In older children and adolescents, less angulation is acceptable because there is less growth and remodeling potential. Active intervention, such as pinning or open reduction, may be necessary.

In fractures of the distal humeral shaft, radial nerve palsy may be present. This should be documented carefully before any manipulation of the fracture. Occasionally, the nerve can become entrapped between the fracture fragments after the manipulation, necessitating surgical exploration.

If a patient has radial nerve function before any manipulation, but loses radial nerve function after the reduction attempt, exploration is warranted. Conversely, if a patient has no radial nerve function on presentation, observation for 8 to 12 weeks is recommended. After this time period has elapsed, nerve exploration should be undertaken if there is no evidence of return of function by clinical examination or nerve conduction studies.[37]

Elbow Fractures

Childhood elbow fractures can be particularly challenging for the orthopedic surgeon. With the various growth centers around the elbow, a large portion of the elbow in the young child is cartilaginous and therefore not visible on radiographs. A child with a swollen tender elbow after trauma should be considered to have a fracture until proven otherwise. Plain radiographs may initially show no fracture, so a high index of suspicion must be maintained. Oblique radiographic views of the injured side can be of great help, as can comparison views of the opposite elbow. Elbow arthrograms and MR images can help to further delineate injury to the cartilaginous growth centers of the elbow.

Supracondylar Humerus Fractures

Of the pediatric elbow injuries, supracondylar humerus fractures tend to produce the most apprehension in the treating

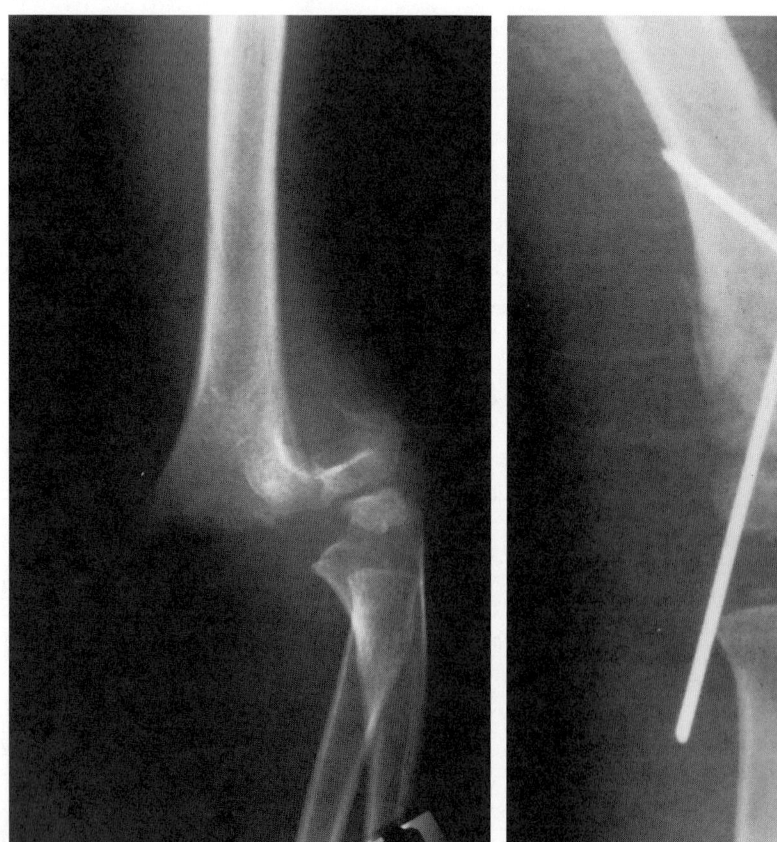
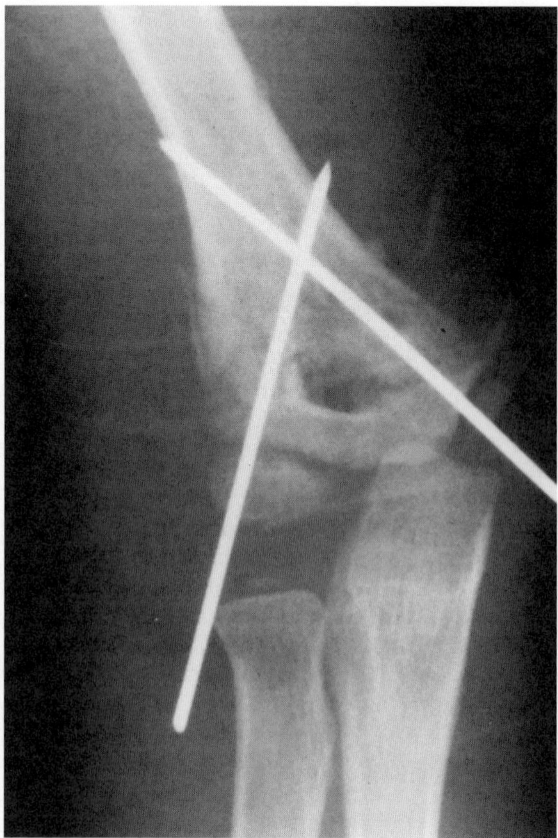

FIG. 25-14. (*A*) Completely displaced supracondylar humerus fracture. (*B*) Alignment after percutaneous fixation.

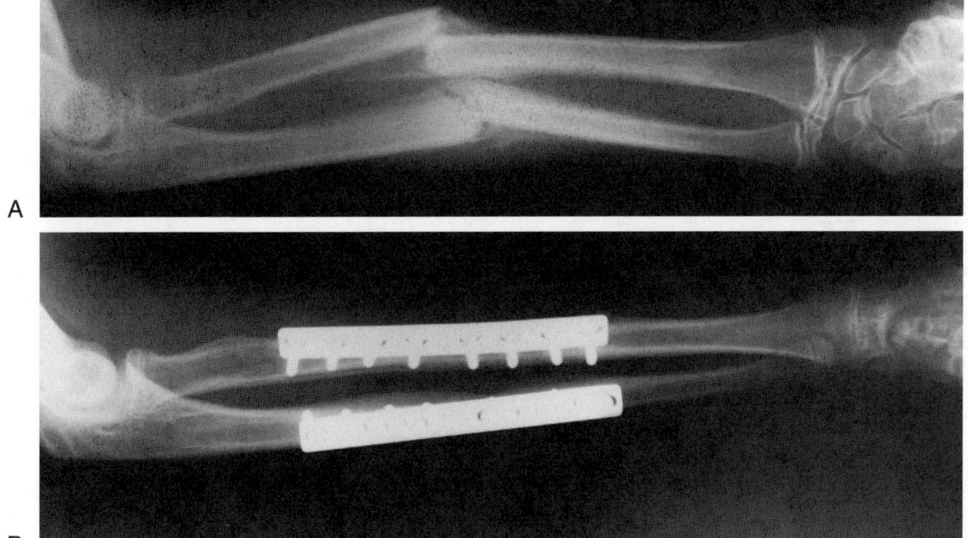

FIG. 25-15. (*A*) Early malunion of radius and ulna fractures. This amount of angulation limits pronation and supination of the forearm and is noticeable. (*B*) After open reduction and internal fixation with plates. The internal fixation obviates the need for a cast in this patient, allowing early rehabilitation to reestablish forearm rotation.

physician. With a displaced supracondylar fracture, there is always impressive swelling around the elbow. To reduce and then maintain an adequate position, the typical extension type of supracondylar fracture of the elbow must be placed in about 120 degrees of flexion. The problem with this position is the potential for vascular compromise in the face of soft tissue swelling. In the past, Volkmann contracture (ischemic necrosis of the forearm musculature from vascular compromise) was a sequela of this fracture.

With the realization that the elbow cannot be held in acute flexion owing to vascular concerns, other methods of treatment have evolved (Fig. 25-14). Percutaneous pinning in conjunction with casting has become the most widely used method. This allows the arm to be placed in an extended position while maintaining fracture alignment.

On presentation, the arm should be carefully checked for radial and ulnar artery pulses as well as for evidence of satisfactory distal perfusion. The brachial artery can be thrombosed, lacerated, or even trapped in the fracture site. If the circulatory status is questionable with the elbow flexed, the arm should be carefully moved to a more extended position to help improve perfusion. If this does not help, the patient should promptly be anesthetized, and a reduction maneuver should be performed. The fracture should be pinned in an acceptable position, and the arm should be extended. If distal perfusion is still inadequate, the brachial artery should be explored.[38] The anteromedial approach to the elbow is straightforward and is extensile, allowing access up the brachium and distally into the forearm.[39]

The mere presence of a distal pulse (radial or ulnar) does not guarantee that there is adequate perfusion of the muscle in the forearm, and a compartment syndrome should be looked for as well. Overall, the incidence of vascular injury with these fractures is about 5%.

Forearm Fractures

The radius is one of the most frequently fractured bones in children. Most of these injuries can be satisfactorily treated with manipulation and casting. The most difficult aspect of treating these injuries can be judging the rotational alignment. If the fracture is allowed to heal in a position of malrotation, significant pronation or supination of the arm can be lost (Fig. 25-15).

Several specific entities should be considered when evaluating the patient. Because the forearm consists of two bones, it is possible to have a fracture of one and a dislocation of the other. A Monteggia fracture is an ulna fracture with a radial head dislocation at the elbow. A Galeazzi fracture is a radius fracture with an ulnar dislocation at the wrist. To avoid missing one of these injuries, it is important to examine both the elbow and the wrist in a patient with a forearm fracture. Good visualization of both the elbow and the wrist on the radiographs is imperative.

In the care of a traumatized patient, much can be learned from a systematic examination of the musculoskeletal system, while paying close attention to the neurovascular status of each extremity. Open fractures, compartment syndromes, spine fractures, and neurovascular compromise are emergent situations and should be dealt with promptly. In the polytrauma patient, musculoskeletal and neurologic injuries are a major cause of morbidity. Orthopedic intervention can improve the acute management of the patient and help to avoid the long-term sequelae of these injuries.

REFERENCES

1. Rockwood CA, Wilkins KE, King RE, eds. Fractures in children. Philadelphia, JB Lippincott, 1991.
2. Marcus RE, Mills MF, Thompson GH. Multiple injury in children. J Bone Joint Surg 1983;65A:1291.
3. Ogden JA. Skeletal injury in the child, ed 2. Philadelphia, WB Saunders, 1990.
4. Albright JA, Brand RA, eds. The scientific basis of orthopaedics. East Norwalk, CT, Appleton & Lange, 1987.
5. Bachulis BL et al. Clinical indication for cervical spine radiographs in the traumatized patient. Am J Surg 1987;153:473.
6. Shaffer MA, Doris PE. Limitation of the cross table lateral view in detecting cervical spine injuries: a retrospective analysis. Ann Emerg Med 1981;10:508.

7. Salter RB, Harris WR. Injuries involving the epiphyseal plate. J Bone Joint Surg 1963;45A:587.

8. Gustilo RB, Anderson JT. Prevention of infection in the treatment of one thousand and twenty five open fractures of long bones: retrospective and prospective analysis. J Bone Joint Surg 1976;58A:453.

9. Matsen FA. Compartmental syndromes. New York, Grune & Stratton, 1980.

10. Hargens AR, Akeson WH, Mubarak SJ. Tissue fluid pressures: from basic research tools to clinical applications. J Orthop Res 1989;7:902.

11. Friedman RJ, Jupiter JB. Vascular injuries and closed extremity fractures in children. Clin Orthop 1984;188:112.

12. Gaspard DJ, Kohl RD Jr. Compartmental syndromes in which the skin is the limiting boundary. Clin Orthop 1975;113:65.

13. Bone L, Bucholz R. The management of fractures in the patient with multiple trauma. J Bone Joint Surg 1986;68A:945.

14. Loder RT. Pediatric polytrauma: orthopaedic care and hospital course. J Orthop Trauma 1987;1:48.

15. Ziv I, Rang M. Treatment of femoral fracture in the child with head injury. J Bone Joint Surg 1983;65B:276.

16. Hoffer M, Garrett A, Brink J, et al. The orthopaedic management of brain injured children. J Bone Joint Surg 1971;53A:567.

17. Aufdermaur M. Spinal injuries in juveniles. J Bone Joint Surg 1974; 56B:513.

18. Evans DL, Bethem D. Cervical spine injuries in children. J Pediatr Orthop 1989;9:563.

19. Lawson JP, Ogden JA, Bucholz RW, et al. Physeal injuries of the cervical spine. J Pediatr Orthop 1987;7:428.

20. McGrory BJ, Klassen RA, Chao EYS, et al. Acute fractures and dislocations of the cervical spine in children and adolescents. J Bone Joint Surg 1993;75A:988.

21. Herzenberg JE, Hensinger RN, Dedrick DK, et al. Emergency transport and positioning of young children who have an injury of the cervical spine. J Bone Joint Surg 1989;71A:15.

22. Pang D, Wilberger JE. Spinal cord injury without radiographic anomalies in children. J Neurosurg 1982;57:114.

23. Bracken M, Shepard MJ, Collins WF, et al. A randomized controlled trial of methylprednisolone or naloxone in the treatment of acute spinal cord injury. N Engl J Med 1990;322:1405.

24. Dearolf WW, Betz RR, Wogel LC, et al. Scoliosis in pediatric spinal cord injured patients. J Pediatr Orthop 1990;10:214.

25. Phillips WA, Hensinger RN. The management of rotatory atlanto-axial subluxation in children. J Bone Joint Surg 1989;71A:664.

26. Fielding JW, Griffin PP. Os odontoideum: an acquired lesion. J Bone Joint Surg 1974;56A:187.

27. Caffey J. The whiplash shaken infant syndrome. Pediatrics 1974;54: 396.

28. Yngve DA, Harris WP, Herndon WA, et al. Spinal cord injury without osseous spine fracture. J Pediatr Orthop 1988;8:153.

29. Weinstein JN, Collalto P, Lehman TR. Thoracolumbar burst fractures treated conservatively: a long-term followup. Spine 1988;13:33.

30. Johnson DL, Falci S. Diagnosis and treatment of pediatric lumbar spine injuries caused by lap belts. Neurosurgery 1990;26:434.

31. Smith WS, Kaufer H. Patterns in mechanisms of lumbar injury associated with lap seatbelts. J Bone Joint Surg 1969;51A:239.

32. Garvin KL, McCarthy RE, Barnes CL, et al. Pediatric pelvic ring fractures. J Pediatr Orthop 1990;10:577.

33. Burgess AR, Eastridge BJ, Young JW, et al. Pelvic ring disruptions: effective classification system and treatment protocols. J Trauma 1990; 30:848.

34. Lombardo SJ, Harvey JP. Fractures of the distal femoral epiphysis. Factors influencing prognosis: a review of thirty-four cases. J Bone Joint Surg 1977;59A:742.

35. Burkhart SS, Peterson HA. Fractures of the proximal tibial epiphysis. J Bone Joint Surg 1979;61A:996.

36. Letts M, Vincent M. The ''floating knee'' in children. J Bone Joint Surg 1986;68B:442.

37. Szalay EA, Rockwood CA. Fractured humerus with radial nerve palsy. Orthop Trans 1982;6:455.

38. Wilkins KE. The management of severely displaced supracondylar fractures of the humerus. Tech Orthop 1989;4:5.

39. Henry AK. Extensile exposure, ed 2. London, Churchill Livingstone, 1957.

Surgery of Infants and Children: Scientific Principles and Practice, edited by
Keith T. Oldham, Paul M. Colombani, and Robert P. Foglia.
Lippincott–Raven Publishers, Philadelphia, © 1997.

CHAPTER 26

Vascular Trauma

Kaj Johansen

At any age, injury to arteries and veins can be worrisome, risking either significant blood loss or organ or tissue ischemia. Because timely management of significant vascular injury is essential, accurate and efficient screening and diagnostic maneuvers are paramount in the trauma setting. In the context of ever more aggressive diagnostic and therapeutic interventions, recognition of the vascular risks of various iatrogenic maneuvers can significantly reduce the toll of such injuries.

This chapter focuses on important general concepts in the recognition and management of vascular trauma in general, emphasizing those anatomic, physiologic, diagnostic, and management features to be considered when the trauma victim is a newborn, infant, or child.

EPIDEMIOLOGY

Vascular injury constitutes about 1% of emergency admissions in a busy adult trauma center, most such trauma victims being young or middle-aged adults. Intended or accidental vascular injury is uncommon in infants and small children. At Harborview Medical Center in Seattle, among 837 vascular injuries managed in a recent 5-year period, only 65 (8%) occurred in patients aged 15 years or younger. Iatrogenic injury, either unintended or deliberate, predominates among cases of vascular trauma in the very young.[1]

Risk factors for traumatic vascular injury in infants and children may vary from those in adults. Blunt and especially penetrating trauma to the extremities or the torso places the axial vessels at risk. Fractures, dislocations, and crush injuries can cause acute or delayed vessel occlusion. Children are less likely to suffer penetrating trauma; likewise, blunt trauma in children is more commonly related to falls, bicycle or playground accidents, or other relatively low–kinetic-energy mechanisms of injury, and are less commonly the result of severe motor vehicular trauma. Although adults who are victims of vehicle–pedestrian accidents more commonly suffer extremity injury, small children in such settings have a higher likelihood of severe central nervous system trauma.

As in adults, the natural history of vascular injury and the long-term results of its repair are poorly documented. Few longitudinal studies are available to characterize outcome in this setting. Whether such stereotypic adult responses to injury as neointimal hyperplasia occur to the same degree in children is unclear. The child's greater collateral vascular reserve likely has an influence not only on the patency of vascular repairs but on whether an injury even initially results in noteworthy symptoms or signs.

ANATOMY AND PHYSIOLOGY

Infants and young children have relatively larger heads and torsos and relatively shorter extremities, which may explain the less common occurrence of extremity vascular trauma in the young. Major long bone fractures, joint dislocations, and their associated traction injuries to nearby vessels are also less common in infants and children. In children, major vessels are closer to the surface, and may be relatively more exposed to external trauma. On the other hand, because their vessels are diminutive, they are a smaller target. In addition, the kinetic energy applied in most pediatric trauma is substantially less than that experienced by adults.

Arteries and veins can sustain damage in multiple different ways. For example, penetrating trauma can partially or completely divide a vessel. Paradoxically, bleeding may be much worse when vessel disruption is incomplete. Total vessel transection often results in vascular constriction, probably mediated by vasoactive factors from the platelet–fibrin thrombus that immediately forms at a site of vascular injury and contraction of the media of the vessel. On the other hand, partial vessel disruption may result only in axial contraction, opening the wound further and permitting even more profuse bleeding.

The histologic structure of arteries provides a hint about how these vessels respond to blunt or penetrating trauma. Although the adventitia and the media contain substantial smooth muscle and elastin and can accommodate to axial, angular, or rotatory stress, the intima is inelastic and frequently fractures under such stresses. Such intimal disruptions, if they occupy a significant proportion of the vessel diameter, can result in partial or complete thrombosis of the vessel.

A particularly noteworthy response of young, healthy arteries, especially to blunt trauma or even the presence of an intralu-

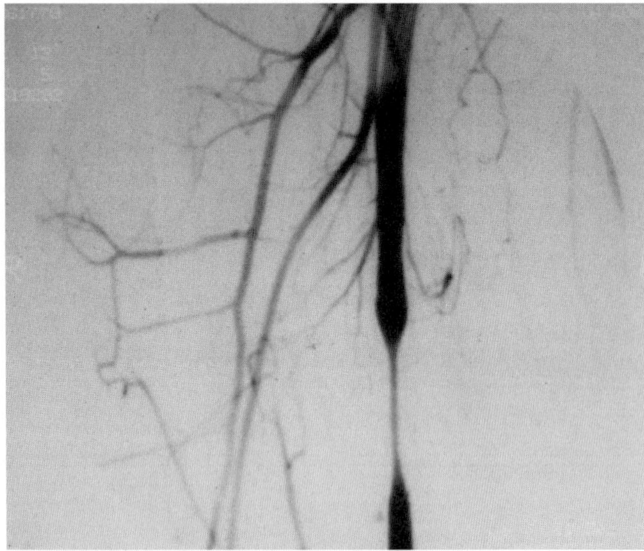

FIG. 26-1. Severe spasm of the superficial femoral artery resulting from a gunshot wound to the thigh in a 14-year-old boy. Repeat arteriography 8 hours later revealed an artery of normal caliber without luminal defect.

minal catheter, is spasm (Fig. 26-1). The physiology underlying arterial spasm remains incompletely understood[2]; its natural history, in the absence of actual structural damage to the artery, is that of gradual resolution over the space of minutes to hours.[3] Spasm is a common cause of reversible ischemic symptoms and signs. Whereas vascular obstruction is almost always caused by thrombus in the adult, an appreciable degree of obstruction in the pediatric population may be caused by reversible spasm.

A well characterized tissue response to ischemia underscores the urgency to restore perfusion in the presence of acute arterial insufficiency. Extensive clinical experience[4] corroborates the experimental observations of Miller and Welch[5] that irreversible tissue loss, most notably to peripheral nerve and skeletal muscle, occurs if severe normothermic ischemia persists beyond 6 hours. The acceptable duration of warm ischemia may be even shorter in circumstances of crush injury, systemic shock, or combined arterial and venous injury. No persuasive data exist to support a conclusion that infantile or juvenile tissues tolerate hypotension or ischemia any better than those of adults.

The degree to which acute arterial insufficiency threatens a limb or organ also is related to the extent to which perfusion can be maintained by collateral circulation. The physiologic basis for the presence and adequacy of collateral circulation is not well defined, and varies by anatomic location. In the adult setting, collateral recruitment is poor around the knee joint, but excellent around the shoulder joint. Thus, limb-threatening ischemia is commonplace after injuries to the popliteal artery (eg, after posterior knee dislocation), yet virtually unheard-of after trauma to the subclavian or axillary arteries (even complete occlusion of which rarely results in significant upper extremity symptoms of arterial insufficiency). Collateral circulation appears to be well developed in infants and children, for example as demonstrated by the observation of minimal or even absent signs of ischemia after axial artery occlusion.

Recognized promptly and managed properly, tissue ischemia

can be reversed and the tissue at risk saved. However, the importance of appreciating the implications of a resultant reperfusion injury have been emphasized. Although the underlying pathophysiology is incompletely understood, ischemia results in a ''leaky'' capillary bed, as well as the generation of oxygen radicals and other cytotoxic products of anaerobic metabolism.[6,7] With reperfusion, a substantial displacement of plasma volume into the extravascular space takes place, resulting in a rise in tissue pressure and potential occlusion of arterioles, venules, and capillaries. If the reperfused tissue is contained within an inelastic envelope (eg, the brain within the calvarium, calf or forearm muscle within an inexpansile fascia), tissue pressures may rise, further obstructing tissue perfusion (compartment syndrome). Besides prolonged or severe ischemia, reperfusion phenomena are worsened by systemic shock and combined arteriovenous injury, and appear to be mitigated by various oxygen radical scavengers, hypothermia, heparin, or partial or gradual reperfusion.[7,8]

CLINICAL PRESENTATION AND DIAGNOSIS

Vascular trauma can present with either overt signs of external or contained hemorrhage or as arterial insufficiency. Alternatively, occult vascular damage may have few, subtle, or no signs and symptoms, and may be discovered only after the passage of time or the performance of various diagnostic studies. Timely diagnosis of vascular damage is important to prevent significant blood loss or irreversible tissue or limb ischemia.

Significant hemorrhage is usually relatively easy to diagnose (Table 26-1). Pulsatile, bright red arterial bleeding from a wound, or a rapidly expanding, sometimes pulsatile hematoma at the site of a closed injury, are diagnostic of significant arterial hemorrhage. Bleeding into closed spaces may be more subtle: substantial blood loss can occur near fractures of the femur or pelvis, or in the retroperitoneum or chest, without significant external signs, and 20% of the circulating blood volume may be lost before hypotension and shock are noted. Central blood pressure is maintained by compensatory physiologic mechanisms, well developed in children, such as peripheral arterial and venous constriction, tachycardia, and central redistribution of blood volume. For these reasons, diagnostic techniques such as peritoneal lavage, ultrasound, or computed tomographic scanning may play a crucial adjunctive role adjunctive role to careful physical examination in young patients in whom the history or clinical setting suggests the potential for major occult hemorrhage.

TABLE 26-1. *Clinical evidence for significant arterial injury*

DEFINITIVE (''HARD'') SIGNS
Pulsatile bleeding from a wound
Rapidly expanding (possibly pulsatile) hematoma
Arteriovenous fistula (bruit, thrill)
Significant evidence for acute arterial insufficiency

SUGGESTIVE (''SOFT'') SIGNS
Unexplained shock or blood loss
Symptoms and signs of accompanying nerve damage
Wound hematoma
Diminished peripheral pulses
Proximity of wound trajectory

Interruption of blood supply results in a series of peripheral symptoms and signs, prompt recognition of which can prevent irreversible tissue ischemia. These clinical stigmata of acute arterial insufficiency are characterized as the "six P's" and include the symptoms of *paresthesia* (nonmyelinated peripheral C nerve fibers are exquisitely sensitive to ischemia) and *pain* (characteristically a dull, aching discomfort found in the most peripheral part of the extremity). Physical findings include *pallor* (the consequences of the loss of arterial blood to the cutaneous circulation), *pulselessness*, and hypothermia ("*polar*" or "*poikilothermia*"). *Paralysis* is a late and ominous finding suggesting advanced neuromuscular dysfunction due to prolonged ischemia.

As noted, the diagnosis of overt hemorrhage or acute arterial insufficiency, especially in the extremities, is relatively straightforward. Substantial interest has accompanied the evolution of diagnostic techniques for occult vascular injury, especially arterial interruption associated with blunt or penetrating trauma. Historically, a low threshold for surgical exploration of vessels at risk from a nearby fracture or gunshot wound was the standard in many trauma centers.[9] However, it became clear that the yield of routine exploration of vessels at risk for trauma but without overt signs of hemorrhage or ischemia is very low.[10] Because physical examination was held to be inadequately sensitive or specific,[9] routine contrast arteriography, highly sensitive and specific for occult arterial damage, became the gold standard for ruling out asymptomatic arterial damage.[11,12]

More recently, however, such screening or exclusion arteriography has been questioned. The technique has a small (2% to 5%) but not negligible incidence of false-positive and false-negative results.[13] It is invasive, time-consuming, and costly. Significantly, several studies have suggested that the clinical yield of routine screening arteriography is low; only 5% to 15% of such studies demonstrate *any* angiographic abnormality, and actual clinical management is significantly altered by such arteriographic screening in as few as 0% to 5% of cases.[13,14]

Since the mid-1980s, efforts to replace exclusion arteriography with various noninvasive diagnostic maneuvers, which may have equivalent accuracy and superior efficiency and cost-effectiveness, have occurred. Most significant has been the resurrection of careful serial physical examination for ruling in or out a significant occult arterial injury.[15] An important adjunct to the careful serial vascular examination has been the demonstration that Doppler arterial pressure measurements are a highly sensitive and specific means of detecting occult extremity arterial injuries. A prospective, contrast arteriography-controlled study suggested that Doppler arterial pressure indices are as accurate as arteriography in detecting occult extremity arterial injuries.[16] This study resulted in construction and validation of a management algorithm that reduced the necessity for screening arteriography by 80% and increased the clinical yield of contrast arteriography to 92% (Fig. 26-2).[17]

Although not yet established by controlled trials, a substantial experience suggests that duplex sonography, like Doppler arterial pressure measurements, offers a reliable noninvasive examination of peripheral vessels, and may well have a significant role to play in diagnosing acute vascular disruptions.[18,19] Duplex sonography can image accurately both arteries and veins. In addition, it can characterize subtle disruptions of the arterial wall as well as pseudoaneurysms and hematomas that might not be demonstrable by contrast arteriography. Because the

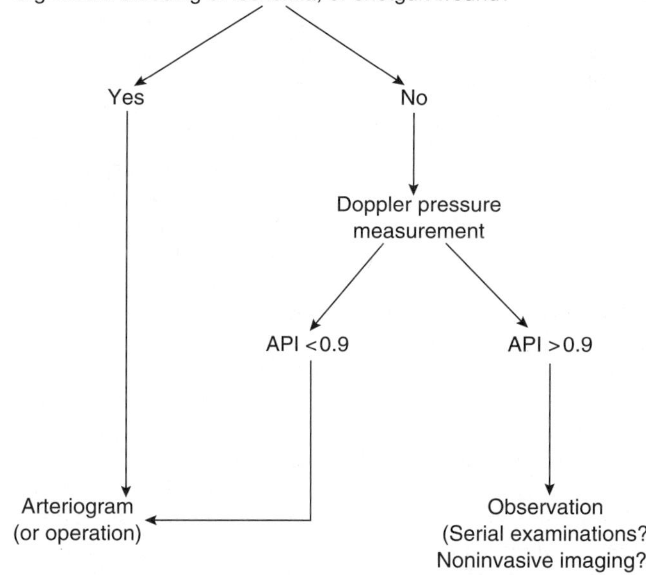

FIG. 26-2. Arteriography-validated management algorithm for patients potentially harboring an extremity arterial injury. API, arterial pressure index. (After Johansen K, Lynch K, Paun M, et al. Non-invasive vascular tests reliably exclude occult arterial trauma in injured extremities. J Trauma 1991; 31:515)

technique combines B-mode ultrasound with continuous-wave Doppler, alterations in the spectral waveform of the Doppler arterial signal can suggest the presence of luminal abnormalities as well. Comparison studies of various experimental canine arterial wounds have demonstrated that duplex scanning is more accurate than contrast arteriography, and markedly more accurate for detecting the presence of arterial laceration.[20] Several large surveys of duplex scanning in trauma victims have demonstrated its speed, accuracy, and cost effectiveness,[18,19,21] especially in corroborating the findings of physical examination or Doppler pressure measurement, or in high-risk or inaccessible areas (eg, the popliteal artery after knee dislocation, or in penetrating blunt or cervical trauma).

In neonates and infants, recognition of arterial occlusion may be hindered by these subjects' excellent collateral reserve, as well as their inability to communicate their symptoms. Femoral pulse palpation is an accurate indicator of aortic or iliac thrombosis after umbilical artery or transfemoral catheterization. Doppler studies may be performed, although the accuracy of Doppler arterial pressure indices for occult arterial injury in youthful trauma victims has not been validated. In settings where noninvasive vascular laboratory techniques are not feasible or not considered credible, arteriography remains the test of choice.

MANAGEMENT

Aggressive intervention after identification of significant vascular injury is usually warranted. The natural history of vascular disruptions, with certain exceptions, is unpredictable and frequently ominous. As emphasized in Chapter 19, it is crucial that the trauma victim be surveyed as "the whole patient" rather than just an ischemic leg or a hemorrhaging neck wound. Proper resuscitative, airway, and general diagnostic and supportive maneuvers always take precedence.

Proximal and distal control of a bleeding site is paramount, and is almost always obtained, in the extremities and in the neck, by direct pressure over the bleeding site (perhaps aided by wadded dressings, towels, or even clothing). Field or emergency room efforts at blind clamping of bleeding sites are usually risky, unnecessary, and inappropriate. Occasionally, bleeding control is obtained by the use of tourniquets or blood pressure cuffs, proximal to or over a wound. This practice is to be discouraged. Although hemorrhage from the bleeding site may be controlled by these techniques, they, unlike direct pressure, also may obliterate collateral arterial flow and therefore worsen distal tissue ischemia.

Operative exposure should be generous in vascular trauma patients, preferably over arteries and veins uninvolved by the injury or by edema, hematoma, splints, or dressings. If the injury is an isolated one and there are no clinical contraindications, heparinization before vessel clamping diminishes the likelihood of small-vessel thrombosis in the ischemic part. In the patient with multiple injuries elsewhere, or with extensive local or regional tissue disruption, systemic heparinization is imprudent, although the local instillation of intraarterial heparin may be useful. Careful distal passage of thrombectomy catheters may frequently remove unexpected amounts of clot.

Management principles for damaged arteries and veins in infants and children do not vary significantly from those observed in adolescents or adults. Arterial injuries that have led to hemorrhage or distal ischemia should almost always be repaired rather than ligated. Occasionally, puncture wounds or lacerations can simply be closed primarily, or short segments of damaged or contused arteries can be excised with restoration of arterial continuity by end-to-end anastomosis. Vascular stenosis after lateral arteriorrhaphy, or end-to-end anastomosis, is a common, morbid, and preventable technical complication. The liberal use of vein patches or interposed segments is encouraged. In adults, such vein interpositions and patches are highly durable and are rarely associated with subsequent complications (although in general, long-term follow-up studies are lacking).

However, several important technical issues that relate to the small size of infants' and children's vessels are worthy of emphasis. For example, because infants and children have small arteries that increase in caliber with growth, avoidance of narrowing vessel anastomoses is particularly important. The use of spatulated anastomoses and microsurgical techniques, including optical magnification, is prudent.[22] To accommodate for vessel growth, repair should be done with interrupted sutures rather than the conventional running sutures commonly used in adult vascular anastomoses. For unclear reasons, interposed venous autografts, at least in certain anatomic sites such as the renal artery in children, have the tendency to become aneurysmal over time. Whether the aneurysmal degeneration that occurs in reversed saphenous vein in the pediatric setting is simply a consequence of the aortic pressure pulse over a prolonged period of time, or to some as-yet-uncharacterized structural inadequacy of pediatric saphenous vein, remains unknown. This phenomenon has led in several centers to the substitution of hypogastric artery for saphenous vein in the treatment of pediatric renal artery occlusive disease.[23] When saphenous vein is

used in the management of pediatric vascular trauma, long-term surveillance (perhaps by duplex sonography) to rule out aneurysmal degeneration of the vein graft seems worthwhile.

Failure of distal revascularization after a technically successful procedure should raise several urgent questions. Is there persistent distal arterial thrombus despite the passage of balloon catheters at the time of the initial reconstruction? Is there kinking or twisting of the vein graft or acute thrombosis at an anastomosis? Is there severe distal spasm in the artery that has been traumatized?[3] The clinician confronted with such problem should maintain a low threshold for reexploring the wound and performing intraoperative contrast arteriography, which may demonstrate a remediable technical defect.

Another important cause of inadequate distal perfusion after technically successful revascularization is the development of *compartment syndrome*. Rapid and complete reperfusion of a severely ischemic capillary bed causes the egress of substantial plasma volume into the soft tissues, usually of the forearm or calf, with a resultant rise in tissue pressure and, if not managed urgently and effectively, permanent nerve and muscle deficits. Muscle necrosis may produce substantial myoglobulinuria, which may result in acute renal failure, acidosis and hyperkalemia, major morbidity, and death. Clinical scenarios suggesting the likelihood of compartment syndrome include circumstances in which peripheral ischemia has been severe or prolonged, in which there may be extensive soft tissue injury secondary to fracture or blunt trauma, or when the patient has been in shock. Early clinical symptoms and signs of compartment syndrome are neurologic rather than vascular, including muscle weakness (resulting in an inability to dorsiflex the foot), pain in the calf muscles with tenderness and tightness on direct compression, and paresthesias and diminished cutaneous sensation over the medial dorsum of the foot. Objective data regarding the presence of compartmental hypertension can be obtained by direct tissue pressure measurements. A tissue pressure over 40 mm Hg, or prolonged pressures over 30 mm Hg, suggests a substantial risk of tissue damage secondary to increased pressure, and warrants operative intervention.

Several techniques for the management of compartment syndrome are used. For the lower extremity, these include four-compartment fasciotomy, either through a single anterior lateral incision or alternatively through lateral and medial longitudinal incisions, and occasionally a fibulectomy. In the upper extremity, a curvilinear volar incision adequately decompresses the two compartments of the forearm.

A low threshold for fasciotomy is warranted when calf or forearm muscle is at risk, and some recommend prophylactic fasciotomy in clinical settings where the risk of developing compartmental hypertension is high (see previous discussion). An elevated index of suspicion should be maintained as well in trauma victims in whom, because they are intubated, intoxicated, or have central or peripheral neurologic injuries, the symptoms of compartment hypertension may not be manifest.

CONTROVERSIES

Several controversies exist in the management of adult vascular trauma, including the proper setting of management priorities for complex or multiple vascular injuries, ligation versus reconstruction of damaged veins, the proper role (if any) for the use of synthetic grafts, and surveillance versus immediate management of certain asymptomatic vascular injuries diagnosed during screening examinations. These dilemmas are present in the management of pediatric vascular trauma as well.

The sobriquet "complex vascular injury" characterizes vascular trauma whose management is complicated by the presence of concurrent injuries whose priority must be established, or (occasionally) other technical or logistic details that complicate an otherwise straightforward management of the vascular wound. Examples include an ischemic extremity due to a lacerated superficial femoral artery associated with a midshaft femur fracture and an impending compartment syndrome, or a severely ischemic extremity in which rapid revascularization cannot be performed because of lack of access to an operating room or a vascular surgeon. Successful management of such injuries requires adherence to Advanced Trauma Life Support principles, and the recognition of the urgency of management of known time-related organ or tissue damage (eg, shock, open fractures, severe limb ischemia, compartment syndrome).

Arterial Injury

Large arteries almost always require repair: the likelihood of irreversible limb and organ ischemia is overwhelmingly high in such circumstances. On the other hand, certain settings in which small or medium-sized paired or multiple arteries are damaged require a determination of what needs to be revascularized and what can simply be ligated. Adult clinical experience has suggested the adequacy of a single tibial artery reaching the foot,[24] and a single wrist artery reaching the hand.[25] Stated another way, an isolated radial or ulnar arterial injury, or a damaged tibial artery, can usually simply be ligated if distal perfusion is intact; collateral perfusion by the remaining undamaged limb arteries is usually adequate to maintain perfusion and function. Although these conclusions have been demonstrable in adult trauma victims, they have not been validated in the setting of equivalent injuries in a pediatric population.

Historically, the presence of any evidence for arterial injury mandated operative exploration and repair.[9] However, a consequence of modern invasive or operative technologies such as transcatheter arteriography, balloon dilatation of intraluminal lesions, and in situ saphenous vein bypass grafting has been the production of large numbers of arterial lesions of ultimately negligible clinical import. Investigations in which surveillance rather than operative management of small, asymptomatic arterial lesions—pseudoaneurysms, low-flow arteriovenous fistulas, diminutive intimal flaps—has been conducted have demonstrated the usually benign and self-limited nature of these lesions.[26,27] Although guidelines distinguishing those lesions that can be observed from those that require operative management have yet to be established, experience at several large trauma centers has suggested that pseudoaneurysms whose dimensions are less than half the diameter of the native vessel, arteriovenous fistulas that are low flow (without palpable thrill or stethoscope-audible bruit), and intimal flaps whose length is less than half the luminal diameter of the native artery, may safely be observed with serial duplex scanning. High-risk problems—a noncompliant patient (or parent), multiple nearby arterial lesions, or a worrisome anatomic location such as the popli-

teal or common femoral artery—warrant a lower threshold for operative intervention.

Venous Injury

Although damaged arteries of any substance require repair, debate continues over the appropriate management of traumatized veins.[28,29] Some have suggested excellent outcomes, including minimal risk of postoperative edema and subsequent venous problems, with simple ligation, even of damaged large veins.[28] However, experimental work evaluating the effect of venous ligation on extremity arterial inflow[30] has confirmed the general clinical impression that venous ligature potentially threatens concurrent arterial repair, increases the risk of compartment syndrome, and results in an elevated risk of later postphlebitic syndrome. A reasonable management policy is to repair large veins (central to the knee or the shoulder), especially if this can be performed by straightforward lateral venorrhaphy or resection and reanastomosis. Veins peripheral to the knee joint or the shoulder can usually simply be ligated (exception: upper extremity revascularization efforts after traumatic amputation. There are no credible data available to detail the natural history of vein ligation or repair in the pediatric population.

It is axiomatic that the best substitute vascular graft tissue is autogenous—for practical purposes, extremity vein or hypogastric artery. However, certain trauma settings may require consideration of alternate graft materials. For example, disruption of the great arteries and veins at the thoracic inlet usually requires graft replacement, yet available autogenous graft material such as the saphenous vein is of inadequate caliber. Another example may be that of severely contaminated and potentially septic open wounds that must be traversed by a vascular graft.

In these settings, "panel" or "spiral" grafts can be fashioned to provide an autogenous conduit of adequate caliber,[31] but this process is tedious and time consuming. Numerous alternative nonautogenous grafts have alternatively been attempted, including cryopreserved homograft vein or artery, preserved human umbilical vein, or bovine carotid artery. Preserved homografts and xenografts are difficult to handle, are expensive, and, most important, are associated with such elevated risks of infection and aneurysmal dilation that they are not currently considered useful.

The use of synthetic grafts may have a preferred role in contaminated wounds, based on certain reports.[32,33] Autogenous grafts in septic wounds have an unpredictable but ominous tendency to become infected and to rupture, threatening resulting exsanguinating hemorrhage. Expanded polytetrafluoroethylene (PTFE; Teflon) grafts have been shown to work very effectively in such settings. If the graft becomes infected, it may develop thrombosis; however, rupture and hemorrhage is a much less common complication.[33] For incompletely understood reasons, PTFE appears to have a mildly antimicrobial propensity. This is not true of Dacron, which is contraindicated in any vascular trauma case in which wound or graft infection is a concern. In addition, prosthetic grafts have an increased likelihood to undergo junctional neointimal hyperplasia compared with autogenous grafts. No long-term follow-up data are available regarding the likelihood of this phenomenon when such grafts are used in the pediatric setting.

IATROGENIC VASCULAR INJURIES IN INFANTS AND CHILDREN

The explosion in vascular diagnostic and therapeutic options has benefited untold numbers of patients. However, each one of them (as well as many other nonvascular interventions) places blood vessels at risk. The clinician must always balance the potential benefits of a vascular diagnostic or therapeutic procedure against the implications of a vascular complication. A series of recognized and predictable iatrogenic vascular complications in newborns, infants, and children warrants discussion.

Vascular damage in neonates and very young infants most commonly arises from complications associated with various monitoring techniques or diagnostic procedures.[34–38] Two important sites of iatrogenic arterial occlusion may develop in the very young—the common femoral artery after diagnostic catheterization,[34–36] or the aorta after umbilical artery cannulation.[37,38] Management of both problems is complicated by the underlying neonatal disease state (congenital heart disease, prematurity, or some other neonatal condition requiring intensive care monitoring). In general, thrombotic occlusion of the aorta, a highly lethal condition, is best managed by distal aortotomy and thrombectomy using small balloon catheters.[38] Common femoral artery thrombosis can usually be treated successfully with localized thrombectomy and repair of the inciting intimal disruption. Vessel thromboses distal to the groin are rarely amenable to operative management because of these vessels' small size. Anticoagulation is effective in preventing proximal and distal thrombus propagation.[39] Thrombolytic therapy is risky and unpredictable in neonates and infants. Prevention is preferable. Heparin administration and the use of microcatheter systems left in situ as briefly as possible may substantially reduce associated thrombotic complications.[39]

Adequate collateral circulation cannot be reliably presumed in newborn or infant children, as demonstrated by occasional upper extremity ischemia after division of the subclavian artery for the purpose of performing subclavian artery–pulmonary artery shunt to treat cyanotic congenital heart disease.[40] The use of extracorporeal membrane oxygenation for neonates with respiratory insufficiency has resulted in a small but unpredictable incidence of cerebrovascular ischemia.[41] Because the common carotid artery is sacrificed for the purpose of arterial outflow from the extracorporeal membrane oxygenation device, the adequacy of collateral cerebral perfusion is challenged, and some authorities now recommend reconstruction of the common carotid artery after successful decannulation.[42]

Iatrogenic causes of vascular trauma are primarily local arterial complications secondary to diagnostic or therapeutic vascular cannulation. Nonvascular conditions undergoing treatment in children have occasionally resulted in treatment-related vascular complications. Tonsillectomy is performed by anatomic necessity very near the carotid artery, and on rare occasion has resulted in inadvertent damage to that vessel, presenting either with profuse arterial hemorrhage or later pseudoaneurysm. Congenital or acquired limb length discrepancy secondary to femoral artery injury is now commonly treated by the osteotomy–distraction technique.[43] Other injuries may include the popliteal artery inadvertently transfixed by a proximal Ilizarov traction pin.[44]

REFERENCES

1. Flanigan DP, Schuler JJ, Meyer JP. Pediatric vascular trauma. In: Flanigan DP, ed. Civilian vascular trauma. Philadelphia, Lea & Febiger, 1992:203.
2. Van Houtte PM, Houston DS. Platelets, endothelium, and basal spasm. Circulation 1985;72:728.
3. Samson R, Pasternak BM. Traumatic arterial spasm: rarity or nonentity. J Trauma 1980;20:607.
4. Malan E, Tattoni G. Physio- and anatopathology of acute ischemia of the extremities. J Cardiovasc Surg 1963;4:2.
5. Miller HH, Welch CH. Quantitative studies on the time factor of arterial injuries. Ann Surg 1949;130:428.
6. Walker PM. Pathophysiology of acute arterial occlusion. Can J Surg 1986;29:340.
7. Perry MO, Shires GT, Albert SA. Cellular changes with graded limb ischemia and reperfusion. J Vasc Surg 1984;1:536.
8. Walker PM. Lindsay TF, Labbe R, et al. Salvage of skeletal muscle with free radical scavengers. J Vasc Surg 1987;5:68.
9. Perry MO, Thal ER, Shires GT. Management of arterial injuries. Ann Surg 1971;173:403.
10. Sirinek KR, Levine BA, Gaskill HV, et al. Reassessment of the role of routine operative exploration in vascular trauma. J Trauma 1981;21:339.
11. Sirinek KR, Gaskill HV, Levine BA, et al. Exclusion angiography for patients with possible vascular injuries of the extremities: a better use of trauma center resources. Surgery 1983;94:598.
12. Snyder WH, Thal ER, Bridges RA, et al. The validity of normal arteriography in penetrating trauma. Arch Surg 1978;113:424.
13. Rose SC, Moore EE. Emergency trauma angiography: accuracy, safety and pitfalls. AJR Am J Roentgenol 1987;148:1243.
14. Weaver FA, Yellin AE, Bauer M, et al. Is arterial proximity a valid indication for arteriography in penetrating extremity trauma? A prospective analysis. Arch Surg 1990;125:1256.
15. Francis H, Thal ER, Weigelt JA, et al. Vascular proximity: is it a valid indication for arteriography in asymptomatic patients? J Trauma 1991;31:512.
16. Lynch K, Johansen KH. Can Doppler pressure measurements replace "exclusion" arteriography in extremity trauma? Ann Surg 1991;214:737.
17. Johansen K, Lynch K, Paun M, et al. Non-invasive vascular tests reliably exclude occult arterial trauma in injured extremities. J Trauma 1991;31:515.
18. Meissner M, Paun M, Johansen K. Duplex scanning for arterial trauma. Am J Surg 1991;161:552.
19. Bynoe WP, Miles WP, Bell RM, et al. Noninvasive diagnosis of vascular trauma by duplex ultrasonography. J Vasc Surg 1991;14:346.
20. Panetta TF, Hunt JP, Buechter KJ, et al. Duplex ultrasonography versus arteriography in the diagnosis of arterial injury: an experimental study. J Trauma 1992;33:627.
21. Fry WR, Dort JA, Smith RS, et al. Duplex scanning replaces arteriography and operative exploration in the diagnosis of potential cervical vascular injury. Am J Surg 1994;168:693.
22. LaQuaglia MP, Upton J, May JW Jr. Microvascular reconstruction of major arteries in neonates and small children. J Pediatr Surg 1991;26:1136.
23. Stanley JC, Fry WJ. Pediatric renal artery occlusive disease and renovascular hypertension: etiology, diagnosis, and operative treatment. Arch Surg 1981;116:669.
24. Ballard JL, Bunt TJ, Malone JM. Management of small artery vascular trauma. Am J Surg 1992;164:316.
25. Johnson M, Ford M, Johansen K, et al. Radial or ulnar artery laceration: repair or ligate? Arch Surg 1993;128:971.
26. Frykberg ER, Crump JM, Dennis JW, et al. Nonoperative observation of clinically occult arterial injuries: a prospective evaluation. Surgery 1991;109:85.
27. Stain SC, Yellin AE, Weaver FA, et al. Selective management of nonocclusive arterial injuries. Arch Surg 1989;124:1136.
28. Timberlake GA, O'Connell RC, Kerstein MD. Venous injuries: to repair or ligate, the dilemma. J Vasc Surg 1986;4:553.
29. Phifer TJ, Gerlock AJ, Vekovius WA, et al. Amputation risk factors in concomitance superficial artery and vein injuries. Ann Surg 1983;199:241.

30. Wright CB, Hobson RW. Hemodynamic effects of femoral venous occlusion in the sub-human primate. Surgery 1974;75:453.
31. Fowl RJ, Martin KD, Sax HC, et al. Use of autologous spiral vein grafts for vascular reconstruction in contaminated fields. J Vasc Surg 1988;8:442.
32. Shah DM, Leather RP, Corson JD, et al. Polytetrafluoroethylene grafts in the rapid reconstruction of acute contaminated peripheral vascular injuries. Am J Surg 1984;148:229.
33. Feliciano DV, Mattox KL, Graham JM, et al. Five-year experience with PTFE grafts in vascular wounds. J Trauma 1985;25:71.
34. Burrows PE, Benson LN, Williams WG, et al. Iliofemoral arterial complications of balloon angioplasty for ischemic obstructions in infants and children. Circulation 1990;92:1697.
35. Flanigan DP, Keifer TJ, Schuler JJ, et al. Experience with iatrogenic pediatric vascular injuries: incidence, etiology, management, and results. Ann Surg 1983;198:430.
36. Klein MD, Coran AG, Whitehouse WM, et al. Management of iatrogenic arterial injuries in infants and children. J Pediatr Surg 1982;17:?933.
37. Vailas GN, Brouilette RT, Scott JB, et al. Neonatal aortic thrombosis: recent experience. J Pediatr 1986;109:101.
38. Flanigan DP, Stolar CJ, Pringle KC, et al. Aortic thrombosis after umbilical artery catheterization: successful surgical management. Arch Surg 1982;117:371.
39. Freed MD, Keane JF, Rosenthal A. The use of heparinization to prevent arterial thrombosis after percutaneous cardiac catheterization in children. Circulation 1974;42:501.
40. Geiss D, Williams WG, Lindsay WK, et al. Upper extremity gangrene: and complication of subclavian artery division. Ann Thorac Surg 1980;30:47.
41. Crombleholme TM, Adzick NS, DeLorimier A, et al. Carotid artery reconstruction following extracorporeal membrane oxygenation. Am J Dis Child 1990;144:872.
42. Moulton SL, Lynch FP, Cornish JD, et al. Carotid artery reconstruction following neonatal extracorporeal membrane oxygenation. J Pediatr Surg 1991;26:794.
43. Taylor LM, Troutman R, Feliciano P, et al. Incidence of later complications following femoral artery catheterization in infants. J Vasc Surg 1990;11:297.
44. Waldhausen J, Mosca V, Johansen K, et al. Delayed presentation of popliteal artery damage during lower extremity Ilizarov distraction. Orthopedics (in press).

Surgery of Infants and Children: Scientific Principles and Practice, edited by Keith T. Oldham, Paul M. Colombani, and Robert P. Foglia.
Lippincott–Raven Publishers, Philadelphia, © 1997.

CHAPTER 27

Drowning and Hypothermia

Madelyn Kahana

DROWNING AND NEAR-DROWNING

In the United States, drowning is the second leading cause of death in children. In 10 states, submersion injuries claim the lives of more children than any other injury or disease process.[1] Preschool-aged children and adolescents are at greatest risk—the former, victims of unprotected backyard swimming pools, the latter, victims of the effects of alcohol-related boating accidents. Male victims outnumber female victims in all age groups and particularly in adolescents, for whom the ratio approaches 10:1. For every child who drowns, four children are admitted to the hospital with significant near-drowning episodes and are evaluated and discharged. For every child evaluated in an emergency department, an estimated 10 others rescued from the water never seek medical attention.

Among children younger than 19 years of age, 1 in 3300 girls drowns, and 1 in 1000 is hospitalized for a near-drowning event. One in 1100 boys drowns, 1 in 300 requires hospital stay for a nonfatal submersion injury,[2] and 1 in 8 is rescued from a perceived water emergency.[1] The magnitude of this problem is truly substantial. In economic terms, the acute and chronic care of these children requires the expenditure of an estimated $400 million annually.[1]

Pathophysiology

Drowning and near-drowning result in multisystem hypoxic injury. The sequence of events during drowning has been investigated extensively in animal models. Initially, there is a period of struggling, during which small amounts of water enter the hypopharynx and produce laryngospasm. Copious amounts of water are then swallowed, followed by gasping and aspiration. In 10% to 15% of animals, laryngospasm persists until death, with no significant aspiration of water into the tracheobronchial tree.[3] Autopsy examinations of the lungs of drowning victims support the notions that pulmonary aspiration is an active process and that trivial quantities of water flow into the trachea passively after consciousness is lost.[4] During resuscitation efforts, gastric contents are almost invariably regurgitated, which complicates the pulmonary injury.

As a result of the period of asphyxia, the drowning victim suffers a global hypoxic injury. No organ system is spared. Although the pulmonary insult is often the focus of discussions of the pathophysiology of drowning and near-drowning, the cerebral injury is the most likely cause of morbidity and mortality in the modern era of pediatric critical care medicine. Other expressions of the hypoxic injury include acute tubular necrosis, loss of gastrointestinal mucosa, depression of myocardial contractility, hepatic necrosis, and disseminated intravascular coagulopathy.[5] In the rare event that large quantities of water are absorbed into the systemic circulation, hemolysis adds to the hematologic pathology and aberrations in serum electrolytes occur.[5]

Much is often made of the differences between the injuries that result from freshwater and saltwater submersions. Only 2% of drowning and near-drowning accidents occur in salt water, so that even if the differences were not trivial, the magnitude of the problem of saltwater drowning is small. In addition, the injury that results from submersion is one of hypoxia. Only in experimental models, when more than 22 mL/kg of water is instilled into the trachea, do the differences between freshwater and saltwater drownings become important. The number of children who absorb that quantity of water during submersion is small.[4]

In theory, saltwater drowning results in rapid diffusion of fluid into the lung from the extravascular space because of the high osmolality of sea water. Protein-rich pulmonary edema results, and surfactant is deactivated. With freshwater aspiration, surfactant is altered, and the lung collapses from the loss of surface tension. In both instances, pulmonary compliance falls, and the work of breathing becomes excessive. In both instances, respiratory failure is inevitable. In both circumstances, the extent and duration of the hypoxic period determine the severity of subsequent global injury.[5]

If there is massive aspiration of fluid at the time of the accident, the victim of saltwater submersion has immediate and profound pulmonary edema. Intravascular volume is contracted, with the potential for severe hypernatremia from the osmotic movement of water from the intravascular space.[3] In the case of the freshwater victim, pulmonary edema is less evident, and the potential for intravascular volume overload is real. Osmotic forces drive water into the intravascular space, and classic water intoxication follows, with the possibility of life-threatening hyponatremia. Fewer than 10% of submersion victims aspirate sufficient fluid to make these differences clinically relevant.

The *diving reflex,* a generally vestigial reflex in humans, active perhaps in 15% of the population, may be important in the recovery from prolonged submersion.[6,7] The diving reflex is responsible for the ability of marine mammals to remain underwater for prolonged periods of time despite their need to respire on the surface. The major factor in their resistance to the consequences of prolonged asphyxia is a set of cardiovascular physiologic adjustments triggered by breath-holding diving, which conserves oxygen for those tissues most sensitive to hypoxia. Cardiac output is markedly reduced secondary to profound bradycardia. Peripheral vasoconstriction limits or arrests blood flow to skeletal muscle, the intestinal tract, and the kidneys. Cerebral blood flow is maintained at or slightly above predive levels. Coronary flow continues at a reduced level. Oxygen consumption drops dramatically to less than half the predive rate. The diving reflex is accentuated by hypothermia, enabling marine mammals to survive up to 70 minutes of submersion. The importance of this reflex in human drowning survivors is still hotly debated.

Treatment Issues

Despite descriptions in the medical literature and the lay press of dramatic recoveries from prolonged submersions, the success of resuscitation therapy for the drowning victim is limited. The extent of the injury inflicted and the potential for recovery are largely predetermined by the duration of the hypoxic period. Prompt prehospital resuscitation is crucial for the child with a potentially reversible process. Delaying initiation of basic or advanced life support in this patient population augments the hypoxic insult. Once the child has suffered a cardiopulmonary arrest, the outcome usually is dismal despite even the best resuscitative efforts—except perhaps in the special circumstance of the cold water drowning victim.

At the time of resuscitation, most submersion victims regurgitate. If gastric contents are aspirated, lung injury can be magnified. In the rare circumstance in which particulate matter is aspirated and the airway is obstructed, the removal of the offending material must precede further resuscitative efforts. Although routine use of the Heimlich maneuver in the near-drowning victim has been widely discussed in the literature, the American Red Cross continues to recommend *not* delaying basic life support to perform this maneuver *except in the case of the patient with an airway obstruction.*[4,8,9] The presence of water in the tracheobronchial tree does not warrant the routine performance of the Heimlich maneuver, which may, in fact, increase the quantity of regurgitated material and hamper efforts at maintaining a patent airway.

If the submersion injury occurs in a contaminated body of water, the pulmonary injury is augmented by the presence of toxic chemicals or bacteria in significant quantities. The presence of chlorine in the concentration used to maintain a residential swimming pool does not substantially alter the lung injury.[10]

As stated previously, the lung injuries that occur as a result of submersion in freshwater and salt water are more alike than they are different.[3,5] Compliance is reduced, surfactant is deactivated, and ventilation–perfusion mismatch produces hypoxemia. In severe injury, endotracheal intubation is mandated by

TABLE 27-1. *Initial ventilator settings for adequate oxygen delivery*

Tidal volume	6–8 mL/kg
Rate	20–30 breaths/min
Positive end-expiratory pressure	5–15 cm H₂O
Inspiratory time	0.8–1.5 s
Inspired oxygen concentration	0.6

blood gas aberrations, the increased work of breathing, and the altered mental status of the patient. The pulmonary injury often rapidly evolves into a pattern consistent with the adult respiratory distress syndrome.

The use of positive end-expiratory pressure (PEEP) to reduce ventilation–perfusion mismatch is the mainstay of successful mechanical ventilation. Efforts to reduce the inspired oxygen concentration to less than 0.6 limit oxygen-related pulmonary injury.[3,5] Allowing hypercapnia is recommended in lieu of the normalization of blood gases in an effort to limit tidal volume and peak inflation pressure and thereby reduce the incidence of airleak syndrome. Instillation of surfactant into the trachea by injection and by nebulization is being investigated. High-frequency oscillation has been used with limited success in the patient with severe lung injury, as has extracorporeal membrane oxygenation.

Conventional ventilation strategies begin with volume- or pressure-limited, time-cycled settings. The goals are twofold. First, the adequacy of oxygen delivery and carbon dioxide removal must be ensured. Second, the injury imposed by the effects of high concentrations of inspired oxygen and excessive tidal volume must be limited. Without attention to the latter, a potentially nonlethal pulmonary injury can evolve into one with mortal characteristics. When concentration of inspired oxygen reaches levels above 0.6, oxygen-related tissue injury is a real danger. To accomplish adequate oxygenation and limit the fraction of inspired oxygen, PEEP therapy should be instituted. Frequently, more than 15 cm H₂O delivered as PEEP is necessary to reduce inspired oxygen to a safe level (Table 27-1).

Adjunctive therapy with steroids and antibiotics has been recommended for the pulmonary injury from near-drowning. Corticosteroids have never been shown to be of benefit. Initially, antibiotics should be reserved for the victim of a contaminated water source. During hospitalization, nosocomial pneumonia certainly occurs in this patient population, and antibiotics should be tailored for the specific infectious agent whenever possible. Broad-spectrum antibiotic use simply predisposes the patient to an infection with a resistant organism or fungus.

The high intrathoracic pressure that results from the use of positive-pressure mechanical ventilation can diminish cardiac output sufficiently to require inotropic support. Should this occur, the placement of a pulmonary artery catheter is instrumental in guiding therapy. Cardiac output and oxygen delivery and extraction can then be measured (Table 27-2). These data facilitate appropriate adjustments in drug selection and dose as well as the manipulation of preload with minimal risk of imposed hydrostatic pulmonary edema.

The intentional elevation of oxygen delivery to supranormal levels in an effort to improve survival has garnered limited enthusiasm, and there is very limited evidence to support this contention. The adequacy of oxygen therapy and delivery in

TABLE 27-2. *Objectives of cardiopulmonary support*

Cardiac index	$\geq$2.5 L/m^2
Oxygen consumption	>125 mL/min
Extraction ratio	20%–30%
Mixed venous oxygen saturation	65%–75%
Arterial oxygen saturation	$\geq$85%
Oxygen delivery	$\geq$450 mL/m^2/min

the child with a severe lung injury is best evaluated with the data acquired from a pulmonary artery catheter. Mixed venous oxygen saturation should be maintained at or above 65% whenever possible. This saturation level requires that the risks of therapy be considered when adjustments are made to achieve this goal. The child with low oxygen consumption may have a favorable mixed venous saturation but is not likely to do well in the long-term (see Table 27-2).

Oxygen delivery can be improved by a number of interventions. Transfusion of red cells, measures to increase cardiac output, and increases in arterial saturation augment oxygen delivery. The optimal hematocrit has not been determined, but in the severely injured child, transfusion to a hemoglobin of 15 g is prudent. Cardiac output can be improved by manipulating preload, contractility, and afterload, as in adults. Optimal variables can be found in Table 27-2. The successful cardiopulmonary support of the pediatric near-drowning patient, although often complex, is almost always possible.

The success of cardiopulmonary support in the drowning victim is offset by the inability of any available therapy to modify the cerebral hypoxic insult. Although methods to reduce cerebral oxygen consumption have been used, no data support that a reduction improves survival. Both hypothermia and barbiturate coma significantly reduce cerebral oxygen consumption, but neither increases the number of neurologically intact survivors. Monitoring intracranial pressure has been recommended to guide therapy, but again, no data support an increase in intact survivors as a result. In fact, data suggest that monitoring intracranial pressure and aggressively treating intracranial hypertension increase the number of *vegetative* near-drowning survivors.[11] Refractory intracranial hypertension certainly predicts poor long-term outcome.

The treatment of the renal insufficiency that accompanies near-drowning is certainly possible because the injury is transient. Should dialysis be required, the duration of acute renal failure is generally between 3 and 6 weeks. Hemodialysis is preferred in the patient with a significant pulmonary insult because peritoneal filling compromises the ability to ensure adequate mechanical ventilation.

The gastrointestinal mucosal injury is also short-lived but demands the use of parenteral nutrition until the mucosa regenerates. Because early and aggressive nutritional support is crucial in the injured child, hyperalimentation is recommended until the gut can support adequate caloric intake. As soon as possible, the enteral route of nutritional support is preferred. Translocation of bacteria is reduced as a result, and the complications associated with intravenous nutrition are avoided. The injury to the liver is also transient and responds to the restoration of adequate circulatory stability. Hepatitis can accompany parenteral hyperalimentation but occurs later in the support of the near-drowning victim.

The hematologic insult in near-drowning injury is a multifactorial one. Disseminated intravascular coagulopathy accompanies hypothermia, hypoxemia, and shock. Hypoxemia injures the bone marrow and results in markedly reduced platelet production that can persist for several weeks. The use of broad-spectrum antibiotics can cause vitamin K deficiency and attendant coagulopathy if replacement therapy is not instituted. Hematologic support of the drowning victim should be tailored to the specific needs of the patient. To avoid hemorrhagic complications, coagulation variables should be normalized whenever possible.

Cold Water Submersions

The circumstance of the cold (ice) water submersion deserves special attention.[12] Cold water locations are implicated in about 2% of all submersion deaths. Because of the protective effects of hypothermia on the brain and other vital organs, intact survival of prolonged submersion is possible, and the absence of vital signs in the victim does not necessarily predict a dismal outcome.

With mild hypothermia (32° to 35°C), oxygen consumption increases as sympathetic output increases and thermogenesis is attempted. At a core temperature below 32°C, shivering ceases and oxygen consumption decreases 7% for each drop in temperature of 1°C. Temperatures below 28°C are associated with severe bradycardia, the presence of a J wave on the electrocardiogram, hypotension, and an increased propensity for spontaneous atrial and ventricular fibrillation. At these temperatures, striated muscular rigidity occurs. At a core temperature of 20° to 22°C, cerebral electrical activity is abolished.

Because cerebral use of oxygen is reduced, dramatic recoveries are possible after prolonged hypothermic submersion and hypoxic insult. The impact of the temperature of the water involved in a submersion injury is particularly crucial in pediatric drowning victims. Children cool quickly because of their large surface area/body weight ratios. They are therefore more likely to benefit from the presence of cold water. Hypothermia must be induced rapidly for maximal beneficial effects. The impact of the increased potency of the diving reflex under hypothermic conditions is yet debated.

Resuscitation of the hypothermic drowning victim must focus not only on the basics of cardiopulmonary resuscitation (CPR) but also on specific efforts to rewarm the patient. Controversy exists with respect to the necessity of cardiac compressions and mechanical ventilation in the hypothermic patient before rewarming. Proceeding with routine CPR measures during rewarming is recommended, unless rewarming is accomplished with cardiopulmonary bypass.[13,14]

From mild or moderate hypothermia (core temperature of more than 30°C), rewarming can be accomplished with a combination of minimally invasive surface and core techniques. From more profound hypothermic injury, the advantages of cardiopulmonary bypass are clear.[13] The dysrhythmia associated with this degree of cold injury can be more easily managed when cardiopulmonary bypass has been instituted.

Using core rewarming techniques, temperature should be raised carefully to avoid profound hypotension as systemic vascular resistance falls. During rewarming, shivering, with an attendant rise in oxygen consumption, should be avoided, and appropriate cardiovascular support should be provided. Although optimal rates of rewarming have been published, the data are scant. Recommendations favor rapid rewarming with careful attention to hemodynamic support during the process.

Regardless of the rewarming technique, resuscitation efforts should continue until the patient's core temperature exceeds 35°C.[15,16] If the child does not respond to resuscitation measures after being rewarmed, it is appropriate to discontinue therapy. Although resuscitation from hypothermic submersion is more likely to succeed, success is certainly not guaranteed.

Outcome Predictors

The ultimate determinant of the quality of a submersion victim's recovery is the duration of the hypoxic injury. Recovery can be modified by hypothermia in ice water drownings. Poor outcome predictors in the pediatric population are divided into those related to the prehospital clinical picture and those that apply to the intensive care unit setting[3,5,17] (Table 27-3). Again, the recovery from pulmonary injury after submersion is the rule. The long-term sequelae of near-drowning relate to the occurrence of hypoxic encephalopathy.

In the prehospital care of children who suffered near-drowning, death or severe neurologic injury was universal when the submersion duration exceeded 10 minutes and when resuscitation efforts to achieve a cardiac rhythm exceeded 25 minutes.[17] In contrast, a good outcome was predictable when the child was responsive at the scene and had reactive pupils and sinus rhythm. Of children who require CPR at the scene of a near-drowning, between 8% and 30% survive neurologically intact. When CPR is required in the emergency department, neurologic recovery is less likely but not impossible.

Ultimate recovery is virtually unheard of in the normothermic patient who reaches the pediatric intensive care unit with a Glasgow coma scale score 5 or lower.[18] Brain-stem auditory-evoked potentials,[19] intracranial pressure monitoring,[20] and sensory-evoked potentials have been examined as outcome predictors in children with hypoxic brain injuries. Only severe aberrations in these tests can accurately predict poor recovery; they add little to the information obtained from careful, sequential neurologic examinations.

In both normothermic and hypothermic patients, neurologic recovery, when it occurs, begins in the first 48 to 72 hours after injury. Children who have made no neurologic recovery in that time frame are unlikely to do so. When some progress has been made, neurologic recovery can proceed slowly for many months and even years.

The neurologic injuries after near-drowning are extremely varied, from minor learning disabilities to a persistent vegetative state. As many as two thirds of children who suffer a near-drowning episode are left with residual neurologic injury. *The impact on the child, the family, and society is substantial.*

TABLE 27-3. *Predictors of death or severe neurologic injury*

Submersion time	>10 min
Resuscitation time	>25 min to sinus rhythm
Glasgow Coma Scale score	≤5 on admission to intensive care unit

Agenda for Prevention

Evidence from both clinical and epidemiologic studies suggests that the most effective means to reduce the physical toll submersion takes on children should focus on prevention rather than on therapy.[16,21–24] The best prevention of the pediatric near-drowning requires adequate supervision of a child at risk. Drownings in residential pools can also be reduced by the installation of complete pool fencing.[1,3,5,10]

Improved supervision of children by their caretakers is the cornerstone of the prevention of near-drowning. Although supervision cannot be replaced by environmental aids, the long history of failed efforts to change the quality of child supervision has led to efforts to restrict access to the most common sites of submersions. Complete pool fencing has the most promise in this regard.[25–29]

For complete pool fencing, a fence should surround the pool and separate it from the house and the yard. It is best constructed to a height of 4.5 feet to prevent scaling by active 4-year-olds. A spring-loaded gate with an automatic lock is mandatory to reduce the opportunity to defeat the fence. In Australia, where legislation mandates regional pool fencing, the number of toddler drownings has been reduced by 80%.[1,26–30] When drownings did occur, the pool fence had almost invariably been defeated by propping open the gate. In the United States, only 15% of in-ground pools are equipped with a complete pool fence.

Pool safety covers have been suggested as an alternative to fencing. The pool cover is much less effective because it is a passive device; that is, it must be repeatedly applied. A soft cover may in fact be a hazard because a small child who attempts to walk on it may become submerged. The pool cover may further obscure the accident. Mechanized hard pool covers, which must be applied repeatedly, are expensive, costing in excess of $6000, substantially more than an adequate pool fence.[16,21–23,30]

Successes with injury prevention have combined legislation with public awareness campaigns.[31] Car seats, bicycle helmets, and seat belts are in widespread use because of these efforts. Drowning now outranks accidental deaths of small children caused by motor vehicles, perhaps because of the safety devices used in vehicles.[16,24–29,32] The data cry out for a similar effort to reduce pediatric submersion deaths and to save about 800 children every year.[1,3,5,10,21–39]

ACCIDENTAL HYPOTHERMIA

Humans are homeothermic mammals well suited to survive in the tropics. They are equipped with a number of physiologic mechanisms to dissipate heat, but to conserve heat, they must rely on intelligent behavior.

Accidental hypothermia is defined as the inadvertent drop in core body temperature below 35°C (95°F). Commonly, hypothermia is classified by severity[33] (Table 27-4). *Mild hypothermia* is defined as a core temperature between 32.2° and 35°C (90° to 95°F). At this body temperature, a child is generally hemodynamically stable, conscious, and when verbal, complains of cold. Except in newborns, shivering is common during mild hypothermia. *Moderate hypothermia* is defined as a core temperature between 26.7° and 32.2°C (80° to 89°F). The child

TABLE 27-4. *Classification of hypothermic states*

Definition	Temperature	Symptoms
Mild	>32.2°–34.4°C (90°–94°F)	Hemodynamic stability Confusion Shivering Complaints of cold Seeks protection
Moderate	26.7°–32.2°C (80°–89°F)	Hemodynamic instability Shivering ceases Combative Dysrhythmias common Dilated pupils Muscle rigidity
Severe	<26.7°C (<80°F)	Coma Flaccidity Ventricular fibrillation or asystole Hemodynamic instability Apnea

with moderate hypothermia is often combative, hemodynamically unstable, and prone to ventricular dysrhythmia. Pupils are dilated, respiratory rate is reduced, and muscles are rigid. In all age ranges, shivering ceases at this body temperature. *Severe hypothermia* is a core temperature of less than 26.7°C (less than 80°F). At this body temperature, a child is comatose, flaccid, apneic, and frequently fibrillates spontaneously or is asystolic.

Pathophysiology

An understanding of the pathophysiology of hypothermia depends on a thorough knowledge of the mechanisms by which the human body loses heat (Table 27-5). Heat loss occurs by four mechanisms: radiation, convection, conduction, and evaporation.[34]

Radiation is the process by which heat energy leaves the skin at the speed of light. It accounts for as much as half of all heat loss, even in a warm environment, and more if the temperature of the surroundings falls. *Conduction* is the transfer of heat to another object by direct contact. When this object is cold water, heat is transferred 32 times faster than it is to air. Wet clothing, cold ground surface, and metal (such as a stretcher or fuselage) also provide excellent heat sinks. *Convection* occurs as warm

TABLE 27-5. *Mechanisms of heat loss and their characteristics*

Mechanism	Characteristics
Radiation	Heat leaves the skin at the speed of light Mechanism for >50% of heat loss
Convection	Warm air is replaced by cold air at the skin surface Mechanism for about 25% of heat loss
Conduction	Transfer of heat by direct contact Increases by a factor of 32 in water
Evaporation	Heat lost by vaporization Mechanism for about 7% of heat loss
Respiration	Combination of mechanisms Accounts for 14% of heat loss at rest

air is replaced by cold air at the skin surface. Even in weather conditions that are still, convection accounts for about 25% of heat loss. In a 12-mph breeze, the rate of heat loss increases by a factor of 5. In a 35-mph wind, heat loss accelerates by a factor of 14. *Evaporation,* the expenditure of heat when water or sweat on the skin surface is vaporized, accounts for 7% of heat loss at rest but, during exertion, can rise to six times the basal metabolic rate. Additionally, by a combination of these mechanisms, heat is lost in warming inhaled air during respiration. At rest, the respiratory system accounts for 14% of heat loss. With exercise, particularly in cold, dry air or at altitude elevation, these losses increase substantially.

Homeothermic responses to cold are integrated and regulated by the hypothalamus. Changes in ambient temperature are detected by thermal receptors in the skin and then transmitted through afferent pathways in the spinal cord to the hypothalamus. From the hypothalamus, a series of signals is sent for heat conservation: muscle tone is increased, and shivering begins. Catecholamines are released, resulting in peripheral vasoconstriction and metabolic thermogenesis. In addition, and perhaps most important, when thermally challenged, the conscious and competent child seeks shelter, increases physical activity, and applies protective clothing.

Children incapable of making intellectual decisions to avoid or protect themselves from a thermal challenge are at increased risk of hypothermia. In a small child, the risk is compounded by the large surface area/mass ratio,[35] which promotes excessive heat loss. The newborn is also compromised by an inability to shiver and generate heat. For thermogenesis, the newborn relies on a sparse supply of brown fat, which is quickly depleted. Once core body temperature falls below 34°C (94°F), protective homeothermic mechanisms are often so blunted that hypothermia progresses rapidly.

Hypothermia affects all organ systems[33,34] (Table 27-6). Cardiac output initially increases and then progressively decreases as hypothermia worsens. Stroke volume, filling pressures, and

TABLE 27-6. *Pathophysiology of hypothermia*

Organ system	Effect
Cardiovascular	J or Osborne wave Atrial and ventricular dysrhythmias Hypotension Hypovolemia
Respiratory	Hypoventilation Bronchorrhea Ciliary dysfunction Loss of airway reflexes
Renal	Cold diuresis Reduction of distal tubular sensitivity to antidiuretic hormone
Central nervous	Loss of judgment Combative behavior Alteration in level of consciousness Coma
Metabolic	Reduced oxygen delivery and consumption Hyperglycemia Hyperkalemia
Gastrointestinal	Ileus Reduced hepatic clearance

heart rate decline. Conduction disturbances are common. In moderate hypothermia, as many as 80% of patients have a characteristic J or Osborne wave (which appears as a hump) at the J point immediately after the QRS complex. As hypothermia deepens, the QRS and ST segments lengthen. When core temperature falls below 30°C, atrial fibrillation, bradycardia, and ventricular extrasystole is common. Below 25°C, asystole in children and fibrillation in adults are common. Hemodynamic instability is promoted by the loss of intravascular volume and vasomotor tone.

As hypothermic injury progresses, so does the depression of the medullary respiratory center. Tracheobronchial ciliary motility is inhibited by cold injury, and production of bronchial secretions (*cold bronchorrhea*) is excessive. The depression of airway-protective reflexes further predisposes the hypothermic patient to the development of bronchopneumonia.

A left shift of the oxyhemoglobin dissociation curve is seen, and oxygen is more tightly bound to hemoglobin, reducing oxygen delivery to tissue. Fortunately, this reduction parallels the decrease in metabolic rate and oxygen consumption. Metabolic rate decreases by 7% for each degree of reduction in core temperature. At 28°C, the basal metabolic rate is 50% of baseline. At a core temperature of less than 30°C, the action of insulin is impaired, uptake of cellular glucose is reduced, and hyperglycemia results. Extracellular potassium can be elevated because of impaired insulin activity and a dysfunctional Na^+-K^+-ATPase pump. Metabolic acidosis is common because of initial increases in lactate production with shivering and reduced lactate clearance by the liver as cold injury becomes severe.

Hypothermia is accompanied by a brisk diuresis, which can result in significant hypovolemia and hyperosmolality. A number of factors contribute to the increase in urine output. As the body attempts to respond to thermal challenge with compensatory vasoconstriction, central blood volume increases, and secretion of antidiuretic hormone decreases. When distal tubular absorption of sodium and water decreases, urine volume rises.

With diuresis, hemoconcentration is common. During hypothermia, blood viscosity increases 2% for each degree that body temperature decreases. Impaired coagulation at modest reductions in body temperature is complicated by the release of tissue thromboplastin and disseminated intravascular coagulopathy as core body temperature continues to fall.[35]

Hypothermia also causes progressive depression of central nervous system activity. Cerebral blood flow decreases 7% for each degree that body temperature decreases. As hypothermia deepens, consciousness is initially clouded, sensible judgment is impaired, and finally, the victim lapses into coma.

Treatment Issues

The treatment of hypothermic children begins in the prehospital setting. The key to successful treatment is recognition. A thermometer that records temperatures below 34°C must be available to measure core temperature. Core temperature is best measured with a flexible probe at the tympanic membrane, distal esophagus, trachea, or bladder. Rectal temperature measurements are often distorted by the presence of stool in the rectal vault.

Once identified, the cold child should be removed from the cold environment as soon as possible. Cold, wet clothing should be removed, and the patient should be wrapped in warm, dry blankets. The specific treatment of hypothermia must coincide with the application of appropriate life support measures.

Although there has been some controversy with respect to the necessity of CPR in the hypothermia victim, the most prudent action is to begin CPR, unless there is a perfusing rhythm and the body temperature is less than 28°C.[33,34] In the latter circumstance, CPR is unnecessary, even in the presence of hypotension, and may provoke ventricular fibrillation. *In all other circumstances, advanced life support measures should be instituted immediately.* Electrical defibrillation is usually unsuccessful at core body temperatures of less than 30°C. Repeated resuscitation efforts should be made as the patient is rewarmed. Resuscitation measures should be continued until the child can be transported to an acute care facility, even if the duration of the resuscitation seems excessive. Dramatic recoveries, although not necessarily the rule, are entirely possible.

In the hospital, the manner in which a patient is rewarmed depends on the severity of the hypothermia and the available technology. Rewarming can be accomplished by passive techniques, active external processes, or core rewarming methods (Table 27-7). Passive rewarming requires that the patient be hemodynamically stable and capable of producing heat spontaneously. The patient is merely removed from the cold environment and wrapped in thermal blankets. This method is reserved for children with mild hypothermia and can cause excessive morbidity and mortality in patients with more severe disease.

Active external rewarming (ie, use of heat packs, environmental heaters, and immersion in warm water) can provide a more rapid return of normothermia. The technical simplicity of these methods makes them widely available. The problems encountered using active surface rewarming are not trivial. When applied to the skin, heating pads or hot water bottles can injure patients with already compromised cutaneous circulation. Unless meticulous attention is given to volume resuscitation, peripheral vasodilation from surface warming can produce dramatic hypotension. Finally, vasodilation can transfer heat from the patient's core, causing a paradoxical decrease in core body temperature, so-called afterdrop.[33,34]

For these reasons, resuscitation efforts, particularly for severely hypothermic children, should use active techniques for core rewarming. These methods range in complexity from heating intravenous fluids to the application of extracorporeal blood

TABLE 27-7. *Rewarming techniques*

Technique	Method
Passive	Warm environment
	Blankets
	Shivering
Active surface	Hot packs
	Immersion in warm water
	Environmental heaters
Active core	Heated intravenous fluids
	Heated inspired respiratory gases
	Gastric lavage
	Colon irrigation
	Peritoneal lavage
	Pleural lavage
	Hemodialysis
	Cardiopulmonary bypass

rewarming. In the emergency department, gastric lavage and colon irrigation with warmed saline can be accomplished easily. Respiratory gases can be heated to 40° to 42°C. Intravenous fluids can and should be warmed to 40°C as well.

Active rewarming of core temperature can be accomplished rapidly using peritoneal lavage with heated saline solutions. When possible, two peritoneal lavage catheters are inserted, and warmed isotonic fluid is allowed to enter the peritoneal cavity passively and then exit by gravity.[33] Lavage rates of 12 L/h can be achieved with this method. Peritoneal lavage should not be performed in the presence of abdominal trauma or when abdominal distention with lavage fluid may impair the patient's respiratory status. In the patient with prior abdominal surgery, placement of the peritoneal catheter should be through a small infraumbilical incision rather than by the percutaneous approach.

In patients with circulatory arrest or intractable ventricular fibrillation, there are significant advantages to rewarming with cardiopulmonary bypass. Extremely rapid rewarming is possible, as is the support of the cardiovascular system. Adequate oxygenation is ensured, hemoconcentration is reversed, and myocardial stress is minimized. Because of the need for systemic anticoagulation, extracorporeal circulation is contraindicated in patients with major traumatic injuries. The complexity of this support system limits its general application.[33,34] Despite the dramatic descriptions of successful resuscitation with cardiopulmonary bypass for rapid warming after prolonged hypothermic arrest,[15,34] this method is *not* a cure-all and does not resuscitate the dead. Successful resuscitation can occur with other core warming methods, and extracorporeal circulation should not be initiated if safer, simpler techniques suffice.

The rate of rewarming should proceed rapidly, particularly if sophisticated life support measures are used.[33,34] Cardiac rhythm becomes stable when warming has produced a core temperature of more than 32°C. Similarly, if cardiac rhythm has not been restored in 30 minutes of resuscitative efforts at 35°C, success is unlikely. During rewarming, *it is imperative to volume-resuscitate the child diligently and to provide the necessary vasoactive pharmacologic support.*

Much discussion can be found in the literature with respect to the interpretation of arterial blood gases during hypothermia. Because of the effects of cold on the dissociation of water, the pH of neutrality increases with decreasing temperature. In addition, hypothermia increases the solubility of carbon dioxide in blood. Therefore, if ventilation is constant, total carbon dioxide is constant, with an ever-increasing dissolved fraction. Even when the P_{CO_2} in the arterial sample decreases, total carbon dioxide is not, in fact, reduced. For these reasons, blood gas interpretation and intervention based on acid–base assessment should be done *without* blood gas temperature correction.[33,34]

Like drowning, hypothermia is a condition that is best prevented. The treatment of the hypothermic child depends on the severity of the cold injury and the available therapeutic resources. The child with mild hypothermia can be treated conservatively with passive techniques and external rewarming. The more challenging patient with moderate or severe hypothermia and hemodynamic instability requires more aggressive invasive methods of rewarming.

Peritoneal lavage should be used promptly, particularly when gastric lavage and heated intravenous fluid therapy have failed. The use of cardiopulmonary bypass should be reserved for the child with severe hypothermia and cardiac standstill or fibrillation. In this circumstance, dramatic recovery is possible.

The rate of rewarming should allow time for adequate volume resuscitation and inotropic support of the circulation to preserve hemodynamic stability. In fact, there is no disadvantage of rapid rewarming if hemodynamic stability is maintained. Slow rewarming can promote morbidity, particularly if protracted cardiac dysrhythmias result. Finally, no patient should be declared dead until resuscitation efforts are unsuccessful at normothermia.

FROSTBITE

Children who present with frostbite injury are often the victims of their enthusiasm for outdoor winter activities. Historically, frostbite was an injury common in wartime efforts, when soldiers were exposed to a cold environment for a prolonged period of time. In fact, more than 7 million active duty days were lost during World War II because of this injury.[33]

Frostnip refers to a minimal injury characterized by pallor and numbness of the affected area. Rewarming the tissue can be accomplished without any risk of tissue loss. *Chilblain,* or *pernio,* is somewhat more severe and involves the face, anterior tibia, or the dorsa of the hands or feet. Repeated exposure to cold can cause vasculitis of the affected area. In *frostbite,* the skin and the subcutaneous tissues are actually frozen. Frostbite commonly occurs after exposure to environmental temperatures of less than 2°C.[33]

Pathophysiology

Until recently, tissue damage from frostbite was thought to be caused by the freezing process. Cellular swelling, the disruption of endothelial integrity, and interstitial and intracellular crystallization were believed to result in irreversible tissue destruction.[36] With greater understanding of reperfusion injury, the pathophysiology of frostbite has been more clearly elucidated. Indeed, it appears as if the bulk of tissue damage from frostbite occurs during rewarming and consequent reperfusion. Arachidonic acid metabolites, platelet aggregates, free radicals, and activated leukocytes have all been implicated.

In a landmark experiment, investigators at the University of Washington[37] demonstrated that the tissue loss after immersion-induced frostbite could be virtually eliminated by treatment before rewarming with an antibody that prevents leukocyte adhesion. In a rabbit model, frostbite was induced by immersion of the hind limb in a saltwater bath of −15°C. Treatment with the leukocyte adhesion antibody at the onset of rewarming effectively eliminated tissue injury. Treatment of the animals at the conclusion of rewarming ameliorated the injury but provided less protection. Control animals suffered typical frostbite injury with extensive deep tissue loss. This new information will certainly affect treatment issues when antibodies against leukocyte adhesion are clinically available.

Treatment Issues

Care of the patient by the prehospital care provider should focus on removing the child from the cold environment and finding appropriate shelter and health care. Aggressive rubbing or other mechanical trauma of the affected area can result in significant tissue damage and should be avoided.

Rewarming of the affected area should be accomplished rapidly by immersion in a warm bath (38° to 40°C) until the area appears flushed. Because of the likelihood of an inadvertent burn injury, dry heat is not recommended. The involved extremity should be elevated. Blisters may be débrided or left intact.[36,38]

Analgesics are required because rewarming produces significant pain. Antibiotics are not routinely recommended and should be reserved for the patient at risk for endocarditis or with clear evidence of infection. A tetanus booster should be administered.

The goal of wound care is the preservation of viable tissue and the prevention of infection. Débridement is facilitated by frequent whirlpool baths in antibiotic solution and application of sterile dressing. Topical antibiotic creams can be used, although aloe has been shown to be equally effective.[39] Amputation should be delayed until demarcation of nonviability is clear, unless uncontrolled wound sepsis intervenes.

Some data indicate that viability can be determined using early radionucleotide angiography. Scintigraphy is performed on days 1 to 3 and on days 5 to 7 to determine vascular sufficiency. Amputation can then be accomplished before mummification. Further clinical experience is required before this approach becomes the standard of care.[33]

Adjuvant therapy holds significant promise for the future. Low-molecular-weight dextran, fibrinolytics,[40] heparin, hyperbaric oxygen, and sympathectomy have been used for frostbite injuries without much success in improving tissue survival. When modifiers of reperfusion events become available for routine clinical use, however, *the results of treatment can be expected to change radically.*

REFERENCES

1. Wintemute GJ. Childhood drowning and near-drowning in the United States. Am J Dis Child 1990;144:663.
2. Wintemute GJ, Drake C, Wright M. Immersion events in residential swimming pools: evidence for an experience effect. Am J Dis Child 1991;145:1200.
3. Orlowski JP. Drowning, near-drowning, and ice-water submersions. Pediatr Clin North Am 1987;34:75.
4. Modell JH. Drowning. N Engl J Med 1993;328:253.
5. Levin DL, Morriss FC, Toro LO, et al. Drowning and near drowning. Pediatr Clin North Am 1993;40:321.
6. Gooden BA. Why some people do not drown: hypothermia versus the diving response. Med J Aust 1992;157:629.
7. Ramey CA, Ramey DN, Hayward JS. Dive response of children in relation to cold-water near drowning. J Appl Physiol 1987;63:665.
8. Werner JZ, Safar P, Bircher NG, et al. No improvement in pulmonary status by gravity drainage or abdominal thrusts after sea water near drowning in dogs. [Abstract] Anesthesiology 1982;57:A81.
9. Heimlich HJ. Subdiaphragmatic pressure to expel water from the lungs of drowning persons. Ann Emerg Med 1981;10:476.
10. Fields AI. Near-drowning in the pediatric population. Crit Care Clin 1992;8:113.
11. Biggart MJ, Bohn DJ. Effect of hypothermia and cardiac arrest on outcome of near-drowning accidents in children. J Pediatr 1990;117:179.
12. Elixson EM. Hypothermia: cold-water drowning. Crit Care Nurs Clin North Am 1991;3:287.
13. Letsou GV, Kopf GS, Elefteriades JA, et al. Is cardiopulmonary bypass effective for treatment of hypothermic arrest due to drowning or exposure? Arch Surg 1992;127:525.
14. Norberg WJ, Agnew RF, Brunsvold R, et al. Successful resuscitation of a cold water submersion victim with the use of cardiopulmonary bypass. Crit Care Med 1992;20:1355.
15. Schissler P, Parker MA, Scott SJ. Profound hypothermia: value of prolonged cardiopulmonary resuscitation. South Med J 1981;74:474.
16. Kemp AM, Sibert JR. Outcome in children who nearly drown: a British Isles study. BMJ 1991;302:931.
17. Quan L, Kinder D. Pediatric submersions: prehospital predictors of outcome. Pediatrics 1992;90:909.
18. Lavelle JM, Shaw KN. Near drowning: is emergency department cardiopulmonary resuscitation or intensive care unit cerebral resuscitation indicated? Crit Care Med 1993;21:368.
19. Fisher B, Peterson B, Hicks G. Use of brainstem auditory-evoked response testing to assess neurologic outcome following near drowning in children. Crit Care Med 1992;20:578.
20. Nussbaum E, Galant SP. Intracranial pressure monitoring as a guide to prognosis in the nearly drowned, severely comatose child. J Pediatr 1983;102:215.
21. Wheatley J, Cass DT. Traumatic deaths in children: the importance of prevention. Med J Aust 1989;150:72.
22. Wintemute GJ, Wright MA. The attitude–practice gap revisited: risk reduction beliefs and behaviors among owners of residential swimming pools. Pediatrics 1991;88:1168.
23. Pearn J. Safety legislation and child mortality. Med J Aust 1991;154:155.
24. Present P. Child drowning study: a report on the epidemiology of drownings in residential pools to children under age five. Washington DC, Directorate for Epidemiology, US Consumer Product Safety Commission, 1987.
25. Pitt WR, Balanda KP. Childhood drowning and near-drowning in Brisbane: the contribution of domestic pools. Med J Aust 1991;154:661.
26. Cass DT, Ross FI, Grattan-Smith TM. Child drownings: a changing pattern. Med J Aust 1991;154:163.
27. Hassall IB. Thirty-six consecutive under 5 year old domestic swimming pool drownings. Aust Pediatr J 1989;25:143.
28. Quan L, Gore EJ, Wentz K, et al. Ten-year study of pediatric drownings and near-drownings in King County, Washington: lessons in injury prevention. Pediatrics 1989;83:1035.
29. Ley P. Isolation fencing and drownings in backyard pools. Med J Aust 1991;154:711.
30. Wintemute GJ. Drowning in early childhood. Pediatr Ann 1992;21:417.
31. Liller KD, Kent EB, Arcari C, et al. Risk factors for drowning and near-drowning among children in Hillsborough County, Florida. Public Health Rep 1993;108:346.
32. Pearn J. The urgency of immersions. Arch Dis Child 1992;67:257.
33. Britt LD, Dascombe WH, Rodriguez A. New horizons in management of hypothermia and frostbite injury. Surg Clin North Am 1991;71:345.
34. Corneli HM. Accidental hypothermia. J Pediatr 1992;120:671.
35. Mann TP, Elliott RIK. Neonatal cold injury. Lancet 1957;229.
36. Edlich RF, Chang DE, Birk KA, et al. Cold injuries. Compr Ther 1989;15:13.
37. Mileski WJ, Raymond JF, Winn RK, et al. Inhibition of leukocyte adherence and aggregation for treatment of severe cold injury in rabbits. J Appl Physiol 1993;74:1432.
38. Granberg PO. Freezing cold injury. Arctic Med Res 1991;6:76.
39. McCauley RL, Heggers JP, Robson MC. Frostbite: methods to minimize tissue loss. Postgrad Med 1990;88:67.
40. Skolnick AA. Early data suggest clot-dissolving drug may help save frostbitten limbs from amputation. JAMA 1992;267:2008.

Surgery of Infants and Children: Scientific Principles and Practice, edited by
Keith T. Oldham, Paul M. Colombani, and Robert P. Foglia.
Lippincott–Raven Publishers, Philadelphia, © 1997.

CHAPTER 28

Stings, Bites, and Poisonings

Charles G. Howell, Robyn M. Hatley, and Diane S. Bairas

During 1992, 1.8 million bites, stings, and poisonings were reported to the nation's poison control centers.[1] More than 90% of these incidents occurred at home, and more than 60% of patients were children younger than 6 years of age.[1] Most of these incidents occur in boys, who tend to explore the environment and its dangerous inhabitants. In most cases, bites, stings, and poisonings are minor incidents; only rarely are they fatal. Most cases are handled over the telephone with the family physician, pediatrician, or an emergency room physician. The more serious incidents can prompt an emergency room visit, hospitalization, and even a stay in the pediatric intensive care unit.

STINGS

Stings covered in this section are those from the venomous families of the order Hymenoptera, including the Apidae (honeybees), Bombidae (bumblebees), Vespidae (wasps, hornets, and yellow jackets), and Formicidae (ants) families.

Epidemiology

Honeybees generally live in hives and are managed commercially to produce honey throughout the United States. Wasps and hornets live in nests that are found under the overhangs of buildings or suspended from branches of trees. Yellow jackets and bumblebees may be found in old tree stumps or in underground tunnels that were previously prepared and inhabited by other animals. The most feared of the Hymenoptera, the so-called killer bees, have slowly migrated north to the United States and can be found in the Southern states. These African honeybees, *Apis mellifera adansonii*, generally travel in swarms, are aggressive, and attack in mass after only minimal provocation. The most destructive of the Hymenoptera, the South African fire ants, were introduced into the United States more than 70 years ago and have slowly migrated to most of the Southern states.

Evaluation

The typical presentation is that of a child with multiple lesions consisting of wheals, flares, and urticaria. Bee stings may simply cause swelling. In some cases this can be followed by an anaphylactic reaction. Fire ants typically produce vesicles within several hours, which may become sterile pustules or secondarily infected. Honeybees may leave the barbed stinger and venom sac in the victim.

Pathophysiology

Hymenoptera venom contains a variety of enzymes, including as phospholipase A and hyaluronidase. It also contains polypeptide toxins, such as mellitin, and kinins. Alkaloids are found in fire ant venom. Antigenic proteins in venom are responsible for the development of the most serious problems from a sting, that is, sensitization and subsequent severe allergic reactions.

Resuscitation

Most stings require little or no treatment. Pruritus can lead to secondary infection. Local measures include removal of the stinger and venom sac if present, cleansing of the site, application of an ice pack, and administration of oral diphenhydramine. The dose of diphenhydramine for children is 5 mg/kg/24 hours, divided every 6 hours, with a maximum dose of 300 mg/24 hours. Large numbers of ant bites on a child can be treated with neutralization of the venom by application of dilute ammonia or bicarbonate. Tetanus prophylaxis is indicated if the child has not been immunized. Systemic allergic reactions generally occur within minutes of the stings, and all occur within several hours. The most severe of these reactions can lead to airway obstruction and death. Delayed systemic reactions are rare.

Severe allergic reactions require prompt emergency treatment and subsequent monitoring and treatment in a well-staffed pediatric intensive care unit. If mild bronchospasm is present, a nebulized bronchodilator should be given. The mainstays of therapy are providing an adequate airway and volume support and administering epinephrine.

Desensitization measures are recommended in patients with severe local reactions or systemic reactions. Specially designed kits and medical alert bracelets are recommended in patients with histories of systemic reactions or anaphylaxis.

Outcome

Nearly 10,000 Hymenoptera bites were reported in children less than 17 years of age in the 1993 Annual Report of the American Association of Poison Control Centers.[1] Sixteen patients suffered major outcomes,[1] and two patients died. More than half of patients did well with little or no treatment and did not require hospitalization. Outcomes are defined as follows:

Minor—minimal symptoms and signs, rapid resolution; limited to skin involvement; no treatment required

Moderate—more serious and prolonged systemic manifestations of toxicity

Major—life-threatening symptoms and signs; residual disability, such as requirement of intubation with mechanical ventilation, cardiac instability, or coma

SNAKE BITES

Pit Vipers

Epidemiology

Pit vipers (rattlesnakes, water moccasins, copperheads) are found throughout the United States. Water moccasin and copperheads are most prevalent in the South and various types of rattlesnakes inhabit all regions. Most bites occur in the summer months, are common in children, and are usually from rattlesnakes. The Southwest is noted for its higher number of rattlesnake bites. The Southeast is noted for bites of the water moccasin and copperhead. Rarely does one encounter a venomous snake bite in the Northeast. The 1993 American Association of Poison Control Centers report[1] of the United States revealed 1265 poisonous snake bites. Seventy-two bites were in children younger than 6 years of age, and 215 bites were in children 6 to 17 years of age.

Evaluation

Pain begins immediately after the bite, followed by progressive swelling. Blisters, ecchymosis, and petechiae may surround the visible bite. When the fang marks are not noted by either the parents or the initial medical team, the child can present a diagnostic enigma if the event was unobserved. Often, in children, the particular type and size of snake is not known.

Pathophysiology

The physiologic response to a venomous snake bite is a consequence of multiple factors. These include the quantity and toxicity of the venom (ie, the degree of envenomation), the size of the child, and the anatomic location of the bite. A child may suffer from multiple bites because of an inability to move away from the snake. A strike to the head and neck is potentially more serious than one to an extremity.[2] Larger snakes inject more venom, and smaller children suffer pronounced effects. The Mojave rattlesnake is the most lethal snake, while the water

moccasin is rarely lethal. Pit viper venom can cause systemic signs of weakness, nausea, diaphoresis, blurred vision and speech, muscle fasciculations, and even convulsions. Cardiovascular effects include hypotension and decreased peripheral vascular resistance. Respiratory effects include decreased respiratory rate and the development of pulmonary edema. Hematologic effects are pronounced and include abnormalities in clotting thought to be due to procoagulants, fibrinolysins, hemorrhagins, and hemolysins in the serum. Actual disturbances in the red-cell morphology have been noted, as has interference in subsequent cross-matching of blood. Nephrotoxic effects of pit viper venom include tubular necrosis and cortical necrosis.

Coral Snakes

Epidemiology

Fewer than 25 of all reported venomous snake bites per year are due to coral snakes. Half of all coral snake bites in the United States are *dry*, which means they do not result in envenomation.[3] Coral snakes are North America's sole representative of the Elapidae family and are a distant relative of the cobras, kraits, and mambas.

Eastern coral snakes range from Florida to Texas, and Western coral snakes range from Texas to Mexico. The coral snake is characterized by a series of red and black bands separated by narrower yellow rings and culminating in a petite black head. They have short anterior fangs and inject their venom with a succession of chewing movements.

Coral snakes are responsible for the widely known rhyme, "red on yellow, kill a fellow; red on black, won't kill Jack." This method of identification removes the confusion about whether the snake in question is a coral snake or nonpoisonous king snake. The three snakes that are considered coral snakes in the United States are the Eastern coral snake (*Micrurus fulvius fulvius*), the Texas or Western coral snake (*Micrurus fulvius tenere*), and the Sonoran coral snake (*Micruroides euryxanthus euryxanthus*). Two species, the Eastern and Western varieties, are responsible for most cases of envenomation by coral snakes in the United States.[4]

The coral snake is timid by nature and normally does not attack unless provoked. Because their jaws are not hinged, they characteristically bite a finger, toe, or fold of skin. They tend to attach to the victim and chew, as opposed to striking and releasing, like a rattlesnake.

Evaluation

Positive identification should be made if at all possible. Coral snake venom is neurotoxic and usually causes only minimal to moderate tissue reaction and pain at the bite area. Coral snake bites are not always followed by envenomation. However, severe envenomation may be present without obvious local tissue reaction.

Symptoms of envenomation usually begin within 8 hours after the bite. If envenomation occurs, symptoms and signs may progress rapidly. A postbulbar paralysis involving the cranial nerves has been observed within a few hours of the bite.

Signs and symptoms may include weakness, nausea, vomiting, excessive salivation, ptosis of the eyelids, dyspnea, abnormal reflexes, seizures, and paralysis, including complete respiratory paralysis.[4] Local signs and symptoms include scratch marks, small puncture wounds, little edema, and paresthesia in the bitten extremity.

Pathophysiology

The venom of the coral snake is a potent neurotoxin that attacks the neuromuscular junction, particularly the cranial nerves. The neurotoxic venom produced by the coral snake is primarily paralytic in action, and respiratory paralysis can result in early death.[5] A time interval of 6 to 8 hours from bite to onset of symptoms may give the victim and physician a false sense of security.[6]

Resuscitation

Prehospital management of the possible envenomation includes the following basic rules:

1. Keep the child as calm and still as possible.
2. Immobilize the involved extremity if possible.
3. Avoid incision and suction unless medical personnel are immediately available.
4. Apply a loose compression wrap to retard lymphatic return.
5. Transport the child to a medical facility as soon as possible.
6. Note the size and type of the snake.

Once the child has arrived at the emergency medical facility equipped to handle the injury, the wound should be evaluated rapidly to determine the presence of pit viper envenomation. Occasionally, the snake has been killed and transported with the victim for identification by appropriate medical personnel. Examination of the involved area reveals the puncture wounds, surrounding erythema, and localized edema. The wound should be cleansed with soap and water while ascertaining the vital signs. An intravenous line should be begun simultaneous with obtaining a complete blood count, platelet count, prothrombin time, partial thromboplastin time, fibrin split products, electrolytes, blood urea nitrogen, creatinine, creatine phosphokinase, blood type and cross-match, and urinalysis. The patient may require fluid resuscitation to expand the intravascular volume and monitoring of vital signs and urine output. Tetanus prophylaxis is indicated. Antivenin should be used in children who have progressively worsening local symptoms or evidence of systemic toxicity. Before administration, a test for hypersensitivity to horse serum should be done, and the appropriate therapeutic agents should be available to treat a severe and immediate anaphylactic reaction.

Controversy persists regarding the use of antivenin and surgical débridement.[7,8,9] A child who has sustained a pit viper envenomation with obvious fang marks and has surrounding erythema and edema extending greater than 12 inches from the bite should receive antivenin, 5 vials initially, and then titrate based on response. Children may require up to 1.5 times the adult dose because of their size in comparison to the amount of envenomation. Table 28-1 lists the guidelines for initial dosage of antivenin. Many bites do not require antivenin, particularly those inflicted by the Pigmy rattler and copperhead and those that have been observed elsewhere for 12 to 24 hours without deterioration of the patient. Because of the potential for serum sickness and even death after the use of antivenin, the physician should be sure that envenomation has occurred before it is used.

Envenomation from coral snakes is lower than that of rattlesnakes, with only about half of coral snake bites resulting in significant envenomation. Surgical intervention normally is not indicated in snake bite victims. Occasionally, digital fasciotomy of the fingers or toes is necessary. A more extensive fasciotomy may be indicated for the treatment of compartment syndrome of an arm or leg identified by clinical examination and compartment pressure monitoring.

Outcome

Most patients who sustain snake bites and are treated appropriately recover without disability. About 8000 poisonous snake bites occur each year in the United States. These bites result in as many as 10 deaths of adults and children each year.[1,10,11] Major and minor soft tissue complications are more common.

MAMMAL BITES

Human

Presentation

The most common site of human bites in children is the upper extremities, followed by the face, neck, and trunk. The potential for serious infection and complications warrants consideration. As with any injury, delay in seeking medical attention increases the probability of infection and complications. Human bites to the hand are more prone to infection than bites on other areas, especially if initially neglected by the patient or family. Bites involving the joint capsule and dorsal tendons, especially if the wound was a puncture, are more likely to lead to serious consequences.

Pathophysiology

The most common pathogens cultured from human bite wounds are *Staphylococcus aureus* and *Staphylococcus epidermidis*. A multitude of other organisms have been reported, including aerobes such as *Streptococcus, Neisseria, Corynebacterium, Proteus, Pseudomonas,* and *Klebsiella* sp as well as *Eikenella corrodens,* and anaerobes such as *Peptostreptococcus, Actinomyces, Fusobacterium,* and *Bacteroides* sp.

One striking difference between human and other mammal bite wounds is the higher number of isolates of bacteria found per wound in human bites. This difference is attributed to the

TABLE 28-1. *Guidelines for initial dosage of antivenin*

Envenomation	Signs	Dose of antivenin
None	No local or systemic signs	0 vials
Minimal	Local swelling, no systemic signs, normal lab data	2–4 vials
Moderate	Swelling beyond site of bite, one or more systemic signs, abnormal lab data (eg, drop in hematocrit or platelet count)	5–9 vials
Severe	Marked local response, severe systemic signs, abnormal lab data	10–15 vials or more

(Data from: Minton S. Venom diseases: snakebite. In: Beeson P, McDermott W, ed. Textbook of medicine. Philadelphia, WB Saunders, 1975:88; Russell F, Carlson RW, Wainschel J. Snake venom poisoning in the United States: experiences with 550 cases. JAMA 1975;233:341; Russell F. Venomous bites and stings: poisonous snakes. In: The Merck manual of diagnosis and therapy, ed 14. Rahway, NJ, Merck, Sharp & Dohme, 1982:2450; and Wingert W, Wainschel J. Diagnosis and management of envenomation by poisonous snakes. South Med J 1975;68:1015)

3:1 ratio of anaerobic bacteria (mostly *Bacteroides* sp) found in human wounds to those found in animal bite wounds.[12] Culture studies for both aerobic and anaerobic organisms should be carried out.

Resuscitation and Management

Most human bites are adequately managed on an outpatient basis by diligent wound care, including pressure irrigation, careful débridement, adequate drainage, excision and suturing in selected cases, and no prophylactic antibiotic therapy.[13] Exploration of the wound should include evaluation for potential crush or tear injuries to tendons, joints, bones, or blood vessels. All devitalized tissue should be removed, including excision of the edges of puncture bite wounds, which are then left open after irrigation. A primary closure may be performed in uninfected wounds after débridement. If a delay in presentation exists, wound closure should be considered only after the infection is eradicated, or by secondary intent.[12] Furthermore, in some bites, such as the closed-fist injury, early aggressive irrigation, débridement, and subsequent antibiotic therapy may be indicated.[13]

The patient's immunization status should be evaluated and updated as necessary for tetanus. A tetanus toxoid booster should be given if the patient has not received a tetanus shot in the past 5 years. If the patient has never been immunized, the tetanus immune globin is given, and active immunization is begun.

Amoxicillin and clavulanate are effective oral agents for the treatment of human bites. If intravenous agents are needed, either cefoxitin, or first-generation cephalosporin plus β-lactamase–resistant penicillin, can be used.[12]

Dog

Presentation

About 1% of emergency department visits are for the treatment of dog bites,[14] and half of all mammal bites, most of which are from dogs, occur in the grammar school age group. Most dog bites are puncture wounds to the hand or arm, except in children younger than 4 years, in whom most of these injuries are to the head and neck. The initial evaluation of a dog bite includes a history of the type of animal and the circumstances surrounding the incident. The wound may initially appear benign until the puncture wounds are noted. The location of the bite is important because bites to the extremities are more likely to become infected than are bites to the head and neck. The physician should look for deep structure involvement, determine the length of time from the injury, and assess the vascular integrity of the extremity.

Pathophysiology

More than 60 species of potentially pathogenic bacteria live in dogs' mouths, and thus it is not surprising that up to 15% of nontrivial dog bite wounds become infected.[14] The usual infecting organisms are staphylococci, streptococci, gram-negative bacilli, and anaerobes. *Pasteurella multocida* is more common when the infection occurs in the first 24 hours.

The incidence of rabies has declined dramatically with legislated of mandatory vaccination of dogs, yet rabies still represents an ever-present threat. Even a house pet must be monitored for abnormal behavior and sacrificed if it exhibits signs of rabies. Any patient who has two or more significant risk factors should have treatment to prevent rabies.[15] The major risk categories are as follows:

- Child younger than 10 years of age
- Deep lacerations
- Head and neck wounds
- An animal whose vaccination status is in doubt

Resuscitation and Management

Rabies postexposure prophylaxis must be considered in every child that is bitten.

Knowledge of the local epidemiology of rabies is important because some locations have no history of rabies cases. The animals predominately responsible for transmitting rabies are dogs, cats, bats, bobcats, foxes, raccoons, skunks, and wild carnivores. Bites from animals such as bats and wild carnivores, unprovoked animal attacks, or unusually aggressive behavior mandate the institution of postexposure rabies prophylaxis. Table 28-2 presents a rabies postexposure prophylaxis guide.

Cat

Presentation

Cat bites and scratches are associated with a variety of diseases, including *Pasteurella multocida,* cat scratch disease,

TABLE 28-2. *Rabies postexposure prophylaxis guide, United States, 1991*

Animal type	Evaluation and disposition of animal	Postexposure prophylaxis recommendations
Dogs and cats	Healthy and available for 10 days' observation	No prophylaxis unless animal develops symptoms of rabies*
	Rabid or suspected rabid†	Immediate vaccination and RIG
	Unknown (escaped)	Consult public health officials for advice
Skunks, raccoons, bats, foxes, most carnivores, and woodchucks	Rapid unless geographic area is known to be free of rabies or until animal is proven negative by lab tests	Immediate vaccination and RIG
Livestock, ferrets, rodents, and rabbits	Consider individually	Consult public health officials; bites of squirrels, hamsters, quinea pigs, gerbils, chipmunks, rats, mice, other rodents, and rabbits almost never require antirabies therapy

* During the 10-day holding period, treatment with RIG and vaccine should be initiated at the first sign of rabies in the biting cat or dog. The symptomatic animal should be killed immediately and tested.
† The animal should be killed and tested as soon as possible. Holding for observation is not recommended. Vaccination is discontinued if immunofluorescent test of the animal is negative. RIG, rabies immune globulin (human).
(American Academy of Pediatrics. Summaries of infectious diseases. In: Peter G, ed. 1994 Red book: report of the Committee on Infectious Diseases, ed 23. Elk Grove Village, IL, American Academy of Pediatrics 1994:391)

ringworm, cutaneous larva migrans, toxoplasmosis, campylobacteriosis, and rabies.[16] Cat scratch disease, formerly attributed to *Afipia felis* and known as *cat scratch bacillus*, is now thought to be secondary to *Rochalimaea henselae*,[16] a fastidious, slow-growing, gram-negative rickettsia. The incidence of cat scratch disease is unknown, but about 80% of cases occur in patients younger than 20 years of age.

Most cat bites are puncture wounds and are prone to develop *Pasteurella multocida* infections. These infections can be detected 24 to 48 hours after the bite and may include swelling, erythema, tenderness, and serous or sanguinopurulent discharge. Regional lymphadenopathy, chills, and fever can occur. Other complications include septic arthritis, osteomyelitis, and tenosynovitis. Subsequently, the patient is at risk for developing cat scratch disease. This disease is manifested by a history of a scratch, followed by the development of regional lymphadenopathy in the drainage area of the innoculation site. Fever, chills, arthralgia, and even an oculoglandular syndrome may be a part of the disease.

Pathophysiology

Most patients who develop cat scratch disease have had a recent contact with a cat, most often a kitten. The organism responsible for the disease is found in the oral flora of 70% to 90% of cats. The infecting agent may be injected through the skin by the thin claws of the cat, allowing the skin lesion to appear deceptively innocuous. Such scratches and puncture wounds must be monitored closely for signs of local infection. The incubation period from the time of the scratch to the appearance of the primary cutaneous lesion is 7 to 12 days, and 5 to 50 days pass from the appearance of the primary lesion to the appearance of lymphadenopathy.[16]

Resuscitation and Management

The drug of choice for the prophylactic treatment of infections from cat bites is penicillin or ampicillin. Antibiotic therapy for cat scratch disease should be considered only for acutely or severely ill patients with systemic symptoms, particularly hepatosplenomegaly. Several reports[16,17,18] suggest the use of oral antibiotics (rifampin, trimethoprim-sulfamethoxazole, or ciprofloxacin) and even intravenous gentamicin for the treatment of the regional lymphadenopathy. Despite these reports of agents that may shorten the duration of the disease, no controlled antimicrobial trials have been performed. Occasionally, excisional biopsy is indicated for diagnostic purposes and may even be indicated for the chronically draining sinus from an infected node.

Outcome

Most patients are treated adequately as outpatients. The overall incidence of infection for human bites is about 10%.[19] Dog bites to the hand warrant special attention owing to anatomy and risk of infection, which can be as high as 30% to 35%.

SPIDER BITES

Brown Recluse Spider

Presentation

Brown recluse spider (*Loxosceles reclusa*) is a medium-sized (1 to 4 cm) spider. It is commonly called a *violin spider* or *fiddleback spider* (because of the unique markings on its thorax).

This spider lives in the Eastern, Southeastern, and Midwestern United States and is commonly found in buildings, cellars, wood piles, and behind or beneath objects in dark areas. The initial indication that a bite has occurred may be the presence of a lesion recognized while changing a child's clothes or bathing. Occasionally, a stinging or burning sensation in areas where clothes may fit tightly, such as the groin, buttocks, or legs, indicates that a bite has occurred. The initial red papule with subsequent vesicle may become dark blue or cyanotic and subsequently develop into a necrotic area of variable size. A more serious reaction in children is systemic loxoscelism manifested by urticaria, a fine maculopapular rash, and fever. These symptoms may progress to coagulopathy, shock, and death.

Pathophysiology

Many different enzymes are identified in the venom of this spider.[20] Hyaluronidase, proteases, esterases, and hemolysins probably lead to the subsequent tissue necrosis, eschar formation, and delayed healing. Histologically, experimental lesions reveal hemorrhage into the dermis, capillary stasis, thrombosis, and subsequent necrosis of all layers within 24 hours.

Treatment

Corticosteroids, phentolamine, immediate wide excision and grafting, hyperbaric oxygen, and oral dapsone with and without excision have all been advocated for therapy. None are demonstrably therapeutic, however, as appropriate prospective trials have not been done. If cellulitis is significant, antibiotic therapy is appropriate. In selected cases, curettage of the early lesion may prevent the spread of the venom and avoid the need for reconstructive surgery.[21]

Outcome

Rare deaths have been reported with the brown recluse spider bite. Occasional bites of the head and neck may require reconstructive surgery with either skin grafts or flaps. The usual wound contracts in 4 to 6 weeks and heals without grafting.

Black Widow Spider (*Lactrodectus mactans, hesperus, and Other Species*)

The female black widow spider is responsible for the envenomation that affects humans. This particular black spider, 1 to 3 cm in length, has a characteristic hourglass abdomen with a red dot.

Presentation

These spiders occur worldwide and particularly like moist conditions, where they may hide under objects. The spider is rarely identified or brought to the examining physician. Therefore, the diagnosis is generally made on the basis of clinical findings. Most children are bitten on the lower extremities.

TABLE 28-3. *Grading scale for* Latrodectus *envenomations*

Grade	Description
1	Asymptomatic
	Local pain at envenomation site
	Normal vital signs
2	Muscular pain in envenomated extremity
	Extension of muscular pain to abdomen if envenomated in lower extremity or chest if envenomated in upper extremity
	Local diaphoresis of envenomation site or involved extremity
	Normal vital signs
3	Generalized muscular pain in back, abdomen, and chest
	Diaphoresis remote from envenomation site
	Abnormal vital signs: hypertension (systolic blood pressure >140 mmHg or diastolic blood pressure >90 mmHg; tachycardia (pulse >100)
	Nausea and vomiting
	Headache

(Clark RF, Wethern-Kestner S, Vance MV, et al. Clinical presentation and treatment of black widow spider envenomation: a review of 163 cases. Ann Emerg Med 1992;21:782)

Symptoms include a known proximity to a spider, a subsequent painful lesion or bite known as a *target lesion* (1 to 2 tiny holes surrounded by pallor and then erythema), and development of skeletal muscle cramping of the affected limb that spreads to the trunk within minutes to one half hour, with resolution within 24 to 48 hours. Abdominal cramps, periorbital edema, diaphoresis, and hypertension are frequent signs in younger children. Priapism has also been noted in children. Laboratory evaluations reveal leukocytosis and occasional increases in creatine phosphokinase levels. Table 28-3 presents a grading scale of envenomation that is useful in evaluating the bites.

Pathophysiology

The venom of the black widow spider bite consists of a multitude of polypeptides that act predominately on the neuromuscular junction as a neurotoxin. This produces spontaneous depolarization with an excessive motor response from acetylcholine release and leads to spasms and cramps in the muscles.[22]

Resuscitation

Initial management depends on the presenting circumstances. Because the spider is rarely recovered and the exact cause of the symptoms may be unknown, the diagnosis can be difficult to establish. Local signs and minimal symptoms may require simple analgesics and reassurance. More serious envenomation may require more intensive evaluation and management (see Table 28-1). Attention to the basic tenets is indicated. Intravenous fluids are begun simultaneous to obtaining blood for routine laboratory evaluation in patients with serious envenomation. Methocarbamol, diazepam, and intravenous calcium have all been recommended for treatment of muscle spasms and abdominal rigidity, with varying results in anecdotal reports. The largest series[22] of black widow spider bites reported no benefit with the use of intravenous calcium. Clark and colleagues[22] recommend the use of intravenous morphine, and benzodiazepines for symptomatic treatment of grade 2 and some grade 3 envenomation cases. When these agents do not control the symptoms, antivenin has been used in children with life-threatening envenomation. The antivenin should be given as a slow intravenous infusion of 1 vial in 50 to 100 mL (relative to size of child) of normal saline. Before administration of antivenin, the physician should determine whether the patient has a known hypersensitivity to horse serum products or has received these types of products in the past. Skin or conjunctival tests for hypersensitivity before administration of antivenin are recommended.

Outcome

In one report of 163 patients, (18 of whom were younger than 13 years of age), the only death was in an adult who developed bronchospasm after receiving the antivenin. In a group of 732 children bitten by black widow spiders, there were six major complications and no deaths.

POISON INGESTION

Epidemiology

Of the nearly 2 million human poison exposure cases reported in 1992, more than 90% occurred in the home,[1] and greater than 60% occurred in children younger than 6 years of age. Of the 705 reported fatalities from poison ingestion in 1992, only 4% occurred in children younger than 6 years.[1] Most children with accidental poisonings present within 2 hours of the incident, whereas most suicide attempts present much later.

The most frequent nonpharmaceutical poisonings involve household cleaners, cosmetics, and personal care items. The most common pharmaceutical exposures are as follows[1]:

- Cough and cold preparations
- Topical preparations
- Acetaminophen
- Antimicrobials
- Psychotropic drugs, such as benzodiazepines

Drugs that may be fatal to a child less than 10 kg if they ingest just one commercially available dose unit (one tablet or capsule) include the following[23]:

- Tricyclic antidepressants
- Phenothiazines
- Camphor
- Chloroquine
- Hydroxychloroquine
- Quinine
- Methyl salicylate
- Theophylline

Evaluation

The most important aspect of an accidental or intentional poisoning is the history. More than 60% of patients have an altered state of consciousness, followed by respiratory depression, arrhythmia, or seizure depending on the agent ingested. About 70% of cases can be confirmed by routine qualitative toxicologic screening.

Resuscitation and Management

Initial management for acute toxic ingestion is the same as with any emergency: attention to the airway, breathing, and circulation. The mainstays of treatment in most cases include the use of syrup of ipecac (10 mL for children 6 months to 1 year of age, 15 mL for children 1 to 12 years of age, and 30 mL for adolescents) or gastric lavage, and activated charcoal (1 to 2 g/kg per dose) with or without a cathartic. The use of whole bowel irrigation for the treatment of serious iron ingestions and cocaine body stuffers and packers has been added to the realm of gastrointestinal decontamination treatment options. This treatment is particularly useful with ingested substances that do not bind to activated charcoal.[24] Golytely, 25 mL/kg/h through a nasogastric tube for up to 6 hours, has been effective in whole bowel irrigation.

Outcome

Most ingestions are handled over the telephone through the local poison control center with no adverse outcome. More serious ingestions are handled in local emergency rooms, and transferred to an intensive care unit if necessary.

REFERENCES

1. Litovitz TL, Holm KC, Clancy C, et al. 1992 Annual Report of the American Association of Poison Control Centers Toxic Exposure Surveillance System. Am J Emerg Med 1993;11:494.
2. Lewis JV, Portera CA. Rattlesnake bite of the face: case report and review of the literature. Am Surg 1999;60:681.
3. Dart RC, Russell FE. Animal poisoning. In: Hall JB, Schmidt GA, Wood L, et al, eds, Principles of critical care, New York, McGraw-Hill, 1992:2163.
4. Banner W. Bites and stings in the pediatric patient. In: Perry PC, Katz SL, Green M, et al, eds. Current problems in pediatrics. Chicago, Yearbook Medical Publishers, 1988:9.
5. Murdock RT, White GL, Pederson DM, et al. Prevention and emergency field management of venomous snakebites during military exercises. Milit Med 1990;155:587.
6. McCollough NC, Gennaro JF. Coral snake bites in the United States. J Fla Med Assoc 1963;99:968.
7. Stewart RM, Page CP, Schwesinger WH, et al. Antivenin and fasciotomy/débridement in the treatment of the severe rattlesnake bite. Am J Surg 1989;158:543.
8. Burch JM, Agarwal R, Mattox K, et al. The treatment of crotalid envenomation without antivenin. J Trauma 1988;28:35.
9. White RR, Weber RA. Poisonous snakebite in central texas. Ann Surg 1991;213:466.
10. Gold BS, Wingert WA. Snake venom poisoning in the US. South Med J 1994;87:579.

11. Parrish HM. Incidence of treated snakebites in the US. Public Health Report 1966;81:269.
12. Brook I. Human and animal bite infections. J Fam Pract 1989;28:713.
13. Callahan M. Controversies in antibiotic choices for bite wounds. Ann Emerg Med 1988;17:1321.
14. Tandberg D, Rusnak R. Mammalian bites. In: Schwartz GR, Safar P, Stone JH, et al, eds. Principles and practice of emergency medicine, ed 2. Philadelphia, WB Saunders, 1986:1618.
15. Robinson DA. Dog bites and rabies: an assessment of risk. Br Med J 1976;1:1066.
16. American Academy of Pediatrics. Summaries of infectious diseases. In: Peter G, ed. 1994 Red book: report of the Committee on Infectious Diseases, ed 23. Elk Grove Village, IL, American Academy of Pediatrics, 1994:151.
17. Bogue CW, Wise JD, Gray GF, et al. Antibiotic therapy for cat-scratch disease? JAMA 1989;262:813.
18. Holley HP. Successful treatment of cat-scratch disease with ciprofloxacin. JAMA 1991;265:1563.
19. Baker MD, Moore SE. Human bites in children. Am J Dis Child 1987;141:1285.
20. Foil LD, Norment BR. Envenomation by Loxoscles reclusa. J Med Entomol 1979;16:18.
21. Hollabaugh RS, Fernandes ET. Management of the brown recluse spider bite. J Pediatr Surg 1989;24:126.
22. Clark RF, Wethern-Kestner S, Vance MV, et al. Clinical presentation and treatment of black widow spider envenomation: a review of 163 cases. Ann Emerg Med 1992;21:782.
23. Koren G. Medications which can kill a toddler with one tablet or teaspoonful. Clin Toxicol 1993;31:407.
24. Phillips F, Gomez H, Brent J. Pediatric gastrointestinal decontamination in acute toxin ingestion. J Clin Pharmacol 1993;33:497.

Surgery of Infants and Children: Scientific Principles and Practice, edited by
Keith T. Oldham, Paul M. Colombani, and Robert P. Foglia.
Lippincott–Raven Publishers, Philadelphia, © 1997.

CHAPTER 29

Burns

Robert L. Sheridan and Ronald G. Tompkins

Management of the seriously burned child is a multifaceted challenge, requiring the exercise of surgical, critical care, rehabilitative, and psychosocial skills. The prognosis of those children suffering such injuries has improved dramatically since the early 1970s, with most not only surviving but enjoying excellent functional and cosmetic outcomes. The objective of this chapter is to review the clinical management of the seriously burned child and to relate progress in this management to the growing understanding of the pathophysiology of burn injury.

EPIDEMIOLOGY AND NATURAL HISTORY

In the developed world, approximately 75% of pediatric burn patients are injured by hot liquid, typically in bathing or cooking accidents. The remaining 25% have suffered flame, contact, chemical, electric, or tar injuries. Although the life-threatening nature of large injuries is often emphasized, the potentially devastating impact of poorly managed smaller burns should not be neglected (Fig. 29-1).

Extensive efforts have been made to diminish the incidence of pediatric burn injury through public education, with mixed effect. Legislation that requires lower temperatures for hot water heaters has been more successful. Such successes, although only locally effective, have been associated with a decreased incidence of hot water injuries in children.[1] Approximately 15% of pediatric burn injuries are attributed to abuse or neglect, and an awareness of this important issue facilitates the prevention of repeated injuries.

Teleologically, our skin envelope has played a crucial role in allowing marine animals to adapt to the land environment. Our survival as individuals continues to depend on the vapor and bacterial barriers provided by normal skin. The epidermal layer provides these two essential functions, whereas the dermis provides the flexibility and strength of the skin. In addition, dermal appendages prevent desiccation of the skin by producing oils, and the reactive dermal microvasculature is responsible for heat dissipation and conservation, allowing us to adapt to changes in environmental temperature. These important functions are compromised or lost when substantial areas of the skin are burned.

An understanding of the natural history of any disease pro-

cess facilitates an understanding of the success of intervention. A burn wound is initially clean, but is rapidly colonized by endogenous bacteria. Because these bacteria multiply in the avascular eschar over the succeeding days, proteases liquefy the eschar, which then separates, leaving a bed of granulation tissue or healing burn depending on the depth of the original injury. If wounds are small, less than 20% of the total body surface, this local infectious challenge is usually tolerated by the child. However, when injuries are larger, systemic infection results, explaining the rare survival of patients with burns in excess of 40% of the body surface in whom this natural history is permitted to unfold.

Children with burns in excess of 20% of the body surface frequently respond to this physiologic challenge with an initial decrease in cardiac output and metabolic rate.[2] Effected by a complex cascade of mediators whose interactions are only beginning to be understood, a hypermetabolic response follows a few hours later, with a near doubling of cardiac output and resting energy expenditure over the subsequent 24 to 48 hours in those who are successfully resuscitated.[3] The magnitude of this response peaks in those with injuries of 60% or more of the body surface at as high as twice the normal basal metabolic rate. This increase in substrate requirements has major implications for the support of burn patients. The etiology of the hypermetabolic response is not entirely understood, but probably involves a combination of factors, including a change in hypothalamic function with coincident rises in glucagon, cortisol, and catecholamines; deficient gastrointestinal barrier function with translocation of bacteria and their by-products; bacterial contamination of the burn wound with systemic release of similar products from this source; and some element of enhanced heat loss by transeschar evaporation of fluid. The hypermetabolic response probably has survival value because it is conserved so broadly over numerous species. An important element of successful management of patients who have sustained large injuries is support of this response through the provision of adequate quantity and quality of substrate. Modification of the response is of unknown value.

MANAGEMENT PHILOSOPHY

The burn management philosophy provides a systematic approach to these patients that includes: 1) an individualized re-

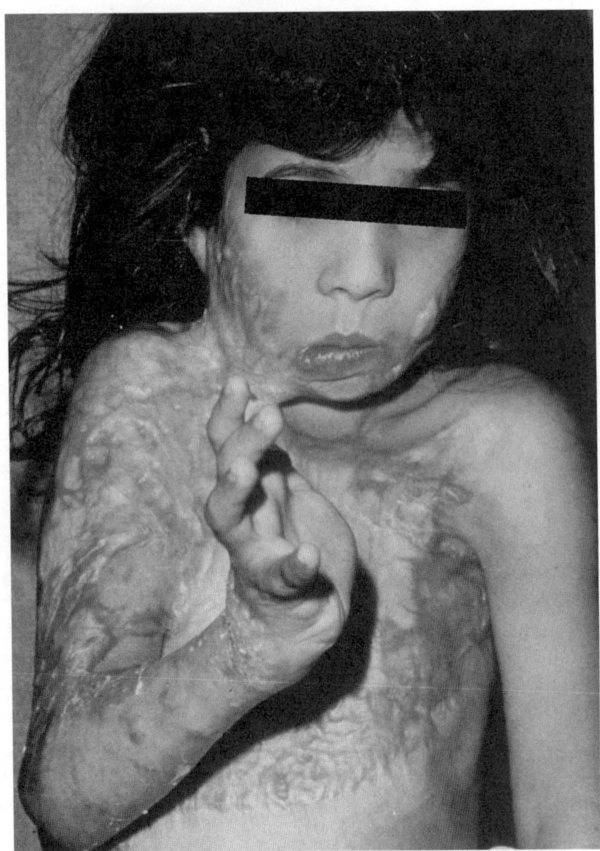

FIG. 29-1. Suboptimal management of small burns can have major adverse functional and cosmetic implications.

chanics are assessed, a rough estimate is made of the circulating volume, the level of consciousness is documented, and the child is completely undressed. This should be done in a warm environment to avoid hypothermia.

Secure airway and vascular access are crucial and should be obtained early during the evaluation. A badly burned face makes tape ineffective to secure the endotracheal tube, and umbilical tape ties should be used. In seriously burned patients, secure venous access is best obtained centrally, although two peripheral intravenous lines are a reasonable option. For venous access in the less severely burned child, peripheral intravenous access is appropriate. Venous access should be obtained through non-burned areas if possible. In the hypovolemic child, intraosseous resuscitation can be lifesaving, although it should be replaced promptly with venous cannulae as soon as practical. All patients should have a nasogastric tube in place, particularly if transported by air, because the child with a gas-filled stomach may vomit and aspirate (Fig. 29-2). A bladder catheter facilitates a smooth fluid resuscitation. Continuous temperature monitoring with rectal, esophageal, or bladder probes and arterial access are helpful in selected patients.

The burn-specific secondary survey (Table 29-1) includes a complete history, vital signs, a detailed physical examination, and laboratory and radiographic studies appropriate for the mechanism of injury. The history, particularly details regarding the mechanism of injury, is important and is ideally obtained from witnesses, rescue personnel, and family members. The mechanism of injury often determines the need for special stud-

suscitation of virtually all children regardless of injury severity, 2) early excision and biologic closure of deep wounds, 3) continuous rehabilitation, 4) judicious use of broad-spectrum antibiotics with early detection and specific treatment of septic foci, 5) intensive patient and family psychosocial support, and 6) long-term follow-up with ongoing rehabilitative and reconstructive support. The acute hospitalization is organized into four phases: 1) initial evaluation and resuscitation, 2) initial wound excision and biologic closure, 3) definitive wound closure, and 4) an intensification of the continuous rehabilitation effort. With this approach, survival with good quality of life can be expected for burn-injured children without anoxic brain injury, virtually regardless of injury size.

INITIAL EVALUATION

Meaningful survival can be expected even in the most severe injuries, and therefore the approach to such patients is aggressive. An organized approach to serious injuries facilitates achieving the optimal outcome and begins with a systematic initial evaluation, which includes a primary survey, effective vascular and airway access, and a systematic secondary survey. Because many burned children have sustained concurrent injuries, the initial evaluation should be approached as in any multiple-trauma patient. After evaluating and securing the airway while maintaining control of the cervical spine, breathing me-

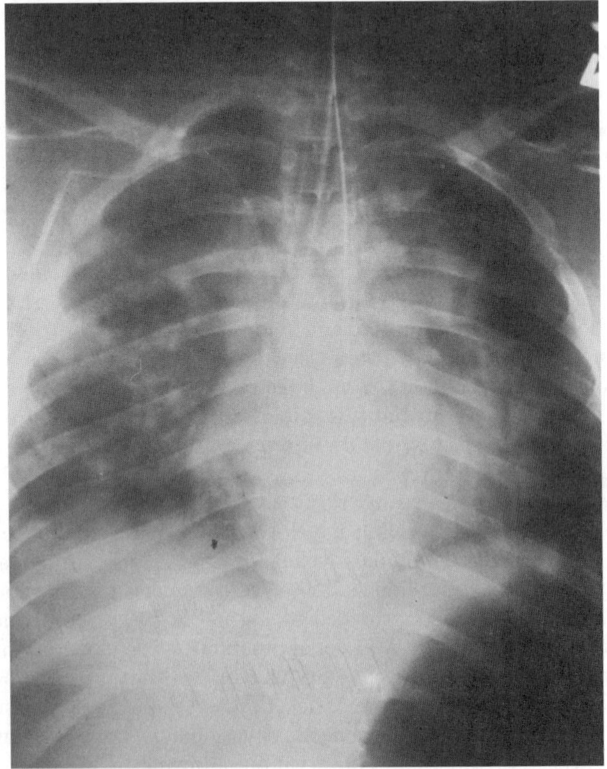

FIG. 29-2. Nasogastric tube function, as well as physical presence, must be regularly verified to minimize the possibility of gastric distention and subsequent aspiration during burn resuscitation.

TABLE 29-1. *Important aspects of the burn-specific secondary survey*

System or modality	Important considerations
History	1. Determine mechanism of injury, closed-space exposure, extrication time, delay in seeking attention, fluid given during transport, and prior illnesses and injuries.
Head, eyes, ears, nose, and throat	1. The globes should be examined and corneal epithelium stained with fluorescein before adnexal swelling makes examination difficult. Adnexal swelling provides excellent coverage and protection of the globe during the first days after injury. Tarsorrhaphy is virtually never indicated acutely. 2. Corneal epithelial loss can be overt, giving a clouded appearance to the cornea, but is more often subtle, requiring fluorescein staining for documentation. Topical ophthalmic antibiotics constitute optimal initial treatment. 3. Signs of airway involvement include perioral and intraoral burns or carbonaceous material and progressive hoarseness. 4. Hot liquid can be aspirated in conjunction with a facial scald injury and result in acute airway compromise, requiring urgent intubation. 5. Endotrachael tube security is crucial and is best maintained with an umbilical tape harness, rather than adhesive tape, on the burned face.
Neck	1. The radiographic evaluation is driven by the mechanism of injury. 2. Rarely, in patients with very deep burns, neck escharotomies are needed to facilitate venous drainage of the head.
Cardiac	1. The cardiac rhythm should be monitored for 24–72 h in those with electrical injury. 2. If intravascular volume and oxygenation are adequately supported, significant arrhythmias are unusual in burned children.
Pulmonary	1. Ensure inflating pressures are less than 40 cm H_2O by performing chest escharotomies when needed. 2. Severe inhalation injury may lead to slough of endobronchial mucosa and thick endobronchial secretions that can occlude the endotracheal tube, so the clinician should be prepared for sudden endotracheal tube occlusions.
Vascular	1. The perfusion of burned extremities should be vigilantly monitored by serial examinations. Indications for escharotomy include decreasing temperature, slowed capillary refill, and diminished Doppler flow in the digital vessels. Do not wait until flow in named vessels is compromised to decompress the extremity. 2. Fasciotomy is indicated after electrical or deep thermal injury when distal flow is compromised on clinical examination. Compartment pressures can be helpful, but clinically worrisome extremities should be decompressed regardless of compartment pressure readings.
Abdomen	1. Nasogastric tubes should be in place and their function verified, particularly before air transport in unpressurized helicopters. 2. An inappropriate resuscitative volume requirement may be a sign of an occult intraabdominal injury. 3. Torso escharotomies may be required to facilitate ventilation in the presence of deep circumferential abdominal wall burns. 4. Immediate ulcer prophylaxis with histamine receptor blockers and antacids is indicated in all children with serious burns.
Genitourinary	1. Bladder catheterization facilitates using urinary output as a resuscitation endpoint and is appropriate in all children who require fluid resuscitation. 2. It is important to ensure that the foreskin is reduced over the bladder catheter after insertion because progressive swelling may otherwise result in paraphimosis.
Neurologic	1. An early neurologic evaluation is important because the child's sensorium is often progressively compromised by medication or hemodynamic instability during the hours after injury. This may require computed tomographic scanning in those suspected of having head trauma. 2. Children who require neuromuscular blockade for transport should also receive adequate sedation and analgesia.
Extremities	1. Extremities that are at risk for ischemia, particularly those with circumferential thermal burns or those with electrical injury, should be promptly decompressed by escharotomy or fasciotomy when clinical examination reveals decreasing temperature and diminished Doppler flow in digital vessels. Limbs at risk should be dressed so they can be frequently examined. 2. The need for escharotomy usually becomes evident during the early hours of resuscitation. Most escharotomies can be delayed until transport has been effected if transport times will not extend beyond 6 h postinjury. 3. Burned extremities should be elevated and splinted in a position of function.
Wound	1. Wounds, although often underestimated in depth and overestimated in size on initial examination, should be evaluated for size, depth, and the presence of circumferential components.
Laboratory	1. Arterial blood gas analysis is important when airway compromise or inhalation injury is present. 2. A normal admission carboxyhemoglobin concentration does not eliminate the possibility of a significant exposure because the half-life of carboxyhemoglobin is 30–40 min in those effectively ventilated with 100% oxygen. 3. Baseline hemoglobin and electrolytes can be helpful later during resuscitation.

continued

TABLE 29-1. *Continued.*

System or modality	Important considerations
Radiography	1. The radiographic evaluation is driven by the mechanism of injury and the need to document placement of supportive cannulas.
Electrical	1. Monitor cardiac rhythm in high- (>1000 V) or intermediate- (>220 V) voltage exposures for 24–72 h.
	2. Low- and intermediate-voltage exposures can cause locally destructive injuries, but uncommonly result in systemic sequelae.
	3. After high-voltage exposures, delayed neurologic and ocular sequelae can occur, so a carefully documented neurologic and ocular examination is an important part of the initial assessment.
	4. Injured extremities should be serially evaluated for intracompartmental edema and promptly decompressed when it develops.
	5. Bladder catheters should be placed in all patients suffering high-voltage exposure to document the presence or absence of pigmenturia. This is treated adequately with volume loading in most patients.
Chemical	1. Irrigate wounds with tap water for at least 30 min. Irrigate the globe with isotonic crystalloid solution. Blepharospasm may require occular anesthetic administration.
	2. Exposures to hydrofluoric acid may be complicated by life-threatening hypocalcemia, particularly exposures to concentrated or anhydrous solutions. Such patients should have serum calcium closely monitored and supplemented. Subeschar injection of 10% calcium gluconate solution is appropriate after exposure to highly concentrated or anhydrous solutions.
Tar	1. Tar should be initially cooled with tap water irrigation and later removed with a lipophilic solvent.

ies, such as computed tomograms (CT) of the head and abdomen, or radiographs of the cervical spine. Other important historical points include past medical and surgical history, time of the last meal, tetanus status, medications and allergies, tap water temperature in hot liquid injuries, and extrication time in closed-space injuries. Vital signs are determined during the secondary survey, and age-specific norms should be known (Table 29-2). It is important to document and maintain a normal body temperature because burned children are especially prone to hypothermia. A complete physical examination should proceed in an organized fashion, not allowing the presence of the burn to distract the examiner from performing a complete assessment.

The patient's neurologic status should be carefully documented early during the evaluation, because many patients become progressively obtunded secondary to the administration of analgesics and sedatives as well as intravascular volume depletion. If injury mechanism is consistent with a head injury, CT should be performed.

Trauma to the head, face, and neck is determined by inspection and palpation. The corneal epithelium and globes should be examined before the development of adnexal edema, which renders the examination more difficult. Major corneal epithelial burns are obvious by the opaque corneal appearance that results. More subtle defects are apparent after staining with topical fluorescein. Upper airway injuries are suspected in the presence of a hoarse voice, burns of the lips or tongue, singed facial and nasal hair, or carbonaceous sputum. Hot liquid aspiration may complicate facial scald burns in small children and should be suspected if there is blistering in or around the mouth. If upper airway compromise is imminent, a clinical judgment based on the suggestion of significant upper airway edema, then endotracheal intubation is mandatory. This is particularly important before committing the child to a long transport. Verification of endotracheal tube security is an important part of the head and neck examination.

The torso should be assessed for compliance, and if ventilation is restricted by overlying circumferential eschar, torso escharotomies should be done promptly with coagulating electrocautery to minimize blood loss. Incisions are typically made axially along the flanks and are connected by one or more horizontal incisions (Fig. 29-3A). The abdomen should be assessed for tenderness or distention. If the mechanism of injury suggests an abdominal injury, CT or peritoneal lavage is appropriate, particularly in the presence of an inappropriate resuscitative volume requirement. Gastric distention is common in distressed children, and nasogastric decompression is routinely recommended during the initial evaluation and transport. Proper nasogastric tube function should be verified regularly. All burned children should receive immediate ulcer prophylaxis with intraluminal antacids and intravenous histamine receptor blockers because the incidence of stress ulceration is unacceptably high if this precaution is not taken. The presence of genital burns should be noted. If the patient is not circumcised, the foreskin should be reduced after placement of the bladder catheter to avoid paraphimosis secondary to progressive edema.

Regular assessment and documentation of peripheral perfusion is crucial during the first postinjury days. Blood flow can be compromised by constricting circumferential eschar as subeschar tissues become progressively edematous, or by progressive intracompartmental edema in patients with electric or deep thermal burns. Both are detected by the development of a progressive increase in the extremity's firmness and a decrease in its distal temperature. Pulsatile Doppler signals in the lower-pressure distal vasculature, such as the palmar arch and digital vessels, should be documented hourly. The loss of pulsatile Doppler signals is consistent with increasing tissue pressure if intravascular volume is adequate. Constricting circumferen-

TABLE 29-2. *Age-specific resuscitation endpoints*

Evaluation	Target
Sensorium	Comfortable, arousable
Urine output	0.5–1.0 mL/kg/h
Base deficit	Less than 2
Systolic pressure	70–90+ mm Hg (twice age in years)

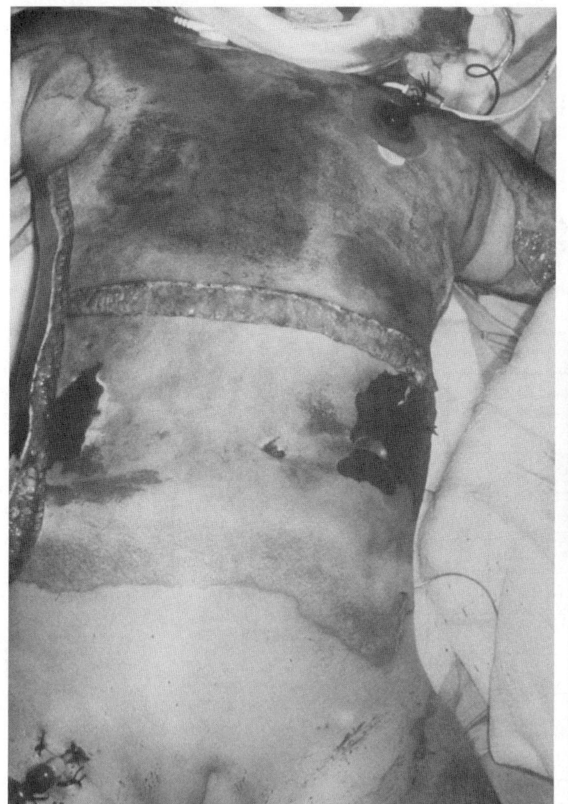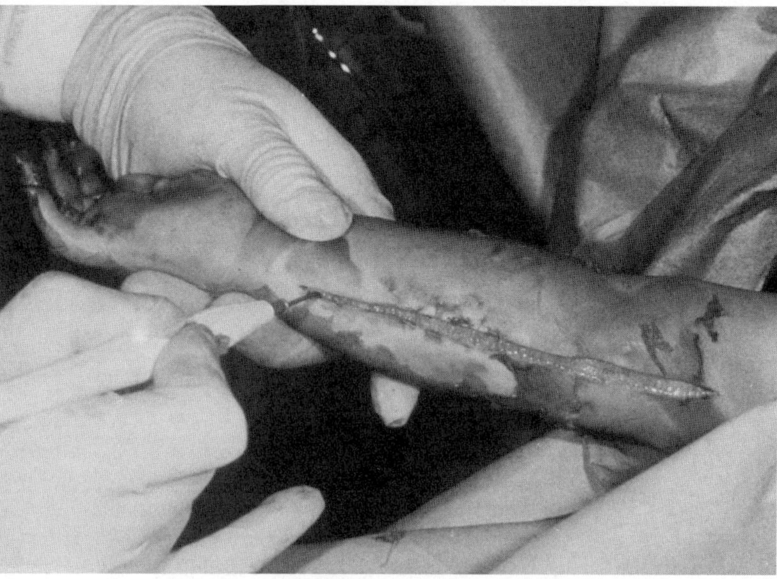

FIG. 29-3. (*A*) Torso escharotomies, done by connecting lateral axial incisions across the midline, facilitate ventilation with low inflating pressures. (*B*) Extremity escharotomies are done using medial and lateral axial incisions.

tial eschar can be divided at the bedside with the coagulating electrocautery using medial and lateral axial incisions (see Fig. 29-3*B*). If the burn is full thickness, it is insensate and no sedation is required. If the burn is partial thickness in depth, light sedation is used. It is important to maintain hemostasis during the procedure and to verify that the procedure has enhanced distal blood flow. Hand escharotomies are often not required once the more proximal upper extremity has been adequately decompressed. If decompression of the arm to the level of the metacarpophalangeal joints has not resulted in adequate digital blood flow, axial digital incisions are made between the extensors and the neurovascular bundles. Ideally, a single incision on the radial aspect of the thumb and the ulnar aspect of the digits suffices. The incisions on the central digits of the hand can be extended proximally between the metacarpals.

Weakness of intracompartmental muscle groups or pain with their passive stretch supports the suspicion of elevated intracompartmental pressures, although such signs can be obscured in many burn patients. The diagnosis of an evolving compartment syndrome in the acutely burned child can be an exceptionally difficult one to make early, and the clinician should decompress such extremities based on clinical suspicion. Compartment pressure measurements can be a useful adjunct in equivocal situations, but clinical judgment should suffice in most cases. If missed, compartment syndromes lead to intracompartmental sepsis or functional deficits later in the patient's course.

Evaluation of the child's wound is deferred until higher-priority evaluations are complete. Important to the initial evaluation are an assessment of the wound depth, size, and circumferential components. Early burn depth estimates are accurate in very deep or very superficial wounds. However, many burns (particularly scald injuries in children) are of indeterminate depth on initial examination. Significant effort has been applied to develop technical aids that accurately gauge burn depth during the initial evaluation,[4] with little clinical success. Fortunately, an accurate determination of depth is not necessary to proceed with initial wound management or fluid resuscitation. In contrast, an accurate assessment of burn size can be made early and is important to initial management because resuscitative fluid administration is primarily determined by overall burn size. Burn size in children is best estimated with an age-specific chart (Fig. 29-4), because the child's body proportions change with growth. The major anthropometric change involves the head and legs. The infant head represents 18% of the total body surface and the legs 14%. In older adolescents and adults, the head represents 9% of the body surface and the legs 18%. It is important to identify circumferential components of the wound because these areas need to be closely monitored for compromise of peripheral perfusion in extremity or neck burns and compromise of ventilation in torso injuries.

Limited laboratory studies are of value during the initial evaluation. Patients with a history of exposure to noxious fumes should have the arterial Pa_{O_2}, Pa_{CO_2}, pH, and carboxyhemoglo-

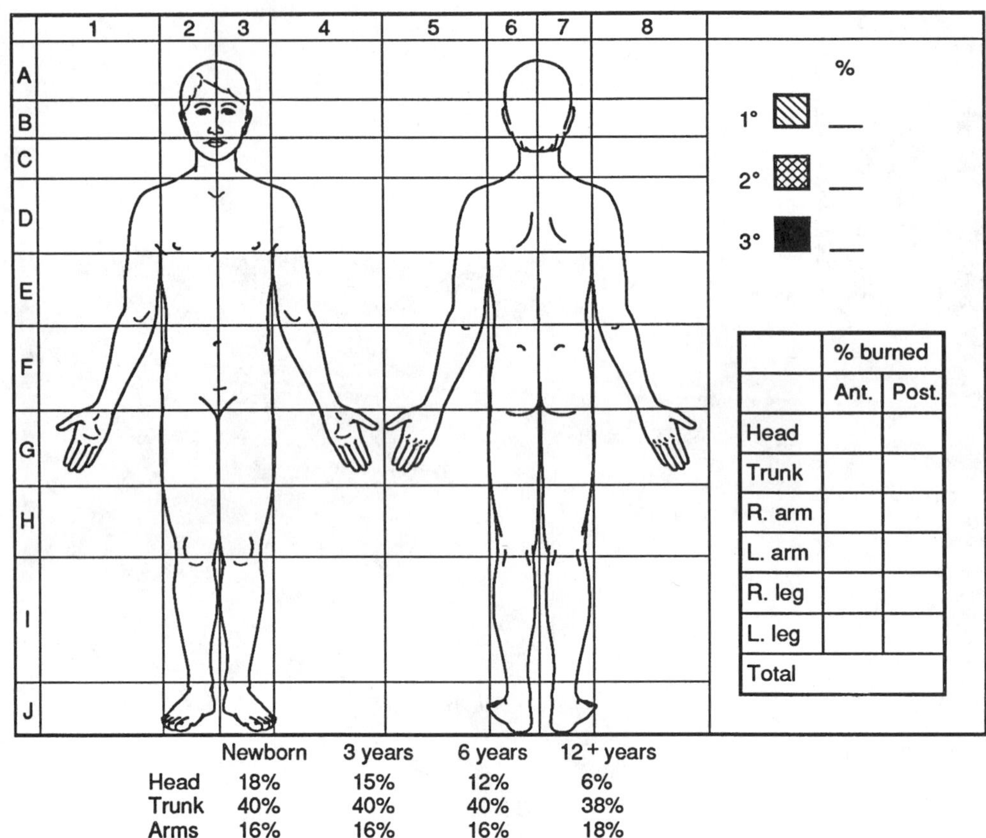

	Newborn	3 years	6 years	12⁺ years
Head	18%	15%	12%	6%
Trunk	40%	40%	40%	38%
Arms	16%	16%	16%	18%
Legs	26%	29%	32%	38%

FIG. 29-4. An age-specific chart facilitates accurate estimation of burn size over a broad range of ages.

bin percentage determined. However, because the half-life of carboxyhemoglobin is 30 to 45 minutes when patients are ventilated with high concentrations of oxygen, a normal carboxyhemoglobin of less than 5% does not preclude significant exposures when patients have been well ventilated with high concentrations of oxygen during transport. Patients with electric or very deep thermal injuries often require blood products during the initial resuscitation, and in such patients a blood bank specimen should be sent. Routine hematology and chemistry profiles are of limited usefulness initially, but do establish a baseline. Urinalysis for occult blood is helpful in patients with electric or very deep thermal burns if gross pigmenturia has been cleared with crystalloid administration. Radiographic evaluation during the initial evaluation is determined in large part by the mechanism of injury and the need to evaluate placement of resuscitative cannulae.

The initial evaluation of patients with electric, chemical, or tar injuries is the same as in those patients with thermal injuries; however, a few additional points require emphasis. Also, children with toxic epidermal necrolysis, purpura fulminans or major soft tissue injuries are well managed in burn units.[5]

Electric

Patients exposed to high voltage (greater than 1000 V) present a combination of deep tissue injury secondary to the passage of current, locally destructive entrance and exit wounds, deep wounds where current arcs across flexed joints, flame burns secondary to clothing ignition, flash burns, axial spine fractures secondary to tetanic contraction of paravertebral mus-

cles, and other injuries related to the fall or blast that so commonly accompanies high-voltage injury. Such patients require a complete trauma evaluation, cardiac monitoring, a bladder catheter to evaluate the urine for pigment, serial monitoring of compartments at risk for pressure elevation, and spine immobilization pending radiographic clearance of the axial spine.

Compartment pressure elevation, secondary to edema of injured muscle, can result in additional ischemic injury if compartments are not promptly released.

Chemical

Patients suffering chemical burns are first managed by at least 30 minutes of copious tap water irrigation. Ocular injuries are irrigated with saline. Topical ophthalmic anesthetics facilitate relief of the blepharospasm that often interferes with effective irrigation of the globe. Life-threatening hypocalcemia can develop in patients exposed to concentrated hydrofluoric acid. This should be anticipated and managed with subeschar injection of 10% calcium gluconate with monitoring and support of the serum ionized calcium before urgent excision of selected extensive wounds. The more common limited exposures to dilute hydrofluoric acid are managed with irrigation and topical calcium gluconate gel.

Tar

Tar is often heated to over 400°F and commonly causes a deep burn. Tar is initially cooled by tap water irrigation to

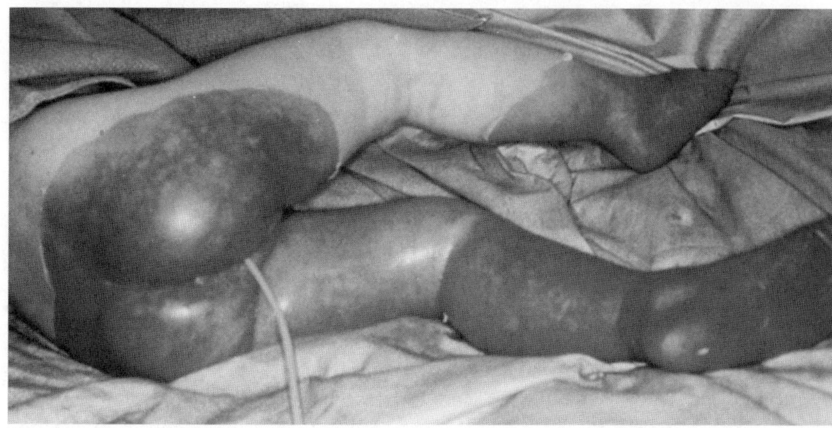

FIG. 29-5. This child's wound is consistent with an intentional immersion in scalding water, demonstrating both flexor sparing and sharply defined margins around a deep burn of very uniform depth.

limit the progression of the injury and is later removed with a lipophilic solvent. After initial irrigation, chemical and tar burns are managed surgically as indicated by depth, which is frequently underestimated on initial examination.

Abuse

All burned children should be evaluated for abuse or neglect. It is an ethical and legal mandate that suspect injuries be filed with the appropriate state agency. Important historical points include tap water temperature, duration of contact, caretakers involved, conflicting reports from involved caretakers, delay in seeking treatment, and prior injuries. Important points of examination (Fig. 29-5) include uniformity of burn depth, absence of splash marks, sharply defined wound margins, porcelain contact sparing, flexor sparing, stocking or glove patterns, dorsal location of contact burns of the hand, and localized very deep contact burns. All such children should be admitted to the hospital regardless of burn size. Suspect cases should be referred to the appropriate state authorities. Radiographic screening of the head and long bones should be considered.

FLUID RESUSCITATION

The large number of fluid resuscitation formulas in common use is a tribute to the fact that no one formula accurately predicts fluid requirements in every child. No formula can replace a physician at the bedside repeatedly evaluating the child's physiology throughout the resuscitative period. The Modified Brooke formula (Table 29-3) is commonly used as a starting point and serves as the basis for this discussion. However, regardless of the formula chosen to initiate resuscitation, subsequent fluid administration is best guided by regular reassessment of resuscitation endpoints, rather than the prediction of any formula.

During the first 24 hours, lactated Ringer (3 to 4 mL/kg/ %burn/24 h) is the primary resuscitative fluid. Children with burns of less than 10% generally do not require a formal fluid resuscitation. Because children weighing less than 10 kg can become hypoglycemic if glucose is not administered, lactated Ringer or half-normal saline with 5% dextrose is added at maintenance rates. Dextrose-containing fluid should not be given as the primary resuscitative fluid because hyperglycemia and

osmotic diuresis result. One half of the calculated 24-hour total should be given during the first 8 hours after injury. These calculations should be based on the time of injury, not on the time that vascular access is achieved. During this first 24-hour period, the resuscitative lactated Ringer infusion should be adjusted up or down in 10% increments every hour based on age-

---

TABLE 29-3. *The Modified Brooke formula**

FIRST 24 H

RESUSCITATIVE FLUID
1. Children >10 kg
    Lactated Ringer: 3–4 mL/kg/% burn/24 h (first half in first 8 h)
    Colloid: none
2. Children <10 kg
    Lactated Ringer: 2–3 mL/kg/% burn/24 h (first half in first 8 h)
    Colloid: none

MAINTENANCE FLUIDS
Lactated Ringer with 5% dextrose
  100 mL/kg for the first 10 kg BW
  50 mL/kg for the second 10 kg BW
  20 mL/kg for BW >20 kg

SECOND 24 H

ALL CHILDREN
  Crystalloid: To maintain urine output. If silver nitrate is used, sodium leaching mandates continued isotonic crystalloid. If other topical is used, free water requirement is significant. Serum sodium should be monitored closely. Nutritional support should begin, preferably by the enteral route.
  Colloid (5% albumin in Lactated Ringer):
    0%–30% burn: none
    30%–50% burn: 0.3 mL/kg/%burn/24 h
    50%–70% burn: 0.4 mL/kg/%burn/24 h
    >70% burn: 0.5 mL/kg/%burn/24 h

BW, body weight.
* The Modified Brooke formula, like all resuscitative formulas, is a helpful starting point. However, a high-quality resuscitation requires the bedside presence of a physician capable of regularly evaluating resuscitation endpoints.

specific resuscitation endpoints such as urine output, sensorium, base deficit, filling pressures, pulse, and blood pressure (see Table 29-2). The importance of an hourly bedside evaluation during this period cannot be overemphasized.

It is important to recognize a failing resuscitation as early as possible because this facilitates salvage of such patients. At any point during a resuscitation, the estimated total fluid administration can be calculated based on the known administered volume and the current rate of infusion. This figure can be divided by the patient's weight and burn size, resulting in a figure that describes the number of milliliters of fluid per kilogram per percent area burned that patient is targeted to receive during the first 24 hours. A failing resuscitation is considered one in which the patient is likely to receive 6 or more mL/kg/%burn during their first 24 postinjury hours. Larger resuscitation fluid volumes are occasionally required by patients whose resuscitations have been delayed, who have suffered inhalation injury, or who have very extensive and deep burns. Such patients may benefit from the early infusion of low-dose dopamine (3 to 5 μg/kg/min), placement of a pulmonary artery catheter, or the early administration of colloid.

Patients who present with gross pigmenturia are at risk for myoglobin-induced acute tubular necrosis. This situation is most commonly seen in patients who have sustained high-voltage electric injury or very deep thermal burns. In such patients, pigment must be cleared promptly. This is ideally accomplished with crystalloid loading, and maintaining a brisk urine output of 2 mL/kg/h. Also helpful is alkalinization of the urine, accomplished by administering 0.12 to 0.5 mEq/kg/h of sodium bicarbonate as a part of the resuscitative fluid. Occasionally, an osmotic diuresis using mannitol is required; however, the administration of osmotic diuretics obscures the urine output as a valid measure of intravascular volume. Therefore, a pulmonary artery or central venous catheter should be placed when mannitol must be used so filling pressures can be used to judge the adequacy of fluid administration.

During the second 24-hour period, colloid administration is appropriate because the diffuse capillary leak that characterizes the first 18 to 24 hours has abated and colloid remains largely intravascular. Colloid, generally 5% or 25% albumin, is administered by infusion at a dose based on burn size (see Table 29-3). During this second 24-hour period, crystalloid requirements markedly diminish, and transeschar free water loss becomes more prominent unless an aqueous topical antimicrobial such as 0.5% silver nitrate, is used. In the former situation, free water administration is commonly required, and in the latter case, transeschar leaching of sodium (350 mEq/m²/24 h) mandates continued administration of isotonic crystalloid. There is major morbidity to aberrations of serum sodium in small children, particularly cerebral edema and seizures or tentorial herniation, so diligent electrolyte monitoring during this period is important. Nutritional support, preferably by an enteral route, should commence during the first 48 postinjury hours.

INITIAL WOUND EXCISION AND BIOLOGIC CLOSURE

Early removal of extensive areas of devitalized tissue with immediate biologic closure of resulting wounds is the primary surgical objective of the first postburn week. This policy of early excision is now widely followed in the United States and is carried out as excision of the entire wound coincident with fluid resuscitation, or, more commonly, by staged excision of all deep partial- and full-thickness components of the wound (less the face, palms, soles, and genitals) over the first 3 to 7 days after injury.[6] The increasing popularity of early excision is based on several documented and theoretic advantages over the traditional approach of allowing eschar to liquefy by bacterial proteases and separate, leaving a bed of granulation tissue that is subsequently autografted. Documented advantages include an improved survival in patients with injuries involving more than 30% to 40% of the body surface, truncated hospital stays, lowered costs, and fewer painful dressing changes. Although not proven, conventional wisdom suggests that a decrease in the duration and intensity of the hypermetabolic and inflammatory response, diminished blood loss, improved immunologic function, and less hypertrophic scarring result from early excision.

Estimation of Burn Depth

In practical terms, only burns that are deep partial or full thickness in depth undergo early excision. Such a policy assumes an ability to determine burn depth accurately during initial examination. Although numerous technical aids, such as laser Doppler flowmeters, intravenous fluorescein, burn wound biopsy, thermography, light reflectance, and fluorescence of intravenous dyes, have been proposed,[4] none has yet equaled in accuracy, reliability, or practicality the eye of an experienced examiner. The differentiation between superficial burns that will heal within 3 weeks with topical antimicrobial treatment and deeper injuries that will require excision can, in general, be made on clinical examination during the first days after injury. Certain patients have a component of their wound the depth of which is difficult to judge on initial examination. If overall wound size is not large, less than 20% of the body surface, then such indeterminate depth wounds can be treated with topical antimicrobials initially until the portion that requires grafting becomes evident. This situation is quite common in children with small injuries from hot liquid. It is practical when managing such injuries to apply topical antimicrobials for 5 to 7 days, limiting excision and grafting to full-thickness components of the wound.

Topical Antimicrobials

Topical antimicrobials play an important supportive role to excision and grafting because they delay the process of wound colonization and infection. There are three topical antibiotics in common use in the United States (Table 29-4). Silver sulfadiazine is the most common because it has a broad spectrum of activity, is simple to apply, has no metabolic or electrolyte implications, and is painless on application. Mafenide acetate, although a carbonic anhydrase inhibitor that causes a moderate metabolic acidosis and is painful on application, is an important element of the topical formulary because it alone reliably penetrates eschar. It is typically applied to eschar at risk for infection and to all deep burns of the external ear. The latter practice

TABLE 29-4. *The three common topical antibiotics in use in the United States and their characteristics*

Silver sulfadiazine	Painless on application, fair to poor eschar penetration, no metabolic side effects, broad antibacterial spectrum
Mafenide acetate	Painful on application, excellent eschar penetration, carbonic anhydrase inhibitor, broad antibacterial spectrum
0.5% Silver nitrate	Painless on application, poor eschar penetration, leaches electrolytes, broad spectrum (including fungi)

has markedly diminished the incidence of auricular chondritis. Silver nitrate, as an aqueous 0.5% solution, is applied to heavy gauze dressings every 2 hours. Although it penetrates eschar poorly and can leach large quantities of sodium and potassium from the wounds, its broad antibacterial and antifungal activity, as well as the flexibility of its use on burns, donor sites, and fresh grafts, make it another alternative topical agent.

Techniques of Excision

A common argument against the policy of early burn wound excision is the prodigious blood loss that has been associated with these procedures. However, modern blood-conserving practices have diminished this concern. Tangential excisions of the torso, neck, and head are done after subeschar injection of dilute epinephrine solutions. Tangential excisions of the extremities are done after exsanguination and inflation of a pneumatic tourniquet. Although substantial experience is required, tissue viability can be readily accessed by color and texture, rather than the presence of diffuse bleeding. Instruments used to excise burned tissue tangentially include hand, compressed gas-powered, and electric dermatomes. When required based on burn depth or extent, fascial excisions are performed with coagulating electrocautery, further diminishing blood loss. Although such procedures have traditionally been limited to 2 hours or 20% of the body surface, far larger procedures can be safely done if blood-conserving practices are rigorously followed and patients are kept warm by maintaining operating room temperatures above 90° or 100°F.

Temporary Wound Closure Alternatives

Once necrotic eschar is excised to a bed of viable tissue, immediate biologic closure is mandatory. Ideally, immediate autografting is performed. When donor sites are insufficient for this purpose, a temporary biologic cover must be chosen, while awaiting healing of donor sites. Such covers should provide a vapor and bacterial barrier over the excised wound. Fresh or cryopreserved human allograft is most appropriate for this purpose. It is placed in a meshed but unexpanded fashion exactly as autograft would be placed. When placed on a viable wound bed, it vascularizes and provides physiologic wound closure until rejected 2 to 4 weeks later, at which time or sooner it is replaced with reharvested autograft. Other temporary covers in common use include porcine xenograft, both fresh and reconstituted, and the synthetic bilaminate Biobrane (Dow Hickman, Sugarland, TX), which has a porous nylon inner layer and a semipermeable outer layer. However, only human allograft will vascularize, and it remains the optimal temporary physiologic wound closure material. A second common use for biologic dressings is as physiologic cover for clean superficial burns as they epithelialize, which minimizes the pain associated with an open partial-thickness burn. Allograft, screened for malignant and infectious diseases, is a precious resource and is not commonly used as a biologic dressing in these circumstances. For this purpose, reconstituted porcine xenograft or Biobrane can be used.

DEFINITIVE WOUND CLOSURE

During the phase of definitive wound closure, allograft is replaced with reharvested autograft and burns of certain specialized areas are addressed. This phase usually begins 1 week after injury and lasts for several weeks thereafter, depending on the extent of burn and the availability of suitable donor sites. Prompt definitive wound closure in patients with large injuries remains an elusive goal despite encouraging early experience with two proposed permanent skin substitutes, artificial skin and cultured epidermal sheets, which are discussed in greater detail subsequently. At the present time, even in patients with extensive injuries, reharvested autograft provides the most practical and durable definitive wound closure material.

Burns of the Face, Ocular Adnexa, and Ears

Because of the thickness and deep appendages of the skin of the central face, relatively deep burns in these areas frequently heal. This is fortunate, because it is difficult to achieve a favorable result with primary excision and grafting of the central face. Unless burns in these areas are of extraordinary depth, they are commonly treated with topical antimicrobial agents for 2 weeks. Areas that remain unhealed are excised and closed with sheet autograft. The face can be considered as consisting of cosmetic units[7] (Fig. 29-6) and it is ideal if full-thickness facial burns can be autografted in cosmetic units if this does not require sacrifice of significant areas of healed burn or unburned skin.

Burns of the ocular adnexa are common management problems. During the first postinjury week, lid edema usually ensures that the underlying globe is adequately protected and lubricated. As wound contracture takes place, exposure and desiccation of the globe occurs with resulting keratitis and corneal ulceration. When this is unresponsive to ocular lubrication, prompt lid release becomes mandatory. Tarsorrhaphy is an ineffective alternative because the forces of wound contracture routinely disrupt the tarsorrhaphy and result in damage to the underlying tarsal plate.

Burns of the external ear are treated with twice-daily cleansing and application of mafenide acetate. It is important to avoid pressure on the burned auricle. Deep burns of the external ear can be complicated by acute suppurative chondritis if topical mafenide acetate is not applied. This complication is recognized

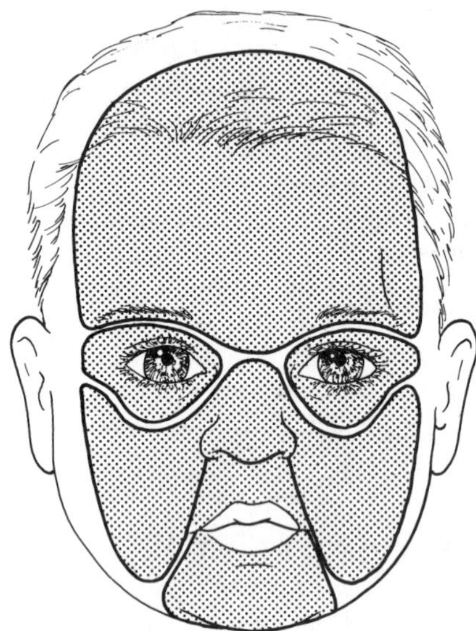

FIG. 29-6. The cosmetic units of the face. It is ideal to autograft the face in cosmetic units if this does not require the sacrifice of significant areas of healed burn or unburned skin.

by progressive auricular edema, erythema, and pain and requires that the infected cartilage be immediately debrided to avoid complete loss of the cartilaginous support of the auricle.

Burns of the Hands and Feet

The increasing survival of patients with large burns has brought into greater focus the importance of the quality of survival after such injuries. A crucial element of postinjury quality of life is hand function; an organized approach to the injuries facilitates optimal functional outcome of hand burns.

The initial evaluation of the burned hand includes screening for other injuries based on mechanism of injury. A complete hand examination is necessary, with particular attention paid to its perfusion by examining the hand for capillary refill, temperature, consistency, and Doppler signals in the palmar arch, digital vessels, and distal pulp. It is not enough to ensure that there is detectable flow in the radial or ulnar arteries. If the hands are cool and firm with circulation impaired in the low-pressure distal circulation by overlying nonelastic eschar, then prompt escharotomies of the upper extremity and hand are performed as described previously. When dealing with high-voltage electric injury or very deep thermal burns, the need for urgent fasciotomy is indicated by progressive firmness of the compartments of the hand and forearm, or progressive neurologic impairment or pain. In equivocal cases, it is most prudent to proceed to decompression promptly, rather than to wait until ischemia has advanced.

Subsequent management of the burned hand is dictated by the depth of the injury. Superficial burns are managed with elevation, topical antimicrobials, and full passive range of motion for each joint twice daily. Splinting the hand in a functional position, with the metacarpophalangeal joints at 70 to 90 degrees, the interphalangeal joints in extension, the thumb in neutral position with the first web space open, and the wrist in 20 to 30 degrees of extension is indicated if there is significant

edema. Healing can be expected within 2 to 3 weeks if injuries are superficial. Deep partial- and full-thickness injuries are best managed with excision and sheet grafting as soon as practical. Hands are immobilized in a functional position for 7 days after surgery before passive and active therapy is resumed. Fourth-degree hand burns, which involve the underlying extensor mechanism, joint capsules, or bone are significantly more difficult management problems; these are managed by staged sheet autografting and often require axial Kirschner wire fixation of open and unstable metacarpophalangeal or interphalangeal joints. Patients with smaller overall burn sizes in association with fourth-degree hand burns are often well served by debridement and groin or abdominal flap coverage. When hand burns are addressed in an organized fashion that stresses continuous hand therapy,[8] most patients with deep partial- and full-thickness hand burns will have normal or near-normal long-term function. Even patients with fourth-degree injuries, although rarely enjoying normal function, can expect to be able to function independently in activities of daily living (Fig. 29-7).

The palmar skin is remarkably thick, even in small children, and thus only approximately 20% of palmar burns require resurfacing. This conservative approach facilitates preservation of the specialized attachment of the palmar skin to the underlying fascia. Full-thickness injuries are grafted with full-thickness or thick split-thickness sheet grafts and splinted in extension to maintain the palm in an open position.

Burns of the feet are managed in a similar fashion. Prompt excision and grafting of deep dermal and full-thickness injuries of the dorsum of the foot usually results in normal function. Fourth-degree injuries, although more difficult management problems, are entirely consistent with a normal functional result. Burns of the plantar surface of the feet are grafted with full- or thick split-thickness sheet grafts if they fail to heal within 3 weeks.

Genital Burns

On initial presentation, it is important to ensure that the burned foreskin is reduced into a normal position because progressive edema may result in paraphimosis. Bladder catheter drainage is not required for the purpose of limiting contamination of perineal wounds with urine. Bladder catheters should be used only to facilitate management of the resuscitation and should be promptly removed when genital edema is resolved and close monitoring of the urine output is no longer required. Likewise, diversion of the intestinal tract is not required to facilitate management of perineal burns. On occasion, contraction of the deeply burned and desiccated foreskin may render the placement of bladder catheters in the acute setting impossible. In these cases, dorsal or ventral incisions through the contracted foreskin will facilitate catheter placement. When debriding the deeply burned foreskin, any viable remnant should be preserved because such tissue may be useful in later reconstruction.

Although there is some enthusiasm for early excision of deep genital burns, our general practice is to manage these limited surface area injuries with topical therapy for a period of 2 to 3 weeks unless the wounds are remarkably deep. Unhealed injuries are debrided and grafted with sheet autograft at this time, with generally excellent cosmetic and functional results.

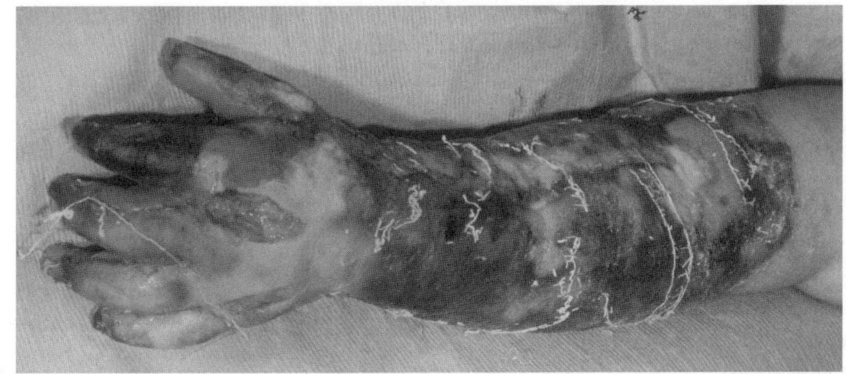

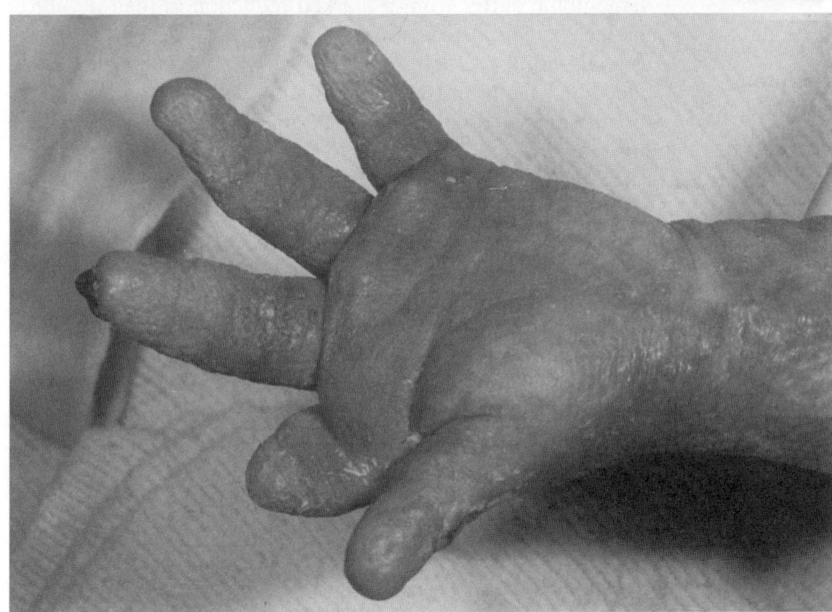

FIG. 29-7. Even highly destructive fourth-degree hand burns can be expected to yield a functional result when managed in an organized fashion that stresses maintenance of functional position and continuous hand therapy.

SELECTED CRITICAL CARE ISSUES

The enhanced survival of patients with large burns has been facilitated by increasingly sophisticated critical care techniques used to support an aggressive surgical approach to wounds, treatment of failing organ systems, and management of the hypermetabolic response to injury. This section reviews some of the important points relevant to the management of inhalation injury and respiratory failure, techniques of arterial and venous access, nutritional support of the hypermetabolic response, and the recognition and management of multiorgan failure in burned children.

Inhalation Injury and Respiratory Failure

The pathophysiology of inhalation injury is complex and varies with the aerosolized toxins particular to the circumstances of individual injuries. However, these such injuries routinely demonstrate the following: 1) upper airway obstruction secondary to progressive edema; 2) reactive bronchospasm from aerosolized irritants; 3) small airway occlusion initially from edema and subsequently from sloughed endobronchial debris and loss of the ciliary clearance mechanism; 4) microatelectasis from

loss of surfactant and alveolar edema; and 5) interstitial and alveolar edema secondary to loss of capillary integrity.[9] The physiologic consequences of these mechanical aberrations are upper and lower airway obstruction with increased airway resistance, decreased compliance, an increase in the dead-space–to–tidal-volume ratio, and intrapulmonary shunting.

The diagnosis of inhalation injury is surprisingly difficult because the components of the smoke to which any individual patient has been exposed are usually unknown. Because current treatment is exclusively supportive, diagnosis provides only prognostic information. Suggestive points in the patient's history include a closed space exposure or prolonged extrication time. Physical signs supporting the diagnosis include singed nasal vibrissae and facial hair, burns of the central face, intraoral burns, carbonaceous debris in the oropharynx, and diffuse wheezing. Bronchoscopy frequently reveals carbonaceous endobronchial debris and mucosal pallor, erythema, or ulceration. Xenon scanning may reveal delayed or asymmetric clearance of the radiotracer secondary to small airway obstruction. Unfortunately, findings at the time of initial evaluation frequently do not correlate with the subsequent clinical course.

The earliest consequence of inhalation injury is upper airway edema, which is commonly seen during the first 6 to 24 hours after injury and is more prominent in patients with large surface area injuries in whom more significant aberrations of capillary integrity and soft tissue edema develop. Although severe steam inhalation can result in direct heat injury to the distal tracheobronchial tree, more distal airway injuries are usually caused by aerosolized toxins rather than thermal energy because the upper airway is a highly effective heat sink. Upper airway obstruction is best managed with prompt endotracheal intubation, which is maintained for 48 to 72 hours, and elevation of the head. In equivocal cases, bronchoscopy is performed and patients with significant upper airway edema are intubated using the bronchoscope as a stylet. Endotracheal tubes are removed when facial edema has largely resolved and there is an audible air leak around the tubes at 40 cm H_2O of inflation with the cuff deflated.

Subsequently, the physiologic consequences of small airway obstruction and intrapulmonary shunting become more prominent, with progressive respiratory failure developing in patients who have sustained significant injuries. Endobronchial debris and the loss of the ciliary clearance mechanism result in a high rate of pneumonia, which is reported to occur in between 20% and 50% of patients who suffer inhalation injury. Successful management of patients with inhalation injury requires aggressive pulmonary toilet, aided by frequent chest physiotherapy and toilet bronchoscopy. Positive-pressure ventilation facilitates management of patients with large shunts or compliance poor enough to result in an excessive work of breathing. Although moderate inflating pressures help to expand recruitable segments, peak inspiratory pressures in excess of 40 cm H_2O should be avoided because they are associated with both overt barotrauma as well as more subtle overpressure injuries to the pulmonary microvasculature and alveoli, which can themselves exacerbate respiratory failure.[10] High inflating pressures are also ineffective in recruiting additional lung because the compliance decrements are not homogeneous, and high pressures simply overdistend more compliant segments. A reasonable approach when ventilating children with poor compliance (Table 29-5) is to use low-volume ventilation and tolerate moderate hypercapnia and respiratory acidosis to facilitate control of inflating pressures (see Chapter 8). This policy has been routinely associated with a low incidence of barotrauma and a high rate of survival.

Carbon Monoxide and Cyanide Exposure

Both carbon monoxide and cyanide are commonly inhaled by victims of closed-space fires. Carbon monoxide is a colorless, odorless gas with an affinity for hemoglobin 200 times that of oxygen. Therefore, patients with significant amounts of carboxyhemoglobin suffer from a marked reduction in their ability to unload oxygen at the peripheral tissue level despite a normal arterial partial pressure of oxygen. Its 2.5-hour half-life is reduced by a factor of five by ventilation with 100% oxygen. Fire victims managed by well trained emergency personnel treated this way from the time of extrication commonly have normal carboxyhemoglobin values (less than 5%) on initial evaluation even after significant exposures to carbon monoxide. Hyperbaric oxygen is appropriate after severe exposures in those patients, who can be safely transported to and treated in the limited access environment of monoplace chambers.

Hydrogen cyanide, which is commonly present in the smoke of structural fires, interferes with oxidative metabolism at the cellular level, resulting in a lactic acidosis. With proper ventilation and fluid resuscitation, the cyanide-induced acidosis corrects in most cases and specific treatment with sodium thiosulfate usually is not required.[11]

Vascular Access Techniques

The successful management of large burns, particularly in the presence of respiratory or other organ failures, depends critically on reliable venous and arterial access, despite the high rates of catheter sepsis traditionally associated with this subpopulation of patients. Peripheral access is often impractical in burn patients and is associated with unacceptable rates of suppurative thrombophlebitis, which can present as sepsis without an obvious focus of infection. For these reasons, in patients with extensive burns, current practice is to use central access almost exclusively, except in those patients with small injuries who require venous access for only a few days.

Arterial access, when required, can be safely maintained through the percutaneous femoral a radical or dorsalis pedis approach.[12] Using small-diameter (2.5 to 3.0 Fr) pressure monitoring catheters. The importance of proper technique cannot be overemphasized if complications are to be avoided. Children intubated for airway protection only, who have no significant shunt or dead space, can be well managed with a transmission oximetry probe and central venous blood gasses.

Because most catheter infections arise from the line tract, rather than the hub, it is thought that strict line care, including a nonocclusive insertion site cleansing every 4 hours, minimizes the risk of both arterial and central venous catheter sepsis. Whenever possible, catheters are inserted through unburned tissue. Using this approach, central venous and arterial catheter sepsis rates approach 3% and 1%, respectively.[12,13]

TABLE 29-5. *A conventional ventilation protocol emphasizing control of peak inflating pressures and associated with a low incidence (<6%) of pulmonary barotrauma*

1. Pressure-controlled ventilation is used in children weighing <8 kg; all others are ventilated with volume-controlled machines.
2. Initial tidal volumes are set between 12 and 15 mL/kg.
3. Peak inspiratory pressure (PIP) is monitored hourly.
4. If PIP exceeds 40 cm H_2O:
   a. Mechanical problems, such as a need for torso escharotomy, are evaluated
   b. Adequate sedation is ensured, the goal being a patient who is lightly asleep but arousable
   c. Tidal volumes are decreased in 10%–20% increments
   d. Respiratory rates are increased as long as auto-positive end expiratory pressure does not occur
   e. Supranormal levels of Pa_{CO_2} are tolerated as long as pH remains >7.2

Nutritional Support

The hypermetabolic response to burn injury is intense until wound closure is complete, and this condition has been considered by some to be detrimental to the patient. However, this assumption must be approached with caution, because this physiologic response has been retained by numerous species over thousands of years, and therefore presumably plays an important role in the recovery from injury. Conventional wisdom indicates that bacteria and their products translocating from an incompetent gut barrier, the burn wound itself, and infectious foci are the ''engines'' driving the hypermetabolic and inflammatory response. Accurate nutritional support of this response is crucial to achieving a favorable outcome.

Accurate support is essential, because underfeeding results in inanition and poor wound healing, whereas overfeeding is associated with hepatic steatosis, leading to hepatic dysfunction and increased CO_2 production, which exacerbates respiratory insufficiency. These factors have led to a plethora of formulas by which nutritional support has been administered. However, patients managed with prompt wound excision and biologic closure have a reduced energy expenditure compared to historic control subjects,[14] and multiple studies have revealed that standard formulas are poorly predictive of actual energy requirements in individual burn patients. For these reasons, indirect calorimetry is commonly used to guide nutritional support of critically burned children. Total energy expenditure can be roughly estimated by using expired gas indirect calorimetry to determine a resting energy expenditure, and then multiplying the resting energy expenditure by a factor of 1.3 to 1.7. Protein loads of 2.5 to 3.0 g/kg/d are recommended to support adequately the amino acid requirements of the seriously burned child.

Multiple Organ Failure and Other Complications of Thermal Injury

It has been said that the successful management of patients with large burns requires identification and management of a series of complications while the wound is progressively closed. Successful clinicians interpret any subtle deterioration as a manifestation of an occult complication until proven otherwise. Common complications of thermal injury are presented in Table 29-6.

The etiology of the multisystem organ failure syndrome likely involves complex cellular and subcellular biology that is only now beginning to be unraveled by investigators using increasing numbers of recombinant products and receptor-blocking antibodies. Our fragmented understanding of this biology, which has been retained in numerous species, makes it clear that we must use caution when considering therapeutic use of these products outside the laboratory.[15] It is widely assumed that development of multiorgan failure is driven by one of several inciting events,[16] including repeated infections, bacteria and their products translocating from an incompetent gut barrier, or the burn wound itself; and that these underlying processes cause multiorgan failure through similar mediator cascades. Prevention of the syndrome would therefore be effected most appropriately by addressing these issues directly, rather than attempting to modify the complex network of mediators that these ''engines'' activate.

The deteriorating burn patient commonly displays early evidence of multiple organ dysfunction in a predictable cascade; increasing obtundation is followed by progressive intrapulmonary shunting with hypoxia, ileus, nonoliguric renal failure, rising cholestatic chemistries, and thrombocytopenia. The most common initiating event is one of the many infections to which burn patients are prone. Certainly, wound sepsis is an obvious potential source. However, this should now be seen infrequently because deep wounds are promptly removed before the onset of infection. The clinical team should search thoroughly for an occult infectious focus when multiorgan dysfunction first becomes evident, because addressing such processes promptly frequently prevents the full development of the syndrome. When an underlying infectious focus can be identified and addressed, organ function improves. If not, failures progress with a predictably fatal outcome. The occult infections that should be considered in such situations (see Table 29-6) include nosocomial sinusitis, which is particularly common in those with nasotracheal tubes; intravascular infections such as endocarditis or suppurative thrombophlebitis, which typically present with fever and bacteremia without localized signs of infection; pneumonia or empyema; intraabdominal infection such as acute cholecystitis or intestinal infarction; osteomyelitis; and infected intravascular devices.

REHABILITATION AND RECONSTRUCTION

With survival after large burns becoming more the rule than the exception, attention has become increasingly focused on the quality rather than the simple fact of survival. Maximizing physical and psychosocial functional recovery is the key to optimizing the overall quality of life after serious burn injury.

Physical function is best optimized by the continuous involvement of dedicated burn occupational and physical therapists, who begin their active involvement with the patient during the acute resuscitation. At this time, their role may be limited to antideformity positioning and splinting of the hands and extremities with twice-daily ranging of all joints. In more stable patients, and in those with large injuries nearing wound closure, therapy sessions may take many hours of each patient's day and involve strengthening, ambulation, active and passive ranging, developing adaptive skills with modified utensils, performing activities of daily living, and, in older adolescents, developing work-related skills. These important activities are continued after discharge.

Psychosocial adaptation after serious burns can be very difficult, particularly if there is serious injury involving the hands or face. Preburn psychiatric illness or family dysfunction may further complicate recovery. The coordinated involvement of psychiatric, psychologic, and social work staff facilitates maximum psychologic recovery and social reintegration. These staff should be actively involved with the patient, family, and local outpatient support services throughout the hospitalization. Planning for discharge and the arrangements and funding for needed outpatient services begins at the time of admission. The expectation for every burned child is a return to family, community life, and mainstream schooling.

TABLE 29-6. *Common complications after burn injury*

System	Complication
Neurologic	1. Transient delirium occurs in up to 30% of patients and usually resolves with supportive therapy when the possibility of anoxia, metabolic disturbance, and structural lesions is eliminated by appropriate studies. 2. Seizures most commonly result from hyponatremia or abrupt benzodiazepine withdrawal. 3. Peripheral nerve injuries occur from direct thermal injury or compression from compartment syndrome, overlying nonelastic eschar, or improper splinting techniques. 4. Delayed peripheral nerve and spinal cord deficits develop weeks or months after high-voltage injury secondary to small vessel injury and demyelinization.
Renal	1. Early acute renal failure follows inadequate perfusion during resuscitation or myoglobinuria. 2. Late renal failure complicates sepsis and multiorgan failure or the use of nephrotoxic agents.
Adrenal	1. Acute adrenal insufficiency secondary to hemorrhage into the gland presents with hypotension, fever, hyponatremia, and hyperkalemia.
Cardiovascular	1. Endocarditis and suppurative thrombophlebitis are intravascular infections that typically present with fever and bacteremia without signs of local infection. 2. Hypertension occurs in up to 20% of children and is best managed with β-adrenergic blockers. 3. Hypotension secondary to sepsis. 4. Venous thromboembolic complications are so infrequent in burned children that routine prophylaxis is not recommended. 5. Iatrogenic catheter insertion complications are minimized by meticulous technique.
Pulmonary	1. Carbon monoxide intoxication, which is best managed acutely with effective ventilatiion with pure oxygen, can be associated with delayed neurologic sequelae. 2. Pulmonary edema due to fluid overload caused by aggressive fluid resuscitation can be potentiated by a capillary leak with fluid shifting into the interstitial space. 3. Pneumonia may occur with or without antecedent inhalation injury and is treated with pulmonary toilet and antibiotics. 4. Respiratory failure may occur early postinjury from inhalation of noxious chemicals, or later in the course secondary to sepsis or pneumonia.
Hematologic	1. Neutropenia and thrombocytopenia, as well as disseminated intravascular coagulation, are common indicators of impending sepsis and should prompt appropriate investigations. 2. Global immunologic deficits associated with burn injury contribute to a high rate of infectious complications.
Otologic	1. Auricular chondritis secondary to bacterial invasion of cartilage results in rapid loss of viable tissue and is prevented by the routine use of topical mafenide acetate on all burned ears. 2. Sinusits and otitis media can be caused by transnasal instrumentation and are treated by relocation of tubes, antibiotics, and judicious surgical drainage. 3. Complications of endotracheal intubation include nasal alar and septal necrosis, vocal cord erosions and ulcerations, tracheal stenosis, and tracheoesophageal and tracheoinominate artery fistulas. The occurrence of such complications is minimized by compulsive attention to tube position, avoidance of oversized tubes, and attention to cuff pressures.
Enteric	1. Hepatic dysfunction, secondary to transient hepatic blood flow deficits and manifested as transaminase elevations, is extremely common during resuscitation from large burns and resolves with volume restitution. Late hepatic failure, beginning with elevations of cholestatic chemistries and progressing through frank failure, complicates sepsis and multiorgan failure. 2. Pancreatitis, beginning with amylase and lipase elevations, and ileus and progressing through hemorrhagic pancreatitis, is usually coincident with splanchnic flow deficits early and sepsis-induced organ failures later in the hospital course. 3. Acalculous cholecystitis, although uncommon in children, can present as sepsis without localized symptoms or signs accompanied by rising cholestatic chemistries. A standard radiographic evaluation can be followed by bedside percutaneous cholecystostomy in unstable patients. 4. Gastroduodenal ulceration, secondary to splanchnic flow deficits that degrade mucosal defenses, is extremely common and often life threatening if routine histamine receptor blockers and antacids are not administered. 5. Intestinal ischemia, which can progress to infarction, is caused by inadequate resuscitation and splanchnic flow deficits.
Ophthalmic	1. Ectropia, from progressive contraction of burned ocular adnexa, results in exposure of the globe. This requires acute eyelid release. Tarsorrhaphy is rarely helpful, more often resulting in injury to the tarsal plate as contraction forces pull out tarsorrhapy sutures. 2. Corneal ulceration, which develops after initial epithelial injury or later exposure secondary to ectropion, can progress to full-thickness corneal destruction if secondary infection occurs. This is prevented by careful globe lubrication with topical antibiotics in the former case and acute lid release in the latter. 3. Symblepharon, or scarring of the lid to the denuded conjunctiva after chemical burns or corneal epithelial defects complicating transcutaneous electrical nerve stimulation are prevented by daily examination and adhesion disruption with a fine glass rod.

TABLE 29-6. *Continued.*

System	Complication
Genitourinary	1. Urinary tract infections are minimized by maintaining bladder catheters only when absolutely required, and are treated with appropriate antibiotics. Neither catheterization nor clonic diversion is required for management of perineal and genital burns.
	2. *Candida* cystitis occurs in those patients treated with bladder catheters and broad-spectrum antibiotics. Catheter change and amphotericin irrigation for 5 d is usually successful. If infections are recurrent, the upper tracts should be screened ultrasonographically.
Musculoskeletal	1. Burned exposed bone is usually debrided with a dental drill until viable cortical bone is reached, which is then allowed to granulate and is autografted. Patients whose overall condition and wounds are appropriate are managed with local or distant flaps.
	2. Fractured and burned extremities are best immobilized with external fixators while overlying burns are grafted. Burn patients with coincident fractures in unburned extremities benefit from prompt internal fixation.
	3. Heterotopic ossification develops weeks after injury, is seen most commonly around deeply burned major joints such as the triceps tendon, and presents with pain and decreased range of motion. Most patients respond to physical therapy, but some require excision of heterotopic bone to achieve full function.
Soft tissue	1. Hypertrophic scar formation is the major cause of the long-term functional and cosmetic deformites seen in pediatric burn patients. This poorly understood process is heralded by a secondary increase in neovascularity between 9 and 13 wk after epithelialization. Management options include grafting of deep dermal and full-thickness wounds, compression garments, judicious steroid injections, topical silicone products, and scar release and resurfacing procedures.

Hypertrophic Scarring and Reconstructive Surgery

Hypertrophic scar formation is a major source of long-term morbidity in burned children (Fig. 29-8). All healed and grafted burns become hypervascular shortly after successful epithelialization. Wounds destined to become hypertrophic have a second surge of neovascularization between 9 and 13 weeks.[17] Additional collagen is formed and contraction occurs over the next 4 to 6 months, at which time the hypervascular tissue involutes, becoming less erythematous and raised over the subsequent 8 to 12 months. Despite the importance of hypertrophic scar formation, our basic understanding of the process remains poor. This lack of understanding is exacerbated by the absence of an animal model of scar hypertrophy.

Wounds that are associated most commonly with hypertrophy are deep dermal burns that heal in 3 or more weeks and full-thickness wounds that heal by contraction and epithelial spread from wound edges. Wounds across flexor surfaces and across the anterior neck and submental area, where there is much tension across the healed wounds, are also subject to scar hypertrophy with increased frequency. However, any wound has the potential to become hypertrophic, and it is often difficult to predict accurately the probability that any individual child will suffer from hypertrophic scar formation.

Our ability to influence the development of hypertrophic scars is limited. Available tools include compression garments, topical silicone sheets, steroid injections, and release or excision and autografting. Compression garments are individually measured and worn beginning within 2 weeks of grafting or wound epithelialization. Compression garments are not advised on the head of children younger than 1 year of age because this may mold the calvarium. Topical silicone has been advocated by some for hypertrophic scar treatment,[18] although the mechanism of action is not clear and the use of topical silicone sheeting is accompanied by frequent skin irritation and rashes. Judicious intradermal steroid injection has been of value in the manage-

ment of limited areas of hypertrophic scarring, usually in cosmetically important areas of small size. These painful intradermal injections require a general anesthetic for proper administration, and it is important to limit the dose to avoid

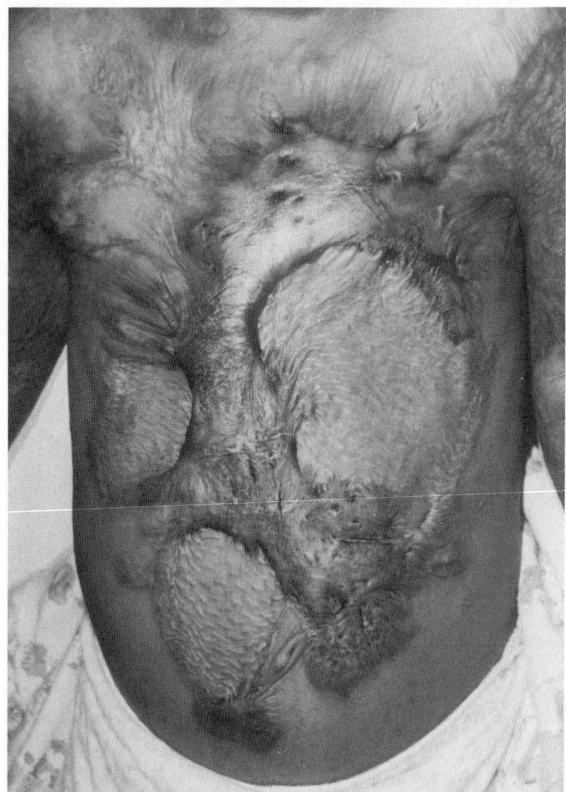

FIG. 29-8. Hypertrophic scar formation has major adverse functional and cosmetic implications.

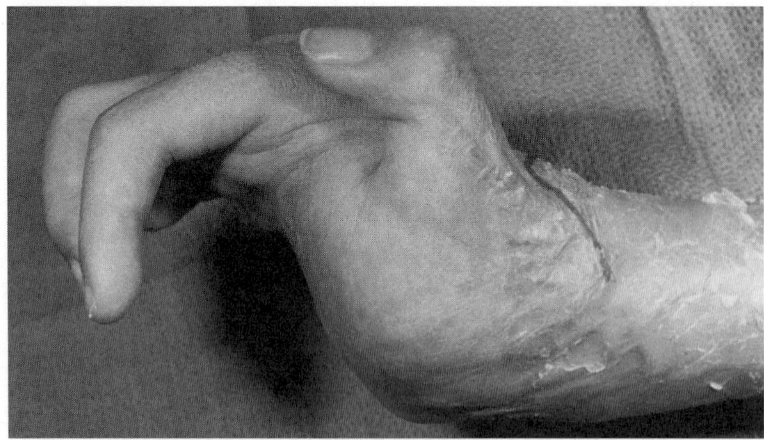

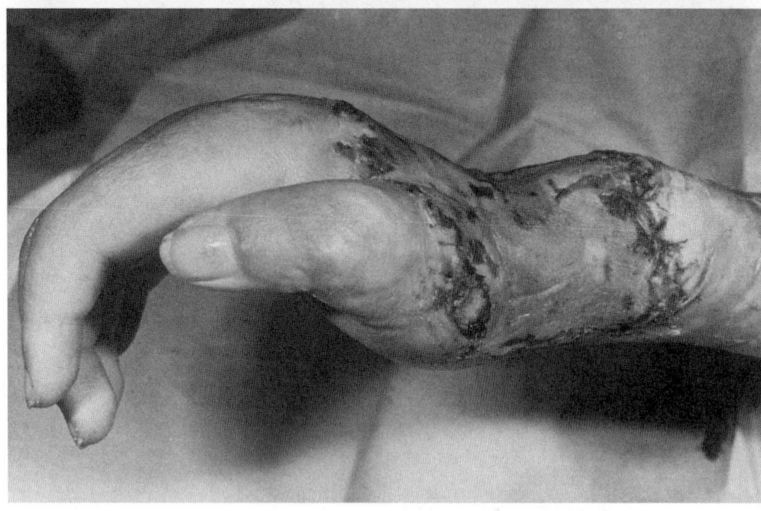

FIG. 29-9. Prompt release and autografting are indicated when hypertrophic scar formation threatens to limit function.

systemic steroid effects. Children with recalcitrant areas of hypertrophic scarring often are best served by release or excision. Resultant wounds are covered with sheet autograft or flaps. Tissue expanders can be of great value, particularly when closing defects of the scalp. When function is not limited, it is ideal to wait 2 years for full scar maturation before embarking on reconstructive procedures. However, when function is threatened, prompt surgery is indicated (Fig. 29-9). Children who survive large injuries commonly require a series of reconstructive procedures over the first few postinjury years to attain optimal cosmetic and functional results.

ON THE HORIZON

There are several exciting potential adjuncts to current burn care that are the topic of frequent discussion and are therefore appropriate to cover here. However, these potential adjuncts are simply supportive and cannot replace excellent clinical care. Indeed, for any such adjunct to be at all effective, it must be used in the setting of optimal clinical care. These potential adjuncts fall into five broad groups: those intended to support or modify the hypermetabolic response, growth factors, innova-

tions in wound management, new critical care technology, and permanent skin substitutes.

It has been demonstrated that although the factors driving the hypermetabolic response may vary from patient to patient, there is a common web of mediators that effect the response. The adverse aspects of the hypermetabolic response are best obviated by minimizing release of inflammatory mediators from the wound by prompt excision and biologic closure; support of gastrointestinal barrier function by ensuring adequate splanchnic blood flow through normalizing hemodynamics and providing enteral nutritional support as soon as possible after injury; and early detection and elimination of infectious foci. These measures are likely to be more effective than attempts to modify the complex cascade of mediators that drive the hypermetabolic response. Although modest modification of the hypermetabolic response, in the form of antipyretics, has become common practice, support rather than major modification of the hypermetabolic response seems most appropriate because our understanding of the basic biology is quite fragmentary. Even β-adrenergic blockade, which has been shown to decrease energy expenditure in burned children,[19] may increase resuscitative fluid requirements without improving cardiac function.[20] Ongoing work with blocking antibodies and recombinant mediators in animal models and in humans promises to enhance our understanding of the hypermetabolic response to injury and to facilitate our support of its beneficial aspects.

Epidermal growth factor and human growth hormone have been associated with shortened donor site healing times in burn patients. However, the differences between control and treated patients have been limited, and any potential benefit should be weighed against the financial and as-yet-undefined long-term physiologic costs of these therapies. Ongoing animal and clinical work with these substances as well as transforming growth factors, platelet-derived growth factors, fibroblast growth factors, and colony-stimulating growth factors promises to enhance our understanding of the biology of wound healing and may lead to improvements in clinical care.

The ability to determine accurately the depth of wounds on initial presentation has the potential to shorten hospital stays by eliminating the period of wound observation commonly used to make accurate predictions of wound healing in children with small burns of indeterminate depth. Although several such technical adjuncts, such as laser Doppler flowmeters and high-resolution ultrasound, have been developed,[4] none has proven of practical clinical utility. The ability of low-power lasers to cause intravenously administered indocyanine green dye to fluoresce is being evaluated and may prove valuable. Bloodless wound debridement using a scanning CO_2 laser has been effective in a porcine model and holds potential promise as a means to decrease the blood loss associated with wound excision. Debriding enzymes have previously been associated with injury to normal tissue, bleeding, pain, infection, and inadequate debridement. New formulations of debriding enzymes that are deactivated by circulating proteases are under development and are designed to liquefy necrotic tissue while causing no injury to healthy tissue. If successful, these substances may also facilitate both wound depth evaluation and blood-conserving removal of eschar.

Critical care technologies under development that may affect burn care include newer modes of ventilation that stress avoidance of high inflating pressures and techniques of extracorporeal support. Nitric oxide, delivered by aerosol into the ventilator circuit, has been shown to decrease intrapulmonary shunt by increasing pulmonary blood flow to well ventilated lung segments, and to decrease pulmonary vascular resistance in patients with respiratory failure.

Definitive wound closure using materials other than autograft is the goal of several ongoing research projects and, if realized, will have an enormous impact on the acute and reconstructive management of burned children. Substitutes under development include epidermal analogs, dermal analogs, and composite substitutes. Of the epidermal analogs, sheets of cultured autologous epithelium is the one in most common clinical use. Although very expensive and associated with low engraftment rates and extreme graft fragility, this technology is of value when managing those patients with truly massive injuries.[21] Patients with smaller injuries are better served by split-thickness autograft. If cultured epidermis becomes fully integrated with a functional dermal analog, its value may rise. Dermal substitutes, designed to be combined with ultrathin autograft, are best represented by the synthetic bilaminate artificial skin developed by Yannas

and Burke that was tested successfully in a large multicenter trial.[22] Although there are allogenic composite substitutes in early clinical trials, none is yet developed to the stage of general clinical use.

As progress in the development of skin substitutes and other innovative aspects of treatment continues, the outlook for the burned child will brighten. Although burn injuries remain a tremendous challenge to the patient, family, and burn unit team, the prognosis for those suffering such injuries continues to improve from both a survival and quality-of-life perspective.

REFERENCES

1. Erdman TC, Feldman KW, Rivara FP, et al. Tap water burn prevention: the effect of legislation. Pediatrics 1991;88:572.
2. Cuthbertson DP. The metabolic response to injury and its nutritional implications: retrospect and prospect. JPEN J Parenter Enteral Nutr 1979;174:270.
3. Youn Y-K, LaLonde C, Demling R. The role of mediators in the response to thermal injury. World J Surg 1992;16:30.
4. Heimbach D, Engrav L, Grube B, et al. Burn depth: a review. World J Surg 1992;16:10.
5. Sheridan RL, Gagnon SW, Tompkins RG. The burn unit as a resource for the management of acute nonburn conditions in children. J Burn Care Rehabil 1995;16:62.
6. Sheridan RL, Tompkins RG, Burke JF. Management of burn wounds with prompt excision and immediate closure. Journal of Intensive Care Medicine 1994;9:6.
7. Gonzalez-Ulloa M. Restoration of the face covering by means of selected skin in regional aesthetic units. Br J Plast Surg 1956;9:212.
8. Sheridan RL, Hurley J, Smith MA, et al. The acutely burned hand: management and outcome based on a ten-year experience with 1047 acute hand burns. Journal of Trauma 1995;38:406.
9. Ruddy RM. Smoke inhalation injury. Pediatr Clin North Am 1994;41:317.
10. Sheridan RL, Kacmarek RM, McEttrick MM, et al. Permission hypercapnia as a ventilatory strategy in burned children: effect on barotrauma, pneumonia, and mortality. Journal of Trauma 1995;39:854.
11. Barillo DJ, Goode R, Esch V. Cyanide poisoning in victims of fire: analysis of 364 cases and review of the literature. J Burn Care Rehabil 1994;15:46.
12. Sheridan RL, Weber JM, Tompkins RG. Prolonged femoral arterial catheterization in pediatric burn patients. Burns 1994;20:451–452.
13. Sheridan RL, Weber JM, Tompkins RG. Low risk of central venous catheter sepsis with weekly catheter change in pediatric burn patients: an analysis of 221 catheters. Burns 1995;21:127.
14. Carlson DE, Cioffi WG, Mason AD, et al. Resting energy expenditure in patients with thermal injuries. Surgery 1992;174:270.
15. Luce JM. Introduction of new technology into critical care practice: a history of HA-1A human monoclonal antibody against endotoxin. Crit Care Med 1993;21:1233.
16. Deitch EA. Multiple organ failure. Adv Surg 1993;26:333.
17. Erlich HP, Kelly SF. Hypertrophic scar: an interruption in the remodeling of repair—a laser Doppler blood flow study. Plast Reconstr Surg 1992;90:993.
18. Ahn ST, Monafo WW, Mustoe TA. Topical silicone gel for the prevention and treatment of hypertrophic scar. Arch Surg 1991;126:499.
19. Breitenstein E, Chiolero RL, Jequier E, et al. Effect of beta-blockade on energy metabolism following burns. Burns 1990;16:259.
20. Horton JW, White DJ, Hunt JL, et al. Effect of propranolol administration on cardiac response to burn injury. J Burn Care Rehabil 1993;14:630.
21. Sheridan RL, Tompkins RG. Cultured autologous epithelium in patients with burns of ninety percent or more of the body surface. Journal of Trauma 1995;38:48.
22. Heimbach D, Luterman A, Burke JF, et al. Artificial dermis for major burns: a multi-center randomized clinical trial. Ann Surg 1988;208:313.

Surgery of Infants and Children: Scientific Principles and Practice, edited by Keith T. Oldham, Paul M. Colombani, and Robert P. Foglia. Lippincott–Raven Publishers, Philadelphia, © 1997.

CHAPTER 30

Principles of Oncology

David N. Korones and Cindy L. Schwartz

Childhood malignancy is a relatively rare event, affecting 1 child in 500 by 15 years of age.[1] Although cancer remains the leading cause of death, after accidents, for children 14 years of age and younger, the past quarter century has seen remarkable advances in treatment, resulting in the survival of more than two thirds of these children. About 1 in 1000 20-year-olds is a survivor of childhood cancer. Much of the early success was achieved with only limited understanding of the pathogenesis of the uncontrolled proliferation of cells that characterizes malignancy. A rapid and ongoing expansion of our understanding of cancer is likely to improve not only rates of cure but also the specificity with which we can halt the growth of malignant cells.

A multidisciplinary approach to the care of the oncology patient is essential. Wilms tumor has been described by D'Angio[2] as a prism through which our knowledge of oncologic principles can be viewed. Pediatric oncologists, surgeons, and radiotherapists tackled the problem of Wilms tumor together and set the stage for our modern era by forming a cooperative group, the National Wilms Tumor Study (NWTS), to investigate treatment approaches. Survival rates soared from 20% with surgery alone to 50% with the addition of radiotherapy and then to 90% with the chemotherapeutic advances of the NWTS. Multiple chemotherapeutic agents were found to be more effective than single agents. Tumor histology was found to predict outcome; the importance of pathologic evaluation of tumor tissue could not be overlooked. Pathologists became increasingly important members of the treatment team. As survival became commonplace, oncologists became aware of long-term problems, such as scoliosis after radiotherapy and cardiotoxicity after treatment with doxorubicin (Adriamycin). Because large numbers of patients were treated by the NWTS groups, relative benefits of components of multimodality therapy could be evaluated and more toxic therapies eliminated in appropriate cohorts. Patients with early-stage disease could be treated with a few weeks of chemotherapy. Radiation could be eliminated, or the dose reduced, in many patients. For patients with stage II disease, intensified two-drug regimens eliminated the cardiotoxicity of the three-drug anthracycline-based regimens. More recently, the NWTS has continued to focus on the ability to shorten treatment duration by intensification of initial therapy.

Although it has been possible to attenuate toxicity by dose modification in some tumors, in other tumors, improvements in survival have been achieved only by dose intensification and increased toxicity. It becomes increasingly clear that treatments must become more specifically designed to kill the abnormal cells, while preserving the normal cells. This can be achieved only with better understanding of the biologic difference between a tumor and a normal cell. Only then will we be able to correct the defect, preferentially killing the tumor cell, or find methods to abrogate the tumor cell's survival advantage.

This chapter explores the principles of tumor cell growth and regulation, the roles of radiotherapy and chemotherapy in treatment, and the causes of treatment failure. Because cytotoxic therapies will remain a major part of our armamentarium for years to come, the long-term effects on normal tissues will continue to plague these patients. Late effects of cancer therapy are discussed at the end of this chapter.

PRINCIPLES OF TUMOR GROWTH

It is ironic that our understanding of the causes and behavior of childhood malignancies lags so far behind our successes in the treatment of these diseases. Until recently, much of what we knew about the biology of tumor growth was derived from older studies of individual tumor cells and aggregates of these cells. With the rapid advances being made in the field of molecular biology, we have begun to understand the behavior of tumors on a more fundamental level. This new knowledge should enable us to design more effective and less toxic regimens than those currently in use.

The biology of tumor growth—the growth cycle, the growth kinetics of tumor masses, and the roles of mutations, differentiation, and metastasis—is explored in this section.

Growth Cycle

The growth cycle is the process by which one cell becomes two. It is arbitrarily divided into five phases, each of which is characterized by a distinct cellular activity related to cell

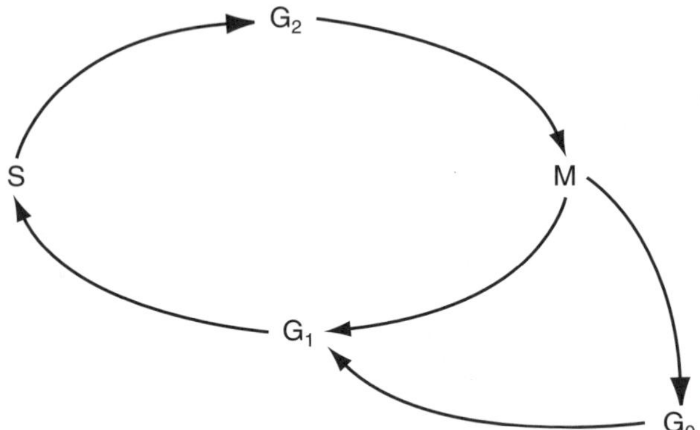

FIG. 30-1. The cell cycle. S, DNA synthesis; M, mitosis; G_0, quiescent phase; G_1, synthesis of enzymes and factors needed for DNA synthesis; G_2, synthesis of enzymes and factors needed for mitosis.

proliferation (Fig. 30-1). The cycle begins on completion of mitosis, when cells enter either G_0 or G_1 (the G stands for gap). Cells that enter G_0 are no longer a part of the growth cycle. Fully differentiated cells, such as hepatocytes or neurons, are in G_0, and under normal circumstances, they remain there to carry out the specific functions of their differentiated phenotypes. Other cells rest in G_0 but can be stimulated to reenter the growth cycle. For example, mature lymphocytes are in G_0, but with the appropriate stimulus, they move into the growth cycle and proliferate. Tumor cells, too, can move in and out of G_0.

Cells can enter G_1 either directly from mitosis or after resting in G_0. G_1 is the gap between completion of mitosis and initiation of DNA synthesis. Enzymes and other factors necessary for DNA synthesis are produced during this phase. The amount of time a tumor cell spends in G_1 is a critical determinant of the doubling time of the tumor. After G_1, cells enter S phase, the period of DNA synthesis during which the entire genome is precisely replicated. Because a relatively high proportion of cancer cells (compared with normal cells) are in S phase, many chemotherapeutic agents are designed to be S-phase specific—that is, they inhibit DNA synthesis. Cells then enter G_2, the period between DNA synthesis and mitosis. Enzymes and other factors necessary for mitosis are synthesized during G_2. G_2 is followed by mitosis, the process by which the two identical sets of chromosomes produced in S phase are divided into each of two daughter cells. After completion of mitosis, the cycle begins anew; cells either drop out of the growth cycle and become quiescent (G_0) or reenter the replication cycle (G_1).

Our understanding of these phases of the growth cycle has been advanced by the discoveries of cyclins and the protein kinase, p34[cdc2], which are critical protein regulators of cell growth.[3] Intracellular levels of cyclins regularly oscillate, peaking just before the cell enters S phase and again just before mitosis. At these peaks, the cyclins complex with a protein kinase, resulting in activation of this enzyme and progression of the cell into the next phase of the cycle. For example, when intracellular levels of cyclin D peak just before S phase, they complex with and activate p34[cdc2].[4] The cell then enters S phase. Similarly, cyclin B peaks and complexes with p34[cdc2] just before mitosis and moves the cell from G_2 into mitosis.[5] Cells do not progress through the cell cycle unless the cyclins peak and complex with and activate p34[cdc2]. A better understanding of these molecular events of the growth cycle may enable us to design therapies that are selectively targeted to interfere with cyclin and p34[cdc2] actions and interactions.

Kinetics of Tumor Growth

Much of what we know about the kinetics of tumor growth is derived from mathematic and animal models developed several decades ago. Skipper[6] established two important principles of tumor growth, known as Skipper's laws, based on observations of the growth of a murine leukemia cell line in mice. The first of these principles is that the doubling time of a given cancer cell or mass of cancer cells is constant. Thus, if it takes 24 hours for one cancer cell to become two, it will take the same amount of time for 1000 cells to become 2000. The second principle is that the percentage of tumor cells killed by a drug is constant, regardless of the number of tumor cells present. For example, if a certain drug kills 90% of a mass of cells, that drug would reduce a tumor burden of 100 cells to 10, or 1,000,000 cells to 100,000.

Although Skipper's laws still apply to growing tumors, they have been substantially modified. The first modification came in 1960, when Mendelsohn[7] introduced the concept of growth fraction. The *growth fraction* is the proportion of a mass of tumor cells that are in the growth cycle (as opposed to G_0). Analysis of tumor cells by flow cytometry or tritiated thymidine labeling has enabled investigators to estimate growth fractions; this percentage of cells in the growth cycle varies from tumor to tumor. The growth fraction ranges from less than 10% in slow-growing tumors, such as low-grade astrocytoma,[8] to 70% to 90% in more aggressive tumors, such as Burkitt lymphoma.[9] Thus, Skipper's laws of cell growth and cell kill do not apply to an entire tumor as originally postulated but only to the fraction of tumor cells in the growth cycle.

When a tumor consists of a few cells, its growth follows Skipper's laws—that is, the growth is exponential, and the tumor rapidly increases in volume. When the tumor is still small, it receives an adequate supply of nutrients and oxygen by direct diffusion and from adjacent or newly developed blood vessels. As the tumor continues to increase in size, however, cells at its center cannot remain viable with simple diffusion of nutrients; furthermore, growth of blood vessels is not always commensurate with tumor growth. Thus, the supply of nutrients and oxygen is diminished. Starved and hypoxic cells drop out of the growth cycle and become quiescent or die. The growth fraction of the tumor is smaller, and as a result, the growth rate of the tumor slows. This phenomenon of exponential growth of a small tumor, followed by slower growth of a large tumor, is referred to as *gompertzian kinetics*. It is an important principle in guiding the treatment of malignancies. Many chemotherapy protocols are based on the rationale that smaller tumors respond better to chemotherapy because they have a higher growth fraction and thus a higher percentage of cells susceptible to the chemotherapy.

Mutations

The behavior of tumor cells is not static: they can become quiescent or differentiate; they can die or grow more rapidly;

and they can acquire features that predispose them to metastasize. These changes in behavior are usually caused by mutations. In vitro studies of proliferating cells show a mutation rate of about one mutation per gene per 10^6 normal cells and about one mutation per gene per 10^5 cancer cells.[10] Thus, there appears to be about a 10-fold increased rate of mutations in malignant cells. Cancer cells not only undergo mutations that convert them from normal to malignant cells but also can undergo a series of mutations that cause them to grow more rapidly and render them less sensitive to chemotherapy. For example, chronic myelogenous leukemia is defined by the presence of a specific mutation: translocation of the short arm of chromosome 9 with the long arm of chromosome 22. Patients can live for years with this low-grade malignancy, but inevitably, the cells become more malignant, proliferate more rapidly, and are refractory to standard therapies. In about 25% of these cases, the tumor progression is associated with a second mutation, loss of function of the tumor suppressor gene, *p53*.[11] Progression of brain tumors and colon cancers has also been associated with mutations in the *p53* gene.[12] Mutations have also been directly implicated in conferring resistance to specific chemotherapeutic agents. For example, resistance of cancer cells to methotrexate is mediated by a genetic alteration called *gene amplification*.[13] This alteration results in the creation of multiple copies of the gene that codes for dihydrofolate reductase, the enzyme blocked by methotrexate. The amplification leads to a tremendous increase in the production of dihydrofolate reductase. The amount produced outpaces the amount of methotrexate available, thus overcoming the inhibitory effect of methotrexate.

Differentiation

Tumor cells are generally characterized by an undifferentiated phenotype. Many pediatric tumors arise as a result of arrest in the normal process of differentiation. This arrest is probably caused by mutations that block differentiation but not proliferation. Because mutations can occur at any point along the pathway of differentiation, a given type of pediatric tumor can be characterized along a spectrum of differentiation. For example, analysis of immunoglobulin gene rearrangements in the lymphoblasts of patients with B-cell acute lymphoblastic leukemia (ALL) reveals that each patient's lymphoblasts are arrested at a specific stage of normal B-cell development.[14] Neuroblastoma cells often have phenotypic characteristics of more mature nervous tissues, such as neurites, neural surface markers, and elaboration of neuropeptides, including vasoactive intestinal peptide. Wilms tumor, neuroblastoma, rhabdomyosarcoma, brain tumors, and germ cell tumors all show varying degrees of differentiation even within a single tumor. Occasionally, the malignant cells of these tumors differentiate spontaneously or in response to therapy. The capacity of some tumor cells to differentiate shows that their relative lack of differentiation is not a fixed defect. Furthermore, because differentiation is associated with growth arrest, investigators are exploring the use of differentiation therapy as a means of treating certain malignancies. The most dramatic advance in this field is the use of all-*trans* retinoic acid for the treatment of acute promyelocytic leukemia (APML). The characteristic t(15,17) of APML encodes for an abnormal mRNA transcript for the retinoic acid α-receptor. This protein appears to block myeloid differentiation. All-*trans* retinoic acid may restore normal differentiation by up-regulation of the normal retinoic acid α-receptor.[15] Most patients with APML treated with this agent achieve remission by induction of differentiation of the promyeloblasts into mature neutrophils.[16]

Metastasis

Metastasis is a major cause of treatment failure and death in children with cancer. In fact, local control of primary tumors with radiation and surgery is so effective for many of the pediatric malignancies that chemotherapy is largely directed toward control of overt or micrometastases. The process of metastasis is an intricate, complex, and incompletely understood phenomenon, requiring the cooperation of tumor cell and host. For a cancer cell to leave a primary tumor and implant and grow at a distant site, it must enter a draining blood vessel from the primary tumor, survive the trip to a distant vascular bed, attach to a specific endothelium, extravasate into host tissue, and find an environment there that is conducive to continued proliferation.

Exciting advances in our understanding of metastasis may lead to therapy specifically designed to prevent it. For example, a critical step in metastasis is the ability of a tumor cell to traverse the basement membrane of adjacent, normal tissue and then adhere to the basement membrane of tissue at distant sites. This may occur as a result of interactions between adhesion molecules on the surface of cancer cells and adhesion molecules on the basement membrane. One such interaction has been explored in studies of the adhesion molecule laminin and its receptor. Increased expression of the laminin receptor on the surfaces of certain carcinoma cells may result in the adherence of these cells to distant, laminin-rich basement membranes. Studies in animals substantiate this hypothesis and open the door to the possibility of metastasis-specific therapy. When animals with tumors expressing laminin receptors are treated with laminin fragments, the receptors on the tumor cells are blocked, and there is a decrease in the number of distant metastases.[17]

Another important aspect of metastasis is tissue invasion. Tumor cells that have active proteases can erode the basement membrane of adjacent, normal tissue. One of the proteases found in tumors, zinc metalloproteinase, is normally inactive. With certain mutations, however, the enzyme becomes active, and the tumor becomes invasive. Administration of metalloproteinase inhibitors to tumor-laden animals with active proteases has resulted in decreased invasion and metastasis.[18]

Each of the pediatric tumors has a fairly characteristic pattern of metastasis. Often, this pattern can be predicted on the basis of mechanical factors; for example, children with osteosarcoma or Ewing sarcoma are most likely to develop lung metastases. Tumor cells dislodge from the primary site and are mechanically detained in small vessels through which the large tumor cells cannot pass. The first small vessels that most circulating tumor cells encounter are the capillary beds of the lungs. Not all pediatric tumors, however, follow this pattern of metastasis. Infants with neuroblastoma develop metastases in the liver, skin, or bone marrow. Clear cell sarcoma of the kidney typically metastasizes to bone and brain. Lymphoma spreads to bone marrow, liver, and spleen. Given the distinct pattern of metastases in these and other tumors, it is apparent that factors other than mechanical ones come into play. The pattern of metastasis may depend on adherence of tumor cells to the peculiar microvasculature of a particular organ. The local milieu also plays a major role; certain organs may be rich in growth factors that the tumor requires for sustained, rapid growth.

Likewise, a tumor can secrete inhibitors of tumor angiogenesis. In some tumor systems, metastases grow when removal of the primary tumor results in lower plasma concentrations of these inhibitors.[19]

PRINCIPLES OF RADIOTHERAPY

DNA damage is responsible for the cytotoxic effects of radiotherapy. Although there is a direct effect on the DNA, the most prominent cytotoxic effect is due to free radicals generated by the ionization of water. Cells are most sensitive to radiotherapy in the early S phase (DNA synthesis) of the cell cycle and in mitosis. Damaged cells manifest injury at the time of cell proliferation. Rapidly dividing cells die rapidly and thus are radiosensitive. More slowly dividing cells are more tolerant to radiation effects, and a response may be seen only months to years after radiotherapy.

The efficacy of radiotherapy is also related to the presence of oxygen in the target tissue and the type of radiation used. Cytotoxicity is more prominent with radiation produced by neutrons, prions, or heavily charged particles than with x-rays, gamma rays, or electrons because of the extent of ionization that is produced along the path of the beam.

Radiation is traditionally administered in small fractions of the total dose. Between radiation doses, sublethal damage may be repaired. There is evidence that normal tissue repairs sublethal damage better than tumors. A technique that has been derived from this that is being investigated is hyperfractionation. Equal total radiation doses are given as small fractions of radiation that are administered more frequently, usually twice daily, as a way either to prevent toxicity to normal tissues or to intensify the dose without increasing toxicity. Fractionation of the radiation also results in prolongation of treatment time. This may allow hypoxic areas of tumor tissue to become reoxygenated. In addition, quiescent cells may be recruited into proliferation, increasing the response rate. Alternatively, for rapidly growing tumors, prolonging treatment time may allow for regrowth of tumor tissue.

The use of radiotherapy requires knowledge of tumor sensitivity and of tolerance to radiation of the normal adjacent tissues. Young children are particularly sensitive to long-term effects of radiotherapy, in part because of their increased growth potential. Although radiotherapy can be used as the sole modality of treatment for tumors such as Hodgkin disease and brain tumors, the use of a single modality for the treatment of malignancy is becoming less common. Combined-modality therapy often offers the possibility of limiting total radiation dose while improving cure rates.

PRINCIPLES OF CHEMOTHERAPY

The ideal drug is one that is targeted to block a specific physiologic process and has little effect on other organs or physiologic processes. Unfortunately, cancer cells are not sufficiently different from normal cells, and many of the drugs designed to kill cancer cells kill normal cells as well. Often, however, enough differences exist between the two cell types to provide a therapeutic window for preferential tumor cell killing, albeit a narrow one. The principles of chemotherapy are based on the relatively rapid growth rate of tumor cells, the gompertzian growth kinetics of tumor masses, and the propensity of tumor cells to undergo mutations and become more resistant to subsequent treatment. These principles provide the rationale for treating cancer promptly with high doses of drugs and with combination chemotherapy.

Chemotherapy Kills Proliferating Cells

Virtually all standard antineoplastic agents interfere with cell proliferation (Table 30-1). At the level of DNA synthesis, antimetabolites, such as methotrexate and 5-fluorouracil, inhibit synthesis of purines and pyrimidines. Alkylating agents, such as cyclophosphamide, mechlorethamine (nitrogen mustard), and carboplatin, covalently bind to DNA and prevent replication and transcription. L-Asparaginase inhibits protein synthesis, and vincristine and paclitaxel (Taxol) interfere with mitotic spindle formation and breakdown. Most of these events occur during G_1, S, G_2, or M phase of the growth cycle. Thus, cells in G_0 are impervious to many of the standard therapies, a phenomenon referred to as *kinetic resistance.*[20] Because a far greater percentage of cancer cells than normal cells are in the growth cycle (as opposed to G_0), drug treatment should favor the destruction of malignant cells over normal cells.

Chemotherapy Guided by Gompertzian Growth Kinetics

According to the gompertzian model of tumor growth, only a fraction of tumor cells in a mass are actively proliferating, and the smaller the tumor, the greater is the proportion of proliferating cells.

Because most chemotherapeutic agents kill proliferating cells, it follows that treatment is most effective in eradicating smaller tumors. This line of reasoning has been successfully applied to the treatment of micrometastases, metastases that are present at diagnosis but are too small to be seen by standard imaging modalities. For example, in the 1970s, the treatment for nonmetastatic Ewing sarcoma, a pediatric bone tumor, was radiotherapy and surgical resection of the primary tumor. Despite excellent local control, most children eventually developed lung metastases.[21] These metastases were probably present at the time of diagnosis but were too small to be seen. In the 1980s, children with nonmetastatic Ewing sarcoma received chemotherapy in addition to local control, and the incidence of lung metastases was dramatically reduced. Similar treatment with chemotherapy for nonmetastatic osteosarcoma, rhabdomyosarcoma, and neuroblastoma reduces the incidence of subsequent metastases and increases cure rates.[21]

The rationale for prolonged intermittent treatment with chemotherapy has its roots in the concept of kinetic resistance. Cells not in the growth cycle at the time of treatment are in G_0 and therefore are likely to be resistant to the effects of growth cycle–specific chemotherapy. These cells can lay dormant for

TABLE 30-1. *Chemotherapeutic agents*

Agents	Mechanism of action	Tumors treated with agent
Dactinomycin	Intercalates in DNA	Wilms tumor, rhabdomyosarcoma, soft tissue sarcoma, Ewing sarcoma, germ cell tumors
Doxorubicin, daunomycin	Intercalates in DNA	Leukemia, lymphomas, solid tumors (except brain)
Bleomycin	Binds DNA	Lymphomas, germ cell tumors (osteosarcoma)
Cisplatin, carboplatin	Alkalating-like agent	Neuroblastoma, brain tumors, germ cell tumors, hepatoblastoma
Cyclophosphamide	Alkylating agent	Leukemia, solid tumors, lymphomas, brain tumors
Ifosfamide	Alkylating agent	Solid tumors, lymphoma, leukemia
Nitrosoureas (CCNU, BCNU)	Alkylating agent	Brain tumors, Hodgkin disease, non-Hodgkin lymphoma
Nitrogen mustard	Alkylating agent	Brain tumors, Hodgkin disease
Dacarbazine	Alkylating agent	Hodgkin disease, sarcoma
Procarbazine	Alkylating agent	Brain tumors, Hodgkin disease
Methotrexate	Antimetabolite	ALL, non-Hodgkin lymphoma, osteosarcoma
6-Mercaptopurine	Antimetabolite	ALL, non-Hodgkin lymphoma
Cytosine arabinoside	Antimetabolite	Leukemias, lymphoma
6-Thioguanine	Antimetabolite	Acute myelogenous leukemia
Prednisone, dexamethasone	Lympholytic agent	ALL, non-Hodgkin lymphoma
Vincristine, vinblastine	Mitotic spindle inhibitor	ALL, lymphomas, solid tumors, brain tumors
Etoposide	Topoisomerase II inhibitor	ALL, lymphomas, solid tumors, brain tumors
L-Asparaginase	Inhibits protein synthesis through asparagine depletion	ALL, non-Hodgkin lymphoma

ALL, acute lymphocytic leukemia.

weeks or even months before reentering the growth cycle. Intermittent pulses of chemotherapy delivered over months increase the likelihood of catching these dormant cells as they reenter the growth cycle and hence are more susceptible to chemotherapy.

Goldie-Coldman Hypothesis

The Goldie-Coldman hypothesis provides the theoretic underpinnings for the simultaneous use of multiple chemotherapeutic agents for the treatment of cancer. According to this hypothesis, proliferating cancer cells are at continued risk of undergoing mutations, and it is possible that some chance mutation will cause the cells to become resistant to certain types of chemotherapy. For example, 1 g of tumor is composed of a billion cells (10^9). If the mutation rate is 1 per 10^5 cells, 1 g of tumor contains 10^4 cells with new mutations, one of which could conceivably confer resistance to treatment with a single drug. If, however, two drugs are used, the chance of a single cell developing two mutations that result in resistance to both drugs is 1 in $10^5 \times 1$ in 10^5 or 1 chance in 10^{10}.[10] Thus, a 1-g tumor is unlikely to contain any cells resistant to two-drug therapy. Although these mathematic calculations are crude and inexact, they illustrate the potential effectiveness of combination chemotherapy. Numerous clinical trials have substantiated the Goldie-Coldman hypothesis. The Dana Farber Cancer Institute protocol for childhood ALL illustrates the dramatic improvements in cure rates with combination chemotherapy.[22] In the 1960s, standard treatment for ALL was vincristine and prednisone. Remission was easily achieved in most children, but most soon relapsed. When doxorubicin was added to the vincristine and prednisone, the survival rate of the children receiving this three-drug combination increased from 38% to 69%. When L-asparaginase was added to the three drugs, survival climbed even higher, to 79%. Now, with a six-drug induction therapy,

remission rates for ALL are 99%, and relapse-free survival rates are as high as 89%.

STRATEGIES FOR TREATMENT WITH CHEMOTHERAPY

During the past 30 years, oncologists have moved from simple, single-agent regimens of chemotherapy to more complex and intensive programs. The new regimens have evolved through clinical trials based not only on the biologic principles described earlier but also on experience. The general strategies employed have included combination chemotherapy, dose intensity, rescue after dose-intensive therapy, and potentiators of chemotherapy.

Combination Chemotherapy

The use of multiple drugs for the treatment of pediatric malignancies is now standard. (Table 30-2 reviews therapies in use for common pediatric malignancies.) These drugs can be administered concomitantly, as in the four- to six-drug regimens employed for remission induction for ALL. They also can be administered sequentially, as in the alternating courses of doxorubicin plus cyclophosphamide and VP-16 plus ifosfamide for Ewing sarcoma. This approach has its origins in the Goldie-Coldman hypothesis. The following principles guide the choices of agents for these combination regimens: (1) the drugs should have documented activity against a given tumor, (2) the drugs should have differing mechanisms of action, (3) there should be as little toxicity overlap as possible, and (4) the drugs should have different patterns of resistance.

TABLE 30-2. *Common chemotherapeutic regimens for specific pediatric tumors*

Tumor	First-line regimens	Second-line regimens
ALL	VCR, Pred, L-asp, MTX, 6-MP ± Doxo/DNR, IT MTX ± Ara-C ± HC	Same, high-dose Ara-C, CY, VP-16, bone marrow transplantation
AML	DNR, Ara-C, 6-TG, VP-16 ± allo BMT	Mitoxantrone/VP-16, Idarubicin, allo BMT
CML	Allo BMT, hydroxyurea, interferon-α	
Hodgkin	RT or MOPP, ABDV, COPP or MOPP/ABDV	Ara-C/cisplatin/etoposide, auto BMT
NHL—large cell	Doxo, Pred, VCR	Ara-C, VP-16, Ifos, CY, MTX, BMT
NHL—B cell	CY, VCR, Doxo, Ara-C, MTX, VP-16, Pred	Ifos, VP-16, BMT
NHL—T cell	Similar to ALL therapy	Reinduction, BMT
Wilms	VCR, Act-D ± Doxo ± CY ± RT	VP-16, Ifos, BMT
Rhabdomyosarcoma	RT, VCR, Act-D ± Doxo ± CY ± VP, ± Ifos	Ifos/VP-16 (BMT)
Soft tissue sarcoma	RT, VCR, Act-D ± Doxo ± CY, ± DTIC ± VP ± Ifos	Ifos/VP-16
Osteosarcoma	HD MTX, Doxo, cisplatin, ± Ifos	Ifos/VP-16, carbo
Ewing sarcoma	RT or surgery, VCR, Act-D, Doxo, CY, Ifos, VP-16	VP-16/Ifos, auto BMT
Neuroblastoma	CY, Doxo ± carbo/cisplatin ± VP-16 ± Ifos ± Auto BMT	Ifos/VP-16/carbo, auto BMT
Germ cell tumor	Cisplatin, VP-16, bleomycin	Ifos, carbo, VCR

ALL, acute lymphocytic leukemia; AML, acute myelogenous leukemia; CML, chronic myelogenous leukemia; NHL, non-Hodgkin lymphoma; RT, radiotherapy; VCR, vincristine; MTX, methotrexate; Pred, prednisone; L-asp, L-asparaginase; 6-MP, 6-mercaptopurine; 6-TG, 6-thioguanine; IT, intrathecal; Ara-C, cytosine arabinoside; Doxo, doxorubicin (Adriamycin); DNR, daunomycin; VP, etoposide (VP-16); CY, cyclophosphamide; Act-D, dactinomycin (Actinomycin D); Ifos, Ifosfamide; carbo, carboplatin; MOPP, nitrogenmustard, vincristine, procarbazine, prednisone; ABDV, doxorubicin, bleomycin, dacarbazine (DTIC), vinblastine; HC, hydrocortisone; allo BMT, allogenic bone marrow transplantation; auto BMT, autologous bone marrow transplantation; COPP, cyclophosphamide, vincristine, prednisone, procarbazine; HD, high-dose.

Dose Intensity

Many antineoplastic drugs have been shown to have steep dose–response curves—that is, the higher the dose, the greater is the tumor cell kill. Numerous clinical studies have demonstrated that increased dose intensity is associated with increased survival.[21] Dose intensity can take the form of higher doses of a drug or more frequent delivery of standard doses of the drug. The importance of the latter is illustrated in a review of children who received varying doses of chemotherapy for ALL and osteosarcoma. The children who received less than 75% of the intended doses of chemotherapy did not fare as well as those who received greater than 75%.[23,24]

One method of safely increasing dose intensity is to provide a ''rescue'' from the toxicity of high-dose chemotherapy after allowing the high doses of the drug to render their antitumor effect. Perhaps the most dramatic example of this is autologous or allogeneic bone marrow transplantation. Such an approach is generally reserved for the patient whose malignancy is not treatable by standard chemotherapy. In this instance, the patient's (or a suitable donor's) bone marrow is harvested and saved. The patient then receives massive doses of chemotherapy (sometimes with total-body irradiation), which ablates the remaining bone marrow. The patient is then rescued from bone marrow aplasia by reinfusion of the patient's own (or the donor's) bone marrow.

High-dose local therapy also increases dose intensity. Examples include intrathecal chemotherapy for cerebrospinal fluid tumors, intraperitoneal therapy for ovarian cancer, and intraarterial administration of chemotherapy in the region of the tumor. Another means of rescue is the use of leucovorin after administration of high doses of methotrexate. Methotrexate inhibits the enzyme dihydrofolate reductase, which plays a critical role in the synthesis of DNA bases. Leucovorin (tetrahydrofolate) is the product of the enzyme; thus, once leucovorin has been given, the enzyme is bypassed, DNA bases are again synthesized, and the severe myelosuppression and mucositis caused by methotrexate are avoided. Finally, safe administration of ifosfamide and high doses of cyclophosphamide were made possible by the concomitant administration of mesna, a compound that prevents cyclophosphamide and ifosfamide-induced hemorrhagic cystitis.

Adjuvant and Neoadjuvant Chemotherapy

Adjuvant chemotherapy is systemic treatment administered in addition to local control of the primary tumor. A large body of experimental and clinical evidence supports this approach to the treatment of pediatric malignancies. For example, as noted earlier, the survival rate for children with nonmetastatic Ewing sarcoma who receive local therapy alone is 5%, compared with 50% to 60% for children who also receive chemotherapy.[21] Children with Wilms tumor or osteosarcoma also have significantly higher survival rates when they receive adjuvant chemotherapy.[21] In the era preceding the routine use of adjuvant chemotherapy for nonmetastatic tumors, most children died of metastases. This suggests that the main contribution of adjuvant chemotherapy is control of micrometastases that were present but not clinically apparent at diagnosis.

Neoadjuvant chemotherapy refers to the administration of chemotherapy before definitive local treatment of the primary tumor. This type of therapy has a number of advantages. Systemic chemotherapy can be started promptly after a biopsy, thus avoiding the 1- to 2-week delays typically required after major surgery. Avoidance of such delays may result in more effective control of micrometastases. Several courses of neoadjuvant therapy may also substantially reduce the size of the primary tumor, converting a previously unresectable tumor into a resectable tumor. No definitive clinical trials prove that the neoadjuvant approach translates into prolonged survival or increased cure rates.

Immunotherapy

Immunotherapy is designed to stimulate the immune system to destroy cancer cells. The strategies for manipulation of the immune system are broad ranging and include the use of tumor vaccines, cytokines such as interferons and interleukin-2, lymphokine-activated killer cells, tumor-infiltrating lymphocytes, activated monocytes, and monoclonal antibodies conjugated to toxins.[25] Although there have been a few trials of immunotherapy in adults, there is little experience with its use in children. The following discussion is confined to three approaches with which there is some experience in the treatment of pediatric malignancies: interferons, activated monocytes, and conjugated antibodies.

The interferons possess a broad range of activities, including activation of cytotoxic T cells, inhibition of cell growth, and inhibition of angiogenesis. The antitumor activity of interferons is well documented for Kaposi sarcoma, hairy cell leukemia, and bladder cancer. Interferons also have proved effective in the treatment of chronic myelogenous leukemia in children and adults. This treatment was investigated in children with recurrent brain tumors; 4 of 21 children responded to interferon-β, including 2 children with brain-stem gliomas. The most frequently encountered toxicity of the interferons is influenza-like symptoms, such as fever, myalgia, and malaise. Bone marrow suppression can also occur and may be dose limiting.

Muramyl tripeptide-phosphatidyl-ethanolamine (MTP-PE) is a monocyte–macrophage activator that has shown promise as an antitumor agent in preclinical studies and in phase I trials. When MTP-PE is encapsulated in liposomes, it is delivered selectively to monocytes and pulmonary macrophages, which in turn become cytotoxic. Animals with metastatic osteosarcoma treated with liposomal MTP-PE had dramatic reductions in the size and number of their pulmonary metastases. Several children with osteosarcoma have been treated with MTP-PE after removal of metastatic lung lesions. Although these children subsequently developed more lung metastases, their tumor nodules were infiltrated with inflammatory cells and surrounded by dense fibrous tissue suggestive of chronic inflammation. It is hypothesized that the MTP-PE–activated macrophages kill or at least contain osteosarcoma micrometastases. MTP-PE is being studied as part of a Pediatric Oncology Group phase III trial for children with newly diagnosed osteosarcoma.

A third example of the potential of immunotherapy is the use of monoclonal antibodies conjugated to cytotoxins. Monoclonal antibodies have been developed that recognize antigens expressed on the surface of tumor cells, but not on host cells. These antibodies are conjugated to potent toxins, such as ricin or radioisotopes. They are then infused systemically and selectively deliver the toxins to the tumor cells. For example, 3F8 is a monoclonal antibody to GD_2, a ganglioside expressed on the surface of neuroblastoma cells. When the 3F8 is radiolabeled with iodine-131 (^{131}I), relatively high doses of this radioisotope can be delivered to the neuroblastoma. Because GD_2 is not found on normal host cells, normal tissues are spared radiation exposure. Children with relapsed neuroblastoma have received infusions of ^{131}I-3F8 in a phase I trial of the immunotoxin; the drug was well tolerated, and a number of children had measurable responses.

Immunotherapy is an innovative approach to the treatment of cancer, but it is still in its infancy. It is a promising method of a more selective, less toxic way of delivering chemotherapy, but it will be some time before it finds its place as a standard part of the treatment of childhood malignancies.

Future Strategies

Exciting and innovative approaches to the treatment of malignancies show promise as gentler and kinder therapies that may be even more effective than the current approaches. A major drawback of standard chemotherapy is the narrow therapeutic window. The goal of many newer therapies is to develop a drug that is targeted more specifically to tumor cells and thus is less toxic to normal cells. One approach is the development of *differentiators*. These are drugs that induce the differentiation of cancer cells and therefore their growth. As previously noted, patients with APML can achieve remission by treatment with all-*trans* retinoic acid, a drug that induces the differentiation of promyeloblasts into mature neutrophils.[13] Interferon-α is a biologic response modifier that inhibits not only angiogenesis but also the growth of certain types of hemangiomas and angiogenic tumors, such as Kaposi sarcoma. Suramin, a polynaphthalene sulfonic urea, blocks the binding of a number of growth factors to their receptors on tumor cells, inhibiting tumor growth. For example, prostate tumors produce, have receptors for, and respond to platelet-derived growth factor. Many patients with advanced prostate carcinoma have responded to suramin,[26] which may be rendering its effect by preventing platelet-derived growth factor from binding to its receptor.

Toxicity

The properties of chemotherapeutic agents that make them effective for treating malignancies make them toxic as well. It follows that therapy targeted at rapidly proliferating cells causes considerable toxicity to the bone marrow and the gastrointestinal tract, the two sites of the most actively proliferating normal cells. Thus, pancytopenia is predictable, and the risk of infection and bleeding is high. Gastrointestinal toxicity includes nausea and vomiting, mouth sores, mucositis, and diarrhea. Loss of integrity of the bowel wall, coupled with profound neutropenia, places these children at high risk for gram-negative bacterial infections. Wound healing requires proliferating cells; thus, such healing is often delayed when the child is on chemotherapy. Furthermore, the risk of infection as a result of treatment with chemotherapy applies to surgical wounds as well. Other toxicities are more specifically related to the agents used: cisplatin causes ototoxicity and renal damage, doxorubicin causes cardiomyopathy, and bleomycin causes pulmonary toxicity. Common toxicities of standard chemotherapeutic agents are shown in Table 30-3.

CAUSES OF TREATMENT FAILURE

Despite the availability of the cytotoxic therapies described earlier, one third of children with pediatric malignancies ulti-

TABLE 30-3. *Toxic effects of common chemotherapy agents**

Agent	Acute effects	Late effects
Dactinomycin (Actinomycin D)	Myelosuppression, hair loss, liver toxicity, pleural effusions, nausea	
Doxorubicin, daunomycin	Myelosuppression, hair loss, nausea, mucositis, heart failure	Cardiomyopathy, arrhythmia
Bleomycin	Pulmonary toxicity	Pulmonary toxicity
Cisplatin	Nausea, hearing loss, renal dysfunction	Renal dysfunction, hearing loss
Carboplatin	Myelosuppression, hair loss, rare ototoxicity and renal dysfunction	
Nitrosoureas, nitrogen mustard	Myelosuppression, hair loss, nausea, pulmonary dysfunction	Sterility, infertility, secondary malignancy, pulmonary dysfunction
Procarbazine	Myelosuppression, hair loss, nausea	Sterility, infertility, secondary malignancy
Cyclophosphamide	Myelosuppression, hair loss, hemorrhagic cystitis, nausea	Secondary malignancy, infertility, sterility, pulmonary fibrosis, bladder carcinoma
Ifosfamide	Myelosuppression, hemorrhagic cystitis, hair loss, nausea, Fanconi syndrome (glucosuria, phosphaturia), renal failure	Fanconi syndrome, secondary malignancy
6-Mercaptopurine, 6-thioguanine	Myelosuppression, hepatotoxicity	
Cytosine arabinoside	Myelosuppression, mucositis, nausea, hepatotoxicity, *Streptococcus viridans* sepsis with high dose	
Methotrexate	Myelosuppression, hair loss, liver toxicity, skin rash, mucositis, nausea, rare pulmonary effects, CNS toxicity with intrathecal or high dose	Leukoencephalopathy, learning disability
Vincristine	Hair loss, peripheral neuropathy, constipation	
Prednisone, dexamethasone	Hypertension, cushingoid facies, GI bleeding, osteoporosis, striae	Osteoporosis
Etoposide	Allergic reaction, hypotension, myelosuppression	Secondary leukemia with translocation involving 11q23
Vinblastine	Myelosuppression, hair loss	
L-Asparaginase	Hives, anaphylaxis, coagulopathy, pancreatitis, transient diabetes mellitus	

* This table does not represent a review of all possible toxicities but rather a compilation of commonly seen effects.

mately succumb to their disease. The growth of tumor cells after intensive treatment can be attributed to a variety of mechanisms by which the tumor cells become able to survive in a harsh environment. Mechanisms of tumor cell resistance to virtually all chemotherapeutic agents have been described and include decreased drug uptake or increased drug removal from the cell, decreased drug-activating or increased drug-inactivating enzymes, increased levels of or altered affinity for an enzyme normally inhibited by the drug, alternative pathways to bypass enzyme inhibition, and increased drug repair. Representative examples of some of these mechanisms are discussed next.

Tumor cells can also reside in the sanctuary sites where chemotherapeutic agents cannot penetrate, that is, the brain and the testes. In these cases, treatment must be devised that can reach these areas by alternative means. For example, in childhood ALL, cranial irradiation, intrathecal medication, and high-dose systemic chemotherapy that penetrates the central nervous system (CNS) have all been used to treat and prevent CNS leukemia.

Radiosensitivity also varies from tumor to tumor. Despite an innate sensitivity of a tumor to radiotherapy, cells that are remote from a vascular supply may be hypoxic. This diminishes the generation of oxygen-derived free radicals and decreases the tumor sensitivity to radiation. A number of experimental approaches to increase oxygen supply to specific tumors are ongoing.

Multiple Drug Resistance

In the early 1970s, a phenomenon was described in which cells with induced resistance to vinblastine simultaneously became resistant to dactinomycin (Actinomycin D) and colchicine, agents that mechanistically had nothing in common with each other or with vinblastine.[27] A cellular change had occurred that prevented these drugs from entering the cell. The resistant cells were found to express a transmembrane protein that was not present in drug-sensitive cells.[28] This transmembrane protein has been identified as a P-glycoprotein (P-gp) with an adenosine triphosphate moiety. Functioning as an efflux pump, P-gp allows cells to eliminate toxic natural substances from the intracellular environment. Substances affected by this pump are commonly hydrophobic or of neutral charge, but bear no other chemical resemblance to each other.[29] P-gp is normally present on body surfaces that are involved in transport, such as the gastrointestinal epithelium, proximal renal tubules, adrenal medulla, and capillary endothelium of the CNS, testis, and placenta. The blood–brain, blood–testis, and fetal–maternal barriers have been attributed to the effect of P-gp on the relevant capillary endothelium.

P-glycoprotein can be detected at the time of diagnosis in some tumors, particularly those that arise in P-gp–expressing organs. A poor prognosis can be predicted for the newly diagnosed patient with P-gp–positive rhabdomyosarcoma and neuroblastoma.[30,31] Similar studies in adults have shown an association between poor prognosis and P-gp expression in acute myelogenous leukemia, myeloma, lymphoma, and breast cancer.[32,33] Expression of P-gp can also be induced by exposure to drugs associated with P-gp–mediated efflux. This pattern of chemotherapy-induced P-gp expression has been described in pediatric osteosarcoma.[34]

This relatively simple explanation of one form of drug resistance suggests an equally simple approach to overcoming this drug resistance. Hydrophobic substances that are preferentially bound by P-gp (eg, verapamil, cyclosporin A, and numerous others) can be used as competitive inhibitors, allowing for increased intracellular accumulation of chemotherapeutic agents, such as anthracyclines, vincristine, and vinblastine.[35] Studies are ongoing to determine whether this approach to chemotherapy is effective in vivo. In the future, it may be possible to down-regulate expression of the *mdr-1* gene, the protein product of which is P-gp. In vitro studies have been performed to determine whether anti–*mdr-1* can be used in this manner, but this research is still in its infancy. Methods may also be devised to prevent the induction of P-gp by specific timing of chemotherapeutic agent exposure.

Resistance to Alkylating Agents

Glutathione (GSH) has been associated with drug resistance to alkylating agents and cisplatin.[36] Cell lines that are resistant to cisplatin and alkylating agents have increased GSH levels compared with sensitive parental cell lines. In addition, these cell lines are often cross-resistant to irradiation. GSH is a nonprotein thiol that appears to play a role in numerous cell processes, including metabolism, transport, and drug detoxification. Increased levels may thus assist in the detoxification of these cytotoxic agents as a result of GSH-linked transferases. Repair of DNA cross-links may be enhanced by GSH. In vitro studies have shown that GSH levels can be lowered with buthionine sulfoximine, an amino acid that inhibits an enzyme necessary for GSH synthesis. Preclinical studies have shown increased survival rates in mice treated with buthionine sulfoximine plus melphalan as compared with mice treated with melphalan alone. Phase I clinical trials are ongoing.

Ability to repair the damage induced by alkylating agents reduces the vulnerability of the target cell. Damage at the O^6 position of guanine in the DNA may be removed by O^6 methylguanine transferase.[37] Repair inhibitors for potential clinical use have not yet been identified, although this strategy is an attractive theoretic approach to enhancing chemotherapy.

Resistance to Antimetabolites

Antimetabolites are agents commonly used in the treatment of pediatric malignancies. Numerous mechanisms of resistance have been described for each of the antimetabolites. Causes of methotrexate resistance are discussed for illustrative purposes.[38]

Dihydrofolate reductase (DHFR) is the target enzyme for methotrexate. Binding of methotrexate to DHFR inhibits tetrahydrofolate formation, required for purine and thymidylate synthesis. Resistant cell lines (and cells from methotrexate-resistant individuals) have increased DHFR activity as a result of gene amplification. Decreased affinity of DHFR for methotrexate is another cause of methotrexate resistance. In either instance, sufficient DHFR activity may be present to abrogate the effects of methotrexate.

Methotrexate is a prodrug that must be polyglutamated on entry into the cell for effective cytotoxicity. Polyglutamation occurs when the free intracellular drug is present in excess of enzyme binding sites. Polyglutamated methotrexate is most effective in inhibiting protein synthesis. As a result of increased intracellular retention of polyglutamated methotrexate, cytotoxicity occurs even after extracellular methotrexate levels have fallen.

All of these causes of methotrexate resistance can be overcome to variable degrees by the use of high-dose methotrexate. High-dose methotrexate has also been used to circumvent abnormal transport mechanisms by relying on passive diffusion. New analogues of methotrexate, such as trimetrexate, may overcome resistance in part by the use of alternate transport mechanisms.

LATE EFFECTS OF CANCER THERAPY

Cytotoxic agents used for the treatment of malignancy are chosen on the basis of the differential sensitivity of tumor cells compared with normal tissue. Nonetheless, normal tissues are affected by these agents. With the cell cycle–specific chemotherapeutic agents, growing tissues are most severely affected. Thus, hair and gastrointestinal mucosa are affected at least as much as the tumor tissue, while the slower-growing tissues are relatively protected. Alkylating agents and DNA intercalating agents can affect the DNA of all body cells. The potential for long-term evidence of tissue injury is increased with these agents. Radiotherapy affects only those body organs that are within the radiation beam but may show even less differential sensitivity between normal and abnormal organs. Combined-modality therapy can result in additive or even synergistic effects, thus enhancing the spectrum of damage.[39]

Although many effects of therapy become apparent while the patient is on chemotherapy or shortly thereafter, other effects become apparent only many years later. Cellular injury that occurs may not become manifest until the tissue in question attempts to grow or divide. For children, this is a profound effect, resulting in significant late effects of cancer therapy.

The types of changes that can be seen are affected by the sensitivity of individual organs to the cytotoxic therapy, the pattern of growth of the individual organs during childhood,[40] and the age of the child who is being evaluated. Organs such as the brain grow rapidly during infancy and preschool years, with slower growth during the rest of childhood and cessation of growth in the teenage years. In contrast, the musculoskeletal system shows two periods of rapid growth: in infancy and again during adolescence. Effects on growth, therefore, are most apparent during these rapid growth spurts. In contrast, the gonads and breasts are not expected to show evidence of development until the teenage years. Thus, gonadal impairment does not become manifest in a prepubertal child.

Understanding the late effects of cytotoxic therapy in a child requires a systematic approach to the evaluation. Cumulative doses of cytotoxic agents and radiotherapy must be calculated, and individual organs must be considered in terms of their likelihood of being affected by the agents used, their sensitivity at the time of treatment, and their likelihood of expressing any effects when the child is first seen.

Central Nervous System

The CNS is affected by both radiotherapy and chemotherapy. Children with brain tumors and ALL who receive cranial irradiation are at highest risk. Because the greatest amount of CNS growth occurs during early infancy, children treated at an early age are most likely to suffer the intellectual consequences. Although cranial irradiation has the most profound effect, chemotherapeutic agents that cross the blood–brain barrier, such as high-dose methotrexate and high-dose cytosine arabinoside, or those that are directly instilled as in intrathecal chemotherapy can exacerbate this problem. Instances of CNS damage have been related to high-dose methotrexate alone. The extreme form of CNS damage is progressive leukoencephalopathy, characterized by dementia, seizures, dysrhythmia, dysphagia, spasticity, ataxia, and coma.[41] More commonly, subtle neurocognitive findings affect school performance and may or may not be associated with computed tomography or magnetic resonance imaging findings, including calcifications, ventricular dilation, and white-matter changes.

Children who are known to be at risk should have neurocognitive testing performed early in the course of their disease and at regular intervals thereafter. Preschool children should be followed closely for acquisition of skills, particularly speech and language development. At the time of school entry, close observation is necessary. Appropriate interventions should be instituted as soon as any evidence of deficits appears. Acquisition of reading skills, mathematic skills, and new languages may be particularly problematic. These children may require more than the usual time to perform daily assignments and to complete tasks in school, particularly tests.

Linear Growth

Children who have undergone irradiation to the hypothalamic–pituitary axis can suffer from abnormalities of growth hormone release or, with higher doses of irradiation, diminished growth hormone synthesis.[42] Often, the growth velocity of these children is in the low-normal range until puberty, when the growth spurt appears substantially impaired. Precocious puberty occurs more commonly after cranial irradiation in early childhood, decreasing the overall interval of growth. To encourage optimal growth potential, some endocrinologists administer growth hormone simultaneously with agents that delay puberty.

Spinal irradiation can compound the effect on ultimate height by the effect on bone growth.

Musculoskeletal Growth

Musculoskeletal hypoplasia is a common late effect in children who have been treated with radiotherapy. *Hypoplasia* refers to the diminished development of bone and soft tissue, including fat, in the area of the radiation field. This is a dose-dependent phenomenon that occurs in virtually all irradiated patients especially if the radiation fields are asymmetric. Asymmetry of radiation fields involving the spine can also result in scoliosis. Although this is often a cosmetic issue, it can affect the psychosocial development of the child.

Gonadal Effects

Children with malignancies are surviving well into the adult period of life. Because most of these patients live in the mainstream of adult society, their goals often include marriage and family. Most long-term survivors of childhood cancer are able to reproduce normal, healthy children. Direct gonadal radiotherapy and specific chemotherapeutic agents, however, particularly the alkylating agents, can affect ovarian and testicular function.

The ovaries are more resistant than the testes to both chemotherapy and radiotherapy. A finite number of ova diminish over the years; gonadotoxic agents hasten the decline. Older women with fewer ova are likely to become amenorrheic from as little as 4 g of cyclophosphamide (Cytoxan) or 400 cGy of radiotherapy; women less than 20 years of age can tolerate more than 20 g/m^2 of cyclophosphamide without cessation of menses.[43] Early menopause remains possible. Women with gonadal injury usually have elevations of luteinizing hormone and follicle-stimulating hormone in addition to inadequate plasma estradiol levels. Attention should be paid to the need for estrogen for pubertal development in young girls and for feminization, bone mineralization, and prevention of coronary artery disease in adult women.

The spermatogonia are more sensitive to the effects of both chemotherapy and radiotherapy than are the Leydig cells. After 10 mg/m^2 of cyclophosphamide or 300 cGy of testicular radiotherapy, a man is likely to be sterile but should have adequate testosterone production to facilitate normal sexual function. Serum FSH is usually elevated, but semen analysis provides the best assessment of ability to father children. Recovery can occur more than a decade after radiotherapy. After more than 12 Gy, Leydig cell damage also occurs. Testosterone supplementation may then be needed both for pubertal development in the prepubertal boy and for continued masculinization and libido in the adult.

Patients who have had significant hypothalamic–pituitary axis irradiation can also suffer from infertility; the gonads are normal but not stimulated by gonadotropic hormones. In these cases, luteinizing hormone and follicle-stimulating hormone levels are low.

Cardiac Effects

The anthracyclines are notorious for their acute and late effects on the myocardium. Early congestive heart failure can occur as the cumulative dose of anthracyclines increases. Many patients show a decrease in their cardiac contractility within 6 months of terminating therapy that later improves. Initially, this was thought to be a good omen, suggesting repair of cardiac injury. We now know that some of these patients, as well as some who appeared well at the end of therapy, experienced late deterioration, manifested by congestive heart failure or dysrhythmia.[44] Steinherz and coworkers[44] described the first cohort of such patients; 14 of 270 presented with overt cardiac symptomatology, 8 of whom died as a result of congestive heart failure or dysrhythmia. Subsequent study of long-term survivors has shown that evidence of myocardial damage can be elicited in virtually all patients treated with anthracyclines. Overt myocardial dysfunction is less common, but the frequency increases with time. Certain initiating factors can result in late decompensation. Weightlifting (which causes increased afterload), pregnancy, and periods of rapid growth (as noted in patients treated with growth hormones) have been reported as initiating factors. The magnitude of this problem has become apparent, and prospective strategies are being devised to prevent cardiac injury. These include the administration of anthracyclines by continuous infusion or concurrently with cardioprotective agents. Afterload reduction is being investigated to prevent progression in patients with early evidence of myocardial damage.

Radiotherapy also has an impact on the myocardium. Soon after direct cardiac radiotherapy, pericardial effusions occur. Valvular damage and pericardial thickening are usually noted later. Penicillin prophylaxis to prevent bacterial endocarditis after operative procedures may then be important. Studies have shown an increased risk of ischemic heart disease after mediastinal irradiation.[45,46] These effects may not become apparent in treated children until several decades after therapy.

Other Organs

The earlier sections included only some of the known risks to long-term cancer survivors. Skin cancer in the radiation field, pulmonary fibrosis after nitrosourea and bleomycin, and hypothyroidism after thyroid irradiation are other notable examples. Interventions, such as the minimalization of oxygen delivered intraoperatively in bleomycin-treated patients or the institution of thyroid hormone replacement with thyroid-stimulating hormone elevation after thyroid irradiation, may prevent the emergence of clinical symptomatology. Long-term survivors of childhood cancer have a 10- to 20-fold increased risk of a second malignancy.[47]

Offspring of patients who are fertile appear to be normal.[48] Although congenital abnormalities have been seen, the frequency does not appear to be greater than in the normal population. Except for those patients for whom there is a genetic predisposition for cancer (eg, von Recklinghausen disease, hereditary retinoblastoma, Wilms tumor), there does not appear to be an excess risk of cancer in offspring.[49,50]

Long-term effects may become apparent in future decades. As long as new agents are being used, or the use of older drugs is redesigned, it will be necessary to continue to care for cancer survivors for years to come.

REFERENCES

1. Ries LA, Hankey BF, Miller BA, et al, eds. Cancer statistics review 1973–88. NIH Publication No. 91-278. Bethesda, NIH, 1991.
2. D'Angio GJ. Oncology seen through the prism of Wilms tumor. Med Pediatr Oncol 1985;13:53.
3. Israel MA. Cancer cell biology. In: Pizzo PA, Poplack DG, eds. Principles and practice of pediatric oncology. Philadelphia, JB Lippincott, 1993:57.
4. Matsushime H, Roussel MF, Ashmun RA, et al. Colony-stimulating factor 1 regulates novel cyclins during the G1 phase of the cell cycle. Cell 1991;65:701.
5. Booker R, Beach D. Interaction between cdc13 + and cdc2 + in the mitosis in fission yeast, dissociation of the G_1 and G_2 roles of the cdc2 + protein kinase. EMBO J 1987;6:344.
6. Skipper HE. Historic milestones in cancer biology: a few that are important to cancer treatment (revisited). Semin Oncol 1979;6:506.
7. Mendelsohn ML. The growth fraction: a new concept applied to tumors. Science 1960;132:1496.
8. Freese A, O'Rourke D, Judy K, et al. The application of 5-bromodeoxyuridine in the management of CNS tumors. J Neurooncol 1994;20:81.
9. Iverson U, Iverson OH, Ziegler JL, et al. Cell kinetics of African cases of Burkitts lymphoma: a preliminary report. Eur J Cancer 1972;8:305.
10. Yarbro JW. The scientific basis of cancer chemotherapy. In: Perry MC, ed. The chemotherapy source book. Baltimore, Williams & Wilkins, 1992:2.
11. Feinstein E, Cimino G, Gale RP, et al. p53 In CML in acute phase. Proc Nat Acad Sci USA 1991;88:6293.
12. Sidransky D, Mikkelsen T, Schwechheimer K, et al. Clonal expansion of p53 mutant cells is associated with brain tumor progression. Nature 1992;335:846-7.
13. Allegra CJ. Antifolates. In: Chabner BA, Collins JM, eds. Cancer chemotherapy principles and practice. Philadelphia, JB Lippincott, 1990:110.
14. Korsmeyer SJ, Hieter PA, Ravetch JV. Developmental hierarchy of immunoglobulin gene rearrangements in human leukemic pre–B cells. Proc Acad Sci USA 1981;78:7096.
15. Chomienne C, Balitrand N, Ballerini P, et al. All-trans retinoic acid modulates the retinoic acid receptor-alpha in promyelocytic cells. J Clin Invest 1991;88:2150.
16. Fernaux P, Castaigne S, Dombret H, et al. All-trans-retinoic acid followed by intensive chemotherapy gives a high complete remission rate and may prolong remissions in newly diagnosed acute promyelocytic leukemia: a pilot study on 26 cases. Blood 1992;80:2176.
17. Barsky SH, Rao CN, Williams JE, et al. Laminin molecular domains which alter metastases in a murine model. J Clin Invest 1984;74:549.
18. Alvarez OA, Carmichael DF, DeClerck YA. Inhibition of collagenolytic activity and metastasis of tumor cells by a recombinant human tissue inhibitor of metalloproteinases. JNCI 1990;82:589.
19. Folkman J, Ingber D. Inhibition of angiogenesis. (Review) Semin Cancer Biol 1992;3:89.
20. Goldie JH. Drug resistance. In: Perry MC, ed. The Chemotherapy source book. Baltimore, Williams & Wilkins, 1992:54.
21. Balis FM, Holcenberg JS, Poplack DG. General principles of chemotherapy. In: Pizzo PA, Poplack DG, eds. Principles and practice of pediatric oncology. Philadelphia, JB Lippincott, 1993:197.
22. Sallan SE, Gelber D, Kimbal V, et al. More is better! Update of Dana Farber Cancer Institute/Children's Hospital childhood acute lymphoblastic leukemia trials. Haematol Blood Transfus 1990;33:459.
23. Gaynon P, Steinherz P, Bleyer WA, et al. Association of delivered drug dose and outcome for children with acute lymphoblastic leukemia and unfavorable presenting features. Med Pediatr Oncol 1991;19:221.
24. Prasad R, Bucco G, Campunacci M, et al. Does drug dose intensity of chemotherapy determine the prognosis of primary high-grade osteosarcoma? (Abstract) Proc Am Soc Clin Oncol 1990;9:311.
25. Cheung NV. Immunotherapy. In: Pizzo PA, Poplack DG, eds. Principles and practice of pediatric oncology. Philadelphia, JB Lippincott, 1993:357.
26. Eisinberger MA, Reyno LM, Jodrell DI, et al. Suramin, an active drug for prostate cancer: interim observations in a phase I trial. J Natl Cancer Inst 1993;86:611.
27. Biedler JL, Riehm H. Cellular resistance to actinomycin D in Chinese hamster cells in vitro: cross resistance radioautographic and cytogenetic studies. Cancer Res 1970;30:1174.
28. Juliano RL, Ling V. A surface glycoprotein modulating drug permeability in Chinese hamster ovary cell mutants. Biochem Biophys Acta 1976;455:152.
29. Pastan I, Gottesman M. Multiple drug resistance in human cancer. N Engl J Med 1987;316:1388.
30. Chan HSL, Thorner PS, Haddad G, et al. Immunohistochemical detec-

tion of P-glycoprotein: prognostic correlation in soft tissue sarcoma of childhood. J Clin Oncol 1990;8:689.

31. Chan HSL, Haddad G, Thorner PS, et al. P-glycoprotein expression as a predictor of the outcome of therapy for neuroblastoma. N Engl J Med 1991;325:1608.

32. Salmon SE, Grogan TM, Miller T, et al. Prediction of doxorubicin resistance in vitro in myeloma, lymphoma, and breast cancer by P-glycoprotein staining. J Natl Cancer Inst 1986;81:696.

33. Holmes J, Jacobs A, Carter G, et al. Multidrug resistance in hematopoietic cell lines, myelodysplastic syndromes and acute myeloblastic leukaemia. Br J Haematol 1989;72:40.

34. Schwartz CL, Rosier R, Willis J, et al. P-glycoprotein (P-GP) expression in osteosarcoma (O.S.) and clinical outcome. Proc ASCO 1992;11:285.

35. Rader M, Scheithauer W. Clinical trials of agents that reverse multidrug resistance. Cancer 1993;72:3553.

36. Hamilton TC, Ozols RF, Dabrow MB. Multidrug resistance to alkylating agents and platinum compounds: state of our knowledge. Oncology 1990;4:101.

37. Yarosh DB, Footer S, Mitra S, et al. Repair of O^6-methylguanine in DNA by demethylation is lacking in MER minus human tumor cell stains. Carcinogenesis 1983;4:199.

38. Bertino JR. Karnofsky memorial lecture: ode to methotrexate. (Review) J Clin Oncol 1993;11:5.

39. D'Angio G, ed. Delayed consequences of cancer therapy: proven and potential. Cancer 1976;37:979.

40. Tanner JM. Physical growth and development. In: Forfar JO, Arniel AC, eds. Textbook of pediatrics. Edinburgh, Churchill Livingstone, 1978:249.

41. Price RA, Jamieson PA. The central nervous system in childhood leukemia. II. Leukoencephalopathy. Cancer 1975;35:306.

42. Sklar CA. Neuroendocrine complication of cancer therapy. In: Schwartz CL, Hobbie WL, Constine LS, et al, eds. Survivors of childhood cancer. St Louis, Mosby–Year Book, 1994.

43. Koyama H, Wada T, Nishizawa Y, et al. Cyclophosphamide-induced ovarian failure and its therapeutic significance in patients with breast cancer. Cancer 1977;39:1403.

44. Steinherz LJ, Steinherz PG, Tan CT, et al. Cardiac toxicity 4–20 years after completing anthracycline therapy. JAMA 1991;266:1672.

45. Hancock SL, Tucker MA, Hoppe RT. Factors affecting late mortality from heart disease after treatment of Hodgkin's disease. JAMA 1993;270:1949.

46. Boivan JF, Hutchison GB, Lubin JH, et al. Coronary artery disease mortality in patients treated for Hodgkin's disease. Cancer 1992;69:1241.

47. Mike V, Meadows AT, D'Angio GL. Incidence of second malignant neoplasm in children: results of an internation study. Lancet 1982;2:1326.

48. Blatt J, Mulvihill JJ, Ziegler JL, et al. Pregnancy outcome following cancer chemotherapy. Am J Med 1980;69:828.

49. Li FP, Fine W, Jaffe N, et al. Offspring of patients treated for cancer in childhood. J Natl Cancer Inst 1979;62:1193.

50. Mulvihill JJ, Myers MH, Connelly RR, et al. Cancer in offspring of long-term survivors of childhood and adolescent cancer. Lancet 1987;2:813.

Surgery of Infants and Children: Scientific Principles and Practice, edited by Keith T. Oldham, Paul M. Colombani, and Robert P. Foglia. Lippincott–Raven Publishers, Philadelphia, © 1997.

CHAPTER 31

Oncogenesis

Ilan R. Kirsch

Cancer is a genetic disease. In every tumor that has been studied in detail, it has been determined that the DNA of the tumor is not the same as the DNA of the nonmalignant cells from which the tumor arose. Tumor cell DNA has undergone one or more point mutations, deletions, insertions, amplifications, or translocations that alter, eliminate, or dysregulate one or more genes involved in the growth or the development of the transformed cell.

For more than a century, physicians and scientists had searched for tumor-specific markers that could distinguish a tumor cell from normal tissue. A number of studies revealed that tumors often share antigens or surface markers reminiscent of fetal development. Some of these developmental or differentiating markers are in fact being used for diagnosis and, rarely, treatment of cancer. In general, however, the search for tumor-specific markers was marked by futility and frustration until the era of recombinant DNA research made possible the molecular, nucleotide-by-nucleotide analysis of tumor cell DNA and the realization that the DNA alterations just described did indeed distinguish cancers from noncancers.

TUMOR-SPECIFIC DNA CHANGES AND THEIR CONSEQUENCES

A small number of consequences of gene alteration are relevant to malignant transformation (Fig. 31-1):

1. The alteration can lead to inappropriate expression of the gene and translation of its product. This is often the result of chromosomal translocation in which the normal regulatory sequence of a gene is left behind during the translocation process and the regulatory control of another locus in the genome is substituted. Viral insertion in proximity to a gene can also alter its regulation, substituting viral promoters or enhancers of transcription for the gene's own.
2. The regulatory process of the gene can remain normal, but the quantity of the gene can be altered by increasing or decreasing its copy number. The gain or loss of the amount of gene product can alter the dynamic equilibrium of interaction of the product with other cellular components. Gene

amplification or deletion leads to this quantitative change. Altering the half-life of an mRNA or protein (by direct mutation of the gene sequence) accomplishes this quantitative change as well.
3. The function of the gene can itself be altered. Point mutations within the coding sequence of the gene can change its catalytic activity or make it less interactive with other proteins that normally act to regulate its function. Chromosomal translocations can change gene function as well by removing entire functional domains from a gene and substituting domains from other loci, such as to create hybrid proteins with novel activities.

These tumor-specific DNA changes are tangible and identifiable (some examples are listed in Table 31-1) and form the basis for emerging strategies for early detection, diagnostic stratification, staging, and even treatment programs for patients with cancer. Cancer need not have been a disease marked by genetic change. For example, it could have been a set-point disease, in which, in certain cells, the levels of various growth-promoting and growth-suppressing functions, while each by itself within a normal range, would combine to provide a particular growth advantage to a particular cell and its subsequent generations. So far, this has not been found to be the case. Our understanding of cancer focuses our attention on two fundamental aspects of biology: genetic instability and cellular proliferation. These two topics form the two broad and intersecting themes of this chapter and the contexts in which the parlance and entities of cancer biology are introduced and discussed.

GENETIC INSTABILITY

Were it not for the inherent instability of DNA, evolution would not have occurred as rapidly, and the normal developmental processes from bacteriophage to humans would be impossible. The processes of DNA replication and cell division are imperfect and error prone and generate novel DNA sequences and gross genomic rearrangements that speed mutagenesis and provide myriad substrates for selection. Bacteriophage integration and excision from a bacterial chromosome, yeast-

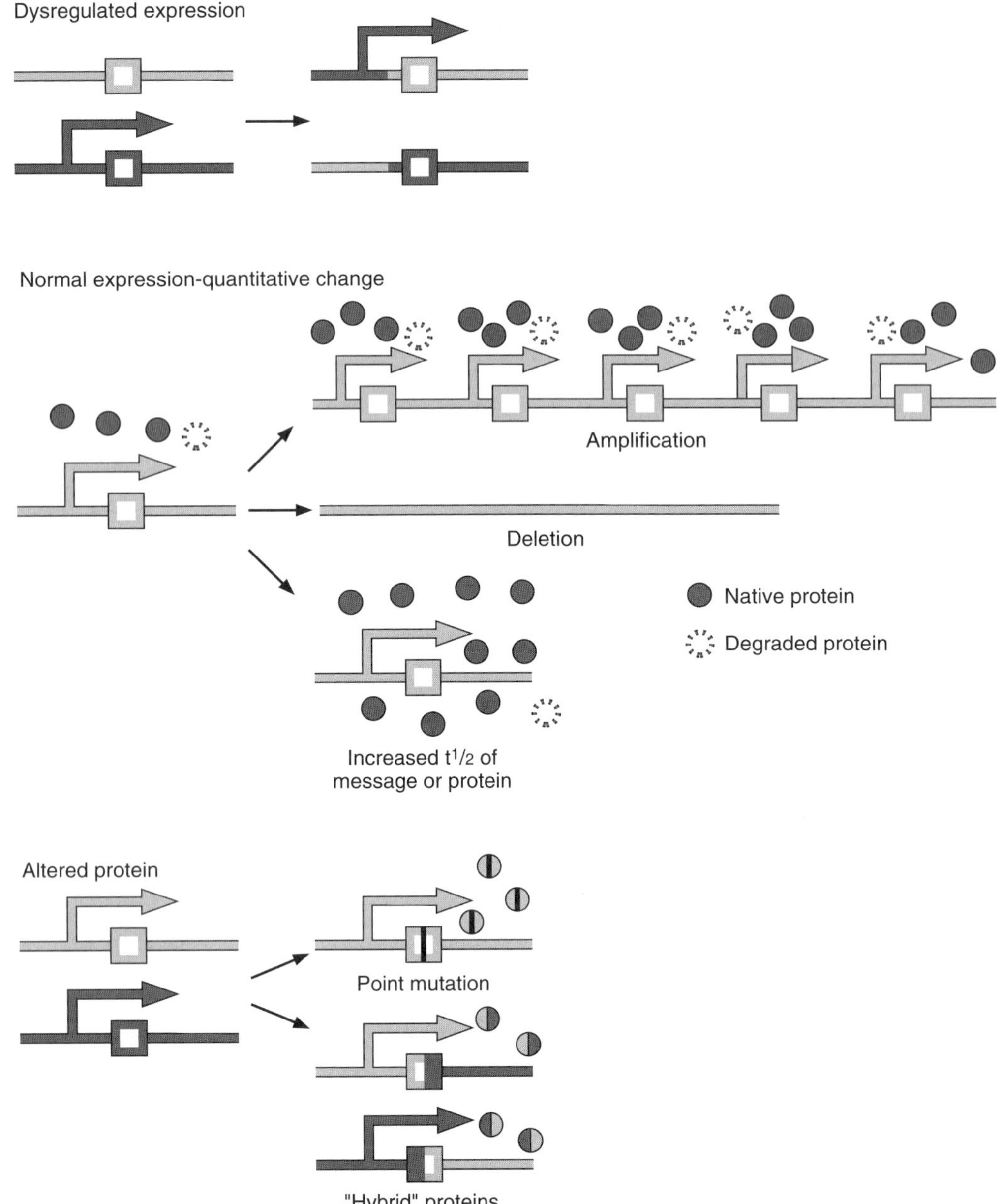

FIG. 31-1. Mechanisms of gene alteration. (*A*) Dysregulated expression. In this example, a chromosomal translocation has replaced the transcriptional regulatory region of one gene (denoted by a box) with that of another. Because of this, a gene formerly quiescent in this cell lineage is now transcribed (indicated by an arrow arising from in front of the gene). (*B*) Normal expression—quantitative change. The product of a gene is altered by amplifying or deleting the gene itself, or by increasing (or decreasing, in an example not shown) the half-life of the gene product. (*C*) Altered protein. The gene product is different from its "wild type" because of a point mutation within the coding sequence of the gene or formation of a "hybrid" protein secondary to chromosomal translocation.

mating–type switching, and the human immune response are each an example of an enzyme-mediated process of DNA reconfiguration that is essential to the normal development and life cycles of these organisms. This normal and inherent instability, however, is also the foundation of carcinogenesis. The programs that have been developed in humans to safeguard the integrity of the genome of individual cells are precisely the targets of alteration or circumvention in randomly occurring malignancies or in cancers induced by carcinogenic exposure. In considering the role of genetic instability in carcinogenesis, a somewhat artificial division can be made between the type of instability that is inherent to every cell in the organism or every cell of a particular cell lineage and that *predisposes* to the development of cancer, versus the type of instability that occurs only in a malignant or premalignant cell and is thus *tumor-specific* and critical to cancer progression or virulence.

TABLE 31-1. *Some examples of possible cancer-contributory gene alterations*

Mechanism	Gene	Malignancy
Dysregulated expression	MYC	Burkitt lymphoma
	SCL	T-cell acute lymphocytic leukemia
	BCL2	Follicular lymphoma
	IGFII	Wilms tumor
Gene amplification	N-MYC	Neuroblastoma
	L-MYC	Lung cancer
Gene deletion	RB	Retinoblastoma
	p53	Many malignancies
Alteration of half-life	p53	Many malignancies
Alteration of protein	p53	Many malignancies
	EWS	Ewing sarcomas
	RAS	Many malignancies

Predisposing Genetic Instability

Risk of developing a mutation that contributes to malignant transformation is a function of a person's inherent genetic instability absent any destabilizing influence and inherent (and in some cases related) ability to prevent, address, and correct damage from carcinogenic exposures. The sorts of cellular functions that contribute to the baseline level of inherent genetic instability include organization of the cellular nucleus; packing of nucleosomes; structural DNA-binding proteins and chromatin structure; DNA breakage, rejoining, and repair enzymes; topoisomerases; DNA polymerases; DNA methylases and methylation recognition enzymes; and others. The sorts of cellular functions that contribute to the inherent ability to address and correct damage from carcinogenic exposures include, again, the DNA breakage, rejoining, and repair enzymes and mismatch recognition and other specific DNA damage–recognizing enzymes (eg, alkyltransferases), detoxifying enzymes, and others.

Syndromes of Genetic Instability

A number of recognized syndromes with onset in childhood are characterized by genetic instability as manifested by relative sensitivity to x-ray or ultraviolet irradiation or certain chemical agents, distinctive chromosomal aberrations seen in karyotypic studies, and predisposition to the development of certain types of cancer. In a later section of this chapter, a second class of cancer-prone syndromes is discussed. The four syndromes highlighted here manifest recognizable genetic instability and are clearly autosomal recessive in inheritance, with the full-blown syndrome being present only in the homozygote. The expression of a demonstrable phenotype and the risk of cancer to the heterozygote carriers for this first group are controversial.

Examples of such instability syndromes are ataxia telangiectasia,[1] Bloom syndrome,[2] Fanconi anemia,[3] and xeroderma pigmentosum.[4] People with ataxia telangiectasia are characterized by progressive cerebellar degeneration, oculocutaneous telangiectasia, radiosensitivity, immunodeficiency, premature aging, a disproportionate increase in lymphoid malignancies, and an increase in the overall frequency of malignancies that are prevalent in the communities or environments in which the patients live. There is an increased frequency of cell-lineage–specific

and nonspecific chromosomal aberrations.[5–9] The genetic defect in these people is still unknown, but the defective gene that governs this disease resides on chromosome 11 band q23[10] and has recently been cloned and characterized.[10a] Patients with Bloom syndrome are characterized by short stature and sun sensitivity. Patients with this syndrome appear to manifest increased sister chromatid exchange. They appear to be at particular risk for the development of acute myelogenous leukemia. The genetic defect in patients with Bloom syndrome may be related to a problem in religation of DNA breaks—perhaps, in particular, those occurring during DNA replication.[11,12] The cloned gene product, BLM, is related to DNA helicases.[12a] Patients with Fanconi anemia manifest skin hyperpigmentation, anatomic defects, problems with growth and development of multiple organ systems, and childhood onset of pancytopenia. Chromosomal analysis reveals numerous aberrations, including fragments, breaks, gaps, rings, and endoreduplications, but not increased sister chromatid exchange.[13,14] These patients are at particular risk for the development of acute myelogenous leukemia, often heralded by a clonal cytogenetic outgrowth.[15] Patients suffering from xeroderma pigmentosum (X-P) have a marked increased incidence of skin cancer in sun-exposed areas. Although the disease is genetically complex, the defects appear to center on a defective mechanism of recognition, excision, and repair of damaged or altered nucleotides. There also seems to be a relation between at least some of the genes whose mutation can cause a xeroderma pigmentosum–like syndrome and the components of the complex of proteins that mediate transcription of DNA into RNA.[16,17] As in the condition of ataxia telangiectasia, the complete phenotype of patients with xeroderma pigmentosum include a variety of neurologic problems whose relation to the sensitivity to irradiation is unclear. Thus, all four of these syndromes are examples of genetic lesions that increase the fundamental propensity of DNA to change or be altered.

Inherent and Acquired Genetic Instability

The four syndromes described earlier are recognized examples of increased genetic instability. Variations on the themes manifested in these syndromes are likely to occur, however, as more subtle manifestations of genetic instability among a normal population. To the ever-present question of a newly diagnosed cancer patient, ''why me?,'' an array of possible answers is beginning to take shape. Randomness and bad luck always play some role. In addition, however, is the comparative innate instability of a person's genome and the comparative ability of that genome to maintain its integrity. If the syndromes described earlier are examples of complete loss of a repair or integrity-monitoring function, the simple presence of the function does not guarantee genomic stability. There can be differences in levels of function even among ''normal'' people—differences in catalytic properties, regulatory capabilities, and so forth. In some cases, these people are ''marked'' by their family histories. For example, some studies have suggested that heterozygotes with ataxia telangiectasia are at increased risk for the development of certain solid tumors.[18] In some cases, the level of destabilizing exposure is so intense that it clearly overwhelms the physiologic safeguards of the genome. Patients whose malignancies can be traced back to atomic bomb exposure[19] or other nuclear accidents are suggestive in this regard. For most cancer patients, however, no clear inherited or acquired influence is obvious. Yet, at some point in time, by definition, a particular cell's inherent instability, combined with an external destabilizing stimulus, results in a mutation or mutations that contribute to malignant transformation. Conversely, genetic predisposition to mutation does not necessarily mean that a person is destined to develop cancer. Only in the presence of the carcinogenic, mutating, or destabilizing influence is a cancer initiated.

GENES INVOLVED IN GROWTH, DEVELOPMENT, AND PROLIFERATION

What are the targets of genetic instability whose mutation or alteration becomes a step toward malignant transformation? This question leads directly to a consideration of the cellular pathway for growth and development. From this consideration emerges an ever-increasing array of genes that have been implicated in one or another type of cancer. The list becomes overwhelming, incomplete, and out-of-date as soon as it is published. The goal of this chapter is not to name every possible growth-affecting gene whose disruption can contribute to malignant transformation. Rather, a framework for viewing the types of genes that affect growth is described. Certain genes are named as examples of a type or class of growth-affecting gene that has been implicated in cancer or whose mechanism of action is instructive or exemplary in terms of understanding a basic principle of carcinogenesis (see Table 31-2 for a list of the genes mentioned in this chapter). Many terms that have achieved common usage in the literature turn out to be more obscuring than revealing. As we become more sophisticated in our understanding of carcinogenesis, certain previously accepted simplistic gene categorizations become problematic. It is important to be familiar with some of the oncologic terminology, while at the same time understanding that much of the terminology, although relatively recent, is already outdated.

Oncogenes, Tumor-Suppressor Genes, Mutator Genes, Death Genes, and Cellular Clocks

Oncogenes

An early view of carcinogenesis was based on an infectious disease model. Cancer was something that was done to a cell by something outside of itself. As cancer-causing viruses were identified for numerous species, this model gained strength.[20] A variety of viruses have been implicated in carcinogenesis, including viruses whose primary genetic material consists of DNA (eg, adenoviruses, papovaviruses, papillomaviruses, hepatitis B virus, and herpesviruses) or RNA (eg, retroviruses). Retroviruses have a distinct stage in their life cycles at which time their genetic material is reverse-transcribed from RNA into a DNA copy and integrated into the host genome. At least two types of cancer-causing retroviruses became apparent, distinguished by the length of time between infection and cancer (Fig. 31-2). Many transmissible retroviruses had a long latent period, and infection was not equivalent to transformation in each infected organism. A second class of viruses had a short

TABLE 31-2. *Genes mentioned in this chapter**

ONCOGENES

SIS
MYC
SRC
RAS
RAF
JUN
FOS
ERBB
ERBB2
FMS
ROS
ERBA
SRC
INT2

TUMOR SUPPRESSORS

p53
RB
APC
DCC

MUTATOR GENES

MSH2
MLH1
PMS1
PMS2

DEATH-AFFECTING GENES

BCL2

CELLULAR CLOCKS

Telomerase (enzyme)

TRANSCRIPTION FACTORS

SCL (TAL1)
LYL1
TAL2
TTG1
TTG2

GROWTH FACTORS

Platelet-derived growth factor
Colony-stimulating factor-1
Epidermal growth factor (EGF)
Transforming growth factor-α
Transforming growth factor-β
Insulin-like growth factor-1
Insulin-like growth factor-2
Fibroblast growth factors

GROWTH FACTOR RECEPTORS

EGF receptor
Thyroid hormone receptor
Steroid hormone receptor

GENES MUTATED IN CANCER SYNDROMES

Neurofibromin
Schwannomin

* Genes are placed in certain categories as a means of convenient inclusion, not exclusion. For example, a gene listed as an oncogene might just as easily have been listed as a growth factor, or receptor, or transducing factor, or transcription factor, depending on its particular function.

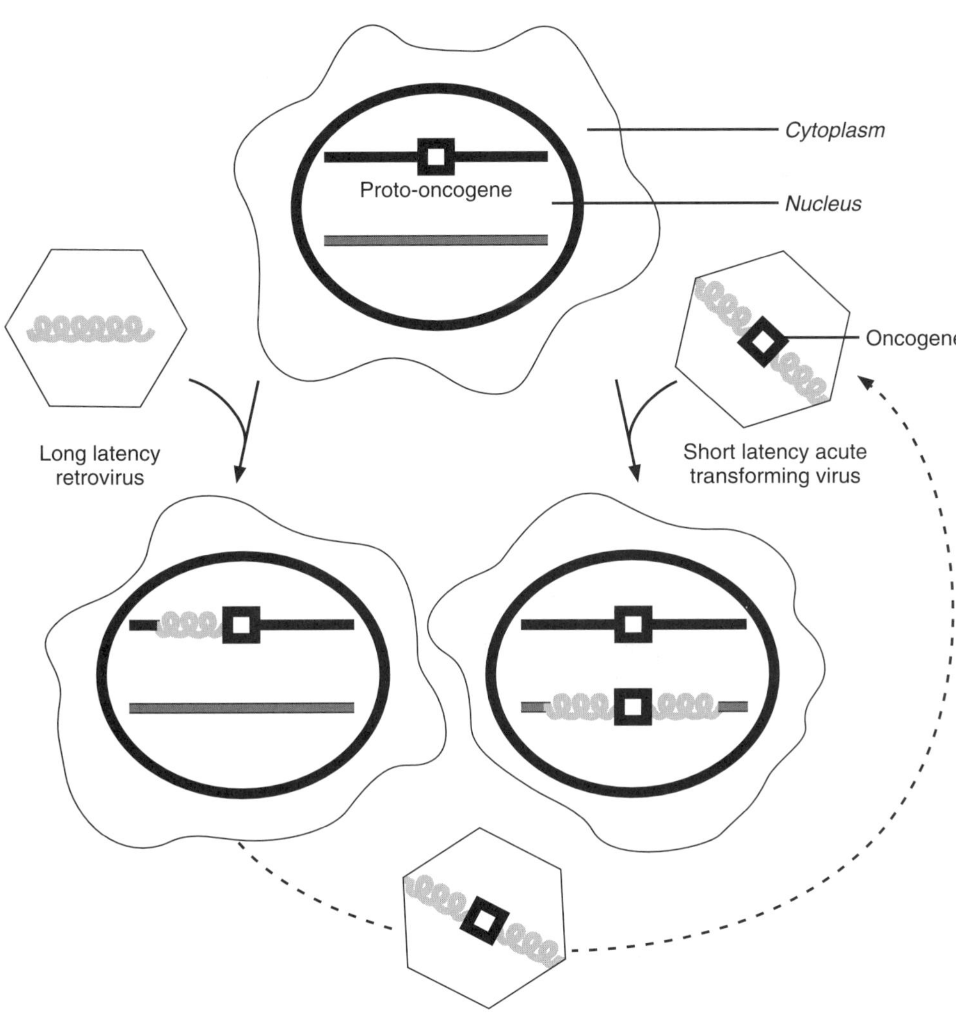

FIG. 31-2. Oncogenes, protooncogenes, and retroviruses. The relation between these elements (and terms) is illustrated. A retrovirus infects cell after cell. It does not cause a cancer until it is integrated next to a growth-affecting gene (protooncogene), causing dysregulated expression of that gene. Rarely, the virus incorporates the growth-affecting gene into its own genome, and in so doing, it carries an acute transforming function (oncogene), which can contribute to cellular transformation at the next cycle of infection.

latency and were much more likely to cause cancer in susceptible organisms. Within the short latency, acute transforming virus, studies were undertaken to identify the acute transforming principle of the viral genome. A variety of cancer-causing oncogenes were thereby identified.[21] In the 1970s, it became apparent that these oncogenes, carried by acute transforming viruses, had normal cellular homologues called *protooncogenes* resident in the genome, where presumably they served a physiologic role in cellular growth and development.[22,23] Some of these genes were further implicated in carcinogenesis with the realization that the onset of cancer in long-latency infection occurred subsequent to sequential rounds of infection and consequent to eventual genomic integration by the DNA copy of the virus next to (and dysregulation, by this mechanism, of) one or another of these protooncogenes (see Fig. 31-2). The names of these genes were originally devised based on the virus in which they were originally identified; for example, *SIS* from *si*mian *s*arcoma virus, *MYC* from avian *my*elocytomatosis, *SRC* from Rous *sarc*oma virus, and so on.

This was the derivation and classic definition of an oncogene: a gene carried by an acute transforming retrovirus that had a normal cellular homologue. The term *oncogene*, as used today, is much less informative and precise, often being applied to any gene that is implicated in growth promotion and carcinogenesis.

This is much less useful conceptually and practically. Cancer is a disease of growth and development. Any gene that functions in a growth pathway, either promoting, regulating, or inhibiting growth, is a potential target for a cancer-inducing event. Thus, understanding the normal functions of these genes and where they fit into a growth-controlling pathway is the key, and grouping them together as oncogenes is less meaningful.

Tumor-Suppressor Genes

Classically, as oncogenes or protooncogenes were viewed as growth-promoting, tumor-suppressor genes were viewed as growth restraining. This view has also been modified with time, but it is worthwhile reviewing the development of the concept of tumor suppression as a way of continuing to build a framework for understanding carcinogenesis.[24–27] In experimental systems in which normal cells are fused with certain tumor cell lines, it is possible to suppress the tumorigenic tendency in the subsequently formed somatic cell hybrid.[28–30] Thus, some products of normal cells can reintroduce growth control to a malignant environment. Furthermore, the tumor-suppressing function can be localized to specific regions of the genome. As normal chromosomes are gradually lost from such hybrids,

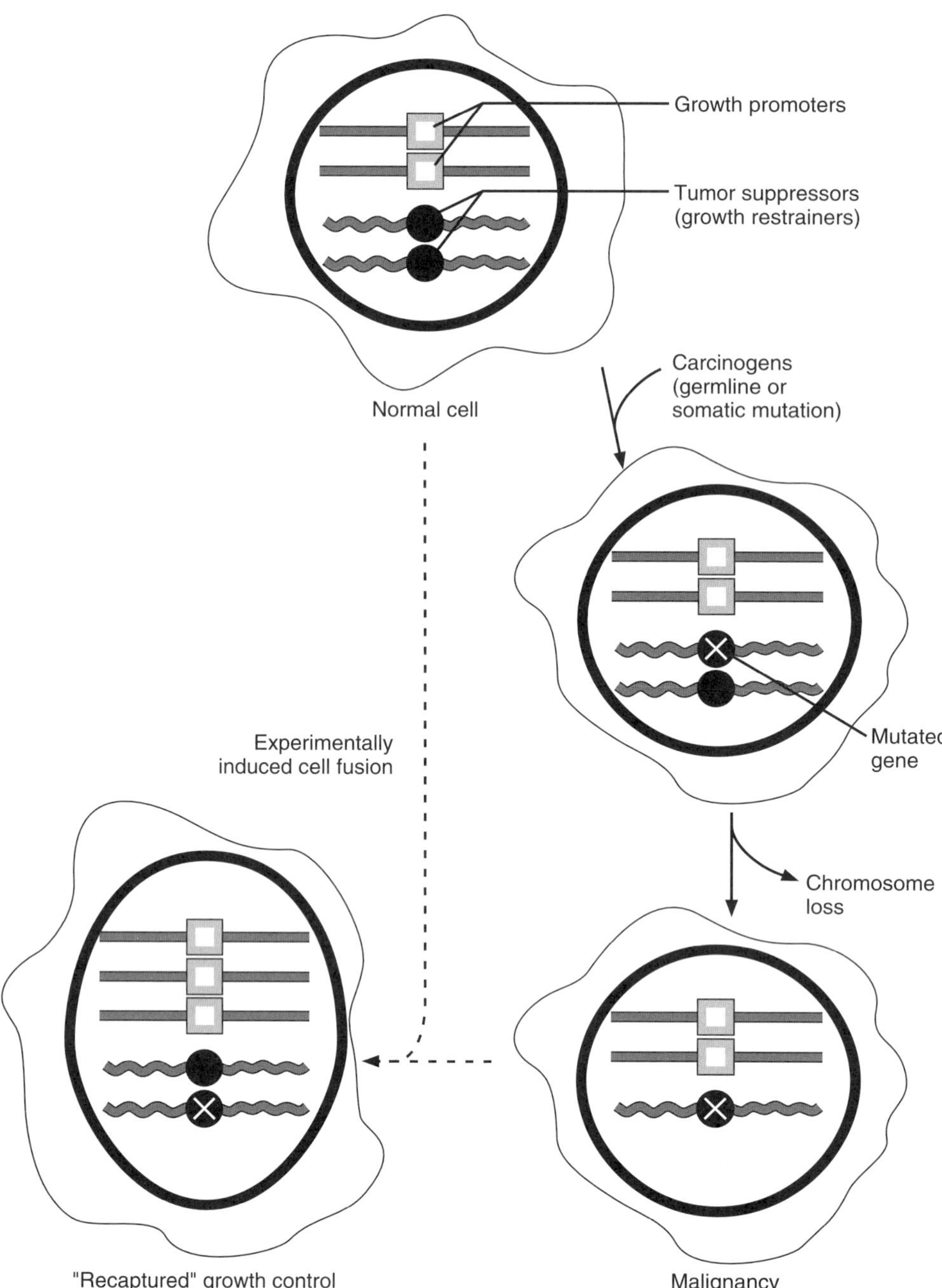

FIG. 31-3. Tumor suppressor genes. A growth-restraining gene is mutated on one allele and lost on the other, leading to uncontrolled proliferation (cancer). If the missing tumor suppressor gene function can be experimentally reintroduced into the cell, growth control is regained.

there comes a point, corresponding to the loss of a certain region, at which the malignant potential of the cell can be reexpressed (Fig. 31-3).

Studies of cancer-prone families (see later) also suggested the existence of genes whose normal function was growth control rather than growth promotion. The inspiration for much of this work began with a statistical study of inherited versus sporadic cases of the rare childhood tumor retinoblastoma.[31] From this analysis, it was suggested that the tumor requires two successive mutations in the genome rather than a single dominant activation of a growth promoting gene. It was postulated that in the familial form of this tumor, one mutated allele of a particular gene was passed in the germline and that only one additional mutation was required for cellular transformation. Thus,

patients with the familial form of retinoblastoma were often younger and more likely to have multiple independent tumors than their counterparts with sporadic malignancies, in whom two rare mutations would be required to occur in each of the two individual alleles in the same cell. Molecular biologic investigation aided by cytogenetic analysis focused attention on a specific region of the genome localized on chromosome 13 as the target for these successive mutations. In occasional retinoblastoma tumors, deletions of a particular region of chromosome 13 were seen.[32] In subsequent studies, it was shown that the normal heterozygosity of this region of chromosome 13 that results from the inheritance of both a paternal and maternal allele was lost in the tumor cells of patients with retinoblastoma.[33] A specific gene, *RB*, was cloned from this region, and it was shown that mutation of both extant copies of this gene in a tumor cell is a prerequisite to the development of retinoblastoma.[34] In other words, *RB* is a tumor-suppressor gene—a functional *RB* gene prevents retinoblast transformation. The study of retinoblastoma has provided a prototype system for evaluating the role of tumor-suppressor genes in various malignancies. Study of the RB gene product has offered a distinctive avenue for exploring the role of these tumor-suppressor genes in regulating cellular growth (see later).

Mutator Genes

We are now entering an area in which the issues of genetic instability and target genes begin to merge. Indeed, it is easy to postulate that one step in oncogenesis would be the mutation of a gene that makes subsequent mutations more likely. As discussed later, most cancers are the result of multiple genetic lesions and therefore require a hypermutable state to be formed. This process is involved in cancer causation and also in cancer progression. Once malignantly transformed, a tumor is a model of accelerated evolution. In these later stages of carcinogenesis, the situation within a tumor cell or tumor cell population becomes genetically complex. The early stages of carcinogenesis are more immediately dissectable.

A certain subclass of colorectal cancers manifests a particular example of genetic instability.[35–38] This instability is the result of mutation in one of a number of genes that combine to recognize and repair nucleotide mismatches that are caused by base alteration or base-pairing errors during DNA replication.[39–41] Among the genes that have been implicated in this process are *MSH2, MLH1, PMS1, PMS2,* and *GTBP*.[42–46b] Some people carry a defective copy of one of these genes in their genomes. A second hit on the other normal allele makes the cell incapable of routine recognition and repair of base mismatches. Mutational events that would normally be discerned and corrected are thereby incorporated into the genetic structure of the cell—the cell is hypermutable. Within the gut, where numerous carcinogens and mutagens can be found, this inability to correct mutational events is particularly likely to result in malignant transformation. It is not just a repair function that is defective, it is also the recognition of the need to repair. There is some evidence that after a certain threshold of DNA damage is reached, a normal cell actually triggers a pathway that leads to its own demise. Thus, defects in the mismatch recognition and repair pathway may increase risk of cancer in at least two ways: by causing an increase in the number of mutational events, and by eliminating the process by which an irreparable excess of mutational events results in elimination of the damaged cell. Although most strongly implicated in a proportion of patients with colorectal cancer, this mechanism is likely to play a role in the causes of other malignancies as well.

Death Genes

Normal development involves programmed cell death. Webs between fingers regress, neurons lacking synaptic connections disappear, thymocytes that are not positively selected are eliminated, and so on. These processes are active, capable of being initiated by internal or external stimuli, and involve the instigation of a genetic program within a cell that leads to its own elimination. As part of this process, the oxidative activity of the cell is altered, the DNA is degraded, and the cell dies and is recycled by phagocytosis. This process is referred to as *apoptosis*[47,48] (from the Greek for falling off, as in a leaf falling off a tree in autumn). One pathway toward carcinogenesis involves the disruption of the normal apoptotic pathway. Cells that would normally die off, live on. This act, by itself, may not make the cells malignant, but it certainly makes them susceptible targets for the accumulation of additional mutations that can result in frank malignancy. One example of this process is the development of follicular lymphoma. Follicular lymphoma is the most common form of non-Hodgkin lymphoma in North America. The malignant cells are usually found to carry a specific karyotypic abnormality, a reciprocal translocation between chromosomes 14 and 18. This juxtaposition of these two chromosomes places the gene *BCL2* (at 18q21) into the context of the immunoglobulin heavy chain locus (at 14q32.3). The result of this contextual change is that *BCL2* is inappropriately expressed in the B cell in which the translocation has occurred.[49,50] Expression of *BCL2* in this situation abrogates the normal apoptotic program for this cell.[51,52] The result is not so much a proliferative advantage for this cell as an indolent increased survivability. It appears that additional steps are needed to convert the cell carrying this translocation into a lymphomatous cell. Such translocation-carrying cells have been discovered in the tonsils and peripheral blood of normal people at frequencies much higher than the incidence of follicular lymphoma.[53] This is just one example of the relation between apoptosis and cancer. Apoptosis is a general phenomenon. *BCL2* is just one of the genes that play a role in inducing or preventing commencement of a programmed cell death pathway.

Cellular Clocks

Different organisms have different, but generally reproducible, life-spans. Similarly, cells taken from animals and placed in culture grow for a certain number of doublings, then go into a crisis period, and then, in general, die out. A fundamental question of biology is what governs this process of senescence and death. How does a cell ''know'' that it has divided a certain number of times and reached its life expectancy? Certainly, this process is another potential target for an oncogenic event. Cells that could not escape their biologic clocks could only divide a finite number of times, no matter what mutations they had incorporated. ''Immortalization'' often accompanies malignant transformation. The process of cellular senescence (and its opposite, immortality) is likely to result from a complex interplay of many different genes and gene products. Among the areas in which some substantive inroads are being made is the relation between a potential clock mechanism and the action of the enzyme telomerase.

Replication of the end of a chromosome presents a particular problem for the DNA polymerase replicative machinery. Starting from the RNA primer, one strand can be copied continuously in a 5′ to 3′ direction, providing the direction of the growing replicative fork, the opposite strand requires successive RNA priming and synthesis as a series of shorter fragments. The 5′ ends of the strands cannot be faithfully replicated (the polymerase cannot extend from nothing [ie, no RNA primer] onto the end of the chromosome). Full genomic replication is accomplished by telomerase. Telomerase is a complex of protein and RNA.[54,55] The RNA recognizes and serves as a template for the particular telomeric DNA sequences (repeated sequences rich in the bases thymine and guanine) that allow the chromosome ends to be "finished." Normal adult human tissues (except for testes continuing to produce sperm), however, do not synthesize much, if any, telomerase. As a result, with each cycle of DNA replication, a bit of the terminal sequences of chromosomes is lost. This event is paralleled in vitro by the gradual diminution of the length of telomere repeats as primary cells continue to be passed in culture. The stepwise reduction in the size of the ends of chromosomes may therefore be envisioned to act as a kind of clock marking the number of replicative cycles that a cell has undergone. The consequences of losing the telomeric repeats may not just be an informational problem. It is also believed that the particular structure of the telomere stabilizes the chromosome and prevents it from undergoing end-to-end fusions with other chromosomes, which has been shown to lead to chromosome breakage, loss, and catastrophic genomic instability. In the rare cell that passes through the crisis stage and becomes immortalized (often seen in murine cell culture, but extremely rare in human cell culture), telomerase has been reactivated. Supportive of the role of telomerase in facilitating cellular immortalization, telomerase activity can be found in certain tumors (eg, ovarian carcinoma) but not in the normal tissue from which the tumors arose.[56–58]

CELLULAR GROWTH–AFFECTING PATHWAY

Normal growth and development involve an intricate system of cellular checks and balances. Dysregulated growth (cancer) occurs when at least one, but usually more than one, component of this system goes awry. Thus, to understand cancer is to understand the control and loss of control of the cellular growth–affecting pathway. This section briefly describes a prototypical growth-controlling pathway and discusses examples of genes and gene classes that function along this pathway and whose alteration contributes to malignant transformation. Description of this prototypical pathway begins outside of the cell with external stimuli to cellular proliferation. From there, the cellular membrane is described, then the cytoplasm and nucleus, where the machinery for DNA replication and cellular division is activated, resulting in the act of proliferation itself. This survey thus divides a growth-affecting pathway into four areas or levels: growth factors, growth factor receptors, cytoplasmic signal–transducing factors, and intranuclear cell cycle and mitosis factors (Fig. 31-4). Classically defined, oncogenes and protooncogenes play roles in each of these areas. Reference to tumor-suppressor genes is most frequently made when the discussion reaches the level of the cell nucleus.

Growth Factors

Extracellular stimuli of cellular proliferation reach the cell by a number of distinct routes. The stimulus can either be incorporated from outside the organism (eg, a foreign antigen) or synthesized within the body (eg, an endocrine hormone) and carried by the circulation to the target cell. The stimulus can be synthesized and secreted within the local environment of the target cell (paracrine stimulation). The stimulus can be synthesized and secreted by the target cell itself (autocrine stimulation). Although certain of these stimuli (particularly of the peptide class) carry the term *growth factor* or *stimulating factor* in their names (eg, platelet-derived growth factor [PDGF], epidermal growth factor [EGF], transforming growth factor [TGF], granulocyte-macrophage colony-stimulating factor), factors that act or bind to the cell surface and that stimulate growth can be a diverse group, structurally and functionally.[59] Many of these factors show specificity for particular cell types or particular cell lineages.[60] This specificity is often conferred by specific receptors elaborated by the target cells for the distinct growth factors (see later).

At least one classically defined oncogene has evolved from a growth factor. The *SIS* gene, the transforming principle of the simian sarcoma virus, has a normal cellular homologue, PDGF. Viruses carrying the *SIS* gene can transform cells that carry the PDGF receptor, suggesting an autocrine loop for growth stimulation that occurs either at the cell surface or within the cell. This process may be mimicked in certain tumors and has been studied in an osteosarcoma cell line that synthesizes both PDGF and the PDGF receptor.[61] Certain tumor cells have been found to release other growth factors (eg, TGF-α and TGF-β), which may also show expression in a limited number of normal tissues, such as placenta. TGF-α is related to EGF and can bind to EGF receptors to stimulate growth. Other examples of growth factors for which some involvement in malignancy has been reported include the insulin-like growth factors (IGF-1 and IGF-2, formerly referred to as *somatomedins* because of their role in mediating the effects of growth hormone).[62] These factors are found in many adult and embryonic tissues. Of possible relevance to carcinogenesis is that IGF-2 is highly expressed in fetal kidney. Wilms tumors express IGF-2 and its receptor. Under experimental conditions, antibodies that block the IGF-2 receptor can inhibit the growth of tumor xenografts in nude mice, suggesting a role for this growth factor in an autocrine loop. The regulation of IGF-2 in Wilms tumor and other pediatric tumors, such as rhabdomyosarcoma, is being investigated. Particular attention is being focused in these studies on the role of differential structure, retention, and expression of the maternal versus the paternal allele on IGF-2 level and consequences of that level to cellular growth. Cultured fibroblasts were an early model for the study of cell growth in vitro and therefore lent themselves to the discovery of a number of fibroblast growth factors (FGFs). Some of these factors are under study, and several have been implicated in one or another aspect of oncogenesis. Several of these factors can be shown to be transforming under experimental conditions. Mouse mammary tumor virus is believed to mediate at least part of its oncogenic function by integrating next to and dysregulating the expression of *INT2*, a member of the FGF family. In addition, acidic and basic FGF (aFGF and bFGF) have been shown to play a critical role in the phenomenon of tumor-induced new blood vessel formation, or *angiogenesis*.[63]

In addition to the defined growth factors described earlier, it is important not to lose track of the fact that a variety of other substances can serve as growth stimulators. Hormones, under certain circumstances, stimulate growth and can be required for oncogenesis. In a dramatic example of the requirement for

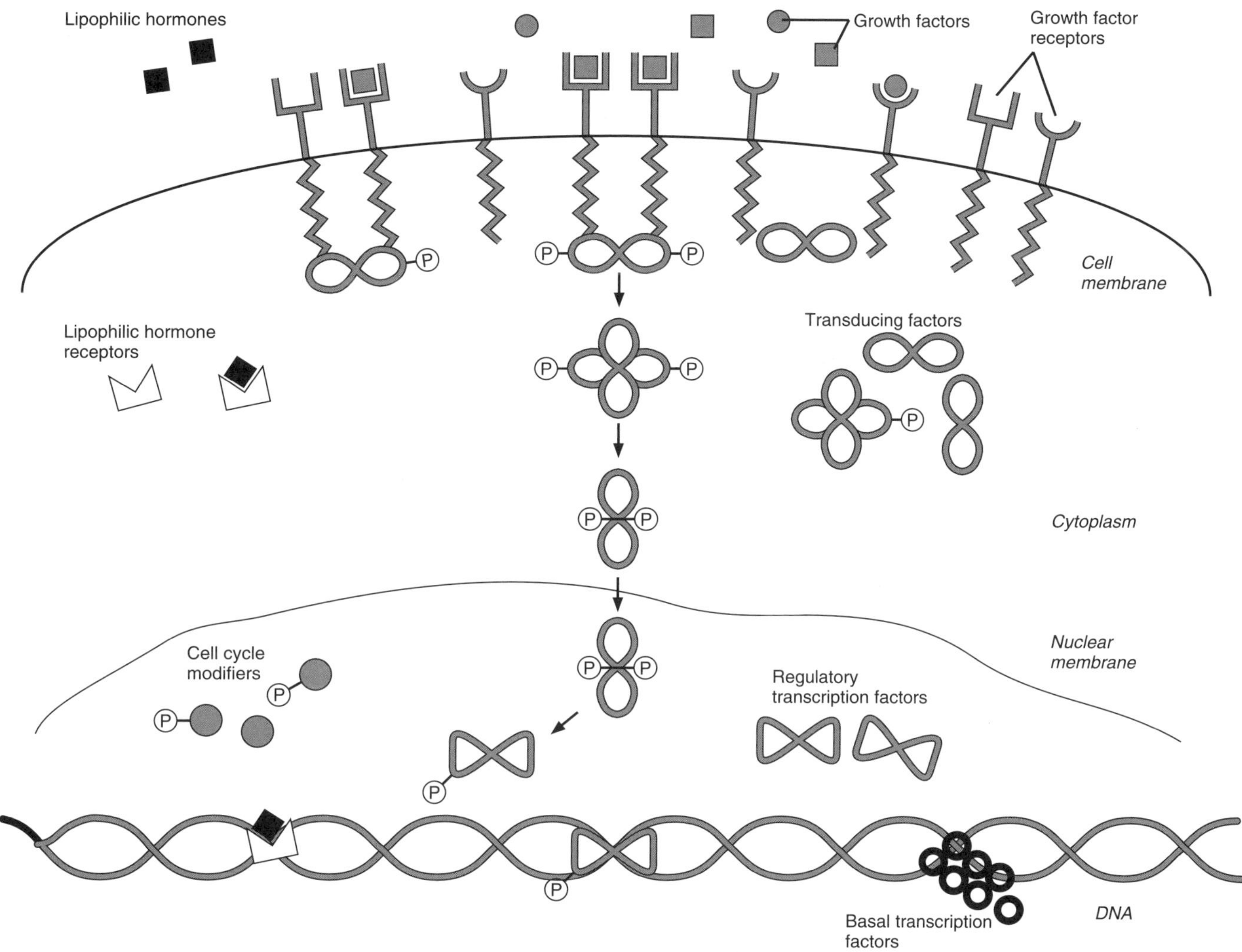

FIG. 31-4. Growth-affecting pathway. A simplified and schematized pathway of growth stimulation starting with the appearance of a growth factor or lipophilic hormone and eventually leading to the triggering of DNA replication and cell division. Components of the pathway include growth factors, hormones, receptors, transducing factors, and nuclear transcription–, cell cycle–, and cell division–regulating factors. Much of the signaling along the course of the pathway can be mediated by sequential targeted phosphorylation (P).

hormonal stimulus in certain oncogenic situations, rats were treated with the mutagen nitroso methylurea and developed mammary tumors that carried mutations of the *RAS* protooncogene (see later for a description of where this oncogene fits in a growth-affecting pathway). The development of these tumors could be prevented by prior oophorectomy, removing the hormonal stimulus to proliferate, but not the mutagenic stimulus.[64] Antigen may, under certain circumstances, act as a growth-stimulatory factor. For certain types of lymphoid malignancies, there appears to be a requirement for the continued expression of an immunoglobulin of a specific antigen-binding capacity, suggesting a continued requirement for antigen-mediated growth stimulation.

Growth Factor Receptors

The activity of growth factors requires that they be recognized by the target cell. Although this can be a nonspecific process, most of the defined growth factors interact with the target cell by binding to specific growth factor receptors. For many polypeptide growth factors, these receptors are membrane-spanning proteins that have an extracellular domain that recognizes the growth factor, a transmembrane domain, and an intracellular domain. With the specific binding of its ligand, the receptor is altered, in many cases involving the activation of phosphorylating or kinase activity of the intracellular domain of the receptor.[65] The activity often leads to the addition of phosphate groups on tyrosine, serine, or threonine residues of other protein substrates, altering their activity in a complex interactional cascade of information[66,67] (see later). The binding of the growth factor to the growth factor receptor is thus communicated from the cell surface into the cell interior. A number of oncogenes have been identified as modified versions of these cell-surface receptors. Among these are the *ERBB* gene, the homologue of the EGF receptor implicated in erythroleukemias in avian systems[68]; *ERBB2 (HER2, NEU)* related to the EGF receptor and relevant at some level to breast cancer; *FMS*, the homologue of the colony-stimulating factor-1 receptor; and *ROS*, related to the insulin receptor. The key to the action of many of these receptors as oncogenes appears to be their alteration to a form that is constitutively active even in the absence of their specific triggering factor or ligand.

Certain hormones, such as retinoic acid, steroids, and thyroxine, are lipid soluble and capable of traversing the plasma membrane without the mediation of a cell-surface receptor.[69] Once inside the cell, the hormones are bound by specific intracellular receptors. These receptors become localized in the nucleus, where they play roles in the regulation of distinct transcriptional programs. The *ERBA* oncogene, which collaborates with *ERBB* on a retrovirus that is implicated in causing avian erythroleukemia, is an altered form of the thyroid hormone receptor.

Cytoplasmic Signal-Transducing Factors

Information is increasing about the pathways by which a mitogenic signal at the cell surface is transduced through the cellular cytoplasm and delivered to the DNA replicative and mitotic enzymatic complexes in the nucleus. Although all the details of the transducing circuit have not been defined, what is known so far lends itself to a vision of a structural cascade of interacting proteins[70] whose sequential activation results in a signaling vector that reaches from the cell surface to the nucleus.[65,71] As mentioned earlier, binding of a growth factor to its receptor leads to an activated state. Different activated receptors interact at the plasma membrane with components of the signal transduction system. At least two (but probably more than two) signal transduction pathways commence at this level, converging further down the cascade in common or related targets (Fig. 31-5).

One pathway commences with the activation of a subset of the large class of G (guanosine triphosphate [GTP] binding) proteins[72] bound to the plasma membrane.[73] Various G proteins have as their downstream effector targets a diversity of molecules, including cyclic adenosine monophosphate–generating enzymes, ion flux channel guardian proteins, and the inositol triphosphate–diacylglycerol second-messenger generating complex. Each of these targets has a widening circle of other targets, effectors, and regulators with which it interacts. For example, diacylglycerol is involved with the activation of a set

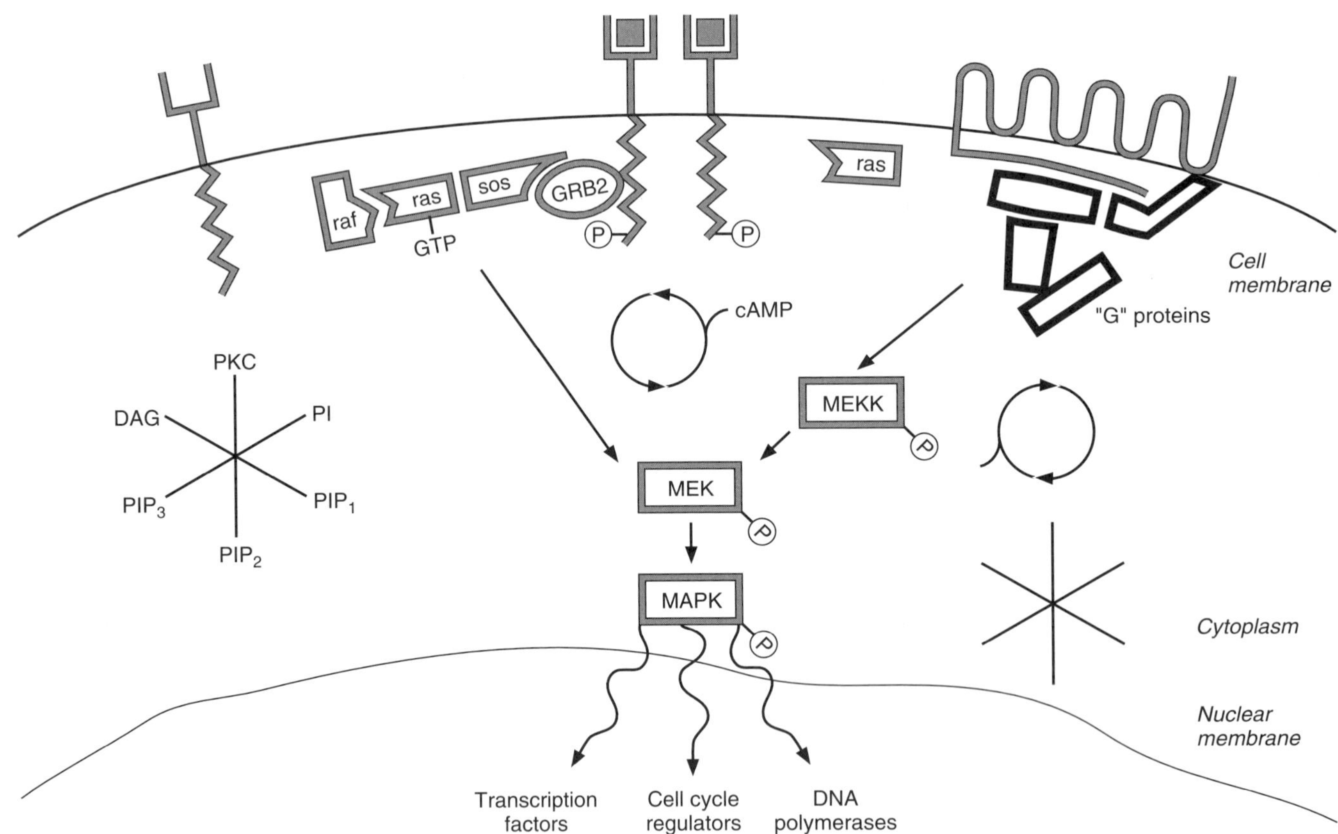

FIG. 31-5. Signal transduction. A simplified and schematized depiction of some of the components relevant to the communication of a stimulus to growth from the cell surface through the cytoplasm to the cell nucleus. A complex and interweaving cascade of energy and phosphate transfers commences at the inner plasma membrane and, for certain pathways (see text), may converge on a sequence of mitogen-activated protein kinases (MEK, MEK kinase [MEKK], and mitogen-activated protein kinase [MAPK] functions). Other relevant functions include cyclic AMP–generating enzymes and the phosphatidyl inositol (PI)–diacyl glycerol (DAG)–protein kinase C (PKC) complex.

of protein phosphorylases termed *protein kinase C* (PKC). PKC subsequently phosphorylates a variety of other cellular proteins. Certain tumor-promoting compounds, such as phorbol esters, also are believed to have their carcinogenicity mediated by activation of PKC. In the enlarging wave that follows, G-protein–involvement regulators of the effect are also brought into play. For example, some phosphatases are capable of mitigating or altering a mitogenic signal by dephosphorylating relevant proteins.[70] Although disruption or mutation of any one of a number of steps along this pathway can contribute to dysregulated growth, certain specifically defined oncogenes appear to be involved at some level of this pathway as well. The *SRC* gene (originally identified as the transforming principle of the Rous sarcoma virus) encodes a tyrosine kinase activity that may feed into the activation of the inositol triphosphate circuitry. The *SRC* gene is capable, however, of phosphorylating a variety of substrates, including some in the alternative pathway discussed later. A whole group of additional oncogenes share homology with this protein kinase catalytic domain of the *SRC* gene and are therefore likely to play related roles in terms of their oncogenicity.

An alternative pathway of signal transduction appears to involve, at an early stage in the cascade, the oncogenes *RAS* and *RAF*.[74] The *RAS* gene is the transforming principle of the Harvey sarcoma virus. It differs by a single amino acid from its cellular homologue. Significantly, mutation of this cellular homologue has been shown to be a prerequisite for transformation in a number of human cancers.[75] The *RAS* gene is similar, but not identical, to the previously mentioned G proteins in that it also is capable of GTP binding and hydrolysis. The mutations that occur in carcinogenic conversion of the cellular *RAS* diminish the inherent GTPase activity of this protein, potentially lengthening the duration of its activated state. It appears that *RAS* is required to become associated with the plasma membrane for its signal transduction role to be realized. The *RAS* gene can interact with the product of another oncogene, *RAF,* to promote intracellular signaling. The *RAS–RAF* (and perhaps additional participants) complex then phosphorylates and activates the protein MEK.[65,66] MEK is also a target of the previously described G protein pathway, where the role of the *RAS–RAF* complex is played by a different protein, MEK kinase. With this convergence of the two pathways on MEK, a possible final common pathway of signal transduction is achieved. MEK phosphorylates mitogen-activated protein kinase, which may have among its targets selected mitogen-activated proteins, including nuclear proteins, that play a role in transcription, cell cycle regulation, DNA replication, and mitosis.[71]

Nuclear Growth–Affecting Genes and Cell Cycle Determinants

The act of cellular proliferation is defined within the nucleus. Here, DNA is replicated. Without DNA replication, cell division is meaningless. After DNA replication, the replicated chromosomes are condensed, the nuclear membrane is dissolved, and mitosis is initiated.

Many gene products localized to the nucleus can contribute to malignant transformation in a tumor system. Some of these products are encoded by classically defined oncogenes or pro-

tooncogenes (eg, *MYC, FOS, JUN*); a large number have been identified because of their dysregulation by cancer-specific chromosomal aberration (eg, *MYC, N-MYC, L-MYC, TTG1, TTG2 (RBTN1, RBTN2), MLL, SCL(TAL1), LYL1, PBX*); some are classically defined tumor-suppressor genes (eg, *p53, RB*), and many have been characterized as a result of in-depth studies of the growth stimulatory and cell cycle processes. Three fundamental types of nuclear-localized gene products have been implicated in oncogenesis: genes that function at nodal points in cell lineage development and differentiation, genes that act as guardians of the integrity of the genome, and genes that rule and regulate the cell cycle from G_0 through G_1, S, G_2, and mitosis. These three fundamental functions are not exclusive of each other, and study of an oncogenic product in one category often spills over into aspects of and interactions with the other two.

The cloning of chromosomal translocations associated with specific types of malignancies has led to the discovery of many DNA-binding transcription factors. The direct line from the dysregulation of these transcription factors to oncogenic transformation has not been definitively shown for any of these genes, but their involvement in some aspect of cellular transformation is compelling.[71] In many cases, their dysregulation by chromosomal translocation appears to be a prerequisite for the occurrence of a specific cancer. In some cases, their oncogenic potentials can be observed by inappropriately expressing them in cell culture systems or by experimentally deregulating them in transgenic mice.

The *MYC* gene is carried by an oncogenic tumor virus.[76] It is invariably translocated and dysregulated in patients with Burkitt lymphoma.[77] It has been shown to be amplified in certain lung cancers. It can cooperate with a mutated *RAS* gene to transform fibroblasts in vitro. When hooked up to a promoter that is active in mammary epithelial cells, it predisposes the transgenic animal to the development of mammary tumors.[78] *MYC* is one of the genes whose expression is induced by the binding of PDGF to its cognate receptor. It is actively expressed in dividing cells and down-regulated in certain model systems in which terminal differentiation can be induced. Its structure has been completely elucidated. Aside from a transcriptional activation domain and a DNA-binding domain, *MYC* also carries two motifs, a helix–loop–helix and a leucine "zipper" that mediate its protein–protein interaction with a host of other positive and negative regulatory transcription factors. The target sequence for its binding to DNA has been defined, at least to some extent. Still, its direct role in oncogenesis, what regulates it, and what it regulates remain inconclusive.

The oncogenes *JUN* and *FOS* are more definitively characterized transcription factors that combine by interaction of their leucine zipper motifs to form AP1.[79] AP1 is a transcription factor that was first observed to bind to an "enhancer of transcription" sequence present in the genome of the tumor virus SV40. AP1 binding sites have been identified in the regulatory regions of many genes, including those that appear to be responsive to the tumor promoter TPA (phorbol ester).

The *SCL(TAL1), LYL1, TAL2, TTG1,* and *TTG2* genes are all examples of genes whose products carry DNA-binding and protein–protein interactive domains and appear to have normal functions in the determination of a cell lineage.[80] For example, *SCL* is normally expressed in early hematopoiesis and then in cells destined for the erythroid, mast, or megakaryocytic lineages. It appears to be a positive regulator of erythroid differentiation.[81] It can form a dimeric complex with *TTG2* during erythroid development.[82,83] It is also the gene most frequently associated by chromosomal aberrations with the development of T-cell leukemia.[84,85] The example of *SCL* underscores a fundamental question in the study of many of these genes: Why does cancer result from dysregulation in one cell lineage of a transcription factor active in determination of a different cell lineage? An ancillary question that arises from these studies is the more fundamental one about the relation between differentiation (or inhibition of differentiation) and cellular proliferation.

Genes That Directly Control the Cell Cycle

All events that are involved in cellular proliferation converge at the level of cell cycle control (Fig. 31-6). The specific proteins that drive a cell into or restrain it from entering G_1, S, G_3, and mitosis are being elucidated. This is fertile ground for the discovery of genes that are critical to tumorigenesis and tumor progression.[86] In mammalian cells, regulation of the cell cycle is believed to be accomplished by sequential and temporally specific activation of a group of proteins called cyclin-dependent kinases (CDKs). Activation of CDKs occurs through their binding with cell cycle–specific cyclins. Together, these complexes drive the cell from one phase of the cell cycle to another.[87–89] For example, the CDK4–cyclin D (there are at least three types of cyclin D—D1, D2, and D3) complex may be essential for recruitment of the cell into the cell cycle or for moving the cell through the *restriction point* in G_1. The cyclins D have short half-lives and are apparent targets for growth factor induction. Cyclin D1 is dysregulated by chromosomal inversion or translocation in parathyroid adenomas and in certain types of lymphoid malignancies. CDK2–cyclin D and

CDK2–cyclin E push the cell into S phase, a phase in which CDK2–cyclin A complexes appear active. Preceding mitosis, CDK1–cyclin B complexes are formed. The whole process is likely initiated by protein phosphorylation and dephosphorylation events, perhaps targeted to a CDK-activating kinase at the end of the signal transduction pathway described earlier.

This system is subject to numerous checks and balances, each of which has potential relevance and offers a potential target in oncogenesis. The tumor-suppressor gene *RB* or one of its closely related family members[26,90] is hypophosphorylated early in G_1. In this underphosphorylated state, the RB protein (pRB) appears to be capable of stopping cell cycle progression. This inhibition is believed to be mediated by the reversible interaction of pRB with other proteins (such as the transcription factor E2F). Phosphorylation of pRB by an activated CDK–cyclin complex (CDK–cyclin D complexes are likely mediators) abrogates the ability of pRB to bind to E2F, which may directly or indirectly release the cell cycle block. Oncogenic DNA tumor viruses are also capable of abrogating the pRB cell cycle blockade by directly binding to (and presumably thereby eliminating from the scene of action) the hypophosphorylated form of the protein. Elimination of pRB by deletion and mutation is the sine qua non of the childhood malignancy retinoblastoma. Mutation of pRB that alters its protein-binding ''pocket'' is an extremely common occurrence in adult carcinomas, such as lung cancer.[91]

The study of the cell cycle is becoming increasingly complex with the realization that there are a host of other proteins (CDK-inhibitory proteins [CKIs])[92,93] that act to inhibit the CDK–cyclin complexes. For example, a protein, p16, can bind to the CDK4–cyclin D complex and inhibit its activity. Mutations in this gene that eliminate its activity occur in patients who suffer from the syndrome of familial melanoma. In those rare lung cancer cell lines with a normal *RB* gene, *p16* gene expression is absent, suggesting that these two genes are likely

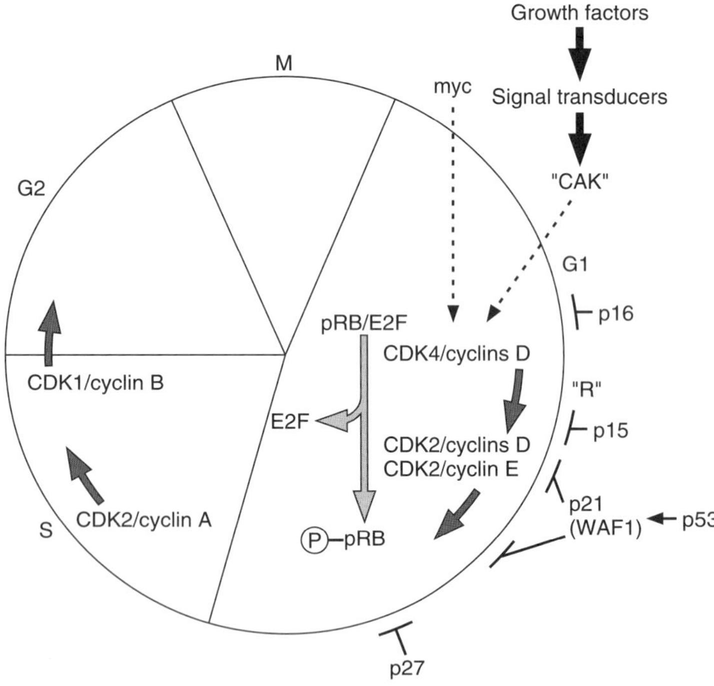

FIG. 31-6. Cell cycle–relevant genes. Some of the genes that are believed to play roles in the stimulation or inhibition of a cell's progress through the cell cycle. These include the cyclin–cyclin-dependent kinase (CDK) complexes that stimulate movement past the restriction (R) point in G_1 and throughout the cell cycle. Also depicted are the *RB* and *p53* genes, the transcription factors *E2F* and *MYC*, and the CDK inhibitors (CKIs) *p16, p15, p21* (eg, *WAF1, PIC1, SDI1*), and *p27*. CAK, CDK-activating kinase.

to have overlapping activity in tumor suppression at a particular point in the cell cycle and that one or the other of them must be eliminated for certain types of cancer to occur or progress.[94] A structurally related gene, *p15,* is induced by agents that cause arrest of the cell cycle in G_1. Another CKI is a 21-kd protein, PIC1 (independently discovered in a variety of systems and called CIP1, CAP20, WAF1, or SDI1), which binds to and inactivates the CDK2–cyclin complexes.[95] Binding to this and other CDK complexes appears to be lost in transformed cells. The tumor suppressor gene *p53* appears capable of increasing the transcription of PIC1, suggesting a possible direct connection between checkpoint control (see later) and cell cycle. In addition to blocking entry of a cell into S phase through this mechanism, it may also directly block DNA replication. Interestingly, this protein is up-regulated in senescent cells, a finding that suggests a linkage among cell cycle control, senescence, and immortalization. Additional CKIs include a 27-kd protein induced by TGF-β that inactivates the CDK2–cyclin E complex and a 24-kd protein that binds in vitro to CDK2 but not CDK4.

Checkpoint Controls, *p53,* and Hyperevolution

Eukaryotic DNA can repair itself when it has undergone structural damage. The process by which this occurs involves not only the myriad of repair enzymes but also other proteins that are capable of recognizing damage when it has occurred. Some damage is the result of occasional nucleotide mismatches that occur during normal DNA replication. Other damage is less the result of a normal (although imperfect) physiologic process than the result of exposure of DNA or chromatin to damaging factors, such as radiation, deranged metabolic pathways, or chemical exposures. Recognition of structural DNA damage is capable of causing growth arrest. The growth arrest can have varying consequences in the affected cell. In some cases, given time, the damage can be repaired, and once repaired, the cell can recommence growth. In other circumstances, depending on the cell type or amount of damage, the growth arrest can give way to a programmed cell death pathway, and the damaged cell can thereby be eliminated.

The time frames within the cell cycle at which DNA damage causes growth arrest are referred to as *checkpoints*[96,97] and are simplistically viewed as moments when the cell checks the integrity of its genetic material and ''decides'' whether to proceed with replication and division. Checkpoints are likely to occur at numerous times within the cell cycle, although the two most easily defined checkpoints are between G_1 and S when the cell ''decides'' whether to commence DNA replication, and between G_2 and M, when the cell ''decides'' whether to proceed with mitosis. Studies in yeast established the conceptual framework of checkpoints and the genes that mediate or control these checkpoints. These genes, when mutated, result in loss of checkpoint control, with a diversity of consequences to the cell. One fundamental consequence, however, is clear. Numerous mechanisms of tumor formation lead to an increased frequency and increased tolerance of mutational events. A tumor is a population of cells constantly being selected for growth advantage. The hypermutable, hyperevolutionary nature of cancer results in an accumulation of mutations within a cell that favor dysregulated growth. Although an argument could be made that it is not in a cell's best interest to be tolerant of mutation, that is

not true for a tumor population. The population is not constrained by a physiologic role or function. The population can sacrifice a high percentage of its individual members to lethal mutation and still continue to grow and spread as a population.

A classic example of a gene that controls a checkpoint in mammalian cells is the *p53* tumor suppressor.[98–102] DNA damage in G_1 results in an increase in the level of *p53* and cell cycle arrest. For severe levels of damage, many types of cells halted in the progression of the cell cycle undergo apoptosis. In the absence of *p53* or in cells carrying mutated *p53,* the cell cycle arrest and apoptosis do not occur, and the checkpoint is abrogated. The gene *p53* is the most commonly mutated gene in oncogenesis. Its gross and refined spectrum of mutations provides insight into its role in cell growth and into the action of carcinogenic compounds. Complete loss of *p53* expression results in loss of checkpoint control and marked predisposition to the development of malignancy. Often, however, *p53* is not deleted but rather is mutated and still expressed. Mutated *p53* can act synergistically with other oncogenes to transform a cell. The level of mutated to wild-type *p53* appears to be crucial in these cases. In situations in which one *p53* allele is mutated but still expressible, malignant transformation is often accompanied by loss of the wild-type allele. A detailed analysis of the exact mutations that occur in tumors of different cell lineages suggests that *p53* is often a direct target of the carcinogens associated with the development of distinct tumors. For example, *p53* mutations in squamous cell carcinoma are most consistent with the formation of thymine dimers by ultraviolet light. Mutations in *p53* in a subgroup of patients with hepatocellular carcinoma are consistent with the experimental evidence for aflatoxin-induced mutations. The spectrum of nucleotide deletions, insertions, transitions (purine-to-purine [G↔A], or pyrimidine-to-pyrimidine [C↔T]), and transversions (G/A↔T/C) in the mutated *p53* genes associated with the development of lung versus colon cancer are distinctly different, suggesting the effects of environmental carcinogens with distinct mutational properties. The crystallized structure of *p53* has been determined,[102a] confirming the experimental suggestions that the mutations that affect this gene alter its DNA-binding capability. This occurs in some cases by direct mutation of the contacting amino acid residues and in other cases by disruption of the protein structure, such as to disrupt protein function. As mentioned, wild-type *p53* can apparently directly up-regulate the transcription of one of the CKIs (eg, p21, WAF1, CIP1) that causes an arrest at the G_1 to S checkpoint. This ability is lost when *p53* is deleted or oncogenically mutated.

MULTISTEP CARCINOGENESIS

As discussed earlier, the act of malignant transformation is usually not the result of a single transforming event. For most cell lineages, however, and particularly as determined for carcinomas and some sarcomas, cancer occurs as the result of the accumulation of multiple mutations that lead to dysregulated growth (Fig. 31-7). Some of these mutations are not oncogenic in themselves but increase the rate of frankly transforming events by disrupting the normal processes of cell cycle progression, checkpoint control, and DNA damage recognition and repair.

The prototype of multistep carcinogenesis is the evolution

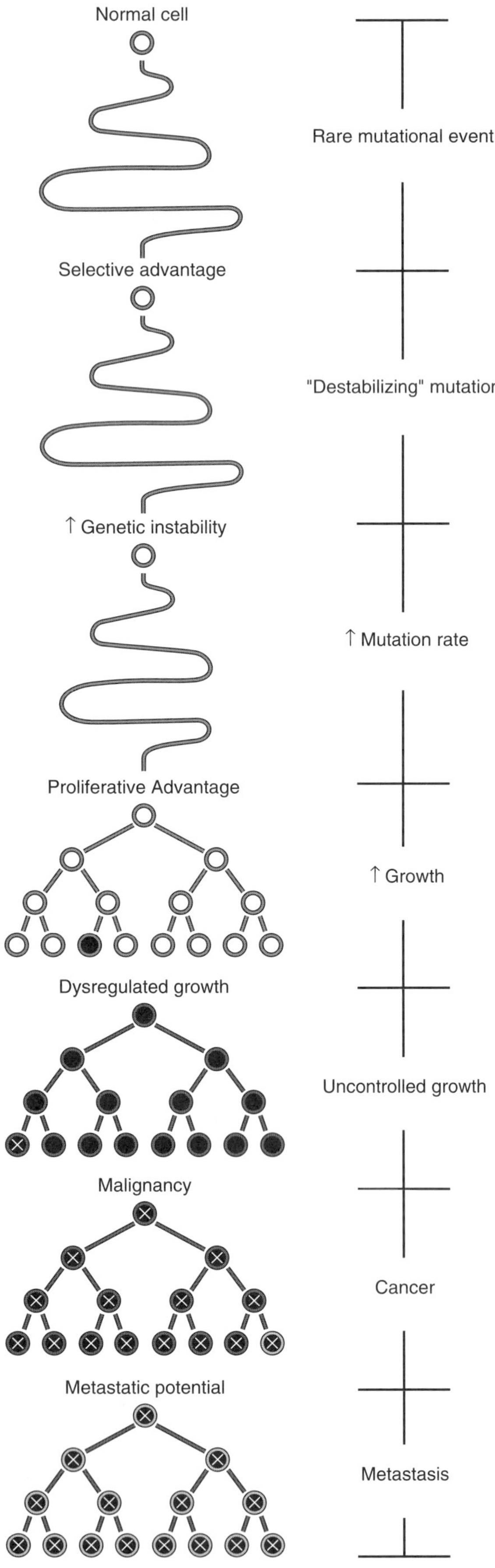

of colorectal cancer; investigators have dissected the histopathologic stages of colonic mucosal epithelial transformation and molecularly characterized each stage in the process.[103–105] This refined analysis suggests that transformation can commence with an increased proliferation within the crypts of the colon of cells carrying a mutated *RAS* gene. A histopathologic progression schema can be drawn from hyperproliferation through early, intermediate, and late adenoma to frank carcinoma and metastatic cancer. Mutations of genes on chromosome 5q (*APC*), 18q (*DCC*), and 17p (*p53*), as well as additional chromosomal aberrations and changes in chromatin methylation patterns, are shown to accumulate corresponding to the progression to frank malignancy. The precise temporal order of acquisition of mutations likely is less relevant than the net accumulation. This is not to suggest, however, that each of these mutations is equivalent. Certain of these mutations may be more relevant to the initiation of the transforming process, while others may be more relevant to its progression.

Most models of multistep carcinogenesis are supported by the obvious epidemiologic fact that cancer is primarily a disease of adults, occurring relatively late in life and often the presumed result of constant or recurrent exposures to an endogenous or environmental destabilizing influence. This argument does not hold for cancer in children, and evidence for the same kind of multistep carcinogenesis for most pediatric malignancies cannot be as clearly delineated as it can for the development of colorectal cancer in adults. Pediatric malignancies, in general, are not characterized by the kind of massive, gross aneuploidy that is seen so often in adult carcinomas. Perhaps, as a corollary, the representational spectrum of malignancies in children is distinct from that in adults, with carcinomas being extremely rare, with leukemias, brain tumors, neuroectodermal tumors, and soft tissue and bone sarcomas predominating. The causes of pediatric malignancies are complex and multifactorial, but certain features of these cancers are distinctive.[106] A subset of pediatric malignancies occurs when their tissue of origin is in a markedly activated and proliferative phase. Pediatric lymphoid malignancies generally involve less mature lymphocytes and occur during the establishment of an immune repertoire, predominantly within the first 10 years of life. Osteosarcoma occurs predominantly during the adolescent growth spurt. Neuroblastoma and Wilms tumor occur at a time related to the formation of the kidney and adrenal and often are clinically detected within the first 2 years of life, as is true of retinoblastoma and retinal development. Brain tumors in children peak within the first 10 years of life and show a predominant relation to the embryonal central nervous system development, as opposed to the pattern of the more supratentorial glial tumors of adults. It is as if, in children, the normal growth and developmental process is on and cannot be turned off, as opposed to in adults, in whom a growth stimulatory circuit that had been

FIG. 31-7. Multistep carcinogenesis. Most cancers are the result of multiple mutational events. The pace of mutation can increase substantially as a result of mutations that make the genome more unstable and that increase the target population by causing certain cells to have a proliferative advantage.

quiescent, or at least tightly controlled, is activated or reactivated.

In addition to the chance occurrence of mutation in a growth-promoting gene, or a genetically determined susceptibility to mutagenic agents (see earlier), there are also distinct syndromes of cancer susceptibility that can manifest in childhood. Clearly, a highly penetrating, familial, childhood-onset cancer syndrome could not have existed during previous generations of human development. Affected children would have died from their malignancies and never reached reproductive age. The previously mentioned example of inherited retinoblastoma is instructive in this regard. Before the advent of ophthalmoscopic examination and ocular enucleation, there was no such thing as familial retinoblastoma. Only when germline *RB* mutations were identified in people with retinal tumors early enough to be surgically cured, so that they reached reproductive age and passed the mutation on to their offspring, did the entity of familial retinoblastoma develop. Essentially, all patients who present with bilateral (or trilateral, affecting the pineal as well) familial retinoblastoma carry a germline *RB* mutation. A distinction can be made, however, between a familial cancer syndrome and inherited cancer predisposition. An inherited predisposition may occur because of a de novo mutation in the sperm or ovum. In these cases, the offspring carries a germline mutation (the mutant gene is present in every cell of the person), but the parent does not. Consequently, it would not be expected that the patient would have a family history of related malignancy.

CANCER-PRONE CONDITIONS

In contrast to the de novo germ cell mutation, there are distinct syndromes of cancer predisposition that affect children and that are familial. In this section, some cancer-prone states for which the altered genes have been identified are described.

Retinoblastoma and Wilms Tumor

True familial retinoblastoma is one example of a cancer-prone condition.[107] Interestingly, although *RB* is pivotal to the cell cycle, carriers of a mutated *RB* gene are at increased risk for a limited number of malignancies. The major risk is for retinoblastoma. Most patients with germline *RB* mutation who survive this ocular malignancy are at increased risk for the development of osteosarcoma, either within or outside of the field of radiation (if radiation is used as part of the treatment of the eye tumor). The germline *RB* mutation is recessive, and a single copy of fully functional RB protein is sufficient for regulation of cell growth. Given normal or elevated mutational frequency, however, it is likely that the other RB allele is mutated or lost in one of the millions of cells that compose the retina or that are involved in bone development. When this happens, a step is taken toward malignant transformation. The likelihood of this second mutational event is such that the risk of tumor formation appears to be dominant in families carrying this gene.

Evidence for a familial predisposition to Wilms tumor is suggested by case reports but is much less well-established than for retinoblastoma.[108–114] In this era, familial Wilms tumor appears to be rare. This probably reflects the more complex genetics of this malignancy; that is, there are at least two separate loci on the short arm of chromosome 11 whose mutations can be associated with the development of Wilms tumor (see relevant chapter). In addition, owing to medical advances, patients with Wilms tumor are surviving into their reproductive years.

Familial Adenomatous Polyposis and Hereditary Nonpolyposis Colorectal Cancer

Patients with familial adenomatous polyposis carry a germline mutation of the *APC* gene located on the long arm of chromosome 5.[105,115] Loss of the other functional *APC* gene is likely to result in the characteristic formation of thousands of benign polyps in the colon. It is as if the normal APC gene acts as a block to proliferation that, when removed, allows dysregulated growth. Within the enlarging benign tumors, additional mutations can occur that result in progression of one or more of the polyps to malignancy. Colorectal cancer is not the only manifestation of inheritance of a mutated *APC* gene; hepatoblastoma is also associated with this germline mutation. Children who survive hepatoblastoma are candidates for screening for *APC* gene mutation and subsequent surveillance for colorectal polyps.

A second syndrome associated with familial incidence of colorectal cancer is hereditary nonpolyposis colorectal cancer,[41,116] a hereditary predisposition, by definition, not preceded by the development of numerous colonic polyps. This syndrome is caused by germline mutation of one of the two alleles of any of the several genes (*MSH2, MLH1, PMS1, PMS2*[42–46]) described earlier, which form an enzymatic complex involved in the recognition and repair of nucleotide mismatches. During persistent colonic mucosal growth and development, the other allele is mutated, and the result is a cell that is particularly susceptible to subsequent mutation. Patients who suffer from this syndrome develop tumors at a younger age (often before 50 years of age, occasionally in adolescence). According to some reports, these tumors are more often right-sided but nonetheless carry a better prognosis. Some sporadic colorectal tumors are also caused by this mismatch repair defect. It is remarkable that this defect is not growth-promoting or does not provide a direct selective advantage to the cell. Rather, its role in oncogenesis appears to be the induction of hypermutability.

Li-Fraumeni Syndrome

While studying the familial clustering of rhabdomyosarcoma, Li and Fraumeni[117,118] observed that one parental branch of the family tree of relevant cohorts showed a marked increased risk for certain types of tumors, including soft tissue sarcomas, breast carcinoma, brain tumors, leukemias, osteosarcomas, and adrenocortical carcinomas. This spectrum of malignancy was distinct from that seen in other familial cancer syndromes and appeared to define a distinct entity referred to as *Li-Fraumeni syndrome* (LFS). Among the affected members of LFS families, the risk of developing a malignancy by 30 years of age may be as high as 50%. The basis for this increased risk of cancer is the presence of one mutated *p53* allele in the germline of the affected family members.[119] As noted, *p53* monitors DNA damage, cell cycle, and programmed cell death. Competition between functional and dysfunctional *p53* can increase the risk of malignant transformation. Subsequent loss of the wild-type *p53* allele can result in an increasingly virulent, anaplastic, and genomically unstable tumor. The spectrum of malignancies suffered by patients with LFS suggests a critical interplay of wild-type and mutated *p53* in certain cell lineages.

Neurofibromatosis Types 1 and 2

Neurofibromatosis types 1 and 2 (NF1 and NF2) are autosomal dominant syndromes characterized by the occurrence of neurofibromas, apparent admixtures of cell types that make up the neurilemmal sheath.[120–123] In NF1, the neurofibromas are found more peripherally. In NF2, the neurofibromas are found more centrally, with a notable occurrence of acoustic nerve involvement. The phenotype of a patient with NF1 includes the classic café au lait skin lesions and Lisch nodules (hamartomas of the iris). Malignancies associated with NF1 include occasional sarcomatous degeneration of a neurofibroma, pheochromocytomas, optic gliomas, glioblastomas, and meningiomas. The mutated gene in NF1, neurofibromin, is found on the long arm of chromosome 17 and encodes a protein with GTPase-activating activity that is postulated to feed into the *RAS* intracellular transducing pathway previously described.[124] The spectrum of malignancies associated with NF2 includes astrocytomas, meningiomas, and melanomas. The gene associated with NF2, schwannomin, is found on the long arm of chromosome 22 and encodes a protein of the MERLIN (moesin, ezrin, radixin-like) family believed to be involved in a linkage of the cellular cytoskeleton to the cellular membrane and in cell–cell and cell–extracellular matrix interactions. The mutations in NF2 result in the formation of a truncated protein. Sporadic meningiomas are often associated with mutation of the schwannomin gene as well. Loss of chromosome 22, which carries the normal schwannomin gene, often accompanies the development of meningiomas.

TUMOR PROGRESSION

Cancers are not static; they continue to evolve. Within a malignancy, internal selective forces favor, over time, the emergence of more rapidly proliferative, more invasive, more metastatic, in sum, more virulent, cells. In addition, in many cases, there is an iatrogenic selection process; chemotherapy selects for cells that are resistant to the drugs being administered. At least four propensities are relevant to a consideration of tumor progression (Fig. 31-8). These are the propensity to grow, to

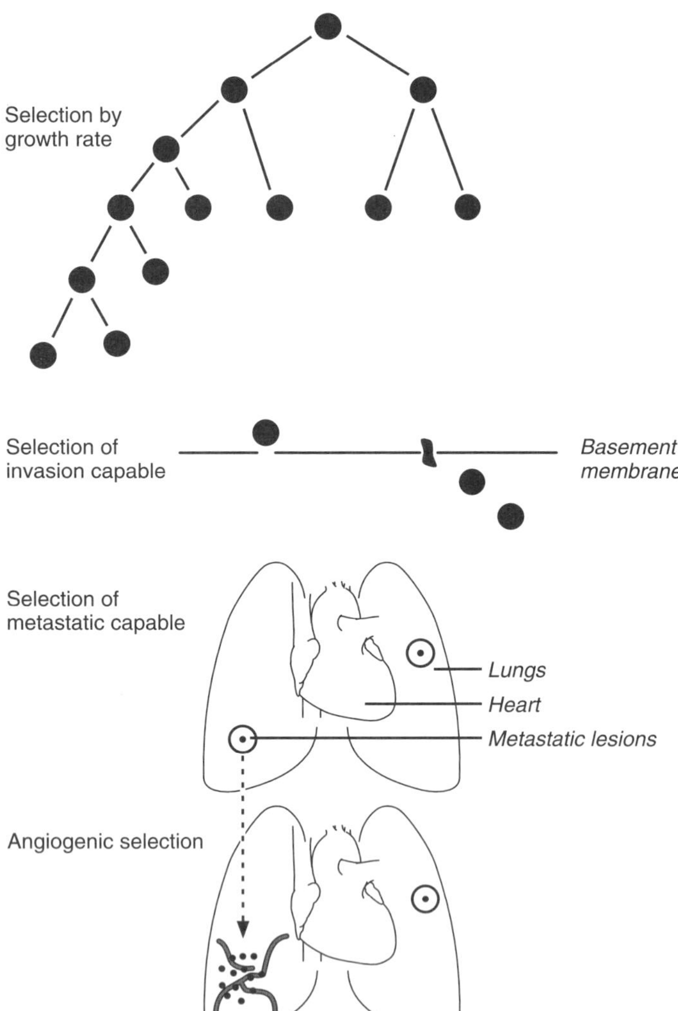

FIG. 31-8. The four components implicated in tumor progression: increased growth rate, the capability to invade through a basement membrane or tissue stroma, the capacity to metastasize, and the ability to recruit a blood supply.

invade, to metastasize, and to recruit a blood supply,[63,125–127] which are elaborated as follows:

1. Faster growing cells, in general, become predominant within a cellular population over time. Thus, up to a certain minimum required time for DNA replication and cell division, mutations that move a cell through a cell cycle, in the absence of other selective factors, are favored.

2. As cells emerge from their "home bases," they encounter a variety of physical barriers to their movement to other parts of the body, in particular, the structures that form tissue boundaries consisting of basement membrane and extracellular stroma. More virulent invasive tumors are capable of elaborating a subpopulation of cells with the ability to bind to, disrupt, or recognize a previously disrupted basement membrane, or to ignore the normal signals that determine tissue boundaries. Once beyond the basement membrane, some tumor cells produce or induce proteases that allow them to carve a path through the tissues into which they have invaded.

3. Certain tumors have a clear predilection to metastasize to certain organs. A component of this predilection is simply geographic. Tumors may be more likely to metastasize into the closest downstream complex vascular bed. At least one other component, however, is involved in organ-specific metastasis. The tumor must find the environment suitable to its growth. It must be able to take advantage of the positive growth factors elaborated by the host tissue and ignore the negative growth factors. Only a small fraction of the malignant cells present in a tumor are successful at becoming metastatic.

4. For continued growth in the site of origination and for new growth at distant sites, tumors must be able to recruit the circulatory system to provide nutrition and remove waste. The angiogenic potential of certain tumors is the topic of Chapter 32.

Human cancer occurs because the human genome is a dynamic, changeable structure, and cellular growth is a complex process in which dozens of genes and their products play a role. Within the past two decades, biomedical research has remarkably advanced the understanding of malignant transformation by delineating in exquisite detail the pathway of cellular growth control, the individual elements (genes) that play roles in one or another part of that pathway, and the processes through which the normal function of these genes are subverted or altered. This perspective on oncogenesis has already led to new approaches to cancer diagnosis, staging, minimal residual disease determination, and prognostic stratification. It is beginning to make inroads into regimens for cancer prevention and has become the focus for the development of logical, targeted combined-modality therapies.

REFERENCES

1. Boder E. Ataxia-telangiectasia: an overview. In: Gatti RA, Swift M, eds. Ataxia-telangiectasia: genetics, neuropathology, and immunology of a degenerative disease of childhood. New York, Alan R Liss, 1985.
2. German J, Bloom D, Passarge E. Bloom's syndrome. XI. Progress report for 1983. Clin Genet 1984;25:166.
3. Fanconi G. Familial constitutional panmyelocytopathy, Fanconi's anemia (F.A.). I. Clinical aspects. Semin Hematol 1967;4:233.
4. Harber LC, Bickers DR. Photosensitivity diseases: principles of diagnosis and treatment. Philadelphia, WB Saunders, 1981.
5. Aurias A, Dutrillaux B, Buriot D, et al. High frequencies of inversions and translocations of chromosome 7 and 14 in ataxia telangiectasia. Mutat Res 1980;69:369.
6. Aurias A, Croquette MF, Nuyts JP, et al. New data on clonal anomalies of chromosome 14 in ataxia telangiectasia: tct(14;14) and inv(14). Hum Genet 1986;72:22.
7. Kohn PH, Whang-Peng J, Levis WR. Chromosomal instability in ataxia telangiectasia. Cancer Genet Cytogenet 1982;6:289.
8. Sparkes RS, Como R, Golde DW. Cytogenetic abnormalities in ataxia telangiectasia with T cell chronic lymphocytic leukemia. Cancer Genet Cytogenet 1980;1:329.
9. Taylor AMR. Cytogenetics of ataxia telangiectasia. In: Bridges BA, Harnden DG, eds. Ataxia-telangiectasia: a cellular link between cancer, neuropathology, and immunodeficiency. New York, John Wiley & Sons, 1982:53.
10. Gatti RA, Berkel I, Boder E, et al. Localization of ataxia-telangiectasia gene to chromosome 11q22-23. Nature 1988;336:577.
10a. Savitsky K, Bar-Shiva A, Gilad S, et al. A single ataxia telangiectasia gene with a product similar to PI-3 kinase. Science 1995;268:1749.
11. Chan JYH, Becker FF, German J, et al. Altered DNA ligase I activity in Bloom's syndrome cells. Nature 1987;325:357.
12. Willis AE, Lindahl T. DNA ligase I deficiency in Bloom's syndrome. Nature 1987;325:355.
12a. Ellis NA, Groden J, Ye T-Z, et al. The Bloom's syndrome gene product is homologous to RecQ helicases. Cell 1995;83:655.
13. Bloom GE, Warner S, Gerald PS, et al. Chromosome abnormalities in constitutional aplastic anemia. N Engl J Med 1966;274:8.
14. Berger R, Bernheim A, Le Coniat M, et al. Chromosomal studies of leukemic and preleukemic Fanconi's anemia patients. Hum Genet 1980;56:59.
15. Butturini A, Gale RP, Verlander PC, et al. Hematologic abnormalities in Fanconi anemia: an International Fanconi Anemia Registry study. Blood 1994;84:1650.
16. Friedberg EC. Xeroderma pigmentosum, Cockayne's syndrome, helicases, and DNA repair: what's the relationship? Cell 1992;71:887.
17. Drapkin R, Sancar A, Reinberg D. Where transcription meets repair. Cell 1994;77:9.
18. Swift M, Morrell D, Massey RB, et al. Incidence of cancer in 161 families affected by ataxia-telangiectasia. N Engl J Med 1991;325:1831.
19. Stram DO, Sposto R, Preston D, et al. Stable chromosome aberrations among A-bomb survivors: an update. Radiat Res 1993;135:29.
20. Rous P. A sarcoma of the fowl transmissible by an agent separable from the tumor cells. J Exp Med 1911;13:397.
21. Bishop JM. Viral oncogenes. Cell 1985;42:23.
22. Bishop JM. Cellular oncogenes and retroviruses. Annu Rev Biochem 1983;52:301.
23. Varmus HE. The molecular genetics of cellular oncogenes. Annu Rev Genet 1984;18:553.
24. Weinberg RA. Tumor suppressor genes. Science 1991;254:1138.
25. Weinberg R. Tumor suppressor genes. Neuron 1993;11:191.
26. Hinds PW, Weinberg RA. Tumor suppressor genes. Curr Opin Genet Dev 1994;4:135.
27. Levine AJ. The tumor suppressor genes. Annu Rev Biochem 1993;62:623.
28. Harris H. The analysis of malignancy by cell fusion: the position in 1988. Cancer Res 1988;48:3302.
29. Stanbridge EJ. Functional evidence for human tumour suppressor genes: chromosome and molecular genetic studies. Cancer Surv 1992;12:5.
30. Anderson MJ, Stanbridge EJ. Tumor suppressor genes studied by cell hybridization and chromosome transfer. FASEB J 1993;7:826.
31. Knudson AG. Mutation and cancer: statistical study of retinoblastoma. Proc Natl Acad Sci USA 1971;68:820.
32. Cowell JK. One hundred years of retinoblastoma research: from the clinic to the gene and back again. Ophthal Paediatr Genet 1989;10:75.
33. Cavenee WK, Dryja TP, Phillips RA, et al. Expression of recessive alleles by chromosomal mechanisms in retinoblastoma. Nature 1983;305:779.

34. Friend SH, Horowitz JM, Gerber R, et al. Deletions of a DNA sequence in retinoblastoma and mesenchymal tumors: organization of the sequences and its encoded protein. Proc Natl Acad Sci USA 1987; 84:9059.

35. Aaltonen LA, Peltomaki P, Leach FS, et al. Clues to the pathogenesis of familial colorectal cancer. Science 1993;260:812.

36. Ionov EL, Peinado MA, Malkhosyan S, et al. Ubiquitous somatic mutations in simple repeated sequences reveal a new mechanism for colonic carcinogenesis. Nature 1993;363:558.

37. Thibodeau SN, Bren G, Schaid D. Microsatellite instability in cancer of the proximal colon. Science 1993;260:816.

38. Liu B, Nicolaides NC, Markowitz S, et al. Mismatch repair gene defects in sporadic colorectal cancers with microsatellite instability. Nature Genet 1995;9:48.

39. Kunkel TA. Slippery DNA and diseases. Nature 1993;365:207.

40. Parsons R, Li G-L, Longley MJ, et al. Hypermutability and mismatch repair deficiency in RER + tumor cells. Cell 1993;75:1227.

41. Service RF. Stalking the start of colon cancer. Science 1994;263:1559.

42. Fishel R, Lescoe MK, Rao MRS, et al. The human mutator gene homolog MSH2 and its association with hereditary nonpolyposis colon cancer. Cell 1993;75:1027.

43. Leach FS, Nicolaides NC, Papadopoulos N, et al. Mutations of a mutS homolog in hereditary nonpolyposis colorectal cancer. Cell 1993;75:1215.

44. Papadopoulos N, Nicolaides NC, Wei Y-F, et al. Mutation of a mutL homolog in hereditary colon cancer. Science 1994;263:1625.

45. Bronner CE, Baker SM, Morrison PT, et al. Mutation in the DNA mismatch repair gene homologue hMLH1 is associated with hereditary non-polyposis colon cancer. Nature 1994;368:258.

46. Nicolaides NC, Papadopoulos N, Liu B, et al. Mutations of two PMS homologues in hereditary nonpolyposis colon cancer. Nature 1994; 371:75.

46a. Palombo F, Gallinari P, Iaccarino I, et al. GTBP, a 160-kilodalton protein essential for mismatch-binding activity in human cells. Science 1995;268:1912.

46b. Papadopoulos N, Nicolaides NC, Liu B, et al. Mutations of GTBP in genetically unstable cells. Science 1995;268:1915.

47. Arends MJ, Wyllie AH. Apoptosis: mechanisms and roles in pathology. Int Rev Exp Pathol 1991;32:223.

48. Wyllie AH. Apoptosis: the 1992 Frank Rose memorial lecture. Br J Cancer 1993;67:205.

49. Tsujimoto Y, Finger LR, Yunis J, et al. Cloning of the chromosome breakpoint of neoplastic B cells with the t(14;18) chromosome translocation. Science 1984;266:1097.

50. Tsujimoto Y, Cossman J, Jaffe E, et al. Involvement of the bcl-2 gene in follicular lymphoma. Science 1985;228:1440.

51. McDonnell TJ, Deane N, Platt F, et al. Bcl-2 immunoglobulin transgenic mice demonstrate extended B cell survival and follicular lymphoproliferation. Cell 1989;57:79.

52. McDonnell TJ, Korsmeyer SJ. Progression from lymphoid hyperplasia to high-grade malignant lymphoma in mice transgenic for the t(14;18). Nature 1991;349.

53. Limpens J, de JOng D, van Krieken JH, et al. Bcl-2/JH rearrangements in benign lymphoid tissues with follicular hyperplasia. Oncogene 1991;6:2271.

54. Greider CW, Blackburn EH. Identification of a specific telomere terminal transferase activity in *Tetrahymena* extracts. Cell 1985;43:405.

55. Greider CW. Chromosome first aid. Cell 1991;67:645.

56. Counter CM, Hairte HW, Bacchetti S, et al. Telomerase activity in human ovarian carcinoma. Proc Natl Acad Sci USA 1994;91:2900.

57. Marx J. Chromosome ends catch fire. Science 1994;265:1656.

58. Kim NW, Piatyszek MA, Prowse KR, et al. Specific association of human telomerase activity with immortal cells and cancer. Science 1994;266:2011.

59. Baserga R. Oncogenes and the strategy of growth factors. Cell 1994; 79:927.

60. Jesse TM, Melton DA. Diffusible factors in vertebrate embryonic induction. Cell 1992;68:257.

61. Beltsholtz C, Westermark B, Ek B, et al. Co-expression of a PDGF-like growth factor and PDGF receptors in a human osteosarcoma cell line: implications for autocrine receptor activation. Cell 1984;39:447.

62. Hirschfeld S, Helman L. Diverse roles of insulin-like growth factors in pediatric solid tumors. In Vivo 1994;8:81.

63. Folkman J, Klagsbrun M. Angiogenic factors. Science 1987;235:442.

64. Sukumar S, Notario V, Martin-Zanca D, et al. Induction of mammary carcinomas in rats by nitroso-methylurea involves malignant activation of H-ras-1 locus by single point mutations. Nature 1983;306:658.

65. Marshall CJ. Specificity of receptor tyrosine kinase signaling: transient versus sustained extracellular signal-regulated kinase activity. Cell 1995;80:179.

66. Crews CM, Erikson RL. Extracellular signals and reversible protein phosphorylation: what to mek of it all. Cell 1993;74:215.

67. Wrana JL, Attisano L, Wieser R, et al. Mechanism of activation of the TGFb receptor. Nature 1994;370:341.

68. Di Fiore PP, Kraus MH. Mechanisms involving an expanding erbB/EGF receptor family of tyrosine kinases in human neoplasia. Cancer Treat Res 1992;61:139.

69. Williams GR. Hormones: solving the specificity puzzle. Nature 1994; 370:330.

70. Hunter T. Protein kinases and phosphatases: the yin and yang of protein phosphorylation and signalling. Cell 1995;80:225.

71. Hill CS, Treisman R. Transcriptional regulation by extracellular signals: mechanisms and specificity. Cell 1995;80:199.

72. Neer EJ. Heterotrimeric G proteins: organizers of transmembrane signals. Cell 1995;80:249.

73. Hepler JR, Gilman AG. G proteins. Trends Biochem Sci 1992;17:383.

74. Lange-Carter CA, Pleiman CM, Gardner AM, et al. A divergence in the MAP kinase regulatory network defined by MEK kinase and raf. Science 1993;260:315.

75. Barbacid M. ras Genes. Annu Rev Biochem 1987;56:779.

76. Marcu KB, Bossone SA, Patel AS. Myc function and regulation. Annu Rev Biochem 1992;61:809.

77. Dalla-Favera R. Chromosomal translocations involving the c-myc oncogene in lymphoid neoplasia. In: Kirsch IR, ed. The causes and consequences of chromosomal aberrations. Boca Raton, FL, CRC Press, 1993.

78. Stewart TA, Pattengale PK, Leder P. Spontaneous mammary adenocarcinomas in transgenic mice that carry and express MTV/myc fusion genes. Cell 1984;38:627.

79. O'Shea EK, Rutkowski R, Kim PS. Mechanism of specificity in the Fos-Jun oncoprotein heterodimer. Cell 1992;68:699.

80. Rabbitts TH. Chromosomal translocations in human cancer. Nature 1994;372:143.

81. Aplan PD, Nakahara K, Orkin SH, et al. The SCL gene product: a positive regulator of erythroid differentiation. EMBO J 1992;11:4073.

82. Warren AJ, Colledge WH, Carlton MBL, et al. The oncogenic cysteine-rich LIM domain protein Rbtn2 is essential for erythroid development. Cell 1994;78:45.

83. Valge-Archer VE, Osada H, Warren AJ, et al. The LIM protein RBTN2 and the basic helix-loop-helix protein TAL1 are present in a complex in erythroid cells. Proc Natl Acad Sci USA 1994;91:8617.

84. Chen Q, Cheng J-T, Tsai L-H, et al. The tal gene undergoes chromosome translocation in T-cell leukemia and potentially encodes a helix-loop-helix protein. EMBO J 1990;9:415.

85. Aplan PD, Lombardi DP, Reaman GH, et al. Involvement of the putative hematopoietic transcription factor SCL in T-cell acute lymphoblastic leukemia. Blood 1992;79:1327.

86. Hartwell LH, Kastan MB. Cell cycle control and cancer. Science 1994; 266:1821.

87. Heichman KA, Roberts JM. Rules to replicate by. Cell 1994;79:557.

88. Nurse P. Ordering S phase and M phase in the cell cycle. Cell 1994; 79:547.

89. Sherr CJ. G1 phase progression: cycling on cue. Cell 1994;79:551.

90. Yuspa SH, Dlugosz AA, Cheng CK, et al. Role of oncogenes and tumor suppressor genes in multistage carcinogenesis. J Invest Dermatol 1994;103:90S.

91. Kaye FJ, Kratzke RA, Gerster JL, et al. A single amino acid substitution results in a retinoblastoma protein defective in phosphorylation and oncoprotein binding. Proc Natl Acad Sci USA 1990;87:6922.

92. Hunter T, Pines J. Cyclins and cancer. II. Cyclin D and CDK inhibitors come of age. Cell 1994;79:573.

93. Pines J. Arresting developments in cell-cycle control. Trends Biochem Sci 1994;19:143.

94. Otterson GA, Kratzke RA, Coxon A, et al. Absence of p16(INK4) protein is restricted to the subset of lung cancer cell lines that retains wildtype RB. Oncogene 1994;9:3375.

95. Peter M, Herskowitz I. Joining the complex: cyclin-dependent kinase inhibitory proteins and the cell cycle. Cell 1994;79:181.

96. Hartwell LH, Weinert TA. Checkpoints: controls that ensure the order of cell cycle events. Science 1989;246:629.

97. Oltvai ZN, Korsmeyer SJ. Checkpoints of dueling dimers foil death wishes. Cell 1994;79:189.

98. Kastan MB, Zhan Q, El-Deiry WS, et al. A mammalian cell cycle checkpoint pathway utilizing p53 and GADD45 is defective in ataxia-telangiectasia. Cell 1992;71:587.

99. Kuerbitz SJ, Plunkett BS, Walsh WV, et al. Wild-type p53 is a cell cycle checkpoint determinant following irradiation. Proc Natl Acad Sci USA 1992;89:7491.

100. Harris DD, Hollstein M. Clinical implications of the p53 tumor-suppressor gene. N Engl J Med 1993;329:1318.

101. Harris CC. p53: At the crossroads of molecular carcinogenesis and risk assessment. Science 1993;262:1980.

102. Lane DP. p53 and human cancers. Br Med Bull 1994;50:582.

102a. Cho Y, Gorina S, Jeffrey PD, et al. Crystal structure of a p53 tumor suppressor–DNA complex: understanding tumorigenic mutations. Science 1994;265:346.

103. Fearon ER, Vogelstein B. A genetic model for colorectal tumorigenesis. Cell 1990;61:759.

104. Vogelstein B. A deadly inheritance. Nature 1990;348:681.

105. Vogelstein B, Kinzler KW. The multistep nature of cancer. Trends Genet 1993;9:138.

106. Pizzo PA, Poplack DG. Principles and practice of pediatric oncology. Philadelphia, JB Lippincott, 1993.

107. Gallie BL. The misadventures of RB1. In: Kirsch IR, ed. The causes and consequences of chromosomal aberrations. Boca Raton, FL, CRC Press, 1993:429.

108. Williamson KA, van Heyningen V. Towards an understanding of Wilms' tumour. Int J Exp Pathol 1994;75:147.

109. Coppes MJ, Haber DA, Grundy PE. Genetic events in the development of Wilms' tumor. N Engl J Med 1994;331:586.

110. Pelletier J. Molecular genetics of Wilms' tumor: insights into normal and abnormal renal development. Can J Oncol 1994;4:262.

111. Coppes MJ, Williams BR. The molecular genetics of Wilms tumor. Cancer Invest 1994;12:57.

112. Koo HP, Hensle TW. Molecular biology of Wilms' tumor. Urol Clin North Am 1993;20:323.

113. Knudson AG Jr. Introduction to the genetics of primary renal tumors in children. Med Pediatr Oncol 1993;21:193.

114. Hastie ND. Wilms' tumour gene and function. Curr Opin Genet Dev 1993;3:408.

115. Schussheim A, Gold D. Isn't it time to rethink familial adenomatous polyposis? Am J Gastroenterol 1994;89:1116.

116. Lynch HT, Smyrk T, Watson P, et al. Hereditary colorectal cancer. Semin Oncol 1991;18:337.

117. Li FP, Fraumeni JFJ. Prospective study of a family cancer syndrome. JAMA 1982;247:2692.

118. Strong LC, Stine M, Norsted TL. Cancer in survivors of childhood soft tissue sarcoma and their relatives. J Natl Cancer Inst 1987;79:1213.

119. Malkin D, Li FP, Strong LC, et al. Germ line p53 mutations in a familial syndrome of breast cancer, sarcomas, and other neoplasms. Science 1990;250:1233.

120. Gutmann DH. New insights into the neurofibromatoses. Curr Opin Neurol 1994;7:166.

121. Ponder BA. Neurofibromatosis: from gene to phenotype. Semin Cancer Biol 1992;3:115.

122. Pykett MJ, Murphy M, Harnish PR, et al. The neurofibromatosis 2 (NF2) tumor suppressor gene encodes multiple alternatively spliced transcripts. Hum Mol Genet 1994;3:559.

123. Viskochil D, White R, Cawthon R. The neurofibromatosis type 1 gene. Annu Rev Neurosci 1993;16:183.

124. Hall A. Signal transduction through small GTPases: a tale of two GAPs. Cell 1992;69:389.

125. Radinsky R, Fidler IJ. Regulation of tumor cell growth at organ-specific metastasis. In Vivo 1992;6:325.

126. Fidler IJ, Ellis LM. The implications of angiogenesis for the biology and therapy of cancer metastasis. Cell 1994;79:185.

127. Stetler-Stevenson WG, Aznavoorian S, Liotta LA. Tumor cell interactions with the extracellular matrix during invasion and metastasis. Annu Rev Cell Biol 1993;9:541.

Surgery of Infants and Children: Scientific Principles and Practice, edited by Keith T. Oldham, Paul M. Colombani, and Robert P. Foglia. Lippincott–Raven Publishers, Philadelphia, © 1997.

CHAPTER 32

Angiogenesis and Hemangiomas

Judah Folkman, John B. Mulliken, and R. Alan B. Ezekowitz

Angiogenesis is the process of new blood vessel growth and is an essential component of reproduction, development, and repair. A hallmark of physiologic angiogenesis is its regulation. It is turned on and off in a predictable manner; in ovulation and wound repair it is activated for only a few days. During angiogenesis, microvascular endothelial cells can migrate rapidly[1] (up to 0.2 to 0.3 mm/d in the rabbit cornea) and can proliferate as rapidly as bone marrow cells, which are among the fastest-growing cells in the body.[2] However, for long periods of time, microvascular endothelial cells are among the most quiescent cells of the body.

A major feature of pathologic angiogenesis is persistent growth of blood vessels. In diseases such as diabetic retinopathy, unabated neovascularization appears to have overcome natural suppressors of blood vessel growth. Angiogenesis that continues for months or years sustains the progression of many other nonneoplastic diseases such as psoriasis, arthritis, and several forms of chronic inflammation.[3] Progressive tumor growth is angiogenesis dependent, and absence of neovascularization or complete blockade of angiogenesis can restrict tumor volume to less than 1 to 2 mm^3 or to a microscopic in situ lesion.[4]

The vascular endothelium is a monolayer of approximately 1000 m^2, an area that would cover a tennis court.[5] An angiogenic focus appears as only a tiny fraction of this area or a small ''hot spot'' of proliferating and migrating endothelial cells that originate from this expanse of resting endothelium. The ultimate goal of antiangiogenic therapy is to return such a neovascular focus to its normal resting state or to prevent its occurrence.

HISTORY OF ANGIOGENESIS RESEARCH

Early Studies of Tumor Blood Vessels

In the first part of this century, most pathologists assumed that simple dilation of existing host blood vessels accounted

for the increased vascularity observed in tumor hyperemia.[6,7] Vasodilation was considered to be a side effect of tumor growth, possibly a result of catabolites released by the tumor. However, a report in 1939 showed that a tumor implant in a transparent chamber in a rabbit ear was associated with accelerated growth of capillary blood vessels in comparison to wound neovascularization, which regressed completely after the wound had healed.[8] Another report in 1945 revealed that new vessels in the neighborhood of a tumor implant arose from host vessels and not from the tumor itself.[9]

Despite these results, which clearly suggested that tumor hyperemia could be related to *new* blood vessel growth (ie, neovascularization) and not solely to vasodilation, a debate continued in the literature for two more decades about whether tumors were supplied by preexisting vessels or by new vessels.[10] Even after a few investigators had begun to accept the notion of tumor-induced neovascularization, a general belief persisted that any vascular response in a tumor was a host inflammatory reaction and was not necessary for tumor growth.[11]

Tumor Growth Depends on Induction of New Microvessels

Tumor Growth Is Angiogenesis-Dependent

In 1971, one of us (J.F.) proposed a different way of thinking about the role of blood vessels in tumor growth in the form of a hypothesis that tumor growth is angiogenesis dependent.[12] I suggested that tumor cells and vascular endothelial cells within a neoplasm ''may constitute a highly integrated ecosystem'' and that endothelial cells may be switched from a resting state to a rapid growth phase by a ''diffusible'' chemical signal from tumor cells. An additional speculation was that angiogenesis could be a relevant target for tumor therapy (ie, antiangiogenic therapy). Because of the confusion between inflammation and angiogenesis that existed then, I attempted to distinguish between the two processes. The experiments that gave rise to these ideas had been carried out in the early 1960s, and revealed that tumor growth in isolated perfused organs was severely restricted in association with absence of vascularization of the tumors.[13–18]

Portions of this chapter were adapted in part from a review in Folkman J, Mulliken JB, Ezekowitz RAB. Antiangiogenic therapy of haemangiomas with interferon A. In: Stuart-Harris R, Penny R, eds. The clinical applications of the interferons. London, Chapman & Hall, 1996 (in press).

These ideas were not accepted at the time. Although a few investigators in the early 1970s had begun to believe that tumors might induce neovascularization, this process was still widely assumed to be an inflammatory host response and possibly detrimental to the tumor. It was also thought that vessels induced by a tumor would become "established" and thus could not undergo involution. Furthermore, compelling evidence that tumors actually depended on neovascularization for their continued growth was lacking. The prevailing wisdom was that tumors could somehow develop around preexisting vasculature. Acceptance of the hypothesis was further hindered because the 1971 report appeared 8 years before it would become possible to grow capillary endothelial cells in vitro,[19] 11 years before the discovery of the first angiogenesis inhibitor,[20] and 13 years before the purification of the first angiogenic protein.[21]

Throughout the 1970s, our laboratory studies were devoted to proving that tumor vessels were new proliferating capillaries; elucidating the sequential steps of the angiogenic process to understand how angiogenesis might be inhibited; developing bioassays so that angiogenesis could be quantified[22]; demonstrating that viable tumor cells released diffusible angiogenic factors that stimulated new capillary growth and endothelial mitosis in vivo,[5,23,24] even when tumor cell proliferation had been arrested by irradiation[25]; and showing that necrotic tumor products were not angiogenic per se (reviewed in Folkman and Cotran[26]). All of these efforts were designed to provide supporting evidence that tumor growth was angiogenesis dependent. Thus, although the field of angiogenesis research originated from an attempt to understand tumor angiogenesis, investigators currently in the field study a wide spectrum of subjects, from developmental biology to molecular genetics, and in a variety of clinical specialties, from cardiology to ophthalmology. Some of the key reports from the Folkman laboratory that form the experimental basis for translation from laboratory to clinical studies are summarized in Table 32-1.

Experimental Evidence Demonstrating That Tumor Growth Is Angiogenesis Dependent

By the mid-1980s, considerable indirect evidence had been assembled to support the hypothesis that tumor growth is angiogenesis dependent. By this time, the idea could be stated in its simplest terms: "Once tumor take has occurred, every further increase in tumor cell population must be preceded by an increase in new capillaries which converge upon the tumor."[5,27] Thus, although neovascularization is necessary but not sufficient for expansion of a tumor, the *absence* of neovascularization prevents expansion of a primary tumor mass beyond 1 to 2 mm³, and may restrict a metastasis to a microscopic, dormant lesion. Most nonneovascularized tumors are not clinically detectable, with the exception of surface lesions on the skin or the external mucous membranes.

Indirect Evidence

Before it was possible selectively or specifically to block the proliferation of tumor blood vessels, indirect experimental evidence was accumulated to support the hypothesis that tumor growth is angiogenesis dependent. The indirect evidence was based on: 1) quantification of the limits to expansion of tumor spheroids in vitro where there is no blood supply; 2) in vivo studies in which a tumor mass is separated from its vascular bed in the rabbit eye; and 3) measurements of tumors still in the prevascular stage of tumor progression.[28–43]

Direct Evidence

By the late 1980s, it was possible to block angiogenesis in a tumor bed without physically separating the tumor from its vascular supply. These experiments provided the first direct evidence that tumor growth was angiogenesis dependent. In some cases a dormant microscopic state was achieved:

1. An angiogenesis inhibitor, TNP-470 (AGM-1470), a synthetic analogue of fumagillin, selectively inhibits proliferating endothelial cells in vitro and in vivo and potently inhibits tumor growth in vivo, but not in vitro.[44]
2. When the cDNA for human basic fibroblast growth factor (bFGF) hybridized to a signal sequence is transfected into normal mouse fibroblasts, the transfected fibroblasts become tumorigenic, export bFGF, and are also angiogenic,[45] When specific antibody against the secreted bFGF is administered to the tumor-bearing mice, there is a dramatic decrease in neovascularization and tumor growth.
3. In a similar experiment, a neutralizing antibody to the angiogenic protein, vascular endothelial growth factor (VEGF), when administered to mice whose tumors use VEGF as a mediator of angiogenesis, results in greater than 90% inhibition of tumor growth.[46]
4. The growth of a brain tumor in nude mice is significantly inhibited or prevented when tumor angiogenesis is suppressed by a strategy in which a dominant-negative mutant of the receptor (*Flk-1*) for the angiogenic peptide VEGF is introduced into host endothelial cells (carried by a retrovirus). When the endothelial cells express this defective receptor, they are unable to respond to VEGF released by the tumor. Thus, they cannot form new capillary blood vessels in response to VEGF released by the tumor.[47]
5. Transformed cells are not tumorigenic until after they have became angiogenic.[48]
6. Specific immunologic inhibition of overexpression of the integrin $\alpha_v\beta_3$ on capillary endothelial cells produces apoptosis of proliferating endothelial cells, blocks neovascularization, and causes tumor regression.[49]
7. The most compelling direct evidence that tumor growth is angiogenesis dependent is based on administration of angiostatin to tumor-bearing mice.[50] Angiostatin is a 38-kD internal fragment of plasminogen, which is a specific inhibitor of proliferating endothelial cells. It does not inhibit tumor cells or other nonendothelial cells in vitro. It is capable of complete blockade of angiogenesis in certain tumors and near-complete blockade in others. When administered systemically to tumor-bearing mice, it holds metastases in a microscopic avascular dormant state of approximately 200 μm diameter.

TABLE 32-1. *Studies from the Folkman Laboratory that have contributed to the development of angiogenesis research*

Year	Development	Reference
NEW CONCEPTS		
1971	Tumors are angiogenesis dependent	12
1972	Antiangiogenic therapy proposed; angiogenesis inhibitors predicted	15
1978	Cell shape regulates cell growth	131
1987	"Angiogenic diseases"	132
1989	Switch to the angiogenic phenotype	40
1995	Unifying mechanisms for presenting patterns of human metastases	133
1995	Tumor dormancy: novel mechanism proposed	134
NEW METHODS		
1963	Tumor growth in isolated perfused organs	13
1972	Organ culture of endothelium in aortic rings	135
1973	Culture of human umbilical vein endothelial cells	136
1974	Rabbit cornea bioassay	33
1974	Chick embryo bioassay	137
1976	Sustained-release polymers for proteins	138
1979	Cloning of capillary endothelial cells	19
1980	Angiogenesis in vitro	139
1989	Biaffinity chromatography for bFGF	140
1994	Quantification of angiogenesis in the chick embryo	141
EXPERIMENTAL FINDINGS		
1971	Isolation of a soluble angiogenic factor (TAF)	23
1972	Indirect evidence that tumor growth is angiogenesis dependent	32
1972	Tumor vessels contain *new* endothelium	142
1975	Tumor angiogenesis activity not inhibited by irradiation	25
1976	Confluent endothelial cells refractory to mitogens	143
1979	Fibrin induces endothelial motility in vitro	144
1979	Elevated angiogenic activity in aqueous fluid of eyes of patients with ocular tumors	145
1980	Administration of an angiogenesis inhibitor to mice and inhibition of tumor growth	146
1980	Demonstration of angiogenic activity in human bladder	147
1980	Heparin potentiates angiogenesis	112
1982	Platelet factor-4 is an angiogenesis inhibitor	20
1984	bFGF, first angiogenic protein purified	21
1985	Angiostatic steroids	148
1987	bFGF is stored in extracellular matrix	149
1990	Healing of duodenal ulcers in rats by oral bFGF	150
1990	Discovery of fungal-derived angiogenesis inhibitor (AGM-1470)	44
1991	Tumor neovascularization is a prognostic indicator in human tumors	151
1992	Clinical study: inhibition of "pure" angiogenesis in children with life-threatening hemangiomas	102
1993	Urinary bFGF level is a diagnostic marker for bladder cancer	152
1993	Betacellulin discovered	153
1993	Vascularization in prostate cancer is a strong prognostic marker	154
1994	Thalidomide is an angiogenesis inhibitor	155
1994	Mediators of angiogenesis in childhood hemangioma are found to be bFGF and VEGF	128
1994	Vascularization in brain tumors and bFGF in cerebrospinal fluid are prognostic markers for risk of recurrence	126
1994	VEGF mediates retinal ischemia	156
1994	Angiostatin discovered	50
1995	Interleukin-12 is an angiogenesis inhibitor	157

bFGF, basic fibroblast growth factor; VEGF, vascular endothelial growth factor.

Lessons Learned About Tumor Angiogenesis

As direct evidence has been assembled to support the essential role of angiogenesis in tumor growth, the angiogenic properties of tumors have become more widely understood.

It is now clear that the presence of angiogenesis does not distinguish between a benign and a malignant tumor.[51] Adrenal adenomas are benign tumors that are highly neovascularized, but appear to lack the growth potential to take advantage of the new blood vessels they have induced. Thus, the onset of angiogenesis *permits* expansion of a tumor mass, but does not guarantee it. In fact, the switch to the angiogenic phenotype may occur independently of other events in tumorigenesis. In most tumors, angiogenesis appears after the expression of the malignant phenotype. However, in carcinoma of the cervix, the preneoplastic stage of dysplasia becomes neovascularized before the malignant tumor appears.[52] This sequence of events also occurs in certain spontaneously arising tumors in animals.[53]

Furthermore, angiogenesis may not be necessary for certain tumor cells that can grow as a flat sheet between membranes (ie, gliomatosis in the meninges). Another observation is that antiangiogenic therapy can bring about involution of growing vessels,[54] which may lead to regression of growing tumors.[55–57] When this result is taken into account with the fact that the replication rate of endothelial cells in tumor capillary vessels is significantly greater than in the endothelial cells of normal tissue (often approaching differences of 100-fold),[2] it is probably inaccurate to think of tumor vessels as "established." It is also not accurate to describe tumors as outgrowing their blood supply. Growing tumors can gradually *compress* their blood supply because of increasing interstitial pressure. These compressed areas become ischemic, but they are not avascular. Necrosis follows. Vessel compression also interferes with the optimal delivery of therapeutic agents.[58] Paradoxically, antiangiogenic therapy can decrease ischemia, apparently as a result of decreased interstitial pressure.

Angiogenic Factors

A family of angiogenic proteins mediates physiologic and pathologic angiogenesis. The known angiogenic factors are listed in Table 32-2. bFGF, acidic FGF, and VEGF are the most commonly identified angiogenic proteins in human tumors as well as in reproductive and developmental angiogenesis.[59] Virtually all of the other angiogenic proteins have been found to be expressed or produced by human tumors.

Endogenous Inhibitors of Endothelial Cell Proliferation

It is becoming recognized that the switch to the angiogenic phenotype by tumors is the result of a net balance between positive and negative regulators of blood vessel growth.[78,79] For many tumors, it is not sufficient that the tumor cells express an angiogenic protein such as VEGF. Natural endothelial inhibitors that were expressed by the normal precursor cell or by neighboring host cells must be down-regulated before the angiogenic switch can occur.[40] This new concept has emerged only since the late 1980s. It has led to a better understanding of the role of endogenous inhibitors of endothelial growth and to a renewed interest in the discovery of other such inhibitors, either in tumors, normal tissues, or in the circulation. Some of the known endogenous inhibitors are listed in Table 32-3.

HEMANGIOMAS OF INFANCY

Hemangiomas that occur in infancy are made up of proliferating capillary blood vessels and represent a form of neovascularization that is not driven by an inflammatory component. Hemangiomas occur in approximately 1 of 100 normal newborns and in 1 of 5 premature infants with a birth weight below 1000 g; they grow rapidly for the first year of life (the proliferating phase), slow down during the next 5 years (involuting phase), and then gradually regress by age 10 to 15 years of age (the involuted phase).[88,89] Most hemangiomas do not need treatment and it is safe to wait for them to undergo natural involution, although during these years of waiting, there is undoubtedly a psychologic burden on the family members. However, approximately 10% of hemangiomas cause serious tissue damage and approximately 1% are life threatening. Thus, hemangiomas in the airway or liver can cause respiratory distress or heart failure, respectively. Large hemangiomas in any location can be the cause of platelet-trapping thrombocytopenic coagulopathy (ie, the Kasabach-Merritt phenomenon). Hepatic hemangiomas may have a high mortality, even without platelet trapping.[89,90]

For more than 25 years, corticosteroids have been the standard therapy world-wide, for serious or life-threatening hemangiomas. However, this therapy leaves much room for improvement. In only 30% of infants do hemangiomas undergo rapid involution (eg, regression of the lesion beginning in 1 week),[89] and these patients are at increased risk for infection, peptic

TABLE 32-2. *Endogenous angiogenic factors*

Growth factor	Molecular weight	Endothelial mitogen (in vitro)	Year reported	Reference
Fibroblast growth factors				
Basic FGF	18,000	+	1984	21
Acidic FGF	16,400	+	1984	60, 61
Angiogenin	14,100	0	1985	62
Transforming growth factor-α	5,500	+	1986	63
Transforming growth factor-β	25,000	$-$*	1986	64, 85
Tumor necrosis factor α	17,000	$-$	1987	65, 66
Vascular endothelial growth factor (VPF/VEGF)	45,000	+	1983 / 1989	67 / 68–70
Platelet-derived endothelial cell growth factor	45,000	DNA synthesis	1989	71
Granulocyte colony-stimulating factor	17,000	+	1991	72
Placental growth factor	25,000	+/0	1991	73
Interleukin-8	40,000	+	1992	74
Hepatocyte growth factor	92,000	+	1992	75, 76
Proliferin	35,000	+	1994	77

* TGF-β inhibits endothelial proliferation in vitro, but a focal injection in vivo stimulates angiogenesis.

TABLE 32-3. *Endogenous negative regulators of endothelial proliferation*

	Inhibits proliferation	Inhibits chemotaxis	In circulation	In extracellular matrix	Reference
Platelet factor-4	+	+	+	−	20, 80, 81, 82
Thrombospondin	+	+	+	+	
Tissue inhibitors of metalloproteinases† (TIMP)	+/0	+	+	+	83, 84
16-kd fragment of prolactin	+				
Angiostatin (38-kd fragment of plasminogen)	+	+			79
Basic fibroblast growth factor (bFGF) soluble receptor‡	+		+		85
Transforming growth factor-β (TGF-β)	+	+	+		64, 85, 86, 87
Interferon-α	+	+	+		96
Placental proliferin-related protein	+				77

* All are angiogenesis inhibitors in vivo except TGF-β.

† TIMP-2 inhibits proliferation and chemotaxis, TIMP-1 and TIMP-3 do not. TIMP-1 and TIMP-2 circulate and TIMP-3 is in the extracellular matrix.

‡ bFGF receptor has not been tested in vivo as an angiogenesis inhibitor.

ulceration, hyperglycemia, poor wound healing, and stunted growth. Few studies have examined the subsequent development of premature babies and newborns treated with corticosteroids for the first 6 months of life. Furthermore, 40% of hemangiomas respond equivocally and 30% do not respond at all.[89] In some cases, corticosteroids have clearly accelerated growth of the hemangioma. When hemangiomas continue to grow despite corticosteroid treatment, there are no satisfactory substitutes, although there are anecdotal reports of favorable outcomes from radiation,[91] cyclophosphamide,[92] and embolization.[93,94]

Discovery of Interferon-α as an Angiogenesis Inhibitor

During the 1980s, a series of in vitro and in vivo experiments revealed that interferon-α had antiangiogenic activity, although this activity is not as potent as that of angiogenesis inhibitors subsequently discovered.[4] Zetter first demonstrated in 1980 that a mixture of mouse interferons could inhibit motility of capillary endothelial cells in vitro.[95] Subsequently, others found that interferon-α inhibited angiogenesis in vivo in experimental animals.[96,97]

On the basis of these laboratory findings, the senior author (J.F.), in response to a call from Carl White in Denver, advised the use of interferon-α in his patient, a 7-year-old boy with pulmonary hemangiomatosis that was unresponsive to corticosteroids. At that time (1988), no angiogenesis inhibitors were in clinical trial and interferon-α was an approved drug, although it had not been previously used as an angiogenesis inhibitor. Administration of interferon-α2a at 3 million U/m^2/d subcutaneously produced regression of the lesions and relief of symptoms in this patient. He was thus the first to be treated with interferon-α because of its antiangiogenic property, and White and colleagues' 1989 report[98] appears to be the first demonstration of antiangiogenic therapy in a human.[99] Other investigators subsequently confirmed the efficacy of interferon-α for sight-, tissue-, and life-threatening hemangiomas.[100–106]

At this writing, interferon-α is considered a second-line drug, most often used for endangering hemangiomas that do not respond to corticosteroids. However, it has been successfully used as a first-line drug by us and by others instead of corticosteroids, for example when corticosteroids are contraindicated or refused by parents. The dose of interferon-α is not well established. The empiric dose is 3×10^6 U/m^2/d, given subcutaneously, but slightly higher doses (eg, 3.5 to 4.0 million U/m^2/d) may be necessary for large hemangiomas, especially if thrombocytopenia is persistent. It appears to be important to administer interferon-α every day; there is a reported failure of interferon-α therapy when given only three times per week.[107] Interferon-α2b has also been used successfully,[108,109] but there is a report of failure of interferon-α2b.[110]

In 1992, we documented accelerated regression in 18 of 20 treated infants and children with either tissue-, sight-, or life-threatening hemangiomas in various cutaneous and visceral locations.[54] Our ongoing experience in another 30 infants with endangering hemangiomas, treated since the 1992 publication, confirms this response. Interferon therapy must be continued, on average, for 6 to 10 months of daily subcutaneous injections. Interferon-α works slowly and regression of a hemangioma is not as rapid as when a hemangioma is a good responder to corticosteroids. Thus, in some situations, for example hemangioma of the upper eyelid, interferon may be too slow to relieve pressure on the cornea to prevent astigmatism. But the complications of local injections of corticosteroid (eg, retinal embolization) are also risky. Therefore, surgical excision is indicated for certain periorbital lesions.[111] Interferon-α has, however, proved to be effective for intraorbital hemangiomas that are refractory to systemic corticosteroids.

Platelet-Trapping Coagulopathy

Thrombocytopenia may be associated with hemangiomas secondary to platelet trapping in the tumor. This is the Kasabach-Merritt phenomenon. In the absence of clinical bleeding, we have learned to avoid the infusion of platelets and blood products for this type of thrombocytopenic coagulopathy. We find that infused platelets are trapped within the hemangioma and cause rapid swelling (within hours) and rebound thrombocytopenia. Transfusions of packed red cells may be required if the hematocrit falls to the low 20% range.

Kasabach-Merritt thrombocytopenia has often been confused with the phenomenon of disseminated intravascular coagulopathy, which sometimes occurs with venous malformations. We find that heparin therapy, a mainstay for the treatment of disseminated intravascular coagulopathy, is contraindicated in infants with Kasabach-Merritt coagulopathy. In experimental studies, heparin potentiates the effect of growth factors on endothelial cells in vitro,[20,112,113] accelerates tumor angiogenesis in vivo,[55] and mobilizes bFGF, a potent angiogenic protein, from extracellular matrix. It may also mobilize other endothelial mitogens such as VEGF. In our early clinical experience with life-threatening Kasabach-Merritt coagulopathy,[54] we observed that heparin, used as conventional treatment of the coagulopathy, accelerated hemangioma growth. Thereafter, we no longer use heparin in infants with hemangiomas and associated thrombocytopenia.

Liver Hemangiomas

For a critically ill infant presenting with a liver mass and congestive failure, the differential diagnosis is hepatic hemangioma versus hepatic arteriovenous malformation (see Folkman and coworkers[87] for review). Mortality rates for hepatic hemangioma (also called hemangioendothelioma) are high,[89] in part because of the difficulty in distinguishing between hepatic hemangioma and arteriovenous malformation.[90,114] In an analysis of a 25-year experience with intrahepatic vascular anomalies, we found 10% of infants had arteriovenous malformation.[115] Hepatomegaly, congestive heart failure, and anemia can be the presenting signs in newborns with either focal hepatic hemangioma or arteriovenous malformation. In contrast, by 1 to 16 weeks of age, a pattern can be seen of multiple hepatic hemangiomas and multiple cutaneous hemangiomas accompanied by hepatomegaly, heart failure, and anemia. Hepatic arteriovenous malformation requires embolization or surgical resection. Interferon-α is not effective therapy for vascular malformations, whether venous or arterial, mainly because these lesions do not contain proliferating capillaries. These errors of vascular morphogenesis appear to involve, at the very least, abnormalities of smooth muscle. For example, venous malformations appear to be deficient in smooth muscle layers.

In our series of 34 liver hemangiomas, the mortality from surgical resection (used exclusively for solitary lesions) was 25% (n = 2/8). Mortality was 43% when hepatic embolization was used for both solitary and multiple hemangiomas (n = 3/7). The mortality was 20% (n = 4/20) when corticosteroids were the first-line therapy. When 11 patients who had failed corticosteroid therapy subsequently received interferon-α therapy, mortality was decreased to 9% (n = 1/11).

Airway Hemangioma

Conventional treatment for airway hemangiomas causing stridor in infants is corticosteroid therapy and excision with CO_2 laser.[116,117] In our institution, members of the Department of Otolaryngology successfully used interferon-α to treat 15 infants with life-threatening subglottic hemangioma who had failed corticosteroid or laser therapy.[106] The mean duration of therapy was 11 months (range, 2 to 31 months).

Kaposi-Like Hemangioma

Kaposi-like infantile hemangioma is rare and is usually unresponsive to therapy, including corticosteroids, embolization, and irradiation.[118–120] There are few reported survivors. The lesion appears later in infancy and is commonly associated with severe Kasabach-Merritt coagulopathy. The unfavorable histologic features are infiltrative sheets and nodules of slender, proliferating endothelial cells admixed with areas of spindle cells surrounded by dilated lymphatic-like spaces. We have given interferon-α to five children with these lethal tumors. Two died from extensively invasive retroperitoneal tumor. A third child is alive at 3 years with a cervicomediastinal tumor, thrombocytopenia, and a tracheostomy, having failed to respond to either corticosteroids, interferon-α, or embolization. Two children are currently receiving interferon-α for large Kaposi-like tumors involving the shoulders and upper arms. They remain thrombocytopenic at this writing.

Cavernous Hemangioma

A histologic section of a vascular lesion that is thought to be a cavernous hemangioma will usually show the lesion to be a venous malformation, especially if the tissue is from a patient older than 10 years of age. Venous malformations consist of large venous structures that resemble varicose veins except for a dearth of vascular smooth muscle. In fact, there may be only one layer of smooth muscle encircling a large lumen that would normally be multilayered. The term ''hemangioma'' is a misnomer for these lesion and may lead to the inappropriate use of interferon. Interferon-α should *not* be used for so-called ''cavernous hemangiomas'' because it could inhibit endothelial growth, which may increase the risk of hemorrhage.

Toxicities of Interferon-α

Most children treated with interferon-α manifest fever up to 39°C during the first 1 to 2 weeks of therapy. Pretreatment with acetaminophen, 1 to 2 hours before injection, ameliorates the febrile response. Daily subcutaneous injection of interferon-α is given in the evening. Toxic side effects of interferon-α are usually reversible. These include an up to fivefold elevation of liver enzymes, transient neutropenia, and anemia. Neutropenia is ascribed to ''margination'' of white cells against the walls of vessels; it is not thought to be caused by suppression of bone marrow. We have not had to terminate therapy prematurely because of these side effects. Most infants on interferon-α gain weight and grow normally, in contrast to infants on prolonged high-dose corticosteroids. Two infants treated with interferon-α had accelerated regression of their lesions, but loss of appetite required discontinuation of therapy. In one patient, a treatment failure, a higher dose of 6 million U/m^2 resulted in hyperactivity for 1 day. A more worrisome possible adverse reaction is the development of long tract signs and increased motor tone in the lower limbs, previously reported in some children receiving interferon-α for laryngeal papillomas.[121] We have observed the development of spastic diaparesis in the lower extremities of 5 infants selected from 55 infants treated with interferon.[121a] The condition is potentially reversible. In 2 infants, recovery occurred after interferon was discontinued. Magnetic resonance imaging showed no significant brain or spinal abnormalities, except minor-to-moderate delayed myelination in 2 patients. Myelination was normal on subsequent radiographic examination in all patients. We recommend careful clinical assessment of neurodevelopmental status during interferon therapy. If signs of diaparesis appear, interferon should be discontinued, or, if the hemangioma continues to be endangering or life-threatening, the dose should be reduced and the risk-benefit ratio be reassessed. "Cotton wool" retinal spots that have occasionally been observed in adults on higher doses of interferon-α therapy[122] have not, to our knowledge, been reported in any children on interferon-α, nor have these spots been seen in any of our patients.

Protocol for Interferon-α Therapy

Infants with hemangiomas that are destructive (eg, deep ulceration of nose or ear), distorting (eg, protrusion of eye), obstructing (eg, airway occlusion), or life threatening (eg, heart failure, thrombocytopenia) are eligible for the interferon protocol. Initially, we try a 2-week course of oral corticosteroids (prednisolone) at a dose of 2 to 3 mg/kg/d. If the tumor displays an obvious response, such as decreased turgor, pallor, arrest of growth, or shrinkage, then corticosteroids are continued for 4 weeks at this concentration. Subsequently, the prednisolone is gradually reduced to a maintenance level of 1 mg/kg and then to 1 to 2 mg/d over a period of 8 to 10 months.

There are at least four indications for interferon treatment of a serious or life-threatening hemangioma:

- Failure to respond to corticosteroids or equivocal response
- Contraindication to long- term corticosteroid therapy (eg, infection, vomiting, or gastrointestinal bleeding)
- Complication of corticosteroid administration (eg, stunted growth or lack of weight gain)
- Parental refusal of corticosteroids

If corticosteroids fail, tapering dosage is begun at or before initiation of interferon therapy. The initial dose for interferon is 1 million U/m^2, and this is increased over 3 to 7 days to 3 million U/m^2 subcutaneously. Interferon-α can be administered during the corticosteroid taper, but we do not recommend coadministration of full therapeutic doses of corticosteroids and interferon. We have no evidence that the two drugs are synergistic. In fact, their combined use may increase toxicity and decrease efficacy.

Our preprotocol evaluation includes complete blood count, liver enzymes, thyroid function tests, photography, and ultrasonography or radiography where indicated, and a urinary level of bFGF (see later).

The most difficult problem experienced by all physicians who care for infants with serious or life-threatening hemangiomas is how to quantify the involution of hemangiomas during a given treatment. Different parameters are required for hemangiomas in different locations. In many situations, a subjective clinical judgment is the only available method, similar to the estimation of "percent pneumothorax" or "percent third-degree burn." Airway hemangiomas require endoscopy for evaluation. Liver hemangiomas can be measured by magnetic resonance imaging, but even this approach is confounded by growth of the child between imaging examinations, and also by conversion of some involuting hemangiomas to fatty tissue. Skin hemangiomas require multiple serial photographs, but description of tissue turgor, warmth over the lesion, and return of function of a limb are just as valuable, regardless of how subjective they may seem.

For infants discharged from the hospital on interferon-α, we have found it helpful to see them approximately every 3 months, if possible. All of the tests are repeated at these intervals whenever possible. (If the lesion has undergone dramatic regression, parents and referring physicians are reluctant to subject the child to blood tests and radiography.) Children are maintained on interferon-α until the lesion is no longer endangering or life threatening, usually in the range of 3 to 12 months. A few infants with large lesions have been treated with interferon-α for more than 1 year. If interferon is discontinued prematurely, there may be rebound growth, necessitating resumption of therapy. Once a hemangioma has undergone accelerated regression on interferon therapy, we have not seen regrowth of a lesion after completion of an adequate course.

Once interferon therapy has been discontinued, the children are assessed again at 3-month intervals and subsequently at yearly intervals.

Cyclophosphamide

A small subgroup of hemangiomas is particularly aggressive and responds slowly to the standard dose of interferon-α of 3 million U/m^2/d. In five cases, biopsy samples were interpreted as histologically unfavorable; they either showed intense mitotic activity in endothelial cells and pericytes above the usual hyperplasia, or they revealed the Kaposi-like histologic appearance as discussed earlier. In some cases, the hemangioma only appears to be responding in a sluggish manner to interferon because the child has outgrown the initial dose; it should then be increased based on a recalculation of body surface area. In some cases, these children have been successfully managed by increasing the dose of interferon-α to 3.5 to 4.0 million U/m^2. If these maneuvers fail, we consider one or two short courses of low-dose cyclophosphamide therapy, based on the report by Hurvitz and colleagues.[92] We have treated three patients with cyclophosphamide in addition to interferon-α. One child had a large liver hemangioma, and the other two had large soft tissue hemangiomas with persistent thrombocytopenia (Kasabach-Merritt phenomenon). An intravenous catheter is placed and these children are hydrated before receiving cyclophosphamide (Cytoxan) 10 mg/kg intravenously over 1 to 2 hours each day for 3 to 4 days. The white blood count is followed closely, but has not been problematic. One child received a second course of cyclophosphamide after 1 month.

Analysis of Basic Fibroblast Growth Factor in Urine

Angiogenic proteins in body fluids can be quantified as an indirect indication of angiogenic activity in patients with tumors. Of the known angiogenic proteins,[123,124] bFGF is among the most potent. We reported that abnormally high levels of bFGF are found in the serum of approximately 10% of a wide spectrum of cancer patients,[125] and in the urine of more than 37% of cancer patients[126] (n = 987 patients). Biologically active bFGF is also abnormally elevated in the cerebrospinal fluid of children with brain tumors, but not in children with hydrocephalus or malignant disease outside of the central nervous system. The bFGF level in cerebrospinal fluid correlates with microvessel density in histologic sections, which itself provides a prognostic indicator of risk of mortality.[127]

Based on these studies, we evaluated the urinary bFGF in infants with hemangiomas, using an enzyme-linked immunosorbent bioassay (R&D Systems, Minneapolis, MN), sensitive to less than 1 pg bFGF/mL and requiring only 2 to 5 mL of fresh urine collected at any time of the day. In this ongoing clinical study, urinary bFGF is elevated up to 25- to 50-fold above normal levels in hemangiomas and returns toward normal with involution of the lesions.[128] Preliminary data suggest that urinary bFGF levels may be useful in the management of hemangiomas in at least two ways:

1. The optimum dosage of interferon-α can be adjusted without having to wait for a change in the size of the hemangioma. Thus, if bFGF remains continuously high on interferon therapy, we consider increasing the dose by small increments until the bFGF level falls.
2. The diagnosis of hemangioma can be distinguished from that of vascular malformation. With few exceptions, the urinary bFGF levels in vascular malformations are in the normal range. This biochemical marker may be helpful because certain vascular malformations, such as those in the liver, are not easy to differentiate from hemangiomas. Furthermore, interferon-α therapy is ineffective and possibly contraindicated in vascular malformations. There are no known drug therapies for vascular malformations.

Proposed Model of the Mechanism for the Antiangiogenic Property of Interferon-α

We reported an immunohistochemical analysis of the proliferating phase, the involuting phase, and the involuted phase of 38 hemangioma specimens from tissue removed by surgical excision in infants and children 3 weeks to 15 years of age, who had not been treated.[128] Of nine independent histochemical markers that correlated with the three stages, the angiogenic proteins bFGF and VEGF were significantly overexpressed in the proliferating phase. During the involuting phase, VEGF had already returned to normal, but the bFGF levels were only half-maximally reduced. By the involuted phase, bFGF levels had decreased to about 20% of their peak values. In contrast, bFGF and VEGF were undetectable or barely detectable in vascular malformations. These results indicate that bFGF and, to a lesser extent, VEGF may act as mediators of the excessive angiogenesis observed in growing hemangiomas.

Singh and associates demonstrated that interferon-α and -β down-regulate the expression of bFGF at the mRNA and protein levels in human carcinomas.[129,130] The mechanism was independent of the antiproliferative effect of the interferons and required long exposure (more than 4 days) of tumor cells to low concentrations of the interferons. Singh and associates also

found that expression of bFGF and subsequent induction of neovascularization by human tumors was inhibited when the tumors were implanted subcutaneously in immunodeficient mice, but not when the tumors were implanted in the subrenal capsule or in the wall of the colon.[130] These studies indicate that in the mouse, interferon-α and -β released by murine skin keratinocytes may, under normal conditions, suppress bFGF production. Fidler has obtained preliminary data to show that keratinocytes from proliferating hemangiomas are deficient in their expression of interferon, in contrast to keratinocytes from normal skin or from involuted hemangiomas, which elaborate normally high levels of interferon (Fidler IJ, Houston, TX, personal communication).

Taken together, these results suggest a hypothetic model of hemangioma in which the angiogenesis suppressor activity of interferon produced by keratinocytes overlying the hemangioma is decreased or deleted. This deficiency of angiogenesis suppressor activity could facilitate the proliferative phase of the hemangioma. In this model, the reappearance of normal interferon production in the overlying skin or neighboring tissue would help to mediate the involuting phase of hemangiomas.

Antiangiogenic Activity of Interferon-α Compared With Other Angiogenesis Inhibitors

Interferon-α is a relatively weak angiogenesis inhibitor compared with others that have entered clinical trial (eg, TNP-470, a synthetic analogue of fumagillin).[44] The ability to make a quantifiable comparison of the antiangiogenic activity of different inhibitors has become possible because of the development of a specific mouse cornea bioassay.[131,153] Murine interferon-α/β has not yet been compared to other angiogenesis inhibitors in this bioassay. However, the antitumor effect of murine interferon-α/β against murine Lewis lung carcinoma has been compared to other angiogenesis inhibitors. The T/C (tumor volume of treated mice divided by tumor volume of untreated, control mice) for interferon shows that it is less effective as an inhibitor of tumor growth than other angiogenesis inhibitors (Table 32-4). Thus, in the future, more potent angiogenesis inhibitors, such as angiostatin,[50] may be added to interferon-α therapy for hemangiomas, or may replace interferon-α.

TABLE 32-4. *Comparison of antitumor activity of different angiogenesis inhibitors against murine Lewis lung carcinoma*

Inhibitor	Treated/control tumor volumes	% Tumor inhibition
Interfereon-α/β	0.75	25%
Platelet factor-4	0.50	50%
AGM-1470 (TNP-470)	0.35	65%
Interleukin-12	0.15	85%
Angiostatin	0.13	87%

O'Reilly MS, Holmgren L, Chen C, et al. Angiostatin induces and sustains dormancy of human primary tumors in mice. Nat Med 1996;2:689.

Future Directions

Hemangiomas represent a form of relatively pure angiogenesis in the human. Our experience in treating them with interferon-α has taught us several important principles of antiangiogenic therapy that may be useful in the future management of patients with cancer or nonneoplastic diseases such as ocular neovascularization.

First, antiangiogenic therapy is directed mainly at a small focus of migrating and proliferating capillary endothelial cells. Thus, a specific angiogenesis inhibitor is less likely to cause bone marrow suppression, gastrointestinal symptoms, or hair loss than a conventional cytotoxic chemotherapeutic agent. This is not to say that drugs that inhibit angiogenesis would have no other actions and would be free of side effects.

Second, because optimal antiangiogenic therapy appears to require continuous treatment for months to a year or more, the design of clinical trials for angiogenesis inhibitors may need to be different than for conventional cytotoxic agents.

Third, resistance to angiogenesis inhibitors has not been a problem in the children receiving long-term interferon-α, nor has drug resistance developed in tumor-bearing animals receiving long-term antiangiogenic therapy. However, most of these angiogenesis inhibitors (eg, TNP-470) act on host endothelial cells and make them refractory to angiogenic stimuli. Because the mutation rate of host cells is low, a high rate of drug resistance would not be predicted. In contrast, when interferon-α is used as a cancer therapy, it may act mainly on the tumor cells to suppress their production of bFGF. In this case, drug resistance could develop, as it does with conventional chemotherapeutic agents, because of the high mutation rate of most tumor cells.

Fourth, in a preliminary, ongoing study that has not yet been published, urinary levels of the angiogenic protein bFGF appear to be useful in distinguishing hemangiomas from vascular malformations. This is an important differential diagnosis, because vascular malformations do not respond to interferon-α therapy. It remains to be seen whether urinary levels of bFGF can be used to select cancer patients who may benefit from interferon-α therapy.

REFERENCES

1. Ausprunk DH, Folkman J. Migration and proliferation of endothelial cells in performed and newly formed blood vessels during tumor angiogenesis. Microvasc Res 1977;15:53.
2. Denekamp J. Vascular attack as a therapeutic strategy for cancer. Cancer Metastasis Rev 1990;3:267.
3. Folkman J, Brem H. Angiogenesis and inflammation. In: Gallin JI, Goldstein IM, Snyderman R, eds. Inflammation: basic principles and clinical correlates, ed 2. New York, Raven Press, 1992:821.
4. Folkman J. Tumor angiogenesis. In: Mendelsohn J, Howley PM, Israel MA, et al, eds. The molecular basis of cancer. Philadelphia, WB Saunders, 1995:206.
5. Folkman J. Angiogenesis. In: Jaffe EA, ed. Biology of endothelial cells. Boston, Martinus Nijhoff, 1984:412.
6. Warren BA. The vascular morphology of tumors. In: Peterson H-I, ed. Tumor blood circulation: angiogenesis, vascular morphology and blood flow of experimental human tumors. Boca Raton, FL, CRC Press, 1979:1.
7. Coman DR, Sheldon WF. The significance of hyperemia around tumor implants. Am J Pathol 1946;22:821.
8. Ide AG, Bake NH, Warren SL. Vascularization of the Brown-Pearce rabbit epithelioma transplant as seen in the transparent ear chamber. AJR Am J Roentgenol 1939;42:891.
9. Algire GH, Chalkely HW, Legallais FY, et al. Vascular reactions of normal and malignant tumors in vivo. I. Vascular reactions of mice to wounds and to normal and neoplastic transplants. J Natl Cancer Inst 1945;6:73.
10. Day ED. Vascular relationships of tumor and host. Prog Exp Tumor Res 1964;4:57.
11. Folkman J. Toward an understanding of angiogenesis: search and discovery. Perspect Biol Med 1985;29:10.
12. Folkman J. Tumor angiogenesis: therapeutic implications. N Engl J Med 1971;285:1182.
13. Folkman J, Long DM, Becker FF. Growth and metastasis of tumor in organ culture. Cancer 1963;16:453.
14. Folkman J, Cole P, Zimmerman S. Tumor behavior in isolated perfused organs: in vitro growth and metastases of biopsy material in rabbit thyroid and canine intestinal segment. Ann Surg 1966;164:491.
15. Folkman J. Anti-angiogenesis: new concept for therapy of solid tumors. Ann Surg 1972;175:408.
16. Folkman J. The vascularization of tumors. Sci Am 1976;234:58.
17. Folkman J, Gimbrone MA Jr. Perfusion of the thyroid. In: Diczfalusy E, ed. Karolinska symposia on research methods in reproduction endocrinology, 4th symposium: perfusion techniques. Stockholm, 1971:237.
18. Folkman J. The intestine as an organ culture. In: Burdette WJ, ed. Carcinoma of the colon and antecedent epithelium. Springfield, IL, Charles C Thomas, 1970:113.
19. Folkman J, Haudenschild CC, Zetter BR. Long-term culture of capillary endothelial cells. Proc Natl Acad Sci U S A 1979;76:5217.
20. Taylor S, Folkman J. Protamine is an inhibitor of angiogenesis. Nature 1982;297:307.
21. Shing Y, Folkman J, Sullivan R, et al. Heparin affinity: purification of a tumor-derived capillary endothelial cell growth factor. Science 1984;223:1296.
22. Folkman J. Antiangiogenesis. In: DeVita VT Jr, Hellman S, Rosenberg SA, eds. Biologic therapy of cancer. Philadelphia, JB Lippincott, 1991:743.
23. Folkman J, Merler E, Abernathy C, et al. Isolation of a tumor factor responsible for angiogenesis. J Exp Med 1971;133:275.
24. Klagsbrun M, Knighton D, Folkman J. Tumor angiogenesis activity in cell grown in tissue culture. Cancer Res 1976;36:110.
25. Auerbach R, Arensman R, Kubai L, et al. Tumor-induced angiogenesis: lack by irradiation. Int J Cancer 1975;15:241.
26. Folkman J, Cotran RS. Relation of vascular proliferation to tumor growth. Int Rev Exp Pathol 1976;16:207.
27. Folkman J, Hochberg M, Knighton D. Self-regulation of growth in three dimensions: the role of surface area limitation. In: Clarkson B, Baserga R, eds. Cold Spring Harbor symposium: control of animal cell proliferation. Cold Spring Harbor, NY, Cold Spring Harbor Laboratory Press, 1974:833.
28. Folkman J, Hochberg M. Self-regulation of growth in three dimensions. J Exp Med 1973;138:745.
29. Adam JA, Maggelakis AA. Diffusion of regulated growth characteristics of a spherical prevascular carcinoma. Bull Math Biol 1990;52:549.
30. Sutherland RM. Cell and environment interactions in tumor microregions: the multicell spheroid model. Science 1988;240:177.
31. Sutherland RM, McCredie JA, Inch WR. Growth of multicell spheroids in tissue culture as a model of nodular carcinomas. J Natl Cancer Inst 1971;46:113.
32. Gimbrone MA Jr., Leapman S, Cotran RS, et al. Tumor dormancy in vivo by prevention of neovascularization. J Exp Med 1972;136:261.
33. Gimbrone MA Jr., Cotran R, Leapman S, et al. Tumor growth and neovascularization: an experimental model using rabbit cornea. J Natl Cancer Inst 1974;52:413.
34. Fujimoto K, Ichimori Y, Kakizoe T, et al. Increased serum levels of basic fibroblast growth factor in patients with renal cell carcinoma. Biochem Biophys Res Commun 1991;180:386.
35. Brem S, Brem H, Folkman J, et al. Prolonged tumor dormancy by prevention of neovascularization in the vitreous. Cancer Res 1976;36:2807.
36. Folkman J. Tumor angiogenesis factor. Cancer Res 1974;34:2109.
37. Tannock IF. Population kinetics of carcinoma cells, capillary endothelial cells, and fibroblasts in a transplanted mouse mammary tumor. Cancer Res 1970;30:2470.
38. Knighton D, Ausprunk D, Tapper D, et al. Avascular and vascular

phases of tumour growth in the chick embryo. Br J Cancer 1977;35:347.

39. Lien W, Ackerman NB. The blood supply of experimental liver metastases. II. A microcirculatory study of normal and tumor vessels of the liver with the use of perfused silicone rubber. Surgery 1970;68:334.

40. Folkman J, Watson K, Ingber D, et al. Induction of angiogenesis during the transition from hyperplasia to neoplasia. Nature 1989;339:58.

41. Thompson WD, Shiach KJ, Fraser RA, et al. Tumors acquire their vasculature by vessel incorporation, not vessel ingrowth. J Pathol 1987;151:323.

42. Skinner SA, Tutton PJ, O'Brien PE. Microvascular architecture of experimental colon tumors in the rat. Cancer Res 1990;50:2411.

43. Folkman J. What is the evidence that tumors are angiogenesis dependent? J Natl Cancer Inst 1990;82:4.

44. Ingber DM, Fujita T, Kishimoto S, et al. Synthetic analogues of fumagillin that inhibit angiogenesis and suppress tumour growth. Nature 1990;348:555.

45. Hori A, Sasada R, Matsutani E, et al. Suppression of solid tumor growth by immuno-neutralizing monoclonal antibody against human basic fibroblast growth factor. Cancer Res 1991;51:6180.

46. Kim KJ, Li B, Winer J, Armanini M, et al. Inhibition of vascular endothelial growth factor-induced angiogenesis suppresses tumour growth in vivo. Nature 1993;362:841.

47. Millauer B, Shawver LK, Plate KH, et al. Glioblastoma growth inhibited in vivo by a dominant-negative Flk-1 mutant. Nature 1994;367:576.

48. Dameron KM, Volpert OV, Tainsky MA, et al. Control of angiogenesis in fibroblasts by p53 regulation of thrombospondin-1. Science 1994;265:1582.

49. Brooks PC, Montgomery AMP, Rosenfeld M, et al. Integrin $\alpha_v\beta_3$ antagonists promote tumor regression by inducing apoptosis of angiogenic blood vessels. Cell 1994;79:1157.

50. O'Reilly MS, Holmgren L, Shing Y, et al. Angiostatin: a novel angiogenesis inhibitor that mediates the suppression of metastases by a Lewis lung carcinoma. Cell 1994;79:315.

51. Ribatti D, Vacca A, Bertossi M, et al. Angiogenesis induced by B-cell non-Hodgkin's lymphomas: lack of correlation with tumor malignancy and immunologic phenotype. Anticancer Res 1990;10:401.

52. Smith-McCune KK, Weidner N. Demonstration and characterization of the angiogenic properties of cervical dysplasia. Cancer Res 1994;54:800.

53. Ziche M, Gullino PM. Angiogenesis and neoplastic progression in vitro. J Natl Cancer Inst 1982;69:483.

54. Mulliken JB, Ohlms LA, Folkman J, et al. Pharmacologic therapy for endangering hemangiomas. Current Opinion in Dermatology 1995:109.

55. Folkman J, Langer R, Linhardt R, et al. Angiogenesis inhibition and tumor regression caused by heparin or a heparin fragment in the presence of cortisone. Science 1983;221:719.

56. O'Reilly MS, Holmgren L, Chen C, et al. Angiostatin induces and sustains dormancy of human primary tumors in mice. Nat Med 1996;2:689.

57. Brooks PC, Clark RAF, Cheresh D. Requirement of vascular integrin $\alpha_v\beta_3$ for angiogenesis. Science 1994;264:569.

58. Jain RK. Delivery of novel therapeutic agents in tumors: physiological barriers and strategies. J Natl Cancer Inst 1989;81:570.

59. Folkman J, Shing Y. Angiogenesis. J Biol Chem 1992;267:10931.

60. Maciag T, Mehlman T, Friesel R, et al. Heparin binds endothelial cell growth factor, the principal endothelial cell mitogen in bovine brain. Science 1994;25:932.

61. Esch F, Baird A, Ling N, et al. Primary structure of bovine pituitary basic fibroblast growth factor (FG) and comparison with the amino-terminal sequence of bovine brain acidic FGF. Proc Natl Acad Sci U S A 1985;82:6507.

62. Fett JW, Strydom DJ, Lobb RR, et al. Isolation and characterization of angiogenin, an angiogenic protein from human colon carcinoma cells. Biochemistry 1985;24:5480.

63. Schreiber AB, Winkler ME, Derynck R. Transforming growth factor-alpha: a more potent angiogenic mediator that epidermal growth factor. Science 1986;232:1250.

64. Roberts AB, Sporn MB, Assoian RK, et al. Transforming growth factor type beta: rapid induction of fibrosis and angiogenesis in vivo and stimulation of collagen formation in vitro. Proc Natl Acad Sci U S A 1986;83:4167.

65. Fràter-Schröder M, Risau W, Hallmann R, et al. Tumor necrosis factor type a, a potent inhibitor of endothelial cell growth in vitro, is angiogenic in vivo. Proc Natl Acad Sci U S A 1987;84:5277.

66. Leibovich SJ, Polverini PJ, Shepard HM, et al. Macrophage-induced angiogenesis is mediated by tumour necrosis factor-alpha. Nature 1987;329:630.

67. Senger DR, Galli SJ, Dvorak AM, et al. Tumor cells secrete a vascular permeability factor that promotes accumulation of ascites fluid. Science 1983;219:983.

68. Ferrara N, Henzel WJ. Pituitary follicular cells secrete a novel heparin-binding growth factor specific for vascular endothelial cells. Biochem Biophys Res Commun 1989;161:851.

69. Connolly DT, Heuvelman DM, Nelson R, et al. Tumor vascular permeability factor stimulates endothelial cell growth and angiogenesis. J Clin Invest 1989;84:1470.

70. Plouet J, Schilling J, Gospodarowicz D. Isolation and characterization of a newly identified endothelial cell mitogen produced by AT-20 cells. EMBO J 1989;8:3801.

71. Ishikawa F, Miyazone K, Hellman U, et al. Identification of angiogenic activity and the cloning and expression of platelet- derived endothelial cell growth factor. Nature 1989;338:557.

72. Bussolino F, Ziche M, Wang JM, et al. In vitro and in vivo activation of endothelial cells by colony stimulating factors. J Clin Invest 1991;87:986.

73. Maglione D, Guerriero V, Viglietto G, et al. Isolation of a human placenta cDNA coding for a protein related to the vascular permeability factor. Proc Natl Acad Sci U S A 1991;88:9267.

74. Koch A, Polverini PJ, Kunkel SL, et al. Interleukin-8 as a macrophage-derived mediator of angiogenesis. Science 1992;258:1178.

75. Rosen EM, Meromsky L, Setter E, et al. Purified scatter factor stimulates epithelial and vascular endothelial cell migration. Proc Soc Exp Biol Med 1990;195:34.

76. Bussolino F, Di Renzo MF, Ziche M, et al. Hepatocyte growth factor is a potent angiogenic factor which stimulates endothelial cell motility and growth. J Cell Biol 1992;119:629.

77. Jackson D, Volpert O, Bouck N, et al. Stimulation and inhibition of angiogenesis by placental proliferin and proliferin-related protein. Science 1994;266:1581.

78. Rastinejad F, Polverini P, Bouck NP. Regulation of the activity of a new inhibitor of angiogenesis by a cancer suppressor gene. Cell 1989;56:345.

79. O'Reilly MS, Holmgren L, Shing Y, et al. Angiostatin: a circulating endothelial cell inhibitor that suppresses angiogenesis and tumor growth. Cold Spring Harb Symp Quant Biol 1994;59:471.

80. Sharpe RJ, Byers HR, Scott CF, et al. Inhibition of murine melanoma and human colon carcinoma by recombinant human platelet factor 4. J Natl Cancer Inst 1990;82:848.

81. Gupta SK, Hassel T, Singh JP. A potent inhibitor of endothelial cell proliferation is generated by proteolytic cleavage of the chemokine platelet factor 4. Proc Natl Acad Sci USA 1995;92:7799.

82. Iruela-Arispe ML, Bornstein P, Sage EH. Thrombospondin exerts an antiangiogenic effect on cord formation by endothelial cells in vitro. Proc Natl Acad Sci USA 1991;88:5026.

83. Murphy A, Unsworth E, Stetler-Stevenson W. Tissue inhibitor of metalloproteinase-2 (TIMP-2) inhibits bFGF induced human microvascular endothelial cell proliferation. J Cell Physiol 1993;157:351.

84. Moses MA, Sudhalter J, Langer R. Identification of an inhibitor of neovascularization from cartilage. Science 1990;248:1410.

85. Baird A, Durkin T. Inhibition of endothelial cell proliferation by type beta-transofrming growth factor: Interactions with acidic and basic fibroblast growth factors. Biochem Biophys Res Commun 1986;138:476.

86. Muller F, Behrens J, Nussbaumer U, et al. Inhibitory action of transforming growth factor beta on endothelial cells. Proc Natl Acad Sci USA 1987;84:5600.

87. Folkman J, Mulliken JB, Ezekowitz RAB. Antiangiogenic therapy of haemangiomas with interferon α. In: Stuart-Harris R, Penny R, eds. The clinical applications of the interferons. London, Chapman and Hall, 1995 (in press).

88. Folkman J. Towards a new understanding of vascular proliferative disease in children. Pediatrics 1984;74:850.

89. Enjolras O, Riche MC, Merland JJ, et al. Management of alarming hemangiomas in infancy: a review of 25 cases. Pediatrics 1990;5:491.

90. Cohen RC, Myers NA. Diagnosis and management of massive hepatic hemangiomas in childhood. J Pediatr Surg 1986;21:6.

91. Schild SE, Buskirk SJ, Frick LM, et al. Radiotherapy for large symptomatic hemangiomas. Int J Radiat Oncol Biol Phys 1991;21:729.

92. Hurvitz CH, Alkalay AL, Sloninsky L, et al. Cyclophosphamide therapy in life-threatening vascular tumors. J Pediatr 1986;109:360.

93. Argenta LC, Bishop E, Cho KJ, et al. Complete resolution of life-threatening hemangiomas by embolization and corticosteroids. Plast Reconstr Surg 1982;70:739.

94. Burrows PE, Mulliken JB, Fellows KE, et al. Childhood hemangiomas and vascular malformations: angiographic differentiation. AJR Am J Roentgenol 1983;141:483.

95. Brouty-Boye D, Zetter BR. Inhibition of cell motility by interferon. Science 1980;108:516.

96. Sidky YA, Borden EC, Wierenga W, et al. Inhibitory effects of interferon-inducing pyrimidinones on the growth of transplantable mouse bladder tumors. Cancer Res 1986;46:3798.

97. Dvorak HF, Gresser I. Microvascular injury in pathogenesis of interferon-induced necrosis of subcutaneous tumors in mice. J Natl Cancer Inst 1989;81:497.

98. White CW, Sondheimer HM, Crouch EC, et al. Treatment of pulmonary hemangiomatosis with recombinant interferon alfa-2a. N Engl J Med 1989;329:1197.

99. Folkman J. Successful treatment of angiogenic disease. N Engl J Med 1989;320:1211.

100. Orchard PJ, Smith CM III, Woods WG, et al. Treatment of haemangioendotheliomas with alpha interferon. Lancet 1989;2:565.

101. White CW, Wolf SJ, Korones DN, et al. Treatment of childhood angiomatous diseases with recombinant interferon alfa-2a. J Pediatr 1991;118:59.

102. Ezekowitz RAB, Mulliken JB, Folkman J. Interferon alfa-2a therapy for life-threatening hemangiomas of infancy. N Engl J Med 1992;326:1456. Errata N Engl J Med 1994;330:300. Errata N Engl J Med 1995;333:595.

103. Spiller JC, Sharma V, Woods GM, et al. Diffuse neonatal hemangiomatosis treated successfully with interferon alfa-2a. J Am Acad Dermatol 1992;27:102.

104. Blei F, Orlow SJ, Geronemus RG. Supraumbilical midabdominal raphe, sternal atresia, and hemangioma in an infant: response of hemangioma to laser and interferon alfa-2a. Pediatr Dermatol 1993;10:71.

105. Blei F, Orlow SJ, Geronemus RG. Interferon alfa-2a therapy for extensive perianal and lower extremity hemangioma. J Am Acad Dermatol 1993;29:98.

106. Ohlms LA, Jones DT, McGill TJI, et al. Interferon alfa-2a therapy for airway hemangiomas. Ann Otol Rhinol Laryngol 1994;103:1.

107. de Castelbajac D, Teillac D, Bodemer C, et al. Hemangiome cephalique tubereux d'evolution fatale; inefficacite du traitment par interferon alpha. Ann Dermatol Venereol 1990;117:821.

108. Loughnan MS, Elder J, Kemp A. Treatment of a massive orbital capillary hemangioma with interferon alfa-2b: short-term results. Arch Ophthalmol 1992;110:1366.

109. Dubois J, Leclerc JBM, Garel L, et al. Radiologic modifications induced by interferon alfa-2b in progressive hemangioma: clinical and CT correlation. (Abstract) In: American Society of Pediatric Radiology, Seattle, Washington, May 12–15, 1993.

110. Teillac-Hamel D, De Prost Y, Bodemer C, et al. Serious childhood angiomas: unsuccessful alpha-2b interferon treatment. A report of 4 cases. Br J Dermatol 1993;129:473.

111. Deans RM, Harris GJ, Kivlin JD. Surgical dissection of capillary hemangiomas: an alternative to intralesional corticosteroids. Arch Ophthalmol 1992;110:1743.

112. Azizkhan RG, Azizkhan JC, Zetter BR, et al. Mast cell heparin stimulates migration of capillary endothelial cells in vitro. J Exp Med 1980;152:931.

113. Sudhalter J, Folkman J, Svahn CM, et al. Importance of size, sulfation and anticoagulant activity in the potentiation of acidic fibroblast growth factor by heparin. J Biol Chem 1989;264:6892.

114. Mulliken JB, Young AE. Vascular birthmarks: hemangiomas and malformations. Philadelphia, WB Saunders, 1988.

115. Boon LM, Burrows PE, Paltiel HJ, et al. Hepatic vascular anomalies in infancy: a twenty-seven year experience. J Pediatr 1995 (submitted J Pediatr (in press).

116. Hawkins DB, Crockett DM, Kahlstrom EJ, et al. Corticosteroid management of airway hemangiomas: long-term follow-up. Laryngoscope 1984;94:633.

117. Healy G, McGill T, Friedman EM. Carbon dioxide laser in subglottic hemangioma: an update. Ann Otol Rhinol Laryngol 1984;93:370.

118. Niedt GW, Greco MA, Wieczorek R, et al. Hemangioma with Kaposi's sarcoma-like features: report of two cases. Pediatr Pathol 1989;9:567.

119. Tsang WYW, Chan JKC. Kaposi-like infantile hemangioendothelioma: a distinctive vascular neoplasm of the retroperitoneum. Am J Surg Pathol 1991;15:982.

120. Zukerberg LR, Nicoloff BJ, Weiss SW. Kaposiform hemangioendothelioma of infancy and childhood. Am J Surg Pathol 1993;17:321.

121. Vesikari T, Nuutila A, Cantell K. Neurologic sequelae following interferon therapy of juvenile laryngeal papilloma. Acta Paediatr 1988;77:619.

121a. Barlow CF, Priebe CJ, Mulliken JB, et al. Adverse effect of interferon alfa-2a in the treatment of hemangiomas of infancy on the early development of the central nervous system: a preliminary report. July, 1996 (submitted for publication).

122. Guyer DR, Tiedeman J, Yannuzzi LA, et al. Interferon-associated retinopathy. Arch Ophthalmol 1993;111:350.

123. Folkman J. Clinical applications of research on angiogenesis. N Engl J Med 1995;333:1757.

124. Watanabe H, Nguyen M, Schizer M, et al. Basic fibroblast growth factor in human serum: a prognostic test for breast cancer. (Abstract) Mol Biol Cell 1992;3:324a.

125. Nguyen M, Watanabe H, Budson AE, et al. Elevated levels of an angiogenic peptide, basic fibroblast growth factor, in the urine of patients with a wide spectrum of cancers. J Natl Cancer Inst 1994;86:356.

126. Li VW, Folkerth RD, Watanabe H, et al. Microvessel count and cerebrospinal fluid basic fibroblast growth factor in children with brain tumours. Lancet 1994;344:82.

127. Folkman J, Mulliken JB, Law T, et al. Unpublished data, 1995.

128. Takahashi K, Mulliken JB, Kozakewich HPW, et al. Cellular markers that distinguish the phases of hemangioma during infancy and childhood. J Clin Invest 1994;93:2357.

129. Singh RK, Gutman M, Bucana CD, et al. Interferons α and β downregulate the expression of basic fibroblast growth factor in human carcinomas. Proc Natl Acad Sci USA 1995;92:4562.

130. Singh RK, Bucana CD, Gutman M, et al. Organ site-dependent expression of basic fibroblast growth factor in human renal cell carcinoma cells. Am J Pathol 1994;145:365.

131. Folkman J, Mascona A. Role of cell shape in growth control. Nature 1978;273:346.

132. Folkman J, Klagsbrun M. Angiogenic factors. Science 1987;235:442.

133. Folkman J. Angiogenesis in cancer, vascular, rheumatoid and other disease. Nature Med 1995;1:27.

134. Holmgren L, O'Reilly MS, Folkman J. Dormancy of micrometastases: balanced proliferation and apoptosis in the presence of angiogenesis suppression. Nat Med 1995;1:149.

135. Sade RM, Folkman J, Cotran RS. DNA synthesis in endothelium of aortic segments in vitro. Exp Cell Res 1972;74:297.

136. Gimbrone MA Jr., Cotran RS, Haudenschild C, et al. Growth and ultrastructure of human vascular endothelium and smooth muscle cells in culture. (Abstract) J Cell Biol 1973;:109a.

137. Auerbach R, Kubai L, Knighton D, et al. A simple procedure for the long-term cultivation of chicken embryos. Dev Biol 1974;41:391.

138. Langer R, Folkman J. Polymers for the sustained release of proteins and other macromolecules. Nature 1976;263:797.

139. Folkman J, Haudenschild C. Angiogenesis in vitro. Nature 1980;288:551.

140. Shing Y, Klagsbrun M, Folkman J. A new method for purifying heparin-binding growth factors. Ann NY Acad Sci 1989;556:166.

141. Nguyen M, Shing Y, Folkman J. Quantitation of angiogenesis and antiangiogenesis in the chick embryo chorioallantoic membrane Microvasc Res 1994;47:31.

142. Cavallo T, Sade R, Folkman J, et al. Tumor angiogenesis: rapid induction of endothelial mitoses demonstrated by autoradiography. J Cell Biol 1972;54:408.

143. Haudenschild CC, Zahniser D, Folkman J, et al. Human vascular endothelial cells in culture: lack of response to serum growth factors. Exp Cell Res 1976;98:175.

144. Kadish JL, Butterfield CE, Folkman J. The effect of fibrin on cultured vascular endothelial cells. Tissue Cell 1979;11:99.

145. Tapper D, Langer R, Bellows AR, et al. Angiogenesis as a diagnostic marker for human eye tumors. Surgery 1979;86:36.

146. Langer RS, Conn H, Vacant J, et al. Control of tumor growth in animals by infusion of an angiogenesis inhibitor. Proc Natl Acad Sci U S A 1980;77:4331.

147. Chodak GW, Haudenschild C, Gittes RF, et al. Angiogenesis as a marker of neoplastic and pre-neoplastic lesions of the human bladder. Ann Surg 1980;192:762.

148. Crum R, Szabo S, Folkman J. A new class of steroids inhibits angiogenesis in the presence of heparin or a heparin fragment. Science 1985;230:1375.

149. Folkman J, Klagsbrun M, Sasse J, et al. A heparin-binding angiogenic protein—basic fibroblast growth factor—is stored within basement membrane. Am J Pathol 1988;130:393.

150. Folkman J. The angiogenic activity of FGF and its possible clinical applications. In: Sara VR, Hall K, Low H, eds. Growth factors: from Genes to clinical application. Karolinska Institute Nobel conference series on growth factors. New York, Raven Press, 1990:201.

151. Weidner N, Semple JP, Welch WR, et al. Tumor angiogenesis correlates with metastasis in invasive breast carcinoma. N Engl J Med 1991;324:1.

152. Nguyen M, Watanabe H, Budson AE, et al. Elevated levels of an angiogenic peptide, basic fibroblast growth factor, in urine of bladder cancer patients. J Natl Cancer Inst 1993;85:241.

152a. Kenyon BM, Voest EE, Chen CC, et al. A model of angiogenesis in the mouse cornea. Invest Ophthalmol Vis Sci 1996;37:1625.

153. Shing Y, Christofori G, Hanahan D, et al. Betacellulin: a novel mitogen from pancreatic B tumour cells. Science 1993;259:1604.

154. Weidner N, Carroll PR, Flax J, et al. Tumor angiogenesis correlates with metastasis in invasive prostate carcinoma. Am J Pathol 1993;143:401.

155. D'Amato RJ, Loughnan MS, Flynn E, et al. Thalidomide is an inhibitor of angiogenesis. Proc Natl Acad Sci U S A 1994;91:4082.

156. Miller JW, Adamis AP, Shima DR, et al. Vascular endothelial growth factor/vascular permeability factor is temporally and spatially correlated with ocular angiogenesis in a primate model. Am J Pathol 1994;145:574.

157. Voest EE, Kenyon BM, O'Reilly MS, et al. Inhibition of angiogenesis in vivo by interleukin 12. J Natl Cancer Inst 1995;87:581.

Surgery of Infants and Children: Scientific Principles and Practice, edited by
Keith T. Oldham, Paul M. Colombani, and Robert P. Foglia.
Lippincott–Raven Publishers, Philadelphia, © 1997.

CHAPTER 33

Renal Tumors

Stephen J. Shochat

Renal tumors represent about 6% of all pediatric cancers, and Wilms tumor (nephroblastoma) accounts for about 97% of all tumors of the kidney in children.[1] This chapter focuses on Wilms tumor and its variants; mesoblastic nephroma and renal cell carcinoma in children are also addressed.

WILMS TUMOR

The eponym *Wilms tumor* was adopted for nephroblastoma after the classic 1899 monogram of Max Wilms described seven cases of mixed malignant tissue tumors of the kidney in children. The first successful nephrectomy for Wilms tumor was performed in 1877, but it was not until the early 1900s that surgery became effective therapy for this tumor. In 1936, Priestley and Schulte reported a 15% 5-year survival rate after nephrectomy. In 1941, Ladd and Gross, using a transabdominal approach to the tumor, reported a survival rate of 24%. Using a therapeutic approach of nephrectomy followed by radiotherapy, Gross and Neuhauser reported a 47% survival rate in 1950. In 1956, Farber introduced systemic chemotherapy to supplement surgery and radiotherapy and in 1964 reported an 89% survival rate in 53 cases.

Because of the rarity of this tumor, further clinical investigation was handicapped until the establishment of the National Wilms Tumor Study (NWTS) in 1969. The first NWTS clearly showed that postoperative abdominal radiotherapy is not necessary for group I children who are less than 2 years old. In addition, the combination of vincristine and actinomycin D was shown to be more effective for the treatment of children in groups II and III than either drug alone. NWTS-2 demonstrated that 6 months of combination chemotherapy with vincristine and actinomycin D is effective treatment for children with group I tumors, none of whom received abdominal radiation. The addition of doxorubicin (Adriamycin) to the combination of vincristine and actinomycin D improved the relapse-free survival rate of children with group II to IV tumors.

Children enrolled in NWTS-1 and NWTS-2 were not stratified according to histology. The separation of Wilms tumor into distinct histopathologic categories based on prognosis was described by Beckwith and Palmer in 1978.[2] In addition to the use of histopathologic categories in NWTS-3, changes were made in inclusion criteria for the various groups, and the present staging system was standardized with the initiation of the NWTS-3 protocol. NWTS-3 established the following results, which are the backbone of present-day conventional therapy:

1. Combination chemotherapy with actinomycin D and vincristine is adequate therapy for children with tumors that are stage I favorable histology or anaplastic variant and stage II favorable histology. Stage I patients are treated for 6 months and stage II patients for 14 months.
2. Postoperative radiotherapy is not required in children with stage I and II favorable histology tumors.
3. Adriamycin is added to actinomycin D and vincristine in patients with stage III favorable histology tumors. These patients also receive 1000 cGy of postoperative radiotherapy. Stage IV patients with favorable histology tumors and children with clear cell sarcoma of the kidney (CCSK) are treated with actinomycin D, vincristine, and doxorubicin plus radiotherapy based on the clinical stage of the primary tumor at the time of resection.

Using the results of the NWTS-3, the NWTS-4 treatment protocol was established in 1986 and recently closed. It is discussed in detail later in this chapter. NWTS-5 is now open for patient accrual.

The basic principle of the NWTS has always been accomplishing a significant improvement in cure rate with reduction in intensity and duration of therapy. Tradition has emphasized establishing for each patient, based on stage and histologic evaluation, the minimum therapy required to achieve maximum therapeutic response. The pathologic classification of Wilms tumor and its effects on therapy and prognosis is used as a guide for the study of other childhood malignancies. In addition, the organization of the NWTS has served as a prototype for other collaborative studies of childhood tumors.

Epidemiology

Wilms tumor is the most common intraabdominal cancer seen in childhood and represents about 6% of all cases of childhood cancer. In the United States, there is an annual incidence of 8 cases per 1 million children younger than than 15 years of age, with the total incidence estimated to be about 350 to 450 cases per year.[3] About 75% of the cases occur in children younger than 5 years of age, with a peak incidence at 2 to 3 years of age. There is an equal sex ratio worldwide, but in the United States, the incidence of Wilms tumor may be slightly higher in girls.

The association of Wilms tumor with specific congenital anomalies and the presence of immature embryonic tissues within this tumor led to the proposal by Knudson[4] of a two-hit mutational model to explain the tumor formation in nephroblastoma. The first step involves either a germinal cell line mutation (a prezygotic event) or a somatic insult (a postzygotic event) for a tumor to occur. The second mutation is usually a somatic insult. The hereditary version of the tumor involves a prezygotic event, and the nonhereditary form involves a postzygotic event, followed by the second somatic insult. Younger patients and patients with aniridia, genitourinary anomalies, bilateral disease, and familial cases have been considered in the hereditary class. The true incidence of hereditary Wilms tumor cases, however, is only about 20% of all Wilms tumors. Hereditary Wilms tumor should not be confused with familial Wilms tumor. Familial Wilms tumor is rare; an evaluation of more than 3000 NWTS patients revealed that only 1% had one or more family members with this tumor.[5]

Multiple congenital malformations and syndromes have been associated with Wilms tumor. The most common anomalies are aniridia, hemihypertrophy, and Beckwith-Wiedemann syndrome. The association of aniridia was first reported in 1964, and associations with mental retardation and genitourinary anomalies were subsequently described.[4] The term *WAGR* (*W*iedemann, *a*niridia, *g*enitourinary malformations, *r*etardation) syndrome was applied to this association. Rarer syndromes are the Denys-Drash syndrome (male pseudohermaphroditism and diffuse glomerular disease) and Perlman syndrome (fetal giantism, renal hamartomas, and nephroblastomatosis). Fifty to 90% of patients with Denys-Drash syndrome develop Wilms tumor.[6] It is important to recognize the association of these syndromes and related malformations so that the appropriate surveillance can be carried out. Hemihypertrophy has been seen in about 3% of Wilms tumor patients and aniridia in 1% of the reported cases. For this reason, patients with sporadic aniridia, hemihypertrophy, and Beckwith-Wiedemann syndrome should be followed by surveillance ultrasonography at 3-month intervals until they are 6 or 7 years of age.

Molecular Genetics

The first clue to the location of a Wilms tumor gene was the detection in patients with WAGR syndrome of a constitutional interstitial deletion on the short arm of chromosome 11 that encompassed part of band 11p13.[6] In patients with WAGR syndrome, inactivation of a tumor-suppressor gene at this locus by a major deletion represents the first of the two hits predicted by Knudson.[4] Further molecular genetic studies demonstrated that inactivation of a gene at the 11p13 locus could also constitute the second somatic hit, leading to tumorigenesis. Investigators have since demonstrated a loss of heterozygosity on the short arm of chromosome 11 in patients with sporadic Wilms tumor. These observations led to the cloning of a specific Wilms tumor gene (*WT1*), which has been isolated from the 11p13

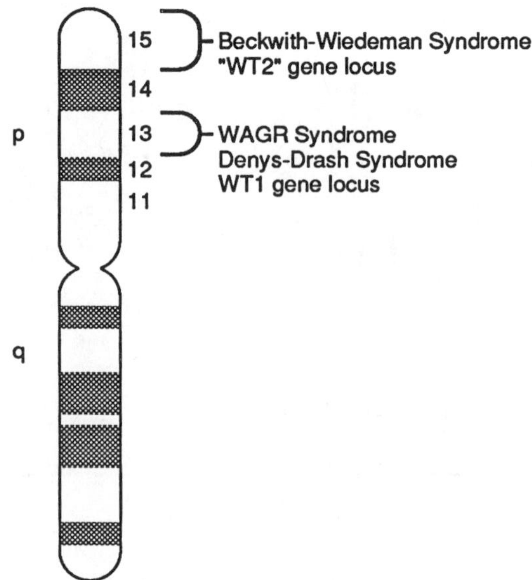

FIG. 33-1. Chromosome 11 Wilms tumor loci.

region[7] (Fig. 33-1). *WT1* has been implicated in the predisposition to develop Wilms tumor, and using sequence analysis, the WT1 protein has been shown to bind DNA at the same site as a growth factor–inducible early gene product (EGR1). The loss of *WT1* DNA-binding activity may contribute to tumor formation. *WT1* has also been shown to be expressed in the developing kidney and urogenital precursors.

A second genetic locus at 11p15 has been identified in patients with familial Beckwith-Wiedemann syndrome. In fact, studies of sporadic Wilms tumors have shown that 11p15 loss of heterozygosity is one of the most common chromosomal deletions. It is possible that genes located at both the 11p15 and the 11p13 regions may be involved in the pathogenesis of Wilms tumor by cooperating with one another. The tumor suppressor gene (*WT2*) at 11p15 has not as yet been cloned. It has been observed that some patients with Beckwith-Wiedemann syndrome have inherited both copies of a region on the short arm of chromosome 11 from the father, an abnormality known as uniparental isodisomy. In this condition, the maternal rather than the paternal allele is lost. This phenomenon of differential genetic contribution of parents to their offspring is called *genomic imprinting*. The loss of the maternal alleles of 11p15 in patients with Beckwith-Wiedemann syndrome and Wilms tumors clearly indicates selection against the maternally derived chromosome during tumorigenesis and thus paternal imprinting of a tumor-suppressor gene (*WT2*) at 11p15. These findings suggest that gene dosage and imprinting may be crucial in the genesis of some Wilms tumors.

An additional Wilms tumor locus at 16q is suggested by loss of heterozygosity for chromosome 16q markers in 20% of Wilms tumors. Loss of heterozygosity at a locus mapping to the distal chromosome 1p has also been found in a small group of patients with Wilms tumor. To determine the incidence of various chromosomal aberrations in patients with Wilms tumor, Grundy and colleagues[8] analyzed 232 patients and found loss of heterozygosity at 11p in 33%, at 16q in 17%, and at 1p in 12%. In addition, these genetic alterations were correlated with outcome. Patients with loss of heterozygosity for chromosome

16q had relapse rates 3.3 times higher and mortality rates 12 times higher than patients without loss of heterozygosity for chromosome 16q. No correlation between relapse and mortality was found with loss of heterozygosity for chromosome 1p or chromosome 11p. New prognostic factors are important if refinements of Wilms tumor therapy are to continue. Therefore, further molecular genetic studies are necessary to identify patients at risk for relapse so that intensification of therapy can be instituted in selected groups of patients. This is the intent of NWTS-5. In the future, molecular genetic characterization of patients with Wilms tumor will likely lead to the identification of subgroups of children with more favorable prognoses who can be managed according to conventional therapy. Patients predisposed to relapse will require more aggressive or new approaches.

Although a number of different genetic loci are linked to Wilms tumor development, the mechanisms underlying altered gene function may be more variable than originally believed. Mutations at different loci or various combinations of genetic lesions could well be responsible for the different categories of Wilms tumors. It has been shown that insertion of an entire chromosome 11 can cause Wilms tumor cells to lose tumorigenicity. Further advances in molecular biology may see new types of cancer therapy develop through manipulation of suppressor genes.

Pathology

One of the major contributions of the NWTS group was the 1978 report by Beckwith and Palmer[2] that separated Wilms tumors into distinct histopathologic categories based on prognosis. An analysis of 427 specimens found that 11% of the patients in this study contributed to 52% of the mortality. Since this report, Wilms tumors have been classified into favorable and unfavorable histologic groups (Fig. 33-2). The *unfavorable* histologic group includes Wilms tumors with anaplasia and two distinct renal tumors, clear cell sarcoma of kidney (CCSK) and malignant rhabdoid tumor of the kidney. Anaplasia can be of

focal or diffuse nature; the focal subtype has a more favorable histology. Anaplasia was present in 4.5% of cases entered on NWTS-3 and is more common in older children, reaching a peak incidence at about 5 years of age. This histopathologic variant is also more frequent in black than in white patients. An interesting feature of the anaplastic variety is that stage I anaplastic Wilms tumors have a biologic behavior similar to favorable histology stage I patients, with similar relapse and cure rates. This suggests that stage I anaplastic tumors are not associated with occult micrometastases in early stages of tumorigenesis. CCSK and rhabdoid tumors of the kidney are now considered separate entities, rather than variants of Wilms tumor; but these two entities continue to be registered on the NWTS. The CCSK (bone-metastasizing renal tumor of childhood) is the most commonly encountered unfavorable histology tumor and was seen in 6% of the patients registered on NWTS-3. The CCSK variant is associated with a high incidence of skeletal metastases, but its site of origin and age distribution are identical to favorable histology Wilms tumors. The tumors are associated with a high incidence of tumor relapse, which suggests that micrometastases occur in an early stage of tumor growth. CCSK may be cystic, and the gross appearance can resemble a multilocular cyst of the kidney. This is important because partial nephrectomy is adequate therapy for multilocular cysts but is inadequate therapy for highly malignant CCSK. CCSK is also a difficult histopathologic entity to characterize, and errors in diagnosis occur. The rhabdoid tumor of the kidney was seen in 2% of NWTS-3 patients, presenting at a median patient age of 13 months. Many cases are also associated with an apparently separate primary neuroectodermal tumor of the brain. These tumors are aggressive and are associated with a mortality rate of about 90%, even in patients with early-stage disease.

Clinical Presentation

Children with Wilms tumor typically present with an asymptomatic abdominal mass. The tumor may be discovered by a

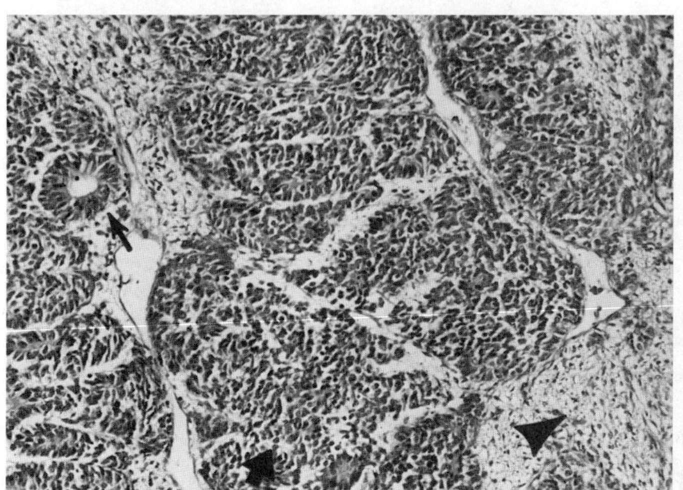
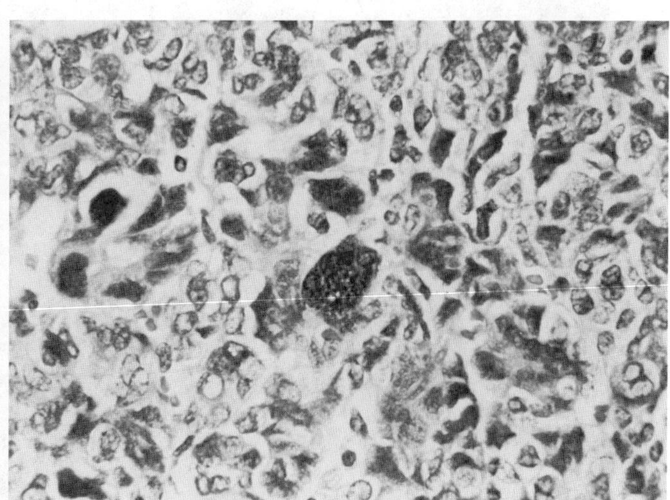

FIG. 33-2. (*A*) Histologic findings of a typical Wilms tumor of favorable histology, including epithelial differentiation (*thin arrow*), blastema morphology (*thick arrow*), and mesenchymal tissue (*arrowhead*). (×170) (*B*) Marked cellular atypia consistent with anaplasia and an unfavorable histology Wilms tumor. This can be either focal or diffuse. (×520) (Courtesy of Kay Washington, MD, Duke University Medical Center, Durham, NC)

parent while bathing the child or by a relative who notices a protuberant abdomen. Associated signs and symptoms, such as malaise, pain, and either microscopic or gross hematuria, are found in about 20% to 30% of patients. Hypertension, presumably due to increased renin activity, is present in about 25% of children with Wilms tumor. Occasionally, a child presents with a rapidly enlarging abdominal mass, anemia, hypertension, and fever. These children usually have a subcapsular hemorrhage within the tumor that leads to the above symptoms. The main differential diagnosis is neuroblastoma. Usually, this distinction is relatively easy because a Wilms tumor is intrarenal, with a characteristic intrinsic abnormality of the urinary collecting system. Neuroblastomas arise within the adrenal gland or the paravertebral sympathetic ganglia, and these masses displace rather than distort the kidney. Benign conditions, such as multicystic kidneys, obstructive uropathy, and renal carbuncles, can lead to confusion and require consideration in the differential diagnosis of an abdominal mass in a child.

A careful physical examination should consider the association of hemihypertrophy, aniridia, or Beckwith-Wiedemann syndrome. The abdominal mass associated with a Wilms tumor is frequently felt in the flank and on the left side and must be distinguished from an enlarged spleen. Tumors that cross the midline are more likely to be neuroblastomas, but large Wilms tumors can present as midline abdominal masses. The presence of bone pain suggests a neuroblastoma, but bony metastases are seen in children with CCSK tumors. Cerebral signs suggesting brain metastases are rare in children with Wilms tumors but can be seen in infants with rhabdoid tumors or CCSK.

The workup of a child with an intraabdominal mass who is suspected of having a Wilms tumor should proceed in a systematic fashion. Imaging studies should be limited to those necessary to establish the presence of an intrarenal lesion. Initially, a real-time ultrasound determines whether the mass is intrarenal or extrarenal and also whether the lesion is cystic or solid (Fig. 33-3). Ultrasonography can also determine the presence and extent of renal vein or inferior vena caval propagation of tumor thrombus. Although ultrasonography also determines the presence of a contralateral kidney, an intravenous pyelogram is necessary to determine the function of the kidneys and to plan radiotherapy, if this is required in the postoperative period. Echocardiography should be performed if there is any suggestion of a tumor thrombus extending into the right atrium. The surgeon, in conjunction with the radiology department, should define the need for preoperative computed tomography (CT) and magnetic resonance (MR) imaging. CT scanning should be performed if the surgeon thinks that additional information is required before proceeding with operative intervention. CT scanning has been found to be superior to ultrasonography in evaluation of Wilms tumor, but CT information is not necessarily essential to the surgeon in the performance of the operative procedure (Fig. 33-4). Although CT scans are helpful in identifying contralateral tumors, an NWTS report found an error rate of 7% in bilateral tumors despite preoperative CT scan. Half of the errors were seen in children with contralateral tumors less than 1 cm in diameter. MR imaging can also provide further information but is frequently not helpful unless there is suspected intravascular extension of tumor, in which case MR imaging is probably the most sensitive imaging study available (Fig. 33-5). Because the lungs are a frequent site of metastatic disease, anteroposterior and lateral chest radiographs should be performed. CT scanning of the chest is not indicated in patients with normal chest radiographs because small nodules detected on CT scan are frequently benign. The NWTS group recommends treatment based on the local stage of the tumor as determined at operation in patients with pulmonary lesions seen on CT only, unless the pulmonary lesions are confirmed by thoracotomy to be metastatic disease. Once the histology of the Wilms tumor is determined, postoperative MR imaging of the brain should be performed in children with rhabdoid and CCSK tumors, and a skeletal survey or bone scan should be carried out in patients with CCSK.[9]

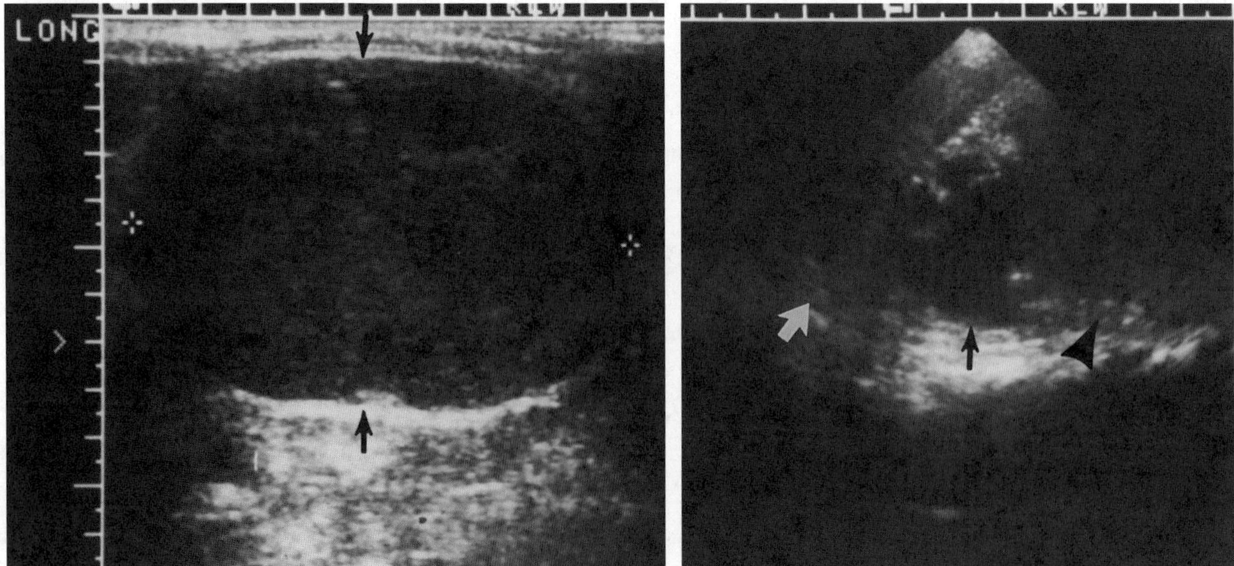

FIG. 33-3. Ultrasound findings of a left-sided Wilms tumor. (*A*) A large, reasonably homogeneous solid mass replaces most of the left kidney (*arrows*). (*B*) The same lesion and its relation to a partially obstructed urinary collecting system (*black arrow*) and spleen (*white arrow*). The Wilms tumor is also indicated (*arrowhead*). (Courtesy of Don Frush, MD, Duke University Medical Center, Durham, NC)

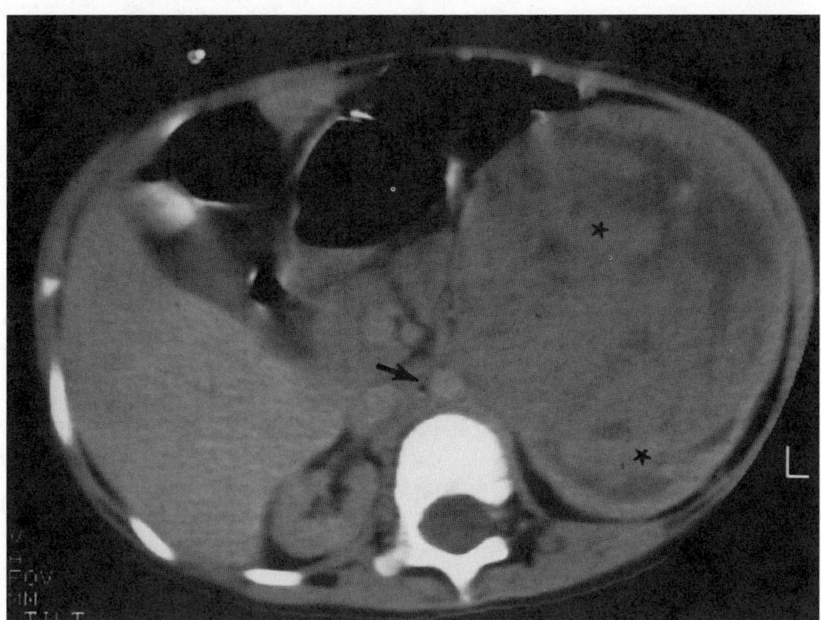

FIG. 33-4. CT image of a left-sided Wilms tumor (*asterisks*). The relations to surrounding viscera and vascular structures are easily seen. The aorta is indicated (*arrow*). This patient has a diminutive contralateral kidney because of co-existing renal disease. (Courtesy of Don Frush, MD, Duke University Medical Center, Durham, NC)

Staging

Accurate staging of patients with Wilms tumors is imperative, and the staging system developed by the NWTS (Table 33-1) has received wide acceptance in the United States. Thorough abdominal exploration should be carried out because the presence of disease beyond the tumor significantly affects therapy and prognosis. Careful investigation of the liver and the contralateral kidney should be performed. The presence of peritoneal implants or bloody peritoneal fluid and the presence or absence of enlarged lymph nodes should be recorded. Careful lymph node sampling is important because the presence of nodal involvement along the periaortic and inferior vena caval lymph node chain is associated with an increased incidence of tumor relapse and a poorer prognosis. A review of lymph node sampling by the NWTS demonstrated a false-negative rate of 31%

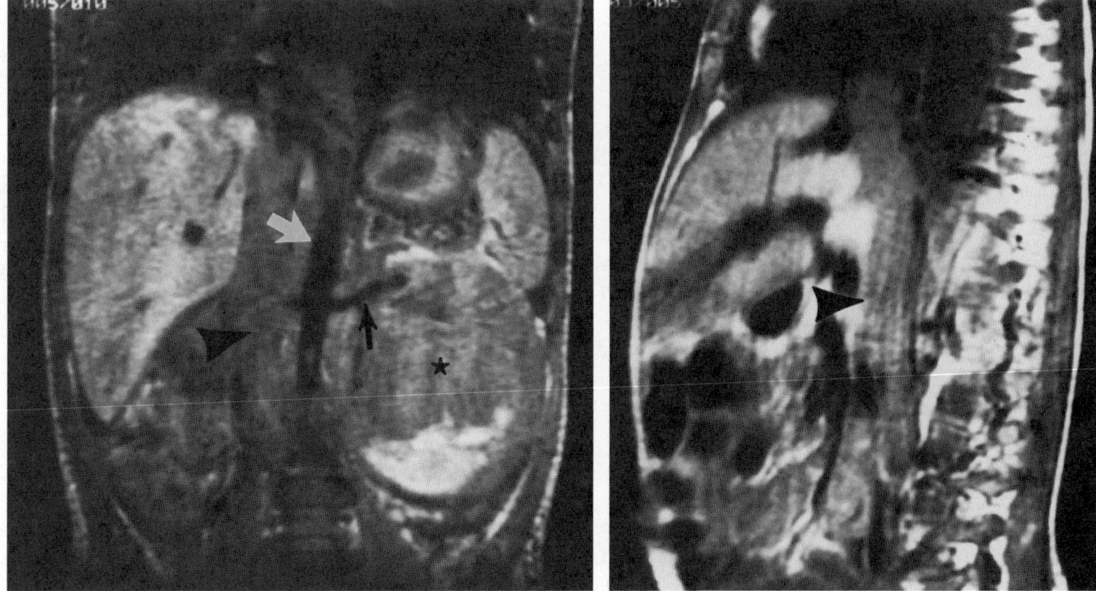

FIG. 33-5. MR image in a patient with a left-sided Wilms tumor and extension of tumor thrombus into the renal vein and inferior vena cava. (*A*) Coronal image showing Wilms tumor (*asterisk*), inferior vena cava thrombus (*arrowhead*), aorta (*white arrow*), and left renal artery (*black arrow*). (*B*) Sagittal image of the same patient. the inferior vena cava is indicated (*arrowhead*). (Courtesy of Don Frush, MD, Duke University Medical Center, Durham, NC)

TABLE 33-1. *Staging system for National Wilms Tumor Study-4 patients*

I	Tumor is limited to kidney and completely excised. The surface of the renal capsule is intact. Tumor was not ruptured before or during removal. There is no residual tumor apparent beyond the margins of excision.
II	Tumor extends beyond the kidney but is completely excised. There is regional extension of the tumor, that is, penetration through the outer surface of the renal capsule into perirenal soft tissues. Vessels outside the kidney substance are infiltrated or contain tumor thrombus. The tumor may have undergone biopsy, or there has been local spillage of tumor contained to the flank. There is no residual tumor apparent at or beyond the margins of excision.
III	Residual nonhematogenous tumor is confined to abdomen. Any one or more of the following occur: 1. Lymph nodes on biopsy are found to be involved in the hilus, the periaortic chains, or beyond. 2. There has been diffuse peritoneal contamination by tumor, such as by spillage of tumor beyond the flank before or during surgery, or by tumor growth that has penetrated through the peritoneal surface. 3. Implants are found on the peritoneal surfaces. 4. The tumor extends beyond the surgical margins either microscopically or grossly. 5. The tumor is not completely resectable because of local infiltration into vital structures.
IV	Hematogenous metastases. Deposits beyond stage III, that is, lung, liver, bone, and brain.
V	Bilateral renal involvement at diagnosis. An attempt should be made to stage each side according to the above criteria on the basis of extent of disease before biopsy.

and a false-positive rate of 18%. Therefore, even clinically negative lymph nodes along the aorta and inferior vena cava should be carefully sampled, as should any suspicious lymph nodes that are detected at operative resection.[10] Formal en bloc lymphadenectomy is not recommended.

Treatment

Surgical Considerations

A meticulous and well-performed operative procedure can accurately determine the stage of disease. A poorly performed procedure can lead to inadequate therapy if the patient is not appropriately staged or to unnecessarily intensive therapy if operative spill of the tumor occurs or if the primary tumor is not resected completely. The leading responsibilities of the surgeon are to remove the primary tumor completely without spillage and to assess the extent of tumor spread.

Radical nephrectomy should be carried out through a generous transperitoneal incision that allows for adequate exposure and complete exploration of the abdomen. Thoracic extension may be necessary but has been associated with a higher complication rate. Any suspicious lesions that may represent metastases should undergo biopsy. The contralateral kidney should be palpated and examined to rule out bilateral involvement. This should be done before resection of the primary tumor if technically feasible. The Gerota fascia should be incised, and the kidney should be palpated and visualized on its anterior and posterior surfaces. Any suspicious lesions should undergo biopsy. Unsuspected small foci of tumor have been reported even in patients with negative imaging studies. Data gathered from the NWTS Bilateral Wilms Tumor Study support this practice; small lesions found in the contralateral kidney at the time of exploration were frequently unfavorable histologic variants. This important information would not have been obtained if the kidney had not been mobilized and biopsy specimens taken. Treatment of patients with bilateral Wilms tumor is discussed later. Isolation of the hilar vessels should be carried out before mobilization of the primary tumor if possible. Initial ligation of the hilar vessels should not be pursued, however, if technically difficult or dangerous because injuries to the mesenteric arteries, celiac vessels, and aorta have been reported. This complication is seen especially with large, left-sided tumors and can be prevented if the tumor is adequately mobilized before ligation of the renal artery and vein. Lymph node sampling is imperative, and any involved or suspicious lymph nodes should be excised. The site of the excised node should be marked with titanium clips. Titanium clips should also be used to mark the tumor bed and any suspicious areas of metastases. The use of titanium metal clips is important because they do not interfere with subsequent CT scanning. Metal clips should not be used for hemostasis, since this confounds subsequent imaging.

Biopsy of the primary tumor should not be carried out before removal, and a meticulous dissection is imperative to avoid rupture of the tumor capsule with spillage of tumor cells. Because staging is affected by the degree of spillage, careful management of the degree of contamination if spillage occurs is essential. Localization of the spillage to the tumor bed allows for a stage II classification rather than stage III in patients with diffuse peritoneal soilage. This distinction is extremely important because stage III patients require total abdominal irradiation and the addition of the cardiotoxic agent doxorubicin to the chemotherapy regimen.

The ureter is ligated and divided as low as possible, but complete removal of the ureter down to the bladder is not necessary. Wilms tumors rarely invade surrounding structures but frequently adhere to adjacent organs. If the tumor cannot be cleanly separated from adjacent structures, excision of the tumor with surrounding structures can be carried out in continuity if the operating surgeon believes that *all* tumor tissue can be completely removed. Because patients with small residual disease respond well to chemotherapy, and because an increased incidence of complications has been associated with tumor resections that include adjacent structures, radical resection is indicated only if all tumor can be removed. In the case of hepatic invasion, a planned wedge resection of the liver, along with the primary tumor, can usually be carried out. Tumor spillage or leaving residual tumor within the liver bed should be avoided, and formal hepatectomy is rarely indicated. Patients with complete resection of adjacent organs usually are classified as stage II, as compared with patients who have residual tumor left within the abdominal cavity, who are stage III. This has significant therapeutic implications because of the intensity of therapy required for stage III patients.

Preoperative tumor rupture is sometimes encountered, and bloody peritoneal fluid should be considered a sign of major soilage within the peritoneal cavity. Rupture posteriorly without hemorrhage or hematoma is classified as stage II, but when a hematoma occurs in association with preoperative rupture, microscopic residual disease is assumed, and the patient is stage III.

Vena caval and atrial involvement by Wilms tumor occurs in about 4% of patients. Survival does not appear to be affected, and the prognosis for this group is comparable stage by stage to children without intravascular involvement. If possible, localization of the thrombus should be determined before operation; this is usually possible using real-time ultrasonography, echocardiography, or MR imaging. Surgical excision of the primary tumor and thrombus is recommended when technically feasible. An intraabdominal approach is sufficient for infrahepatic lesions, with extraction of the caval thrombus after proximal and distal control of the vena cava are obtained. Use of a Fogarty or Foley catheter balloon may be required. Free-floating thrombi that are easily removed are classified as stage II, but thrombi that invade the vessel or that adhere to the wall of the vessel are classified as stage III. Exposure of the inferior vena cava as it enters the atrium is obtained through a thoracoabdominal incision or through the membranous portion of the diaphragm in cases in which the tumor thrombus extends to the hepatic veins or superiorly to the atrium. The inferior vena cava is isolated and occluded at the atrium, and the tumor thrombus is removed through an infrahepatic caval incision. Patients with atrial extension of tumor thrombus require cardiopulmonary bypass for thrombus removal. In these patients, a midline abdominal incision with a median sternotomy should be considered.

A complication rate of about 20% is seen after primary nephrectomy for Wilms tumor.[11] The most frequent complication is small bowel obstruction, followed by major intraoperative hemorrhage, wound infection, vascular injury, and injury to other organs. Nine deaths occurred in a series of 1910 NWTS patients after nephrectomy for Wilms tumor; there was one intraoperative death, and eight deaths were related to peritonitis and sepsis secondary to bowel obstruction or bowel injury. Factors associated with an increased incidence of complications were advanced local tumor stage at diagnosis, intravascular tumor extension, resection of other visceral organs at the time of nephrectomy, and thoracoabdominal incision. Critical intraoperative judgment concerning radical resection with contiguous organs versus biopsy, postoperative chemotherapy, and second-look surgery may be required to decrease the risk of complications. Because invasion of adjacent organs is rarely seen in Wilms tumor patients, radical resection is infrequently indicated.

Most cases of small bowel obstruction in this series were due to adhesions, followed by intussusception and internal hernia. Most cases occurred within the first 3 months after nephrectomy, and 16 of the 17 cases of intussusception were observed within the first 3 weeks after nephrectomy. The incidence of small bowel obstruction did not appear to be increased in children who received postoperative radiotherapy.

Postoperative Therapy

As mentioned earlier, the postoperative treatment of Wilms tumor has gradually evolved since the inception of the NWTS in 1969. The present therapy of Wilms tumor is based on the findings of NWTS-3 and NWTS-4. The treatment scheme for NWTS is outlined in Figure 33-6. It compared conventional therapy with a pulse-intensive chemotherapy regimen administered for different lengths of time. One of the main questions in the NWTS-4 randomized trial was socioeconomic: can a 1-day continuous infusion of actinomycin D reduce costs, discomfort to the patient, and inconvenience to the family? The data are being analyzed. The outcome of the NWTS-4 determined that the pulse-intensive regimens produce less hematologic toxicity than the standard regimen while maintaining an excellent, relapse-free survival. The pulse-intensive regimens are now recommended as standard therapy in NWTS-5. Children who are less than 24 months of age with stage I favorable histology Wilms tumors that weigh less than 550 g will not receive adjuvant chemotherapy or radiotherapy after surgery in NWTS-5. The conventional therapy is as follows:

1. Combination chemotherapy with actinomycin D and vincristine is adequate therapy for children with tumors that are stage I favorable histology or anaplastic histology and stage II favorable histology. Stage I patients are treated for 6 months and stage II patients for 15 months.
2. Postoperative radiotherapy is not required in children with stage I and stage II favorable histology tumors and stage I anaplastic histology tumors.

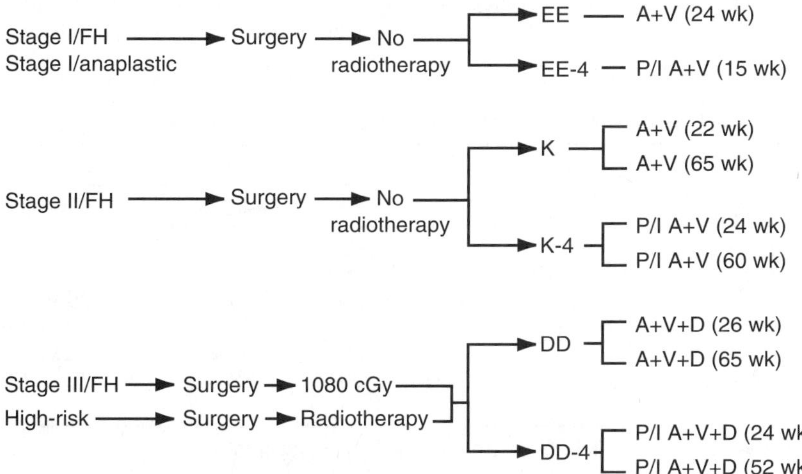

FIG. 33-6. Treatment protocol from the National Wilms Tumor Study-4. The high-risk category includes stage IV/FH and patients with clear cell sarcoma of any stage. Clear cell sarcoma patients are given 1080 cGY radiotherapy, as are patients in stage IV/FH if the primary tumor would qualify as stage III were there no metastases. A, actinomycin; V, vincristine; D, doxorubicin (Adriamycin); P/I, pulse-intensive; FH, favorable histology.

3. Doxorubicin is added to actinomycin D and vincristine in patients with stage III favorable histology tumors. These patients also receive 1000 cGy of postoperative radiation.
4. Stage IV patients with favorable histology tumors and children with CCSK histology are treated with actinomycin D, vincristine, and doxorubicin plus radiotherapy based on the clinical stage of the primary tumor at the time of resection.

The following recommendations have been suggested for patients with unfavorable histology anaplastic tumors. Patients with stage I focal or diffuse anaplasia continue to be treated with actinomycin D and vincristine without abdominal irradiation. Because patients with stage II to IV tumors with focal anaplasia have an excellent prognosis, treatment with vincristine, actinomycin D, and doxorubicin plus abdominal irradiation is recommended. The 4-year survival in this subgroup of children is 100%. The addition of cyclophosphamide to the three-drug treatment regimen of actinomycin D, vincristine, and doxorubicin in children with stage II to IV tumors with diffuse anaplasia improved the 4-year relapse-free survival rate from 27% to 52%. Despite the benefit seen by the addition of cyclophosphamide to the treatment regimen, the results of therapy in children with stage III to IV diffuse anaplastic tumors requires intensification of treatment, possibly by the addition of etoposide. Rhabdoid tumors have not responded to any of the standard regimens and were excluded from NWTS-4. Various multiagent chemotherapy protocols have been suggested, and the combination of carboplatin, etoposide, and cyclophosphamide will be studied in these difficult patients in the future.

The overall survival statistics for NWTS-3 are shown in Table 33-2. The 4-year survival rate was 75% for patients with CCSK.[12] Unfortunately, the 4-year survival rate for malignant rhabdoid tumors was 25%. The survival statistics for patients with stage II to IV focal anaplastic tumors was 100%, but this represented a small fraction of the total group of patients with anaplasia. Patients with stage II to IV diffuse anaplastic tumors had a 4-year survival rate (mentioned earlier) of 27% with three-drug chemotherapy versus 52% with actinomycin D, vincristine, doxorubicin, and cyclophosphamide.

Although the survival rate of patients with Wilms tumor in general is favorable, adverse side effects are associated with therapy. Second malignant neoplasms have been reported, with a cumulative risk at 10 years of 1%. Most second malignancies occur in irradiated areas. Although no significant cardiovascular problems have been reported in NWTS patients treated with doxorubicin, this drug is a cardiotoxic agent, and cardiac abnormalities in patients with long-term survival have been reported after doxorubicin therapy in other patient groups. The concerns remain. Refinements in radiotherapy have significantly decreased posttreatment musculoskeletal abnormalities, but scoliosis and musculoskeletal abnormalities in patients with early-stage disease who do not receive postoperative radiotherapy are about seven times less frequent than in patients who receive postoperative radiotherapy.[13]

Preoperative Chemotherapy

One of the main controversies in the treatment of children with Wilms tumor is whether to embark on a course of preoperative chemotherapy, as suggested by the International Society of Pediatric Oncology. The surgeon considering the use of preoperative chemotherapy should realize that there can be significant adverse affects on staging and histologic evaluation in children who receive preoperative chemotherapy, which could lead to either overtreatment or undertreatment. Evidence to support the dangers of undertreatment is derived from an International Society of Pediatric Oncology study that showed an increased incidence of infradiaphragmatic relapses in patients who did not receive postoperative radiotherapy. Obviously, patients with lymph node involvement were missed owing to preoperative chemotherapy. If this problem is to be avoided in patients receiving preoperative therapy, radiotherapy will have to be given to all of these children, or the potential cardiotoxic drug doxorubicin will have to be added to the postoperative chemotherapy regimen. Side effects of radiotherapy are well recognized, as are the toxic side effects of the various chemotherapeutic agents. In addition, the occurrence of second malignant neoplasms must be considered in patients who are receiving combined-modality therapy. Another potential hazard of preoperative therapy is that the histologic appearance of the primary tumor may be altered after therapy and can resemble unfavorable anaplastic histology at the time of nephrectomy. This would lead to unnecessary intensification of therapy. Proponents of preoperative therapy suggest that the tumor is easier to resect, with a decreased incidence of tumor spill and lower mortality and morbidity rates. Morbidity and mortality rates after tumor resection in NWTS were extremely low, however, and the incidence of tumor spill was about 10%. In addition, local tumor spill alters therapy little because these patients are classified as stage II according to NWTS protocols. Another argument used for preoperative therapy is that renal units can be spared and the so-called hyper-

TABLE 33-2. *Survival results in randomized patients from the National Wilms Tumor Study-3*

Stage	Histology	Regimen	No.	Relapse-free	Overall
				2-Year survival (%)	
I	Favorable	AMD + VCR, 10 wk vs 6 mo	469	90 vs 93	98
II	Favorable	15 mo AMD + VCR vs AMD + VCR + ADR (±RT)	262	91 vs 90	99 vs 93
II	Favorable	AMD + VCR ± ADR (No RT vs 2000 cGy)	262	90 vs 91	95 vs 96
III	Favorable	AMD + VCR vs AMD + VCR + ADR (15 mo + RT)	264	77 vs 88	88 vs 95
III	Favorable	AMD + VCR ± ADR 1000 vs 2000 cGy	264	82 vs 83	92 vs 91
Any IV	Any unfavorable	AMD + VCR + ADR vs AMD + VCR + ADR + CPM (15 mo + RT)	291	63 vs 69	78 vs 80

AMD, dactinomycin (Actinomycin D); VCR, vincristine; ADR, doxorubicin (Adriamycin); CPM, cyclophosphamide; RT, radiotherapy.

filtration syndrome can be prevented. There is little evidence to support the concept that preoperative therapy allows for partial nephrectomy in a significant number of patients treated in this manner, and hyperfiltration injury after unilateral nephrectomy in children is rare and poorly documented.

Despite these arguments against the use of preoperative therapy, specific patient groups can be identified who would appear to benefit from preoperative chemotherapy. These are patients with bilateral tumors, patients with inferior vena caval and intraatrial involvement, and patients with massive tumors considered by the operating surgeon to be nonresectable without undue risk to the patient. If preoperative therapy is considered, a biopsy to confirm the diagnosis of Wilms tumor is imperative because an error rate of between 5% and 9% has been reported in the absence of this information. In children with bilateral Wilms tumors, biopsy must be performed on both sides because the histology may be favorable on one side and unfavorable on the other. The number of patients with truly inoperable tumors is hard to ascertain because only 5% of patients registered on NWTS-3 were classified as inoperable. The potential danger of preoperative chemotherapy in patients with inferior vena caval and intraatrial involvement has not been borne out by studies, and no cases of tumor emboli have been reported. A significant finding in several reports is the excellent response to preoperative therapy in patients with atrial extension of tumor. Ritchey and colleagues[14] reported a complete response of the atrial component in 10 of 14 cases, and Oberholzer and associates[15] were able to avoid thoracotomy in 4 cases. The adoption of preoperative chemotherapy for all patients with Wilms tumor is not recommended by the NWTS group. This certainly can be questioned, however, because of the excellent results obtained in an enormous number of patients entered on the NWTS whose tumor stage and histology were confirmed by carefully performed nephrectomy before further therapy. This course of action has allowed therapy to be modified for each child, with the hope that the complications of therapy can be minimized without altering long-term disease-free survival.

Treatment of Bilateral Wilms Tumor

Bilateral Wilms tumors occur in about 5% of children with Wilms tumors. These children tend to present at any early age, and there is an increased frequency of genitourinary anomalies and hemihypertrophy. Despite sophisticated diagnostic techniques, the contralateral lesion is not diagnosed preoperatively in about one third of the patients. Unfavorable histology is seen in about 10% of cases, and there is discordant histology in a significant number of cases. The larger tumor does not necessarily contain the unfavorable histologic type. This finding underscores the importance of biopsy of both lesions before therapy. In a review by Blute and colleagues,[16] the 3-year survival rate of 145 patients with bilateral Wilms tumor registered on NWTS-2 and NWTS-3 was 76%. This finding was despite the fact that only 38% of the patients had all tumor resected at one or more operations. The best prognosis was seen in patients younger than 3 years of age at the time of diagnosis, patients with low-stage individual lesions, patients with favorable histologies, and patients with negative lymph nodes.

The NWTS recommendations for the treatment of bilateral Wilms tumors stresses the importance of preserving renal units. A transperitoneal operation is carried out, and nephrectomy is avoided. The histologic subtype and stage of both tumors are determined by bilateral biopsy and lymph node sampling. Complete excision of both tumors can be considered if two thirds or more of the total renal parenchyma can be preserved. Postoperative chemotherapy with actinomycin D and vincristine is administered according to the NWTS-4 protocols. The response to therapy should be evaluated about 2 months after initiating chemotherapy. CT should be performed at this time to assess the reduction in tumor volume and the feasibility of partial resection. A laparotomy should be carried out if resection appears feasible. At the time of this procedure, partial nephrectomy or wedge resection of the tumors should be performed if possible. This should be carried out if it does not compromise the tumor resection and if negative margins can be obtained. If extensive tumor involvement precludes partial resection of one kidney, complete excision of the tumor from the least involved kidney is performed. If this procedure leaves a viable and functioning kidney, radical nephrectomy is performed to remove the kidney with the extensive involvement. If a persistent viable tumor remains after the second laparotomy, doxorubicin should be added to the chemotherapeutic regimen. The patient should be reevaluated in about 3 months to assess the feasibility of further resection. If evidence of persistent tumor remains, a third procedure should be performed and all residual tumor removed if possible. If abdominal exploration confirms the presence of persistent disease that cannot be resected, the areas of disease should be marked using titanium clips, and the patient should receive radiotherapy. Bench surgery and renal autotransplantation can be considered in difficult cases and can be combined with intraoperative radiotherapy. Bilateral nephrectomy should be considered as a last resort because renal transplantation has been associated with a high tumor recurrence rate within the 2 years that follow resection of the tumor. In patients with unfavorable histology, more aggressive chemotherapy and radiotherapy should be considered after the initial procedure, and a more radical operation should be performed at the second procedure with an aim at removing all tumor tissue. Patients with bilateral Wilms tumors require long-term follow-up because relapses have occurred as late as 5 years after treatment, and renal failure has been seen in about 5% of patients.

Treatment of Metastatic Disease

In patients with Wilms tumors, the treatment of metastatic disease depends on the time at which metastases are diagnosed and on the pathology of the primary tumor. Patients with stage IV favorable histology tumors at diagnosis have a good prognosis, while unfavorable histology patients and patients who relapse with metastatic disease have a grave prognosis. About 12% of patients with Wilms tumors have evidence of hematogenous metastases at diagnosis, and 20% of favorable histology tumors relapse after therapy.[17]

Eighty percent of stage IV patients have pulmonary metastases, and most relapses are also pulmonary (Fig. 33-7). Patients with pulmonary metastases usually can be managed by combined chemotherapy and radiotherapy. Pulmonary resection is rarely indicated. Pulmonary injury associated with lung irradiation is significant; 13% of patients developed diffuse interstitial

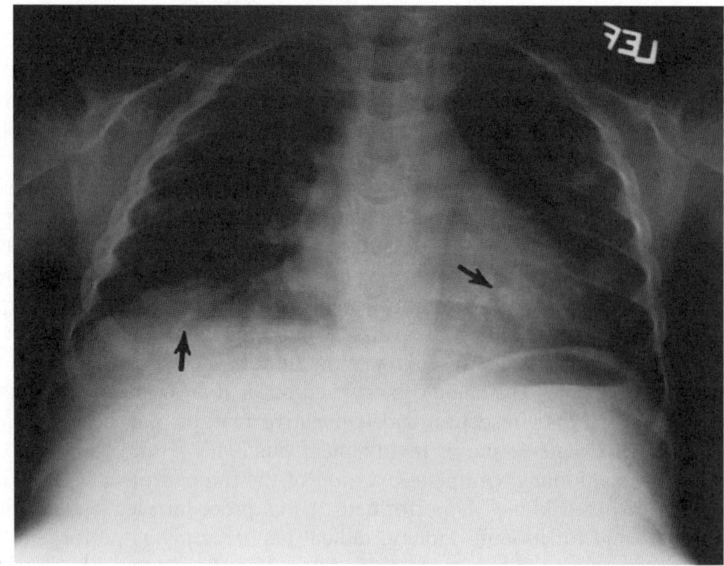
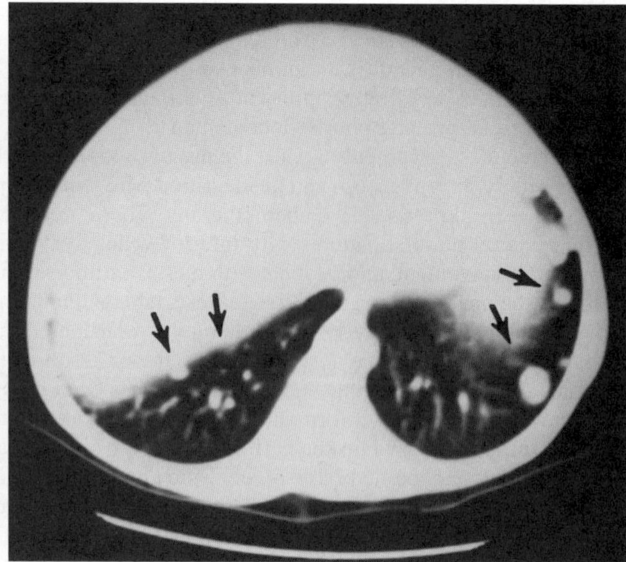

FIG. 33-7. Plain chest radiograph (*A*) and corresponding thoracic CT image (*B*) in a child with multiple bilateral pulmonary metastases (*arrows*) from Wilms tumor.

pneumonitis in NWTS-3. In an attempt to avoid pulmonary irradiation, de Kraker and colleagues[18] treated patients with preoperative chemotherapy followed by pulmonary resection for residual disease (5 of 36 patients), with a survival rate of 83%. Twenty-six of the 36 patients did not receive pulmonary irradiation. Further studies with a larger patient base are required to define an optimal treatment plan. Green and associates[19] reviewed 211 patients from NWTS-1, NWTS-2, and NWTS-3 with recurrent Wilms tumors defined by lung metastases. They found no difference in the 4-year survival rates of patients with and without surgical removal of pulmonary metastases in addition to pulmonary irradiation and chemotherapy. Although histologic confirmation of pulmonary relapse may be indicated, these data suggest that complete removal of pulmonary metastases at relapse does not increase survival.

Hepatic involvement associated with Wilms tumors has been considered to be a poor prognostic sign (Fig. 33-8), but a review of NWTS-1, NWTS-2, and NWTS-3 does not support this contention. Overall survival of patients with liver invasion and patients with liver metastases at initial diagnosis compares favorably with the overall NWTS experience. Based on this experience, the presence of multiple liver metastases should not alter the therapy of the primary tumor. As mentioned earlier, major hepatic lobectomy in conjunction with radical nephrectomy is rarely required and should be reserved for selected cases. Despite the favorable prognosis seen with liver metastases at diagnosis, relapse to the liver carries a grave prognosis with or without hepatic resection. If an isolated relapse to the liver is detected without evidence of other metastases, hepatic resection should be considered. This is a rare occurrence.

Future Directions

The future treatment of Wilms tumors will continue to be refined in the tradition of the NWTS, so that the morbidity of treatment is decreased without sacrificing relapse-free survival.

Previous NWTS studies have identified a subgroup of stage I patients younger than 2 years of age with tumors weighing less than 550 g who have an excellent prognosis. Selection of these patients, combined with microstaging of stage I patients as described by Weeks and Beckwith,[20] suggests that it may be possible to omit postoperative adjuvant therapy in these children. A carefully performed nephrectomy with staging is imperative if adjuvant chemotherapy is to be eliminated in this group of patients. A small number of patients treated in this manner have been reported by Larson and colleagues[21] to have excellent survival statistics.

Depending on the outcome of ongoing genetic studies, high-risk patients may be identified in the future in whom more intensive therapy can be administered. NWTS-5 was designed

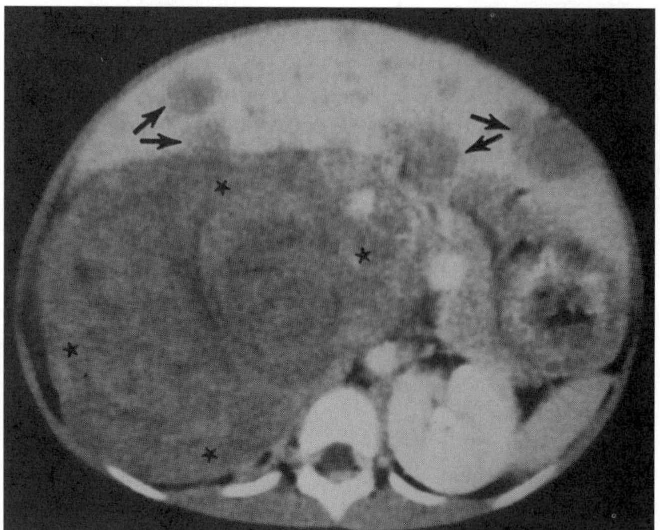

FIG. 33-8. CT image of a right-sided Wilms tumor (*asterisks*) with multiple liver metastases (*arrows*).

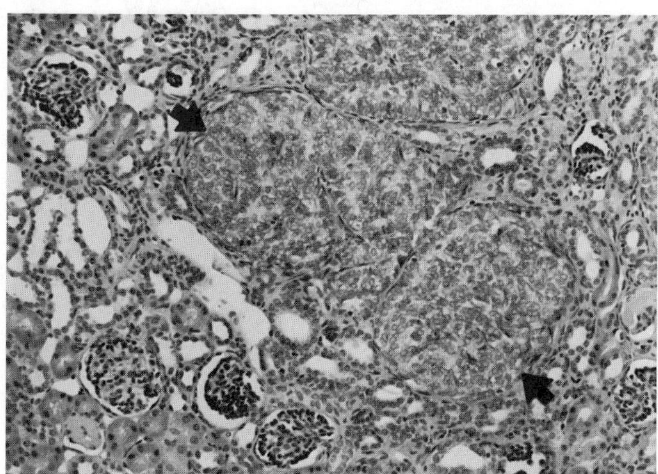

FIG. 33-9. Histologic specimen of a kidney reveals a perilobar nephrogenic rest (*arrows*). (×170.) (Courtesy of Kay Washington, MD, Duke University Medical Center, Durham, NC)

with this in mind. NWTS-5 is newly opened for patient entry with the following objectives:

- To determine whether loss of heterozygosity for chromosome 16q markers in tumor tissue is associated with a poor prognosis for children with Wilms tumors of favorable histology
- To determine whether loss of heterozygosity for chromosome 1p markers in tumor tissue is associated with a poor prognosis for children with Wilms tumors of favorable histology
- To determine whether increased DNA content in tumor cells is associated with a poor prognosis
- To improve the survival and disease-free interval of patients with Wilms tumors of unfavorable histology with diffuse anaplasia and CCSK by using a new treatment regimen that includes etoposide and cyclophosphamide
- To improve the disease-free survival of patients with malignant rhabdoid tumors of the kidney by using a new treatment regimen that includes carboplatin, etoposide, and cyclophosphamide

Stage II and III patients may be classified by the loss of heterozygosity of 16q into groups that require more intensive or less intensive therapy. For example, stage III patients without lymph node metastases or loss of heterozygosity of 16q may be able to have radiotherapy and the cardiotoxic agent doxorubicin eliminated from their regimens.

Further refinement of cytogenetic technology and the use of nuclear morphometric studies to predict response to therapy may be forthcoming. Several biologic markers have been described in patients with Wilms tumors that may be helpful in diagnosis and monitoring for recurrent disease. The most prominent of these markers are serum renin, hyaluronidase, and hyaluronic acid–stimulating activity.

NEPHROBLASTOMATOSIS

The term *nephroblastomatosis* has been in use for some time, but Beckwith and associates[22] proposed a new classification based on materials submitted to the NWTS pathology center. These researchers suggest that the term *nephrogenic rest* be used for foci of abnormal nephrogenic cells that appear to be precursors to Wilms tumor. Nephrogenic rests are considered *intralobar* or *perilobar,* depending on their location within the kidney. The term nephroblastomatosis should be used for cases in which there is diffuse or multifocal presence of nephrogenic rests. Perilobar nephrogenic rests do not appear to be precursor lesions of Wilms tumor (Fig. 33-9), but intralobar nephrogenic rests are rarely seen except in association with Wilms tumor. Forty-one percent of cases of unilateral Wilms tumor are associated with nephrogenic rests, and almost all cases of bilateral Wilms tumor are associated with nephrogenic rests. Nephrogenic rests were found in 94% of the kidneys resected in unilateral cases that went on to develop metachronous contralateral Wilms tumors. For this reason, any child with nephrogenic rests within the resected specimen after removal of unilateral Wilms tumor should be monitored carefully with imaging studies for the development of subsequent tumor in the contralateral kidney.

The treatment of children with nephroblastomatosis is not clearly established. Bilateral biopsies should be performed in children suspected of having nephroblastomatosis, and biopsy specimens should be carefully reviewed by experienced pathologists. Children with nephroblastomatosis should be followed carefully with imaging studies (ultrasound, CT) to determine the status of the lesions within the kidneys (Fig. 33-10). A second-look procedure should be reserved for children with progressive lesions. The surgical approach to these lesions should be similar to the guidelines outlined for treatment of bilateral Wilms tumor. All efforts to preserve renal units should be considered in the management of these children.

CONGENITAL MESOBLASTIC NEPHROMA

Congenital mesoblastic nephroma is a relatively benign renal tumor, usually occurring in infants younger than 3 months of age. Although true Wilms tumors do occur in infants, they are extremely rare. A review of the NWTS between 1969 and 1984 revealed 18 cases of mesoblastic nephroma, four cases of favorable histology Wilms tumor, and one rhabdoid tumor. The treatment of mesoblastic nephroma should be total excision using the same surgical guidelines as described for Wilms tumor. Chemotherapy of congenital mesoblastic nephroma should be reserved for cases of incomplete resection or intraoperative rupture. The chemotherapy protocol used for these children should follow the recommendations for favorable histology stage I Wilms tumor.

RENAL CELL CARCINOMA

Renal cell carcinomas in children are rare, representing 1.8% to 6.3% of the malignant renal tumors of childhood.[23] Only 3% to 5% of all renal cell carcinomas occur in patients younger than 20 years of age. In children, the average age at presentation is between 9 and 12 years, but one case was reported in an infant 10 months of age. In adults, there is a male predominance, but no sex predilection has been found in children. Pediatric patients usually present with an abdominal mass; adults most

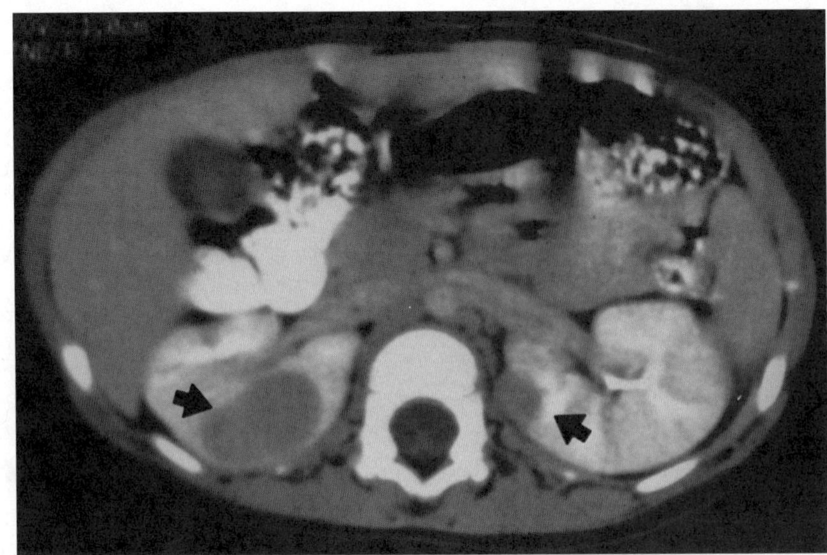

FIG. 33-10. CT image in a child with nephroblastomatosis showing small bilateral Wilms tumors (*arrows*). (Courtesy of Don Frush, MD, Duke University Medical Center, Durham, NC)

commonly present with hematuria. Hematuria occurs in half of the pediatric patients, and calcification is seen on abdominal radiographs in one fourth of the patients. Hypertension is a rare finding. Various staging systems have been used in children with renal cell carcinoma, but in general, prognosis correlates best with evidence of metastatic disease, vascular invasion, and histologic grading. The overall 5-year survival rate of children with renal cell carcinoma is about 64%. Because effective adjuvant therapy has not been found, most children who survive have localized disease without vascular invasion and low histologic grades. Radiotherapy has not been found to improve the prognosis in patients with renal cell carcinoma. Although a number of chemotherapeutic agents have been tried, no effective protocol has been established. Isolated case reports showing response to recombinant interleukin-2 and α-interferon have been made. Definition of an optimal therapeutic strategy awaits a multiinstitution study on a larger cohort to determine whether adjuvant therapy after radical nephrectomy is efficacious.

REFERENCES

1. Li FP. Cancers in children. In: Schottenfeld D, Fraumeni JF Jr, eds. Cancer epidemiology and prevention. Philadelphia, WB Saunders, 1982:1012.
2. Beckwith JB, Palmer NF. Histopathology and prognosis of Wilms' tumor. Cancer 1978;41:1927.
3. D'Angio GJ, Beckwith JB, Breslow N, et al. Wilms' tumor (nephroblastoma, renal embryoma). In: Pizzo PA, Poplack DG, eds. Principals and practice of pediatric oncology. Philadelphia, JB Lippincott, 1989:583.
4. Knudson AG. Introduction to the genetics of primary renal tumors in children. Med Pediatr Oncol 1993;21:193.
5. Breslow NE, Beckwith JB. Epidemiological features of Wilms' tumor: results of the National Wilms' Tumor Study. J Natl Cancer Inst 1982;68:429.
6. Coppes MJ, Haber DA, Grundy PE. Genetic events in the development of Wilms' tumor. N Engl J Med 1994;331:586.
7. Koo HP, Hensle TW. Molecular biology of Wilms' tumor. Urol Clin North Am 1993;20:323.
8. Grundy PE, Telzerow PE, Breslow N, et al. Loss of heterozygosity for chromosomes 1 bq and 1p in Wilms tumors predicts an adverse outcome. Cancer Res 1994;54:2331.
9. D'Angio GJ, Breslow N, Beckwith JB, et al. Imaging studies for followup of patients with primary renal tumor of childhood: a report from the National Wilms' Tumor Study. Med Pediatr Oncol 1989;17:313.
10. Othersen HB Jr, deLorimer A, Hrabousky E, et al. Surgical evaluation of lymph node metastases in Wilms' tumor. J Pediatr Surg 1990;25:330.
11. Ritchey, ML, Kelalis PP, Breslow NB, et al. Surgical complications after nephrectomy for Wilms' tumor: a report from the National Wilms' Tumor Study-3. Surg Gynecol Obstet 1992;175:507.
12. D'Angio GJ, Breslow N, Beckwith JB, et al. Treatment of Wilms' tumor: results of the third National Wilms' Tumor Study. Cancer 1989;64:349.
13. Evans, AE, Norkool P, Evans MS, et al. Late effects of treatment of Wilms' tumor: a report from the National Wilms' Tumor Study. Cancer 1991;67:331.
14. Ritchey ML, Kelalis PP, Haase GM, et al. Preoperative therapy for intracaval and atrial extension of Wilms' tumor. Cancer 1993;71:4104.
15. Oberholzer HF, Falkson G, DeJager LC. Successful management of inferior vena cava and right atrial nephroblastoma tumor thrombus with preoperative chemotherapy. Med Pediatr Oncol 1992;20:61.
16. Blute ML, Kelalis PP, Offord KP, et al. Bilateral Wilms' tumor. J Urol 1987;138:968.
17. Breslow NE, Sharples K, Beckwith JB, et al. Prognostic factors in nonmetastatic, favorable histology Wilms' tumor. Cancer 1991;68:2345.
18. de Kraker J, Lemerle J, Voute PA, et al. Wilms' tumor with pulmonary metastases at diagnosis: the significance of primary chemotherapy. J Clin Oncol 1990;8:1187.
19. Green DM, Breslow N, Ii Y, et al. The role of the surgical excision in the management of Wilms' tumor patients with pulmonary metastases: a report from the National Wilms' Tumor Study. J Pediatr Surg 1991;26:728.
20. Weeks DA, Beckwith JB. Relapse-associated variables in stage I favorable histology Wilms' tumor. Cancer 1987;60:1204.
21. Larson E, Prez-Atayde AR, Green DM, et al. Surgery only for the treatment of patients with stage I (Cassady) Wilms' tumor. Cancer 1990;66:264.
22. Beckwith JB, Kiviat NB, Bonadio JF, et al. Nephrogenic rests of nephroblastomatosis and the pathogenesis of Wilms' tumor. Pediatr Pathol 1990;10:1.
23. Eckschlager TE, Kodet R. Renal cell carcinoma in children: a single institution's experience. Med Pediatr Oncol 1994;23:36.

Surgery of Infants and Children: Scientific Principles and Practice, edited by Keith T. Oldham, Paul M. Colombani, and Robert P. Foglia. Lippincott–Raven Publishers, Philadelphia, © 1997.

CHAPTER 34

Neuroblastoma

Eisuke Nagabuchi and Moritz M. Ziegler

Neuroblastoma is the most common solid tumor in childhood, often associated with spontaneous regression. Infants with neuroblastomas, even with disseminated disease, have a far better prognosis than children older than 1 year of age. Because of these unique characteristics, this disease has been of great clinical and experimental interest. Progress in molecular, cellular, and immune biology in the past 10 years has greatly contributed to promoting further understanding of the nature and behavior of neuroblastoma. It is now clear that it is a heterogenesis disease process.[1] Factors such as chromosomal abnormalities, protooncogene expression, and biochemical markers have been extensively studied for categorizing groups of patients with different prognoses.[2] These achievements in our understanding of neuroblastoma, however, have not had as significant an impact on the clinical management of the disease as they have had on our knowledge about the process of oncogenesis at molecular and cellular levels.

The outcome for patients with advanced-stage neuroblastomas has improved considerably in this decade, but long-term survival is still limited. Although the improvement has been attributed in part to better and more aggressive operative techniques, the treatment of neuroblastoma is a good example of the benefit of multimodality therapies. Most treatment regimens are provided by national cooperative groups, such as the Children's Cancer Study Group (CCG) and the Pediatric Oncology Group (POG).

The surgeon provides but one element of the modern multimodal treatment. Pediatric oncologists, radiotherapists, and bone marrow transplantation (BMT) specialists are among the members of the pediatric oncology team. Surgical procedures for neuroblastoma are undertaken for both diagnostic and therapeutic purposes. The goals of operative treatment include sampling tumor tissue for diagnosis; primary, delayed primary, and second-look tumor resection; cytoreduction or debulking; resection of metastatic lesions; and palliative resection.

Concomitant with advances in the study of neuroblastoma, new strategies based on risk groups have been proposed, and clinical trials of future therapies are being intensively investigated. Such future therapies may be included in treatment protocols for high-risk neuroblastoma patients strongly resistant to present multimodality therapies. This chapter reviews the principles and practices that apply to the modern care of the child with neuroblastoma.

DEFINITION AND EPIDEMIOLOGY

Neuroblastoma is a tumor derived from the sympathogonia, cells found at the site of neural crest tissue anywhere in the body. The tumor is characterized by several unique behaviors, including the secretion of catecholamine products, the potential to spontaneously, or with stimulation, mature to a benign ganglioneuroma, and a high incidence of spontaneous regression.

According to a population-based study in North America,[3] the annual incidence of neuroblastoma is 10.95 per 1 million children younger than the age of 15 years and 27.75 per 1 million children between the ages of 0 and 4 years. The annual mortality rate from neuroblastoma is 4.89 per 1 million and 9.10 per 1 million for the age groups 0 to 14 years and 0 to 4 years, respectively. More than half of neuroblastomas are associated with advanced-stage disease (III or IV), and about 40% of patients have disseminated disease (Table 34-1). The 10-year survival rates for patients with Children's Cancer Study Group (CCG) stage I to IV and IV-S disease are 88%, 90%, 63%, 21%, and 81%, respectively. (Unless otherwise indicated, stages given in this chapter are according to the CCG staging system.)

Neuroblastoma is slightly predominant in boys; however, correlation between gender and prognosis remains controversial.[4]

Reports have been made of familial neuroblastomas and of neuroblastoma in a family with pheochromocytomas. Neuroblastoma has been reported in infants with Beckwith-Wiedemann syndrome, Hirschsprung disease, and fetal alcohol syndrome and in the offspring of mothers taking phenylhydantoin for seizure disorders.

PATHOLOGY

Classic Histopathology

The gross appearance of the tumor depends on its location, degree of maturation, and whether it has developed hemorrhage or necrosis. The tumor is classically purple, highly vascular, and friable; however, it becomes more nodular and frequently fleshy white with maturation or in response to therapy. Larger

TABLE 34-1. *Percentage distribution of neuroblastoma cases by age and stage*

Area	Age (y)	Stage					Total
		I	II	III	IV	IV-S	
Quebec	<1	7.7	7.7	6.9	7.7	7.7	37.7
	>1	7.7	6.9	10.8	36.9	0	62.3
Greater Delaware Valley	<1	12.8	11.0	3.7	11.0	7.3	45.7
	>1	6.7	9.8	7.3	30.5	0	54.3
Total	<1	10.5	9.5	5.1	9.5	7.5	42.2
	>1	7.1	8.5	8.8	33.3	0	57.8
		17.7	18.0	13.9	42.9	7.5	

(Bernstein ML, Leclerc JM, Bunin G, et al. A population-based study of neuroblastoma incidence, survival, and mortality in North America. J Clin Oncol 1992;10:323)

tumors frequently have hemorrhage and necrosis, resulting in intratumor calcification.

Neuroblastomas typically have a rosette formation microscopically. They may also have scattered ganglion cells or immature chromaffin cells. Histopathologic characteristics, such as the degree of differentiation, maturation, lymphoid infiltration, calcification, anaplasia, necrosis, mitotic activity, neurofibrillary material (neuropil), and multinucleate cells, have been evaluated to predict the patient's prognosis.

Shimada Classification

Shimada and colleagues[5] developed an age-linked classification system based on morphology of the primary tumor. Characteristics such as the degree of cellular differentiation, nuclear morphology of neuroblastic cells, and organizational pattern of the stromal tissue were used. These researchers divided neuroblastomas into two prognostic subgroups: favorable histology and unfavorable histology[6] (Table 34-2). This classification has been widely accepted and has proved to be useful for predicting disease outcome.

Joshi and colleagues[7] proposed a new histologic grading system defined by calcification and mitotic rate, in which patients are divided into two risk groups by grades (Tables 34-3 and 34-4). Convenience and reproducibility of this grading system compared with the Shimada classification was emphasized in

TABLE 34-2. *Shimada classification system*

	Favorable histology	Unfavorable histology
Stroma-rich	Well-differentiated or intermixed	Nodular
Stroma-poor		
Age <1.5 y	MKI <200/5000	MKI >200/5000
Age 1.5–5 y	MKI <100/5000 and differentiating	MKI >100/5000 or undifferentiated
Age >5 y	None	All

MKI, mitotic–karyorrhectic index.
(Chatten J, Shimada H, Sather HN, et al. Prognostic value of histopathology in advanced neuroblastoma: a report from the Children's Cancer Study Group. Hum Pathol 1988;19:1187)

their report from the POG. In a follow-up study, they also reported a correlation between histologic grades and nonmorphologic factors, such as DNA index, *N-myc* oncogene amplification, and serum lactate dehydrogenase (LDH) levels.[8] The superiority of this system, however, has not yet been confirmed by other investigators.

IMMUNOBIOLOGY

Spontaneous Regression

Neuroblastoma is the most common human tumor to undergo spontaneous regression. The maximum incidence of spontaneous regression as estimated in a Danish survey is about 10%.[9] This phenomenon frequently occurs in infants with stage IV-S (International Staging System [INSS] stage 4S) neuroblastomas. It may be explained by an immune defense mechanism.[10] Beckwith and Perrin[11] reported that, at autopsy, the adrenal glands of stillborn babies contained ''nests'' of neuroblastomas at a frequency much higher than the incidence of clinical neuroblastoma. This suggested that most tumor nests disappear and fail to develop into clinical tumors. In addition, several studies[12,13] have suggested that patients with neuroblastomas are likely to have lymphocytes with specific antitumor activity, and that serum obtained from neuroblastoma patients contains factors capable of blocking cellular antitumor activity. Further linkage of an immune mechanism to spontaneous regression of neuroblastoma was reported by Squire and colleagues,[14] who found that archival human neuroblastoma cells from patients with stage I to IV disease expressed low levels of class I major histocompatibility complex (MHC) antigen, while cells from stage IV-S patients expressed normal levels. Furthermore, surviving patients had tumors of higher class I antigen expression than did nonsurvivors from the same stage.

An alternate explanation for the spontaneous regression of neuroblastoma is known as the *two-hit theory* of oncogenesis by Knudson and Meadows.[15] In this hypothesis, the initial neuroblastoma is thought to be a hyperplastic lesion and not a true neoplasm (first hit). Without a second mutation, the hyperplastic process would eventually cease, and the tumor would disappear. Malignant behavior in this scenario is confirmed by the second event. This concept quickly became accepted, especially with regard to children younger than 1 year of age (typical INSS stage 4S neuroblastoma). Preliminary observations of children

TABLE 34-3. *Histologic grade*

Grade	Mitotic rate*		Calcification
1	Low	and	+
2	Low	or	+
3	High	and	−

* Low is 10 or fewer per 10 high-power fields; high is more than 10 per 10 high-power fields.

(Joshi VV, Cantor AB, Altshuler G, et al. Age-linked prognostic categorization based on a new histologic grading system of neuroblastomas. Cancer 1992;69:2197)

with stage IV-S disease have shown an interesting relation between tumor regression and *N-myc* oncogene amplification. It appears that at an early stage, the tumor-suppressor mechanism functions more strongly. Later, this diminishes, and *N-myc* oncogene amplification becomes overt.[16] Thus, *N-myc* expression may be related to a second-hit mutation, but this relation has not been fully defined.

Studies on signal transduction and nerve growth factor (NGF) can be helpful in understanding the mechanism of tumor regression. Kogner and colleagues[17] have shown that neuroblastomas coexpressing mRNA for both the *TRK* gene and the low-affinity NGF receptor (*LNGFR*) are favorable tumors likely to differentiate or regress spontaneously (see *TRK* Genes and Neurotrophin Receptors). This study also supports a functional role for NGF in differentiation or regression of neuroblastoma in vivo. The process of neuroblastoma regression, however, remains an enigma.

Host–Tumor Immunobiology

T-Cell–Mediated Antitumor Immune Activity

Neuroblastoma cells are resistant to T-cell–mediated tumor lysis. An in vitro study[18] demonstrated that human neuroblastoma cell lines weakly express class I MHC surface antigens and β_2-microglobulin, factors necessary for an effective interaction of T lymphocytes with specific tumor cell antigens. Most human neuroblastomas also express low levels of class I MHC antigens. A notable exception is stage IV-S disease, as mentioned earlier.[14] This poor expression of class I MHC antigens may account for the resistance to T-cell–mediated antitumor activity.

In an attempt to correlate molecular cytogenetic events with immunobiologic activities, it was hypothesized that the *N-myc* protooncogene down-regulates the expression of class I MHC antigens. In fact, the findings in rat neuroblastoma tissue suggested possible down-regulation of class I MHC genes by *N-*

TABLE 34-4. *Risk groups linked with histologic grade*

	Grade 1	Grade 2	Grade 3
Low-risk group	All ages	≤1 y of age	None
High-risk group	None	>1 y of age	All ages

(Joshi VV, Cantor AB, Altshuler G, et al. Age-linked prognostic categorization based on a new histologic grading system of neuroblastomas. Cancer 1992;69:2197)

myc transfection.[19] *N-myc* and class I MHC expression, however, are not necessarily inversely related in human neuroblastoma cells.[18]

Tumor Lysis by Natural Killer Cells and Lymphokine-Activated Killer Cells

Despite minimal class I MHC antigen expression by neuroblastoma cells, more antitumor activity is found in a subset of T lymphocytes recognized as natural killer (NK) cells. NK cell activity in children with nonmetastatic stage III neuroblastomas is significantly greater than in children with localized stage I and II disease or in healthy children.[20] This increased NK cell activity may result from exposure to cellular products from the tumor. Similarly, metastatic stage IV disease is associated with impaired NK cell function, perhaps secondary to NK cell suppression mediated by host monocytes.[10]

In vitro observations suggest that recombinant interferon-α (IFN-α) and recombinant interleukin-2 (IL-2) induce lymphokine-activated killer (LAK) cell activity against neuroblastoma.[20] A report analyzing IL-2–activated tumor-infiltrating lymphocytes (TILs) from patients with neuroblastomas revealed more cytotoxicity to neuroblastoma than that produced by IL-2–activated peripheral blood lymphocytes. Furthermore, these TILs had a high proportion of NK cells. This observation suggests a potential role for TILs as a tool for adoptive immunotherapy[21] (see Adoptive Immunotherapy With Tumor-Infiltrating Lymphocytes).

Antibodies to Neuroblastoma

Neuroblastoma cells are sensitive to antibody-dependent cell-mediated cytotoxicity as well as complement-dependent cytotoxicity.[22] Although a particular neuroblastoma antigen has not been defined, monoclonal murine antibodies have been raised to both the neural cell adhesion molecule (NCAM) and ganglioside G_{D2}. NCAM is uniformly expressed in neuroblastoma tumors and is also preferentially expressed in human NK cells. Because of the importance of host NK cells to antitumor activity, the potential role of NCAM in NK–tumor cell adhesion and cytotoxicity has been studied. NCAMs, however, probably do not play a major role in the cytolytic interaction between NK cells and NCAM-positive tumor cells.[23]

L1, a member of the NCAM family, is another molecule of interest. Studies using mouse antibodies to human L1 have shown that an association between NCAM and L1 may play an important role in cell–cell adhesion.[24] Expression of the L1 molecule, in addition to NCAM, has been demonstrated in a cell line established from a patient with advanced neuroblastoma associated with *N-myc* amplification.[25] Results from mouse neuroblastoma studies may be consistent with these reports. In vivo and in vitro, more metastatic and invasive mouse neuroblastoma cell lines revealed more L1 expression that was directly correlated with expression of *N-myc* mRNA[26] (Fig. 34-1). Enhanced expression of the L1 molecule in more aggressive cell lines has been observed in mouse melanoma, another tumor of neural crest origin.

Ganglioside G_{D2} is the predominant antigen in neuroblastoma cells. The antibodies 3F8,[22] murine immunoglobulin G_3 (IgG$_3$),

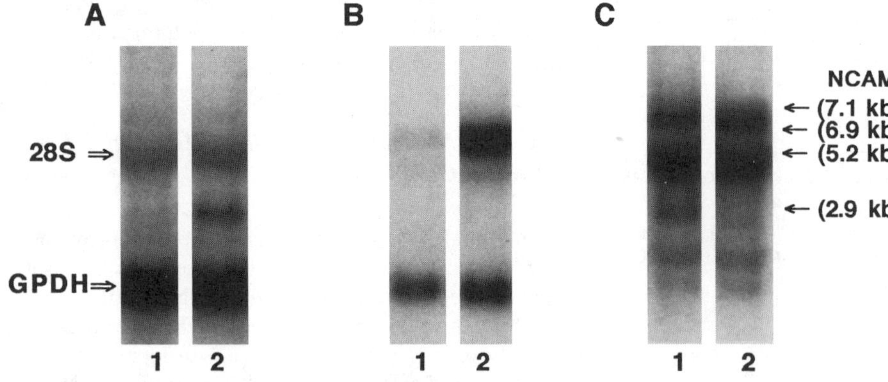

FIG. 34-1. Northern blot analysis of N-*MYC*, L1, and neural crest adhesion molecule (NCAM) mRNA in murine neuroblastoma cell lines C1300-NB (*lane 1*) and TBJ-NB (*lane 2*). (*A*) N-*MYC* mRNA (2.9 kb). (*B*) L1 mRNA (6 kb). (*C*) NCAM mRNA (2.9, 5.2, 6.9, and 7.1 kb).

murine IgG$_{2a}$, 14G2a,[27] and human and mouse chimeric antibody ch14.18[28] bind the ganglioside G$_{D2}$ antigen with exquisite specificity. These antibodies are able to alter both complement and cell-mediated cytotoxicity of neuroblastoma cells by effector cells, such as peripheral blood mononuclear cells or granulocytes. The chimeric antibody ch14.18 is more potent than the murine antibody 14G2a in this regard. Granulocytes mediate the lysis of neuroblastoma cells with ch14.18 more effectively than peripheral blood mononuclear cells.[28] Induction of antibody-dependent cell-mediated cytotoxicity with anti–ganglioside G$_{D2}$ antibodies is enhanced by cytokines such as granulocyte-macrophage colony-stimulating factor[22,29] and IL-2.[30] Based on these in vitro findings, clinical studies using anti–ganglioside G$_{D2}$ antibodies for selective tumor targeting have been developed for both diagnostic and therapeutic purposes.

CD44 is a cell-surface glycoprotein expressed in most normal tissues. Its function includes a role in lymphocyte homing, cell–matrix attachment, and tumor metastasis. Studies have indicated a possible use of this protein as a prognostic marker for neuroblastoma. In these studies, the expression of CD44 in neuroblastoma patients was associated with a favorable outcome.[31] Furthermore, CD44 expression showed a negative relation with *N-myc* amplification, suggesting another important role for the *N-myc* products.[32] The overall function of CD44 in tumor progression and metastasis is still unclear.

MOLECULAR BIOLOGY

Tumor-Suppressor Genes and Loss of Heterozygosity

Chromosomal studies have demonstrated that specific deletions may contribute to oncogenesis. For example, the *RB* gene in retinoblastoma and the *WT1* gene in Wilms tumor may be tumor-suppressor genes in whose absence malignant neoplastic growth occurs. Deletion of the short arm of chromosome 1 (chromosome 1p) is the most characteristic genetic abnormality in neuroblastoma, occurring in 77% of clinical cases.[33] Analysis of the chromosomal DNA has demonstrated that the chromosome band 1p36 is the common region of loss of heterozygosity. Although a neuroblastoma-suppresser gene has yet been cloned, chromosome 1p36 is considered to be the site of a suppressor gene crucial for tumor development.

A helix-loop-helix encoding gene located in region 1p36 has been identified and isolated. The expression of the gene, termed *heir-1*, has shown a clear inverse correlation with *N-myc* oncogene expression in neuroblastoma tumors and in embryonic tissue. This suggests that both genes may be regulated in the same pathway.[34] It may also indicate that *heir*-1 plays a significant role in the malignant transformation of neuroblastoma. Thus, *heir*-1 may have a suppressing effect on *N-myc*.

The *p53* gene is a tumor-suppressor gene located on the short arm of chromosome 17. Frequent mutations of this gene have been reported in many adult malignancies. Studies in neuroblastoma cell lines and clinical tumors have revealed a low frequency of *p53* gene aberrations,[35] indicating that *p53* gene mutations do not play an important role in malignant transformation and progression of neuroblastoma. It may be possible that other genes located on 17p play a major role in the tumorigenesis of neuroblastoma.[36]

Tumor Cell Ploidy

With flow cytometric measurement of nuclear DNA content, patients with neuroblastomas of lower stages show hyperploidy, a pattern that has been confirmed to be an unfavorable prognostic factor in many adult malignancies. In contrast, a diploid pattern appears to be associated with advanced stages of the disease. These latter patients with normal tumor cell DNA content may have elusive genetic abnormalities undetectable by flow cytometry.[33]

Protooncogenes

Amplification of N-myc

Cytogenetic abnormalities, such as extrachromosomal double-minute chromatin bodies and chromosomally integrated homogeneously staining regions, frequently occur in neuroblastomas, indicating amplification of oncogenes. Amplification of the *N-myc* oncogene has been identified in neuroblastomas carrying these two cytogenetic abnormalities.[37] The normal single-copy locus of this protooncogene is mapped to chromosome 2p. It is assumed that the function of *N-myc* in normal cells of neural crest origin is to regulate cell growth and differentiation. Although the mechanism of promoting *N-myc* amplification has not been explained, amplification of *N-myc* is a prognostic factor of clinical significance when present. More than 30% of

TABLE 34-5. *Clinical features and genetic types of neuroblastoma*

Feature	Type 1	Type 2	Type 3
Age	Usually <12 mo	Usually >12 mo	Usually >12 mo
INSS stage	Usually 1, 2, 4S	Usually 3, 4	Usually 3, 4
Ploidy	Hyperploid or triploid	Near-diploid or near-tetraploid	Near-diploid or near-tetraploid
Chromosome 1p	Normal	±1pLOH	±1pLOH
N-*MYC* copy	Normal	Normal	Amplified
Survival rate (%)	~95	25–50	~5
TRK-A	High	High to low	Low to none

INSS, International Staging System.
(Modified from Brodeur GM, Castleberry RP. Neuroblastoma. In: Pizzo PA, Poplack DG, eds. Principles and practice of pediatric oncology. Philadelphia, JB Lippincott, 1993:739)

neuroblastoma patients with advanced disease had *N-myc* amplification and poor disease outcomes.[33] Because patients with less advanced disease rarely show *N-myc* amplification, additional cytogenetic factors, such as DNA ploidy and *TRK* gene expression, should lead to a better prediction of prognosis (Table 34-5).

TRK *Genes and Neurotrophin Receptors*

Neurotrophic peptides include NGF, brain-derived neurotrophic factor (BDNF), neurotrophin-3 (NT-3) and NT-4/5. Each has a specific high-affinity receptor: *TRK-A* for NGF, *TRK-B* for BDNF and NT-4/5, and *TRK-C* for NT-3. *LNGFR* also binds nonspecifically to the four neurotrophins noted. NGF is crucial for the growth and differentiation of nerve cells. Therefore, a variety of attempts to use NGF to regulate human neuroblastoma cell growth in vitro have been made. Unfortunately, none offers clear evidence of therapeutic potential.

TRK-A gene expression in human neuroblastomas has been intensively investigated. The expression of *TRK-A* mRNA is associated with an absence of *N-myc* amplification, lower disease stage, lower patient age, and a more favorable outcome.[38] In addition, tumor cells overexpressing *TRK-A* mRNA showed NGF-dependent differentiation. Depletion of NGF caused cell death in these tumors, suggesting susceptibility to differentiation into benign ganglioneuroma or regression as a result of programmed cell death (apoptosis).[39] Univariate analysis indicates that *TRK-A* gene expression and *N-myc* amplification are powerful prognostic factors in human neuroblastoma patients.

Expression of *LNGFR* has also been shown in a subset of neuroblastoma patients with better outcomes. The best survival rate is found in neuroblastoma patients coexpressing both *TRK-A* and *LNGFR* mRNA.[17] A potential response to NGF may explain the high susceptibility to spontaneous regression in this group. The functional role and prognostic significance of *LNGFR* expression, however, remain unclear.

The expression and function of *TRK-B* and BDNF has been examined in both neuroblastoma cell lines and primary tumors. In contrast to *TRK-A*, *TRK-B* is expressed exclusively in aggressive neuroblastomas with *N-myc* amplification.[40] In vitro data from human neuroblastoma cell lines also support the importance of the *TRK-B*–BDNF pathway for growth and differentiation of *N-myc*–amplified neuroblastomas. BDNF is likely to promote cell survival and induce neurite growth; however, the role of BDNF in tumor progression in advanced neuroblastomas with *TRK-B* expression has not been clarified. Another role of BDNF has been proposed in an in vitro study,[41] in which BDNF-treated cell lines demonstrated less accumulation of vinblastine. This suggests that BDNF may induce drug resistance in neuroblastoma and that the multidrug-resistance gene, *mdr-1*, may not be involved in this event.

Other Protooncogenes

Overexpression of *Ha-ras*[42] and *c-src*[43] genes is associated with lower clinical stage neuroblastomas and prolonged patient survival. *Ha-ras* and *c-src* may become useful tools for predicting the outcome of neuroblastomas without *N-myc* amplification.

Studies on the *nm23* gene have demonstrated that robust expression of *nm23* is associated with significant reductions in neuroblastoma patient survival.[44] Aggressive neuroblastomas also present molecular alterations to *nm23*.

In an attempt to find other genetic factors in addition to *N-myc*, the *bcl-2* protooncogene has been investigated in untreated neuroblastomas. The *bcl-2* gene specifically blocks apoptosis, an active form of cellular demise that usually occurs in neurogenesis. The expression of *bcl-2* is strongly associated with unfavorable histology and *N-myc* amplification.[45] Results from single gene transfection experiments also reveal that *bcl-2* inhibits chemotherapy-induced apoptosis.[46] The *bcl-2* gene may promote progression of neuroblastoma by inducing tumor resistance to chemotherapeutic agents.

Multidrug Resistance

The *MDR1* gene and its product P-glycoprotein probably play important roles in the development of resistance to chemotherapeutic agents in a large number of human malignancies. The role of the *MDR1*–P-glycoprotein pathway in human neuroblastoma is still controversial. Bourhis and colleagues[47] reported a significant correlation of *MDR1* mRNA expression with chemotherapy and the presence of disseminated disease that was independent of *N-myc* amplification. An inverse correlation between expression of *MDR1* and *N-myc* was demonstrated by Nakagawara and colleagues.[48] To link the clinical chemoresistance frequently observed in advanced neuroblastomas to *MDR1* and P-glycoprotein expressions requires further study. Other mechanisms also may exist for neuroblastoma cells to acquire multidrug resistance after chemotherapy.

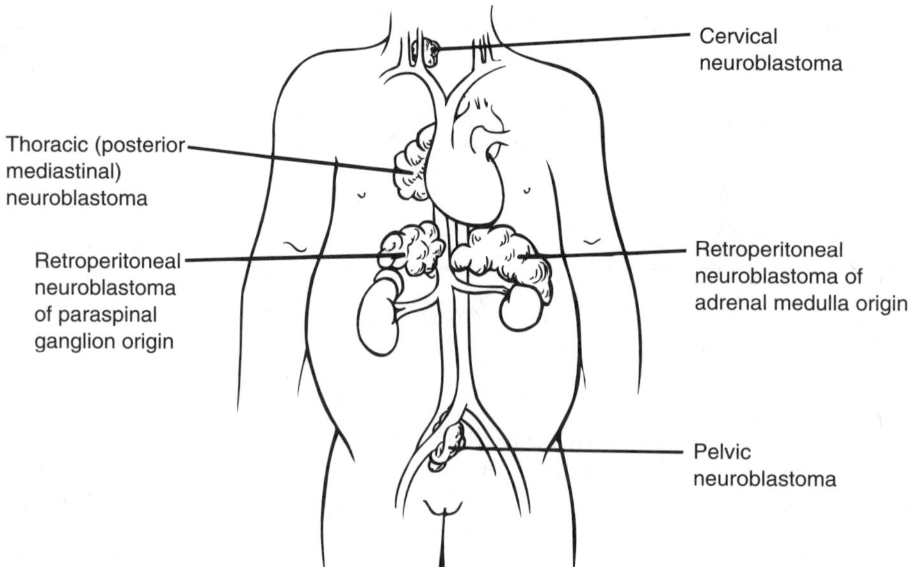

FIG. 34-2. Primary sites of neuroblastoma.

DIAGNOSIS

Anatomic Features

Neuroblastoma usually occurs in the abdominal cavity. Abdominal mass is the most common clinical feature, presenting in 50% to 70% of reported cases. Primary sites of the tumor in these cases are the retroperitoneum (75%), either adrenal medulla (50%; Fig. 34-2), or paraspinal ganglia (25%). In 20% of cases, the tumor originates in the posterior mediastinum. Fewer than 5% of neuroblastomas present as a cervical or pelvic tumor.

Signs and symptoms of neuroblastoma often reflect its primary site. A palpable abdominal mass, abdominal pain, or vomiting may indicate a tumor in the abdomen. Respiratory distress or dysphagia may be a reflection of a thoracic tumor. Altered defecation or urination may be caused by mechanical compression of a pelvic tumor or by spinal cord compression of a paraspinal tumor. Spinal cord compression may also present with an altered gait. A tumor in the neck or upper thorax can produce Horner syndrome (ptosis, miosis, and anhydrosis), enophthalmos, and heterochromia of the iris. Acute cerebellar ataxia has also been observed. This is characterized by the dancing-eye syndrome, which includes opsoclonus, myoclonus, and chaotic nystagmus. Two thirds of these cases occur in infants with mediastinal primary tumors and favorable prognoses.

Additional signs and symptoms that reflect excessive catecholamine or vasoactive intestinal polypeptide secretion include diarrhea, weight loss, and hypertension.

Metastatic Patterns

Neuroblastomas characterized by diffuse metastatic spread were first described in children by Pepper in 1901. Infants in this group usually have stage IV-S disease (INSS stage 4S) and are younger than 1 year of age. Patients with stage IV-S disease may present with "blueberry muffin" cutaneous lesions, respiratory distress secondary to massive hepatomegaly, bone marrow disease, and a primary tumor. Neuroblastomas in older patients have a different pattern of metastatic disease, in which skeletal, bone marrow, and lymph node metastases are predominant. The brain, spinal cord, heart, and lungs are rare sites of metastases, except with advanced disease. Advanced disease may be associated with "black eyes" as a result of retroorbital venous plexus spread. This is an ominous physical sign in a child without a history of head trauma.

Laboratory Findings

Screening for Neuroblastoma

Using its unique catecholamine synthesis and catabolism properties, mass screening of neuroblastoma by quantitating urinary vanillylmandelic acid (VMA) and homovanillic acid (HVA) was first started in Japan,[49] followed by Quebec,[3] north England, and Austria. The sensitivity for detecting neuroblastomas is 96% using high-performance liquid chromatography when both VMA and HVA levels are used.[49]

Studies on neonatal mass screening in these countries strongly suggest that there are at least two types of neuroblastomas: neuroblastomas with a good prognosis (aneuploid, no *N-myc* amplification, catecholamine secretion, and detectable by screening) and neuroblastomas with a poor prognosis (diploid, *N-myc* amplification, less catecholamine secretion, and less detectable by screening). Based on this hypothesis, the improvement in outcome for patients with neuroblastoma by mass screening in Japan[50] could be due to selection of a large number of neuroblastomas with a favorable prognosis that, if not detected, might spontaneously regress. Reports have been made, however, of deaths from tumor progression,[49] a case of progressive tumor with unfavorable histologic features,[51] and a case associated with *N-myc* amplification[52] among positive neuroblastomas found by mass screening. These cases indicate the potential for detecting neuroblastomas with poor prognoses by mass screening. Mass screening at later ages[52–54] has also been proposed to detect neuroblastomas with an unfavorable prognosis that would be missed at the 6-month screening. If these tumors could be detected in earlier stages by late-age screening, therapeutic strategies and presumably mortality rates associated with neuroblastomas would be greatly improved.

Tumor Markers for Clinical Monitoring

Catecholamine Metabolites

A urine specimen is of clinical value for monitoring disease outcome and for screening purposes. This is done by measuring products of tyrosine breakdown and catecholamine synthesis. Dihydroxyphenylalanine is metabolized by a decarboxylase enzyme to vanillactic acid; dopamine is metabolized by an oxidase to HVA; and norepinephrine is metabolized by a transferase to VMA. High levels of urine VMA or HVA (VMA or HVA 3 standard deviations or more above the mean per creatinine, corrected for age[2]) are important as markers for tumor progression in those neuroblastomas characterized by nonamplified *N-myc*. The levels also serve as a prognostic indicator. Neuroblastomas with *N-myc* amplification tend to be dopaminergic with normal VMA and norepinephrine. The measurement of urinary dopamine can be recommended for detecting a so-called nonsecretory neuroblastoma.[54] Follow-up monitoring of urinary catecholamine secretion can detect a relapse of neuroblastoma, whereas mild elevations of the products may indicate remission or maturation of residual elements.[55] Random urine samples are preferable to 24-hour urine estimations for younger children.[56]

Lactate Dehydrogenase

Despite its nonspecificity, LDH can have great prognostic significance. As an independent prognostic factor, high serum levels of LDH reflect high proliferative activity or large tumor burden.[57] Elevated serum LDH greater than 1500 IU/L is associated with a poor prognosis.[8] LDH can be used as a marker to monitor disease activity or the response to therapy. Elevated serum LDH levels have been reported in stage IV-S infants with *N-myc* amplification accompanied by poor outcome.[16]

Serum Ferritin

Elevated serum ferritin levels (more than 150 ng/mL) are often seen in advanced-stage neuroblastomas, indicating a poor prognosis.[58] Levels return to normal during clinical remission. High levels of serum ferritin may be a reflection of large tumor burden or rapid tumor progression. Despite a large tumor burden, stage IV-S neuroblastomas demonstrate serum ferritin levels within normal ranges.

Neuron-Specific Enolase

Neuron-specific enolase (NSE) is considered to be a useful prognostic marker for advanced neuroblastomas. The incidence of elevated NSE levels increases with stage.[59] Serum levels of NSE greater than 100 ng/mL are associated with a poor outcome. NSE has been reported to correlate with the tumor burden,[60] suggesting its reliability as a marker to monitor disease course. The significance of NSE after relapses is controversial. High serum levels of NSE are rarely seen in stage IV-S neuroblastomas.

Circulating Tumor-Derived Ganglioside G_{D2}

Ganglioside G_{D2}, a molecule predominantly expressed in neuroblastoma, is shed from the tumor surface and is easily detected in the plasma of patients with neuroblastomas. A decrease of circulating tumor-derived ganglioside G_{D2} in response to therapy and an increase with relapse[61] have been reported, indicating the value of ganglioside G_{D2} in monitoring the clinical course of the disease. It has also been reported that high levels of ganglioside G_{D2} at diagnosis are associated with rapid tumor progression and low survival rates in advanced-stage neuroblastomas. Ganglioside G_{D2} may play a crucial role in tumor formation and progression by modulating tumor–host interactions.[62]

Circulating Neuroblastoma Cells

Using a highly sensitive reverse transcriptase–polymerase chain reaction (RT-PCR), neuroblastoma cells in the peripheral blood have been recognized.[63] This assay is able to detect a single neuroblastoma cell in 10^7 peripheral blood mononuclear cells. When this analysis becomes available as a daily laboratory measurement, it will be useful for predicting disease outcome, monitoring tumor relapse, and screening peripheral stem cell harvests before autologous transplantation.

Radiographic Imaging

Standard Radiographs

Chest radiography is a useful tool for the diagnosis of thoracic neuroblastoma. A POG study[64] demonstrated that a mediastinal mass was discovered on incidental chest radiograph in almost half of patients with thoracic neuroblastoma who had symptoms unrelated to their tumors (Fig. 34-3).

Abdominal radiography is less useful, but as many as half of abdominal neuroblastomas are detectable as a mass with fine calcification.

Ultrasonography

Ultrasonography is essential for the initial assessment of a suspected abdominal mass, although its sensitivity and accuracy are less than computed tomography (CT) and magnetic resonance (MR) imaging.[65] Ultrasound can delineate major vessels and organs that may be involved by the tumor, and it can provide real-time three-dimensional information regarding to their relation to the tumor. Color Doppler can supply further information about vascular engulfment within the tumor.[66] Doppler ultrasound scanning may also offer a better understanding of the

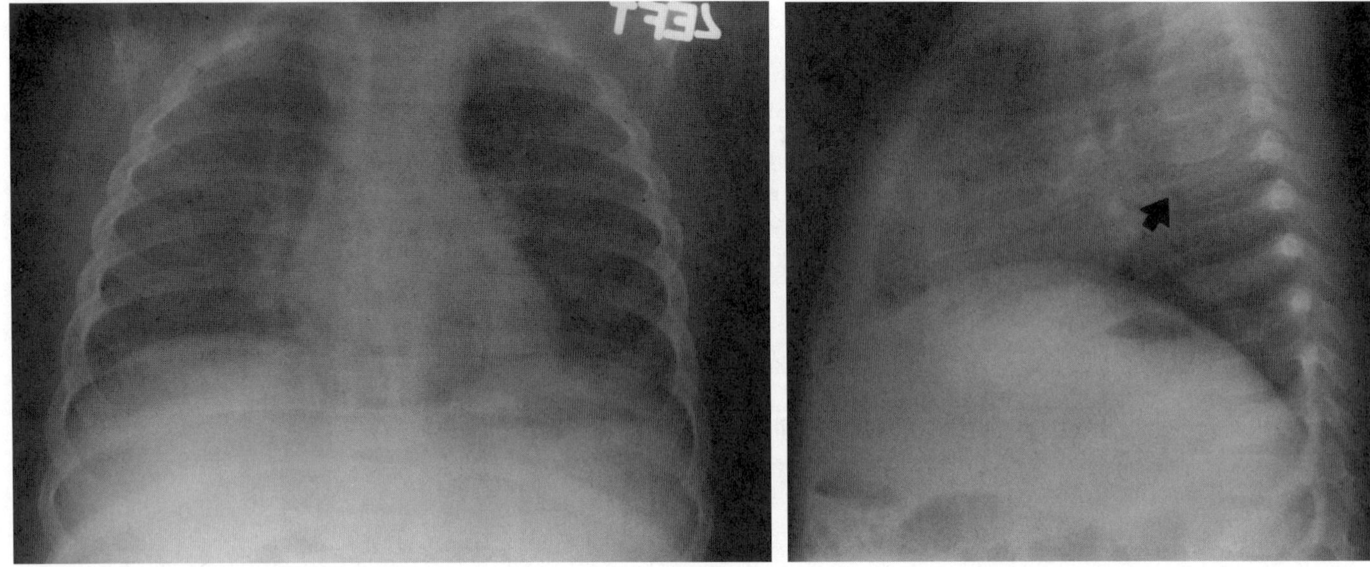

FIG. 34-3. Chest radiographs of a 1-year-old with mild respiratory symptoms. (*A*) Anteroposterior image, which was initially interpreted as normal. (*B*) Lateral image showing a posterior mediastinal mass (*arrow*) of moderate size.

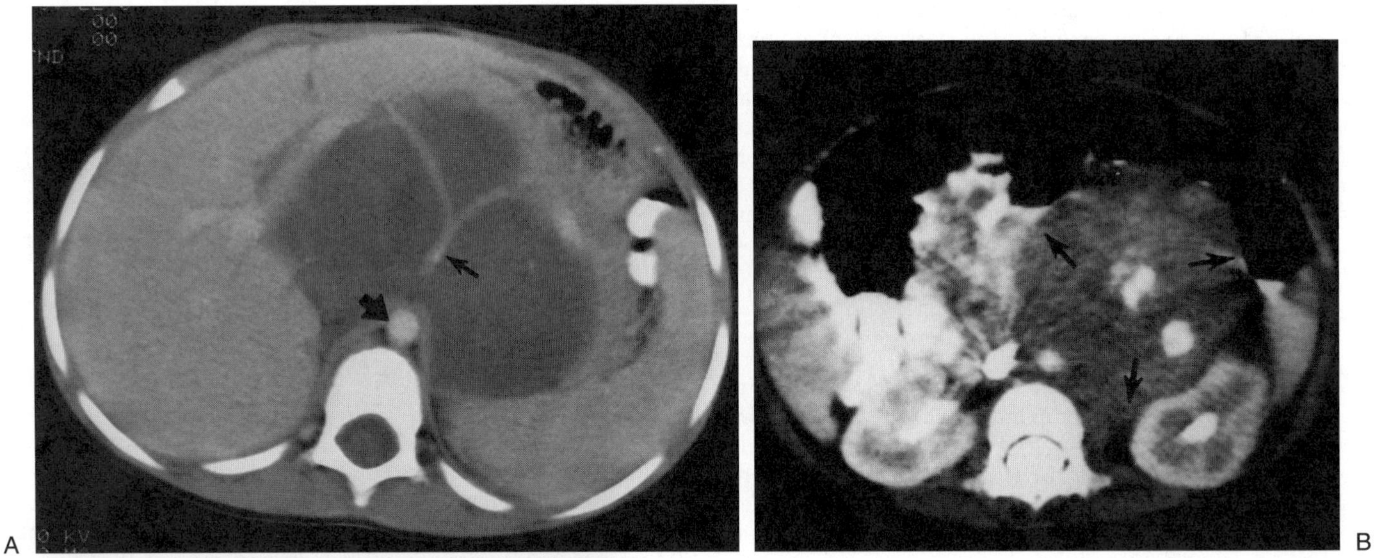

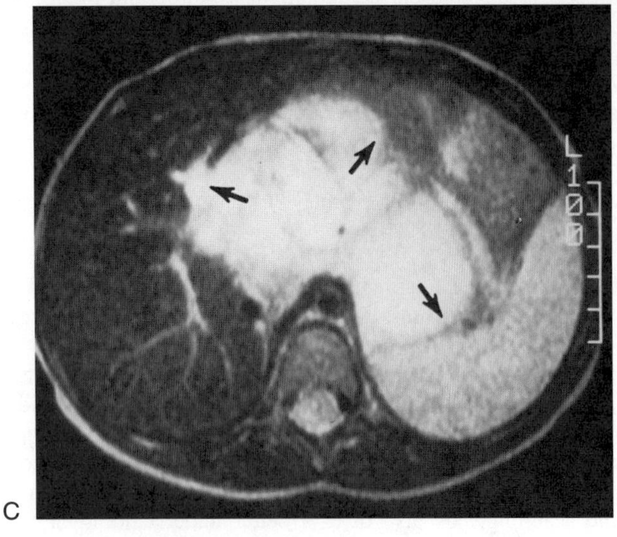

FIG. 34-4. Abdominal neuroblastomas often present with advanced disease, particularly when the aorta and its major branches are involved. (*A*) A large homogeneous abdominal neuroblastoma surrounding the aorta (*thick arrow*) and the celiac artery (*thin arrow*) on CT. (*B*) A similar but heavily calcified neuroblastoma (*arrow*) on CT. (*C*) T2-weighted MR image of a neuroblastoma (*arrows*) similar to those shown in *A* and *B*.

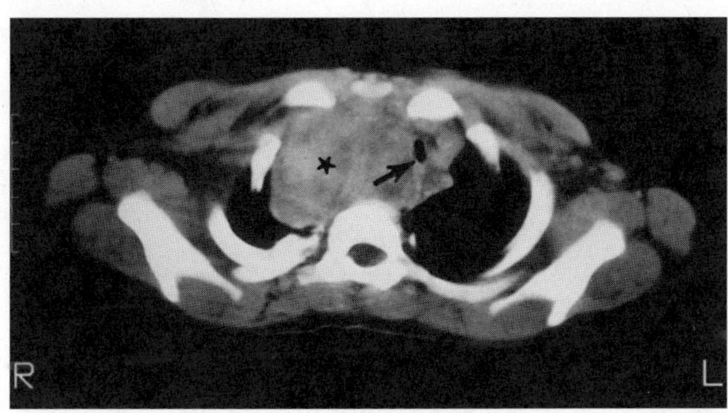

FIG. 34-5. CT scan illustrating severe compression and displacement of the trachea (*arrow*) by a thoracic inlet neuroblastoma (*asterisk*). This child was severely dyspneic on presentation.

biologic behavior of the tumor by analyzing malignant neovasculature.[67]

Computed Tomography

Computed tomography remains a useful modality to evaluate neuroblastoma. CT can demonstrate calcification in almost 85% of neuroblastomas. Intraspinal extension of the tumor can be determined on contrast-enhanced CT.[68] Intravenous contrast may demonstrate vascular encasement. CT and MR imaging enable three-dimensional measurements of the tumor with more accuracy than ultrasound (Figs. 34-4 and 34-5).

Magnetic Resonance Imaging

Magnetic resonance imaging is the most useful and most sensitive imaging modality for the diagnosis and staging of neuroblastoma[65] (Fig. 34-6). On T1-weighted images, the signal intensity of neuroblastoma is higher than that of the liver but equal to that of the kidney. The tumor has a strong signal intensity, visualized as a bright lesion on T2-weighted images, brighter than the liver or muscle but a little less bright than the kidney. In mass-screened infants, the simultaneous examination of T1- and T2-weighted images[65] has demonstrated 100% sensitivity for the detection of neuroblastomas. Encasement of major vessels can be better defined by MR imaging than CT. Bone marrow metastases may also be detectable by MR imaging. It more accordingly depicts intraspinal extension than contrast-enhanced CT. The advent of MR imaging may have replaced the role of myelography in examining such intraspinal extension. MR imaging in the coronal plane is suitable for routine assessment of the whole body from the neck to pelvis and is also helpful for evaluating abdominal tumors, especially in the renoadrenal location. Evaluation of neuroblastomas by contrast-enhanced MR imaging with Gd-DTPA may provide more accurate differential diagnoses and anatomic views.[69] Further studies are necessary to confirm the value of this enhancement agent.

Metaiodobenzylguanidine Imaging

Metaiodobenzylguanidine (MIBG) is transported to and stored in the distal storage granules of chromaffin cells in the same way as noradrenaline. MIBG has been used for scintigraphic imaging of neuroblastoma. The MIBG scintiscan is the imaging study of choice in evaluating bone and bone marrow involvement by neuroblastoma (Fig. 34-7A), although its availability is limited in the United States. Iodine-131 (^{131}I) or iodine-123 (^{123}I) is used to label MIBG. ^{123}I-MIBG is becoming more widely available and supplies a reduced absorbed radiation dosage and superior spatial resolution.[70] The reported sensitivity and specificity of MIBG in the detection of neuroblastomas with bone and bone marrow metastases are 82% and 91%, respectively. Primary tumors and lymph node metastases are also detectable (see Fig. 34-7B). MIBG can demonstrate more sites of tumor involvement in bone and bone marrow than either technetium-99m methylene diphosphonate (^{99m}Tc-MDP) bone

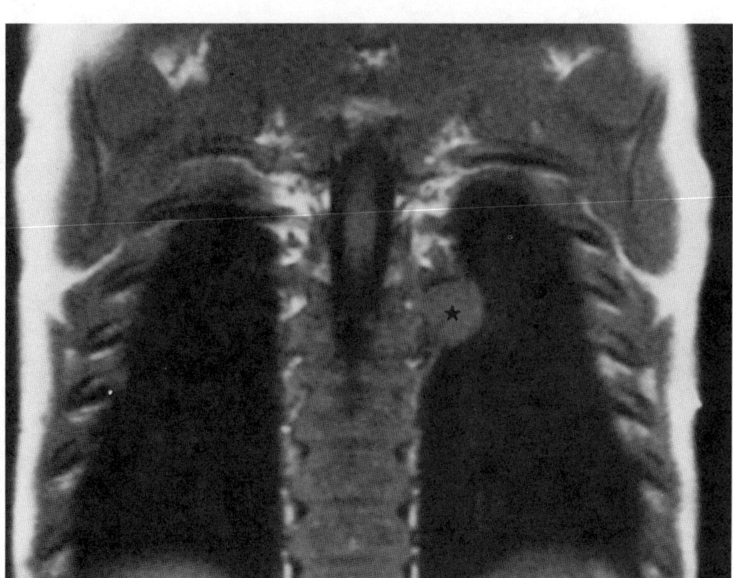

FIG. 34-6. This sagittal MR image is the same neuroblastoma shown in Figure 34-4B (*asterisk*). The relation to the spine and other structures can be demonstrated in three dimensions.

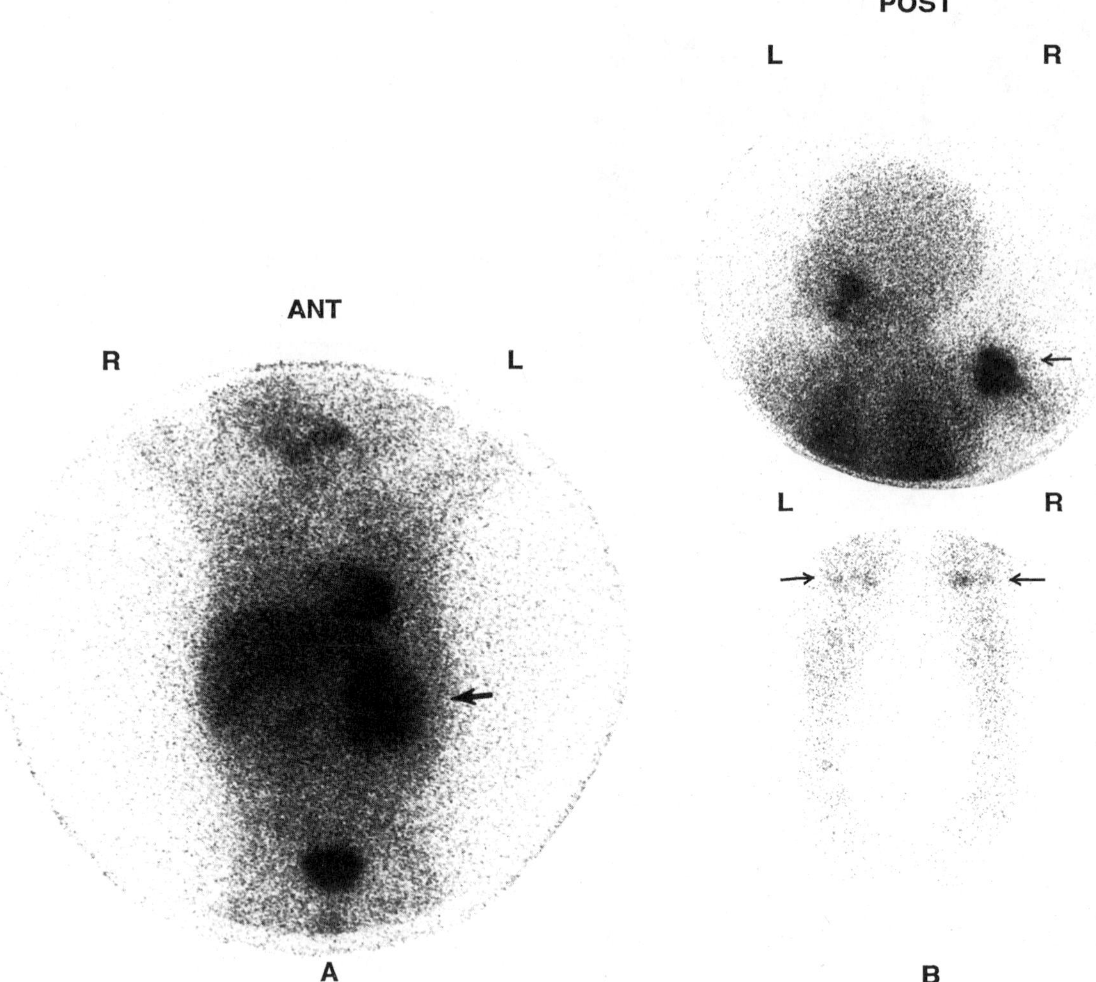

FIG. 34-7. Iodine-123 (^{123}I) MIBG scan. (*A*) A 23-month-old patient with a left upper quadrant neuroblastoma (*arrow*). There is intense uptake of ^{123}I MIBG in the primary tumor. Uptake in the liver, myocardium, and oral salivary glands is normal. Bladder activity is due to excretion of ^{123}I and metabolites. (*B*) A 3-year-old patient with metastatic neuroblastoma. Abnormal ^{123}I MIBG uptake indicative of tumor is present in both proximal tibial metaphyses, in the left distal tibial metaphysis, and in the right shoulder (*arrows*). (Courtesy of M.J. Gelfand, MD, Children's Hospital Medical Center, Cincinnati)

scan or plain radiography.[71] Reports have been made, however, of false-negative cases with MIBG scan that were positive on bone scintigraphy.[72] MIBG is also useful for monitoring the response to therapy, and it may be able to identify a specific group of neuroblastomas that require more aggressive treatment. MIBG uptake indicates better prognoses in infants younger than 1 year of age with metastatic neuroblastoma.[73]

Radiolabeled Anti–Ganglioside G$_{D2}$ Antibody Imaging

The murine monoclonal antibody 3F8 radiolabeled with ^{131}I has a higher tumor uptake than ^{131}I-MIBG in neuroblastomas. The sensitivity and specificity of ^{131}I-3F8 are superior to those of ^{131}I-MIBG, especially in the detection of bone or bone marrow metastases.[74] The complementary role of ^{131}I-14G2a plus ^{123}I-MIBG has also been reported for the scintigraphic detection of neuroblastomas.[27] Despite this superiority, the clinical appli-

cation of ^{131}I anti–ganglioside G$_{D2}$ antibody imaging is still limited. One obstacle is the induction of human antimouse antibody (HAMA), which precludes the multiple use of the radiolabeled antibodies by impairing their specificity to tumor antigens, accelerating their clearance, and decreasing their antitumor activity. A study in a small group of patients with stage IV disease demonstrated that myeloablative chemotherapy and autologous BMT after ^{131}I-3F8 imaging strongly suppressed the HAMA. This suggests a correlation between low levels of HAMA and long-term survival.[75] ^{131}I-3F8 imaging may be of diagnostic value before autologous BMT.

Bone Scintigraphy

Technetium-99m–MDP bone scanning is inferior to MIBG in detecting neuroblastomas with skeletal or extraskeletal involvement. Monitoring MDP-avid neuroblastomas by bone scintigraphy often results in false-positive imaging for months after tumor remission. Nevertheless, [99mTc]-MDP bone scanning is the second choice if MIBG imaging is not available or is negative.[2,72]

Bone Marrow Examination

Bone marrow biopsy has been regarded as a routine and important method for detection of bone marrow involvement with neuroblastoma. Both aspiration and trephine biopsy are available, the latter having better diagnostic value. To collect more accurate information, taking specimens from multiple sites is recommended. Immunohistochemical staining with antibodies such as anti–ganglioside G_{D2}, S-100, NSE, and ferritin is also useful for reducing the number of false-negative cases.[76] Because biopsy is invasive and painful, noninvasive alternatives have been tested. Studies have suggested the superiority of MR imaging[77] and MIBG[78] over bone marrow biopsy in detecting marrow infiltration by neuroblastoma, although the specificity of these studies requires further evaluation. Immunocytologic analyses of bone marrow samples from advanced neuroblastoma detected a large population of CD10 cells in a group of patients with advanced-stage disease. This group of patients is associated with a better prognosis.[79] An expanded population of CD10 cells may have prognostic value and add yet another diagnostic parameter to conventional bone marrow biopsy.

Tumor Staging

Two major staging systems have been used for neuroblastoma: the Evans classification (CCG)[80] and the surgicopathologic staging (POG)[81] (Table 34-6). Both staging systems have prognostic value and have been accepted by several foreign study groups. The Committee on Tumor Registration of the Japanese Society of Pediatric Surgeons and the Study Group on Neuroblastoma have adopted the CCG system. The Italian Cooperative Group for Neuroblastoma (ICGNB) has employed the POG system. Some differences and discrepancies between the two systems present obstacles to a population study of neuroblastomas. In an attempt to incorporate elements from both of these widely accepted systems, international criteria for a common neuroblastoma staging system (the INSS) were presented in 1987. The INSS has been revised, and some modifications and clarifications have been made[2] (Table 34-7).

Evaluation of the primary tumor and the metastatic sites in the INSS system largely depends on CT or MR imaging and on bone marrow biopsy (Table 34-8). MIBG scanning is also recommended for monitoring response to therapy and for evaluating new patients.

Differential Diagnosis

Undifferentiated small blue round cell neuroblastomas may be misinterpreted as rhabdomyosarcoma, primitive neuroectodermal tumors, Ewing sarcoma, non-Hodgkin lymphoma, or acute megakaryoblastic leukemia. The use of a panel of specific antibodies[77] is helpful to facilitate such histologic differentiation. Electron microscopy can be useful for seeing both neurosecretory dense-core granules in the peripheral cytoplasm and neural processes containing microtubules. The criteria for diagnosis of neuroblastoma recommended in the INSS staging system emphasizes histology as well as urine or serum catecholamine products (Table 34-9).

Urinary catecholamines and their metabolites, such as VMA,

TABLE 34-6. *Tumor staging systems for neuroblastoma*

Children's Cancer Study Group*		Pediatric Oncology Group†	
I	Tumor confined to the organ or structure of origin	A	Complete gross resection of primary tumor, with or without microscopic residual disease. Intracavitary lymph nodes, not adhered to and removed with primary (nodes adhered to or within tumor resection may be positive for tumor without upstaging patient to stage C), histologically free of tumor. If primary in abdomen or pelvis, liver histologically free of tumor
II	Tumor extends in continuity beyond the organ or structure of origin but does not cross the midline. Regional lymph nodes on the homolateral side may be involved.	B	Grossly unresected primary tumor. Nodes and liver same as stage A
III	Tumor extends in continuity beyond the midline. Regional lymph nodes may be involved bilaterally.	C	Complete or incomplete resection of primary tumor. Intracavitary nodes not adhered to primary tumor are histologically positive for tumor. Liver as in stage A
IV	Remote disease involving skeleton, organs, soft tissues, or distant lymph note groups	D	Any dissemination of disease beyond intracavitary nodes, such as to extracavitary nodes, liver, skin, bone marrow, bone
IV-S	Patients who would otherwise be stage I or II, but who have remote disease confined only to one or more of the following sites: liver, skin, or bone marrow (without radiographic evidence of bone metastases on complete skeletal survey)	D(S)	Same as Evans IV-S; would be Evans stage I or II except for metastatic tumor in liver, bone marrow, or skin

* Evans AE, D'Angio GJ, Randolf J. A proposed staging for children with neuroblastoma: Children's Cancer Study Group A. Cancer 1971;27:374.

† Nitschke R, Smith EI, Shocat S, et al. Localized neuroblastoma treated by surgery: a Pediatric Oncology Group study. J Clin Oncol 1988;6:1271.

TABLE 34-7. *International staging system for neuroblastoma*

1	Localized tumor with complete gross excision, with or without microscopic residual disease; representative ipsilateral lymph nodes negative for tumor microscopically (nodes attached to and removed with the primary tumor may be positive)
2A	Localized tumor with incomplete gross excision; representative ipsilateral nonadherent lymph nodes negative for tumor microscopically
2B	Localized tumor with or without complete gross excision, with ipsilateral nonadherent lymph nodes positive for tumor. Enlarged contralateral lymph nodes must be negative microscopically.
3	Unresectable unilateral tumor infiltration across the midline,* with or without regional lymph node involvement; or localized unilateral tumor with contralateral regional lymph node involvement; or midline tumor with bilateral extension by infiltration (unresectable) or by lymph node involvement.
4	Any primary tumor with dissemination to distant lymph nodes, bone marrow, liver, skin, or other organs (except as defined for stage 4S)
4S	Localized primary tumor (as defined for stage 1, 2A, or 2B), with dissemination limited to skin, liver, or bone marrow† (limited to infants <1 year of age)

* The midline is defined as the vertebral column. Tumors originating on one side and crossing the midline must infiltrate to or beyond the opposite side of the vertebral column.

† Marrow involvement in stage 4S should be minimal, that is, <10% of total nucleated cells indentified as malignant on bone marrow biopsy or on marrow aspirate. More extensive marrow involvement would be negative if considered to be stage 4. The MIBG scan (if performed) should be negative in the marrow.

(Brodeur GM, Pritchard J, Berthold F, et al. Revisions of the international criteria for neuroblastoma diagnosis, staging, and response to treatment. J Clin Oncol 1993;11:1446)

TABLE 34-8. *Assessment of extent of disease*

Tumor sites	Recommended tests
Primary tumor	CT or MR imaging* with 3D measurements; MIGB scan, if available
Metastatic sites†	
Bone marrow	Bilateral posterior iliac crest marrow aspirates and trephine (core) bone marrow biopsies required to exclude marrow involvement. A single positive site documents marrow involvement. Core biopsies must contain at least 1 cm of marrow (excluding cartilage) to be considered adequate.
Bone	MIGB scan; ^{99m}Tc scan required if MIGB scan is negative or unavailable, and plain radiographs of positive lesions are recommended.
Lymph nodes	Clinical examination (palpable nodes) confirmed histologically. CT scan for nonpalpable nodes (3D measurements)
Abdomen and liver	CT or MR imaging* with 3D measurements
Chest	AP and lateral chest radiographs. CT and MR imaging are necessary if chest radiograph positive, or if abdominal mass or nodes extend into chest.

* Ultrasound is considered suboptimal for accurate 3D measurements.

† The MIBG scan is applicable to all sites of disease.

(Brodeur GM, Pritchard J, Berthold F, et al. Revisions of the international criteria for neuroblastoma diagnosis, staging, and response to treatment. J Clin Oncol 1993;11:1446)

HVA, and dopamine, have no diagnostic value in nonsecretory neuroblastomas, which account for 2% to 25%[82] of these tumors. On the other hand, catecholamine production and high urine levels of its products have been reported in some ganglioneuromas.

Clinically, the diverse symptoms at presentation with neuroblastoma can confuse the diagnosis. Acute cerebellar ataxia with opsoclonus and myoclonus can be confused with a neurologic disease that occurs primarily in the spinal cord. This type of neuroblastoma is most often found in the mediastinum. Widespread bone involvement may resemble nonneoplastic bone disease associated with systemic inflammatory changes, such as osteomyelitis or rheumatoid arthritis. Symptoms of vasoactive intestinal polypeptide secretion can be misinterpreted as symptoms of infectious or inflammatory bowel disease.

TREATMENT PLAN

Despite the favorable enigmatic characteristics of neuroblastoma—the most common tumor to undergo spontaneous regression and a tumor with a tendency for differentiation to a benign mature form—disease outcome remains dismal. Modern multimodal therapy has not yet improved the outcome of neuroblastoma to the same extent it has for other childhood malignancies. Therapies based on new strategies that reflect achievements in molecular and immunobiologic fields have been launched, however, and clinical trials are underway. These therapies alone or in combination with conventional modalities, such as surgery, chemotherapy, or radiotherapy, are expected to improve survival of advanced neuroblastomas with poor prognoses.

Operative Therapy

Although complete resection of the tumor offers the best survival rate in patients with localized neuroblastomas, opera-

TABLE 34-9. *Diagnosis of neuroblastoma*

Established if:
(1) Unequivocal pathologic diagnosis is made from tumor tissue by light microscopy (with or without immunohistology, electron microscopy, increased urine or serum catecholamines or metabolites); *or*
(2) Bone marrow aspirate or trephine biopsy contains unequivocal tumor cells (eg, syncytioma or immunocytologically positive clumps of cells) and increased urine catecholamines or metabolites.

(Brodeur GM, Pritchard J, Berthold F, et al. Revisions of the international criteria for neuroblastoma diagnosis, staging and response to treatment. J Clin Oncol 1993;11:1446)

tive therapy is likely to play a subordinate role in the curative treatment of most neuroblastomas.[83] The value of complete tumor removal in localized neuroblastomas may be overestimated because of the propensity for spontaneous regression observed in localized neuroblastomas. In addition, more than half of patients present with advanced local or metastatic disease, which requires intensive multimodal therapy. Operation is required for cytoreduction or debulking at primary or delayed procedures. Furthermore, up-to-date findings in molecular cytogenetics strongly support the concept of heterogeneity among neuroblastomas, identifying at least two types of neuroblastoma: one with a good prognosis, the other with a poor prognosis. The role of operation must take into consideration the cytogenetic recognition of the heterogeneity of neuroblastomas, identifying tumor types with good or bad prognoses.

Operative Augmentation of the Host–Tumor Relation

Surgical stress can be immunodepressive, and in that circumstance, the antitumor immune response holds in check tumor progression. Operation alone can be detrimental to the host–tumor relation. Some animal studies suggest that both electrocauterization and laser therapy of the tumor may increase the host antitumor immune response to neuroblastoma. Partial tumor electrocoagulation in the murine model impaired the growth of both residual local and distant tumor, compared with sharp excision of the tumor.[84] A similar antitumor effect was demonstrated by the use of a carbon dioxide laser in the same murine model.[85] Studies confirming the same clinical effect on patients have not been done.

Operative Technique

Incision

More than half of neuroblastomas arise in the abdominal cavity.[86] Tumor size, the extent of vascular engulfment, and tumor location should be considered in selecting the approach for abdominal neuroblastoma. Options available for the abdominal incision include a transverse incision, bilateral subcostal incisions with a thoracic extension, a midline incision with or without intercostal extension, or a transthoracic, transdiaphragmatic incision with an abdominal extension into a paramedian position, staying in an extraperitoneal plane. This latter incision is especially useful for excision of neuroblastomas with thoracoabdominal extension or with periaortic or celiac axial encasement (Fig. 34-8).

Operative Principles

The tumor should be carefully exposed, clarifying the relation between the tumor and normal organs and vessels. One of a pair of viscera, such as an adrenal gland or a kidney, can be sacrificed to accomplish complete tumor resection. In most cases, however, deliberate dissection of the tumor from the renal vessels can salvage the kidney. En bloc dissection is ideal for removal of the neuroblastoma unless vital parenchymal organs or vascular structures are involved. Simultaneous resection of

the liver, spleen, pancreas, or intestine with the tumor generally should not be considered. If engulfment of major vessels such as the aorta, vena cava, or their branches is found, tumor dissection must be performed to free the vessels completely. This frequently results in piecemeal division and excision of the tumor. Because of fragility of the highly vascularized tumor capsule, much more attention has to be paid to malignant neuroblastomas than to mature ganglioneuroblastomas or ganglioneuromas to avoid tumor rupture.

Use of the Cavitron ultrasonic aspirator in selected patients allows better skeletonization of the major vessels, with less blood loss and fewer complications.[87] Use of the argon beam coagulator and lasers[88] also helps to achieve complete or near-complete resection[89] and reduces operative complications.

For the primary operation, life-threatening procedures should be avoided because the second-look operation is frequently effective in obtaining cytoreduction and local tumor control. Reduction of the tumor burden by adjuvant chemotherapy or radiotherapy may lead to a safer second-look operation or to a delayed primary operation.

Laparoscopy usually provides enough tissue for both staging and biologic marker studies, with minimal invasiveness and low morbidity.[90] The laparoscopic approach is used for exploratory laparotomy, retroperitoneal node dissection, and tumor biopsy.

Dumbbell-Type Neuroblastomas

Dumbbell-type neuroblastomas expand intraspinally, and unique treatment may be required. Laminectomy as a primary intraspinal operation or the alternative of primary chemotherapy is used to treat symptom-producing intraspinal tumors. Primary chemotherapy, rather than initial laminectomy or radiotherapy, effectively controls the tumor and preserves spinal cord function.[91] Excision of the residual primary tumor from its thoracic, abdominal, or sacral site should be done. Care should be taken to minimize surgical complications, such as leakage of cerebrospinal fluid or uncontrollable intraspinal bleeding. Because residual foraminal disease rarely regrows to a symptom-developing size, the importance of conservative therapy in this circumstance should be emphasized.

Surgical Treatment by Stages

Operative therapy for neuroblastoma is stage related. The management of neuroblastomas in this section has been designed based on the CCG staging system. Considering the significance of a globally acceptable staging system, however, INSS stages have been applied to replace CCG stages (Fig. 34-9). The INSS stage of disease cannot be determined before operation because resectability plays an essential role in this staging system.[2,88] For the initial assessment and planning of the primary treatment, therefore, the CCG classification may be preferable.

INSS Stage 1 (CCG Stage I or POG Stage A)

A complete resection of localized neuroblastoma may be the only therapy required.[81] Regional lymph nodes should be excised during operation for accurate staging, but adjacent normal

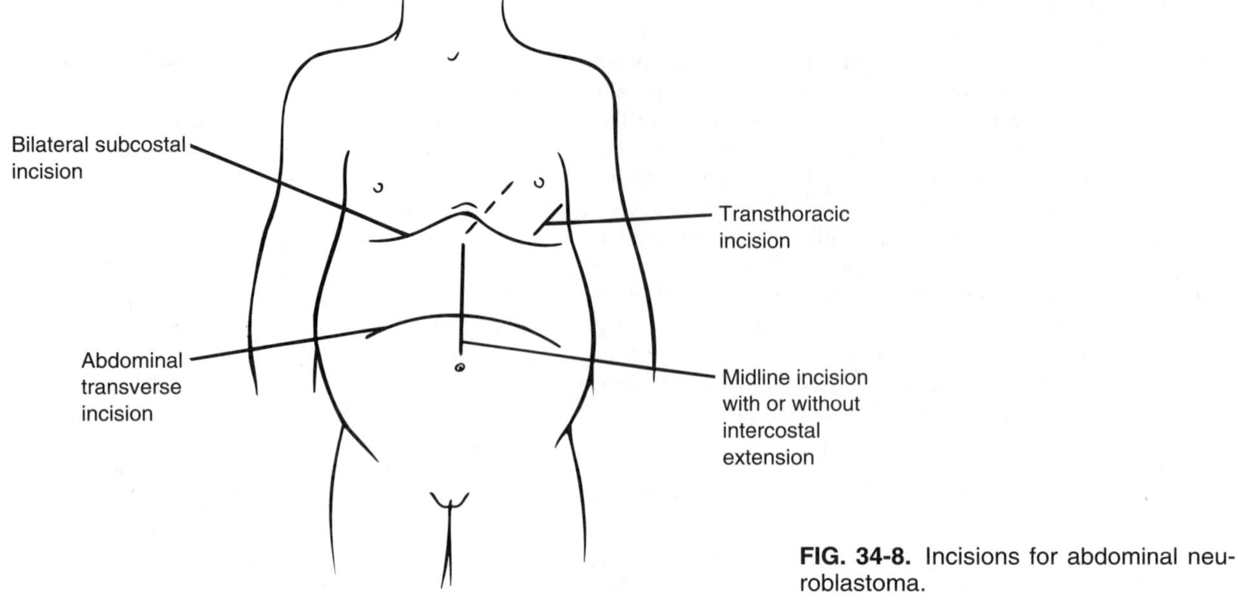

FIG. 34-8. Incisions for abdominal neuroblastoma.

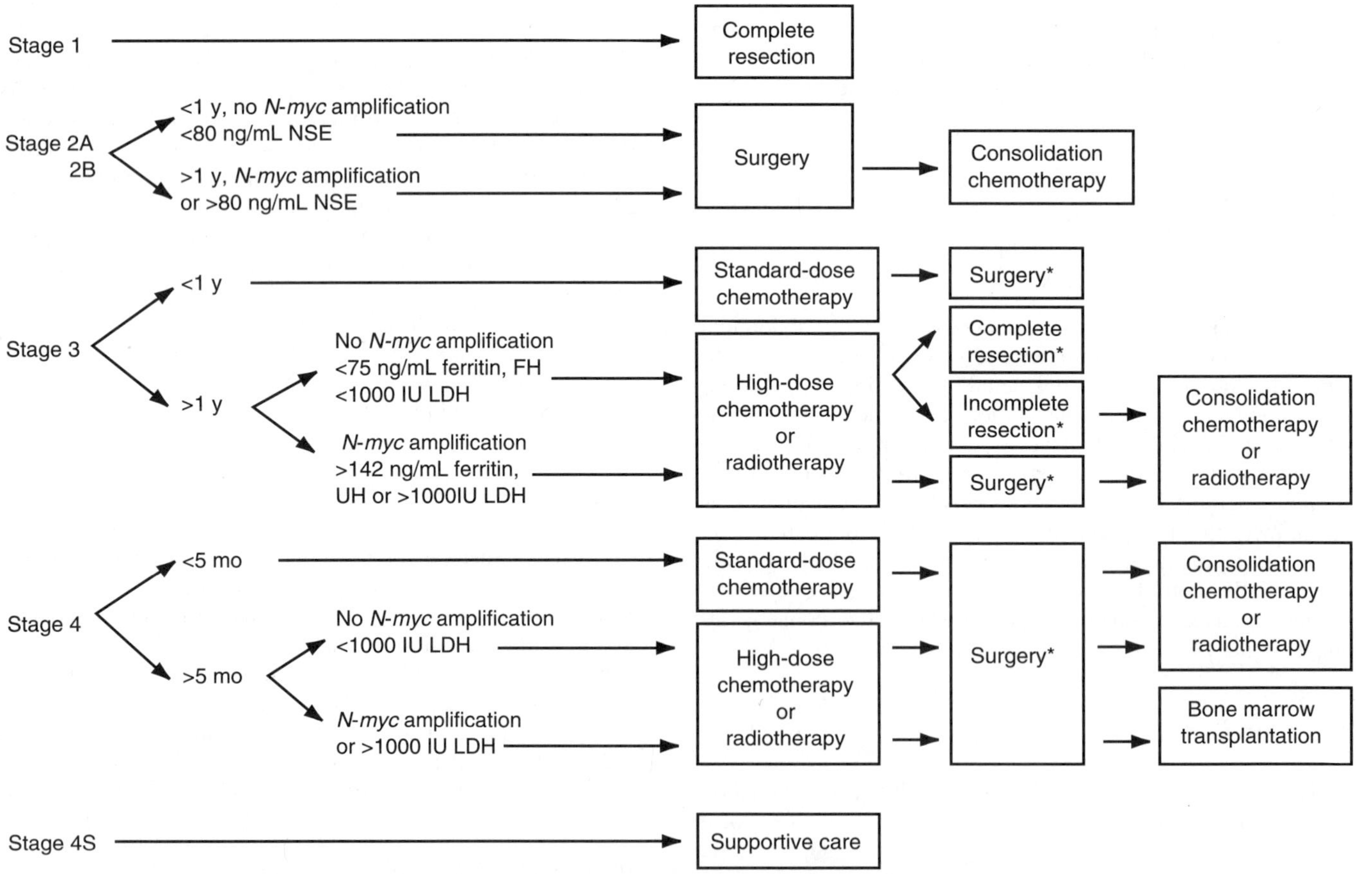

FIG. 34-9. Management of neuroblastomas. *Second-look or delayed primary surgery. (After Ishizu H, Ziegler MM. Neoplasms. In: Levine BA, Copeland EM, Howard RJ, et al, eds. Current practice of surgery, vol 3, sect 7. New York, Churchill Livingstone, 1992:1)

organs should be spared. Regardless of the presence of microscopic residual disease, only close observation follows operative resection.

INSS Stages 2A and 2B (CCG Stage II or POG Stage B)

Localized neuroblastomas are usually associated with a good prognosis even without a complete resection.[57,92] Adjuvant therapy, however, should be taken into account in this group of neuroblastomas, depending on the risk factors, such as age, N-myc copy number, histology, ferritin, and NSE. Primary operative resection alone may be chosen for stage 2A and 2B neuroblastomas if all risk factors are prognostically favorable. Second-look or delayed primary operation may be planned after reduction of tumor size by chemotherapy or radiotherapy. Lymph node resection is beneficial for reducing the tumor burden as well as for precise staging of the disease. Because significant differences have not been observed in the survival of patients with stage 2A and 2B disease, especially patients younger than 1 year of age,[2] patients with stage 2A and 2B disease can be treated the same.

INSS Stage 3 (CCG Stage III or POG Stage C)

Chemotherapy or radiotherapy is often the first treatment for unresectable nonmetastatic neuroblastomas. Delayed primary or second-look resection may be scheduled after adjuvant therapy. These secondary procedures not only may enable total tumor removal but also are important to reassess the extent of the disease and to evaluate the histologic response to adjuvant therapy. Aggressive multimodality therapy is likely to induce the best outcome of the disease.[93] The ICGNB reported complete tumor resection in 73% of patients with localized but unresectable neuroblastomas who underwent operation after induction chemotherapy. This suggests the importance of complete tumor removal achieved by late operation for favorable outcome disease.[94] The report also indicated that age, primary tumor site, and LDH level could be defined as risk factors. No further consolidation therapy may be needed if complete tumor excision is accomplished after adjuvant therapy.

INSS Stage 4 (CCG Stage IV or POG Stage D)

Aggressive multimodality therapy has been done in an attempt to improve the otherwise poor outcome for patients with metastatic neuroblastomas. Operative therapy after intensive chemotherapy or radiotherapy usually is adopted as the combination, but the role of operation in this tumor stage is controversial. A favorable influence of complete resection of the tumor[89] and regional lymph nodes[95] has been reported. Others suggest that complete operative excision does not improve survival in comparison with incomplete excision.[96] Cytoreduction by surgical resection, however, regardless of whether it is complete or incomplete, is preferable to biopsy. Surgical resection may be of particular benefit to remove as much gross tumor as possible for patients who receive autologous or allogeneic BMT in combination with high-dose chemotherapy and total body irradiation (TBI).[88] In addition to resectability, serum LDH, histology,[97] and age[98] may indicate prognostic significance in this group.

INSS Stage 4S (CCG Stage IV-S or POG Stage D[S])

Only supportive therapy has been recommended for this stage of neuroblastoma because of the high incidence of spontaneous regression and the resultant good prognosis.[99] Limited chemotherapy, local irradiation,[88] or minimal resection can be applied to infants with life-threatening symptoms from hepatomegaly. Operative placement of a Silastic pouch as a temporary abdominal wall may be a choice for those who demonstrate rapid liver extension that causes either respiratory compromise secondary to diaphragmatic elevation or an obstruction of the inferior vena cava. This procedure may help to avoid life-threatening events until reduction of the extended liver is achieved by either spontaneous regression or adjuvant therapy. A retrospective study of CCG stage IV-S neuroblastomas indicated that extirpation of the primary tumor is both safe and effective in this stage, even when associated with massive hepatomegaly.[100] The limited number of patients and lack of information about new tumor markers, however, have made it difficult to accept this approach as the initial therapy. Although heterogeneity of INSS stage 4S neuroblastoma has been reported,[101] factors useful to detect heterogeneous subtypes with different prognoses remain debatable. N-myc amplification[98,101] and age[98,100] as markers with prognostic significance are controversial. The site of the primary tumor may be of prognostic value; massive abdominal tumors are at high risk of progression,[98] while extraadrenal primary tumors have a favorable prognosis.[100] Aggressive therapy, such as operative resection, chemotherapy, or radiotherapy, may be another option for a subset of INSS stage 4S patients with poor prognoses. The actual impact of these modalities on this group of patients has not yet been confirmed.

Chemotherapy and Bone Marrow Transplantation

Chemotherapy

For patients with advanced neuroblastomas, chemotherapy has been the mainstay of multimodality treatment. Various agents, including cyclophosphamide,[102] doxorubicin, vincristine,[103] teniposide, peptichemio,[104] and cisplatin[103] have demonstrated efficacy in neuroblastoma response (Table 34-10). Generally, combinations of multiple drugs are adopted as first-line chemotherapy in the expectation of synergic effects, different cytotoxicity, and a reduction of side effects. No regimen has had a significant impact on the long-term survival of advanced neuroblastoma in children older than 1 year of age. In an attempt to improve the poor prognosis of advanced neuroblastoma, newer agents, such as ifosfamide,[105,106] etoposide, carboplatin,[107] iproplatin,[108] and desferrioxamine,[109] have been applied in phase II trials (see Table 34-10). Furthermore, phase I studies of trimetrexate[110] and topotecan[111] in pediatric solid tumors have revealed treatment potential for refractory neuroblastoma. Efficacy of time-dependent drugs may be further improved by continuous infusion instead of bolus injection.

TABLE 34-10. *Chemotherapy for neuroblastoma*

Agent	Standard dose (mg/m^2)	High dose (mg/m^2)	References
Cyclophosphamide	600	6000	102, 108
Doxorubicin	35	160	91, 104
Vincristine	3	12	103, 104
Teniposide	150	375	104,112
Peptichemio	180	450	104
Melphalan	—	180	112
Cisplatin	60	400–720	103, 104, 112
Ifosfamide	9000	54,000	105, 106
Etoposide	250	500–1600	102, 103, 107
Carboplatin	100	1600	107, 109
Iproplatin		325	108
Deferoxamine		4500	109

Bone Marrow Transplantation

High-dose chemotherapy may produce better responses than conventional chemotherapy. Severe bone marrow suppression often follows and disturbs the further administration of myelosuppressive drugs. BMT may be the way to avoid such myelotoxicity during intensive chemotherapy. High-dose melphalan,[112] with or without total body irradiation, is used as a myeloablative preparation before BMT. Other myelotoxic agents are also used in combination with high-dose melphalan. Some studies have reported the impact of BMT after high-dose chemotherapy on tumor remission in patients with refractory neuroblastoma. The value of this modality, however, has not been well established.[113] Questions remain unsolved regarding criteria of patient selection, superiority between autologous and allogeneic BMT, and the necessity of purging the marrow of putative tumor cells.[114] A randomized study conducted by the European Neuroblastoma Study Group demonstrated that high-dose melphalan followed by autologous BMT significantly prolongs the median progression-free duration but does not improve the long-term cure rate because of the convergence of the survival curves.[112] A case-control study using the European Bone Marrow Transplant Solid Tumor Registry found that allogenic and autologous BMT patients do not show significant differences in progression-free survival (41% and 35% at 2 years, respectively).[115] Several randomized studies being conducted by the POG and CCG[114] may provide clear answers to these controversies.

Cytokines for Bone Marrow Support

Colony-stimulating factors may be feasible alternatives in patients with severe bone marrow suppression after intensive chemotherapy. A study of granulocyte colony-stimulating factor demonstrated that the intravenous administration of this cytokine significantly shortens the duration of neutropenia and may lead to fewer infections in children with advanced neuroblastoma.[116] The LMCE (Lyon, Marseille, Institut Curie, East of France) group reported that after megatherapy and during induction chemotherapy, granulocyte-macrophage colony-stimulating factor shortens the periods of bone marrow aplasia.[117] Pharmacokinetic studies indicate that subcutaneous administration is preferable in granulocyte colony-stimulating factor therapy.[118]

Radiotherapy

Total body irradiation is often used as part of the myeloablative therapy for bone marrow infusion.[114] Local irradiation is also given in combination with chemotherapy and surgery for local tumor control in children with lymph node metastases, especially those older than 1 year of age.[119]

^{131}I-MIBG has been used for the treatment of refractory neuroblastoma, taking advantage of its high tumor uptake.[71] In an investigation of patients with advanced chemoresistant neuroblastomas, response rates approached 33%.[120] ^{125}I-MIBG may be another option for neuroblastomas with micrometastases or bone marrow infiltration.[121] Studies on the diagnostic use of ^{131}I-MIBG suggest that MIBG therapy can be used as first-line therapy, followed by chemotherapy, without significant hematologic toxicity.[122]

Haase and colleagues[123] reported on low-dose electron-beam intraoperative radiotherapy with aggressive surgical resection. In this study, local tumor control was achieved in 72% of children with stage III or IV neuroblastomas. A controlled prospective study of intraoperative radiotherapy in the treatment of pediatric neoplasms is being conducted by the CCG.

Immunotherapy

Significant evidence suggests a linkage between the immune response and neuroblastoma. Two basic problems, however, remain unsettled for a clinical application of host antitumor immunity: (1) no neuroblastoma-specific antigen has been identified, and (2) neuroblastomas fail to express class I MHC antigens, limiting effective T cell–mediated cytotoxicity. IFN-α or IFN-γ, IL-2, LA cells, and TILs alone or in combination have been tested clinically to improve the outcome of disease by inducing class I MHC antigens on tumor cells or by enhancing the non–MHC-restricted antitumor response, such as occurs with NK or LAK cell activity.

Early studies using recombinant IFN-γ in children with refractory neuroblastomas demonstrated increased expression of class I antigens without any measurable impact on patient outcome. This result is possibly explained by the vast residual tumor burden and the immunocompromised status after primary intensive therapy.[10]

Clinical efficacy in IL-2 treatment with or without LAK cells in advanced-stage neuroblastoma therapy is still controversial, despite evidence of immunomodulation in vivo.[124] Favrot and associates[125] reported an objective response to IL-2 after high-dose chemotherapy and autologous BMT in children with refractory neuroblastoma, achieving a 50% response rate (one complete response and one partial response in four patients). To investigate the impact of IL-2 after autologous BMT, a prospective study designed by the LMCE group is underway.[126]

Protocol Therapy

The strategy for the treatment of advanced-stage neuroblastoma is based on multimodality therapy. To establish effective

TABLE 34-11. *Protocol therapy for neuroblastoma*

Study group	Disease stage	Regimen	Survival rate	Reference
CCG (CCG-321P3)	Stage II with amplified N-*myc* amplification; stage III with UH, N-*myc* amplification, or elevated serum ferritin; or stage IV	IC: CPM/CDDP/Doxo/VP-16 Delayed surgical resection Local irradiation MC: CDDP/VP-16/L-PAM + TBI Purged autologous BMT	3-y PFS: 44%	127
POG (POG 8441)	Stage D (1 y or older)	IC, MC: CDDP/VM-26/CPM/ Doxo Delayed surgical resection and MC Second-look surgical resection and MC (CR or PR after POG 8441)	4-y OS: 24%	128
(POG 8340)		MAT: L-PAM/TBI Purged autologous BMT		
ICGNB (AIEOP NB85)	Stage 3 (localized but unresectable)	IC, MC: PTC/VCR/CPM/ CDDP/Doxo/VM-26	5-y OS: 68% (stage 3)	92
		Delayed surgical resection with or without (for CR) MC	5-y OS: 27% (stage 4)	97
	Stage 4 (1 y or older)	MAT: VCR/FTBI/L-PAM Unpurged autologous BMT (IT: Chemoradiotherapy ± surgery)		
LMCE (LMCE2)	Refractory stage 4 Stage 3 or 4 in relapse	MC: VP-16/CDDP or CBDCA MAT1: VM26/BCUN/CDDP or CBDCA Purged BMT1 MAT2: VCR/L-PAM/TBI Purged BMT2	5-y OS: 33%	129

IC, induction chemotherapy; MC, maintenance chemotherapy; MAT, myeloablative therapy; TBI, total body irradiation; FTBI, fractionated TBI; UH, unfavorable histology; CR, complete remission; PR, partial remission; PFS, progression-free survival; OS, overall survival; CPM, cyclophosphamide; CDDP, cisplatin; Doxo, doxorubicin; VP-16, etoposide; L-PAM, L-phenylalanine mustard; BMT, bone marrow transplantation; VM-26, teniposide; PTC, peptichemio; VCR, vincristine; CBDCA, carboplatin; CCG, Children's Cancer Study Group; POG, Pediatric Oncology Group; ICGNB, Italian Cooperative Group for Neuroblastoma; LMCE, Lyon, Marseille, Institut Curie, East of France.

therapy, a number of clinical trials have been generated by various study groups, including the CCG,[127] POG,[128] European Neuroblastoma Study Group, ICGNB, and LMCE.[129] Protocols in these studies include intensive chemotherapy, radiotherapy, operation, or BMT, or some combination of these (Table 34-11). Although some of the studies are retrospective, nonrandomized, or small in sample size, the results from various regimens are relatively consistent and encouraging.

Assessment of Therapeutic Response

Precise evaluation of the therapeutic response of primary and metastatic sites to treatment is essential for confirming the efficacy of therapy, predicting disease outcome, and planning the next therapeutic modality. The International Neuroblastoma Response Criteria[2] was presented in 1988 and has since been revised (Table 34-12). The determination of response should be based on the volume of the primary tumor and large metastases measured by three-dimensional imaging, such as CT or MR imaging (see Table 34-8). Normalization of urinary catecholamines is included in the determination of the response of metastatic sites.

TREATMENT OUTCOME

Tumor Outcome

Tumor stage,[130] patient age,[98] and various biochemical and oncogenic markers have demonstrated their usefulness in predicting the outcome of neuroblastoma. These tumor markers include serum LDH, NSE, and ferritin,[131] N-*myc* amplification, DNA ploidy, and *TRK-A* gene expression. Histopathology of the tumor using the Shimada classification has also been useful (Table 34-13). In addition, disease outcome can be affected by treatment; intensive therapy may improve the poor outcome of children with advanced metastatic neuroblastoma (see Table 34-11). A few studies that compare multiple prognostic factors have selected powerful markers to separate patients into

TABLE 34-12. *International neuroblastoma response criteria*

Response	Primary tumor*	Metastatic sites*
Complete	No tumor	No tumor; catecholamines normal
Very good partial	Decreased by 90%–99%	No tumor; catecholamines normal; residual ^{99m}Tc bone changes allowed
Partial	Decreased by >50%	All measurable sites decreased by >50%. Bones and bone marrow: number of positive bone sites decreased by >50%; no more than one positive bone marrow site allowed.†
Mixed		No new lesions; >50% reduction of any measurable lesion (primary or metastases) with <50% reduction of any other; <25% increase in any existing lesions
No		No new lesions; <50% reduction but <25% increase in any existing lesion
Progressive disease		Any new lesion; increase of any measurable lesions by >25%; previous negative marrow positive for tumor

* Evaluation of primary and metastatic disease as outlined in Table 34-8.

† One positive marrow aspirate or biopsy allowed for partial response if this represents a decrease from the number of positive sites at diagnosis.

(Brodeur GM, Pritchard J, Berthold F, et al. Revisions of the international criteria for neuroblastoma diagnosis, staging, and response to treatment. J Clin Oncol 1993;11:1446)

subgroups with significant prognostic differences. The INSS has plans to evaluate three or four risk groups of factors that categorize patients into several unequivocal groups. These risk groups include: neuroblastomas with spontaneous regression without therapy, neuroblastomas with curable disease with mild therapy, possibly curable neuroblastomas treated with high-intensity therapy, and neuroblastomas with a poor prognosis resistant to even highly intensive chemo(radio)therapy and BMT.[2] Then, stage-oriented multimodality therapy will be reorganized by risk group, providing appropriate intensity of therapy to each subcategory.

Potential for New Treatment Strategies

Differentiating Agents

Retinoids such as 13-*cis*-retinoic acid (*cis*-RA) and all-*trans* retinoic acid have been clinically tested because of their attractive characteristics that induce cell differentiation and growth arrest. Reynolds and colleagues[132] applied *cis*-RA to a small number of patients with stage IV neuroblastomas without *N-myc* amplification and reported a reduction of tumor content in the bone marrow. A CCG group report, however, demonstrated no significant response to *cis*-RA treatment in patients with

refractory metastatic neuroblastoma.[133] Because retinoids are tumoristatic rather than tumoricidal, tumor shrinkage may not be the optimal response to assess. Retinoids may be better applied to patients with minimal residual disease after BMT to prevent relapse.[134] Indeed, a Japanese study reported an improved 72% 3-year disease-free survival rate in children with advanced neuroblastoma treated with intensive therapy and BMT followed by *cis*-RA.[134] Retinoids have milder clinical toxicities than chemotherapeutic agents. Hypercalcemia may be the dose-limiting toxicity for *cis*-RA,[135] and the central nervous system toxicity of pseudotumor cerebri may occur with retinoic acid.[136]

Target Therapy

Targeted immunotherapy using anti–ganglioside G_{D2} antibodies may be a promising approach for the treatment of advanced neuroblastomas. Antibody-dependent cell-mediated cytotoxicity and probably complement-dependent cytotoxicity, are possible mechanisms for killing neuroblastoma cells in vivo with these antibodies. In a phase II trial, the mouse monoclonal antibody 3F8 induced a tumor response in 40% of patients with stage IV neuroblastoma resistant to chemotherapy.[137]

Phase I studies of 14G2a have demonstrated significant re-

TABLE 34-13. *Prognostic factors for neuroblastoma*

Prognostic factor	Stage	Survival (%)	Reference
Evans stage	I	5-y OS:100	130
	II	85	
	III	44	
Age			
<1 y	3	5-y PFS:72	92
≥1 y		39	
<5 mo	IV	5-y PFS:100	97
≥5 mo		57	
Lactate dehydrogenase			
Normal	3	5-y PFS:70	
<1000 IU/L		48	92
≥1000 IU/L		24	
Normal	IV	6-y EFS:36	96
Elevated		10	
Neuron-specific enolase			
<80 ng/mL	I–III	5-y EFS:69	59
≥80 ng/mL		0	
Ferritin			
<75 ng/mL	III	2-y PFS:79	131
≥142 ng/mL		31	
N-*myc*			
Not amplified	A–D(S)	4-y OS:87	8
Amplified		44	
DNA index			
>1	A–D(S)	6-y OS:99	8
1		74	
Histology			
Favorable	III	3-y OS:85	6
Unfavorable		33	
TRK-A			
High-level mRNA	I–IVS	6-y OS:86	39
Low-level mRNA		14	

OS, overall survival; PFS, progression-free survival; EFS, event-free survival.

sponses in patients with refractory stage IV neuroblastomas.[138] High levels of HAMA have also been observed in most patients.[139] This modality may be most effective when applied to a group of patients with minimal residual disease,[135] and to avoid relapse, repeated administration of the antibody may be necessary. Furthermore, combination therapy with IL-2 and 14G2a is being evaluated in a phase I protocol of the CCG.[30] Preliminary results indicate that in vivo cell-mediated killing of neuroblastoma cells can be effectively induced by this treatment regimen.

Correlation between HAMA and antitumor response associated with murine anti–ganglioside G_{D2} antibodies has not yet been clinically confirmed. HAMA may jeopardize the frequent administration of murine anti–ganglioside G_{D2} antibodies, however, and may limit clinical efficacy of such therapy. Recombinant DNA technology may offer an alternative to bypass HAMA by producing a human and mouse chimeric antibody, ch14.18. Superiority of ch14.18 over 14G2a in antibody-dependent cell-mediated cytotoxicity to neuroblastoma cells in vitro was supported by a phase I trial of the chimeric antibody, in which a durable response was achieved in children with refractory neuroblastoma.[140] Combination therapy of ch14.18 with cytokines such as granulocyte-macrophage colony-stimulating factor and IL-2 will be included in future trials.[138]

Adoptive Immunotherapy With Tumor-Infiltrating Lymphocytes

Encouraged by the higher cytotoxicity of TILs than that of LAK cells in vitro,[20] adoptive immunotherapy using TILs and cytokines is undergoing clinical trial. Preliminary results from the POG trial of TILs in combination with IFN and IL-2 have indicated an objective response in patients with refractory neuroblastoma.[141] Preliminary data also suggest that the 14G2a antibody, in combination with IL-2, may enhance TIL growth.[139] Difficulty in culturing and expanding TILs, however, is limiting further clinical application of this therapy.[142]

Gene Therapy

Clinical trials of neuroblastoma treatment by gene transfer have been launched in several institutions. A phase I study is underway at St Jude's Children's Research Hospital, in which patients with relapsed or refractory neuroblastomas are treated with a subcutaneous injection of IL-2 gene-transduced autologous neuroblastoma cells.[143] The impact on the host antitumor response of immune modulation by cytokine gene transfer will be evaluated in this treatment regimen.

Another gene transfer technique, transducing marker genes into tumor cells, is also being tested. The protocol has been designed to evaluate the clinical significance of marker gene–transferred neuroblastoma cells. The goals are to predict relapse and assess efficacy of marrow purging in patients with disseminated neuroblastoma treated with intensive therapy followed by antibody BMT. Preliminary results indicated that transduction efficiency is sufficient for detecting relapse from the transplanted marrow.[144,145]

REFERENCES

1. Brodeur GM, Nakagawara A. Molecular basis of clinical heterogeneity in neuroblastoma. Am J Pediatr Hematol Oncol 1992;14:111.
2. Brodeur GM, Pritchard J, Berthold F, et al. Revisions of the international criteria for neuroblastoma diagnosis, staging, and response to treatment. J Clin Oncol 1993;11:1446.
3. Bernstein ML, Leclerc JM, Bunin G, et al. A population-based study of neuroblastoma incidence, survival, and mortality in North America. J Clin Oncol 1992;10:323.
4. Hale G, Gula MJ, Blatt J. Impact of gender on the natural history of neuroblastoma. Pediatr Hematol Oncol 1994;11:91.
5. Shimada H, Chatten J, Newton WAJ, et al. Histopathologic prognostic factors in neuroblastic tumors: definition of subtypes of ganglioneuroblastoma and an age-linked classification of neuroblastomas. J Natl Cancer Inst 1984;73:405.
6. Chatten J, Shimada H, Sather HN, et al. Prognostic value of histopathology in advanced neuroblastoma: a report from the Children's Cancer Study Group. Hum Pathol 1988;19:1187.
7. Joshi VV, Cantor AB, Altshuler G, et al. Age-linked prognostic categorization based on a new histologic grading system of neuroblastomas. Cancer 1992;69:2197.
8. Joshi, VV, Cantor AB, Brodeur GM, et al. Correlation between morphologic and other prognostic markers of neuroblastoma: a study of histologic grade, DNA index, N-myc gene copy number, and lactic dehydrogenase in patients in the Pediatric Oncology Group. Cancer 1993;71:3173.
9. Carlsen NLT. How frequent is spontaneous remission of neuroblastomas? Implications for screening. Br J Cancer 1990;61:441.
10. Ziegler MM. Immunobiology of neuroblastoma. Pediatr Surg Int 1991;6:2.
11. Beckwith JB, Perrin EV. In situ neuroblastomas: a contribution to the natural history of neural crest tumors. Am J Pathol 1963;43:1089.
12. Hellstrom I, Hellstrom KE, Bill AH, et al. Studies on cellular immunity to human neuroblastoma cells. Int J Cancer 1970;7:172.
13. Bill AH. Immune aspects of neuroblastoma. Am J Surg 1971;122:142.
14. Squire R, Fowler CL, Brooks SP, et al. The relationship of class I MHC antigen expression to stage IV-S disease and survival in neuroblastoma. J Pediatr Surg 1990;25:381.
15. Knudson AGJ, Meadows AT. Regression of neuroblastoma IV-S: a genetic hypothesis. N Engl J Med 1980;302:1254.
16. Nakagawara A, Sasazuki T, Akiyama H, et al. N-myc oncogene and stage IV-S neuroblastoma. Cancer 1990;65:1960.
17. Kogner P, Barbany G, Dominici C, et al. Coexpression of messenger RNA for TRK protooncogene and low affinity nerve growth factor receptor in neuroblastoma with favorable prognosis. Cancer Res 1993;53:2044.
18. Cooper MJ, Hutchins GM, Mennie RJ, et al. β_2-Microglobulin expression in human embryonal neuroblastoma reflects its developmental regulation. Cancer Res 1990;50:3694.
19. Van't Veer LJ, Beijersbergen RL, Bernards R. N-myc suppresses major histocompatibility complex class I gene expression through down-regulation of the p50 subunit of NF-χB. EMBO J 1993;12:195.
20. Alvarado CS, Findley HW, Chan WC, et al. Natural killer cells in children with malignant solid tumors. Cancer 1989;63:83.
21. Kataoka Y, Matsumura T, Yamamoto S, et al. Distinct cytotoxicity against neuroblastoma cells of peripheral blood and tumor-infiltrating lymphocytes from patients with neuroblastoma. Cancer Lett 1993;73:11.
22. Cheung NKV. Immunotherapy: neuroblastoma as a model. Pediatr Clin North Am 1991;38:425.
23. Lanier LL, Chang C, Azuma M, et al. Molecular and functional analysis of human natural killer cell–associated neural cell adhesion molecule (N-CAM/CD56). J Immunol 1991;146:4421.
24. Kemshead JT, Patel K, Phimister B. Neuroblastoma in the very young child: biological considerations. Br J Cancer 1992;18:S102.
25. Melino G, Vernole P, Annicchiarico-Petruzzelli M, et al. An inducible cell line (Natasha), from a neuroblastoma patient with circulating HRS-positive blasts, expressing neurohormones. Anticancer Res 1992;12:1199-1206.
26. Nagabuchi E, Kunikane H, Krishan A, et al. In vitro invasiveness in comparison with the expression of MHC-1 antigen in murine neuroblastoma. (Abstract) Proc Am Assoc Cancer Res 1994;35:62.

27. Reuland P, Handgretinger R, Smykowsky H, et al. Application of the murine anti–Gd-2 antibody 14.Gd-2a for diagnosis and therapy of neuroblastoma. Nucl Med Biol 1991;18:121.

28. Barker E, Mueller BM, Handgretinger R, et al. Effect of a chimeric anti-ganglioside G_{D2} antibody on cell-mediated lysis of human neuroblastoma cells. Cancer Res 1991;51:144.

29. Baker E, Reisfeld RA. A mechanism for neutrophil-mediated lysis of human neuroblastoma cells. Cancer Res 1993;53:362.

30. Hank JA, Surfus J, Gan J, et al. Treatment of neuroblastoma patients with antiganglioside G_{D2} antibody plus interleukin-2 induces antibody-dependent cellular cytotoxicity against neuroblastoma detected in vitro. J Immunol 1994;15:29.

31. Favrot MC, Combaret V, Lasset C. CD44: a new prognostic marker for neuroblastoma. N Engl J Med 1993;329:1965.

32. Gross N, Beretta C, Peruisseau G, et al. CD44H expression by human neuroblastoma cells: relation to *MYCN* amplification and lineage differentiation. Cancer Res 1994;54:4238.

33. Brodeur GM. Patterns and significance of genetic changes in neuroblastomas. In: Pretlow TG II, Pretlow TP, eds. Biochemical and molecular aspects of selected cancers. San Diego, Academic, 1991:251.

34. Aguzzi A, Ellmeier W, Weith A. Dominant and recessive molecular changes in neuroblastomas. Brain Pathol 1992;2:195.

35. Vogan K, Bernstein M, Leclerc JM, et al. Absence of *p53* gene mutations in primary neuroblastomas. Cancer Res 1993;53:5269.

36. Hosoi G, Hara J, Okamura T, et al. Low frequency of the p53 gene mutations in neuroblastoma. Cancer 1994;73:3087.

37. Schwab M. Human neuroblastoma: amplification of the N-*myc* oncogene and loss of a putative cancer-preventing gene on chromosome 1p. In: Wiestler OD, Schlegel U, Schramm J, eds. Molecular neuro-oncology and its impact on the clinical management of brain tumors. Berlin, Springer-Verlag, 1994:7.

38. Nakagawara A, Arima M, Azar CG, et al. Inverse relation between *trk* expression and N-*myc* amplification in human neuroblastoma. Cancer Res 1992;52:1364.

39. Nakagawara A, Arima-Nakagawara M, Scavarda NJ, et al. Association between high levels of expression of the TRK gene and favorable outcome in human neuroblastoma. N Engl J Med 1993;328:847.

40. Nakagawara A, Azar CG, Scavarda NJ, et al. Expression and function of *TRK*-B and *BDNF* in human neuroblastoma. Mol Cell Biol 1994;14:759.

41. Valle P, Scala S, Lucarelli E, et al. Brain-derived neurotrophic factor (BDNF) expression alters vinblastine (Vbl) toxicity in neuroblastoma (NB). (Abstract) Proc Am Assoc Cancer Res 1994;35:322.

42. Matsunaga T, Takahashi H, Ohnuma N, et al. Expression of *N-myc* and c-*src* protooncogenes correlating to the undifferentiated phenotype and prognosis of primary neuroblastomas. Cancer Res 1991;51:3148.

43. Matsunaga T, Shirasawa H, Tanabe M, et al. Expression of alternatively spliced *src* messenger RNAs related to normal differentiation in human neuroblastomas. Cancer Res 1993;53:3179.

44. Leone A, Seeger RC, Hong CM, et al. Evidence for *nm23* RNA overexpression, DNA amplification and mutation in aggressive childhood neuroblastomas. Oncogene 1993;8:855.

45. Castle VP, Heidelberger KP, Bromberg J, et al. Expression of the apoptosis-suppressing protein *bcl*-2, in neuroblastoma is associated with unfavorable histology and *N-myc* amplification. Am J Pathol 1993;143:1543.

46. Dole M, Nuñez G, Merchant AK, et al. Bcl-2 inhibits chemotherapy-induced apoptosis in neuroblastoma. Cancer Res 1994;54:3253.

47. Bourhis J, Bénard J, Hartmann O, et al. Correlation of MDR1 gene expression with chemotherapy in neuroblastoma. J Natl Cancer Inst 1989;81:1401.

48. Nakagawara A, Kadomatsu K, Sato S, et al. Inverse correlation between expression of multidrug resistance gene and N-myc oncogene in human neuroblastoma. Cancer Res 1990;50:3043.

49. Sawada T. Past and future of neuroblastoma screening in Japan. Am J Pediatr Hematol Oncol 1992;14:320.

50. Naito H, Sasaki M, Yamashiro K, et al. Improvement in prognosis of neuroblastoma through mass population screening. J Pediatr Surg 1990;25:245.

51. Bernstein ML, Azouz EM, Woods W, et al. Persistence and possible progression of a pelvic neuroblastoma detected by mass screening during 19 months. Am J Pediatr Hematol Oncol 1994;16:164.

52. Kerbl R, Urban C, Starz I, et al. Neuroblastoma with *N-myc* amplification detected by urine: mass screening in infants after the sixth month of life. Med Pediatr Oncol 1993;21:625.

53. Hayashi Y, Hanada R, Yamamoto K. Biology of neuroblastomas in Japan found by screening. Am J Pediatr Hematol Oncol 1992;14:342.

54. Nakagawara A, Zaizen Y, Ikeda K, et al. Different genomic and metabolic patterns between mass screening-positive and mass screening-negative later-presenting neuroblastomas. Cancer 1991;68:2037.

55. Horn M, Blatt J. Continued remission in children with neuroblastoma despite elevations of urinary catecholamine metabolites. Am J Pediatr Hematol Oncol 1992;14:202.

56. Fitzgibbon MC, Tormey WP. Paediatric reference ranges for urinary catecholamines/metabolites and their relevance in neuroblastoma diagnosis. Ann Clin Biochem 1994;31:1.

57. Berthold F, Kassenböhmer R, Zieschang J. Multivariate evaluation of prognostic factors in localized neuroblastoma. Am J Pediatr Hematol Oncol 1994;16:107.

58. Silber JH, Evans AE, Fridman M. Models to predict outcome from childhood neuroblastoma: the role of serum ferritin and tumor histology. Cancer Res 1991;51:1426.

59. Berthold F, Engelhardt-Fahrner U, Schneider A, et al. Age dependence and prognostic impact of neuron specific enolase (NSE) in children with neuroblastoma. In Vivo 1991;5:245.

60. Tsuchida Y, Honna T, Iwanaka T, et al. Serial determination of serum neuron-specific enolase in patients with neuroblastoma and other pediatric tumors. J Pediatr Surg 1987;22:419.

61. Valentino L, Moss T, Olson E, et al. Shed tumor gangliosides and progression of human neuroblastoma. Blood 1990;75:1564.

62. Ladisch S, Li R, Olson E. Ceramide structure predicts tumor ganglioside immunosuppressive activity. Proc Natl Acad Sci USA 1994;91:1974.

63. Mattano LAJ, Moss TJ, Emerson SG. Sensitive detection of rare circulating neuroblastoma cells by the reverse transcriptase-polymerase chain reaction. Cancer Res 1992;52:4701.

64. Adams GA, Shochat SJ, Smith EI, et al. Thoracic neuroblastoma: a Pediatric Oncology Group study. J Pediatr Surg 1993;28:372.

65. Tanabe M, Yoshida H, Ohnuma N, et al. Imaging of neuroblastoma in patients identified by mass screening using urinary catecholamine metabolites. J Pediatr Surg 1993;28:617.

66. Goldstein I, Gomez K, Copel JA. The real-time and color Doppler appearance of adrenal neuroblastoma in a third-trimester fetus. Obstet Gynecol 1994;83:854.

67. Campenhout IV, Patriquin H. Malignant microvasculature in abdominal tumors in children: detection with Doppler US. Radiol 1992;183:445.

68. NG YY, Kingston JE. The role of radiology in the staging of neuroblastoma. Clin Radiol 1993;47:226.

69. Kornreich L, Horev G, Kaplinsky C, et al. Neuroblastoma: evaluation with contrast enhanced MR imaging. Pediatr Radiol 1991;21:566.

70. Paltiel HJ, Gelfand MJ, Elgazzar AH, et al. Neural crest tumors: I-123 MIBG imaging in children. Radiol 1994;190:117.

71. Gelfand MJ. Meta-iodobenzylguanidine in children. Semin Nucl Med 1993;13:231.

72. Turba E, Fagioli G, Mancini AF, et al. Evaluation of stage 4 neuroblastoma patients by means of MIBG and ^{99m}Tc-MDP scintigraphy. J Nucl Biol Med 1993;37:107.

73. Labreveux de Cervens C, Hartmann O, Bonnin F, et al. What is the prognostic value of osteomedullary uptake on MIGB scan in neuroblastoma patients under one year of age. Med Pediatr Oncol 1994;22:107.

74. Yeh SDJ, Larson SM, Burch L, et al. Radioimmunodetection of neuroblastoma with iodine-131-3F8: correlation with biopsy, iodine-131-metaiodobenzylguanidine and standard diagnostic modalities. J Nucl Med 1990;32:769.

75. Cheung NKV, Cheung IY, Canete A, et al. Antibody response to murine anti-G_{D2} monoclonal antibodies: correlation with patient survival. Cancer Res 1994;54:2228.

76. Wirnsberger GH, Becker H, Ziervogel K, et al. Diagnostic immuno-histochemistry of neuroblastic tumors. Am J Surg Pathol 1992;16:49.

77. Corbett R, Olliff J, Fairley N, et al. A prospective comparison between magnetic resonance imaging, meta-iodobenzylguanidine scintigraphy and marrow histology/cytology in neuroblastoma. Eur J Cancer 1991;27:1560.

78. Osmanagaoglu K, Lippens M, Benoit Y, et al. A comparison of iodine-123 meta-iodobenzylguanidine scintigraphy and single bone marrow

aspiration biopsy in the diagnosis and follow-up of 26 children with neuroblastoma. Eur J Nucl Med 1993;20:1154.

79. Mandel M, Rechvi G, Neumann Y, et al. CD10$^+$ cell population in the bone marrow of patients with advanced neuroblastoma. Med Pediatr Oncol 1994;22:115.

80. Evans AE, D'Angio GJ, Randolph J. A proposed staging for children with neuroblastoma: Children's Cancer Study Group A. Cancer 1971; 27:374.

81. Nitschke R, Smith EI, Shochat S, et al. Localized neuroblastoma treated by surgery: a Pediatric Oncology Group study. J Clin Oncol 1988;6:1271.

82. Huddart SN, Muir KR, Parkes S, et al. Neuroblastoma: a 32-year population-based study—implications for screening. Med Pediatr Oncol 1993;21:96.

83. Ziegler MM. Pediatric surgical oncology. Curr Opin Pediatr 1990;2: 580.

84. Ziegler MM, Vega A, Koop CE. Electrocoagulation induced immunity: an explanation for regression of neuroblastoma. J Pediatr Surg 1980;15:34.

85. McCormack CJ, Naim JO, Rogers DW, et al. Beneficial effects following carbon dioxide laser excision on experimental neuroblastoma. J Pediatr Surg 1989;24:201.

86. Ishizu H, Ziegler MM. Neoplasms. In: Levine BA, Copeland EM, Howard RJ, et al, eds. Current practice of surgery, vol 3. New York, Churchill Livingstone, 1992:3.

87. Loo R, Applebaum H, Takasugi J, et al. Resection of advanced stage neuroblastoma with the Cavitron ultrasonic surgical aspirator. J Pediatr Surg 1988;23:1135.

88. Azizkhan RG, Haase GM. Current biologic and therapeutic implications in the surgery of neuroblastoma. Semin Surg Oncol 1993;9:493.

89. Haase GM, O'Leary MC, Ramsay NKC, et al. Aggressive surgery combined with intensive chemotherapy improves survival in poor-risk neuroblastoma. J Pediatr Surg 1991;26:1119.

90. Lobe TE. The applications of laparoscopy and lasers in pediatric surgery. Surg Ann 1993;25:175.

91. Plantaz D, Hartmann O, Kalifa C, et al. Localized dumbbell neuroblastoma: a study of 25 cases treated between 1982 and 1987 using the same protocol. Med Pediatr Oncol 1993;21:249.

92. Matthay KK, Sather HN, Seeger RC, et al. Excellent outcome of stage II neuroblastoma is independent of residual disease and radiation therapy. J Clin Oncol 1989;7:236.

93. West DC, Shamberger RC, Macklis RM, et al. Stage III neuroblastoma over 1 year of age at diagnosis: improved survival with intensive multimodality therapy including multiple alkylating agents. J Clin Oncol 1993;11:84.

94. Garaventa A, Bernardi BD, Pianca C, et al. Localized but unresectable neuroblastoma: treatment and outcome of 145 cases. J Clin Oncol 1993;11:1770.

95. Tsuchida Y, Yokoyama J, Kaneko M, et al. Therapeutic significance of surgery in advanced neuroblastoma: a report from the Study Group of Japan. J Pediatr Surg 1992;27:616.

96. Kiely EM. The surgical challenge of neuroblastoma. J Pediatr Surg 1994;29:128.

97. Berthold F, Trechow R, Utsch S, et al. Prognostic factors in metastatic neuroblastoma. Am J Pediatr Hematol Oncol 1992;14:207.

98. De Bernardi B, Pianca C, Boni L, et al. Disseminated neuroblastoma (stage IV and IV-S) in the first year of life. Cancer 1992;70:1625.

99. Seeger RC, Reynolds CP. Neuroblastoma. In: Holland JF, Frei E III, Bast RCJ, et al, eds. Cancer medicine. Philadelphia, Lea & Febiger, 1993:2172.

100. Martinez DA, King DR, Ginn-Pease ME, et al. Resection of the primary tumor is appropriate for children with stage IV-S neuroblastoma: an analysis of 37 patients. J Pediatr Surg 1992;27:1016.

101. Wilson PCG, Coppes MJ, Solh H, et al. Neuroblastoma stage IV-S: a heterogeneous disease. Med Pediatr Oncol 1991;19:467.

102. Méresse V, Vassal G, Michon J, et al. Combined continuous infusion etoposide with high-dose cyclophosphamide for refractory neuroblastoma: a phase II study from the Société Française d'Oncologie Pédiatrique. J Clin Oncol 1993;11:630.

103. Pearson ADJ, Craft AW, Pinkerton CR, et al. High-dose rapid schedule chemotherapy for disseminated neuroblastoma. Eur J Cancer 1992; 28A:1654.

104. De Bernardi B, Carli M, Casale F, et al. Standard-dose and high-dose peptichemio and cisplatin in children with disseminated poor-risk neuroblastoma: two studies by the Italian Cooperative Group for Neuroblastoma. J Clin Oncol 1992;10:1870.

105. Lowis SP, Pearson ADJ, Reid MM, et al. Prohibitive toxicity of a dose-intense regime for metastatic neuroblastoma containing ifosfamide, doxorubicin and cisplatin. Cancer Chemother Pharmacol 1993; 31:415.

106. Pinkerton CR, Zucker JM, Hartmann O, et al. Short duration, high dose, alternating chemotherapy in metastatic neuroblastoma (ENSG 3C induction regimen). Br J Cancer 1990;62:319.

107. Frappaz D, Michon J, Hartmann O, et al. Etoposide and carboplatin in neuroblastoma: a French Society of Pediatric Oncology phase II study. J Clin Oncol 1992;10:1592.

108. Nitschke R, Pratt C, Harris M, et al. Evaluation of CHIP (iproplatin) in recurrent pediatric malignant solid tumors: a phase II study (Pediatric Oncology Group). Invest New Drugs 1992;10:93.

109. Donfrancesco A, Deb G, Angioni A, et al. D-CECaT: a breakthrough for patients with neuroblastoma. Anticancer Drugs 1993;4:317.

110. Pappo AS, Vats T, Williams TE, et al. Phase I trial of trimetrexate in pediatric solid tumors: a Pediatric Oncology Group Study. Med Pediatr Oncol 1993;21:280.

111. Pratt CB, Stewart C, Santana VM, et al. Phase I study of topotecan for pediatric patients with malignant solid tumors. J Clin Oncol 1994; 12:539.

112. Pinkerton CR. ENSG1-randomized study of high-dose melphalan in neuroblastoma. Bone Marrow Transplant 1991;7(Suppl 3):112.

113. Simone JV. Autologous bone marrow transplantation in childhood cancer. J Clin Oncol 1993;11:1439.

114. Graham-Pole JR. Myeloablative treatment supported by marrow infusions for children with neuroblastoma. In: Armitage JO, Antman KH, eds. High-dose cancer therapy: pharmacology, hematopoietins, stem cells. Baltimore, Williams & Wilkins, 1992:735.

115. Ladenstein R, Lasset C, Hartmann O, et al. Comparison of auto versus allografting as consolidation of primary treatments in advanced neuroblastoma over one year of age at diagnosis: report from the European Group for Bone Marrow Transplantation. Bone Marrow Transplant 1994;14:37.

116. Housholder SE, Rackoff WR, Goldman J, et al. A case-control retrospective study of the efficacy of granulocyte-colony-stimulating factor in children with neuroblastoma. Am J Pediatr Hematol Oncol 1994; 16:132.

117. Ladenstein R, Favrot M, Lasset C, et al. Indication and limits of megatherapy and bone marrow transplantation in high-risk neuroblastoma: a single centre analysis of prognostic factors. Eur J Cancer 1993;29A:947.

118. Stute N, Santana VM, Rodman JH, et al. Pharmacokinetics of subcutaneous recombinant human granulocyte colony-stimulating factor in children. Blood 1992;79:2849.

119. Castleberry RP, Kun LE, Shuster JJ, et al. Radiotherapy improves the outlook for patients older than 1 year with Pediatric Oncology Group stage C neuroblastoma. J Clin Oncol 1991;9:789.

120. Lashford LS, Lewis IJ, Fielding SL, et al. Phase I/II study of iodine 131 metaiodobenzylguanidine in chemoresistant neuroblastoma: a United Kingdom Children's Cancer Study Group investigation. J Clin Oncol 1992;10:1889.

121. Hoefnagel CA, Smets L, Voûte PA, et al. Iodine-125-MIBG therapy for neuroblastoma. J Nucl Med 1991;32:361.

122. Mastrangelo R, Lasorella A, Iavarone A, et al. Critical observations on neuroblastoma treatment with 131-I-metaiodobenzylguanidine at diagnosis. Med Pediatr Oncol 1993;21:411.

123. Haase GM, Meagher DPJ, McNeely LK, et al. Electron beam intraoperative radiation therapy for pediatric neoplasms. Cancer 1994;73: 740.

124. Ribeiro RC, Rill D, Roberson PK, et al. Continuous infusion of interleukin-2 in children with refractory malignancies. Cancer 1993;72: 623.

125. Favrot MC, Michon J, Floret D, et al. Interleukin 2 immunotherapy in children with neuroblastoma after high-dose chemotherapy and autologous bone marrow transplantation. Pediatr Hematol Oncol 1990;7:275.

126. Negrier S, Michon J, Floret D, et al. Interleukin-2 and lymphokine-activated killer cells in 15 children with advanced metastatic neuroblastoma. J Clin Oncol 1991;9:1363.

127. Matthay KK, Atkinson JB, Stram DO, et al. Patterns of relapse after

autologous purged bone marrow transplantation for neuroblastoma: a Children's Cancer Group pilot study. J Clin Oncol 1993;11:2226.

128. Shuster JJ, Cantor AB, McWilliams N, et al. The prognostic significance of autologous bone marrow transplant in advanced neuroblastoma. J Clin Oncol 1991;9:1045.

129. Philip T, Ladenstein R, Zucker JM, et al. Double megatherapy and autologous bone marrow transplantation for advanced neuroblastoma: the LMCE2 study. Br J Cancer 1993;67:119.

130. Evans AE, D'Angio GJ, Sather HN, et al. A comparison of four staging systems for localized and regional neuroblastoma: a report from the Children's Cancer Study Group. J Clin Oncol 1990;8:678.

131. Hann HWL, Evans AE, Siegel SE, et al. Prognostic importance of serum ferritin in patients with stage III and IV neuroblastoma: the Children's Cancer Study Group experience. Cancer Res 1985;45: 2843.

132. Reynolds CP, Kane DJ, Einhorn PA, et al. Response of neuroblastoma to retinoic acid in vitro and in vivo. In: Evans AE, D'Angio GJ, Knudson AG, et al, eds. Advances in neuroblastoma research 3. New York, Wiley-Liss, 1991:203.

133. Finklestein JZ, Krailo MD, Lenarsky C, et al. 13-cis-Retinoic acid (NSC 122758) in the treatment of children with metastatic neuroblastoma unresponsive to conventional chemotherapy: report from the Children's Cancer Study Group. Med Pediatr Oncol 1992;20:307.

134. Mugishima H, Iwata M, Okabe I, et al. Autologous bone marrow transplantation in children with advanced neuroblastoma. Cancer 1994;74:972.

135. Villablanca JG, Khan AA, Avramis VI, et al. Hypercalcemia: a dose-limiting toxicity associated with 13-cis-retinoic acid. Am J Pediatr Hematol Oncol 1993;15:410.

136. Smith MA, Adamson PC, Balis FM, et al. Phase I and pharmacokinetic evaluation of all-trans-retinoic acid in pediatric patients with cancer. J Clin Oncol 1992;10:1666.

137. Cheung NKV, Burch L, Kushner BH, et al. Monoclonal antibody 3F8 can effect durable remissions in neuroblastoma patients refractory to chemotherapy: a phase II trial. In: Evans AE, D'Angio GJ, Knudson AG, et al, eds. Advances in neuroblastoma research 3. New York, Wiley-Liss, 1991:395.

138. Handgretinger R, Baader P, Dopfer R, et al. A phase I study of neuroblastoma with the anti-ganglioside GD2 antibody 14.G2a. Cancer Immunol Immunother 1992;35:199.

139. Murray JL, Cunningham JE, Brewer H, et al. Phase I trial of murine monoclonal antibody 14G2a administered by prolonged intravenous infusion in patients with neuroectodermal tumors. J Clin Oncol 1994; 12:184.

140. Yu AL, Gillies SD, Reisfeld RA. Phase I clinical trial of ch14.18 in patients with refractory neuroblastoma. (Abstract) Proc Am Soc Clin Oncol 1991;10:318.

141. Wexler L, Thiele C, McClure L, et al. Adoptive immunotherapy (AI) of refractory neuroblastoma (NB) with tumor-infiltrating lymphocytes (TIL), interferon-gamma (IFN-γ), and interleukin-2 (IL-2). (Abstract) Proc Am Soc Clin Oncol 1992;11:368.

142. Rivoltini L, Arienti F, Orazi A, et al. Phenotypic and functional analysis of lymphocytes infiltrating paediatric tumours, with a characterization of the tumour phenotype. Cancer Immunol Immunother 1992;34: 241.

143. Brenner MK, Furman WI, Santana VM, et al. Clinical protocol: phase I study of cytokine-gene modified autologous neuroblastoma cells for treatment of relapsed/refractory neuroblastoma. Hum Gene Ther 1993;3:665.

144. Bushle RM, Foreman NK, Bartholomew C, et al. Retrovirus-mediated gene transfer as an approach to analyze neuroblastoma relapse after autologous bone marrow transplantation. Hum Gene Ther 1992;3: 129.

145. Brenner M, Santana V, Bowman L, et al. Clinical protocol: use of marker genes to investigate the mechanism of relapse and the effect of bone marrow purging in autologous transplantation for stage D neuroblastoma. Hum Gene Ther 1993;4:809.

Surgery of Infants and Children: Scientific Principles and Practice, edited by Keith T. Oldham, Paul M. Colombani, and Robert P. Foglia. Lippincott–Raven Publishers, Philadelphia, © 1997.

CHAPTER 35

Rhabdomyosarcoma and Nonrhabdomyomatous Sarcomas

Michael P. LaQuaglia

The study of soft tissue malignant tumors arising from mesenchyme has been revolutionized by developments in molecular embryology, cytogenetics, and gene cloning. Advances in these fields have in some cases eliminated total reliance on light microscopic histology and immunohistochemistry for correct diagnosis. As knowledge evolves, the prospect of molecular staging and use of genetic analysis for determination of risk status will become a reality.

This chapter organizes the soft tissue sarcomas by cell of origin. It begins with a discussion of relevant scientific developments, which is followed by an analysis of diagnoses, staging, and treatment. Finally, future developments in treatment are explored.

CLINICAL PROBLEM

Soft tissue sarcomas are the sixth most common malignancy of childhood, with rhabdomyosarcoma by far the most frequent. In the United States, about 250 new rhabdomyosarcomas are diagnosed each year, for a yearly incidence of about 4.35 per 1 million children younger than 14 years of age. In comparison, other sarcomas occur with the following incidence: 0.80 for fibrosarcoma, 0.55 for neurogenic sarcoma, 0.37 for tenosynovial sarcoma, 0.37 for primitive neuroectodermal tumor (PNET), 0.37 for hemangiopericytoma, and 0.18 for leiomyosarcoma.[1–3] The incidence of desmoplastic small round cell tumors (DSRCT), malignant rhabdoid tumors, alveolar soft parts sarcoma, and liposarcomas is nearly zero in childhood, although small series have been reported. The incidence of osteosarcoma is 2.82, and that of Ewing sarcoma is 2.76, but these are primarily lesions arising from bone. Extraosseous osteosarcoma and Ewing sarcoma are rare. Each histopathologic subtype has characteristic biologic, clinical, and prognostic parameters that influence treatment. Figure 35-1 shows the relative percentages of sarcomas presenting to a major cancer center during a 10-year period. Figure 35-2 is a breakdown of rare soft tissue sarcomas by histologic subtype. Figure 35-3 depicts the age distributions and Figure 35-4 shows the primary tumor size distributions for four histologic types of soft tissue sarcoma at

diagnosis. The principal therapeutic problem in all soft tissue sarcomas is matching treatment intensity to prognostic risk. Important to this consideration are underlying biologic factors and clinical prognostic variables.

RHABDOMYOSARCOMA

Epidemiology

Soft tissue sarcomas are the sixth most common childhood malignancy, and rhabdomyosarcoma is the most common soft tissue sarcoma of childhood. It accounts for 5% to 8% of cases of childhood cancer and for about 70% of the sarcomas. The incidence in African-American children is about half that in whites. Rhabdomyosarcoma of the bladder, vagina, and head and neck region usually occurs in infants and small children; extremity and truncal lesions predominantly occur in later childhood and adolescence.[4]

Pathology

Rhabdomyosarcomas are malignant tumors arising from the ubiquitously distributed primitive mesenchyme found in the fetus. These tumors display characteristics of striated muscle, including immunohistochemical expression of skeletal muscle myosin and actin, desmin, myoglobin, and Z-band protein. Electron microscopy may show actin and myosin bundles or Z-band material. Expression of the DNA-binding protein MYOD1 has been shown to be a lineage marker for rhabdomyosarcoma.[5,6]

Based on classic pathology, rhabdomyosarcoma is divided into four main histopathologic subtypes: embryonal, alveolar, botryoid, and pleomorphic. The most common type in children is embryonal, the microscopic characteristics of which are illustrated in Figure 35-5. Botryoid tumors are really of the embryonal subtype but grow into a hollow space (ie, vagina, bladder), so that they develop a characteristic grapelike gross morphology. Alveolar tumors are so named because of a resem-

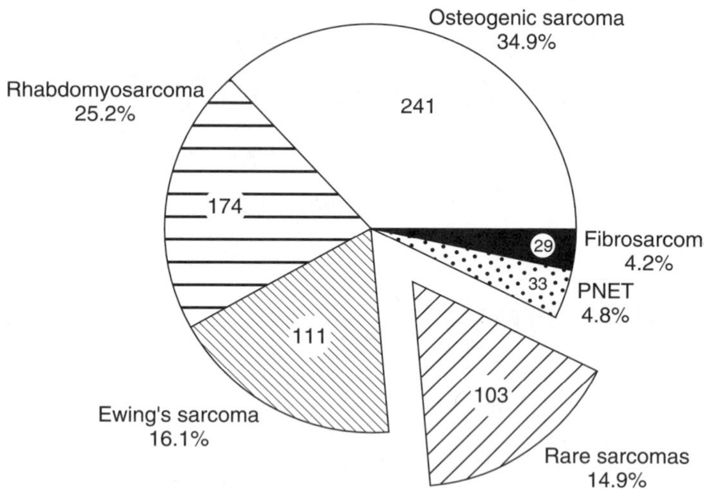

FIG. 35-1. Relative proportions of childhood sarcomas diagnosed at the Memorial Sloan-Kettering Cancer Center during a 10-year period. PNET, peripheral primitive neuroectodermal tumor.

blance to the microscopic structure of the lung (Fig. 35-6). Rhabdomyosarcomas are identified as alveolar if *any* alveolar elements are found in the tumors. Pleomorphic tumors usually occur in adults. For all cell types, sites of occurrence include the head and neck (orbit, infratemporal fossa); genitourinary tract, including perineum and perianal area; extremities; trunk (chest wall, paraspinal area); retroperitoneum; and biliary tract.

Biology

Myogenic cell differentiation can be arbitrarily divided into three broad stages: (1) commitment of a multipotent stem cell to a monopotent myoblast, (2) differentiation of a monopotent myoblast into a multinucleated myofiber expressing muscle-specific genes, and (3) maturation, during which the expression of specific cellular proteins progresses through embryonic, fetal, neonatal, and adult patterns.[7] A simplified schema for myoblast differentiation is depicted in Figure 35-7. Genetic determinants of the first stage of myogenic cell differentiation were identified initially. It was observed that fibroblasts briefly exposed to 5-azacytidine developed a myoblastic phenotype

(presence of myotubes). Genomic DNA transfection experiments verified that myoblast but not fibroblast DNA could convert fibroblasts into stably determined myoblasts. The frequency of conversion was consistent with a single genetic locus. This allowed the first identification of a myogenic determination gene, *MYOD1*.[8] *MYOD* is expressed exclusively in skeletal muscle and in myoblasts derived from 5-azacytidine–treated fibroblasts. When this gene is transfected, under the control of a viral promoter, into a variety of cell types (ie, fibroblast, melanoma cells, neuroblastoma, hepatic cells, and adipocytes) expression of the *MYOD* cDNA induces myogenesis with expression of muscle-specific structural genes. It was also determined that a second myogenic regulatory gene, *MYD*, induces *MYOD* expression. Thus, *MYD* and *MYOD* are genetic determinants of the first phase of myogenic differentiation.

Wright and colleagues[9] showed that the gene *myogenin*, which was induced in rat myoblasts about 30 hours after exposure to the differentiating agent 5-bromodeoxyuridine, was capable of converting mesenchymal stem cells to myosin-positive cells in a transfection assay. Another muscle-associated protein, desmin, was also induced. These data support a regulatory role for myogenin in the differentiation of myoblasts to multinucle-

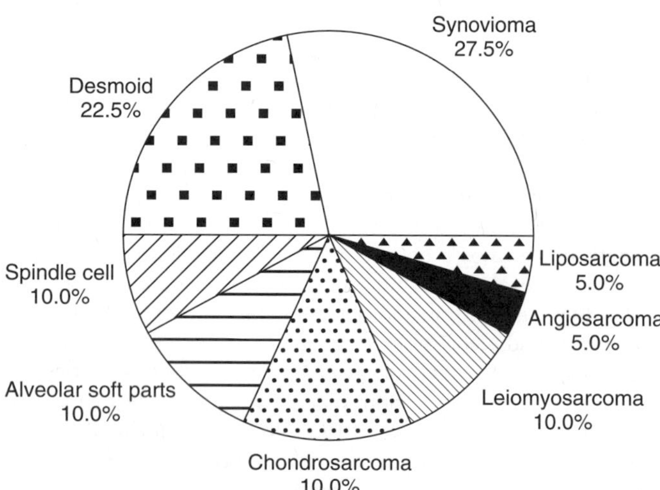

FIG. 35-2. Relative proportions of rare childhood soft tissue tumors observed during a 10-year period.

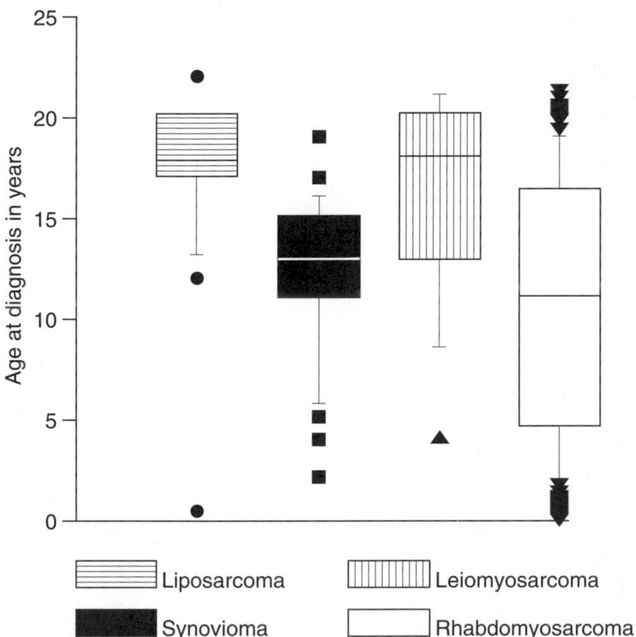

FIG. 35-3. Age distributions at diagnosis of four types of soft tissue sarcomas diagnosed in childhood and adolescence.

ated myofibers. Interestingly, myogenin has significant homology to *MYOD1*, although they are different genes by Southern analysis. Also, retinoic acid induced myogenin synthesis and myogenic differentiation in a rat rhabdomyosarcoma cell line.

Analysis of rhabdomyosarcoma cell lines, as well as lines from other embryonal tumors, has shown that *MYOD1* is always expressed, whereas myogenin is selectively expressed in more differentiated clones. Strong myogenin expression was observed in a cell line that immunostained for desmin, α-sarcomeric actin, and skeletomuscular myosin. The same line exhibited thick and thin filaments and Z-line materials. These data support *MYOD1* as a lineage marker and myogenin as a marker of differentiation in human rhabdomyosarcoma.

Scrable and associates[5] used *MYOD1* expression as part of an algorithm to determine the differential pathology of rhabdomyosarcoma. The investigators first analyzed 45 embryonal tumors for *MYOD1* expression. Of these, 35 were straightforward diagnostic problems, and in these, *MYOD1* expression occurred in all rhabdomyosarcomas but in no case of another histologic type (eg, Ewing sarcoma, neuroepithelioma, non-Hodgkin lymphoma, neuroblastoma). Thus, the researchers showed that *MYOD1* can be used as a marker for rhabdomyosarcoma. Next, the tumors were analyzed for loss of heterozygosity on the short arm of chromosome 11 (11p) using Southern blots probed with chromosomal markers. The data showed that embryonal but not alveolar rhabdomyosarcoma was associated with a loss of heterozygosity at chromosome 11p. This loss of heterozygosity was not associated with discernible cytogenetic abnormalities on chromosome 11p. Furthermore, cytogenetic analyses of alveolar tumors frequently demonstrated a characteristic t(2;13)(q37;q14) translocation. These findings taken together allowed the investigators to establish a diagnostic schema for rhabdomyosarcoma based on molecular and cytogenetic findings. A suspected rhabdomyosarcoma would first be analyzed

by Northern blot or immunohistochemistry, or both, for the expression of *MYOD1*. If positive, this would establish that the tumor is derived from a myoblastic lineage. Cytogenetic analysis would then support a diagnosis of alveolar subtype if the characteristic translocation was identified. If no cytogenetic abnormalities were seen, loss of heterozygosity at chromosome 11p would establish that the tumor is an embryonal subtype. The role of myogenin in this schema has not been evaluated, but presumably expression of this gene should be observed in more differentiated tumors. Improved prognosis for myogenin-positive tumors remains speculative.

Presentation and Diagnostic Evaluation

The incidence of rhabdomyosarcoma is biphasic, with one peak in infancy followed by a second in adolescence. Presentation is site dependent. Head and neck lesions can cause facial or cervical swelling and associated pain or skin discoloration. Sinusitis or middle ear infections can occur because the tumor blocks the normal drainage from these sites (ie, sinusoidal ostia, eustachian tubes). Epistaxis, proptosis, or cranial nerve palsies may also be evident in head and neck lesions. Genitourinary tumors present with gross or microscopic hematuria, a suprapubic mass, or urinary tract infection or obstruction. Vaginal and cervical primary tumors often prolapse through the vaginal orifice as a friable polypoid mass and may hemorrhage. Paratesticular lesions are most often observed in adolescence, and a hard mass above the testis that is separable by physical examination from the testis is observed. Extremity tumors present as painless or painful expanding masses, and there may be an associated limp or overlying skin change. Local bony invasion may result in pathologic fractures.

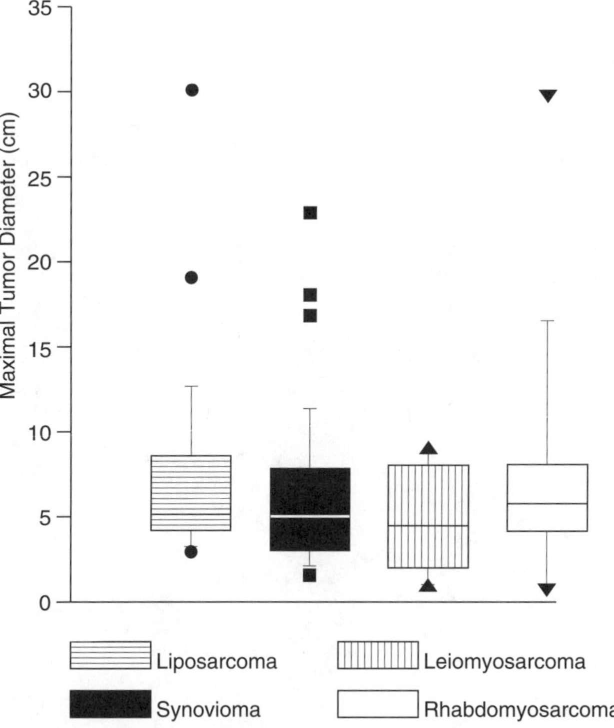

FIG. 35-4. Size distributions at diagnosis of four types of soft tissue sarcomas diagnosed in childhood and adolescence.

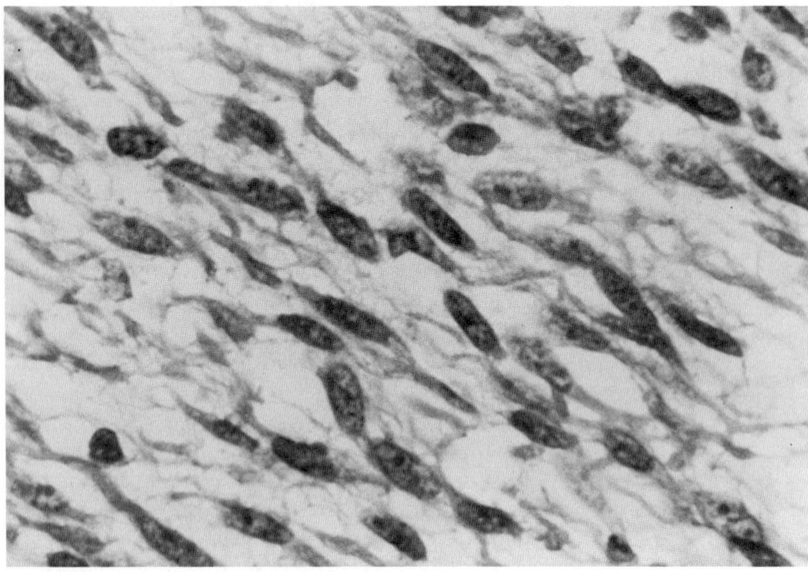

FIG. 35-5. Photomicrograph of a specimen of embryonal rhabdomyosarcoma.

Rational management depends on a thorough pretreatment workup that defines completely local tumor extent as well as evaluating regional and distant sites of metastases. Table 35-1 lists the standard workup for pediatric sarcoma patients. An extensive history, including family history of breast cancer or other forms of sarcoma, and thorough physical examination are elementary. Radiographic staging has been markedly facilitated by modern imaging methods. Even greater progress in this area is promised by efforts in the field of positron emission scanning, which allows determination of the metabolic activity of a tumor mass. The T2-weighted magnetic resonance image appearance of a large rhabdomyosarcoma arising in the buttock of a 3-year-old is shown in Figure 35-8.

Staging

An evolution has occurred in sarcoma staging during the past 10 years, with most groups adopting the TNM system defined by the International Union Against Cancer.[10] This staging system and its approximate correlation with the older Intergroup Rhabdomyosarcoma Study (IRS) classification is listed in Table 35-2. The TNM schema attempts to divide stage into definable clinical components. It is applied before any therapeutic interventions, although a second staging based on histologic findings of the primary tumor and regional lymph nodes can also be performed after resection.

Local tumor invasion is the consequence of cellular and molecular phenotypic properties, which are rapidly being defined by molecular analyses. The ability of cells to invade surrounding basement membranes depends on manufacture of a spectrum of lytic enzymes and on cellular motility. Furthermore, regional or distant metastases are not possible without initial cellular invasion. The gross invasion assessed for TNM staging is a rough measure of these cellular events. In this sense, the TNM system begins to relate macroscopic tumor behavior to the properties and interactions of individual tumor cells. Future direc-

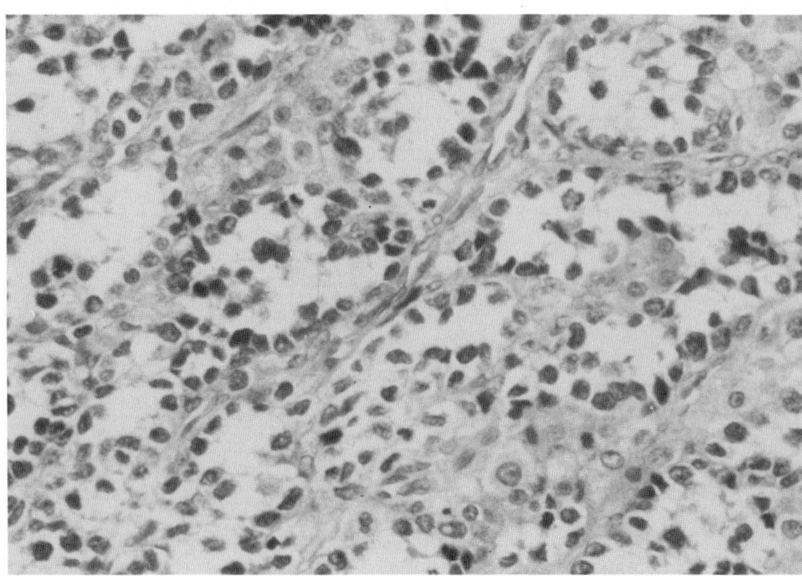

FIG. 35-6. Photomicrograph of a specimen of alveolar rhabdomyosarcoma illustrating the lunglike cytoarchitecture.

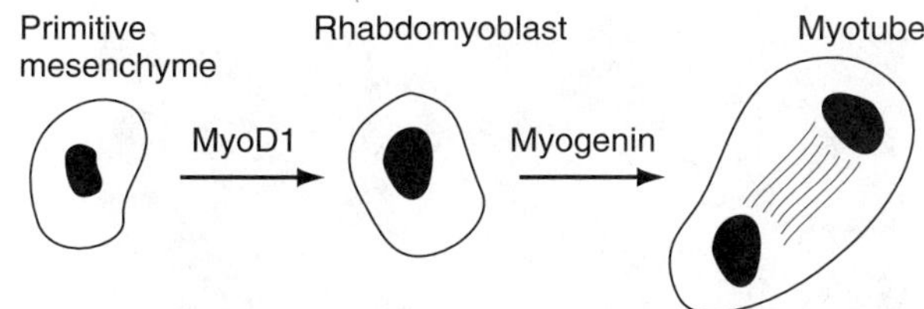

FIG. 35-7. Simplified schema of myoblastic differentiation illustrating the roles of MyoD1 and myogenin.

tions include more precise definitions of the process of tumor cell invasion. Assays of collagenolytic activity and growth and invasion in nude mice are intermediate steps in this regard. Eventually, genetic determinants of invasion and metastasis that are the final determinants of prognosis will be identified.

Using the TNM system, the reported overall percentage of patients with tumors greater than 5 cm ranges from 50% to

TABLE 35-1. *Diagnostic evaluation for suspected rhabdomyosarcoma*

Examination or test	Rationale
History and physical examination	Search for nodes, size of primary mass, general condition, underlying conditions
Complete blood cell count	Bone marrow replacement associated with anemia or thrombocytopenia; bone marrow toxicity is the major side effect of chemotherapy.
Electrolytes, renal and hepatic functions tests	Renal toxicity associated with cisplatin and other alkylators; genitourinary tumors may obstruct ureters; hepatic toxicity with dactinomycin
Four-site bone marrow aspirations, two-site bone biopsies	Bone marrow metastases reported in up to 6% of patients at diagnosis (29% of stage 4 patients have marrow involvement); bone marrow assessment before chemotherapy
Bone scan	Possibility of bone and bone marrow metastases
CT of the primary site	Evaluation of tumor size, invasiveness, enlargement of regional nodes, and complicating ureteral, biliary, bowel, or airway obstruction
CT of possible metastatic sites	CT scan of the lungs and liver should be done to rule out parenchymal metastases.
MR imaging	MR imaging is done for the same rationale as CT scanning. It may give more detailed information regarding the extent of viable tumor (T2-weighted imaging) and the presence of hepatic disease.
Gallium scanning	Both the primary tumor and metastatic deposits may be identified by gallium scanning.

68%. The proportions of other staging variables include: invasive tumors, 37% to 71%; regional nodal involvement, 7% to 28%; and distant metastases at diagnosis, 20% to 23%.

A sarcoma is adequately staged when the following criteria are met:

1. The primary tumor pathology and histopathologic subtype have been determined by biopsy.
2. All components in the TNM staging system are known with reasonable certainty.

Biopsy should be done on metastatic regional lymph nodes, but extensive nodal dissections are not indicated. In the special case of paratesticular rhabdomyosarcoma, a limited dissection of ipsilateral, periaortic nodes is used as a determinant of the need for nodal irradiation. The use of prechemotherapy nodal sampling in paratesticular rhabdomyosarcoma is controversial. Many European groups favor chemotherapy along with radical orchiectomy as sole primary treatment. Most North American groups favor lymph node biopsy with consequent periaortic nodal irradiation if N1 status is proved. Laparoscopic biopsy is adequate.

Small, accessible primary lesions should undergo excisional biopsy. The surgeon should attempt to obtain a clear microscopic margin. Larger infiltrating lesions or those whose removal causes debilitation or deformity (ie, amputation or cystectomy) should undergo limited incisional or endoscopic biopsy. It is acceptable to perform transperineal needle-core biopsies for bladder neck or perineal primary tumors. Enough biopsy material for light and electron microscopic analysis, immunohistochemistry, and cytogenetics should be obtained. It is preferable to freeze extra tissue to facilitate further specialized studies. Even though such investigations do not have direct, short-term benefit for the patient, they are crucial in expanding knowledge concerning rhabdomyosarcoma. Tissue should be frozen in liquid nitrogen as soon as possible after biopsy.

Treatment

The modern treatment of rhabdomyosarcoma is multidisciplinary and includes multiagent chemotherapy, judicious resection, and radiotherapy. Common chemotherapeutic agents used in rhabdomyosarcoma treatment are listed in Table 35-3 along with their response rates when used as single agents in the treatment of rhabdomyosarcoma. The intensity of therapy should be tailored to the risk of subsequent relapse, which is a function of TNM stage. In general, agents are combined to limit drug resistance while attaining a synergistic antitumor effect. A major surgical responsibility during chemotherapy is maintenance of adequate vascular access both for administration of medications and for blood sampling. An external or implanted vascular access device usually can be inserted at the time of diagnostic biopsy.

Surgical resection of the primary tumor was the mainstay of treatment 30 years ago but resulted in overall survival rates in the range of 20%. This improved to 50% with the addition of chemotherapy, resulting in a period when the role of tumor resection in rhabdomyosarcoma was questioned. It is difficult to prove that surgical removal of the primary tumor alters survival probability. A major reason is that a significant proportion of

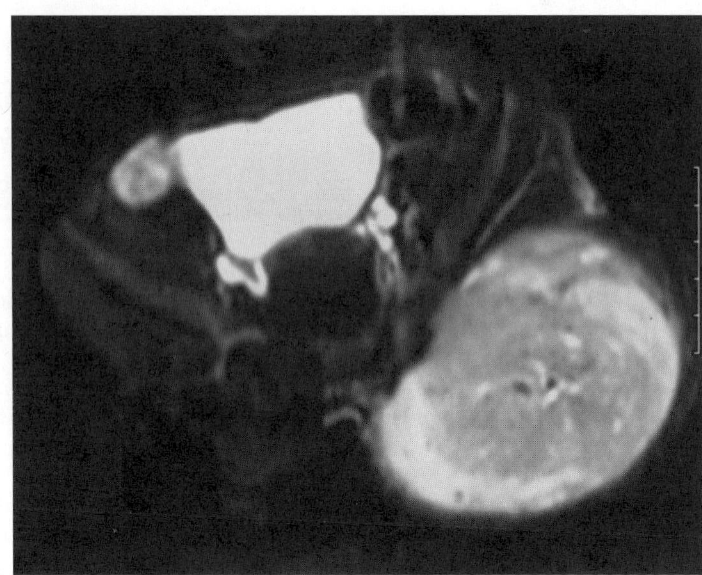

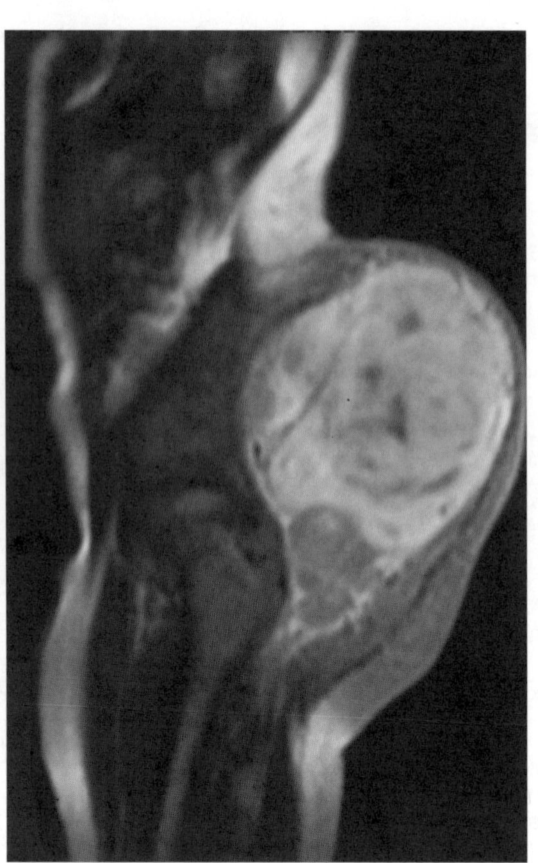

FIG. 35-8. (*A*) T2-weighted axial MR image showing a large rhabdomyosarcoma of the left buttock in a 3-year-old child. The indistinct border suggests local invasiveness. (*B*) Sagittal view of the same tumor.

patients have distant metastases at the time of presentation, and this so profoundly influences survival that the effect of other variables is obscured. In addition, most tumors that can be readily removed without serious disfigurement or disability are resected. Thus, the effect of leaving a tumor in situ cannot readily be evaluated. With present survival rates, it would be unethical to randomize patients with nonmetastatic, resectable tumors to a nonsurgical arm. It is recommended that complete resection of primary tumors should be undertaken either before chemotherapy for small noninvasive lesions or after documented response with more formidable primary tumors. In certain situations in which chemotherapy results in complete or very good tumor regression, external-beam radiotherapy can be used as a

TABLE 35-2. *Comparison of two staging stytems*

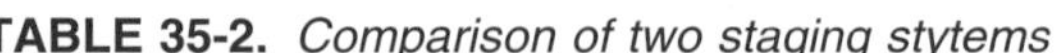

TNM STAGING SYSTEM

Clinical stage	Invasiveness	Size	Status of lymph nodes	Distant metastases
I	T1	a or b	N0	M0
II	T2	a or b	N0	M0
III	T1	a or b	N1	M0
IV	T1–2	a or b	N0–1	M1

INTERGROUP RHABDOMYOSARCOMA CLINICAL GROUPS

Group	Criteria
I	Localized completely resected disease
A	Confined to organ or muscle of origin
B	Infiltration outside organ or muscle of origin but no regional nodal involvement
II	Compromised or regional resection
A	Gross resection with microscopic residual
B	Regional disease, completely resected, but nodes may be involved or there is extension into adjacent organs
C	Regional disease, nodes involved, microscopic residual disease after resection
III	Incomplete resection or biopsy alone with gross residual disease
IV	Distant metastases at diagnosis

T1, noninvasive; T2, invasive; Ta, ≤5 cm; Tb, >5 cm; N0, regional nodes negative; N1, nodes positive; M0, no distant metastases at diagnosis; M1, metastases present.

TABLE 35-3. *Response rates of rhabdomyosarcoma to chemotherapeutic agents*

Chemotherapy agent	Response rate (%)
Cisplatin	21
Cyclophosphamide	13
Dactinomycin	14
Doxorubicin	40
Etoposide	6
Ifosfamide	14
Melphalan	4
Vincristine	42
Paclitaxel	—

(La Quaglia MP. Extremity rhabdomyosarcoma: biological principles, staging, and treatment. Semin Surg Oncol 1993; 9:510)

primary means of local control. Even in these circumstances, biopsy is important to document complete tumor eradication. Debilitating or disfiguring surgery should only be performed if residual tumor is present after both chemotherapy and therapeutic radiotherapy. Amputation for extremity rhabdomyosarcomas does not enhance cure and should be performed only when lesions are bulky, invade bone or neurovascular structures, or are recurrent. Similarly, radical cystectomy is reserved for situations in which complete tumor eradication has not been accomplished by chemotherapy and external-beam radiotherapy. The guiding principle of rhabdomyosarcoma surgery is complete tumor resection; however, removal of large amounts of adjacent normal tissue (ie, muscle group resection, amputation) does not, in itself, affect outcome.

External-beam radiotherapy of the primary site or involved regional nodal echelons has contributed to locoregional control. Clinical data suggest that control of microscopic rhabdomyosarcoma can be accomplished with doses of 4000 cGy, whereas gross deposits require more than 5400 cGy for sterilization.[11]

Outcome

Table 35-4 lists the results of studies analyzing the effects of various prognostic factors on outcome in rhabdomyosarcoma.[12–17] As expected, the presence of distant parenchymal metastases at diagnosis has an overwhelming, adverse effect on survival. Because of this, some groups have analyzed the effects of prognostic parameters in nonmetastatic subsets. Site and invasiveness of the primary tumor have also been independent predictors of outcome in some studies. Regarding site, most researchers agree that orbital, paratesticular, and vaginal primary tumors are associated with improved outcome, whereas extremity, parameningeal, and truncal or retroperitoneal tumors carry a worse prognosis. Survival is stage dependent, as mentioned earlier. This is illustrated in Figure 35-9, which graphs overall 5-year survival rates by IRS clinical group. When all cases (both high and low risk) are included, the overall survival from rhabdomyosarcoma is about 50%.

Most studies conclude that overall and disease-free survival in rhabdomyosarcoma are equivalent. This means that salvage after initial relapse is negligible, making primary therapy for rhabdomyosarcoma crucial for long-term survival. This suggests that, after risk assessment by staging, therapy should be as intense as possible to eradicate the tumor. This may mean use of myeloablative therapy with autologous or peripheral stem cell rescue for high-risk patients. The effects of this intense therapy on survival are unknown.

Future Directions

The results of myeloablative regimens with bone marrow or peripheral stem cell rescue are being analyzed. In addition, work is being done to refine the use of surgery and radiotherapy to maximize individual efficacy while diminishing morbidity. Interstitial brachytherapy and intraoperative radiotherapy are two areas of collaboration between the surgeon and radiation oncologist that are being evaluated. Biologic or immunologic therapy for rhabdomyosarcoma is not available. It has been shown, however, that retinoids have a differentiating influence on rhabdomyosarcoma cells in culture. These agents have been used clinically for certain forms of leukemia and neuroblastoma, so it is possible that they have some therapeutic effect on muscle tumors. Also, because insulin-like growth factor-2 is required for growth of rhabdomyosarcoma cells in vitro, strategies to inhibit this stimulus using the pharmacologic agent suramin may prove fruitful. These are areas of ongoing clinical and laboratory research.

NONRHABDOMYOMATOUS SOFT TISSUE SARCOMAS

Rhabdomyosarcoma is the predominant malignant soft tissue tumor encountered in infancy, childhood, and adolescence. The other soft tissue sarcomas comprise a heterogeneous group. These are listed in Table 35-5 along with incidence, present therapy, and reported overall survival rates. Primary surgical resection is more important in these tumors and may be sufficient.

Fibrosarcoma

Epidemiology

Fibrosarcomas, although rare, are the most common nonrhabdomyomatous sarcomas of infancy, childhood, and adolescence. A biphasic age incidence similar to that observed with rhabdo-

TABLE 35-4. *Significant prognostic factors for rhabdomyosarcoma in multivariate analyses*

Institution	Number of patients	Date	Independent predictors of outcome
Memorial Sloan-Kettering Cancer Center	290	1994	Age at diagnosis, invasion, metastases, histology, regional lymph nodes
Italian Cooperative Group[13]	145	1991	Site, size, alveolar histology, clinical group
International RMS Workshop[14*]	951	1991	Invasiveness, site, interaction between invasiveness and site
Cooperative Soft Tissue Sarcoma study (CWS-81)[15*]	131	1986	Site, degree of tumor regression after 7 wk of four-drug chemotherapy
International Society of Pediatric Oncology[16*]	253	1988	Site, stage, sex
International Rhabdomyosarcoma Study[17]	505	1987	Invasiveness, size, metastases, alveolar histology

* Series includes patients without distant metastases at diagnosis (M0).

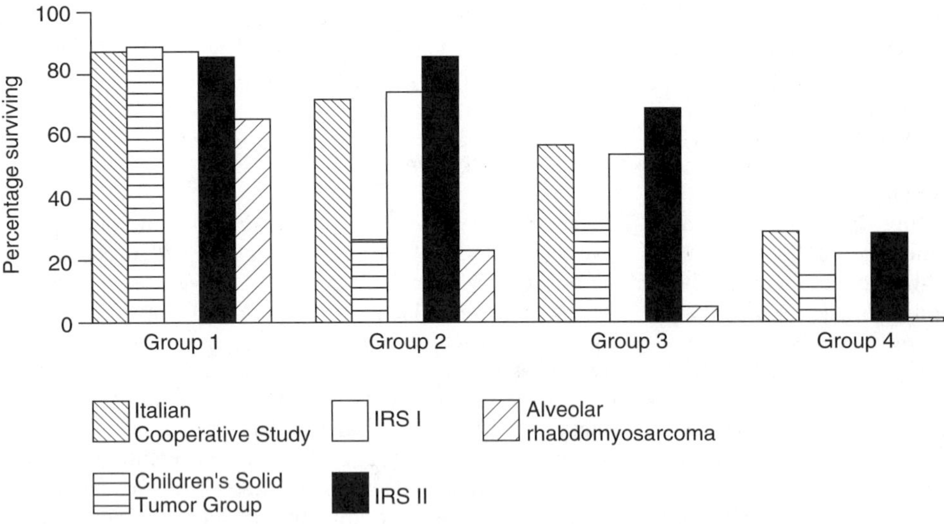

FIG. 35-9. Overall survival rates 5 years after diagnosis reported by Intergroup Rhabdomyosarcoma Study (IRS) I and II as well as two European cooperative groups. A report limited to alveolar primary tumors is included for comparison.

myosarcoma is characteristic, with one peak in children younger than 5 years of age and a second between 10 and 15 years of age. They are most frequently encountered on extremities, with 70% of congenital fibrosarcomas occurring distally. Cases are equally distributed between boys and girls. Most reports suggest that prognosis is better in younger children.[18,19]

Pathology

Fibrosarcomas are spindle cell tumors characterized by a herringbone or interweaving pattern of tumor cells, with a large amount of stromal collagen putatively arising from a fibroblastic lineage. Fibrosarcoma can be difficult, if not impossible, to distinguish histologically from desmoids or aggressive fibromatoses. For practical purposes, desmoids, fibromatoses, and low-grade fibrosarcomas can be thought of as a spectrum of similar and related neoplasms. Important characteristics of ma-

lignancy include nuclear pleomorphism, mitotic index, and basophilia. The tumor must be distinguished from undifferentiated rhabdomyosarcoma, neurofibrosarcoma, nodular fasciitis, myositis ossificans, and inflammatory pseudotumor.

Biology

Microcell-mediated transfer of human chromosome 1q into the human fibrosarcoma cell line HT1080 resulted in these cells attaining a more flattened morphology and a reduced tumorigenic potential in nude mice. A similar reduction in tumorigenicity was observed after transfer of chromosome 11 but not chromosome 2, 7, or 12. These data suggest the possibility of a fibrosarcoma tumor-suppressor activity on human chromosomes 1q and 11. This has been disputed by cDNA transfection experiments using the tumor-suppressor gene $p53$.[20]

In other experiments using HT1080 cells, increased expres-

TABLE 35-5. *Incidence, therapy, and survival rates for soft tissue sarcomas*

Sarcoma	Incidence* (M:F) White	Incidence* (M:F) Nonwhite	Primary therapy	Reported 5-y survival rate (%)
Rhabdomyosarcoma	4.8:3.9	5.5:2.8	C, S, R	50 overall
Fibrosarcoma	0.7:0.9	2.2:0.6	S, ?R	>90 (M0)
Synoviosarcoma	0.5:0.3	0.6:0	S	60–70
Peripheral primitive neuroectodermal tumor			C, S, R	20 overall
Leiomyosarcoma	0:0.4	0:0.6	S	75 stage I, 25 overall
Neurofibrosarcoma	0.5:0.6	0:1.1	S, ?C	
Alveolar soft parts sarcoma	0.2:0.2	—	S	62 at 5 y; 18 at 20 y
Liposarcoma	0.6:0.4	0.6:1.1	S, ?R	65
Hemangiopericytoma	0.4:0.4	1.1:0.6	S	30–70
Malignant fibrous histiocytoma	Very rare, most commonly secondary tumor	—	S, R(+ margin)	—
Rhabdoid tumor	1.9% of renal tumors in infancy	—	S, C	Very poor

M0, no distant metastases at diagnosis. S, surgery; C, chemotherapy; R, radiotherapy.

* Incidence per million patients 14 years old and younger, per year.

sion of mutated (one base-pair) *N-ras* was associated with maintenance of the transformed state in culture. In mouse fibrosarcoma systems, expression of *C-myc* was inversely correlated with class I major histocompatibility complex (MHC) expression, and *C-fos* expression was directly correlated.

Finally, the metastatic potential of 3-methylcholanthrene–induced fibrosarcomas in mice has been correlated with class I MHC expression. Transfection of highly metastatic T10 cells with cloned class I genes (*H-2kb, H-2Kk*) abolished metastasis formation and reduced tumorigenicity in syngeneic mice. Also, treatment of murine fibrosarcoma cells with interferon-γ causes up-regulation of class I MHC molecules.

A number of publications have dealt with the correlation of metastability and class I human leukocyte antigen expression in mouse fibrosarcoma models.[21]

Presentation and Diagnostic Evaluation

Congenital fibrosarcomas and those diagnosed in early childhood are usually located on the distal upper or lower extremity. The trunk is a secondary site. A hard, often infiltrating mass is appreciated, and there may be fixation to the skin or deep structures. Fibrosarcomas of the head and neck may be associated with esophageal or tracheal obstruction, so that dysphagia and respiratory distress or stridor are also occasionally observed. High-grade lesions may invade bony or neural structures and metastasize to lung and liver. Multifocal lesions with multiple primary tumors affecting an extremity are sometimes seen. Bone marrow metastases do not develop. Evaluation is similar to that for rhabdomyosarcoma, except that bone marrow aspiration and biopsy are not required.

Staging

The TNM schema previously outlined is used, although lymph node metastases from fibrosarcoma are uncommon unless high-grade lesions are involved. An adequate incisional or excisional biopsy, depending on the extent and invasiveness of the primary lesion, should be obtained.

Treatment

The primary treatment of fibrosarcoma is surgical resection with negative microscopic margins if this can be done without significant debilitation or deformity. Occasionally, patients present with rapidly progressive or extensive lesions. Under these circumstances, an initial trial of systemic chemotherapy can result in gratifying tumor regression. In young children (usually younger than 5 years), these tumors can be indolent and sometimes regress spontaneously. In these cases, if complete resection requires mutilating surgery, such as amputation or laryngectomy, a plan of simple observation may be best. Often, the tumor mass is dormant for years, allowing growth of the affected part and the possibility of a less debilitating or deforming resection later. This is illustrated by the magnetic reso-

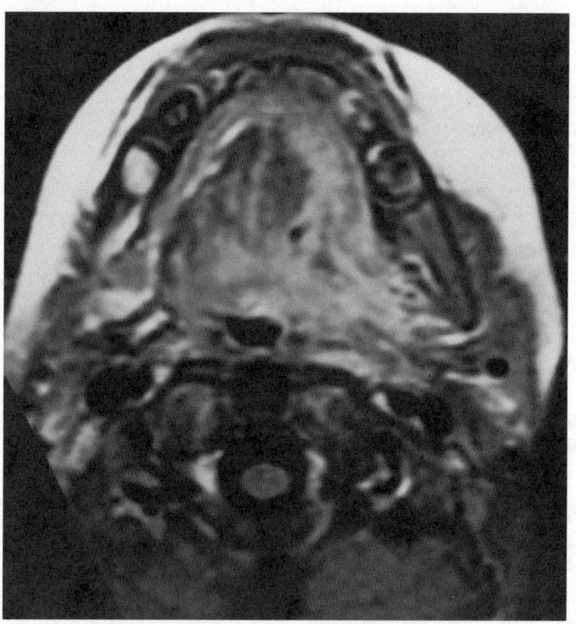

FIG. 35-10. Axial T2-weighted MR image of an infiltrating low-grade fibrosarcoma in the oropharynx of a 2-year-old child. The tumor was unresponsive to systemic chemotherapy but remained stable.

nance image in Figure 35-10, which shows an extensive, low-grade fibrosarcoma of the base of the tongue in a 2-year-old child. The pharynx and hypopharynx were involved, and resection would have resulted in devastating deformity and disability. Systemic chemotherapy had no effect. This child has been simply observed for 2 years, with stable disease. Limited experience with other, similar patients has yielded comparable results. Heroic resections should only be performed if the tumor is progressive or otherwise causing severe symptoms.

Systemic chemotherapy has no defined role in treatment of fibrosarcomas. Occasionally, high-grade lesions, especially in very young children, respond to a variety of agents. Chemotherapy may be appropriate for unresectable, symptomatic, and progressive lesions.[22] Effective chemotherapeutic agents include doxorubicin, actinomycin D, vincristine, and cyclophosphamide, in various combinations. The combination of ifosfamide and etoposide is effective in the treatment of metastatic fibrosarcoma. In summary, systemic chemotherapy can be useful for extensive or progressive lesions. A common initial regimen includes actinomycin D and vincristine because these are generally less toxic than alkylating agents.

External-beam radiotherapy was associated with a lower local recurrence rate for margin-positive, low-grade sarcomas, including fibrosarcomas, in the only prospective randomized trial to date. Interstitial brachytherapy has been shown to lower local recurrence rates with margin-positive or margin-negative, high-grade lesions. Despite this, most patients should initially be treated by wide surgical excision.

Outcome

The survival rate for low-grade, nonmetastatic fibrosarcomas occurring in infancy is over 90%. Patients with metastatic disease have a guarded prognosis and require multidisciplinary therapy.

Future Directions

Because of the association of fibrosarcoma virulence with class I MHC expression, future attempts at immune modulation of these antigens may be effective in preventing or treating metastases. Possibilities include treatment with MHC-modulating agents like tumor necrosis factor-α or interferon-γ, or gene transfection strategies aimed at increasing class I MHC expression.

Tenosynovial Sarcoma

Epidemiology

Tenosynovial sarcoma is the third most common malignant pediatric soft tissue tumor. In large combined adult and pediatric series, tenosynovial sarcomas compose about 8% of all soft tissue sarcomas. In a report of nonrhabdomyomatous soft tissue sarcomas, this histology was identified in 29% of patients.[23] The male/female ratio of distribution is 1:1.2 to 1:1.6. Most patients present in early adolescence, but there is also a small incidence spike at 5 years of age, giving the familiar bimodal age distribution observed with other sarcomas.

Pathology

Tenosynovial sarcomas arise from the synovial tissue, which is ubiquitous in the body and helps comprise tendons, joint membranes, and bursae. Synonyms include *synovioma* or *tenosynovioma, pseudoglandular synovial sarcoma, clear cell sarcoma,* and *chordoid sarcoma.* The lower extremity is the most common site of origin, with an equal distribution between the thigh, foot, and posterior knee. The shoulder and forearm are also relatively common areas of involvement. Tenosynovial sar-

comas close to bone may incite a periosteal reaction. Other possible primary sites include the abdominal wall and trunk and the head and neck, with the tongue and retropharyngeal or hypopharyngeal areas being the most common.

The most common metastatic sites are lungs and pleura. Tenosynovial sarcomas are known to relapse in lung even decades after resection of the primary tumor. Metastasis to regional lymph nodes and subcutaneous sites has been described, but this is rare. Terminal metastasis to diffuse organs is possible.

Microscopically, tenosynovial sarcoma is divided into two subtypes—monophasic and biphasic. In the biphasic form, epithelioid cells and stromal spindle cells are observed. The epithelioid component is arranged in glandlike structures resembling true epithelial cells but devoid of basement membrane (Fig. 35-11). The ratio of spindle to pseudoepithelioid components varies, but in most cases, the stromal element is much more abundant than the pseudoglandular element. The biphasic subtype has been associated with a better prognosis, but newer studies have not verified this finding. The monophasic variant is the most common and consists of sheets and parallel cords of spindle-shaped cells with little cytoplasm and cigar-shaped nuclei. Outcome is generally worse with monophasic histology.

Biology

Tenosynovial sarcomas, although composing 10% of soft tissue sarcomas, have not undergone the intense study devoted to rhabdomyosarcomas. No known genetic factors can be used as lineage or differentiation markers, and no prognostic factors beyond clinical and light microscopic parameters have been established. A specific cytogenetic abnormality, t(X;18)(p11.2; q11.2), has been characterized, and this can be helpful in differentiating this tumor from other childhood sarcomas.[24] The karyotypic profiles do not differ between monophasic and biphasic tumors.

Presentation and Diagnostic Evaluation

Most patients present with an enlarging extremity mass. Pain may be prominent if bony or neural invasion is present. Re-

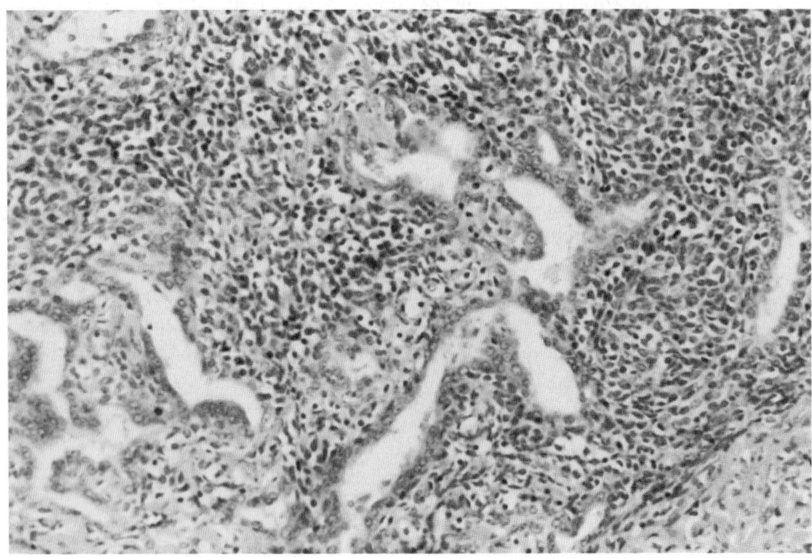

FIG. 35-11. Photomicrograph of a specimen of biphasic tendosynovial sarcoma illustrating the pseudoglandular morphology.

gional lymph node metastases occur in 3% and distant metastases (lung) in 6% of patients at diagnosis. Evaluation similar to that described for rhabdomyosarcoma is appropriate. Adequate radiographic imaging of the primary site is crucial because of the impact of complete resection on outcome.

Treatment

Chemotherapy has historically been ineffective, and the primary treatment of tenosynovial sarcoma is surgical. The goal is clear microscopic margins, and every effort should be made to accomplish this, including the use of amputation. Limb-sparing procedures are acceptable if complete resection is accomplished. Incomplete removal results in a high rate of local recurrence.

Rosen and associates[25] reported on the use of high-dose ifosfamide in the treatment of metastases from tenosynovial sarcoma. All of 13 treated patients were reported to have had an objective response. Chemotherapy is reserved for patients presenting with metastatic disease or those in whom complete resection with clear microscopic margins cannot be accomplished.

Outcome

Overall survival rates are in the range of 43% to 75%. Important prognostic indicators are large primary tumor size and high nuclear grade with extensive tumor necrosis (high grade) as well as the presence of metastases at diagnosis. Diminished survival is observed with tumors more than 10 cm in diameter at diagnosis compared with those less than 5 cm, with 5-year survival rates of 86% and 22%, respectively. Some series showed no effect of monophasic versus biphasic histology on outcome.[26,27]

Future Directions

A better understanding of tenosynovial sarcoma biology is required before new clinical therapies can be initiated. Because a unique translocation has been identified, cloning of the breakpoint region is feasible and may give biologic insight.

Peripheral Primitive Neuroectodermal Tumor

Epidemiology, Pathology, and Clinical Presentation

Peripheral primitive neuroectodermal tumors (peripheral neuroepithelioma, Askin tumor, peripheral neuroblastoma) are small, round, blue cell malignancies only recently distinguished from Ewing sarcoma by ultrastructural and immunocytochemical features. These tumors share the t(11;22)(q24;q12) translocation with Ewing sarcoma and esthesioneuroblastoma. The incidence is low, with 54 patients treated during a 20-year period reported from one major cancer center. About two thirds of patients are 19 years of age or younger at diagnosis, and 57% are male. The disease affects predominantly white patients, and 82% of tumors are localized at diagnosis. Common sites of involvement include the following locations: chest wall (33%), pelvis (22%), paraspinal area (13%), retroperitoneum (11%), limbs (9%), and abdomen (7%). Epidural extension from the primary tumor was reported in 24% of patients at diagnosis, and 18% had distant metastases.[28] None of the patients in this series with chest wall primary tumors had distant metastases at diagnosis. All primary tumors were greater than 5 cm in diameter in at least one dimension. Urinary catecholamines are *not* elevated in PNET. There is no familial or sex predilection.

Light microscopic criteria include fairly uniform, poorly differentiated round cells arranged in cords, nests, or clusters; no spindle cells with fine reticular or collagenous processes; no ganglionic or schwannian differentiation; and positive immunostaining for neuron-specific enolase. Ultrastructurally, neurosecretory-like granules and tapering ''neuritic'' cytoplasmic processes are evident.

Treatment

Outcome of PNET has been historically poor, although survival rates for Ewing sarcoma, which is a related neoplasm sharing the typical translocation (11;22), approach 60% to 65% in reported series of patients presenting without distant metastases. There may be underlying differences in fundamental biology, but the data also suggest that the multidisciplinary approach used for Ewing sarcoma, which includes multiagent chemotherapy, may have utility in the treatment of PNET. Diagnosis should be established by incisional biopsy, and the patient should be quickly started on an intensive multiagent chemotherapy regimen. A dose–response effect of cyclophosphamide has been observed. Occasionally, the tumor can be completely resected before chemotherapy, and this should be done if feasible without an extensive procedure or the requirement for complicated reconstructive techniques. In most cases, definitive resection should be deferred until after administration of several cycles of systemic treatment. In general, surgery is required because complete responses to chemotherapy do not occur. External-beam radiotherapy (4500 to 6000 cGy) can shrink but not cure macroscopic tumors. Radiation may be effective in improving local control after resection, especially if margins are microscopically positive.

Outcome and Future Directions

In patients with localized PNET at diagnosis, complete resection of all gross disease within 3 months resulted in an improved progression-free survival ($P = .0003$). The effect of myeloablative therapy with autologous bone marrow rescue is being evaluated.

Desmoplastic Small Round Cell Tumor

Epidemiology

The DSRCT is a distinctive malignant neoplasm. Eighty percent of patients present before the age of 30 years, and about half are between 5 and 20 years of age at diagnosis. There is

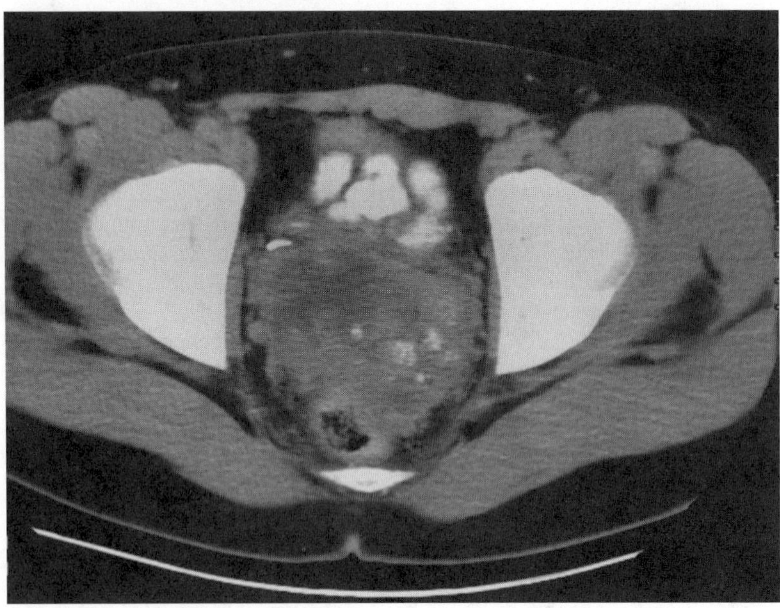

FIG. 35-12. CT scan of a large pelvic desmoplastic small round cell tumor partially encircling the rectum.

a striking male predominance (male/female ratio, 4.1:1) and most of the patients are white.[29]

Pathology

Most patients tumor localized to the abdominal cavity, often with multiple peritoneal implants. In some cases, a major tumor mass in the retroperitoneum, pelvis, omentum, or peripancreatic region is identified. Figure 35-12 is a CT scan illustrating a large pelvic DSRCT that partially encircled the rectum in a teenage boy. Multiple extrapelvic serosal implants were identified at laparotomy. There have been two reports of extraabdominal disease: one in lung and another in the anterior mediastinum. In both cases, the tumor was in contact with pleura. Initially, the tumor remains localized to the abdominal cavity, but distant metastases may occur with progression.

A striking feature is the frequent occurrence of divergent, multilineage differentiation with expression of epithelial, neural, and myogenic immunophenotypes. On light microscopy, variably sized and shaped, sharply outlined nests of tumor cells are separated by a cellular desmoplastic stroma (Fig. 35-13). Central necrosis and cystic degeneration are common. A distinctive ultrastructural feature is the presence of intermediate-sized cytoplasmic filaments.

Biology

Cytogenetic analyses of these tumors have shown a t(11; 22)(p13;q11.2-12) translocation. Band 22q12 is the site of the *EWS* (Ewing sarcoma) gene, and 11p13 contains the *WT1* (Wilms tumor gene) site. The *EWS* and *WT1* genes are fused in DSRCT. The consequences of this translocation and the

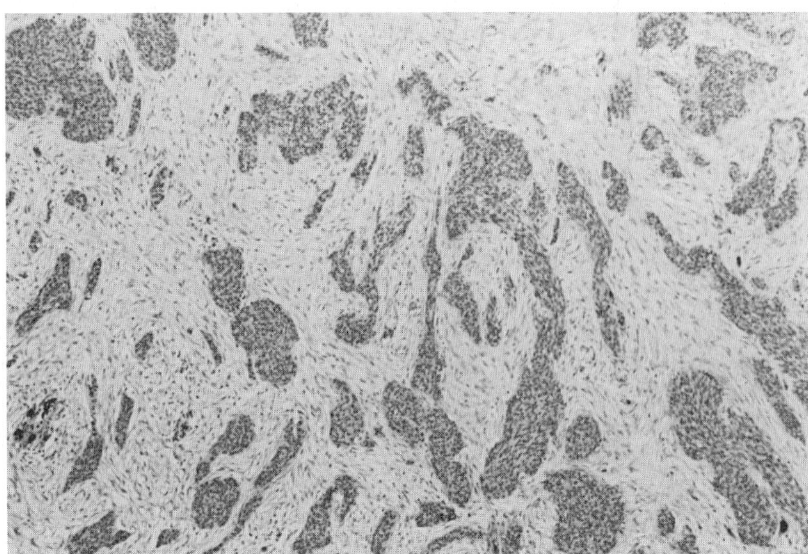

FIG. 35-13. Photomicrograph of a specimen of desmoplastic small round cell tumor. Nests of tumor cells are separated by a cellular desmoplastic stroma.

mechanism by which it might contribute to the malignant phenotype remain to be elucidated.[30]

Presentation and Diagnosis

Common presenting complaints include abdominal or back pain, abdominal distention or mass, acute abdomen, and bowel, biliary, or ureteral obstruction. Small nodules found in hernia sacs during repair have been the first indication of disease. CT of the chest and abdomen using both gastrointestinal and intravascular contrast is the most useful diagnostic procedure. Initial laparoscopic biopsy is adequate to establish the diagnosis and assess the extent of abdominal disease. Small serosal nodules not detected by imaging studies can be identified using laparoscopic magnification. A careful pelvic and serosal inspection should be carried out. Adequate tissue for immunohistochemistry, electron microscopy, and molecular biologic studies should be obtained.

Treatment

Because DSRCT is a diffuse serosal malignancy, systemic chemotherapy using a dose-intensive sarcoma regimen is the initial treatment. Serial abdominal CT scans can be followed to judge response, remembering that small mucosal implants may escape detection with these imaging studies. After 4 to 7 cycles of chemotherapy, exploratory laparotomy with resection of all gross disease is attempted. Consolidation chemotherapy and external-beam radiotherapy to the primary site are then employed. If diffuse peritoneal seeding is identified either at diagnostic or second-look laparotomy or laparoscopy, total abdominal irradiation is required. Myeloablative chemotherapy with autologous marrow reconstitution may also be necessary.

Outcome

Of 19 reported patients with adequate follow-up, only 2 were disease-free 2 and 3.5 years after diagnosis. The other 17 died from progressive disease between 6 months and 4 years after presentation.

Future Directions

Clinical trials investigating the role of dose-intensive chemotherapy with alkylators and myeloablation with autologous marrow reconstitution are ongoing. The historically dismal prognosis observed with DSRCT justifies aggressive measures in selected patients.

Neurofibrosarcoma

Epidemiology

Neurofibrosarcomas (neurogenic sarcoma, malignant schwannoma, malignant nerve sheath tumor, malignant neurilemoma) compose 5% to 10% of nonrhabdomyomatous soft tissue sarcomas in childhood. About 20% of all patients (children and adults) with neurofibrosarcoma have von Recklinghausen disease (neurofibromatosis type I [NF1]), and 5% to 16% of patients with NF1 have neurofibrosarcomas. The incidence of NF1 in children with neurofibrosarcomas is as high as 66%.[31] Neurofibrosarcomas have been reported as secondary tumors after external-beam radiotherapy.

Pathology

The most common sites in children are extremity (42%), retroperitoneum (25%), and trunk. Fewer than 10% of patients present with metastatic disease. Microscopically, the tumor resembles fibrosarcoma but is differentiated by the presence of schwannian elements. Whorllike, storiform, and tactile body-like formations are observed, and the S-100 stain is positive in about 60% of cases. Ultrastructural findings are important distinguishing criteria, and in all suspected cases, a specimen should be sent for electron microscopy. Ultrastructural findings include the presence of schwannian differentiation with cytoplasmic concavities lacking neurites. The tumors may have a melanocytic (pigmented) component. Primary neurofibrosarcoma of skin and subcutaneous tissues has also been described.

Biology

The gene for NF1 has been identified and is thought to have tumor-suppressor properties, although this remains to be proved. A somatic deletion in the *NF1* gene (chromosome 17) was observed in a neurofibrosarcoma specimen from a neurofibromatosis patient, supporting the tumor-suppressor concept. Others have reported a deletion at chromosome 22q12 in neurofibrosarcoma.[32]

Presentation and Diagnosis

Two thirds of patients have associated NF1. Aggressive diagnostic procedures, including biopsy, are warranted when enlarging extremity or truncal masses are observed. Depending on location, pain may be prominent. Radicular or sciatic pain is reported with paraspinal or retroperitoneal tumors causing sciatic pressure. Spontaneous hemothorax has been reported with chest wall primary tumors. Pelvic tumors may present as a perineal or perianal mass.

Treatment

The primary treatment of neurofibrosarcoma is wide local excision. In one series of 20 patients (14 with neurofibromatosis), there was local recurrence in 8 of 12 patients undergoing local tumor excision plus radiotherapy or chemotherapy but only in 1 of 6 patients treated with radical excision as well as chemotherapy or irradiation.[33] Unfortunately, a significant number of those patients had distant metastases despite local control. Patients with intermediate or high-grade neurofibrosarcomas should undergo radical local excision followed by chemotherapy and irradiation.

Leiomyosarcoma

Epidemiology, Pathology, and Clinical Presentation

Leiomyosarcoma accounts for 7% of soft tissue sarcomas in adults but less than 2% of childhood sarcomas. The gastrointestinal (oropharynx to anus) or genitourinary tract, retroperitoneum, lungs, pulmonary artery, vascular wall (ie, middle third of the inferior vena cava, saphenous or femoral vein), popliteal artery, sinonasal area, and peripheral soft tissue (ie, extremities) are reported sites of involvement.[34,35] Most cases are gastrointestinal in origin. The lungs are the most common site for metastases. Regional lymph node involvement occurs in 14% of gastric (perigastric nodes) and in 5% of small intestinal leiomyosarcomas at diagnosis. Dissemination to liver and brain has also been reported. Also, tumors arising from gastrointestinal structures can disseminate throughout the peritoneal cavity. Leiomyosarcoma has been reported in patients with von Recklinghausen disease and coincident with the occurrence of neurofibrosarcoma.

Pathologically, most muscle-like tumors in childhood are variants of rhabdomyosarcoma. True leiomyosarcomas are derived from smooth muscle and are often pseudoencapsulated and cytologically demonstrate uniform elongated cells with cigar-shaped nuclei. An epithelioid variant with more aggressive behavior is reported to arise in up to 40% of cases. Leiomyosarcoma can arise diffusely and can be accompanied by leiomyoblastomas, which are benign smooth muscle tumors. It is difficult to distinguish leiomyoblastoma from leiomyosarcoma. Usual criteria for determination of malignancy include cellular atypia, necrosis, gross tumor size, the presence of one mitosis per two high-power fields (one per five high-power fields in cases of epithelioid leiomyosarcoma), or the finding of lymph node, peritoneal, or parenchymal metastases. Bone marrow metastases are not reported.

The usual presentation is local pain (up to 80%) or gastrointestinal bleeding (60%). There are also reports of presentation with intussusception and perforation of a Meckel diverticulum. Some researchers state that intussusception secondary to this lesion does not occur in childhood. Congenital leiomyosarcoma associated with hydrops fetalis has also been reported. Double-contrast CT scans, gastrointestinal contrast studies, and endoscopy can aid in diagnosis.

Treatment and Outcome

The most effective treatment for leiomyosarcoma is complete surgical resection. This should be accomplished even when resection requires amputation or results in other disability because chemotherapy and radiotherapy are ineffective. There are reports of long-term survival with resection for cases with hepatic and cerebral metastases. It is recommended that, for gastrointestinal tumors, a 10-cm margin of bowel be obtained along with a wide mesenteric resection. For gastric primary tumors, omentectomy is advised as well.

Overall, about half of gastrointestinal primary tumors can be resected for cure at diagnosis. In these cases, the survival rate is 50% at 5 years, falling to 35% at 10 years. In a series of gastrointestinal leiomyosarcomas reported by Ng,[36] overall survival was stage dependent, with the following survival rates: stage I, 75%; stage II, 52%; stage III, 28%; stage IV, 7% to 12%. Important determinants of disease-free survival in multivariate analysis include tumor rupture ($P = .002$), contiguous organ invasion ($P = .02$), and high tumor grade ($P = .02$).[36] Size (more than 5 cm) and location were predictive of outcome in other analyses. Pediatric colorectal leiomyosarcomas, although extremely rare, are reported to have a relatively favorable prognosis.

Liposarcoma

Epidemiology, Pathology, and Clinical Presentation

Liposarcomas are one of the most common soft tissue sarcomas in adults but are extremely rare in childhood. The peak incidence is in the second decade of life, and there is equal distribution between the sexes. Most pediatric tumors are of the myxoid histopathologic subtype and are low grade. The most common sites are, in order, the lower extremity, upper extremity, and retroperitoneum. Head and neck and genitourinary primary tumors have also been described. The usual presenting complaint is a mass that is often painless. Metastases are uncommon, and the lung is the most common site. Lymph node metastases are possible but extremely rare, and their presence casts doubt on the diagnosis.

Treatment and Outcome

The treatment of choice is complete surgical excision with negative microscopic margins. In a pediatric and adolescent series, two patients with microscopic residual tumors were disease-free at 2 and 11.8 years from diagnosis after adjuvant use of external-beam radiotherapy.[37] This suggests that external-beam radiotherapy may be useful for control of residual microscopic disease. In the same report, all four patients with gross residual disease died from progression despite adjuvant treatment.

Alveolar Soft Parts Sarcoma

Epidemiology and Pathology

Alveolar soft parts sarcoma is a rare tumor, with only 102 cases reported during a 50-year period. Because the cell of origin is unknown, however, this malignancy has sparked considerable interest, with a large number of publications in the pathology literature. The tumor is associated with skeletal muscle and fascia. The thigh and buttocks are the most common sites (39.5%), followed by abdominal and chest walls and other sites. About one third of patients have metastases at diagnosis, which occur most frequently in lung, bone, and brain, in that order. Microscopically, the tumor consists of a mass or ball of cells with a necrotic center that mimics an alveolar space.[38] Ultrastructurally, there are well-developed Golgi apparatus and associated small granules or vesicles.

Treatment and Outcome

The primary treatment is surgical and the roles of chemotherapy and radiotherapy remain undefined. Most patients experience relapse in distant sites and die from progressive disease, although this can take 20 years or more. In one large series, the median survival was 11 years for patients free of metastases at diagnosis, falling to 3 years for those presenting with distant metastases. Because ultimate disease progression is likely, future investigation of the role of adjuvant therapy in completely resected, nonmetastatic disease is reasonable but will require a collaborative group effort.

Hemangiopericytoma

Epidemiology and Pathology

Childhood hemangiopericytomas are rare, composing about 3% of all soft tissue sarcomas in this group. In one report, 5 of 62 (8%) nonrhabdomyogenic soft tissue sarcomas were classified as hemangiopericytomas.[23] The tumor arises from pericytes, which in themselves are multipotent and can be precursors of endothelial cells, smooth muscle, rhabdomyoblasts, or fibroblasts. Hemangiopericytomas may have either a benign or malignant phenotype. Histologic criteria of malignancy include hypercellularity, high mitotic index, and intratumoral hemorrhage and necrosis. Malignant endothelial cell sarcomas (angiosarcomas or hemangiosarcomas) are not observed in childhood. Hemangiopericytomas can arise anywhere in the body, including the head and neck (especially tongue), lacrimal glands, chest wall, retroperitoneum, prostatic area and pelvis, liver, central nervous system, temporal bone, and extremities (thigh, hand). The most common sites are the extremities, followed by retroperitoneum. Metastases are hematogenous, usually affecting lungs and bone.

Infantile hemangiopericytomas have histologic characteristics that are similar to the adult form but follow a more benign course. These tumors are usually localized to the subdermal layers, although extensive local infiltration has been observed.

Treatment and Outcome

The surgical principle is to obtain complete surgical resection with negative microscopic margins. Resection alone controls disease in 30% of patients. External-beam radiotherapy has been effective against microscopic residual disease and may also cause regression of gross tumor deposits.[39] In general, external-beam radiotherapy is more effective against microscopic levels of tumor. Some tumors have also responded to systemic chemotherapy, although no standard regimen has been employed and response rates have been variable. Standard treatment for a malignant tumor includes complete local excision if possible, or excision plus external-beam radiotherapy of residual disease. This is usually followed by a course of adjuvant chemotherapy because of the observation that half of tumors recur. Agents that have been employed in the treatment of hemangiopericytoma include continuous infusion doxorubicin, ifosfamide, etoposide, cyclophosphamide, vincristine, metho-

trexate, dactinomycin, and mitoxantrone. My institution uses a combination of ifosfamide and etoposide for systemic treatment of metastatic hemangiopericytoma.

Benign tumors are curable with complete surgical resection. Most infantile hemangiopericytomas follow this course and are adequately treated by wide local excision. The reported survival rates for malignant forms of the disease range from 30% to 70%, and at least half of tumors recur.[40]

Malignant Fibrous Histiocytoma

Epidemiology and Pathology

Malignant fibrous histiocytoma is the most common soft tissue sarcoma observed in adults but composes 8% to 10% of nonrhabdomyomatous sarcomas in childhood. Cytogenetic analysis shows abnormalities at chromosomes 19p13, 11p11, 3p12, and 1q11.[41] Also, tumors exhibiting the 19p + abnormality are more likely to recur locally or systemically. Microscopically, the tumor resembles fibrosarcoma but can be differentiated by the absence of a herringbone pattern and the presence of cellular pleomorphism and a variety of cell types. Certain childhood recurrent fibrosarcomas[42] and sometimes aggressive fibromatosis can have the appearance of malignant fibrous histiocytoma. Also, this is one of the most common radiation-induced sarcomas, and several cases of orbital occurrence after radiotherapy for retinoblastoma have been reported.

The extremities (lower to upper) are most commonly affected, followed by the trunk, scalp, and viscera. Pulmonary metastases are observed most frequently, followed by brain and other sites. Systemic symptoms include fever, chills, and weight loss. Hypergammaglobulinemia and amyloidosis may occur.

Treatment and Outcome

The accepted primary treatment for malignant fibrous histiocytoma is wide surgical excision. It has been demonstrated that limb salvage is feasible with addition of external-beam irradiation of the tumor bed in certain small, extremity lesions with close margins. In a series of nine patients with malignant fibrous histiocytoma, there were six survivors 20 months to 8 years after surgical resection.[43] Two children experienced pulmonary metastases and died despite the use of adjuvant multiagent chemotherapy and radiotherapy. Poor outcome was associated with large, deep, and proximal tumors as well as with the storiform and pleomorphic histologic subtype with atypical mitoses.

In a second report, seven patients with malignant fibrous histiocytomas, ranging in age from 6 months to 11 years, were treated.[44] Anatomic sites included head and neck (3), chest wall (2), pelvis (1), and buttock (1). The two patients with chest wall tumors underwent initial complete excision, and biopsy alone was performed in the others. All patients received vincristine, dactinomycin, and cyclophosphamide, and some also were treated with doxorubicin. Patients with residual disease were also treated with 1500 to 5000 cGy of external-beam radiotherapy. The two patients with chest wall lesions who had undergone complete excision were continuously disease-free 1.4 and 9 years after initiation of treatment. Of the five with residual disease, three had a complete response to chemotherapy and radiotherapy, and two were free of recurrence at 4 and 5 years. Tumor dissemination to lungs, the central nervous system, liver, and subcutaneous tissues was observed in the remaining three children.

In summary, complete surgical excision is the key to successful treatment of childhood malignant fibrous histiocytoma. Systemic chemotherapy combined with external-beam radiotherapy can induce complete responses and long-term remissions in patients with residual disease.

Rhabdoid Tumor

Epidemiology and Pathology

Rhabdoid tumors are rare, highly malignant neoplasms usually observed in the kidney. They were once thought to be a variant of Wilms tumor. Although the cell of origin remains unknown, rhabdoid tumors are now considered sarcoma-like in their biologic behavior and are usually treated with chemotherapy protocols designed for soft tissue sarcomas. As mentioned, this neoplasm is likely to present in the kidney, but other sites, such as the brain, mediastinum, forehead, liver, and paravertebral region, have also been described. An IRS report identified 26 rhabdoid tumors among 3000 childhood sarcomas in the database.[45] Eleven of the patients were infants younger than 1 year of age. The tumors affected predominantly the soft tissues of the proximal extremities, trunk, retroperitoneum, abdomen, and pelvis.

Histologically, the growth pattern is predominantly solid or solid and trabecular. The cells are polygonal with vesicular nuclei and prominent nucleoli, and cytoplasmic intermediate filament inclusions are observed with electron microscopy or immunohistochemistry. The tumor exhibits mesenchymal as well as subtle epithelial differentiation.

Treatment and Outcome

The tumor is resistant to both chemotherapy and radiotherapy, and has a poor outcome. Most treatment regimens combine all three modalities. As noted, sarcoma chemotherapy protocols (ie, ifosfamide and etoposide) are usually used. The surgical goal is complete excision if feasible. In the report from the IRS, 19 of 26 patients died from disease within 1 to 82 months (median, 6 months), but 5 more were alive with residual disease for 2 to 13 years. Rhabdoid tumor patients had a significantly worse survival when compared with patients with rhabdomyosarcoma ($P < .001$). This poor prognosis despite multidisciplinary therapy supports the use of new, intensive protocols in the management of rhabdoid tumor. These may include marrow ablation with autologous marrow reconstitution.

Gastrointestinal Autonomic Nerve Tumors

Epidemiology and Pathology

Gastrointestinal autonomic nerve tumors are extremely rare stromal tumors of the intestinal tract or retroperitoneum, first described by Herrera in 1984. Twenty-four cases have been reported, mostly in adults but including patients as young as 10 years of age. Distinction from other gastrointestinal tumors is based on electron microscopic findings, which include neuron-like cells with long axonal cytoplasmic processes ending in bulbous synapse-like structures that contain dense-core neurosecretory granules and clear vesicles. The liver is the primary reported site of dissemination.

Treatment and Outcome

In a report of 12 cases,[46] 7 patients (58%) relapsed at the primary site or in liver, and 4 patients died. Aggressive tumor behavior was correlated with size (more than 10 cm) and mitotic count (at least 5 mitoses per high-power field).

Secondary Sarcomas

Epidemiology and Pathology

As the survival of pediatric malignancies has improved with the use of multidisciplinary therapy, the incidence of secondary malignancies has increased. These secondary tumors are associated with the use of mutagenic treatments (radiotherapy, chemotherapy) and predisposing genetic traits in the patient (ie, retinoblastoma gene or *p53* deletions or mutations). Tucker and colleagues[47] reported on 9170 cancer patients with 2-year or longer follow-up and a mean age at diagnosis of 7 years. They identified 48 cases of secondary bone cancer in this cohort when the expected incidence was calculated to be 0.4 cases. This translated into a relative risk (RR) of secondary bone cancer in these treated patients of 133 (95% confidence interval, 98 to 176). This risk was highest among retinoblastoma (RR, 999) and Ewing sarcoma (RR, 649) patients. The RR of bone sarcoma after treatment of other primary tumors was 297 for rhabdomyosarcoma, 127 for Wilms tumor, and 106 for Hodgkin disease. In all instances, the risk of a second primary tumor rose with time, with an overall cumulative risk of secondary bone malignancy of $5.5 \pm 2.1\%$ 30 years after chemotherapy and radiotherapy. Within 30 years, $14.1 \pm 4.3\%$ of retinoblastoma patients had secondary bone tumors. Other reports have documented the occurrence of secondary soft tissue sarcomas after chemotherapy or external-beam irradiation.[48] The most commonly observed secondary soft tissue sarcomas are malignant fibrous histiocytomas, followed by undifferentiated sarcomas. Secondary tumors can arise in areas adjacent rather than directly within a radiation portal.

Treatment and Outcome

The treatment of secondary soft tissue sarcomas should follow guidelines established for primary tumors of the same phenotype. For instance, wide excision should be performed for secondary malignant fibrous histiocytoma, and chemotherapy can be used for metastatic disease. Because these patients underwent previous therapy, there may be limitations to total chemotherapy (ie, doxorubicin) and radiation dose.

REFERENCES

1. Miller RW, Dalager NA. U.S. childhood cancer deaths by cell type. J Pediatr 1974;85:664.
2. Kramer S, Meadows AT, Jarrett P, et al. Incidence of childhood cancer: experience of a decade in a population-based registry. J Natl Cancer Inst 1983;70:49.
3. Stiller CA, Parkin DM. International variations in the incidence of childhood soft-tissue sarcomas. Paediatr Perinatol Epidemiol 1994;8:107.
4. La Quaglia MP. Extremity rhabdomyosarcoma: biological principles, staging, and treatment. Semin Surg Oncol 1993;9:510.
5. Scrable H, Witte D, Shimada H, et al. Molecular differential pathology of rhabdomyosarcoma. Genes Chromosom Cancer 1989;1:23.
6. Dias P, Parham DM, Shapiro DN, et al. Myogenic regulatory protein (MyoD1) expression in childhood solid tumors: diagnostic utility in rhabdomyosarcoma. Am J Pathol 1990;137:1283.
7. Buckingham M. Molecular biology of muscle development (meeting review). Cell 1994;78:15.
8. Davis RL, Weintrub H, Lassar AB. Expression of a single transfected cDNA converts fibroblasts to myoblasts. Cell 1987;51:987.
9. Wright WE, Sassoon DA, Lin VK. Myogenin, a factor regulating myogenesis has a domain homologous to MyoD. Cell 1989;56:606.
10. Harmer MH, ed. TNM classification of pediatric tumors. Geneva, International Union Against Cancer, 1982:23.
11. Mandell L, Ghavimi F, Peretz T, et al. Radiocurability of microscopic disease in childhood rhabdomyosarcoma with radiation doses less than 4000 cGy. J Clin Oncol 1990;8:1536.
12. La Quaglia MP, Heller G, Ghavimi F, et al. The effect of age at diagnosis on outcome in rhabdomyosarcoma. Cancer 1994;73:109.
13. Carli M, Guglielmi M, Sotti G, et al. Prognostic factors in children with rhabdomyosarcoma (RMS), results of the Italian cooperative study RMS-79. (Meeting abstract) Med Pediatr Oncol 1991;19:398.
14. Rodary C, Gehan EA, Flamant F, et al. Prognostic factors in 951 children with non-metastatic rhabdomyosarcoma: a report from the international rhabdomyosarcoma workshop. Med Pediatr Oncol 1991;19:89.
15. Suder J, Stienen U, Kaatsch P, et al. Analysis of prognostic factors in rhabdomyosarcoma: preliminary univariate and multivariate results of the soft tissue sarcoma study (CWS-81). Klin Padiatr 1986;198:218.
16. Rodary C, Rey A, Rezvani A, et al. Prognostic factors in rhabdomyosarcomas in childhood: study carried out with 253 children registered by the International Society of Pediatric Oncology. Bull Cancer 1988;75:213.
17. Lawrence W Jr, Gehan EA, Hays DM, et al. Prognostic significance of staging factors of the UICC staging system in childhood rhabdomyosarcoma: a report from the Intergroup Rhabdomyosarcoma Study (IRS-II). J Clin Oncol 1987;5:46.
18. Exelby PR, Knapper WH, Huvos AG, et al. Soft tissue fibrosarcoma in children. J Pediatr Surg 1973;8:415.
19. Soule EH, Pritchard DJ. Fibrosarcoma of infants and children: a review of 110 cases. Cancer 1977;40:1711.
20. Anderson MJ, Casey G, Fasching CL, et al. Evidence that wild-type TP53, and not genes on either chromosome 1 or 11, controls the tumorigenic phenotype of the human fibrosarcoma HT1080. Genes Chromosom Cancer 1994;9:266.
21. Shiloni E, Karp SE, Custer MC, et al. Retroviral transduction of interferon-gamma cDNA into a nonimmunogenic murine fibrosarcoma: generation of T cells in draining lymph nodes capable of treating established parental metastatic tumor. Cancer Immunol Immunother 1993;37:286.
22. Ninane J, Gosseye S, Pantion E, et al. Congenital fibrosarcoma. Cancer 1986;58:1400.
23. Horowitz ME, Pratt CB, Webber BL, et al. Therapy of childhood soft tissue sarcomas other than rhabdomyosarcoma: a review of 62 cases treated at a single institution. J Clin Oncol 1986;4:559.
24. Knight JC, Reeves BR, Kearney L, et al. Localization of the synovial sarcoma t(X;)(p11.2•1.2) breakpoint by fluorescence in situ hybridization. Hum Mol Genet 1992;1:633.
25. Rosen G, Forscher C, Lowenbraun S, et al. Synovial sarcoma: uniform response of metastases to high dose ifosfamide. Cancer 1994;73:2506.
26. Brodsky JT, Burt ME, Hajdu SI, et al. Tendosynovial sarcoma: clinicopathologic features, treatment and prognosis. Cancer 1992;70:484.
27. Oda Y, Hashimoto H, Tsuneyoshi M, et al. Survival in synovial sarcoma: a multivariate study of prognostic factors with special emphasis on the comparison between early death and long-term survival. Am J Pathol 1993;17:35.
28. Kushner BH, Hajdu SI, Gulati SC, et al. Extracranial primitive neuroectodermal tumor. Cancer 1991;67:1825.
29. Gerald WL, Rosai J. Desmoplastic small round cell tumor with multiphenotypic differentiation. Zentrabl Pathol 1993;139:141.
30. Ladanyi M, Gerald W. Fusion of the EWS and WT1 genes in the desmoplastic small round cell tumor. Cancer Res 1994;54:2837.
31. Riccardi VM, Powell PP. Neurofibrosarcoma as a complication of von Recklinghausen neurofibromatosis. Neurofibromatosis 1989;2:152.
32. Legius E, Marchuk DA, Collins FS, et al. Somatic deletion of the neurofibromatosis type 1 gene in a neurofibrosarcoma supports a tumour suppressor gene hypothesis. Nat Genet 1993;3:122.
33. Storm FK, Eilber FR, Mirra J, et al. Neurofibrosarcoma. Cancer 1980;45:126.
34. Angerpointer TA, Weitz H, Haas RJ. Intestinal leiomyosarcoma in childhood: case report and review of the literature. J Pediatr Surg 1981;16:491.
35. Lack EE. Leiomyosarcoma in children: a clinicopathologic study of 10 cases. Pediatr Pathol 1986;6:181.
36. Ng EH, Pollock RE, Munsell MF, et al. Prognostic factors influencing survival in gastrointestinal leiomyosarcomas: Implications for surgical management and staging. Ann Surg 1992;215:68.
37. La Quaglia MP, Spiro SA, Ghavimi F, et al. Liposarcoma in patients younger than or equal to 22 years of age. Cancer 1993;72:3114.
38. Lieberman PH, Brennan MF, Kimmel M, et al. Alveolar soft-part sarcoma: a clinico-pathologic study of half a century. Cancer 1989;63:1.
39. Velasco A, Mora X, Baeza R, et al. Hemangiopericytoma: report of 4 cases. Rev Med Chil 1993;121:1305.
40. Auguste LJ, Razak MJ, Sako K. Hemangiopericytoma. J Clin Oncol 1982;20:260.
41. Sreekantaiah C, Rao UN, Karakousis CP, et al. Cytogenetic findings in a malignant fibrous histiocytoma of the gallbladder. Cancer Genet Cytogenet 1992;59:30.
42. Salloum E, Caillaud JM, Flamant F, et al. Poor prognosis infantile fibrosarcoma with pathologic features of malignant fibrous histiocytoma after local recurrence. Med Pediatr Oncol 1990;18:295.
43. Cole CH, Magee JF, Gianoulis M, et al. Malignant fibrous histiocytoma in childhood. Cancer 1993;71:4077.
44. Raney RB Jr, Allen A, O'Neill J, et al. Malignant fibrous histiocytoma of soft tissue in childhood. Cancer 1986;57:2198.
45. Kodet R, Newton WA Jr, Sachs N, et al. Rhabdoid tumors of soft tissues: a clinicopathologic study of 26 cases enrolled on the Intergroup Rhabdomyosarcoma Study. Hum Pathol 1991;22:674.
46. Lauwers GY, Erlandson RA, Casper ES, et al. Gastrointestinal autonomic nerve tumors: a clinicopathological, immunohistochemical, and ultrastructural study of 12 cases. Am J Pathol 1993;17:887.
47. Tucker MA, D'Angio GJ, Boice JD, et al. Bone sarcomas linked to radiotherapy and chemotherapy in children. N Engl J Med 1987;317:588.
48. Kushner BH, Zauber A, Tan CTC. Second malignancies after childhood Hodgkin's disease. Cancer 1988;62:1364.

Surgery of Infants and Children: Scientific Principles and Practice, edited by
Keith T. Oldham, Paul M. Colombani, and Robert P. Foglia.
Lippincott–Raven Publishers, Philadelphia, © 1997.

CHAPTER 36

Hepatoblastoma and Hepatocellular Carcinoma

Edward P. Tagge and Derya U. Tagge

Tumors of the pediatric liver, although relatively rare, pose a considerable diagnostic and therapeutic challenge. About 60% of hepatic tumors in children are malignant, representing 15% of all pediatric solid tumors. The epithelial tumors hepatoblastoma and hepatocellular carcinoma (HCC) make up most of these malignant tumors. Total surgical excision offers the only realistic chance for a positive outcome, but unfortunately, less than half of tumors are resectable at diagnosis. However, new preoperative chemotherapeutic regimens have increased the number of liver tumors that ultimately can be resected. In addition, total hepatectomy with orthotopic liver transplantation may improve the survival rates of patients with tumors not amenable to extirpation by partial hepatectomy.

EPIDEMIOLOGY

Overall, hepatic malignancies are the 10th most frequent childhood tumor, representing between 0.5% and 2% of all pediatric tumors. The annual incidence of malignant hepatic tumors in the United States is 1.6 per million children, with hepatoblastoma accounting for 0.9 and HCC for 0.7. Both hepatoblastoma and HCC demonstrate a male predominance in North America, with ratios of 2:1 and 1.4:1, respectively. The median age at diagnosis of hepatoblastoma is 1 year, with most patients diagnosed within the first 18 months of life. On the other hand, HCC has a median age of diagnosis of 12 years, with a much wider age range.

Hepatoblastoma is the third most common intraabdominal malignant tumor in childhood, after neuroblastoma and Wilms tumor. Congenital abnormalities appear to be relatively common in children with hepatoblastoma. Beckwith-Wiedemann syndrome (BWS) is an autosomal dominant syndrome consisting of macrosomia, macroglossia, abdominal wall defects, visceromegaly, neonatal hypoglycemia, and occasional hemihypertrophy. BWS is associated with an elevated risk of embryonal neoplasia, particularly hepatoblastoma and Wilms tumor. Occasionally,deletions on the short arm of chromosome 11 are noted in patients with BWS and hepatoblastoma. This loss of somatic heterozygosity has been implicated as a possible patho-

genic mechanism. Although the true incidence of hepatoblastoma in BWS patients is difficult to determine, one study noted that in about 250 patients with complete and incomplete forms of BWS, 4 patients had hepatoblastoma (1.6%), a significantly higher proportion than the 1:100,000 incidence of hepatoblastoma in the general population.

Other reported congenital defects in children with hepatoblastoma include both hemihypertrophy and Wilms tumor without BWS, precocious puberty, polycystic disease of the kidneys, Meckel diverticulum, urogenital system anomalies, and congenital absence of the adrenal gland.

A significantly increased frequency of hepatoblastoma has been noted in kindreds harboring familial adenomatous polyposis (FAP), a dominantly inherited disorder predisposing to multiple colonic adenomas and early-onset carcinomas. This association was first reported in 1983, when five children with hepatoblastoma were noted to have a family history of polyposis coli. Based on numerous case reports plus the results of an international survey of FAP registries, 2 of 470 (0.42%) children born to 241 FAP patients had hepatoblastoma. Although this figure is significantly higher than the general 1:100,000 incidence, an empiric risk of less than 1% for hepatoblastoma can be cited to people with FAP, for genetic counseling purposes. One British study, however, estimated that 1 in 20 patients with hepatoblastoma is likely to be associated with FAP and that survivors are at increased risk of developing adenomatous polyps at a very young age. Supporting this statement was a series examining 11 hepatoblastoma survivors, in which adenomatous colonic lesions were sought in 7 and detected in 6 patients between 7 and 25 years of age.

Childhood HCC in the United States is associated with cirrhosis in 5% of cases, significantly less than its adult counterpart. Significant geographic variation does exist, however, and large series of childhood HCC from the Far East are closely related to both cirrhosis and hepatitis B virus (HBV) surface antigen positivity. This association between chronic HBV infection and HCC suggests an etiologic mechanism, but several epidemiologic observations (relatively low life-time risk, non–HBV-associated tumors, anecdotal familial clustering) indicate that additional factors are necessary to explain observed patterns of HCC incidence. For instance, 47 HCC tumors in an Alaskan population were analyzed, and neither chronic HBV infection nor inherited susceptibility alone were sufficient to explain the HCC distribution in those Alaskan families.

Children with the chronic form of hereditary tryrosinemia who survive beyond 2 years of age have a strikingly high incidence of HCC, 16 of 43 patients in one series. Biliary cirrhosis secondary to extrahepatic biliary atresia has also been associated with HCC in patients who survive longer than 3 years, as has biliary cirrhosis secondary to prolonged parenteral nutrition. Other associated conditions include glycogen storage disease, cystinosis (de Toni–Fanconi syndrome) and Wilson disease.

ANATOMY

The major contribution of 20th century liver anatomists was the demonstration that the liver is a segmental organ, based on the distribution of the bile duct, portal vein, and hepatic artery branches to the liver substance. This segmentation is not apparent on external examination of the liver. The division between right and left lobes of the liver lies along a plane that runs from the gallbladder fossa inferiorly to the suprahepatic inferior vena cava superiorly. This plane is not avascular, however, because it contains the middle hepatic vein. Each major lobe is divided into two segments on the basis of the second-order branching of the portal vein, hepatic artery, and bile ducts. The right lobe contains an anterior and posterior segment divided by a plane in which the orientation is nearly coronal. The left lobe is divided into medial and lateral segments along the plane of the ligamentum venosum and ligamentum teres.

This division of the liver does not take into account the caudate lobe, which lies on the posterior aspect of the liver along the left side of the retrohepatic inferior vena cava. The caudate lobe is conveniently thought of as an entity separate from the four major segments; it receives its portal vein, hepatic artery, and bile duct supply directly from both the right and left main branches of those structures. The hepatic venous drainage of the caudate lobe empties directly into the retrohepatic cava through short, independent hepatic veins.

Knowledge of hepatic anatomy is essential to extirpate hepatic tumors safely, as this can be a significant technical challenge. Up to three of these four hepatic segments can routinely be resected, because of the liver's remarkable ability to regenerate. As much as 85% of the liver can be removed, with subsequent complete regeneration of liver cell mass within 1 to 3 months after surgery. Mortality from hepatic lobectomy historically has ranged from 10% to 25%, although modern surgical techniques and careful preoperative and postoperative management can substantially reduce those percentages.

PATHOLOGY

Until the mid-1960s, it was generally assumed that all epithelial hepatic tumors in the pediatric age range were morphologically and behaviorally similar. In 1967, Ishak and Glunz[1] not only stressed the histologic differences of hepatoblastoma and HCC, but for the first time noted an overall better survival for hepatoblastoma as well as the potential importance of histologic subtypes of these tumors.

Hepatoblastoma

Hepatoblastoma is one of the solid embryonic neoplasms of childhood, and thus many of its histologic manifestations recapitulate the developmental phases of the liver. The gross appearance of a hepatoblastoma is that of a lobulated, bulging, tan mass, often punctuated by areas of necrosis and surrounded by a pseudocapsule. Hepatoblastoma is most often unifocal, with the right lobe affected 60% to 70% of the time. Microscopic vascular spread, however, may be found beyond an apparently encapsulated tumor, making it important to review the gross specimen with the pathologist so that blocks for microscopic examination are obtained from resection margins.

Two basic histologic patterns of hepatoblastoma have been delineated by Ishak and Glunz[1]: pure epithelial and mixed epithelial–mesenchymal. The pure epithelial type contains either fetal or embryonal cells, or admixtures of the two (Fig. 36-1). Fetal cells are slightly smaller than normal hepatocytes and have a relatively low nucleocytoplasmic ratio. The cells are extremely uniform, mitotic activity is sparse, and cords of tumor cells arranged in two-cell plates can produce canalicular bile. These cells correspond in size and configuration to fetal hepatocytes, and extramedullary hematopoiesis is often prominent. Embryonal cells have a more primitive histologic appearance than the fetal pattern, with marked cellular atypia, mitotic activity, and necrosis.

When a neoplastic mesenchymal component accompanies the epithelial elements, the tumor is characterized as a mixed hepatoblastoma. Osteoid is the most common expression of mesenchymal differentiation in the hepatoblastoma (Fig. 36-2). The mesenchymal elements generally lack overtly malignant features and are found in hepatoblastomas that are predominantly fetal and embryonal. Other differentiated tissues that can occur as minor components of a hepatoblastoma include squamous epithelium (Fig. 36-3), cartilage, skeletal muscle, renal tubules, and ganglion cells. About 30% of hepatoblastomas are mixed tumors.

Attempts have been made to correlate predominant histologic patterns with outlook, analogous to the clinicopathologic results

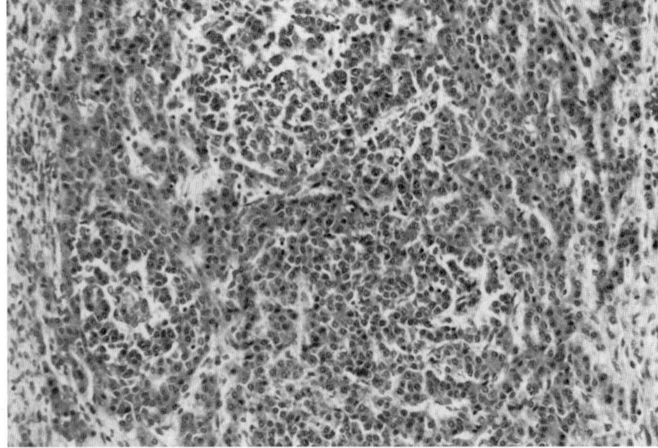

FIG. 36-1. Pure epithelial hepatoblastoma, with mixture of embryonal and fetal tumor cells. (×100) (Photomicrograph courtesy of Dr. Eduardo J. Yunis, Director of Pathology, Children's Hospital of Pittsburgh)

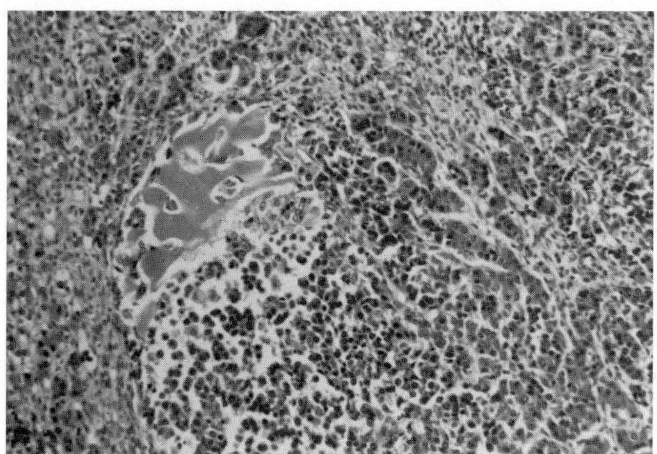

FIG. 36-2. Osteoid deposits in a mixed hepatoblastoma form circumscribed globular masses surrounded by fetal and embryonal hepatocytes. (×200) (Photomicrograph courtesy of Dr. Eduardo J. Yunis, Director of Pathology, Children's Hospital of Pittsburgh)

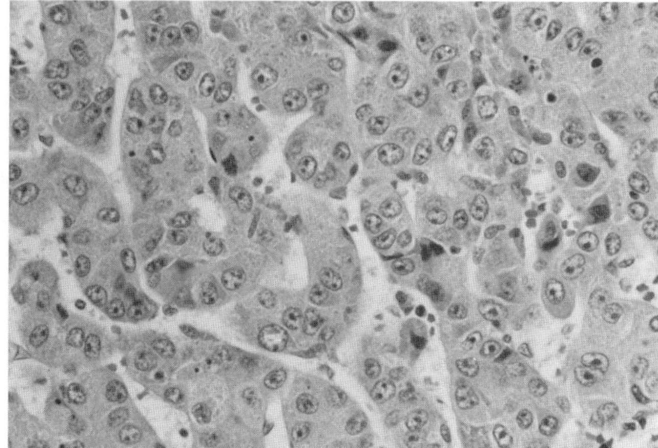

FIG. 36-4. Hepatocellular carcinoma, characterized by relatively large cells with a high nucleocytoplasmic ratio, mild nuclear pleomorphism, and increased nucleolar prominence. (×450) (Photomicrograph courtesy of Dr. Eduardo J. Yunis, Director of Pathology, Children's Hospital of Pittsburgh)

of the National Wilms' Tumor Study. The epithelial component of hepatoblastoma appears to be the most important histologic determinant of prognosis. In a large Pediatric Oncology Group (POG) and Children's Cancer Study Group (CCSG) intergroup study of 168 patients with totally resected hepatoblastomas, pure fetal histology bestowed a survival advantage compared with all other histologies (24-month survival rate of 92% versus 57%; $P = .02$). In that same study, however, fetal histology was not predictive in more advanced disease. Other data suggest that the malignant potential of a hepatoblastoma is more dependent on the presence of any embryonal or undifferentiated cells than on the predominance of either epithelial cell type.

Hepatoblastoma appears to have other distinctive morphologic patterns. A macrotrabecular, or differentiating, hepatoblastoma resembling HCC has been described. Kasai and Watanabe[2] described tumors that contain sheets of small, undif-

ferentiated cells that resemble neuroblastoma cells. They called these tumors *anaplastic hepatoblastomas,* although the tumor cells may be fetal, embryonal, or indistinguishable from adult hepatocarcinoma. Some have described a worse prognosis for this group.

Hepatocellular Carcinoma

The gross and microscopic features of HCC in childhood are similar to those of its adult counterpart, except in the lack of underlying cirrhosis in most pediatric patients. HCC may be either nodular or diffuse, and both major lobes of the liver are involved in at least 50% to 80% of cases, making resection and thus cure rates low. Associated severe fibrosis or cirrhosis from an underlying chronic liver disease is more often encountered

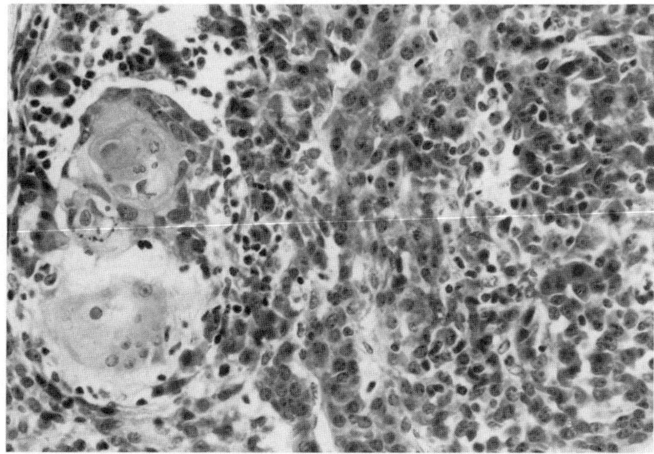

FIG. 36-3. Mixed hepatoblastoma with an island of squamous epithelium. (×450) (Photomicrograph courtesy of Dr. Eduardo J. Yunis, Director of Pathology, Children's Hospital of Pittsburgh)

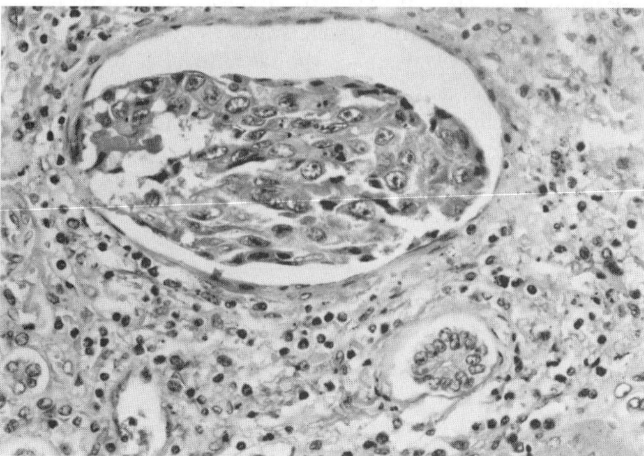

FIG. 36-5. Tumor thrombus graphically demonstrating vascular invasion in hepatocellular carcinoma. (×200) (Photomicrograph courtesy of Dr. Eduardo J. Yunis, Director of Pathology, Children's Hospital of Pittsburgh)

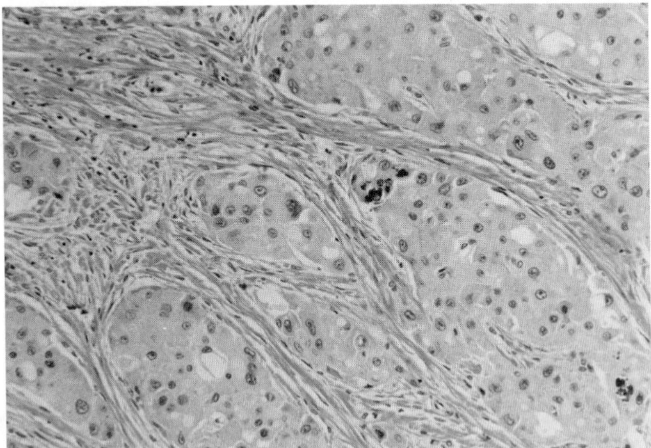

FIG. 36-6. Fibrolamellar carcinoma characterized by abundant cytoplasm and prominent fibrous stroma. Note the nuclear pseudoinclusions. ($\times$200) (Photomicrograph courtesy of Dr. Eduardo J. Yunis, Director of Pathology, Children's Hospital of Pittsburgh)

than in children with hepatoblastoma, and is secondary to a variety of diseases: tyrosinemia, α_1-antitrypsin deficiency, familial cholestatic cirrhosis, parenteral hyperalimentation, or extrahepatic biliary atresia. HCC is distinguished from hepatoblastoma microscopically by the presence of cells larger than normal hepatocytes, broad trabeculae, considerable nuclear pleomorphism, nucleolar prominence, tumor giant cells, and the absence of hematopoiesis (Fig. 36-4). Cytologic atypia, mitotic activity, and vascular invasion clearly identify the cords and nests of cells as malignant; tumor thrombi are noted frequently (Fig. 36-5).

A distinctive variant of HCC occurs in the noncirrhotic livers of older children and young adults. This tumor, termed *fibrolamellar carcinoma,* potentially has a more favorable prognosis than does the usual HCC. It is characterized by plump, deeply eosinophilic hepatocytes encompassed by an abundant fibrous stoma composed of thin parallel fibrous bands that separate the epithelial cells into trabeculae or large nodules (Fig. 36-6). Fibroblasts separate hepatocytes from the encompassing collagen. The abundant fibrous tissue, which is unusual for HCC, may impart a gross appearance similar to focal nodular hyperplasia. The tumor is often very large at presentation. It frequently occurs in the left lobe of the liver, and is not associated with hepatitis B infection or cirrhosis. α-Fetoprotein levels are not usually elevated, tumors are suitable for resection in up to half of cases, and there is some evidence that this variant may have a better prognosis.

GENETICS AND BIOLOGY

Hepatoblastoma

Beckwith-Wiedemann Syndrome

More than 10% of children with the BWS develop hepatoblastoma, rhabdomyosarcoma, or Wilms tumor. Koufos and colleagues[3] reported on two patients with hepatoblastoma who

were constitutionally heterozygous (ie, displayed both parental alleles in their peripheral leukocytes) at two specific loci on chromosome 11. In both of these patients, one of the alleles at each of these loci was missing in the primary hepatoblastoma tissue. This tumor-specific loss of heterozygosity (LOH) is the sine qua non of a tumor-suppressor gene, suggesting that these tumors were caused by the expression of a mutant allele on chromosome 11 that was unmasked by the elimination of the balancing wild-type allele at that same locus. Koufos and colleagues[3] hypothesized that the normal gene at that locus was responsible for the orderly progression of normal differentiation, suggesting that human embryonal tumors reflect abnormalities in genes important to normal organogenesis. This hypothesis linked two previously disparate observations: the relatively frequent association between rare tumors and congenital malformation syndromes, and the specific loss of constitutional heterozygosity in embryonal cancers. Interestingly, no specific cytogenetic finding has been identified in BWS patients at risk for the development of hepatoblastoma, suggesting that this LOH is below the resolution of normal karyotyping. Cytogenetic abnormalities have been inconsistently reported, including triplication of the 11p15 region and a constitutional interstitial deletion of 11p11 with pericentric inversion of chromosome 9.

Familial Adenomatous Polyposis

Familial adenomatous polyposis has been shown to result from germline mutations in the adenomatous polyposis coli (APC) tumor-suppressor gene, which maps to chromosome 5q. Although the exact role of the APC gene is unknown, immunoprecipitation experiments have linked it to α- and β-catenin, which are proteins that bind to the cell adhesion molecule E-cadherin. This suggests that the APC gene is involved in cell adhesion, although it is unknown how cell adhesion abnormalities and hepatic tumor initiation are related.

DNA Content

Analyzing cellular DNA content using flow cytometry allows correlation with a tumor's malignant potential. Of 29 cases of hepatoblastoma studied with flow cytometry, 23 (79.9%) tumors were diploid, and 6 (20.7%) were aneuploid (hyperploid). Diploid tumors were almost equally distributed among all clinical stages, whereas aneuploid tumors tended to occur in higher stages. Children with diploid tumors showed higher survival rates than those with aneuploid tumors (71% versus 31% at 6 years). Although these differences were not statistically significant, the authors thought that larger numbers of patients would probably yield statistically significant results, making DNA content analysis potentially an important part of therapy planning.

Hepatocellular Carcinoma

The molecular puzzle of HCC pathogenesis has not been solved, but many potential pieces have been identified; HBV, p53 tumor-suppressor gene, aflatoxin B_1 (AFB), and human papillomavirus are among the most prominent considerations.

Hepatitis Virus

Model systems of hepatocarcinogenesis have demonstrated that oncogenesis requires both mitotic activation and a transformation event. It has been speculated that HBV may promote mitotic activation as a result of hepatocytic necrosis and may also initiate DNA alterations as a direct result of viral disruption of the host genome by integration or excision. Because the integration of viral regulatory sequences near cellular genes crucial for growth and differentiation rarely occurs, insertional mutagenesis does not appear to be an important mechanism of hepatocyte transformation. On the other hand, evidence suggests that transcriptional transactivation of cellular protooncogenes by viral products could be a more important process.

The causal relation of HBV infection with childhood HCC has been less certain than that in adult HCC. Certain children with HCC, for instance those in Africa and Asia, appear to share the same strong association with HBV as is seen in adults. Of particular epidemiologic interest in these populations is the possibility of vertical HBV transmission. A report from Malaysia in 1990 noted six cases of childhood HCC; hepatitis B surface antigen (HBsAg) seropositivity was confirmed in five cases, and tissue HBsAg was shown in four.[4] An associated maternal HBsAg seropositivity was shown in two of the seropositive children, including the mother of the youngest seropositive patient who developed HCC at 7 years of age. If one ascribed vertical (perinatal) HBV transmission as the causative factor in these two cases, then the maximum incubation period between the time of infection and the development of malignancy in the 7 year old was at most 8 years. This contrasts markedly to the 20-year incubation period that is a minimum before the development of adult HCC. However, if vertical HBV transmission is determined to be an important cause of HCC in these populations, then prevention through vaccination programs could significantly reduce the prevalence of this lethal malignancy.

The relatively low life-time risk associated with chronic HBV infection suggests that infection alone is not sufficient for HCC development. Additional factors have been implicated that may act either independently or as cofactors; these are (1) genetic susceptibility, and (2) environmental variables, such as AFB, drinking water source, alcohol use, and tobacco exposure. Variation in risk may also be attributable to coinfection with other hepatitis viruses. Accumulating data on hepatitis C virus (HCV) infection suggests that it is a significant risk factor for HCC. In Japan, more than 70% of patients with HCC are positive for HCV antibody, and HCV RNA has been identified in tumor tissue by reverse transcription polymerase chain reaction in more than half of 20 HCC cases.[5]

Tumor-Suppressor Gene

Evidence also exists that a tumor-suppressor gene may be responsible for HCC oncogenesis. LOH has been frequently shown for many chromosomes in HCC, including 1p, 4q, 5q, 10q, 11p, 13q, 16q, and 17p. A group from Kyoto University in Japan examined 56 cases of human HCC for LOH at 13 loci on 5 chromosomes.[6] Allelic losses were most commonly detected on chromosomes 13q (47%), 16q (40%), and 17p (64%), whereas losses on chromosome 4p and 11p were observed in less than 22% of cases. The common region of allelic loss on chromosome 13q was mapped to the region that includes the retinoblastoma gene, and the 17p loss was mapped to the p53 tumor-suppressor gene site. Chromosomal losses were more frequently associated with portal vein thrombosis, intrahepatic metastasis, increased tumor size, a poorly differentiated phenotype, and advanced clinical stage. Cumulative losses of 13q, 16q, and 17p were significantly more common in clinical stage IV patients or histologically poorly differentiated tumors. If these data are reproducible, the finding of LOH may help predict prognosis and determine therapy in the future.

Aflatoxin B_1

Molecular genetic studies have speculated that a causal link exists between AFB exposure in HCC and the p53 tumor-suppressor gene.[7] Studies in high AFB exposure areas have found that half of HCC tumors have an identical p53 mutation, involving an AGG to AGT mutation at codon 249, resulting in an arginine to serine amino acid substitution. In a study from Fox Chase Cancer Center,[8] however, only 2 of 107 (1.9%) tumors demonstrated this codon 249 mutation. To further investigate the relation of AFB and p53 mutations in hepatocarcinogenesis, normal liver samples from the United States, Thailand, and Qidong, China (where AFB exposures are negligible, low, and high, respectively) were examined. The frequency of the AGG to AGT mutation at codon 249 paralleled the level of AFB exposure, supporting the hypothesis that this fungal toxin has a causative role in hepatocarcinogenesis.

To further elucidate the relation between p53 mutations, high AFB exposure, and HBV infection in HCC, another study examined 43 HCC specimens, 23 from Qidong, China, and 10 each from the National Institutes of Health and the Kuakini Medical Center in Hawaii.[9] Mutant p53 protein was detected in 61% of HCC specimens from China, 30% from the National Institutes of Health samples, and 60% of the samples from Hawaii. A statistically significant association between detection of mutant p53 protein and detection of HBsAg in hepatocytes of the adjacent nontumorous liver tissues was observed in patients from China and the United States considered together ($P \leq .01$). These results suggested two possible mechanisms by which HBV could be involved in this mutation. Chronic HBV infection when established by vertical transmission could cause a perinatal mutation in one p53 allele, with the other p53 allele undergoing mutation later in life. It is also possible that HBV could cause a dominant negative mutation in a single allele of the p53 gene in some patients, resulting in the loss of tumor suppression.

These observed differences in p53 mutations suggests that HCC has varied underlying genetic causes in different regions of the world. Alternatively, p53 mutations observed may not represent primary oncogenic effects, but instead may reflect genetic changes due to tumor progression facilitated by AFB exposure.

Miscellaneous Pathogenetic Factors

DNA analysis by flow cytometry has not been particularly helpful in HCC. In one series of 50 patients from China, 78% of tumors were found to be aneuploid, and 22% were diploid. No cytometric correlation between DNA distribution and HBsAg positivity, the presence of liver cirrhosis, or tumor size was seen. In addition, no correlation between the DNA pattern and survival rates in patients who underwent hepatic resection was identified.

Expression of the CD15 antigen, one of the cell adhesion molecules, was found in 29% of 56 HCC tumors studied, while nonmalignant hepatocytes did not express CD15. Patients with CD15-positive HCC had histologic intrahepatic metastasis more often than did those with CD15-negative HCC ($P < .02$). The 3-year survival rate of patients with CD15-negative HCC (36%) was better than that of patients with CD15-positive HCC (13%), although the difference was not statistically significant. The authors hypothesized that CD15-positive tumor cells would more easily reattach to sinusoidal endothelial cells, thus establishing intrahepatic metastases and leading to a worse outcome. In another study, the *nm23* gene, a tumor suppressor gene related to metastatic potential, was investigated in 25 HCC tumors. An similar relation between *nm23*-H1 expression and intrahepatic metastases of HCC was seen.

Proliferating cell nuclear antigen (PCNA) is a nuclear protein synthesized in G_1–S phase of the cell cycle and therefore related to cell proliferative activity. Seventy-two HCC patients were studied for PCNA activity, and this was found to be significantly and positively associated with a positive margin ($P = .003$), direct liver invasion by tumor ($P = .02$), and venous penetration ($P = .02$).[10] It had no significant association with tumor size, cellular differentiation, or HBsAg status.

CLINICAL ISSUES

Presentation

Hepatoblastoma

Hepatoblastoma most frequently presents as an asymptomatic abdominal mass in children younger than 2 years, although some tumors are detected in the neonatal period. Anorexia, weight loss, vomiting, and abdominal pain are seen less frequently than in HCC. About 10% of cases are first noted on routine physical examination. Jaundice and splenomegaly are rare. Features of BWS, hemihypertrophy, or isosexual precocity can also be seen in these children. Osteopenia is present in a number of cases and is occasionally severe; patients present with back pain, refusal to walk, and pathologic fractures of weight-bearing bones.

Hepatocellular Carcinoma

Abdominal distention and right upper quadrant mass are the most common presentations of HCC, and they may be superimposed on the symptomatology of preexisting liver disease. Abdominal pain occurs in about half of patients, and nausea and vomiting are common. The duration of symptoms is relatively short (mean, 1 to 2 months), although the mean duration of symptoms is considerably longer in the fibrolamellar type (11 months). Hemoperitoneum with an acute abdominal crisis is a rare and dramatic initial presentation. Jaundice is more frequent in HCC than in hepatoblastoma, occurring in about 25% of cases. Splenomegaly may be present when there is coexisting cirrhosis, and polycythemia is occasionally present due to the extrarenal production of erythropoietin.

Differential Diagnosis

About 60% of abdominal hepatic masses in children are malignant (Table 36-1). Of the primary malignancies, hepatoblastoma is the most common, followed closely by HCC. Other, less common primary hepatic malignancies include sarcomas (rhabdosarcoma, leiomyosarcoma, angiosarcoma, and undifferentiated sarcoma) as well as lymphoma, malignant teratoma, and endocrine tumors. Most of the benign tumors are vascular tumors (hemangiomas), with other possibilities including mesenchymal hamartoma, focal nodular hyperplasia, and adenoma.

Diagnostic Evaluation

Blood Values

Laboratory abnormalities potentially found in children with hepatic tumors include anemia, hypoglycemia, and occasionally thrombocytosis. The most valuable laboratory test for both the diagnosis and monitoring of hepatic tumors is α-fetoprotein (AFP). This fetal protein is a single-chain sialated glycoprotein with a molecular weight of 67.5 kd. Its synthesis, which begins at 28 days of fetal life, occurs initially in the yolk sac and the liver, but by 11 weeks' gestation, it is made exclusively in the liver. Peak levels are reached at 14 weeks' gestation, at which time it is the dominant serum protein. Thereafter, a rapid decline in concentration occurs until term, when levels are normally between 20,000 and 120,000 ng/mL. Levels continue to fall

TABLE 36-1. *Differential diagnosis of liver tumors in children*

Tumor type	Percentage of all liver tumors
Malignant	64
Hepatoblastoma	35
Hepatocellular carcinoma	20
Sarcoma	9
Benign	36
Vascular	17
Mesenchymal hamartoma	9
Focal nodular hyperplasia	3
Adenoma	2
Other	5

(Adapted from Dehner LP, Pediatric surgical pathology, ed 2. Baltimore, Williams & Wilkins, 1987:480)

until 1 year of age, when they reach adult levels: 2 months (20 to 400 ng/mL), 6 months (30 ng/mL), and 1 year (3 to 15 ng/mL). The normal serum half-life of AFP is 5 to 7 days, but it is longer in younger infants.

AFP levels are elevated in 70% to 90% of patients with hepatoblastoma and in at least 50% of children with HCC. AFP is an excellent marker for primary hepatic tumors, although it can be elevated in germ cell tumors (endodermal sinus component) and occasionally in benign vascular lesions. Even more importantly, AFP levels provide an excellent marker for monitoring therapy. After complete tumor resection, an exponential fall to the normal range can be expected. Failure to achieve normal levels implies residual disease, whereas secondary elevation suggests disease recurrence. Non-AFP producing metastases have been reported, however, after resection of AFP-secreting tumor.

Other potentially useful laboratory values include the vitamin B_{12}–binding protein, which can be found in the serum of patients with the fibrolamellar variant of HCC. The level of this unsaturated vitamin B_{12}–binding protein is significantly elevated in patients with HCC, rising with disease progression. Other diagnostic tests include serologic evaluation for HBV in older children and β-human chorionic gonadotropin levels in children with precocious puberty.

Diagnostic Imaging

Plain radiographs of the abdomen invariably demonstrate the presence of a right upper quadrant mass, and calcification is seen in about 10% of malignant tumors. Ultrasonography is particularly useful in establishing the presence of a mass within an enlarged liver and in differentiating solid from cystic masses. Ultrasonography has thus become the preferred screening test because it is effective, inexpensive, and noninvasive, and does not involve ionizing radiation. Both hepatoblastoma and HCC demonstrate diffuse hyperechoic areas, whereas benign lesions are poorly echogenic, with scattered internal echoes. Ultrasound may also reveal involvement of the inferior vena cava, hepatic veins, and portal veins.

Computed tomographic (CT) scanning of the liver is particularly important for defining the extent of tumor involvement, the anatomic landmarks, and the tumor's operability (Fig. 36-7). The presence or absence of tumor in the anatomic lobes of the liver usually can be determined by CT scan, but this is not necessarily definitive. Hepatoblastoma and HCC are characteristically of lower attenuation than the surrounding normal hepatic tissue, although rarely the tumor may be isodense and difficult to visualize. Intravenous contrast injection results in patchy enhancement throughout the tumor mass. Intravenous contrast studies are particularly helpful in identifying vascular tumors (hemangiomas), which may be difficult to differentiate on unenhanced scans.

The role of hepatic angiography in the diagnosis and management of hepatic tumors has been debated for some time. Angiography identifies the anatomy of the hepatic vasculature and occasionally can give useful information on tumor resectability (Fig. 36-8). This modality has been improved by the introduction of digital subtraction angiography, which has the advantage of providing excellent images of the portal venous system with low-dose arterial injection. Some groups feel that CT and angiography together provide the most useful investigations for defining the extent and the resectability of hepatic malignant disease. Arteriography using an iodized oil, Lipiodol, which is selectively retained by tumor tissue for many days after administration, has been advocated as more sensitive than standard arteriography (Fig. 36-9). Generally however, the role of angiography, in the present era of magnetic resonance imaging (MRI) and spiral CT scanners appears limited.

MRI is increasingly used in the evaluation of hepatic masses. It can provide detailed information not only on the segmental anatomy of a hepatic tumor but also on the vascular anatomy of the liver. With increasing experience, MRI appears to be

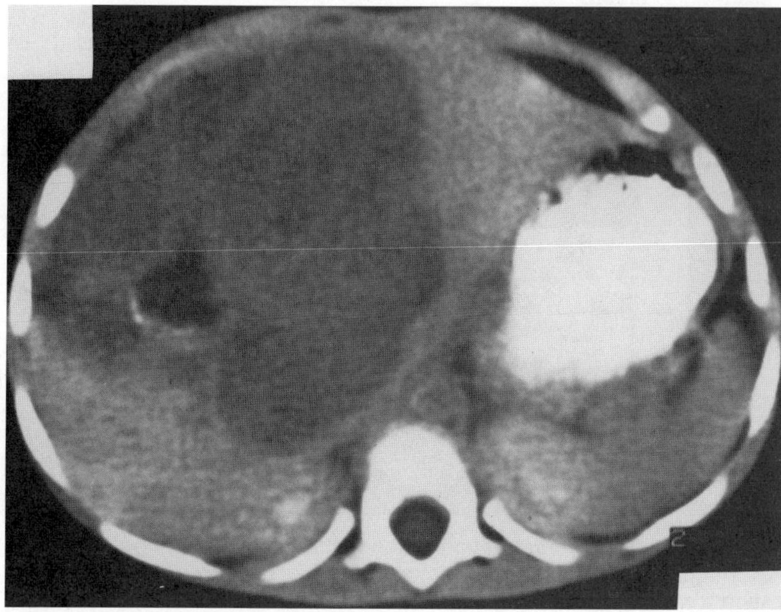

FIG. 36-7. Abdominal CT scan of a large hepatoblastoma, occupying most of the liver, other than the left lateral segment. Note the lower attenuation signal of the tumor, as compared with the surrounding normal liver.

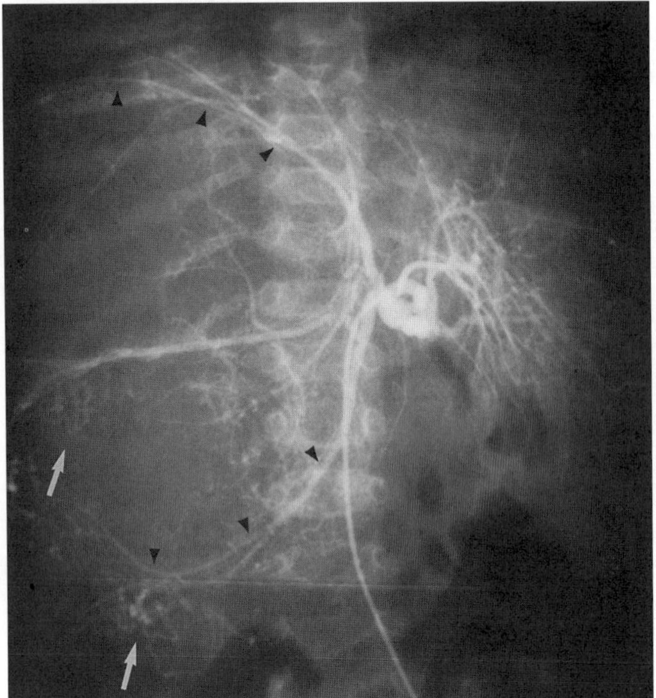

FIG. 36-8. Hepatic angiography performed for the tumor noted in Figure 36-7. Celiac arterial injection demonstrated a large mass effect, with splaying of the branches of the right hepatic artery (*dark arrowheads*) as well as irregular tumor vascularity (*light arrows*).

superior to the modalities mentioned earlier for imaging hepatic tumors because it defines more accurately parenchymal involvement and tumor margins. Delineation of tumor involvement of important vascular structures, in particular the hepatic and portal veins, is reliable even in the smallest patients.

Percutaneous liver biopsy is controversial; some authors have reported rupture of a hepatoblastoma as well as isolated cases of tumor seeding along the biopsy tract. These authors reserve this technique for tumors that are obviously not amenable to primary resection. For those who believe that primary chemotherapy should be given to all hepatic tumors, percutaneous needle biopsy has a definite role in confirming the diagnosis before medical therapy. Cytologic and ultrastuctural features of fine-needle biopsy specimens from children with hepatoblastoma and HCC have provided reliable information for accurate diagnoses.

Staging

A clinical grouping schema is essential for formulating prognoses and interpreting data from clinical trials. Although there is no universally accepted system, the most widely used approach is that of the CCSG, based on the extent of the tumor and the results of surgical resection:

Group I—complete tumor resection as initial treatment
Group IIA—complete tumor resection after initial chemotherapy or radiotherapy
Group IIB—residual disease confined to one lobe after resection
Group IIIA—disease involving both lobes of the liver
Group IIIB—regional nodal involvement
Group IV—distant metastases, regardless of extent of tumor

The Japanese Society for Pediatric Surgery has attempted to establish a classification based on the TNM (tumor, node, metastasis) system, using tumor size, number of lobes involved, regional node involvement, and presence of metastatic spread. Because both of these systems are clinical groupings dependent on operative findings, however, they are of little value in identifying patients who would benefit from presurgical chemotherapy. Thus, the International Society of Pediatric Surgical Oncology (SIOP), with a strong emphasis on preoperative chemotherapy, has recently generated a preoperative staging system based on radiologic imaging. Its utility is under investigation.

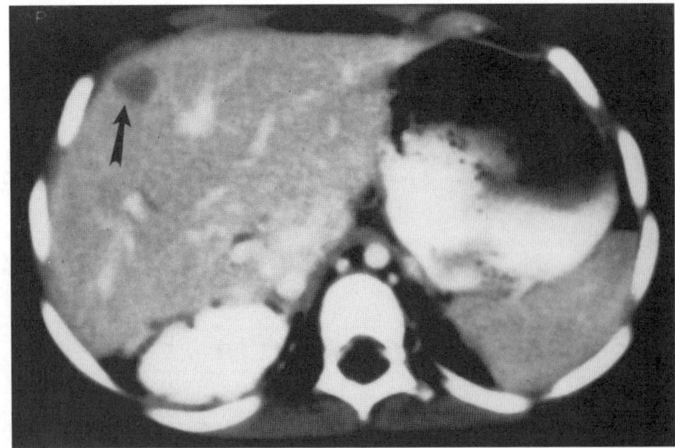
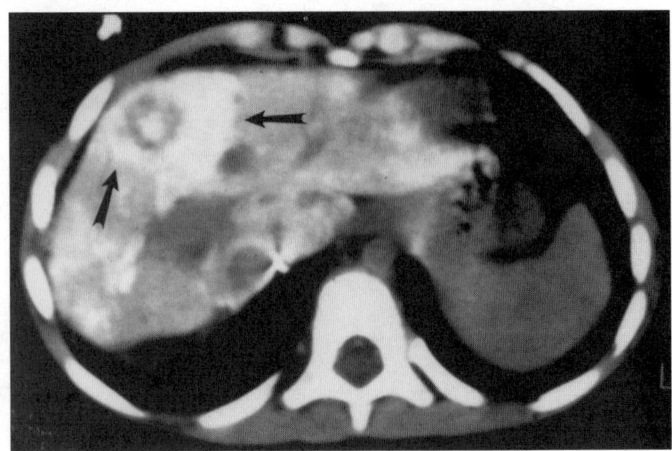

FIG. 36-9. (*A*) Abdominal CT scan demonstrating a small, low-attenuation lesion in the right lobe of the liver. (*B*) Abdominal CT scan performed 24 hours after arteriographic injection using Lipiodol. The Lipiodol is retained in the tumor, demonstrating a much larger lesion than originally appreciated.

Treatment

Surgery

Historical data indicate that cure of malignant liver tumors in children is not possible without complete resection of the primary tumor. With some exceptions, this dictum holds true today. In a recently completed CCSG protocol, 85% of patients with completely resected tumors were disease free at 2 years, as compared with 12% of those with incompletely or unresectable tumors. Until recently, operative staging for all hepatic tumors was thought to be mandatory because imaging studies were not consistently able to determine resectability. With better anatomic definition by CT and MRI and the use of preoperative chemotherapy in a growing number of patients, this dictum has been called into question. Many clinicians now evaluate resectability solely with diagnostic imaging and perform needle biopsy in unresectable tumors to determine a precise histologic diagnosis before instituting chemotherapy.

Most agree that tumors should be removed along anatomic planes, with at least 2 cm of tumor-free margin if possible. Standard anatomic resections include left lateral segmentectomy, right lobectomy, and left lobectomy. Left lateral segmentectomy includes the liver substance to the left of the falciform ligament, while right and left lobectomies involve removal of the liver tissue on either side of the anatomic plane that runs from the gallbladder bed to the suprahepatic vena cava. Right trisegmentectomy is the complete removal of the right lobe plus the medial segment of the left lobe, while left trisegmentectomy is the complete removal of the left lobe plus the anterior segment of the right lobe.

Hepatic tumor resection in children can be accomplished either transabdominally or thoracoabdominally. The liver is mobilized by dividing its diaphragmatic attachments, exposing the suprahepatic vena cava. Some authors recommended passing tapes around the vena cava above and below the liver to ensure control vascular. The porta hepatis is dissected, and the vessels and bile ducts to the involved lobe are ligated and divided. The liver capsule is then incised in an area demarcated by division of the hepatic artery and portal vein. Intraoperative ultrasonography allows accurate identification of tumors and their relation to segmental vessels and bile ducts, facilitating accurate liver dissection with maximal preservation of normal liver parenchyma. The liver substance can be divided in a number of ways: finger fracture, suction knife, ultrasonic dissector, or contact neodymium-YAG laser. All these techniques expose the bridging vessels so they can then be ligated as they are encountered. The ultrasonic surgical dissector (CUSA), developed from the work of Hodgson and Delguerico, may be useful. The tip of the hand piece is a vibrating device that oscillates with a frequency of 23,000 cycles/second. The effect is a preferential destruction of parenchymal cells in a radius of 1 to 2 mm around the tip of the instrument, while the blood vessels and bile ducts, which contain relatively larger volumes of elastic tissue and collagen, are preserved. The coaxial suction and irrigation built into the hand piece allow a clean dissection and accurate placement of clips or ligatures unto the ducts and blood vessels.

Because of the short extrahepatic length of the hepatic veins in children, these vessels may be better approached by dissection through the liver substance rather than at their exit from the liver. After removal of the lobe, hemostasis and bile drainage are controlled. Intraoperative cannulation and irrigation of the biliary tract to identify any possible biliary leaks may be useful. T-tube drainage is not used because stricture in the small bile duct of an infant is a significant risk, and there is no conclusive evidence that ductal drainage decreases the incidence of postoperative bile leak.

Large hepatic tumors can be difficult to remove safely, and adjunctive measures have been developed for their intraoperative management. Profound hypothermia with circulatory arrest and cardiopulmonary bypass has been used. With the core temperature cooled to 20°C, circulatory arrest for as long as 60 minutes can be performed, allowing tumor resection and repair of vascular structures to be performed in a bloodless operative field. Another technique involves the use of hemodilutional anesthesia. Major liver resections are begun by phlebotomy of the patient's whole blood and replacement with lactated Ringer solution. Surgery is then performed at 32°C with halothane-induced hypotension to reduce metabolic demand and red-cell loss, with retransfusion of the patient's whole blood at the conclusion of the liver resection. Another technique includes normothermic total vascular exclusion, interrupting the hepatic circulation for as long as 1 hour by clamping the porta hepatis and the vena cava above and below the liver. Finally, ex situ surgery is possible, which involves removal of the entire liver, perfusion with a cooled preservation solution, resection of the tumor, and reanastomosis of the liver. However, no childhood hepatic tumor resection using these techniques has been reported.

Chemotherapy

In the early 1970s, it became evident that hepatoblastoma was potentially a chemoresponsive tumor, with cisplatin and doxorubicin the most effective single agents. Clinical and radiologic response of the primary tumor was often dramatic, and even complete disappearance of lung metastases or multinodular tumor foci within the liver were documented (Fig. 36-10). Initial efforts using chemotherapy to increase the percentage of children able to undergo resection were not encouraging. Subsequently, Weinblatt reported in 1982 that 7 of 8 (87%)[11] unresectable childhood hepatic malignancies treated with chemotherapy exhibited a pronounced clinical response: four hepatoblastoma children were able to have complete surgical excision of residual disease, and one HCC patient had complete disappearance of all disease without surgery.

With this ability to shrink hepatic tumors (particularly hepatoblastoma) with chemotherapy, some authors, particularly in Europe, have advocated preoperative chemotherapy for all hepatic tumors, believing that chemotherapy renders the tumors smaller and less friable. Tumor shrinkage is almost always accompanied by clinical improvement, so the patient may be in better general condition for subsequent surgery. In the United States and Germany, however, patients treated on national protocols have had initial surgical exploration to ascertain tumor resectability. For patients able to undergo complete primary resection, less intensive and shorter adjuvant chemotherapy treatments have been used. For instance, an ongoing POG study is investigating the role of single-drug therapy (doxorubicin

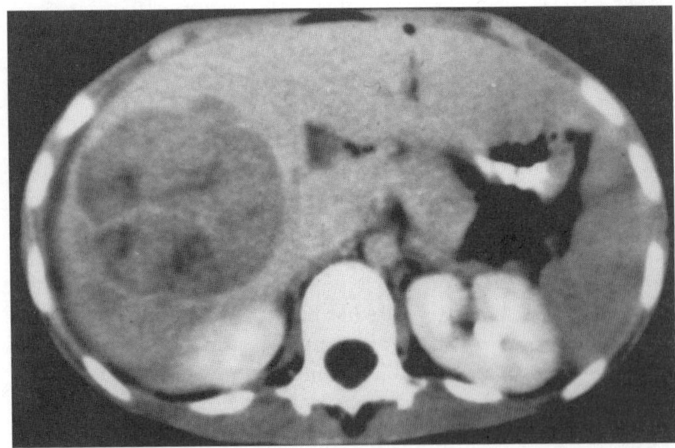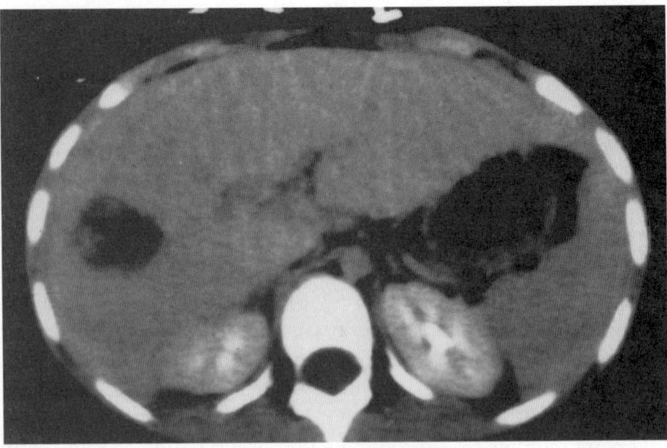

FIG. 36-10. (*A*) Abdominal CT scan of large hepatoblastoma occupying the right lobe of the liver and encroaching on the medial segment of the left lobe. (*B*) Abdominal CT scan of same hepatoblastoma after preoperative chemotherapy with doxorubicin and cisplatin.

[Adriamycin]) in stage I (initial complete resection) hepatoblastoma patients with fetal histology. In addition, several reports have documented an increase in operative morbidity associated with delayed resections after chemotherapy, compared with primary resection. The reasons for this remain unclear, but cardiac toxicity from doxorubicin plays a definite role.

Several series have noted that preoperative chemotherapy can reduce hepatoblastoma tumor sizes by 35% to 95% and convert about 65% of hepatoblastoma tumors from unresectable to resectable. The CCSG protocol 823F (1986 to 1989) treated 22 hepatoblastoma patients with four cycles of preoperative doxorubicin and cisplatin; there were 12 complete responders and 8 partial responders. Eighteen of these patients underwent second-look operations, and 15 patients were able to undergo complete excision (68%). Dose-limiting toxicity, mainly cardiac and hematopoietic, was seen with doxorubicin, although more recent evidence suggests that continuous infusion doxorubicin is less toxic and as effective as bolus administration. The POG and CCSG intergroup protocol 8881 (1989 to 1992) compared two preoperative chemotherapy regimens: cisplatin and doxorubicin versus cisplatin, 5-fluorouracil (5-FU), and vincristine. This randomized study demonstrated no difference in survival rates, but the combination of cisplatin and doxorubicin was much more toxic than the cisplatin, 5-FU, and vincristine regimen. Of 173 total patients treated in this study, there were 7 deaths related to drug toxicity, all in the cisplatin plus doxorubicin group: 3 deaths from sepsis, 1 from hepatitis, 2 from cardiomyopathy, and 1 from multiorgan failure. In addition, severe neutropenia, thrombocytopenia, and the need for parenteral nutrition were seen much more commonly in patients receiving the regimen with doxorubicin.

Preoperative chemotherapy has not been as effective for children with HCC. Doxorubicin, etoposide, and 5-FU have all been reported to produce partial remission in a small percentage of HCC cases, but the remissions have been short-lived. Also, because of the multicentric origin of HCC, it is less likely that preoperative chemotherapy will contribute significantly to subsequent successful resection. Thus, in the case of a suspected HCC, complete primary removal of the tumor should be aggressively attempted, even using extended resections if needed. Un-

fortunately, only one third of HCC cases are amenable to aggressive resection, and only one third of those patients are long-term survivors. Several phase I and II studies are evaluating the effectiveness of different chemotherapeutic agents, particularly paclitaxel (Taxol), in patients with unresectable HCC.

In an attempt to render more tumors resectable, Japanese investigators have used preoperative intrahepatic arterial chemotherapy, with or without Lipiodol, with success in rendering certain inoperable tumors operable. The role for this invasive technique is still under investigation.

Adjuvant chemotherapy has also been effective for hepatoblastoma patients. In one study, only 1 of 16 patients who underwent complete resection followed by adjuvant chemotherapy developed distant metastases, compared with 7 of 11 historical controls who did not receive adjuvant chemotherapy. Recommended adjuvant chemotherapy has to this point included cisplatin with doxorubicin, instituted about 4 weeks after hepatic resection, with treatment cycles administered 3 to 4 weeks apart for a total of six cycles.

Radiotherapy

Even though the role of radiotherapy in hepatoblastoma or HCC has not been formally evaluated, there is circumstantial evidence from the Villejuif (Paris) group that radiation may improve local control in unresected tumors, particularly hepatoblastoma. Only the SIOP study has used radiotherapy to treat residual "miniscopic" disease after incomplete resection; local control of tumor was attained in 3 of 4 patients with residual microscopic disease and in 7 of 10 patients with gross residual disease. Dosages of radiation used to treat hepatic tumors have ranged from 1200 to 2000 cGy. Although radiotherapy has resulted in tumor regression, such treatment has not been curative, and as with chemotherapy, radiation to the liver immediately after resection may potentially limit regeneration.

Liver Transplantation

The presence of unresectable tumor in the liver, without metastatic disease, would appear to provide an ideal opportunity for cure by orthotopic liver transplantation. Review of more than 600 liver transplantations performed for both primary and metastatic liver malignancies in adults and children revealed poor results overall. Several subsets of patients were defined, however, that may benefit from this therapy, including children with hepatoblastoma and fibrolamellar HCC. The initial reported American experience with liver transplantation for hepatoblastoma comprised 12 cases managed in nine centers, with varying preoperative and postoperative chemotherapy regimens. There was a 50% disease-free survival at 24 to 70 months after transplantation. Three patients died from recurrent hepatoblastoma, and three patients died from transplant-related complications. In an even larger series, Tagge and colleagues reported 15 children with either stage III or IV HCC or hepatoblastoma who were treated with total hepatectomy and orthotopic liver transplantation.[12] At a mean follow-up of 1.9 years, 5 of 6 children with hepatoblastoma and 4 of 9 children with HCC were alive without evidence of disease. All these children were treated with both preoperative and postoperative chemotherapy. Although longer follow-up is needed, these data tend to support the concept that total hepatectomy and orthotopic liver transplantation may improve survival for selected children with advanced disease. Because of the shortage of available donor organs and the unanswered questions regarding tumor recurrence, however, liver transplantation for childhood hepatic malignancy should only be performed on protocol at major transplantation centers.

Outcome

In their 1967 monograph, Ishak and Glunz noted that none of 12 HCC children and 10 of 35 (29%) hepatoblastoma patients survived, and that 9 of 10 (90%) survivors had undergone tumor resection. Subsequently, a 1974 survey of the Surgical Section of the American Academy of Pediatrics reported survival rates of 35% (45 of 129) for hepatoblastoma and 13% (12 of 98) for HCC, with no patient surviving without resection.

The CCSG-8881 intergroup study (August 1989 to December 1992) included a total of 139 patients: 108 patients with hepatoblastoma and 31 with HCC. Primary resection could be performed in only 37% and 10% of patients, respectively. Although exact data have not yet been reported, preoperative chemotherapy converted a large percentage of unresectable hepatoblastomas to resectable tumors, although many patients required trisegmentectomies to accomplish tumor removal. Initial 3-year survival rates were 70% for hepatoblastoma and 25% for HCC patients.

In Europe, two studies are examining the treatment of childhood hepatic neoplasms: the SIOP study (SIOPEL 1) and the German Society of Pediatric Oncology study (HB-89). Both studies reflect the bias of most European surgeons that preoperative chemotherapy is beneficial for all patients. In the SIOPEL 1 study, no tumor is primarily resected without preoperative chemotherapy; in the HB-89 study, only small tumors are primarily resected. The HB-89 study was closed in December 1992. Of the 64 patients with hepatoblastoma, 30% (19) underwent primary tumor resection, and 88% (30 of 34) of those treated with chemotherapy subsequently had their tumors resected. Histologic subclassifications and vascular invasion portended a poor prognosis only in advanced stage (III and IV) hepatoblastomas. No patient without complete surgical removal of all tumor after chemotherapy remained in remission. The overall probability for disease-free survival was 100% for patients with stage I, 75% for stage II, 67% for stage III, and 0% for stage IV tumors.

Patients with the fibrolamellar variant of HCC have been reported to have a better prognosis than those with standard HCC. Several small series have reported 2- and 5-year survival rates of more than 50%. However, the combined CCSG, POG, and Southwest Oncology Group study demonstrated no difference in survival rates between among patients with fibrolamellar HCC and regular HCC, stage for stage.

REFERENCES

1. Ishak KG, Glunz PR. Hepatoblastoma and hepatocarcinoma in infancy and childhood: report of 47 cases. Cancer 1967;20:396.
2. Kasai M, Watanabe I. Histologic classification of liver cell carcinoma in infancy and childhood and its clinical evaluation: a study of 70 cases collected in Japan. Cancer 1970;24:551.
3. Koufos A, Hansen MF, Copeland NG, et al. Loss of heterozygosity in three embryonal tumours suggests a common pathogenetic mechanism. Nature 1985;316:330.
4. Cheah PL, Laoi LM, Lin HP, et al. Childhood primary hepatocellular carcinoma and hepatitis B virus infection. Cancer 1990;65:174.
5. Kobayashi S, Hayashi H, Itoh Y, et al. Detection of minus-strand hepatitis C virus in tumor tissues of hepatocellular carcinoma. Cancer 1996;73:48.
6. Mishida N, Fukuda Y, Kokurya H, et al. Accumulation of allelic loss on arms of chromosomes 13q, 16q, and 17p in the advanced stages of human hepatocellular carcinoma. Int J Cancer 199251:862.
7. Bressac B, Kew M, Wands J, et al. Selective G to T mutations of p53 gene in hepatocellular carcinoma from southern Africa. Nature 1991;350:429.
8. Aguilar F, Harris C, Sun T, et al. Geographic variation of p53 mutational profile in nonmalignant human liver. Science 1994;264:1317.
9. Hsai CC, Kleiner DE Jr, Axiotis CA, et al. Mutations of p53 gene in hepatocellular carcinoma: roles of hepatitis B virus and aflotoxin in the diet. JNCI 1992;84:1638.
10. Ng IO, Lai EC, Fan ST, et al. Prognostic significance of proliferating cell nuclear antigen expression in hepatocellular carcinoma. Cancer 1994;73:2268.
11. Weinblatt ME, Siegel SE, Siegel MM, et al. Preoperative chemotherapy for unresectable primary hepatic malignancies in children. Cancer 1982;50:1061.
12. Tagge EP, Tagge DU, Reyes J, et al. Resection, including transplanation, for hepatoblastoma and hepatocellular carcinoma: Impact on survival. J Pediatr Surg 1992;27(3):292.

Surgery of Infants and Children: Scientific Principles and Practice, edited by
Keith T. Oldham, Paul M. Colombani, and Robert P. Foglia.
Lippincott–Raven Publishers, Philadelphia, © 1997.

CHAPTER 37

Leukemias and Lymphomas

Barbara A. Duffy and Curt I. Civin

Acute leukemias and lymphomas constitute about 40% of all childhood malignancies. Accurate and sophisticated classification of pediatric leukemias and lymphomas is based on extensive evaluation by standard morphologic, immunophenotypic, cytochemical, and cytogenetic techniques. Classification has guided improvements in disease-specific therapy that have resulted in improved disease-free survival and cure rates. Several reviews of the treatment of pediatric hematologic malignancies have been published. Pediatric Oncology Group (POG) protocols form the basis for the illustrations of therapy in this chapter, although similar protocols are in use for other cooperative groups.

ACUTE MYELOGENOUS LEUKEMIA

Acute myelogenous leukemia (AML) accounts for 15% to 20% of childhood leukemias. AML, like all leukemias, is the final result of a leukemic transformation of a single early hematopoietic cell. All the blast cells in a given patient are the clonal progeny of this one cell of origin. Acquired chromosomal abnormalities can be demonstrated in nearly all cases of AML. A chromosomal abnormality can result in a differentiation stage–associated regulatory element controlling the expression of a cellular protooncogene. Overexpression of this protooncogene can lead to leukemogenesis. A structurally abnormal oncoprotein may be produced by a chromosomal abnormality. The BCR-ABL protein involved in the t(9;22) translocation that characterizes chronic myelogenous leukemia and the fusion gene of the t(15;17) translocation of acute promyelocytic leukemia (FAB M3 AML), which includes a retinoic acid receptor, are examples of structurally abnormal oncoproteins caused by chromosomal translocations. Although it is hoped that such information will translate rapidly into more effective treatment for AML (as may be the case with all-*trans* retinoic acid therapy for FAB M3 AML), pediatric AML therapy is not as successful as that for childhood acute lymphoblastic leukemia (ALL).[1]

Treatment Phases

Therapy for AML is best divided conceptually into two phases: an induction phase, followed by an intensive consolidation phase. With intensive myelotoxic induction chemotherapy, remission is achieved in about 85% of children with AML. This remission induction chemotherapy rapidly reduces the total body leukemic burden so that no clinically detectable disease is apparent by the end of the (successful) induction phase. In addition, induction therapy allows for the regrowth of normal hematopoietic progenitor cells that were previously displaced from the marrow space by the expanding leukemia. Once remission is achieved, consolidation therapy is aimed at eliminating minimal residual disease, with the premise that treatment must be myelotoxic to kill AML blasts effectively.

Supportive Care

Integral to any chemotherapeutic regimen for AML is effective supportive care. The most serious chemotherapy-induced problems in AML are bleeding, infection, tumor lysis syndrome, and leukostasis.

Bleeding usually results from profound thrombocytopenia and can be corrected with leukocyte-poor platelet transfusions. Disseminated intravascular coagulation (DIC) must also be suspected, especially in patients with acute promyelocytic leukemia (FAB M3 AML). With the initiation of chemotherapy, DIC may worsen because cell lysis releases intracellular thromboplastin. When DIC is present, patients may benefit from the administration of fresh frozen plasma or prophylactic low-dose heparin, 50 U/kg every 6 hours, in addition to concentrated platelet transfusions.

Children with AML frequently present with fever and infection during treatment. Because induction therapy for AML is severely myelosuppressive, the resulting neutropenia is often of long duration and is frequently complicated by bacterial or fungal infections. Febrile neutropenic patients require an immediate extensive clinical evaluation with multiple cultures of blood and other sites of specific concern. They should be treated promptly with empiric broad-spectrum antibiotics that cover both gram-positive and gram-negative bacteria. There should be a low threshold for the administration of antifungal therapy in patients with persistent neutropenic fevers. Treatment with acyclovir is strongly recommended for all active varicella-zoster virus (VZV) infections (eg, chicken pox, herpes zoster, herpes simplex) during therapy. Children with AML require prophylactic antibiotic therapy against *Pneumocystis carinii* pneumonia. A regimen of trimethoprim-sulfamethoxazole taken 3 days per week is effective for prophylaxis and generally does not add to the chemotherapy-induced myelosuppression. For patients who are sensitive or allergic to trimethoprim-sulfamethoxazole, dapsone or pentamidine can be substituted.

Patients with very high white blood cell (WBC) counts (more than 200,000/mL) are at risk for leukostasis, especially in the lungs and brain. In patients with symptoms, exchange transfusions or leukapheresis may be indicated to lower the WBC count rapidly. When performed, these measures should be followed promptly by the administration of chemotherapy; otherwise, the blast cell count rises again rapidly. The treatment for patients with high WBC counts may be complicated simultaneously by leukostasis and tumor lysis syndrome.

Tumor lysis syndrome, with hyperkalemia, hyperuricemia, hyperphosphatemia, and hypocalcemia, results from a rapid lysis of leukemic cells. With the administration of allopurinol and aggressive hydration, life-threatening electrolyte abnormalities can usually be avoided. Patients who experience oliguria (urine output below 1 mL/kg/h) may require emergency dialysis, especially if cytoreductive therapy must be initiated before achieving the full effects of preventive measures.

Remission Induction

Prognostic factors have not been identified consistently in childhood AML. A high WBC count at diagnosis, myelodysplastic presentations, or cytogenetic abnormalities associated with myelodysplastic syndromes have been generally accepted as poor prognostic factors.

Remission induction therapy in AML must be intensive enough to induce bone marrow hypoplasia. An exception to this rule may be FAB M3 AML, which may not require bone marrow hypoplasia for remission induction. Many pediatric AML induction regimens use a 7-day course of cytarabine with a 3-day course of an anthracycline, usually daunomycin. POG AML protocols include 6-thioguanine in this first induction course.[2] The second induction course includes high-dose cytarabine administration.[3] In the POG experience, about 85% of children with AML achieve remission after these two induction chemotherapy courses.

Intensive Consolidation Chemotherapy

Consolidation chemotherapy begins after remission induction. Patients with AML who have an HLA-identical sibling are generally offered allogeneic bone marrow transplantation (BMT) as the preferred consolidation therapy. For patients in first remission who undergo allogeneic transplants for AML, 50% to 70% long-term disease-free survival rates have been demonstrated in several BMT trials. In a POG AML study, patients without HLA-identical siblings were randomized to one of two consolidation therapies. Autologous BMT and intensive conventional consolidation chemotherapy were studied for their rates of disease-free survival. Patients who were assigned to the chemotherapy arm received seven cycles of conventional continuation chemotherapy. Many clinical trials that employed similar consolidation chemotherapy protocols reported 30% to 40% disease-free survival rates. Patients who underwent autologous BMT were prepared with a busulfan and cyclophosphamide regimen. Hematopoietic rescue from this myeloablative chemotherapy was achieved with their own autologous marrow that had been purged with the cyclophosphamide derivative, 4-hydroperoxycyclophosphamide.[4] Forthcoming results of this POG trial are expected to confirm prior suggestions that autologous BMT provides intermediate results, better than standard chemotherapy but inferior to allogeneic BMT.[5]

Central Nervous System Therapy

As many as 20% of children with AML have leukemic blasts in their cerebrospinal fluid cytology at diagnosis. Central nervous system (CNS) disease in AML, however, has not been demonstrated to be an independent poor prognostic factor. Patients with AML and asymptomatic CNS leukemia at diagnosis have a failure pattern similar to most patients without cerebrospinal fluid blast cells at diagnosis. In the POG AML protocol trial, intrathecal cytarabine was administered for four or six doses during induction chemotherapy, depending on the absence or presence of CNS leukemia at presentation.

Treatment of Relapse

A challenge in pediatric oncology is to design effective therapy for recurrent AML. Relapsed AML is frequently difficult to reinduce into remission, especially if the relapse occurs during active chemotherapy. Remission can be reinduced in about half of patients by various regimens. For patients with recurrent promyelocytic leukemia (FAB M3 AML), all-*trans* retinoic acid may provide a remission. Regimens, such as etoposide plus 2-chlorodeoxyadenosine, high-dose cytarabine with or without asparaginase or an anthracycline, and mitoxantrone with etoposide and cyclosporine, provide successful reinduction chemotherapy for a significant number of AML patients. For patients with early bone marrow relapse and an HLA-identical donor, prompt allogeneic BMT without preceding chemotherapy may be an effective salvage therapy.

For patients who achieve second remission and who have HLA-identical siblings, allogeneic BMT is the treatment of choice. For the remaining patients, autologous BMT with a purged marrow is also effective consolidation therapy.

Complications of Therapy

The complications of AML therapy are most often the results of intensive chemotherapy-induced bone marrow hypoplasia. Symptomatic anemia and bleeding can be controlled with transfusions of leukocyte-poor blood products (ie, packed red blood cells and platelets). As discussed earlier, all neutropenic fevers need to be evaluated extensively and treated aggressively with broad-spectrum antibiotics and, if required, with the early addition of antifungal (eg, amphotericin) and antiviral (eg, acyclovir) agents. Mucositis, vomiting, and diarrhea are common gastrointestinal toxicities. Typhlitis is a severe and potentially life-threatening complication that can result in ileus, lower gastrointestinal bleeding, abdominal pain, perforation, and septic shock. Treatment involves bowel rest, broad-spectrum antibiotics, and intravenous hydration. Surgical intervention during periods of profound neutropenia (less than 250 neutrophils/mL) is reserved for perforation, septic shock, intractable hemorrhage, and acidosis.

CHRONIC MYELOGENOUS LEUKEMIA

Chronic myelogenous leukemia occurs rarely in children and adolescents. It is primarily the same disease with the same genotype [t(9;22)] in the pediatric population as it is in adults. Juvenile chronic myelogenous leukemia is a unique and rare leukemia that occurs mainly in infants and small children and lacks the t(9;22) characteristic. A discussion of these two rare chronic leukemias is beyond the scope of this chapter.

ACUTE LYMPHOBLASTIC LEUKEMIA

The therapy for childhood ALL is highly successful, with an overall disease-free rate of over 70%. Clinical trials have strikingly improved the prognosis of ALL during the past 30 years. In addition, these trials have enhanced the understanding of the biologic heterogeneity of ALL. The identification of diagnostic features that predict high or standard risk for treatment failure has guided treatment selection for subgroups of ALL patients.

Initial Prognostic Subgroups

The POG, Children's Cancer Study Group, and other cooperative clinical trial groups, as well as single institutions, have analyzed clinical and laboratory findings present at diagnosis that are predictive of treatment failure. Three strong prognostic findings are the patient's age, WBC count, and leukemic blast DNA index at diagnosis. A low WBC count at initial diagnosis, patient age near the median age for the incidence of ALL (3 to 4 years), and a DNA index higher than 1.16 define the best prognostic group of patients with ALL. Although quantitative predictors of prognosis operate on a continuum, clinical trials define prognostic risk groups of patients in an absolute fashion. For example, in POG studies, 3- to 5-year-old children with an initial WBC count of less than 100,000/μL can be included in the standard-risk group, but patients who are 1 to 3 or 6 to 10 years old must have WBC counts of less than 10,000/mL to be included. Infants, children older than 10 years, and adolescents are in the high-risk group, as are patients with overt CNS disease at diagnosis. Patients who, by age or WBC count at diagnosis, would be segregated into the high-risk category can be downgraded to the standard-risk group if their leukemic blasts have a favorable DNA index. The POG is studying the treatment for children with ALL according to three risk strata: lesser, standard, and high risk for treatment failure.

Immunophenotype and Cytogenetics

For patients treated on POG B-lineage ALL protocols, the leukemias must have cell surface markers consistent with non-B, non-T lymphoid immunophenotype. Lymphoid leukemias with cell-surface markers consistent with mature B-cell (ie, surface immunoglobulin–positive, Burkitt leukemia; less than 1% of childhood ALL cases) or T-lymphoid immunophenotype (15% to 20% of childhood ALL) behave aggressively and relapse early and frequently when treated by chemotherapy protocols that are highly effective for the most common childhood B-lineage ALL phenotypes. With the design of intensive regimens aimed at these aggressive leukemias, the prognosis for patients with T-cell leukemias and mature B-cell leukemias has improved greatly. Treatment of T-cell and mature B-cell leukemias is discussed later in the section on lymphomas.

Within the group of childhood ALL cases, expression of the CD10 antigen (CALLA) and lack of cytoplasmic immunoglobulin were once thought to be associated with a favorable long-term prognosis. Later studies, however, did not confirm the prognostic power of these leukemia cell immunophenotypes. In addition, leukemia cell expression of the CD34 hematopoietic progenitor cell antigen has been demonstrated to be a good prognostic feature in B-lineage ALL.[6]

Leukemia cell cytogenetic features make powerful contributions to prognostic information. The presence of more than 50 chromosomes in the leukemic blast (ie, DNA index higher than 1.16) predicts favorably for outcome. The prognostic influence of hyperdiploidy is so strong that a child who is otherwise considered at high risk for relapse by age or WBC count can be reclassified and treated successfully in the standard-risk group if the blast cells are hyperdiploid.

Specific chromosomal translocations predict a high risk for relapse in childhood ALL. The Philadelphia chromosome, t(9;22)(q34;11), has been consistently associated with a poor outcome. In ALL, this translocation leads to the creation of a fusion gene, *bcr-abl*. This fusion gene encodes for leukemia-specific mRNA and protein with tyrosine kinase activity, which is strongly associated with malignant transformation. The t(1;19)(q23;q13) chromosomal translocation occurs in a subset of the cytoplasmic immunoglobulin–positive (pre–B-cell) ALL cases. It is the decisive factor in the poorer prognosis previously associated with pre–B-cell ALL. The t(8;14)(q24;q23) translocation is associated with a poorer outcome because it is highly associated with the mature B-cell immunophenotype. These translocations identify poor prognostic groups of children with ALL for whom usually effective therapy often fails. Consequently, the hope is that further understanding of the effects of these and other translocations will lead to enhanced understanding of malignant cell growth and differentiation and to improved therapies.

Investigative Therapy

With the imperfect nature of therapy and the rapidly expanding biologic information base, it is not yet appropriate for a consensus on standard therapeutic regimens for childhood ALL. Although one goal in pediatric oncology is to return much of the care of these patients to the primary pediatrician, all children with leukemia now should be treated according to either a cooperative group protocol or a large, single-institution clinical research protocol. As previously mentioned, appropriate evaluation of the child with newly diagnosed ALL requires sophisticated laboratory techniques to characterize the leukemia thoroughly. Many aggressive treatment protocols mandate the rapid availability of a pediatric intensive care unit. Furthermore, continued clinical research is still needed to improve therapy toward the goal of a uniformly effective standard of care. Children with ALL, for now and in the near future, should be referred for treatment to pediatric cancer centers in which there are concentrations of relevant expertise and clinical research protocols.

Although the detailed approaches to the management of various risk categories may be somewhat different, all treatment regimens for childhood B-lineage ALL include the following components: supportive care, remission induction, consolidation, maintenance therapy, and CNS prophylaxis.

Initial Supportive Therapy

Each newly diagnosed child with ALL should be examined and evaluated carefully for complications of leukemic infiltration in the bone marrow. Symptomatic anemia and thrombocytopenia demand transfusions with leukocyte-poor irradiated blood components. As in AML, fevers in a neutropenic patient require a complete evaluation and prompt empiric therapy with broad-spectrum antibiotics that cover both gram-negative and gram-positive pathogens. The addition of an antifungal antibiotic, such as fluconazole, may prevent the development of clinical fungal infections in patients who have neutropenic fevers before or during induction chemotherapy.

Tumor lysis syndrome often occurs with treatment of ALL. As discussed previously, hyperuricemia, hyperkalemia, hyperphosphatemia, and hypocalcemia must be prevented or controlled with the administration of intravenous fluids, allopurinol, alkalinization, and careful electrolyte management. Emergency renal dialysis is required when the patient has oliguria.

Each patient should have titers for VZV and, if indicated, human immunodeficiency virus measured before receiving blood products and chemotherapy. Patients who have not previously had VZV should receive VZV immunoglobulin within 72 hours of each VZV exposure while on therapy. All active VZV infections that occur while the patient receives chemotherapy should be treated with acyclovir.

Problems with hyperleukocytosis are relatively rare in ALL and are restricted to patients with WBC counts higher than 200,000/mL. The treatment of hyperleukocytosis was discussed in the section on supportive care of AML.

Induction, Consolidation, and Maintenance Therapy for Standard-Risk Acute Lymphoblastic Leukemia

The goal of induction chemotherapy in ALL is to reduce rapidly the total body burden of leukemic cells and thus achieve a complete remission. This remission, during which no leukemia is clinically detectable, allows for growth and development of normal bone marrow progenitor cells. For patients at standard risk for relapse, a 98% complete response rate has been obtained with the three-drug remission induction regimen of prednisone, vincristine, and asparaginase. Even in remission, however, these patients may have a total body burden of up to 10^9 residual leukemic cells.

Consolidation therapy aims to achieve several more logs of leukemic cell kill in the next several weeks to months of therapy. A POG trial of a consolidation regimen involved 12 biweekly infusions of intermediate-dose methotrexate and 6-mercaptopurine (6-MP), alternating with intramuscular methotrexate and daily oral 6-MP. In the pilot phase of this protocol, only 5 of 59 standard-risk patients experienced leukemia relapse, suggesting highly effective therapy. Toxicity from this regimen remains minimal and transient (mainly stomatitis), with the exception that seizures have been observed.

At the completion of the consolidation period, patients receive maintenance therapy to complete a total of 2.5 years of ALL therapy. Maintenance therapy consists of daily oral 6-MP and weekly intramuscular methotrexate injections. The goal of maintenance therapy is to eradicate the last leukemic cells while the child resumes normal activities.[7]

High-Risk Therapy

For patients at high risk for relapse, a four-drug remission induction regimen of prednisone, vincristine, asparaginase, and an anthracycline (usually daunomycin) is used. The addition of daunomycin increases the remission induction rate to about 97% in these patients. Daunomycin, however, also increases the myelosuppression and the risk of neutropenic fevers.

A POG pilot trial explored the feasibility of using the biweekly intravenous methotrexate and 6-MP infusions for consolidation therapy for high-risk patients. This regimen demonstrated efficacy in standard-risk patients, as previously mentioned. A favorable continuous complete remission rate has been obtained thus far in the POG high-risk pilot study using this consolidation regimen. An alternative regimen attempts to prevent the emergence of leukemic cellular drug resistance by including non–cross-resistant chemotherapeutic agents, including cytarabine, daunomycin, and teniposide.[8] A POG randomized study will determine the more effective consolidation regimen.

Maintenance therapy for high-risk patients is identical to that for standard-risk patients. Weekly intramuscular methotrexate injections with daily doses of oral 6-MP continue until 2.5 years of antileukemic therapy is completed.

Central Nervous System Prophylaxis

In the context of systemic chemotherapy, intrathecal chemotherapy with or without cranial irradiation can prevent the emergence of overt CNS leukemia in 90% to 95% of children with ALL. Children with B-lineage ALL treated on POG protocols receive age-adjusted doses of triple intrathecal chemotherapy with cytarabine, hydrocortisone, and methotrexate on day 1 of induction chemotherapy. Both standard-risk and high-risk patients receive periodic triple intrathecal injections during consolidation and maintenance therapy. POG protocols do not use cranial irradiation for prophylactic therapy. Other groups, however, are similarly successful in preventing overt CNS leukemia with CNS irradiation (1800 cGy). After intrathecal injections, children commonly experience vomiting and headache. Arachnoiditis is less frequently seen. Occasionally, children experience focal or generalized seizures associated with intrathecal chemotherapy and methotrexate infusions. Evaluations of these children have revealed generally normal neurologic examinations, with computed tomography (CT) scans of the brain that are either normal or demonstrate mild white matter changes and patchy calcifications. For these patients, anticonvulsant therapy is usually given until antileukemic therapy is completed. The long-term neurodevelopmental effects of intrathecal chemotherapy without cranial irradiation remain to be determined.

Treatment of Central Nervous System Acute Lymphoblastic Leukemia

Children with B-lineage ALL who have more than 5 blast cells/mL cerebrospinal fluid (ie, definite CNS leukemia) receive more frequent intrathecal chemotherapy during induction and consolidation therapy. These patients also receive craniospinal irradiation, with a total dose of 2400 cGy delivered to the brain and 1500 cGy to the spinal cord. Toxicities from this therapy include somnolence syndrome, neurodevelopmental impairment, and secondary brain tumors.

Remission

At the end of induction, consolidation, and maintenance therapy, the patient is evaluated for remission status. *Remission* is defined as less than 5% blasts in a bone marrow examination, with normal peripheral blood counts and no extramedullary disease. New techniques of DNA analysis that detect 1 malignant cell among 100,000 to 1,000,000 normal marrow cells are being clinically tested to investigate their predictive powers for relapse.[9] If the predictive powers of these techniques are confirmed, patients found to have minimal residual disease after having received ALL therapy for a specified time will receive intensified treatment, including BMT, before they relapse overtly.

Treatment of Relapse

As in AML, the primary goal of therapy for recurrent ALL is to reinduce remission. Generally, remission induction therapy consists of the intensive four-drug combination with triple intrathecal chemotherapy described earlier for high-risk patients at initial diagnosis. Most patients with recurrent ALL achieve a second remission. The frequency of successful reinduction overall, however, has been decreasing with intensified first-remission treatment. Children who experience relapse while on chemotherapy or shortly after the completion of chemotherapy have a low probability of ultimate cure. For patients who have relapses more than 1 year after the completion of chemotherapy, intensive chemotherapy can lead to a 30% to 50% long-term disease-free survival. For children with HLA-identical siblings, an allogenic BMT with a preparatory regimen, such as cyclophosphamide with total body irradiation, may offer the best option for long-term disease-free control. Even allogeneic BMT, however, does not cure most children with recurrent ALL. Thus, prevention of relapse is the preferred strategy.

Autologous BMT (using marrow purged in vitro by monoclonal antibodies or chemotherapeutic agents) or matched unrelated donor BMT provide hope and potential salvage therapy for children without HLA-identical siblings. Research continues into novel conditioning regimens and purging strategies because most patients with relapsed ALL relapse again, even after BMT.

Complications

Most of the complications seen during ALL therapy result from chemotherapeutic side effects. With prednisone administration during induction chemotherapy, most patients develop a cushingoid appearance. Less commonly, symptomatic hypertension and hyperglycemia develop. Rarely, children experience avascular necrosis of the femoral head. After vincristine administration, nerve conduction abnormalities (eg, wrist or foot drop, vocal cord dysfunction, and facial nerve palsies) may develop. In a minority of patients, repetitive administration of methotrexate produces sustained elevations of hepatic transaminases. No correlation has been demonstrated, however, between the level of transaminase elevation and the degree of hepatic fibrosis in liver biopsy specimens. Frank cirrhosis is rare.

As in AML therapy, the prophylactic use of trimethoprim-sulfamethoxazole has virtually eliminated *P carinii* infection from this population. Administration of trimethoprim-sulfamethoxazole 3 days per week is effective in prophylaxis for *P carinii* pneumonia and generally does not produce myelosuppression.

Fortunately, most children with ALL experience no major side effects during treatment. The improved survival of patients with ALL has focused attention on the late effects of antileukemic therapy. Late effects include CNS sequelae, such as intellectual and neurodevelopmental impairment, which can result from intensive CNS therapy or repeated CNS prophylaxis after relapse. CNS irradiation can also lead to neuroendocrine abnormalities, such as short stature and delayed puberty. For patients with ALL, gonadal function is generally normal. The occurrence of secondary malignancies appears to be low, with brain tumors and AML seen most frequently.

PEDIATRIC NON-HODGKIN LYMPHOMA

Non-Hodgkin lymphoma (NHL) accounts for about 10% of pediatric malignancies. NHL in children differs from that in adults. Whereas adult NHL is predominantly nodal in origin, childhood lymphomas are generally extranodal. In addition, childhood NHL is often a generalized disease at diagnosis. These differences may be due to age-related differences in immune system development. These age-related differences may result in variations in the lymphoid cell types at greatest risk for malignant transformation.

Histologic and Cytogenetic Features

The histologic subtypes of pediatric NHL are limited to lymphoblastic lymphoma (generally of T-lymphoid lineage), noncleaved cell lymphoma (including Burkitt lymphoma), and large cell lymphoma (of T-lymphoid or B-lymphoid origin). Well-differentiated lymphoma and chronic lymphocytic leukemia are rarely diagnosed in childhood. NHL results from the malignant transformation of a lymphoid cell that retains self-renewal capacity with an apparent maturation arrest. Also, as in leukemia, chromosomal abnormalities have been identified, and their relation to the malignant transformation is partially elucidated. This includes the classic t(8;14) translocation of Burkitt lymphoma.

Patient Evaluation

Histologic diagnosis and disease extent determine the therapy for childhood NHL.[10] It is extremely important that pathologic specimens be handled properly, so that microscopic, cytochemical, cytogenetic, immunophenotypic, and molecular diagnostic studies can be done. Extensive or mutilative surgical resection is not required with childhood NHL because most cases are responsive to chemotherapy and radiotherapy. Easily resectable low-stage disease should be excised.

The evaluation of the child with suspected NHL begins with a complete physical examination, with all masses and adenopathy measured in at least two dimensions. Radiographic diagnostic tests should include a skeletal survey, chest radiography, CT or magnetic resonance imaging (MRI) of the chest, abdomen, and pelvis, and if indicated, the brain. Blood work should include a complete blood count, serum chemistries with uric acid and lactate dehydrogenase, blood urea nitrogen and creatinine, and liver function tests. Because of the increasing incidence of acquired immunodeficiency syndrome–associated lymphomas, human immunodeficiency virus serologies should be included in a complete evaluation.

Advanced-Stage Lymphoblastic Lymphoma

Patients with advanced-stage lymphoblastic lymphoma or T-cell leukemia present a therapeutic challenge. Many of the children have large mediastinal masses. They often present with superior mediastinal syndrome, with superior venal caval compression, tracheal deviation or compression, and respiratory compromise. Because of the rapid response of these lymphomas to chemotherapy, these patients often benefit from 24 to 48 hours of steroid therapy before subsequent chemotherapy. The steroid therapy is used to shrink the mediastinal mass and to begin cancer cell lysis with less rapid kinetics. Emergency radiotherapy is almost never required, given the rapid response of these lymphomas to chemotherapy. Airway management in this group of patients can be a difficult issue, and it is prudent to reduce the size of large masses before instrumentation. If possible, diagnostic biopsies are done under local anesthesia. These children require careful fluid and electrolyte management to control the often present tumor lysis syndrome.

A POG protocol study of advanced-stage T-cell lymphomas and T-cell leukemias employed an intensive regimen consisting of a 3-month induction consolidation period, followed by a 10-cycle maintenance period, with or without a 20-week course of asparaginase. Triple intrathecal chemotherapy provided CNS prophylaxis. For patients with overt CNS disease at diagnosis, additional triple intrathecal chemotherapy with craniospinal irradiation was given.

Advanced-Stage Large Cell Lymphoma

Most children with advanced-stage large cell lymphoma can be treated successfully with about 1 year of chemotherapy. Intensive induction chemotherapy consists of vincristine, prednisone, doxorubicin, and intrathecal methotrexate, with or without cyclophosphamide. Unless the patient has CNS disease at diagnosis or has residual nodal disease at the completion of induction chemotherapy, radiotherapy is not offered. In the regimen that includes cyclophosphamide, maintenance therapy consists of vincristine, cyclophosphamide, doxorubicin, and prednisone pulses alternating with 6-MP, methotrexate, and prednisone pulses. The maintenance therapy consists of repetitive cycles of vincristine, doxorubicin, and prednisone.[11]

Advanced-Stage Diffuse Undifferentiated Lymphoma

Patients with stage III and IV diffuse undifferentiated (Burkitt type) lymphoma and B-cell leukemia have traditionally had disease that is difficult to cure. Therefore, therapy has intensified, with consequent complications of profound bone marrow hypoplasia, infections, and the need for blood product transfusions. Total B therapy for advanced mature B-cell lymphomas and leukemias consists of four courses of intensive chemotherapy.[12] Each course of therapy consists of two cycles. Cycle 1 includes methotrexate, cytarabine, cyclophosphamide, vincristine, and doxorubicin. Cycle 2 includes a 24-hour infusion of methotrexate with leucovorin rescue, a 48-hour infusion of cytarabine, and CNS prophylaxis provided by intrathecal methotrexate. Pulses of chemotherapy are delivered as soon as the absolute phagocytic count reaches 500/mL and the platelet count reaches 100,000/mL, to avoid rapid tumor regrowth between chemotherapeutic cycles. Hematopoietic growth factors are used to shorten the duration between chemotherapy cycles by enhancing bone marrow recovery. With such intensive chemotherapy, about half of patients achieve long-term disease-free remissions.

Patients with limited-stage (I and II) disease, unlike patients with advanced-stage NHL, may require only induction and short, relatively gentle consolidation chemotherapy for long-term, disease-free survival. Induction and consolidation chemotherapy consists of pulses of vincristine, prednisone, doxorubicin, and cyclophosphamide. Radiotherapy is not employed in these patients because it does not notably improve long-term disease-free survival.[13] The POG is shortening maintenance therapy to less than 3 months of total chemotherapy in certain disease classifications.

HODGKIN DISEASE

Hodgkin disease is primarily the same disease in children and adolescents as it is in adults. Because of growth issues, however, the therapy of Hodgkin disease in children relies more heavily on chemotherapy than radiotherapy.

Histology

It is generally agreed that the malignant cell of Hodgkin disease is the Reed-Sternberg cell. The normal counterpart to this cell is yet to be identified. Unlike leukemias and NHL, no consistent chromosomal abnormality has been identified.

Histologically, Hodgkin disease specimens are often an admixture of apparently normal reactive cells (ie, lymphocytes, plasma cells, and eosinophils) along with the Reed-Sternberg cells. In the Rye classification, Hodgkin disease is divided into the following subgroups: lymphocyte predominance, lymphocyte depletion, mixed cellularity, and nodular sclerosis. With lymphocyte predominance, cellular proliferation in the lymph node often involves benign-appearing lymphocytes with or without histiocytes. In contrast, with lymphocyte depletion, there is a relative scarcity of lymphocytes with a predominance of abnormal cells. Reed-Sternberg cells predominate with an effacement of the lymph node in mixed cellularity Hodgkin disease. Finally, with nodular sclerosis, the lacunar variant of the Reed-Sternberg cell is seen. In addition, involved lymph nodes are often divided by a proliferation of thick collagenous bands.[14]

Patient Evaluation

The clinical evaluation of the child with suspected Hodgkin disease is similar to that for NHL. A complete history of the presenting illness with attention to the presence or absence of constitutional symptoms should begin the evaluation. A detailed physical examination with special emphasis on all nodal areas, including the Waldeyer ring, is essential. All enlarged nodes should be measured in two dimensions. Radiographic diagnostic tests include chest radiography; CT or MRI scans of the high neck, chest abdomen, and pelvis; and gallium scan. Blood work should include that recommended for NHL plus a sedimentation rate, serum copper, and baseline thyroid function studies. A bone marrow aspirate and biopsy should be done.

The diagnosis of Hodgkin disease rests on the lymph node biopsy. As in NHL, it is extremely important that pathologic specimens be handled properly so that lymph node architecture and subtyping can be evaluated. With the high-resolution images obtained by MRI scans, the traditional staging of abdominal laparotomy is an elective procedure that is of greatest value in adolescent patients in whom radiotherapy alone is being considered for treatment. Foregoing a splenectomy greatly reduces the small but finite risk of sepsis that is seen in splenectomized patients.

Staging

The Ann Arbor Staging classification (Table 37-1) is used both in Hodgkin disease and in NHL.[15] It is based on the strong evidence that Hodgkin disease generally spreads from one adjacent nodal area to another until late in the disease course. In the Ann Arbor system, the absence or presence of three signs (temperature higher than 38°C for 3 consecutive days, drenching night sweats, and unexplained loss of over 10% of body weight) are indicated by the suffix letter A or B, respectively. This system bases disease classification on the gross distribution of lymphatic involvement with respect to the diaphragm and, in advanced stages, the presence of organ involvement.

TABLE 37-1. *Ann Arbor staging classification for Hodgkin disease*

Stage*	Definition
I	Involvement of a single lymph node region (I) or of a single extralymphatic organ or site (I$_E$)
II	Involvement of two or more lymph node regions on the same side of the diaphragm (II) or localized involvement of an extralymphatic organ or site and one or more lymph node regions on the same side of the diaphragm (II$_E$)
III	Involvement of lymph node regions on both sides of the diaphragm (III), which may be accompanied by involvement of the spleen (III$_S$) or by localized involvement of an extralymphatic organ or site (III$_E$) or both (III$_{SE}$)
IV	Diffuse or disseminated involvement of one or more extralymphatic organs or tissue with or without associated lymph node involvement

* The absence or presence of temperature over 38°C for 3 consecutive days, drenching night sweats, or unexplained loss of 10% or more of body weight in the 6 months preceding admission are to be denoted in all cases by the suffix A or B, respectively.

Treatment

The treatment of all stages of Hodgkin disease is highly successful, with 75% to 85% of all patients achieving long-term disease-free survival. POG is studying the addition of adjuvant doses of radiotherapy to multiagent chemotherapy, with the goal of improving the long-term disease-free survival and reducing late effects of therapy. Therapeutic doses of radiation can inhibit the growth of immature bones and tissues and contribute to the development of secondary malignancies in patients with Hodgkin disease. If long-term disease-free survival could be maintained, it would be highly desirable to minimize or totally eliminate radiotherapy in the growing child with Hodgkin disease.

The chemotherapy used in young patients with Hodgkin disease also has potential late effects. Bleomycin can cause pulmonary fibrosis that may be exacerbated by pulmonary radiotherapy. Anthracycline use, with or without chest irradiation, may result in myocardial damage and ultimately heart failure. The administration of six cycles of nitrogen mustard, vincristine, procarbazine, and prednisone causes uniform male sterility, while sparing the hormonal activity of the testes. Menarcheal women may experience infertility, irregular menses, and early menopause after effective Hodgkin disease therapy. The alkylating agents used in chemotherapeutic regimens are thought to be responsible, along with radiotherapy, for the increased risk for secondary malignancies in children with Hodgkin disease. The childhood survivors are at increased risk for AML and its precursor, myelodysplastic syndrome.

REFERENCES

1. Grier H, Civin C. Acute and chronic myeloproliferative disorders and myelodysplasia. In: Nathan DG, Oski FA, eds. Hematology of infancy and childhood, ed 4. Philadelphia, WB Saunders, 1993:1288.

2. Steuber C, Krischer J, Culbert S. Prognostic factors and treatment outcome in childhood acute myeloid leukemia (AML): the POG experience. In: Gale R, ed. Acute myelogenous leukemia: progress and controversies. New York, Wiley-Liss, 1990:193.

3. Ravindranath Y, Steuber CP, Krischer J, et al.: High-dose cytarabine for intensification of early therapy of childhood acute myeloid leukemia: a Pediatric Oncology Group study. J Clin Oncol 1991;9:572.

4. Yeager AM, Kaizer H, Santos GW, et al. Autologous bone marrow transplantation in patients with acute nonlymphocytic leukemias, using ex vivo marrow treatment with 4-hydroperoxycyclophosphamide. N Engl J Med 1986;315:141.

5. Zittoun R, Mandelli F, Willemze R, et al. Autologous or allogeneic bone marrow transplantation compared with intensive chemotherapy in acute myelogenous leukemia. N Engl J Med 1994;332:217.

6. Pui CH, Behm FG, Crist WM. Clinical and biologic relevance of immunologic marker studies in childhood acute lymphoblastic leukemia. Blood 1993;82:343.

7. Pochedly C, Civin C. Childhood acute lymphoblastic leukemia, parts I and II. Hematol Oncol Clin North Am 1986;4,5.

8. Camitta B, Leventhal B, Lauer S. Intermediate dose methotrexate and 6-mercaptopurine therapy for non-T, non-B acute lymphocytic leukemia in childhood: a Pediatric Oncology Group study. J Clin Oncol 1989;7:1539.

9. Campana D, Pui CH. Detection of minimal residual disease in acute leukemia: methodologic advances and clinical significance. Blood 1995;85:1416.

10. Hvizdala E, Berard T, Callihan T. Nonlymphoblastic lymphoma in children—histology and stage related response to therapy: a Pediatric Oncology Group Study. J Clin Oncol 1991;9:1189.

11. Weinstein H, Lack E, Cassady J. APO therapy for malignant lymphoma of large cell ''histiocytic'' type of childhood: analysis of treatment results of 29 patients. Blood 1989;64:422.

12. Murphy S, Bowman W, Abromowitch M. Results of treatment of advanced-stage Burkitt's lymphoma and B-cell (Slg +) acute lymphoblastic leukemia with high-dose fractionated cyclophosphamide and coordinated high-dose methotrexate and cytarabine. J Clin Oncol 1986;4:1732.

13. Link M, Donaldson S, Berard C. Results of treatment of childhood localized non-Hodgkin's lymphoma with combination chemotherapy with or without radiotherapy. N Engl J Med 1990;322:1169.

14. Leventhal B, Donaldson S. Hodgkin's disease. In: Pizzo P, Poplack D, eds. Principles and practice of pediatric oncology. Philadelphia, JB Lippincott, 1993:577.

15. Carbone P, Kaplan H, Husshoff K. Report of the committee on Hodgkin's disease staging classification. Cancer Res 1971;31:1860.

Surgery of Infants and Children: Scientific Principles and Practice, edited by
Keith T. Oldham, Paul M. Colombani, and Robert P. Foglia.
Lippincott–Raven Publishers, Philadelphia, © 1997.

CHAPTER 38

Germ Cell Tumors

Michael A. Skinner

One of the great mysteries of human embryology is how the single-cell pluripotential zygote, formed by the union of two germ cells, is able to differentiate into the multiplicity of different tissues seen in the fully developed human. This genetic versatility is in contrast to the equally fascinating notion that in the fully developed organism, while each cell in the body contains every gene, relatively few of these genes are actually expressed within a particular tissue type. Clearly, at some point during embryonic development, a regulatory process is initiated to ensure the expression of only those genes actually necessary for the formation and function of a particular organ.

This genetic regulation is circumvented in tumors that arise from primitive germ cells. These neoplasms appear to recapitulate some aspects of embryonic development, so that they can be composed of a mixture of tissue types representative of many different organs in various stages of maturity. This fascinating aspect of germ cell neoplasms distinguishes them from other pediatric tumors.

Although germ cell tumors most commonly arise in the germ cells located within the gonads, they can originate in other sites as well. In this chapter, emphasis is placed on extragonadal germ cell neoplasms; tumors of the ovaries and testes are discussed in greater detail elsewhere in this volume.

EPIDEMIOLOGY

Germ cell tumors account for about 3% of neoplasms in children and adolescents. Because of the bias in pediatric centers toward the treatment of malignant tumors, it has been difficult to determine the overall incidence of these neoplasms; the number of benign lesions has typically been underrepresented in large published series. Based on recent population-based studies, germ cell tumors in all locations have been estimated to occur at an incidence of about 4 to 6 cases per 1 million children.[1] The report from the Children's Tumor Registry in Manchester, England, noted that the incidence of these tumors has significantly increased during the past three decades.[2]

About 25% to 33% of germ cell neoplasms are malignant, and the ratio of female patients to male patients is roughly 3:1 in children younger than the age of 15 years. In large population-based studies, the mean age of the patients at the time of diagno-

sis varies according to the anatomic location.[3,4] Ovarian tumors are diagnosed in girls at a mean age of about 10 to 12 years, while testicular lesions in children occur at a mean age of roughly 2 years. Most sacrococcygeal tumors are seen in early infancy, but they rarely can develop as late as adolescence. Most mediastinal and retroperitoneal germ cell tumors are diagnosed after the age of 2 years.

Risk factors for the development of gonadal germ cell neoplasms include the presence of dysgenetic gonads, a family history of the disease, and cryptorchid testes.[1] Most germ cell neoplasms, however, occur in the absence of these findings. Klinefelter syndrome has been strongly associated with the presence of extragonadal tumors, especially of the mediastinum. There has been speculation about the possibility that germ cell tumors may be a rare manifestation of the Li-Fraumeni syndrome. Although no firm data link any maternal factors with the subsequent formation of germ cell tumors, the presence of an infection during pregnancy has been implicated.[2] Also, there appears to be a higher incidence of these tumors among twins.

EMBRYOLOGY, PATHOLOGY, AND ANATOMY

Germ cell neoplasms are thought to originate from the primordial germ cells. Embryologically, these cells become visible during the fourth week of gestation as they form in the yolk sac near the origin of the allantois. As the craniocaudal fold of the embryo forms, the dorsal portion of the yolk sac is internalized. During this process, the primitive germ cells migrate through the dorsal mesentery of the hindgut to rest in the gonadal ridges, where they ultimately reside in the developing gonad. For unknown reasons, these cells occasionally miss their proper destination and, if transformed, can multiply in an extragonadal location. These locations are usually somewhere in the midline, ranging from the sacrococcygeum to an intracranial site.

The histologic classification of pediatric germ cell tumors follows:

- Germinoma
- Teratoma
  Mature
  Immature

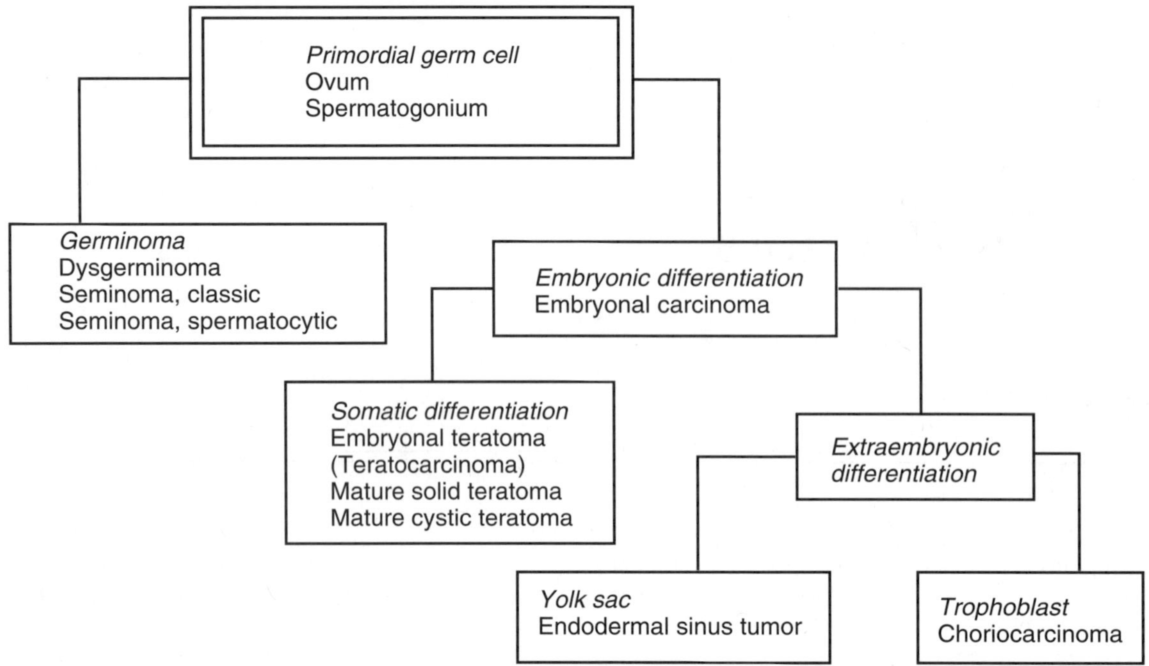

FIG. 38-1. Diagram showing the derivation of different germ cell tumor subtypes. (After Dehner LP, ed. Pediatric pathology, ed 2. Baltimore, Williams & Wilkins, 1987:764)

- Embryonal carcinoma
- Yolk sac tumor (endodermal sinus tumor)
- Choriocarcinoma
- Gonadoblastoma
- Mixed germ cell tumor

An understanding of the various differentiation pathways available to the pediatric germ cell is helpful in comprehending the nomenclature of these pathologic subtypes. First, recall that the embryo is not the only product of gestation. Rather, three separate types of gestational tissue are derived from the embryonic zygote, which is itself formed by the fusion of the male and female germ cells. These three tissue types are the yolk sac, the placenta and its chorionic membranes, and the fetus. A germ cell neoplasm can recapitulate any of these organ systems.

For example, as illustrated in Figure 38-1, a primordial germ cell can become transformed before undergoing any further differentiation, resulting in a pure germ cell tumor. Such a lesion is called a *seminoma* if in the testes, *dysgerminoma* in the ovary, or *germinoma* if arising in an extragonadal site. Alternatively, the primordial germ cell can exhibit some differentiation into one of the three gestational elements before transformation. In cases in which differentiation into somatic elements occurs, tissue from one or more of the embryonic somatic cell layers exists, and a teratoma is seen. Cells that differentiate along extraembryonic lines can recapitulate tissue reminiscent of trophoblast, leading to the formation of a choriocarcinoma. Finally, a yolk sac tumor, also called an *endodermal sinus tumor,* can result from the malignant transformation of a germ cell into the yolk sac gestational elements. The yolk sac tumor is the most common form of malignant germ cell neoplasm found in children.

Historically, pathologists have demanded that tissues from each of the three somatic cell layers be recognized before a tumor is classified as a teratoma. This requirement has been relaxed, and most pathologists now require the presence of only two embryonic layers in these tumors. In rare cases, teratomas contain elements from only one somatic layer. Histologically, teratomas are further classified according their stage of immaturity, which is the degree to which they recapitulate undifferentiated fetal tissues as opposed to mature somatic tissue. A commonly used grading system is shown in Table 38-1. In general, the more immature the cells are, the more aggressively the tumor behaves. Overall, most teratomas below grade 3 act benignly, but it is impossible to predict precisely how individual tumors will behave. In very young patients, such as newborns, the presence of immature fetal tissue is to be expected and is of little prognostic significance. The malignant potential and clinical behavior of a teratoma are related less to the histologic maturity than to the presence of adjacent frankly malignant germ cell elements within the tumor; such tissue is from one of the other malignant subtypes listed earlier.

TABLE 38-1. *Histologic grading of teratomas*

Grade	Characteristics
0	All mature tissues with absent or rare mitotic activity
1	Some immaturity with absent or very limited neuroepithelium (1 focus per slide)
2	Greater immaturity than in grade 1 with small amount of neuroepithelium (2–3 per 40× microscopic fields per slide)
3 (immature)	Greater immaturity than in grade 2 with more neuroepithelium

(Norris HJ, Zirkin HJ, Benson WL. Immature [malignant] teratoma of the ovary: a clinical and pathological study of 58 cases. Cancer 1976;37:2359)

TABLE 38-2. *Site and histologic distribution of 170 pediatric germ cell tumors from the Federal Republic of Germany pediatric tumor registry, 1966–1984*

Site	Pathologic subtype						Number of tumors	Percentage of tumors germ cell
	Teratoma	YST	EC	Germ	Mixed	Chorio		
Ovary	27	7	0	9	7	0	50	29
Testicle	14	18	1	1	8	0	42	25
Sacrococcygeum	20	10	0	0	8	0	38	22
Cervix	9	0	0	0	1	0	10	6
CNS	0	1	0	5	1	2	9	5
Retroperitoneum	4	2	1	0	1	0	8	5
Mediastinum	5	1	0	1	0	0	7	4
Other	3	1	2	0	0	0	6	4
TOTAL	82	40	4	16	26	2	170	100

YST, yolk sac tumor; EC, embryonal carcinoma; germ, germinoma; mixed, mixed germ cell tumor; chorio, choriocarcinoma.
(Data from Harms D, Janig U. Germ cell tumors of childhood. Virchows Arch [A] 1986;409:223)

The pathologic subtypes and sites of origin in 170 germ cell tumors from the Federal Republic of Germany Tumor Registry are shown in Table 38-2.[5] As shown in this population-based series, teratomas are the most common histologic subtype among extragonadal germ cell tumors. These lesions usually arise in the sacral region, the mediastinum, peritoneum, and intracranially. Rarely, these neoplasms appear in the stomach, the liver, or within the urinary tract. About 25% of teratomas are malignant; a histologic example is shown in Figure 38-2. Although any form of germ cell malignancy can be seen in association with a teratoma, the yolk sac or endodermal sinus tumor is present most frequently.

The unequivocally malignant germ cell tumors, as shown in Figure 38-3, range from the usually well-behaved germinomas to the very aggressive choriocarcinomas. In about 11% of malignant germ cell tumors, excluding teratomas, more than one pathologic subtype is seen. Germinomas occur most frequently within gonadal sites or in the pineal region of the central nervous system. Pure yolk sac tumors are found most frequently in the ovaries, testes, or sacral region. This pathologic subtype also is commonly seen with sacrococcygeal teratomas. Embryonal carcinomas are rare and usually arise in the testes. Gonadoblastoma, which acts like a benign lesion, occurs almost exclusively in dysgenetic gonads in association with the XY genotype.[1] In about 25% of these cases, there is an associated focus of malignant germinoma.

GENETIC ASPECTS AND SERUM MARKERS

As with any neoplasm, the primary initiating factor in the formation of germ cell tumors is a genetic one; one or a number of genes are abnormally expressed to cause unchecked growth of the tumor. Alternatively, there is the absence of some gene expression that would normally serve to control cellular replication. In many tumors, alterations in the chromosomes have provided valuable clues for determining which genes may be important in the genesis or progression of the neoplasm. For example, tumor-suppressor genes have been located in regions of the genome that are absent in the tumor when compared with

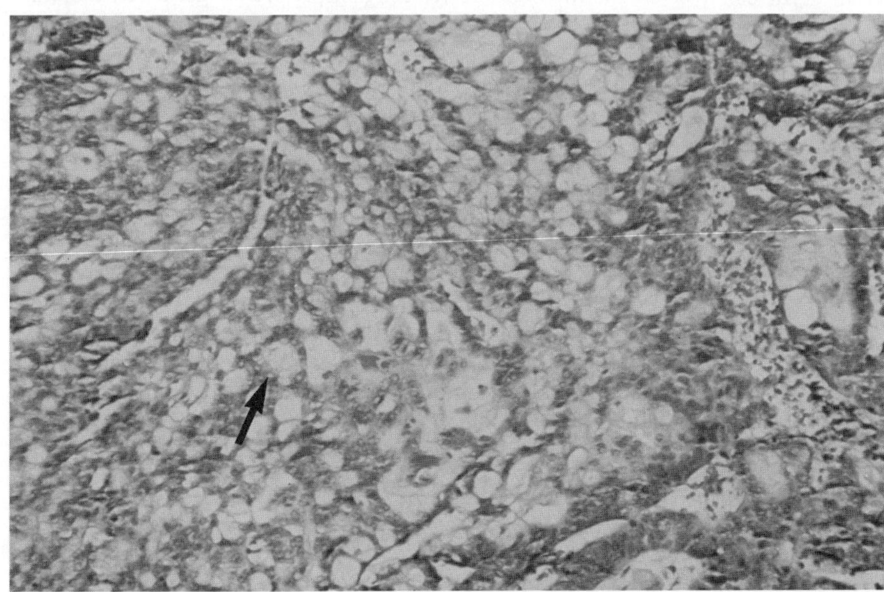

FIG. 38-2. Histologic section demonstrating malignant yolk sac (endodermal sinus tumor elements within a teratoma). This is the microcystic histologic subtype, and the arrow indicates a characteristic hyaline globule. (Courtesy of M. Collins, MD, Department of Pathology, Indiana University School of Medicine, Indianapolis)

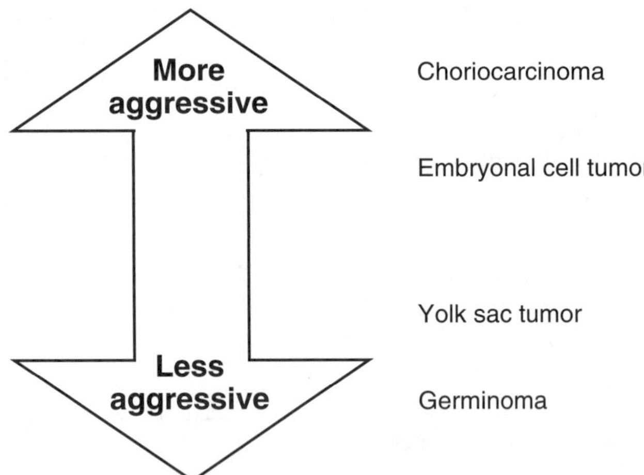

FIG. 38-3. The relative aggressiveness of germ cell tumor pathologic subtypes.

TABLE 38-3. *Normal infant serum α-fetoprotein (AFP) levels at various ages*

Age	Mean AFP (ng/mL)
Premature	134,000
Newborn	48,000
Newborn to 2 wk	33,000
2 wk–1 mo	9,500
2 mo	323
3 mo	88
4 mo	74
5 mo	47
6 mo	13
8 mo	8.5

(Data from Wu JT, Book L, Sudar K. Serum α-fetoprotein [AFP] levels in normal infants. Pediatr Res 1981;15:50)

normal tissue. Usually, a region of one chromosome is missing, leading to the loss of heterozygosity, as demonstrated by informative genetic markers. In other cases, there is the amplification, or an increase in the copy number, of a particular gene in the tumor. This is the case in some neuroblastomas, in which the amplification of the *N-myc* oncogene is a marker of more aggressive tumor biology.

Investigators have examined the chromosomes of germ cell tumors in the hope of finding clues to the molecular pathogenesis of this disease. In cultured cell lines, nonrandom abnormalities of chromosomes 1 and 12 have been observed. Further, in studies of resected gonadal and extragonadal germ cell tumors, gains of genetic material in chromosomes 1, 7, 12, 21, 22, or 6 were seen in more than of 70% of cases.[6] Other investigators have found consistent genetic rearrangements of chromosomes 1, 12, and 17 in seminomas. Further, loss of heterozygosity has been reported on chromosome 12. In assays of known oncogenes, no consistent abnormalities have been seen in germ cell tumors.

The most consistent cytogenetic abnormality in germ cell neoplasms is amplification in a region of the short arm of chromosome 12. This finding has been termed an *isochromosome,* designated i(12p), and was seen in more than 80% of tumors in some series.[7] Isochromosomes have been noted in tumors of all cell types, and it has been suggested that increased i(12p) copy number may be associated with more aggressive tumors. Further, the abnormality appears to be a relatively specific cytogenetic marker for germ cell tumors because it is seen infrequently in other neoplasms. The high frequency of i(12p) in these tumors provides strong evidence that a gene important in the differentiation or growth of germ cells resides on chromosome 12. How the abnormalities in this segment of the genome influence the initiation or progression of germ cell tumors is unknown.

Some germ cell tumors produce and secrete protein products that can be measured in the serum. For example, yolk sac tumors often produce α-fetoprotein (AFP) because the yolk sac is the source of this factor during early embryogenesis. The serum level of this product can also be elevated in patients who have embryonal carcinoma. After complete resection of an AFP-pro-

ducing tumor, the serum level of the protein should drop at a rate reflecting its normal half-life, which is about 4 days.[8] The AFP level can then be measured serially to monitor for recurrence of the tumor. In newborns, the use of AFP in this manner is somewhat complicated because the AFP is normally high in neonates. Reference values for AFP at various ages are shown in Table 38-3.

Another important serum factor produced by germ cell neoplasms is β-human chorionic gonadotropin (β-hCG). Normally produced by the placenta after the successful implantation of the fertilized egg, β-hCG is a marker for germ cell neoplasms that have trophoblastic elements. Choriocarcinomas invariably produce this protein, and the marker is useful both in making the initial diagnosis and in follow-up after surgical treatment. The serum marker placental alkaline phosphatase level has been reported to be elevated in about 60% of patients with stage I testicular seminoma and in 100% patients with stage II or III disease.[9] The levels normalize after orchiectomy, suggesting that this marker may be useful in the early detection of disease recurrence. The usefulness of placental alkaline phosphatase levels in the clinical management of extragonadal germinomas has not been well studied. Finally, another serum marker that is often elevated in germinomas is lactate dehydrogenase, but this is finding is relatively nonspecific for germ cell tumors.

CLINICAL ASPECTS OF EXTRAGONADAL GERM CELL TUMORS

Germ cell tumors arise from pluripotential germ cells located throughout the body. Anatomically, the tumors can occur either within the gonads or extragonadally. In clinical series in which pediatric germ cell tumors of all locations and pathologic subtypes were tabulated, about 45% to 50% of the lesions were gonadal in location; the remainder occurred within the soft tissues in various other parts of the body[1,3,5] (see Table 38-2). The focus of this chapter is on extragonadal germ cell tumors; tumors arising from the ovaries and testes are discussed elsewhere.

Sacrococcygeal Germ Cell Neoplasms

The sacrococcygeum is the most common location for nongonadal germ cell tumors, accounting for 32% to 66% of the total in various large clinical series. Furthermore, this is the most common tumor in the newborn period, occurring in about 1 in 35,000 births. These tumors generally present clinically as a large exophytic midline mass located posterior to the sacrum (Fig. 38-4). The anus is usually displaced anteriorly, depending on the size of the tumor. In a report by Altman and associates,[10] in which the members of the Surgical Section of the American Academy of Pediatrics (AAP) were surveyed, data from 405 cases were tabulated. The most commonly used anatomic classification system for sacrococcygeal teratomas was first presented in this report (Fig. 38-5). The percentage of tumors presenting in each class, as reported in this study and in a much smaller population-based study from Sweden, are tabulated in Table 38-4.

The differential diagnosis for masses in the sacral region of the newborn includes teratoma, lipoma, meningocele, dermoid cyst, and a host of other tumors or malformations. It is important to distinguish a tumor from lesions that can communicate with the spinal canal, such as meningoceles and lipomeningoceles. These malformations can arise proximal to the sacrum along the spine and are often covered with a dural membrane rather than skin. Plain spine radiographs may reveal a bony defect, suggesting a dural communication.

Associated congenital anomalies are seen in about 20% of patients who have sacrococcygeal teratomas.[2,4,10] The anomalies are usually musculoskeletal in origin, but also present are abnormalities of the kidneys, central nervous system, heart, and alimentary tract. In addition, the Currarino triad can be associated with a teratoma.[11] This syndrome, inherited in an autosomal dominant manner, consists of a presacral tumor, anorectal stenosis, and sacral bony abnormalities (Fig. 38-6). The Currarino triad is rare; fewer than 100 patients have been reported. In about one third of cases, the presacral mass is a teratoma; also seen are lipomeningoceles, meningoceles, and epidermoid cysts. Typically, the patients present with severe constipation, which may resolve after removal of the tumor. The author saw

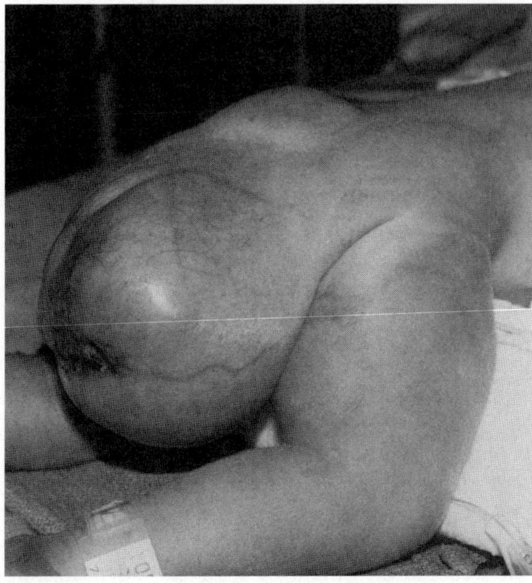

FIG. 38-4. Typical sacrococcygeal teratoma, demonstrating a large mass with anterior deviation of the anus. This very large tumor also exhibits ulceration of the overlying skin.

this syndrome in a patient who was initially referred for evaluation of presumed Hirschsprung disease. This underscores the importance of a digital rectal examination in these children to evaluate the presacral region. In some of these children, anal atresia or stenosis requiring surgical treatment is the presenting diagnosis.

In the AAP survey, 60% of sacrococcygeal teratomas were diagnosed at birth, and only about 6% came to clinical attention after the age of 2 years.[10] Aside from the obvious tumor, other associated signs and symptoms are high-output heart failure due to vascular shunting through the tumor and, rarely, evidence of disseminated intravascular coagulation in infants with large, bleeding lesions. In these cases, an emergency operation may be necessary to remove the tumor and prevent exsanguination. Finally, birth dystocia occasionally is seen owing to the tumor bulk, and some investigators have reported that as many as 25% of sacrococcygeal teratomas are discovered on antenatal sonogram.[12] This is a potentially important indication for cesarean delivery. AAP anatomic class II and IV tumors, with their reduced external bulk, are usually among the later diagnosed lesions. Symptoms of neoplasms located entirely within the pelvis or abdomen are often indirect and can include constipation, urinary retention, decreased appetite, and failure to thrive.

Radiologic evaluation should begin with anteroposterior and lateral radiographs of the pelvis and spine. Calcifications are a frequent finding in teratomas; these can be diffuse and stippled or dense and recognizable as a partially formed bone or tooth. In general, calcifications are less common in frankly malignant lesions. The sacral spine may reveal a defect, suggesting invasion of the spinal canal by the tumor or that the lesion is not a teratoma but rather some anomaly of the spinal cord. Ultrasonography, computed tomography, or magnetic resonance imaging can be useful in determining the pelvic and abdominal extent of the tumor as well as its anatomic relation to adjacent structures (Fig. 38-7). Magnetic resonance imaging is particularly useful in evaluating infiltration into the spinal canal.

In most large clinical series of sacrococcygeal teratomas, about 80% of the tumors are benign.[3,4,5,12,13] About 20% to 25% of these benign tumors contain immature elements. Malignant tumors are slightly more common in boys, and as with teratomas in other locations, the malignancy stems from other germ cell elements residing with the teratoma. These are most commonly of the yolk sac (endodermal sinus tumor) but can also be composed of embryonal carcinoma or undifferentiated germ cell malignancy. Elements of germinoma or choriocarcinoma are rare. Occasionally, a pure sacrococcygeal yolk sac tumor is seen, with no associated teratoma. The presence of a malignant component is commonly associated with elevated serum AFP levels.

The incidence of tumor malignancy is significantly related to the age of the patient at the time of diagnosis.[10] When the tumor is found before the age of 1 month, the risk of malignancy is about 5%. Between 1 and 12 months of age, the malignancy rate is about 60%, and in children older than 1 year of age, over 75% of germ cell tumors of the sacral region are malignant. The increasing frequency of malignancy with age parallels the higher AAP anatomic class seen in older children (Table 38-5).

In most cases, surgery is the principal mode of treatment for sacrococcygeal teratomas. In neonates, every attempt should be made to remove the lesion completely within the first week of

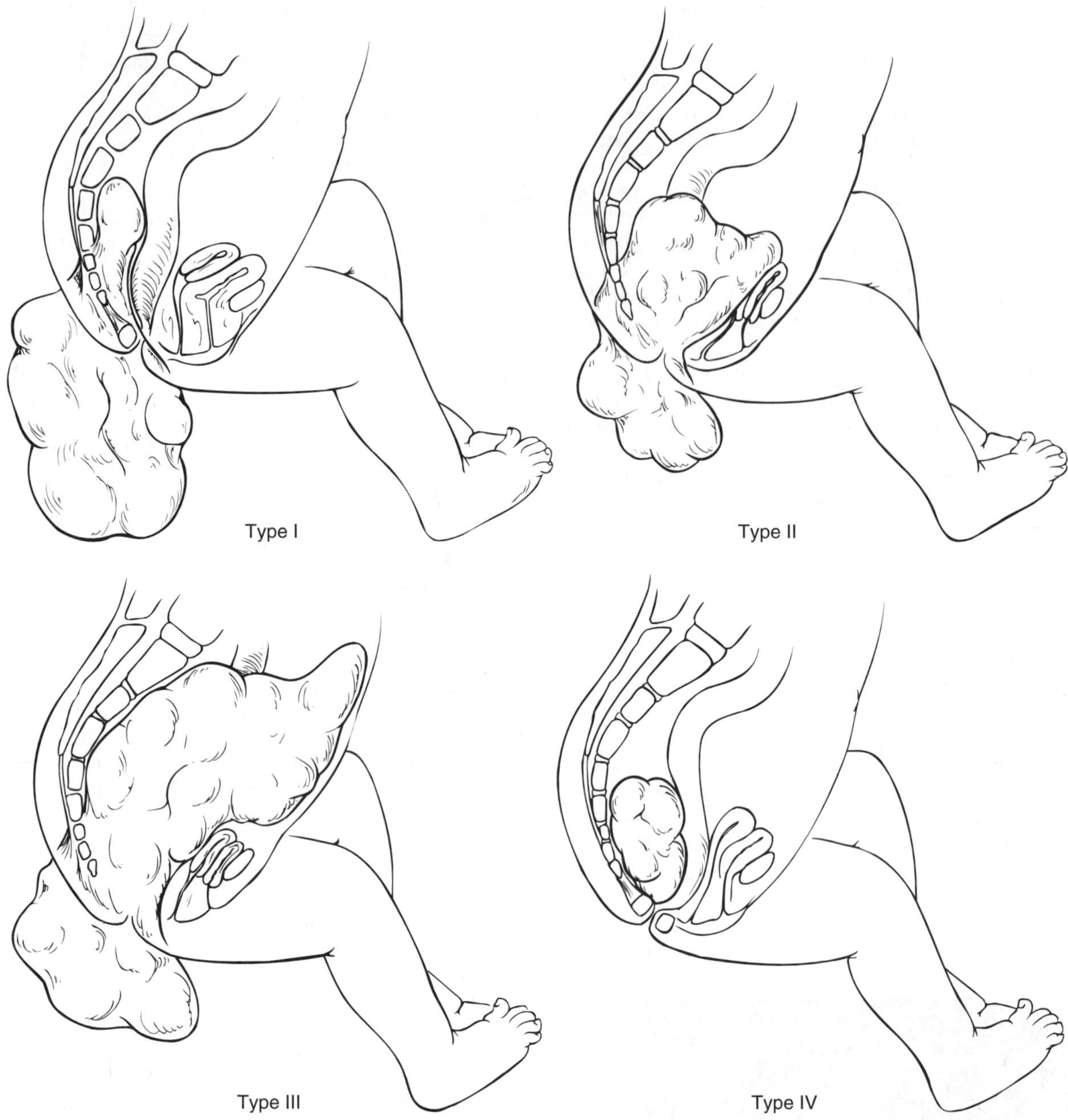

FIG. 38-5. Anatomic classification of sacrococcygeal teratomas. (After Altman RP, Randolph JG, Lilly JR. Sacrococcygeal teratoma: American Academy of Pediatrics surgical section survey—1973. J Pediatr Surg 1974;9:391)

life. For tumors whose major component is located outside the pelvis and abdomen, the patient should be placed in the prone position. A chevron type of incision is made (Fig. 38-8) to allow resection of an amount of skin appropriate for a cosmetically acceptable closure. The tumor is removed after raising skin flaps around the mass superiorly and inferiorly. The sacral artery should be ligated early to reduce blood loss, and the coccyx should be removed. Failure to remove the coccyx results in a local tumor recurrence rate of about 37%. Care should be taken to avoid injury to the anus and rectum, and a surgical sponge can be placed into the anus at the beginning of the operation to aid in the recognition of the rectum during the dissection.

After removal of the tumor, the levator anatomy is reconstructed by suturing the rectum to the presacral fascia. Most pediatric surgeons place drains under the skin flaps to prevent fluid accumulation.

About half of sacrococcygeal teratomas have a significant pelvic or abdominal component (AAP classes II and III), and about 15% of such lesions are entirely presacral, with no external component (AAP class IV).[10] In these cases, it may be preferable to begin the operation with the patient in the supine position, and to start the dissection in the abdomen. The sacral artery can be easily ligated at its origin, and the tumor can be mobilized in the pelvis before beginning the external portion

TABLE 38-4. *Frequency of sacrococcygeal teratoma presentation and the American Academy of Pediatrics anatomic classifications*

Anatomic classification	Frequency (%)	
	AAP survey	Swedish study
I	47	28
II	34	44
III	9	16
IV	10	12

(Data from Altman RP, Randolph JG, Lilly JR. Sacrococcygeal teratoma: American Academy of Pediatrics Surgical Section survey—1973. J Pediatr Surg 1974;9:389; and Havranek P, Rubenson A, Guth D, et al. Sacrococcygeal teratomas in Sweden: a 10-year retrospective study. J Pediatr Surg 1992; 27:1447)

of the operation. In large clinical series, more than 90% of class I sacrococcygeal neoplasms have been successfully removed at the initial operation. Primary surgical resection has been less successful when there is a large abdominal component (AAP classes II, III, and IV). This reflects the increased frequency of malignant histology in these lesions, which may be related to a delay in diagnosis. In any case, most malignant sacrococcygeal neoplasms with extension into the pelvis exhibit local invasion into the sacrum or other structures that precludes complete resection. Moreover, about 5% of patients with sacrococcygeal neoplasms have metastatic disease at the time of diagnosis. Sites of spread include lung, liver, brain, and peritoneum.[10] Metastasis is far more likely in the older child and is rare in the newborn.

As expected, the outcome for children with sacrococcygeal neoplasms is related to the presence of malignancy within the lesion and the stage of disease at diagnosis:

Stage I—complete tumor resection with negative tumor margins; positive markers fall to normal; negative lymph nodes

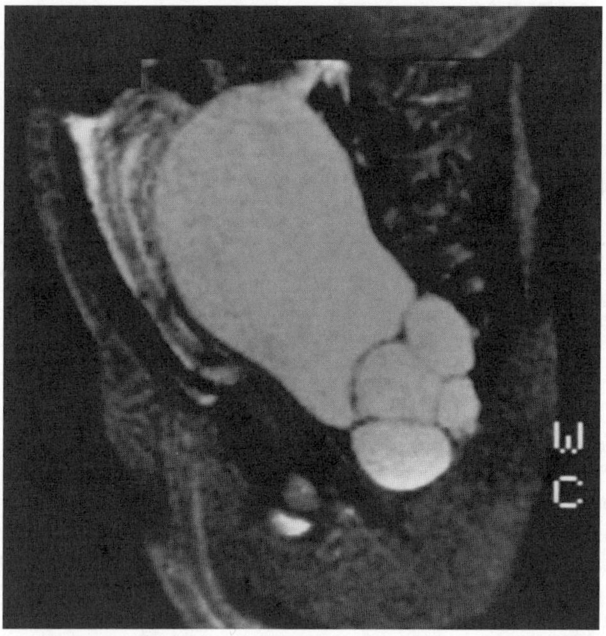

FIG. 38-7. MR image showing the abdominal extent of a presacral teratoma.

Stage II—microscopic residual disease; negative lymph nodes; positive or negative tumor markers
Stage III—gross residual disease or biopsy only; nodes positive or negative
Stage IV—distant metastases

Surgical resection is curative in most benign tumors. The long-term survival rate of neonates after surgery is 92% to 95%; most of the mortality relates to coincident birth anomalies or to hemorrhage during the operation. Because malignancy is uncommon, mortality related to the recurrence of disease is unu-

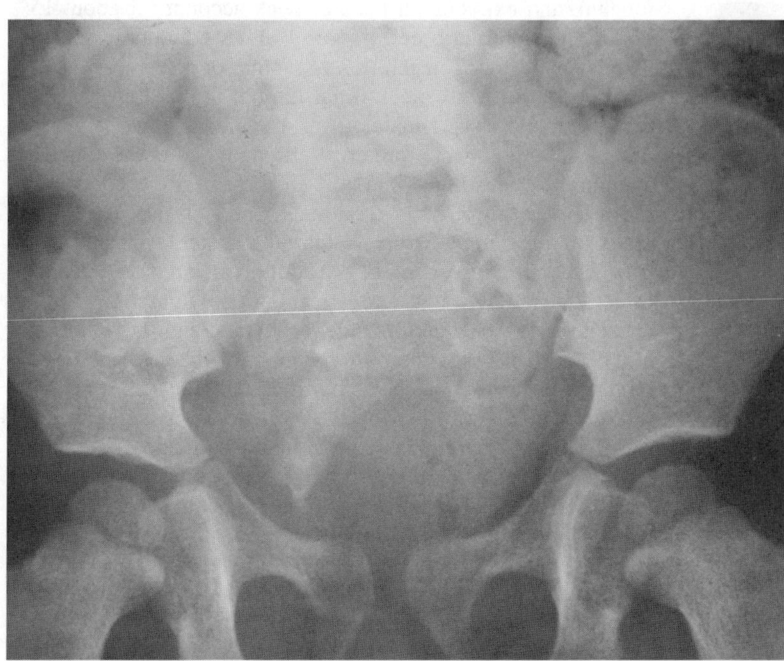

FIG. 38-6. Spinal radiograph of a patient who has the Currarino triad, demonstrating the typical sacral bony abnormality. (Courtesy of L.D. Narla, MD, Medical College of Virginia, Richmond)

TABLE 38-5. *Incidence of sacrococcygeal teratoma malignancy at different American Academy of Pediatrics anatomic classifications*

AAP classification	Percentage malignant
I	8
II	21
III	34
IV	38

(Data from Altman RP, Randolph JG, Lilly JR. Sacrococcygeal teratoma: American Academy of Pediatrics Surgical Section survey—1973. J Pediatr Surg 1974;9:389)

sual. In older children, there is a higher incidence of malignancy, and the survival rate decreases. In the AAP survey, only 45% of patients older than 2 years of age at diagnosis survived long-term. In another review of malignant tumors, the survival rate was a dismal 20%.[14] The patients in these studies, however, were treated before the routine use of multiagent chemotherapy; the use of adjuvant modalities in the treatment of germ cell tumors appears to improve survival and is discussed later.

As many as 23% of immature teratomas recur after surgical resection.[14,15] These recurrences usually are local, but distant metastases may be seen. Risk factors for recurrence include age greater than 1 year and an elevated serum AFP level at the time of diagnosis. In one study, three of four patients with elevation of this serum factor had tumor recurrence, while no recurrence was seen in eight patients whose immature teratomas were associated with normal serum AFP levels.[15] Elevation of AFP is probably an indicator of malignancy, and patients with this finding may benefit from multiagent chemotherapy even if extensive histologic sampling of the tumor fails to reveal malignant elements.

Finally, it is well known that in rare cases, an unequivocally benign sacrococcygeal teratoma can recur as a malignancy after

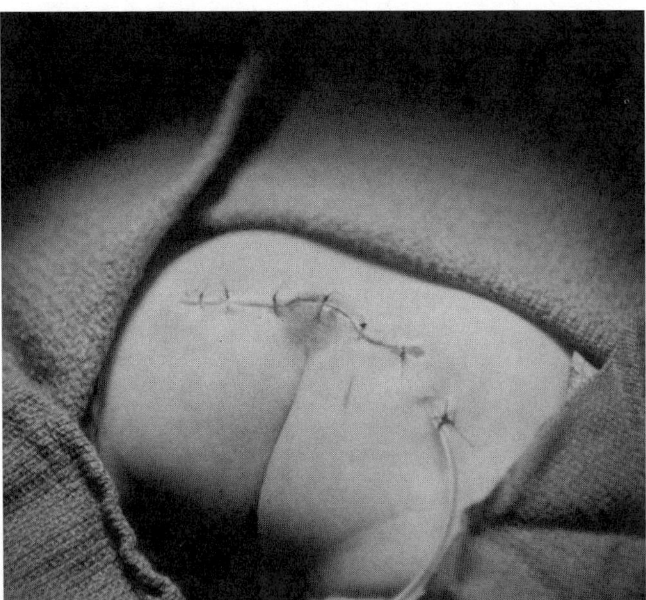

FIG. 38-8. Wound closure after resection of a sacrococcygeal teratoma.

successful removal. This occurs in about 3% to 10% of cases and usually is noted 6 to 33 months after the initial resection.[16] Case reports have documented this event as late as adulthood. Unfortunately, the recurrent tumor can be metastatic to distant sites when discovered, which underscores the importance of clinical follow-up in these patients. Serum AFP should be monitored and frequent rectal examinations performed to detect presacral recurrence as early as possible. Close follow-up of is especially important in patients with immature teratomas, which have an increased recurrence rate. If possible, the recurrent tumor mass should be resected surgically, and the patient should be treated with multiagent chemotherapy.

Functional complications can be seen after the successful removal of a sacrococcygeal tumor. In one population-based report, about 25% of the children older than 3 years of age experienced fecal soiling.[17] Some of these children demonstrated abnormalities when they were studied anomanometrically. Also, 16% of the patients had urinary incontinence, and a minority of these required intermittent clean catheterization to excrete urine. In another report, urodynamic studies were performed on children who had urinary tract dysfunction after removal of the sacrococcygeal neoplasm.[18] A neurogenic cause of the dysfunction was demonstrated in 82% of these children; the authors attributed this to pelvic nerve injury during the surgical dissection. Finally, these children rarely exhibit lower limb weakness from sciatic nerve palsy. Although each of these functional problems theoretically should be more common after resection of tumors with large intrapelvic components, this has not consistently been the case. Some of these problems were seen in patients after the otherwise uncomplicated removal of class I sacrococcygeal teratomas. These complications underscore the fact that children should be followed for several years after surgery to ensure normal bowel and bladder development.

Germ Cell Neoplasms in Other Sites

Germ cell neoplasms that arise in the mediastinum, retroperitoneum, and extracranial head or neck account for about 15% of extragonadal germ cell tumors.[3,5] Less commonly seen are neoplasms in the stomach, liver, vagina, or elsewhere.

About 20% of all mediastinal tumors in children are germ cell tumors; in large clinical series, the mediastinum is the second most common site for germ cell tumors, after the sacrococcygeum.[19] Occurring principally in the anterior mediastinum, these lesions are usually teratomas, and only about 20% are malignant. Rarely, they originate in the posterior mediastinum. They can present from infancy to adulthood, but most childhood tumors are diagnosed at 1 to 3 years of age. Symptoms usually relate to the airway and include dyspnea, coughing, wheezing, and chest pain. As with any large anterior mediastinal mass in children, the airway can be compromised by the loss of negative intrathoracic pressure during the induction of general anesthesia. Therefore, careful assessment of the trachea is essential before surgery. As with sacrococcygeal neoplasms, the benign lesions are usually cured with surgery alone; this usually entails an anterior thoracotomy. Malignant tumors usually contain yolk sac elements. If they are not successfully resected, the outcome is dismal, unless there is a good response to chemotherapy.

About 5% of germ cell tumors in children arise in the retroperitoneum. These tumors occur more frequently in girls than in boys, and they usually are diagnosed before the patient is 4 years of age, with a mean age of 18 months.[20] Patients often present with abdominal pain, and a large mass is evident on physical examination. About 75% of these lesions are benign teratomas; the remainder are either pure yolk sac tumors or a mixture of these two histologies. The differential diagnosis of these masses includes the other, more common abdominal tumors of childhood, such as Wilms tumor and neuroblastoma. Radiographic findings, such as calcifications suggestive of bone or tooth formation, can help to establish the diagnosis preoperatively. The treatment of choice is surgical; as in other sites, successfully resected mature teratomas are associated with a good outcome, and malignant tumors that are unresectable have a guarded prognosis. The use of chemotherapy must be individualized; in general, however, the same principles should be used in the treatment of retroperitoneal tumors as in tumors in other sites.

Finally, about 5% of germ cell tumors arise in the extracranial head and neck region. They are usually located in the anterior or lateral neck but can occur on the face, in the mouth, in the nasopharynx, or in the orbit. These tumors often present in infancy and can be congenital. Tumors obstructing the pharynx can present antenatally with maternal polyhydramnios or nonimmune fetal hydrops. Clinically, these lesions can look similar to lymphangiomas or cystic hygromas. Pathologically, they are usually teratomas, and it is uncommon for them to contain any malignant elements. The rare malignancies are either pure yolk sac tumors or mixed germ cell tumors containing yolk sac elements. Benign lesions are easily treated with surgical resection.[4]

Choriocarcinoma is a rare and particularly aggressive variant of germ cell tumors and presents most often in one of two age ranges. Gestational choriocarcinoma is a true congenital tumor—the lesion arises from the placenta and spreads to the fetus.[21] These children often present with the *infantile choriocarcinoma syndrome*. The constellation of findings in this syndrome includes presentation from birth to 6 months of age with anemia, hepatomegaly, and possibly a history of hematemesis or melena. Central nervous system symptoms also may be seen, and patients may exhibit signs of precocious puberty, owing to the elevated serum β-hCG levels. The most commonly involved organ is the liver, but multiple sites are usually involved, including the lung and subcutaneous tissues. Because the tumor is so rare, diagnosis is often delayed, and the outcome is poor. A report was made, however, of a survivor of the infantile choriocarcinoma syndrome after aggressive surgery and chemotherapy.[22] In this case, an important clue to the diagnosis was the presence of an elevated β-hCG level.

In older children, choriocarcinoma presents most often in the pineal region. The median age of these patients is about 12 years, and the outcome is generally poor.

Adjuvant Treatment of Nongonadal Germ Cell Tumors

Although there are few prospective trials, the outcome in children with sacrococcygeal malignancies and other nongonadal germ cell tumors is thought to be improved with the use of multiagent chemotherapy. This is reasonable, given the progress that has been made in the treatment of tumors arising from the testes and ovaries. The introduction of cisplatin has been especially important in this regard. Other agents that have been used to treat malignant germ cell tumors include etoposide, bleomycin, cyclophosphamide, and doxorubicin; several clinical trials are underway comparing various chemotherapy regimens.

In a Children's Cancer Group study investigating the usefulness of chemotherapy in malignant germ cell tumors, the 4-year survival rate of patients with nongonadal tumors was 54%.[23] Most of these lesions were sacrococcygeal, and only frankly malignant tumors were included; immature teratomas were excluded. The results were independent of the particular histologic subtype. The most important factor in determining survival was the local extent of the tumor. When the lesion was isolated to one structure or organ, there was a 70% survival rate, and patients who did not have the entire lesion removed were eight times more likely to suffer an adverse event than children who were rendered tumor-free by surgery. In this report, the presence of microscopic residual disease was associated with only a slight improvement in outcome compared with patients with gross residual disease. In general, these results for the outcome of malignant nongonadal germ cell tumors treated with chemotherapy are similar to results from other studies.

Although unproved, there may be benefit to second-look surgery to remove disease remaining after chemotherapy.[24] These procedures should probably be limited to cases in which a potentially resectable mass remains after therapy or in which there is continued elevation of an informative serum marker. In one study, surgeons were able to find residual tumor in children who had elevated serum tumor markers, although the radiographic imaging studies were negative.[25]

The successful use of radiotherapy as the primary mode of therapy for localized gonadal and nongonadal germinomas is well described. In other types of germ cell tumors, the indications for this therapy are less well-defined, but there have been isolated reports of the usefulness of radiotherapy in the local control of unresectable malignant tumors.

REFERENCES

1. Hawkins EP. Pathology of germ cell tumors in children. Crit Rev Oncol Hematol 1990;10:165.
2. Birch JM, Marsden HB, Swindell R. Pre-natal factors in the origin of germ cell tumours of childhood. Carcinogenesis 1982;3:75
3. Marsden HB, Birch JM, Swindell R. Germ cell tumours of childhood: a review of 137 cases. J Clin Pathol 1981;34:879
4. Billmire DF, Grosfeld JL. Teratomas in childhood: analysis of 142 cases. J Pediatr Surg 1986;21:548.
5. Harms D, Janig U. Germ cell tumours of childhood: report of 170 cases including 59 pure and partial yolk-sac tumours. Virchows Arch [A] 1986;409:223
6. Ilson DH, Bosl GJ, Motzer R, et al. Genetic analysis of germ cell tumors: current progress and future prospects. Hematol Oncol Clin North Am 1991;5:1271.
7. Suijkerbuijk RF, Sinke RJ, Meloni AM, et al. Overrepresentation of chromosome 12p sequences and karyotypic evolution in i(12p)-negative testicular germ-cell tumors revealed by fluorescence in situ hybridization. Cancer Genet Cytogenet 1993;70:85.
8. Wu JT, Book L, Sudar K. Serum alpha fetoprotein (AFP) levels in normal infants. Pediatr Res 1981;15:50
9. Koshida K, Nishino A, Yamamoto H, et al. The role of alkaline phosphatase isoenzymes as tumor markers for testicular germ cell tumors. J Urol 1991;146:57.
10. Altman RP, Randolph JG, Lilly JR. Sacrococcygeal teratoma: American Academy of Pediatrics surgical section survey—1973. J Pediatr Surg 1974;9:389.

11. Currarino G, Coln D, Votteler T. Triad of anorectal, sacral, and presacral anomalies. AJR 1981;137:395.
12. Havranek P, Rubenson A, Guth D, et al. Sacrococcygeal teratoma in Sweden: a 10-year national retrospective study. J Pediatr Surg 1992;27:1447.
13. Tapper D, Lack EE. Teratomas in infancy and childhood: a 54-year experience at the Children's Hospital Medical Center. Ann Surg 1983;198:398.
14. Ein SH, Mancer K, Adeyemi SD. Malignant sacrococcygeal teratoma—endodermal sinus, yolk sac tumor—in infants and children: a 32-year review. J Pediatr Surg 1985;20:473.
15. Malogolowkin MH, Ortega JA, Krailo M, et al. Immature teratomas: identification of patients at risk for malignant recurrence. J Natl Cancer Inst 1989;81:870.
16. Hawkins E, Issacs H, Cushing B, et al. Occult malignancy in neonatal sacrococcygeal teratomas: a report from a combined pediatric oncology group and children's cancer group study. Am J Pediatr Hematol Oncol 1993;15:406.
17. Havranek P, Hedlund H, Rubenson A, et al. Sacrococcygeal teratoma in Sweden between 1978 and 1989: long-term functional results. J Pediatr Surg 1992;27:916.
18. Boemers TML, van Gool JD, de Jong TPVM, et al. Lower urinary tract dysfunction in children with benign sacrococcygeal teratoma. J Urol 1994;151:174.
19. Azarow KS, Pearl RH, Zurcher R, et al. Primary mediastinal masses: a comparison of adult and pediatric populations. J Thorac Cardiovasc Surg 1993;106:67.
20. Lack EE, Travis WD, Welch KJ. Retroperitoneal germ cell tumors in childhood: a clinical and pathologic study of 11 cases. Cancer 1985;56:602.
21. Shitara T, Oshima Y, Yugami S, et al. Choriocarcinoma in children. Am J Pediatr Hematol Oncol 1993;15:268.
22. Belchis DA, Mowry J, Davis JH. Infantile choriocarcinoma: re-examination of a potentially curable entity. Cancer 1993;72:2028.
23. Ablin AR, Krailo MD, Ransay NKC, et al. Results of treatment of malignant germ cell tumors in 93 children: a report from the Children's Cancer Study group. J Clin Oncol 1991;9:1782.
24. Nichols CR, Fox EP. Extragonadal and pediatric germ cell tumors. Hematol Oncol Clin North Am 1991;5:1189.
25. Marina NM, Rao B, Etcubanas E, et al. The role of second-look surgery in the management of advanced germ cell malignancies. Cancer 1991;68:309.

Surgery of Infants and Children: Scientific Principles and Practice, edited by Keith T. Oldham, Paul M. Colombani, and Robert P. Foglia. Lippincott–Raven Publishers, Philadelphia, © 1997.

CHAPTER 39

Transplant Immunology

Rita A. Kostecke, Barbara A. Gaines, and Suzanne T. Ildstad

HISTORY

The field of immunology is undergoing vigorous and exciting growth. It is on the discoveries of the past that present developments are built. In her review article, "Concepts of Infection and Resistance: A History of Immunology Until the Time of Louis Pasteur," Antoinette Stettler states that the term *immunis* was originally used to describe the medieval Church's freedom from a ruler's control. Later, this concept became subsumed into the modern definition of legal immunity from prosecution.

The first time the term *immunis* was formally associated with medicine and disease was in 1878, when Littre included it in his *Dictionnaire de Médecine*. Stettler, however, quotes an earlier use in an ancient writer's response to surviving a plague epidemic: "*Equibus Dei gratia ego immunis evasi.*"[1] Even if this use was not truly in a modern sense, the sentiment is one that has surely echoed down the years and with which we can even now identify.

It is difficult, however, to determine the true beginning of immunology. Was it in 1798, when Edward Jenner developed the cowpox vaccine? In 1880, when Louis Pasteur elucidated his "germ theory of disease?" We could point to Emil von Behring's Nobel Prize in 1901 for "work on serum therapy," that is, his discovery of antibody and passive immunity, as the beginning of modern immunology. However, the work of his predecessors surely deserves some mention, as well as an acknowledgment that science and medicine build on all that came before.

The early healers, following the teachings of Hippocrates and Galen, and under the influence of Aristotle, held that disease was caused by an imbalance of humors (blood, phlegm, yellow bile, and black bile) and that health could be restored by bringing these back into balance. Although this view may seem primitive to today's physicians, it was important in the early development of immunology, and in fact the terminology persists today in our division of the immune system into "cellular" and "humoral" components.

In the 1850s, there were two main schools of thought that purported to explain the theories of immunity: the *cellularists* and the *humoralists*. This division was both intellectual and sociopolitical; most of the cellularists were French (or franco-

philes), whereas the humoralists were German. The cellularists believed that "the chief defense of the body against infection resided in the phagocytic and digestive powers of the macrophage and the microphage (today's polymorphonuclear leukocyte), while the humoralists (with the weight of tradition behind them) claimed that only the soluble substances of the blood and other body fluids could immobilize and destroy invading pathogens."[2] Both groups were correct in modern terms because both cellular and humoral components contribute to immunity.

In 1858, Robert Virchow first elucidated the cellularist's position by claiming that pathology was due to a malfunction of cells rather than an imbalance of humors. This view was not widely accepted, and it was not until 1884 that the Russian zoologist Elie Metchnikoff reintroduced it by suggesting that phagocytic cells, which were known to be involved in inflammatory responses, in fact represented a valuable defense against invading organisms. The humoralist camp was quick to attack such contrary notions, and by 1888 the observations of George Nuttall that serum from normal animals possessed a natural toxicity for some organisms set the stage for much scholarly disagreement. The discovery in 1890 by Emil von Behring and Shibasaburo Kitasato that immunity to diphtheria and tetanus is caused by a substance they termed *antikörper* ("antibody") seemed to settle the battle in favor of the humoralists. Research then turned almost entirely toward the humoral view, and the antibody became of central importance.

The next major advance in immunology was Paul Ehrlich's side chain theory of antibody formation. In this, he stated that antibodies were components of the cell surface, and that an antigen selected the specific side chain (one of many present on each antibody) to which it fit and was internalized into the cell, leading to the production of more of that specific antibody. This theory, of course, necessitated that each antibody possess an almost infinite number of side chains, which rapidly became a tenuous position.

The instruction theory, in which the antigen was seen as a template, was advanced to answer this problem; perhaps its best known proponent was Linus Pauling, who, in the 1940s, applied his Nobel Prize-winning theory of interatomic and intramolecular forces to the investigation of antibody–antigen interactions. F. MacFarlane Burnet, in 1941, proposed the adaptive enzyme theory in which antigen is viewed as a stimulus to the enzymes necessary for globulin synthesis (and thus antibodies). In 1949, Burnet and Frank Fenner followed this with their indirect template theory, wherein they stated that each antigen is able to impress the information for its specific determinant on the genome, thus creating antibody specificity during protein formation (remember that the 1950s were when Francis Crick formalized his "central dogma" of genetics, that information on protein structure flowed from DNA to RNA to protein). In 1955, Niels Jerne revived and expanded Ehrlich's concepts of antibody formation, stating that antigen would interact with a specific antibody and then be transported to cells to be reproduced; this was the beginning of the *selective* (rather than instructive) view of the immune system. In this view, antibody functioned as a selective carrier of antigens, and hence the name.

In 1957, Burnet and David Talmadge hypothesized that each lymphocyte has antibody on its cell surface that recognizes only one antigen. This is known as the *clonal theory of the immune response*. The next year, Joshua Lederberg and Sir Gustav J. V. Nossal demonstrated the reality of this thesis. After this, in 1959, Burnet and Talmadge postulated the *clonal selection theory of antibody formation*, suggesting that interaction of antigen with antibody receptor on B lymphocytes triggered a signal for both antibody production and the proliferation of a clone of cells with complementary receptors for that antigen. Shortly thereafter, Gerald Edelman and Rodney Porter determined that antibody comprised two identical light and two identical heavy protein chains, and, in 1963, suggested the structure of antibody, for which they received a Nobel Prize in 1972. Almost 70 years after Ehrlich first theorized about antibody, Edelman (in 1970) finally described immunoglobulin as a combination of subunit chains of different functional domains, and stated that the heavy chain defined the function of the different immunoglobulin classes. At this time, isotyping could be performed, and the five classes of immunoglobulins—IgA, IgD, IgE, IgG, and IgM—were identified. T. T Wu and Elvin Kabat continued the characterization of antibody by localizing the hypervariable regions of light and heavy chains and suggesting that these regions were involved in defining the binding site for antigen. Finally, in 1987, Susumu Tonegawa received the Nobel Prize for demonstrating how the different segments of immunoglobulin genes (V, D, J, and C) combine to result in the multiplicity of immunoglobulins.

Hence, information gathered by basic research in many different areas has allowed the field of immunology to develop and advance. As a result of this understanding, clinical improvements have occurred, among the most important of which is the capacity for successful solid organ and cellular transplantation (Fig. 39-1).

COMPONENTS OF THE IMMUNE SYSTEM: OVERVIEW AND TERMINOLOGY

All of the cells of the immune system derive from a single pluripotent hematopoietic stem cell. This precursor, under the influence of various cytokines and growth factors, produces at least nine cell lineages, including T lymphocytes, B lymphocytes, natural killer (NK) cells, the monocyte–macrophage lineage, erythrocytes, platelets, eosinophils, basophils, neutro-

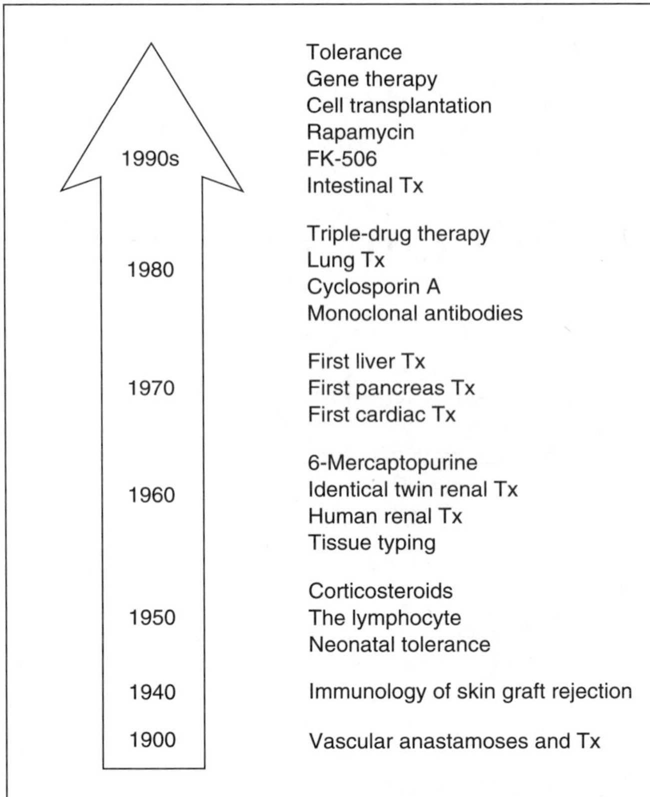

FIG. 39-1. The explosion in knowledge due to basic science research in diverse fields has led to an equivalent increase in clinical applications. Tx, transplantation. (After Conrad BG, Ildstad ST. Chimerism and tolerance: the myth becomes a reality. In: Sher LS, Makowka L, eds. Intra-abdominal organ transplantation 2000. Austin, RG Landes, 1994:82)

phils, mast cells, glial cells, and dendritic cells (Fig. 39-2). The major components of the immune system comprise T cells, B cells, NK cells, and cells of the monocyte–macrophage lineage, including dendritic cells, plus cytokines and adhesion molecules.

Cytokines are soluble messenger proteins that can function in an *autocrine* fashion (on the cell that releases the factor) or in a *paracrine* fashion (on nearby cells). In structure, they are low–molecular-weight proteins and are often glycosylated. Functionally, they allow communication between cells and play a primary role in "spreading the word" about immune activation.

The major division of the immune system is into a *humoral* and a *cellular* arm. B lymphocytes, which produce antibody, are the main components of the humoral aspect of the immune system, whereas T lymphocytes, which produce various cytokines to stimulate other cells in the immune system, as well as directly functioning to destroy cells, comprise the cellular arm. In short, the lymphocyte, whether T or B, is the specifically reactive cell of the immune system.

Before each cell type can be discussed in detail, an appreciation of the general concepts in an immune response is necessary (Fig. 39-3 and Table 39-1) (see also Chapters 11 and 12).

The immune response itself can be divided into several

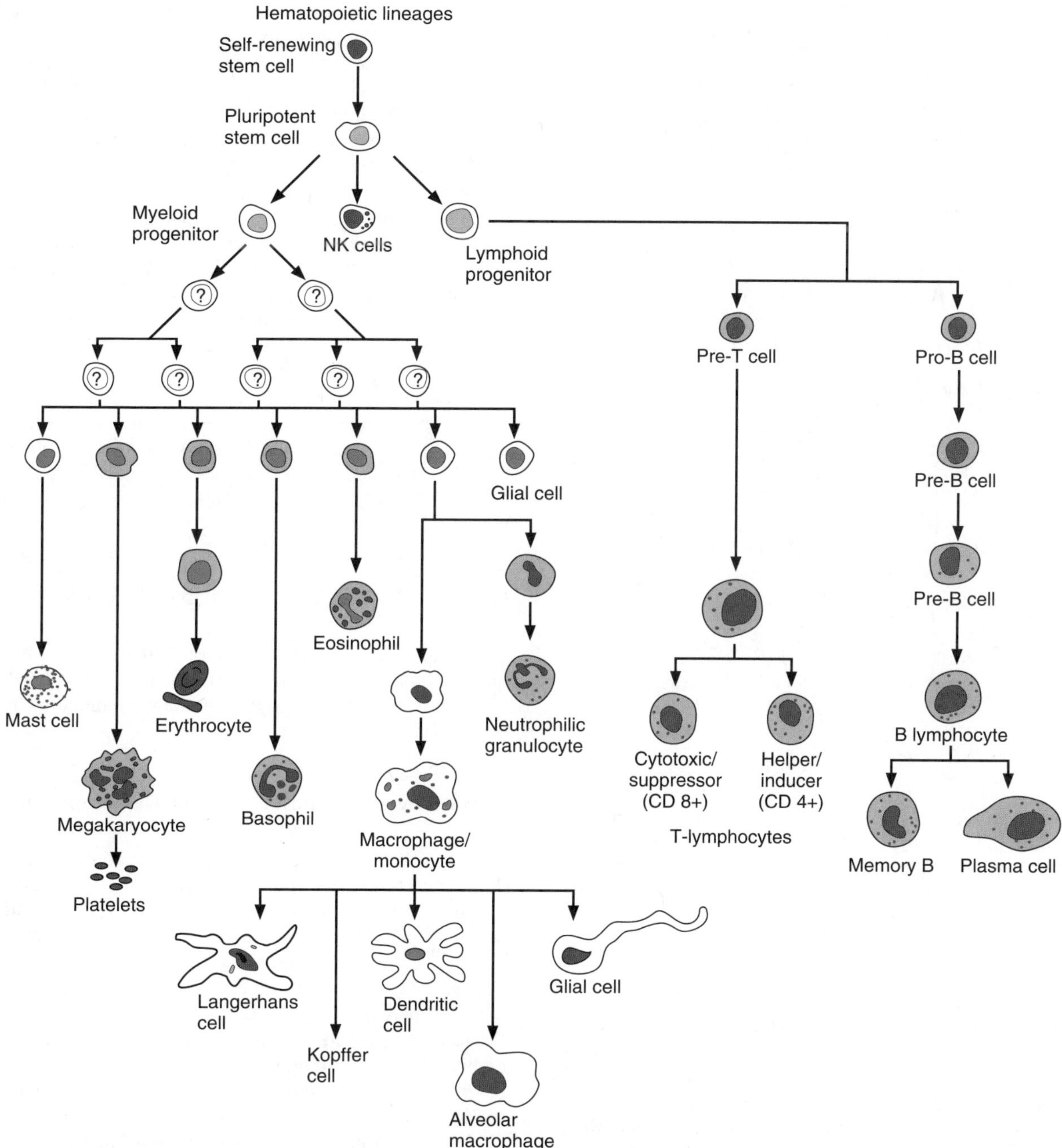

FIG. 39-2. All cells of the immune system arise from a common, pluripotent stem cell. The initial division is into the lymphoid and myeloid progenitor cells. Most early myeloid and lymphoid development in the adult occurs in the bone marrow; final maturation occurs in the peripheral blood and lymph organs after cell exposure to antigen. The major exception to this is the T lymphocyte, whose maturation occurs in the thymus. NK, natural killer. (After Ildstad ST, Simmons RL. Biology of organ transplantation and immunosuppression. In: Starzl TE, Shapiro R, Simmons RL, eds. Atlas of organ transplantation. New York, Gower Medical Publishers, 1992:1.3)

stages. First, the antigen must be *recognized* by the effector cell. In adaptive immune responses, this occurs as follows: antigen-presenting cells (APC) internalize and digest a foreign protein (*antigen*) into small fragments known as epitopes. These epitopes, 5 to 15 amino acids in length, in association with other molecules, are displayed on the surface of the APC to a specifically reactive T or B lymphocyte. Only those lympho-

cytes that have the correct receptor for an antigen can bind and recognize that antigen. This is known as the clonal nature of the immune response.

Next, activation of either the T- or B-cell subset occurs. This is the *response* phase, and occurs when antigen binds to the receptors of effector cells and the cells receive the appropriate accessory signal. Finally, in the *removal* phase, the B cells pro-

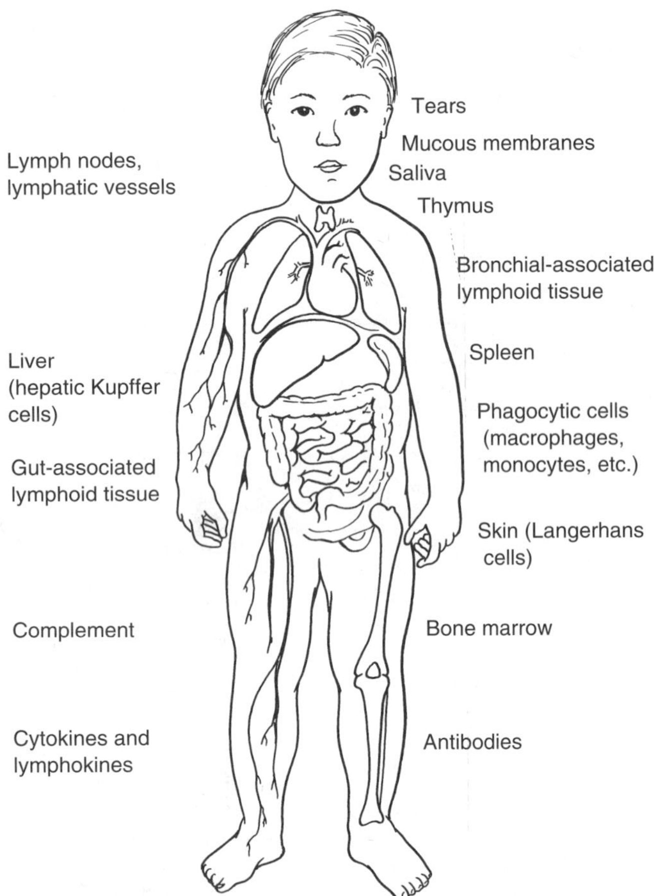

FIG. 39-3. The human immune system is a complex, interrelated system of both active and passive, acquired and innate defenses. The thymus and bone marrow are central immune organs, whereas the lymph nodes, skin, gut-associated lymphoid tissue, bronchial-associated lymphoid tissue, and spleen are peripheral lymphoid tissues.

duce antibody specific for the stimulating antigen, while the T cells mediate a cellular inflammatory response culminating in the destruction or removal of cells.

The activated lymphocytes are deployed to the site of infection or, as in the case of a transplant, foreign tissue, where they discriminate between self and nonself and mediate their specific

TABLE 39-1. *Components of the immune system*

Cell type	Role
B cells	Antibody production
T cells	Cytotoxic T cells (CD8)
	Helper T cells (CD4)
Antigen presenting cells	Antigen processing and delivery to effector cells of immune system
	Necessary co-stimulatory factors
Cytokines	Communication
	Activation
	Inhibition
Adhesion molecules	Stablize cell-to-cell interactions

immune activity. The extent of an immune response is regulated by positive and negative feedback loops.

T lymphocytes (or thymus-derived lymphocytes) arise from the yolk sac, fetal liver, and bone marrow precursor cells that migrate to the thymus during fetal and early postnatal life, whereas *B lymphocytes* (or bone marrow-derived lymphocytes) arise and mature in the bone marrow. In the past, B cells were also called ''bursal equivalent cells'' because, in chickens, this cell matures in the bursa of Fabricius. It is now known that, in humans, the bone marrow is equivalent to the bursa.

Commitment to a particular fate, that is, to a particular cell type, occurs very early in hematopoietic differentiation. The earliest point of differentiation is between those progenitors committed to lymphoid lineages and those of the myeloid lineages. The lymphoid lineages comprise the T and B lymphocytes, as well as the NK cells. After maturation, these cells migrate to and populate the peripheral lymphoid tissues, including the spleen, lymph nodes, gut-associated lymphoid tissue (the GALT system), and bronchial-associated lymphoid tissue (the BALT system). The myeloid lineages include all other cell types.

ONTOGENY OF THE IMMUNE SYSTEM

Any discussion of the ontogeny of the immune system requires a thorough understanding of hematopoietic development in general, and the biology of the hematopoietic stem cell in particular.

The Yolk Sac: Earliest Source of Hematopoietic Cells

Human hematopoiesis can first be detected in the yolk sac during the third week of gestation, when simple diffusion of nutrients is no longer sufficient to provide for the nutritional needs of the embryo (Fig. 39-4). Blood cells form extravascularly in the yolk sac endoderm and then migrate into the mesenchymal layer and, from there, into the vascular network (Fig. 39-5). A network of endodermal tubules also appears to play a role in the migration of blood cells from the yolk sac to the embryo. The developing yolk sac vasculature serves as a means of transport of the primitive hematopoietic cells from the yolk sac to the embryo, and is the forerunner of the placenta.

Yolk sac blood island cells have multilineage potential and are required for intraembryonic hematopoiesis. In the late 1960s, it was shown that cells from the yolk sac could rescue lethally irradiated adult mice from radiation-induced aplasia, confirming that these cells had stem cell capability. Yolk sac cells form erythroid, megakaryocytic, granulocytic, and mixed colonies in vitro. In addition, organ culture experiments demonstrated that early–gestational-age embryos cultured in the absence of the yolk sac failed to undergo hematopoiesis, even when growth factors were added to the medium. Maximum numbers of yolk sac stem cells are present at 4.5 to 5 weeks' gestational age, and after this time, yolk sac hematopoietic activity begins to decline.[3,4] No progenitors are detectable in the yolk sac after 60 days' gestation. It is believed that this represents the migration of hematopoietic progenitors from the yolk sac to the liver, which becomes the next major site of embryonic and fetal hematopoiesis.

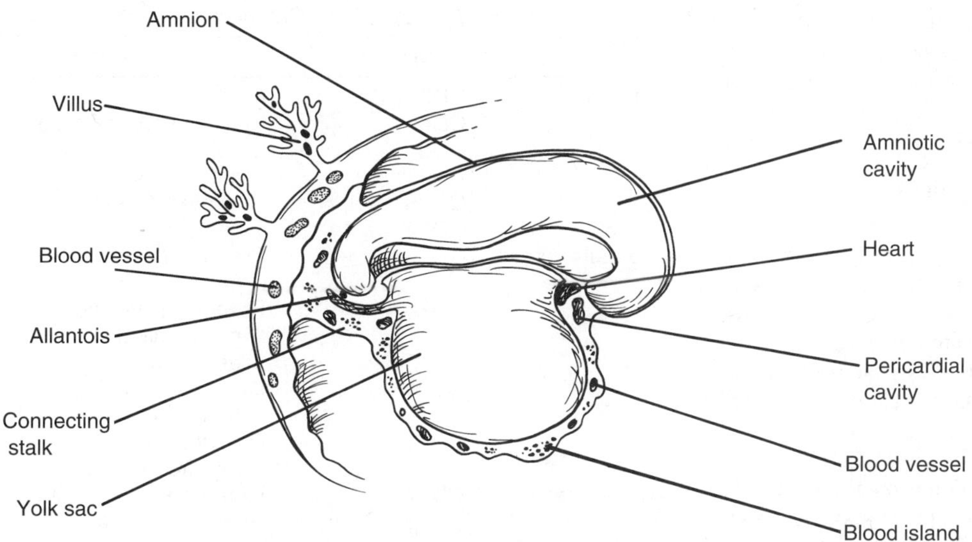

FIG. 39-4. The main site of initial hematopoiesis in the human embryo is the yolk sac. Extraembryonic blood island and blood vessel formation in the 19-day-old embryo are illustrated. (After Sadler TE. Lagman's medical embryology, ed 5. Baltimore, Williams & Wilkins, 1984:69)

Regulation of the early events in hematopoiesis is not clearly defined, but *hematopoietic growth factors*, or cytokines, are likely to play an important regulatory role. Stem cell factor (SCF) has received considerable attention. This cytokine is a "survivor" cytokine that induces a profound proliferative response in cultured hematopoietic stem cells when combined with other early-acting cytokines such as interleukin (IL)-1, IL-3, and IL-6.[5,6] Bone marrow cultured under SCF-enriched conditions has also been shown to engraft more efficiently in mice. Mice with a mutation in the gene for SCF (the Steel locus) demonstrate a series of defects that suggest that this factor is important during embryogenesis. These defects include sterility and severe anemia, with decreased numbers of cells from all the hematopoietic lineages.[7]

Modern techniques of molecular biology have been used to study the expression of the gene for SCF. Expression of any gene begins with the transcription of the double-stranded DNA into single-stranded messenger RNA (mRNA). The mRNA is then transported from the nucleus to the cell's cytoplasm, where it is translated into protein by the ribosome. The presence of a particular mRNA in a cell indicates that the gene of interest has been activated. Assaying for SCF mRNA transcription has revealed that this cytokine is present in both the mesoderm and the endoderm of the yolk sac.[7] mRNA for SCF is also found in the fetal liver and in the mesoderm around the dorsal aorta and the genital ridges. The distribution of SCF expression seems to indicate that it may have a role in the migration of hematopoietic and germ cells, as well as in their proliferation and differentiation.

Role of Fetal Liver in Hematopoiesis

The fetal liver is the site of hematopoiesis during most of gestation. In the human, the liver primordium is first apparent by the middle of the third week of gestation. By the tenth week of development, the liver comprises approximately 10% of the embryo, and there are large areas of hematopoiesis intermingling with the hepatocytes and sinusoids. During the last 2 months of human gestation, hepatic hematopoiesis decreases and the bone marrow compartment assumes this responsibility.[8]

Stem cells from the fetal liver have been demonstrated to possess both a capacity for self-renewal and the ability to differentiate into any of the multiple hematopoietic lineages.[9–11] Labeling studies have been used to follow the fate of individual fetal liver stem cells and conclusively demonstrate that these

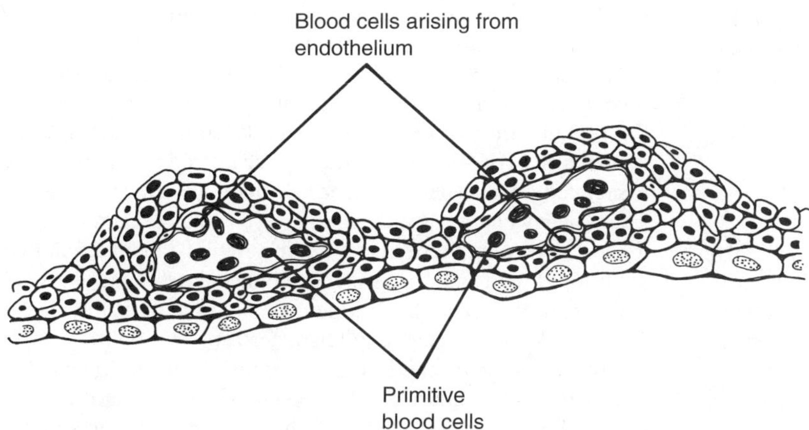

FIG. 39-5. Blood cells arise from the blood islands of the yolk sac; the developing vasculature is thought to be responsible for transport of these cells from the yolk sac to the developing embryo. (After Moore KL, Persaud TVN. The developing human, ed 5. Philadelphia, WB Saunders, 1993:64)

cells are multipotent.[6] Moreover, there are preliminary data to suggest that fetal stem cells have enhanced proliferative and self-renewal abilities compared with stem cells derived from cord blood or adult bone marrow.[11]

Role of Bone Marrow in Hematopoiesis

During the third trimester of human gestation, the liver gradually loses its hematopoietic function and the bone marrow assumes the supremacy in this role that it will maintain throughout adult life. During times of severe hematologic stress, however, even in adults, extramedullary hematopoiesis can occur in both the liver and spleen. This indicates that the adult hepatic environment is not completely inhospitable to hematopoiesis.

Initially the marrow cavities in most bones are involved in hematopoiesis, but gradually this function becomes restricted to the flat bones. By early adulthood, most hematopoietic activity occurs in the sternum, vertebral bodies, iliac crest, and ribs. The microenvironment of the marrow cavity consists of bony spicules surrounded by a rich stroma of fat cells, supporting cells, and hematopoietic precursors. It is believed that the stem cell is adherent to bony cortex and that more differentiated progenitors are more centrally located.

CLUSTER OF DIFFERENTIATION ANTIGENS

The cells in the immune system are characterized by their surface molecules. These surface markers are now recognized (and thus defined) by specific monoclonal antibodies and can be used to classify cells phenotypically and functionally as belonging to a specific lineage. A surface marker on a cell that identifies a particular lineage, or a particular differentiation stage of a lineage, that has a defined structure, and that is recognized by a specific group of monoclonal antibodies, is known as a member of a *cluster of differentiation (CD). CD antigens* are defined by a numeric system. Homologous markers in different species are referred to by the same CD marker number, and monoclonal antibodies developed in different laboratories are assigned to preexisting CD numbers.

Each individual cell type expresses a number of CD antigens, and as more cell surface proteins are identified, the CD markers "found" on a particular cell can increase. For example, T lymphocytes that in the recent past might have been known merely as CD4 + cells (that is, a cell with a surface protein recognized by a monoclonal antibody designated "CD4") might now be described as a CD4 + /$\alpha\beta$-TCR + /CD3 + /class I + lymphocyte. Table 39-2 lists some of the more frequently encountered CD markers.

THE MAJOR HISTOCOMPATIBILITY COMPLEX

The *major histocompatibility complex (MHC)* is a highly polymorphic region of genes located on the short arm of chromosome 6 (Fig. 39-6). The proteins encoded by these genes, the *human leukocyte antigens (HLA)*, are the most important determinants of acceptance or rejection of allografts. Other histocompatibility antigens are found outside the MHC and are termed *minor antigens*. These are less strongly antigenic than

TABLE 39-2. *CD markers*

Cell type	Marker	Distribution
T cells	CD3	All T cells
	CD4	Helper/inducer T cells
	CD8	Cytotoxic/supressor T cells
	CD25	Activated T cells
	CD28	T cell subset
B cells	CD19	Precursor B cells, B cells
	CD20	Precursor B cells, B cells, follicular dendritic cells
	CD21	Precursor B cells, mature B cells
	CD22	Precursor B cells, mature B cells
Stem cells	CD34	Hematopoietic precursor
Natural killer cells	CD16/FCRIII	All resting NK cells
	CD56	Pan NK marker
Monocytes	CD14	Most monocytes

the MHC antigens but are sufficient to function in graft-versus-host disease (GVHD) and graft rejection.

The MHC (or HLA region) is divided into three classes based on functional differences in the gene products. These regions produce HLA class I, II, and III proteins. For transplantation, class I and II antigens are of primary importance. These loci are spatially organized such that the class I genes are at the telomeric end of chromosome 6, the class II genes are at the centromeric end, and the class III genes are in between. All cells, except mature erythrocytes, express class I antigens. However, only certain cells, notably the APCs, also express class II antigens. Products of both class I (HLA-A, HLA-B, and HLA-C) and class II (HLA-DR, HLA-DQ, and HLA-DP) are involved in antigen presentation. Class I molecules are recognized by CD8 + cytotoxic T cells and class II molecules by CD4 + T helper (TH) cells. Class III proteins comprise the complement system.

The HLA class I region was the first of the HLA regions to be identified. The most common class I loci are A, B and C, whereas the less predominant are E, F, G, and H. Only the first three (A, B, and C) are clearly involved in antigen presentation. The other loci appear to have other functions.[12] Each of these loci has multiple allelic expression (identified by number, eg, HLA-A2), inherited in a codominant fashion from each parent.

Although each individual's HLA region is genetically unique, and produces a unique combination of class I proteins, the proteins themselves are structurally similar. Each protein contains an MHC-encoded α (heavy) chain and a noncovalently associated, non–MHC-encoded β chain (β_2-microglobulin). The α heavy chain has three domains (α1, α2, α3) and includes a short, hydrophobic transmembrane region (about 25 amino acids long) with an intracellular (cytoplasmic) tail and an extracellular portion. The three-dimensional structure of the class I molecule has been elegantly characterized.

Most receptors in the immune system are heterodimers, and the MHC class I and class II molecules follow this rule. The extracellular region of the two light (α1 and α2) chains of the

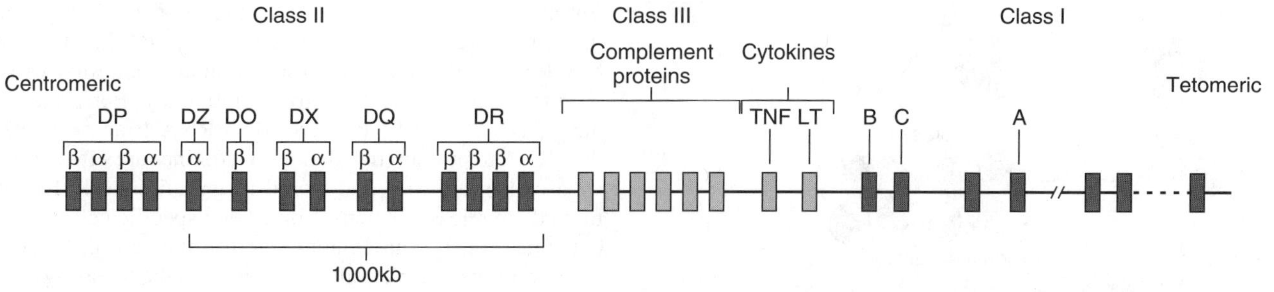

FIG. 39-6. The major histocompatibility region can be divided into several classes based on functional differences of the proteins produced by the different genes. The human leukocyte antigen class I genes are found at the telomeric end of the short arm of chromosome 6, whereas the class II genes are found at the centromeric end. Also found in this region are the genes for the class III (complement) proteins and some cytokines. TNF, tumor necrosis factor; LT, leukotriene. (After Abbas AK, Lichtman AH, Pober JS. Cellular and molecular immunology. Philadelphia, WB Saunders, 1991:110)

class I molecule forms a cleft (*antigen-binding site*) that can accept a 10- to 20-amino-acid fragment. The size of the antigen-binding site requires that, before binding to the class I antigen-binding site, a foreign protein must first be processed into smaller fragments. Successful binding between an antigen fragment (or epitope) and the class I protein expressed on an APC's surface is necessary for recognition and interaction with a CD8+ cytotoxic T cell. This interaction between class I molecules and the CD8+ T cell plus antigen is essential to allow for host recognition of foreign antigen.

The class II genes of the MHC were identified subsequent to the class I genes. The first of these genes to be mapped was designated the HLA-D-related gene (HLA-DR). The major HLA class II region comprises the DR, DP, and DQ isotypes, as well as the less important DN and DO. As with the class I antigens, all MHC class II molecules are structurally similar. Unlike the class I antigens, the class II proteins are formed by two different, noncovalently linked chains (α and β) and are not associated with β_2-microglobulin. Both the chains are divided into two segments ($\alpha1$, $\alpha2$, and $\beta1$, $\beta2$) and have a hydrophobic transmembrane region and an intracellular (cytoplasmic) region. The three-dimensional structure of the class II molecule has been characterized. As with class I molecules, both the α and β chains are involved in binding foreign peptides, and this interaction is, as before, of relatively low affinity.

MHC genes are inherited according to classic Mendelian genetics. Each child receives one chromosome 6 from each parent, and the genes encoded by that chromosome are codominant with the other chromosome 6. Inheritance of class I genes is relatively straightforward because only one copy of each class I gene is expressed within the cell. However, class II genes may be multiply expressed within a single individual. Practically, this means that an individual inherits three HLA class I alleles (A, B, and C) from each parent and therefore expresses six different class I proteins. Six class II genes are also inherited (three from each parent), but because there is variable gene expression, up to 10 to 20 different proteins can be generated by an individual.

Tissue Typing for Transplantation

There are two main rules that govern the immunogenicity of the MHC. First, the antigenic specificity of a given MHC locus is determined by one (structural) gene, and, second, individuals can respond to any MHC alloantigen (an antigen other than self) that they *do not* express, but cannot respond to an alloantigen that they *do* express.

HLA differences between individuals have traditionally been identified using serologic techniques. Donor lymphocytes are incubated with a panel of pooled sera containing defined anti-HLA antibodies, and complement is added. Complement causes lysis of those cells with attached antibody, and only those cells that express an HLA antigen present in the panel combine with that antibody and are lysed. The number of cells lysed is measured either visually or with radioactive labels. This method allows determination of the antigenic expression of the donor. Serologic HLA typing is useful in identifying the class I expression of an individual, but does not readily distinguish the class II antigens.

Until the late 1980s, class II typing was performed using a functional assay. This assay, known as a *mixed lymphocyte reactivity (MLR) assay*, measures lymphocyte proliferation in response to stimulation. In the simplest form of this assay (the two-way MLR), lymphocytes from the recipient are placed into culture with donor lymphocytes that have been inactivated by irradiation. After 5 days, the recipient cells are examined for proliferation, which is measured by incorporation of tritiated thymidine (Fig. 39-7). Thymidine uptake (positive response) indicates recognition of class II molecules on the donor lymphocytes as foreign. A lack of proliferation (negative response) would imply that both the donor and recipient lymphocytes share the same class II molecules.

Advances in molecular biology have revolutionized the practice of tissue typing, and are particularly useful for class II genes because the MLR assay is time consuming, expensive, and relatively nonspecific. The molecular technique of *polymerase chain reaction (PCR)* has been applied to HLA typing with great success, increasing both the specificity of typing and the speed of the procedure. In PCR analysis, primers are constructed against portions of the actual HLA gene under investigation. If the target gene is present in the donor, this DNA sequence is amplified and can be detected.

In clinical practice, potential bone marrow transplant recipients and some solid organ transplant recipients are HLA typed

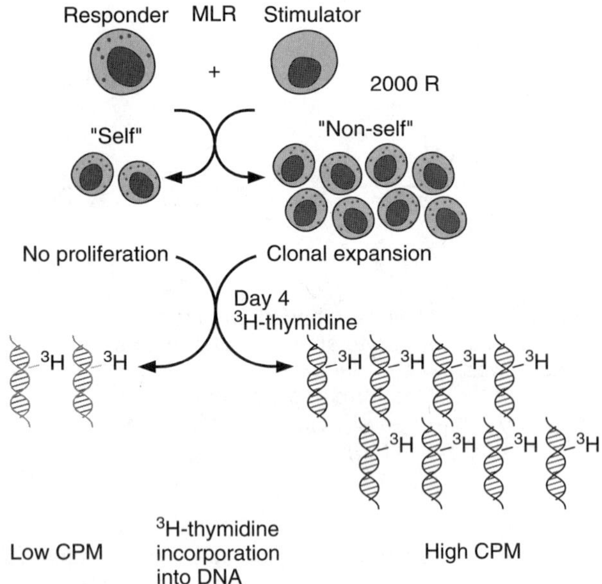

FIG. 39-7. In mixed lymphocyte reactivity (MLR) typing, lymphocytes from the recipient are cocultured with irradiated donor lymphocyte cells. Proliferation, as measured by uptake of tritiated (³H) thymidine, reflects activation of the cells. CPM, counts per minute. (Courtesy of Rich James, University Surgical Associates, Pittsburgh, PA)

for both class I and class II antigens. In the case of kidney transplantation, when a donor is identified, HLA typing is performed and attempts are made to match donor and recipient as closely as possible. Even when there is an excellent match, before transplantation cells from the donor must be incubated in serum from the potential recipient to test for the presence of preformed cytotoxic antibody in the recipient's serum. Preformed antibody, found most frequently in patients who have rejected a previous transplant, have been been multiply transfused, or are multiparous, is responsible for *hyperacute* rejection. In the case of liver, heart, lung, and small intestine transplantation, HLA matching is less important.

HLA typing is critical for bone marrow transplantation (BMT). It is important to match the donor and recipient as closely as possible because the incidence and severity of GVHD is highly correlated to the degree of disparity between donor and recipient.

CYTOKINES

Overview

Cytokines are very small glycoproteins that mediate and regulate communication between various cells of the immune system. They can be membrane bound or soluble, and are central to the immune response. Table 39-3 lists some of the more widely recognized cytokines and their functions. Lymphocytes and monocytes produce most of the cytokines, which may also be referred to as *lymphokines* and *monokines*, respectively. A number of other cells can secrete these mediators, including NK cells, mast cells, dendritic cells, keratinocytes, granulocytes,

fibroblasts, and epithelial cells. Cytokines perform a myriad of functions, often acting synergistically to elicit the maximal effect. Release of cytokines is a self-limited event. Most cytokine production is regulated posttranscriptionally. For protein synthesis, DNA must be transcribed to RNA (transcription) and then RNA to protein (translation). Cytokines are often produced by a cell in advance and stored in granules ready for nearly immediate release on activation of that specific cell type. Most cytokines function in an autocrine (on the cell itself) or paracrine (on surrounding cells) fashion, with the releasing cell and target cell in proximity. Target specificity is determined by the presence of a receptor unique for a particular cytokine on the cell surface. Receptor density on resting cells is low. Regulation of receptor expression, however, is an important mechanism controlling cellular activation and susceptibility to cytokine stimulation. Considerable functional redundancy exists among the cytokines, providing a protective mechanism if one system is malfunctioning.

Several general categories of function for cytokines can be determined. Cytokines can function as T-cell growth factors, B-cell activators, mediators of inflammation, and hematopoietic stem cell growth regulators. Most, if not all, cytokines have more than one effect on different cell types.

Mediators of Inflammation

Cytokines function systemically to provide protection against viral infection and initiate the inflammatory response to bacteria. The most important proteins in inflammation are the type I interferons (IFN-α, IFN-β), tumor necrosis factor (TNF), and IL-1. IFN-α and IFN-β are small polypeptides released from mononuclear cells and fibroblasts in response to viral infection. They bind to the same cell surface receptor, inducing an antiproliferative response and up-regulating MHC class I expression. Type I interferons also enhance NK activity.

TNF, referred to as "cachexin" in earlier literature, is the primary mediator of the response to gram-negative sepsis. It is released from macrophages that have been stimulated by the bacterial cell wall toxin lipopolysaccharide (LPS). Virtually all cells have receptors for TNF, indicating the wide-ranging properties of this cytokine. Soluble forms of the TNF receptor also exist, and serve to regulate the bioavailability of soluble TNF by competing with the cell surface receptors for TNF binding. At low levels, TNF functions locally and induces effects designed to protect the host from invading bacteria. It activates neutrophils and enhances their adhesive properties, allowing for local accumulation of these phagocytes. In addition, TNF stimulates macrophages to release cytokines, including IL-1, IL-6, and TNF itself, and induces up-regulation of class I expression. In the face of overwhelming bacterial infection, however, these locally beneficial properties of TNF become systemically toxic and lead to shock. In this setting, TNF causes a decrease in myocardial contractility, capillary leakage, disseminated intravascular coagulation, fever, and disturbances in metabolic control, leading first to hyperglycemia and then hypoglycemia. In addition, TNF has been associated with adult respiratory distress syndrome and acute tubular necrosis. Anti-TNF monoclonal antibodies have been investigated as a potential therapeutic agent in the treatment of sepsis. Initial results suggest that this therapy prolongs sur-

TABLE 39-3. *Cytokines and their functions*

Cytokine	Primary cell that secretes	Principal action
Interleukin 1	Macrophages	Activates T helper cells, initiates the cellular immune response, inflammatory mediator
Interleukin 2	CD4 T cells	T cell growth factor, stimulates proliferation and differentiation of T lymphocytes, enhances cytolytic activity of NK cells
Interleukin 3	CD4 T cells	Stimulates proliferation and differentiation of hematopoietic progenitors
Interleukin 4	CD4 T cells (TH2 subset)	B cell stimulating factor, induces differentiation of naive CD4 T helper cells into TH2 subset
Interleukin 5	CD4 T cells	B cell stimulating factor, eosinophil activation, proliferation and differentiation
Interleukin 6	CD4 T cells	T and B cell growth and differentiation
	Macrophages	Activates hematopoietic precursors, stimulates production of acute phase proteins
Interleukin 7	Bone marrow stromal cells	Differentiation of B cell precursors
Interleukin 8	Monocytes	Neutrophil, T cell and basophil chemotaxtic factor, activates neutrophils
Interleukin 9	CD4 T cells	Supports hematopoietic cell growth in long-term cultures
Interleukin 10	CD4 T cells (TH2 subset)	Cytokine synthesis inhibitory factor, suppresses differentiation of naive CD4 T helper cells into TH1 subset, enhances B cell growth and differentiation
Interleukin 11	Bone marrow stromal cells	Enhances early hematopoietic growth and differentiation in synergism with IL-3 and IL-4, stimulates synthesis of hepatic acute phase proteins
Interleukin 12	B cells, macrophages	NK stimulatory factor enhances cell mediated cytotoxicity of NK and CD8 T cells, promotes differentiation of naive CD4 T helper cells into TH1 subset
Interleukin 13	T cells	Similar in action to IL-4
Interleukin 14	T cells	B cell growth factor
Stem cell factor	Bone marrow stromal cells Fetal liver cells Yolk sac	Synergizes with other primitive cytokines to stimulate proliferation of early myeloid, erythroid and lymphoid cell lineages, and primitive germ cells
Granulocyte stimulating factor (G-CSF)	Monocytes	Enhances granulocyte differentiation
Granulocyte-macrophage stimulating factor (GM-CSF)	Activated T cells Macrophages	Stimulates granulocytes, macrophages and eosinophil growth
Erythropoietin	Kidney	Stimulates erythrocyte production
Interferon-gamma (INF-γ)	Activated T cells	Induces MHC class I and class II expression on cells Enhances NK cytotoxicity Activates macrophages and endothelial cells
Tumor necrosis factor	Macrophages	Mediates response to sepsis, induces IL-1 secretion

vival in animals challenged with a lethal inoculum of bacteria.[13,14]

The functional properties of *IL-1* are similar to those of TNF. It is a potent mediator of inflammation and serves to protect the host from invading bacteria and virus. IL-1, like TNF, is principally released from activated macrophages; however, other cells, including lymphocytes, NK cells, and endothelial cells, also produce this cytokine. Release of IL-1 by macrophages is stimulated by LPS, TNF, IL-1 itself, or contact with CD4+ T cells. Once released, IL-1 has many of the same biologic effects as TNF, although it does not directly cause tissue injury and even at very high doses is not lethal. One important difference between the two cytokines, however, is the effect of IL-1 on lymphocyte activation. IL-1 serves to enhance the proliferation of CD4+ cells and to stimulate B-cell growth.

Hematopoietic Stimulatory Factors

Cytokines also play a major role in production of the immune system by the bone marrow stem cell. It has long been recognized that stem cells isolated from adult bone marrow are unable to proliferate and differentiate in the absence of a stromal layer.[15] Considerable work has focused on defining the components of the stroma that are essential to support stem cell survival. As a result, the hematopoietic growth factors have been identified.

Conceptually, two categories of cytokines have been described: those that are active early in differentiation, inducing the initially quiescent stem cell to divide, and those that are lineage specific. Examples of early-acting hematopoietic cytokines include IL-3, IL-6, IL-11, IL-12, SCF, leukemia inhibitory factor, and granulocyte–macrophage colony-stimulating factor

(GM-CSF).[16] Cytokines that seem to stimulate lineage-specific differentiation include erythropoietin, monocyte colony-stimulating factor (M-CSF), and IL-5. Considerable functional overlap is apparent, however, and many cytokines appear to be important throughout the differentiation process. In addition, the most pronounced effects occur when multiple cytokines are added to stem cells, emphasizing the importance of synergy and the underlying complexity of the system.

Clinically, the characterization of these hematopoietic growth factors has had profound impact. Patients rendered neutropenic from trauma, sepsis, chemotherapy, BMT, and other causes often respond to GM-CSF or granulocyte colony–stimulating factor (G-CSF). Patients with a deficiency of erythropoietin due to renal failure no longer require transfusion therapy if exogenous erythropoietin is provided. Until the early 1990s, the cytokine for platelet production has remained elusive. However, two groups simultaneously identified this cytokine (thrombopoietin), and the gene for it has been cloned and sequenced.[17]

T CELLS

Overview

T cells are classically divided into *CD4+ helper* and *CD8+ cytotoxic* subsets. TH cells *influence* the activity of other cells, whereas cytotoxic T cells act directly to *destroy* other cells. Although these categories were once thought to be mutually exclusive, it is now known that a subset of CD4+ cells may also function as cytotoxic effector cells, and that some CD8+ cells may behave similarly to helper cells.

Each of these types of T cells expresses a structurally similar T-cell receptor (TCR) on the cell surface. The TCR is a complex of proteins that includes the antigen-specific receptor itself, a CD3 molecule, and associated invariant chains γ, δ, and ϵ (Fig. 39-8).

T-Cell Receptors

There are two types of TCRs, those that express $\alpha\beta$ chains, and those that express $\gamma\delta$. Most T cells in the blood and peripheral lymphoid tissues are $\alpha\beta$ TCR positive ($\alpha\beta$-TCR), whereas a few T lymphocytes are $\gamma\delta$ TCR positive ($\gamma\delta$-TCR). In mice, most of the T cells found in the epithelium are $\gamma\delta$-TCR cells, whereas in humans the $\gamma\delta$ TCR subset is distributed among other tissues as well.

The $\alpha\beta$-TCR is a heterodimer consisting of two α chains and two β chains. This protein is associated with a CD3 molecule, which itself is associated with the invariant chains γ, δ, and ϵ. This, taken together, is referred to as the *TCR complex*. When an antigen binds to the $\alpha\beta$-TCR, the conformation of the CD3 molecule changes and it transmits a message into the cell to activate the genetic machinery leading to an immune response.

The TCR does not recognize soluble antigen alone. CD4+ cells must recognize antigen in association with MHC class II molecules and CD8+ cells must recognize antigen in association with class I MHC present on the APC presenting the antigen to the T cell.

T-Helper Cell Subsets

Although all TH cells, as their name implies, recruit and stimulate other cells of the immune system in response to antigens, they do not all perform this function in the same way. TH lymphocytes can be further subdivided into at least two different groups: *TH1* and *TH2*. Whereas TH1 cells support cellular immune responses, TH2 cells support humoral responses.

The different TH cell subsets were first defined in a panel of mouse CD4+ clones; based on differential cytokine secretion, these cells were divided into TH1 and TH2 subsets.[18] TH1 cells secrete IL-2 and IFN-γ, whereas TH2 cells secrete IL-4, IL-5, IL-6, and IL-10. In addition, both subtypes also produce several lymphokines in common, namely, IL-3, GM-CSF, TNF, and preproenkephalin.[19] Both TH1 and TH2 subsets are believed to arise from a TH0 cell.

There appears to be an inhibitory feedback loop between the TH1 and TH2 subsets that may explain why most immune responses are predominantly cellular or predominantly humoral. Specifically, IFN-γ, secreted by TH1 cells, inhibits activation of TH2 cells, whereas IL-10, secreted by TH2 cells, inhibits TH1 proliferation[20] (Fig. 39-9).

The TH1 and TH2 cell subsets have also been characterized in humans. Differential cytokine secretion was demonstrated in CD4+ human T cells stimulated by either purified protein derivative (PPD) from *Mycobacterium tuberculosis* or the *Toxocara canis* excretory stimulatory antigen (TES). The PPD-stimulated cells produced IL-2 and IFN-γ, but not IL-4 or IL-5, whereas the TES-stimulated cells produced IL-4 and IL-5, but not IFN-γ or IL-2.[21] Based on this finding (and other data), it appears that bacterial antigens preferentially expand TH1 clones, whereas helminthic antigens and atopic allergens expand TH2 clones.[22] The importance of this is that a specific antigen induces the secretion of specific cytokines, or, conversely, through antigenic stimulation the aspect of the immune system (humoral vs. cellular) most appropriate to a particular antigen is recruited.

The existence of subtypes of CD8+ T cells has not yet been conclusively proven, but differential cytokine production between antigen-stimulated CD8+ clones has been demonstrated, and thus the presence of functional differences in these cells also seems likely.

T-Cell Development

T-cell development involves a series of complex steps involving genetically programmed acquisition of various cell surface markers. Most $\alpha\beta$-TCR+ T cells are believed to mature in the thymus. Fewer than 1% of all pre-T cells that enter the thymus emerge as phenotypically and functionally mature T cells. The pluripotent stem cell, which produces at least 11 different cell types or lineages, produces a precursor T lymphocyte that is TCR−/CD4−/CD8− but CD44+. This cell migrates to the thymus, where it undergoes a series of complex events resulting in maturation. During T-cell maturation, potentially autoreactive clones are removed by negative selection, an active process involving apoptosis (Fig. 39-10). The rearrangement and expres-

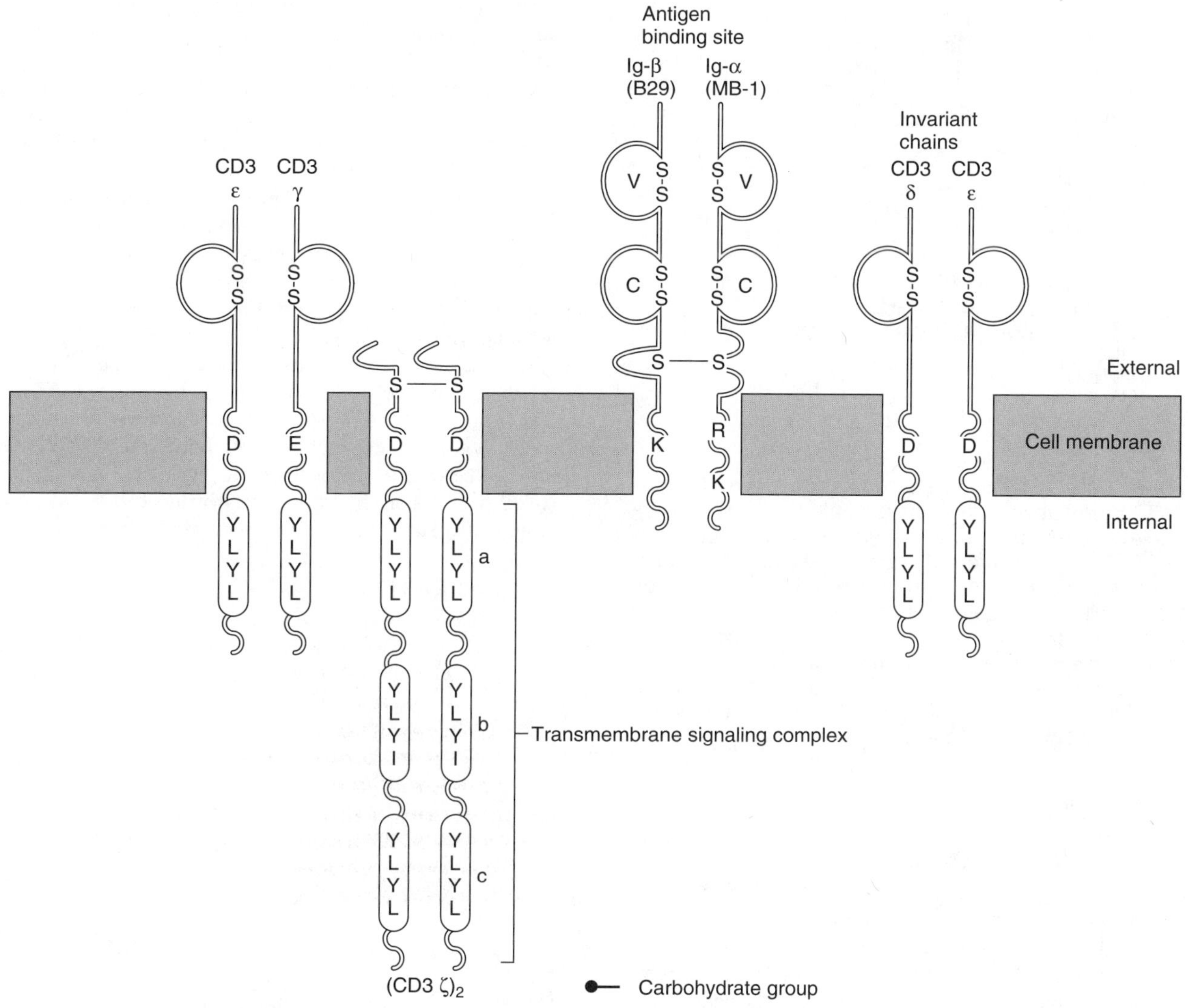

FIG. 39-8. The T-cell antigen receptor complex comprises four polypeptide dimers (TCR $\alpha\beta$, CD3 $\gamma\epsilon$, CD3 $\delta\epsilon$, and CD3 $\zeta\zeta$). As shown in this schematic, the antigen binding site itself is formed from the variable regions of the $\alpha\beta$ TCR heterodimer (or the $\gamma\epsilon$ TCR heterodimer). The associated CD3 protein is an important cytoplasmic signaling component of the TCR complex, and through interaction with intracellular tyrosine kinases, translates the signals generated by antigen binding into functional changes in cellular activity. C, constant region; V, variable region. (After Malissen B, Schmitt-Verhulst AM. Transmembrane signalling through the T-cell receptor–CD3 complex. Curr Opin Immunol 1993;5:324)

sion of the TCR α and β chains occurs at the same time that the CD44 marker is lost. At this time, CD4 and CD8 are coexpressed and the CD3/$\alpha\beta$-TCR complex is created. This phenotype is referred to as the *double-positive stage*. At the double-positive stage, each cell expresses $\alpha\beta$ TCR+/CD3+/CD4+/CD8+. This is a critical point in T-cell development. After double-positive cells have been generated, the developing T cells undergo both positive and negative selection events. During *positive selection*, those T cells whose TCRs have the capacity to recognize antigen in association with self-MHC survive, whereas those that cannot fail to develop further. The mechanism for positive selection is unclear, but protein kinases have been implicated. *Negative selection* (or *clonal deletion*) occurs by apoptosis (programmed cell death) to delete thymocytes with TCRs that strongly respond to self-antigens. As a result, those cells that would mediate autoimmunity are deleted.

Positive selection is mediated through interactions of developing thymocytes with non–bone-marrow-derived host stromal thymic epithelial cells in the thymic cortex, and negative selection is mediated by bone–marrow-derived dendritic cells in the corticomedullary junction and medulla. The small number of cells that survive this process of negative and positive selection (see later) leave the thymus as mature, single-positive (CD4+ or CD8+) T lymphocytes with rearranged TCR genes. The full phenotypic designation of these mature T lymphocytes is $\alpha\beta$-TCR+/CD3+/CD8+ or $\alpha\beta$-TCR+/CD3+/CD4+. Each TCR is a unique product of gene recombination, providing the specificity of the immune response.

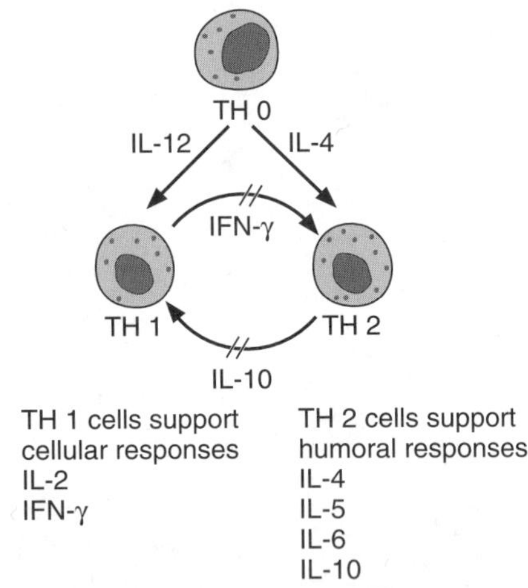

FIG. 39-9. Differential cytokine production determines T-helper (TH) cell subset differentiation. Interleukin-12 (IL-12), released by macrophages after stimulation by bacteria, protozoa, or viruses, and interferon-γ (IFN-γ), released by natural killer cells and $\gamma\epsilon$ T cells, cause the naive (TH0) cell to develop into a TH1 cell. Conversely, helminthic pathogens stimulate $\gamma\epsilon$ T cells, basophils, or mast cells and perhaps another, unknown, cell type to release IL-4. This IL drives TH0 cells to differentiate into the TH2 subset. TH2 cells produce IL-10, which inhibits the activation of TH1 cells. TH1 cells produce IFN-γ, which inhibits TH2 activity.

Apoptosis

Apoptosis, or programmed cell death, is an active process of cellular destruction or cell suicide that occurs by activation of an endogenous intracellular endonuclease. It is a default mechanism that proceeds if the T cell is autoreactive and encounters its ligand, or antigen, during development. Cells undergoing apoptosis demonstrate specific morphologic changes; their cellular DNA becomes fragmented and cell shrinkage is seen. Interestingly, those cells that undergo apoptosis do not incite an inflammatory response in the surrounding tissue. Teleologically, this would have substantial advantages.

There are several functions of apoptosis as it relates to immune function. This process acts to remove cells with nonfunctional receptors. Apoptosis also is responsible for deleting autoreactive T cells in the thymus to achieve "central tolerance," and in the peripheral lymphoid organs to remove both T and B cells to achieve "peripheral tolerance." One view of apoptosis is that it ensures self-tolerance and down-regulates excessive immune response.[23] Apoptosis plays a major role in fetal development and in T-cell development. For example, it is the mechanism by which digits are formed (by resorption of interdigital webs) during development of the hand. Finally, if apoptosis could be selectively triggered in cancer therapy, it could be a major benefit.

Both T and B lymphocytes undergo apoptosis. The molecular mechanism for apoptosis has been elegantly defined. The genes implicated in central T-cell apoptosis have been identified and include *p53*, *c-myc*, *nur-77*, *pim-1*, the *bcl-2* family, and *APO-1/Fas*. Most is known about the last two. *APO-1/Fas* and the *bcl-2* gene family appear to have reciprocal roles. The bcl-2

protein prevents cells from undergoing apoptosis, whereas the APO-1/Fas receptor may be essential to eliminate excess T cells[24] (Fig. 39-11).

A great deal is now known about the genetics of apoptosis. The *bcl-2* gene, originally isolated from the t(14;18) chromosomal breakpoint in follicular B-cell lymphoma, has been identified as an important regulator of apoptosis. This gene, which functions to rescue cells from programmed death without causing cell proliferation, is now known to be one of the *bcl-2*–related gene family.[25] Other genes in this family include *Bax*, *Bcl-x*, and *Mcl-1*. This family shares two highly conserved regions: *bcl-2* homology 1 (BH1) and *bcl-2* homology 2 (BH2) domains. Mutations in either BH1 and BH2 results in loss of cell death suppression activity. The mechanism used to activate mature resting T cells (that of signaling by the CD3–TCR complex) is the same as that which triggers apoptosis in developing T cells, but how these reciprocal activities are regulated is unknown. The critical factor that determines cell fate (activation vs. self-destruction) is dramatically influenced by stage in development (mature vs. immature, respectively).

$\alpha\beta$ T-Cell Receptors

The $\alpha\beta$ TCR comprises two α and two β chains. They are associated with a CD3 molecule, and together comprise the

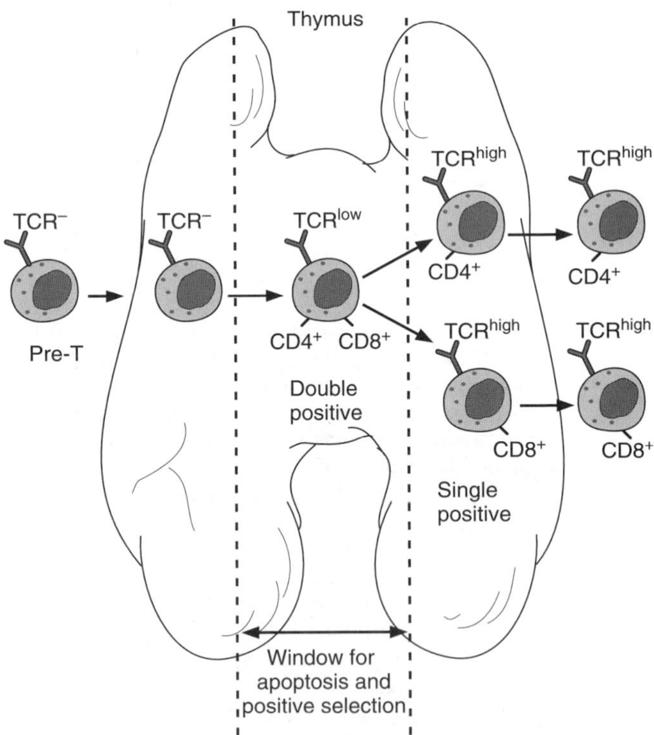

FIG. 39-10. The pre-T cell homes to the thymus after early development in the bone marrow. In the thymus, the T cell undergoes a complex maturation whereby it gains the TCR receptor and both the CD4 and CD8 receptors (the double-positive stage). At this stage, the cell undergoes both positive and negative selection to remove potentially autoreactive as well as nonfunctional T cells by apoptosis. Later, the T cell loses either the CD4 or the CD8 receptor (the single-positive stage) and leaves the thymus as a fully mature T cell.

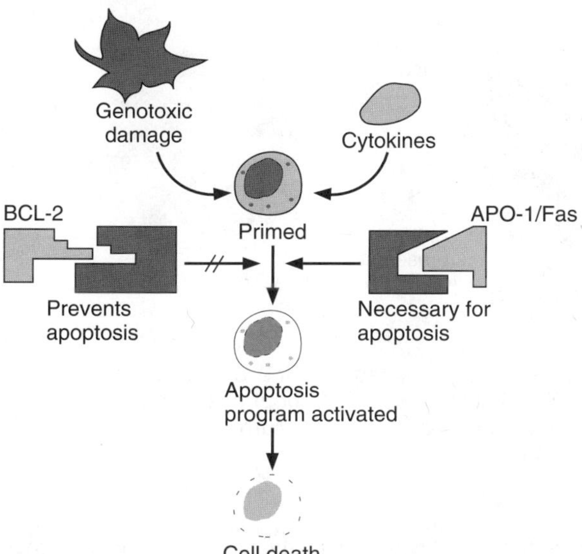

FIG. 39-11. Apoptosis, or programmed cell death, is an active process of cell suicide that occurs by the production of an endogenous intracellular endonuclease. In effect, the cell causes its own destruction by enzymatic cleavage of the DNA. Apoptosis is important in many ways. It removes nonfunctional and autoreactive cells during development, both in the thymus (central tolerance) and in the periphery (peripheral tolerance). During fetal development, the resorption of tissues (as in the digital web spaces) is also caused by apoptosis. (After Wylie A. Death gets a brake. Nature 1994;369:272)

TCR complex. The CD3 molecule itself is associated with the invariant chains γ, δ, and ϵ. When an antigen binds to the TCR, the conformation of the CD3 molecule changes and it transmits a message into the cell to activate the genetic machinery leading to an immune response (Fig. 39-12).

The TCR does not recognize soluble antigen by itself; CD4+ cells require that the antigen be presented in association with MHC class II molecules for recognition, and CD8+ cells require that it be presented in association with MHC class I.

$\tau\delta$-T Cells: Gut- and Bronchial-Associated Lymphoid Tissue

$\tau\delta$ T-cell receptor-positive T cells are located at areas of interface between the internal and the external milieu. These

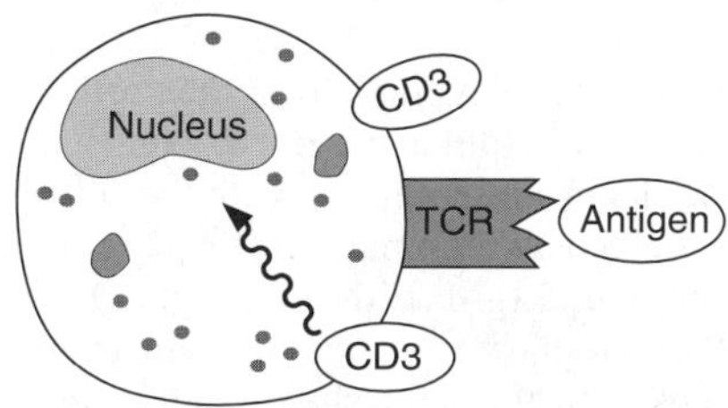

FIG. 39-12. Binding of a receptor by either an antigen or a cytokine (or both) leads to many changes in cellular activity. (After Swain SL, Wreth M. Editorial overview. Lymphocytes: the ultimate computers? Curr Opin Immunol 1994;6:355)

cells are thought to be particularly important in host resistance to infection. There are several different subsets of $\tau\delta$ TCR+ cells, and these are distributed in different locations. Each subset may express different cell surface proteins.

These cells are believed to develop independently of the thymus. Each of these subsets may differ in origin, selection, and function. The two most widely recognized compartments are the *GALT* and *BALT*. Cell trafficking to "spread the word" has been observed between the two compartments.

T-Cell Activation

When the T cell encounters its antigen, activation results (Fig. 39-13A). After a number of complex steps, cytokine synthesis, granule exocytosis, clonal expansion, and cell differentiation occur. Activation of a T cell requires more than a simple interaction between the antigen and the TCR. It has been demonstrated that the APC not only physically delivers the antigen to the TCR, but that specific ligands on the APC bind with T-cell surface molecules to provide *costimulatory signals* necessary for maximal T-cell activation and IL-2 secretion. In the absence of these complex requirements, T-cell activation cannot occur, and *anergy*, or functional inactivation, may result (see Fig. 39-13B).

The antigen–MHC complex must first bind the TCR of the naive (inactive) T cell, or, in some cases, the activated T cell, and then the accessory cell must provide a second, costimulatory signal. Without this interaction, CD8+ cytotoxic T cells will be inhibited (anergic) after antigen binding. Similarly, TH1 CD4+ lymphocytes that undergo TCR binding without accessory cell stimulation become anergic.

This second costimulatory signal occurs when a molecule on the T cell (CD28) interacts with a ligand (B7) on the APC surface. CD28 is a T-cell surface glycoprotein made of two identical disulfide-linked subunits. All human CD4+ cells and approximately half of CD8+ cells express CD28. A second, closely related antigen known as cytolytic T-lymphocyte–associated antigen (CTLA-4) is a cell surface protein that resembles CD28 and that also binds B7. Unlike CD28, which is expressed on T cells in the inactive state, CTLA-4 is expressed on T cells only after activation. The ligand found on the APC is B7 (also known as BB-1 or CD80). B7 is a highly glycosylated membrane protein that is constitutively expressed on APCs.

In CD4+ lymphocytes, the activation cascade is as follows: antigen, presented by an APC, binds to the specifically reactive TCR. As the interaction occurs, CD4 binds to class II and CD28 binds to B7 to stabilize the antigen–TCR interaction. As a result, increased amounts of mRNA encoding IL-2 in the T cell are produced. This mRNA is transcribed into the protein IL-2, which acts, in a paracrine fashion, to up-regulate the IL-2 receptors on the surface of nearby T lymphocytes. Resting T cells do not express the IL-2 receptor. Within hours after antigen binds to the cell, IL-2 receptors appear, and $\alpha\beta$-TCR as well as CD3 expression is decreased.

Although CD8+ T cells do not produce IL-2 themselves after TCR stimulation and CD28–B7 interaction, they become responsive to the presence of IL-2 and up-regulate and activate their IL-2 receptors.

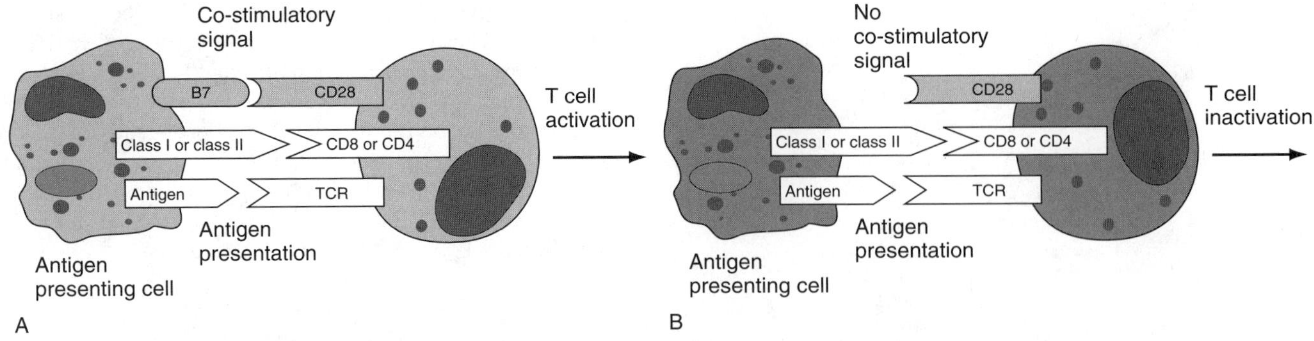

FIG. 39-13. (*A*) Interaction of an antigen with its specific T-cell receptor requires the presence of a costimulatory signal (B7 and CD28 interaction) to achieve T-cell activation. (*B*) Without this signal the same events (antigen and receptor interaction) result in T-cell inactivation. (After Murphy DB. T-cell mediated immunosuppression. Curr Opin Immunol 1993;5:411)

Cytokines That Function as T-Cell Growth Factors

The most important cytokine that functions as T-cell growth factor is *IL-2*. IL-2 is produced by CD4+ T cells and has both autocrine and paracrine activity. Stimulation by IL-2 causes T lymphocytes to begin proliferation. Resting T cells do not express IL-2 receptors. In the presence of IL-2, the number of IL-2 receptors on the cell is up-regulated. T-cell activation, then, is initiated when an antigen is presented to a CD4+ T cell by an APC with MHC class II molecule expression. IL-2 up-regulates both further IL-2 release and the expression of IL-2 receptors on the cell surface, leading to an amplification of the immune response. This cytokine–receptor interaction results in a clonal proliferation of T cells, as well as an increased production of both IL-2 and IL-2 receptors. Increased IL-2 results in further recruitment and proliferation of specifically reactive T cells. Once antigen is no longer present, the IL-2 receptors are down-regulated, and the activation cascade is halted. IL-2 has proven useful in a number of clinical trials to enhance the response of patients with various malignancies to their own tumor.

On the APC side of the T-cell–APC interaction, engagement of the APC class I or class II molecules with CD4 or CD8 and the TCR with antigen results in production of increased quantities of IL-1, which acts further to stimulate the immune response.

B CELLS

Overview

Whereas T lymphocytes function in cellular immunity, B lymphocytes are involved in humoral immunity. The primary function of B cells is to produce antibody in response to antigenic stimulation. Like T cells, B lymphocytes are clonal in nature; that is, each B cell can produce one (and only one) antibody in response to a specific antigen. The antigen-specific receptor for the B cell is the immunoglobulin itself. The B-cell receptor is a heterodimer composed of two light chains and two heavy chains. Similar to T cells, the membrane-bound immunoglobulin that functions as the B-cell antigen receptor is associated with several transmembrane glycoproteins (Ig-α; Ig-β) that

are the functional equivalents of CD3 on the T cell. Associated with this complex are coreceptor proteins such as CD19-CR2-TAPA-1, which interact with cytoplasmic signaling molecules (Fig. 39-14).

B-Cell Development

In the bone marrow, B lymphocytes differentiate from the hematopoietic stem cell into either mature, immunoglobulin-secreting plasma cells or stable peripheral B cells. The stage of maturation of a B cell can be determined from the expression of surface markers, the status of gene rearrangement, or the rate and type of immunoglobulin secretion. Maturation of B lymphocytes is both antigen independent and antigen dependent.

Bone marrow is the site of *antigen-dependent B-cell development*, whereas the peripheral lymphoid tissues are the site of *antigen-dependent maturation*, which occurs later when the mature B cell encounters its specific antigen.

The *pro–B-cell stage* is the first stage in development of the pluripotent hematopoietic stem cell into the B-cell lineage. In the pro-B cell, the B-lymphocyte immunoglobulin genes remain in a germline configuration (unrearranged), but the cell is committed to the B-cell lineage (Fig. 39-15*A*). The pro-B cell then undergoes heavy chain V(D)J recombination with subsequent expression of the cytoplasmic μ (heavy) chain. Once gene arrangement has occurred the cell is termed a pre-B cell. The μ (heavy) chain then associates with the surrogate light chains (ω and ι) produced by the early B-cell genes $\lambda5$ and *VpreB*, or can remain unassociated in the cytoplasm. The pre-B cell can neither recognize nor respond to antigen, despite the presence of this receptor.

The immature B cell develops from the pre-B cell while still in the bone marrow. Unlike the pre-B cell, which expresses cytoplasmic μ chains and receptors with the μ heavy chain and surrogate light chains, the immature B cell is characterized by true membrane-bound IgM. Either the light chain λ or κ gene rearranges, the cytoplasmic μ heavy chain from the previous stage associates with the light chain, and an immunoglobulin heterodimer is formed that is then expressed on the cell surface. Although immature B cells express membrane-bound IgM, unlike mature B cells, they do not proliferate or differentiate in response to antigen.

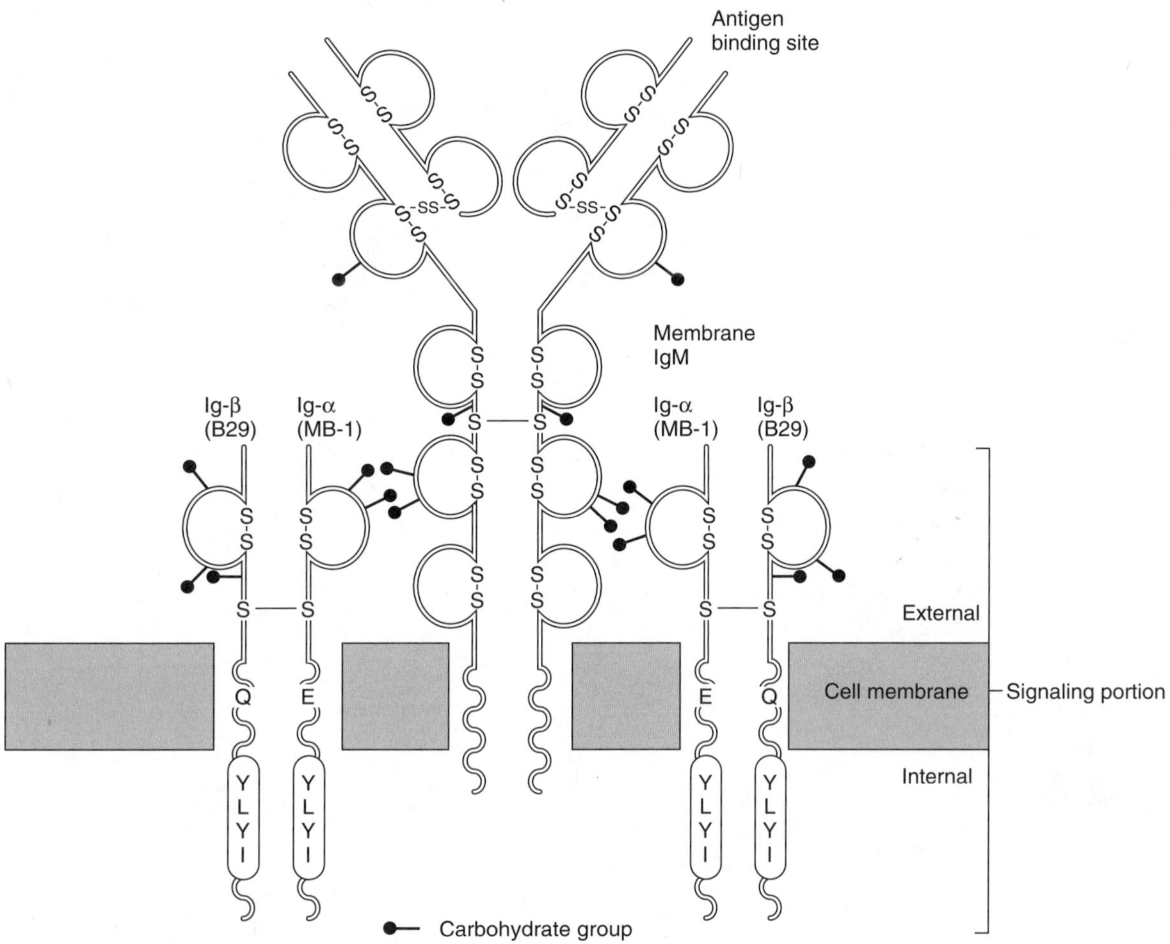

FIG. 39-14. B-cell receptor complex. Each receptor is composed of the immunoglobulin itself and two associated α and β chains whose transmembrane portions function to transduce signals to the inside of the cell. (After Malissen B, Schmitt-Verhulst AM. Transmembrane signalling through the T-cell receptor–CD3 complex. Curr Opin Immunol 1993;5:324)

Once immature B cells express a complete immunoglobulin receptor, they migrate from the bone marrow to the peripheral lymphoid tissues and circulate through the bloodstream. Even in the absence of further antigenic stimulation, these cells continue to mature. Phenotypically, the mature cells exhibit coexpression of μ and δ heavy chains associated with the original κ or λ light chain. Mature B cells are capable of responding to antigenic stimulation. Most of the resting peripheral B lymphocytes are IgM + or IgM + /IgD + . The antigen-specific receptor is the immunoglobulin itself. They require stimulation by their specific antigen for the final stage of maturation to occur. Without stimulation, they persist as senescent, mature B lymphocytes in the periphery.

Antigen-Dependent B-Cell Maturation

T helper cells and APCs are critical to activation of B cells by their specific antigen. Dendritic cells and macrophages (APCs) digest or process the antigen and transport it to other dendritic cells in the lymph nodes. Activated CD4 + TH cells express a cell surface molecule (variously called T-BAM, p39, or the CD40 ligand CD40L) that binds to CD40 on the surface of a B cell. This binding, plus secreted cytokines, leads to B-cell proliferation, class switching, and the development of *memory B cells*.

With activation, B cells proliferate and differentiate further into antibody-producing *plasma cells*. This is the primary antibody response. At the early stage of antibody response, the activated B cell has a low rate of immunoglobulin secretion. Later, antibody response with a higher rate of immunoglobulin secretion occurs. It is at this stage that the B cell can undergo *isotype switching*, an active process that involves gene rearrangement. Activated B cells that undergo isotype switching produce IgA, IgE, or IgG of the same antigenic specificity (with the same V region) as the previously expressed IgD and IgM. Some of these cells may not secrete antibody, but become, instead, memory B cells with persistent membrane-bound immunoglobulin (see Fig. 39-15B). Later stimulation of memory cells by the appropriate antigen results in a rapid secondary antibody response. Memory B cells produce antibody of higher affinity to antigen due to affinity maturation (point mutations of the genome during the resting phase, also known as somatic hypermutation).

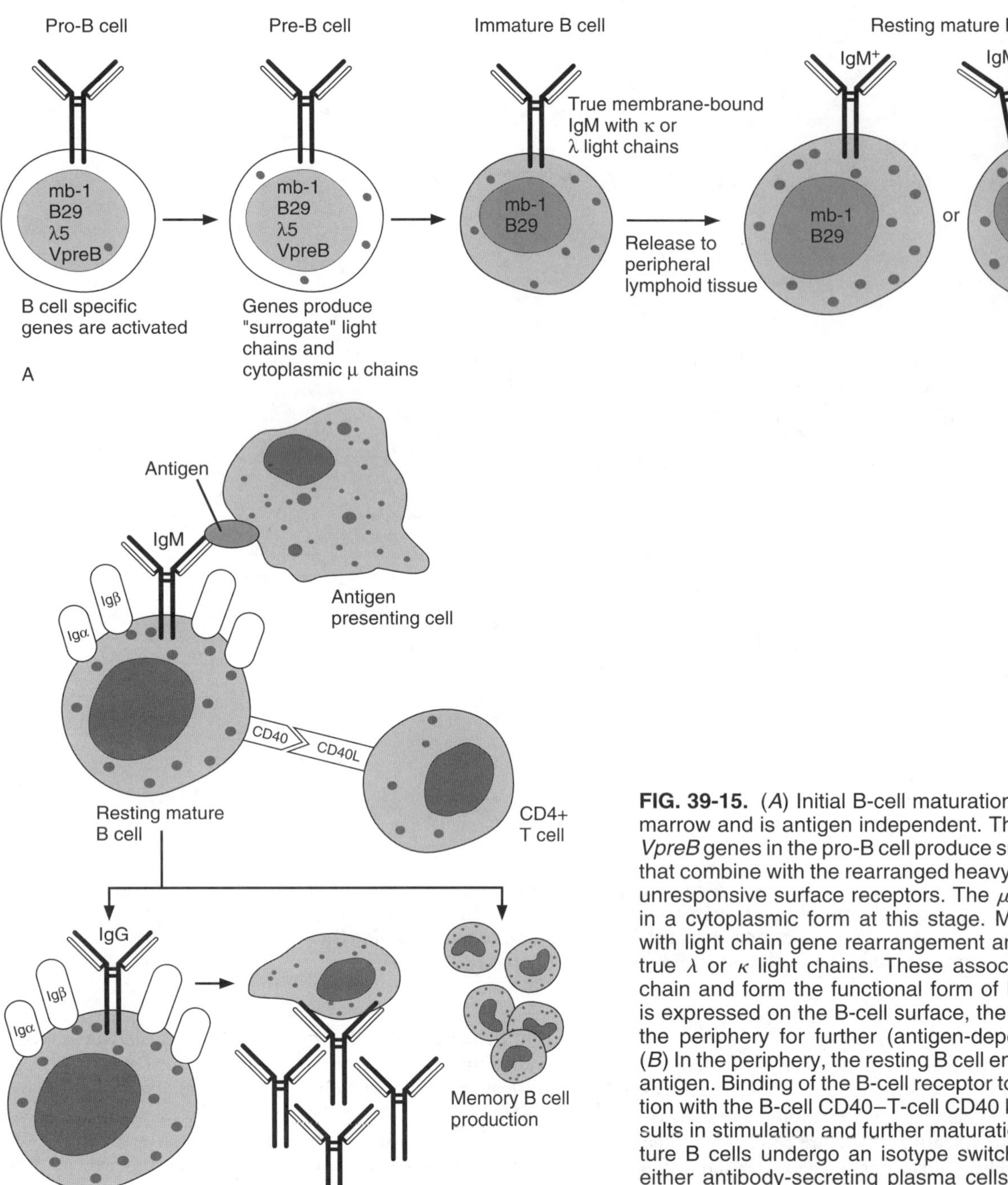

FIG. 39-15. (*A*) Initial B-cell maturation occurs in the bone marrow and is antigen independent. The activated *M5* and *VpreB* genes in the pro-B cell produce surrogate light chains that combine with the rearranged heavy μ chain as antigen-unresponsive surface receptors. The μ chain is also found in a cytoplasmic form at this stage. Maturation continues with light chain gene rearrangement and the production of true λ or κ light chains. These associate with the heavy chain and form the functional form of IgM. When this IgM is expressed on the B-cell surface, the cell is released into the periphery for further (antigen-dependent) maturation. (*B*) In the periphery, the resting B cell encounters its specific antigen. Binding of the B-cell receptor to antigen in association with the B-cell CD40–T-cell CD40 ligand interaction results in stimulation and further maturation of the B cell. Mature B cells undergo an isotype switch and then become either antibody-secreting plasma cells or resting memory cells. (*A* after Hogman J, Grossschedl R. Regulation and gene expression at early stages of B-cell differentiation. Curr Opin Immunol 1994;6:220)

Thus, antibody-secreting plasma cells can arise from either a primary antibody response due to stimulation of mature B cells by antigen or from a secondary antibody response due to stimulation of memory B cells by antigen.

Immunoglobulins

Immunoglobulins are glycoproteins produced primarily by plasma cells in response to foreign antigens. They are hetero-dimers and consist of two identical light (L) and two identical heavy (H) chains. Each of these chains contains both variable (VH and VL) and constant (CH and CL) regions. There are two L chain subclasses (κ and λ), with four known subtypes of λ. The *variable* region of the antibody is the antigen-binding site, whereas the *constant* portion contains a complement-binding site (Fc) and determines the immunoglobulin class, or isotype. The variable regions are at the amino-terminal end of the immunoglobulin molecule, whereas the constant regions are at the carboxy-terminal end (Fig. 39-16).

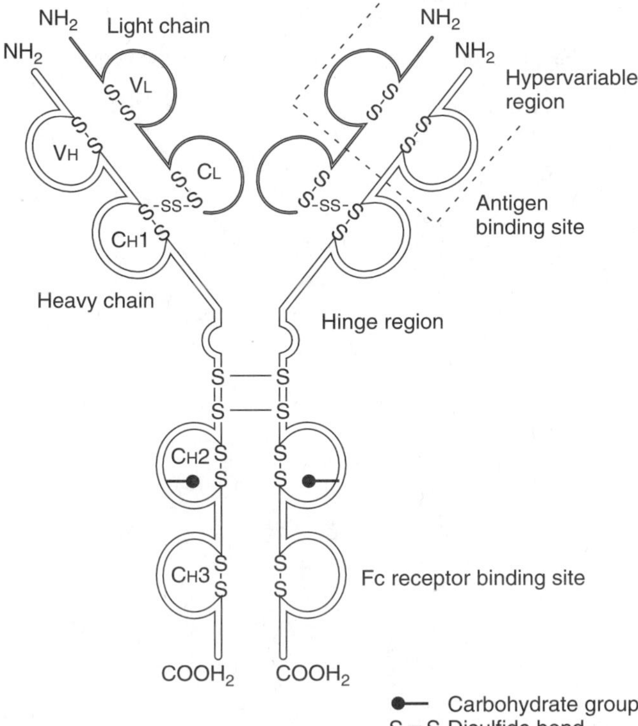

FIG. 39-16. The immunoglobulin is composed of two heavy and two light chains. The heavy chain constant region determines the isotype of the molecule, whereas the heavy and the light chain variable regions constitute the receptor or antigen-binding portion of the immunoglobulin. CH, heavy chain constant region; CL, light chain constant region; VH, heavy chain variable region; VL, light chain variable region. (After Abbas AK, Lichtman AH, Pober JS. Cellular and molecular immunology. Philadelphia, WB Saunders, 1991:39)

The heavy chain constant region determines the *isotype* of an immunoglobulin, whereas the hypervariable region, with the variable region, comprises the antigen-binding site (Fab). The immunoglobulin also contains a hinge region between the first and second constant domains (C1 and C2).

The functional regions of antibodies were originally described using enzymatic digestion. Papain digestion of the immunoglobulin results in the production of three similar-sized peptide fragments, one Fc and two Fab regions. The Fab region has the antigen-binding–associated activity, and the Fc comprises the effector functions (eg, complement binding). Pepsin digestion results in one (Fab)2 region comprising the two Fab units plus the hinge region, and random peptides from the digested Fc region (Fig. 39-17A). The two chains are held together by the intermolecular disulfide bonds, which also help to impart the molecular shape.

Classes of Immunoglobulins

The five immunoglobulin classes are IgM, IgD, IgG, IgA, and IgE (Fig. 39-18). Each of these is differentiated from the other by heavy chain structural differences and by functional differences in activity. Each immunoglobulin is composed of two heavy and two light chains; in addition, some immunoglobulins are also found as more complex molecules, such as pentamers (five immunoglobulin molecules) and dimers (two immunoglobulins).

IgM (a pentamer) is expressed on resting B cells and is the first antibody to appear in a primary antibody response. It is also the first antibody made in the neonatal period. IgM is effective in fixing complement, which leads to eventual phagocytosis or lysis of microorganisms. IgM is also found in immune complexes in autoimmune disease.

IgG, a monomer with multiple subtypes (IgG1, IgG2, IgG3, and IgG4), appears in a primary immune response after isotype switching. IgG is the most prevalent antibody; 75% of human immunoglobulin is of this isotype. IgG is the only immunoglobulin that crosses the placenta to provide protection to the fetus and neonate. Similar to IgM, IgG binds to receptors on phagocytic cells to facilitate the destruction of microorganisms.

IgG and IgM function in internal host defenses, whereas the next subtype, IgA, is responsible for external host defenses.

IgA exists in two subtypes, IgA1 and IgA2. The monomer IgA1 is a serum antibody, whereas the dimer sIgA (IgA2) is a secretory form of IgA connected by the J (or joining) chain plus a glycoprotein ''secretory piece.'' Mucosal IgA is secreted locally, is found on mucous membranes, and has potent antiviral activity. It provides the primary defense against locoinvasive infections because of its location at these sites of interface between the internal and external systems. The principal function of sIgA may, in fact, be as simple as providing a physical barrier preventing absorption and adherence of antigens to mucosal surfaces.

Studies have suggested two additional functions for sIgA. The first of these is to neutralize intracellular pathogens (eg, viruses) within epithelial cells, and the second is to bind antigen within the lamina propria and excrete this antigen into an adjacent lumen. IgA also fixes complement by the alternative pathway. IgA is found in greatest concentration in saliva, tears, bronchial fluid, mucus, and the small intestine. Serum IgA is the second most common antibody and comprises about 15% of the total. Secretory IgA, on the other hand, is synthesized in a greater amount than all the other types of immunoglobulins combined.

IgE functions in type I hypersensitivity responses, also known as IgE-mediated or anaphylactoid responses. In this reaction, the mediators released from mast cells and basophils result in increased vascular permeability and smooth muscle contraction. IgE also functions in the destruction of parasites.

IgD is found in minute quantities in the serum and, with IgM, is the predominant antibody found on the immature B lymphocyte.

Immunoglobulin Gene Rearrangement and Class Switching in B Cells

The development of B cells from the stem cell to the mature B cell can be described in terms of rearrangement of the heavy and light chain genes. Rearrangement is responsible for the tremendous antigenic diversity of antibodies. The usual antibody repertoire is described as 10^9 to 10^{11} different specificities. Without the ability to rearrange genes, each specific immunoglobulin would need to be encoded by a distinct gene sequence.

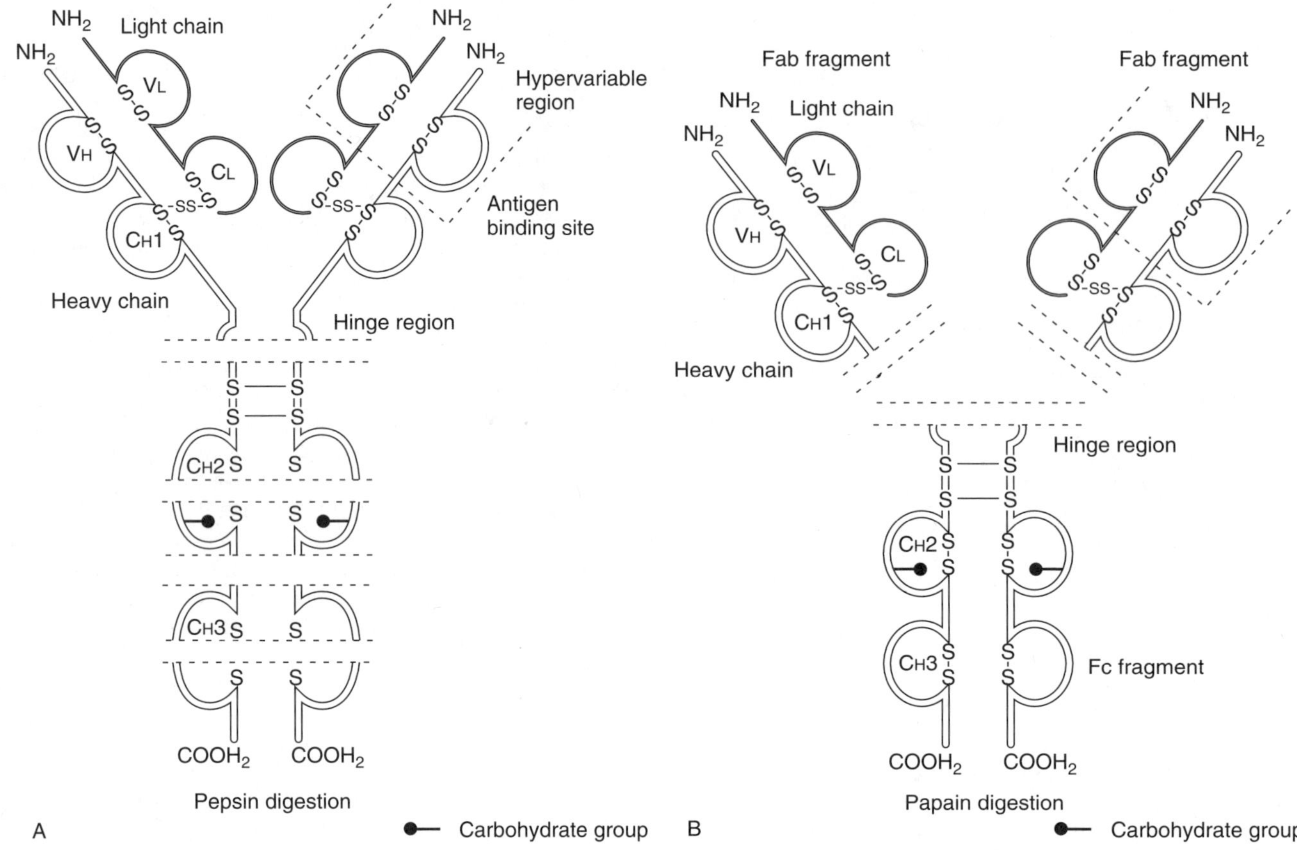

FIG. 39-17. The functional domains of the immunoglobulins were originally defined using enzymatic digestion. Pepsin cleaves the molecule into one (Fab)2 region (*A*), whereas papain digestion results in two Fab segments and one Fc segment (*B*). The Fab segment is the antigen binding site, and the Fc region has effector functions such as complement binding. CH, heavy chain constant region; CL, light chain constant region; VH, heavy chain variable region; VL, light chain variable region. (After Abbas AK, Lichtman AH, Pober JS. Cellular and molecular immunology. Philadelphia, WB Saunders, 1991:39)

This would require a prohibitively large amount of genetic material.

The unrearranged light and heavy chain genes are known as *germline DNA*. The recombination system that enables the rearrangement of the germline DNA is the *VDJ recombinase system*. VDJ recombinase mediates rearrangement of both the B-cell immunoglobulin genes and the T-cell TCR variable region genes. The sequence of gene rearrangements is highly regulated; in the immunoglobulin gene system, the heavy chain genes are always rearranged before the light chain genes, although the particular gene segments recombined on a chromosome are random.

The first rearrangement occurs on the heavy chain chromosomes during the stem cell to pre–B-cell development phase through the association of a *DH* gene (ie, *h*eavy chain, *d*iversity gene) with a *JH* gene (*h*eavy chain, *j*oining gene). Then, the DJ segment (or DHJH segment) is associated with a *VH* gene (*h*eavy chain, *v*ariable gene) and the complete VDJ (or VHDHJH segment) is formed. After this occurs, the pre-B cell can produce cytoplasmic μ chains (but not surface IgM, because there is no associated light chain production). The diversity that can be obtained by this rearrangement depends on random selection from among the several V, D, and J gene segments

available and also on junctional changes (addition of N regions) catalyzed by terminal deoxynucleotidyl transferase.

Next, light chain rearrangement occurs. Only one light chain isotype is expressed on the surface of a mature B cell (isotype exclusion). During light chain rearrangement, the κ locus is manipulated before the λ locus in the mouse (and presumably the human). Ninety-five percent of mature B cells have a κ light chain, whereas only 5% have a λ light chain. After a complex rearrangement, the B cell expresses surface IgM, composed of two identical rearranged heavy and two identical rearranged light chains. With expression of the surface IgM receptor, the B cell can now migrate into the peripheral blood and lymphoid tissues for final, antigen-dependent maturation.

Affinity Maturation

Antibodies produced in a secondary (memory) response have higher antigenic affinity than those produced in a primary response. This is termed *affinity maturation*. There are two possible causes of this. First, there may be a shift in the repertoire of the germline genes used in primary and secondary (memory) responses. Second, there may be a diversification of this pri-

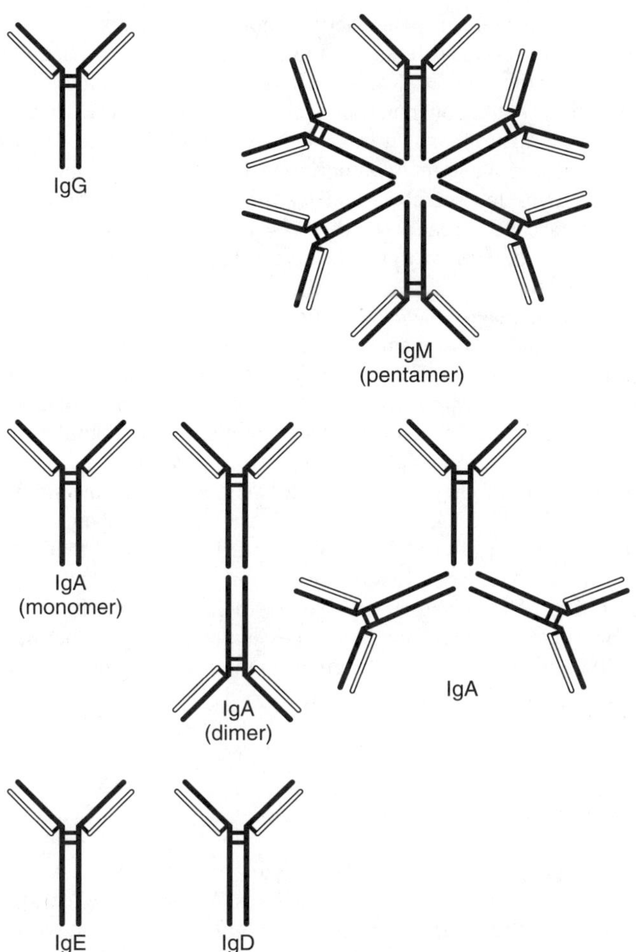

FIG. 39-18. The different immunoglobulin classes comprise varied arrangements of the same molecule.

mary response by *somatic hypermutation*, a process whereby apparently random changes in heavy and light chains result in development of clones with greater or lesser affinity for an antigen. Those clones with higher affinity for an antigen are selected and enter the pool of memory cells. Some support for the latter method as the main mechanism can be seen in the fact that specific "key mutations" that increase the affinity of antigen for antibody become disseminated throughout the gene pool within 2 weeks after activation of B cells. This prevalence of a specific clone is probably the result of both positive selection of cells with high-affinity receptors and negative selection of those with low-affinity receptors.

B-Cell Receptors and Signaling

The mechanism by which binding of antigen to the cell surface immunoglobulin receptor of the B cell is translated into intracellular signals has been difficult to characterize. B-cell receptor-associated proteins that resemble the CD3 complex of the TCR have been identified.[26] This complex is characterized as a disulfide-linked heterodimer of two transmembrane glycoproteins, Ig-α (encoded by the gene *mb-1*) and Ig-β (encoded by the gene *B29*). Together, these comprise the B-cell receptor

complex. The immunoglobulin functions as the antigen receptor, whereas the heterodimer functions as the signal transduction mechanism. Presumably, the first event in signal transduction is cross-linking of the B-cell receptor complex. Internalization of antigen leads to activation of various tyrosine kinases within the cell. These, in turn, signal the induction of transcription of the genes necessary for proliferation and differentiation of cells. Potentially, cross-linkage of surface Ig receptors by antigen would initiate a signal cascade involving guanosine triphosphate-binding proteins, protein serine kinases, and protein tyrosine kinases and phosphatases. The final product is an activated B lymphocyte.

B-Cell Growth Factors: IL-4

IL-4 is the prototypic B-cell growth factor. It is produced by CD4 + T cells and is responsible for inducing resting B cells to proliferate. It also stimulates the up-regulation of expression of MHC class II molecules. IL-4 is secreted by the TH2 subtype of CD4 + T cells and activates B cells and mast cells, while down-regulating macrophage function. It is a mast cell growth factor. In addition, IL-4 plays an important regulatory role in the interaction between TH1 and TH2 cells (see earlier). IL-4 also negatively affects TH1 cellular function, decreasing the release of such TH1 cellular products as IL-2 and IFN. Other cytokines involved in B-cell growth and differentiation include IL-5, IL-6, and IL-7.

NATURAL KILLER CELLS

Natural killer cells are cytotoxic lymphocytes that, unlike T cells, do not require interaction with an APC of self-origin to respond to antigen. Their activation response is immediate and does not require "priming." Phenotypically, NK cells are large, granular lymphocytes and, like other cells of the immune system, they arise from the pluripotent hematopoietic stem cell. In humans, their cell surface phenotype is CD16 + /CD56 + . The main function of the NK cells is to kill tumors or virally infected cells through a nonspecific mechanism that does not involve MHC restriction.

A subset of NK cells has been demonstrated that has the ability selectively to destroy allogeneic cells. This ability may be clonally distributed and involve the same MHC class I antigens used by cytotoxic T lymphocytes (CD8 + T cells).[27] These and further studies show that there is heterogeneous population of NK cells in each individual, and that the different NK cell clones can recognize and selectively lyse normal allogeneic cells but do not react against autologous cells.[28]

Other work has indicated that NK cells secrete immunoregulatory cytokines, including IFN-γ, TNF-α, IL-1β, GM-CSF, and transforming growth factor (TGF)-β.[29,30] The ability of NK cells to secrete IFN-γ enables them to activate host macrophages before antigen-specific T-cell presentation.

NK cell activity is regulated by cytokine secretion by macrophages and T cells. The best known of these regulatory cytokines are IL-2, IFN-α/β, TGF-1β, IFN-γ, and IL-4. In addition, IL-10 (cytokine synthesis inhibitory factor) and IL-12 (NK stimulatory factor) have been found to be important in NK regulation. IL-10, originally identified as a product of TH2 cells, inhibits IFN-γ secretion from TH1 and NK cells through the inhibition of macrophage derived cofactors TNF-α and IL-12, and possibly by direct action on NK cells. IL-12, conversely, enhances the cytolytic activity and proliferation of both NK and T cells; this lymphokine directly and indirectly (by IL-2 and TNF-α) induces IFN-γ secretion. Finally, evidence is accumulating that NK cells themselves may influence whether TH1 or TH2 CD4+ subsets predominate.

MONONUCLEAR PHAGOCYTE SYSTEM: THE ANTIGEN-PRESENTING CELLS

The monocyte–macrophage family was previously known as the reticuloendothelial system. It is now termed the mononuclear phagocyte system, and includes tissue macrophages such as alveolar macrophages, tissue histiocytes, peritoneal macrophages, dendritic cells, hepatic Kupffer cells, Langerhans cells in the skin, osteoclasts, and microglia. These cells can mediate effector functions such as destruction of *opsonized* (antibody-coated) bacteria (ie, extracellular pathogens) as well as intracellular pathogens. Macrophages also have an antibody-independent NK-like activity. They express surface receptors, including those for the Fc region of IgG, activated complement, and lymphokines. The most important role for macrophages in the immune response is antigen presentation. Macrophages and monocytes, as well as dendritic cells, are known collectively as *APCs* because they play a critical role in sampling the environment for foreign antigen. They are scavenger cells that function to phagocytose antigen, digest it into sequences 5 to 15 amino acids in length, and present these fragments, known as epitopes, on the cell surface. This displayed epitope is then recognized by the effector cell (lymphocyte) with the appropriate HLA class marker and a complementary receptor.

The two most recognized APCs are *macrophages* and *dendritic cells*. Both are bone marrow-derived cells. Dendritic cells are a hundred times more efficient at presenting antigen than macrophages. During antigen exposure, dendritic cells move into peripheral lymph nodes, where they mature, up-regulate their MHC class II expression, and become specialized at activating T cells. For a primary immune response, a naive T cell must be selected and stimulated. Because these naive cells are in the peripheral lymphoid tissues, the antigen responsible for stimulation must be transported to those tissues by the dendritic cells.

Macrophage Activation

The immune system is highly integrated and interdependent. The binding of a specifically reactive T cell to a macrophage presenting the antigen initiates a series of events that ultimately results in an amplification of the immune response. Conversely, activated T lymphocytes release macrophage-activating lymphokines, which activate macrophages so that they become multinucleated giant cells.

The first cytokine identified was *migration inhibitory factor*, which causes macrophages to increase expression of IL-6 and TNF-α. IFN-γ and TNF-α are critical components of macrophage activation. In vitro, LPS is a potent stimulator of many early events in macrophage activation leading to the production of TNF-α, IL-1, and IL-6, but requires that the macrophage be prestimulated with IFN-γ. That is, IFN-γ causes induction of TNF-α receptors on macrophages, and then the TNF-α produced by macrophages in response to LPS stimulation can act on the macrophage in an autocrine fashion, thereby amplifying further cytokine secretion and leading to the production of a signal cascade. Creation of this cascade in vitro using LPS is thought to be similar to the in vivo inflammatory response of tissue in sepsis.

In vivo, macrophage activation can be divided into three routes. First, macrophages can be activated by the release of soluble TNF-α and IFN-γ from TH1 CD4+ T cells (resulting in antitumor and antimicrobial activity). Second, macrophages may be activated by soluble IFN-γ and membrane-bound TNF-α. Finally, macrophages may be activated by TH2 CD4+ T lymphocytes if they are preprimed with IFN-γ from another source. The TH2 cells can then activate the macrophages, presumably as a result of CD28–B7 interaction. Without this IFN-γ priming, TH2 cells function to inhibit macrophages through secretion of IL-4 and IL-10 (which, themselves, inhibit TNF-α production). Therefore, it may be the macrophage rather than TH0 cells that determine whether a response is predominantly TH1 (cellular) or TH2 (humoral).

Granulocytes

The polymorphonuclear leukocytes are nonspecific amplifiers and effectors of immune responses. *Neutrophils* exert their activity through surface receptors for IgG, C3d, and C3b, *basophils* through surface receptors for IgE, C3a, and C5a, and *eosinophils* through receptors for IgE as well as direct cytotoxic effects on parasites.

Eosinophils are terminally differentiated leukocytes found in submucosal tissues. They are recruited to sites of specific immune reactions, including allergies. These cells elaborate leukotriene C4, platelet-activating factor, lipoxins, cationic proteins from cytoplasmic granules that result in local tissue damage and dysfunction, as well as the cytokines GM-CSF, IL-3, IL-5, IL-1α, IL-6, IL-8, TNF-α, TGF-α, and TGF-β. Functionally, IL-3 and GM-CSF promote eosinophil survival and enhance eosinophil effector responses, and IL-5 antagonizes apoptosis. The four cationic basic proteins—major basic protein, eosinophil-derived neurotoxin, eosinophil-cationic protein, and eosinophil peroxidase—contribute to the acute and late inflammatory effects.[31]

Neutrophils, also called polymorphonuclear leukocytes, are large granular cells with a multilobed nucleus. They are the most numerous of the white blood cells and play a major role in host defense against invading microorganisms and in the acute inflammatory response. Foreign antigen encountered by the neutrophil is phagocytized and degraded within the cell by microbicidal enzymes within the granules and reactive oxygen metabolites generated on the cell surface. Patients deficient in polymorphonuclear leukocytes are highly susceptible to bacterial infection. This protective function of neutrophils, however, is tempered by the relatively nonspecific nature of the reaction. Evidence now suggests that neutrophils, and the enzymatic products they produce, are important mediators in such inflammatory disorders as rheumatoid arthritis and adult respiratory distress syndrome.

Mast cells release cytokines after activation by antigen. The main cytokines released by the mast cell include TNF-α, IL-4, IL-5, and IL-6. TNF-α stimulates endothelial leukocyte adhesion molecule (ELAM-1) expression by endothelial cells and integrins on Langerhans cells, and helps to recruit neutrophils. Because they release IL-4 after stimulation, both mast cells and basophils (another cell type that releases IL-4) may function to influence the development of the TH2 subset of CD4+ T lymphocytes.[32]

COMPLEMENT

In 1901, Jules Bordet discovered that serum that had been heated to nonphysiologic temperatures was no longer able to lyse bacteria, despite the fact that the antibody present was still able to agglutinate bacteria. Bordet postulated the presence of a separate, heat-labile component of serum that "complemented" antibody function in cell lysis. Although he conceptualized this as a single agent, we now know that the complement system is a complex, interrelated system of proteins.

The principal functions of the complement system include *complement-mediated cytotoxicity* or *cytolysis* (by the C5b-9 membrane attack complex [MAC]), *opsonization and phagocytosis* (which depend on the ligands C3b and iC3b and their receptors CR1 and CR3), and *inflammatory responses* (due to the proinflammatory mediators C3a, C4a, and C5a; Table 39-4). The complement system is important in modulating the adaptive immune responses, including antigen presentation, T-cell activation, B-cell activation, antibody response, and immunologic memory. For example, the breakdown products of this cascade can be the proinflammatory mediators C5a, C4a, and C3a, which lead to smooth muscle contraction, vasoactive amine release, and increased vascular permeability. C5a is the most biologically significant of these. It also functions as a potent chemoattractant for neutrophils and macrophages, stimulates neutrophil and macrophage responses (such as cytokine secretion), and stimulates IL-6 synthesis.[33]

The schema of the complement system is similar to the coagulation cascade. In both of these, previously activated proteins (known as zymogens) act on the next protein in the system to effect its activation. In this fashion, an amplification of response is obtained.

The complement system is divided into classic and alternative pathways. The *classic pathway* depends on specific interaction between an immunoglobulin and complement. The C1q subunit of complement factor C1 is activated by interacting with IgG or IgM, which in turn activates C1r and C1s (two other subunits of C1). IgM is more efficient at activating the complement cascade than IgG. The activated C1 then cleaves C4 into C4b and C4a, and C2 into C2a and C2b. C4b then binds to an activating surface, functions as an acceptor for C2a, and forms the classic C3 convertase C4b2a. This convertase then cleaves C3 into C3b and C3a. C3b can have two different functions. It can continue as part of the classic pathway, combining with C4b to produce the classic C5 convertase C4b3b2a, or it can act to amplify alternate pathway activation. The classic C5 convertase cleaves C5 into C5a and C5b, and C5b then initiates the terminal pathway to produce MAC C5b6-9.

TABLE 39-4. *Complements and their functions*

Complement	Function
C1q, Clr, Cls	Forms a CA^{+2} linked complex (C1qClr$_2$Cls) which binds to Ig and initiates the classic complement pathway
C4, C2	Classic pathway; w/Cls forms C3 convertase (C4b2b)
C3	Active C3 (C3b) is an opsonin that activates the alternative pathway, C3a causes mast cell degranulation and smooth muscle contraction; other breakdown products are C3bi, C3d, C3e and C3g
C5	Active, membrane-bound C5 (C5b) activates the alternative pathway, C5a is chemotactic for macrophages and neutrophils, causes smooth muscle contraction, mast cell degranulation, increased capillary permeability
C6, C7, C8, C9	With C5b assembles into membrane attack complex
B, D	Binds with C3 and is then cleaved by D to form C3 convertase (C3bBb) for alternative pathway
P	Stabilizes C3bBb
C4bp, H(β_1H)	C4bp binds C4b, H binds C3b; these act as cofactors to cleave and inactivate C3b and C4b

The immunoglobulins IgG and IgM use the classic pathway, whereas IgA and IgD use the *alternative pathway*. The alternative pathway, also known as the slow pathway, does not depend on the presence of antibody. Small amounts of activated C3 (C3.H$_2$O), which functions like C3b, are continuously formed in the fluid phase. This C3.H2O attaches to the amino or hydroxyl groups of surrounding surfaces, binds to factor B, and is cleaved by factor D to form the alternate C3 convertase C3bBb. This complex cleaves C3 into C3b and C3a; the C3b is added to the previous convertase to form the alternate C5 convertase C3bBb3b. This alternate C5 convertase, like the classic C5 convertase, cleaves C5 into C5a and C5b and leads into the terminal pathway that forms MAC C5b6-9.

TYING IT ALL TOGETHER: THE REJECTION RESPONSE

Classically, organ rejection is divided into three categories that differ in both time of occurrence and mechanics.

Hyperacute rejection occurs immediately after the transplanted organ becomes vascularized. This type of rejection is mediated by preformed antibodies present in the recipient's serum against antigens expressed on the cells of the donor. It causes immediate destruction of the graft and is usually termed "white rejection." The preformed antibodies bind to antigens present on donor endothelial cells, activating complement and resulting in direct destruction of the donor tissue. In kidney transplantation, this type of rejection is seen after transplantation of ABO-incompatible grafts. Preformed anti-donor antibodies are also found in the serum of patients who have previously rejected an organ or been multiply transfused, and in multiparous women who have been exposed to foreign antigens from the fetus during pregnancy. Incubating patient serum with splenocytes or lymph nodes from the donor before transplantation is an effective means of screening for this potentially catastrophic event. This type of antibody-mediated rejection is also responsible for the initial events in the rejection of most xenografts. In this case, antibodies against other species are found naturally in the recipient's serum. Control of hyperacute rejection is one of the major challenges in experimental xenotransplantation.

Acute rejection characteristically occurs during the first 6 months after transplantation and can result whenever clinical immunosuppression is inadequate. This type of rejection is cellularly mediated and results in a lytic destruction of the donor tissue. The transplantation of a foreign organ or tissue into a patient exposes the host to the histocompatibility antigens present on the donor cells. All cells express class I, whereas APCs and some other cell types also express class II. Host CD4+ cells become activated when their TCR complex (CD3-$\alpha\beta$TCR in association with CD4) is exposed to an alloantigen in combination with an MHC class II molecule. Either donor endothelial cells or the so-called "passenger lymphocytes" (the APCs) in the graft can carry out this antigen-presenting function. In addition to stimulating the CD4+ cells with antigen, APCs that present the antigen are activated to produce IL-1, which causes proliferation of cells. Activation by the association of TCR and alloantigen stimulates a clonal proliferation of the CD4+ cells by inducing the production of both IL-2 and the expression of the IL-2 receptor on the cell surface. These CD4+ cells help to initiate the cascade of events that results in graft rejection. CD8+ cytotoxic T cells in the vicinity are also stimulated to proliferate by the paracrine effects of IL-2. Activated CD8+ cells are the primary effector cells in the acute rejection response, directly lysing the donor cells. The CD8+ cells recognize donor class I antigen. Other cells, including B cells and macrophages, are also activated by the cytokines (IL-5 and IL-6 in the case of B cells) secreted by the proliferating CD4+ cells. Histologic examination of tissues undergoing acute rejection reveals a dense cellular infiltrate with both CD4+ and CD8+ cells present.

The third type of rejection is *chronic rejection*, which is characterized by a gradual replacement of the transplanted organ by fibrous tissue, leading to an eventual loss of function. The mechanism of chronic rejection is less well understood than that of acute rejection, but it is believed to be antibody mediated. One hypothesis is that chronic deposition of antibody–antigen complexes in the blood vessels of the transplanted organ induces an ischemic tissue injury that is repaired by fibrosis. Vanishing bile duct syndrome in liver transplants, coronary atherosclerosis in heart transplants, and bronchiolitis obliterans in lung transplants are all believed to represent a form of chronic rejection. Unfortunately, available immunosuppressive agents fail to treat chronic rejection. Clinically, only 20% of cadaveric renal allografts are functional at 10 years.[34]

The terms "acute rejection" and "chronic rejection" are misnomers of sorts. Both types of rejection can occur at any time after transplantation, and the two conditions can coexist. The terminology does, however, provide a useful framework for conceptualizing rejection in that acute rejection is readily treatable if diagnosed early (although graft function does not usually return to prerejection levels), whereas chronic rejection is an insidious, gradual, and relatively untreatable form of the disease. As the mechanism responsible for chronic rejection becomes better understood, new strategies in intervention may become available.

THE PRESENT AND THE FUTURE: BONE MARROW TRANSPLANTATION, CHIMERISM, AND TOLERANCE

The immunosuppression agents used in clinical transplantation are usually successful in preventing acute graft rejection. They are nonspecific in function and induce a delicate balance in which the host immune system is rendered relatively unresponsive to permit allograft survival. In addition to the considerable end-organ toxicities of the individual drugs, the immunosuppression places the transplant recipient at risk for life-threatening infection because of an inability to respond to pathogens. Generalized immunosuppression is also associated with an increased risk of malignancy, approaching 30 times that of the normal population.[35] Moreover, chronic rejection remains a major limitation. For these reasons, achieving a drug-free state in which allograft survival could be maintained without artificial immunosuppression is the goal of immunologists working in transplantation.

In experimental models, such a state of permanent, donor-specific tolerance has been achieved using BMT. The successful engraftment of donor bone marrow has been shown to render the host tolerant to future tissue or organ transplants from the same donor. Tolerance was permanent and donor specific; grafts from a third party were rejected normally. Animals treated in such a way are called *chimeras*.

Unfortunately, conventional BMT is not a benign procedure. First, the patient's native hematopoietic system must be "conditioned" to provide space for the donor cells. Conditioning incorporates a combination of total-body irradiation and high-dose chemotherapy. In the treatment of hematologic malignancies, this conditioning is in itself part of the anticancer therapy, and patients treated with supralethal doses of chemotherapy or radiation therapy are rescued by the transplantation of bone marrow. In the case of organ transplantation, however, the toxicity of the preparative therapy cannot be justified. The second major limitation of BMT is GVHD, in which the transplanted mature donor cells see the host as foreign. Post-BMT GVHD is a major cause of morbidity and morality.

Studies have demonstrated that full host ablation is not required for the induction of tolerance. The coengraftment of bone marrow from both host and donor is sufficient to permit permanent survival of transplanted organs and tissues. Such mixed chimeras have several advantages over fully ablated recipients.[36] First, they demonstrate superior immunocompetence because APCs of both host and donor are present.[37] Second, mixed chimeras in both experimental models and clinical reports are resistant to GVHD. Finally, low levels of donor cell engraftment can be achieved using nonlethal conditioning regimens. Clinical trials are underway in several centers to evaluate combined bone marrow and solid organ transplantation for the induction of permanent, drug-free tolerance.

Another approach that was investigated was the removal of GVHD-inducing cells from the donor bone marrow before transplantation. T-cell depletion (TCD) was performed in a number of clinical BMT trials in the 1980s.[38] The results of these studies demonstrated a decreased occurrence of GVHD in patients who received TCD bone marrow. Unfortunately, however, this favorable outcome was tempered by a prohibitively high rate of engraftment failure, an essentially lethal complication in aggressively conditioned patients. It was concluded that T cells were essential for engraftment of stem cells, and approaches for TCD were abandoned. More recently, a novel cell type in bone marrow that permits engraftment without GVHD has been identified. This cell expresses some T-cell markers and therefore would have been removed by classic TCD regimens. In a murine model, such a *facilitating cell* has been identified and purified.[39] This cell permits engraftment of purified allogeneic stem cells without GVHD. Large-scale purification of stem cells and facilitating cells may in the future allow for a component type of BMT, with minimal conditioning and little or no risk of GVHD. As a result, BMT could be more readily justified in chronic disease states known to be treatable by BMT in which the morbidity and mortality from conventional BMT could not be justified.

Autologous BMT is another means to avoid the risks of GVHD and graft failure. Studies evaluating the mobilization and isolation of stem cells from peripheral blood in donors treated with various hematopoietic growth factors are underway. Several clinical trials have been instituted to evaluate autologous peripheral blood stem cell transplantation as a salvage therapy for metastatic breast cancer. Other trials using allogeneic donors are underway, but have been limited by GVHD.

Graft-Versus-Host Disease

Graft-versus-host disease is a potentially lethal disorder in which mature T cells in the donor tissue or organ perceive the host as foreign. In effect, immunocompetent donor cells attempt to reject the host. Although in the past GVHD was believed to be associated only with BMT, it has become recognized as a relatively frequent occurrence in recipients of hepatic transplants as well as after donor-directed transfusions.[38] This antigen-specific recognition activates the donor T cells, resulting in the release of cytokines, including IL-1 and TNF, which serve to amplify the response further. The end result is tissue damaged mediated, at least in part, by cytotoxic T cells. Further investigation has suggested that the NK cell has an important role in the pathogenesis of GVHD, particularly in the production of the proinflammatory cytokines IFN-γ and TNF-α.[40] Clinically, GVHD tends to affect tissues of epithelial origin, including the skin, gastrointestinal tract, and liver. In transfusion and solid organ GVHD, the bone marrow itself is also a target. Patients suffering from GVHD have pancytopenia, skin rashes, elevated liver function test results, and often diarrhea. They are also at risk for severe infections because of the overall immuno-

suppressive nature of the disease and the drugs used in its treatment. Histologically, GVHD is marked by necrosis and degeneration of the epidermis, intestinal villi, hepatocytes, and bile ducts, with a moderate inflammatory infiltrate. Treatment consists of glucocorticoids and other immunosuppressive agents used to suppress the donor T-cell response.

GVHD is a well known complication of BMT,[41] and virtually all patients who undergo this procedure receive some type of prophylaxis. Regimens including cyclosporin or methotrexate have been successful in both reducing the likelihood of development of GVHD and lessening the severity of the disease once it has become evident.[42] Another prophylactic strategy in BMT involves the removal of T cells from the bone marrow allograft before transplantation. Unfortunately, grafts treated in this manner have an increased risk of failure of engraftment. As discussed earlier, application of the facilitating cell may provide a means of performing allogeneic BMT without the potential complications of GVHD.

Transfusion Graft-Versus-Host Disease

Although GVHD is most frequently associated with BMT, it can develop in several other clinical situations as well. Transfusion-associated GVHD is a well characterized syndrome first noted in the mid-1960s in immunodeficient children who received blood transfusions. Symptoms of the disorder include pancytopenia, dermatitis, and diarrhea. The mortality approaches 90% in some reports. Other clinical syndromes associated with this disorder include patients with hematologic malignancies and infants with erythroblastosis fetalis. In nations with a relatively homogeneous gene pool, there is a significant incidence of transfusion GVHD in immunocompetent patients undergoing surgical procedures who receive transfusions of fresh whole blood. The major risk factor for the disease is a general state of immunodeficiency, either intrinsic or iatrogenically induced through radiation or chemotherapy protocols. Immunocompetent transfusion recipients who share an HLA haplotype with an HLA-homozygous donor (eg, a parent-to-child transfusion) are also at high risk. Transfusion GVHD is usually suspected on clinical grounds in patients who are at risk. A classic histologic picture on skin biopsy is the hallmark for diagnosis.

Transfusion GVHD is readily preventable. Irradiation of blood products with between 15 to 20 Gy of γ radiation effectively decreases the proliferative response of donor lymphocytes, while maintaining the viability of other blood components, particularly the platelets. Other techniques of lymphocyte depletion have been less successful at preventing transfusion GVHD, although there continues to be active investigation of depletion techniques that avoid irradiation. It is recommended that all patients who are undergoing BMT, are immunocompromised either because of a primary disease process or as the result of iatrogenic interventions, or are receiving transfusion from family member donors, should receive irradiated blood.

Immunocompetence of the Fetus

The thymus is believed to be central to development of mature T cells. An important question in the development of the immune system is at what point during gestation the thymus becomes functional. In other words, when are fully immunocompetent T cells, capable of discriminating self from nonself, present in the fetal circulation? Indirect evidence of fetal immunocompetence can be derived from phenotypic examination of T-cell subsets within the fetus. Acquisition of the $\alpha\beta$-TCR occurs in the thymus under normal conditions. In human fetuses, $\alpha\beta$-TCR + cells are detectable in the fetal liver toward the end of the first trimester, suggesting that some degree of self–nonself discrimination is probably operational at that point. In vitro assays of immune function provide an interesting picture of fetal immunoreactivity. The MLR, a measure of lymphocyte proliferation in response to antigenic stimuli, is clearly reactive at 15 to 22 weeks of gestation. On the other hand, the cell mediated lympholysis (CML), which measures the cytotoxic effector function of lymphocytes, is blunted, suggesting some degree of immaturity in the cell-mediated immune responses.[43] Coincident with appearance of $\alpha\beta$-TCR + T lymphocytes is the loss of the privileged period during which bone marrow stem cells can engraft without cytoreduction.

Tolerance During Development

The concept that the fetus and neonate are immunologically privileged, in that they demonstrate decreased reactivity to foreign antigen, has been present since the beginning of the transplantation era. In the mid-1950s, Billingham and colleagues noted that neonatal mice that received an inoculum of bone marrow and spleen cells from a genetically different strain of mouse developed permanent, donor-specific tolerance to skin grafts, but they effectively rejected third-party grafts. This work was seminal in establishing the concept that the immune system could be manipulated in such a way as to induce tolerance, and introduced the principle that hematopoietic chimerism was a potent means to achieve a tolerant state. In addition, the idea that the neonatal period is one of immunologic privilege was first advanced. Since that time, the model of neonatal tolerance induction in the mouse has been used extensively to define the mechanism of self–nonself discrimination. In mice, neonatal tolerance is strain dependent and is closely associated with class II of the MHC. The explanation for this phenomenon is complex. First, there is the general immaturity of the immune system, with alloreactive host cells found in the thymus, but not in the periphery. After an infusion of donor cells, a state of chimerism in the lymphoid organs is created. In the thymus, donor reactive cells are eliminated by the process of clonal deletion (elimination of self-reactive cells by apoptosis). Mature cells that escape to the periphery can be rendered nonfunctional by clonal anergy (rendering the cells unable to respond to antigen), ultimately resulting in a state of tolerance.[44] This has been referred to as *peripheral tolerance*. Animals that become tolerized neonatally permanently accept skin grafts from their bone marrow donor, but reject third-party grafts. Similar donor-specific tolerance and chimerism has been achieved in adult recipients. However, in adult recipients, some degree of myeloablation is required to make space for stem cells to engraft. Unfortunately, human neonates do not appear to be immunologically privileged, and demonstrate the ability to reject both solid organ and tissue grafts.

Cord Blood and Fetal Liver Transplantation: New Frontiers

Umbilical cord blood has been identified as an enriched source of early hematopoietic progenitors and has been investigated as a possible source of stem cells for both autologous and allogeneic transplantation. There are two potential advantages of cord blood for transplantation. First, most T lymphocytes isolated from cord blood have a naive phenotype (CD45RA +) and may be less likely to induce GVHD. Second, cord blood appears to be greatly enriched in stem cells and early progenitors compared to adult peripheral blood.[45] The clinical application of cord blood transplantation has thus far been limited to children. HLA-matched sibling cord blood transplants have been successfully performed in children suffering from Fanconi anemia and juvenile chronic myelogenous leukemia.

Cryopreserved cord blood stem cells have been suggested as a potential source of cells for autologous transplantation as well. Umbilical cord blood harvested at the time of delivery is cryopreserved and stored. If the patient should contract a life-threatening hematologic disorder or a malignancy treatable by BMT later in life, the stored autologous cells could be used for BMT, thereby avoiding GVHD. Application of this technology is still in its infancy, and it has yet to be definitively determined whether a single collection of cord blood contains sufficient stem cells to repopulate an adult recipient. In the next 10 years, many of these unknowns will be answered.

Fetal hematopoietic tissue has also been used as a source of transplantable hematopoietic cells. The fetus is particularly attractive given the immaturity of the fetal thymus and lack of mature T lymphocytes. In 1975, it was reported that a child with severe combined immunodeficiency syndrome had been successfully treated by transplantation of fetal liver cells from an unrelated donor.[46] Immunocompetent T and B lymphocytes of donor origin developed in the child. However, he died a year after transplantation because of GVHD. In France, Touraine's group has performed over 200 fetal liver transplants for patients suffering from inborn errors of metabolism, aplastic anemia, and immunodeficiency diseases. Fifty percent of their patients with immunodeficiency diseases and 77% of those with inborn errors of metabolism are alive with at least partial improvement in the underlying disease state.[47] No HLA matching was performed in these cases. The results of these initial fetal liver transplants indicate that the fetal liver can provide a source of hematopoietic progenitors capable of functioning in an allogeneic environment, at least under highly specific host conditions.

The fetus has also been examined as the recipient of hematologic transplants. In theory, transplantation of the hematopoietic precursors before the development of immunocompetence may overcome the traditional barriers associated with allogeneic BMT. In newborn mice, bone marrow can be successfully transplanted without conditioning within 72 hours of birth. In humans, this privileged time for engraftment without conditioning disappears sometime early in the second trimester of gestation. Touraine and colleagues have reported on four patients transplanted at 17 to 28 weeks of gestation with fetal liver cells to treat thalassemia major, severe combined immunodeficiency syndrome, and bare lymphocyte syndrome.[48,49] Three of the four patients demonstrated graft take and improvement in clinical condition, although graft function was not immediate and the infants required further hematologic therapy for a period after birth. The fourth patient, however, became bradycardic and died in utero during the liver stem cell infusion, underscoring that this therapy is still experimental and is associated with considerable risk to the fetus.

REFERENCES

1. Stettler A. Die Vorstellungen von Ansteckung and Abwehr: zur Geschichte der Immunitätslehre bis zur Zeit von Louis Pasteur. Gesnerus 1972;29:255.
2. Silverstein AS. A history of immunology. San Diego: Academic Press, 1989:39.
3. Migliaccio G, Migliaccio AR, Petti S, et al. Human embryonic hemopoiesis: kinetics of progenitors and precursors underlying the yolk sac → liver transition. J Clin Invest 1986;78:51.
4. Dommergues M, Aubeny E, Dumez Y, et al. Hematopoiesis in the human yolk sac: quantitation of erythroid and granulopoietic progenitors between 3.5 and 8 weeks of the development. Bone Marrow Transplant 1992;9(Suppl 1):23.
5. Brugger W, Mocklin W, Heimfield S, et al. Ex vivo expansion of enriched peripheral blood CD34$^+$ progenitor cells by stem cell factor, interleukin 1β (IL-1β), IL-6, IL-3, interferon-γ, and erythropoietin. Blood 1993;81:2579.
6. de Vries P, Brasel KA, Eisenman JR, et al. The effect of recombinant mast cell growth factor on purified murine hematopoietic stem cells. J Exp Med 1991;173:1205.
7. Matsui Y, Zsebo KM, Hogan BL. Embryonic expression of a haematopoietic growth factor encoded by the *Sl* locus and the ligand for c-kit. Nature 1990;347:667.
8. Sadler TW. Langman's medical embryology, ed 5. Baltimore, Williams & Wilkins, 1985.
9. Sanhadj K, Touraine JL, Aitouche A, et al. Fetal liver cell transplantation in various murine models. Bone Marrow Transplant 1992;9(Suppl 1):77.
10. Jordan CT, McKearn JP, Lemischka IR. Cellular and developmental properties of fetal hematopoietic stem cells. Cell 1990;61:953.
11. Lansdorp PM, Dragowski W, Mayani H. Ontogeny-related changes in proliferative potential of human hematopoietic cells. J Exp Med 1993;178:787.
12. Trowsdale J. Genomic structure and function in MHC. Trends Genet 1993;9(4):117.
13. Abbas AK, Lichtman AH, Pober JS. Cellular and molecular Immunology. Philadelphia, WB Saunders, 1991.
14. Tracey KJ, Cerami A. Tumor necrosis factor: an updated review of its biology. Crit Care Med 1993;21(Suppl):S415.
15. Dexter TM, Allen TD, Lajtha LG. Conditions controlling the proliferation of hematopoietic stem cells in vitro. J Cell Physiol 1977;91:335.
16. Ogawa M. Differentiation and proliferation of hematopoietic stem cells. Blood 1993;81:2844.
17. Lok S, Kaushansky K, Holly RD, et al. Cloning and expression of murine thrombopoietin cDNA and stimulation of platelet production in vivo. Nature 1994;369:565.
18. Mosmann TR, Cherwinski H. Bond MW, et al. Two types of murine T helper cell clones. I. Definition according to profiles of lymphokine activities and secreted proteins. J Immunol 1986;136:2348.
19. Street NE, Schumacher JH, Fong TA, et al. Heterogeneity of mouse helper T cells: evidence from bulk cultures and limiting dilution cloning for precursors of Th1 and Th2 cells. J Immunol 1990;144:1629.
20. Trinchieri G. Interleukin-12 and its role in the generation of TH1 cells. Immunology Today 1993;14:335.
21. Del Prete CF, De Carli M, Mastromauro C, et al. Purified protein derivative of *Mycobacterium tuberculosis* and excretory-secretory antigens of *Toxocara canis* expand in vitro human T cells with stable and opposite (type 1 T helper or type 2 T helper) profile of cytokine production. J Clin Invest 1991;88:346.
22. Romagnani S. Human TH1 and TH2 subsets: regulation of differentiation and role in protection and immunopathology. Int Arch Allergy Immunol 1992;98:279.
23. Krammer PH, Behrman I, Daniel P, et al. Regulation of apoptosis in the immune system. Curr Opin Immunol 1994;6:279.
24. Hockenberry DM, Oltvai ZN, Win XM, et al. Bcl-2 functions in an antioxidant pathway to prevent apoptosis. Cell 1993;75:241.
25. Vaux DL, Cory S, Adams JM. Bcl-2 gene promotes haemopoietic cell survival and cooperates with c-myc to immortalize pre-B cells. Nature 1988;335:440.
26. Van Noesel CJ, Brouns GS, Van Scijndel GM, et al. Comparison of human B-cell antigen receptor complexes: membrane-expressed forms of immunoglobulin (Ig)M, IgD and IgG are associated with structurally related heterodimers. J Exp Med 1992;175:1511.
27. Moretta L, Ciccone E, Moretta A, et al. NK cells: nonself or no self? Immunology Today 1992;13:300.
28. Ciccone E, Pende D, Viale O, et al. Evidence of a natural killer (NK) cell repertoire for (allo) antigen recognition: definition of five distinct NK-determined allospecificities in humans. J Exp Med 1992;175:709.
29. Perussia B. Lymphokine-activated killer cells, natural killer cells, and cytokines. Curr Opin Immunol 1991;3:49.
30. Bancroft GJ. The role of natural killer cells in innate resistance to infection. Curr Opin Immunol 1993;5:503.
31. Weller PF. Eosinophils: structure and functions. Curr Opin Immunol 1994;6:85.
32. Schwartz LB. Mast cells: function and contents. Curr Opin Immunol 1994;6:91.
33. Tomlinson S. Complement defense mechanisms. Curr Opin Immunol 1993;5:83.
34. Takemoto S. Terasaki PI, Maruya E, et al. Molecular matching for clinical kidney transplantation. Transplant Proc 1993;25:206.
35. Penn I. The price of immunotherapy. Curr Probl Surg 1981;18:716.
36. Ildstad ST, Sachs DH. Reconstitution with syngeneic plus allogeneic or xenogeneic bone marrow leads to specific acceptance of allografts or xenografts. Nature 1984;307:168.
37. Singer A, Hathcock KS, Hodes RJ. Self recognition in allogeneic radiation bone marrow chimeras: a radiation resistant host element dictates the self specificity and immune response gene phenotype of T helper cells J Exp Med 1981;153:1286.
38. Ferrar JL, Deeg, JH. Mechanisms of disease: graft versus host. N Engl J Med 1991;324:667.
39. Kaufman CK, Colson YC, Wren SM, et al. Phenotypic characterization of a novel bone marrow derived cell that facilitates engraftment of allogeneic bone marrow stem cells. Blood 1994;84:2436.
40. Xun C, Brown SA, Jennings CD, et al. Acute graft versus host like disease induced by transplantation of human activated natural killer cells into SCID mice. Transplantation 1993;56:409.
41. Armitage JO. Bone marrow transplantation. N Engl J Med 1994;330:827.
42. Martin PJ, Schoch G. Fisher L, et al. A retrospective analysis of therapy for acute graft-versus-host disease: initial treatment. Blood 1990;76:1464.
43. Elk S, Ringden O, Markling L, et al. Immunological capacity of human fetal liver cells. Bone Marrow Transplant 1994;14:9.
44. Streilein JW. Neonatal tolerance of H-2 alloantigens: procuring graft acceptance the "old fashioned" way. Transplantation 1991;52:110.
45. Broxmeyer HE, Douglas GW, Hangou G, et al. Human umbilical cord blood as a potential source of transplantable hematopoietic stem/progenitor cells. Proc Natl Acad Sci USA 1989;86:3828.
46. Keightley RG, Lauton AR, Cooper MD. Successful fetal liver transplantation in a child with severe combined immunodeficiency syndrome. Lancet 1975;2(7940):850.
47. Touraine JL. Rationale and results of in utero transplants of stem cells in humans. Bone Marrow Transplant 1992;10(Suppl 1):121.
48. Touraine JL, Raudrant D, Royo C, et al. In utero transplantation of stem cells in bare lymphocyte syndrome. Lancet 1989;1(8651):1382.
49. Touraine JL, Raudrant D, Rabaud A, et al. In utero transplantation of stem cells in humans: immunological aspects and clinical follow-up of patients. Bone Marrow Transplant 1992;9(Suppl 1):98.

Surgery of Infants and Children: Scientific Principles and Practice, edited by
Keith T. Oldham, Paul M. Colombani, and Robert P. Foglia.
Lippincott–Raven Publishers, Philadelphia, © 1997.

CHAPTER 40

Clinical Immunosuppression

Paul M. Colombani

Much of the success of clinical transplantation since the 1970s is directly attributable to advances in immunosuppressive therapies. These advances have come from a variety of different areas, including drug development for cancer and antimicrobial therapies as well as more specific immune therapies based on an increased knowledge of the immune reaction to solid organ transplants.

Systemic immunosuppression has been required in solid organ transplantation since the first transplants were done between people who were not identical twins. The absence of human leukocyte antigen (HLA) identity, resulting in alloreactivity, makes immunosuppression necessary, as outlined in detail in Chapter 39. The overall goal of clinical immunosuppression is to provide specific nonreactivity on the part of the organ recipient to the antigens of the donor. Although some gains have been made in providing specific donor unreactivity to transplant recipients, most of the progress in clinical immunosuppression has not been in the area of donor-specific suppression of the immune alloreaction. Newer agents have narrower but nonspecific target sites of action on the immune system. In theory, more precise immunosuppression that targets activated immune cells stimulated against the donor organ results in fewer complications for the organ recipient.

The overall goal for all forms of clinical immunosuppression is to prevent or treat rejection and render the transplant recipient unreactive to donor alloantigens. This goal is balanced by the need to avoid the inherent toxicities of these immunosuppressive regimens, as well as avoiding the infectious complications and long-term threat of malignancy engendered by long-term immunosuppression. Strategies based on these goals have tended to increase the number of agents used in an attempt to decrease the overall dose of each agent and thereby decrease the toxicity of each drug. In addition, in stable patients, doses frequently are reduced and agents withdrawn to decrease the incidence of long-term complications. In the pediatric population, which by nature is looking at decades of immunosuppression, it is important to actively minimize long-term toxicity, particularly because of the risk of secondary malignancy in these patients. In addition, the pediatric patient, who is immunologically naive to a variety of bacterial, fungal, infectious, and viral agents, is at greater risk than the adult transplant recipient for opportunistic infectious complications after therapeutic immunosuppression.

This chapter covers the classification of immunosuppressive agents in clinical use for solid organ and bone marrow transplantation as well as for treatment of autoimmune diseases. The specific agents approved for clinical use and a number of investigational agents under development are discussed. A general strategy of treatment is outlined, and the short- and long-term complications associated with immunosuppression are reviewed.

CLASSIFICATION OF AGENTS

A variety of antimetabolites, bacterial- or fungal-derived antibiotics, and alkylating agents that have been used for cancer chemotherapy also provide clinical immunosuppression. This discussion, however, is limited to those agents in clinical use or undergoing development and testing.

Immunosuppressive drugs may be classified by a variety of methods; a common method divides them into specific and nonspecific agents. The nonspecific agents include antiinflammatory drugs such as corticosteroids; antiproliferative agents such as azathioprine (6-mercaptopurine), methotrexate, and cyclophosphamide; and new antiproliferative agents such mycophenolate mofetil, brequinar sodium, and mizorabine. Nonspecific agents that inhibit cell maturation include 15-deoxyspergualin. Agents that provide more specific immunosuppression can be divided into the anticytokine synthesis agents, which include cyclosporine, FK506 (tacrolimus), and rapamycin; agents that blockade antigen recognition, which include many of the monoclonal antibodies; and agents that are specifically cytotoxic to T cells or that remove them from the circulation. This last group includes graft irradiation, ultraviolet light, thoracic duct drainage, total lymphoid radiation, and thymectomy. Table 40-1 summarizes this classification of immunosuppressive drugs. In general, this drug classification is arbitrary and there may be considerable overlap of category for some of these drugs (eg, corticosteroids). As outlined in Table 40-1, only a few of the agents listed are currently approved by the Food and Drug Administration (FDA) for clinical use. Much of the advances made since the 1970s have been attributed to just a few of these agents. It is hoped that the almost bewildering number of new

691

TABLE 40-1. *Immunosuppressive drugs*

Agent	Mechanism of Action
NONSPECIFIC AGENTS	
Anti-inflammatory	
Corticosteroids*	Inhibit gene activation
Antiproliferative agents (antimetabolites)	
Azathioprine (6-mercaptopurine)*	Inhibits phosphoribosylpyrophosphate aminotransferase
Methotrexate	Inhibits dihydrotolate dihydrogenase
Mycophenolate mofetil (RS-61443)*	Inhibits IMP dehydrogenase
Mizoribine	Inhibits IMP dehydrogenase
Brequinar sodium	Inhibits DITO dehydrogenase
Alkylating agents	
Nitrogen mustard	Blocks DNA transcription
Cyclophosphamide	Blocks DNA transcription
Cell maturation inhibitors	
15-deoxyspergualin	Inhibits antigen presentation
SPECIFIC AGENTS	
Anticytokine synthesis	
Cyclosporine and derivatives*	Inhibits early T-cell activation (calcium dependent)
Tacrolimus*	Inhibits early T-cell activation (calcium dependent)
Rapamycin	Blocks calcium-dependent and -independent cell activation
Leflunomide (HWA486)	Inhibits tyrosine kinases
Receptor antagonist/antigen recognition	
15-Deoxyspergualin	Receptor agtagonist
Antilymphocyte globulin*	Receptor antagonist
Antithymocyte globulin*	Receptor antagonist
Monoclonal antibodies	
OKT3	T-cell receptor antagonist
Anti-TAC	IL-2 receptor antagonist
Anti–LFA-1	Lymphocyte adhesion molecule antagonist
Anti–ICAM-1	Cell adhesion molecule antagonist
Cytokine inhibitors	
Soluble IL-1	Receptor antagonist
Anti-tumor necrosis factor	Receptor antagonist
NONSPECIFIC METHODS	
Ultraviolet irradiation	Lymphocyte depletion
X-irradiation	
Graft	Lymphocyte depletion
Total lymphoid	Lymphocyte depletion
Thoracic duct drainage	Lymphocyte depletion
Thymectomy	Lymphocyte depletion

IMP, inositol monophosphate; IL, interleukin.
* Approved by the Food and Drug Administration for clinical use.

agents on the horizon will provide further improvements in clinical immunosuppressive strategies.

CLINICALLY APPROVED AGENTS

A growing number of immunosuppressive agents are in clinical use. These agents have specific mechanisms of action that sometimes overlap. Figure 40-1 depicts the cellular sites of action of a number of these clinically used and investigational agents.[1] The following descriptions of these agents also delineate potential toxicities, common routes of administration, and dosages.

Corticosteroids

The corticosteroids, both methylprednisolone and prednisone, have been a mainstay of clinical immunosuppression since the 1950s. Corticosteroids have potent antiinflammatory effects, as well as providing a general inhibition of anabolic activities and significant inhibition of gene activation. There may also be a direct cytotoxic effect on lymphocytes with higher doses. Steroids are used both for induction therapy as well as the treatment of rejection.[2,3] Pediatric patients are usually pulsed with higher steroid doses (10 mg/kg/d), with tapering over time. Maintenance therapy is usually in dose ranges between 0.1 and 0.3 mg/kg/d. With the availability of other immunosuppressive agents for use in combination with corticosteroids, the use of high-dose steroids has been abandoned because of extremely high morbidity and mortality secondary to opportunistic infections. In addition to the infection risks, the acute toxicity effects of steroids include potent sodium and water retention with secondary hypertension. Chronic use of steroids may lead to decreased bone mineralization with osteoporosis, and effects on gastric acidity and gastritis.

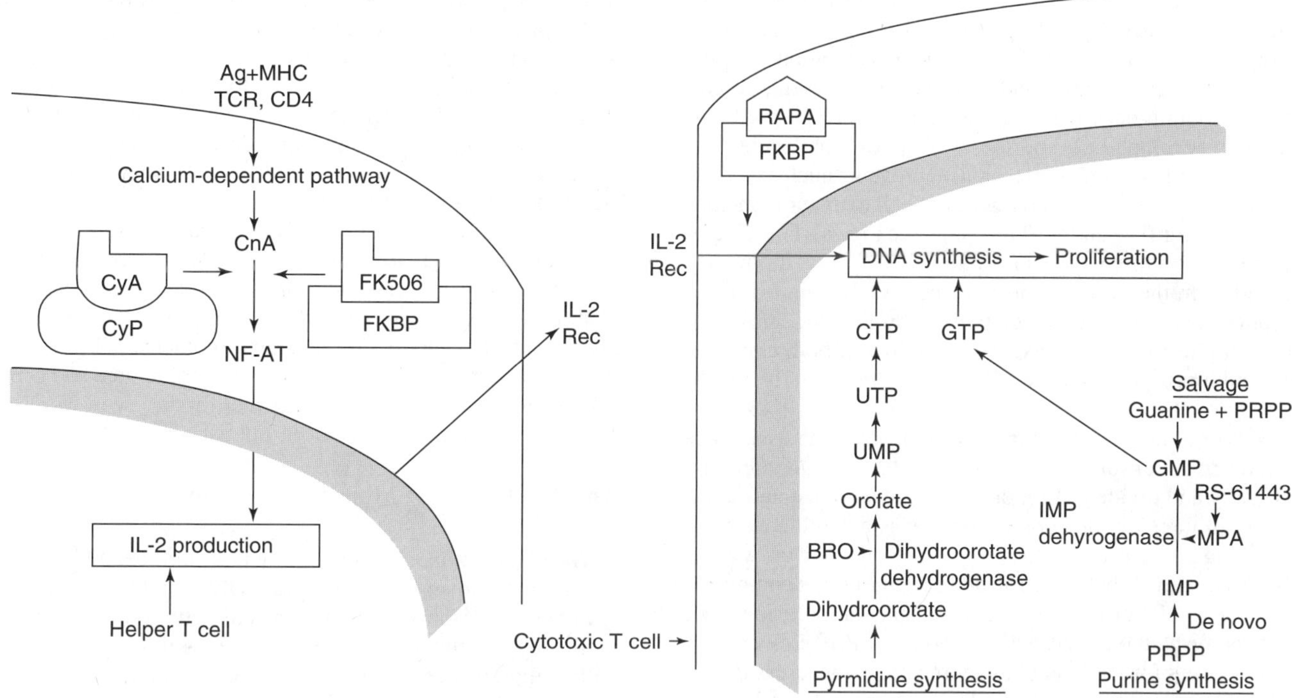

FIG. 40-1. Site of action of immunosuppressant drugs. Ag, antigen; BRO, ; CnA, ; CTP, ara-cytidine triphosphate; CyA, cyclosporine A; CyP, ; FKBP, FK binding protein; GMP, guanosine monophosphate; GTP, guanosine triphosphate; IL-2, interleukin-2; IMP, inosine monophosphate; MHC, major histocompatibility complex; MPA, ; NF-AT, ; PRPP, phosphoribosylpyrophosphate; RAPA, rapamycin; Rec, receptor; RS-61443, mycophenolate mofetil; TCR, T-cell receptor; UMP, uridine monophosphate; UTP, uridine triphosphate.

Azathioprine (Imuran)

Azathioprine and its metabolic end-product 6-mercaptopurine are used clinically as purine analogs to inhibit DNA synthesis. Both of these agents compete for enzymes involved in purine biosynthesis. The end result is fewer purines available for DNA synthesis and a secondary failure of DNA synthesis and cell division. Azathioprine is the most commonly used agent in clinical organ transplantation. It is well absorbed orally but can also be given intravenously. Dosing of azathioprine is usually 1 to 2 mg/kg in a single daily dose. The major toxicity seen with azathioprine is bone marrow suppression. All precursors in the bone marrow may be affected, with neutropenia, anemia, and thrombocytopenia seen. Most commonly, neutropenia develops first in patients. Early in the course of azathioprine administration, white blood cell counts should be followed and dose adjustments made for patients whose white blood cell counts fall below 5000/mm^3. Late toxicity of azathioprine is occasionally seen, and includes red cell aplasia, hepatitis, and pancreatitis.[4]

Mycophenolate Mofetil (Cellcept)

Mycophenolate mofetil is an antimetabolite approved for clinical use in 1995.[5,6] It competitively inhibits inositol monophosphate dehydrogenase, which is a critical enzyme in the purine salvage pathway. The fact that the purine salvage pathway is absolutely critical for purine biosynthesis in lymphocytes is exploited by the use of mycophenolate mofetil. Other mammalian cells are able to synthesize purines de novo and thus undergo little or no inhibition, but DNA synthesis and cell division of T and B lymphocytes are markedly inhibited by mycophenolate. Like azathioprine, mycophenolate is well absorbed orally, and the usual dose for adults is 1 to 2 g/d divided in two doses (q12h). In the pediatric population, little is known concerning adequate dosing and pharmacokinetics. Currently, children are given 25 mg/kg/d in divided doses for clinical immunosuppressive regimens. Alternative dosing using body surface area is also utilized: 1200 mg/m^2/d in divided doses. The principal toxicities of mycophenolate are gastrointestinal (GI), with anorexia, nausea, vomiting, and diarrhea. Patients also may have crampy abdominal pain, and at high doses, bone marrow suppression with anemia and neutropenia may develop.

Cyclosporine

Cyclosporine is an intracellular fungal metabolite whose immunosuppressive activity was identified in 1976. It was quickly brought to clinical use and approved by the FDA in 1984 for transplantation. Cyclosporine is a cyclic peptide comprising 11 amino acids. The native compound is extremely hydrophobic and easily partitions into lipid membranes. Cyclosporine appears to impart specific immunosuppression by inhibiting T-lymphocyte activation events.[7,8] This inhibition of early activation events results in a failure of helper T cells to synthesize and release interleukin (IL)-2, a potent cytokine and inducer of cytotoxic T-cell activity.[9] It appears that the site of action of cyclosporine is along the calcium-dependent activation pathway from the T-cell receptor, and involves calcineurin, a calcium–calmodulin-dependent phosphatase, a cyclosporine-binding protein (cyclophilin), and the cyclosporine molecule.[10–12] This cytoplasmic inhibition mechanism prevents nuclear activation and the expression of early genes of cell activation, including the genes for IL-2 and IL-2 receptor (see Fig. 40-1).[13] Cyclosporine may be administered intravenously or orally. It is poorly absorbed from the GI tract and must be dissolved in oil. After absorption, cyclosporine is metabolized by the cytochrome P-450 system, resulting in an extensive number of both clinically active and inactive metabolites. Drugs that are similarly metabolized by or that alter the activity of cytochrome P-450 also alter cyclosporine pharmacokinetics and levels. The usual dose for solid organ transplantation patients is 10 mg/kg/d, administered orally and divided q12h, or 5 mg/kg/d administered intravenously in three divided doses (q8h) or as a continuous infusion. Trough levels of cyclosporine are followed on a daily basis. Trough levels between 150 and 500 ng/mL are commonly acceptable levels for clinical organ transplantation, depending on the assay method used and the donor organ. Lower dose ranges are used for heart and kidney recipients, whereas higher ranges are reserved for liver transplant recipients. Neoral, a new microemulsion preparation of cyclosporine, was approved for clinical use in 1995 and may offer improved oral absorption and simpler dosing.[14,15] Pharmacokinetic analysis of Neoral demonstrates an improved area under the curve. Better oral absorption may provide improved immunosuppression but may also increase toxicity. Toxic side effects of cyclosporine include neurologic symptoms (tremor, seizures), hypertension, hirsutism, hypercholesterolemia, hepatotoxicity, and nephrotoxicity. All these toxic side effects are dose related and many are alleviated with dose reduction.

Tacrolimus (Prograf)

Tacrolimus, formerly named FK506, is a macrolide antibiotic derived from bacteria (*Streptomyces tsukabiensis*). It has been shown to have potent immunosuppressive activity, apparently 100-fold more potent than cyclosporine's. Tacrolimus, like cyclosporine, inhibits early T-cell activation events.[16 18] It appears that tacrolimus also affects the calcium–calmodulin–calcineurin axis, but has its own unique binding peptide to form a molecular complex with these compounds in the cytoplasm.[19] For all practical purposes, both cyclosporine and tacrolimus have the same mechanisms of action, although there are subtle differences in their spectra of activity. Tacrolimus may be administered intravenously or given orally. It is rapidly absorbed from the GI tract with good pharmacokinetic activity. Given this easy absorption even with postoperative ileus, most transplant centers rarely use intravenous tacrolimus. Both adult and pediatric patients are administered tacrolimus orally beginning at 0.15 mg/kg/dose q12h. Occasionally a patient requires intravenous administration, and this is given either by continuous infusion or intermittent doses of 0.05 mg/kg/d divided q12h. Trough levels of tacrolimus are followed daily until stable. Individual pediatric patients can have widely disparate levels on standard dosing and, as a result, levels are required for optimal management. Trough levels between 5 and 10 ng/mL are initial targets, with higher levels obtained during rejection treatment and lower levels tolerated in stable patients. Tacrolimus is metabolized by the cytochrome P-450 system in the liver, and dose adjustments should be made in patients with significant liver insufficiency. Patients may require a single daily dose or doses held for high trough levels or early liver dysfunction. As with cyclosporine, significant dose adjustments of tacrolimus may be necessary when used with other drugs that affect cytochrome P-450 activity. The principal toxicities of tacrolimus are neurologic (tremor, nervousness, sleeplessness, and nightmares); hypertension; gastric upset with nausea, vomiting, and diarrhea; hyperglycemia and hyperkalemia; and nephrotoxicity. Like cyclosporine, most of these toxic side effects are dose related and usually respond to dose adjustment. Guidelines for the use of tacrolimus in pediatric recipients have been published.[20]

Anti-CD3 (OKT3) Monoclonal Antibody

The OKT3 monoclonal antibody is a murine antibody raised against the human T-cell receptor (OKT3, CD3) on human T lymphocytes.[21] This antibody binds directly to the T3 receptor on the T lymphocyte. After binding, cross-linking of receptors with complement deposition and direct cytotoxicity may occur. Alternatively, capping and internalization of the receptor after antibody binding may also serve to inhibit the activity of the affected T lymphocyte. This is a nonspecific action on all T lymphocytes because the T-cell receptor is present on all mature T lymphocytes. The usual dose for OKT3 is 2.5 mg/d intravenously for patients under 20 kg body weight and 5 mg/d intravenously for patients weighing more than 20 kg. The white blood counts of patients are followed and circulating T3 cells assessed in the blood. The percentage of T3 lymphocytes in the blood should be less than 2% to 3% to achieve the therapeutic goal. Patients may require higher doses of OKT3 to achieve an adequate drop in circulating T3 lymphocytes. Dose escalation to 7.5 or even 10 mg daily may occasionally be necessary. Patients who have had previous exposure to the OKT3 antibody may express anti-murine antibodies, which block OKT3 activity directly. In this situation, supernormal intravenous doses of OKT3 may be necessary to overcome these inhibitory antibodies. The principal toxicity of OKT3 is directly related to the intravenous administration of foreign protein. Fever, myalgia, stiff neck, and headache are all seen, particularly during the first few days of administration. With the rapid lysis of T cells after the first doses of OKT3, a cytokine release syndrome also may develop, with secondary reactive pulmonary edema and respiratory distress. Patients may occasionally have a meningitis-like syndrome that requires cessation of treatment. Before OKT3 administration, patients are given corticosteroids, diphenhydramine, and acetaminophen. Patients are also assessed for fluid overload. Patients who are hypervolemic with early pulmonary edema should undergo dialysis before receiving the first dose of OKT3. Fluid restrictions, dialysis, antiinflammatories, antipyretics, and antihistamines all serve to minimize patient symptoms.

Antithymocyte Globulin (ATGAM)

Antithymocyte globulin is a polyclonal antibody derived from rabbit sera that is specific for human T lymphocytes.[22–24]

This agent is given intravenously to effect a rapid destruction of T lymphocytes. The dosage is 15 mg/kg/d given as a single intravenous dose. Significant side effects are related to the administration of a foreign protein, and patients are pretreated and treated in a way similar to those receiving OKT3.

NEW AGENTS

As seen in Table 40-1, a host of new agents is under development for clinical use in organ transplantation. Many of these agents have only been through animal experimental trials or clinical trials with adults.

New Drugs

Mizoribine (Bredinin) is a purine analog similar to mycophenolate that inhibits inositol monophosphate dehydrogenase.[25,26] This agent has both GI and marrow toxicity and is in clinical trials for transplantation.

Brequinar sodium (DUP-785) is a pyrimidine analog that inhibits a dihydroorate dehydrogenase.[27,28] Potential toxicity includes bone marrow and mucosal epithelium effects.

Cyclosporine G and Sandoz IMM125 are *cyclosporine analogs.*[20,29,30] Both of these agents appear to have less renal and central nervous system toxicity than native cyclosporine. The mechanisms of action of these agents are presumably the same as for cyclosporine and tacrolimus.

Rapamycin is a macrolide antibiotic similar to tacrolimus but derived from a different bacterial species. Rapamycin, although it binds to FK binding protein and inhibits calcium–calmodulin–calcineurin, also is a potent inhibitor of late activation events. More specifically, rapamycin may have effects on T-cell maturation and may inhibit calcium-independent cell activation events.[31–33]

Leflunomide (HWA486) is another agent under development that has a specific action on T-cell activation events. This agent specifically inhibits tyrosine kinases, and is undergoing clinical trials.[34]

15-Deoxyspergualin inhibits cell growth and maturation.[35] It may also function as a receptor antagonist to inhibit antigen presentation.[36] Its major toxicities are bone marrow suppression and GI upset.

Other Monoclonal Antibodies

A number of specific monoclonal antibodies have been developed that affect different aspects of the T-cell repertoire. Anti-CD5, like OKT3, is a monoclonal antibody that specifically binds CD5 + cells. Anti-TAC is a monoclonal antibody specific to the IL-2 receptor that specifically binds to cells expressing the IL-2 receptor (ie, activated T-effector cells).[37,38] Anti–LFA-1 and anti–ICAM-1 are monoclonal antibodies that have been raised against cellular adhesion molecules. LFA-1 is the adhesion molecule (receptor) on T lymphocytes that recognizes ICAM-1, which is an adhesion molecule on T-lymphocyte target cells.[39,40] Other monoclonal antibodies under investigation include Campath-IH, Campath-IM, anti-CD2, anti-OKT4A, anti-TNF, anti–IL-10, and anti–IL-1.[41]

TREATMENT STRATEGIES

All of the agents described previously can be used alone or in combination to provide an adequate strategy to maintain a graft in the transplant recipient with the goal of reduced rejection or toxicity. Treatment strategies for clinical immunosuppression may be divided into three groups: induction, maintenance, and treatment of rejection.

Induction Therapy

Induction therapy may be thought of as the immunosuppression provided to the patient before the implantation of the graft and for the first few weeks after transplantation. Induction therapy may simply be the initiation of maintenance immunosuppressive therapy with a high-dose steroid pulse and taper after implantation of the transplanted organ. More commonly, induction therapy consists of administration of an antithymocyte preparation (antilymphocyte globulin or OKT3 monoclonal antibody) to provide potent T-cell inhibition or elimination at the initiation of the transplant procedure and engraftment. Table 40-2 outlines common pediatric induction protocols for clinical transplantation immunosuppression. The advantage of induction therapy is that it provides potent and specific T-cell immunosuppression before sensitization of the recipient to the engrafted alloantigens. Induction therapy is not universally

TABLE 40-2. *Common immunosuppressive protocols in children*

INDUCTION	
Corticosteroids:	10 mg/kg/d × 2–3 d then decrease 2 mg/kg/d q.o.d. until 1 mg/kg/d
	or
ATGAM:	15 mg/kg/d IV × 5–7 d
	or
OKT3:	2.5 mg (<20 kg) to 5.0 mg (>20 kg) IV q.d. × 5–7 d
MAINTENANCE	
Cyclosporine:	10 mg/kg/d divided q12h PO 5 mg/kg/d divided q8h IV or continuous infusion
	or
Tacrolimus:	0.3 mg/kg/d divided q12h PO (0.15 mg/kg/dose) 0.05 mg/kg/d divided q12h IV
Azathioprine:	1–2 mg/kg/d IV or PO
	or
Mycophenolate mofetil:	25 mg/kg/d divided q12h (1200 mg/m² BSA/d div q12⁰)
REJECTION	
Corticosteroids:	Pulse as above, then taper; may repeat × 1
ATGAM:	Dose as above; treat 10–14 d Monitor CD2 and CD 11 levels in blood
	or
OKT3:	Dose as above; treat 10–14 d Monitor CD3 levels in blood

ATGAM, antithymocyte globulin.

practiced in pediatric transplant recipients because of the potential complications that may attend the use of such potent immunosuppression. The incidence of opportunistic infections (viral, fungal, and protozoal) and secondary malignancies (posttransplant lymphoproliferative disease) appears to be higher in patients who have received treatment with ATGAM or the OKT3 monoclonal antibody.[42,43] Short courses of induction, however, may not place the recipient at increased risk for these complications. In addition, as clinical experience with antithymocyte preparations increases, dose reductions will most likely be made. These reductions may serve to increase safety while preserving efficacy.

Maintenance Therapy

After induction therapy, whether it be high-dose steroids and a taper or an antithymocyte preparation, maintenance therapy involves maintaining the program of conventional immunosuppression to prevent graft rejection. Conventional maintenance therapy has evolved over the years and includes multiple immunosuppressive agents given in nontoxic doses. Table 40-2 outlines the commonly used maintenance immunosuppressive regimens for clinical transplantation. Historically, corticosteroids such as prednisone and azathioprine were used to maintain grafts after induction therapy. With FDA approval in 1984, cyclosporine was added to the armamentarium for maintenance therapy. Triple-drug therapy is cyclosporine-based immunosuppression using cyclosporine, azathioprine, and prednisone, and is the most common regimen for many transplant recipients. Triple-drug therapy permits lower doses of cyclosporine and azathioprine to be given, as well as allowing for use of low-dose steroids or every-other-day steroid therapy. Since 1995, mycophenolate mofetil has been available for substitution for azathioprine in clinical immunosuppressive protocols. In stable renal transplant patients, cyclosporine may be discontinued and the recipient maintained on azathioprine and every-other-day steroids. Alternatively, patients have been maintained on cyclosporine monotherapy with complete withdrawal of azathioprine and steroids.

After the 1994 FDA approval of tacrolimus, this agent rapidly gained in popularity in maintenance therapy for solid organ transplant recipients. Tacrolimus-based therapy may include tacrolimus and prednisone, but also may use azathioprine or mycophenolate. The potent activity of tacrolimus allows more rapid steroid withdrawal, and many patients can be maintained off steroids completely with the use of tacrolimus.

With the availability of other agents in the future, further drug combinations will be used to provide the least possible short- and long-term toxicity with the lowest possible rejection rates.

Antirejection Strategy

A number of strategies are available for the patient who undergoes an acute rejection episode. For typical patients, alteration in clinical graft function prompts a sampling for biopsy and pathologic evaluation of the graft for rejection. The first line of rejection treatment is a high-dose corticosteroid pulse (10 mg/kg/d for 2 to 3 days) and taper using methylprednisolone.

Patients who fail to respond adequately to a steroid pulse may undergo a second steroid pulse or be placed on an antithymocyte preparation. Both the OKT3 monoclonal antibody and antithymocyte polyclonal antibody preparations are available and provide potent treatment for rejection. Greater than 90% of patients respond to corticosteroid pulse or antithymocyte preparations.

With the availability of tacrolimus, a number of pediatric and adult patients have been treated for steroid- and cyclosporine-resistant rejection without the need for repeated steroid pulses and antithymocyte preparations.[44] Similarly, mycophenolate mofetil also makes it possible to attempt treatment of rejection without the use of antithymocyte preparations.[45] In general, a combination of these approaches adequately treats an acute rejection episode in most patients.

For the patient with chronic rejection, newer agents may be on the horizon to slow or reverse the rejection process. In the liver transplant recipient whose organ has significant regenerative abilities, the use of high-dose tacrolimus appears to have some effect on reversing chronic rejection, if the patients are seen early in their course. With potent inhibitory action on B lymphocytes, mycophenolate mofetil may play a future role in the treatment of chronic rejection.[46–48] For the heart or kidney transplant, in which the target organ has little regenerative capability, significant chronic rejection cannot go on for any length of time before there is irreversible organ damage, which may require retransplantation or resumption of dialysis.

GENERAL COMPLICATIONS OF IMMUNOSUPPRESSION

As stated at the beginning of the chapter, clinical immunosuppressive strategies entail striking a balance between freedom from rejection episodes and freedom from the toxicity and complications of immunosuppression. In simple terms, the more potent the immunosuppressive regimen, the fewer the rejection episodes, but the greater the chances for opportunistic infection, late malignancy, and drug toxicity. Table 40-3 summarizes the general complications of immunosuppression.

TABLE 40-3. *Some complications of immunosuppression*

OPPORTUNISTIC INFECTIONS
Fungus (*Candida* spp, *Aspergillus* spp)
Protozoa (*Pneumocystis carinii*, *Cryptosporidium* spp)
Viruses (cytomegalovirus, herpes simples virus, varicella-zoster virus, Epstein-Barr virus)

SECONDARY MALIGNANCY
Posttransplant lymphoproliferative disease
Kaposi sarcoma
Non-Hodgkin lymphoma, Hodgkin disease
Skin, cervical, lung, ovarian, breast, gastrointestinal malignancies

DRUG TOXICITIES
Corticosteroids: osteoporosis, avascular necrosis of hip, gastritis, Cushing syndrome
Azathioprine: hepatitis, pancreatitis, red cell aplasia
Cyclosporine: nephrotoxicity, hypertension, elevated cholesterol
Tacrolimus: nephrotoxicity, hypertension hepatotoxicity (?), diabetes (?)

The specific toxicities of the immunosuppressive drugs are described in the sections pertaining to each drug. In general, the goal of multidrug therapy is to decrease the individual toxicities of the drugs used. In addition, the more severe the toxicities seen with higher doses of these agents, the greater the chance for poor patient compliance with drug regimens, or more general difficulties with patients.

Opportunistic infections are problematic in patients undergoing significant chronic clinical immunosuppression. As the potency of the agents and the number of drugs used increase, so does the likelihood of opportunistic infections. These infections are particularly problematic for the pediatric recipient. The pediatric recipient, overall, has a naive immune system, has not been exposed to a variety of bacterial, fungal, or viral agents, and cannot develop specific immunity to many of these agents. As a result, the pediatric recipient is at risk for significant opportunistic infection, particularly from parasitic and viral pathogens. In the peritransplantation period, both bacterial and fungal infections have higher frequency rates than in the adult population.[49,50] Aggressive surveillance and vigilance for enteric pathogens and fungi is important. In addition, these patients are at risk for development of *Pneumocystis carinii* pneumonia. It is recommended that patients undergoing induction immunosuppression or rejection treatment with monoclonal or polyclonal antibodies receive *Pneumocystis* prophylaxis with trimethoprim-sulfamethoxazole.

Viral infections are also problematic for the pediatric recipient. The typical pediatric organ transplant recipient is usually seronegative for cytomegalovirus (CMV) and other herpesviruses such as herpes simplex virus type 1 (HSV-1), varicella-zoster virus (VZV), and Epstein-Barr virus (EBV). All four of these viral pathogens can wreak havoc on the pediatric transplant recipient. Pediatric patients who receive a CMV-seropositive donor organ should undergo CMV prophylaxis with a specific anti-CMV immunoglobulin, intravenous gancyclovir, or both. Fortunately, the clinical prophylactic use of immunoglobulins and gancyclovir has markedly decreased the incidence of life-threatening CMV infections in pediatric organ transplant recipients. Similarly, patients undergoing induction therapy or being treated for rejection with antithymocyte preparations should receive acyclovir prophylaxis for HSV-1 and VZV. Both of these herpesviruses can either produce a primary infection in naive recipients or reactivate infection in seropositive individuals. Treatment with intravenous acyclovir for HSV-1 and VZV is required with initial primary infections. EBV infection is also problematic in the management of the posttransplantation organ recipient. Although 80% of the adult population is seropositive for EBV, few children are. EBV infection causes the mononucleosis syndrome. In addition to causing this clinical syndrome of lymphadenopathy, hepatosplenomegaly, sore throat, and fever, EBV directly targets and transfects B lymphocytes. The infected B lymphocyte is "transformed" in these patients to a state of continuous division, like a lymphoma or leukemia cell.[51,52] In the immunologically normal patient in whom mononucleosis develops, there is a secondary effector T-cell response that eliminates these clones of immortalized B cells. In the immunosuppressed patient, the EBV-transformed B lymphocyte may continue to grow unchecked because the T-cell arm of the immune system is compromised by the drugs. The EBV-negative transplant recipient who gets either an EBV-positive donor organ or acquires EBV from the community may contract a significant EBV infection. The first phase is a mononucleosis syndrome, characterized by typical features of mononucleosis including fever, chills, hepatosplenomegaly, and lymphadenopathy. At this stage, patients should be treated with acyclovir or gancyclovir and immunosuppression tapered, if possible. Patients may go on to manifest a polyclonal lymphoproliferative disorder secondary to the EBV transformation of B lymphocytes and their unchecked proliferation. At this point, immunosuppression should be discontinued in these patients. Finally, a monoclonal lymphoproliferative syndrome may develop in these patients, which is essentially a lymphoma or leukemia. With the development of an overt monoclonal lymphoproliferative syndrome, immunosuppression is withdrawn, and if patients do not immediately respond, they should receive chemotherapy to treat the lymphoma or leukemia. With active drug withdrawal, there is always a risk of loss of the organ from rejection. Renal transplant recipients may need to go back on dialysis, and liver, heart, and lung transplant recipients may need to be retransplanted if they go on to develop chronic rejection.

In addition to the posttransplantation lymphoproliferative disease, other malignancies may develop in patients, as discussed later.

LATE EFFECTS OF IMMUNOSUPPRESSION

The long-term survival of solid organ transplant recipients requires lifelong treatment with immunosuppressive drugs. Despite the use of multiple agents in small doses, significant toxicities, both specifically and nonspecifically related to the immunosuppression, occur. The primary long-term effects of corticosteroids include Cushing syndrome, osteoporosis, avascular necrosis, cataracts, glaucoma, cardiovascular disease, and gastritis–peptic ulcer disease. The long-term effects of azathioprine include hepatitis, pancreatitis, and red cell aplasia. The long-term effects of cyclosporine include hypercholesterolemia, arteriosclerosis, hypertension, and nephrotoxicity. The long-term effects of tacrolimus may be hypertension and nephrotoxicity, but it is too early to determine what other side effects may develop over time.

The most serious long-term effects of immunosuppression are the late malignancies that may be seen in these patients. Kaposi sarcoma may develop, as well as the posttransplantation lymphoproliferative diseases that are specific to chronically immunosuppressed patients.[53–55] In addition, patients are at higher risk for common malignancies seen in nonimmunosuppressed patients. The most common cancer seen in immunosuppressed patients is skin cancer, which mimics its frequency in the general population. Slightly higher incidences of Hodgkin disease, non-Hodgkin lymphoma, and breast, colon, lung, uterine, and ovarian cancer have been seen in transplant recipients.[56] For this reason, patients should undergo yearly cancer surveillance, including chest radiography to look for lymphoma and Hodgkin disease, Pap smear and pelvic examination for women, and a general physical examination to look for skin lesions or any other problems.

DRUG COMBINATIONS

As more immunosuppressive agents are approved by the FDA for clinical use, these drugs will most likely be rolled into already existing drug regimens. As described earlier, cyclosporine- and tacrolimus-based therapies are the mainstays of clinical immunosuppression. The introduction of mycophenolate may replace azathioprine as the drug of choice to inhibit both T- and B-cell proliferation. Other drugs may be added that have different sites of action on the immune system. New drug combination therapies will continue to benefit the transplant recipient by using combinations of drugs at lower concentrations for fewer individual drug toxicities.

Pharmacologically, drug combination therapies provide three different end results. First, synergized inhibitory action results if two drugs that act along the same metabolic pathway are used; the two drugs potentiate each other's effect by magnifying the response of each because the metabolic pathway end-product is markedly diminished with both drugs in use. Second, drugs that act on different metabolic pathways usually have additive effects, in which each metabolic pathway is inhibited to a certain degree by each drug and the end-result is an enhanced effect on cell function. Last, drugs that act at the same site of action actually antagonize each other because they usually compete for the same receptor and block each other's action.[57,58]

For practical purposes, it is therefore best to select drugs to be used in combination that act at different sites, either along the same metabolic pathway (synergy) or different metabolic pathways (additive).

IMMUNOSUPPRESSIVE DRUG WITHDRAWAL

The alternative to multiple low-dose drug combinations is the use of more potent single immunosuppressive agents to allow for the gradual withdrawal of other agents. This procedure is a common practice and will continue to be used as more potent agents are developed. At present, multiple drugs are used early in the transplantation patient's postoperative course. These combination drugs allow for a significant rejection-free stabilization period, as well as possible accommodation of the patient's immune system to the new organ. Over time, stable patients may have some of their immunosuppressive drugs withdrawn. In the pediatric age group, steroid withdrawal has been used clinically with success. Both cyclosporine- and tacrolimus-based therapies allow for every-other-day steroids and potential steroid withdrawal.[51] A certain percentage of patients who have steroids completely withdrawn have a late rejection episode, but these are usually well treated with reinstitution of pulse-and-taper steroids. Patients may subsequently undergo successful steroid withdrawal if cyclosporine and tacrolimus are maintained at reasonable serum levels.

Similarly, cyclosporine has been withdrawn from stable renal patients who are then maintained on azathioprine and low-dose steroids indefinitely. This avoids the long-term nephrotoxic effects of cyclosporine, as well as resulting in reduced costs related to maintenance on this immunosuppressive agent.

Patients have also had their azathioprine and steroids withdrawn, to be maintained on cyclosporine or tacrolimus alone as the sole immunosuppressive agent. This cyclosporine or tacrolimus monotherapy requires slightly higher dosing with cyclosporine or tacrolimus. Although monotherapy avoids the use of steroids or long-term azathioprine, it may lead to long-term

hypertension and nephrotoxicity related to the use of these drugs at higher levels.

IMMUNOLOGIC ACCOMMODATION

As outlined in Chapter 39, in some patients there appears to be a change in the immune system that allows the organism to accommodate the alloantigenic transplanted organ. A number of theories have been proposed for this immunologic accommodation, or induction of tolerance. First, there may be clonal deletion of alloreactive cytotoxic T cells, removing cells from circulation that would reject the transplanted organ. Second, suppressor T cells may be generated that down-regulate the effector cytotoxic T-cell immune response to the transplanted organ. Third, the identification of long-lived donor lymphocytes in transplanted organs or in the draining lymph nodes from the area of transplanted organs has led to the concept of microchimerism as a mechanism of immunologic accommodation.[59] In this scenario, there is a two-way process in which competent immune cells are transplanted with the organ and interact with the recipient, essentially establishing a graft-versus-host reaction. On the other side, the recipient immune system infiltrates the transplanted graft and establishes a rejection process. This two-way process may eventually lead to a stand-off between the competing competent lymphocytes, and may be the basis for immunologic accommodation. This theory has prompted one center systematically to withdraw immunosuppression in stable patients 5 to 10 years after their liver transplant procedure (Starzl TE, personal communication).

DONOR AND RECIPIENT MODIFICATION

To achieve immunologic accommodation without the use of long-term immunosuppressive agents, methods are being devised that attempt to modify the donor organ before harvesting or during cold preservation. These methods include removal of passenger lymphocytes or dendritic cells, blockade and down-regulation of the major histocompatibility antigen complex, and down-regulation of adhesion molecules.

The recipient's immune repertoire can also be modified before transplantation. Methods include clonal deletion of alloreactive cells and up-regulation of autoregulatory cells. Historically, recipient modification has also been performed in living related donor kidney transplantation with the use of donor-specific transfusions of aliquots of red blood cells and passenger lymphocytes in the presence of either azathioprine or cyclosporine (immunologic enhancement). These repetitive, small doses of antigen appear to down-regulate or remove the alloreactive recipient lymphocytes from the circulation. Similarly, the use of T-cell–depleted bone marrow transplanted from the donor to the recipient at the time of organ transplantation is another method to introduce and spur the process of immunologic accommodation or microchimerism. Both of these methods have been shown to be useful in liver and kidney allografts.[60,61] The future may see further attempts to promote tolerance in the transplant recipient, allowing, it is hoped, for the complete removal of immunosuppressive drugs and their attendant toxicities.

REFERENCES

1. Groth C-G, Ohlman S, Gannedahl F, et al. New immunosuppressive drugs in transplantation. Transplant Proc 1993;25:281.
2. Billingham RE, Krohn PL, Medawar PB. Effect of cortisone on survival of skin homografts in rabbits. Br Med J 1951;1:476.
3. Starzal TE, Marchioro TL, Waddell WR. The reversal of rejection in human renal allografts with subsequent development of homograft tolerance. Surg Gynecol Obstet 1963;117:385.
4. Murray JE, Merrill JP, Harrison JH, et al. Prolonged survival of human-kidney homografts by immunosuppressive. Ann Plast Surg 1984;12:70.
5. Sollinger HN, Belzer FO, Deierhoi MH, et al. RS61443 (mycophenolate mofetil): a multicenter study for refractory kidney transplant rejection. Ann Surg 1992;216:513.
6. Ensley RD, Bristow MR, Olsen SL, et al. The use of mycophenolate mofetil (RS61443) in human heart transplant recipients. Transplantation 1993;66:75.
7. Borel JF, Feurer C, Gubler HU, et al. Biological effects of cyclosporin A: a new antilymphocytic agent. Agents Actions 1976;6:486.
8. Calre RY, White DJG, Thiru S, et al. Cyclosporine A in patients receiving renal allografts from cadaveric donors. Lancet 1978;2:1323.
9. Bloemerra E, VanOers RHJ, Weinreich S, et al. The influence of cyclosporine A on the alternative pathways of human T cell activation in vitro. Eur J Immunol 1989;19:943.
10. Colombani PM, Robb A, Hess AD. Cyclosporine binding to calmodulin: a possible site of action on T-lymphocytes. Science 1985;228:337.
11. Harding MW, Galat A, Uehling DE, et al. A receptor for the immunosuppressant FK506 is a cis-trans peptidyl-propyl isomerase. Nature 1989;341:758
12. Siekierka JJ, Sigal NH. FK506 and cyclosporin A: immunosuppressive mechanism of action and beyond. Curr Opin Immunol 1992;4:548.
13. Colombani PM, Hess AD. Cyclosporine as calmodulin inhibitor: a commentary. J Biochem Pharmacol 1987;36:3789.
14. Kahan BD, Dunn J, Fitts C, et al. Reduced inter- and intrasubject variability in cyclopharmacokinetics in renal transplant recipients treated with a microemulsion formula in conjunction with fasting, low fat meals or high fat meals. Transplantation 1995,59:505.
15. Kovarik JM. Cyclosporine pharmacokinetics and variability from a microemulsion formulation: a multicenter investigation in kidney transplant patients. Transplantation 1995;58:658.
16. Tocci MJ, Matkovich DA, Collier KA, et al. The immunosuppressant FK506 selectively inhibits expression of early T-cell activation genes. J Immunol 1989;143:718.
17. Kino T, Hatanaka H. Miyata S, et al. FK506, a novel immunosuppressant isolated from a *Streptomyces* II immunosuppressive effect of FK506 in vitro. J Antibiot (Tokyo) 1987;40:1256.
18. Johansson A, Miller E. Evidence that the immunosuppressive effects of FK506 and cyclosporine are identical. Transplantation 1990;50:1001.
19. Siekierka JJ, Hung SHY, Poe M, et al. A cytosolic binding protein for the immunosuppressant FK506 has peptidyl-propyl isomerase activity but is distinct from cyclophilin. Nature 1989;341:755.
20. Esquivel FO, So SK, McDiarmid SV, et al. Suggested guidelines for the use of tacrolimus in pediatric liver transplant patients. Transplantation 1996;61:845.
21. Parlevliet KJ, Schellekens PTA. Monoclonal antibodies in renal transplantation: a review. Transpl Int 1992;5:234.
22. Hardy MA, Nowygrod R, Elberg A, et al. Use of ATG in treatment of steroid-resistant rejection. Transplantation 1980;29:162.
23. Wechter WJ, Morrell RN, Bergan J, et al. Extended treatment with antithymocyte globulin (ATGAM) in renal allograft recipients. Transplantation 1979;28:365.
24. Kahan BD. Immunosuppressive therapy. Curr Opin Immunol 1992;4:553.
25. Kokado Y, Kanno N, Yoshioka T, et al. Herpes simplex esophagitis in a renal transplant patient treated with OKT3 and deoxyspergualin. Clin Transpl 1989;298:189.
26. Mita K, Akiyama N, Nagao T, et al. Advantages of mizoribine over azathioprine in combination with cyclosporine from renal transplant. Transplant Proc 1990;22:1679.
27. Jaffe BD, Jones EA, Loveless SE, et al. The unique immunosuppressive activity of brequinar sodium. Transplant Proc 1993;25:19.
28. Makowka L, Chapman F, Cramer DV. Historical development of brequinar sodium as a new immunosuppressive drug for transplantation. Transplant Proc 1993;25:2.
29. Henry ML, Elkhammas EA, Tesi RJ, et al. A randomized prospective trial of OG37-325 versus cyclosporine in cadaveric renal transplantation: a one year follow-up. In: The annual meeting of the American Society of Transplant Physicians, Houston, Texas, May, 1993, abstract 74.
30. Leichtman A, Adams M, Berrnett W, et al. Normal liver function values in human renal transplant recipients treated with OG 37-325. In: The annual meeting of the American Society of Transplant Physicians, Houston, Texas, May, 1993, abstract 66.
31. Kimball PM, Kerman RH, Kahen BD. Rapamycin and cyclosporine produce synergistic but nonidentical mechanisms of immunosuppression. Transplant Proc 1991;23:1027.
32. Dumont FJ, Melino MR, Staruch MJ, et al. The immunosuppressive macrolides FK506 and rapamycin act as reciprocal antagonists in murine T-cells. J Immunol 1990;144:1418.
33. Stepkowski SM, Chen H, Daloze P, et al. Rapamycin, a potent immunosuppressive drug for vascularized heart, kidney and small bowel transplantation in the rat. Transplantation 1991;51:22.
34. Lang R, Wagner H, Heeg K. Differential effects of the immunosuppressive agents cyclosporine and leflunomide in vivo. Transplantation 1995;59:382.
35. Yuh DD, Morris RE. The immunopharmacology of immunosuppression by 15-deoxyspergualin. Transplantation 1993;55:578.
36. Amemiya H, Suzuki S, Ota K, et al. Effect of a novel immunosuppressive agent, deoxyspergualin on rejection in kidney transplant recipients. Transplant Proc 1990;22:1606.
37. Carpenter CB, Kirkman RL, Shapiro ME, et al. Prophylactic use of monoclonal anti-IL-2 receptor antibody in cadaveric renal transplantation. Am J Kidney Dis 1989;14:54.
38. Kirkman RL, Shapiro ME, Carpenter CB, et al. A randomized prospective trial of anti-TRC monoclonal antibody in human renal transplantation. Transplantation 1991;51:107.
39. Cosimi AB, Conti D, Delmonico FL, et al. In vivo effects of monoclonal antibody to ICAM-1 (CD54) in non-human primates with renal allografts. J Immunol 1990;144:4604.
40. Stoppa AM, Maraninchi D, Blais D, et al. Anti-LFA 1 monoclonal antibody (25.3) for treatment of steroid-resistant grade III-IV acute graft vs. host disease. Transpl Int 1991;4:3.
41. Friend PJ, Hale G, Waldmann H, et al. Campath-IM prophylactic use after kidney transplantation: a randomized controlled clinical trial. Transplantation 1989;48:248.
42. McDiarmid SV, Busittil RN, Terasaki P, et al. OKT3 treatment of steroid resistant rejection in pediatric liver transplant recipients. J Pediatr Gastroenterol Nutr 1992;14:86.
43. Renard TH, Andrew WS, Foster ME. Relationship between OKT3 administration, EBV seroconversion and the lymphoproliferative syndrome in pediatric liver transplant recipients. Transplant Proc 1991;23:1473.
44. Egawa H, Esquivil CO, So SK, et al. FK506 conversion therapy in pediatric liver transplantation. Transplantation 1994;57:1169.
45. Sallinger HW, Belzer FO, Dererhoi MH, et al. RS-61443 (mycophenolate mofetil): a multicenter study for refractory kidney transplant rejection. Ann Surg 1992;216:513.
46. European Mycophenolate Mofetil Cooperative Study Group. Placebo-controlled study of mycophenolate mofetil combined with cyclosporin and corticosteroids for prevention/acute rejection. Lancet 1 1995;345:1321.
47. Morris RE, Hoyt EG, Murphy MP. Mycophenolic acid morpholinoethylester (RS-6134) is a new immunosuppressant that prevents and halts heart allograft rejection by selective inhibition of T and B cell purine synthesis. Transplant Proc 1990;22:1659.
48. Platz KP, Sollinger HW, Hullett DA, et al. RS-61443, a new, potent immunosuppressive agent. Transplantation 1991;51:27.
49. Hibberd PL, Rubin RH. Prevention of cytomegalovirus infection in the pediatric renal transplant recipient. Pediatr Nephrol 1991;5:112.
50. Saint-Vil D, Luks FI, Lebel P, et al. Infections complications of pediatric liver transplantation. J Pediatr Surg 1991;26:908.
51. Ellis D. Clinical use of tacrolimus (FK506) in infants and children with renal transplants. Pediatr Nephrol 1995;9:487.
52. Kuo PC, Dafoe DC, Alfrey EJ, et al. Post-transplant lymphoproliferative disorders and Epstein-Barr virus prophylaxis. Transplantation 1995;59:135.

53. Lubowitz D. Epstein-Barr virus: an old dog with new tricks. N Engl J Med 1995;332:55.

54. Cho J, Chachoua A. Kaposi's sarcoma. Curr Opin Oncol 1992;4:667.

55. Hanto DW, Firizzera G, Gajl-Peczalska KJ, et al. Epstein-Barr virus, immunodeficiency and B-cell lymphoproliferation. Transplantation 1985;39:461.

56. Penn I. The changing pattern of post-transplant malignancies. Transplant Proc 1991;23:1101.

57. Zhang P, Colombani PM. Drug–drug interactions between Diterpene, T_{11}, and agents affecting T-lymphocyte immunosuppressive drugs. Present at FASEB annual meeting, Los Angeles, California, April, 1992.

58. Kaham BD, Gibbons S, Tejpal N, et al. Synergistic effect of the rapamycin–cyclosporine combination: median effect analysis of in vitro immune performances by human T lymphocytes in PHA, CD3 and MLR proliferative and cytotoxic assay. Transplant Proc 1991;23:1090.

59. Starzl TE. Liver allo- and xenotransplantation. Transplant Proc 1993;25:15.

60. Ilstead ST, Wren SM, Bluestone JA, et al. Characterization of mixed allogeneic chimeras immunocompetency in vitro reactivity and genetic specificity of tolerance. J Exp Med 1985;162:231.

61. Barber WH, Mankin JA, Laskow DA, et al. Long-term results of a controlled prospective study with transfusion of donor-specific bone marrow in 57 consecutive renal allograft recipients. Transplantation 1991;51:70.

Surgery of Infants and Children: Scientific Principles and Practice, edited by Keith T. Oldham, Paul M. Colombani, and Robert P. Foglia. Lippincott–Raven Publishers, Philadelphia, © 1997.

CHAPTER 41

Organ Donation, Procurement, and Preservation

Frederick C. Ryckman

Organ transplantation has created unique ethical, social, and health care allocation issues as the demand for transplantation has outpaced the supply of donor organs. This critical donor organ shortage has prompted efforts within the medical and nonmedical community to increase organ donation, required the development of complex systems to distribute available resources, and prompted research to improve organ recovery and preservation techniques. The organ shortage has also stimulated review of current donor criteria, leading to an expanding tolerance of donor age ranges, stability, and aggressive surgical organ recovery techniques. This chapter reviews the critical issues of organ donation, procurement, and preservation.

DONOR IDENTIFICATION

Early recognition of possible donors, rapid and accurate assessment of brain death, and proper physiologic management are necessary to meet the increased needs for organ transplantation.

Recognition of Possible Organ Donors

Multiple studies have estimated that in the 1990s, 12,000 to 27,000 potential organ donors die each year in the United States. Only 15% to 30% of the potential donors reach successful donation.[1–3] Health care professionals are the most critical link in this organ procurement process. Suitable candidates must be recognized, and the organ acquisition process begun. Head injury represents the most common etiology of brain death, representing 77% of all organ donors.[4,5] In experienced trauma centers, 75% of these potential donors were recognized at the time of admission; 92% had Glasgow Coma Scale (GCS) scores of 5 or less, and 84% had GCS scores of 3 to 4.[5] People with nontraumatic brain death are less frequently identified. In the Pennsylvania study, the medical community missed between 25% and 34% of potential donors.[3] These were more often older than the age of 45 years, of minority races, and in the hospital

for at least 5 days. Intracranial hemorrhage or anoxic brain death were the more common causes of death. A broader application of expanded donor age criteria and increased professional education would allow their inclusion in this critical donor pool.

Although recognition of potential donors is the initial step to increasing organ availability, securing consent for donation from the responsible family member is unfortunately often unsuccessful. In 1990, United Network for Organ Sharing (UNOS) statistics reviewed 15,000 eligible donors, and confirmed that only 30% of families consented to donation.[1,6] A separation of the discussion related to brain death, and the issues surrounding organ donation, increased donation rates from 18% to 57%. In addition, trained transplant procurement coordinators experienced much greater success in seeking successful donation then did the physician responsible for declaring brain death.[1]

Ethnic minorities have infrequently participated in organ donation in the past. Recent efforts at community education and broadening the ethnic diversity of transplant procurement professionals have attempted to address this disparity. Using this approach, consent rates increased from 12% in 1989 to 31% in 1990.[7] The importance of stressing organ donation in the pediatric population cannot be overestimated.

Families of pediatric patients may be more willing to agree to donation than families of adult patients.[8] In a study conducted at Vanderbilt University, several key factors were identified: 1) the presence of an attending pediatric surgeon who was aware of both the acute donor organ shortage, and had experienced first-hand the benefit of organ transplantation in their practice; 2) improved rapport and trust between the parents and hospital team, achieved through extended periods of bedside care and discussion; 3) concentration of the decision-making responsibility in the hands of the child's parents; 4) a desire by parents of potential donors to help another child, and prevent similar feelings of loss in other parents; and 5) younger parents with greater overall donor awareness.[8] The extreme need for pediatric donor organs and the frequent willingness of the patients to consider donation mandate that all potential pediatric donors be recognized, and the parents offered the opportunity to donate.

The importance of rapid recognition of potential donors is emphasized by their often precipitous neurologic decline after

TABLE 41-1. *Laboratory screening before organ donation*

Hematology
  Complete blood count, prothrombin and partial thrombo-
    plastin time, platelet count
Chemistry
  Electrolytes, blood urea nitrogen, creatinine liver function
    tests, calcium, phosphate, urine analysis
Microbiology
  Blood urine, and sputum culture, sputum gram stain, results
    of prior cultures if patient febrile while hospitalized
Serology
  VDRL, hepatitis B surface antigen, human immonodefi-
    ciency virus, cytomegalovirus, ABO blood type, human
    leukocyte antigen tissue typing
Respiratory
  Chest radiograph, arterial blood gas
Cardiovascular (heart donor)
  Electrocardiogram, echocardiogram

TABLE 41-2. *Criteria for declaration of brain death*

Identified and *irreversible* etiology of brain death despite max-
  imum medical therapy
Absence of hypothermia, drug intoxication, metabolic en-
  cephalopathy, shock
Clincal presence of *brain death* by examination
  Cerebral unresponsiveness
  No spontaneous motor activity
  Absent pupillary, corneal, and oculocephalic/oculovestibu-
    lar reflexes
  Absent cough reflex with deep tracheal suctioning
  No increase in heart rate in response to intravenous admin-
    istration of atropine
  No respiratory efforts on apnea testing ($Paco_2$ >60 mm
    Hg)
Persistent absence of all brain function after period of obser-
  vation acceptable for age of patient:

Age of Patient	Interval between Examinations
0–1 wk	No period defined
1 wk– 2 mo	48 h
2 mo–1 y	24 h
1–2 y	12–24 h
>2 y of age	12 h

admission. Twenty percent of potential organ donors die within 6 hours of hospital admission, and 50% die within 24 hours despite intensive care.[4] Prompt recognition and referral to the Organ Procurement Organization (OPO) is essential to preserve organ function in these unstable patients.

Minimal acceptable criteria for assessing possible organ donors include 1) local criteria for brain death met, 2) patient age younger than 65 years, 3) absence of malignancy with metastatic potential, and 4) absence of sepsis or other communicable disease. Based on these inclusive criteria, all potential donors should be referred to the OPO for further evaluation. Cadaveric donors require a screening history, physical examination, blood screening tests, and specific tests of target organ function to ensure donor organ acceptability (Table 41-1). Contraindications include the following:

- Uncontrolled infection of any etiology
- Acquired immunodeficiency syndrome
- Viral hepatitis
- Malignancy (except primary brain tumor)
- Intravenous drug abuse

Arbitrary age restrictions used to exclude potential donors in the past have been reevaluated, expanding donor ages up to 70 years. The physiologic function of the organ, rather than the donor's age, is often a better determinant of acceptability. Specific functional testing and direct organ biopsy allow identification of physiologically acceptable organs from older potential donors. Experience has indicated that when organ function is acceptable, these people make good organ donors.

Declaration of Brain Death

Brain death criteria are determined by each state; however, many have now adopted the criteria in the President's Commission for the Study of Ethical Problems in Medicine and Biomedical and Behavioral Research, defining by physical examination the absence of all cerebral and brain stem function.[9] Confirmation by reexamination after a 12-hour waiting period is usually acceptable for final declaration in children older than 2 years of age and adults. In infants 7 days to 2 months of age, a 48-

hour waiting period between examinations is recommended. The interval between examinations is abbreviated to 24 hours in the 2-month- to 1-year-old potential donor, and 12 to 24 hours is acceptable in a patient older than 1 year (Table 41-2). Brain death can also be identified by demonstrating the absence of cerebral blood flow on a radionuclide scan or cerebral arteriographic study. When cerebral blood flow is absent, brain death is established and no waiting period is necessary. The electroencephalograph (EEG) is not necessary to establish brain death. However, if an EEG is obtained and is equivocal, it cannot be ignored. A cerebral blood flow study is the next logical step in these cases.

DONOR MANAGEMENT

Donor management principles include restoration and maintenance of hemodynamic stability, maximizing tissue perfusion and oxygen delivery, and treatment of direct complications associated with brain death.[10]

Intravenous Fluid Management

Reestablishment of the circulating blood volume is the first priority. Most donors are hypovolemic secondary to fluid restriction, diuretic use, and diabetes insipidus. Fluid is administered to restore central venous pressure to 10 cm H_2O, using lactated Ringer solution to prevent further hypernatremia. Red blood cells are administered to reach a hematocrit of 35%. Cytomegalovirus-negative or micropore-filtered blood products are recommended when possible. Systemic release of plasminogen activator from necrotic brain can also cause a diffuse coagulopathy. Inappropriate bleeding should be treated by specific blood coagulation component therapy. Administration of epsilon aminocaproic acid should be avoided because of its microvascular thrombotic effects.

The autonomic nervous system dysfunction associated with increased intracranial pressure often precipitates severe hypertension and bradyarrhythmias. Progressive brain stem infarction later causes decreasing sympathetic tone and loss of neurohumoral circulatory control, leading to hypotension. If restoration of blood volume does not achieve a normal systolic pressure, vasopressors are necessary. Dopamine (2 to 10 μg/kg/min, 20 μg/kg/min maximum) is the vasopressor of choice because it encourages both renal and mesenteric vasodilatation. Dobutamine and isoproterenol cause associated vasodilatation, whereas phenylephrine, norepinephrine, and epinephrine can contribute to hypoperfusion secondary to vasoconstriction. These agents are used only for refractory hypotension. The goal of adequate fluid resuscitation is sufficient urine output. In most cases, a urine output of 0.5 to 2.0 mL/kg/h implies sufficient renal perfusion. If blood volume reconstitution and low-dose vasopressor support are unsuccessful, pulmonary artery catheter placement with cardiac output monitoring is essential to guide further resuscitation and vasopressor therapy. Persistent oliguria, despite adequate resuscitation, suggests intrinsic renal disease or excessive vasopressin administration.

Additional Hormonal Therapy

Investigation has shown a significant fall in serum cortisol, insulin, and thyroid hormone levels with brain death. A 50% fall in free triiodothyronine (T_3) and thyroxine levels occurs within 1 hour of brain death, and no thyroid hormone may be detectable by 16 hours. Administration of thyroid hormone has been associated with improved myocardial performance and tissue metabolism.[11] The following recommendations for additional hormone therapy in adults can be made: 1) T_3, 2 μg/h intravenously (IV), 2) cortisol, 100 mg/hr IV, and 3) insulin, 10 to 20 U/h IV. These should be administered until anaerobic metabolism is corrected as documented by normal serum lactate production. These dosages must be appropriately diminished in pediatric donors. The use of agents to prevent oxygen free radical damage, such as mannitol, superoxide desmutase, allopurinol, and steroids, is experimental and further research is necessary to document their specific benefits to donors.

Diabetes Insipidus

Hypothalamic–pituitary axis destruction leads to decreased secretion of antidiuretic hormone. This neurogenic diabetes insipidus is seen in 50% to 75% of patients with brain death. Insufficient antidiuretic hormone leads to decreased renal tubular water absorption, yielding voluminous amounts of dilute urine and precipitating severe electrolyte loss, hypernatremia, hypocalcemia, hypophosphatemia, and hypomagnesemia. Treatment is instituted using aqueous vasopressin administered IV at 0.5 to 1.0 μg/h until the urine output is 2 to 3 mL/kg/h. Excessive dosages can cause mesenteric and renal vascular vasoconstriction. Arginine vasopressin (desmopressin, DDAVP), administered IV or as a nasal spray, has lower vasopressive effects and a longer duration of action, and is the drug of choice for treating neurogenic diabetes insipidus.[12]

Temperature Regulation

Initial periods of hyperthermia usually progress to hypothermia. Heated blankets, intravenous fluids, and ventilator gases are usually sufficient to stabilize the temperature above 34°C.

Pulmonary Care

Ventilator settings of 10 to 15 mL/kg tidal volume and F_{IO_2} as needed should be used to achieve a Pa_{O_2} of 100 mm Hg. Elevated positive end-expiratory pressure (PEEP) is preferable to increased F_{IO_2}. Endotracheal suctioning, positional therapy, and routine surveillance cultures should be undertaken. Pulmonary edema can occur secondary to fluid overload, increased vascular permeability associated with adult respiratory distress syndrome, or neurogenic causes. Treatment of each is supportive, using PEEP. When increased PEEP and F_{IO_2} are required, a pulmonary artery catheter is helpful.

DONOR AGE CRITERIA

The need to expand the donor organ pool is emphasized by the rapid growth of recipient waiting lists for solid organ transplantation, while 3.6% of patients listed for renal transplantation, 11.4% of patients listed for heart transplantation, and 8% of patients listed for liver transplantation die awaiting organ availability without the benefit of transplantation.[13] It has been feared that organs from older-aged donors would not be suitable for transplantation because of physiologic deterioration within the organ. Arbitrary age limits were initially imposed on potential donors in an attempt to ensure the quality of the donor organs. However, strict age restriction also carries the risk of excluding organs from potentially suitable donors. More recent studies have reevaluated the policy of routinely excluding older donors. In kidney transplant recipients, organs from older donors do just as well as organs from the "ideal"-aged donor, assuming the potential donor had normal renal function at the time of harvest. The use of routine biopsy and histologic evaluation is helpful in ensuring adequate allograft potential for transplantation.[14] Similar results have been reported in liver and heart transplant recipients, although the experience is not as extensive. Liver allograft function after transplantation was not significantly different between donors older than 50 years of age and younger, "ideal" donors. Patient survival was also equivalent. In addition, atherosclerosis is relatively uncommon in the distal abdominal visceral vessels, and therefore rarely complicates hepatic artery anastomosis at the time of transplantation.[14] Heart donation from people older than 45 years of age has also been shown to be acceptable, with graft survival and complication rates similar to those with younger donors.[14] These studies indicate that age itself should not be a barrier to organ donation, and that organ donors could be selected more appropriately on the basis of organ function. The aggressive use of biopsy to identify diseased organs will help to increase the use of suitable older donors.

Non–Heart-Beating Cadaver Donors

Renewed interest in the use of non–heart-beating cadaver donors (NHBD) has also emerged as a route to overcome the persistent shortage of organ donors.[15] These donors have not met conventional brain death criteria because of retained brain stem reflexes, or the next of kin has requested formal withdrawal of life support and documented cardiac arrest before donor organ procurement.

After detailed consent explaining the format of donation is obtained, patients are administered heparin and α-adrenergic blocking agents to prevent thrombosis and terminal ischemic vasospasm. Life support is terminated. After the cessation of heart beat and respiration, and declaration of brain death, hypothermic perfusion of the abdominal viscera is undertaken through a previously placed femoral artery cannula, or through a cannula placed at the aortic bifurcation through a rapid midline sternotomy–laparotomy. Organs are cooled and harvested en bloc, separated while maintaining hypothermic conditions, and reperfused with preservation solution.

Kidney, liver, pancreas, and lung allografts have been harvested using these techniques. Organ function using these techniques has been acceptable. Kidney function after transplantation has been equivalent to that of the traditional cadaveric organ experience. Liver preservation has been good when warm ischemic times were minimal. In donors in whom prolonged agonal periods existed, organ function can be significantly compromised.[16,17] This preliminary experience suggests that NHBDs are acceptable donor organ sources as long as a carefully controlled harvest is undertaken.

Unrelated Living Donors

Unrelated living-donor kidney transplantation has become generally accepted as a highly successful means of treating patients with end-stage renal disease. Good results have been reported with and without the use of donor-specific blood transfusions. The consensus is that unrelated living donors should be emotionally related to the recipient (eg, spouse, stepparent, stepchild). Long-term results in the recipients need to be carefully evaluated.[18,19]

ORGAN RECOVERY OPERATIVE TECHNIQUES

The extreme shortage of donor organs makes it essential to consider every potential donor as a multiorgan donor. Multiple studies have demonstrated that organs harvested from multiorgan donors function equally well as organs from single-organ donors.[20] Successful multiorgan harvest requires the simultaneous identification of potential organ recipients so that careful and systematic plans can be made to provide for optimal recovery of all usable organs by the procurement surgical team. Each member of that team should possess knowledge of the multiorgan procurement procedures, and be willing to cooperate and communicate to ensure the mutual success of all operating teams.

Anesthesia

Significant neurologic injury in most donors results in the loss of normal neuroregulatory function. Support for the 2 to 4 hours required for multiorgan procurement requires careful anesthetic monitoring and management. Core temperature should remain above 35°C until all preparations for harvest are completed, requiring heated humidifiers on the anesthetic circuit, and warming blankets. Hemodynamic stability is essential, but is often compromised by the fluid restrictions imposed by the prior treatment of head injury and the massive urinary losses of diabetes insipidus. Central blood volume monitoring, the judicious use of systemic arginine vasopressin, and transfusion to maintain a hemoglobin greater than 9 g/dL should be undertaken. Inotropic drugs are often necessary. Anesthetic support should be maintained until in situ hypothermic perfusion of the organs is begun.

Surgical Procedures

The procedure for multiorgan procurement is carried out through a midline incision extending from the suprasternal notch to the pubis. A small opening in both pleural spaces prevents the development of an unexpected tension pneumothorax, and the midline diaphragmatic attachments of the diaphragm are divided to allow access to the entire abdomen and chest.

Multiorgan procurement most often includes donation of the liver, kidneys, and heart, but may also include pancreas, small intestine, heart–lung, or lung donation as well. Tissue donation of cornea, skin, bone, bone marrow, or heart valves can be completed after termination of life support and solid organ recovery. General principles of organ recovery include 1) identification and preservation of all blood supply to the donor organs until the time of organ removal, 2) minimal mobilization and handling of the donor tissue until hypothermic preservation has begun, and 3) sequential harvest of organs to allow continuous hypothermic perfusion of the remaining in situ donor organs—heart first, then liver–pancreas, and then kidneys. Hypothermic organ perfusion is achieved through a cannula inserted into the distal aorta, using retrograde perfusion after the aorta is cross-clamped at the level of the diaphragmatic aortic hiatus. Portal venous perfusion is provided through cannulation of the splenic vein if the pancreas is not procured, or through the superior or inferior mesenteric veins at the root of the mesentery during pancreatic donation. Venous decompression occurs through the suprahepatic vena caval–atrial junction, which is divided during heart procurement. When heart harvest is not undertaken, a separate inferior vena caval drainage catheter is placed to decompress the abdominal viscera during hypothermic perfusion. The specific steps of multiorgan procurement are summarized in Table 41-3.[20]

Most procurement teams prefer stepwise, meticulous dissection of the vascular structures before in situ perfusion, local topical cooling, and organ harvest. However, in donors who are hemodynamically unstable, a long operative procedure may not be tolerated. An acceptable alternative technique is the ''rapid flush technique,'' described by Starzl and associates, in which vena cava and aortic cannulation immediately precedes cardiectomy, with no mobilization of the abdominal viscera.[21] During cardiac harvest, the donor organs are flushed with 15 L of 4°C solution. The abdominal organs are then dissected after hypothermic perfusion in a bloodless field.

Either procurement method is acceptable, and both allow the retrieval of normal organs.

TABLE 41-3. *Outline of heart, liver, pancreas, and kidney recovery*

INITIAL LIVER DISSECTION

1. Free gallbladder from peritoneal attachments
2. Identify the blood supply to the liver, checking for left gastric branch to left lobe and for SMA branch to right lobe
3. Divide common bile duct at the duodenum, flush by way of gallbladder
4. Trace common hepatic artery to celiac axis, ligate right gastric artery and gastroduodenal arteries
5. Divide splenic and left gastric and gastroduodenal arteries*
6. Free splenic vein and SMV, ligate distally, and divide
7. Encircle supraceliac aorta
8. Free and encircle distal aorta and vena cava

INITAL HEART DISSECTION

1. Open pericardium, tack-up
2. Free aorta and vena cava from pulmonary artery
3. Place cardioplegia needle after heparinization

INITIAL KIDNEY DISSECTION

1. Mobilize right colon
2. Free ureters, divide, and culture
3. Identify, ligate, and divide SMA†
4. Encircle suprarenal aorta
5. Minimal freeing up of kidneys

INITIAL PANCREAS DISSECTION

1. Mobilize pancreas/spleen en bloc from retroperitoneum
2. Instill antibiotic solution in duodenum, staple and divide proximal and distal duodenal segment
3. Preserve gastroduodenal and splenic artery perfusion until harvest
4. Portal cannula into distal SMV/IMV

IN-SITU HYPOTHERMIC PERFUSION

1. Heparinize patient 3 mg/kg (200–400 U/kg)
2. Ligate distal aorta and vena cava and cannulate
3. Ligate SMV, precool until donor temperature 28°–31°C or bradycardia develops
4. Staple SVC, clamp infrainnominate aorta
5. Start cardioplegia, clamp supraceliac aorta
6. Start aortic and portal flush with UW solution
7. Discontinue anesthesia support

FINAL HEART DISSECTION

1. Divide inferior vena cava at right atrium
2. Divide left pulmonary vein

3. Divide main pulmonary artery at bifurcation
4. Superior vena cava divided proximal to the staple line
5. Right pulmonary veins divided
6. Left atrium freed from pericardium
7. Aortic clamp removed and aorta stapled and divided
8. Heart removed, prepared for implantation, and packaged

FINAL LIVER DISSECTION

1. Aortic flush continues
2. Slow portal flush after 0.5–1.0 L infused
3. Identify proximal end of SMA, cross-clamp aorta at orifice of SMA†
4. Continue kidney flush with UW solution
5. Divide aorta between aortic cross-clamps, preserving celiac axis origin
6. Divide vena cava above renal veins
7. Free suprahepatic vena cava from diaphragm
8. Remove liver with wide cuff of diaphragm
9. Free liver from retroperitoneal attachments
10. Reflush portal vein, aorta, and bile duct with UW solution
11. Package liver on back table in UW solution
12. After kidneys are removed
   a. Iliac artery and vein harvested for grafts
   b. Lymph nodes and piece of spleen removed for matching

FINAL RENAL DISSECTION

1. Aorta and vena cava divided below cannulas
2. Assistant holds up ureters and aortic and vena caval cannulas
3. Dissecting on vertebral column, kidneys removed en bloc
4. Kidneys separated on the back table, packaged individually
5. Lymph nodes and piece of spleen removed for matching

FINAL PANCREAS DISSECTION‡

1. Ligate and divide splenic, gastroduodenal artery
2. Divide IMV, SMV below pancreas
3. Divide portal vein just above duodenal pancreatic junction
4. After kidneys are removed
   a. Iliac artery and vein harvested for grafts
   b. Lymph nodes and piece of spleen removed for matching

SMA, superior mesenteric artery; SMV, superior mesenteric vein; IMV, inferior mesenteric vein; UW, University of Wisconsin (preservation solution).
* Only if no left gastric branch to liver; preserve splenic artery/vein if pancreas harvest planned.
† Only if no SMA branch to liver, and not pancreas donor.
‡ Carried out simultaneously with final liver dissection.
Modified from Wood RP, Shaw BW. Multiple organ procurement. In: Cerilli GJ, ed. Organ transplantation and replacement. Philadelphia, JB Lippincott, 322.

ORGAN PRESERVATION TECHNIQUES

Organ preservation has the following goals: 1) maintaining adequate organ function throughout the ischemic period; 2) providing time for organ distribution, including tissue typing, transportation, and recipient preparation; and 3) providing time for unique surgical procedures to allow maximum use of the donor organs (eg, reduced-size liver transplantation). Each tissue preserved has unique metabolic requirements, and therefore optimal preservation techniques vary between organs. There is also a variable tolerance to cold ischemic preservation among the individual organs; the heart has the least tolerance, the pancreas and liver have somewhat greater tolerance, and the kidney has the greatest tolerance. Nevertheless, all organs begin to suffer progressive cellular damage after removal from the intact circulatory system. Organ preservation retards but does not prevent this process.[22–27]

Organ preservation requires maintenance of hypothermic conditions and prevention of cellular swelling.

The two primary ways to preserve solid organs for transplantation, simple cold storage and continuous hypothermic perfusion, both depend on hypothermia.[22,24,28] Rapid hypothermia is achieved in large solid organs through combined surface cooling and core cooling using hypothermic vascular flush-out procedures. The primary contribution of hypothermia is the suppression of adenosine triphosphate (ATP) loss and pH decrement that occur in ischemic tissues. Hypothermic preservation suppresses mitochondrial function, and decreases ATP consumption to adenosine diphosphate, its conversion to adenosine monophosphate, and the subsequent loss of the oxypurines. This substantially contributes to the maintenance of adequate energy stores within the cell. At the temperatures used for simple storage (4° to 5°C), oxygen demands are decreased by 95%, and acellular perfusates supply sufficient oxygen to the tissue to meet the decreased energy demands.[22–25,28]

Prevention of cellular swelling depends on plasma membrane activity and the sodium–potassium (Na-K) pump. Hypothermia depresses the activity of the Na-K pump, leading to rapid exchange of extracellular sodium for intracellular potassium, and a decrease in the cellular membrane potential. Chlorine passively enters the cell, following its concentration and electrical gradients. Increasing cellular osmolarity leads to water entry and subsequent cellular swelling. Swelling can be minimized by the addition of impermeable osmolar agents to the preservation solutions, such as mannitol, sucrose, or glycols, and substitution of impermeable anionic species such as phosphate, sulfate, or gluconate for chlorine. These are commonly added to preservation fluids and appear to be essential components of hypothermic storage solutions.[22–25]

There have been many modifications in the preservation solutions used in organ transplantation since the mid-1960s. The components of the two most commonly used solutions, Euro-Collins solution and University of Wisconsin preservation solution (UW solution), are shown in Table 41-4. Although both have been used successfully for short-duration static hypothermic storage, the superiority of UW solution for extended solid organ preservation has been documented in many studies. The components of UW solution were selected in an effort to develop a solution that would prevent hypothermia-induced cell swelling in all transplantable organs. This was achieved using lactobionic acid, a relatively large–molecular-mass anion; raffinose, a trisaccharide;, and hydroxyethyl starch, a colloid. In addition, specific metabolites or inhibitors of organ injury were added to establish an appropriate biochemical environment to facilitate rapid restoration of normal metabolism. To achieve this goal, the UW solution contains adenosine, to stimulate ATP synthesis on reperfusion; glutathione, as an antioxidant to suppress reperfusion injury caused by the generation of oxygen free radicals; and allopurinol, to suppress one source of oxygen free radicals, xanthine oxidase. Antibiotics to prevent bacterial contamination and dexamethasone to suppress lysosomal enzyme release during ischemia and to stabilize plasma membranes were also added.[23,26,27]

Isolated cell perfusion and animal transplant models have suggested the following conclusions concerning the effective-

TABLE 41-4. *Composition of cold storage solutions*

Substance	Concentration (mmol/L) Euro-Collins	University of Wisconsin
Na$^+$	9.3	
K$^+$	107	
Cl$^-$	14	
HCO$_3^-$	9.3	
PO$_4^{2-}$	93	
K$^+$ lactobionate		100
KH$_2$PO$_4$		25
MgSO$_4$		5
Glucose	182	
Raffinose		30
Hydroxyethyl starch (g/L)		50
Glutathione		3
Adenosine		3
Insulin (mg/L)		40
Dexamethasone (mg/L)	8	
pH	7.0	7.4
Osmolarity (mOsm/L)	325	320

ness of these components. Lactobionate is an essential component, both as a osmotic agent to suppress cell swelling and as a chelating agent for calcium and iron. Glutathione functions as an important antioxidant for the metabolism of superoxide anions in the mitochondria, and is an essential component for long-term preservation. Adenosine may increase available purine precursors for the regeneration of ATP, and it may also play a role in long-term preservation. Raffinose does not appear to be essential, and it can be replaced by other saccharides, or possibly even omitted. The colloid hydroxyethyl starch is not essential for liver and kidney preservation, but seems beneficial for heart and pancreas preservation.[23,27]

Prevention of reperfusion injury is an important aspect of successful transplantation. Reperfusion injury occurs through a variety of mechanisms, including 1) activation of enzyme systems that produce oxygen free radicals in parenchymal cells, endothelial cells, or circulating macrophages and neutrophils; 2) activation of arachidonic acid metabolism, producing prostaglandins, leukotrienes, and thromboxane; and 3) direct endothelial cell damage.[27] These lead to platelet activation, vasoconstriction, and inhibition of effective cellular reperfusion. Efforts to prevent reperfusion injury using oxygen free radical scavengers, calcium channel blockers, and inhibitors of phospholipase metabolism have not been particularly successful. The value of administering vascular flush solutions containing adenosine or albumin and antioxidants just before reperfusion in humans is still unclear, although these have proved beneficial in experimental settings.[27]

The benefits of modification or simplification of the UW solution do not outweigh the advantage it affords as the single best perfusion solution for all organs during multiorgan harvest. Identification of further factors responsible for extended organ preservation is difficult in human transplantation studies. The need for donor organs stimulates the use of donors previously unacceptable because of issues of age, stability, and extended preservation times. Because these factors adversely affect organ function, further laboratory investigation will be needed to define subsequent modifications in preservation solutions and their application.

ORGAN DISTRIBUTION

In the mid-1960s, improved survival in cadaveric donor kidneys transplanted into genetically matched recipients stimulated the formation of regional organ sharing agreements between transplant centers. Expansion of this concept, and the need for coordination of a national organ distribution network, led to the formation of UNOS in 1977. Expansion beyond kidney transplantation to include recipients awaiting other organ transplants occurred in the late 1970s. The complexity of this service, and the explosion of transplant services, caused UNOS to join with histocompatibility laboratories to develop a national "Organ Center," and this organization was awarded the federal contract to operate the national Organ Procurement and Transplantation Network (OPTN) in 1986. Membership in the national OPTN was mandated in the Omnibus Budget Reconciliation Act in 1986, requiring all transplant centers to join UNOS if they wished access to Medicare/Medicaid funding. UNOS policy is reviewed by the Department of Health and Human Services, but UNOS policy does not have the force of law. The regulations developed by the transplant community through UNOS representation concerning the quality of transplantation care, represent the voluntary efforts of these health care providers to supply optimal ethical and medical services to the public.[28]

The organ distribution system is based on 11 geographic regions of the United States, defined by population size and organ sharing concerns. However, improved preservation and distribution systems and changing population demographics have stimulated review of this distribution mechanism. Potential organ recipients are stratified by "status" codes reflecting the urgency of need. Organ donors are registered through UNOS, and organs are distributed to the patient with the greatest need, giving priority to local, then regional, and finally national waiting list registrants. The decision to accept any donor organ offered through this system rests with the patient's transplantation physicians and surgeons. The management of the donor, the coordination of the procurement process, and the distribution of donor organs is undertaken by the local OPO serving the donor's community.

REFERENCES

1. Randall T. Too few human organs for transplantation, too many in need . . . and the gap widens. JAMA 1991;265:1223.
2. First WH, Fanning WJ. Donor management and matching. Cardiol Clin 1990;8:55.
3. Nathan HM, Jarrell BE, Broznik B, et al. Estimation and characterization of the potential renal organ donor pool in Pennsylvania. Transplantation 1991;51:142.
4. Mackersie RC, Bronsther OL, Shackford SR. Organ procurement in patients with fatal head injuries: the fate of the potential donor. Ann Surg 1991;213:143.
5. Mygaard CE, Townsend RN, Diamond DL. Organ donor management and organ outcome: a 6 year review from a Level I trauma center. J Trauma 1990;30:728.
6. Alexander JW, Vaughn WK, Carey MA. The use of marginal donors for organ transplantation: the older and younger donors. Transplant Proc 1991;23:905–909.
7. First MR. Transplantation in the nineties. Transplantation 1992;53:1.
8. Morris JA Jr, Wilcox TR, Frist WH. Pediatric organ donation: the paradox of organ shortage despite the remarkable willingness of families to donate. Pediatrics 1992;89:411.
9. Task Force for the Determination of Brain Death in Children. Guidelines for the determination of brain death in children. Neurology 1987;37:1077.
10. Darby JM, Stein K, Grenvik A, et al. Approach to management of the heartbeating "brain dead" organ donor. JAMA 1989;261:2222.
11. Powner DJ, Hendrich A, Lagler RG, et al. Hormonal changes in brain dead patients. Crit Care Med 1990;18:702.
12. Debelak L, Pollak R, Reckard C. Arginine vasopressin versus desmopressin for the treatment of diabetes insipidus in the brain dead organ donor. Transplant Proc 1990;22:351.
13. UNOS Update. 1994;10(5):230.
14. Alexander JW, Vaughn WK. The use of "marginal" donors for organ transplantation: the influence of donor age on outcome. Transplantation 1991;51:135.
15. Anaise D, Smith R, Ishimaru M, et al. An approach to organ salvage from non-heartbeating cadaver donors under existing legal and ethical requirements for transplantation. Transplantation 1990;49:290.
16. Casavilla A, Ramirez C, Shapiro R, et al. Experience with liver and kidney allografts from non-heart-beating donors. Proc 1995;28(5):2898.
17. D'Alessandro AM, Hoffman RM, Knechtle SJ, et al. Successful extrarenal transplantation from non-heart-beating donors (NHBD's). Transplantation 1995;59(7)977.
18. Sollinger HW, Kalayoglu M, Belzer FO. Use of the donor specific transfusion protocol in living-unrelated donor-recipient combinations. Ann Surg 1986;204:315.
19. Sanfilippo F, Thacker L, Vaughn WK. Living-donor renal transplantation in SEOPF. Transplantation 1990;49:25.
20. Wood RP, Shaw BW. Multiple organ procurement. In: Cerilli GJ, ed. Organ transplantation and replacement. Philadelphia, JB Lippincott, 1988:322.
21. Yanaga K, Kakizoe S, Ikeda T, et al. Procurement of liver allografts from non-heart beating donors. Transplant Proc 1990;22:156.
22. Southard JH, Belzer FO. Organ preservation. In: Flye MW, ed. Principles of organ transplantation. Philadelphia, WB Saunders, 1989:194.
23. Southard JH, Belzer FO. The University of Wisconsin organ preservation solution: components, comparisons, and modifications. Transplantation Reviews 1993;7:176.
24. Collins GM. Kidney preservation by cold storage. In: Cerilli GJ, ed. Organ transplantation and replacement. Philadelphia, JB Lippincott, 1988:312.
25. Belzer FO. Evaluation of preservation of the intra-abdominal organs. Transplant Proc 1993;25:2527.
26. Southard JH, van Gulik TM, Ametani MS, et al. Important components of the UW solution. Transplantation 1990;49:251.
27. Southard JH, Belzer FO. New concepts in organ preservation. Clin Transpl 1993;7:134.
28. Southard JH, Belzer FO. Kidney preservation by perfusion. In: Cerilli GJ, ed. Organ transplantation and replacement. Philadelphia, JB Lippincott, 1988:296.

Surgery of Infants and Children: Scientific Principles and Practice, edited by Keith T. Oldham, Paul M. Colombani, and Robert P. Foglia. Lippincott–Raven Publishers, Philadelphia, © 1997.

CHAPTER 42

Kidney

Philip C. Guzzetta, Jr.

CAUSES OF RENAL FAILURE IN CHILDREN

The "usual" child with renal failure is a white teenage boy with congenital kidney disease. The North American Pediatric Renal Transplant Cooperative Study (NAPRTCS) is a cooperative group that gathers data on children with renal failure from 83 centers in North America. Since 1987, NAPRTCS has evaluated almost 4000 children and 3400 kidney transplants. NAPRTCS has listed the most common causes of renal failure in its patient population to be aplastic/hypoplastic/dysplastic kidneys, obstructive uropathy, focal segmental glomerulosclerosis, and reflux nephropathy (Table 42-1). Almost half of the children who require a renal transplant in the first 5 years of life have either aplastic/hypoplastic/dysplastic kidneys or obstructive uropathy, both of which are more common in boys, resulting in a male predominance (60%) in NAPRTCS patients.

The racial distribution of renal failure is similar to the U.S. population as a whole, with two thirds of the patients being white, 15% black, 13% Hispanic, and 5% other races. Previously, patients were entered into NAPRTCS only after receiving a kidney transplant, but since 1992 patients have been entered when they were placed on any form of dialysis or they received a preemptive (without ever requiring dialysis) transplant. This change of entry criteria may result in the renal failure population appearing younger than previously. The percentages of children entered into NAPRTCS by age category are 0 to 1 years, 6%; 2 to 5 years, 17%; 6 to 12 years, 36%, 13 to 17 years 39%; and 18 to 20 years, 2%. Twenty-five percent of children are receiving a preemptive transplant, and 60% of those on dialysis are using peritoneal dialysis.

PRETRANSPLANTATION ASSESSMENT OF THE CHILD WITH RENAL FAILURE

Urologic Evaluation

Many of the children with renal failure have structural abnormalities of the urinary tract and thus have already been evaluated and treated for those problems. The indications for extirpation of the native kidneys and ureters are discussed later. The evaluation of the bladder requires a voiding cystourethrogram and may require cystometrogram studies as well, particularly in those patients with neurogenic bladders or vesicoureteral reflux and a high-pressure bladder. It is preferable to have the urinary tract repair completed well in advance of the transplantation because of the potential complications from immunosuppressive medications after major bladder reconstructive surgery. Patients with bladder augmentation with intestine may have difficulties posttransplantation with urinary tract infection, mucus plugging, and electrolyte disturbances.

In the patient who has never had good urine output, or who had bilateral nephrectomies early in life, the bladder may be very small and noncompliant. Nonetheless, as long as the musculature is normal, the bladders will dilate rather quickly once the transplant is producing urine, and there usually is no need to prepare the bladder with irrigations pretransplantation, which may predispose the child to urinary tract infections.

Bilateral Nephrectomies

Approximately 25% of children undergo removal of all native renal tissue before transplantation. The most common indications for removal are severe hypertension or dilated, chronically infected urinary tracts. Patients with nephrotic syndrome may also require nephrectomies to control protein loss and lessen the risk of thrombotic complications because of the hypercoagulable state seen with nephrosis. Infants with congenital polycystic kidneys may warrant bilateral nephrectomies to reduce the large kidneys impinging on the diaphragm, restricting respiration and compressing the gastrointestinal tract, making feeding difficult. The decision to perform bilateral nephrectomies for hypertension is affected by the high incidence of hypertension in children after renal transplantation. If the hypertension requires multiple medications to control or it seems to be increasing in severity as the date of transplantation nears, it is safest to recommend pretransplantation nephrectomies. Posttransplantation bilateral nephrectomy is an option when hypertension worsens after surgery and other causes of hypertension have been ruled out.

When nephrotic syndrome or a chronically infected urinary tract is the indication for nephrectomies, the surgery should be performed at least 6 weeks before living, related donor (LRD)

TABLE 42-1. *1994 North American Pediatric Renal Transplant Cooperative Study data on the causes of renal failure in that patient population (N = 3176)*[*]

Diagnosis	No. of patients (%)
Aplastic/hypoplastic/dysplastic kidneys	540 (17.0)
Obstructive uropathy	532 (16.8)
Focal segmental glomerulosclerosis	364 (11.5)
Reflux nephropathy	180 (5.7)
Systemic immunologic disease	149 (4.7)
Chronic glomerulonephritis	138 (4.3)
Congenital nephrotic syndrome	97 (3.1)
Syndrome of agenesis of abdominal musculature	97 (3.1)
Polycystic kidney disease	89 (2.8)
Hemolytic uremic syndrome	88 (2.8)
Medullary cystic disease/juvenile nephronophthisis	84 (2.6)
Cystinosis	86 (2.7)
Familial nephritis	71 (2.2)
Pyelonephritis/interstitial nephritis	69 (2.2)
Membranoproliferative glomerulonephritis type I	68 (2.1)
Renal infarct	66 (2.1)
Idiopathic crescentic glomerulonephritis	54 (1.7)
Membranoproliferative glomerulonephritis type II	31 (1.0)
Oxalosis	24 (0.8)
Drash syndrome	17 (0.5)
Membranous nephropathy	17 (0.5)
Wilms tumor	16 (0.5)
Sickle cell nephropathy	4 (0.1)
Diabetic glomerulonephritis	1 (0.0)
Other	176 (5.5)
Unknown	118 (3.7)

[*] Subgroup totals may be less than 3176 because of missing data.

transplantation is scheduled or the patient is listed for a cadaver kidney. When the indication is hypertension, or a grossly dilated system without infection, the nephrectomies are preferentially done at the time of transplantation. Performing the nephrectomies at the time of transplantation lengthens the operative time, but not the recovery time, and spares the child a separate operation.

In the patient with small kidneys and nonrefluxing ureters, the kidneys can be removed through a posterior approach (Fig. 42-1), which is less painful and faster than bilateral flank incisions. When the entire ureter must be excised, bilateral flank incisions are used to do the nephroureterectomies. Because most children with renal failure are on peritoneal dialysis, the transperitoneal route for nephrectomies is avoided.

Preemptive Transplant

One quarter of children receiving a renal transplant do so without having been placed on pretransplantation dialysis. Because renal disease in children is usually slowly progressive and many patients have been followed for years with a diagnosis of renal dysfunction, there is an opportunity to perform the transplantation without the expense, inconvenience, and potential complications of peritoneal dialysis or hemodialysis. The timing for transplantation in these patients must be individualized and usually depends on growth and development, rate of deterioration of renal function, and the nephrologist and family agreeing that the child should receive a transplant before dialysis is required.

Ideally, the preemptive transplantation is done using a LRD kidney so that the likelihood of success is greatest. When there is delayed function of the allograft, the blood urea nitrogen (BUN) may rise in response to steroid administration sufficiently to require dialysis despite the fact that the patient did not require it before transplantation. The success rate for preemptive transplantations is slightly better than for transplantations done when the patients are on dialysis.[1]

Living, Related Donor or Cadaver Donor

The improvement in cadaver allograft survival with cyclosporine has led some adult transplant surgeons to question the need for LRD renal transplants. In children, the LRD allografts continue to have a significantly better function rate than cadaver grafts. The high rate of immediate function of the LRD kidneys allows a short period of induction therapy and rapid transition to maintenance immunosuppression with prednisone, azathioprine, and cyclosporine. Although the incidence of rejection is the same in LRD and cadaver kidneys in the first 15 days posttransplantation, there is a significant difference thereafter, with the cadaver grafts having a higher rejection incidence.

The age of the donor of the cadaver kidney also affects the function of the allograft, with grafts from donors younger than 10 years of age, and particularly those younger than 5 years of age, having a poorer function rate than those from older donors (Fig. 42-2). This problem of young donors is not an issue with LRD kidneys.

The scarcity of cadaver grafts is another incentive for the families to consider LRD kidney transplant. The rapid increase in the number of patients on the waiting list for a cadaver kidney, from 11,822 in 1987 to 25,720 in July, 1994,[2] has created a special problem for the pediatric renal failure patient, who tends to have a shorter time on the waiting list and low preformed antibody titers (panel reactive antibodies), because those factors, plus the human leukocyte antigen matching, determine which recipient is offered the kidney.

The United Network for Organ Sharing (UNOS) has been responsive to the needs of children, for whom a long delay on the waiting list may translate into lifelong growth and development impairment. UNOS has assigned two additional preference points to patients younger than 19 years of age, with those younger than 11 years receiving three rather than two points. Nonetheless, the prospect of a lengthy wait for a cadaver graft that has a lower likelihood of long-term function has encouraged many families to opt for LRD kidney transplant.

Psychosocial Readiness for Transplantation

Proper preparation of the patient and family for life after renal transplantation cannot be overemphasized. The expectations of

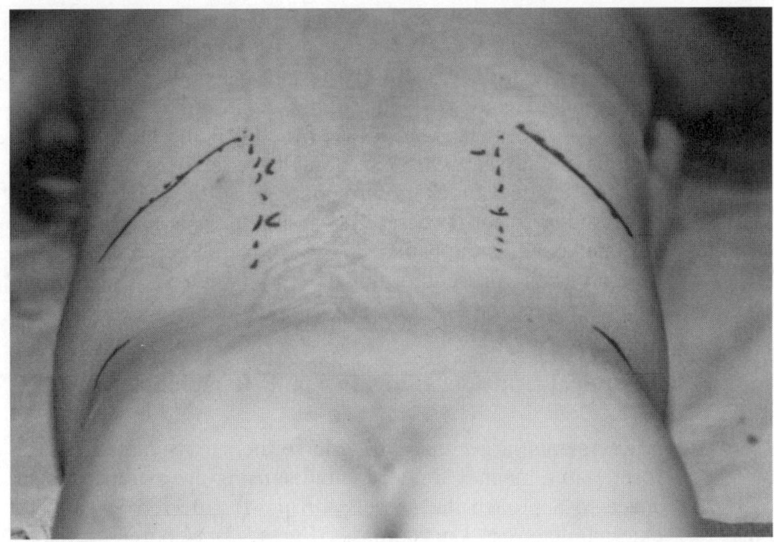

FIG. 42-1. Intraoperative photograph showing incisions used for posterior approach for bilateral nephrectomy.

a miracle, which have been fostered by the lay press, must be tempered by the reality of a 25% (LRD) to 40% (cadaver donor) graft failure rate at 5 years and the complications of lifelong immunosuppression. The patients who have never been on dialysis and undergo preemptive renal transplant may find it very difficult to understand postoperative complications and the value of their new organ.

Forty percent of children receiving kidney transplants are teenagers, and this is the group at greatest risk for noncompliance to medication orders. Once the excitement of the operation is over and the teenager is expected to take control of their life and care, the danger of discontinuing the immunosuppressive medications is highest. Just as children of this age desire independence from authority figures normally, they also look to gain independence from their transplant team. Unfortunately, despite many efforts to inform the patients and work closely with their families, this continues to be a substantial cause of graft loss in teenagers.

Patient and family sentiments about transplantation need to be discussed in detail before the patient is listed for a cadaver kidney or scheduled for an LRD. The financial commitment for posttransplantation medications and multiple outpatient visits also needs to be fully understood to prevent a feeling of betrayal on the part of the patient and family when they are faced with those burdens, in spite of a well functioning transplant. These children are patients for life, and a clear under-

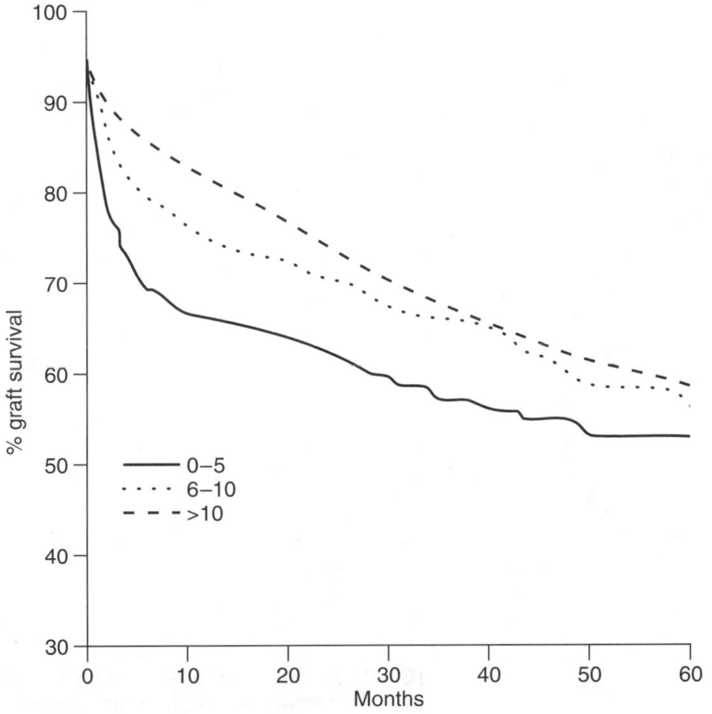

FIG. 42-2. 1994 North American Pediatric Renal Transplant Cooperative Study data showing the effect of donor age on graft function in cadaver renal transplants. (Cohn RA, Chavers B, Sullivan EK, et al. Renal transplatation and chronic dialysis in children and adolescents. The 1994 annual report of the North American Pediatric Renal Transplant Cooperative Study. Pediatric Nephrology (in press) 1996.)

standing of that fact is mandatory to ensure the best chance for long-term graft function with minimal long-term complications.

OPERATIVE PROCEDURE

Intraoperative Management of Fluids and Medications

Once the patient has been anesthetized, a Foley catheter is placed into the urinary bladder and antibacterial solution is used to fill the bladder under gravity. In the patient with a small, unused bladder, it is important not to overdistend the bladder, which may lead to mucosal disruption or bladder rupture. Venous access usually consists of a subclavian central venous double-lumen catheter and a large-bore peripheral intravenous (IV) line. The subclavian location is preferred over the internal jugular site because the patients retain that line while receiving antithymocyte globulin (ATG), it is an easy access for phlebotomy for the first week, and children are more comfortable with the catheter not exiting the neck for that period of time. Use of an arterial line depends on the size of the patient, the preoperative blood pressure, and preference of the anesthesiologist. For routine transplantations in patients weighing more than 10 kg, an arterial line is not necessary.

All patients are given prophylactic antibiotics in the perioperative period; we prefer a second-generation cephalosporin, with the first dose given immediately before surgery. Methylprednisolone, 2.5 mg/kg, and azathioprine, 2.5 mg/kg, are given IV before implantation of the kidney. Fluid replacement is by normal saline or albumin using blood sparingly unless the hematocrit is less than 25% or there has been a significant blood loss during the transplant.

Mannitol, 1 g/kg up to 50 g, is given to the recipient just before releasing the vascular clamps. The central venous pressure (CVP) should be greater than 12 cm H_2O when the clamps are released. The critical factor in assessing the volume status is to palpate the kidney after it has been perfused for several minutes. The kidney should be turgid and pink. If the kidney is soft and there is no evidence of a vascular problem, additional volume is necessary, regardless of the CVP and the amount of volume already administered. Some have advocated the use of calcium channel blockers intraarterially in these patients, but that usually is not necessary if careful attention is paid to the volume status. If the patient is not producing copious urine by the end of the procedure, dopamine is begun at 3 μg/kg/min and continued for 24 hours.

Technical Considerations in Small Recipients

Recipients larger than 20 kg have their transplantation performed in a manner similar to adults, using the extraperitoneal space to approach the vessels for end-to-side renal vessel to external iliac vessel anastomoses (Fig. 42-3). Neoureterocystostomy is accomplished by means of a Lich extravesical antirefluxing anastomosis[3] (Fig. 42-4).

In the recipient weighing less than 20 kg, there are several unique technical problems. Many of these patients require bilateral nephrectomies for dilated urinary tracts with infection or significant nephrotic syndrome at least 6 weeks before transplantation. Nonetheless, a right retroperitoneal approach to the vessels can be accomplished despite a previous right nephrectomy. As with older children, if the nephrectomies can be safely done at the time of transplantation, that is preferable and the kidneys are removed through bilateral extraperitoneal flank incisions. The transplanted kidney is then placed into the right retroperitoneal space. It is easy to expose the inferior vena cava and aorta from the right retroperitoneum so that the renal vessels can be sutured end-to-side to the inferior vena cava and the aorta (Fig. 42-5). An adult kidney can be placed into that space even in a child smaller than 10 kg, although in those very small

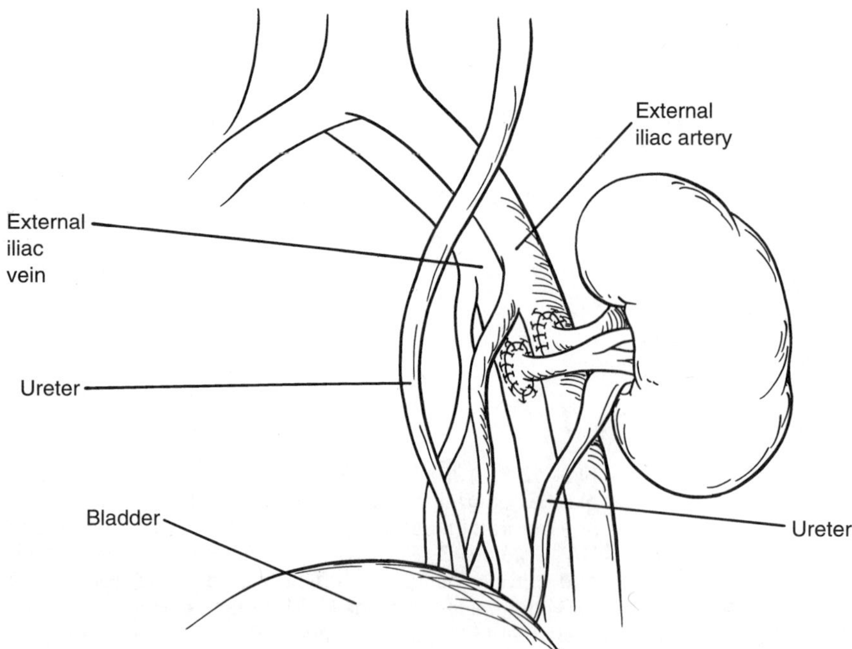

FIG. 42-3. Renal artery-and-vein to external iliac artery-and-vein anastomoses.

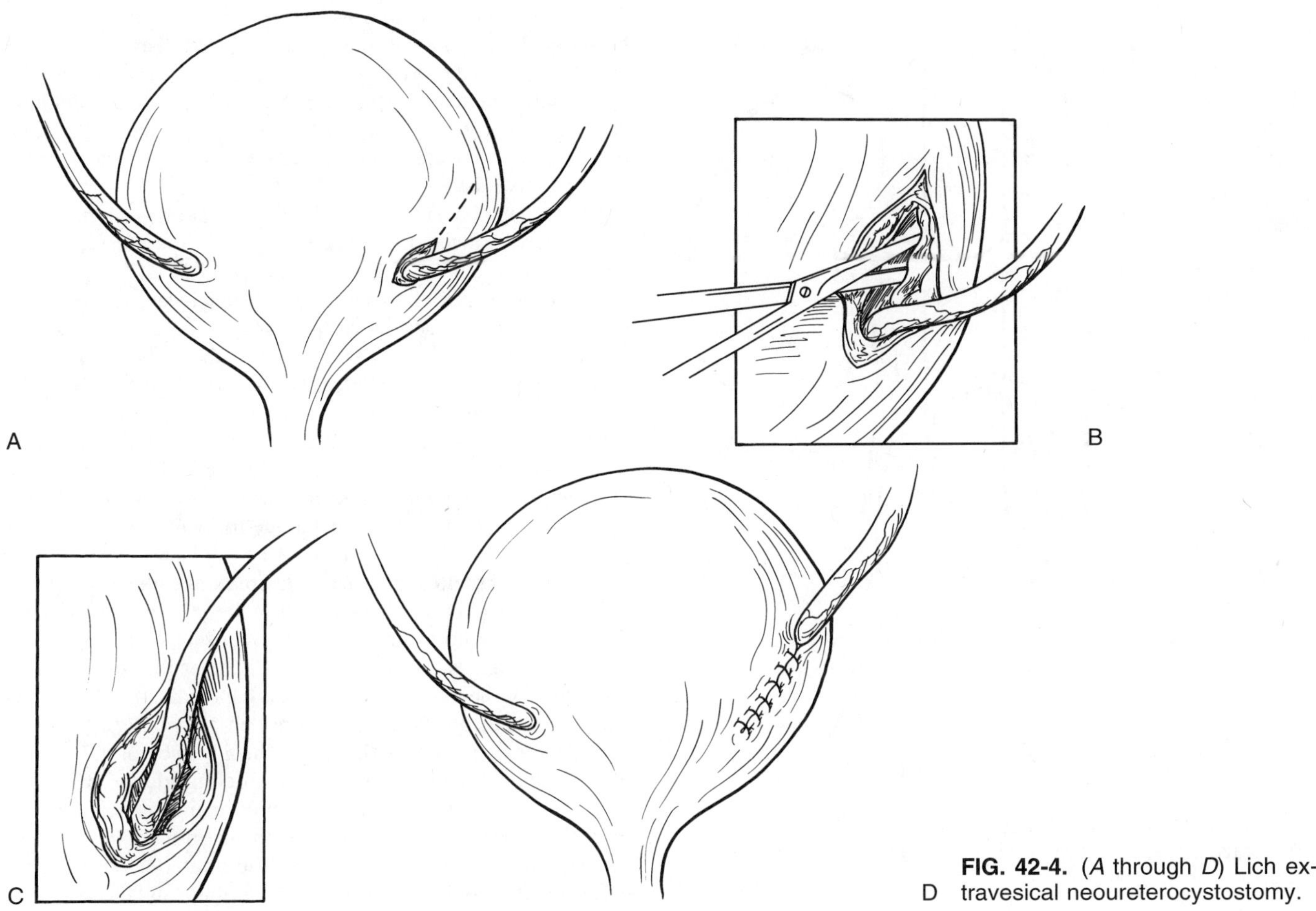

FIG. 42-4. (*A through D*) Lich extravesical neoureterocystostomy.

children, only the external oblique muscle is closed to prevent compression of the allograft.

Although transperitoneal placement of the kidney in the recipient weighing less than 20 kg has been advocated,[4] the retroperitoneal approach allows immediate peritoneal dialysis if needed, decreases postoperative ileus, and allows for easy percutaneous renal biopsy. The ureteral anastomosis to the bladder is usually the Lich extravesical type, as in the older child.

POSTOPERATIVE MANAGEMENT

Patient Monitoring and Fluid and Electrolyte Management

The child is placed in the intensive care unit for at least 1 day to monitor urinary output and be given fluid replacement based on that output on an hourly basis. The patient with native kidneys in place and some urine output pretransplantation and the child with poor urine output in the first hour after surgery should have an immediate DTPA (diethylaminetriamine pentaacetic acid) renal scan to ensure good perfusion of the transplanted kidney. Delaying the renal scan until the next day and finding the kidney is not being perfused ensures allograft loss. Doppler ultrasound examination may give similar information in those circumstances and can be performed at the bedside.

The patients are not placed on stringent isolation status while moderately immunosuppressed, but good hand washing and avoiding contact with people with respiratory tract or skin infections are stressed. After the first few days, patients are allowed outside the room as long as they wear a mask.

It is most important to monitor urine output, CVP, creatinine, potassium, and phosphorus in the immediate posttransplantation period. If the patient has not had nephrectomies, urine output may be a poor measure of allograft function. Use of CVP measurement as a guide to fluid administration must be done in the context of the urine output, so that with an excellent urine output and a low CVP (less than 5 cm H_2O), urine replace with normal saline is all that is necessary. With good urine output and a high CVP, diuretic therapy or slightly less than volume-for-volume urine replacement is appropriate. When urine output is poor, low CVP should prompt aggressive volume expansion with colloid or blood (if needed), and high CVP should be treated with diuretics.

If the patient has a prompt diuresis, as do most LRD recipients, it is important to be attentive to hypokalemia and hypophosphatemia, which can develop within 6 to 8 hours when the urine output is greater than 4 mL/kg/h and is being replaced with normal saline without potassium or phosphorus added. Levels of electrolytes, BUN, and serum creatinine should be obtained at least every 6 hours in the immediate posttransplantation period. If the serum creatinine is dropping quickly and the urine output is greater than 4 mL/kg/h, replacement of the urine

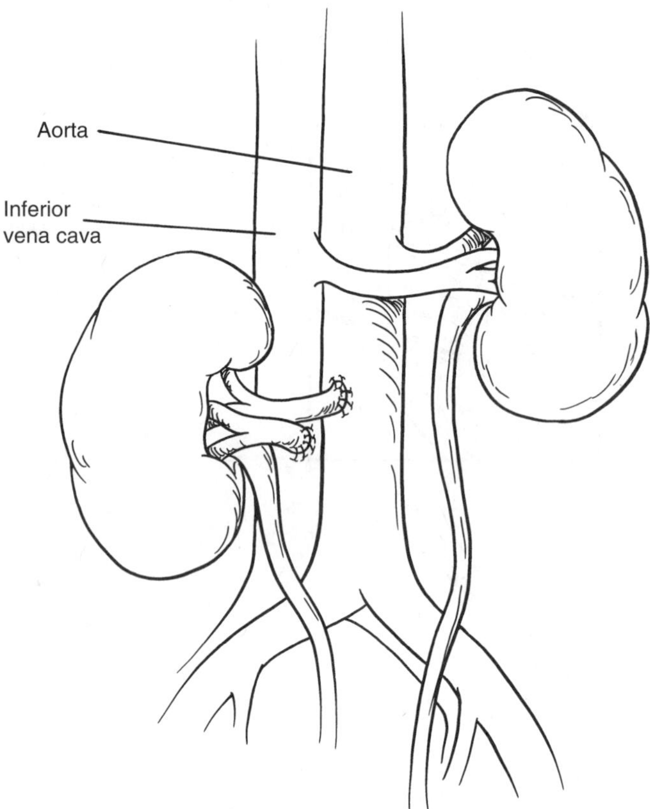

FIG. 42-5. Renal artery-to-aorta and renal vein-to-inferior vena cava anastomoses used in small renal transplant recipients.

output above that amount should be with 0.75 mL replacement/ 1.0 mL urine to prevent volume overload and hypokalemia. Most important, the patient needs to be evaluated repeatedly in the first 24 hours, with fluid management tailored to the whole patient picture rather than just one factor, such as the urine output or CVP measurement.

Pain Control

Great advances have been made in the postoperative pain management for all children since the mid-1980s. Although there are many techniques to accomplish analgesia after renal transplantation, the most important factor is that the patient should be given enough medication to be comfortable, and rigid adherence to a predetermined dose or frequency schedule is discouraged in favor of individualization of analgesia to the patient needs. The two most popular and effective pain management techniques are epidural catheter analgesia and patient-controlled analgesia (PCA).

The epidural catheter technique has many positive features for the transplantation patient. The analgesia infused may be a long-acting narcotic, a local anesthetic, or a combination of the two. When the epidural catheter is placed at the start of the transplantation procedure, the amount of anesthetic agents given during the operation can be lessened considerably. For those patients with bilateral flank incisions, the amount of epi-

dural anesthetic is similar to that given for a single incision because of the regional analgesia produced. The patients are able to breath comfortably and ambulate with assistance with an epidural catheter in place. We usually leave the epidural catheter in place when the patients are transferred to the floor from the intensive care unit, and remove it on the third or fourth postoperative day.

On the negative side, the epidural medication is administered exclusively by the pain management team of the anesthesiology department in our hospital, and thus the nurse and surgeon depend on another group to administer the analgesic agents. Often the patients cannot sense that their bladder is full with the epidural catheter in place, so the Foley catheter is left in place until after the epidural catheter is removed. If a local anesthetic is part of the epidural medication, numbness of the lower extremities may occur, which limits ambulation and also seems to have a disquieting effect on the younger children. Despite these negatives, epidural catheter analgesia is the preferred postoperative pain management technique for pediatric renal transplants.

PCA is an excellent alternative to epidural catheter analgesia in the older patient. For patients to use the PCA pump properly, they must be able to understand the concept of giving themselves the analgesic medication in a manner that prevents the formation of the peaks and valleys in the medication level seen when the medication is administered on a 4-hourly basis. The use of PCA by parents is flawed by the tendency of the parents to keep the children asleep rather than comfortable. It is clear that just as in adults, children use more pain medication with PCA than with traditional 4-hourly dosing of narcotics, but obtain significantly better pain relief. The limitations of PCA include that it is not best for very small children, and the analgesia may not be as good as that with an epidural catheter without giving doses of narcotics that cause serious side effects.

Immunosuppression

The basis of immune suppression in the transplantation patient is discussed in detail in Chapter 40. At the Children's Medical Center of Dallas, the immunosuppressive protocol is adjusted depending on whether the kidney is from a cadaver donor or a LRD, and whether the child is determined to have statural growth potential. The cadaver kidney recipients all receive induction therapy with ATG, beginning within 24 hours of the transplantation, combined with methylprednisolone and azathioprine, which are given IV in the operating room. The ATG is given until the transplanted kidney is clearly functioning well, and the cyclosporine level is therapeutic (trough level greater than 350 ng/mL by TDx). The ATG is begun at a dose of 15 mg/kg and is used for a minimum of 5 days in these patients and for as long as 14 days if needed. Adequacy of immunosuppression with ATG is estimated by the percentage of lymphocytes in the complete blood count differential each day, and if this exceeds 5%, the dose is increased to 20 mg/kg.

When the creatinine is less than 2.0 mg/dL, cyclosporine is given concurrently with the ATG until the cyclosporine level is therapeutic, at which time the ATG is stopped. The cyclosporine dose is started at 15 mg/kg/d divided into two doses and adjusted to reach the therapeutic level desired. Children are notoriously variable in their absorption of cyclosporine, but usually require higher doses than adults on a per kilogram basis to attain the same levels. Some children have more predictable levels when the drug is administered three times a day. New formulations of oral cyclosporine may enhance the absorption, which in the usual form is only about 30% absorbed. Regardless of growth potential, the cadaver kidney recipients are managed identically until 3 months after transplantation, when the patients with potential for statural growth begin an alternate-day prednisone dosing that eventually leads to prednisone administration QOD. A protocol for immunosuppression in the child receiving a cadaver kidney without statural growth potential is given in Table 42-2.

The LRD recipients are either begun on cyclosporine pretransplantation, or induction therapy with ATG is used in a method similar to that in the cadaver kidney recipients. The unpredictability of cyclosporine levels in the early postoperative period and the relatively high risk of early rejection in LRD recipients has encouraged us to use ATG induction in our small LRD recipients. A protocol for immunosuppression in the child receiving an LRD kidney without statural growth potential is given in Table 42-3.

COMPLICATIONS

Technical Problems

There may be problems with the vascular or urologic component of the renal transplant. One of the most distressing complications of renal transplantations in children is the high rate of graft loss from vascular thrombosis. In the 1994 NAPRTCS report, vascular thrombosis was responsible for 13% of the failed grafts and occurred in about 3% of all children receiving a kidney transplant, which is a much higher rate than seen in adults. The cause of vascular thrombosis is not clear, and may not be a technical problem in many patients. Young recipients, particularly those receiving an LRD as a preemptive transplant, young donors for cadaver kidneys, and prolonged cold ischemia times (greater than 24 hours) are associated with an increased risk of vascular thrombosis.[5] Although the use of cyclosporine was suggested as a possible cause of vascular thrombosis, that has not been proven. There is an association of transplant renal artery stenosis and vascular thrombosis if the patient becomes hypovolemic or blood pressure control is obtained using angiotensin-converting enzyme inhibitors.[6]

Transplant renal artery stenosis occurs in between 5% and 10% of children, as opposed to about 2% in adult series. The stenosis may result from technical problems at the anastomosis or from immunologic causes, such as chronic rejection, which are usually seen within the main renal artery. Because most children require some antihypertensive medication after transplantation, deciding which child should be studied for renal artery stenosis may be difficult. If the hypertension is increasing in severity and requiring additional medications for control, or the renal function is deteriorating as the hypertension is controlled, the child should be investigated for renal artery stenosis.

Doppler ultrasound examination may suggest stenosis of the transplant renal artery. The DTPA renal scan performed without and with pretreatment with captopril may also be helpful; a decrease in renal function after captopril administration is consistent with renal artery stenosis. Neither a negative Doppler ultrasound nor a negative captopril-pretreated renal scan is sensitive enough to exclude transplant renal artery stenosis,[6] and the definitive test remains selective angiography, which has the added advantage of being the method of treatment with percutaneous transluminal angioplasty (PTA). If the patient is at least 1 month posttransplantation, correction of the stenosis, regardless of its location, by PTA is recommended. If the PTA is unsuccessful, surgical correction has a high rate of success with preservation of renal function. Patients with an identified transplant renal artery stenosis should have the condition corrected by PTA or surgery.

Urologic complications include urinary leak, ureteral obstruction, and vesicoureteral reflux. Urinary leak may be caused by disruption of the neoureterocystostomy or necrosis of the distal ureter. The diagnosis is usually made by renal scan, but may be suggested by a rising BUN and serum creatinine, perinephric fluid, and a pleural effusion on the same side as the kidney. Operative correction is mandatory. Care must be taken in the construction of the neoureterocystostomy that the tunnel is long enough to prevent reflux and leak, but not so long and tight that the blood supply to the distal ureter is compromised.

Obstruction of the ureter may be another sign of distal ureter necrosis or that the bladder tunnel is too tight. It is particularly important in the small patient receiving an adult kidney that the ureter be free from compression or twisting to prevent obstruction. Formation of a lymphocele may also compress the ureter, but with careful ligation of the perivascular tissues when the vessels are mobilized for anastomosis, lymphoceles are rare except in the patients retransplanted on the same side. Surgical correction of the obstruction must be done promptly.

Vesicoureteral reflux depends on the type of neoureterocystostomy, the condition of the patient's bladder before transplantation, and voiding habits of the patient posttransplantation. Use of the Lich anastomosis has a low incidence of symptomatic reflux; however, the true incidence of reflux in these patients is unknown. Recurrent urinary tract infections prompt the investigation for reflux, which occurs most commonly in children with dysfunctional voiding patterns or abnormal bladders. If the urinary tract infections are recurrent and the reflux is significant, reimplantation of the transplanted ureter is indicated.

Rejection

Despite significant improvements in the overall care of the renal transplant patient, rejection remains the most common cause of graft loss in the pediatric patient. In the 1994 NAPRTCS report, 51% of the kidneys that failed were lost to some form of rejection. The definition of rejection in that study was any clinical or pathologic data that caused the physician to treat the patient with antirejection therapy. Rejection is suspected in those patients with rising serum creatinine, fever, and graft enlargement or tenderness. In patients on high doses of immunosuppressive medications, the clinical signs may be very subtle or absent, and a minor rise in creatinine may be the first evidence of rejection.

In the NAPRTCS study, the diagnosis of rejection was made on biopsy about half the time, and slightly more than half the kidneys lost to rejection were lost to chronic rejection. As was mentioned previously, rejection within the first 2 weeks occurs in the same percentage of LRD and cadaver donor transplants,

TABLE 42-2. *Children's Medical Center of Dallas protocol for immunosuppressive medication after cadaver renal transplantation in a child without statural growth potential*

Time post-transplantation	Date	Weight	ALG	Prednisone			Azathioprine	Cyclosporine
On call to operating room				Methylprednisolone 2.5 mg/kg IV = mg			2.5 mg/kg/d IV = mg	
Day 0			15 mg/kg* =	Methylprednisolone 1 mg/kg @ 7 h postop.			Wt > 25 kg = 25 mg/d IV/po Wt ≤ 25 kg = 12.5 mg/d	Begin on day 5 or creatinine ≤2 mg/
1, 2			15 mg/kg =	2 mg/kg ÷ bid = ___ mg ___ mg/dose			When ALG stopped, increase 2.5 mg/kg/d p.o.	dL† @ 15 mg/kg bid = mg bid
3, 4			15 mg/kg =	1.75/kg =	mg ÷ bid =	/ ↓‡		
5, 6			15 mg/kg† =	1.6/kg =	mg ÷ bid =	/ ↓‡		Adjust dose to give a
7, 8, 9				1.5/kg =	mg ÷ bid =	/ ↓‡	2.5 mg/kg/d p.o. (max. dose	TDx trough level of
10, 11, 12				1.25/kg =	mg ÷ bid =	/ ↓‡	150 mg/d)	400–475
13, 14, 15				1.0 mg/kg/d =	mg		↓	
16, 17, 18				0.75 mg/kg/d =	mg		↓	
19–29				0.6 mg/kg/d =	mg		↓	
30–89				0.5 mg/kg/d =	mg		↓	↓ Dosage to give trough level of 350 ± 25
Day 90–4 mo				0.4 mg/kg/d =	mg		↓	
4–5 mo				0.35 mg/kg/d =	mg		↓	
5–6 mo				0.3 mg/kg/d =	mg		↓	
6–10 mo				0.25 mg/kg/d =	mg		↓	
10–12 mo				0.2 mg/kg/d =	mg		↓	↓ At 12 mo, dosage to give trough level of 200–300
≥12 mos				0.15 mg/kg/d =	mg		↓	

ALG, antilymphocyte globulin; WT, weight; ↓, decrease.

* Give day 0 ALG on evening of transplantation day.

† If poor graft function due to acute tubular necrosis persists delay cyclosporine and continue ALG until days 10 and 12, respectively, or until creatinine is ≤2.0 mg/dL, whichever comes first. Always continue ALG for 2 days after starting cyclosporine. Do not delay cyclosporine beyond day 10, regardless of graft function.

‡ Decrease PM dose only.

TABLE 42-3. *Children's Medical Center of Dallas protocol for immunosuppressive medication after living, related donor renal transplantation in a child without statural growth potential*

Time post-transplantation	Date	Weight	TMP/SMX	Prednisone	Azathioprine	Cyclosporine
5 d Pretransplantation					2.5 mg/kg/d = ____ mg	Begin on d −5
On call to operating room				Methylprednisolone 2.5 mg/kg IV = ____ mg	2.5 mg/kg/d IV	@ 15 mg/kg ÷ bid = ____
Day 0				Methylprednisolone 1 mg/kg @ 7 h postop.	Continue; change to p.o. when tolerated	(____ mg bid)
1,2			5–10 mg/kg/d TMP	2 mg/kg ÷ bid = ____ mg = ____ mg/dose		Adjust dose to give
3, 4			↓	1.75/kg = mg ÷ bid = / ↓*	↓	a TDx trough
5, 6			↓	1.6/kg = mg ÷ bid = / ↓*	↓	level of 400–475
7, 8, 9			↓	1.5/kg = mg ÷ bid = / ↓*	2.5 mg/kg/d p.o.	
10, 11, 12			↓	1.25/kg = mg ÷ bid = / ↓*	(max dose 150 mg/d)	
13, 14, 15			↓	1.0 mg/kg d = mg	↓	
16, 17, 18			↓	0.75 mg/kg/d = mg	↓	
19–29			↓	0.6 mg/kg/d = mg	↓	
30–89			↓	0.5 mg/kg/d = mg	↓	↓ Dosage to give
Day 90–4 mo			↓	0.4 mg/kg/d = mg	↓	trough level of 350 ± 25
4–5 mo			↓	0.35 mg/kg/d = mg	↓	
5–6 mo			↓	0.3 mg/kg/d = mg	↓	
6–10 mo			↓	0.25 mg/kg/d = mg	↓	At 12 mo, dosage
10–12 mo			↓	0.2 mg/kg/d = mg	↓	to give trough
≥12 mo			↓	0.15 mg/kg/d = mg	↓	level of 200–300

TMP/SMX, trimethoprim–sulfamethoxazole (Bactrim); ↓, decrease.
* Decrease PM dose only.

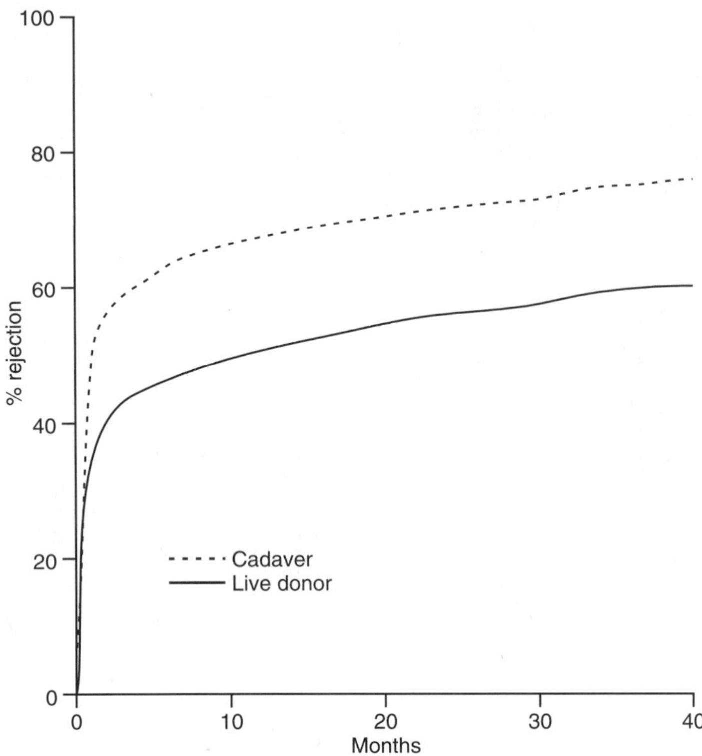

FIG. 42-6. 1994 North American Pediatric Renal Transplant Cooperative Study data on time to first rejection in living related donor and cadaver kidney recipients. (Cohn RA, Chavers B, Sullivan EK, et al. Renal transplantation and chronic dialysis in children and adolescents. The 1994 Annual Report of the North American Pediatric Renal Transplant Cooperative Study. Pediatric Nephrology; in press, 1996).

but thereafter, rejection is much more likely to occur in recipients of cadaver grafts (Fig. 42-6). Recipient age does not affect the incidence of or time to acute rejection; however, recipients of cadaver kidneys from donors younger than 6 years of age have a higher incidence of rejection at 1 year than those receiving kidneys from older donors.

Regardless of kidney source, patients with better human leukocyte antigen matching have lower rates of rejection. The rejection incidence is lower in recipients treated with early ATG, antilymphocyte globulin, or OKT3 (induction therapy) than in those without. The benefit of the antilymphocyte induction therapy is most pronounced in the cadaver kidney recipients, but also is seen in the LRD kidney recipients. Treatment of rejection is by pulsing the steroid dose, usually to 20 mg/kg of methylprednisolone, for a 3-day period. If there is significant improvement of renal function with the steroid bolus, the patient is weaned down to the prerejection steroid dose over a several-day period. If the response to the steroid bolus is incomplete, OKT3 is given over a 10-day period. Combining steroid pulse and OKT3 in this fashion reverses acute rejection in more than 85% of patients.[7]

In the 1994 NAPRTCS study, approximately half the patients treated for acute rejection had complete reversal of the rejection, with a return to baseline creatinine. The LRD recipients had a slightly higher rate of complete rejection reversal than the cadaver recipients (56% vs. 48%). Partial reversal of rejection occurred in 40% of the LRD recipients and 44% of the cadaver recipients. Therefore, 4% of the LRD and 8% of the cadaver kidneys were lost for each treated rejection episode.

Chronic rejection remains a serious problem that is probably multifactorial in etiology. Acute rejection clearly sets the stage for chronic rejection, but perfusion injury, cyclosporine toxic-ity, and hypertension may also play a role. There is some evidence that ''silent'' acute rejection may be ongoing in some patients with stable graft function, which may explain the development of chronic rejection in patients without a history of acute rejection.[8] There is no effective therapy for chronic rejection, and once renal function is significantly compromised, such children should be reconsidered for another transplant even before they are placed on dialysis. Severe hypertension may mandate transplant nephrectomy at the time of or before the next transplantation. As induction therapy and treatment of acute rejection have improved, chronic rejection has become the leading cause of graft loss in pediatric patients, and thus new strategies for prevention and treatment of chronic rejection are necessary.

Infection

Renal transplant recipients are at increased risk for infection from many organisms, but clinically the most problematic are the viruses, particularly cytomegalovirus (CMV), Epstein-Barr virus (EBV), hepatitis B or C, and human immunodeficiency virus (HIV).[9] Posttransplantation viral infection may result from transmission of the virus within the kidney, from blood product administration, or from recrudescence of the recipient's own indolent infection. The risk of clinically significant CMV and EBV infections correlates with the degree of immunosuppression given, and there is a higher incidence of those infections when patients receive polyclonal or monoclonal antilymphocyte agents.

With all the viral infections, symptomatic disease usually develops more than 1 month posttransplantation. CMV infection may range from asymptomatic elevation of serum viral titers to lethal pneumonia. The recipients who are CMV negative before transplantation and receive a CMV-positive kidney are at very high risk for CMV infection. The use of acyclovir and hyperimmune globulin prophylactically in the patient at high risk for CMV infection decreases the risk of symptomatic infection with minimal side effects, but is expensive. Ganciclovir is much more effective against CMV, but its high incidence of toxicity limits its use to patients with symptomatic disease or to a short course with low doses when the patient is receiving maximum immunosuppression, such as during OKT3 therapy. There has been much evidence to link CMV infection with an increased risk of allograft dysfunction that may be partially immune regulated and partially caused by direct damage of the kidney by the virus.

EBV infection is important because of its strong association with lymphoproliferative disease (LPD). Although malignancies of many types are more common in the transplantation patient, LPD is most commonly seen in the highly immunosuppressed patients with EBV infection. LPD may occur within months of the transplantation or not for years thereafter. The patient may present with asymptomatic lymphadenopathy or splenomegaly. Reduction of immunosuppression is often adequate treatment; however, the immunosuppression may have to be completely stopped, resulting in kidney rejection and loss.

Hepatitis C infection in the transplant recipient is serious because it is difficult, if not impossible, to eradicate and long-term infection leads to severe liver disease. Because there is no effective treatment, we do not accept kidneys from donors that are hepatitis C antibody positive. In the future, hepatitis vaccines may help to alleviate this problem.

HIV infection is a significant risk in the transplant patient and has led to screening of all potential donors for HIV antibodies. Many centers, ours included, refuse kidneys from donors who are HIV antibody negative but have a life-style consistent with a high risk for acquiring HIV, such as IV drug abusers.

OUTCOME

The patient survival for renal transplantations in children is similar to that in adults, with a 2-year survival rate of 95%. The survival rate for LRD recipients is 96.5%, and for cadaver kidney recipients, 94.0% (Fig. 42-7). The most common cause of death was infection. The patients younger than 2 years of age had a 15% mortality rate, which is significantly greater than that in older children. The kidney transplant was functioning in 43% of the patients who died. A malignancy has developed after transplantation in approximately 1% of patients enrolled in the 1994 NAPRTCS study, and that is with a relatively short follow-up period. The most common malignancy was LPD.

Kidney transplant function at 2 and 5 years, respectively, was 86% and 74% for LRD and 72% and 58% for cadaver grafts (Fig. 42-8). For LRD grafts, graft function rate is worse if the recipient is younger than 2 years of age, black, had received more than five prior transfusions, and had not received an antilymphocyte agent on day 0 or 1. For cadaver grafts, graft function was worse if any of the risk factors of poor outcome for

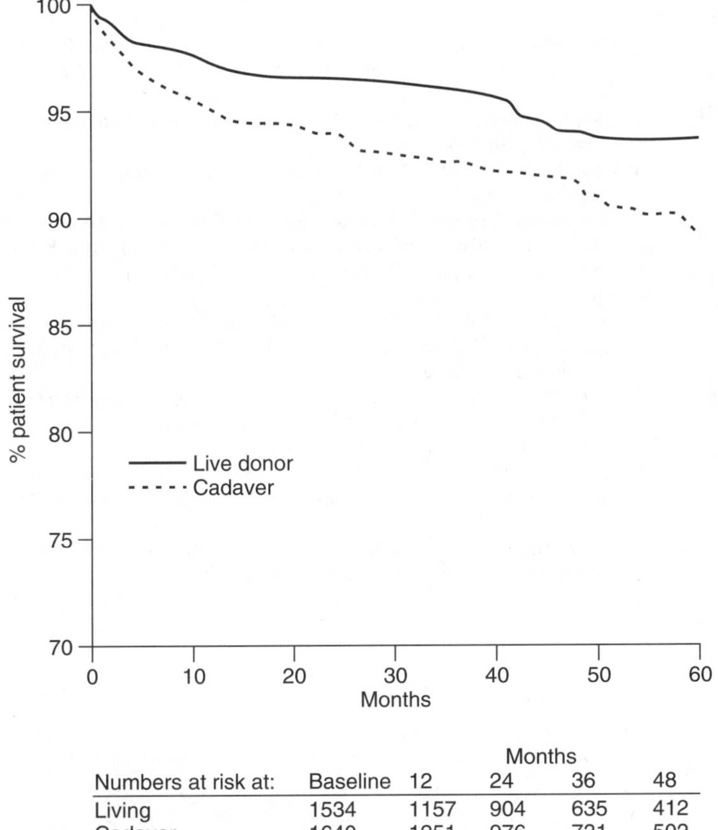

Numbers at risk at:	Baseline	12	Months 24	36	48
Living		1534	1157	904	635	412
Cadaver		1640	1251	976	731	502

FIG. 42-7. 1994 North American Pediatric Renal Transplant Cooperative Study data on patient survival after living related donor and cadaver kidney transplants. (Cohn RA, Chavers B, Sullivan EK, et al. Renal transplantation and chronic dialysis in children and adolescents. The 1994 North American Pediatric Renal Transplant Cooperative Study. Pediatric Nephrology; in press, 1996).

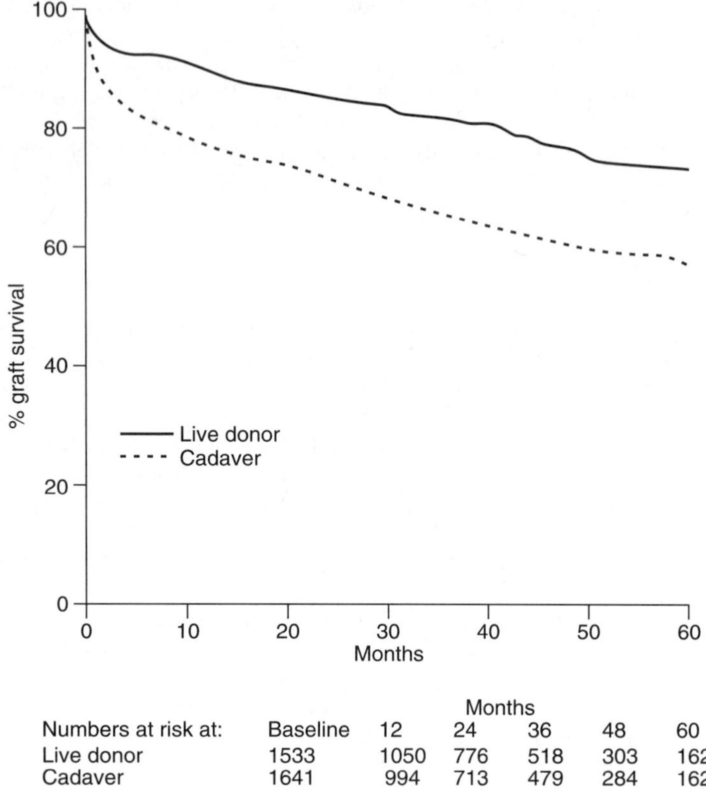

FIG. 42-8. 1994 North American Pediatric Renal Transplant Cooperative Study data on graft survival after living related donor and cadaver kidney transplants. (Cohn RA, Chavers B, Sullivan EK, et al. Renal transplantation and chronic dialysis in children and adolescents. The 1994 North American Pediatric Renal Transplant Cooperative Study. Pediatric Nephrology; in press, 1996).

Numbers at risk at:	Baseline	12	24	36	48	60
Live donor	1533	1050	776	518	303	162
Cadaver	1641	994	713	479	284	162

LRD existed or the donor was younger than 6 years of age, the recipient had received a prior transplant, there were no HLA-DR matches, or the transplantation was performed in 1987 compared to 1991.

Acute tubular necrosis (ATN), defined as use of dialysis within a week of transplant, developed in 5.6% of LRD grafts and 19.7% of cadaver grafts. The rate of ATN in cadaver grafts decreased from 22.3% in 1987 to 16.2% in 1993. Most significantly, at 3 years posttransplantation, 73% of cadaver grafts without ATN were functioning, compared to only 49% of those with ATN.

Despite efforts to minimize steroid administration, growth retardation remains a significant problem, particularly in the older child. For the children younger than 6 years of age, accelerated growth is anticipated with a functioning allograft. For the recipients older than 6 years of age, the growth is stable at a rate similar to that of the normal population, but they do not tend to have catch-up growth, and thus remain small compared to age-matched control subjects. Graft function is important to growth; a poorly functioning kidney or one being treated with high doses of steroids for rejection has a negative impact on the child's growth.

REFERENCES

1. Cohn RA. Preemptive transplantation. In: Tejani AH, Fine RN, eds. Pediatric renal transplantation. New York, Wiley-Liss, 1994:87.
2. UNOS Update. 1994;10(7):37.
3. Lich R, Howerton LW, Davis LA. Recurrent urosepsis in children. J Urol 1961;86:554.
4. Najarian JS, Frey DJ, Matas AJ, et al. Renal transplantation in infants. Ann Surg 1990;212:353.
5. Harmon WE, Stablein D, Alexander SR, et al. Graft thrombosis in pediatric renal transplant recipients: a report from the North American Pediatric Renal Transplant Cooperative Study. Transplantation 1991;51: 406.
6. Glicklich D, Tellis VA, Quinn T, et al. Comparison of captopril scan and Doppler ultrasound as screening tests for transplant renal artery stenosis. Transplantation 1990;49:217.
7. Ortho Multicenter Transplant Study Group. A randomized clinical trial of OKT3 monoclonal antibody for acute rejection of cadaver renal transplants. N Engl J Med 1985;313:337.
8. Rush DN, Henry SF, Jeffrey JR, et al. Histological findings in early routine biopsies of stable renal allograft recipients. Transplantation 1994;57:208.
9. Rubin RH, Tolkoff-Rubin NE. The impact of infection on the outcome of transplantation. Transplant Proc 1991;23:2068.

Surgery of Infants and Children: Scientific Principles and Practice, edited by
Keith T. Oldham, Paul M. Colombani, and Robert P. Foglia.
Lippincott–Raven Publishers, Philadelphia, © 1997.

CHAPTER 43

Liver

Walter Andrews

Liver transplantation is now considered a reasonable therapeutic option for the treatment of end-stage liver disease. Achieving this goal, however, has been the result of the work of many distinguished physicians. In the United States, Thomas Starzl[1] is credited with the development of the surgical technique for transplantation. He published his first successful series of liver transplants, all of which were pediatric, in 1963. After this series, Starzl[2] reported on another child who was well 26 years after liver transplantation. Sir Roy Calne[3,4] in London, England, was among the first to investigate the use of azathioprine and later cyclosporine as effective immunosuppressants. Rudolph Pichlmayr[5–7] in Hanover, Germany, pioneered the use of anti-lymphocyte serum as an effective immunosuppressant and also initiated investigation into the techniques of reduced-size and "split" liver transplantation. Christoph Broelsch[8] developed the technique and successfully argued for the use of living, related liver transplantation.

The modern era of pediatric liver transplantation in the United States began in 1984 when cyclosporine began to be used as the standard immunosuppressive agent. Before this time, the 1-year survival rate after liver transplantation was 19%, but with the use of cyclosporine, this survival rate increased to 65%. These improved results led to a rapid rise in the number of liver transplantations performed in the United States. According to statistics from the United Network for Organ Sharing (UNOS),[9] in 1995 there were 101 centers performing liver transplants. Sixty-nine of these centers also were engaged in pediatric liver transplantation. As an illustration of this growth, Table 43-1 shows the number of children and adults who have undergone liver transplants in the United States from 1988 to 1993. Approximately 20% of all the liver transplant procedures performed in the United States are in pediatric patients.

INDICATIONS FOR LIVER TRANSPLANTATION

The complications of end-stage liver disease that govern the necessity and timing for pediatric liver transplantation, although similar, are not identical to those in adults (Table 43-2).

The development of *hepatic encephalopathy* is considered an absolute indication for transplantation. The diagnosis of hepatic encephalopathy is made by clinical examination. Hepatic encephalopathy is divided into four clinical grades. Grade IV is defined as a child who has only signs of brain stem activity. Grade III includes children who are in a coma but respond to deep pain. Grade II patients are somnolent, but arouse easily with appropriate responses. Grade I children are irritable, difficult to console, and or have shortened attention spans with difficulty concentrating. There are no reliable diagnostic tests that can make this diagnosis in advance of clinical symptoms.

Medically unmanageable *complications of portal hypertension* also necessitate a new liver. Bleeding from esophageal or gastric varices is common in children with end-stage liver disease. Initially, these varices are managed by obliterative techniques such as sclerotherapy or banding. However, if breakthrough bleeding occurs, if gastric varices develop that are not amenable to direct treatment, or if a complication from sclerotherapy or banding occurs, then liver transplantation is indicated. Ascites is initially managed with salt and fluid restriction. If this fails, then diuretics are added along with albumin infusions if the serum albumin is less than 2.5 g/dL. With progressive liver dysfunction, ascites tends to become increasingly resistant to medical management, leading to respiratory compromise and thereby necessitating transplantation. Care must be exercised in the management of ascites because aggressive treatment can lead to the development of the hepatorenal syndrome.

Decreasing synthetic function, as evidenced by a falling serum albumin or a rising prothrombin time, is indication for transplantation. There can be several reasons for a decline in the serum albumin, including progressive ascites, poor nutrition, or decreased liver production. If the serum albumin remains low despite aggressive nutritional management and control of the ascites, the most likely reason for the decline is failing synthetic function. The prothrombin time is a vitamin K–dependent function. Because vitamin K is a fat-soluble vitamin, the initial rise in the prothrombin time can be caused by poor absorption rather than declining hepatic function. However, when a fixed coagulopathy that no longer responds to intravenous vitamin K therapy develops, liver transplantation is indicated. In addition, a patient who exhibits a fixed coagulopathy in the *absence* of other liver abnormalities must be evaluated for the presence of a hepatic metabolic disease.

TABLE 43-1. *Number of patients receiving liver transplants, by year*

	1988	1989	1990	1991	1992	1993
Pediatric	408	453	513	500	493	524
Adult	1305	1748	2176	2452	2569	2919

United Network for Organ Sharing.

Pruritus, although not life threatening, can be an absolute indication for transplantation. Pruritus is a common complication of cholestasis that is difficult to control. Multiple therapies have been tried for this condition, including antihistamines, bile salt resin binders, and phototherapy. None is completely effective, and some patients are refractory to all management. Severe excoriations can develop in these patients, including exposure of the cartilage over the nose and ears. These patients require constant watching to prevent these complications, which totally disrupts the patient's and family's life-style, leading to sleep disruption and loss of concentration. When pruritus has progressed to this level, transplantation is indicated.

An indication for liver transplantation that is unique to pediatric patients is *growth failure*. Growth failure is defined as a marked decline in or complete lack of growth. Sex, ethnic background, and genetic predisposition are taken into account when evaluating growth rates. Growth failure is an indication of a failing liver, but is not an indication for transplantation until the patient has failed an aggressive dietary management program. This program includes increasing the caloric density of the child's formula, followed by nighttime or continuous tube feedings. In addition, these children need aggressive fat-soluble vitamin support (A, D, E, and K). Children with severe vitamin D or E deficiency that is not responsive to supplementation should also be considered for early transplantation because of the potential for permanent bone or neurologic damage.

Liver transplantation can be a rational treatment for *hepatoblastoma*. At our center, these patients must meet several strict pretransplantation criteria. The cancer must not be resectable, it must be confined to the liver without any local or distant metastases, it must have a demonstrated a response to chemotherapy, and the patient must be able to tolerate at least two more cycles of chemotherapy after the transplantation. The true success of liver transplantation for hepatoblastoma is difficult to determine. Koneru and associates,[10] in a summary of the U.S. experience, reported a 1-year survival rate of 58%. Unfortunately, none of the reported patients in this series had the

same pretransplantation or posttransplantation treatment. Although the survival rate is inferior to an overall 1-year survival rate of 71% for noncancer patients, it is superior to the reported 20% to 30% survival rate after transplantation for hepatocellular carcinoma.

Poor quality of life or social invalidism can be indications for liver transplantation. Chronic fatigue is a debilitating problem that can prevent young children from reaching developmental milestones or cause older children to fall behind academically because of a lack of concentration or an inability to attend school. Social invalidism occurs when children can no longer participate in the usual social activities that are appropriate for their age. This is especially true for teenagers. For example, a teenager with Crigler-Najjar syndrome was unable to attend any after-school functions or spend the night or weekend away from home because she had to spend 14 hours a day under bilirubin lights. This led to severe depression and threats of suicide. In smaller children with biliary atresia, recurrent episodes of cholangitis that require repeated, prolonged hospital stays for intravenous antibiotics not only impair normal family routines but can delay the child's social development. When life has deteriorated to this level of nonfunction, transplantation is a reasonable alternative.

Objective Indications

Several retrospective studies have been done to determine if there are any objective indicators of liver function that may be used to determine the appropriate timing of a liver transplant. Malatack and colleagues,[11] using a multivariate model, identified four variables as possible determinants of early mortality before transplantation: history of ascites, indirect bilirubin, cholesterol level, and partial thromboplastin time. These variables were then given a numeric score and weighted so that a total score could be determined. Using this system, they were able to predict patients who would be at high risk for death in the ensuing 6 months. Shaw and coworkers[12] also developed a preoperative risk score based on the clinical criteria of ascites, malnutrition, serum bilirubin, age, number of transfusions, the presence of coagulopathy, and the presence of hepatic encephalopathy. Patients with a high risk score were more likely to die before surgery than those patients with a low score.

Caffeine clearance has been proposed as a measure of liver functional capacity. However, in a study of liver regeneration after liver resection, caffeine clearance did not show any correlation to the amount of remaining hepatic mass or the rate of regeneration.[13] The hepatic clearance and metabolism of lidocaine to its metabolite, MEGX, has also been described as a possible technique to assess the amount of functional hepatic mass. Chiffon and colleagues,[14] in a study of patients with chronic liver disease, noted that patients with a low lidocaine clearance were at higher risk for development of hepatic decompensation. A similar study has not yet been performed in children.

TABLE 43-2. *Indications for pediatric liver transplantation*

Hepatic encephalopathy
Complications of portal hypertension
   Uncontrollable variceal bleeding
   Medically unmanageable ascites
Decreasing synthetic function
   Rising prothrombin time despite adequate parenteral vitamin K
   Declining serum albumin despite adequate nutrition
Severe pruritus
Growth failure
Hepatoblastoma
Poor quality of life or social invalidism

Contraindications

In the early years of liver transplantation, the contraindications to the procedure were strict and absolute. However, as experience was gained with the procedure, established contraindications were challenged and the undoable became possible. Few absolute contraindications remain. Metastatic liver cancer and cancer metastatic to the liver are still considered absolute contraindications. Although the presence of any active infection is still considered an absolute contraindication, patients have been successfully transplanted with a resolving acute varicella infection without complications. Patients with limited long-term survival were traditionally not considered candidates for transplantation; however, our center's positive experience with liver transplantation in patients with cystic fibrosis has made us reexamine this policy.

Psychosocial problems can compromise a patient's immediate and long-term postoperative course. If significant psychosocial problems arise before surgery, the child may not be approved for transplantation if these problems could interfere with the child's obtaining the appropriate long-term posttransplantation care. Noncompliance on the part of the family with pretransplantation medical regimes, despite a clear understanding of the consequences, is considered a contraindication to transplantation at our center. Kennard and associates[15] identified a variety of potential psychosocial variables that may identify families who are at risk for posttransplantation dysfunction. These variables include financial stress, including limited insurance coverage, patients with severe developmental delays, and patients with lengthy postoperative stays. Once these factors are identified, extra support and intervention can be initiated to alleviate or prevent the psychosocial complications that could sabotage an otherwise successful outcome.

PEDIATRIC LIVER DISEASE REQUIRING TRANSPLANTATION

A variety of diseases can lead to end-stage liver disease in children. Table 43-3 lists the diseases that have required liver transplantation at our center. Biliary atresia is the most common diagnosis in children that leads to end-stage liver disease. Although the Kasai procedure (portoenterostomy) is the appropriate initial surgical procedure for infants with biliary atresia, this procedure, unfortunately, often only delays rather than prevents the need for a liver transplant. Recurrent episodes of cholangitis, growth failure, and the development of portal hypertension all lead to the need for transplantation in these patients. Genetic metabolic disorders are the second most common indication for transplantation, and of these, α_1-antitrypsin deficiency is the most common. Rather than presenting with pulmonary disease, these children present with severe cirrhosis, portal hypertension, and eventually hepatic failure. Other, more common metabolic diseases that require liver transplantation include tyrosinemia, Wilson disease, and glycogen storage disease type 4.

Acute hepatic failure can lead to liver transplantation in the pediatric population. In our series, a variety of etiologic agents have been identified, including hepatitis A, hepatitis B, cytomegalovirus (CMV) hepatitis, Wilson disease, autoimmune hepatitis, and acetaminophen toxicity. Since 1990, we have noted an increase in the number of cases of acute hepatic failure for which no etiology could be identified other than a histologic diagnosis of ''hepatitis'' or ''massive hepatic necrosis.'' Autoimmune hepatitis and chronic active hepatitis can also progress to chronic liver disease. These diseases tend to occur in older children and have highly variable courses. Hepatitis B and C are rare causes for chronic liver disease in children because of the long time between infection and development of cirrhosis and the relative rarity of hepatitis B in pediatric patients in the United States.

PREOPERATIVE ASSESSMENT

Elective Transplantation

The preoperative evaluation of a potential candidate is focused on two areas. The first is to determine if the patient is a candidate for a transplant, and the second concerns when the patient will need transplantation. Because there are no reliable methods to determine how much remaining functional liver is present, an idea of the patient's overall condition is obtained by the evaluation of a variety of factors.

Liver function is evaluated by determining the total and direct bilirubin and the hepatic enzyme levels. In chronic liver disease, these results are not predictive, but they are helpful for establishing a baseline. More important are the serum albumin and clotting factors. A persistent, low serum albumin despite good nutritional intake, or clotting factors that remain persistently elevated despite adequate vitamin K replacement, are both highly suggestive of declining hepatic function. Evidence of portal hypertension is determined by physical examination (ascites, splenic enlargement, caput medusae, hemorrhoids) and serial

TABLE 43-3. *Diseases leading to pediatric liver transplantation*

Biliary atresia
Intrahepatic cholestasis syndromes
   Alagille syndrome
   Byler syndrome
   Biliary hypoplasia
   Familial cholestasis
Metabolic diseases
   α_1-Antitrypsin deficiency
   Tyrosinemia
   Glycogen storage disease type I
   Wilson disease
   Cystic fibrosis
Hepatitis
   Chronic active hepatitis
   Neonatal hepatitis
   Rubella hepatitis
   Cytomegalovirus hepatitis
Structural biliary diseases
   Choledochal cyst
   Sclerosing cholangitis
   Caroli disease
Acute hepatic failure
   Hepatitis A
   Hepatitis B
   Non-A, Non-B, Non-C hepatitis
Overdoses
   Acetaminophen
   Depocane
Cryptogenic cirrhosis
Histiocytosis X
Hepatoblastoma

complete blood counts that demonstrate a declining white cell count or a decreasing platelet count. Some centers have reported the use of galactose, caffeine, or lidocaine clearances to evaluate the liver's metabolic capacity. These tests, however, have not been widely used by most pediatric transplantation centers.

Imaging studies include an abdominal ultrasound to determine the patency of the portal, splenic, and superior mesenteric veins and the inferior vena cava. Bone films are obtained to screen for vitamin D deficiency (rickets) and in some patients establish bone age to confirm growth failure.

Nutritional status is evaluated by anthropometric studies, a careful dietary history, and an evaluation of fat-soluble vitamin levels as well as zinc and copper levels. The patient's immune status is evaluated by determining antibody titers to hepatitis A, B, and C, varicella, CMV, Epstein-Barr virus (EBV), and herpes virus. A careful immunization history is also obtained. Every attempt should be made to have the child completely immunized (as appropriate for age) before transplantation. It is unknown how well the child will respond to an immunization after immunosuppression has been initiated. In addition, after transplantation, the child should not receive any live virus vaccines.

Patients and their families are evaluated by both psychology and social service. Through these interviews, insights are obtained regarding potential family problems that might affect their ability to cope with the stresses of the transplantation process. The only significant social or psychological problem what would eliminate a patient from candidacy would be a recurrent history of noncompliance with medical therapy despite repeated counseling.

After the evaluation is completed, the patient's candidacy and urgency are determined by a transplant committee. Recommendations are then made to the referring doctor regarding any alterations in the child's current medical management that may improve their pretransplantation clinical condition. The most common suggestion is an increase in caloric intake. In an infant who is eating well, the formula can be concentrated up to 30 calories per ounce. In an older child, liquid dietary supplements are recommended. If oral intake is poor, tube feedings are usually recommended. These feedings usually start with nighttime feeds, but if necessary move to continuous 24-hour tube feeding. Fat-soluble vitamins usually need to be supplemented, especially vitamin E, which has been shown to be critical in neural development. Pruritus can be a debilitating problem for which there is no good treatment. Antihistamines are usually the first-line treatment, as well phototherapy. If these are not successful, rifampin often has a beneficial effect. A difficult problem can be the management of recurrent variceal hemorrhage. The first line of therapy is endoscopic treatment either with sclerotherapy or banding. This often requires several sessions for adequate control. If endoscopic control fails and the patient has excellent synthetic function and is not considered an early transplant candidate, the use of a portosystemic shunt may be considered. Surgically, we favor the use of a distal splenorenal shunt. A transjugular intrahepatic portal shunt has been used effectively as a temporizing measure in adults with end-stage liver disease, but the stents are too large for smaller children.

Emergent Liver Transplantation

The most common reason for an emergent liver transplantation is acute hepatic failure. These children can, without warning, rapidly become hemodynamically and neurologically unstable. Children with an episode of acute hepatic injury and prolonged clotting times must be carefully observed for the development of hypoglycemia and neurologic deterioration.

When these patients are initially seen, an aggressive search should be undertaken to determine the cause of hepatic failure. Viral, toxin, and metabolic screens are indicated. If the patient is stable, and not coagulopathic, a liver biopsy should be obtained (percutaneous or open) for histologic study and viral culture. Careful, serial neurologic evaluations are required and the degree and progression, if any, of hepatic coma must be carefully followed. When a patient reaches stage III or IV coma, an intracranial pressure (ICP) monitor is recommended. Cerebral perfusion pressures must be carefully followed, with efforts directed toward maintaining both an adequate systolic blood pressure and a low ICP. Acute renal failure, in the form of hepatorenal syndrome, may occur, requiring the use of hemofiltration to prevent systemic volume overload and its deleterious effects on ICP. Pulmonary decompensation is frequent, due either to volume overload or neurogenic pulmonary edema. Ventilator support is required when either pulmonary decompensation occurs or the child's coma progresses to the point that the child can no longer protect his or her airway. Fever is common in the population and an aggressive surveillance for infection should be maintained. If fever occurs, we recommend broad-spectrum antibiotic coverage.

Patients who present with acute hepatic decompensation should be immediately listed for transplantation. If the patient is in stage III or IV coma or if the factor V level is less than 15% of normal levels, transplantation is required. Transplantation is not indicated if the patient has evidence of sepsis or has progressed neurologically to brain death. Despite all efforts, once patients have progressed to stage IV coma, their chances for a complete neurologic recovery are substantially reduced.

OPERATIVE PROCEDURE

Anesthesia

Most patients who arrive for liver transplantation do not have the luxury of a long NPO status. In addition, hypoglycemia develops in most pediatric patients with end-stage liver disease when they are fasted for longer than 6 hours. Therefore, anesthesia is induced with a rapid-sequence technique and cricoid pressure. Anesthesia is maintained with inhalational agents and intravenous paralytic and narcotic drugs. Arterial and central venous monitoring lines and large-bore lines for blood and plasma administration are placed after induction. In our experience, a flow-directed pulmonary catheter has not been helpful unless the patient has a history of cardiac problems.

Management of Intraoperative Blood Loss and Coagulopathy

Factors that increase the amount of bleeding that occurs during the dissection of the native liver include two or more upper abdominal operations, two or more episodes of cholangitis or peritonitis, or severe coagulopathy (prothrombin longer than 20 seconds). Monitoring of intraoperative blood loss is a combination of an evaluation of the patient's filling pressure (central venous pressure) and the amount of losses recorded from the sponges and the suction catheter. Volume loss early in the procedure is replaced with crystalloid, fresh frozen plasma, and leukocyte-filtered packed red blood cells. Because of the ongoing blood loss, during the dissection of the native liver, the use of fresh frozen plasma and packed red blood cells is kept to a minimum. However, it is incumbent on the surgeon to use meticulous technique to keep these ongoing losses at a minimum. Most blood products, including platelets, are given after revascularization of the graft, when blood losses are much lower and adequate clotting is necessary.

Clotting status is monitored every 1 to 2 hours by the prothrombin time and the partial thromboplastin time. In addition, some centers rely heavily on the intraoperative use of the thromboelastograph. This machine measures the integrity of the coagulation process by tracking clot formation, clot integrity, and clot lysis.

After revascularization of the new liver, the initial bleeding is surgical, from vascular anastomoses or from the cut surface of the liver if a reduced-size graft is used. After this bleeding is controlled, a second phase of bleeding can occur that has been ascribed to premature fibrinolysis (presumably because of the new liver's inability to metabolize profibrinolytic proteins). This process is confirmed with the thromboelastograph and can be treated with ϵ-aminocaproic acid. In our experience, however, maintenance of a platelet count during the revascularization phase of greater than 100,000 virtually eliminates this second phase of bleeding. Those patients who have had this second phase of bleeding despite an adequate platelet count must be carefully evaluated for the presence of true disseminated intravascular coagulation or a severely compromised graft (primary nonfunction)

Surgical Techniques

Whole-Organ Transplantation

The procedure for whole-organ transplantation begins, as with all transplantations, with the new organ. We preserve all grafts with University of Wisconsin solution at 4°C. This solution allows for hepatic preservation times of at least 24 hours. Increased biliary complications, however, have been reported in grafts that have cold storage times greater than 12 hours. The new organ is prepared for implantation by the removal of any excess tissue from the graft so that the vessels are adequately exposed for suturing. Because of the precarious nature of the blood supply to the bile duct, it is not trimmed or cleaned. If a right hepatic artery originating from the superior mesenteric artery is present, this is connected end to side to the common hepatic artery, taking extreme care not to twist either vessel.

Recipient Hepatectomy

While the organ is being prepared on the back table, the dissection of the recipient's liver is begun. The patient's abdomen is prepped from nipples to the groin and side-to-side down to the operating table. This area is widely draped and the towels are secured in place with either staples or skin sutures. Several types of incisions can be used. In general, every attempt should be made to incorporate any previous abdominal incisions into the transplantation incision. In small children, a bilateral subcostal incision is adequate, with the right side of the incision extending almost to the 12th rib. In larger children with less pliable costal margins, an upper midline extension is often required. In children with a very low previous right-sided transverse incision, a midline incision is made starting at the xiphoid with subsequent incorporation of the right transverse incision. Electrocautery is extensively used for the division of the subcutaneous tissues. Large collateral veins are often present in the subcutaneous tissue that can bleed extensively if not adequately controlled. The muscle layers are divided with electrocautery and the peritoneal cavity is entered. Ascites fluid is aspirated and cultured. The ligamentum teres is divided and ligated. In patients without prior surgery, the hilum of the liver is dissected and the portal tract structures are identified and isolated. The common bile duct is divided, if possible, just below the insertion of the cystic duct. Care must be taken not to disturb extensively the distal blood supply of the duct during the dissection. The hepatic artery can easily be palpated in the left side of the porta, especially after opening the gastrohepatic ligament. The common hepatic artery is dissected proximally to its right and left bifurcation. Distally, the gastroduodenal artery is ligated and an additional 1 to 2 cm of hepatic artery proximal to this point is exposed. During the hepatic artery dissection, two arterial aberrancies can be discovered. A right hepatic artery can originate from the superior mesenteric artery; this vessel is found posterior to the portal vein. A left hepatic artery can arise from the left gastric artery and travel into the liver by way of the gastrohepatic ligament. The left gastric vessel is rarely large enough to supply the donor organ; however, occasionally a right hepatic artery off the superior mesenteric can be larger than the main hepatic artery and should be initially preserved for possible use in the hepatic artery anastomosis. After the bile duct and the hepatic artery are exposed, the portal vein is easily seen in the posterior portion of the porta and cleaned circumferentially. During the portal vein dissection, the coronary vein is identified and ligated. The hepatic artery and portal vein are usually not divided until the recipient's liver is ready for removal. If the patient weighs less than 15 kg and does not have a previously constructed Roux-en-Y limb, or if the recipient bile duct is too small for a duct-to-duct biliary reconstruction, it is best to construct the Roux-en-Y limb before clamping the portal vein. If the patient has had previous biliary surgery, the right upper quadrant can be encased in adhesions. These adhesions are best divided with the judicious use of electrocautery. Extreme care must be taken not to injure the bowel. If a cautery injury occurs, even if it appears to be only serosal, it should be immediately repaired. As the bowel that is adherent to the underside of the liver is freed, the previously constructed Roux-en-Y limb will be encountered. The Roux-en-Y will be anterior to the hilar vessels, but the right branch of the hepatic artery often is close to the right edge of the loop. The Roux-en-Y is encircled and divided with a gastrointestinal stapler close to the liver hilum to preserve maximum length for its reuse in the biliary reconstruction of the donor liver. After the Roux-en-Y limb is divided, the dissection continues as described previously. After the hilar dissection is completed and before removal of the old liver, the proximal portion of the Roux-en-Y is examined to make sure that it is at least 20 to 45 cm in length and that it enters the proximal jejunum no further than 15 cm from the ligament of Treitz. A Roux-en-Y that is an inappropriate length or inserts greater than 20 cm from the ligament of Treitz can significantly affect the postoperative absorption of immunosuppressive medications. Because the lysis of adhesions in the lower abdomen is often necessary to identify these landmarks, and because this often results in increased blood loss, this dissection may be more appropriately done after the new liver is revascularized. The Roux-en-Y can be placed either antecolic or retrocolic, depending on the best fit with the least amount of tension. After the hilar dissection is completed, the gastrohepatic, coronary, and triangular ligaments are divided with electrocautery. The caudate lobe is mobilized and a sponge is placed posterior to the caudate to help in the identification of the proper position for the retrocaval dissection. The liver can now be mobilized anteriorly and to the left. This exposes the inferior vena cava (IVC). The peritoneum overlying the IVC if often highly vascular and should be divided with incontinuity ligatures. The sponge can now be palpated through the tissue below the vena cava at the level of the diaphragm above the right adrenal vein. This area is opened with electrocautery, which exposes the sponge and thereby creates an opening in the retroperitoneum below the IVC. This retrocaval dissection is carried inferiorly to the level of the IVC using incontinuity ligatures. The infrahepatic and suprahepatic venae cavae are then cleaned circumferentially.

This completes the recipient liver dissection. Before implantation of the new liver, the hepatic artery is examined for adequate size to support the arterial blood flow of the new liver. If the artery appears to be of sufficient size, the hepatic artery is divided high in the hepatic hilum, preserving the bifurcation of the right and left hepatic arteries (Fig. 43-1*A*). A Carrel patch of the donor celiac axis can then be anastomosed to the splayed bifurcation of the right and left hepatic arteries of the recipient (see Fig. 43-1*B*). If this is not possible, then a Carrel patch of the donor celiac artery is used (see Fig. 43-1*C*). If the artery is thought to be of insufficient caliber or have poor flow, then an iliac artery graft from the donor is used. The aortic end of the graft is then sewn end to side to the recipient's aorta just below the left renal vein or to the supraceliac aorta. In the infrarenal position, the graft is routed through the base of the transverse mesocolon, through the lesser sac, over the pancreas, and out the lesser sac at the lesser curve of the stomach. These arterial anastomotic modifications are made before removing the recipient liver to minimize the warm ischemic time of the donor organ.

Bleeding during the recipient liver dissection can be significant. Bleeding is worst in patients with prior surgery because of the large raw surfaces left on the liver, bowel, and diaphragm. This bleeding is best controlled as it occurs rather than waiting until completion of the dissection. Bleeding can almost always be controlled with a combination of electrocautery, suture liga-

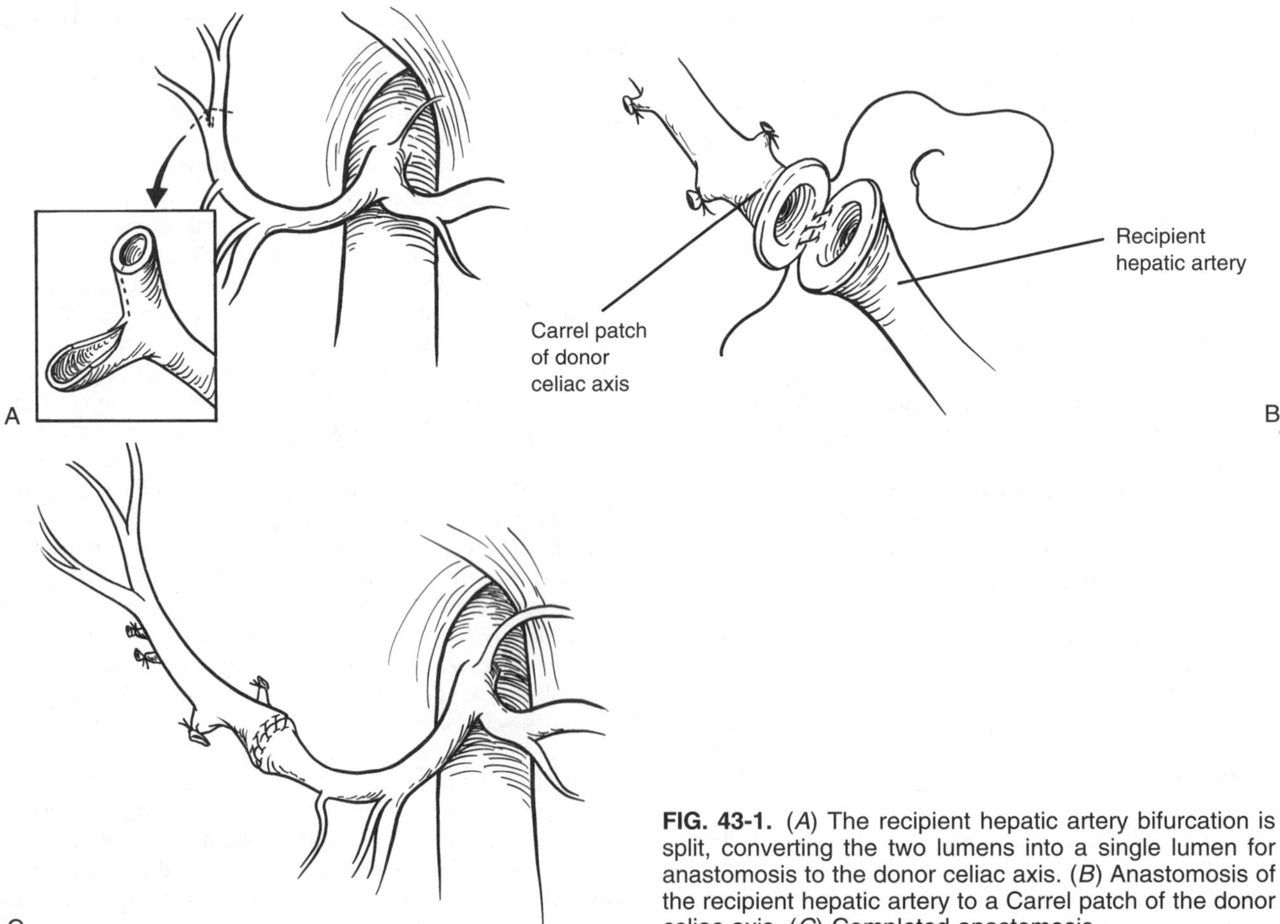

FIG. 43-1. (*A*) The recipient hepatic artery bifurcation is split, converting the two lumens into a single lumen for anastomosis to the donor celiac axis. (*B*) Anastomosis of the recipient hepatic artery to a Carrel patch of the donor celiac axis. (*C*) Completed anastomosis.

tures, and argon beam coagulation. Further hemostasis is then accomplished in the retroperitoneum after the liver is removed.

Venovenous bypass is a technique that has gained significant popularity in the adult transplant programs. Before removal of the recipient's liver, catheters are placed in the left femoral vein and portal vein. Blood is then pumped from these vessels by a centrifugal pump to a catheter that has been placed in the left axillary vein. This method bypasses the IVC and portal vein obstruction that occurs when the liver is removed. Venovenous bypass can improve patient stability and can decrease blood loss by decreasing the pressure in the portal and retroperitoneal veins. However, we have found that children with end-stage liver disease have sufficient retroperitoneal collaterals that when the IVC is clamped, there is minimal bowel edema and any systematic hypotension is easily corrected by volume replacement. Therefore, we believe that venovenous bypass is indicated only in children with acute hepatic failure and hepatic coma. These patients have not had sufficient time for collateral formation, and excessive fluid loading can be detrimental to cerebral function.

Anhepatic Phase

The recipient liver is removed by the ligation of the portal vein and hepatic artery in the hilum of the liver, the placement of a cross-clamp on the suprahepatic cava at the diaphragm, and the placement of a cross-clamp on the infrahepatic cava just above the takeoff of the right renal vein. Care is taken to divide the suprahepatic cava at the level of the hepatic veins, to ensure an adequate suprahepatic cuff. The infrahepatic cava is also divided deep in the liver to achieve maximum length. After the liver is removed, the suprahepatic cuff is enlarged by transversely dividing the hepatic veins so they form one large opening. The infrahepatic cava is carefully trimmed to provide maximum length. The donor liver is then removed from its ice bath and the anastomotic timer started. The liver should be reperfused within 1 hour and 20 minutes. If all four vascular anastomoses cannot be completed in this time, then the cava anastomoses and the portal vein anastomoses should be completed and the clamps released on these vessels. The arterial anastomoses can be completed after reperfusion. All anastomoses are performed using an intima-to-intima imbricating technique with a monofilament, nonabsorbable running suture.

Implantation begins with end-to-end suprahepatic and infrahepatic caval anastomoses. Before completion of the infrahepatic anastomoses, the portal vein and the hepatic artery of the donor liver are flushed with 10 mL/kg of 4°C lactated Ringer solution with 5% albumin to remove the preservation solution and to fill the liver with fluid, which displaces any air in the liver and thereby decreases the chance of an air embolus on reperfusion. The portal vein is then clamped at its junction with the pancreas and carefully opened to remove any clot that may have formed during its occlusion. Sponges are then placed posterior to the right lobe of the liver, moving it toward the donor portal vein. An end-to-end anastomosis is then performed, which becomes taut when the sponges are removed. The hepatic arterial anastomoses are last, and performed as previously described.

Reperfusion and Biliary Reconstruction

The suprahepatic and infrahepatic clamps are removed, restoring caval flow. The arterial clamp is removed, starting hepatic reperfusion. The portal vein clamp is then slowly removed. During reperfusion, the new liver can absorb a significant amount of the circulating blood volume. This, in combination with bleeding from the cut surface of a reduced-size graft, can require the need for rapid volume infusion. Controlling portal vein flow gives the anesthesiologist an opportunity to stay ahead of the volume loss. Once the clamps are removed, the suprahepatic cava must be carefully checked for any bleeding from small phrenic veins. These must be carefully ligated; otherwise, they can lead to significant postoperative bleeding. The liver should resume its normal color in 10 to 20 minutes. Once the patient is hemodynamically stable, further enhancement of hepatic perfusion can be achieved by the injection of 0.15 mg/kg of verapamil through the hepatic artery.

After adequate homeostasis is achieved, attention is turned to the biliary system. Two types of biliary reconstructions are used: duct-to-duct direct biliary anastomoses or an end-to-side Roux-en-Y choledochojejunostomy (Fig. 43-2). At our center, the duct-to-duct reconstruction is performed with interrupted absorbable sutures over the largest T tube that the distal duct will accommodate. The Roux-en-Y anastomosis is performed with interrupted absorbable sutures over an indwelling stent without external drainage. The integrity of both of these procedures is checked during surgery with a cholangiogram. Figure 43-3 depicts all of the completed vascular and biliary anastomoses.

After the biliary anastomosis is completed, final hemostasis is obtained, the abdomen is irrigated with an antibiotic solution, and three closed suction drains are placed (in both subphrenic spaces and the subhepatic space). The abdomen is closed with absorbable PDS suture using running technique.

Reduced-Size Transplantation

Unfortunately, there are insufficient whole livers for transplantation in pediatric recipients. This has led to the development of techniques for reducing a liver from a larger donor to a pediatric recipient. The necessity for reducing a liver can be roughly estimated by the donor-to-recipient weight ratio. If this ratio is greater than 3 : 1, a left lobe graft is required, and if the ratio is greater than 5 : 1, a left lateral segment graft is necessary. Significant pretransplantation ascites, however, can stretch the abdominal wall, allowing the placement of a larger graft. At our center, we believe that the best determinant of an appropriately sized graft is to compare the distance between the xiphoid and the umbilicus in the recipient to the maximum craniocaudal dimension of the new graft. The graft must be less than the xiphoid–umbilicus distance in the recipient for it to fit and the recipient's abdomen to be primarily closed. In cases of living, related transplants, the volume of the graft must be greater than 1% of the recipient's weight, or, by using computed tomography scan liver volumetrics, the volume of the donor segment to be used should be less than the whole volume of the recipient liver.

The technical problems with either left lobe or left lateral segment grafts have centered on how to control bleeding or bile

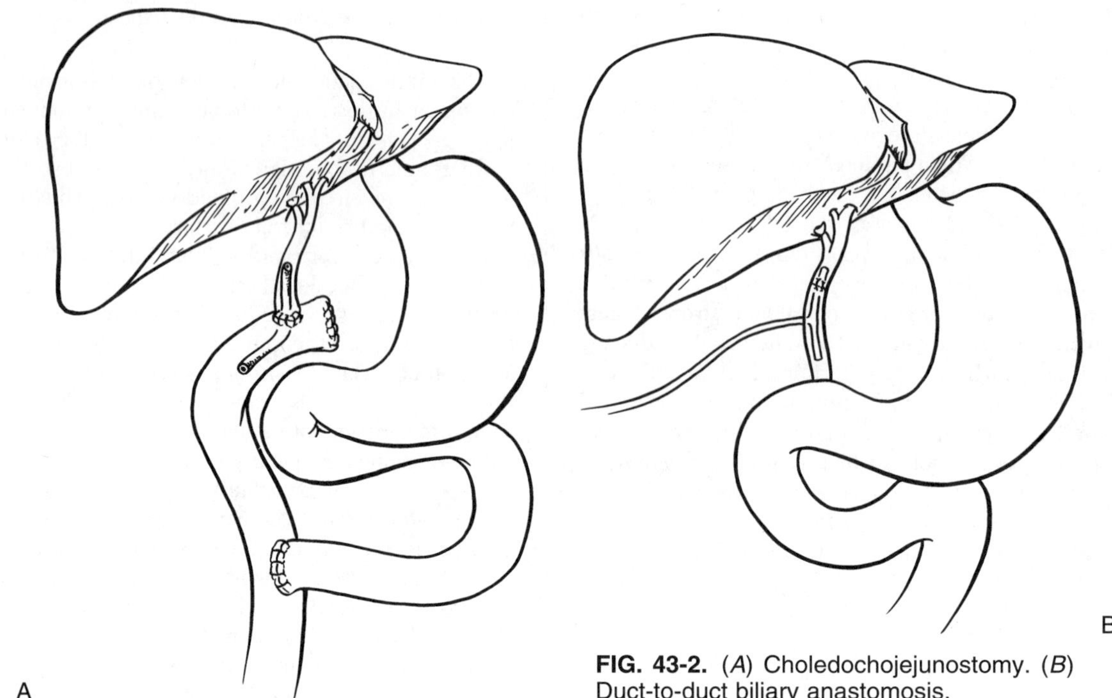

A

FIG. 43-2. (*A*) Choledochojejunostomy. (*B*) Duct-to-duct biliary anastomosis.

B

leaks from the cut surface of the liver, and how to reconstruct the vena cava of the donor liver to fit the smaller vena cava of the recipient.[16]

The donor liver reduction is carried out on the back table and consists of either a right lobectomy for a left lobe graft

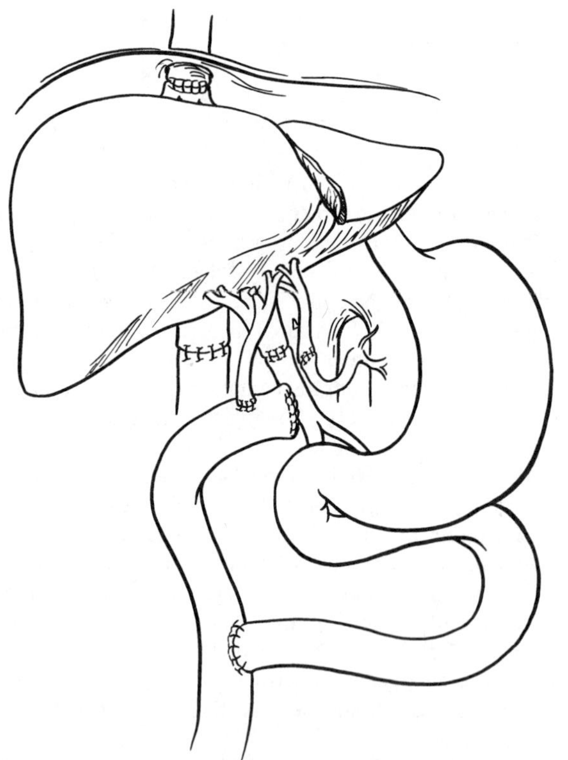

FIG. 43-3. Completed vascular and biliary anastomoses.

(segments 2, 3, and 4) or a right trisegmentectomy for a left lateral segment graft (segments 2 and 3) (Fig. 43-4). The donor hilar vessels are preserved with the graft (segments 2 and 3) for implantation into the recipient. The key to the dissection of the biliary system is to stay below and to the right of the common bile duct at all times. If both the right and left sides of the duct are dissected to identify the hilar anatomy, the common bile duct can be devascularized, with the potential for a biliary leak or stricture. The liver parenchyma is divided with finger fracture technique, ligating vessels and biliary structures as they are encountered. The donor vena cava is retained in the left lobe graft and, if necessary, tapered throughout its length to fit the recipient vena cava (Fig. 43-5A). For a left lateral segment graft, a right trisegmentectomy is performed, but the cava is totally removed and a Carrel patch is taken from the suprahepatic cava around the left hepatic vein (see Fig. 43-4B). To decrease bleeding from the cut surface of the graft, Vicryl mesh is sewn across it under tension.

For a left lobe graft, the recipient vena cava is removed with the recipient liver. In the left lateral segment graft, the recipient vena cava is left intact. This requires the ligation of multiple vena caval perforators originating from the caudate lobe. The recipient hepatic veins are then converted to a single opening, and the donor left hepatic vein is sewn end to side to the recipient hepatic vein cuff. Usually, in both left lobe and left lateral segment grafts, the graft is rotated about 90 degrees so the cut surface faces the hepatic recess normally occupied by the right hepatic lobe. The donor hepatic artery, if sufficiently long, is directly anastomosed to either the supraceliac or infrarenal aorta. If this is not possible, an iliac artery graft is run from the infrarenal aorta to the donor hepatic artery. The donor portal vein is anastomosed end to end to the recipient portal vein. This can be difficult because the final position of the graft almost always requires the portal vein to travel a circuitous route. The bile duct reconstruction is always a Roux-en-Y choledochoju-

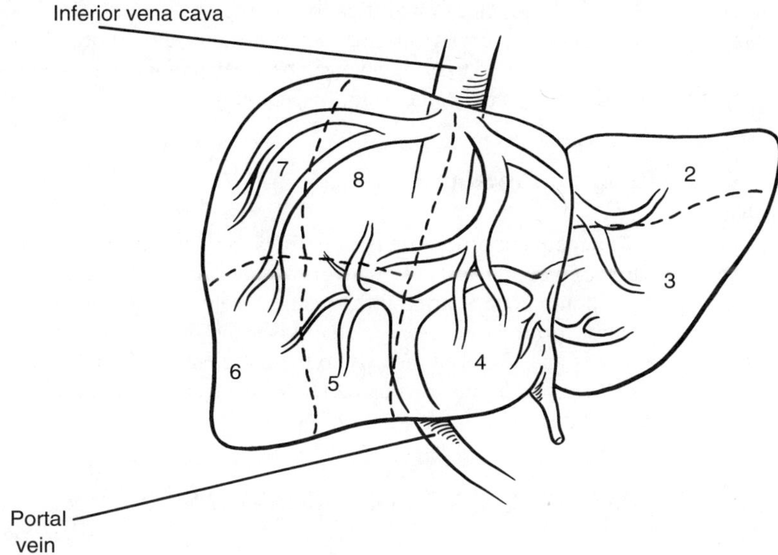

FIG. 43-4. Segmental anatomy of the liver.

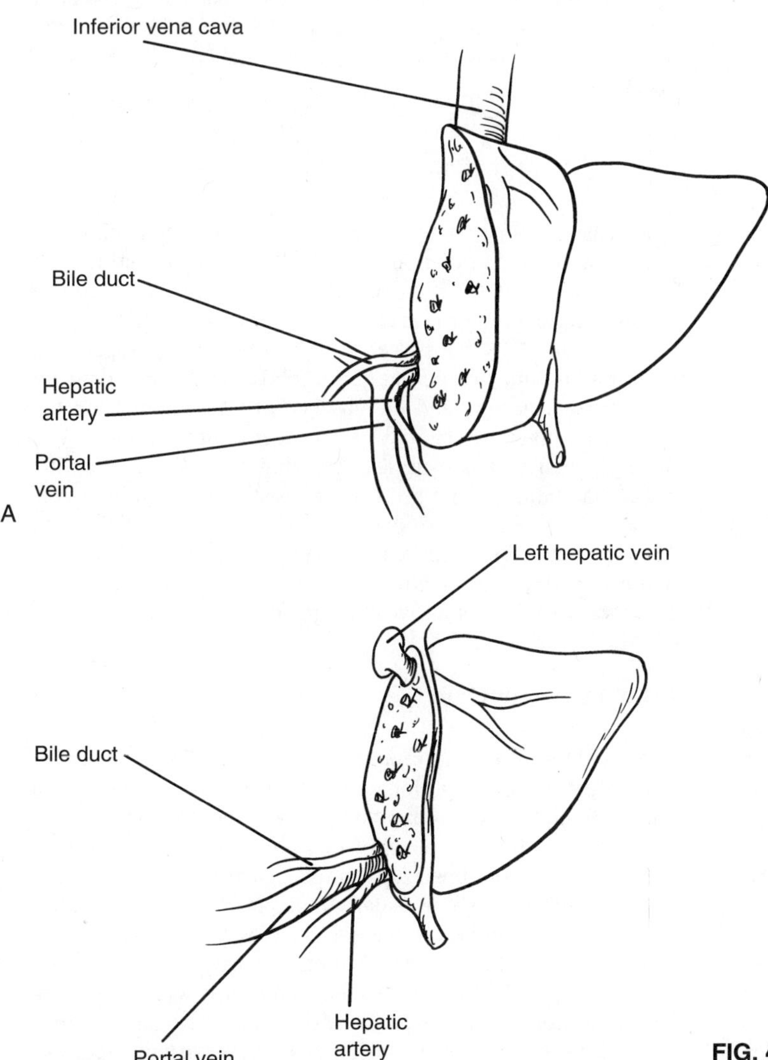

FIG. 43-5. (*A*) Left lobe graft consisting of segments 2 to 4. (*B*) Left lateral segment graft consisting of segments 2 and 3.

nostomy. Bleeding from the cut surface is controlled by direct suture ligation of bleeders through the mesh and by argon coagulation.

Split-Liver Transplantation

One unfortunate aspect of reduced-size transplantation is that a large portion of viable donor liver is discarded. With the ever-increasing shortage of livers, it was logical to attempt to use both parts of the donor liver to transplant two patients. The technique for split-liver transplantation is still in evolution.[17,18] Early experience was less than satisfactory because of complications related to the viability of segment 4 when it was retained with the left lobe graft. Removal of segment 4 has decreased these problems, but the variability of the anatomy of the hepatic artery and biliary system has led to the recommendation that before splitting a liver, both a cholangiogram and a hepatic arteriogram should be performed. Several studies have made recommendations regarding where the arterial, venous, and biliary systems should be divided to minimize postoperative complications.[19]

LIVING, RELATED DONATION

Living, related donor (LRD) liver transplantation was a natural outgrowth of the developments of reduced-size transplantation and split-liver transplantation. Its development was spurred by the need to expand further the donor pool for children weighing less than 10 kg. Reduced-size transplantation has not been as advantageous in children because the relative excess of adult donors has disappeared, and split livers continue to have technical problems. The use of LRDs also increases the potential overall risk to the family by adding a procedure in an otherwise healthy parent or other family member. The ethical issues surrounding LRD transplantation have been extensively debated and, at present, the utility of the procedure outweighs the observed complications. This procedure was first performed in 1989 and has since been expanded in the United States and Japan.[19,20] LRD is now being successfully performed in a number of centers around the world.

Donor Procedure

A bilateral subcostal incision in used. The left triangular and gastrohepatic ligaments are divided. The recommended technique is to remove the left lateral segment (segments 2 and 3) from the donor (Fig. 43-5B). The left hepatic artery is exposed at its bifurcation from the common hepatic artery and the left portal vein is exposed posteriorly. Length is obtained on the left portal vein by ligating the branches to the caudate lobe. The left bile duct is ligated distal to the branch that drains segment 4 (see Fig. 43-5A). The liver is then divided within or on the falciform ligament using finger fracture technique. The left portal vein, left hepatic artery, and hepatic vein are then clamped and divided and the segment is rapidly flushed with University of Wisconsin solution (see Fig. 43-5B). Segments of donor saphenous vein and inferior mesenteric vein are then removed for lengthening of the hepatic artery and portal vein,

which is done under magnification on the back table. Alternatively, cryopreserved autologous saphenous and iliofemoral veins may be used to bridge the gap between donor and recipient hepatic artery and portal vein, respectively.

Recipient Procedure

The recipient procedure is essentially the same as the implantation of the left lateral segment graft from a reduced-size donor. If the donor hepatic arterial flow comes from the aorta, an interposition graft is necessary; otherwise, the donor left hepatic artery is anastomosed directly to the recipient's hepatic artery. The biliary system is reconstructed with a Roux-en-Y choledochojejunostomy.

POSTOPERATIVE COMPLICATIONS

Postoperative complications after liver transplantation can happen for a variety of reasons. The preoperative condition of the patient is strongly associated with the probability of development of a complication. The sicker the patient at the time of transplantation, the greater the chance that there will be a complication, and the longer will be the hospital stay. In the following sections, several of these potential complications are discussed.

Primary Nonfunction

Primary nonfunction is a poorly understood complication that occurs in about 5% of grafts. Basically, primary nonfunction is the absence of function of the new liver despite adequate perfusion. The diagnosis is clear in 72 to 96 hours after surgery and is manifest by the presence of hepatic encephalopathy, a prothrombin time greater than 25 seconds and uncorrectable by fresh frozen plasma, and the absence of bile output from the liver. This diagnosis should be considered intraoperatively if there is persistent nonsurgical bleeding that occurs after the revascularization of the graft. Postoperatively, the initial liver enzymes are often high (alanine aminotransferase of 5000 to 15,000), indicating significant hepatocellular injury. This is a nonrecoverable complication and the patient will die. The only effective treatment is early retransplantation.

Primary Dysfunction

An additional 15% of recipients may suffer from a period of initial dysfunction or prolonged cholestasis. These patients can be differentiated from those with primary nonfunction. Patients with graft dysfunction are not encephalopathic, even though they may have poor bile output or persistently elevated clotting studies. Unfortunately, it usually requires 48 to 72 hours after the transplantation before the two diagnoses can be separated. Primary dysfunction is related to organ harvest injury. A liver biopsy usually shows disordered hepatic cords with ballooning of the hepatocytes and hepatocyte dropout. The clinical course of these patients is often characterized by a persistent hyperbilirubinemia despite normalization of the liver enzymes and coagulation factors. Most of these patients eventually normalize their hepatic function, but it may take 3 to 6 months. A few patients remain persistently cholestatic and require eventual retransplantation. Several factors that seem to carry an increased risk for the development of primary dysfunction include prolonged donor hospitalization (greater than 3 days), older age (greater than 49 years), extended preservation time (greater than 18 hours), fatty changes in the donor liver biopsy specimen, reduced-size liver grafts, and a younger recipient age.[21] Primary dysfunction can also be difficult to separate from rejection. Primary dysfunction patients should have serial liver biopsies to ensure that persistent laboratory abnormalities are not from concomitant rejection.

Vascular Complications

Vascular complications are know to occur with the vena cava, portal vein, and particularly the hepatic artery anastomoses. Complications of the hepatic vein or venal caval anastomoses primarily cause outflow obstruction.[22] This obstruction leads to the clinical symptoms of graft swelling, medically uncontrollable ascites, and poor urine output, mimicking Budd-Chiari syndrome. These suprahepatic or infrahepatic caval obstructions usually are caused when either a whole graft that is small for a recipient or a reduced-size graft rotates into the right upper quadrant recess, thereby torquing the caval anastomosis. This can be confirmed in the early postoperative period by abdominal ultrasound. Vena caval obstruction in the early postoperative period requires reoperation for correction. When implanting small whole livers or reduced-size livers, the graft must be rotated 90 degrees to prevent an obstruction. In addition, the technique for triangulating the caval anastomosis has been described to be associated with a reduced incidence of obstruction. Stricture at the anastomotic site, which causes late outflow obstruction, may be documented by venography and pressure measurements, and can usually be treated by balloon dilatation.

Thrombosis of the portal venous anastomoses is an infrequent complication, occurring in 2% to 3% of transplants. This complication is usually technical and occurs particularly when there is a size disparity between vessels, as noted in reduced-sized grafts. The diagnosis is made by abdominal duplex Doppler ultrasound. If the portal vein clots immediately after surgery and is not corrected, the graft undergoes necrosis and is lost. Therefore, prompt reoperation with declotting of the vein and repair of the technical problem that caused the thrombosis is required to salvage the graft.[23]

Hepatic artery thrombosis (HAT) is the most frequently encountered vascular complication. The hepatic artery is an "end artery" that supplies nutrition predominantly to the extrahepatic and intrahepatic biliary system. If HAT occurs, several potential problems can follow: rarely, submassive to massive hepatic necrosis with intrahepatic abscess formation; necrosis of the extrahepatic biliary system with a bile leak; or necrosis of a portion of the intrahepatic biliary system with formation of infected intrahepatic bilomas and biliary strictures. The incidence of HAT in the pediatric age group has been reported to be as high as 25%, versus 5% in adult series. At our center, the overall incidence of HAT is 8%.

HAT is a difficult diagnosis to make on clinical grounds alone. The classic presentation of HAT is fever beginning 10 days to 2 weeks posttransplantation. The fever occasionally is associated with parenchymal enzyme changes. Graft enlargement with increased firmness may also be present. Confirmation of the diagnosis requires a hepatic arteriogram that shows the absence of hepatic arterial flow to the liver.

The treatment of HAT has undergone substantial changes since the mid-1980s. Initially, it was thought that the only therapy for HAT was immediate retransplantation. Later, it was discovered that these patients could be effectively treated with percutaneous, transhepatic drainage of the intrahepatic bilomas. This was then followed by transhepatic dilation and stenting of the subsequent intrahepatic biliary strictures. This therapy was effective in preventing the need for retransplantation in most of our HAT patients, but it required multiple transhepatic procedures over the ensuing months to years. The development of transabdominal color duplex Doppler ultrasound allowed for the frequent noninvasive monitoring of the hepatic artery. This has prompted the rethinking of the management of HAT. At our center, we follow hepatic artery flow with daily transabdominal Doppler studies for 2 weeks. If a change occurs in the Doppler signal, the patient immediately undergoes an arteriogram. If the arteriogram shows a thrombosis, then urokinase is directly infused into the artery. This dissolves the clot and restores arterial flow to the liver. The patient then is taken to the operating room, where the hepatic artery is reexplored and the arterial anastomosis is revised, either by simple revision or by improving arterial inflow by adding an iliac arterial graft from the recipient aorta to the donor hepatic artery. We have been using this aggressive approach to HAT since 1992, and have had four children follow this protocol. None of these children has required retransplantation, and only one (the first) has had any biliary complications. The early detection and aggressive treatment of HAT can effectively eliminate the traditional complications associated with it. In addition to close monitoring of the hepatic artery flow, some centers routinely use additional pharmacologic methods to decrease the thrombosis rate. These regimens include one or more of the following: low-dose aspirin, dipyridamole, low–molecular-weight dextran, heparin, and prostaglandin E_1. It is not clear if any of these manipulations make a difference because there are no randomized studies. In our pediatric transplants, we only use low–molecular-weight dextran and aspirin in those patients in whom the anastomosis was technically difficult (approximately one third of the cases). Pharmacologic therapy, however, cannot compensate for poor surgical technique. Several additional factors have been reported to be associated with HAT: cyclosporine use, small recipient size (less than 16 kg), a recipient hepatic artery that is less than 3 mm, edema of the graft that occurs as a complication of rejection, and a hypercoagulable posttransplantation state that has been associated with diminished protein C, protein S, and antithrombin 3 levels.[24,25]

Biliary Complications

The biliary anastomosis in transplantation has been called the Achilles' heel of the procedure. The reported incidence of biliary complications ranges from 2.3% to 38%.[26,27] The best method for biliary reconstruction in the absence of a usable recipient bile duct is the end-to-side Roux-en-Y choledochojejunostomy and, when a suitable recipient bile duct is available, an end-to-end choledocho-choledochochostomy.

In a review of our biliary complications, we noted an overall rate of 14%. There was a large preponderance of strictures, with only 12% of the grafts having bile leaks. Most of the early (less than 1 year posttransplantation) biliary complications were associated with HAT. Our initial approach to the biliary complications related to HAT was retransplantation; however, these patients experienced a 60% mortality and a 20% rethrombosis rate. Our next approach was to deal directly with the biliary complications of intrahepatic bilomas and biliary strictures. This was accomplished using transhepatic drainage of abscesses and transhepatic balloon dilatation of strictures. With this aggressive approach, 64% of the grafts with acute biliary complications from HAT were salvaged, and 50% of these patients remain free of biliary complications. Unfortunately, the transhepatic approach is not a panacea, usually requiring more than one procedure and a duration of therapy ranging from 1 to 14 months. During catheter drainage, the patient is at risk for cholangitis, especially during catheter manipulations or contrast studies. Two patients died in our series from biliary catheter-related gram-negative sepsis. It is imperative that broad-spectrum antibiotics be started before and continued for at least 24 hours after any biliary procedure, including contrast studies.

Little data exist regarding late (more than 1 year posttransplantation) biliary strictures. In our series, late biliary strictures occurred in six (4%) patients; two were in duct-to-duct anastomoses and four were in Roux-en-Y reconstructions. Their onset was insidious, occurring from 18 to 51 months after transplantation, with only one patient presenting with symptoms of biliary stasis. Most of theses patients were initially treated for rejection as outpatients, and further work-up with an abdominal ultrasound was initiated only after they failed to respond to therapy. A mechanical problem with the biliary tract must be considered in the differential diagnosis of late hyperbilirubinemia or transaminase elevations. Strictures of the hepatic duct bifurcation were a particularly difficult management problem. Five such strictures occurred in the early group and two in the late group. A transhepatic approach was unsuccessful in treating all of the late strictures and two of the early strictures. Operative revision was performed in three grafts (one early and two late). At each exploration, dense fibrous tissue was noted at the site of the strictures. This type of biliary injury could be explained by either an ischemic insult or trauma to the area.[28] However, the long time to the development of these strictures makes an injury that occurred at the time of transplantation unlikely. We use indwelling stents for biliary reconstruction. It has been suggested that the stent could be a source of of chronic irritation to the biliary system, causing stricture formation.[29]

Retained biliary stents deserve additional mention. We have encountered two patients in whom the surgically placed biliary stent failed to pass 4 and 26 months after transplantation. In both cases, the stent served as a nidus for biliary stone formation, resulting in biliary tract obstruction. Both patients required stent removal followed by transhepatic biliary lithotripsy to remove the impacted stones. We have also seen one patient in whom a retained stent perforated the Roux-en-Y limb. If, after 4 months, a stent is still found in either the biliary system or the Roux-en-Y limb, serious consideration should be given to its removal.

Infection

Infection from bacterial, viral, or fungal causes continues to be the single largest complication after liver transplantation. Bacterial infections have predominated at our center. Most of these are related to central lines. We change all intraoperative central lines within 5 days, and if longer central access is necessary, cuffed central lines are inserted. Intraabdominal bacterial infections are not as frequent now as they were in the past. Several factors have contributed to this decrease: intraoperative bacterial and fungal cultures are taken of both subhepatic spaces and patients are immediately treated for any positive bacterial or fungal results; intraabdominal hematomas are surgically evacuated to remove them as a potential culture medium; and fungal cultures of the Roux-en-Y lumen are taken and the patient immediately treated if they are positive. Despite these measures, a persistent problem is bacterial and fungal infections at the cut edge of a reduced-size liver graft. All patients with a reduced-size graft have a fluid collection at the cut surface, and in our series 54% (13/24) of these were of a significant size. Of these, 62% (8/13) became infected, and of these, three were fungal. Bacterial infections were readily diagnosed by percutaneous aspiration followed by percutaneous drainage of the abscess. If the abscess at the cut surface contains fungus (*Candida* sp), operative drainage with Penrose drains is necessary.

CMV is a common pathogen in postoperative liver transplant patients.[30] CMV infection can be either primary (liver graft of transfused blood as source) or reactivated. An additional risk factor for CMV infection is the aggressive use of immunosuppression and, in particular, the use of antilymphocyte globulin.[8] Intravenous ganciclovir is the treatment of choice. A variety of prophylactic protocols for the prevention of CMV infection have been published. All have centered around the use of intravenous γ-globulin (regular or CMV hyperimmune), oral acyclovir, intravenous ganciclovir, or oral ganciclovir.

EBV infections are important in children because of their association with posttransplantation lymphoproliferative disorder (PTLD).[31] Evidence of EBV activation should prompt a reduction in immunosuppression. At our center, we use a polymerase chain reaction (PCR) technique as a marker for an acute EBV infection. PTLD may present as focal nodal disease, as an extranodal mass, or as an infiltrative process. A confirmed diagnosis of PTLD is initially treated with either reduction or withdrawal of immunosuppression and the initiation of antiviral therapy with either acyclovir or ganciclovir. Extensive disease or PTLD that is resistant to withdrawal of immunosuppression requires additional treatment with either interferon-α or chemotherapy.

Rejection

Despite improvements in immunosuppressive regimens, rejection continues to be a significant problem after liver transplantation. To minimize the effects of rejection, the diagnosis must be made promptly and early treatment initiated. Rejection after liver transplantation can be divided into three categories: hyperacute (humoral), acute, and chronic.

Hyperacute rejection is most commonly seen in kidney transplantation where there is a positive antibody cross-match, and occurs within minutes after the graft is reperfused. In liver transplantation, even with a positive cross-match, hyperacute rejection is rare. Even in the face of an ABO-incompatible (ABO-I) transplant (eg, A donor into O recipient), elevations in the donor antibody titer do not occur until the fifth to seventh postoperative day. In addition, the major site of injury in the liver from an ABO-I transplant is not the endothelium, but rather the biliary epithelium.

Acute cellular rejection is the most common form of rejection after liver transplantation, and it occurs in 50% to 70% of all patients. The clinical diagnosis of rejection in children can be difficult. Rejection usually occurs between the 7th and 14th posttransplantation days, but it can occur any time. Commonly, the parents note that the child is not as active or playful as normal. Occasionally, fever can be present along with an increase in graft size and firmness. Increased white blood cell counts can also occur. The most common diagnostic criterion is an increase in the liver function tests, primarily in the γ-glutamyl transferase and, to a lesser extent, in the alanine and aspartate aminotransferases. Unfortunately, none of these clinical criteria is absolutely diagnostic of rejection. Infections such as CMV or EBV can mimic the clinical pattern of rejection. The best diagnostic tool for rejection is the liver biopsy. Histologically, rejection is defined as a mixed lymphoid infiltrate (lymphocytes, neutrophils, eosinophils) that is concentrated in the portal areas, with associated bile duct injury. Endothelial injury, especially around the central veins, is a variable component of this pattern. The utility of the liver biopsy is not only to diagnose rejection, but, often as important, to rule out other causes of liver dysfunction.

Chronic rejection after liver transplantation is often suspected but difficult to prove. The generally recognized definition of chronic rejection is histologic. There is a loss of the bile ducts from greater than 50% of portal triads when at least 15 to 20 portal triads are counted, there is occlusion of the medium-sized arterioles with "foam cells," and there is little or no portal infiltrate. Another term for chronic rejection is the "vanishing bile duct syndrome." It is not clear what the mechanism is for this process, but it is thought to be a combination of humoral and cell-mediated processes. Chronic rejection is suspected when a rising γ-glutamyl transferase and total bilirubin develop in the absence of biliary obstruction. This pattern can gradually appear or it can occur after the treatment of a severe rejection episode. The diagnosis of chronic rejection requires multiple liver biopsies from different sites so a sufficient number of portal areas can be obtained.

The treatment of rejection is a stepwise process. If humoral rejection is suspected, as in an ABO-I transplant, plasmapheresis is initiated to decrease the antibody level. A liver biopsy is also obtained to determine if there is the coexistence of cellular rejection. Acute cellular rejection can be treated a variety of ways, and treatment tends to be center specific. In general, the initial therapy is a steroid (methylprednisolone) boost. If this is not effective, additional treatment with antilymphocyte preparations such as OKT3 (mouse monoclonal antibody to the CD3 receptor on the T lymphocyte) or an antithymocyte preparation (polyclonal antibody preparation, usually made by injecting horses with a human thymus cell preparation). More recently, additional antirejection medications, including tacrolimus and mycophenolate mofetil, have become available for use in acute rejection.

The treatment for rejection, if it is diagnosed and treated promptly, is over 95% effective. It is rare for a pediatric patient to lose a graft because of acute rejection alone. Chronic rejection is a very difficult process to treat. Until relatively recently, there has been no effective therapy except for retransplantation. If caught early, before there is widespread bile duct loss, and the total bilirubin is less than 4, treatment with tacrolimus has been able gradually to restore the liver function studies to normal in 60% to 70% of cases. However, once there is widespread bile duct loss, there is no effective therapy. In a few anecdotal cases, bile ducts have been reported to reappear if the patient remains clinically well except for jaundice. Unfortunately, these reports stated that at least a year elapsed from the original diagnosis of chronic rejection to the time that the bile ducts reappeared. Most patients with chronic rejection do not remain well for this period of time, and retransplantation is necessary.

IMMUNOSUPPRESSIVE MANAGEMENT

Our immunosuppressive management has evolved over time. We now use a tacrolimus-based immunosuppressive regimen along with steroids (Table 43-4). Immediately after transplantation, the child is treated only with a polyclonal antithymocyte preparation (ATGAM) and methylprednisolone. Because both cyclosporine and tacrolimus are nephrotoxic, the use of the ATGAM allows time for the liver and kidneys to recover from the transplantation. Once the patient has an adequate urine output and the prothrombin time has decreased to normal (usually by the second to fourth day after transplantation), cyclosporine or tacrolimus therapy is initiated.

Acute rejection is confirmed with a liver biopsy and treated with three daily boluses of steroids (10 mg/kg/d of methylprednisolone) and an increase in the tacrolimus level to 15 to 20 ng/mL. If this is not effective, the steroid boluses are repeated. If this is not effective, a repeat liver biopsy is performed. If this still shows rejection, mycophenolate mofetil is added to the steroids and tacrolimus. Patients who are on a cyclosporine-based regimen in whom rejection develops are also treated with three steroid boluses. If this is not effective, the boluses are repeated. If this fails, then the patient is converted to tacrolimus, with target levels of 15 to 20 ng/mL. If this fails, a repeat liver biopsy is performed, and if rejection is still present, the patient is treated with either OKT3 or the addition of mycophenolate mofetil.

RESULTS

We have reviewed our results after 10 years of pediatric liver transplantation, during which time 225 transplants were performed in 202 patients. It must be remembered, however, that transplantation over the last decade has undergone a revolution. Sacred dictums have become old wives' tales, and procedures that were thought impossible are now commonplace. Any retrospective analysis in this type of environment is immediately flawed because experience, and therefore clinical practice, is constantly changing. Since the mid-1980s, our immunosuppressive protocols have changed, we have improved and expanded our surgical techniques, new antiviral and antibacterial agents have been developed, and the care of the critically ill child has improved. In reviewing our experience, it would be inappropriate to interpret our 10-year survival rates as an indicator

TABLE 43-4. *Immunosuppression in the pediatric liver transplant recipient*

Year	Induction	Maintenance
1984–1987	None	Prednisone — 10 mg/kg in operating room >40 kg — 200–20 mg in 5 d <40 kg — 100–20 mg in 5 d Cyclosporine — Start postoperative d1 at 6 mg/kg/d IV. Start PO when tolerating diet at 20 mg/kd/d. Target level of 300–400 ng/mL by whole-blood HPLC
1987–1990	None	Same as above, with the addition of azathioprine, 1–2 mg/kg/d
1990–1992	Antithymocyte preparation 15–20 mg/kg/d for 3–5 d in patients with pretransplantation renal dysfunction	Same as above: triple therapy with prednisone, azathioprine, and cyclosporine. Target levels 350–400 ng/mL by whole-blood TDX assay.
1992–1994	Antithymocyte preparation (ATGAM) 15–30 mg/kg/d for a minimum of 3 d	Methylprednisolone 1 mg/kg IV qd × 3 d; 0.75 mg/kg IV qd × 2, then prednisone 2 mg/kg/d tapered to 1 mg/kg/d in 2 wk, then to 0.25 mg/kg/d at 1 mo, and 0.1 mg/kg/d by 3 mo. Cyclosporine and azathioprine as above.
1994–1996	As above, with ATGAM limited to 3–5 d for renal sparing	Steroids as above. Tacrolimus started when prothrombin time has normalized at 0.3 mg/kg/d. Dose adjusted to level of 12–15 ng/mL. No azathioprine

HPLC, high-pressure liquid chromatography.

of the potential for pediatric liver transplantation. Rather, they should serve as a baseline from which improvements can be made.

Our overall patient survival rates for the entire series of children at 1, 5, and 10 years were 76%, 70%, and 61%, respectively, and the overall graft survival rates for 1, 5, and 10 years were 71%, 63%, and 59%, respectively (Fig. 43-6). The pretransplantation diagnosis of a metabolic disease positively affected 10-year survival (90%), and the pretransplantation diagnosis of acute hepatic failure adversely affected survival (43%; Fig. 43-7). This is not surprising, because most patients with metabolic liver disease are in good nutritional and physiologic condition except for their metabolic defect. Patients in acute hepatic failure who require transplantation, however, require intensive care management, are in either stage III or stage IV hepatic coma, and often have renal compromise. Therefore, the preoperative condition of the patient, at least at the extremes, does have an influence on outcome. These same conclusions were reached by Burdelski and colleagues,[32] in a discussion of outcomes after pediatric liver transplantation for metabolic

diseases, and by Hanid and coworkers[33] and Lidofsky and colleagues,[34] who reported a 50% to 70% survival rate after transplantation for acute hepatic failure. The survival of patients with biliary atresia (62% at 10 years) closely approximated the survival of the total group (61% at 10 years; see Fig. 43-7). This is important because, before transplantation, these patients often are in poor nutritional condition, have a coagulopathy, and have had previous surgery. Because posttransplantation survival was not decreased in the biliary atresia group, and because the Kasai operation yields a 20% to 30% chance of long-term bile drainage, it would appear to be logical to proceed with a Kasai procedure before liver transplantation. In addition, even though the Kasai procedure may fail, it may function long enough for the patient to experience some linear growth, thereby increasing the potentially available donor pool. Otte and associates[35] also reported excellent survival rates with liver transplantation in 198 children with biliary atresia (82% at 1 year and 78% at 5 years), and these data also support the use of the Kasai procedure before transplantation.

Age less than 1 year has been reported to yield poorer out-

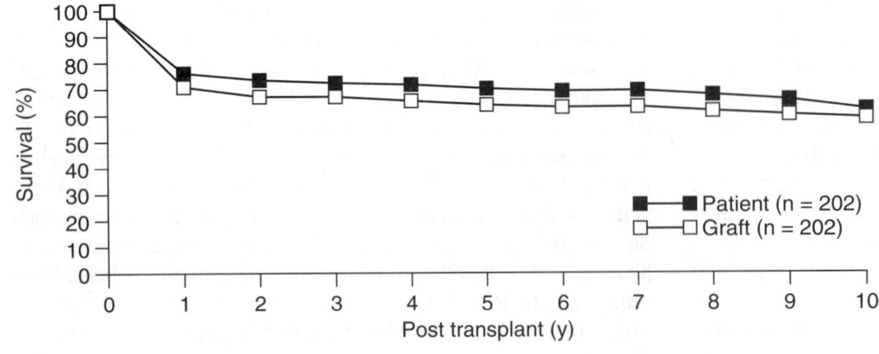

FIG. 43-6. Actuarial patient and liver graft survival for 10 years.

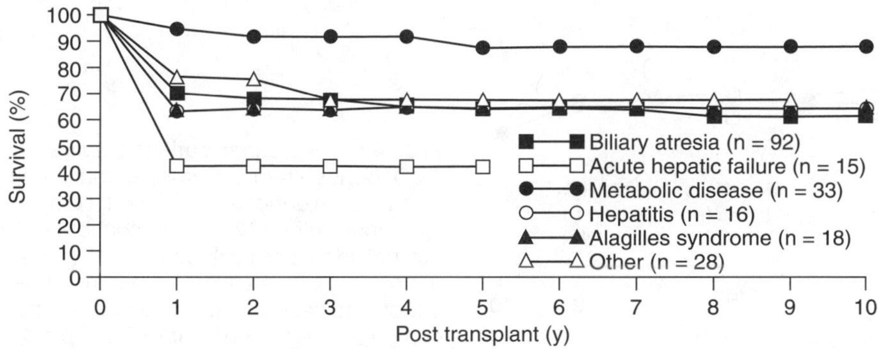

FIG. 43-7. Actuarial patient survival by pretransplantation diagnosis.

come after liver transplantation.[36] In our series, age below 1 year did not adversely effect outcome. The most likely explanation for this is that the less than 1-year-old group did not experience a higher incidence of hepatic artery thrombosis or biliary complications compared to the patients older than 1 year of age.

Our 5-year patient survival rate after retransplantation was worse than with a primary graft (72% vs. 50%). This is not surprising, because 76% of the retransplanted patients were UNOS status 4 patients at the time of retransplantation. Even though 50% of the patients were ultimately salvaged with retransplantation, its avoidance would obviously be beneficial. One of the significant causes for retransplantation was HAT. Our protocol for the detection and management of HAT has substantially decreased the morbidity from this problem. Rejection was responsible for one quarter of the graft losses that required retransplantation, and two thirds of these were from chronic rejection. The chronic rejection graft losses were seen early in our experience. In the last 5 years, chronic rejection has not been a significant problem. Primary nonfunction occurred in 1% of our patients and always required retransplantation for survival.

Patient survival has been reported to be adversely affected by a poor preoperative status.[12] To evaluate this, we compared patient and graft survivals between groups based on their pretransplantation UNOS status (Fig. 43-8). Patient and graft survival rates at 5 and 9 years were 10% to 15% poorer in the UNOS status 4 patients, but this was not statistically significant. These data support our current policy that, once accepted for transplantation, a patient would be excluded only for an acute systemic infection or irreversible brain injury.

One of the more recent technical advances has been the use of reduced-size grafts in pediatric patients.[37] This technique was developed because of the shortage of size-matched cadaveric donors, and during its development (1986 to 1988) there was an apparent excess in adult and older child donors. Initially, we used this technique only in our sickest patients, with a subsequent high mortality that was unrelated to the procedure (49% 5-year survival). With additional experience, our patient and graft survival is now comparable to that in whole-organ transplants, and we routinely use this technique. Unfortunately, with the expansion of both the indications and the ages for potential adult liver transplant recipients, the relative excess of these donor organs has disappeared and the waiting time for a pediatric recipient has again increased.

There has been controversy surrounding graft survival in the black transplant population.[38,39] This prompted us to evaluate our patient and graft survivals stratified by race. Our black recipients had better 5-year patient and graft survival rates (76% and 76%) than the other races (70% and 63%). There were no retransplantations in the black population. The poorest 5-year patient and graft survival rates were noted in the Latin American population (65% and 59%). None of these survival differences was statistically significant, and there are no obvious explanations for these differences.

Our center has been interested in the use of ABO-I livers for transplantation since 1987. The use of ABO-I transplants is controversial, and the literature gives conflicting results.[40–42] We have transplanted 23 ABO-I transplants with a 5-year patient survival rate that is comparable to the total group (61% vs. 69% P = ns; Fig. 43-9). Graft survival, however was decreased at 7 years (44% vs. 62%). The reason for this discrepancy is that the first three patients who received an ABO-I graft received conventional immunosuppressive management. They

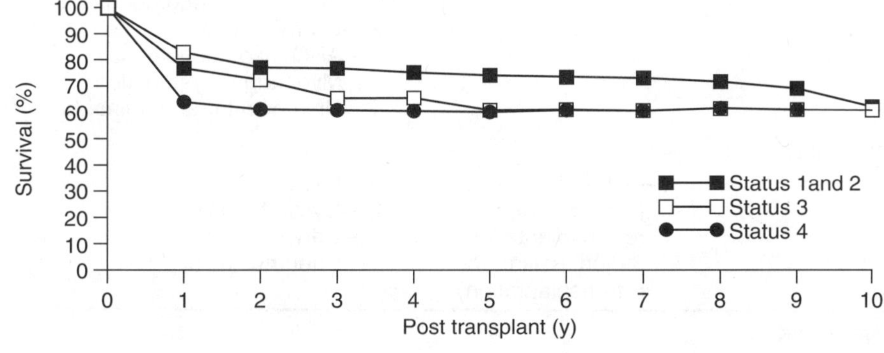

FIG. 43-8. Actuarial patient survival by United Network for Organ Sharing status. Status 1, home doing well; status 2, in and out of the hospital; status 3, requires continuous hospitalization; status 4, requires continuous intensive care.

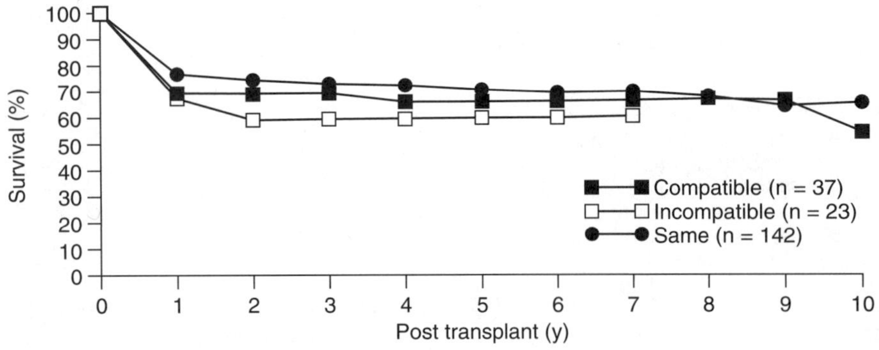

FIG. 43-9. Actuarial patient survival by ABO donor status. Same, same blood type for both donor and recipient; compatible, donor blood type is compatible with but not identical to the recipient (eg, O donor into A recipient); incompatible, donor and recipient blood types are not compatible (eg, A donor into O recipient).

all lost their grafts, and two subsequently died. The remaining patients were treated under a prospective protocol that uses plasmapheresis to decrease the donor ABO titer in the recipient. With the prospective use of this protocol, the 3-year patient and graft survival rates have increased to 67% and 59%, respectively. These numbers are not significantly different from the 3-year patient and graft survival rates for the ABO compatible group (70% and 67%). We reserve ABO-I transplants for UNOS status 3 and 4 patients.

The direct results of improvements in techniques and knowledge are best illustrated by our improvements in patient and graft survival. Between 1993 and 1995, our patient survival rate was 88% and our graft survival rate was 82%. This improved survival was associated with a substantial decrease in the number of days the patients stayed in the hospital after transplantation (less than 14 days).

The best way to improve survival, obviously, is to prevent the complications that lead to patient death. As a model, we reviewed the methodology proposed by Shaw and colleagues.[12] Deaths were stratified into four categories according to possible antecedent causes. After their analysis of 21 adult and 23 pediatric deaths, Shaw and colleagues concluded: 1) poor preoperative physiologic status results in a poor transplantation outcome; 2)

surgical errors played a minor role in deaths; 3) aggressive rejection therapy can lead to immunocompromise and death; and 4) seemingly successful transplants can be lost for a variety of unexpected reasons.

In our series, after evaluating the deaths that occurred less than 6 months posttransplantation, we modified our protocols (Table 43-5). To decrease the deaths attributed to Shaw and colleagues' category 1, we now are using ICP monitoring in patients with stage 4 hepatic coma to manage increased ICP better.[34,43] We are attempting to decrease our category 2 deaths by our new management protocol for HAT. Infections at the cut surface of a reduced-size liver, as discussed previously, are a problem. With our current management program, these infections have been readily controlled. The deaths caused by accelerated rejection have not be seen in the last 5 years. In the last category, the causes of eight technical deaths have been addressed and corrective measures instituted. The septic and pulmonary complications have been diminished by the introduction of effective therapy for CMV infections and improved critical care management. PTLD remains a perplexing problem, but the advent of an EBV PCR has allowed earlier detection of an infection so that immunosuppression can be rapidly lowered or discontinued. High-dose acyclovir prophylaxis and im-

TABLE 43-5. *Deaths after pediatric liver transplantation, from a total series of 202 patients*

Category 1	Category 2	Category 3	Category 4
DEATHS <6 MO AFTER TRANSPLANTATION (43 PATIENTS)			
7—Acute hepatic failure with stage IV coma	3—Hepatic artery thrombosis 2—Massive blood loss 1—Infected liver cut surface 1—Prolonged portal vein occlusion 1—Cardiac arrest 1—Lung hemorrhage	3—Accelerated rejection	8—Technical problems 4—Lung infections (2 viral, 2 bacterial) 3—PTLD 2—Lung hemorrhage 2—Pulmonary decompensation 2—Gram-negative sepsis 1—ABO incompatible 1—Myocardial dysfunction 1—Unknown intrabdominal bleed
DEATHS >6 MO AFTER TRANSPLANTATION (17 PATIENTS)			
0	1—Hepatic artery thrombosis	7—Chronic rejection (4 died after retransplantation, 3 died waiting for retransplantation)	5—PTLD 2—Cystic fibrosis 1—Cancer 1—Pneumonia

PTLD, posttransplantation lymphoproliferative disorder.

munoglobulin therapy has been used since 1994 for CMV and potentially EBV prophylaxis. It is still too early to assess the effectiveness of this approach on the development of PTLD. The remaining four deaths remain disturbingly unexplained (two pulmonary hemorrhages, one myocardial dysfunction, and one late intraabdominal bleed).

Over 40% of the late deaths were related to a failure of immunosuppression, with subsequent chronic rejection and retransplantation. A variety of new immunosuppressive agents are under investigation, and the real potential for a decrease in chronic rejection exists in the near future.[44] The other major cause of late deaths was the diffuse form of PTLD.[45,46] Most disturbingly, all of these episodes occurred without any antecedent rejection therapy or increased immunosuppression. Two patients died before therapy could be instituted, and three failed to survive with treatment. We are exploring a modification of a Hodgkin disease chemotherapy protocol that may have some promise in these difficult patients.

In summary, except for the cases of acute hepatic failure, the patients' antecedent physiologic condition did not contribute directly to posttransplantation death. Surgical complications continue to cause morbidity, but only rarely lead to posttransplantation mortality. To decrease mortality, any complication must be rapidly detected and aggressively corrected. It is hoped that acute and chronic rejection will become less of a problem with the advent of newer immunosuppressive agents. PTLD is currently our greatest threat to long-term survival. The release of the newer and more powerful immunosuppressive agents may decrease the incidence of chronic rejection, but the price may be overimmunosuppression with the development of PTLD. Pediatric liver transplantation is a successful therapeutic modality for children with end-stage liver disease. A reasonable long-term posttransplantation survival is possible, and with ongoing medical advances, this survival can only be expected to increase.

The main limitation in the application of this life-saving therapy is the availability of donors. Pediatric patients are already at a disadvantage because major trauma in small children is infrequent and declining with the wide application of car seat, seat belt, swimming pool, and helmet laws. Therefore, each potential pediatric donor becomes an even more precious resource. Education of our medical and surgical colleagues about the success of pediatric liver transplantation can be an effective approach to increasing organ donation.

ALTERNATIVES TO TRADITIONAL TRANSPLANTATION

Unfortunately, in situations of either acute or chronic hepatic decompensation, a liver may not be readily available. There are few alternatives that can be used to stabilize a patient until an organ becomes available. Three techniques are undergoing investigation. One involves the use of a cartridge that contains hepatocytes (either porcine or human hepatoblastoma cells) suspended in a matrix that surrounds semipermeable hollow fibers. As the recipient's blood passes through these hollow fibers, the hepatocytes clear the toxins. The second technique involves the extracorporeal use of a liver (either porcine or human) that is hooked directly to a recipient. This is not a new technique, but it has been revived as a bridge to transplantation. The use of porcine livers for extracorporeal perfusion has had limited clinical success because of hyperacute vascular rejection. Finally, direct hepatocyte transplantation into the spleen has been investigated. This technique has been promising in animals, but its usefulness for humans is unknown.

REFERENCES

1. Starzl TE, Groth CG, Bretteshneider L, et al. Orthotopic homotransplantation of the human liver. Ann Surg 1968;168:392.
2. Starzl TE, Iwatsuki S, Van Theil DH, et al. Evolution of liver transplantation. Hepatology 1982;2:614.
3. Calne RY, Murray JE. Inhibition of the rejection of renal homografts in dogs by Burroughs Wellcome 57-222. Surg Forum 1961;12:118.
4. Calne RY, Rolles K, White DJG, et al. Cyclosporin A initially as the only immunosuppressant in 34 recipients of cadaveric organs: 32 kidneys, 2 pancreases, and 2 livers. Lancet 1979;2:1033.
5. Pichlmayr R, Brendel LJ, Zenker R. Production and effect of heterologous anticanine lymphocyte serum. Surgery 1967;61:774.
6. Ringe B, Pichlmayr R, Burdelski M. A new technique of hepatic vein reconstruction in partial liver transplantation. Transplant Int 1988;1:30.
7. Pichlmayr R, Ringe B, Gubernatis G, et al. Transplantation einer Spenderleber auf zwei Empfanger (Splitting-Transplantation): Eine neue Methode in der Weiterenteicklung der Lebersegmenttransplantation. Langenbecks Arch Chir 1988;373:127.
8. Broelsch CE, Whitington PF, Emond JC, et al. Liver transplantation in children from living related donors: surgical techniques and results. Ann Surg 1991;214:428.
9. United Network for Organ Sharing OPTN/Scientific Registry. June 24, 1994.
10. Koneru P, et al. Liver transplantation for hepatoblastoma: the American experience. Ann Surg 1990;213:118.
11. Malatack J, et al. Choosing a pediatric recipient for orthotopic liver transplantation. J Pediatr 1987;111:479.
12. Shaw B, Wood P, Stratta R, et al. Stratifying the causes of death in liver transplant recipients: an approach to improving survival. Arch Surg 1989;124:895.
13. Farinati F, et al. Serum and salivary caffeine clearance in cirrhosis: any role in the selection for surgery and timing for transplantation? J Hepatol 1993;18:135.
14. Shiffman M, et al. Hepatic lidocaine metabolism and complications of cirrhosis. Transplantation 1993;55:830.
15. Kennard B, et al. Soc Work Health Care 1990;15:19.
16. Emond JC, Whitington PF, Thistlethwaite JR, et al. Reduced-size orthotopic liver transplantation: use in the management of children with chronic liver disease. Hepatology 1989;10:867.
17. Emond JC, Whitington PF, Thistlethwaite JR, et al. Transplantation of two patients with one liver. Ann Surg 1990;212:14.
18. Rat P, Paris P, Friedman S, et al. Split-liver orthotopic liver transplantation: how to divide the portal pedicle. Surgery 1992;112:522.
19. Emond JC. Clinical application of living-related liver transplantation. Gastroenterol Clin North Am 1993;22:301.
20. Mori K, Nagata I, Yamagata S, et al. The introduction of microvascular surgery to hepatic artery reconstruction in living-donor liver transplantation: its surgical advantages compared with conventional procedures. Transplantation 1992;54:263.
21. Ploeg RJ, D'Alessandro AM, Knechtle SJ, et al. Risk factors for primary dysfunction after liver transplantation: a multivariate analysis. Transplantation 1993;55:807.
22. Edmond JC, Heffron TG, et al. Reconstruction of the hepatic vein in reduced size hepatic transplantation. Surg Gynecol Obstet 1993;176:11.
23. Moreno Gonzalez E, Garcia Garcia I, et al. Liver transplantation in patients with thrombosis of the portal, splenic or superior mesenteric venin. Br J Surg 1993;80:81.
24. Hennein HA, Mendeloff EN, et al. Aortic revascularization of orthotopic liver allografts: indications and long-term follow-up. Surgery 1993;113:379.
25. Mor E, Schwartz ME, et al. Prolonged preservation in University of Wisconsin solution associated hepatic artery thrombosis after orthotopic liver transplantation. Transplantation 1993;56:1399.

26. Evans RA, Ruby ND, O'Grady JG, et al. Biliary complications following orthotopic liver transplantation. Clin Radiol 1990;41:190.
27. Ringr B, Oldhafer K, Bunzendahl H, et al. Analysis of biliary complications following orthotopic liver transplantation. Transplant Proc 1989; 21:2472.
28. Li S, Stratta RJ, et al. Diffuse biliary tract injury after orthotopic liver transplantation. Am J Surg 1992;164:536.
29. Rouch DA, Emond JC, Thistlethwaite JR, et al. Choledochocholedochostomy without a T-tube or internal stent in transplantation of the liver. Surg Gynecol Obstet 1990;170:239.
30. Stratta RJ, Shaeffer MS, et al. Cytomegalovirus infection and disease after liver transplantation: an overview. (Review) Dig Dis Sci 1992; 37:673.
31. Sokal EM, Caragiozoglou T, et al. Epstein-Barr virus serology and Epstein-Barr virus-associated lymphoproliferative disorders in pediatric liver transplant recipients. Transplantation 1993;56:1294.
32. Burdelski M, Rodeck B, Latta A, et al. Treatment of inherited metabolic disorders by liver transplantation. J Inherit Metab Dis 1991;14:604.
33. Hanid M, Davies M, Mellon P, et al. Clinical monitoring of intracranial pressure in fulminant hepatic failure. Gut 1980;21:866.
34. Lidofsky S, Bass N, Prager M, et al. Intracranial pressure monitoring and liver transplantation for fulminant hepatic failure. Hepatology 1992;16:1.
35. Otte JB, de Ville de Goyet J, Reding R, et al. Sequential treatment of biliary atresia with Kasai portoenterostomy and liver transplantation: a review. Hepatology 1994;20:415.
36. Esquivel C, Koneru B, Karrer F, et al. Liver transplantation before 1 year of age. J Pediatr 1987;110:545.
37. Broelsch C, Emond J, Thistlethwaite JR, et al. Liver transplantation, including the concept of reduced-size liver transplants in children. Ann Surg 1989;208:410.
38. Cecka J, Ghertson D, Cho Y, et al. HLA polymorphisms, ethnicity, and graft survival. Transplant Proc 1993;25:2446.
39. Greenstein S, Schechner R, Tellis V, et al. Twenty-five year review of race and transplantation at a single institution. Transplant Proc 1993; 25:2448.
40. Renard TH, Shimaoka S, Le Bherz D, et al. ABO-incompatible liver transplantation in children: a prospective approach. Transplant Proc 1993;25:1953.
41. Lo C, Shaked A, Busuttil R. Risk factors for liver transplantation across the ABO barrier. Transplantation 1994;58:543.
42. Tanaka A, Tanaka K, Kital T, et al. Living related liver transplantation across ABO blood groups. Transplantation 1994;58:548.
43. Keays R, Potter D, O'Grady J, et al. Intracranial and cerebral perfusion pressure changes before, during, and after orthotopic liver transplantation for fulminant hepatic failure. QJM 1991;79:425.
44. Ferraresso M, Kahan B. New immunosuppressive agents for pediatric transplantation. Pediatr Nephrol 1993;7:567.
45. Ho M, Jaffe R, Miller G, et al. The frequency of Epstein-Barr virus infection and associated lymphoproliferative syndrome after transplantation and its manifestations in children. Transplantation 1988;45:719.
46. Makatack J, Gartner C, Urback A, et al. Orthotopic liver transplantation, Epstein-Barr virus, cyclosporine, and lymphoproliferative disease: a growing concern. J Pediatr 1991;118:667.

Surgery of Infants and Children: Scientific Principles and Practice, edited by Keith T. Oldham, Paul M. Colombani, and Robert P. Foglia. Lippincott–Raven Publishers, Philadelphia, © 1997.

CHAPTER 44

Heart and Lung

Theodore C. Koutlas and Thomas L. Spray

Since the mid-1980s, thoracic organ transplantation has become successfully established in the pediatric patient population. Transplantation is now an important option in the treatment of congenital heart and lung disease, as well as the end-stage diseases of those organs. Unfortunately, despite the clinical success in heart and lung transplantation in children, problems with donor availability, especially for infant recipients, have severely limited this form of treatment. Pediatric heart and lung transplant recipients make up only about 6% to 8% of all thoracic transplant patients. In addition, problems such as chronic rejection, graft coronary artery disease (CAD), bronchiolitis obliterans, and the infectious and neoplastic complications of current methods of immunosuppression pose serious questions regarding the long-term utility of thoracic organ transplantation. This chapter focuses on the clinical aspects of heart, lung, and heart–lung transplantation in infants and children, including indications, preoperative evaluation, operative techniques, postoperative management, and outcome.

HEART TRANSPLANTATION

Early experimental work in heart transplantation was reported by Carrel in 1905, then by Demikhov from the Soviet Union in 1946. After extensive research by Lower and Shumway at Stanford in the early 1960s, Barnaard performed the first successful orthotopic heart transplantation in South Africa in 1967. Over the next year, over 100 transplants were performed throughout the world, but the results were extremely poor because of allograft rejection or opportunistic infection. The introduction of cyclosporine immunosuppression in the early 1980s, combined with the development of endomyocardial biopsy techniques and a uniform method of grading rejection, drastically improved recipient survival. Although a number of heart transplantations were performed on older children in the early years of heart transplantation, it was not until 1985 that the first successful neonatal cardiac transplantation was performed, by Bailey at Loma Linda. This was preceded by his unsuccessful attempt at cardiac xenotransplantation in a newborn.

Over 1600 heart transplantations have been performed worldwide on patients younger than 18 years of age, and approxi-

mately 150 are performed yearly in the United States.[1] There is a bimodal age distribution among heart transplant recipients (Fig. 44-1); a large group of patients are infants with complex congenital heart disease, most of these younger than 2 months of age, whereas another group is scattered about the early teenage years as a result of the impact of cardiomyopathy on that age group (Fig. 44-2).

The primary indication for heart transplantation in infancy is complex congenital heart disease without a reasonable corrective or palliative surgical option. The most common congenital anomaly treated by neonatal heart transplantation is hypoplastic left heart syndrome (HLHS), a group of defects characterized by aortic or mitral atresia/stenosis with a diminutive left ventricle. Although several centers have had success with a staged palliative approach to HLHS, this has not been widespread, and the mortality rates for this approach have remained high at many centers that have otherwise good results with other forms of congenital heart disease. This has led many centers such as Loma Linda to consider orthotopic heart transplantation as the primary treatment for this anomaly. Long transplant waiting lists have led some institutions to advocate performing a stage I palliation (Norwood procedure) to help stabilize the patient and discontinue the prostaglandins, then listing the patient for heart transplantation.[2] Other forms of congenital heart disease treated by cardiac transplantation during infancy include unbalanced atrioventricular canal, single ventricle, complex truncus arteriosus, double-outlet right ventricle, Ebstein anomaly, L-transposition of the great arteries, and pulmonary atresia with intact ventricular septum.[3] Congenital cardiomyopathy is also an uncommon indication for heart transplantation in infancy.

Children with congenital heart disease who have undergone previous corrective or palliative procedures may exhibit residual or progressive cardiac dysfunction that ultimately requires cardiac transplantation. This group makes up approximately 30% of pediatric heart transplantations from ages 1 to 18 years.[1] Cardiac dysfunction is often related to atrioventricular or semilunar valvar insufficiency, which then results in a dilated cardiomyopathy. A small subgroup of these patients have postcardiotomy cardiac failure requiring extracorporeal membrane oxygenation (ECMO) or a ventricular assist device to maintain life. Even the most complex forms of congenital heart disease, such as heterotaxy syndromes and other anomalies of systemic

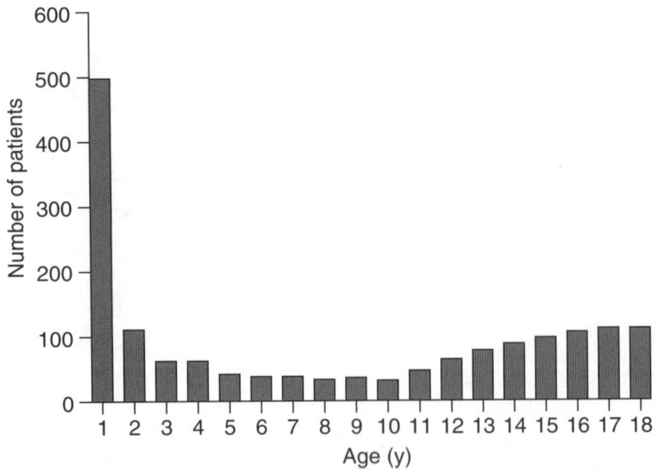

FIG. 44-1. The distribution of pediatric heart transplant recipients by age.

and venous drainage, are amenable to cardiac transplantation with suitable reconstruction.[4,5] Multiple previous palliative procedures, including those involving the pulmonary arteries, do not preclude successful transplantation.[6]

Most pediatric heart transplantations outside infancy are for cardiomyopathy, over half of which are idiopathic in nature. Other etiologies of cardiomyopathy include viral, familial, and hypertrophic. Other, less common indications for cardiac transplantation are doxorubicin-induced cardiotoxicity from chemotherapy for malignancy, and obstructive cardiac tumors such as fibromas and rhabdomyomas that are not amenable to surgical resection.

Preoperative Evaluation

The pretransplantation evaluation is a multidisciplinary screening process that is a vital aspect of successful organ transplantation programs. Potential recipients undergo a thorough physical and psychosocial evaluation. The presence of an adequate family support system is of paramount importance; parents must demonstrate the ability and resources to comply with the complex medical regimens transplant recipients require, and cope with the potential for long or frequent hospitalizations. In addition to this multidisciplinary evaluation, patients undergo screening laboratory tests, including a viral serology panel (eg, human immunodeficiency virus, cytomegalovirus (CMV), Epstein-Barr virus, hepatitis). The cardiac evaluation is performed by echocardiography and cardiac catheterization. The anatomy of systemic and pulmonary venous connections of the heart and the pulmonary arteries is precisely identified. Important hemodynamic data obtained at catheterization include the systemic cardiac output (Qs) and pulmonary vascular resistance (PVR$_i$), both indexed to the patient's body area:

$$\text{Cardiac Index (L/min/m}^2) = \frac{\text{O}_2 \text{ consumption}}{\text{Systemic Arterial O}_2 \text{ content} - \text{Mixed Venous O}_2 \text{ content}}$$

$$\begin{array}{l}\text{Pulmonary Vascular} \\ \text{Resistance, indexed} \\ \text{(mm Hg/L/min/m}^2)\end{array} = \frac{\begin{array}{c}\text{mean PA pressure} \\ - \text{ mean LA pressure}\end{array}}{\text{Pulmonary flow, indexed}}$$

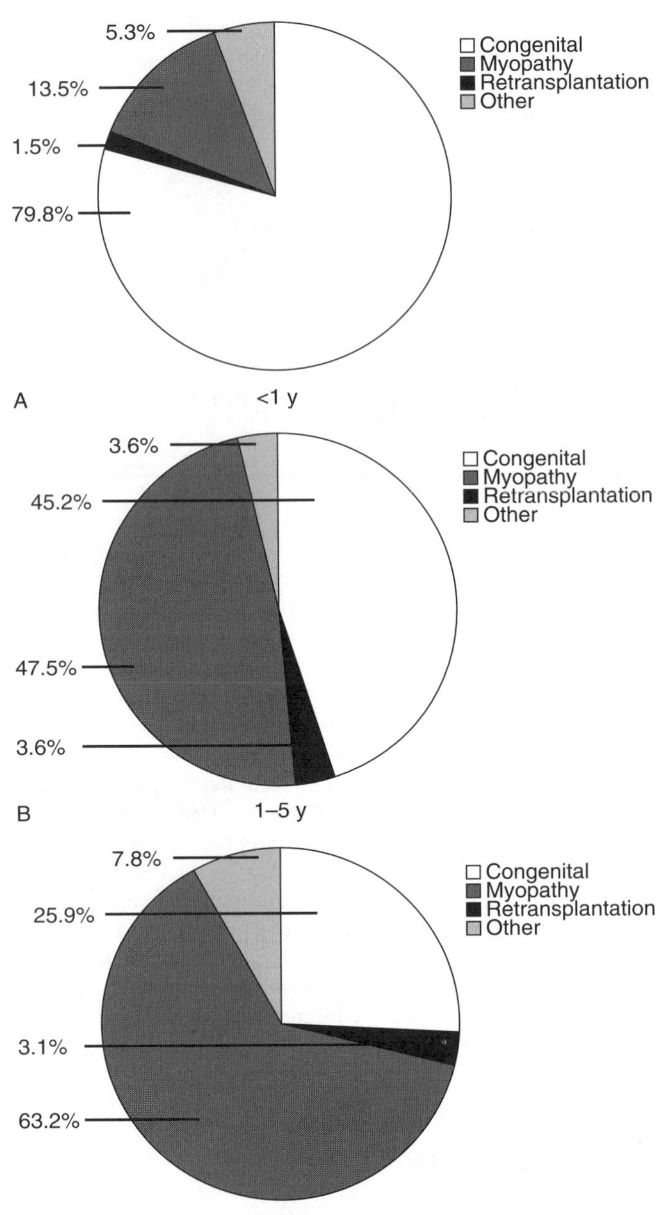

FIG. 44-2. Indications for pediatric heart transplantation by age: (*A*) younger than 1 year, (*B*) 1 to 5 years, (*C*) 6 to 18 years.

Patients with elevated PVR$_i$ (greater than 4 to 6 Wood units) are tested with pulmonary vasodilators, including sodium nitroprusside, oxygen (F$_{IO_2}$ 100%), and inhaled nitric oxide to establish whether the pulmonary vascular bed is reactive. In general, the presence of a fixed PVR$_i$ in excess of 6 to 8 Wood units is a contraindication to orthotopic heart transplantation. Patients who demonstrate improvement with vasodilators may be transplanted with a survival rate comparable to that in patients with normal resistance.[6] Although patients with fixed pulmonary hypertension have been successfully transplanted, they have a much higher mortality rate, usually because of postoperative right ventricular failure. Other contraindications to cardiac transplantation include multiple noncardiac congenital anomalies, active malignancy, infection, severe metabolic disease (ie, diabetes mellitus), multiple organ failure, and the lack of an adequate family support system.

Children with cardiomyopathy are referred for cardiac transplantation for chronic congestive heart failure that limits activity, or arrhythmias that are difficult to control. The mortality for idiopathic dilated cardiomyopathy in children is highest in the first year after diagnosis. Patients with left ventricular shortening fractions of less than 15% by echocardiography and no improvement on follow-up echocardiography have the lowest survival rates, and should be referred for transplantation early.[7] The timing for transplantation in children with hypertrophic cardiomyopathy is less clear, because some patients may improve with medication. Those patients with poor diastolic function, despite medical therapy, or recurrent arrhythmias, should be recommended for cardiac transplantation.

Children listed for heart transplantation should be closely monitored until their transplantation, either as outpatients if their condition permits, or while hospitalized. Good nutritional status should be maintained, and supplementation such as tube feedings used as needed. A close watch for infectious complications is important, and any subtle indications of infection should be thoroughly investigated. Major infections require patients to have their transplantation status put on hold until they are treated adequately. Anticongestive therapy should be optimized, using digoxin, diuretics, and afterload reduction with captopril or other angiotensin-converting enzyme inhibitors. If heart failure worsens, hospitalization may be required for inotropic support with dobutamine or phosphodiesterase inhibitors such as amrinone or milrinone. Long-term therapy may require the placement of an intravenous access device such as a broviac catheter. The use of ECMO as a bridge to cardiac transplantation in critically ill children has been limited, mostly to children with postcardiotomy ventricular failure. Although survival rates of up to 50% have been reported, in general, results have been poor.[8]

The infant or neonate referred for cardiac transplantation requires several other considerations. Infants with complex congenital heart disease such as HLHS are commonly confined to a neonatal intensive care unit, and usually maintained on a continuous infusion of prostaglandin E_1 to prevent closure of the ductus arteriosus if there is ductal-dependent physiology. Balloon atrial septostomy may be helpful if there is a restrictive patent foramen ovale, to improve mixing of saturated and desaturated blood and decompress the left atrium. Other important issues are the maintenance of adequate nutritional support, avoidance of renal and metabolic complications, and the prompt and thorough treatment of any infectious complications, especially line sepsis, in these fragile infants. Common neonatal problem such as seizures, necrotizing enterocolitis, and intraventricular hemorrhage are also seen in these patients. At the minimum, 10% to 20% of infants die while awaiting a donor heart.[4] As mentioned earlier, initial palliative procedures such as the Norwood procedure for HLHS, or Blalock-Taussig shunt for lesions with ductal-dependent pulmonary blood flow, can be performed in the face of a prolonged wait for a donor.

In 1988, the United Network for Organ Sharing developed a classification for patients awaiting heart transplantation. Status I applies to all infants younger than 6 months of age, and older children and adults who require stay in an intensive care unit, inotropic or ventilatory support, or intraaortic balloon pump or ventricular assist device support. All other patients with less acuity are classified status II. A patient's status may change depending on changes in their clinical condition, or the patient may be placed on hold because of infection or other complication, then later reactivated.

Donor Organ Procurement

Criteria for an ideal donor organ are as follows:

- Meets requirement for brain death
- Consent from next of kin
- ABO compatibility
- Weight compatibility
- Normal echocardiogram
- Age younger than 35 years
- Normal heart by visual inspection at time of harvest

The shortage of suitable organ donors, especially for neonatal recipients, has led to many attempts at expanding the donor pool. Hearts from donors requiring prolonged cardiopulmonary resuscitation or significant inotropic support, or with moderately impaired ventricular function by echocardiogram (left ventricular shortening fraction greater than 25%, without major wall motion abnormalities), have been successfully transplanted in infant recipients.[4] Donor-to-recipient weight ratios of up to 4 : 1 have been used in infants, and ischemic times have been successfully extended upward of 9 hours. Deviations from the "ideal" donor criteria should be individualized, and although the use of a marginal donor for a dying infant on ECMO may be justified, the use of the same heart for a child stable as an outpatient would not.

Good donor management is a vital part of successful organ transplantation. The main goals are maintenance of normothermia, euvolemia, adequate tissue perfusion, and prevention of infection. Often, donors with poor cardiac function on initial evaluation will respond to volume loading and low-dose inotropic support with a significant improvement in function. A recent chest radiograph, blood counts, and cultures for febrile episodes should be obtained to screen for evidence of infection in the donor. Diabetes insipidus is common in organ donors after brain death, and should be treated with vasopressin to prevent severe volume depletion.

Once the donor is in the operating room, heparin and antibiotics are given. The heart is approached through median sternotomy, and suspended in a pericardial cradle. The aorta is mobilized as distal to the head vessels as possible, especially if the recipient has HLHS. Once the venae cavae are sufficiently mobilized, the proximal superior vena cava is ligated, and the ascending aorta is cross-clamped (Fig. 44-3A). Cold crystalloid cardioplegia is infused in the aortic root, and the heart is vented by dividing the inferior vena cava and either a right pulmonary vein or the tip of the left atrial appendage (see Fig. 44-3B). After the cardioplegia is infused, the heart is excised by lifting the apex superiorly and dividing the pulmonary veins posteriorly, either separately, or leaving a small cuff of left atrium, depending on whether the lungs are being procured for transplantation as well (see Fig. 44-3C). The superior vena cava is

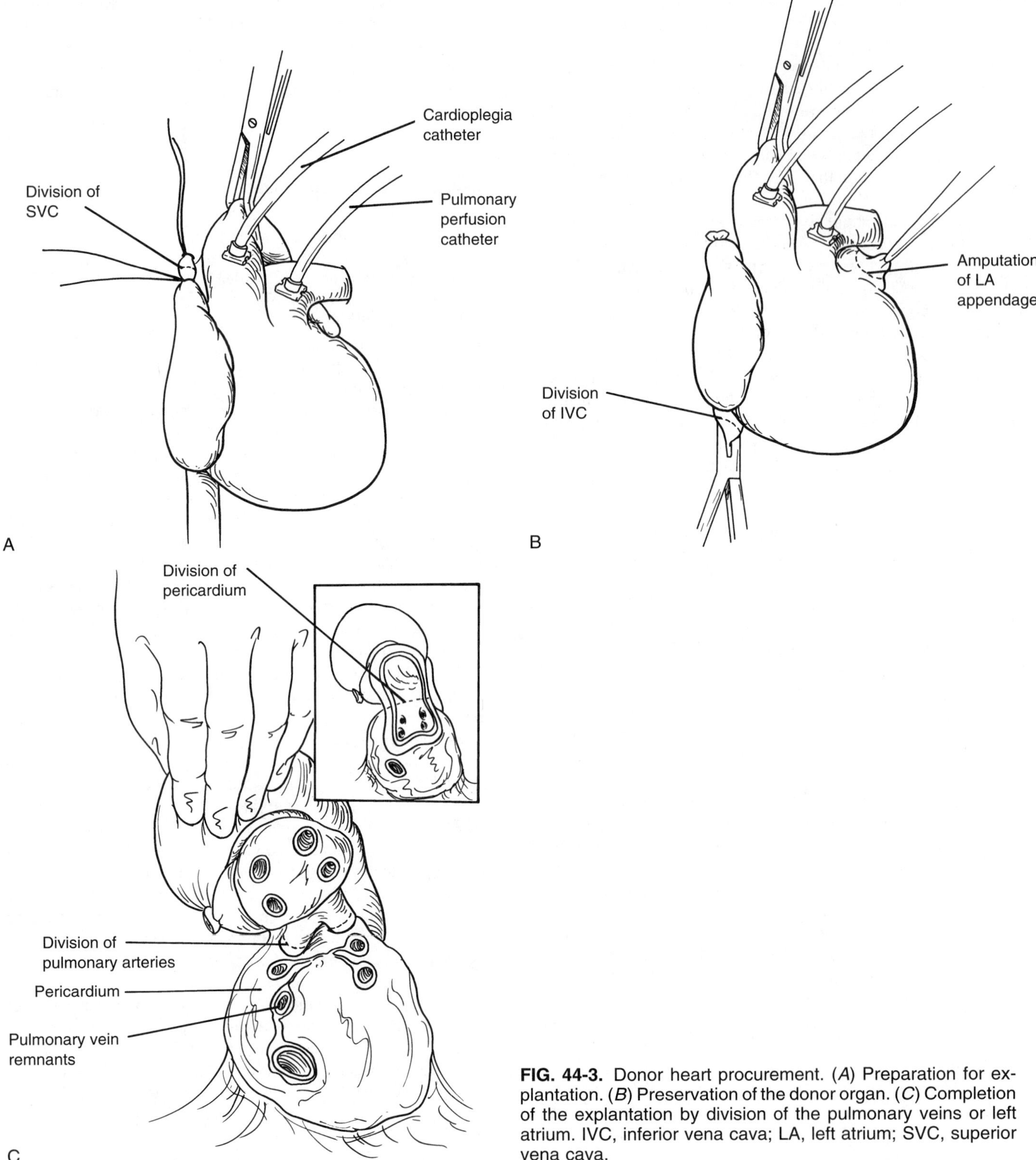

FIG. 44-3. Donor heart procurement. (*A*) Preparation for explantation. (*B*) Preservation of the donor organ. (*C*) Completion of the explantation by division of the pulmonary veins or left atrium. IVC, inferior vena cava; LA, left atrium; SVC, superior vena cava.

then divided proximal to its ligation point, and the aorta divided as far distal as possible. Excess tissue such as venae cavae or pulmonary veins is taken if needed for implantation because of recipient anomalies. The donor heart is placed in cold (4°C), sterile saline, then triple bagged in a sterile manner for transport. Preparing the organ by removing excess tissue is reserved for just before implantation, to prevent the potential discard of any important tissue. In general, cold ischemic time is limited to a maximum of 4 to 5 hours.

Recipient Procedure

Once adequate hemodynamic monitoring is in place and the recipient is properly anesthetized, a median sternotomy is performed, and the heart is suspended in a pericardial cradle. If there have been previous sternotomies, appropriate precautions should be taken, including the groins in the sterile field for access for femoral bypass, and the use of an oscillating sternal saw. Once in the chest, the main pulmonary artery is dissected off the aorta past the bifurcation, and the pericardial reflection is mobilized off the aortic arch. In the case of a recipient with HLHS, the aortic arch vessels are mobilized proximally and controlled with snares, and the descending thoracic aorta is dissected to a level 2 to 3 cm below the insertion of the ductus arteriosus. The right and left pulmonary arteries are mobilized and controlled with snares in preparation for cardiopulmonary bypass. After heparinization, the main pulmonary artery is cannulated for arterial inflow, and a single venous cannula is placed in the right atrium because circulatory arrest will be used (Fig. 44-4A). Immediately on instituting cardiopulmonary bypass, the pulmonary arteries are snared tight, perfusing the body through a patent ductus arteriosus. The recipient is cooled to 18°C for circulatory arrest. Once the donor organ is available in the operating room (cardiopulmonary bypass is usually not commenced until the procurement team arrives in the operating room) and the patient has been adequately cooled, circulatory arrest is established, the arch vessels are snared tightly, and the patient is exsanguinated into the venous reservoir. The aorta is divided just above the valve and incised longitudinally along the lesser curve of the aortic arch to a level 1 to 2 cm below the ductal insertion site on the descending aorta (see Fig. 44-4B). The ductus is ligated next to the pulmonary artery and divided, then the main pulmonary artery is transected just below the bifurcation. The right atrial incision is started superiorly at the base of the appendage. This incision is then carried down into the coronary sinus and across the atrial septum into the left atrium (see Fig. 44-4C). The superior aspect of the right atrial incision is then carried across the septum, opening the roof of the left atrium. The lateral wall of the left atrium is the incised above the left pulmonary veins, including the left atrial appendage with the specimen (see Fig. 44-4D).

While the recipient heart is explanted, the donor organ is prepared on the back table in a cold saline solution. The right atrium is incised from the inferior vena cava laterally to the base of the appendage, avoiding the area of the sinoatrial node. The pulmonary vein confluence is excised off the back of the left atrium, leaving an opening comparable in size to the recipient left atrial cuff. The pulmonary artery is transected just below the bifurcation to provide a wide anastomosis. The aorta is trimmed depending on the level required in the recipient. Care

must be taken to check for and adequately close a patent foramen ovale, which is frequently present, especially in infant hearts. Failure to do so may result in significant postoperative right-to-left shunting in the face of pulmonary hypertension.

The implantation is begun by anastomosing the lateral wall of the left atrium, from the level of the left atrial appendage inferiorly (see Fig. 44-4E). Monofilament absorbable suture is used for all anastomoses to provide potential for long-term anastomotic growth. A left ventricular vent is placed through the right superior pulmonary vein, and the left atrial anastomosis is completed by reconstructing the intraatrial septum. The arch of the aorta is then reconstructed (see Fig. 44-4F). The right atrial anastomosis is begun at the inferior vena cava orifice, then taken superiorly along the intraatrial septum (see Fig. 44-4G). Once the right atrial anastomosis is completed, the ligature is removed from the donor superior vena cava, and the venous cannula is placed through the vena caval stump. The ascending aorta is then cannulated by a new pursestring, air is evacuated, and cardiopulmonary bypass resumed. The snares are released from the head vessels and warming is commenced. The pulmonary anastomosis is then performed in an end-to-end fashion. If time permits, this may be done during circulatory arrest in a drier field. After adequate warming, the patient is weaned from cardiopulmonary bypass and the cannulas removed (see Fig. 44-4H). Right atrial, left atrial, and occasionally pulmonary artery pressure catheters are placed before discontinuing bypass, and brought out through the skin below the incision.

In older children with cardiomyopathy or infants without aortic arch abnormalities, the recipient procedure is similar to that performed on adults. The ascending aorta is mobilized to the pericardial reflection and is used for arterial cannulation. The child is cooled to 26° to 28°C only, because the implantation is done under aortic cross-clamp, not circulatory arrest. After the atrial anastomoses, the aortic anastomosis is performed in an end-to-end fashion in the mid-ascending aorta. The pulmonary artery anastomosis may or may not be performed during aortic cross-clamp, depending on the amount of time the implant takes.

There are numerous other variations of the implantation procedure, depending on the recipient anatomy present. Modifications accounting for a persistent left superior vena cava, prior cavopulmonary shunt or Fontan procedure, corrected transposition of the great arteries, and situs inversus totalis have all been described, but are beyond the scope of this chapter.[4,5]

Postoperative Management

The recipient is returned from the operating room to an isolation room in the intensive care unit. Mechanical ventilation is required initially, but is weaned as rapidly as possible. Antibiotics are continued until all monitoring lines and chest tubes have been removed. In older patients, early ambulation is encouraged.

Some level of inotropic support is required in virtually all heart transplant recipients. Isoproterenol is often an ideal choice because of the inotropic and chronotropic effects, because many patients have a slower-than-optimal heart rate initially. Dobutamine and dopamine, especially at ''renal dose,'' are also frequently used. Epinephrine and norepinephrine are usually reserved for poor graft function. Sodium nitroprusside infusion

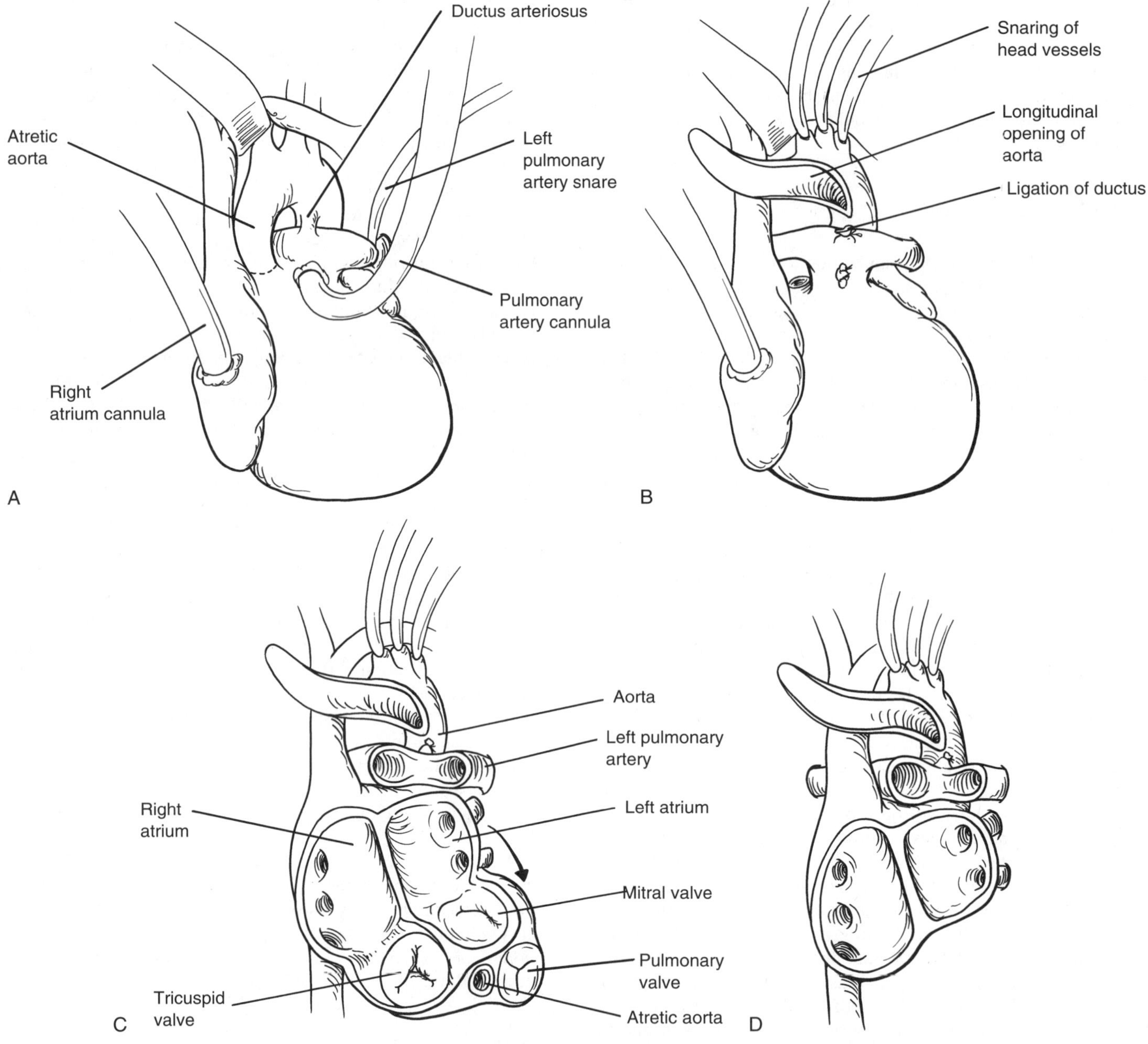

FIG. 44-4. Recipient procedure. (*A*) Cannulation of the recipient with hypoplastic left heart syndrome. (*B*) Longitudinal incision in the recipient aortic arch. (*C*) Excision of the recipient heart, preserving right and left atrial cuffs. (*D*) Explantation of recipient heart completed. (*E*) Implantation of the donor organ beginning at the left atrial anastomosis. (*F*) Aortic arch reconstruction for the recipient with hypoplastic left heart syndrome. (*G*) Completion of the right atrial anastomosis. (*H*) Implantation complete, with decannulation after weaning from cardiopulmonary bypass. (*continued*)

is used for afterload reduction in the early postoperative period. Right ventricular dysfunction due to pulmonary hypertension may respond to phosphodiesterase inhibitors such as amrinone or milrinone. Inhaled nitric oxide has been shown to be an effective selective pulmonary vasodilator with few systemic side effects, and is useful in cardiac transplant recipients with pulmonary hypertension.

Standard triple-drug (prednisone, cyclosporine, azathioprine) immunosuppression therapy has been successfully used in pediatric cardiac transplant recipients.[9] The induction and maintenance doses of medications used for immunosuppression at the Children's Hospital of Philadelphia are listed in Table 44-1. Because of the adverse effects of corticosteroids on somatic growth in children, withdrawal from prednisone is usually at-

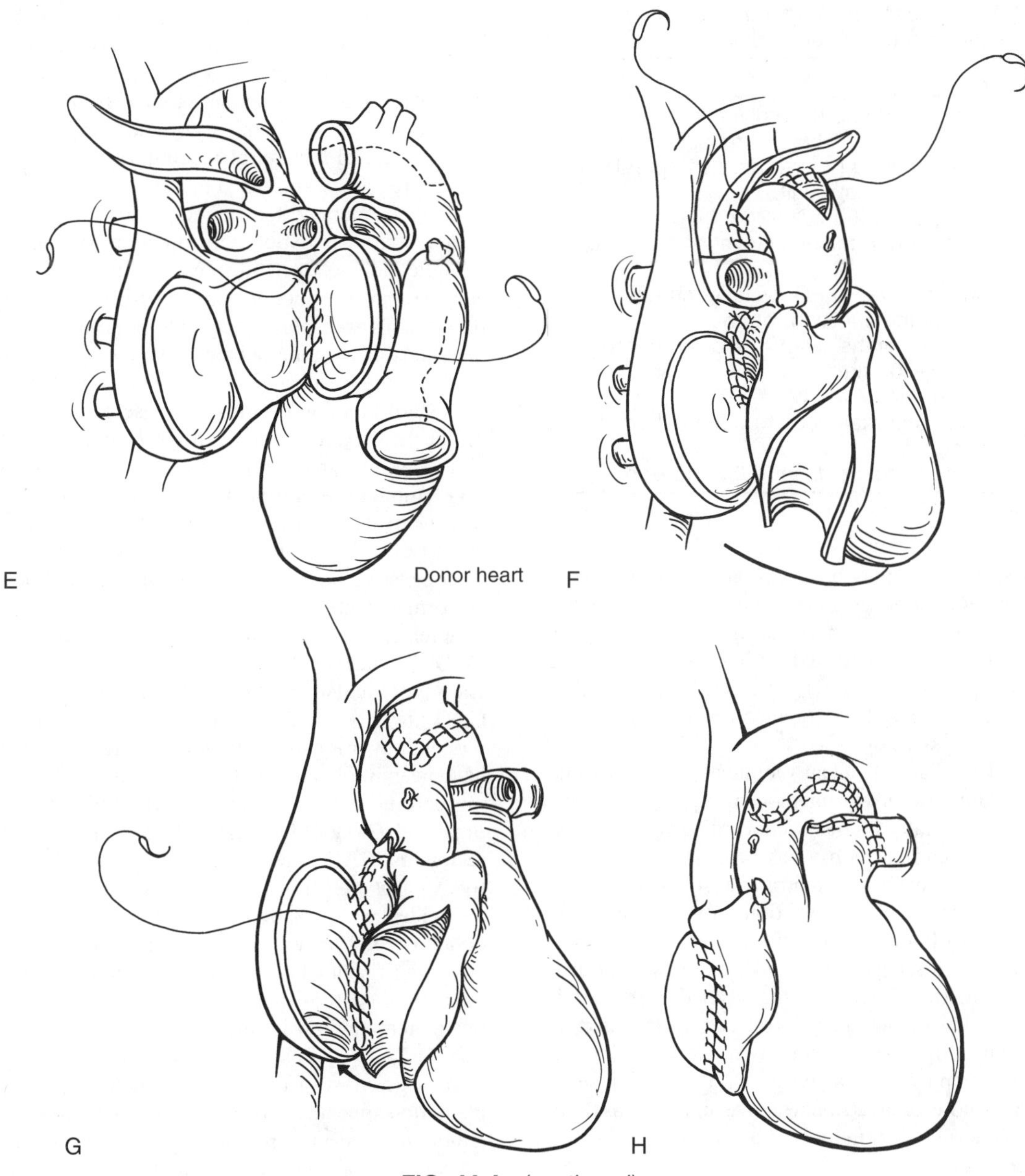

FIG. 44-4. *(continued)*

tempted at 6 months posttransplantation. It has been shown that up to 80% of patients may be successfully weaned from steroids; only one fourth of these patients have an episode of rejection in the first 6 months.[10] Some cardiac centers recommend the use of OKT3 (a murine monoclonal CD3 antibody) or antithymocyte globulin induction therapy for 2 weeks posttransplantation.[11] Although this appears to be well tolerated by most recipients, there has been concern linking the use of these agents with an increased incidence of posttransplantation lymphoproliferative disease. Tacrolimus (formerly called FK-506) has been shown by the Pittsburgh group[12] to be an effective immunosuppressive agent in children. Unfortunately, limited availability has prevented more widespread use of the drug. Recipients with significant cyclosporine side effects such as hirsutism and gingival hyperplasia, however, may benefit from switching to tacrolimus.

Infectious prophylaxis includes oral nystatin for fungal prophylaxis, and oral trimethoprim-sulfamethoxazole three times per week. Pentamidine inhalation treatment is an effective alternative to trimethoprim-sulfamethoxazole for *Pneumocystis carinii* prophylaxis if bone marrow suppression is a problem. Routine CMV prophylaxis is not used in cardiac transplant recipients at our institution.

Complications

Acute rejection and infection are the most common complications after cardiac transplantation. Nearly 60% to 75% of patients have at least one episode of rejection, and it should be expected that about a third will have an episode in the first 3 months, 50% within the first year posttransplantation.[13] Some

TABLE 44-1. *Heart and lung transplantation immunosuppression regimen*

Drug	Dosage
Azathioprine	2–3 mg/kg/d; one dose given in the operating room, before transplantation
Cyclosporine	0.25–0.5 mg/kg IV over 3 h postoperatively in intensive care unit
	Then, 1.5–2.5 mg/kg/24 h by continous infusion to maintain level of 300–350 ng/mL
	Change over to PO cyclosporine as intestinal function returns
	After 6 months, level is allowed to drop to 200–300 ng/mL
Prednisone	1 mg/kg/d for 2 wk, IV or PO
	Then decrease dose to 0.5 mg/kg/d for 6 mo
	Then decrease dose to 0.2 mg/kg/d

studies suggest that infants may be less prone to rejection than older children.[4,13] Rejection episodes have also been shown frequently to correlate with low cyclosporine levels. Episodes of acute rejection are usually treated with a 3-day course of intravenous methylprednisolone (10 mg/kg). OKT3 and antithymocyte globulin are reserved for an incomplete response or rejection refractory to steroids.

Unlike in adult cardiac transplant recipients, there is some controversy regarding the proper method of rejection surveillance in children, especially infants. Echocardiography-guided transjugular endomyocardial biopsy has been shown to be an effective means of monitoring pediatric transplant recipients for rejection.[14] The protocol for rejection surveillance at the Children's Hospital of Philadelphia includes routine endomyocardial biopsy before discharge, at 3 and 6 months posttransplantation, and again after the recipient is weaned from prednisone. Biopsy procedures are also performed if rejection is suspected clinically. Signs and symptoms of cardiac rejection include changes in appetite or activity, fever, or increase in resting heart rate more than 20 bpm above normal baseline. The international grading system for cardiac transplant rejection is shown in Table 44-2.

Although infectious complications are common in cardiac

TABLE 44-2. *The international grading system for cardiac transplant rejection*

Grade	Description
0	No rejection
1	
A	Focal (perivascular or interstitial) infiltrate without necrosis
B	Diffuse but sparse infiltrate without necrosis
2	One focus only with aggressive infiltration or focal myocyte damage
3	
A	Multifocal aggression infiltrate or myocyte damage
B	Diffuse inflammatory process with necrosis
4	Diffuse, aggressive, polymorphous ± infiltrate, ± edema, ± hemorrhage, ± vasculitis, with necrosis

transplant recipients, infection-related deaths do not appear to be. Bacterial infections are most common in the early posttransplantation period, but can occur late after transplantation, and usually respond to proper antibiotic therapy. Of viral infections, CMV appears to be the most common, and is treated with intravenous ganciclovir. Viral respiratory infections usually occur with a frequency similar to that in normal children, and appear to be well tolerated by the recipient.

Aside from rejection and infection, the main postoperative complications after heart transplantation are hypertension, seizures, renal dysfunction, or liver dysfunction. Nearly 10% of infant heart transplant recipients require perioperative peritoneal dialysis. Among neonates, 10% to 15% require phenobarbital therapy for postoperative seizures, which may result from the use of circulatory arrest in these patients.[4]

The primary late complications of pediatric cardiac transplant recipients are chronic rejection, graft CAD, and posttransplantation lymphoproliferative disease. Rejection may account for up to 25% of deaths after cardiac transplantation.[15]

The onset of graft CAD may be suggested by symptoms of congestive heart failure in recipients. Echocardiograms are performed routinely during follow-up visits of heart transplant recipients, and worsening ventricular function is a sign of graft CAD. The new onset of arrhythmias after transplantation, especially ventricular, may be an indication of underlying CAD.[16] CAD may also be found on routine follow-up catheterization, without any prior suggestion of disease. A number of etiologies have been implicated in the development of graft CAD, including chronic cellular rejection, hyperlipidemia, vascular rejection, and CMV infection. Unlike in adult cardiac transplant recipients, CAD appears to develop in pediatric patients relatively early after transplantation, with one series demonstrating an incidence of 35% by 2 years after transplantation.[17] A review of 815 pediatric transplantation patients found nearly 8% to have significant CAD by angiogram or autopsy findings.[18] The mean time posttransplantation to diagnosis was 2.2 years, with one patient having significant CAD 2 months after transplantation. Only 20% of patients diagnosed with graft CAD were still alive, with most of the deaths sudden or unexpected. Retransplantation appears to be the only viable option for these patients, although the results are not especially encouraging, with 1- and 3-year survival rates of 71% and 47%, respectively, and with CAD developing in the second grafts in 20% of retransplantation patients.[19]

Neoplastic disease is seen in 3% to 7% of long-term transplantation survivors.[15] Most have a lymphoproliferative disorder, most often B-cell but occasionally T-cell in type. Most of these patients have evidence of an exposure to Epstein-Barr virus infection. As mentioned previously, there may be a correlation between the use of OKT3 or antithymocyte globulin and the late onset of lymphoproliferative disease.[20] Most cases of lymphoproliferative disease respond to a reduction in immunosuppression and treatment with acyclovir. Other malignancies seen much less frequently include squamous cell carcinomas and hepatocellular carcinoma.[15]

Results

The largest group of infant cardiac transplant recipients reported in the literature is from Loma Linda, where over 140 heart transplantations in infants younger than 1 year of age have been performed.[4] Nearly 70% of these were for HLHS, and the rest were for other complex congenital anomalies (20%) or cardiomyopathy or tumor (8%). The operative (30-day) survival rate was 89%, with the primary causes of mortality primary graft failure, technical problems, pneumonia, or acute rejection. The average postoperative hospitalization was 2 to 3 weeks. There were nine late deaths, most of these resulting from either acute or chronic rejection. The overall survival rate was 83%, with 5-year actuarial survival rate of 80%, with the neonatal recipients having a slightly better outcome compared to older infants.

Stanford[15] reported their series of 72 patients younger than 18 years of age who have undergone heart transplantation since 1977. Only 25% were younger than 1 year of age (mean, 9 years), and nearly two thirds had cardiomyopathy unrelated to congenital heart disease. The operative survival rate was 87.5%, with deaths mainly caused by pulmonary hypertension/right ventricular failure, and acute rejection. There were 20 late deaths, 24% due to rejection, and 17% due to graft CAD. Actuarial survival rates at 1, 5, and 10 years were 75%, 60%, and 50%, respectively. There was no survival difference between age groups demonstrated in this series.

At St. Louis Children's Hospital from 1983 to 1993, 45 heart transplantations were performed, over half for infants with HLHS.[21] The infant group had a survival rate (92%) similar to that of the Loma Linda series, whereas the pediatric group (older than 1 year of age) had an 80% early survival rate.

Results from the Registry of the International Society for Heart and Lung Transplantation contrast to those of Loma Linda and St. Louis Children's Hospital. The operative mortality rate was higher for infants than for older children (ages 1 to 18 years; 25% vs. 15%).[1] In addition, 1- and 2-year survival rates are also lower for infants (65% and 60%, respectively) than older children (80% and 75%, respectively).

Aside from survival, it has been demonstrated that transplanted hearts in children appear to grow normally, and the left ventricle increases muscle mass to maintain the normal left ventricular mass–volume ratio over time.[22] Exercise testing in older children has shown peak heart rate and oxygen consumption to be consistently two thirds that predicted in heart transplant recipients.[23] Somatic growth appears to be normal in infants after heart transplantation, and neurologic development generally preserved, although some neurologic abnormalities may be seen in up to 20% of neonatal recipients on long-term follow-up.[4]

Despite vast improvements in immunosuppression, rejection surveillance, technical aspects, and perioperative management, long-term results with pediatric heart transplantation have been disappointing, with the 10-year survival rate at best 50%. Chronic rejection, graft CAD, and the long-term effects of immunosuppression on growth continue to cloud the development of cardiac transplantation as the primary treatment of complex congenital heart disease.

LUNG TRANSPLANTATION

The first experimental work in lung transplantation was reported by Demikhov in the 1940s, using canine lobar allografts. Subsequently, Metras from France in the 1950s described experimental techniques in canine orthotopic lung transplantation. The first human lung transplantation was performed in 1963 by James Hardy at the University of Mississippi, but the patient died postoperatively from renal failure and sepsis. Nearly 50 lung transplantations was performed in the next 20 years without success, usually because of pulmonary failure or complications with the bronchial anastomosis. Improved bronchial anastomotic techniques, including the use of the omental wrap, as well as the advent of cyclosporine, helped pave the way for the first successful single-lung transplantation in 1983 by Cooper. The successful use of en bloc double-lung transplantation in cystic fibrosis patients was pioneered by the Toronto group, but this technique was soon abandoned when the complication was found to be approximately 75%. They subsequently introduced the technique of bilateral sequential lung transplantation, which is commonly used today. Refinements in the surgical techniques and improved results in adult lung transplantation have subsequently led to their application in pediatric patients, including infants.

As of January 1995, 278 lung transplant recipients younger than 20 years of age had been included in the St. Louis International Lung Transplant Registry.[24] Unlike adult lung transplant recipients, most of whom receive single-lung transplants, usually for emphysema or pulmonary fibrosis, only 20% of pediatric lung transplantations are single lung. Most pediatric lung transplantations are bilateral, and there is a much higher proportion for pulmonary vascular disease. Early pediatric lung transplantations were usually on older teenagers with either cystic fibrosis or pulmonary hypertension. As experience in lung transplantation has grown, the indications for lung transplantation have been broadened, and infants as young as 3 months of age have successfully undergone lung transplantation (Fig. 44-5).

There are a number of disease processes that are successfully treated by lung transplantation (Table 44-3). Primary indications for transplantation in infancy include bronchopulmonary dysplasia, congenital surfactant deficiencies, congenital diaphragmatic hernia, and pulmonary vein stenosis. Infants with pulmonary fibrosis are usually referred for lung transplantation because of ventilator dependence.

Most older children who are referred for transplantation have either cystic fibrosis or pulmonary hypertension (primary or secondary). Although most patients with cystic fibrosis survive beyond childhood before lung function deteriorates enough to require transplantation, a small number may progress rapidly enough to require intervention. Indications include progressive hypercapnea and oxygen dependence, worsening exercise tolerance, FEV_1 (forced expiratory volume in 1 second) less than 30% predicted, and an increasing frequency of hospitalizations for infectious episodes or poor weight gain despite adequate nutritional supplementation. Pediatric patients with end-stage cystic fibrosis are often extremely debilitated and their tracheobronchial tree is frequently colonized with multiple resistant organisms, particularly pseudomonal species, making postoperative management of these patients difficult.

Primary pulmonary hypertension also usually affects young adults, but a small percentage of patients with primary pulmonary hypertension present earlier in life and become rapidly symptomatic. Children with secondary pulmonary hypertension due to cardiac defects (Eisenmenger syndrome) may also reach adulthood before symptoms progress, but more commonly have

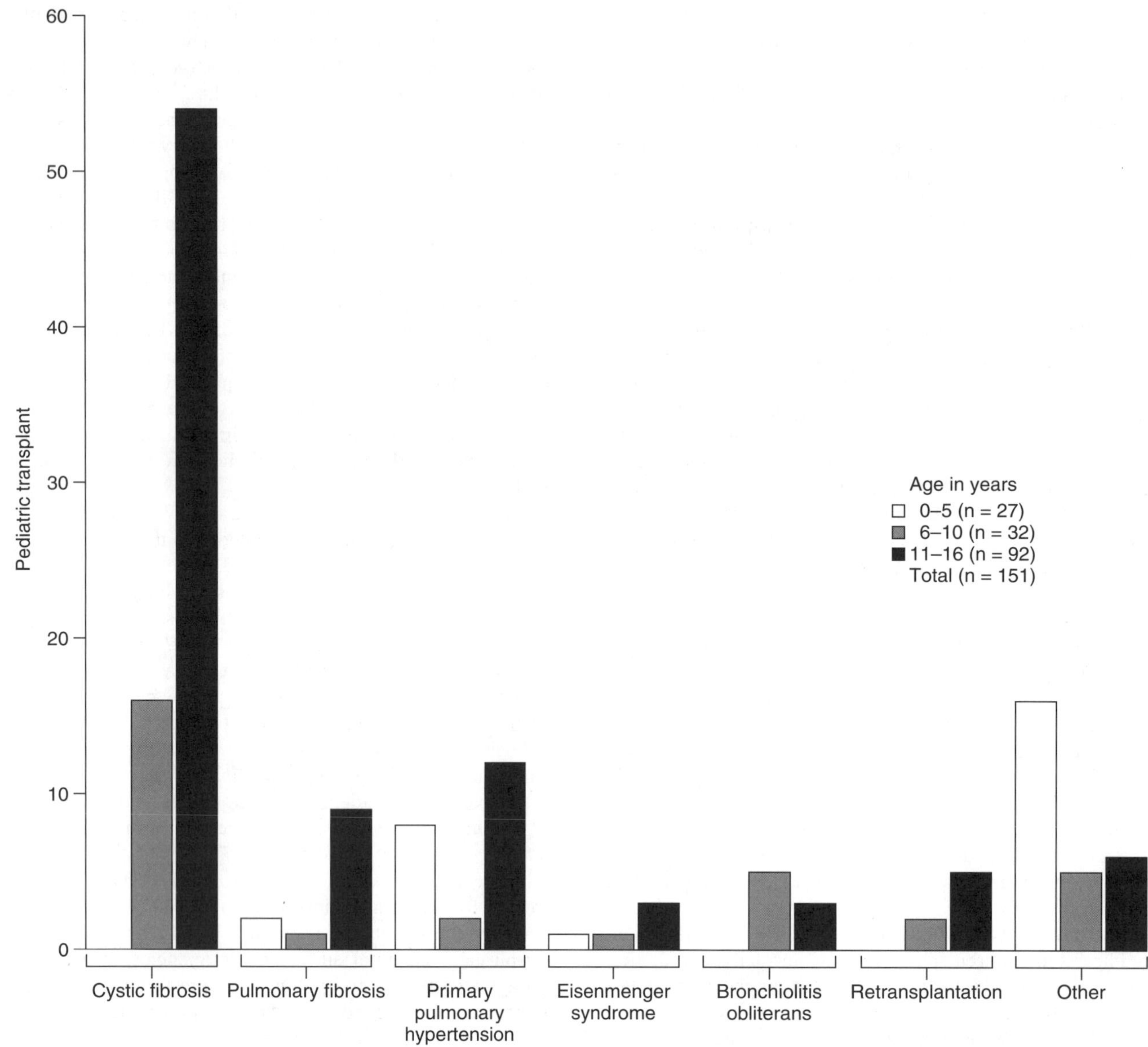

FIG. 44-5. Indications for pediatric lung transplantation by age group. (St Louis International Lung Transplant Registry. 1995 report. St Louis, St Louis International Lung Transplant Registry, 1995)

difficulties at an earlier age. Although patients with primary or secondary pulmonary hypertension may retain stable cardiopulmonary function for extended periods of time, symptoms such as syncope or right heart dysfunction develop late in the disease course, and sudden death may be imminent at this point. Early referral for transplantation is recommended if PVR_1 is fixed (greater than 10 Wood units) with evidence of increased right atrial pressure (greater than 8 mm Hg) and decreased cardiac output (less than 2.2 L/min/m^2). A general indication for lung transplantation in end-stage pulmonary disease is an estimated survival of 12 to 18 months without transplantation.

Unlike in adults, the choice of whether to perform a single or bilateral lung transplantation is often a complicated issue in pediatric patients. Certainly, septic lung diseases such as cystic fibrosis require bilateral lung transplantation to prevent subsequent infecting of the transplanted lung from the contralateral

native lung. Other forms of pulmonary fibrosis in pediatric patients may be successfully treated with single-lung transplantation, but, in general, bilateral organs are preferred in children to allow for better lung function during growth, and possibly to provide greater stability during episodes of acute or chronic rejection. Single-lung transplantation, bilateral lung transplantation, single or bilateral transplantation with intracardiac repair, or heart–lung transplantation are all options for patients with pulmonary hypertension, depending on the cardiac and pulmonary anatomy, function, and donor organ availability. The use of single-lung transplantation for pulmonary hypertension is controversial. Management of the early postoperative course can be difficult as a result of reperfusion edema because most of the cardiac output is directed to the transplanted single lung. Operative mortality is somewhat higher for single-lung transplantation in pulmonary hypertension. Many surgeons believe

TABLE 44-3. *Indications for pediatric lung transplantation*

PULMONARY FIBROSIS
Usual interstitial fibrosis
Desquamative interstitial fibrosis (rare)
Pulmonary alveolar proteinosis
Idiopathic pulmonary alveolar microlithiasis
Cystic fibrosis
Radiation-induced pulmonary fibrosis
Bronchiolitis obliterans
Bronchopulmonary dysplasia
Congenital surfactant deficiencies
Collagen vascular disease

PULMONARY VASCULAR DISEASE
Primary pulmonary hypertension
Pulmonary hypertension after corrected congenital heart disease
Pulmonary hypertension and correctable congenital heart disease (Eisenmenger syndrome)
Pulmonary vein stenosis
"Inadequate" pulmonary vascular bed
Pulmonary atresia, ventricular septal defect, no central pulmonary arteries

CONGENITAL DIAPHRAGMATIC HERNIA

that the onset of bronchiolitis obliterans after single-lung transplantation creates a severe $\dot{V}/\dot{Q}$ mismatch, with most of the cardiac output going through the poorly ventilated transplanted lung. Thus, bilateral lung transplantation for pulmonary hypertension is preferred if donor organs are available, although if a patient's deteriorating condition requires, single-lung transplantation can be safely performed. The use of combined intracardiac repair with lung transplantation has been described in children with secondary pulmonary hypertension and may obviate the need for heart–lung transplantation in many patients.[25] Repairs may include closure of atrial and ventricular septal defects, patent ductus arteriosus ligation, and repair of right ventricular outflow tracts. Contraindications to this approach include poor ventricular function, significant atrioventricular or semilunar valvar insufficiency, and complex forms of congenital heart disease, including single-ventricle physiology.

Preoperative Evaluation

In general, the preoperative evaluation process is similar to that in the cardiac transplant recipient. Again, psychosocial evaluation of these patients is important, and a compliant, willing family with adequate support systems is crucial to success. A nutritional assessment is performed, particularly in cystic fibrosis patients, who are often quite malnourished. Pulmonary function tests are included in the evaluation of patients old enough to cooperate with their performance. Echocardiography and cardiac catheterization are required for all patients with pulmonary hypertension. Absolute contraindications to lung transplantation include severe cardiac dysfunction, active collagen vascular disease, poorly controlled diabetes mellitus, malignancy, multiple organ system failure, and infection not confined to the respiratory tract. Sepsis originating from the respiratory tract, particularly in cystic fibrosis patients, is not a contraindi-

cation to lung transplantation per se, unless the tracheobronchial tree is colonized with virulent, multiple-drug resistant organisms such as *Pseudomonas cepacia*. Children on active ventilatory support or high-dose steroids must be individually considered for lung transplantation because of the probability of significant postoperative complications. In addition, a small subgroup of recipients have been maintained on ECMO before lung transplantation.[25] Although the use of ECMO in stabilizing critically ill pulmonary patients until donor lungs become available may be appealing, its widespread use as a bridge to lung transplantation has not been firmly established because waiting times may be prolonged. Other relative contraindications to lung transplantation include severe malnutrition, chest wall deformities or scoliosis, which may affect postoperative ventilatory function, or a history of pleurodesis or pleurectomy. Cyanotic patients with previous thoracotomies for palliative cardiac procedures should be carefully considered for transplantation because of the high risk of significant hemorrhage from the numerous collaterals that are formed in the chest adhesions of these patients.

Donor Organ Procurement

It is estimated that only 10% to 20% of solid organ donors have lungs suitable for procurement.[26] Many donors require a significant period of ventilatory support before the declaration of brain death, and this frequently results in bacterial colonization of the tracheobronchial tree or pneumonia. In addition, a significant smoking history or evidence of chest trauma may preclude the use of lungs from an organ donor. The requirements for a satisfactory lung donor are listed in Table 44-4. On initial evaluation, the most important aspects of the donor are the oxygenation of the patient (Po_2 greater than 300 mm Hg on 100% Fio_2) and compliance of the lungs (tidal volumes of

TABLE 44-4. *Criteria of donor lung suitability (ideal donor)*

PRELIMINARY
Age <55 y
ABO compatibility
Chest roentenogram clear
Adequate size match to recipient
History
    Smoking ≤20 pack-years
    No significant thoracic trauma (blunt, penetrating)
    No aspiration/sepsis
    Gram stain and culture data if prolonged intubation
    No prior cardiac/pulmonary operation
Oxygenation
    Arterial oxygen tension ≥300 mm Hg on inspired oxygen fraction of 1.0
    5 cm H_2O positive end-expiratory pressure

FINAL ASSESSMENT
Chest roentgenogram shows no unfavorable changes
Oxygenation has not deteriorated
Bronchoscopy shows no aspiration, purulence, or mass
Visual/manual assessment
    Parenchyma satisfactory
    No adhesions or masses
    Further evaluation of trauma

15 mL/kg should be maintained with minimal elevations in the peak inspiratory pressures). The chest radiogram should be clear without evidence of contusions or infiltrates. Bronchoscopy is performed on evaluation and there should be minimal clear secretions without purulence, blood, or evidence of bronchitis. In the operating room, the lungs are inspected for masses or evidence of trauma and gently palpated. Donors and recipients are matched by ABO compatibility and size. Unlike in adult lung transplantation, matching lung size in children should be fairly close because there is little room for oversizing. Matching donor and recipient height appears to be the most accurate method of size-matching the lungs.

In an attempt to expand the limited donor pool for lung transplant recipients, some studies have focused on the use of ''marginal'' donors for lung transplantation.[27] It appears that liberalizing donor radiographic, bronchoscopic, and hemodynamic criteria has produced equivalent survival rates.

Donor lung procurement is usually performed in conjunction with heart procurement. After median sternotomy, the inferior pulmonary ligaments are divided bilaterally and the pulmonary arteries are mobilized from bifurcation to the hilum. Just before aortic cross-clamping, prostaglandin E_1 is infused by needle catheter in the main pulmonary artery. Once the cross-clamp is placed, the inferior vena cava and the left atrial appendage are divided to vent the heart and lungs, then either cold Euro-Collins or University of Wisconsin solution is infused into the pulmonary artery cannula simultaneously while cardioplegia is given. The heart is then explanted, dividing the right and left pulmonary arteries at the bifurcation, and leaving a small (5 mm) cuff of left atrium on the pulmonary veins. Either the trachea or mainstem bronchus, depending on whether a single lung or both lungs are being used by the same institution, is then stapled with the lungs partially inflated (Fig. 44-6A). For single-lung procurement, the hilum is then dissected from the mediastinal tissue and the lung is removed. For bilateral lung transplantation, the lungs are removed en bloc by stapling and transecting the distal esophagus and the descending thoracic aorta, then dissecting the entire tissue bloc off the posterior mediastinum to the level of the trachea (see Fig. 44-6B and C). Once the trachea is divided, the bloc is removed and the lungs are placed in cold sterile saline and triple bagged for transport. Division of the lung bloc and back table dissection are reserved for just before transplantation, preserving any excess vessel length. Maximum cold ischemic time for transplanted lungs is approximately 8 to 9 hours.

Recipient Procedure

The technique for pediatric pulmonary transplantation is similar to that used in adults. A bilateral transverse (clam-shell) thoracotomy is preferred for bilateral transplantation (Fig. 44-7A); if a single-lung transplantation is combined with intracardiac repair, the incision is not extended as far on the contralateral side (see Fig. 44-7B). For single-lung transplantation alone, a posterolateral thoracotomy is used. Unlike in adult lung transplantation, where cardiopulmonary bypass is used sparingly, cardiopulmonary bypass is used in nearly all pediatric lung transplantations. This improves exposure, facilitates dissection of the hilum, and provides access to the heart in the event that the transplantation is combined with intracardiac repair. The ascending aorta and either the right atrial appendage or the venae cavae are cannulated for cardiopulmonary bypass. Once the donor organs are immediately available and on inspection are adequate, cardiopulmonary bypass is commenced. The recipient lungs are excised, dividing the pulmonary arteries and veins at their major divisions, and then the mainstem bronchus is stapled and divided just proximal to the takeoff of each upper lobe bronchus (see Fig. 44-7C). In cystic fibrosis patients with heavy contamination of the tracheobronchial tree, antibiotic irrigation of the blind tracheal segment through the endotracheal tube is performed before implantation of the donor lungs. The donor lung is positioned in the chest and bronchial anastomosis is begun. A simple end-to-end anastomosis with monofilament absorbable suture is used. The membranous portion of the bronchus is anastomosed in a continuous fashion, with interrupted sutures placed in the cartilaginous segment. A telescoping anastomosis is used only in the event of a significant bronchial size mismatch. Surrounding excess mediastinal tissue may be used to cover the bronchial anastomosis, but omental or pericardial wraps usually are not necessary. The pulmonary artery anastomosis is then performed, followed by anastomosing the donor pulmonary veins to the recipient left atrium, both using monofilament suture in a continuous fashion. Although tension on the suture line should be avoided, oversizing the length of the pulmonary vessels may produce kinking, which is equally undesirable.

The contralateral lung is then implanted in a similar fashion. If intracardiac repair is required (closure of atrial or ventricular septal defects), this is carried out under a hypothermic cardioplegic arrest before the lung implantation (see Fig. 44-7D). In more complex cases such as ventricular septal defect closure with right ventricular outflow tract reconstruction after implantation of the lungs, closure of the ventricular septal defect and the outflow tract reconstruction may be performed under cardioplegic arrest.

After the lung implantation, the suture lines are inspected for hemostasis and the patient is weaned from cardiopulmonary bypass. Aprotinin is frequently used, especially in reoperations, to reduce postoperative bleeding problems. The chest is closed in standard fashion, with two or three sternal wires used to approximate the sternum. Two chest tubes are placed on each side, one at the base and one extended to the apex. A broviac intravenous catheter is commonly placed, if time allows at the end of the procedure, for postoperative venous access.

Postoperative Management

Like cardiac transplantation patients, the lung transplant recipient requires a reverse isolation intensive care unit room. Ventilatory support is maintained to provide adequate oxygenation while minimizing airway pressure and the inspired oxygen concentration. In general, 3 to 5 cm of positive end-expiratory pressure is acceptable with peak airway pressures below 35 mm Hg. Judicious fluid management is used with restriction of fluid intake early to help limit reperfusion edema. Pulmonary hypertension may be treated with hyperventilation or infusions such as sodium nitroprusside or prostaglandin E_1. Inhaled nitric oxide has been shown to be a potent selective pulmonary vasodilator, and is useful in controlling postoperative pulmonary hypertension, and may also improve $\dot{V}/\dot{Q}$ matching. ECMO has been

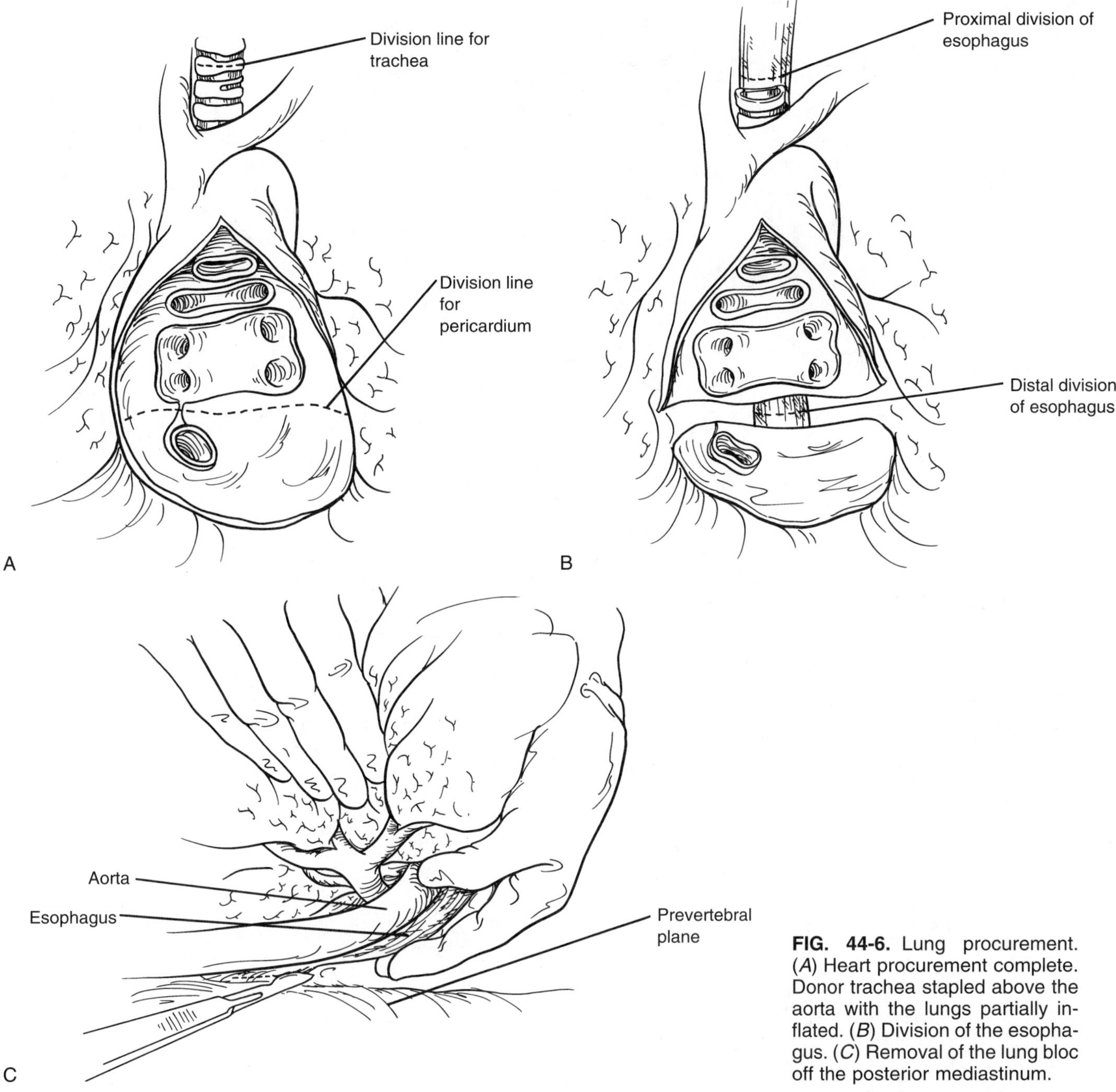

FIG. 44-6. Lung procurement. (*A*) Heart procurement complete. Donor trachea stapled above the aorta with the lungs partially inflated. (*B*) Division of the esophagus. (*C*) Removal of the lung bloc off the posterior mediastinum.

successfully used in some cases of severe reperfusion edema or graft failure in pediatric patients.[25]

Reperfusion injury of the transplanted lung is typically evidenced by poor lung compliance, hypoxia, and perihilar infiltrates, usually occurring immediately after transplantation. This responds to prolonged ventilatory support, with gradual resolution in most cases. Other causes of hypoxia and poor lung compliance in the immediate postoperative period include acute rejection, graft failure, or overwhelming viral or bacterial infection of the transplanted lungs.

In general, the goal is to extubate lung transplant recipients 24 to 48 hours after surgery. Patients with pulmonary hypertension are paralyzed and sedated for a slightly longer period of time to avoid a potential acute pulmonary hypertensive crisis. Cystic fibrosis patients may need to be maintained longer on the ventilator as well because of copious airway secretions, malnutrition, or chronic respiratory muscle fatigue. Before extubation, a thoracic epidural catheter is placed for pain relief and fiberoptic bronchoscopy is performed, inspecting the integrity of the bronchial anastomosis and removing any blood or secretions from the airways. Bronchoscopy is used liberally in the postoperative period for pulmonary toilet or evaluation of chest radiography changes. Chest tubes often need to remain in place for an extended period of time in lung recipients because of increased fluid transudation in the pleural spaces. Despite this, ambulation should be encouraged early, and the use

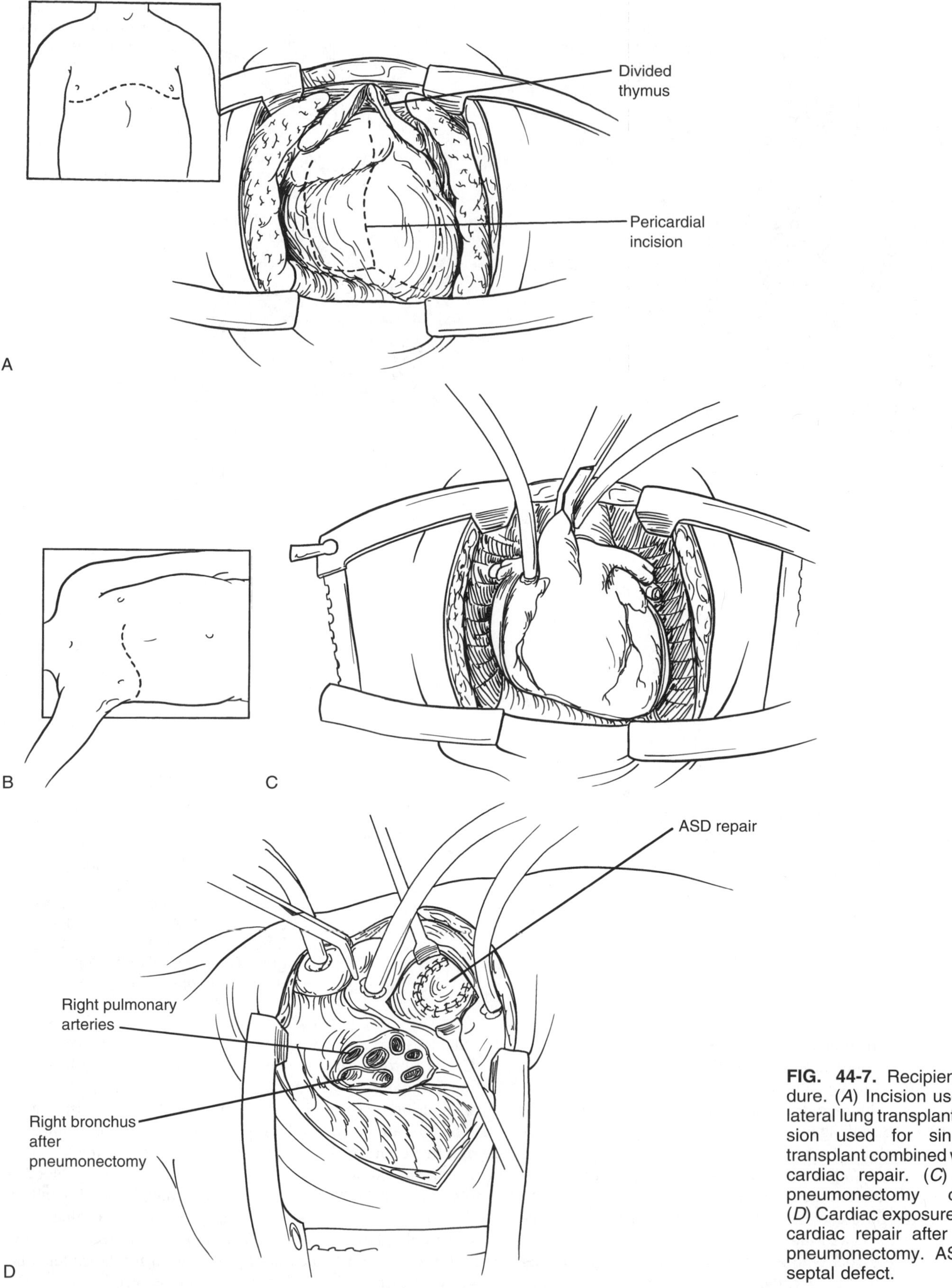

FIG. 44-7. Recipient procedure. (*A*) Incision used for bilateral lung transplant. (*B*) Incision used for single lung transplant combined with intracardiac repair. (*C*) Bilateral pneumonectomy complete. (*D*) Cardiac exposure for intracardiac repair after recipient pneumonectomy. ASD, atrial septal defect.

of epidural analgesics is useful for this. Adequate nutritional support is of vital importance and the diet is rapidly advanced if possible, with nutritional supplements or nasojejunal feeds used as needed. Vancomycin and cefoxitin are used as perioperative antibiotic coverage and continued until all invasive lines and tubes are removed. Cystic fibrosis patients require antibiotics tailored to sensitivity patterns of resistant pseudomonal species that often colonize their airways. Frequent surveillance samples of blood, urine, and sputum are sent for bacterial and viral culture, and bronchioalveolar lavage is obtained for viral cultures and viral immunohistochemistry.

Immunosuppression for lung transplant patients at the Children's Hospital of Philadelphia is the same as that outlined in the guide on heart transplantation. In addition to *P carinii* and fungal prophylaxis, 6 weeks of CMV prophylaxis—ganciclovir, 5 mg/kg bid $\times$ 2 weeks, then qd $\times$ 4 weeks—is used in all patients because of the high incidence of CMV pneumonia in lung transplant recipients. Rejection surveillance is performed by fiberoptic bronchoscopy and transbronchial biopsy in addition to bronchioalveolar lavage.[28] A useful technique for infant lung transplant recipients where the endotracheal tube is too small to admit an adequate-sized bronchoscope for biopsy is to place a suction catheter fluoroscopically in a lobar bronchus through the endotracheal tube, then pass the biopsy forceps through it. Recipients undergo fiberoptic bronchoscopy and biopsy sampling before discharge and at 3-month intervals over the first year after transplantation. Biopsies allow for the evaluation of rejection and provide samples for immunohistochemistry for evidence of viral infection, including CMV and adenovirus. Open-lung biopsy is used in the event of progressive lung parenchymal changes without an adequate diagnosis obtained from transbronchial biopsy.

Complications

In contrast to heart transplant recipients, rejection is common in lung transplant recipients, with usually at least one episode in the first month posttransplantation.[25,26] Most rejection episodes occur in the first 3 months after transplantation. Transplant recipients are treated for rejection either based on a high clinical suspicion, or if rejection is demonstrated by transbronchial biopsy (Tables 44-5 through 44-7). Rejection episodes are treated with methylprednisolone pulse therapy, 10 to 15 mg/kg $\times$ 3 days, with a dramatic clinical response in most instances. Incomplete responses or persistent rejection may require antithymocyte globulin or OKT3 therapy. Early death from acute rejection is uncommon in lung transplant recipients, occurring in less than 10% of patients.

TABLE 44-5. *Clinical criteria for the diagnosis of rejection*

Parameter	Indication
Temperature	Rise >5°C above stable baseline
Oxygenation	Fall >10 mm Hg below stable baseline
Radiograph	New or changing infiltrates
Spirometry	Fall in FEV_1 >10% below stable baseline
Infection	Excluded
Drug therapy	Response to treatment with methylprednisolone

TABLE 44-6. *Histologic grading system for acute pulmonary rejection*

Grade	Description
Normal (A0)	No significant abnormality
Minimal acute rejection (A1)	Infrequent perivascular infiltrates
Mild acute rejection (A2)	Frequent perivascular infiltrates around venules and arterioles
Moderate acute (A3)	Dense perivascular infiltrates with extension into alveolar septa
Severe acute rejection (A4)	Diffuse perivascular, interstitial, and air-space infiltrates; alveolar pneumocyte damage; possibly parenchymal necrosis, infarction, or necrotizing vasculitis

Infectious complications are a major cause of morbidity and death among lung transplant recipients. Over 25% of deaths in recipients less than 90 days after transplantation result from infection, with most infectious complications originating in the transplanted lungs. Bacterial infections are most common, occurring in 20% to 25% of patients, and primarily in cystic fibrosis patients. The most common organisms in these patients are pseudomonal species. Panresistant *P cepacia* is such a particularly virulent organism that some centers will not transplant cystic fibrosis patients colonized with this organism. As might be expected in a pediatric population, viral respiratory infections are common. Etiologies include CMV, Epstein-Barr virus, parainfluenza virus, and respiratory syncytial virus. CMV pneumonia is particularly common, occurring in nearly 25% of transplant recipients, particularly in CMV-seronegative recipients

TABLE 44-7. *Working formulation for classification and grading of pulmonary rejection*

GRADE A: ACUTE REJECTION

Minimal acute rejection
Mild acute rejection
Moderate acute rejection
Severe acute rejection
    With evidence of bronchiolar inflammation
    Without evidence of bronchiolar inflammation
    With large airway inflammation
    No bronchioles are present

GRADE B: ACTIVE AIRWAY DAMAGE WITHOUT SCARRING

Lymphocytic bronchitis
Lymphocytic bronchiolitis

GRADE C: CHRONIC AIRWAY REJECTION

Bronchiolitis obliterans, subtotal
Bronchiolitis obliterans, total
    Active
    Inactive

GRADE D: CHRONIC VASCULAR REJECTION

GRADE E: VASCULITIS

receiving lungs from CMV-positive donors.[25,29] Transbronchial biopsy and bronchioalveolar lavage are useful in the diagnosis of CMV pneumonia and other viral infections of the lung. Fungal infections also make up a number of infectious complications. Candidal colonization of the airways occurs frequently, but invasive pneumonitis is uncommon and may be treated with fluconazole or amphotericin B. Aside from *Candida* species, the most frequent fungal organism is *Aspergillus*, which may colonize or infect up to 5% to 15% of transplant recipients.[29] Colonization alone may be observed, but evidence of invasive infection on bronchoscopy or biopsy should be treated with itraconazole, with amphotericin B added if there is evidence of disease progression.

As expected, bronchial complications may be a source of morbidity in transplant recipients, affecting approximately 10% to 15% of bronchial anastomoses at risk.[25,26,29] Stenosis at the anastomotic site is the most frequent complication, and is usually treated by bronchoscopic dilatation and placement of silicone (Silastic) stents in severe cases. Postoperative bronchial disruption is uncommon and is usually associated with underlying infection or prolonged ventilatory support, both of which interfere with healing of the bronchial anastomosis. Most bronchial disruptions are contained and heal spontaneously if adequately drained.

The primary long-term complication of lung transplantation, as in cardiac transplantation, is chronic rejection. In lung transplant recipients, however, chronic rejection may take the form of bronchiolitis obliterans. This complication has been reported in 25% to 40% of long-term survivors and can occur within 6 months of transplantation.[25,26] Like posttransplantation CAD in the cardiac transplant recipient, the etiology of bronchiolitis obliterans is unknown, but presumed to be either of viral origin or caused by underimmunosuppression of the recipient. Some patients respond to an increase in immunosuppression with stabilization of pulmonary function, but at best this is usually maintained at a level below their initial postoperative pulmonary function. Occasionally, bronchiolitis obliterans may be rapidly progressive. Retransplantation for end-stage bronchiolitis obliterans is controversial and the results have been poor, with relatively few survivors. Bronchiolitis obliterans is the cause of approximately 25% of late deaths of lung transplant recipients.[26]

Lymphoproliferative disease occurs in 5% to 22% of pediatric lung transplantation long-term survivors. Etiologies may include CMV, Epstein-Barr virus, or overimmunosuppression. Although patients may respond to a decrease in their immunosuppression, approximately 5% of late deaths after lung transplantation are caused by malignancy.[25,29]

Results

In general, the results for pediatric lung transplantation have paralleled the adult experience, considering the much higher proportion of bilateral lung transplantations in children. St Louis Children's Hospital[25] reported their results in 33 children with a mean age of 10 years, 25% of whom required preoperative mechanical ventilation, 10% of whom were on ECMO at the time of transplantation. Operative survival and 1-year survival rates were 78% and 62%, respectively. Thirteen of these patients had concomitant intracardiac repairs. Sepsis and acute

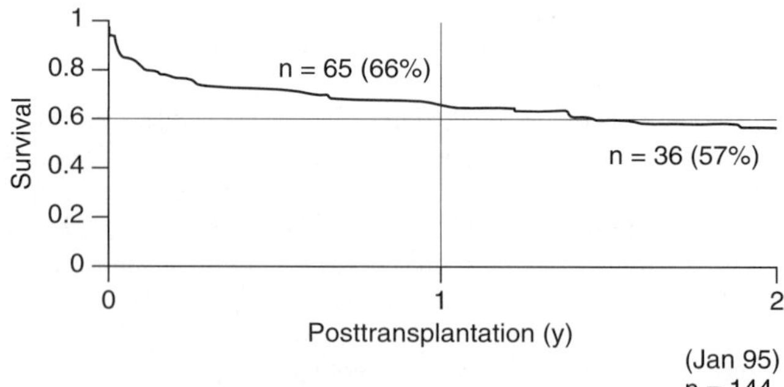

FIG. 44-8. Two-year actuarial survival rate for pediatric lung transplant recipients. (St Louis International Lung Transplant Registry. 1995 report. St Louis, St Louis International Lung Transplant Registry, 1995)

graft failure were the most common causes of death early, and bronchiolitis obliterans and posttransplantation lymphoproliferative disease were the late causes of death.

The Marseilles/Montreal lung transplantation group[30] reported excellent results in 20 children, with no operative mortality and 85% and 75% 1- and 2-year survival rates. In this study, however, 19 of the transplantations were for cystic fibrosis and almost exclusively in older children.

The 1995 St. Louis Lung Transplant Registry[24] reports a 66% 1-year survival rate and a 57% 2-year survival rate for 144 pediatric lung transplantation patients younger than 16 years of age (Fig. 44-8). Cystic fibrosis patients appear to have a better survival rate (70%, 65%, 1- and 2-year) than pulmonary hypertension patients (62%, 55%, 1- and 2-year). Pulmonary hypertension patients with bilateral lungs have a slightly higher survival rate than single-lung recipients (61% vs. 53% in 2 years).

Starnes and colleagues[31] have addressed the critical issue of the donor shortage by using lobar transplantation with grafts taken from either cadavers or living, related donors. In an early report of six patients, the operative survival rate was 83%, demonstrating that in an urgent situation such as acute deterioration requiring mechanical ventilation on ECMO, this option is surgically feasible. Wider application of this technique awaits further follow-up, however.

HEART–LUNG TRANSPLANTATION

Reitz performed the first successful heart–lung transplantation at Stanford in 1981. The use of heart–lung transplantation enjoyed brief popularity in the mid- to late 1980s, primarily for the treatment of pulmonary hypertension and cystic fibrosis. In cystic fibrosis patients, the recipient heart was often used for a separate cardiac transplant recipient (so-called ''domino'' procedure). The success of single and bilateral lung transplantation since 1990 and the shortage of suitable donors has severely curtailed the use of heart–lung transplantation in thoracic organ transplantation.

Over 250 patients younger than 18 years of age have undergone heart–lung transplantation worldwide.[1] Almost half of these were for congenital heart disease, another 15% for pulmonary hypertension, and 10% of these were retransplantations

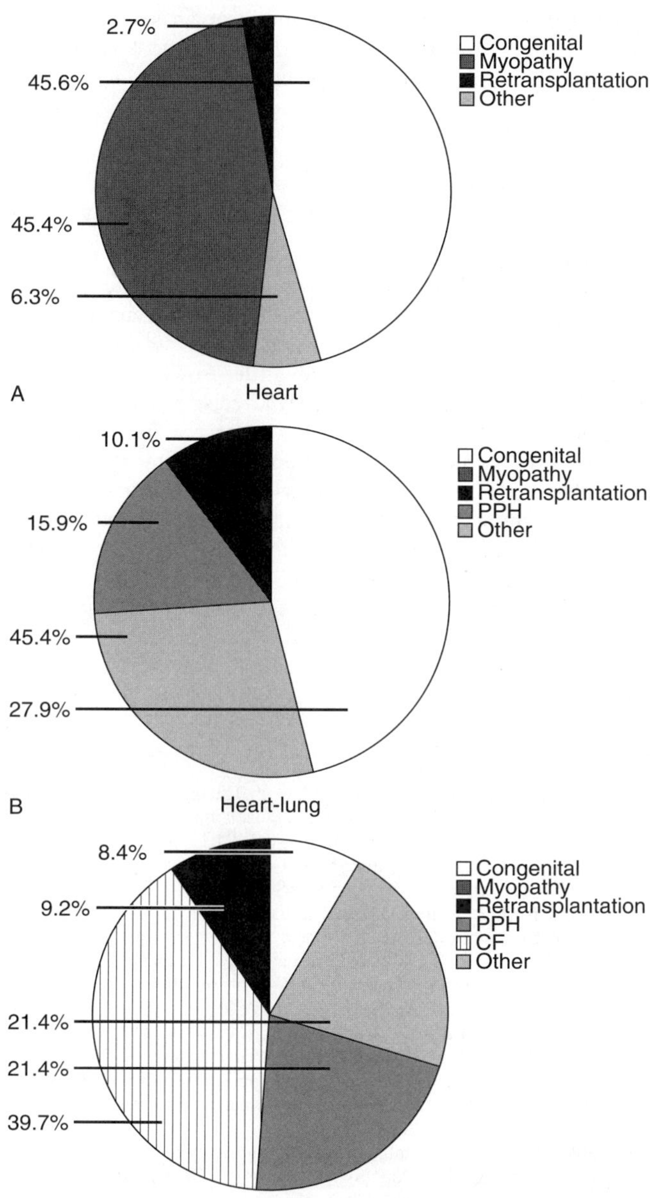

FIG. 44-9. Indications for pediatric transplantation: (*A*) heart, (*B*) heart–lung, (*C*) lung. CF, cystic fibrosis; PPH, primary pulmonary hypertension.

(Fig. 44-9). Heart–lung transplantation is reserved for patients with pulmonary hypertension or parenchymal disease and either poor ventricular function, significant valvar insufficiency, or complex, uncorrectable congenital heart disease. The pretransplantation evaluation is similar to that in heart and lung transplantation candidates, and includes echocardiography and cardiac catheterization. Pulmonary hypertension and the nature of the cardiac disease should be well documented; an isolated heart or lung transplant is preferable because of lower operative mortality and shorter waiting periods. Indications for transplantation include class III to IV congestive heart failure, syncope, hemoptysis, and right heart failure. Evidence of significant pulmonary hypertension on cardiac catheterization includes right atrial pressures greater than 8 mm Hg, cardiac index less than 2.2 L/min/m^2, and PVR$_i$ greater than 10 Wood units.

Donor Organ Procurement

Suitable donor criteria for heart–lung transplantation are the same as those mentioned previously. Again, a clear chest radiograph, normal fiberoptic bronchoscopy, good lung oxygenation and compliance, and an echocardiogram demonstrating adequate wall motion, ventricular thickness, and valve function are required. A median sternotomy is used, and after dissection of the ascending aorta and venae cavae, the donor bloc is flushed with crystalloid cardioplegia in the aortic root and Euro-Collins solution in the pulmonary artery after a prostaglandin E$_1$ infusion. The heart is vented by dividing the inferior vena cava and the left atrial appendage. The venae cavae are then divided and the esophagus is stapled and transected near the diaphragm and in the superior mediastinum. The bloc is then dissected off the posterior mediastinum. After dividing the aorta, the trachea is stapled and divided well above the carina with the lungs partially inflated. The heart–lung bloc is then placed in cold saline and packaged for transport. A cold ischemic time of less than 4 to 5 hours is recommended for optimum postoperative graft function.

Recipient Operation

The recipient operation is begun by either a median sternotomy or a transverse thoracotomy (clam-shell) incision. The transverse thoracotomy incision is preferred because this provides better exposure to the pulmonary hila. The ascending aorta and individual venae cavae are then cannulated for cardiopulmonary bypass. An aortic cross-clamp is placed and the aorta is divided, and the heart is then explanted, leaving a right atrial cuff. This is followed by sequential lung removal, preserving the phrenic nerves on a pedicle of pericardium. Meticulous hemostasis of the posterior mediastinum is of the utmost importance. The intraoperative use of aprotinin has helped significantly to lower bleeding complications. Once the recipient's organs are removed, the heart–lung bloc is placed in the chest by passing the lungs under the pericardial pedicles containing the phrenic nerves. The tracheal anastomosis is performed with a continuous monofilament suture followed by the right atrial anastomosis. The left atrium is vented through the right superior pulmonary vein and the aortic anastomosis is performed in a continuous end-to-end fashion using monofilament suture. The cross-clamp is removed and the heart and lungs are reperfused. The patient is weaned from cardiopulmonary bypass, hemostasis is obtained, and the incision is closed.

Postoperative Management

In general, the management of heart–lung transplantation patients parallels that of other thoracic organ transplant recipients. Fluid intake and ventilator support are minimized. Isoproterenol may be useful as an inotrope because it has a chronotropic effect on the donor heart, as well as decreasing pulmonary vascular resistance. Again, early extubation and ambulation are encouraged. Immunosuppression and infection prophylaxis are identical to that in the lung transplant recipient.

One key point of management of the heart–lung recipient is that rejection may affect the heart and lungs at separate times. Children undergo echocardiography routinely to follow myocardial function. Both endomyocardial biopsy and transbronchial biopsy are carried out on routine basis; however, clinical suspicion of rejection of the lungs may require early intravenous methylprednisolone therapy. Isolated lung rejection occurs commonly, and the incidence of isolated cardiac rejection after heart–lung transplantation appears to be lower than in cardiac transplantation alone.

Results

Although heart–lung transplantation is performed at many medical centers and the world experience with pediatric patients is considerable, most major series in heart–lung transplantation do not separate results for the pediatric age group. The International Society for Heart Lung Transplantation in 1994 demonstrated an operative survival of approximately 75% for pediatric heart–lung transplant recipients, with 1- and 2-year survival rates of 60% and 55%, respectively.[1] The actuarial survival rate for patients older than 6 years of age was 45%, but only 25% to 30% for patients younger than 5 years of age (Fig. 44-10).

The Stanford University experience consisted of 109 patients with an average age of 39 years.[32] Approximately 75% of these patients were transplanted for some form of pulmonary hypertension. Actuarial survival rates at 1, 5, and 10 years were 68%, 43%, and 23%, respectively. The operative mortality rate was 13%. Although lung rejection occurred frequently and isolated heart rejection less frequently, simultaneous heart and lung rejection was uncommon. Although graft CAD seemed to develop less frequently than in patients after isolated heart transplantation, bronchiolitis obliterans was a major cause of morbidity and mortality in the long term after heart–lung transplantation.

Yacoub's group[33] from Great Britain reported their results with 303 consecutive heart–lung transplantation patients in 1991. Half of these procedures were for pulmonary vascular disease and the other half for parenchymal lung disease, most of these cystic fibrosis. Actuarial survival rates 1 and 2 years after surgery were 61% and 51%, respectively. The operative (30-day) mortality rate was approximately 30%, with the most frequent causes of early death multiple organ system failure, bleeding, and infection. Late deaths were most commonly caused by bronchiolitis obliterans, bacterial infection, or CMV infection.

FUTURE TRENDS

Pediatric thoracic transplantation has evolved into an effective treatment modality for heart and pulmonary failure, as well as unrepairable congenital anomalies of those organs. Unfortunately, the success of transplantation has led to a remarkable growth in the recipient pool with little growth in the donor pool. The donor shortage particularly affects neonatal and infant recipients, for whom suitable donors are scarce. In addition, the long-term follow-up on thoracic transplant recipients has been particularly disappointing, with survival at 10 years less than 50%. Extensive ongoing research in the areas of xenotransplantation and modulation of the human immune system lends promise to the idea of a limitless supply of organs and a reduction of the long-term effects of our current immunosuppression techniques.

REFERENCES

1. Hosenpud JD, Novick RJ, Breen TJ, et al. The registry of The International Society for Heart and Lung Transplantation: eleventh official report—1994. J Heart Lung Transplant 1994;13:561.
2. Bove EL. Transplantation after first-stage reconstruction for hypoplastic left heart syndrome. Ann Thorac Surg 1991;52:701.
3. Boucek MM, Bernstein D. Heart transplantation in infancy. Progress in Pediatric Cardiology 1993;2(4):20.
4. Bailey LL, Gundry SR, Razzouk AJ, et al. Bless the babies: one hundred fifteen late survivors of heart transplantation during the first year of life. J Thorac Cardiovasc Surg 1993;105:805.
5. Spray TL. Pediatric heart transplantation. In: Flye MW, ed. Atlas of organ transplantation. Philadelphia, WB Saunders, 1995:259.
6. Cooper MM, Fuzesi L, Addonizio LJ, et al. Pediatric heart transplantation after operations involving the pulmonary arteries. J Thorac Cardiovasc Surg 1991;102:386.
7. Lewis AB. Prognostic value of echocardiography in children with idiopathic dilated cardiomyopathy. Am Heart J 1994;128:133.
8. del Nido PJ, Armitage JM, Fricker FJ, et al. Extracorporeal membrane oxygenation support as a bridge to pediatric heart transplantation. Circulation 1994;90(pt 2):II-66.
9. Canter CE, Saffitz JE, Moorhead S, et al. Early results after pediatric cardiac transplantation with triple immunosuppression therapy. Am J Cardiol 1993;71:971.
10. Canter CE, Moorhead S, Saffitz JE, et al. Steroid withdrawal in the pediatric heart transplant recipient initially treated with triple immunosuppression. J Heart Lung Transplant 1994;13:74.
11. Shaddy RE, Bullock EA, Morwessel NJ, et al. Murine monoclonal CD3 antibody (OKT3)-based early rejection prophylaxis in pediatric heart transplantation. J Heart Lung Transplant 1993;12:434.
12. Armitage JM, Fricker FJ, del Nido P, et al. A decade (1982 to 1992) of pediatric cardiac transplantation and the impact of FK 506 immunosuppression. J Thorac Cardiovasc Surg 1993;105:464.
13. Braunlin EA, Canter CE, Olivari MT, et al. Rejection and infection after pediatric cardiac transplantation. Ann Thorac Surg 1990;49:385.
14. Canter CE, Appleton RS, Saffitz JE, et al. Surveillance for rejection by echocardiographically guided endomyocardial biopsy in the infant heart transplant recipient. Circulation 1991;84(Suppl III):III-310.
15. Sarris GE, Smith JA, Bernstin D, et al. Pediatric cardiac transplantation: the Stanford experience. Circulation 1994;90(5 pt 2):1151.
16. Park JK, Hus DT, Hordof AJ, et al. Arrhythmias in pediatric heart transplant recipients: prevalence and association with death, coronary artery disease, and rejection. J Heart Lung Transplant 1993;12:596.

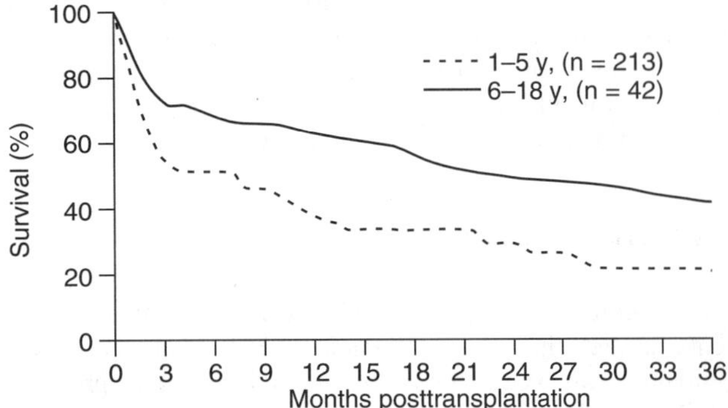

FIG. 44-10. Actuarial survival rates for heart–lung transplantation by age.

17. Braulin EA, Hunter DW, Canter CE, et al. Coronary artery disease in pediatric cardiac transplant recipients receiving triple-drug immunosuppression. Circulation 1991;84(Suppl III):III-303.

18. Pahl E, Zales VR, Ficker FJ, et al. Posttransplant coronary artery disease in children: a multicenter national survey. Circulation 1994;9(pt 2):II-56.

19. Michler RE, Edward NM, Hsu D, et al. Pediatric retransplantation. J Heart Lung Transplant 1993;12:S319.

20. Dresdale AR, Lutz S, Drost C, et al. Prospective evaluation of malignant neoplasms in cardiac transplant recipients uniformly treated with prophylactic antilymphocyte globulin. J Thorac Cardiovasc Surg 1993;106:1202.

21. Spray TL. Transplantation of the heart and lungs in children. Annu Rev Med 1994;45:139.

22. Zales VR, Wright KL, Pahl E, et al. Normal left ventricular muscle mass and mass/volume ratio after pediatric cardiac transplantation. Circulation 1994;90(pt 2):II-61.

23. Nixon PA, Fricker FJ, Noyes BE, et al. Exercise testing in pediatric heart, heart-lung, and lung recipients. Chest 1995;107:1328.

24. St. Louis International Lung Transplant Registry. 1995 report. St Louis, St Louis International Lung Transplant Registry, 1995.

25. Spray TL, Mallory GB, Canter CE, et al. Pediatric lung transplantation: indications, techniques and early results. J Thorac Cardiovasc Surg 1994;107:990.

26. Davis RD Jr, Pasque MK. Pulmonary transplantation. Ann Surg 1995;221:14.

27. Sundaresan S, Semenkovich J, Ochoa L, et al. Cardiac and pulmonary replacement. J Thorac Cardiovasc Surg 1995;109:1075.

28. Kurland G, Noyes BE, Jaffe R, et al. Bronchoalveolar lavage and transbronchial biopsy in children following heart-lung and lung transplantation. Chest 1993;104:1043.

29. Armitage JM, Kurland G, Michaels M, et al. Critical issues in pediatric lung transplantation. J Thorac Cardiovasc Surg 1995;109:60.

30. Métras D, Shennib H, Kreitmann B, et al. Double-lung transplantation in children: a report of 20 cases. Ann Thorac Surg 1993;55:352.

31. Starnes VA, Barr ML, Cohen RG. Lobar transplantation. J Thorac Cardiovasc Surg 1994;108:403.

32. Sarris GE, Smith JA, Shumway NE, et al. Long-term results of combined heart-lung transplantation: the Stanford experience. J Heart Lung Transplant 1994;13:940.

33. Madden B, Radley-Smith R, Hodson M, et al. Medium-term results of heart and lung transplantation. J Heart Lung Transplant 1992;11:S241.

Surgery of Infants and Children: Scientific Principles and Practice, edited by Keith T. Oldham, Paul M. Colombani, and Robert P. Foglia. Lippincott–Raven Publishers, Philadelphia, © 1997.

CHAPTER 45

Bone Marrow

Mark J. Mogul, Curtis W. Turner, and Andrew M. Yeager

Clinical bone marrow transplantation (BMT) epitomizes the application of basic scientific principles of immunobiology and stem cell biology to effective therapeutic interventions. Conversely, observations in clinical BMT settings greatly contribute to our understanding of basic transplantation biology. Since the mid-1960s, BMT has evolved and expanded into an intensive therapy that is increasingly applied with curative intent to various hematologic, neoplastic, immunologic, and genetic disorders of childhood and adolescence. Largely as a result of advances in supportive care and in the "bench-to-bedside" clinical application of basic research findings in transplantation immunobiology, post-BMT survival and quality of life have improved substantially since the mid-1980s. Despite these major advances, several procedure-related complications remain responsible for morbidity and mortality associated with pediatric BMT.

As the application of transplantation of bone marrow and other sources of lymphohematopoietic stem cells in childhood diseases expands, both pediatric surgeons and pediatric surgical subspecialists will become acquainted with children who may require or may have received a marrow or stem cell transplant. This chapter reviews the scientific principles and clinical procedures of marrow and stem cell collection and transplantation, selected transplant-associated complications, and the results of BMT in children with neoplastic and nonneoplastic diseases.

IMMUNOBIOLOGIC PRINCIPLES OF BONE MARROW TRANSPLANTATION

After BMT, the lymphoid and hematopoietic systems of the recipient are repopulated by normal donor-derived cells, which arise from a common primitive pluripotential stem cell (Fig. 45-1). This cell expresses the CD34 antigen (CD34+) and does not express other immunophenotypic markers of myeloid (CD33) or lymphoid (CD3) differentiation. Strong evidence suggests that the bone marrow stromal cells also arise from the pluripotent CD34+ lineage-negative stem cell. Unlike committed lymphoid and hematopoietic cells, the stem cell is capable of self-renewal and provides a sustained source of its own cell population.

In normal individuals, CD34+ cells account for only 0.5%

to 1.0% of the total nucleated marrow cells. CD34+ cells are found with higher frequencies in placental (umbilical cord) blood, which has been used as a source of stem cells for successful allogeneic transplantation into related and, more recently, unrelated fully or partially histocompatible recipients. CD34+ cells can be mobilized from the marrow into the peripheral blood circulation by administration of cytokines such as granulocyte colony-stimulating factor (G-CSF), chemotherapy such as cyclophosphamide, or a combination of both, and these cells can then be collected by leukapheresis procedures through large-lumen central venous catheters and used for transplantation. Infusion of CD34+ cells isolated from autologous (the patient's own) bone marrow or cytokine-mobilized peripheral blood progenitor cells restores normal hematopoiesis in patients with solid tumors (breast cancer, lymphoma, and neuroblastoma) after they have received marrow-lethal antineoplastic therapy (Table 45-1).

Allogeneic BMT presents an immunologic "double barrier." The immune system of the recipient may mediate rejection of the donor cells, as may occur after allotransplantation of solid organs (eg, kidneys, liver, or heart). Rejection phenomena are decidedly uncommon in children with neoplastic diseases who have received transplants of histocompatible bone marrow from related allogeneic donors. Patients with severe aplastic anemia who are heavily transfused with blood products and then undergo BMT from histocompatible, related donors are at higher risk for graft rejection than their untransfused counterparts, likely because of the development of host cellular immune reactivity against minor transplant antigens on donor cells. Extensive lymphocyte depletion from the bone marrow graft in an effort to reduce the risks of acute graft-versus-host disease has also been associated with failure of sustained engraftment in some patients. There is a greater risk of graft rejection in recipients of BMTs from fully or partially matched unrelated donors, or from related allogeneic donors mismatched with the recipient for two or more human leukocyte antigen (HLA) loci.

The second aspect of the double barrier in allogeneic BMT is acute graft-versus-host disease, which occurs with much greater frequency than graft rejection. This reaction of donor lymphocytes against host organs and tissues can occur even after BMT from a genotypically HLA-identical sibling donor, where the risk of some clinical acute graft-versus-host disease is 30% to

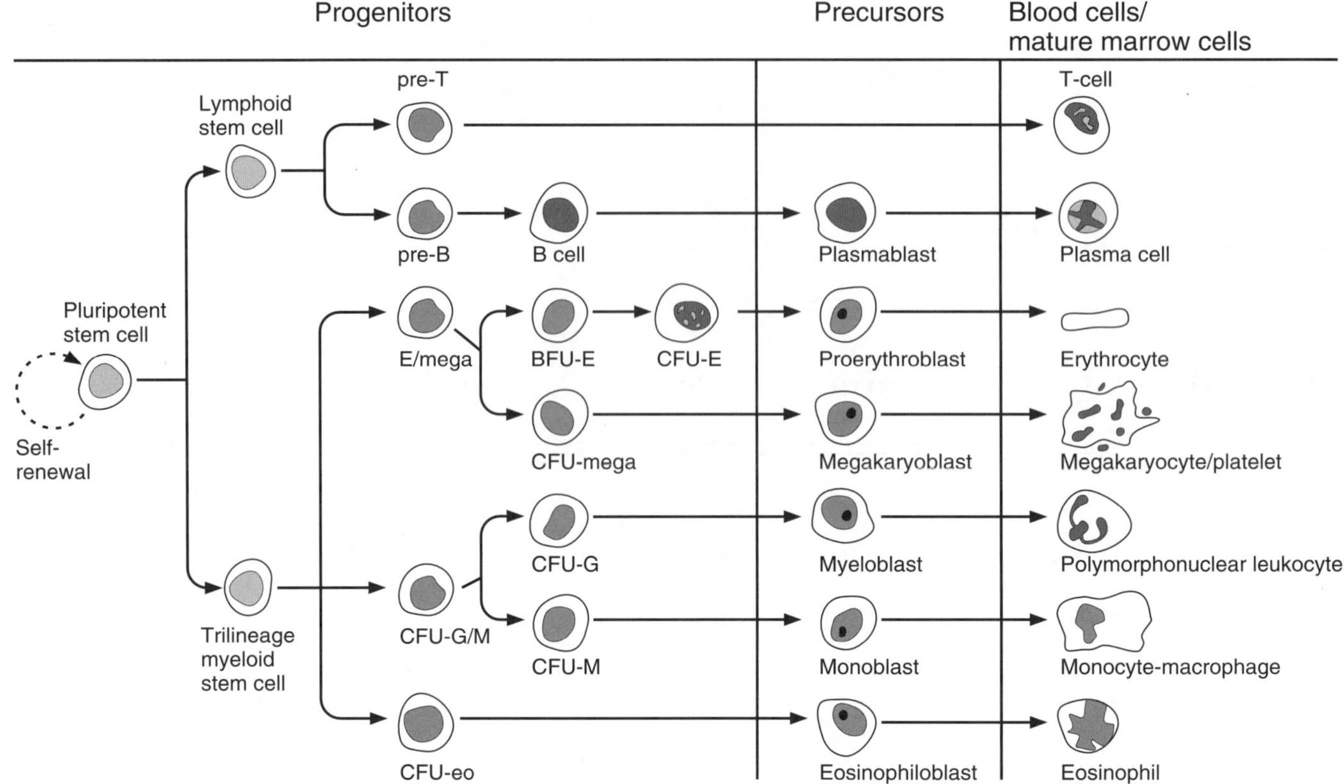

FIG. 45-1. Hematopoietic cell generation and differentiation. All lymphoid and hematopoietic cells arise from a stem cell, which bears the CD34 antigen and which is also capable of self-replication. BFU, burst-forming unit; CFU, colony-forming unit; E, erythrocyte; eo, eosinophil; G, granulocyte; M, monocyte–macrophage; mega, megakaryocyte.

50%. The overall risk of occurrence of any degree of acute graft-versus-host disease is similar in children and adults, but the risk of severe (grades III to IV) acute graft-versus-host disease is lower in pediatric patients.

Before receiving an infusion of bone marrow or other source of stem cells, the patient must first undergo a preparative regimen that provides both intensive immunosuppression (to prevent rejection of the allogeneic marrow graft) and marrow-lethal therapy (to eliminate residual tumor cells or defective stem cells). Preparative regimens include intensive combination chemotherapy, with or without total-body irradiation. Most preparative regimens include high-dose cyclophosphamide, which has both immunosuppressive and antineoplastic properties, and may include total-body irradiation. Many other preparative regimens have been developed, relying on the addition

or substitution of chemotherapeutic agents such as cytosine arabinoside or etoposide, by modification of radiation therapy doses and schedules, or by use of intensive polychemotherapy without total-body irradiation. For example, the combination of high-dose oral busulfan and intravenous cyclophosphamide has been used extensively for allogeneic and autologous BMTs in children with acute myeloid leukemia. Busulfan is highly toxic to normal as well as neoplastic hematopoietic stem cells, and the busulfan–cyclophosphamide regimen has been used before bone marrow grafting for thalassemia, infantile osteopetrosis, lysosomal storage diseases, and cellular immunodeficiency syndromes to displace or eradicate the ineffective host lymphohematopoietic cell populations. Because studies have suggested that the pharmacokinetics of high-dose busulfan differ in patients younger than 6 years of age, use of busulfan dosing based on body surface area rather than body weight has been recommended in younger children.

After allogeneic BMT, the recipient becomes a "chimera," a word taken from Greek mythology describing a beast with the head of one animal and the body of another, because his or her blood cells are of foreign (donor) origin. BMT or stem cell transplantation leads to repopulation of the circulating erythrocytes, leukocytes, platelets, and lymphocytes of the recipient with donor-derived cells, as well as the monocyte- and macrophage-derived phagocytic cells (hepatic Kupffer cells, pulmonary alveolar macrophages, osteoclasts, fixed tissue macrophages, and cutaneous Langerhans cells). Evidence also

TABLE 45-1. *Sources of stem cells*

Source	Potential recipient
Bone marrow	Allogeneic, syngeneic, or autologous
Peripheral blood (mobilized from marrow with cytokines or chemotherapy)	Autologous ? Syngeneic ? Allogeneic
Placental ("cord") blood	Allogeneic ? Autologous (gene therapy)

suggests that some of the central nervous system macrophages, or microglia, are also repopulated by donor allogeneic cells after BMT; this may have implications for treatment by stem cell transplantation of genetic diseases affecting the central nervous system.

RATIONALE FOR BONE MARROW TRANSPLANTATION

There are two different rationales for BMT in human diseases. The first is the use of BMT from a normal donor to replace deficient or defective lymphoid or hematopoietic cells (or both) by providing normal stem cells. This is the basis for BMT in aplastic anemia, selected cytopenias, cellular immunodeficiency states such as severe combined immunodeficiency and Wiskott-Aldrich syndrome, infantile osteopetrosis (a disorder of osteoclast function), and lysosomal storage diseases such as the mucopolysaccharidoses and sphingolipidoses. In these diseases, the normal stem cells must come from healthy, related or unrelated allogeneic donors, or, if there is one, a healthy, unaffected identical twin (syngeneic) donor. As the patient's own stem cells are either inadequate (eg, aplastic anemia) or affected with the defect that the BMT is designed to correct (eg, genetic diseases), autologous BMT is not an option in these conditions. In theory, however, single-gene defects causing some of these conditions ultimately may be corrected by gene-insertion therapy at the stem cell level, and this represents one of the exciting new areas of research in stem cell transplantation.

The second rationale for BMT is to replace normal stem cells that have been intentionally destroyed as a result of intensive antineoplastic therapy. This is the basis for BMT in leukemia, lymphoma, and selected solid tumors in childhood and adolescence. The stem cell transplant serves as a treatment for a planned iatrogenic complication of the very intensive antitumor therapy (ie, acquired severe aplastic anemia). The patient receives intensive antineoplastic therapy, consisting of combination high-dose chemotherapy with or without total-body irradiation; the major dose-limiting adverse effect of such intensive antitumor treatment is the eradication of normal bone marrow stem cells, and an infusion of stem cells counteracts the otherwise fatal aplasia. In theory, stem cell rescue after intensive myeloablative therapy for neoplastic diseases may be obtained from allogeneic, syngeneic, or autologous sources. However, for children with leukemia and some lymphomas or solid tumors such as neuroblastoma, there is concern that occult tumor may be present in the autologous marrow and may lead to recurrence of disease after infusion. A great deal of interest has centered on so-called "negative selection" methods for ex vivo treatment, or "purging" of autologous marrow to eliminate tumor cell contamination. Immunologic methods (eg, monoclonal antibodies with complement, or conjugated with toxins or magnetic beads) and pharmacologic methods (eg, cyclophosphamide congeners such as mafosfamide and 4-hydroperoxy-cyclophosphamide) have been used for this purpose. More recently, "positive selection" methods have been developed to obtain purified CD34+ cells from autologous bone marrow, and to reinfuse these cells into patients with solid tumors. This approach has been used in adults undergoing autologous transplantation for solid tumors like breast cancer and in some children with solid tumors. Positively selected stem cell transplants cannot be used routinely in patients with acute leukemias because of the likelihood that CD34 is expressed on these malignant cells.

The antileukemic effect of allogeneic BMT may extend beyond the repopulation of hematopoiesis by donor-derived cells. The relapse rates after allogeneic BMT for acute leukemia are significantly lower than after syngeneic (identical twin) BMT in similar groups of patients, suggesting an immunologic graft-versus-leukemia effect that is similar to but discernible from the graft-versus-host disease discussed later in this chapter. This effect is most apparent in adults with chronic myelogenous leukemia, where high relapse rates have been associated with infusion of allogeneic marrow depleted of lymphocytes in an attempt to decrease graft-versus-host disease, and appears to be operative after allogeneic BMT for acute myeloid leukemia. The contribution of a graft-versus-leukemia effect after allogeneic BMT for acute lymphocytic leukemia, however, is controversial.

TYPES OF BONE MARROW TRANSPLANTS

There are three different sources of bone marrow for clinical transplantation: allogeneic, syngeneic, or autologous (Table 45-2). Most BMTs have been carried out from allogeneic donors, usually healthy siblings with whom the recipient is genotypically histocompatible at both the class I (HLA-A and -B) and class II (HLA-D) regions, both donor and recipient having received the same HLA haplotypes (located on chromosome 6) from each parent. Therefore, there is only a 25% chance that a BMT candidate will be genotypically HLA-identical to any sibling; in practice, the chance that siblings are histocompatible is approximately 40% because of ethnic and racial clustering of various HLA antigens. The disease-free survival in patients given BMTs from related donors mismatched at up to one HLA locus (HLA-A, -B, or -D), however, is comparable to that in recipients of fully matched allogeneic transplants.

In children without suitably histocompatible, related donors, BMT from phenotypically histocompatible, unrelated allogeneic donors (matched for recipients at most or all of the HLA-A, -B, and -D antigens) identified through national or international registries, may be considered. Results of these unrelated allogeneic transplants are encouraging in children and adolescents with acute or chronic leukemia, aplastic anemia, or genetic storage diseases who lack histocompatible, related marrow donors.

Syngeneic grafts are obtained from identical twins. It is un-

TABLE 45-2. *Sources of bone marrow grafts*

Type of graft	Source
Allogeneic	Related donors (usually siblings; occasionally parents or other phenotypically histocompatible relatives)
	Unrelated, volunteer donors (identified through registries; fully or partially histocompatible)
Autologous	Patient (cannot be used in the case of bone marrow failure or in neoplastic diseases with obvious marrow involvement by tumor)
Syngeneic	Identical twin

common to have both a child needing a BMT and a healthy identical twin donor, but syngeneic BMTs serve as an important standard against which to measure the effectiveness of autologous marrow rescue. Syngeneic marrow transplantation is associated with substantially lower risks of transplant-related complications like graft-versus-host disease and opportunistic infections such as viral pneumonitis. However, the decrease in transplant-related mortality after syngeneic BMT is offset by an increased risk of leukemic relapse; the absence of significant graft-versus-host disease is accompanied by a loss of the graft-versus-leukemia effect observed after allogeneic transplantation.

In some patients with acute leukemia or lymphoma who lack suitable histocompatible, related or unrelated allogeneic donors, autologous stem cell transplants may be considered, in which the patients serve as their own donors. This approach is not feasible in bone marrow failure states such as aplastic anemia or in patients with intrinsic disorders of hematopoiesis, cellular immunity, or cellular metabolism (eg, storage diseases) because of the lack of adequate quantity or quality of the autologous stem cells. Autologous stem cell grafting has been most successful in patients with acute myeloid leukemia, Hodgkin disease, non-Hodgkin lymphomas, and selected solid tumors, such as neuroblastoma. Encouraging relapse-free survival has been reported after autologous BMT in children with acute lymphoblastic leukemia whose initial remission durations exceeded 36 months. Because of the concern that occult tumor cell contamination might contribute to relapse of disease after autologous transplant, the bone marrow is usually collected in remission and often treated with monoclonal antibodies, chemotherapeutic agents, or combinations thereof to purge the sample of tumor cells without undue damage to the normal residual stem cells. The stem cells are then cryopreserved (usually in liquid nitrogen), and then infused into the patient after completion of intensive antineoplastic therapy.

Studies in both adults and children have suggested that CD34+ progenitor cells, mobilized by administration of cytokines such as G-CSF, chemotherapy (cyclophosphamide or 5-fluorouracil), or both agents, and collected from the peripheral blood circulation by apheresis procedures analogous to those used for collection of platelets or leukocytes, may be used as a source of stem cells for autologous transplantation in lymphoma, Hodgkin disease, and solid tumors (eg, neuroblastoma, rhabdomyosarcoma, Ewing sarcoma). Methods for therapeutic apheresis of mobilized peripheral blood progenitor cells have been successfully applied in pediatric patients as small as 7 or 8 kg, using central venous catheters with or without additional radial arterial catheters. Early studies also suggest that peripheral blood progenitor cells may be obtained from allogeneic histocompatible, related donors in sufficient quantities to reconstitute hematopoiesis after marrow-lethal therapy in pediatric patients with lymphohematopoietic malignancies.

Finally, an often overlooked source of stem cells is placental, or umbilical cord, blood. The content of CD34+ cells in placental blood is high, and the number of cells obtained from one delivery has been sufficient to reconstitute hematopoiesis in pediatric recipients. Placental blood transplants from HLA-identical, related donors have been successfully administered to children with neoplastic and hematologic diseases, and regional placental blood cell banks have been developed to provide a source of unrelated, histocompatible stem cells, from which several successful transplants have now been conducted. Because placental blood cells are thought to be excellent targets for insertion of exogenous functional genes, the future application of gene therapy may rely on introduction of the appropriate genetic material into autologous placental blood cells and infusion into the patient, with (or possibly without) preceding marrow-lethal treatment.

BONE MARROW COLLECTION AND ADMINISTRATION

Bone marrow collection (Fig. 45-2) is carried out under sterile conditions in an operating room suite. The donor, who in autologous transplantation is also the patient, receives general (or, less commonly, epidural) anesthesia, and multiple bone marrow aspirates are obtained from both posterior iliac crests. On occasion, marrow is also collected from the anterior iliac crests. Approximately 3×10^8 nucleated bone marrow cells per kilogram of recipient weight is obtained for an allogeneic BMT. The bone marrow is collected in sterile, heparinized tissue culture medium, filtered through a series of stainless-steel mesh screens to remove bone particles and fat and to make a single-cell suspension, and placed in a sterile plastic transfer pack identical to that used for clinical blood banking. The bone marrow may be infused directly into the recipient or may be processed further; for example, incompatible allogeneic erythrocytes may be removed by centrifugation, or autologous marrow may be treated ex vivo and cryopreserved. The bone marrow is given to the recipient intravenously through an indwelling central venous catheter, which is routinely used for administration of chemotherapy and hydration before transplantation and for antibiotics, immunosuppressive agents, blood products, and parenteral alimentation after transplantation. The risks of bone marrow collection are minimal to a healthy donor and are usually related to the risks of anesthesia. The marrow donor has some soreness at the aspirate sites for 1 to 3 days after the procedure, but is usually discharged from the hospital within 24 hours after bone marrow collection.

CLINICAL RESULTS OF BONE MARROW TRANSPLANTATION

Table 45-3 lists some of the diseases curable by BMT.

Immunodeficiency States

Severe combined immunodeficiency syndrome, Wiskott-Aldrich syndrome, and other cellular immunodeficiencies have been cured with allogeneic BMT. For example, allogeneic bone marrow grafting is associated with at least a 50% to 60% chance of long-term disease-free survival and restoration of cellular immune function by normal donor cells in infants who have severe combined immunodeficiency. Because they lack the cellular immune responses to reject histocompatible marrow grafts, infants with severe combined immunodeficiency usually do not require a pretransplantation conditioning regimen. In cellular immunodeficiencies associated with hematopoietic abnormalities (eg, the thrombocytopenia in Wiskott-Aldrich syndrome), pretransplantation cytoreduction is administered to eradicate the dysfunctional lymphoid and hematopoietic stem cells.

Hematopoietic Disorders

Allogeneic marrow transplantation from a healthy, histocompatible sibling is the treatment of choice for children with severe aplastic anemia and leads to complete hematologic reconstitution. The cure rate after allogeneic transplantation in severe aplastic anemia is 80% to 90%, which is superior to immunosuppressive therapy (steroids or antithymocyte globulin) alone. Other disorders of stem cells or selective hematopoietic lineages, such as Fanconi pancytopenia syndrome, congenital red cell aplasia (Blackfan-Diamond-Josephs syndrome), congenital neutropenia (Kostmann syndrome), and amegakaryocytic thrombocytopenia, have been successfully treated with allogeneic BMT. Children who have Fanconi syndrome are at higher risk for more severe treatment-related toxicity after transplantation because of defective cellular DNA repair mechanisms, and require modified pretransplantation preparative regimens (decreased doses of cyclophosphamide or total-body irradiation). Allogeneic BMT has been successfully carried out in the case of leukocyte metabolic abnormalities such as chronic granulomatous disease. Hemoglobinopathies may also be cured with allogeneic BMT. The results of transplantation in children with β-thalassemia major are impressive, and early results of allogeneic transplantation in children with high-risk sickle cell anemia

(eg, recurrent cerebrovascular events, recurrent pulmonary crises) are also encouraging.

An instructive example of the versatility of clinical BMT is seen in infantile, or ''malignant'' osteopetrosis. Infants affected with this condition die with marrow failure (secondary to obliteration of marrow cavities) and massive hepatosplenomegaly (because of extramedullary hematopoiesis), and with profound neurologic deficits because of encroachment of the cranial foramina on cranial nerves and from hydrocephalus due to narrowing of the foramen magnum. Infantile osteopetrosis is caused by abnormal osteoclasts, leading to failure of normal bone remodeling and resorption. Because osteoclasts are derived from the monocyte–macrophage axis, BMT is curative in infantile osteopetrosis by repopulating the entire hematopoietic system with normal donor-derived cells, including functional osteoclasts.

Lysosomal Storage Diseases and Other Metabolic Diseases

Bone marrow transplantation from a healthy, enzymatically normal donor may provide a self-renewing cellular source of replacement lysosomal hydrolase in infants and children with genetic storage diseases. This innovative application of BMT is highly controversial, and studies are in progress to determine the long-term effects of transplantation on neurologic and psychological function in children thus treated. Allogeneic transplantation has been used for several lysosomal storage diseases,

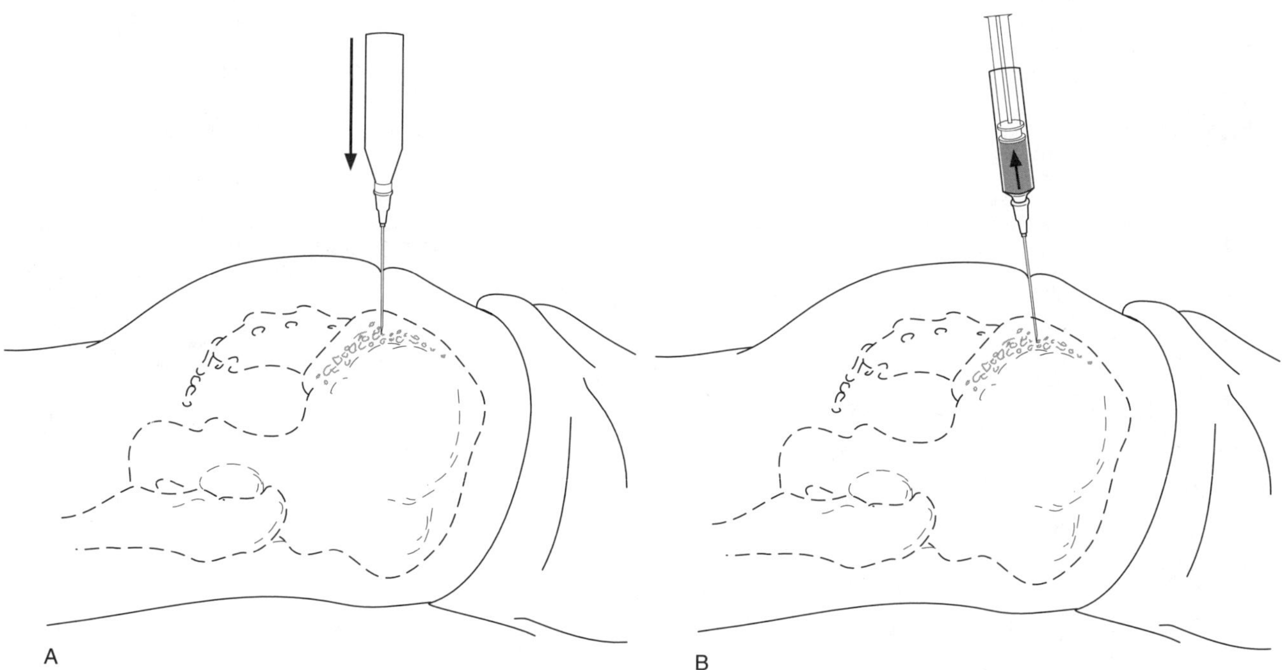

A

B

FIG. 45-2. Marrow collection procedure. Multiple bone marrow aspirates are obtained from each posterior iliac crest through one or two cutaneous puncture sites and redirection of the needle along the crest (*A* and *B*). A limited amount of marrow may be obtained in similar fashion from the anterior iliac crests of larger patients. Marrow is collected in heparinized tissue culture medium or saline and filtered to prepare a single-cell suspension (*C*), which is then processed further or infused directly into the recipient through a central venous access device (*D*). (*continued*)

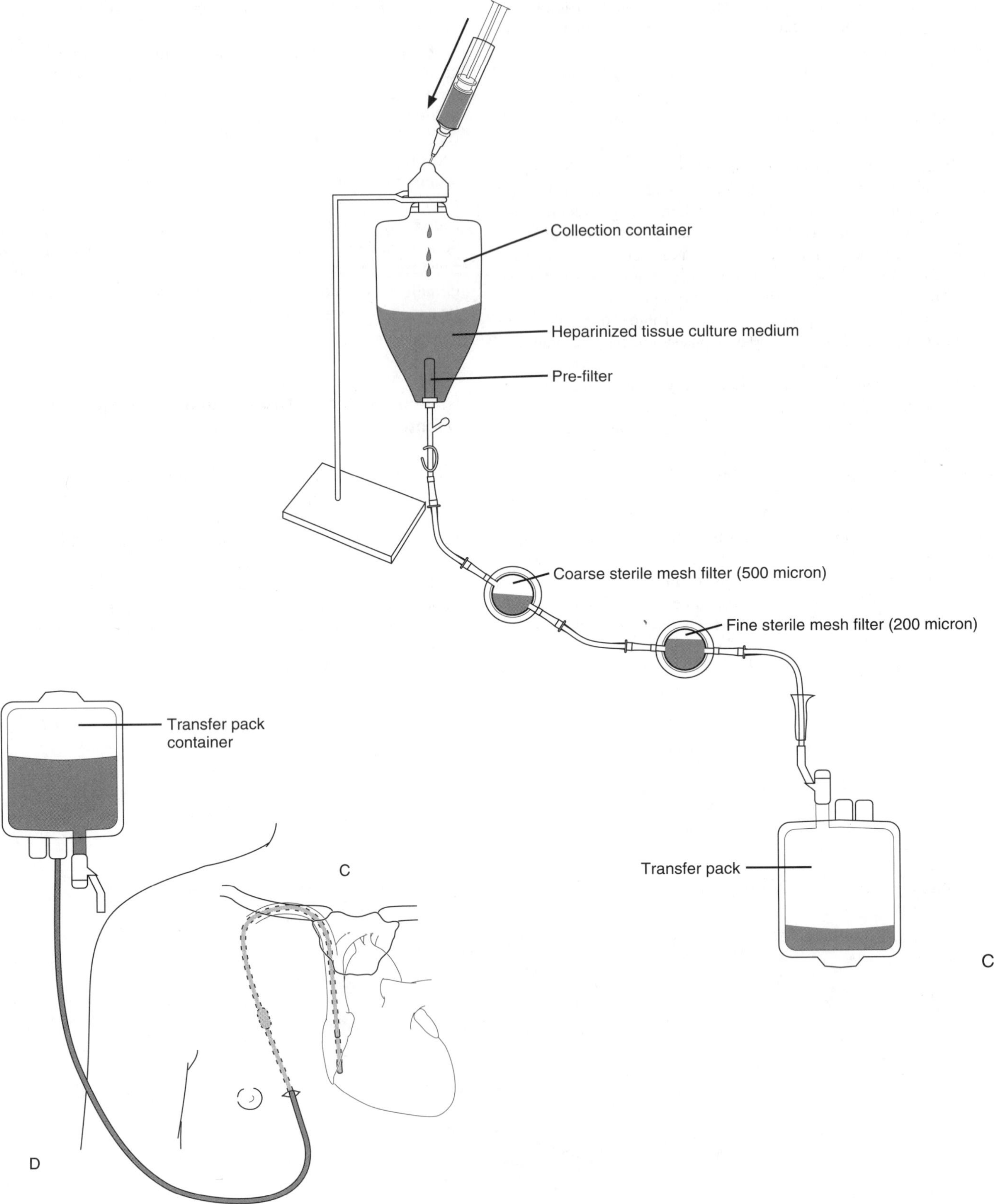

FIG. 45-2. *(continued)*

TABLE 45-3. *Diseases curable by bone marrow transplantation**

Immunodeficiency states
  Severe combined immunodeficiency
  Reticular dysgenesis
  Wiskott-Aldrich syndrome
Hematopoietic disorders
  Amegakaryocytic thrombocytopenia
  Aplastic anemia
  β-Thalassemia major
  Chronic granulomatous disease
  Congenital agranulocytosis
  Congenital hypoplastic anemia (Blackfan-Diamond-Josephs syndrome)
  Fanconi pancytopenia syndrome
  Infantile osteopetrosis
  Sickle cell hemoglobinopathy
Genetic diseases (limited to presymptomatic or asymptomatic patients)
  Sphingolipidoses (metachromatic leukodystrophy, Gaucher disease, Krabbe disease)
  Mucopolysaccharidoses (especially Hurler, Hunter, Maroteaux-Lamy syndromes)
  Adrenoleukodystrophy
Neoplastic diseases
  Acute lymphocytic leukemia (in second remission or high-risk first remission)
  Acute myeloid leukemia (in first or second remission or in untreated first relapse)
  Chronic myelocytic leukemia (in chronic or accelerated phase)
  Hodgkin and non-Hodgkin lymphoma (in second remission or responding first relapse)
  Neuroblastoma (in first remission)
  Selected nonhematopoietic malignancies (Ewing sarcoma, rhabdomyosarcoma, Wilms tumor)

* List is not exhaustive.

including the mucopolysaccharidoses (such as the Hurler and Maroteaux-Lamy syndromes) and the sphingolipidoses (metachromatic leukodystrophy, Krabbe leukodystrophy), and in adrenoleukodystrophy, a disorder of lipid metabolism by peroxisomes. Results strongly suggest that the optimal therapeutic benefit of BMT in these disorders occurs when the procedure is performed on asymptomatic or minimally symptomatic patients.

Neoplastic Diseases

Acute Lymphocytic Leukemia

Many children with acute lymphocytic leukemia are cured with initial induction and maintenance therapy. However, children with specific subtypes of acute lymphocytic leukemia (eg, Philadelphia chromosome-positive, or infant leukemia with the 4;11 chromosomal translocation) are at high risk for relapse and may benefit from allogeneic BMT in first remission. Pediatric patients with acute lymphocytic leukemia who relapse have a very small chance for cure with chemotherapy alone and should be considered for allogeneic transplantation in second remission, which has been shown to be superior to chemotherapy in

children with both short (less than 24 months) and long (greater than 24 months) durations of first remission. Relapse-free survival rates of 35% to 55% and relapse rates of 20% to 40% have been reported in children receiving allogeneic BMT for second-remission acute lymphocytic leukemia. If transplantation is delayed until third or later remissions, the risk of posttransplantation leukemic relapse increases to greater than 50%, suggesting that second remission may be the optimal time to proceed with this intensive therapy.

Acute Myeloid Leukemia

With conventional-dose chemotherapy alone, the chance for long-term leukemia-free survival of children who have acute myeloid leukemia is 25% to 40%, depending on the antileukemic regimens used. Some patients are at higher risk for leukemic relapse by virtue of karyotypic abnormalities identified at the time of diagnosis, specific cytopathologic classification (eg, FAB class M4, M5, M6, or M7), or failure to attain remission after initial intensive induction chemotherapy; these patients may benefit from allogeneic BMT during first remission. Other children who have acute myeloid leukemia may have better survival after bone marrow grafting during first remission if the chance for cure with the chemotherapeutic regimen used is lower than 30%. Because studies suggest that 40% to 65% of children who receive allogeneic transplants for acute myeloid leukemia during first remission are long-term relapse-free survivors, there is a trend toward proceeding with allografting in children with first-remission myeloid leukemia if a histocompatible, related donor can be identified. Children who relapse with acute myeloid leukemia cannot be cured with conventional chemotherapy, and BMT provides the only chance for long-term disease-free survival. Survival rates of 25% to 40% have been reported in children who undergo allogeneic BMT in first untreated relapse or second remission of acute myeloid leukemia.

Autologous Bone Marrow Transplantation in Acute Leukemia

Autologous BMT may serve as an alterative source of stem cells in children with acute leukemia who might benefit from transplantation but lack a suitable related or unrelated donor. As indicated earlier, a concern with autologous transplantation is the possibility that occult leukemic cells may be reinfused with the normal autologous stem cells, thus leading to disease recurrence. Elegant studies using gene-marked autologous marrow have demonstrated that leukemic cells from an untreated autologous marrow graft can be detected at posttransplantation relapse; however, residual leukemia in the patient may also have contributed to the recurrence of disease. Because of these concerns, many investigators believe that some method for ex vivo marrow purging should be used to eliminate occult tumor from the autologous ''remission'' marrow collected in remission. In acute lymphocytic leukemia, the most encouraging studies of autologous transplantation have used immunotoxins or monoclonal antibodies directed against specific lymphoid leukemia cell antigens. In children with lymphocytic leukemia in second or subsequent remission, disease-free survival rates of

20% to 45% have been reported after intensive chemoradiation therapy and immunologically purged autografts, but relapse rates of 30% to 70% have been observed in these series. It appears that relapse-free survival is highest in patients with long (over 3 or 4 years) durations of first remission. In acute myeloid leukemia, disease-free survival is encouraging in recipients of autologous marrow chemopurged with congeners of cyclophosphamide (mafosfamide or 4-hydroperoxycyclophosphamide); patients undergoing autologous transplantation with chemopurged marrow for second- or third-remission myeloid leukemia have a disease-free survival rate of 30%, with a relapse rate of approximately 50%, similar to that observed after syngeneic transplantation. Clearly, the greatest reason for failure of autologous transplantation in acute leukemias is relapse, and methods to decrease posttransplantation relapse by administration of immunomodulatory agents are under investigation. Interleukin-2, interferon, or cyclosporine, or immunostimulatory agents such as linomide may provide an immunologic antitumor effect after autologous transplantation

Neuroblastoma

Children older than 12 months of age who have disseminated or stage IV neuroblastoma have a very unfavorable prognosis, with a disease-free survival rate of less than 10% with combination chemotherapy alone. When carried out during the first complete remission, allogeneic or autologous BMT in children with this disease is associated with cure rates of 25% to 40%, but children who undergo transplantation during partial or second complete remissions have much poorer disease-free survival. The possible contamination of the autograft with occult tumor cells has led to the use of ex vivo bone marrow autograft purging, especially with monoclonal antibodies directed at neuroblastoma-specific antigens, typically coupled to immunomagnetic beads.

Other Malignancies

Patients who have relapsed Hodgkin and non-Hodgkin lymphoma may be cured with allogeneic or autologous BMT; the best results (35% to 50% cure rate) are observed when patients have minimal residual disease or are in a second complete remission. Patients who have bulky residual lymphoma or progressive drug-resistant disease at the time of transplantation are at very high risk for tumor recurrence. More intensive pretransplantation preparative regimens need to be developed that effectively eradicate a resistant or bulky residual tumor with acceptable toxicity. For example, multiagent pretransplantation chemotherapy, including combinations of busulfan, cyclophosphamide, etoposide (VP-16), or cytosine arabinoside may be useful for these patients. Preliminary experience with autologous transplantation as part of the treatment of other solid tumors of childhood (eg, rhabdomyosarcoma, Ewing sarcoma, neuroectodermal tumors, Wilms tumor, and possibly central nervous system tumors) has also been encouraging, particularly when used before disease progression. Again, the observation that patients with refractory disease or large tumor burdens at the time of transplantation are at especially high risk for relapse underscores the suggestion that intensive cytoreductive therapy

with bone marrow stem cell rescue should be applied during states of minimal residual disease (eg, first or second complete remission) in children at high risk for recurrence of solid tumors.

TRANSPLANT-ASSOCIATED COMPLICATIONS

Table 45-4 lists the complications associated with allogeneic BMT.

Infections

The stem cell transplant recipient is aplastic for several weeks after the cells are infused, and during this time is at risk for bacterial and fungal sepsis. The most common gram-positive bacterial organisms encountered are *Staphylococcus aureus*, *Staphylococcus epidermidis*, and *Streptococcus viridans*, and the most common gram-negative pathogens are *Pseudomonas aeruginosa*, *Klebsiella pneumoniae*, and *Escherichia coli*. Fungal pathogens, including *Candida* and *Aspergillus* species, may cause focal or disseminated infections. Empiric broad-spectrum antibiotics during febrile aplastic episodes decreases the risk of fatal posttransplantation sepsis, and prophylaxis with antifungal agents such as low-dose amphotericin B or fluconazole may be of value.

In the patient with severe acute graft-versus-host disease, there is an increased risk of infections related to both the immunosuppressive therapy (eg, steroids, antithymocyte globulin, cyclosporine) and the immune dysregulation that results from this disease process. These infections occur in the context of the nonneutropenic patient. For example, invasive fungal disease such as focal or disseminated aspergillosis may occur. Patients with a history of acute graft-versus-host disease are also at significantly higher risk for development of opportunistic viral infections, chiefly pneumonitis caused by cytomegalovirus.

Graft-Versus-Host Disease

Acute graft-versus-host disease is caused by an immunologic attack of donor cytotoxic T lymphocytes on various target organs and tissues of the allogeneic BMT recipient. It is now appreciated that a cytokine cascade involving at least interleukin-1 and tumor necrosis factor occurs during the acute graft-

TABLE 45-4. *Complications of allogeneic bone marrow transplantation*

Graft rejection (uncommon)
Infections during aplasia (bacterial or fungal)
Graft-versus-host disease
    Acute (target areas: skin, liver, gastrointestinal tract)
    Chronic
Hepatic venoocclusive disease
Interstitial pneumonitis (especially due to cytomegalovirus)
Late effects
    Cataracts
    Growth retardation
    Pulmonary fibrosis
    Sterility

versus-host process, and that natural killer cells also contribute to the pathophysiology of this condition. The initial clinical manifestations of acute graft-versus-host disease occur 2 to 3 weeks after transplantation and may involve the skin, the liver, the gastrointestinal tract, or combinations of these sites. Although mild cases of acute graft-versus-host disease usually respond to therapy, severe, multisystem acute graft-versus-host disease is associated with substantial morbidity and mortality.

Cutaneous manifestations of acute graft-versus-host disease represent a spectrum of severity based on extent and type of involvement. Erythematous macular and papular eruptions may be limited or may progress to confluent erythema or, in severe cases, vesiculobullous lesions and extensive desquamation; in these, manifestations resemble those of toxic epidermal necrolysis. The ears, palms, and soles are commonly affected. Cutaneous acute graft-versus-host disease may be pruritic or painful, and some patients describe sensations similar to those of a severe sunburn. Skin biopsies are used to document the diagnosis of acute graft-versus-host disease and to provide a histopathologic grading of the process. Vacuolar changes in the basal cell layer (dermal–epidermal junction), dyskeratotic cells, and inflammatory cell infiltration are all characteristics of the cutaneous histopathology of acute graft-versus-host disease.

Hepatic manifestations of acute graft-versus-host disease are those of obstructive jaundice: conjugated hyperbilirubinemia and elevation of alkaline phosphatase without striking aberration of transaminases. Liver dysfunction after BMT may be caused by other conditions, such as venoocclusive disease (VOD), viral or toxic hepatitis, or drug-associated cholestasis; to differentiate the etiology of these conditions, liver biopsy may be required. The histopathologic hallmark of hepatic graft-versus-host disease is bile duct necrosis with lymphocytic infiltration.

Gastrointestinal acute graft-versus-host disease is characterized by profuse, secretory diarrhea and abdominal cramps. In severe cases, extensive mucosal sloughing occurs with hemorrhagic enteritis and risk of infection with enteropathic viruses (eg, rotavirus, adenovirus, or coxsackievirus). Gastroduodenoscopic or rectal suction biopsies of the mucosa can be used for histopathologic assessment of gut damage by graft-versus-host disease (eg, crypt cell necrosis, ''exploding'' crypts, and epithelial loss).

Cyclosporine, alone or in combination with a course of corticosteroids or intravenous methotrexate, is the mainstay for prevention of acute graft-versus-host disease because it suppresses the development of donor cytotoxic T cells that mediate the acute graft-versus-host reaction, thereby enhancing immunologic tolerance of graft to host. Initially, cyclosporine is administered intravenously to the allogeneic BMT recipient; when the patient is able to take oral medications and adequate absorption of oral dosing is documented, cyclosporine is then given orally. Unlike recipients of solid organ transplants who must remain on cyclosporine for their entire lifetimes, recipients of allogeneic BMT typically remain on cyclosporine for only 6 to 12 months. After that time, the medication is discontinued because a state of tolerance is achieved between donor lymphoid cells and recipient histocompatibility antigens. The major dose-limiting toxicity of cyclosporine is renal impairment, occasionally leading to reversible acute renal failure.

Several methods have been explored to prevent or decrease acute graft-versus-host disease by ex vivo treatment of the donor bone marrow graft to deplete T lymphocytes, including incubation with anti–T-cell monoclonal antibodies or immunotoxin conjugates, separation with soybean lectin, incubation with high-dose corticosteroids, and counterflow centrifugal elutriation. These methods may decrease the incidence and severity of acute graft-versus-host reactions but have also been associated with both failure of sustained engraftment and increased relapse rates. The challenge remains selectively to deplete donor lymphocytes—or their precursors—that mediate the graft-versus-host effect, but to retain those cell populations that provide a graft-versus-leukemia effect and facilitate allogeneic stem cell engraftment.

Hepatic Venoocclusive Disease

Hepatic VOD is characterized by tender hepatomegaly, hyperbilirubinemia, excessive weight gain, and ascites, with an onset at 1 to 2 weeks after BMT. Patients with extensive previous chemotherapy and those with abnormal hepatic blood chemistries at time of transplantation are at highest risk for development of this complication. The pathophysiology of this condition is not fully understood, but it is likely that the intensive pretransplantation conditioning regimen damages the endothelium, causing fibrin depositions in the hepatic venules and ultimately leading to ischemic hepatic failure. VOD may occur in up to 15% of BMT patients and has a case-fatality rate of 50%. There is no definitive therapy for VOD. Some advocate low-dose heparin, and observations of low antithrombin III levels in some patients with VOD suggest that administration of antithrombin III may be of value in this disease.

Interstitial Pneumonitis

Interstitial pneumonitis due to cytomegalovirus infection has historically been a major cause of mortality after allogeneic BMT. Characteristically occurring 2 to 3 months after transplantation, its manifestations include fever, tachypnea, dyspnea, and hypoxemia. The striking lack of substantial auscultatory findings (eg, rales and rhonchi) contrasts with impressive radiographic findings of bilateral interstitial infiltrates. Although cytomegalovirus is associated with most cases of posttransplantation interstitial pneumonitis, other infectious agents (usually viral pathogens such as adenovirus or parainfluenzavirus) may also cause this disease, or the process may be idiopathic. It is therefore important to establish the etiology of interstitial pneumonitis by bronchoscopy with bronchoalveolar lavage or, in some cases, by open or thoracoscopic lung biopsy. In the past, the therapy of this difficult complication was limited to symptomatic supportive care, but more recent approaches to combination therapy with an antiviral agent (ganciclovir or foscarnet) and intravenous immunoglobulin G with high anti-cytomegalovirus titer have shown promising results, potentially decreasing the case-fatality rate of cytomegalovirus pneumonia by 50% or more. In patients who are undergoing transplantation without previous exposure to cytomegalovirus infection and whose allogeneic bone marrow donors are also negative for anti-cytomegalovirus antibodies, prevention of introduction of cytomegalovirus infection is important. Because blood products such as platelets can transmit cytomegalovirus, administration of exclusively cytomegalovirus-negative blood products to these patients can prevent the development of cytomegalovirus infection. A new approach that may be promising is the ex vivo expansion of donor-derived cytotoxic T-cell clones directed against viral pathogens, such as cytomegalovirus, and infusion of these cells into the recipient as treatment for or prevention of infection by these agents.

Late Effects

The quality of life is excellent for most children who have undergone BMT. Late transplant-related toxicities may include sterility, cataracts, growth failure, and chronic pulmonary fibrosis with restrictive lung disease. The etiology of these adverse effects is multifactorial: prior chemotherapy and radiation therapy for the underlying neoplastic disease, pretransplantation preparative regimens, and graft-versus-host disease and its treatment (eg, high-dose, long-term corticosteroids) may all contribute to late organ system failure in the patient who has had a transplant. After BMT for acute leukemia, most cases of significant growth failure or endocrine dysfunction have occurred in the context of regimens containing total-body irradiation added to local (eg, craniospinal) radiation therapy; most of these patients have had systemic chronic graft-versus-host disease as well.

BIBLIOGRAPHY

Beatty PG. Results of allogeneic bone marrow transplantation with unrelated or mismatched donors. Semin Oncol 1992;19:13.

Burdach S, Jürgens H, Peters C, et al. Myeloablative radiochemotherapy and hematopoietic stem-cell rescue in poor-prognosis Ewing's sarcoma. J Clin Oncol 1993;11:1482.

Horowitz MM, Bortin MM. Results of bone marrow transplants from human leukocyte antigen-identical sibling donors for treatment of childhood leukemias. Am J Pediatr Hematol Oncol 1993;15:56.

Johnson FL, Pochedly C, eds. Bone marrow transplantation in children. New York, Raven Press, 1990.

Jones RJ, Lee KSK, Beschorner WE, et al. Venoocclusive disease of the liver following bone marrow transplantation. Transplantation 1987;44:778.

Kernan NA, Bartsch G, Ash RC, et al. Analysis of 462 transplantations from unrelated donors facilitated by the National Marrow Donor Program. N Engl J Med 1993;328:593.

Kolb HJ, Bender-Götze C. Late complications after allogeneic bone marrow transplantation for leukaemia. Bone Marrow Transplant 1990;6:61.

Rowe JM, Ciobanu N, Ascensao J, et al. Recommended guidelines for the management of autologous and allogeneic bone marrow transplantation. Ann Intern Med 1994;120:143.

Seeger RC, Reynolds CP. Treatment of high-risk solid tumors of childhood with intensive therapy and autologous bone marrow transplantation. Pediatr Clin North Am 1991;38:393.

Sullivan KM, Agura E, Anasetti C, et al. Chronic graft-versus-host disease and other late complications of bone marrow transplantation. Semin Hematol 1991;28:250.

Vogelsang GB, Wagner JE. Graft-versus-host disease. Hematol Oncol Clin North Am 1990;4:625.

Yeager AM. Pediatric bone marrow transplantation. Pediatr Rev 1991;12:364.

Surgery of Infants and Children: Scientific Principles and Practice, edited by Keith T. Oldham, Paul M. Colombani, and Robert P. Foglia. Lippincott–Raven Publishers, Philadelphia, © 1997.

CHAPTER 46

Uncommon and Experimental Pediatric Transplant Procedures

Paul M. Colombani and Dennis Lund

The previous chapters in this transplant section have described the individual operative procedures and results for the various solid organ and bone marrow transplants. This chapter discusses the more uncommon pediatric transplant procedures including combinations of solid organs and bone marrow, multivisceral and abdominal cluster transplantation, small intestinal transplantation, and whole pancreas transplantation. In addition, this chapter discusses future directions for transplantation including xenotransplantation and cellular transplants for metabolic diseases.

COMBINATION TRANSPLANTS

With rapid advances in clinical solid organ and bone marrow transplantation since the 1970s, transplant centers have been extending the indications for transplantation to include multiple organ transplants in the same patient. These combinations first began when a kidney transplant was performed on a heart transplant recipient in renal failure. Liver transplants have also been combined with heart transplants, and the kidney has been transplanted with the liver in patients with end-stage liver disease and prolonged renal failure from hepatorenal syndrome.[1] With the advent and popularization of whole pancreas transplantation, the combination of a pancreas with a kidney for the diabetic patient with end-stage renal disease has been quite successful.[2] All of these transplants are essentially two independent operations; each of which has been discussed above. The complications posed by these combination transplants are also independent and appear to be similar to those posed by single organ transplants. Rejection rates, however, appear to be lower when the liver is combined with either heart or kidney transplant. Similarly, the combination of kidney and pancreas transplants has resulted in improved pancreatic graft survival. This protective effect that occurs when liver transplantation is combined with other organs has been applied to the use of liver–small bowel transplantation, which is discussed later in this chapter.

Using techniques outlined in Chapter 39, donor bone marrow has also been used in combination with kidney and liver transplant procedures to attempt to improve graft acceptance and decrease rejection rates. In general, transplants that include the combination of solid organs and the addition of donor bone marrow have resulted in improved graft and patient survival compared with liver or kidney transplants alone.[3,4]

MULTIVISCERAL TRANSPLANTS

The first multivisceral transplant was performed in 1981 by Reitz et al with an en bloc heart–lung transplant.[5] The initial indications for a heart–lung transplant were lung disease and advanced pulmonary hypertension. Following the initial success of this approach, the indications for en bloc heart–lung transplant were extended to include patients with primary pulmonary diseases such as cystic fibrosis. This approach required the removal of an often perfectly normal lung. This prompted the ''domino procedure'' in which a cystic fibrosis patient underwent a heart–lung transplant and his ''normal'' lung was then transplanted into a lung-only recipient (as a living-unrelated lung transplant). With the advent of single and double lung transplants as discussed in Chapter 44, the use of en bloc heart and lung transplantation for pulmonary indications has largely disappeared.

Since the late 1980s, abdominal multivisceral transplants have been attempted. With the use of newer immunosuppressive agents, such as Tacrolimus (FK506), these multivisceral transplants have been more successful.[6,7] The most common multivisceral transplant is a combined en bloc liver and small intestine transplant which is discussed later. Some patients have received multiple upper abdominal viscera in what is termed a *cluster transplant*. A series of these cluster transplants was performed in Pittsburgh for a variety of indications, most commonly benign pancreatic tumors or pancreatic tumors metastatic to the liver.[8] These upper abdominal cluster transplants included the duodenum and pancreas, portions of the stomach, small intestine, colon, and liver (Fig. 46-1). In general, cluster transplants have not been convincingly successful. High morbidity and mortality has resulted from complications related to the patients' underlying malignant disease, a high incidence of Ep-

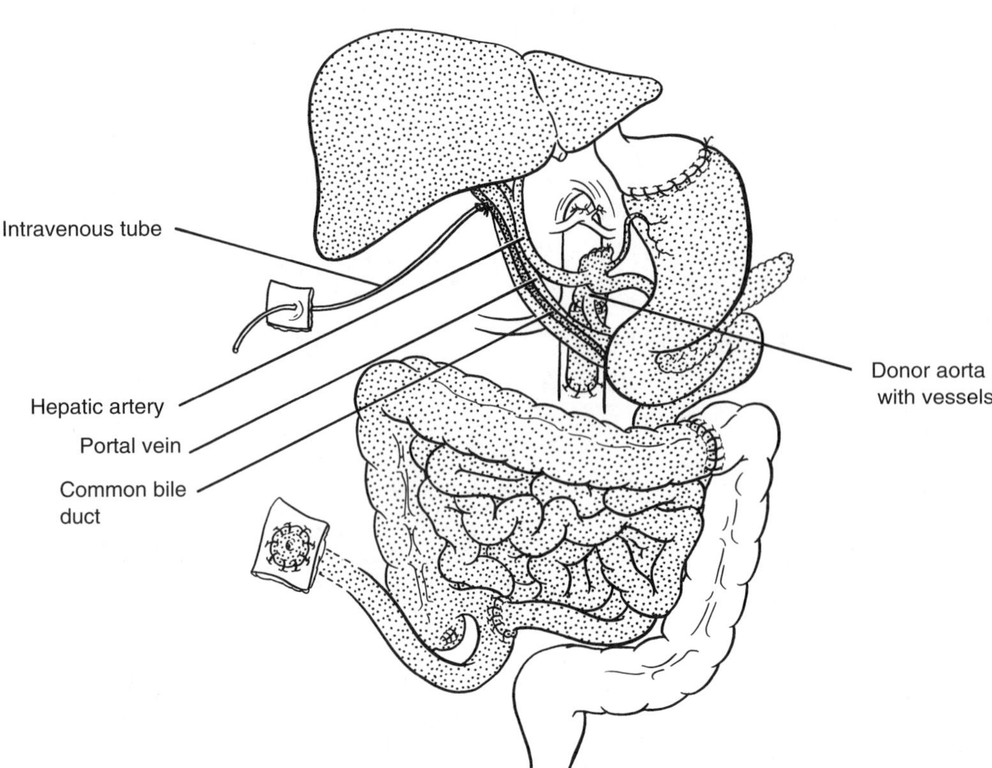

FIG. 46-1. Multivisceral transplantation. The stomach, pancreas, duodenum, and small and large bowel were transplanted with the liver in this instance. The donor suprahepatic vena cava was anastomosed end to side to the donor inferior vena cava.[8] Stippled areas indicate donor grafts.

stein-Barr virus (EBV)-related lymphoproliferative disease, and other serious viral infectious complications.

SMALL INTESTINE

Transplantation of the bowel remains one of the true challenges in transplantation. Despite more than 30 years of clinical attempts at intestinal transplantation, it remains an experimental therapy. During most of this period, the clinical pressure to provide a satisfactory nutrient-absorptive organ for patients with short bowel syndrome has remained despite our advances in parenteral nutrition, long-term central venous access, and procedures to improve gut length and absorptive surface. The recent availability of potent immunosuppressive agents (cyclosporine and Tacrolimus) has allowed transplant surgeons to overcome recipients' vigorous immune response against this complex immune target (small intestine). These agents, however, have also increased potential immunosuppressive complications, often leading to graft or patient loss. Many difficult clinical problems remain, but experience with small bowel transplants has vastly increased, particularly in the past 8 years. Twenty-five transplant centers worldwide are now active in clinical intestinal transplantation. The area is particularly important to pediatric specialists since children are more likely to have difficulties with long-term intravenous hyperalimentation due to problems associated with venous access or the development of liver disease.

Indications for Intestinal Transplantation

Virtually any child with intestinal failure who has an unrecoverable prognosis may be a candidate for intestinal transplan-

tation. Potential causes of intestinal failure in children include the following:

- Jejunoileal atresia
- Necrotizing enterocolitis
- Gastroschisis with associated volvulus or atresia
- Midgut volvulus due to intestinal malrotation
- Intestinal pseudoobstruction
- Total intestinal Hirschsprung disease
- Microvillus inclusion disease
- Intestinal polyposis

Patients with total intestinal neuropathy or myopathy are difficult to diagnose, but once the diagnosis is accurately made, the prognosis can be quite certain. Predicting the outcome of patients with short-gut syndrome is more difficult because both the length of the bowel as well as its quality and the presence or absence of a colon or ileocecal valve determine whether the bowel can successfully adapt (see Chapter 69 on short bowel syndrome).

For patients with intestinal failure, the indications for transplantation include loss of central venous access that makes parenteral nutrition impossible, short bowel syndrome and failure of the remaining bowel to adapt, and inability to be fed enterally with the development of hyperalimentation-induced liver disease.

Clinical Experience with Intestinal Transplants

Before the introduction of cyclosporine, multiple attempts at both cadaveric and living-related small intestinal transplants were performed at several institutions. Immunosuppression regimens included azathioprine, high-dose steroids, and antilymphocyte preparations.[9,10] These regimens proved inadequate to prevent rejection and graft loss. The widespread availability of parenteral nutrition after 1970 reduced some of the pressure on clinicians to attempt transplantation in patients with short bowel syndrome.[11] As time passed, however, the limitations of hyperalimentation became more apparent, particularly in children. These included problems with chronic intravenous access, such as infection and thrombosis, as well as the appearance of liver disease associated with chronic use of intravenous feedings.

In 1984, the Food and Drug Administration approved cyclosporine, with dramatic impact on the success of liver transplantation. The first attempted intestinal transplant using cyclosporine was performed in Toronto in 1985, 15 years after the first human leukocyte antigen (HLA)-identical bowel transplant was performed in New York.[12,13] The intriguing result had a profound influence on subsequent attempts at bowel transplantation. The donor was a blood group O cadaver; the recipient was a young woman with Gardener syndrome who was blood group A and who had a desmoid tumor leading to intestinal loss. The transplant was placed in heterotopic position with systemic venous drainage. Immunosuppression consisted of cyclosporine and steroids. Six days postoperatively, the patient developed severe hemolytic anemia associated with anti-A antibodies, that is, graft versus host disease. She ultimately succumbed to neurologic complications, although the graft when removed on posttransplant day 10 showed only mild rejection. Since this experience, virtually all subsequent cases of intestinal transplantation have involved only blood-group–identical donors and recipients, despite the fact that some liver transplants have been successful with different donor and recipient blood types.

Other isolated intestinal grafts were tried with primary cyclosporine immunosuppression during the late 1980s. One of the largest experiences was in Paris, where nine grafts were performed in seven patients. All donors were cadavers, and all were HLA-mismatched.[14] In one case, the donor was blood group O and the recipient was group A. The grafts were placed in heterotopic position with aortic inflow and inferior vena cava outflow, and proximal bowel continuity was established with distal stomas for surveillance biopsies. Induction immunosuppression consisted of antithymocyte globulin for 15 days and was maintained with cyclosporine and steroids. Rejection was treated with a variety of antibodies, including OKT3, antilymphocyte globulin, and anti-IL2 receptor antibodies.

Two grafts were lost in the operating room, one from patient death and another due to infarction. The ABO-mismatched patient developed severe hemolytic anemia. Four other grafts were lost to early rejection requiring graft removal. One grafts survived for 6 months and another for 17 months. One patient, who received her graft from a premature anencephalic donor, is alive and well and free of intravenous feedings almost 7 years since her transplant. Whether or not the immaturity of the donor played a role in the success of this graft is open to speculation.[15]

The concept of multivisceral cluster transplants in dogs was first presented in 1960 by Starzl at the Surgical Forum and is covered in a previous section.[16]

Until 1988, intestinal transplantation had not been shown much success. In that year, Grant and his coworkers in London, Ontario performed the first truly successful liver–bowel transplant.[17] The recipient was a 41-year-old woman who had lost her intestine due to mesenteric artery thrombosis associated with antithrombin III deficiency. Her liver was otherwise normal. She underwent liver–small bowel transplantation with the arterial supply from the aorta via a conduit. This was made from the donor aorta and the native portal vein which were anastomosed to the side of the donor portal vein to create an orthotopic graft (Fig. 46-2). The proximal bowel was connected to the donor duodenum, and the distal ileum was exteriorized. The donor was pretreated with OKT3 and antilymphocyte serum. The recipient received induction immunosuppression with OKT3 for 10 days followed by cyclosporine and prednisone. Enteral feedings were begun early, 5 days postoperatively, and the patient was weaned off of parenteral nutrition by 2 months posttransplant. This patient survived for more than 5 years and ultimately succumbed to recurrent mesenteric thrombosis.

Grant's group performed five transplants through 1991: three liver–small bowel grafts, of which two were successful (both patients survived approximately 5 years), and two multivisceral grafts in patients who developed lymphoma at 210 and 320 days, respectively. The one nonsurviving liver–bowel graft patient died at 90 days from complications of intraoperative hypotension due to extensive venous thrombosis and poor venous return.[18]

Grant's success, particularly with the two liver–bowel grafts, supported the theory that the liver protects bowel grafts, allowing them to be accepted with cyclosporine immunosuppression when isolated bowel transplantation failed. Much experimental animal evidence also supported this hypothesis,[19] and Grant's clinical experience led to a relative explosion of interest in clinical intestinal transplantation.

Tacrolimus (FK506), a more powerful drug for immunosuppression, debuted in the late 1980s. This drug works via the same mechanism as cyclosporine but is much more potent. The seminal work with FK506 was done at the University of Pittsburgh by Starzl's group,[20] and they began a large clinical experience with this drug in intestinal transplant patients. Over 5 years, 41 children and 30 adults underwent intestinal transplants with FK506 at the University of Pittsburgh.[21,22] This is the largest single institution experience with intestinal transplantation in the world and represents 42% of all of the intestinal transplants done to date. The children received a total of 44 grafts, including 10 isolated small bowel grafts (Fig. 46-3), 27 liver–bowel grafts, and 7 multivisceral grafts (see Fig. 46-1). All grafts were from ABO-identical donors. Graft preservation was done with cold University of Wisconsin solution, and donors were not pretreated to deplete the lymphocyte population of the grafts. These grafts were typically placed in orthotopic position with portal drainage of intestinal venous blood. Immunosuppression was induced with intravenous FK506 and prostaglandin E_1. It was maintained with enteral FK506, steroids (which were rapidly weaned), and low-dose azathioprine.

The children in this group who received isolated intestinal grafts had the longest survival and the least complicated postoperative hospital courses. As of 1995, the graft survival rate for the pediatric patients was 52%, and 58% of these patients were still alive. Of the four children who received retransplants, only one is alive.

The second largest experience of transplanting intestine in children was at the University of Nebraska, where Langnas and his group[23] had performed intestinal transplants in 26 children

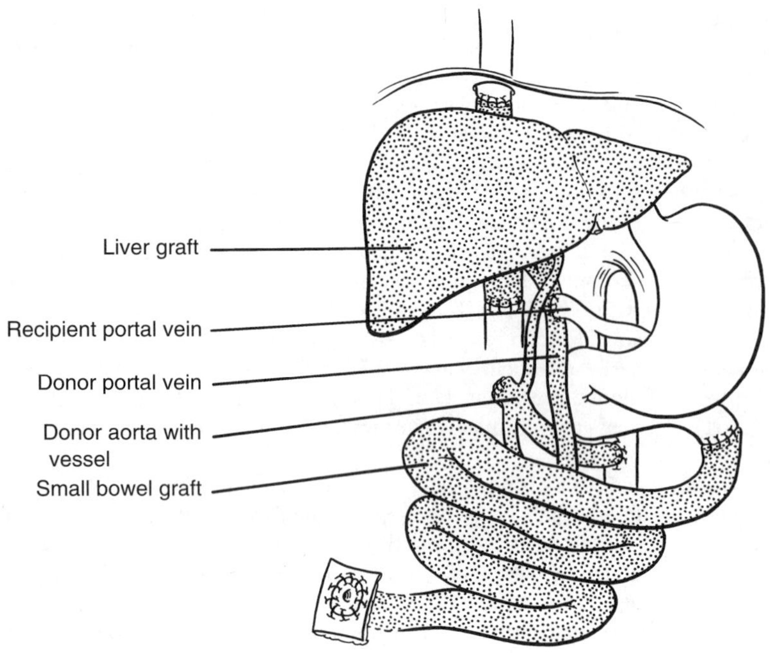

FIG. 46-2. Anatomy of combined liver–intestine graft as performed by Grant.[17] Arterial reconstruction was by means of an aortic conduit from the donor anastomosed to the recipient's infrarenal aorta. The donor portal vein was connected end to side to the recipient portal vein. Stippled areas indicate engrafted liver and small intestine.

as of 1995. Donors were pretreated with antithymocyte globulin and OKT3, and recipient immunosuppression was with enteral FK506 and steroids. Eight patients received isolated intestinal grafts, one of which was removed for hyperacute rejection. Of the 18 patients who received liver–bowel grafts, the 1-year survival rate was 63%.

Grant compiled the world's experience for his presentation at the Fourth International Symposium on Small Bowel Transplantation in Pittsburgh in October 1995. As of June 1995, 180 intestinal transplants had been performed in 170 patients. Of these, 69 (38%) were transplants of isolated intestine, 83 (46%) were liver–intestine, and 28 (16%) were multivisceral grafts. A total of 25 transplant centers have performed clinical intestinal transplants, and 55% of all the intestinal transplants have been

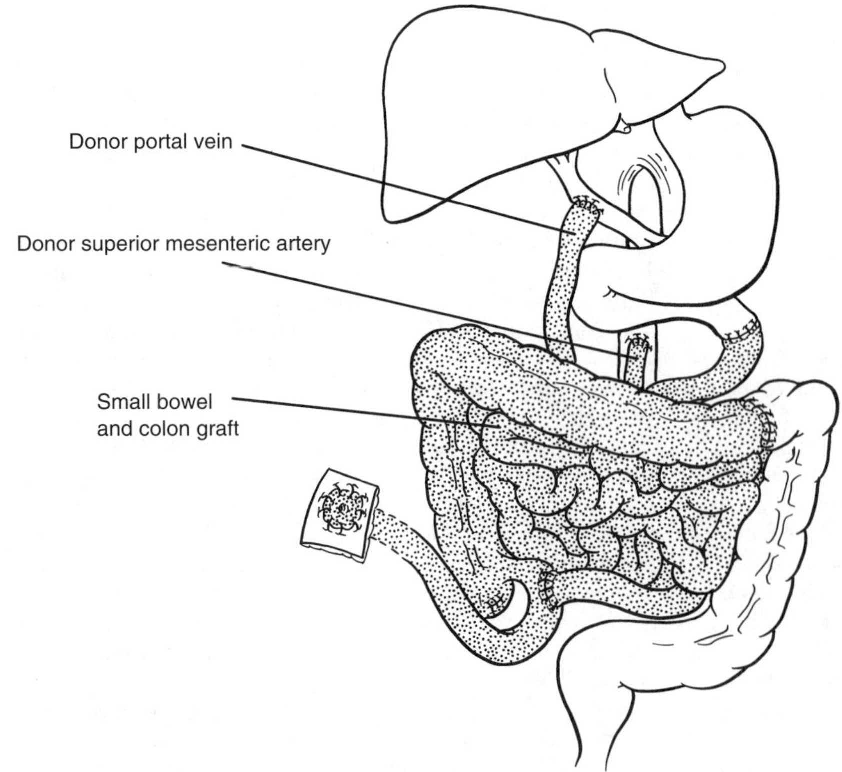

FIG. 46-3. Isolated intestinal transplant, including the right and transverse colon, as performed at the University of Pittsburgh. Portal venous outflow was through the recipient portal vein. A Bishop-Koop type of ileostomy was used to provide access to the bowel for biopsies.[21,22] Stippled areas indicate small bowel graft.

performed in children younger than 10 years. In general, the results have been better with FK506 than with cyclosporine. Patients receiving isolated intestinal grafts also had better outcomes.

In patients who received isolated intestinal grafts with FK506 through June 1995, 1-year and 3-year graft survival rates were 70% and 50%, respectively. The 3-year graft survival rate with cyclosporine was 10% in isolated grafts. In patients who received liver–bowel grafts, 1- and 3-year graft survival rates with FK506 were 65% and 40%, respectively, and with cyclosporine, they were 45% and 30%, respectively. Multivisceral graft recipients had about a 50% 1-year graft survival rate and a 40% 3-year graft survival rate with either drug. The grafts were functioning in 55% of the patients who died, which highlights the problem of potential overimmunosuppression.

The most optimistic data collected by Grant, however, was that among the 86 patients surviving with functioning intestinal transplants, 78% had full graft function and were free of intravenous hyperalimentation. Children who received intestinal grafts have had slightly better graft survival rates at 3 years than have the adults (52% versus 42%) in the University of Pittsburgh experience.[21,22] the mortality rate for children on waiting lists for liver–bowel grafts, however, is approximately 50%. Furthermore, in the Pittsburgh experience, the patient survival of those children who received grafts while on life support was negligible, and patients who were in the hospital awaiting transplants did not fare as well as children who were waiting at home until a donor graft became available.[21]

Technical Considerations

HLA matching of the donor and recipient has generally not been used in liver or intestinal transplants, although ABO-identical donors should be used. Although long-term graft survival can be achieved with HLA mismatch and a positive crossmatch, theoretic HLA advantages may be associated with using living-related donors. To date, however, the evidence for this is sparse.

Likewise, the role of donor pretreatment for preventing graft versus host disease (GVHD) is unknown. GVHD is a common complication associated with bone marrow transplantation, but has not been a frequent problem in patients who have received ABO-identical intestinal grafts. There is evidence of donor lymphocytes in the recipient blood stream after intestinal transplantation, but this is not accompanied by clinical GVHD.[24]. Intestinal transplant patients may appear septic in the first days after transplant, which may be mediated by cytokines associated with the allogeneic mixed lymphocyte reaction. It also occurred however, in one patient who received an intestinal graft from an identical twin after resection of an abdominal desmoid tumor on posttransplant day four.[25]

A variety of techniques have been used to vascularize these grafts. It is generally thought that portal drainage of the blood from the intestine is better and may provide trophic factors for the liver as well as confer a slight immunologic advantage.[26,27] This is, however, technically more difficult than draining the portal blood into the inferior vena cava. Arterialization of the graft is usually achieved by using a conduit of aorta from the donor and anastomosing this to the recipient's infrarenal aorta. Typically, the proximal intestine is placed in continuity with the recipient bowel to allow early enteral feeding and also enteral administration of FK506, where it is well absorbed early after surgery. Some type of distal stoma is used to provide access for surveillance biopsies, and total intestinal continuity is restored after the patient is stable and has shown good graft acceptance.

Complications of Intestinal Transplantation

Rejection is the most frequent complication of intestinal transplantation. Intestinal rejection is a patchy process and may be subtle; therefore, multiple random biopsies are usually taken of the intestinal graft at preset intervals or when clinical conditions, such as fever or diarrhea, warrant them. Even severely damaged intestinal mucosa can recover if the rejection is controlled, but clearly early diagnosis is beneficial. To achieve this, measures of intestinal permeability, which are somewhat nonspecific,[17] may help as well the use of electron microscopy or immunohistochemical technique when processing the biopsies.[28]

Septic episodes are also frequent in intestinal transplant patients, and the dilemma for the clinician is whether an ill patient has infection, rejection, or both. Viral, fungal, and bacterial infections can all occur in these immunosuppressed patients, particularly in patients receiving large amounts of immunosuppression due to frequent bouts of rejection. The group at the University of Pittsburgh has used selective bacterial decontamination in their patients, but the data does not suggest that this diminishes episodes of sepsis.[29]

Lymphoproliferative disease (LPD) remains a life-threatening problem for patients receiving intestinal transplants. It is associated with EBV, and EBV particles can be identified with immunohistochemical probes in the cells of these tumors.[30] In the data collected by Grant, the incidence of grafts lost to LPD was 12% in 180 intestinal transplants. Children may be particularly prone to this complication with a reported incidence of 31% in 41 children receiving intestinal grafts at the University of Pittsburgh.[21] The initial treatment for LPD is to withdraw the immunosuppression as much as tolerated and to administer immunoglobulin. Acyclovir, Gancyclovir, and gamma-interferon may also be beneficial. Assessing peripheral blood with a probe for EBV using polymerase chain reaction may detect LPD early and allow intervention before clinical disease develops.[31]

Cytomegalovirus (CMV) disease has also been a problem in children receiving intestinal transplants. Some programs now avoid using donors who have positive antibody titers to CMV, but this further reduces the available donor pool for these patients who have a high waiting list mortality. The incidence of CMV disease was 30% in the Pittsburgh intestinal transplant children if either the donor or the recipient or both were CMV positive, but no CMV disease occurred in cases in which both the donor and recipient were CMV negative.[25] Treatment of symptomatic CMV disease is with Gancyclovir and reduction of the immunosuppression, if possible.

The future for children with intestinal failure who need transplants is getting brighter. Tremendous clinical experience has been obtained, and many hurdles have been overcome. Some theoretic problems, such as GVHD which is frequently seen with animal intestinal transplants, have not appeared with regularity in clinical intestinal transplantation. Clearly, the availability of FK506 was a major breakthrough, allowing isolated intestinal transplants to succeed for the first time.

New immunosuppressive agents will undoubtedly become available. Improved techniques for identifying rejection and LPD and for preventing and treating are actively being sought. One of the most difficult aspects of caring for these patients is to balance the immunosuppression to avoid overimmunosuppression with its attendant risks of infection and development of LPD. This will require further clinical experience.

One of the potentially exciting areas in transplantation immunology is the manipulation of the biologic response to transplantation. Recently, Starzl's group has found evidence for the establishment of long-term chimeric states in recipients of stable allografts.[32] This has led to efforts in Pittsburgh and Miami to enhance the development of long-term chimerism in intestinal transplant recipients by infusing donor bone marrow along with intestinal grafts.[33,34]

Despite the great improvement in outcome of intestinal transplantation, the survival data and clinical results suggest that this modality remains experimental and should be reserved for patients who have no other alternative. As outcomes improve with experience, new drugs, and possibly with biologic manipulation of the immune response, intestinal transplantation will become one of the standard treatments of children with irreversible intestinal failure.

WHOLE-ORGAN PANCREATIC TRANSPLANTS

Since the mid-1980s, solitary pancreas transplantation and combined kidney pancreas transplantation for patients with diabetes mellitus has gained in popularity and success.[35–37] Only a handful of children, however, have received pancreas transplant for diabetes mellitus for a number of reasons. First, no definitive data shows that a successful pancreas transplant prevents the long-term complications of diabetes mellitus. Second, most pediatric juvenile-onset diabetes mellitus patients have not developed any of of these side effects. Third, the risks of long-term immunosuppression in the pediatric population have outweighed the benefit of freedom from insulin administration and dietary restriction. For the adult diabetic, with or without diabetes complications, there are a number of incentives for pancreas transplantation, including no daily insulin injection requirement, relief from dietary restrictions, and the potential reversal or alleviation of retinopathy, neuropathy, arterial disease, and renal failure associated with long-term diabetes mellitus. Although dramatic improvement has occurred over the last decade in patient and graft survival following pancreas transplantation, there are still significant failure rates and complications related to solitary pancreas transplants.[38] These transplants either do nothing to reverse complications of long-term diabetes are either or may accelerate them. Only diabetic neuropathy has the potential for some improvement following successful pancreas transplantation.

For the diabetic patient who already has developed end-stage renal disease and will undergo a renal transplant, the posttransplant immunosuppression may provide a reasonable risk umbrella to perform a simultaneous pancreas transplant to free the patient from daily insulin injections and severe dietary restrictions. Pancreas graft survival in patients receiving kidney transplants is more than double that of patients receiving pancreas transplants alone.[39] Although pancreas graft survival is improved with the addition of the renal transplant, the overall number and severity of complications in patients undergoing combined kidney–pancreas transplantation is consistently higher than those receiving a kidney transplant alone. Candidates for combined kidney–pancreas transplantation include those with overt secondary complications of diabetes mellitus including end-stage renal disease. The ideal candidate is a patient with minimal secondary complications outside the kidneys and good general clinical condition. Patients also must be able to understand the posttransplant requirements for their care and be aware of the potential morbidity associated with adding the pancreas transplant.

The technical aspects of pancreas transplantation have significantly evolved, providing improved results. Whole-organ pancreas transplants are superior to segmental transplants. Including donor duodenum for anastomosis is associated with fewer complications than direct anastomosis of the pancreas to the bowel or bladder. Bladder anastomosis appears to be the preferred choice to handle exocrine function over intestine, stomach, peritoneal cavity, or duct ablation (ligation or injection). Other controversial technical considerations include peritoneal versus extraperitoneal placement and systemic versus splanchnic venous drainage for insulin delivery.

The pancreas is procured along with other intraabdominal organs. The pancreas can be removed en bloc with other organs after crossclamping and cold perfusion with University of Wisconsin solution, or the pancreas and spleen can be removed separately from the liver. Occasionally, vascular anomalies may preclude the use of the pancreas since priority is given to the liver, which is a life-saving organ. The principles of preparing the pancreas for placement into the recipient include adequate mobilization of the portal vein and superior mesenteric and splenic arteries. A Y-donor iliac graft is sewn to the superior mesenteric and splenic arteries. The splenic vessels are ligated, and the spleen is removed. The duodenal segment is trimmed, and a small duodenal cuff around the ampulla of Vater is used for anastomosis to the bladder. Finally, the mesenteric bundle of lymphatic and small vessels is ligated prior to implantation. The iliac Y graft is used to connect the splenic and superior mesenteric arteries prior to implantation. The pancreas is placed in the right iliac fossa, anastomosing the portal vein to the iliac vein and the Y-graft to the iliac artery.[36] The cuff of duodenum is anastomosed side-to-side directly to the bladder. Alternatively, the duodenum can be anastomosed to a defunctionalized Roux-en-y loop of small intestine. This bladder anastomosis is currently the first choice of connection to handle exocrine function from the pancreas and Roux-en-y small intestinal connection reserved for those patients having complications from their bladder hook-up. Most commonly, a kidney transplant is also placed in the left iliac fossa, anastomosing the renal artery and vein to the iliac artery and vein, respectively. The ureter is then placed in the bladder using a standard ureteroneocystostomy. Figure 46-4 is a diagram of the pelvic placement of the kidney and pancreas transplants.

Patients are followed closely in an intensive care unit postoperatively. Immunosuppression regimens vary, but usually involve triple therapy with cyclosporine or FK506 or quadruple therapy with induction of antilymphocyte globulin or OKT3 monoclonal antibodies. Early and late graft rejection episodes are common and require aggressive therapy. Other postopera-

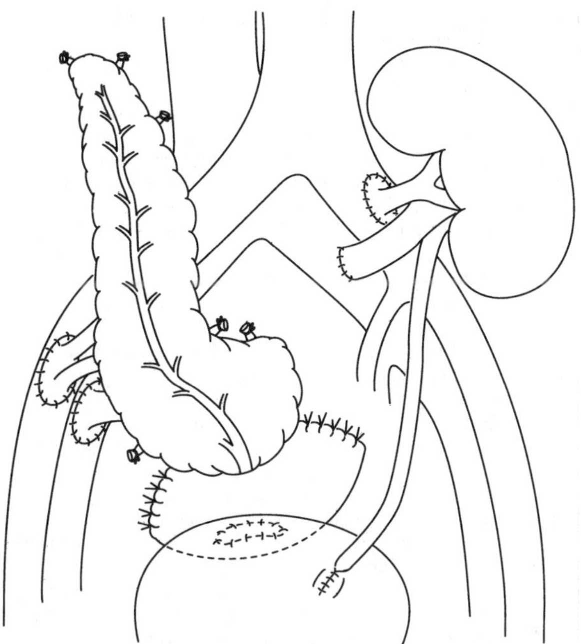

FIG. 46-4. Diagrammatic representation of vascular and bladder anastomoses and placement for pancreas and kidney transplants. (After Terasaki PI, ed. Clinical transplantation 1989. Los Angeles, UCLA Tissue Typing Laboratory, 1989)

tive complications include graft nonfunction, thrombosis, bleeding, infection or problems with the bladder. Bladder complications would include leaks, fistula formation, infection, hematuria, chronic urethritis, balanitis, cystitis, and urethral strictures. Patients also can have significant sodium and bicarbonate losses from pancreatic exocrine secretions into the bladder which can lead to significant dehydration. Patients with intestinal anastomoses may develop obstruction, perforation, or fistula. Recurrent pancreatitis can occasionally occur posttransplant.[40,41] Patients may also redevelop diabetes mellitus, presumably on an immune basis.

The diabetic patient who receives either a solitary pancreas or pancreas–kidney seems to gain little improvement or reversal of the complications of long-term diabetes mellitus. Diabetic retinopathy, nephropathy, and arteriosclerosis do not seem to improve with successful pancreas transplant. There does, however, seem to be some modest improvement in diabetic neuropathy following successful pancreas transplantation.

The overall results at centers performing large numbers of pancreas and combined kidney–pancreas transplants show very good patient and allograft survival. The best results appear to be in patients who receive combined kidney–pancreas transplants. Patient survival rates are between 87% and 100%, kidney survival rates between 75% and 95%, and pancreas survival rates between 62% and 92%. Mean follow-up for some these studies has ranged from 12 to 24 months. In general, the results for pancreas alone or pancreas after kidney transplant have been less successful. Similarly, when compared with kidney transplants alone, for both diabetic and nondiabetic patients, although graft and patient survival rates are comparable to those with pancreas transplants alone, the patients who receive a pan-

creas transplant have a much higher morbidity as discussed earlier.[42–44]

FUTURE DIRECTIONS: CELLULAR TRANSPLANTATION

Unlike bone marrow transplantation, which involves a complete restructuring of the immune system along with the transplanted organ, transplantation of cellular elements has had limited clinical success. Primarily, there has been experimental and clinical progress in islet cell transplantation to provide a cellular substitute for whole-organ pancreas transplantation.[45] Experimental hepatocyte transplantation for metabolic diseases may be a substitute for whole liver transplantation.[46] A variety of experimental techniques has been used including graft (cell) modification as well as the altering and provision of a protected environment for the transplanted cells. The latter process, known as *microencapsulation*, has been somewhat successful for pancreatic islet and hepatocyte experimental transplants.[47,48] In coming years, pancreatic islet, adult and fetal hepatocytes may be used to provide necessary peptides or enzymes for a number of medical diseases. Obviously, if gene transfer techniques come to fruition, whole-organ and cellular transplantation for the metabolic diseases may become of historic interest.

Islet Transplantation

Transplantation of insulin-producing cells without exocrine pancreatic tissue would be the ideal treatment for diabetic patients, given that the complications of pancreas transplantation are principally those related to the exocrine gland. A reliable delivery method for a sufficient number of islet transplants early in the patient's disease may alter the natural history of diabetes. Clinical islet cell transplant programs to date, however, have not been able to provide sufficient numbers of islets to maintain long-term glucose homeostasis; loss of islet numbers may occur from fibrosis, rejection, or recurrent autoimmunity. Research directions for islet transplantation now include improvements in harvest techniques, multiple pooled donors to increase islet numbers, graft modification to theoretically decrease allogenicity or to create a privileged environment for transplanted islets, and xenotransplantation.[49,50]

Xenotransplantation

The continued cadaveric organ and tissue donor shortage and the inherent limitations in securing healthy, living-related donors have continued to create pressure to develop successful xenotransplantation program. A number of technical, ethical, and immunologic barriers have made this approach impractical in the past.[51,52] Rapid advances in molecular biology and molecular immunology with an emerging ability to provide graft modification may herald a new era in transplantation when xenotransplantation may not be beyond our technical capabilities. Xenotransplants are divided into discordant and concordant grafts. *Discordant grafts* are those from species against which the recipient has preformed natural antibody. Discordant species for humans include all nonprimate mammals. *Concordant species* are those against which the donor does not have pre-formed natural antibody. Concordant species for humans are the primates.[53]

There appear to be four important barriers to successful xeno-transplantation: immunologic, ethical, infectious, and metabolic. The immunologic barriers to xenotransplantation vary depending on the species match, whether concordant or discordant. Discordant species undergo immediate humoral rejection due to preformed natural antibody deposition in the graft with complement activation, destruction of the endothelium, and graft thrombosis. Although concordant xenotransplants do not have this aggressive initial humoral response, both discordant and concordant species xenotransplants would be expected to have accelerated and severe cellular rejection because of the dissimilarity of tissue antigens between the species. The experimental use of soluble complement receptor and plasmapheresis may overcome humeral hyperacute rejection and allow for discordant xenotransplantation.[54,55]

The second barrier to xenotransplantation is an ethical one, particularly concerning concordant species such as human–primate xenotransplants. Currently, most large primates endangered species, and animal rights activists are extremely concerned about using endangered species for human transplantation. For discordant species, such as swine, of which hundreds of thousands are raised and slaughtered for human consumption, there are fewer ethical concerns.

The third barrier is technical and relates to the possibility of infection from transmitting an animal pathogen to the human species. The large number of viral pathogens among primates for which there is no effective treatment (especially retroviruses) makes the use of donor primates problematic. Other mammalian species, such as swine, are less likely to transmit viral illnesses to humans.[56] In any event, careful studies must be performed on donor animals before transplantation and on patients who have received xenografts to determine if any animal infections have been transmitted.

The fourth barrier is the important question of whether the new organ from a lower mammalian or primate species will be satisfactory to perform the complex series of metabolic tasks required by the human recipient. The new organ must provide the wide variety of enzymes and peptides required for normal human function, and also, the human must make antibodies to these new circulating proteins and peptides. If complexing antibodies are created, the patient may cease to have a functioning organ. Again, these controversial questions must be carefully addressed for patients receiving whole-organ xenografts.

REFERENCES

1. Belle SH, Beringer KC, Murphy JB, et al. The Pitt-UNO liver transplant registry. In: Terasaki P, and Cecka T, eds. Clinical transplants 1992. Los Angeles, UCLA Tissue Typing Laboratory, 1992:17.
2. Sullinger HW. Current status of simultaneous pancreas–kidney transplantation. Transplant Proc 1994;26:375.
3. Fontes P, Rao AS, Demetris AJ, et al. Augmentation with bone marrow of donor leukocyte migration for kidney, liver, lung and pancreas islet transplantation. Lancet I 1994;344:151.
4. Barber WH, Mankin JA, Laskow DA, et al. Long-term result of a controlled prospective study with transfusion of donor specific bone marrow in 57 cadaveric renal allograft recipients. Transplantation 1991;51:70.
5. Reitz BA, Wallwork JL, Hunt SA, et al. Heart–lung transplantation: successful therapy for patients with pulmonary vascular disease. N Engl J Med 1982;306:557.
6. Todo S, Tsakis A, Kareem AE, et al. Abdominal multivisceral transplantation. Transplantation 1995;59:234.
7. Williams JW, Sankary HN, Foster PF, et al. Splanchnic transplantation: an approach to the infant dependent on parenteral nutrition who develops irreversible liver disease. JAMA 1989;261:1458.
8. Starzl TE, Rowe M, Todo S, et al. Transplantation of multiple abdominal viscera. JAMA 1989;261:1449.
9. Merrill JP, Murray JR, Harrison JH, et al. Successful homotransplant of a human kidney between identical twins. JAMA 1956;160:277.
10. Olivier CL, Retorri R, Olivier CH, et al. Homotransplantation orthotopique de l'intestin grele et des colon droit et transverse chez l'homme. J Chir (Paris) 1969;98:323.
11. Dudrick SJ, Wilmore DW, Vars HM, et al. Long-term total parenteral nutrition with growth, development, and positive nitrogen balance. Surgery 1968;64:134.
12. Fortner JG, Sichuk G, Litwin SD, et al. Immunological responses to an intestinal allograft with HLA identical donor–recipient. Transplantation 1972;14:531.
13. Cohen Z, Silverman RE, Wassef R, et al. Small intestinal transplantation using cyclosporine: report of a case. Transplantation 1986;42:613.
14. Goulet OJ, Revillon Y, Jan D, et al. Small-bowel transplantation in children. Transplant Proc 1990;22:2499.
15. Goulet O, Jan D, Sarnacki S, et al. Isolated and combined small bowel–liver transplantation in Paris: 1987 to 1995. In: Proceedings of the Fourth International Symposium on Small Bowel Transplantation. Transplant Proc. In press.
16. Starzl TE, Kaupp HA Jr. Mass homotransplantation of abdominal organs in dogs. Surg Forum 1960;11:28.
17. Grant D, Wall W, Mimeault R, et al. Successful small bowel–liver transplantation. Lancet I 1990;335:181.
18. McAlister VC, Grant DR. Clinical small bowel transplantation. In: Grant DR, Wood RFM, eds. Small bowel transplantation. London, Edward Arnold Press, 1994:121.
19. Kamada N. Experimental liver transplantation. Boca Raton, CRC Press, 1988.
20. Hoffman AL, Makowka L, Banner L, et al. The use of FK-506 for small intestine allotransplantation. Transplantation 1990;49:483.
21. Reyes J, Todo S, Bueno J, et al. Intestinal transplantation in children: five year experience. In: Proceedings of the Fourth International Symposium on Small Bowel Transplantation. Transplant Proc. In press.
22. Furukawa H, Abu-Elmagd K, Reyes J, et al. Intestinal transplantation in 30 adults. In: Proceedings of the Fourth International Symposium on Small Bowel Transplantation. Transplant Proc. In press.
23. Langnas AN, Antonson DL, Kaufman SS, et al. Preliminary experience with intestinal transplantation in infants and children. In: Proceedings of the Fourth International Symposium on Small Bowel Transplantation. Transplant Proc. In press.
24. Iwaki Y, Starzl TE, Yaihashi A, et al. Replacement of donor lymphoid tissue in small bowel transplants. Lancet I 1991;337:818.
25. Morris J, Johnson D, Rimmer J, et al. Identical twin small bowel transplant after resection of abdominal desmoid tumor. In: Proceedings of the Fourth International Symposium on Small Bowel Transplantation. Transplant Proc. In press.
26. Schraut WH, Abraham VS, Lee KK. Portal versus systemic venous drainage for small bowel allografts. Surgery 1985;98:579.
27. Shaffer D, Diflo T, Love W, et al. Metabolic effects of systemic versus portal venous drainage or orthotopic small bowel isografts. Transplant Proc 1989;21:2872.
28. Sonnino RE, Riddle JM, Besser AS. Small bowel transplantation in the rat: ultrastructural changes during early phases of rejection. J Invest Surg 1988;3:181.
29. Reyes J, Abu-Elmagd K, Tzakis A, et al. Infectious complications after human small bowel transplantation. Transplant Proc 1992;24:1249.
30. Klein G. Epstein-Barr virus strategy in normal and neoplastic B cells. Cell 1994;77:791.
31. Green M, Reyes J, Jabbour N, et al. Use of quantitative PCR to predict onset of Epstein-Barr viral infection and post-transplant lymphoproliferative disease after intestinal transplantation in children. In: Proceedings of the Fourth International Symposium on Small Bowel Transplantation. Transplant Proc. In press.
32. Starzl TE, Demetris AJ, Murase N, et al. Cell migration, chimerism, and graft acceptance. Lancet I 1992;339:1579.

33. Todo S, Reyes J, Furukawa H, et al. Outcome analysis of 71 clinical intestinal transplantations. Ann Surg 1995;222:270.

34. Tzakis A, Webb M, Nery J, et al. Experience with clinical intestinal transplantation at the University of Miami. In: Proceedings of the Fourth International Symposium on Small Bowel Transplantation. Transplant Proc. In press.

35. Sollinger HW, Stratta RJ, D'Alessandro F, et al. Experience with simultaneous pancreas kidney transplant. Ann Surg 1988;208:475.

36. Taylor RJ, Byron JS, Stratta RJ. Kidney/pancreas transplantation: a review of the current status. Urol Clin North Am 1994;21:343.

37. Remuzzi G, Ruggenenti P, Mauer S. Pancreas and kidney/pancreas transplants: experimental medicine or real improvement. Lancet I 1994; 343:27.

38. Sutherland DER. Pancreatic transplantation: an update. Diabetes Rev 1993;1:1.

39. Sollinger HW, Knechtle SJ, Reed A, et al. Experience with 100 consecutive simultaneous kidney–pancreas transplants with bladder drainage. Ann Surg 1991;214:703.

40. Rosen CB, Frohnert PP, Velosa JA, et al. Morbidity of pancreas transplantation during cadaveric renal transplantation. Transplantation 1991; 51:123.

41. Shaffer D, Madras PN, Sahyoun AI, et al. Combined kidney and pancreas transplantation: a three year experience. Arch Surg 1992;127: 574.

42. Sutherland DER, Dunn LD, Goetz FC, et al. A 10 year experience with 290 pancreas transplants at a single institution. Ann Surg 1989;210: 274.

43. Cheung AHS, Sutherland DER, Gillingham KJ, et al. Simultaneous pancreas–kidney transplant versus kidney transplant alone in diabetic patients. Kidney Int 1992;41:924.

44. McDonald JC. In search of the Holy Grail (actively acquired immunologic tolerance). Ann Surg 1995;221:439.

45. Warnock GL, Rajotte RV. Human pancreatic islet transplantation. Transplant Rev 1992;6:195.

46. Zhang H, Miescher-Clemens E, Drugas G, et al. Intrahepatic hepatocyte transplantation following subtotal hepatectomy in the recipient: a possible model in the treatment of hepatic enzyme deficiency. J Pediatr Surg 1992;27:312.

47. Sullivan SJ, Maki J, Borland KM, et al. Biohybrid artificial pancreas: long term implantation studies in diabetic pancreatectomized dogs. Science 1991;252:718.

48. Lanza RP, Borland KM, Lodge P, et al. Treatment of severely diabetic pancreatectomized dogs using a diffusion-based hybrid pancreas. Diabetes 1992;41:886.

49. Soon-Shiong P, Feldman E, Nelson R, et al. Long term reversal of diabetes by the injection of immunoprotected islets. Proc Natl Acad Sci USA 1993;90:5843.

50. Posselt AM, Barker CF, Tomaszewski JE, et al. Induction of donor-specific unresponsiveness by intrathymic islet transplantation. Science 1990;249:1293.

51. Bach FH, Turman MA, Vercellotti GM, et al. Accommodation: a working paradigm for progressing toward clinical discordant xenografting. Transplant Proc 1991;23:205.

52. Bach FH, Robson SC, Winkler H, et al. Barriers to xenotransplantation. Nature Med 1995;1:869.

53. Leventhal JR, Ranjet J, Fryer JP, et al. Removal of baboon and human antiporcine IgG and IgM natural antibodies by immunoabsorption. Transplantation 1995;59:294.

54. Alexandre G, et al. Plasmapheresis and splenectomy in experimental renal xenotransplantation. In: Hardy MA, ed. Xenograft 25. New York, Elsevier, 1989:25.

55. Platt JL, Bach FH. The barrier to xenotransplantation. Transplantation 1991;52:1037.

56. Auchincloss H. Xenogeneic transplantation. Transplantation 1988;46: 1.

Surgical Practice

SECTION A

Head and Neck

Surgery of Infants and Children: Scientific Principles and Practice, edited by Keith T. Oldham, Paul M. Colombani, and Robert P. Foglia. Lippincott–Raven Publishers, Philadelphia, © 1997.

CHAPTER 47

Ophthalmology

Michael X. Repka

The human visual system is an important yet often poorly understood subject in a physician's education. A large percentage of the afferent and efferent connections of the brain relate to the eye and its functions. This chapter attempts to impart a basic understanding of the diagnosis and initial management of common ocular problems seen in children.

OCULAR DEVELOPMENT

Embryologic Development

The eye begins its development during the fourth week of pregnancy as a thickening of the neural tube called the optic placode. This evaginates from the prosencephalon to form the optic vesicle. During the fifth week, the optic vesicle invaginates to form the optic cup. This occurs at the same time that the branchial pouches are reaching the surface ectoderm. This temporal relation is important in understanding the frequent occurrence of malformations of the globe and structures derived from the branchial arches. The classic developmental malformation is the Goldenhar syndrome. This syndrome is also known as the oculo-auriculvertebral syndrome. Other problems that result from defects in the structures derived from the branchial arches include ocular malformations (limbal choristomas), preauricular appendages or sinuses, hearing disorders, and vertebral defects.

The ocular lens forms during the sixth week of pregnancy. The optic nerve axons sprout from the retinal ganglion cells and enter the optic stalk during the seventh week. By the eighth week, retinal differentiation begins. At the ninth week, the eyeball is 1 mm in diameter.

The eyelids open and the retina completes differentiation during the eighth month. At full term, the fetus' eye is 16 mm in diameter and the optic nerve has completed myelination. Children born prematurely complete retinal differentiation and vascularization postnatally. Because of the anomalous influences of the preterm environment, retinopathy of prematurity can develop as discussed later in this chapter.

Postnatal Ocular System Development

At birth, an infant's visual system is capable of formed vision. The retinal fovea completes development during the first year. This portion of the retina is used for straight-ahead vision. The globe grows to 22 mm in diameter during the third year and to 24 mm in diameter by the end of adolescence. Likewise, the occipital cortex undergoes tremendous elaboration and growth during the first 7 years of life.

Visual Development

The development of vision is a dynamic process during childhood. For normal vision to develop, focused, clear visual input is required. If visual input is adversely affected—for instance, by scarring, a cataract, or even a refractive error—normal vision does not develop.

Visual development begins shortly before term, proceeding rapidly through the first 2 years of life, then more slowly for the rest of the first decade. After this time, a child's visual ability remains largely unchanged into adulthood. Thus, any injury or event that affects visual input, even temporarily, has life-long adverse consequences.

Amblyopia

Amblyopia, which occurs in 2% of the population, is a reduction in visual acuity due to deprivation during the period of visual development. Amblyopia has no structural effect on the retina, optic nerve, and lateral geniculate. Nearly all the changes occur in the multiple layers of gray matter in the occipital lobe. When the development of vision in one eye is deprived, the cells in the occipital lobe layers that receive information from that eye are markedly reduced in number and size, whereas the layers that correspond to the opposite eye are enlarged.

In general, visual acuity is less than 20/40 in the affected eye. Amblyopia may occur in one or both eyes. In many cases, the problem is not detected until the patient's vision is tested, usually upon entering school. At this late point, visual development is not correctable with current interventions. Amblyopia has become the largest morbidity following eye trauma in children, especially now that more sophisticated surgical techniques allow severely damaged eyes to be preserved.

The treatment of amblyopia consists of correcting any refractive error with glasses or contact lenses. Then, the patient must use the poor amblyopic eye. This is most commonly accomplished by occluding the sound eye with a patch. Other methods include using drops or special blurring glasses. Such treatment may last for 1 year or longer. Treatment loses its effectiveness as the occipital cortex matures and is generally ineffective after age 8 years.

DETERMINATION OF VISUAL ACUITY

The visual system accounts for a large proportion of the sensory input that the central nervous system receives. The ability to quickly assess a patient's visual function is an important part of physical diagnosis for all physicians. The approach to measuring visual acuity differs based on the patient's age.

Preverbal Children

Acuity in preverbal children during the first year of life is assessed in terms of what age they would be following what would have been a term delivery. In other words, visual development is not accelerated by preterm delivery.

Acuity testing of preverbal children is performed at a distance of 0.5 m using an attractive, colorful toy. A handlight is not used because it is an aversive stimulus for some patients and a too easily seen stimulus for others. Testing is performed monocularly, covering the opposite eye with a patch, hand, or a piece of 2-inch tape. By 6 weeks of life, an infant should fixate the target quickly. By 3 months, the patient should be able to follow the target as it moves before the eyes in a 40-degree arc. Many infants can perform these tasks even earlier. Visual function that does not meet these guidelines requires a thorough evaluation. Abnormalities may be present anywhere within the visual system from eye to occipital lobe. A few children have primary delayed visual maturation and eventually become normal. Children with cortical visual impairment respond more favorably to brightly colored objects rather than black and white targets. They may also adopt unusual head positions to place their remaining visual field in the forward direction.

The evaluation of a toddler's vision should include an assessment of behavior during unstructured play as well as visual function when patched. Children with normal vision appear unimpaired when using either eye after a few moments of distress from the patch. Children who have impaired vision often cry uncontrollably or become withdrawn when trying to use an impaired eye.

Verbal Children

Around the age of 3 years, children can read one of the pediatric eye charts. These tests involve picture recognition or detection of the orientation of a test figure (eg, tumbling ''E''). Though such testing is best performed using a distance target, pediatric near cards are useful for inpatient and intensive care situations. In the United States, acuity is reported as a Snellen fraction, with 20 as the numerator. A denominator of 30 or less indicates normal acuity. Denominators greater than 30 denote vision poorer than normal. Any child found to have vision less than 20/30 deserves a complete ophthalmologic examination.

An important part of the examination of visual function is an assessment of the peripheral visual field. Such fields are notoriously unreliable in this age group. Usually, it is better to assess fields by observing the patient's behavior. A patient with hemianopia may ignore part of the visual environment.

THE RED EYE

After refraction, the most common reason that a patient seeks ophthalmologic consultation is for a red eye. The redness is caused by dilated vessels in both the conjunctiva and deeper ocular tissues. There may or may not be associated pain. The causes of a red eye include conjunctivitis, iritis, glaucoma, corneal exposure and abrasion, and endophthalmitis. The symptoms and signs to evaluate are the amount and type of ocular discharge, pain, shape and clarity of the iris, the quality of the red reflex, the presence of fluorescein staining of the cornea, and the visual acuity.

Conjunctivitis

Conjunctivitis is the most common cause of a red eye in the pediatric patient. Pain in usually mild. Conjunctivitis, unlike other causes of red eye, is associated with copious discharge. Health care providers are often the unwitting vector of epidemics of viral conjunctivitis. Following contact with a patient with a red eye, hands must be washed and the areas of the office or clinic visited by the patient must also be thoroughly cleaned.

Viral Etiology

The most common etiology of conjunctivitis is viral. Many different viruses are implicated, but the most common are the adenoviruses. These are responsible for numerous outbreaks in the spring and summer. The conjunctiva is pink and slightly thickened, especially the palpebra conjunctiva which is the back surface of the eyelid. This tissue often loses its smooth surface, becoming bumpy and resembling a cobblestone road. There is intense photophobia. The discharge is usually clear, and often there is a prominent painless preauricular lymph node.

Though many cases of conjunctivitis are isolated, some types are associated with fever, pharyngitis, and other symptoms of an upper respiratory infection. The disease is self-limited, usually resolving in 7 to 10 days. Cultures usually are not necessary.

Supportive therapy includes cool compresses, artificial tears, topical and systemic antihistamines, and topical mast-cell stabilizers (eg, ketorolac, levocabastine, lodoxamide). There is temptation to use topical corticosteroids since they greatly ameliorate symptoms; however, these should not be used without ophthalmologist supervision because they adversely affect a herpetic infection.

Herpetic Etiology

Herpes simplex virus produces a viral conjunctivitis indistinguishable from any other type of viral conjunctivitis. This infection is self-limited. The presence of clear vesicles on the eyelids is usually secondary to a herpes simplex infection and confirms the diagnosis without the need for culture.

Unlike the other causes of viral conjunctivitis, this virus becomes latent in the trigeminal nerve ganglion. Once there, the herpes simplex virus is responsible for recurrent keratitis, a major cause of blindness in the United States. The recurrent inflammation and ulceration of the cornea leads to scarring and vascularization. These changes in the cornea reduce clarity and eventually reduce vision. Many patients eventually require corneal transplantation in an attempt to restore vision.

When the diagnosis of a herpes simplex infection—whether primary or secondary—is made, a topical antiviral agent is administered (eg, trifluridine). Many clinicians even suggest systemic acyclovir for treating infant herpetic ocular disease or any case involving the eyelids or cornea because of the high frequency of systemic infection.

Patients with herpetic disease or its history should be treated cautiously with topical steroids because the disease dramatically worsens. Such a deleterious effect may also be seen with the use of systemic corticosteroids. For this reason, the use of topical steroids should be avoided by nonophthalmologists in treating conjunctivitis and all other causes of a red eye. Ophthalmologic consultation is advised when such drugs are considered, especially when there is a history of ocular herpes or recurrent ocular inflammation. A patient with the history of prior ocular herpes infection needs to be treated with topical antiviral drugs during the time steroids are required. Such coverage appears to prevent a recurrence of the ocular disease.

Bacterial Etiology

The signs of bacterial conjunctivitis include an injected conjunctiva, both bulbar and palpebral, associated with a purulent discharge. There is no preauricular lymphadenopathy. The causative organisms include *Neisseria*, *Haemophilus*, *Staphylococcus*, and *Streptococcus*. The latter two are probably the most frequent. A Gram stain and culture should be performed to assist in selecting the appropriate antibiotic therapy. A broad-spectrum topical agent (eg, Polytrim, a conbination of trimethoprim and polymyxin B sulfate) is used initially if the Gram stain does not suggest *Neisseria gonorrhea*. Patients who wear contact lenses need special attention. *Pseudomonas* can have a devastating effect on the cornea in these patients due to its quick invasion, and sometimes even perforation, of the cornea. Many organisms are resistant to common topical antimicrobials. Redness or pain in a contact lens wearing patient should elicit emergent ophthalmologic consultation, removal of the lens, and culture of any discharge.

Chlamydial Etiology

Conjunctival infection and destruction from chlamydia is one of the most common causes of preventable blindness in the world. This form of the disease is trachoma. In the United States, the disease presents as either neonatal (see later) or inclusion conjunctivitis. These forms of the disease are not associated with visual loss.

Inclusion conjunctivitis presents as a prolonged follicular conjunctivitis with mild mucopurulent discharge. The diagnosis is made by Giemsa stain, culture, or most rapidly by fluorescent antibody test of conjunctival swab. The diagnosis of chlamydia in older children suggests child abuse and should be appropriately reported. Therapy is systemic.

Ophthalmia Neonatorum

The ophthalmia neonatorum form of conjunctivitis is seen in the first 2 weeks after birth. With the discontinuation of silver nitrate drops, the single topical application of erythromycin or tetracycline ointment has replaced silver nitrate in the delivery room. Despite this treatment, ophthalmia neonatorum is seen due to bacteria, chlamydia, and herpes simplex.

One of the common causes of ophthalmia neonatorum is *N gonorrheae*. Though the incidence has been reduced through the use of postnatal prophylaxis, the disease still occurs and can lead to blindness if untreated. Unlike other bacteria that require an epithelial defect to infect the cornea, *N gonorrheae* may invade an intact epithelium. Infections with this pathogen must be treated with systemic antibiotics, usually ceftriaxone. Topical therapy, such as erythromycin ointment, can be used but is much less important to the success of the therapy.

Chlamydia trachomatis conjunctivitis is probably the most common cause of neonatal conjunctivitis, occurring in 4 of every 1000 births. It involves a moderate mucopurulent conjunctivitis with onset 7 to 14 days after vaginal delivery. Diagnosis is made with a fluorescent antibody test or a Giemsa stain of a conjunctival swab. Cultures can also be obtained. Treatment is a 10-day course of oral erythromycin. Topical agents are not necessary.

Glaucoma

Glaucoma, a disease characterized by elevated intraocular pressure, is an infrequent cause of a red eye in childhood. Compared with conjunctivitis, an eye with glaucoma is minimally injected. The triad of ocular signs that should alert the physician to the diagnosis of congenital or infantile glaucoma include red conjunctiva of the bulbar surface, enlarged and cloudy cornea, and tearing. There may also be photophobia and blepharospasm. Older children may present with pain in the eye and vomiting.

Most patients present within the first year of life. Ocular involvement is often bilateral. The congenital disease may present alone, as part of an ocular syndrome, or as part of a systemic syndrome. The systemic syndromes include aniridia, the congenital rubella syndrome (cataract, hearing, cardiac), Lowe syndrome (renal, cataract), Sturge-Weber syndrome, and neurofibromatosis type 1. Glaucoma may also occur following ocular injuries, especially blunt trauma to the eye, and as a postoperative complication following intraocular ophthalmologic surgery.

The elevated pressure within the eye that causes congenital, infantile, and juvenile forms of glaucoma is usually produced by impaired drainage of fluid from the eye. The pressure is responsible for producing the enlargement of the eye and the destruction of the optic nerve. Prompt institution of pressure reducing treatment may prevent optic nerve damage. Emergent treatment includes acetazolamide, β-blockers, and filtration surgery. Therapy is life-long, and many of these patients suffer severe visual impairment.

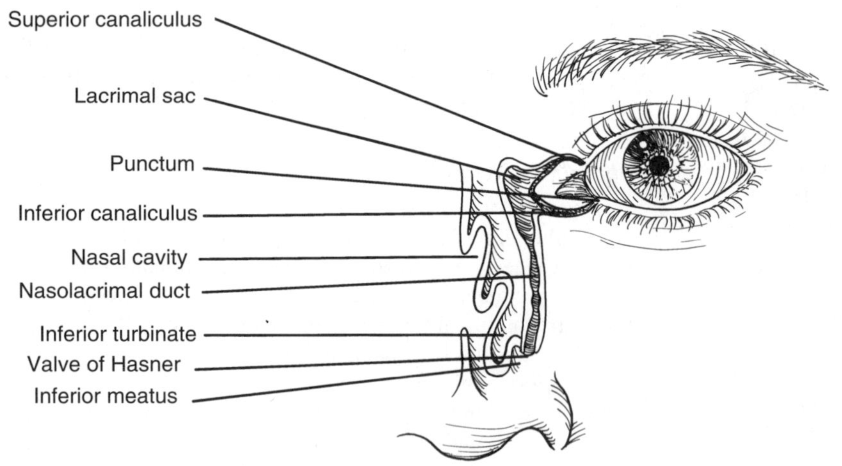

FIG. 47-1. Anatomy of the lacrimal drainage system. Tears pass through the lacrimal puncta, located in both eyelids into the lacrimal canaliculi. Tears then pass into the lacrimal sac, move down into the nasolacrimal duct, and finally into the nasopharynx below the inferior turbinate.

Iritis

Childhood iritis, or inflammation of the iris, may follow trauma, be associated with juvenile rheumatoid arthritis, or be idiopathic. The most common cause is blunt trauma to the eye. The patient presents with a red eye, pain, photophobia, and reduced vision. Iritis is treated with a cycloplegic and steroid drops.

Any patient with iritis in the absence of trauma should be tested for rheumatoid arthritis and antinuclear antibodies. Most cases are idiopathic, but a few patients have arthritis. The morphology of the inflammation may suggest the etiology. Patients with juvenile rheumatoid arthritis should be carefully followed for the development of glaucoma and cataract. The iritis may precede or follow the diagnosis of the arthritis. Once the diagnosis is made, life-long ophthalmologic observation is recommended.

NASOLACRIMAL ABNORMALITIES

Tearing is nearly the only symptom produced by abnormalities of the nasolacrimal system in children. The lacrimal drainage system begins at the nasal aspect of the eyelids (Fig. 47-1). The small openings in the margins of the lids are the lacrimal puncta. These are situated about 3 mm from the medial canthus. Tears flow through these 0.5-mm openings into the canaliculi, which are 5-mm ducts leading to the lacrimal sac. The lacrimal sac is located between the lacrimal bone and the medial canthus and tendon of the eyelids. Tears drain from the lacrimal sac along the nasolacrimal duct into the nose beneath the inferior turbinate. The tears are then swallowed.

The lacrimal drainage system is subject to a variety of congenital problems and are frequently damaged by facial trauma. The most common congenital problem is simple obstruction. The nasolacrimal duct is blocked in about 10% of neonates. Many of these cases spontaneously remit, while others need surgical intervention at about 1 year of age.

Trauma to the eye, lids, or nasal bone is another important cause cause of blockage. Such an injury can easily be missed when accompanied by more severe injuries and can go undiscovered for days or weeks. This problem is much easier to repair in the acute setting, however, when scarring of the damaged structures has not occurred. In addition, the physician should consider the possibility of globe injury in any patient who has sustained a facial injury that has damaged the lacrimal drainage. Ophthalmologic consultation is obtained to assure there has been no disruption to the eye, even if the patient is not sufficiently stable for lacrimal treatment.

Diagnosis

Blockage should be suspected in the presence of an unremitting ocular discharge despite the use of topical antibiotics. An intermittent discharge likely represents a partial obstruction. This can occur when there is mild swelling of the nasal mucosa. The discharge can be clear or purulent.

Simple testing of the drainage system may be performed by adding a drop of 2% fluorescein to each eye. Normally, all traces of the dye disappear in 5 minutes. If the dye remains in the tear film, this is good evidence for an obstruction. Comparison of a symptomatic eye with an asymptomatic eye is very reliable. Alternatively, a cotton applicator can be placed under the inferior turbinate. If it is stained yellow from the dye, patency is confirmed. This test is understandably difficult to perform on most patients.

More complex testing involves computerized tomographic (CT) views with contrast, a study rarely obtained.

Treatment

The general approach to treating a patient with a congenital obstruction is observation and lacrimal sac massage with judicious use of topical antibiotics when the discharge becomes purulent. Blockages in most patients open spontaneously during the first year of life. If the problem does not resolve by age 1 year, the child should undergo a probing of the nasolacrimal duct. For patients who need to undergo some other surgical procedure, the probing should be performed at the same time rather than waiting the full year.

The probing procedure involves passing a thin flexible wire through the nasolacrimal system from the lacrimal puncta to the nose. Patency is confirmed by irrigating the system with fluorescein colored saline, which is recovered from the nose.

This procedure is successful in more than 95% of cases. For those that fail, the procedure is usually repeated. If it fails again, the probing is combined with the placement of a temporary silicone stent. Occasionally, an otolaryngologist may assist in retrieving the stent using nasal endoscopy. The stent is removed in about 8 weeks. For patients with trauma in this region, a stent is always placed in an attempt to achieve healing.

Some patients with a more extensive lacrimal drainage malformation cannot be successfully probed. For these patients an osteotomy of the lacrimal bone is made, directly linking the lacrimal sac with the nasopharynx, thus bypassing the nasolacrimal duct.

INTRAOCULAR INFECTION

Endophthalmitis refers to an infection of the interior of an eye. Bacterial endophthalmitis, though rare, usually follows ocular surgery or trauma. Endogenous endophthalmitis is uncommon and is usually associated with sinus disease from *Haemophilus influenza* or *Streptococcus pneumoniae*. The eye becomes extremely red and painful, the patient may be febrile and develop leukocytosis, the red reflex is lost, and vision is reduced or absent. The prognosis for vision is poor because of the virulence of the typical infection and the difficulty of the diagnosis. The earlier an accurate diagnosis can be made, the better the visual outcome for the patient.

Fungus and Cytomegalovirus

Of special concern to the pediatric surgeon are the opportunistic intraocular infections associated with immunosuppression and debilitation, but not the dramatic symptoms of bacterial endophthalmitis. Usually, the eye is not markedly uncomfortable, the sclera is white, and the vision is not reduced until the condition is very advanced.

Fungal endophthalmitis occurs in debilitated patients, oncology patients, and preterm infants. Infection is usually associated with an in-dwelling catheter, positive blood cultures for *Candida albicans*, and invasive fungal disease. Screening studies of the at-risk population have found from 10% to 30% have fungal endophthalmitis.[1] Though it is recommended that children undergo serial examinations, the ocular infection is nearly always evident during the first examination. Unlike with bacterial infections, the eye with a fungal infection appears quiet. One clue that indicates a problem is a reduction in the quality of the red reflex observed during direct ophthalmoscopy. Indirect ophthalmoscopy of the retina in these cases demonstrates multiple 1-mm diameter whitish, fluffy accumulations in the preretinal vitreous. Direct culture of these lesions is rarely necessary since the diagnosis would have already been made from blood cultures.

Effective treatment includes systemic antifungal therapy with amphotericin B, already being used for the systemic infection. A few clinicians have used intravitreal injections of antifungal drugs in conjunction with a surgical vitrectomy. One approach has not proved to be superior to another. Generally, the fungal lesions disappear slowly with parenteral therapy, leaving little residual damage in the eye.

Cytomegalovirus (CMV) produces a characteristic retinitis, readily diagnosed with the indirect ophthalmoscope. This retinitis consists of a hemorrhagic inflammation of patches of the retina. The lesions are fluffy and white with multiple hemorrhages. Laboratory support of the diagnosis from cultures of other sites corroborates the diagnosis. If CMV retinitis develops, the treatment consists of ganciclovir, foscarnet or both drugs. These agents appear capable of arresting the retinal infection

OCULAR AND ADNEXAL TUMORS

Many different benign and malignant tumors of the eye and the adnexa occur during childhood.[2] These may lead to loss of vision, the eye, or even life.

Retinoblastoma

Retinoblastoma is the most common intraocular malignancy of children. It has an estimated incidence of 1 in 15,000 live births, is seen equally among boys and girls, and affects all races. Unilateral involvement occurs in about 70% of cases and bilateral involvement in 30%. Most cases are diagnosed before age 4 years.

The tumor is highly malignant and, when untreated, is uniformly fatal. The tumor arises from primitive retinal cells and is an undifferentiated neuroblastic tumor.

Approximately 90% of retinoblastomas are sporadic; 40% are due to germinal mutations. These mutations are present in every cell and are thus hereditary. These patients are identified by a positive family history, or more commonly by the presence of multiple tumors in one eye, bilateral ocular tumors, or the concomitant occurrence of a pinealoma.

The genetics of retinoblastoma have been the subject of intense scrutiny and serve as a model of oncogenesis. The retinoblastoma locus is on the long arm (q) of chromosome 13. Varying sizes of chromosomal deletions of this area have been shown to produce the tumor. These observations coupled with the observed genetics of the malignancy led to the current understanding of the etiology of this tumor. A patient must suffer two mutations of this region, according to the "two hit hypothesis" formulated by Knudson in 1971. Patients who have the hereditary form of the tumor likely had a germinal mutation, which is represented in every cell of the body. A second mutation in the complementary chromosome of a retinal cell is necessary to cause tumor development.

Evaluation

The diagnosis of retinoblastoma is usually precipitated by the detection of leukocoria (white retinal reflex). The abnormality is noted in a photograph or observed by the patient's parent or physician. Less often the precipitating diagnosis is strabismus or even visual loss. The ocular misalignment prompts an ophthalmologic examination, at which time the tumor is typically detected. For these reasons, the onset of strabismus or an unusual red reflex should always lead to an urgent ophthalmologic consultation, including a complete fundus examination. Generally the tumor is readily identified by ophthalmoscopy. Supplementary evaluations include ultrasound and CT scanning of the globe to look for evidence of calcification. Additional oncologic work-up involves neuroimaging, bone marrow aspiration, and a lumbar puncture.

Therapy

A fundamental part of treatment for children with retinoblastoma is family genetic counseling. If there is no family history of the tumor, the risk for a second affected child varies from 1% to 6%. If the family history is positive, the risk for a second affected child is 40%.[3]

The appropriate therapy for the condition varies depending on the extent of involvement within an eye and also on whether one or both eyes are involved. The goals of therapy are to save the patient's life, to save vision in at least one eye, and to save the eyes themselves.

Enucleation, or removal of the entire eyeball, is the time-honored method of managing retinoblastoma. This treatment is effective if the tumor has not escaped the confines of the eye; enucleation remains the preferred treatment of unilateral retinoblastoma. Eye-sparing therapies, such as radiotherapy, cryotherapy, or photocoagulation (laser therapy), are also popular, but retinal tumors usually present when they are too large to be successfully treated by these methods. Patients with bilateral tumors often undergo enucleation of the poorer eye and one of the other therapies in the opposite eye. Enucleation is also performed for an eye that has not responded to these alternative therapies.

Enucleation in the young patient leads to a slowing of orbital and eyelid growth on the treated side, producing an asymmetric facial appearance as the patient ages, often requiring surgical repair. In addition, tumor may recur in the eye socket of enucleation patients. Protrusion of an implant or pain in the socket should prompt neuroimaging of the orbit to search for tumor recurrence.

Among the eye-saving treatments, radiation therapy may be applied to the tumor using an external beam or an implantable plaque. The latter technique is useful only for small tumors. Radiation therapy has been implicated in the development of secondary orbital tumors; however, such tumors also occur outside of the field of radiation, suggesting that these patients are genetically predisposed to developing secondary tumors.

Available focal treatments are cryotherapy, photocoagulation, and thermodestruction. These techniques, like brachytherapy, are valuable only for the smallest, localized lesions.

Chemotherapy has no proven role for intraocular disease. Such therapy is used for metastatic and orbital disease. It is used after as a final attempt to save an otherwise insalvageable eye. For these patients the prognosis is extremely poor.

Prognosis

The survival of patients with retinoblastoma now exceeds 90%. If there are distant metastases or orbital invasion, the prognosis is grim. Most deaths occur within 3 years of the diagnosis.

Patients with the hereditary form of retinoblastoma, having survived the initial tumor, are vulnerable throughout their lives to develop secondary malignancies. These tumors may occur within the radiation treatment field or in untreated locations. Reported tumors include osteogenic sarcoma of the skull and femur, spindle-cell sarcoma, chondrosarcoma, rhabdomyosarcoma, astrocytoma, neuroblastoma, leukemia, sebaceous-cell carcinoma, and malignant melanoma. Of particular note is the pinealoblastoma, a tumor that appears identical to the retinoblastoma. The development of this tumor should precipitate an ophthalmoscopic examination. The 35-year cumulative rate for the development of secondary malignancies is about 35% for those receiving external beam irradiation.

Rhabdomyosarcoma

Rhabdomyosarcoma, which originates from undifferentiated mesenchyme, is the most common intraorbital malignant tumor of childhood. The disease most often presents as a rapidly developing proptosis before the age of 10 years.

This presentation should lead to an emergent neuroimaging study, a biopsy of the mass, and a metastatic evaluation, including chest radiograph, blood counts, bone scans, and bone marrow biopsy.

Rhabdomyosarcomas are differentiated on the basis of histologic features, which correlate with prognosis.

Treatment

Surgery, once the mainstay of treatment of this tumor, is now generally restricted to the diagnostic biopsy, which on occasion may be excisional. Radiation therapy, applied to the entire orbit and the surrounding orbital bones, controls 90% of orbital disease. Chemotherapy is used to treat metastatic disease and as adjuvant therapy for orbital disease. These therapies lead to visual loss in nearly every treated eye and to facial asymmetry.

Prognosis

The 3-year survival of orbital disease has improved to 93%. Even patients with meningeal disease have survival rates exceeding 60%. Future studies will likely refine the chemotherapy regimen used for this tumor.

Periocular Hemangioma

Capillary hemangiomas, or infantile periocular hemangiomas, are the most common orbital tumors of childhood.[4] These benign neoplasms arise from the rapid proliferation of endothelial cells. These tumors may be small "birthmarks" or very large disfiguring masses. They undergo proliferative, intermediate, and involutional phases of growth during childhood. The most important effects are opthalmologic.

The tumors present as a superficial strawberry nevus, as a subcutaneous dark blue hemangioma, or as an orbital tumor. The first two presentations may be readily diagnosed on clinical inspection. The third requires neuroimaging and often biopsy. The most important differential diagnosis of this last form is rhabdomyosarcoma.

There are occasional systemic associations. The most important is thrombocytopenia from platelet entrapment within the tumor. Other coagulation disorders and anemia have been reported. High output congestive heart failure may develop if there is substantial tumor volume. Airway compromise from similar tumors located in the trachea or bronchi may result.

Treatment

Therapy is recommended whenever there is a suspicion of either occlusion amblyopia or refractive amblyopia. The former occurs if the eyelid is so full of tumor that a ptosis results. The patient cannot see from the affected eye, and visual development is adversely affected. The tumor may also exert pressure on the cornea, reshaping the cornea, and producing significant astigmatism. This would defocus all incoming images. Neither situation is compatible with the development of sound vision.

The treatment of these lesions is controversial. Surgery and radiation therapy have been attempted, but are usually ineffective. Most practitioners today use systemic corticosteroids or intralesional injections of corticosteroids to reduce the tumor mass. Rapid resolution has been reported with each of these therapies. Interferon alpha-2a and laser therapy have also been used with limited success. Laser therapy is helpful with the more superficial lesions, which are usually not associated with amblyopia. Treatment today often combines a number of these therapies to obtain the best therapeutic index.

Prognosis

If given sufficient time, with or without therapy, these tumors regress. Visual loss is the most important complication, affecting 50% of the patients. Regression of the tumor often leaves some structural abnormalities of the affected tissue.

Orbital and Eyelid Dermoid

Dermoid cysts of the periorbital and orbital regions are common in childhood. These cysts are congenital choristomas, representing ectoderm that is trapped during development of the orbit. The tumors are generally identified as solitary, firm, nodules attached to the orbital margin. Diagnosis generally occurs within the first year or two of life. These benign tumors slowly expand. With rupture, they elicit a chronic inflammatory reaction. Less often, dermoid tumors arise deep within the orbit. Such tumors present as proptosis or as difficulty with eye movement. The differential diagnosis includes rhabdomyosarcoma. These patients present in later childhood or adolescence.

If the posterior extent of the tumor can be determined from the clinical examination, no additional work-up is needed. Otherwise, a CT scan of the orbit is needed to assess the posterior extent of the tumor within the orbit. Similarly, if there is proptosis, neuroimaging is crucial to complete preoperative planning. Ultrasound is an alternative diagnostic modality.

Treatment

These dermoid lesions are benign and slow-growing. Observation is an acceptable therapy until the patient can receive general anesthesia. Surgical excision is the sole treatment for these tumors. For periorbital lesions, total excision is curative, and recurrences are very uncommon. Incomplete excision may lead to a chronic inflammatory reaction. Orbital lesions are usually extensive. Careful preoperative planning is needed to ensure that the entire tumor is excised without compromising other ocular structures. Chronic inflammation from residual tumor within the orbit produces a frozen, immobile globe.

RETINOPATHY OF PREMATURITY

Retinopathy of prematurity (ROP) is the abnormal development of retinal blood vessels in the preterm infant, especially affecting very low birthweight infants (less than 1000 g). Retinal blood vessels first grow into the eye at the optic nerve during the last 16 weeks of pregnancy and normally finish their growth at term. The preterm infant is delivered with actively growing retinal blood vessels, which are subjected to the numerous stresses of the preterm infant. Implicated factors include nutrition, light, oxygen, carbon dioxide, acidosis, and numerous others. These influences produce an anomaly of vascular growth, recognized as ROP. About 1000 patients are blinded annually, and many more suffer lesser degrees of visual loss from ROP.

Threshold Disease

Almost every patient with a birthweight less than 900 g develops ROP as do some infants who weigh between 900 and 1200 g. In most cases, the abnormal vasculature disappears, leaving little or no trace of its existence; however, when the amount of disease reaches a critical threshold, the chance of an unfavorable visual outcome reaches 50%. At this stage, surgical intervention has been shown to be effective. This stage usually occurs at about term. Babies who were sicker during the neonatal course (eg, bronchopulmonary dysplasia, necrotizing enterocolitis, intraventricular hemorrhage) seem to be at greater risk for achieving the more severe stages of ROP than generally well babies of the same birthweight.

Treatment

The value of ablative therapy for ROP was suggested and eventually proved during the 1980s. Initially, therapy was administered by transscleral cryotherapy to the avascular portion of the retina. Since 1991, laser photoablation has become standard treatment for ROP because of its equivalent efficacy with far less discomfort and tissue trauma. Laser treatment is administered to the sedated patient usually in the nursery.

Even with these treatments, more than 25% of these patients have poor vision in the affected eye. The visual impairment results from distortion of the retina, retinal detachment, glaucoma, and even loss of the eye. For patients who fail ablative therapy, advanced interventions, including scleral buckling and vitrectomy, are offered. The value of these procedures in maintaining a functional eye is not yet established.

TRAUMA

The most common cause of preventable yet permanent vision loss is trauma. Many accidents leading to eye damage can be prevented by wearing safety glasses made with polycarbonate lenses. This plastic, found in typical sport glasses, does not shatter and deflects the energy of any impact to the frame of the glasses and to the bony orbit, structures more capable of sustaining an impact without suffering irreparable damage. All physicians should remind their young patients of the value of such protection, especially when playing ball sports.

The eyes are largely protected from minor facial trauma by their position in the bony orbit. Ocular trauma occurs either as part of major head trauma or from direct trauma to the eye by a projectile (eg, tennis ball) or by direct penetration from a sharp object (eg, stick). The latter can cause substantial ocular and periocular damage without any observable facial or cranial damage and, in some cases, no externally obvious damage. Penetrating trauma to the globe is nearly always associated with a poor visual and cosmetic outcome.

The evaluation of a patient with a potential ocular injury begins with an assessment of the globe, followed by the optic nerve, and lastly the periocular structures (eyelids, orbital bones, eye muscles, lacrimal drainage system). Even a small wound of the eyelid can hide a devastating injury of the globe. Whenever these assessments can not be performed conclusively and safely by the emergency physician, the patient should be evaluated by an ophthalmologist before or during the initial surgical interventions. There are numerous examples of patients having an ocular problem undetected for days after an injury. Early intervention is more successful in preserving ocular structure and function than treatment provided days after an accident. A rigid shield should be secured over the eye, without an underlying patch, to prevent any pressure on the eyeball.

The trauma examination requires an assessment of the anterior segment of the eye, direct ophthalmoscopy, and visual acuity. Care must be taken to avoid putting any pressure on the globe. This is often difficult in children, who develop blepharospasm when the physician attempts to open the eyelids. If the examination cannot be performed without forcing the lids open, it should be deferred until the patient is asleep in the operating room. There is too great a risk of prolapsing ocular contents from finger pressure.

The physician tests the function of the eye simply by testing visual acuity. For the unresponsive patient, an assessment of direct pupillary reactions to light is sufficient. If the pupil of the traumatized side reacts as well as the unaffected side, the afferent or visual sensory system is probably unaffected. The examination of the anterior segment should search for evidence of blood and irregularities in the shape of the pupil. The blood may be inside the eye in front of the iris (hyphema). Subconjunctival hemorrhage suggests as well as obscures a rupture of one of the walls of the eyeball.

Corneal Abrasion

Corneal abrasions are one of the most common ocular complaints to present to an emergency room. The corneal epithelium is scraped from the surface of the cornea, producing intense pain. Visual acuity is often reduced. The instillation of a single drop of anesthetic (eg, proparacaine HC1 0.5%) allows complete examination. Detecting a corneal abrasion is aided by instilling fluorescein dye. This orange coloring agent binds to exposed basement membrane. When illuminated with a cobalt blue light source, the dye fluoresces an easily detectable bright green. A careful search of the conjunctiva and upper lid should be made for a retained foreign body.

Treatment is aimed at promoting healing of the surface. This includes patching the eye or immobilizing the upper lid with tape. In addition, topical lubricants and antibiotics are used. Topical steroids should be avoided because they can retard epithelial healing and ignite a latent herpes infection.

Hyphema

Blunt trauma to the eyeball from a fist, ball, or other concussive force, such as an automobile airbag, may lead to bleeding inside the eye without rupturing the eye. Blood within the anterior chamber is termed a hyphema. Such blood lies between the posterior surface of the cornea and the anterior surfaces of the iris and lens. The patient presents in one of two ways. The first occurs several hours after an accident manifest by cloudy or smoky vision, produced by unclotted blood circulating in the anterior chamber. The second presentation occurs 1 or 2 days after the trauma with pain in the eye due to a secondary glaucoma. The blood clots in the outflow channels, blocking aqueous flow through the anterior chamber and out of the eye.

Hyphema is diagnosed by identifying blood in the anterior chamber with a penlight or a slit lamp. The blood settles to the inferior portion of the anterior chamber, clotting and obscuring the iris behind it. The clot may fill a variable portion of the anterior chamber, anywhere from a small portion up to the entire anterior chamber. Circulating blood, unless very dense, can be seen only with the aid of a slit lamp biomicroscope. The amount of blood is directly related to the risk of complications from this injury.

There are two important complications of hyphema. The major risk is an elevation of the the intraocular pressure because the blood blocks the outflow channels of the eye. The pressure may become so high that perfusion of the central retinal artery may cease, leading to retinal ischemia and infarction with irreversible visual loss. Lesser pressure elevations can compromise the vascular supply to the optic nerve, leading to its infarction and consequent permanent visual loss. Each of these unfavorable outcomes is more common in patients with sickle hemoglobin. Every patient evaluated for hyphema should be specifically asked about history of sickle cell disease. Where there is inadequate history, hemoglobin electrophoresis should be obtained. The second important complication is staining of the cornea with blood components, which can lead to long-term visual impairment.

Treatment

The management of hyphemas is individualized. In the past, patients were patched and hospitalized at bed rest. Today, most patients are treated at home; however, if daily follow-up is difficult or the hemorrhage is large, admission for several days is recommended.

The pharmacologic treatment of hyphema is controversial. For many patients, topical corticosteroids and atropine are administered to the affected eye. For patients with large hemorrhages or sickle cell hemoglobin, hospitalization and parenteral administration of the antifibrinolytic agent, aminocaproic acid, for 3 days is appropriate. Aminocaproic acid prevents rebleeding, which can be a major cause of morbidity in these patients. Some clinicians have reported similar success with oral corticosteroids. Increased intraocular pressure may result from damage to the aqueous drainage system or from clogging of that system by red blood cells or hemoglobin. This can be controlled with ocular pressure-reducing medications.

In most patients, the clot begins to retract and resorb quickly and the intraocular pressure is readily controlled with medication. For some, however, serious complications that demand clot removal develop. The major indication for surgical intervention is increased unresponsive intraocular pressure. As mentioned earlier, persistent clot eventually stains the cornea with significant sequela of amblyopia.

Ruptured Globe

The structural integrity of the eye may be compromised following both blunt and perforating trauma. This trauma may be isolated to the eye or part of multiple system damage. Trauma from a tennis ball striking the orbit or similar cause can make the eye wall rupture much as a balloon would split. The break usually occurs at the corneal limbus or under the scleral attachments of the extraocular muscles. Most often, vision is reduced and the diagnosis readily made with a cursory examination of the anterior and posterior segments. There can be an occult rupture even with good visual acuity and little discomfort. Even in the patient with multiple trauma, an eye examination should be performed in the operating room once the patient is stabilized.

If there is a history of a projectile or other object striking the eye or possibly penetrating the orbit, a CT scan of the orbit is needed. Magnetic resonance imaging is particularly useful for vegetable matter within the orbit. The radiologist should search for a foreign body, both in the globe and the orbit. The middle cranial fossa should also be included in the examination as objects have been known to pass through the orbit into the brain. Ophthalmologic ultrasound can also be useful, particularly in a patient unable to complete a CT scan. This study can be performed in the operating room or intensive care unit with minimal disruption of the patient's care.

Treatment

The initial surgical approach is a primary closure of the eye wall with suture. When primary closure is impossible because of loss of tissue, tissue adhesive or autologous sclera from an eye bank can be used. Once the eye is closed, the state of the ocular contents can be assessed. Frequently, the lens is damaged or extruded. The retina may be detached or also extruded. Definitive treatment can be deferred for a few days to stabilize the patient or to schedule a referral to an ocular trauma center. Systemic antibiotics are used because of the high risk of endophthalmitis following an open globe or perforation.

For patients with substantial intraocular disruption, an attempt is made to restore the outer structure of the eye during the first posttrauma week. If no useful vision is detectable, the injured eye even, when cosmetically acceptable, must be removed. Retention of a damaged eye 2 weeks after an injury has been associated with triggering an intense, possibly blinding inflammation in the uninjured eye. This response, known as sympathetic ophthalmia, represents an autoimmune response to a retinal antigen. The risk for developing this condition is lifelong. Patients who maintain some useful vision from the damaged eye must be monitored for this uveitis and treated with systemic corticosteroids.

Despite the devastating injury many patients sustain, modern ophthalmic surgical techniques save many eyes that might have been lost. Many adult patients retain useful vision with the help of contact lenses and intraocular lens implants. In children, however, the injury places the damaged eye at a disadvantage compared with the opposite eye. The children may spend months with occlusion or poor refractive correction while the ocular structures heal. Thus, the risk of amblyopia and consequent life-long poor vision is extremely high.[5]

Eyelid Injuries

Most blunt injuries to the eyelids lead to only soft tissue damage without functional disruption and heal spontaneously. Every eyelid injury, however, carries the risk of an occult ocular rupture. The examiner must confirm the integrity of the eyeball and the visual function must be assured. A small, innocuous penetrating injury through the eyelid (eg, from a coat hanger wire) can also rupture the globe.

Emergency treatment of an eyelid laceration should include placement of a shield to protect the wound and the globe until it has been examined and found to be intact. Swelling of the easily distensible eyelid tissue should be treated with cold compresses and subsequently with warm compresses.

Lacerations can usually be closed primarily, even when a third of the eyelid tissue has been lost. Larger defects require tissue transfer grafts from the other lid. The repair is performed by first closing the lid margin with three sutures, then the tarsus, and finally the skin. A laceration through the nasal aspect of the lid typically damages the nasolacrimal drainage system. Such lacerations must be managed with reanastamosis of the lacrimal drainage system followed by the lid closure. The lacrimal system is then stented with silicone tubes.

Orbital Trauma

The orbit is composed of nine bones (Fig. 47-2) and serves to protect the globe from injury as well as to provide rigid fixation for the muscles that move the eye. Still, these bones and the structures within the orbit are at risk from penetrating and blunt trauma.

Following orbital trauma, visual acuity needs to be assessed and then monitored because a fracture of the deep orbit could compromise the optic nerve as a result of the fracture or an associated hemorrhage. The external examination should note any lid lacerations, particularly those located nasally. These may disrupt the lacrimal drainage system (discussed in the next

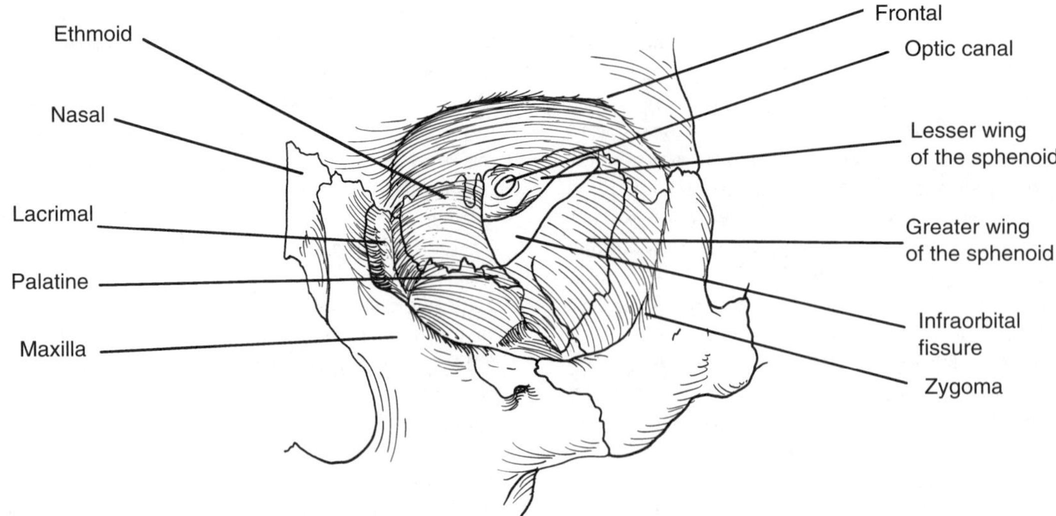

FIG. 47-2. Anatomy of the orbit. The nine bones (greater and lesser wings of the sphenoid, temporal, frontal, zygoma, nasal, ethmoid, maxilla, and palatine) that constitute the orbit are shown. These provide protection for the eye as well as a firm anchoring point for the extraocular muscles.

section). The examiner should also assess ocular rotations and the orbital rim, feeling for any discontinuity or depression, which would suggest a fracture.[6] The position of the globe should be assessed. Protrusion suggests a retrobulbar hemorrhage, edema, or air. A sunken appearance or endophthalmos is likely due to a blow-out fracture of one or more orbital walls with protrusion of orbital contents into the maxillary or ethmoidal sinuses or the anterior cranial fossa. Crepitance of the skin or air seen during an imaging study is consistent with orbital emphysema, which is seen with any orbital wall fracture. Other signs of a medial wall fracture include epistaxis and tearing. An orbital roof fracture may also be associated with rhinorrhea. The examiner then assesses ocular motility. When the ocular movements are impaired, orbital edema, hemorrhage, or muscle entrapment is likely. A CT scan is the best way to assess each of the orbital structures and should be obtained whenever there is significant orbital trauma. Orbital x-rays are inadequate.

Patients with orbital wall fractures should be initially treated with cold compresses, antitussives, and a broad-spectrum antibiotic. Surgical management is reserved for patients with significant dystopia or endophthalmos, prolapse of much orbital tissue into a sinus, or extraocular muscle entrapment. This surgery is often delayed for several days and need not be performed at the time of presentation. Complicated fractures of the orbital rim, wall, and other facial bones require the involvement of ophthalmologic and otolaryngologic consultants.

Retrobulbar Hemorrhage

A large orbital hemorrhage usually occurs after trauma, but may occur spontaneously or after surgery of the orbit and eyelids. The eye is proptotic, and the conjunctiva is displaced forward with blood. The spontaneous occurrences are associated with a blood dyscrasia, malnutrition, alcoholism, ophthalmic aneurysm, and tumor. In addition to proptosis, there is pain, nausea, vomiting, subconjunctival hemorrhage, and loss of vi-

sion. This is a true ophthalmologic emergency. If the circulation to the retina and the optic nerve is compromised, orbital decompression is needed to preserve vision. A lateral canthotomy is performed and acetazolamide therapy instituted. Occasionally, orbital wall surgery is emergently needed to reduce the orbital pressure.

Lacrimal Drainage Disruption

The lacrimal or tear drainage system extends from the medial aspect of both the upper and lower eyelids, through the lacrimal bone, into the nasopharynx below the inferior turbinate. Disruption from a laceration or blunt trauma leads to chronic tearing. Patients with injuries in this area should be examined to determine the patency of the drainage system. A CT scan with instillation of contrast material into the tear highlights the drainage system well. Similarly, recovery of fluorescein-colored saline from the nose after placement in the tear confirms patency but does not localize a blockage.

CATARACT

Cataracts are opacities of the lens of the eye. These are associated with substantial permanent visual loss in children. Even with optimum treatment, more than 30% of affected patients remain legally blind in that eye. The most important factor in controlling the visual outcome is early, prompt treatment.

Cataracts occur in both healthy children and in children with other systemic disorders. All physicians should be able to examine the red reflex of the undilated pupil using the direct ophthalmoscope. Possible etiologies and associations include metabolic disorders, intrauterine infections, chromosomal abnormalities, craniofacial malformations, skeletal disorders, skin disorders, and muscle disease. In general, most cataracts are found during physical examination of otherwise healthy patients. Antibody

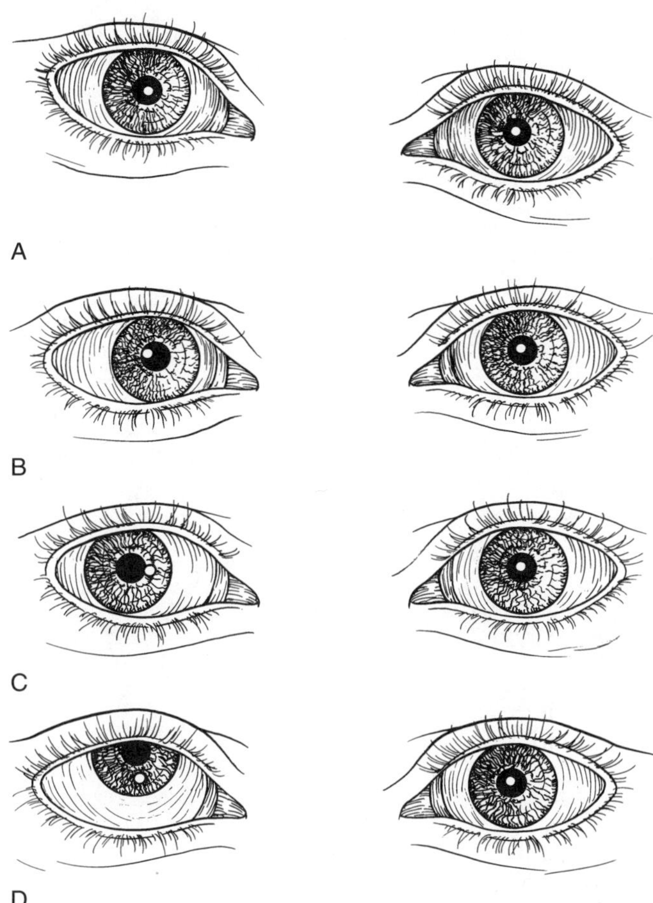

FIG. 47-3. Normal eye alignment (*A*) and the three basic deviations of strabismus, including esotropia, in which the eyes turn in (*B*); exotropia, in which the eyes turn out (*C*); and hypertropia, in which the eyes deviate vertically (*D*).

titers for rubella and urine analysis for reducing substances (galactose) should be obtained.

STRABISMUS

The term *strabismus* describes any misalignment of the eyes and has largely replaced the term *squint.* The treatment of strabismus is varied. Selected cases may be observed, others are treated with glasses or eyedrops, and many require surgery. Such surgery represents the vast majority of pediatric ophthalmologic surgery, although many patients are offered visual training as an alternative to surgery. In most cases, such training is not curative and should be discouraged.

There are three types of strabismus (Fig. 47-3). *Esotropia* is the term for crossed eyes, *exotropia* for eyes that turn out, and *hypertropia* for eyes that are vertically misaligned. Strabismus may be idiopathic, myopathic, or neuropathic.

Treatment

Strabismus surgery has three basic goals.[7] First and most important is to restore single binocular vision and to eliminate diplopia. Second, the peripheral visual field for patients with esotropia must be expanded. This has been correlated with improved development, particularly of fine motor skills in younger patients and driving ability in older patients. Third, surgery is undertaken to dramatically improve patients' psychosocial functioning since strabismus has been shown to have an adverse effect on performance throughout life. Each of these goals can be achieved with accurate surgical realignment of the eyes.

Treatment is divided among two distinct methods, conventional surgery and extraocular muscle chemodenervation. Incisional surgery has been practiced for well over a century and is performed under anesthesia. The extrocular muscles are either weakened in a procedure termed a *recession* or strengthened with a *resection* procedure. As an alternative, chemodenervation has been used since the mid-1980s. In this technique, a series of injections of botulinum neurotoxin A are administered to one or more of the extraocular muscles, temporarily weakening the muscle. This technique has met with widespread acceptance for treating esotropia secondary to a sixth cranial nerve palsy and some acceptance for infantile esotropia. Its role for treating other strabismic conditions remains to be established.

REFERENCES

1. Enzenauer RW, Calderwood S, Levin AV, Elder JE, et al. Screening for fungal endophthalmitis in children at risk. Pediatrics 1992;90:451.
2. Shields JA, Carol CL. Ocular tumors in childhood. Pediatr Clin North Am 1993;40:805.
3. Musarell MA, Gallie BL. A simplified scheme for genetic counseling in retinoblastoma. J Pediatr Ophthalmol Strabismus 1987;24:124.
4. Haik BG, Karicioglu ZA, Gordon RA, et al. Capillary hemangioma (infantile periocular hemangioma). Surv Ophthalmol 1994;38:399.
5. Lavrich JB, Goldberg DS, Nelson LB, et al. Visual outcome of severe eye injuries during the amblyopiagenic years. Binocular Vision Eye Muscle Q 1994;9:39.
6. Dutton JJ, Manson PN, Iliff N, et al. Management of blow-out fractures of the orbital floor. Surv Ophthalmol 1990;35:279.
7. Keltner JL. Strabismus surgery in adults: functional and psychosocial implications. Arch Ophthalmol 1994;112:599-600.

Surgery of Infants and Children: Scientific Principles and Practice, edited by Keith T. Oldham, Paul M. Colombani, and Robert P. Foglia. Lippincott–Raven Publishers, Philadelphia, © 1997.

CHAPTER 48

Craniofacial Anomalies

Jeffrey L. Marsh

Congenital deformities of the skull and face, or craniofacial anomalies,[1] differ from anomalies of other regions of the body in several important ways:

1. Craniofacial anomalies usually are overt at birth.
2. Parents and health care professionals alike can recognize an error of in utero craniofacial development without the aid of specialized physical examination or diagnostic medical imaging.
3. Craniofacial dysmorphology has major psychosocial consequences in most cultures.

In contrast, cavitary anomalies (eg, intracranial, intrathoracic, or intraabdominal) usually do not present perinatally, generally require ancillary diagnostic maneuvers for definition, and are rarely recognized by the the child's parents or society at large.

The delivery room personnel may be the first to share the shock of a newborn's craniofacial anomaly with the parents. Although delivery room personnel may take a positive approach in informing the parents, misinformation, fear, and confusion are often conveyed. Furthermore, there is a pervasive prejudice within our society that facial deformity implies impaired cognitive function; this is false in most cases. Facial deformity is often associated with evil or dysfunctional persons in Western art and literature. Consider the disfigured faces of Christ's tormentors in Flemish Renaissance paintings or the *Phantom of the Opera*. Parents of a child with congenital defects that are not visible may not consider impaired social integration, but to parents of a craniofacially deformed infant, how the child will function with peers, get a job, and find a mate are paramount questions shortly after birth.

This chapter is not meant to teach surgical management of craniofacial anomalies. Rather, it is intended to be a guide for health care professionals who may be confronted with a child with a craniofacial anomaly and who wish to better understand the nature of the anomaly, its physical and psychological consequences, and the ability of contemporary interdisciplinary team care to habilitate affected people.

CRANIOFACIAL DEVELOPMENT

Normal Development

The development of the head is a complex process that has been studied in detail over the past century with increased comprehension thanks to technological advances in investigative tools. Excellent reviews of current knowledge and hypotheses have been published.[2-4] This brief section focuses on the key features of normal development that are thought to be implicated in the expression of craniofacial anomalies.

Fetal and postnatal craniofacial growth and development are well characterized. The cranium and upper face reflect the early maturation of the central nervous system, whereas the middle and lower face require dental eruption and puberty to reach definitive form and size. The term infant is born with one quarter of the adult brain volume. By age 2 years, three quarters of adult brain volume has developed. The eyes follow the brain's growth pattern and reach almost adult size by age 4 years. This rapid growth is responsible for the dominance of the cranium and prominence of the eyes in the child's head. Craniofacial proportions change with the onset of puberty. The midface and lower face elongate and protrude producing the definitive adult face with its sexual dimorphism. Aging from infancy to adulthood is, therefore, associated not only with enlargement of the head but also changes in shape and proportions of its components; this is called *allometric growth*.

Contemporary developmental research focuses on cellular processes, including proliferation, degeneration, differentiation, migration, and the extracellular matrix. Although the cellular dynamics of the progression from zygote to embryonic germ layers are poorly understood, the importance of interplay among neurectoderm, surface ectoderm, mesoderm, and endoderm in the development of the head is appreciated. Cephalic neural crest is thought to be the source of most craniofacial mesenchyme, a process that requires migration and loss of epithelial configuration. Early craniofacial embryonic development is characterized by the formation of headfolds, which are outgrowths that form and surround cavities or grooves, which then close either totally or partially by the continued enlargement of the outgrowths. In addition, surface ectoderm placodes develop, which contribute to the eyes (optic placode), nose (nasal placode), ear (acoustic placode), and branchial arches (epibranchial placode). Outpouching of the ventral foregut creates pharyngeal pouches that interact with overlying surface ectoderm and mesenchymal cells at the site of the developing branchial grooves.

As the adjacent branchial arches enlarge, the grooves deepen. Five branchial arches, separated by four grooves, arise in the human embryo. The middle and lower face arise from these arches with the first arch being dominant. The central portion of the face arises from the frontonasal process and then fuses with the paired maxillary processes of the first branchial arches. Where facial swellings contact each other, an epithelial plate develops, which either degenerates or persists as an epithelial lines structure, for example, the nasolacrimal duct, depending on location. Facial muscles develop by interaction between specific nerves and focal mesenchyme. The craniofacial skeleton arises from a number of discrete ossification centers with one or, in a few cases, two centers per definitive named bone. Two types of bone develop in the head—membranous and endochondral. Membranous bone comprises most of the cranial vault and facial bones; endochondral bones comprise most of the cranial base.

Current Concepts Regarding Abnormal Development

There are two types of craniofacial anomalies—malformations and deformations. *Malformation* means that the part never formed correctly; *deformation* means that the part formed correctly but was secondarily deformed. Neither term indicates the process whereby the malformation or deformation occurred. Some craniofacial anomalies are hereditary and, in an increasing number of cases, the abnormal chromosome has been identified. Some result from recognized teratogens, and some are thought to be the result of intrauterine constraint, vascular accidents, or amniotic bands. Most are sporadic and their induction factors unknown.[1,5]

Disorders of cell proliferation, degeneration, differentiation, and migration as well as in the composition of the extracellular matrix have been postulated as the mechanism whereby malformations occur. Although there is no consensus on classification of either of the etiologies of craniofacial anomalies or their dysmorphology, several used schemes have been proposed. Based on current concepts of embryology, Vermeij-Keers[6] proposed three different groups of malformations: cerebrocranial dysplasia (malformations of the brain and cranium); cerebrocraniofacial dysplasia (facial defects involving the brain or eyes and the cranium); and craniofacial dysplasias (defects of the face and cranium alone). These groupings help us in understanding specific anomalies in light of current concepts of embryology. In contrast, Tessier[7] has proposed a topographic soft and hard tissue map for classifying craniofacial anomalies, which has been widely adopted to facilitate communication about rare defects.

The dysmorphology of some craniofacial anomalies seems to document arrest of embryogenesis (Fig. 48-1A). Others seem to portray failures of fusion (see Fig. 48-1B), and in others, a gross disruption of spatial processes (see Fig. 48-1C). The similarity between an anomaly and an embryonic stage, however, does not necessarily mean that the two are directly related. Current research on homeobox genes,[4] the ''blueprint'' for anatomic organization, and the biochemical aspects of genetic expression should yield additional understanding of the origin and expression of craniofacial anomalies. It is possible that such understanding will eventually permit treatment based on etiol-

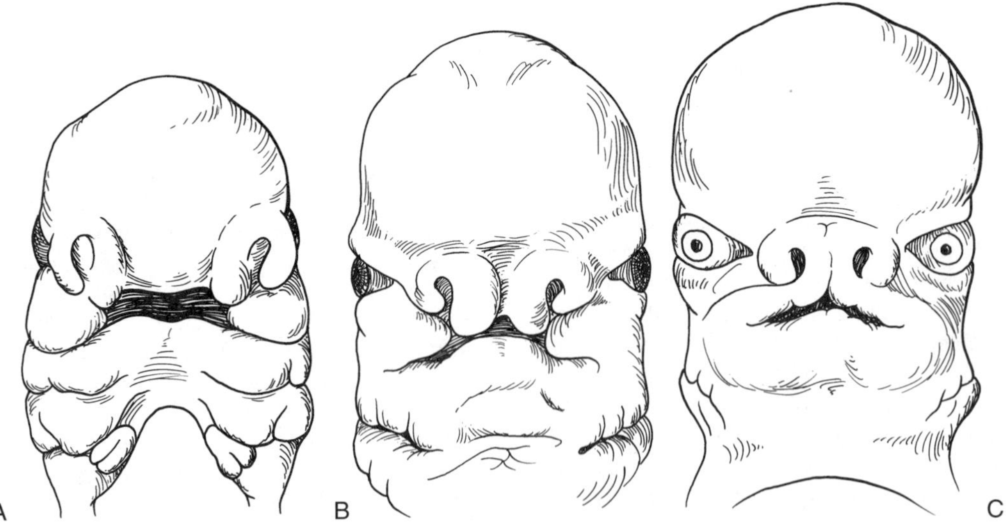

FIG. 48-1. (*A*) At 5 weeks' gestation, the human embryo has developed grooves between the central and lateral portions of the face. Figure 48-10 depicts a child in whom a midline cleft suggests the right and left medial elements have not completely fused. (*B*) At 6 and a half weeks, the embryo has widely spaced eyes. When orbital migration toward the midline does not subsequently occur, ocular hypertelorism results, as in Figure 48-4. (*C*) By 7 weeks' gestation, the primordial external ear begins to form in the neck. An absence of the external ear and auditory meatus, as depicted in Figure 48-11, suggests either a basic regional anatomic error in the genome or disruption of a cellular differentiation/migration process.

ogy and abnormal process. That possibility remains a distant hope at this time. Contemporary treatment of craniofacial anomalies consists of managing their manifestations rather than their causes.

THE CRANIOFACIAL DEFORMITIES TEAM: INTERDISCIPLINARY CARE

Craniofacial anomalies affect both the skull and the face; however, some major facial anomalies without cranial abnormalities are also categorized as craniofacial anomalies because of the extent of involvement. No single health care discipline has all of the expertise necessary for evaluating, treating, and following a patient with a craniofacial anomaly. For this reason, the standard for contemporary care of craniofacial anomalies involves a craniofacial interdisciplinary team. The craniofacial deformities team developed from the cleft lip and palate team by adding the neurosciences and ancillary services necessary to execute complex operations. The team approach has been endorsed by a consensus conference on clefts and other craniofacial anomalies conducted by the American Cleft Palate/Craniofacial Association and funded by the US Department of Maternal and Child Health.[8] A directory of craniofacial teams is maintained by the American Cleft Palate/Craniofacial Association, 1218 Grandview Avenue, Pittsburgh PA 15211 and can be obtained by phoning 1-800-24CLEFT.

The disciplines represented by the craniofacial team usually include audiology, genetics, neurosurgery, nursing, ophthalmology, orthodontics, oral–maxillofacial surgery, otolaryngology, pediatric dentistry, pediatrics, plastic/craniofacial surgery, prosthodontics, psychology/psychiatry, social services, and speech/language pathology.[9] Anesthesiology, computer services, neurology, and radiology are important components of surgical planning and execution but usually do not participate as regular team members. At the St. Louis Children's Hospital at the Washington University Medical Center, we conduct full craniofacial team evaluations of these patients on an annual basis from 1 to 4 years of age, every 2 years from age 4 through 14 years, and then at ages 17 and 20 years, when the patients are then graduated from the program. Patients with new or persistent problems are seen more frequently by whichever providers are appropriate.

The primary purposes of the craniofacial team are to formulate and update a long-term care plan, to coordinate recommendations with primary and secondary local providers, and to provide tertiary services. Although details of craniofacial team function vary from center to center, standard elements include:

- Regularly scheduled ambulatory multidisciplinary patient evaluations
- Collation of individual provider recommendations into a coherent, efficient, comprehensive care plan;
- Production of a written report for the patient's primary and secondary care providers
- Production of a written interpretive letter for the parents and patient, if of appropriate age
- Monitoring of status of treatment recommendations;
- A program of quality assurance
- Maintenance of permanent records with standard documentation at regular intervals using text, photographs, and diagnostic medical imaging

Coordinating the interventions of separate providers minimizes the consumption of time and resources, disruption of daily life, and psychological distress.

DIAGNOSTIC AND OUTCOME CRANIOFACIAL EVALUATION

As with all congenital disorders, diagnosis begins with a complete history and physical examination. This evaluation should include the parents and, when possible, any family members who are suspected of having similar disorders. If a positive family history for craniofacial deformities is elicited, referral to a medical geneticist versed in dysmorphology is indicated.

Craniofacial clefts, aplasias, and severe hypoplasias are usually recognized at birth. Abnormalities of head shape and mild to moderate hypoplasia may initially be interpreted as the result of the birthing process and not be appreciated as anomalies until several months after birth when they have not normalized.

A complete physical examination of the head and neck should be performed regardless of how focal the anomaly seems since many seemingly isolated anomalies have subtle associated findings. The general appearance of the patient with respect to alertness, ease of respiration, age-appropriateness of behavior, and nutritional status should be noted. The head is assessed for symmetry and proportion. Function of cranial nerves II through VIII and XII is discretely tested as are the combined functions of IX through XI for swallowing and speech. The scalp is inspected for hair pattern, alopecia, and masses. With respect to the cranium, perimeter shape, status of the fontanelles, osseous integrity, presence or absence of sutural ridges, and forehead, supraorbital, and nasofrontal configurations are recorded. The eyes are examined for the relation between the globes and the orbits, the distance between the pupils in central conjugate gaze, the medial canthal distance, the palpebral fissure orientation, eyelid continuity and function, eyelash orientation, lacrimal function, globe motion, and visual status. Examining the midface, the physician should note the orientation of the nasal dorsum and its height, the configuration of the nasal tip and its projection, the placement of the nasal septum, the status of the intranasal mucosa, the patency of each nasal airway, and the soft and hard tissues of the cheeks. The ears, including the external auditory meati, are evaluated for placement, shape, and size. The lips are inspected for clefts, cysts, or pits, and the labial competency at rest and during speech and eating is evaluated. The intraoral examination includes temporomandibular joint function, the physical and occlusal dental status, the dentoskeletal maxillary–mandibular relationship, lingual and palatal anatomic integrity and function, and the oropharyngeal lymphoid tissues. The range of motion of the neck is tested, spontaneously and provocatively, and the neck is palpated for restrictive muscles and masses. An experienced craniofacial examiner can conduct this evaluation in a brief period and then focus on the pathology detected.

Diagnostic medical imaging is an important part of evaluating a patient with a craniofacial anomaly. Increasingly, craniofacial anomalies are being indentified antenatally on ultrasound. Counseling is provided to the parents antenatally as well as perinatally in such cases. After birth, routine skull x-rays are useful for identifying premature fusion of cranial sutures (craniosynostosis), ultrasound for identifying hydrocephalus, computed tomography (CT) scans for osseous anomalies, and magnetic resonance (MR) scans for intracranial and extracranial soft tissue anomalies. The development of software to produce surface-shaded and volumetric three-dimensional skeletal and soft tissue images from CT or MR digital data has greatly increased our knowledge of craniofacial anomalies and our ability to plan complex operations, to assess the execution of surgical plans, and to evaluate the outcome longitudinally.[10,11]

SURGICAL MANAGEMENT OF CRANIOFACIAL ANOMALIES

Intracranial and Extracranial Procedures

Cranium

The two major categories of cranial anomalies that demand the attention of the craniofacial surgeon are shape and masses. Deformation of cranial shape is a common consequence of birth and should correct to a normal shape within the first few weeks of life. Persistence of an abnormal cranial shape beyond the second month of life is cause for evaluation and management as appropriate. Although a cranial mass noted perinatally may be an innocent cephalohematoma that will resolve over time, those that persist need to be evaluated for intracranial extension.

Premature fusion of cranial sutures, known as *craniosynostosis,* causes abnormal cranial shape due to a combination of growth restraint, secondary to the synostosis, and compensatory deformation, secondary to pressure exerted by the growing brain on cranial bones not restricted by synostosis (Fig. 48-2). In addition to cranial abnormality, craniosynostosis may also produce deformity of the orbit, midface, or lower face. For most of this century, surgical intervention has sought to ablate the synostotic suture. It was thought that craniosynostosis produced increased intracranial pressure, hydrocephalus, blindness, and mental retardation. These dire prognostications seem to be excessive in light of contemporary experience. Few patients with craniosynostosis have such associated morbidity, and most who do experience syndromic synostosis involving multiple sutures. In some cases of single-suture nonsyndromic craniosynostosis and in many cases of multiple-suture synostosis, low-grade increased intracranial pressure has been documented.[12] The neurologic significance of this finding remains a subject of debate. Over the past several decades, operative correction of calvarial and superior orbital deformities and an attempt to prevent subsequent secondary facial deformation have become surgical goals in treating craniosynostosis. Collaboration between craniofacial surgeons and neurosurgeons has led to more normal outcomes than were achieved earlier.

The relation between cranial abnormality, specifically asymmetry or plagiocephaly, and restriction of head/neck mobility is of interest to craniofacial, pediatric, and orthopedic surgeons, as well as pediatricians and physical therapists. It has long been recognized that limited head/neck motion in an infant results in cranial deformity, such as occipital flattening (brachycephaly) secondary to papoose board swaddling, anteroposterior elongation and bitemporal narrowing (scaphocephaly) secondary to prematurity, and asymmetry (plagiocephaly) secondary to torticollis. Cranial deformity with limited neck motion is not always a case in which the cranial problem follows the cervical one, however. A common type of plagiocephaly, known as plagiocephaly without synostosis, is present at birth and can produce a secondary neck dysfunction due to asymmetric brain mass. The uneven distribution of intracranial mass about the midsagittal axis means that the infant's head consistently falls to the heavier side rather than falling right and left with equal chance. In turn, the contralateral neck muscles are stretched and the ipsilateral ones contract. If the process is not interrupted with physical therapy or correction of the plagiocephaly, the neck dysfunction progresses to fixed limitation in range of motion which in turn aggravates the plagiocephaly. Although physical therapy can improve the neck range of motion, it does not correct the skull deformity. Plagiocephaly without synostosis can be identified by the history, physical examination, and the documentation of radiolucent sutures on screening skull x-rays. For patients younger than 12 months, plagiocephaly without synostosis is managed with cranial molding helmets (Fig. 48-3).[13] After 1 year of age, the child's skull is too hard to respond, and the only option is surgical cranial reconstruction. The infant with true torticollis, in contrast, presents with a history of a normal-appearing head and a perinatal mass in the sternocleidomastoid muscle, which is followed by tightening and shortening of the affected muscle. As the range of neck motion diminishes, secondary cranial and, at times, facial deformity develops progressively. Neck therapy for these patients usually resolves the limited range of motion and restores normal craniofacial configuration.

Differentiation between extracranial and combined intracranial–extracranial masses is necessary for masses that persist beyond the perinatal period or that are associated with craniofacial dysmorphology. The most common extracranial mass is a dermoid cyst. Dermoid cysts usually are identifiable on physical examination by their location along facial embryologic fusion lines, such as the superolateral orbit and nasal dorsum, their subcutaneous position, their immobility, their firmness and lack of compressibility, and the integrity of adjacent bone. Since orbital dermoids rarely extend intracranially, they can be excised without diagnostic imaging. Nasal dermoids may be contiguous with intracranial extensions. Some authors recommend CT or MR imaging of all patients with nasal dermoids before excision to preclude the inadvertent amputation of a transcranial connection with subsequent cerebrospinal fluid leak or intracranial infection. It is appropriate to perform such imaging for patients with nasal masses and abnormally wide interorbital spaces (interpupillary distance, medial canthal distance, and bony interorbital distance greater than 97%). If intracranial extension is suspected, dermoid excision is performed in conjunction with neurosurgery, and craniotomy is anticipated. If intracranial extension is not suspected, simple excision is performed under general anesthesia on an outpatient basis.

Masses associated with craniofacial dysmorphology are most often *encephaloceles*. Encephaloceles can present cranially, orbitally, nasally, or intraorally. Computer-assisted medical imaging (CT and MR) is used to define the aberrant anatomy and to formulate a surgical plan. Combined intracranial–extracranial resection of the encephalocele with synchronous reconstruction of cranial or facial deformities is the preferred treatment. Although two-stage management, involving transcranial resection followed metachronously by extracranial resection and reconstruction, was preferred historically to minimize postoperative

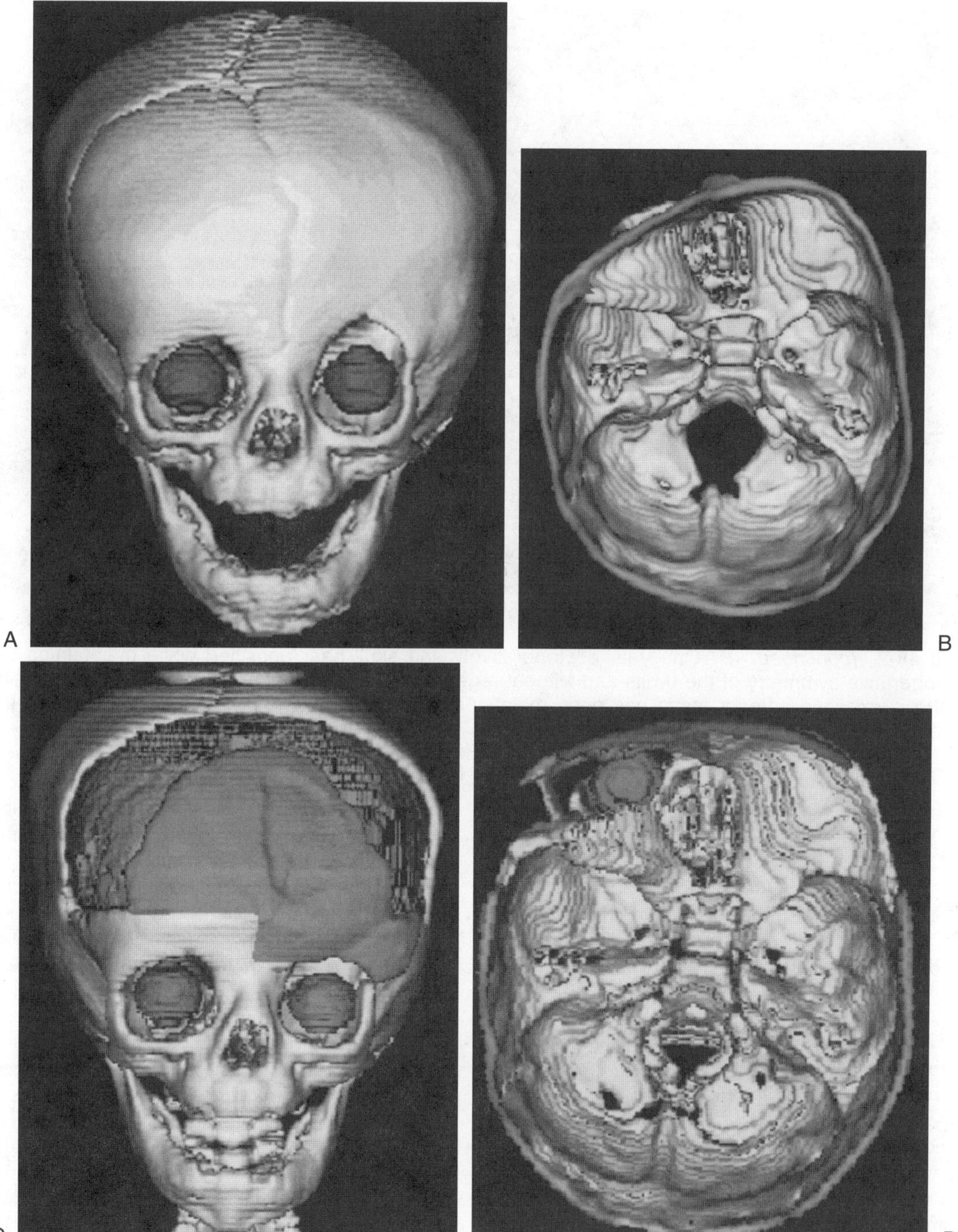

FIG. 48-2. Three-dimensional CT osseous reformations with globe opacification of a child with cranio-synostosis that caused abnormal cranial shape. (*A*) Preoperatively, there is a ridge where the left coronal suture should be, the orbital rims are asymmetric, and the left orbit is vertically elongated. (*B*) The view of the endocranial base preoperatively shows that the anterior hemicranial fossa ipsilateral is compressed against the synostosis and that the contralateral has expanded, "unroofing" the ipsilateral globe. (*C*) Perioperatively, the reshaped and repositioned frontal bones and right superolateral orbit appear in green. The gray brain is seen through the bicoronal craniectomy defect. (*D*) The basal view perioperatively shows that the right frontal bone and superolateral orbital rim (*green*) have been moved ventrally and the left frontal bone moved dorsally to achieve anterior fossa symmetry and appropriate orbital roof depth. The globe (*red*) is visible through the ventral enlargement of the orbital roof. The placement of an autologous calvarial graft (*orange*) maintains the orbital rim advancement. *(continued)*

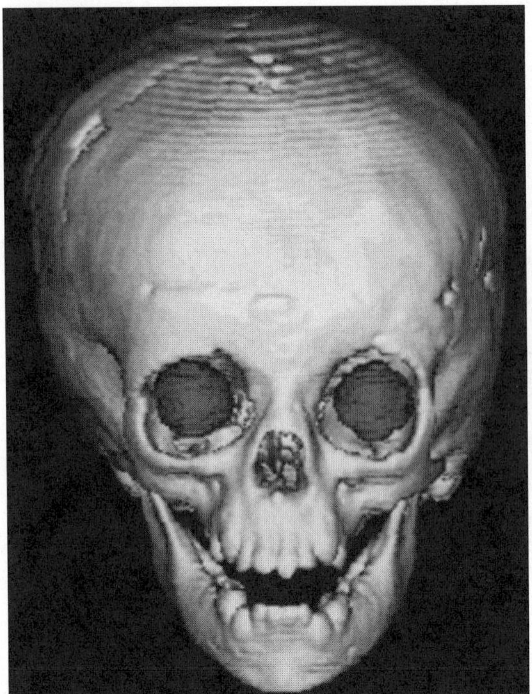

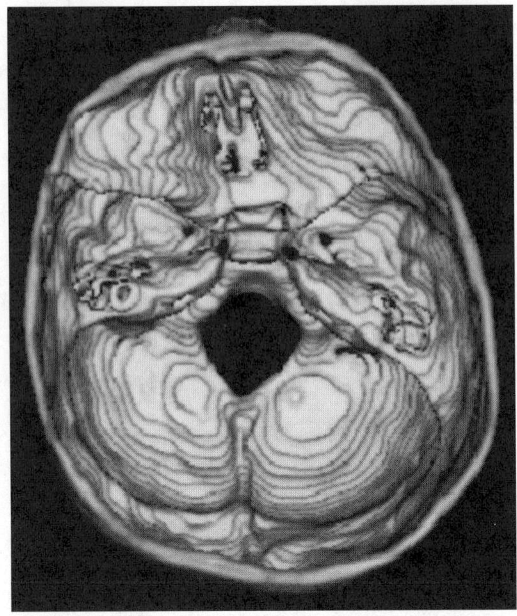

E   F

FIG. 48-2. *(continued)* *(E)* One year postoperatively, the skull has reossified while maintaining the perioperative symmetry of the orbits and without regenerating a left coronal suture. *(F)* The symmetry of the normalized anterior fossa has been maintained. The asymmetric posterior fossa remains the same as seen preoperatively. (See Color Fig. 48-2*C* and *D.*)

infection, contemporary craniofacial surgical techniques make one-stage management safe and effective.[14]

Ocular Globes and Orbits

The cranial and orbital cavities are separated by thin bones superiorly, laterally, and medially. The orbital roof is the floor of the anterior cranial fossa; the posterolateral wall of the orbit is the anterior wall of the middle cranial fossa; and the superomedial wall of the orbit is the floor of the cribriform fossa. The bone structure that surrounds the orbital contents is referred to as the *orbit.* Operations on the caudal half of the orbit usually can be performed extracranially without concern for damage to the brain. In contrast, operations on the cephalic half of the orbit frequently require craniotomy to dissect the dura off the bone to be manipulated and to protect the brain from surgical instruments.

The ocular globe can be anomalous due to one of several possibilities: abnormal globe size with normal extraocular orbital contents, orbit size, and location; abnormal extraocular contents volume with normal globe size, orbit size and location; abnormal orbit size or location with normal globe and extraocular contents size; or combinations of these.

Macroophthalmia refers to a globe that is larger than normal, *microophthalmia* is a globe that is smaller than normal, and *anophthalmia* refers to a globe that is congenitally absent. Of these, microophthalmia is most common. If the microophthalmic globe has normal vision, no intervention is indicated. If the microophthalmic globe does not have useful vision, it can be covered with a cosmetic painted scleral conformer to achieve a symmetric facial appearance. Although true anophthalmia is very rare, marked microophthalmia often is misdiagnosed as anophthalmia. In the infant, surgical insertion of an inflatable custom orbital expander into the orbit can induce orbital expansion similar to that which occurs normally in response to the rapid growth of the globe in the first few years of life.[15] If tissue-expanding orbital expansion has not been performed, surgical orbital expansion can be done in older patients to facilitate insertion of an age-appropriate ocular prosthesis size.

The volume of the extraocular contents may be higher or lower than normal. When it is higher, the process may be diffuse, as with thyrotoxic proptosis, or discrete, as with an intraorbital tumor. Surgical expansion of the osseous orbit to increase orbital volume can allow the globe to return to a more normal relation with respect to the orbital rim when direct or complete excision of the pathologic process is not feasible. Reduced volume of the extraocular contents results in enophthalmos. Enophthalmos can be corrected by augmenting the orbital contents with either autogenous or alloplastic material; autogenous bone and cartilage are preferred.

Abnormally small orbit size usually is the consequence of inadequate growth of the orbital contents either from congenital hypoplasia–aplasia or as a consequence of radiotherapy in the young child. Intracranial–extracranial orbital expansion is performed to achieve facial symmetry and to allow placement of an appropriate ocular prosthesis.

Abnormally large orbital size usually is the consequence of an intraorbital mass such as an orbital encephalocele, neurofibromatosis, or hemangioma. Management of the etiologic process must precede or be synchronous with surgical reduction of the orbit.

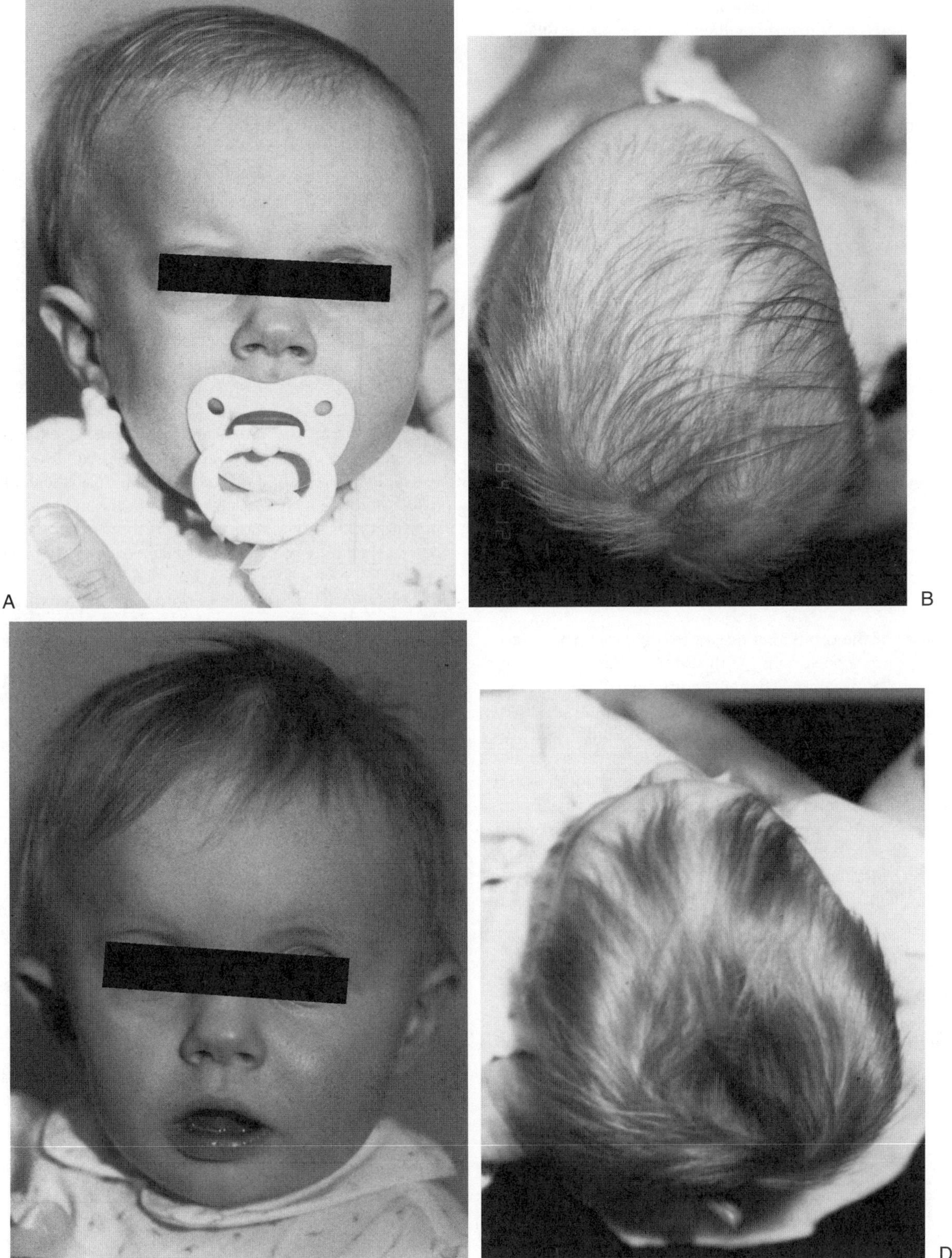

FIG. 48-3. (*A* and *B*) Five-month-old girl with plagiocephaly without synostosis. Note the flattened left occiput and protruding right occiput. (*C* and *D*) Four months after cranial-molding helmet therapy, cranial and facial symmetry is significantly improved.

Assessment of spatial malposition of the globe requires the physician to separate illusory malposition due to strabismus from actual malposition due to anomalous orbital location. The globe and orbit can be malpositioned with respect to the horizontal, cephalad–caudad, or anteroposterior planes. Horizontal malposition may be lateral, which is called *hypertelorism* (Fig. 48-4), or medial, known as *hypotelorism.* Cephalad–caudad malposition is refereed to as *dystopia.* There are no specific terms for orbital anteroposterior malposition. The major neural structures, vasculature, and the origin of five of the six extraocular muscles are concentrated at the apex of the orbit. Neither the apex nor the structures it contains is relocatable. The ventral two thirds of the orbit can be separated from the apex with osteotomies and repositioned with respect to any of the six degrees of freedom (x, y, z, pitch, roll, yaw). Repositioning the ventral, or "useful," orbit repositions the globe and the extraocular orbital contents as well.[16] The movement of the globe does not coincide perfectly with that of the bone and cannot be accurately predicted. Synchronous or, more commonly, secondary modification of the periorbital soft tissues is often necessary following orbital repositioning.

Subcranial Procedures

Ocular Globes and Orbits

Deformities of the orbits that do not involve the orbital roof and do not require repositioning of the circumferential orbit are treated without craniotomy. The most common of such anomalies is hypoplasia or aplasia of the inferolateral orbital rim associated with Treacher Collins syndrome (mandibulofacial dysostosis).[1] The osseous deficiency is reflected in the overlying soft tissues with caudal displacement of the lateral canthi, eyelid clefts (coloboma), and caudal globe displacement (dystopia). Reconstruction of these deformities requires repair of the eyelid coloboma, soft tissue transfer from the upper eyelid to the lower, augmentation of the bony deficit with autogenous bone graft or alloplastic implant, and reinsertion of the lateral canthus (lateral canthoplasty).

Bulging eyes (proptosis or exorbitism) is sometimes corrected by a subcranial procedure. This usually is in conjunction with ventral movement of the midface but, in unusual circumstances, can be performed as an isolated procedure. This is performed more commonly in adults than children to treat hyperthyroid exophthalmos that is unresponsive to medical management.

Midface

The *midface* denotes the region of the head between the orbits and the mandible. With respect to soft tissue, it includes the cheeks, the nose, and the upper lips. With respect to skeleton, it includes the maxilla and the maxillary dentition, the bones that comprise the nose, the zygomas (cheek bones), and the inferior orbital rims. The midface contains the nasal and paranasal sinus cavities and is bordered superiorly by the orbital cavities, inferiorly by the oral cavity, superoposteriorly by the cranial cavity, and inferoposteriorly by the nasal pharyngeal cavity.

The midface may be anomalous with respect to size, position, or both. Maxillary hypoplasia is associated with a number of syndromes. The major consequences of maxillary hypoplasia are abnormal dental occlusion, with the maxillary dentition within the mandibular dentition (complete crossbite) rather than the normal reverse relation; a concave midface appearance ("dish face"); impaired nasal airway, secondary to both the constriction of the nasal cavity within the small maxilla and the retroposition of the maxilla which narrows the velopharyngeal space (the connection between the nasal and oral pharynges); and shallow inferior orbits producing proptosis (Figs. 48-5 and 48-6).

Several constellations of congenital anomalies—which include premature fusion of cranial sutures (*craniosynostosis*), midface retrusion, and a variety of acral deformities (ranging from mild thumb anomalies to complex syndactyly)—are known as the craniosynostosis syndromes. These include the following eponymic syndromes: Apert, Crouzon, Saethre-Chotzen, Pfeiffer, and Carpenter.[1] The combination of cranial base deformity, which results from the cranial synostosis, and the midface retrusion produces a shallow orbit that cannot adequately contain the globe and other orbital contents. As discussed earlier, the cranial and superior orbital dysmorphology is usually corrected in infancy. Although surgical advancement of the midface has been performed in infancy, resulting in high morbidity and some mortality, it is more commonly performed before the child begins primary school or during middle to late adolescence when there is a complete adult dentition. Midface advancement is performed to normalize the maxillary–mandibular dentoskeletal relation, to improve the nasal airway, to enlarge the orbital volume, and to destigmatize facial appearance.[17] When midface advancement is performed in childhood, exact correction of the dental occlusion is not possible since this requires a combination of orthodontics and orthognathic (jaw) surgery, which is possible only when the permanent teeth have erupted. Advancement of the midface can benefit a compromised nasal airway in two ways: by enlarging the nasal cavity through nasal septal realignment and turbinate outfracture or resection, and by enlarging the nasopharynx and velopharynx after ventral displacement of the soft palate. Midface advancement can increase orbital volume by ventral displacement of the caudal two thirds of the osseous orbit. Eliminating or minimizing the stigmata of midface retrusion, such as sunken midface, upper lip posterior to the lower lip, relative lower jaw prominence, and bulging eyes, can improve psychosocial function.

Not all patients with maxillary deformities require advancement of the entire midface. In fact, most patient undergo maxillary advancement surgery primarily for dentoskeletal problems. These patients may have a congenital maxillary deficiency or the maxillary problem may be associated with another anomaly, such as cleft lip or palate. Treatment for these patients is deferred until the adult dentition has erupted and pubertal growth is decelerating, which occurs at about 14 years of age for the average female and 16 to 18 years for the average male. The jaw surgery is preceded by a presurgical phase of orthodontics, usually lasting 12 to 18 months, which aligns the teeth for the best possible occlusion following the operation. A postoperative phase of orthodontic treatment follows, with 6 to 12 months of hardware and then several years of retainers, to detail the result of surgery. The use of rigid internal fixation has simplified the postoperative management of jaw surgery patients by avoiding the need for intermaxillary fixation (wiring the jaws together) (Fig. 48-7).

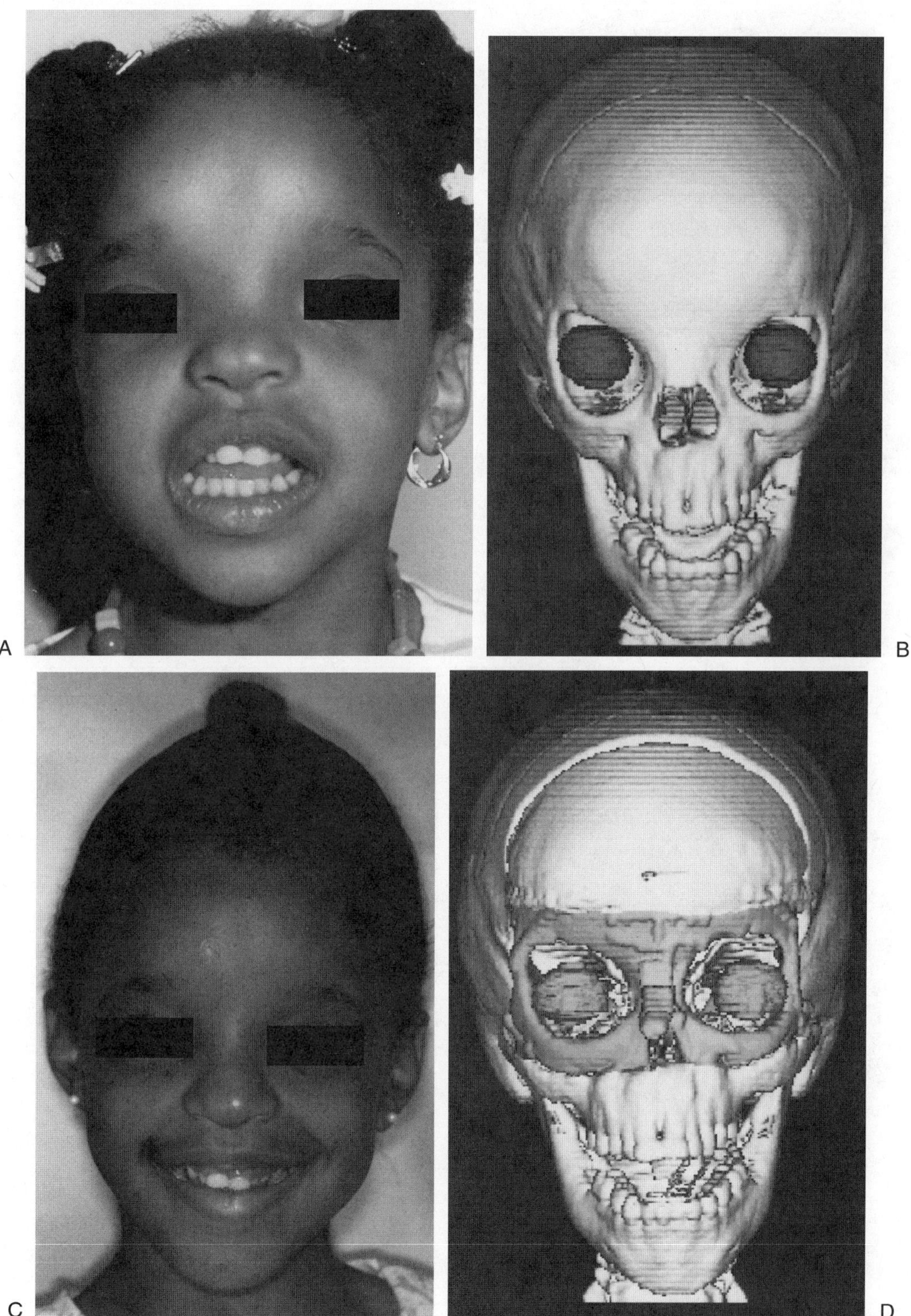

FIG. 48-4. (*A*) Three-year-old girl with hypertelorism, wide nasal bridge, and bifid nasal tip. (*B*) Preoperative three-dimensional CT osseous reformation with globe opacification. Note the superolateral elongation and rotation of the orbital rims and the excessively wide interorbital space. (*C*) Two years after intracranial and extracranial mesial repositioning of the orbits and nasal reconstruction. (*D*) The perioperative three-dimensional CT reformation following frontal craniotomy to protect the frontal lobes during orbital osteotomies, resection of the excess interorbital bone, mesial repositioning and rotation of both orbits, and nasal reconstruction with titanium-plate rigid internal fixation. (See Color Fig. 48-4*D*.)

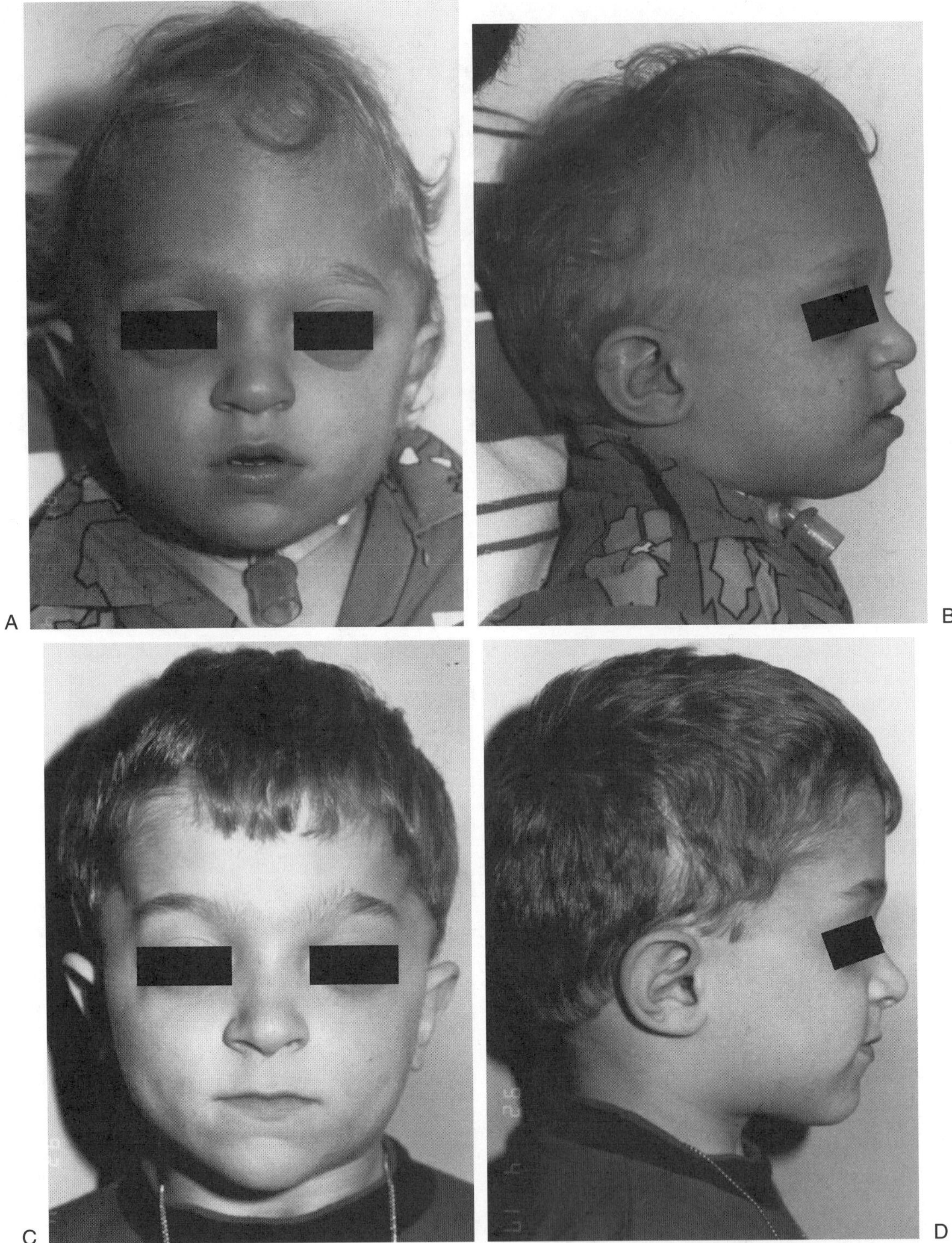

FIG. 48-5. (*A* and *B*) Two-year-old boy with cranial dysmorphology (acrocephaly), bulging eyes (proptosis), and midface retrusion secondary to Crouzon syndrome (craniofacial dysostosis). Tracheotomy was necessary to stabilize the upper airway due to the midface retrusion. (*C* and *D*) Three years after calvarial reconstruction and frontofacial advancement, the boy is 3 years, 8 months old. Cranial configuration is normalized as is the upper-to-lower lip relation. The airway has been stabilized and the tracheostomy eliminated. There is residual proptosis.

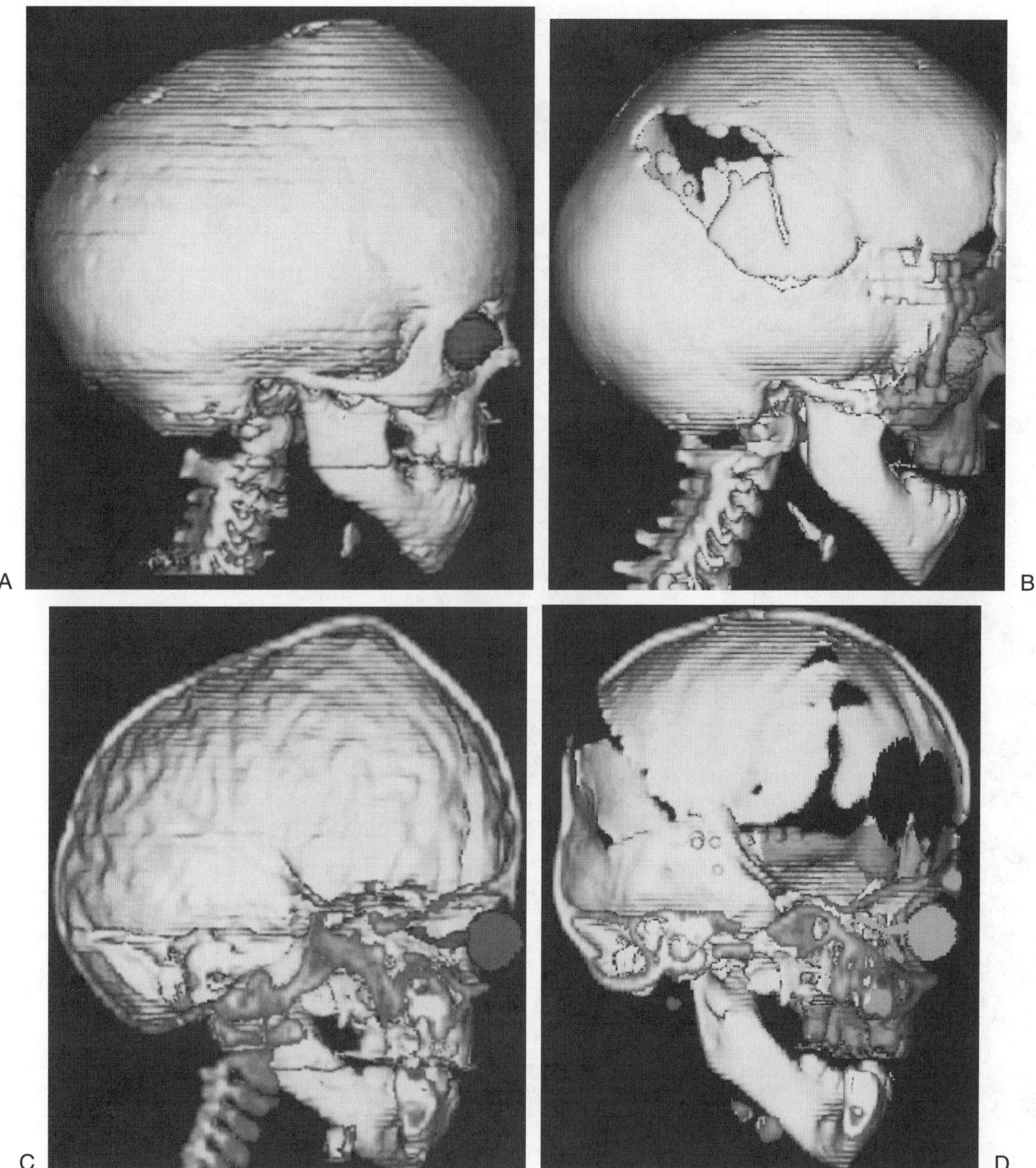

FIG. 48-6. Lateral three-dimensional osseous reformation with globe opacification of a child with shallow orbits. (*A*) The preoperative image shows AP cranial elongation and ventral towering with maxillary retrusion and anterior open bite. (*B*) The postoperative image, which does not include the ventral-most portion of the skull, shows cranial reshaping, calvarial defects due to cranial volume expansion, and titanium-plate rigid internal fixation at the superolateral orbit and along the zygomatic arch to maintain the midface advancement. Longitudinal orbital three-dimensional osseous reformation of the same patient with globe and optic nerve opacification. (*C*) The preoperative image shows the globe protruding because of the shallow orbit. (*D*) The postoperative image shows an improved globe–orbit relation after the orbit has been expanded through ventral displacement of both the superior and inferior orbital rims and adjacent bones. The reconstructed calvaria is displayed in yellow, the advanced midface in green, and the globe and optic nerve in red. (See Color Fig. 48-6*B* and *D*.)

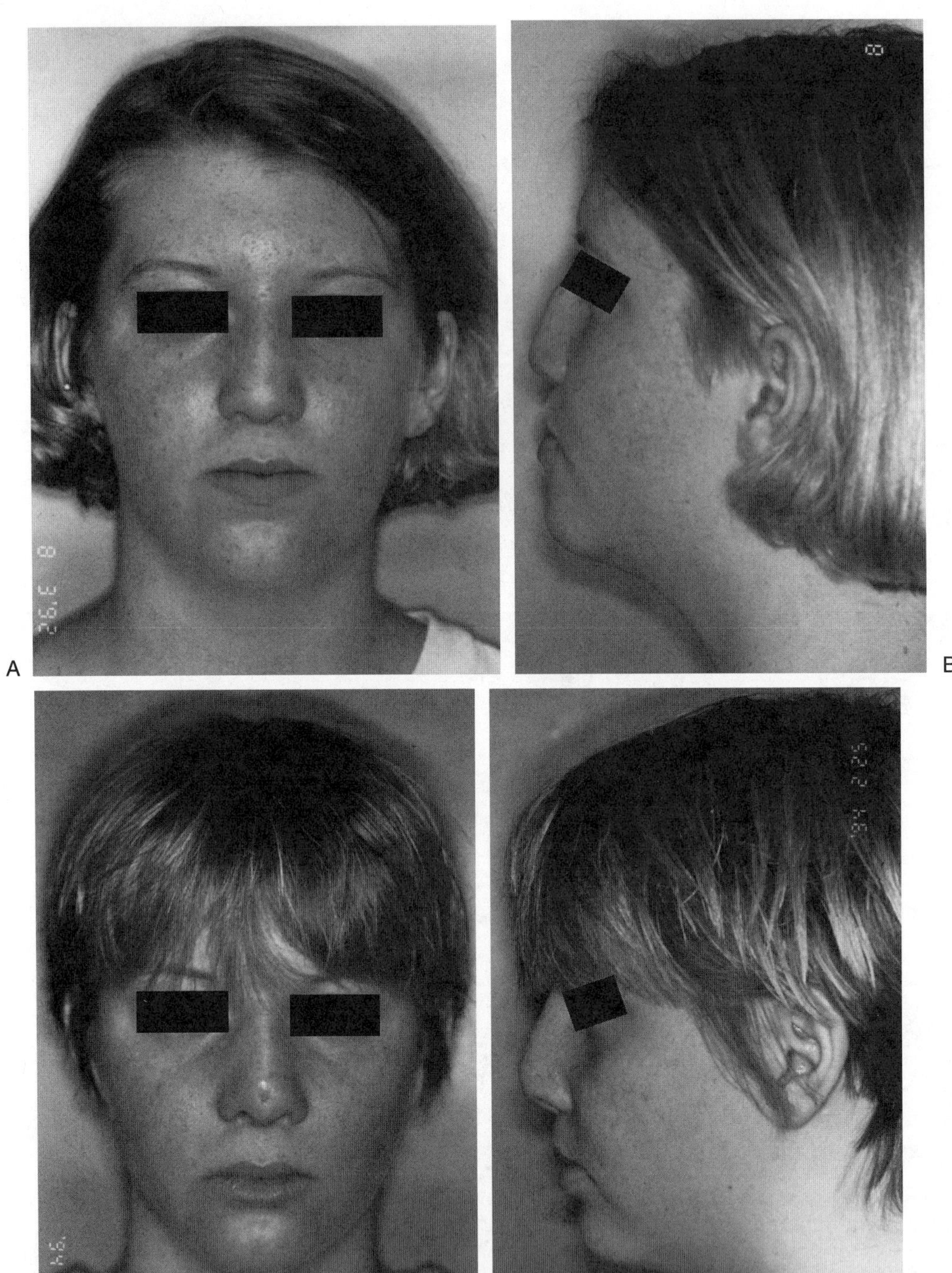

FIG. 48-7. (*A*) Thirteen-year-old girl with congenital nasomaxillary retrusion (Binder syndrome). (*B*) Note the sunken midface appearance, the posterior position of the upper lip compared with the lower, and the lack of lower nasal projection. (*C* and *D*) One and a half years after Le-Fort I type midface advancement and 6 months after nasal reconstruction with autogenous rib graft, the appearance is improved.

Mandible

The mandible may be deficient (*micrognathia*) or excessive (*prognathia*) in the sagittal plane or three dimensionally asymmetric due to unilateral hypoplasia or hyperplasia. Ventral mandibular protrusion is rarely identified until late childhood or adolescence since mandibular prognathia usually develops during the pubertal growth spurt. Other than affecting appearance and occasionally mastication, mandibular prognathism does not endanger vital functions. In contrast, posterior displacement of the mandible (*retrognathia*), secondary to symmetric micrognathia or asymmetric hypoplasia, can present a perinatal emergency if the tongue obstructs the airway (*glossoptosis*). The constellation of micrognathia/retrognathia, glossoptosis, and respiratory obstruction is known as the *Robin sequence.*[18] Many, but not all, infants with Robin sequence also have a cleft palate. The inability to breath freely precludes the ability to feed effectively. Management of the Robin sequence proceeds through a hierarchy beginning with prone positioning and special feeding techniques and culminating in tracheotomy and feeding gastrostomy. Only a small minority of infants with Robin sequence actually require surgical airway and feeding management.

Hypoplasia or aplasia of the hemimandible, unilaterally or bilaterally, occurs in about 1 of every 5000 births, often in conjunction with anomalies of the cranium, orbit and globe, midface, external and middle ears, cervical and thoracic vertebrae, and ribs. This constellation of anomalies is currently known as *hemifacial microsomia* (Figs. 48-8 and 48-9).[19] (It was previously referred to as first and second branchial arch syndrome since many of the involved structures derive from those arches.) With complete aplasia of the hemimandible, the upper airway may be unstable at birth due to lingual obstruction.

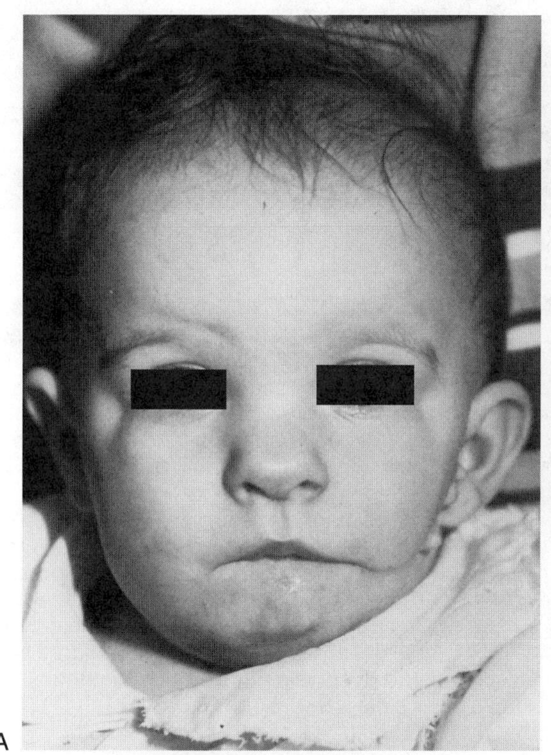

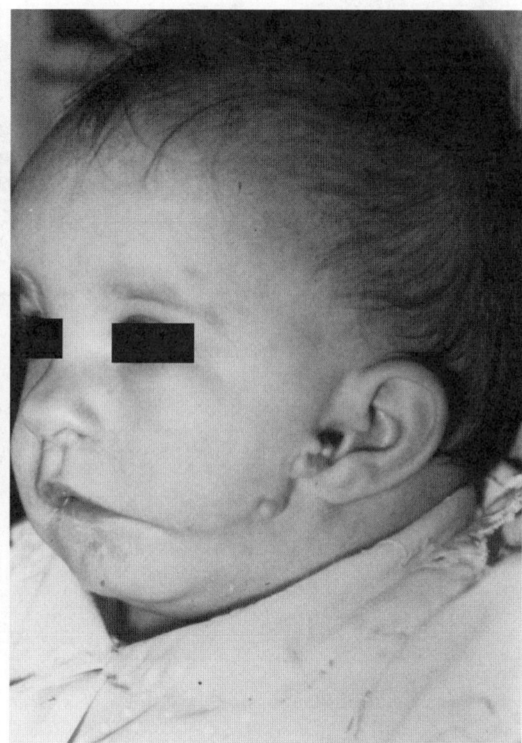

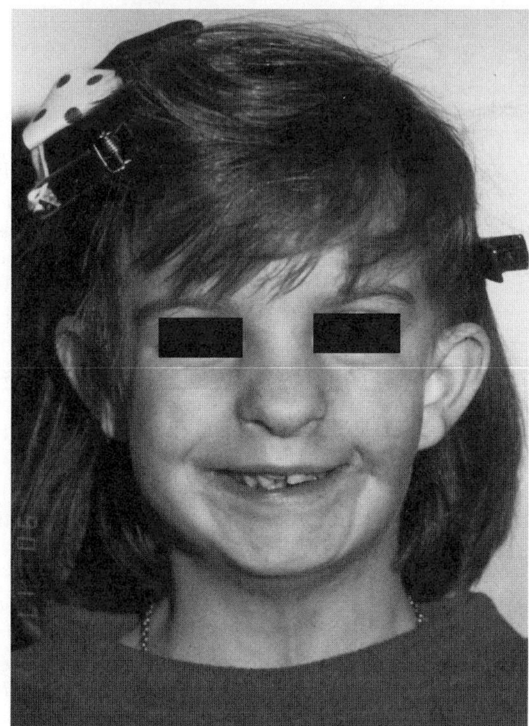

FIG. 48-8. (*A* and *B*) Five-month-old girl with left hemifacial microsomia. The lower face is deviated to the left because of mandibular hypoplasia. Soft tissue hypoplasia of the left face aggravates the asymmetry. The left oral commisure is displaced laterally as a cleft (macrostomia) with subdermal continuation to the ear (Tessier no. 5). Chondrocutaneous tags are present along the path of the cleft. (*C*) The same patient at age 6 years after removal of preauricular tags at age 1 year, repair of macrostomia at age 3 years, mandibular osteotomy for repositioning at 4 years, and microvascular transfer of parascapular dermofat free flap for soft tissue augmentation of the left cheek at age 6 years.

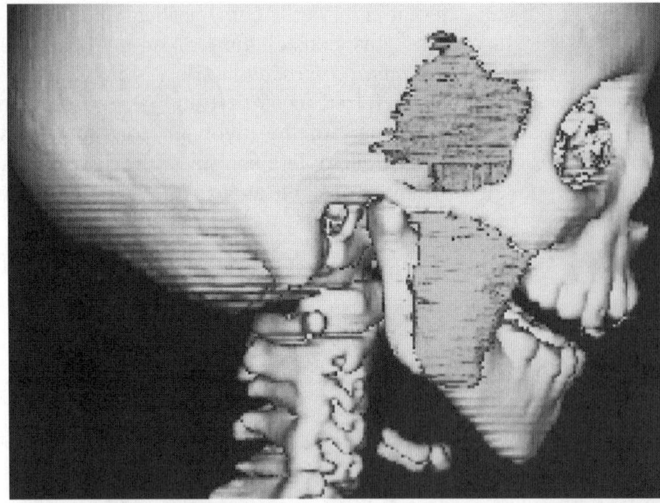

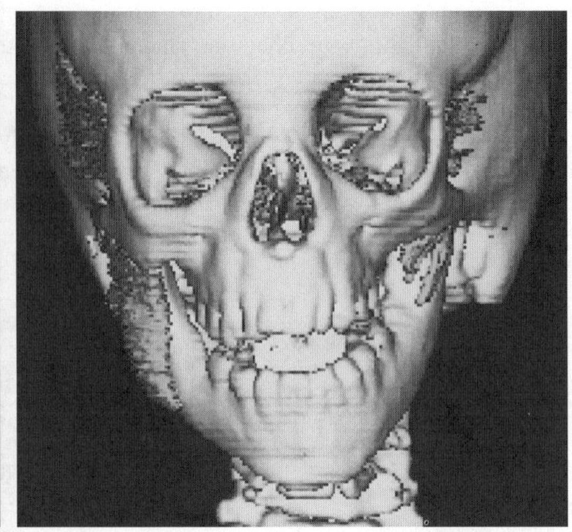

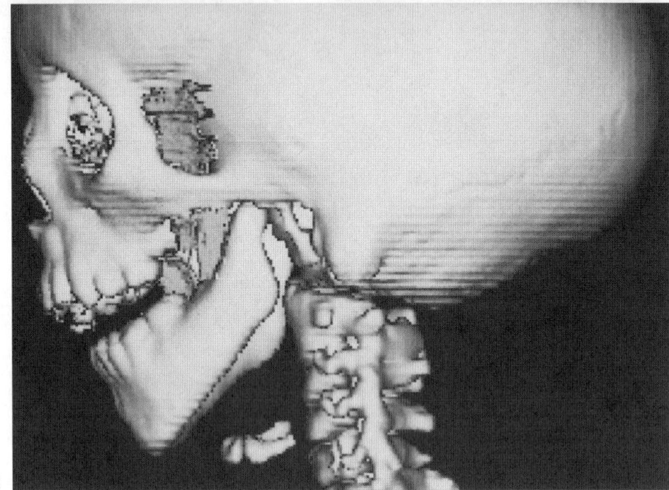

FIG. 48-9. (*A*) In a case involving mandibular hypoplasia, three-dimensional CT osseous surface reformations with opacification of the temporalis (*top*) and masseter muscles (*bottom*) in the unaffected right side of the face. Note normal osseous anatomy and bulk and normal origin and insertion of both muscles. (*B*) The lower face midline is deviated to the left, and the left mandibular angle is displaced medially. Muscular hypoplasia is also evident. (*C*) On the affected side, the temporalis is hypoplastic but relatively normal in origin and insertion sites. The masseter, however, is not only hypoplastic but also has an aberrant insertion. Hypoplasia and dysplasia of the left hemimandible are also visible. (See Color Fig. 48-9.)

Tracheotomy is necessary in such neonates. Decannulation often is not possible for such children until the absent mandible has been reconstructed, usually with an autogenous costochondral graft. Neonates with lesser degrees of mandibular agenesis/ hypoplasia may require prone positioning or may even be stable lying supine. Neonates with unstable airways due to mandibular dysmorphology often also have difficulties with feeding and may require a feeding gastrostomy. Mandibular reconstruction is considered beginning at 4 years of age. If the airway is still unstable or there is significant maxillary and mandibular asymmetry with tilt (*cant*) of the dental occlusal plane, mandible reconstruction is performed with or without bone graft as needed. Additional jaw surgery during the teen years after completion of pubertal growth should be anticipated in about half of the patients. The remainder are treated with orthodontics alone. Hypoplastic soft tissue augmentation with microvascular transfer of a parascapular dermofat free flap, external ear reconstruction (see later discussion on microtia), and reanimation of congenital facial palsy follow airway stabilization and management of dentoskeletal deformity. Although there is a broad phenotype spectrum in hemifacial microsomia, many patients require multiple operations beyond infancy, violating the ideal of completing craniofacial normalization before the child is aware of the anomaly and the intervention required to reconstruct it.

Nose

Congenital nasal deformity often accompanies major anomalies of the cranium, orbits, or midface. Nasal anomalies may consist of enlargement or diminution of otherwise normal structures, clefting, duplication, gross malformation, and agenesis. Any type of nasal anomaly may also include malposition. Although anomalies of the external nose are the most easily recognized, bilateral obstruction to the nasal airway, whether external or internal, presents a perinatal emergency since the neonate is an obligate nasal breather. Endotracheal intubation is usually necessary to establish a secure airway. Such obstruction usually is due to choanal atresia, and the diagnosis of this is made clinically by the inability to pass a small catheter or feeding tube through the nares into the oropharynx and is confirmed with CT scan of the head. Surgical opening of the choanae (the space which connects the nasal cavities with the nasopharynx) and placement of internal stents is successful in some infants, depending on the nature (soft tissue versus bone) and extent of the atresia. In patients for whom it fails, tracheotomy is required for airway stabilization.

Nasal reconstruction is an integral part of the management of eyes that are too far apart along the horizontal plane (*hypertelorism*) and of cleft lip. Autogenous bone, calvaria, or rib, is used during the intracranial–extracranial correction of the hypertelorism to reconstruct the hypoplastic nasal dorsum, and soft tissue redundancy is resected at that time or subsequently. The nasal tip is deformed in both unilateral and bilateral cleft lip patients. The tip deformity is often addressed at the time of initial lip repair in infancy and subsequently, as indicated, in association with other cleft-related operations. Regardless of the etiology, surgeons do not have the skill to reconstruct a satisfactory nose during infancy or early childhood that will grow into a satisfactory adult nose during puberty. All parents are informed that additional nasal surgery should be anticipated in the midteens (Fig. 48-10). At that time, the nose is examined and the desires of the patient discussed. If the patient wishes additional nasal revision, it is performed. If not, surgery is deferred until desired.

Ears

Ear anomalies range from trivial, such as preauricular tags, to physiologically significant, such as complete agenesis (microtia) with loss of air-conduction hearing. Patients with ear anomalies should be screened for three additional problems: hearing loss, mandibular anomalies, and renal anomalies. Hearing loss is rarely associated with tags and lesser auricle deformations, but it is always associated with major auricular malformations. Hearing is assessed with evoked response audiometry in neonates and by age-appropriate audiometry in older infants and children. When bilateral hearing loss of a magnitude expected to interfere with normal speech is detected, hearing aids are placed in infancy. While unilateral hearing loss does not require an augmentative device, hearing conservation tips and school seating guidelines are provided to the parents, and regular audiograms are obtained to monitor the status of the normal hearing ear. Because much of the auricle and middle ear is derived from the first branchial arch, external and middle ear anomalies are often associated with mandibular anomalies. The relation between ear and mandible anomalies is inconsistent, however, with respect to both incidence and magnitude. While agenesis of the mandibular condyle or marked hypoplasia of the hemimandible is diagnosable on physical examination and radiologic imaging in the infant, lesser degrees of mandibular asymmetry may not become manifest until the complete primary dentition has erupted or even the pubertal growth spurt and eruption of the permanent dentition has occurred. Patients with external ear anomalies without overt mandible deformity should be evaluated on a routine schedule into the teen years to identify and manage dentoskeletal deformity when it becomes evident. A few patients with ear anomalies also have renal anomalies. While the risk is low, it is finite and often is not diagnosed clinically until urinary stasis has resulted in infection and deformation of the urinary excretory system. Screening abdominal ultrasound, a minimally risky and low-cost procedure, should be done for all patients with ear anomalies to identify those with renal anomalies who can benefit from early interceptive therapy.

Although preauricular tags can be ligature amputated in the nursery, the base of the tag should first be carefully palpated for a cartilagenous internal component. If a cartilagenous core is present and not surgically excised, recurrence of the mound can be expected with growth. When a cartilagenous core is present, formal surgical excision should be performed.

Protruding ears may be noted in the nursery. Considerable success has been reported from Japan with using binding and ear molds in the perinatal period to correct excessive ear protrusion. When the child presents as a toddler or older, as is common in America, surgical correction is necessary. The ear is examined to determine the cause of the protrusion, which is either absence of the antihelical fold, excess caval cartilage, an obtuse auriculocephalic angle, or a combination of these. A procedure is selected that addresses the dysmorphology responsible for the protrusion. Protruding ears are preferentially corrected after 6 years of age since the external ear is almost adult size at that time and the cartilage is formed enough to preclude recurrence. Correction is usually performed when the protrusion becomes of psychosocial significance for the child.

Both excessive protrusion and diminution may occur with constricted ears. Constricted ears are often referred to as ''cup'' or ''lop'' ears due to the circular constriction of the helical rim, which resembles a cup, or the folding over of the superior helical rim, which resembles a rabbit's lop ear. The timing for correcting constricted ears is similar to that for outstanding ears except in the more marked cases which require reconstruction similar to that for microtia (see later). In mild cases, there is adequate tissue in the affected ear for rearrangement reconstruction. In moderately and severely affected cases, additional cartilage from the contralateral ear or rib and skin from the mastoid or groin are necessary to correct the dysmorphology and reconstruct an ear of similar size to the opposite normal ear.

Microtia is the term used to describe reduction anomalies of the external ear. Microtia is graded from I, designating marked reduction in auricle size with preservation of general ear shape, to III, designating negligible ear remnants with no resemblance to a normal ear. Regardless of the grade of microtia, reconstruction of a normal sized and shaped auricle requires transfer of local or distant tissues (Fig. 48-11).[20] Auricle reconstruction requires at least two and often three operations over a minimum of 6 months. Although a few surgeons still use alloplastic materials for the absent cartilagenous framework, most ear reconstruction is performed using an autogenous costal cartilage framework. This framework is placed under glabrous skin where the auricle should have developed. Preoperative or intraoperative tissue expansion is a useful adjunct to obtain sufficient skin for covering a three-dimensional framework. In rare cases of microtia associated with other marked craniofacial anomalies, such as hemifacial miscrosomia, there may not be adequate local glabrous skin. A temporalis fascial flap surfaced with skin graft is used to cover the cartilage framework. After the cartilage framework has been successfully imbedded into the mastoid-region pocket, a minimum of 3 months postoperatively, an auriculocephalic sulcus (the space between the medial surface of the normal auricle and the head in which eyeglass temples rest) is created. The surgically created sulcus is lined with groin full-thickness skin graft, and the microtic remnants are rotated to create an ear lobe. A final stage of reconstruction is chosen by many patients and their families to achieve as much similarity of detail between the reconstructed and the unaffected normal auricle as possible. Auricle reconstruction is usually initiated at age 7 years when the child has large enough costal cartilages to construct an adult-size framework and an adult-size ear can

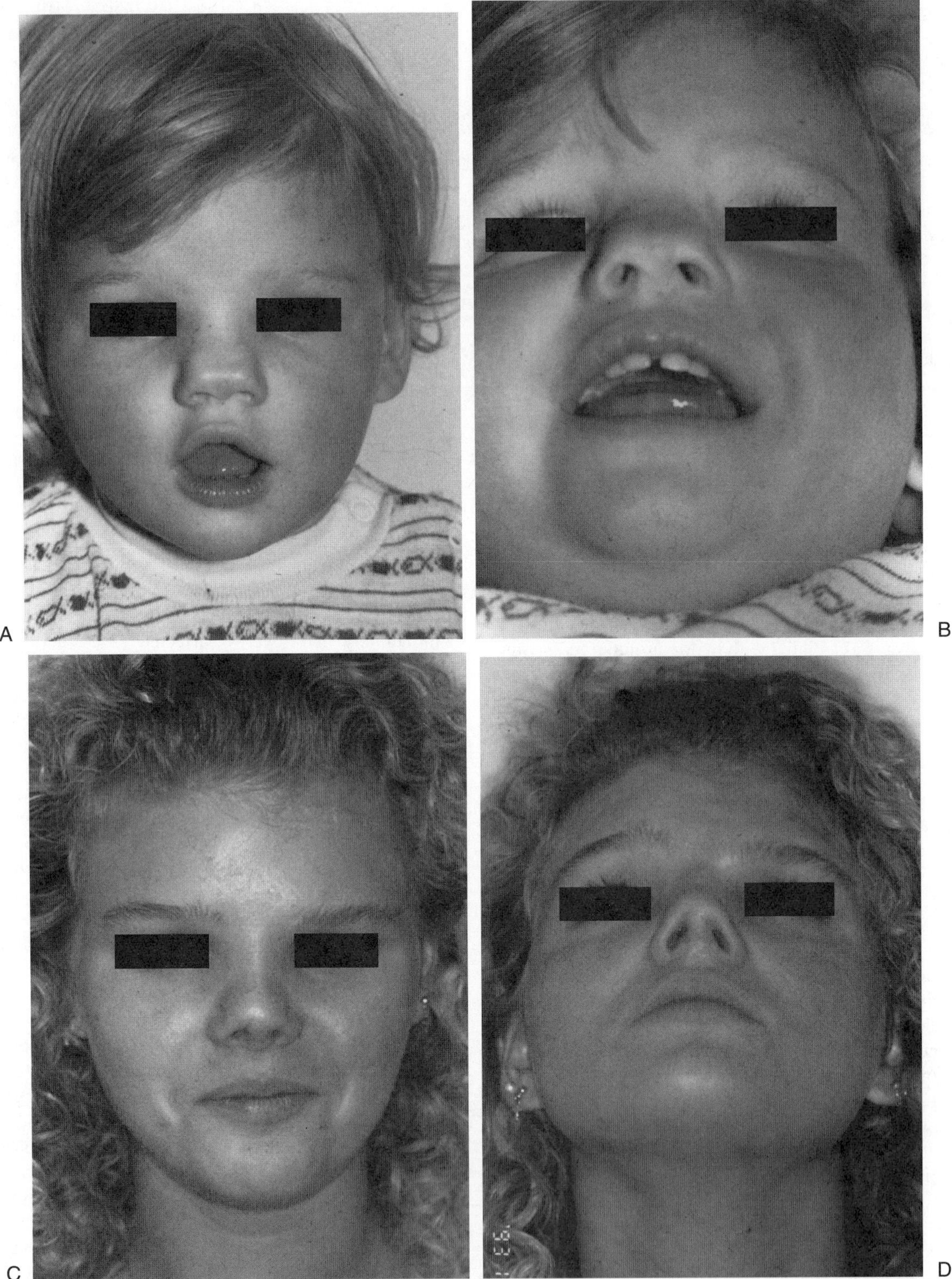

FIG. 48-10. (*A*) A 19-month-old girl with bifid nose and grade I hypertelorism secondary to incomplete midline craniofacial cleft (Tessier nos. 0 through 14). (*B*) The basilar view demonstrates diastasis of the nasal alar cartilages with a broad, boxy nasal tip and wide alar base. (*C* and *D*) The result at age 17 years, after nasal reconstruction in childhood and adolescence.

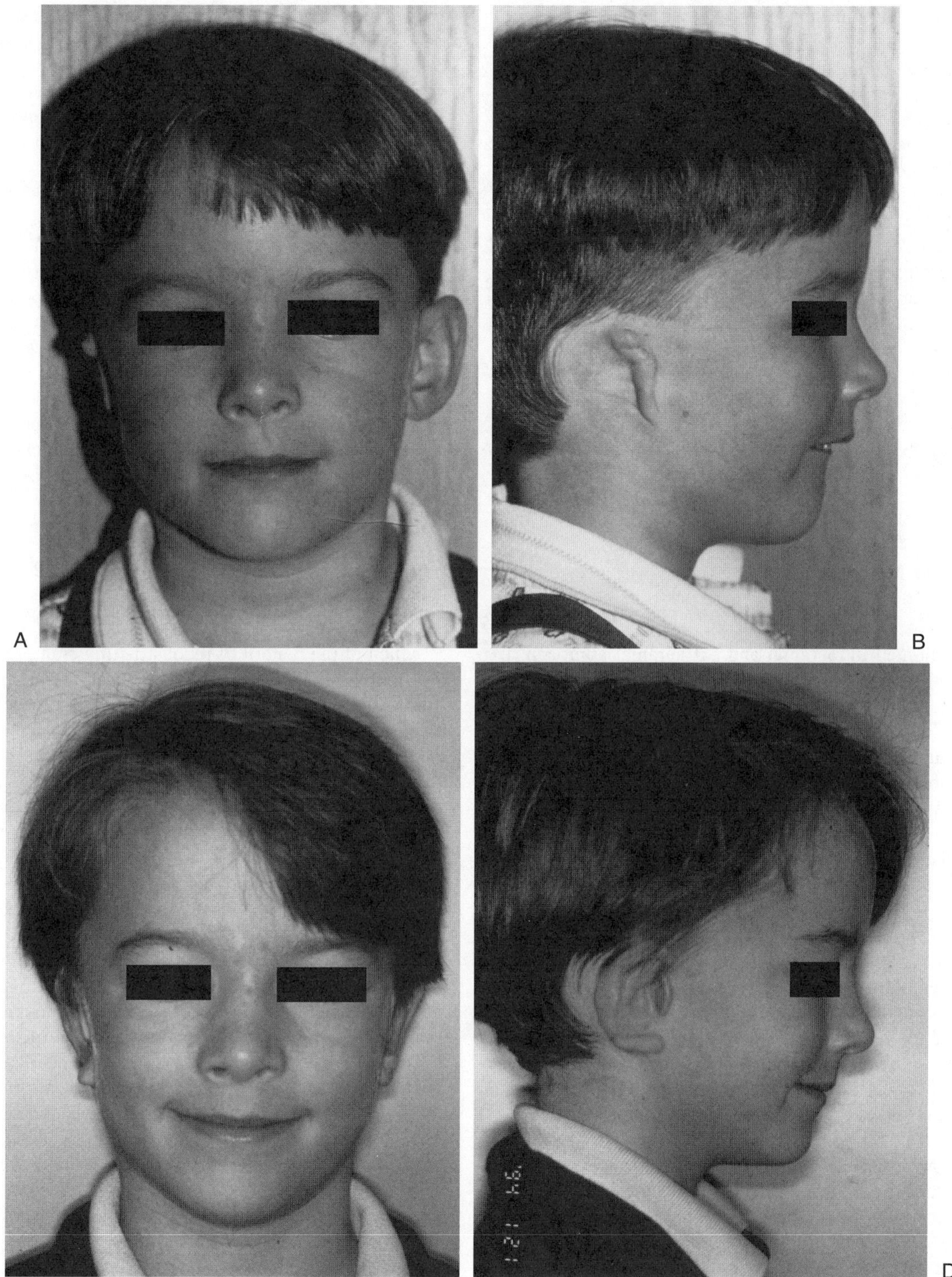

FIG. 48-11. (*A* and *B*) Five-year-old boy with right microtia and protruding left ear. (*C* and *D*) The result 3 years after reconstructing the right auricle with local skin, an autogenous rib cartilage graft and groin skin graft, and tragal reconstruction with left ear composite chondrocutaneous graft.

be reconstructed without appearing excessively large for the child's face.

As noted earlier, the major concern with ear anomalies is the status of hearing. All patients with microtia lack air-conduction hearing. Although most patients with microtia have intact inner ears, some also have a sensorineural hearing loss as well. The feasibility of restoring air-conduction hearing depends on the integrity of the middle ear. If a middle ear cavity is present and the ossicles do not appear too deformed on a temporal bone CT scan, surgical construction of an external auditory canal, ossicular reconstruction, and tympanoplasty are possible. These procedures can endanger the facial nerve, however, and when all goes well, the quality of hearing is still lower than normal. For these reasons, we do not recommend attempting restoration of air-conduction hearing unless there is bilateral hearing loss or the patient is old enough, at least in the middle teens, to understand the benefits and risks of the attempt to make the decision.

OUTCOME OF CRANIOFACIAL MANAGEMENT

Morbidity and Mortality

Definitive skeletal correction of major craniofacial anomalies requires a combined intracranial and extracranial approach. It required untethered vision, a willingness to take risk, and advances in surgical technique to initiate and then develop such operations [21]. A major inhibition to developing the intracranial–extracranial approach was fear of lethal infection following elective communication between the nasooral and cranial cavities. This fear was clearly not unfounded according to the early morbidity and mortality reports of such procedures. Individual[22] and multicenter[23] reports documented significant infections in 2% to 7% of intracranial–extracranial cases and death in 0.2% to 2%. As experience with craniofacial surgery was accrued, the associated morbidity and mortality diminished. The most recent published data reports 2% infection and 0.5% death in 355 procedures between 1980 and 1989.[24]

This reduction in morbidity and mortality may be related to mastery of the technique, modifications of technique, and improvements in ancillary activities. Mastery of technique develops from specialized training in craniofacial surgery fellowships, concentration of cases at craniofacial centers, and performance of sufficient operations per annum to maintain competence. Modifications of technique include separation of the cranial from the nasooral cavities with a galeal–frontalis flap and anterior fossa bone grafts, avoidance of intracranial "dead space" in older children and adults, diminished blood loss via elective hypotensive anesthesia, use of autologous and directed donor blood when transfusion is necessary, and avoidance of elective tracheotomy in most cases. Improvements in ancillary activities include advances in computer-assisted medical imaging, including three-dimensional CT and MR scans, to define the aberrant anatomy, to plan surgery, and to evaluate perioperative and long-term results,[10,11] as well as specially designed facial rigid internal fixation devices to eliminate perioperative osseous fragment mobility, to minimize postoperative relapse, and to avoid intermaxillary fixation.[25]

Combining these factors has significantly reduced operative time from more than 12 hours for complex procedures to less than 6 hours in most cases, has reduced the duration of intensive care stay from multiple days to overnight or not at all, has reduced the duration of hospitalization from 7 to 10 days to 3 to 5 days, and has allowed patients to resume normal daily activities, excluding head contact sports, in about 1 week rather than several.

Physical Function

Although craniofacial operations obviously improve patients' physical functions by improving corneal protection, upper airway patency, and the ability to chew, rigorous documentation of such improvements is lacking. Objective outcome data are available for visual acuity and extraocular mobility[26] as well as dental occlusion and maxillary and mandibular position, using cephalometric measurements.[27] An attempt to document olfaction following orbital repositioning surgery, which usually involves interrupting at least some of the olfactory fibers, yielded confusing results due to inconsistency of subjective and objective assessments.[28]

Psychosocial Function

Much of the benefit of reconstructing craniofacial anomalies is thought to be improved psychosocial function. Although some authors have attempted to document the effect of major facial deformity on psychosocial development and the subsequent effect of surgical reconstruction, the validity of the hypothesis remains to be established.[29,30] Generalizations are difficult because of the small numbers of cases, a range of facial disfigurement and surgical outcomes, varied ages at operation, as well as differing family units, socioeconomic and residential experiences, and support and educational services.

The family's coping ability and the residential locus seem to be the most useful indicators of the child's success at social integration. Families that move beyond the initial shock of a deformed face and focus on the child as an individual with other assets and liabilities seem to nurture a child who is self-confident and able to effectively deal with teasing and other untoward social experiences. Children who live in rural environments, where their self-identity is based more on their extended family relationships than on their appearance, seem to cope better than children in urban areas who are more often confronted by inquisitive and, at times, offensive strangers. As a group, people with craniofacial deformities have better psychosocial function than was anticipated when study of their function began several decades ago.

A second hypothesis that underlies decisions regarding the timing of treatment for craniofacial anomalies is that it is better to normalize young children's deformities before they develop a full psychosocial awareness, even if multiple operations that may intrude into the age of awareness are required. While this hypothesis is intuitively sensible, it also remains to be validated.

One benefit of dedicated craniofacial centers has been the establishment of patient registries and the standardization of long-term follow-up. Data is now becoming available for patients treated with contemporary treatments as infants and children who are now young adults. Although the limited numbers of affected people and other limiting factors enumerated earlier preclude rigorous comparative studies, reference to historic controls should shed some light on this subject.

REFERENCES

1. Gorlin RJ, Cohen MM Jr, Levin LS. Syndromes of the head and neck. New York, Oxford University Press, 1990.
2. Enlow D. Facial growth, ed 3. Philadelphia, WB Saunders, 1990.
3. Sperber GH. Craniofacial embryology, ed 4. London, Wright, 1989.
4. Thorogood P, Ferretti P. Heads and tales: recent advances in craniofacial development. Br Dent J 1992;173:301.
5. Cohen MM Jr. Etiopathogenesis of craniosynostosis. Neurosurg Clin North Am 1991;2:507.
6. Vermeij-Keers C. Craniofacial embryology and morphogenesis: normal and abnormal. In: Stricker M, et al. Craniofacial malformations. Edinburgh: Churchill Livingstone, 1990:27.
7. Tessier P. Anatomic classification of facial, cranio-facial and laterofacial clefts. J Maxillofac Surg 1976;4:69.
8. American Cleft Palate—Craniofacial Association. Parameters for the evaluation and treatment of patients with cleft lip/palate or other craniofacial anomalies. Cleft Palate Craniofac J 1993;30(suppl 1).
9. Marsh JL, Vannier MW. Comprehensive care for craniofacial deformities. St Louis, CV Mosby, 1985.
10. Lo LJ, Marsh JL, Vannier MW, et al. Craniofacial computer assisted surgical planning and simulation. Clin Plast Surg 1994;21:501.
11. Marsh JL, Vannier MW. Three-dimensional surface imaging from CT scans for the study of craniofacial dysmorphology. J Craniofac Genet Dev Biol 1989;9:61.
12. Gault DT, Renier D, Marchac D, et al. Intracranial pressure and intracranial volume in children with craniosynostosis. Plast Reconstr Surg 1992;90:377.
13. Clarren SK. Plagiocephaly and torticollis: etiology, natural history, and helmet treatment. J Pediatr 1981;98:92.
14. David DJ. Cephaloceles: classification, pathology, and management—a review. J Craniofac Surg 1993;4:192.
15. Elisevich K, Bite U, Colcleugh R. Microorbitalism: a technique for orbital rim expansion. Plast Reconstr Surg 1991;88:609.
16. Tessier P, Guiot G, Derome P. Orbital hypertelorism. II. Definite treatment of orbital hypertelorism (OR.H.) by craniofacial or by extracranial osteotomies. Scand J Plast Reconstr Surg 1973;7:39.
17. Tessier P. Total osteotomy of the middle third of the face for faciostenosis or for sequelae of Le Fort III fractures. Plast Reconstr Surg 1971; 48:533.
18. Shprintzen RJ. The implications of the diagnosis of Robin sequence. Cleft Palate Craniofac J 1992;29:205.
19. Vento A, LaBrie RA, Mulliken JB. The O.M.E.N.S. classification of hemifacial microsomia. Cleft Palate Craniofac J 1991;28:68.
20. Brent B. Auricular repair with autogenous rib cartilage grafts: two decades of experience with 600 cases. Plast Reconstr Surg 1992;90: 355.
21. Tessier P. Orbital hypertelorism. I. Successive surgical attempts: material and methods, causes and mechanisms. Scand J Plast Reconstr Surg 1972;6:135.
22. Munro IR, Sabatier RE. An analysis of 12 years of craniomaxillofacial surgery in Toronto. Plast Reconstr Surg 1985;76:29.
23. Whitaker LA, Munro IR, Salyer KE, et al. Combined report of problems and complications in 793 craniofacial operations. Plast Reconstr Surg 1979;64:198.
24. Stieg PE, Mulliken JB. Neurosurgical complications in craniofacial surgery. Neurosurg Clin North Am 1991;2:703.
25. Beals SP, Munro IR. The use of miniplates in craniomaxillofacial surgery. Plast Reconstr Surg 1987;79:33.
26. Newman SA. Ophthalmic features of craniosynostosis. Neurosurg Clin North Am 1991;2:587.
27. Marsh JL ed. Long-term results of craniofacial surgery. Cleft Palate J 1986;23(suppl):1.
28. McCathy JG. A study of gustatory and olfactory function in patients with craniofacial anomalies. Plast Reconstr Surg 1979;64:52.
29. Eder RA, ed. Developmental perspectives on craniofacial deformities. New York, Springer-Verlag, 1995.
30. Pertschuk MJ, Whitaker LA. Social and psychological effects of craniofacial deformity and surgical reconstruction. Clin Plast Surg 1982;9: 297.

Surgery of Infants and Children: Scientific Principles and Practice, edited by Keith T. Oldham, Paul M. Colombani, and Robert P. Foglia. Lippincott–Raven Publishers, Philadelphia, © 1997.

CHAPTER 49

Cleft Lip and Cleft Palate

Peter D. Witt

THE IMPORTANCE OF TEAM CARE

Facial cleft deformities are among the most common birth defects encountered in pediatric practice. One infant in every 700 live births has a cleft lip (25% of all clefts), cleft palate (25%), or both (50%). Excluded from these incidence data are babies born with clefts that are part of a complex syndrome or the various trisomies.

The surgical treatment of a child with cleft lip, cleft palate, or both follows a carefully planned sequence of staged procedures. The order of the stages is dictated by the priority of preserving function. The cleft lip is repaired first, the cleft palate second, and secondary management for velopharyngeal dysfunction is then undertaken if indicated. Bone grafting of the alveolar ridge defect is performed during the mixed-dentition stage. During adolescence, nasal reconstructive surgery, including augmentative tip rhinoplasty, or septoplasty is performed as indicated. Orthognathic jaw surgery for complex dentoskeletal deformities is usually last in the treatment sequence.

In the past, the timing of cleft lip repair was dictated by a child's weight (10 pounds), age (10 weeks), and hemoglobin level (10 g). This scheme was predicated on a commitment to avoid anesthetic complications, particularly when ether was the main agent used. Accordingly, improvements in anesthesia have allowed earlier intervention.

The existence of a facial cleft in a child calls for a long-term treatment plan. Both therapy and rehabilitation begin soon after birth, and most patients continue therapy of some sort until they reach their late teens or early twenties. Current standards of cleft care include comprehensive multidisciplinary management by the cleft palate team. The concept of an organized team evolved to address the fragmented care provided by independent specialists. The fundamental principle driving this approach involves sharing information and cultivating a global perspective about a given patient's needs.

Once health professionals recognized the confusing array of problems that an infant with a facial cleft might develop, the concept of team care for such children arose. Specialists from the three major areas of cleft care include medical/surgical (plastic surgery, pediatrics, nursing, social services), dental (pedodontics, prosthodontics, orthodontics, and oral surgery), and speech/hearing (otolaryngology, audiology, and speech therapy). This comprehensive team approach gives the child with a cleft the greatest opportunity for a pleasing appearance, healthy teeth, intact hearing, and intelligible speech. Additionally, this approach allows any problems to be identified early and limits any negative consequences of facial cleft deformities.

Problems With Feeding

Many infants with cleft lip and palate cannot generate enough suction to draw milk from the breast or bottle. The cleft palate nurser (a special bottle with a cross-cut nipple) can be used to deliver formula or pumped breast milk to these children. Before this feeding method is used, a physician must determine that the infant has a normal cough and gag reflex. Cross-cut nipples allow a slow, steady drip of milk to an infant held in an upright position. Infants with a cleft lip and palate require frequent burping because they swallow more air.

EMBRYOLOGY: NORMAL AND ABNORMAL DEVELOPMENT OF THE LIP AND PALATE

Data from human populations suggest many factors are involved in the etiology of cleft lip and palate. It is generally accepted that facial tissues, including the lip and palate, arise from cranioneural crest cells.[1] These cells migrate from their original positions at the margins of the neural fold. Normally, the facial prominences (the medial nasal, lateral nasal, and maxillary prominence) meet to fuse with each other below the nasal pit and thus separate the nasal from the oral cavities. Failure of the facial prominences to fuse leads to cleft lip, whereas failure of the palatal shelves (medial extensions of the maxillary prominences) to fuse leads to cleft palate (Fig. 49-1).

The secondary palate arises as bilateral outgrowths from the maxillary processes. These shelves initially grow vertically down the side of the tongue, then elevate at a precise time to a horizontal position above the dorsum of the tongue, and fuse with each other to form an intact palate. Palatal shelf elevation may be the result of an intrinsic shelf-elevating force, chiefly generated by the progressive accumulation and hydration of

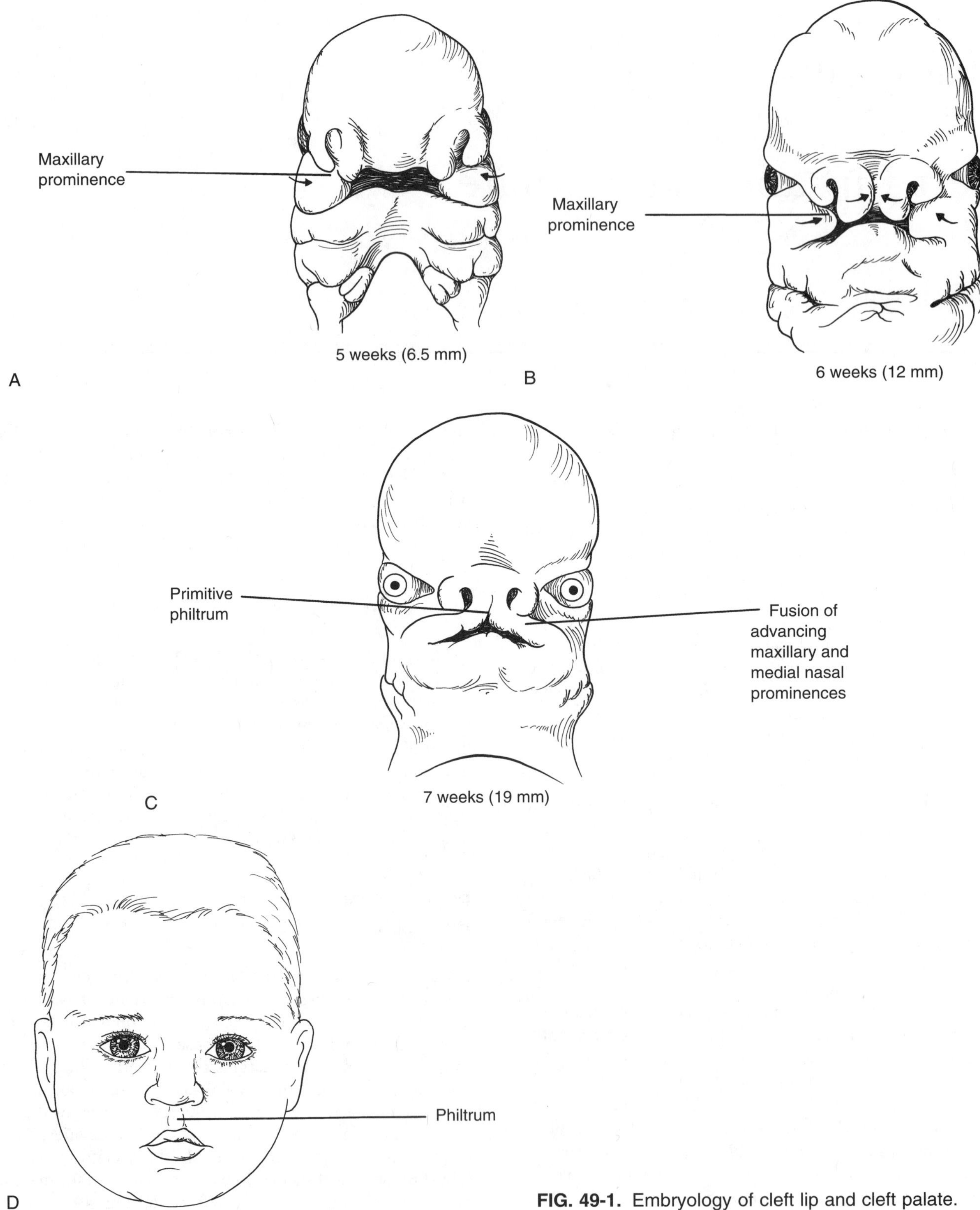

FIG. 49-1. Embryology of cleft lip and cleft palate.

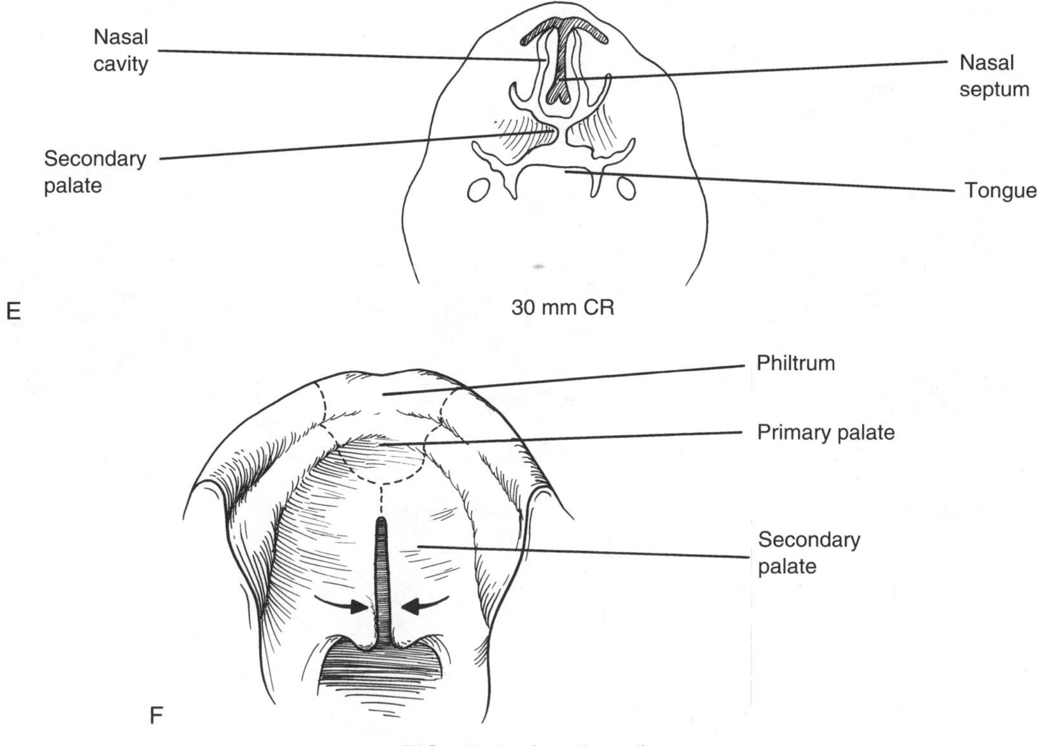

FIG. 49-1. *(continued)*

hyaluronic acid. Interference with shelf elevation is the putative mechanism by which most cases of human cleft palate arise. Cleft palate may also result from disturbances in shelf growth, defective shelf fusion, failure of medial edge cell death, postfusion rupture, and failure of mesenchymal consolidation and differentiation.

Agents that can negatively affect the growth and development of the primary palate (that is, a cleft extending ventrally from the incisive foramen) include Dilantin (phenytoin), alcohol, hypoxia, retinoids (member of the vitamin A family), and possibly dietary factors such as vitamin deficiency.

The multifactorial ''threshold'' hypothesis was described in 1963 to explain the phenomenon of facial clefting.[2] It states that genetic and environmental factors affecting a person determine the liability for a particular disease process. Cleft lip and palate occur when the cumulative liability crosses a certain threshold, for instance, failure of the embryonic facial process to make sufficient contact for fusion. Increasing liability would indicate that the development of an individual embryo is affected by additional factors that increase the likelihood that the embryo will be unable to make sufficient contact for fusion.

Cleft lip, with or without cleft palate, should be thought of as a unique anomaly distinct from clefts of the secondary palate (traditionally known as isolated cleft palate). The normal process of a palatal closure occurs during much of the last half of the first trimester. Because the lip usually closes by the end of the sixth week and then palatal fusion proceeds posteriorly during the next several weeks, isolated cleft palate usually arises from different morphogenic events than does cleft lip with or without cleft palate.

The incidence of isolated cleft palate is quite similar in different racial groups. In contrast, the incidence of cleft lip with or without cleft palate varies widely, with rates being highest in Native Americans and lowest in African-Americans. Twice as many males are affected by cleft lip than females, whereas both sexes are equally affected by isolated cleft palate.

Associated Anomalies

Associated anomalies occur frequently in patients with cleft lip, cleft palate, or both. While data regarding frequency of associated anomalies have been inconsistent historically, recent data suggest that associated anomalies occur in up to 63% of this population. About half of all patients with multiple anomalies have recognized syndromes, sequences, or associations. The high frequency of associated anomalies has obvious implications for the genetic counseling offered to all patients at cleft palate and craniofacial centers. The need for a thorough evaluation of children with congenital orofacial clefts is essential and should include a medical and genetic history, a physical examination, and phenotype analysis, including anthropometric measurements. When the causal factors are identified, the patient and family can receive appropriate counseling, including a description of prognosis and recurrence risk.

REPAIR OF THE UNILATERAL AND BILATERAL CLEFT LIP

Unilateral Cleft Lip

The Millard rotation-advancement cheiloplasty is the single most popular operative procedure in the world for repairing the unilateral cleft lip (Fig. 49-2). This technique can be applied

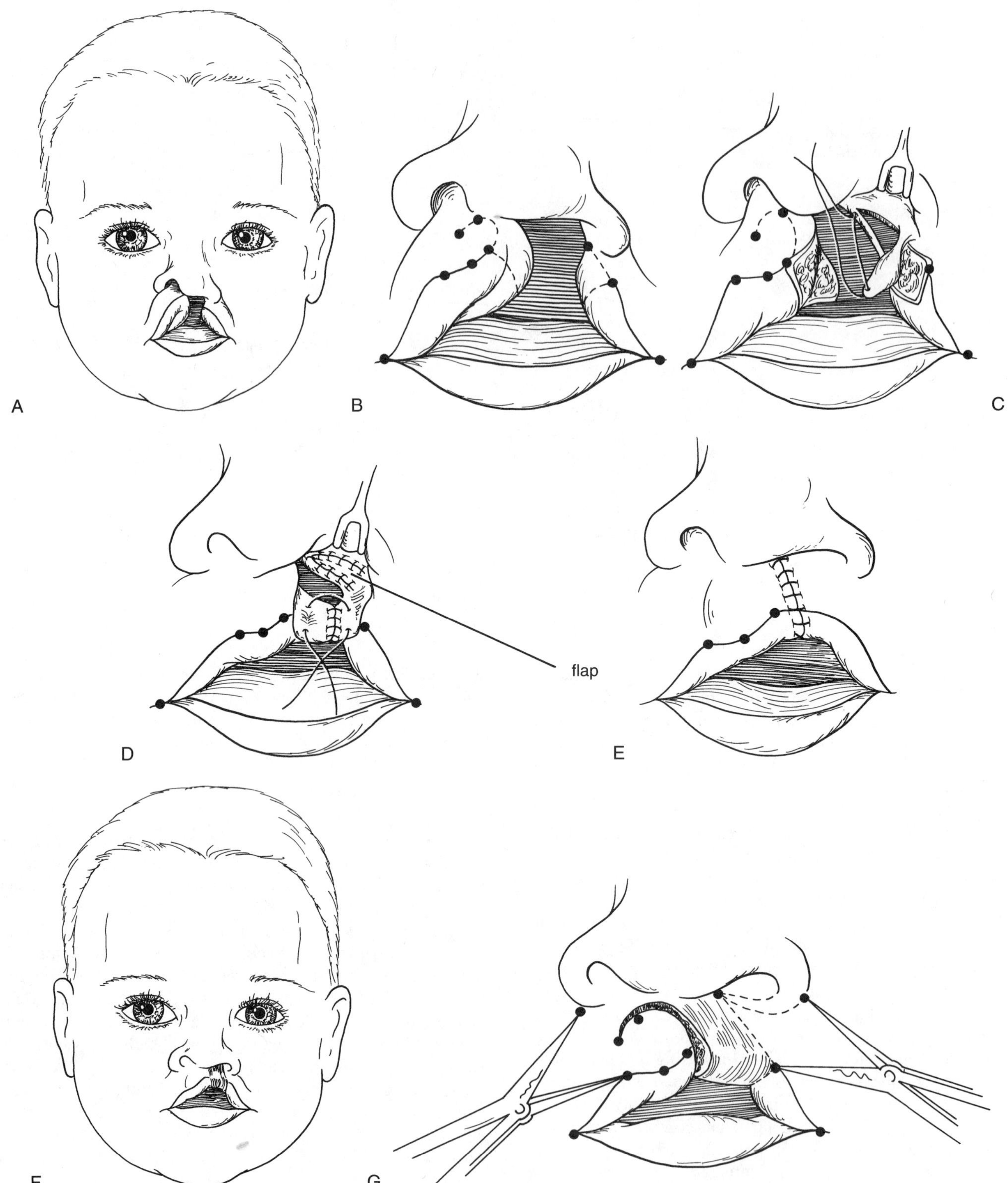

FIG. 49-2. Unilateral cleft lip repaired by rotation-advancement cheiloplasty. (*continued*)

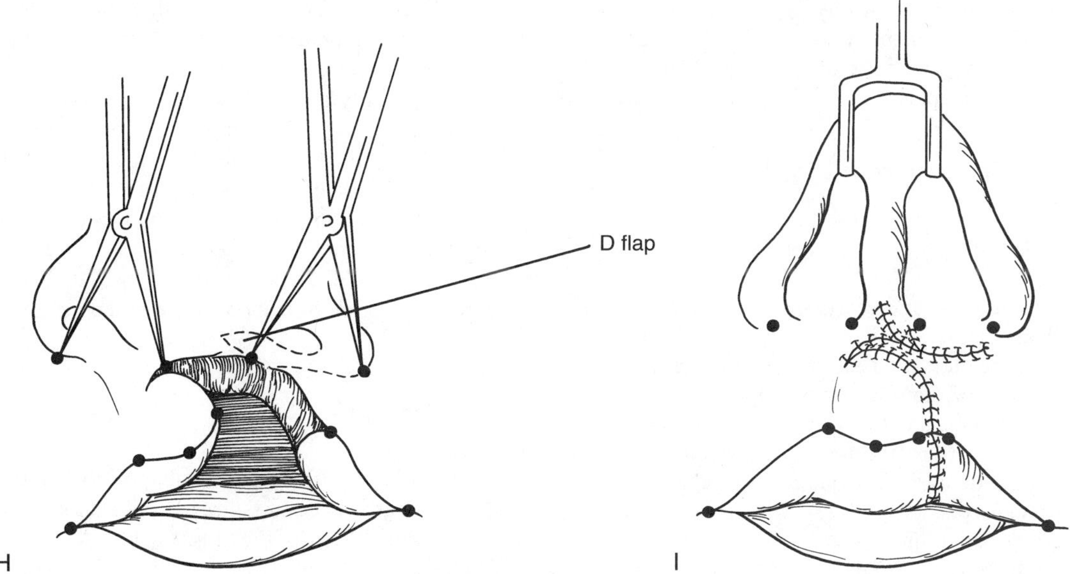

FIG. 49-2. *(continued)*

effectively to essentially all unilateral cleft lip deformities including wide, complete forms.[3]

Infants with isolated cleft lip are divided into two subsets: those with and those without alveolar clefts. If there is no alveolar cleft or if there is an alveolar cleft, but minimal deformity of the alveolus, a definitive Millard rotation-advancement cheiloplasty is performed any time after 6 weeks of age. If there is deformity of the alveolus with ventral protrusion of the premaxilla, a preliminary soft tissue closure (lip adhesion) with placement of a passive alveolar molding appliance is performed at 6 weeks of age. Definitive cheiloplasty is performed 6 months later at an average age of about 7 months.

The advantages of the Millard repair include:

1. Favorable scar position. The technique ensures preservation of the cupid's bow complex with construction of a symmetric, unviolated philtral column and retention of the central dimple hollow.
2. Easy access to repair accompanying nasal deformities. The classic cleft nasal deformity can be addressed at primary cheiloplasty. The technique provides direct access to the nasal cartilages through the lateral advancement incision and the basilar columella through which the alar cartilages can be completely mobilized for repositioning.
3. Flexibility. The design of the operation can be altered, and the surgeon is not forced to accept a predetermined, inflexible plan, dependent on accurate inviolate measurements, such as those inherent to the triangular flap repair.

Increasingly, surgeons use a passive, nonpinned, self-retained maxillary appliance, which delivers no force, but acts as a palatal stabilizer in which the force is generated by initial cleft lip adhesion. This orthopedic appliance provides guiding forces to contour and mold the alveolar segments. Obturation of the palatal cleft through the molding appliance enhances the feeding mechanism, tongue positioning, and swallowing. Following alignment of the alveolar ridge, its integrity can be fixated at a later time with bone grafting, usually from the iliac crest.

Bilateral Cleft Lip

Treating the patient with bilateral complete cleft lip and palate is a more complex problem. The goals of achieving normal appearance, speech, and dentition in these patients are elusive at best. One of the basic problems associated with bilateral cleft lip is the fixation of the alar bases to the relatively retroposed lateral maxillary segments. The alar–facial junction must be freed if it is to come forward and rest medially without tension in front of the premaxilla and adjacent to the columella. This maneuver, freeing the lip and alar base from the facial surface of the maxilla and from the frontal process of the maxilla on both the facial and nasal sides, is crucial.

Complications

Acute complications of either unilateral or bilateral cleft lip repair are fortunately rare and can be avoided by using good technique. Early complications include bleeding and infection, which reportedly occur in 1% to 2% of cases. Wound disruption following cleft repair ranges from 1% to 7% and is usually limited to cases of bilateral cleft lip. If the patient is seen soon after a traumatic disruption, surgical reclosure is indicated. More commonly, the cause of the disruption is doubtful or related to improper technique (ie, failure to release tension in the wide complete clefts). For these cases, a conservative course of management is indicated, using topical antibiotics followed by delayed surgical reclosure.

Nasal airway obstruction can result from surgical rearrangement of tissue that narrows one or both nostrils and from immediate postoperative edema. This complication is noted particularly in repair of bilateral clefts. Generally, the infant adapts quickly to a change from nasal breathing to mouth breathing without incident, but occasionally gentle insertion of a short nasal cannula can ameliorate respiratory distress.

Late deformities include deformities of the lip (including vermilion irregularities, muscle deformity, objectionable external scars) and of the nose. Treatments vary, require the surgeon to have command of a large repertoire of techniques, and are beyond the scope of this chapter.

REPAIR OF THE CLEFT PALATE

Normal Anatomy

The hard palate is static and serves as a wall between the oral and nasal chambers. It is covered by mucoperiosteum, and there is a clear delineation between the mucosa of the hard palate and the mucosa of the alveolar process.

The soft palate is mobile and functions as a valve to dynamically separate the nose from the mouth for swallowing and speaking. Soft palate function is required to produce English vowels and consonants, except for ''m'',''n'', and the combination ''ng''. The soft palate must be capable of rapid and very responsive action. Its function depends on the levator veli palatini muscles arising on each side of the base of the skull from the apex of the petrous portion of the temporal bone. These muscles elevate the soft palate and draw it posteriorly, and they are responsible for medial movement of the lateral pharyngeal wall. The superior constrictor muscle of the pharynx and the uvular muscle may assist in velopharyngeal closure by increasing the bulk of the nasal surface of the soft palate as it contracts in the posterior direction.

Abnormal Anatomy

Clinically, most palatal clefts that accompany clefts of the lip tend to appear long and relatively narrow, whereas isolated clefts of the secondary palate are frequently U-shaped or broadly V-shaped. A complete cleft of the secondary palate extends ventrally to the incisive foramen.

The timing of operative repair of the palate is a subject of controversy. It is generally accepted that palatal repair should be accomplished before meaningful speech develops and, in all instances, before age 18 months to optimize the speech results. For our patients at St. Louis Children's Hospital, palatoplasty is performed at 12 and 14 months of age.

The outstanding problem in the speech of children with cleft palate is hypernasality or escape of sound into the nasal cavity. Maladaptive articulatory patterns can make speech completely unintelligible. Speech therapy is usually indicated for children with cleft lip and palate, generally between ages 4 and 10 years.

Primary Palatoplasty

Closure of the hard palate by elevating mucoperiosteal flaps was first described in the mid-19th century. During the 20th century, efforts have been directed toward making the palate as long as possible. The primary reason for repairing a cleft palate is to provide a mechanism for normal speech. This goal must be weighed against the repair's effect on facial growth, specifically maxillary growth. Statistically significant data concerning these issues are not available in the literature.

Additional problems affecting patients with cleft palate include hearing loss, presence of articulation errors, delayed intellectual development, and cultural and educational deprivation. These factors must be considered in the total patient assessment which is readily accomplished by a multidisciplinary team.

There are three distinct approaches for handling the mucoperiosteum in cleft palate repair. They include bipedicle mucoperiosteal flaps, bilateral peninsular flaps with skeletonization of the greater palatine neurovascular bundles to optimize tissue mobilization, and a double-opposing Z-plasty repair, which does not include lateral relaxing incisions, but rather depends on the medial mobilization of the mucoperiosteum.

Complications

Delayed complications of palatoplasty include fistulas and mid-facial growth disturbances. A palatal fistula may occur anywhere along the site of the original cleft. A fistula may represent a failure of technique or a problem in wound healing, which in turn usually is the result of excessive tension on the suture line. The reported incidence of fistulization varies widely, ranging from 0% to 34% of all patients with repaired clefts. A palatal fistula may result in symptoms of audible nasal air escape during speech and the perception of hypernasality.

There is controversy concerning accurate identification of a symptomatic fistula, the extent of the effects on speech, and decisions regarding surgical management. Most speech pathologists agree, however, that a symptomatic fistula may cause a deterioration in speech quality and intelligibility, and it can lead to significant communication impairment. Surgical repair of palatal fistulas can be technically difficult in many cases, because of a paucity of virgin local tissue for closure or excessive scarring. Therefore, in clinical practice, many surgeons repair only fistulas they believe are likely to be most symptomatic.

The relationship between palatal fistulas and hypernasality, nasal air emission, and diminished oral pressure should be studied in each patient. In many cases, it is wise to repair a symptomatic palatal fistula before further evaluating and managing velopharyngeal (VP) function. Admittedly, this approach may require a patient to undergo two separate operations: one to repair the palatal fistula and the other to manage the velopharynx. This management algorithm is rational, however, since some patients show complete elimination of VP symptoms following fistula repair alone.

Analysis of Results

Prospective comparative studies of palatoplasty techniques are lacking in the literature. Success in achieving VP closure following primary palatoplasty varies considerably and symptoms of persistent VP dysfunction (VPD) range from 5% to 38%. This variability in occurrence most likely is due to differences in definitions and opinions regarding what constitutes VPD. Randomized controlled studies with combined evaluation methods, in which speech and VP function are judged by independent raters with known intrarater and interrater reliability, are needed to evaluate the efficacy of specific interventions.

SECONDARY SURGERY FOR CLEFT PALATE CASES: VELOPHARYNGEAL DYSFUNCTION

The main objective of primary palatoplasty is to achieve adequate VP function and normal oral–nasal resonance. It is well-known that a sizable proportion of children who undergo cleft palate repair develop speech production disorders. Traditionally, surgeons have focussed on the symptom of hypernasality and have attributed it to inadequate palatal length. Accordingly, operations have been devised to address these structural deficits. These procedures attempt to lengthen the palate (eg, V–Y pushback, double-opposing Z-plasty) or to reduce the static opening between the nasal and oral pharynges (eg, pharyngeal flap, sphincter pharyngoplasty). Additionally, posterior pharyngeal wall augmentation is designed to obturate the VP in situations in which the VP gap is minimal or when VPD occurs in the presence of "touch closure."

Historically, surgeons have believed that abnormalities in static palatal anatomy were responsible etiologically for postpalatoplasty speech disorders. As a result, earlier attention was concentrated on maximizing palatal length or minimizing fistulization; however, there was little or no understanding that the VP mechanism is a complex sphincter, one that requires more than anatomic integrity for its dynamic, temporally sensitive function.

The relation between perceptual, anatomic, and physiologic variables has not been appreciated until relatively recently. Thus, to believe that hypernasality generally is the result of inadequate anatomy alone represents a simplistic view of VP function. Instrumental assessment modalities have shown that palatal length is not the only variable necessary for achieving normal closure of the VP port. It is possible to have a long but immobile velum which cannot effect closure. It is also possible to have a short velum with normal resonance due to active function of the lateral and posterior pharyngeal walls. Conversely, the capacity for adequate VP function does not guarantee normal resonance.

The advent of increasingly sophisticated means of assessing the VP mechanism has enabled the identification of discrete pathologic entities. Direct visualization such as nasoendoscopy and multiview videofluoroscopy of the velum and lateral and posterior pharyngeal walls, coupled with other instrumental assessment techniques, have allowed correlation of anatomic, physiologic, and perceptual information.[4]

Pharyngeal Flap

The pharyngeal flap has been the most popular method for secondary management of VPD over the past three decades. With this procedure, tissue from the posterior pharyngeal wall is attached to the soft palate, creating a midline obstruction of the oral and nasal cavities with two patent small lateral openings or ports, which ideally remain patent during respiration and nasal speech production and stay closed for oral consonant phonemes.

Sphincter Pharyngoplasty

Sphincter pharyngoplasty (SP) is an alternative therapy designed to tighten the central orifice and occlude the lateral ports.

The SP described by Jackson is the most commonly used today. The SP is constructed from the posterior tonsillar pillars, which are elevated to include the palatopharyngeal muscles at the top of the tonsillar fossa and are sutured end-to-end.

This technique allows for dynamic sphincter closure as the result of retained neuromuscular innervation. Putative advantages of SP include technical ease of execution, superior speech results, few complications, reduced anesthesia time, low financial cost, nonobstruction of the nasal airway, and no violation of the velum. Most reports promoting SP have not been subjected to critical analysis, however.[5]

Palatal Lengthening

Palatal lengthening has been used to eliminate small VP gaps. This concept has significant theoretical appeal for secondary palatal management as it attempts to lengthen the palate without violating the remainder of the dynamic function of the VP mechanism and would appear to be more physiologically normal than the pharyngeal flap or various sphincter pharyngoplasties. Historically, the V–Y pushback procedure was designed to create a retrodisplacement of the palatal mucoperiosteum and velar musculature. The primary goal is to lengthen the palate during initial palatoplasty and thereby lower the recurrence of postoperative VPD.

Wound healing, postoperative contraction, and scarring have made it impossible to predict the ultimate length gained with the so-called lengthening maneuver. Since the 1980s, the advent of the double-opposing Z-plasty procedure has become accepted as a means of gaining palatal length and restoring anatomy of the velar musculature. Again, reports concerning the efficacy of the procedure have been documented at primary palatoplasty only; however, this procedure appears to benefit patients with unrepaired submucous cleft palate and with small residual central VP gaps. Its use as a secondary procedure is currently under investigation.

Posterior Wall Augmentation

Surgeons may be reluctant to perform VP surgery for patients with mild symptoms of VPD. The risk–benefit ratio must be thoroughly considered in arriving at treatment recommendations in these cases. For some patients, posterior wall augmentation would have several advantages. The goal is to achieve VP closure without altering the function of the velum or lateral wall. This alternative concept is attractive since it offers less chance of obstructing the airway; it may offer more precise control of the size of augmentation, and it is theoretically reversible.

Many materials have been used for anterior displacement of the posterior pharyngeal wall. These include autogenous pharyngeal tissue, petroleum jelly, paraffin, cartilage, adjacent soft tissue, silastic, fat, Teflon, and proplast.

Prosthetic Management

Prosthetic appliances are used as a nonsurgical intervention for VPD. These include the speech bulb and the palatal lift prosthesis. Prosthetic treatment has been available for many decades. The speech bulb is an acrylic mass which is used for obturating residual VP gaps to achieve closure when there is inadequate tissue to do so. The palatal lift is generally reserved for patients who have adequate tissue but poor control of coordination and timing of VP movements. The speech bulb often is used for the patient with VPD when surgical intervention is contraindicated. It is also appropriate as a trial treatment method for patients with variable VP closure when it is unclear whether surgical management of the velopharynx alone will provide a noticeable or significant improvement in speech quality. In these patients, a trial of prosthetic management may provide the diagnostic information needed to help establish an appropriate management plan.

In another diagnostic capacity, a prosthesis can be used to determine whether dynamic VP activity can be stimulated or improved. Prosthetic management may facilitate motion of the velum, posterior pharyngeal wall, or lateral walls in some patients. A trial of prosthetic management may be appropriate for some patients in whom little or no VP movement is observed. In such instances, surgical intervention would require near or complete obstruction of the nasopharyngeal airway. If improved muscle or structural function can be demonstrated, the information might be useful in altering an existing diagnosis or management plan.

The goal of all secondary surgical management is to treat hypernasality and nasal emission and to create a mechanism that allows appropriate VP function. It is increasingly clear that what is heard does not necessarily correlate with what is seen. The VP sphincter is a highly complex and only partially understood mechanism. While it is not always possible to match a particular surgery to the complexities of this mechanism, it is hoped that ultimately, differential diagnosis will lead to differential management.

CLEFT LIP NASAL DEFORMITY

The achievement of nasal symmetry in patients with cleft lip is still a fascinating challenge, despite a century of increasing understanding of the underlying pathology and sophistication of surgical technique. Valid assessment of operative results requires a study of a large number of patients over time, and a surgeon's lifetime may be barely adequate for evaluating such data. Meaningful conclusions regarding techniques are conspicuously absent from the literature because objective comparative studies are difficult to undertake and data collection may require many years to collect.

Increasing numbers of cleft surgeons are undertaking nasal correction, at least in part, during primary cheiloplasty. This evolution has likely attenuated the severity cleft nasal deformity seen in the not-too-distant past.

Many surgeons now undertake tip rhinoplasty in infancy coincident with normalization of the nostril sill, nasal base, alar–facial junction, and the ventral floor of the nose. Alar cartilages are manipulated only to the extent that they are repositioned after wide undermining, from the piriform rim to the medial crus. Submucosal freeing of the alar cartilage alone without extensive intranasal incisions can produce excellent results and does not intensify the risk of vestibular stenosis. Nasal septal deflection is a consistent finding among patients with complete unilateral and bilateral cleft lip and palate. In such instances, nasal revisional surgery with attention to the septum may be indicated to facilitate breathing or to normalize appearance.

THE ROLES OF ORTHODONTICS, ORTHOGNATHIC SURGERY, AND ALVEOLAR BONE GRAFTING

Orthodontics and Orthognathic Surgery

Surgical expansion and consolidation of the maxillary arch followed by maxillary advancement and subsequent lip and nose soft tissue revisions are necessary in about 10% of combined cleft lip and palate cases. Patients undergoing surgery involving the jaws and dental arches benefit from orthodontic planning and treatment preoperatively and in the postsurgical stabilization phase. This is necessary because there are almost always dental compensations for the jaw variations observed. The positional changes of the teeth may not be stable or desirable if the jaws are realigned surgically. Thus, orthodontic treatment preoperatively for the patient who will undergo osteotomy involves decompensating the dentition, that is, realigning the teeth over each bone to which they are attached. Surgical correction of jaw position would then not only align the jaws, but would also place the teeth in a stable configuration with one jaw properly related to the other. The orthodontist working with the orthognathic surgery candidate must know where the jaws are intended to be pre-positioned before planning any treatment as a part of the total therapy. If the jaws are going to be tipped, impacted, rotated, or reduced in any way, the position of the teeth must be considered. An orthodontist prepares the patient by using models set on a metal articulator.

The school-age child or adolescent with a unilateral complete cleft of the lip and palate tends to develop a mandibular prognathic appearance. This is the result of a combination of mandibular excess and maxillary deficiency. Dental study models of the teeth are necessary so that the relation of the maxillary to mandibular dentition can be accurately assessed in three dimensions. Cephalometric (standardized, life-sized skull x-ray) analysis and prediction tracings provide information for deciding whether a patient can be treated by orthodontics alone or in combination with a surgical orthognathic procedure.

Management of complex dentoskeletal deformities requires team interaction, involving combined orthodontic and orthognathic surgical specialists. The orthodontist and surgeon must coordinate formulation of a treatment plan and cooperate in its implementation. Deciding to delay orthodontic or surgical treatment until growth is stabilized may reflect sound judgment but may not be in the patient's best interest, especially when psychosocial concerns are weighed. Occasionally, skeletal surgery may be indicated before growth is completed if an additional procedure may be necessary should the patient outgrow the correction.

Approximately 12 to 18 months of orthodontics are usually necessary to align the teeth, correct any midline discrepancy, and localize space for prosthetic replacement of teeth. Providing space for surgical osteotomies between both the crown and roots of the adjacent teeth is an important part of surgical preparation. The effect of surgery on speech is a consideration for the patient with a cleft. The patients who have borderline VP competency presurgically are at greatest risk of developing incompetency following maxillary advancement.

Another role the orthodontist plays in planning for jaw surgery is in the construction of an acrylic splint that is wired between the teeth during surgery to stabilize the surgically created position of the jaws. Applying a splint ensures there is little guess work in surgery as to the desired position of the jaws and teeth or the proper position of the skeletal and dental midlines. Work done preoperatively in the orthodontic laboratory can provide the surgeon with specific information about the amount of bone to be removed or added and about the direction of movement of the jaws. In this sense, dental study models, facial and intraoral photographs, panoramic radiographs of the teeth, and frontal and lateral cephalometrics can provide useful information.

A general dictum in orthognathic surgery states that any movements of the maxilla greater than 8 mm should probably involve both jaws. It is usually better to accomplish some movement of the maxilla and some in the opposite direction of the mandible rather than to risk vascular and other problems, such as relapse inherent in attempting to move a cleft maxilla further than 8 mm.

Orthodontic treatment may be necessary before definitive alveolar bone grafting for several reasons. First, if there is a posterior crossbite, orthodontic expansion of the segments preoperatively improves the occlusion but may widen an existing fistula. In most cases, the larger fistula is favorable because it provides better access with respect to surgical visualization and manipulation. Simultaneous closure of the palatal and vestibular fistulas is performed when the bone graft is placed. Retention of the corrected crossbite with an orthodontic appliance postsurgically is indicated because the bone graft alone does not maintain the expansion.

Second, alignment of the teeth adjacent to the cleft is limited by the available bone into which the roots of the teeth can be moved. Early movement of the roots into the grafted bone appears to consolidate the alveolar bone and improve the crest height.

Third, eruption of the maxillary canine usually occurs through the grafted bone following surgery. With orthodontic movement, enough space is opened to create an unobstructed path for eruption of the cuspid. Often, the canine erupts rapidly once bone is available. If the lateral incisors are malformed or absent, especially in patients with bilateral clefts, the canine is manipulated to erupt adjacent to the central incisors. This situation is advantageous in closing space and avoiding prosthetic replacement of the absent lateral incisor.

Alveolar Bone Grafting

There are several reasons for alveolar bone grafting. The provision of bone support for unerupted teeth and the teeth adjacent to the cleft may be the most important reason. If the bone graft is placed after eruption of the canine, however, the bone does not improve the crestal height of support and quickly resorbs to its original level.

The second benefit of alveolar bone grafts is the closure of oral–nasal fistulas. By using the three-layer closure technique with the graft sandwiched between the two soft tissue planes, the success rate of fistula closure is routinely high.

A third benefit is the support and elevation of the alar base on the cleft side. This helps to improve nasal tip and lip symmetry and provides a stable platform to support the nasal structures. The alveolar bone grafts aid in construction of a continuous arch form and alveolar ridge. This can help the prosthodontist by enabling a more aesthetic and hygienic prosthesis to be placed when and if teeth are missing. Finally, bone grafts help to stabilize the premaxilla in the bilateral cleft patient.

FUTURE PERSPECTIVES

Recently, a class of regulatory genes that influence several of the growth-related cell behaviors has been characterized. They are known as *homeobox genes* and may prove to be key elements in controlling developmental abnormalities, cancers, and perhaps even regenerating the mature vertebrate animal including humans. Homeobox genes are so-named because they all contain a similar segment of bases called the homeobox, the rest of the gene varies in composition. These genes encode a class of regulatory peptides which specifically bind DNA and then induce transcription of genes downstream from the binding site. The DNA-binding sequence of the homeobox protein is known as the *homeodomain* and is highly conserved across the phylogenetic spectrum.

In terms of their distribution, many homeobox genes are found in several tissues during development, but may be more important in regional gradients specifying vertebrate pattern formation, such as craniofacial or limb development. They are found in embryogenesis, but are also expressed in the adult animal, perhaps inappropriately during human carcinogenesis. Additionally, they are expressed at higher levels, such as in the salamander limb amputation blastema.

Homeobox genes regulate growth-related behaviors and have been isolated and characterized with respect to chromosomal location, localization of gene transcripts, and mRNA products. These genes have been induced and their products blocked, resulting in morphogenetically visible changes. They may prove to be extremely important modulators, whose dysfunction may ultimately explain the cellular behavior response for facial clefting processes.

There is mounting interest in the possibility of treating cleft lip in utero. Intrauterine fetal surgery may emerge as the next frontier in the advancement of cleft lip and palate surgery. The principal advantage of intrauterine repair is the absence of typical adult scar formation observed during specific phases of fetal wound healing. Although factors responsible for scarless fetal wound healing have yet to be determined precisely, a variety of features unique to the fetal environment may be influential. Possible factors include reduced oxygen tension in fetal tissues, composition of the dermal extracellular matrix (ie, hyaluronic acid), growth factors in the amniotic fluid, and inhibited immune response.

The feasibility of intrauterine cleft lip repair has already been explored in animal models including mice, rabbits, sheep, and monkeys. All of these models have demonstrated excellent wound healing characteristics involving skin, muscle, and bone, in a fashion reminiscent of the process of regeneration. Experience with fetal surgery in human populations, however, is limited and has been restricted to a narrowly defined group of life-threatening problems such as diaphragmatic hernia. Many issues remain unresolved, such as the optimal gestational age for which fetal interventions are efficacious and safe. Additionally, much speculation exists concerning the real benefits of fetal surgery when compared with the risks to mother and child for non–life-threatening malformations. These risks include premature labor, spontaneous abortion, and maternal infectious complications.

Although the prospects for fetal cleft lip and palate repair are promising, extensive research comparing the risks and benefits must be undertaken before its widespread implementation. Confounding the scenario is the issue regarding the fetus as a person with rights, which raises enormous ethical questions. History has taught us repeatedly about the havoc wrought by rapidly burgeoning technology that outstrips the emergence of an appropriate philosophic base to accompany those changes. In this sense, it must be remembered that every good idea has as many disadvantages as advantages.

We are on the verge of major changes in the treatment of congenital craniofacial deformities. The increasing use of microsurgery, minimal invasive surgery laboratories, application of molecular biology, and possibly intrauterine fetal surgery will play important roles in our understanding of the pathogenesis and treatment of cleft lip and cleft palate deformities.

REFERENCES

1. Ferguson MWJ. Palate development. Development 1988;103 (suppl): 41.
2. Falconer DS. The inheritance of liability to certain diseases estimated from incidence among relatives. Ann Hum Genet 1965;29:51.
3. Witt PD, Hardesty RA. Rotation-advancement repair of the unilateral cleft lip: one center's perspective. Clin Plast Surg 1993; 20:633.
4. Witt PD, D'Antonio LL. Velopharyngeal insufficiency and secondary palatal management: a new look at an old problem. Clin Plast Surg 1993; 20:707.
5. Witt PD, D'Antonio LL, Zimmerman GJ, et al. Sphincter pharyngoplasty: a preoperative and postoperative analysis of perceptual speech characteristics and endoscopic studies of velopharyngeal function. Plast Reconstr Surg 1994;93:1154.

Surgery of Infants and Children: Scientific Principles and Practice, edited by
Keith T. Oldham, Paul M. Colombani, and Robert P. Foglia.
Lippincott–Raven Publishers, Philadelphia, © 1997.

CHAPTER 50

Otolaryngologic Disorders

David E. Tunkel and Bevan Yueh

Pediatric otolaryngology encompasses the diagnosis and treatment of childhood head and neck disease. This expanding discipline includes the management of acquired and congenital cervicofacial masses, inflammatory and neoplastic diseases of the upper aerodigestive tract (including pharynx, nose, sinuses, larynx), and otologic disease.

The broad scope of pediatric otolaryngology cannot be covered in a single chapter. Recent advances in the management of laryngotracheal disorders and inflammatory sinus disease are described comprehensively, and several other topics within pediatric otolaryngology are briefly discussed.

PEDIATRIC LARYNGOTRACHEAL DISORDERS

Pediatric upper airway disease can be congenital or acquired. Prominent symptoms include impaired ventilation, stridor, and voice abnormalities. The following section details an approach to evaluating the young child with stridor.

The Evaluation of Stridor

The infant with stridor requires a systematic evaluation dictated by the severity of airway compromise. When airway obstruction is severe or rapidly progressive, the evaluation often consists of immediate endoscopy in the operating suite with stabilization of the airway. Subacute or chronic stridor without airway compromise can be evaluated with an orderly history and physical examination, airway endoscopy, and radiographic studies.[1]

The etiology of stridor can be suggested by history, and attention is placed on the time of onset, the duration of stridor, and any aggravating or alleviating factors. Stridor that starts at or near the time of birth suggests the presence of a congenital laryngotracheal anomaly such as laryngomalacia, vocal cord paralysis, congenital subglottic stenosis, or a compressive vascular ring. A history of endotracheal intubation is associated with acquired subglottic stenosis. The details of intubation, such as tube size, duration of intubation, and the reasons for intubation should be documented. Hoarseness or absent cry are symptoms of glottic lesions, such as vocal cord paralysis, laryngeal

papillomatosis, or a glottic web. Low- pitched barky cough associated with stridor suggests a subglottic lesion, such as subglottic stenosis, edema, or hemangioma.

When stridor occurs suddenly in a previously asymptomatic child, foreign body aspiration must be considered. A negative history does not rule out this possibility. Acute inflammatory laryngotracheal disease such as viral laryngotracheobronchitis (croup) or bacterial epiglottitis also should be considered.

Examination of the child with stridor involves a full head and neck evaluation, looking for head and neck masses and stigmata of craniofacial syndromes. Stridor should be defined in regard to the portion of the respiratory cycle involved with noisy breathing. Inspiratory stridor usually suggests obstruction above the level of the glottis, either in the supraglottic larynx or pharynx. Biphasic stridor (both inspiratory and expiratory) occurs with glottic or subglottic lesions. Expiratory stridor accompanies airway obstruction in the intrathoracic tracheobronchial tree. Changes in stridor with positioning, agitation, or feeding may suggest the type of airway lesion present. Stridor from laryngomalacia usually worsens in the crying child and improves with prone positioning.

Examination of the larynx can be performed with indirect mirror techniques in cooperative older children, but most young children require fiberoptic laryngoscopy to visualize the dynamic larynx. This technique is performed on awake children with topical anesthesia and allows an assessment of the airway from the nasal vestibule to the glottis. The supraglottic larynx can be seen during all phases of breathing. True vocal cord anatomy and motion is documented.

Soft tissue lateral and anteroposterior neck radiographs are useful in outlining epiglottis size, retropharyngeal profile, and subglottic and tracheal anatomy. Chest radiographs can suggest vascular-ring compression of the trachea and can rule out concomitant pulmonary disease. Mediastinal masses, an uncommon but serious cause of childhood stridor, can be seen on chest radiographs (Fig. 50-1). Inspiratory–expiratory and lateral decubitus chest radiographs can display air trapping that suggests bronchial foreign-body aspiration.

Airway fluoroscopy, usually combined with barium esophagography, can image changes in airway caliber during active respiration. A barium esophagram can be diagnostic for a compressive vascular ring (Fig. 50-2). Gastroesophageal reflux or

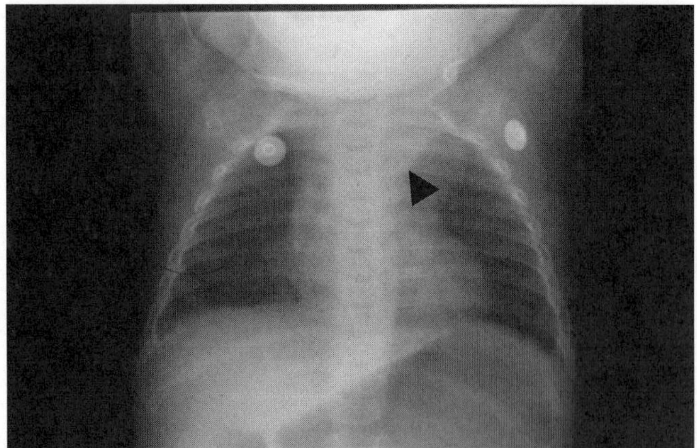

FIG. 50-1. Chest radiograph of a 9-month-old child with stridor for 2 days. Note mediastinal mass with tracheal compression and shift to right (*arrow*). Biopsy was diagnostic for neuroblastoma.

aspiration can also be detected. Computed tomography (CT) and magnetic resonance imaging are used when a neck or chest mass that needs anatomic definition is found.

The most definitive evaluation of static airway anatomy is obtained with direct laryngoscopy and rigid bronchoscopy performed in the operating room under general anesthesia. Rigid telescopes combined with operative laryngoscopes or bronchoscopes provide a magnified assessment of hypopharyngeal, laryngeal, and tracheobronchial anatomy. Direct palpation of laryngeal structures, assessment of airway diameters, biopsy of masses, and even electromyography of laryngeal muscles can be performed intraoperatively. The operating

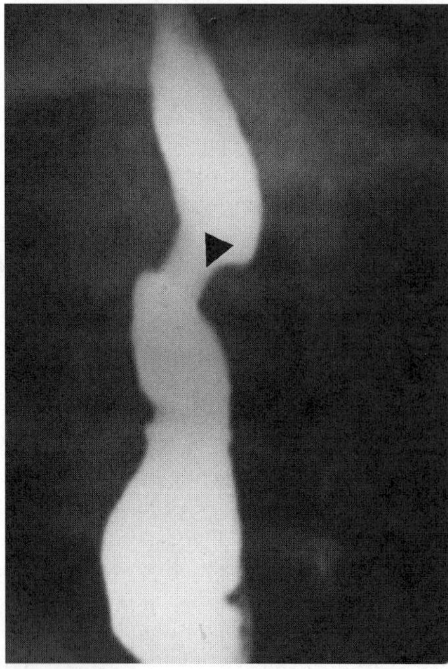

FIG. 50-2. Barium esophagram of a 5-week-old child with stridor, demonstrating indentation of the esophagus (*arrow*) by a vascular ring (double aortic arch).

microscope and suspension laryngoscopes provide a unique magnified assessment of laryngeal structures with stereoscopic vision (Fig. 50-3).

Some laryngeal lesions can be treated endoscopically at the time of assessment using general anesthesia. They include draining laryngeal cysts or removing laryngeal masses such as papilloma. The carbon dioxide (CO_2) laser or conventional microlaryngeal surgical techniques are used in these cases. Table 50-1 outlines the usefulness of several radiographic and endoscopic tests for diagnosing the most common pediatric laryngeal disorders. Operative direct laryngoscopy and bronchoscopy is the gold standard for diagnosing fixed laryngotracheal lesions, whereas flexible awake fiberoptic laryngoscopy is more useful for dynamic processes.

Differential Diagnosis of Stridor in Infants

Laryngomalacia is the most common congenital laryngeal anomaly, comprising about 60% of all laryngeal problems in neonates. Coarse, high-pitched, inspiratory stridor is caused by supraglottic obstruction from flaccid laryngeal structures. Inward prolapse of the aryepiglottic folds and arytenoids with curling of the epiglottis is seen on awake fiberoptic laryngoscopy. Additional sites of airway pathology have been found in up to 20% of infants with laryngomalacia; hence, a complete airway evaluation is advisable even after this diagnosis is made. Laryngomalacia usually resolves spontaneously by age 2 years. In some children, feeding problems, cyanosis, apnea, or failure to thrive from this condition may warrant surgical intervention.

Vocal cord paralysis is the second most common cause of neonatal stridor. Vocal cord motion abnormalities can be either unilateral or bilateral. Bilateral paralysis is the most common cause of severe upper airway obstruction at birth. Vocal cord paralysis can be either congenital or acquired, and diagnosis is best made by observing vocal cord motion with the flexible laryngoscope in awake, spontaneously breathing children. Stridor from vocal cord paralysis is usually inspiratory or biphasic, and in unilateral paralysis, it can be accompanied by a weak, breathy cry. The inability of vocal cords to abduct leads to airway obstruction with stridor. The inability of the vocal cords to completely adduct and close the glottis can cause hoarseness and aspiration. Congenital unilateral vocal cord paralysis can be associated with intrathoracic congenital abnormalities, whereas bilateral vocal cord paralysis can be associated with central nervous system abnormalities (ie, Arnold-Chiari malformation). Acquired vocal cord paralysis can occur following traumatic injury to the larynx and following surgical procedures to the chest or neck where the laryngeal nerve is injured.

Unilateral vocal cord paralysis is usually well compensated for in children, and only conservative feeding intervention and airway monitoring are necessary. Occasionally, the unilateral paralysis significantly impairs the airway in young infants, and tracheotomy may be necessary to stabilize respiratory function. Bilateral vocal cord paralysis in infants usually causes severe respiratory compromise, and tracheotomy is necessary until vocal cord motion returns spontaneously or until a surgical procedure is performed to improve the glottic airway.

Subglottic stenosis is a congenital or acquired narrowing of the subglottic airway. Biphasic stridor and barky cough, often with apparent crouplike illnesses, is a common presenta-

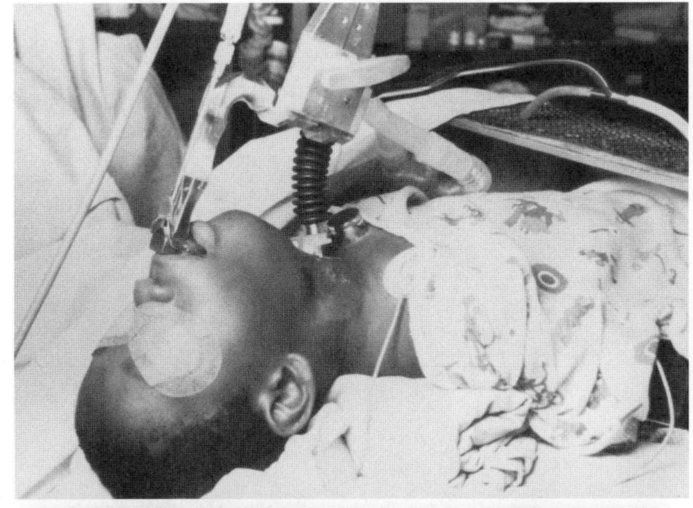

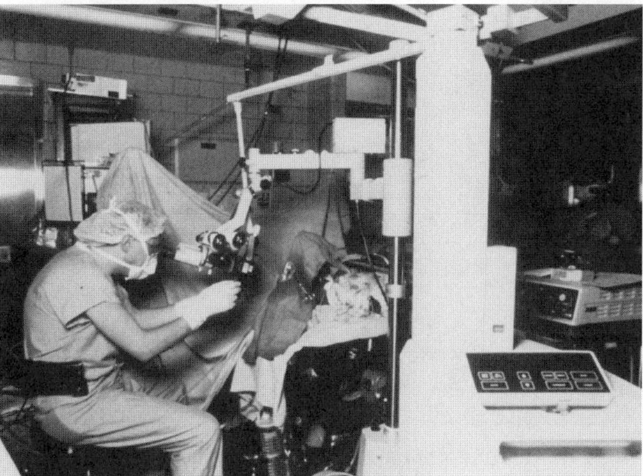

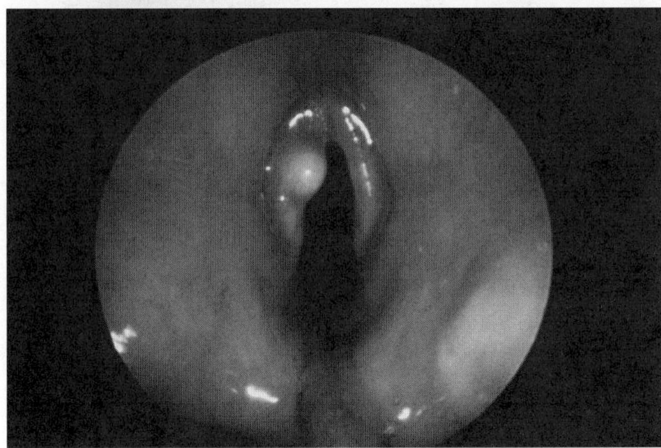

FIG. 50-3. The use of suspension microlaryngoscopy equipment. (*A*) Operative laryngoscope and suspension bar. (*B*) Operating microscope with CO_2 laser allows magnification, depth perception, and precise endolaryngeal surgery. (*C*) A laryngeal examination with suspension laryngoscope. The benign left vocal cord cyst caused hoarseness in this 12-year-old boy.

tion. In the neonatal intensive care unit, subglottic stenosis usually presents as extubation failure. Congenital subglottic stenosis is characterized by abnormal shape and size of the cricoid cartilage and the associated soft tissues. Acquired subglottic stenosis, with subglottic scarring secondary to la-

ryngeal injury from endotracheal intubation, is more common and usually more severe.

The diagnosis of subglottic stenosis is suggested by neck radiographs and confirmed by direct laryngoscopy and bronchoscopy in the operating room (Fig. 50-4). Severe cases require

TABLE 50-1. *Usefulness of various diagnostic tests for children with stridor*

Disorder	Neck/airway films	Airway fluoroscopy	Barium esophagram	Fiberoptic laryngoscopy	Operative laryngoscopy/ bronchoscopy
Laryngomalacia	−	−	−	**	+
Tracheomalacia	−	+	−	−	**
Vocal cord paralysis	−	−	−	**	+
Subglottic stenosis	+	+	−	−	**
Vascular ring	−	+	+	−	**
Laryngeal web	−	−	−	**	**
Laryngeal cleft	−	−	+	−	**
Subglottic hemangioma	+	+	−	−	**
Epiglottitis	**	X	X	X	**
Laryngotracheo-bronchitis	**	**	−	−	**
Papilloma	−	−	−	**	**

− Usually not diagnostic
+ Often suggests diagnosis
** Diagnostic procedure of choice
X Dangerous/not recommended

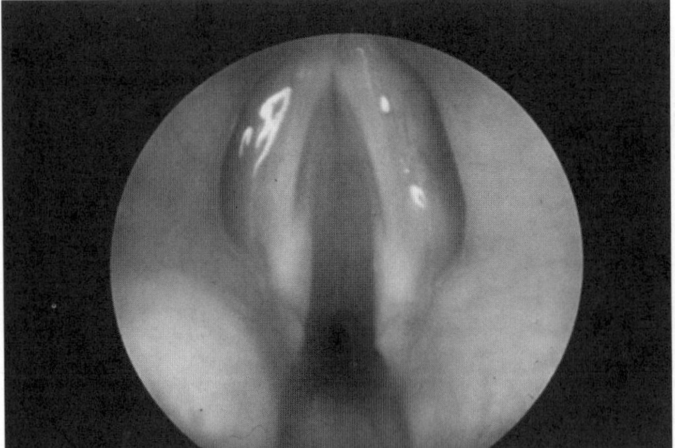

FIG. 50-4. Circumferential subglottic stenosis in a 15-month-old child. The infant required tracheotomy during the first week of life for this severe congenital lesion.

tracheotomy and subsequent laryngotracheal reconstruction. Moderate airway obstruction from subglottic stenosis can be relieved by endoscopic methods or anterior cricoid split. Mild cases can be observed with hope of further laryngeal growth and resolution of symptoms.

Subglottic hemangioma is an uncommon benign lesion that causes biphasic stridor, usually presenting within the first 3 to 6 months of life. Cutaneous hemangiomas are found in half of these infants. A submucosal mass is seen in the subglottis at direct laryngoscopy. Tracheotomy is performed for severe airway compromise. Intralesional and systemic steroids and endoscopic laser excision can play a role in management. These lesions usually regress during the second year of life. Recent literature has suggested the use of interferon to enhance hemangioma regression.[1a]

Recurrent respiratory papillomatosis (RRP) is the most common pediatric laryngeal tumor. Papillomas are typically confined to the larynx, but in severe cases they can extend throughout the tracheobronchial tree and pharynx (Fig. 50-5). Hoarseness and stridor are common symptoms, and presentation almost always occurs before age 3 years. A maternal history of genital papilloma exists for 60% of patients with RRP. Diagnosis is made by laryngoscopy (Fig. 50-6). Laryngoscopic removal of papilloma, usually by CO_2 laser vaporization, is necessary to prevent severe airway compromise. Repeated surgery is the rule, and periods of rapid papilloma growth are intermittent and unpredictable. Tracheotomy should be avoided, as it has been associated with tracheobronchial dissemination of papilloma in RRP patients.

SURGICAL TREATMENT OF CHILDHOOD LARYNGOTRACHEAL DISORDERS

Laryngomalacia

Most children with laryngomalacia require no treatment, but some children experience episodic cyanosis or apnea, feeding difficulties, or failure to thrive. Although tracheotomy has been performed for airway obstruction due to laryngomalacia, epig-

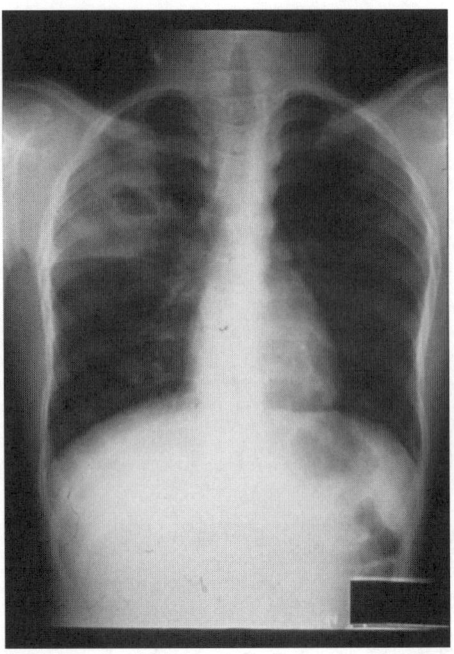

FIG. 50-5. Chest radiograph of a 13-year-old child with papillomatosis involving pulmonary parenchyma.

lottoplasty techniques developed in the past decade can improve respiratory function without tracheotomy.[2] Operative endoscopy is performed, and redundant supraglottic soft tissues in the region of the aryepiglottic folds are trimmed using microlaryngeal scissors or the CO_2 laser. These patients have less stridor, improved feeding, and less obstruction according to postoperative sleep studies.[2a–c]

Vocal Cord Paralysis

Infants with bilateral vocal cord paralysis usually require tracheotomy for airway stabilization. If spontaneous movement does not return after 12 months, surgery to improve the glottic

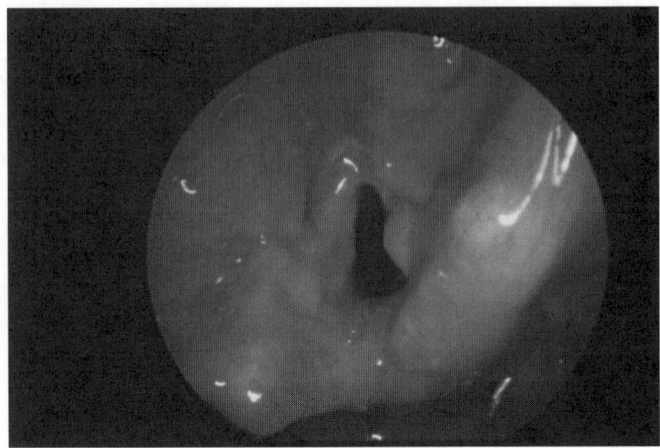

FIG. 50-6. Direct laryngoscopy of a papilloma of the larynx with prominent supraglottic involvement.

airway is considered. These procedures include: removal of the arytenoid, detachment of the vocal ligament, or lateralization of the vocal cord to increase the airway size between the two immobile vocal cords.[3] These procedures can be done endoscopically (transverse laser cordotomy, laser arytenoidectomy) or through open laryngofissure or lateral pharyngotomy approaches (arytenoidectomy, lateralization).

Unilateral vocal cord paralysis rarely requires surgical intervention in children because compensation for glottic closure deficit occurs even when the affected cord does not regain innervation. In older children who have troublesome aspiration or hoarseness after acquired unilateral vocal cord paralysis (post-CNS injury, post cardiothoracic surgery), however, procedures are performed to medialize the immobile vocal cord to allow complete glottic closure during phonation and swallowing. This can be accomplished by endoscopic injection of Gelfoam (Upjohn, Kalamazoo, MI), fat, or Teflon into the paraglottic space as well as by external placement of implants into the space between the thyroid cartilage and its inner perichondrium.

Surgery for Subglottic Stenosis

Corrective surgical procedures for subglottic stenosis have been refined to allow successful decannulation of many children with tracheotomy. These techniques avoid the need for tracheotomy altogether in some children.

Endoscopic methods of enlarging the narrowed subglottis have involved dilatation, serial laser excisions, and most recently, the microsurgical creation of mucosal flaps combined with scar excision. These methods have been most useful in treating adults with subglottic stenosis. Children usually have extensive lesions with mature scar and long lengths of stenosis, and open laryngotracheal reconstruction is the mainstay of their surgical treatment.[4]

The anterior cricoid split was developed by Cotton and Seid in 1980 to avoid tracheotomy in neonates with acquired subglottic stenosis who had failed extubation. This procedure (Fig. 50-7) involves incising the lower portion of the anterior thyroid cartilage, the anterior cricoid cartilage, and the upper two to three tracheal rings to allow anterior laryngeal expansion.[5] Stenting with an upsized endotracheal tube is performed for 5 to 14 days. This procedure should not be performed on patients with severe pulmonary disease or severe subglottic stenosis, but when used in appropriate cases, tracheotomy can be avoided in more than 70% of these infants. Anterior cricoid split has also been used for infants with recurrent crouplike illnesses from mild subglottic stenosis. Since the early 1990s, auricular and costal cartilage grafts have been used to augment the laryngeal expansion achieved with the anterior cricoid split.

Laryngotracheal reconstruction (LTR) for severe subglottic stenosis has several underlying principles: the cricoid cartilage is split to allow expansion; laryngeal skeletal support is preserved or restored with cartilage grafts; scars are not excised; and raw areas are allowed to resurface with muscosa. Costal cartilage is the most versatile graft material for laryngeal expansion. The outer perichondrium is left attached to the cartilage to be used intraluminally to reduce granulation. The grafts are carved with flanges or bevels to prevent prolapse into the lumen (Fig. 50-8). Grafts are secured with absorbable sutures. Various stents, most commonly Teflon, have been used for LTR.[6] When peristomal airway narrowing is present, a tracheotomy tube can be wired to a long Teflon stent to provide fixed support into the upper thoracic trachea.

LTR procedures are tailored to the subglottic anatomy, which is determined by endoscopic examination. The larynx can be split anteriorly and posteriorly, and cartilage grafts can be placed in one or both of these locations to expand to the stenotic sites. For severe stenosis, lateral cricoid splits without grafts may allow additional expansion of the subglottic diameter. These advances have allowed 85% to 90% success in decannulation of children with tracheotomy for severe subglottic stenosis.[4]

Single-stage LTR allows for decannulation at the time of laryngeal reconstruction and avoids the need for tracheotomy to treat subglottic stenosis in symptomatic young children. In

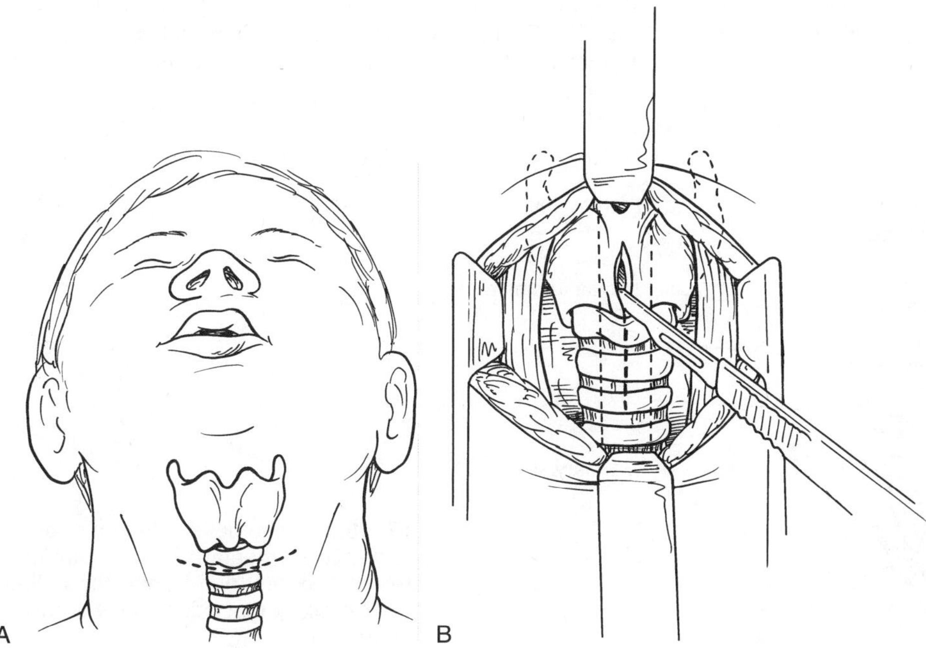

FIG. 50-7. Anterior cricoid split involves dividing the lower thyroid cartilage, the cricoid ring, and the upper two tracheal rings in the anterior midline and then stenting with an endotracheal tube.

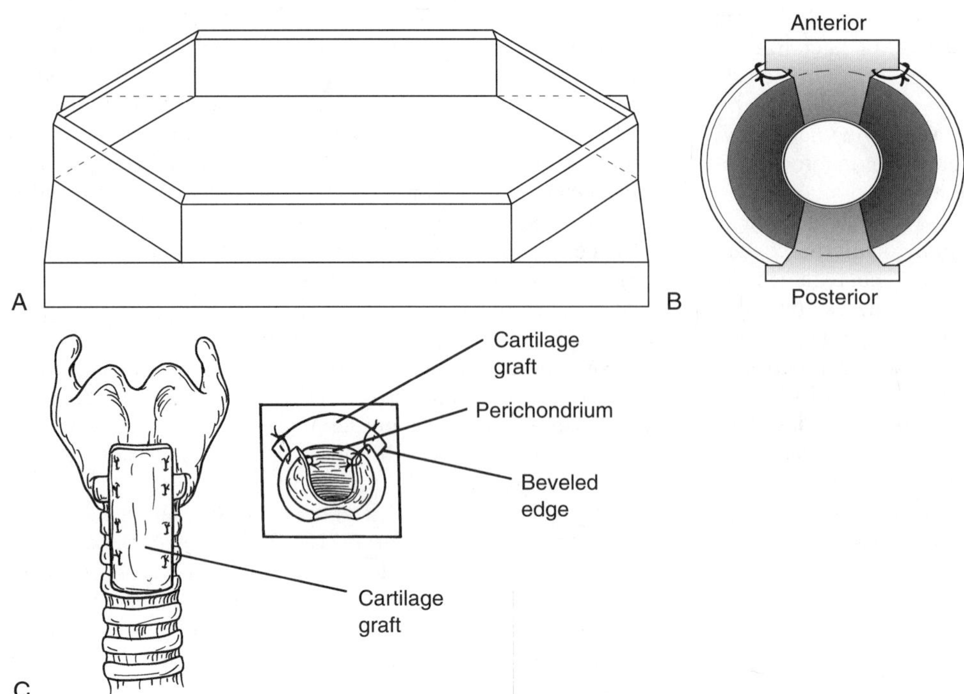

FIG. 50-8. A costal cartilage graft is carved with beveled sides and flanges to avoid intraluminal collapse. This schematic of a cross section of subglottis shows the flanged anterior and posterior grafts in place.

this procedure, children with mild or moderate (usually anterior) subglottic stenosis have costal grafts sewn into the anterior larynx over an age-appropriate endotracheal tube.[7,8] The endotracheal tube serves as a short-term stent, and extubation is attempted when airway edema has receded several days after surgery.

Partial cricoid resection with thyrotracheal anastomosis has been recently described as a method to excise high-grade subglottic stenosis of short length.[9] This procedure involves isolation of the recurrent laryngeal nerves, resection of the cricoid and intrinsic subglottic scar, and primary closure of the upper trachea to the lower thyroid cartilage. This technique is not widely used, probably because of the technical challenge of nerve preservation in infants.

NOSE AND SINUSES

Chronic Sinusitis in Children

The use of CT scans and rigid endoscopes have been the center of recent advances in diagnosing and treating inflammatory paranasal sinus disease. These methods help to determine the anatomic and physiologic factors involved in impairment of paranasal sinus drainage in children. Sinusitis primarily develops in the anterior ethmoid–middle meatal area. Mucosal inflammation at this site impairs clearance of secretions from the maxillary sinus and frontal sinuses. This ''ostiomeatal complex'' is the focus of surgery in children with sinusitis that is refractory to conventional medical therapy (Fig. 50-9).[10]

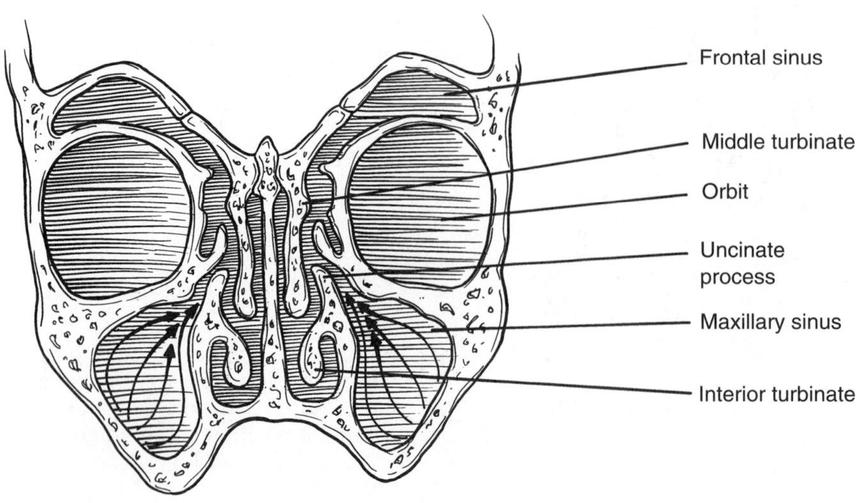

FIG. 50-9. Schematic of the anterior ethmoid–middle meatal ("ostiomeatal unit") area of maxillary and frontal sinus drainage. Maxillary mucociliary flow is toward this area.

The medical management of chronic sinusitis in children consists of long courses of antibiotics, topical nasal steroid sprays, nasal irrigations, and decongestants and antihistamines. The efficacy of these regimens for pediatric chronic sinusitis has not been well documented. With the advent of CT scan and endoscopic examination to document the presence of inflammatory mucosal disease and bony sinus abnormalities, a subset of children with refractory sinusitis are being identified as surgical candidates. Functional endoscopic sinus surgery (FESS) has been used to enhance sinus drainage and to allow secondary resolution of mucosal disease within the ethmoid, maxillary, frontal, and sphenoid sinuses.

Various systemic and local anatomic factors can predispose to ostiomeatal obstruction and sinusitis in children. Allergic factors, humoral immune deficiency, and primary ciliary dyskinesia can predispose to ostiomeatal mucosal disease. Anatomic factors associated with sinusitis in children include nasal septal deviation, pneumatization of the middle turbinate (concha bullosa), development of ethmoid cells along the maxillary roof occluding the maxillary ostia (Haller cells), and other bony abnormalities. Children with cystic fibrosis usually have chronic sinonasal inflammation, including nasal obstruction and polyposis, or even maxillary and ethmoid mucocele formation. Sinus surgery aimed at removing nasal polyps, draining obstructed sinuses, and marsupializing mucoceles is often successful in relieving nasal symptoms in these patients.

The diagnostic evaluation for children with refractory chronic sinusitis includes serologic and functional tests of the immune system and delineation of sinus anatomy. In addition to the usual otolaryngologic evaluation, a thorough immunologic and allergy assessment is performed on children being considered for endoscopic sinus surgery. In children with refractory pansinusitis, mucocele formation, or nasal polyposis, sweat chloride testing should be performed to exclude cystic fibrosis. Endoscopic assessment of the intranasal anatomy is performed after thorough vasoconstriction with topical agents, and this is usually done in the office. For young children, this is performed at the time of endoscopic surgery under general anesthesia. Attention is focused on anatomy of the middle meatus and the presence of drainage or mucosal disease in this area. Coronal CT of the paranasal sinuses is performed to assess the extent of sinus mucosal disease and to define the bony sinus anatomy.

FESS has been used to treat refractory pediatric sinusitis in children for since the mid-1980s. The keystone of the successful endoscopic approach is the ability to surgically address the ostiomeatal disease that interferes with mucociliary clearance in other sinuses. FESS involves telescopic-guided dissection of the anterior ethmoid and maxillary ostia to marsupialize part or all of the ethmoid cells and to increase the size of the sinus outflow tracts. The extent of surgical dissection is tailored to the extent of disease evident on preoperative CT scans and intraoperative endoscopic assessment. In children, surgery always involves exenteration of the anterior ethmoid area with enlargement of the natural ostium of the maxillary sinus because anterior ethmoid and maxillary mucosal disease is nearly universal in children with chronic sinusitis.

FESS can be used to treat posterior ethmoid, sphenoid, and frontal inflammatory disease, when necessary, by extending dissection to include these areas. Anatomic bony abnormalities, which predispose to sinusitis in some children, can be treated with endoscopic sinus surgery. FESS has also been useful in treating refractory sinusitis in children, including children with underlying systemic disease such as cystic fibrosis.[11] About 75% of the 31 children undergoing such procedures had marked improvement in symptoms 1 year after surgery according to parent interviews.[12] Surgical control of refractory sinusitis is particularly helpful for children with concomitant pulmonary disease.

Complications of endoscopic sinus surgery are infrequent. FESS in children requires thorough understanding of endoscopic sinus anatomy because of the proximity of the ethmoid complex to the orbit and the anterior skull base. Orbital hematoma, blindness from optic nerve injury, and cerebrospinal fluid leak from dural penetration are rare but morbid complications of paranasal sinus surgery.[13]

The role of ancillary surgical modalities such as adenoidectomy, tonsillectomy, antral lavage, and inferior meatal nasoantral windows in treating pediatric sinusitis is not clear. The results of these traditional techniques for childhood sinusitis have been variable. Children with nasal obstruction and rhinorrhea from adenoidal enlargement or infection can benefit from adenoidectomy. The distinction between diseased adenoids and chronic sinusitis can be difficult in young children.

Antral puncture is useful for culture of maxillary sinus contents. Inferior meatal windows have a theoretical disadvantage since ostiomeatal mucosal disease is not removed, and mucociliary clearance of the maxillary sinuses direct secretions away from these openings and toward the middle meatus.

Complications of Sinusitis

Complications of acute and chronic sinusitis can be local, intraorbital, or intracranial spread of infection from a paranasal sinus source. The incidence of these highly morbid complications can be markedly decreased by prompt diagnosis and treatment with antibiotics and surgery.

Orbital complications of sinusitis are still seen in children. They are usually due to spread of infection from the ethmoid sinuses across the lamina papyracea (the thin medial orbital wall) via congenital dehiscences, retrograde thrombophlebitis, or direct bone erosion from infection. These complications include preseptal cellulitis (inflammation of the eyelids), true intraorbital abscesses, and cavernous sinus thrombosis (Table 50-2). Treatment of orbital extension of sinus infection requires both otolaryngologic and ophthalmologic evaluation to assess

TABLE 50-2. *Complications of sinusitis*

Local	Recurrent infection
	Mucocele/mucopyocele
	Osteomyelitis
Orbital	Preseptal/periorbital cellulitis
	Orbital cellulitis
	Subperiosteal abscess
	Orbital abscess
	Cavernous sinus thrombosis
Intracranial	Meningitis
	Epidural abscess
	Subdural empyema
	Parenchymal brain abscess
	Dural sinus thrombosis

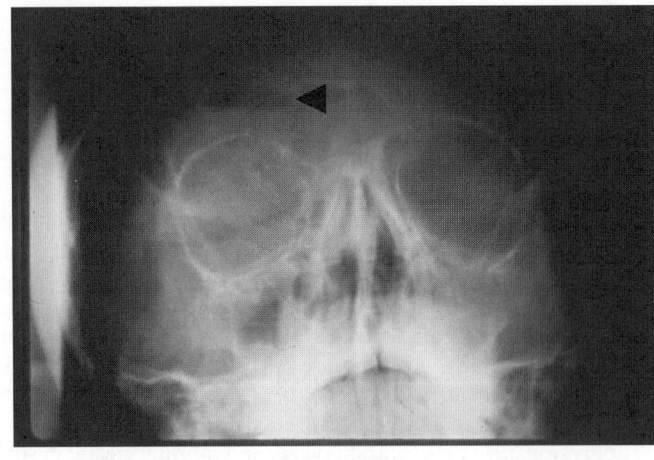
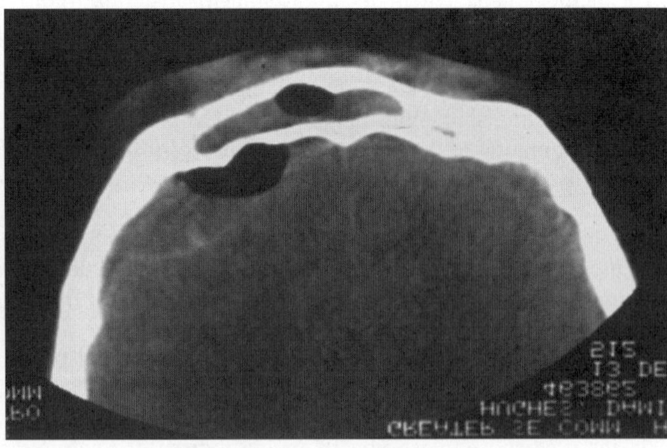

FIG. 50-10. A Caldwell sinus radiograph of a 16-year-old (*A*) with frontal sinusitis (air–fluid level)(*arrow*) and epidural abscess. A CT scan (*B*) confirms air–fluid level in the epidural space (*arrow*).

and preserve vision and ocular motion. Parenteral antibiotics are used to treat cellulitis, and orbital abscesses are drained. External and endoscopic approaches are designed to decompress the orbit, to drain loculated abscesses, to drain infected sinuses, and to remove infected mucosa from the offending sinuses.

Intracranial infections secondary to sinusitis occur from direct infectious extension or hematogenous seeding. Sphenoiditis has been associated with meningitis. Acute infection of the frontal sinus can extend posteriorly through congenital pathways or via valveless veins to cause intracranial infections. Adolescent boys with acute frontal sinusitis are particularly susceptible to intracranial complications (Fig. 50-10). Medical therapy consists of parenteral antibiotics that achieve high cerebrospinal fluid levels directed against the broad spectrum of sinus pathogens. Surgical drainage through combined neurosurgical and otolaryngologic efforts are used to drain subdural and epidural collections. Sinus drainage may be performed at the time of neurosurgical drainage or secondarily in unstable patients.

Choanal Atresia

Choanal atresia is a congenital obstruction between the posterior nasal cavity and the nasopharynx. Unilateral choanal atresia is more common, but bilateral atresia can present as neonatal respiratory distress. About 90% of choanal atresia consists of bony atresia plates, and the remainder are membranous obstructions. Associated congenital anomalies are found in about 50% of infants with choanal atresia, most notably in children with CHARGE association. Initial management of bilateral choanal atresia requires oral airway use to stabilize respiratory function in neonates who are obligate nasal breathers. The inability to pass catheters from the nose to the pharynx suggests the diagnosis of choanal atresia, and this diagnosis is confirmed by direct telescopic examination with rigid and flexible telescopes. The bony and membranous anatomy of the atresia plate is detailed by high resolution axial CT scan of the midface (Fig. 50-11).

Surgical treatment of choanal atresia involves removing the atresia plate while preserving the mucosal flaps.[14] Stents are used for 6 to 12 weeks. Unilateral choanal atresia repair is

performed electively in preschool-age children. Bilateral atresia repair is attempted in infancy, with the understanding that revision choanal enlargement may be necessary later in childhood. Transpalatal approaches to the choana offer the best exposure for removing extensive bony atresia plates, but they may predispose to maxillodental growth abnormalities. Transnasal approaches include microscopic visualization, rigid telescopic visualization, and external rhinoplasty approaches.[15] CO_2 and KTP lasers have been used to vaporize atresia plates.

OTOLOGY

Otitis Media

Otitis media is the most frequent diagnosis made by pediatricians, and placement of tympanostomy tubes is the most commonly performed surgical procedure in the United States. Medical therapy for acute otitis media consists of antibiotics directed

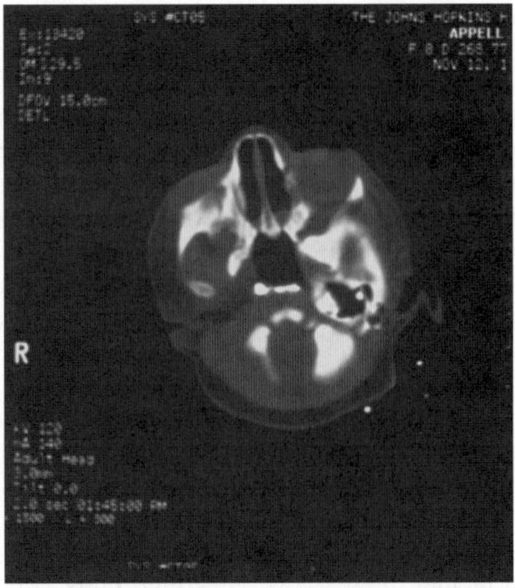

FIG. 50-11. Axial CT scan of a neonate with CHARGE association and bilateral bony choanal atresia (*arrows*).

against the most commonly cultured middle ear pathogens.[16] Indications for surgical therapy of otitis media include recurrent infections refractory to prophylactic antibiotics; persistent middle ear effusions, especially when associated with conductive hearing loss or tympanic membrane structural changes; and development of intratemporal or intracranial suppurative complications of otitis media. Myringotomy, usually with placement of an indwelling tympanostomy tube, allows middle-ear fluid to drain (with opportunity to send cultures) and improves hearing by ventilating the middle-ear space. Recent literature supports the use of adenoidectomy as an adjunctive surgical measure for otitis media with effusion, particularly for children ages 4 to 8 years and for children who have recurrent middle- ear disease after one set of tympanostomy tubes.[17]

Chronic Otitis Media/Cholesteatoma

Chronic suppurative otitis media is a condition marked by long-standing purulent otorrhea, usually through a tympanic membrane perforation or a tympanostomy tube. Gram-negative organisms predominate, and medical therapy consists of aural toilet (suctioning and irrigations), ototopical antibiotics, and intravenous antibiotics. Oral quinolone antibiotics have been used successfully, but these agents are usually avoided in young children because of theoretical concerns about cartilage growth effects.

Cholesteatoma is a collection of keratinizing squamous epithelium within the temporal bone, usually involving the middle ear. Cholesteatoma can be congenital, arising from embryonic rests of squamous epithelium. Acquired cholesteatoma is more common, developing from tympanic membrane retraction pockets or perforations associated with eustachian tube dysfunction or chronic otitis media. Cholesteatoma can cause ossicular erosion, facial palsy, and other intratemporal complications by local expansion (pressure necrosis), secretion of osteolytic enzymes, and by harboring chronic infection. Cholesteatoma requires surgical removal with a variety of tympanomastoid techniques beyond the scope of this chapter. Even with modern microsurgical techniques, recurrence of childhood cholesteatoma is common, and long term follow-up is crucial.

Advances in the treatment of chronic suppurative otitis media/cholesteatoma include middle-ear endoscopy using rigid telescopes to visualize early recurrences of cholesteatoma, facial nerve monitoring devices that allow safer operation within the temporal bone, and high-resolution temporal bone CT scans to precisely display temporal bone anatomy.

Surgery for Hearing Loss

Conductive hearing loss occurs when the middle-ear acoustic transfer mechanism is disrupted by infection, trauma, or other disease processes that affect the continuity and mobility of the ossicular chain. Large tympanic membrane perforations, usually from prior infection or trauma, can be associated with conductive hearing losses. Tympanoplastic techniques using autologous tissue grafts to recreate an intact tympanic membrane can correct this hearing loss.

Ossicular chain discontinuity can result from chronic middle-ear infection or from trauma. The articulation between the incus and the stapes is the most common site of ossicular erosion or disruption, but the chain can be damaged at any point. These conductive hearing losses can be improved by microsurgical ossiculoplasty, using repositioned autologous ossicles, homograft ossicles, or prosthetic materials. The ossicular prostheses used most frequently today are constructed of hydroxylapatite, allowing restoration of ossicular continuity with improved hearing.

The treatment of sensorineural hearing loss in children centers around amplification (hearing aids), educational efforts, and medical testing to rule out treatable or progressive forms of sensorineural loss. The cochlear implant is a new treatment of profound hearing loss in children who have not benefited from amplification. This implant is an electrode which is surgically implanted into the scala tympani of the cochlea, usually through the round window. The electrode is coupled to a microprocessor which converts external acoustic energy to directly stimulate the auditory nerve. Clinical trials have documented improvements in speech recognition and hearing threshold levels.[18,19] About 60% of deaf children with cochlear implants have improved speech intelligibility.[20]

TONSILLECTOMY AND ADENOIDECTOMY

Adenotonsillectomy is still performed for recurrent pharyngitis refractory to medical treatment. Guidelines for the use of this procedure continue to evolve based on frequency of infection and severity of each episode. Outpatient tonsillectomy has been performed successfully in selected patients.

The treatment of obstructive sleep apnea (OSA) in children has centered around adenotonsillectomy. Adenotonsillar hypertrophy is the usual cause of OSA in children without craniofacial syndrome or neuromotor disease. These patients require careful monitoring of respiratory function after surgery.[21]

SIALORRHEA

Sialorrhea, or drooling, is a problem of children with disordered oromotor function as seen in cerebral palsy. Drooling is almost always caused by impaired oral clearance and not from increased saliva production. Oromotor physical therapy is useful for some neurologically impaired children with sialorrhea. Medical therapy using anticholinergic agents is associated with troublesome side effects such as blurred vision, constipation, and urinary retention. Surgery for sialorrhea involves combinations of salivary gland removal, duct ligation, duct rerouting, and interruption of parasympathetic innervation to salivary glands.

The most successful surgical approach for drooling is bilateral submandibular gland excision combined with bilateral parotid-duct ligation.[22] Transient parotid swelling occurs in most patients but resolves over several days. Xerostomia has not been a problem, but meticulous dental care is required to prevent caries. Submandibular glands are excised through small upper cervical incisions, and the parotid ducts are ligated transorally near the Stenson duct orifice in the buccal mucosa adjacent to the maxillary second molars.

REFERENCES

1. Tunkel DE, Zalzal GH. Stridor in infants and children: ambulatory evaluation and operative diagnosis. Clin Pediatr 1992;31:48-55.

1a. MacArthur CJ, Senders CW, Katz J. The use of interferon alpha-2a for life-threatening hemangiomas. Arch Otolaryngol Head Neck Surg 1995;121:690.

2. Zalzal GH, Anon JB, Cotton RT. Epiglottoplasty for the treatment of laryngomalacia. Ann Otol Rhinol Laryngol 1987;96:72.

2a. Holinger LD, Konior RJ. Surgical management of severe laryngomalacia. Laryngoscope 1989;99:136.

2b. Marcus CL, Crockett DM, Davidson-Ward SL. Evaluation of epiglottoplasty as treatment for severe laryngomalacia. J Pediatr 1990;117:706.

2c. Kelly SM, Gray SD. Unilateral endoscopic supraglottoplasty for severe laryngomalacia. Arch Otolaryngol Head Neck Surg 1995;121:1351.

3. Grundfast KM, Harley E. Vocal cord paralysis. Otolaryngol Clin North Am 1989;22:569.

4. Cotton RT. The problem of pediatric laryngotracheal stenosis: a clinical and experimental study on the efficacy of autogenous cartilaginous grafts placed between the vertically divided halves of the posterior lamina of the cricoid cartilage. Laryngoscope 1991;101(suppl 56):1.

5. Cotton RT, Myer CM, Bratcher GO, et al. Anterior cricoid split (1977-1987): evolution of a technique. Arch Otolaryngol Head Neck Surg 1988;114:1300.

6. Zalzal GH. Use of stents in laryngotracheal reconstruction in children; indications, technical considerations, and complications. Laryngoscope 1988;98:849.

7. Seid AB, Pransky SM, Kearns DB. One-stage laryngotracheoplasty. Arch Otolaryngol Head Neck Surg 1991;117:408.

8. April MM, Marsh BR. Laryngotracheal reconstruction for subglottic stenosis. Ann Otol Rhinol Laryngol 1993;102:176.

9. Monnier P, Savry M, Chapuis G. Partial cricoid resection with primary tracheal anastomosis for subglottic stenosis in infants and children. Laryngoscope 1993;103:1273.

10. Kennedy DW, Zinreich SJ, Rosenbaum AE. Functional endoscopic sinus surgery: theory and diagnostic evaluation. Arch Otolaryngol 1985;111:576.

11. Duplechain JK, White JA, Miller RH. Pediatric sinusitis: the role of endoscopic sinus surgery in cystic fibrosis and other forms of sinonasal disease. Arch Otolaryngol Head Neck Surg 1991;117:422.

12. Lusk RP, Muntz HR. Endoscopic sinus surgery in children with chronic sinusitis; a pilot study. Laryngoscope 1990;100:654.

13. Stankiewicz JA. Complications of endoscopic intranasal ethmoidectomy. Laryngoscope 1987;97:1270.

14. Richardson MA, Osguthorpe JD. Surgical management of choanal atresia. Laryngoscope 1988;98:915.

15. Stankiewicz JA. The endoscopic repair of choanal atresia. Otolaryngol Head Neck Surg 1990;103:931.

16. Kempthorne J, Giebink GS. Pediatric approach to the diagnosis and management of otitis media. Otolaryngol Clin North Am 1991;24:905.

17. Bluestone CD. Indications for tonsillectomy, adenoidectomy, and tympanostomy tube insertion: results of randomized trials as applied to clinical practice. Adv Otolaryngol-Head Neck Surg 1991;5:193.

18. Staller SJ, Beiter AL, Brimacombe JA, et al. Pediatric performance with the Nucleus 22-channel cochlear implant system. Amer J Otology 1991;12:126.

19. Kveton J, Balkany TJ. Status of cochlear implantation in children. J Pediatr 1991;118:1.

20. Tobey EA, Angelette S, Murchison C, et al. Speech production performance in children with multichannel cochlear implants. Amer J Otology 1991;12:165.

21. McColley SA, April MM, Carroll JL, et al. Respiratory compromise after adenotonsillectomy in children with obstructive sleep apnea. Arch Otolaryngol Head Neck Surg 1992;118:940.

22. Shott SR, Myer CM, Cotton RT. Surgical management of sialorrhea. Otolaryngol Head Neck Surg 1989;101:47.

Surgery of Infants and Children: Scientific Principles and Practice, edited by Keith T. Oldham, Paul M. Colombani, and Robert P. Foglia. Lippincott–Raven Publishers, Philadelphia, © 1997.

CHAPTER 51

Neck

Mary E. Fallat

Although the neck is a small portion of the total body area, it accounts for a relatively large amount of pathology encountered by pediatric surgeons in clinical practice (Table 51-1). The neck is often the focus of abnormalities that require a working knowledge of embryology, anatomy, and clinical diagnosis to effectively formulate a treatment plan. Because the rich lymphatic supply in the neck offers a medium for both benign and malignant disease, good judgment is critical to determine the difference. Diagnosis might involve a formal surgical procedure or a less invasive test, such as fine-needle aspiration (FNA) or a radiographic study. A treatment plan might involve surgery or a conservative approach, depending on the diagnosis. The need for surgery may be complicated by antecedent infection. Few other operative sites require as much skill and judgment to determine the timing of, need for, and anatomic approach to an operation.

EMBRYOLOGY

Pharyngeal development commences during the first few weeks of embryonic life and precedes that of the other organs of the foregut. The pharyngeal primordium relevant to this chapter is the branchial apparatus, consisting initially of five paired endodermal pharyngeal pouches and four corresponding ectodermal branchial clefts with mesodermal branchial arches between consecutive pairs.[1]

Of the four branchial clefts visible in the fifth week of gestation, only the most dorsal portion of the first cleft persists as the external auditory canal. The eustachian tube and cavity of the middle ear are formed from the corresponding portion of the first pharyngeal pouch, and the closing plate between pouch and cleft is represented by tympanic membrane. The remaining branchial clefts obliterate during the sixth and seventh weeks. The approximate location of obliterated embryonic clefts, arches, and pouches that may have clinical significance is outlined in Table 51-2, and is relevant to the origin of the epithelium-lined cysts, sinuses, and fistulas encountered in clinical practice. The minute pits, sinuses, and cysts seen in the skin near the anterior border of the ascending helical limb of the ear are believed to represent ectodermal folds sequestered during fusion of the six hillocks that form the pinna, rather than

branchial defects. Midline cervical clefts occur because of imperfect midline fusion of the paired branchial arch tissue during early gestation.

The thyroid gland is formed by the median thyroid anlage (origin marked by foramen cecum) and the lateral thyroid anlage (the fourth and fifth branchial pouch complex). A median stalk is attached to the future foramen cecum of the tongue which usually has a lumen. Elongation of the embryo leaves the thyroid gland caudal to its point of origin. In the fifth week of development, the attenuated stalk (thyroglossal duct) loses its lumen and fragments, leaving a pit at the ultimate location of the foramen cecum and a distal remnant attached to the thyroid isthmus which often persists as a pyramidal lobe. Mesodermal anlage of the body of the hyoid bone usually appear soon after, and if the thyroglossal duct is not yet obliterated, a persistent thyroglossal duct related to the hyoid bone results.

The thymus develops as bilateral sacculations from the ventral aspects of the third pharyngeal pouches during the sixth week of life. The sacculations elongate and separate from the pouches during gestational weeks seven and eight, becoming increasingly cellular as they fuse in the midline and migrate into the mediastinum. The thymus primordia retain a lumen, called the thymopharyngeal duct, which obliterates after medial fusion of its two halves. A cervical thymic cyst is thought to result from arrest of the normal embryonic migration of the thymic primordia, by the persistence of the thymopharyngeal tract or by cystic degeneration of Hassall corpuscles and other thymic components.

ANATOMY

Surface Anatomy

In the anterior neck, the superior border of the manubrium of the sternum demarcates the inferior extent of the suprasternal space (jugular notch), limited laterally by the sternal heads of the sternocleidomastoid muscles. In the midline anterior neck, midway between the suprasternal space and the chin, the laryngeal prominence (Adam's apple) is formed by the V-shaped thyroid cartilage of the larynx. At the superior border of the prominence, the laryngeal notch is palpable. Above the laryn-

TABLE 51-1. *Differential diagnosis of neck masses in children*

CONGENITAL MASSES
Cystic hygroma
Hemangioma
Branchial cleft cyst
Thyroglossal duct cyst
Dermoid cyst
Laryngocele
Teratoma

NONINFLAMMATORY BENIGN MASSES
Epidermoid inclusion cyst
Lipoma
Fibroma
Neurofibroma
Neurilemmoma
Ranula
Torticollis
Thyroid nodule
Fibrous tissue tumors

INFLAMMATORY MASSES
Reactive lymphadenopathy
Suppurative adenitis (abscess)
Mononucleosis
Sialadenitis
Tuberculosis
Granulomatous lymphadenopathy
Cat-scratch disease

NONINFLAMMATORY MALIGNANT MASSES
Hodgkin disease
NonHodgkin lymphoma
Leukemia
Rhabdomyosarcoma
Thyroid malignancies
Salivary gland malignancies
Neuroblastoma
Germ-cell neoplasms
Metastatic nodules

geal prominence, the hyoid bone can be palpated. The chin is formed by the mental protuberance of the mandible, and at the posterior border of the jaw, the prominent angle is continued superiorly as the ramus.

The root of the neck is the junctional area between the neck proper and the thorax. It is limited laterally by the first rib, anteriorly by the manubrium of the sternum, and posteriorly by the first three thoracic vertebrae. It transmits all the structures passing between the neck and thorax.

Fasciae of the Neck

The superficial fascia of the head and neck is continuous with the superficial fascia of the pectoral, deltoid, and back regions. The deep fasciae consist of the outer investing layer, the middle cervical layer, the prevertebral, and the pretracheal fasciae. The outer investing layer (external cervical fascia) completely surrounds the neck like a stocking, extending from the clavicle over the mandible to the zygoma. Posteriorly, this layer fuses with the ligamentum nucha. In the anterior triangle, this layer is bound to the hyoid bone and is subdivided into suprahyoid and infrahyoid portions. The middle cervical fascia, composed of two layers, encloses the strap muscles of the neck.

The prevertebral fascia covers the anterior aspect of the cervical vertebrae. It continues in the axilla as the cervical axillary sheath which surrounds the brachial plexus and axillary artery, then continues inferiorly as the endothoracic fascia of the thoracic cavity, and expands over the lung apex as the cervical diaphragm or Sibson fascia at the cervicothoracic aperture. A potential cleft between the prevertebral fascia and the fascia of the pharynx, the retropharyngeal space, is limited superiorly by the base of the skull and laterally by the attachment of prevertebral to middle cervical fascia. Inferiorly, the retropharyngeal space communicates with the posterior mediastinum.

The visceral component of the neck is located between the prevertebral and middle cervical fascia. It contains the major arteries and nerves in the neck, the cervical portions of the digestive and respiratory systems, and the thyroid and parathyroid glands. The visceral (pretracheal) fascia is a tubular projection into the neck of the visceral fascia of the mediastinum, where it is continuous with the fibrous pericardium. It encloses the esophagus, trachea, pharynx, and larynx and contributes laterally to the formation of the carotid sheath.

Lymph Nodes

Lymph nodes that drain lymph from the head and neck are arranged symmetrically on both sides of the neck (Fig. 51-1). Node groups, drainage areas, and anatomic location of the groups are listed in Table 51-3. In addition to the groups noted, vertical chains of nodes are present along the entire length of the carotid sheath and receive most of the lymphatic drainage from the head and neck. Additional lymphoid tissue pertinent to this chapter is located in the Waldeyer ring, which includes the nasopharynx, tonsils, base of the tongue, and oropharyngeal wall.

Triangles of the Neck

The neck is divided into three main triangles—the anterior, the posterior, and the suboccipital. The anterior triangle of the neck is bounded posteriorly by the anterior border of the sternocleidomastoid muscle and anteriorly by the midline of the neck. The base is formed by the lower border of the mandible, and the apex is at the sternum. This triangle can be subdivided into three paired and one common triangle—the muscular, carotid, and submandibular (digastric) triangles and the unpaired submental triangle. The posterior triangle of the neck is divided by the posterior belly of the omohyoid into a small subclavian and a large occipital triangle. The suboccipital triangle is located in the posterior midline. The major boundaries and contents of the individual triangles are listed in Table 51-4, and anterior and posterior triangles are depicted in Fig. 51-2.

DIAGNOSTIC APPROACH

The initial evaluation of infants and children with head and neck complaints begins with a complete history and physical examination. Eighty percent of neck masses in children are benign. Important historical points to consider include site and

TABLE 51-2. *Relationship of embryonic derivatives to clinical abnormalities*

Embryonic derivative	Anatomic course	Remnant or result of abnormal development
CLEFT OR POUCH		
First Cleft	Ostium lies below mandible and above hyoid bone; tract extends in direction of external auditory canal and relates to the facial nerve, often traveling within the parotid gland	External sinus tract or fistula connecting to external auditory canal or eustachian tube. Cystic mass in front of, behind, or below ear lobe or in submandibular region
Second Cleft	Ostium lies at anterior border of sternocleidomastoid muscle, usually at junction of lower and middle thirds; tract ascends between branches of internal and external carotid arteries to tonsillar fossa	External sinus tract or fistula along lower anterior border of sternocleidomastoid muscle. Cystic mass deep to anterior border of sternocleidomastoid muscle at level of carotid bifurcation
Third Pouch	Ostium (if present) should lie anterior to anterior border of clavicular head of sternocleidomastoid muscle and track cephalad through or around left thyroid lobe toward pyriform sinus	External sinus tract or fistula along lower anterior border of sternocleidomastoid muscle. Cystic mass adjacent to left lobe of thyroid gland, often communicating with left pyriform sinus
Fourth Pouch	Ostium (if present) lies in anterior cervical triangle and passes inferiorly to the aorta (left) or subclavian artery (right) in upper mediastinum; ascends with recurrent laryngeal nerve to enter esophagus	Sinus tract in anterior cervical triangle
ARCH		
Third Arch	Anterior neck bounded laterally by sternocleidomastoid muscles (entrapment of epithelium of arch origin)	Midline dermoid cyst

duration of symptoms, systemic signs of illness such as unexplained fever or weight loss, associated illnesses such as otitis media or streptococcal pharyngitis, and exacerbating or ameliorating factors. An inflammatory lesion usually has a short duration or may recur. A lesion of long duration, or one identified at or soon after birth, is more likely to be congenital, benign, or both. A painless, rapidly enlarging mass is often malignant.

The initial symptoms of a solid tumor in the head and neck area are often nonspecific and caused by the effect of the mass on surrounding tissues.

Physical examination of the child includes careful inspection and palpation of the neck abnormality, as well as examination of the face, scalp, ears, and oral cavity, which may yield the initiating source of the neck pathology. A general physical ex-

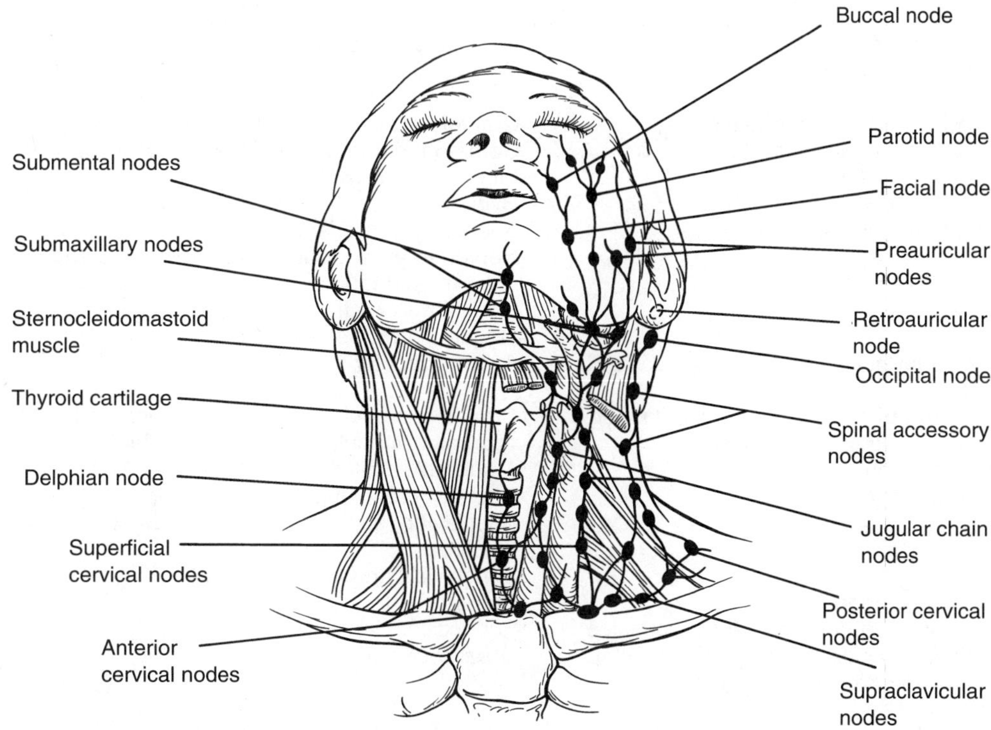

FIG. 51-1. Lymphatics and lymph nodes of the head and neck.

TABLE 51-3. *Lymph node drainage of the head and neck*

Lymph node group	Anatomic location	Drainage area
Anterior auricular	Located anterior to tragus	Pinna Scalp
Posterior auricular	Located on mastoid process under deep fascia	Back of the pinna External auditory meatus Temporal area
Occipital	Located between external occipital protuberance and mastoid process under deep fascia	Posterior scalp
Parotid	Lie within substance of parotid gland under deep fascia	Nasopharynx External auditory canal Eyelids Inner ear
Submaxillary	Located within fascia of submaxillary gland	Cheek Angle of the mouth Side of the nose Upper portion of the lower lip Gum Side of the tongue
Facial	Located superficial and deep to anterior facial and internal maxillary vessels	Face Pharynx Mucous membranes of the cheek
Superficial cervical	Located along external jugular vein	Parotid Lower portions of the external ear
Submental	Located lateral to midline of submental triangle	Lower lip Floor of the mouth Apex of the tongue
Anterior cervical	Lie in midline of neck with a superficial and deep group	Thyroid gland Larynx Trachea

TABLE 51-4. *Triangles of the neck*

Triangle	Boundaries	Contents
Muscular	Superior belly of omohyoid muscle Sternocleidomastoid muscle Midline of neck	Infrahyoid muscles Thyroid gland
Carotid	Superior belly of omohyoid muscle Posterior belly of digastric muscle Sternocleidomastoid muscle	Cranial nerves X and XII Common, external, and internal carotid arteries Internal jugular vein Hyoid bone
Submandibular (digastric)	Two bellies of the digastric muscles Mandible	Submandibular gland Nerves to anterior belly of the digastric and mylohyoid muscles Cranial nerve XII Lingual and facial arteries
Submental	Between anterior bellies of digastric muscle Hyoid bone	Anterior jugular veins
Posterior (subclavian and occipital)	Posterior border of sternocleidomastoid muscle Anterior border of trapezius muscle Superior nuchal line Middle third of clavicle	Cranial nerve XI, phrenic, lesser occipital, greater auricular, transverse cervical, supraclavicular nerves Roots of brachial plexus Subclavian, suprascapular, transverse cervical arteries Subclavian and external jugular veins
Suboccipital	Rectus capitis posterior major muscle Obliquus capitis superior and inferior muscles Semispinalis and longissimus capitis muscles Posterior atlantooccipital membrane Posterior arch of the atlas	Vertebral artery Suboccipital nerve Greater occipital nerve

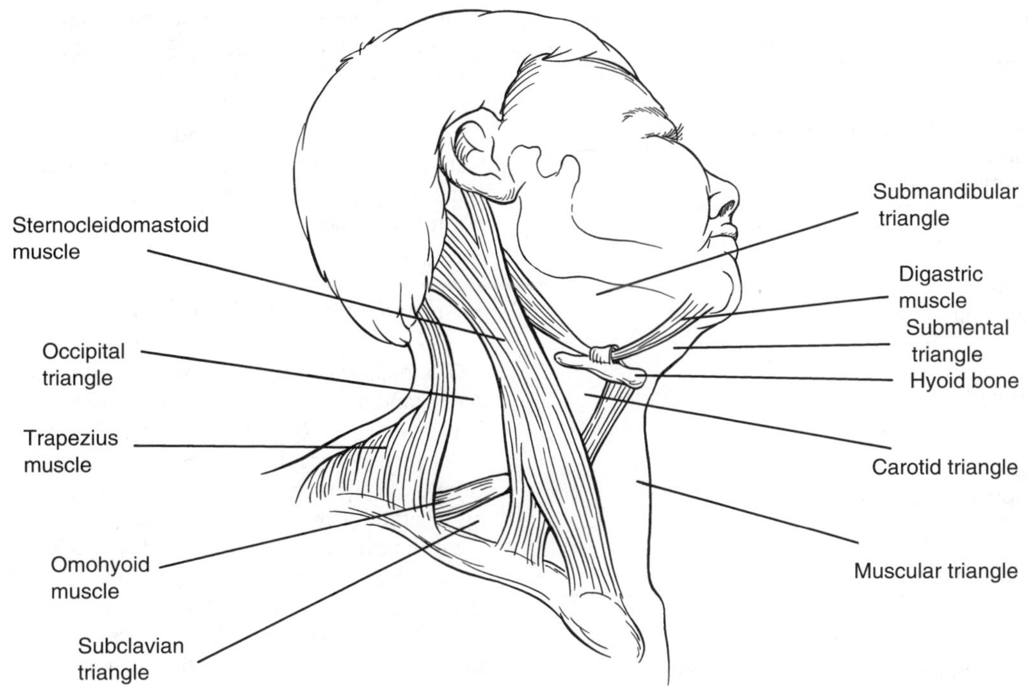

FIG. 51-2. Triangles of the neck.

amination including the chest, abdomen, genitalia, and extremities completes the evaluation. Subsequent diagnostic work-up is guided by the preliminary history and physical examination.

In some situations, such as a case of presumedly benign lymphadenopathy, the surgical consultant may decide that no work-up is necessary. A simple complete blood count with a peripheral smear may help define an acute infection. If the diagnosis is questionable, an ultrasound, computed tomographic (CT) scan, magnetic resonance imaging (MRI), or FNA often guide the need for therapeutic surgical intervention.

Radiographic Studies

Ultrasound is particularly helpful in distinguishing solid from cystic masses or in determining maturation of a deep cervical abscess. Doppler ultrasound can distinguish a vascular mass, such as a hemangioma, from an avascular lesion. A CT scan is more useful when a tumor is diagnosed or suspected, and this modality also helps delineate thoracic extensions of neck masses. Using intravenous contrast (enhancement) defines vascular structures and highlights tumor boundaries including the extent of any bony invasion. CT scan is also extremely sensitive and accurate for localizing deep fascial space infections in the neck. MRI provides three-dimensional anatomic detail, but has drawbacks including high cost and the need to sedate younger patients to prevent motion artifact. It is particularly useful if spinal cord or intracranial extension of a tumor is suspected. T_2-weighted imaging identifies areas of increased vascularity, and T_1-weighted images enhanced with gadolinium allow precise localization of central nervous system tumors. A good quality T_2-weighted image can also delineate the position of the facial nerve with respect to a parotid tumor.

Gallium 67 scanning is useful in the initial staging and monitoring of disease response or recurrence in high-grade non-Hodgkin lymphomas. The metal ion gallium 67 has characteristics similar to those of the ferric ion, and its uptake in tumors is mediated when gallium 67–transferrin complex formed in the plasma binds to transferrin receptors in the tumor. Gallium isotope uptake occurs in the liver, spleen, bone, nasal passages, lacrimal and salivary glands, and thymus in normal children.

Additional radiographic studies that may be needed to evaluate a neck mass are chest radiograph, bone scan, and CT scans of the abdomen, chest, or brain as part of a metastatic work-up if a malignant tumor is suspected or diagnosed. A chest x-ray can rule out pulmonary involvement in tuberculosis or a potentially systemic fungal disease.

Fine-Needle Aspiration

The use of aspiration cytology using FNA was first advocated as a diagnostic tool in the early 1930s, but has only recently gained popularity for pediatric patients.[2] The procedure is generally done by a pediatric pathologist with an ''aspiration gun,'' which allows the dominant hand to control needle direction while using the other hand to stabilize the mass. The gauge of needle varies from 20 to 25, depending on the type of mass being aspirated. The technique appears to be safe with only occasional bruising or minor hematomas as complications. In about 10% of cases, the amount of material obtained is inadequate for diagnosis. The accuracy rate in the remainder is approximately 98%.

The advantages of FNA over excisional biopsy include the ability to perform the procedure in an office or clinic setting, no need for general anesthesia, lower cost than open biopsy, diagnosis within 24 hours, and no subsequent scar. Enough material can usually be generated for cytology as well as culture,

TABLE 51-5. *Pathologic processes in the neck potentially diagnosed with FNA*

BENIGN
Reactive lymphadenitis (lymphadenopathy)
Lymph node abscess
Granulomatous lymphadenitis
Pilomatrixoma (calcifying epithelioma of Malherbe)
Lymphangioma
Hemangioma
Branchial cleft cyst
Thyroglossal duct cyst
Fibromatosis coli
Sialadenitis
Pleomorphic adenoma

MALIGNANT
Hodgkin disease
NonHodgkin lymphoma
Leukemic infiltrate
Rhabdomyosarcoma
Papillary thyroid carcinoma

flow cytometry, chromosome analysis, or electron microscopy as indicated by the pathologist. Table 51-5 lists some of the processes amenable to diagnosis with FNA. A lymph node that persists or grows for longer than 6 weeks and does not respond to antibiotics should be considered for biopsy by FNA.

The information obtained on FNA can be either reassuring to the child's physician and child's parents or can lead to more rapid treatment for another entity. Because of the possibility of sampling error, excisional biopsy should be considered if a lymph node or neck mass continues to enlarge over 2 to 3 weeks or persists in size for 3 months after FNA.

BENIGN LESIONS

Lymphadenopathy

Benign cervical lymphadenopathy accounts for most neck masses in children, the causes of which are protean. Although viral and bacterial etiologies are most common, atypical mycobacteria infections, mononucleosis, and cat-scratch disease are other frequent diagnoses. Tuberculosis and fungal diseases are occasionally encountered. If the underlying cause is evident, treatment is usually directed toward the etiologic agent or watchful waiting is advocated. Under these circumstances, the lymphadenopathy often regresses, although frequently, it does not totally disappear.

Viral and Bacterial Etiologies

The pediatric surgeon is often asked to evaluate a child with long-standing cervical lymphadenopathy. Careful questioning may reveal a history of frequent upper respiratory infections, otitis media, tonsillitis, sinusitis, or allergies associated with rhinitis. The lymphadenopathy may fluctuate in size, depending on whether or not the child has an active infection. The nodes are ordinarily mobile and located in the upper anterior cervical areas. They may be bilateral and may be slightly tender in the presence of active infection. In most cases, this adenopathy can be treated conservatively. An associated identified bacterial infection is treated with antimicrobial agents. Bacterial lymphadenitis most typically involves penicillin-resistant staphylococcal or Group A β-hemolytic streptococcal etiologies. If biopsy seems indicated, an FNA can be done and usually reveals reactive lymphadenopathy, allowing continued observation and alleviating parental anxiety. An aspirate can also be obtained for culture, although culture proves positive in only about 15% of cases.[2]

Bacterial infections may instead be characterized by rapid nodal enlargement followed by slow evolution to an abscess or suppurative lymphadenitis with overlying skin erythema and fluctuance (Fig. 51-3). Young children tend to have associated fever until the abscess matures and can be drained, despite appropriate antimicrobial therapy. Ultrasound may help to plan optimal timing of the surgical drainage.

The timing and approach to surgical therapy of a probable phlegmon or abscess is dictated by suspected etiology and the need for diagnosis versus therapy. Not all surgical procedures need to be done under general anesthesia. Small neck abscesses

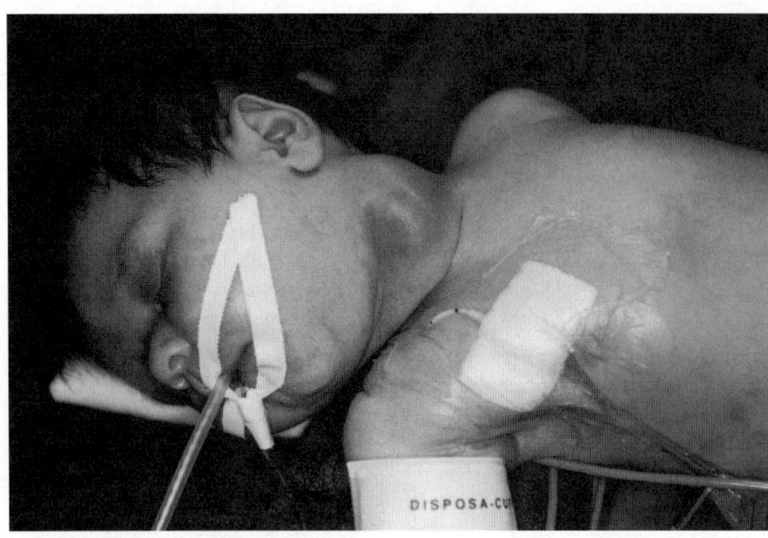

FIG. 51-3. Large cervical abscess in an infant.

may be drained in a treatment room with conscious sedation and appropriate monitoring; large or multiloculated abscesses are better drained in the operating room. A transverse incision is made over the main area of fluctuance unless this is inappropriate for cosmetic reasons, and it should be long enough to enable the surgeon to probe the abscess cavity and break up any loculations. This ensures adequate drainage and allows placement of a passive drain, such as a Penrose, or packing material. Incisions made very high or very low in the neck should be made parallel to the mandible or clavicle, respectively, and at least 1 or 1.5 cm away from these bony landmarks to preclude significant scarring.

Adequate surgical drainage in combination with appropriate antimicrobial therapy usually resolves simple suppurative processes. Identification of an unusual organism such as *Pseudomonas* or an abscess recurrence may indicate an underlying immunosuppressive illness or congenital anomaly and should prompt an appropriate work-up.

Tuberculosis, Atypical Mycobacteria, and Fungal Etiologies

Atypical mycobacteria (AMB) can be cultured from soil, water, and some food products. It is likely, however, that the oropharynx and respiratory tract act as the reservoir for these infections, since AMB can also be cultured from these sites in asymptomatic patients. The most common organisms causing infection in humans are *Mycobacterium avium*, *Mycobacterium intracellularis*, and *Mycobacterium scrofulaceum*. The collective group is now known as *M avium* complex (MAC). Unlike *Mycobacterium tuberculosis* (TB), person-to-person transmission of MAC has not been documented.[3,4]

Uncomplicated cases of AMB often present as a group of upper cervical nodes located close to the mandible which are initially rubbery, firm, and nontender. They later become matted together to form a confluent mass which may be several centimeters in diameter. The child is usually otherwise well, whereas cases of TB are more common in immunocompromised children and are accompanied by symptoms or signs of illness such as fever and respiratory complaints. An occasional patient has a superimposed pyogenic infection with fever, and an acid-fast stain and culture for mycobacteria at the time of abscess drainage may prove helpful in diagnosis if the wound later fails to heal properly.

An intradermal skin test with standard tuberculin antigens may be helpful because there is a cross-reactivity between AMB and TB. Reactions to intermediate-strength purified protein derivative (5 tuberculin units) are usually 5 to 10 mm in diameter in cases of AMB, and significantly greater than 10 mm in TB cases. FNA or incisional biopsy in cases of both AMB and TB reveals granulomatous lymphadenopathy with central caseous necrosis, aggregates of histiocytes, or Langerhan giant cells (Fig. 51-4).

If the child is in a high-risk group for *M tuberculosis* infection, a trial of anti-TB chemotherapy is appropriate. Atypical mycobacteria infections respond poorly to chemotherapy. Incision and drainage or incomplete nodal excision of AMB invariably leads to recurrence or cutaneous draining sinuses, and complete excision is needed and ordinarily curative.

Fungal infections are less frequent and more often seen in immunocompromised patients. *Candida albicans* is the most frequently reported pathogen.

Mononucleosis (Epstein-Barr Virus Infection)

The lymphadenopathy associated with mononucleosis is usually bilateral and more common in the adolescent than the child. Hepatosplenomegaly may be present, and a monospot or Epstein-Barr virus (EBV) titers are positive. The lymphadenopathy resolves within weeks.

An occasional patient with a history of mononucleosis later develops Hodgkin disease or nonHodgkin lymphoma, but the association is not common enough to warrant routine node biopsy in every patient with mononucleosis. Cervical node biopsy is warranted in patients who have persistent or recurrent lymphadenopathy in the face of normal or declining EBV titers following a documented case of mononucleosis.

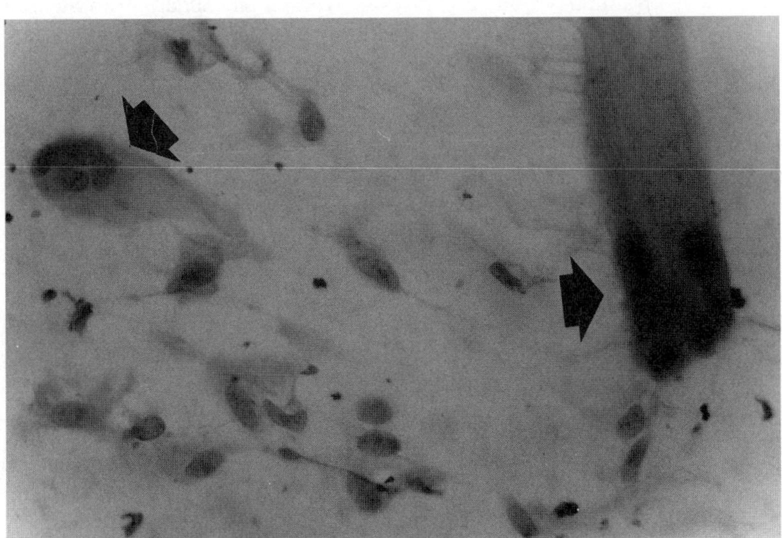

FIG. 51-4. Photomicrograph of a smear from a fine-needle aspiration of a child with cervical lymphadenopathy. Aggregates of histiocytes as seen here were scattered throughout the smears giving a diagnosis of granulomatous lymphadenitis. (PAP, ×400.)

Cat-Scratch Disease

The classic features of cat-scratch disease (CSD) include self-limited, regional lymphadenopathy occurring in healthy people following a cat scratch or bite distal to the affected node. Common sites of node enlargement other than the neck are the axilla, elbow, and groin. Recently, it has been determined that affected persons are more likely to have been scratched, licked in the face, or bitten by a kitten younger than 1 year and to have been exposed to a kitten with fleas.[5] Other animals, such as dogs and monkeys, and inanimate objects have also been implicated in transmission.[6]

Historically, a noncommercial skin test prepared from lymph node aspirates from patients with this disease was used to help confirm the diagnosis, but this test was never standardized or approved for general use. The Warthin-Starry silver stain defined pleomorphic organisms in lymph node biopsy specimens, and *Afipia felis* was felt to be a causative organism. More recently, the role of the organism *Bartonella* (formerly *Rochalimaea*) *henselae*, and *quintana*, members of the Rickettsiaceae family, has been implicated as the etiologic agent.[5,7] Preliminary results using a *B henselae*-based serologic indirect fluorescent-antibody test, which appears to be both a sensitive and specific diagnostic tool, have suggested that the disease may be more prevalent than previously suspected. The domestic cat is a major persistent reservoir for the organism, and the cat flea (*Ctenocephalides felis*) is a potential vector.

The most common constitutional symptoms associated with CSD are fever and malaise, although most children have mild symptoms and a benign clinical course. Severe complications including encephalitis, follicular conjunctivitis, and neuroretinitis have also been described. A papule may form at the site of primary inoculation. In most cases, the disease resolves spontaneously within a couple of months. Lymph node biopsy reveals multiple microabscesses or granulomas.

Other Agents

Other unusual causes of cervical lymphadenitis have been reported and include actinomyces, toxoplasmosis, tularemia, Kawasaki disease, *Yersinia enterocolitica*, *Nocardia* species, and Kikuchi disease.

Surgical Management of Lymphadenitis

In cases of cervical lymphadenitis that do not respond to a course of standard antimicrobial therapy or TB therapy, or lymphadenitis that is persistent or enlarges after diagnosis of mononucleosis or CSD, surgical excision for diagnosis is the recommended treatment. Similarly, in cases of cervical lymphadenitis that fit the diagnosis of AMB infection clinically, surgical excision without drainage is the recommended treatment.[3] Definitive surgery in the latter circumstance should involve complete excision of all involved sinus tracts and nodes if feasible. Cases of parotid involvement treated with superficial parotidectomy, or that have neural involvement that precludes complete resection of involved nodes, usually heal normally.[4] Adjunctive antimicrobial therapy with trimethoprim-sulfamethoxazole, rifampin, or gentamicin has occasionally been used in cases of AMB or CSD. There are no case-controlled studies comparing the use of these drugs to treatment without antibiotics, and their use should probably be reserved for disseminated or problematic disease.

Enlarged cervical nodes may require biopsy in almost any site in the neck. A small transverse incision made in a skin crease overlying the node is usually sufficient for biopsy. Nodes in the posterior triangle are usually superficial and easily excised, with careful avoidance of the spinal accessory nerve. In most cases, nodal tissue can be directly approached and then teased away from surrounding tissue using blunt dissection to avoid damage to important structures.

To approach the supraclavicular area, an incision is made over the lateral edge of the sternocleidomastoid muscle. After incising the platysma, the nodal tissue between the omohyoid muscle superiorly, external jugular vein laterally, carotid sheath medially, and clavicle inferiorly are dissected free. The anterior scalene muscle, brachial plexus, and phrenic nerve can be visualized at the base of the dissection. Submandibular node excision requires careful avoidance of the mandibular branch of cranial nerve VII.

INFLAMMATORY PROCESSES AND SERIOUS INFECTIONS

Salivary Glands

Sialadenitis, or inflammation of a salivary gland, is one of the most common benign entities affecting children and can usually be distinguished from neoplasia by the presence of episodic pain and swelling.[8] The process may be due to a bacterial suppurative infection, a viral infection, a chronic process without determined cause, or a granulomatous process. It is more common in boys, and the parotid gland is the salivary gland most often involved. Acute suppurative sialadenitis is usually a disease of infants due to *Staphylococcus aureus*. The process progresses to abscess formation in many cases, requiring formal incision and drainage which are curative in conjunction with antibiotics.

In older infants and children without proper immunization, the etiologic agent of sialadenitis may be the mumps virus. Mumps is a bilateral process, without an exudate from Stensen duct, and it is associated with neutropenia and an elevated serum amylase.

Chronic sialadenitis or recurring parotitis is often an idiopathic process. Simultaneous bilateral involvement is rare. Implicated etiologies include drug sensitivity, iodide, food intolerances, and opioids. It may be associated with pharyngitis, recurring tonsillitis, or poor oral hygiene. Serum amylase is normal, and there is an associated leukocytosis. Culture of material expressed from the parotid duct is of little value because only nonpathogenic organisms are recovered. Rarely, patients with cystic fibrosis develop parotitis, and many of these patients also have chronically enlarged submandibular glands.

The most common inflammatory processes involving the salivary glands are CSD, AMB infection, and reactive hyperplasia of periparotid and intraparotid lymph nodes. More remote causes of chronic parotitis include an autoimmune process, EBV infection, sarcoidosis, tuberculosis, or occult lymphoma. Attacks of chronic parotid sialadenitis are characterized by recurring, painful swelling and tenderness of the involved gland lasting 1 to 7 days and aggravated by chewing and swallowing. Attacks occur approximately every 3 to 4 months. The site of involvement seems to be random. The orifice of the Stensen duct may appear red and pouting.

Salivary gland infections are unusual and often self-limited.[8] If a salivary duct is obstructed with a stone, infection is controlled with antibiotics and stone removal. If the gland undergoes necrosis, excision is necessary. Operation in the presence of infection or marked inflammation makes facial nerve dissection and preservation extremely difficult.

Fascial Space Infections

Life-threatening infections of the neck most commonly originate from suppurative complications of dental, oropharyngeal, or otorhinolaryngeal infections.[9] From these sites, infection can extend along natural fascial planes into deep cervical spaces or vascular compartments. These infections can be fatal if they obstruct the local airway or directly extend to vital structures, such as the mediastinum or carotid sheath.

Typical deep infections of the neck are polymicrobial, reflecting the microflora of the contiguous mucosal surfaces from which the infections originate. Invasiveness is often influenced by synergistic interactions among multiple microbes. Immunocompromised hosts and people with otogenic infection associated with chronic otitis media or mastoiditis may also develop invasive infections with enteric gram-negative bacilli and *S aureus*.

Deep fascial-space infections of the head and neck are often odontogenic in origin. Potentially life-threatening infections may involve the submandibular, lateral pharyngeal, and retropharyngeal spaces.

It is imperative that clinical specimens obtained for the diagnosis of deep head and neck infections are not contaminated by resident oronasopharyngeal flora.[9] This is best accomplished using a needle and syringe to aspirate loculated pus extraorally. Localization can be accomplished with ultrasound guidance. After the skin is cleansed, pus is aspirated into the syringe and all air carefully expressed. If a swab is used, it should be saturated with purulent material and inserted into a tube specifically designed for anaerobic conditions.

Ludwig Angina

The prototype submandibular space infection is Ludwig angina, which is an aggressive and rapidly spreading "woody" cellulitis, which commonly occurs following infection of the second or third mandibular molars (70% to 85% of cases). The submylohyoid space is initially involved, followed by contiguous extension of infection to involve the entire submandibular space in a symmetrical manner. Once established, infection can evolve very rapidly, with the tongue enlarging 2 to 3 times its normal size. Cellulitis of the submandibular space may spread directly into the lateral pharyngeal space and then to the retropharyngeal space and mediastinum through a connection between submandibular and lateral pharyngeal spaces known as the buccopharyngeal gap. Clinically, the patient has fever and complains of mouth pain, stiff neck, drooling, and dysphagia.

Posterior extension of the process directly involves the epiglottis, and the patient must lean forward to maximize the diameter of the airway. A tender indurated area of swelling, sometimes with palpable crepitus, is present in the submandibular area. Respiratory efforts may be compromised, leading to stridor and cyanosis. A radiographic view of the teeth may indicate the source of infection, and lateral views of the neck demonstrate soft-tissue swelling around the airway and the presence of submandibular gas.

The therapy for Ludwig angina includes maintaining an adequate airway. Although this may necessitate urgent tracheostomy, endotracheal intubation can be tried under controlled conditions using a flexible fiberoptic bronchoscope. Blind oral or nasotracheal intubation is both traumatic and unsafe because of the potential for inducing severe laryngospasm.

Penicillin G is the antibiotic of choice, but immunocompromised patients require a broader spectrum of coverage against organisms such as facultative gram-negative rods and *S aureus*. If the patient does not respond adequately to therapy with antibiotics alone after 36 to 48 hours or if fluctuance is detected, needle aspiration or definitive incision and drainage should be performed. Additionally, the implicated infected teeth should be extracted.

Infection of the Lateral Pharyngeal Space

Infections of the lateral pharyngeal space are potentially life-threatening because they involve vital structures within the carotid sheath. Anatomically, the lateral pharyngeal space is divided into anterior and posterior compartments. The anterior compartment contains no vital structures and is the compartment close to the tonsillar fossa. The posterior compartment, however, contains cranial nerves IX through XII, the carotid sheath and its contents, and the cervical sympathetic trunk. Infections of the lateral pharyngeal space may arise from sources throughout the neck. Dental infections are the most common, followed by peritonsillar abscess and parotitis, otitis, or mastoiditis. Infection of the anterior compartment is often suppurative. Cardinal clinical features include trismus, induration and swelling below the angle of the mandible, systemic sepsis, and medial bulging of the pharyngeal wall. Suppuration may advance to the retropharyngeal space and the mediastinum or may spread to involve the posterior compartment of the lateral pharyngeal space. Timely surgical incision and drainage is mandatory.

Infection of the Retropharyngeal Space

The retropharyngeal space is bound anteriorly by the constrictor muscles of the neck and their fascia and posteriorly by the deep cervical fascia extending from the base of the skull to the level of the superior mediastinum, where the two fascial layers fuse. In young children, infection usually reaches the space via lymphatics as a complication of suppurative adenitis. Onset may be insidious with fever, irritability, drooling, or possibly nuchal rigidity. More acute symptoms include dysphagia due to a local mass effect or secondary to laryngeal edema. Bulging of the posterior pharyngeal wall is usually observed, but careful palpation may be necessary to appreciate this sign.

The main dangers associated with this infection are severe laryngeal edema and consequent airway obstruction or rupture of the abscess with aspiration or asphyxia. Retropharyngeal infections are best managed by surgical drainage through the posterior wall of the pharynx in conjunction with appropriate intravenous antimicrobial therapy.

Peritonsillar Abscess

Peritonsillar abscess or quinsy is a suppurative complication of acute tonsillitis involving the peritonsillar space. The peritonsillar space consists of loose areolar tissue overlying the tonsil and surrounded by the superior pharyngeal constrictor muscle and the anterior and posterior tonsillar pillars. Peritonsillar abscesses are most common in late adolescence and young adulthood. Symptoms include fever, sore throat, dysphagia, trismus, pooling of saliva, and a muffled voice. The abscess is usually unilateral and associated with cervical lymphadenitis. Examination of the pharynx reveals swelling of the anterior pillar and soft palate with possible swelling of the middle or lower pole of the tonsil. Spontaneous rupture with aspiration of purulent material, particularly while the patient is sleeping, is the main hazard. Airway obstruction or dissection into the lateral pharyngeal space are more serious but unusual complications. High doses of penicillin usually result in a rapid response. If pus is present, incision and drainage is done via a transoral approach with an incision along the anterior tonsillar pillar allowing the abscess to drain intraorally. If the abscess is so large that it compromises the airway, tracheostomy may be necessary before it is safe to drain the abscess. Peritonsillar abscesses frequently recur and are an indication for tonsillectomy.

EMBRYONIC REMNANTS AND CYSTIC DISEASE

Branchial Derivatives

A wide array of congenital abnormalities may be seen in the neck of young children including sinuses, cysts, fistulas, and cartilaginous rests. Many are remnants of the embryonic branchial apparatus. Sinuses, fistulas, and cartilaginous remnants are usually present at birth and noticed early in life. Cysts are more often recognized later in childhood when they fill with secretions and produce a mass. All of these abnormalities except for cartilage may become infected and present as an abscess or with drainage and surrounding erythema.

Table 51-2 relates the embryonic derivative (cleft, arch, or pouch) to a potential anatomic course in the child and the type of embryologic remnant or abnormal developmental process likely to be seen in that location. Second branchial cleft anomalies are the most common anomaly in this category followed by first branchial cleft abnormalities. Anomalies of the third and fourth branchial clefts or pouches are rare. What some authors have considered pouch III internal sinuses are considered by others to be of pouch IV origin.[10,11] Interestingly, almost all reported cases have occurred on the left side. The lesion usually becomes symptomatic before age 10 years, often presenting as suppurative thyroiditis. Contrast esophagogram may

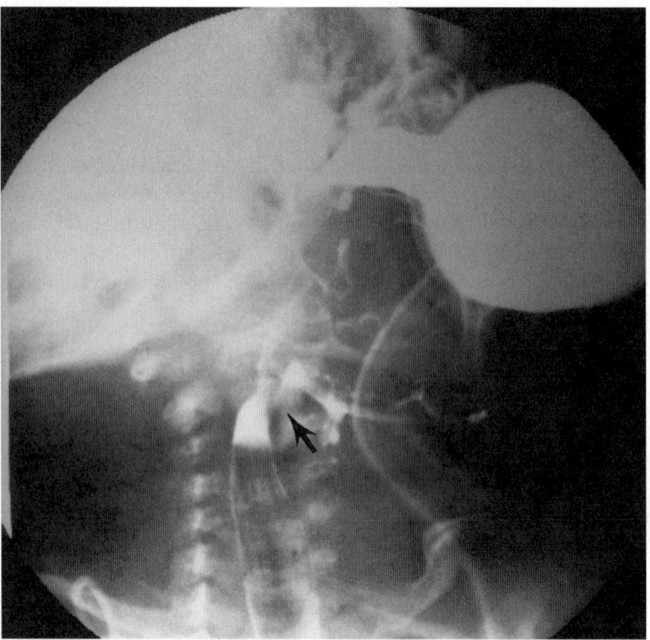

FIG. 51-5. Esophagogram demonstrating the sinus tract from pyriform sinus (*arrow*) consistent with branchial pouch anomaly.

demonstrate a fistula between pyriform sinus and neck (Fig. 51-5).

A cartilaginous remnant at the anterior border of the sternocleidomastoid muscle is usually not associated with a tract or cyst and requires only simple local excision. An elliptical incision is made around a preauricular sinus, and dissection is carried out in the pretragal groove to the cartilage of the external auditory canal. Branchial cleft remnants associated with fistulas require complete excision of the ostium and dissection of the tract up to its origin in the external auditory canal, pharynx, or pyriform sinus, where it is ligated. Inserting a small probe may help to identify the tract at surgery. An elliptical incision should be made around the ostium, followed by location of the tract with precise dissection on the wall of the tract to minimize injury to adjacent structures.

First branchial cleft sinus tracts may course through the parotid gland in proximity to the facial nerve (Fig. 51-6A). The patient's face is turned up on the involved side, and draping should be done to allow visualization of the lateral aspect of the eye and corner of the mouth. Muscle relaxants should be avoided; a nerve stimulator should be available to avoid injury to the facial nerve branches. The incision adjacent to the mandible should be parallel and at least 1 cm inferior to the lower border of the ramus to avoid an unsightly scar. The incision should extend in front of the ear as necessary to dissect out the entire tract. The superficial lobe of the parotid gland may need to be reflected upward to expose the tract or excised in cases of chronic infection. The tract needs to be followed to its eventual termination in the external auditory canal where it is ligated with absorbable suture.

Second branchial cleft anomalies should be excised with the neck positioned in slight hyperextension and turned away from the lesion (see Fig. 51-6B). These sinus tracts often require a ''stepladder'' counter incision to visualize and dissect out the

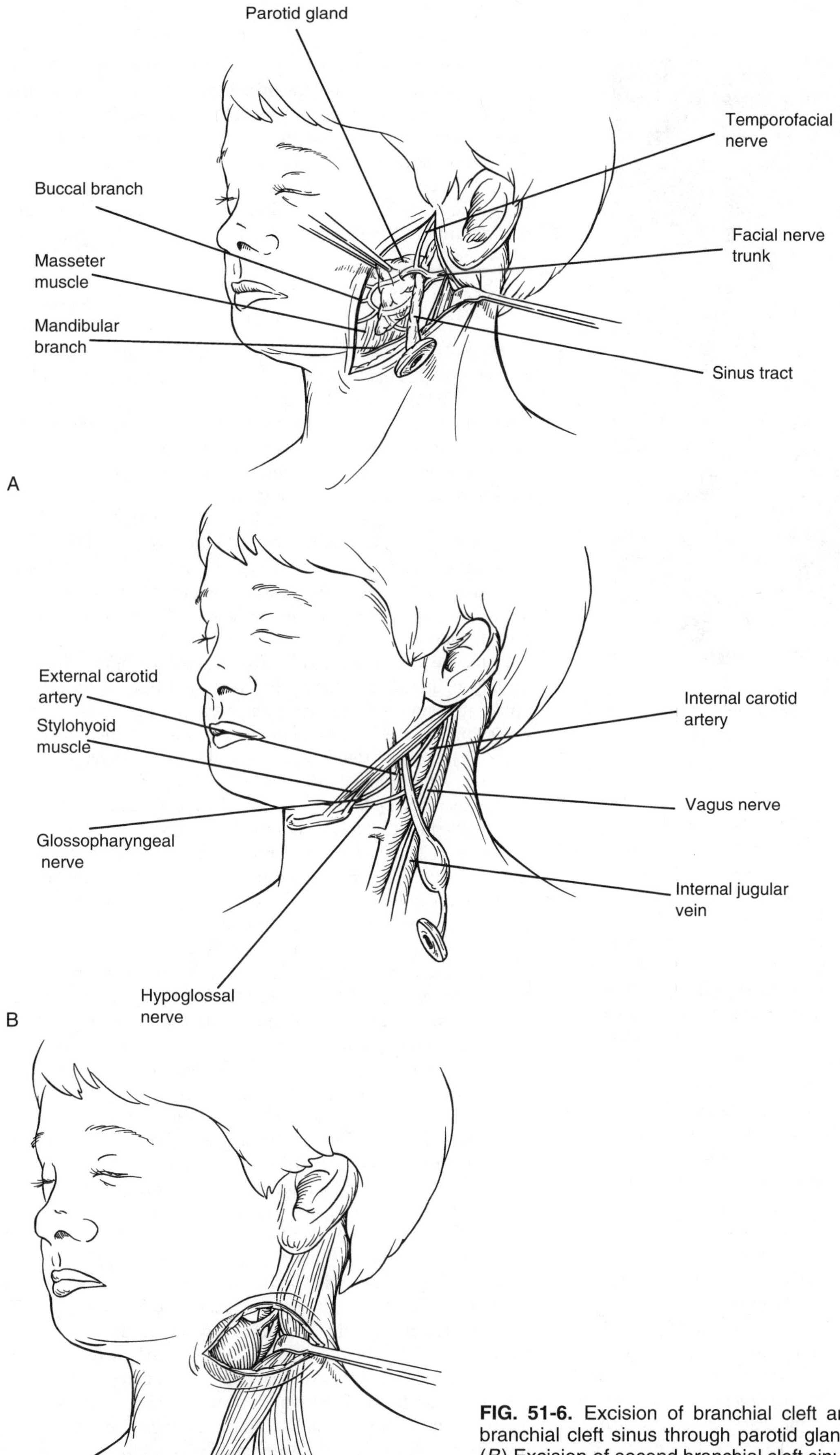

FIG. 51-6. Excision of branchial cleft anomalies. (*A*) Excision of first branchial cleft sinus through parotid gland to external auditory meatus. (*B*) Excision of second branchial cleft sinus through carotid bifurcation to tonsillar fossa. (*C*) Branchial cyst with pedicle posterior to jugular vein.

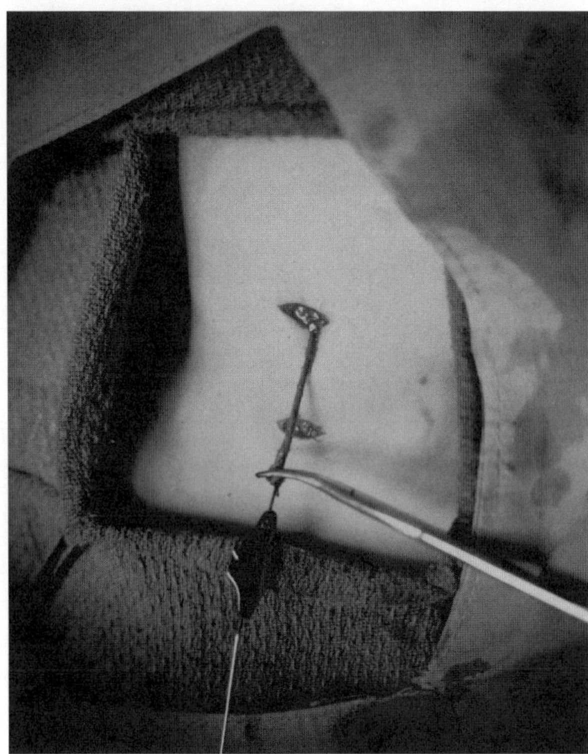

FIG. 51-7. Operative photograph illustrating stair-step incision used in excising a second branchial cleft sinus. A probe has been introduced into the sinus tract to aid in dissection.

entire tract (Fig. 51-7). The tract courses between internal and external carotid arteries, ultimately terminating in the tonsillar fossa. Care should be taken to avoid injury to the hypoglossal and glossopharyngeal nerves, which are deep to the tract. The tract is dissected as far as possible followed by ligation with absorbable suture. Drainage is reserved for wounds complicated by previous infection. Isolated branchial cysts in the neck are approached through a transverse neck incision made in a skin crease in proximity to the cystic enlargement (see Fig. 51-6C). A tract leading to the pharynx should always be looked for to prevent a recurrence. The spinal accessory, hypoglossal, and vagus nerves may be in proximity to this type of cyst.

Third or fourth branchial cleft anomalies can be difficult to both recognize and treat. They almost always occur on the left side. In an older child or adolescent, the tract entering the pyriform sinus can sometimes be recognized endoscopically and cannulated with a Fogarty catheter before operating on the neck. A left hemithyroidectomy is usually needed as part of the en bloc dissection of the anomaly, since the tract travels through or in proximity to the upper left lobe of the thyroid gland. After it leaves the thyroid gland, the tract travels cephalad in proximity to the superior laryngeal nerve and the hypoglossal nerve then deviates medially to the pyriform sinus. Complete excision requires that the tract be followed to the pyriform sinus, where it is ligated in proximity. The incision is closed over the drainage. The procedure may be complicated by a leak at the site of pyriform sinus closure, and the patient is best treated in this instance with a nasogastric or nasojejunal feeding tube for 2 weeks until the area closes spontaneously.

For remnants of the embryologic branchial apparatus, the goal of therapy is complete excision. If infection is evident when the child first presents, initial incision with drainage or antimicrobial therapy is needed. Surgical extirpation should be delayed for several weeks following the surgical drainage procedure. Recurrence is likely if any portion of the congenital tract or cyst is left behind. Malignant degeneration has been reported in branchial remnants persisting to adulthood.

Ranula

A ranula is a sublingual cyst or mucocele and is a benign retention cyst in the floor of the mouth originating from salivary glands.[12] It can appear as a pea-sized swelling to the right or left of the midline adjacent to the frenulum, as a submandibular swelling, or as a large cystic swelling extending from the base of the tongue bilaterally or unilaterally from the dental arch to the hypopharynx, producing airway obstruction.

There are two varieties of ranula—simple and plunging. Each has a different clinical behavior and appearance and requires a different treatment. Simple ranulas are true retention cysts of the unnamed but numerous salivary glands lying in proximity to the lining of the mucous membrane of the oral cavity. They arise from ductal obstruction with secondary cyst formation in the blocked duct and have a true epithelial lining. They are usually painless, unilateral, fluctuant, and have a translucent bluish appearance. With increasing size, they can cross the midline submucosally resulting in tongue deviation. Plunging ranulas are cysts that extend beyond the mucous membrane of the oral cavity through the mylohyoid muscle into the fascial planes of the neck. They may appear as a mass in the neck without any visible intraoral lesion and can be confused with other cysts of the neck. They arise as a consequence of ductal obstruction, lack an epithelial lining and are pseudocysts. Definitive diagnosis rests on the anatomic relation of the cyst and pathologic evaluation of the cyst wall following excision.

A simple ranula should be unroofed into the oral cavity. A probe is placed in the Wharton duct to avoid unintentional injury to this structure, and the dome of the cyst is circumscribed, with the oral mucous membrane sutured to the margin of the cyst with a running interlocking stitch of absorbable suture. The ranula cavity obliterates over 1 to 2 weeks after the procedure.

Plunging ranulas should be treated by meticulous dissection of the cyst and excision in continuity with the sublingual salivary gland of origin. The sublingual glands lie in the floor of the mouth on either side of the lingual frenulum in the sublingual depression on the inner surface of the mandible. The glands are covered by the mucous membrane of the floor of the mouth and lie on the mylohyoid muscle inferiorly and are bounded by the submandibular glands laterally. A sublingual gland is generally approached intraorally by making a linear incision lateral to the lingual frenulum or adjacent to the sublingual fold. The submandibular duct is cannulated before dissection, and the course of the lingual nerve is noted where it passes deep to the duct. Blunt dissection of the sublingual gland is then performed as far as the submandibular gland. If the cyst is large, the dissection is carried along the lateral border to the mylohyoid muscle into the submandibular region of the neck, and an external incision is made to ensure complete excision of the cyst.

Thyroglossal Duct Cyst, Dermoids, and Midline Cervical Clefts

A thyroglossal duct cyst may be found from the foramen cecum of the tongue to the normal position of the thyroid gland. Ectopic thyroid tissue may be associated with the cyst or sinus tract. The cyst is generally located overlying the hyoid bone in the midline and is always within 2 cm of the midline. Although the lesion may be noted at any age, thyroglossal duct cysts are usually recognized by age 5 years.[13] This cyst moves with protrusion of the tongue and swallowing. Thyroglossal cysts never have natural fistulas to the neck because the embryologic thyroglossal tract does not reach the surface of the neck. An external draining sinus may be the result of spontaneous or surgical drainage of an infected cyst.

Congenital dermoid inclusion cysts are superficial and located in proximity to the hyoid bone. They are epithelial-lined cysts with variable skin appendages in a mesodermal stroma. These masses do not move with swallowing or tongue protrusion. On occasion, a dermoid cyst ruptures, resulting in an intense granulomatous inflammatory reaction. In contrast to thyroglossal duct cysts, dermoid cysts rarely become infected.

A midline cervical cleft presents as a vertically oriented patch of thinly epithelialized tissue in the low anterior midline of the neck, several centimeters in length and 4 to 6 mm wide. It may have a raw and reddish moist surface or may be adorned by skin tabs, short sinuses that end blindly, or cartilaginous remnants.

A thyroglossal duct cyst complicated by infection should first be managed by incision and drainage and antimicrobial agents. When the infection has resolved, definitive operation is performed. The patient is positioned with the neck extended, and a transverse incision is made overlying the cyst or around a sinus tract which may have formed to the skin (Fig. 51-8A). The cyst has a tract that penetrates the platysma muscle and leads to the hyoid bone (see Fig. 51-8B). A wide total excision of the tract to include the mid-portion of the hyoid bone should be done.[14] The muscular attachments to the superior and inferior aspects of the body of the hyoid bone are divided (see Fig. 51-8C). The tract usually coarses through the hyoid bone and extends to the foramen cecum. The dissection is continued, removing a core of tissue at the base of the tongue (see Fig. 51-8D). To determine proximity to the foramen cecum, the surgeon can ask the anesthesiologist to depress the base of the tongue with a gloved finger, which aids in recognizing the most proximal portion of the tract. The tract is ligated where it meets the base of the tongue. Closure is accomplished over a small penrose drain which usually is removed the morning after surgery.

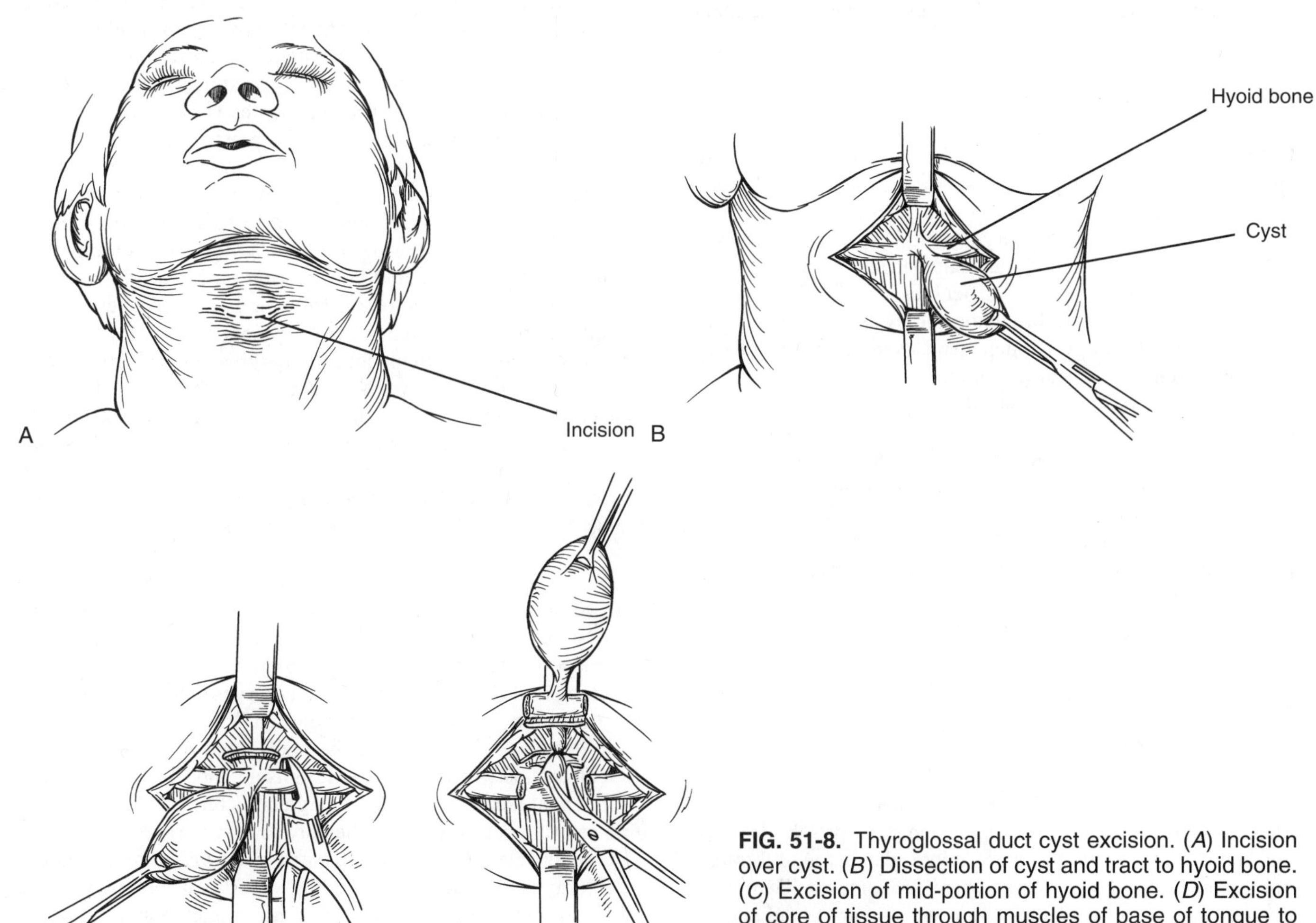

FIG. 51-8. Thyroglossal duct cyst excision. (*A*) Incision over cyst. (*B*) Dissection of cyst and tract to hyoid bone. (*C*) Excision of mid-portion of hyoid bone. (*D*) Excision of core of tissue through muscles of base of tongue to foramen cecum and ligation of duct.

Complete initial excision of a thyroglossal duct cyst as described is generally curative. Recurrences are usually associated with prior history of infection or inadequate surgical excision. Thyroid neoplasia has been described in ectopic thyroid tissue, both associated and unassociated with thyroglossal duct cysts.

Dermoid cysts are treated with simple excision and do not recur if the entire cyst wall is excised. Excision of a midline cervical cleft is of cosmetic importance only and is treated electively. Excision is done with a series of Z-plasty incisions to prevent a linear contracture that interferes with extension of the head.

Thymic Cyst

A thymic cyst can present as a firm, nontender cystic swelling in the lower third of the lateral neck. These cysts often appear anterior to the sternocleidomastoid muscle but can extend beneath it.[15] Approximately half have a mediastinal extension. Chest radiographs help diagnose those with mediastinal components. A thymic cyst occupies the anterior mediastinum and lies anterior to the trachea, and it may be associated with parathyroid tissue. A cervical thymic cyst can usually be completely removed via a transverse cervical incision centered over the mass. If a mediastinal extension precludes complete excision by this approach, it may be necessary to split the upper sternum for exposure of the anterior upper mediastinum. The wound is not drained unless the thoracic duct is injured. Diagnosis is made by the identification of thymic tissue in the cyst wall.

Other Cystic Masses

Additional cystic masses that can be seen in the neck include epidermoid cysts, laryngoceles, and duplication cysts. Epidermoid cysts are epithelial-lined cysts without skin appendages or mesodermal elements. A laryngocele is a cyst that arises as a dilation of the sac of the laryngeal ventricle, usually causing inspiratory stridor or feeding difficulties. Duplication cysts of the esophagus or ectopic bronchogenic cysts can occasionally be found low in the neck. Bronchogenic cysts indent the trachea, causing stridor or tracheal deviation.

Epidermoid cysts require simple excision. If the cyst is ruptured, care should be taken to remove the entire cyst wall to prevent a recurrence. Treatment of a laryngocele requires airway control followed by needle aspiration or surgical excision of the cyst. Resection of the entire cyst usually is not required. Esophageal duplication cysts are treated by resection or marsupialization. Bronchogenic paratracheal cysts characteristically do not connect to the tracheal lumen and can be dissected cleanly away from the trachea or adjacent great vessels.

BENIGN TUMORS

Salivary Glands

The salivary glands can be subdivided into three major glands—including the parotid, submandibular or submaxillary, and sublingual—as well as many minor glands found throughout the oral cavity, pharynx, and paranasal sinuses. There is an inverse relation between the size of the salivary gland and the likelihood that a tumor within that gland is malignant.

The most common benign neoplasm affecting the major salivary glands is a benign vascular lesion, such as a hemangioma or lymphangioma.[8] Typical hemangiomatous lesions are first noticed within a few weeks or months of birth and are usually confined to the intracapsular portion of the gland. A surface sentinel lesion occasionally provides the clue to diagnosis. Diagnosis can be made by ultrasonography, especially with Doppler.

Pleomorphic or mixed tumors of the parotid gland in children are next in frequency and are the most common epithelial tumors. Most are benign and occur in the superficial lobe. Other benign epithelial tumors that occur in children include Warthin tumors and cystadenomas. Warthin tumors (papillary cystadenoma lymphomatosum) usually occur in males, approximately 10% are bilateral, and they are composed of lymphoid tissue containing germinal centers.

Salivary gland pathology that requires surgical intervention in infancy or childhood is unusual, with the parotid gland being the most commonly affected. The operative strategies are often challenging because of the need to dissect the facial nerve.[8,16] Benign processes are more common than malignant, and inflammatory processes are more common than neoplasms.

Treatment of hemangiomas, hemangioendotheliomas, and mixed lesions of the salivary glands is generally conservative as involution of vascular components is expected by age 4 to 6 years. This is in spite of an often rapidly expanding lesion in infancy. Operation is fraught with a high risk of bleeding and facial nerve injury. Patients with primary or residual juxtaparotid lymphangioma may ultimately require one or several staged excisions. The goal of any procedure requiring a direct approach to the parotid gland is to achieve as complete an excision as possible with dissection and preservation of the facial nerve.

Surgical treatment of pleomorphic or mixed tumors of the parotid gland consists of superficial or total parotidectomy to include a margin of normal tissue in all directions around the tumor with dissection and preservation of the facial nerve. Recurrences are fairly common following surgical excision if a limited approach is taken or tumor spillage occurs. For recurrent tumors or tumors with inadequate margins, postoperative radiotherapy effectively prevents further recurrences. If the diagnosis of a tumor in the parotid gland by cell type is not made preoperatively and there is a solid mass in the parotid, parotid lobectomy is indicated. If the diagnosis of a Warthin tumor is made preoperatively, enucleation suffices to treat the tumor, but patients must be followed to observe the contralateral gland.

Operations on the parotid gland are performed without muscle relaxants and with the nerve stimulator available. The facial nerve runs between the two anatomic lobes of the parotid gland and should be preserved unless involved by tumor. The incision is made in the preauricular area and carried inferiorly toward the angle of the mandible, where it curves anterior but parallel to the ramus and at least 1 cm below it (Fig. 51-9A). The digastric muscle is exposed, and the main trunk of the facial nerve identified between the digastric muscle and the external auditory canal (see Fig. 51-9B). The gland is retracted superior and anteriorly because all branches of the nerve are identified until the superficial lobe is removed (see Fig. 51-9C). If a deep parotidectomy should also be done, the superficial lobe is removed first. Branches of the facial nerve are retracted and protected. If branches of the facial nerve or the main trunk itself require

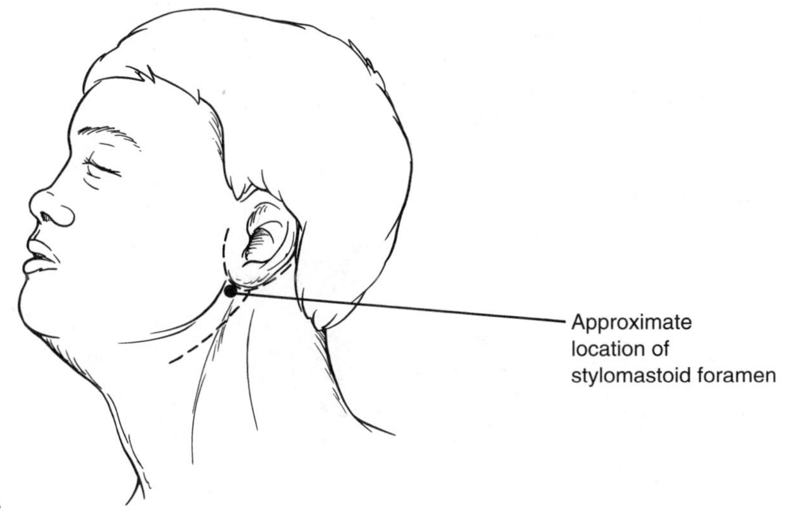

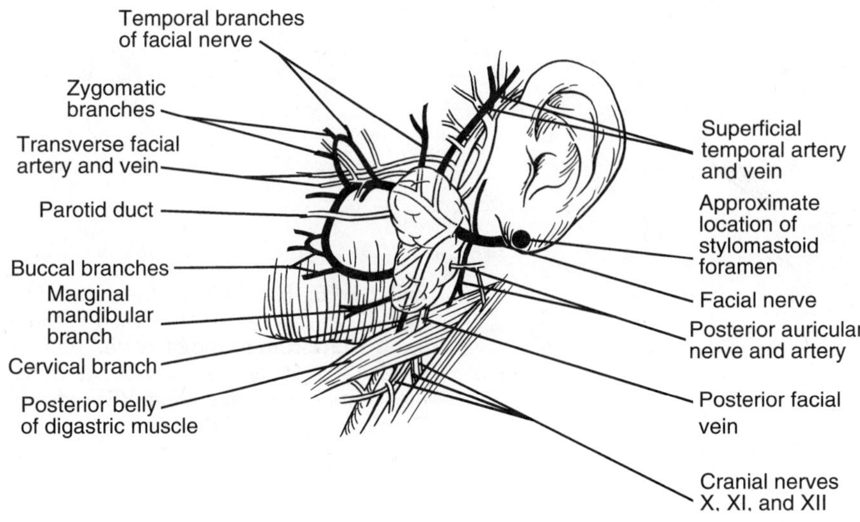

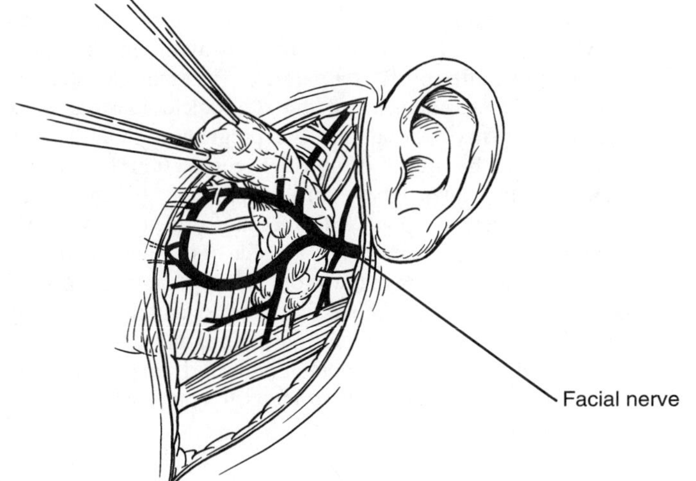

FIG. 51-9. Superficial parotidectomy. (*A*) Incision. (*B*) Relation of the branches of facial nerve and vessels to the parotid gland. (*C*) Dissection and elevation of the superficial lobe exposes the facial nerve's main trunk.

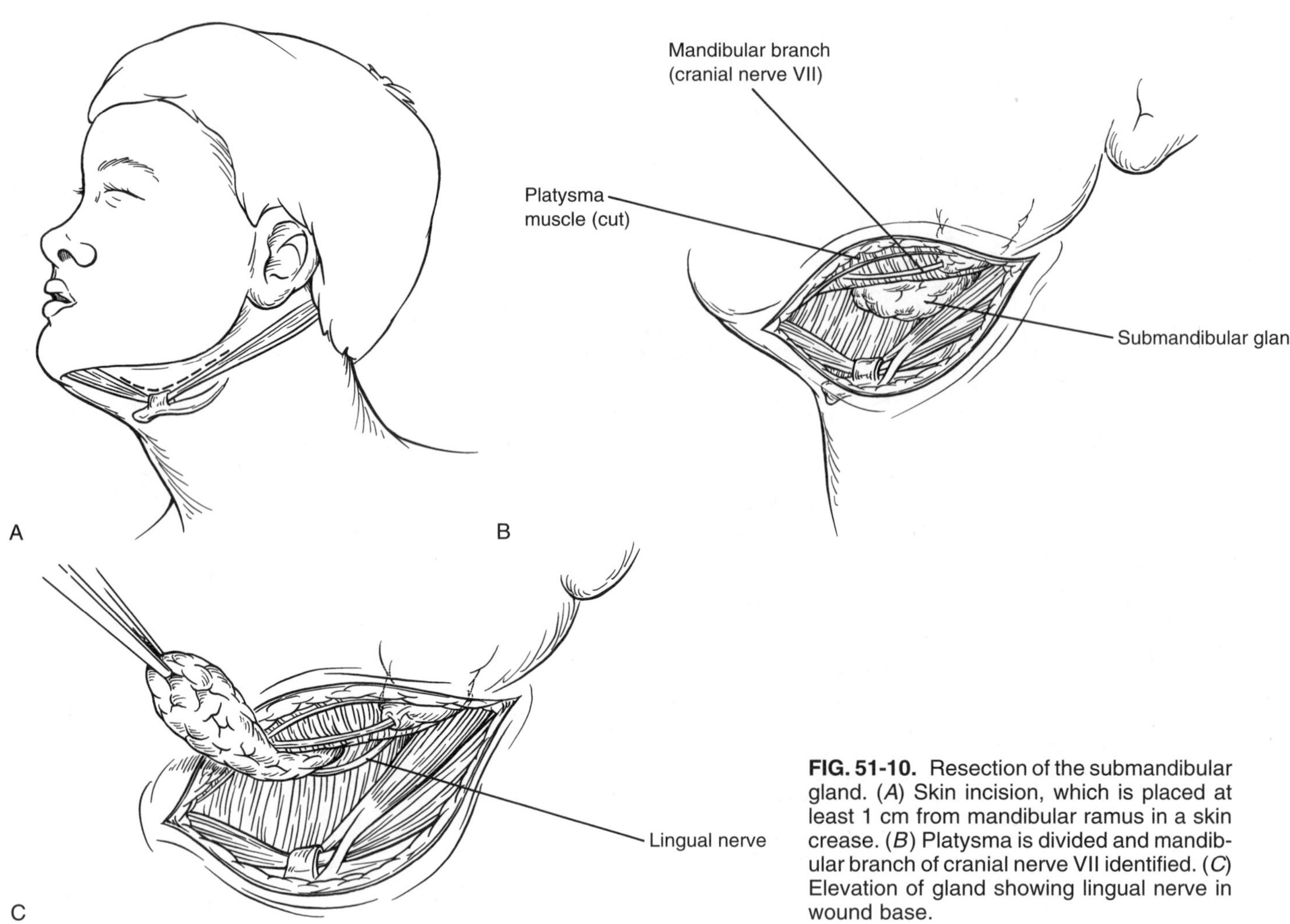

FIG. 51-10. Resection of the submandibular gland. (*A*) Skin incision, which is placed at least 1 cm from mandibular ramus in a skin crease. (*B*) Platysma is divided and mandibular branch of cranial nerve VII identified. (*C*) Elevation of gland showing lingual nerve in wound base.

resection, nerve grafting is often used. The sural nerve and the greater auricular nerve are considered to be acceptable conduits. The facial nerve has the highest success rate (about 90%) for peripheral nerve grafting. It may take 6 months or more for function to be restored following grafting.

Resection of the submandibular gland is usually performed through a submandibular incision carried through the subcutaneous tissue and platysma (Fig. 51-10*A*). The most important structure to identify and to avoid is the mandibular branch of cranial nerve VII, which controls the ability to raise the commissure of the lip on the ipsilateral side (see Fig. 51-10*B*). The lingual nerve is deep to the submandibular gland and must be identified before dividing the deep blood supply to the gland (see Fig. 51-10*C*). Damage to this nerve results in loss of taste. The chorda tympani nerve extends off of the lingual nerve and is divided during resection of the submandibular gland. The hypoglossal nerve is deep to the gland also, but usually is not seen during excision and should not be damaged during resection of the gland.

Torticollis

Torticollis or fibromatosis colli is a fibromatosis of childhood and the only fibromatosis with exclusive localization to a single anatomic site. It involves tightness of one sternocleidomastoid muscle following an idiopathic inflammatory process in the newborn period. It typically is noticed by the infant's parents a few weeks after birth as a painless, firm mass located in the body of the sternal head of the sternocleidomastoid muscle. Questioning may reveal that the pregnancy or delivery was characterized by breech or unusual presentation, forceps assistance, or prolonged labor. On examination, the child usually has a characteristic pose with the chin tipped away from the lesion and head pulled down to the side of the mass. In instances where the diagnosis is in question, an FNA can be helpful (Fig. 51-11). A combination of passive exercise and massage usually enhances spontaneous resolution of torticollis. Surgical treatment by dividing the sternocleidomastoid muscle is reserved for recalcitrant cases in which facial hypoplasia results on the involved side.

Fibrous Tissue Tumors

Although generally considered benign, the fibrous tissue tumors are a group of histologically aggressive-looking tumors of mesenchymal origin that have no tendency to distant spread.[17] Their behavior tends to vary with the patient's age. Aggressive fibromatoses often arise around the mandible and

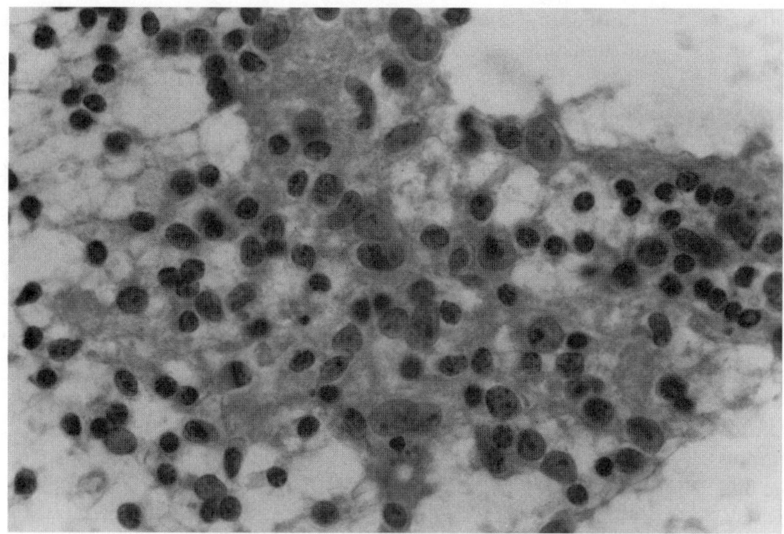

FIG. 51-11. Photomicrograph of smear from a fine-needle aspiration of a child with a right neck mass at the head of the sternocleidomastoid muscle. An admixture of degenerating, multinucleated myocytes (*arrows*) and fibroblasts confirm the clinical diagnosis of fibromatosis colli. (PAP, × 400.)

may grow rapidly. The prognosis is best if the tumor is diagnosed during the first 2 years of life. A favorable response to chemotherapy is also age-dependent; children older than 7 years and adolescents respond poorly. Most fibrous tissue tumors can be removed by simple surgical excision, but some recur. If the lesion cannot be totally excised or recurs soon after surgical excision, chemotherapy is indicated followed by reexcision of residual or recurrent disease.

Neurofibroma

Plexiform neurofibroma is the most frequently occurring benign tumor of the peripheral nerves. It is a form of von Recklinghausen disease, which is nonmetastasizing but locally invasive. Neurofibromas of this type become symptomatic early and exhibit progressive growth throughout the patient's life. A mass effect is caused by abnormal tumor tissue and by simultaneous growth of surrounding mesenchymal soft tissues. Plexiform neurofibromas are not premalignant, but total removal of abnormal tissue usually cannot be accomplished without cosmetic deformity. Surrounding bone responds by remodeling and absorption. Surgical procedures are designed to relieve symptoms or improve cosmesis.

Arteriovenous Malformations

Arteriovenous malformations are benign complex vascular lesions of congenital origin. Primary neck arteriovenous malformations are unusual, but may present as a pulsatile mass in the neck. High-output congestive heart failure can occur with very large symptomatic arteriovenous malformations. A more superficial mass is recognized by increased local warmth associated with pulsating varicosities under or within the skin. Examination with the Doppler can reveal a continuous bruit. The diagnosis may be suggested by Doppler ultrasound and confirmed by angiography, which reveals arterial dilation and tortuosity, arteriovenous connections, early venous filling, and associated dilation of venous channels.

The approach to managing congenital arteriovenous malformations depends on the extent of the lesion, its location, and whether there are associated physiologic derangements. A cure can only be obtained by total resection of the entire malformation, and this is often not feasible in the neck. Transarterial selective embolization may be needed to stem the progressive growth of the malformation. Embolization can be used alone or as a preoperative adjuvant to surgical resection.

MALIGNANT LESIONS

Cancer is the second leading cause of death in children aged 1 to 14 years, after traumatic injuries. Approximately 5% of the malignancies involve the head and neck, but 27% of pediatric cancer deaths are due to primary tumors in this region. Many of these tumors are rare. Table 51-1 lists tumors that may present in the cervical area. The benign nature of a tumor may often be predicted by mass location, appearance, and definition from surrounding structures. Most malignant lesions do not present until childhood or in the teenage years; few present at birth. Most midline lesions are benign.

MALIGNANT LYMPHOMAS

Malignant lymphomas are the third most common malignant tumor in children. Of all childhood lymphomas, approximately 60% are nonHodgkin lymphomas (NHL) and 40% are Hodgkin disease (HD). These are discussed in detail in Chapter 37.

NonHodgkin Lymphoma

Approximately 10% of all NHL in children aged birth to 15 years in the United States arise in the head and neck.[18] There are three major histopathologic subtypes of NHL in children: small-cell noncleaved (Burkitt or nonBurkitt); lymphoblastic lymphoma; and large-cell lymphoma. Most of the NHL presenting in the neck are of the small-cell noncleaved histologic subtype and predominantly B-cell origin, and they arise from lymphoid tissue around or near facial bones including the mandible, Waldeyer ring, maxillary sinus, thyroid gland, salivary glands, or lymph nodes in the neck. The endemic Burkitt-type of NHL, which has a predilection for the mandible and maxillary antrum, is relatively rare in the United States. Lymphoblastic lymphoma is a T-cell lymphoma that is usually supradiaphragmatic and commonly presents as a mediastinal mass. The diffuse large-cell lymphoma can present in a variety of locations but often is extranodal. Follicular (nodular) lymphomas that remain localized to nodes or nodal change are very rare during childhood. The skin of the head and neck is also the most common location for cutaneous lymphoma in childhood. The median age of presentation is 6 to 8 years, and the most common histopathologic subtype is lymphoblastic.

The incidence of NHL in childhood increases with age (mean 8 to 10 years) and has a male predominance of nearly 3 to 1. The tumors usually grow rapidly causing neck swelling in almost half of patients or a visible mass associated with pain due to pressure or invasion of nerves or bony structures. The diagnosis is often made within a month of symptom onset.

In nonendemic localities, the mandible is the most common head and neck site for Burkitt lymphoma, followed by the Waldeyer ring and the maxillary sinus. Tumors affecting the mandible may result in loosening of teeth or toothache-like complaints, localized swelling, and lip numbness. A cervical swelling or mass representing metastases may be seen with tonsillar and base of tongue lesions.

No studies specific to childhood head and neck lymphomas are available for determining independent prognostic factors in multivariate analysis. Data from existing adult and pediatric studies suggest that extent of disease at diagnosis is the most important predictor of outcome, with bone marrow involvement and intracranial extension associated with poor prognosis.

Hodgkin Disease

Hodgkin disease is relatively uncommon in children, particularly those younger than 5 years. In children, HD has a male-to-female predilection of approximately 2 to 1. The cervical lymph nodes are most commonly involved, and the most common histologic subtype is nodular sclerosing (65%), followed by mixed cellularity (22%), and lymphocyte predominant (9%). Lymphocyte-depleted Hodgkin disease is unusual in children.

When a tumor with primary or nodal involvement in the neck is suspected, a tissue diagnosis can be obtained by incisional biopsy of enlarged or matted neck nodes in the neck. Biopsies should be performed with preservation of neurovascular structures. Initial frozen sections should be done to clarify the diagnosis. If the tumor suggests HD or NHL, tumor resection should not be attempted and the surgical excision should be confined to the minimum required to establish the diagnosis.[18] Adequate tissue must be obtained for diagnostic and specialized studies. There should be good communication between surgeon and pathologist before the procedure regarding the amount of tissue

required, and biopsy material should be sent fresh and sterile for standard hematoxylin–eosin staining, immunophenotyping, cytogenetics, and gene rearrangements. A portion of the specimen should be frozen in the event other studies are required later. If preoperative CT scan identifies mediastinal involvement with impending airway compromise, the biopsy may require local anesthesia because of the risk of cardiorespiratory arrest due to cardiovascular collapse during general anesthesia. Staging, treatment, and prognosis of NHL and HD is discussed elsewhere in this textbook.

Salivary Glands

Malignant tumors of the salivary glands may occur at any age, and congenital lesions have been reported.[8,16] An association of head and neck irradiation with subsequent development of salivary gland malignancy has also been described. Approximately half of all epithelial tumors of the salivary glands in children are malignant, and they occur more commonly in females. Asymptomatic swelling is the most common presenting symptom. Fixation to skin or deep tissues or weakness or paralysis of the facial nerve invariably indicates that a tumor is malignant. The parotid is the most common salivary gland involved, and tumors of minor salivary gland origin are almost unheard of before puberty.

Mucoepidermoid carcinoma (MEC) is the most common childhood salivary gland malignancy (50%), and prognosis correlates with pathologic grading. This tumor contains both epidermoid and mucus-containing cells and can be low-grade or high-grade. Approximately two thirds of the tumors are low-grade, have a low incidence of recurrence and infrequent cervical node metastasis, and have an excellent prognosis.

Acinic cell carcinoma is the next most common epithelial salivary gland malignancy, most of which are low-grade neoplasms. Next in frequency are adenocarcinomas and then undifferentiated carcinoma. Adenoid cystic carcinomas and malignant mixed tumors occur infrequently in children.

Epithelial salivary gland tumors may present in the neonatal period, are usually of major salivary gland origin, and occur predominantly in the parotid gland. They have been termed *embryomas* or *sialoblastomas*, and approximately 25% are malignant, variously classified as low-grade basaloid adenocarcinomas or adenoid cystic carcinomas.

The presence of nodal enlargement is another strong presumption of malignancy, with squamous carcinoma, MEC, adenocarcinoma, and malignant mixed tumor showing the highest incidence of regional node involvement. Distant metastases are uncommon.

Childhood NHL occurs rarely in the salivary glands, and the parotid is most commonly involved. Most patients present with an enlarging mass, which may be painful if the tumor has invaded bone. Rhabdomyosarcoma of the parotid gland has been reported with the usual presentation of a mass at the angle of the mandible. Involvement of one or more cranial nerves or concomitant cervical adenopathy is not uncommon, and many patients present with advanced disease.

For malignant salivary gland pathology, surgery is the primary treatment modality.[16] Operative therapy and results vary with location of the tumor, stage of disease, and histologic type.

Small tumors require wide excision. For the parotid, this usually involves conservative superficial parotidectomy or lateral parotidectomy with seventh nerve preservation. For the submandibular gland, the excision involves resecting the gland. Total parotidectomy may be indicated in conjunction with conservative node dissection in the presence of palpable regional lymph nodes. Controversy exists regarding neck dissection in patients with no palpable nodes.

Mucoepidermoid carcinoma frequently metastasizes to regional neck nodes but rarely disseminates. For this reason, conservative node dissection at the time of parotidectomy is usually done. This dissection includes the nodes in the subdigastric area, the nodes above the spinal accessory nerve, and all of the periparotid lymph nodes. If grossly or histologically positive nodes are present in the operative specimen, the operation can be extended into a radical or modified neck dissection.

Adenocarcinomas and malignant mixed tumors are treated by wide excision, and some surgeons advocate prophylactic radical neck dissection. Acinic cell carcinoma is a slow-growing, low-grade tumor treated by local excision. The adenoid cystic carcinoma (cylindroma) is a slow-growing tumor that spreads along nerve sheaths and is difficult to eradicate surgically. High-dose radiotherapy is often effective in controlling local disease, but late metastases are common. In patients presenting with unresectable parotid disease, surgical treatment is usually limited to biopsy or tumor debulking, followed by appropriate adjuvant therapy.

Surgical therapy is individualized for tumors of intermediate malignancy or invasiveness. The seventh nerve is sacrificed only if it is found to be adhering to or invaded by tumor. In some cases, resection of submandibular or malignant minor salivary tumors or radical parotid gland resection also involves removing the adjacent zygoma, temporal bone, mandibular ramus, or masseter muscle. Adjunctive radiation therapy seems to enhance locoregional tumor control, particularly with high-stage, high-grade malignancies. Lymphomas and sarcomas that arise within salivary glands are treated like similar tumors elsewhere in the body.

Neuroblastoma

Neuroblastoma only rarely presents as a primary tumor in the neck, and an enlarged neck node may be the first sign of disseminated retroperitoneal or intrathoracic disease.[19] Congenital neuroblastoma is known to occur in the neonate, presenting externally in the lateral neck or internally in the retropharyngeal space. In the infant, the mass is usually a painless, firm, smooth lesion. Physical signs and symptoms may include dysphasia, cough, hoarseness, or stridor. In older children, a fullness of the lateral oropharyngeal wall can be detected, with advanced cases associated with earache and facial paralysis. Rarely, symptoms caused by increased levels of circulating catecholamines or cutaneous manifestations may occur. Primary cervical neuroblastoma often originates in the cervical autonomic chain and has a favorable prognosis, particularly in infants.

Primary cervical neuroblastomas are treated with surgical excision if possible. Staging to ascertain the site of origin as well as dissemination should be done. Surgical intervention is not recommended in the presence of dissemination.

Sarcomas

Rhabdomyosarcoma is the most common sarcoma occurring in children, as well as the most common sarcoma occurring in the neck.[20] The nasopharynx is the second most common site in the head and neck region, and primary involvement of the soft tissues of the neck is possible but uncommon. Approximately 80% to 85% of head and neck rhabdomyosarcomas are the embryonal type, and most others are the alveolar type. Primary rhabdomyosarcomas of the salivary glands also occur but are seldom seen in children. Staging of rhabdomyosarcoma is based on clinical findings and takes into consideration the adequacy of tumor removal. Fibrosarcomas, malignant fibrous histiocytomas, myosarcomas, liposarcomas, sarcomas of peripheral nerve origin, and vascular sarcomas are uncommon in children.

Primary rhabdomyosarcomas of the nasopharynx are treated with biopsy followed by multiagent chemotherapy and radiation. Primary rhabdomyosarcomas or soft tissue sarcomas of the neck are widely excised if possible followed by adjuvant chemotherapy with or without irradiation. Wide resection margins in the head and neck are anatomically difficult to achieve, and high local recurrence rates are expected if the tumor is not removed with wide margins. Routine elective neck dissection is generally believed to be unwarranted.

Germ-Cell Neoplasms

Germ-cell neoplasms diagnosed in the first two decades of life are often found in extragonadal sites, with approximately 5% to 6% involving the head and neck region.[21] Many are present in the newborn, occurring most commonly in the midline or lateral neck (Fig. 51-12). They may also originate in or around the oropharynx (epignathi) and nasopharynx and typically present in the newborn with respiratory obstruction or feeding difficulties. Most germ-cell tumors in the head and neck of children are composed predominantly of teratomas, but some, such as endodermal sinus tumors, have other admixed

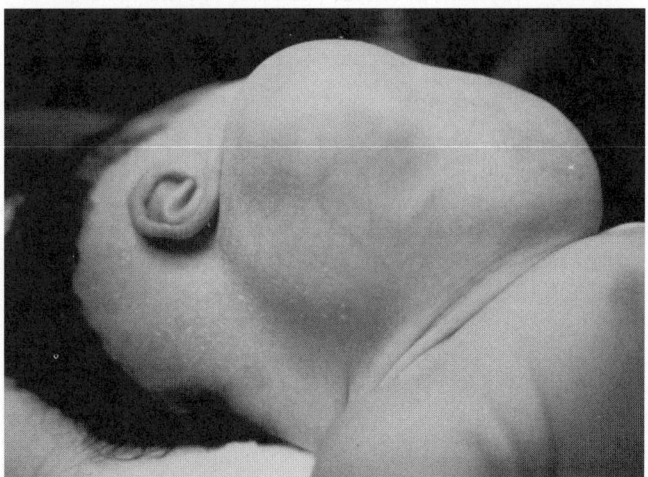

FIG. 51-12. Newborn infant with large cervical teratoma.

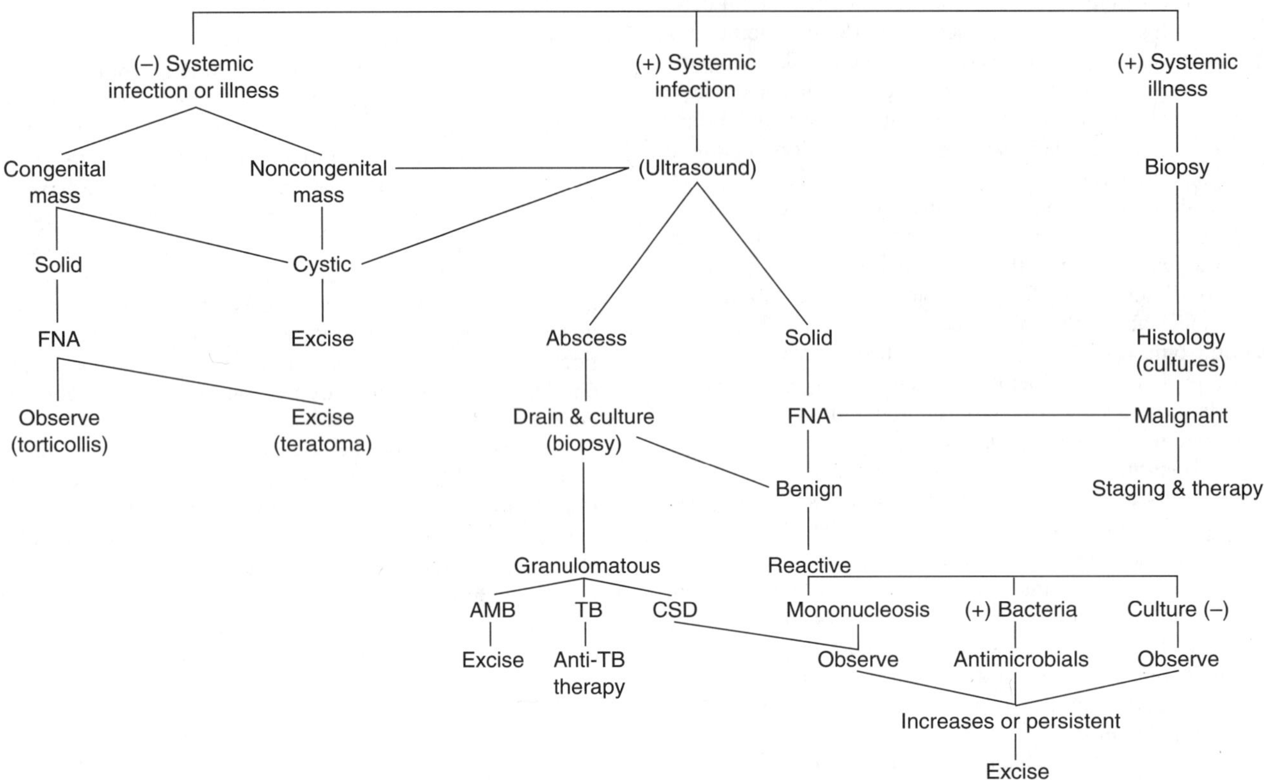

FIG. 51-13. Algorithm for the evaluation and treatment approach to neck masses in children. FNA, fine needle aspiration; AMB, atypical mycobacteria; TB, tuberculosis; CSD, cat scratch disease.

germ-cell components. True teratomas are lesions derived from all three germ-cell layers. The components of endodermal sinus tumor that present in a cervical teratoma usually behave aggressively, often leading to death. Serum alpha-fetoprotein is a helpful marker for both endodermal sinus tumors and teratomas.

The cervical region is the location of less than 10% of all teratomas in children. The mother may have polyhydramnios, and cesarian section is recommended if the diagnosis is made prenatally. Generally, cervical teratomas present as large submental or submandibular masses at birth. Most affected infants have respiratory distress or obstruction. The teratomas commonly are immature, but almost always behave in a benign fashion.

Management of cervical and pharyngeal teratomas begins with airway maintenance because mortality is related primarily to airway compromise. Excision is accomplished soon after birth. Nasopharyngeal teratomas must be differentiated from encephaloceles and gliomas, and intracranial extension must be excluded.

THERAPEUTIC AND SURGICAL CONSIDERATIONS

A general algorithm for the approach to neck masses in children is outlined in Figure 51-13.

REFERENCES

1. Skandalakis JE, Gray SW, Todd NW. The pharynx and its derivatives. In: Skandalakis JE, Gray SW, eds. Embryology for surgeons, ed 2. Baltimore, Williams & Wilkins, 1994:17.
2. Buchino JJ, Jones VF. Fine needle aspiration in the evaluation of children with lymphadenopathy. Arch Pediatr Adolesc Med 1994;148: 1327.
3. Taha AM, Davidson PT, Bailey WC. Surgical treatment of atypical mycobacterial lymphadenitis in children. Pediatr Infect Dis J 1985;4: 664.
4. Sigalet D, Lees G, Fanning A. Atypical tuberculosis in the pediatric patient: implications for the pediatric surgeon. J Pediatr Surg 1992;27: 1381.
5. Zangwill KM, Hamilton DH, Perkins BA, et al. Cat scratch disease in Connecticut: epidemiology, risk factors, and evaluation of a new diagnostic test. N Engl J Med 1993;329:8.
6. Committee on Infectious Diseases. Summaries of infectious diseases. In: Peter G, Halsey NA, Marcuse EK, et al, eds. Red Book, ed 23. Elk Grove Village, IL, American Academy of Pediatrics, 1994:150.
7. Koehler JE, Glaser CA, Tappero JW. *Rochalimaea henselae* infection: a new zoonosis with the domestic cat as reservoir. JAMA 1994;271: 531.
8. Welch KJ. The salivary glands. In: Welch KJ, Randolph JG, Ravitch MM, et al, eds. Pediatric surgery, ed 4. Chicago, Year Book Medical Publishers, 1986:487.
9. Chow AW. Life-threatening infections of the head and neck. Clin Infect Dis 1992;14:991.
10. Lin J-N, Wang K-L. Persistent third branchial apparatus. J Pediatr Surg 1991;26:663.
11. Godin MS, Kearns DB, Pransky SM, et al. Fourth branchial pouch

sinus: principles of diagnosis and management. Laryngoscope 1990; 100:174.

12. Quick CA, Lowell SH. Ranula and the sublingual salivary glands. Arch Otolaryngol 1977;103:397.

13. Telander RL, Filston HC. Review of head and neck lesions in infancy and childhood. Surg Clin North Am 1992;72:1429.

14. Ein SH, Shandling B, Stephens CA, et al. The problem of recurrent thyroglossal duct remnants. J Pediatr Surg 1984;19:437.

15. Wagner CW, Vinocur CD, Weintraub WH, et al. Respiratory complications in cervical thymic cysts. J Pediatr Surg 1988;23:657.

16. Spiro RH, Spiro JD. Salivary gland tumors. Head and neck cancer. II. Site-specific problems. Prob Gen Surg 1988;5:217.

17. Goepfert H, Cangir A. Head and neck tumors in infants and children. In: Head and Neck Cancer. I. General Considerations. Prob Gen Surg 1988;5:71.

18. LaQuaglia MP. Non-Hodgkin lymphoma of the head and neck in childhood. Semin Pediatr Surg 1994;3:207.

19. Haase GM. Head and neck neuroblastoma. Semin Pediatr Surg 1994; 3:194.

20. Wiener ES. Head and neck rhabdomyosarcoma. Semin Pediatr Surg 1994;3:203.

21. Filston HC. Hemangiomas, cystic hygromas, and teratomas of the head and neck. Semin Pediatr Surg 1994;3:147.

Surgery of Infants and Children: Scientific Principles and Practice, edited by
Keith T. Oldham, Paul M. Colombani, and Robert P. Foglia.
Lippincott–Raven Publishers, Philadelphia, © 1997.

CHAPTER 52

Thyroid and Parathyroid

Michael A. Skinner

Diseases of the thyroid and parathyroid glands are relatively unusual in children. In one population-based study of schoolage children in the western United States, the point prevalence of thyroid disease was 36.7 per 1000 children.[1] In about half of these cases, the diagnosis of diffuse gland hypertrophy (goiter) was made, and thyroiditis was the second most common abnormality. Thyroid nodules and disorders of altered thyroid hormone level were less common, and malignant neoplasms were exceedingly rare; only two cases of papillary thyroid carcinoma were found in this population of nearly 5000 children observed clinically for 3 years.

Surgical evaluation or treatment of thyroid disease may be necessary in patients exhibiting a physiologic abnormality, such as increased hormone secretion, or in cases of benign or malignant neoplasia. Rarely, a congenital anatomic anomaly of the thyroid necessitates surgery.

EMBRYOLOGY

The thyroid gland is the first endocrine organ to mature in fetal development. It arises as an outpouching of the embryonic alimentary tract at about 24 days' gestation. The structure originates as a thickening of the primitive pharyngeal floor just caudal to the median tongue bud, and soon elongates inferiorly to form the thyroid diverticulum. As the embryo enlarges, the developing thyroid gland descends into the neck from the base of the tongue. The organ passes ventral to the hyoid bone and the laryngeal cartilages, while maintaining a tubular connection to the tongue known as the *thyroglossal duct.* The opening of this duct into the base of the tongue is called the *foramen cecum.* Typically, the thyroglossal duct changes from a hollow structure to a solid diverticulum, and divides. The original opening into the oropharynx usually remains as a blind pit at the base of the tongue.

Histologically, the primordial thyroid cells begin to form discrete cords that further differentiate to form small cellular groups at about 10 weeks' gestation. In the 11th week, colloid begins to form, and thyroxine (T_4) can then be demonstrated in the embryo. Early in the development of the thyroid gland,

the ventral portions of the fourth pharyngeal pouches develop into the ultimobranchial bodies. These structures contain neural crest cells that migrate into the branchial arches and fuse with the embryonic thyroid gland. Subsequently, they diffuse through the gland to form the parafollicular cells or C cells.

The thyroid gland has usually reached its final location in the neck by 7 weeks' gestation. In about half of the population, there is a pyramidal lobe of the thyroid gland, which is the inferior portion of the thyroid diverticulum persisting as a cranial extension of the gland in the midline. Congenital malformations of the thyroid gland include thyroglossal ducts and sinuses, which are discussed elsewhere in this volume. Furthermore, accessory thyroid tissue originating from remnants of the thyroglossal duct may appear in the tongue or anywhere along the course of caudal migration during development. Rarely, but of occasional surgical importance, the gland fails to descend altogether, resulting in a lingual thyroid. Incomplete descent results in the gland appearing high in the neck or near the hyoid bone.

The parathyroid glands are derived from the third and fourth pharyngeal pouches. This process begins at about 5 weeks' gestation, when the epithelium in the dorsal portions of the pouches begins to proliferate, forming small nodules on the dorsal aspect of each pouch. During the 6th week of development, the parathyroid glands associated with the third pair of pharyngeal pouches migrate caudally with the thymic primordium, finally coming to rest on the dorsal surface of the thyroid gland low in the neck. The parathyroid glands arising from the fourth pharyngeal pouches also descend in the neck, but they ultimately come to rest at a position superior to the glands derived from the third pouches. Functioning chief cells are active during fetal development to assist in regulating calcium metabolism.

PHYSIOLOGY

The synthesis of thyroid hormones occurs within the thyroid gland at the interface between the follicular cell and the thyroglobulin. Recognized histologically as colloid, thyroglobulin is a glycoprotein that functions as a scaffold for hormone produc-

857

tion and storage. The first step in thyroid synthesis production is the iodination of tyrosine molecules to form either monoiodotyrosine, if there is one iodine molecule attached, or diiodotyrosine, if two iodine molecules are bound. These iodinated tyrosine molecules are then coupled to form the definitive thyroid hormones triiodothyronine (T_3) and T_4. If monoiodotyrosine is attached to diiodotyrosine, T_3 results. Two diiodotyrosines bound together constitute a T_4 molecule.

The thyroid gland secretes primarily T_4; about 80% of the T_3 in the circulation represents metabolized T_4 that has been partially deiodinated in the liver, kidney, or other peripheral tissues. In the circulation, most of the thyroid hormones are protein bound, increasing their solubility in the plasma. The most abundant hormone carrier is thyroid-binding globulin (TBG); other carriers include prealbumin and albumin. Because the only physiologically active thyroid hormone is that which is free in the plasma, the plasma levels of these proteins must be considered when patients are being evaluated for abnormalities of thyroid function. Moreover, there are rare inherited defects in thyroid carrier proteins in which the avidity of hormone binding is altered. In these patients, the total plasma and bound fractions may be abnormal, but the free T_3 and T_4 are normal, and the patients are clinically euthyroid. Although T_4 is nearly 50-fold more concentrated in the plasma than T_3, the latter moiety binds much more avidly to the thyroid receptor and therefore accounts for most of the physiologic effect of thyroid hormone.

When free thyroid hormone reaches the target cell, the hormone molecule initially crosses the cell membrane and is transported to the nucleus of the cell, where most of the physiologic effects of thyroid hormone occur. Here, the T_3 molecule interacts with the nuclear receptors, and the receptor–T_3 conjugate binds to DNA to regulated genetic transcription.[2] The structure of the T_3 receptors has been defined and is known to possess a ''zinc finger'' domain that determines the specific DNA sequence bound by the molecule. There at least four different T_3 receptor subtypes, and these molecules exhibit specificity with regard to both tissue type and the stage of embryonic development.

Thyroid hormone produces many effects within the cell, including an increase in the number of sodium pumps at the cell membrane, an increase in adenosine triphosphate production by the mitochondria, as well as other gene-regulating effects occurring within the nucleus. Overall, thyroid hormone increases cellular oxygen consumption and basal metabolic rate, stimulates protein synthesis, and influences carbohydrate, lipid, and vitamin metabolism. Although many of the genes regulated by thyroid hormone remain to be elucidated, it is known that the enzymes responsible for lipolysis and lipogenesis are produced in response to thyroid hormone. Thus, the fatty acids released from adipose tissue by thyroid hormone are the principal energy source for the calorigenesis induced by the hormone.

The production and secretion of T_3 and T_4 by the thyroid gland are chiefly controlled by thyroid-stimulating hormone (TSH). This protein is secreted by the anterior pituitary gland, principally in response to thyrotropin-releasing hormone, which is secreted by the hypothalamus. In addition, peptides present within the thyroid gland may assist in the production and secretion of thyroid hormones.[3] Among these are neuropeptide Y, substance P, cholecystokinin, and vasoactive intestinal peptide. It is thought that these peptides interact to further modulate thyroid function, but the exact mechanisms are unknown, and this is a topic of investigation. Under the influence of TSH, thyroid follicular cells form pseudopods that extend into the colloid encircling the thyroglobulin, and they form vesicles that then fuse with protease-containing lysosomes. The thyroglobulin is then subjected to hydrolysis and proteolysis, resulting in the release of free T_4 into the circulation.

NONNEOPLASTIC THYROID CONDITIONS

The evaluation of a child suspected of having thyroid disease should begin with a physical examination of the neck. The size of the gland and its consistency should be assessed. Diffuse enlargement makes the diagnosis of simple colloid goiter more likely, or if the child is hyperthyroid, Graves disease should be suspected. Chronic lymphocytic (Hashimoto) thyroiditis is classically associated with a gland that feels granular or pebbly in nature. Firmness in the gland suggests an infiltrative process; a hard gland may suggest neoplasia. Tenderness in the thyroid gland is most commonly associated with an acute inflammatory process. Finally, the presence of enlarged neck lymph nodes should be recorded; thyroid carcinoma may be associated with local metastases before the primary tumor can be palpated.

Laboratory tests are essential in the evaluation of altered thyroid function. The TSH is elevated in hypothyroid states and is an extremely sensitive measure of this condition. The plasma free T_4 level is an accurate measure of the biologically active hormone and is generally unaffected by the amount of protein binding in the circulation. When plasma total T_3 and T_4 are measured, an evaluation of TBG may be necessary to gauge the level of biologically active (unbound) hormone. Plasma levels of TBG are altered in a number of conditions, affecting the level of total T_4. In particular, TBG is increased in the neonatal period and decreased in the presence of exogenous glucocorticoids, androgens, and anabolic steroids. Other medications that affect T_4 metabolism include phenytoin and phenobarbital, which induce hepatic degradation of T_4 and decrease hormone binding to TBG. Finally, rare conditions exist in which the TBG level is congenitally altered.

Several radiologic modalities are available to assist in imaging the thyroid gland. Radionuclide scintigraphy is probably the most commonly used test. The three nuclides usually available for diagnostic imaging include iodine-123 (^{123}I), iodine-131 (^{131}I), and technetium 99m (^{99m}Tc). The radioiodines are most effective in detecting ectopic thyroid tissue or metastatic thyroid carcinoma, and ^{99m}Tc-pertechnetate is thought by some radiologists to enable superior imaging of thyroid gland nodules or tumors. Increasingly, ultrasound is being used to aid in the evaluation of thyroid gland lesions.

Hypothyroidism

Although rare, some children are afflicted with acquired or congenital diseases of thyroid hormone production, resulting in either increased or decreased hormone production and secretion. Disorders of hypothyroidism are rarely treated surgically and may result from a defect anywhere in the hypothalamic–pituitary–thyroid axis. The differential diagnosis of hypothyroidism in childhood is listed here:

- Hypothalamic failure
- Pituitary failure
- Thyrotropin gene mutation
- Thyroid dysgenesis or agenesis
- Inborn errors of thyroid hormone synthesis
- Iodine deficiency
- Medications (iodide, propylthiouracil, methimazole, amiodarone)
- Hashimoto thyroiditis
- TSH-blocking antibody
- TSH-receptor defect
- Neck irradiation

Moreover, a hypothyroid state may be seen in conditions of hormone unresponsiveness, such as when there is a defect in the thyroid receptor gene; in such cases, the plasma T_4 level is elevated.

Thyroid gland dysgenesis is the most common cause of hypothyroidism diagnosed in neonatal screening programs, accounting for about 90% of these patients. In about one third of these babies, no thyroid tissue is seen on radionuclide scanning; in the rest of these patients, a rudimentary gland may be found in an ectopic location, such as at the base of the tongue. Often, there has been enough transplacental thyroid hormone present through development so that even children with complete thyroid agenesis do not have symptoms at birth. In some cases, ectopically located thyroid tissue may supply a sufficient amount of T_4 for many years, or it may fail in childhood. These conditions may come to clinical attention with the development of a sublingual or midline neck mass. Surgeons should be mindful of this possibility when evaluating children with neck masses, and consideration should be given to performing radionuclide thyroid scanning before removing any unusual neck mass to ensure that all the functioning thyroid tissue is not accidentally resected.

Goiter and Thyroiditis

When children are specifically surveyed for abnormalities of the thyroid gland, a goiter is found in about 3% of the population.[1] This prevalence rate has decreased markedly with the increased use of iodized table salt. Indeed, early in this century, the incidence of thyroid enlargement was as high as 70% in children living in iodide-poor regions of the country. Goiters can be classified as either diffusely enlarged or nodular; they may be associated with increased hormone secretion (thyrotoxicosis), or the patient may be euthyroid. Physiologically, diffuse goiters may be related to autoimmune diseases, a response to a nonautoimmune inflammatory condition, or compensation for some defect in hormone production. The differential diagnosis of diffuse thyroid enlargement is as follows:

- Autoimmune mediated
    Chronic lymphocytic (Hashimoto) thyroiditis
    Graves disease
    Simple colloid goiter
- Compensatory
    Iodine deficiency
    Medications
    Goitrogens
    Hormone or receptor defect
- Inflammatory conditions
    Acute suppurative thyroiditis
    Subacute thyroiditis

Most children with goiters are euthyroid, and surgical resection is rarely indicated.

In a study of 5462 Croatian schoolchildren, 152 subjects (2.78%) had thyromegaly.[4] The various causes of thyroid enlargement in this population are presented in Table 52-1. As in other studies of populations with adequate dietary iodine intake, most of these patients had simple colloid goiter, which is frequently called *adolescent goiter* or *nontoxic goiter*. Studies have suggested that this disease may be part of the spectrum of autoimmune thyroid diseases, and in up to 90% of patients, there may be circulating thyroid-stimulating antibodies present.[5] The measurement of such antibodies is not particularly useful in making the diagnosis of simple colloid goiter; rather, the diagnosis is established by excluding the other known causes of thyroid enlargement.

The laboratory evaluation of thyroid enlargement should start with plasma free T_4 and TSH levels to determine whether the patient is euthyroid. Normal levels of TSH and thyroid hormone should be documented, and the diffuse nature of the goiter can be documented scintigraphically or by ultrasound. Usually, no specific treatment is recommended for simple colloid goiter. The natural history of the condition is not well known, but in one study in which adolescents with diffuse colloid goiter were reevaluated some 20 years later, nearly 60% of the glands were judged to be normal in size.[1] This spontaneous rate of colloid goiter resolution was not significantly different than the response rate in children treated with exogenous thyroid hormone. Thus, simple colloid goiters generally should not undergo any specific treatment. In rare cases, a trial of thyroid hormone may be done. Surgical resection of the gland is indicated infrequently when symptoms are related to the size of the goiter, when there is a suspicion of neoplasia, or for cosmetic reasons.

Another common cause of diffusely enlarged thyroid glands in children is chronic lymphocytic thyroiditis, also know as *Hashimoto thyroiditis*. Occurring most frequently in adolescent girls, this condition is part of the spectrum of autoimmune thyroid disorders. Indeed, the condition is associated with the presence of other autoimmune disorders, such as juvenile rheumatoid arthritis, Addison disease, and type I diabetes mellitus. Patients are usually euthyroid and slowly progress to become hypothyroid. About 10% of these patients, however, are hyperthyroid; this condition has been termed *hashitoxicosis*. Patients

TABLE 52-1. *Causes of thyroid gland enlargement in 5462 Croatian schoolchildren*

Diagnosis	Frequency (%)
Simple goiter	2.3
Chronic lymphocytic thyroiditis	0.35
Graves disease	0.07
Benign adenoma	0.04
Cyst	0.02
TOTAL	2.78

(Adapted from Jaksic J, Dumic M, Filipovic B, et al. Thyroid disease in a school population with thyromegaly. Arch Dis Child 1994;70:103)

with chronic lymphocytic thyroiditis are characterized by high titers of the circulating antithyroglobulin and antimicrosomal autoantibodies, which are presumably responsible for the B-lymphocytic infiltrate found in the thyroid gland on histologic evaluation.

Children with chronic lymphocytic thyroiditis generally come to clinical evaluation because of thyroid gland enlargement. On palpation, the gland is generally pebbly or granular in texture and may be mildly tender. Diagnosis generally no longer requires a thyroid biopsy and may be established by the discovery of high-titer antithyroid antibodies in association with the proper clinical and laboratory circumstances. Plasma thyroid hormone levels are generally not useful, but the TSH level may be elevated in 70% of patients. Thyroid ultrasound demonstrates a diffuse hypoechogenicity, and scintigraphy shows a patchy uptake of the tracer. In rare cases, autoantibodies cannot be detected, and fine-needle aspirate of the gland may be needed to confirm the diagnosis. Treatment is usually expectant; in as many as one third of adolescent patients, the chronic lymphocytic thyroiditis resolves spontaneously, with normalization of gland size and disappearance of the antithyroid antibodies. Administration of thyroid hormone to euthyroid patients has been shown to be ineffective in reducing the size of the goiter and is thus probably not indicated.[6] Thyroid function studies should be obtained every 6 months, and exogenous hormone should be administered if hypothyroidism develops.

Subacute (de Quervain) thyroiditis is rarely seen in children. This condition is caused by viral infection and is characterized by tender, painful swelling of the gland. Typically, there is mild thyrotoxicosis owing to injury to the thyroid follicles with leakage of thyroid hormone into the circulation. This may be reflected by elevated T_3 and T_4 levels and decreased TSH level. Radioactive iodine uptake is decreased as a result of thyroid follicular cell dysfunction; this finding distinguishes subacute thyroiditis from Graves disease. Histologically, granulomas and epithelioid cells may be seen. Treatment is symptomatic and generally consists of nonsteroidal antiinflammatory agents or steroids. The disease usually lasts 2 to 9 months, and complete recovery can be expected.

Acute suppurative thyroiditis is caused by a bacterial infection of the gland. On examination, the patient may have evidence of sepsis, with an acutely inflamed thyroid gland. Patients are usually euthyroid. The offending organisms are usually staphylococci or mixed aerobic and anaerobic flora. There may be a congenital pharyngeal sinus tract predisposing to infection. Treatment consists of antibiotics; if an abscess develops, incision and drainage may be necessary. The thyroid gland can be expected to recover completely.

Hyperthyroidism

With rare exceptions, hyperthyroidism of childhood is caused by Graves disease, or diffuse toxic goiter. Other possible causes include the following:

- Graves disease (diffuse toxic goiter)
- Toxic nodular goiter
- Subacute thyroiditis
- Chronic lymphocytic thyroiditis
- Neonatal thyroiditis
- TSH-secreting pituitary tumor
- McCune-Albright syndrome

The McCune-Albright syndrome is the association of bony fibrous dysplasia, skin pigmentation abnormalities, and abnormally increased hormone secretion by the endocrine organs, including the thyroid, parathyroid, and adrenal glands. Hyperthyroidism occurs congenitally in about 1% of babies born to women with active Graves disease. In these patients, the onset of the condition may be delayed until 2 to 3 weeks after birth.

Graves disease is seen in girls about 5 times more commonly than in boys, and the incidence steadily increases throughout childhood and peaks in the adolescent years. The onset is usually insidious, and the condition develops over several months. Initial symptoms include nervousness, emotional lability, and declining school performance. Then, weight loss becomes manifest, and increased sweating, palpitations, heat intolerance, and malaise may develop. True exophthalmos is an unusual finding in children, but a conspicuous stare is commonly seen. A goiter is evident on physical examination in more than 95% of cases. The thyroid gland is smooth, firm, and nontender. A bruit may be heard on auscultation. Laboratory evaluation generally reveals elevated free T_4 and decreased TSH levels. In 10% to 20% of patients, there is only elevation of T_3, a condition know as T_3 *toxicosis*. The diagnosis of Graves disease is further supported by the presence of TSH-stimulating immunoglobulins.

Graves disease is an autoimmune disease caused by the presence of TSH-receptor antibodies. These autoantibodies stimulate the thyroid follicles to increase iodide uptake and cyclic adenosine monophosphate production, inducing the production and secretion of increased thyroid hormone. As with many other autoimmune diseases, the inciting event to elicit the antibody response against the TSH receptor is unknown. Reports have suggested that the TSH-binding proteins are present in a number of gram-positive and gram-negative bacteria. It is possible that infection with these organisms elicits an antibody response that reacts with the TSH receptor.[7] In addition, an infectious cause of Graves disease is further supported by some epidemiologic reports of disease clustering.[8]

Methods for treating Graves disease include antithyroid medications, radioactive ^{131}I, and surgical resection.[9] Most pediatric endocrinologists begin therapy with antithyroid medications. The most commonly used drugs are methimazole and propylthiouracil, which act principally by inhibiting follicle cell organification of iodide and the coupling of iodotyrosines to reduce thyroid hormone production. Further, there may be some immunosuppressive activity because there is usually a reduction in antithyroid antibodies. Because of its longer half-life and increased potency, methimazole is usually preferred. The initial dose is 30 mg once daily, which should be reduced if the patient is younger than an adolescent. The TSH level should be monitored carefully; rising levels signal overtreatment and can cause further increase in the goiter size. When the patient is euthyroid, as determined by normal T_3 and T_4 levels, the dose of methimazole should be reduced to 10 mg once daily and maintained at a level to ensure normal thyroid hormone levels.

Side effects of methimazole are unusual but include nausea, minor skin reactions, urticaria, arthalgia, arthritis, and fever. The most serious reaction is an idiosyncratic agranulocytosis. This can occur at any time during the course of treatment or even during a second course of the drug. The onset of a sore throat with fever should raise concern, and a neutrophil count should be obtained. Typically, the granulocyte count rises 2 to 3 weeks after stopping the drug, but in rare cases, fatal opportunistic infections have been reported. Treatment with parenteral antibiotics during the recovery period has been recommended.

The duration of medical treatment is controversial, but the goal is to treat long enough to allow for resolution of the disease. In general, treatment should be continued for 3 to 4 years. The remission rate is about 25% after 2 years of treatment, and the continuing remission rate is about 25% every 2 years. In most children, the remission of Graves disease occurs within 6 months of discontinuing antithyroid therapy. The resolution rate is decreased in children who have persistence of their TSH-receptor antibodies during and after treatment. Interestingly, in one report, it was observed that the addition of T_4 to methimazole for treating patients with Graves disease resulted in a significantly lower incidence of disease recurrence.[10] In this study of adults, T_4 administration significantly reduced the levels of TSH antibodies, which is postulated to account for the improvement in clinical outcome. Although these results are provocative, they need to be confirmed before this treatment can be recommended. In children, moreover, the effects of T_4 in managing Graves disease are unknown.

In patients with Graves disease resistant to treatment with antithyroid medications, or in those who have a severe reaction to the medication, the thyroid gland must undergo definitive ablation. Methods of definitively treating Graves disease include either surgical resection or ablation with radioactive ^{131}I. Neither of these modalities is without complications. Although ^{131}I therapy is effective, and the disease remission rate is low, patients have a 50% to 80% incidence of long-term hypothyroidism after treatment.[11] Furthermore, although radioiodine has become the treatment of choice in young adults, its use in children and adolescents has been controversial. Despite a lack of evidence, concerns have been raised about the possibility of teratogenic or carcinogenic effects in these younger patients.[12] Thus, surgical treatment is recommended in rare cases for children with Graves disease refractory to medical treatment.

When surgery is indicated, subtotal thyroidectomy is the procedure of choice for the treatment of Graves disease and is appropriate treatment for patients who refuse radioiodine treatment, fail medical management, or have thyroids so large that they have compression symptoms. Patients should be rendered euthyroid before undergoing surgery. Methimazole should be used to decrease T_3 and T_4 levels into the normal range. Alternatively, β-blocking agents such as propranolol can be used to ameliorate the adrenergic symptoms of hyperthyroidism. Finally, iodine in the form of Lugol solution, 5 to 10 drops per day, should be administered for 4 to 7 days before surgery to reduce the vascularity of the gland. In large studies of adults treated with subtotal thyroidectomy for Graves disease, the rate of recurrent hyperthyroidism is about 6% to 10% at 10-year follow-up.[11] Patients continue to relapse even later, and 30% of patients exhibit recurrent hyperthyroidism 25 years after their subtotal thyroidectomy.[9] There is also a significant risk of permanent hypothyroidism in these patients, which affects about 5% of patients 1 year after surgery, increasing to as high as 50% of patients who are observed for 25 years. The incidence of hyperthyroidism or hypothyroidism is even higher when abnormal TSH levels are considered, which suggest subclinical abnormalities in hormone production. These findings underscore the importance of carefully following these patients postoperatively to monitor thyroid status. The long-term outcome in children with surgically managed Graves disease is unknown.

NEOPLASTIC THYROID CONDITIONS

Thyroid Nodules

Thyroid nodules are uncommon in children, but their importance stems from a relatively high likelihood of associated cancer. In pediatric studies, the incidence of malignancy in thyroid nodules has been about 20%.[13,14] This is a much lower incidence of cancer than was reported in previous decades and is thought to reflect the decreased number of children who have been exposed to neck radiation for trivial reasons. Proper evaluation and treatment of these lesions is essential because the cancer may be at an easily curable stage. A summary of pathologic results of several large series of children who underwent surgery for thyroid nodules is presented in Table 52-2.

The differential diagnosis of solitary thyroid nodules is as follows:

- Adenoma
- Carcinoma
- Thyroid cyst
- Ectopic thyroid gland
- Cystic hygroma

TABLE 52-2. *Diagnoses in children treated for thyroid nodules*

	Patient series		
	Desjardins, 1987	Hung, 1992	Yip, 1994
Patients	58	71	122
Malignant nodules	12 (21%)	14 (20%)	16 (13%)
Histologic subtype			
Papillary	8	9	12
Follicular	3	0	3
Mixed	0	2	0
Anaplastic	0	2	0
Medullary	1	1	0
Benign nodules (%)	46 (79%)	57 (80%)	106 (87%)
Diagnosis			
Follicular adenoma	27	48	26
Thyroiditis	6	4	17
Thyroglossal cyst	2	3	0
Colloid nodule	0	2	57
Branchial cyst	5	0	0
Other	6	0	6

* One patient in this series had lymphoma of the thyroid gland.
(Data from Desjardins JG, Khan AH, Montupet P, et al. Management of thyroid nodules in children: a 20-year experience. J Pediatr Surg 1987;22:736; Hung W, Anderson KD, Chandra RS, et al. Solitary thyroid nodules in 71 children and adolescents. J Pediatr Surg 1992;27:1407; and Yip FWK, Reeve TS, Poole AG, et al. Thyroid nodules in childhood and adolescence. Aust NZ J Surg 1994;64:676)

- Thyroglossal duct remnant
- Germ cell tumor

In most large pediatric series, girls with nodules outnumber boys by a ratio of about 2:1.[15] Most patients come to clinical attention because of masses in their necks; thyroid dysfunction (an abnormal hormone level) is unusual. A careful neck examination should be performed, with special attention directed to determine whether there are enlarged cervical lymph nodes. Such a finding is suggestive of locally advanced carcinoma but may occur in patients with benign disease as well. In general, it is impossible to differentiate benign from malignant lesions on clinical grounds. The serum TSH level should be measured to identify patients with unsuspected thryotoxicosis resulting from an autonomously functioning nodule. Although imaging studies are often performed early in the evaluation process, they are unreliable at distinguishing benign from malignant nodules. Malignant nodules can be either functioning or nonfunctioning on thyroid scintiscan. Similarly, ultrasonography is usually non-diagnostic; malignant nodules can be either solid or cystic. Thus, these imaging studies should be deferred in the evaluation of thyroid nodules in children. A therapeutic trial of exogenous thyroid hormone to induce nodule regression, as is often pre-scribed in adults, is not recommended for children.

The use of fine-needle aspiration cytology to evaluate thyroid nodules is well established in adults, and the use of this technique has significantly decreased the incidence of thyroidectomy for benign conditions. Further, this has doubled the number of surgical patients whose pathologic evaluation reveals carcinoma.[16] The overall reduction in surgery has resulted from the practice of observing benign lesions, rather than removing them. Although this practice is safe in adults, the incidence of false-negative cytology with an attendant delay in the diagnosis of thyroid cancer is about 1% to 6%.

In children, the usefulness of fine-needle aspiration cytology in the evaluation of thyroid nodules has not been well defined. Children may be somewhat more difficult to evaluate than adults, owing to the smaller size of the nodule and the frequent need to sedate the patient to allow safe and accurate aspiration. Moreover, few pediatric pathologists have sufficient experience in interpreting thyroid cytology. For these reasons, pediatric surgeons have historically recommended the removal of thyroid nodules in virtually all cases. Thus, there have been few large studies defining the natural history of cytologically benign nodules in children. In one study of 57 children with thyroid nodules evaluated with aspiration, the incidence of malignancy was 18%.[17] There was one papillary carcinoma initially misdiagnosed as a benign lesion, which was eventually recognized as a malignancy after clinical follow-up. As shown in Table 52-2, about 80% of pediatric thyroid nodules are benign. If the safety of treating these lesions nonoperatively is demonstrated, the potential savings in operative morbidity and cost may be significant.

The pattern of thyroid disease in adolescents differs from that in younger children and is similar to that in adults. In one large series, the incidence of malignancy in thyroid nodules from patients 13 to 18 years old was only 11%.[15] For this reason, in centers where an experienced thyroid cytopathologist is available, it may be acceptable to initiate the evaluation of thyroid nodules in adolescent patients with aspiration cytology. The results indicate either unequivocal cancer, a benign lesion, or a lesion suspicious for carcinoma. If the nodule is judged to be benign, it can be followed up with serial physical examinations and ultrasound studies. Surgical resection should be performed if the nodule is malignant or suspicious, or if a benign nodule is shown to increase in size. Some endocrinologists recommend that benign thyroid nodules be suppressed with exogenous thyroid hormone, but this has not been show to alter the natural history of such nodules. If a cystic lesion disappears after aspiration, surgery can be deferred. The lesion should be removed if it recurs. Although cyst fluid can be sent for cytologic analysis, the sensitivity of this test for determining the presence of cancer is unknown.[16]

In prepubertal children, there is increased difficulty in obtaining aspiration cytology, and the pattern of benign disease is different than in adults. Thus, the natural history of these lesions is unknown, and the safety of nonoperative treatment has not been demonstrated. Therefore, it is recommended that all thyroid nodules be removed in children younger than 13 years. Some surgeons obtain preoperative ultrasound examination and thyroid scintigraphy as an aid in determining the anatomy.[13,18] The recommendations for evaluation of thyroid nodules in children are summarized in Figure 52-1. It cannot be overstated

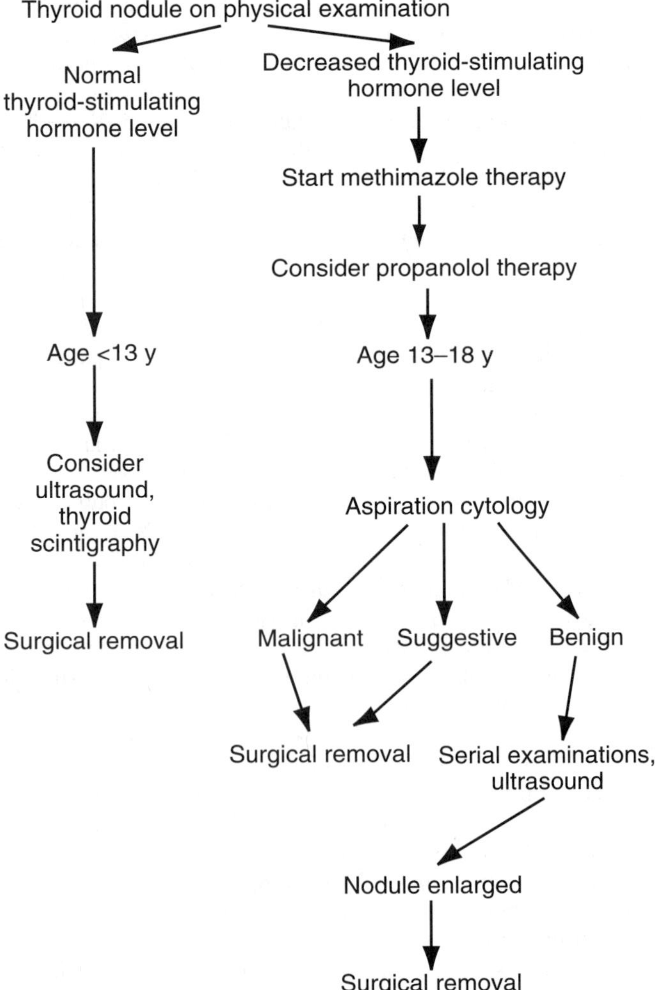

FIG. 52-1. Algorithm for the management of a solitary thyroid nodule in childhood.

that if there is any question about the reliability of the cytologic evaluation, excisional biopsy of all thyroid nodules irrespective of patient age should be performed.

Thyroid Carcinoma

Carcinoma of the thyroid gland is relatively unusual in children, occurring in the United States at an incidence of about 1 case per 1 million children each year, representing only about 3% of all childhood malignancies. In most large clinical series, the peak incidence is in children between 10 and 18 years of age, and girls usually outnumber boys by a ratio of 2:1. About 10% of all malignant thyroid tumors occur in children.

The importance of radiation as an etiologic factor in thyroid carcinoma is undisputed, and the incidence of thyroid tumors in children has decreased during the past two decades owing to the reduced use of radiation to treat benign diseases. Historically, external radiation was used to "treat" enlarged thymuses in neonates, enlarged adenoids and tonsils, and various skin conditions. More recently, the importance of radiation as a cause of thyroid cancer has been reemphasized since a marked increase in the incidence of these tumors has been observed in the Republic of Belarus after the 1986 Chernobyl nuclear power plant catastrophe.[19] The latency period for the development of thyroid cancer after radiation exposure is about 4 to 6 years, and in the Belarus population, there has been a 62-fold increase in thyroid tumor incidence since the Chernobyl accident.

Thyroid carcinoma also occurs at an increased incidence after treatment for a previous childhood malignancy. As more children are successfully treated for cancer, the carcinogenic effects of chemotherapy and radiation used in such treatment have become evident. In one study, thyroid cancers constituted about 9% of second malignancies occurring after treatment for childhood tumors.[20] Hodgkin lymphoma was the most common first malignancy associated with the subsequent development of thyroid cancer. About 71% of such thyroid neoplasms followed the use of radiation to the neck, but alkylating agents alone also predispose to thyroid cancer. The mean age at diagnosis of the thyroid tumors in this study was 20 years, underscoring the importance of careful surveillance for second tumors in children who are being observed after the successful treatment of cancer.

Research has helped to elucidate some of the genetic events that may be responsible for the neoplastic process in thyroid tumors. The *RAS* protooncogene has been shown to exhibit activating mutations in human thyroid cancers.[21] Interestingly, this genetic mutation was found in only 20% of tumors with papillary histology but was present in 80% of follicular tumors. Other studies have demonstrated that *RAS* is frequently activated in benign follicular adenomas, which suggests that this genetic event occurs early in the transformation process.[22] The different genetic events operating in the histologic subtypes of thyroid cancer may account for the disparity in their biologic behavior.

In about 35% of papillary thyroid cancers, an activating mutation of the *RET* protooncogene is found.[23] The RET protein is a receptor tyrosine kinase molecule that probably functions within the cell to regulate proliferation or differentiation. The ligand to the receptor has not yet been discovered. In these affected thyroid tumors, the gene is activated by the fusion of the tyrosine kinase region of *RET* to another gene. This may occur through a chromosomal inversion involving the 10th chromosome, where *RET* is located; or in some cases, a translocation event may fuse a gene from another chromosome to *RET* to form the chimeric transforming gene.[24] The expression of this chimeric gene has been shown to cause transformation of cell lines in vitro, and this is probably one of the steps in transformation of thyroid cells to form papillary carcinomas.

The *RET* protooncogene is also important in the genesis of medullary thyroid carcinoma (MTC). Various mutations in *RET* are associated with the multiple endocrine neoplasia type II syndromes (MEN IIa and IIb) and with familial MTC. MTC is usually the first tumor to develop in these patients. In addition, as many as 40% of sporadic nonfamilial MTCs possess *RET* mutations.[25] Although the specific functions of the normal or mutated *RET* protooncogene are unknown, it is thought that the mutations perturb the intracellular signaling pathways to alter the proliferation or differentiation of the neural crest derived tissues involved in the MEN II syndromes.

The nature of the specific *RET* mutations responsible for the MEN II syndromes can provide some clues to the pathogenesis of the diseases. For example, the mutations that have been seen in the MEN IIa syndrome all exist in the region of the gene that codes for the extracellular portion of the protein, thought to be part of the ligand-binding domain.[26,27] These mutations may increase the tyrosine kinase activity of the protein, which in turn may confer ligand-independent growth on the cell, presumably causing increased proliferation and, ultimately, transformation of the target cells. Thus, it is likely that the *RET* mutations causing MEN IIa alter receptor substrate specificity in some way, working through an intact intracellular signaling pathway. In contrast, patients with MEN IIb have *RET* mutations located in the intracellular tyrosine kinase domain of the protein and therefore may exhibit unrestrained kinase activity along a different signal transduction pathway than is normally activated.[25,28,29] This newly activated signal pathway may trigger increased cellular proliferation and transformation. The genetic difference may account for the phenotypic differences seen between the MEN IIa and IIb syndromes, such as earlier presentation of the MTC in patients with MEN IIb.

Carcinoma of the thyroid gland typically presents as a thyroid mass, as enlarged cervical lymph nodes, or with both of these findings. In one large clinical study of thyroid carcinoma in children, the more recently diagnosed patients were somewhat less likely to have enlarged regional lymph nodes at their initial presentation.[30] In this study, 63% of children diagnosed from 1936 to 1971 had palpable adenopathy at diagnosis; this rate decreased to 36% in children seen after 1971. The incidence of cervical lymph node metastasis found during pathologic evaluation of the surgical specimen was 88% in each of the two groups. A compilation of the clinical aspects of several large clinical series of children with differentiated thyroid carcinoma is presented in Table 52-3.

The pathologic diagnosis can be established either by thin-needle aspiration cytology, if an experienced cytopathologist is available, or by frozen-section analysis of a biopsy specimen at the time of surgery. As shown in Table 52-3, most of these patients have papillary thyroid carcinoma, which can usually be differentiated from benign conditions by either of these techniques. Before surgery, most children should have a thyroid scan to determine whether the thyroid mass contains functioning thyroid tissue. Some investigators also recommend an ultra-

TABLE 52-3. *Clinical aspects of differentiated thyroid cancer in children from six large series*

	Clinical series*					
	A	B	C	D	E	F
Total patients	89	59	58	100	49	72
Mean age	12.8	NA	11.9	13.3	14.0	11
Percentage female	81	66	69	71	69	71
Histology						
Papillary	83	37	58	87	44	50
Follicular	6	19	0	7	4	21
Medullary	0	1	0	0	1	0
Other	0	2	0	6	0	0
Percentage with metastasis	88	50	90	71	73	75
Surgical procedure						
Total thyroidectomy	79	49	21	46	0	29
Subtotal thyroidectomy	5	†	22	†	49	0
Lobectomy or other	5	0	15	54	0	43
Lymph node procedure	75	NA	49	89	73	83
Percentage receiving radiotherapy	82	71	17	22	98	42
Median follow-up (y)	NA	11	28	20	7.7	13
Cancer mortality rate (%)	2.2	3.4	3.4	0	2.0	17

NA, data not available.

*Data from the following series:

  A. Harness JA, Thompson NW, McLeod MK, et al. Differentiated thyroid carcinoma in children and adolescents. World J. Surg 1992;16:547

  B. Samuel AM, Sharma SM. Differentiated thyroid carcinomas in children and adolescents. Cancer 1991;67:2186

  C. Zimmerman D, Hay ID, Gough IR, et al. Papillary thyroid carcinoma in children and adults: long-term follow-up of 1039 patients conservatively treated at one institution during three decades. Surgery 1988;104:1157

  D. La Quaglia MP, Corbally MT, Heller G, et al. Recurrence and morbidity in differentiated thyroid carcinoma in children. Surgery 1988;104:1149

  E. Ceccarelli C, Pacini F, Lippi F, et al. Thyroid cancer in children and adolescents. Surgery 1988; 104:1143

  F. Schlumberger M, DeVathaire F, Travagli JP, et al. Differentiated thyroid carcinoma in childhood: long term follow-up in 72 patients. J Clin Endocrinol Metab 1987;65:1088

† In these studies, the children who had a total or near-total thyroidectomy were not subgrouped.

sound study to determine whether the lesion is cystic and to serve as a guide during the surgical procedure.[18] Because of the relatively high incidence of pulmonary metastasis in children with thyroid carcinoma, a preoperative chest radiograph should be obtained.

The surgical management of thyroid cancer in children is controversial. Unfortunately, there have been no clinical trials comparing the various surgical management options. As seen in Table 52-3, the long-term outcome is usually good, irrespective of the particular surgical procedure employed. Surgeons advocating aggressive thyroid resections argue that total thyroidectomy, with lymph node dissection if the regional nodes are involved with cancer, is the most successful method of obtaining local control of the tumor.[30–32] Moreover, removing the entire thyroid gland makes radioiodine ablative therapy more effective because there is less functioning endocrine tissue to take up the radionuclide. Those who argue that lesser thyroid gland resection is indicated hold that differentiated thyroid carcinoma in children is a relatively indolent disease and that survival is apparently not a function of the extent of gland removal.[33,34] Further, there is a significant incidence of major surgical complications associated with total thyroidectomy in children. For example, the reported incidence of recurrent laryngeal nerve injury is 0% to 24%,[30] and the reported frequency

of permanent hypocalcemia is 6% to 27%.[30,33,35] These complications are reported to occur less commonly in the more recent clinical series.[30]

In one retrospective review of many children treated for differentiated thyroid cancer, there was multivariate analysis of the factors that were predictive of early disease recurrence.[33] In this study of 93 patients followed up for a median of 20 years, the tumor recurrence rate after treatment was 34%. The only factors significantly predictive of early recurrence were a lower age at diagnosis and the tumor histology. In particular, children older than 12 years at diagnosis were less likely to experience tumor recurrence than younger children. Further, follicular tumors were more likely than papillary tumors to be cured at the initial procedure. Thus, it appears that tumor factors may be more important than treatment factors in determining the clinical outcome in children with differentiated thyroid cancer. Another important finding in this study was the significant association between major surgical complications and the extent of the surgical procedure. Also, these complications occurred significantly more frequently in younger children than in older patients.

Thus, because of opposing viewpoints and in the absence of controlled trials, it is difficult to make firm recommendations regarding the surgical management of differentiated thyroid cancer in children. Some surgeons suggest that if the tumor is clearly isolated to one lobe of the gland, lobectomy with isthmus resection may be sufficient.[32] In one clinical series, however, 66% of patients had bilateral tumors, and 81% of tumors exhibited multifocality.[32] Therefore, most surgeons believe that more aggressive thyroid gland resections are usually indicated, and recommend that either total or near-total thyroidectomy be performed for the treatment of endocrine thyroid cancer. The recurrent laryngeal nerve should be identified and care taken to prevent accidental injury. The parathyroid glands should be protected; probably the safest means of preserving parathyroid gland function is to identify and autotransplant one or two of the glands into the sternocleidomastoid muscle or into the nondominant forearm.[36] Tumor involving the recurrent laryngeal nerves probably should not be aggressively resected; ^{131}I may successfully eradicate residual tumor. Moreover, if there are enlarged lymph nodes suggestive of regional metastasis, a node dissection is recommended. In patients with locally advanced disease, it is especially important to remove as much of the thyroid gland as possible, to allow subsequent radioiodine scanning and treatment should the tumor recur. After surgery, most investigators recommend that all patients with endocrine thyroid cancer be treated with exogenous thyroid hormone to suppress TSH-mediated stimulation of the gland.

In most studies, the incidence of pulmonary metastases at diagnosis of thyroid cancer in childhood is about 6%.[34,37] This almost never occurs in the absence of significant cervical lymph node metastases. Pulmonary metastases require treatment with radioiodine. Furthermore, plain chest radiographs demonstrate the pulmonary disease in only about 60% of cases.[37] Thus, scanning with radioiodine is necessary to detect these metastatic deposits, and this scan may be falsely negative if there is significant residual thyroid gland remaining in the neck. It seems reasonable to remove as much of the gland at the initial operation as can be done safely, to decrease the need for a riskier repeat dissection if the tumor should recur in the thyroid bed.

The recurrence rate of thyroid cancer in patients followed up for 20 years is about 30%, and late deaths from persistent or recurrent disease are not uncommon.[32,33] This underscores the importance of aggressive, early treatment and relatively frequent, long-term follow-up. An ^{131}I whole body scan should be performed about 6 weeks after the thyroid resection to detect residual tumor remaining in the neck and in the lungs. If positive, therapeutic doses of the radionuclide should be administered and repeated as necessary to treat residual metastatic disease.[30] Diagnostic radioiodine scans should be repeated yearly to assay for recurrence of the neoplasm. Thyroglobulin has been shown to be a useful marker of residual or metastatic thyroid cancer; the plasma level of this protein should be measured yearly, and an elevated value should raise the suspicion for recurrent disease.[38] The diagnostic accuracy of this test is significantly decreased in children who have residual thyroid tissue and in those who are receiving thyroid hormone supplementation.

About 5% of thyroid neoplasms in children are medullary carcinomas, arising from the parafollicular C cells. MTC can be either familial or sporadic. Familial tumors occur in patients who have MEN IIa or IIb or the familial MTC syndrome. MTC is usually the first tumor to develop in MEN patients and is the most common cause of death in this group. The neoplasm is particularly virulent in patients with MEN IIb and has been

reported to occur in infancy.[39] As with other thyroid neoplasms, the clinical diagnosis of MTC is often made after there is significant spread of tumor to the adjacent cervical lymph nodes or to distant sites.[40] The only effective treatment for MTC is surgical resection, underscoring the importance of early diagnosis and therapy before metastasis occurs. For this reason, management of MTC in children from families with MEN II relies on the presymptomatic detection of the *RET* protooncogene mutation responsible for the disease. Children with MTC and MEN IIa should undergo total thyroidectomy at about 5 years of age, before the cancer spreads beyond the thyroid gland.[41] Indeed, as exemplified in Figure 52-2, about 80% of children who undergo thyroidectomy based on the presence of the *RET* mutation already have foci of MTC within the thyroid gland.[42] Because of the increased virulence of MTC in children with MEN IIb, it may be preferable to remove their thyroid glands in infancy. Because of the high incidence of bilateral disease, complete removal of the thyroid gland is the recommended procedure for surgical management of MTC in children.[43] In addition, the lymph nodes in the central compartment of the neck, medial to the carotid sheaths and between the hyoid bone and the sternum, should be removed.

In patients with MEN IIa, the risk of hyperparathyroidism is about 30%.[44] In view of this, and because of the risk of permanent hypoparathyroidism after total thyroidectomy, the parathyroid glands should be identified, removed from the neck, and autotransplanted into the nondominant forearm.[42] If hyperparathyroidism develops, it is easier and safer to remove a portion of the heterotopic tissue from the forearm than to reexplore the neck to find the hyperplastic parathyroid gland. In my experience, the parathyroid tissue has uniformly grafted successfully, with no incidents of permanent hypoparathyroidism.[41] Most children treated in this way experience a transient period of hypocalcemia that requires temporary calcium and vitamin D supplementation.

PARATHYROID GLANDS

The parathyroid glands are responsible for maintaining calcium and phosphate homeostasis. Parathyroid hormone (PTH) is secreted as an 84–amino acid protein, which is rapidly cleaved in the liver and kidney into the carboxy-terminal, amino-terminal, and mid-region fragments. The target organs of PTH include the kidney and the bones, which possess specific receptors for the hormone. In the kidney, PTH stimulates enzymes responsible for the production of the active vitamin D metabolite 1,25-dihydroxycholecalciferol, which then acts on the intestinal mucosa to increase calcium absorption. Mobilization of calcium from the bones is directly stimulated by PTH, a process that also requires vitamin D.

The biologic activity of PTH resides in the amino-terminal segment, but because of its short half-life in the circulation, the plasma level of this moiety is low. The C-terminal fragment levels are 50- to 500-fold those of the N-terminal fragment, and most clinical assays of PTH measure C-terminal levels of the hormone. These assays are usually effective for the evaluation of hyperparathyroidism, but the C-terminal fragment is cleared in the kidney, and plasma levels of the protein may therefore be selectively elevated if there is a component of renal failure. The laboratory hallmark of hyperparathyroidism is the finding

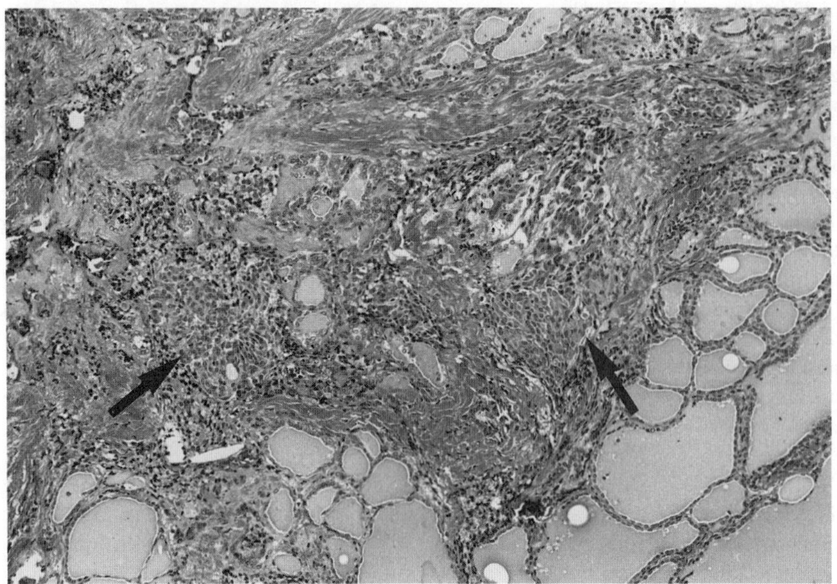

FIG. 52-2. Photomicrograph of thyroidectomy specimen demonstrating microscopic foci of medullary thyroid carcinoma. The prophylactic thyroidectomy was performed in a 10-year-old child who had a *RET* protooncogene mutation associated with MEN IIa.

of an elevated plasma PTH level with hypercalcemia. Radiographic evaluation is useful in patients who have had chronically elevated PTH levels, but the characteristic bone findings are not seen acutely.

In evaluating the child for hyperparathyroidism, a 24-hour measurement of urinary calcium should be performed to rule out familial hypocalciuric hypercalcemia. Also known as familial benign hypercalcemia, this condition usually comes to clinical attention in a child with an elevated serum calcium level but without other symptoms. Serum levels of magnesium may also be elevated, and the condition may affect other family members. The disease is inherited as an autosomal dominant disorder and is caused by a heterozygous mutation in the Ca^{2+}-sensing receptor gene.[45] The PTH level and the parathyroid glands are normal; there is usually no benefit to parathyroidectomy. In rare cases, a neonate born to affected parents presents with severe hypercalcemia. These infants have inherited mutations in both copies of the Ca^{2+}-sensing receptor gene, often have hyperplasia of the parathyroid glands, and benefit from parathyroidectomy.

The differential diagnosis of hypercalcemia in childhood is as follows:

- Elevated PTH level
    Primary hyperparathyroidism
    Secondary hyperparathyroidism
    Tertiary hyperparathyroidism
    Ectopic PTH production
- Hypervitaminosis D
- Sarcoidosis
- Subcutaneous fat necrosis
- Familial hypocalciuric hypercalcemia
- Idiopathic hypercalcemia of infancy
- Thyrotoxicosis
- Hypervitaminosis A
- Hypophosphatasia
- Prolonged immobilization
- Thiazide diuretics

Unlike adults, children rarely have abnormal serum calcium levels related to neoplasms. In exceedingly rare cases, however, tumors secrete a parathyroid-related polypeptide that elevates the calcium level. Neoplasms in which this has been reported include malignant rhabdoid tumor, mesoblastic nephroma, rhabdomyosarcoma, neuroblastoma, and lymphoma. In these patients, the PTH level is generally normal or decreased.

Primary hyperparathyroidism in childhood most commonly results from a solitary hyperfunctioning adenoma, and more rarely from diffuse hyperplasia of all four glands.[46] Hyperparathyroidism resulting from hyperplasia in all four glands is a feature of MEN I. Furthermore, as stated previously, about 30% of patients with MEN IIa experience hyperparathyroidism.[44] Primary hyperparathyroidism of infancy is a rare disorder that is often fatal.[47,48] In about half of reported cases, there is a familial component to the disease. The condition usually develops within the first 3 months of life, and presenting signs include hypotonicity, respiratory distress, failure to thrive, lethargy, and polyuria. Pathologically, there is usually diffuse parathyroid gland hyperplasia. Early recognition and treatment of primary hyperparathyroidism of infancy is essential to allow normal growth and development of the baby.

Once the diagnosis of hyperparathyroidism is established, the offending parathyroid tissue should be resected. There is no place for medical management of primary hyperparathyroidism in children. During the procedure, all four of the parathyroid glands should be identified and biopsy performed. If one gland is clearly enlarged and adenomatous, it should be removed. If the other glands are normal, they should be marked with a nonabsorbable suture and left in place. In familial cases, there is propensity for hyperplasia to develop, and these patients should probably be treated as if there were diffuse parathyroid hyperplasia, irrespective of the biopsy results.

Some disagreement exists regarding the preferred surgical management of parathyroid gland hyperplasia involving all of the glands. Some surgeons recommend three and one half–gland parathyroidectomy, while others prefer to remove all of the glands and heterotopically transplant some tissue into the nondominant forearm.[47] The latter approach has the advantage of avoiding repeated neck exploration if hyperparathyroidism should recur and has been shown to be safe in infants and children.[42] Moreover, total parathyroidectomy with heterotopic autotransplantation has been shown to result in improved survival in infants with severe hypercalcemia.[47] As mentioned, patients with total parathyroidectomy and autotransplantation require a short period of vitamin D and calcium supplementation until the heterotopic tissue begins to function.

Secondary hyperparathyroidism occurs when the parathyroid glands are stimulated to increase PTH secretion in response to decreased calcium. This is usually seen in children with renal insufficiency but also can be associated with malabsorption syndromes. These patients typically respond to medical treatment to decrease intestinal phosphorus absorption, but in rare cases, they severe renal osteodystrophy manifested by skeletal fractures and metastatic calcifications develps. These children are candidates for total parathyroidectomy with autotransplantation.[46] Some patients with chronic renal failure and secondary hyperparathyroidism who undergo renal transplantation have persistent hyperfunction of the glands even after the inciting stimulus (hypocalcemia from renal failure) is removed. This is termed *tertiary hyperparathyroidism* and results from four-gland hyperplasia. Children with this condition are also candidates for total parathyroidectomy with autotransplantation.

REFERENCES

1. Rallison ML, Dobyns BM, Meikle AW, et al. Natural history of thyroid abnormalities: prevalence, incidence, and regression of thyroid diseases in adolescents and young adults. Am J Med 1991;91:363.
2. Epstein FH. The molecular basis of thyroid hormone action. N Engl J Med 1994;331:847.
3. Ahren B. Regulatory peptides in the thyroid gland: a review on their localization and function. Acta Endocrinol 1991;124:225.
4. Jaksic J, Dumic M, Filipovic B, et al. Thyroid disease in a school population with thyromegaly. Arch Dis Child 1994;70:103.
5. Fisher DA, Pandian MR, Carlton E. Autoimmune thyroid disease: an expanding spectrum. Pediatr Clin North Am 1987;34:907.
6. Rother KI, Zimmerman D, Schwenk WF. Effect of thyroid hormone treatment on thyromegaly in children and adolescents with Hashimoto disease. J Pediatr 1994;124:599.
7. Tomer Y, Davies TF. Infection, thyroid disease, and autoimmunity. Endocr Rev 1993;14:107.
8. Phillips DI, Barker DJ, Rees Smith B, et al. The geographical distribution of thyrotoxicosis in England according the presence or absence of TSH-receptor antibodies. Clin Endocrinol 1985;23:283.
9. Franklyn JA. The management of hyperthyroidism. N Engl J Med 1994;330:1731.
10. Hashizume K, Ichikawa K, Sakurai A, et al. Administration of thyroxine in treated Graves' disease: effects on the level of antibodies to thyroid-stimulating hormone receptors and on the risk of recurrence of hyperthyroidism. N Engl J Med 1991;324:947.
11. Berglund J, Christensen SB, Dymling JF, et al. The incidence of recurrence and hypothyroidism following treatment with antithyroid drugs, surgery, or radioiodine in all patients with thyrotoxicosis in Malmo during the period 1970–1974. J Intern Med 1991;229:435.
12. Klein I, Becker DV, Levey GS. Treatment of hyperthyroid disease. Ann Intern Med 1994;121:281.
13. Hung W, Anderson KD, Chandra RS, et al. Solitary thyroid nodules in 71 children and adolescents. J Pediatr Surg 1992;27:1407.
14. Desjardins JG, Khan AH, Montupet P, et al. Management of thyroid nodules in children: a 20-year experience. J Pediatr Surg 1987;22:736.
15. Yip FWK, Reeve TS, Poole AG, et al. Thyroid nodules in childhood and adolescence. Aust N Z J Surg 1994;64:676.
16. Mazzaferri EL. Management of a solitary thyroid nodule. N Engl J Med 1993;328:553.
17. Raab SS, Silverman JF, Elsheikh TM, et al. Pediatric thyroid nodules: disease demographics and clinical management by fine needle aspiration biopsy. Pediatrics 1995;95:46.
18. Newman KD. The current management of thyroid tumors in childhood. Semin Pediatr Surg 1993;2:69.
19. Nikiforov Y, Gnepp DR. Pediatric thyroid cancer after the Chernobyl disaster: pathomorphologic study of 84 cases (1991–1992) from the Republic of Belarus. Cancer 1994;74:748.
20. Smith MB, Xue H, Strong L, et al. Forty-year experience with second malignancies after treatment of childhood cancer: analysis of outcome following the development of the second malignancy. J Pediatr Surg 1993;28:1342.
21. Lemoine NR, Mayall ES, Wyllie FS, et al. Activated ras mutations in human thyroid cancers. Cancer Res 1988;48:4459.
22. Lemoine NR, Mayall ES, Wyllie FS, et al. High frequency of ras oncogene activation in all stages of thyroid tumorigenesis. Oncogene 1989;4:159.
23. Bongarzone I, Butti MG, Coronelli S, et al. Frequent activation of *ret* protooncogene by fusion with a new activating gene in papillary thyroid carcinomas. Cancer Res 1994;54:2979.
24. Sozzi G, Bongarzone I, Miozzo M, et al. A t(10;17) translocation creates the RET/PTC2 chimeric transforming sequence in papillary thyroid carcinoma. Genes Chrom Cancer 1994;9:244.
25. Eng C, Smith DP, Mulligan LM, et al. Point mutation within the tyrosine kinase domain of the RET proto-oncogene in multiple endocrine neoplasia type 2B and related sporadic tumours. Hum Mol Genet 1994;3:237.
26. Mulligan LM, Kwok JBJ, Healey CS, et al. Germ-line mutations of the RET protooncogene in multiple endocrine neoplasia type 2A. Nature 1993;363:458.
27. Donis-Keller H, Dou S, Chi D, et al. Mutations in the RET proto-oncogene are associated with MEN 2A and FMTC. Hum Mol Genet 1993;2:851.
28. Hofstra RMW, Landsvater RM, Ceccherini I, et al. A mutation in the RET proto-oncogene associated with multiple endocrine neoplasia type 2B and sporadic medullary thyroid carcinoma. Nature 1994;367:375.
29. Carlson KM, Dou S, Chi D, et al. Single missense mutation in the tyrosine kinase domain of the RET protooncogene is associated with multiple endocrine neoplasia type 2B. Proc Natl Acad Sci 1994;91:1579.
30. Harness JA, Thompson NW, McLeod MK, et al. Differentiated thyroid carcinoma in children and adolescents. World J Surg 1992;16:547.
31. Ceccarelli C, Pacini F, Lippi F, et al. Thyroid cancer in children and adolescents. Surgery 1988;104:1143.
32. Schlumberger M, De Vathaire F, Travagli JP, et al. Differentiated thyroid carcinoma in childhood: long term follow-up in 72 patients. J Clin Endocrinol Metab 1987;65:1088.
33. La Quaglia MP, Corbally MT, Heller G, et al. Recurrence and morbidity in differentiated thyroid carcinoma in children. Surgery 1988;104:1149.
34. Zimmerman D, Hay ID, Gough IR, et al. Papillary thyroid carcinoma in children and adults: long-term follow-up of 1039 patients conservatively treated at one institution during three decades. Surgery 1988;104:1157.
35. de Roy van Zuidewijn DBW, Songun I, Kievit J, et al. Complications of thyroid surgery. Ann Surg Oncol 1995;2:56.
36. Wells SA Jr, Farndon JR, Dale JK, et al. Long term evaluation of patients with primary parathyroid hyperplasia managed by total parathyroidectomy and heterotopic autotransplantation. Ann Surg 1980;192:451.
37. Vassilopoulou-Sellin R, Klein MJ, Smith TH, et al. Pulmonary metastases in children and young adults with differentiated thyroid cancer. Cancer 1993;71:1348.
38. Kirk JM, Mort C, Grant DB, et al. The usefulness of serum thyroglobulin in the follow-up of differentiated thyroid carcinoma in children. Med Pediatr Oncol 1992;20:201.
39. Samaan NA, Draznin MB, Halpin RE, et al. Multiple endocrine syndrome type IIb in early childhood. Cancer 1991;68:1832.
40. Gorlin JB, Sallan SE. Thyroid cancer in childhood. Endocrinol Metab Clin North Am 1990;19:649.
41. Wells SA, Jr, Chi DD, Toshima K, et al. Predictive testing and prophylactic thyroidectomy in patients at risk for multiple endocrine neoplasia type 2a. Ann Surg 1994;220:237.
42. Skinner MA, DeBenedetti MK, Moley JF, et al. Medullary thyroid

carcinoma in children with multiple endocrine neoplasia types 2A and 2B. J Pediatr Surg (in press).

43. Telander RL, Zimmerman D, van Heerden JA, et al. Results of early thyroidectomy for multiple endocrine neoplasia type 2. J Pediatr Surg 1986;21:1190.

44. Howe JR, Norton JA, Wells SA, Jr. Prevalence of pheochromocytoma and hyperparathyroidism in multiple endocrine neoplasia type 2A: results of long-term follow-up. Surgery 1993;114:1070.

45. Pollak MR, Brown EM, Chou YH, et al. Mutations in the Ca(2 +)-sensing receptor gene cause familial hypocalciuric hypercalcemia and neonatal severe hyperparathyroidism. Cell 1993;75:1297.

46. Ross AJ III. Parathyroid surgery in children. Prog Pediatr Surg 1991; 26:48.

47. Ross AJ III, Cooper A, Attie MF, et al. Primary hyperparathyroidism in infancy. J Pediatr Surg 1986;21:493.

48. Kulczycka H, Kaminski W, Wozniewicz B, et al. Primary hyperparathyroidism in infancy: diagnostic and therapeutic difficulties. Klin Padiatr 1991;203:116.

Thorax

Surgery of Infants and Children: Scientific Principles and Practice, edited by Keith T. Oldham, Paul M. Colombani, and Robert P. Foglia. Lippincott–Raven Publishers, Philadelphia, © 1997.

CHAPTER 53

Chest Wall and Breast

Jessica Kandel and J. Alex Haller

The most common congenital abnormality of the chest wall is *pectus excavatum*, a concave depression of the lower sternum. This problem accounts for at least 90% of surgical consultations for infants and children with chest wall abnormalities. Another 7% of patients with chest wall abnormalities have a convex deformity, *pectus carinatum*. The remainder have rare and unusual chest wall deformities, such as Poland syndrome or Cantrell syndrome. Rarely, a newborn infant has missing portions of the chest wall, such as a cleft sternum or deficient ribs. Of all the chest wall deformities, very few are associated with any known genetic or chromosomal abnormalities. Exceptions to this are children with Marfan syndrome or cartilaginous dystrophies such as Jeune syndrome.[1,2]

FORMATION OF STERNAL DEFECTS

The human sternum first appears as a vertical pair of embryonic bars during the sixth week of fetal development. These are derived from somatic mesoderm. Sternal defects probably represent a failure of midline fusion, which normally takes place during the seventh gestational week.[3] When midline fusion does not occur, varying degrees of cleft sternum result. It is usually the upper one third or one half of the sternum that does not fuse, but rarely, the whole sternum may remain separated, in which case the heart may be displaced through this defect. Although the clefts may be isolated anomalies, ectopia cordis is an important association. The sequence of embryologic events that result in ectopia cordis is not clear, but may be related to the maldevelopment of the heart itself since the incidence of associated intracardiac defects is high. Cantrell syndrome, defined as the association of a cleft lower sternum, high omphalocele, anterior diaphragmatic hernia, pericardial deficiency, and congenital heart defect, is also a related problem.[4] No distinct genetic defect has been associated with any of these sternal defects.

A small sternal cleft, which does not expose the contents of the mediastinum, does not necessarily require intervention. Larger defects and completely bifid sternums require repair to protect mediastinal structures and to correct paradoxical chest wall motion. Various operative techniques have been described. If the chest wall is sufficiently compliant, as in a neonate, the sternal bars can be directly reapproximated. If direct approximation is not tolerated by the patient because of the loss of intrathoracic volume and cardiac compression, costal chondrotomies can be performed to allow apposition of the sternal halves without tension. Postoperative results in these rare patients have been reportedly satisfactory. Normal growth and development appear to be limited only by associated anomalies.[5,6]

PECTUS EXCAVATUM

Embryology and Development

Newborns with pectus excavatum are thought to have an overgrowth of costal cartilages during chest wall development in utero. These cartilages appear to have excessive longitudinal growth and as a consequence, the sternum is depressed into a more posterior position than normal. When the lungs inflate at birth, the sternum does not come forward into normal position because the elongated costal cartilages hold it in an aberrant dorsal position. Children with pectus excavatum at birth have paradoxical movement of the sternum; that is, with inspiration the sternum retracts while the lateral portions of the chest wall expand. Although the costal cartilage abnormality begins in utero, the deformity is not necessarily obvious in the endomorphic infant. Generally, the chest wall deformity, if significant, is apparent by 2 to 3 years of age.

If the growth deformity persists or increases in severity during childhood, there may be further progression with pubertal growth. Because the heart may be displaced into the left hemithorax in moderate and severe defects, the left side of the sternum may be elevated, causing the sternum to rotate toward the right; thus, the deformity may become asymmetric.

No genetic or chromosomal abnormalities are known to correspond with the development of pectus excavatum. However, an increased incidence of these abnormalities has been noted in some families.

Physiology and Pathophysiology

The magnitude and significance of the physiologic consequences of pectus excavatum have been extensively debated, and the issue remains controversial. Most reports suggest that quantitative respiratory mechanics, as measured by pulmonary function tests done at rest or maximal exercise, are normal or mildly restricted in children with these abnormalities.[7–9] The data are confounded by the difficulty of obtaining meaningful pulmonary function studies in young children. In older children with pectus excavatum, resting pulmonary function studies have always been found to be normal. Exercise pulmonary function studies in older children and adolescents with severe pectus excavatum deformities have demonstrated statistically significant lower lung volumes than for normal patients. The functional significance remains controversial. The evidence with regard to cardiac function is conflicting,[10,11] but there is consistent suggestion that right ventricular filling may be impaired in some patients with severe pectus deformities. Measured exercise tolerance is generally normal in these children, however.

Small children with pectus excavatum rarely, if ever, have clinical symptomatology of note. Older children and adolescents may be brought for evaluation with complaints of limited ability to participate in competitive sports. While there are many potential explanations for these kinds of symptoms, and while the anatomic defect may be severe, the available objective data do not offer support for the concept that substantial physiologic

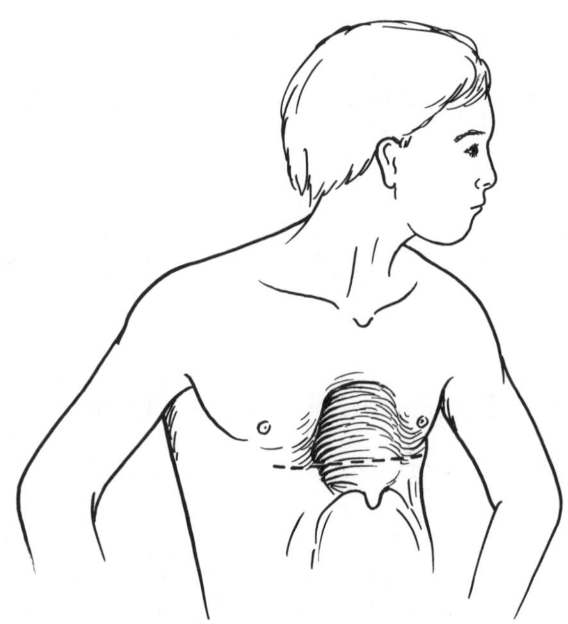

FIG. 53-2. A transverse inframammary incision is placed across the mid-portion of the excavatum defect.

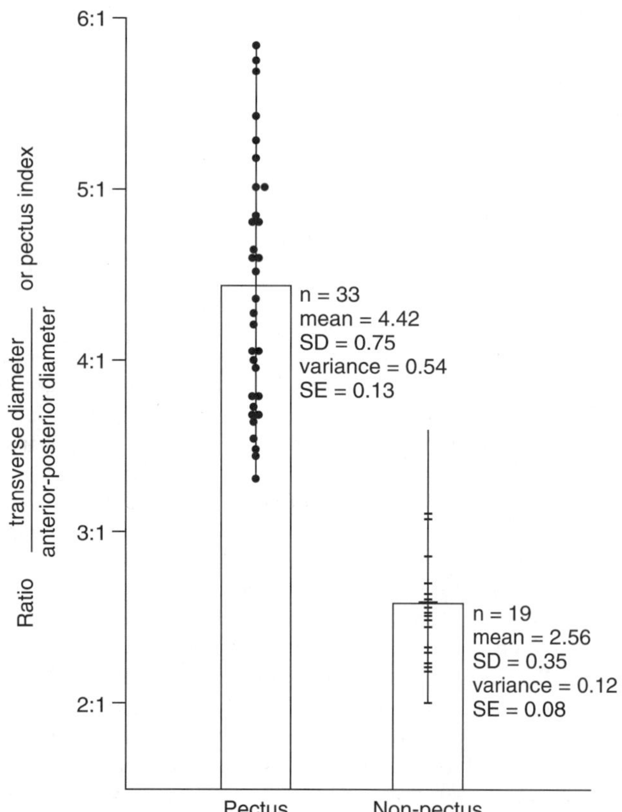

FIG. 53-1. The ratios of transverse to AP thoracic diameter in 33 operated pectus excavatum patients and 19 unoperated control patients are shown. While such quantitative data show substantial differences in the two groups, correlation with physiologic and clinical abnormalities is difficult to demonstrate. (After Haller JR, Kramer SS, Lietman SA. Use of CT scans in selection of patients for pectus excavatum surgery: a preliminary report. J Pediatr Surg 1987;22:904)

improvement in cardiorespiratory function is likely to occur postoperatively. Studies evaluating this question have shown conflicting results.[7–14] Further complicating this evaluation is the fact that different authors have used a variety of surgical techniques, making the comparisons more difficult. One recent prospective study of exercise pulmonary function and exercise performance was done in teenage patients with pectus excavatum. They underwent evaluation before and after surgical repair by one group and were compared to age-matched normal control patients.[15] Preoperatively, the pectus excavatum subjects had a significantly lower forced vital capacity than the normal control patients (81 +/-14% of predicted versus 98 +/-9% predicted, $P < 0.001$). The degree of deformity as measured by chest computed tomography (CT) correlated with total lung capacity. Postoperatively, operated patients were found to have modestly increased exercise tolerance and higher hemoglobin oxygen saturations as measured by pulse oximetry during exercise.[15]

No long-term actuarial data about the health risks of unoperated (or operated) pectus excavatum have yet been collated; however, both parents and physicians commonly offer subjective, retrospective reports of improved respiratory function or exercise tolerance following surgical repair. Most clinicians believe that the degree of pulmonary dysfunction associated with pectus excavatum is minor if present at all, and this physiologic abnormality rarely presents a compelling surgical indication.

From the presently available evidence, it seems reasonable to conclude that most children with pectus excavatum experience relatively minor physical limitations. An exception may be the competitive athlete in whom modest improvement in exercise tolerance with pectus excavatum repair is important. The degree of benefit to the average person who rarely exercises at maximal levels appears to be limited. The benefit is likely attributable to more normal cardiac function rather than to changes in respiratory mechanics.

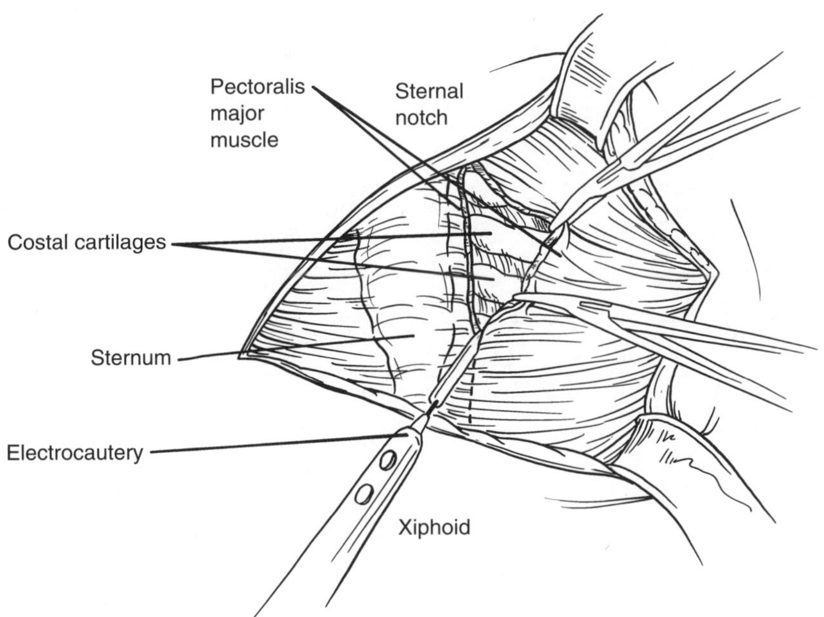

FIG. 53-3. Skin flaps are elevated at the level of the pectoral fascia using electrocoagulation to decrease blood loss. The pectoral muscles are reflected by incising the fascia in the midline and sweeping muscle flaps laterally to the costochondral junctions.

Clinical Presentation

Children with pectus excavatum are generally active, apparently healthy children brought for evaluation of the visible anatomic deformity. Occasionally, nonspecific pain is the presenting complaint. Adolescents and older children may present for evaluation driven by cosmetic concerns about the appearance of the chest wall. The physical findings are generally obvious. The deformity is most often a symmetric one involving the lower sternum that ranges from mild to severe. This stratification is subjective and is best documented radiographically at the initial visit for longitudinal assessment as a child grows and develops. The children have a characteristic stoop shouldered posture with a protuberant abdomen. The heart is also displaced into the left hemithorax due to compression from the depressed sternum, and the point of maximal impact may be lateral to the areola.

A variety of anatomic measurements have been recom-

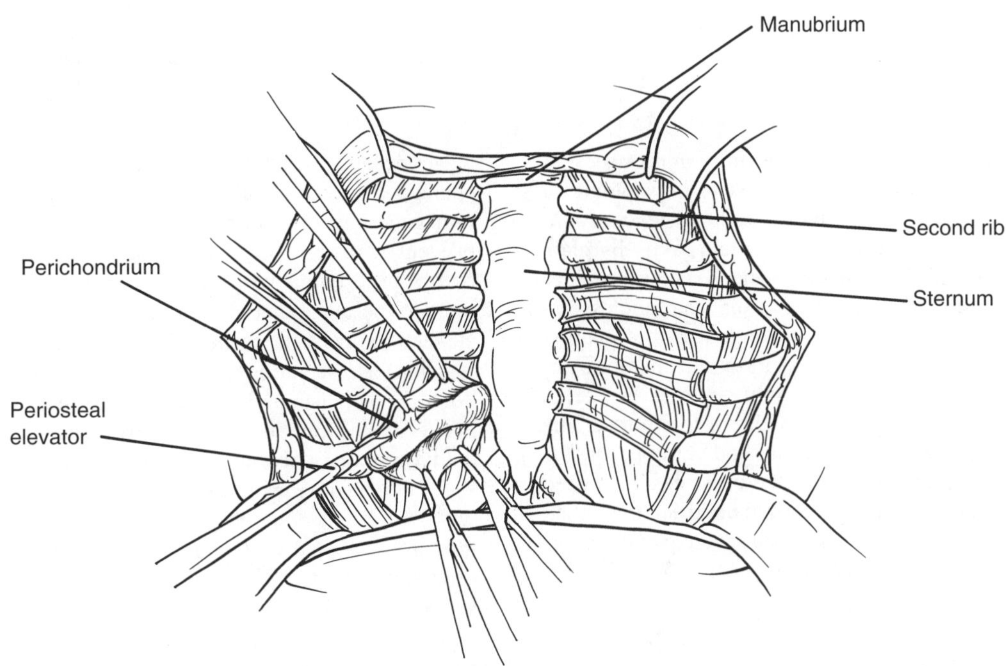

FIG. 53-4. With exposure of the entire defect (usually ribs 3 through 7) accomplished, the perichondrium is incised and elevated sharply from each abnormal costal cartilage. Care is taken with the posterior portion of the dissection to avoid penetration of the pleura causing a pneumothorax.

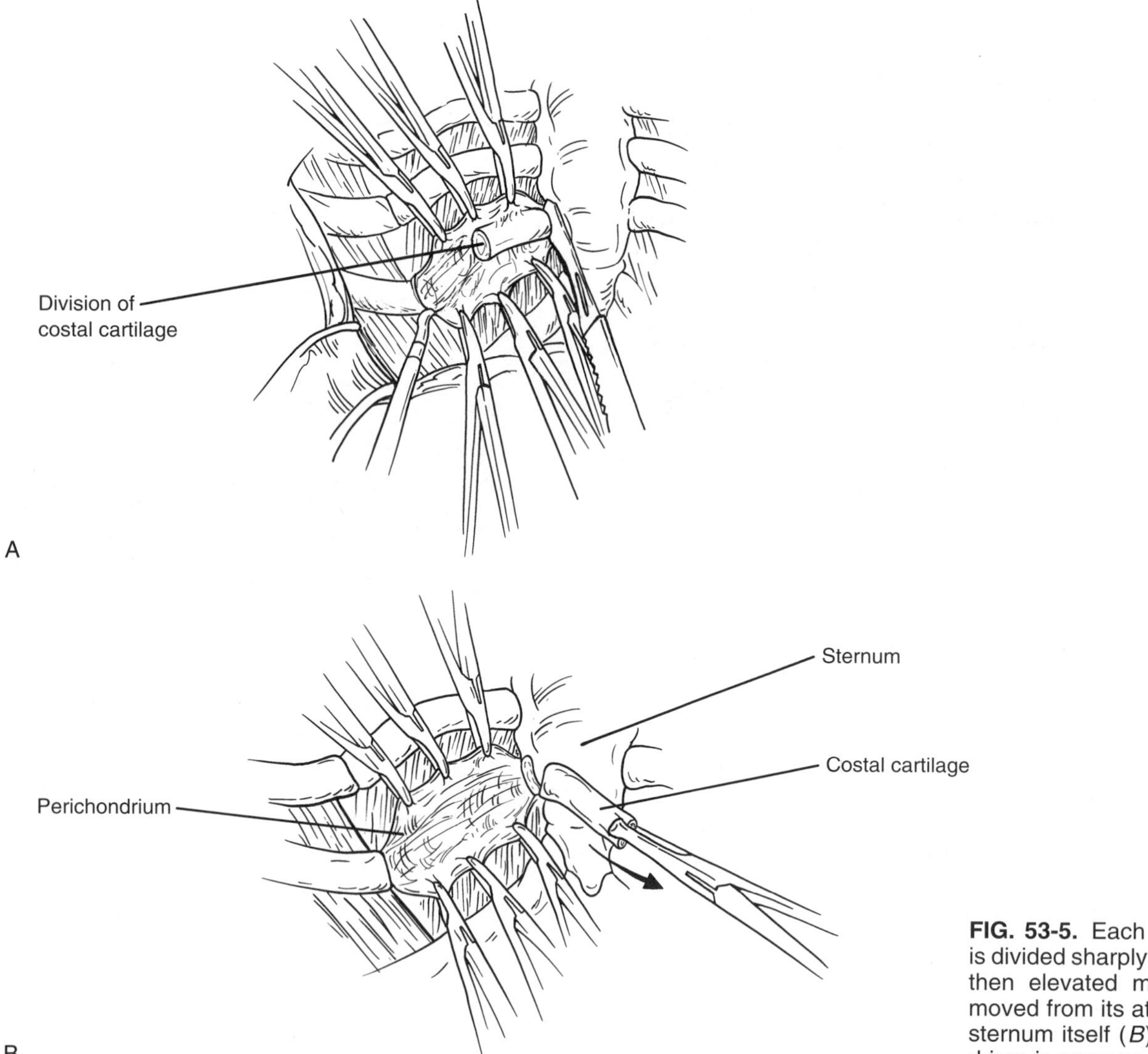

FIG. 53-5. Each costal cartilage is divided sharply laterally (*A*) and then elevated medially and removed from its attachment to the sternum itself (*B*). The perichondrium is preserved.

mended over the years to document the severity of pectus excavatum and to potentially relate the problem to physiologic or clinical abnormalities. These measurements have generally involved evaluating the geometry of the thoracic cavity by plain radiographic films or CT.[16,17] Of these, the CT scan provides more precision regarding displacement of the heart and assessment of abnormal lung volumes. With regard to the imaging evaluation, one reasonably simple measure of the anatomic abnormality can be obtained by measuring the depth of the sternal defect and relating this to the overall width of the thorax. The ratio of the distance between the sternum and vertebral bodies and the overall transverse diameter of the chest has been used to calculate an index of severity. In normal children, this index is never greater than 2.5. In patients with a severe pectus deformity, this index exceeds 3 and may be as great as 5 or 6[17] (Fig. 53-1).

Operative Indications

Candidates for repair of pectus excavatum should be carefully selected. Although measurements of sternal depression appear to correlate with the degree of restrictive pulmonary changes,[9,17] even a child with a relatively deep pectus excavatum generally has normal exercise tolerance. It is, therefore, prudent to assess both physiologic and anatomic parameters before proceeding with surgery. Indications for surgery may include the questions of exercise limitation mentioned earlier, cosmetic concerns, cardiac abnormalities, significant psychological distress, and a future requirement for median sternotomy, such as a patient with Marfan syndrome who has both pectus excavatum and aortic insufficiency.[18] The timing of operative repair is also a subject of substantial controversy and should vary with the indication. Good results have been reported with operations done both in school-age children and after the growth associated with puberty. If the patient has Marfan syndrome, the incidence of recurrence may be reduced by delaying surgery until maximal growth has been obtained.[19] It is noteworthy that preferred practice has shifted in the last two decades from operating in small children to performing the repair in older children and adolescents. One theoretical basis for this is concern about recurrence in small children since the costal cartilage growth in a 4- or 5-year-old child is incomplete and

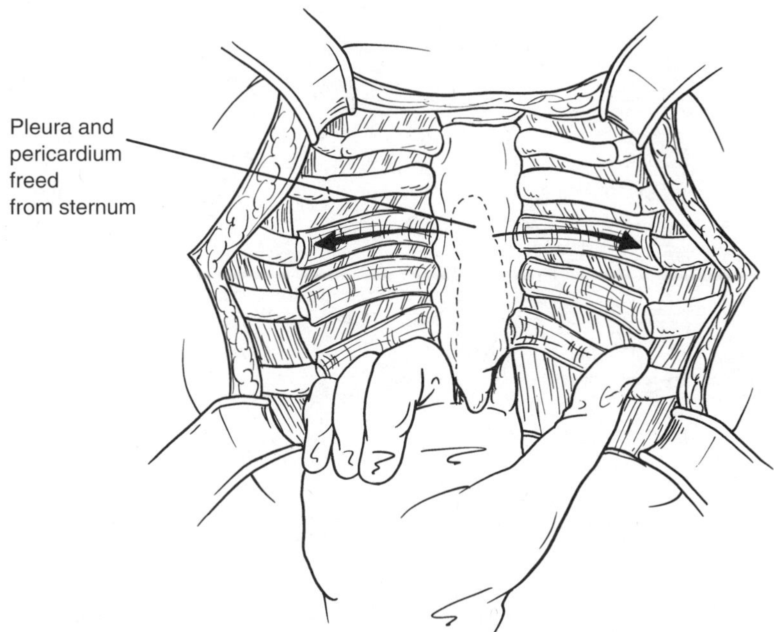

FIG. 53-6. After each pair of costal cartilages is resected for the length of the entire deformity, the sternum itself is mobilized. This is begun by creating a subxiphoid tunnel with blunt dissection. The pleura is swept laterally away from the sternum to minimize the possibility of a pneumothorax.

there is virtually never a compelling physiologic need for operative repair at this age. In addition, acquired thoracic dystrophy has been reported in young children undergoing pectus excavature repair and this is discussed below.

Operative Technique

The operative technique most commonly used to repair pectus excavatum is based on the principles articulated by Ravitch[20] (Figs. 53-2 to 53-11). These are derived from the fundamental concept that the involved costal cartilages are abnormal and must, therefore, be excised. The sternum itself is usually normal but displaced. A transverse or a vertical incision is centered over the point of maximum sternal depression; the transverse incision is generally preferred because it is more appealing cosmetically. With the transverse incision, subcutaneous flaps are raised superiorly and inferiorly. The pectoralis muscles are then dissected laterally exposing the costal cartilages over their entire length. A normal costal cartilage is exposed cephalad and caudad as well unless the deformity extends to the xiphoid, as is usual, in which case the entire lower sternum and xiphoid must be exposed. The deformed lower costal cartilages are then resected subperichondrially to their junction with the sternum. The xiphoid is elevated and a retrosternal plane developed bluntly, with care taken to sweep the pleura off of the posterior sternum. The perichondrial bundles are detached from the lower sternum. An anterior transverse osteotomy of the sternum is

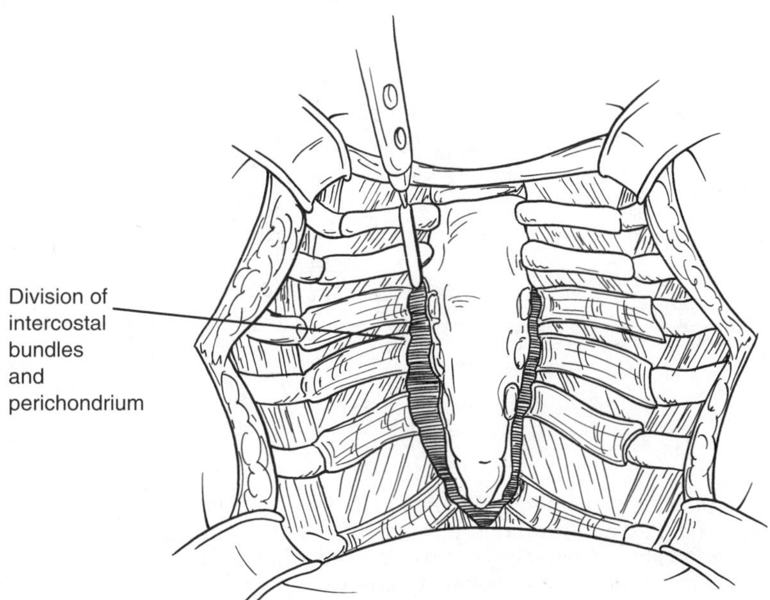

FIG. 53-7. The intercostal bundles and the perichondrium are detached from the sternum bilaterally to permit full mobility of the sternum.

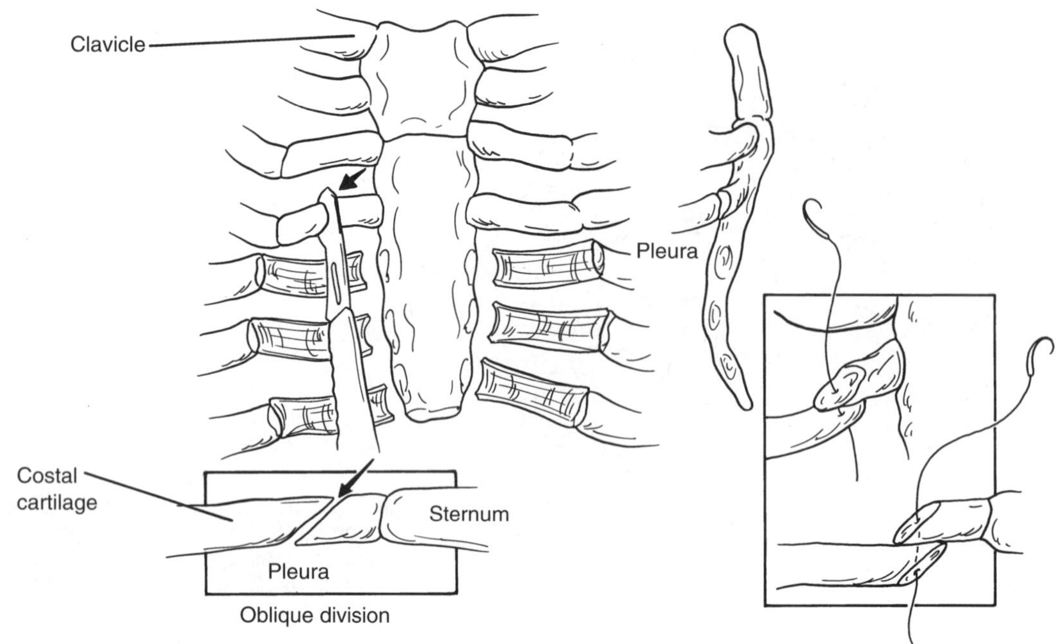

FIG. 53-8. The costal cartilage immediately above the most cephalad abnormal costal cartilage is divided obliquely from medial to lateral as shown. This is often at the level of the second costal cartilage, at the manubrial–sternal junction. The divided normal costal cartilages are then allowed to overlap, the medial portion being anterior and the lateral portion being posterior. Suture fixation of the transected cartilage provides immobilization and thus ensures sternal support at this level (*inset*).

then performed at a level just above the most cephalad of the resected cartilage segments. The sternum is then lifted anteriorly into a neutral position. It can be supported in this position by obliquely dividing the lowest of the intact costal cartilages medial to lateral so that the medial portion is displaced anteriorly by the lateral portion. Additional support is usually provided by placing a strut posterior to the sternum. Many techniques have been used successfully, but perhaps the most simple is the use of a stainless steel orthopedic bar or pin. Lateral support for the strut is provided by securing it to the medial

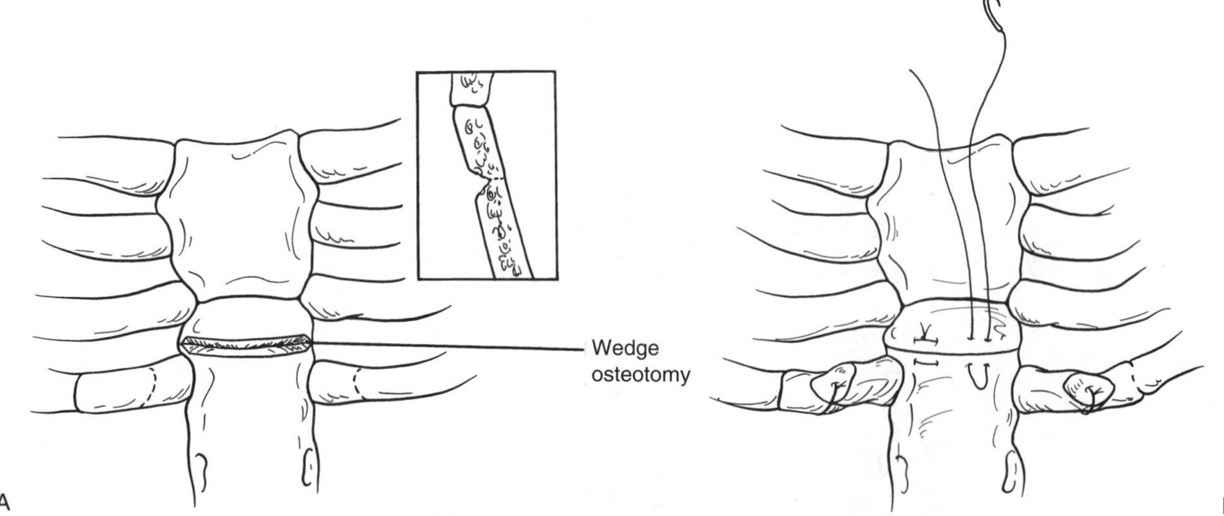

FIG. 53-9. The sternum is stabilized in a neutral position by a variety of techniques. (*A*) This technique involves creating an anterior wedge osteotomy. (*B*) A wedge of bone is removed, then sutures are placed to elevate and fix the sternum in neutral position. Posterior or multiple osteotomies may be necessary depending on the individual deformity. The principle is to obtain a neutral, stable position of the sternum.

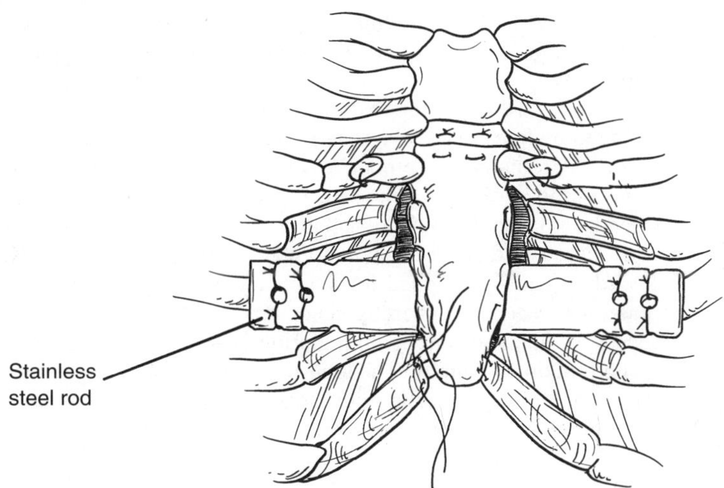

FIG. 53-10. The sternum is further supported in neutral position by a substernal stainless steel rod secured to appropriate ribs. The defect is closed with approximation of the intercostal bundles to the sternum.

ends of an appropriate rib. Typically, the costal cartilages regenerate in 6 to 8 weeks, and once reattached to the sternum, it is fixed in a normal position for subsequent growth and development.

After this process is complete, the strut can be removed. Substernal and subcutaneous drains are placed to prevent postoperative fluid collections. The requirement for transfusion should be extremely rare. Postoperatively, a brief course of antibiotics is often given. Potential early complications include pneumothorax; fluid accumulation in the pleural space, mediastinum, or subcutaneous tissue; and wound infection. Late complications include migration of the substernal bar and recurrence. The incidence of the latter should be less than 5%.[16,21] The patient is typically hospitalized for 4 to 6 days and can

return to full activity after 6 to 8 weeks when the costal cartilages have fixed the sternum in its new neutral position.

Results of Operation

Most patients should obtain a satisfactory cosmetic and technical result. As noted previously, the physiologic consequences of the repair of pectus excavatum have not been clearly demonstrated. Some investigators have noted modest improvements in exercise tolerance postoperatively.[12,15] In other series, pulmonary function either did not change or declined slightly.[13] The latter finding was attributed to scarring of the chest wall and the consequent diminution of compliance and may reflect

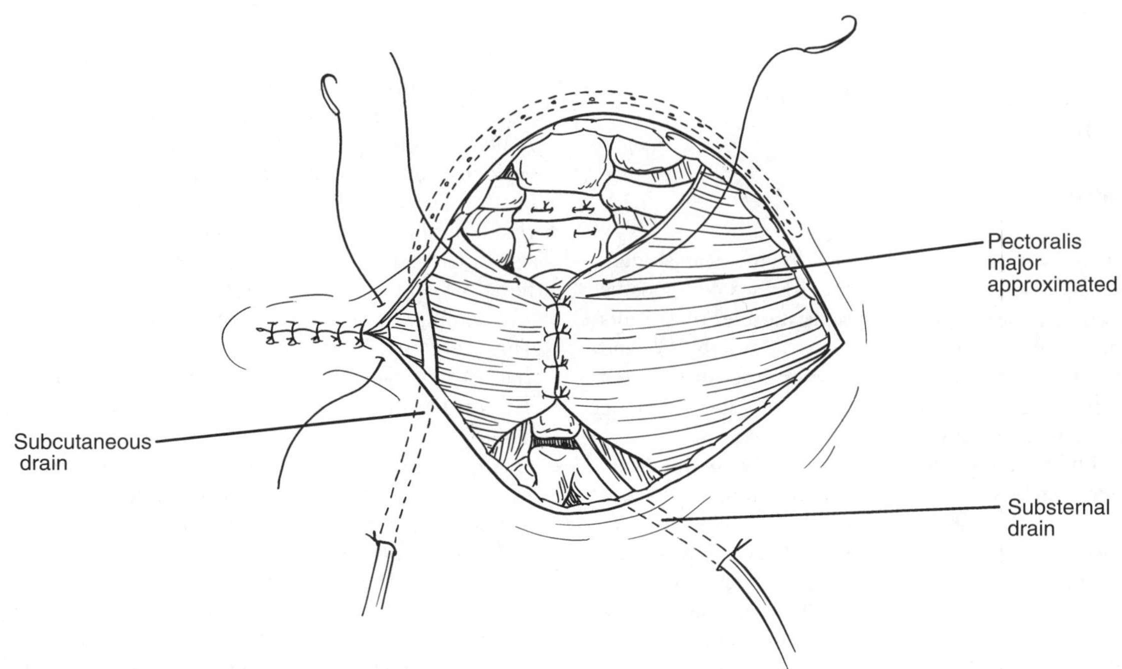

FIG. 53-11. The sternum is now fully stabilized, and the pectoralis muscle flaps are closed. Small closed-suction drains are typically placed in the subcutaneous and substernal spaces to prevent postoperative fluid accumulation.

differences in operative technique. An acquired thoracic chondrodystrophy syndrome is also reported postoperatively; this is discussed later in the section on Jeune syndrome. The psychological benefits of repair have not specifically been studied, but may contribute significantly to the enhanced sense of well-being noted by many patients postoperatively.

PECTUS CARINATUM

Pectus carinatum refers to anterior displacement of the sternum that is caused by overgrowth of the costal cartilages. Unlike the pectus excavatum deformity, the cartilaginous overgrowth in this case causes protrusion rather than depression of the sternum. This is a much less common deformity than the excavatum deformity as previously noted. These deformities arise later in childhood than do excavatum malformations, typically becoming prominent during adolescent growth. It is predominantly a symmetric defect, but can be unilateral leading to considerable asymmetry. No specific genetic defects have been associated with pectus carinatum, and the developmental events responsible for its appearance are unknown.

Children with pectus carinatum deformities have not been found to have any physiologic abnormalities. Hence, the principal indication for surgical repair is cosmetic. Operative intervention should be delayed until after adolescent growth is complete or nearly complete. The procedure is similar to that described earlier for correcting pectus excavatum: the involved costal cartilages are resected subperichondrially and a transverse sternal osteotomy is performed, allowing the sternum to be placed and secured in a neutral position. Potential complications include pneumothorax, subcutaneous fluid collections, and wound infection and should be relatively rare.[22,23] Perioperative care is similar to that discussed with regard to pectus excavatum.

RARE AND UNUSUAL CHEST WALL DEFORMITIES

Poland Syndrome

This anomaly was initially described by medical student Alfred Poland in 1841. In this syndrome, various components of the chest wall may be deficient or absent: muscles (pectoralis major and minor, serratus anterior), ribs two through five, and soft tissue (including breast or nipple). Deformities of the hand or vertebrae may also be seen. The embryologic or genetic events responsible for Poland syndrome are unknown.[24]

Children with Poland syndrome present early in childhood if the chest wall defects cause lung herniation that is apparent with crying or coughing. The underlying lung in patients with Poland syndrome is normal. If the bony defect is relatively large, the child may have a functional flail chest with respiratory compromise, and prompt operative intervention may be required. If the primary problem is one of muscular and soft tissue deficiency, the problem becomes increasingly obvious with exercise, although the involved shoulder function is normal and most patients do not have a decrease in strength of the shoulder musculature. The different components of this syndrome are quite varied in their presentation. When the problem is principally cosmetic, as it often is, reconstruction can be planned electively.

With regard to treatment, bony defects of the thorax may be bridged by free rib grafts harvested from the contralateral chest wall.[25] Alternatively, composites of synthetic mesh and autologous tissue have also been used. These techniques can be combined with a latissimus dorsi flap to correct the muscular and soft tissue defects.[26,27] Submuscular or subcutaneous breast prostheses may be added for symmetry when female patients enter adolescence. Generally, reconstruction for all of these aspects of the syndrome is done during adolescence since there is no functional penalty. The long-term results following reconstruction have been good with regard to both function and appearance.

Cantrell Syndrome

Cantrell syndrome is defined as the association of a cleft lower sternum, high omphalocele, anterior diaphragmatic hernia, pericardial defect, and a congenital heart anomaly, as noted earlier. The first case reported by Cantrell had apparent ectopia cordis but upon close inspection, the heart was actually found to be present in an omphalocele sac over the upper abdomen and was easily placed into the thorax. Urgent repair of the abdominal defect with closure of the abdominal wall and protection of the exposed heart is indicated. Frequently, it is possible to correct the anterior diaphragmatic defect at the same operation. In a few instances, the associated congenital heart abnormality has also been corrected simultaneously, but this is rare. Long-term surgical results have been excellent in survivors.

Jeune Syndrome

This syndrome is also known as newborn asphyxiating thoracic chondrodystrophy. It is generally lethal at birth or shortly after. The abnormality results from failure of chest wall growth in utero, resulting in secondary pulmonary hypoplasia which is typically severe. As noted, the result is generally prompt with death following delivery. Some infants have survived for a period of months, and the rare patient may present in later infancy with increasing dyspnea and respiratory failure secondary to failed growth of the thoracic cavity.

Attempts at chest wall expansion have been undertaken. These are typically individualized efforts at sternotomy and chest wall expansion with a variety of struts and skin coverage. The results are too limited for a consensus recommendation regarding therapy.

An acquired form of Jeune syndrome has recently been recognized in patients who have undergone elaborate operative procedures for pectus excavatum correction in infancy. Apparently, these infants were subjected to operation before the age of 2 to 3 years and underwent such extensive resection of the chest wall cartilage that subsequent chest wall growth never occurred. Consequently, these children developed dyspnea in childhood or adolescence and were found to have substantially diminished pulmonary function related to the restrictive chest wall. This is an important concern with regard to premature pectus excavatum repair. These children represent a form of acquired thoracic dystrophy and a number have undergone operative release with chest wall expansion. Early results appear satisfactory but long-term results are lacking and the numbers are small.

Traumatic Chest Wall Deformities

Traumatic chest wall deformities in children are rare since most trauma in children is blunt trauma. Traumatic chest wall defects generally result from penetrating or explosive injuries. These may require operative correction using the basic principles of rib grafting and soft tissue coverage with adjacent or transferred muscle. The immediate effect of chest wall disruption can be catastrophic in infants and young children because of the great mobility of the mediastinum. This is considered in detail in the discussion of thoracic trauma. (Chapter 23)

TUMORS OF THE CHEST WALL

Benign Tumors

Benign soft tissue tumors of the chest wall occur as commonly as they do elsewhere in the body, and include lipomas, hematomas, cystic hygromas, hemangiomas, and desmoid tumors. Most should be treated by excision. In contrast, benign lesions of the bony thorax are relatively rare in children. These may be isolated lesions, such as enchondromas, osteochondromas, eosinophilic granulomas, bone cysts, or manifestations of a systemic process, such as neurofibromatosis. Isolated lesions may be difficult to distinguish from malignant tumors radiographically; excisional biopsy is therefore generally required to rule out a malignant process.[28]

Malignant Tumors

The most common malignant tumor of the chest wall in children is Ewing sarcoma, usually originating in a rib. Clinical manifestations include pain at the site of the chest wall mass, fever, and pleural effusion. Treatment should begin with biopsy of the mass and excision if feasible at the time of diagnosis. Patients whose lesions are initially deemed unresectable often demonstrate significant tumor shrinkage after chemotherapy. Children whose primary tumors can be completely resected and who receive postoperative radiotherapy and chemotherapy have a survival rate of approximately 50%. In contrast, children presenting with metastatic Ewing sarcoma have a very poor prognosis.

Histologically, Ewing sarcoma is similar to Askin tumor (or malignant small-cell tumor of the thoracopulmonary region); both are small round-cell tumors of neuroectodermal origin. Some authors group them together as primitive neuroectodermal tumors. However, Askin tumors as originally described are relatively rare, have a female predominance, originate in the soft tissue rather than the bony skeleton, and may have a worse prognosis despite similar treatment.[29–31]

Rhabdomyosarcomas are the most common soft tissue malignancy of the chest wall in children. Children with these lesions tend to present with more advanced disease than those with Ewing sarcoma, but the strategy for treatment is similar. Tumors that are resectable should be completely excised. Postoperative combined radiotherapy and chemotherapy are generally used. Survival even with completely resected chest wall rhabdomyosarcoma is probably less than 50%; children presenting with metastatic disease have a dismal prognosis.[32,33]

BREAST DISORDERS

Congenital Anomalies

In the sixth week of gestation, an ectodermal ridge appears (the milk line), which runs from each axilla to the inguinal region. The breasts develop from this primordium.[3] The most common congenital anomaly of the breast, accessory nipples (polythelia), usually appears along the thoracic portion of the milk line; accessory breasts (polymastia) are similarly located. However, both types of accessory breast tissue have been noted in ectopic sites (eg, buttock, back, thigh). Congenital absence of the breast (amastia) is comparatively rare.

Accessory and ectopic breast tissue, which contains glandular structures, responds to hormonal stimulation, and thus may cause periodic discomfort after menarche. Supernumerary nipples and breasts have been reported to undergo malignant transformation. Accordingly, these structures should be removed when diagnosed.[34] Amastia in girls should be treated with augmentation mammoplasty.

Breast Disorders in Prepubertal Children

Infections of breast tissue may occur in the neonatal period (mastitis neonatorum), probably because these structures have been stimulated by exposure to maternal hormones. Treatment should be with antibiotics and drainage of abscesses when they occur. Precocious breast growth in prepubertal girls (premature thelarche) is a common and benign condition. The examiner should seek out and exclude other signs of precocious puberty, since these may signal an underlying endocrine disorder or syndrome. In general, breast masses in prepubertal girls should be followed by careful clinical examinations. Given the risk of injury to the breast bud and the exceedingly low incidence of malignancy, biopsy should be reserved for clearly suspicious masses.

Breast Disorders in Adolescent Boys

Breast enlargement with puberty (gynecomastia) is very common in boys and generally resolves in the early teenage years. Persistent gynecomastia is also usually a benign physical condition, associated with otherwise normal maturation. It is rarely a manifestation of abnormal sex hormone production. If it causes significant psychological distress, operative treatment should be considered. Discrete breast masses are uncommon, but probably should be biopsied. Both subcutaneous mastectomy (for gynecomastia) and breast biopsy can generally be performed in an outpatient setting through a partial circumareolar incision.

Breast Disorders in Adolescent Girls

Breast masses in adolescent girls are overwhelmingly likely to be benign.[35] Because the possibility of breast carcinoma does exist, however, and because these tumors may be harder to detect and more aggressive than in older women, such masses should be carefully evaluated. A family history should be taken. Mammography is not, in general, a useful screening tool in women younger than 30 years of age because of the relative density of their breasts. Instead, adolescent girls should be followed by physical examination and should be taught breast self-examination. Masses that are difficult to evaluate by palpation can be better defined by ultrasound.

Fibrocystic Changes

Fibrocystic changes are so common that they probably do not represent a disorder. Adolescents may give a history of breast pain increasing with menses. Findings on physical exam may vary from discrete cysts to diffusely lumpy breasts. Cysts can be aspirated in the office or under ultrasound guidance. Only cyst fluid that is bloody or serosanguineous requires cytopathologic examination. If the cyst does not recur after 2 or 3 months, the patient can simply be followed by serial physical examinations. Occasionally, the examiner may find a single dominant lump that persists over several months and is not clearly a fibroadenoma. In such cases, excisional biopsy may be required. Histologic findings in fibrocystic breast tissue have been divided into three prognostic categories: nonproliferative, proliferative changes with no atypia, and proliferative changes with atypia. Most young women with fibrocystic changes have nonproliferative histology and are at no increased risk for breast cancer. Only patients with both proliferative changes and atypia appear to have a clearly increased risk of breast cancer.[36]

Fibroadenomas

Solid breast masses that are smooth, round, mobile, and rubbery in texture are likely to be fibroadenomas. As with fibrocystic changes, adult women with some histologic subtypes of this benign lesion have been shown to be at risk for the subsequent development of carcinoma at another site.[37] In adolescent girls, whose overall risk of carcinoma is very low, it appears reasonable to treat these lesions conservatively.[38,39] Therefore, masses that have the characteristics of fibroadenomas by palpation and that are stable should probably be followed by careful, serial physical examinations. If the mass is ill-defined, irregular, or enlarging, an excisional biopsy should be performed.

Cystosarcoma Phyllodes

Most cystosarcoma phyllodes tumors are benign, but about 25% may be malignant. Because of the rarity of infiltrating ductal carcinoma in adolescent girls, cystosarcoma phyllodes may represent the most common form of primary breast cancer in this age group. These tumors present clinically as bulky, irregular, rapidly enlarging breast masses. Like fibroadenomas, which they resemble histologically, they are of fibroepithelial origin. Benign phyllodes tumors are distinguished from fibroadenomas on microscopic examination by stromal overgrowth and cellularity, but there may be considerable overlap. Hence, on occasion it may be difficult to distinguish benign cystosarcoma phyllodes from fibroadenoma. Histologically malignant tumors, with high mitotic indices and microscopic local invasion, are more likely to recur after excision; metastasis is very rare. Treatment should include wide local excision and close clinical follow-up.[40,41]

Breast Biopsy

Most breast masses should be accessible through a partial circumareolar incision oriented toward the quadrant in which the mass is found. These incisions generally result in cosmetically acceptable scars, and importantly, do not interfere with the design of skin flaps should a mastectomy be required later. They may be closed with absorbable sutures; drains are generally not required. Part of the fresh specimen should be reserved for determining estrogen and progesterone receptors if malignancy is found.

Malignant Tumors

Risk factors for breast cancer in adolescent girls seem to parallel those for adult women and include a family history of breast cancer, some benign breast lesions (fibrocystic changes with proliferation or atypia, complex fibroadenomas), and possibly previous radiation to the neck or chest.[37,42] The acceptable surgical options for treating infiltrating ductal carcinoma in adolescent girls should include modified radical mastectomy or wide local excision combined with axillary dissection and postoperative radiotherapy. Although younger women with breast carcinoma tend to have more aggressive disease, their prognosis does not appear to be adversely affected by the choice of breast conservation surgery. Systemic adjuvant chemotherapy should probably be considered in almost all young women with breast cancer, given their increased risks of recurrence and progression of disease.[43]

REFERENCES

1. Golladay ES, Char F, Mollitt DL. Children with Marfan's syndrome and pectus excavatum. South Med J 1985;78(11):1319.
2. Ayres JG, Pope FM, Reidy JF, Clark TJ. Abnormalities of the lungs and thoracic cage in the Ehlers-Danlos syndrome. Thorax 1985;40(4):300.
3. Skandalakis JE, Gray SW, Ricketts R, Skandalakis LJ. The anterior body wall. In: Skandalakis JE, Gray SW, eds. Embryology for surgeons: the embryological basis for the treatment of congenital defects, ed 4. Baltimore, Williams & Wilkins, 1994:541.
4. Cantrell JR, Haller JA, Ravitch MM. A syndrome of congenital defects involving the abdominal wall, sternum, diaphragm, pericardium, and heart. Surg Gynecol Obstet 1958;107:602.
5. Ravitch MM. Congenital deformities of the chest wall and their operative correction. Philadelphia, WB Saunders, 1977.
6. Sabiston DC Jr. The surgical management of congenital bifid sternum with partial ectopia cordis. J Thorac Surg 1958;35:118.
7. Morshuis W, Folgering H, Barentsz J, et al. Pulmonary function before surgery for pectus excavatum and at long-term follow-up. Chest 1994;105(6):1646.

8. Morshuis WJ, Folgering HT, Barentsz JO, et al. Exercise cardiorespiratory function before and one year after operation for pectus excavatum. J Thorac Cardiovasc Surg 1994;107(6):1403.

9. Kaguraoka H, Ohnuki T, Itaoka T, et al. Degree of severity of pectus excavatum and pulmonary function in preoperative and postoperative periods. J Thorac Cardiovasc Surg 1992;104(5):1483.

10. Peterson RJ, Young WG Jr, Godwin JD, et al. Noninvasive assessment of exercise cardiac function before and after pectus excavatum repair. J Thorac Cardiovasc Surg 1985;90(2):251.

11. Beiser GD, Epstein SE, Stampfer M, et al. Impairment of cardiac function in patients with pectus excavatum, with improvement after operative correction. N Engl J Med 1972;287(6):267.

12. Cahill JL, Lees GM, Robertson HT. A summary of preoperative and postoperative cardiorespiratory performance in patients undergoing pectus excavatum and carinatum repair. J Pediatr Surg 1984;19:430.

13. Derveaux L, Clarysse I, Ivanoff I, et al. Preoperative and postoperative abnormalities in chest x-ray indices and in lung function in pectus deformities. Chest 1989;95:850.

14. Wynn SR, Driscoll DJ, Ostrom NK, et al. Exercise cardiorespiratory function in adolescents with pectus excavatum: observations before and after operation. J Thorac Cardiovasc Surg 1990;99:41.

15. Quigley PM, Haller JA, Laughlin GM, et al. Cardiorespiratory function before and after corrective surgery in pectus excavatum. J Peds 1996;178(5Ptl):638.

16. Shamberger RC, Welch KJ. Surgical repair of pectus excavatum. J Pediatr Surg 1988;23(7):615.

17. Haller JR, Kramer SS, Lietman SA. Use of CT scans in selection of patients for pectus excavatum surgery: a preliminary report. J Pediatr Surg 1987;22(10):904.

18. Shamberger RC, Welch KJ, Castaneda AR, et al. Anterior chest wall deformities and congenital heart disease. J Thorac Cardiovasc Surg 1988;96(3):427.

19. Arn PH, Scherer LR, Haller JA Jr, et al. Outcome of pectus excavatum in patients with Marfan syndrome and in the general population. J Pediatr 1989;115(6):954.

20. Ravitch MM. The operative treatment of pectus excavatum. Ann Surg 1949;129:929.

21. Haller JA Jr, Scherer LR, Turner CS, et al. Evolving management of pectus excavatum based on a single institutional experience of 664 patients. Ann Surg 1989;209(5):578.

22. Pickard LR, Tepas JJ, Shermeta DW, et al. Pectus carinatum: results of surgical therapy. J Pediatr Surg 1979;14(3):3228.

23. Shamberger RC, Welch KJ. Surgical correction of pectus carinatum. J Pediatr Surg 1987;22(1):48.

24. Clarkson P. Poland's syndactyly. Guy's Hospital Rep 1962;3:335.

25. Ravitch MM. Atypical deformities of the chest wall—absence and deformities of the ribs and costal cartilages. Surgery 1966;59:438.

26. Urschel HC Jr, Byrd HS, Sethi SM, et al. Poland's syndrome: improved surgical management. Ann Thorac Surg 1984;37(3):204.

27. Haller JA Jr, Colombani PM, Miller D, et al. Early reconstruction of Poland's syndrome using autologous rib grafts combined with a latissimus muscle flap. J Pediatr Surg 1984;19:423.

28. Franken EA Smith JA, Smith WL. Tumors of the chest wall in infants and children. Pediatr Radiol 1977;6:13.

29. Shamberger RC, Tarbel NJ, Perez-Atayde AR, et al. Malignant small round cell tumor (Ewing's PNET) of the chest wall in children. J Pediatr Surg 1994;29(2)ķ9.

30. Askin FB, Rosai J, Sibley RK, et al. Malignant small cell tumor of the thoracopulmonary region in childhood. Cancer 1979;43:2438.

31. Grosfeld JL. Primary tumors of the chest wall and mediastinum in children. Semin Thorac Cardiovasc Surg 1994;6(4):235.

32. Mahesh Kumar AP, Green A, Smith JW, et al. Combined therapy for malignant tumors of the chest wall in children. J Pediatr Surg 1977;12(6):991.

33. Raney RB Jr, Ragab AH, Ruymann FB, et al. Soft tissue sarcoma of the trunk in childhood. Cancer 1982;49:2612.

34. Martin VG, Pelletteiere EV, Gress D, et al. Paget's disease in an adolescent arising in a supernumerary nipple. J Cutan Pathol 1994;21(3):283.

35. Neinstein LS, Atkinson J, Diament M. Prevalence and longitudinal study of breast masses in adolescents. J Adolesc Health 1993;14(4):277.

36. Fiorica JV. Fibrocystic changes. Obstet Gynecol Clin North Am 1994;21(3):445.

37. Dupont WD, Page DL, Parl FF, et al. Long-term risk of breast cancer in women with fibroadenoma. N Engl J Med 1994;331(1):10.

38. Simmons PS. Diagnostic considerations in breast disorders of children and adolescents. Obstet Gynecol Clin North Am 1992;19(1):91.

39. Siegal A, Kaufman Z, Siegal G. Breast masses in adolescent females. J Surg Oncol 1992;51(3):169.

40. Leveque J, Meunier B, Wattier E, et al. Malignant cystosarcoma phyllodes of the breast in adolescent females. Eur J Obstet Gynecol Reproduc Biol 1994;54:197.

41. Grimes MH. Cystosarcoma phyllodes of the breast: histologic features, flow cytometric analysis, and clinical correlations. Mod Pathol 1992;5(3):232.

42. Green DM, Edge SB, Penetrante RB, et al. In situ breast carcinoma after treatment during adolescence for thyroid cancer with radioiodine. Med Pediatr Oncol 1995;24(2):82.

43. Fowble BL, Schultz DJ, Overmoyer B, et al. The influence of young age on outcome in early stage breast cancer. Int J Radiat Oncol Biol Phys 1994;30(1):23.

Surgery of Infants and Children: Scientific Principles and Practice, edited by
Keith T. Oldham, Paul M. Colombani, and Robert P. Foglia.
Lippincott–Raven Publishers, Philadelphia, © 1997.

CHAPTER 54

Congenital Diaphragmatic Hernia

Charles J.H. Stolar

HISTORY

The earliest English language description of the gross anatomy and pathophysiology associated with congenital diaphragmatic hernia (CDH) was presented by Dr. George McCauley, an associate of Dr. John Hunter, in 1754[1]:

The child was born in the lying-in-hospital in Brownlow Street on the 24th of August, 1752: and was a fully grown boy, remarkably fat and fleshy. He was the fifth child of a healthy young woman who was well during her pregnancy. The child, when first born, started and shuddered; so that the nurse apprehended his going into fits. He breathed also with difficulty and it was some time before he could cry; which when he did, there was something peculiar in its note. He seemed to revive a little in about half an hour and breathed more freely: but soon relapsed and died before he was quite an hour and a half old. Being informed of these particulars by the mother, the matron, and the nurse, I was desirous of examining the body . . . I laid open the abdomen and found none of the intestines were contained in that cavity except part of the colon which was distended with meconium. Before I proceeded further with the dissection I sent to acquaint my ingenious friend, Dr. Hunter. We together dissected and examined this curious subject: and at the same time committed to writing the most remarkable appearances.

When the sternum was raised, the stomach with the greatest part of the intestines, with the spleen, and part of the pancreas were found in the left cavity of the thorax; having been protruded through a discontinuation, or rather an aperture of the diaphragm, about an inch from the natural passage of the esophagus.

From the extraordinary bulk of the parts contained in the left side of the thorax, the mediastinum, the heart, the esophagus, and the descending aorta were forced a considerable way to the right side of the thorax; because there was not the least mark of rupture or inflammation about the edges of the chasm: and because it is probable that the diminished size of the left lobes of the lungs, and the heart and mediastinum being pushed to the right side, were gradually affected by the bulk and increase of the viscera.

As the esophagus was pushed to the right side by the stomach and the bowels, in the cavity of the thorax it kept the same course and pierced the diaphragm not in the usual place, but considerably further to the right side: and the aperture through which it passed was backwards and to the right side with respect to that for the vena cava.

I have preserved the heart and lungs to show the disproportioned sizes of the lobes. And I have dried and prepared the diaphragm with its connections to the vertebrae and sternum to show the preternatural aperture through which the bowels passed into the thorax; as also the passage of the esophagus to the right side of the diaphragm.

Although other physicians contributed a variety of insights,[2-4] little changed from this scenario until very recently. Bochdalek[5] speculated that the hernia resulted from a posterolateral rupture of the membrane separating the pleuroperitoneal canal into two cavities. He also speculated incorrectly that the best way to repair the defect was through the bed of the twelfth rib. Whether this was actually ever attempted is unclear. The earliest, although unsuccessful, efforts to repair CDH were by Nauman[6] in 1888 and O'Dwyer[7] in 1890. The first reports of successful repair were by Aue[8] in 1901, involving an adult patient, and by Heidenhain[9] in 1905, involving a child. The groundwork for treating CDH in the newborn period was laid by Hedblom[10] whose review of the reported cases as of 1925 showed that 75% of 44 cases diagnosed in the newborn period died. He suggested that earlier intervention might improve survival. Successful repair of CDH remained rare until 1940 when Ladd and Gross[11] reported the survival of 9 of 16 patients, the youngest being 40-hours-old. It was not until 1946 that Gross[12] reported the survival of an infant less than 24-hours-old after operative repair of the defect. Until the safety net of extracorporeal membrane oxygenation (ECMO) was established in the 1980s, the standard of care remained emergent surgery and hopeful postoperative resuscitation.

EPIDEMIOLOGY OF CONGENITAL DIAPHRAGMATIC HERNIA

The reported incidence of CDH is estimated between 1 in 2000 to 5000 births.[12-15] In 1987, the National Maternity Hospital of Dublin reported an incidence of 1 in 2107 births after reviewing 90,000 patient records.[16] The incidence in stillborns is less well documented. Records confirm a number of stillborn

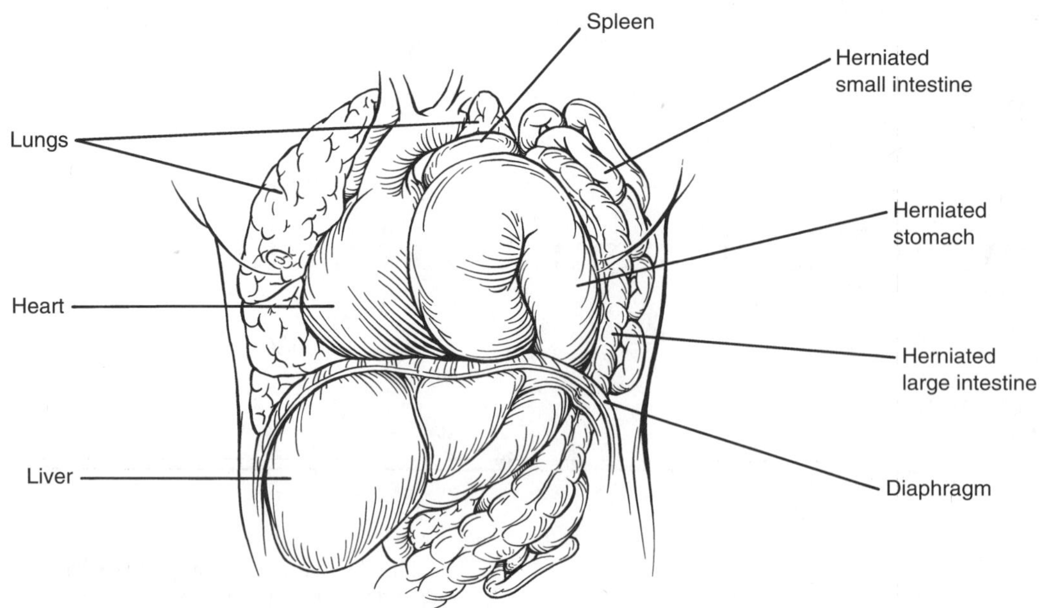

FIG. 54-1. Left-sided congenital diaphragmatic hernia demonstrating translocation of the abdominal viscera into the left hemothorax and displacement of the mediastinum to the contralateral side.

fetuses with CDH, but their deaths are usually due to an associated fatal congenital anomaly.[17,18] The hernia is left-sided in 80% of patients and right-sided in 20%. Rare cases are bilateral. Although there are scattered occurrences of familial CDH reported, there is no known genetic cause. CDH is thought to represent a sporadic developmental anomaly.[19,20] Certain drugs and insecticides, such as phenometrazine, thalidomide, quinine, and nitrofen, as well as vitamin A deficiency, have been associated with an increased incidence of CDH.[21,22]

GROSS ANATOMY

The more common left-sided CDH features a 2- to 4-cm posterolateral defect in the diaphragm through which the abdominal viscera have been translocated into the hemithorax. This can include the left lobe of the liver, the spleen, and the entire gastrointestinal tract. The stomach is often in the chest, causing some degree of obstruction of the gastroesophageal junction. This, in turn, causes dilation and ectasia of the esophagus. On the right side, the large right lobe of the liver can occupy much of the hemithorax in addition to abdominal viscera. The hepatic veins can drain ectopically into the right atrium complicating reduction of the hernia. The defect usually features open communication between the chest and abdomen, although some infants have a membrane of parietal pleura and peritoneum separating the two. This must be distinguished from an eventration of the diaphragm, which results from phrenic nerve or anterior horn-cell degeneration with muscle fibers of the diaphragm usually remaining. On occasion, the kidney is located in the chest of an infant with CDH as well, tethered by the renal vessels in a more cephalad location. Regardless of the side on which the hernia is located, there is generally a scaphoid abdomen with loss of abdominal domain (Figs. 54-1 and 54-2).

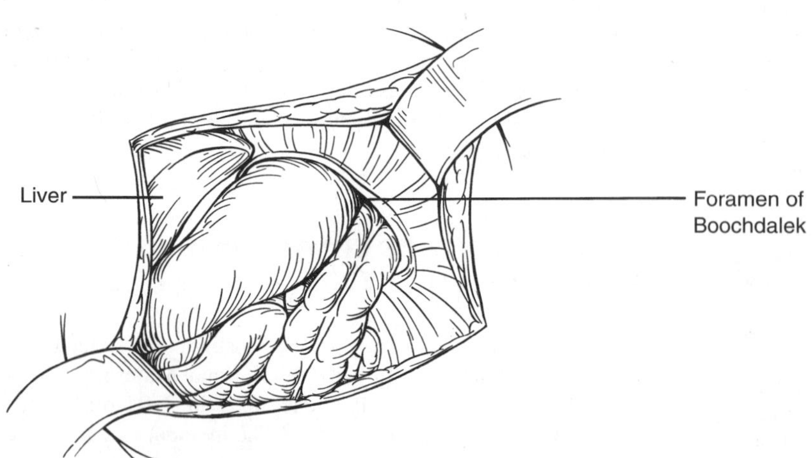

FIG. 54-2. Left-sided congenital diaphragmatic hernia viewed from a left subcostal incision showing herniation of intestine through the aperture (foramen of Bochdalek) in the diaphragm.

ASSOCIATED ANOMALIES

A newborn with one major congenital anomaly has an increased incidence of an additional malformation when compared with the general population. Infants with CDH are no different. Associated defects were observed in 28% of babies with CDH reported to the Iowa Birth Defects Registry (1988–1991)[23] and 28% reported to the Minnesota State Registry (1985–1989).[18] This incidence was 31% in a recent report from Boston Children's Hospital (1985–1993).[24] An additional major anomaly is usually associated with a worse prognosis than if the CDH is an isolated problem. Less the 6% of such infants survive. The reported incidence of associated anomalies ranges between 40% and 57%, whereas autopsy reports on stillborns with CDH report a 95% incidence of associated defects.[25] The stillborn defects are usually anencephaly, myelomeningocele, hydrocephalus, encephalocele, ventricular–septal defects, vascular rings, coarctation of the aorta, trisomy, esophageal atresia, omphalocele, and cleft palate.[3,18,21] The cardiovascular anomalies are especially common and important.

EMBRYOLOGY

The normal diaphragm is derived from several components. The central tendon is formed from the septum transversum; small dorsolateral portions are from pleuroperitoneal membranes; the dorsal crura are from the esophageal mesentery; and the posterior lateral muscle is derived from the intercostal muscle groups. Development of the diaphragm begins at week four in human gestation with formation of the septum transversum, which separates the thoracic and abdominal cavities of the embryonic coelom leaving two pleuroperitoneal canals dorsolaterally. The pleuroperitoneal folds extend from the lateral body wall and grow medial and ventral until week seven, when they fuse with the septum transversum and the mesentery of the esophagus. Muscularization then ensues, either as a result of myoblasts migrating from the cervical myotomes or of burrowing of the primitive lungs, which causes the innermost layer of intercostal muscle to be incorporated into the diaphragm. At the junction of the lumbar and costal muscle groups posterolaterally, the fibrous lumbocostal trigone remains as a small remnant of the pleuroperitoneal membrane, relying for its strength on the fusion of the two muscle groups in the final stages of development. Delay or failure of muscular fusion leaves this area weak, perhaps predisposing to herniation. Though his understanding of the embryogenesis was not correct, Bochdalek first described this vulnerable area of the posterolateral diaphragm in 1848, and the most common site for diaphragmatic hernia bears his name.

The etiology of CDH is uncertain, but its developmental consequences are well documented. During the early development of the diaphragm, the midgut is herniated into the yolk sac. If closure of the pleuroperitoneal canal has not occurred by the time the midgut returns to the abdomen (weeks 9 through 10), the abdominal viscera herniate through the lumbocostal trigone into the ipsilateral thorax. This prevents the normal counterclockwise rotation and fixation of the midgut. No hernia sac is present if the herniation occurs before complete closure of the pleuroperitoneal canal, but a nonmuscularized membrane forms a hernia sac in 10% to 15% of CDH patients.[26] Although some authors claim the herniation can occur late in gestation or be intermittently present as a dynamic process,[25] in most cases

the defect is established by weeks 10 to 12, and the postnatal problems relate to the effects of the herniated viscera on the developing lungs and heart.[27]

Development of the lungs begins between the third and fourth weeks of gestation as a ventral outpouching in the foregut. The primitive bronchi undergo a process of successive branching until week 16 after which the number of alveolar air spaces begins to increase. This process continues from week 24 until 8 years of age[28] and is discussed in detail in Chapters 8 and 57. Because CDH occurs during the process of bronchial subdivision, it is at this stage that lung development is compromised. Although all major bronchial buds are present at birth, the number of bronchial branchings in the affected lungs is greatly reduced. The number of alveoli per acini may be normal or increased in these lungs, but the absolute number of alveoli is decreased because of the reduced number of alveolar divisions. In addition, the alveoli can be small and lined by immature cuboidal epithelium not usually seen after the 13th week of gestation (Fig. 54-3). Animal studies have suggested that these alveoli also feature overgrowth of type II pneumocytes,[29,30] but this observation is controversial.[31] Importantly, the pulmonary vascular bed is abnormal as well. The development of the pulmonary arterial tree follows in parallel the development of the airways and is similarly compromised (Fig. 54-4). In addition, the small preacinar and intraacinar arterioles feature inappropriate and significant medial muscular hyperplasia. Although this is more pronounced on the ipsilateral side, the contralateral side is affected as well in all regards as a consequence of the shifted mediastinum in utero. The heart may be smaller than normal in infants with CDH as well. Recent animal studies[32] and human ultrasound observations[33,34] suggest this, although the clinical implications are unclear.[34]

Other embryologic concepts are worth mentioning. Some suggest that CDH is due to an instrinsic abnormality in the lungs with the diaphragmatic defect being secondary rather than primary.[35,36] The hypothesis is that primary pulmonary hypoplasia allows abdominal viscera to herniate into the chest through a diaphragm made vulnerable by a paucity of myoblasts. This notion has been enhanced by work using a rat model of CDH induced by nitrofen, showing that the diaphragm forms abnormally only after lung development is altered by the teratogen.[37,38]

The role of fetal breathing in lung development in general and in diaphragmatic hernia in particular is a subject of increasing interest. Early work by Alcorn et al[39] showed that selective bronchial ligation in fetal animals created lung growth in rats. This concept has been explored more recently by Wilson et al,[40,41] who showed similar results in lambs with and without fetal diaphragmatic hernias. Preliminary reports by Adzick et al describe an experience with CDH where surgical obstruction of the trachea appeared to cause lung growth.[41a] At this writing, one of three fetuses treated in this manner survived.[42] Santin and colleagues[43] have proposed the presence of pulmonary growth peptides released into the amniotic fluid of fetal sheep from the kidney. Pulmonary hypoplasia in the presence of altered renal development may result from decreased production of these peptides.[43]

DIAGNOSIS

The diagnosis of CDH is often made on a prenatal ultrasound examination and is accurate about 90% of the time with an

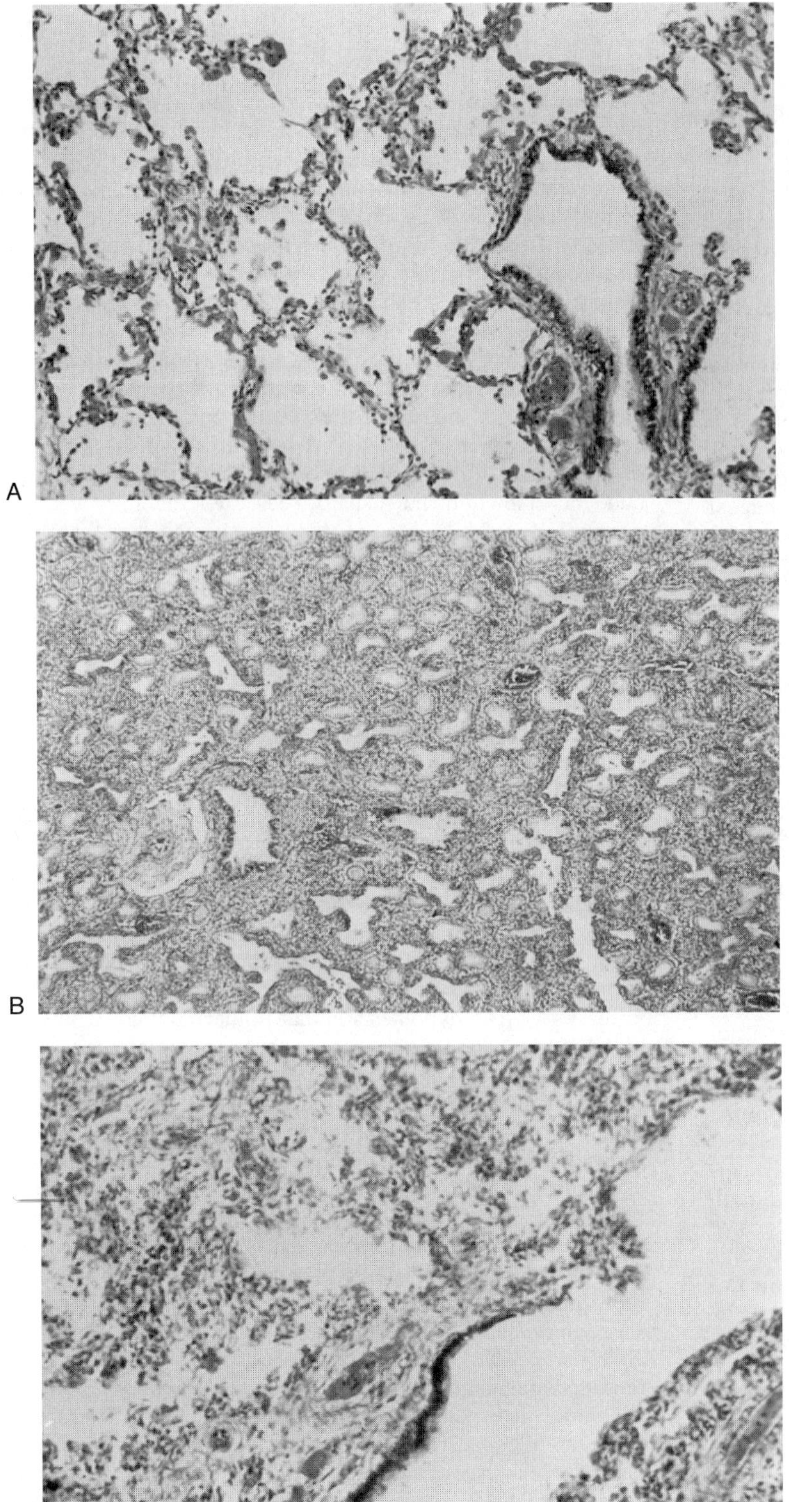

FIG. 54-3. (*A*) Normal microscopic anatomy of the lung with fully developed alveoli and mature, flattened alveolar epithelial cells. (*B*) Photomicrograph at 20 weeks' gestation of normal fetal cuboidal epithelium within incompletely formed alveoli. (*C*) Hypoplastic lung from an infant with a congenital posterolateral diaphragmatic hernia. Alveoli are absent; this microscopic anatomy is similar to that of the normal fetal lung. Although the lung is a heterogeneous organ and the spectrum of diaphragmatic hernia is broad, the histologic abnormalities illustrated are typical of the problem. (Coran AG, Oldham KT. The pediatric thorax. In: Greenfield LG, Mulholland MW, Oldham KT, et al, eds. Surgery: scientific principles and practice. Philadelphia, JB Lippincott, 1993:1827)

experienced observer. The ultrasound is usually obtained for routine obstetric care or because of concerns aroused by the development of polyhydramnios. Polyhydramnios is thought to result from distortion of the gastroesophageal junction by translocation of the stomach into the thorax with resultant foregut obstruction. The ultrasound diagnosis is suggested by observing the stomach or fluid-filled loops of intestine in the same cross-sectional view as the heart. Other signs include the absence of a stomach in the abdomen, the liver within the thorax, or often abdominal viscera in the chest. Children with CDH may have microgastria because of interference with fetal swallowing of amniotic fluid. On the right, the liver may functionally

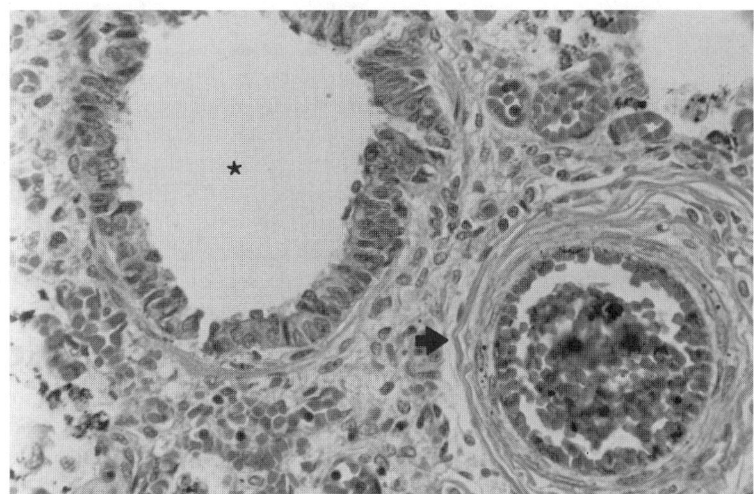

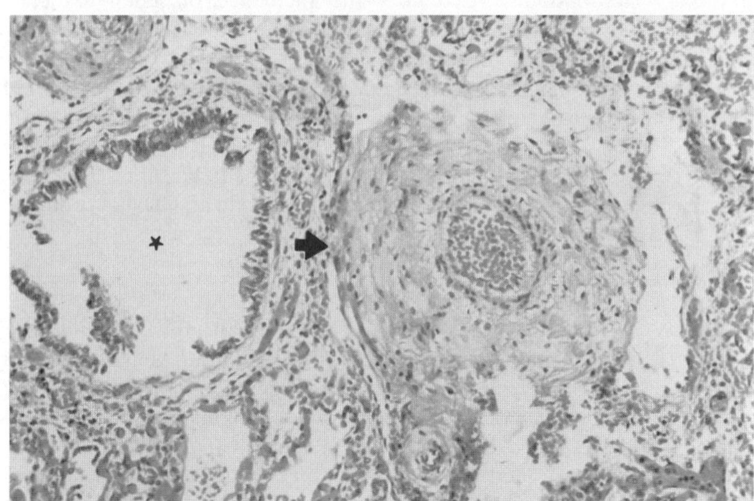

FIG. 54-4. Histology of the pulmonary artery. Pulmonary artery branches of similar size and location are shown in a normal infant (*A*) and in an infant a with Boochdalek diaphragmatic hernia (*B*). In particular, there is increased muscle mass associated with the arterial wall (*arrows*) in the latter case. The conducting airways shown (asterisks) are of similar size. The vascular smooth muscle can be exquisitely sensitive to chemical, hormonal, and paracrine mediators in the neonatal period. Pulmonary artery vasospasm is an important cause of persistent fetal circulation and respiratory failure. (Coran AG, Oldham KT. The pediatric thorax. In: Greenfield LG, ed. Surgery: scientific principles and practice. Philadelphia, JB Lippincott, 1994:1827)

close the diaphragm and obscure the diagnosis before or after birth. Functional information concerning fetal breathing can be obtained by duplex Doppler examination of amniotic flow at the fetal nares. A fetal "tidal volume per minute of ventilation" can be determined, which may have some bearing on prognosis.[44] Interpreting the fetal ultrasound requires experience because other diagnoses, such as esophageal atresia or cystic lung-bud anomalies, can result in similar images.

The diagnosis of CDH is suggested in a newborn with respiratory distress within the first 24 hours of life. Classically, these infants have a scaphoid abdomen and an asymmetric, distended chest. The chest may become more distended as swallowed air passes into the intestines. Breath sounds may or may not be heard on the ipsilateral side. Shifting of the mediastinum may move the trachea away from the side of the hernia and obstruct venous blood return to the heart, causing hypotension and venous hypertension of the head and neck. The stigmata of respiratory distress are commonly present.

The diagnosis of CDH is confirmed typically by a plain chest radiograph which demonstrates air-filled loops of intestine in the chest (Fig. 54-5). The rare infant with bilateral CDHs can have a confusing radiograph. On occasion, the diagnosis is not clear on plain chest radiograph because of similarities to congenital lung-bud abnormalities. If the nasogastric tube is posi-

tioned with its tip in a thoracic stomach, this confirms the diagnosis of CDH, although some infants need a contrast upper gastrointestinal series. Once the diagnosis of CDH is confirmed, anomalies of the cardiovascular, central nervous, and renal systems should be sought by ultrasound examinations.

Although most infants with CDH present in the first 24 hours of life, some can appear later. These children have a variety of presentations including mild respiratory distress, an incidental finding in chest radiograph, chronic pulmonary disease, pneumonia, pleural effusion, empyema, or gastric volvulus. Presentation with gastric volvulus is worthy of emphasis because it is an indication for emergent surgical intervention.

DIFFERENTIAL DIAGNOSIS

The prenatal and neonatal diagnosis of CDH can be confused with a variety of other lesions including eventration of the diaphragm, pentalogy of Cantrell, Morgagni hernia, congenital axial hiatus hernia, congenital cystic disease of the lung, and primary agenesis of the lung. Diaphragmatic eventration has many causes, but in the newborn, it commonly results from birth trauma or Wernig-Hoffman anterior horn-cell disease. The eventuated diaphragm can rise as high as the third intercostal

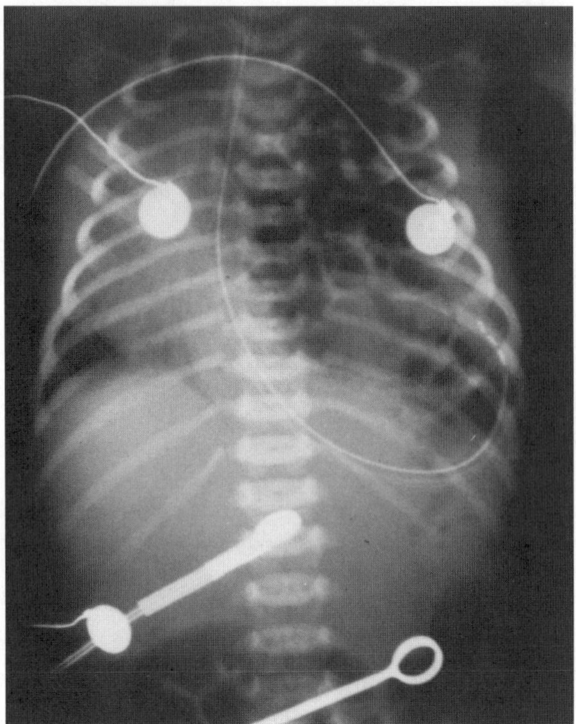

FIG. 54-5. Plain chest radiograph of an infant with a left posterolateral congenital diaphragmatic hernia.

space. The physiologic consequences are quite variable, ranging from asymptomatic infants to acute respiratory distress. The diagnosis can be made generally by fluoroscopy or real-time ultrasound demonstrating paradoxical movement of the diaphragm with breathing.

Morgagni hernias occur in the anterior muscular diaphragm at the hiatus for the internal mammary artery and are rarer than the Bochdalek hernias. Affected infants can present with gastrointestinal crisis because of incarceration and need emergent surgery; however, most are asymptomatic.

Success in managing CDH has improved dramatically from the time when virtually all of these symptomatic newborns were considered doomed.[45]

TREATMENT

Prenatal Care

The diagnosis of CDH is being made with increasing frequency by prenatal ultrasound examination. The prenatal diagnosis of CDH should be complimented by a careful search for other congenital anomalies, particularly those of the cardiovascular and nervous systems. Evaluation of fetal karyotype should be accomplished by amniocentesis, chorionic villous, or fetal blood sampling. The current standard of care is to ensure the health of the mother and fetus, while bringing the neonate to delivery as close to term as possible. The advantage of prenatal diagnosis is not so much for surgical preparation as it is for educating parents about possible treatments and outcomes. It also allows the fetus and mother to be referred safely to an appropriate level III tertiary perinatal center where the full array of respiratory care expertise and strategies, including inhaled nitric oxide, oscillating ventilators, and extracorporeal membrane oxygenation, are immediately available. Anything less compromises the best possible outcome. As a matter of principle, a spontaneous vaginal delivery is preferred unless obstetric issues supervene. The mere diagnosis of CDH is not an indication for elective cesarean section.

Fetal intervention is a source of considerable controversy. As discussed later in the Outcome section, the prognosis for isolated CDH is not as grave as once thought, and hence, the rationale for operating on the mother and fetus simultaneously may be ill founded. In published reports, 17 fetuses have undergone in utero correction of a CDH with 4 initial survivors reported and 2 long-term survivors.[45a] The natural history of the fetus into CDH is highly controversial, and this of course must be known if patients for fetal intervention are to be selected appropriately. Likewise, the incidence of lethal associated anomalies is not clearly known, and this too is relevant to selecting therapy.

Animals with induced CDHs have been shown to respond to antenatal treatment with dexamethasone and thyroid-releasing hormone by increasing functional alveolar maturity, but there was no effect on the numbers of bronchiolar units. Experience using this treatment in the human fetus with CDH is pending.[46]

Preoperative Care

Once the CDH diagnosis is made, all efforts should be directed toward stabilizing the brittle cardiorespiratory system while inducing a minimum of iatrogenic injury. It is essential to consider that CDH is a physiologic, not a surgical, emergency.

Resuscitation begins with endotracheal and nasogastric intubation to facilitate ventilation and gastrointestinal decomposition. Ventilation by mask or ambubag is contraindicated to avoid distention of the bowel. Arterial and venous access can be acquired through the umbilicus. If the umbilical venous catheter can be passed across the liver into the right atrium, it is useful for mixed venous blood gas analysis. Although the postductal umbilical artery is appropriate for blood pressure monitoring, it is essential to monitor arterial oxygen saturation in a preductal location as well. An important part of the treatment decision algorithm is to estimate whether the infant has enough lung for adequate gas exchange. Although controversial and the subject of continuing debate, our experience as well as other authors' shows that an infant unable to fully saturate the preductal hemoglobin with oxygen as well as achieve a pCO_2 level less than 50 mmHg in the face of maximal conventional therapy probably has pulmonary hypoplasia to a degree incompatible with life.[47,49] It is important to make this estimation before embarking on an emotionally difficult and expensive course of therapy that will be ultimately unsuccessful.

The definition of conventional treatment is the subject of controversy. While a strategy based on muscle paralysis and induced alkalosis with hyperventilation is widespread, others advocate a strict avoidance of all muscle paralysis. More recent experience suggests that it is appropriate to take advantage of native respiratory effort with ventilator support only to move the chest wall adequately. For this strategy, sufficient supplemental oxygen is administered to maintain preductal oxygen saturation at higher than 80%. The postductal values are virtually disregarded other than as an index of right-to-left shunting. Because oxygen delivery, not oxygen saturation, is the goal, this approach requires adequate circulating hemoglobin levels (consider fetal versus adult forms) and adequate arterial perfusion pressure. Hypercapnea is permitted to avoid iatrogenic barotrauma, and this is discussed in detail in Chapter 8. Blood and crystalloid administration and cardiotonic drugs in appropriate doses are important adjuncts. Because some infants with CDH may have associated cardiac hypoplasia, cardiotonic drugs may compromise oxygen consumption in the myocardium. Agents such as tolazoline, while sometimes effective in ameliorating pulmonary hypertension, often precipitate systemic hypotension and tachyphylaxis develops predictably. Systemic hypotension may be the result of inadequate circulating blood volume in this circumstance, and this is to be avoided. Tolazoline is an alpha-adrenergic antagonist with inotropic and chronotropic effects on cardiac muscle. It has a histamine-like effect on gastrin and pepsin secretion.[50] The usual approach is to administer an intravenous bolus of 1 to 2 mg/kg, and if there is an improvement in the postductal oxygen saturation, a continuous infusion is initiated.

New agents such as inhaled nitric oxide (NO) may also have a role in the preoperative management of pulmonary hypertension in the infant with CDH. Because NO is rapidly bound to and inactivated by hemoglobin, it has virtually no systemic effects when inhaled. Its effects are apparently limited to the smooth muscle in the pulmonary arteriole. Although theoretically appealing, the clinical efficacy of inhaled NO in CDH patients has been difficult to demonstrate in the initial limited trials. A principal reason is that CDH patients are heterogeneous, and the differences are further modified by the variety of treatments in use. Lungs unsullied by iatrogenic injury respond differently than those that are not. More than one center has reported some CDH infants whose pulmonary hypertension was controlled by inhaled NO[51]; however, this experience has been difficult to transfer from one infant to another.

It may be that the infant with CDH is surfactant deficient, although this too is an area of controversy. Pringle et al[29] showed that lambs with CDH had hypertrophy of type II pneumocytes. Subsequent animal work by Glick et al suggests otherwise.[30] Clinical attempts to learn whether the human infant with CDH is surfactant deficient are limited to comparative amniotic fluid examinations. Some data suggest that the human CDH neonate is surfactant deficient at birth[31] while others do not.[52] Regardless, aggressive positive pressure ventilation strategies can injure the type II pneumocyte and alter the infant's ability to maintain normal surfactant production. Consequently, exogenous surfactant administration has been advocated for neonates with CDH, and there is anecdotal support for this approach. Prospective human trials have not been conducted to date.

Hypoplastic lungs are subject to inordinate airway pressures in the effort to achieve adequate ventilation. Air frequently extravasates along the tracheobronchial tree and ruptures into the pleural space resulting in a pneumothorax. The contralateral lung is usually more vulnerable than the ipsilateral lung because it is more compliant. Tube thoracostomy or needle aspiration is indicated promptly if pneumothorax is suspected. Delay in obtaining emergency chest radiograph is not a reason to delay decompression of the chest if pneumothorax is suspected. A high index of suspicion is always warranted. The goal of the tube thoracostomy is to decompress the chest and to equalize the intrathoracic–extrathoracic pressures. Negative pressure application to the chest tube is not routinely indicated. Suction applied to a hypoplastic lung results in overdistention and exacerbation of the pulmonary hypertension. The use of prophylactic chest tubes in preparation for surgery has been advocated in the past, but current data do not support this approach.

The type of mechanical ventilation provided for the infant with a CDH is largely a matter of personal preference. Most infants can be successfully treated with a simple pressure-cycled ventilator using a combination of high respiratory rates (up to 100 bpm) and modest peak airway pressures (18 to 22 cm H_2O with no positive end expiratory pressure [PEEP]), or using lower rates (20 to 40 bpm) and higher pressures (22 to35 cm H_2O, 3 to 5 cm PEEP). In selected refractory infants with inordinate CO_2 retention or poor preductal oxygenation, support can be provided with a high frequency oscillating ventilator. In this mode, volumes of air less than the anatomical dead space are provided at 2400 cycles/min (40 Hz). Gas exchange is thought to occur by diffusion from laminar air flow currents rather than bulk oxygen delivery under pressure. The symmetrical sine wave associated with the oscillations is thought to cause less barotrauma than conventional pressure-controlled ventilation. Tidal volume can be controlled without large changes in mean airway pressure. This strategy often affords excellent ventilation, although the effect on oxygenation is less predictable. Experience with infants with CDH is reasonably limited, and no prospective trials have defined its role. Other new strategies are also under investigation. Currently, this is best considered in the individual context of one's own institutional experience.

Timing of Surgery

Historically, CDH has been considered a surgical emergency. Infants were rushed to the operating room as soon as possible after birth in the hope that reducing the abdominal contents from the chest would relieve the compression of the lungs. It was thought that to delay was to entertain disaster. However, this approach neglects the embryology of CDH, whereby the damage to the developing lung occurs weeks before birth and the primary problems relate to intrinsic deficiencies of the lung itself, not to simple extrinsic compression. It now appears clear that emergency surgery only adds surgical and anesthetic morbidity to an unstable patient without reversing the underlying physiologic problem.

As stated earlier, CDH is now considered a physiologic rather than surgical emergency. Current data suggest that prolonged preoperative stabilization with delayed repair may be an important key to treating the infant with CDH. Repair of the hernia does not increase the surface area available for gas exchange in hypoplastic lungs. The alveoli are not atelectatic and do not expand upon decompression of the chest. If adequate gas exchange is achieved perinatally, it is possible that anesthesia or surgery may induce recurrent, refractory, or unstable pulmonary vasospasm. An ill-timed operation can initiate this process and may lead to the demise of the infant.

A consensus has developed recently that surgery be performed when pulmonary vascular tone is maximally stabilized. This is followed by preductal–postductal oximetry and serial cardiac echocardiography with duplex Doppler examinations. Recent reports on infants with CDH studied by whole-body plethysmography during prolonged preoperative resuscitation demonstrate that infant minute ventilation improves with decreased mechanical support over the first several days of life with concomitant improvement in blood gas parameters.[53] A timely operation can often be performed after 100 hours with minimal supplemental oxygen and airway pressure requirements, particularly if therapy is guided primarily by preductal oxygen saturation. It is speculated that the hypertrophied muscle in the intraacinar arterioles is undergoing remodeling at a slower rate than usually seen at the time of birth. It appears that this type of preoperative stabilization can allow the diameter of these vessels to increase over time and that the sensitivity to vasospasm will similarly diminish.

Treating the infant who cannot be stabilized with this approach is controversial. It is, however, clear that an unstable infant is not made more stable by an operation. Assuming that no iatrogenic insults occur, it is entirely possible that an infant who cannot be stabilized preoperatively has pulmonary hypoplasia to a degree incompatible with life. Bohn et al[48] report an approach whereby an infant who cannot be controlled by their conventional care is not considered an operative candidate. Over the past 12 years, this author has treated 9 infants with CDH from birth who were never able to achieve a preductal arterial blood hemoglobin saturation greater than 90% or be ventilated to a pCO_2 less than 60 mmHg. All nine infants died and, at autopsy, had lung weight and radial alveolar counts less than the fifth percentile, consistent with the most severe pulmonary hypoplasia. Other reports suggest that no therapy, especially ECMO, should be withheld from refractory infants because of an inability to establish the history from arterial blood gases. These reports appear to depend on postductal rather preductal blood gas assessments.

Anesthesia

The conventional ventilators used with anesthesia machines are too compliant and have too much dead space for efficient ventilation of CDH infants. Consequently, the use of an infant ventilator, either conventional pressure-cycled or oscillating, is favored for surgery for CDH. Anesthesia is achieved by intravenous narcotic and muscle relaxant techniques. Nitrous oxide is to be avoided because of the associated bowel distention.

Surgery

As discussed later, some infants with CDH require ECMO for resuscitation either before or after surgery. Because of the heparin requirement, ECMO alters the manner in which the operation is conducted. Specifically, any cut surface may bleed.

Most surgeons approach the defect through an appropriate subcostal incision. The viscera are gently reduced and eviscerated from the abdomen for adequate visualization (Fig. 54-6). The spleen on the left and the liver on either side can be difficult to reduce, but this must be done without injury. Cephalad placement of the hepatic veins can make reduction of the liver difficult. On the right side, the kidney and adrenal gland may be found in the chest as well. On either side, the posterolateral defect is best seen after visceral reduction is complete. When there is a true hernia sac with a membrane of parietal pleura and peritoneum, this should be resected to achieve adequate healing. Usually the anterior rim of the diaphragm is better developed than the posterior component. The variable posterior rim is rolled up like a window shade in the retroperitoneum (Fig. 54-7). When tissue is adequate, a primary repair approximating anterior and posterior elements is accomplished with nonabsorbable suture material. Although it is possible to anchor some of the anterior diaphragm to a rib posteriorly, inordinate efforts should not be made to achieve a primary repair. It is safer, in these circumstances, to place prosthetic material to complete the closure. Procedures for nonrotation of the midgut as well as appendectomy are not needed and potentially dangerous because of the risk for hemorrhage. For the same reason, muscle flaps or thoracoplasty to close the diaphragm are not indicated (Figs. 54-8 and 54-9).

With loss of abdominal domain, abdominal wall closure may not be possible or excessive intraabdominal pressure on the vena cava and viscera may result. In this case the skin only

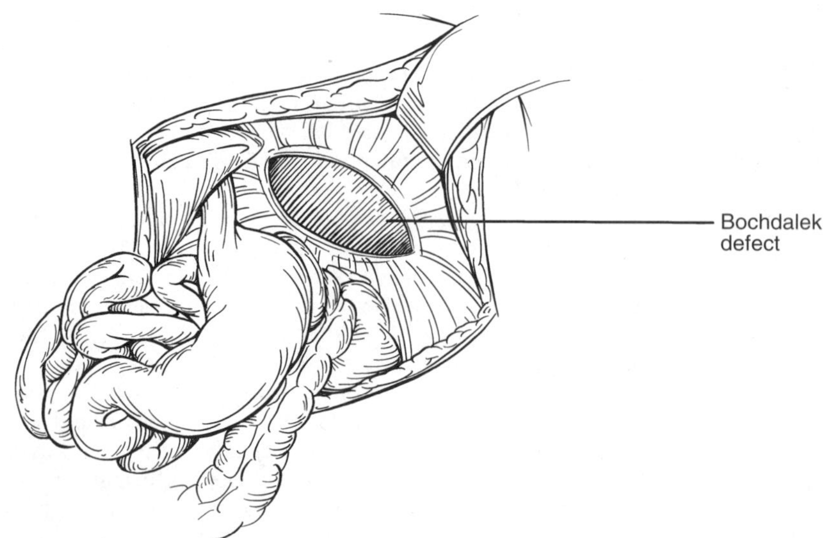

FIG. 54-6. The abdominal contents have been reduced from the thorax, clearly demonstrating the defect.

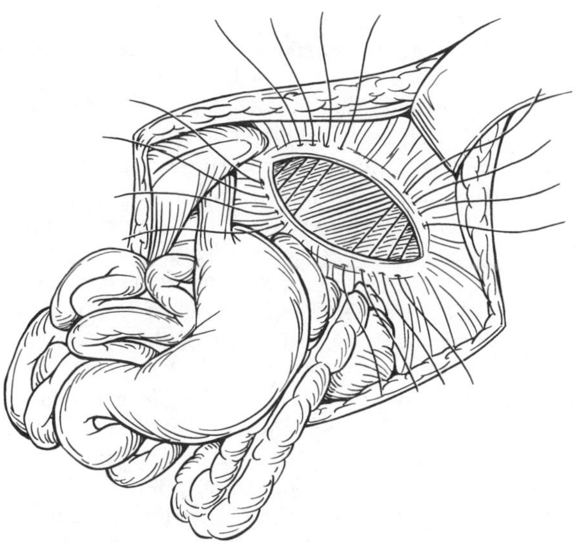

FIG. 54-7. The posterior rim of the defect has been unrolled like a window shade before being closed by primary repair.

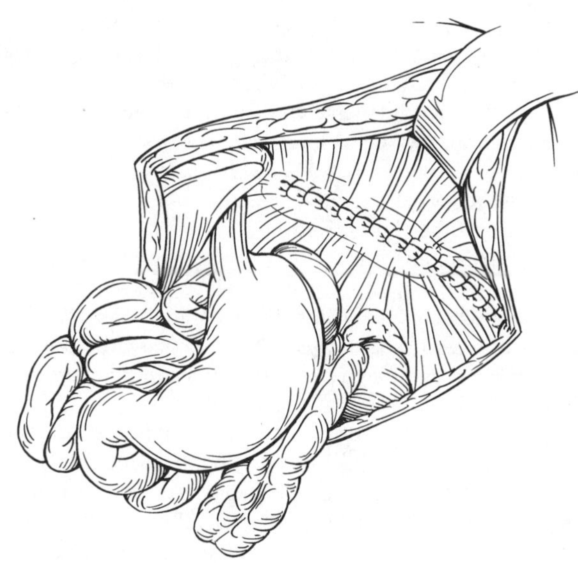

FIG. 54-9. Appearance of the congenital diaphragmatic hernia defect after primary repair.

can be closed over the viscera or the abdominal wall can be augmented with a prosthetic sheet. If used, a prosthetic pouch is managed much like the patient with an abdominal wall defect and removed in a timely fashion.

A tube thoracostomy is generally not needed in either hemithorax for the CDH infant, unless there is a pneumothorax, a bronchopleural fistula, bleeding, or some other specific indication. The ipsilateral lung is hypoplastic and hence smaller than that hemithorax. Because the pleural space is driven to obliterate itself, and because the lung is not yet capable of filling it, the remaining space will be filled with pleural fluid. Unless there is active bleeding or an air leak, this will not compromise the function of that lung. An unnecessary chest tube will only deny the pleural space its biologic imperative.

Extracorporeal Membrane Oxygenation in the Infant With CDH

ECMO is a form of partial cardiopulmonary bypass designed to use biomedical organs for extracorporeal life support with the goal of maintaining oxygen delivery for an extended period during which the pathologic processes that led to acute respiratory failure resolve and the tasks of oxygen delivery are returned to the biologic organs. ECMO was introduced in 1977 as a treatment for neonates with overwhelming respiratory failure unresponsive to conventional respiratory care.[54] The first report of infants being treated with ECMO for CDH was in 1982 (see Chapter 8). ECMO for CDH is currently administered by

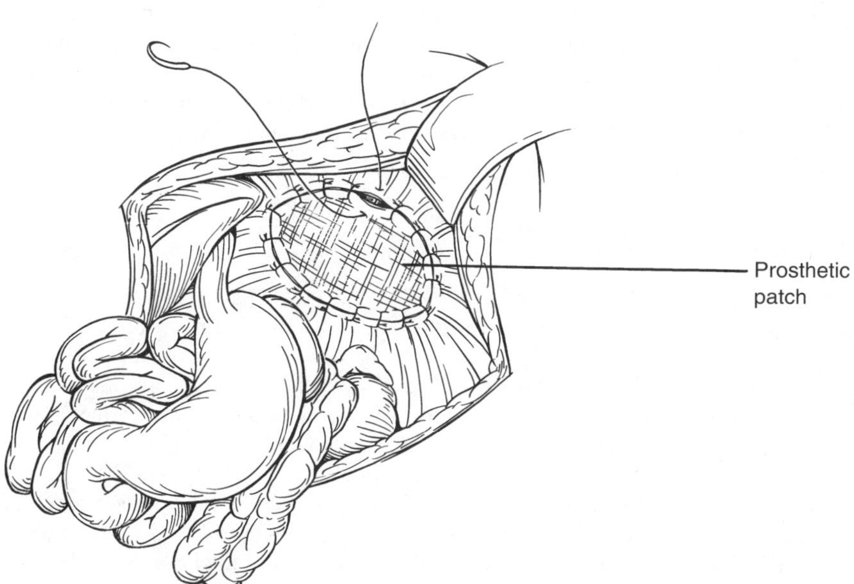

FIG. 54-8. This large defect has been repaired with a prosthetic material.

venoarterial access obtained through the right internal jugular vein and right common carotid artery. This allows access to the right atrium and ascending aorta with an operation that can be done in the neonatal intensive care unit under local anesthesia. Increasing numbers of CDH infants are being successfully supported with venovenous ECMO.[55] This technique uses a single cannula with a double lumen which allows blood to be drained and returned to the right atrium via the internal jugular vein. This technique requires that the heart be pumping effectively and that the mediastinum not be displaced so as to preclude safe cannula placement. With either technique, the goal of the therapy is to meet tissue oxygen requirements while providing a period of heart and lung rest during which pulmonary hypertension abates. ECMO can treat reversible pulmonary hypertension in the infant with CDH as outlined, but it is not a treatment for pulmonary hypoplasia. ECMO support is feasible for the days or weeks it requires for the neonate to escape from the period of vulnerability related to the transitional circulation and pulmonary vasospasm. To the best of our knowledge, infants cannot be kept on ECMO long enough for significant lung growth to occur. While on ECMO, the pulmonary vasculature undergoes the usual perinatal increases in compliance but at a much slower pace than normal. In addition, the ability of ECMO to treat and prevent the problems of barotrauma and oxygen toxicity is very important.

Criteria for the institution of ECMO were developed to ''rescue'' newborns with a projected mortality risk of at least 80% in the face of maximal conventional therapy. It has proved difficult to reach consensus on what constitutes conventional care and what criteria accurately predict an 80% mortality rate. For ethical reasons, it has been difficult to test the criteria in a randomized way when 80% of the control group would be expected to die. Regardless, we favor a physiologic approach to identifying an ECMO candidate rather than one that relies on calculated score or numerical index. Remembering that the goal of all therapy is to maintain oxygen delivery sufficient for tissue oxygen requirements, the following indication for ECMO in neonates with CDH is used: inadequate oxygen delivery despite adequate volume resuscitation, circulating hemoglobin content, pharmacologic support, and ventilation. Inadequate oxygen delivery becomes manifest by mixed venous hemoglobin desaturation, progressive metabolic acidosis, and multiple organ dysfunction. PaO_2, $PaCO_2$, a calculated oxygenation index, and determination of the alveolar–arterial oxygen gradient can help the clinician identify ECMO candidates, but there is no substitute for the overall clinical judgment about oxygen delivery. This requires frequent bedside assessment.

The issue of pulmonary hypoplasia that is incompatible with life must be considered in this discussion of ECMO and CDH infants. Such an infant can be supported with ECMO and appear quite healthy on bypass. The situation is untenable, however, if there is not a reversible disease process. We favor assessment of the arterial blood in a preductal location as a reasonable measure of the lungs' potential for meaningful gas exchange. We embraced this concept based on reports from Boix-Ochoa et al and Bohn et al as well as our own experience.[56] As noted, an infant with CDH who is unable to fully oxygenate its preductal blood or to achieve a $PaCO_2$ less than 50 mmHg with maximal conventional therapy has a high likelihood of having pulmonary hypoplasia to a degree incompatible with life. ECMO for such an infant creates unrealistic expectations. One must be mindful that right-to-left shunting through the ductus arteriosus alters the blood gas measurements in a postductal umbilical artery sample. This can lead to misleading assessments of the infant's condition and result in precipitous use of ECMO. The notion of relying on preductal blood gas analysis has not been reported by others for this purpose. All other reports use postductal blood gas measurements and have the above noted limitations. Some clinicians have opted to treat all infants with CDH who are failing conventional therapy without regard to extent of pulmonary hypoplasia. In the Registry of the Extracorporeal Life Support Organization, there are no reports of survivors who failed to meet the previously noted preductal arterial blood gas criteria.[57]

Because ECMO is potentially needed for any infant with CDH, the conduct of the surgical repair must be modified accordingly. The possible need for systemic heparinization is responsible for most of these modifications. Because any cut surface may bleed, dissection is kept to a minimum and use of the electrocautery is emphasized. No effort is made to correct the nonrotation of the midgut or to do an appendectomy. Meticulous hemostasis is the rule with liberal use of fibrin glue. Thrombocytopenia or other medical causes of coagulopathy must be anticipated and corrected.

An occasional CDH infant demonstrates adequate lung parenchyma during the preoperative resuscitation, but subsequently becomes unstable and refractory to conventional therapy for a variety of reasons. Such infants may deteriorate from persistent or recurrent pulmonary hypertension and are excellent ECMO candidates. ECMO can be a potent resuscitative tool for this preoperative stabilization. Once stable, the infant can undergo repair of the hernia either while on ECMO or after it is complete. The optimal timing of surgery in this circumstance is not clear since some surgeons prefer to do it early and others prefer a later time. Current data do not allow definitive conclusions in this regard. The ongoing heparinization and consumptive thrombocytopenia does, of course, require special considerations if repair is performed while in ECMO. It may be that the use of Σ-aminocaproic acid as an antifibrinolytic agent decreases the hemorrhagic complications.[58] If an infant has CDH repair while on ECMO, it is extremely important to be aware of potential for bleeding in any body space including the abdomen, either thorax, and the pericardium. Bleeding in each site creates its own unique clinical picture that is often masked by the ongoing ECMO perfusion until very late. A high index of clinical suspicion is mandatory.

OUTCOMES

The survival rate for infants with CDH is unknown. The concept of a hidden mortality is, to some degree, correct. Specifically, we do not know how many fetal deaths occur with CDH. In reported series, however, most such fetuses have major associated anomaly which contributes to the poor outcome.[24] Survival rates for live born infants with CDH also require careful analysis because therapy is evolving rapidly and the reported results do not involve controlled trials. In the last decade, CDH treatment has evolved from what was considered a dire surgical emergency to an operation done electively. It may be that ECMO as a safety net has given the clinician a sense of security to challenge conventional wisdom and to test other treatment strategies.

An important concept is the notion that the infant with CDH benefits from an extended period of preoperative stabilization. Recent reviews of survival data with delayed repair of CDH depend on small patient populations and often consist of experience gathered from heterogeneous treatment strategies, but the outcomes are encouraging nevertheless. Comparing 33 CDH infants, Cartlidge et al[59] reported a survival rate of 12.5% for those treated early compared with a survival rate of 52.5% for those who were stabilized for later repair. West et al[59a] reviewed 111 children from five ECMO centers. When delayed repair (5 to 72 h) was compared with emergent surgery, the survival rate improved from 43% to 67.4% with delayed surgery. In this series, an 80% overall survival rate was achieved for infants requiring ECMO support and having delayed repair. Breaux et al reported an increase in survival from 20% to 55% with delayed repair, regardless of whether ECMO was required. In this series, the average time of surgery was 26.5 hours. In 1991, Price et al[57] reported the evolution of ph directed therapy over a 10-year period. It was notable that as surgery was delayed longer and longer, right-to-left shunting was minimized, ventilator support could be diminished, and the need for ECMO decreased while survival increased.

In the Registry of the Extracorporeal Life Support Organization, 63% of all infants with CDH treated with ECMO since 1976 have survived regardless of the timing of surgical repair. This collective data from more than 100 participating centers reflect survival of the most desperately ill infants born live with CDH. It is a reasonable assumption that most children not treated with ECMO also survived, suggesting a hopeful prognosis for infants with CDH.

FOLLOW-UP

The human lung continues to grow after birth, and the number of alveoli multiply during the first several years of life to achieve a normal number of alveoli per bronchiole. Because the total number of airways is reduced in the infant with CDH, a normal number of alveoli is never achieved. However, the number of alveoli per acinus may, as a compensation, actually be increased. The alveoli may also become overdistended to fill the hemithorax on the ipsilateral side while the contralateral lung may herniate across the mediastinum. Kitagawa et al[60] and Koumbourlis et al[61] found that most survivors lead unaffected lives.

An element of mild restrictive small airway disease exists in some of these infants. Although most infants have diminished compliance in addition to this restrictive defect, serial pulmonary function testing demonstrates improving compliance and real lung growth with time.[61] Exercise tolerance tests as well as oxygen uptake and capillary blood gas measurements are generally normal in surviving CDH patients. Wohl et al[62] studied survivors over 18 years of age and found that total lung capacity and vital capacity were 99% of predicted values. In this study, the diffusion coefficient was normal, and the forced expiratory volume and vital capacity were 89% and 80% of predicted values at 1 second, respectively. Xenon 133 radiospirometry showed equal lung volumes bilaterally, but blood flow to the ipsilateral side was reduced in all patients, suggesting

that vascular growth never matches alveolar growth. Lund et al[63] report a significant incidence of chronic lung disease in survivors, but this may be related to iatrogenic lung injury or the late pulmonary consequences of gastroesophageal reflux.

A high incidence of gastroesophageal reflux and foregut dysmotility has been documented in CDH survivors.[64] The problem is seen with similar frequency in both ECMO and non-ECMO patients. Upper gastrointestinal series show a generally dilated and ectatic esophagus, a football-shaped stomach, and delayed gastric emptying. These findings may be a consequence of the hernia itself causing foregut obstruction and polyhydramnios. Many infants with CDH and foregut dysmotility have feeding difficulties. Most can be managed by one of a variety of feeding regimens and prokinetic agents. Some patients require antireflux and gastric emptying surgery.

Roye and colleagues report that almost 15% of CDH survivors over 4 years old have evidence of scoliosis, many with a chest wall deformity that resembles pectus excavatum (personal communication). In this experience, spine surgery has not yet been needed, but 30% of these children are using braces. A smaller number have had their pectus deformity corrected.

Neurocognitive outcome and follow-up is accruing as more of these children live longer. There are scant data on this subject for CDH survivors except for those who are part of ECMO follow-up studies. Stolar et al[65] reported neurocognitive follow-up at 3 years (mean) and showed that ECMO treated infants with CDH fared worse than all other ECMO entry diagnoses. In that aggregate experience, three of five children had normal cognitive function, whereas two of three had normal motor function. The etiology of this morbidity may be related to the ECMO treatment and reflect also the grave illness these infants faced.

FUTURE THERAPIES

In a lamb model, lungs made hypoplastic by the creation of a fetal diaphragmatic hernia grow in utero if the defect is repaired before birth. With this background and an estimation of a 70% hidden mortality for CDH, Harrison and his colleagues have attempted open fetal correction of CDH in the human. Although a small number of fetuses have survived this procedure, most have died.[66] The role of associated anomalies, patient selection, disagreement concerning the real mortality for this diagnosis, maternal risk, and the issue of preterm labor make fetal intervention tantalizing but a highly controversial approach at present.

Hirschl et al[67] recently reported the first infants with CDH who were treated with partial liquid ventilation using perflubron while simultaneously supported on ECMO. Oxygen delivery via a liquid in the airway is a novel concept. Because of both surfactant-like activity and antiinflammatory properties, perflurocarbons may hold special promise for selected infants.

NO is a potent inhaled pulmonary vasodilator that also holds promise for pulmonary hypertension in neonates, regardless of etiology. Current reports of NO used for infants with CDH are quite small and inconsistent, suggesting that efficacy is unpredictable and other factors such as exogenous surfactant therapy may contribute to their utility.[68]

Finally, for the infant with severe pulmonary hypoplasia who is truly refractory to all forms of therapy, lung transplantation may be an option. Technical problems, donor availability, and long-term concerns are substantial obstacles at present. A small number of centers are studying this possibility in animals,[69] while two human infants have been transplanted with reduced-volume lungs from parental donors.[70]

REFERENCES

1. Macaulay G. An account of viscera herniation. Phil Trans Roy Coll Phys 1754;6:25.
2. Cooper AP. The anatomy and surgical treatment of abdominal hernia. London, Longman, Rees, Orme, Brown, and Green, 1827.
3. Ravitch MM. Congenital diaphragmatic hernia. In: Nyhus LM, ed. Hernia. Philadelphia, JB Lippincott, 1964.
4. Bowditch HI. Peculiar case of diaphragmatic hernia. Buffalo Med J 1853;9:65.
5. Bochdalek VA. Einige Betrachtungen uber die Enstehung des angeborenen Zwerfekkbruches. Als Bietrag Zur pathologischen Anatomie der Hernien vjscher Prakt Heilk 1848;18:89.
6. Nauman G. Hernia diaphragmatica: laparotomie dod. Hygeia 1888;50:524.
7. O'Dwyer J. Operation for relief of congenital diaphragmatic hernia. Ann Surg 1890;11:124.
8. Aue O. Uber angeborenen Zwerfellhernien. Dtsch Z Chiu 1920;160:14.
9. Heidenhain L. Gesichte eines Falles von chronisher Incarceration des Mageus in einer angeborenen Zwerchfellhernien welcher durcher Paparotomie geheilt wurde, mitansheissenden Bermerkungen uber die Moglichkeit, das Kardiacarconom der Speisehre zzu reseciren. Dtsch Z Chiu 1905;76:394.
10. Hedblom CA. Diaphragmatic hernia: a study of 378 cases in which an operation was performed. JAMA 1925;85:947.
11. Ladd W, Gross RE. Congenital diaphragmatic hernia. N Engl J Med 1940;223:917.
12. Gross RE. Congenital hernia of the diaphragm. Am J Dis Chil 1946;71:579.
13. Chinn DH, Filly RA, Callen PW, et al. Congenital diaphragmatic hernia diagnosed prenatally by ultrasound. Radiology 1983;126:119.
14. Falconer AR, Brown RA, Helms P, et al. Pulmonary sequellae in survivors of congenital diaphragmatic hernia. Thorax 1990;45:126.
15. Gleeson F, Spitz L. Pitfalls in the diagnosis of congenital diaphragmatic hernia. Arch Dis Child 1988;66:670.
16. Puri P, Gorman WA. Natural history of congenital diaphragmatic hernia: implications for management. Pediatr Surg Inst 1987;2:327.
17. Wenstrom KD, Weiner CP, Anderson KD, et al. A five year statewide experience with congenital diaphragmatic hernia. Am J Obstet Gynecol 1991;165:838.
18. Green PW, Reismer PT. Registry of fetal defects in Minnesota, incidence of congenital diaphragmatic hernia. Presented at annual meeting of The Extracorporeal Life Support Organization; Breckenridge, Colorado September 1990.
19. Butler NR, Claireaux AE. Congenital diaphragmatic hernia as cause of perinatal mortality. Lancet 1962;1:659.
20. Greenwald HM, Steiner M. Diaphragmatic hernia in infancy and childhood. Am J Dis Child 1929;38:361.
21. David TJ, Illingsworth CF. Diaphragmatic hernia in the southwest of England. J Med Genet 1976;13:253.
22. Wakarny J, Roth CB. Congenital malformations induced in rats by maternal Vitamin A deficiency. J Nutr 1948;35:1.
23. Sharland GK, Lockhart SM, Heward AJ, et al. Prognosis in fetal diaphragmatic hernia. Am J Obstet Gynecol 1992;166:9.
24. Wilson JM, Fauza DO, Lund DP, et al. Antenatal diagnosis of congenital diaphragmatic hernia is not an indicator of outcome. J Pediatr Surg 1994;29:815.
25. Adzick NS, Harison MR, Glick PL, et al. Diaphragmatic hernia in the fetus: prenatal diagnosis and outcome in 94 cases. J Pediatr Surg 1985;20:357.
26. Lewis WH. The development of the muscular system. In: Keibel F, Mall FP, eds. Manual of human embryology. Philadelphia, JB Lippincott, 1910:455.
27. Areechon W, Reid L. Hypoplasia of the lung with congenital diaphragmatic hernia. Brit Med J 1963;1:230.
28. Dunhill MS. Postnatal growth of the lung. Thorax 1962 17:329.
29. Pringle KC, Turner JW, Schofield JC, et al. Creation and repair of diaphragmatic hernia: lung development and morphology. J Pediatr Surg 1984;19:131.
30. Glick PL, Stannard VA, et al. Pathophysiology of congenital diaphragmatic hernia. II. The fetal lamb model is surfactant deficient. J Pediatr Surg 1992;27:382.
31. Wilcox DT, Holm BA, Glick PL. Surfactant deficiency in the lamb model. J Pediatr Surg, 1993;28:757.
32. Karamanoukian HL, Wilcox DT, Glick PL. The missing link in congenital diaphragmatic hernia: fetal cardiac dysfunction J Pediatr Surg 1994;29:1370.
33. Crawford DC, Drake DP, Allan LD. Prenatal diagnosis of reversible cardiac hypoplasia associated with congenital diaphragmatic hernia: implications for postnatal management. J Clin Ultrasound 1987;14:718.
34. Crawford DC, Wright VM, Drake DP, et al. Fetal diaphragmatic hernia: the value of fetal echocardiography in the prediction of postnatal outcome. Br J Obstet Gynaecol 1989;96:705.
35. Gattone VH, Morse DE, A scanning electron microscopic study of congenital diaphragmatic hernia. J Submicrosc Cytol Pathol 1982;14:483.
36. Irritani I. Experimental study of the embryogenesis of congenital diaphragmatic hernia. Anat Embryol 1984;169:133.
37. Kluth D, Kanagah P, Reich P, et al. Nitrofen induced diaphragmatic hernias in rats: an animal model. J Pediatr Surg 1990;25:850.
38. Tenbrinck R, Tobboel D, Gaillard JLJ. Experimentally induced congenital diaphragmatic hernia in rats. J Pediatr Surg 1990;25:426.
39. Alcorn D, Adamson T, Lambert J, et al. Morphological effects of chronic tracheal ligation and drainage in the fetal lamb lung. J Anat 1976;122:649.
40. DiFiore JW, Wilson JM. Lung liquid, fetal lamb lung growth, and congenital diaphragmatic hernia. Pediatr Surg Int 1995;10:2.
41. DiFiore JW, Fauza DO, Slavin R, et al. Experimental fetal tracheal ligation and congenital diaphragmtic hernia: a pulmonary vascular morphometric analysis. J Pediatr Surg 1994;29:248.
41a. Hedrick MH, Estem JM, Sullivan KM, et al. Plug the lung until it grows: a new method to treat CDH in utero. J Pediatr Surg 1994;29:612.
42. Bealer, JF, Skarsgard, ED, Hedrick, MH, et al. The "PLUG" odyssey: adventures in fetal tracheal occlusion. J Pediatr Surg 1995;30:361.
43. Sawin RW, Wilcox DT, Karamanoukian HL, et al. Increased peptide growth factors in the amniotic fluid of sheep with congenital diaphragmatic hernia. Presented at the 11th Annual CNMC Symposium on ECMO and Advanced Therapies for Respiratory Failure; February 1995; Keystone, Colo.
44. Badalian SS, Fox HE, Stolar CJH, et al. Fetal breathing characteristics and postnatal outcome in cases of congenital diaphragmatic hernia. Am J Obstet Gynecol 1994;171:970.
45. Greenwald HM, Steiner M. Diaphragmatic hernia in infancy and childhood. Am J Dis Child 1929;38:361.
45a. Evans MI, Adzick MS, Johnson MP, et al. Fetal therapy—1994. Curr Opin Obstet Gynecol 1994;6:58.
46. Losty PD, Suen HC, Manganaro TF, et al. Prenatal hormone therapy improves pulmonary compliance in nitrofen induced congenital diaphragmatic hernia rat model. J Pediatr Surg 1995;30:420.
47. Stolar CJH, Dillon PW, Reyes C, et al. Selective use of extracorporeal membrane oxygenation in the management of congenital diaphragmatic hernia. J Pediatr Surg 1988;23:207.
48. Bohn D, Masanori T, Perrin D, et al. Ventilatory predictors of pulmonary hypoplasia in congenital diaphragmatic hernia, confirmed by morphometric assessment. J Pediatr 1987;111:423.
49. Aronoff MD, Molik K, Wiley A, et al. Effect of ECMO entry criteria on mortality of infants with congenital diaphragmatic hernia. Presented at The 11th CNMC Symposium on ECMO and Advanced Therapies for Respiratory Failure; February 1995; Keystone, Colo.
50. Ford WDA, Sudipta S, Barker AP, et al. Pulmonary hypertension in lambs with congenital diaphragmatic hernia: vasodilator prostaglandins, isoprenaline, and tolazoline. J Pediatr Surg 1990;25:487.
51. Karamanoukian HL, Glick PL, Zayek M. Clinical experience with inhaled nitric oxide in congenital diaphragmatic hernia and congenital hypoplasia of the lungs. Pediatrics 1994;94:1.
52. Sullivan KM, Hargood S, Flake A, et al. Amniotic fluid phospholipid

analysis in the fetus with congenital diaphragmatic hernia. J Pediatr Surg 1994;29:1020.

53. Moffitt S, Schultz K, Stolar CJH, et al. Preoperative cardiorespiratory trends in infants with congenital diaphragmatic hernia. J Pediatr Surg 1995;30:604.

54. Barlett RH, Gazzaniga AB, Fong SW, et al. Extracorporeal membrane oxygenation for cardiopulmonary failure, experience with 28 cases. J Thorac Cardiovasc Surg 1977;73:375.

55. Cornish JD, Heiss KF, Clark RH, et al. Efficacy of venovenous extracorporeal membrane oxygenation for neonates with respiratory and circulatory compromise. J Pediatr 1993;122:105.

56. Wun JT, Sahni R, Stolar CJH. Congenital diaphragmatic hernia: survival treated with very delayed surgery, spontaneous respiration and no chest tube. J Pediatr Surg 1995;30:406.

57. Price MR, Galantowicz ME, Stolar CJH. Congenital diaphragmatic hernia, extracorporeal membrane oxygenation, and death: a spectrum of etiologies. J Pediatr Surg 1991;26:1023.

58. Wilson JM, Bower LK, Fackler JT, et al. AMICAR decreases the incidence of intracranial hemorrhage and other hemorrhagic complications of ECMO. J Pediatr Surg 1993;28:536.

59. Cartlidge PT, Mann NP, Kapila L. Preoperative stabilization in congenital diaphragmatic hernia. Arch Dis Child 1986;61:1226.

59a.West KW, Bengston K, Rescorla FJ, et al. Delayed surgical repair and ECMO improves survival in CDH. Ann Surg 1992;216:454.

60. Kitagawa M, Hislop A, Boyden EA, et al. Lung hypoplasia in congenital diaphragmatic hernia: a quantitative study of airway, artery, and alveolar development. Brit J Surg 1971;58:342.

61. Koumbourlis AC, Stolar CJH, and Stylianos S. Lung function in infants after repair of congenital diaphragmatic hernia. Am Rev Respir Dis 1994;148:A548.

62. Wohl MB, Griscom NT, Streider DJ, The lung following repair of congenital diaphragmatic hernia. J Pediatr 1977;90:405.

63. Lund DP, Mirchell J, Karasch V, et al. Congenital diaphragmatic hernia: the hidden morbidity. J Pediatr Surg 1994;29:258.

64. Stolar CJH, Dillon PW, Levy J. Anatomic and functional abnormalities of the esophagus in infants surviving congenital diaphragmatic hernia. Am J Surg 1990;159:204.

65. Stolar CJH, Crisafi M, Driscoll Y. Neurocognitive outcome for infants treated with extracorporeal membrane oxygenation: are infants with congenital diaphragmatic hernia different? J Pediatr Surg 1995;30:366.

66. Harrison MR, Adzick S, Flake AW, et al. Correction of congenital diaphragmatic hernia in utero. VI: hard earned lessons. J Pediatr Surg 1993;28:1411.

67. Hirschl R, Pranikoff T, Bartlett RH, et al. Congenital diaphragmatic hernia supported by liquid ventilation and extracorporeal membrane oxygenation. J Pediatr Surg. In press.

68. Karamanoukian HL, Glick PL, Wilcox DT, et al. Pathophysiology of congenital diaphragmatic hernia. VIII: inhaled nitric oxide requires exogenous surfactant therapy in the congenital diaphragmatic hernia lamb model. J Pediatr Surg 1995;30:1.

69. Weinstein S, Lazar EL, Stolar CJH, et al. Acute hemodynamic evaluation of reduced lung transplant. Transplantation. In press.

70. Starns V. Reduced volume lung transplantation in two infants with congenital diaphragmatic hernia. Presented at the Tenth Annual CNMC ECMO Symposium; February 1994; Keystone, Colo.

Surgery of Infants and Children: Scientific Principles and Practice, edited by Keith T. Oldham, Paul M. Colombani, and Robert P. Foglia. Lippincott–Raven Publishers, Philadelphia, © 1997.

CHAPTER 55

Subglottic Airway

Richard G. Azizkhan and Michael G. Caty

Children with respiratory distress often present with symptoms of airway obstruction that rapidly progress and become life-threatening. Many different types of airway lesions cause airway obstruction in children, and knowledge of these is essential to establish a precise diagnosis. The physician must rapidly determine the precise anatomic problem and institute the appropriate therapy. The evaluation of an infant with respiratory distress begins with a review of the history of the child's symptoms because they may provide important clues to the underlying etiology of the problem. The history should also focus on the circumstances around the onset of the respiratory compromise in addition to the rapidity of symptom progression. The nature of the child's cry, a history of associated dysphagia or feeding problems, as well as the possibility of foreign-body aspiration should be evaluated. A previous history of endotracheal intubation, trauma, or underlying cardiopulmonary abnormalities should also be carefully reviewed.

The degree of respiratory insufficiency can be partially determined by physical findings. Cyanosis, severe suprasternal and intercostal retractions, tachypnea, and lethargy indicate severe respiratory compromise. In some patients, only subtle findings may be present, including irritability, restlessness, tachycardia, and feeding difficulties. With upper airway obstruction, stridor is the most important physical sign and can be present in either the expiratory or inspiratory phase of the respiratory cycle or in both.[1,2] Stridor is an adventitial respiratory noise created by airway turbulence. The characteristics of stridor as well as its relationship to the respiratory cycle may be useful in establishing a differential diagnosis and setting the priorities for diagnostic evaluation.[2] Several anatomic features of the airway in infants differ from those of older children or adults.[3,4] The caliber of the airway is small and can be readily obstructed by secretions or mucosal swelling. The larynx is cephalad and anterior, making visualization more difficult for the inexperienced clinician. The length of the trachea is very short (approximately 4 to 5 cm), thus increasing the risk of unplanned extubation or right mainstem intubation during flexion or extension of the infant's head and neck.

Congenital lesions causing airway obstruction may not always manifest as respiratory compromise in the immediate neonatal period but may present later once inflammation or edema creates a critical airway problem. In any patient with airway compromise, control of the airway is imperative and the first order of business. Once airway and ventilatory control has been obtained, a thorough evaluation should be initiated to delineate the structural or functional airway abnormalities and any associated malformations.

The major focus of postoperative management is on maintaining a secure airway. For patients whose airway obstruction has been relieved, careful monitoring of the patient and hemoglobin saturation may be all that is required. Those children undergoing more complex procedures may require an indwelling endotracheal tube or a laryngeal–tracheal stent for postoperative airway control. Sedation, pain control, and paralysis should be considered to maintain the airway until the patient can be safely decannulated.

TRACHEOBRONCHOSCOPY

Tracheobronchoscopy, the visual, instrument-aided examination of the airways, has been increasingly used for both diagnostic and therapeutic purposes in infants and children.[5-7] Bronchoscopy is indicated when it is the safest, most effective, and most appropriate method to obtain information that is needed to care for the patient or when it is the best way to accomplish specific therapeutic goals. The advent of the flexible bronchoscope considerably expanded the traditional indications for bronchoscopy, most of which were therapeutic (eg, foreign-body extraction). Endoscopy can reveal airway structure, airway dynamics, and airway contents, as well as provide access to foreign bodies, secretions, and washings from the lower airways. If the child has stridor at the time of the examination, the vibrating structures should be seen, unless the examiner is looking in the wrong place. A significant percentage of children with stridor have more than one airway lesion, thus the entire upper and lower airway should be examined unless there is a good reason not to do so (ie, critical tracheal stenosis).[5]

Rigid Bronchoscopes

Rigid (''open tube'') bronchoscopes range in diameter from approximately 2.5 to 8.5 mm, and in length from 20 to 50 cm.[1]

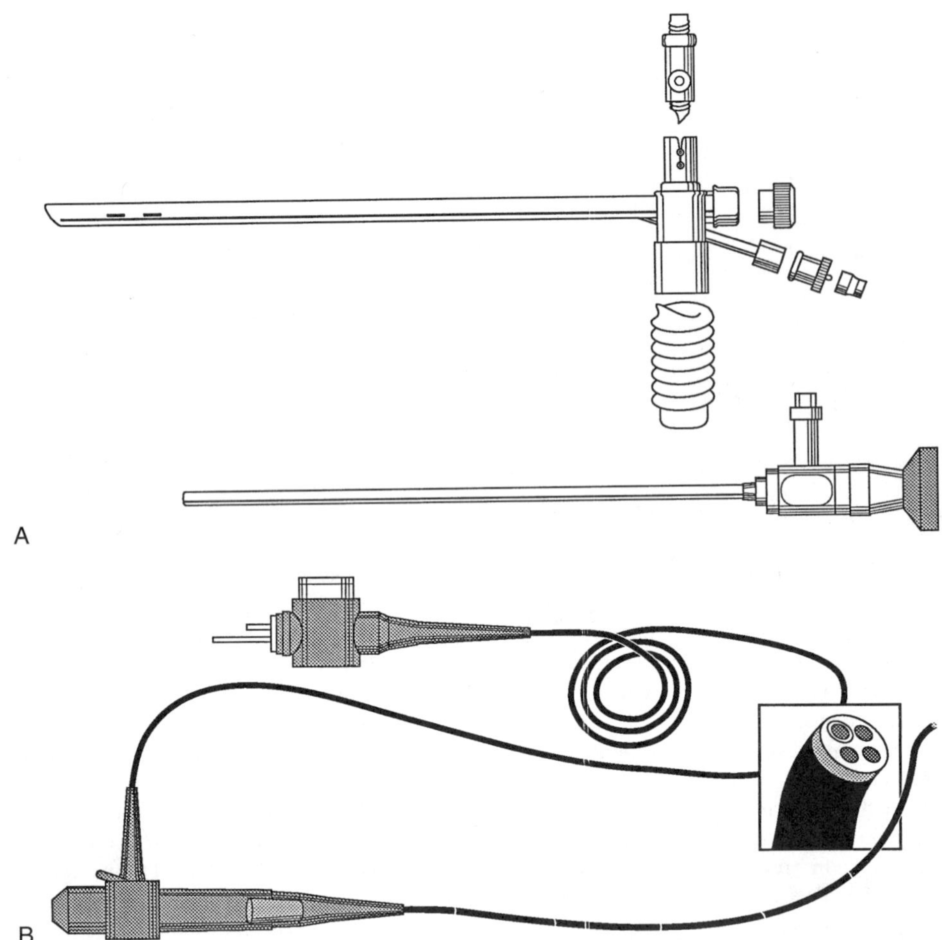

FIG. 55-1. (*A*) A Storz pediatric ventilating bronchoscope (*top*) and a Hopkins rod lens telescope (*bottom*). (*B*) Flexible pediatric bronchoscope.

The most salient feature of the rigid bronchoscope is that it is sufficiently large to function as an endotracheal tube; the patient ventilates through the rigid bronchoscope. The airways distal to the tip of the bronchoscope are illuminated either with a prism inserted partially into the lumen or by fiberoptics through the glass rod telescope (Fig. 55-1). The optical characteristics of rigid bronchoscopes when used with the glass rod telescope are spectacular and are unequaled by any other bronchoscopic device (Fig. 55-2). When the prism is used with the open tube,

visualization may be difficult through the bronchoscope; however, this mode is often necessary while manipulating instruments passed through the bronchoscope.[5]

The large lumen of the rigid bronchoscope makes it relatively simple to pass a variety of instruments, including forceps, suction catheters, snares, and retrieval baskets, into the airways. Since a large part of the bronchoscope lumen is occupied by the glass rod telescope, special instruments have been designed for use with the telescope. These include the optical forceps,

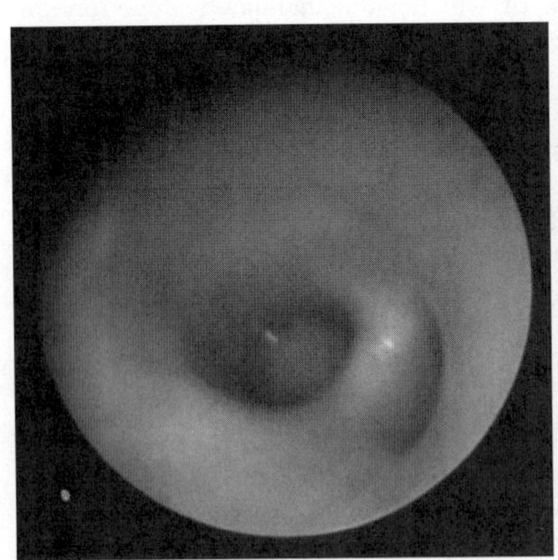

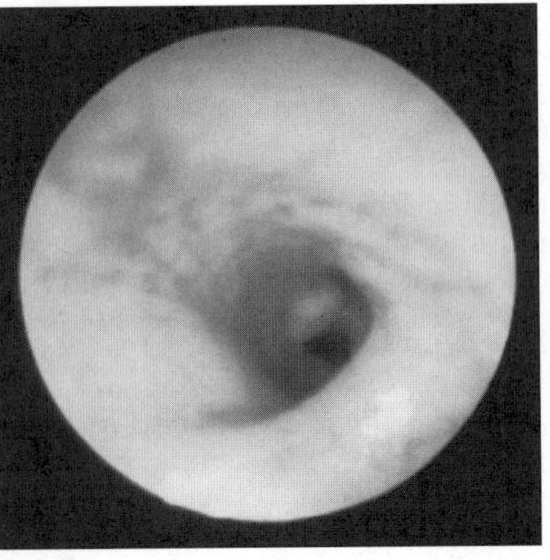

FIG. 55-2. (*A*) The bronchus intermedius of a 600-g premature neonate who required prolonged ventilatory support and failed extubation is seen through a rigid bronchoscope. The right upper lobe orifice is seen at the 3-o'clock position and an obstructing granuloma is present in the bronchus intermedius itself. (*B*) After forceps extraction of the obstructing lesion, the airway was patent. The patient was rapidly weaned from the ventilator and successfully extubated. (See Color Fig. 55-2.)

which operates in conjunction with the telescope, and ultrathin forceps, which can be passed along side the telescope.[5] Other tools, such as suction catheters, balloon-tipped catheters, and laser fibers, also can be passed through the bronchoscope in parallel with the telescope.

The use of a rigid bronchoscope does not guarantee that the patient will ventilate easily because glass rod telescopes significantly reduce the functional lumen of the endoscope and increase airway resistance.[5] For example, the bronchoscope most commonly used in infants has a 3.5-mm internal diameter, while the diameter of the corresponding telescope is 2.5 mm. Therefore, it is essential that the patient's hemoglobin-oxygen saturation and ventilation be carefully monitored during rigid bronchoscopy. It is often important to evaluate airway dynamics in infants and children. Airway dynamics may be altered by anesthesia or sedation, depending on the type and level used. It is important to examine the airway with the patient spontaneously breathing because dynamic airway collapse can easily be missed during positive-pressure ventilation. The bronchoscope itself can also alter dynamics, either by stenting the airway or by changing airway resistance and therefore the pressure relationships.[5]

Flexible Bronchoscopes

Flexible bronchoscopes differ from rigid bronchoscopes in several ways. The flexible bronchoscope is distinguished by its ability to flex the distal end to as much as 180 degrees (Fig 55-1B). They are essentially solid and relatively small so that the patient breathes around the flexible endoscope, rather than through the rigid endoscopes.[8] The standard pediatric flexible bronchoscope is approximately 3.5 mm in outer diameter and incorporates a suction channel that is only 1.2 mm in diameter. Adult flexible instruments range up to 6 mm in diameter, with a 2.7-mm suction channel. Because the trachea of a newborn infant is only about 5 to 5.5 mm in diameter, however, such instruments are clearly not suitable for pediatric use. Flexible bronchoscopes as small as 2.2 mm in diameter are available. The flexible bronchoscope can be easily guided into the upper lobes or other locations that are difficult to reach with a rigid endoscope.[5-8] In general, a rigid bronchoscope allows direct visualization of segmental bronchi, but the standard pediatric flexible bronchoscope can be inserted several generations further. Flexible bronchoscopes are usually inserted through the nose rather than through the mouth and can also be passed through endotracheal or tracheostomy tubes of appropriate size. The image produced by a flexible bronchoscope is composed of several thousand points of light, each representing the color and light intensity transmitted by a single glass fiber. The resolution of this image is inherently inferior to that obtained with the glass rod telescope discussed earlier. In practice, however, the perceived image quality is quite good because the operator's eye rapidly compensates for the lower resolution.[5]

Atelectasis is a relatively common indication for bronchoscopy and can be caused by a variety of lesions that obstruct the airways. Flexible bronchoscopes are useful for diagnostic evaluation, which routinely includes cytologic and microbiologic evaluation of washings from the affected area. Occasionally, lavage with mucolytic agents may be necessary, and rarely, a rigid bronchoscopy with forceps extraction must be used in patients who have discrete mucous plugs (Fig. 55-3).[5] If the

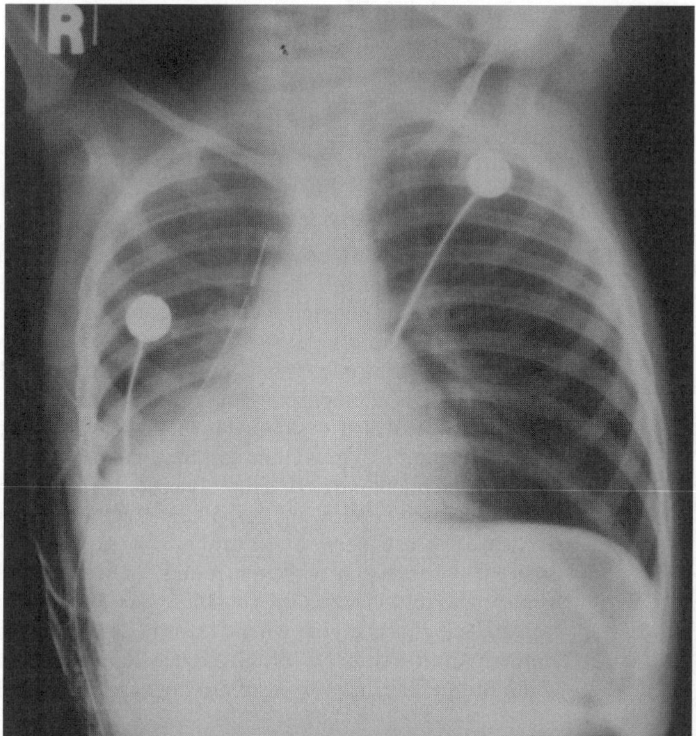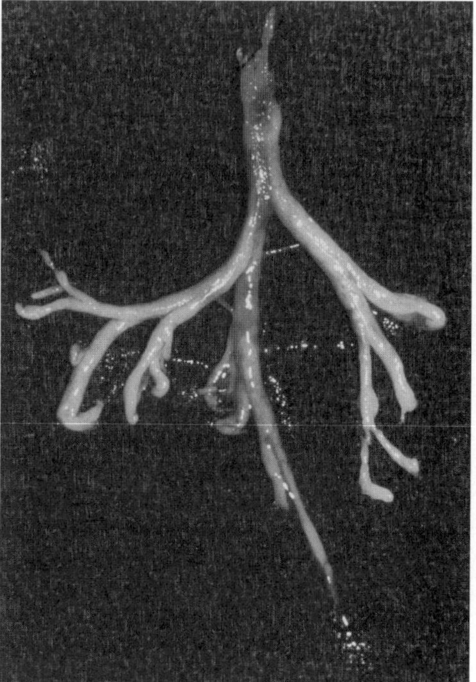

FIG. 55-3. (*A*) Chest radiograph of an 11-year-old boy with chronic right lower lobe atelectasis and pneumonia. (*B*) A large mucus plug with an arborized configuration corresponding to the segmental airway anatomy was removed from this patient with a rigid bronchoscope.

atelectasis is due to an impacted foreign body or a tissue mass, then rigid bronchoscopy is needed.

Endoscopic techniques can also be useful during extubation in selected patients. When a child has previously failed extubation, direct examination of the airway may define the problem (see Fig. 55-2). The lower airways are initially examined through the endotracheal tube, and then the nasopharynx and larynx are examined with a flexible bronchoscope which has been passed through an appropriate sized new endotracheal tube. The existing indwelling endotracheal tube is withdrawn after the tip of the bronchoscope is positioned just above the glottis. The bronchoscope is withdrawn if the anatomy and function appear favorable after several minutes of observation. If the child has evidence of obstruction or severe respiratory dysfunction, the bronchoscope is advanced into the trachea, and the fresh endotracheal tube is subsequently passed. Subglottic edema that is significant enough to prevent successful extubation may not become apparent for 5 to 10 minutes after extubation; therefore, the airway should be examined leisurely.[5]

Complications of Bronchoscopy

Bronchoscopy is not a procedure that can be taken lightly regardless of the technique used. The patient must be properly prepared and monitored before, during, and after the procedure. The endoscopist must be well trained and prepared to recognize and deal with any complication that may arise. The consequences of direct or indirect tissue trauma are the most commonly observed complications and include mucosal trauma, hemoptysis or epistaxis, pneumothorax, subglottic edema, tracheal or bronchial perforation, and trauma to the vocal cords.[5] These complications occur more commonly with rigid instruments than with flexible ones, partially because of the nature of the instruments and partially because of the types of procedures selected.[5] For example, flexible bronchoscopes are rarely if ever used for foreign-body extraction, a situation in which mucosal tears or bronchial perforation may occur.

Physiologic complications of bronchoscopy include hypoxia, hypercarbia, bradycardia or other cardiac arrhythmias, laryngospasm, and bronchospasm. Hypoxia and hypercarbia may occur because a flexible instrument obstructs the airway or because prolonged manipulation of an instrument through the open channel of a rigid endoscope interrupts positive-pressure ventilation. Cardiac arrhythmias and laryngospasm can result from direct vagal stimulation often as a consequence of inadequate topical anesthesia.[5] Inadequate sedation or topical anesthesia can result in mechanical trauma from coughing. If the patient's stomach is not empty, aspiration may result from induced regurgitation or gastroesophageal reflux. Passage of a bronchoscope and the associated anesthesia or sedation alter the patients' ability to breathe, placing them at risk for other complications as well. Therefore, it is essential that patients be monitored appropriately throughout the procedure.

TRACHEOSTOMY

Indications

The surgeon treating infants and children with tracheobronchial abnormalities must be comfortable with the technique and postoperative care of tracheostomies. Emergency tracheostomy for airway obstructions secondary to infection was the most common indication for tracheostomy in the past. Currently, tracheostomy is most commonly performed on infants and children with congenital or acquired structural abnormalities of the airway.[9] Long-term meticulous care of the tracheostomy is necessary to avoid complications.

There are multiple indications for tracheostomy in infants and children. These include central nervous system problems, craniofacial anomalies, vocal cord paralysis, and the following congenital and acquired structural airway abnormalities[9]:

- Bilateral choanal atresia
- Severe micrognathia (eg, Pierre Robin syndrome)
- Oropharyngeal tumors (eg, lymphangioma, teratoma, hemangiopericytoma)
- Cervical masses obstructing larynx or trachea
- Bilateral vocal cord paralysis
- Anomalies of the larynx (eg, atresia, webs, laryngomalacia)
- Subglottic obstruction (eg, stenosis, hemangioma)
- Central apnea
- Chronic respiratory failure and support
- Chronic aspiration risk (eg, severe oropharyngeal dysmotility, prolonged coma)
- Acute obstruction from infection (eg, epiglottitis)
- Significant craniofacial trauma
- Laryngeal trauma (eg, fractured larynx)
- Inability to achieve oral airway during resuscitation

Children with structural abnormalities of the airway often need a tracheostomy as an adjunct to airway reconstruction. Placement of a tracheostomy for airway protection is often beneficial in children with craniofacial anomalies such as the Pierre Robin syndrome. Other indications include the former premature infant with parenchymal lung disease and the infant with central apnea, both indications for long-term mechanical ventilatory support.[9–11]

Cricothyroidotomy

Occasionally, orotracheal intubation is not feasible during a life-threatening acute airway obstruction episode. Immediate tracheal access can be obtained using a needle cricothyroidotomy with a 14- gauge intravenous cannula percutaneously inserted through the cricothyroid membrane. High-flow plastic tubing with 100% oxygen is connected to this cannula. Since this technique is a temporizing maneuver, a more secure surgical or orotracheal airway should be obtained as soon as possible, preferably within 15 to 20 minutes. Surgical cricothyroidotomy is also an excellent method of rapidly securing a difficult airway in an emergency. Following this, a larger and more stable endotracheal tube can be inserted through the cricothyroid membrane. This approach is better suited for older children and teenagers as it has caused irrevocable injury to the cricoid cartilage and subglottic region when performed in infants and small children. Conversion to a formal tracheostomy is recommended within a few days if prolonged airway support is likely.

Tracheostomy Technique

The technique of tracheostomy in infants and children has evolved as posttracheostomy complications have been identified. Important principles include the preservation of tracheal tissue by not excising a window or flap and by not performing the procedure on an infant without a secured airway.[9] The infant or child should be anesthetized in the operating room with an airway in place. A small roll is placed under the child's shoulders and the neck prepped. A transverse cervical skin incision is done. The cervical fascia is incised vertically and the thyroid isthmus retracted. Traction sutures made of prolene are placed on both sides of the trachea, and a vertical tracheotomy is performed through the third and fourth tracheal rings. Communication with the anesthesiologist is established, and the tracheostomy tube is placed as the endotracheal tube is withdrawn. The traction sutures are taped to the neck for use in emergently replacing the tube in the event of accidental dislodgment.

Postoperative Care

Those caring for the child postoperatively should be comfortable with emergent replacement of the tracheostomy tube. Physicians and nurses need to be able to rapidly correct an unexpected loss of the airway in an infant with a recent tracheostomy. Ideally, the steps and life-saving maneuvers should be rehearsed with the team each and every time a new tracheostomy is placed. These steps include: suctioning the airway; establishing ventilation by bag-masking the child until the airway can be secured by experienced people; reintubating the child through the glottis if feasible; or replacing the tracheostomy using a small suction tube to cannulate the trachea through the stoma and sliding the tracheostomy tube over the catheter. An attempt to blindly reinsert the tracheostomy tube at the bedside can be disastrous if the tube enters the anterior mediastinum or perforates the posterior trachea. Until the first tracheostomy tube change, an intubation set and appropriate endotracheal tube as well as suction catheters that fit through the tracheostomy must be readily available.

Complications can occur early or late. Early complications include accidental decannulation, tracheal obstruction, bleeding, and pneumothorax.[9] Late complications include formation of granulation tissue, tracheal obstructions, tube occlusion, and tracheoinnominate fistula.[9]

Tracheostomy Home Care

If a child is to return home with a tracheostomy, a systematic approach to educating and supporting the home caregivers must be established. Parents or other caregivers must be given intensive hospital training on tracheostomy care and replacement. They should also be well versed in emergency procedures and have CPR training before the child is discharged. Most children benefit from home apnea monitors. Home nursing is also an integral part of the care of children with tracheostomies. Finally, the hospital-based resources must be immediately available for parents to contact. An expanded treatment of this aspect of tracheostomy care can be found in several of the references.[10,11]

Tracheostomy Decannulation

When appropriate, the child is prepared for decannulation. Before tracheostomy decannulation, flexible laryngotracheo-

bronchoscopy is performed in all children to assess the proximal and distal airway for either intraluminal or extrinsic obstructing lesions. Recognizing and treating pathologic lesions, such as peristomal tracheal collapse or obstructing granulomas, is essential for a complication-free and safe extubation. Most children tolerate decannulation well. Approximately 10% of infants with long-standing tracheostomies (more than 1 year) have significant cricoid collapse or severe peristomal tracheomalacia.[12] A simple one-stage procedure can be used to close the tracheocutaneous fistula and alleviate the cricoid collapse in these children.[12] Under orotracheal general anesthesia, the tracheostomy stoma is excised in a horizontal ellipse down to the tracheal wall, removing excessive scar involving the skin and subcutaneous tissue. A small portion (1 mm) of the tracheal opening is circumferentially excised along with any peristomal tracheal granulation tissue. The tracheal opening is closed transversely with interrupted absorbable 4-0 or 5-0 monofilament sutures. The anterior cricoid suspension is performed by the extraluminal placement of three to four absorbable 3-0 monofilament sutures from the adherent tissue overlying the anterior trachea and cricoid ring through the musculofascial insertions of the cervical strap muscles adjacent to the sternum. Once tied, these sutures significantly elevate the anterior cricoid and peristomal trachea by pulling the airway ventrally and inferiorly. The strap muscles cover the tracheal suture line, and the skin and soft tissue are closed in a transverse fashion. Most patients can be extubated in the immediate perioperative period.

AIRWAY FOREIGN BODIES

Airway obstruction due to foreign bodies is common and potentially fatal. Although foreign-body aspiration can occur at any age, approximately 80% of the children who aspirate foreign objects are under age 3 years, and two thirds are boys. Children at this age lack molar teeth and cannot effectively chew their ingested food. Nuts, particularly peanuts, account for over half of all inhaled objects followed by vegetable fragments, such as seeds, popcorn, and an array of toys and other small objects. A careful history should be obtained, but in many cases, the sudden onset of coughing may be the only notable event. Some patients actually cease coughing by the time they reach medical facilities because sensory receptors of the respiratory tract physiologically adapt. During this quiet interval, the child may lack any symptoms, conveying a false impression to parents and physicians that the object has been coughed out or swallowed. Classic physical findings of foreign-body aspiration include the unilateral presence of decreased breath sounds because of of decreased ventilation of the affected lung as well as unilateral bronchi from partial occlusion of the bronchus. Approximately 75% of the patients have at least one element of the classic triad of wheezing, coughing, and diminished or absent breath sounds.[5]

Radiographic Imaging

A chest radiograph with inspiration and expiration films should be obtained for any child with a history compatible with foreign-body aspiration. Approximately 10% of aspirated foreign bodies are radiopaque. Thus, in most patients, indirect find-

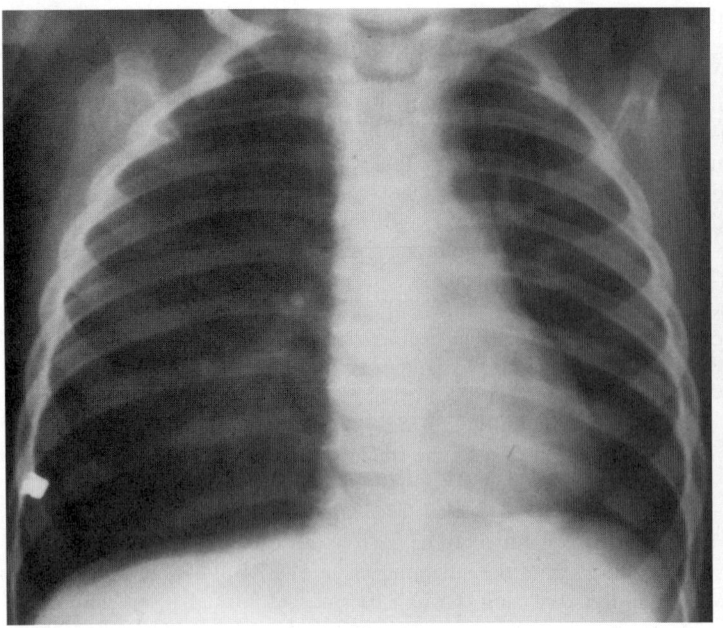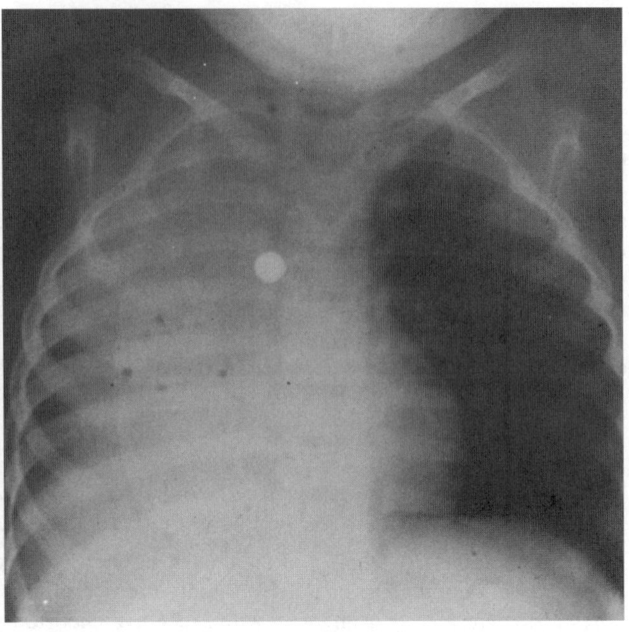

A

B

FIG. 55-4. (*A*) Radiographic appearance of unilateral emphysema and air trapping secondary to a partial occlusion of the right main bronchus from a foreign-body aspiration. Mediastinal shift toward the contralateral hemithorax is common. (*B*) Total occlusion of the right main bronchus by a radiopaque foreign body has produced atelectasis and mediastinal shift toward the affected right side.

ings secondary to unilateral obstruction of the airway are required to make the diagnosis. Unilateral emphysema with air trapping secondary to a high grade partial occlusion of the main bronchus is the classic radiographic finding for a foreign body (Fig 55-4*A*). In these patients, air may enter the affected lobe or lung on inspiration, but subsequently, expiratory air trapping leads to focal alveolar overinflation. Chest fluoroscopy and decubitus views of the chest may also demonstrate air trapping. In approximately one fourth of the patients, total occlusion of a bronchus may produce atelectasis or pneumonic infiltrates rather than emphysema (Fig 55-4*B*). It is important to appreciate that the chest radiograph and physical examination may be normal in the presence of an aspirated foreign body if it is lodged in the larynx or the trachea.[13] Migration of foreign bodies may cause changing physical and radiographic findings.

Endoscopic Foreign-Body Retrieval

Children, especially infants, who have the sudden onset of wheezing or pneumonia that does not respond to treatment should be considered for bronchoscopy to rule out foreign-body aspiration. Approximately 15% of all pediatric aspirations occur without an adult witness. The presence of normal physical findings and normal chest radiographs in a child with a history of aspiration does not negate the need for endoscopic evaluation.[5] Rigid bronchoscopy should be performed by an experienced pediatric surgical endoscopist and an anesthesiologist experienced in the care of the pediatric airway. If a foreign body has been lodged in the airway for more than 24 hours, a parenteral antibiotic (ampicillin or penicillin) is usually administered. Modern pediatric ventilating bronchoscopes coupled with a Hopkins rod lens and appropriate extraction devices, including

alligator, peanut, and fine foreign-body forceps, Fogarty catheters, Dormia baskets, and other endoscopic equipment are essential for successfully extracting a variety of foreign bodies. Preendoscopy knowledge of the shape, size, and composition of the aspirated foreign body (ie, pieces of toys, screws, spherical objects) is extremely helpful in planning for extraction. We have found it useful to practice grasping a similar or identical object ex vivo to be sure that the instrumentation and technique are appropriate for successful extraction. Direct laryngoscopy is performed using a small laryngoscope with a straight blade. Instillation of a small amount of 1% lidocaine around the vocal cords and in the subglottis diminishes vagal reflexes during the procedure. Careful visualization of the subglottic and tracheal area is performed first. As the bronchoscope is advanced towards the carina, the foreign body is usually visualized in one of the mainstem bronchi. The right mainstem bronchus is the most common site as the orientation is straight and dependent, resulting in deposition by gravity. Before the foreign body is extracted, the contralateral main bronchus is visualized to be sure the area is normal and free of any additional foreign bodies. The optimal instrument for extraction depends on the type and shape of the foreign body. Flat foreign objects with an edge are easily extracted by forceps. Spherical foreign bodies such as peanuts, marbles, and round seeds may require Fogarty catheter, peanut forceps, or a Dormia basket for successful extraction. The use of optical telescopic forceps has improved the visualization and removal of certain foreign bodies (Fig. 55-5).[5] Once a foreign body has been grasped, the endoscopist generally manipulates the foreign body to the tip of the bronchoscope. The bronchoscope forceps and foreign body are then removed as an entire assembly from the airway. The endoscopist carefully watches the extraction procedure to ensure that the foreign body does not fall back into the airway. Excellent communication

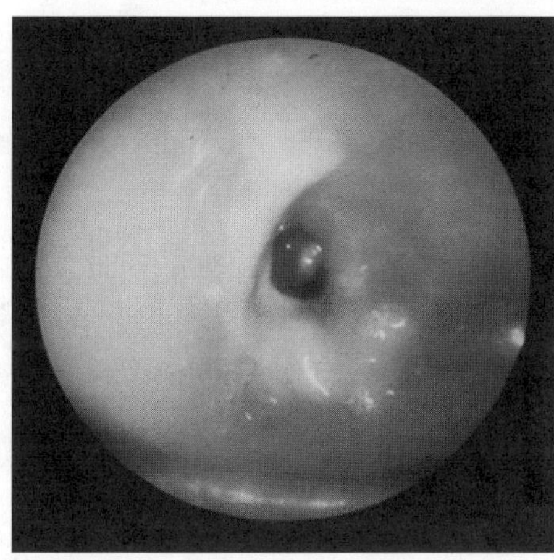

FIG. 55-5. Metallic foreign body lodged in the bronchus intermedius as seen through a rigid bronchoscope using a Hopkins lens system. (See Color Fig. 55-5.)

must be maintained between the endoscopist and the anesthesiologist during the entire procedure. Occasionally, the foreign body is dislodged as it comes through the vocal cords and may lodge in the back of the pharynx or in the piriform sinuses. Direct laryngoscopy and the use of McGill forceps is usually successful in removing the foreign body from these areas. At the completion of the procedure, a repeat endoscopy is performed to rule out the presence of other foreign bodies or retained fragments, and bacterial cultures are obtained from the affected bronchus as well. In patients who have had vegetable material impacted in a main bronchus, an area of inflamed mucosa with granulation tissue is often present. Usually, this granulation tissue contracts and heals once the foreign body has been extracted. Generally, fulguration is not needed. Purulent secretions obstructing a main bronchus following extraction of a foreign body should be carefully suctioned and submitted for appropriate cultures.

Foreign bodies occasionally migrate to a more distal segmental bronchus beyond the reach of a rigid bronchoscope. They can be dislodged with 2F or 3F Fogarty catheter or the passage of a pediatric flexible bronchoscope, with a Dormia basket through the ventilating bronchoscope.[5] The flexible bronchoscope allows only a limited choice of instruments to be passed to the foreign body, obstructs more of the airway, and is generally not as well suited as the rigid bronchoscope for this purpose. Nevertheless, in selected circumstances, the flexible bronchoscope can be very helpful. Specifically, when a foreign body is suspected but not proven, a flexible examination can definitively rule on the presence of a foreign body.[5,7] In older children, examination of airways distal to the range of the rigid bronchoscope may reveal foreign bodies not otherwise seen. The flexible instruments have also proved useful in the follow-up examination of patients who have had a foreign body extracted earlier because examination may not require general anesthesia as it would for rigid bronchoscopy.

Following endoscopic removal of foreign bodies, most children and infants experience hoarseness from edema of the vocal cords and the subglottic region. This typically resolves in 24 to 48 hours. The patient is usually placed on humidified oxygen and is observed either in the pediatric intensive care unit or in some other monitored environment. Patients must remain well hydrated and occasionally require racemic epinephrine and bronchodilators. Chest physiotherapy and postural drainage also may be helpful in clearing purulent secretions from affected lobes. A chest radiograph following bronchoscopy is obtained. Patients who have persistent symptoms may require repeat bronchoscopy after 1 week of intensive physiotherapy and antibiotics. Radiographic abnormalities occasionally persist and are also an indication for repeat endoscopy.

Operative Retrieval

Rarely, a foreign body may need to be extracted by a thoracotomy and bronchotomy or even a lobectomy. When foreign bodies are too large to be brought through the vocal cords, a tracheotomy should be performed over the bronchoscope and the foreign body removed in that fashion. Tracheostomy decannulation can be done within 48 hours if the airway is otherwise normal. A foreign body that has been impacted for weeks is typically surrounded by a dense inflammatory action and granulation tissue. In some patients, bronchiectasis and abscess formation may have occurred. Occasionally, a history of hemoptysis has been present and should be considered a red flag to alert the surgeon because some of these patients may develop massive hemorrhage during extraction. These patients occasionally require segmental lung resection or lobectomy.

EMBRYOLOGY

The laryngotracheal groove arises from the ventral surface of the foregut during the third and fourth gestational weeks (Carnegie stages 10 to 13).[14] Concurrently, cells lining the coelomic cavity divide to become a proliferating primitive mesenchyme and, eventually, pulmonary muscle, cartilage, and connective tissue. During the fifth week (stages 14 and 15), caudal progression of the embryonic trachea is followed by bifurcation and the appearance of lung buds (Fig. 55-6). During the sixth week (stages 16 and 17), the lobar bronchi lengthen and abut the esophagus. These asymmetric (right larger than left) buds rapidly divide into lobar, and by the seventh week (stages 18 and 19), into tertiary bronchi. At this stage, pseudostratified epithelium lines the larger airways. Differentiation and branching of the epithelial bronchial tree depends on the presence of the mediastinal mesenchyme.[14,15] The formation of new smaller bronchi continues through the 16th week. Bronchial subdivisions continue until the 17th order is established between the sixth and seventh month. At that time, alveolar differentiation occurs at the site of the distal terminal bronchi and continues until well after birth. The initial vascular supply of the differentiating bronchial buds develops from the splanchnic plexus that originates from the dorsal aorta and drains into the plexus of cardinal veins.[16] The bronchial arterial blood supply develops from gradual interconnection with the sixth aortic arch, leaving the bronchial vasculature as a remnant of the embryonic vascular system. The tracheal bifurcation is initially high in the cervical region and descends to the level of the T1 vertebra by 8 weeks' gestation and to T3 or T4 at birth. Cartilage appears in the trachea during the 10th gestational week (stage 20) and bronchial cartilage is present by the 16th week.[14,15] After about

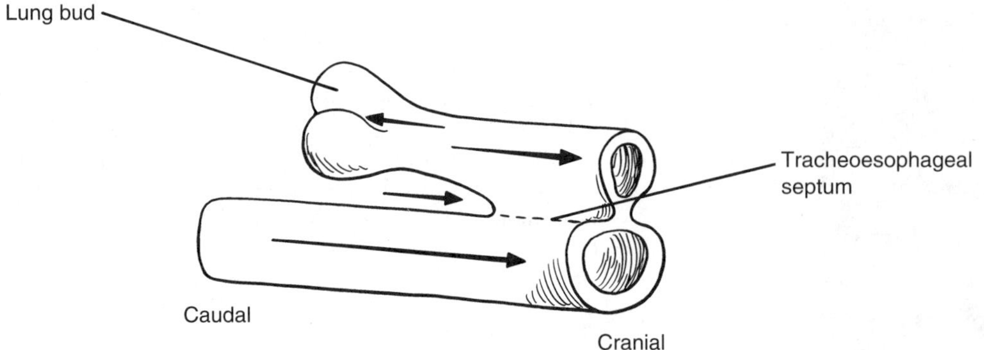

FIG. 55-6. Division of the foregut and trachea into trachea and esophagus during the fifth week of gestation. Arrows represent the direction of morphogenesis.

16 weeks, the primary events in fetal lung development are related to the successive generation of terminal airways and alveoli.

Congenital anomalies of the respiratory system are relatively uncommon and can occur along the entire tracheobronchopulmonary axis. Associated extrapulmonary anomalies are frequently present and may be part of a syndrome or association. Nearly 45% of the children with congenital airway obstruction have associated congenital anomalies.[1,2,4] Some of these anomalies have a significant impact on the child's prognosis.[4] Although the cause of these various malformations is usually unknown, each constellation of abnormalities likely results from causal mechanisms that differ in time, mode of action, and the embryonic region affected. Thus, the various congenital abnormalities are failures of normal growth and differentiation of different parts of the embryonic respiratory system. For example, defective mesodermal development in early embryogenesis may be responsible for the VACTERL association (V, vertebral anomalies; A, anal anomalies; C, cardiac defects; T, tracheoesophageal fistula; E, esophageal atresia; R, renal anomalies; and L, limb anomalies). In addition, experimental evidence suggests that vitamin A may play an important role in the development of the airway and lungs. Vitamin A deficiency in animal embryos causes a keratizing metaplasia of the tracheobronchial tree and pulmonary agenesis.[17] Retinoic acid appears to be important for embryonic cell differentiation in many organ systems and is currently the object of intense scientific investigation.[14] Primary abnormalities of the developing lung bud itself may lead to a variety of abnormalities including congenital lobar emphysema, bronchogenic cysts, sequestrations, and cystic adenomatoid malformation. In most of these lesions, there is an abnormality in the bronchial relation to the lung and the foregut.[14] Gestational teratogens may have selected effects on specific organ development. Huot and colleagues[18] described a relation between the maternal use of valproic acid and tracheomalacia and laryngeal hypoplasia in their offspring. Severe congenital tracheal stenosis has also been reported in infants of diabetic mothers.[19]

TRACHEAL ANOMALIES

Tracheal Stenosis: Congenital and Acquired

The etiologies of most congenital airway obstructions are not known. It is presumed that interference with tracheobronchial organogenesis by teratogens, embryonic vascular accidents, ge-

netic or other environmental stresses at a critical stage of airway development is responsible for these abnormalities.[14] The different forms of tracheal stenosis, especially the funnel-like stenosis or generalized tracheal hypoplasia, represent failure of normal growth and development. In more than 50% of these infants, a segmental stenosis is found in which the cartilaginous rings are abnormal in shape and form complete rings.[20] Experimentally induced tracheal agenesis occurs in young chick embryos when silver clips are placed in the neck region.[21] The clinical manifestations of congenital tracheal stenosis vary from life-threatening respiratory distress at birth to subtle symptoms of airway compromise in older children. The most significant symptoms are pathologic sound abnormalities, including stridor and alterations of cry and cough.[22] Other symptoms frequently seen in these patients include atypical and persistent bronchiolitis, bronchitis, respiratory distress, and sudden death.

Introducing an endotracheal tube into the airway may compound these patients' problems. An endotracheal tube may cause inflammation and swelling at the stenosis site, leading to progresive airway obstruction. Congenital obstructing lesions of the trachea or distal airway may also become life-threatening after the onset of a respiratory infection. The cross-sectional area of the airway can be decreased by one third to one half its normal diameter with as little as 1 mm of edema in an infant or in a child with an abnormal trachea. This accounts for the rapid progression of symptoms in some children who have acute inflammatory conditions superimposed on preexisting tracheal narrowing.

Diagnostic Evaluation

Expeditious diagnostic evaluation to define the tracheobronchial anatomy is required following the onset of airway symptoms. Anatomic localization of tracheal narrowing is now best achieved by endoscopic techniques, although careful radiologic studies can provide significant clues as to the location of the obstruction.[5,23]

High-contrast radiographs (high KV) and fluoroscopy in two projections can give an accurate assessment of the child's airway (Fig. 55-7A). Computed tomography (CT) scans provide a rapid and more precise method of measuring the extent and length of airway narrowing or displacement (Fig. 55-7B). Visualization of the anatomic relations of the airways to surrounding structures such as the great vessels can be enhanced with intravascular contrast. Three-dimensional image reconstruction is also possible with newer computer software and is helpful in

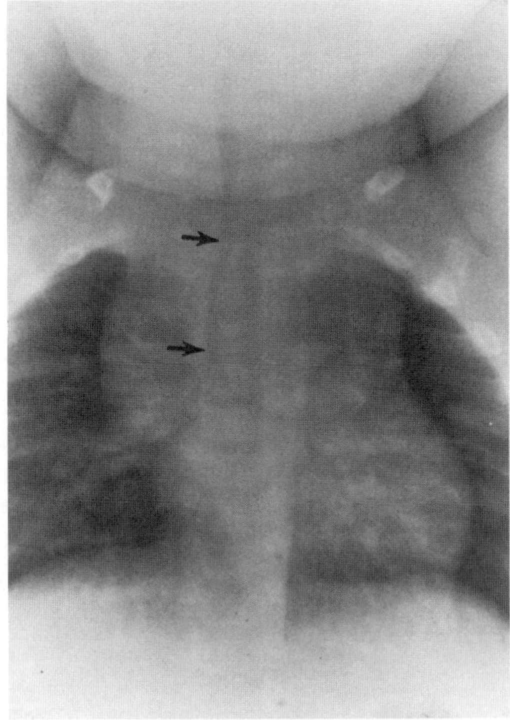

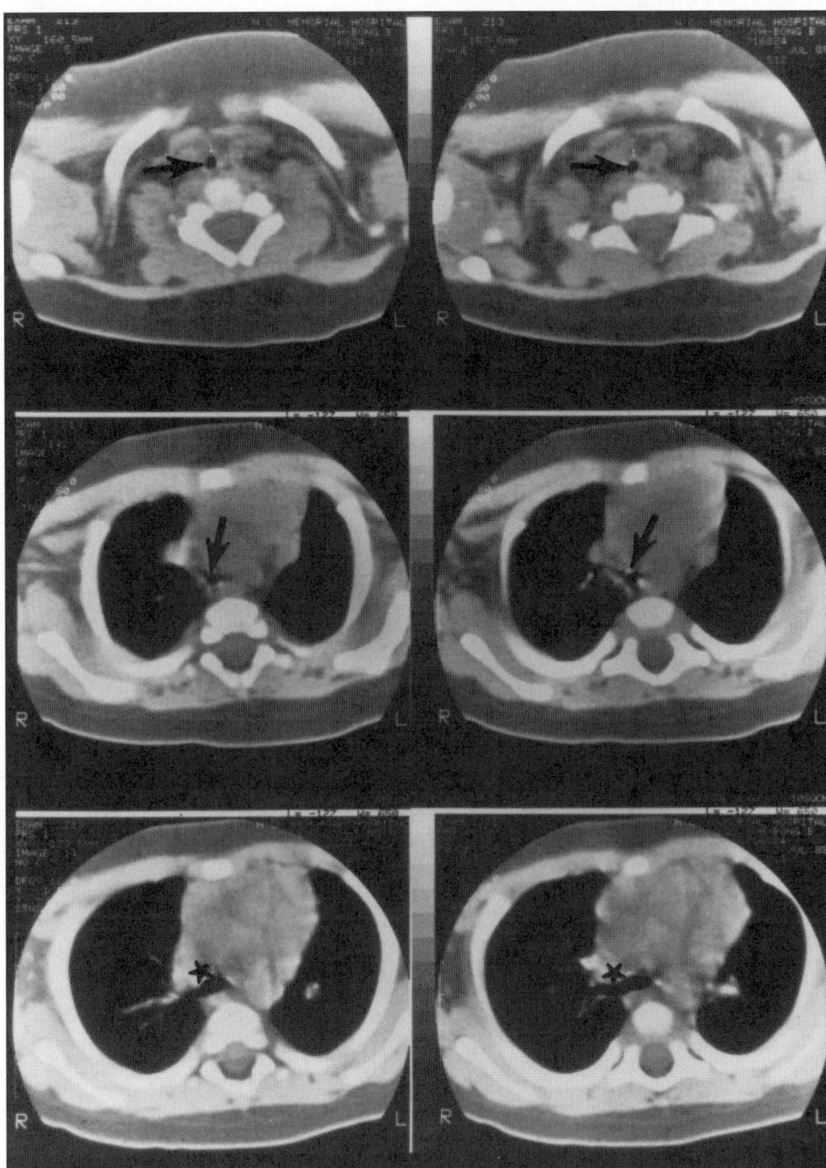

FIG. 55-7. (*A*) Chest radiograph demonstrating cervical and mediastinal tracheal stenosis in a 4-month-old (*arrows*). (*B*) Chest CT scan in the same patient delineating the length and nature of this airway anomaly. Note the diminutive trachea (*arrows*) with narrowing to the carina (*stars*).

planning surgical reconstruction. Magnetic resonance imaging (MRI) has the intrinsic advantage of not using ionizing radiation and has been useful in some patients. Unfortunately, the images take longer to obtain and are therefore more prone to patient motion artifact.

Bronchography is generally avoided because of its risks; however, in selected patients, water soluble isosmolar contrast agents may provide excellent definitions of lesions in larger airways.[5] The barium esophagogram is a useful preliminary study to look for evidence of esophageal and airway compression from a vascular lesion. Echocardiography and angiography may be indicated for suspected vascular ring or pulmonary artery sling abnormalities. Fifty percent of children with congenital tracheal stenosis have an associated vascular malformation. These anomalies must be identified prior to tracheal reconstruction. In older children, pulmonary function studies include inspiratory–expiratory flow volume curves to provide informa-

tion regarding tracheal air movement. However, most patients with these lesions are too young for this to be helpful.

Tracheal Resection

The treatment of tracheal stenoses must be individualized based on the extent of the process, the site of the lesion, and the age of the patient (Fig. 55-8). Several techniques to correct tracheal stenosis have been used with varying success.[24–28] Segmental tracheal resection with end-to-end anastomosis is considered the treatment of choice for short-segment tracheal stenosis secondary to complete tracheal rings.[24] Segmental resection beyond five rings is generally possible only with bilateral release of the pulmonary hila through the pericardium.[29]

Several surgical principles govern the technical aspects of tracheal reconstruction. The trachea can be readily exposed

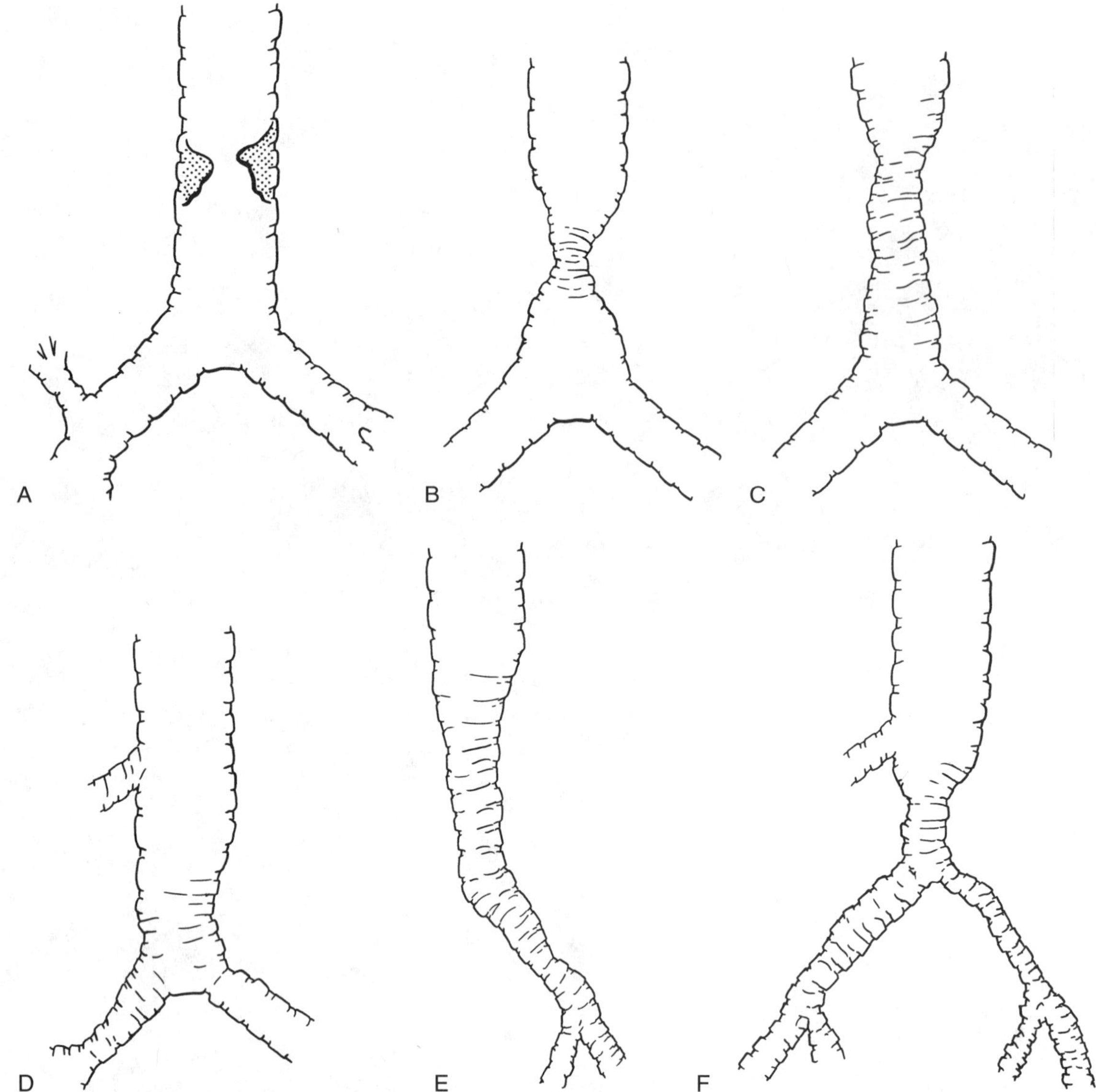

FIG. 55-8. A variety of anatomic abnormalities of the trachea are seen in children with complete tracheal rings. Some of the possibilities are illustrated.

from the cricoid to the carina through a sternotomy incision. Preserving the lateral blood vessels to the trachea is critically important, and therefore, circumferential dissection is limited to approximately 1 to 2 cm proximal and distal to the stenosis. Posterior and lateral dissections should be adjacent to the tracheal wall to avoid recurrent laryngeal nerve injury. The trachea should be divided as close as possible to the stenosis, leaving good cartilaginous rings both proximally and distally for the anastomosis. Insufficient excision of the stenosis leads to a prompt recurrence. Ventilation can be maintained through a separate anesthesia circuit or through jet cannulas placed translaryngeally through the endotracheal tube and distally across the area of resection into each main bronchus.[28] Once the anastomosis is complete, the jet cannulas or distal circuit can be removed and the translaryngeal endotracheal tube can be advanced across the anastomotic site. A molded prosthetic brace to maintain head and neck flexion postoperatively is preferred

in children. Laryngeal release is associated with postoperative dysphasia and aspiration in children and is therefore avoided. Tracheostomy is also avoided if possible. Patch tracheoplasty without resection is a safer technique for a longer stenosis.[26,29]

Tracheoplasty

An anterior patch tracheoplasty usually involves incising the length of the tracheal stricture by interpositioning a supporting tissue, such as cartilage graft, dura, or pericardium, to enlarge the tracheal lumen.[25,26] Posterior incision of the tracheal rings has also been attempted with sutured interposition of the anterior wall of the esophagus to fill the gap. Only one of three such patients has survived long term.[23]

The first successful reconstruction of subtotal tracheal stenosis with complete tracheal rings was reported in a 12-month-old

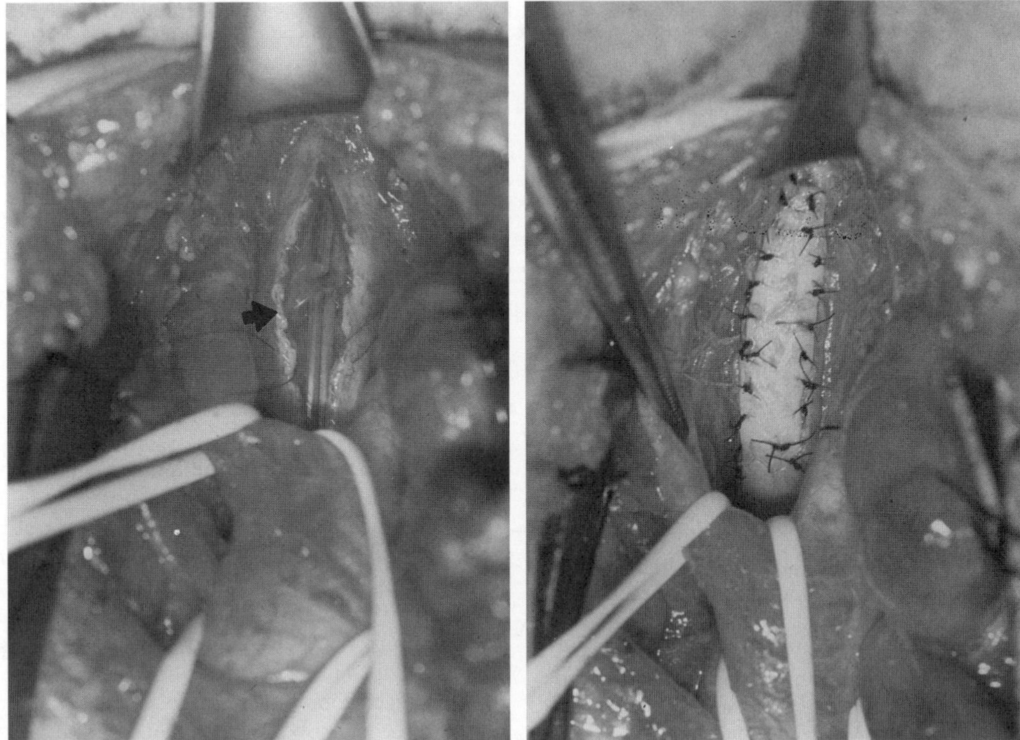

FIG. 55-9. (*A*) Operative view of the opened trachea in an infant with tracheal stenosis from complete tracheal rings. Note the endotracheal tube with two jet ventilation cannulas that have been positioned into each main bronchus. (*B*) A patch tracheoplasty with autogenous cartilage graft was sutured in place.

infant in 1982.[26] Since that time, other patients have undergone successful reconstruction with either cartilage or pericardial graft techniques (Fig. 55-9). Intraoperative airway control has been successfully managed with conventional and high-frequency jet ventilation or cardiopulmonary bypass.[25,28] In some patients, postoperative symptoms of airway collapse have been minimized by suspending a cartilage graft from the innominate artery. The cartilage graft can be sealed with a vascularized pedicle of pericardium.

Postoperative Management

Following reconstructive tracheal surgery, infants require endotracheal intubation for several days to 2 weeks. Airway edema can be significant enough to cause obstruction in the perioperative period. Furthermore, the endotracheal tube acts as a stent, keeping the airway open and facilitating repair and healing of the reconstructed trachea. Nasotracheal intubation is used preferentially because the endotracheal tube can be stabilized in position more securely. Unnecessary movements of the endotracheal tube or unplanned extubation must be avoided to minimize the risk of damage to the newly reconstructed airway. These patients also require continuous monitoring, careful pulmonary toilet, and endoscopic removal of any obstructing granulation tissue. Fiberoptic endoscopy may be required through the endotracheal tube prior to extubation. Granulation tissue at the suture line may need to be ablated with endoscopic cauterization using a potassium titanyl phosphate (KTP-532) or argon

laser.[20] Recurrent tracheal stenosis following tracheoplasty has been successfully treated with balloon dilatation.[30]

The use of systemic steroids or intralesional steroid injections to prevent local inflammation and edema postoperatively remains controversial for this group of patients.[31] Epithelial regeneration, migration, and therefore healing are delayed with steroids, which supports the argument against their use. However, postoperative edema of the airway and glottis can be significantly reduced following a short course of high-dose steroids. Furthermore, in some patients, abundant granulation tissue and associated inflammation within the airway dramatically improve with steroid administration. The selective and judicious use of steroids is primarily supported by anecdotal experiences.

To date, no one has reported clinical experience using prosthetic tracheal replacement in children. Vacanti et al[32] used a novel matrix scaffolding and cell culture to construct a tracheobioprosthesis. These have been implanted in animal models with limited success. It is too early to ascertain if this technology can be expanded and applied to congenital tracheal stenosis in humans.

Tracheal Bronchus and Tracheal Diverticulum

Anomalies of tracheal budding occur during the third and fourth gestational weeks when the trachea bifurcates and differentiates. Tracheal diverticula resemble a bronchus and typically originate from the trachea to end blindly or to communicate with a rudimentary lung. Tracheal bronchi are relatively common with the right upper lobe bronchus most commonly affected. In addition, a tracheal bronchus may connect to an isolated intrathoracic lung segment or to the apical segment of an upper lobe.[33] Symptoms generally occur only in patients who have a stenosis of the bronchus or other lung anomaly. Resection is usually curative in symptomatic patients. Common symptoms include pneumonia and neonatal respiratory distress. A variety of associated anomalies, such as dextrocardia, must be recognized. In a series by McLaughlin et al,[33] 14 of 18 patients had other congenital anomalies including Down syndrome and multiple fused ribs.

Tracheomalacia and Bronchomalacia

Airway malacia denotes a softening or weakening of the trachea. Tracheomalacia is a condition in which the structural integrity of the trachea is diminished and the cartilaginous rings are not rigid enough to prevent airway collapse during expiration. Tracheomalacia may occur in localized segments or diffusely throughout the airway.[34–37] Although a precise embryonic explanation for tracheomalacia is lacking, extrinsic pressure or compression of the embryonic cartilaginous rings may cause gradual and progressive erosion of the structural elements of the airway. Vascular rings, for example, circumferentially entrap the trachea, preventing normal growth. Constant pulsatile impingement may also injure the tracheal wall in these patients. Tracheobronchomalacia may also be acquired. Children who have bronchopulmonary dysplasia or chronic indwelling cuffed endotracheal or tracheostomy tubes are at particular risk. Important causes of tracheomalacia include the following:

- Idiopathy
- Vascular rings or slings
- Esophageal atresia or tracheoesophageal fistula
- Aberrant innominate artery
- Mediastinal masses
- Prolonged intubation for interstitial lung disease
- Bronchopulmonary dysplasia

Diagnostic Evaluation

Although anteroposterior and lateral chest radiographs can show airway compression, cinefluoroscopy better demonstrates the dynamics of airway movement with tracheal expansion and collapse during inspiration and expiration. Esophageal contrast agents enhance the visualization of swallowing and define whether esophageal distention compresses the airway. Bronchoscopy with the patient breathing spontaneously is the best method of demonstrating dynamic distortion and compression of the trachea (Fig. 55-10).[5,9] In segmental tracheomalacia, the rigid bronchoscope can be easily passed through the region of compression. Vascular anomalies such as a vascular ring can be seen as a characteristic pulsating compression through the tracheal wall. Continuous monitoring of oxygen saturation during the endoscopic procedure is essential.

Tracheal Suspension

Mild tracheomalacia is common and does not require surgical intervention. Diffuse tracheobronchomalacia that is not amenable to surgical correction has been successfully managed with prolonged positive-pressure respiratory support. Operation is clearly indicated when life-threatening airway obstruction and reflex apnea occur in infants with tracheomalacia.[35] Vascular rings require division of the constricting vessels with retraction and suspension of the vessels to ensure that the tracheal lumen is no longer compressed. Infants with an aberrant innominate artery or tracheomalacia associated with esophageal atresia are treated by suturing the aortic arch and origin of the innominate artery to the underside of the sternum to suspend the anterior tracheal wall and to relieve the collapse.[35] Our preference is to approach this procedure extrapleurally through the left third interspace, although a sternal approach is also effective. The lobes of the thymus are first separated or partially removed. To distribute the tension equally along the wall of the great vessels, a patch made of polytetrafluoroethylene (PTFE) or Dacron is first sutured to the origin of the innominate artery and the arch of the aorta with fine 5-0 nonabsorbable sutures. Additional 2-0 nonabsorbable sutures are placed from the graft through the sternum and tied on the ventral surface. Dissection between the trachea and the aorta must be avoided to prevent disrupting the connective tissue link between these two structures. Intraoperative endoscopy is necessary to verify that the tracheal collapse has been alleviated once the suspension has been performed. Results have been quite satisfactory in properly selected patients.

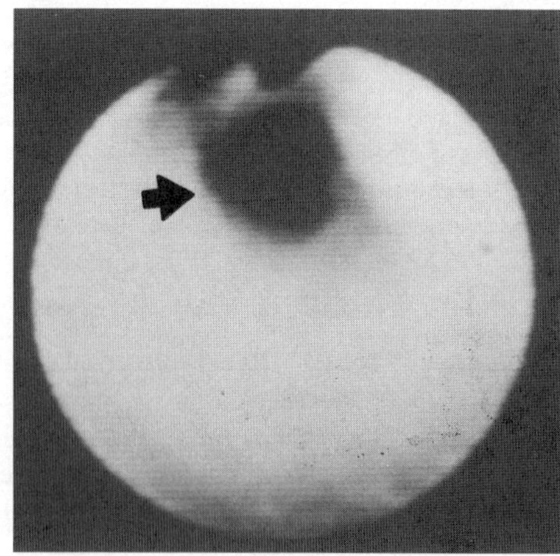
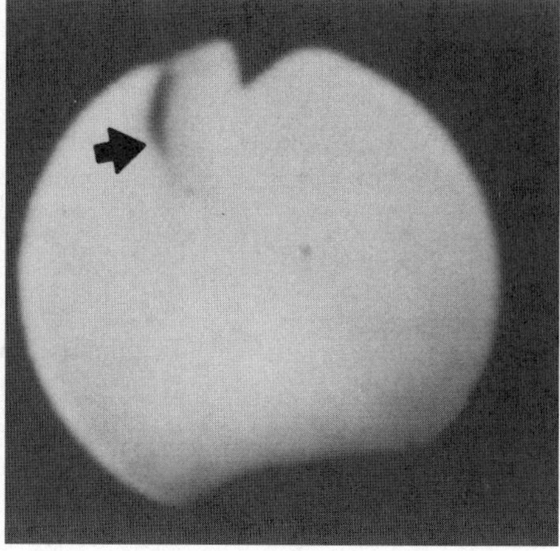

FIG. 55-10. (*A*) Endoscopic view of the left main bronchus on inspiration in a child with severe tracheobronchial malacia (*arrow*). (*B*) The same view during expiration demonstrating the collapsed airway (*arrow*).

Endobronchial Stents

Endoscopic placement of endobronchial stents for localized stenosis or severe tracheomalacia or bronchomalacia is now a relatively well-established technique in adult patients. There have been a few reports of using stents for nonmalignant disease in children.[36,37] The relatively small diameter of the pediatric airways is a serious impediment to this form of therapy, however, and long-term results are unclear. Nevertheless, it is an attractive possibility for some children with severe tracheomalacia or bronchomalacia, especially if localized.

BRONCHOPULMONARY FOREGUT ANOMALIES

The embryonic esophagus and trachea become distinct with the initiation of septation 22 to 24 days after conception and is complete at 34 to 36 days.[15] Disorders of development of the embryonic foregut give rise to a number of related congenital malformations including the following[15]:

- Esophageal atresia or tracheoesophageal fistula
- Esophageal duplication
- Esophageal bronchus
- Bronchobiliary fistula
- Bronchogenic cyst
- Pulmonary sequestration
- Related anomalies (eg, cystic adenomatoid malformation, tracheal bronchus)

Tracheoesophageal Fistula and Esophageal Atresia

The separation of the esophagus from the trachea during the fourth week of gestation is a major developmental milestone. Significant and related malformations arise if there is any perturbation of normal cell division at that stage. Esophageal atresia results from the faulty separation of the trachea and esophagus and is described in detail in Chapter 61.[15,39–44]

Esophageal Bronchus

Bronchial connection between the esophagus and the airway is an extremely rare anomaly.[45,46] This malformation putatively develops from a supernumerary lung bud arising from the esophagus. Most often, a lower lobe is aerated by this ectopic bronchus, but occasionally an entire main bronchus and lung may be involved.[47] In addition, the pulmonary vasculature may be abnormal with the arterial supply coming off the aorta and the venous drainage going into either the systemic or pulmonary veins. These anatomic features may cloud the distinction between this anomaly and extralobar sequestration. As with other tracheoesophageal malformations, associated anomalies are common, and these include cardiac, genitourinary, vertebral, and diaphragmatic defects.[48] Esophageal bronchus malformations are found twice as often in females as in males.

Symptoms of recurrent pulmonary infection because of inadequate bronchial drainage usually occur early in childhood with a bronchoesophageal fistula. In rare cases, the abnormality is not discovered until adolescence or adulthood. Associated malformations can also overshadow the pulmonary manifestations of this anomaly. Roentgenographic findings of an esophageal bronchus are somewhat inconsistent because of the spectrum of anatomic defects. If an entire lung is involved, changes in the pulmonary parenchyma are usually identified in early infancy[49]; however, isolated segments or lobes can retain a near-normal radiographic appearance for months or years. Collapse, consolidation, cavitation, and cyst formation within the pulmonary parenchyma are some of the typical radiographic patterns possible. Aggressive pulmonary toilet and antimicrobial therapy may improve the radiographic appearance, yet return to normal is unusual. The diagnosis is best confirmed by carefully done contrast studies of the esophagus; however, false-negative studies do occur. Excision of the abnormal lung and closure of the bronchoesophageal fistula is the treatment of choice and is usually well tolerated. Prognosis depends on early diagnosis and treatment as well as the severity of any associated anomalies.

Bronchobiliary Fistula

Congenital tracheobronchial–biliary fistulas are extremely rare anomalies among the bronchopulmonary foregut malformations.[50] Virtually all of these infants have significant respiratory problems in early infancy. The cardinal symptom, bile-stained sputum, should lead to bronchoscopy or bronchography to establish the diagnosis. These fistulas may arise from the distal trachea or either mainstem bronchus. Surgical division of the fistulous tract is the only effective therapy for this condition.[50–52]

Bronchogenic Cyst

Bronchogenic cysts arise from abnormal buds from the embryonic tracheobronchial tree that occur proximal to the region of alveolar differentiation. The timing of the separation influences the anatomic locations of these cysts. Early separation (carinal, first order bronchi) results in a subcarinal or mediastinal bronchogenic cyst, whereas later separation (distal bronchi) may result in an intraparenchymal lesion. Bronchogenic cysts may or may not communicate with the airways.[53,54]

Bronchogenic cysts most commonly occur along the posterior membranous trachea at the level of the carina, although paratracheal, hilar, and periesophageal locations are also common (Fig. 55-11). Extrinsic tracheobronchial compression can result in obstructive emphysema, pneumonia, and pulmonary abscess. In infants, mediastinal and peribronchial cysts may cause partial bronchial obstruction with air trapping, which can be indistinguishable from congenital lobar emphysema. The symptomatology of lesions arising in the lung and of those arising in the airway overlap significantly. Seventy percent of the treated patients develop infectious complications, most often due to partial bronchial obstruction.[55] Delay in diagnosis remains common and frequently occurs only after a pneumonic process incompletely resolves with appropriate therapy.

The radiographic appearance of bronchogenic cysts is somewhat variable depending on the location of the cyst and degree of bronchial obstruction.[54] The presence of persistent pneumonia, air-fluid levels, air-filled cyst under tension, pneumothorax,

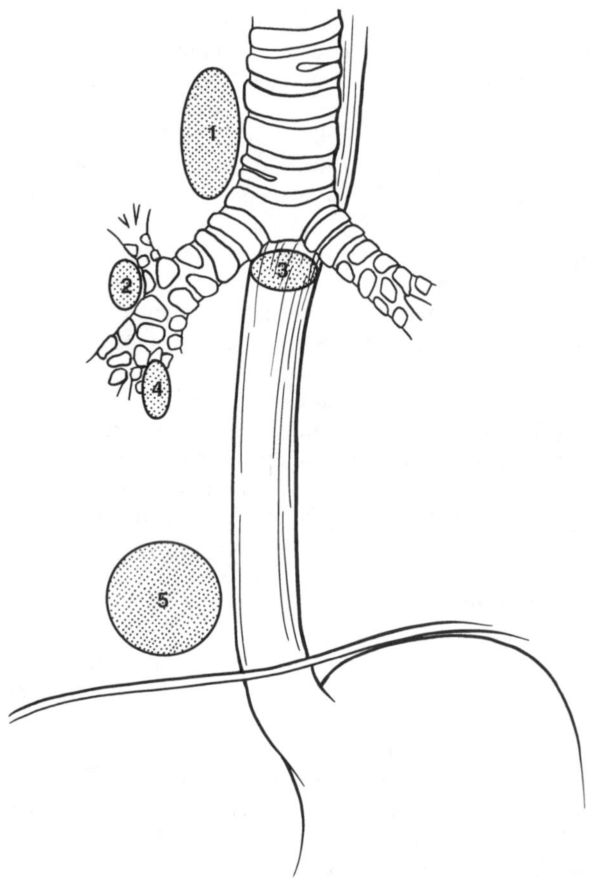

FIG. 55-11. Anatomic location of bronchogenic cysts in the mediastinum: (1) paratracheal, (2) hilar, (3) subcarinal, (4) intraparenchymal, and (5) inferior mediastinal.

lobar emphysema, and mediastinal mass warrant further investigation. CT and MRI scans are useful in differentiating cystic from solid masses and may identify other abnormalities.[55] Barium esophagography occasionally demonstrates esophageal compression by a cyst. Local resection is indicated for all bronchogenic cysts, even if they are asymptomatic.[53] Thoracoscopic resection may be appropriate for selected lesions in perihilar and periesophageal regions.[55] Intraparenchymal bronchogenic cysts are often associated with superimposed infection in the surrounding lung. Despite aggressive preoperative antimicrobial and supportive therapy, segmental lung resection may not be possible and lobectomy may be required. Bronchogenic and lung cysts are discussed in detail in Chapter 57.

INTRALUMINAL LESIONS

Hemangiomas

Intraluminal hemangiomas are congenital vascular malformations causing inspiratory stridor and significant airway obstruction due to their critical anatomic location.[31] The subglottic location is most common, although vascular malformations can be seen anywhere within the tracheobronchial tree. The degree of obstruction varies and can be exacerbated by certain positions

or crying, which increase venous pressure and lead to vascular engorgement. Most patients present in the first 6 months of life, and more than half of these patients also have cutaneous hemangiomas, providing a useful clue to the diagnosis. Female infants are twice as likely to be affected as males.

Hemangiomas are best diagnosed by endoscopy. The lesions are typically asymmetric and may be covered by a normal smooth mucosa. Biopsy of vascular lesions is discouraged because of the risk of significant hemorrhage.[5] Treatment varies with the degree of symptomatology. Although spontaneous involution occurs, most subglottic hemangiomas require definitive treatment. In 1984, Healy and McGill[56] reported on the successful treatment of 31 children with subglottic hemangiomas using the CO_2 laser coupled with an operating microscope. More recent reports confirm the utility and low complication rate of the CO_2 laser for this problem.[57] The argon and KTP-532 lasers are also particularly well suited to treating hemangiomas and other vascular lesions within the airway because of the hemoglobin absorbs their respective laser light exceptionally well.[31,58]

Tracheobronchial Tumors

Primary tumors of the tracheobronchial tree are rare in children. Benign neoplasms of the tracheobronchial tree are mesenchymal lesions that include granular cell tumors, chondroma,

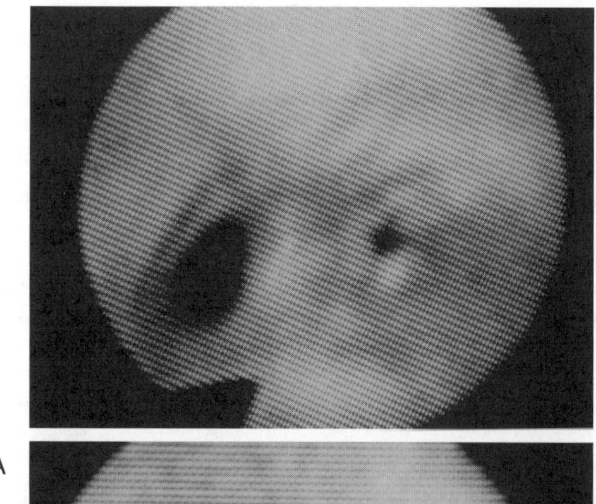
A

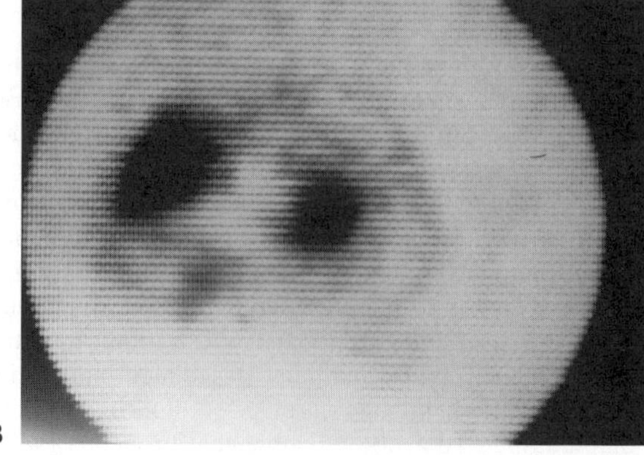
B

FIG. 55-12. (A) Acquired bronchial stenosis involving the right mainstem bronchus in a 1300-g infant. (B) The airway 1 month after endoscopic laser ablation of the endobronchial cicatrix.

leiomyoma, mucus gland adenoma, teratoma, lipoma, hemangioma, and lymphangioma.[59] Local bronchial resection and, in some cases, endobronchial ablation are usually effective techniques for small lesions. Larger and more distally located lesions may require an appropriate anatomic pulmonary resection. Preserving the normal distal lung is one of the primary goals of surgical therapy.

Primary bronchogenic carcinomas, bronchial neoplasms with salivary gland features, and carcinoid tumors are the main categories of primary epithelial neoplasms with malignant behavior. The most frequently encountered tumors are bronchial adenomas, including mucoepidermoid carcinomas, adenoid cystic carcinomas, and carcinoids. Carcinoids predominate in children. These tumors usually present with hemoptysis, cough, or symptoms of bronchial obstruction. Diagnosis is occasionally made with a CT scan, but the definitive diagnosis is best obtained with bronchoscopy showing a polypoid endobronchial mass or a peribronchial infiltrating tumor. Segmental bronchial resection is preferred for polypoid lesions as endoscopic ablation may result in local recurrence. In addition, about 10% of these lesions metastasize. Anatomic lung resection may be necessary, especially for locally infiltrating tumors. Lung tumors are discussed in detail in Chapter 57.

Tracheal Webs

Tracheal webs or stenoses that are not associated with gross deformity of the underlying cartilage may be amenable to effective laser treatment. Lesions in the proximal trachea can be satisfactorily approached with the CO_2, argon, or KTP lasers.[56,57,60] Lesions in the distal trachea and bronchi are more easily and safely treated with the argon or KTP laser, especially in small children.[61] Children with a stenosis longer than 1 to 2 cm or in whom the airway cartilage is either deficient or structurally abnormal may not be good candidates for laser treatment alone. Segmental tracheal resection or a cartilage interposition graft may be necessary in these situations.[23,25,26]

Bronchial Atresia

Localized bronchial atresia is a rare anomaly, which may simulate lobar emphysema, or a mediastinal mass. The atretic bronchus obstructs the flow of secretions and air from the distal lung to the main tracheobronchial tree. At birth the obstructed lung retains fluid but eventually the affected lobe or segment becomes hyperaerated as air enters through the pores of Kohn.[62] These patients accumulate secretions proximal to the atresia and a mucocele forms.[63,64] Emphysema of the segment may cause compression of the normal lung tissue and may be associated with wheezing and stridor. Plain chest radiographs often demonstrate a hilar mass with radiating solid channels surrounded by hyperaerated lung. A cystic central mucocele can be visualized by chest tomography. This can help to differentiate bronchial atresia from a bronchogenic cyst or lobar emphysema. These patients are at risk for serious pulmonary infection when entrapped secretions become infected. Although these children may be asymptomatic for long intervals, resection is indicated.[65]

Bronchial Stenosis

Acquired bronchial stenosis is a major cause of morbidity and mortality in infants who require prolonged intubation and respiratory support. Repeated endobronchial injury from suction catheters is a common and preventable cause of this problem, which occurs in approximately 1% of chronically intubated infants.[61,66] Treatment with endoscopic-guided forceps resection, electroresection, or dilatation has resulted in mixed success. The recent development of small quartz fiberoptic cables (300 to 600 μm) for the argon laser has made it possible to successfully treat distal bronchial lesions even in small premature infants (Fig. 55-12). Fiberoptic cables can be passed through either rigid or flexible bronchoscopes (Fig. 55-13). The argon and KTP lasers are also particularly useful for removing tracheal or endobronchial granulomas in children following repair of tracheal stenosis. The fiberoptic cables used for the neo-

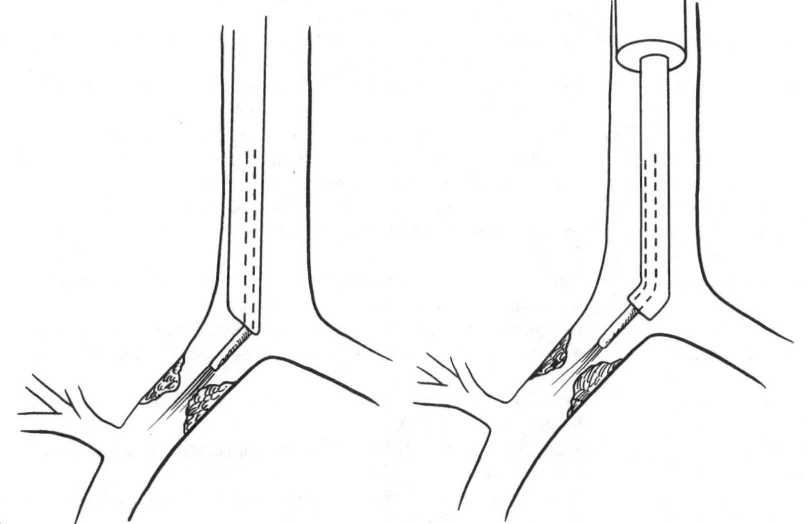

FIG. 55-13. (*A*) A quartz fiberoptic laser cable is passed through the suction channel of a flexible bronchoscope and is positioned parallel to the bronchial wall and nearly perpendicular to the lesion. (*B*) The laser is fired with the laser cable tip positioned less than 1 mm from the target tissue. The obstructing lesion is outlined by the shaded areas.

dymium:yttrium-aluminum-garnet (Nd:YAG) laser are too large relative to the airway of infants and small children, as are the lesions created. In addition, the laser energy's depth of penetration is less controlled and often extends deeply into the tissues, making the Nd:YAG laser more dangerous to use in small children.[61]

REFERENCES

1. Holinger LD. Etiology of stridor in the neonate, infant and child. Ann Otol Rhinol Laryngol 1980;89:397.
2. Ryckman FC, Rodgers BM. Obstructive airway disease in infants and children. Surg Clin North Am 1985;65:1663.
3. Backofen JE, Rogers MC. Upper airway disease. In: Rogers MC, ed. Textbook of pediatric intensive care. Baltimore, Williams & Wilkins, 1987:171.
4. Holinger LD. Clinical aspects of congenital anomalies of the larynx, trachea, bronchi, and esophagus. J Laryngol Otol 1961;75:1.
5. Wood RE, Azizkhan RG. Bronchoscopy and endobronchial procedures. In: Holcomb GW, ed. Pediatric endoscopic surgery, ed 1. Norwalk, Conn., Appleton & Lange, 1993:135.
6. Wood RE. Clinical applications of ultrathin flexible bronchoscopes. Pediatr Pulmonol 1985;1:244.
7. Wood RE, Azizkhan RG, Lacey SR, et al. Surgical applications of ultrathin flexible bronchoscopes in infants. Ann Otol Rhinol Laryngol 1991;100:116.
8. Wood RE. Spelunking in the pediatric airways: exploration with a flexible bronchoscope. Pediatr Clin North Am 1984;31:785.
9. Johnson DG. Lesions of the larynx and trachea: tracheostomy. In: Welch KJ, Randolph JG, Ravitch MM, et al, eds. Pediatric surgery, ed 4. Chicago, Year Book Medical Publishers, 1986:622.
10. Duncan BW, Howell LJ, deLorimer AA, et al. Tracheostomy in children with emphasis on home care. J Pediatr Surg 1992;27:432.
11. Magrath HL. A practical guide to home care of the child with a tracheostomy. In: Othersen HB, ed. The pediatric airway. Philadelphia, WB Saunders, 1991:197.
12. Azizkhan RG, Lacey SR, Wood RE. Anterior cricoid suspension and tracheal stoma closure for children with cricoid collapse and peristomal tracheomalacia following tracheostomy. J Pediatr Surg 1993;28:169.
13. Johnson DG. Bronchoscopy. In: Welch KJ, Randolph JG, Ravitch MM, et al, eds. Pediatric surgery, ed 4. Chicago, Year Book Medical Publishers, 1986:619.
14. Tibboel D, Kluth D. Embryology of congenital lesions of the tracheobronchial tree. In Lobe TE, ed. Tracheal reconstruction in infancy. Philadelphia, WB Saunders, 1991:1.
15. Gray SW, Skandalakis J. Embryology for surgeons; Philadelphia, WB Saunders, 1972:293.
16. Congdon ED. Transformation of the aortic arch system during development of the human embryo. Contrib Embryol Carnegie Inst 1922;14:47.
17. Chythil F. Vitamin A and lung development. Pediatr Pulmonol 1985;1:115.
18. Huot C, Gauthier M, Lebel M, et al. Congenital malformations associated with the maternal use of valproic acid. Can J Neurol Sci 1987;14:290.
19. Tack E, Perlman J. Tracheal stenosis. Lethal malformation in two infants of diabetic mothers. Am J Dis Child 1987;141:77.
20. Lobe TE, Hayden CK, Nicholas D, et al. Successful management of congenital tracheal stenosis in infancy. J Pediatr Surg 1987;22:1137.
21. Lemez L. Sites for experimental production of tracheal and/or esophageal malformations in 4 day old chick embryos. Folia Morphol (Praha) 1980;28:52.
22. Hirschberg J, Lellei I. Stenose, respectivement of obstruction de la trachee des nourrissons et des petits enfants. Therapeutische Umschau/Revue Therapeutique 1982;12:997.
23. Lobe TE. Operative technique and considerations for the reconstruction of congenital stenoses of the trachea in infants. In Lobe TE, ed. Tracheal reconstruction in infancy. Philadelphia, WB Saunders, 1991:79.
24. Grillo HC, Zannini P. Management of obstructing tracheal disease in children. J Pediatr Surg 1984;19:414.
25. Idriss FS, DeLeon SY, Ilbawi MN et al. Tracheoplasty with pericardial patch for extensive tracheal stenosis in infants and children. J Thorac Cardiovasc Surg 1984;88:527.
26. Kimura K, Mukohara N, Tsugawa C, et al. Tracheoplasty for congenital stenosis of the entire trachea. J Pediatr Surg 1982;17:869.
27. Cohen M, Weber T, Rao C. Balloon dilatation of tracheal and bronchial stenosis. Am J Radiol 1984;142:477.
28. Schur MS, Maccioli GA, Azizkhan RG, et al. High frequency jet ventilation in the management of congenital tracheal stenosis. Anesthesiology 1988;68:952.
29. Tsugawa C, Kimura K, et al. Congenital stenosis involving a long segment of the trachea: further experience in reconstructive surgery. J Pediatr Surg 1988;23:471.
30. Philippart AI, Long JA, Greenholz SK. Balloon dilatation of postoperative tracheal stenosis. J Pediatr Surg 1988;23:1178.
31. Strunk CL. Laser treatment of congenital lesions of the tracheobronchial tree. In Lobe TE, ed. Tracheal reconstruction in infancy. Philadelphia, WB Saunders, 1991:111.
32. Vacanti CA, Paige KT, Kim WS, et al. Experimental tracheal replacement using tissue-engineered cartilage. J Pediatr Surg 1994;29:201.
33. McLaughlin FJ, Streider DJ, Harris GB, et al. Tracheal bronchus: associations with respiratory morbidity in childhood. J Pediatr 1985;106:751.
34. Harrison MR, Hendren WH. Agenesis of the lung complicated by vascular compression and bronchomalacia. J Pediatr Surg 1975;10:813.
35. Schwartz MZ, Filler RM. Tracheal compression as a cause of apnea following repair of tracheoesophageal fistula: treatment by aortopexy. J Pediatr Surg 1980;15:842.
36. Vinograd I, Filler R, Bahoric A. Long-term functional results of prosthetic airway splinting in tracheomalacia and bronchomalacia. J Pediatr Surg 1987;22:38.
37. Mair CE, Parsons CD, Lally MK. Treatment for severe bronchomalacia with expanding endobronchial stents. Arch Otolaryngol Head Neck Surg 1990;116:1087.
38. Azizkhan RG, Grimmer DL, Askin FB, et al. Acquired lobar emphysema (overinflation): clinical and pathological evaluation of infants requiring lobectomy. J Pediatr Surg 1992;27:1145.
39. Randolph JG. Esophageal atresia and congenital stenosis. In: Welch KJ, Randolph JG, Ravitch MM, et al, eds. Pediatric surgery, ed 4. Chicago, Year Book Medical Publishers, 1986:682.
40. Martin LW, Alexander F. Esophageal atresia. Surg Clin North Am 1985;65:1099.
41. Randolph JG, Newman KD, Anderson KD. Current results in repair of esophageal atresia with tracheoesophageal fistula using physiological guide to therapy. Ann Surg 1989;209:526.
42. Azizkhan RG. Esophageal atresia and distal tracheoesophageal atresia in a neonate. Postgrad Gen Surg 1992;4:1.
43. Grosfeld JL, Ballantine TVN. Esophageal atresia and tracheoesophageal fistula: effect of delayed thoracotomy on survival. Surgery 1978;84:394.
44. Filston HC, Chitwood WR, Schkolne B, et al. The Fogarty balloon catheter as an aid to management of the infant with esophageal atresia and tracheoesophageal fistula complicated by severe RDS or pneumonia. J Pediatr Surg 1982;17:149.
45. Gans SL, Potts WJ. Anomalous lobe of lung arising from the esophagus. J Thorac Surg 1951;21:313.
46. John S, Gopinath N, McPhall C. Congenital esophagobronchial fistula. Br J Surg 1965;52:941.
47. Nikaido H, Swenson O. The ectopic origin of the right main bronchus from the esophagus: a case of pneumonectomy in a neonate. J Thorac Cardiovasc Surg 1971;62:151.
48. Toyama W. Esophageal atresia and tracheoesophageal fistula in association with bronchial and pulmonary abnormalities. J Pediatr Surg 1972;7:302.
49. Hanna EA. Broncho–esophageal fistula with total sequestration of the right lung. Ann Surg 1964;159:599.
50. Kalayoglu M, Olcay I. Congenital bronchobiliary fistula associated with esophageal atresia and tracheoesophageal fistula. J Pediatr Surg 1976;11:463.
51. Sane SM, Sieber WK, Girdany BR. Congenital bronchobiliary fistula. Surgery 1971:69:599.
52. Wagget J, Stool S, Bishop JC, et al. Congenital bronchobiliary fistula. J Pediatr Surg 1970;5:566.
53. Ramenofsky ML, Leape LL, McCauley RGK. Bronchogenic cyst. J Pediatr Surg 1979;14:219.

54. Rogers LF, Osmer JC. Bronchogenic cysts: a review of 46 cases. Am J Roentgenol. 1964;91:273.
55. Azizkhan RG. Congenital pulmonary conditions in childhood. Chest Clin North Am 1993;3:547.
56. Healy GB, McGill T. Carbon dioxide laser in subglottic hemangioma: an update. Ann Otol Rhinol Laryngol 1984;93:370.
57. Bagwell CE. CO_2 laser excision of pediatric airway lesions. J Pediatr Surg 1990;25:1152.
58. Tan OT, Carney JM, Margolis R, et al. Histological responses of port wine stains treated by argon, carbon dioxide and tunable dye lasers. Arch Dermatol 1986; 122:1016.
59. Dehner LP. Mediastinum, lungs and cardiovascular system. In Dehner LP. Pediatric surgical pathology, ed 2. Baltimore, Williams & Wilkins, 1987:229.
60. Gans SL, Austin E. The use of lasers in pediatric surgery. J Pediatr Surg 1988;23:695.
61. Azizkhan RG, Lacey SR, Wood RE. Acquired symptomatic bronchial stenosis in infants: successful management utilizing an argon laser. J Pediatr Surg 1990;25:19.
62. Schuster SR, Harris G, Williams A, et al. Bronchial atresia: a recognizable entity in the pediatric age group. J Pediatr Surg 1978;13:682.
63. Cohen AM, Solomon EH, Alfidi RJ. Computed tomography in bronchial atresia. Am J Radiol 1980;135:1097.
64. Oh K, Dorst J, White JJ. Syndrome of bronchial atresia or stenosis with mucocele and focal hyperinflation of the lung. Johns Hopkins Med J 1976;138:48.
65. Haller JA, Tepas JJ, White JJ, et al. The natural history of bronchial atresia: serial observations of a case from birth to operative correction. J Thorac Cardiovasc Surg 1980;79:868.
66. Greenholz SK, Hall RJ, Lilly JR, et al. Surgical implications of bronchopulmonary dysplasia. J Pediatr Surg 1987;22:1131.

Surgery of Infants and Children: Scientific Principles and Practice, edited by Keith T. Oldham, Paul M. Colombani, and Robert P. Foglia. Lippincott–Raven Publishers, Philadelphia, © 1997.

CHAPTER 56

Mediastinum and Pleura

Bradley M. Rodgers and Eugene D. McGahren III

THORACIC EMBRYOLOGY

Most of the important embryologic events in the development of the thorax are completed by the eighth or ninth week of gestation. The thoracic cavity fully separates from the abdominal cavity by closure of the pleuroperitoneal folds of the diaphragm during the eighth week of gestation.[1] Failure of complete closure results in congenital diaphragmatic hernia. Diaphragmatic muscularization occurs principally by the ingrowth of muscle from the lateral chest wall. Arrest of this process may produce anomalies such as congenital eventration of the diaphragm. The paired pleural cavities begin to form by the invagination of the lung buds into the paired pericardioperitoneal canals, connecting the primitive pericardial and peritoneal cavities. The pleural cavities are isolated by the development of the pleuropericardial and pleuroperitoneal membranes, a process completed by the sixth week of gestation[2] (Fig. 56-1). During the sixth week of development, the lateral thoracic wall begins to form by extensions of the lateral vertebral processes, which forms the ribs. During this same interval, the sternum forms anteriorly as a pair of bands of condensed mesenchyme. By the seventh week, these sternal bands begin to fuse cranially, displacing the heart caudally. Fusion of the sternum and its junction with the developing ribs is complete by the ninth week of gestation.[3] Abnormalities of development at this stage may result in sternal clefts and complex abnormalities of chest wall development such as Poland syndrome.

During the third week of gestation, the laryngotracheal groove forms at the cranial end of the foregut, giving rise to the primitive trachea. At the same time, proliferation of mesenchyme of the foregut mesentery leads to the development of the cartilage, muscle, and connective tissue of the lungs. By the fourth week of gestation, the elongating trachea has bifurcated into right and left mainstem bronchi, and by the 16th week, segmental bronchi have begun to form.[4] Abnormalities of this segmentation may lead to forms of pulmonary agenesis or tracheal branching abnormalities such as bronchogenic cysts. The close timing of parallel embryologic events occurring in the trachea and the esophagus during this interval often leads to complementary abnormalities in these two structures.

The pulmonary arteries begin as a capillary network extending caudally from the aortic sac. By the sixth week of gestation, there are bilateral sixth aortic arches carrying blood to the developing pulmonary mesenchyme. By the seventh week, the right arch has involuted, leaving the left sixth arch which is the primordium of the main pulmonary artery. Abnormalities occurring during this interval may lead to defects of pulmonary vascular development such as pulmonary sequestration. The details of bronchopulmonary development are outlined in greater detail in Chapter 54.

Between the sixth and eighth week of gestation, the jugular lymphatic sacs are connected with the cisterna chyli through bilateral systems of thoracic lymphatic channels, which are interconnected by numerous branches.[5] The inferior portion of the right channel and the superior portion of the left, together with a diagonal channel at the level of the fourth thoracic vertebra, persist to form the definitive thoracic duct by the ninth week of gestation. Abnormalities of this process explain the high incidence of anatomic variation of the thoracic duct system. The thymus arises from the third pharyngeal pouch in the fifth week of gestation. Between the seventh and eighth week, the thymus elongates caudally until, by the end of the eighth week, the left and right primordia have fused at the level of the aortic arch.[6] By the end of the ninth week, the mesenchyme of the thymus begins to be populated with lymphoid cells, probably of systemic origin.

POSTNATAL THORACIC DEVELOPMENT

Structurally, the chest and mediastinum are almost fully developed at the time of birth; however, a few changes take place later. The first and most dramatic change is the shift from fetal to adult circulation. During the infant's first breaths, its pulmonary vascular resistance falls dramatically. This allows the pulmonary vasculature to accept the entire cardiac output, thereby facilitating closure of various fetal shunts, particularly the foramen ovale and the ductus arteriosus. The ductus functionally closes shortly after birth through contraction of its muscular wall, and its anatomic closure is accomplished over 1 to 3 months by proliferation of the intimal layer.[7,8]

The lungs continue their development after birth in a more subtle manner. Initially, in the postnatal period, the number of

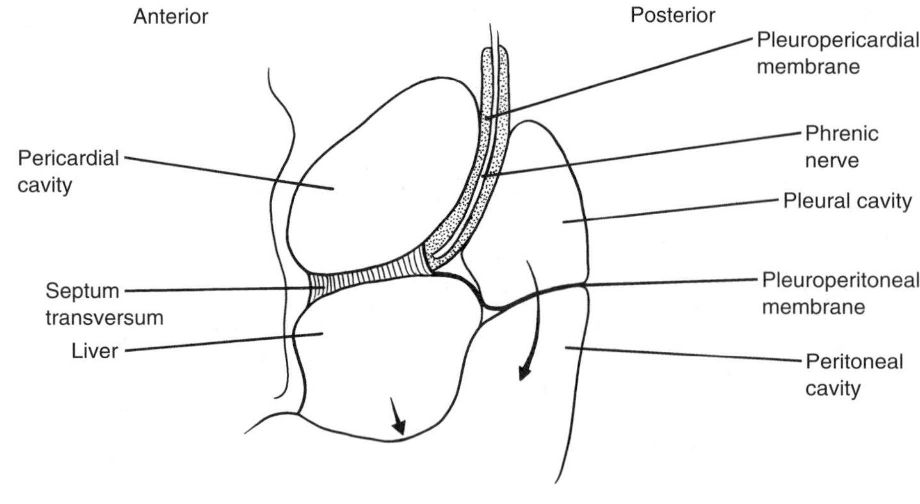

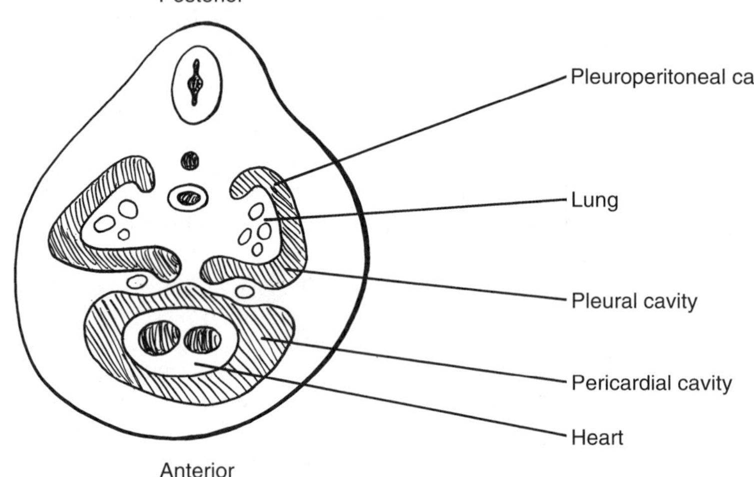

FIG. 56-1. Formation of the pleural cavities. The pleura are separated from the pericardial cavity by the formation of the pleuropericardial membrane. The phrenic nerve descends through this membrane to meet the septum transversum, a major component of the diaphragm. The final step in isolation of the pleural cavities is completion of the pleuroperitoneal membrane with obliteration of the pleuroperitoneal canal. The lung buds project laterally into the pleural cavities, forming the separate visceral and parietal pleuras. (After O'Rahilly R, Müller F. Human embryology and teratology. New York, Wiley-Liss, 1992;172)

immature alveoli increases, and these alveoli are able to generate new immature alveoli which subsequently enlarge into mature alveoli. Consequently, the area of the air–blood interface continues to increase as the alveoli and capillaries multiply. These changes continue through at least the eighth year of life. Only about 50 million, or one sixth of the adult number of alveoli, are present at birth.[9] The structural integrity of the airway improves after birth as the flexible cartilage of the infant's larynx and trachea becomes more rigid.

ANATOMY

Fully developed, the mediastinum and the pleural spaces represent a collection of complex organs interacting in a constant and literally fluid manner. The mediastinum represents the central portion of the thoracic cavity. Its boundaries are the sternum anteriorly, the vertebral column posteriorly, and the medial parietal pleural surfaces of the right and left lungs laterally. The mediastinum contains four compartments: the superior, anterior, middle, and posterior (Fig. 56-2). The superior mediastinum lies in the thoracic space cephalad to a plane joining the fourth thoracic vertebra and the sternomanubrial junction. The

anterior mediastinum is bounded superiorly by the superior mediastinum, inferiorly by the diaphragm, anteriorly by the sternum, and posteriorly by the pericardium. The middle mediastinum is bounded by the anterior and posterior limits of the pericardium. The posterior mediastinum is bounded superiorly by the superior mediastinum, inferiorly by the diaphragm, anteriorly by the pericardium, and posteriorly by the vertebral column.

The right and left pleural spaces are separate entities which extend from the lateral aspects of the mediastinum as they envelope each lung. The parietal pleura lines the thoracic wall while the visceral pleura adheres intimately to the pulmonary surface. A thin layer of mesothelial cells separates the two surfaces.[10] In some areas, the parietal pleura may fold onto itself until the lung intercedes during inspiration. These areas are found inferiorly along the edges of the diaphragm, in the costodiaphragmatic sinus, and in a small cleft behind the sternum known as the costomediastinal sinus.[10] The blood supply of the parietal pleura is derived from the intercostal, internal mammary, superior phrenic, and anterior mediastinal arteries. Corresponding veins drain the parietal pleura into the systemic veins. The visceral pleura is supplied by bronchial and pulmonary artery radicals; however, venous drainage is only to the pulmo-

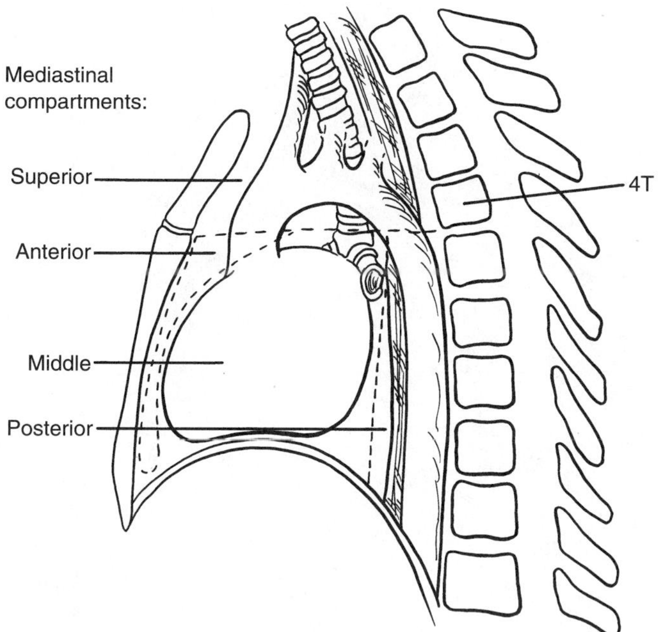

FIG. 56-2. Anatomic division of the mediastinum into superior, anterior, middle, and posterior compartments.

nary circulation.[10] The parietal pleura receives sensory innervation from the intercostal and phrenic nerves. This results in relatively precise sensory localization. The visceral pleura receives vagal and sympathetic innervation and has far less precise sensory localization.[10]

Ongoing dynamics between the systemic and pulmonary vascularity and the lymphatic circulation maintain a relatively constant amount of pleural fluid, which is evenly distributed within the pleural space.[11,12] Most pleural fluid is formed from the systemic circulation and, in turn, mostly absorbed by the parietal pleura. Fluid travels along pressure gradients in the pleural space until it is primarily resorbed by parietal pleural lymphatics. Elevation of systemic venous pressure or lymphatic pressure results in excessive accumulation of pleural fluid either by increased production (venous congestion) or decreased absorption (lymphatic congestion). Normally, therefore, there is little interchange between pleural and pulmonary fluids. Pulmonary edema can disturb this balance by presenting a greater amount of fluid to the visceral pleura from the pulmonary parenchyma itself.[13]

PHYSIOLOGY

The anatomy of the pleural space plays a significant role in respiratory physiology. During quiet respiration, the intrapleural pressure is -8 to -9 mmHg during inspiration and -3 to -6 mmHg during expiration. A positive gradient exists between the intrabronchial pressure and intrapleural pressure throughout the respiratory cycle, thus holding the pleural surfaces together.[10] During inspiration, the lung is expanded by the negative pressure generated by the movement of the diaphragm and thoracic wall. In normal breathing, the diaphragmatic excursion is only about 2 cm. If the diaphragm is para-

lyzed, as seen in eventration of the diaphragm, it moves paradoxically upward during inspiration in response to the fall in intrathoracic pressure, interfering with ventilation of the ipsilateral lung (Fig. 56-3). The major accessory muscles of inspiration include the scalene and sternocleidomastoid muscles. These are usually quiescent during normal breathing, but may be quite active during exercise or respiratory insufficiency.[14] Expiration is usually a passive event, but may become active during exercise and hyperventilation. The abdominal wall muscles are the most important muscles in active expiration, but are aided by intercostal muscles.[14]

Various factors influence the efficiency of ventilation. First, the chest wall is quite elastic. There is an ongoing tension between the lung, which naturally tends to recoil inward, and the thoracic wall which tends to recoil outward. This tension helps to keep the lung expanded. At rest, the upper lung is relatively more expanded than the lower lung, because the intrathoracic pressure is less negative at the base than at the apex due to gravity. During inspiration, however, the lower lung expands more, relative to the upper lung, demonstrating a greater compliance.[15] Gravity is not the lone determinant of this vertical gradient. The shapes of the intrathoracic organs, the chest wall orientation, and the tendency of the structures to resist displacement or deformation contribute to this gradient.[16,17] In fact, the two lungs can function almost as separate structures with different mechanical properties.[16] The position of the patient may also affect the distribution of ventilation within the lung. For example, experimental studies have shown an improvement in oxygenation in animals placed in the prone versus the supine position because small airway patency is better maintained in the prone position.[18]

The foregoing section has described the respiratory status of the child and the adult, but there are special considerations in the infant. Anatomic and physiologic dynamics are not fully developed in the neonate. The overly compliant chest wall is easily distorted during respiratory efforts. This is especially true during sleep because intercostal muscle activity is reduced, resulting in decreased lung dynamic compliance. Neonatal lung tissue is more viscous, peripheral airways offer more resistance, and mismatches of ventilation and perfusion are more marked than in the older child and adult. The upper airway is quite pliable and can close at pressures of 4 mmHg. Neck extension can enhance airway patency while flexion can hinder it. In addition, the functional residual capacity (FRC) in the neonate comprises a relatively higher proportion of lung capacity due to a decreased expiratory phase. This helps in the absorption of intrapulmonary fluid and the maintenance of a more uniform airway expansion, but leaves the infant vulnerable to atelectasis.[19]

OPERATIVE PRINCIPLES

Anesthetic considerations are extremely important for infants and children undergoing thoracic surgery. The normal cardiopulmonary physiology in these young patients may compromise their ability to respond to the changes induced by general anesthesia. Infants and children have a relatively small FRC compared with tidal volume. In newborns, the FRC actually overlaps the closing volume of the lung.[20] Thus, newborns are especially prone to alveolar collapse during open chest anesthesia. The use of positive end expiratory pressure (PEEP) may

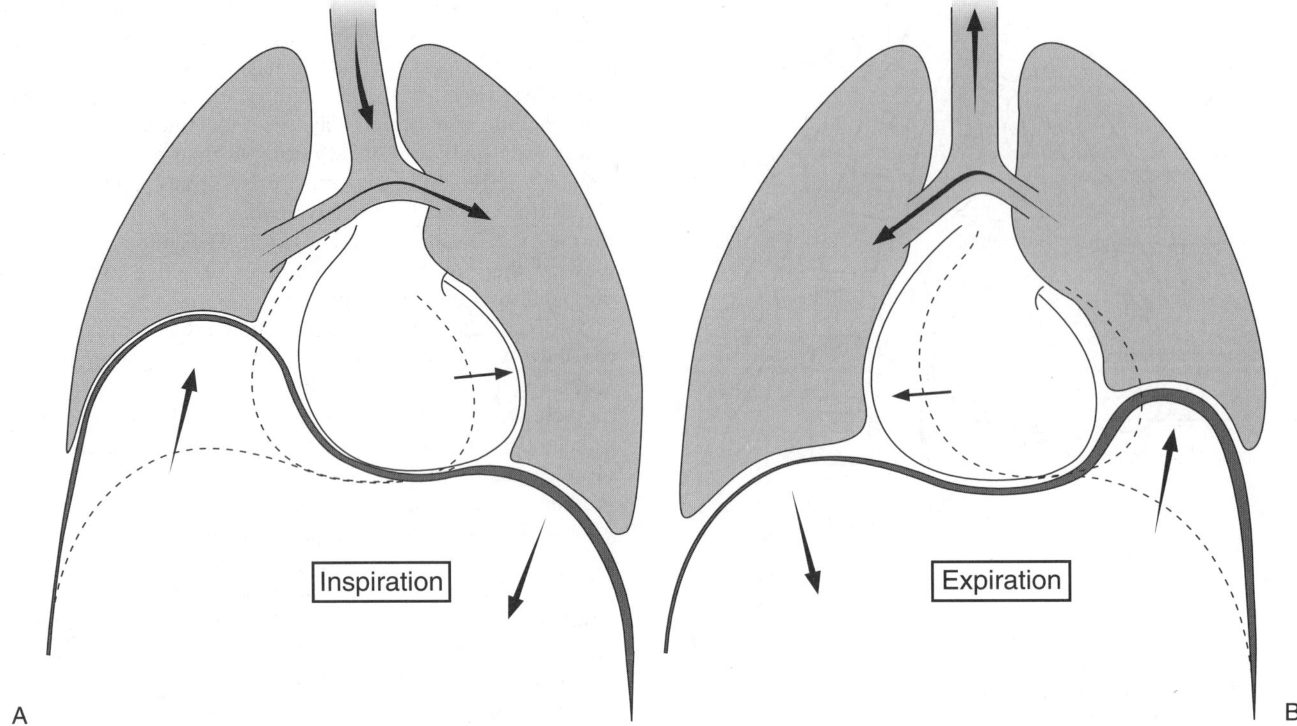

FIG. 56-3. Pathophysiologic changes with paralysis of the right hemidiaphragm. (*A*) During inspiration, the normal left hemidiaphragm descends, increasing intraabdominal pressure. This elevates the right hemidiaphragm and shifts the mediastinal structures to the left. Gas in the right lung is forced into the left lung, increasing dead-space ventilation. (*B*) During expiration, the normal left diaphragm elevates, reducing intraabdominal pressure and allowing the right diaphragm to descend. The mediastinal structures move back toward the right side. Gas in the left lung is forced into the right lung. The movement of air from one lung to the other during the respiratory cycle is dead-space ventilation, termed *Pendelluft*. (After Rodgers BM, McGahren ED. Congenital eventration of the diaphragm. In: Modern problems in pediatrics, vol 24. Basel: S Karger, 1989:121)

prevent atelectasis and eliminate clinically significant hypoxia. The infant's myocardium is relatively less sensitive to the positive inotropic effects of isoproterenol and dopamine and relatively more sensitive to the negative inotropic effects of propranolol.[21] The infant's myocardium is also less compliant than that of the older child. Because of this different physiology, the cardiac output in infants is augmented by increasing heart rate at a relatively constant stroke volume. As the heart rate increases, however, there is less time for ventricular filling. A point is reached at which the infant can no longer increase cardiac output and shock ensues. Shock may develop rapidly in infants, and is often heralded only by a progressive increase in heart rate rather than a gradual decline in blood pressure. If the response to positive inotropic support is inadequate, vigorous volume resuscitation is necessary to support the peripheral circulation.

Pulmonary physiology in the lateral decubitus position has been thoroughly studied in adult patients but poorly evaluated in children. Gravity increases the pulmonary blood flow to the dependent lung as compared with the nondependent lung. Conversely, ventilation is superior in the nondependent lung because of elevation of the dependent diaphragm and gravitational shifts of the mediastinum[22] (Fig. 56-4). These changes in ventilation may be even more significant in children because the mediastinum is more mobile and the abdominal organs are relatively larger. An anesthetized, paralyzed child in the lateral decubitus position, therefore, may experience significant ventilation–perfusion mismatch. The reduction of regional ventilation in the child's dependent lung may precipitate alveolar collapse and systemic hypoxia. This ventilation–perfusion mismatch may be further exacerbated by one-lung ventilation techniques like those used for many thoracoscopic procedures. In this instance, all blood flow to the nondependent and nonventilated lung becomes shunt flow, creating an obligatory right-to-left shunt. Many infants and children become significantly hypoxic under these conditions and can not tolerate one-lung ventilation in this position. Increasing the FIO_2 and respiratory rate may be enough to compensate for this shunt fraction and to allow the procedure to be completed. The use of positive-pressure ventilation with positive and expiratory pressure prevents alveolar collapse and maximizes ventilation of the dependent lung.

Maintaining the fluid and glucose balance in children undergoing thoracic surgery is critical. Fluid overload in neonates may open a previously closed ductus arteriosus, creating a significant shunt. Likewise, excessive administration of crystalloids during an operative procedure may precipitate interstitial pulmonary edema, further aggravating the potential for systemic hypoxia. Infants undergoing thoracic surgery should receive no more than 75% of their calculated maintenance fluid volume in the first 24 to 48 hours postoperatively. Reductions

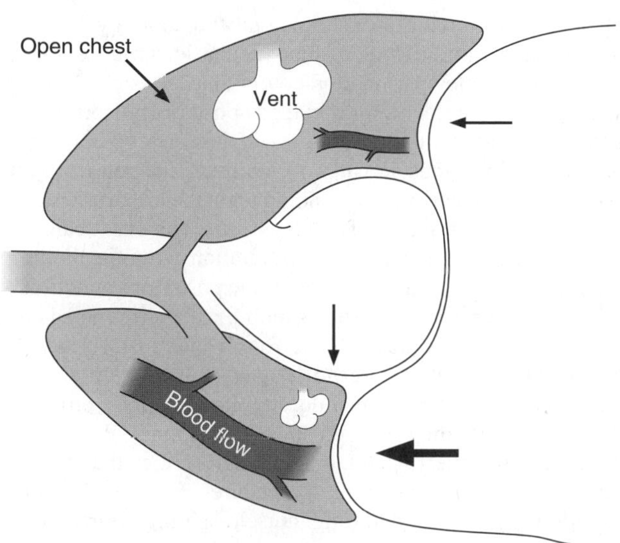

FIG. 56-4. Pathophysiologic changes in the pleura and mediastinum in the lateral decubitus position during anesthesia with an open chest. Ventilation in the nondependent lung is superior to that in the dependent lung because of elevation of the dependent diaphragm and gravitational shifts of the mediastinum. Perfusion, on the other hand, is superior in the dependent lung because of gravitational forces. Both ventilation and perfusion in the nondependent, operated lung may be further impaired by compression during surgery.

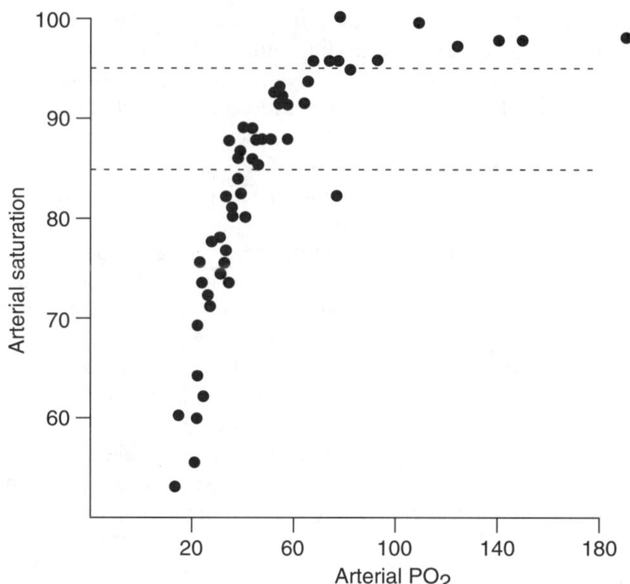

FIG. 56-5. Measured relationship between Pao$_2$ (in mmHg) and percent of transcutaneous oxygen saturation in human neonates. An oxygen dissociation curve for this patient population is generated. Maintaining saturation levels between 85% and 95% avoids Pao$_2$ levels higher than 100 or less than 50 mmHg. Arterial saturation levels higher than 95% are associated with unacceptable levels of Pao$_2$ for premature human infants.

in fluid intake are usually accompanied by reductions in glucose intake. Thus, careful glucose monitoring is important during this interval.

Intraoperative and perioperative monitoring of cardiac and respiratory function is essential in infants and children since their clinical condition may change rapidly. In the past, the size of these patients often made sophisticated monitoring of cardiopulmonary function difficult or impossible, but modern equipment has largely overcome these difficulties. As a minimum, all children undergoing thoracic surgery should have continuous monitoring of heart rate, blood pressure, electrocardiogram, oxygen saturation, and temperature. Blood pressure monitoring is facilitated by Doppler equipment, such as the Dinamap. This instrument can repeatedly measure systolic, diastolic, and mean blood pressure at preset time intervals in patients of all sizes. Automated blood pressure readings correlate closely with intraarterial readings if appropriate sized cuffs are used.[23]

Oxygen saturation can be continuously measured with transcutaneous sensors. This equipment can be used on patients of all ages, and the readings are not adversely affected by the percentage of fetal hemoglobin in the circulation. Because of the shape of the oxyhemoglobin curve, oxygen saturation provides a better method for detecting levels of hypoxia than for detecting hyperoxia. This is not of practical importance except in small premature infants, in whom persistent excessive oxygenation can affect retinal circulation. When oxygen saturations are maintained at or below 95%, the PaO$_2$ is not likely to exceed 100 mmHg[24] (Fig. 56-5). Maintaining saturation levels between 85% and 95% assures a safe range of partial pressure of oxygen for premature infants. The ability to continuously monitor oxy-

gen saturation has provided a sensitive method for detecting mechanical anesthetic complications, such as mainstem intubation or obstruction of the endotracheal tube. Using these devices in the postoperative period has greatly reduced the need for arterial blood gas sampling. Two oxygen-saturation sensors can be used to detect right-to-left shunting through the ductus arteriosus. One sensor is placed proximal (right arm), and one is placed distal (legs) to the ductus arteriosus. A difference of greater than 5% saturation indicates significant shunting. Recent advances in technology have created accurate and practical end tidal CO$_2$ monitors. These devices are connected to the endotracheal tube and sample expired gas concentrations. They provide an accurate correlation with arterial PCO$_2$, except in infants who weigh less than 4 kg. In these small patients, sampling errors of the small tidal volume may lead to inaccurate readings.[25]

Catheters are available for measuring pulmonary capillary wedge pressure and calorimetric cardiac output in pediatric patients. In infants, these catheters (4F) must usually be inserted by cutdown techniques, but in older children they may be placed percutaneously. Percutaneous arterial catheters (22F and 24F) can be used in infants and children. Usually, these are placed in the radial artery, although the femoral artery may be used in small infants for short-term monitoring.

Certain relatively common thoracic surgical procedures in children require special anesthetic considerations. Airway endoscopy is frequently performed in children to evaluate stridor or to remove airway foreign bodies. Most of these procedures are performed under general anesthesia using a rigid ventilating bronchoscope. Insertion of this instrument in small children, even under general anesthesia, may precipitate laryngospasm. Applying topical anesthesia (lidocaine 4%) on the cords before introducing the bronchoscope reduces the hazard of laryngospasm and eliminates much of the discomfort of the procedure. Positive-pressure ventilation through the bronchoscope is contraindicated in many of the bronchoscopic procedures performed in children. For example, positive pressure used in patients with airway foreign bodies may impact the foreign body onto the carina or into a distal bronchus. In addition, patients with pulmonary air trapping, such as children with lobar emphysema, who are undergoing bronchoscopy for selective airway aspiration may experience sudden respiratory collapse with positive-pressure ventilation because of the rapid enlargement of the involved lobe or development of a pneumothorax. Rah documented the inadequacies of ventilation with the smallest bronchoscopes (2.5 to 3 mm) when the rod lens telescope is in place.[26] The lumen available for ventilation under these circumstances is small, and expiration of gas from the lung is impeded. When using these bronchoscopes, the surgeon is advised to remove the telescope intermittently, allowing periods of ventilation to avoid severe hypercarbia or pneumothorax.

Pain relief in children undergoing thoracic surgery is important to minimize respiratory complications. Intrapleural catheters inserted after the operation is complete provide excellent postoperative analgesia with intermittent or continuous infusion of bupivacaine.[27,28] Regional anesthetic techniques, including local infiltration of the surgical wound and intercostal nerve blocks, may also help. Older children can be safely treated with patient- controlled analgesia (PCA) pumps that allow intravenous infusion of measured doses of analgesics.[29]

The standard operative approach for most pediatric thoracic procedures has traditionally been the posterolateral thoracotomy. This incision divides a portion of the latissimus dorsi muscle and the serratus anterior muscle beneath it. For many years, a rib resection was advocated for the retropleural dissection used in correcting esophageal atresia with tracheoesophageal fistula. Currently, however, an intercostal approach is preferred in an effort to avoid growth disturbances of the chest wall. Chetcuti et al reviewed a series of 302 patients who had survived esophageal atresia repair for four decades.[30] Of patients who underwent a rib resection thoracotomy, 38% developed either anterior chest wall asymmetry, scoliosis, or both. However, 25% of patients who underwent an intercostal thoracotomy without rib resection developed similar skeletal abnormalities. These deformities appeared to be progressive, since their incidence increased with longer follow-up. Their incidence also increased significantly when more than one thoracotomy was necessary. The authors felt that the major factor that produced anterior chest wall asymmetry was partial denervation of the serratus anterior with subsequent atrophy of this muscle, rather than the rib resection itself. The development of scoliosis was more common in patients who had congenital vertebral anomalies, but was thought to be secondary to interference with intercostal muscle function in patients with normal spines. Jaureguizar et al followed 89 patients after correction of esophageal atresia.[31] Of these patients, 24% developed shoulder elevation on the side of the thoracotomy and 20% were found to have chest wall deformities, including asymmetric breast growth in female patients. Denervation of the serratus anterior muscle was also felt to be responsible for these abnormalities. Goodman et al recently reported atrophy of both the serratus anterior and latissimus dorsi muscles in computed tomography (CT) studies

of patients following a posterolateral thoracotomy.[32] Because of these and similar studies, many pediatric surgeons advocate the of use muscle-sparing thoracotomy incisions.[33–35] The incision for these thoracotomies extends posteriorly from the midaxillary line to avoid interference with breast development. The latissimus dorsi muscle can be mobilized and retracted either posteriorly or anteriorly, depending upon the exposure required. With anterior retraction of the latissimus, the chest can be entered through the triangle of auscultation without dividing or mobilizing the serratus muscle. With posterior retraction, the inferior border of the serratus is mobilized and retracted anteriorly to allow entry through the fourth intercostal space (Fig. 56-6). Although there are no long-term follow-up studies of chest wall development in children following these procedures, it is felt that avoiding division and denervation of these muscles minimizes the chest wall and spinal deformities that occur following standard thoracotomy procedures. Ponn et al evaluated 62 adult patients undergoing muscle-sparing thoracotomy 6 months after surgery. In these patients, forced vital capacity was significantly better preserved than in patients undergoing standard muscle-splitting thoracotomies.[36]

THORACOSCOPY

The desire for a minimally invasive and minimally deforming thoracotomy has naturally led pediatric surgeons to explore thoracoscopy for many intrathoracic procedures. In thoracoscopy, the pleural cavity is accessed by instruments placed through trocars that are inserted through the intercostal space. The intercostal muscles are not divided, and the muscles of the chest wall are left undisturbed. Initially proposed in 1976 as a technique for obtaining pulmonary biopsies in immunocompromised children, thoracoscopy has now been applied to a diverse range of thoracic disorders in children.[37] With the development of sophisticated dissecting and retracting instruments, many therapeutic procedures can now be performed in the thoracic cavity through these trocars (Fig. 56-7). The success of thoracoscopy depends on the ability to establish a sufficient pneumothorax that allows visualization of the area of pathology. Very small patients and those with pleural symphysis are thus not good candidates for thoracoscopic procedures. Careful preoperative imaging is essential for planning appropriate patient position and trocar location. Most thoracoscopy procedures are best performed in a full lateral decubitus position, although procedures involving lesions in the anterior or posterior mediastinum may be more easily accomplished by placing the patient in a 45-degree lateral position or an exaggerated lateral position, respectively.

Procedures involving retraction of the lung or extensive dissection within the mediastinum are best performed under general anesthesia using either tracheal or selective mainstem ventilation. Positive-pressure ventilation in patients with tracheal ventilation may inferfere with maintenance of a pneumothorax, reducing the visibility in the operated chest. Whenever possible, these patients should be allowed to breath spontaneously during the procedure. This can usually be accomplished by using regional anesthetic techniques in addition to inhalation agents. Simple procedures, such as pleurodesis or pulmonary biopsy, can be performed under regional anesthesia using an intercostal block with additional intravenous sedation as needed.[38] Selective mainstem intubation has the advantage of allowing com-

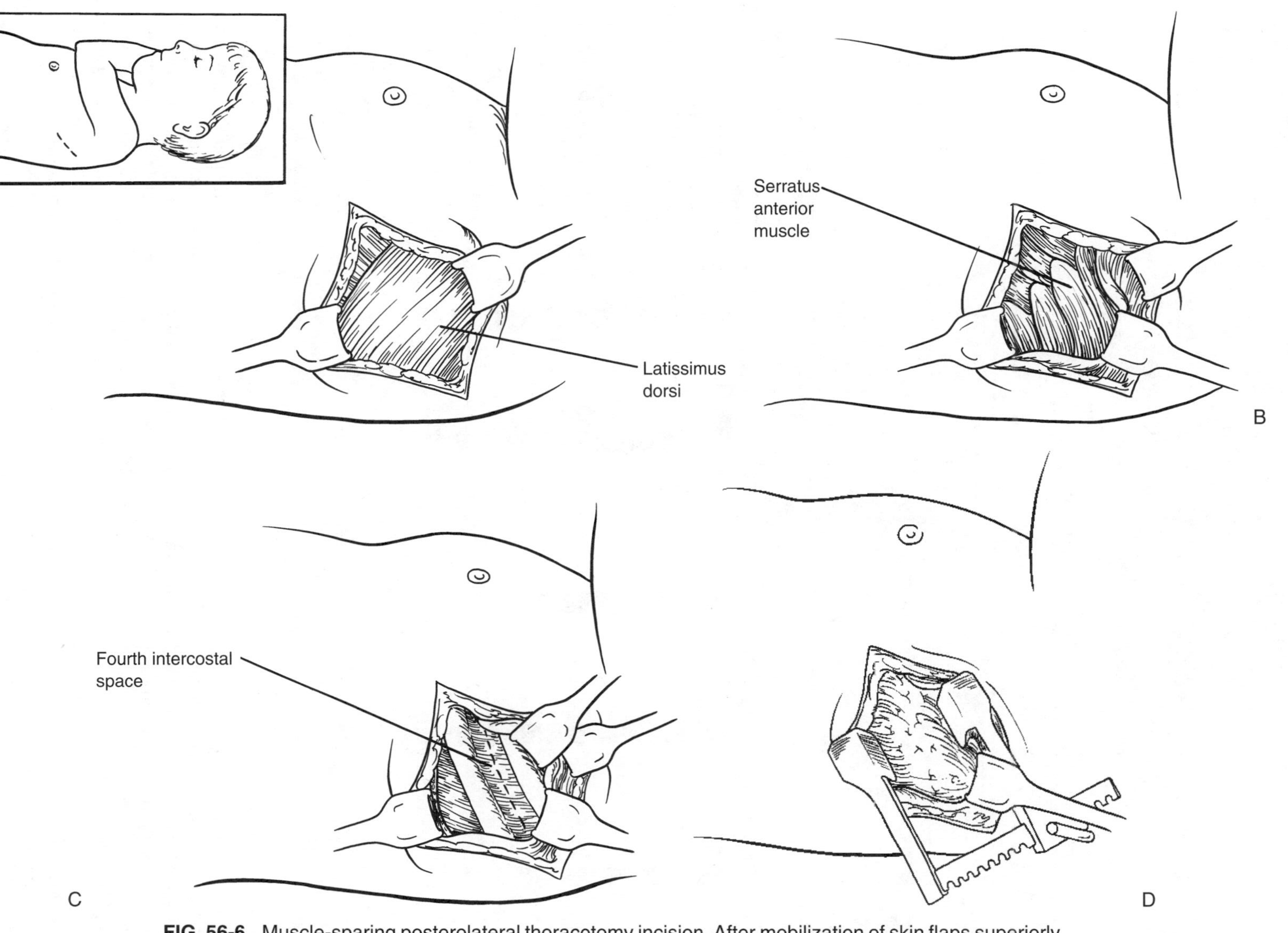

FIG. 56-6. Muscle-sparing posterolateral thoracotomy incision. After mobilization of skin flaps superiorly and inferiorly (*A*), the latissimus dorsi muscle is retracted posteriorly to expose the serratus anterior muscle (*B*). (*C*) The serratus anterior muscle is mobilized superiorly to expose the intercostal space. Entry into the thorax may either be transpleural (*D*) or retropleural.

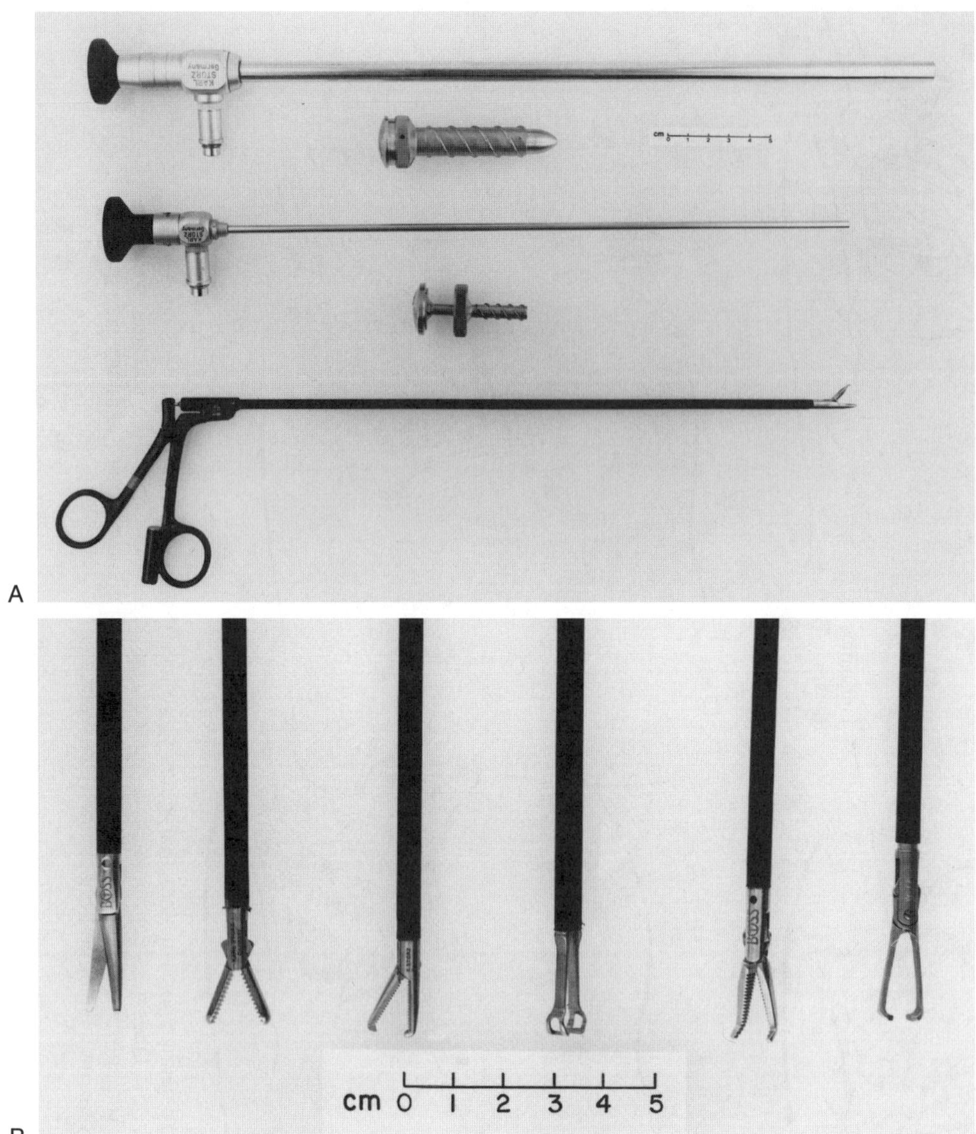

FIG. 56-7. Examples of 10- and 5-mm thoracoscope telescopes and trocars. The trocars are straight, rigid sleeves through which telescopes and instruments can be passed. They contain no valves so that an open pneumothorax can be maintained. The trocars are secured by twisting them into the intercostal space. (*A; top to bottom*) The 10- and 5-mm telescopes are forward viewing (0 degrees); the cup biopsy forceps are useful for simple biopsy. (*B*) The 5-mm instruments include (*left to right*) Metzenbaum scissors, nontoothed and toothed grasping forceps, Babcock clamp, right-angled dissector, and Alyce forceps. These instruments have insulated shafts so they can be used with the electrocautery.

plete collapse of the ipsilateral lung, thus avoiding the need for retraction. After insertion of the initial trocar and telescope, the entire hemithorax is evaluated for areas of unsuspected pathology. Planning is then completed for insertion of the trocars for dissecting and retracting instruments. The lesion is then dissected entirely from its surrounding structures or biopsied. Hemostatis can be achieved either with the insulated electrocautery or by applying metallic clips. A chest tube is inserted through one of the trocar tracts, and the remaining tracts are closed in layers.

In pediatric patients, thoracoscopy is most commonly used for biopsy or excision of mediastinal lesions, for pulmonary biopsy in patients with diffuse or localized interstitial infiltrates, for pleurodesis in treatment of pneumothorax, and for treatment of chylothorax. Thoracoscopy biopsy or excision of mediastinal lesions has been successful in more than 95% of the children reported, and there have been no significant complications when using the technique for this purpose.[39] Preoperative imaging is especially important for these patients to ensure they are appropriately positioned to allow access to the area of pathol-ogy. Cross-sectional scans are particularly helpful to define the relation of the lesion to vital structures in the mediastinum. For simple biopsy of the mediastinal lesions, two trocars are usually sufficient—one for the telescope and one for the biopsy forceps. Additional trocars are necessary if excision of the lesion is anticipated. Retracting and dissecting instruments can be passed through these trocars to allow complete removal of the lesion. Several authors have described complete excision of bronchogenic cysts in children using the thoracoscope.[39–41] Aspiration of the cyst under direct vision these patients facilitates its removal through the trocar tract. The use of thoracoscopy to biopsy mediastinal lymphadenopathy has proved particularly helpful in children. Patients with bulky lesions with some element of tracheal compression can be biopsied under regional anesthesia, reducing the anesthetic hazard of the procedure. In addition to superficial biopsies of these lymph nodes, deeper biopsies can be obtained by direct incision or by core biopsy needles passed through the chest wall under direct vision.

The use of thoracoscopy to provide accurate tissue diagnosis in children with diffuse or localized pulmonary infiltrates has been successful in nearly 100% of the patients reported.[42] These biopsies can be obtained using cup biopsy forceps, although the endoscopic stapling device provides better pneumostasis. This device must be passed through a 12-mm trocar and must be able to be passed at least 5 cm into the chest to open the anvil. It is therefore not applicable in smaller patients, usually those younger than 4 years. Most complications of thoracoscopy in children have occurred in patients undergoing lung biopsy who are immunosuppressed and on mechanical ventilation.[42] Problems in obtaining hemostasis or pneumostasis after these procedures may lead to serious complications, including bleeding and bronchopulmonary fistulas. Many of these children should be biopsied by open techniques that provide better control. Watine et al described complete excision of an extralobar pulmonary sequestration in a young girl.[43]

Thoracoscopic treatment of pneumothorax can be accomplished by various methods, including talc pleurodesis, mechanical pleural abrasion, and pleurectomy. Talc pleurodesis and pleurectomy have been successful in virtually 100% of the patients in whom they have been used.[44] Mechanical pleural abrasion is successful in 90% to 95%.[45] Talc pleurodesis is simple to perform and can be completed under regional anesthesia. With any of these techniques, blebs or cysts can be excised using the endoscopic stapler. Thoracoscopy can be used to treat chylothorax, either by occluding the thoracic duct with metallic clips or by spraying the mediastinum with fibrin glue.[46]

As pediatric surgeons have become more comfortable with the technique of thoracoscopy, they have applied it to many innovative clinical situations. Thoracoscopy has been used to evaluate and to repair traumatic diaphragmatic hernias and to perform a dorsal sympathectomy to treat axillary and palmar hyperhidrosis.[47–49] Laborde et al first described the use of thoracoscopy for interrupting the patent ductus arteriosus in 1993, and their successful results have been duplicated by others.[50,51] Burke et al extended this technique to the thoracoscopic division of a vascular ring.[52] Pellegrini et al performed esophagomyotomy with the thoracoscope to treat esophageal achalasia.[53]

PNEUMOTHORAX

A pneumothorax is an accumulation of air within the pleural space. It may occur spontaneously or as the result of trauma, surgery, or a therapeutic intervention. If the air accumulates under pressure, a tension pneumothorax ensues. A pneumothorax decreases pulmonary volume, compliance, and diffusing capacity. If the pneumothorax is greater than 50% of chest volume, hypoxia may result secondary to ventilation–perfusion mismatch. This can often be compensated for by a normal lung. Children with underlying chronic pulmonary disease may suffer relatively smaller pneumothoraces secondary to diminished elastic recoil of their lungs, but the symptomatic consequences may be more significant because of their small margin of pulmonary reserve.[54,55] Spontaneous pneumothorax may occur in children with no known underlying disease or may result from or, in fact, reveal an underlying condition, such as a congenital bleb, pneumonia with pneumatocele or abscess, tuberculosis, or cystic adenomatoid malformation. Traumatic pneumothorax may result from a tear in the pleura, esophagus, trachea, or bronchi. Iatrogenic causes include mechanical ventilation, thoracentesis or central venous catheter insertion, bronchoscopy, or cardiopulmonary resuscitation.[54,56–58]

The most common presenting symptoms of pneumothorax are ipsilateral chest pain and dyspnea.[54,57] Severe dyspnea should alert the surgeon to the presence of a tension pneumothorax. Physical examination may reveal diminished breath sounds on one side of the chest or a shift of the trachea from the suprasternal notch. A pneumothorax is usually detectable on a chest radiograph and is enhanced if the radiograph is taken at end expiration. It is common practice for the size of a pneumothorax to be described as a proportion of the chest field on an upright radiograph. Of course, the actual volume loss of the lung is greater than such a description since pulmonary volume is lost in three dimensions. The following formula is used to more accurately estimate this loss:

$$\frac{\text{diameter of lung}^3}{\text{diameter of hemithorax}^3} \times 100 = \% \text{ pneumothorax}$$

Other authors have developed a nomogram for this same purpose[59] (Fig. 56-8).

A number of factors determine the proper management of a pneumothorax. These include the initial size, symptomatology, ongoing expansion, presence of tension, and any contributing underlying condition. A spontaneous unilateral pneumothorax that is asymptomatic and less than 15% to 20% of the chest volume can usually be followed by observation alone.[54,58] Pleural air reabsorbs at a rate of 1.25% per day, but this can be hastened by breathing 100% oxygen.[54] Classically, such a pneumothorax occurs in an ectomorphic, adolescent male. If there is no known underlying pathology, the chances are that

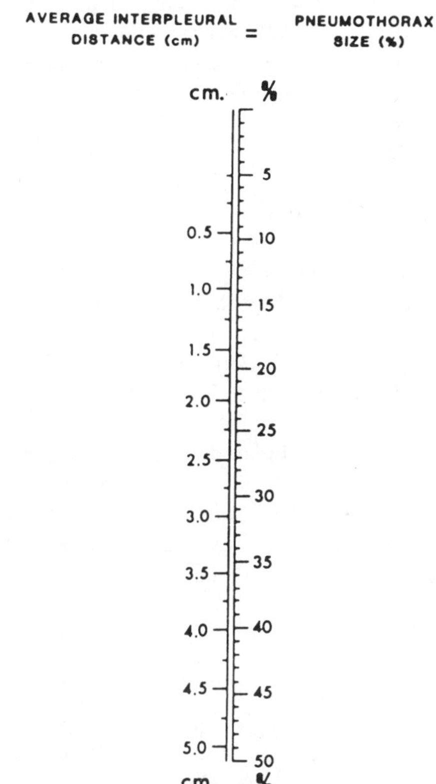

FIG. 56-8. A nomogram for predicting the percentage of involvement with a pneumothorax in larger children and adolescents.

such an episode represents the rupture of a subpleural bleb or cyst, the manifestation of a familial tendency, or perhaps even the presence of undetected tuberculosis.[60] Pneumothorax recurs with a frequency of 50% after the first episode, 62% after the second, and 83% after the third.[54,61]

Symptomatic or large pneumothoraces usually require intervention. Thoracentesis can be attempted in a relatively small pneumothorax, but if air is continuously aspirated or if the pneumothorax recurs, a chest tube must be inserted. A tension pneumothorax poses a surgical emergency, and a chest tube should be placed immediately. If a tube is not immediately available or if the patient's condition deteriorates during preparation for placement, a large-bore (14-gauge) needle should be placed in the second intercostal space anteriorly to relieve the tension. If the pneumothorax recurs after tube thoracostomy, or if the air leak persists, further intervention is necessary. The choice of intervention is determined by the cause of the condition. In a posttraumatic pneumothorax, large or persistent air leaks may indicate damage to the airway or the esophagus. Appropriate diagnostic studies using esophagograms, bronchoscopy, esophagoscopy, thoracoscopy, or thoracotomy should be undertaken and direct repair of the injury performed. In a nontraumatic pneumothorax, the persistence of an air leak may accompany a chronic underlying condition, such as cystic fibrosis, bronchopulmonary dysplasia, lung cysts, or blebs. Treatment of these patients usually requires resection of the local pathology or pleurodesis.

Pleurodesis can be undertaken by instilling chemical agents into the pleural space through a chest tube, by thoracoscopy, or by thoracotomy. In the past, agents such as silver nitrate, quinacrine, iodized oil, and hypertonic glucose have been used, but currently, talc or tetracycline derivatives, such as doxycycline, or fibrin sealant are more commonly used.[44,62–65] Talc is less painful and more uniformly successful than doxycycline. Treatment with talc has been shown to be particularly effective in treating pneumothoraces in children with cystic fibrosis.[44]

Traditionally, thoracotomy has been used for more aggressive interventions such as mechanical pleurodesis, pleurectomy, or resection of lung blebs or cysts; however, thoracoscopy is emerging as the preferred technique for all of these interventions.[66,67] It allows excellent visualization of the entire pleural space with a low surgical morbidity. It also allows use of a wider range of anesthetic techniques since older children can often undergo thoracoscopic pleurodesis under sedation with intercostal nerve block. Pleurodesis can be accomplished by thoracoscopy using either a talc spray, mechanical pleural abrasion, or pleurectomy.[68] The results of thoracoscopic pleurodesis for pneumothorax have been excellent, and complications of the technique are very uncommon.[66,67,69]

CHYLOTHORAX

Chylothorax is an accumulation of lymphatic fluid in the pleural space. The main causes of chylothorax in children are idiopathic chylothorax of infancy, injury to lymphatic channels as a result of an operative procedure or trauma, malignancy, and miscellaneous diseases. Idiopathic chylothorax presents in infancy and is thought to be secondary to congenital defects of the thoracic lymphatics or to birth trauma; however, congenital pulmonary lymphangiectasis or lymphangiomatosis may be more frequent causes than appreciated. The most common traumatic chylothorax is due to operative injury, usually following cardiac surgical procedures. The incidence of chylothorax following thoracic surgery in children ranges from 0.25% to 0.9%.[70] Traumatic injury to the thoracic duct has been reported secondary to either blunt or penetrating thoracic trauma. Chylothorax secondary to malignancy is seen in older children and is usually due to obstruction of the thoracic duct by lymphoma. The occurrence of chylothorax with neuroblastoma has also been reported.[71] If an older child presents with chylothorax but has no history of trauma or operation, an intrathoracic tumor should be suspected and investigated with chest CT or magnetic resonance imaging (MRI). Miscellaneous diseases causing chylothorax may include benign tumors, lymphangiomatosis, or superior vena cava thrombosis.

Chylothorax usually presents with significant respiratory insufficiency, although it may present as the incidental finding of a pleural effusion on an imaging study of the chest. Prenatal ultrasound may detect chylothorax in the fetus. The diagnosis of chylothorax is confirmed by evaluating the pleural fluid. Chyle is usually milky in color, but may be serosanguinous or straw colored in children who are receiving no enteral fats, such as those who have just undergone surgery. Chyle generally contains a total fat content of more than 400 mg/dL, triglycerides of more than 220 mg/dL, a protein content that is half that of plasma, and a specific gravity greater than 1.012. On Gram stain of the fluid, more than 90% of the cells seen are lymphocytes, and Sudan red stain may demonstrate chylomicrons.[72,73]

Treatment of chylothorax has traditionally been nonoperative, with 70% to 80% of patients responding.[72,74] Lymphatic flow through the thoracic duct can be diminished by feeding the patient a diet that principally contains medium-chain triglycerides. These fats are absorbed directly into the portal venous system unlike long-chain fatty acids which are absorbed through the intestinal lymphatics. If chyle drainage persists, the patient can be placed on total parental nutrition with no oral intake. The pleural space is drained by thoracentesis or tube thoracostomy. Loss of significant volumes of chyle from the pleural space represents a considerable loss of protein and lymphocytes to these children. These losses must be monitored closely and

FIG. 56-9. Placement of a subcutaneous pleuroperitoneal shunt. (*A* and *B*) The thoracic end of the shunt is placed at an angle through the intercostal space in a dependent position. (*C*) The pumping chamber is drawn into a subcutaneous pocket from a counterincision in the abdomen. (*D*) Free flow of chyle through the system is confirmed by compressing the pump chamber. (*E*) The peritoneal catheter is placed through a pursestring in the posterior rectus fascia. (After Murphy MC, Newman BM, Rodgers BM. Pleural peritoneal shunts in the management of persistent chylothorax. Ann Thorac Surg 1989; 48:1995)

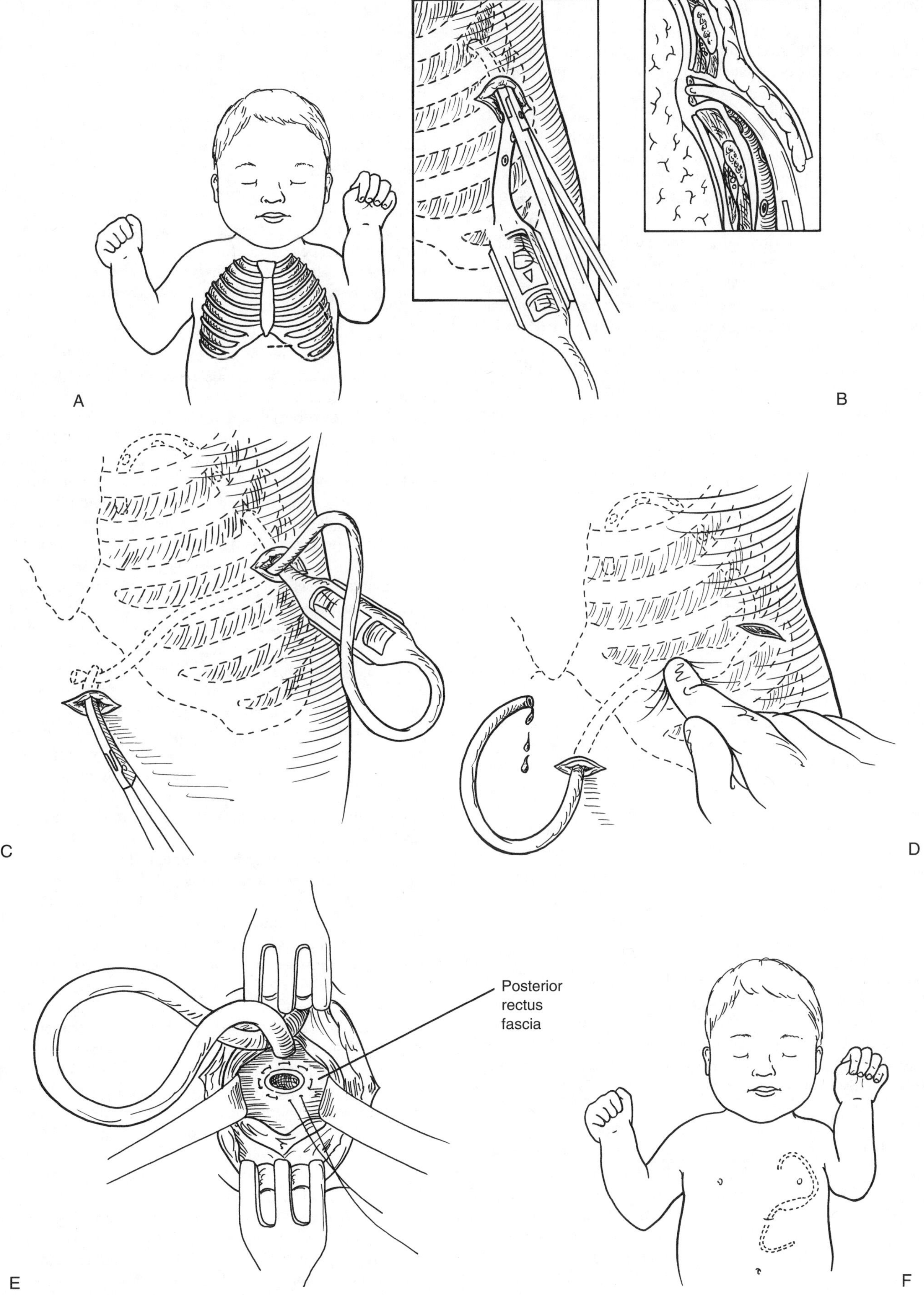

Posterior
rectus
fascia
A
B
C
D
E
F

replaced to avoid severe nutritional deficits. If nonoperative treatment fails to eliminate the lymphatic drainage, surgical therapy can be attempted to obliterate the thoracic duct or area of leakage or to create a pleurodesis.[75] These objectives can be accomplished either by thoracotomy or by thoracoscopy.[46,74] Covering the area of leakage with fibrin glue has been effective in eliminating chyle drainage. Recent reports have described the use of a pleuroperitoneal shunt to treat chylothorax. This shunt can be placed completely subcutaneously or the pumping chamber can be exteriorized to facilitate its compression (Fig. 56-9). These shunts are simple to place and are highly effective, eliminating drainage in 85% to 95% of these patients.[47,76] The timing of surgical intervention has been a matter of some debate. An early report by Randolph and Gross recommended surgical intervention if the chylothorax does not respond to nonoperative treatment by 21 days.[77] However, recent reports recommend intervention at as early as 5 to 7 days, particularly if less invasive procedures such as thoracoscopy or a pleuroperitoneal shunt are to be used.[46,76] This is especially true if the child has elevated right-heart pressures or central venous thrombosis. Such children are unlikely to respond to nonoperative treatment.[72,76] Ultimately, the results of treatment, either nonoperative or operative, are excellent.

EMPYEMA

Empyema refers to the accumulation of infected fluid in the pleural space. In children, this is usually the result of severe pneumonia[78]; however, empyema may also result from infection of the retropharyngeal, mediastinal, or paravertebral spaces.[79] Thoracic trauma or an immunocompromised state may also lead to empyema,[78] and children who are immunocompromised are more susceptible to it. Empyema may develop in a loculated hemothorax occurring subsequent to trauma. In 1962, the American Thoracic Society described what is now the three classic stages of empyema.[80] The first stage, or the *exudative stage*, is characterized by an accumulation of thin pleural fluid with few cells. The pleura and lung are mobile, and this fluid is amenable to drainage by thoracentesis. This stage may last only 24 to 72 hours. The second stage is the *fibrinopurulent stage*. Consolidation of infected pleural fluid results in an accumulation of fibrinous material, formation of loculations, and loss of lung mobility. This stage lasts 7 to 10 days. The third stage is the *organizing stage*. A pleural peel forms secondary to fibroblast proliferation and resorption of fibrin. The lung becomes entrapped, and capillary proliferation extends from the fibrinous peel into the visceral pleura itself. This usually occurs 2 to 4 weeks after the initial development of the empyema.

Before the widespread use of antibiotics, empyema was caused principally by infections of *Streptococcus pneumoniae*, *Streptococcus pyogenes*, *Staphylococcus aureus*, and *Hemophilus influenzae*. The introduction of sulfapyridine and penicillin decreased the overall incidence of empyema, but *S aureus* emerged as the primary offending pathogen. In the past 20 years, effective therapy for *S aureus* has allowed the emergence of a variety of bacterial organisms, including anaerobic bacteria, as causes of empyema in children[81]:

MORE COMMON
- *Streptococcus pneumoniae*
- *Staphylococcus aureus*
- *Hemophilis influenzae*

LESS COMMON
- Bacteroides species
- Other streptococcal species
- *Pseudomonas aeruginosa*

Contemporary series report a preponderance of *H influenza* and streptococcal species in children.[82–85] However, some series still report *S aureus* as the most common pathogen.[81,86,87] Interestingly, two of these latter series are from developing countries.[86,87]

Children with empyema generally present with fever, cough, respiratory insufficiency, and chest pain.[81,86,88] Physical signs may include dullness on chest percussion, tactile and vocal fremitus, decreased breath sounds, rales, and a pleural friction rub.[81,88] A chest radiograph reveals a thickened pleura in addition to the primary pneumonic process and pleural fluid. Transthoracic ultrasound may further delineate the pleural fluid collection; however, CT scan is the most accurate method of assessing the degree of pleural thickening, fluid loculation, and lung consolidation.[82–84] The diagnosis of empyema is confirmed by thoracentesis. The fluid is characteristically turbid and may be thick during the later stages of the infection. Laboratory analysis reveals a specific gravity greater than 1.016, protein greater than 3 g/dL, LDH greater than 200 U/L, pleural fluid protein/serum protein ratio greater than 0.5, pleural fluid LDH/serum LDH ratio greater than 0.6, and white blood cell count higher than 15,000/mm^3. Fibrin clots may also be present.[88] Once the diagnosis of empyema is made, appropriate antibiotics should be administered based on Gram stain and culture of the pleural fluid or sputum. Complete drainage of the empyema should be accomplished either by thoracentesis or tube thoracostomy.[89] Some children present with such advanced disease that the pleural involvement has passed the exudative stage. In these patients, thoracentesis or even tube drainage may not be adequate to obtain a clinical response. In general, the longer the prehospital or pretreatment illness has persisted, the more likely further interventions will be needed.[90]

A suboptimal clinical response of the patient to antibiotics and drainage determines the need for additional intervention. Most patients are free of fever and residual pleural fluid within 3 to 5 days following institution of therapy. Persistence of fever or loculation of the pleural fluid requires the surgeon to consider further intervention.[82,83,89,90] The nature and timing of this intervention has remained a subject of debate. The primary surgical objective must be to remove all of the residual infected pleural fluid, to break up any loculations, and to free the lung to expand and to fill the pleural space. Many pediatric surgical series have discussed decortication for this objective, either through a formal thoracotomy or a mini-thoracotomy. Properly used, the term *decortication* refers to the removal of a thick, fibrotic visceral peel that is restricting the underlying lung.[91] In fact, the procedure actually described in most series is better termed *pleural debridement* since fluid and fibrinous peel from the visceral and parietal pleural surfaces are removed to extract truly infected material. This can be accomplished without the trauma and blood loss usually associated with true decortication procedures, and pleural debridement should be considered ear-

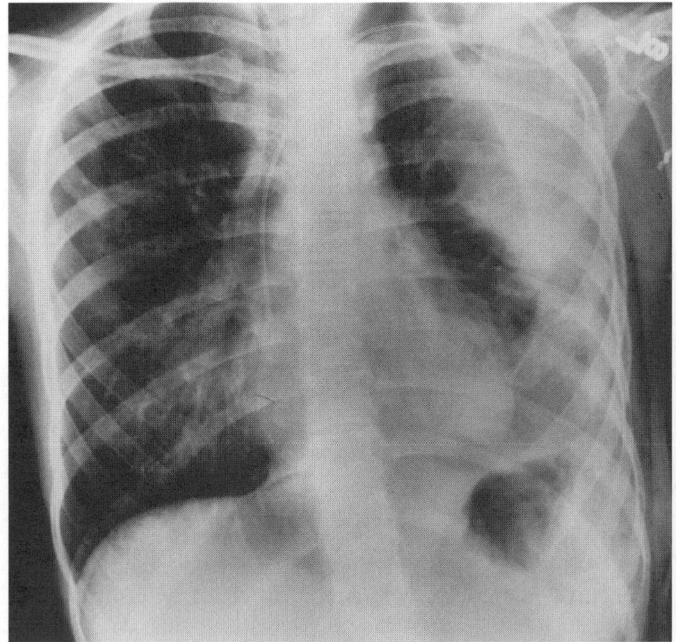
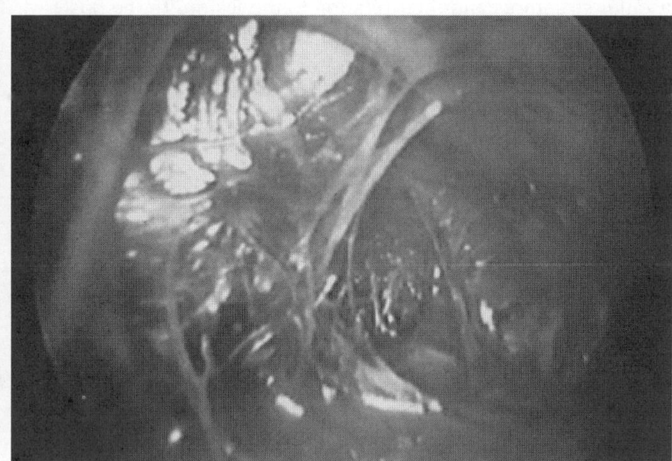

FIG. 56-10. (*A*) Frontal chest radiograph of a 15 year-old boy who developed a posttraumatic empyema in the left hemithorax. A culture of chest tube drainage grew *Staphylococcus aureus*. (*B*) At the time of thoracoscopic pleural debridement, there were multiple thin pleural adhesions, which were completely lysed with blunt and sharp dissection. A single chest tube was left in place and removed 3 days later.

lier in the course of the empyema. Pleural loculations in some patients can be lysed by instilling urokinase or streptokinase through existing chest tubes before resorting to surgical intervention. The pleural space can be debrided by thoracoscopy, mini-thoracotomy with or without partial rib resection, or full thoracotomy.[82,83,89,92] Kern et al have described excellent clinical response using thoracoscopic pleural debridement in 12 children with refractory empyema.[92] Generally, prompt clinical recovery was the rule. Although controversial, some believe that this procedure is indicated if there is not complete clinical response after 5 to 7 days of antibiotic therapy (Fig. 56-10). In the event that a lung abscess develops, treatment may require pneumonostomy, wedge resection, or lobar resection.[93,94] Radiographic findings often lag behind clinical response; therefore, they should not be used alone as indications for further intervention. With prompt and adequate treatment, the overall outcome for children with empyema is excellent. Pulmonary function after recovery is usually clinically normal, although some investigators have found mild restrictive or obstructive disease on follow-up spirometry.[85,86,95]

MEDIASTINAL MASSES

The mediastinum is the most common location of intrathoracic masses in children. The large number of structures within the mediastinum creates a vast array of potential diagnoses. Dividing the mediastinum into arbitrary anatomic compartments has significantly helped to limit the differential diagnoses and to plan diagnostic studies. Although several schema have been proposed, this section discusses one that divides the mediastinum into four compartments: superior, anterior, middle, and posterior as delineated on the lateral chest radiograph (see Fig. 56-2).

The superior mediastinal compartment contains the great vessels and most of the thymus gland. Tumors of the thymus, such as thymomas or germ-cell tumors, may present in this compartment. Lymphangiomas are usually found in the superior mediastinum. The anterior mediastinum contains the lower portion of the thymus and scattered lymphatic tissue. In addition to thymic tumors, lymphomas may develop in this compartment. Bronchogenic cysts in the hilum occur within the middle mediastinum. The posterior mediastinum contains the esophagus, the descending aorta, and the sympathetic nerves and ganglia. The posterior compartment is the site of most neurogenic tumors, such as neuroblastomas and ganglioneuromas. Esophageal cysts also present within this compartment. Most mediastinal masses in children are found in the posterior compartment.

Most mediastinal masses in children are confined to a single compartment, although large masses may extend into adjacent compartments. Certain lesions, such as mediastinal lymphangiomas and hemangiomas, may primarily involve more than one compartment. Most mediastinal masses discovered in children younger than 6 years are benign, whereas masses diagnosed in older children are more likely to be malignant tumors. Almost half of the children with mediastinal masses are asymptomatic at the time of diagnosis.[96] Those with symptoms may present either with respiratory symptoms or chest pain.

The principles of the diagnostic evaluation of a mediastinal mass in a child are to determine its primary location, to define its morphology, and to delineate its involvement of surrounding structures.[97] Conventional chest radiographs are the primary radiologic examination and guide subsequent imaging. The presence and character of calcification noted on this study may help to establish the diagnosis. Cross-sectional imaging is used to further define the location and extent of the mass. CT studies are most commonly used for lesions in the anterior and middle compartments. MRI may have significant advantages in evaluating lesions in the superior and posterior mediastinal compartments. In the superior mediastinum, the MRI can delineate the vascular structures and their relation to the lesion. In the posterior compartment, the MRI allows determination of intraspinal involvement of neurogenic tumors.[98] The MRI in both areas has the distinct advantage of allowing multiplanar imaging.[99] Transthoracic ultrasound may be helpful in differentiating between loculated pleural fluid and pleural masses as well as in differentiating cystic from solid lesions in the anterior or posterior compartments.[100]

GERM-CELL TUMORS

The mediastinum is the most common location for extragonadal germ-cell tumors, including teratomas, dysgerminomas, choriocarcinomas, endodermal sinus tumors, and dermoid cysts. Most of these lesions arise in the superior or anterior mediastinal compartments. These tumors are thought to arise from germ cells that have stopped migrating during embryogenesis and have persisted within the region of the thymus.[101] Teratomas comprise 80% of primary germ-cell tumors found in the mediastinum.

The mediastinum is the second most common location for teratomas in children, next to the sacrococcygeal area. Mediastinal teratomas comprise approximately 10% to 20% of mediastinal tumors and approximately 10% of all teratomas.[102,103] Most are located in the anterior or superior mediastinum, although they may occur within the pericardium or the posterior mediastinum.[102–104] The rate of malignancy of these lesions varies from 10 to 25%.[102–104] Males and females are equally affected. Characteristically, mediastinal teratomas are primarily, although not always entirely, cystic and are derived from more than one germinal layer. Ectodermal components predominate, and calcifications may be present.[102,104]

Mediastinal teratomas may present in various ways. They may be detected on prenatal ultrasound and be associated with fetal hydrops and polyhydramnios.[105] The most common presenting symptom is respiratory insufficiency secondary to airway compression, compression of the pulmonary parenchyma, or intrapleural rupture of the teratoma.[106,107] Interestingly, only a minority of mediastinal teratomas present with respiratory symptoms in the newborn period.[108] Most of these tumors do not present until adolescence. Tissue within the teratoma may be functioning in a physiologic manner causing symptoms related to the particular hormone or enzyme secreted.[109,110] Some teratomas may become infected, resulting in a febrile presentation.[111] There have been reports of intrapericardial teratomas presenting with cardiac tamponade.[112] Teratomas may also present as incidental findings on chest imaging studies.[108] Once suspected, imaging of a mediastinal teratoma is best accomplished by CT or MRI. CT is particularly useful for evaluating these lesions, since it allows for the identification of fat and calcifications.[99] If a teratoma is intrapericardial or within the posterior mediastinum, angiography may be helpful to define the vascular anatomy. Laboratory evaluation should include measurement of serum alpha-fetoprotein, carcinoembryonic antigen, and human chorionic gonadotrophin to assist in patient follow-up if the lesion appears malignant.

Treatment of mediastinal teratomas is surgical excision either by thoracotomy or sternotomy. Usually, the lesions are well encapsulated with minimal vascularity, although pericardial and posterior mediastinal tumors may have significant vascular supply from the aorta. Malignant teratomas often envelope adjacent structures. The outcome for these malignant tumors is poor despite adjunctive chemotherapy and radiation therapy.[102,103] Malignancy may be difficult to determine histologically at initial resection, and occasionally, patients present with malignant recurrence after removal of a teratoma initially thought to be benign[103]; therefore, long-term follow-up is required for all children after removal of a mediastinal teratoma.

THYMOMA

Thymomas are the most common neoplasms of the anterior mediastinum in adults, but they are rare in children.[113–115] Although thymomas are commonly associated with myasthenia gravis in adults, only a single patient less than 19 years of age has been reported with both a thymoma and myasthenia gravis.[113] Thymomas represent neoplasms of epithelial or lymphocytic origin.[115] Malignant potential is determined by the presence and extent of microscopic or macroscopic invasion beyond the capsule of the gland.[114] Malignant thymomas are histologically similar to lymphoblastic lymphoma and must be differentiated from that disease.[104,113] The treatment of these lesions is complete surgical excision. Radiation therapy and chemotherapy may be required for advanced stages of malignancy or partially resected or unresectable disease.[115,116]

THYMIC CYSTS

Thymic cysts are uncommon lesions that may present as either mediastinal or neck masses in children.[55,104,117,118] Mediastinal thymic cysts are generally asymptomatic and are found incidentally. Their origin has been a subject of debate, with some authors arguing that they are congenital in nature, while others suggest they are secondary to inflammation.[117,118] Regardless, they are uniformly benign in children.[118] Thymic cysts are lined by ciliated epithelium with components of lymphocytes, thymic tissue, cholesterol crystals, and Hassall corpuscles within the wall.[118] When a thymic cyst is suspected, transthoracic ultrasound, CT scan, or fine-needle aspiration may help confirm the diagnosis. Thymic cysts rarely involve adjacent structures and are generally easily resected. Successful resection of a thymic cyst by thoracoscopy has recently been described.[119]

BRONCHOGENIC CYSTS

Bronchogenic cysts are part of a spectrum of anomalies that arise from abnormalities of ventral foregut budding. Gerle proposed the term *bronchopulmonary–foregut malformations* to encompass the anomalies of bronchogenic cysts, pulmonary sequestrations, and abnormalities of tracheal budding.[120] Most bronchogenic cysts are located in the middle mediastinum close to the trachea or mainstem bronchi. They may also be located more peripherally within the lung parenchyma itself.[121] These are discussed in Chapter 57. Mediastinal cysts are typically lined with ciliated columnar epithelium and contain thick mucous. The walls of the cysts are usually thin and may contain hyaline cartilage, scattered smooth muscle, mucous glands, and nerve fibers. The walls never contain the well-developed muscle layers and nerve plexuses characteristic of enteric cysts. Bronchogenic cysts rarely communicate with the airway, but they may densely adhere to it. The cysts may, however, communicate with the gastrointestinal tract, usually below the diaphragm.[120] There may be associated vertebral anomalies.[122] Bronchogenic cysts often cause symptoms ranging from stridor to frank respiratory distress. This is particularly true for cysts in infants and for cysts located near the carina.[122] These cysts, however, are often discovered as incidental findings on chest radiographs. If the cyst itself is not always evident, associated findings of compression of the trachea or bronchi or atelectasis may lead to the diagnosis. If a bronchogenic cyst is suspected, a contrast-enhanced CT scan of the chest should be obtained to confirm the diagnosis and to delineate the regional anatomy. MRI may be equally as helpful in this regard but avoid the risks of radiation.[123]

Once detected, bronchogenic cysts should be excised. This is usually accomplished by thoracotomy. Recent reports have demonstrated that these cysts can be completely excised using thoracoscopic techniques, and this is the preferred technique for centrally located lesions.[39–41] Peripheral bronchogenic cysts can be excised by thoracoscopy if they are not completely encompassed by the pulmonary parenchyma. Cysts which are asymptomatic at the time of diagnosis should still be removed because they are prone to causing airway obstruction, infection, and although rarely, even cancer with the passage of time.[121,123,124] If the cyst cannot be completely excised, the epithelium should be fulgurated. These children must be monitored for recurrence.[125]

LYMPHOMA

Lymphoma, both Hodgkin and nonHodgkin, is the most common cause of anterior and middle mediastinal masses in children.[126] Hodgkin disease tends to have a predisposition to the cervical or mediastinal regions and may present as local or disseminated disease. NonHodgkin lymphomas are assumed to be disseminated when first discovered.[126] Most nonHodgkin tumors found in the mediastinum are of a lymphoblastic T-cell origin.[126]

A mediastinal lymphoma may present as an incidental finding on a chest radiograph or by causing respiratory distress or superior vena cava syndrome.[126,127] NonHodgkin lymphomas grow quickly and tend to be more severe in their respiratory manifestations, with 50% to 70% having associated pleural effusions.[126,128] A chest CT scan determines the size and location of the tumor and the degree of airway compression.[129,130] Hodgkin lymphoma may present with fever or systemic symptoms.

The diagnosis of lymphoma is established by tissue biopsy. In some instances, a lymph node can be biopsied, a chest effusion can be sampled, or a bone marrow aspirate can be obtained for diagnosis.[131] However, when the mediastinal mass represents the only available tissue or when symptomatology does

not allow delay in diagnosis, direct biopsy of the mediastinal mass is necessary.[132,133] Fine-needle aspirates are unsuccessful in obtaining diagnostic material up to 50% of the time.[134] Therefore, more aggressive procedures are usually needed. These include core-needle biopsies, thoracoscopic biopsy, or anterior thoracotomy.[128,135] Local anesthesia can be used for needle aspirations or for biopsies requiring limited incisions.

If general anesthesia is needed, it is best induced in a partial or total upright position with the patient breathing spontaneously. Airway collapse may ensue if muscle relaxants are used. In cases where complete anesthesia and relaxation are required, however, a rigid bronchoscope should be available to access and to support the lower airway should difficulties arise.[132] It is difficult to know ahead of time which patient will not tolerate anesthesia. Traditionally, it has been believed that the more significant the respiratory symptoms, the greater the risk of anesthesia. Shamberger et al attempted to quantify this risk by measuring the cross-sectional area of the compressed trachea by CT. A tracheal cross-sectional area that is larger than 50% of expected suggests an uneventful anesthesia according to this study[130] (Fig. 56-11).

If respiratory symptoms truly prohibit manipulation of the patient, mediastinal radiation, perhaps supplemented by steroids, can rapidly shrink the tumor and relieve symptoms. However, this may also destroy any hope of obtaining reliable tissue to provide a precise diagnosis of the type of lymphoma.[130,132,133,136] Therefore, the surgeon should try to obtain tissue before treatment if possible.

MEDIASTINAL LYMPH NODES

Mediastinal lymph nodes may become enlarged as part of several nonmalignant conditions. These include sarcoidosis, Castleman's disease, histoplasmosis, coccidiomycosis, tuberculosis, and rarely, bacterial and viral infections.[137,138] Lymph node enlargement may result in respiratory symptomatology, dysphagia, or superior vena cava syndrome. A chest CT scan may be required to delineate the extent of mediastinal nodal pathology. Evaluation of these patients may ultimately require nodal biopsy if other diagnostic tests are inconclusive. Modalities commonly used for tissue sampling include needle biopsy, thoracoscopy, or thoracotomy.

PERICARDIAL CYSTS

Pericardial cysts result when the mesodermal lacunae fail to coalesce in the developing pericardium.[117] These cysts are typically thin-walled, contain a flat mesothelial lining, and are generally found at the cardiophrenic angle in the middle mediastinum.[55] These patients are usually asymptomatic, and the cysts present as incidental findings on chest images. They are uniformly benign.[55,118] Ultrasound and CT scan usually confirm the diagnosis. Surgical excision is uncomplicated, and some pericardial cysts have been removed by thoracoscopy.[119,139] Because of the benign and asymptomatic nature of these cysts, some authors feel that observation may be justified.[117]

LYMPHANGIOMA

Lymphangiomas are congenital lesions that contain abnormal proliferation of lymphatic and vascular tissue. They can be com-

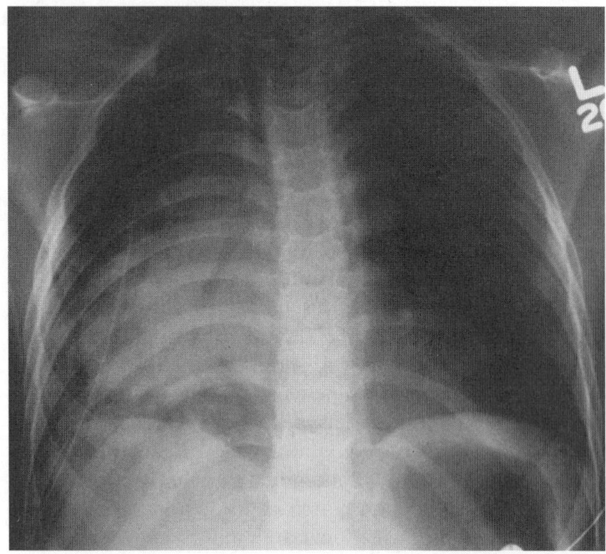
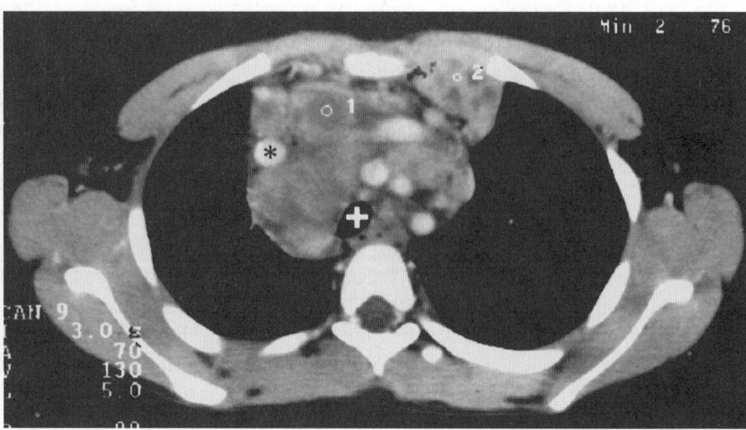

FIG. 56-11. (*A*) Frontal chest radiograph of a 14-year-old girl with respiratory symptoms secondary to a large anterior mediastinal mass. (*B*) Chest CT scan demonstrates a bulky mediastinal lesion displaying the trachea (*plus sign*) posteriorly and to the right and compressing the tracheal lumen approximately 50%. The superior vena cava (*asterisk*) is displaced laterally. A percutaneous needle biopsy was nondiagnostic. Biopsy obtained by thoracosocpy under local anesthesia confirmed nodular sclerosing Hodgkin disease.

prised principally of large lymphatic cysts, and thus bear the name *cystic hygroma*, or they can consist of denser tissue with more prominent vascular elements and be termed *lymphangiomas*. Lymphangiomatous tissue consists of vessels with a thin endothelial lining and some smooth muscle.[140] There are several theories regarding the formation of lymphangiomas, but the most commonly accepted one suggests that lymphangiomas represent the failure in part of the embryonic lymph sacs to establish adequate drainage into the venous system.[104,140]

Lymphangiomas occur in 1 in 6000 births. Isolated mediastinal lymphangiomas represent only about 1% of these cases.[141–143] Large cervical lymphangiomas, however, may extend into the mediastinum in 2% to 10% of cases.[55,104,140] Isolated mediastinal lymphangiomas are usually found in the anterior mediastinum, although they can be found in other compartments of the mediastinum as well.[104] Cervical lymphangiomas often extend into the posterior mediastinum. Lymphangiomas of the neck and axilla usually present by 2 years of age and are readily apparent on physical examination; however, mediastinal lymphangiomas often are incidental findings on chest imaging or first come to the physician's attention with the onset of respiratory symptoms. Prenatal ultrasound may detect a mediastinal lymphangioma.[143]

The presenting symptoms of mediastinal lymphangiomas are the result of their impingement upon the airway, lungs, or other mediastinal structures. Infection or collections of chyle in the pleura or pericardium may occur. Hemorrhage into a lymphangioma with rapid enlargement and sudden onset of symptoms has been described.[142–145] Mediastinal lymphangiomas appear as homogeneous masses on chest radiograph. Ultrasonography reveals their primarily cystic nature, sometimes containing debris. CT reveals the cystic nature of the lesion as well as the extent of its involvement with other mediastinal structures. Calcifications are usually not present unless there is a significant vascular component.[142,144]

There have been reports of spontaneous regression of lymphangiomas, but these are sporadic and not part of the natural course of this lesion. The optimal therapy of mediastinal lymphangiomas is total excision by thoracotomy or sternotomy, but it is widely agreed that vital structures should not be sacrificed during attempts at total excision.[55,104,140,141] Because tissue must often be left behind and because some lesions are simply not resectable due to their extensive involvement of vital structures, alternative strategies for therapy have been advanced.[141] Recent reports suggest intralesional bleomycin or OK-432 injection as primary therapy.[146,147] Bleomycin, in particular, has been successful in shrinking some large lymphangiomas to resectable size.[147] Injections of glucose, iodine, and tetracycline, or dexamethasone have been used for sclerosis of residual tissue after resection with varying results.[141,145] Irradiation of these lesions is discouraged.[140]

The most common postoperative complication after resection of a lymphangioma is development of lymph accumulation. Repeated aspiration of the fluid often resolves this difficulty. Fibrin glue or chemical sclerosis with doxycycline may be helpful if aspiration fails.[140] In some cases, resection of all or part of the residual tissue may be necessary. Lymphangiomas recur in at least 10% to 15% of cases if resection has not been complete; therefore, close long-term follow-up of these children is necessary.

NEUROFIBROMA

Mediastinal neurofibromas may occur as isolated tumors or may be manifestations of von Recklinghausen's disease. They often have a dumbbell shape and may extend from or along spinal nerve roots, intercostal nerves, the sympathetic chain, or the vagus nerve. Neurofibromas are often detected incidentally on chest radiographs. The presence of scoliosis, widened intervertebral foramina, or disruption of the costovertebral angle may suggest the diagnosis. A chest MRI scan can delineate the extent of the tumor and can detect any extension of the tumor into the spinal canal.[148] Large tumors are known to undergo malignant change. Excision is recommended, although it may not be possible to completely resect portions extending deep within vertebral foramina or costovertebral junctions. Thoracic laminectomy may be required to completely excise some of these tumors. Occasionally, total excision may not be possible and subsequent attempts at resection may be required.[148]

REFERENCES

1. Wells LJ. Development of the human diaphragm and pleural sacs. Embryology 1954;35:107.
2. Bremer JL. The diaphragm and diaphragmatic hernia. Arch Pathol 1943;36:539.
3. Chen JM. Studies of the morphogenesis of the mouse sternum. J Anat 1952;86:373.
4. Wells LJ, Boyden EA. The development of the bronchopulmonary segments in human embryos of horizons XIVV to XIX. Am J Anat 1954;95:163.
5. Davis HK. A statistical study of the thoracic duct in man. Am J Anat 1915;17:211.
6. Weller GL. Development of the thyroid, parathyroid and thymus glands in man. Embryology 1933;24:93.
7. Adams FH, Lind J. Physiologic studies on the cardio-vascular status of the normal newborn infant (with special reference to the ductus arteriosus). Am J Dis Child 1957;93:13.
8. Joger VV, Wollerman OJ. An anatomical study of the closure of the ductus arteriosus. Am J Pathol 1942;18:595.
9. Dunnill MS. Postnatal growth of the lung. Thorax 1962;17:329.
10. Davis RD, Oldham HN, Sabiston DC. The mediastinum. In: Sabiston DC, Spencer FC, eds. Surgery of the chest, ed 5. Philadelphia, WB Saunders, 1990:444.
11. Agostoni E, D'Angelo E. Pleural liquid pressure. J Appl Physiol 1991;71:393.
12. Wang PM, Lai-Fook SJ. Upward flow of pleural liquid near lobar margins due to cardiogenic motion. J Appl Physiol 1992;73:2314.
13. Wiener-Kronish JP, Broaddus VC. Interrelationships of pleural and pulmonary interstitial liquid. Annu Rev Physiol 1993;55:209.
14. West JB. Mechanics of breathing. In: West JB, ed. Respiratory physiology: the essentials, ed 4. Baltimore, Williams & Wilkins, 1990:87.
15. West JB. Ventilation. In: West JB, ed. Respiratory physiology: the essentials, ed 4. Baltimore, Williams & Wilkins, 1990:11.
16. Hubmayr RD, Margulies SS. Effects of unilateral hyperinflation on the interpulmonary distribution of pleural pressure. J Appl Physiol 1992;73:1650.
17. Lai-Fook SJ, Rodarte JR. Pleural pressure distribution and its relationship to lung volume and interstitial pressure. J Appl Physiol 1991;70:967.
18. Mutoh T, Guest RJ, Lamm WJE, et al. Prone position alters the effect of volume overload on regional pleural pressures and improves hypoxemia in pigs in vivo. Am Rev Respir Dis 1992;146:300.
19. Gross I. Respiratory diseases: developmental considerations. In: Oski FA, ed. Principles and practice of pediatrics, ed 1. Philadelphia, JB Lippincott, 1990:329.
20. Smith CA, Nelson NM. The physiology of the newborn infant. Springfield, IL, Charles C. Thomas, 1976:207.
21. Driscoll DJ. Use of inotropic and chronotropic agents in neonates. Clin Perinatol 1987;14:931.
22. Benumof JL. Physiology of the lateral decubitus position, the open chest, and one-lung ventilation. In: Kaplan JA ed. Thoracic anesthesia, ed 2. New York, Churchill-Livingstone, 1991:193.
23. Darnall RA. Noninvasive blood pressure measurement in the neonate. Clin Perinatol 1985;12:31.
24. Solimano AJ, Smyth JA, Mann TK, et al. Pulse oximetry advantages in infants with bronchopulmonary dysplasia. Pediatrics 1986;78:844.
25. McEvedy BAB, McLeod ME, Kirpalani H, et al. End-tidal carbon dioxide measurements in critically ill neonates: a comparison of sidestream and mainstream capnometers. Can J Anaesth 1990;37:322.
26. Rah KH, Salzberg AM, Boyan CP, et al. Respiratory acidosis with small Storz-Hopkins bronchoscopes: occurrence and management. Ann Thorac Surg 1979;27:197.
27. McIlvaine WB, Chang JHT, Jones M. The effective use of intrapleural bupivacaine for analgesia after thoracic and subcostal incisions in children. J Pediatr Surg 1988;23:1184.
28. Tobias JD, Martin LD, Oakes L, et al. Postoperative analgesia following thoracotomy in children: interpleural catheters. J Pediatr Surg 1993;28:1466.
29. Rodgers BM, Webb CJ, Stergois D, et al. Patient controlled analgesia in pediatric surgery. J Pediatr Surg 1987;23:259.
30. Chetcuti P, Myers NA, Phelan PD, et al. Chest wall deformity in patients with repaired esophageal atresia. J Pediatr Surg 1989;24:244.
31. Jaureguizar E, Vazquez J, Murcia J, et al. Morbid musculoskeletal sequelae of thoracotomy for tracheoesophageal fistula. J Pediatr Surg 1985;20:511.
32. Goodman P, Balachandran S, Guinto FC. Postoperative atrophy of posterolateral chest wall musculature: CT demonstration. J Comput Assist Tomogr 1992;17:63.
33. Goh DW, Brereton RJ. Triangle of auscultation thoracotomy for esophageal atresia. J Thorac Cardiovasc Surg 1992;103:14.
34. Karwande SV, Rowles JR. Simplified muscle-sparing thoracotomy for patent ductus arteriosus ligation in neonates. Ann Thorac Surg 1992;54:164.
35. Rothenberg SS, Pokorny WJ. Experience with a total muscle-sparing approach for thoracotomies in neonates, infants, and children. J Pediatr Surg 1992;27:1157.
36. Ponn RB, Ferneini A, D'Agostino RS, et al. Comparison of late pulmonary function after posterolateral and muscle-sparing thoracotomy. Ann Thorac Surg 1992;53:675.
37. Rodgers BM. Thoracoscopic procedures in children. Semin Pediatr Surg 1993;2:182.
38. McGahren ED, Kern JA, Rodgers BM. Anesthetic techniques for pediatric thoracoscopy. Ann Thorac Surg. 1995;60:927.
39. Kern JA, Daniel TM, Tribble CG, et al. Thoracoscopic diagnosis and treatment of mediastinal masses. Ann Thorac Surg 1993;56:92.
40. Dillon PW, Cilley RE, Krummel TM. Video-assisted thoracoscopic excision of intrathoracic masses in children: report of two cases. Surg Laparosc Endosc 1993;3:433.
41. Lobe TE. Pediatric thoracoscopy. Semin Thorac Cardiovasc Surg 1993;5:298.
42. Rodgers BM. Pediatric thoracoscopy: where have we come and what have we learned. Ann Thorac Surg 1993;56:704.
43. Watine O, Mensier E, Delecluse P, et al. Pulmonary sequestration treated by video-assisted thoracoscopic resection. Eur J Cardiothorac Surg 1994;8:155.
44. Tribble CG, Selden RF, Rodgers BM. Talc poudrage in the treatment of spontaneous pneumothoraces in patients with cystic fibrosis. Ann Surg 1986;204:677.
45. Urschel JD, Chan WKY. Technical report: thoracoscopic pleural abrasion for pneumothorax. J Laparosc Surg 1993;3:351.
46. Graham DD, McGahren ED, Tribble CG, et al. Use of video-assisted thoracic surgery in the treatment of chylothorax. Ann Thorac Surg 1994;57:1507.
47. Graeber GM, Jones DR. The role of thoracoscopy in thoracic trauma. Ann Thorac Surg 1993;56:646.
48. Kern JA, Tribble CG, Spotnitz WD, et al. Thoracoscopy: a potential role in the subacute management of patients with thoraco-abdominal trauma. Chest 1993;104:942.
49. Kao MC, Lee WY, Yip KM, et al. Palmar hyperhidrosis in children: treatment with video endoscopic laser sympathectomy. J Pediatr Surg 1994;29:387.
50. Laborde F, Hoirhomme P, Karam J, et al. A new video-assisted thoracoscopic surgical technique for interruption of patent ductus arteriosus in infants and children. J Thorac Cardiovasc Surg 1993;105:278.
51. Förster R. Thoracoscopic clipping of patent ductus arteriosus in premature infants. Ann Thorac Surg 1993;56:1418.
52. Burke RP, Chang AC. Video-assisted thoracoscopic division of a vas-

cular ring in an infant: A new operative technique. J Cardiovasc Surg 1993;8:537.

53. Pellegrini CA, Leichter R, Patti M, et al. Thoracoscopic esophageal myotomy in the treatment of achalasia. Ann Thorac Surg 1993;56:680.

54. DeMeester TR, Lafontaine E. The pleura. In: Sabiston DC, Spencer FC, eds. Surgery of the chest, ed 5. Philadelphia, WB Saunders, 1990:444.

55. Ravitch MM. Mediastinal cysts and tumors. In: Welch KJ, Randolph JG, Ravitch MM, et al, eds. Pediatric Surgery, ed 4. Chicago, Year Book Medical Publishers, 1986:602.

56. Benteur L, Canny G, Thorner P, et al. Spontaneous pneumothorax in cystic adenomatoid malformation. Chest 1991;99:1292.

57. Davis AM, Wensley DF, Phelan PD. Spontaneous pneumothorax in pediatric patients. Respir Med 1993;87:531.

58. Kemp JS, Seilheimer DK. Diseases of the pleura. In: Oski FA, ed. Principles and practice of pediatrics, ed 1. Philadelphia, JB Lippincott, 1990:1378.

59. Rhea JT, DeLuca SA, Greene RE. Determining the size of pneumothorax in the upright patient. Radiology 1982;144:733.

60. Kjaergaard H. Spontaneous pneumothorax in the apparently healthy. Acta Med Scand Suppl 1932;43:1.

61. Gaensler EA. Parietal pleurectomy for recurrent pneumothorax. Surg Gynecol Obstet 1956;102:293.

62. Austin EH, Flye MW. The treatment of recurrent malignant pleural effusion. Ann Thor Surg 1979;28:190.

63. Spector ML, Stern RC. Pneumothorax in cystic fibrosis: a 26-year experience. Ann Thorac Surg 1989;47:204.

64. Stephenson LW. Treatment of pneumothorax with intrapleural tetracycline. Chest 1985;88:803.

65. Thorsrud GK. Pleural reaction to irritants. Acta Chir Scand 1965;355:1.

66. Hazelrigg SR, Landreneau RJ, Mack M, et al. Thoracoscopic stapled resection for spontaneous pneumothorax. J Thorac Cardiovasc Surg 1993;105:389.

67. Cannon WB, Vierra MA, Cannon A. Thoracoscopy for spontaneous pneumothorax. Ann Thorac Surg 1993;56:686.

68. Inderbitzi RGC, Furrer M, Striffeler H, et al. Thoracoscopic pleurectomy for treatment of complicated spontaneous pneumothorax. J Thorac Cardiovasc Surg 1993;105:84.

69. Rodgers BM, McGahren ED. Endoscopy in children. Chest Surg Clin North Am 1993;3:405.

70. Allen EM, Van Heeckeren DW, Spector ML, et al. Management of nutritional and infectious complications of postoperative chylothorax in children. J Pediatr Surg 1991;26:1169.

71. Easa D, Balaraman V, Ash K, et al. Congenital chylothorax and mediastinal neuroblastoma. J Pediatr Surg 1991;26:96.

72. Bond SJ, Guzzetta PC, Snyder ML, et al. Management of pediatric postoperative chylothorax. Ann Thorac Surg 1993;56:469.

73. Telander RL, Moir CR. Acquired diseases of the lung and pleura. In: Ashcraft KW, Holder TM, eds. Pediatric Surgery, ed 2. Philadelphia, WB Saunders, 1993:188.

74. Ferguson MK. Thoracoscopy for empyema, bronchopleural fistula, and chylothorax. Ann Thorac Surg 1993;56:644.

75. Valentine VG, Raffin TA. The management of chylothorax. Chest 1992;102:586.

76. Rheuban KS, Kron IL, Carpenter MA, et al. Pleuroperitoneal shunts for refractory chylothorax after operation for congenital heart disease. Ann Thorac Surg 1992;53:85.

77. Randolph JG, Gross RE. Congenital chylothorax. Arch Surg 1957;74:405.

78. Fajardo E, Chang MG. Pleural empyema in children: a nationwide retrospective study. South Med J 1987;80:593.

79. Bartlett JC, Gorbach SL, Thadepalli HT, et al. Bacteriology of empyema. Lancet 1974;1:338.

80. American Thoracic Society. Management of nontuberculous empyema. Am Rev Respir Dis 1962;85:935.

81. Chonmaitree T, Powell KR. Parapneumonic pleural effusion and empyema in children. Clin Pediatr 1983;22:414.

82. Foglia RP, Randolph J. Current indications for decortication in the treatment of empyema in children. J Pediatr Surg 1987;22:28.

83. Gustafson RA, Murray GF, Warden HE, Hill RC. Role of lung decortication in symptomatic empyemas in children. Ann Thorac Surg 1990;49:940.

84. Hoff SJ, Neblett WW, Heller RM, et al. Postpneumonic empyema in childhood: selecting appropriate therapy. J Pediatr Surg 1989;24:659.

85. McLaughlin FJ, Goldmann DA, Rosenbaum DM, et al. Empyema in children: clinical course and long-term follow-up. Pediatrics 1984;73:587.

86. Goeman A, Kipur N, Toppare M, et al. Conservative treatment of empyema in children. Respiration 1993;60:182.

87. Mangete ED, Kombo BB, Legg-Jack TE. Thoracic empyema: a study of 56 patients. Arch Dis Child 1993;69:587.

88. Lewis KT, Bukstein DA. Parapneumonic empyema in children: diagnosis and management. Am Fam Physician 1992;46:1443.

89. Kosloske AM, Carwright KC. The controversial role of decortication in the management of pediatric empyema. J Thorac Cardiovasc Surg 1988;96:166.

90. Hoff SJ, Neblett WW, Edwards KM. Parapneumonic empyema in children: decortication hastens recovery in patients with severe pleural infections. Pediatr Infect Dis J 1990;10:194.

91. Hendren WH, Haggerty RJ. Staphylococcic pneumonia in infancy and childhood. JAMA 1958;168:6.

92. Kern JA, Rodgers BM. Thoracoscopy in the management of empyema in children. J Pediatr Surg 1993;28:1128.

93. Kosloske AM, Ball WS, Butler C, et al. Drainage of pediatric lung abscess by cough, catheter, or complete resection. J Pediatr Surg 1986;21:596.

94. Lacey SR, Kosloske AM. Pneumonostomy in the management of pediatric lung abscess. J Pediatr Surg 1983;18:625.

95. Redding GJ, Walund L, Walund D, et al. Lung function in children following empyema. Am J Dis Child 1990;144:1337.

96. Azarow KS, Pearl RH, Zurcher R, et al. Primary mediastinal masses. J Thorac Cardiovasc Surg 1993;106:67.

97. Merten DJ. Diagnostic imaging of mediastinal masses in children. Am J Radiol 1992;158:825.

98. Meza MP, Benson M, Slovis TL. Imaging of mediastinal masses in children. Radiol Clin North Am 1993;31:583.

99. Link KM, Samuels LJ, Reed JC, et al. Magnetic resonance imaging of the mediastinum. J Thorac Imaging 1993;8:34.

100. Rosenberg HK. The complementary roles of ultrasound and plain film radiography in differentiating pediatric chest abnormalities. Radiographics 1986;6:427.

101. Grosfeld JL, Billmire DF. Teratomas in infancy and childhood. Curr Probl Cancer 1985;IX:9.

102. Grosfeld JL, Skinner MA, Rescorla FJ, et al. Mediastinal tumors in children: experience with 196 cases. Ann Surg Oncol 1994;1:121.

103. Lakhoo K, Boyle M, Drake DP. Mediastinal teratomas: review of 15 pediatric cases. J Pediatr Surg 1993;28:1161.

104. Pokorny WJ. Mediastinal tumors. In: Ashcraft KW, Holder TM, eds. Pediatric surgery, ed 2. Philadelphia, WB Saunders, 1993:218.

105. Kuller JA, Laifer SA, Martin JG, et al. Unusual presentations of fetal teratoma. J Perinatol 1991;40:294.

106. Ashour M, Hawass NE, Adam KAR. Spontaneous intrapleural rupture of mediastinal teratoma. Respir Med 1993;87:69.

107. Mogilner JG, Fonseca J, Davies MRQ. Life-threatening respiratory distress caused by a mediastinal teratoma in a newborn. J Pediatr Surg 1992;27:1519.

108. Siebert J, Marvin J, Rose EF, et al. Mediastinal teratoma: a rare cause of severe respiratory distress in the newborn. J Pediatr Surg 1976;11:253.

109. Honicky RE, dePapp EW. Mediastinal teratoma with endocrine function. Am J Dis Child 1973;126:650.

110. Sommerland BC, Cleland WP, Yong NK. Physiological activity in mediastinal teratoma. Thorax 1975;30:510.

111. Sidani AH, Oberson R, Délèze G, et al. Infected teratoma of lower posterior mediastinum in a six-year-old boy. Pediatr Radiol 1991;21:438.

112. Aldousany AW, Joyner JC, Price RA, et al. Diagnosis and treatment of intrapericardial teratoma. Pediatr Cardiol 1987;8:51.

113. Copper JD. Current therapy for thymoma. Chest 1993;103:3345.

114. Couture MM, Mountain CF. Thymoma. Semin Surg Oncol 1990;6:110.

115. Pokorny WJ. Thymomas. In: Oski FA, ed. Principles and practice of pediatrics, ed 1. Philadelphia, JB Lippincott, 1990:1613.

116. Pollack A, Komaki R, Cox JD, et al. Thymoma: treatment and prognosis. Int J Radiat Oncol Biol Phys 1992;23:1037.

117. Rice TW. Benign neoplasms and cysts of the mediastinum. Semin Thorac Cardiovasc Surg 1992;4:25.

118. Wick MR. Mediastinal cysts and intrathoracic thyroid tumors. Semin Diagn Pathol 1990;7:285.

119. Hazelrigg SR, Landreneau RJ, Mack MJ, et al. Thoracoscopic resection of mediastinal cysts. Ann Thorac Surg 1993;56:659.

120. Gerle RD, Jaretzki A, Ashley CA, et al. Congenital bronchopulmonary–foregut malformation: pulmonary sequestration communicating with the gastrointestinal tract. New Engl J Med 1968;278:1413.

121. St. Georges R, Deslauriers J, Duranceau A, et al. Clinical spectrum of bronchogenic cysts of the mediastinum and lung in the adult. Ann Thorac Surg 1991;52:6.

122. Lazar RH, Younis BT, Bassila MN. Bronchogenic cysts: a cause of stridor in the neonate. Am J Otolaryngol 1991;12:117.

123. Suen GC, Mathisen DJ, Grillo HC, et al. Surgical management and radiological characteristics of bronchogenic cysts. Ann Thorac Surg 1993;55:476.

124. Olsen JB, Clemmensen O, Andersen K. Adenocarcinoma arising in a foregut cyst of the mediastinum. Ann Thorac Surg 1991;51:497.

125. Read CA, Moront M, Carangelo R. Recurrent bronchogenic cyst: An argument for complete surgical excision. Arch Surg 1991; 126:1306.

126. Mauch PM, Kalish LA, Kaden M, et al. Patterns of presentation of Hodgkin disease: implication for etiology and pathogenesis. Cancer 1993;71:2062.

127. Ingram L, Rivera GK, Shapiro DN. Superior vena cava syndrome associated with childhood malignancy: analysis of 24 cases. Med Pediatr Oncol 1990;1 8:476.

128. Shorter NA, Fiston HC. Lymphomas. In: Ashcraft KW, Holder TM, eds. Pediatric surgery, ed 2. Philadelphia, WB Saunders, 1993;863.

129. Azizkhan RG, Dudgeon DL, Buck JR, et al. Life-threatening airway obstruction as a complication to the management of mediastinal masses in children. J Pediatr Surg 1985;20:816.

130. Shamberger RC, Holyman RS, Griscom NT, et al. CT quantitation of tracheal cross-section area as a guide to the surgical and anesthetic management of children with anterior mediastinal masses. J Pediatr Surg 1991;26:138.

131. Kurtyberg J, Graham ML. Non-Hodgkin's lymphoma. Biological classification and implication for therapy. Pediatr Clin North Am 1991;38:443.

132. Ferrari LR, Bedford RF. General anesthesia prior to treatment of anterior mediastinal masses in pediatric cancer patients. Anesthesiology 1990;72:991.

133. Halpern S, Chatten J, Meadows AT, et al. Anterior mediastinal masses: anesthesia hazards and other problems. J Pediatr 1983;102:407.

134. King MR, Telander RL, Smithson WA, et al. Primary mediastinal tumors in children. J Pediatr Surg 1992;17:512.

135. Carr TF, Lockwood L, Stevens RF, et al. Childhood B cell lymphomas arising in the mediastinum. J Clin Pathol 1993;46:513.

136. Loeffler JS, Leopold KA, Recht A, et al. Emergency prebiopsy radiation for mediastinal masses: impact on subsequent pathologic diagnosis and outcome. J Clin Oncol 1986;4:716.

137. Lemonine G, Montupet P. Mediastinal tumors in infancy and childhood. In: Fallis JC, Filler RM, Lemoina G, eds. Pediatric thoracic surgery. New York, Elsevier, 1991:258.

138. Sills RH. The spleen and lymph nodes. In: Oski FA, ed. Principles and practice of pediatrics. Philadelphia, JB Lippincott, 1990:1540.

139. Szinicz G, Taqxer F, Riedlinger J, et al. Thoracoscopic resection of a pericardial cyst. Thorac Card Surg 1992;40:190.

140. Glasson MJ, Taylor SF. Cervical cervico-mediastinal and intrathoracic lymphangioma. Prog Pediatr Surg 1991;27:62.

141. Hancock JF, St-Vil D, Luka FI, et al. Complications of lymphangiomas in children. J Pediatr Surg 1992;27:220.

142. Kostopoulos GK, Fessatidis JT, Hevas AL, et al. Mediastinal cystic hygroma: Report of a case with review of the literature. Eur J Cardiothorac Surg 1993;7:166.

143. Zalel Y, Shalev E, Ben-Ami M, et al. Ultrasonic diagnosis of mediastinal cystic hygroma. Prenat Diagn 1992;12:541.

144. Gupta AK, Bery M, Raghav B, et al. Mediastinal and skeletal lymphangiomas in a child. Pediatr Radiol 1991;21:129.

145. Pokorny WJ. Congenital malformation of the lymphatic system In: Oski FA, ed. Principles and practice of pediatrics, ed 1. Philadelphia, JB Lippincott 1990:1612.

146. Ogita S, Tsuto T, Deguchi E, et al. OK-432 therapy for unresectable lymphangiomas in children. J Pediatr Surg 1991;26:263.

147. Okada A, Kubota A, Fukuzawa M, et al. Injection of bleomycin as a primary therapy of cystic lymphangioma. J Pediatr Surg 1992;27:440.

148. Lee CW, Shulman K, Morecki R, et al. Malignant degeneration of thoracic neurofibroma. N Y State J Med 1975;75:347.

Surgery of Infants and Children: Scientific Principles and Practice, edited by Keith T. Oldham, Paul M. Colombani, and Robert P. Foglia. Lippincott–Raven Publishers, Philadelphia, © 1997.

CHAPTER 57

Lung

Keith T. Oldham

Infants and children manifest an extraordinary diversity of congenital and acquired abnormalities of the lung. Although none is truly common, all the surgical conditions presented in this chapter are important since physiologic lung dysfunction is a potential consequence. Because impaired respiratory gas exchange can be life-threatening, it is of fundamental importance that those who care for infants and children be familiar with these lesions. A full understanding of respiratory physiology requires consideration of the chest wall, diaphragm, and airways in addition to the lungs. This text considers each component separately for reasons of organizational and educational expediency. The reader is referred to other chapters for these specific related discussions, and also to Chapter 8, which considers respiratory physiology in detail.

EMBRYOLOGY AND ANATOMY

Lung Development

By the end of the third weeks of gestation, the laryngotracheal groove is discernible in the ventral aspect of the proximal foregut in human embryos. This groove develops into a tracheal diverticulum, a primordium that elongates caudally and lies ventral and parallel to the dorsal foregut, the primitive esophagus. By the middle of week 6 of gestation, the trachea has undergone symmetric distal division into the left and right main-stem bronchi. Mesenchymal proliferation follows in the adjacent mediastinum and is necessary for normal lung organogenesis. This mesoderm is ultimately the source of cartilage, smooth muscle, and connective tissue to the developing lungs. Progressive bronchial branching follows, and by the seventh gestational week, three to five orders of bronchi are present. Tracheal and esophageal separation are normally complete at this time[1] (Fig. 57-1). All major bronchial beds are present by 8 to 9 weeks' gestation, when closure of the pleural peritoneal canal completes formation of the diaphragm. By this time, segmental and lobar lung development is complete. After about 16 weeks' gestation, the primary events in fetal lung development are related to the successive formation of terminal airways and alveoli—the critical sites for respiratory gas exchange. This process is of profound importance in understanding the physiologic

consequences of mass lesions in the fetal thorax[2] (see Chaps. 8 and 54). With regard to understanding the specific physiologic response to pulmonary surgery in infants, several points bear reiteration. Alveoli undergo highly significant maturation and development during the third trimester and during early postnatal life. Both the number and size of alveoli increase during this time. Most of this process is completed by 2 to 4 years of age,[2–5] although it continues until about age 8. Because of this age-related potential for compensatory lung growth, the tolerance of pulmonary resection in infants and children is generally good.

Normal Anatomy

The normal lobar and segmental anatomy of mature lungs and some key anatomic relations to adjacent structures are summarized in Figures 57-2 and 57-3.[6] Although a detailed review of lung anatomy is beyond the scope of this text, several points of particular clinical relevance are emphasized next.

The right lung is normally larger than the left, with an upper, middle, and lower lobe each supplied by its respective bronchus. The left lung is formed by upper and lower lobes similarly situated, and the lingula is analogous to the right middle lobe. The tracheal bifurcation is at the fourth or fifth vertebral body by the time of birth. The right main-stem bronchus is normally larger, more vertical, and about half the length of the left. These anatomic features account for the preferential drainage of endobronchial material or foreign bodies into the right lung, particularly the right lower lobe.

The circulation on which respiratory gas exchange depends is derived from the pulmonary artery and its branches. The circulation that provides nutritive support for the lung parenchyma and the bronchi, however, is systemic. The main left bronchus and its dependent airways are supplied by two bronchial arteries that arise from the anterior surface of the descending thoracic aorta. On the right, a single bronchial artery is usually present and is derived from either the third right intercostal artery or the more superior of the two left bronchial arteries. Intramural collateral flow from the trachea to the bronchi is derived from the inferior thyroid arteries, which are supplied by the thyrocervical trunks of the subclavian arteries. Venous

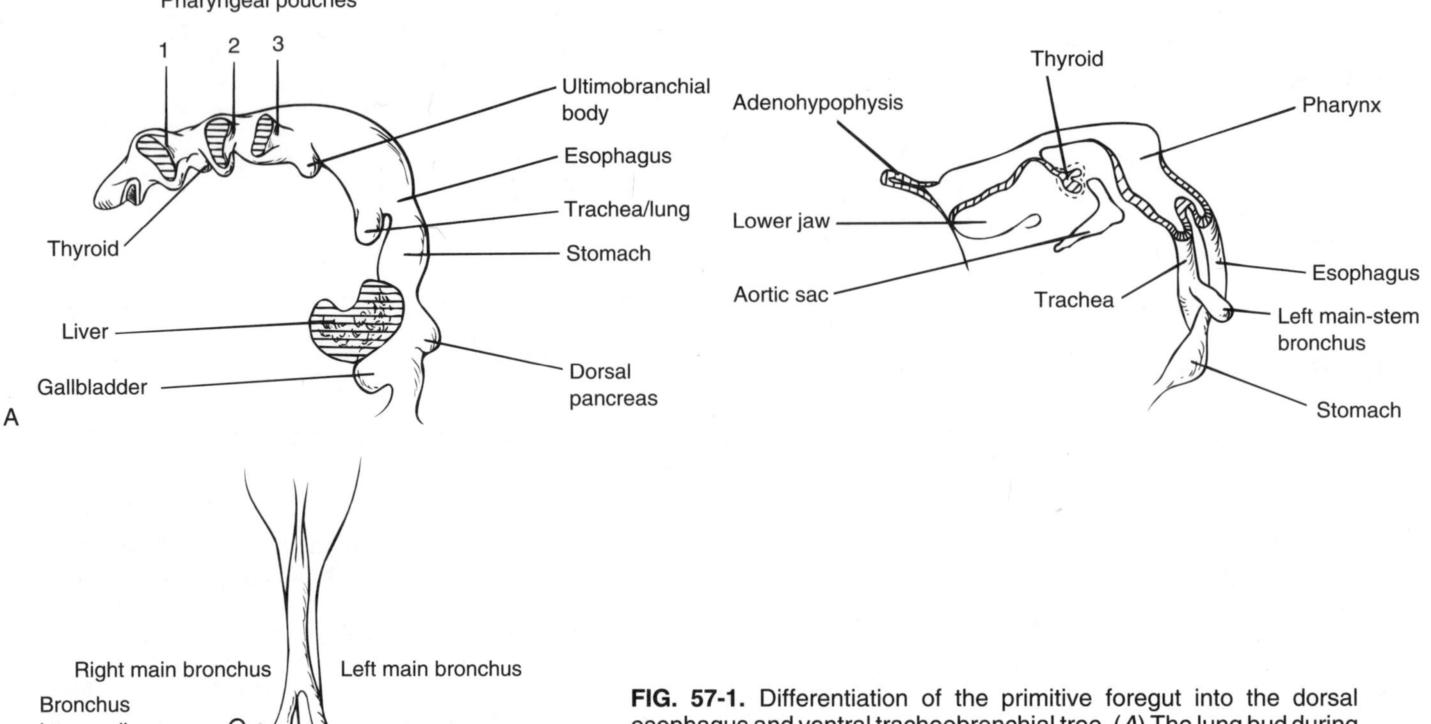

FIG. 57-1. Differentiation of the primitive foregut into the dorsal esophagus and ventral tracheobronchial tree. (*A*) The lung bud during the fifth gestational week. (*B*) Lateral view during the middle of the sixth gestational week. (*C*) Front view of the bronchial tree at the start of the seventh gestational week. (After Gray SW, Skandalakis JE. The trachea and lungs. In: Embryology for surgeons: the embryological basis for the treatment of congenital defects, ed 2. Baltimore, Williams & Wilkins, 1994:416)

bronchial drainage is into the azygous and hemiazygous systems. Generally, both arteries and veins follow the segmental and lobar architecture of the bronchi. These points assume substantial importance in the discussions that follow.

At the microscopic level, several features deserve specific comment. A normal bronchus is demonstrated in Figure 57-4*A*.[7] The epithelium is ciliated, pseudostratified, columnar epithelium. Smooth muscle demarcates the basal extent of the mucosa. Mucus-producing glands are apparent in the submucosa. Parasympathetic ganglion cells are abundant, and by definition, cartilage is present. Cartilage is an essential structural element for maintaining expiratory patency of the major conducting airways. Proceeding distally in the tracheobronchial tree, luminal size diminishes, and certain features are lost. In particular, as the bronchus becomes a bronchiole, cartilage is lost, the glands disappear, and the epithelium becomes simple, columnar, and ciliated. Smooth muscle and elastic tissues remain. More distally, these elements drop out of the terminal bronchiole as the need to conduct large volumes of air diminishes. Eventually, at the level of the respiratory bronchiole and the alveoli, where gas exchange occurs, capillaries and epithelial cells are juxtaposed intimately (see Fig. 57-4*B*). Most oxygen and carbon dioxide diffusion actually occurs across a membrane composed only of thin cytoplasmic extensions of the type I epithelial cell and the capillary endothelial cell bound by a common basement membrane. This is only nanometers in thickness.

Parenchymal lung lesions in infants and children are divided in the following discussion into those that are congenital and those that are acquired. Anomalies that result from disordered organogenesis during foregut development are reviewed in detail[8–10] (Fig. 57-5). Certain conditions, such as cystic fibrosis (CF) and bullous disease, may have both congenital and acquired features, and these individual aspects are reviewed in context.

CONGENITAL DISORDERS

Congenital Lobar Emphysema

Congenital lobar emphysema, or congenital lobar overinflation, refers to the abnormal postnatal collection of air within a lobe of the lung that is otherwise anatomically normal. This condition is characterized by expiratory air-trapping within the affected lobe, resulting in lobar parenchymal distention. Compression of adjacent normal lung and mediastinal structures is expected, and physiologic impairment of gas exchange is common. The process is classically the result of developmental deficiency of the cartilage that supports the bronchus to the involved lobe, resulting in focal bronchial collapse and obstruction to expiratory air flow. This specific defect, however, is demonstrable in only one third to two thirds of surgically resected emphysematous lobes.[11] The remainder of these infants and children have a variety of partially obstructing bronchial

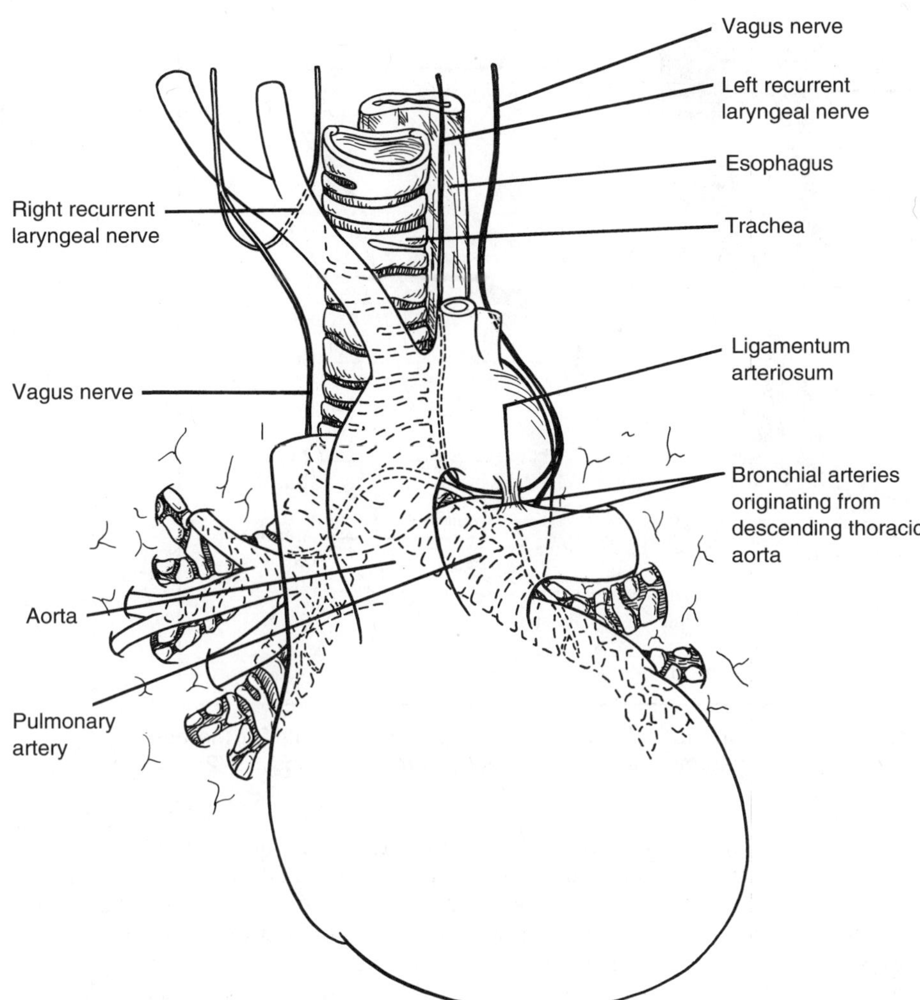

FIG. 57-2. Key anatomic relations of the structures of the pulmonary hilum.

lesions. Some are endobronchial and potentially reversible (eg, viscid secretions, mucous plugs, or granulation tissue). Some are the result of extrinsic compression with partial obstruction from mediastinal lymphadenopathy, adjacent vascular structures such as an aberrant or enlarged pulmonary artery or ductus arteriosus, mediastinal cysts or tumors that are bronchogenic in origin, or other congenital or acquired mediastinal lesions with an intimate hilar relation. For these reasons, preresection bronchoscopic evaluation is routinely done with the expectation that reversible bronchial obstruction be corrected before sacrificing a lung lobe that is otherwise normal.

In addition, developmental abnormalities of the alveoli or the terminal airways may be associated with the clinical findings of congenital lobar emphysema. Of note in this regard is the finding of *polyalveolar morphology,* a descriptive histologic term that refers to a substantial and abnormal increase in the number of alveoli present. In this circumstance, postnatal air-trapping occurs within these many alveoli.

Congenital lobar emphysema is a rare lesion, with a 2:1 or 3:1 male predominance. It is most common in the white population. Unilobar involvement is the rule, with affected sites distributed in the following manner: left upper lobe, 40% to 50%; right middle lobe, 30% to 40%; right upper lobe, 20%; lower lobes, 1%; and multiple sites the remainder[10,11] (Fig. 57-

6). Congenital lobar emphysema is associated with congenital heart disease or abnormalities of the great vessels in about 15% of infants.[12-15] Indeed, extrinsic bronchial compression from vascular structures appears to be a common etiologic problem in this circumstance. For this reason, screening echocardiography is appropriate in all infants with congenital lobar emphysema.

Affected infants usually do not have symptoms at birth. With the onset of extrauterine life and spontaneous respiration, air-trapping and progressive lobar distention develop. Initial clinical symptoms are generally tachypnea and dyspnea, followed by cyanosis if oxygenation is sufficiently impaired. A cough or wheezing may also be present, but this is of little specificity. About half of affected infants develop symptoms in the first few days of life; the remainder develop symptoms within the first 6 months. Older infants and children may have few or no symptoms. Infants may have rapidly progressive respiratory failure, with up to 10% to 15% of patients requiring emergency thoracotomy. Generally, the clinical progression is slower, and some patients remain without symptoms.

The clinical presentation may be one of progressive respiratory distress; therefore, an affected infant may become increasingly agitated, anxious, and tachypneic. These normal responses to hypoxemia exacerbate the air-trapping phenomenon as the

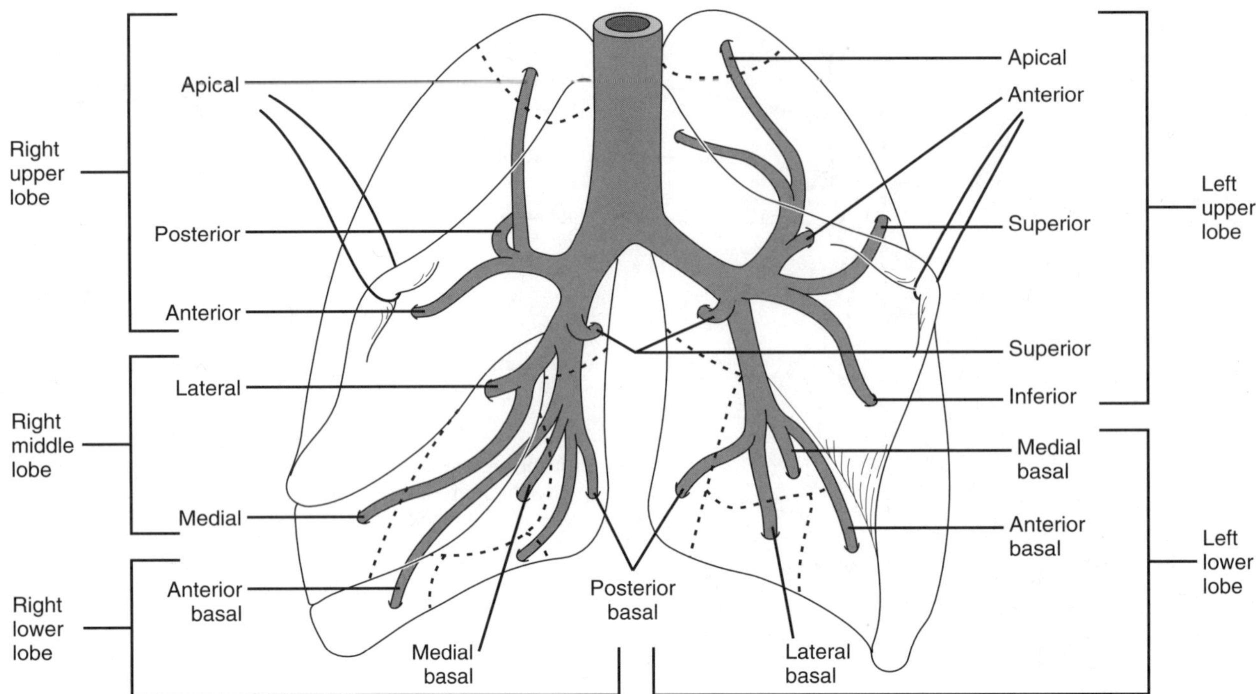

FIG. 57-3. The segmental bronchi and their corresponding bronchopulmonary segments for the right and left lungs. (After Grant JCB. An atlas of anatomy, ed 6. Baltimore, Williams & Wilkins, 1972)

peak inspiratory and expiratory pressures escalate. In particular, focal bronchial collapse occurs with excessive expiratory effort; as this develops, the lobar emphysema worsens, and further compromise in gas exchange results. Likewise, positive-pressure ventilation can induce acute lobar distention with potentially catastrophic respiratory decompensation or mediastinal displacement. The physiologic derangements may be indistinguishable from those of tension pneumothorax. This is an important consideration during endoscopic evaluation of the endobronchial tree. Particularly in infants with preoperative symptoms, the surgeon must be prepared to decompress the thorax by emergent thoracotomy and then to proceed with definitive lobectomy.

Congenital lobar emphysema is typically found in term infants, but acquired emphysematous disease in preterm infants is common.[16] Generally, this latter problem results from lung injury related to positive-pressure mechanical ventilation and is often seen in conjunction with bronchopulmonary dysplasia. Unlike congenital lobar emphysema, multiple areas of focal hyperinflation and interstitial emphysema are often present. Unilobar right lower lobe involvement is also common, probably as a consequence of endotracheal tube positioning, which selectively ventilates the right main-stem bronchus. These characteristics help differentiate congenital and acquired disease.

Physical findings of congenital lobar emphysema may include an asymmetric thorax, a shift in the apical cardiac impulse to the contralateral side, and focal hyperresonance and diminished breath sounds over the affected lobe. None of these findings, however, has the necessary sensitivity and specificity to demonstrate the precise nature of the problem.

The diagnosis is best established by plain chest radiograph (see Fig. 57-6). Typical findings include lobar hyperinflation, contralateral shift of the mediastinum and trachea, compression or even lobar atelectasis of adjacent lung, and flattening of the ipsilateral hemidiaphragm. If these findings are all present, there is no need for additional imaging studies. Differentiating this presentation from tension pneumothorax is essential. The latter is characterized by collapse of the entire affected lung into the hilum. In contrast, although lobar emphysema can be dramatic in its radiographic appearance, adjacent compressed lung can almost always be discerned, most often the lower lobe at the base of the thorax. In addition, the occasional congenital cystic adenomatoid malformation (CCAM) with a single large cystic component can be mistaken for lobar emphysema. Because lobar emphysema rarely involves the lower lobes, this is an important differentiating feature. Nonetheless, the surgical management of these latter two lesions is similar, so that preoperative differentiation is less important than for tension pneumothorax, for which the treatment is different. As with most mass lesions in the chest, computed tomography (CT) and magnetic resonance (MR) imaging provide excellent anatomic information for infants with congenital lobar emphysema. These procedures are most helpful in elective situations when the diagnosis is in doubt. In addition, ventilation–perfusion scans have been employed to evaluate infants with lobar emphysema, particularly when the areas of involvement are multiple or the disease acquired.[17] In this setting, specific areas of nonfunctional lung can be identified and resected if they appear to compromise adjacent normal lung.

Because the natural history of congenital lobar emphysema is often progressive and includes potentially life-threatening respiratory insufficiency, prompt surgical lobectomy is the treatment of choice for infants and young children. Because the underlying lesion is structural, nonspecific treatment can be considered only a supportive adjunct in patients with symptoms. In patients without symptoms, particularly older children, this

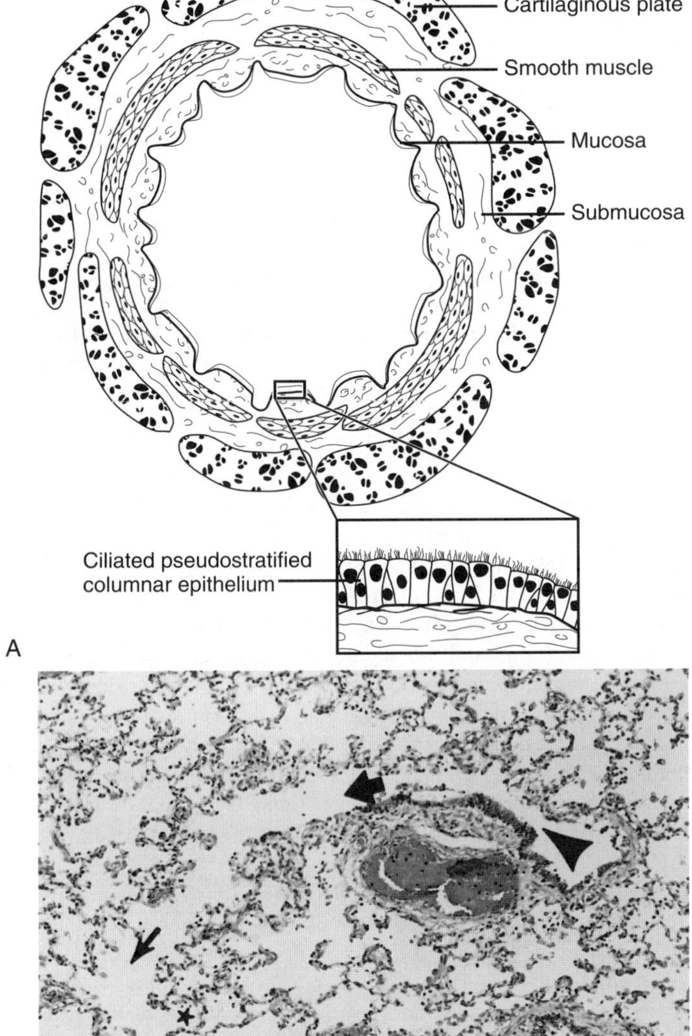

FIG. 57-4. (*A*) A normal bronchus. Cartilaginous plates are present circumferentially. Smooth muscle is at the boundary between mucosa and submucosa. Ciliated pseudostratified columnar epithelium is present. (*B*) A normal terminal bronchiole (*arrowhead*) lined by cuboidal to columnar epithelium, progresses to a respiratory bronchiole (*thick arrow*), which in turn leads to alveolar ducts (*thin arrow*). The alveolar ducts have incomplete walls and open into numerous alveoli (*asterisks*). A bronchiole that contains slips of smooth muscle in the wall is shown in cross section (*lower right*). (Hematoxylin–eosin, ×100) (*A* after Reith EJ, Ross MA. Atlas of descriptive histology, ed 2. New York, Harper & Row, 1970; *B* courtesy of Kay Washington, MD, Duke University Medical Center; Durham, NC)

approach may be tempered reasonably because the likelihood of sudden decompensation in this circumstance is low. The necessity for routine endoscopic evaluation of the affected bronchus has been noted. The purpose is to identify and eliminate reversible endobronchial obstructions from secretions, mucous plugging, or granulation tissue. Clearly reversible endobronchial problems should be corrected without parenchymal lung resection.

Extrinsic bronchial compression is associated generally with a focal cartilaginous defect of the affected bronchus that is not adequately relieved by simple decompression. Although congenital lobar emphysema results from a specific anatomic defect, reconstructive procedures, such as bronchoplasty or segmental bronchial resection and anastomosis, are generally inappropriate. The diminutive size of the infant bronchus and the possibility of nonfocal cartilaginous tracheobronchial defects present important technical obstacles to successful local reconstructive procedures. In addition, there is little reason to select this approach because the clinical results of lobectomy are generally excellent for this lesion.[12–15,18]

Acquired emphysema is often seen in preterm infants with a multitude of other problems. Treatment is generally medical and supportive, with the natural history being one of slow resolution over a number of months. In the acute phase, selective ventilation of nonemphysematous areas of lung or the use of alternative strategies such as high frequency oscillatory or jet ventilation can minimize the peak airway pressure, which is directly correlated to the formation of emphysema. These approaches can also help infants with congenital lobar emphysema if prolonged transport is necessary or there is delay in reaching the operating suite.

As noted, infants and children have an excellent response to lobectomy for congenital lobar emphysema[12–15,18] (see Fig. 57-6*B*). Even in those who are critically ill and require emergency thoracotomy, the physiologic response is a predictably prompt and dramatic return to normal after resection of the affected lobe. Mortality for this specific lesion is rare in a modern pediatric surgical environment. The general risks of thoracotomy and lung resection include morbidity related to anesthesia, empyema, pneumothorax, infection, bleeding, and bronchopleural fistula. These are not different than for any other neonatal thoracotomy and lobectomy and are presented in detail in the section that deals with outcomes after lung resection. The cumulative incidence of these types of complications is about 5% to 10% in most modern pediatric surgical practices, although it has been as high as 20% to 40% in recent decades.[10,12–15] Long-term pulmonary function is also predictably excellent after lobar resection, and this is discussed separately later. For infants with coexisting congenital heart disease, acquired pulmonary emphysema, or additional medical problems, the outcome is generally dictated by these other conditions.

In follow-up studies by Frenckner and Freyschuss,[19] actual lung volumes—residual volume, vital capacity, total lung capacity, and forced expiratory volume in 1 second (FEV_1)—in patients who had undergone neonatal lobectomy for congenital lobar emphysema were 90% of predicted values, and no long-term functional impairment was reported. Infants who had undergone neonatal lobectomy for congenital lobar emphysema were followed as adults by McBride and colleagues in 1980.[18] Ipsilateral and contralateral lung volumes were found to be equal despite the previous lobectomy. This appeared to be the result of compensatory tissue growth, not simply distention of residual lung parenchyma. In this latter study, perfusion was found to be equally distributed between the operated and nonoperated lungs. These patients demonstrated diminished respiratory flow rates compared with expected values (FEV_1, 72% of predicted; maximal mid-expiratory flow, 45% of predicted).

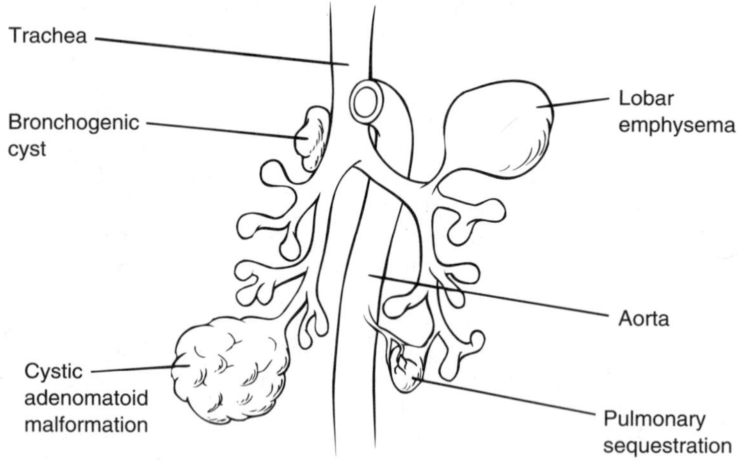

FIG. 57-5. Classic developmental abnormalities of the tracheobronchial tree. (After Haller JA Jr, Golladay ES, Pickard LR, et al. Surgical management of lung bud anomalies: lobar emphysema, bronchogenic cyst, cystic adenomatoid malformation, and intralobar pulmonary sequestration. Ann Thorac Surg 1979;28:34)

These findings appear to result from disproportional growth between the conducting and the terminal airways during infancy. This concept does not diminish the excellent clinical prognosis for these infants, and is presented in detail in the outcome summary at the end of this chapter.

Congenital Cystic Adenomatoid Malformation

Congenital cystic adenomatoid malformation is a term applied to a spectrum of lobar hamartomatous abnormalities of the lung. The pathologic definition requires an increase in terminal respiratory structures, usually bronchioles, in a glandular or adenomatoid pattern that is normally seen during organogenesis. It is suggested that developmental control of the lobar lung bud and the surrounding mediastinal mesenchyme is lost between 16 and 20 weeks' gestation, giving rise to a lesion that is composed of multiple interconnected cysts that are disorganized and variably sized.[20] Involvement is generally unilobar, and communication with the tracheobronchial tree is usually present. Three types of CCAM lesions were described by Stocker and colleagues[21] in 1977 and are illustrated in Figures 57-7 and 57-8.

Subsequently, others used the terms *cystic, intermediate,* and *solid* to categorize the different lesions observed with this malformation. Most recently, Adzick and colleagues[22] defined these lesions as either macrocystic (greater than 5-mm cyst diameter) or microcystic (solid or less than 5-mm cyst diameter), by use of prenatal ultrasound examination to differentiate between the two. Because the natural history is dependent on morphologic type, the distinctions have more than semantic import. Clinical treatment and outcomes are presented later.

Both before and after parturition, the important physiologic consequences of CCAM result from mediastinal or normal lung compression by the mass lesion. Lesions of great size, particularly those that are microcystic or solid in composition, are potentially associated with in utero mediastinal displacement, hydrops fetalis, and fetal death. As many as one third of all newborns with CCAM have evidence of fetal hydrops at delivery. It is now routine to establish the diagnosis of CCAM by prenatal ultrasound. The data for the fetus diagnosed with CCAM are more limited and controversial, but it appears that as many as half of cases result in fetal death.[21,22] Adzick and

colleagues[23] suggested that the appearance of anasarca or hydrops in fetuses with microcystic CCAM is an indication of impending fetal demise; they reported neonatal survival after fetal lobectomy in four selected patients. Macrocystic lesions appear less threatening in utero, and although some have been managed with prenatal thoracoamniotic shunting or aspiration, most of these infants can be successfully treated after delivery at term. In addition, it appears that a substantial number of macrocystic lesions, perhaps one third, diminish in size during fetal development.[24,25] This is an important area of active investigation. Appropriate selection of patients for prenatal therapy depends on accurate information defining the natural history of CCAM.

Postpartum physiologic problems related to CCAM generally result from either pulmonary hypoplasia in newborns or inadequate tracheobronchial drainage with secondary infection in older infants and children. The former problem appears related to in utero compression and developmental arrest of the ipsilateral lung by the CCAM mass. In addition, some degree of contralateral pulmonary hypoplasia resulting from the shifted mediastinum is common. Pulmonary parenchymal hypoplasia and persistent pulmonary hypertension can result in acute respiratory failure in newborns. Severely affected infants with CCAM may have all the ventilatory instability of infants with congenital diaphragmatic hernias. This includes the potential need for conventional mechanical ventilation, high-frequency or jet ventilation, or extracorporeal life support. These issues are discussed in detail in Chapters 8 and 54. Although the spectrum of physiologic derangement includes both acute life-threatening respiratory failure and progressive newborn respiratory insufficiency, only about 30% of live-born infants with CCAM present in these ways.[26] Most present with infectious pulmonary problems related to the persistent communication of the CCAM with the tracheobronchial tree. The abnormal lung parenchyma is exposed to environmental organisms but lacks normal clearance mechanisms. This leads to a variety of infectious problems, such as recurrent pneumonia or lung abscess, or to more subtle chronic problems, such as failure to thrive.

CCAM lesions are uncommon, representing about 30% to 40% of developmental lung bud anomalies in most reports. There is a slight male predominance and no apparent racial or

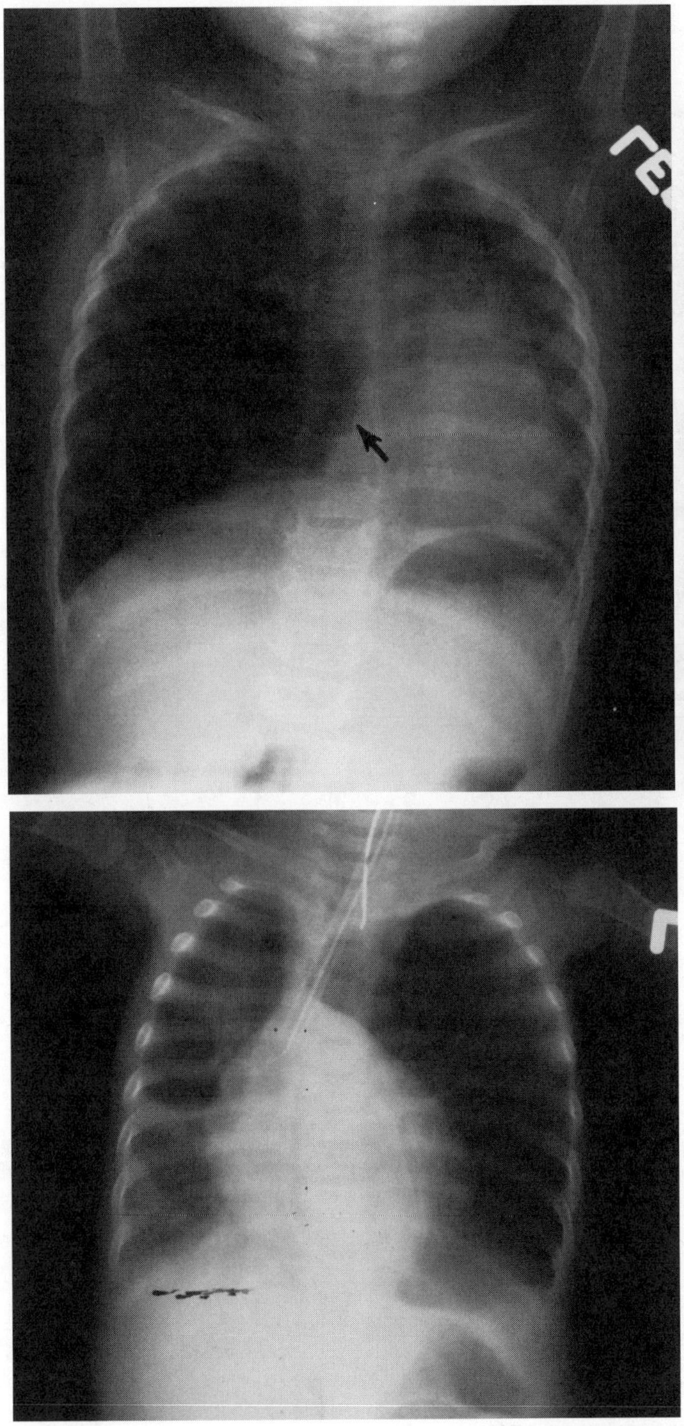

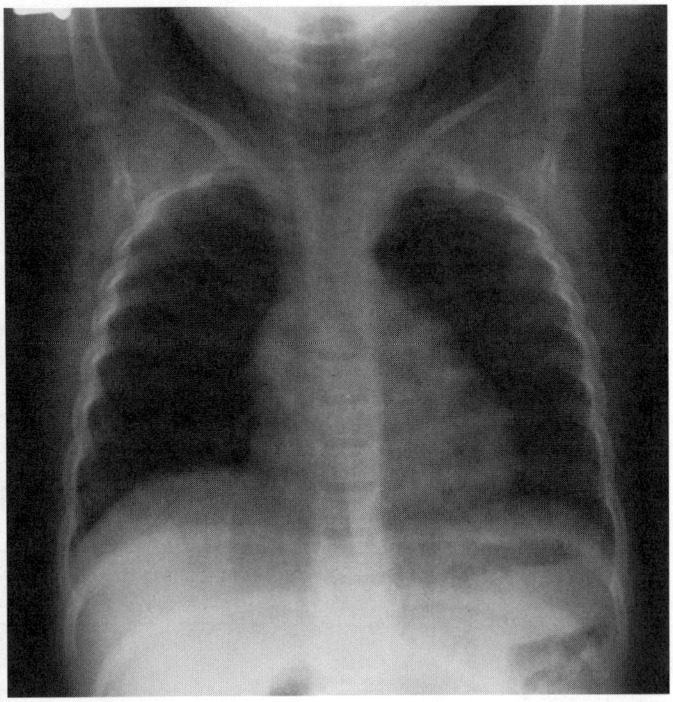

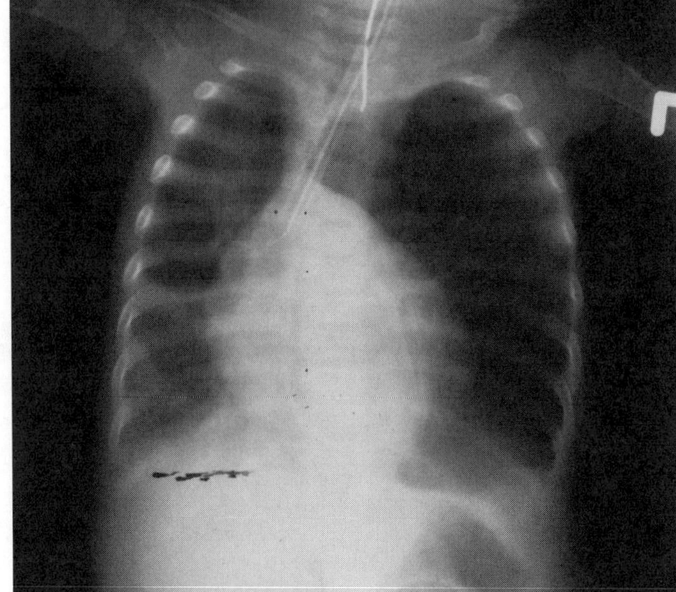

FIG. 57-6. Congenital lobar emphysema involving the right middle lobe. (*A*) Herniation of the affected lobe across the midline has occurred (*arrow*), with compression of the adjacent right upper and right lower lobes. Mediastinal shift into the contralateral thorax is also apparent. (*B*) Essentially normal appearance of this child's chest radiograph shortly after right middle lobe resection. (*C*) Similar abnormalities in a 4-month-old girl with involvement of the left upper lobe, the most common site of congenital lobar emphysema.

geographic predilection. CCAM lesions are equally distributed between the left and right lobes, with bilateral disease being rare. Unilobar involvement is most common, with any lobe at risk, although there appears to be slight predilection for the lower lobes in most reports. Fortunately, multilobar disease tends to be unilateral, so that surgical resection can be achieved by pneumonectomy if necessary. A maternal history of polyhydramnios is common, and preterm delivery occurs in as many as half of these infants. Therefore, the many problems of preterm delivery may be superimposed. Depending on the institutional

environment, half or more of these lesions are detected and referred based on prenatal ultrasonography findings. As outlined earlier, about one third of newborns with CCAM develop symptoms of tachypnea, dyspnea, cyanosis, or overt respiratory insufficiency in the first month of life. The remainder present with the consequences of pulmonary infection—half of these within the first year of life and the remainder at periods up to and including adulthood. Later presentations include recurrent or persistent pneumonia, lung abscess, pneumothorax, reactive airway disease, and failure to thrive, but not usually progressive

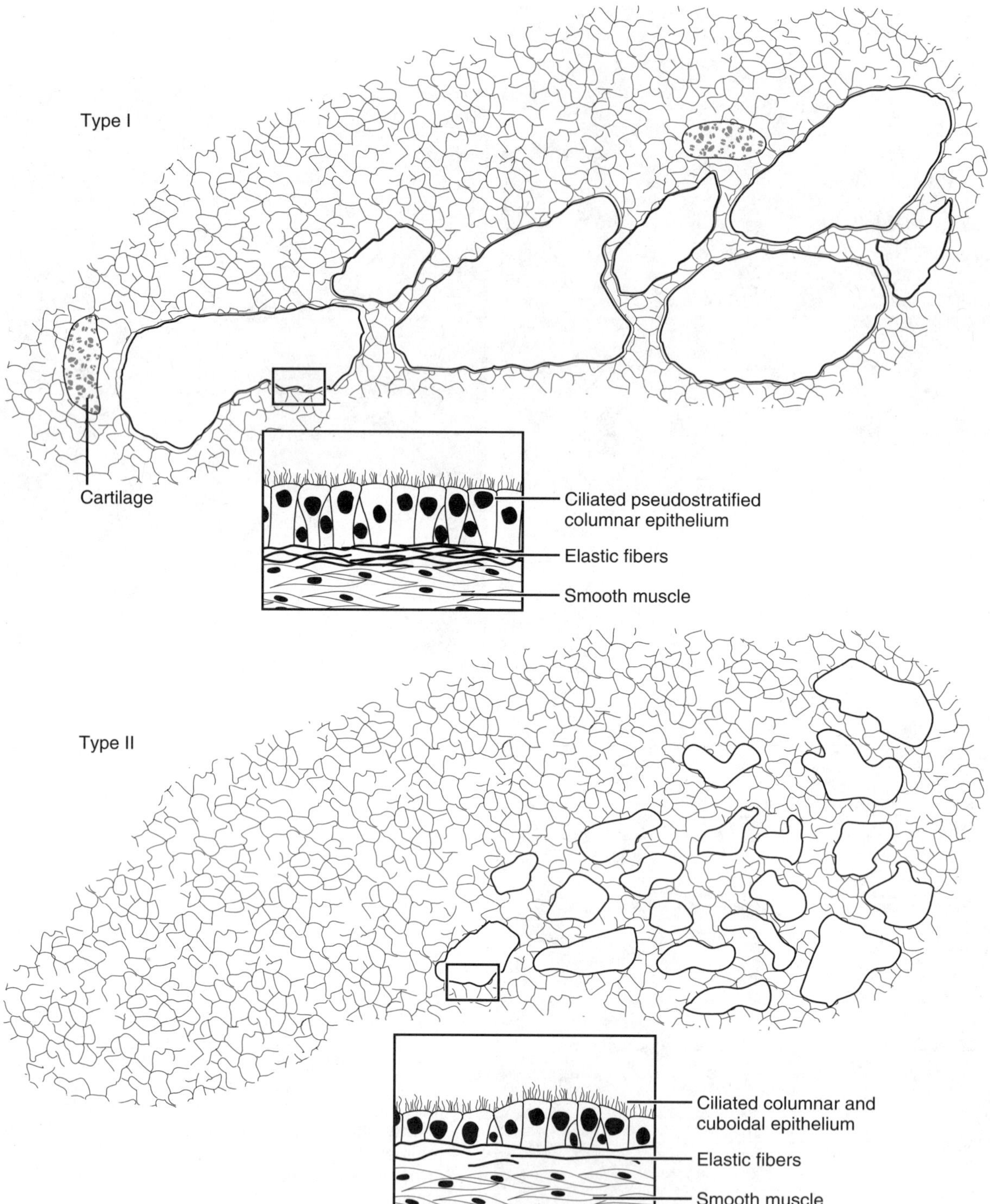

FIG. 57-7. Congenital cystic adenomatoid malformation (CCAM) types. Type I lesions are composed of irregular cysts larger than 2 cm in diameter; elastic tissue is regularly present; and cartilage is present in 10% of lesions. The epithelium is ciliated, pseudostratified columnar epithelium. Relatively normal alveolar structures are adjacent to or interspersed with these cysts. Type II lesions have more and smaller cysts, less than 1 cm in diameter. The epithelium is ciliated cuboidal or columnar; there is less elastic tissue and no cartilage. The lesions blend into relatively normal lung parenchyma with large alveolus-like structures. Type III lesions occupy the entire affected lobe, and despite the CCAM nomenclature, there are no cystic spaces. Rather, masses of cuboidal epithelium line alveolus-like structures where no gas exchange can occur. (After Stocker JT, Madewell JE, Drake RM. Congenital cystic adenomatoid malformation of the lung. Hum Pathol 1977;8:155) (*Figure continues.*)

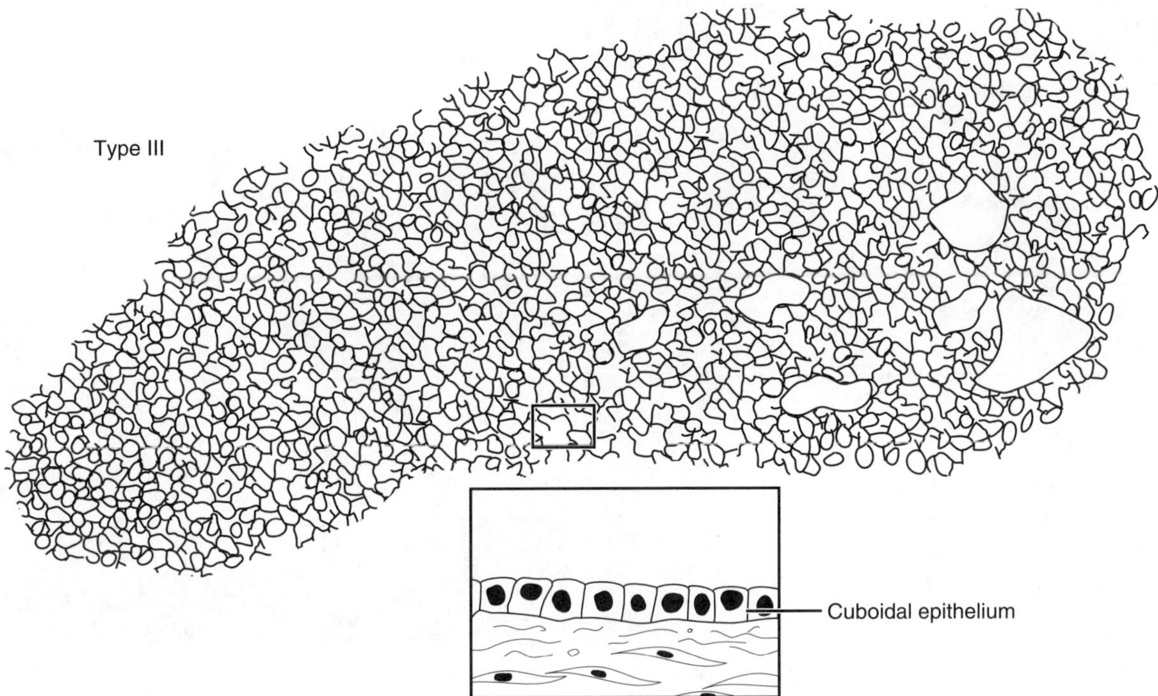

FIG. 57-7. *Continued.*

respiratory insufficiency in older patients. Associated anomalies, including congenital heart disease, pectus excavatum, renal agenesis, skeletal anomalies, jejunal atresia, and others, have been reported, but the incidence is variable and may be no more than for the normal population.[9,10]

The issues related to prenatal diagnosis have been discussed. The postnatal evaluation of infants with nonspecific respiratory symptoms is best begun with a plain chest radiograph. In infants with CCAM, however, the radiographic findings are variable. Images obtained shortly after birth may show retained fetal lung

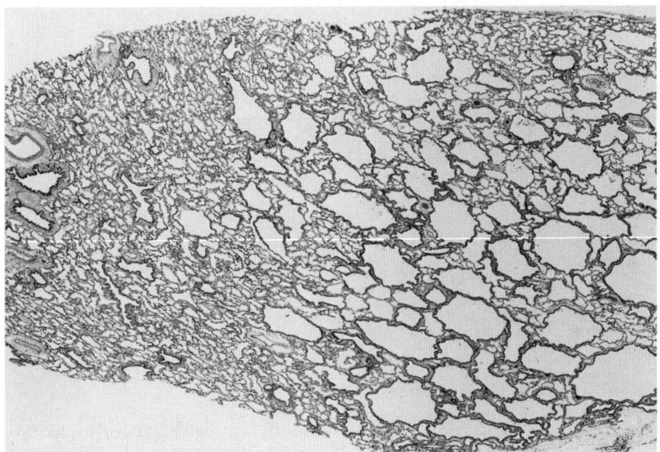

FIG. 57-8. Congenital cystic adenomatoid malformation type II. Numerous small cysts are separated by alveolar-like spaces and merge with normal parenchyma. (Hematoxylin–eosin, ×12.) (Courtesy of Kay Washington, MD, Duke University Medical Center, Durham, NC)

fluid within the lesion, and if it is a microcystic or solid lesion, this may not change with time. Macrocystic lesions tend to become aerated with ventilation, and the chest radiograph then has an area of air-filled cysts within the thorax. In infants, this appearance must be distinguished from congenital diaphragmatic hernia, particularly when the left side is involved. Although plain films alone are generally adequate, passage of a nasogastric tube into the stomach or an upper or lower gastrointestinal tract contrast study showing intrathoracic intestine may be helpful in distinguishing the two. Because the surgical approach is generally different for these two lesions, prospective distinction is important. Mediastinal displacement, compression of adjacent normal lung, and flattening of the intact ipsilateral diaphragm are also typical plain chest radiograph findings for CCAM. In older children with infectious complications, the findings are often less clear, and either CT with intravenous contrast or MR evaluation is necessary to provide definitive anatomic detail of the lesion (Fig. 57-9). Angiography has little or no role in the diagnosis of CCAM and other thoracic mass lesions in the modern environment because it has demonstrable risks and the information derived is available by less invasive means.

The principal goal of treatment for CCAM is to resect the area of abnormal lung promptly. Some carefully selected fetuses may benefit from prenatal intervention; however, concerns remain about the natural history of the lesions, appropriate patient selection, and the risk of preterm labor. Experience with this approach is limited and is insufficient to be definitive. Generally, an in utero diagnosis and macrocystic disease are indications for sequential observation and delivery in a tertiary care environment where prompt thoracotomy and state-of-the-art critical care support are available. For the infant, treatment most often requires a thoracotomy with lobectomy. This can be life-

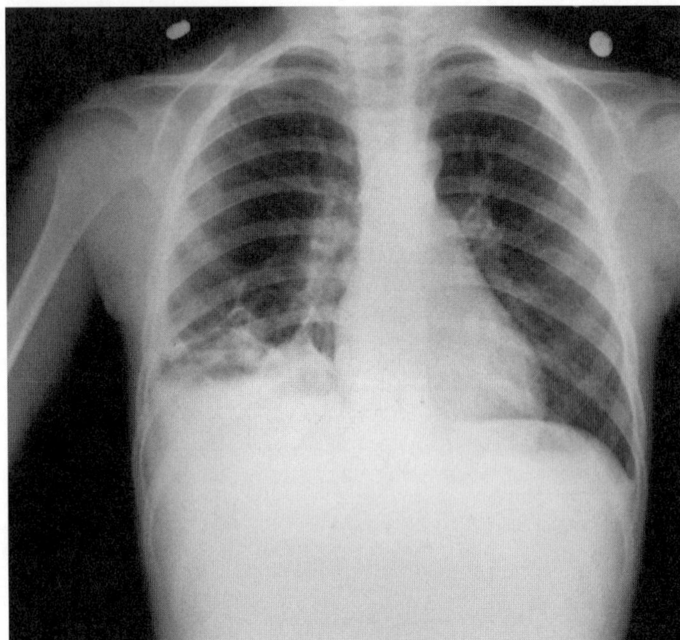

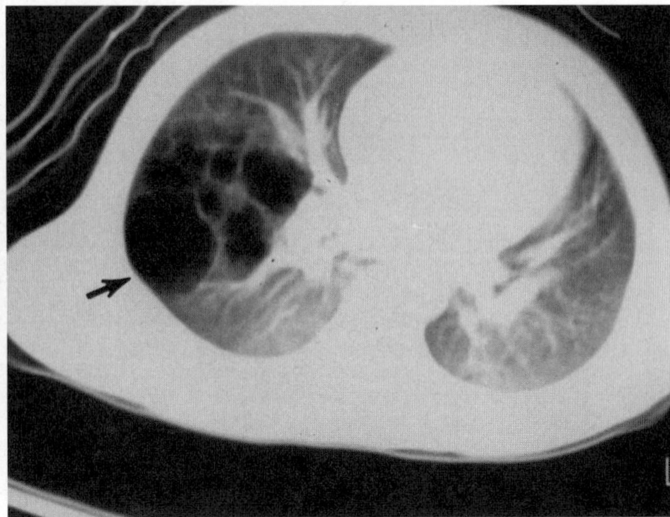

FIG. 57-9. (*A*) Plain chest radiograph of a 9-year-old child who presented with fever, pleuritic chest pain, and cough. The lesion is an infected cystic adenomatoid malformation of the right lower lobe. (*B*) The lesion in *A* is shown on chest CT scan after treatment with antibiotics and before surgical resection of the right lower lobe (Coran AG, Oldham KT. The pediatric thorax. In: Greenfield LJ, Mulholland MW, Oldham KT, et al. Surgery: scientific principles and practice. Philadelphia, JB Lippincott, 1993:813)

saving in critically ill newborns with mediastinal shift and normal lung compression from a ventilated and expanding CCAM. Figure 57-10 demonstrates the relative size of a right lower lobe CCAM deliberately delivered from the thorax of an infant in extremis. The normal adjacent lung was allowed to ventilate, providing immediate physiologic relief before lobar resection. Because of the long-term risk of infectious complications, surgical resection is considered standard in older patients and in patients without symptoms. It is appropriate in the setting of an acute infectious process to treat a child preoperatively with systemic antibiotics to reduce acute inflammation. Long-term medical management, however, is not appropriate. At least 14 reports of malignancy occurring within these and other congenital cystic lung lesions add further rationale for surgical resection.[27–29] Pulmonary blastoma and rhabdomyosarcoma are the most common of these.

Pneumonectomy is required in as many as 15% to 20% of affected patients to achieve complete resection of a complex or multilobar CCAM.[9,10,13] For the limited and well-demarcated CCAM, formal segmental resection has been reported, but data suggest that operative morbidity may be greater with this approach, and there is little or no apparent long-term benefit.

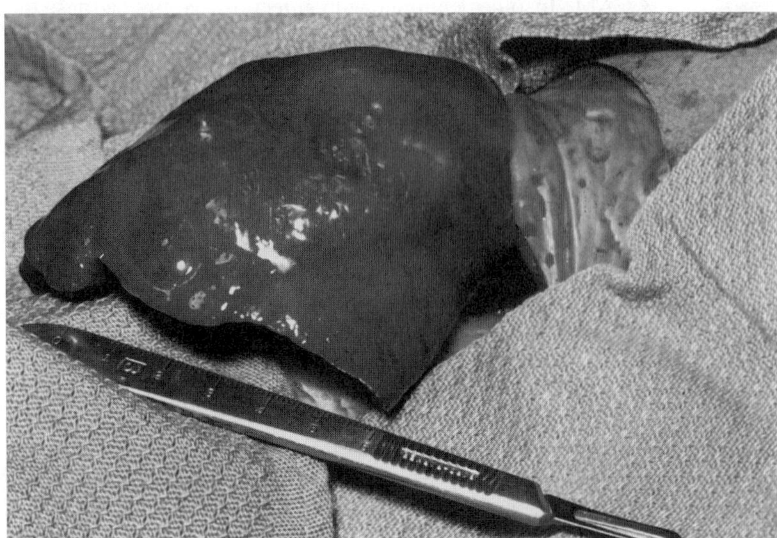

FIG. 57-10. Right lower lobe cystic adenomatoid malformation that led to acute respiratory distress in a neonate. The size of the lobe after delivery from the thorax is much larger than the volume of the infant thoracic cavity. Delivery of such a space-occupying mass lesion from the thorax can lead to profound and immediate physiologic relief.

Outcome after surgical resection of CCAM is generally good. Adzick and colleagues[23] reported survival in four of six selected fetuses with microcystic CCAM after in utero thoracotomy and lobectomy between 24 and 32 weeks' gestation. For infants who are found at birth to have CCAM, the survival probability with resection is between 80% and 100% in most reports.[9,10,13] When it occurs, death is usually the result of respiratory failure in newborns. In older children with infectious presentations, death is rare. The potential complications of neonatal lobectomy for CCAM are not different than for other similar lesions. Although many complications are possible, the overall incidence is less than 10%, and most can be readily managed. Most children have excellent long-term pulmonary function after lobectomy for CCAM. The experience after pneumonectomy is more limited and perhaps less optimistic given the larger extent of the resected lung (see discussion of outcomes after lung resection at the end of this chapter).

Pulmonary Sequestration

Pulmonary sequestration is a form of bronchopulmonary–foregut malformation that gives rise to a mass of lung tissue that is not normally related to the functional lung. In particular, the sequestration can reside outside of the lung and be invested with its own visceral pleura (extralobar sequestration; Fig. 57-11), or it can be located within the visceral pleura of the normal lung (intralobar sequestration).[30,31] The incidence of the two forms is roughly equal. In either case, a sequestration does not communicate with the tracheobronchial tree through a normal bronchus, and the blood supply is derived from one or more anomalous systemic arteries, most often rising from the descending thoracic aorta. The arterial blood supply for an extralobar sequestration, however, is derived from an infradiaphragmatic source in up to 20% of patients.[9,10,30–32] Venous

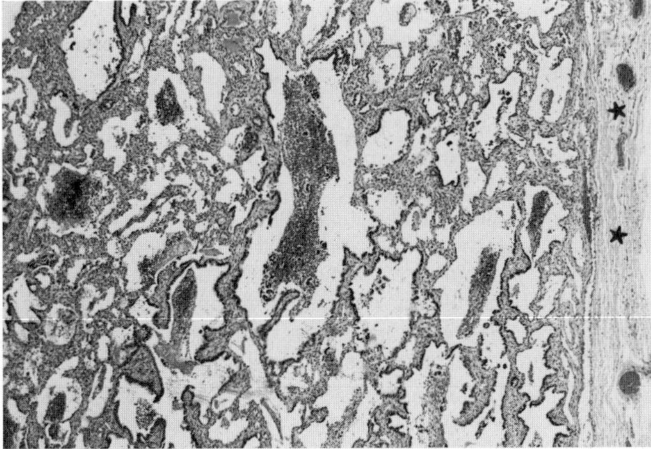

FIG. 57-11. Extralobar sequestration. This lesion was resected from the left lower thorax. It was invested in a separate visceral pleura (*asterisks*) with arterial blood supply from the descending thoracic aorta. The chest radiograph is shown in Figure 57-12. Microscopically, this lesion consists of uniformly dilated bronchioles and alveoli. (×40.) (Courtesy of Kay Washington, MD, Duke University Medical Center, Durham, NC)

drainage can be through either the appropriate pulmonary vein, which is typical for intralobar sequestration, or the azygous system, which is typical for extralobar sequestration. Because of the foregut derivation, occasional communication with the esophagus or stomach is found. An extralobar sequestration may be located within the diaphragm or even in a subdiaphragmatic position.

Many anatomic variations occur with regard to location, the relation to the normal lung, and the systemic arterial blood supply. Conflicting theories of embryogenesis have been offered by way of explanation, distinguishing between disordered budding of the normal tracheobronchial tree and accessory budding from the primitive foregut. The developmental events remain unknown, but the spectrum of bronchopulmonary foregut malformations is broad. The surgeon who treats these lesions simply must be prepared for variations in the blood supply and relations to the lungs and esophagus. The most important technical concern here is the need to identify the arterial blood supply. Infradiaphragmatic arteries to a pulmonary sequestration are typically elastic and possibly atherosclerotic vessels found within the inferior pulmonary ligament. These require precise surgical control to avoid retraction below the diaphragm and occult intraoperative hemorrhage. Communication between the esophagus or stomach and a pulmonary sequestration occurs in about 10% of patients and must be specifically sought, either intraoperatively or possibly preoperatively by contrast study of the gastrointestinal tract.

Prenatal diagnosis by maternal ultrasound screening is a common mode of discovery of pulmonary sequestrations, particularly for extralobar lesions.[33] Typically, a posterior mediastinal or infradiaphragmatic solid mass is observed. The anomalous arterial blood supply may be demonstrable with Doppler ultrasound techniques. Some of these fetuses are vulnerable to the same in utero risks seen with CCAM and congenital diaphragmatic hernia. A large intrathoracic mass lesion can lead to mediastinal compression, hydrops fetalis, and fetal demise. Although relatively uncommon, this is an important possibility to consider in the perinatal care of these fetuses and mothers.

Most extralobar sequestrations are diagnosed within the first months or years of life. About 10% to 15% of infants with congenital diaphragmatic hernias have one or more extralobar sequestrations, and this relation accounts for their frequent discovery.[30–32] Physiologic derangements in infants with pulmonary sequestration include hemorrhage, respiratory distress, feeding intolerance, and congestive heart failure.[30–32,34] The latter problem results from substantial arteriovenous shunting that can occur within the sequestered lobe, leading to high-output cardiac failure.

Intralobar pulmonary sequestrations generally present with infectious sequelae related to inadequate tracheobronchial drainage from the lesion or from the adjacent atelectatic lung. Recurrent or persistent pneumonia, lung abscess, and hemoptysis are among the more common presentations. Because these symptoms require temporal evolution, intralobar sequestration usually presents in childhood or adult life, but not infancy. Half of patients with intralobar sequestrations present after the second decade of life.[35–38]

Pulmonary sequestrations are uncommon lesions but represent about 20% to 40% of the congenital lung bud anomalies in most reports.[9,10,13] The male predominance is as high as 3:1 in some reports, particularly for extralobar sequestration. No racial or geographic influence on incidence is known. Newborns

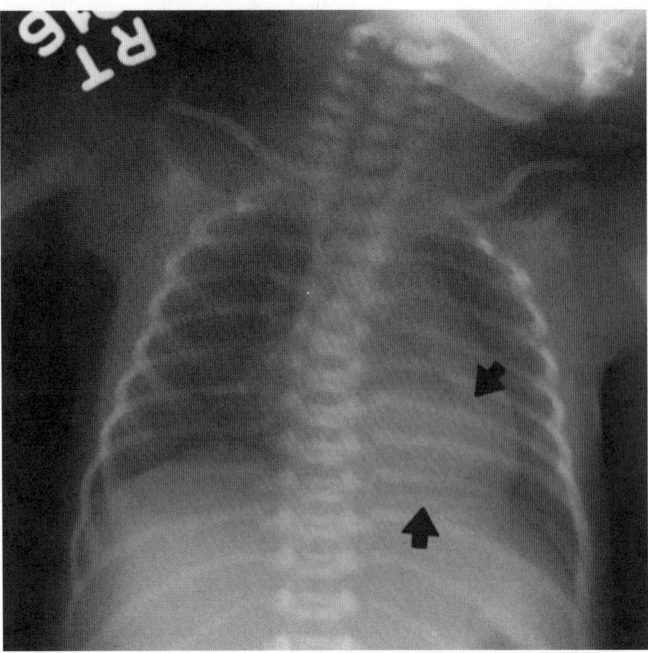

FIG. 57-12. Chest radiograph of an extralobar pulmonary sequestration (*arrows*) in the left lower thorax. The contour of the retrocardiac left hemidiaphragm has been obliterated. This was a newborn with no symptoms whose lesion was first noticed on prenatal maternal ultrasound.

have a broad spectrum of presentations. These include respiratory distress, pneumonia, feeding intolerance, congestive heart failure, and hemorrhage. Some pulmonary sequestrations are discovered as asymptomatic posterior mediastinal or abdominal masses. Intralobar sequestrations generally become infected given sufficient time. Other congenital anomalies are present in up to 40% of infants and children with extralobar sequestrations, while intralobar sequestration appears to occur in otherwise normal infants. Among the defects reported with extralobar sequestrations are ipsilateral diaphragmatic defects, chest wall and vertebral deformities, hindgut duplications, congenital heart disease, and a variety of others.[9,10,13]

The imaging evaluation of pulmonary sequestration is relatively straightforward. Prenatal ultrasound discovery is routine and has been mentioned. For newborns with respiratory symptoms, a plain chest radiograph is the standard initial investigation. Ninety percent of extralobar sequestrations appear as posterior mediastinal mass lesions in the left hemithorax. Most commonly, they appear as triangular retrocardiac density on the anteroposterior view (Fig. 57-12). On lateral view, they are posterior to the left lower lobe at or near the level of the diaphragm. Although many anatomic variations are possible, this appearance is nearly diagnostic on plain radiograph.

Sixty percent of intralobar sequestrations occur on the left, typically involving the posterior and basal segments of the left lower lobe[9,10,13] (Fig. 57-13). The appearance is generally that of lobar pneumonia and atelectasis. Air–fluid levels may be present if an abnormal communication with the tracheobronchial tree is patent. The intralobar mass, however, may be obscured and the plain films nondiagnostic. Although any lobe can be involved with a sequestration, upper lobe involvement

is present in only 10% to 15% of cases, and bilateral sequestrations are rare.

Particularly for intralobar sequestrations, additional imaging is required to establish the diagnosis. Ultrasound, contrast-enhanced CT (see Fig. 57-13*B*), and MR imaging (Fig. 57-14) all provide excellent anatomic detail, including identification of the systemic vascular blood supply.[39] Ultrasound has the potential advantage of Doppler blood flow assessment to identify the arterial supply. Particularly when prenatal ultrasound is the discovery tool, this provides gratifying, correlative data. Angiography, although emphasized in the past, is not required for either diagnosis or operative planning given the modern capabilities of less invasive imaging techniques.

Generally, resection is recommended for both intralobar and extralobar pulmonary sequestrations. Although extralobar sequestrations may be incidental autopsy findings in the elderly, diagnostic uncertainty about the nature of a posterior mediastinal mass, as well as low but real risks of hemorrhage, infection, and malignancy over a lifetime, must be weighed against the risks of a relatively straightforward surgical resection. Certainly, any symptomatic extralobar pulmonary sequestration requires resection. Simple excision is generally straightforward. By definition, the lesion can be resected without the need to disturb the normal lung. The needs to establish vascular control and to rule out foregut communication have been noted.

Patients with intralobar sequestrations are more likely to present with infection or hemorrhage; therefore, preoperative treatment with systemic antibiotics may be necessary. In the absence of this problem, prompt lobar resection is indicated. The principle for surgical management of an intralobar sequestration is to remove the affected area. In the face of acute or chronic inflammation, this generally requires a formal lobectomy. Although limited segmental resection is feasible in the absence of infection and when the surrounding lung parenchyma is normal, it is practical in only about 25% of patients. Most series report a predominance of lobectomies for intralobar sequestration.[12,13] As with extralobar sequestrations, attention must be directed to the systemic arterial blood supply because all the technical issues are similar for intralobar and extralobar lesions. Although standard practice has been thoracotomy and appropriate resection, limited experience with thoracoscopic resection of extralobar sequestrations has been successful, and this approach appears to be appropriate in selected patients.

As with other pulmonary resections in a modern pediatric surgical environment, the survival rate approaches 100% for pulmonary sequestration in the absence of other medical problems. Likewise, the complications and postoperative morbidity are generally minimal. In particular, extralobar resections do not involve removal of normal lung parenchyma, so these children can be expected to have normal pulmonary function and excellent functional outcomes. Reports of intraoperative exsanguination from the loss of control of the systemic arterial blood supply have received considerable attention in the literature historically. This is an important but straightforward technical concern that does not diminish the expectation for an excellent outcome today.

Bronchogenic Cysts and Lung Cysts

A developmental cyst arising from the trachea or a bronchus is referred to as a *bronchogenic cyst*. These account for about

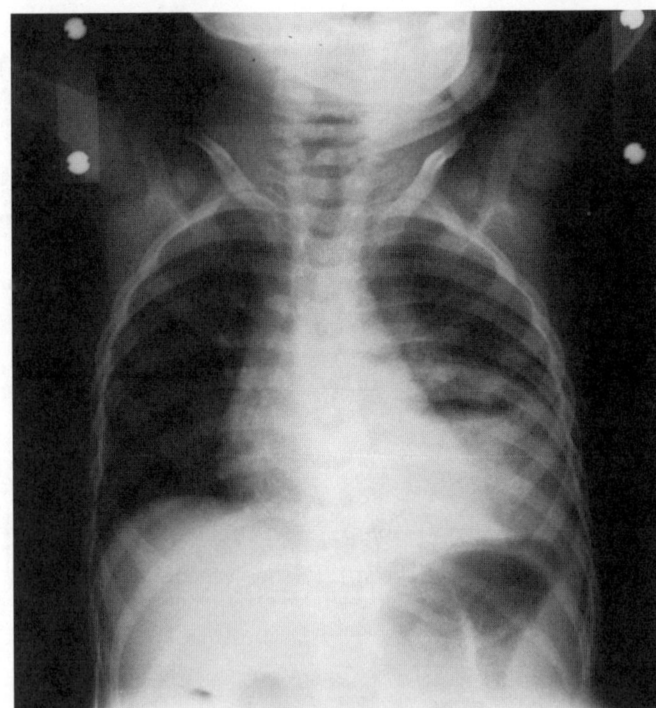

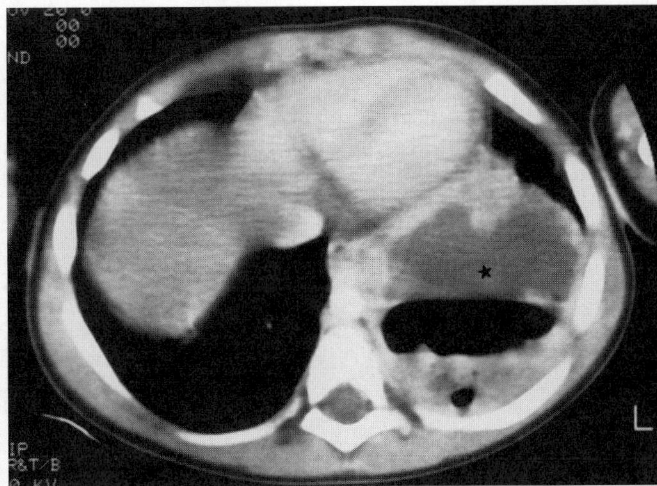

FIG. 57-13. (*A*) Plain chest radiograph of a child with fever and cough who has an infected intralobar sequestration of the left lower lobe. (*B*) CT scan of the same lesion (*asterisk*).

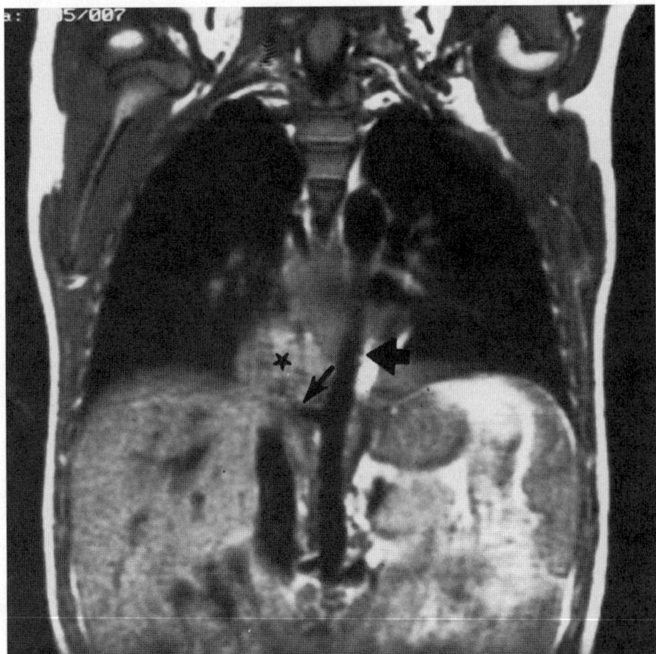

FIG. 57-14. MR image of a right lower lobe extralobar pulmonary sequestration (*asterisk*), with the descending aorta visualized (*thick arrow*) and clear demonstration of the systemic arterial blood supply to the sequestration (*thin arrow*). (Courtesy of George Bissett, MD, Duke University Medical Center, Durham, NC)

20% to 30% of congenital bronchopulmonary–foregut cystic malformations.[12,13] Potential locations include the cervical or thoracic trachea, the hilar bronchi, or the more distal intraparenchymal bronchi. It has been reported that about 70% of thoracic bronchogenic cysts are located within the lung parenchyma, and the remainder are in the mediastinum; but this distribution varies considerably among different reports.[8–10,13,40] Ectopic bronchogenic cysts, including those in paravertebral, paraesophageal, pericardial, subcarinal, and subcutaneous locations, have been reported.

Bronchogenic cysts are typically unilocular mucus-filled lesions arising from the posterior membranous portion of the airway. They do not usually communicate with the functional tracheobronchial tree. Many anatomic variations, however, have been described. By definition, the cyst has structural elements of the airway, including cartilage, smooth muscle, mucous glands, and respiratory epithelium. Likewise, these lesions have a normal bronchial arterial blood supply. The character of the epithelium depends on the site of origin; ciliated columnar, cuboidal, and squamous epithelium are all found within the tracheobronchial tree and therefore within these cysts (Fig. 57-15).

This section also considers cystic lung lesions that result from abnormal development of the more distal airways, alveoli, or pleural or lymphatic tissue. Even collectively, these true lung cysts are rare congenital lesions. They constitute a heterogeneous group of lung parenchymal cystic lesions with histologic features representative of their sites of origin. The spectrum is varied and can overlap with cysts that are bronchogenic in origin. Differentiation of the tissue of origin for simple lung cysts is principally of pathologic interest because the presentations are similar and clinical management is generally straightforward with a good outcome. One important exception is when the developmental abnormality is lymphatic in origin. The result

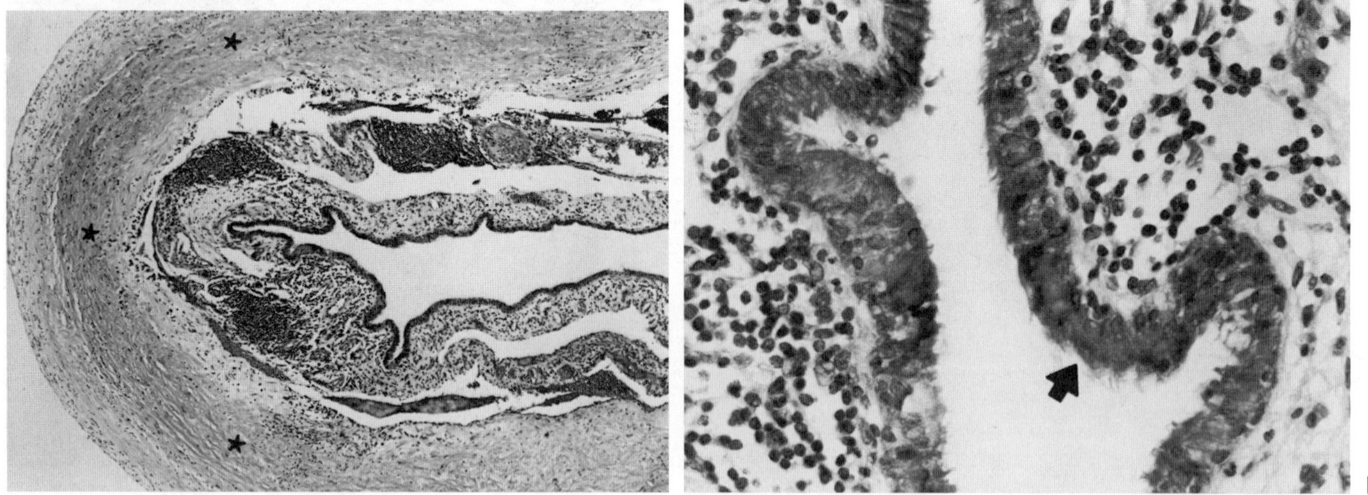

FIG. 57-15. (*A*) Bronchogenic cyst. The wall of this bronchogenic cyst consists of dense fibrous tissue (*asterisks*). Cartilage and seromucinous glands were also present (not shown). (Masson trichrome, ×52.) (*B*) The cyst is lined by ciliated pseudostratified columnar epithelium (*arrow*). (Masson trichrome, ×400.) (Courtesy of Kay Washington, MD, Duke University Medical Center, Durham, NC)

then may be pulmonary lymphangiectasis. This is typically characterized by diffuse bilateral pulmonary cystic disease, and the outcome is often lethal because resection is not feasible.

The discussion of bronchogenic and other lung cysts is consolidated because of the overlap in their clinical presentations and the similarity in their embryologic origins. As with other congenital cystic lung lesions, physiologic injury from bronchogenic and lung cysts generally results from either compression of adjacent hollow viscera, such as the airway or esophagus (Fig. 57-16), or inadequate drainage of secretions with secondary infection. Malignancies have been reported within these lesions as well; both rhabdomyosarcoma and bronchogenic carcinoma have been described.[27–29] In newborns with cysts adjacent to the trachea or proximal airways, respiratory distress or air-trapping with lobar emphysema are important and potentially life-threatening problems. More distal lesions may be asymptomatic or may present with evidence of infection. The latter usually occur in older children because time is necessary for the development of infection. Clinical presentations range from no symptoms to life-threatening respiratory distress, although the latter is rare. Infection and nonspecific respiratory symptoms, such as cough, dyspnea, tachypnea, wheezing, or chest pain, are typical. The usual chest radiographic appearance of a bronchogenic cyst is that of a smooth, roughly spherical, paratracheal, or hilar solid mass without calcification (Fig. 57-17). Displacement of the adjacent airway and distal air-trapping are relatively frequent, even in patients without symptoms. Air–fluid levels suggest communication with the tracheobronchial tree or foregut, and this is a particularly likely finding in the presence of acute infection.

True lung cysts can occur anywhere. They are typically single, unilocular lesions. One example of a small subpleural lung cyst is shown in Figure 57-18. These can be large, however, and difficult to distinguish from a lung abscess or macrocytic CCAM on chest radiograph. Discovery of a bronchogenic or true lung cyst after slow or incomplete radiographic resolution of acute pneumonia also has been well described. As with other

thoracic mass lesions, CT and MR imaging provide both diagnostic accuracy and excellent definition of the anatomic relations of these lesions (see Figs. 57-17 and 57-18). In the patient with dysphagia and a paraesophageal bronchogenic cyst, a contrast esophagogram may demonstrate extrinsic compression at

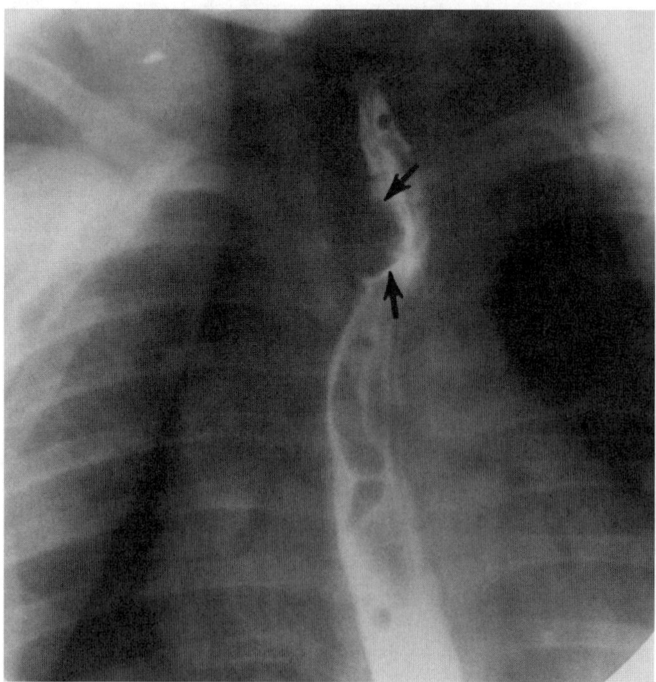

FIG. 57-16. Esophogram demonstrating extrinsic compression (*arrows*) from a foregut-derived cystic lesion that caused symptomatic tracheal obstruction in an infant. At time of excision, this lesion had both esophageal and tracheal elements, consistent with a shared embryologic origin. Simple excision relieved the symptoms.

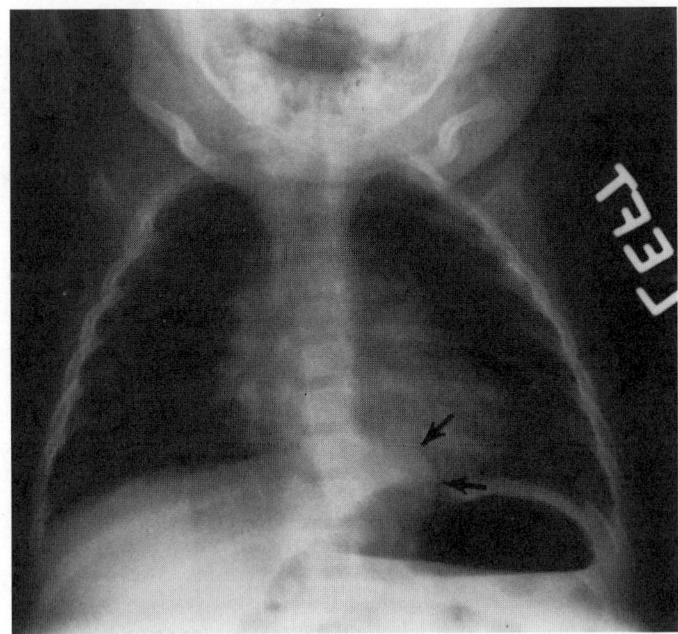

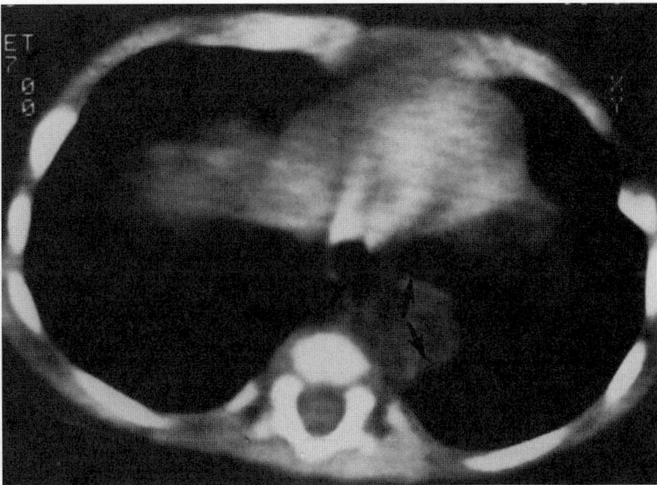

FIG. 57-17. (*A*) Plain chest radiograph of a child with a mediastinal bronchogenic cyst (*arrows*). (*B*) CT of the same lesion (*arrows*). (Courtesy of Don Frush, MD, Duke University Medical Center, Durham, NC)

the site of the lesion (see Fig. 57-16). Likewise, endoscopic examination of the tracheobronchial tree or esophagus may show extrinsic compression. Neither of the latter two examinations is specific for a bronchogenic cyst, but other possibilities are relatively few. Notable among these are mediastinal lymphadenopathy or tumor, particularly lymphoma.

Resection of the cystic abnormality is standard treatment for virtually all bronchogenic and lung cysts, even if asymptomatic. The risk of infection appears to be high, although no prospective data exist. Generally, simple local resection is easily accomplished and definitive. Occasionally, however, limited parenchymal lung resection or even lobectomy may be required. Pre-

operative treatment of pneumonia is helpful in diminishing perioperative morbidity and in minimizing the magnitude of parenchymal resection. Preservation of adjacent normal parenchyma is an important operative principle. Wedge resection, segmentectomy, and lobectomy have all been reported for individual circumstances. As with many other thoracic lesions, thoracoscopic resection of bronchogenic and lung cysts is feasible for selected patients. It is essential to establish precise anatomic relations preoperatively if a thoracoscopic approach is planned because bronchogenic cysts are often beneath the mediastinal pleura and therefore require pleural incision and mediastinal exploration to localize the lesion. Mediastinal exploration is

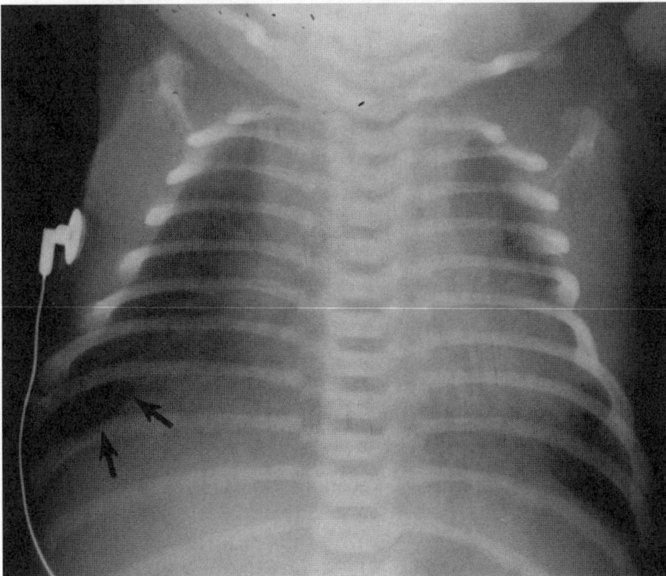

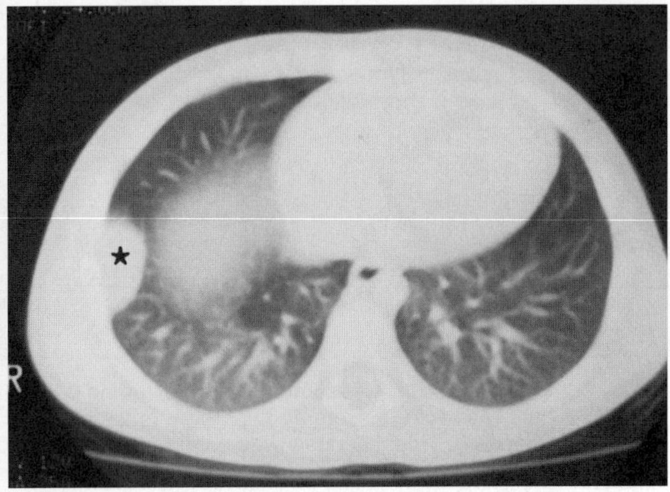

FIG. 57-18. (*A*) Small peripheral true congenital lung cyst that was air filled in the neonatal period (*arrows*). (*B*) CT appearance (*asterisk*) at 5 years of age, when the lesion was fluid filled and the child presented with pleuritic chest pain on the right. Surgical excision was curative.

important for infants with lobar emphysema because an occult bronchogenic cyst may be responsible, and relief is occasionally possible without lobar lung resection.

The long-term outcome for infants and children with bronchogenic and true lung cysts is excellent because they generally do not require sacrifice of significant normal lung parenchyma. Likewise, perioperative morbidity is low and mortality rare, particularly for mediastinal lesions without tracheobronchial communication. If lung resection is required, outcome is not different than for patients with other lung lesions, such as lobar emphysema or CCAM, and these outcomes are presented later in detail.

Pulmonary Agenesis, Aplasia, and Hypoplasia

Pulmonary Agenesis

Pulmonary agenesis refers to the unilateral or bilateral absence of the entire lung and bronchial tree. Bilateral pulmonary agenesis is rare enough to be reportable and is inconsistent with survival. Unilateral pulmonary agenesis is rare, with several hundred cases reported in the world literature, and is considered briefly.[10,41] Involvement of the right and left sides is roughly equal, and no gender-related propensity is apparent. The pathogenesis is unknown, although it is presumed that agenesis represents a failure of bronchial budding from the trachea during early organogenesis. Associated anomalies are present in more than half of patients.[42] Congenital abnormalities of the heart and the great vessels; esophageal abnormalities, including tracheoesophageal fistula; skeletal anomalies; genitourinary malformations; imperforate anus; cleft palate; asplenia; and many others have been reported.[10,42,43] For unknown reasons, these anomalies are more commonly associated with right-sided agenesis; hence, left-sided involvement carries a considerably better long-term prognosis. Children with pulmonary agenesis present in one of three categories: (1) patients without symptoms for whom the finding is incidental, (2) patients with specific respiratory symptoms, or (3) patients with associated problems who come to medical attention. Among the latter, infants with congenital heart disease or tracheoesophageal fistula are notable and can present difficult joint management issues (Fig. 57-19). Respiratory symptoms may include an entire spectrum of nonspecific complaints. Dyspnea, tachypnea, cyanosis, exercise intolerance, wheezing, cough, and failure to thrive are among these. Recurrent pneumonia and bronchitis are the most common clinical problems. The physiologic basis for this vulnerability to pulmonary infection is unclear, although it has been suggested that the sole remaining bronchus is functionally abnormal and thus unable to clear secretions effectively. Regardless, infection in the single lung must always be considered a life-threatening problem, and aggressive nonoperative management is indicated.

The diagnosis of unilateral pulmonary agenesis is rarely obtained by history and physical examination alone. In older children, asymmetry of the chest or scoliosis may be present, although these are not often apparent in infants. Because the ipsilateral hemithorax is occupied by herniated contralateral lung and the heart, absent or diminished breath sounds and shifted heart sounds are predictable physical findings. These are relatively insensitive and nonspecific findings.

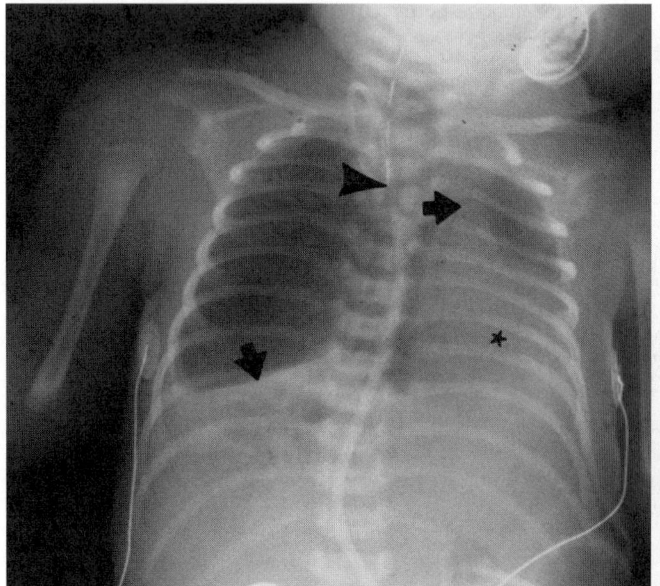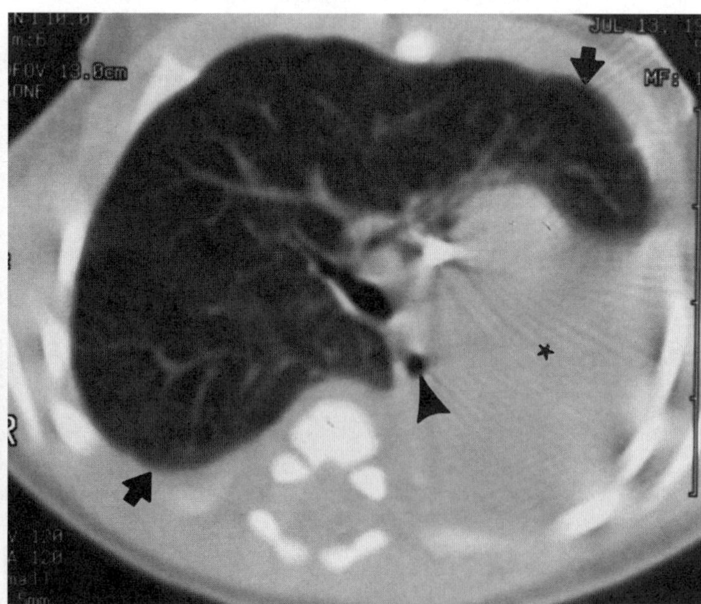

FIG. 57-19. (*A*) Chest radiograph illustrating unilateral left pulmonary agenesis. The right lung is overinflated, and the ipsilateral diaphragm is flattened (*thick arrows*). The mediastinum is shifted to the left (*asterisk*). This diagnosis was confirmed endoscopically through the absence of a left main-stem bronchus. A confounding issue here is the presence of esophageal atresia with a distal tracheal esophageal fistula. On this radiograph, the nasoesophageal tube is positioned at the distal end of the proximal esophageal pouch (*arrowhead*). (*B*) CT scan of the chest for this lesion. The normal right lung is overinflated (*arrow*), with shift of the heart into the left hemithorax (*asterisk*). The distal esophageal fistula is visible here as well (*arrowhead*).

A plain chest radiograph is abnormal but generally not definitive. The diagnosis is most simply confirmed by bronchoscopy. A normal trachea and contralateral main-stem bronchus with complete absence of the ipsilateral bronchus is diagnostic. CT, ultrasound, and MR imaging may be helpful as well, although none of these is routinely required. Figure 57-19 illustrates both plain chest radiographic and CT findings in an infant with unilateral pulmonary agenesis. In children with congenital heart disease, angiography or echocardiography shows complete absence of the ipsilateral pulmonary artery, and this too is pathognomonic. Contrast bronchography has been abandoned for this diagnosis because it has substantial risks to the single normal lung and is essentially unnecessary with modern imaging and endoscopic techniques.

Standard treatment for unilateral pulmonary agenesis consists of nonoperative respiratory support, particularly aggressive antibiotic treatment for recurrent infections. Lung transplantation has not been reported for this indication. The major surgical issues relate to the management of associated anomalies. The principles are to limit operative interventions to those that are physiologically essential and to time anesthesia for occasions when maximal lung function can be anticipated. Intrathoracic procedures that involve compression of the single lung, such as tracheoesophageal fistula repair, are particularly hazardous, although they can be accomplished by a coordinated and experienced surgical team without cardiopulmonary bypass.

Historically, about one half to one third of children with unilateral pulmonary agenesis failed to survive beyond the first 5 years of life.[10,41] Most of this mortality is related to perinatal death, problems of associated anomalies, or recurrent pulmonary infections. In recent years, the prognosis for these patients appears to be improving.

Pulmonary Aplasia and Hypoplasia

Pulmonary aplasia results from the interrupted development of the normal bronchial tree with either absence of or reduction in the number of normal alveoli. Pulmonary hypoplasia refers to the reduction in size of an entire lung and its individual components. Although these lesions generally arise for different reasons, the former as a primary defect in organogenesis and the latter secondary to extrinsic compression from an intrathoracic mass lesion, they are physiologically similar and are therefore presented jointly here. Although primary pulmonary hypoplasia does occur spontaneously (Fig. 57-20), this problem is more often the result of lesions such as congenital diaphragmatic hernia or CCAM, which limit alveolar development in utero. These children present with newborn pulmonary hypertension, persistent fetal circulation, and respiratory failure. These physiologic problems and their treatment are covered in detail in Chapter 54 and are not repeated here.

Several forms of congenital thoracic dystrophy produce acute or chronic asphyxiation related to pulmonary hypoplasia. All are rare; Jeune thoracic dystrophy is the least rare.[44] The physiologic problem, pulmonary hypoplasia, results from in utero restriction of lung development by an abnormal chest wall. Most affected infants have many other problems and do not survive. The only circumstance in which surgical intervention appears rational is in potentially nonlethal forms of the disease. In this circumstance, procedures designed to enlarge the thorax have been attempted. Median sternotomy and several individualized forms of thoracoplasty have been described. Insufficient data are available for any meaningful clinical analysis of these approaches.

ACQUIRED LUNG DISEASE

Infectious and inflammatory conditions of the lung share certain physiologic and morphologic features. It has become apparent that many of the humoral and cellular events which regulate acute lung injury are endogenous components of the host inflammatory response. Although this response is an essential component of the normal host defense system, extraordinary stimuli that result in exuberant systemic activation generate a variety of end-organ injuries. The lungs appear to be uniquely vulnerable, and the interaction between host phagocytic cells and the pulmonary microvascular endothelial cell is fundamental. Whether the initial stimulus is barotrauma, oxygen toxicity, pneumonia, acid aspiration, sepsis, thermal injury, or some other proinflammatory stimulus, the inflammatory response is

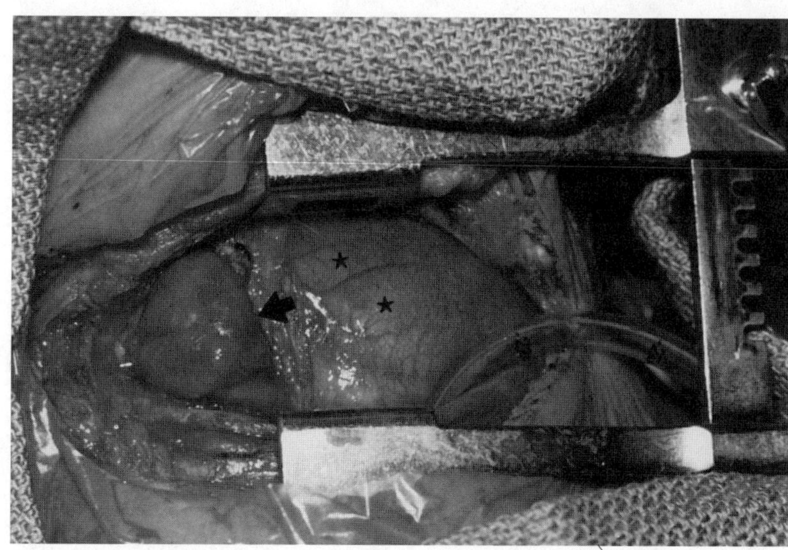

FIG. 57-20. Operative photograph showing primary pulmonary hypoplasia. This child had no underlying intrathoracic mass lesion. The diminutive right lung is seen (*arrow*) in contrast to the normal pericardium (*asterisks*).

similar. This response regulates the progression of both adult and pediatric acquired lung disease.

The acute phase of microvascular lung injury results from neutrophil (polymorphonuclear leukocyte [PMN]) induced alveolar endothelial cell injury, and this is regulated by both humoral and local factors. Oxygen-derived free radicals, proteases, cytokines, eicosanoids, endotoxin, complement-activation products, and probably platelet-activating factor and nitric oxide are involved as either signaling or effector molecules. Activated neutrophils are recruited to the pulmonary vascular bed by chemotactic factors, such as C5a and LTB$_4$. Carefully orchestrated PMN binding by a succession of adhesion receptors leads sequentially to neutrophil rolling, static binding, and then transvascular migration. The initial step in this process is dependent on selectin-carbohydrate binding (see Chap. 11). Selectin-mediated rolling of the neutrophil in the microvasculature allows sampling of the endothelial cell microenvironment until secondary, relatively firm integrin-dependent binding occurs. Data suggest that the unique phenotypic characteristics of the pulmonary capillary endothelial cell and its singular anatomic location are important factors in this process of targeting the lung microvasculature. It appears that tumor necrosis factor-α, interleukin-1, interleukin-6, and interleukin-8 have significant regulatory capabilities with regard to both adhesion-receptor and ligand expression during these events. Nitric oxide has been implicated as a regulator of PMN–endothelial cell binding. Adherence of the activated neutrophils to the endothelium creates a microenvironment in which PMN-derived oxidants, proteases, and cationic proteins are discharged under conditions that lead to acute endothelial cell injury. In particular, activated neutrophils release NADPH oxidase–derived oxygen metabolites and cytoplasmic proteases. In this microenvironment, there is relative isolation from circulating antioxidants and antiproteases. Endothelial cell injury results and is characterized by adenosine triphosphate depletion, cytoskeletal disassembly, and cell membrane disruption with cytolysis. Loss of microvascular integrity results, and pulmonary dysfunction follows[45] (Figs. 57-21 and 57-22). If the patient survives the acute injury, mononuclear cell infiltration, chronic inflammation, and repair follow. Repair after severe injury leads to collagen deposition and possibly chronic lung disease. This scenario is common to many if not all forms of inflammatory and infectious lung disease in children and adults.

Every physician who cares for neonatal patients is familiar with the infant respiratory distress syndrome. Although this process is principally the result of preterm delivery and pulmonary surfactant deficiency, a key additional contribution is derived from the type of inflammatory response and lung injury outlined earlier. This response is triggered by the need for oxygen therapy and positive-pressure mechanical ventilation, both potentially proinflammatory stimuli. Although the management of infant respiratory distress syndrome has improved substantially in the last decade with the introduction of exogenous surfactant replacement, acute microvascular lung injury still occurs with disturbing frequency in these infants. Depending on the clinical course, chronic lung injury and fibrosis can result. Clinicians refer to this result as *bronchopulmonary dysplasia;* it was described by Northway and colleagues[46] and is shown in Figures 57-23 and 57-24. Its occurrence and progression appear to be determined largely by the inflammatory response detailed earlier. Bronchopulmonary dysplasia is a common problem of substantial clinical importance.

The fundamental processes of lung injury and healing are the focus of enormous investigative efforts in many laboratories around the world. Our understanding of these events is evolving rapidly. A detailed review of the clinical management of the acute respiratory distress syndromes and bronchopulmonary dysplasia is beyond the scope of this text, but several excellent reviews are available.[47–50]

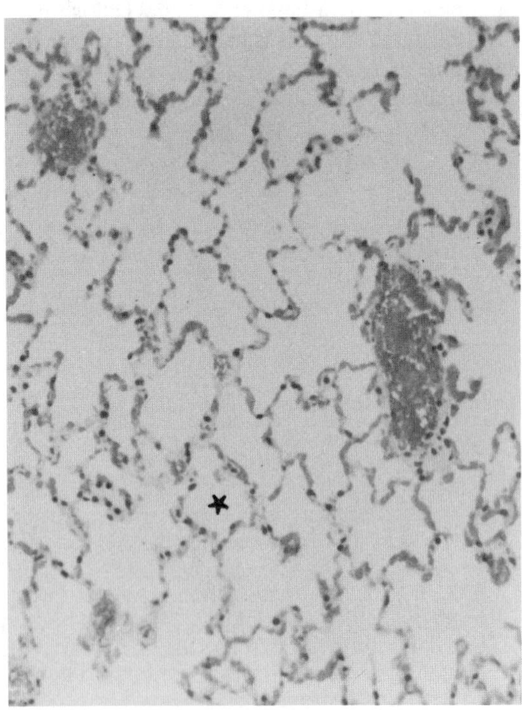
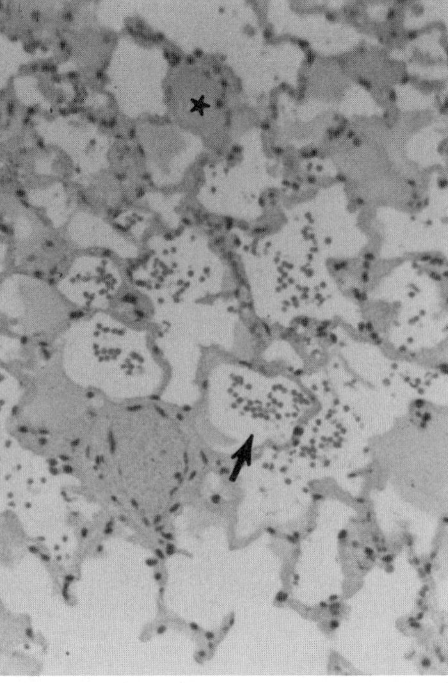

FIG. 57-21. Photomicrographs of lung after experimental microvascular injury. (*A*) Normal lung histology with normal alveoli (*asterisk*). (*B*) Neutrophil infiltration, alveolar edema (*asterisk*), intraalveolar hemorrhage (*arrow*), and acute lung injury. (Turnage RH, Guice KS, Oldham KT. Pulmonary microvascular injury following intestinal reperfusion. New Horizons 1994;2:463)

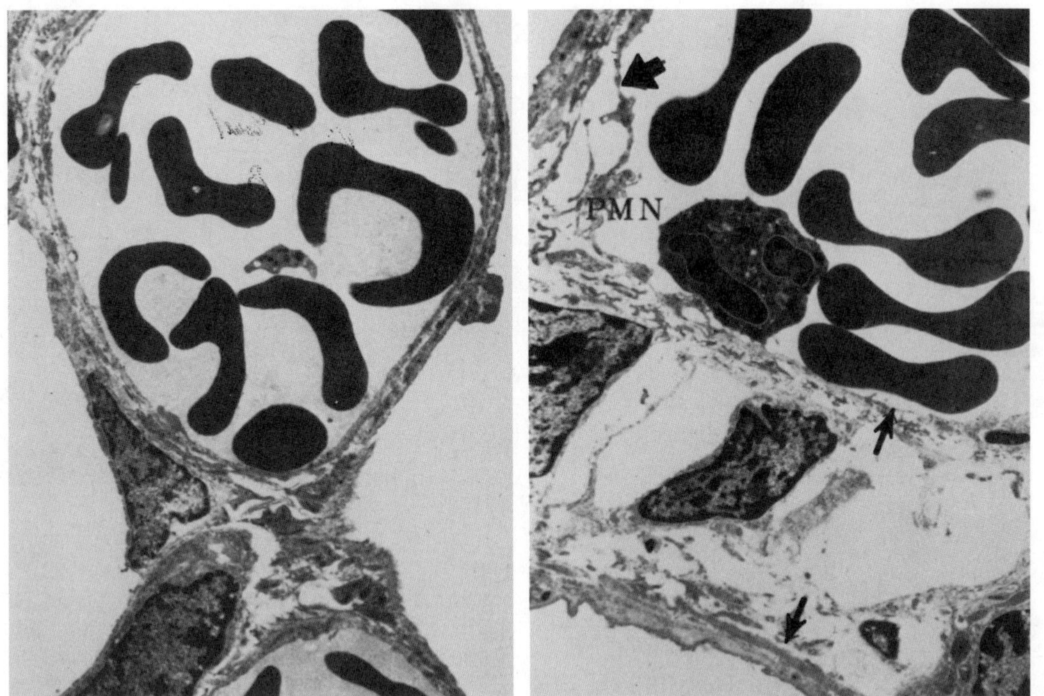

FIG. 57-22. Electron photomicrographs of lung after experimental microvascular injury. This figure is similar to Figure 57-21, except that magnification is greater. (*A*) Normal lung aveolar capillary. (*B*) Endothelial cell separation from the basement membrane (*thick arrow*), interstitial edema formation (*thin arrows*), and neutrophil (PMN) sequestration following experimental acute lung injury. Intraalveolar edema, hemorrhage, and fibrin deposition are also important features of this type of injury. (Turnage RH, Guice KS, Oldham KT. Pulmonary microvascular injury following intestinal reperfusion. New Horizons 1994;2:463)

Lung Abscess

Generally, a lung abscess develops when at least one of two fundamental problems exist: (1) a primary failure of host defenses is present, or (2) repeated aspiration of oral or intestinal bacteria into the tracheobronchial tree occurs. Some of the relevant deficiencies are provided in Table 57-1. As elsewhere, the abscess results from tissue necrosis related to pyogenic, toxin-producing bacterial organisms and to phagocytic cells that generate cytotoxic oxidants and proteases. Both cellular lung elements and the extracellular lung matrix are destroyed; tissue necrosis and cavitation within the lung parenchyma follow. The involved area is surrounded by atelectasis and pneumonia. A chronic lung abscess develops with varying degrees of circumferential fibrosis and may involve substantial destruction of parenchyma, usually in a lobar distribution. Typically, the abscess cavity communicates with the normal tracheobronchial tree, and this relation has important diagnostic and treatment implications.

Lung abscesses that form without underlying structural abnormalities are now uncommon in infants and children, although they are still potentially serious. In the modern medical environment, infants and children at particular risk are those who are iatrogenically immunocompromised.

As noted, the other major contributing factor to the development of lung abscess is aspiration of oral and gastric secretions. Although aspiration is a common event in infants and children, lung abscesses do not ordinarily follow. Certain groups of children, however, appear to be at particular risk. Among these are children with cerebral palsy or other causes of neurologic dysfunction who may be unable to protect the airway adequately. Repetitive, incompletely cleared aspiration events result. Institutionalized children with periodontal and dental disease and patients who have been treated with antibiotics for some other reason may be at high risk as well, presumably because of the presence of a larger than normal proximal reservoir of potentially pathogenic bacteria.

Lung abscesses are typically polymicrobial, with both anaerobic and aerobic bacteria. Since the 1970s, when anaerobic cultures became routine, oral anaerobic organisms have predominated in epidemiologic reviews of causative organisms. *Bacteroides* sp, group B β-hemolytic streptococci, *Escherichia coli, Pseudomonas* sp, *Proteus* sp, and *Aerobacter aerogenes* are all important and relatively frequent pathogens in this setting.[51,52] This is in contrast to *Staphylococcus aureus* and *Klebsiella pneumoniae,* which were the most common and important causes of lung abscesses in Western countries two decades ago. It remains important, however, to recognize that the latter organisms are both associated with substantial parenchymal lung destruction and are still important pathogens. Both require long-term and aggressive antibiotic treatment.

Secondary and even primary pulmonary infection with a variety of fungal and other organisms may lead to the development of a lung abscess as well. *Aspergillus*, *Actinomyces*, and *Nocardia* sp are among these pathogenic organisms. Cavitary tuberculosis was once an important risk factor for the development of

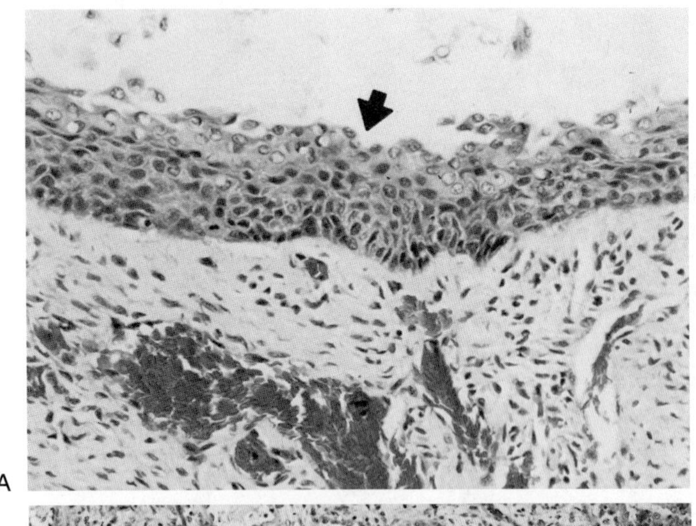

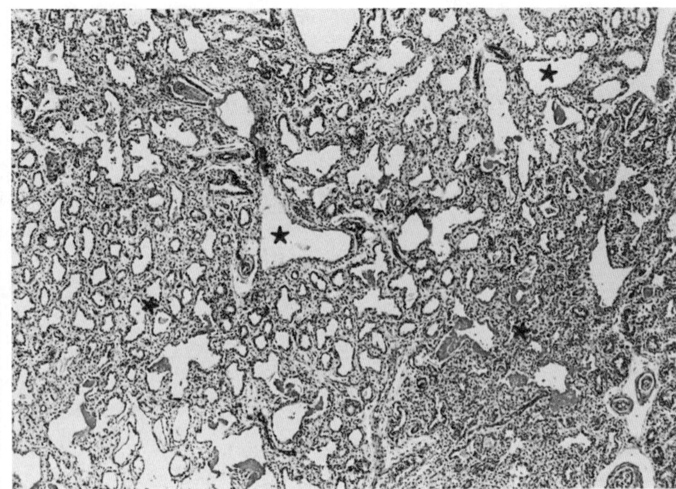

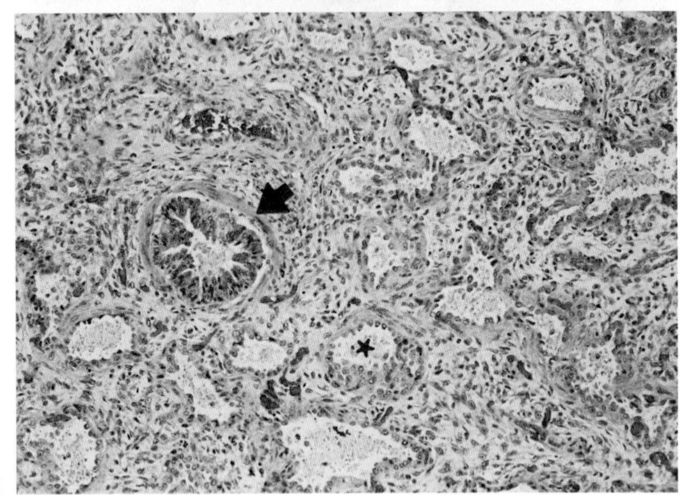

FIG. 57-23. Bronchopulmonary dysplasia (BPD). (*A*) Squamous metaplasia (*arrow*) of the trachea and larger bronchi can be seen in the reparative phase of BPD and may persist focally in long-standing BPD. The submucosa is fibrotic, with loss of submucosal glands. (Hematoxylin–eosin ×250.) (*B*) Variability in distention of airspaces (*asterisks*) is a feature of the reparative phase of BPD. The alveolar walls are thickened by edema and early fibrosis. (Hematoxylin–eosin, ×52.) (*C*) In later stages of BPD, as reparative changes give way to chronic changes, the alveolar walls contain more fibrous tissue and there is early smooth muscle hyperplasia in the wall of a bronchiole (*arrow*). The air spaces (*asterisk*) are lined by cuboidal cells. (Hematoxylin–eosin, ×100.) (Courtesy of Kay Washington, MD, Duke University Medical Center, Durham, NC)

secondary pyogenic lung abscesses in adults. Given the worldwide resurgence of tuberculosis, including that among children in the United States (see later), it may be worthwhile to recall this experience in coming years.

The clinical presentation of a patient with a lung abscess commonly includes systemic complaints, such as fever, chills, night sweats, anorexia, and weight loss. Nonspecific respiratory symptoms, such as coughing and wheezing, are frequent as well. More specific and alarming symptoms, such as a productive cough, fetid sputum, or hemoptysis, are later events associated with suppurative disease and cavitation. These latter findings in particular should lead to a prompt laboratory and imaging evaluation because the physical examination generally yields only nonspecific signs of pulmonary consolidation. The most important examination is generally a plain chest radiograph. A single cavity in a dependent location with an air–fluid level is classic (Fig. 57-25). Predictably, lung abscesses occur in areas of the lung that are dependent. Two thirds are found in the right lung; the superior segment of the lower lobe and the posterior segment of the upper lobe are most common.[51–52] An ambulatory patient is more likely to have involvement of basal segments of the lower lobes because these are dependent in the upright position. Areas of surrounding consolidation, pneumonia, and a thick fibrous wall are all typical but variable in appearance. It may be impossible to differentiate a lung ab-

scess from an infected cystic lung lesion on radiographs obtained at a single point in time. This is apparent in the radiographs in Figures 57-9, 57-12, and 57-25, each of which represents a different lesion. Generally, sequential films demonstrate resolution of pneumonia or an abscess, while congenital cystic lesions remain and become conspicuous. A pneumatocele may develop after treatment of necrotizing pneumonia or a lung abscess and may have a residual cystic appearance; however, these air-filled cavities typically do not have air–fluid levels (Fig. 57-26). In addition, patients generally improve clinically or have no symptoms after treatment when the typical air-filled cavity becomes apparent. CT and MR imaging are both excellent techniques for evaluating intrathoracic mass lesions such as a lung abscess; however, their routine use is not required, and their expense can be substantial.

A lung abscess, like any other abscess, requires prompt drainage and treatment with appropriate antibiotics. Drainage may occur spontaneously into the tracheobronchial tree, and this is a time at which large amounts of purulent, malodorous sputum may be expectorated. Postural drainage and appropriate suctioning are simple yet fundamental aspects of care at this time. Infants, small children, and others who cannot eliminate sputum effectively may require more aggressive endoscopic or surgical drainage.

Endoscopic drainage of a lung abscess into the tracheobron-

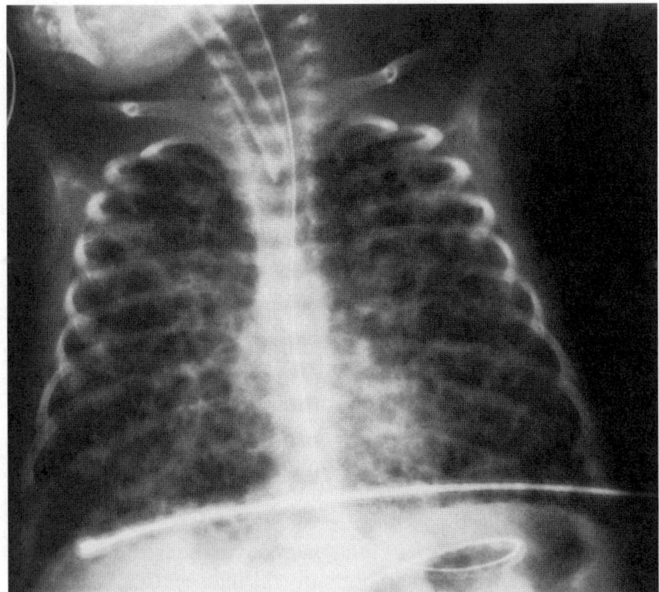

FIG. 57-24. Plain radiograph showing the appearance of an infant with severe bronchopulmonary dysplasia. This particular pattern is consistent with the histologic appearance of Figure 57-23B and C. There is variability in the distention of the air spaces, focal air-trapping, and fibrosis. (Courtesy of Herman Grossman, MD, Duke University Medical Center, Durham, NC)

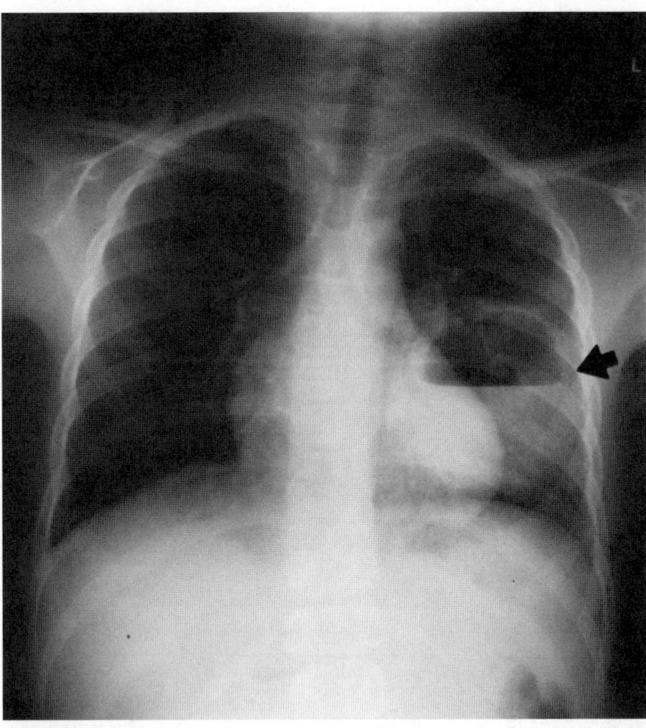

FIG. 57-25. Plain chest radiograph showing the classic appearance of a thick-walled pulmonary parenchymal abscess with an obvious air–fluid level (*arrow*). (Courtesy of Don Frush, MD, Duke University Medical Center, Durham, NC)

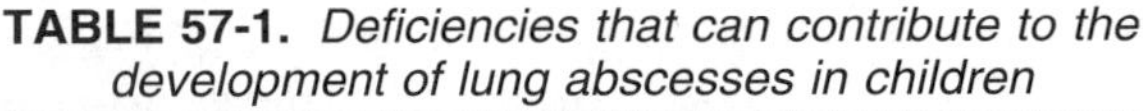

TABLE 57-1. *Deficiencies that can contribute to the development of lung abscesses in children*

INADEQUATE MECHANICAL CLEARANCE MECHANISMS

Structural abnormalities
  Retained endobronchial foreign body
  Tracheostomy
  Underlying cystic disease of the lung
Cystic fibrosis
α_1-Antitrypsin deficiency
Any cause of partial bronchial obstruction
Ineffective cough (neurologically impaired patients)
Immotile cilia (Kartagener syndrome)

INADEQUATE CELLULAR HOST DEFENSES

Transplantation, oncology, or other patients who are iatrogenically immunosuppressed by chemotherapy or antirejection regimens
Severe combined immunodeficiency syndrome
Chronic granulomatous disease
Other hereditary granulocyte deficiencies

INADEQUATE HUMORAL HOST DEFICIENCIES

Hereditary complement deficiencies
Agammaglobulinemia
Immunoglobulin A deficiency
Iatrogenic manipulation of humoral defenses (monoclonal antibodies, receptor antagonists, and other strategies to alter the humoral component of the inflammatory response are currently in preclinical trials)

chial tree can be achieved with a variety of needles, catheters, or other instruments passed through rigid or flexible instruments. If possible, this is preferred to other methods of surgical drainage. Intraoperative control of the airway is essential when endoscopic drainage of a lung abscess is done because the decompression of purulent material into an adjacent bronchus or the contralateral lung may be life-threatening if the abscess is sizable. The contralateral lung is best protected either by positioning the involved lung dependently or by selective intubation and balloon exclusion of the normal main-stem bronchus. A flexible endoscope has the advantage of better access to the peripheral airways, while a rigid bronchoscope allows the use of larger instruments and provides better visualization and control of the trachea and primary bronchi. The choice is best individualized. Most infants and children require general anesthesia for the initial endobronchial drainage procedure because of the absolute need for control of the airway. Fluoroscopy or ultrasound may provide valuable guidance in localizing the lesion intraoperatively if necessary. Subsequent drainage or aspiration procedures may be needed, depending on the clinical response.

Transpleural diagnostic aspiration and both open and closed external drainage are all described and appropriate for selected high-risk patients. The risks of pleural contamination and empyema, however, make these approaches desirable only in circumstances in which the abscess is peripheral in location and chronic enough that the visceral and parietal pleura are adherent. These approaches are best reserved for specific indications in complex abscesses after failure of initial drainage and antibiotics. Regardless of the drainage technique selected, the abscess contents require microbiologic evaluation to identify the organ-

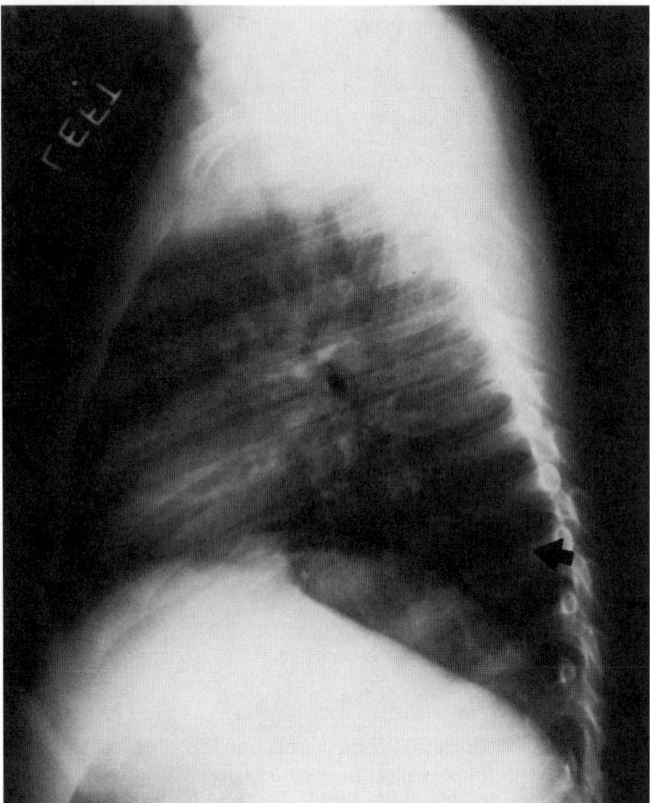

FIG. 57-26. Lateral radiograph of the chest taken after treatment for *Staphlococcus aureus* bacteremia showing the typical appearance of an air-filled postpneumonic pneumatomacele (*arrow*).

isms involved and to direct subsequent antibiotic therapy. Empiric initial therapy should cover anaerobic organisms as well as gram-negative organisms and *S aureus*. Clindamycin rather than penicillin G is recommended because increasing numbers of resistant oral anaerobes and resistant *S aureus* organisms make penicillin therapy prone to failure.[53] Antibiotic therapy is generally required for 6 to 12 weeks, although this depends on the patient's response and the rate at which the chest radiograph clears.[50–53] Most patients with lung abscesses are successfully treated with drainage and antibiotics alone. Patients with underlying immunodeficiences that can be corrected or modified should have this done. Modulation of immunosuppression drugs in transplant recipients, delay in chemotherapy for oncology patients, treatment with granulocyte colony-stimulating factor, and other similar approaches are appropriate when possible.

Operative management of a lung abscess is reserved for patients with specific related complications. Failure to control the initial infection or recurrent infection, massive or recurrent hemoptysis, bronchopleural fistula, and a persistent cavitary lesion are indications for operative resection of the affected lung. Immunosuppressed patients are at particular risk for these complications. Although a trial of medical therapy is appropriate in immunosuppressed patients, failure is much more probable, and prompt parenchymal resection is often required. The surgical principle that governs management of the complicated lung abscess is that resection of the involved parenchyma is required. This generally takes the form of a formal lobectomy; if done

in the face of acute inflammation, this can be a formidable technical challenge. In this circumstance, the bronchial stump closure requires particular care to avoid an air leak and a bronchopleural fistula.

Pulmonary Surgery in Cystic Fibrosis

The molecular basis of CF has been defined in the past several years. With regard to CF pulmonary disease, dysfunction of the adenosine triphosphate–dependent regulatory domain in the chloride channel of respiratory epithelial cell membranes results in the elaboration of abnormally viscid secretions that are chloride and water deficient.[54,55] This is reviewed in some detail in Chapter 71. Bacterial clearance from the airways is impaired, and colonization by pathogenic organisms, particularly *Pseudomonas aeruginosa*, results. Chronic and recurrent respiratory infections follow, with a wide range of secondary pulmonary problems. All these complications are the result of chronic infection, inflammation, and lung parenchymal destruction; most are adequately treated without surgical intervention.

Most affected patients are cared for in multidisciplinary centers with specific CF programs. Standard treatment for the pulmonary disease of CF includes many supportive measures, such as the use of mucolytic agents, physiotherapy, and aggressive antibiotic therapy, particularly aerosolized and systemic aminoglycosides. In addition, several new therapies are emerging. DNAase has been approved for clinical use.[56] This enzyme degrades neutrophil-derived DNA in respiratory secretions, making the mucus less viscid and therefore more easily cleared. Pharmacologic blockade of neutrophil elastase, a cytoplasmic protease, is undergoing preclinical evaluation. Most exciting is the realistic prospect of specific human gene therapy. Insertion of the *CFTR* (cystic fibrosis transmembrane regulator) gene has been accomplished in deficient mammalian cells.[57] The overall approach to the medical care for CF patients has been reviewed in detail.[58] The combined effect of these approaches is that the mean life expectancy for patients with CF is now about 28 years.

The pulmonary complications of CF that require surgical management are diminishing in frequency. It is not likely, however, that these will disappear in the near future because a substantial number of patients with chronic CF lung disease will exist for decades. Although none of these surgical problems is common, they are all potentially serious, and all physicians and surgeons who deal with CF patients must be familiar with them.

Bronchiectasis

Bronchiectasis refers to the structural and functional destruction of the bronchi by chronic or recurrent infection. Although many causes exist, CF is among the most common and important of these in childhood. Bronchiectasis results from recurrent pyogenic bacterial infection that injures and then destroys the cartilage, elastin, smooth muscle, and other structural elements of the airways, replacing them with collagen (Fig. 57-27). Epithelial metaplasia also occurs, so ciliated respiratory epithelium is replaced by squamous epithelium. These structural changes in the conducting airways exacerbate the underlying problem with the clearance of secretions that characterizes CF. Therefore, successive pyogenic bronchial infections and additional

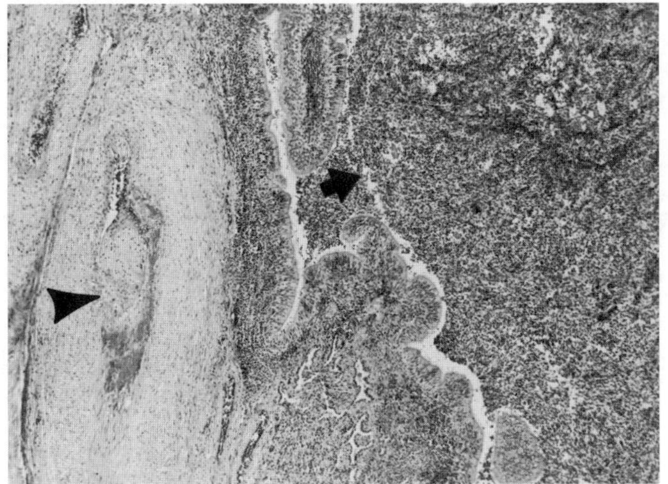

FIG. 57-27. Cystic fibrosis. A dense mucopurulent exudate (*arrow*) is present in the bronchial lumen of an adolescent with cystic fibrosis. Bronchiectasis is the result of repeated episodes of mucus plugging, followed by infection, necrotizing inflammation, and destruction of the structural elements of the airway. The adjacent vessel contains a recent thrombus (*arrowhead*). (Hematoxylin–eosin, ×52.) (Courtesy of Kay Washington, MD, Duke University Medical Center, Durham, NC)

injury occur. The pattern of bronchial destruction has a variety of morphologic features that have been termed *cylindrical, saccular,* or *tubular*.[59] Although they are of pathologic and historic interest, these distinctions are largely irrelevant now with regard to both pathogenesis and therapy.

Areas of bronchiectasis may be either localized or diffuse. Patients with CF have a systemic disease, and diffuse lung disease is always present. Bronchiectasis, however, tends to occur in specific lobar distributions; the lower lobes are more frequently involved.[60,61] Symptoms of bronchiectasis in patients with CF are exceedingly difficult to differentiate from those of the underlying disease. Generally, the problem occurs in older children and adolescents because it requires a number of years for the bronchial destruction to occur. Discovery usually results from increasingly frequent bouts of infection and chronic cough, particularly with the expectoration of larger amounts of sputum, which may be fetid. Chest radiographs with persistent findings of focal pneumonia are also a harbinger of bronchiectasis. Plain radiographs are inadequate to evaluate the disease process in this circumstance. Historically, contrast bronchography was used to localize the disease and define its extent, but this is no longer necessary and has significant hazards. Likewise, bronchoscopy is of limited value because the distal airways must be evaluated and the pathology is often beyond the view of conventional instruments. Chest CT provides excellent definition of the areas of involvement, and MR imaging provides similar information.[62] If surgical management is under consideration, ventilation–perfusion scans are of substantial value as well because they identify areas of little or no gas exchange.[9,61] Because correlation of anatomic disease with the site of physiologic dysfunction is possible, these data are potentially helpful in preoperative resectional planning. Pulmonary function studies are helpful as well because these patients are generally old enough to cooperate, and the information obtained can help to anticipate tolerance for thoracotomy and lung resection.

The initial and often only treatment necessary for CF patients with bronchiectasis is nonoperative. Indications for resectional therapy for bronchiectasis, whether it results from CF or some other cause, all relate to specific complications of the process[63]:

- Specific respiratory symptoms that progressively limit daily life, growth, or development, *and*
- Severe localized disease, *and*
- Evidence that parenchymal resection will not be physiologically limiting, *or*
- Recurrent or life-threatening hemorrhage

All are subjective and none are absolute. The number of children with CF who require resectional therapy for bronchiectasis has steadily diminished during the past two decades as their nonoperative care has improved. Decisions regarding the necessity for resection, the timing of resection, and the extent of resection require mature clinical judgment and substantial experience with CF patients.

The surgical principle that guides resectional therapy for bronchiectasis is to remove specific areas of severe involvement while preserving normal or less diseased areas of adjacent lung tissue. Generally, this means that segmental or lobar resection is performed. It is preferable to resect areas of disease that are known to be stable rather than those that are still evolving. It is essential to plan the resectional procedure preoperatively in detail by correlating areas of severe radiographic bronchiectatic change with zones of physiologic dysfunction on ventilation–perfusion scan. Patients with diffuse lung disease from CF are intolerant of the loss of functional lung parenchyma. Furthermore, the intraoperative assessment of the lung is generally unhelpful in CF patients because the parenchyma is all abnormal to some extent.

The most comprehensive study of outcomes for CF patients after surgical resection for bronchiectasis was published in 1979.[63] Despite improvements in medical care, this review remains relevant. After parenchymal lung resection for bronchiectasis, 61% of CF patients had substantially improved symptoms, 21% had some improvement, and 18% had no improvement or worsened. The authors reported no operative deaths in the last decade of the review. Similar experience has been repeated on a smaller scale at other institutions.[64]

Hemoptysis is an important complication in CF patients with bronchiectasis. The chronic inflammatory and infectious destruction of the airways leads initially to exposure and then to erosion of the bronchial arteries. Pseudoaneurysm formation and hemorrhage can follow (Fig. 57-28). Most of these patients with hemoptysis have relatively minor bleeding that is self-limiting and that can be managed with the same general supportive approaches discussed earlier. For recurrent or refractory hemoptysis, angiographic localization and embolization of a bleeding site is the preferred method of management. For life-threatening bleeding, lobar resection is appropriate, with two technical requirements: (1) before parenchymal resection, it is essential to localize the site of hemorrhage to at least the lobe that is bleeding; and (2) control of the airway must be achieved, preferably with selective intubation of the nonbleeding main-stem bronchus. In addition, balloon exclusion of the bleeding bronchus is desirable because the nonbleeding lung will be dependent intraoperatively and therefore at risk for obstruction from blood clot during the course of the thoracotomy and lung resection.

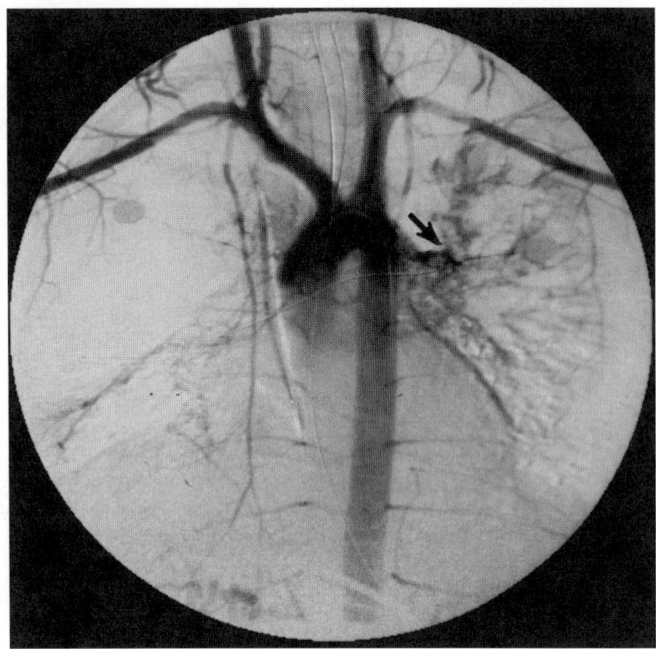

FIG. 57-28. Angiogram in an adolescent with cystic fibrosis and refractory life-threatening pulmonary hemorrhage from the left upper lobe showing active bronchial arterial bleeding (*arrow*). Emergency left upper lobe resection was required, because angiographic embolization was of only transient benefit.

Pneumothorax

The subject of spontaneous pneumothorax is presented elsewhere in detail (see Chap. 56). With specific regard to patients who have CF, spontaneous pneumothorax is often a relatively late event in the course of the disease. Adolescents and young adults with advanced disease are at highest risk, and these patients also have significantly diminished physiologic tolerance. They may develop local infection with bleb formation and rupture, or alveolar rupture from localized air-trapping may occur. This diagnosis is rarely obscure in CF patients because the resulting chest pain and dyspnea are not well tolerated. The diagnosis is ordinarily confirmed by plain chest radiograph. As with any pneumothorax, the treatment objective is prompt evacuation of the air with approximation of the visceral and parietal pleura to seal the air leak. In patients with symptoms, conventional tube thoracostomy with sealed drainage to reexpand the lung is the safest and most effective therapy. Lesser maneuvers, such as needle aspiration, small catheter drainage, or oxygen therapy for transpleural air absorption, are of limited value in this population. In patients without symptoms, however, a therapeutic trial of these less morbid alternatives may be appropriate.

A major question in regard to surgical therapy in patients with spontaneous pneumothorax secondary to CF is whether pleurodesis should be done. The recurrence rate in these patients is about 50% in the absence of definitive treatment.[63,65] Furthermore, the risks of pneumothorax may be substantial. For these reasons, it may be appropriate to offer pleurodesis to CF patients at the time of an initial pneumothorax. Sclerosing agents placed into the pleural cavity through a chest tube can accomplish

this, although the procedure is tedious and can be painful.[65] In addition, if unsuccessful, subsequent entry into the pleural space may be hazardous. Open pleurodesis or pleurectomy through a limited thoracotomy is predictably successful and can be done without mortality, although the morbidity is substantial.[66] Thoracoscopic pleurodesis with talc poudrage also has been reported.[67,68] This combines the advantages of excellent, direct visualization with a procedure that is highly successful, predictable, and has limited morbidity. Although the experience is limited, this appears to be an excellent approach. In CF patients, it is important to consider that the major additional disadvantage to pleurodesis is the increased difficulty of lung transplantation. Given that lung replacement is feasible, this potential need must be weighed carefully because some consider pleurodesis a contraindication to lung replacement.

Therapeutic Bronchoscopy

Endobronchial toilet is effectively achieved routinely in patients with CF without the need for bronchoscopic suction or lavage. A 1982 trial demonstrated that although the technique of endoscopic lavage and mucolytic agents is effective, the response is transient and short-lived.[69] Therefore, this approach has been abandoned for routine use, although it is periodically useful in selected patients with specific exacerbations of their disease. When it is done, cultures can be obtained to direct specific antibiotic therapy.

Lung Replacement

Lung replacement has become feasible as a treatment for the ultimate complication of CF, chronic and irreversible respiratory failure. The September 1994 summary of the St Louis Lung Transplant Registry reported that 466 of the 3160 lung transplantations recorded worldwide to that time were for patients with CF.[70] Of the 133 lung transplantations done in patients younger than the age of 16 years, 64 were for CF, mainly in teenagers, and all in patients older than 5 years of age. All but one CF patient received a bilateral lung transplantation because the risk of leaving a diseased contralateral lung in an immunosuppressed patient is deemed prohibitive. The 3-year actuarial survival rate is 57% for CF patients, with a disease-specific survival rate ranging from 62% (chronic emphysema) to 49% (pulmonary hypertension) among lung transplant recipients. A specific discussion of lung transplantation in children is presented in Chapter 44. Although definitive medical treatment for CF is likely in the future, so that this need will eventually disappear, many patients with chronic CF lung disease will require lung replacement for years to come.

Bullous Lung Disease

Bullae or blebs are saccular areas of subpleural air within the lung that are thought to result from an air leak from an adjacent alveolus. Generally, the term *bleb* refers to a smaller air collection and *bulla* to a larger one, although there are no specific numeric thresholds to distinguish between the use of the two terms. The important functional distinction is that the grossly apparent lesions (bullae) are associated with the loss of adjacent lung parenchyma, while this is not true of blebs. Blebs and bullae are not associated with normal alveoli or capillaries; hence, no gas exchange occurs within them, although they do communicate with the tracheobronchial tree.[71]

Bullae and blebs are either congenital or acquired. Acquired lesions are usually a consequence of chronic infection related to a problem such as CF, α_1-antitrypsin deficiency, or another similar condition. Bullous emphysema is a common form of acquired adult chronic obstructive pulmonary disease, but this is rarely seen in children. Congenital bullae and blebs apparently result from disordered development of alveoli and terminal airways during organogenesis. The discussion that follows deals principally with blebs and bullae rather than the underlying pulmonary diseases.

The clinical symptoms of blebs and bullae are generally the result of either spontaneous pneumothorax from rupture into the pleural space or exercise intolerance because of diminished lung volumes and inadequate respiratory reserve. The latter problem is generally associated with underlying diffuse lung disease. Plain chest radiographs and CT are usually adequate for definitive imaging. Apical disease is most common, and bilateral disease is frequent. α_1-Antitrypsin deficiency is unique in its propensity to form basal blebs.[72]

The management of blebs and bullae is dependent on the degree of symptomatology and the underlying lung problem. Treatment of smaller lesions is usually limited to problems that result from air leak, specifically pneumothorax. Generally, tube thoracostomy is the appropriate treatment for the first spontaneous pneumothorax. Recurrent pneumothorax occurs in 20% to 50% of patients with congenital bullous disease, and this incidence increases significantly with each additional pneumothorax.[73] It is therefore appropriate to consider definitive operative treatment after a first recurrent pneumothorax associated with congenital bullous disease. The details of this approach are discussed in Chapter 56 and in the CF section of this chapter.

The principles for operative management of lung bullae are to remove the area of involvement, to conserve all possible normal lung tissue, and to obtain a secure, airtight closure of the lung. The resections, therefore, generally are not segmental or lobar, but rather nonanatomic in nature.[73,74] Resection of bullae with or without pleurodesis is highly effective. Closure of the bleb margin can present problems, but modern stapling devices confer more security and efficiency to this procedure than do traditional suture closure techniques. Therefore, stapled resections are considered routine for this problem. Resection of bullae can be done through either a thoracoscopic approach or an open thoracotomy, with limited morbidity and mortality[73–75] (Fig. 57-29). The thoracoscopic approach appears to be highly effective, rapid, and less morbid than open thoracotomy. Potential problems with air leak are best prevented by concurrent pleurodesis or pleurectomy.

The outcome after bleb resection is dependent on the amount of remaining lung and the extent of underlying disease. For congenital blebs with a large portion of the normal lung retained, the outcome is predictably excellent. For extensive local disease or for blebs acquired as a consequence of systemic disease, this is more problematic. Specifically, if preoperative evaluation shows that the bullae occupy more than one third of the ipsilateral thorax, if ventilation–perfusion scan shows little or no function in the area of the bullae, and if pulmonary function studies indicate tolerance for thoracotomy and lung resection, the outcome is much more favorable postoperatively.[73]

Bronchiectasis

Bronchiectasis was discussed in some detail in the presentation of surgical problems associated with CF. The pathogenesis and treatment of the process are generally similar in patients without CF and are not repeated in detail here, although a number of other causes exist. Collectively, these conditions are relatively common, yet the complication of bronchiectasis is not. Those of particular importance in childhood are retained endobronchial foreign bodies, bronchial stenosis after a bout of pneumonia or acute bronchitis, endobronchial tumors, α_1-antitrypsin deficiency, Kartagener (immotile cilia) syndrome, structural lung lesions, chronic aspiration, and a variety of immunodeficiencies.[9,76,77] In addition, congenital bronchiectasis can occur without an underlying cause. The fundamental lesion is one of chronic distal airway infection with loss of structural integrity of the conducting airways, inadequate clearance of secretions and bacteria, and sequential bouts of destructive inflammation and infection. Although many different bacterial and viral organisms can initiate the bronchiectatic process, specific pathogens of note include measles and pertussis, both of which have undergone a resurgence in the United States because of inadequate childhood immunization practices. Likewise, tuberculosis is an important and increasing cause of concern.

In previously healthy patients, the development of persistent respiratory symptoms and chronic, productive cough with fetid sputum or hemoptysis is highly suggestive of bronchiectasis. Unlike CF patients, these symptoms are easily identified in otherwise normal patients. The evaluation, treatment, and surgical principles are similar to those presented for bronchiectasis associated with CF. Bronchoscopy is essential because clearly reversible lesions, such as endobronchial tumors or foreign bodies, must be corrected. Otherwise, the approach is to define the extent of disease and provide nonoperative treatment, principally in the form of antibiotics specific for oral bacterial pathogens. CT scanning is an excellent diagnostic technique[62] (Fig. 57-30). The underlying disease is treated if possible. The spread of bronchiectasis to new areas of previously normal lung is unlikely with appropriate treatment, although progression at the site of previously injured lung occurs in about 25% of patients, even with appropriate treatment.[9] Operative indications are related either to substantial disability or hemorrhage that is directly attributable to focal disease. Generally, segmental or lobar lung resection via thoracotomy is the procedure of choice. Conservation of uninvolved lung is a fundamental surgical principle, and in otherwise normal patients, this approach yields an excellent outcome. Using these principles, Wilson and Decker[78] reported that 75% of patients with focal bronchiectasis did not have symptoms or substantially improved postoperatively, while virtually none worsened. As expected, the prognosis in the presence of systemic or diffuse lung disease is substantially diminished.

Echinococcal Lung Disease

Echinococcus granulosus and *Echinococcus multilocularis* are parasites responsible for hydatid cystic lung disease in chil-

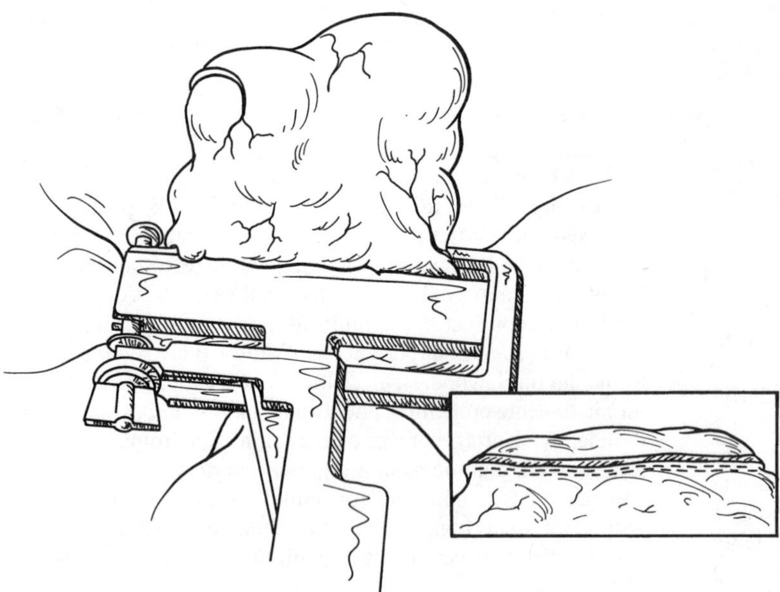

FIG. 57-29. Stapled resection of congenital apical bullous disease of the lung. (After Nohl-Oser HC, Nissen R, Schreibe HN. Surgery of the lung. New York, Theime-Stratton, 1981)

dren. Echinococcal infection is endemic but rare among native populations of the Southwest United States, Northwestern Canada, and Alaska. The predominant vector in North America is the dog; in the Middle East, Australia, and most other regions, exposure to sheep or cattle appears responsible for transmission to the human intermediate host. Humans become infected by eating food contaminated by the scoleces of these parasites. Liver involvement is most common, followed by lung, brain, spleen, and other organs.[79] The presentation of pulmonary disease includes patients without symptoms as well as those with cough, dyspnea, fever, and chest pain. Those who do not have

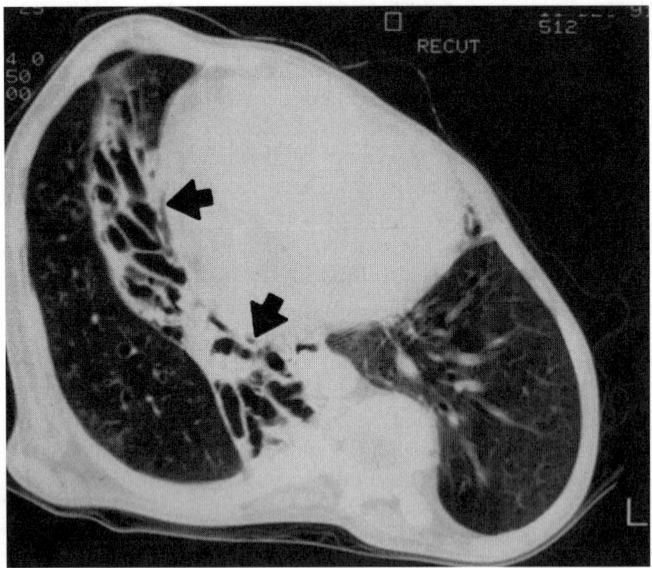

FIG. 57-30. CT image of the chest showing severe bronchiectasis secondary to gastroesophageal reflux. This child had involvement of the right lower and the right middle lobes (*arrows*). Lesser involvement of the left lower lobe also was present. Substantial clinical improvement followed right middle and lower lobectomy.

symptoms are thought to have been infected more recently because the hydatid cyst requires time to develop. Solitary lung cysts are often large, and air–fluid levels may be seen on chest radiograph. Calcification may be present as well. The diagnosis can be confirmed with an accuracy of 80% or more with one or more of the following serologic tests: indirect hemagglutination, complement fixation, dot immunobinding, or enzyme-linked immunosorbent assay.[79] Transpleural aspiration is also diagnostic, demonstrating *Echinococcus* sp hooklets and protoscoleces. Lamy and colleagues[80] advocated this latter approach for the Canadian and Alaskan variety of *E granulosus*, based on a small clinical series suggesting a relatively benign natural history of self-limiting disease not associated with anaphylaxis and generally not requiring operative intervention. Conventional therapy for disease in patients from other geographic locations, however, calls for perioperative mebendazole treatment and prompt surgical resection of the thick-walled cyst, with care taken to avoid pleural contamination.[73] The risks of anaphylaxis and local implantation of scolices appear low with lung disease, but most surgeons experienced with this disease argue against pleural spillage whether at the time of diagnosis or treatment. Antibiotic therapy alone is insufficient to eliminate the thick-walled cyst. Because of the risk of secondary bacterial infection, surgical resection of the cyst is recommended. Simple wedge resection is appropriate without scolecidal agents, such as hypertonic saline or ethyl alcohol, because the risk is substantial if drainage of these agents into the tracheobronchial tree occurs.

Opportunistic Lung Infections

The number of infants and children who have opportunistic pulmonary infections produced by mycobacterial, protozoan, viral, fungal, and bacterial pathogens is steadily growing because of progressive increases in the numbers of immunocompromised hosts. Transplant recipients, oncology patients, human immunodeficiency virus victims, and others offer a burgeoning population at risk. Typically, at-risk patients develop

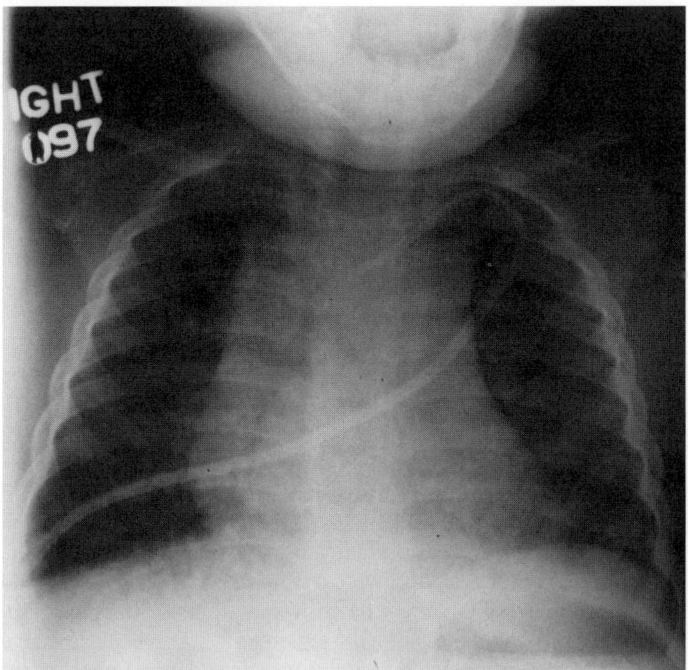

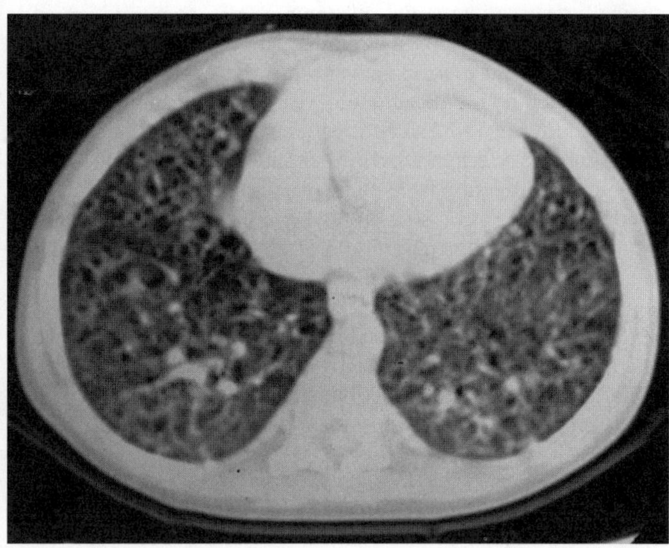

A

B

FIG. 57-31. Child with acquired immunodeficiency syndrome and a bilateral interstitial pneumonitis. (*A*) Plain chest radiograph showing a relatively subtle reticular pneumonitis. (*B*) Appearance on CT. Open lung biopsy is often necessary for definitive diagnosis in these circumstances. (Courtesy of Cindy Miller, MD, Duke University Medical Center, Durham, NC)

diffuse interstitial pneumonitis with clinical symptoms that range from cough and fever to life-threatening respiratory distress (Fig. 57-31). Depending on the underlying disease, many receive empiric antibiotic therapy with trimethoprim-sulfamethoxazole or other agents to treat possible pathogens such as *Pneumocystis carinii* (Fig. 57-32). A definitive tissue diagnosis becomes necessary for progressive or refractory disease. The most common surgical requirement for these immunosuppressed patients with interstitial lung disease is to provide tissue samples for histopathology and microbiologic analysis to direct specific therapy. Both transbronchial biopsy and percutaneous lung biopsy yield small tissue samples that may be helpful in differentiating among infectious, neoplastic, rejection-related, and inflammatory lung processes. Bronchoalveolar lavage is likewise helpful in identifying some pathogens in immunosuppressed children with pneumonia.[81] Formal lung biopsy, however, whether by limited open thoracotomy or thoracoscopic means, is often preferred because of the larger specimen and its definitive nature. Although the surgical procedure is generally well-tolerated, its combination with the underlying disease process yields substantial perioperative morbidity and mortality. In one review of open lung biopsies among childhood bone marrow transplant recipients with interstitial lung disease, the 30-day mortality rate was 45%, and the overall mortality rate was 74%.[82] A definitive diagnosis results from open lung biopsy in between 50% and 90% of immunosuppressed patients with interstitial lung disease, although the incidence of treatable disease is substantially lower.[82,83]

From a technical standpoint, the thoracoscopic approach with use of a stapled wedge resection has rapidly gained acceptance in children with diffuse lung disease who are of sufficient size to use the commercially available stapling devices within the thorax (about 15 kg).[68] Smaller children are also appropriate for thoracoscopic lung biopsy, although suture closure or coagulation of the lung may be needed. Conventional open biopsy remains an appropriate alternative, although the operative morbidity may be greater.

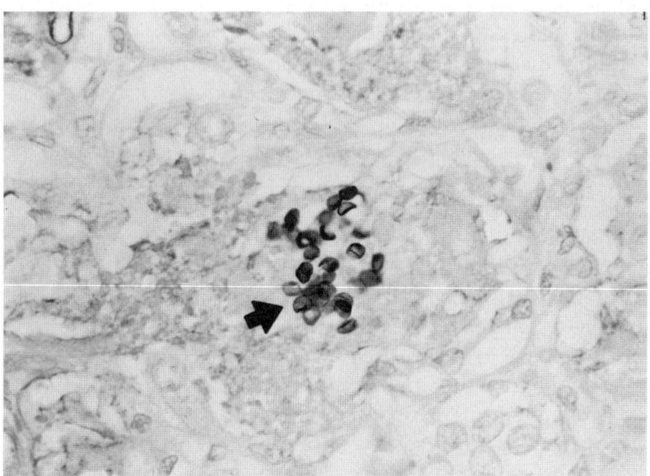

FIG. 57-32. *Pneumocystis carinii* pneumonia. The 4- to 6-μm encysted form of *P carinii* is round or helmet-shaped (*arrow*). These organisms are generally found within the intraalveolar transudative froth. (Methenamine silver, $\times$60.) (Courtesy of Kay Washington, MD, Duke University Medical Center, Durham, NC)

Pneumocystis carinii

Pneumocystis carinii is the most common protozoan lung infection that occurs in the immunocompromised host.[81–83] It typically causes interstitial pneumonia, hypoxemia, fever, and tachypnea. Acute respiratory failure may follow. Bronchoalveolar lavage may be diagnostic, but the organisms are best demonstrated by methenamine silver staining of lung tissue, as shown in Figure 57-32. Identification of these organisms is one of the diagnostic criteria for differentiating human immunodeficiency virus infection from clinical acquired immunodeficiency syndrome (see Chap. 10). Prophylaxis in high-risk patients or treatment for presumed or mild disease is initially with trimethoprim-sulfamethoxazole. If the disease is refractory or progressive, however, pentamidine isethionate is required.[84] *Toxoplasma gondii* is a protozoan infection that can cause clinical pneumonitis indistinguishable from *P carinii* except by pathologic evaluation. The distinction is important because the latter infection requires treatment with pyrimethamine sulfadiazine.

Fungi

Fungal infection, in particular, is an important and increasing source of pulmonary infection among immunocompromised children. Nosocomial infection with *Candida albicans* and other *Candida* species in critically ill hospitalized patients is quite common. Candidal pulmonary disease is often associated with sepsis and life-threatening systemic disease. Prophylaxis with oral antifungal agents (see later) is appropriate for high-risk patients to prevent pulmonary or systemic infection. This approach includes oral nystatin and topical amphotericin B bladder irrigation to prevent urinary tract colonization. Systemic amphotericin B is standard therapy for invasive or intracavitary candidal infection. Oral agents may be appropriate for airway colonization, but intravenous treatment with amphotericin B is necessary for candidal pneumonitis.[84] Combination therapy with 5-fluorocytosine, ketoconazole, fluconazole, or other agents may be useful as well, although no prospective studies address this question.

Fungi that are endemic pulmonary human pathogens in the United States include *Histoplasma capsulatum* in the Mississippi and Ohio River Valleys, *Blastomyces dermatitides* in the South and East, and *Coccidioides immitis* in California and the Southwest. Many people in these regions demonstrate serologic evidence of exposure, but few have clinical evidence of disease. Although any organ can be affected, lung involvement is common, particularly for blastomycosis and coccidioidomycosis. Histoplasmosis may be associated with massive mediastinal lymphadenopathy. For all three of these organisms, a common clinical scenario is the discovery of a single lung nodule on a chest radiograph in an otherwise healthy patient who does not have symptoms. This may present a diagnostic dilemma that necessitates wedge resection for a definitive pathologic evaluation. In patients for whom the diagnosis is clear from the history and serology, this is not necessary. Typically, affected patients require no further treatment if they do not have symptoms.

Healthy people rarely develop fungal pneumonia or disseminated disease, but this is a particular risk in the immunosuppressed host. In the latter instance, the diagnosis should be established and systemic antifungal treatment initiated. The appropriate diagnosis may be established if substantial elevations in acute complement fixation titers occur, but this is a time-consuming process because specimens obtained 4 to 6 weeks apart are required for comparison. Sputum, tracheobronchial aspirates, and lung tissue for culture are all useful as well. Amphotericin B is the treatment of choice for these organisms if the patient has systemic disease, has specific pulmonary symptoms, or is immunocompromised. Less serious disease can be treated with one of the azole class of antifungal agents, such as miconazole, ketoconazole, fluconazole, or itraconazole. Once the diagnosis is established, operation is indicated only for specific pulmonary complications, and these are rare.

Aspergillosis, mucormycosis, and other fungal infections are seen in immunocompromised hosts as well. These are potentially life-threatening when pulmonary infection is involved, and essentially all these infections require systemic amphotericin B treatment. Aspergillosis, in particular, is associated with cavitary tuberculosis and, in this setting, often requires resection because it is difficult to eradicate the aspergilloma within the sequestered lung cavity. Mucormycosis is an aggressive and often lethal fungal infection resulting from the *Rhizopus* sp, which can occur anywhere. If a patient is to survive this invasive necrotizing infection, aggressive surgical débridement of involved tissue is necessary.

Mycobacteria

Childhood pulmonary infection from *Mycobacterium tuberculosis* and atypical mycobacterial forms is a substantial public health issue in the United States.[85] The acquired immunodeficiency virus epidemic and concurrent resurgence of tuberculosis in the adult population appear to be important causes. The natural history of the disease does not appear fundamentally different in children than adults, but the emergence of atypical and antibiotic-resistant strains of mycobacteria is an increasingly important problem. Transmission is generally through a respiratory route, and the lung is the most common site of involvement. The initial treatment is always medical with multidrug antibiotic regimens, including combinations of isoniazid, rifampin, ethambutol, streptomycin, paraaminosalicylic acid, and pyrazinamide.[84] Common atypical organisms include *M avium*, *M intracellulare*, and *M kansasii*. These organisms all require treatment with rifampin and at least two additional agents, usually for 6 to 12 months or longer.

The goal of surgery in these patients is generally to obtain lung or lymph node tissue to establish the diagnosis or to deal with specific complications. Among these complications are bronchiectasis and cavitary disease with a secondary lung abscess, both of which were discussed earlier. Other operative indications for pulmonary tuberculosis include recurrent or persistent hemorrhage, refractory nodular disease with resistant organisms, empyema with a restrictive component, irreversible lung destruction, and residual cavitary or caseous disease after 6 months of therapy.[86] The surgical principle is to perform a minimal resection of the affected lung parenchyma, conserving lung that is normal or reversibly involved. The disease can be controlled or eradicated in most circumstances by appropriate concurrent antibiotic therapy, and the outcome is generally good.[51]

Viral Infection

Herpes viruses, particularly the cytomegalovirus (CMV), are the most common pulmonary viral pathogens in immunosuppressed patients. Ebstein-Barr virus, the herpes simplex viruses, and varicella-zoster virus are among this group. CMV infection in solid organ transplant recipients is especially common; evidence of infection is present in 30% or more of these patients. This is in part because of its transmission through the transplanted organ. In some series, CMV is the most common infectious pathogen among immunosuppressed children with diffuse alveolar and interstitial lung disease.[81–83] Diagnosis by culture, polymerase chain reaction, or a rise in anti-CMV antibody titers is often too slow to be of clinical utility. The development of fluorescent anti-CMV monoclonal antibodies has allowed diagnosis to be established by direct staining of tissue or other specimens within 24 hours.[84] In addition, specific antiviral therapy is available for CMV in the form of ganciclovir. Acyclovir is effective against other herpes viruses, and hyperimmune immunoglobulin G also appears to be beneficial in the treatment of clinical herpes infection.

LUNG TUMORS

Primary Lung Tumors

The definitive contemporary review of primary pulmonary neoplasms in children was by Hartman and Shochat in 1983.[87] They found that of 230 primary tumors, 151 were malignant and 79 benign. Their findings are summarized in Table 57-2. Since this represents the entire English language literature to that date, it is clear that all the lesions are rare.

TABLE 57-2. *Classification by cell type of 230 primary lung tumors in children*

Type of tumor	Patients
BENIGN	79
Inflammatory pseudotumor	45
Hamartoma	15
Neurogenic tumor	9
Leiomyoma	6
Mucous gland adenoma	2
Myoblastoma	2
MALIGNANT	151
Bronchial adenoma	65
Bronchogenic carcinoma	47
Pulmonary blastoma	14
Leiomyosarcoma	9
Rhabdomyosarcoma	6
Hemangiopericytoma	3
Lymphoma	3
Teratoma	2
Plasmacytoma	1
Myxosarcoma	1

(Hartman GE, Shochat SJ. Primary pulmonary neoplasms of childhood: a review. Ann Thorac Surg 1983;36:108)

Malignant Tumors

Bronchial Adenoma

The most common primary lung tumors in children are a heterogeneous group of low-grade adenocarcinomas incorrectly but irrevocably termed *bronchial adenomas*. These lesions have a variety of histologic features that have led to the use of several descriptive names: *carcinoid, mucoepidermoid carcinoma,* and *adenoid cystic carcinoma (cylindroma)*. In reality, all have the potential for metastatic spread, although this incidence is low, about 5% to 10%.[87]

Endobronchial carcinoid tumors are the most common of these, generally representing 80% to 85% of this group. These lesions, like other carcinoid tumors, are derived from neural crest stem cells and retain their potential for serotonin and peptide hormone synthesis. Plasma serotonin and urine 5-hydroxyindoleacetic acid levels may be elevated in these patients, and they are therefore potentially useful tumor markers. The carcinoid syndrome has been reported in a single child with an endobronchial carcinoid tumor.[88]

The clinical presentation is typically one of recurrent or persistent pneumonia because of partial or complete bronchial obstruction. Because of the critical anatomic location, the tumors generally become symptomatic while relatively small, although it appears that the rate of growth is slow. Radiographic imaging is generally nondiagnostic (Fig. 57-33). Bronchoscopic findings are, however, unique and compelling. The lesion is best described as a pink, friable mulberry. Although biopsy can be done, it is inadvisable for several reasons: (1) hemorrhage can be substantial or even life-threatening, (2) the histopathology is difficult to evaluate with a small specimen and limited time (Fig. 57-34), (3) the gross appearance is predictable from a diagnostic standpoint, and (4) obstructing bronchial adenomas require resection, the nature of which is generally dictated by anatomic rather than pathologic features.

Careful endoscopic mapping under direct vision is essential to planning operative management. Endoscopy and video systems have evolved rapidly and offer substantial improvement in this aspect of care. Although endoscopic resection is reported, it is considered ill advised because of the risks of hemorrhage, bronchial stenosis, local recurrence, and the inability to examine regional lymph nodes. In older children and those with small tumors without lymphatic spread, successful segmental bronchial resection has been done.[89] Most patients with endobronchial carcinoid tumors, however, require lobectomy or pneumonectomy, depending on the specific location of the tumor. Regional lymph node sampling, particularly in the presence of clinically suspicious nodes, is also appropriate. These carcinoid tumors are radiosensitive, and this may be an appropriate therapy for nonresectable disease, although available data are too limited for definitive guidelines. The 10-year survival rate in children after surgical resection for endobronchial carcinoid tumor is about 90%.[87]

Endobronchial mucoepidermoid carcinomas represent 10% to 15% of bronchial adenomas. Their clinical features in childhood are similar to those of endobronchial carcinoid tumors, particularly with regard to presentation, diagnostic evaluation, and surgical treatment. The principal difference involves the histopathology. These lesions have both mucus-secreting and

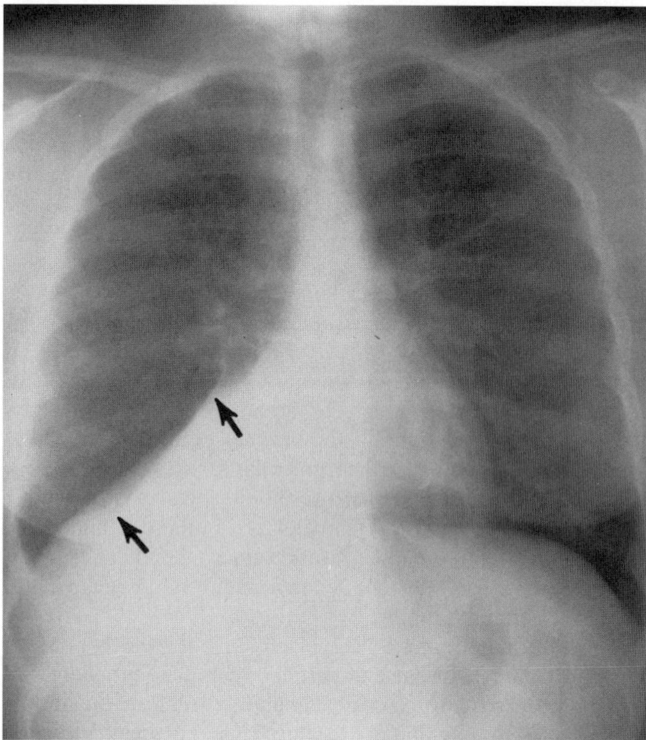

FIG. 57-33. Chest radiograph of a 15-year-old girl with a 3-week history of refractory penumonia. Right middle and right lower lobe collapse is obvious (*arrows*). At bronchoscopy, this patient was found to have a nearly completely obstructing carcinoid of the bronchus intermedius.

epidermoid cells. Only one child is reported to have had malignant spread of this lesion, and this tumor was characterized by a predominance of epidermoid cellular elements.[87] The postoperative survival rate approaches 100%.

Adenoid cystic carcinoma (cylindroma) is the least common form of bronchial adenoma in childhood. The important distinction for this tumor is the observation that it is an indolent malignancy with a propensity for submucosal spread and late recurrence.[90] Intraoperative frozen-section evaluation of the surgical margin of the bronchus is therefore appropriate when resecting a bronchial adenoma. These lesions are otherwise clinically indistinguishable from other forms of bronchial adenomas.

Bronchogenic Carcinoma

Primary bronchogenic carcinoma is rare in children; about 50 cases have been reported in the world's literature.[87] Only 10% of these were squamous cell carcinomas, and the remainder were adenocarcinomas or undifferentiated carcinomas. Although rare, persistent case reports suggest an important etiologic association with preexisting cystic bronchopulmonary–foregut abnormalities.

The unfortunate experience with this lesion is that patients often have hemoptysis, cough, dyspnea, chest pain, anemia, weight loss, or bone pain when diagnosed, and most have nonresectable or disseminated disease. The average survival in this circumstance is 7 months.[87] For children with localized disease who undergo complete resection, a small Japanese experience suggests that about half have long-term survival.[91]

Pulmonary Blastoma

Pulmonary blastoma is a rare tumor that is seen in both adults and children. About 25% of the patients are younger than 16 years of age at presentation, and 60% of these are younger than 4 years of age.[87] The distinctive pathologic feature of pulmonary blastoma is that it is composed of cells that resemble fetal lung and that have metastatic potential. Most patients present with symptoms of cough, chest pain, hemoptysis, or frank hemorrhage, and the lesion is identified on plain chest radiograph. These are generally peripheral lesions, and lobar resection is the most common surgical procedure. Forty to 50% of patients have long-term survival with this approach. The roles of chemotherapy and irradiation have not been prospectively evaluated.

Other Malignant Neoplasms

The inventory of other rare primary lung malignancies is summarized in Table 57-2. In addition, neurofibrosarcoma, fibrosarcoma, mesothelioma, and other lung malignancies have been reported. The general clinical approach to these was detailed earlier. Radiographic imaging is best obtained for all primary lung neoplasms with either CT or MR imaging. The operative goal is to resect all gross disease and to conserve as much normal lung parenchyma as possible. The limited experience for each of these lesions precludes meaningful statistical analysis of adjuvant therapy, and treatment is generally individualized.

Benign Lung Tumors

Inflammatory Pseudotumor

Inflammatory pseudotumor is a rare lesion that presents as a solitary lung nodule in children. As the term suggests, it is not malignant, nor is it truly neoplastic. The histopathology typically shows a variety of inflammatory cells, including lymphocytes and fat-laden macrophages, as well as other lung parenchymal cell types. Descriptive pathologic names are abundant in the literature and reflect the fact that there is considerable variety in the appearance of the participant inflammatory cells.[92] Among these names are *plasma cell granuloma, histiocytoma, xanthofibroma,* and *lung adenoma.* The pathogenesis of this unique local inflammatory process is unknown.

Inflammatory pseudotumor is the most common benign lung mass in infants and children. Seventy-five percent of the children are older than 5 years of age; 30% do not have symptoms when discovered; and 20% have a history of previous pulmonary infection.[87] Other presentations include cough, fever, chest pain, hemoptysis, and airway obstruction. Pneumonia is diagnosed in about 10% of these children. Large inflammatory pseudotumors have resulted in esophageal obstruction and death from extrinsic compression of mediastinal structures.

The imaging approach is not different than for other mass lesions in the thorax. Plain chest radiographs are followed by either CT or MR imaging. The lesions appear as solid parenchy-

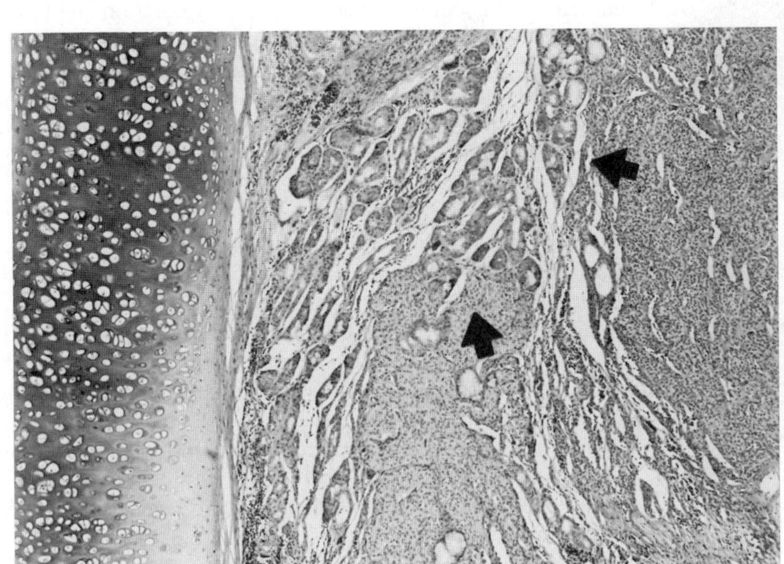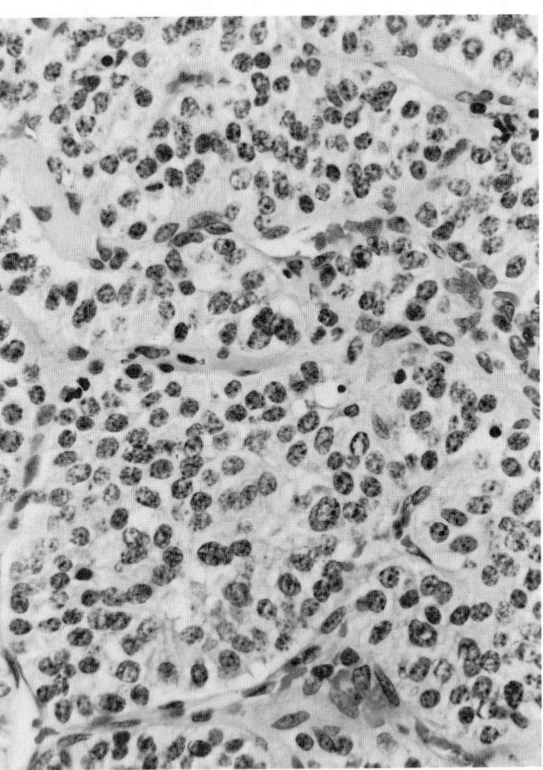

FIG. 57-34. The child whose chest radiograph is seen in Figure 57-33 underwent resection of the endobronchial lesion with the right middle and right lower lobes. The right upper lobe was preserved. The pathology was consistent with an endobronchial carcinoid. (*A*) The carcinoid tumor arises in the submucosa of the bronchus and infiltrates among submucosal glands (*arrows*). (Hematoxylin–eosin, ×52.) (*B*) This carcinoid tumor consisted of uniform cells with round or oval nuclei and abundant pale or eosinophilic cytoplasm. The cells are arranged in nests, and trabeculae are separated by a fine vascular network. This is a typical carcinoid appearance. (Hematoxylin–eosin, ×400.) (Courtesy of Kay Washington, MD, Duke University Medical Center, Durham, NC)

mal nodules or larger masses that may be indistinguishable from neoplasms. Calcification can be dramatic (Fig. 57-35). The natural history of the process is generally one of either slow growth or spontaneous resolution. Metastatic spread has not been observed. If the diagnosis is clear, urgent surgical resection is not required because the lesion may resolve. In reality, the lesion is often indistinguishable from a primary malignancy with both preoperative imaging and intraoperative biopsy. Hence, surgical resection is often done for diagnosis, and this is appropriate. Formal lobectomy or local resection is required, depending on the level of diagnostic uncertainty and the anatomic relations involved.

Hamartomas

Hamartomatous lung nodules are seen commonly in adults but are rarely discovered in children. They are considered congenital in origin, presumably because most are asymptomatic and therefore escape childhood detection. They may occur in either endobronchial or parenchymal lung sites and are characterized by the presence of cartilage, respiratory epithelium, and collagen.[93] Endobronchial lesions cause clinical symptoms at a relatively small size. Lung parenchymal lesions in children may be large, however, and can produce symptoms of respiratory distress or mediastinal compression. Death in the neonatal period has been reported. Older children fare well after local resection. Most adults have small asymptomatic peripheral lesions readily excised by open or thoracoscopic wedge resection.

Other Benign Tumors

A number of primary benign lung tumors have been reported in children. Table 57-2 summarizes a number of these. The clinical approach detailed earlier is applicable in these tumors as well because prospective differentiation between benign and malignant lesions is often not possible. When feasible, limited local resection of these tumors is done. This is usually to establish the diagnosis because many of these patients do not have symptoms.

Mucous gland adenomas require particular mention. These benign endobronchial tumors are often included in the group of potentially malignant bronchial adenomas because their clinical

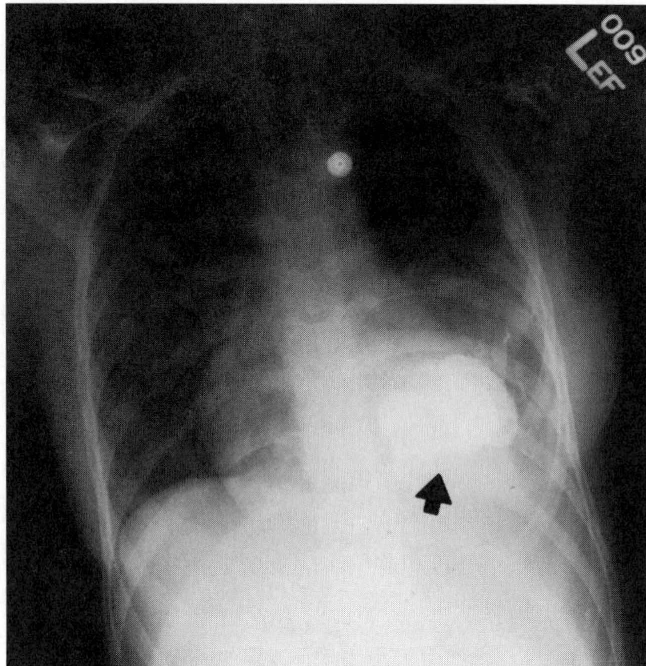

FIG. 57-35. Radiograph illustrating a calcified pulmonary parenchymal lesion, which proved to be an inflammatory pseudotumor (*arrow*). This degree of calcification is unusual. The predominant histologic cell type involved was a plasma cell. (Courtesy of Don Frush, MD, Duke University Medical Center, Durham, NC)

presentation is virtually indistinguishable. These are truly benign entities, however, without known metastatic potential.[87] This is important largely for prognostic purposes because their removal generally requires lobar resection, as detailed earlier in the discussion of endobronchial carcinoid tumors.

Metastatic Lung Tumors

The approach to children with metastatic lung tumors is considerably different than for adults with similar lesions because it is clear that patient survival is much more likely in the younger population. The most common causes of metastatic lung tumors in children are Wilms tumor and osteogenic sarcoma.[94] The approach to the child with metastatic Wilms tumor in the lung involves standard initial surgical management, including radical nephrectomy and regional lymphadenectomy. In addition, the treatment includes systemic chemotherapy and bilateral lung irradiation (see Chap. 33). Surgical resection of lung metastatic lesions is generally done for persistent or new metastases after the initial course of treatment is complete. About half of the children with pulmonary metastases from Wilms tumor can be saved with this approach.[94,95]

Adjuvant chemotherapy has reduced the incidence of metastatic lung lesions secondary to osteogenic sarcoma from about 80% to 30% during the past 10 to 15 years[94] (Fig. 57-36). National protocols in the United States include an aggressive surgical approach to pulmonary metastases after adequate chemotherapy and after appropriate resection of the primary

tumor. With a combination of chemotherapy and sometimes multiple or bilateral pulmonary resections, about 40% of patients with metastatic lung disease from osteogenic sarcoma can be saved.[94,96] The surgical principles are to perform limited wedge resections and conserve normal parenchyma because the lesions tend to be small, subpleural nodules, and they may be numerous. It is common that operative exploration and bimanual palpation reveal lesions not discernible on preoperative imaging studies. This is a compelling argument for open thoracotomy rather than thoracoscopy in these particular patients, because with the closed approach, the surgeon surrenders the tactile input that is so important for detection of small metastases.

A host of other metastatic lung tumors have been treated surgically in children. The general principles are that the lesions must be stable, the primary disease controlled, the metastatic disease isolated to the lungs, and an aggressive effort endorsed by all participants. Generally, these patients first require adjuvant chemotherapy and receive irradiation for radiosensitive tumors. The surgical approach is to limit parenchymal resection to the metastatic sites and the immediately adjacent parenchyma, although lobectomy has been advocated both to diminish the risk of recurrence and to resect larger metastatic deposits. These patients require individualized care, and the experience is too limited for meaningful statistical analysis.

PULMONARY RESECTION IN CHILDREN

Techniques

A detailed description of the technical aspects of lung resection and pulmonary surgery is beyond the scope of this text. Several noteworthy thoracic surgical atlases are available.[73,74] There are few anatomic or technical differences between children and adults other than those related to overall size. Although technical precision is required for pulmonary surgery regardless of age or size, small infants in particular have little margin for

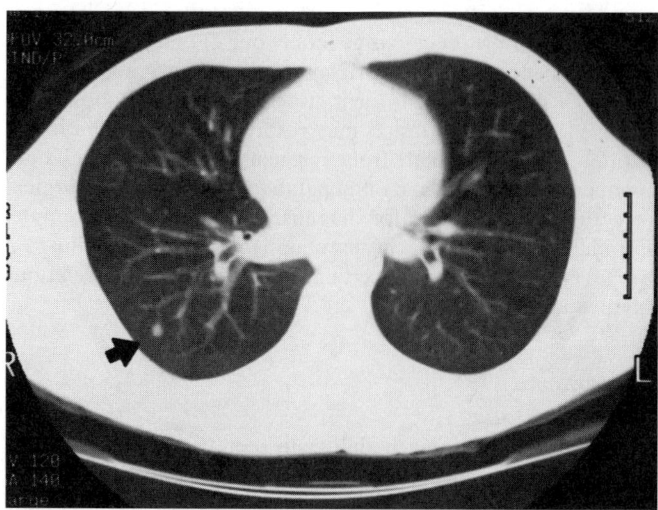

FIG. 57-36. CT scan of the chest showing an obvious metastatic lung nodule in an adolescent with primary osteogenic sarcoma (*arrow*).

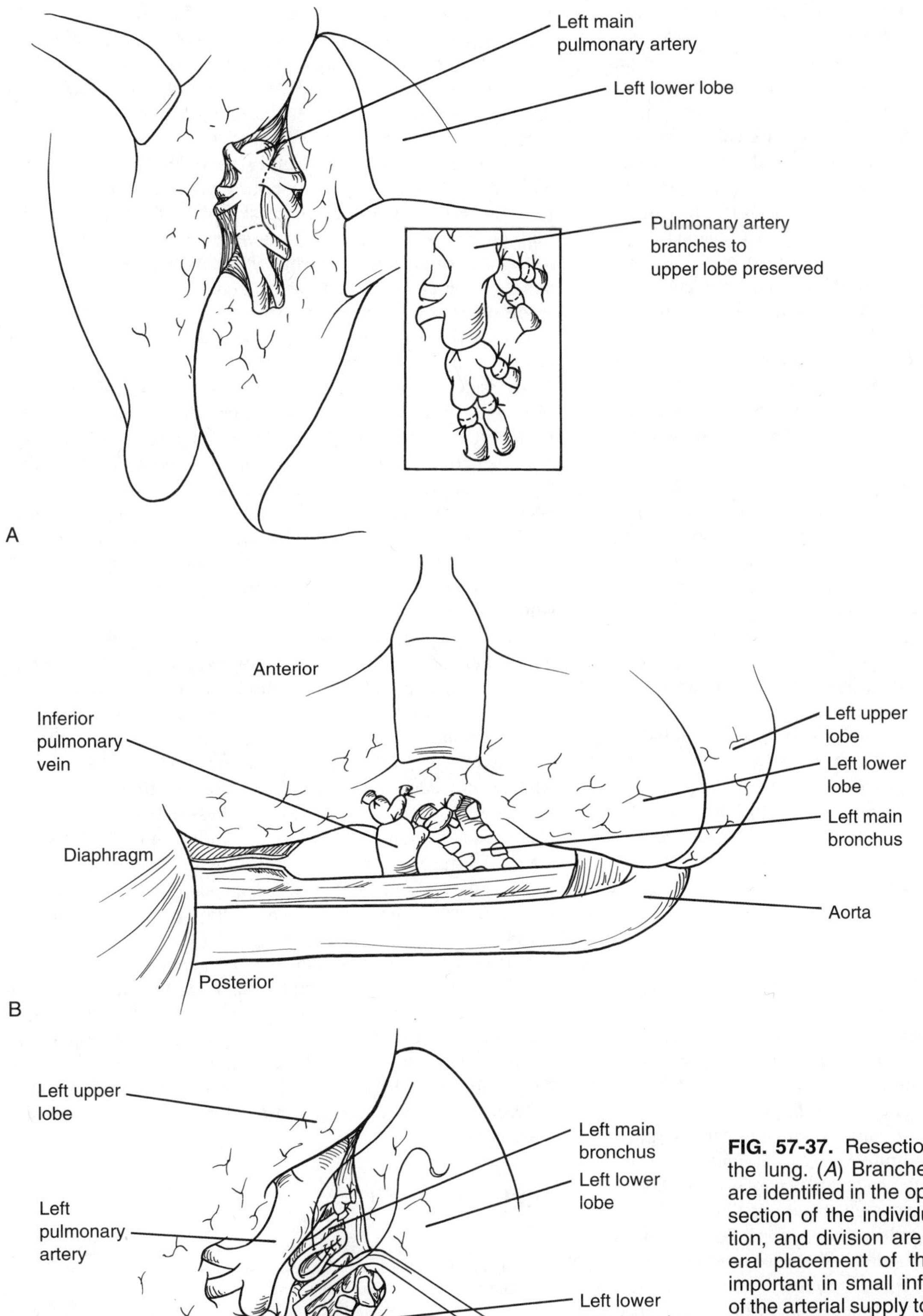

FIG. 57-37. Resection of the left lower lobe of the lung. (*A*) Branches of the pulmonary artery are identified in the open fissure. Meticulous dissection of the individual arterial branches, ligation, and division are illustrated. (*Inset*) Peripheral placement of the ligatures is particularly important in small infants to avoid compromise of the arterial supply to the remaining upper lobe. Appropriate sites for arterial division are indicated. (*B*) The inferior pulmonary vein is controlled, ligated, and divided after the inferior pulmonary ligament is opened. (*C*) The left lower lobe bronchus is controlled and divided. Bronchial stump closure is best done with a handsewn closure in infants and small children. (After Nohl-Oser HC, Nissen R, Schreibe HN. Surgery of the lung. New York, Theime-Stratton, 1981)

error. One of the common lung resections, left lower lobectomy, is illustrated in Figure 57-37. The principles of complete hilar dissection, meticulous vascular control, and bronchial stump closure are illustrated and apply to all lobar or whole lung resections. Bronchial stump closure is easily and reliably done in adults and older children with commercial surgical stapling devices. In infants and small children, this is undesirable because the size of the instrument may make its application insufficiently precise. When working with small airways, the difference between an acceptable and compromised residual bronchus can be exceedingly small. In addition, some staples may be too large for the secure closure of an infant bronchus. For these reasons, a carefully hand-sewn bronchial closure is preferable in infants and small children.

Wedge resections of peripheral lung lesions are common in pediatric thoracic surgery, and this is generally straightforward from a technical standpoint. Stapling devices can be used on lung parenchyma, even in small infants. These are more efficient and possibly more reliable than hand-sewn lung closures. One application is shown in Figure 57-29, with multiple bullae resection. Segmental lung resections are sometimes appropriate as well, although a review of the literature suggests that the perioperative morbidity secondary to air leak and hemorrhage may be greater than for formal lobectomy.[9] When appropriate, these more limited resections are individualized to follow the segmental anatomy of the lung, and this was reviewed briefly in the introductory portion of this chapter. The principles of proximal and distal vascular control and bronchial closure are not different than for formal lobectomy.

Thoracoscopy in children has developed rapidly with the introduction of new instruments and particularly microelectronic video camera systems. Its applications are expanding rapidly, and with prudent use, the technique offers the possibility of equivalent outcomes for a variety of selected intrathoracic procedures without the morbidity of a thoracotomy incision. It therefore has considerable appeal. This procedure is presented in detail in Chapter 56.

Outcomes After Lung Resection

In the absence of diffuse lung disease or pulmonary hypoplasia, pulmonary resection up to and including unilateral pneumonectomy is well tolerated by infants and children.[18,19,97–99] Preservation of normal lung tissue is a fundamental surgical principle in pediatric thoracic surgery, although the surgeon must balance the need to definitively treat the underlying pathology. The age at which lung resection occurs is also relevant to outcome.[18,19] It appears that adults have fixed lung volumes and pulmonary capacities, with little functional compensation after pulmonary resection. As detailed earlier, normal infants and children continue to undergo lung growth and alveolar development through much of the first decade of life. Their compensatory potential is inversely related to age during this time.

Although nonanatomic peripheral lung resections are common for diagnostic efforts, lobectomy is the most common resectional surgical procedure for primary lung pathology. McBride and colleagues performed a clinical follow-up and spirometry on 15 patients between 8 and 32 years of age who had undergone pulmonary resection for congenital lobar emphysema in early childhood.[18] The volume of lung parenchymal

tissue lost was estimated to be 8% to 45%. At follow-up, 11 of these children were without respiratory symptoms of any kind, 2 had reactive airway disease, and 2 had mild dyspnea on exertion. Height, weight, and chest radiographs were all within normal range. Lung volumes (total lung capacity and vital capacity) were within the range considered normal, although the mean value for each was slightly lower than expected (93% and 94%, respectively). The volume compensation was thought to be the result of unilateral increase in the volume of remaining lung on the ipsilateral side. Pulmonary artery blood flow after lobectomy was equal and normally distributed, suggesting compensatory growth of the vascular bed as well. At the cellular level, others have shown compensatory increases in the DNA, protein, collagen content, and weight of residual lung parenchyma after pulmonary resection.[100]

McBride and colleagues[18] showed decreased expiratory flow rates and airway conductance after childhood lobectomy. This is consistent with some degree of persistent airway obstruction. Together, these findings suggest mild disproportion between the compensatory growth of airways and that of the alveoli. This is consistent with the observation that structural and functional maturation of the conducting airways occurs before similar maturation of the terminal airways and alveoli. Despite these findings, children generally have good or excellent functional results after lobectomy.[19,97,98]

Childhood pneumonectomy is followed by contralateral lung overinflation and age-dependent compensatory growth, as outlined earlier. The affected hemithorax is occupied by a shift of the mediastinum, elevation of the hemidiaphragm, and serous fluid accumulation, which eventually evolves into a fibrothorax. The mediastinal shift in a newborn or infant may be dramatic whether it occurs rapidly or over a period of time. Diminished venous return to the heart and compression of the trachea or residual main-stem bronchus by the aorta can be life-threatening.[101] This problem has been treated with a variety of tracheal and vascular reconstructive and suspension procedures and by the placement of an intrathoracic balloon prosthesis. This risk appears to diminish with age.

Spirometry shows predictable decrease of lung volumes after pneumonectomy as well as higher than normal pulmonary arterial pressures, particularly with exercise. Significantly, however, even with this degree of parenchymal resection, functional outcomes are good or excellent in most children.[102] Little or no restriction in lifestyle is to be expected in children who undergo major pulmonary resection in the absence of other lung disease.

REFERENCES

1. Gray SW, Skandalakis JE. The trachea and lungs. In: Embryology for surgeons: the embryological basis for the treatment of congenital defects. Philadelphia, WB Saunders, 1972:293.
2. DiFiore JW, Wilson JM. Lung development. Semin Pediatr Surg 1994;3:221.
3. Thurlbeck WM. Postnatal growth and development of the lung. Am Rev Respir Dis 1975;111:803.
4. Davies GM, Reid L. Growth of the alveoli and pulmonary arteries in childhood. Thorax 1970;25:669.
5. Dunhill MS. Postnatal growth of the lung. Thorax 1962;17:329.
6. Grant JCB. An atlas of anatomy, ed 6. Baltimore, Williams & Wilkins, 1972.
7. Reith EJ, Ross MH. Atlas of descriptive histology, ed 2. New York, Harper & Row, 1970.

8. Haller JA Jr, Golladay ES, Pickard LR, et al. Surgical management of lung bud anomalies: lobar emphysema, bronchogenic cyst, cystic adenomatoid malformation, and intralobar pulmonary sequestration. Ann Thorac Surg 1979;28:33.

9. Ryckman FC, Rosenkrantz JG. Thoracic surgical problems in infancy and childhood. Surg Clin North Am 1985;65:1423.

10. DeLorimer AA. Congenital malformations and neonatal problems of the respiratory tract. In: Welch KJ, Randolph JG, Ravitch MM, et al, eds. Pediatric surgery, ed 4. Chicago, Year Book Medical Pub, 1986: 631.

11. Murray GF. Congenital lobar emphysema. Surg Gynecol Obstet 124: 611, 1967.

12. Buntain WL, Isaacs H Jr, Payne VC Jr, et al. Lobar emphysema, cystic adenomatoid malformation, pulmonary sequestration, and bronchogenic cyst in infancy and childhood: a clinical group. J Pediatr Surg 1974;9:85.

13. Wesley JR, Heidelberger KP, DiPietro MA, et al. Diagnosis and management of congenital cystic disease of the lung in children. J Pediatr Surg 1986;21:202.

14. Hendren WH, McKee DM. Lobar emphysema of infancy. J Pediatr Surg 1966;1:24.

15. Jones JC, Almond CH, Snyder HM, et al. Lobar emphysema and congenital heart disease in infancy. J Thorac Cardiovasc Surg 1965; 49:1.

16. Cooney DR, Menke JA, Allen JE. ''Acquired'' lobar emphysema: a complication of respiratory distress in premature infants. J Pediatr Surg 1977;12:897.

17. Markowitz RI, Mercurio MR, Vahjen GA, et al. Congenital lobar emphysema. Clin Pediatr 1989;28:19.

18. McBride JT, Wohl MEB, Strieder DL, et al. Lung growth and airway function after lobectomy in infancy for congenital lobar emphysema. J Clin Invest 1980;66:962.

19. Frenckner B, Freyschuss U. Pulmonary function after lobectomy for congenital lobar emphysema and congenital cystic adenomatoid malformation: a follow-up study. Scand J Thorac Cardiovasc Surg 1982; 16:293.

20. Miller RK, Sieber WK, Yunis EJ. Congenital adenomatoid malformation of the lung: a report of 17 cases and review of the literature. Pathol Annu 1980;15:387.

21. Stocker JT, Madewell JE, Drake RM. Congenital cystic adenomatoid malformation of the lung. Hum Pathol 1977;8:155.

22. Adzick NS, Harrison MR, Glick PL, et al. Fetal cystic adenomatoid malformation: prenatal diagnosis and natural history. J Pediatr Surg 1985;20:483.

23. Adzick NS, Harrison MR, Flake AW, et al. Fetal surgery for cystic adenomatoid malformation of the lung. J Pediatr Surg 1993;28:806.

24. Budorick NE, Pretorius DH, Leopold GR, et al. Spontaneous improvement of intrathoracic masses diagnosed in utero. J Ultrasound Med 1992;11:653.

25. Revillon Y, Jan D, Plattner V, et al. Congenital cystic adenomatoid malformation of the lung: prenatal management and prognosis. J Pediatr Surg 1993;28:1009.

26. Wolf SA, Hertzler JH, Philippart AI. Cystic adenomatoid dysplasia of the lung. J Pediatr Surg 1980;15:925.

27. Hedlund GL, Bisset GS, Bove KE. Malignant neoplasms arising in cystic hamartomas of the lung in childhood. Radiology 1989;173:77.

28. Shariff S, Thomas JA, Shetty N, et al. Primary pulmonary rhabdomyosarcoma in a child, with a review of literature. J Surg Oncol 1988; 38:261.

29. Domizio P, Liesner RJ, Dicks-Mireaux C, et al. Malignant mesenchymoma associated with a congenital lung cyst in a child: case report and review of the literature. Pediatr Pathol 1990;10:785.

30. Landing BH. Congenital malformations and genetic disorders of the respiratory tract (larynx, trachea, bronchi and lungs). Am Rev Respir Dis 1979;120:151.

31. Sade RM, Clouse M, Ellis FH Jr. The spectrum of pulmonary sequestration. Ann Thorac Surg 1974;18:644.

32. Savic B, Birtel FJ, Tholen W, et al. Lung sequestration: report of seven cases and review of 540 published cases. Thorax 1979;34:96.

33. Dolkart LA, Reimers FT, Helmuth WV, et al. Antenatal diagnosis of pulmonary sequestration: a review. Obstet Gynecol Surv 1992;47: 515.

34. Levine MM, Nudel DB, Gootman N, et al. Pulmonary sequestration causing congestive heart failure in infancy: a report of two cases and review of the literature. Ann Thorac Surg 1982;34:581.

35. Buntain WL, Woolley MM, Mahour GH, et al. Pulmonary sequestration in children: a 25-year experience. Surgery 1977;81:413.

36. Carter R. Pulmonary sequestration: collective review. Ann Thorac Surg 1969;7:68.

37. Smith RA. Some controversial aspects of intralobar sequestration of the lung. Surg Gynecol Obstet 1962;114:57.

38. Samji FM, Sachs HJ, Perkins DG. Cystic disease of the lungs. Surg Clin North Am 1988;68:581.

39. Stein SM, Cox JL, Hernanz-Schulman M, et al. Pediatric chest disease: evaluation by computerized tomography, magnetic resonance imaging, and ultrasonography. South Med J 1992;85:735.

40. Weichert RF, Lindsey ES, Pearce CW. Bronchogenic cyst with unilateral obstructive emphysema. J Thorac Cardiovasc Surg 1970;59:287.

41. Booth JB, Berry CL. Unilateral pulmonary agenesis. Arch Dis Child 1967;42:361.

42. Osborne J, Masel J, McCredie J. A spectrum of skeletal anomalies associated with pulmonary agenesis: possible neural crest injuries. Pediatr Radiol 1989;19:425.

43. Hoffman MA, Superina R, Wesson DE. Unilateral pulmonary agenesis with esophageal atresia and distal tracheoesophageal fistula: report of two cases. J Pediatr Surg 1989;10:1084.

44. Finegold MJ, Katzew H, Genieser NB, et al. Lung structure in thoracic dystrophy. Am J Dis Child 1971;122:153.

45. Turnage RH, Guice KS, Oldham KT. Pulmonary microvascular injury following intestinal reperfusion. New Horizons 1994;2:463.

46. Northway WH Jr, Rosan RC, Porter DY. Pulmonary disease following respiratory therapy of hyaline-membrane disease. N Engl J Med 1967; 276:357.

47. Northway WH Jr. Bronchopulmonary dysplasia: twenty-five years later. Pediatrics 1992;89:969.

48. Escobedo MB, Gonzalez A. Bronchopulmonary dysplasia in the tiny infant. Clin Perinatol 1986;13:315.

49. Northway WH Jr, Moss RB, Carlisle KB, et al. Late pulmonary sequelae of bronchopulmonary dysplasia. N Engl J Med 1990;323:1793.

50. Kollef MH, Schuster DP. Medical progress: the acute respiratory distress syndrome. N Engl J Med 1995;332:27.

51. Kosloske A. Infections of the lungs, pleura, and mediastinum. In: Welch KJ, Randolph JG, Ravitch MM, et al, eds. Pediatric surgery, ed 4. Chicago, Year Book Medical Pub, 1986:657.

52. Alexander JC, Wolfe WG. Lung abscess and empyema of the thorax. Surg Clin North Am 1980;60:835.

53. Scott SS. Pulmonary infections. In: Sabiston DC Jr, ed. Textbook of surgery: the biological basis of modern surgical practice, ed 14. Philadelphia, WB Saunders, 1991:1709.

54. Riordan J, Rommens JM, Kerem BS, et al. Identification of the cystic fibrosis gene: cloning and characterization of complementary DNA. Science 1989;245:1066.

55. Widdicombe JH, Wine JJ. The basic defect in cystic fibrosis. Trends Biochem Sci 1991;16:474.

56. Gutteridge C, Kuhn RJ. Pulmozyme: dornase alfa. Pediatr Nurs 1994; 20:278.

57. Drumm H, Pope H, Cliff W, et al. Correction of the cystic fibrosis defect in vitro by retrovirus-mediated gene transfer. Cell 1990;62: 1227.

58. Rosenstein BJ, Zeitlin PL. Recent advances in cystic fibrosis. Curr Opin Pediatr 1991;3:392.

59. Gross RE. Bronchiectasis. In: The surgery of infancy and childhood: its principles and techniques. Philadelphia, WB Saunders, 1953:785.

60. Sanderson JM, Kennedy MCS, Johnson MF, et al. Bronchiectasis. Results of surgical and conservative management: a review of 393 cases. Thorax 1974;29:407.

61. Lewiston NJ. Bronchiectasis in childhood. Pediatr Clin North Am 1984;31:865.

62. Herman M, Michalkova K, Kopriva F. High-resolution CT in the assessment of bronchiectasis in children. Pediatr Radiol 1993;23:376.

63. Schuster SR, Schwartz MZ. Surgical management of the pulmonary complications of cystic fibrosis. In: Ravitch MM, Welch KJ, Benson CD, et al, eds. Pediatric surgery, ed 3. Chicago, Year Book, 1979.

64. Marmon L, Schidlow D, Palmer J, et al. Pulmonary resection for complications of cystic fibrosis. J Pediatr Surg 1983;18:811.

65. Luck SR, Raffensperger JG, Sullivan HJ, et al. Management of pneu-

mothorax in children with chronic pulmonary disease. J Thorac Cardiovasc Surg 1977;74:834.

66. Stowe SM, Boat TF, Mendelsohn H, et al. Open thoracotomy for pneumothorax in cystic fibrosis. Am Rev Respir Dis 1975;111:611.

67. Tribble CG, Selden RF, Rodgers BM. Talc poudrage in the treatment of spontaneous pneumothoraces in patients with cystic fibrosis. Ann Surg 1986;204:677.

68. Rodgers BM. Thoracoscopy. In: Holcomb GW III, ed. Pediatric endoscopic surgery. Norwalk, Appleton & Lange, 1994:103.

69. Rothman BF, Stone RT, Walker LH, et al. Bronchoscopic lavage for cystic fibrosis patients: an adjunct to therapy. Ann Otol Rhinol Laryngol 1982;91:641.

70. St Louis International Lung Transplant Registry. September 1994 Report. Barnes Hospital, Washington University, St Louis.

71. Miller WS. A study of the human pleura pulmonalis: its relation to the blebs and bullae of emphysema. AJR 1926;15:399.

72. Fitzgerald MX, Keelan PJ, Cugell DW, et al. Long-term results of surgery for bullous emphysema. J Thorac Cardiovasc Surg 1974;68:566.

73. Nohl-Oser HC, Nissen R, Schreiber HW. Surgery of the lung. New York, Theime-Stratton, 1981.

74. Ravitch MM, Steichen FM. Atlas of general thoracic surgery. Philadelphia, WB Saunders, 1988.

75. Nathanson LK, Shimi SM, Wood RA, et al. Videothoracoscopic ligation of bulla and pleurectomy for spontaneous pneumothorax. Ann Thorac Surg 1991;52:316.

76. Eliasson R, Mossberg B, Camner P, et al. The immotile-cilia syndrome. N Engl J Med 1977;297:1.

77. Scott JH, Anderson CL, Shankar PS, et al. Alpha1-antitrypsin deficiency with diffuse bronchiectasis and cirrhosis of the liver. Chest 1977;71:535.

78. Wilson JF, Decker AM. The surgical management of bronchiectasis. Ann Surg 1982:195:354.

79. Lucy MR. Hepatic infection. In: Greenfield LJ, Mulholland MW, Oldham KT, et al, eds. Surgery: scientific principles and practice. Philadelphia, JB Lippincott, 1993:867.

80. Lamy AL, Cameron BH, LeBlanc JG, et al. Giant hydatid lung cysts in the Canadian Northwest: outcome of conservative treatment in three children. J Pediatr Surg 1993;28:1140.

81. Winthrop AL, Waddell T, Superina RA. The diagnosis of pneumonia in the immunocompromised child: use of bronchoalveolar lavage. J Pediatr Surg 1990;25:878.

82. Snyder CL, Ramsay NK, McGlave PB, et al. Diagnostic open-lung biopsy after bone marrow transplantation. J Pediatr Surg 1990;25:871.

83. Bonfils-Roberts EA, Nickodem A, Nealon TF Jr. Retrospective analysis of the efficacy of open lung biopsy in acquired immunodeficiency syndrome. Ann Thorac Surg 1990;49:115.

84. Dunn DL. Infection. In: Greenfield LJ, Mulholland MW, Oldham KT, et al, eds. Surgery: scientific principles and practice, ed 2. Philadelphia, JB Lippincott, 1996.

85. Menzies D, Fanning A, Yuan L, et al. Current concepts: tuberculosis among health care workers. N Engl J Med 1995;332:92.

86. Welch KJ. Pulmonary tuberculosis. In: Ravitch MM, et al, eds. Pediatric surgery, ed 3. Chicago, Year Book Medical Pub, 1979.

87. Hartman GE, Shochat SJ. Primary pulmonary neoplasms of childhood: a review. Ann Thorac Surg 1983;36:108.

88. Lack EE, Harris GB, Eraklis AJ, et al. Primary bronchial tumors in childhood. Cancer 1983;51:492.

89. Verska JJ, Connolly JE. Bronchial adenomas in children. J Thorac Cardiovasc Surg 1968;55:411.

90. Conlan AA, Payne WS, Woolner LB. Adenoid cystic carcinoma (cylindroma) mucoepidermoid carcinoma of the bronchus: factors affecting survival. J Thorac Cardiovasc Surg 1978;76:369.

91. Niitu Y, Kubota H, Hasegawa S, et al. Lung cancer (squamous cell carcinoma) in adolescence. Am J Dis Child 1974;127:108.

92. Cohen MC, Kaschula RO. Primary pulmonary tumors in childhood: a review of 31 years' experience and the literature. Pediatr Pulmonol 1992;14:222.

93. Fudge TL, Ochsner JL, Mills NL. Clinical spectrum of pulmonary hamartomas. Ann Thorac Surg 1980;30:36.

94. Filler RM. Tumors of the lung. In: Welch KJ, Randolph JG, Ravitch MM, et al, eds. Pediatric surgery, ed 4. Chicago, Year Book Medical Pub, 1986:673.

95. Simone JV, Cassady JR, Filler RM. Cancers of childhood. In: DeVita VT Jr, Hellman S, Rosenberg SA, eds. Cancer: principles and practice of oncology. Philadelphia, JB Lippincott, 1982:1254.

96. Schaller RT Jr, Haas J, Schaller J, et al. Improved survival in children with osteosarcoma following resection of pulmonary metastases. J Pediatr Surg 1975;10:545.

97. Brandesky G. Long-term results of pulmonary resections in childhood. Prog Pediatr Surg 1977;10:267.

98. Giammona ST, Mandelbaum I, Battersby JS, et al. The late cardiopulmonary effects of childhood pneumonectomy. Pediatrics 1966;37:79.

99. Buhain WJ, Brody JS. Compensatory growth of the lung following pneumonectomy. J Appl Physiol 1973;35:898.

100. Cowan MJ, Crystal RG. Lung growth after unilateral pneumonectomy: quantitation of collagen synthesis and content. Am Rev Respir Dis 1975;3:267.

101. Szarnicki R, Maurseth K, deLaval M, et al. Tracheal compression by the aortic arch following right pneumonectomy. Ann Thorac Surg 1978;25:231.

102. Szots I, Toth T. Long-term results of the surgical treatment for pulmonary malformations and disorders. Prog Pediatr Surg 1977;10:277.

Surgery of Infants and Children: Scientific Principles and Practice, edited by Keith T. Oldham, Paul M. Colombani, and Robert P. Foglia. Lippincott–Raven Publishers, Philadelphia, © 1997.

CHAPTER 58

Congenital Heart Disease

Ross M. Ungerleider, Mark D. Plunkett, and J. William Gaynor

In the 1990s, it is becoming standard practice to repair many congenital heart defects in early infancy as a one-stage procedure. The preference for palliation, as opposed to correction, is related less to age and size of the patient than to the presence of unrepairable anatomy or severe associated defects that increase the risk of exposure to cardiopulmonary bypass (CPB). The ability to stabilize patients and obtain accurate diagnostic information before surgical intervention has improved decision making and has sparked the evolution of neonatal cardiac surgery as a true subspecialty within the field of cardiac surgery. All of this progress is related to the development of cardiac surgery during the past four decades, and many of the techniques that enable safe infant cardiac repair represent improvements of some of the earlier techniques.

HISTORICAL PERSPECTIVE

Although cardiac surgery was performed before 1950, it was essentially limited to treatment of traumatic injury. Elective repair of intracardiac defects could only be accomplished with the use of indirect methods that had limited application and acceptance. Diagnostic capabilities were limited as well.

Several important developments in the 1950s allowed cardiac surgery to develop. Bigelow and colleagues[1] made the important observation that mild hypothermia significantly lowers basal metabolism and substantially increases the time that the body, particularly the brain, can tolerate periods of little or no perfusion. When mild hypothermia was created by placing the patient in an ice water bath and lowering core temperature to about 30° to 32°C, a period of circulatory arrest could be extended to 7 to 9 minutes. This provided surgeons with the time to perform more intricate intracardiac repairs. Hypothermia combined with caval occlusion was reported to lead to safe outcomes for aortic and pulmonary valvotomy as well as for closure of simple atrial septal defects (ASDs).[2–5] There are still a few excellent centers in the 1990s that report the use of this technique for occasional patients for whom the risk of CPB might be increased.[6,7] More importantly, the experience accrued by this technique taught surgeons that they could safely repair intracardiac defects under direct vision in a bloodless field. This technique is still applied, in a more modern sense, with the use

of core cooling to profoundly low temperatures (15° to 18°C) using CPB. CPB is then stopped, and the bypass cannulas are removed, leaving the patient in circulatory arrest. At these profoundly low temperatures, surgeons can probably extend the safe period of operative intervention to as long as 45 to 60 minutes.[8–14] This technique of deep hypothermic circulatory arrest is commonly employed for the correction of numerous heart defects in neonates and small infants and is clearly based on experiences from the earliest days of cardiac surgery.

In 1953, Gibbon[15] performed the first successful open cardiac procedure using an artificial heart–lung machine (pump oxygenator) when he closed an ASD in a young girl. The clear advantage was the ability to perform open heart surgery in a bloodless and stationary operative field without severe restriction on the available time. Intricate repairs of complex congenital heart defects became feasible. By the mid-1950s, several types of artificial oxygenators were becoming available, and it was possible to begin direct-vision cardiac surgery using extracorporeal life support on a routine basis.

The entire technology was different from what is currently available. Although it is now safe to place small infants on CPB for extended periods of time,[16–18] CPB in 1955 was only available at great risk for older and larger patients (generally older than 5 years). As we now appreciate, these are often the patients who, by virtue of having survived with congenital heart disease for so long, have developed physiologic adaptation to their abnormalities and are least likely to tolerate a sudden operative change in their compensated physiology. Therefore, the early attempts to provide corrective heart surgery for many defects were met with limited success.[19]

The first step, therefore, seemed to be backward, as surgeons recognized the need to retain techniques of palliation developed before the availability of the pump oxygenator. This approach to congenital heart surgery has permeated surgical thinking for so long that many in the field still believe that the best policy for treatment of most congenital heart lesions should be initial palliation followed by eventual correction. Palliation was easy in the respect that it required little knowledge of cardiac anatomy and only a moderate understanding of physiology. For this reason, training acquired a distinctive differential diagnosis format. Patients with congenital heart defects were placed into two basic groups—cyanotic and noncyanotic. Patients within each category were distinguished by a number of features unique to each possible diagnosis. For example, cyanotic heart defects were remembered by the clinician as the T lesions (eg, tetralogy of Fallot, transposition of the great arteries, tricuspid atresia, total anomalous pulmonary venous return, terrible pulmonary atresia (stenosis), truncus arteriosus). The clinician would then examine the patient for subtleties of auscultation, evaluate the chest radiograph, and review the laboratory parameters to determine the most likely diagnosis. The patient would then undergo cardiac catheterization to confirm the diagnostic impression. If the patient was found to have cyanosis from reduced pulmonary blood flow, a systemic pulmonary artery shunt to increase pulmonary blood flow was placed. Patients with noncyanotic lesions usually had too much pulmonary blood flow and presented in congestive heart failure. In an infant, this is usually manifested by tachypnea and failure to thrive because the tachypnea interferes with eating. These patients would often undergo pulmonary artery banding to reduce pulmonary blood flow. In the era of palliation, a pediatric cardiac surgeon could get by with these two procedures: a shunt to treat reduced pulmonary blood flow, or a pulmonary artery band to treat increased pulmonary blood flow. It was not necessary to have a detailed understanding of the intracardiac anatomy because palliation rather than reconstruction was the objective.

Although palliation has been the mainstay for successful heart surgery in children for several decades, it provided a framework for thinking about the management of congenital heart lesions that may no longer be appropriate. A number of changes have occurred during the past several years that justify an entirely different approach.

The first of these was the ability to stabilize patients who have ductal-dependent lesions with prostaglandins, specifically prostaglandin E_1 (PGE_1). PGE_1 is infused intravenously (into the central circulation) and maintains patency of the ductus arteriosus.[8,20] The importance of this discovery relates to initial management of the patient. There are two types of ductal-dependent lesions: (1) lesions that require a patent ductus arteriosus for pulmonary blood flow, for example, pulmonary atresia; and (2) lesions that require a ductus arteriosus for systemic blood flow. Examples of the latter are seen in infants with an interrupted aortic arch, severe aortic coarctation, or the hypoplastic left heart syndrome (Fig. 58-1). Patients who depend on the ductus arteriosus for pulmonary blood flow become cyanotic when the ductus artcriosus begins to close shortly after birth. The degree of cyanosis is dependent on other sources of pulmonary blood flow. When the ductus is the only source of pulmonary blood flow, the cyanosis can become intense. The lesion is considered ductal dependent if there is insufficient blood flow to sustain life without flow through the ductus. Infants who depend on the ductus for systemic blood flow become extremely acidotic as the ductus begins to close and they lose perfusion to the lower body. In addition, these infants usually have pulmonary hypertension and overperfusion of the lungs, resulting in tachypnea and heart failure. Before the use of prostaglandins, these infants required emergent surgery. Patients in the first group would receive a systemic pulmonary shunt— usually performed under duress because these infants often had severe cyanosis and associated acidosis. Infants with severe coarctation required urgent repair, and their mortality risk was increased because they also presented in unstable condition with pulmonary hypertension and systemic acidosis. PGE_1 has essen-

tially enabled surgeons to convert these emergency operations into elective procedures. By restoring and maintaining ductal patency, PGE_1 allows these critically ill infants to be stabilized.[21,22] For patients who require the ductus for pulmonary blood flow, the systemic pulmonary shunt is reopened. This is all the initial treatment needed. For patients with interrupted aortic arch or severe coarctation, distal perfusion is restored, acidosis is corrected, and the infant is in far less critical condition at the time of operation. In both cases, time is provided for the pediatric cardiac team (cardiologists, surgeons, anesthesiologists, and intensive care specialists) to diagnose the condition and stabilize the patient before any surgical intervention. Outcomes have improved substantially.

With the advent of two-dimensional echocardiography augmented by Doppler color flow imaging, it has become possible to diagnose rapidly, accurately, and thoroughly the nature and extent of cardiac lesions.[23–25] A critically ill infant with a ductal-dependent lesion can be stabilized with the infusion of PGE_1. Echocardiography is performed, and a complete anatomic diagnosis is provided. Occasionally, cardiac catheterization is helpful to answer any remaining questions regarding the diagnosis or plans for management.

Parallel growth has occurred in pediatric critical care and in the understanding of how to best care for the variety of complex defects that these infants can present.[26] Most important has been an understanding of the importance of ventilator management in stabilizing these patients.[26–28] This is especially true for patients with defects that can lead to excessive pulmonary blood flow, such as hypoplastic left heart syndrome or interrupted aortic arch. These patients usually present in heart failure with excessive pulmonary blood flow. Although there is a tendency to place these infants on mechanical ventilation with high oxygen concentrations and rapid ventilation, they are actually more appropriately cared for by hypoventilation on low oxygen concentrations. This increases pulmonary vascular resistance and may help to enhance systemic perfusion, rather than pulmonary perfusion, across the ductus. Advances in technology have resulted in better catheters that can be easily inserted into the small central veins and arteries of infants. A variety of pharmacologic agents are available to help optimize the hemodynamics in these infants.

MANAGEMENT OF CARDIAC DEFECTS

The result of these advances is that infants born with complex cardiac abnormalities can be quickly diagnosed and medically stabilized. Management can be directed at providing the optimal procedure for each specific lesion, and surgical decision making is related to determining which of three categories the patient best fits: (1) patients who have defects for which there is no palliation and for which repair is the only option to treat symptoms; (2) patients who have defects for which repair is not possible and for whom palliation is the only option; and (3) patients who have defects that can be completely repaired or palliated in infancy.

Defects That Require Repair

Heart defects that must be repaired when they present in infancy include the following:

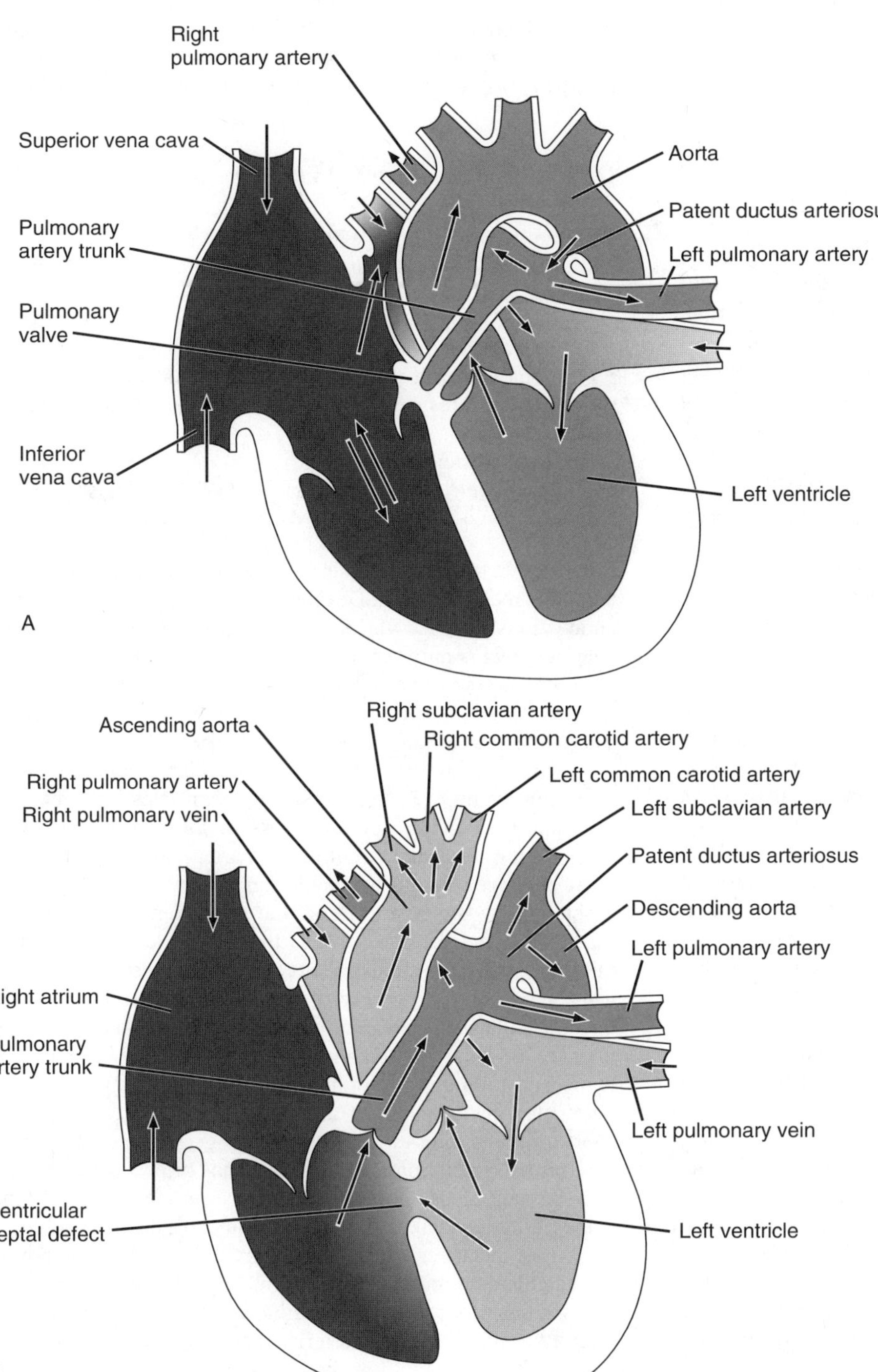

FIG. 58-1. Dependence on the patent ductus arteriosus can occur in two ways. (*A*) Ductal dependency for pulmonary blood flow. In this schematic of a patient with pulmonary valvular atresia, the ductus arteriosus must be open for blood to enter the pulmonary arteries. As the ductus arteriosus closes, pulmonary blood flow is lost, and the patient becomes cyanotic. (*B*) Example of dependence on the ductus arteriosus for perfusion of the distal aorta. In this schematic of a patient with interrupted aortic arch, left ventricular blood (which is oxygenated) is able to cross the ventricular septal defect and enter the pulmonary artery, where it mixes with right ventricular blood. All of this flow is then distributed to the branch pulmonary arteries as well as across the ductus arteriosus to the descending aorta. Patients with this type of ductal dependence can have differential cyanosis because the blood in the pulmonary artery has lower saturation than blood in the aorta. When the ductus arteriosus begins to close in these patients, the flow to the descending aorta is lost, and the patient becomes severely acidotic. Furthermore, these patients have a tendency to overperfuse their pulmonary vascular bed because pulmonary vascular resistance is usually lower than systemic resistance. Management of these patients requires ventilator manipulation to increase pulmonary resistance and pharmacologic therapy (systemic afterload reduction) to enhance systemic perfusion.

- Patent ductus arteriosus
- Atrial septal defect
- Cor triatriatum
- Total anomalous pulmonary venous return
- Critical aortic stenosis
- Aortic coarctation
- Aortopulmonary window
- Truncus arteriosus

These are characterized by anatomic defects suitable for correction and for which there is no reasonable physiologic palliation. In patients with patent ductus arteriosus, ligation is curative and far more simple than any imaginable palliation. Patients with ASDs are rarely symptomatic in infancy, but when they fail to thrive or develop heart failure, the lesions are best treated with surgical closure. Catheter device closure of ASDs is not currently an option for infants, although this technology may be available in the near future. ASDs are easily diagnosed with echocardiography. Cardiac catheterization is not usually necessary to determine the need for surgical closure. In a previous era, ASDs were not closed if cardiac catheterization disclosed a shunt fraction of less than 1.5:1. Because of the current safety of CPB and the ongoing risk of paradoxical emboli with resultant neurologic injury from small ASDs, the mere presence of an ASD can be considered an indication for closure, making the need for catheterization and measurement of the shunt fraction unnecessary. Most clinicians consider an ASD to be hemodynamically significant if the right ventricle appears enlarged on echocardiography. Cor triatriatum, a narrowed connection between the pulmonary venous confluence and the left atrium, produces obstruction of pulmonary venous drainage into the left atrium and requires urgent decompression. The only palliation for these patients is to place them on CPB (eg, extracorporeal membrane oxygenation) to prevent blood from traversing the pulmonary vasculature and contributing to the blockage.[29] The only possible palliation is the first step in the repair of this defect. These infants require relief of the left atrial obstruction before they can be removed from bypass. Likewise, infants with total anomalous pulmonary venous return require repair. If they have obstruction to their pulmonary venous drainage as a component to their anatomic lesions, then they are similar to infants with cor triatriatum and may be initially stabilized with extracorporeal membrane oxygenation bypass.[29] Infants with critical aortic stenosis or coarctation may be initially stabilized with prostaglandins, and this provides time to evaluate more completely the extent of the defect. Many of these infants have severe associated cardiac defects that impact significantly on management options. There is no palliative way to treat the symptoms produced by the aortic stenosis or coarctation. Relief of these symptoms is best obtained by aortic valvotomy or by coarctation repair. Infants with aortopulmonary windows have symptoms similar to those seen with a large patent ductus arteriosus. Although repair is more complicated than patent ductus arteriosus ligation, obliteration of the aortopulmonary window with the patient on CPB is preferable to palliation, which would require banding of the distal pulmonary arteries.[30] Truncus arteriosus is a severe congenital heart defect that produces excessive pulmonary blood flow. Because the main pulmonary artery arises from the side of the aorta, flow is similar to that seen in a ductus arteriosus in that it persists throughout systole and diastole. Although there have been reports of banding the branch pulmonary arteries to palliate these patients, mortality rates with this have been high, and it is probably more proper to repair this defect completely in infancy[31,32] (Fig. 58-2).

Defects That Require Palliation

Some infants present with heart defects that cannot be repaired in infancy and that must be palliated. Defects initially treatable only with palliation include the following:

- Single ventricle anatomy
- Pulmonary atresia with intact ventricular septum
- Pulmonary atresia with multiple aortopulmonary collateral arteries
- Neonatal Ebstein anomaly
- Multiple ventricular septal defects (VSDs; "Swiss cheese" septum)

For a defect to be repairable, it must have the components for anatomic reconstruction. Despite intracardiac holes or abnormal connections between various portions of the cardiac anatomy, a heart defect is only repairable if the heart has two atria or has the potential for septating a common atrium such that there is a separate chamber for systemic and pulmonary venous return. There must be two atrioventricular (AV) valves or the possibility of constructing two AV valves from a large common valve. Most importantly, there must be two ventricles, each capable of supporting their respective parts of the circulation. There must be an aorta and a pulmonary artery. Each great vessel must be large enough to enable unimpeded flow to its distal vascular bed. By these criteria, the most common reason that a heart defect is unrepairable is that a ventricular chamber is missing (such as in tricuspid atresia or hypoplastic right or left heart syndrome). A variety of cardiac anomalies present with univentricular anatomy, and palliation may be necessary when they are associated with an imbalance of flow between the systemic and pulmonary circulations. Whenever palliation is required for management of a congenital heart defect, both the short-term and long-term goals of management must be clearly determined. Palliation should be a means of best achieving the ultimate goal. It is short-sighted to treat immediate symptoms if the palliation makes the ultimate outcome less desirable.

In most instances, palliation is provided to infants with noncorrectable anatomy when the ultimate goal is a Fontan procedure. In this procedure, the systemic venous return is connected directly to the pulmonary arteries, and pulmonary flow occurs in a passive fashion.[33] For the Fontan procedure to be successful, the pulmonary arteries must grow without distortion to an adequate size, which is usually obtained when the patient is 1 to 2 years old. Furthermore, the patient's single ventricle must remain undamaged by excessive and chronic volume loading (from too large a shunt)[34] or pressure loading (from obstructed outflow).[35] Therefore, palliation for these patients must protect the pulmonary arteries from distortion and the ventricle from progressive damage. Shunts should be performed for infants who are cyanotic and ductal dependent for pulmonary blood flow. These shunts should be performed preferably to the more central pulmonary arteries to prevent the chance of stenosis at a peripheral site that might interfere with the success of a later Fontan procedure.

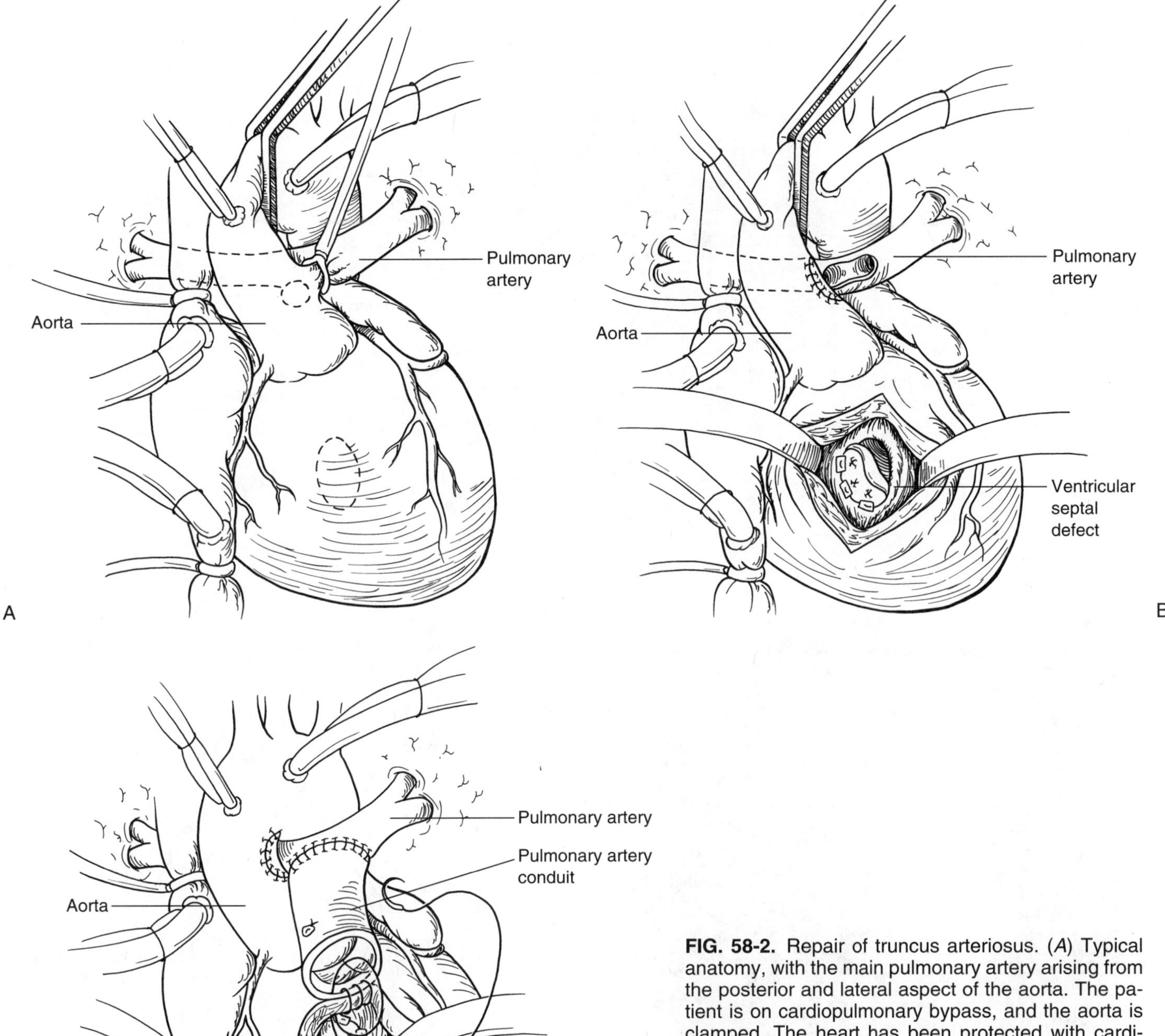

FIG. 58-2. Repair of truncus arteriosus. (*A*) Typical anatomy, with the main pulmonary artery arising from the posterior and lateral aspect of the aorta. The patient is on cardiopulmonary bypass, and the aorta is clamped. The heart has been protected with cardioplegia solution. (*B*) The main pulmonary trunk has been removed from the aorta, and the defect in the aorta has been repaired with a patch. Through a ventriculotomy, the ventricular septal defect is exposed and closed with a patch of prosthetic material. (*C*) Continuity between the right ventricle and the pulmonary artery is then established with a valved conduit, such as a pulmonary artery homograft, as shown here. (Mavroudis C, Backer CL. Truncus arteriosus. In: Mavroudis C, Backer CL, eds. Pediatric cardiac surgery. St Louis, CV Mosby, 1994)

Infants with excessive pulmonary blood flow may be treated simply by a pulmonary artery band. More often, these infants have complex defects that require reconstruction of the entire left ventricular (LV) outflow tract and a variety of more involved palliative procedures (such as a Damus-Kaye-Stansel or Norwood procedure).[35–37] The best procedure is determined by the long-term goal of management for each patient (Fig. 58-3).

Occasionally, a patient with potentially repairable anatomy may require palliation in infancy. These patients include those with pulmonary atresia with an intact septum as well as those

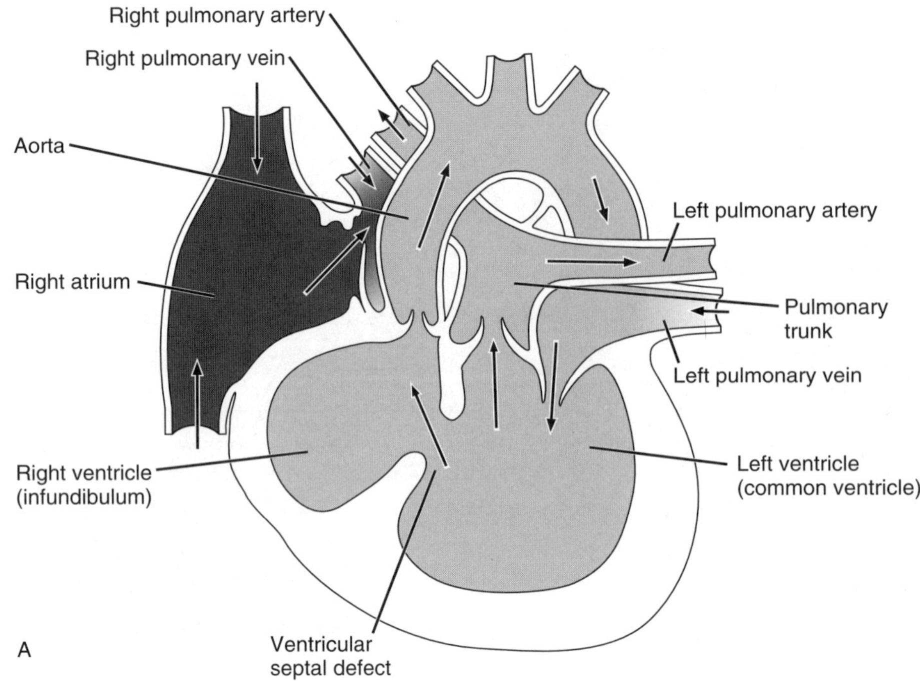

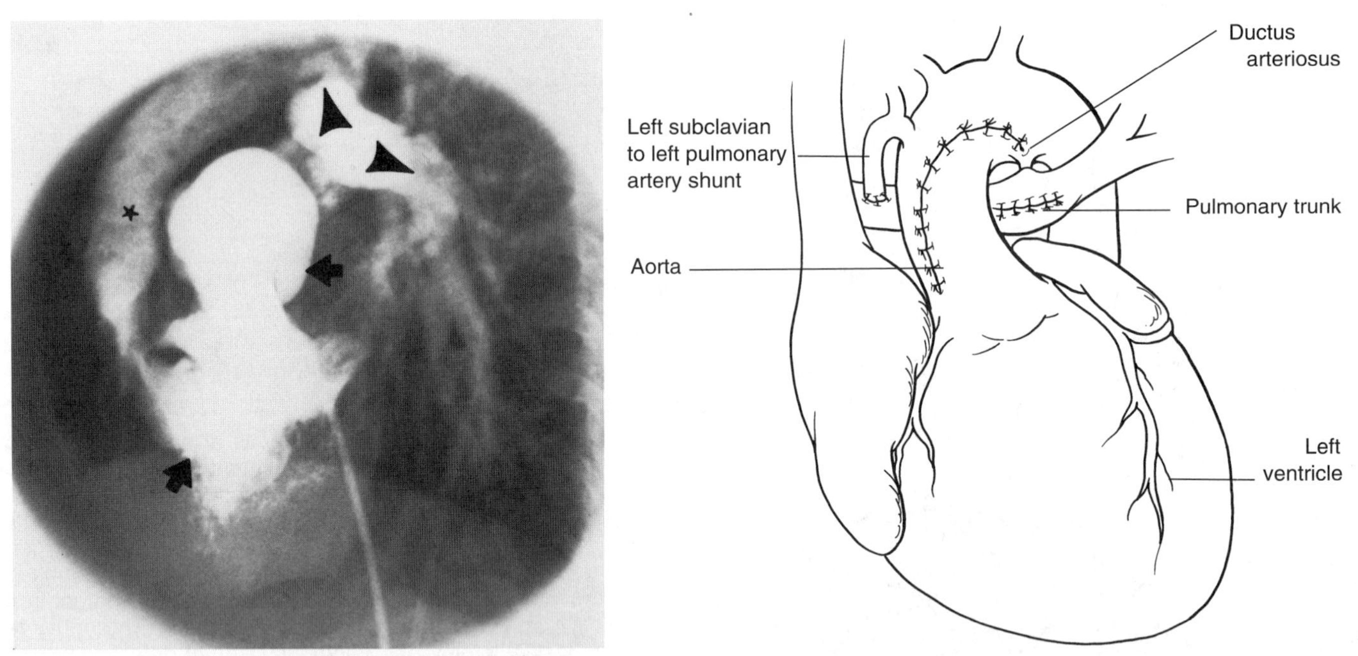

FIG. 58-3. In staging patients for a Fontan procedure, aggressive forms of palliation are sometimes necessary. (*A*) Schematic of the typical anatomy in tricuspid atresia with transposition of the great arteries. In these cases, the aorta, which arises from the small right ventricle, may have restricted inflow from subaortic stenosis that can occur at the valve as well as at the ventricular septal defect leading into the infundibular chamber. (*B*) Angiogram obtained from a patient with this anatomy who received a previous pulmonary artery band. Aorta (*asterisk*) left ventricle (*arrows*), pulmonary arteries (arrowheads). The left ventricle in this patient has obstruction at both outlets and will undergo damaging changes before the Fontan procedure. (*C*) A more appropriate solution for these patients is anastomosis of the pulmonary artery to the aorta to form a single outflow tract (Norwood-type procedure). The pulmonary blood supply is provided by a shunt (shown as a subclavian to pulmonary anastomosis). These patients will have unobstructed outflow and ultimately be better candidates for a Fontan procedure.

with pulmonary atresia associated with a VSD and multiple aortopulmonary collateral arteries supplying the pulmonary vasculature. Palliation for these infants is designed to provide adequate pulmonary blood flow through a shunt for a specific time. During this period, the right ventricle and tricuspid valve may grow to a size that enables a two-ventricle repair (in pulmonary atresia with an intact ventricular septum), or the pulmonary arteries may grow to a size that allows them to be connected to the right ventricle (pulmonary atresia with multiple aortopulmonary collateral arteries). Likewise, patients with multiple VSDs (Swiss cheese septum) may be best treated with a pulmonary artery band to control heart failure from excessive pulmonary blood flow. Many of these VSDs may close spontaneously,[38] and the ultimate plan is to remove the band at a later time and close a single remaining VSD if necessary. In these latter cases, palliation actually helps to stage initially unrepairable anatomy to complete repair. Nevertheless, the choice of palliation used is influenced by the expectations for the patient's outcome.

Transplantation

Heart, lung, or heart–lung transplantation is sometimes indicated for children with cardiomyopathies, for children who have failed previous attempts at palliation or correction of complex congenital heart lesions, and for children with certain uncorrectable cardiac lesions.[39] The immediate morbidity and mortality of transplantation in infants and children has been considerably reduced in recent years.[40] Short-term and medium-term survival after transplantation, however, remains lower for infants and children than for adults. The long-term results (20 years or more) of cardiac and pulmonary transplantation in children are unknown. Children undergoing transplantation remain at risk for rejection and the long-term complications of immunosuppression, including growth retardation, graft atherosclerosis, posttransplantation lymphoproliferative disease, cyclosporine-induced nephrotoxicity, and hypertension.

In neonates and infants, the most common indication for cardiac transplantation is the hypoplastic left heart syndrome. Results of transplantation compare favorably with alternative methods of treatment such as the Norwood procedure.[40,41] In older children, the most common indications for cardiac transplantation are cardiomyopathy or failure of previous attempts to palliate or repair complex congenital heart disease. Factors that increase the risk and difficulty of transplantation include (1) multiple previous operations, (2) elevated pulmonary vascular resistance, (3) a need for pulmonary artery reconstruction, and (4) some systemic venous anomalies. Despite these difficulties, transplantation is an increasingly attractive option for some children with congenital heart disease and offers the opportunity for increased exercise tolerance, improved life-style, and increased life expectancy.

Specific Defects

For many years, the ability to repair heart defects completely in infants was limited by the size of the patient. In many instances, it was believed to be safer to perform palliation in infancy and to delay complete repair until the child grew. Studies have since examined the outcomes for patients receiving staged repair versus early infant correction.[42–44] Along with the

TABLE 58-1. *Defects that can be repaired or palliated in infancy*

Defect	Palliaton
Ventricular septal defect	Band
Atrioventricular canal	Band
Transposition of the great arteries	Atrial septostomy
Tetralogy of Fallot	Shunt
Pulmonary atresia and ventricular septal defect	Shunt
Double-outlet right ventricle	Shunt or band
Interrupted aortic arch	Arch repair and band

excellent results being reported for correction of heart defects in infancy, there is now a strongly held bias by many authorities that early infant correction is often preferable to palliation. The increasing safety of neonatal CPB has also encouraged this approach. Table 58-1 lists some of the defects affected by this evolution.

Ventricular Septal Defects

VSDs can occur in a variety of locations (Fig. 58-4). Depending on their size, nature, and location, they may have a high incidence of spontaneous closure.[45,46] For this reason, they are usually treated with medical management in the hope that surgical closure will not be required. In infants with symptoms, however, surgical intervention may be required shortly after birth. VSDs that continue to produce significant shunts should be surgically repaired if they have not spontaneously closed by 1 year of age. As for ASDs, cardiac catheterization plays a decreasing role in determining the need for VSD closure. Cardiac catheterization allows calculation of pulmonary vascular resistance; more than 8 wood units can be considered a contraindication to VSD closure. It is unlikely, however, that pulmonary vascular resistance of this magnitude will be encountered if VSDs are repaired when the infant is younger than 6 months of age. Therefore, large VSDs (including AV canal defects) can usually be safely repaired without preliminary catheterization before 6 months of age. Cardiac catheterization should be performed in older patients (older than 1 year) or in any patient in whom pulmonary hypertension is a concern, before closure of the VSD. In these patients, pulmonary vascular resistance should be calculated with and without oxygen to evaluate the reactivity of the pulmonary vasculature. Although some surgeons still prefer to band the pulmonary artery in infants who weigh less than 3 kg, VSD repair can be safely accomplished in small infants, including those who weigh less than 2 kg. Occasionally, surgical repair is assisted by using the technique of profound hypothermia with total circulatory arrest.[47,48] For this technique, the patient is placed on CPB, and core temperature is cooled to 18°C. CPB is then stopped, and the cannulas used for CPB are removed so that the surgeon can close the VSD in a bloodless field. Cannulas are then reinserted, and the patient is warmed to a normal temperature before being separated from CPB. Barratt-Boyes and colleagues[47,48] initially reported this technique for the closure of VSDs in infants, and refinements in the technique have enhanced its safety as an

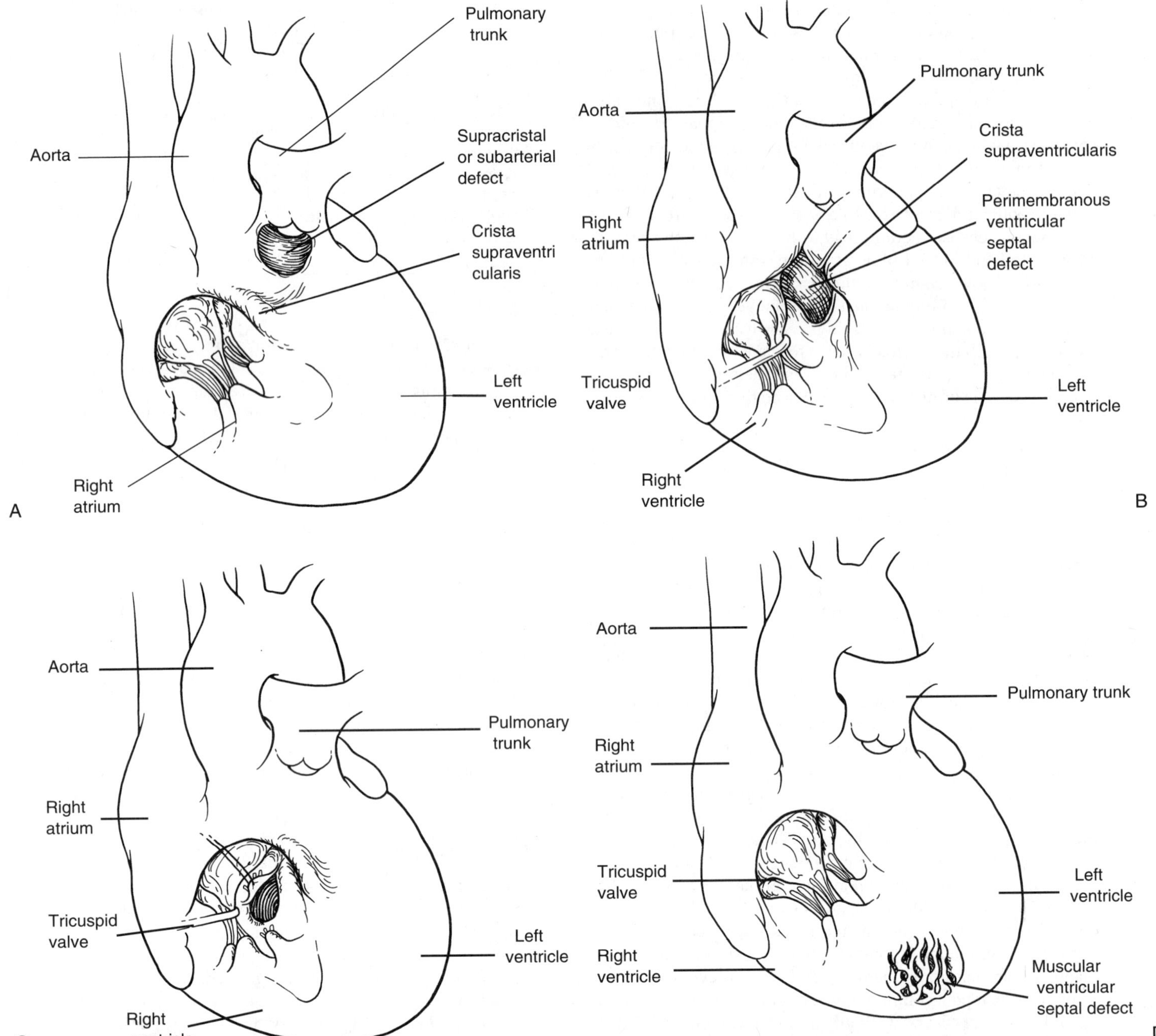

FIG. 58-4. Classic anatomic types of ventricular septal defects. (*A*) A supracristal or subarterial defect. This defect occurs in the infundibular septum and is a deficiency of the conal septum. This defect is best exposed through the right ventricle or pulmonary artery. (*B*) A perimembranous ventricular septal defect occurs below the crista supraventricularis and can be easily approached through the tricuspid valve (transatrial) or through a small ventriculotomy. (*C*) An AV canal or inlet type ventricular septal defect occurs in the septum immediately adjacent to the septal leaflet of the tricuspid valve. Exposure for this type of ventricular septal defect is best obtained through the tricuspid valve using a transatrial approach. (*D*) A muscular ventricular septal defect occurring near the ventricular apex with flow directed around numerous trabecula. (After Mavroudis C, Backer CL, Idriss FS. Ventricular septal defect. In: Mavroudis C, Backer CL, eds. Pediatric cardiac surgery. St Louis, CV Mosby, 1994)

option for intracardiac repair in even very small infants.[13] Most single VSDs present the surgeon with an opportunity to repair an infant's cardiac defect completely, enabling the child to grow and develop normally without cardiac limitations.

Atrioventricular Canals

AV canal (complete AV septal) defects present a more complex surgical challenge and also produce a more disturbing physiologic alteration to the infant. The combination of the significant left-to-right shunt from the large intracardiac defect and valvular insufficiency from the abnormal AV valve can lead to substantial heart failure and failure to thrive in early infancy. Although a pulmonary artery band can limit the amount of pulmonary blood flow, it does not address the problems created by the AV valve insufficiency. This defect often can be repaired using hypothermic circulatory arrest, even in very small infants, with excellent results.[13,49] Repair involves creating a new ventricular and atrial septum, and then suspending the common AV valve from this in a manner that divides it into *tricuspid* and *mitral* components (Fig. 58-5). Elective repair of AV canal should be performed before 6 months of age. Cardiac catheterization before repair is usually not necessary.

Transposition of the Great Arteries

Transposition of the great arteries has undergone the greatest evolution in management during the past decade. This defect is characterized by abnormal connection between the ventricles and the great vessels such that the aorta arises from the right ventricle and the pulmonary artery arises from the left ventricle. To survive, these infants require a mixing of oxygenated blood in their left atrium with blood on the right side of the heart so that it can be ejected into the aorta. Occasionally, these infants have a VSD that can serve this function, but most often, an atrial septostomy is created in infancy. This is achieved either by surgical resection or, more commonly, in the catheterization laboratory by pulling an inflated balloon catheter across the atrial septum—called a *Rashkind balloon septostomy*. With this palliation, infants historically survived until 3 to 4 months of age. At that time, an operation would be performed to redirect blood flow within the heart such that the systemic venous return would be baffled into the mitral valve (and thus into the pulmonary artery) and the pulmonary venous return would be directed into the tricuspid valve (and thus out the aorta). These atrial switch procedures (Mustard or Senning procedures) were the mainstays of surgical treatment for years.[50,51] Unfortunately, even with atrial septostomy to allow mixing, transposition of the great arteries carries about a 10% mortality rate in the first month of life. Patients who survived to undergo a Mustard or Senning procedure received an operation that committed the right ventricle and tricuspid valve to systemic afterload for life. The long-term results were variable and unpredictable.

Advances in neonatal cardiac repair have produced the techniques and technology that have led most surgeons to prefer anatomic repair of this defect shortly after birth by arterial switch. In this procedure, the great arteries (including the coronary arteries) are transferred to their appropriate ventricular connections (Fig. 58-6). If this procedure is performed early in life, before the left ventricle loses its ability to pump against systemic afterload (first 2 weeks after birth), the outcome can be exceptional, with nearly perfect short-term and long-term results.[52–55] Transposition of the great arteries has become an outstanding example of how complete neonatal repair offers an option that provides patients with advantages not achievable by early palliation followed by later repair.

Tetralogy of Fallout

The controversy regarding the best management strategy for tetralogy of Fallot continues to the present time, but it is becoming increasingly apparent that early complete repair is preferable to palliation (shunting) in infancy, followed by later anatomic correction. Numerous reports document outstanding results with complete repair of tetralogy of Fallot in the neonatal and early infant period without the need for preliminary palliation.[13,56–59] Some studies have even suggested a disadvantage to a protocol that includes palliation if surgery is required before a certain age.[44,60] Palliation can carry its own mortality and morbidity, including problems that may preclude the possibility of ever performing complete repair of the defect. Furthermore, recent examination of the cost of early one-stage repair versus two-stage repair (palliation followed by eventual correction) documents a significant cost savings accrued by early infant repair of tetralogy of Fallot.[61] Furthermore, primary repair before 6 months of age can be accomplished with low risk and avoids the potential problem of cyanotic spells, which may increase mortality rates.[61,62] Repair requires closure of the VSD and enlargement of the outflow tract between the right ventricle and the pulmonary artery (Fig. 58-7). In extremely severe forms of tetralogy of Fallot, the connection between the right ventricle and the pulmonary artery may be atretic (tetralogy of Fallot with pulmonary atresia; pulmonary atresia with VSD). These infants are always ductal dependent for their pulmonary blood flow, and the standard management for these patients has been placement of an aortopulmonary shunt in infancy followed by repair (with VSD closure and a right ventricle–pulmonary artery conduit) in early childhood. It is an option, however, to perform primary repair of this extreme form of tetralogy of Fallot in early infancy. The authors have repaired nine infants with this defect without hospital mortality. In three of these infants, the connection between the right ventricle and the pulmonary artery was created without the need for a conduit, suggesting another possible advantage of early infant repair.

Double-Outlet Right Ventricle

Double-outlet right ventricle includes a variety of defects that have in common a VSD and an origin of both great arteries, for the most part, from the right ventricle. Depending on the location of the VSD relative to the great vessels, the physiology of these defects can be similar to (1) a large VSD, (2) tetralogy of Fallot, or (3) transposition of the great arteries.[63] In some instances, there is an associated coarctation of the aorta. Despite the complexity of some of these defects, they all meet criteria for complete repair because all the necessary components are present and normal anatomy can be constructed. This always entails closure of the VSD. In some instances, repair may also

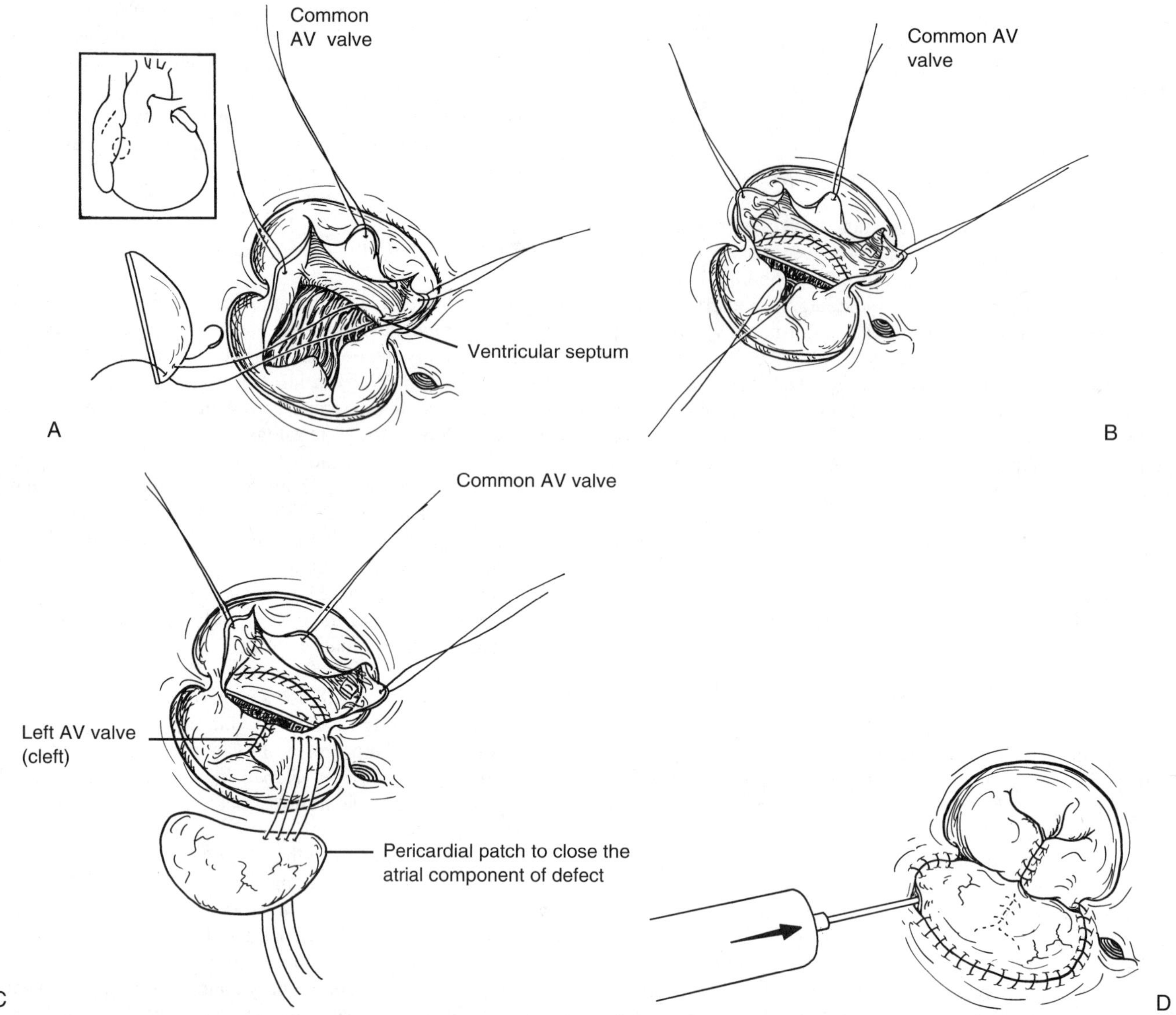

FIG. 58-5. Repair of an AV canal (complete atrioventricular septal) defect. (*A*) The defect is viewed through an atrial incision, and the ventricular septum is repaired with a patch of prosthetic material that is placed with continuous suture so that it underlies the common AV valve. (*B*) The edges of this patch are secured to the edges of the ventricular defect, with the suture brought through the substance of the common AV valve. (*C*) The cleft in the newly formed mitral valve (left AV valve) is repaired with interrupted sutures, and then the atrial component of the defect is repaired with a patch of pericardium so that the AV valve is sandwiched between two patches. (*D*) Before completing the atrial closure, the left atrium is filled with saline.

include an arterial switch or simultaneous repair of aortic coarctation through a median sternotomy.[63]

Interrupted Aortic Arch

Infants with an interrupted aortic arch usually present with dependency on the ductus (and therefore the need for prostaglandins) (see Fig. 58-1) to maintain perfusion of the lower body. These patients almost invariably have a VSD. Although these patients can be managed by reconnection of the aorta and banding of the pulmonary artery through a left thoracotomy, they have an easily repairable defect if approached through a median sternotomy and CPB. The aortic arch can be repaired using a short period of circulatory arrest, and the VSD can be closed while the patient is being rewarmed for removal from CPB.

Occasionally, a patient with a repairable heart defect requires palliation because the heart defect coexists with other serious medical conditions that preclude safe use of CPB. In addition, an infant may require urgent surgical intervention. For example, if a patient cannot be stabilized before obtaining complete diagnostic information because the ductus arteriosus is not responding to PGE$_1$, palliation may be appropriate. These patients may also be best managed by initial palliation. Therefore, the defects listed in Table 58-1 can be managed with a flexible approach,

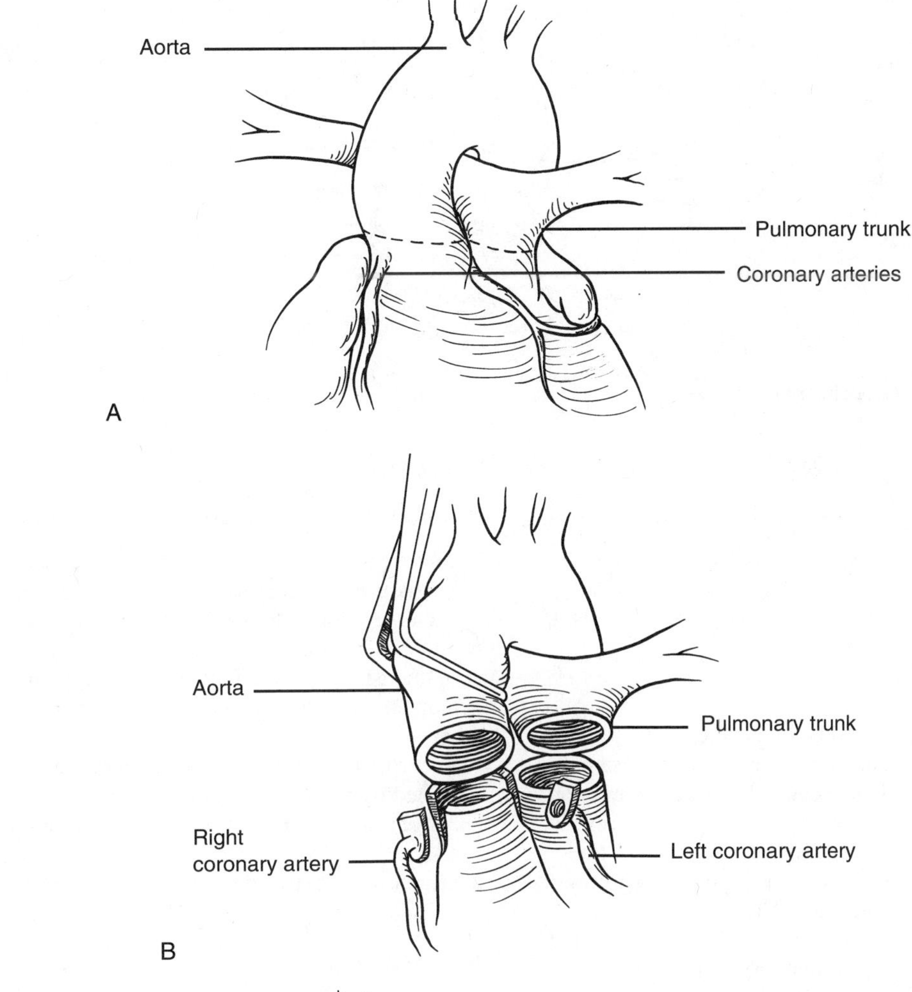

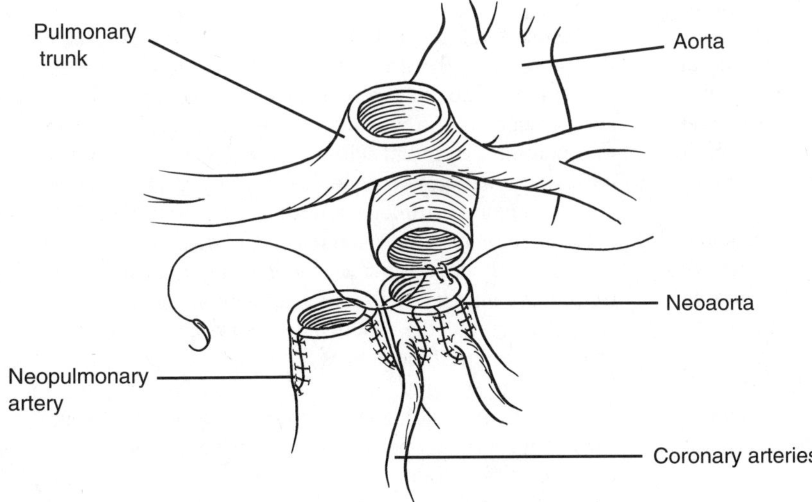

FIG. 58-6. (*A*) The typical anatomy of transposition of the great vessels is shown, with the aorta anterior and slightly to the right of the pulmonary artery. The coronary arteries can be seen arising from the aorta. (*B*) Repair is best accomplished by an arterial switch procedure in infancy. The great vessels are transsected, and the coronary arteries are removed from the aorta and placed into the proximal pulmonary artery (neoaorta). (*C*) The distal aorta is then brought behind the pulmonary artery bifurcation (Lecompte maneuver), and the neoaorta anastomosis is completed. (*D*) The defects in the neopulmonary artery (previous aorta) are repaired with pericardium, and the pulmonary artery repair is then completed (*continued*).

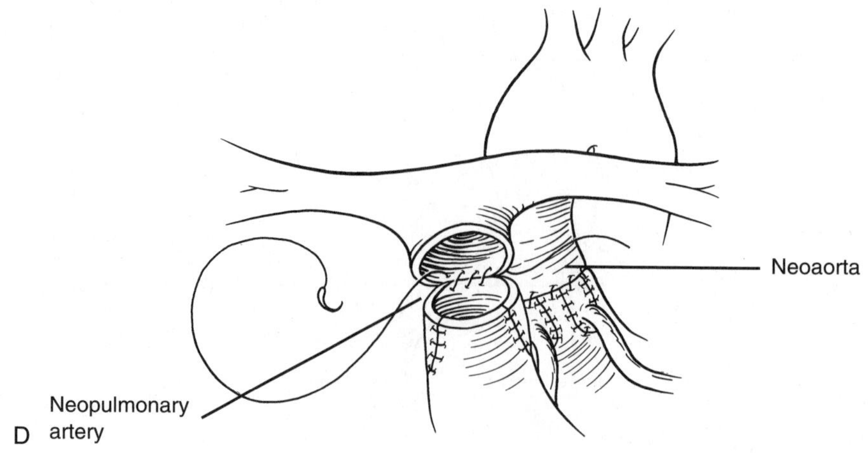

FIG. 58-6. *(continued)*

and the surgical team should attempt to individualize care to obtain the best results.

TIMING OF SURGERY

An additional issue that needs to be considered is the timing for surgical intervention. Patients need intervention in the neonatal period if they are ductal dependent and require the infusion of prostaglandins. Patients need timely intervention in certain defects (eg, transposition of the great arteries, double-outlet right ventricle with subpulmonary VSD) to avoid deconditioning of important cardiac structures (eg, the left ventricle) to a point that options for repair are altered. Conditions associated with a high risk for developing pulmonary hypertension (eg, large VSD, AV canal) should be repaired before its development, usually by 6 months of age. Patients who are candidates for a Fontan procedure need carefully planned procedures at various stages to protect the ventricle and to optimize pulmonary artery growth. Patients with cyanotic heart defects should undergo a repair procedure by 2 years of age if possible to limit the impact of cyanosis on neurologic and myocardial development.

It is best to understand congenital heart disease from the anatomic perspective of what is and what is not repairable, and then to design a management plan accordingly. Repairable lesions are best repaired without initial palliation, and in some instances, no palliative options exist. When palliation is an option, primary repair of correctable defects, even in tiny infants, should be given consideration because outcomes are generally better when repair is performed by teams experienced in neonatal cardiac repair.

POSTOPERATIVE CONVALESCENCE

Postoperative patients are best managed in a pediatric intensive care unit by a team of specialists (including surgeons, anesthesiology and critical care specialists, cardiologists, and nurses) who are dedicated to and have experience with neonates and young infants after cardiac surgery. No single component of this team should attempt to dominate every aspect of care because successful management of the neonate after cardiac repair is truly a team effort that requires constant surveillance and cooperation. The difference between good and excellent results is dependent on the development of an outstanding pediatric intensive care unit with experienced, skilled, and dedicated personnel who communicate and collaborate well with one another.

In the ideal environment, postoperative convalescence is determined by three factors: (1) the existence of any residual defects, (2) the effect on the heart and the infant of the systems used for repair, and (3) the physiologic adaptation required by the heart to adjust to the repair.

Residual Defects

Residual defects include associated malformations that limit the capacity of the infant to survive. These may be cardiac or noncardiac, and they reflect anatomic abnormalities that the surgeon cannot correct and that impact on the infant's recovery. For example, an infant with DiGeorge syndrome and immunodeficiency may not convalesce normally after a technically excellent repair of truncus arteriosus. Likewise, a patient with distal pulmonary artery stenosis (beyond reach of the surgeon) may have elevated right ventricular pressure after repair of tetralogy of Fallot, and this may hamper convalescence. The detrimental effect of the distal pulmonary stenosis may be made more prominent if the patient has significant pulmonary insufficiency from a right ventricular outflow patch. This may all relate to the patient's anatomic deformity and the requirements for an appropriately performed repair. Nevertheless, these residual defects can produce disturbing problems in the postoperative period that the surgeon may need to address. In the example given, one residual defect can be eliminated by placing a pulmonary valve to limit the impact of the distal pulmonary artery stenoses. It is important to understand that any aspect of the anatomy that is not or cannot be made normal may contribute to difficulties during convalescence. All residual problems and their relation to each other must be carefully evaluated postoperatively. Occasionally, careful analysis of these various problems can help the team arrive at an appropriate recommendation that might help a patient who is convalescing poorly.

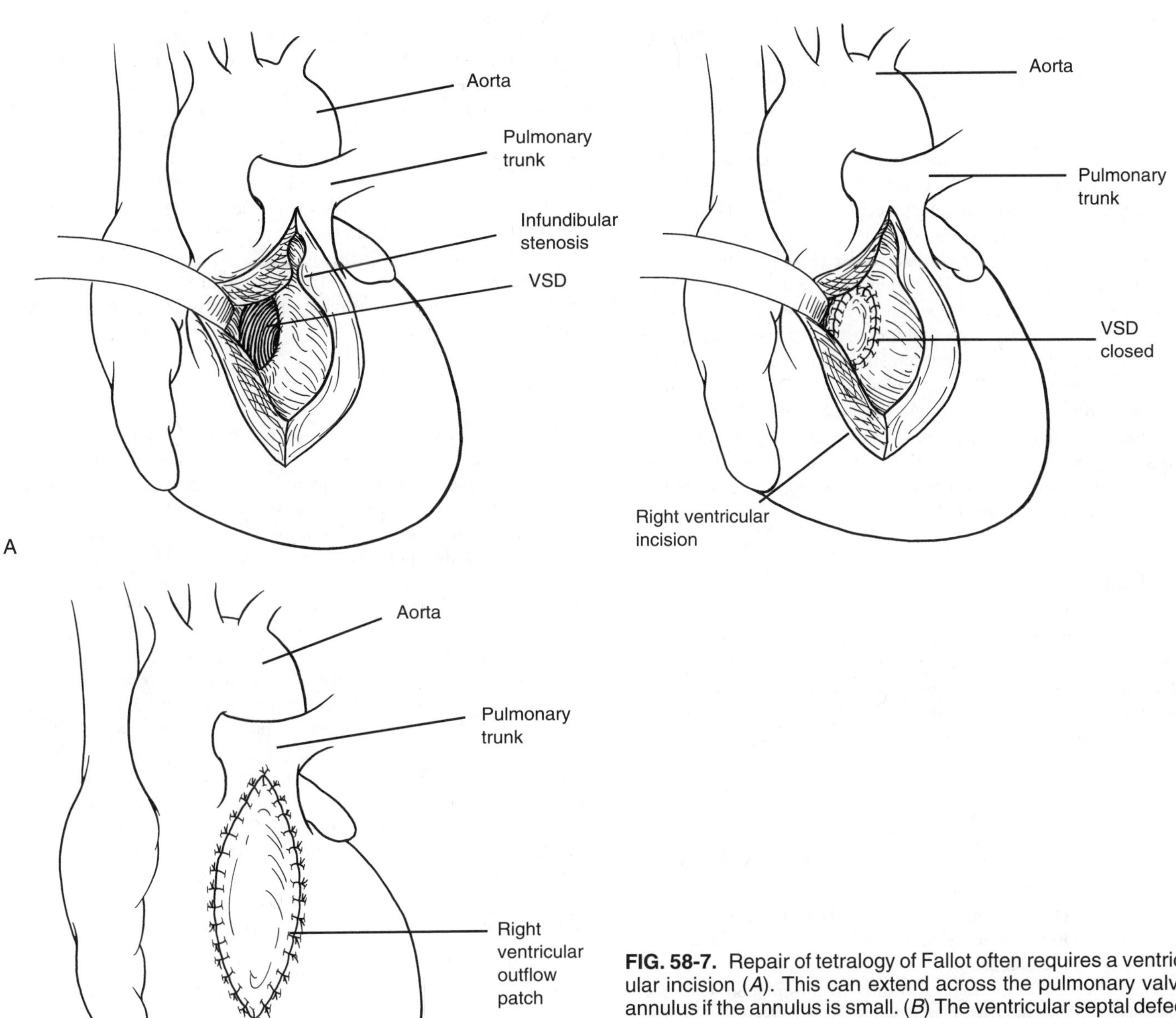

FIG. 58-7. Repair of tetralogy of Fallot often requires a ventricular incision (*A*). This can extend across the pulmonary valve annulus if the annulus is small. (*B*) The ventricular septal defect is then closed with a patch. (*C*) The ventricular incision is likewise closed with a patch to enlarge the right ventricular outflow. (Repair of tetrology through a right atrial incision has recently become favored in selected patients.)

A second type of residual defect is one that the surgeon leaves by performing an inadequate repair. An example would be a residual shunt along the edge of a VSD patch where a suture has torn or has been placed in an imperfect location. A significant residual defect in the surgical repair can have a major impact on outcome, with prolonged intensive care unit convalescence, the need for another operation, or even death. The use of echocardiography in the operating room to evaluate the surgical repair before removing the patient from the operating room has virtually eliminated the likelihood that a patient will be brought to the intensive care unit with a residual surgical defect that requires further intervention.[38,64–68] If patients are convalescing abnormally and intraoperative echocardiography was not performed, then echocardiography should be performed in the intensive care unit to identify any residual surgical defect that may require revision to enhance the patient's recovery.

Effect of the Systems Used for Repair

The effect of the systems used for repair can play an important role in the first several days after infant cardiac repair. These systems usually include CPB with variable degrees of hypothermia, aortic cross-clamping with cardiac ischemia, the use of cardioplegia solution, and periods of low flow or no flow. Exposure of a patient to CPB results in activation of a variety of humoral substances[13,69] (complement, vasoactive amines, and others), alteration of coagulation and hematologic factors, and changes in lymphocyte and immune function. How these factors affect convalescence after cardiac surgery is not entirely clear, but some commonly observed problems with fluid retention, decreased pulmonary compliance (or increased pulmonary vascular resistance with pulmonary hypertension), and hypothyroidism (low circulating triiodothyronine) may all be related to exposure to the CPB circuit. Cardiac recovery after repair may also relate to whether the myocardium was ischemic at any time during repair and how the heart was protected during this period of ischemia. Alterations in ventricular function may reflect recovery of injured muscle, and it is not uncommon for infants to require inotropic support for a short period after cardiac repair. When ventricular dysfunction is observed after neonatal cardiac repair, it is important to consider its relation to the systems necessary for cardiac repair. This is usually a recoverable injury, but it may be a significant factor in the postoperative period. Finally, when periods of deep hypothermic circulatory arrest have been employed for part of the repair, the entire body may manifest some degree of ischemic injury. This may manifest as renal insufficiency, hepatic insufficiency, pulmonary insufficiency, or neurologic injury.[9–11,14] Although none of these problems are common, any of them may be observed and should be understood in relation to the CPB strategy employed. Some of these alterations can play an important role in the postoperative recovery.

Physiologic Adaptation

Finally, the postoperative recovery is affected by the physiology of the defect before and after repair. This is especially true after palliative procedures, when one abnormality is exchanged for another, and it is sometimes difficult to predict accurately how the heart and circulation will adapt. Palliated congenital heart disease can present an enormous challenge to those involved with the infant's postoperative care.[26] An excellent example of this is the management of shunt physiology in infants who have shunts performed to palliate defects presenting with ductal-dependant distal aortic perfusion and pulmonary overcirculation (eg, hypoplastic left heart syndrome, univentricular heart with interrupted aortic arch). In these patients, cardiac output is distributed to the systemic and pulmonary circulations, depending on the balance between systemic and pulmonary resistance. Excessive shunt flow results in diminished systemic perfusion with hypotension and acidosis. Excessive systemic perfusion results in inadequate pulmonary blood flow with hypoxemia. Anyone who has cared for these patients can attest to how difficult it is to achieve and then maintain the proper balance in the face of dynamically changing compliance of the pulmonary and systemic vascular beds in the recovery period. Pulmonary resistance can be manipulated in these patients with alterations in ventilation that generate hypercarbia with low inspired oxygen (to increase pulmonary resistance and increase systemic blood flow) or to hypocarbia and high inspired oxygen (to decrease pulmonary resistance and increase pulmonary blood flow). Variable resistance between the two circuits is also affected by chest wall compliance, peak inspiratory pressures, systemic afterload, and the effects of pharmacologic agents on the peripheral and pulmonary vasculature.[70] Palliation may be the best option for the surgical management of a particular heart defect, but palliation by no means indicates that the postoperative care will be easier. In fact, because the circulation is still abnormal, it is sometimes more difficult to care for the palliated patient.

In patients who undergo complete repair, the physiologic alteration imposed on the heart by the new circulation often is an important factor in the postoperative convalescent pattern. It is critical that the team understand the impact of these changes. For example, closure of a VSD significantly increases afterload to the left ventricle by removing a low-resistance outlet for LV ejection. The acute change in LV afterload may be reflected as diminished LV ejection and low cardiac output. An afterload reduction agent is an ideal choice of therapy in these instances. After repair of an AV canal defect, there is an increase in LV afterload not only by closing the VSD but also by making the left AV valve more competent. These patients can also have right ventricular dysfunction from pulmonary hypertension that may be treated with ventilator manipulation or inhaled nitric oxide.

Timing

Timing is also a factor in this process. The longer a heart has been abnormal, the more likely it is that there will be some difficulty related to sudden physiologic alteration. The best example of this is in infants with transposition of the great arteries. Arterial switch in the first 10 days of life is usually well tolerated. Beyond this period, the left ventricle becomes progressively less prepared to adapt suddenly to systemic afterload, and an arterial switch performed at 4 weeks of life risks severe LV dysfunction from which the patient may not survive without temporary LV support (Fig. 58-8). In this circumstance, however, if the pulmonary artery is banded for as few as 5 days before arterial switch, the left ventricle can recondition so that arterial switch has an excellent chance of success without the need for postoperative LV assist.[71] The preoperative physiologic adaptation of the heart and how the new anatomy created by surgery will be tolerated should be considered for every congenital heart defect. It is likely that the emphasis on early neonatal repair will diminish the importance of this consideration because hearts will be physiologically reconstructed before developing adaptive compensatory responses to abnormal loading conditions. In addition, this a time when they should be

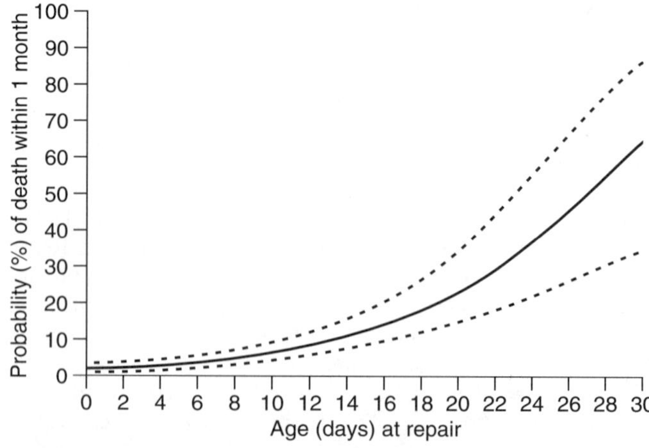

FIG. 58-8. The estimated probability of death within 1 month after an arterial switch repair for simple complete transposition as a function of age in days at repair. The risk is higher when age at operation is 8 days or older, as compared with the survival rate if repair is done in the first week of life. *Solid line*, mena; *dotted lines*, ± standard deviation. (After Kirklin JW. Surgical repair for complete transposition, vol 1. Cardiol Young 1991:19)

TABLE 58-2. *Approximate Hospital mortality rates for congenital heart repair**

Defect repaired	Mortality rate (%)
Patent ductus arteriosus	<0.5
Atrial septal defect	0.5
Cor triatriatum	2
Total anomalous pulmonary venous return	5–10†
Critical aortic stenosis	10–30†
Aortic coarctation	5
Aortopulmonary window	1–3
Truncus arteriosus	10
Ventricular septal defect	2
AV canal	5–10
Transposition of the great arteries	5–10
Tetralogy of Fallot	5
Double-outlet right ventricle	5–12
Interrupted aortic arch	10–20
Single ventricle (shunts)	5
Single ventricle (bands)	5–10

* Considers defects only as primary defect without other significant anomaly.

† Outcome is greatly and variably affected by associated cardiovascular problems.

most capable of supporting normal physiology. Conversely, cardiac repair on previously palliated patients or on older children who have not had prior surgery can produce dramatic effects related to the physiology of adaptation.

Using an approach based on this philosophy, patient outcomes have improved with respect to hospital and long-term survival as well as with respect to quality of life. In most programs with dedicated pediatric cardiac surgical services, overall hospital survival is between 88% to 95% and is most influenced by the type of defects seen in the patient population. Table 58-2 indicates the expected hospital mortality rates for the various lesions discussed in this chapter when repaired using modern technology and surgical techniques.[13,72–74]

More detail regarding specific techniques, outcomes, and complications for surgical repair of each of the lesions listed in Table 58-2 is beyond the scope and intention of this chapter. Readers who are interested in this level of detail are encouraged to refer to one of the several texts dealing with pediatric cardiac surgery.[13,72–74]

Pediatric cardiac surgery is becoming far simpler with the advent of newer and better technology that improves diagnosis and initial stabilization of the patient. The surgeon has the opportunity to determine the optimal treatment of each specific defect. Our improved understanding of the effects of CPB and of the systems employed to enable cardiac reconstruction has made it is easier to prevent related postoperative problems. The technology available makes possible intricate and precise repair of complex defects in the neonatal period. Decision making for the surgical management of congenital heart defects has never been easier—repairable defects can be safely corrected at virtually any age and size. The limitations to repair are imposed more by anatomy and associated problems than by limitations in technology or surgical abilities. Dedicated and knowledgeable postoperative care by a team of specialists can further optimize outcomes, and the future for infants born with congenital heart disease has never been brighter.

REFERENCES

1. Bigelow WG, Callaghan JC, Hopps JA. General hypothermia for experimental intracardiac surgery. Ann Surg 1950;132:531.
2. Lewis FJ, Taufic M. Closure of atrial septal defects with the aid of hypothermia: experimental accomplishments and the report of one successful case. Surgery 1953;33:52.
3. Swan H, Zeavin I. Cessation of circulation in general hypothermia. III. Techniques of intra-cardiac surgery under direct vision. Ann Surg 1954;139:385.
4. Swan H, Zeavin I, Blount SG Jr, et al. Surgery by direct vision in the open heart during hypothermia. JAMA 1953;153:1081.
5. Ungerleider RM. Direct vision aortic valvotomy: predecessor to modern aortic surgery. Ann Thorac Surg 1994;57:1351.
6. de Leval M. Surgery of the left ventricular outflow tract. In: Stark J, de Leval M, eds. Surgery for congenital heart defects, ed 2. Philadelphia, WB Saunders, 1994:511.
7. Sink JD, Smallhorn JF, Macartney FJ, et al. Management of critical aortic stenosis in infancy. J Thorac Cardiovasc Surg 1984;887:82.
8. Graham TP, Atwood GF, Boucek RJ Jr. Pharmacologic dilation of the ductus arteriosus with prostaglandin E1 in infants with congenital heart disease. South Med J 1978;71:1238.
9. Greeley WJ, Kern FH, Ungerleider RM, et al. The effect of hypothermic cardiopulmonary bypass and total circulatory arrest on cerebral metabolism in neonates, infants, and children. J Thorac Cardiovasc Surg 1991;101:783.
10. Greeley WJ, Ungerleider RM. Assessing the effect of cardiopulmonary bypass on the brain. Ann Thorac Surg 1991;52:417.
11. Greeley WJ, Ungerleider RM, Kern FH, et al. Effects of cardiopulmonary bypass on cerebral blood flow in neonates, infants, and children. Circulation 1989;80:1209.
12. Griepp EV, Griepp RB. Cerebral consequences of hypothermic circulatory arrest in adults. J Cardiac Surg 1992;7:134.
13. Kirklin JW, Barratt-Boyes BG. Cardiac surgery, ed 2. New York, Churchill Livingstone, 1993:1779.
14. Mault JR, Ohtake S, Klingensmith ME, et al. Cerebral metabolism and circulatory arrest: effects of duration and strategies for protection. Ann Thorac Surg 1993;55:57.
15. Gibbon JH. Application of a mechanical heart and lung apparatus to cardiac surgery. Minn Med 1954;37:171.
16. Bartlett RH, Andrews AF, Toomasian JM. Extracorporeal membrane oxygenation for newborn respiratory failure: 45 cases. Surgery 1982;92:425.
17. Bartlett RH, Gazzaniga AB, Toomasian JM, et al. Extracorporeal membrane oxygenation (ECMO) in neonatal respiratory failure: 100 cases. Ann Surg 1986;204:236.
18. Bartlett RH, Roloff DW, Cornell RG. Extracorporeal circulation in neonatal respiratory failure: a prospective randomized study. Pediatrics 1985;76:479.
19. Mustard WT, Chute AL, Keith JD, et al. A surgical approach to transposition of the great vessels with extracorporeal circuit. Surgery 1954;36:39.
20. Neutze JM, Starling MB, Elliot RB, et al. Palliation of cyanotic congenital heart disease in infancy with E-type prostaglandins. Circulation 1977;55:238.
21. Donahoo JS, Roland JM, Kan J, et al. Prostaglandin E1 as an adjunct to emergency cardiac operation in neonates. J Thorac Cardiovasc Surg 1981;81:227.
22. Freed MD, Heyman MA, Lewis AB, et al. Prostaglandin E1 in infants with ductus arteriosus–dependent congenital heart disease. Circulation 1981;64:899.
23. Kisslo JA. Doppler color flow imaging. In: Kisslo JA, Adams DV, Belkin RN, eds. New York, Churchill Livingstone, 1988.
24. Kisslo JA, Ramm OT, Thurstone FL. Cardiac imaging using a phased array ultrasound system. II. Clinical technique and application. Circulation 1976;53:262.
25. Silverman NH. Pediatric echocardiography. Baltimore, Williams & Wilkins, 1993.
26. Meliones JN, Ungerleider RM, et al. Perioperative management of congenital heart disease. In: Moylan JA, ed. Surgical critical care. St Louis, CV Mosby, 1994:205.
27. Kocis K, Meliones JN, Dekeon MK, et al. High-frequency jet ventilation for respiratory failure after congenital heart surgery. Circulation 1992;86:II127.

28. Meliones JN, Bove EL, Dekeon MK, et al. High frequency jet ventilation improves cardiac function after the Fontan procedure. Circulation 1991;84(Suppl III):364.

29. Klein MD, Shaheen KW, Whittlesey GC, et al. Extracorporeal membrane oxygenation for the circulatory support of children after repair of congenital heart disease. J Thorac Cardiovasc Surg 1990;100:498.

30. Gaynor JW, Ungerleider RM. Aortopulmonary window. In: Mavroudis C, Backer CL, eds. Pediatric cardiac surgery. St Louis, CV Mosby, 1994:237.

31. Bove EL, Beekman RHI, Snider AR, et al. Repair of truncus arteriosus in the neonate and young infant. Ann Thorac Surg 1989;47:499.

32. Mavroudis C, Backer CL. Truncus arteriosus. In: Mavroudis C, Backer CL, eds. Pediatric cardiac surgery. St Louis, CV Mosby, 1994:237.

33. Fontan F, Baudet E. Surgical repair of tricuspid atresia. Thorax 1971;26:240.

34. Kuroda O, Sano T, Matsuda H, et al. Analysis of the effects of the Blalock-Taussig shunt on ventricular function and the prognosis in patients with single ventricle. Circulation 1987;76(Suppl III):24.

35. Rothman A, Lang P, Lock JE, et al. Surgical management of subaortic obstruction in single left ventricle and tricuspid atresia. J Am Coll Cardiol 1987;10:421.

36. Norwood WI, Lang P, Hansen D. Physiologic repair of aortic atresia–hypoplastic left heart syndrome. N Engl J Med 1983;308:23.

37. Norwood WI, Pigott JD. Recent advances in cardiac surgery. Pediatr Clin North Am 1985;32:1117.

38. Gussenhoven EJ, van Herwerden LA, van Suylen RJ, et al. Recognition of residual ventricular septal defect by intraoperative contrast echocardiography. Eur Heart J 1989;10:801.

39. Spray TL. Transplantation of the heart and lungs in children. Annu Rev Med 1994;45:139.

40. Tweddell JS, Canter CE, Bridges ND, et al. Predictors of operative mortality and morbidity after infant heart transplantation. Ann Thorac Surg 1994;58:972.

41. Starnes VA, Griffin ML, Pitlick PT, et al. Current approach to hypoplastic left heart syndrome: palliation, transplantation, or both? J Thorac Cardiovasc Surg 1992;104:189.

42. Castaneda AR, Mayer JE Jr, Jonas RA. Repair of complete atrioventricular canal in infancy. World J Surg 1985;9:590.

43. Kirklin JW, Blackstone EH, Jonas RA, et al. Morphologic and surgical determinants of outcome events after repair of tetralogy of Fallot and pulmonary stenosis: a two institution study. J Thorac Cardiovasc Surg 1992;103:706.

44. Vobecky SJ, Williams WG, Trusler GA, et al. Survival analysis of infants under age 18 months presenting with tetralogy of Fallot. Ann Thorac Surg 1993;56:944.

45. Hoffman JIE, Rudolph AM. The natural history of ventricular septal defects in infancy. Am J Cardiol 1965;16:634.

46. Mavroudis C, Backer CL, Idriss FS. Ventricular septal defect. In: Mavroudis C, Backer CL, eds. Pediatric cardiac surgery. St Louis, CV Mosby, 1994:201.

47. Barratt-Boyes BG, Neutze JM, Clarkson PM, et al. Repair of ventricular septal defect in the first two years of life using profound hypothermia-circulatory arrest techniques. Ann Surg 1976;184:376.

48. Barratt-Boyes BG, Simpson M, Neutze JM. Intracardiac surgery in neonates and infants using deep hypothermia with surface cooling and limited cardiopulmonary bypass. Circulation 1971;43(Suppl I):25.

49. Ungerleider RM. Atrial septal defects, ostium primum defects, and atrioventricular canals. In: Sabiston DC Jr, ed. Textbook of surgery: the biological basis of modern surgical practice, ed 14. Philadelphia, WB Saunders, 1991:1873.

50. Mustard WI, Keith JD, Trusler GA, et al. The surgical management of transposition of the great vessels. J Thorac Cardiovasc Surg 1964;48:953.

51. Senning A. Surgical correction of transposition of the great vessels. Surgery 1959;45:966.

52. Castaneda AR, Norwood WI, Jonas RA, et al. Transposition of the great arteries and intact ventricular septum: anatomical repair in the neonate. Ann Thorac Surg 1984;38:438.

53. Kirklin JW. The surgical repair for complete transposition. Cardiol Young 1991;1:13.

54. Lupinetti FM, Bove EL, Minich LL, et al. Intermediate-term survival and functional results after arterial repair for transposition of the great arteries. J Thorac Cardiovasc Surg 1992;103:421.

55. Quagebeur JM, Rohmer J, Ottenkamp J, et al. The arterial switch operation: an eight-year experience. J Thorac Cardiovasc Surg 1986;92:361.

56. Castaneda AR, Freed MD, Williams RG, et al. Repair of tetralogy of Fallot in infancy: early and late results. J Thorac Cardiovasc Surg 1977;74:372.

57. Castaneda AR, Mayer J. Tetralogy of Fallot. In: Stark J, de Leval M, eds. Surgery for congenital heart defects, ed 2. Philadelphia, WB Saunders, 1994:405.

58. Di Donato RM, Jonas RA, Lang P, et al. Neonatal repair of tetralogy of Fallot with and without pulmonary atresia. J Thorac Cardiovasc Surg 1991;101:126.

59. Groh MA, Meliones JN, Bove EL, et al. Repair of tetralogy of Fallot in infancy: effect of pulmonary artery size on outcome. Circulation 1991;84:(Suppl III):206.

60. Castaneda AR. Invited commentary to article by Vobecky et al. Ann Thorac Surg 1993;56:949.

61. Ungerleider RM, Gaynor JW, Meliones JN, et al. Primary one-stage repair of TOF in infants is cost effective and may decrease mortality associated with palliation or late presentation. Unpublished data.

62. Uva MS, Lacour-Gayet F, Komiya T, et al. Surgery for tetralogy of Fallot at less than six months of age. J Thorac Cardiovasc Surg 1994;107:1291.

63. Ungerleider RM, Sabiston DC Jr, eds. Double outlet right ventricle. Philadelphia, Hanley & Belfus, 1989:91.

64. Muhiudeen IA, Roberson DA, Silverman NH, et al. Intraoperative echocardiography in infants and children with congenital cardiac shunt lesions: transesophageal versus epicardial echocardiography. J Am Coll Cardiol 1990;16:1687.

65. Ungerleider RM. The use of intraoperative epicardial echocardiography with color flow imaging during the repair of atrioventricular septal defects. Cardiol Young 1992;2:56.

66. Ungerleider RM, Greeley WJ, Kanter RJ, et al. The learning curve for intraoperative echocardiography during congenital heart surgery. Ann Thorac Surg 1992;54:691.

67. Ungerleider RM, Greeley WJ, Sheikh KH, et al. The use of intraoperative echo with Doppler color flow imaging to predict outcome after repair of congenital cardiac defects. Ann Surg 1989;210:526.

68. Ungerleider RM, Greeley WJ, Sheikh KH, et al. Routine use of intraoperative epicardial echocardiography and Doppler color flow imaging to guide and evaluate repair of congenital heart defects. J Thorac Cardiovasc Surg 1990;100:297.

69. Finn A, Dreyer WJ. Neutrophil adhesion and the inflammatory response induced by cardiopulmonary bypass. Cardiol Young 1993;3:244.

70. Ohtake S, Mault JR, Lilly MK, et al. Effect of a systemic–pulmonary artery shunt on myocardial function and perfusion in a piglet model. Surg Forum 1991;42:200.

71. Jonas RA, Giglia TM, Sanders SP, et al. Rapid, two-stage arterial switch for transposition of the great arteries and intact ventricular septum beyond the neonatal period. Circulation 1989;80(Suppl I):203.

72. Castaneda AR, Mayer JEJ, Jonas RA, et al. Cardiac surgery in the neonate and infant. Philadelphia, WB Saunders, 1994.

73. Mavroudis C, Backer C, eds. Pediatric cardiac surgery. St Louis, CV Mosby, 1994.

74. Stark J, de Leval M. Surgery for congenital heart defects, ed 2. Philadelphia, WB Saunders, 1994.

Surgery of Infants and Children: Scientific Principles and Practice, edited by
Keith T. Oldham, Paul M. Colombani, and Robert P. Foglia.
Lippincott–Raven Publishers, Philadelphia, © 1997.

CHAPTER 59

Pericardium and Great Vessels

Walter Pegoli, Jr.

PERICARDIUM

Embryology

The pericardial sac begins to take shape early in the 4th week of gestation. Clefts in the embryonic mesoderm develop and ultimately separate the somatic and splanchnic components. These individual clefts coalescence and form a single cavity. The central region of this cavity becomes the pericardial space, and the lateral aspects eventually form the pleural cavities. The floor of the pericardial cavity contains a layer of splanchnopleure that develops into the cardiogenic plate. This plate ultimately forms the myocardium and the visceral pericardium.

Early in gestation, the pericardial cavity is large, and the pleural cavities are relatively small. With development of the fetal lungs, the size of the pleural cavities increases rapidly. Abnormalities in the formation of the pleuropericardial membrane result in pericardial defects. These defects are attributable to abnormal organogenesis during the 5th week of gestation. Most abnormalities are located on the left side.

Anatomy

The pericardium surrounds the heart and is lined by simple squamous epithelium or mesothelium. It has both visceral and parietal layers. The visceral pericardium is intimately associated with the heart; the parietal pericardium forms the outer layer of the pericardial cavity. The area between the visceral and parietal pericardia is the pericardial space. The pericardial space is filled with a small volume of serous fluid that acts as a lubricant. The two components of the pericardium are contiguous at the sites where great vessels enter and exit the heart.

The anterior pericardium separates the heart from the sternum. The posterior pericardium is adjacent to the esophagus and thoracic aorta. Superiorly, the pericardium separates the heart from the thymus; the inferior aspect of the pericardium is integrated into the central tendon and anterior aspect of the diaphragm. Laterally, the pericardium and the parietal pleura are in intimate contact.

The blood supply to the pericardium is derived from branches of the internal thoracic arteries and the descending thoracic aorta. The venous drainage is through the azygous system. The sympathetic trunks and the phrenic and vagus nerves innervate the pericardium. Lymph drains through the thoracic duct and the right lymphatic duct. The absorptive capacity of the pericardium is limited. Therefore, situations that increase fluid formation, such as inflammatory states, can lead to pericardial effusions.

Physiology

Understanding pericardial function in both normal and diseased states is critical for physicians who treat children with cardiac disorders. The pericardium performs several important functions. It fixes the heart anatomically within the thorax, it minimizes the friction between the heart and surrounding structures during the cardiac cycle, it prevents mechanical distortion of the great vessels, and it helps to prevent spread of infection from contiguous sites. The parietal pericardium is composed of connective tissue. Because collagen is the major structural component, the pericardium has a limited ability to distend acutely. When the contents of the pericardial sac exceed a particular volume, a point of pericardial nonextensibility is reached, and the pericardium limits cardiac filling and therefore cardiac output. This is the physiologic basis for tamponade (Fig. 59-1). Clinical evidence for tamponade includes the Beck triad: (1) elevated central venous pressure (distended neck veins); (2) a small, quiet heart (diminished QRS-complex amplitude); and (3) systemic hypotension. A paradoxical pulse may be demonstrated on physical examination. Experiments in dogs have shown that hydrostatic distending pressures of 3 to 8 mmHg can produce a noncompliant pericardium and result in tamponade.[1] In children, the most frequent condition that produces a pericardial effusion that exceeds pericardial reserve volume is a viral infection. Chronic pericardial effusions of considerably greater size can be tolerated without physiologic decompensation because the pericardium is capable of modest distention without hydrostatic pressure increases under these conditions.

Anatomic Defects

Anatomic defects in the pericardium are uncommon and usually occur on the left side. These defects communicate with the

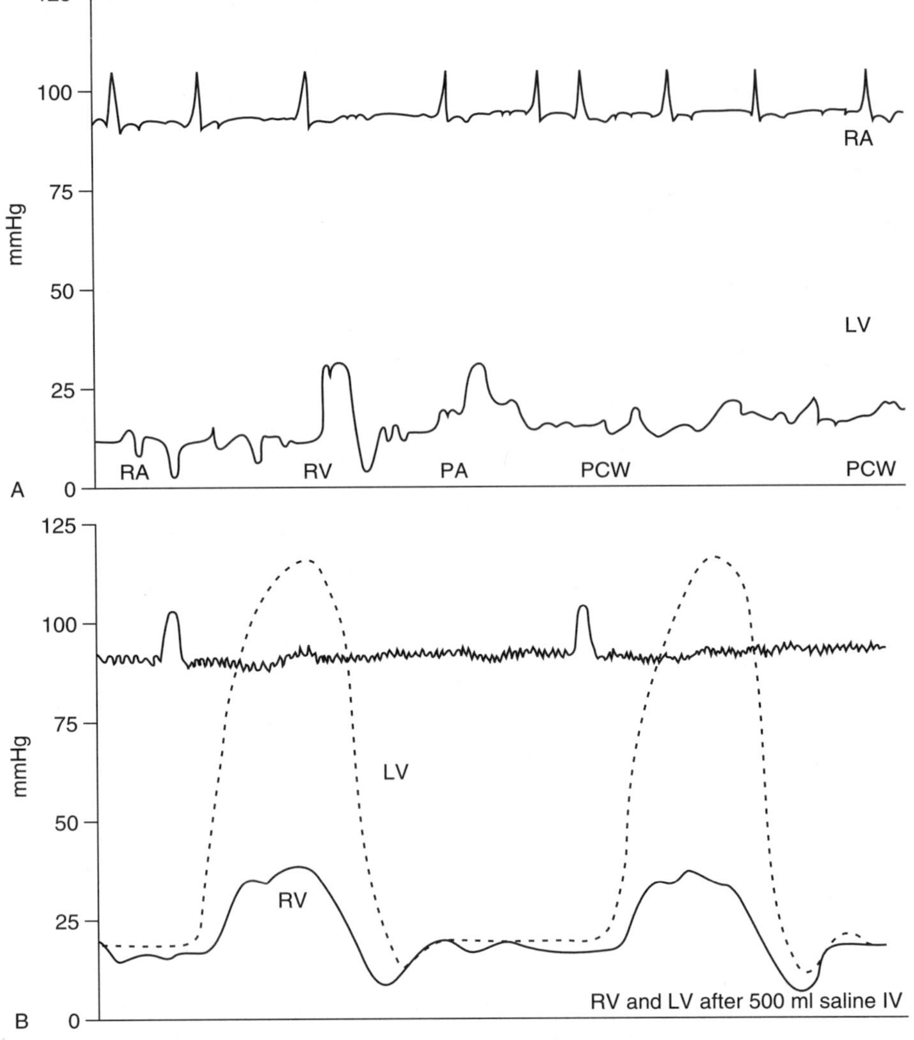

FIG. 59-1. Pressure recordings from a patient with constrictive pericarditis. (*A*) The right atrial (RA) tracing shows elevated pressure and prominent *y* descent. The right ventricular (RV) tracing exhibits the typical dip and plateau pattern, or "square root sign." There is equalization of the RA, RV diastolic, pulmonary artery (PA) diastolic, pulmonary capillary wedge (PCW), and left ventricular (LV) diastolic pressures. (*B*) RV and LV diastolic pressures increase and equalize after administration of 500 mL of saline. (After Brockington GM, Zebede J, Pandian NG. Constrictive pericarditis. Cardiol Clin 1990;8:649)

ipsilateral pleural space. If the defect is large, segments of the heart or the entire heart can be located within the pleural space. More often, a small portion of the heart is herniated into the pleural space, most commonly the auricular appendage. The phrenic nerve usually courses along the anterior margin of these smaller defects.

Pericardial defects are often associated with cardiac anomalies; the most common are the tetralogy of Fallot, patent ductus arteriosus (PDA), mitral valve prolapse, and mitral stenosis. Bronchogenic cysts and enteric cysts are also associated with these defects. The Cantrell pentalogy is present when pericardial defects are associated with diaphragmatic defects, abdominal wall defects, lower sternal defects, and intracardiac abnormalities.

Most patients with pericardial defects do not have symptoms. Chest pain, shortness of breath, dizziness, and hemoptysis can occur with cardiac displacement, however, and sudden death with cardiac herniation and strangulation has been described.

On physical examination, patients exhibit a systolic murmur, accompanied by a shift of the point of maximal cardiac impulse to the side of the defect. Electrocardiographic findings can include right-axis deviation, incomplete right bundle branch block, or right ventricular hypertrophy. On plain chest radiograph, there is elongation of the left heart border. Echocardiography is routinely done but is relatively nonspecific. The finding of a left atrial aneurysm should raise the possibility of a partial pericardial defect. The diagnosis of a pericardial defect is most reliably established with computed tomography (CT) or magnetic resonance (MR) imaging.

Patients with large or complete pericardial defects have little or no potential for herniation and strangulation and are not considered for surgical intervention. Patients with partial defects are at risk for cardiac herniation and sudden death. These patients should undergo surgical reconstruction by enlarging the defect, resecting the pericardium, or patching the defect with prosthetic material or local tissue transfer (Fig. 59-2).

Pericardial Cysts and Diverticula

Diverticula or cystic sequestrations of the pericardium typically occur at the cardiophrenic angle. Like the pericardium itself, they are lined by simple squamous epithelium and filled with serous fluid. These anomalies result from failure of the

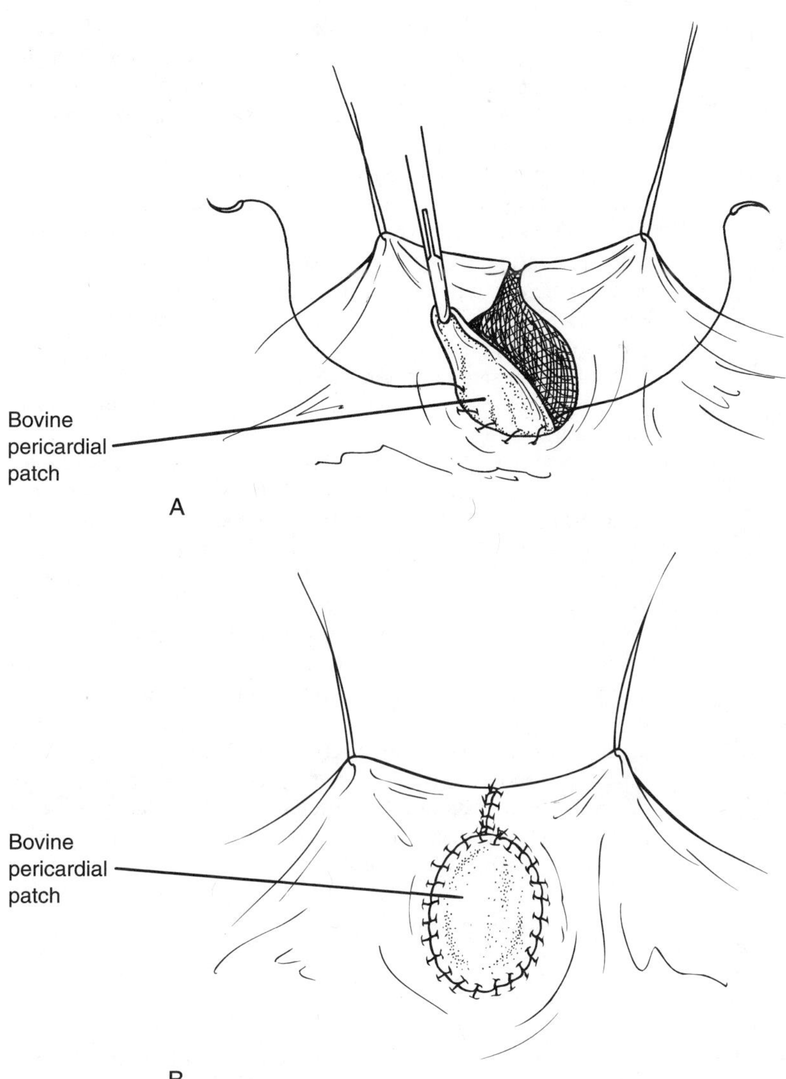

FIG. 59-2. Schematic depictions before (*A*) and after (*B*) bovine patch closure of pericardium. (After Miller PL, Katz NM, Kulkarni PK. Right congenital pericardial defects. Am Heart J 1993;126:1235)

ventral parietal recess of the pericardium to regress. Complete persistence leads to a diverticulum; partial distal persistence is associated with the development of a pericardial cyst.

Pericardial cysts and diverticula have a male predominance and are twice as likely to occur on the right side. Ninety percent are unilocular; the remainder are multilocular. Although most patients with these findings do not have symptoms, precordial or substernal chest pain, dyspnea, and chronic nonproductive cough have been noted. Complications of pericardial cysts are rare. As with any benign cystic lesion, infection, rupture, and compression of adjacent structures from local enlargement can occur. Malignancy is rare. These cysts are not known to regress spontaneously.

On plain chest radiograph, the typical pericardial cyst appears as a smooth, rounded mass in the region of the cardiophrenic angle. The differential diagnosis includes foramen of Morgagni hernia, mediastinal cystic hygroma, and mediastinal teratoma. As for most thoracic structural anomalies, contrast-enhanced CT is a sensitive diagnostic tool. The lesion is seen as a thin-walled oval or tubular structure filled with fluid. It typically displaces rather than infiltrates surrounding structures.

Surgical excision is advised for these lesions. This is both diagnostic and prophylactic. When symptomatic, cysts should certainly be removed. The blood supply is limited, so the cyst can be excised without difficulty. Diverticula require ligation and removal. This is technically straightforward and either a conventional transthoracic or a thoracoscopic approach can be used. Aspiration has been done in high-risk patients, using either fluoroscopic or ultrasonographic guidance; however, recurrence is an important concern with this approach. In one 3-year follow-up of a small group of patients who underwent aspiration, no recurrences were reported.[2]

Infections

The classic clinical triad for acute pericarditis includes chest pain, pericardial friction rub, and electrocardiographic abnormalities. The most common causes of acute pericarditis in children are viral infection, bacterial infection, uremia, and trauma. Precordial pain is characteristic of the acute condition. The onset usually coincides with fever but can follow a shaking chill. The pain is usually intensified by respiration, coughing, swallowing, or the supine position. In some patients, the pain is diminished by the assumption of an upright position.

Specific Forms of Viral Pericarditis

Acute viral pericarditis can follow infection with the coxsackievirus B, echovirus 8, mumps, Ebstein-Barr virus, influenza, poliomyelitis, or varicella virus. Patients with infectious mononucleosis can present with acute pericarditis and cardiac tamponade followed by progressive pericardial restriction. Viral pericarditis evokes significant inflammation. The inflammatory process can be serous, serofibrinous, fibrinous, suppurative, hemorrhagic, or some combination of these. Viral pericarditis is usually of the fibrinous or serofibrinous variety; suppurative pericarditis is often the result of bacterial infection. With resolution of the acute process, the fibrin either undergoes fibrinolysis or becomes organized to obliterate the pericardial space. The latter outcome is more frequent after severe infections. Intense inflammation leads to chronic injury due to the deposition and organization of fibrin, visceral and parietal pericardial adhesion, calcification, and progressive pericardial constriction.

Patients with viral pericarditis usually have an antecedent history of an upper respiratory tract infection. Seventy percent of patients have temperatures as high as 39°C. Pleuritic chest pain, a pericardial friction rub, cough, and a pericardial effusion are common. The pericardial fluid typically is clear and serous, resolving spontaneously in most cases.

A specific virus rarely can be retrieved from pericardial fluid, stool, or blood. The diagnosis is commonly established by demonstrating a four-fold increase in serial neutralizing antibody titers in serum. The electrocardiogram may demonstrate sequential ST-T–segment and T-wave changes. Sinus tachycardia is often present.[3] Atrial and ventricular arrhythmias result from inflammation of the underlying myocardium. In otherwise healthy children, the differential diagnosis should include blunt chest trauma, systemic lupus erythematosus, rheumatic pericarditis, and bacterial endocarditis.

Patients with viral pericarditis have no symptoms for about 1 to 2 weeks. Those with coxsackievirus or echovirus infections are at particular risk for myocarditis with cardiac insufficiency and cardiomegaly. The cardiac dysfunction can resolve completely or result in persistent physiologic dysfunction that can take the form of chronic ventricular failure or even sudden death. Patients with coxsackievirus infections are at risk for the development of coronary artery aneurysms and therefore require vigorous and regular follow-up.

The basic treatment for patients with acute viral pericarditis is bed rest and analgesics. Specific antiviral agents are not available for the responsible pathogens. During the acute phase, patients should be observed for evidence of cardiac tamponade, myocarditis, and heart failure. Patients with significant pain are treated with a 3- to 7-day course of systemic steroids. In patients with mild symptoms, aspirin or indomethacin are adequate. This therapy generally results in the rapid resolution of symptoms within 12 to 24 hours.

Bacterial Pericarditis

Children who present with bacterial pericarditis commonly have a history of acute pharyngitis, pneumonia, meningitis, otitis media, anemia, impetigo, or purulent arthritis. The most common organism is *Staphylococcus aureus,* followed in frequency by *Haemophilus influenzae* type B, *Neisseria meningitidis,* other gram-negative organisms, *Streptoccocus pneumoniae,* and β-hemolytic streptococcal organisms.

Bacterial pericarditis presents as an acute illness with high fever, shaking chills, dyspnea, night sweats, and cough. Chest pain is an uncommon symptom. Patients can manifest tachycardia, a pericardial friction rub, pulsus paradoxicus, and in severe cases, systemic hypotension. The white blood cell count usually exceeds 17,000 cells/μL, with a shift toward immature forms on the differential count.

A plain chest radiograph may show findings that correlate with the cause. In particular, pulmonary parenchymal disease, pneumonia, pleural effusion, or mediastinal widening may be evident radiographically. Nonspecific ST-T–wave changes are present on electrocardiogram. The leukocyte count of the pericardial fluid is usually greater than 50,000 cells/μL, consisting mostly of polymorphonuclear leukocytes; the glucose level is usually less than 35 mg/dL; and the protein content is more than 3 g/dL.[4]

Antibiotic therapy alone is inadequate treatment for acute bacterial pericarditis. Mortality rates are reduced by surgical drainage combined with appropriate antibiotic treatment. The initial antibiotic coverage should include an agent effective against *S aureus* and an aminoglycoside. Patients with a penicillin allergy should receive systemic vancomycin. Either closed or open drainage should be instituted as outlined later, and early pericardiectomy should be considered to prevent the development of constrictive pericarditis.

Surgical Intervention

Pericardiocentesis

Aspiration of pericardial fluid can be a life-saving maneuver in patients with cardiac tamponade regardless of the cause. In addition, it is an indispensable adjunct to the diagnosis and treatment of idiopathic pericardial effusions. The most common approach is a subxiphoid route. The procedure is optimally done with full cardiac monitoring. A long needle is attached to a syringe and electrocardiograph lead. The needle is usually inserted to the left of the xiphoid and directed to the ipsilateral shoulder posteriorly at a 45-degree angle. The needle is slowly advanced until fluid is retrieved or until electrocardiographic changes occur (Fig. 59-3). An adjunct to this procedure is to use this needle as a guide for placing a catheter into the pericardial space. This can be done by threading a catheter through the needle or by placing a wire through the needle and using the wire to direct a larger catheter. This latter technique is especially valuable in patients who had recurrent effusions requiring repeated pericardiocentesis.

The potential risks of pericardiocentesis include pneumothorax, myocardial or coronary artery injury, and arrhythmias. The use of sonographic guidance techniques has lessened the incidence of these potentially life-threatening complications.

Pericardiostomy

Open drainage of the pericardium is most commonly required in cases of malignant effusions or acute pyogenic pericarditis.

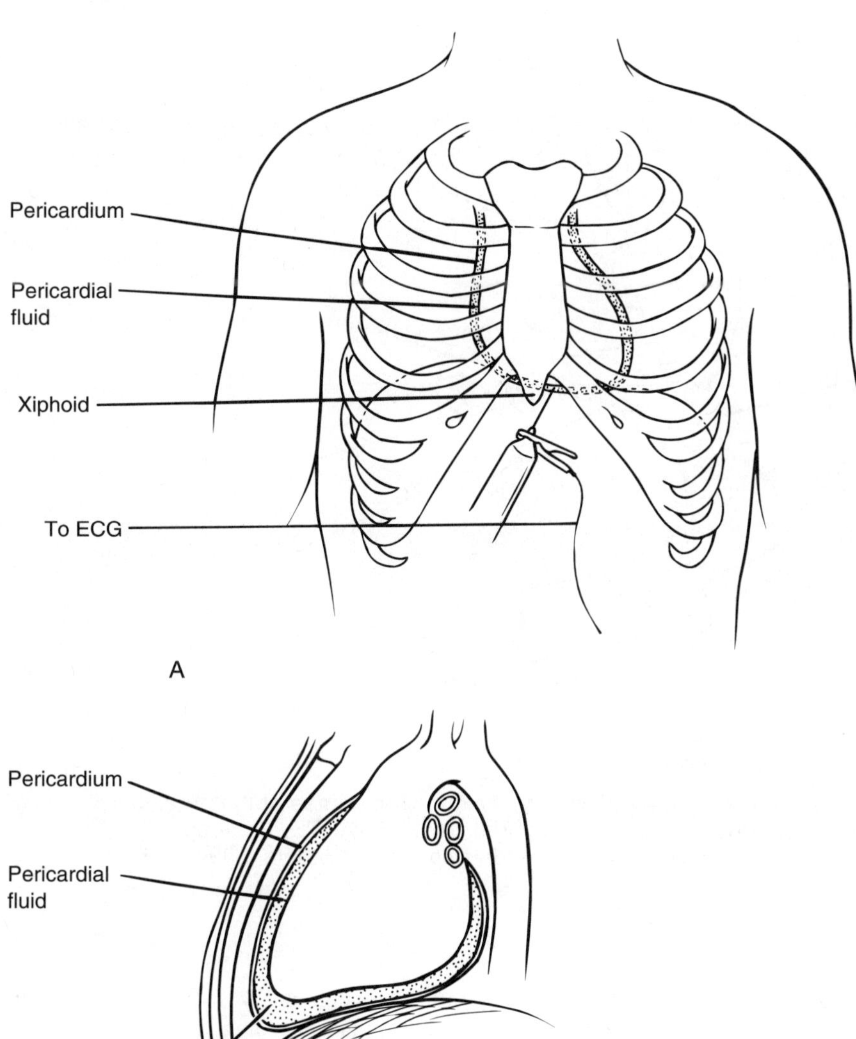

FIG. 59-3. Technique of pericardiocentesis. Needle is inserted to the left of the xiphoid and directed toward the ipsilateral shoulder, posteriorly at a 45-degree angle. The electrocardiographic lead is attached to the needle. (After Ebert PA, Najafi H. The pericardium. In: Sabiston DC Jr, Spencer FC, eds. Gibbons' surgery of the chest, ed 5. Philadelphia, WB Saunders, 1990:1234)

The former is rare in children. For the latter, this procedure may be necessary if the effusion is fibrinous or fibrinopurulent and has multiple loculations. Classically, this procedure was done through an open subxiphoid approach that allowed dependent drainage while avoiding contamination of the pleural space.

Pericardiostomy recently has been performed using thoracoscopic techniques. The patient is positioned supine at 45 degrees to allow the lung to fall posteriorly after pneumothorax has been achieved. Access ports are placed in the seventh intercostal space, mid-axillary line; fourth intercostal space, mid-clavicular line; and sixth intercostal space, anterior axillary line (Fig. 59-4). The thoracoscope is inserted through the port in the seventh intercostal space. Dissection using monopolar current is avoided because it can fibrillate the heart and result in cardiac arrest if used in proximity to the myocardium. The laser or bipolar cautery is recommended for hemostasis. Segments of the lateral pericardium can be excised under direct vision. During dissection, it is important to identify the vagus and phrenic nerves on the pericardial surface. An advantage of the thoracoscopic approach is complete visualization of the pericardium. The ability to identify both the phrenic and vagus nerves, improved cosmesis, and less postoperative discomfort are additional benefits. The major disadvantage is that drainage is into the pleural cavity; when this is an undesirable clinical outcome, such as with bacterial pericarditis, an alternative route is indicated.

Pericardiectomy

Resection of the pericardium is performed for patients with constrictive pericarditis. The procedure can be performed

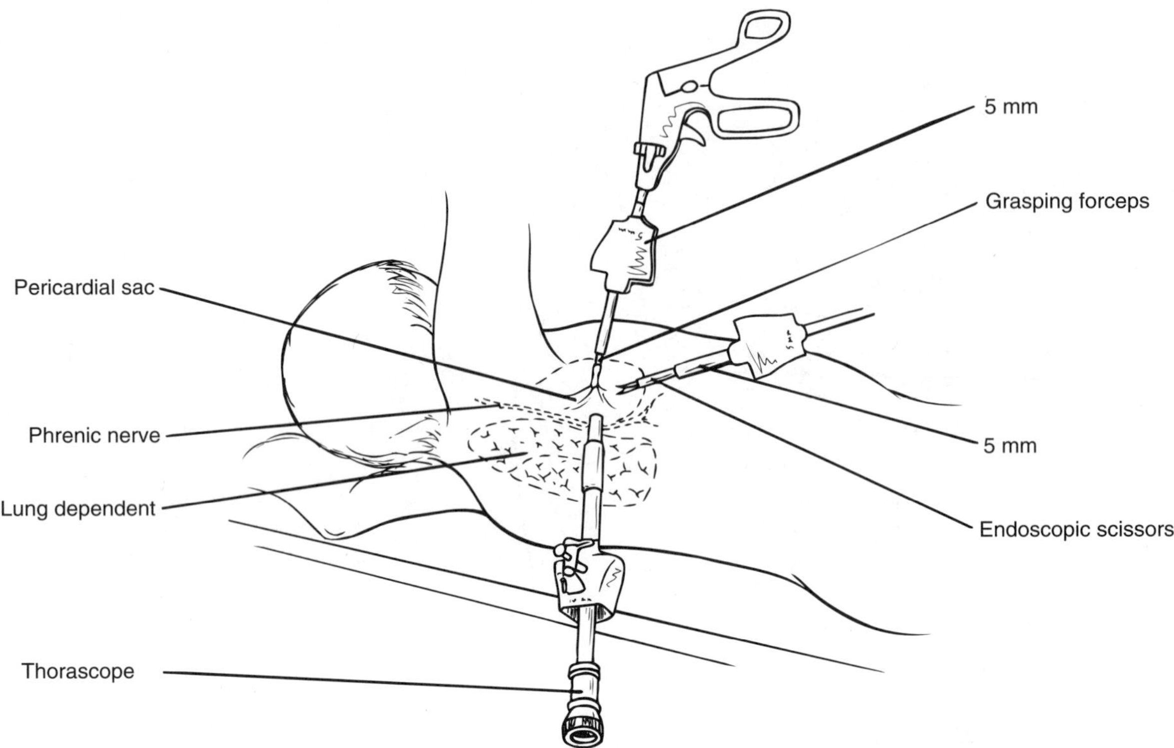

FIG. 59-4. Thoracoscopic pericardiostomy using three-puncture technique. The course of the phrenic nerve can been seen along anterolateral surface of the pericardium. (After Lobe TE, Schropp KP. Pericardiectomy. In: Pediatric laparoscopy and thoracoscopy. Philadelphia, WB Saunders, 1994:239)

through either a median sternotomy or an anterolateral thoracotomy. Cardiopulmonary bypass may be an advantage in that the heart can be manipulated to a greater degree. Additionally, the posterior, lateral, and diaphragmatic aspects of the pericardium can be resected, which is difficult with conventional thoracotomies (Figs. 59-5 and 59-6). The major risks in the use of cardiopulmonary bypass are systemic heparinization and concomitant bleeding. The principal alternative approach is the anterolateral thoracotomy, usually through the left fifth intercostal space (Fig. 59-7). The advantage is that cardiopulmonary bypass is not required and the risk of bleeding is therefore diminished.

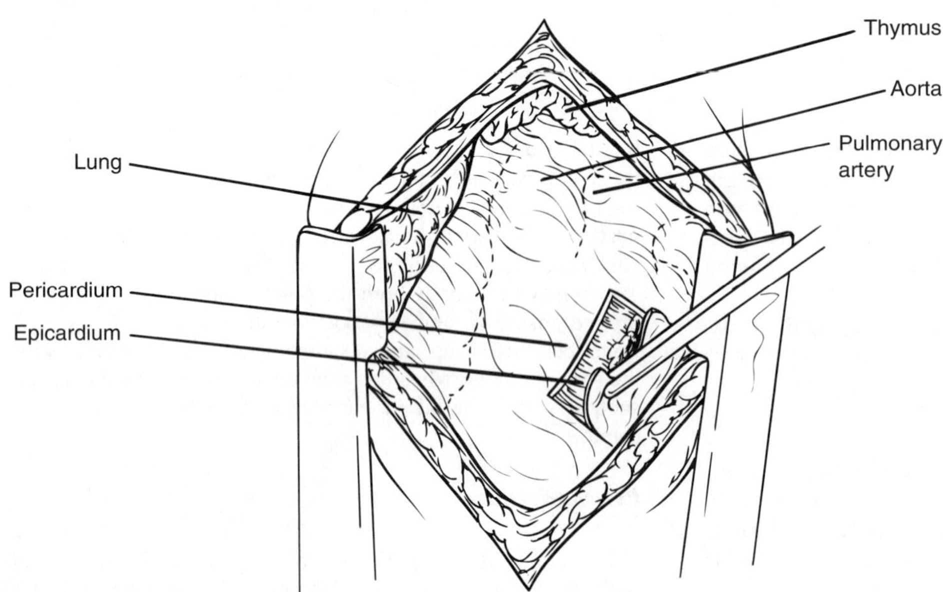

FIG. 59-5. Pericardium exposed through median sternotomy. Incision and dissection in proepicardial plane. (After Ebert PA, Najafi H. The pericardium. In: Sabiston DC Jr, Spencer FC, eds. Gibbons' surgery of the chest, ed 5. Philadelphia, WB Saunders, 1990:1242)

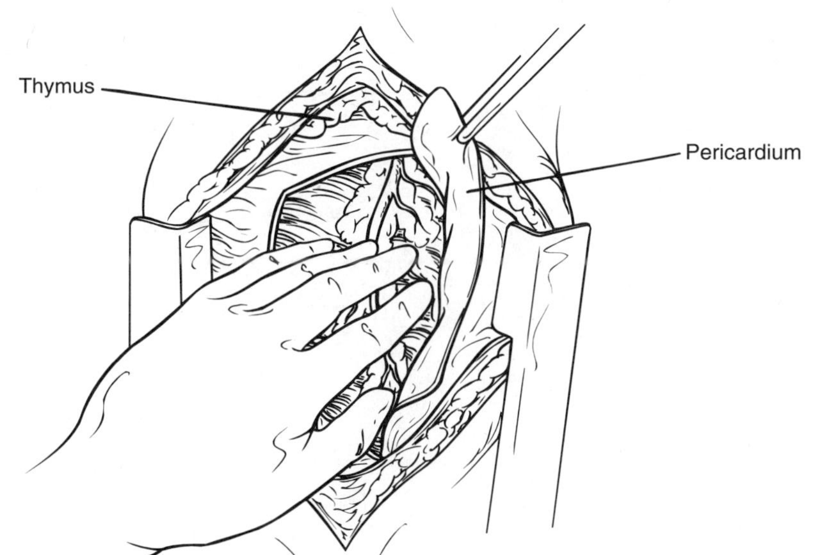

FIG. 59-6. Anterior pericardiectomy through median sternotomy. Excision extends from the right and left phrenic nerves. (After Ebert PA, Najafi H. The pericardium. In: Sabiston DC Jr, Spencer FC, eds. Gibbons' surgery of the chest, ed 5. Philadelphia, WB Saunders, 1990:1242)

GREAT VESSELS

Embryology

The earliest embryonic blood vessels develop from yolk sac mesoderm. These take the form of arborizing cords of angioblasts. The heart forms ventral to the foregut. Paired aortic arches pass laterally from the ventral heart, around the gut, eventually uniting to form the dorsal aorta. During the 5th week of development, a series of paired vessels that supply the six branchial clefts form, segments of which develop into the aortic arch and its major branches. Nearly all important anomalies of the aorta and its branches can be explained by the abnormal growth and involution of one or more portions of the primitive arch system. The six pairs of arches are not all present simultaneously (Fig. 59-8). The first and second arches develop initially, and most segments undergo involution. The remnants of the first branchial arch form part of the mandibular artery. Remnants from the second arch form the hyoid artery and arteries of the inner ear. A large portion of the third arch remains and eventually forms part of the common carotid artery and the internal carotid artery. The right fourth arch forms the proximal portion of the right subclavian artery, and the distal segment is derived from a portion of the right dorsal aorta. A remnant of the left fourth arch forms the segment of the aorta between the origin of the left common carotid artery and the left subclavian artery. The fifth aortic arch pairs are transient and regress early. The right sixth arch forms the proximal right pulmonary artery; the proximal left sixth arch develops into the proximal left pulmonary artery, and the distal portion remains as the ductus arteriosus (Fig. 59-9).

In the embryo, the heart and great vessels begin as cervical structures that later migrate caudally. On rare occasions, the aortic arch fails in this migration and remains in the cervical position, forming a *cervical aortic arch*. This structure is an anatomic curiosity and typically produces no symptoms, but this possibility should be considered in the evaluation of a pulsatile neck mass.

Critical events in the embryologic development of the great vessels occur during the 8th week of gestation. A double aortic arch results if the left and right fourth arches both persist. If the left fourth arch regresses and the right fourth arch persists, a right aortic arch results. Abnormal segmental regression of the left fourth arch results in abnormalities in the aorta that range from coarctation to complete interruption of the aortic arch.

Anatomy

The ascending aorta originates at the heart and travels through the pericardium, where it emerges to become the aortic arch. The superior vena cava lies to the right, and the pulmonary artery crosses posterior to the ascending arch. The aortic arch passes anterior to the trachea, giving rise to the brachiocephalic trunk or innominate artery, the first of three great arteries originating from the aortic arch. The brachiocephalic artery divides promptly into the right common carotid artery and the right subclavian artery. The second great branch of the aortic arch is the left common carotid artery, which runs almost vertically cephalad between the left pleural sac and the trachea to the base of the neck. The third and most distal artery arising from the aortic arch is the left subclavian artery, which passes along the cephalad aspect of the left pleural sac. As it gives rise to its three great branches, the anterior aspect of the arch of the aorta is covered by the left brachiocephalic vein. The aorta normally passes to the left of the trachea. The left phrenic nerve and the vagus nerve cross the anterior aspect of the aorta. On the right, at the level where the vagus nerve lies directly anterior to the subclavian artery, the nerve gives rise to the right recurrent laryngeal nerve, which passes posterior and then cephalad, thereby encircling the right subclavian artery. At about the level of the origin of the left subclavian artery, the aortic arch is joined on its inferior border by the ligamentum arteriosum extending from the left pulmonary artery. The vagus nerve on the left side courses anterior to the arch of the aorta in the vicinity of the ligamentum arteriosum and gives off the left recurrent laryngeal nerve, which

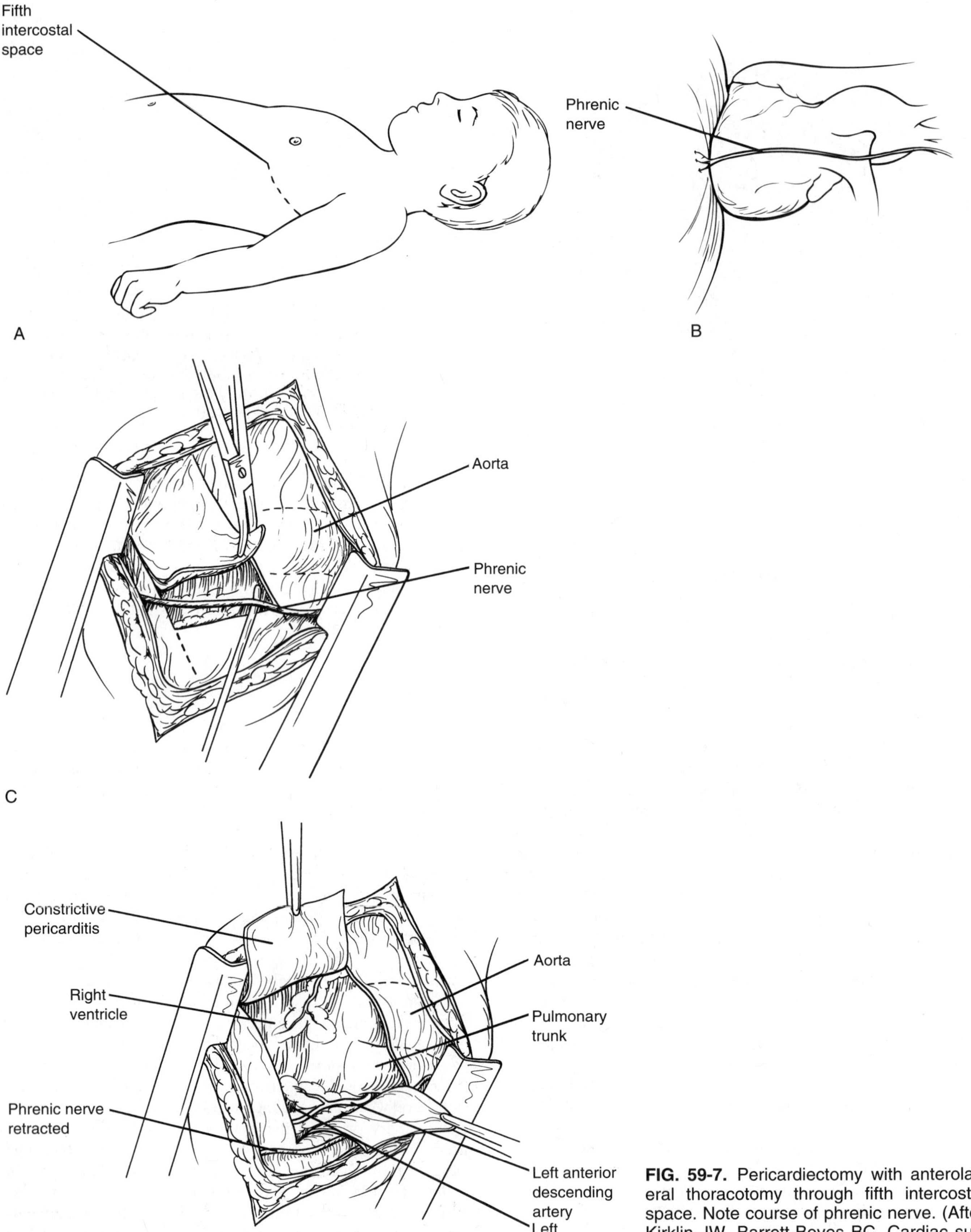

FIG. 59-7. Pericardiectomy with anterolateral thoracotomy through fifth intercostal space. Note course of phrenic nerve. (After Kirklin JW, Barrett-Boyes BC. Cardiac surgery. New York, John Wiley & Sons, 1986:1438)

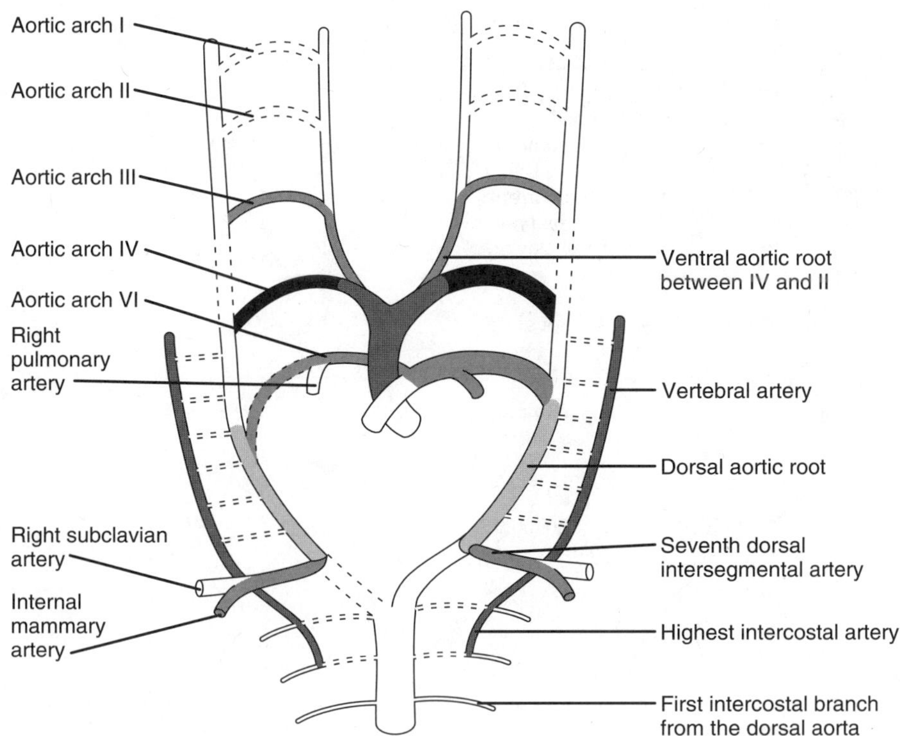

FIG. 59-8. Schematic depiction of primitive aortic arch system. Dashed lines depict structures that normally involute. (After Barry A. The aortic arch derivatives in the human adult. Anat Record 1951;111:221)

passes around the arch in intimate contact with the junction of the aorta and ligamentum arteriosum (Fig. 59-10).

Anomalies of the Aortic Arch

During the past several decades, surgical correction of the major anomalies of the aortic arch has become routine. Although some malformations are asymptomatic, patients with potentially life-threatening obstruction of the trachea or esophagus can be offered a predictably curative surgical procedure in most instances.[5,6]

Double Aortic Arch

The most common type of symptomatic aortic arch abnormality is the double aortic arch. It is derived embryologically

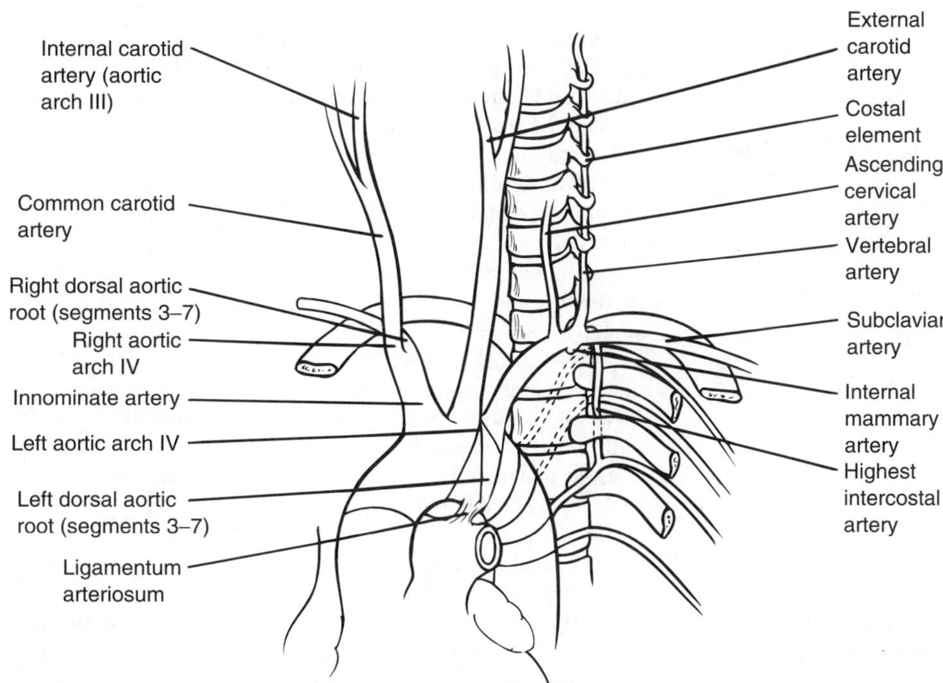

FIG. 59-9. Anterior view of normal aortic arch anatomy. Origins of embryonic arch system are indicated. (After Barry A. The aortic arch derivatives in the human adult. Anat Record 1951;111:221)

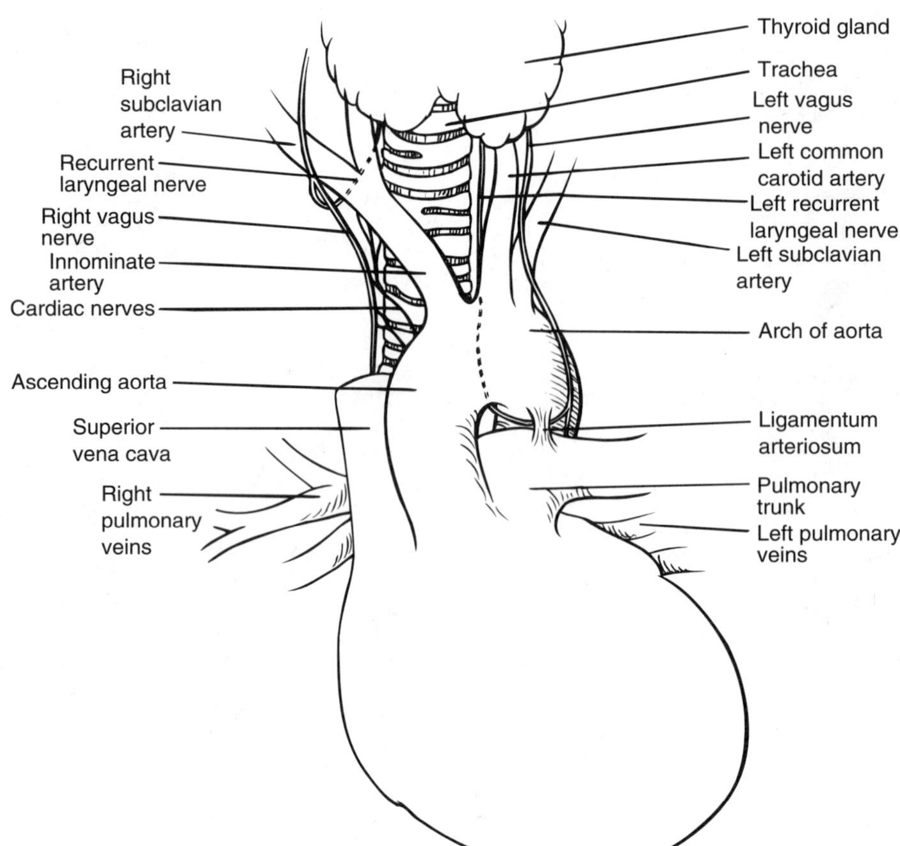

FIG. 59-10. Anterior view of normal aortic arch anatomy and its relation to the aerodigestive tract and major nerves.

from persistence of the paired aortic arches and presents anatomically as a bifurcation of the ascending aorta. The right and left arches encircle the trachea and esophagus and then join posteriorly to form the descending aorta (Fig. 59-11). In its most usual form, each common carotid artery and subclavian artery arises independently from its respective arch. This liga-

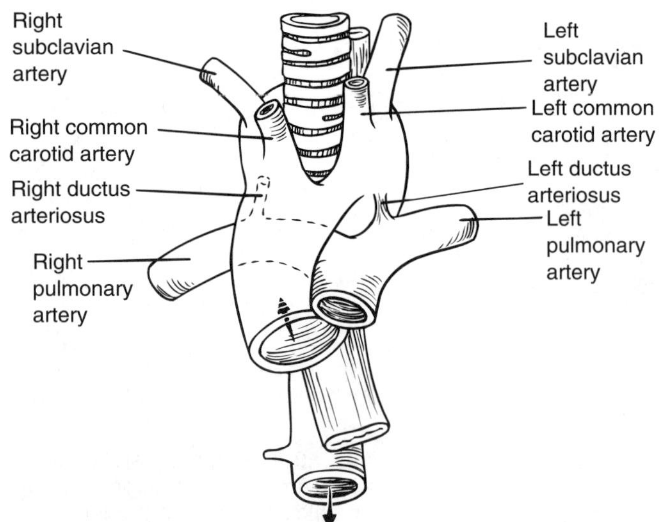

FIG. 59-11. Schematic illustration of double aortic arch encircling esophagus and trachea.

mentum arteriosum can be found on either or both arches. Usually the right (posterior) arch is larger than the left (anterior) arch, although the arches can be equal in size or asymmetric with a dominant anterior arch.

Seventy-five percent of patients with these anatomic variations have symptoms. Physiologically limiting tracheal compression leads to inspiratory stridor, dyspnea, and wheezing. The presentation is generally during infancy, and the urgency can be great. Because of concurrent esophageal obstruction and the risk of aspiration, symptoms are often exacerbated by feeding; dysphagia may be the presenting symptom. About 20% of these infants have associated cardiac anomalies, with ventricular septal defects and tetralogy of Fallot being most common.

On plain chest radiograph, a vascular shadow to the right of the trachea and esophagus is noted (Fig. 59-12). If a vascular anomaly is suspected, the next step in the evaluation is a barium esophagogram (Fig. 59-13). On anteroposterior view, there is bilateral compression of the esophagus. Lateral projections show anterior and posterior indentation as the arch crosses the midline. Historically, angiography was routine for evaluation of these patients. Today, MR imaging and contrast-enhanced CT have replaced angiography for the definitive evaluation of vascular rings (Fig. 59-14). MR imaging depicts vascular and tracheobronchial anatomy with a high degree of spatial resolution without the need for intravascular contrast agents.

Treatment for a symptomatic double aortic arch is surgical. The aim of surgery is to relieve tracheal and esophageal compression and their attendant symptoms by dividing the con-

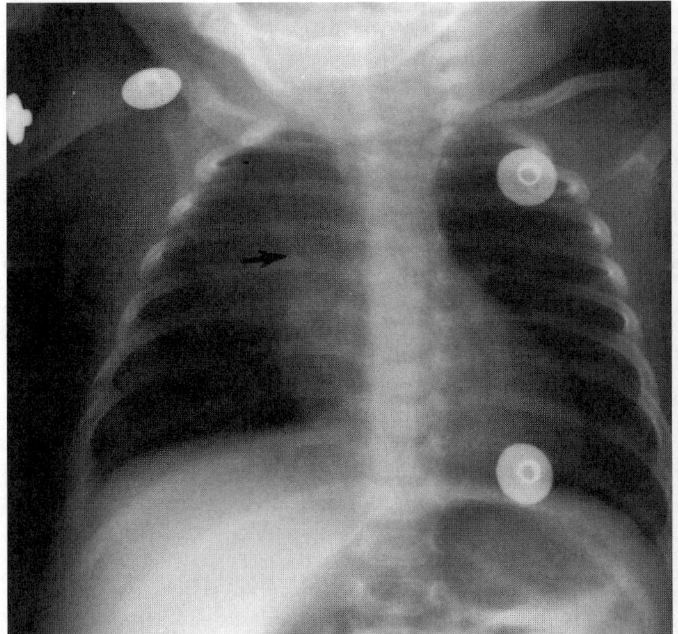

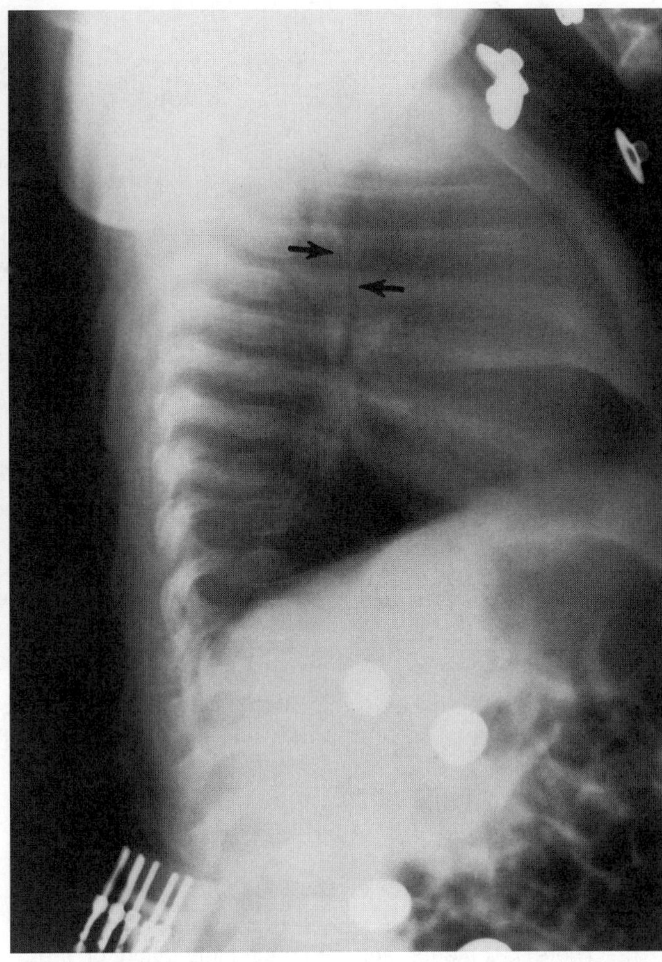

FIG. 59-12. Anteroposterior (*A*) and lateral (*B*) chest radiographs of a 6-week-old child with stridor and dysphagia. The AP view shows a right aortic knob (*arrow*), and the lateral view exhibits narrowing of the tracheal air column (*arrows*). The findings are consistent with a vascular ring.

stricting vascular ring while preserving distal perfusion. As with all vascular rings, exposure is achieved through a left posterolateral thoracotomy incision through the third or fourth intercostal space. All major vascular structures are dissected and definitively identified. The nondominant arch is then divided; this usually means that the anterior arch is divided and oversewn at its junction with the descending aorta distal to the left common carotid and subclavian arteries. When the right (posterior) arch is dominant or equal in size, it is preferentially divided near the origin of the descending aorta. It is prudent to ensure that radial and carotid pulses are preserved during temporary vascular clamp occlusion at the planned site of arch interruption before surgical division for this and other vascular ring corrections, regardless of the anatomic configuration. It is also essential to divide any residual fibrous tissue meticulously around the trachea and esophagus after the vascular ring is divided. During this portion of the procedure, great care must be taken to avoid injury to the recurrent laryngeal nerve. If a diverticulum of Kommerell is present at the origin of the aortic portion of the ligamentum arteriosum, it should be sewn to the prevertebral fascia to prevent the possibility of future recurrence. If persistent tracheal compression by the anterior arch remains after the vascular ring has been divided, sutures can be placed through the undersurface of the sternum and tied to suspend and open the trachea and esophagus.

Right Aortic Arch

Three abnormalities of clinical significance are related to a persistent right aortic arch. The most common is an independent right aortic arch that is a mirror image of the normal left arch. This abnormality is associated with situs inversus. The second variation is a right aortic arch associated with a right thoracic descending aorta. This type is not associated with situs inversus but may be associated with a double superior vena cava and a retroesophageal left subclavian artery. The third type is a right-sided aortic arch that courses behind the esophagus into a normal left descending thoracic aorta. Compression of the trachea and esophagus by a vascular ring mechanism can occur if a right aortic arch is associated with a left ligamentum arteriosum. The ring is formed by the aorta and the pulmonary artery to the right and anterior; the left ligamentum arteriosum completes the ring around the trachea and esophagus (Fig. 59-15). These anomalies occur in less than 1% of the population. The most common associated defect is congenital heart disease. Tetralogy of Fallot, double-outlet right ventricle, pulmonary atresia, and ventricular septal defect have been described.[7,8]

Patients who have isolated right aortic arches without structural cardiac anomalies usually have neither symptoms nor evidence of esophageal or tracheal obstruction. Patients with restrictive vascular rings exhibit progressive respiratory symp-

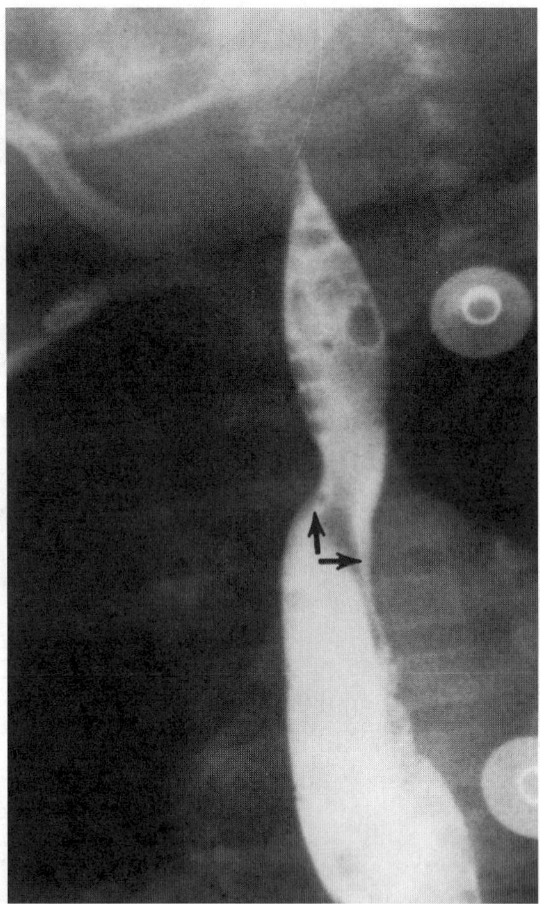

FIG. 59-13. Barium esophagogram of the patient in Figure 59-12. There is anterior and posterior indentation of the esophagus at the sites of encirclement by the left and right aortic arches. This is consistent with compression by a vascular ring, in this case, a double aortic arch.

toms. Stridor and wheezing can be absent in the infant, but these symptoms develop over time because normal growth of the aorta results in symptomatic tracheal compression. These children generally present within the first several years of life, but not in the neonatal period. Evaluation of these lesions is the same as that described for a double aortic arch. A plain chest radiograph commonly identifies a right aortic arch. Thereafter, echocardiography and MR imaging further elucidate the anatomy.

Patients with symptoms require surgical division of this vascular ring. The approach is through a left posterior lateral thoracotomy. It is important to identify the arch and its branches as well as the ligamentum arteriosum. The ligamentum is then doubly ligated and divided, taking care not to injure the recurrent laryngeal nerve. It is occasionally necessary to divide the left subclavian artery at its origin to achieve adequate release of the entrapped esophagus and trachea.

Anomalous Right Subclavian Artery

In about 0.5% of the population, the right subclavian artery originates as the terminal branch from a normal left aortic arch

and passes posterior to the esophagus and trachea but anterior to the vertebral column. This results from the embryologic persistence of a portion of the distal right fourth aortic arch. This anomaly is associated with the classic presentation of interference with swallowing (*dysphagia lusoria*), described by Bayford in 1787.[5] Because this form of vascular ring is incomplete, however, most of these patients do not have symptoms. Plain chest radiographs usually are nondiagnostic. If the index of suspicion is high, barium esophagogram shows a shallow oblique posterior indentation slanting upward from left to right, which is caused by the impression of the right subclavian artery. Evaluation and treatment are undertaken as outlined earlier for other vascular rings. Patients with symptoms should undergo surgical correction. The aortic arch and the aberrant right subclavian artery are identified. On occasion, the anomalous subclavian artery arises from a bulbous diverticulum that is a remnant of the right distal fourth arch. The classic treatment for this anomaly is ligation and division of the right subclavian artery at its anomalous origin. During this segment of the dissection, it is important to identify the recurrent laryngeal nerve that normally encircles the portion of the subclavian artery derived from the right fourth arch. As described earlier, the ligamentum arteriosum is also divided.

Pulmonary Artery Sling

The pulmonary artery sling is not truly related to aortic arch abnormalities, but it is in this clinical context that the lesion is generally encountered. The distal trachea, right main-stem bronchus, or both are compressed by an aberrant left pulmonary artery. This is an important diagnosis to establish prospectively because it is best approached by median sternotomy with the

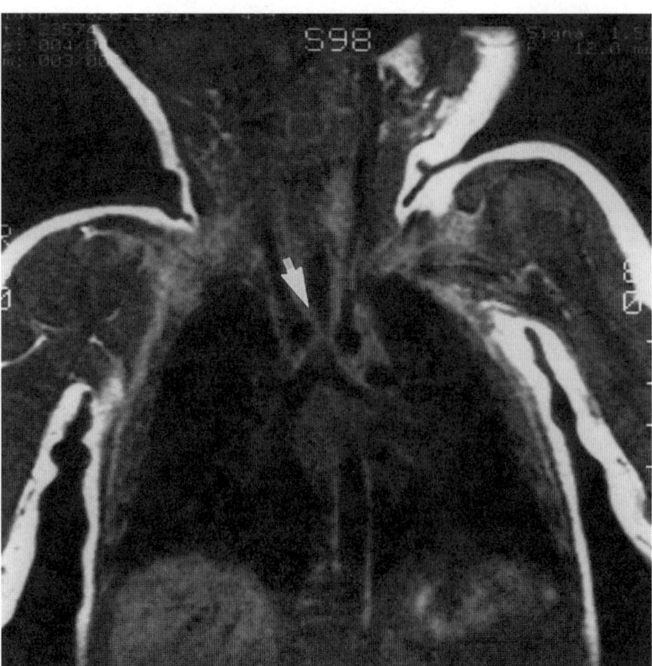

FIG. 59-14. Magnetic resonance image of double aortic arch. Note the symmetry of cephalic vessels and compression of the trachea (*arrow*).

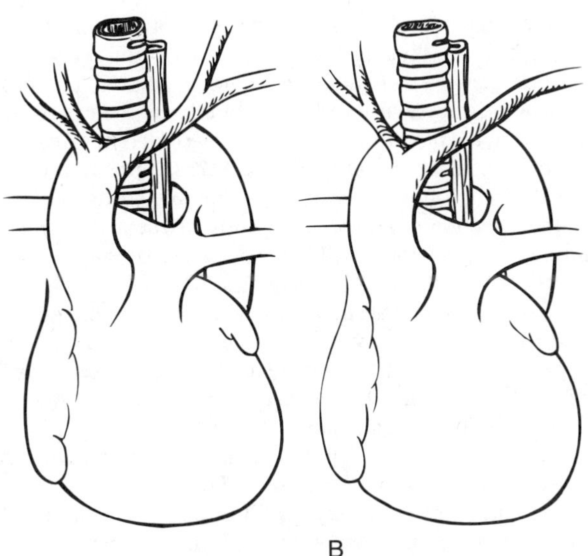

FIG. 59-15. Anomalies of the aortic arch and its branches. (*A*) Right aortic arch with left ligamentum arteriosum, left descending aorta, and left innominate artery. (*B*) Right aortic arch with left ligamentum arteriosum, left descending aorta, and left subclavian and carotid arteries. (After Haryle HRS. The development and anomalies of the aortic arch and its branches. Br J Surg 1959;46:561)

option of cardiopulmonary bypass. The principles of management previously articulated apply here as well, although division of the left pulmonary artery and release of the vascular ring must be followed by repositioning of the pulmonary artery anterior to the trachea and surgical reconstruction. In addition, segmental resection of the trachea or right main-stem bronchus may be necessary to relieve intrinsic tracheobronchial stenosis. Endoscopic assessment of the airway is essential for this purpose.

Treatment Results

The prognosis for patients with symptomatic vascular rings who undergo surgical release is excellent. Relief of esophageal and tracheal compression is predictable and immediate. Modern imaging and surgical techniques make unexpected findings and intraoperative complications unusual. Coexisting conditions, however, particularly congenital heart disease, impose important attendant morbidity. Tracheomalacia can follow the surgical release of a vascular ring, and this is one specific indication for aortopexy. These issues are discussed elsewhere in this text.

Coarctation of the Aorta

Coarctation of the aorta is a constriction of the lumen that results in obstruction to blood flow. The lesion is either focal or elongated, and the site is categorized as *preductal*, proximal to the ductus arteriosus, or *postductal*, distal to this landmark

(Fig. 59-16). Postductal coarctation is the most common type, and typically the ductus arteriosus involutes normally. In patients with preductal coarctation, the ductus arteriosus is usually patent.

When coarctation of the aorta is classified as a type of congenital cardiac lesion, it is the third most common type of congenital heart disease in infants, ranking behind ventricular septal defect and PDA in frequency. This lesion accounts for about 10% of cases of congenital heart disease. Ninety percent of patients with aortic coarctation have associated intracardiac anomalies; the most common are ventricular septal defects, aortic and mitral valve abnormalities, and PDA.[9] Twenty percent of infants admitted to the hospital with congestive heart failure have coarctation of the aorta. There is 3:1 male predominance, and the autopsy incidence is about 1 in 4000. Coarctation is also relatively common in a number of noncardiac conditions, such as Turner syndrome and congenital lobar emphysema.

The cause of the lesion is unknown. It has been suggested that there may be an abnormally large extension of the ductus arteriosus into the wall of the adjacent aorta. If so, it is feasible that this tissue contracts and undergoes fibrosis during the transition to extrauterine life, and that this process leads to coarctation. There is histologic evidence to support this concept. In patients with aortic coarctation, the media is abnormally prominent, and there is evidence of intimal hyperplasia. Another theory is that the coarctation results from a transient reduction in aortic blood flow during the neonatal period. Compensatory increases in flow through the ductus may produce a jet effect, leading to aortic intimal injury opposite the ductus and generating fibrosis, narrowing, and classic coarctation.[10]

The symptoms in patients with coarctation depend on the site. Patients with preductal coarctation often present during the neonatal period or infancy with failure to thrive and congestive heart failure. The latter problem may be exacerbated by associated intracardiac defects. Patients with postductal coarctation have much more diverse symptoms that depend on the degree of obstruction to blood flow. In infants, the nonspecific findings of as failure to thrive, poor feeding, and irritability can result from minor narrowing. In contrast, high-grade obstructions to distal flow can present as an acute emergency with all of the

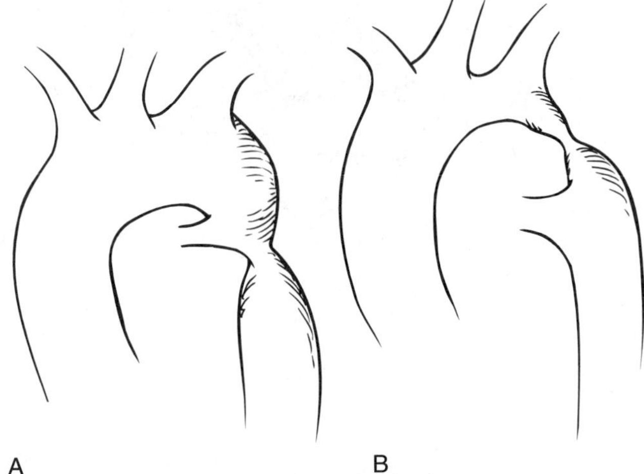

FIG. 59-16. Schematic representations of coarctation of the aorta. (*A*) Postductal. (*B*) Preductal.

end-organ consequences of inadequate regional perfusion, oliguria, lactic acidosis, and multisystem organ failure.

On physical examination, a harsh systolic murmur over the back or left lateral chest is classic. A blood pressure gradient between the upper and lower extremities in a child is highly suspicious. Proximal hypertension is expected, with lower extremity hypotension. Likewise, bounding upper extremity pulses with diminished femoral and lower extremity pulses raise the possibility of coarctation. Aortic coarctation should always be considered in the evaluation of a infant or child with hypertension. As in older patients, evidence of collateral flow through the intercostal and internal thoracic arteries is often present. This finding is supported by notching of the inferior rib margins by enlarged intercostal arteries on plain chest radiograph.

The diagnosis can be confirmed using a number of different modalities. Duplex Doppler echocardiography gives excellent and noninvasive resolution of the lesion and provides additional information about associated intracardiac anomalies. With advanced technology, this evaluation can yield physiologic information as well, by estimating the pressure gradient across the lesion. Angiography, however, remains the gold standard for diagnosis. It provides definitive information concerning the anatomy and associated cardiac anomalies and precise measurement of the pressure gradient across the obstruction. Angiography routinely is obtained before surgery.

The surgical management of coarctation of the aorta began in the 1940s. The procedure described by Gross consisted of resection of the area of aortic narrowing with a primary end-to-end aortic anastomosis. This concept was elegant and simple. Although its implementation was initially complex, it is now routine. Through a posterolateral thoracotomy, the aortic arch, descending aorta, and great vessels are identified. The aorta and the ligamentum arteriosum are then controlled (Fig. 59-17). The lig-

amentum is then divided and the area of aortic coarctation resected. If the lesion is elongated, proximal and distal aortic mobility can be enhanced by ligating and dividing adjacent intercostal vessels. A primary end-to-end anastomosis is then performed using interrupted monofilament suture. The outcome is excellent in this circumstance. In one series, a 92% success rate was reported at 5-year follow-up with this technique.[11] Advantages include the resection of all abnormal aortic tissue and restoration of normal aortic anatomy without prosthetic material.

In patients for whom a primary anastomosis is not possible because of inadequate aortic arch length, an interposition graft is used. In 1961, Gross reported the use of aortic homografts in 70 patients. Although there were no deaths noted and complication rate was minimal,[12] subsequent experience with these and other similar patients suggests important long-term risks related to degenerative changes and aneurysm formation. Others subsequently described the use of Dacron, polytetrafluoroethylene, and other prosthetic grafts in patients with complex lesions, with recurrent coarctation after primary repair, and with aneurysmal changes after homograft placement.

During the past 15 years, a technique was developed to avoid the potential problems of prosthetic conduits and the real problems of aortic anastomosis under tension—the subclavian patch aortoplasty. In this procedure, the origin of the left subclavian artery is dissected to its first branch, and the vertebral artery is ligated to prevent subclavian steal. The subclavian artery is then ligated and divided just proximal to its first branch. The aorta is incised longitudinally through the area of coarctation into the subclavian artery. The resultant subclavian flap is then rotated downward and sutured into place with a series of fine interrupted monofilament sutures, providing autologous arterial tissue for reconstruction. Advantages include the use of autologous tissue, a limited dissection, and a relatively short operative time. Because spinal cord ischemia injury is a risk in all operations on the thoracic aorta, this latter advantage is potentially significant. Campbell and associates[13] performed this technique in 53 infants, with a mortality rate of 4%. Concerns remain, however, about long-term growth and development of the left upper extremity, because decreased limb lengths and mass in children after flap aortoplasty have been described.[14]

Regardless of technique, postoperative complications after coarctation repair are relatively infrequent but potentially serious. These consist of hemorrhage, hemothorax, recurrent laryngeal nerve paralysis, infection, thrombosis, late stenosis, and spinal cord injury. A complication particular to coarctation repair is postoperative paradoxical hypertension. This problem occurs in 7% to 28% of patients and initially presents within the first 24 hours after surgery as an elevation in systolic blood pressure.[15] This is generally amenable to pharmacologic control in an intensive care or other hospital setting and lasts a few days. Subsequently, longer-lasting diastolic hypertension can develop. This is thought to be due to aberrant activation of the sympathetic nervous system. The late phase can be prolonged, and there is evidence that it is renin dependent.[16]

Patients with postcoarctation hypertension can develop splanchnic vasoconstriction and mesenteric ischemia. Abdominal pain, ileus, and lactic acidosis can lead to presentation as an acute abdominal crisis. Histologic examination of mesenteric blood vessels shows necrotizing mesenteric arteritis.[17] The most successful treatment of postcoarctectomy syndrome is that of prevention by aggressive medical intervention when hypertension becomes evident. Sodium nitroprusside, propanolol, and reserpine are among the most useful agents.

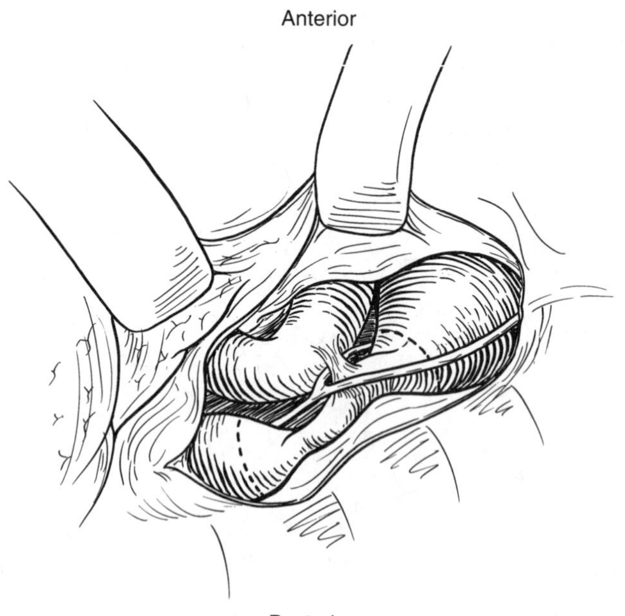

FIG. 59-17. Illustration of the operative view of preductal coarctation as seen through a left thoracotomy. Dotted lines depict sites of aortic transection. Note courses of vagus and recurrent laryngeal nerves with regard to the aorta and the ligamentum arteriosum.

The least common but most disabling complication after co-arctation repair is paraplegia, which occurs in 0.7% to 1.5% of patients.[15] In an attempt to avoid this complication, some have monitored distal aortic pressure during cross-clamping to ascertain the efficacy of collateral circulation, with the concept that if the distal aortic perfusion pressure falls below 50 mmHg, bypass perfusion should be instituted. An alternative approach is to monitor electromyographic evoked potential in the lower extremities because these are reliably maintained at perfusion pressures above 60 mmHg.[18] In this instance, shunting is instituted to maintain distal aortic pressures of more than 60 mmHg during surgical repair.

Although the management of coarctation remains fundamentally surgical, interventional radiographic techniques have been developed with a balloon angioplasty approach.[19] Since the introduction of these techniques in the early 1980s, several studies have compared the results of angioplasty and classic surgical repair. Early results with angioplasty were good, with comparable rates of postprocedure morbidity and mortality. Long-term follow-up, however, has identified unacceptably high rates of both stenosis (14% to 80%) and aneurysmal dilation (9% to 40%) at the angioplasty site.[20] Therefore, angioplasty should be considered only as an alternative to conventional surgical

techniques in patients who have prohibitive risks for conventional surgical repair.

The overall mortality rate using classic surgical techniques is about 10%. Comparable results are described using either a subclavian flap or a primary anastomotic technique. Stenosis at the coarctation site can occur and is thought to be due to either failure of anastomotic growth or an inadequate aortic resection. These patients present with similar signs and symptoms as de novo patients. If hypertension cannot be controlled readily by medical management, angiography with gradient determination should be undertaken and reoperation considered. Reoperation is made difficult by scarring at the previous operative site, and as with all reoperations, morbidity and mortality rates are higher.[21]

Patent Ductus Arteriosus

The ductus arteriosus is indispensable to the maintenance of fetal circulation. It is a conduit that shunts most of the right ventricular outflow from the pulmonary artery and developing lung into the descending thoracic aorta and systemic circulation (Fig. 59-18). Normally, this vessel closes within days of birth

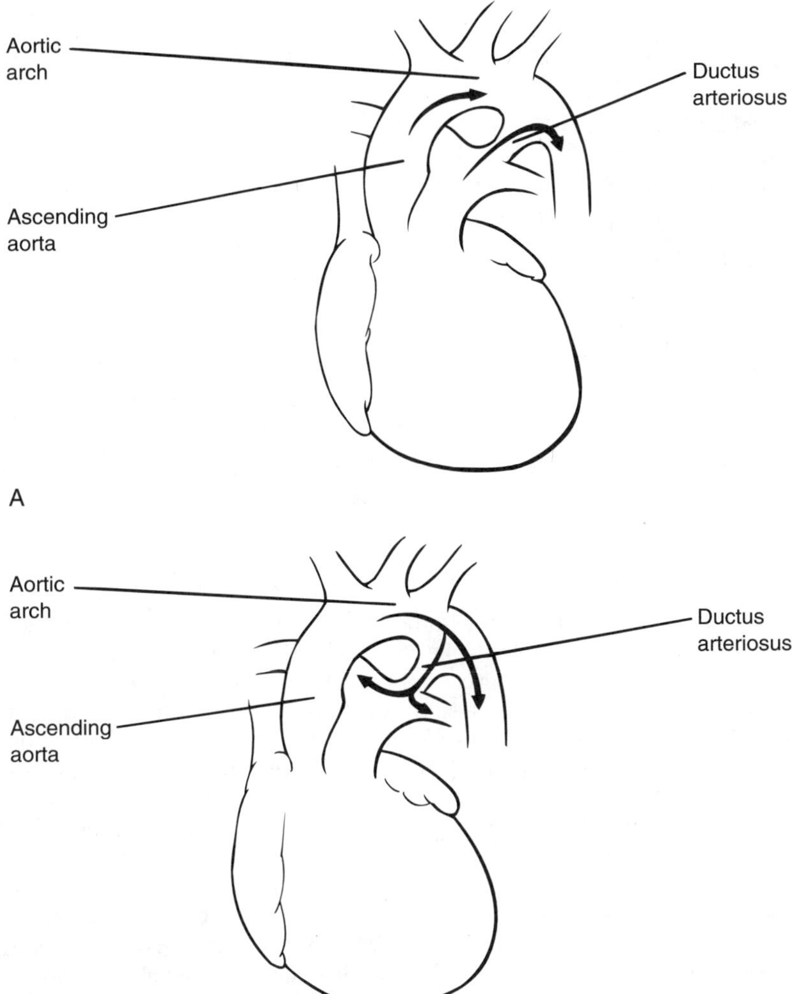

FIG. 59-18. Drawing of circulatory patterns through the ductus arteriosus before (*A*) and after (*B*) birth.

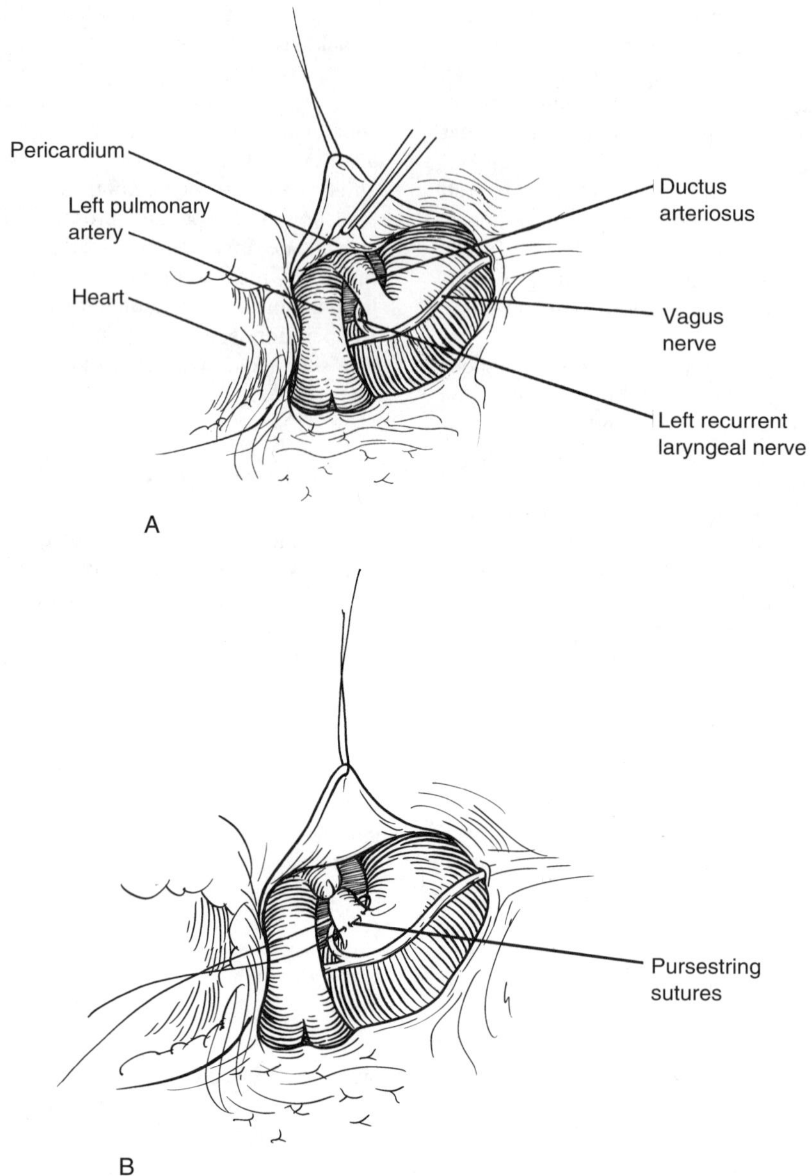

FIG. 59-19. Operative view of ligation of ductus arteriosus. (*A*) Normal anatomy depicted through left posterolateral thoracotomy. (*B*) Suture ligation using large multifilament nonabsorbable sutures. Several alternative techniques for closure are also commonly used.

and is obliterated during the first year of life. It is then referred to as the *ligamentum arteriosum*. Failure of closure should be considered an anomalous condition and is associated with significant morbidity and mortality. PDA is the most common type of extracardiac shunt.

The ductus arteriosus is derived from the dorsal aspect of the left sixth aortic arch and forms a circuit between the pulmonary artery and the descending thoracic aorta just distal to the origin of the left subclavian artery. Structurally, the normal ductus arteriosus is 5 to 7 mm in diameter and 7 to 10 mm in length. It has a conical shape, with a smaller pulmonary orifice. Ductal closure occurs as a natural part of the transition from fetal to adult circulation. Closure occurs in two phases. The first phase is functional, and the second is anatomic. In utero, ductal patency is maintained by low oxygen tension and autocrine regula-

tion of endogenous prostaglandin synthesis.[22] Functional closure occurs when the vascular smooth muscle in the wall of the ductus constricts and the intimal cushions become opposed. The functional closure usually occurs within the first day of life in normal full-term infants. Anatomic closure marked by fibrosis occurs much later. Cristie[23] reported that 88% of infants had an anatomically closed ductus arteriosus after 60 days of extrauterine life, and this rate was 99% at 1 year of age.

Patency of the ductus arteriosus is clinically significant in about 1 in 5000 live full-term births, but is much more common in premature infants. A direct relation exists between gestational age and the incidence of PDA. Histologic analysis of the ductus arteriosus in operated infants has shown altered architecture of the medial smooth muscle cells as well as an abnormality of the intimal endothelial cushions.[24] The defect is often associated

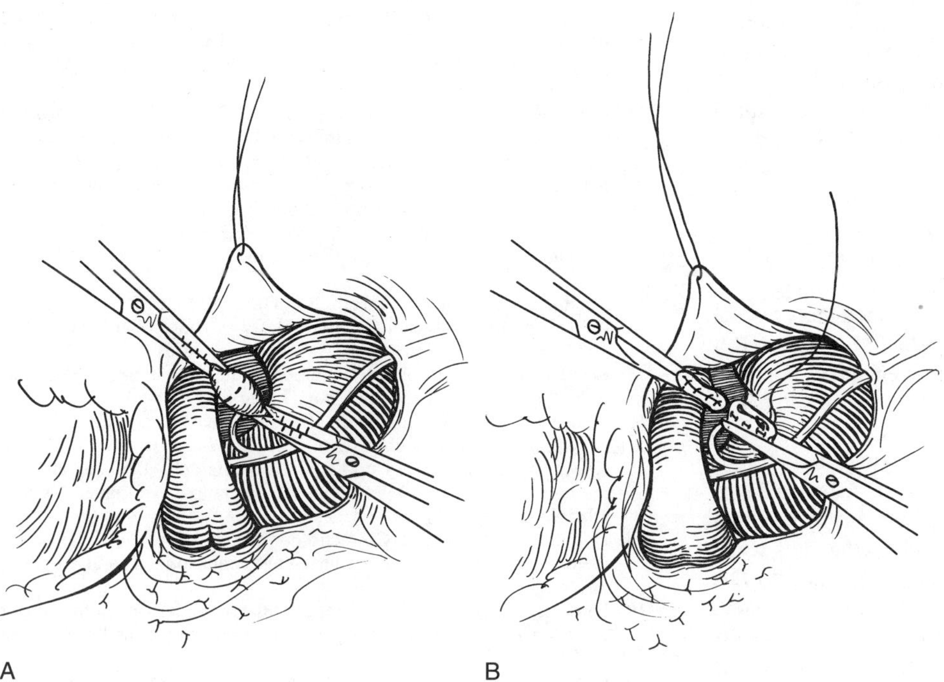

FIG. 59-20. The ductus arteriosus can be divided, particularly in older infants and children. The ductus is viewed here through a left posterolateral thoracotomy. (*A*) Proximal and distal control is obtained by vascular clamps. (*B*) Double-suture ligation of both proximal and distal ends before division.

with other congenital abnormalities. Among these, cardiac malformations are common, and certain conditions, such as pulmonary hypertension, are predictable. Infants with severe pulmonary hypertension, such as that with congenital diaphragmatic hernia and pulmonary hypoplasia, often depend on a PDA to sustain cardiac function. For reasons that are unknown, PDA is twice as frequent in girls as in boys.

The natural history of a PDA is well documented. Untreated, ductal patency in the infant has significant morbidity and a mortality rate as high as 30%.[9] The usual cause of death in untreated patients is congestive heart failure. In patients more than a year old, bacterial endocarditis is a common cause of morbidity. Aneurysmal dilation of the ductus arteriosus, left to right shunting, and pulmonary hypertension can occur in patients who survive to adulthood.[25]

In preterm infants with respiratory distress syndrome, the incidence of PDA is as high as 80%. Symptoms in these patients include intolerance of feeding and high-output cardiac failure. Bounding peripheral pulses, tachypnea, and tachycardia are characteristic. The physical examination typically reveals a classic ''machinery'' murmur over the left upper sternal border. Doppler ultrasonography has shown a marked reduction in splanchnic blood flow in patients with PDA, and an important clinical correlation with neonatal necrotizing enterocolitis exists.[26]

The diagnosis of PDA can be made using several modalities. Chest radiography can show cardiomegaly and pulmonary congestion. Doppler echocardiography is routinely used for screening. It is highly accurate, noninvasive, and portable. Shunt flow can be quantitated with Doppler echocardiography, and the diagnosis of associated cardiac anomalies often can be made. Doppler is often sufficient to make management decisions, but cardiac catheterization can be used as an adjunct to elucidate complex intracardiac anomalies.

As noted earlier, certain circumstances require that ductal patency be maintained to preserve cardiac function and aortic blood flow. This is most successfully accomplished pharmacologically using prostaglandin E_1 or E_2[27] (see Chap. 58).

In most normal infants, persistent ductal patency leads to significant morbidity and mortality. Generally, the presence of prolonged or symptomatic ductus arteriosus patency is an indication for closure. Since 1939, the traditional therapy for PDA has been surgical ligation[28]; however, nonoperative management has been successful in selected term infants. Indomethacin, by means of inhibition of prostaglandin synthesis, is effective in closing a PDA in most preterm infants.[29] Its use, however, has been associated with necrotizing enterocolitis, bowel perforation, reduced renal function, and delayed closure. Indomethacin is contraindicated in infants with renal impairment, sepsis, coagulopathy, intracranial hemorrhage, liver failure, or a physiologically urgent need for closure.

For infants who are inappropriate for or nonresponsive to pharmacologic treatment, surgical PDA ligation is indicated. The procedure is done through a left posterior lateral thoracotomy using either a transpleural or an extrapleural approach. The pulmonary artery, aorta, ductus arteriosus, and left recurrent laryngeal nerve require identification. This is often facilitated by identifying the origin of the left subclavian artery, which is easily found; the ductus arteriosus is close by on the inferior medial aspect of the aorta at this point. Proximal and distal control of the ductus is obtained, taking care not to injure the recurrent laryngeal nerve. In certain instances, the ductus can be as large or larger than the descending thoracic aorta. Care must be taken to differentiate the ductus and the left pulmonary artery. The ductus is then either simply ligated or ligated and divided. The ductus can be ligated with large multifilament nonabsorbable sutures or surgical clips (Fig. 59-19). It can be divided between vascular clamps and oversewn with monofilament nonabsorbable sutures (Fig. 59-20), although this is potentially hazardous in preterm infants. Postoperative complications are minimal but include hemorrhage, infection, pneumothorax, pneumonia, hemothorax, and injury to the recurrent laryngeal nerve. Outcome is determined by other medical conditions. In patients undergoing simple ligation, there have been occasional reports of recanalization requiring reoperation with division and oversewing of the proximal and distal ends of the ductus.[30]

Transcatheter embolization closure of the PDA has been described. Closure rates of up to 92% using prosthetic sponges or metal coils have been reported.[31] In the past several years, thoracoscopic PDA ligation has been attempted. Although it is technically feasible, the advantages are not immediately apparent, and the risk of hemorrhage is of substantial concern. Reports on the long-term follow-up of these patients have not been published. Therefore, these procedures have not achieved broad acceptance.

In infants with asymptomatic PDA, treatment is not recommended unless signs of cardiovascular compromise become evident. Initially, fluid restriction and diuretic therapy are all that is required. If these modalities fail, then indomethacin is used. Given intravenously, indomethacin results in a permanent PDA closure rate of 70% to 90%.[32] Infants in whom indomethacin therapy fails should undergo surgical PDA closure. The results of surgical closure are excellent. In infants, the mortality rate is less than 1%. In older children with evidence of pulmonary hypertension and right ventricular dysfunction, the mortality rate is substantially greater.

REFERENCES

1. Freeman G, LeWinter MM. Pericardial adaptations during cardiac dilatation in dogs. Circ Res 1984;54:294.
2. Klatte EC, Yune HY. Diagnosis and treatment of pericardial cysts. Radiology 1972;104:541.
3. Surawicz B, Lassiter KC. Electrocardiogram in pericarditis. Am J Cardiol 1970;26:471.
4. Rubin RH, Moellering RC Jr. Clinical, microbiologic, and therapeutic aspects of purulent pericarditis. Am J Med 1975;59:68.
5. McNally PR, Rak KM. Dysphagia lusoria caused by persistent right aortic arch with aberrant left subclavian artery and diverticulum of Kommerell. Dig Dis Sci 1992;37:144.
6. Gross RE. Surgical relief for tracheal obstruction from a vascular ring. N Engl J Med 1945;233:586.
7. Moës CA. Vascular rings and anomalies of the aortic arch. In: Keith JD, Rowe RD, Vlad D. Heart diseases in infancy and childhood, ed 3. New York, Macmillan, 1978:869.
8. Paris M. Retrecissement considerable de laorte paetorale observe a la Hotel Dieu de Paris. J Chir Desault 1791;2:107.
9. Gaynor JW, Sabiston DC. Patent ductus arteriosus, coarctation of the aorta, aortopulmonary window, and anomalies of the aortic arch. In: Sabiston DC, Spenser FC, eds. Surgery of the chest. Philadelphia, WB Saunders, 1990.
10. Nugent EW, Plauth WH Jr, Edwards JE, et al. The pathology, abnormal physiology, clinical recognition, and medical and surgical treatment of congenital heart disease. In: Hurstt JW, ed. The heart, ed 7. New York, McGraw Hill, 1990.
11. Cobanoglu A, Teply JF, Gronkemeier GL, et al. Coarctation of the aorta in patients younger than three months: a critique of the subclavian flap operation. J Thorac Cardiovasc Surg 1985;89:121.
12. Schuster SR, Gross RE. Surgery for coarctation of the aorta: a review of 500 cases. J Thorac Cardiovasc Surg 1962;43:54.
13. Campbell DB, Waldhausen JA, Pierce WS, et al. Should elective repair of coarctation of the aorta be done in infancy? J Thorac Cardiovasc Surg 1984;88:979.
14. Todd DJ, Dangerfield DH, Hamilton DI, et al. Late effects of the left upper limb of subclavian flap aortoplasty. J Thorac Cardiovasc Surg 1983;85:678.
15. Lerberg DB, Hardesty RL. Coarctation of the aorta in infants and children: 25 years of experience. Ann Thorac Surg 1982;33:159.
16. Leandro J, Balfe JW, Smallhorn JF, et al. Coarctation of the aorta and hypertension. Child Nephrol Urol 1992;12:124.
17. Kawanchi M, Tada Y, Asano K, et al. Angiographic demonstration of mesenteric arterial changes in post coarctation syndrome. Surgery 1985;98:602.
18. Hughes RK, Reemsta K. Correction of coarctation of the aorta: manometric determination of safety during test occlusion. J Thorac Cardiovasc Surg 1971;62:31.
19. Perry SB, Zeevi B, Keane JF, et al. Interventional catheterization of left heart lesions, including aortic and mitral stenosis and coarctation of the aorta. Cardiol Clinic 1989;7:341.
20. Rao PS, Chopra PS. Role of balloon angioplasty in the treatment of aortic coarctation. Ann Thorac Surg 1991;52:621.
21. Footer ED. Re-operation for aortic coarctation. Ann Thorac Surg 1984;38:81.
22. Barst RJ, Garsony WM. The pharmacologic treatment of patent ductus arteriosus. Drugs 1989;38:249.22.
23. Cristie A. Normal closing time of the foramen ovale and the ductus arteriosus: anatomic and statistical study. Am J Dis Child 1930;40:323.
24. Slaup J, van Monsteron JC, Poelmann RE, et al. Formation of intimal cushions in the ductus arteriosus as a model for vascular intimal thickening: an immunohistochemical study of changes in extracellular matrix components. Atherosclerosis 1992;93:25.
25. Colermyer DS, Shoker GF, Hughes CF, et al. Persistent ductus arteriosus in adults: a review of surgical experience with 25 patients. Med J Aust 1991;155:233.
26. Wong SN, Lor NS, Hui PW. Abnormal neural and splanchnic arterial Doppler pattern in premature babies with symptomatic patent ductus arteriosus. J Ultrasound Med 1990;9:125.
27. Buck ML. Prostaglandin E1 treatment of congenital heart disease: use prior to neonatal transport. Drug Intell Clin Pharm 1991;25:408.
28. Gross RE, Hubbard JP. Surgical ligation of a patent ductus arteriosus: reports of first successful case. JAMA 1939;112:729.
29. Bhatt V, Nahata MC. Pharmacologic management of patent ductus arteriosus. Clin Pharmacol 1989;8:17.
30. Ghani SA, Hashima R. Surgical management of patent ductus arteriosus: a review of 413 cases. J R Coll Surg Edinb 1989;34:33.
31. Hoskinig MCK, Benson LN, Musewe N, et al. Transcatheter occlusion of the persistently patent ductus arteriosus: forty month follow-up and prevalence of residual shunting. Circulation 1991;84:2313.
32. Hammerman C, Aramburo MJ. Prolonged indomethacin therapy for the prevention of recurrences of patient ductus arteriosus. J Pediatr 1990;117:771.

Surgery of Infants and Children: Scientific Principles and Practice, edited by Keith T. Oldham, Paul M. Colombani, and Robert P. Foglia. Lippincott–Raven Publishers, Philadelphia, © 1997.

CHAPTER 60

Esophagus

Bradley M. Rodgers and Eugene D. McGahren III

EMBRYOLOGY

The esophagus is differentiated from the primitive foregut during the fourth week of gestation. A diverticulum of this foregut also gives rise to the trachea. The two structures are separated as the tracheal groove develops and subsequently by the process of esophagotracheal septation. Separation proceeds from caudad to cephalad and is complete by 5 weeks' gestation[1] (Fig. 60-1). Aberrations during this stage of development result in esophageal atresia and tracheoesophageal fistulas. Although initially short, the esophagus elongates with the growth and descent of the lung and the heart. It reaches its full length, relative to the size of the developing fetus, during the seventh week of gestation.[1] At this point, the intraabdominal portion of the esophagus is relatively longer than it will ultimately be during adulthood.

The epithelial lining of the esophagus is derived from the primitive endoderm. The muscular coat of the upper third of the esophagus is striated muscle and arises from the mesoderm of the branchial arches, while the smooth musculature of the distal two thirds is derived from splanchnic mesenchyme.[2] The lumen of the esophagus is nearly obliterated during the seventh and eighth weeks of gestation secondary to rapid proliferation of mucosal epithelial cells. A single lumen is restored by the 10th week, with growth of the muscular wall.[3] The epithelial lining of the esophagus is ciliated at this point, but a stratified, nonkeratinizing, squamous epithelium begins replacing the ciliated epithelium at about the fourth month of gestation. Some regions of ciliated epithelium may persist along the length of the esophagus until birth.[4]

By 8 weeks' gestation, muscle and immature neurons are identifiable within the wall of esophagus.[5] These layers gradually mature until fetal swallowing commences at 16 weeks' gestation.[6] This activity precedes the onset of respiratory activity in the fetus. The ability to swallow amniotic fluid is important to normal fetal development, and by late gestation, the fetus swallows between 500 and 1100 mL/d.[7] Failure of this function results in delayed fetal growth and polyhydramnios.[8]

ANATOMY

The fully developed esophagus is a highly specialized muscular tube extending from the pharynx and cricopharyngeus

sphincter in the neck to the lower esophageal sphincter and gastroesophageal junction in the abdomen. The muscular wall of the esophagus develops in a manner similar to that of the rest of the gastrointestinal tract and consists of an outer longitudinal layer and an inner circular layer. The longitudinal muscle layer of the esophagus is more highly developed than the circular one, although it develops slightly later in gestation. The longitudinal muscle layer develops in the ninth week, while the circular layer develops during the sixth week of gestation.[2] The fibers of the longitudinal muscle diverge in the upper portion of the esophagus to attach to the posterior surface of the cricoid cartilage. This decussation exposes the circular muscle posteriorly, producing an area of relative weakness in the esophageal wall at the level of the cricopharyngeus sphincter (the area of Laimer; Fig. 60-2). This area is particularly vulnerable to perforation during rigid esophagoscopy or other instrumentation. The muscle fibers of the upper third of the esophagus are striated, while those of the lower third are smooth muscle. The middle third contains a mixture of both muscle types. Therefore, diseases of smooth muscle, such as scleroderma, principally affect the lower portion of the esophagus. The epithelium of the mature esophagus is a nonkeratinizing stratified squamous epithelium. The thick muscularis mucosa and elastic fibers in the submucosa produce prominent longitudinal mucosal folds in the nondistended esophagus. Small glands of mucus and bicarbonate-secreting cells with ducts opening onto the surface of the epithelium are scattered throughout the length of the esophagus, particularly in the lower third.[9] The esophagus lacks a serosa except in the abdominal portion.

The blood supply of the esophagus is segmental. The upper esophagus is supplied by branches descending from the inferior thyroid artery, which are closely approximated to the longitudinal muscle layer. The middle and lower thirds of the esophagus are supplied by branches arising directly from the bronchial vessels or descending thoracic aorta. The abdominal and lower thoracic esophagus also receive blood supply from the left gastric and inferior phrenic arteries.[2] The innervation of the esophagus is derived from both parasympathetic and sympathetic fibers. The cervical sympathetic trunks send fibers along the inferior thyroid artery to the upper third of the esophagus, while the middle and lower thirds are supplied by branches from the greater splanchnic nerves. The thoracic esophagus is supplied

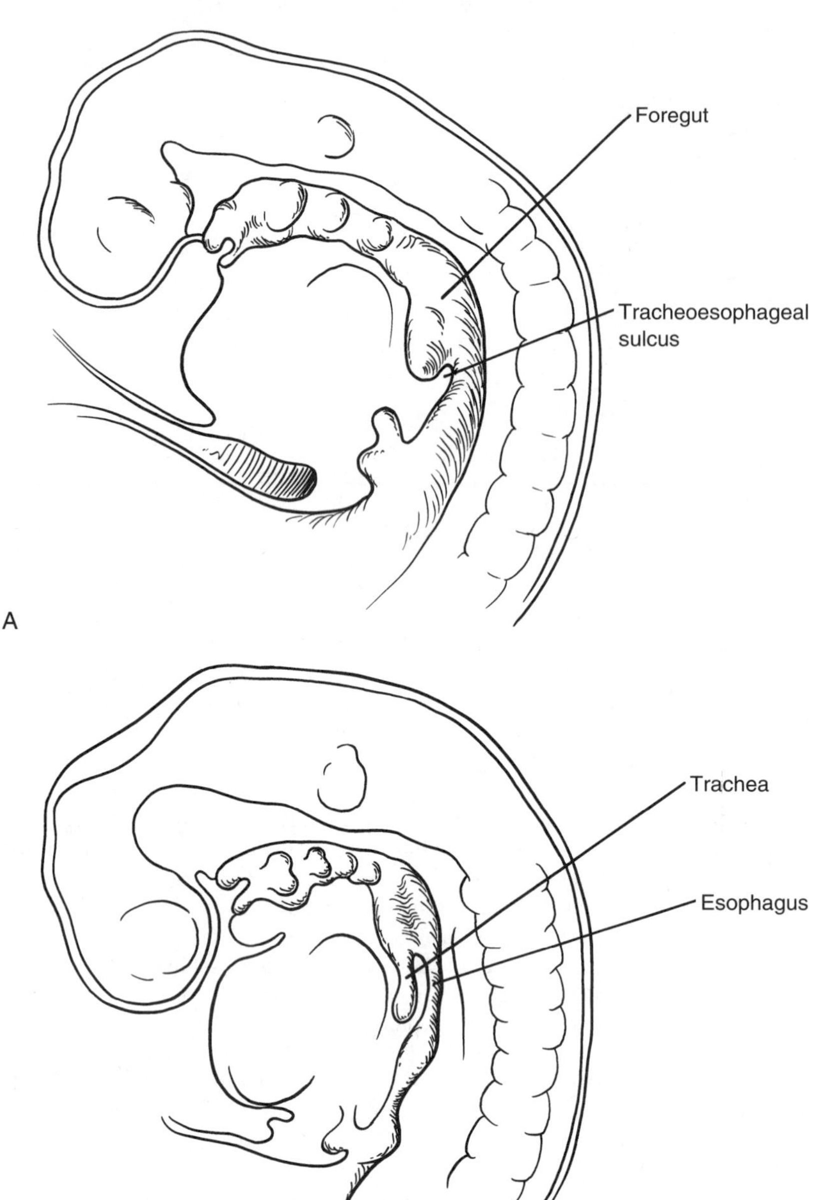

FIG. 60-1. Separation of the trachea and the esophagus. (*A*) By the fourth week of gestation, the tracheoesophageal septum is evident, initiating the division of the trachea, anteriorly, from the foregut, posteriorly. (*B*) The septum remains at about the same level in the fetus when the trachea elongates, forming separate respiratory and gastrointestinal tracts, a process that is complete by 6 weeks' gestation. (After Sutliff KS, Hutchins GM. Septation of the respiratory and digestive tracts in human embryos: crucial role of the tracheoesophageal sulcus. Anat Rec 1994;238:237)

by branches of the esophageal vagal plexus, arising directly from the vagus trunks in the chest.[10]

The esophagus varies in length from 13 to 25 cm, depending on the age and height of the patient.[11] It begins as a midline structure at the level of the cricoid cartilage in the lower cervical region and descends through the chest, slightly to the left of the midline. The lower thoracic esophagus returns to the midline as it curves anteriorly to pass through the diaphragm at the level of the 10th thoracic vertebra. Anteriorly, it is adjacent to the trachea and recurrent laryngeal nerves; posteriorly, it crosses the thoracic duct at the level of the fourth thoracic vertebra. There are four areas of natural anatomic constriction of the esophagus: at the level of the cricopharyngeus sphincter; as the aortic arch crosses anteriorly; as the left main-stem bronchus crosses anteriorly; and at the level of the lower esophageal sphincter. Foreign bodies of the esophagus tend to lodge at one of these areas of constriction, and burns from caustic ingestion tend to be more severe in these regions.

The act of swallowing is initiated by impulses from the swallowing center, an area in the reticular formation of the rostral medulla where the nuclei of cranial nerves IX and X are located.[10] The peristaltic wave begins in the pharynx and passes through the cricopharyngeus sphincter into the body of the esophagus and through the gastroesophageal junction without interruption. The opening of the cricopharyngeus sphincter is coordinated with contraction of pharyngeal muscles. The initial event in esophageal peristalsis is stimulation of the longitudinal muscle layer, followed by segmental activation of the circular muscle and relaxation of the lower esophageal sphincter. Although primary esophageal stripping waves are initiated by impulses from the swallowing center, secondary peristalsis is mediated by local intramural pathways and serves to return material that refluxes into the lower esophagus to the stomach.[10]

The upper esophageal sphincter is a high-pressure zone 1.5 to 3 cms in length, corresponding to the anatomic location of the cricopharyngeus muscle. The resting tone of this sphincter is significantly higher than that in the lower esophageal sphincter. Measurements in adults have revealed pressures of 50 to 130 mmHg in this area.[12] Although there is no morphologic distinction in the muscular wall of the lower esophagus, there is a functional sphincter in this region, known as the *lower esophageal sphincter*. Manometric studies have demonstrated a high-pressure zone in this region, with intraluminal pressures ranging from 10 to 40 mmHg, extending for 2 to 4 cm along the distal esophagus. The primary role of the lower esophageal sphincter is the prevention of reflux of gastric contents back into the lower esophagus. The lower esophageal sphincter relaxes as the primary peristaltic wave traverses the esophageal body and remains open until the peristaltic wave enters the sphincter and closes it. Lower esophageal sphincter pressure is responsive to several influences, including intraabdominal pressure, intragastric protein, the gastrointestinal hormones gastrin and secretin, and caffeine, narcotics, theophylline derivatives, benzodiazepines, and alcohol.[13,14] The position of the lower esophageal sphincter is maintained by the phrenoesophageal ligament. This ligament is derived from fascia of the abdominal diaphragm

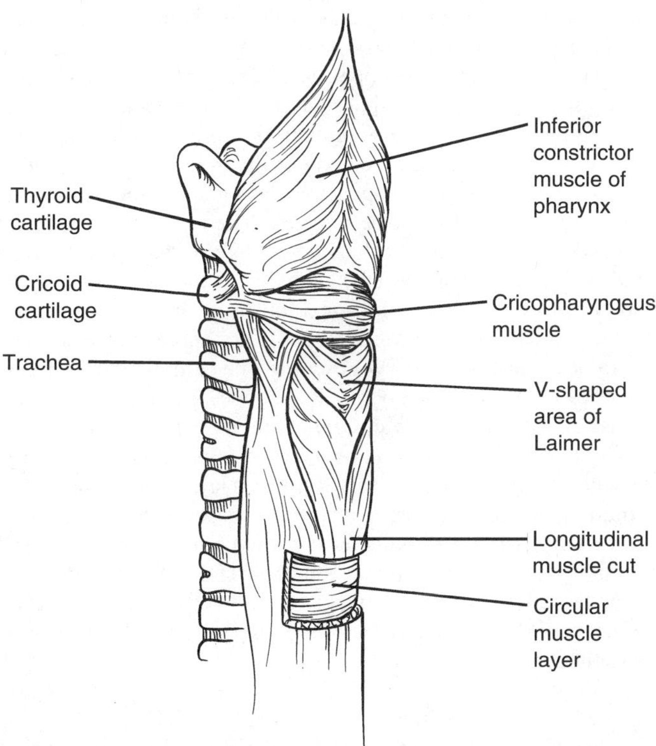

FIG. 60-2. The muscular wall of the pharynx and esophagus. The longitudinal muscle fibers decussate superiorly to produce an area of weakness, the area of Laimer. This represents the location of most instrumental esophageal perforations. (After Netter FH. Ciba collection of medical illustrations, vol 3, part I sec II, plate 3. I. Upper digestive tract. West Caldwell, NJ: Ciba Pharmaceutical Co., 1983.)

and is divided into ascending and descending leaves. The ascending leaf passes through the hiatus to attach to the esophagus 2 to 3 cm above the diaphragm, while the descending leaf inserts below the gastroesophageal junction.[7] In the interdeglutitory phase, the esophageal lumen is kept empty by lower sphincter and cricopharyngeal tone, preventing gastroesophageal reflux and ingestion of air with respiration.

ESOPHAGOSCOPY

The radiologic evaluation of most esophageal disorders begins with a contrast esophagogram or a chest computed tomographic (CT) or magnetic resonance imaging scan. The definitive diagnosis, however, of many of the disorders in childhood depends on direct observation by esophagoscopy. The earliest use of the esophagoscope in children was for the removal of foreign bodies, but it is used increasingly to evaluate symptoms of dysphagia or gastroesophageal reflux, to evaluate and dilate congenital or acquired esophageal strictures, to evaluate the esophagus after trauma, and for sclerotherapy for bleeding esophageal varices.[15–17] Before the performance of esophagoscopy, an evaluation of the child should be undertaken that is appropriate for the condition being addressed. A frontal and lateral chest radiograph and possibly a CT scan should be obtained to look for any unusual intrathoracic anatomy or any other abnormality, such as scoliosis, that may create hazards during the performance of the procedure. A contrast esophagram may be obtained, depending on the patient's symptoms and clinical condition.

Both flexible and rigid esophagoscopes are available that are suitable for use in children. The earliest generation of flexible esophagogastroscopes for children have an outside diameter of 7.2 mm, but are limited to two-way deflection of the tip. These endoscopes may be passed into the esophagus of a full-term newborn infant and larger children, but they are not suitable for smaller infants. The newest generation of flexible esophagogastroscopes have the capability of four-way tip deflection, but an outside diameter of 9.2 mm.[15] Each of these instruments has a suction channel through which 5F biopsy forceps, foreign body instruments, or sclerotherapy injection needles may be passed. The advantage of the flexible esophagoscope is that it may be used with topical anesthesia and sedation for routine diagnostic endoscopy in children. The disadvantages of this instrument are that the biopsy and foreign body instruments that pass through the operating channel are relatively small, and therapeutic esophagoscopy can be impractical.

Rigid esophagoscopes are available in sizes suitable for use in any infant or child. These range from 2.5 to 6 mm internal diameter with a length of 20 or 30 cm. These instruments employ the same Hopkins rod-lens telescope used for rigid bronchoscopy and provide superior visualization to flexible instruments. Foreign body and biopsy instruments may be passed through a separate channel of the esophagoscope, or larger instruments may be coupled to the telescope and passed directly through the lumen of the scope (Fig. 60-3). In addition to the availability of a broader range of sizes of endoscopes, the rigid esophagoscope allows passage of larger instruments, thus facilitating therapeutic esophagoscopy.

Diagnostic esophagoscopy with the flexible gastroscope may be performed under topical anesthesia with intravenous sedation. Pretreatment with atropine is used to reduce oral secretions

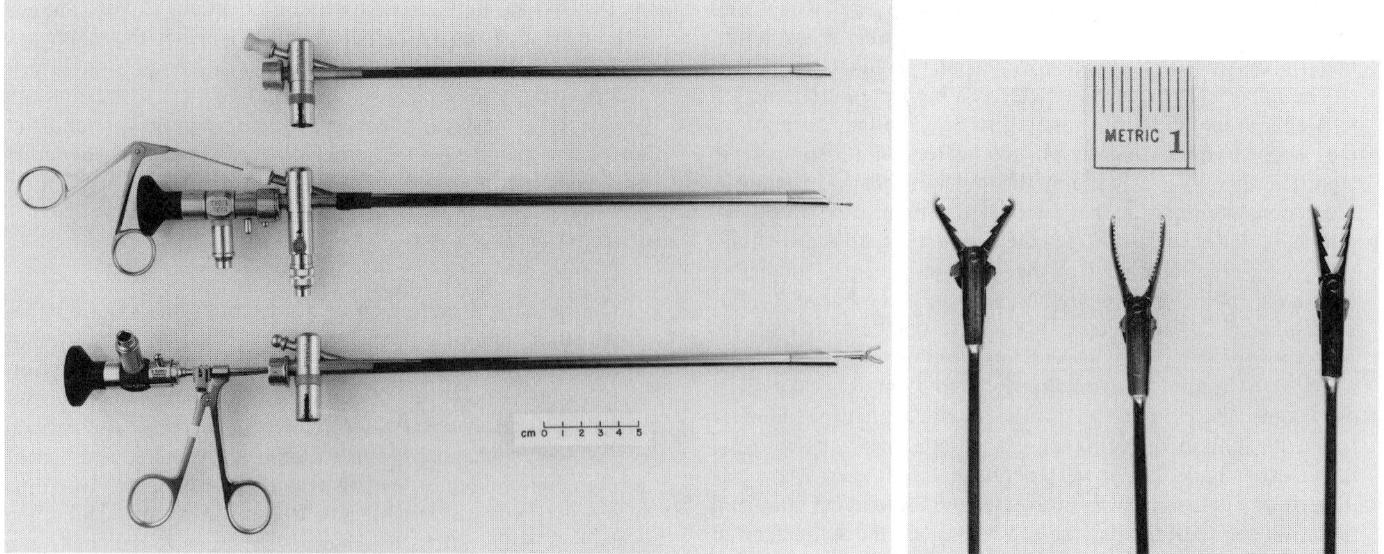

FIG. 60-3. Rigid pediatric esophagoscopes. (*A*) The 3 mm × 30 cm rigid esophagoscope (*top*) is suitable for use in infants. The 5 mm (*center*) and 6 mm (*bottom*) × 30 cm esophagoscopes can be used in older children. Each of these esophagoscopes accepts the Hopkins Rod-Lens telescope. Foreign body and biopsy instruments can be passed directly through the lumen of the esophagoscope (*bottom*) or through the offset instrument channel (*center*). (*B*) Specialized foreign body forceps used through these esophagoscopes include grasping forceps (*left* and *right*) and peanut forceps (*center*).

and block reflex bradycardia. These children should be observed with cardiac and oxygen saturation monitors during the procedure. The child is placed in the left lateral position with the neck slightly extended. A plastic mouth guard may be used in older children but is not needed for infants without teeth. The esophagoscope is passed gently over the tongue, and a slight deflection is placed in the tip as the patient is induced to swallow. With gentle pressure, the scope is pushed through the cricopharyngeus sphincter into the upper esophagus. It is then passed through the length of the esophagus, keeping the lumen under direct vision. The gastroesophageal junction may be visualized from below by passing the instrument into the stomach and retroflexing. Care must be taken not to insufflate excessive air because many smaller children experience respiratory distress with gastric distention. The region of the cricopharyngeal sphincter is more carefully examined as the esophagoscope is withdrawn.

The technique of rigid esophagoscopy is more difficult to learn and may carry a significant incidence of complications in inexperienced hands. Rigid esophagoscopy is performed under general anesthesia in children. Because of the flexibility of the larynx and upper airway, these children should be intubated for airway control before insertion of the esophagoscope. The patient is placed supine, and a soft roll is placed under the shoulders to extend the cervical spine. The appropriate-sized esophagoscope is passed gently along the right border of the tongue into the right piriform sinus under direct vision. The scope is then moved medially to visualize the right arytenoid cartilage and the posterior wall of the larynx. The tip of the scope is gently insinuated behind the posterior laryngeal wall and directed anteriorly to expose the circopharyngeus sphincter. Under general anesthesia, this sphincter is usually relaxed and open, and the esophagoscope can be passed under direct vision

into the upper esophagus. If the sphincter is in spasm, a small filiform dilator or a nasogastric tube can be passed through the esophagoscope into the upper esophagus and used as a guide. The esophagoscope is supported and manipulated by the surgeon's left hand, which also protects the child's teeth. The endoscope is passed through the body of the esophagus under direct vision. To pass the esophagoscope through the esophagogastric junction, the head must be hyperextended and the instrument passed to the left, anteriorly. It should be possible to visualize the entire length of the esophagus from the cricopharyngeus sphincter to the gastroesophageal junction with this equipment.

Complications of esophagoscopy are more common than with bronchoscopy or laryngoscopy. The complications of passage of either the rigid or flexible scopes are usually encountered at the level of the cricopharyngeus.[18] Perforation of the cricopharyngeus occurs in about 0.03% of patients with flexible esophagoscopy, but mucosal lacerations are not unusual.[19] Perforation of the piriform sinus or the posterolateral aspect of the cricopharyngeus sphincter is more common with the rigid esophagoscope and occurs in about 0.1% of patients.[19] Perforation of the body of the esophagus is rare and occurs principally when biopsy specimens are taken or in patients with esophageal stricture.

Iatrogenic perforation of the esophagus is the most common cause of perforation encountered in children. The diagnosis is suspected with the development of a spiking fever or pain and crepitation in the cervical region after esophagoscopy. The diagnosis is confirmed by demonstration of mediastinal or cervical emphysema on plain radiograms and extravasation of contrast on esophagogram.[20] Most iatrogenic perforations are small and well contained. These may be treated with intravenous antibiotics, with the child receiving nothing by mouth.[21] Larger perforations and those communicating with a pleural space need open drainage and attempts at closure.[22] Pleural flaps or intercostal muscle flaps may be used to secure the esophageal closure.

FOREIGN BODY INGESTION

Foreign body ingestion in children continues to be a common problem and occasionally result in significant morbidity and even mortality.[23] More than half of children with foreign body ingestion are younger than 4 years of age. In most cases, the patient admits to the ingestion or the episode is witnessed by an adult. In younger children, with unwitnessed ingestion, the diagnosis is suspected on the basis of the sudden onset of symptoms. Coins continue to be the most common objects ingested, but with the increasing prevalence of electronic equipment in the home, button battery ingestion is frequently encountered.[24,25] Most ingested foreign bodies that reach the stomach successfully pass through the gastrointestinal tract without causing further symptoms. About 20% of all ingested foreign bodies lodge in the esophagus, presumably because of the relatively weak peristalsis of the esophageal musculature and the lack of room in the chest in small children for distention of the esophagus.[26]

Most of these children have symptoms of dysphagia, excessive salivation, choking, or neck pain, although about 10% of patients with esophageal foreign body entrapment do not have symptoms at the time of presentation.[27] This percentage is high enough to warrant radiologic surveillance of all patients with clinical suspicion of foreign body ingestion. Most children with esophageal foreign bodies have no previous history of esophageal disease, although patients who have undergone tracheoesophageal fistula repair are somewhat more prone to suffer esophageal foreign body impaction, especially with certain types of meat.[28] Neurologically impaired or psychotic patients are at risk for foreign body ingestion as well. In the absence of a previous operation, foreign bodies tend to lodge in areas of physiologic constriction of the esophagus: the cricopharyngeus; the mid-esophagus, where the aorta and left main-stem bronchus cross; and at the lower esophageal sphincter. Most esophageal foreign bodies impact in the region of the cricophyarngeus in children.[28] Foreign bodies of the proximal and middle third of the esophagus may produce respiratory symptoms by dilation of the proximal esophagus or direct compression of the membranous trachea, which lies immediately anterior to this portion of the esophagus. Foreign bodies anywhere along the length of the esophagus may produce pain with local mucosal erosion or may erode completely through the wall of the esophagus, resulting in mediastinitis. Chronic foreign bodies may present with esophageal obstruction from a large inflammatory mass.[29]

Foreign bodies entrapped in the proximal and middle thirds of the esophagus are unlikely to pass spontaneously and should be removed at the time of diagnosis. In contrast, at least 60% of coins in the distal esophagus pass spontaneously.[30] A period of waiting in these patients may be justified, allowing some liquids by mouth. Other authors have suggested that food impaction in the distal esophagus can be washed into the stomach by encouraging ingestion of liquids or solids.[31] Some have advocated the use of a bougie, under sedation, to force a smooth foreign body in the distal esophagus into the stomach.[32] Continued entrapment of a foreign body in the esophagus, however, increases the risk for respiratory symptoms, aspiration, and

esophageal perforation. Therefore, retained esophageal foreign bodies should be extracted. All foreign bodies with sharp edges and those that might fragment on removal should be removed endoscopically. Endoscopic removal of foreign bodies in children is performed under general anesthesia with endotracheal intubation to protect the patient's airway. In most cases, the rigid esophagoscope should be employed because the foreign body instruments that can be used through the flexible endoscopes are too small. It is critical that appropriate foreign body instruments are available before initiating this procedure (see Fig. 60-3). Smooth foreign bodies, such as coins, particularly those in the upper esophagus in somewhat older children, may be safely removed with balloon catheter techniques within 24 hours of ingestion. Removal of an esophageal foreign body with a balloon catheter is usually performed under sedation in the radiology suite.[33,34] Monitoring of the procedure, under fluoroscopy, allows controlled removal and retrieval of the foreign body. Chronic esophageal foreign bodies, which have eroded into or through the wall of the esophagus, must be removed by thoracotomy, unless a portion of the foreign body can be visualized from within the esophageal lumen by endoscopy.[28,34] Complications of either of these techniques of foreign body extraction are rare in children, and successful removal is accomplished in virtually 100% of patients.

Late complications of impacted esophageal foreign bodies in children are uncommon. Stricture formation is infrequent unless the foreign body has been neglected or has eroded through the esophageal wall. Complications from ingested button batteries appear to be more common than from other esophageal foreign bodies. Leakage of the potassium hydroxide contained within these batteries may lead to local esophageal burns and the development of scarring and stenosis.[25]

CAUSTIC ESOPHAGEAL INJURY

Caustic injuries of the esophagus in children continue to be a significant problem despite federal legislation limiting the concentration of alkaline agents sold for household use and requiring prominent labeling of toxic products.[35] Anderson and colleagues[36] estimated that 17,000 children a year in the United States are seen for caustic ingestion. Most of these cases represent accidental ingestion in children younger than 5 years of age, although suicide attempts in adolescent patients are occasionally encountered. Most, and the most severe, esophageal caustic injuries are seen as a result of ingestion of alkaline products distributed for household cleaning.[37] The extent and severity of the esophageal injury is dependent on the amount and nature of the caustic material ingested. The distribution of ingested solid caustic agents tends to be less uniform along the length of the esophagus than is seen after ingestion of liquid agents. Contact with the esophageal surface by concentrated alkali leads to liquefaction necrosis and edema. These lesions tend to be deep or transmural. Extensive vascular thrombosis may result in gangrene and perforation or severe contracture of the esophagus. Acid ingestion, on the other hand, tend to produce a superficial eschar, which often protects the deeper tissues from injury.

Children with any form of caustic ingestion usually present with symptoms of pain and irritability. Excess salivation and dysphagia are common. Respiratory distress, usually secondary to laryngeal burns, occurs in about 15% of these patients.[38] However, 20% of children with caustic ingestion present with no symptoms, and half of these patients have significant esophageal injury.[39,40] In general, it is difficult to correlate the severity or extent of esophageal injury with symptoms at presentation, but the presence of epigastric pain or respiratory symptoms correlates strongly with significant esophageal injury.[40]

The initial management of children with caustic ingestion should be aimed at determining the extent and severity of injury.[41] It is particularly important to determine the presence of burns beyond the level of the upper esophageal sphincter. All patients with suspected caustic ingestion should undergo endoscopic evaluation of the esophagus under general anesthesia, preferably with the rigid esophagoscope, although the flexible instrument can be used.[42] Preoperative chest and abdominal radiographs should be obtained, examining for mediastinal or abdominal free air, which would indicate full-thickness necrosis with perforation. Endoscopic examinations should be performed within 24 hours of the ingestion to avoid the interval of maximal edema and friability. The esophagoscope should be passed only as far as the first burn beyond the cricopharyngeus to minimize the risk of iatrogenic injury. The degree and extent of the burn are noted. Patients with respiratory symptoms should also undergo direct laryngoscopy and bronchoscopy.

Patients with first-degree injuries characterized by mucosal erythema and edema rarely develop sequelae and require no specific therapy for their injuries. Patients with second-degree injuries have mucosal ulceration with noncircumferential fibrin plaques and should be observed closely in the hospital. Patients with third-degree injuries have circumferential mucosal slough and require more aggressive management.[43] The treatment of second- and third-degree esophageal injuries is controversial. Most authors favor treatment of these patients for 3 weeks with prednisone, 2 to 2.5 mg/kg/d, and antibiotics such as ampicillin, 50 mg/kg/d, to attempt to minimize the inflammatory response and subsequent stricture formation.[41] In a randomized, prospective trial of the use of steroids in 131 children suspected of having caustic injury, 60 were found to have an injury at endoscopy.[36] Twenty-one of these children (35%) developed strictures, evenly divided between those receiving and not receiving steroids. Only a single patient with second-degree injury developed a stricture (Table 60-1). On the basis of these data, there

is no benefit to treatment of these children with steroids. Nonetheless, until other studies confirm these findings, steroids and antibiotics are widely considered to be appropriate treatment for second- and third-degree burns. Patients with frank perforation or severe hemorrhage require emergent thoracotomy and esophagectomy with subsequent esophageal replacement. Twenty to 30% of children with second- and third-degree injury of the esophagus progress to develop strictures. These patients require repeated esophageal dilation and may benefit from direct injection of steroids such as triamcinolone, 40 mg/mL, into the stricture.[44] Failure of the stricture to resolve after 6 to 12 months of dilation is an indication for esophagectomy and esophageal replacement with a gastric tube or colonic interposition. Long-term follow-up of all these patients is important because they have an increased incidence of esophageal carcinoma later in life.[45]

ESOPHAGEAL STENOSIS

Stenoses of the esophagus are classified as acquired or congenital. Acquired stenosis may be caused by caustic ingestion or chronic foreign body entrapment, as already discussed. The most common cause of acquired esophageal stenosis in children, however, is chronic esophagitis secondary to gastroesophageal reflux. Isolated true congenital esophageal stenosis is uncommon. Five percent of patients with tracheoesophageal fistula have congenital narrowing of the distal esophagus, often presenting with symptoms of dysphagia after successful surgical repair of the esophageal atresia.[46] Unlike stenosis secondary to gastroesophageal reflux, which is common in these patients, this type of stenosis tends to be fusiform in character and usually involves the middle or distal esophagus, above the esophagogastric junction (Fig. 60-4). These stenoses usually respond to esophageal dilation, although resection has occasionally been recommended.

Congenital esophageal stenosis also occurs in conjunction with rests of embryonic tissue within the wall of the esophagus.[47] These stenoses are localized and most often found in the distal third of the esophagus. They also may be associated with esophageal atresia anomalies. These patients usually do not have symptoms while breastfed or on infant formula, but they begin to have symptoms of dysphagia when they are introduced to soft or solid foods. The diagnosis is suggested by barium esophagogram and confirmed by pathologic evaluation of the resected esophageal specimen. There is usually no abnormality noted at esophagoscopy because the overlying mucosa is normal. These stenoses are localized but do not respond to dilation. Segmental resection of the area of stenosis completely relieves symptoms in these children. Congenital webs and diaphragms are extremely rare in children. They tend to occur in the middle and lower third of the esophagus. These lesions usually respond to vigorous dilation or endoesophageal resection and rarely require esophageal resection for relief of symptoms.[48] Traditionally, dilation of esophageal stenoses has been performed with tapered, mercury-weighted bougies (Maloney or Savary dilator). More recently, dilation with balloon catheters (Grüntzig) under fluoroscopic guidance has been described.[49,50] This procedure is usually performed with the child sedated or anesthetized. Significant complications have rarely been reported, and the success rate approximates 95%.[50]

Barrett esophagus is a condition in which specialized colum-

TABLE 60-1. *Relation of steroid treatment to stricture formation and the need for esophageal replacement, according to the degree of esophageal injury*

Degree of burn	No. of burns	Stricture	Replacement
Steroid group			
First	6	0 (0%)	0 (0%)
Second	15	1 (7%)	1 (100%)
Third	10	9 (90%)	3 (33%)
All	31	10 (32%)	4 (40%)
Control group			
First	13	0 (0%)	0 (0%)
Second	5	0 (0%)	0 (0%)
Third	11	11 (100%)	7 (64%)
All	29	11 (38%)*	7 (64%)*

* *P*>.05 for the comparison of steroid and control groups.
(Anderson KD, Rouse TM, Randolph JG. A controlled trial of corticosteroids in children with corrosive injury of the esophagus. N Engl J Med 1990;323:637)

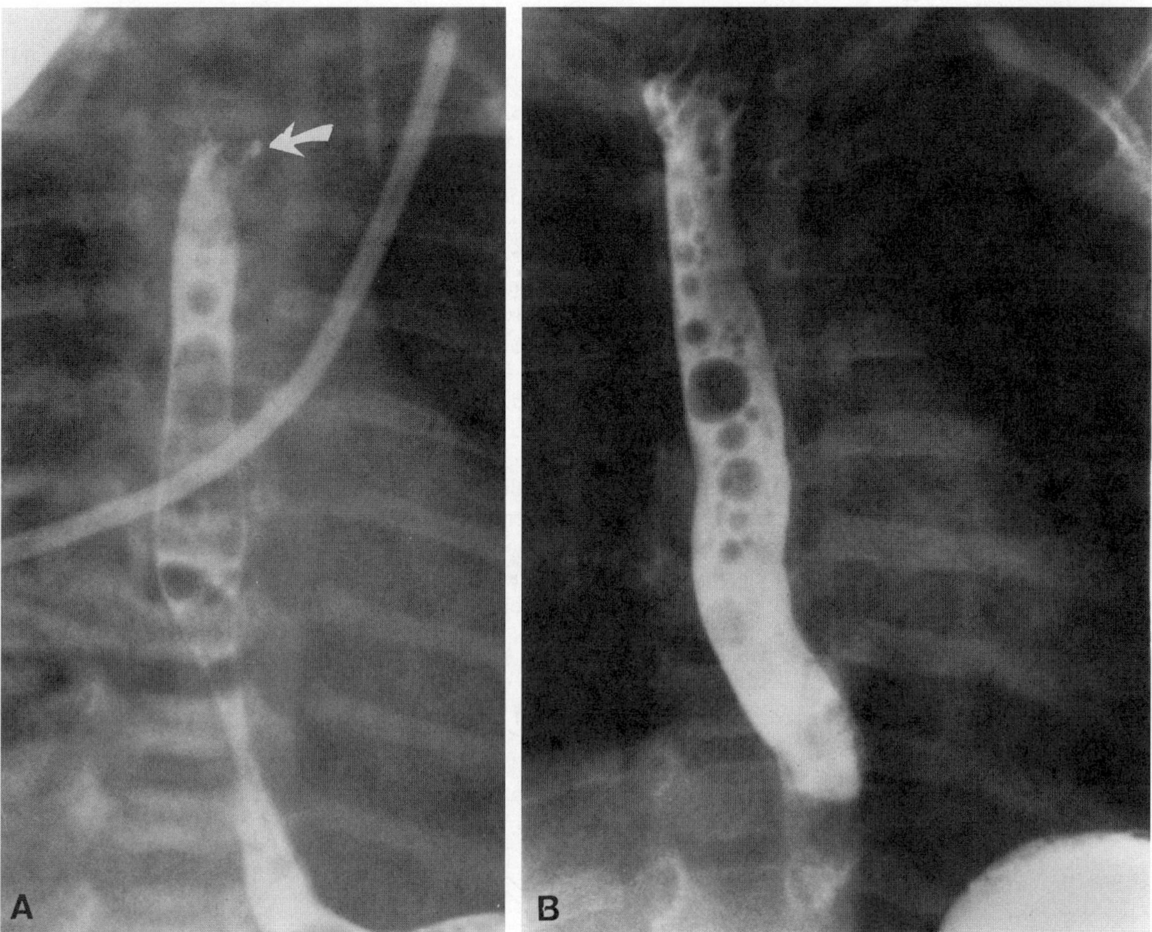

FIG. 60-4. Esophageal stenosis associated with esophageal atresia and tracheoesophageal fistula. (*A*) Barium esophagogram obtained 1 week after repair of a type C esophageal fistula. The level of the esophageal anastomosis is identified by a small amount of leakage of the contrast (*arrow*). A fusiform stricture of the distal third of the esophagus is noted, with mild proximal dilation. (*B*) After a single antegrade dilation of the distal stricture, the patient experienced no further dysphagia. A barium esophagogram at 3 months of age revealed no residual stricture and a widely patent anastomosis.

nar epithelium extends for more than 3 cm above the top of the lower esophageal sphincter. Whereas islands of normal appearing gastric epithelium are relatively common in the esophagus, Barrett goblet epithelium is specialized in nature and contains cells that stain positive with Alcian blue at a pH of 2.5.[51] The age range of patients with Barrett epithelium appears to be bimodal, with the pediatric peak in the interval between 0 and 15 years.[52] Barrett epithelium is frequently associated with severe and unrelenting strictures of the esophagus, often in the proximal and middle thirds.[53] Although Barrett esophagus was at one time thought to be a congenital condition, most now agree that this disorder is acquired. Gastroesophageal reflux is thought to be the major precursor to the development of Barrett epithelium in children.[54,55] In addition to gastroesophageal reflux, other predisposing conditions include esophageal atresia, lye ingestion, and mental retardation. The incidence of Barrett epithelium appears to be exceptionally high in the esophagus just proximal to the cervical anastomosis in gastric tube reconstruction of the esophagus.[56] Children with Barrett esophagus

usually present with symptoms of severe gastroesophageal reflux in the first year of life. Often, these patients have significant dysphagia secondary to esophagitis or esophageal strictures.[53] They may first present to the physician with a food impaction at the level of the stricture. Hematemesis and respiratory symptoms secondary to chronic aspiration are often seen. The diagnosis of Barrett esophagus requires multiple biopsy specimens of the esophageal mucosa, obtained well proximal to the lower esophageal sphincter. Unlike adult patients, most children with Barrett epithelium do not show any gross changes on endoscopic observation, and these specimens must be obtained in blind fashion.[55] The diagnosis of Barrett esophagus is made on demonstration of the specialized metaplastic epithelium characteristic of this disorder, although many pediatric series have described patients with Barrett esophagus in whom only normal-appearing gastric mucosa was identified at biopsy.[54] The true frequency of Barrett epithelium in children is therefore unknown.

Stein and associates[57] demonstrated other functional foregut abnormalities in adult patients with Barrett esophagus. These patients have a higher incidence of duodenogastric reflux producing alkaline exposure of the esophagus. They also appear to have reduced amplitude of contraction of the peristaltic wave in the distal third of the esophagus, perhaps interfering with esophageal clearance of refluxed material. Gastric acid analysis in adults with Barrett esophagus demonstrates high basal and stimulated gastric acid secretion, as compared with control patients with esophagitis in the absence of Barrett epithelium. The rate of gastric emptying in these two groups of patients, however, appeared unaffected by Barrett esophagus. Similar studies in children with Barrett esophagus have not been reported.

Treatment of patients with Barrett esophagus focuses on the elimination of the gastroesophageal reflux and chronic esophagitis. Treatment with histamine-2–blocking agents, proton-pump inhibitors, and antacids may eliminate the acid reflux but does nothing for the alkaline reflux characteristic in these patients. Most authors believe that the alkaline reflux is primarily responsible for the development of esophagitis and perhaps dysplasia of this epithelium. For this reason, the surgical elimi-

nation of gastroesophageal reflux is universally recommended.[52,53,55] Even with successful operation, however, the Barrett epithelium rarely completely regresses in children with this disorder.[58]

Barrett epithelium of the special columnar variety is a premalignant condition. Patients with Barrett epithelium have a 30- to 125-fold increased incidence of adenocarcinoma of the esophagus.[59] Hassall and colleagues[59] reported the case of a 17-year-old boy with Barrett esophagus and severe dysphagia who was found to have an adenocarcinoma of the esophagus on esophagoscopy. They reviewed nine additional cases of adenocarcinoma developing in young patients with Barrett epithelium reported in the literature. The prognosis of these patients appears to be particularly poor, even after esophageal resection. Children with Barrett esophagus require careful long-term follow-up with esophageal biopsies to detect the development of dysplasia within this epithelium. Younes and colleagues[60] demonstrated accumulation of p53 protein, as well as intraepithelial adenocarcinoma, in patients with dysplastic Barrett epithelium. This analysis may prove helpful in differentiating those patients who are likely to develop malignancy, thus allowing earlier treatment.

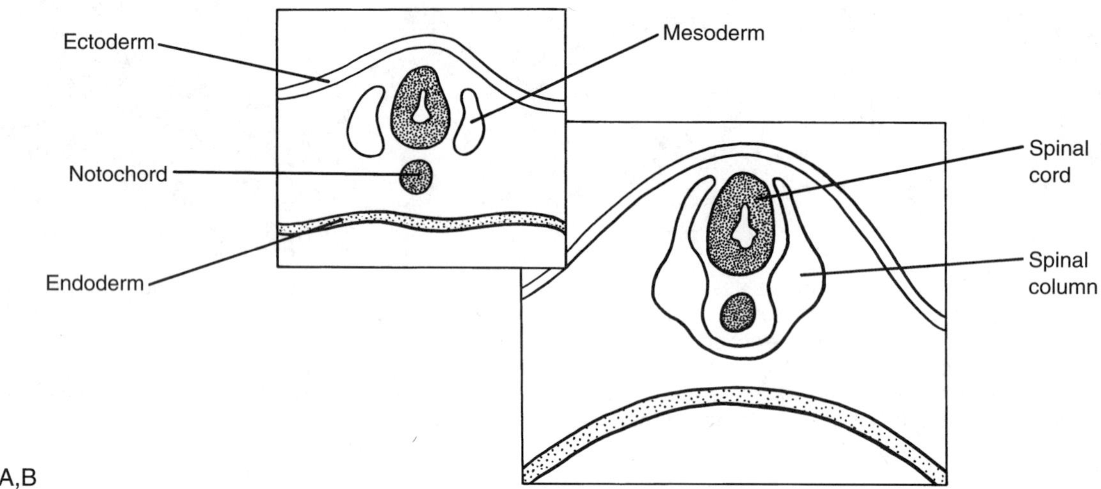

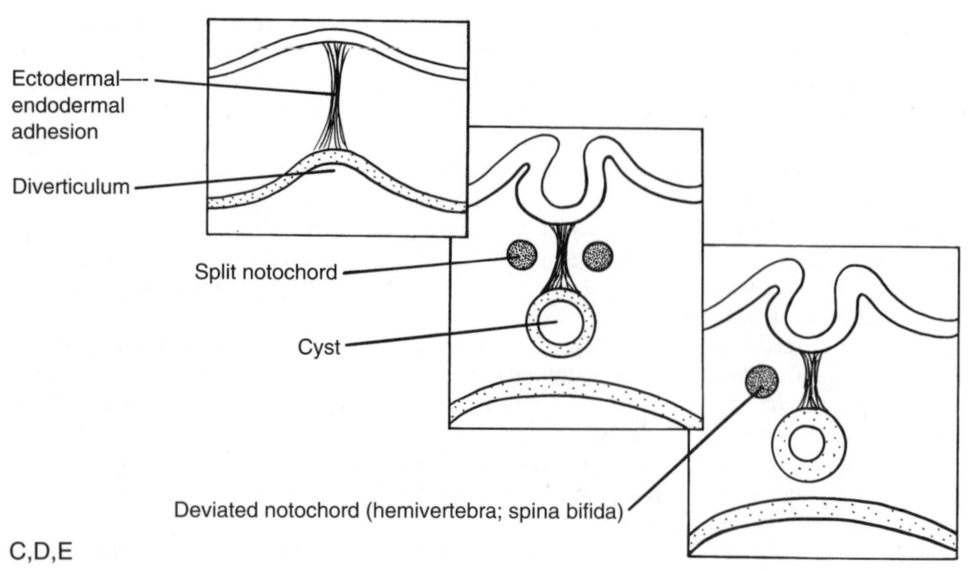

FIG. 60-5. Development of the split notochord syndrome. (*A* and *B*) The normal process of enclosure of the spinal cord and notochord by the paraxial mesodermal cell mass to form the vertebral body. (*C* through *E*) In the cephalic end of the embryo, the ectoderm and endoderm are in close proximity. Adhesions between the two can interfere with the cephalad growth of the notochord. A split notochord can result in the development of spina bifida, and deviation of the notochord can result in hemivertebra formation. (After Beardmore HE, Wiglesworth FW. Vertebral anomalies and alimentary duplications. Pediatr Clin North Am 1958;5:457)

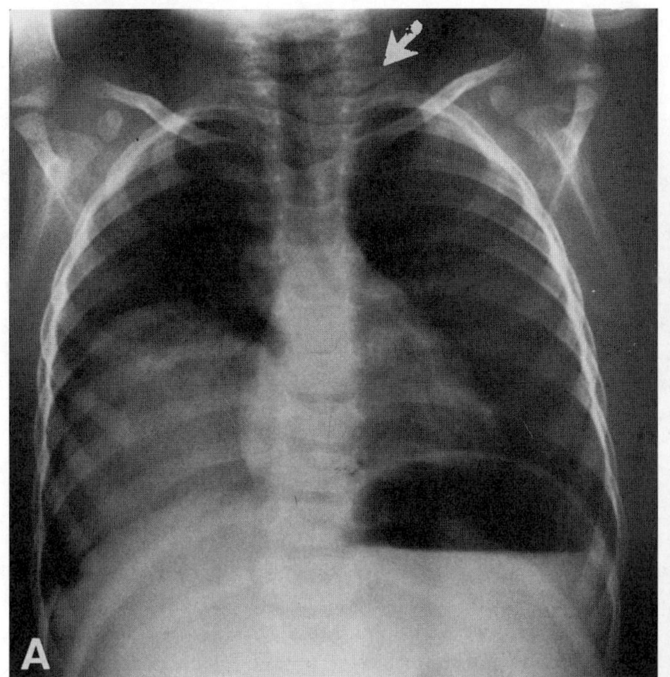

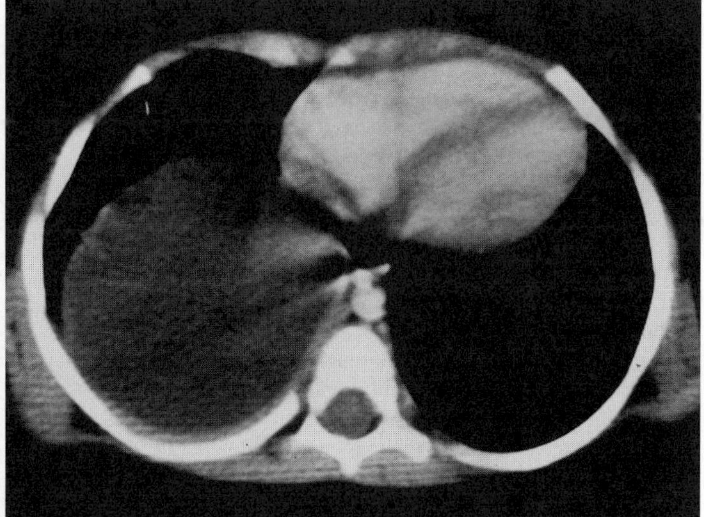

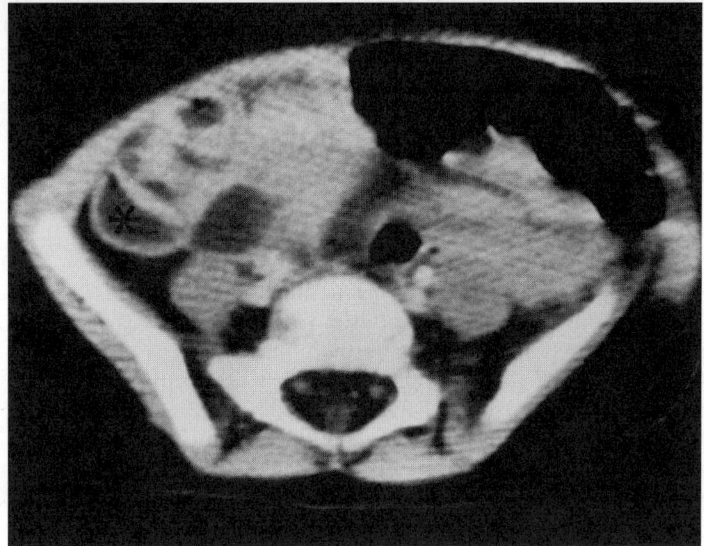

FIG. 60-6. (*A*) Frontal chest radiograph of a 3-year-old girl with symptoms of dyspnea and cough. A well-circumscribed mass is evident projecting into the right hemithorax. A hemivertebra is noted at C-7 (*arrow*). (*B*) The chest CT scan demonstrates a well-circumscribed, homogeneous, posterior mediastinal mass extending into the right hemithorax. (*C*) The abdominal CT scan suggests the presence of a tubular duplication (***) in the right abdomen. Thoracotomy revealed an enteric cyst, separate from the wall of the true esophagus, but connected to the prevertebral fascia in the thoracic inlet by a fibrous cord. Subsequent laparotomy revealed a long tubular duplication of the proximal jejunum, which was treated by excising the mucosa and most of the muscular wall.

ENTERIC CYSTS

Enteric cysts of the mediastinum are uncommon anomalies and compose only 10% of all intestinal duplication cysts. The nomenclature used to characterize these cysts has been confusing and reflects uncertainty about their embryologic origin. Fallon and associates[61] suggested the designation of two classes of esophageal cysts: intramural esophageal cysts and enteric cysts. Intramural esophageal cysts occur within the wall of the esophagus and are thought to represent defects of vacuolation of the primitive esophagus. During the fourth week of development, the esophageal mucosa proliferates to obliterate the esophageal lumen completely. At 6 weeks' gestation, vacuoles begin to form within this solid mass of epithelial cells, gradually coalescing to reestablish an esophageal lumen. Disruptions of

this process presumably leave epithelial cells within the wall of the esophagus, which can lead to development of intramural esophageal cysts.[62] These cysts are lined by columnar or pseudostratified columnar epithelium with cilia, which is consistent with the foregut epithelium of a 4- to 6-week embryo. These lesions have also been referred to as *true duplications of the esophagus* and *archenteric cysts*, although the term *intramural esophageal cysts* seems most appropriate. The embryology of enteric cysts is more controversial, but most authors believe they are caused by abnormalities of separation of the endoderm from the notochord. It has been proposed that they represent a distortion of the cephalic portion of the notochord by adhesions between the endoderm and ectoderm, which are in close proximity in this region of the embryo.[63] Traction on these adhesions with growth of the embryo results in posterior displacement of rests of endoderm as well as deformity of the notochord, producing the so-called split notochord syndrome[64] (Fig. 60-5). Enteric cysts are characterized by their posterior location within the mediastinum and attachment to the anterior vertebral bodies. They contain well-developed muscular layers in the wall and a variety of embryonic epithelia.[62] Half of enteric cysts are associated with vertebral anomalies, usually spina bifida or hemivertebrae, reflecting the embryologic distortion of the notochord.[61] These cysts usually move caudally as the embryo grows and the intrathoracic viscera descend, and often the vertebral anomalies encountered are in the lower cervical spine.[63] A high percentage of these patients have an associated abdominal intestinal duplication cyst[64] (Fig. 60-6). Enteric cysts have a spectrum of anatomic presentation, ranging from isolated posterior mediastinal cysts to fistulas from the proximal gastrointestinal tract to the dorsal thoracic skin, passing through the vertebral column and spinal canal. Bajpai and Mathur[65] demonstrated intraspinal anomalies by myelography in three of four patients with enteric cysts and vertebral abnormalities.

One third of patients with esophageal cysts remain asymptomatic in childhood, and the cysts are not detected until adulthood. The remaining children present with symptoms of dysphagia or respiratory distress. Intramural esophageal cysts are more likely to present with symptoms of dysphagia because of their close proximity to the wall of the esophagus. Enteric cysts may present with dysphagia or respiratory distress, depending on the size of the cyst. Most esophageal cysts contain some gastric epithelium. Thus, ulceration with bleeding and rapid expansion of esophageal cysts has been described.[63,66,67] The diagnosis of an esophageal cyst is suspected by findings on frontal and lateral chest radiographs. Most of these lesions project into the right hemithorax, presumably as a result of changes occurring during intestinal rotation.[63,68] The presence of vertebral anomalies in the cervical or thoracic spine strongly suggests the diagnosis of an enteric cyst. Transthoracic sonography may be helpful in confirming the cystic nature of these lesions and in differentiating them from posterior mediastinal tumors.[69] A contrast esophagogram may demonstrate distortion of the esophagus, either by an intramural or enteric cyst. CT scanning may help in defining the relation of the cyst to surrounding structures and in evaluating for associated vertebral defects. Thoracic magnetic resonance imaging studies may provide all this information as well as detect intraspinal abnormalities.[67,70] Therefore, this is the preferred method of confirming the diagnosis. Esophagoscopy has little to offer in this evaluation because the esophageal mucosa is normal, even overlying the intramural esophageal cysts. Abdominal radiographic studies may be helpful in detecting an abdominal intestinal duplication, often associated with an enteric cyst.

Esophageal cysts found in children should be surgically excised. Patients who present with severe respiratory symptoms secondary to rapid expansion of a cyst may be temporarily relieved by decompression by transthoracic aspiration, although this is rarely necessary. An intramural esophageal cyst may be enucleated by division of the esophageal musculature overlying the cyst and careful dissection of the cyst from the esophageal wall. Usually, this can be accomplished without violation of the esophageal lumen. A patient with multiple intramural esophageal cysts has been described, and this possibility must be kept in mind when reviewing preoperative radiographs and while performing the surgical procedure.[71] An enteric cyst is totally

separate from the true esophageal wall but usually has a fibrous connection to the anterior vertebral body, which should be removed with the cyst. Often, this connection may pass cephalad, out of the thorax, to communicate with a lower cervical vertebra. Small esophageal cysts of either type are potentially resectable by thoracoscopic techniques, thus avoiding some of the morbidity of a formal thoracotomy. Although complications are rarely reported in children after resection of esophageal cysts, there can be a high incidence of gastroesophageal reflux in adults.[72] This suggests that careful follow-up of these patients is necessary.

ACHALASIA

Neuromuscular abnormalities of the esophagus present as a spectrum of disorders from diffuse esophageal spasm to vigorous achalasia and, finally, to achalasia. Achalasia of the esophagus is a motor disorder affecting virtually the entire length of the esophagus. The cause of achalasia is obscure. Histologic findings in the esophageal wall have been variable but often include degeneration of the ganglion cells in the myenteric plexus, chronic inflammatory changes of the inner circular muscle layer,[73] and a paucity of vasoactive intestinal polypeptide containing nerve fibers in the distal esophagus.[74] Studies have suggested that nitric oxide may have an important role in the relaxation of the lower esophageal sphincter muscle.[75]

Achalasia is relatively uncommon in the population at large

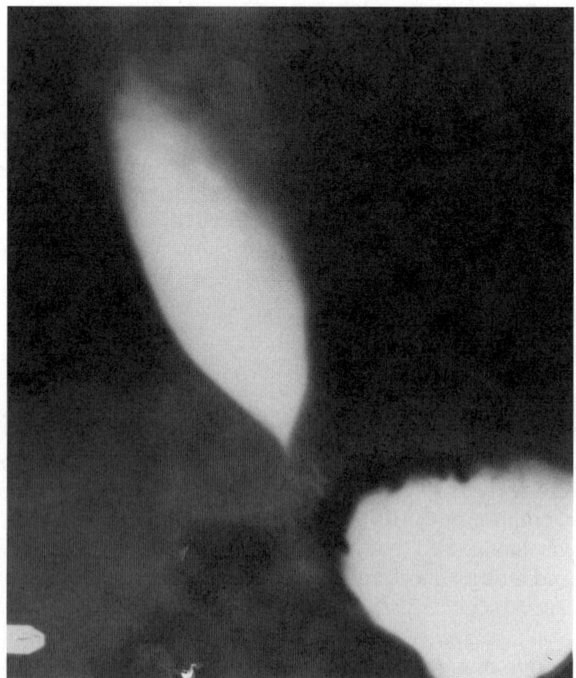

FIG. 60-7. Barium esophagogram obtained in a 3-month-old boy with esophageal achalasia. This study demonstrates marked dilation of the esophagus with a characteristic "bird's beak" at the esophagogastric junction. (Moazam F, Rodgers BM. Infantile achalasia: brief clinical report. J Thorac Cardiovasc Surg 1976;72:809)

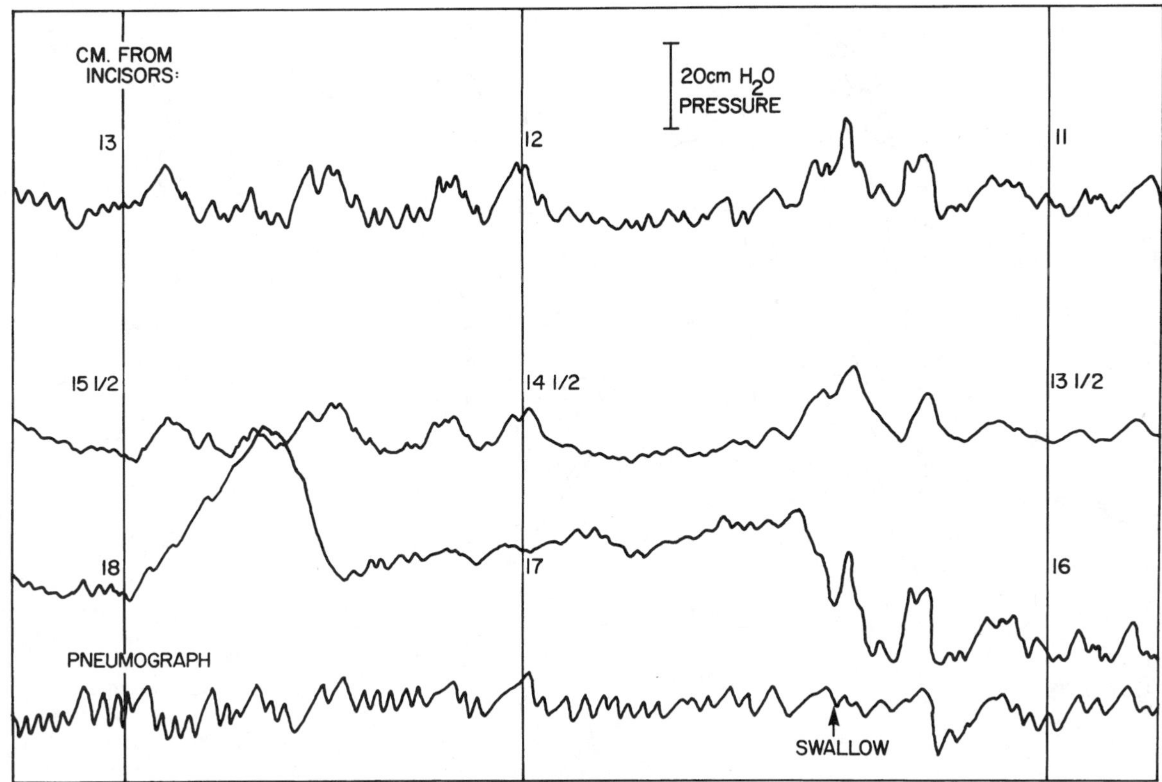

FIG. 60-8. Esophageal manometric tracing from a 3-month-old boy with esophageal achalasia. There is a high-pressure zone in the region of the lower esophageal sphincter extending from 18 cm to 16.5 cm from the incisors. There is poor esophageal contractility and lack of progression of esophageal peristalsis with swallowing. (Moazam F, Rodgers BM. Infantile achalasia: brief clinical report. J Thorac Cardiovasc Surg 1976;72:809)

and rare in childhood. Only about 4% of patients afflicted with achalasia present with symptoms before the age of 15 years.[76] Two thirds of children with achalasia are boys. Familial occurrence of esophageal achalasia has been reported in a small number of patients and appears to be inherited as an autosomal recessive trait.[77] Esophageal achalasia appears to be a component of a few genetic syndromes, including Sjögren syndrome and the so-called AAA syndrome, consisting of achalasia, adrenal insufficiency, and alacrima.

The symptoms of achalasia consist primarily of dysphagia and respiratory complaints. In very young children, respiratory symptoms often are predominant. A history of chronic cough, recurrent wheezing, and frequent pneumonia is common in these patients. The absence of a classic history of dysphagia in these children often delays the establishment of a diagnosis of achalasia. In older children, swallowing symptoms are more obvious, and regurgitation of undigested food, dysphagia, and weight loss are seen in most patients.[78] The diagnosis of esophageal achalasia may be suspected by an upright chest radiograph, which often demonstrates a widened mediastinum, with an air–fluid level in the posterior mediastinum. Barium esophagogram demonstrates dilation of the body of the esophagus with narrowing at the gastroesophageal junction in the form of a bird's beak (Fig. 60-7). Retained secretions within the esophageal lumen and poor peristaltic activity may be noted. The definitive diagnosis of achalasia, however, rests on manometric evaluation of the esophagus. Characteristically, there is an absence of coordinated peristaltic contractions in the body of the esophagus and failure of complete relaxation of the lower esophageal sphincter in response to swallowing. The resting sphincter pressure is elevated, and high-amplitude contractions may be noted sporadically within the body of the esophagus (Fig. 60-8).

The treatment of esophageal achalasia is controversial. The symptoms of dysphagia in some patients may respond to pharmacologic therapy using calcium-channel blocking agents such as nifedipine or verapamil. In a double-blind study of adults,[79] both agents reduced resting sphincter pressure, but only nifedipine reduced the amplitude of contractions in the body of the esophagus. Neither agent consistently resulted in significant clinical improvement. Similar findings have been reported in a small number of adolescents,[80] but there were no changes noted in the peristaltic activity in the body of the esophagus, and the relief of symptoms, when it occurred, was transient. Others have suggested that these agents be reserved for patients at high risk for surgery or to provide temporary relief of symptoms until definitive surgery can be performed.[81]

In adult patients, pneumatic dilation of the sphincter has been used to relieve esophageal obstruction and dysphagia.[82] Balloon dilation of the sphincter in pediatric patients has been less successful, however.[83] The incidence of postdilatation gastroesophageal reflux appears to be higher in children, and the procedure is technically more difficult in younger patients. For this reason, most children with esophageal achalasia require an esophagomyotomy for the long-term relief of symptoms. These

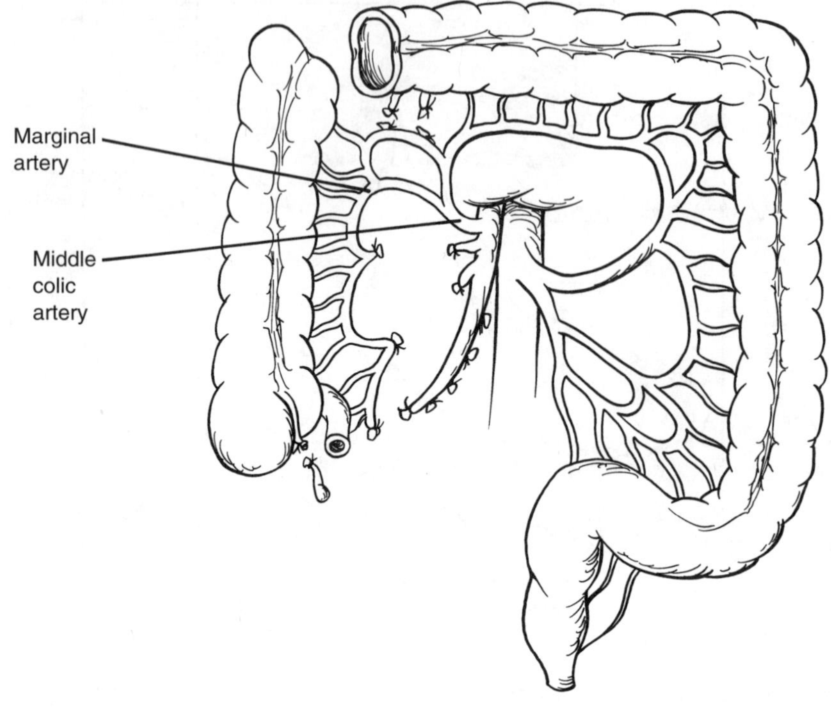

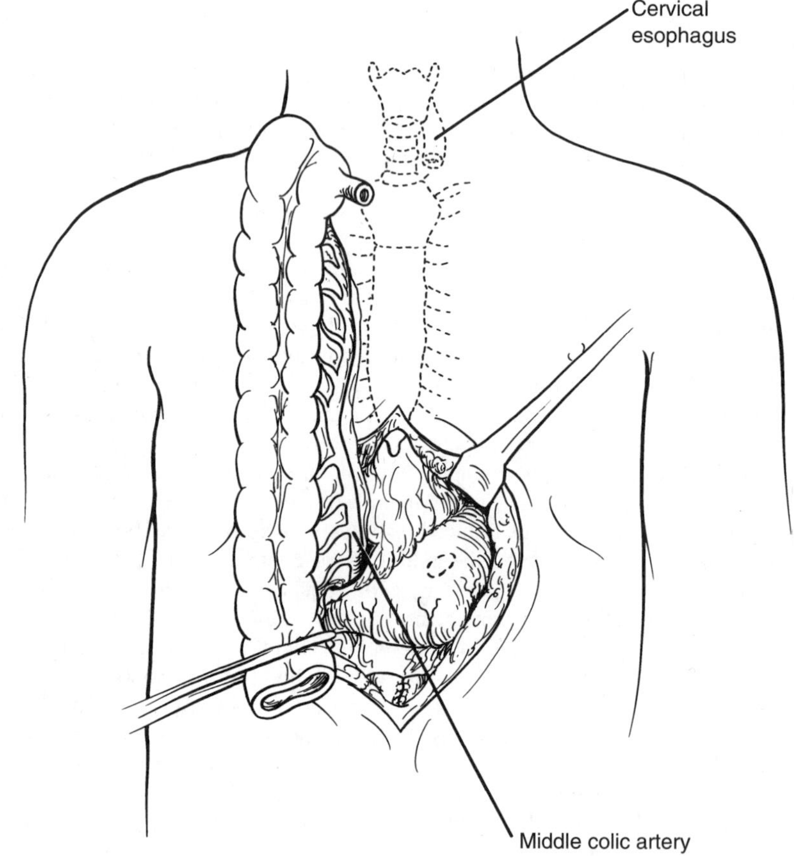

FIG. 60-9. Esophageal replacement using a right colon interposition in a retrosternal position. *(continued)*

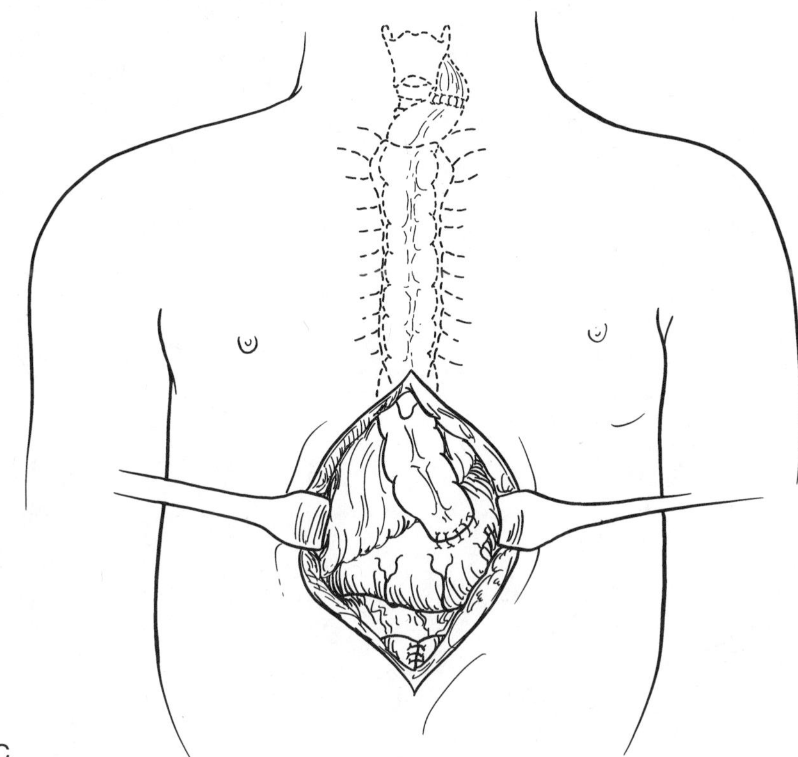

C

FIG. 60-9. *(continued)*

patients may have considerable retained secretions in the esophagus and should have overnight decompression of the esophagus before the induction of general anesthesia to minimize the risk of aspiration. The myotomy should extend less than 1 cm onto the gastric wall in children to reduce the incidence of postoperative gastroesophageal reflux.[84] A similar esophageal myotomy can be performed using thoracoscopic techniques.[85] Nonetheless, about 20% of children have symptomatic gastroesophageal reflux after simple myotomy, and many surgeons routinely recommend the addition of an antireflux procedure to the operation. Because of the poor esophageal motility in patients with esophageal achalasia, a complete fundic wrap should be avoided. A partial wrap or a very loose circumferential wrap is preferable in these patients.[86] Successful relief of symptoms appears to be possible in 90% to 95% of children using these surgical principles.[76,78,83] Deterioration of the initial excellent clinical results can occur 15 to 20 years after esophagomyotomy.[87] Achalasia is also recognized as a predisposing factor for the development of esophageal cancer.[88] These children, therefore, should have close long-term follow-up.

Although classic esophageal achalasia principally involves the lower esophageal sphincter, primary cricopharyngeal achalasia occasionally is encountered in children.[89] In this disorder, there is a persistent high-pressure zone in the region of the cricopharyngeus muscle, although the associated motor disorders of the body of the esophagus, as seen in classic achalasia, are less common. These patients exhibit symptoms of intermittent cervical dysphagia, primarily manifested by choking and coughing with attempts at swallowing. Occasionally, these children complain of pain in the neck during these intervals. Definitive diagnosis of cricopharyngeal achalasia is difficult because manometric studies of the proximal esophageal sphincter are difficult to perform. Lateral projections of the barium esophagogram may show thickening of the cricopharyngeus muscle posteriorly. Many patients with cricopharyngeal achalasia respond to forceful dilation of the upper esophageal sphincter under general anesthesia. This appears to be successful enough to warrant its use for initial therapy. If dilation fails to provide prolonged symptomatic relief, a cricopharyngeal myotomy may be performed and usually has excellent long-term results.

ESOPHAGEAL REPLACEMENT

Contemporary management of pediatric esophageal lesions has substantially diminished the need for esophageal replacement surgery. However, a variety of complex and refractory problems still necessitate this procedure for occasional infants and children. The major indications for esophageal replacement include the following:

1. Esophageal atresia, particularly long-gap esophageal atresia without a tracheoesophageal fistula. Although many of these children can undergo primary esophagoesophagostomy, this remains a difficult lesion, and esophageal replacement is sometimes necessary as a secondary approach.
2. Complex gastroesophageal reflux, usually when associated with a refractory esophageal stricture. Contemporary medical therapy with histamine-2–receptor antagonists, proton-pump inhibitors, prokinetic agents, and antacids, combined with the aggressive use of surgical antireflux procedures, has nearly eliminated these patients from the group who still require esophageal replacement.
3. Complex corrosive injury with esophageal stricture or dysfunction. Despite legislated safety standards for a variety

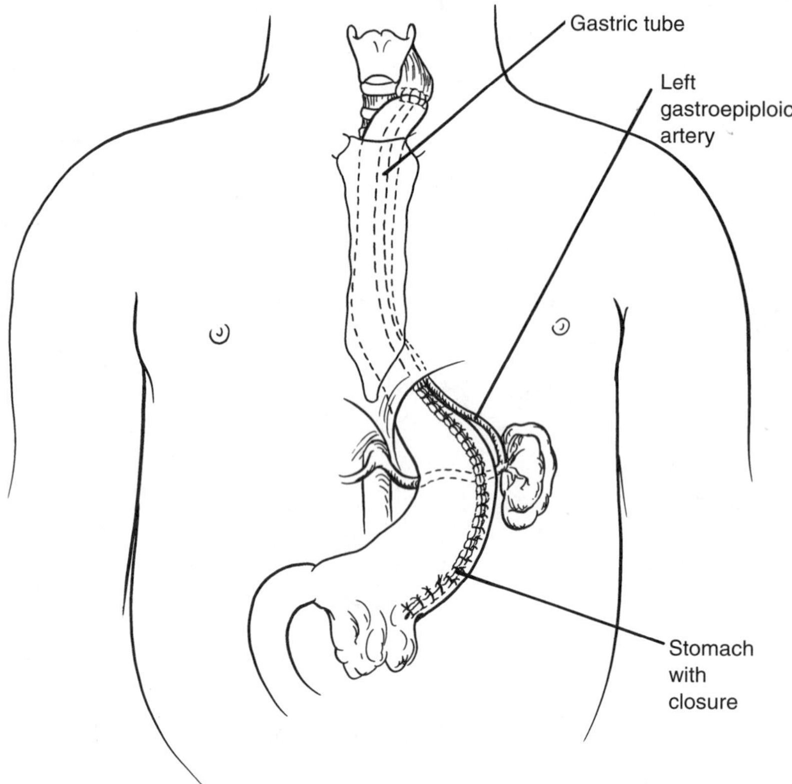

FIG. 60-10. The reverse gastric tube esophageal substitute.

of household products and their containers, children continue to be victims of accidental corrosive injury. Therapy is nonspecific and may be ineffective. This remains an uncommon but persistent indication for esophageal replacement.

4. A variety of inflammatory and infectious conditions, perhaps most notably, candidal esophagitis. This group includes patients with a variety of underlying conditions, and it may be the one population under discussion that is increasing in size. Immunosuppressed oncology patients, transplant recipients, and other similar patients are at particular risk for acquired opportunistic infections and inflammatory conditions that may be refractory and result in esophageal injury.

5. Patients with other rare esophageal conditions, including perforation, trauma, complex foreign bodies, operative complications, tumors, congenital esophageal stenosis, and achalasia, have periodic need for esophageal substitution. Esophageal varices are essentially removed from this inventory because of the effectiveness of alternative sclerotherapy and shunting strategies.

The selection of a particular form of esophageal replacement remains a controversial subject for which the surgeon's personal experience and preference are of great importance. Several anatomic reconstructions provide roughly equivalent outcomes. All are less perfect than the native esophagus. The goals to which all substitutes aspire include the following principles:

1. The conduit should bridge the defect through a course that is short and straight and that encourages dependent drainage, because none of the conduits empty effectively by active peristalsis.

2. As much native esophagus as possible should be preserved, particularly the cricopharyngeus and lower esophageal sphincter regions.

3. Gastric acid reflux should be minimized, possibly with an antireflux procedure.

4. Because all the options are complex, and technical complications are therefore relatively common, simplicity is desirable.

Alternatives include the staged construction of a skin tube, usually in an antethoracic position. These are generally of limited interest because this approach has been replaced by better conduits. The colon has been used most extensively for esophageal replacement.[90–94] Virtually all anatomic arrangements have been advocated: the right colon with a middle colic artery vascular pedicle (Fig. 60-9), the left colon based on the left colic artery, the transverse colon, and the right colon with the ileocecal valve preserved to minimize acid reflux. All are roughly equivalent in terms of technical difficulty and outcome.

The conduit is generally placed in either an anterior (retrosternal) or posterior (left retrohilar) mediastinal position. The retrosternal position is technically simpler, but the course of the conduit compromises the principles of short, straight, and dependent drainage. Although the retrohilar position is better with regard to these concerns, it is more complex technically and requires a thoracotomy in addition to the cervical and abdominal incisions. Operative mortality is rare. Morbidity is common. Short-term morbidity is often related to technical complications, most commonly ischemia. This may result in a cervical anastomotic leak in up to 30% of patients. Anastomotic strictures and infarction of the entire conduit are also well described. Long-term problems are related principally to acid reflux, pulmonary dysfunction, and the development of functional emptying problems. As indicated, the collective worldwide experience is greatest with colon substitutes, and despite periodic enthusiasm for the alternatives, none has been proved superior to colon interposition.

The small bowel has also been used as an esophageal conduit, both as a pedicle-based interposition and as a free graft with vascular supply provided by microsurgical techniques.[95,96] The pedicle graft has more technical problems than the colon substitute, without clear advantage. The free graft may be of substantial utility for relatively short segment esophageal replacement, particularly in the cervical and upper thoracic esophagus.

The stomach may be used for esophageal replacement, either as a reverse gastric tube interposition or by transposition of the whole organ into the thorax. These two approaches have been the subject of considerable attention. The gastric pull-up has been advocated in children because of the large and favorable palliative experience with adults who have esophageal carcinoma. Noteworthy success has been reported in children.[97] Concerns remain about acid reflux and pulmonary dysfunction, particularly in smaller children, in whom the volume of the postprandial stomach in the thorax may substantially restrict ventilation. The reverse gastric tube is a viable approach that reduces this particular problem, but this has generally similar complication rates and long-term results to other techniques[98,99] (Fig. 60-10). A variety of synthetic esophageal conduits have been designed for experimental use, but none has achieved clinical use.

The outcomes for these complex procedures are difficult to compare objectively because of their relative infrequency and their many variations. Most children can have a functional esophageal conduit constructed if necessary. Both technical and functional complications are common, but operative mortality is rare. No substitute approaches ideal native esophageal function.

REFERENCES

1. Sutliff KS, Hutchins GM. Septation of the respiratory and digestive tracts in human embryos: crucial role of the tracheoesophageal sulcus. Anat Rec 1994;238:237.
2. DeNardi FG, Riddell RH. The normal esophagus. Am J Surg Pathol 1991;15:296.
3. Johns BAE. Developmental changes in the oesophageal epithelium in man. J Anat 1952;86:431.
4. Grand RJ, Watkins JB, Torti FM. Development of the human gastrointestinal tract: a review. Gastroenterol 1976;70:790.
5. Hitchcock RJ, Pemble MJ, Bishop AE, et al. Quantitative study of the development and maturation of human oesophageal innervation. J Anat 1992;180:175.
6. Sherman DJ, Ross MG, Day L, et al. Fetal swallowing: correlation of electromyography and esophageal fluid flow. Am J Physiol 1990;258:R1386.
7. Bombeck CT, Dillard DH, Nyhus LM. Muscular anatomy of the gastroesophageal junction and the role of phrenoesophageal ligament: autopsy study of sphincter mechanism. Ann Surg 1966;164:643.
8. Fuino Y, Agnew CL, Schreyer P, et al. Amniotic fluid volume response to esophageal occlusion in fetal sheep. Am J Obstet Gynecol 1991;165:1620.
9. Goldstein JL, Schlesinger PK, Mozwecz HL, et al. Esophageal mucosal resistance. Gastroenterol Clin North Am 1990;19:565.
10. Kutchai HC. Gastrointestinal motility. In: Berne RM, Levy MN, eds. Physiology, ed 3. St Louis, Mosby Year Book, 1993:38.
11. Strobel CT, Byrne WJ, Ament ME, et al. Correlation of esophageal length in children with height: application to the Tuttle test without prior esophageal manometry. J Pediatr 1979;94:81.
12. Welch RW, Luckmann K, Ricks PM, et al. Manometry of the normal esophageal sphincter and its alteration in laryngectomy. J Clin Invest 1979;63:1036.
13. Behar J, Field S, Marin C. Effect of glucagon, secretin and vasoactive intestinal peptide on the feline lower esophageal sphincter: mechanisms of action. Gastroenterol 1977;77:1001.
14. Cohen S, Lipshutz W. Hormonal regulation of human esophageal sphincter competence: interaction of gastrin and secretin. J Clin Invest 1971;50:449.
15. Ament ME, Christie DL. Upper gastrointestinal fiberoptic endoscopy in pediatric patients. Gastroenterology 1977;72:1244.
16. Gans SL. Pediatric endoscopy, ed 9. New York, Grune and Stratton, 1983:55.
17. Stiegmann GV. Techniques for endoscopic obliteration of esophageal varices. Surg Ann 1991;23:175.
18. Pasricha PJ, Fleischer DE, Kalloo AN. Endoscopic perforations of the upper digestive tract: a review of their pathogenesis, prevention and management. Gastroenterology 1994;106:787.
19. Katz D. Morbidity and mortality in standard and flexible gastrointestinal endoscopy. Gastrointest Endosc 1967;14:134.
20. Panzini L, Burrell MI, Traube M. Instrumental esophageal perforation. Am J Gastroenterol 1994;89:367.
21. Cameron JL, Kieffer RF, Hendruf TF, et al. Selective non-operative management of contained intra-thoracic esophageal perforations. Ann Thorac Surg 1979;27:404.
22. Michell, Grillo HC, Malt RA. Operative and non-operative management of esophageal perforations. Ann Surg 1981;94:57.
23. Lyons MF, Tsuchida AM. Foreign bodies of the gastrointestinal tract. Med Clin North Am 1993;77:1101.
24. Binder L, Anderson WA. Pediatric gastrointestinal foreign body ingestions. Ann Emerg Med 1984;13:112.
25. Litovitz T, Schmitz BF. Ingestion of cylindrical and button batteries: an analysis of 2382 cases. Pediatrics 1992;89:747.
26. Nandi P, Ong GB. Foreign body in the oesophagus: review of 2394 cases. Br J Surg 1978;65:5.
27. Paul RI, Christoffel K, Binns HJ, et al. Foreign body ingestions in children: risk of complication varies with site of initial health care contact. Pediatrics 1993;91:121.
28. Crysdale WS. Esophageal foreign bodies in children: 15-year review of 484 cases. Ann Otol Rhinol Laryngol 1991;100:320.
29. Burton DM, Stith JA. Extraluminal esophageal coin erosion in children: case report and review. Int J Pediatr Otol 1992;23:187.
30. Conners GP, Chamberlin JM, Ochsenschlager DW. Symptoms and spontaneous passage of esophageal coins. Arch Pediatr Adolesc Med 1995;149:36.
31. Robbins MI, Shortsleeve MJ. Treatment of acute esophageal food impaction with glucagon, an effervescent agent, and water. AJR 1994;162:325.
32. Webb WA. Management of foreign bodies of the upper gastrointestinal tract. Gastroenterology 1988;94:204.
33. Kelley JE, Leech MH, Carr MG. A safe and cost-effective protocol for the management of esophageal coins in children. J Pediatr Surg 1993;28:898.
34. Schunk JE, Harrison AM, Corneli HM, et al. Fluoroscopic Foley catheter removal of esophageal foreign bodies in children: experience with 415 episodes. Pediatrics 1994;94:709.
35. Walton WW. An evaluation of the poison prevention packaging act. Pediatrics 1982;69:363.
36. Anderson KD, Rouse TM, Randolph JG. A controlled trial of corticosteroids in children with corrosive injury of the esophagus. N Engl J Med 1990;323:637.
37. Scott JC, Jones B, Eisele DW, et al. Caustic ingestion injuries of the upper aerodigestive tract. Laryngoscope 1992;102:1.
38. Vergauwen P, Moulin D, Buts JP, et al. Caustic burns of the upper digestive and respiratory tracts. Eur J Pediatr 1991;150:700.
39. Gaudreault P, Parent M, McGuigan MA, et al. Predictability of esophageal injury from signs and symptoms: a study of caustic ingestion in 378 children. Pediatrics 1983;71:767.
40. Gorman RL, Khin-Maung-Gyi MT, Klein-Schwartz W, et al. Initial symptoms as predictors of esophageal injury in alkaline corrosive ingestions. Am J Emerg Med 1992;10:189.

41. Haller JA, Andrews HG, White JJ, et al. Pathophysiology and management of acute corrosive burns of the esophagus: results of treatment in 285 children. J Pediatr Surg 1971;6:578.

42. Costanzo JD, Noirclerc M, Jouglard J, et al. New therapeutic approach to corrosive burns of the upper gastrointestinal tract. Gut 1980;21:370.

43. deGoyet J, Moulin D, Otte JD. Indications for and means of surgical treatment of corrosive esophagitis in children. In: Follis JC, Filler RM, Lemoine G, eds. Pediatric thoracic surgery. New York, Elsevier Science Publishing, 1991.

44. Holder TM, Ashcraft KW, Leape L. The treatment of patients with esophageal strictures by local steroid injections. J Pediatr Surg 1969;4:646.

45. Hopkins RA, Postlethwait RW. Caustic burns and carcinoma of the esophagus. Ann Surg 1981;194:146.

46. Margarit J, Castanön M, Ribó JM, et al. Congenital esophageal stenosis associated with tracheoesophageal fistula. Pediatr Surg Int 1994;9:577.

47. Yeung CK, Spitz L, Brereton RJ, et al. Congenital esophageal stenosis due to tracheobronchial remnants: a rare but important association with esophageal atresia. J Pediatr Surg 1992;27:852.

48. Bremner CG. Benign strictures of the esophagus. Curr Prob Surg 1992;19:401.

49. Goldthorn JF, Ball WS, Wilkinson LG, et al. Esophageal strictures in children: treatment by serial balloon catheter dilatation. Radiology 1984;153:655.

50. Lindor KD, Ott BJ, Hughes RW. Balloon dilatation of upper digestive tract strictures. Gastroenterology 1985;89:545.

51. Hassall E. Barrett's esophagus: congenital or acquired? Am J Gastroenterol 1993;88:819.

52. Snyder JD, Goldman H. Barrett's esophagus in children and young adults. Dig Dis 1190;35:1185.

53. Hassall E, Weinstein WM, Ament ME. Barrett's esophagus in childhood. Gastroenterology 1985;89:1331.

54. Hassall E. Barrett's esophagus: new definitions and approaches in children. J Pediatr Gastroenterol Nutr 1993;16:345.

55. Othersen HB, Ocampo RJ, Parker EF, et al. Barrett's esophagus in children. Ann Surg 1993;217:676.

56. Lindahi H, Rintala R, Sariola H, et al. Cervical Barrett's esophagus: a common complication of gastric tube reconstruction. J Pediatr Surg 1990;25:446.

57. Stein HJ, Hoeft S, DeMeester TR. Functional foregut abnormalities in Barrett's esophagus. J Thorac Cardiovasc Surg 1993;105:107.

58. Cheu HW, Grosfeld Jl, Heifetz SA, et al. Persistence of Barrett's esophagus in children after antireflux surgery: influence on followup care. J Pediatr Surg 1992;27:260.

59. Hassall E, Dimmick JE, Magee JF. Adenocarcinoma in childhood Barrett's esophagus: case documentation and the need for surveillance in children. Am J Gastroenterol 1993;88:281.

60. Younes M, Lebovitz RM, Lechago LV, et al. p53 Protein accumulation in Barrett's metaplasia, dysplasia, and carcinoma: a followup study. Gastroenterology 1993;105:1637.

61. Fallon M, Gordon ARG, Lendrum AC. Mediastinal cysts of foregut origin associated with vertebral abnormalities. Br J Surg 1954;41:520.

62. Kirwan WO, Walbaum PR, McCormack RJM. Cystic intrathoracic derivatives of the foregut and their complications. Thorax 1973;28:424.

63. Beardmore HE, Wiglesworth FW. Vertebral anomalies and alimentary duplications. Pediatr Clin North Am 1958;5:457.

64. Bentley JFR, Smith JR. Developmental posterior enteric remnants and spinal malformations. Arch Dis Child 1960;35:76.

65. Bajpai M, Mathur M. Duplications of the alimentary tract: clues to the missing links. J Pediatr Surg 1994;29:1361.

66. Ladd WE, Scott HW. Esophageal duplications or mediastinal cysts of enteric origin. Surgery 1944;16:815.

67. Ruffin WK, Hansen DE. An esophageal duplication cyst presenting as an abdominal mass. Am J Gastroenterol 1989;84:571.

68. Pokorny WJ, Goldstein R. Enteric thoracoabdominal duplications in children. Thorac Cardiovasc Surg 1984;878:821.

69. Fitch SJ, Tonkin ILD, Tonkin AK. Imaging of foregut duplication cysts. Radiographics 1986;6:189.

70. Lupetin AR, Dash N. MRI appearance of esophageal duplication cyst. Gastrointest Radiol 1987;12:7.

71. Robison RJ, Pavlina PM, Scherer LR, et al. Brief communications. J Thorac Cardiovasc Surg 1987;94:144.

72. Salo JA, Ala-Kulju KV. Congenital esophageal cysts in adults. Ann Thorac Surg 1987;44:135.

73. Csendes A, Smok G, Braghetto I, et al. Histological studies of Auerbach's plexuses of the oesophagus, stomach, jejunum, and colon in patients with achalasia of the oesophagus: correlation with gastric acid secretion, presence of parietal cells and gastric emptying of solids. Gut 1992;33:150.

74. Aggestrup S, Uddman R, Sundler F, et al. Lack of vasoactive intestinal polypeptide nerves in esophageal achalasia. Gastroenterology 1983;84:924.

75. Murray J, Du C, Ledlow A, et al. Nitric oxide: mediator of nonadrenergic noncholinergic responses of opossum esophageal muscle. Am J Physiol 1991;6:G401.

76. Nichoul-Fékété C, Bawah F, Lortat-Jacob S, et al. Achalasia of the esophagus in childhood: surgical treatment in 35 cases with special reference to familial cases and glucocorticoid deficiency association. Hepatogastroenterology 1991;38:510.

77. Monnig PJ. Familial achalasia in children. Ann Thorac Surg 1990;49:1019.

78. Myers NA, Jolley SG, Taylor R. Achalasia of the cardia in children: a worldwide survey. J Pediatr Surg 1994;29:1375.

79. Triadafilopoulos G, Aaronson M, Sackel S, et al. Medical treatment of esophageal achalasia: double-blind crossover study of oral nifedipine, verapamil, and placebo. Dig Dis Sci 1991;36:260.

80. Maksimak M, Perlmutter DH, Winter HS. The use of nifedipine for the treatment of achalasia in children. J Pediatr Gastroenterol Nutr 1986;5:883.

81. Short TP, Thomas E. An overview of the role of calcium antagonists in the treatment of achalasia and diffuse oesophageal spasm. Drugs 1992;43:177.

82. Tack J, Janssens J, Vantrappen G. Non-surgical treatment of achalasia. Hepatogastroenterology 1991;38:498.

83. Emblem R, Stringer MD, Hall CM, et al. Current results of surgery for achalasia of the cardia. Arch Dis Childhood 1993;68:749.

84. Ellis FH. Esophagomyotomy by the thoracic approach for esophageal achalasia. Hepatogastroenterology 1991;38:498.

85. Pellegrini CA, Leichter R, Patti M, et al. Thoracoscopic esophageal myotomy in the treatment of achalasia. Ann Thorac Surg 1993;56:680.

86. Allen KB, Ricketts RR. Surgery for achalasia of the cardia in children: the Dor-Gavriliu procedure. J Pediatr Surg 1992;27:1418.

87. Malthaner RA, Todd TR, Miller L, et al. Long-term results in surgically managed esophageal achalasia. Ann Thorac Surg 1994;58:1343.

88. Meijssen MAC, Tilanus HW, Van Blankenstein M, et al. Achalasia complicated by oesophageal squamous cell carcinoma: a prospective study in 195 patients. Gut 1992;33:155.

89. Skinner MA, Shorter NA. Primary neonatal cricopharyngeal achalasia: a case report and review of the literature. J Pediatr Surg 1992;27:1509.

90. Gross RE, Firestone FN. Colonic reconstruction of the esophagus in infants and children. Surgery 1967;61:955.

91. German JC, Waterston DJ. Colon interposition for the replacement of the esophagus in children. J Pediatr Surg 1976;11:227.

92. Freeman NW, Cass DT. Colon interposition: a modification of the Waterston technique using the normal esophageal route. J Pediatr Surg 1982;17:17.

93. Kelly JP, Shackelford GD, Roberts CL. Esophageal replacement with colon in children: functional results and long-term growth. Ann Thorac Surg 1983;36:634.

94. Campbell JR, Webber BR, Harrison MW, et al. Esophageal replacement in infants and children by colon interposition. Am J Surg 1982:144:29.

95. Saeki M, Tsuchida Y, Ogata T, et al. Long-term results of jejunal replacement of the esophagus. J Pediatr Surg 1988;23:483.

96. Coleman JJ, Tan KC, Searles JM, et al. Jejunal free autograft: analysis of complications and their resolution. Plast Reconstr Surg 1989;84:589.

97. Spitz L, Kiely E, Sparnon T. Gastric transposition for esophageal replacement in children. Ann Surg 1987;206:69.

98. Cohen DH, Middletown AW, Fletcher J. Gastric tube esophagoplasty. J Pediatr Surg 1974;9:451.

99. Anderson KD, Randolph JG. The gastric tube for esophageal replacement in infants and children. J Thorac Cardiovasc Surg 1973;66:33.

Surgery of Infants and Children: Scientific Principles and Practice, edited by
Keith T. Oldham, Paul M. Colombani, and Robert P. Foglia.
Lippincott–Raven Publishers, Philadelphia, © 1997.

CHAPTER 61

Esophageal Atresia and Tracheoesophageal Fistula

Spencer W. Beasley

Esophageal atresia is a congenital abnormality in which the mid-portion of the esophagus is absent. Its estimated live birth incidence is 1 in 3570[1] to 1 in 4500.[2] Most patients have an additional abnormal communication between the trachea and lower esophageal segment called a *distal tracheoesophageal fistula*. The remainder of patients have either no fistula or a fistula between the trachea and upper esophageal segments. A history of maternal polyhydramnios and prematurity is common. More than half of patients with esophageal atresia have other major congenital anomalies, of which congenital heart disease, urinary tract abnormalities, and gastrointestinal tract abnormalities are the most common. Esophageal atresia and tracheoesophageal fistula are correctable surgically, with generally good results. The diagnosis should be suspected in any newborn infant who appears to have excessive mucus or saliva at birth, with or without respiratory distress.

EMBRYOLOGY

Abnormal Development of the Esophagus

The esophagus develops from the primitive foregut immediately distal to the pharynx. Fusion of the caudal ends of the laryngotracheal grooves, which develop on either side of the proximal part of the esophagus during the fourth week of gestation, separates the laryngotracheal tube from the esophagus. It is likely that the insult that causes esophageal atresia occurs before 32 days' gestation.

Theories of Embryogenesis

The morphologic changes that occur during embryogenesis have been well described, but their interpretation and causes are poorly understood[3] (Table 61-1). The following summarizes the main theories of embryogenesis in esophageal atresia.

Intraembryonic Pressure

Some workers have suggested that esophageal atresia may result from excessive intraembryonic pressure, due to an enlarged embryonic heart, abnormal vessels, the pneumatoenteric recesses, or embryonic hyperflexion. During the critical phase of development, however, it is difficult to see how the embryo could be rigid enough to exert sufficient pressure on any one part to prevent its development.

Epithelial Occlusion

The epithelial occlusion theory proposes that esophageal atresia results from failure of recanalization after physiologic occlusion of the esophageal lumen. This explanation has been discounted because esophageal atresia has been observed in embryos well before the period when physiologic narrowing occurs. Total occlusion of the esophageal lumen has never been reported.

Vascular Accident

The theory that esophageal atresia is caused by an in utero disturbance of the regional microcirculation has little support. In segmental bowel atresia, it is a relatively late occurrence, whereas in esophageal atresia, it would have to occur much earlier, at a time when it is hard to imagine that there could be areas of hypoxia. Moreover, it is unlikely that this mechanism would produce a tracheoesophageal fistula.

Differential Growth

Theories proposing that esophageal atresia is the result of abnormalities of differential growth rate are in vogue (Fig. 61-1). Concepts of dysfunction of active cellular proliferation include faulty development of the tracheoesophageal septum,

TABLE 61-1. *Theories of embryogenesis of esophageal atresia*

INTRAEMBRYONIC PRESSURE
Pressure from an enlarged embyonic heart
Pressure from abnormal vessels
Pressure by the pneumatoenteric recesses
Embyonic hyperflexion

EPITHELIAL OCCULUSION

VASCULAR ACCIDENT

ABNORMALITIES OF DIFFERENTIAL GROWTH RATES
Faulty development of tracheoesophageal septum
Overgrowth of lateral esophageal ridges
Ventral displacement of the dorsal fold of foregut
Disturbance of the mesenchymal control of differentiation

overgrowth of the lateral esophageal ridges, ventral displacement of the dorsal fold of the foregut, and disturbance of the mesenchymal control of differentiation. These various models probably represent different interpretations of the same process and are not necessarily mutually exclusive. The exact mechanism of deformity remains uncertain.

Unifying Concept

It appears that some (as yet unrecognized) factor alters the rate and timing of cell proliferation and differentiation in the region of the esophagus and developing lung bud before 34 days' gestation. Proliferative cellular activity of the ventral side of the foregut at the beginning of the third week is followed immediately by a rapid increase in the length of both the esophagus and trachea. Failure of esophageal growth to keep pace during this period produces a prominent dorsal fold or posterior deviation of the lateral esophageal groove. This latter occurrence would explain the tracheoesophageal fistula as well as tracheal remnants within the fistula.

ANATOMIC AND PHYSIOLOGIC CONSIDERATIONS

Anatomic Variations

Esophageal atresia with a distal tracheoesophageal fistula is by far the most common type of abnormality (Fig. 61-2). The length of the upper esophageal segment is variable but usually reaches within 1 cm of the level of the arch of the azygos vein. The length of the upper esophagus can be estimated preoperatively by the length of tube that can be introduced through the mouth into the esophagus, or by air in the esophagus on plain radiography; at operation, this length can be estimated when the anesthetist introduces a stiff catheter into the esophagus. The lower esophageal segment commences from the posterior wall of the trachea, usually just proximal to the carina. The level of the tracheoesophageal fistula can be assessed by identifying the carinal air shadow, knowing that the distal esophagus extends at least that far superiorly into the mediastinum. Al-

though the upper esophageal segment is relatively thick walled as a result of hypertrophy from obstruction in utero, the lower segment has a smaller caliber. At thoracotomy, however, the lower segment may be seen to expand with air during assisted ventilation. Vagal fibers coursing over its surface assist in its identification at operation.

The most important varieties of esophageal atresia and tracheoesophageal fistula are summarized in Figure 61-2. Various systems of classification have been used, of which the Vogt[4] (1929) and Gross[5] (1953) systems have been the most popular. Confusion with other classifications and difficulties in their application to unusual variants have gradually lead to their abandonment in favor of descriptive terms.

Surgical Approach

The approach employed for any thoracotomy in a neonate is determined by the need for good exposure and the effect the incision will have on subsequent growth and function of the chest wall. An intercostal approach offers little morbidity and satisfactory exposure.

Rib resection is not employed, and the posterior fibers of serratus anterior are either retracted anteriorly or divided low at their origin off the chest wall to preserve their innervation.

Many years ago, multiple thoracotomies were performed deliberately as part of staged repairs and in the management of major esophageal complications. It is now evident that multiple thoracotomies increase the likelihood and severity of anterior chest wall deformity, scoliosis, decreased total lung capacity, and decreased vital capacity. In part, this may be a consequence of the reasons for which multiple thoracotomies were performed, such as anastomotic dehiscence or empyema.[6] Improvements in neonatal care and surgical technique have meant that staged procedures for repair of esophageal atresia are now performed rarely.

Vascular Supply of the Esophagus and Its Influence on Esophageal Mobilization

The cervical portion of the esophagus is supplied by the inferior thyroid artery, which gives off esophageal branches. These branches run vertically downward to the level of the arch of the aorta, where they anastomose with esophageal branches that come directly from the aorta and bronchial arteries (Fig. 61-3). The remainder of the thoracic esophagus, particularly that part below the tracheal bifurcation, is supplied by segmental branches from the aorta, but these are of relatively small caliber. They form anastomoses with adjacent vessels, including branches from the intercostal arteries. The distal esophagus is supplied by the ascending branch of the left gastric artery, with some assistance from branches of the inferior phrenic artery. In esophageal atresia, the blood supply to the esophagus is believed to follow the same pattern.[7]

The surgical significance of the vascular supply of the esophagus is that the cervical and abdominal portions are supplied by vessels that run along the esophagus, whereas the thoracic portion is supplied segmentally, and has the most tenuous connections. There is a risk that excessive mobilization of the thoracic esophagus may render it ischemic. In esophageal atresia

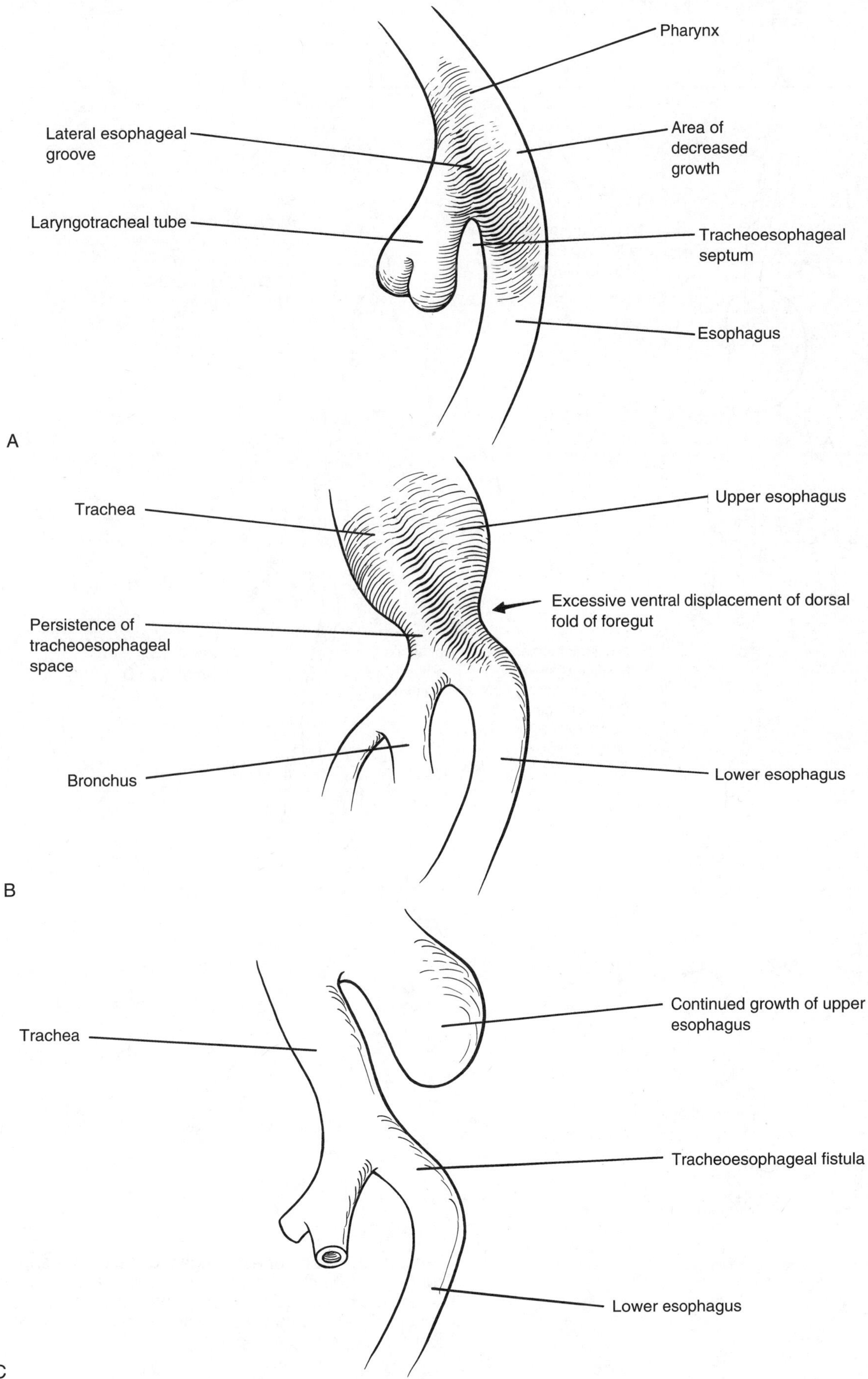

FIG. 61-1. Embryogenesis of esophageal atresia.

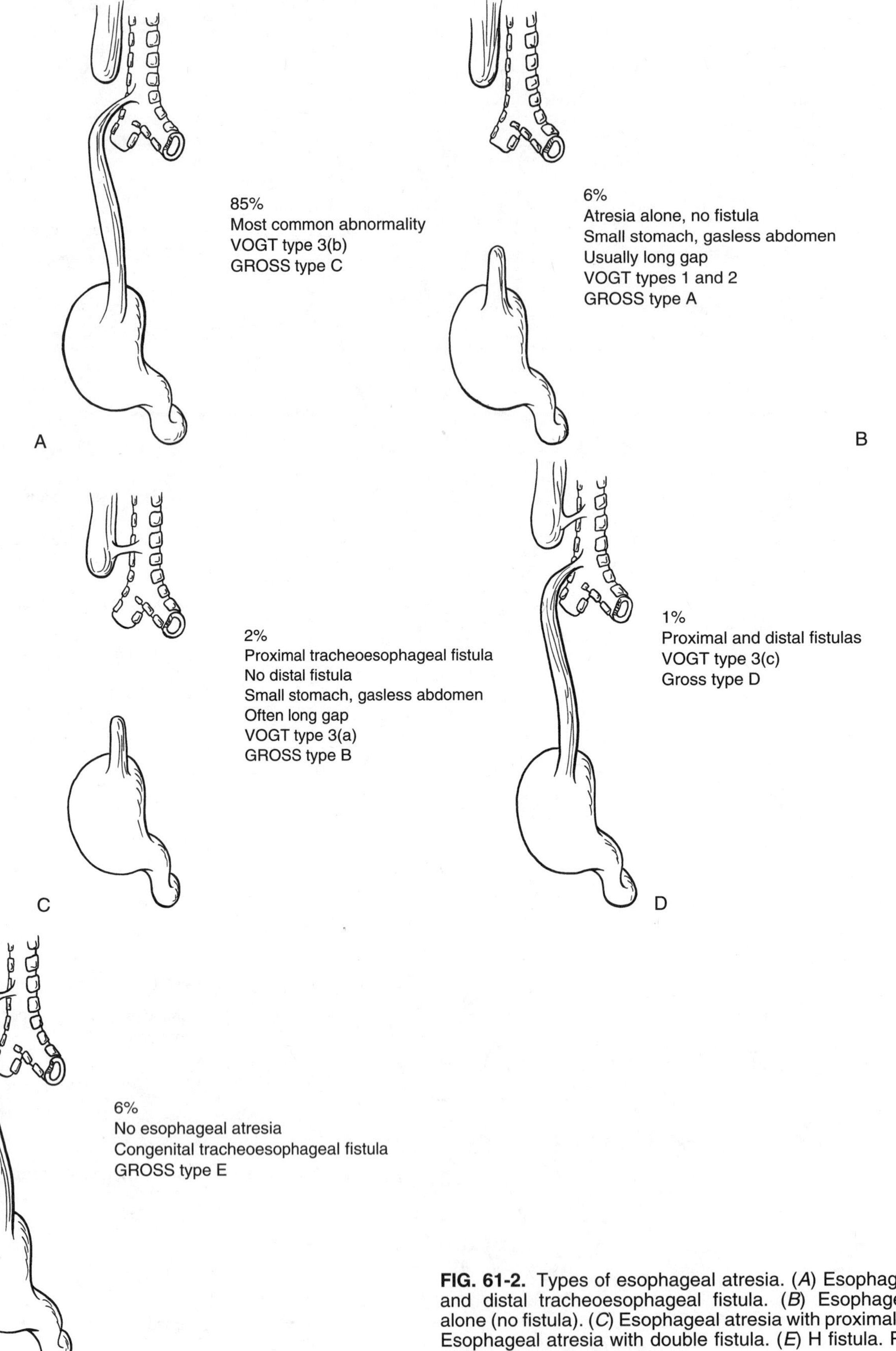

FIG. 61-2. Types of esophageal atresia. (*A*) Esophageal atresia and distal tracheoesophageal fistula. (*B*) Esophageal atresia alone (no fistula). (*C*) Esophageal atresia with proximal fistula. (*D*) Esophageal atresia with double fistula. (*E*) H fistula. Percentage reflects approximate incidence.

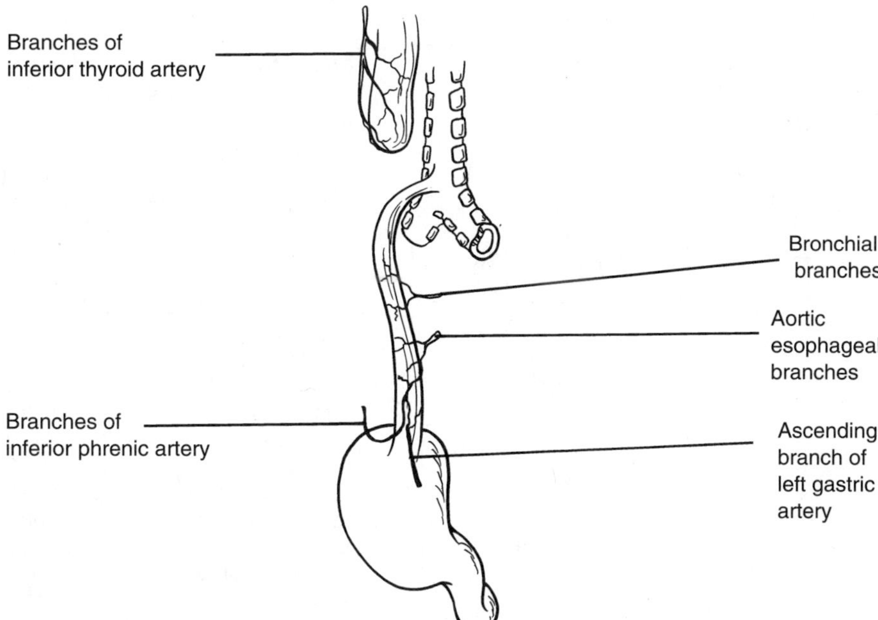

FIG. 61-3. Vascular supply of esophagus in esophageal atresia.

with an extensive gap between the two esophageal segments (so-called long-gap esophageal atresia), an anastomosis may only be achievable after mobilization of both segments. Knowledge of the vascular anatomy enables the surgeon to be confident of the blood supply; even when mobilization of the upper esophagus is extensive and continues well up into the neck, there is little risk of ischemia. On the other hand, extensive mobilization of the lower esophageal segment by disrupting its segmental supply is more likely to devascularize it. This influences the approach to long-gap esophageal atresia: the upper segment is fully mobilized first, after which the lower segment is mobilized only as much as is required to achieve an end-to-end anastomosis without excessive tension.

Circular or spiral myotomies may further compromise the blood supply of the esophagus, which explains their high complication rate. They may also compromise the innervation of the esophagus, adversely affecting its motility.

Innervation of the Esophagus

The esophagus is supplied by the autonomic nervous system. The sympathetic supply comes from preganglionic neurons in the thoracic and upper lumbar spinal cord. Postganglionic fibers enter the esophagus by way of visceral branches of the sympathetic trunks and greater splanchnic nerves.

Parasympathetic neurons located in the nuclei of the vagus have preganglionic fibers that pass with the vagus nerves. They synapse with short postganglionic neurons situated within the intramural myenteric and submucosal plexuses. These innervate the smooth muscle and secretory cells. An inherent abnormality of the parasympathetic supply in esophageal atresia and the vulnerability of vagal fibers during surgical dissection and mobilization of the esophagus may be responsible for the abnormalities of esophageal function seen in repaired esophageal atresia (see later).

Esophageal Dysmotility

Esophageal motility is abnormal both before and after repair of esophageal atresia. Evidence of inherent congenital motor dysfunction has come from preoperative manometric studies, including studies in patients with H-type tracheoesophageal fistulas. Postoperative manometric studies after repair of esophageal atresia have shown that almost the entire length of the esophagus has abnormal motility, regardless of the extent of dissection or tension at the anastomosis.

The surgical procedure may further adversely affect esophageal motility if the fine vagal fibers are injured during mobilization of the esophagus. Patients tend to improve gradually with age but often need to drink with their meals. Abnormal esophageal motility may contribute to tracheal aspiration. Poor esophageal clearance allows acidic gastric juice to remain in the lower esophagus for a longer period of time than is normal, which may explain the observation that children with esophageal atresia are more likely to suffer complications of gastroesophageal reflux. Anastomotic stricture, recurrent tracheoesophageal fistula, and tracheal instability from tracheomalacia all contribute to disordered esophageal motility.

Gastroesophageal Reflux

Gastroesophageal reflux is common in infants with esophageal atresia. Esophageal dysmotility, poor esophageal clearance, and anastomotic narrowing make gastroesophageal reflux more significant and hazardous in esophageal atresia patients than in normal infants. Esophageal dilatation alone is not effective as definitive treatment for an esophageal stricture secondary to gastroesophageal reflux because ongoing reflux causes the stricture to recur rapidly, often within weeks. The appropriate treatment for such strictures is fundoplication to prevent further

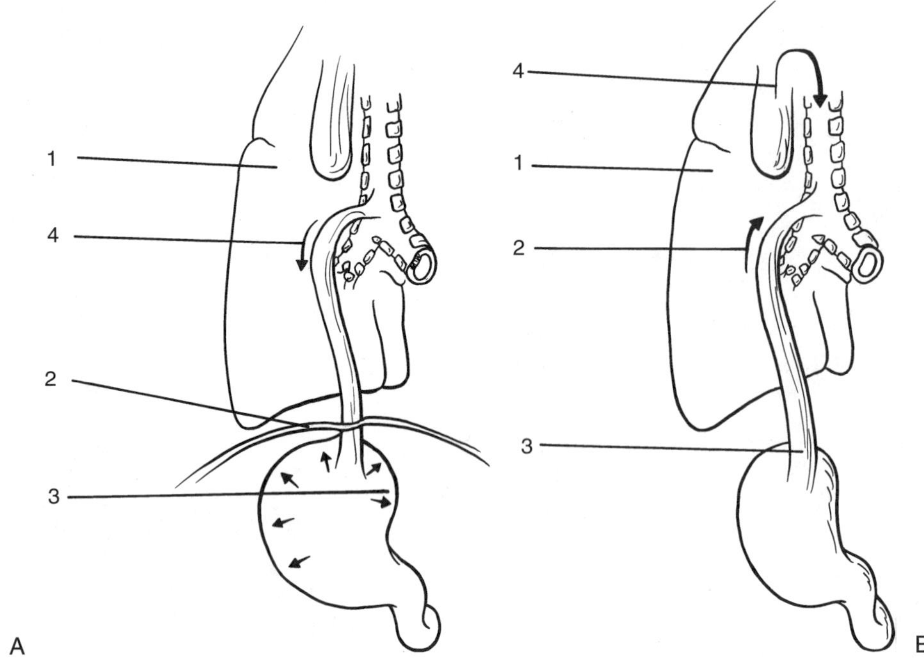

FIG. 61-4. Physiologic effects of a distal tracheoesophageal fistula. (*A*) 1. Hyaline membrane disease may necessitate higher ventilatory pressures, which encourage air to pass through the distal fistula. 2. A distended abdomen elevates and "splints" the diaphragm. 3. Gastric distention may result in gastric rupture and pneumoperitoneum. 4. Passage of air through a distal tracheoesophageal fistula diminishes the effective tidal volume. (*B*) 1. Aspiration of gastric juice leads to soiling of the lungs and pneumonia. 2. Gastroesophageal reflux. 3. Direction of gastric fluid proximally through distal fistula. 4. Overflow of secretions or inadvertent feeding may contribute to aspiration and contamination of the airway.

reflux, at which time esophageal dilatation may also be appropriate. After this procedure, most strictures resolve spontaneously.

Tracheoesophageal Fistula

A distal tracheoesophageal fistula can compromise an infant in two ways. First, escape of air down the tracheoesophageal fistula into the stomach and beyond results in gaseous distention of the abdomen, causing elevation of the diaphragm (so-called splinting of the diaphragm) and restriction of ventilation (Fig. 61-4*A*). The neonate depends almost entirely on diaphragmatic movement for effective ventilation because the transverse (rather than oblique) configuration of the neonatal ribs means that intrathoracic volume increases little with intercostal contraction (Fig. 61-5). Clinically, the infant is observed to be in respiratory distress, with tachypnea and abdominal distention.

Secondly, in the presence of gastroesophageal reflux (which is common), gastric juice may ascend the esophagus and enter the airway through the fistula (see Fig. 61-4*B*). The frequency with which this mechanism causes contamination of the airway in esophageal atresia is unclear, but in isolated tracheoesophageal fistula (H-fistula), passage of food through the fistula accounts for the recurrent chest infections so often seen. In esophageal atresia, pneumonia is perhaps more likely to occur from overflow of secretions from the blind upper esophageal segment or by inadvertent feeding before diagnosis.

Tracheomalacia

Some degree of structural and functional weakness of the trachea is expected in esophageal atresia, but in some patients, it may be severe enough to cause respiratory obstruction.[8] There is a deficiency in cartilage and an increase in the length of the transverse muscle of the posterior tracheal wall.[9] The cartilage is unable to support the tracheal wall, which has a perimeter greater than normal. The section of the trachea most affected is at the level of the blind-ending proximal esophageal segment. The lower half of the trachea and, occasionally, the whole trachea may also be involved. When the abnormality is confined to the intrathoracic trachea, the signs are those of expiratory obstruction. Conditions that increase intrathoracic pressure, such as lower respiratory infection, exacerbate the degree of tracheal collapse. The usual signs of tracheomalacia are those of intermittent expiratory obstruction and normal inspiration. There may be feeding difficulties and vomiting. An esophageal stricture predisposes to inhalation of saliva and food. Distention

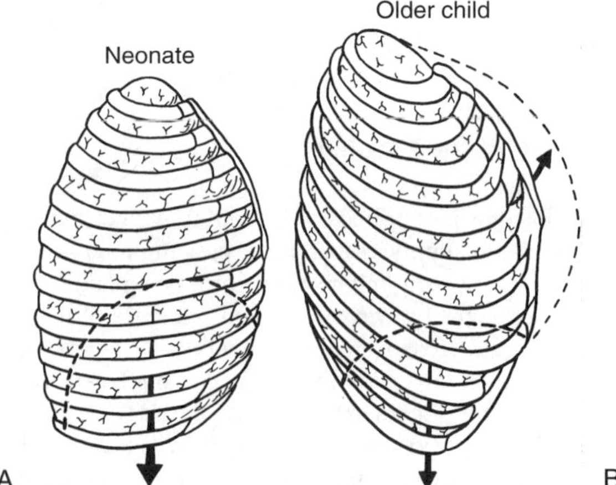

FIG. 61-5. Neonate's dependency on diaphragmatic movement for ventilation. (*A*) In neonates, horizontal ribs cannot enlarge the thorax, and diaphragmatic contraction increases intrathoracic volume. (*B*) In older children, elevation of ribs increases intrathoracic volume, which is assisted by contraction of diaphragm.

of the proximal esophagus may compress the trachea and worsen the obstruction of tracheomalacia. In turn, the expiratory obstruction promotes gastroesophageal reflux by increasing intraabdominal pressure. Gastroesophageal reflux, therefore, may be both a cause and result of the tracheomalacia.

The natural history of tracheomalacia is spontaneous improvement with time. When symptoms are mild, no active intervention is necessary, although the seal-bark cough may persist into adult life. When tracheomalacia is more severe, careful attention must be paid to feeding. The infant should be offered small amounts of soft foods until late in the first year. Associated gastroesophageal reflux should be managed initially by positioning with the head 30° upright and thickening of feeds. If respiratory symptoms persist, or an esophageal stricture develops, a fundoplication should be performed. If there is no gastroesophageal reflux, any esophageal stricture should be dilated. Aortopexy (tracheopexy) is employed when these measures have failed and the child has recurrent cyanotic episodes due to expiratory obstruction. The rationale for aortopexy relies on the observation that there are fibrous connections between the posterior surface of the aorta and the anterior wall of the trachea. Drawing the ascending arch of the aorta anteriorly and suturing it to the body of the sternum holds the tracheal lumen open by tightening these fibrous connections.

Prematurity

The combination of hyaline membrane disease in premature infants and splinting of the diaphragm from preferential entry of air through the fistula may produce respiratory embarrassment severe enough to necessitate ventilatory support. This may exacerbate the problem of air passing through the fistula, further compromising ventilation. For this reason, management should be directed at maintaining the lowest possible ventilatory pressures to achieve adequate oxygenation, followed by early division of the tracheoesophageal fistula.[6,10] Because hyaline membrane disease takes 24 to 48 hours to develop, there is time to divide the fistula before the respiratory distress becomes fully established and the complications of inadequate ventilation against an elevated diaphragm or ruptured stomach occur. The earlier practice of performing an emergency gastrostomy in infants with major escape of air through a distal tracheoesophageal fistula has been abandoned. This is because the massive air leak often continued after gastrostomy and made ventilation even more ineffective as the air continued to pass preferentially through the fistula.

Closure of the fistula improves the ease of ventilation because (1) there is no further escape of air down the distal fistula; (2) there is no diaphragmatic splinting interfering with ventilation; and (3) soiling of the lungs with gastric secretions is prevented. In most infants, esophageal continuity can be achieved at the time of thoracotomy to divide the fistula.

DIAGNOSIS OF ESOPHAGEAL ATRESIA

Clinical Diagnosis

Any excessively drooling infant should be assumed to have esophageal atresia until proved otherwise. The diagnosis is made when a stiff 10-gauge French catheter introduced through the mouth (Fig. 61-6A) becomes arrested at about 10 cm from the alveolar ridge. Failure to pass the catheter into the stomach, demonstrated by radiograph, confirms the diagnosis of esophageal atresia. Fluid aspirated up the catheter does not usually turn blue litmus pink, as would be expected with gastric aspirate. A tube of smaller caliber may curl up in the proximal pouch and give a misleading impression of esophageal continuity[11] (see Fig. 61-6B). The tube should not be introduced through the nose because it may injure the nasal passages. Contrast studies, on the rare occasions that they are required, should be performed by an experienced pediatric radiologist, or after transfer to the tertiary institution, and with the use of a small amount (0.5 to 1 mL) of water-soluble contrast.

Diagnosis of Anatomic Type

Determination of definitive treatment is dependent on the anatomic variant. It is necessary to know whether there is a fistula between the trachea and one or other esophageal segment. It is also useful to have information about the distance between the esophageal ends when there is no distal fistula. Plain chest radiograph with a tube in place shows the blind upper pouch in the upper mediastinum. The lateral view may display an open fistula and air in the lower esophagus. Visualization of the tracheal bifurcation shows the level of the tracheoesophageal fistula.

The Gasless Abdomen

Absence of gas in the abdomen suggests that the patient has either atresia without a fistula or atresia with a proximal fistula only (see Fig. 61-2B or 2C). A carefully performed upper-pouch contrast study or bronchoscopy demonstrates the presence of a proximal fistula in about 20% of cases. If no upper-pouch fistula is found, then esophageal atresia without fistula is assumed, and the patient can proceed to gastrostomy. The length of the lower esophagus can be demonstrated at that time by passing a metal bougie from the stomach through the gastroesophageal junction. Simultaneous insertion of a catheter into the upper pouch enables an estimation of the length of gap between the esophageal ends.

Distal Tracheoesophageal Fistula

If there is gas below the level of the diaphragm on plain radiographs of the abdomen, then it can be safely assumed that there is a distal tracheoesophageal fistula. Only a small proportion of these patients have an upper-pouch fistula, and this becomes evident at the time of thoracotomy. Some surgeons, however, prefer to perform a preoperative upper contrast study or bronchoscopy routinely.

H-Fistula

The presenting features of an infant with an isolated tracheoesophageal fistula is different because the esophagus is intact.

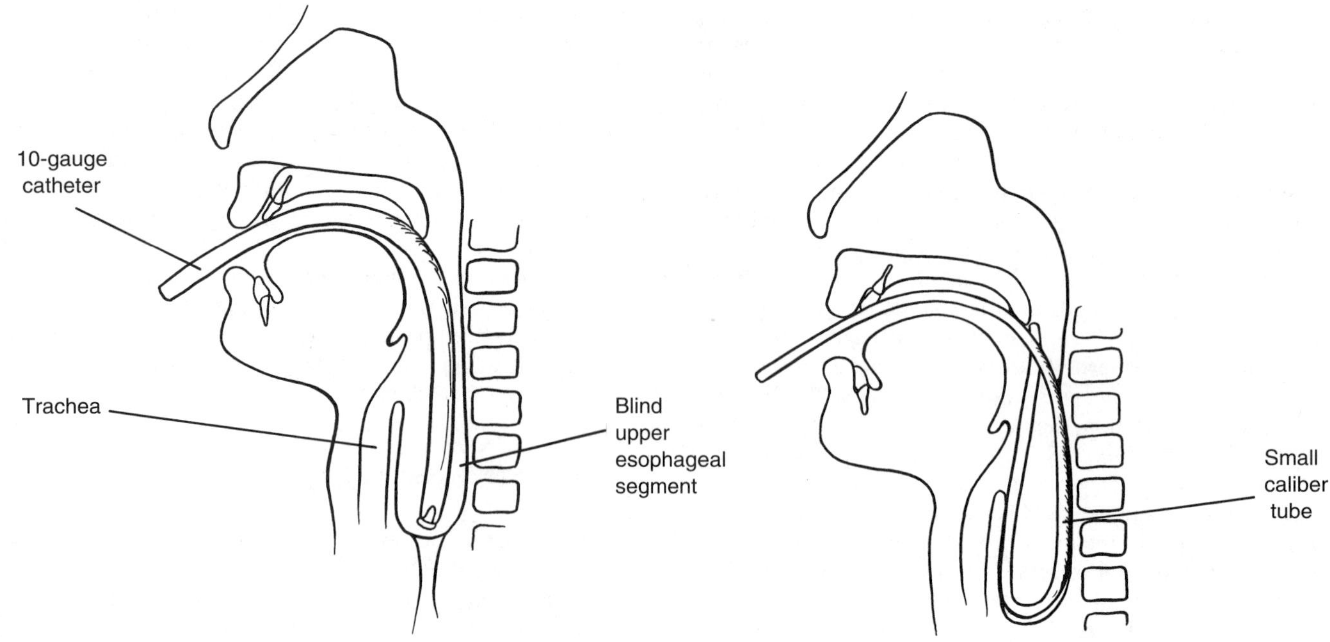

FIG. 61-6. (*A*) The diagnosis of esophageal atresia is confirmed when a 10-gauge (French) catheter cannot be passed beyond 10 cm from the gums. (*B*) A smaller-caliber tube is not used because it may curl up in the upper esophageal segment, giving a false impression of esophageal continuity.

These infants can swallow but may choke and cough when eating. When air escapes through the fistula, they may present with abdominal distention. Recurrent aspiration from food may lead to repeated chest infections. The diagnosis is confirmed on mid-esophageal contrast study or endoscopy.[12]

Associated Abnormalities

More than half of infants born with esophageal atresia have one or more associated congenital abnormalities (Table 61-2). Not all affect the management of esophageal atresia, and not all require treatment with the same urgency (Table 61-3). Those who require treatment should be diagnosed early. The VATER association describes a commonly encountered spectrum of associated anomalies: *v*ertebral, *a*norectal, *t*racheoesophageal, *r*adial, and renal abnormalities, as well as congenital heart disease, duodenal atresia, and a number of other abnormalities. It is best to regard the VATER or VACTERL association as encompassing a spectrum of anomalies that frequently occur at the same time.

Trisomy 18 and 21 occur more commonly in patients with esophageal atresia than might be expected (in about 5% of patients in one series). When trisomy 18 is suspected clinically, the chromosomes should be analyzed immediately and surgery postponed until the results are available. Where there are features of Down syndrome, the possibility of associated duodenal atresia, congenital heart disease, and Hirschsprung disease must be considered.

CHARGE association is seen in about 2%. The outlook in

TABLE 61-2. *Incidence of associated anomalies in 84 patients with esophageal atresia*

Anomaly	Frequency (%)
Congenital heart disease	20
Urinary tract	22
Orthopaedic	15
Gastrointestinal	22
Chromosomal	4.8
Total	58

TABLE 61-3. *Relevance of associated anomaly to esophageal atresia*

Anomalies	Relevance
Meckel diverticulum	Interesting but not relevant in
Duplex kidney	relation to management
Vertebral anomalies	Relevant because of frequency of association (treatment may be required)
Pelviureteric junction obstruction	Demands treatment, but not urgently, and esophageal atresia
Vesicoureteric reflux	takes undisputed priority
Duodenal atresia and anorectal anomaly	Demands early treatment: Needs to be coordinated with treatment of esophageal atresia
Congenital dislocation of the hip	Does not need to be coordinated with treatment of esophageal atresia
Duct-dependent congenital heart disease	May take priority over complete repair of esophageal atresia
Trisomy 18	Incompatible with survival
Bilateral renal agenesis	Incompatible with survival

these children is better than previously believed: up to one third are mentally normal or only mildly retarded.

MANAGEMENT OF ESOPHAGEAL ATRESIA

Initial Management

Handling of the infant should be kept to a minimum because excessive disturbance may lead to crying, increases the infant's oxygen consumption, exposes the infant to cold stress, and may cause dramatic cardiovascular responses in an unstable newborn. Crying tends to fill the stomach with air; this increases the likelihood of regurgitation of gastric contents into the trachea and increases abdominal distention, which in turn impedes ventilation. Care must be taken to avoid excessive cooling in the delivery room and during subsequent stabilization and transport (Table 61-4).

A number of infants with esophageal atresia have respiratory distress because of prematurity, other congenital abnormalities, aspiration pneumonia, or diaphragmatic splinting caused by excessive escape of air through the distal fistula into the stomach. If blood gas monitoring facilities are not available, the infant must be kept pink at all times; a short period of hypoxia is more dangerous than several hours of hyperoxia.

Aspiration is prevented by maintaining a partly upright position and by repeated suction of the upper esophageal pouch. This keeps the proximal esophagus empty and reduces the likelihood of overflow of saliva into the lungs. The upper esophagus should be suctioned every 10 minutes, or more often if the child appears to have excessive mucus or air bubbles.

On no account must infants with esophageal atresia be fed. Any material swallowed is likely to end up in the lungs and cause aspiration pneumonia. Attending staff must be aware that the only thing to be introduced through the mouth should be the suction catheter.

Resuscitation by vigorous ''bagging'' may force air through the distal fistula and cause abdominal distention. The stomach may distend rapidly and cause elevation and splinting of the diaphragm, increasing the respiratory difficulty.

Transfer to a major tertiary pediatric institution is best not delayed. The Neonatal Emergency Transport Service, or regional equivalent, should be notified early, and arrangements should be made to continue suctioning of the upper esophageal pouch before and during transport. In general, the infant should be positioned in a partly upright position with the head elevated to allow emptying of the proximal blind-ending pouch.[13] This position minimizes regurgitation of gastric contents up the distal tracheoesophageal fistula, decreases the work of breathing, and improves oxygenation.

Management of Associated Abnormalities

Congenital Heart Disease

Antenatal ultrasonography often identifies congenital cardiac abnormalities. Irrespective of this, preoperative echocardiography should be performed routinely in all infants with esophageal atresia. An echocardiogram defines any significant congenital heart disease and determines the position of the aortic arch.

Infants with non–duct-dependent conditions should have early repair of the esophageal atresia while pulmonary vascular resistance is high, and the cardiac condition should be treated definitively later.[14]

Infants with severe right or left heart obstructive lesions, in whom either the pulmonary or systemic circulation is duct dependent, deteriorate rapidly when the duct closes. Most of these patients present in the first day of life because of their heart disease; others deteriorate during repair of the esophageal atresia, or early in the postoperative period if the diagnosis was not made preoperatively. They should be supported hemodynamically with a prostaglandin E_1 infusion (to keep the duct open), and the esophagus should be repaired when the clinical condition is stable. Any palliative or reparative cardiac surgery is performed subsequently.

Urinary Tract Abnormalities

Most urinary tract abnormalities are not life-threatening but are best detected early, before irreversible damage to the kid-

TABLE 61-4. *Prevention of excessive heat loss in esophageal atresia*

Cause of heat loss	Mechanism	Intervention
High surface area/body volume ratio	Evaporation	Place in incubator.
Prematurity	Thin skin	Place in incubator.
	Small size	
	Immature thermoregulating center in hypothalamus	
Attachment of monitoring devices and intravascular lines	Opening incubator is requirement for access	Keep handling to minimum. Use heat lamp.
Anaesthetic drugs		
Halothane	Peripheral vasodilation	Use heating blanket on operating table.
Muscle relaxants	Prevent shivering	Use overhead heat lamp until fully draped. Warm operating room. Use rectal probe to monitor temperature. Use warmed humidified inspired gases. Infuse patient with warmed intravenous solutions. Ensure adequate circulating volume.
Thoracotomy	Evaporative heat loss	Keep duration of surgery to minimum.

neys has occurred. Reflux-associated nephropathy occurs in about 5% of patients with esophageal atresia. It is worthwhile to identify patients with bilateral renal agenesis or severely cystic dysplastic kidneys before operation because repair of the esophageal atresia in these patients is probably inappropriate. When kidneys cannot be found on ultrasound examination, a nuclear renal scan confirms the absence of functioning renal tissue. Patients with bilateral renal agenesis may not have features of Potter syndrome in the presence of esophageal atresia because there is no oligohydramnios.

A renal sonogram should be performed before surgery, unless the infant has been observed to pass urine. A micturating cystourethrogram should be performed if the renal ultrasound is abnormal, but this can be delayed for some weeks after repair of the esophageal atresia.

Gastrointestinal Abnormalities

All children with esophageal atresia should have careful examination of the anorectal region. When an anorectal anomaly is identified, the esophageal atresia is repaired first, after which the anorectal anomaly is treated, either by anoplasty, colostomy, or primary neonatal anorectoplasty, depending on its nature. When esophageal atresia occurs with duodenal atresia and high imperforate anus, a thoracotomy is performed first to correct the esophageal atresia, followed by a duodenostomy and then colostomy.

Chromosomal Aberrations

It is important to recognize trisomy 18 early because its poor prognosis represents a contraindication to surgical repair of the esophageal atresia.

Orthopedic Abnormalities

Congenital vertebral anomalies (eg, hemivertebrae) may produce progressive scoliosis, for which later surgical stabilization of the spine is required in about 15% of patients. Limb abnormalities include radial club hand, absent thumb, and isolated thumb abnormalities. Congenital dislocation of the hip and congenital talipes equinovarus also occur more frequently than might be expected.

Anterior chest wall deformity and secondary scoliosis were common when the rib was resected at thoracotomy, when staged procedures were employed, and when intrathoracic sepsis was common. The current intercostal approach in esophageal atresia makes this late complication infrequent.

Summary of Preoperative Investigations

A plain radiograph of the torso provides information on the lungs (evidence of aspiration), the pneumonitis vertebral column (hemivertebrae form part of the VATER association), and most importantly, the presence of gas in the bowel below the diaphragm. Absence of gas signifies that there is no distal tracheoesophageal fistula. Most of these infants have a wide gap between the esophageal ends and no fistula at all, while a few have a proximal tracheoesophageal fistula. This can be demonstrated by endoscopy or a careful esophageal contrast study performed in the tertiary center. In some centers, bronchoscopy is performed routinely in all infants with esophageal atresia. Renal ultrasonography and echocardiography are routine preoperative investigations.

Operative Repair of Esophageal Atresia

Operation is performed promptly after the preoperative evaluation is concluded. If the infant has evidence of respiratory compromise (ie, pneumonitis or lobar collapse), especially if this involves the left lung, operation should be delayed 1 to 2 days to optimize the pulmonary status before repair.

In patients in whom ventilation with positive pressure is difficult because of air passing down the tracheoesophageal fistula into the stomach, major morbidity can occur because of gastric perforation, pneumoperitoneum, and elevation of the diaphragm, which worsens ventilation. In these cases, urgent laparotomy to control the air leakage is required. The technique involves insertion of a Foley catheter into the lower esophagus via the gastric perforation. This occludes the distal tracheoesophageal fistula and allows thoracotomy to proceed to surgically divide the distal tracheoesophageal fistula.

In preparation for thoracotomy, the infant is placed with the right side uppermost and a towel folded underneath the left chest to give lateral flexion. A transverse incision centered on the inferior angle of the scapula allows a fourth intercostal extrapleural approach. The extrapleural approach is favored because, if there is an anastomotic leak, an empyema is less likely to develop. The azygos vein is ligated and divided.

The connection of the distal esophagus to the trachea is identified. Transfixion sutures close the fistula, which is then divided. Care is taken to avoid damage to the vagal fibers and blood supply to the distal esophageal segment.

The upper esophagus is mobilized enough to allow an end-to-end, one-layer, interrupted esophageal anastomosis between the upper pouch and lower esophageal segment (Fig. 61-7). On occasion, the lower esophagus may require mobilization to prevent undue tension on the anastomosis. If an anastomosis cannot be done without undue tension, despite extensive mobilization of the two esophageal segments, an esophageal myotomy can be done. This can be performed using a circular myotomy or a spiral myotomy; in selected cases, a second myotomy can be performed proximal to the first one. A chest drain may be placed at the discretion of the surgeon.

Esophageal Atresia Without Fistula

This variant of esophageal atresia presents some specific problems that may be difficult to overcome. When there is no distal tracheoesophageal fistula, there is almost always a substantial gap between the esophageal ends. Sometimes, there is virtually no lower esophageal segment above the level of the diaphragm.

The length of the upper esophageal segment can be demonstrated by the contrast study performed to exclude a proximal fistula and can be confirmed at the time of gastrostomy by the passage of a radioopaque catheter through the mouth into the esophagus. The lower esophageal segment is also evaluated at the time of gastrostomy by introducing a metal bougie through

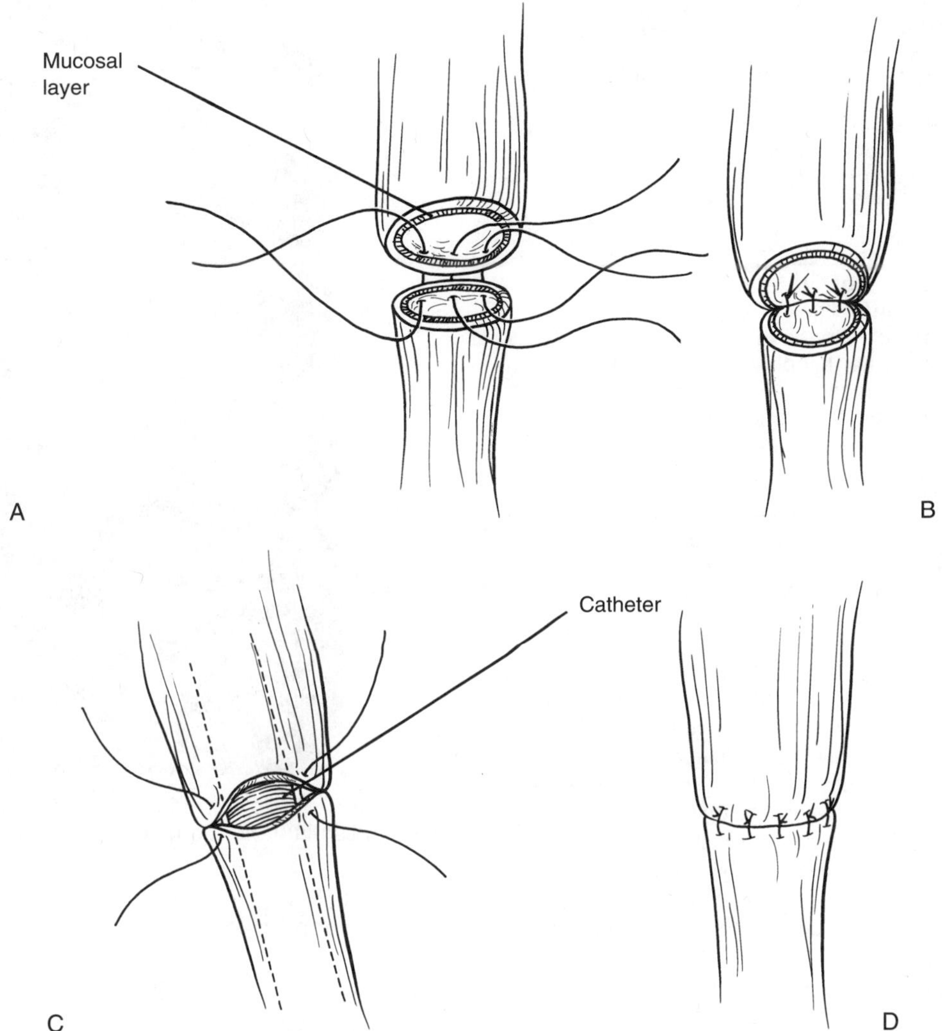

FIG. 61-7. The esophageal anastomosis. (*A*) Three or four interrupted all-layered sutures are inserted in the far wall of the esophageal segments. It is important to ensure that each suture includes mucosa because the mucosal layer tends to retract out of view. (*B*) The sutures are ligated with the knots tied on the mucosal side, drawing the esophageal ends together. (*C*) A catheter is introduced through the upper pouch into the lower esophageal segment. (*D*) The end-to-end all-layered interrupted 5-0 absorbable anastomosis is completed. On the near wall, the knots are tied on the outside.

the gastroesophageal junction into the lower esophagus and observing its position using an image intensifier.

Primary esophageal anastomosis is often delayed for 3 months, which may allow time for bougienage of the upper pouch. It can be facilitated by the maneuvers outlined in Table 61-5. It is usually possible to obtain esophageal continuity without resorting to esophageal replacement.

Isolated Tracheoesophageal Fistula (H-Fistula)

Tracheoesophageal fistula without atresia presents an entirely different clinical spectrum from esophageal atresia. The esophagus is intact and patent, but there is an oblique fistula running downward from the trachea to the esophagus, usually at the level of T1 to T3. Apart from gastroesophageal reflux, other congenital abnormalities are less common than in patients with esophageal atresia.

Most fistulas are in the root of the neck, at about the level of the second thoracic vertebra. This means that a cervical approach usually provides the best access to the fistula. The recurrent laryngeal nerves, which lie in the grooves between the esophagus and trachea, are closely related to the fistula and may be vulnerable to damage during operative dissection.

The obliquity of the fistula and the close apposition of the trachea and esophagus mean that the fistula is occluded for much of the time. Pressure changes and the upward movement of the esophagus during swallowing may open the fistula, allowing air from the trachea to enter the esophagus, or esophageal contents to enter the trachea. The symptoms produced by an H-fistula or N-fistula result from this "two-way traffic" through the fistula. The usual symptoms suggestive of a congenital tracheoesophageal fistula include choking and cyanotic attacks with feeding, aspiration pneumonia, and abdominal distention with air. A few patients appear to have excessive

TABLE 61-5. *Maneuvers to achieve esophageal anastomosis in long-gap esophageal atresia*

Full mobilization of upper esophageal segment (to level of cricopharyngeus)
Dissection of lower esophageal segment to (or through) esophageal hiatus
Myotomy (usually of upper pouch)
  Circular
  Spiral
Mobilization of stomach into chest
  Through esophageal hiatus
  Division of lesser curve[15]
If the above measures fail, esophagostomy and gastrostomy may be required, with later esophageal replacement using one of the following options:
  Isoperistaltic gastric tube or reversed gastric tube
  Gastric transposition
  Jejunal interposition
  Esophagocoloplasty

* Spitz L. Gastric replacement of the esophagus. In: Spitz LV, Nixon HH. Robb & Smith's operative surgery, pediatric surgery, ed 4. London, Butterworth, 1988:142.

secretions; this is presumably related to irritation of the respiratory tract from the passage of saliva and milk through the fistula. Unfortunately, choking with or without cyanotic episodes may be attributed to other causes, leading to diagnostic delay of the fistula. The clinical picture may be further confused if the patient at times has no symptoms. When the diagnosis is suspected on clinical grounds, the fistula can be identified by radiology or bronchoscopy. A mid-esophageal tube introduces barium, which is viewed on continuous fluoroscopy and recorded on video (Fig. 61-8). When the initial barium swallow is negative, or when barium appears in the trachea but the route is obscure, the examination should be repeated with barium introduced through a mid-esophageal catheter.[12]

The fistula should be divided surgically. This may be delayed in some patients with severe pneumonia, who may first require resuscitation and several days of antibiotic treatment. Bronchoscopic cannulation of the fistula to assist in its identification at surgery is not always easy to achieve.

The fistula is usually best approached through a right-sided supraclavicular incision 1 to 1.5 cm above the clavicle; this minimizes the possibility of injury to the thoracic duct. Dissection may be facilitated by division of the sternomastoid muscle. The strap muscles are retracted medially, and the dissection is continued medial to the carotid sheath. The fistula should be divided, rather than ligated, to reduce the likelihood of recurrence. Placement of a muscle flap between the divided fistula ends may decrease the likelihood of recurrence. A contrast esophagogram is usually obtained 1 week after repair. This assesses the presence of an anastomotic leak, any stricture, and the amount of gastroesophageal reflux. Drainage of the wound is not normally necessary, and gastrostomy is not used. At completion of the operation, the anesthetist inspects the vocal cords.

COMPLICATIONS OF REPAIR OF ESOPHAGEAL ATRESIA

A variety of complications can occur after repair of esophageal atresia; these are listed in Table 61-6 and described in more detail next.

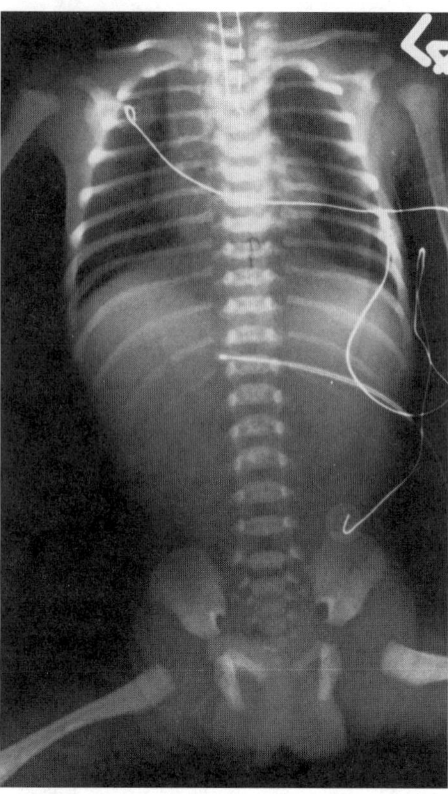

FIG. 61-8. Radiologic diagnosis of an esophageal atresia without fistula; note the gasless abdomen.

Anastomotic Leak

Anastomotic leakage can vary enormously in significance, from a minor radiologic leak in an otherwise well infant to complete anastomotic disruption with mediastinitis, empyema, pneumothorax, and septicemia (Fig. 61-9A). Factors that contribute to anastomotic leakage include insecure or incorrectly placed sutures, excessive tension at the anastomosis, ischemia of the esophageal ends, and sepsis. The extent of the esophageal dissection undertaken is the balance between that required to

TABLE 61-6. *Esophageal complications after repair of esophageal atresia*

Anastomotic leaks
  Incidental—small radiological leak, no clinical symptoms
  Minor leakage—saliva in chest drain (if used), but infant clinically well
  Major leakage
    Mediastinitis or abscess
    Pneumothorax or empyema
    Radiologically confirmed major esophageal disruption
Recurrent tracheoesophageal fistula
Anastomotic stricture
Motility problems: delayed esophageal clearance
Esophageal pseudodiverticulum after leakage or circular myotomy
Shelf at site of anastomosis (secondary to eccentric anastomosis)
Gastroesophageal reflux

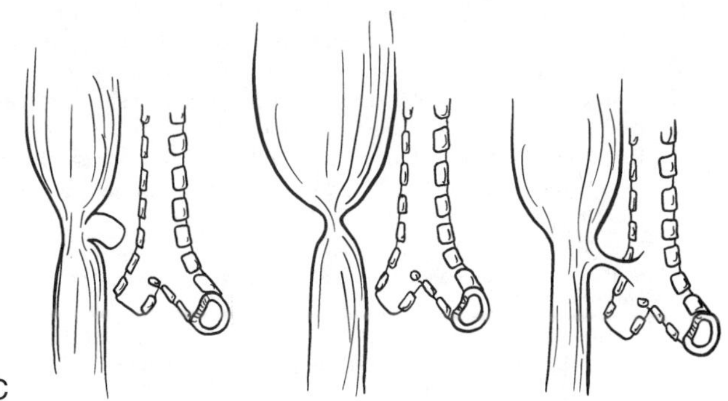

FIG. 61-9. Esophageal complications of repaired esophageal atresia and tracheoesophageal fistula. (*A*) Anastomotic leak; (*B*) anastomotic stricture; (*C*) recurrent tracheoesophageal stricture.

gain adequate length to avoid excessive tension at the anastomosis, and that resulting in potential injury to the blood supply of both esophageal ends, which may occur when the esophagus is mobilized extensively or when esophageal myotomy is performed. An interrupted one-layer, end-to-end esophageal anastomosis using absorbable sutures appears to have the lowest rates of leakage, stricture, and recurrent fistula.

Most leaks are successfully managed nonoperatively. Total parenteral nutrition enables oral feeding to be ceased. Antibiotics are commenced, and the leak usually closes spontaneously. A long-standing leak may require gastrostomy to allow continuation of enteral feeding. Cervical esophagostomy is necessary only rarely, when supportive therapy has been unsuccessful and when ongoing major sepsis has proved difficult to control.

Anastomotic Stricture

Anastomotic stricture is the most common reason for further surgery after repair of esophageal atresia (see Fig. 61-9*B*). Factors that predispose to stricture formation include rough handling of the esophagus at the time of repair, ischemia of the esophageal ends, excessive tension of the esophageal anastomosis, the choice of suture material (eg, silk), anastomotic leak or dehiscence, the use of a two-layer anastomosis, and gastroesophageal reflux. Gastroesophageal reflux is the most common cause of late stricture development.

Infants with a stricture develop feeding difficulties and dysphagia. The first symptom may be that the infant appears to eat slowly with excessive regurgitation, with or without cyanotic episodes. Older children present with foreign body impaction of food in the esophagus, most commonly between 1 and 5 years of age. The diagnosis of a stricture is confirmed by barium swallow or esophagoscopy.

In patients with mild narrowing of the esophagus, one or two dilatations may be all that is required. An antireflux operation usually is necessary when there is associated gastroesophageal reflux.

Recurrent Tracheoesophageal Fistula

A recurrent tracheoesophageal fistula is a severe and potentially dangerous complication (see Fig. 61-9*C*). Failure to close the fistula adequately at the time of initial thoracotomy, and an anastomotic leak with local infection and abscess formation, may contribute to the development of a recurrent fistula.

Coughing, gagging, choking, cyanosis, apnea, and recurrent chest infections are symptoms suggestive of a recurrent tracheoesophageal fistula. The typical presentation is that of an infant who coughs and splutters with each feed. The most reliable method of confirming the diagnosis is cineradiographic tube esophagography with the patient prone. A nasogastric tube is introduced into the esophagus, and the esophagus is filled with barium while the tube is gradually withdrawn. Bronchoscopy is an alternative method. Spontaneous closure of a recurrent fistula is unlikely. When the child is in optimal respiratory and general condition (usually after a period of intravenous nutrition), thoracotomy is performed through the original incision. The fistula is divided using a transpleural approach.

Gastroesophageal Reflux

Radiographically demonstrable reflux can be seen in almost all infants after tracheoesophageal fistula repair. If there has been mobilization of the distal esophageal segment, the angle of His may be altered. The degree of functional consequence of the reflux is variable. The combination of reflux and poor esophageal motility means that acid can bathe the esophagus for protracted periods of time. This can cause dysphagia when an esophagitis stricture forms at the anastomosis or in the distal esophagus. About 25% of infants subsequently require an antireflux operation.

OUTCOME

A steady decline in mortality rates has been seen in patients with esophageal atresia. In the past, most deaths resulted from respiratory failure, inadequate resuscitation, and complications of prematurity. The other major causes of mortality related to the complications of the esophageal atresia, particularly those related to dehiscence of the esophageal anastomosis and prolonged poor nutrition.

The current major causes of mortality are the associated major congenital abnormalities.[15] Infants no longer die from prematurity or esophageal complications; consequently, the previously used Waterston classification has little relevance today.

It is possible that long-term survival in repaired esophageal atresia patients may be limited by the effects of gastroesophageal reflux and poor esophageal clearance; there is some concern that dysplastic changes in the lower esophageal mucosa may predispose to esophageal carcinoma.

REFERENCES

1. Bankier A, Brady J, Myers NA. Epidemiology and genetics. In: Beasley SW, Myers NA, Auldist AW, eds. Esophageal atresia. London, Chapman & Hall Medical, 1991:19.
2. Myers NA. Esophageal atresia: the epitome of modern surgery. Ann Roy Coll Surg 1974;54:277.
3. Beasley SW. Embryology. In: Beasley SW, Myers NA, Auldist AW, eds. Esophageal atresia. London, Chapman & Hall Medical, 1991:31.

4. Vogt EC. Congenital esophageal atresia. AJR 1929;22:463.
5. Gross RE. Surgery of infancy and childhood. Philadelphia, WB Saunders, 1953:76.
6. Beasley SW. Influence of anatomy and physiology on the management of esophageal atresia. Prog Pediatr Surg 1991;27:53.
7. Lister J. The blood supply to the esophagus in relation to esophageal atresia. Arch Dis Child 1964;39:131.
8. Spitz L, Phelan PD. Tracheomalacia. In: Beasley SW, Myers NA, Auldist AW, eds. Esophageal atresia. London, Chapman & Hall Medical, 1991:331.
9. Wailoo MP, Emergy JL. The trachea in children with tracheoesophageal fistula. Histopathology 1979;3:329.
10. Holmes SJK, Kylie EM, Spitz L. Tracheoesophageal fistula and the respiratory distress syndrome. Pediatr Surg Int 1987;2:16.
11. Beasley SW, Auldist AW, Myers NA. Current surgical management of esophageal atresia and/or tracheoesophageal fistula. Aust NZ J Surg 1989;59:707.
12. Beasley SW, Myers NA. The diagnosis of congenital tracheoesophageal fistula. J Pediatr Surg 1988;23:415.
13. Roy RND. Transport of the neonate with esophageal atresia. In: Beasley SW, Myers NA, Auldist AW, eds. Esophageal atresia. London, Chapman & Hall Medical, 1991:93.
14. Mee RBB, Beasley SW, Auldist AW, et al. Influence of congenital heart disease on management of esophageal atresia. Pediatr Surg Int 1992;7:90.
15. Scharli AF. Esophageal reconstruction in very long atresia by elongation of the lesser curvature. Pediatr Surg Int 1992;7:101.

Surgery of Infants and Children: Scientific Principles and Practice, edited by Keith T. Oldham, Paul M. Colombani, and Robert P. Foglia. Lippincott–Raven Publishers, Philadelphia, © 1997.

CHAPTER 62

Gastroesophageal Reflux

Robert P. Foglia

Gastroesophageal reflux (GER) is a major cause of morbidity in children. In a number of children's hospitals, related operations are the most common intraabdominal procedures performed. Its incidence is difficult to quantitate because the definition and evaluation vary among institutions. GER is a relatively newly described disease entity. Research in the 1960s generally ascribed GER to the presence of a partial thoracic stomach and identified a hiatal hernia as a prominent component of the pathophysiology. The 1960s and 1970s saw progressive improvement in diagnostic studies used to assess GER. The first large report of surgically treated infants with GER opened the modern era of the evaluation and treatment of this entity in the pediatric population in 1974.[1]

GER is defined as the presence of gastric contents in the esophagus. Virtually all humans have this occur regularly; the clinical objective is to differentitate those individuals with pathologic GER who are at risk for complicatios related to this event. The presentation of pathologic GER can vary, and not all children with reflux have emesis. Clinically significant GER can be categorized in three broad patterns of presentation. The first is characterized by overt emesis. The other two presentations are referred to as *silent reflux* because emesis is absent. The second involves reflux to the level of the epiglottis, with gastric contents spilling into the tracheobronchial tree and causing acid aspiration with respiratory symptoms. The third type of reflux involves the esophagus alone.

Infants normally have some degree of emesis, ranging from a wet burp to regurgitation of a significant amount, if not all, of a recent feeding. Children with pathologic GER, however, often regurgitate larger volumes more frequently. The differential diagnosis of children with emesis should take into account the character of the emesis. Bilious emesis in young children is considered to be caused by obstruction until proved otherwise. The emesis with GER is nonbilious and typically occurs during a feeding or just after. Often, the parent finds the crib sheet or pillow stained by the vomited material. In the child who is several weeks of age, the major differential diagnosis is pyloric stenosis. If the GER is severe, weight loss and failure to thrive can occur. Parents may describe the number of times the child's clothes must be changed each day. In older children, the repeated emesis can lead to social problems and poor self-esteem. The presence of emesis makes the diagnosis of reflux

easy to identify; however, the lack of emesis does not rule out this problem.

Aspiration of gastric contents into the tracheobronchial tree can cause apnea, pneumonia, bronchitis, and asthma.[2] Gastric contents can be a potent trigger for apnea and bradycardia owing to reflex laryngospasm. A decrease in esophageal pH can be associated with the simultaneous development of respiratory symptoms. These respiratory symptoms can be as mild as coughing or as critical as apnea, which can be a mechanism for sudden infant death syndrome.[3] In infants and children with recurrent episodes of pneumonia thought to be aspiration related, the association with GER may be relatively straightforward. Conversely, a number of patients with reflux may have asthma or bronchitis for many years, and this may be the primary or even sole symptom of the GER.

Symptoms related solely to acid bathing the esophagus include poor feeding, dysphagia, and Sandifer syndrome. Findings may include esophagitis, esophageal ulceration, stricture formation, melena, bleeding, anemia, and Barrett esophagus.

ASSOCIATED ANOMALIES

Children with esophageal atresia are likely to have reflux for several reasons. Because of the discontinuity of the esophagus, there is not the normal innervation into the area of the lower esophageal sphincter. In addition, at the time of repair of esophageal atresia, there may be a need to mobilize the distal esophageal segment to achieve sufficient length to carry out an anastomosis without tension. This can change the configuration of the angle of His, thereby disrupting one anatomic antireflux mechanism. Extensive mobilization of the distal esophagus can actually pull part of the stomach up through the diaphragm, creating a hiatal hernia. This may be true in the typical tracheoesophageal fistula repair with the distal esophageal segment attached to the trachea, and is of even more concern in children with pure esophageal atresia and a long gap between the two esophageal segments. If GER is present, its sequelae may be more severe in these patients because of esophageal dysmotility and ineffective acid clearance from the distal esophagus. In this event, the gastric acid contents remains in contact with the esophagus longer, causing further inflammation of the distal esophagus.

After repair of a diaphragmatic hernia, patients are more likely to have pathologic GER, with an incidence as high as 35%.[4,5] Closure of the diaphragmatic defect can place tension on the esophageal crura, pulling the left crus laterally and altering the anatomy of the gastroesophageal (GE) junction. Hiatal hernia is uncommon in children with GER, but when present, this confers a high likelihood that the reflux will not respond to medical therapy. Finally, there is a high incidence of GER in neurologically impaired patients. It is unclear whether this is due to a central mechanism or whether chronic retching in some of these children causes reflux.

ANATOMY AND PHYSIOLOGY

The anatomy and physiology of GER can be considered in terms of the dynamic events occurring in three distinct areas: the esophagus, the GE junction, and the stomach (Fig. 62-1). The esophagus functions as a conduit to transport material from the pharynx to the stomach. The initial propulsion of food into the esophagus is under skeletal muscle control. After the bolus begins to descend in the esophagus, propulsion is due to smooth muscle function. In the normal circumstance, a coordinated primary esophageal stripping wave moves the food through the esophagus. A secondary esophageal wave serves to clear any

residual material not moved distally by the primary wave, or any gastric contents that reflux into the esophagus.

Normally, there is an intraabdominal segment of the distal esophagus below the diaphragm. Although there is not a true anatomic sphincter present, the lower esophageal segment at the level of the diaphragm functions as a physiologic sphincter. Factors contributing to the GE junction function include the length of the intraabdominal esophagus, the relative difference in the diameters of the intraabdominal portion of the esophagus and the fundus of the stomach, and the presence of a high-pressure zone at the GE junction.[6]

The stomach acts a reservoir, and the competency of the GE junction prevents a pathologic reflux. If there is an obstruction to gastric emptying, either from a true mechanical problem or a physiologic abnormality, the contents remain in the stomach for a protracted period, and intragastric pressure increases within the stomach. If there is concomitant dysfunction at the GE junction, acid reflux can occur.

Lower esophageal sphincter pressure (LESP) is controlled by several mechanisms. With a primary esophageal peristaltic wave, LESP decreases, and this opens the GE junction to allow the bolus of material to pass from the esophagus into the stomach. In the pathologic circumstance, LESP decreases in the absence of a peristaltic wave, and the GE junction opens. This allows gastric contents to reflux into the esophagus. It appears that relaxation at the GE junction is controlled by both a central mechanism and an enteric neurotransmitter. Vasoactive intestinal peptide is one candidate for this mediator.[7]

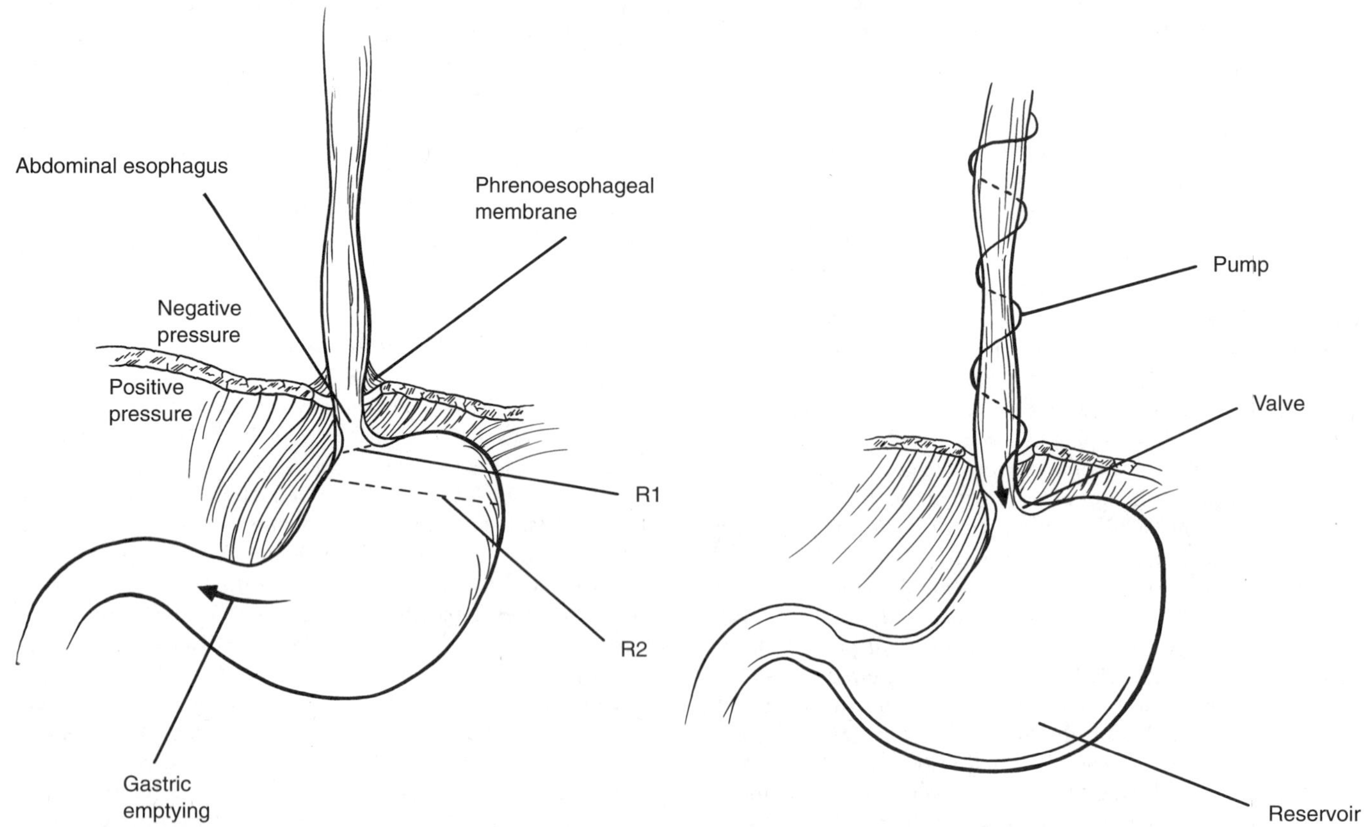

FIG. 62-1. (*A*) Anatomic and physiologic factors that influence gastroesophageal competency. (*B*) Schematic representation of the interaction of the esophagus, gastroesophageal junction, and stomach. R1 and R2 designation illustrate the diameters of the distal esophagus and fundus, respectively.

PATHOPHYSIOLOGY

Initially, pathologic GER was thought to result from a hiatal hernia and was described as a partial thoracic stomach. In adult screening tests, about half of people 50 years of age have a radiographically demonstrable hiatal hernia. Most of these individuals do not have significant symptoms of GER. In children with pH probe-proven pathologic GER, the incidence of a hiatal hernia is 3% to 6%.

GER may be of marked significance or of little or no functional consequence. If a patient has brief episodes of acid reflux into the lower esophagus, but has no clinical symptoms, this is considered physiologic. An understanding of the elements that allow for a greater degree and amount of GER helps to explain both the process and the strategies that can be used to correct the reflux (see Fig. 62-1). The normal position of an intraabdominal segment of esophagus allows for the development of a high-pressure zone. The acute angle (angle of His) between the intraabdominal portion of the esophagus and the cephalad of the greater curvature of the stomach allows for a marked difference in the diameter of the intraabdominal portion of the esophagus and the superior portion of the stomach. The law of LaPlace states that the tension in two areas that are in continuity is inversely related to their radii. Thus, if the diameter (or radius) of the stomach at the level of the fundus (R2) is five times longer than the diameter (or radius) of the intraabdominal portion of the esophagus (R1, see Fig. 62-1), then the tension is five times greater in the esophagus than in the stomach, and this tends to prevent reflux. If the angle of His is not present, the relation of the distal esophagus and the proximal stomach becomes more like the shape of a funnel. The difference in the esophageal and gastric diameters is smaller, and the pressure differential between the two areas is less; affording a greater potential for reflux. This problem is seen in patients with hiatal hernias, in whom a portion of the stomach is above the diaphragm and the angle of His may be absent. This is also prevalent in patients after repair of esophageal atresia or tracheoesophageal fistula.

LESP is affected by a number of factors:

ANATOMIC
- Status Post (S/P) esophageal atresia repair
- S/P diaphragmatic hernia repair
- Hiatal hernia

PHARMACOLOGIC
- Narcotics
- Alcohol
- Benzodiazepines
- Theophylline
- Others

Endogenous hormones, such as gastrin, secretin, and cholecystokinin, modulate LESP. Inflammation of the distal esophagus decreases LESP. Several pharmacologic agents affect LESP. Metoclopramide both increases LESP and acts as a prokinetic agent. Conversely, alcohol, narcotics, benzodiazepines, and theophylline derivatives decrease LESP. In the evaluation a patient with suspected GER, it is important to identify whether the child is receiving any medication that might adversely alter LESP. A classic situation is a premature infant who is receiving theophylline as treatment for apnea and bradycardia. The medication is given to increase the respiratory drive; however, the apnea and bradycardia might result from silent reflux, and the theophylline may actually be exacerbating GER.

The esophagus can be considered to be a type of pump that moves liquids and solids into the stomach. In the semiupright or upright position, esophageal motility and gravity transport food down the esophagus into the stomach and clear the esophagus of refluxed material (see Fig. 62-1*B*). The lower esophageal sphincter and the GE junction function as a physiologic valve and depend on an intraabdominal length of esophagus and a high-pressure zone. The GE junction is highly influenced by medications and inflammation. A mechanically inadequate lower esophageal sphincter can be due to inadequate sphincter pressure, inadequate intraabdominal esophageal length, or decreased abdominal pressure.[8] The final component of this mechanical model is the stomach, which functions as a reservoir. Gastric abnormalities that can result in GER include increased gastric pressure caused by decreased or delayed gastric emptying, and increased acid secretions. Likewise, gastric dilation and retching can alter the anatomy in the area of the cardia and fundus and afford greater likelihood of reflux. In addition, reflux of duodenal contents into the stomach and subsequent duodenogastric reflux may affect the distal esophagus and the GE junction and may cause more pathology than acid reflux alone.

In some patients, GER is a component of a foregut motility disorder and can be associated with dyscoordinate esophageal peristalsis and motility and delayed gastric emptying. GER can be quantitated by the number of times that acid is noted in the esophagus on a pH probe study. Fifteen to 20 brief episodes of incompetency of the GE junction occur normally daily (referred to as *eructation* or *burping*). If there is prompt esophageal clearance, this is not of functional significance. The combination of acid reflux and poor esophageal motility causes the esophagus to be bathed in acid for a protracted period. Patients with associated tracheoesophageal fistulas often have dyscoordinate esophageal peristalsis, thus, they are at high risk for the development of pathologic acid reflux. These children can develop an anastomotic stricture due to technical problems with the anastomosis, such as tension and a marginal blood supply, combined with the subsequent effect of acid at the anastomosis. They also are at risk for esophagitis and stricture formation in the distal esophagus.

Strategies to correct GER should address abnormalities of the esophageal motility, ineffective LESP due to anatomic or pharmacologic causes, and gastric anomalies, especially delayed gastric emptying.

DIAGNOSIS

The evaluation of the infant or child with suspected pathologic GER begins with a detailed history and physical examination. In the young child, pyloric stenosis and GER can be confused. The pattern of emesis, both in terms of frequency and severity, often allows for differentiation. The patient may have a history of recurrent upper respiratory infections, bronchitis, pneumonitis, pneumonia, or asthma. Any of these can be indicative of GER. Poor feeding can be due to repetitive bouts of reflux and subsequent esophagitis or esophageal stricture formation.

Physical examination can reveal obvious emesis, a cough related to GER, pneumonia, or Sandifer syndrome. In the latter circumstance, the child repetitively turns his or her head to one side to improve peristalsis in the esophagus. This can be confused with torticollis. In some patients, a period of hospitalization may ascertain whether there is a significant feeding problem. Specific questions about the amount of food the infant is taking can help define failure to thrive and potential causes of emesis. A period of observation also allows for identification of the frequency and severity of GER and assessment of the effect of treatment strategies.

The diagnostic tests available to evaluate the patient with suspected GER include an esophagogram, esophageal pH probe measurement, scintigraphy, esophageal manometry, esophagoscopy, and biopsy. Each of these tests has advantages and disadvantages, and most are not performed in every patient.

Esophagogram

The esophagogram is the most commonly used diagnostic test in the evaluation of GER. It is an excellent screening test, is arguably the easiest test to perform, and provides information about the anatomy of the esophagus, stomach, and duodenum as well as their function. Fluoroscopy can identify the presence of GER and whether the refluxed material remains in the esophagus alone or results in aspiration of acid into the tracheobronchial tree. Abnormalities of the esophagus, such as esophagitis, ulceration, stricture, dilation, and twisting, are identified (Figs. 62-2 through 62-6). The presence of normal peristalsis in the

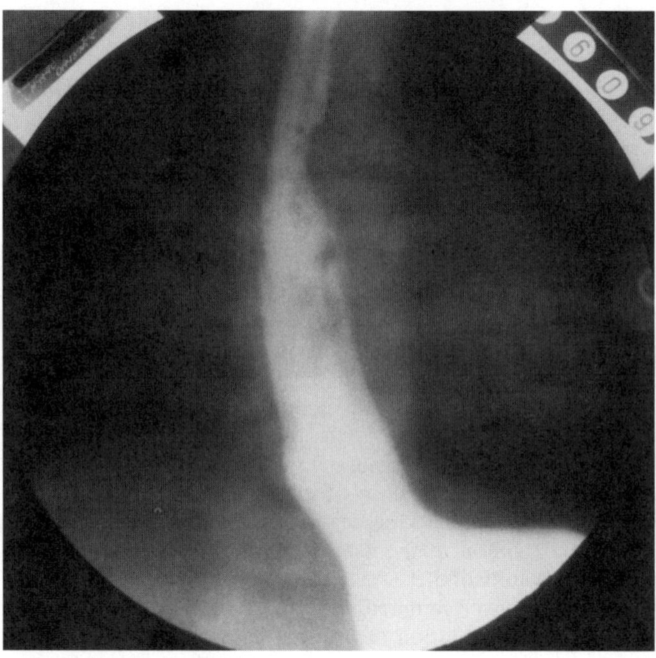

FIG. 62-3. Contrast esophagogram showing significant gastroesophageal reflux.

esophagus and stomach can be evaluated. The presence of a hiatal hernia, the position of the GE junction, the configuration of the stomach, and the angle of His can also be evaluated. In addition, a number of abnormalities that cause a delay in gastric emptying, such as pyloric stenosis, malrotation, or a duodenal web, can be identified. The esophagogram is reviewed with spot films and cinefluoroscopy. The latter gives a representation of the dynamic process of swallowing and GER. Another point of evaluation in this study is the rapidity of esophageal clearance of refluxed gastric contents. In the esophagus with poor peristalsis, refluxed contrast may remain for a lengthy period of time. In the patient who has had repair of esophageal atresia, the esophagogram can identify abnormal esophageal motility, an anastomotic stricture, a more distal stricture, and GER. The overall sensitivity of the esophagogram in the evaluation of GER is about 85%.[9] A major limitation is the short interval used to evaluate the subject. If reflux is noted during the deglutition of barium, or if it is noted when the stomach is filled with contrast, a positive diagnosis is made. The absence of reflux during the relatively short evaluation, however, does not rule out its presence.

The esophagogram is also valuable in patients who have a clinical history of reflux and who have had an antireflux procedure. In these patients, the study allows for an evaluation of the GER and determination of whether a fundoplication is still intact, its position, any difficulty with esophageal peristalsis delivering contrast through the area of the fundoplication, and any delay in gastric emptying.

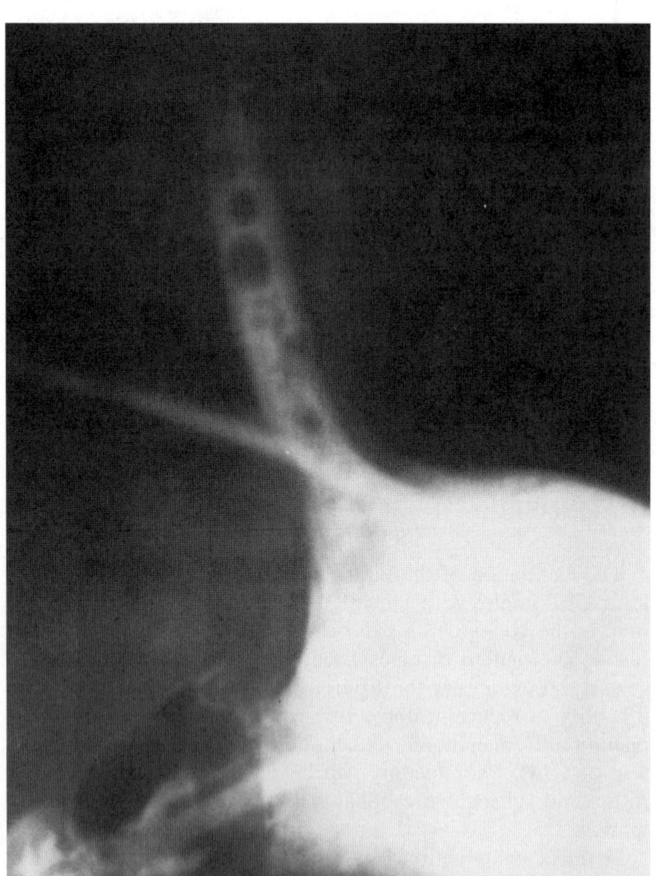

FIG. 62-2. Radiograph demonstrating the loss of the angle of His. The angle between the greater curvature and the esophagus is larger than usual. This decreases the disparity in diameter between the esophagus and stomach. See also Fig. 62-1.

Esophageal pH Monitoring

During the past 20 years, the prolonged monitoring of esophageal pH has become the standard for evaluation of GER.[10,11]

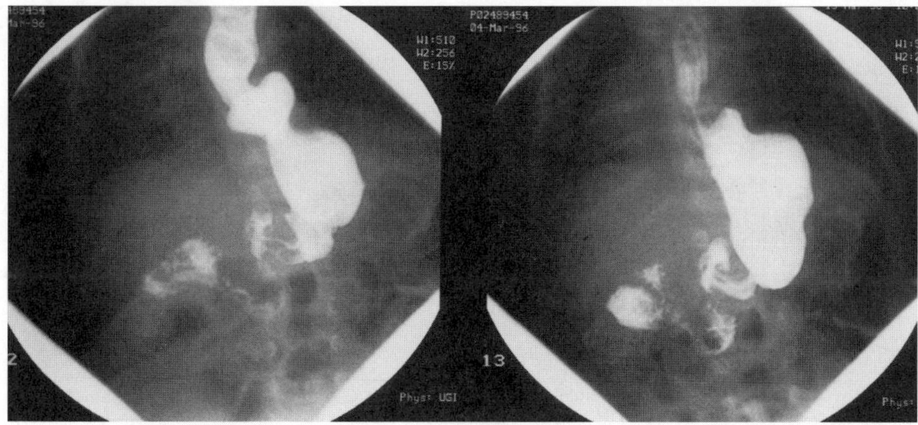

FIG. 62-4. Esophagogram of a 4-month-old patient with dextrocardia, marked gastroesophageal reflux, hiatal hernia, and malrotation.

The test consists of placing a 2F probe through the nose into the distal esophagus. Continuous pH monitoring is performed during the following 24 hours. The study measures the presence of acid in the distal esophagus, the number of reflux episodes, and typically reports the length of time acid is present for each episode, the total amount of time that acid is present in the esophagus, and the longest continuous periods of time that acid is present in the esophagus. Evaluation is carried out while the child is awake, asleep, supine, sitting, or upright. It is important to feed the child during the study. NPO status throughout the study may give a false-negative result because the stomach is not filled. Associated problems, such as cough, choking, cyanosis, oxygen desaturation, or apnea, can be recorded. Because the esophageal pH monitoring test is performed for a protracted period, it is a much more representative study for the presence of pathologic GER than an esophagogram. Shortening the length of the study can cause difficulties in interpretation. For example, 12-hour monitoring does not identify up to 20% of patients with pathologic reflux.[12]

The data are recorded by computerized telemetry in a nearly physiologic setting and can be combined with an apnea study.

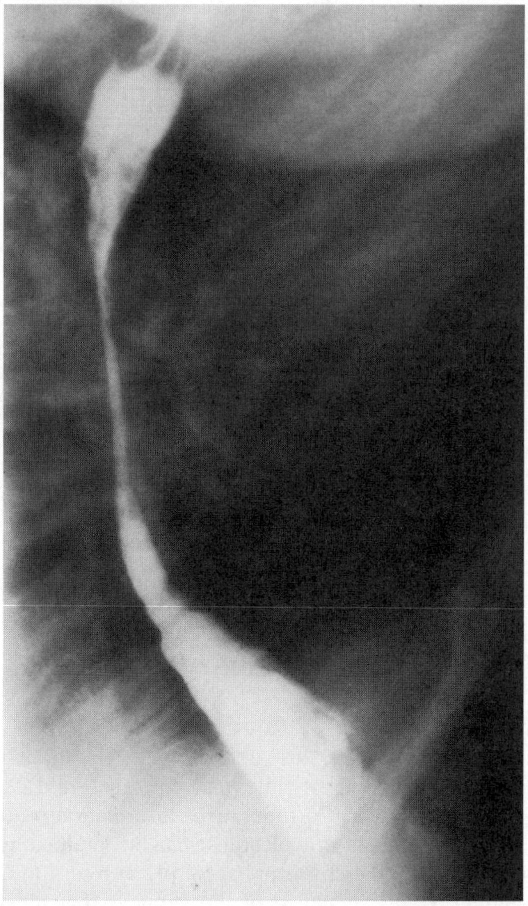

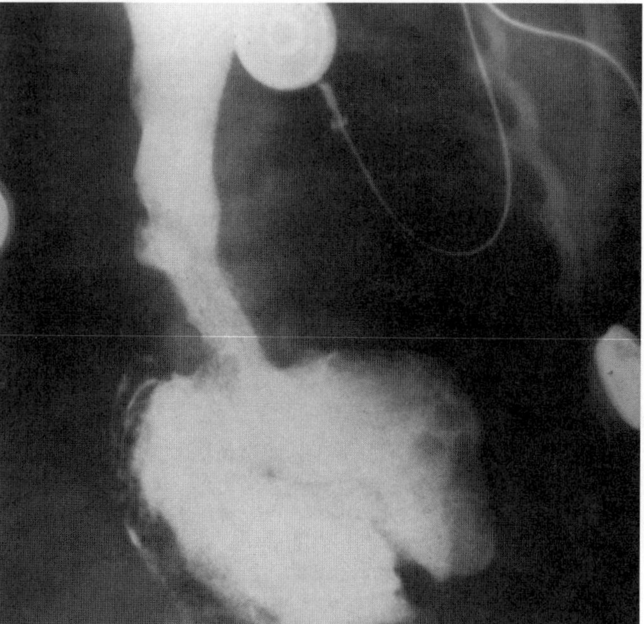

FIG. 62-5. Esophagogram showing a long narrow esophageal stricture secondary to gastroesophageal reflux.

FIG. 62-6. Esophagogram showing a large esophageal ulcer induced by pathologic acid GER.

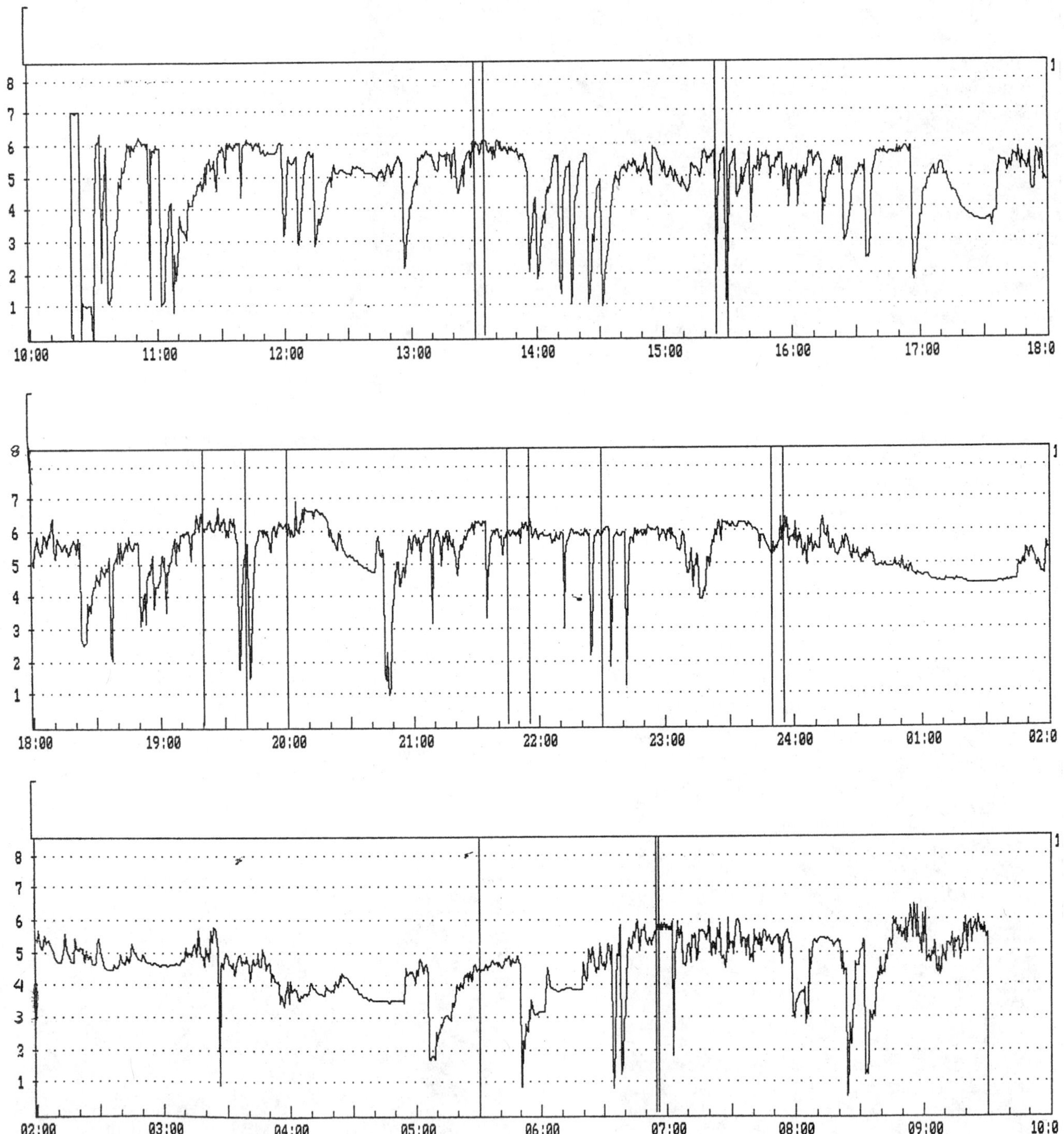

FIG. 62-7. Graph of a 24-hour pH probe study demonstrating gastroesophageal reflux. The ordinate lists esophageal pH and the abscissa indicates the time of day.

Figure 62-7 shows a typical 24-hour pH probe study. Table 62-1 gives a breakdown of this pH probe study, identifying the findings of clinical interest.

The major advantages of the pH probe study are that it has a 98% specificity for the identification of GER and that it is carried out under normal conditions (no sedation or anesthesia), over an extended length of time, and with the child carrying out normal activities. Corroborative information regarding esophageal motility and acid clearance can be obtained by analysis of the time it takes for esophageal pH to return to normal after feeding. A disadvantage of the study is that most food buffers the gastric pH to a level near that of the esophageal pH.

TABLE 62-1. *Esophageal pH probe data listing the number of episodes of reflux, number of episodes longer than 5 minutes, and fraction of time with pH less than 4.0**

Acid reflux > 0 min postprandial	Total	Upright	Supine	Asleep	Awake	Gas	Cry
Duration (h:min)	21:52	07:56	13:56	16:01	05:51	00:03	00:40
Reflux episodes	49	22	29	26	25	1	3
Reflux episodes > 5 min	9	1	8	5	4	0	0
Longest reflux episode (min)	46	10	43	43	10	1	1
Total time pH <4.0 (min)	189	35	154	125	63	1	1
Fraction time pH <4.0 (%)	14.4	7.3	18.4	13.0	18.0	31.1	3.5

* This study shows acid in the esophagogram 14.4% of the time, which is an abnormal result.

A false-negative evaluation of GER may be assumed during the postprandial period. To avoid this problem, feeding times should be recorded. Feeding with a highly acidic liquid, such as apple juice, can be done if necessary to clarify this.

Radionuclide Scan

Scintigraphy for GER involves the ingestion of a radionuclide-labeled liquid or semisolid material; alternatively, the material is administered through a tube in the stomach. Semisolids are now used more frequently than liquids alone. The patient is subsequently placed under a gamma counter, and for 90 minutes, the amount of the nuclide leaving the stomach is measured. This study serves two major purposes: (1) it identifies the presence of GER and the aspiration of gastric contents into the tracheobronchial tree by the presence of the nuclide in the lungs; (2) it provides physiologic information regarding the efficacy of gastric emptying. The norm is that half of the meal passes out of the stomach into the small intestine within 1 hour of its ingestion.

Advantages of the radionuclide study include the quantitative measurement of gastric emptying, which can be used for subsequent comparison. The study is more accurate than an upper gastrointestinal series in identifying a delay in gastric emptying. As such, it is an important test in the identification of a foregut motility disorder.

Disadvantages of the radionuclide study include low-dose radiation exposure, the necessity for the patient to remain under the gamma counter for a lengthy period, and the potential difficulty obtaining an accurate assessment of gastric emptying if the patient has significant pathologic GER and loses a portion of the nuclide label with emesis.

Esophageal Manometry

Measurement of the intraluminal pressures in the esophagus and at the GE junction gives useful physiologic information about GER and esophageal motility. It provides information regarding LES function, pressure, and length. Normal LESP is considered to be 15 mmHg or more. When properly performed, the study has a sensitivity for detecting pathologic GER of about 70%. Esophageal manometry is more useful and has better developed normal standards in adults than in children. It is gener-ally considered the most difficult of the studies available to assess GER, and, in children, is used infrequently.

Endoscopy and Biopsy

Esophagoscopy allows visualization of the distal esophagus, the GE junction, and the stomach and affords the opportunity to obtain biopsy specimens. A biopsy can help to identify the presence and degree of esophagitis. An important related finding is that of Barrett esophagus (see Chapter 60). Esophagoscopy can also provide a baseline for following the patient postoperatively, especially if a distal esophageal stricture is present. Bronchoscopy can be helpful in patients with pulmonary symptoms and suspected GER. The bronchoscopy can allow for aspiration of material from the bronchial segments with analysis for the presence of lipid-laden macrophages, which correlate with GER and aspiration.[13,14]

MEDICAL TREATMENT

Management of the infant or child with GER should take into account whether there is an anatomic cause for the reflux and also the severity of the reflux. Concomitant anatomic anomalies may contribute to severe reflux that is difficult to obviate without operative intervention. Patients who have undergone esophageal atresia or diaphragmatic hernia repair, and those with a hiatal hernia may be more recalcitrant to nonoperative management. Patients with these associated anatomic problems, however, make up only a small number of all patients with GER. In patients with pathologic reflux, the goal of treatment is to decrease the amount of reflux and to relieve symptoms. Overall, nonoperative treatment of GER is successful in 80% or more of children. The patients most likely to respond well are those with mild to moderate reflux. Children with moderate to severe reflux are less likely to do well without surgical intervention. Other factors that influence the prognosis of GER are patient age, the presence of a significant neurologic deficit, and whether the GER is part of a foregut motility disorder.

Infants without complications related to their GER are likely to do well with medical treatment. There appears to be physiologic maturation of the LES during the first 4 to 6 months of age. As infants begin to sit up and stand, gravity helps minimize the reflux as well. Also, this time usually corresponds with the beginning of solid feedings. These factors work together to decrease the amount of GER in most infants. In contrast, children with dysfunctional esophageal peristalsis, GER, and significant delay in gastric emptying are likely to have synergism of these factors, limiting the probability of a good response to medical treatment.

GER in neurologically impaired patients can be particularly difficult to treat. The reflux in many of these patients may be potentiated by hypertonicity, which raises intraabdominal and intragastric pressures. In addition, many of these patients have behavioral retching. This is difficult to stop and often contributes to reflux. GER to the level of the epiglottis is a particular problem in neurologically impaired children who cannot protect the airway and thus are at higher risk for aspiration-related problems.

Symptomatic GER in patients beyond 6 to 8 years of age may not be associated with spontaneous improvement seen in infants and younger children. These children are already upright and eating solid food.

The major medical components of GER treatment, especially in young children, include upright positioning, frequent and low-volume feedings, thickened feedings, and pharmacologic treatment with antacids and prokinetic agents. Placing the child in an upright position exploits gravity and promotes better clearance from the esophagus. The infant seat has been advocated for many years for this purpose. Young children tend to slide downward in this device, however, and it is not always effective in achieving semiupright position for any length of time. During the past 10 to 15 years, the use of the prone position with the head upright 30 degrees has proven to be a significant improvement in the therapy of GER.[15] This position should be kept for at least 60 minutes after feedings. The major disadvantage of this technique is that it can be difficult to maintain for an older, more mobile infant.

A second important consideration is the frequency and character of the feedings. More frequent, smaller-volume feedings distend the stomach less. Thickening the milk or formula with rice cereal and similar substances also decreases the amount of GER. The combination of frequent, smaller, and thickened feedings is a mainstay in the management of these children.

LESP is decreased by inflammation, as seen with peptic esophagitis. Medications that reduce gastric acid production have become integral in the medical treatment of GER. An array of pharmacologic agents can have a salutary effect. H_2-antagonists, such as ranitidine, and proton pump inhibitors, such as omeprazole, have demonstrated efficacy.[16,17] Their mechanism of action is likely from antiinflammatory effects on the distal esophagus via decreased gastric acidity. This causes an increase in LESP and thus ameliorates GER. Prokinetic agents, such as metoclopramide and cisapride (Propulsid), improve peristalsis and gastric emptying. Treatment with cisapride not only aids in gastric emptying but also improves esophageal peristalsis and helps clear gastric contents from the distal esophagus. In addition to improving peristalsis, metoclopramide increases LESP.

In patients with mild reflux, strategies to decrease acid production and to improve motility are effective. In patients with more severe GER, the response to nonoperative treatment usually is not as satisfying. Because long-term pharmacologic treatment can pose additional problems, there comes a point when other options, such as surgery, should be considered. These pharmacologic agents have associated side effects, including extrapyramidal reactions, sedation, and diarrhea.[18] A fundamental consideration with the use of pharmacologic agents is whether they are modifying the symptoms of pathologic reflux or actually decreasing the reflux itself. If they primarily modify the symptoms, then a management strategy that deals with the causes of reflux and by prevents the event is appealing.

SURGICAL CORRECTION

Gastroesophageal reflux should be corrected surgically if the symptoms cannot be controlled medically or if an anatomic abnormality is contributing significantly. In addition, if a patient has significant GER and cannot protect the airway (eg, a neurologically impaired patient), then operative intervention is indicated.

Indications for operative intervention in the treatment of GER include the following:

- Unremitting emesis
- Failure to grow adequately
- Recurrent pneumonitis
- Apnea
- Refractory reactive airway disease
- Esophagitis
- Esophageal stricture
- Hiatal hernia

The child with multiple episodes of emesis each day often fails to thrive because of a lack of appropriate nutrition. Parents and physicians are hard pressed to miss the bouts of emesis, the need to have clothes changed, and the associated lack of appropriate weight gain. The decision to perform an operative procedure to correct GER is straightforward in the patient with recurrent emesis who has not improved with medical management. Many patients have silent reflux and primarily respiratory symptoms. If, despite medical therapy, the child is having repetitive bouts of pneumonitis, aspiration pneumonia, or apneic spells, it is clear that nonoperative management is not achieving the desired result. Other patients may have evidence of long-standing lung disease manifested by chronic bronchitis or asthma-like symptoms.[19] Personal experience with a group of pediatric lung transplant recipients indicates that GER is not uncommon in this setting. Acid reflux with aspiration into the tracheobronchial tree can cause life-threatening pulmonary infection in this immunocompromised group. Pulmonary symptoms due to GER that are unresponsive to medical therapy are well treated by an antireflux operation.[19]

Operation is indicated also for chronic esophagitis. This can lead to a cycle of acute and chronic inflammation, fibrosis, and stricture formation. The inflammation can progress to the point of chronic bleeding and can cause iron deficiency anemia. Patients may develop hematemesis or melena. Chronic esophagitis is associated with the development of Barrett esophagus (see Chapter 60).

In the older child who can verbalize, the complaint of persistent lower chest discomfort or persistent dysphagia is an indication for operation. In the younger child, there may be a significant aversion to food. This poor appetite may improve markedly after the reflux is obviated.

The principles for surgical treatment of GER include the establishment of an intraabdominal portion of the esophagus and the development of a lower esophageal sphincter that resists the passage of gastric contents from the stomach to the esophagus. The mechanical model of the esophagus, GE junction, and stomach (see Fig. 62-1) allows for an understanding of the goals of operation. The surgeon creates an antireflux valve around a portion of the intraabdominal esophagus by bringing a portion of the fundus of the stomach around the esophagus. An important tenet is that the 360-degree fundoplication should never be tight or snug but floppy. The goal is not to have the fundoplication impinge on or constrict the esophagus during the resting state. Before operation, if intragastric pressure increases, gastric contents can easily pass from the stomach into the esophagus because no effective antireflux mechanism is in place. After an antireflux procedure, an increase in intragastric pressure temporarily causes the portion of the stomach positioned around the intraabdominal esophagus to act as a pinchcock valve (Fig. 62-8). As soon as intragastric pressure decreases, the enfolded stomach around the esophagus collapses and does not impinge on the esophagus. The floppy characteristic of the fundoplication is integral to the repair. It should not function as an impediment to passage of food from the esophagus to the stomach. If there is esophageal dysmotility and the fundoplication is tight, liquids or solids may not be able to pass from the esophagus into the stomach. Likewise, material refluxed into the esophagus may not be able to clear easily. This problem is particularly significant in patients with previous esophageal atresia repair because they have predictably poor peristalsis. In these cases, nothing should be done to create a further impediment to the prograde passage of material from esophagus to stomach.

The pump function of the esophagus depends on peristalsis. The valve mechanism is created by the fundoplication around the intraabdominal portion of the esophagus. The third component of a successful repair relates to the function of the stomach itself. Malrotation, pylorospasm, and idiopathic causes of delayed gastric emptying all create an increase in the reservoir capacity of the stomach. Dilation causes an increase in gastric pressure, which can lead to retching. In this case, the fundoplication prevents egress of material retrograde into the esophagus. Retching can disrupt or displace the fundoplication into the mediastinum. Correction of GER by an antireflux procedure in the presence of continued poor gastric emptying is contraindicated. If there is objective evidence of delayed gastric emptying, the fundoplication should be combined with a gastric emptying procedure.

Operative Technique

Pediatric surgeons generally prefer an abdominal approach for operation. The Nissen fundoplication is the most commonly performed procedure, but many recommend a partial anterior (modified Thal) or a partial posterior (Toupet) antireflux procedure. Each of these procedures includes the principles of creating an intraabdominal segment of esophagus, creating a high-pressure zone in this portion of the esophagus, and preserving the angle of His. The procedure can be performed with equally good results via either an open technique or laparoscopically.

In a Nissen fundoplication, the intraabdominal esophagus is circumferentially encircled. If a hiatal hernia is present, the stomach is reduced from the chest, and mobilization is carried out so that the distal esophagus is below the diaphragm. The esophageal hiatus is assessed. If it is patulous posterior to the esophagus, several nonabsorbable sutures are used to reapproximate the crura (Fig. 62-9A). This decreases the likelihood of a displacement of the fundoplication, cranially through the hiatus. The upper fundus is then brought posterior and to the right side of the esophagus. The anesthesiologist passes a bougie through the mouth, down the esophagus, and into the stomach. The largest bougie that easily passes through the esophagus should be used. The fundoplication is then carried out over the bougie,

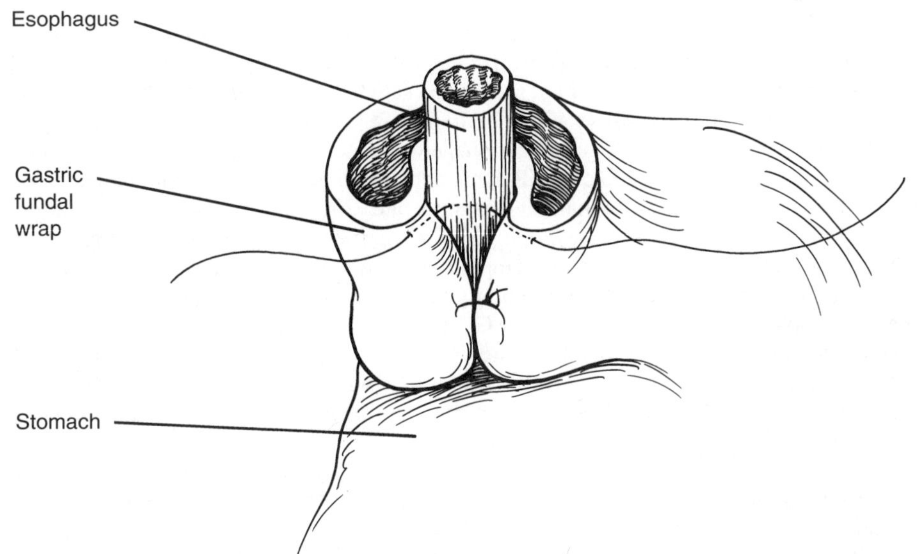

FIG. 62-8. Formation of an antireflux valve around the intraabdominal esophagus. As intragastric pressure increases, it presses inward on the esophagus. As intragastric pressure returns to normal, there is no impingement on the esophagus.

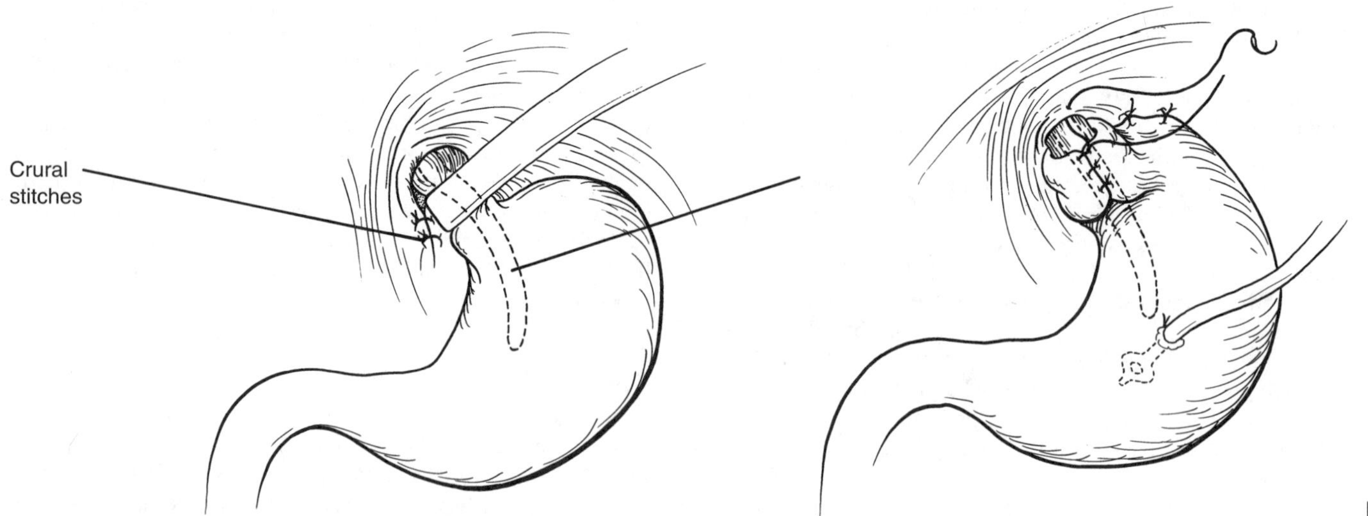

FIG. 62-9. Creation of a 360-degree Nissen fundoplication. (*A*) The esophageal hiatus is closed. (*B*) The completed fundic wrap is secured to the diaphragm and a gastrostomy tube is placed.

wrapping the esophagus within the fundus. A series of interrupted nonabsorbable sutures are placed in the fundus to the left of the esophagus, superficially through the anterior wall of the esophagus, and then to the portion of the fundus brought to the right of the esophagus. When these sutures are tied, a 360-degree fundoplication results (see Fig. 62-9B). A loose fundoplication is created by performing the operation with a large bougie in place in the esophagus. The most superior suture of the fundoplication is used to secure it to the esophagus just ventral to the esophageal hiatus. This also helps prevent movement of the fundoplication. Several nonabsorbable sutures are used to secure the fundus to the left of the fundoplication to the diaphragm. This tends to reform a normal angle of His. The bougie is then removed. In children younger than 2 years of age, in neurologically impaired children, and in those requiring tube feedings, a gastrostomy tube is placed. In patients with a significant delay in gastric emptying, a gastric emptying procedure is carried out. This can consist either of a pyloroplasty, pyloromyotomy, or antroplasty.[20]

Some surgeons contend that the 360-degree wrap significantly inhibits the child's ability to clear material from the esophagus. Gas bloat syndrome is seen in about 3% of these patients.[21] A postoperative patient with a small bowel obstruction who cannot vomit and may develop massive gastric dilation. Because of these problems, some surgeons favor a fundoplication in which the fundus is not brought circumferentially around the entire esophagus. Instead, the esophagus is wrapped with the stomach for 180 to 270 degrees. In patients with a short esophagus, such as can occur after repair of esophageal atresia, a partial fundoplication may diminish the risk of distal esophageal obstruction.

A number of complications can be related to the technical aspects of the operative repair.These include problems with the esophageal hiatus. If this is widely patent, appropriate reapproximation of the crura needs to be done to prevent migration of a portion of the fundoplication above the diaphragm. If an insufficient portion of the abdominal esophagus is mobilized, the fundoplication and therefore the functional LES may be inadequate. Another problem in the patient with insufficient potential intaabdominal esophagus mobilized is the inadvertent wrapping of the stomach rather that the lower esophagus. If the fundoplication is too tight around the esophagus, it may impede passage of food into the stomach. Care must be taken to bring the fundus loosely around the esophagus. The fundus can also be twisted as it is brought posterior to the esophagus, which causes malfunction of the wrap. Other technical considerations include avoidance of vagal nerve injury. This can be a particular problem in the patient with a previously failed fundoplication. Placing the gastrostomy tube in the antrum of the stomach and directing it toward the pylorus can lead to partial gastric outlet obstruction, often with the balloon of the gastrostomy tube.

Results

Many centers report 80% to 90% good to excellent results with an antireflux operation for the infant or child with GER who has not responded satisfactorily to medical therapy. These results include both the Nissen fundoplication and various partial fundoplications, either anterior or posterior.[21–24] The treatment of GER in patients without associated anomalies has a more than 90% success rate. Children with symptoms of failure to thrive often show a significant compensatory weight gain, pulmonary symptoms improve, and esophagitis and strictures can be substantially resolved. Further, the use of multiple medications to treat GER often can be stopped.

Operative intervention often results in improvement in the overall health of children with congenital heart disease who have failure to thrive and GER. Almost all pediatric reports have a high incidence of associated anomalies in patients with GER. The outcomes in these patients are more disparate.

In a combined study from two institutions, 1200 consecutive patients who underwent fundoplication for GER were reviewed.[9] Similar to other reports, many (39%) of patients were neurologically impaired. At the time of these initial operations, 871 patients underwent a fundoplication alone, while 286 children underwent both fundoplication and a gastric emptying procedure. A significant neurologic abnormality was present in 25% of the children who had fundoplication alone; in contrast, 75% of patients who had a gastric emptying procedure added to the fundoplication were neurologically impaired. The most common symptoms in the children operated on were repeated emesis (75%), feeding disorders in neurologically impaired children (39%), failure to thrive (32%), and respiratory problems, including repeated pneumonia (29%), asthma, or reactive airway disease (10%). Esophageal pH probe studies identified GER in 99% of the patients, and barium esophagogram with slight abdominal pressure applied showed GER in 86% of 1147 patients studied. A hiatal hernia was present in only 6% of the children. Manometry was used in a small number of children, and LESP was less than 15 mmHg in 61% of patients studied. Endoscopy and biopsy showed histologic evidence of esophagitis in 65% of the patients thus evaluated.

This study showed relief of emesis in essentially 100% of patients, and weight gain in almost all patients as well. There was cessation or marked improvement of pulmonary symptoms in 91% of the children. Operation is generally considered to result in improvement in more than 90% of patients who have significant esophagitis or stricture.

The results of antireflux procedures for the treatment of GER in neurologically impaired children vary. Indications for surgical intervention include the common problems related to GER and the concommitant need for gastrostomy tube placement to aid in feeding. Controversy exists regarding whether an antireflux procedure should be done routinely at the time of gastrostomy tube placement in these children, whether evaluation for GER should be carried out, or whether the gastrostomy tube placement should be done alone.

Central nervous system disorders, both congenital and acquired, are associated with GER.[25] Because gastrostomy tube placement can result in a decrease in LESP, which can add to the likelihood of reflux, we believe it is appropriate to evaluate the neurologically impaired child for GER before gastrostomy tube placement. If GER is identified, further evaluation to identify the presence of delayed gastric emptying is done. If the patient has evidence of reflux, an antireflux procedure is done concurrent with the gastrostomy tube placement. If the child also has delayed gastric emptying, a gastric emptying procedure is added to the gastrostomy tube placement and antireflux procedure.

Complications

The incidence of death after fundoplication in most large series is about 1% to 2%. It is largely skewed to patients who have major associated problems and is usually not related directly to the operation. A variety of complications can be seen after an antireflux procedure. These include:

- Pulmonary dysfunction
- Wound infection
- Gas bloat syndrome
- Herniation of fundoplication
- Intestinal obstruction
- Dysphagia
- Gastrostomy tube problems

Atelectasis or pneumonia is seen in 3% to 5% of patients, and wound infection is seen in about 1% to 2% of patients. The gas bloat syndrome is seen in about 3% of patients after a Nissen fundoplication. It is usually transient in nature, lasting several weeks, and usually is avoided by forming a floppy wrap. It can be dealt with effectively by venting through a gastrostomy tube or button.

During the past decade, increasing evidence has shown a strong association between pathologic GER and delayed gastric emptying. The failure of a fundoplication, either with disruption or slippage of the fundoplication into the mediastinum, is often related to delayed gastric emptying. The incidence of delayed gastric emptying in patients with pH-proven GER has been reported to be 22%.[26] This association is more common in neurologically impaired children.

Recurrent GER recurs in about 10% of all patients and in about 25% of neurologically impaired children after fundoplication.[27] In children with clinical evidence of emesis or regurgitation after fundoplication, evaluation should include an esophagogram to assess for GER and to evaluate the presence and position of the fundoplication. If GER is present, a gastric emptying study should be done to ensure that delayed gastric emptying is not contributing. This may be a major issue if the patient cannot empty the stomach in a prograde manner and therefore retches. If this is the case, reconstruction of the fundoplication be done with a gastric emptying procedure. The addition of the gastric emptying procedure decreases the failure rate of the fundoplication and is not usually associated with dumping problems or alkaline reflux.[28] Some believe that because of the possibility of injury to the vagal nerve trunks at the time of the reconstruction of the fundoplication, a gastric emptying procedure should be performed even without obvious evidence of delayed gastric emptying in the reoperative setting.[9]

Dysphagia is seen infrequently in patients after fundoplication. It is associated with esophagitis, stricture formation, a tight fundoplication, and poor esophageal peristalsis. Typically, esophagitis resolves in patients promptly after successful fundoplication. A stricture, however, may take some time and several esophageal dilations before appreciable improvement is noted (Fig. 62-10). Dysphagia can be caused by a snug fundoplication. This is best avoided by performing the wrap over an appropriate-sized bougie so that the fundal wrap does not collapse or constrict the esophagus. Dysphagia is almost nonexistent in patients who have had a partial fundoplication. Attention to the laxity of the circimferential fundoplication is especially important in patients with poor or discoordinate esophageal motility. In these children, the passage of a bolus of semisolid or solid food through the esophagus may be largely dependent on gravity. Any esophageal obstruction due to the fundic impingement on the esophagus can cause obstruction and dysphagia.

Intestinal obstruction develops in 1% to 10% of patients after fundoplication. The likelihood of its occurrence appears to be lessened if additional intaabdominal procedures are limited, if handling of the small intestine is kept to a minimum, and if the dissection involves only the stomach and adjacent structures.

Potential gastrostomy site problems include excoriation at

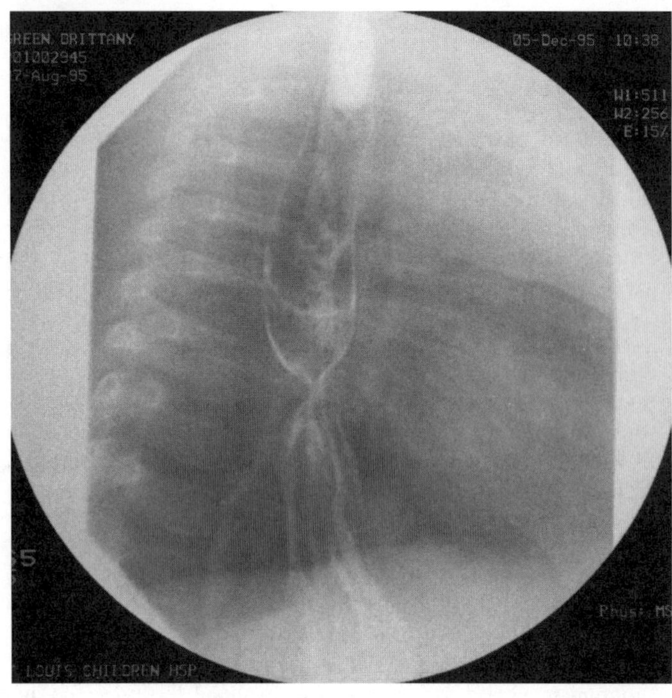
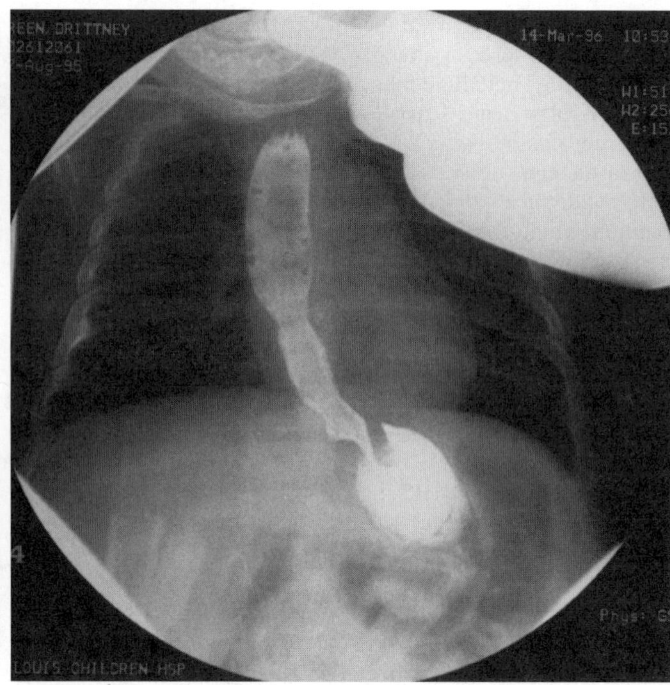

FIG. 62-10. (*A*) Esophagogram showing a tight esophageal stricture in a child after repair of a pure esophageal atresia. This patient had severe gastroesophageal reflux. (*B*) In the same patient 2 months after a Nissen fundoplication and two esophageal dilations, there is resolution of the stricture. In addition can see the fundal wrap around the intraabdominal esophagus.

the exit site on the skin and obstruction of the gastric outlet or proximal small intestine. These are primarily related to the gastrostomy tube not being well secured. If the balloon or bulbous end of the catheter is not pulled up against the anterior gastric wall, gastric juice can leak out along the gastrostomy tract and cause skin irritation. If the tube is not anchored well, a balloon can migrate to the pylorus and cause obstruction, or it can pass into the duodenum and become a source of obstruction there. One of the common causes of emesis in a child with a gastrostomy tube in place is malposition of the tube. The development of the gastrostomy button has largely resolved these problems.

REFERENCES

1. Randolph JG, Lilly JR, Anderson KD. Surgical treatment of gastroesophageal reflux in infants. Ann Surg 1974;180:479.
2. Berquist WE, Rachelefsky GS, Kadden M, et al. Gastroesophageal reflux, associated recurrent pneumonia and chronic asthma in children. Pediatrics 1981;68:29.
3. Jolley SG, Halpern LM, Tunell WP, et al. The risk of sudden infant death from gastroesophageal reflux. J Pediatr Surg 1991;26:691.
4. Stolar CJH, Levy JP, Dillon PW, et al. Anatomic and functional abnormalities in the esophagus in infants surviving congenital diaphragmatic hernia. Am J Surg 1990;159:204.
5. Koot VC, Bergmeijer JH, Bos AP, et al. Incidence and management of gastroesophageal reflux after repair of congenital diaphragmatic hernia. J Pediatr Surg 1993;28:48.
6. Skinner DB. Pathophysiology of gastroesophageal reflux. Ann Surg 1985;202:546.
7. Hillemeier AC. Reflux and esophagitis. In: Walker WA, Durie PR, Hamilton JR, et al, eds. Pediatric gastrointestinal disease. Philadelphia, BC Decker, 1991.
8. DeMeester TR, Dunnington GL. Esophageal anatomy and physiology. In: Greenfield LJ, Mulholland MW, Oldham KT, et al, eds. Surgery: scientific principles and practice. Philadelphia, JB Lippincott, 1993.
9. Fonkalsrud EW, Ellis DG, Shaw A, et al. A combined hospital experience with fundoplication and gastric emptying procedure for gastroesophageal reflux in children. J Am Coll Surg 1995;180:449.
10. Jolley SG, Johnson DG, Herbst JJ, et al. An assessment of gastroesophageal reflux in children by extended pH monitoring of the distal esophagus. Surgery 1978;84:16.
11. DeMeester TR, Wang CI, Wernly JA, et al. Technique, indications and clinical use of 24 hour esophageal pH monitoring. J Thorac Cardiovasc Surg 1980;79:665.
12. Friesen CA, Holder TM, Ashcraft KW, et al. Abbreviated esophageal pH monitoring as an indication for fundoplication in children. J Pediatr Surg 1992;27:776.
13. Nussbaum E, Maji JC, Mathis R, et al. Association of lipid-laden alveolar macrophages and gastroesophageal reflux in children. J Pediatr 1987;110:190.
14. Collins KA, Geisinger KR, Wagner PH, et al. The cytologic evaluation of lipid laden alveolar macrophages as an indicator of aspiration pneumonia in young children. Arch Pathol Lab Med 1995;119:229.
15. Meyers WF, Herbst JJ. Effectiveness of positioning therapy for gastroesophageal reflux. Pediatrics 1982;79:768.
16. Gunasekeran TS, Hassall E. Efficacy and safety of omeprazole for severe gastroesophageal reflux in children. J Pediatr 1993;123:148.
17. Hassall E. Wrap session: is the Nissen slipping? Can medical treatment replace surgery for severe gastroesophageal reflux in children? Am J Gastroenterol 1995;90:1212.
18. Harrington RA, Hamilton CW, Brogden RN, et al. Metoclopramide: an updated review of its pharmacologic properties and clinical use. Drugs 1983;25:451.
19. Foglia RP, Fonkalsrud EW, Ament ME, et al. Gastroesophageal fundoplication for the management of chronic pulmonary disease in children. Am J Surg 1980;140:72.
20. Fonkalsrud EW, Ament ME, Vargas J. Gastric antroplasty for the treatment of delayed gastric emptying and gastroesophageal reflux in children. Am J Surg 1992;164:327.
21. Ashcraft KW. Gastroesophageal reflux. In: Ashcraft KW, Holder TM, eds. Pediatric surgery, ed 2. Philadelphia, WB Saunders, 1993.

22. Bliss D, Hirschl R, Oldham K, et al. Efficacy of anterior gastric fundoplication in the treatment of gastroesophageal reflux in infants and children. J Pediatr Surg 1994;29:1071.

23. Bensoussan AL, Yazbeck S, Carcellar-Blanchard L. Results and complications of Toupet partial posterior wrap: 10 years experience. J Pediatr Surg 1994;29:1215.

24. Randolph JG. Experience with the Nissen fundoplication for correction of gastroesophageal reflux in infants. Ann Surg 1983;198:579.

25. Halpern LM, Jolley SG, Johnson DG. Gastroesophageal reflux: a significant association with central nervous system disease in children. J Pediatr Surg 1991;26:171.

26. Fonkalsrud EW, Foglia RP. Operative treatment for the gastroesophageal reflux syndrome in children. J Pediatr Surg 1989;24:525.

27. Martinez DA, Ginn-Pease ME, Caniano DA. Sequelae of antireflux surgery in profoundly disabled children. J Pediatr Surg 1992;27:267.

28. Buchmiller TL, Curr M, Fonkalsrud EW. Assessment of alkaline reflux in children after Nissen fundoplication and pyloroplasty. J Am Coll Surg 1994;178:1.

Abdomen and Abdominal Wall

Surgery of Infants and Children: Scientific Principles and Practice, edited by Keith T. Oldham, Paul M. Colombani, and Robert P. Foglia. Lippincott–Raven Publishers, Philadelphia, © 1997.

CHAPTER 63

Clinical Principles of Abdominal Surgery

George W. Holcomb, III

PERITONEUM

The peritoneal cavity is divided into two separate cavities connected by the epiploic foramen. This opening connects the lesser sac behind the stomach and liver with the greater peritoneal cavity. Anatomically, the general peritoneal sac is divided into several spaces, owing to the fixed visceral attachments to the retroperitoneum. The right and left subphrenic spaces are common locations for abscess formation. The left and right subhepatic spaces are located between the liver and transverse mesocolon and are separated by the epiploic foramen. The right subhepatic space is a common site for inflammatory processes arising from the biliary system, the head of the pancreas, and the duodenum. Located to the right of the small bowel mesentery, the right infracolic space has direct communication with the right subhepatic space. Viscera included in this space are the appendix, cecum, and right female adnexa. Because of its location, inflammatory processes from the right infracolic sac may spread to the lesser sac. Similarly, the left infracolic space is located left of the obliquely oriented small bowel mesentery and contains the sigmoid colon and left female adnexa. The remaining spaces include the pelvis and lateral paracolic gutters. Inflammatory processes tend to remain localized to these spaces if host defense mechanisms are effective.

The peritoneum is the serous membrane that encloses the abdominal cavity and is reflected onto its associated viscera. This monolayer lining consists of mesothelial cells in a continuous layer resting on a basement membrane constructed from a collagen lattice. The apical surfaces of the mesothelial cells are lined with microvilli so that the entire surface area of the peritoneum is approximately equal to that of the skin.

A complex circulation system present within the peritoneum provides a small volume of fluid for lubricating purposes that promotes mobility between visceral organs. Excess fluid accumulates in the subdiaphragmatic spaces and is actively pumped into the thoracic duct with diaphragmatic contraction. Although clearance of excess peritoneal fluid is effective, this process may also promote entry of bacteria into the systemic circulation, causing bacteremia. An additional fluid transfer mechanism is the lymphatic system. The diaphragmatic and peritoneal lymphatics are large and do not have valves or occlusive junctions.

With certain diseases and during peritoneal dialysis, these lymphatics play an important part in transport of fluids. In addition to clearance through the above-mentioned transport mechanisms, the peritoneum contains macrophages, mast cells, basophils, and eosinophils, which respond to inflammation and infection.

In response to injury, peritoneal healing differs from skin. The entire peritoneal defect becomes endothelialized simultaneously, not from the borders, as occurs with epidermalization of skin wounds.[1,2] Moreover, the granulation and contraction that occurs around the edges of skin wounds does not occur during peritoneal healing. Reepithelialization of the parietal peritoneum occurs within 5 to 6 days of injury with complete repair by 8 days. Healing of the visceral peritoneum does not differ significantly from that of the parietal peritoneum, but it may occur 1 to 2 days earlier.[3] Several studies have confirmed that reepithelialization from peritoneal injury appears to occur faster in immature versus mature rats. In two studies, mesothelial regeneration was complete by 5 days in the immature rat compared with 7 days in the adult rat.[4,5]

Innervation

The parietal peritoneum is derived from the somatopleural mesoderm, while the splanchnopleural mesoderm gives rise to the visceral peritoneum. Because of this different derivation, the parietal peritoneum shares its neurovascular and lymphatic connections with the musculoskeletal abdominal wall, while the visceral peritoneum shares its connections with its associated visceral organs. For this reason, perception of painful stimuli is markedly different between the visceral and parietal peritoneum.

Visceral pain is perceived through neuronal pathways from the lower thoracic and lumbar splanchnic nerves and from the parasympathetic pathways of the vagus and sacral plexus. As such, visceral pain is usually dull and aching, and it may be poorly localized. A steady, vague pain usually occurs after inflammation of the visceral peritoneum, whereas severe, intermittent, colicky pain results from hollow visceral obstruction. Moreover, nausea, vomiting, and sweating commonly occur with visceral inflammation.

Generalized discomfort in the epigastric, periumbilical, and hypogastric regions may correspond with foregut, midgut, and hindgut inflammation. Inflammatory processes in the stomach, pancreas, duodenum, and biliary system may initially be manifested with vague epigastric discomfort. Similarly, small bowel and right and transverse colon inflammation is sensed as periumbilical discomfort, while left colon, sigmoid, and rectal pain is perceived as lower abdominal pain.

Because neuronal innervation to the parietal peritoneum is derived from the somatic nerves supplying the adjacent abdominal wall structures and skin, inflammatory stimulation is usually more localized, intense, and constant than with visceral pain. Stimulation of the parietal peritoneum is usually responsible for localization of the disease process. An example of the difference between recognition of visceral and parietal stimuli is found with appendicitis. Early appendiceal distention may be manifested by a periumbilical dull or cramping discomfort. With inflammation of the overlying parietal peritoneum, localization of the pain to the right lower quadrant typically develops, leading to the diagnosis of appendicitis.

Adhesions

Peritoneal adhesions occur as a by-product of laparotomy and inflammation. A number of drugs, including corticosteroids, nonsteroidal antiinflammatory agents, and dextran, have been used to decrease postoperative adhesions. Although corticosteroids have not been found to be useful, ibuprofen and dextran have proved to be of some benefit.[6–10] Barrier agents, such as polytetrafluoroethylene and oxidized regenerated cellulose, have also been used in gynecologic studies.[11–13] With intact hemostasis, these agents have been observed to be effective in localized peritoneal injury. Instillation of crystalloid solution has also been tried to decrease postoperative adhesions, but this isolated agent has not been effective.[10,14]

Controversy exists whether peritoneal closure to cover areas denuded by previous dissection is beneficial. A large number of animal studies demonstrate enhanced adhesion formation to suture lines when the peritoneum is closed over denuded tissue.[15] Experimental evidence indicates that areas stripped of peritoneum heal satisfactorily.[16,17] Moreover, suturing of the peritoneum may actually increase the formation of adhesions.[16,17–19] It has been postulated that one way to reduce postoperative adhesions is through the use of laparoscopic surgery. In a prospective multicenter trial, second-look laparoscopy and adhesiolysis were performed.[20] Of the areas where laparoscopic adhesiolysis had been previously performed, 67% contained adhesions at second-look laparoscopy. De novo adhesion formation, however, was substantially reduced by the laparoscopic surgery—new adhesions were noted in only 16% of the patients. Reduced adhesions were also found by Garrard and colleagues[21] in an experimental study comparing laparotomy and laparoscopy. Therefore, it appears that laparoscopic surgical techniques may reduce de novo adhesion formation, although reformation of old adhesions that have been lysed continues to be a major problem.

ACUTE ABDOMINAL CONDITIONS

Acute abdominal diseases in infants, children, and adolescents are often different from those conditions found in adults.

Congenital abnormalities are usually the cause for abdominal symptoms in infants and young children. As the child grows older, diseases and symptoms common to adults become more prevalent.

The approach to the patient depends largely on the patient's age. Historical data may be lacking in infants and children too young to verbalize their complaints specifically. Often, young parents are not as perceptive as grandparents in detailing an accurate history of the young child's symptoms. Moreover, children may be placed in daycare centers, and a detailed history may actually be unknown to the parents.

Physical examination is most important and often difficult in determining the cause of a child's illness. The young child may be frightened and apprehensive, thus precluding an accurate examination. It may be helpful to examine an infant or young child in the parent's lap where they feel secure and comfortable, allowing a more accurate evaluation. In addition, abdominal palpation may be easier to perform and more information may be gained with the use of a stethoscope rather than the physician's hand. Often, children relax their abdominal muscles if they believe the physician is merely trying to listen to abdominal sounds rather than attempting to elicit tenderness. It is usually best to examine the region of suspected abdominal pathology last to get a more accurate interpretation of the abdominal examination. When examining the location of symptoms first, the child may become apprehensive and sense that the remainder of the examination also will be painful. When examining young children and adolescents, another helpful maneuver is to distract the child from the examination through talking. Questions about school, play, siblings, family, and so forth may distract the child from the palpation and permit a more accurate evaluation.

The rectal and pelvic examination in infants and children may not be as helpful as in adults. Rectal examination is not necessary in every case of abdominal discomfort. When indicated, however, it may be useful in eliciting a cause for the symptoms. Similarly, rarely do prepubescent girls need a pelvic examination. Rectal examination may serve the same purpose by documenting the presence of a cervix, uterus or pelvic abscess and other masses. External genitalia examination, however, is an important component to evaluation of the child with abdominal symptoms because vaginal atresia, imperforate hymen, or foreign bodies can cause abdominal symptoms.

Laboratory data can be useful in children with abdominal symptoms. Hematocrit, leukocyte count, and urinalysis should be helpful in most children with these complaints. Other, more specific tests, such as serum amylase, sedimentation rate, liver function tests, and clotting tests, may be reserved for investigation of suspected organ cause. Sometimes, radiographic tests are the most helpful in evaluating abdominal symptoms in infants and children. These may be especially advantageous in infants who present with abdominal distention, nausea, and vomiting. In general, supine and upright radiographs should be performed when plain films are requested. In infants, a left decubitus radiograph serves the same purpose as an upright and may demonstrate evidence of pneumoperitoneum and obstruction. A prone cross-table lateral radiograph is helpful in documenting the presence or absence of air in the rectum. The absence of rectal gas may be useful in diagnosing conditions, such as small bowel obstruction, intestinal atresia, and meconium ileus. Chest radiographs may also be helpful because pneumonia can cause upper abdominal discomfort, particularly with pleurisy. When evaluating a child with fever and abdominal complaints, it is important to realize that pneumonia may not be apparent if the child is dehydrated but will be evident on subsequent chest radiographs after rehydration. Ultrasound examination can be useful in evaluating abdominal symptoms as well. Most pediatric radiologists are adept at imaging both solid and hollow intestinal viscera and frequently can determine the cause of a child's complaints. It is important, however, to provide the ultrasonographer with as much information as possible relating to the history and examination so that the study is directed toward the suspected organ. Computed tomography (CT) examination may also be employed in cases in which plain radiographs and sonographic studies have failed to determine the diagnosis. Moreover, CT and even magnetic resonance imaging (MRI) may be required when a neoplasm is suspected.

Specific abdominal conditions are addressed in individual chapters. In general, however, certain diseases are more frequent in infants than in older children and adolescents. Acute abdominal symptoms in infants may occur from incarceration of an inguinal hernia, intestinal obstruction from intussusception, or intestinal volvulus and from necrotizing enterocolitis (NEC) or meconium ileus. Peculiar to infancy is pyloric stenosis with forceful vomiting.

Prepubertal children can have abdominal symptoms from appendicitis, mesenteric adenitis, urinary tract infection, and viral syndromes. In addition, constipation is commonly seen in young children and often mimics symptoms of acute abdominal disease. Moreover, abdominal symptoms may be seen in diseases such as sickle cell crisis, hemolytic uremic syndrome, Henoch-Schönlein purpura, and pneumonia. In older children, diseases seen in adults become more common. Included in this group are gallstones, pancreatitis, inflammatory bowel disease, salpingitis, and appendicitis. Ovarian neoplasms, cysts, and torsion also occur in adolescent girls. Traumatic abdominal injury may occur in children of all ages and requires special investigation.

SURGICAL TECHNIQUES

Laparoscopy

Although Stephen Gans[22,23] described diagnostic laparoscopy for a contralateral inguinal hernia and laparoscopy for other diseases in 1973, few pediatric surgeons were quick to incorporate laparoscopy into their practices. Before 1987, most laparoscopic procedures in adults were performed by gynecologists. After the initial report of laparoscopic cholecystectomy by Dubois and colleagues in 1989,[24] and the sentinel article by Reddick and Olsen in 1989,[25] a revolution in endoscopic surgery began. Now, a large number of open procedures in adults have an endoscopic counterpart. Application of this new endoscopic approach has been less rapid in children, however, primarily because the advantages of the endoscopic route, such as decreased hospitalization, reduced discomfort, improved cosmesis, and a faster return to work, may not be as relevant to children as to adults. Moreover, small incisions are already employed for a variety of pediatric surgical procedures, and use of several small incisions for endoscopic surgery may not be more beneficial. Nevertheless, certain pediatric operations lend

themselves to an endoscopic approach, and this may become the preferred approach in some of these in the future.

Although the principles of the laparoscopic technique for children are similar to those used in adults, several unique differences require special attention. Because of the smaller abdominal cavity in children, especially infants, it is important to separate the cannulas as widely as possible to provide adequate working space for efficient performance of the operation. Placement of the ports too closely hinders the operation and most likely diminishes the advantages of this approach. As an example, for cholecystectomy in adults, the epigastric cannula is usually positioned in the midline of the epigastrium, and the right lower port is often placed just below the level of the umbilicus. In a young child, however, the epigastric incision should be situated more to the patient's left, and the right lower port may be placed in the inguinal crease, which separates the cannulas sufficiently for an adequate working space.

Infants and young children have pliable abdominal walls. Therefore, it is necessary to advance the trocar cautiously as it penetrates the peritoneum to prevent injury to the underlying viscera and intestine. Once the sharp trocar has penetrated the peritoneum, it is prudent to direct it anteriorly above the underlying intestine, viscera, and major vessels as the trocar and cannula are inserted deeper into the abdominal cavity. In addition, use of the Veress needle in children and, in particular, infants is discouraged for creation of pneumoperitoneum. A much safer technique is an umbilical cutdown with insertion of the umbilical cannula into the peritoneal cavity under direct vision. This cutdown technique should prevent serious injury related to a blind puncture of the peritoneal cavity with the Veress needle.

Another special concern in children is excessive abdominal insufflation. In a research model, Liem and associates[26] demonstrated a direct correlation between insufflation pressure using CO_2 and hypercapnea. In addition, there was marked acidemia, hypoxia, and increased exhaled CO_2 with higher insufflation pressures. The authors recommended using insufflation pressures of less than 15 mmHg. Many pediatric surgeons, however, continue to use 15 mmHg as the maximum inflating pressure without apparent adverse clinical sequelae.

Absolute contraindications to laparoscopy include abdominal wall sepsis at the cannula site, an uncorrectable bleeding disorder, and the inability to create a pneumoperitoneum. The most important relative contraindication is severe inflammation of the target organ, such as the appendix or gallbladder, particularly when perforated.

Diagnostic and Procedural Laparoscopy

Laparoscopy can be employed for diagnostic purposes or for performance of a definitive operation. Diagnostic laparoscopy can be valuable in infants and children. Indications for diagnostic laparoscopy include evaluation of a nonpalpable testis, determination of the presence or absence of a contralateral patent processus vaginalis (CPPV) in a child with a known unilateral inguinal hernia, evaluation for chronic abdominal pain, diagnostic assessment for the presence of appendicitis, evaluation of traumatic injury, and in children with cancer.

A thorough preoperative conference is arranged with the parents and child, if age appropriate, at which time the procedure, risks, and benefits are discussed. General endotracheal anesthesia is usually preferred, but mask anesthesia is possible for short cases.[27] An orogastric tube is inserted for genetic decompression, and the bladder is emptied using a Credé maneuver. The bladder is generally not catheterized, especially in young boys, to avoid iatrogenic urethral injury.

The abdomen is prepared and draped widely. An umbilical cutdown is performed for visual access to the abdominal cavity. Use of the Veress needle for initial insufflation is discouraged owing to the risk of injury to the abdominal viscera and vasculature. For brief diagnostic laparoscopy, especially in infants, a 3-mm cannula and telescope may be sufficient. For more extensive visualization and in older patients, either a 5-mm or 10-mm cannula and telescope are preferred. When operative laparoscopy is required, additional ports can be inserted as needed. Insufflation pressures up to 15 mmHg have not caused significant adverse clinical sequelae in the authors' experience with more than 500 laparoscopies.

Evaluation for a Nonpalpable Testis

The use of laparoscopy in boys with nonpalpable testes has a number of advantages and few disadvantages. Some surgeons who do not favor this approach argue that a complete examination of the inguinal region and abdominal cavity can be performed through an inguinal approach and that it is rarely necessary to resort to a two-stage procedure for orchiopexy.[28,29] Proponents of the laparoscopic approach emphasize two valid points. First, some intraabdominal testes are not identified at the time of inguinal exploration and are even missed by experienced surgeons.[30,31] Second, a laparoscopic approach allows the surgeon to defer the second-stage Fowler-Stephens orchiopexy, when indicated, preventing disruption of the vasal collateral vessels that might occur with extensive dissection using an initial inguinal incision. With a two-stage approach for the abdominal testis (initial laparoscopy with vascular ligation followed later by Fowler-Stephens orchiopexy), the success rate should be greater than a one-stage approach, although the reported data are described in only a few small series with short follow-up evaluations.[32–34]

The present concept of a two-staged approach for a nonpalpable testis began in 1959 when Fowler and Stephens[35] described the role of the testicular vascular anatomy and the salvage of high undescended testes. Until 1984, however, a single-stage approach was used by most surgeons. Ransley and colleagues[36] described the preliminary ligation of the gonadal vessels before orchiopexy for an intraabdominal testis in 10 patients. Although it was difficult for the authors to quantify successful augmentation of the vasal collateral circulation with the initial ligation, it was their subjective opinion that the increased vascularity was significant. Moreover, the enlarged bulk of the vascular pedicle containing the vas and vessels greatly facilitated dissection during subsequent orchiopexy. The first use of laparoscopy to locate an impalpable testis was described by Cortesi and associates in 1976.[37] Others also have reported the use of endoscopy for this purpose, but Bloom[32] was the first to describe a planned two-step approach with initial pelviscopic clip ligation of the spermatic vessels followed several months later by an open Fowler-Stephens orchiopexy. Since that report, others have described their experiences with this two staged procedure when the testis is visualized in an intraabdominal position.[31,34,37–40] Moreover, laparoscopic orchiectomy has been advocated in teenagers and in younger children with an atrophic testis or ambiguous external genitalia.[41–44]

Under general anesthesia before laparoscopy, a final examination is performed to ensure that the testicle is not palpable. When the testis is located in the inguinal canal or scrotum with the patient under anesthesia, then laparoscopy is not necessary. When the testis is not palpated, however, laparoscopy is performed, and the findings help the surgeon determine whether

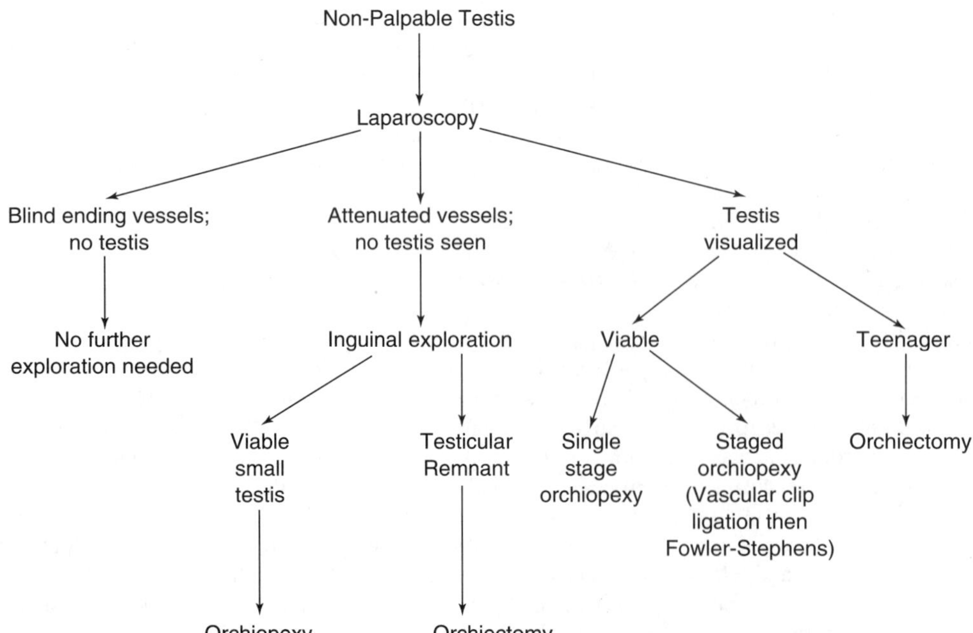

FIG. 63-1. Algorithm depicting the operative management of patients with nonpalpable testes undergoing initial diagnostic laparoscopy. The next operative step depends on the findings at diagnostic laparoscopy.

vascular clip ligation, orchiectomy, or an inguinal exploration is indicated (Fig. 63-1).

At diagnostic laparoscopy for the nonpalpable testis, several findings may be apparent. If a testis is found intraabdominally and the vascular leash appears short, then initial endoscopic clip ligation can be performed laparoscopically. A 5-mm ipsilateral lower abdominal incision is made for placement of a cannula, as is a 3-mm suprapubic incision. A 3-mm grasping forceps is inserted through the suprapubic cannula for dissection and elevation of the vascular leash. A 5-mm endoscopic clip applier is directed through the 5-mm port, and the vascular pedicle is ligated at least 1 cm from the testicle (Fig. 63-2). Great care should be taken to ensure that the ureter is not incorporated in the vascular ligation. The operation is then terminated, incisions are closed, and the patient is awakened from anesthesia. Six to 9 months later, the patient returns for a Fowler-Stephens orchiopexy, with the testicle then being nourished by collateral vessels surrounding the vas deferens.

If the testis is identified to be high in the inguinal canal, but not truly intraabdominal (so-called peeping testis), then usually a one-stage orchiopexy is possible (Fig. 63-3). On occasion, however, it may not be possible to relocate this testicle in the scrotum, thus requiring a staged procedure.

If there is no evidence of a testis, but a normal vascular pedicle and vas deferens are seen entering a closed internal ring, then inguinal exploration is probably indicated. Although the vas deferens and testicular vessels are likely to lead the surgeon to an atrophic testicular remnant, Turek and colleagues[45] found 6% of such specimens to have seminiferous tubules with germal elements. They recommended excision of these testicular remnants because of increased malignant potential. On occasion, however, a small, but viable, testis is found, and orchiopexy is possible.

At laparoscopy, if the testicular vessels are noted to end blindly and do not enter the internal ring, then inguinal explora-

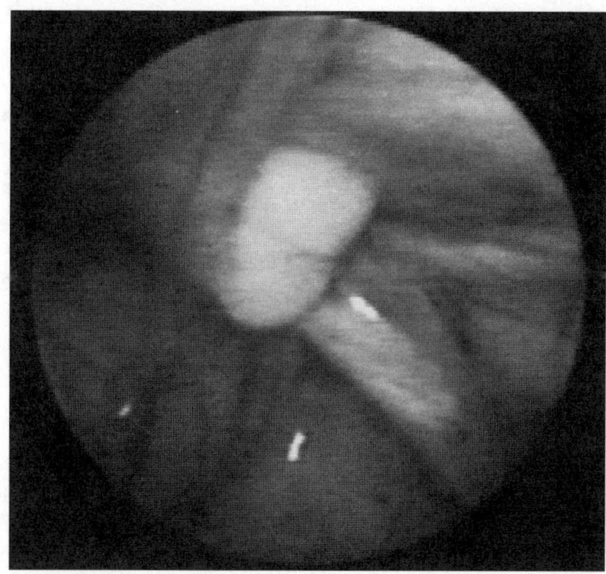

FIG. 63-3. Laparoscopic view depicting a "peeping testis," which resides in the inguinal canal and is pushed into the abdominal cavity with external manual pressure. This accounts for the fact that the testis is not palpable on examination. Most of these testes can be brought into the scrotum using conventional orchiopexy. (Holcomb GW III, Brock JW III, Neblett WW III, et al. Laparoscopy for the nonpalpable testis. Am Surg 1994;60:143)

tion is not indicated. In a study from Children's Hospital at Vanderbilt University Medical Center (CH-VUMC), no tissue submitted at the end of blind-ending testicular vessels, whether documented laparoscopically or at surgical exploration, was found to have viable testicular tissue.[46]

In teenagers with intraabdominal testes or in younger children with atrophic intraabdominal testes, orchiectomy can be performed laparoscopically or though a separate inguinal incision. Laparoscopic orchiectomy is accomplished in a similar fashion to clip ligation, as previously described. The peritoneum overlying the vessels and vas deferens is incised, and the vascular pedicle and vas deferens are ligated using endoscopic clips. Using the cautery, the remaining tissue around the intraabdominal testis is severed, and the testis is removed (Fig. 63-4).

Between 1988 and 1992, 287 infants and children were evaluated for an undescended testis at CH-VUMC.[34] In 35 boys, the testis was not palpable, and these boys underwent initial diagnostic laparoscopy. In 11 boys, the testis was visualized at endoscopy. In 7 patients, it was found in an inguinal hernia sac, and a single-stage conventional orchiopexy was performed in each of these boys. In 4 boys, an intraabdominal testis was seen, and 3 infants underwent laparoscopic clip ligation of the testicular vessels. An initial orchiectomy was required in 1 teenage patient. The 3 infants with initial laparoscopic clip ligation subsequently had a second-stage Fowler-Stephens procedure, with clinical success determined 1-year postoperatively. In 21 of the remaining 24 boys, small attenuated testicular vessels were noted to pass into the inguinal canal, thus requiring an inguinal exploration. A small atrophic testicular remnant was excised in 15 patients, but orchiopexy was possible in 6 patients because an adequate-sized testicle was found.

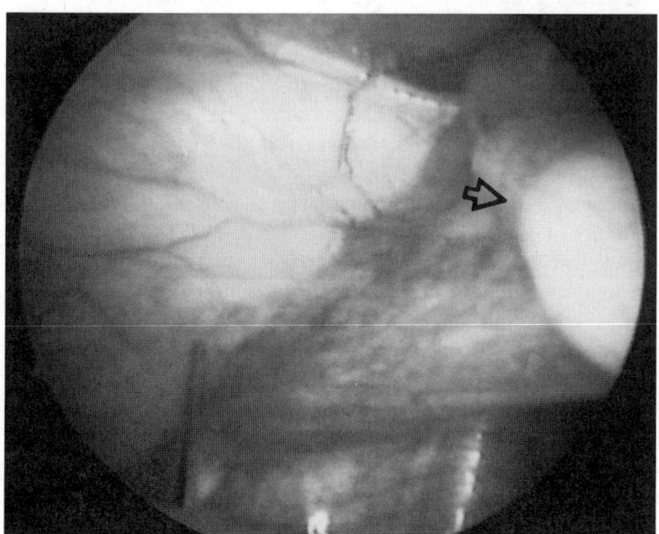

FIG. 63-2. An endoscopic clip has been placed across the testicular vessels as the first stage of a two-stage Fowler-Stephens procedure for an intraabdominal testis (arrow). (Holcomb GW III, Brock JW III, Neblett WW III, et al. Laparoscopy for the nonpalpable testis. Am Surg 1994;60:143)

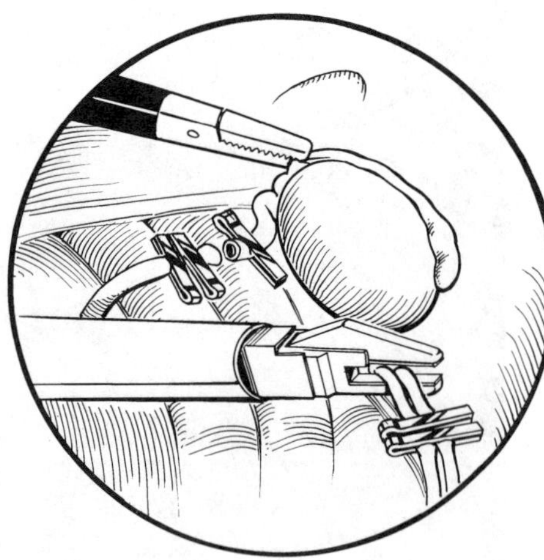

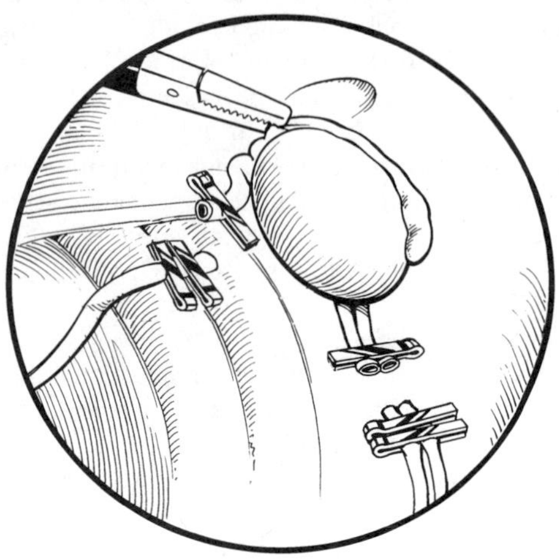

FIG. 63-4. Drawing depicting laparoscopic orchiectomy for an intraabdominal testis in a teenager or younger child with an atrophic abdominal testis. (Holcomb GW III, Brock JW III, Neblett WW III, et al. Laparoscopy for the nonpalpable testis. Am Surg 1994;60:143)

Laparoscopy for Contralateral Patent Processus Vaginalis

A controversial subject among pediatric surgeons continues to be whether to perform a contralateral exploration under the same anesthesia in an infant or child with a known unilateral inguinal hernia. Advocates of routine bilateral exploration note that between 40% and 60% of children have a CPPV, and bilateral exploration prevents the need for a repeat operation with hernia repair in the future. A second anesthesia and the cost of a second procedure are avoided using this approach.[47–50] Proponents for repair of the unilateral hernia alone argue that only 10% to 30% of children undergoing unilateral hernia repair return with a symptomatic contralateral hernia; therefore, in most children, an unnecessary contralateral operation would be avoided.[51,52] Moreover, there is a small risk of injury to the testicle and vas deferens during inguinal exploration, which also would be avoided. One report of 313 children undergoing inguinal herniorrhaphy documented segments of vas deferens in five specimens (1.6%).[47] In another review, 160 infants with unilateral or bilateral repair were followed for up to 20 years and were discovered to have a 2% incidence of testicular atrophy.[51]

Attempts at documenting whether a CPPV exists are not new. In 1967, Kramer and Davis[53] described passing a Bake dilator through the known inguinal hernia sac to probe the contralateral side to see if a patent processus existed. Kiesewetter and Oh[50] found herniography to be an accurate way to reduce the incidence of unnecessary contralateral explorations, although they noted disadvantages such as pain with injection, gonadal radiation, and the requirement of an experienced radiologist. Harrison and coworkers[54] and Powell[55] described diagnostic pneumoperitoneum for detecting a clinically occult processus vaginalis.

With the increased use of diagnostic laparoscopy, a study was undertaken at CH-VUMC to ascertain whether laparoscopy would be beneficial in the evaluation of a CPPV in a child with a known unilateral inguinal hernia.[56] After induction of general endotracheal anesthesia, the patient was examined and the surgeon asked to document if a CPPV was present on clinical examination. Diagnostic peritoneoscopy was then performed through the umbilicus using a 3-mm cannula and telescope. Pneumoperitoneum was created to a pressure of 15 mmHg, and the inguinal canal and scrotum were inspected to see if insufflation alone would be sufficient for the diagnosis of CPPV. Diagnostic peritoneoscopy was then performed (Fig. 63-5). Three hundred and ninety-three consecutive patients were evaluated between May 1, 1992 and December 31, 1993. The patients ranged in age from 1 month to 10 years, with a mean of 19.9 months and median of 11 months. Three hundred and forty-three patients were boys, and 54 were girls. Of the 393 patients, 57 had known bilateral inguinal hernias, leaving 336 patients with unilateral inguinal hernias. Two hundred and ninety-six were boys and 40 were girls. Based on physical examination under anesthesia, the surgeon indicated that he would explore the contralateral side in 122 patients; however a CPPV was noted at laparoscopy in only 57 patients (47%). The surgeon determined that he would not explore the contralateral side in 214 patients; however, 78 children (36%) had a CPPV at laparoscopy. Insufflation was not reliable in determining the presence of a CPPV because an inguinal or scrotal bulge was only visualized on the side of the known unilateral inguinal hernia in 219 patients (65%). On the contralateral side documented to have a CPPV, it was present in only 34 patients (25%). Of the 336 patients undergoing laparoscopy, 131 were found to have a unilateral hernia and a CPPV (39%), whereas 205 patients were noted to have a unilateral hernia alone (61%). When added to the 57 patients with known bilateral inguinal hernia, 188

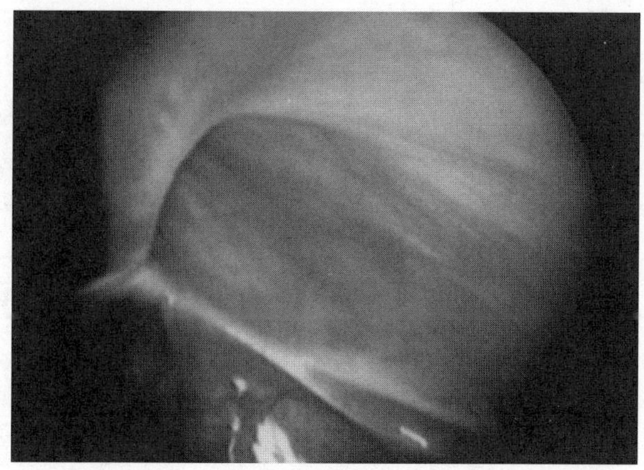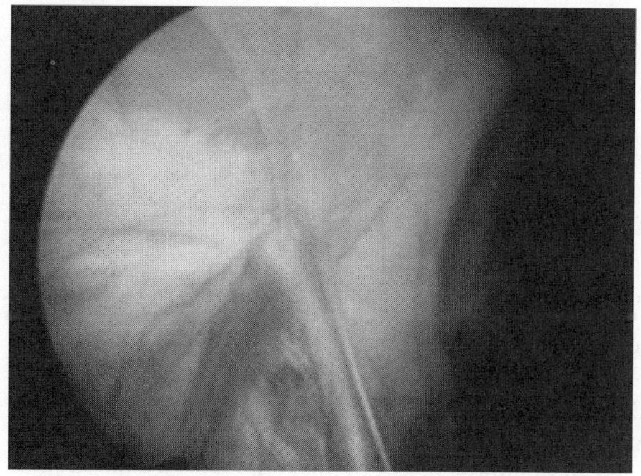

FIG. 63-5. Diagnostic laparoscopy, through the umbilicus is performed in a 6-month-old patient with a known right inguinal hernia (*A*). There is no evidence of a left patent processus vaginalis (*B*), and unnecessary left inguinal exploration is avoided.

(48%) underwent bilateral repair, and 205 patients (52%) underwent unilateral repair.

Complications were minimal in this series. One patient developed an inguinal wound infection managed by antibiotics. No patient has returned with a missed contralateral hernia to date. In one patient, there was a negative exploration on the contralateral side because the CPPV was less than 2 cm in length at exploration, which was the criteria used. This study confirmed previous reports that neither physical examination, abdominal insufflation, patient sex, nor patient age are reliable for determining the need for contralateral exploration. Moreover, it also confirmed that diagnostic laparoscopy can be performed safely even in infants and young children. In comparison with other techniques for determining a CPPV, laparoscopy appears to be the most accurate means of achieving this goal. Another question relates to the method of laparoscopy. The author is exploring whether laparoscopy through the known inguinal hernia sac using a 70-degree telescope will yield similar results.[57]

Other Indications

Evaluation for chronic abdominal pain is another valid indication for diagnostic laparoscopy in children. Despite multiple radiographic studies, laboratory tests, and physical examinations, an open laparotomy is often necessary in selected circumstances when abdominal pain persists. Laparoscopy has been used in children to document the causes of recurring episodes of pain. Telander reported an incidence of positive findings in 60% of 40 cases using laparoscopy for evaluation of chronic abdominal pain (personal communication). Moreover, 30% of these 40 patients had an abnormal appendix on pathologic examination. In a recent presentation, Stafford[58] described his experience with 10 patients. Seven of 10 children improved and became pain free after laparoscopy, which consisted of peritoneal lavage, appendectomy, and lysis of congenital bands or adhesions primarily involving the right colon. The other three children were subsequently found to have systemic mastocytosis, generalized idiopathic myositis, and regional enteritis, respectively. All patients were discharged from the hospital by the third postoperative day. Only one child has required read-

mission for persistent pain and fever, and he was subsequently found to have regional enteritis on repeat colonoscopy. At 7 to 12 months follow-up, Stafford reports that nine children are pain free, and a single child is improving with antiinflammatory medication. Schier and Waldschmidt[59] have also employed peritoneoscopy for this condition with success.

Diagnostic laparoscopy also may be useful in children with suspected appendicitis. In addition, this technique can be used to direct the best location for an open incision when the surgeon for any reason is not comfortable with continuation of the laparoscopic approach. Moreover, it can be used in evaluation of traumatic injuries in children in whom the radiographic and other noninvasive evaluations are equivocal. Also, infants with ambiguous genitalia are ideal candidates for diagnostic laparoscopy for determination of their internal status.[60]

Diagnostic laparoscopy is also being used for evaluation for resectability and for staging purposes in children with cancer when the radiographic evaluations are not diagnostic. Using an initial endoscopic approach, if resectability appears possible, then an open procedure is performed. If resectability is not feasible, however, then biopsy can be performed endoscopically followed by appropriate adjuvant therapy. Second-look laparoscopy may be useful after adjuvant therapy when indicated. In a review of institutions participating in the Children's Cancer Group, 24 children were documented to have undergone laparoscopy as part of their surgical management.[61] Indications included evaluation for possible metastatic tumor or recurrent disease, consideration of a new mass for suspected cancer, and evaluation of hepatoblastoma for resectability. Five patients underwent diagnostic staging laparoscopy, including four with Hodgkin disease. No complications were noted in this group of patients.

Procedural Laparoscopy

Cholecystectomy

Laparoscopic cholecystectomy is the preferred technique for cholecystectomy of many pediatric surgeons.[62–66] Advantages of the laparoscopic route include a shorter postoperative hospitalization, reduced discomfort, and improved cosmesis.[67] Whether the children actually have a faster return to routine activities such as school and play has not been documented, although it is suspected that this is also a benefit.

The indications for laparoscopic cholecystectomy are similar to those for the open procedure. Contraindications to the laparoscopic approach were mentioned earlier.

A four-cannula technique is employed in children. The epigastric port should be placed more to the patient's left in smaller children, and the right lower port should be placed in the inguinal crease in young children. The two right-sided 5-mm cannulas are used for retraction during the procedure. The final port is either 5 or 10-mm and located in the umbilicus. The telescope is introduced through this cannulua. In children younger than 10 years, a 5-mm umbilical port is sufficient because the optics of the 5-mm telescope are sufficient in these patients. The epigastric port is either 5 mm or 10 mm, depending on the surgeon's preference. It is probably necessary to have at least one 10-mm port so that the gall bladder can be extracted through this cannula. Therefore, if a 5-mm epigastric cannula is inserted, the umbilical port should be 10-mm. This is the author's usual preference as 5-mm endoscopic clip appliers are now available for use through the epigastric port. The gall bladder is removed through the umbilical site.

The principles of the technique are similar to those described in adults and in other reports.[25,63,67,68] After mobilization of the cystic duct, cholangiography is performed in all patients to define the anatomy and help prevent inadvertent common bile duct injury. A Kumar clamp is the author's preferred instrument; this is placed across the infundibulum of the gallbladder (Fig. 63-6). A 23-gauge sclerotherapy needle is inserted down the side arm of the clamp and into the infundibulum. With this technique, lateral incision of the cystic duct is not required in very

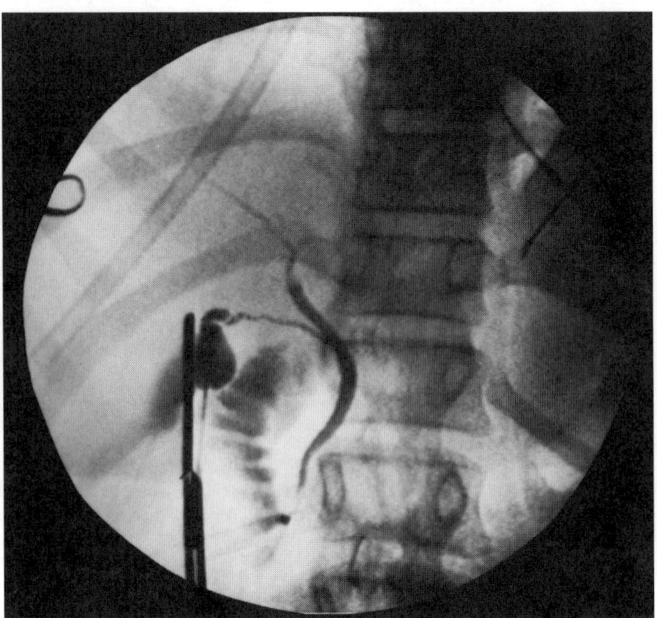

FIG. 63-7. Intraoperative cholangiogram demonstrating free flow through the cystic duct into the common bile duct and duodenum in an 8-year-old patient. Opacification is also seen in the right hepatic duct and in a portion of the left duct.

small children (Fig. 63-7). After cholangiography and with accurate identification of the cystic duct, the duct and cystic artery are divided between clips, and the gallbladder is removed in a retrograde fashion. Several instruments can be employed for retrograde dissection of the gallbladder, including the curved cautery, spatula cautery, and dissecting scissors with cautery attached. Before complete detachment of the gallbladder from the liver, it is important to inspect the gallbladder bed for bleeding. Once the gallbladder is completely detached, this visualization becomes more difficult. The gallbladder can be extracted through a 5-mm incision in very small children but usually requires a 10-mm port in larger children. It is safer to keep children in the hospital overnight for observation, but most can be discharged the day after the procedure on oral analgesics. Occasionally, a child may require 2 postoperative days of hospitalization because of persistent discomfort.

Thirty-five children aged 25 months to 19 years underwent laparoscopic cholecystectomy at CH-VUMC between June 1990 and June 1994. The mean age was 12.3 years, and the median age was 13 years. Seven patients had hemolytic disease, 5 had sickle cell disease, 2 had hereditary spherocytosis, and 21 had idiopathic gallstones. Four patients had undergone a previous procedure; three were gastrostomies, and one was for insertion of a ventriculoperitoneal shunt. Cholangiography was attempted in 33 patients and was successful in 25 patients. In 17 of 19 patients, cholangiography was successful using the Kumar clamp and sclerotherapy technique (Table 63-1).

The mean operative time for elective laparoscopic cholecystectomy was 110 minutes, and the mean time for laparoscopic removal of an acutely inflamed gallbladder was 150 minutes in five patients.

No complications have been noted in the postoperative period. Specifically, there have been no wound infections, biliary leaks, bile duct strictures, retained common duct stones, reoperations, or conversions to an open procedure.

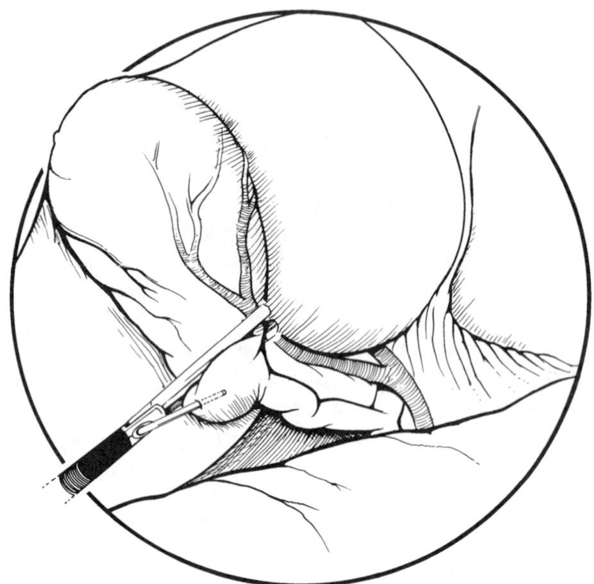

FIG. 63-6. For cholangiography, a Kumar clamp is placed across the infundibulum of the gallbladder. Through the side arm of the clamp, a 23-gauge sclerotherapy needle is advanced into the infundibulum, and cholangiography is performed. With this technique, difficulty advancing a cholangiocatheter into a small cystic duct is avoided.

TABLE 63-1. *Techniques used for laparoscopic cholangiography*

Technique, instruments	Attempted cholangiography	Successful cholangiography
Kumar clamp, sclerotherapy needle	19	17
Olsen clamp, taut cholangiocatheter	9	5
Endoclip, ureteral catheter	4	2
Endoscopic retrograde cholangio-pancreatography, nasobiliary catheter	1	1
TOTALS	33	25

Appendectomy

In 1980, Leape and Ramenosky[69] employed diagnostic laparoscopy to reduce the number of appendectomies performed in which a noninflamed appendix was removed. Three years later, Semm[70] described incidental laparoscopic appendectomy during gynecologic procedures but did not think that laparoscopy should be employed for the acutely inflamed appendix. As procedural laparoscopy has become refined, however, an increasing number of pediatric surgeons are using the laparoscopic approach for appendectomy.[71–76]

The author prefers to use clip ligation. Therefore, the size and position of the cannulas is dependent on whether the endoscopic stapler is utilized. A 10-mm cannula is inserted in the left lower abdominal quadrant and a 5-mm cannula in the umbilicus and suprapubic region. A grasping forceps is placed through the suprapubic port and the appendix retracted inferiorly. With the 5-mm camera in the umbilicus, the working port is the left lower quadrant port through which the dissection is accomplished and the endoscopic clips placed across the mesoappendix. After clip ligation of the mesoappendix, the base of the appendix is ligated with two chromic pretied ligatures, and the appendix is divided distal to the second ligature.

If the endoscopic stapler is preferred, a change in the placement of the cannulas is necessary. A 12-mm cannula is inserted after umbilical cutdown, and a 5-mm port is placed in the left lower quadrant and suprapubic region (Fig. 63-8). The endoscopic stapler is inserted through the umbilical port and employed for ligation and division of the mesoappendix and appendix (Fig. 63-9).

Whether all children should undergo laparoscopic appendectomy for acute appendicitis is debatable. In many patients, especially young, thin children, a 2-cm right lower quadrant incision is sufficient for appendectomy and is usually followed by an early postoperative discharge. Moreover, the laparoscopic approach in a patient with an abscess is also controversial. Laparoscopy does allow irrigation and débridement of the generalized peritoneal cavity with suction evacuation of the infected material under direct visualization. On the other hand, reduced hospitalization has not been shown to be a benefit of the laparos-

copic approach in this situation because most children require prolonged hospitalization for antibiotics and ileus. Moreover, the operative time is increased for the laparoscopic approach for appendicitis with abscess compared with that for appendicitis without abscess.[73,77]

A selective approach to laparoscopic appendectomy may be preferable (Table 63-2). Children older than 8-10 years of age, particularly adolescent girls in whom the diagnosis is unclear regarding either a gynecologic or appendiceal cause for unexplained low abdominal pain and chronic right lower quadrant discomfort, may constitute sufficient indications for the laparoscopic approach. It may be preferable in the moderately obese and obese child in whom larger incisions are needed and the potential for wound infection is increased. In addition, an athlete who desires early return to athletic participation may be a patient in whom laparoscopy is better suited. At this time, there does not appear to be an advantage to the laparoscopic technique for appendicitis with abscess in children.

Using this selective approach, a small group of 65 patients underwent laparoscopic appendectomy at CH-VUMC. Four children had developed abscesses from perforation, but the abscess cavity was opened laparoscopically and appendectomy accomplished in 3 of these patients. One patient required conversion to an open appendectomy. In the remaining 61 patients, 58 had acute nonperforated appendicitis. Of the 3 patients without appendicitis, 1 child had terminal ileitis, and the other 2 patients failed to exhibit any pathology to account for the symptoms. No intraoperative or postoperative complications have developed in this series.

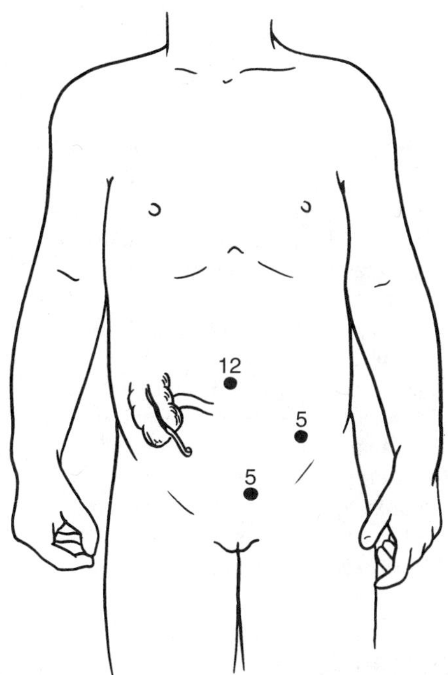

FIG. 63-8. Diagram depicting the preferred locations for the cannulas in the three-port technique for laparoscopic appendectomy. A 12-mm cannula is inserted through the umbilicus. A 5-mm cannula is then placed in the left lower abdominal quadrant and another one in the suprapubic region.

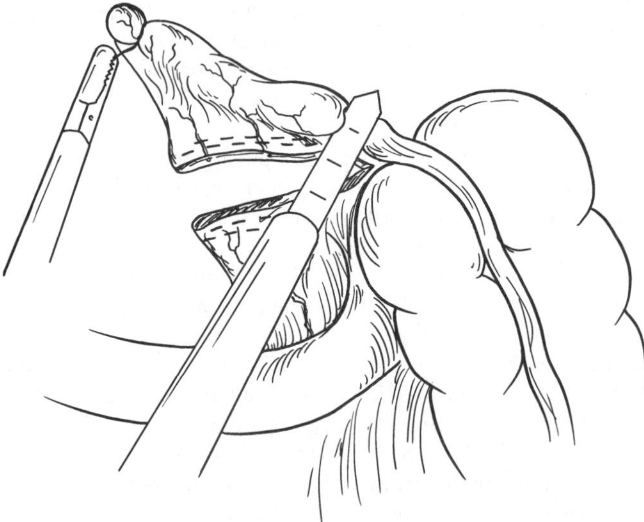

FIG. 63-9. Ligation and division of the mesoappendix and appendix is performed in two separate steps using the endoscopic stapler.

Fundoplication and Splenectomy

The laparoscopic approach is an alternative to the open operation for fundoplication and splenectomy in children. Advantages of the laparoscopic technique for these two procedures include reduced discomfort compared with that of an upper abdominal incision, reduced respiratory complications, and rapid return of pulmonary function.[78–80] In addition, there may be a reduced postoperative ileus as well. Although these advantages have been proposed, there has not been a prospective study between the open and the laparoscopic approaches to these two surgical procedures.

A number of investigators[79–81] have described an early experience with laparoscopic fundoplication. The basic principles of the laparoscopic operation are similar to those of the open procedure. Four or five cannulas are usually employed for the endoscopic procedure. The diaphragmatic crura are approximated, the gastric fundus is mobilized, and a 360-degree Nissen fundoplication is performed using either silk sutures or staples. Alternative techniques, such as the Thal anterior fundoplication, can also be performed laparoscopically. Because most children undergoing fundoplication require gastrostomy, this can be performed either laparoscopically or by use of percutaneous endoscopic gastrostomy. Moreover, pyloromyotomy may be performed laparoscopically, or a pyloroplasty may be accomplished in an open fashion by enlarging one of the upper abdominal laparoscopy incisions.

TABLE 63-2. *Selective approach to laparoscopic appendectomy*

1. Children older than 8–10 years
2. Adolescent girls
3. Obese children
4. Laparoscopy for chronic abdominal pain
5. Athletes

Georgeson[80] reviewed the first 60 children to undergo laparoscopic Nissen fundoplication with and without gastrostomy at the Children's Hospital of Alabama and compared these patients with a similar group of 60 consecutive children undergoing the open operation. The median postoperative stay was 3 days shorter for the laparoscopic group, and these patients also were able to receive feedings sooner than those in the open group.

Successful laparoscopic splenectomy has also been described in children.[82–84] Several important steps are required for completion of the laparoscopic operation. The lienocolic ligament is divided using electrocautery, and the short gastric vessels are ligated with clips, then transected. Sometimes, the most superior short gastric vessel is not divided until after the spleen is mobilized. The lienorenal ligament is then divided, if not done previously, and the spleen is mobilized. The vascular pedicle is then dissected, ligated, and divided. Division of the vascular pedicle can be accomplished in several ways. An endoscopic stapler is preferred by some authors for ligation, followed by division of the entire pedicle. Although mass vascular ligation would not be elected by most pediatric surgeons using the open approach, no complications have been reported to date with this technique. An alternative is careful separation of the artery and vein with individual ligation using suture ligatures followed by division.

After complete mobilization, the spleen is placed into an endoscopic retrieval bag and is then ready for extrusion. A previously used commercial morcellator can be used to dice the specimen into small pieces for removal. An alternative technique is manual morcellation. If the spleen is small, enlarging one of the cannula sites is an alternative technique, and complete extraction is accomplished in this manner. Experienced pathologists can evaluate morcellated tissue, and the adoption of this technique should not interfere with the proper staging and histologic evaluation of the spleen or of other solid pediatric tumors.[83]

Lobe and colleagues[83] described their experience with seven patients. Successful laparoscopic splenectomy was accomplished in six, and one was converted to the open technique because of bleeding from a short gastric vessel. The median operative time was 3.5 hours, and the median postoperative discharge was 2 days. No other complications were described.

Other Indications

A number of additional laparoscopic procedures have been reported in children, including gastrostomy without fundoplication, assistance with insertion and removal of ventriculoperitoneal shunts, gonadectomy for intersex anomalies, ovarian cystectomy, and testicular vein ligation for management of varicocele.[60,85–87] Moreover, increasing experience is being gained with the laparoscopic approach for intestinal resection. Georgeson[88] described his experience with the laparoscopic Soavé operation for correction of Hirschsprung disease in children and neonates without colostomy. In addition, laparoscopic Duhamel and Swenson procedures have been successfully performed. A two-stage approach for ulcerative colitis may be advantageous in the future, with an initial laparoscopic colectomy and ileostomy followed by open mucosal proctectomy and ileoanal anastomosis as a second stage. Advantages would include an early discharge from the hospital after the initial laparoscopic colectomy and reduced operating time for the ileoanal procedure. Other described laparoscopic procedures include guided gastropexy for intermittent gastric volvulus, laparoscopic Meckel diverticulectomy, and laparoscopy for the diagnosis of biliary atresia.[89–91] Laparoscopic nephrectomy has also been reported in children.[92,93]

Laparoscopic pyloromyotomy was initially described by Alain.[94] It has also been reported by Tan[95] with favorable results. Whether the laparoscopic approach will supplant the traditional open procedure is unknown at this time; however, several ongoing prospective trials might answer this question.

A final indication for laparoscopy is in the area of fetal surgery. Researchers at the Fetal Treatment Program at the University of California, San Francisco have developed a technique for endoscopic fetal surgery. With this approach, the risk for preterm labor should be minimized. Studies have progressed in primates, with the ultimate future goal of human application.[96,97]

Complications

A number of reports on laparoscopic procedures in adults have documented complications from specific procedures.[98–102] Little has been written about complications in infants and children, although they are most likely to occur with introduction of the Veress needle and trocars. Because of potential complications with the Veress needle, the authors no longer employ this technique but rather use an umbilical cutdown with direct visual insertion of the umbilical cannula into the peritoneal cavity. As previously mentioned, careful attention is given to introduction of a sharp trocar to prevent underlying intestinal, visceral, and vascular injuries in a child with a pliable abdominal wall. Also, misidentification of the cystic or common duct during laparoscopic cholecystectomy is another hazard, but this rarely occurs when a cholangiogram is performed before ligation of any structure believed to be the cystic duct.

Other complications include inadvertent cautery injury to the intestine during dissection or coagulation because the electrical current may arc outside the visualized field. With careful and constant attention to use of the cautery, however, this rarely occurs. Moreover, use of the bipolar instrument should assist in prevention of this complication.

Two other possible complications are bleeding and infection. One reason to use the laparoscopic approach with small incisions is reduction in postoperative wound infection. Therefore, this complication should not occur often. Excessive bleeding may develop, particularly with procedures such as splenectomy or nephrectomy, but these operations should not be performed by inexperienced surgeons. Therefore, most bleeding complications should be controllable in experienced hands. Conversion to an open procedure should be accomplished without hesitation if bleeding becomes excessive during laparoscopy.

Vanderbilt Children's Hospital Experience

Patients undergoing either diagnostic or procedural laparoscopy between January 1990 and October 1993 at Vanderbilt

Children's Hospital were reviewed (Table 63-3). Three hundred and ninety-two patients underwent a diagnostic procedure alone. The most common indication was evaluation of a CPPV in 323 children. One hundred and ninety-five of these patients were reported in a prospective review of this technique.[56] Fifty-six patients underwent laparoscopy alone for evaluation of a nonpalpable testis. Four patients had diagnostic laparoscopy for chronic abdominal pain, and four underwent laparoscopy for evaluation of a recurrent hernia. Other indications included evaluation for possible appendicitis (1), investigation for a traumatic injury (1), differentiation of a duplication versus ovarian cyst (1), evaluation of a persistent postoperative hydrocele (1), and evaluation of a 46XY infant with ambiguous genitalia (1).

Procedural laparoscopy included cholecystectomy (31), appendectomy (18), ligation of testicular vessels for an intraabdominal testis (13), ligation of the testicular vein for management of varicocele (2), gastrostomy (4), insertion and removal of ventriculoperitoneal shunt (5), nephrectomy (1), splenectomy (1), fundoplication (2), gonadectomy (2), insertion of dialysis catheter (1), and ovarian cystectomy (1).

In this series, complications have been minimal. One patient had mild symptoms of postcholecystectomy syndrome after laparoscopic cholecystectomy. A previously mentioned patient who underwent laparoscopic appendectomy was converted to an open procedure, and one undergoing fundoplication was also converted. One patient undergoing removal of a ventriculoperitoneal shunt required conversion to an open procedure because of a small bowel obstruction around the shunt.

Incisions

The location of the abdominal incision for entry into the peritoneal cavity should be individualized according to the pro-

TABLE 63-3. *Laparoscopic experience with 473 patients at Children's Hospital, Vanderbilt University Medical Center, January 1990 through October 1993*

DIAGNOSTIC (392 PATIENTS)	
Evaluation of contralateral processus vaginalis	323
Evaluation of nonpalpable testis	56
Chronic abdominal pain	4
Evaluation of recurrent hernia	4
Diagnostic for appendicitis	1
Evaluation for possible traumatic injury	1
Duplication versus ovarian cyst	1
Evaluation of chronic postoperative hydrocele	1
Evaluation of 46XY infant with ambiguous genitalia	1
PROCEDURAL (81 PATIENTS)	
Cholecystectomy	31
Appendectomy	18
Vascular ligation of abdominal testis	13
Insertion or removal of ventriculoperitoneal shunt	5
Gastrostomy	4
Ligation of testicular vein (varicocele)	2
Gonadectomy	2
Fundoplication	2
Splenectomy	1
Nephrectomy	1
Ovarian cystectomy	1
Insertion of dialysis catheter	1

posed operation. Other factors include the experience and training of the surgeon, the size and age of the patient, and the possibility of previous abdominal operations. In general, a laparotomy is performed through a transverse incision in the newborn, as compared with a midline incision used in adolescents. In newborns, the transverse incisions are usually either supraumbilical or infraumbilical and usually are located on the right side of the abdomen because of diseases specific to newborns. A supraumbilical transverse incision is usually preferred for correction of malrotation, repair of duodenal stenosis or atresia, and biliary exploration. Some pediatric surgeons prefer the supraumbilical approach for NEC as well. A right infraumbilical transverse incision may be used for exploration for NEC and for exploration for intussusception, distal intestinal atresia, or obstruction and meconium ileus.

For some neonatal conditions, stomas are required as a temporary measure if the infant is critically ill, is too small for primary anastomosis, or has NEC. Although location of the stoma is an individual decision, the author prefers placement through the lateral or medial aspect of the incision. Because the abdominal cavity is usually explored through a transverse right lower quadrant incision for most diseases requiring a stoma, the stoma may be exteriorized either medially or laterally through that incision. A side-by-side double-barreled enterostomy is the preferred technique because, at subsequent closure, a formal laparotomy is not required. Also, access to the distal bowel is preferred in some circumstances for radiographic evaluation of obstruction or distal strictures. An alternative technique, however, is a single functioning stoma with closure of the distal end, which is positioned just beneath the peritoneum.

A controversial issue among pediatric surgeons is drainage of appendiceal abscesses after appendectomy. If drainage is desired and Penrose drains are employed, these can be placed in the right pelvis and right paracolic subhepatic region, then exteriorized through the lateral aspect of the incision. If a closed-suction drain is preferred, it may be exteriorized separately from the abdominal incision, but the incision itself is not drained. Drainage through the incision allows the surgeon to close the remainder of the wound in a subcuticular fashion, which leaves a small amount of the skin open at the drain site. An improved cosmetic appearance results with this subcuticular closure.

Stomas

Stomas are frequently required in pediatric surgery. Most are temporary, although in selected cases, a permanent ostomy is necessary.

Gastrostomy

Gastrostomies are often performed in infants and children for nutritional supplementation either in conjunction with fundoplication or as an isolated procedure. The most common site for placement is along the greater curvature of the stomach, with tube exteriorization in the left upper abdominal quadrant. If a lesser curvature gastrostomy site is selected, exteriorization may be preferable in the right upper abdominal quadrant. Regardless of site selection, it is important to position the stoma

away from the costal margin because the stoma tends to rise superiorly as the child grows, which can cause complications later. A Janeway gastrostomy may also be employed, although it has the disadvantage of possible leakage of gastric contents, with resulting skin irritation and breakdown. It is entirely satisfactory, however, if leakage does not occur.

Enterostomy

In infants too small for primary anastomosis or in those with large discrepancies between proximal and distal intestines, a temporary enterostomy is often required. Several different techniques are available for creation of an enterostomy in infants and children. In 1957, Bishop and Koop[103] described an end-to-side Roux-en-Y anastomosis between proximal and distal ileum for intestinal obstruction due to meconium ileus. The distal ileum is brought out as a single ileostomy stoma. The advantage of this technique is that a small catheter may be inserted through the ileostomy into the distal bowel with instillation of liquefying solutions for passage of the remaining tenacious meconium. Moreover, ileostomy closure can often be accomplished by oversewing the cutaneous stoma, leaving the patent functional end-to-side anastomosis intact. A disadvantage of this technique is the creation of an intraabdominal anastomosis usually between bowel of widely disparate size, which may leak causing peritonitis. Santulli and Blanc[104] described a reverse of the Bishop-Koop stoma for management of this problem. Using this technique, the proximal dilated intestine is exteriorized as a single stoma, and the narrow distal intestine is anastomosed end-to-side just below the peritoneum. Irrigation can also be accomplished using this single stoma, but a formal ileostomy closure is usually required.

Another stomal technique is exteriorization of the two limbs of intestine side to side, either through the laparotomy incision or through a separate incision (Fig. 63-10). The advantage of this technique is the absence of an intraabdominal anastomosis. Formal closure is usually required, however, although it is often a procedure confined to the area of the stoma without general abdominal exploration and an accompanying ileus. This is the preferred technique in very small or very sick infants.

A loop ileostomy is often used for intestinal diversion in children after colectomy and mucosal proctectomy with ileoanal anastomosis for ulcerative colitis. The intent of diversion is prevention of leakage of the ileoanal anastomosis with resulting pelvic sepsis. This stoma is usually closed within 2 months after the original procedure.

A final technique for ileostomy is end-ileostomy with closure of the distal segment. This is certainly acceptable in cases in which access to the distal bowel is not required. In patients with NEC, however, when radiographic examination of the distal ileum is desired before stomal closure, it is usually preferable to exteriorize the two limbs of bowel side by side. With this technique, a prograde study for stricture evaluation is possible through the mucous fistula.

Colostomy

Three techniques for colostomy are employed in infants and children, in contrast to adults, in whom an end-colostomy is

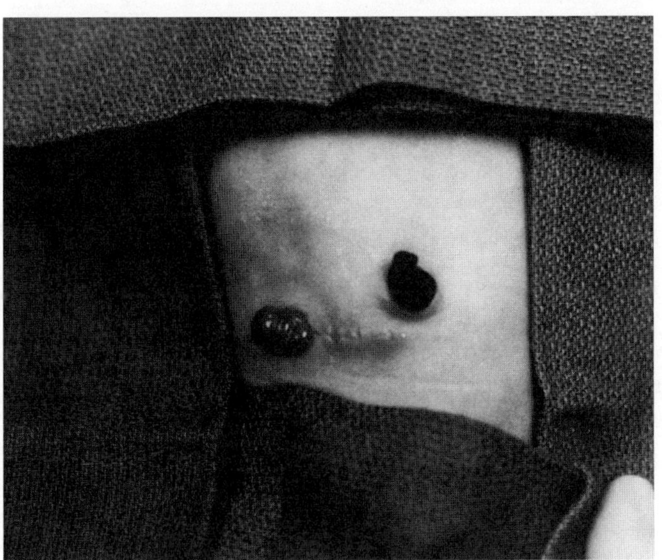

FIG. 63-10. Photograph of a 2200-g infant before enterostomy closure. This patient underwent side-by-side exteriorization through the right lateral aspect of the incision after intestinal resection, which was required for necrotizing enterocolitis.

used almost exclusively. Colostomy is usually required in newborns with Hirschsprung disease and is preferred by most surgeons, although experience is increasing with a primary pullthrough procedure without diversion. For classic rectosigmoid Hirschsprung disease, one of three options is available. A loop colostomy brought through the incision works well, as does an end-colostomy with closure of the distal colon. A divided colostomy is another technique. Because the anus is patent in infants with Hirschsprung disease, spillover from the functioning ostomy to the distal limb is not a significant concern. In cases of high anorectal atresia, however, it is important to separate the proximal and distal fecal streams, and a divided colostomy is preferred. It is important to allow urine to drain from the distal orifice because of the bladder fistula; this tends to prevent hyperchloremic acidosis. The functioning stoma is usually brought out through the lateral aspect of the left lower quadrant incision and the distal stoma exteriorized through the medial aspect of the incision. Regardless of the type of colostomy, it is important to secure the anterior and posterior fascial layers to the bowel to prevent herniation of small intestine with resulting obstruction. Use of silk sutures for fascial attachment is also preferred because visualization of the sutures at subsequent takedown makes fascial dissection easier and helps prevent entry into the colon.

Appendicovesicostomy

Appendicovesicostomy is a stoma unique to pediatric practice. The appendix is used as a catheterizable conduit after bladder augmentation.[105,106] It can be positioned either in the lower abdominal quadrant or in the perineum to provide easy access for bladder catheterization.[107] Because of this potential use, incidental appendectomy should not be performed in patients who

may need bladder augmentation, such as children with spina bifida.

The umbilicus merits special emphasis as a site for placement of intestinal stomas. Cameron[108,109] has recommended the use of the umbilicus for temporary ostomies in infants and children and has reported his experience in 47 patients. Advantages include its convenience for placement of appliances and cosmesis after closure.

Complications

Complications from stomas are not infrequent but can be minimized with careful attention to technique.[110] Mild complications include skin irritation from contact with intestinal contents. This usually occurs because the caregiver is not able to place a tight seal with the appliance around the stoma. The likely reason is that the stoma is flush with the skin and not elevated for easy placement of the appliance. Another reason is that the stoma may be positioned in a place that does not lend itself well to placement of an appliance. For instance, if a colostomy is placed too low in the left or right lower quadrant areas, the appliance may not sit well and may leak because of the contour of the underlying pelvis and hip elevations.

Other complications include stomal prolapse, which is usually confined to the distal colon with a loop or divided colostomy. Small bowel obstruction may develop either around the stoma or from herniation of small bowel loops if the fascial approximation to the colon not properly sutured. As previously mentioned, it is important to secure the colon to the anterior and posterior layers of the fascia with a number of interrupted silk sutures to prevent this complication. In infants with an ileostomy for NEC, it is often not necessary to secure the ileum to the fascia because the dense inflammatory reaction within the abdominal cavity does not allow the small intestine sufficient mobility for herniation. The inflammatory response also helps the ileostomy to attach to the fascial stoma. An important concept to remember is that rarely is a stoma too elevated above the skin in an infant, but a stoma that is flush with the skin usually causes several complications.

SPECIFIC SURGICAL PROBLEMS

Small Bowel Obstruction

Congenital lesions causing small intestinal obstruction usually present in the neonatal period. Examples include intestinal malrotation and other anomalies of rotation, small intestinal atresia, meconium ileus, intestinal aganglionosis, and intestinal duplication anomalies. Detailed discussions of these lesions are presented in other sections of this book.

Acquired causes of small intestinal obstruction include inguinal hernia, intussusception, inflammatory strictures from NEC, appendiceal abscess or Crohn disease, and neoplastic disorders. Lymphoma is the most frequent malignant neoplasm that causes obstruction of the small intestine, and polyps are the most common benign tumor in children. These conditions are also discussed in other chapters.

Small intestinal obstruction may also occur after laparotomy, usually from adhesions. An incidence of 2.2% was reported by

Festen[111] in 1476 laparotomies. Seventy percent of the obstructions in this series were due to a single adhesion.

Any child who has had a previous laparotomy is at risk for adhesive small bowel obstruction. Early symptoms include crampy abdominal pain, anorexia, nausea, and vomiting. Lethargy and reduced activity often occur as well, but usually later. Bowel sounds may be hyperactive initially and high pitched. Occasionally, borborygmi are present. As intestinal distention increases, the intermittent peristaltic discomfort disappears and is replaced by constant pain from peritoneal irritation and intestinal distention. Pain is greater with a lower intestinal obstruction because of increased abdominal wall and intestinal distention. In fact, with a proximal small bowel obstruction, abdominal distention may not be apparent because vomiting may empty the obstructed loops. Indications of intestinal ischemia and necrosis include fever, a rapid pulse, leukocytosis, and peritonitis.

Evaluation initially should include supine and upright abdominal films for evaluation of air–fluid levels and free intestinal air. A prone cross-table lateral film is useful in infants to determine if air is present in the rectum. Rectal gas is usually indicative of partial rather than complete obstruction unless the film has been taken so soon after the onset of complete obstruction that the air has not been evacuated. Initial treatment is directed toward rehydration and electrolyte correction. A nasogastric tube should be placed for decompression and antibiotics administered. Operative intervention should be reserved for a complete bowel obstruction or failure of nonoperative management by 24 hours. In general, if the original incision was made transversely in one of the abdominal quadrants, then the midline approach is preferable because intestinal loops may have adhered to the old scar, making access to the peritoneal cavity difficult and hazardous.

Akgür and colleagues[112] recently reviewed 230 adhesive small bowel obstructions in 181 children. Immediate operation was performed for 81 episodes that presented with fever, leukocytosis, abdominal tenderness, or complete obstruction. Of the remaining 149 episodes, 110 were successfully managed conservatively; however, 39 of these subsequently required surgical intervention. The recurrence rate after surgical management was 18.75% and for nonoperative treatment was 36.47% ($P <$ .01). Using a conservative approach in selected patients, 40% were spared operation without any adverse consequences.

Postoperative intussusception is a problem unique to pediatric patients.[113] The diagnosis is often delayed owing to the protean manifestations of the disorder (distention, nausea, and vomiting) that, when encountered shortly after an abdominal operation, usually result in a low index of suspicion because these symptoms are confused with the frequent occurrence of postoperative ileus. Most patients with postoperative intussusception develop symptoms within 1 to 2 weeks after operation.[114] This is in contrast to adhesive obstruction, in which most patients present 2 weeks or more after surgery. Therefore, a high index of suspicion is required for an early diagnosis in the postoperative period, particularly if nasogastric suction has been instituted. In that situation, abdominal distention and cramping pain are minimized, but the real clue is a marked increase in the volume of gastric suction. Surgical exploration is required in all cases of postoperative intussusception (Fig. 63-11).

Ascites

Although many causes for the development of ascites are known, only a few conditions account for most childhood cases. Ascites can develop as a result of congenital cardiovascular disease and cardiac failure, hepatorenal syndrome, lymphatic and urinary obstruction, prenatal bowel perforation with meconium peritonitis, and pancreatic, biliary, and ovarian conditions. In some instances, the development of ascites is expected, such as in infants with biliary atresia with failed surgical portoenterostomy. In other cases, the reason is unclear, and paracentesis is important for diagnosis and relief of tension. After paracentesis, the cause is usually apparent. A large mesenteric or omental cyst may be mistaken for ascites.

Ascitic chylous fluid may be clear in newborns but is usually cloudy and turbid after feedings have been initiated. There is an

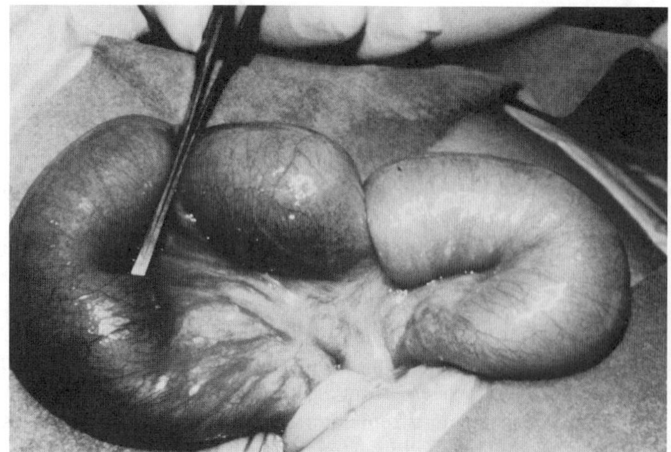
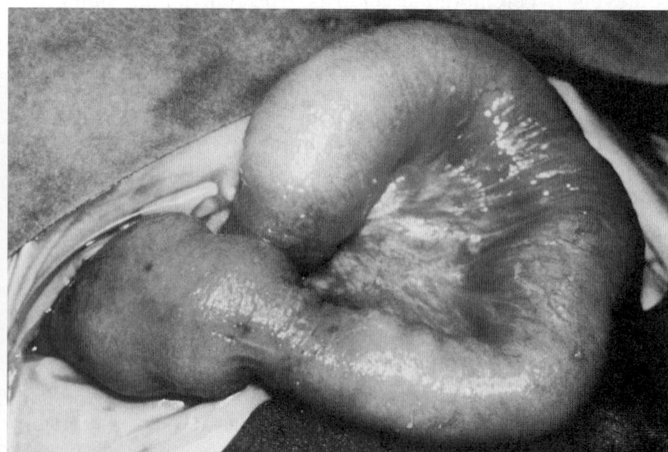

FIG. 63-11. Postoperative jejunojejunal intussusception (*top*) found at laparotomy is manually reduced (*bottom*). There is no lead point for the postoperative small bowel intussusception. (Holcomb GW III, Ross AJ III, O'Neill JA Jr. Postoperative intussusception: increasing frequency or increasing awareness? South Med J 1991;84:1334)

increase in the total fat and triglyceride content and a decrease in protein. Leukocytosis usually occurs with lymphocyte predominance. In a review of 59 children with chylous ascites, Vasko and Tapper[115] found congenital malformation in 39%, unknown in 31%, inflammation in 15%, and neoplasm in 3%. Most infants and children respond to nonoperative therapy directed toward reducing the fat and elevating the protein content in diets. Medium-chain triglycerides are often employed for this purpose. Total parenteral nutrition may also be used. If identifiable causes are present, such as abdominal cyst, trauma, or malrotation, those conditions should be corrected. Exploration is reserved for failure of nonoperative therapy for 4 to 6 weeks. Preoperative feedings of cream with a lipophilic dye may help identify the site of the leak at operation. On occasion, a peritoneal venous shunt is required when repeated attempts at nonoperative and operative therapy have failed.

Ascites may also develop secondary to spontaneous or traumatic biliary tract perforation.[116,117] In a review of 50 cases of biliary ascites in infancy, laparotomy was required in all cases, and biliary tract drainage was performed in 45 patients. Thirty-six patients survived local drainage alone without repair of the biliary perforation. With traumatic injuries in older children, drainage, possible cholecystectomy, and ductal repair are sometimes indicated. Biliary ascites may also occur after failed therapy for biliary atresia, neonatal hepatitis, or cytomegalovirus. Paracentesis reveals biliary fluid with a bilirubin content usually greater than 400 mg/mL.

Pancreatic ascites in children is usually related to traumatic injury. Most cases are related to the development of a pancreatic pseudocyst. The major reason for delayed or incorrect preoperative diagnosis of pancreatic ascites appears to be the failure to analyze the acidic fluid for amylase.[118] Pancreatic ascites usually resolves after pseudocyst drainage. Persistent ascites requires surgical correction.

Ovarian ascites may occur after birth, rarely develops in older children, and may be related to large cysts in neonates. In adolescent girls, ascites may accompany ovarian tumors, such as thecoma, and it may be a part of Meigs syndrome.

Urinary ascites usually results from mechanical obstruction of the urinary tract. Causes reported include posterior urethral valves, urethrocele, urethral atresia, neurogenic bladder, and bladder neck obstruction.[119,120] Bladder perforations have also been reported as the cause for ascites.[121,122] The infant usually develops abdominal distention, sometimes with extensive ascites. An elevated serum creatinine and urea may result from peritoneal absorption of urine. Urinary function, however, may be relatively normal. A voiding cystourethrogram and intravenous urography can detect urinary leakage in most cases.

Meconium Peritonitis

Meconium peritonitis is an aseptic peritonitis secondary to the spillage of meconium in the abdominal cavity due to intestinal perforation in the fetus. Perforation usually results from intestinal obstruction due to atresia, stenosis, meconium ileus, intussusception, or gastroschisis. Massive abdominal distention may be evident at birth or may develop shortly after birth, sometimes with associated abdominal wall erythema and edema. Abdominal radiographs may demonstrate evidence of obstruction, and scattered calcifications also may be seen. Neonatal abdominal calcification has been reported without associated meconium peritonitis.[123]

When intestinal obstruction or bowel perforation are evident, operation is required; however, patients with abdominal calcifications who are asymptomatic do not need operative intervention. Abdominal laparotomy may be difficult and may involve significant blood and fluid loss. All devitalized tissue should be removed, although it is important to preserve an adequate intestinal length. Primary anastomosis may be accomplished after intestinal resection if infection is not present within the abdominal cavity. Nevertheless, a temporary stoma should be performed if extensive bacterial contamination has occurred.

With modern technology and appropriate critical care, the prognosis for children has greatly improved. The present survival rate generally depends on the underlying cause; the size, maturity, and stamina of the patient; and early intervention when indicated.

REFERENCES

1. Rodgers KE, DiZerega GS. Modulation of peritoneal re-epithelialization by postsurgical macrophages. J Surg Res 1992;53:542.
2. DiZerega GS. The peritoneum and its response to surgical injury. Prog Clin Biol Res 1990;358:1.
3. Raftery AT. Regeneration of parietal and visceral peritoneum: an electron microscopical study. J Anat 1973;115:375.
4. Ellis H, Harrison W, Hugh TB. The healing of peritoneum under normal and pathological conditions. Br J Surg 1965;52:471.
5. Raftery AT. Regeneration of parietal and visceral peritoneum in the immature animal: a light and electron microscopical study. Br J Surg 1973;60:969.
6. Liao SK, Suehiro GT, McNamara JJ. Prevention of postoperative intestinal adhesions in primates. Surg Gynecol Obstet 1973;137:816.
7. Pfeffer WH, Wheeler JE, Tschoepe RL, et al. The effect of dexamethasone and promethazine administration on adhesion formation, tubal function and ultrastructure following microsurgical anastomosis of rabbit oviducts. Fertil Steril 1980;34:162.
8. Siegler AM, Kontopoulos V, Wang CF. Prevention of postoperative adhesions in rabbits with ibuprofen, a nonsteroidal anti-inflammatory agent. Fertil Steril 1980;34:46.
9. Nishimura K, Nakamura RM, DiZerega GS. Ibuprofen inhibition of postsurgical adhesion formation: a time and dose response biochemical evaluation in rabbits. J Surg Res 1984;36:115.
10. Adhesion Study Group. Reduction of postoperative pelvic adhesions with intraperitoneal 32% dextran 70: a prospective, randomized clinical trial. Fertil Steril 1983;40:612.
11. Interceed (TC7) Adhesion Barrier Study Group. Prevention of postsurgical adhesions by INTERCEED (TC7), an absorbable adhesion barrier: a prospective, randomized multicenter clinical study. Fertil Steril 1989;51:933.
12. Interceed (TC7) Adhesion Barrier Study Group II. Pelvic sidewall adhesion reformation: microsurgery alone or with Interceed absorbable adhesion barrier. Surg Gynecol Obstet 1993;177:135.
13. Surgical Membrane Study Group. Prophylaxis of pelvic sidewall adhesions with Gore-Tex surgical membrane: a multicenter clinical investigation. Fertil Steril 1991;57:921.
14. Jansen RPS. Failure of intraperitoneal adjuncts to improve the outcome of pelvic operation in young women. Am J Obstet Gynecol 1985;153:363.
15. DiZerega GS, Rodgers KE. The peritoneum. New York, Springer-Verlag, 1992.
16. Hubbard TB, Khan MZ, Carag VR, et al. The pathology of peritoneal repair: its relation to the formation of adhesions. Ann Surg 1967;165:908.
17. Singleton AO Jr, Rowe Jr, Rowe EB, et al. Failure of reperitonealization to prevent abdominal adhesions in the dog. Am J Surg 1952;18:789.
18. Thomas JW, Rhoades JE. Adhesions resulting from removal of serosa

from an area of bowel: failure of "oversewing" to lower incidence in the rat and the guinea pig. Arch Surg 1950;61:565.

19. Trimpe HD, Bacon HE. Clinical and experimental study of denuded surfaces in extensive surgery of the colon and rectum. Am J Surg 1952;34:596.

20. Operative Laparoscopy Study Group. Postoperative adhesion development after operative laparoscopy: evaluation at early second look procedures. Fertil Steril 1991;55:700.

21. Garrard LC, Nanney L, Richards WO. Adhesion formation is reduced after laparoscopic surgery. (Abstract) SAGES 1994, Complications of Laparoscopy and Flexible Endoscopy. Nashville, April 16–19, 1994.

22. Gans SL, Berci G. Peritoneoscopy in infants and children. J Pediatr Surg 1973;8:399.

23. Gans SL. Historical development of pediatric endoscopic surgery. In: Holcomb GW III, ed. Pediatric endoscopic surgery. Norwalk, CT, Appleton & Lange, 1993:1.

24. Dubois F, Berthelots G, Levard H. Cholecystectomy par coelioscopie. Presse Med 1989;18:980.

25. Reddick EJ, Olsen DO. Laparoscopic laser cholecystectomy. Surg Endosc 1989;3:131.

26. Liem TK, Applebaum H, Herzberger B. Hemodynamic and ventilatory effects of abdominal CO_2 insufflation at various pressures in the young swine. J Pediatr Surg 1994;29:966.

27. Tobias JD, Holcomb GW III, Brock JW III, et al. General anesthesia by mask with spontaneous ventilation during brief laparoscopic inspection of the peritoneum in children. J Laparoendosc Surg 1996;6: 175–180.

28. Duckett JW. Pediatric laparoscopy: prudence please. (Editorial) J Urol 1994;151:742.

29. Hazebroek FWJ, Molenaar JC. The management of the impalpable testis by surgery alone. J Urol 1992;148:629.

30. Elder JS. Laparoscopy for the non-palpable testis. Semin Pediatr Surg 1993;2:168.

31. Bloom DA, Ritchey ML, Manzoni G. Laparoscopy for the nonpalpable testis. In: Holcomb GW III, ed. Pediatric endoscopic surgery. Norwalk, CT, Appleton & Lange, 1993:41.

32. Bloom DA. Two-step orchiopexy with pelviscopic clip ligation of the spermatic vessels. J Urol 1991;145:1030.

33. Elder JS. Two-stage Fowler-Stephens orchiopexy in the management of intra-abdominal testes. J Urol 1992;148:1239.

34. Holcomb GW III, Brock JW III, Neblett WW III, et al. Laparoscopy for the nonpalpable testis. Am Surg 1994;60:143.

35. Fowler R Jr, Stephens FD. The role of testicular vascular anatomy in the salvage of high undescended testes. Aust NZ J Surg 1959;29:92.

36. Ransley PG, Vordermark JS, Caldamone AA, et al. Preliminary ligation of the gonadal vessels prior to orchidopexy for the intra-abdominal testicle: a staged Fowler-Stephens procedure. World J Urol 1984; 2:266.

37. Cortesi N, Ferrari P, Zambarda E, et al. Diagnosis of bilateral abdominal cryptorchidism by laparoscopy. Endoscopy 1976;8:33.

38. Holcomb GW III. Laparoscopic evaluation for a contralateral inguinal hernia or a non-palpable testis. Pediatr Ann 1993;22:678.

39. Diamond DA, Caldamone AA. The value of laparoscopy for 106 impalpable testes relative to clinical presentation. J Urol 1992;148: 632.

40. Castilho LN. Laparoscopy for the nonpalpable testis: how to interpret the endoscopic findings. J Urol 1990;144:1215.

41. Naslund MJ, Gearhart JP, Jeffs RD. Laparoscopy: its selected use in patients with unilateral nonpalpable testis after human chorionic gonadotropin stimulation. J Urol 1988;142:108.

42. Thomas MD, Mercer LC, Saltzstein EC. Laparoscopic orchiectomy for unilateral intra-abdominal testis. J Urol 1992;148:1251.

43. Castilho LN, Ferreira U, Netto NR Jr, et al. Laparoscopic pediatric orchiectomy. J Endourol 1992;6:155.

44. Gililland J, Cummings D, Hibbert ML, et al. Laparoscopic orchiectomy in a patient with complete androgen insensitivity. J Laparoendosc Surg 1993;3:51.

45. Turek PJ, Ewalt DH, Snyder HM, et al. The absent cryptorchid testis: surgical findings and their implications for diagnosis and etiology. J Urol 1994;151:718.

46. Miller D, Pope JC IV, Brock JW III, Holcomb GW III. Management of the absent testicle: Expertease and review. Abstract presented to southern section. American Urologic Association Meeting, Puerto Rico, 1996.

47. Sparkman RS: Bilateral exploration in inguinal hernia in juvenile patients. Surgery 1962;51:393.

48. Holcomb GW Jr. Routine bilateral inguinal hernia repair. Am J Dis Child 1965;109:114.

49. Gilbert M, Clatworthy HW. Bilateral operations for inguinal hernia and hydrocele in infancy and childhood. Am J Surg 1959;97:255.

50. Kiesewetter WB, Oh KS. Unilateral inguinal hernias in children: what about the opposite side? Arch Surg 1980;115:1443.

51. McGregor DB, Halverson K, McVay CB. The unilateral pediatric inguinal hernia: should the contralateral side be explored? J Pediatr Surg 1980;15:313.

52. Surana R, Puri P. Is contralateral exploration necessary in infants with unilateral inguinal hernia? J Pediatr Surg 1993;28:1026.

53. Kramer SG, Davis SE. Transperitoneal detection of occult inguinal hernia. Milit Med 1967;132:512.

54. Harrison CB, Kaplan GW, Scherz HC, et al. Diagnostic peritoneoscopy for the detection of the clinically occult contralateral hernia in children. J Urol 1990;144:510.

55. Powell RW. Intraoperative diagnostic pneumoperitoneum in pediatric patients with unilateral inguinal hernias: the Goldstein test. J Pediatr Surg 1985;20:418.

56. Holcomb GW III, Brock JW III, Morgan WM III. Laparoscopic evaluation for a contralateral patent processus vaginalis. J Pediatr Surg 1994;29:970.

57. Holcomb GW III, Morgan WM III, Brock JW III: laparoscopic evaluation for an antralateral patent processus vaginalis II. Journal of Pediatric Surgery 1996;31:000.

58. Stafford PW. The evaluation of chronic abdominal pain in children: a role for diagnostic laparoscopy? (Abstract) Third International Congress on Endoscopy and Laparoscopy in Children. Münster, Germany, February 1–2, 1994.

59. Schier F, Waldschmidt J. Laparoscopy in children with ill-defined abdominal pain. Surg Endosc 1994;8:97.

60. Powell DM, Newman KD. Laparoscopy for intersex abnormalities. In: Holcomb GW III, ed. Pediatric endoscopic surgery. Norwalk, CT, Appleton & Lange, 1993.

61. Holcomb GW III, Tomita SS, Haase GM, et al. Minimally invasive surgery in children with cancer. Cancer 1995;76:121–128.

62. Holcomb GW III, Olsen DO, Sharp KW. Laparoscopic cholecystectomy in the pediatric patient. J Pediatr Surg 1991;26:1186.

63. Holcomb GW III. Laparoscopic cholecystectomy.In: Holcomb GW III, ed. Pediatric endoscopic surgery. Norwalk, CT, Appleton & Lange, 1993:29.

64. Newman KD, Marmon LM, Attorri R, et al. Laparoscopic cholecystectomy in pediatric patients. J Pediatr Surg 1991;26:1184.

65. Moir CR, Donohue JH, VanHeerden JA. Laparoscopic cholecystectomy in children: initial experience and recommendations. J Pediatr Surg 1992;27:1066.

66. Davidoff AM, Branum GD, Chong WK, et al. The technique of laparoscopic cholecystectomy in children. Ann Surg 1992;215:186.

67. Holcomb GW III, Sharp KW, Neblett WW III, et al. Laparoscopic cholecystectomy in infants and children: modifications and cost analysis. J Pediatr Surg 1994;29:900–904.

68. Holcomb GW III. Laparoscopic cholecystectomy. Semin Pediatr Surg 1993;2:159.

69. Leape LL, Ramenosky ML. Laparoscopy for questionable appendicitis: can it reduce the negative appendectomy rate? Ann Surg 1980; 191:410.

70. Semm K. Endoscopic appendectomy. Endoscopy 1983;15:50.

71. Holcomb GW III. Laparoscopic appendectomy in children. Laparosc Surg 1993;1:145.

72. Valla JS, Limonne B, Valla V, et al. Laparoscopic appendectomy in children: report of 465 cases. Surg Laparosc Endosc 1991;1:166.

73. Gilchrist BF, Lobe TE, Schropp KP, et al. Is there a role for laparoscopic appendectomy in pediatric surgery? J Pediatr Surg 1992;27: 209.

74. Naffis D. Laparoscopic appendectomy in children. Semin Pediatr Surg 1993;2:174.

75. Schropp KP, Lobe TE. Laparoscopic appendectomy.In: Holcomb GW III, ed. Pediatric endoscopic surgery. Norwalk, CT, Appleton & Lange, 1993:21.

76. Miller J. Laparoscopic appendectomy. Pediatr Ann 1993;22:663.

77. Holcomb GW III, Georgeson KE, Lobe TE, et al. Pediatric laparoscopy and thoracoscopy. (Symposium) Contemp Surg 1994;44:183.

78. Lobe TE, Presbury GJ, Smith BM, et al. Laparoscopic splenectomy. Pediatr Ann 1993;22:671.

79. Lobe TE, Schropp KP, Lunsford K. Laparoscopic Nissen fundoplication in childhood. J Pediatr Surg 1993;28:358.

80. Georgeson KE. Laparoscopic gastrostomy and fundoplication. Pediatr Ann 1993;22:675.

81. Rothenberg S. Laparoscopic Nissen fundoplication in children Nashville, TN. Presented, SAGES, April 1994.

82. Tulman S, Holcomb GW III, Karamanoukian HL, et al. Pediatric laparoscopic splenectomy. J Pediatr Surg 1993;28:689.

83. Lobe TE, Schropp KP, Joyner RE, et al. The suitability of automatic tissue morcellation for the endoscopic removal of large specimens in pediatric surgery. J Pediatr Surg 1994;29:232.

84. Smith BM, Schropp KP, Lobe TE, et al. Laparoscopic splenectomy in childhood. J Pediatr Surg 1994;29:975.

85. Holcomb GW III. Wherein lies the future? Semin Pediatr Surg 1993; 2:195.

86. Holcomb GW III. Future applications in children.In: Holcomb GW III, ed. Pediatric endoscopic surgery. Norwalk, CT, Appleton & Lange, 1993:173.

87. Moir CR. Laparoscopy for the female patient.In: Holcomb GW III, ed. Pediatric endoscopic surgery. Norwalk, CT, Appleton & Lange, 1993:51.

88. Georgeson KE. Laparoscopic Soavé procedure in infants. Nashville, TN Presented, SAGES, 1994.

89. Cameron BH, Blair GK. Laparoscopic-guided gastropexy for intermittent gastric volvulus. J Pediatr Surg 1993;28:1628.

90. Huang CS, Lin LH. Laparoscopic Meckel's diverticulectomy in infants: report of three cases. J Pediatr Surg 1993;28:1486.

91. Waldschmidt J, Schier F. Laparoscopical surgery in neonates and infants. Eur J Pediatr Surg 1991;1:145.

92. Koyle MA, Woo HH, Kavoussi LR. Laparoscopic nephrectomy in the first year of life. J Pediatr Surg 1993;28:693–695.

93. Kerbl K, Clayman RV, Kavoussi LR. Laparoscopic nephrectomy. In: Holcomb GW III, ed. Pediatric endoscopic surgery. Norwalk, CT, Appleton & Lange, 1993:93.

94. Alain JL. Laparoscopic treatment of pyloric stenosis. Presented at the Symposium on Endoscopic Surgery in Children, Berlin, December 1992.

95. Tan HL. Laparoscopic pyloromyotomy versus open operation: which is better? (Abstract) Third International Congress on Endoscopy and Laparoscopy in Children. Münster, Germany, February 1–2, 1994.

96. Estes JM, Adzick NS, Harrison MR. Fetoscopic surgery.In: Holcomb GW III, ed. Pediatric endoscopic surgery. Norwalk, CT, Appleton & Lange, 1993:155.

97. Estes JM, MacGillivray TE, Hedrick MH, et al. Fetoscopic surgery for the treatment of congenital anomalies. J Pediatr Surg 1992;27: 950.

98. Kane MG, Krejs GJ. Complications of diagnostic laparoscopy in Dallas: a 7-year prospective study. Gastrointest Endosc 1984;30:237.

99. Katz M, Beck P, Tanger ML. Major vessel injury during laparoscopy: anatomy of two cases. Am J Obstet Gynecol 1979;135:544.

100. Oshinsky GS, Smith AD. Laparoscopic needles and trocars: an overview of designs and complications. J Laparoendosc Surg 1992;2:117.

101. Davidoff AM, Pappas TN, Hilleren DJ, et al. Mechanisms of major biliary injury during laparoscopic cholecystectomy. Ann Surg 1992; 215:196.

102. Peters JH, Gibbons GD, Innes JT, et al. Complications of laparoscopic cholecystectomy. Surgery 1991;110:769.

103. Bishop HC, Koop CE. Management of meconium ileus: resection, Roux-en-Y anastomosis and ileostomy irrigation with pancreatic enzymes. Ann Surg 1957;145:410.

104. Santulli TV, Blanc WA. Congenital atresia of the intestine: pathogenesis and treatment. Ann Surg 1961;154:939.

105. Duckett JW, Lotfi AH. Appendicovesicostomy (and variations) in bladder reconstruction. J Urol 1993;149:567.

106. Issa MM, Oesterling JE, Canning DA, et al. A new technique of using the in situ appendix as a catheterizable stoma in continent urinary reservoirs. J Urol 1989;141:1385.

107. Holcomb GW III, Murphy P, Snyder HM III, et al. Continent urinary reconstruction in ischiopagus tripus conjoined twins. J Urol 1989; 141:100.

108. Cameron GS, Lau GYP. The umbilicus as a site for temporary colostomy in infants. J Pediatr Surg 1982;17:362.

109. Fitzgerald PG, Lau GYP, Cameron GS. Use of the umbilical site for temporary ostomy: review of 47 cases. J Pediatr Surg 1989;24:973.

110. Festen C, Severijnen RSVM, vdStaak FHJM. Enterostomy complications in infants. Acta Chir Scand 1988;154:525.

111. Festen C. Postoperative small bowel obstruction in infants and children. Ann Surg 1982;196:580.

112. Akgür FM, Tanyel FC, Büyükpamukçu N, et al. Adhesive small bowel obstruction in children: the place and predictors of success for conservative treatment. J Pediatr Surg 1991;26:37.

113. Holcomb GW III, Ross AJ III, O'Neill JA Jr. Postoperative intussusception: increasing frequency or increasing awareness? South Med J 1991;84:1334.

114. Mollitt DL, Ballentine TV, Grosfeld JL. Postoperative intussusception. in infancy and childhood: analysis of 119 cases. Surgery 1979; 86:402.

115. Vasko JS, Tapper RI. Surgical significance of chylous ascites. Arch Surg 1967;95:355.

116. Prevot J, Rickham PP. Acute biliary peritonitis. Prog Pediatr Surg 1971;1:196.

117. Hansen RC, Wasnich RD, DeVries PA, et al. Bile ascites in infancy: diagnosis with ^{131}I-rose bengal. Pediatrics 1974;84:719.

118. Rubin SZ, Ein SH. The unusual presentation of pancreatitis in infancy. J Pediatr Surg 1979;14:146.

119. Unger SW, Chandler JG. Chylous ascites in infants and children. Surgery 1983;93:455.

120. Mann CM, Leape LL, Holden TM, et al. Neonatal urinary ascites: a report of 2 cases of unusual etiology and a review of the literature. J Urol 1974;111:124.

121. Cywes S, Wynne J, Louw JH, et al. Urinary ascites in the newborn, with a report of two cases. J Pediatr Surg 1968;3:350.

122. Tank ES, Davis R, Hoit JF, et al. Mechanisms of trauma during breech delivery. Obstet Gynecol 1971;38:761.

123. Miller JP, Smith SD, Newman B, et al. Neonatal abdominal calcifications: Is it always meconium peritonitis? J Pediatr Surg 1988;23:555.

Surgery of Infants and Children: Scientific Principles and Practice, edited by Keith T. Oldham, Paul M. Colombani, and Robert P. Foglia. Lippincott–Raven Publishers, Philadelphia, © 1997.

CHAPTER 64

Hernias and Umbilicus

Frederick J. Rescorla

INGUINAL HERNIA

Embryology

Most inguinal hernias in infants and children are indirect inguinal hernias due to patent processus vaginalis. The pertinent embryology of the inguinal region relates to the development and descent of the testes and their relation to the processus vaginalis.

The gonads develop near the kidney as a result of migration of primitive germ cells from the yolk sac to the genital ridge, which is completed by 6 weeks' gestation. Differentiation into testes or ovary occurs by 7 or 8 weeks' gestation under hormonal influences. The gubernaculum forms from the caudal end of the mesonephros and is attached to the lower pole of the testes. The lower portion of the gubernaculum has several thin, cordlike structures that appear to guide the testes into the scrotum. These occasionally pass to ectopic locations (perineum *or* femoral region) outside the line of normal scrotal descent. Downward retroperitoneal migration of the gonads starts at about 3 months' gestation. The ovary reaches the pelvic brim at about 12 weeks' gestation and remains at this level. The remnant of the gubernaculum in girls forms the ovarian and uterine ligaments. The testes continue to descend, reaching the level of the internal ring by 7 months' gestation.

The peritoneum bulges into the inguinal canal as the processus vaginalis before testicular descent. The gubernaculum precedes the testes. As it reaches the bottom of the scrotal sac, it begins to shorten, and the testes complete the scrotal descent. The testis passes through the inguinal canal in a few days but takes about 4 weeks to migrate from the external ring to the lower scrotum. As the testis evaginates the abdominal wall, the layers of the spermatic cord are formed from the layers of the abdominal wall. The internal spermatic fascia forms from the transversalis fascia, the cremasteric fascia from the internal oblique and transversus abdominis, and the external spermatic fascia from the fascia of the external oblique.

The processus vaginalis normally closes during the last few weeks of term gestation after the completion of testicular descent. It obliterates initially both at the level of the internal inguinal ring and just above the testes. The portion adjacent to the testes becomes the tunica vaginalis. In girls, the canal of Nuck corresponds to the processus vaginalis, opens into the labium majus, and usually obliterates earlier than the processus vaginalis, at about 7 months' gestation.

Failure of closure of the processus vaginalis accounts for nearly all of the inguinoscrotal abnormalities seen in infancy and childhood. Although reason for failure of closure is unknown, it is more common in cases of testicular nondescent and prematurity. In addition, persistent patency is twice as common on the right side (probably related to later descent of the right testis).

Pathology

An indirect inguinal hernia occurs when intestinal contents enter the inguinal region through a patent processus vaginalis. Depending on the degree of patency of the distal processus, the hernia may be confined to the inguinal region or pass down into the scrotum (Fig. 64-1). A communicating hydrocele occurs when the opening is narrow, allowing fluid but not intestinal structures to pass into the inguinoscrotal region. A scrotal hydrocele occurs when the proximal portion of the processus vaginalis obliterates and the tunica vaginalis fills with fluid. Hydrocele can also occur along the cord because the processus may obliterate proximal and distal to an isolated cystic dilation. In little girls, the processus (canal of Nuck) may remain patent and may fill with fluid or allow the ovary and fallopian tube to enter the inguinal region.

Clinical Presentation and Initial Management

Presenting Symptoms

A *hernia* is generally identified as a bulge in the area of the lower abdominal crease, with varying degrees of extension from the area of the internal inguinal ring down along the path of the cord structures to the hemiscrotum. The differential diagnosis includes a communicating hydrocele, which usually has a history of size fluctuation, transilluminates on examination, and is usually not reducible on physical examination. Other, less

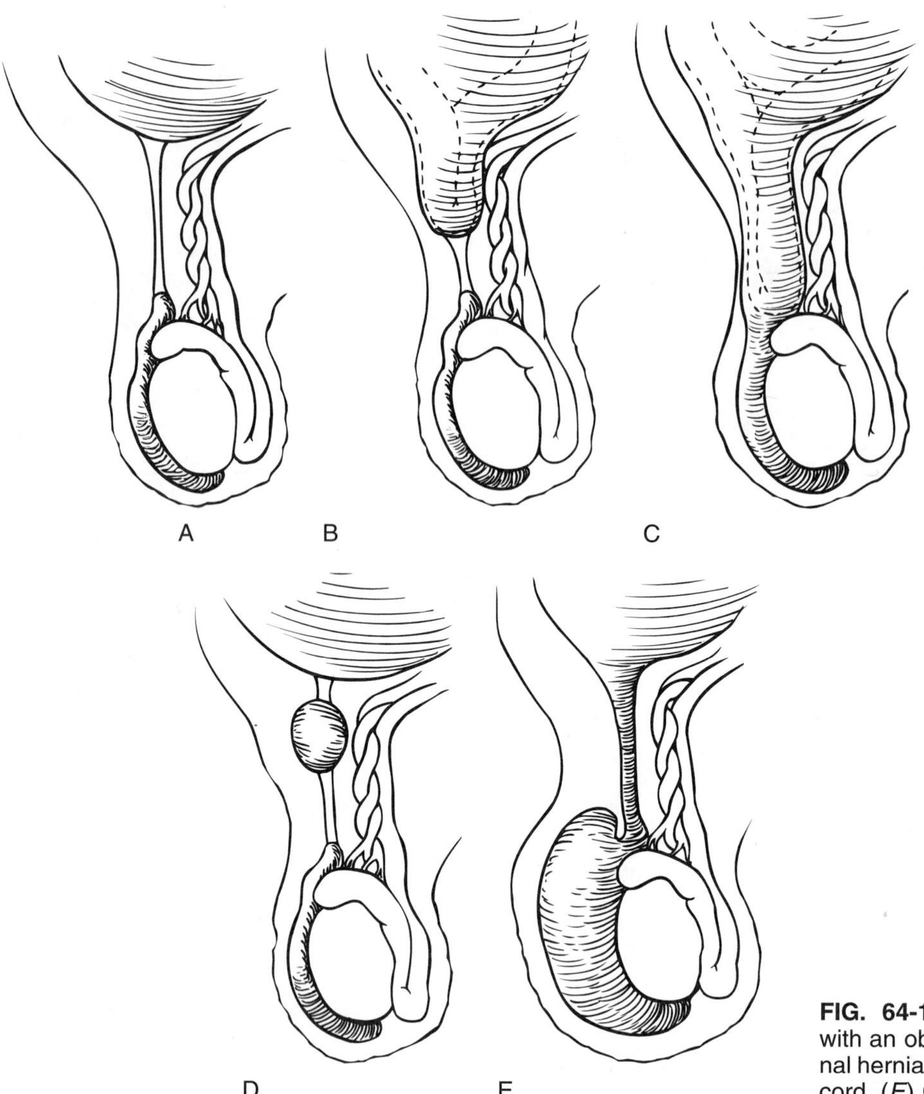

FIG. 64-1. (*A*) Normal inguinoscrotal anatomy with an obliterated processus vaginalis. (*B*) Inguinal hernia. (*C*) Scrotal hernia. (*D*) Hydrocele of the cord. (*E*) Communicating hydrocele.

common abnormalities include torsion of the testes and inguinal lymphadenopathy. In addition, a retractile testis frequently is felt as a mass just below the external ring. In girls, an asymptomatic labial mass is frequently identified. If not repaired, this can lead to torsion and strangulation of the ovary and fallopian tube. In most patients, the hernia reduces either spontaneously or with gentle pressure by the parent or physician.

Conditions associated with an increased occurrence of inguinal hernias include prematurity, undescended testes, epispadias, bladder exstrophy, ambiguous genitalia, and a positive family history. Inguinal hernias are more common in children with increased intraabdominal pressure secondary to abdominal wall defects and in children in whom ventriculoperitoneal shunts or peritoneal dialysis is used.

At initial examination, an attempt should be made to reduce the hernia. This can be facilitated with one hand applying gentle pressure on the lowest aspect of the hernia and the other hand forming an inverted V at the level of the internal inguinal ring to force the hernia contents back through and not superficial to the external inguinal ring (Fig. 64-2). If reduction is not possible, the hernia is incarcerated.

Incarceration

Incarceration represents the most common complication associated with inguinal hernias. Incarceration is reported in 6% to 18% of patients in several large series,[1–3] and several researchers have reported rates of about 30% for infants less than 2 months of age.[1,4] Contained structures can include small bowel, appendix, omentum, colon, or, rarely, Meckel diverticulum. In girls, the ovary, fallopian tube, or both are usually incarcerated. Rarely, the uterus is drawn into the sac along with the fallopian tube.

It is essential at the time of the initial evaluation to attempt reduction of an incarcerated hernia. The only exception to this is a long-standing incarceration with evidence of peritoneal irritation. Reduction can be attempted in the presence of uncomplicated clinical and radiographic bowel obstruction. An attempt by the surgeon with several minutes of gentle pressure is usually successful. If unsuccessful, sedation administered intramuscularly or intravenously may allow adequate relaxation to allow reduction.

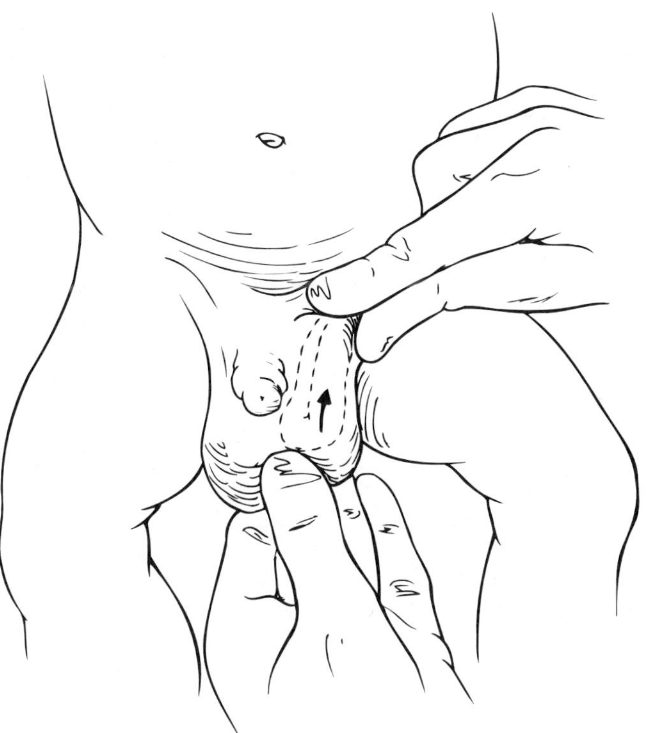

FIG. 64-2. Manual reduction of an inguinal hernia. Two fingers form an inverted V to allow reduction through the external inguinal ring.

Indications for Surgery

Due to the high rate of complications associated with inguinal hernias, repair is generally recommended shortly after the diagnosis is established. In an otherwise healthy child with an easily reducible hernia, outpatient surgery is scheduled within a few weeks at the convenience of the parents and surgeon. If reduction is moderately difficult, repair should be performed within a few days and the parents advised to return if incarceration occurs. If reduction is difficult or requires sedation, most surgeons admit the child for close observation and perform the procedure within the next 24 hours. The child with one episode of incarceration may have another and should be observed closely. An irreducible hernia requires immediate exploration.

In girls, hernias frequently appear as asymptomatic labial masses that can be difficult to reduce. The ovary is usually not strangulated, and the question arises as to the urgency of repair of an irreducible structure that is not compromised and that may have been incarcerated for days or weeks. The occurrence of strangulation of ovaries in this location is well documented, so that same day or next day repair is probably the most prudent.

Premature infants diagnosed with hernias while in the neonatal units can be safely repaired before discharge. The neonatal staff can observe these patients, and as long as reduction is easy, repair can be delayed. Premature infants with inguinal hernias diagnosed after discharge may have surgery delayed to allow a general anesthetic on an outpatient basis if the hernia is easily reducible. Because the natural history of communicating and noncommunicating hydrocele can result in spontaneous closure and resolution, a period of observation until 1 year of age is generally warranted.

Contralateral Side

Few topics in pediatric surgery have drawn as much attention or generated more controversy than the management of the contralateral side in children presenting with a unilateral hernia. The only purpose of a contralateral exploration is to avoid the occurrence of a hernia on that side at a later date. The advantages of routine contralateral exploration are related to avoiding the issues associated with the development of a contralateral hernia, including parental anxiety, cost, anesthesia, and risk of contralateral incarceration. The disadvantages include potential injury to the vas deferens and testes, increased operative time, and the fact that in many infants it is an unnecessary procedure. The relevant issues in the debate revolve around the frequency of occurrence of contralateral hernias and the relation of this to age, gender, and side of the clinically apparent hernia.

Rothenberg and Barnett[5] in 1955 reported that bilateral hernias occurred in all of the infants in their study who were younger than 1 year and in 65% of those older than 1 year. Kiesewetter and Parenzan[6] attempted to determine the role of contralateral exploration in children younger than 2 years. They performed contralateral exploration in 100 infants with clinical unilateral hernias and identified a contralateral patent processus vaginalis in 61% of cases. A second group of 237 infants underwent unilateral repair only, and 31% went on to have contralateral hernias. In view of these data, Kiesewetter and Parenzan recommended bilateral repairs for children younger than 2 years.

A similar study by Sparkman[7] in 1962, involving 918 infants and children, identified a contralateral patent processus vaginalis in 57%. A second group of 1944 children underwent unilateral repair only, and 15.8% had subsequent contralateral hernias. In a review of 2764 patients undergoing routine contralateral exploration, Rowe and colleagues[8] reported a decreasing patency rate with advancing age. Patent processus vaginalis was seen in 63% of infants younger than 2 months, gradually decreasing to an incidence of about 40% after 2 years of age.

Two more recent reports of unilateral repairs at all ages observed a somewhat lower incidence of contralateral hernias but also focused on the side of recurrence. A 20-year follow-up study reported an overall contralateral hernia occurrence rate of 22%, with a 41% occurrence rate of a right hernia after an initial left hernia repair and a 14% occurrence rate of a left hernia after an initial right repair.[9] In a review of 904 unilateral repairs, Given and Rubin[10] reported a contralateral occurrence rate of 6.8%, with subsequent occurrence of a right hernia in 9.6% of patients and left hernia in 5.4%. This study may be somewhat flawed in that the mean delay between hernia repairs was 26.8 months and the follow-up period of the study patients was only 9 to 32 months.

Several series of unilateral repairs have also reported low rates of development of contralateral hernias, although the accuracy of follow-up is questionable. The occurrence rates of a contralateral hernia were 5.8% in Kobe, Japan,[11] 3.7% in Jakarta, Indonesia,[12] and 2% in Karachi, Pakistan.[13] These investigators found no significant prediction for occurrence based on the original side or gender.

In an attempt to focus on infants, Surana and Puri[14] reviewed infants between 1 week and 6 months of age (excluding premature infants who underwent bilateral exploration) undergoing unilateral repair. Ten percent of those with long-term follow-up (5 to 17 years) had contralateral hernias. Of those with initial right hernias, left hernias developed in 8.7%; of those with initial left hernias, right hernias developed in 16.6%. Only 1 of 12 girls had a contralateral hernia.

The case for premature infants is less clear, with several of the previously mentioned series including routine bilateral explorations for premature infants younger than 6 months. In a review of 222 very-low-birthweight (less than 1500 g) neonates with hernias, 61% had bilateral presentation.[15] Many researchers reporting on premature infants have observed bilateral rates exceeding 80%, but many consider a patent processus vaginalis equivalent to a hernia.[4,16,17] Misra and associates,[18] in a follow-up study of 251 infants younger than 6 months who underwent unilateral repair, observed that contralateral hernias developed in 8%. Only 13% of the premature infants in this group experienced contralateral hernias. In general, these studies appear to draw into question the routine bilateral management of premature and young infants.

The issue of young girls with hernias is also controversial. In one study of 117 girls with hernias, the rates of significant contralateral sacs (more than 1 cm) was 60% for patients younger than 1 year, 28% for patients 1 to 7 years of age, and 33% for patients older than 7 years.[19] Although these rates are similar to those for boys, the rate of contralateral hernia occurrence is unknown in girls compared with boys or with advancing age among girls. Several studies have reported a similar 2:1 ratio for right-sided and left-sided hernias but a more even distribution of hernias in older girls than in older boys.[19,20] In addition, if unilateral repairs are performed, the contralateral hernia rate is between 8% and 25% and appears unrelated to age or the original side of repair.[19,20]

Although many articles have been written on this subject, the actual percentages are within the ranges presented in this chapter. The basic questions remain: How many infants and children have a contralateral patent processus vaginalis, and what percentage of these have a subsequent hernia? The initial data by Rowe and colleagues[8] of contralateral patency rates of 63% in infants younger than 2 months decreasing to 40% after 2 years of age appear secure, with subsequent hernias developing in about 25% to 50% of these patients.

The pediatric surgeon is then left with three options: (1) never exploring the contralateral side, (2) exploring up to a certain age (eg, premature infants, 6 months, 1 or 2 years), or (3) attempting to determine contralateral patency and thus avoid negative explorations. If the other side is to be explored, it may be more reasonable to operate on the clinically uninvolved right sides more often or to an older age than the uninvolved left sides owing to the 2:1 ratio for occurrences of contralateral right hernias compared with left hernias. If a reliable and safe method were available to determine patency, negative contralateral explorations could be eliminated, but even with this approach, at least two contralateral repairs would be performed to prevent one clinical hernia.

Several methods have been used in an attempt to avoid negative contralateral explorations. The use of a Bakes dilator through the hernia sac to evaluate the contralateral side has been advocated[21] but has been difficult and unreliable in other reports.[22] Herniography has also been used but has disadvantages, including pain with injection, radiation, and time and cost

of a radiologist. As a result, this technique has not been widely accepted. Pneumoperitoneum also has been used. In a series of 64 children, only 5 (8%) had contralateral patent processus vaginalis, although one later developed a contralateral hernia.[23] This technique was shown to be unreliable for determining patency of the processus vaginalis in a study using pneumoperitoneum followed by laparoscopy.[24] The use of ultrasound of the contralateral groin was reported to have an accuracy of 91% for detecting a contralateral patent processus vaginalis.[25]

The introduction of laparoscopy into pediatric surgery has allowed diagnostic visualization of the opposite side. Several reports have documented initial diagnostic laparoscopy in children presenting with unilateral hernias.[24,26,27] The incidence of contralateral patent processus vaginalis detected by this method ranges from 30% to 53%, again consistent with previous reports on intraoperative patency determinations. Of interest, the incidence of patent processus vaginalis does not decrease with advancing age during the first 5 years of life.[24,26] A more reasonable approach is to evaluate the other side by passing a 30-degree or 70-degree oblique scope through the open hernia sac. This technique appears attractive in that it may avoid negative contralateral exploration in cases in which it would routinely be performed by the surgeon. It appears to have little advantage in older children who would normally undergo unilateral repair only. If performed in the latter setting, laparoscopy may actually lead to an increased rate of contralateral exploration, although it should reliably eliminate the occurrence of any subsequent indirect inguinal hernias.

From the preceding discussion it is clear that this topic remains controversial. My preferred method in boys less than 2 years old and girls younger than 5 or 6 years old who present with unilateral hernias is to examine the contralateral side by passing a 70-degree angled scope through the open hernia sac (Fig. 64-3). To minimize cost, this should be performed with nondisposable materials. The bladder is emptied with a crede maneuver before the procedure. A 5-mm reusable trocar is passed under direct vision through the open hernia sac into the peritoneal cavity. A silk tie is passed around the sac and trocar above the level of the internal ring and secured to maintain the pneumoperitoneum. This trocar does not have a side port for CO_2 insufflation, which is therefore accomplished by attaching the CO_2 tubing to a suction catheter placed into the trocar. After low-pressure insufflation, the 70-degree angled telescope is passed through the trocar and the contralateral side examined (Fig. 64-4). If a contralateral patent processus vaginalis is identified, contralateral exploration is performed. Because of the angle of approach, it is not possible to determine the length of the patent processus vaginalis. At facilities where laparoscopy is not available, the preferred method is to perform routine contralateral exploration in boys younger than 1 year and girls younger than 5 or 6 years.

Operative Management

The operative procedure for repair of an indirect inguinal hernia involves high ligation of the hernia sac at the level of the internal ring. A transverse incision is placed in the lowest inguinal crease. Scarpa fascia is incised and the external oblique fascia identified. Dissection is continued laterally just above the external oblique to the inguinal ligament, which is then

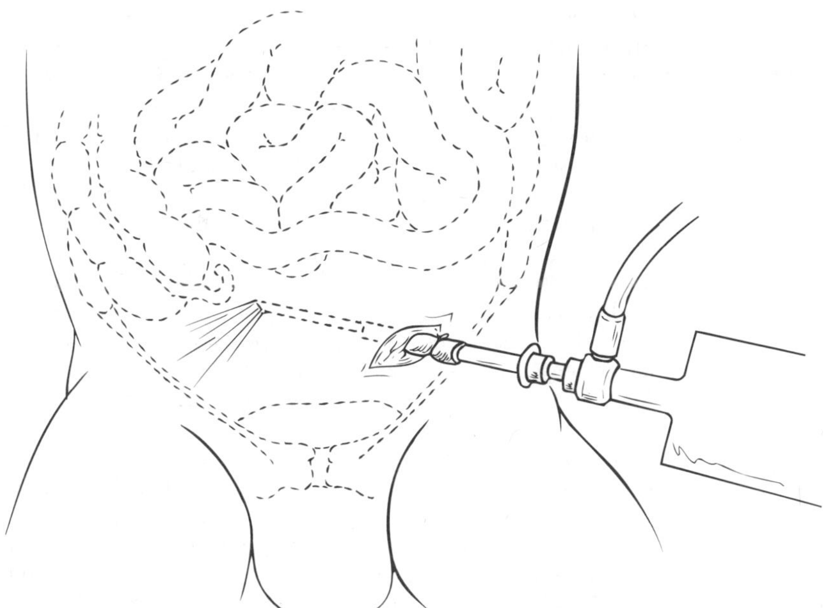

FIG. 64-3. Nonpuncture laparoscopy. A 70-degree oblique, 4-mm diameter telescope through a 5-mm nondisposable cannula is used to visualize the contralateral internal inguinal ring.

followed inferiorly to expose the external inguinal ring. The external oblique fascia is opened in the direction of its fibers, taking care to avoid injury to the ilioinguinal nerve. Some surgeons prefer to perform the repair in young infants without opening the external oblique (Mitchell-Banks technique).[28] The rationale for this modification is based on the proximity of the external and internal inguinal rings in neonates. The cremaster muscle fibers are gently dissected in a direction perpendicular to the axis of the cord structures. This exposes the hernia sac on the anteromedial surface of the cord. The sac is gently elevated, and the spermatic vessels and vas deferens are separated from the sac. When the sac is free, it is divided between clamps.

The proximal sac is gently elevated and the cord structures dissected free to the level of the internal ring where the sac is ligated. The distal sac is examined and if short may be left in place. If the sac extends into the scrotum, the anterior aspect can be excised. If a hydrocele is present, it should also be excised, taking care to avoid injury to the testes and epididymis. In addition, the testes should not be separated from the scrotal attachments. If the testis is undescended or retractile and will not remain in the scrotum, an orchiopexy is performed. The external oblique is then closed. Local anesthetic can be placed in the area of the ilioinguinal nerve and in the subcutaneous tissue to provide postoperative pain relief. The remaining layers

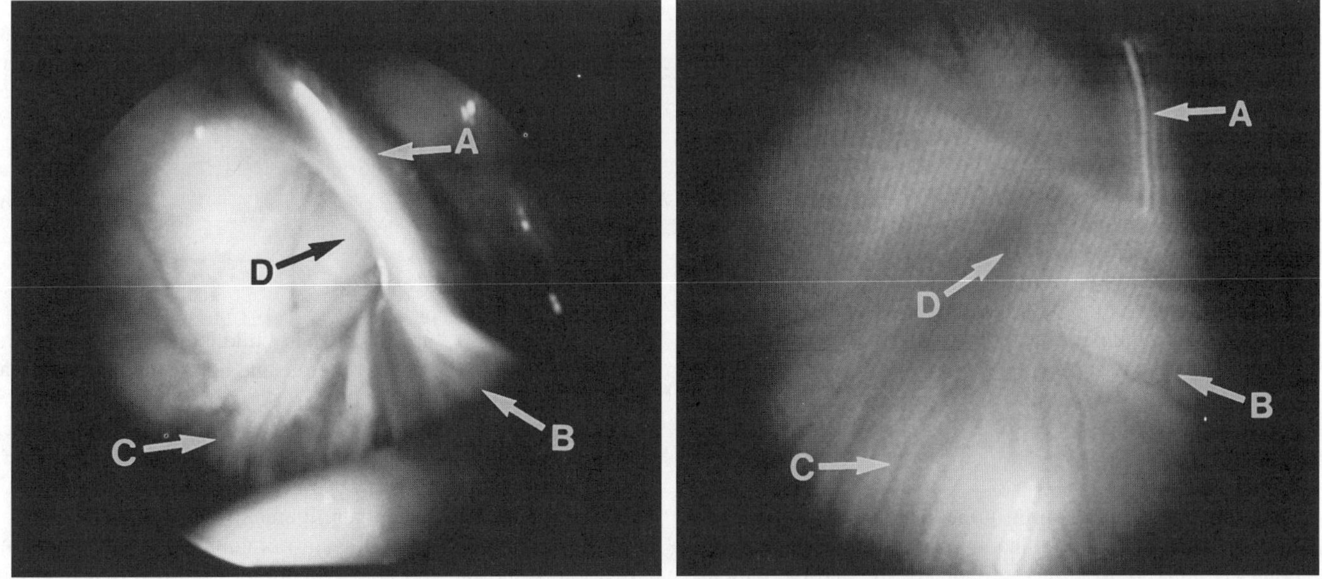

FIG. 64-4. Photographs of left internal inguinal ring showing lateral umbilical fold (A), vas deferens (B), testicular vessels (C), and patent processus vaginalis (D).

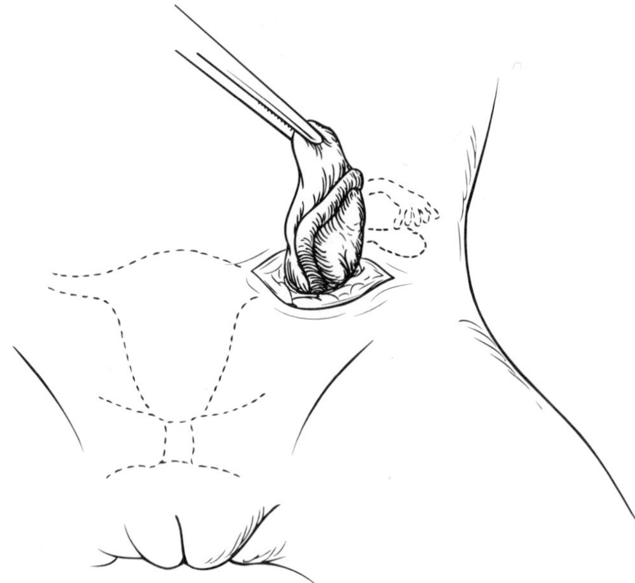

FIG. 64-5. Sliding hernia in a girl with the fallopian tube in the wall of the sac.

are closed, and a collodion topical dressing is placed over the wound in infants. A standard dressing is used for older children.

This procedure is adequate for nearly all indirect inguinal hernias. Occasionally, particularly in neonates with large hernias, the internal ring appears excessively dilated. In these cases, the internal ring can be closed along its medial aspect, below the cord structures.

In girls, the initial exposure is identical. The hernia sac and round ligament are dissected free, and the distal attachments are divided. The sac is then mobilized to the level of the internal ring. The fallopian tube is frequently within the wall of the hernia sac as a sliding hernia (Fig. 64-5). This can occasionally be identified by looking through the sac to ensure that the ligature is placed distal to the fallopian tube. I prefer to open the sac, gently pull on the round ligament until the fallopian tube is identified, and if a slider is not present, to simply ligate the sac. The internal ring is closed, and the remainder of the closure is identical to that in boys. If a slider of the fallopian tube is present, the sac can be ligated distal to the fallopian tube, divided, and invaginated into the peritoneal cavity, with closure of the internal ring. Another method, described by Goldstein and Potts,[20] involves incising the sac along the borders of the fallopian tube to the level of the internal ring. A pursestring suture is then placed in the remainder of the sac at the level of the internal ring. The tube with the attached portion of the sac is then placed into the peritoneal cavity, the suture is tied, and the internal ring is closed.

Incarceration

An irreducible hernia requires immediate exploration. Occasionally, the hernia reduces on induction of anesthesia. Nonviable bowel is unlikely to reduce spontaneously, and the patient in this setting can undergo a standard exploration. The sac should be opened, and if cloudy or bloody fluid or foul odor

is encountered, the previously entrapped bowel should be identified. This can usually be accomplished through the open sac but may require a lateral extension of the internal ring or a separate abdominal incision to allow visualization.

If the bowel remains entrapped, the sac is opened and the bowel inspected. Clearly viable bowel is returned to the abdominal cavity. This may require gentle retraction at the level of the internal ring or actual lateral extension of the internal ring. If the entrapped bowel is ischemic or discolored, it should be delivered further into the wound so that clearly viable bowel is identified. This may also require enlargement of the internal ring. The bowel is then covered with a warm, saline-soaked laparotomy pack for several minutes. The bowel is examined for signs of viability, such as color, antimesenteric pulsations, and peristalsis. If viability is questionable or if it is clearly necrotic, a resection with an end-to-end anastomosis is performed. A standard hernia repair is performed after return of the bowel to the abdominal cavity. Separation of the sac from the cord structures is frequently difficult in these cases, and care should be taken to avoid injury to the vas deferens and gonadal vessels as well as to ensure complete ligation of the sac at the level of the internal ring. Some researchers have advocated a transperitoneal approach with closure of the internal ring in infants with irreducible hernias to avoid this difficult dissection.[29]

A discolored or blue testis may be seen at the time of exploration in irreducible cases or in situations of recent reduction of an incarcerated hernia. If the testis is clearly necrotic, it may be removed, but if questionable, it should be left in place. Several infants with blue testes observed intraoperatively have had normal-sized testes on follow-up examination.[30]

Direct Inguinal Hernia

Although rare in children, an initially observed direct inguinal hernia should be repaired with a standard direct hernia repair. The conjoined tendon can be secured to the inguinal ligament in a Bassini repair. If there is concern about a possible femoral hernia, the surgeon can proceed with a Cooper ligament (McVay) repair. Many direct hernias present as recurrent hernias and may represent direct hernias missed at the original procedure or a direct occurrence due to disruption of the floor at the initial procedure.[31,32] A Cooper ligament repair is preferred in this setting.

Femoral Hernia

Femoral hernias are unusual in childhood. They present as masses lateral to the pubic tubercle and below the inguinal ligament. They are also reported in some series after an initial inguinal exploration, which may be due to an original missed femoral hernia or iatrogenic disruption of the femoral canal.[33] Repair can be accomplished by three methods. A standard inguinal approach with a Cooper ligament (McVay) repair is the most common repair. A low infrainguinal approach involves ligation of the sac and approximation of the inguinal ligament to the Cooper ligament. A suprainguinal (transperitoneal or extraperitoneal) approach occasionally is useful in incarcerated cases to allow easier intestinal repair, although incarcerated femoral hernias are extremely rare in childhood.

Complications

Complications after inguinal hernia repair are unusual. The data on complications are inherently deficient because patients with complications may not seek follow-up at the original institutions. Some complications are related to technical factors (recurrence, iatrogenic cryptorchidism), while others are related to the underlying process, such as bowel ischemia, gonadal infarction, and testicular atrophy related to an incarcerated hernia. Wound infection occurs in less than 1% of all reported series and is disproportionately represented in cases that progress to irreducible hernias.

Recurrent Hernia

The occurrence rate of recurrent inguinal hernias after uncomplicated inguinal hernia repairs is generally reported at 0.5% to 1%,[3,34,35] with rates as high as 2% for premature infants.[16,18] The rate of recurrence after repair of an incarcerated hernia has been reported at 3% to 6%.[3,36] The true incidence, however, is probably unknown owing to problems of accurate long-term follow-up. Recurrence generally occurs in 50% of the patients within 1 year of the original repair; this rate is over 75% by 2 years.[32,34]

Recurrent hernias have a number of causes. Indirect recurrences can result from failure to identify the sac at the original procedure, failure to ligate the sac at the level of the internal ring, or a tear in the sac in which a strip of peritoneum remains along the cord structures. Direct recurrences are the result of damage to the floor at the original procedure or a missed direct hernia at the original exploration. Wright,[34] in a review of 13 recurrent hernias from an original group of 1600 hernia repairs, observed that 5 were indirect, 7 direct, and 1 both direct and indirect. In a review of 71 recurrent hernias, Grosfeld and colleagues[32] reported that 51 were indirect and 20 direct. In this series, 15 of the patients had increased abdominal pressure (ventriculoperitoneal shunts, ascites), which may predispose to recurrence.

Technical ways to avoid a recurrence were discussed earlier. Management of recurrent hernias can usually be accomplished through an inguinal approach. An indirect sac is managed with high ligation at the level of the internal inguinal ring. If the internal ring is large, it may be partially closed medial to the cord structures. If a direct hernia is present, the posterior wall of the inguinal canal should be repaired, bringing the transversalis fascia to the inguinal ligament or Cooper ligament (McVay repair). The preferred method is the Cooper ligament repair. Some researchers advocate a transperitoneal approach if an immediate recurrent hernia develops. This allows easier visualization of the hernia sac, enabling the surgeon to avoid injury to the cord structures.[29]

Iatrogenic Cryptorchidism

Iatrogenic cryptorchidism can occasionally result after hernia repair, although it is a preventable problem.[37,38] If an unde-

scended testis is observed preoperatively, an orchiopexy should be performed at the time of hernia repair. In addition, at the conclusion of a routine herniorrhaphy, the testis should be placed in an intrascrotal position. The presence of a retractile testis associated with a hernia may predispose to this owing to disruption of the cremasteric fibers. If the testis will not remain in a scrotal position, an orchiopexy should be performed at the time of hernia repair.

Incarceration

Intestinal complications requiring bowel resection are relatively unusual, occurring exclusively with incarcerated hernias. Intestinal resections have been reported in about 1.4% to 1.8% of the total group of incarcerated hernias and in 4% to 7% of the irreducible cases.[1,3]

The reported incidence of testicular infarction and subsequent atrophy with incarceration ranges from 4% to 12%,[1,36] with higher rates among the irreducible cases. This presumably occurs from compression of the gonadal vessels by the irreducible hernia, although some atrophic testes develop as a result of damage incurred during repair of a difficult incarcerated hernia. In their series of 351 incarcerated hernias, Rowe and Clatworthy[1] reported that 8 of 68 irreducible cases (22.8%) were associated with vascular compromise of the testes. Others have also observed an increased rate of gonadal atrophy with irreducible cases.[39] Many of these testes are atrophic on follow-up, although there have been several cases of blue testes that are normal in size at long-term follow-up.[30] Young infants are at higher risk, with testicular infarction rates of 30% to 33% reported in infants younger than 2 or 3 months.[30,39] These problems underscore the need for prompt reduction of incarcerated hernias and avoidance of repeat episodes of incarceration.

Preoperative and Postoperative Care

The anesthetic management of neonates with inguinal hernias is also controversial. The main issues involve the risk of apnea relative to: (1) the postconceptional age (PCA) for premature and term infants, and (2) the risk of apnea based on the type of anesthetic (general versus spinal or epidural).

One of the initial studies by Steward[40] reported that 18% of preterm infants developed apnea after general anesthesia for herniorrhaphy, compared with zero episodes in term infants. Of those who developed apnea, all were 8 weeks old or younger and therefore, based on inclusion criteria, less than 47 weeks PCA. Liu and colleagues[41] documented a 40% incidence of postoperative apnea in preterm infants with a PCA of less than 44 weeks. Gregory and Steward[42] subsequently recommended 18 hours of postoperative monitoring for preterm infants less than 44 weeks PCA. Welborn and colleagues[43] confirmed these recommendations in another study, in which periodic breathing occurred in premature infants with a PCA of less than 44 weeks. Kurth and colleagues,[44] however, in 1987 reported a 37% incidence of apnea in 47 preterm infants less than 60 weeks PCA and therefore extended the recommendation to 60 weeks. Unfortunately, several infants in this study had more extensive procedures. Apnea was seen in three healthy outpatients with PCAs of 43, 52, and 54 weeks, although only the 43-week-old infant had apnea past the recovery room period (12 hours).

More recent studies have questioned the need for extended monitoring of these neonates. In 1991, Melone and colleagues[45] presented a series of 124 premature infants (average gestational age, 32.7 weeks; average PCA, 45.3 weeks) who underwent herniorrhaphy with general anesthesia. They reported one early apneic episode and one episode identified on a home monitor in a child with a prior history of apnea. One patient required ventilatory support in the recovery room and another for 24 hours. They concluded that these patients could be managed safely as outpatients, although this conclusion was later criticized by Peutrell and Hughes.[46] Naylor and colleagues[47] stratified a group of term and premature infants by gestational age as well as risk factors defined as history of apnea and bradycardia, anemia (hemoglobin less than 10 g/dL), chronic respiratory disease, or need for theophylline. They reported a 34.5% incidence of postoperative apnea and bradycardia for those younger than 40 weeks PCA. The incidence was much lower for those 40 weeks PCA or older, and all of these could be identified by their preoperative risk factors. In addition, no episodes of postoperative apnea and bradycardia occurred in term infants. The researchers therefore recommended outpatient management at 40 weeks PCA or older in the absence of risk factors.

Although these two studies favor outpatient management of premature infants, they must be balanced against some of the earlier reports. In addition, a 1993 report by Gollin and colleagues[48] on hospitalized premature infants who underwent herniorrhaphy before discharge reported a high rate of complications (23% had apnea or bradycardia). Although these neonates were hospitalized, they had a mean PCA of 38.9 weeks (range, 33 to 47 weeks), and if at home, some may have been candidates for outpatient management at other medical centers. The researchers reported that a history of respiratory distress syndrome or bronchopulmonary dysplasia, history of patent ductus arteriosus, and low absolute weight were independent risk factors for postoperative complications.

The management of term infants is also somewhat unclear. Several studies have failed to demonstrate any apnea in term infants,[43,47] but there have been several case reports of postoperative apnea in term infants (PCA, 41.5 to 44.5 weeks).[49–51] Two of the episodes occurred within 1 hour of anesthetic administration, but one episode involving a 44.5-week PCA child occurred 6 hours after the end of anesthesia.[50]

Several other groups have reported on the use of spinal anesthesia to decrease the risk of apnea in high-risk infants. In a study of 84 high-risk infants (mean PCA, 41.5 weeks; range, 27 to 60 weeks) who underwent inguinal hernia repair under spinal anesthesia, Veverka and colleagues[52] observed no occurrences of postoperative apnea. Sartorelli and colleagues[53] reported on 140 high-risk infants (PCA, 44.8 ± 7.8 weeks), with only one case of apnea occurring in a child who received a supplemental dose of midazolam. Webster and colleagues,[54] in a report on spinal anesthesia in 44 premature infants (PCA, 40.54 ± 2.18), observed 5 with postoperative apnea (4.5 to 29 hours after surgery), although all 5 infants had received supplemental mask inhalation anesthesia. In all of these series and others reviewed, a small percentage of patients required supplementation with intravenous or inhalation agents, thus increasing the risk of apnea. The use of caudal epidural catheters in awake expremature babies is another technique with advantages of longer action and postoperative pain relief.[55] In addition, many centers use a caudal epidural to supplement the general anesthesia.

Anesthetic management at a given institution is primarily determined in conjunction with an anesthesiologist. An unsupplemented spinal anesthetic is preferable, but these have limited duration. If supplemental agents are required, patients may be at risk for postanesthetic apnea. In a comparative review of all of these techniques, Gallagher[56] recommended 12-hour postoperative apnea monitoring for all preterm infants with PCAs of less than 44 to 46 weeks. His practice was to monitor all preterm infants with PCAs of less than 60 weeks. On review of the literature, he recommended monitoring all term infants with PCAs of less than 44 weeks and all premature infants with PCAs of less than 51 to 54 weeks for at least 12 to 18 hours.

DISORDERS OF THE UMBILICUS

Embryology and Pathology

Disorders of the umbilical region are due either to persistence of structures, which usually obliterate before birth, or failure of closure of the umbilical ring. The umbilicus in early gestation is formed as the result of a fusion of the body stalk containing the umbilical vessels and allantois with the extracoelomic yolk stalk containing the vitelline (omphalomesenteric) duct and vessels.

The vitelline or omphalomesenteric duct normally obliterates at 7 or 8 weeks' gestation. Failure of obliteration results in persistence of remnants, which can lead to a wide variety of disorders depending on the stage of arrest. Persistence of the omphalomesenteric duct most frequently leads to a Meckel diverticulum with no connection to the umbilicus; however, the omphalomesenteric duct can occasionally have a vessel extending to the umbilicus (Fig. 64-6A). In addition, the omphalomesenteric duct may remain attached to the umbilicus as an umbilical fistula (see Fig. 64-6B). Other disorders include an umbilical polyp (see Fig. 64-6C) and a sinus or an enteric cyst located below the umbilicus.

Urachal anomalies occur when the allantois fails to involute into the usual cordlike urachus. Early in development, the allantois and cloaca are in communication. As the bladder forms from the ventral portion of the cloaca, it descends toward the pelvis with the urachus, the apical connection of the bladder to the umbilicus. The urachus is located between the peritoneum and transversalis fascia in the space of Retzius, and this investment usually limits extension of urachal disorders. The urachus normally becomes a fibrous cord at 4 or 5 months' gestation and is identified as the median umbilical ligament. Failure of this process may result in several anatomic abnormalities. A patent urachus (Fig. 64-7A) represents a total lack of involution. A urachal sinus (see Fig. 64-7B) occurs when the cephalad portion of the urachus remains open, and a urachal cyst (see Fig. 64-7C) occurs when the central portion fails to involute. An alternating sinus can drain into the umbilicus and bladder. A vesicourachal diverticulum represents a remnant at the top of the bladder, but this does not affect the umbilicus. Various theories have attempted to explain urachal abnormalities. Although an association with obstruction of the lower urinary tract has been reported, it is unusual.

The fetal midgut normally returns to the abdominal cavity by 10 to 12 weeks' gestation, and the abdominal wall proceeds

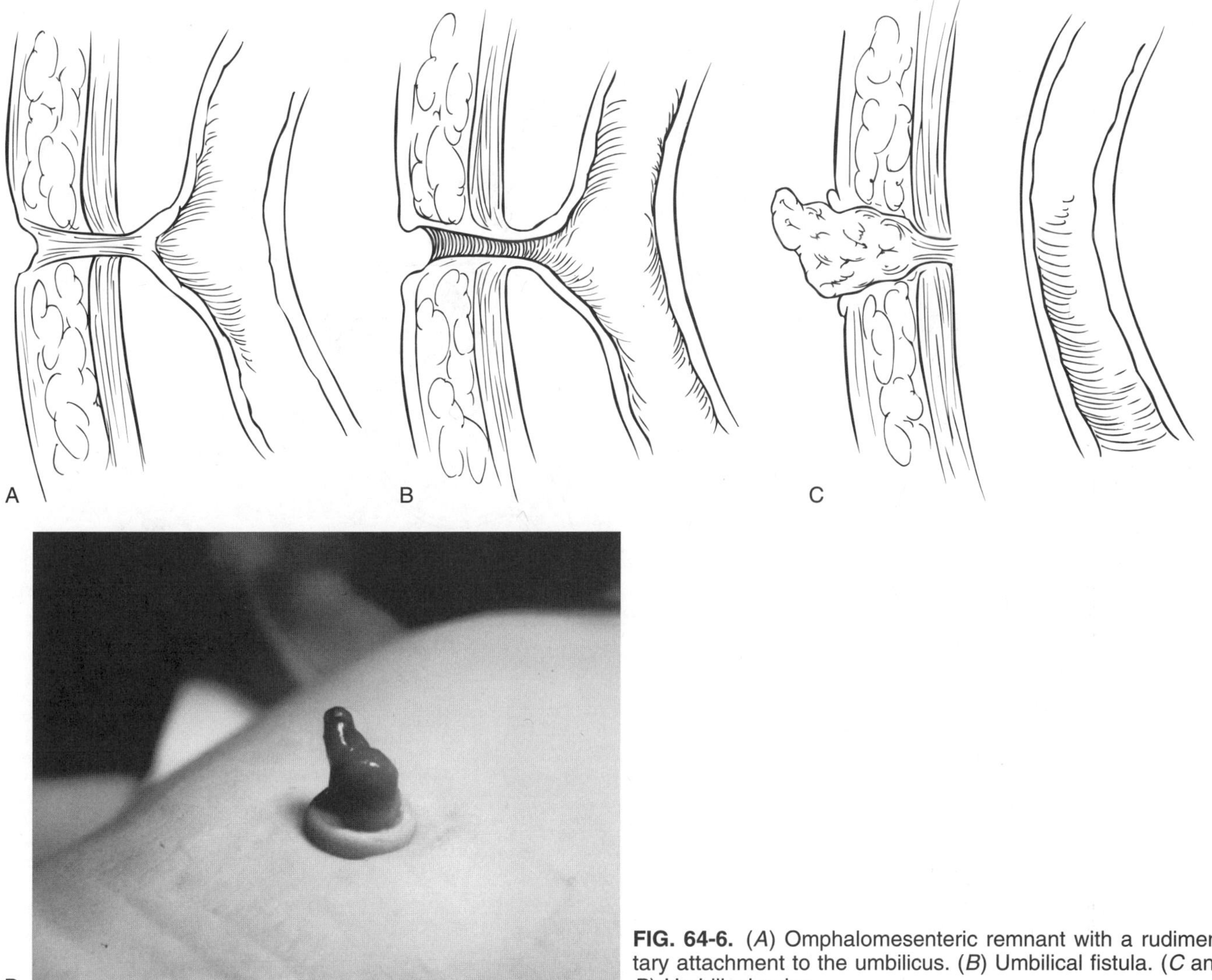

FIG. 64-6. (*A*) Omphalomesenteric remnant with a rudimentary attachment to the umbilicus. (*B*) Umbilical fistula. (*C* and *D*) Umbilical polyp.

to close. The umbilicus closes as mesoderm migrates in to form the abdominal wall. Failure of this closure can lead to an omphalocele, hernia of the umbilical cord, or an umbilical hernia. The first two present at delivery as abdominal wall defects and are discussed in other chapters. The umbilical ring continues to close until birth as the linea alba narrows and the rectus muscles approach the midline. The round ligament and a thickening of the transversalis fascia (umbilical fascia) also protect this area. The round ligament usually crosses the ring to insert on the inferior margin, but it can instead attach to the superior ring. In addition, the umbilical fascia can be absent or incompletely cover the umbilical ring, predisposing to defects.

Urachal Abnormalities

Clinical Presentation and Diagnosis

The patent urachus accounts for about half of anomalies and generally presents in the newborn period with urine draining from the umbilicus. The umbilical cord in these infants is often enlarged and edematous. The diagnosis can be confirmed by catheterization of the tract. A lateral voiding cystourethrogram demonstrates the opening, and intravesical methylene blue confirms the diagnosis.

Urachal cysts account for about 30% of cases that occur primarily in the lower third of the urachus. They are usually asymptomatic, and only one third of cases are identified in infancy or childhood.[57] Most present in older children and adults as urachal abscesses. These patients have a tender infraumbilical mass that may drain into the umbilicus or bladder. Intraperitoneal rupture has also been reported,[58] but some patients have only umbilical erythema.[59] A urachal sinus (15% of cases) usually presents with intermittent periumbilical pain and tenderness. This can usually be diagnosed either by probing the tract or with a lateral contrast injection study of the sinus. A vesicourachal diverticulum is a remnant at the top of the bladder and accounts for about 5% of urachal abnormalities.

The location of the urachus allows excellent evaluation by

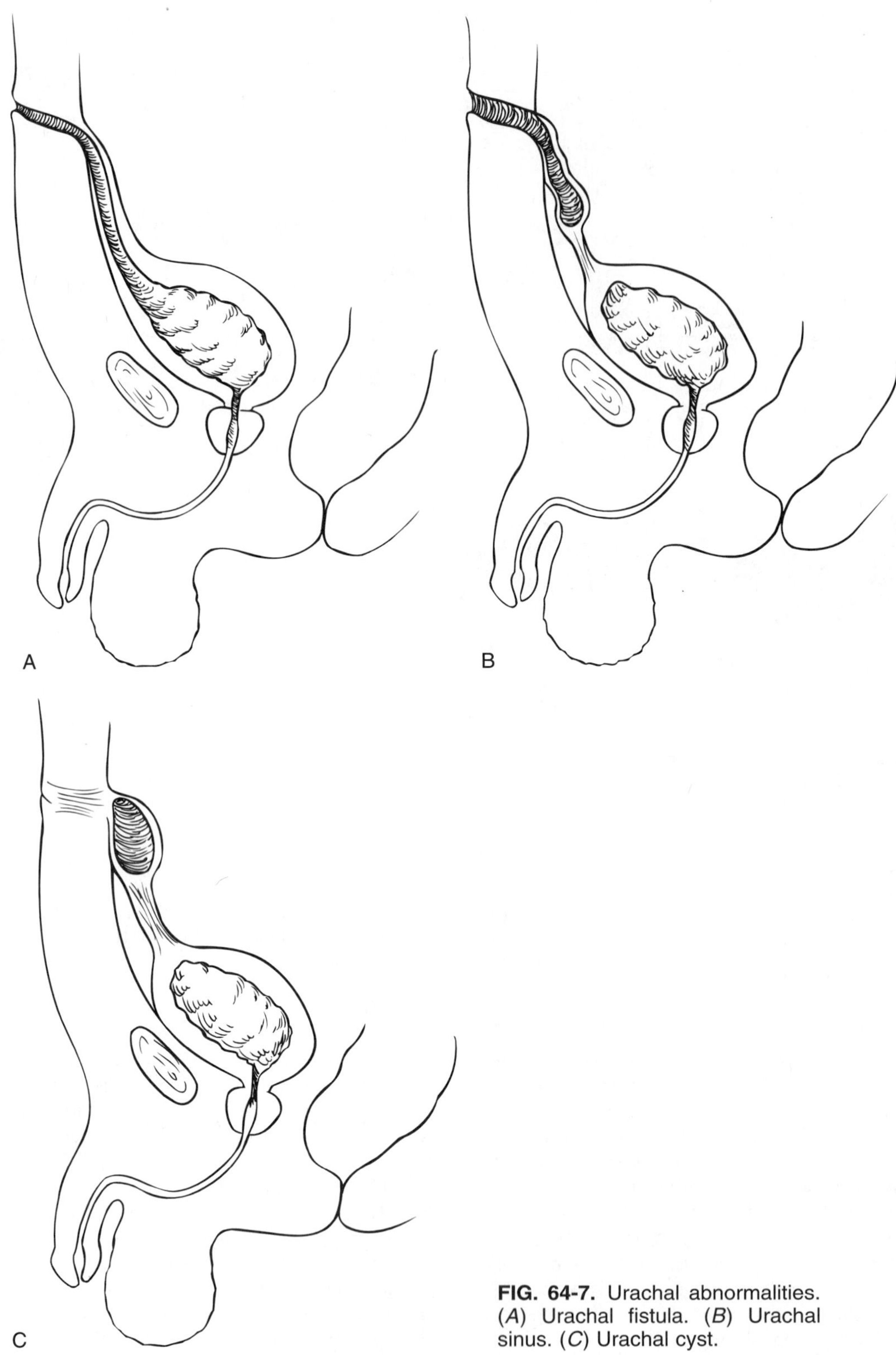

FIG. 64-7. Urachal abnormalities. (*A*) Urachal fistula. (*B*) Urachal sinus. (*C*) Urachal cyst.

ultrasound or computed tomography. Routine ultrasound, however, demonstrates a small elliptical, hypoechoic structure above the bladder in up to 62% of children given the test, and these should not be mistaken for pathologic processes.[60] Rich and colleagues[61] recommend an intravenous pyelogram to evaluate for concomitant urinary anomalies, although others have suggested that a voiding cystourethrogram may be more useful to aid in identification of a urachal cyst and to allow evaluation of vesicoureteral reflux.[57] An ultrasound of the urachal region, kidney, and bladder and a voiding cystourethrogram are usually adequate.

Treatment

If lower urinary tract obstruction is identified, it should be managed before the urachal anomaly. The standard of treatment for urachal anomalies consists of complete excision of the urachus, generally with a cuff of bladder. The rationale for excision of a cuff of bladder is based on the risk of malignancy, and so long as the distal margin of the mucosa of a urachal sinus or cyst is excised, excision of a portion of bladder is not necessary.[58,59]

The management of an infected urachal cyst may occasionally merit initial incision and drainage or percutaneous drainage with antibiotic therapy followed by delayed excision. Resection of the urachus can be achieved through a transverse or vertical incision. In addition, laparoscopic excision of an infected urachal cyst has been reported.[62]

Umbilical Hernia

Incidence and Natural History

Umbilical hernia is one of the more common pediatric surgical problems. The factors of interest center on the incidence based on age and race as well as spontaneous closure rates. Several older observational studies provide most of the available data. The actual incidence is unknown, but in one large infant clinic (consisting of only 1% black infants), umbilical hernia was identified in 18.5% of infants younger than 6 months.[63] The incidence of umbilical hernia has been observed to be higher in black children. In a large comparative study, Evans[64] reported an incidence of 24.7% among black infants and 3% among white infants. The cause for the racial difference is unknown, but the most likely factors are related to differences in the incidence of umbilical fascia defects.

The incidence of umbilical hernias decreases with advancing age in all races. In a study evaluating a large black population, Crump[65] reported an incidence of umbilical hernias of 41.6% in those younger than 1 year, declining to 15.9% at 4 years, 9.3% at 5 years, and 0% between 8 and 16 years of age. Crump also reported a higher incidence among premature infants. Walker[66] performed a 6-year follow-up study of 314 black infants younger than 3 months. He observed that 96% of initial fascial defects of less than 0.5 cm closed spontaneously, but no defects greater than 1.5 cm closed during the 6-year observation period. Spontaneous closure of defects greater than 1.5 cm in internal diameter has been reported, although at a lower rate than smaller defects.[67]

The increased incidence of umbilical hernias in premature

children was mentioned already. In one follow-up study,[68] 75% of very-low-birthweight infants (501 to 1500 g) had hernias at 3 months of age, with resolution occurring during the next 12 months to a 0% incidence at 12 months.

Clinical Presentation and Management

Most infants present with asymptomatic umbilical hernias. Incarceration and strangulation remain the only absolute indicators for surgical repair, and both of these are rare, occurring not at all in several large series[63,66] and as scattered occurrences in other reports.[67,69,70] Haller and colleagues[70] reported incarceration in 6 children and 102 adults during a 15-year period and recommended childhood repair to prevent adult incarceration. Others have observed that adult umbilical hernias generally do not result from unrepaired childhood hernias.

It appears that the low rate of incarceration and strangulation does not support a policy of early repair. Although some have recommended repair of large defects (more than 1.5 cm in diameter) at 1 to 2 years of age, spontaneous closure does occur in some of these defects.[71] Based on a review of the available data on closure rates, umbilical hernias that persist at 5 years of age should be repaired.

Surgical Management

Operative repair is accomplished through an infraumbilical curvilinear incision. The fascia inferior to the hernia sac is identified and the sac encircled at the level of the fascia. The fascial closure can be open or closed. In the former, the sac is excised and the fascia closed. In the closed technique, the sac is sharply detached from the umbilicus and inverted, and the fascia is closed over the sac. The dermis underlying the center of the umbilicus is secured to the fascia to restore the normal umbilical contour.

OMPHALOMESENTERIC DUCT ANOMALIES

An umbilical fistula (see Fig. 64-6B) usually presents with intestinal contents draining from the umbilicus after cord separation and needs no other formal diagnostic studies. An umbilical polyp (see Fig. 64-6C and D) can appear similar to a granuloma but does not respond to silver nitrate. It can contain small bowel or gastric mucosa. An enteric cyst can be asymptomatic or can present as an umbilical mass as the cyst fills with fluid.

Excision of these structures can usually be achieved with an intraumbilical incision. If the opening in the fascia is inadequate, a vertical extension allows adequate exposure. Complete excision is performed, and if a connection to the ileum is present, it is delivered into the wound and closed in a transverse fashion.

Umbilical Granuloma

An umbilical granuloma typically appears after cord separation as a mass of pink granulation tissue at the base of the umbilicus. Successful treatment consists of one or more applications of silver nitrate. If the lesion persists after several treatments. it should be excised because it may actually represent an umbilical polyp.

Periumbilical Necrotizing Fasciitis

Necrotizing fasciitis is a rare soft tissue infection that occurs in neonates. These cases usually start as omphalitis, which itself is rare with routine umbilical care. In the largest reported series, 7 of 8 patients died.[72] Most cases present with progressive erythema, abdominal wall induration, and discoloration of the umbilicus. One successful case report[73] emphasized the need for débridement and wide excision as well as excision of the umbilical vessels and urachal remnant to a point where they appear normal. A temporary Silastic patch is usually necessary for closure of the abdominal wall.

REFERENCES

1. Rowe MI, Clatworthy HW. Incarcerated and strangulated hernias in children. Arch Surg 1970;101:136.
2. DeBoer A. Inguinal hernia in infants and children. Arch Surg 1957; 75:920.
3. Farrow GA, Thompson S. Incarcerated inguinal hernia in infants and children: a five year review at the Hospital for Sick Children, Toronto, 1955–1959 inclusive. Can J Surg 1963;6:63.
4. Rescorla FJ, Grosfeld JL. Inguinal hernia repair in the perinatal period and early infancy: clinical considerations. J Pediatr Surg 1984;19:832.
5. Rothenberg RE, Barnett T. Bilateral herniotomy in infants and children. Surgery 1955;37:947.
6. Kiesewetter WB, Parenzan L. When should hernia in the infant be treated bilaterally? JAMA 1959;171:127.
7. Sparkman RS. Bilateral exploration in inguinal hernia in juvenile patients. Surgery 1962;51:393.
8. Rowe MI, Copelson LW, Clatworthy HW. The patent processus vaginalis and the inguinal hernia. J Pediatr Surg 1969;4:102.
9. McGregor DB, Halverson K, McVay CB. The unilateral pediatric inguinal hernia: should the contralateral side be explored? J Pediatr Surg 1980;15:313.
10. Given JP, Rubin SZ. Occurrence of contralateral inguinal hernia following unilateral repair in a pediatric hospital. J Pediatr Surg 1989;24:963.
11. Muraji T, Noda T, Higashimoto Y, et al. Contralateral incidence after repair of unilateral inguinal hernia in infants and children. Pediatr Surg Int 1993;8:455.
12. Wardhani H, Arianto A, Halimun EM. Inguinal hernia in children in Indonesia. Pediatr Surg Int 1993;8:464.
13. Hasan N. Management of inguinal hernia of childhood as practiced in Karachi, Pakistan. Pediatr Surg Int 1993;8:462.
14. Surana R, Puri P. Is contralateral exploration necessary in infants with unilateral inguinal hernia? J Pediatr Surg 1993;28:1026.
15. Rajput A, Gauderer MWL, Hack M. Inguinal hernias in very low birth weight infants: incidence and timing of repair. J Pediatr Surg 1992;27:1322.
16. Krieger NR, Shochat SJ, McGowan V, et al. Early hernia repair in the premature infant: long-term follow-up. J Pediatr Surg 1994;29:978.
17. Moss RL, Hatch EI. Inguinal hernia repair in early infancy. Am J Surg 1991;161:596.
18. Misra D, Hewitt G, Potts SR, et al. Inguinal herniotomy in young infants, with emphasis on premature neonates. J Pediatr Surg 1994;29:1496.
19. Wright JE. Inguinal hernia in girls: desirability and dangers of bilateral exploration. Aust Paediatr J 1982;18:55.
20. Goldstein IR, Potts WJ. Inguinal hernia in female infant and children. Ann Surg 1957;148:819.
21. Kramer SG, Davis SE. Transperitoneal detection of occult inguinal hernia. Milit Med 1967;132:512.
22. Kiesewetter WB, Oh KS. Unilateral inguinal hernias in children. Arch Surg 1980;115:1443.
23. Harrison CB, Kaplan GW, Scherz HC, et al. Diagnostic pneumoperitoneum for the detection of the clinically occult contralateral hernia in children. J Urol 1990;144:510.
24. Holcomb GW III, Brock JW III, Morgan WM III. Laparoscopic evaluation for contralateral patent processus vaginalis. J Pediatr Surg 1994;29:970.
25. Erez I, Kovalivker M, Schneider N, et al. Elective sonographic evaluation of inguinal hernia in children: an effective alternative to routine contralateral exploration. Pediatr Surg Int 1993;8:415.
26. Wolf SA, Hopkins JW. Laparoscopic incidence of contralateral patent processus vaginalis in boys with clinical unilateral inguinal hernias. J Pediatr Surg 1994;29:1118.
27. Chu CC, Chou CY, Hsu TM, et al. Intraoperative laparoscopy in unilateral hernia repair to detect a contralateral patent processus vaginalis. Pediatr Surg Int 1993;8:385.
28. Kurlan MZ, Wels PB, Piedad OH. Inguinal herniorrhaphy by the Mitchell Banks technique. J Pediatr Surg 1972;7:427.
29. Misra D, Hewitt G, Potts SR, et al. Transperitoneal closure of the internal ring in incarcerated infantile inguinal hernias. J Pediatr Surg 1995;30:95.
30. Slowman JG, Mylius RE. Testicular infarction in infancy: Its association with irreducible inguinal hernia. Med J Aust 1958;1:242.
31. Wright JE. Direct inguinal hernia in infancy and childhood. Pediatr Surg Int 1994;9:161.
32. Grosfeld JL, Minnick K, Shedd F, et al. Inguinal hernia in children: factors affecting recurrence in 62 cases. J Pediatr Surg 1991;26:283.
33. Wright JE. Femoral hernia in childhood. Pediatr Surg Int 1994;9:167.
34. Wright JE. Recurrent inguinal hernia in infancy and childhood. Pediatr Surg Int 1994;9:164.
35. Zhang JZ, Li XZ. Inguinal hernia in infants and children in China. Pediatr Surg Int 1993;8:458.
36. Clatworthy HW, Thompson AG. Incarcerated and strangulated inguinal hernia in infants: a preventable risk. JAMA 1954;154:123.
37. Puri P, Guiney EJ, O'Donnel B. Inguinal hernia in infants: the fate of the testis following incarceration. J Pediatr Surg 1984;19:44.
38. Kaplan GW. Iatrogenic cryptorchidism resulting from hernia repair. Surg Gynecol Obstet 1976;142:671.
39. Fasching G, Hollwarth ME. Risk of testicular lesions following incarcerated inguinal hernia in infants. Pediatr Surg Int 1989;4:265.
40. Steward DJ. Preterm infants are more prone to complications following minor surgery than are term infants. Anesthesiology 1982;56:304.
41. Liu LMP, Cote CJ, Goudsouzian NG, et al. Life threatening apnea in infants recovering from anesthesia. Anesthesiology 1983;59:506.
42. Gregory GA, Steward DJ. Life threatening perioperative apnea in the ex-"premie." Anesthesiology 1983;59:495.
43. Welborn LG, Ramirez N, Oh TH, et al. Postanesthetic apnea and periodic breathing in infants. Anesthesiology 1986;65:658.
44. Kurth CD, Spitzer AR, Broennle AM, et al. Postoperative apnea in preterm infants. Anesthesiology 1987;66:483.
45. Melone JH, Schwartz MZ, Tyson KRT, et al. Outpatient inguinal herniorrhaphy in premature infants: is it safe? J Pediatr Surg 1992;27:203.
46. Peutrell JM, Hughes DG. To the editor. J Pediatr Surg 1992;27:1487.
47. Naylor B, Radhakrishnan J, McLaughlin D. Postoperative apnea in infants. 1992;27:955.
48. Gollin G, Bell C, Dubose R, et al. Predictors of postoperative respiratory complications in premature infants after inguinal herniorrhaphy. J Pediatr Surg 1993;28:244.
49. Tetzlaff JE, Annand DW, Pudimat MA, Nicodemus HF. Postoperative apnea in a full-term infant. Anesthesiology 1988;69:426.
50. Karayan J, LaCoste L, Fusciardi J. Postoperative apnea in a full-term infant. Anesthesiology 1991;75:375.
51. Cote CJ, Kelly DH. Postoperative apnea in a full-term infant with a demonstrable respiratory pattern abnormality. Anesthesiology 1990;72:559.
52. Veverka TJ, Henry DN, Milroy MJ, et al. Spinal anesthesia reduces the hazard of apnea in high-risk infants. Am Surg 1991;57:531.
53. Sartorelli KH, Abajian JC, Kreutz JM, et al. Improved outcome utilizing spinal anesthesia in high-risk infants. J Pediatr Surg 1992;27:1022.
54. Webster AC, McKishnie JD, Kenyon CF, et al. Spinal anaesthesia for inguinal hernia repair in high-risk neonates. Can J Anaesth 1991;38:281.
55. Peutrell JM, Hughes DG. Epidural anaesthesia through caudal catheters for inguinal herniotomies in awake expremature babies. Anaesthesia 1993;47:128.

56. Gallagher TM. Regional anaesthesia for surgical treatment of inguinal hernia in preterm babies. Arch Dis Childhood 1993;69:623.
57. MacNeily AE, Koleilat N, Kiruluta HG, et al. Urachal abscesses: protean manifestations, their recognition and management. Urology 1992;40:530.
58. Iuchtman M, Rahav S, Zer M, et al. Management of urachal anomalies in children and adults. Urology 1993;42:426.
59. Newman BM, Karp MP, Jewett TC, et al. Advances in the management of infected urachal cysts. J Pediatr Surg 1986;21:1051.
60. Cacciarelli AA, Kass EJ, Yang SS. Urachal remnants: sonographic demonstration in children. Radiology 1990;174:473.
61. Rich RH, Hardy BE, Filler RM. Surgery for anomalies of the urachus. J Pediatr Surg 1983;18:370.
62. Siegel JF, Winfield HN, Valderrama E, et al. Laparoscopic excision of urachal cyst. J Urol 1994;151:1631.
63. Woods GE. Some observations on umbilical hernia in infants. Arch Dis Child 1953;28:450.
64. Evans A. The comparative incidence of umbilical hernias in colored and white infants. J Natl Med Assoc 1941;33:158.
65. Crump EP. Umbilical hernia. I. Occurrence of the infantile type in Negro infants and children. J Pediatr 1952;40:214.
66. Walker SH. The natural history of umbilical hernia: a six-year follow-up of 314 Negro children with this defect. Clin Pediatr 1967;6:29.
67. Sibley WL, Lynn HE, Harris LE. A 25-year study of infantile umbilical hernia. Surgery 1964;55:462.
68. Vohr BR, Rosenfeld AG, Oh W. Umbilical hernia in low birth weight infants (less than 1500 grams). J Pediatr 1977;90:807.
69. Lassaletta L, Fonkalsrud EW, Tovar JA, et al. The management of umbilical hernias in infancy and childhood. J Pediatr Surg 1975;10:405.
70. Haller JA Jr, Morgan WW, Stumbaugh S, et al. Repair of umbilical hernias in childhood to prevent adult incarceration. Am Surg 1971;37:246.
71. Neblett WW III, Holcomb GW III. Umbilical and other abdominal wall hernias. In: Ashcraft KW, Holder TM, eds. Pediatric surgery, ed 2. Philadelphia, WB Saunders, 1993:557.
72. Lally KP, Atkinson JB, Woolley MM, et al. Necrotizing fasciitis: a serious sequela of omphalitis in the newborn. Ann Surg 1984;199:101.
73. Kosloske AM, Bartow SA. Débridement of periumbilical necrotizing fasciitis: importance of excision of the umbilical vessels and urachal remnant. J Pediatr Surg 1991;26:808.

Surgery of Infants and Children: Scientific Principles and Practice, edited by Keith T. Oldham, Paul M. Colombani, and Robert P. Foglia. Lippincott–Raven Publishers, Philadelphia, © 1997.

CHAPTER 65

Abdominal Wall Defects

Thomas F. Tracy, Jr.

Abdominal wall defects are similar to most newborn congenital disorders that are linked to defects in development and triggered either by chromosomal or environmental and teratogenic alterations. This chapter examines the embryologic relations required for normal abdominal wall development and evaluates the evidence for specific fetal events leading to the newborn presentation of gastroschisis or omphalocele. As pediatric surgeons will more frequently find, the management and care of these defects will not only remain a surgical challenge in the newborn period but also will become a diagnostic and therapeutic concern for prenatal fetal management.

It remains traditional for both malformations to be presented together topically because of the common clinical presentation of a ventral abdominal defect and the common surgical treatment goal of closure of that defect. Distinctions between gastroschisis and omphalocele have, in the past, been generated only through general anatomic and embryologic definitions. A number of recent experimental and clinical observations, however, have provided exciting insights into potential genetic and teratogenic causes as well as distinct cellular and molecular alterations that are the foundation of each malformation.

PATHOLOGY

Omphalocele is a central abdominal defect through which both hollow and solid abdominal viscera can pass. These defects are uniformly covered by a membrane of amnion externally and peritoneum internally. The umbilical cord inserts into the membrane. The central defect can range in size from a few centimeters in diameter to defects that extend to the lower chondral margins. These latter defects, known as *giant omphaloceles*, contain liver, small and large bowel, and occasionally other organs. Smaller defects may have only a few loops of bowel and can be more realistically viewed as hernias of the umbilical cord.

Gastroschisis is a different lesion from omphalocele. The ventral defect is uniformly small (4 cm or less) and is found to the right of an intact, central umbilical cord. There have been rare reports of left-sided defects, which may in fact represent true ruptured omphaloceles. The external appearance of uncov-

ered loops of bowel may be either clearly discerned or hidden owing to foreshortening of the bowel and an extensive reactive inflammatory peel on the bowel serosa. The liver and other solid organs remain within the abdomen, but the gonads may also be found externally. Distinct vascular changes in the amniotic epithelium have been described in gastroschisis. Ultrastructural analysis has demonstrated numerous lipid droplets within the epithelial cells of the placenta that are distinctly different from the appearance of meconium in the underlying chorion. The amniotic epithelial cells are otherwise intact.

These are clearly two distinct definitions of the pathology of both ventral defects. Before further examinations of their divergence, each should be understood relative to its common departure from normal embryologic and fetal development of the anterior abdominal wall.

ABDOMINAL WALL DEVELOPMENT

General Features and Relation to Gut Development

The embryologic anterior body wall develops first from the somatopleure and tail folds of the embryo with an open midgut and body stalk. Simultaneous cranial, caudal, and lateral closure of embryonic folds leads to anterior fusion at the umbilical ring by 28 days' postconception. Before the sixth week of development, the somatopleure of the abdominal wall is composed of fused mesoderm and ectoderm. After that, the somatopleure is invaded by mesodermal components of myotomes situated lateral to the vertebral column.

In normal development, the leading edges of mesoderm differentiate into the rectus muscle bodies that eventually fuse in the midline. Before fusion, the lateral mesodermal components divide into the three layers destined to be the muscle bodies of the lateral abdominal wall. Abdominal visceral development proceeds in parallel with its closure. Fusion of lateral folds mentioned previously occurs at about 20 days' postconception, at the same time as foregut division. During embryologic days 28 to 35, the midgut elongates and by necessity extrudes through the umbilical ring 2 weeks later. During the 7th week, the rectus muscles are separated with a long body stalk holding the midgut.

Approximation from cranial and caudal ends is complete by the 12th week as the midgut returns to within the abdomen. Boundaries of the abdomen are then formed cranially by the septum transversum and caudally by inversion of secondary mesoderm separating the cloaca from the abdomen.

Suspected Causes of Ventral Defects

In an attempt to suggest an etiologic mechanism for ventral defects, some studies have examined the potential relation of innervated migratory mesenchyme to the completion of abdominal wall closure. Bands of mesenchyme, along with spinal segmental and cutaneous terminal nerves, are thought to be critical to sternal, abdominal, and limb development. Embryologists have been encouraged to focus on this question by the finding that experimental absence of the innervation has led to failed limb development.

The relation of migrating mesenchyme and associated cutaneous nerves to abdominal wall closure has been demonstrated in embryologic studies of normal thoracic and abdominal wall development. From those observations, it is apparent that the sternum is formed from condensations of mesenchyme from the dorsolateral body wall, labeled *sternal bands*. Similar well-innervated bands have been also noted during abdominal wall development in mice and rats. Although the requirement for innervation of these mesenchymal bands on limb development in mice has been demonstrated, the same is only assumed and remains unproved for the anterior body wall. Indeed, no significant alterations in sensation through dermatomes of the anterior body wall have been found clinically in either gastroschisis or omphalocele.

Without any observed changes in abdominal wall innervation in clinical practice, it seems more likely that ventral defects follow a failure of fusion of cranial, lateral, and caudal folds that occurs before mesenchymal migration and innervation. A single study of fetuses with abdominal wall defects and associated anal and urologic malformations suggests that a failure in the embryologic cell deposition process takes place, during which ectodermal cells are not added to the mesodermal compartment of the embryo. This process of cell deposition normally occurs in the neural crest and in the body wall placode. Failure of ectodermal deposition may therefore be the basis of a constellation of embryologic events related to the neural crest, and it may also have a role in ventral defects. Specific factors that can be mechanistically linked to the causes of these defects remain elusive. Through attempts to uncover etiologic agents or cellular alterations, however, the first clear distinctions between both entities emerge.

Because of the absence of multiple associated anomalies (discussed later), gastroschisis as an isolated malformation has been investigated the most extensively for the presence of environmental risk factors and potential teratogenic links. The position of the anomaly to the right of the umbilicus lends itself to the possibility that gastroschisis results from a vascular disruption of the omphalomesenteric artery. This, coupled with its most frequently associated anomaly, intestinal atresia, would indicate an attractive embryologic link to other vascular disruptions (see Associated Anomalies). Early investigations, therefore, sought to find a link to prenatal ingestion of vasoconstrictive agents.

Throughout all previous epidemiologic studies, maternal age and positive smoking history have been identified as important historical factors, with a particular risk noted for smoking in women younger than 20 years old. One initial clinical survey found mothers of affected infants had a higher incidence of aspirin ingestion or oral contraceptive use. A higher incidence of cocaine use was also clearly demonstrated.

The largest case-controlled surveillance program was first undertaken by the Sloan Epidemiology Unit of Boston University to examine the use of drugs during the first trimester in relation to gastroschisis. No increased risk was found for antihistamines, antibiotics, oral contraceptives, or spermicides. Significant risk, however, was associated with the use of ibuprofen, salicylates, phenylpropanolamine, propanolamine, pseudoephedrine, and other decongestants. Additionally, acetaminophen was associated with gastroschisis, eliminating an isolated specific class of drugs with vasoactive side effects. This pattern of drug use may alternately reflect an underlying maternal illnesses rather than the drugs themselves, which would be taken for symptomatic relief.

This possibility of maternal illness or exposure is further suggested by a study of Washington State residents that showed a greater risk of gastroschisis for infants born in January, February, or March. This implies a cluster of defects that follow from a possible seasonal environmental exposure.

An alternative etiologic theory proposes that gastroschisis follows an in utero disruption of an omphalocele. The ability to follow abdominal wall defects by prenatal ultrasound (discussed later) has offered some credence to that theory by clearly demonstrating one fetus with an omphalocele that appeared to undergo rupture of the membrane late in gestation. A classic defect of gastroschisis was then found at term.

New multicenter registries for gastroschisis may provide a more specific set of causes along the lines of fetal vascular disruption or links to maternal illness and drugs. A single case report of gastroschisis associated with arthrogryposis multiplex congenita, consisting of intestinal atresia, Moebius anomaly, and selective skeletal muscle hypoplasia, further underscores the potential of intrauterine vascular occlusion as a reasonable cause. The extensive volume of prenatal diagnosis and fetal monitoring would most likely have offered more evidence of omphalocele rupture if it were obviously causally related to gastroschisis.

Unfortunately, the same interest in finding a potential teratogenic relation in gastroschisis has not been sought after or described for omphalocele. Studies of that defect have alternatively looked for chromosomal alterations that account for the patterns of associated anomalies linked to omphalocele.

INCIDENCE

The largest epidemiologic studies have found that generally omphalocele occurs in 1 in 4000 births and gastroschisis in 1 in 6000 to 10,000 births. Both occur in males and females equally. A surprising finding has come from a large registry in Scotland that determined by prenatal ultrasound that the incidence of abdominal wall defects was as frequent as 1 in 2500 fetuses.

In a review of more than 500,000 live births, the prevalence of omphalocele was found to be 0.21 in 1000, and gastroschisis was 0.08 in 1000. Combining stillbirths and live births, another study found a prevalence of 0.19 and 0.14 in 1000 for omphalocele and gastroschisis, respectively.

PATHOPHYSIOLOGY

The physiologic impact of an omphalocele is directly related to its size and more significantly to any associated anomalies. Whether pulmonary hypoplasia that accompanies giant omphalocele is related to the omphalocele or a true associated anomaly is unknown. One would anticipate that a large ventral defect, which could be considered the reverse of congenital diaphragmatic hernia, would not interfere therefore with lung development. The presence of a large defect does appear to direct the development of a globular liver that conforms to its extracolonic position rather than its normal lobular architecture. To date, no specific alterations in the fetal intestine have been determined microscopically. Only in cases of ruptured omphalocele has there been any evidence of serosal inflammation. Normal motility and function have been almost universally observed, and surprisingly, there have been few cases of delayed complications from associated malrotation.

In contrast to the absence of any detrimental effects on the fetal gut by an omphalocele, gastroschisis results in severe abnormalities of fetal bowel function. Studies by Langer and colleagues have attempted to use experimental fetal models to elucidate the cause of the fetal intestinal response to extraperitoneal amniotic exposure. Previous experiments implicated changes in fetal urine and in amniotic fluid composition, resulting in progressive acidity (pH $<$ 6.9) and increased epidermal growth factor late in gestation. Using fetal rabbits with relatively short gestational periods, experimental intraperitoneal injections of amniotic fluid failed to duplicate serosal inflammatory changes seen in gastroschisis. Experimental formation of gastroschisis, however, resulted in fetal and intestinal growth retardation, mesenteric shortening, and a small peritoneal cavity.

Fetal sheep have been used to induce experimental gastroschisis, and this results in a thick inflammatory "peel" on the bowel surface, mucosal villous atrophy, and abnormalities of the myenteric nervous system. All alterations were directly related to the length of exposure to the amniotic fluid. Further experiments found that fetal bowel compression resulted in bowel wall thickening and mucosal edema, whereas the fibrinous, inflammatory peel on the serosa occurred only with amniotic fluid exposure. The effects of amniotic fluid were found to be reversible with fetal repair late in gestation. To test whether vascular disruption was part of the pathophysiology, intestinal blood flow was measured and found to be identical between experimental gastroschisis and the control fetuses. Hence, the current concept is that fetal intestinal injury with abdominal wall defects is related to amniotic fluid exposure and partial intestinal obstruction in utero.

One of the best studies of the human fetal response to gastroschisis comes from Amoury and colleagues. Histologic studies of intestinal samples have found the fibrinous peel to be a feature that begins at 30 weeks' gestation. This peel consists of type I collagen. Changes in the mucosa, submucosa, or muscularis were related to the degree of intestinal infarction. No ab-

normalities were seen in myenteric ganglion cells to account for the related neonatal hypomotility. Villous atrophy was identified as the structural basis for the clinical problem of altered nutrient uptake in the newborn.

ASSOCIATED ANOMALIES

Few associated abnormalities are found in infants with gastroschisis compared with those with omphalocele. Obligate malrotation, intestinal atresia, polyhydramnios, and Meckel diverticulum represent 75% of the associated problems in patients with gastroschisis. An international survey by Moore and Nur in 1986 revealed that only 21% of 203 cases of gastroschisis had an associated malformation. In contrast, 54% of 287 patients with omphalocele had associated malformations.

In a large study of fetal karyotypic abnormalities in children with abdominal wall defects, more than 40% of fetuses with omphalocele were abnormal, compared with no fetuses with gastroschisis. As expected, abnormal karyotypes were encountered in fetuses with multiple anomalies compared with isolated defects. Abnormal karyotypes include trisomy 18, 13, and 21 as well as Turner syndrome and Klinefelter syndrome. One population-based study found that while there were significant differences in maternal age for infants with isolated omphalocele or gastroschisis, no differences in maternal age could be demonstrated among those with associated anomalies. In familial cases of single defects, an autosomal recessive pattern of inheritance was found. Multiple defects appeared sporadic, however, and they did not correspond to any known genetic pattern of inheritance. Up to 72% of patients with omphalocele have anomalies within the cardiovascular, genitourinary, and central nervous systems. The most common cluster of abnormalities is found in Beckwith-Wiedemann syndrome, composed of omphalocele, macroglossia, pancreatic hyperplasia resulting in hypoglycemia along with other elements of visceromegaly, and craniofacial abnormalities. This syndrome has been mapped to chromosome 11pter-p15.4.

As mentioned previously, gastroschisis is primarily associated with jejunoileal atresia. Perhaps the most disturbing complication of the malformation is the potential for in utero midgut volvulus. This catastrophic complication can also occur postnatally owing to failure to recognize a fragile, compromised vascular pedicle to the extruded gut.

Several studies have shown that up to 30% of newborns with gastroschisis have significant growth retardation. Most newborns with gastroschisis are below the 50th percentile in weight and commonly have low serum levels of albumin, immunoglobulin G, transferrin, and total serum proteins. Potential reasons for the development of intrauterine growth retardation include diminished uterine blood flow, abnormal fetal nutrient balance, or specific growth factor deficiencies. In a study of 21 cases of prenatally diagnosed gastroschisis, more than half of the fetuses were prenatally growth retarded, and seven patients in this group had birthweights that were less than the 10th percentile. Three newborns not identified with ultrasound to have intrauterine growth retardation were subsequently born with growth retardation. An interesting observation from this study was the finding that early primary closure was accomplished in growth-retarded newborns with gastroschisis, resulting in a shorter hospitalization and fewer complication. Thus, it appears that intrauterine growth retardation does not negatively affect outcome in this circumstance.

PRENATAL DIAGNOSIS

Prenatal Ultrasound

The ability to diagnose most abdominal wall defects through uterine prenatal ultrasound has immediate consequences for subsequent treatments. The diagnosis of omphalocele or gastroschisis can be made after 14 weeks' gestation when the fetal midgut has normally returned to the abdominal cavity. If an abdominal wall defect is identified on screening maternal ultrasound, a follow up examination should be done, with special emphasis on the search for associated malformations, especially in cases of omphalocele.

A detailed examination must be performed, beginning with measurement of biparietal skull diameter and femur length, which provides information about the extent of growth retardation. The size of the abdominal defect should be determined, especially in cases of gastroschisis, in which a small defect may be associated with the development of bowel dilation later in gestation. Measurements of the abdominal diameter and estimates of the volume of herniated viscera may establish parameters predictive of the need for staged repair versus primary closure. Associated malformations should be sought initially and followed through the course of pregnancy.

The accuracy of detecting concurrent malformation in fetuses with omphalocele was studied in 43 fetuses; 67% had additional malformations, and of these, 23 were considered major and 6, minor. In this study, there were a significant number of terminated pregnancies, which provided autopsy data. Fetal ultrasound correctly identified 29 of 58 (50%) individual anomalies; 7 of 7 in the central nervous system, 8 of 14 cardiac anomalies, and 1 of 5 craniofacial abnormalities. Anomalies missed by ultrasound included renal dysplasia, esophageal atresia with tracheoesophageal fistula, congenital diaphragmatic hernia, pulmonary hypoplasia, and Beckwith-Wiedemann syndrome. Results from other large regional surveys have found the diagnosis of associated anomalies to be accurate in greater than 70% of cases.

Serial ultrasound examinations should concentrate on the appearance of eviscerated bowel in gastroschisis, noting the presence of bowel dilation and the development of a fibrotic peel. Both are late gestational manifestations of bowel atresia, owing to constriction at the point of the abdominal wall defect and exposure of the gut to amniotic fluid. In clinical studies of the development of gut dilation, there is good correlation with fetal distress but no correlation with surgical outcome. The presence of a bowel diameter greater than 18 mm in one series of 24 fetuses was associated with significant delay in oral feeding and also with a high likelihood of bowel resection. The clinical significance of a finding of bowel dilation in a fetus with an abdominal wall defect is not yet clear. It is premature to initiate or alter fetal or obstetric therapy on the basis of these findings in infants with gastroschisis.

Questions remain in some centers regarding the sensitivity and specificity of fetal ultrasound for the diagnosis of abdominal wall defects. One early review of a group of 20 patients with gastroschisis and 20 patients with omphalocele found a false-negative rate of 35% and 22% for ultrasound in patients with gastroschisis and omphalocele, respectively. Fortunately, the failure of screening ultrasound had no effect on newborn outcome. Larger general population studies have determined that up to 66% of infants with omphalocele and 70% of those with gastroschisis are diagnosed prenatally. Further improvement is likely.

Fetal Markers

Fetal markers have had some usefulness in the diagnosis of ventral defects. The most studied and understood marker has been the presence of elevated maternal α-fetoprotein (AFP) in serum indicating either a neural tube or ventral defect. Ninety percent of cases of omphalocele and 100% of gastroschisis cases are associated with elevated AFP. Amniotic fluid acetylcholinesterase (ACHE) has been used to evaluate neural tube defects and has also been identified in one study of the amniotic fluid of 16 pregnancies with gastroschisis. ACHE was negative in the cases of omphalocele. With immunoassay methods for ACHE, it is possible to distinguish open neural tube defects from abdominal wall defects. In addition, levels of ACHE have been found to be greater for neural deficits than for gastroschisis.

Screening for elevated maternal AFP is the most direct indication for a fetal ultrasound examination to determine the presence of a ventral defect. In a search for other potential biologic markers, the maternal serum human chorionic gonadotropin level has also been found to be elevated during the second trimester when an abdominal wall defect was demonstrated on ultrasound. No prospective study of human chorionic gonadotropin levels has been performed. A demonstration of the complementarity of these tests is found in cases of equivocal sonographic findings in which a normal maternal AFP and negative ACHE would be most compatible with the prenatal diagnosis of omphalocele.

PRENATAL MANAGEMENT

Initial Consideration

With the diagnosis of either gastroschisis or omphalocele, amniocentesis for karyotype should be performed to determine whether other lethal anomalies are present. Because of the low rate of aneuploidy with gastroschisis, some centers reserve karyotype analysis for confirmed cases of omphalocele but not for clearly defined gastroschisis. This is a critical time for the resources of a fetal management team or multidisciplinary perinatal center. Decisions incorporating medical, ethical, moral, and religious data need to be made regarding the termination of pregnancy in cases of defined and confirmed lethal anomalies. Counseling about ventral abdominal defects and any identified associated anomalies must begin once the specific diagnoses are made.

One approach has been to introduce families at the point of diagnosis to all the components of a fetal management group, including the high-risk perinatal center, the newborn intensive care unit, neonatologists, the pediatric surgical staff, and clinical nurse specialists. Based on the diagnosis of gastroschisis or omphalocele, the exact nature of the defect, pathophysiology, expected fetal course, and potential complications are first introduced. The parents are familiarized with the individual events and attending physicians. Fellows and residents from each clinical service play an important role in patient care and bimonthly follow-up.

As discussed previously, the associated conditions of growth retardation, respiratory distress, and potential preterm delivery prompt important follow up and delivery at a complete perinatal center. For gastroschisis, studies have demonstrated a greater rate of primary closure, with significantly less postoperative assisted ventilation for prenatally transferred newborns. Trends toward earlier enteral feeding and discharge have been noted.

In infants with omphalocele, it has become apparent that the morbidity and mortality is directly related to associated congenital anomalies. In infants with giant omphalocele, cesarean section may become necessary with growing concerns for dystocia rather than for protection of the viscera or drainage of the membrane.

The controversies in perinatal management of abdominal wall defects primarily revolve around the infant with gastroschisis. In the absence of complicating anomalies, such as intestinal atresia, improving the quality of the eviscerated bowel usually improves outcome. A relevant issue then becomes the source of injury to the bowel (see Pathophysiology). This can be prenatal (exposure to amniotic fluid), intrapartum (decreased perfusion, visceral compression with uterine contractions), or postnatal (increased distention secondary to ingestion of air, exposure to pathogens, heat and fluid losses). Each scenario then provides possibilities for potential interventions, such as earlier delivery, avoidance of labor and vaginal delivery, and intrauterine rather than postnatal transfer to tertiary-level care centers. No prospective, randomized study has provided a definitive answer to these issues. Contemporary studies, at best, seek to understand the individual issues. The outcome variables measured are ability to achieve primary closure, time on ventilator, time to enteral feedings, and duration of hospitalization.

Early delivery has been proposed on theoretic grounds, with anticipated improvement for those infants who had bowel dilation in utero. The impact of mode of delivery on outcome in the absence of fetal distress or maternal complications has been reviewed by several authors. Most centers have concluded that cesarean section is not indicated except for obstetric concerns. There has been no significant benefit in terms of the outcome variables for infants with gastroschisis delivered by cesarean section. Further studies have examined whether postnatal transport or delay in time to surgery adversely affect the infant. In a study by Novotny and colleagues, 32 infants were delivered by cesarean section. Elective delivery was performed with the pediatric surgical team in an adjacent room for immediate repair of gastroschisis. The authors remarked that the peel and edema were much less prominent and that reduction with primary repair occurred more easily. Nonelective cesarean section infants required transfer for operation that averaged about 6 hours of life. When infants less than 34 weeks' estimated gestational age with a second anomaly were excluded, then the ability to accomplish primary repair in the delivery room was higher (8 of 9), than that for transferred infants (5 of 13). Time to extubation, time to enteral feeding, and length of hospital stay were all significantly shorter for the immediate surgery group. These findings are consistent with those from a London series in which 40 infants with gastroschisis were treated at a tertiary referral center after either in utero transfer (9 patients) or postnatal transfer (31 patients). Primary closure was accomplished in 78% of the former group versus 55% of the latter. In utero transfers also had a tendency toward shorter ventilator support, total parenteral nutrition (TPN), and hospital stay. The question of whether there is an advantage to delivery in a regional versus peripheral obstetric center if postnatal transport is necessary was addressed by a group in Birmingham, England. They demonstrated that if patients came to operation within the same period of time postnatally, then primary closure rates of 89% to 94% could be achieved for each group. A 23-day period of TPN was the average for both groups, which simply states that good results can be achieved even with postnatal transfer of patients.

NEWBORN MANAGEMENT

Common principles of newborn resuscitation and preoperative management mentioned elsewhere apply to these defects. Specific considerations for omphalocele relate to a close newborn examination for the integrity of the defect and an appreciation of any associated pulmonary disease that might accompany giant omphalocele. Endotracheal intubation, ventilation, and arterial and venous access may all need to be provided, based on an initial survey that identifies other severe cardiac or urologic anomalies. If transport is anticipated, the membrane should be covered with sterile saline-soaked gauze, and a protective barrier to prevent heat loss should be applied. Plastic wrap is ideal for omphalocele coverage and protection. Broad-spectrum antibiotics should be started.

Consideration of associated anomalies should have priority over concern for surgical repair. An exception to this might occur with disruption of the membrane and evisceration. Most disruptions are minor, however, and usually can be sealed with sterile petrolatum-impregnated gauze while secondary evaluations are underway.

The initial approach to gastroschisis is different owing to its relative freedom from associated anomalies. Inappropriate or careless coverage of the eviscerated bowel may induce torsion of the vascular pedicle containing the mesenteric vessels. If this is covered with nontransparent dressings, progressive intestinal ischemia may develop. The use of transparent surgical bowel bags along with manual stabilization during transport should be emphasized. Nasogastric decompression is essential and should begin immediately after birth.

The optimal goal of surgical treatment for both defects is skin, fascia, and muscle coverage, which ultimately restores the form and normal muscular function of the anterior abdominal wall. In considering both defects, only omphalocele might qualify for nonoperative management. In that case, a covered ventral hernia can be established by the use of agents that initially provide a bacteriostatic eschar, followed by progressive epithelialization. Many topical agents have been applied and discarded because of associated toxicity. Current practices include the application of silver nitrate, silver sulfadiazine cream, povidone-iodine (Betadine) solution, and triiodomethane–petrolatum (Iodoform) gauze. Any prolonged use of iodinated compounds is accompanied by the risk of thyroid suppression.

Nonoperative management for giant omphalocele does not preclude reduction of viscera into the abdomen. Significant success has been achieved by repeated wrapping of the omphalocele in a figure-of-eight fashion using semielastic gauze dressing. This material, when changed daily with increased tension, has allowed for progressive reduction of liver and bowel in the face of resolving pulmonary disease or cardiac stabilization.

OPERATIVE MANAGEMENT

Omphalocele

Small and medium-sized defects can usually be handled with primary fascial closure with appropriate monitoring of intraabdominal pressure (Fig. 65-1). Elevation of abdominal pressure at abdominal wall closure results in decreased venous return, decreased cardiac output, decreased pulmonary compliance, decreased ventilation, and decreased splanchnic perfusion. Pressure monitoring may be aided by arterial and central venous lines as well as by nasogastric tubes and Foley catheters. When transduced continuously, the latter two give excellent indicators of elevated intraabdominal pressure. Two studies prospectively examined the usefulness of intragastric and bladder pressure measurements during attempted primary repair. Using bladder pressure monitoring to maintain intraabdominal pressure at less than 20 mmHg, the decision to perform staged repair was influenced in 7 of 13 patients with gastroschisis in whom primary repair was thought to have been possible. Intragastric pressures of less than 20 mmHg and increases in central venous pressure of less than 20 mmHg have both been parameters that have successfully guided staged repair of omphalocele and gastroschisis. With these guidelines, there appear to be no complications of increased intraabdominal pressure.

Patients should be uniformly intubated for anesthesia and assisted ventilation during paralysis. Controversy has sometimes arisen over whether the sac should be removed, and many reports and experiences have presented both sides. Generally, the smaller the defect, the easier removal of the sac before fascial closure. As the size of the defect increases, the sac remains attached to larger areas of the liver. The improved benefits of the removal of the portion of amnion and peritoneum is overshadowed by the risks of laceration of the newborn liver and hemorrhage.

If the sac is removed, the umbilical vessels must be identified and ligated. No specific intraabdominal maneuvers are necessary. If approximation can be accomplished within specific pressure limits, skin flaps are created by sharp dissection away from the fascia. Interrupted sutures are then placed in the fascia from the superior portion of the defect to the inferior edge. These are sequentially tied while intraabdominal pressure is monitored and care is taken to prevent extensive compression or decreased ventilation (Fig. 65-2) Creative methods for skin closure of smaller defects have been described to enable formation of a false umbilicus. Subcuticular absorbable sutures placed in a pursestring fashion have yielded excellent results.

Considerable experience, judgment, and art are required in the management of larger defects and giant omphaloceles. Treatment options can take the following courses: (1) short-term (up to 14 days) silo reduction, followed by closure using fascia or prosthetic materials when adequate skin coverage for both is available; (2) long-term (2 to 6 weeks) silo reduction, followed by the same maneuvers; or (3) a staged reduction closing skin flaps over the amnion, followed by delayed (6 to 12 months) closure of the ventral hernia.

If short-term reduction is attempted, a Dacron-reinforced Silastic membrane is attached to the right and left edges of the fascia after raising a minimal edge of skin (Fig. 65-3). Aggressive skin flap formation should not be performed because it leads to skin retraction that is detrimental to subsequent closure. The Silastic sheets are sutured or stapled closed at the superior and inferior margins, with closure in the middle by any material, noting that progressive closure will be accomplished by progressive tightening at the mid-portion. Numerous materials and devices have been described for this purpose; the most cost-effective methods are sutures and umbilical tape. There is no need to remove the amniotic membrane because this is a perfect bacteriostatic peritoneal layer over which the Silastic sheets can be applied.

Gastroschisis

Three major concerns dominate the operative management of gastroschisis. The first is the recognition of significant in

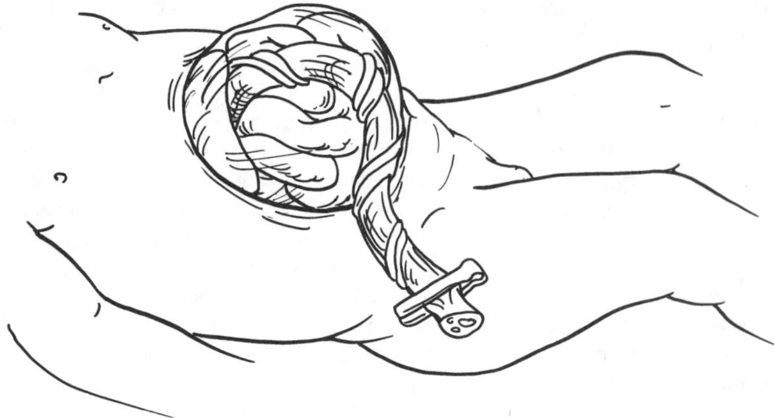

FIG. 65-1. Small to moderate sized omphalocele.

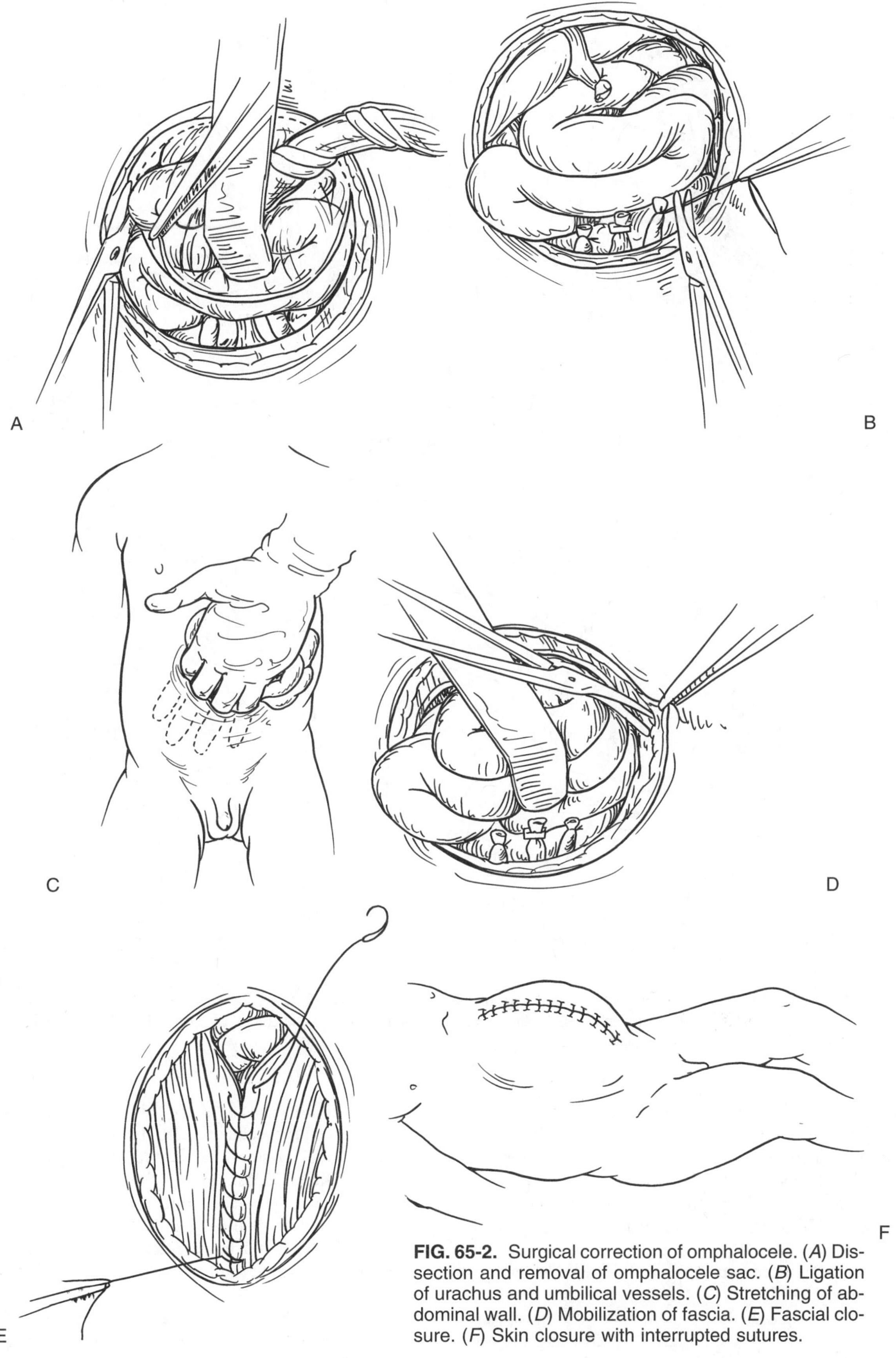

FIG. 65-2. Surgical correction of omphalocele. (*A*) Dissection and removal of omphalocele sac. (*B*) Ligation of urachus and umbilical vessels. (*C*) Stretching of abdominal wall. (*D*) Mobilization of fascia. (*E*) Fascial closure. (*F*) Skin closure with interrupted sutures.

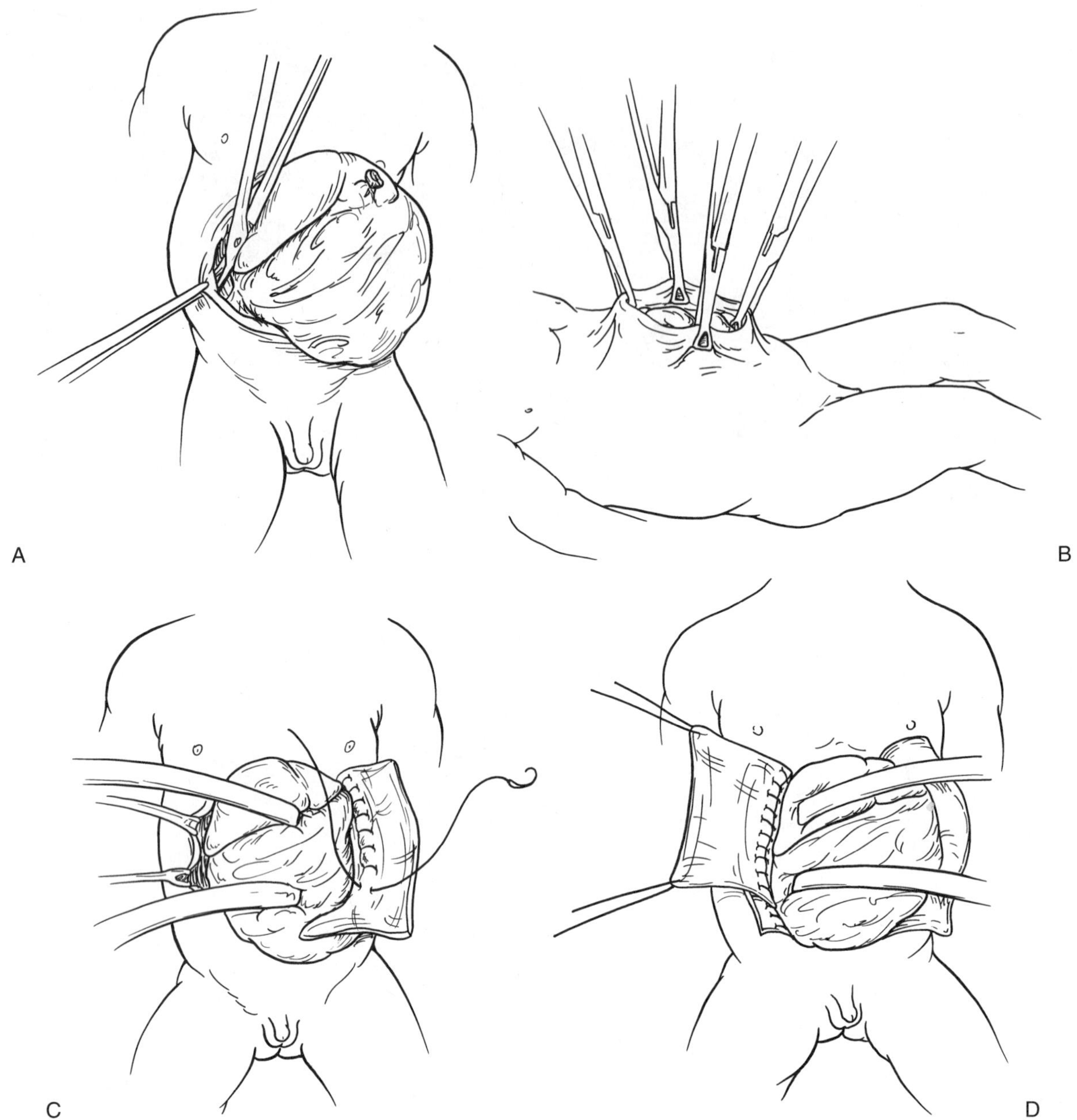

FIG. 65-3. Surgical management of large (giant) omphalocele. (*A*) Dissection and removal of omphalocele sac. (*B*) Stretching and extension of abdominal wall. (*C*) Application of Gore-Tex patch to left abdominal wall. (*D*) Application of patch to right abdominal wall. *(continued)*

utero complications, which include growth retardation, midgut volvulus, segmental bowel infarction, and intestinal perforation. Eviscerated abdominal contents should be examined after establishing mechanical support and maintaining vascular integrity to identify any of the listed complications. No attempt should be made to decompress the bowel or to remove the reactive peel.

Second, with heightened concerns for fluid replacement appropriate for increased losses, venous lines are placed, and at least 125 to 175 mL/kg/d of fluid is administered. Appropriate conductive (water blanket) or convective (BAIR-Hugger, Augustine Medical, Eden Prairie, MN) warming is mandatory during the procedure.

After the abdomen is prepared, the umbilicus is identified and preserved for reconstruction. In as many as 75% of infants, the eviscerated contents can be reduced into the abdomen. Extension of the defect should continue superiorly to open a narrow defect and allow for reduction (Fig. 65-4*A* and *B*).

A third major challenge is the management of infarcted bowel, which should be resected, with the open bowel ends oversewn. Interrupted sutures may be placed in areas of perforation, and no attempt should be made for primary anastomosis in areas of segmental infarction or identified atresia. The intraoperative management of atresia has frequently been an area of concern based on earlier unsuccessful attempts to establish continuity. It was argued that proximal decompression by an

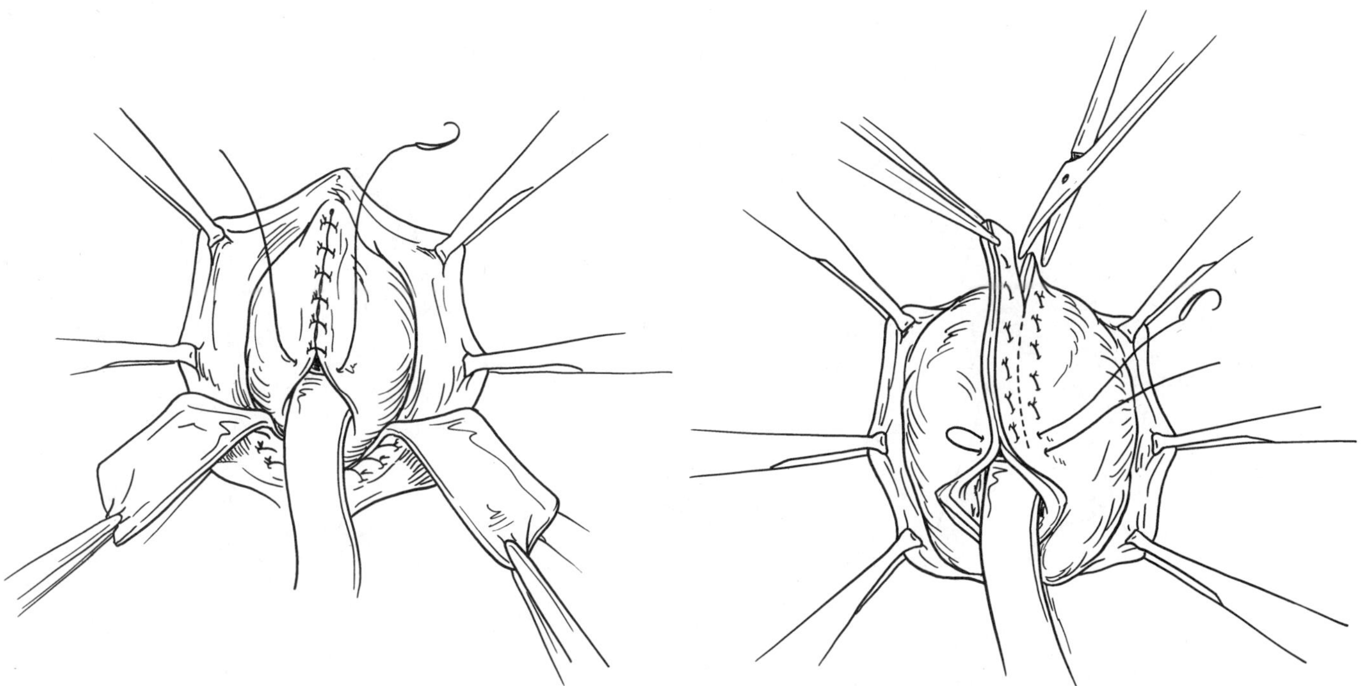

E

F

FIG. 65-3. *Continued.* (*E*) Approximation and creation of Gore-Tex silo. (*F*) Secondary shortening of silo and staged closure of abdominal wall.

enterostomy could then be followed by delayed anastomosis 2 to 6 weeks after intestinal coverage and resolution of the peel. Recent experience indicates that decompressive ostomies are not required. Bowel atresia can be successfully managed by nasogastric decompression for 2 to 4 weeks after abdominal wall closure, allowing for precise anastomosis of even multiple atretic segments with ancillary tapering enteroplasties. Delays in reanastomosis for 2 weeks result in resolution of the peel, but extension to 4 weeks may be necessary to allow for nutritional optimization. This may occur at the expense of further bowel dilation; however, tapering should eliminate any further negative impact.

Once the abdominal contents (which may include small and large bowel, stomach, bladder, ovaries, uterine tubes, and testes) have been reduced, interrupted absorbable sutures are placed in the fascia. Closure is then accomplished, with monitoring of intraabdominal pressure, as for omphalocele. The skin is then closed over the defect, allowing the umbilicus to come to its normal central position.

The inability to accomplish complete reduction should prompt consideration of the use of skin flaps for coverage or, more appropriately, the use of Dacron-reinforced Silastic sheeting as a silo. The fascial defect is enlarged as for primary repair, and the Silastic is sewn with nonabsorbable sutures in a running fashion to either edge. The remaining edges of this silo are also closed with sutures (see Fig. 65-4*C* and *D*). Progressive reduction without vascular compromise or perforation due to pressure can be accomplished by various means; the most simple and accessible is umbilical tape and heavy suture (see Fig. 65-4*E* and *F*). Reduction to fascial approximation may be reached in several days or up to 2 weeks later.

In the face of a large defect that allows for reduction but difficult closure of the fascia, Gore-Tex patches are an alterna-

tive if skin flaps can then be brought over the Gore-Tex. A durable closure is provided, which may or may not require further operative revision, owing to excellent regrowth of fibrous tissue into the patch. Long-term follow-up of patients undergoing this method of repair has shown that many of these patches are extruded as the infant grows.

POSTOPERATIVE MANAGEMENT AND COMPLICATIONS

The major immediate postoperative concerns are for respiratory insufficiency, nutritional support, and wound care. For both omphalocele and gastroschisis, TPN via a central should be initiated immediately. Paralysis and heavy sedation may be necessary to aid ventilatory support initially, but prolonged use is at the cost of increased peripheral and abdominal wall edema. Flaps should be examined for evidence of ischemia, cellulitis, or fascitis. After repair of both defects, significant erythema of the abdominal wall can appear through the first 72 hours postoperatively. Surgeons must carefully examine the wound to differentiate the response from early wound infection. Oral or nasogastric decompression is maintained.

An association of gastroschisis with necrotizing enterocolitis (NEC) has been identified after repair. The presentation of NEC was reported in 10 of 54 patients, with a mean of 2.1 instances of pneumatosis per patient. Only one episode of pneumoperitoneum required operation, and no perforation was found. Episodes of NEC occurred later in the hospital course or patients were readmitted with NEC. TPN-associated cholestasis, delayed enteral feedings, and other intestinal anomalies had a positive correlation with NEC. This high incidence of a relatively benign atypical form of NEC should not, therefore, preclude

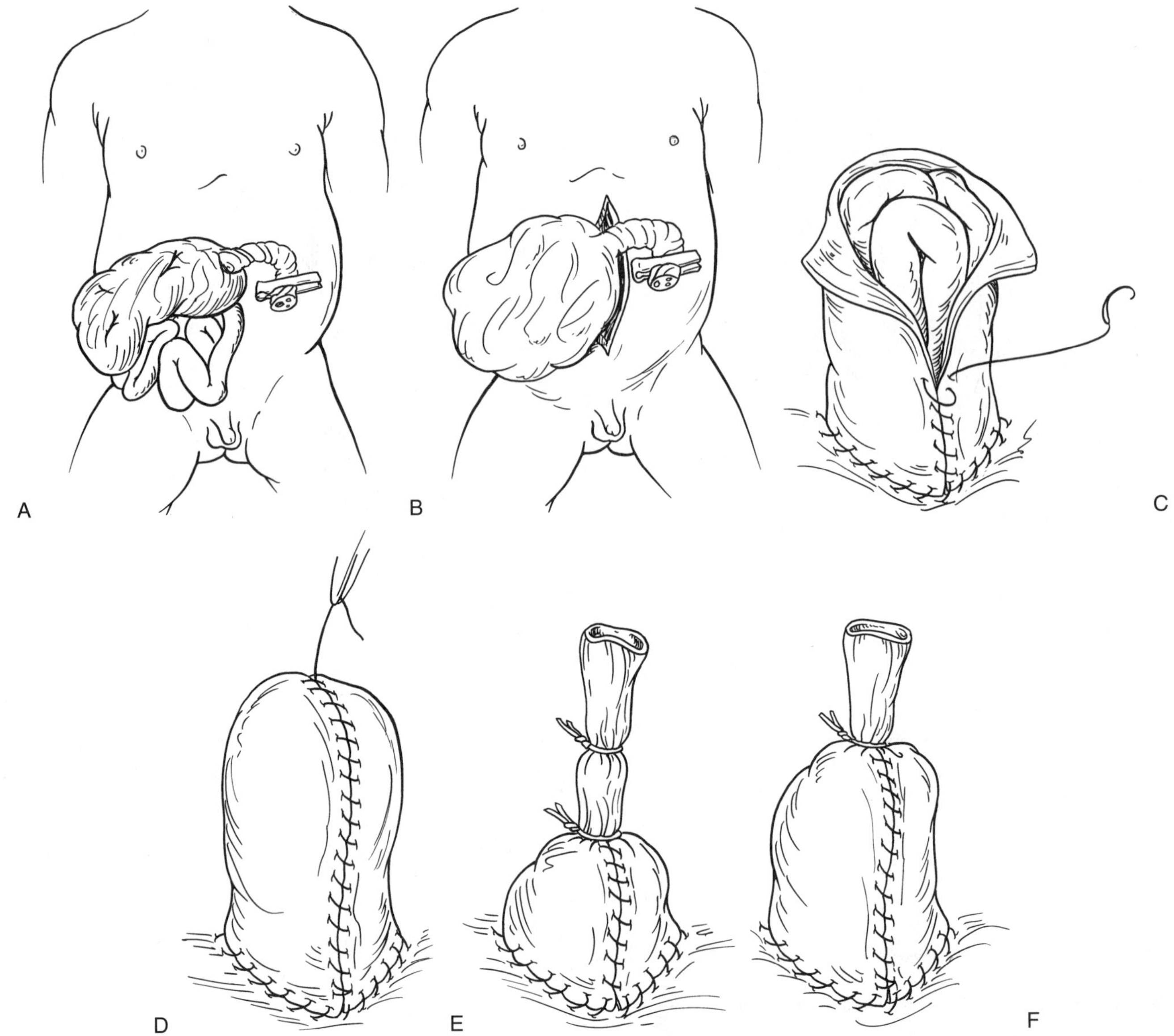

FIG. 65-4. Management of gastroschisis. (*A*) Gastroschisis defect. (*B*) Extension of opening with midline incision (optional). (*C*) Use of silo if primary closure is not possible. (*D*) Finished silo. (*E* and *F*) Staged ligation of silo with reduction of silo contents into abdominal cavity proper.

initiation of the enteral feedings as soon as possible. There is no direct evidence that earlier feeding is protective against postoperative NEC.

Delayed intestinal motility has been one of the central postoperative concerns in patients with gastroschisis. One of the first clinical studies of this problem found that patients who underwent primary reduction and closure had a clear advantage with respect to earlier institution of enteral feedings and discharge. The conclusions of the report on patients treated during the 1970s have been echoed in a recent study of prenatally diagnosed fetuses with gastroschisis. For infants who underwent primary repair either immediately or in the delivery room, earlier enteral feeding, shorter ventilator dependency and more rapid discharge were observed.

For both gastroschisis and omphalocele, the duration of mechanical ventilation postoperatively may be directly related to the degree of pulmonary compromise created by the repair. Although several methods of intraoperative intraabdominal pressure monitoring have been described, only recently have real time flow–volume curves been found to be helpful in postoperative respiratory management.

In one study of preoperative and postoperative flow–volume curves, closure of the abdominal defect resulted in decreases to 50% of normal for forced vital capacity and respiratory system compliance. In this series of 17 patients, forced vital capacity approached normal 4 weeks after operation, while compliance remained 50% lower than controls. In a study with slightly longer follow-up, functional residual capacity measured from 1 to 10 months postnatally for a group of six infants with omphalocele and seven with gastroschisis showed a significant decrease from mean control values of 30 to 25 mL/kg. Thus, ventral defects may result in impaired lung growth.

SECONDARY SURGICAL REPAIR

Most secondary reconstructions are required for patients with giant omphaloceles. Ideally, eventual fascial repair is the goal. Fascial substitutes that have been described include Marlex and Prolene mesh, Gore-Tex and lyophilized dura mater. The latter material was used as an adjunct for abdominal wall closing in three children without complications.

Experimentally, one of the most attractive options has been the use of an inner Gore-Tex patch reinforced externally by Prolene or Marlex mesh. Few adhesions to the inner Gore-Tex were found, whereas dense fibrinous tissue readily infiltrated the external mesh.

Several reports of primary fascial closure after abdominal placement of tissue expanders show good long-term results. Another successive technique of tissue expansion involves placement of saline-filled expanders within the rectus sheath. If this technique provides enough fascial coverage, skin coverage can be provided by the use of subcutaneous tissue expanders. Excessive intraabdominal pressure during tissue expansion, however, must be avoided.

The long-term results of patients repaired gastroschisis and omphalocele appear to be good, but late surgical problems should be anticipated. When followed for a mean of 5 years, postoperative ventral hernia developed in 25% of patients with omphalocele and in equal percentage of gastroschisis patients. Intestinal obstruction was more common after omphalocele repair. Complications occurred whether closure was primary or delayed.

In most cases of omphalocele, early termination of pregnancy owing to chromosomal abnormalities or early newborn death are the major sources of mortality. Morbidity for the remaining 20% to 50% of newborns rests in ongoing problems with associated malformations or secondary reconstructions. Evidence of prolonged pulmonary compromise has been provided. Secondary infection of synthetic prosthetic materials may be anticipated and may require removal before final attempts at fascial closure. Recurrent small bowel obstructions due to adhesion and gastric outlet obstruction from excessive splenic or hepatic compression have been reported. Inguinal hernias and gastroesophageal reflux appear with greater frequency in these patients.

In a review of patients with gastroschisis, the ability to perform primary fascial closure ranged from 31% to 81% of patients. A critical review of patient parameters showed no differences with respect to patient weight, gestational age, and associated fetal complications and abnormalities. In contemporary reports, survival is expected for infants with gastroschisis or omphalocele who do not have other anomalies. When considering all patients, gastroschisis patients have a surgical rate of approximately 85% and omphalocele patients somewhat less, depending upon the nature of other problems.

Life-long concerns of short gut syndrome, respiratory compromise, and developmental delay in nearly 20% of children require continued attention. Although clinical management has significantly diminished newborn morbidity and mortality rates, the potential remains to ameliorate earlier fetal injury and associated problems.

BIBLIOGRAPHY

Allen RG, Wrenn EL. Silon as a sac in the treatment of omphalocele and gastroschisis. J Pediatr Surg 1969;4:3.

Coughlin JP, Drucker DE, Jewell MR, et al. Delivery room repair of gastroschisis. Surgery 1993;114:822.

deVries PA. The pathogenesis of gastroschisis and omphalocele. J Pediatr Surg 1980;15:245.

Grosfeld JL, Dawes I, Weber TR. Congenital abdominal wall defects: current management and survival. Surg Clin North Am 1981;61:1037.

Grosfeld JL, Weber TR. Congenital abdominal wall defects: gastroschisis and omphalocele. Curr Probl Surg 1982;19:159.

Knight PJ, Buckner D, Vassy LE. Omphalocele: treatment options. Surgery 1981;89:332.

Langer JC, Khanna J, Caco C, et al. Prenatal diagnosis of gastroschisis: development of objective sonographic criteria for predicting outcome. Obstet Gynecol 1993;81:53.

Lewis DF, Towers CV, Garite TJ, et al. Fetal gastroschisis and omphalocele: is cesarean section the best mode of delivery? Am J Obstet Gynecol 1990;163:773.

Mollitt DL, Ballantine TV, Grosfeld JL, et al. A critical assessment of fluid requirements in gastroschisis. J Pediatr Surg 1978;13:217.

Moretti M, Khoury A, Rodriquez J, et al. The effect of mode of delivery on the perinatal outcome in fetuses with abdominal wall defects. Am J Obstet Gynecol 1990;163:833.

Nicholls G, Upadhyaya V, Gornall P, et al. Is specialist centre delivery of gastroschisis beneficial? Arch Dis Child 1993;69:71.

Novotny DA, Klein RL, Boeckman CR. Gastroschisis: an 18-year review. J Pediatr Surg 1993;28:650.

Pryde Pg, Bardicel M, Treadwell MC, et al. Gastroschisis: can antenatal ultrasound predict infant outcomes? (Review) Obstet Gynecol 1994;84:505.

Sakala EP, Erhard LN, White JJ. Elective cesarean section improves outcomes of neonates with gastroschisis. Gynecol Obstet 1993;169:1050.

Schuster SR. A new method for the staged repair of large omphaloceles. Surg Gynecol Obstet 1967;125:837.

Schuster SR. Omphalocele and gastroschisis. In: Welch KJ, Randolph JG, Ravitch MM, et al, eds. Pediatric surgery, ed 4. Chicago, Year Book, 1986:740.

Schwartz MZ, Tyson KR, Milliorn K, et al. Staged reduction using a Silastic sac is the treatment of choice for large congenital abdominal wall defects. J Pediatr Surg 1983;18:713.

Sipes SL, Weiner CP, Sipes II DR, et al. Gastroschisis and omphalocele: does either antenatal diagnosis or route of delivery make a difference in perinatal outcome? Obstet Gynecol 1990;76:195.

Stringer MD, Brereton RJ, Wright VM. Controversies in the management of gastroschisis: a study of 40 patients. Arch Dis Child 1991;66:34.

Wesley JR, Drongowski R, Coran AG. Intragastric pressure measurement: a guide for reduction and closure of the Silastic chimney in omphalocele and gastroschisis. J Pediatr Surg 1981;16:264.

Surgery of Infants and Children: Scientific Principles and Practice, edited by Keith T. Oldham, Paul M. Colombani, and Robert P. Foglia. Lippincott–Raven Publishers, Philadelphia, © 1997.

CHAPTER 66

Bladder, Cloacal Exstrophy, and Prune Belly Syndrome

Steven G. Docimo, Robert D. Jeffs, and John P. Gearhart

BLADDER EXSTROPHY

Incidence

Exstrophy of the urinary bladder is a rare but potentially devastating anomaly. A study of 6.3 million births worldwide revealed an incidence of bladder and cloacal exstrophy of 3.3 per 100,000, with a male/female ratio of 1.5 to 1.[1] The incidence of isolated epispadias was 2.4 per 100,000 live births. Most series have documented a higher male/female ratio, on average 2.3:1.[2]

Embryology

The normal cloacal membrane is a bilaminar structure that occupies an infraumbilical position on the developing abdominal wall. Mesenchymal elements invade the membrane to unite the lower abdominal musculature, and genital folds fuse superiorly to form the genital tubercle. The normal cloacal membrane is situated on the ventral side of the developing phallic structure. The classic explanation for the occurrence of exstrophic anomalies, based on experimental studies in chick embryos,[3] is an overgrowth or persistence of the cloacal membrane on the lower anterior abdominal area, preventing the normal mesenchymal ingrowth.[4] This causes divergence of the lower abdominal muscular structures and forces the genital ridges to fuse caudal to the cloacal membrane.[5] The various manifestations of the exstrophy–epispadias complex come about when the cloacal membrane ruptures. The stage of ingrowth of the urorectal septum at the time of rupture determines whether the result is an exstrophic urinary tract alone (classic bladder exstrophy or epispadias) or a cloacal exstrophy with the hindgut interposed between the hemibladders. Thomalla and associates[6] produced cloacal exstrophy in a chick embryo after injuring the area of the cloacal membrane with a laser. They proposed that premature rupture of the membrane alone, without an abnormal wedge effect, might produce exstrophy. An alternative explanation based on rat studies has been proposed by Mildenberger and

associates.[7] In their view, the "glandular hillock," referring to the genital tubercle, does not form in the infraumbilical region. For this reason, the cloacal membrane remains immediately caudal to the umbilicus. The body stalk, therefore, does not migrate cranially, preventing ingrowth of mesenchyme into the midline.

Predisposing Factors

Some evidence exists for a genetic predisposition to exstrophy and epispadias. According to an international survey conducted by Shapiro and associates,[8] the risk for recurrence of exstrophy or epispadias in a given family is 1 in 275 births. The likelihood of an exstrophic parent producing a child with exstrophy or epispadias is about 1 in 70, or 500 times the risk for the general population. Ives and associates[9] looked at the families of 102 patients with exstrophy and found no recurrences among their 162 siblings. They estimated the incidence of recurrence to be less than 1% based on a review of the literature. Smith and associates[10] reported the occurrence of nontwin siblings with cloacal exstrophy and other elements of the complex consisting of omphalocele, exstrophy, imperforate anus, and spinal defects.

No definite medical or environmental factors predispose to the development of exstrophy. The international clearinghouse of birth defects noted a slightly increased risk of exstrophy or epispadias in children of mothers younger than 20 years of age.[1] An increased risk of bladder exstrophy after the use of maternal progestins has been postulated.[11] A single case of bladder exstrophy in the child of a user of lysergic acid diethylamide was reported in 1970,[12] but there have been no other reports of this association to the knowledge of the authors.

Presentation

As opposed to other, more common congenital urinary tract abnormalities, exstrophy of the bladder is relatively rarely diagnosed prenatally.[13,14] This is probably because of the more subtle nature of the sonographic findings and the rarity of the disorder. Jaffe and associates[15] described a case diagnosed prenatally and suggested several criteria for the diagnosis of exstrophy of the bladder. First, there is no bladder filling even after diuretic, with or without a lower abdominal wall mass. In addition, a low-set umbilicus, normal scrotum, and a small phallus are generally present. Retrospective reviews suggest that the diagnosis should be suspected on the basis of nonvisualization of the bladder and a low-set umbilicus.[16–18]

At birth, the diagnosis of classic bladder exstrophy is usually easily made. The characteristic findings in boys include the bladder plate protruding just beneath the umbilical cord. On either side of the bladder, the rectus muscles are divergent, leading to the separated pubic bones. This separation is caused by an outward rotation of the innominate bones, eversion of the pubic rami, and, in the most severe cases, lateral separation of the inferior innominate bones.[19] The male infant exhibits a short phallus with a dorsal urethral plate, a splayed glans, and dorsal chordee. The phallic length is influenced by the separation of the pubic bones, but there may also be a true deficiency of corporal length.[20] Despite these abnormalities, the phallus in bladder exstrophy can generally be reconstructed to be cosmetically and functionally acceptable. Rarely is it necessary to consider sex reassignment owing to an inadequate phallus.[2] The scrotum is generally normally developed, although the testicles are often located in the distal inguinal canal.[17] Commonly, bilateral inguinal hernias are seen at birth. This is due to the large internal and external rings and the lack of obliquity of the inguinal canals. In a retrospective review, Husmann and associates[21] found that 56% of boys and 15% of girls with exstrophy have inguinal hernias; this was confirmed by Peppas and associates,[22] who reported that 82% of boys and 11% of girls had inguinal hernias, respectively. Ten to 53% of the patients presenting with hernia within 1 year of primary closure were incarcerated at presentation, and both groups recommend hernia repair at the time of primary closure. Hernia repair requires both excision of the hernia and repair of the muscular defect to prevent recurrence.[17,22]

In girls, the genital defect is analogous to that in boys but is more easily reconstructed. The mons pubis, clitoris, and labia are separated, and the vaginal orifice is displaced anteriorly.[23] The pelvic floor defect predisposes to uterine prolapse, especially after pregnancy and delivery.[24] Uterine prolapse is less common after early pelvic closure with osteotomy.[2]

The anus may be anteriorly placed and is sometimes patulous. It represents the posterior extent of the myofascial defect. Anal continence may be affected by the divergence of the pelvic musculature, and this should be assessed before consideration of diversion of urine to the rectosigmoid. Rectal prolapse occurs frequently in untreated patients, possibly due to straining in response to irritation of the bladder mucosa. Prolapse virtually always disappears after bladder closure or cystectomy and represents an indication for surgical management of the exstrophied bladder.[2]

Pathophysiology of the Exstrophied Bladder

The pathophysiology of the bladder wall in exstrophy is only beginning to be understood. It appears that the bladder muscula-

ture contains a normal complement of muscarinic receptors for contractile stimulus.[25] Tissue/matrix ratios of normal and exstrophied bladders have been compared. In urologically normal children, this ratio was found to be 0.33 ± 0.11, and in children with classic bladder exstrophy closed in the first week of life, it was 0.83 ± 0.46. Although the tissue/matrix ratio is increased in exstrophied bladders, the impact on capacity and eventual urinary continence is unknown. Other factors clearly play a role in the functional characteristics of the exstrophied bladder. Studies are underway to document the effect of collagen content and type in the bladder wall and the impact of the clinical course on outcome.[26]

Evaluation at Birth

The appearance of the exstrophic neonate can be grotesque to both the parents and the delivery room staff, who likely have seen nothing similar. The pediatrician or family practitioner is unlikely to have experience with more than one or two cases of bladder exstrophy. It is essential that the child be seen by a pediatric genitourinary surgeon with special interest and experience in this problem who can realistically counsel the parents and determine initial therapy. The impact of a major birth defect can be made significantly worse by conjectural advice or inappropriate initial management.

The bladder mucosa is easily injured and inflamed. The umbilical cord should be ligated with suture to avoid mucosal abrasion, which can be caused by an umbilical clamp. The bladder should not be covered with moistened gauze or petrolatum-coated gauze; it is best protected with a clear plastic wrap. Each time a diaper is changed, the bladder surface should be irrigated with sterile saline and the plastic wrap replaced. General and cardiopulmonary assessment should be completed as per routine but with an eye toward the likelihood of major surgery in the neonatal period. The kidneys should be examined by ultrasound for hydronephrosis, and a radionuclide scan should be performed to assess function. Intravenous urography is an alternative but is often suboptimal in the newborn period.

The parents should be reassured at this stage. In general, the child with classic bladder exstrophy is a healthy, robust infant. The parents need to be aware that, with the proper care, their baby has the prospect of a normal life.[27] Ambulation, sexual function, and renal function are likely to be preserved. An effective reconstruction to allow urinary storage, drainage, and control can be expected, with an acceptable cosmetic appearance. The support of social workers, nurses, and parents of other children with exstrophy is invaluable, and is usually available at a large medical center with an interest in this problem.[17,28]

Initial Management

Closure of the pelvic ring is an important adjunct to the eventual attainment of urinary continence. If operation can be carried out within the first 72 hours of life, the pelvic ring can sometimes be closed effectively without the need for osteotomy.[29] When the pubic separation is wide, or when surgery cannot be accomplished until the child is older, osteotomy is essential to the closure of the pelvic ring. Osteotomy should be performed at the same time as the bladder surgery. This requires a well-coordinated surgical and anesthesia team to avoid undue blood loss and risk of prolonged anesthesia.

Two approaches to pelvic osteotomy for exstrophy have predominated: posterior bilateral iliac osteotomy and anterior bilateral transverse innominate osteotomy. Both approaches provide improved symphyseal approximation, making the midline abdominal closure easier and decreasing the likelihood of dehiscence.[30,31] Closing the bladder neck within the pelvic ring allows approximation of the levators and the puborectal sling and provides an improved eventual continence rate.[30,31]

The authors' preference is for an anterior approach to osteotomy, dividing the innominate bone above the acetabulum.[32–34] Initially, the anterior approach was used in patients who had failed an initial attempt at closure.[32] The results were so satisfactory that, at this institution, this approach is used in essentially all cases of bladder exstrophy. The technique is similar to that of a Salter osteotomy. Both sides of the innominate are exposed simultaneously, and a horizontal osteotomy is performed using a Gigli saw or an oscillating saw. The osteotomy extends from 5 mm above the anteroinferior iliac spine to the most cranial part of the sciatic notch. A vertical iliac osteotomy is also performed at the same time using rongeurs and leaving the posterior table intact. This appears to give better pelvic contour and more mobility at the pubis. Pins for an external fixator are inserted before wound closure. The infant is already in position and prepared so that the bladder closure can begin immediately.

Posterior iliac osteotomy is performed through vertical incisions close to the sacroiliac joints. Satisfactory results can be obtained with this approach, as demonstrated by a review of 100 patients who underwent the procedure. For patients who achieved a pubic diastasis of less than 2 cm, the eventual continence rate was significantly higher.[35] Other forms of osteotomy are used less commonly. Using a three-dimensional cast of a tomographically reconstructed exstrophied pelvis, McKenna and colleagues[36] compared various osteotomies. Their preference was for an anterior, mid-ilium diagonal osteotomy performed through the same incision as the exstrophy closure. Although there are some concerns about this approach, specifically the risk of infection in the incision made next to the colonized bladder, long-term follow-up of greater numbers will define the role of this idea. Osteotomy of the superior ramus of the pubis is another technique that has been used, although its anatomic benefits are not as readily apparent[37]; its application will probably by limited to those patients with a minimal diastasis.

Patients undergoing exstrophy closure without osteotomy and those who have a posterior osteotomy are maintained in modified Bryant traction for 4 weeks. The hips are kept in 60 degrees of flexion, and the knees are straight. If anterior osteotomy is performed, the external fixator is left in place for 4 to 6 weeks (Fig. 66-1), and light Buck traction is maintained for at least 2 weeks, with the legs supported only on a pillow.

Bladder and Urethral Closure

The various steps in primary bladder closure are illustrated in Figure 66-2. A strip of mucosa, 2 cm wide, extending from the distal trigone to below the verumontanum in boys and to the vaginal orifice in girls, outlines prostatic and posterior urethral construction. The male urethral groove is usually of adequate

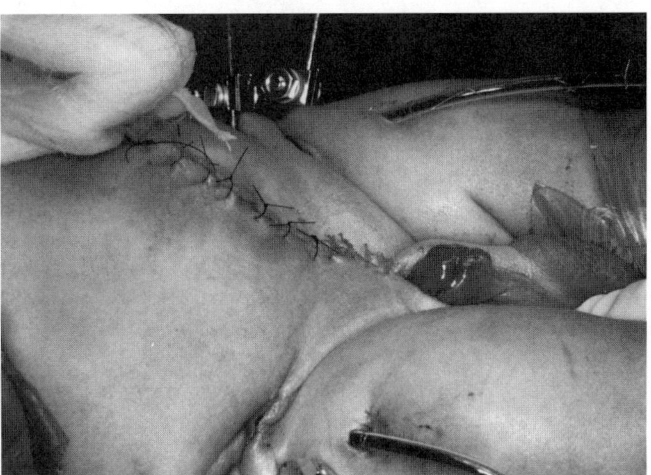

FIG. 66-1. Initial bladder closure is completed. The rods are visible laterally for attachment to the external fixator.

length to allow for primary closure. If necessary, the groove can be elongated using paraexstrophy skin flaps as described by Duckett.[38] In a review of 78 patients who had paraexstrophy skin flaps as part of their initial reconstruction, there was a 40% complication rate, most commonly urethral stricture.[39] For this reason, the use of such flaps is significantly decreased at the authors' institution. When they are needed, great care should be exercised to follow plastic surgical principles of rotational flaps.[40]

An incision is made outlining the bladder mucosa and the prostatic plate. The urethral groove is transected distal to the verumontanum only if paraexstrophy flaps are to be used. It is no longer necessary to free the corpora extensively or to join them in the midline because of the preference for later epispadias repair as described by Ransley and associates.[41] The urethra in the female patient does not require lengthening at the time of initial bladder closure.

The umbilical area is dissected free and discarded. The bladder muscle is freed from the rectus sheath on each side. The peritoneum is exposed above the bladder, and a careful extraperitoneal dissection reveals the retropubic space on each side. The wide band of fibers and muscle representing the pelvic diaphragm is detached subperiosteally from the pubis bilaterally. This dissection must be carried onto the inferior ramus to allow the bladder neck the mobility to fall within the pelvic ring. The mucosa and muscle of the bladder are closed in the midline. The urethra is also closed proximally, and this opening should accommodate a 14F sound. The opening should allow enough resistance to stimulate bladder growth and prevent bladder prolapse, but not enough to cause upper tract changes. The posterior urethra and bladder neck are buttressed with a second layer of local tissue if possible.

The bladder is drained by a suprapubic Malecot catheter for 3 to 4 weeks. The urethra is not stented to avoid pressure necrosis and prevent accumulation of infected secretions. Ureteral stents provide urinary drainage for the first 10 days to 2 weeks to avoid ureteral obstruction and hypertension. After the bladder and urethra have been closed and all drainage tubes are in place, the pelvis is closed by placing pressure on both greater trochanters. Horizontal mattress sutures are placed in the pubis, with

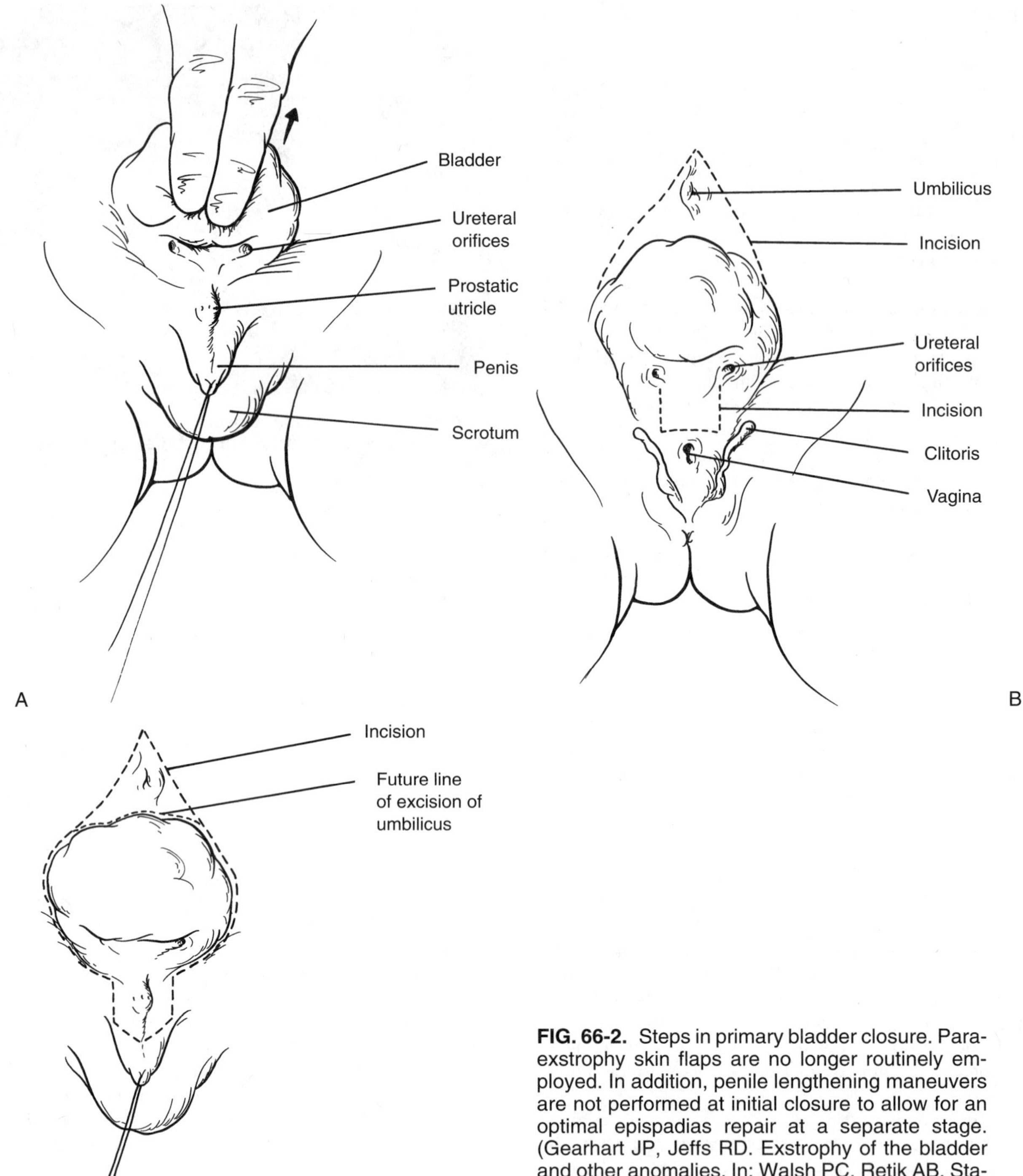

FIG. 66-2. Steps in primary bladder closure. Para-exstrophy skin flaps are no longer routinely employed. In addition, penile lengthening maneuvers are not performed at initial closure to allow for an optimal epispadias repair at a separate stage. (Gearhart JP, Jeffs RD. Exstrophy of the bladder and other anomalies. In: Walsh PC, Retik AB, Stamey JA, et al. Campbell's urology, ed 6. Philadelphia, WB Saunders, 1992) (*continued*)

the knot away from the neourethra. A simple umbilicoplasty is performed with a V-shaped skin flap, and the drainage tubes are brought out through this site.

Broad-spectrum antibiotics are administered before and during the procedure to convert a contaminated area into a clean surgical wound. These antibiotics are continued postoperatively, then converted to low-dose oral prophylactic antibiotics.

The factors in achieving successful primary closure have been well documented. Husmann and associates[42] found that urethral catheters, abdominal distention, infection, and poor nutrition appear to be associated with bladder prolapse or dehiscence. Along the same lines, a review of patients treated at Johns Hopkins Hospital stressed the importance of the osteotomy; avoidance of urethral tubes; use of postoperative antibiotics, pelvic immobilization, and ureteral stenting catheters; and maintenance of patient comfort.[43]

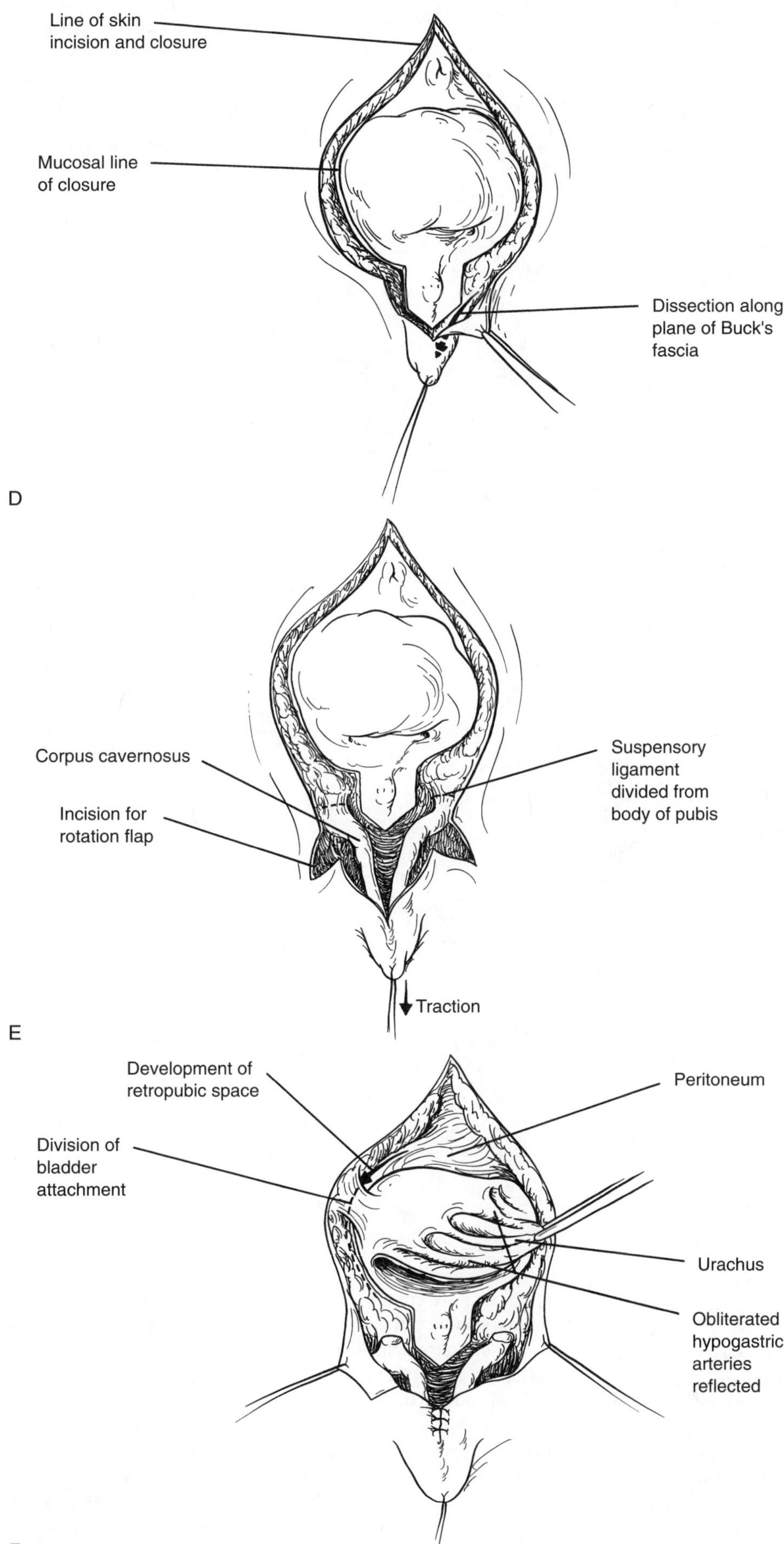

FIG. 66-2. *Continued.*

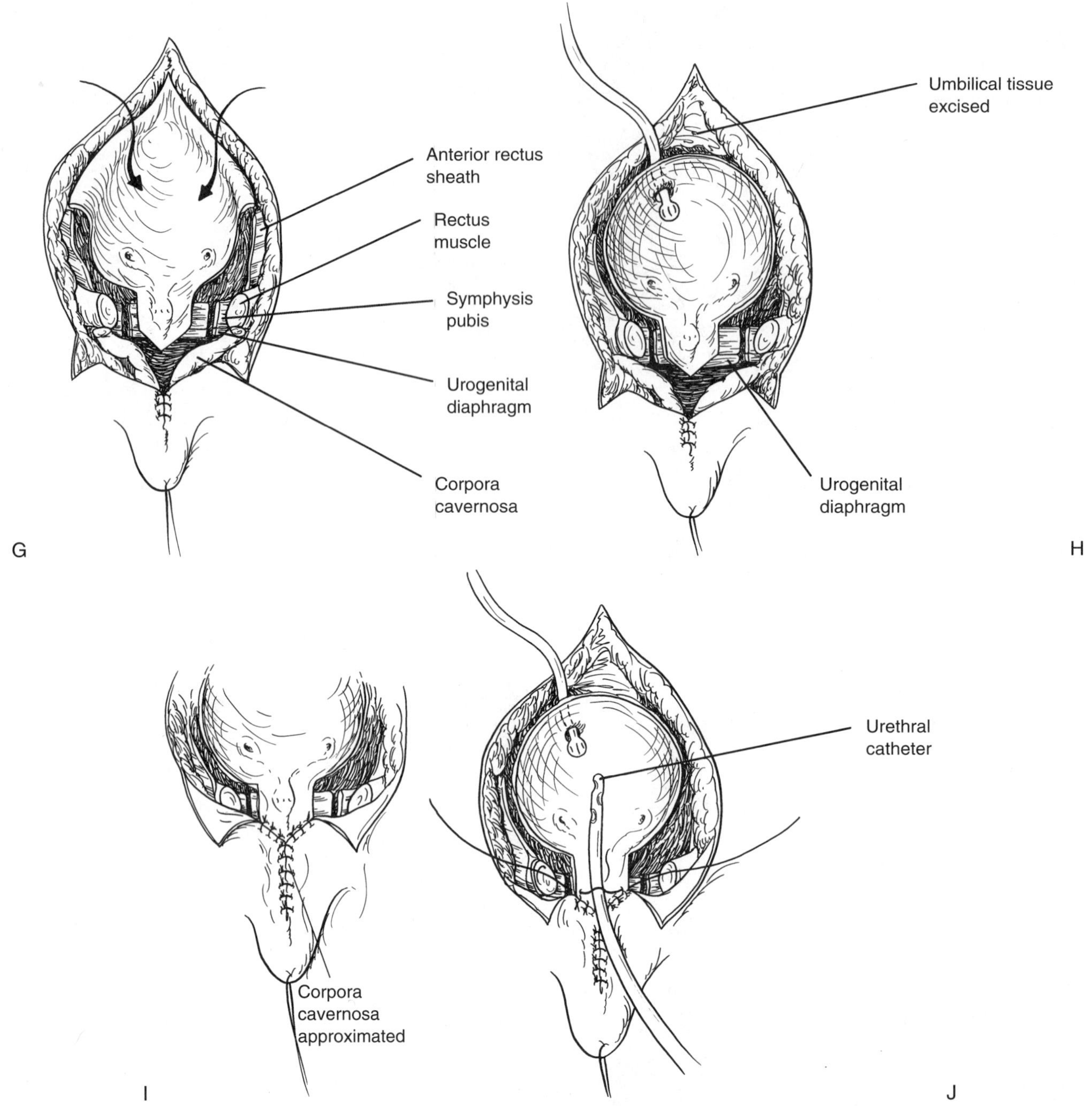

FIG. 66-2. *Continued.*

Postoperative Care

The initial closure of bladder exstrophy creates complete epispadias with incontinence. The bladder outlet is calibrated with a sound or catheter 4 weeks after closure, and if adequate, the suprapubic tube is removed. An intravenous pyelogram is obtained to assess the status of the upper tracts. Residual urine is estimated by catheterization, and urine culture is obtained before the patient leaves the hospital. If the initial pyelogram shows good drainage, the upper tracts are followed with ultrasound examinations every 6 months to 1 year. Prophylactic antibiotics are continued for at least 6 months. Urethral dilation or intermittent catheterization may be necessary if urinary retention and hydronephrosis or urinary infection develop. An antireflux procedure is occasionally performed within the first year after closure if the residual urine and dilation persist. Because it is unusual to have a useful continent interval after initial bladder closure, this should be immediately investigated with a renal ultrasound and urethral calibration, cystoscopy, or both.

The bladder eventually increases in capacity, and this can be estimated by performing cystograms under anesthesia at 2 to 3 years of age. Nearly all patients demonstrate reflux on this

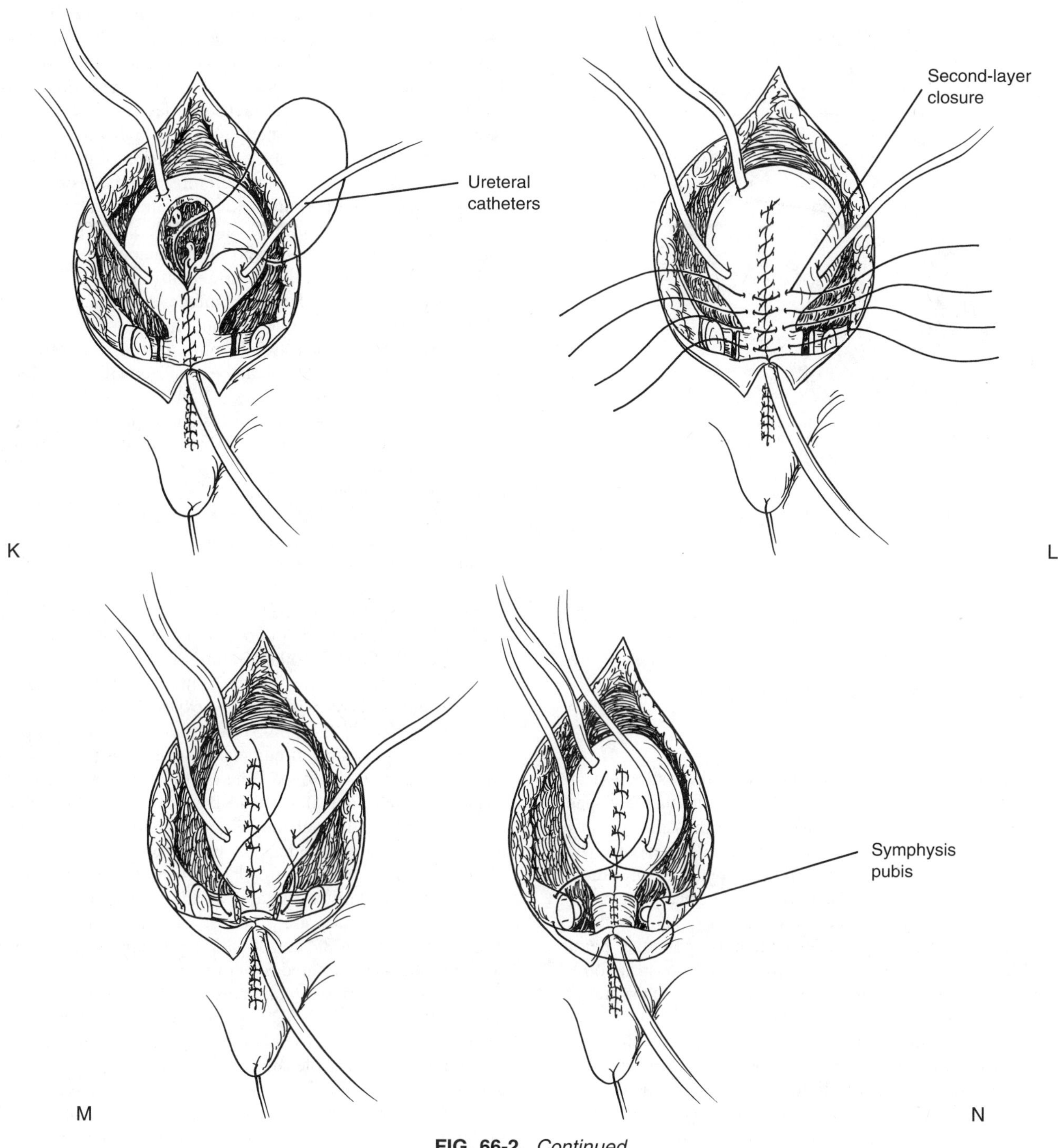

FIG. 66-2. *Continued.*

examination. Ideally, the bladder capacity gradually increases to at least 60 mL before a continence procedure, which in some cases can take 4 to 5 years. Some believe that a bladder capacity of 100 mL is necessary for a successful functional result.[44]

If uncontrollable hydronephrosis develops, revision of the bladder outlet, possibly requiring advancement skin flaps, should be considered. Rarely, a child requires urinary diversion, usually to a nonrefluxing colon conduit,[45] to preserve renal function.

Epispadias Repair

Repair of the penis and urethra was formerly the last step of the staged reconstruction of bladder exstrophy in boys. This is no longer the case because it has been shown that the repair of epispadias can contribute significantly to the development of bladder capacity. A median increase in bladder capacity of 54.5 mL was achieved after initial epispadias repair in boys with exstrophied bladders smaller than 60 mL. Twenty-two of 25 of

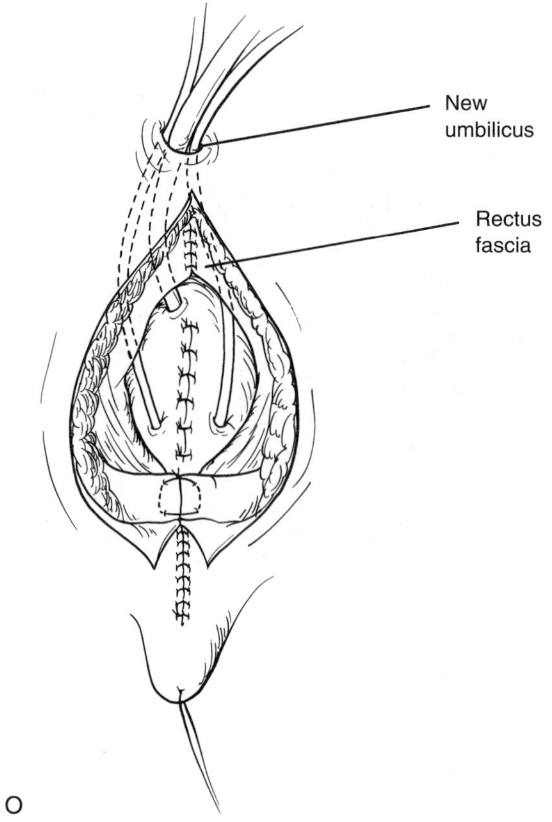

FIG. 66-2. *Continued.*

these patients evaluable after bladder neck reconstruction are acceptably continent. An even larger increase in bladder capacity has been noted in epispadias patients.[46] Epispadias repair is carried out at 2 to 3 years of age. Because most boys with exstrophy have a small penis and little extra penile skin, stimulation with parenteral testosterone precedes surgical repair.[47]

The five goals of penile reconstruction in patients with exstrophy–epispadias are (1) achievement of potential penile length, (2) correction of dorsal chordee, (3) reconstruction of the penile urethra, (4) reconstruction of the glans penis, and (5) adequate skin coverage.

Penile lengthening has been described as a key component in initial bladder exstrophy closure. The authors limit their attempts at penile lengthening initially to facilitate a thorough corporal dissection at the time of epispadias repair. Techniques for achieving penile length vary, but all have in common the release of a portion of corporal tissue from the inferior pubic ramus, preservation of the neurovascular bundles, and achievement of maximal urethral length. All residual suspensory tissue must be taken down. The corpora are then dissected off of the inferior pubic rami. Kelley and Eraklis[48] described a technique involving complete removal of the corpora from the bone, leaving the neurovascular structures intact. Most consider this too risky, and a limited dissection is generally carried out, as described by Johnston.[49] The urethra is freed from underlying cavernosal tissue, taking care not to dissect to the verumontanum, possibly damaging the ejaculatory ducts.[50] Usually, significant length is obtained by this maneuver alone, without division of the urethral plate, although urethral lengthening occasionally

must be carried out. Some believe that the urethral plate should be divided or discarded and replaced in nearly all cases to achieve maximal penile length. The urethra can be reconstructed or lengthened using a free skin graft[50] or a vascularized preputial graft.[51] Kramer and Jackson[52] described a comprehensive technique for penile lengthening employing an inverted V incision, mobilization of the corpora, division of the distal urethral plate, tubularization of the urethra, and extension using a free or vascularized preputial skin tube and rhomboid flaps to bring hair-bearing skin into the suprapubic area. This approach can be useful in the patient who has not undergone osteotomy and has a wide intrapubic area to reconstruct.

Correction of dorsal chordee involves several steps. First, the release of all tethering penile skin and the release of the urethral plate provide significant straightening. Corporal disproportion is nearly always present and can be managed either by elongating the dorsum with dermal grafts[53] or by ventral plication or rotation.[54] The intersymphyseal distance appears to influence both penile length and chordee, and consideration may be given to osteotomy and pelvic closure as an aid in achieving satisfactory length and release of chordee.[53,55]

As alluded to earlier, there are several approaches to the reconstruction of the urethra. If adequate tissue is available, the urethral plate can be tubularized, as in a modified Young urethroplasty,[17] or tubularized and transferred to the ventral side of the corpora, as in the Cantwell-Ransley approach.[41] The urethra can be lengthened or completely replaced with free skin grafts, pedicle flaps, or other techniques.[50,51]

The preferred technique at the authors' institution for epispadias repair in boys with bladder exstrophy is the Cantwell-Ransley approach[56] (Fig. 66-3). A Prolene stay suture is placed in the glans. A ventral circumcising incision is made, and the ventral corpora is degloved. The central leash of vascularized tissue that leads dorsally to the base of the urethral plate is carefully spared. An incision is made on either side of the urethral plate, leaving an adequate width for tubularization. The corporal bodies are then freed completely from the urethral plate from the glans to the area of the proximal urethra. The neurovascular bundles are protected bilaterally. The urethra is tubularized over an 8F or 10F silicone urethral stent, then the corporal bodies are rotated inward over the urethra and sutured together with 5-0 polydioxanone suture, with or without creating windows in the tunica albuginea of the dorsal corpora.

In any repair, reapproximation of the glans is important both to function and to a pleasing cosmetic appearance. The area corresponding to the urethral meatus tends to have a dorsal orientation and can be advanced by making a vertical incision in the midline and closing it horizontally. The lateral glans on either side is completely denuded of skin to create broad, raw surfaces. These are reapproximated with layered absorbable sutures. The glans skin may be closed with small absorbable sutures or with small nylon sutures, which are removed after 7 to 10 days to avoid scarring.

The final challenge to epispadias repair is penile skin coverage. If the urethra is reconstructed without preputial skin, coverage may be obtained by transferring the ventral prepuce to the dorsum of the penis. This can be accomplished by dividing the prepuce in the midline and bringing it around as paired flaps. A buttonhole can be made in the prepuce through which the glans is delivered. The ventral preputial skin can also be brought

(*text continues on page 1105*)

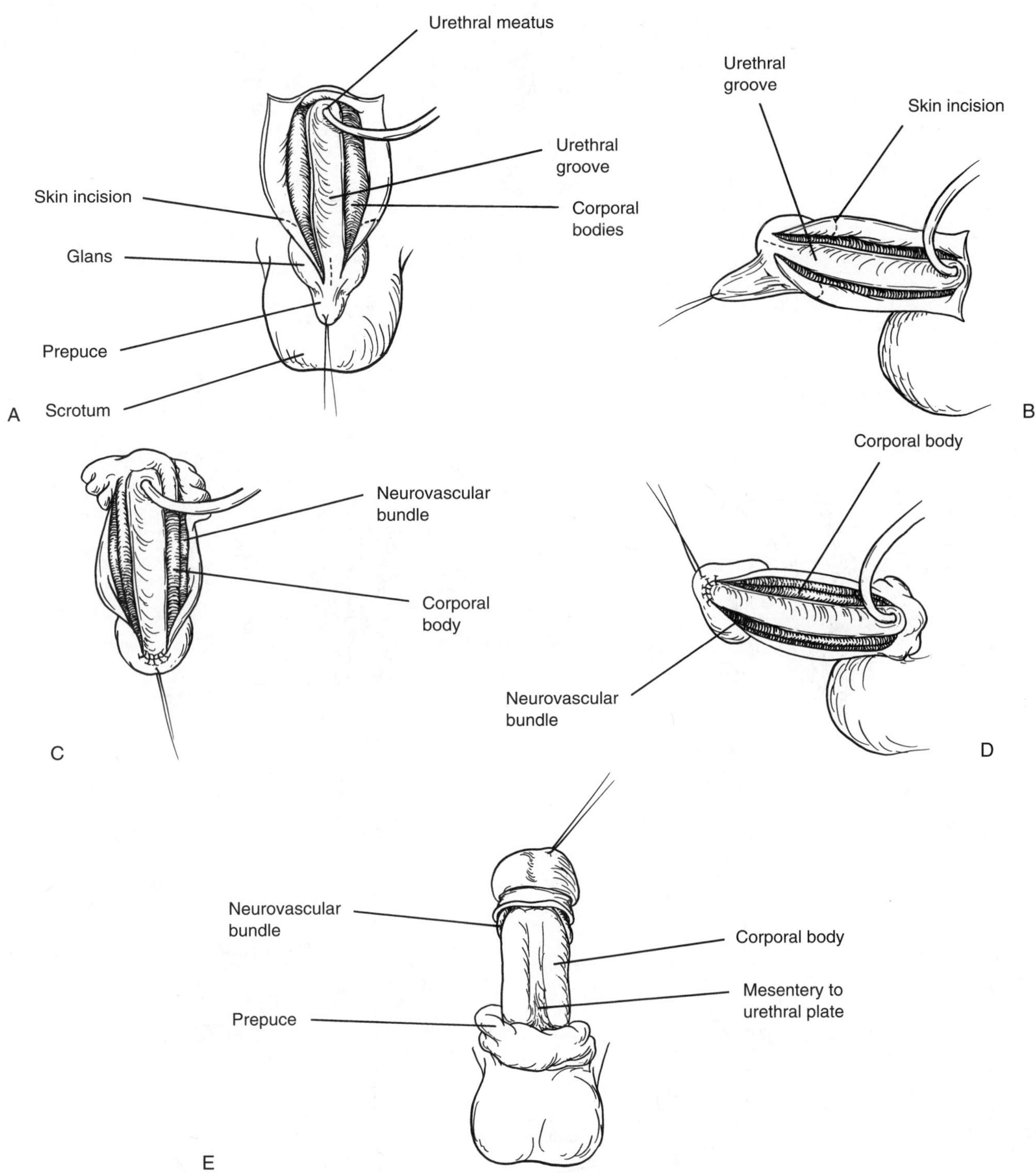

FIG. 66-3. The Cantwell-Ransley epispadias repair. (Gearhart JP, Jeffs RD. Exstrophy of the bladder and other anomalies. In: Walsh PC, Retik AB, Stamey JA, et al. Campbell's urology, ed 6. Philadelphia, WB Saunders, 1992) (*continued*)

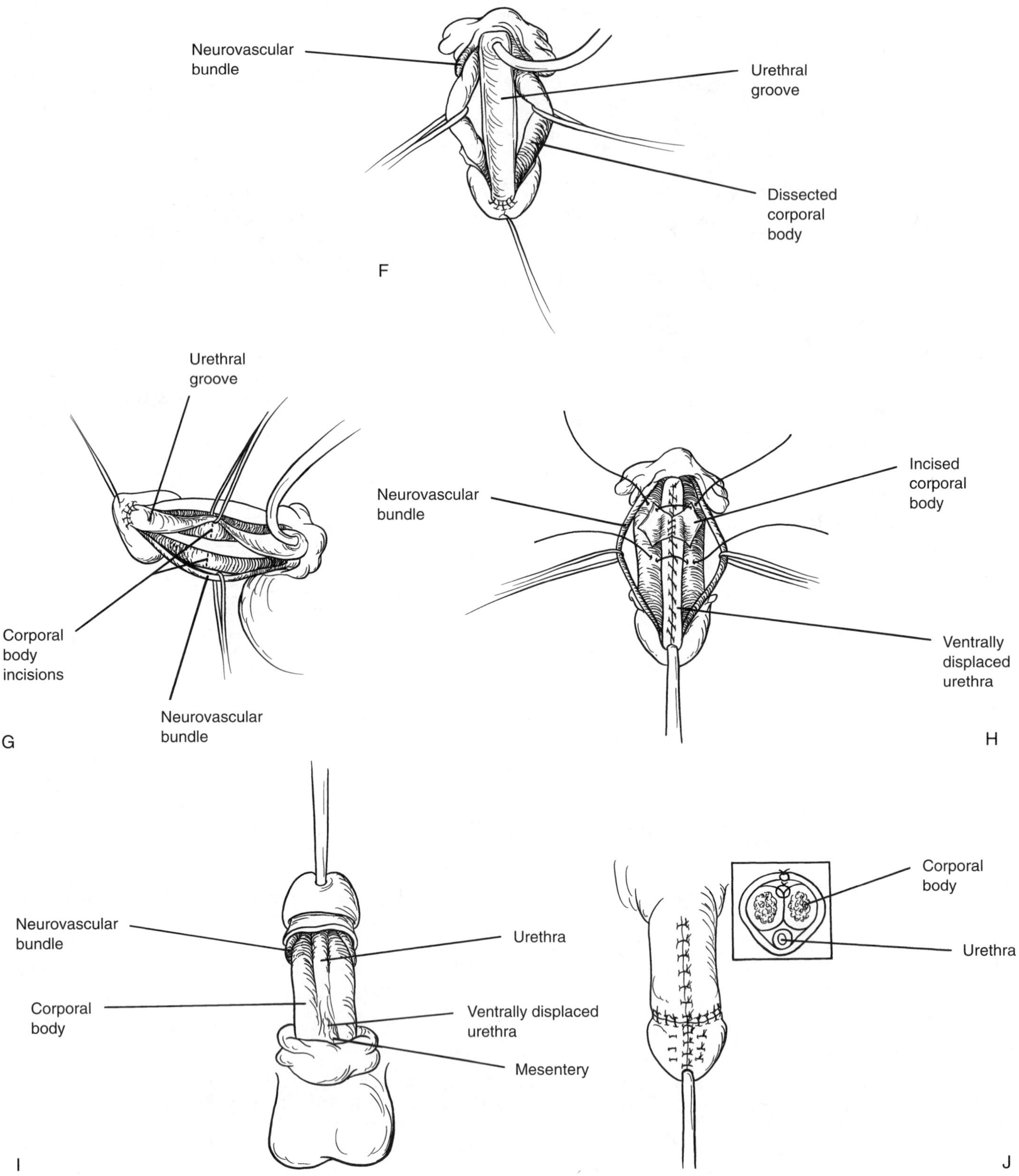

FIG. 66-3. *Continued.*

around as a vascularized pedicle flap.[41] Options for penile coverage when the prepuce has been used to reconstruct the urethra are more limited. If there is not enough remaining preputial skin to cover the dorsal phallus, lower abdominal skin flaps can be rotated in for proximal shaft coverage, or split-thickness skin graft can be used.[51,52]

Bladder Neck Reconstruction

Timing is crucial to the success of bladder neck reconstruction. An adequate bladder capacity is an absolute prerequisite for success. The patient must old enough to cooperate with toilet training. Under anesthesia, the bladder capacity is measured after the child reaches the age of 3 to 4 years. If the capacity is 60 mL or greater, bladder neck reconstruction can be considered. Nearly all of these children exhibit vesicoureteral reflux, and an antireflux procedure is required at the time of bladder neck reconstruction. The bladder is exposed and opened using a lower transverse incision (Fig. 66-4). This is extended vertically in the midline, and vertical closure of this incision narrows the area of the bladder neck at the end of the procedure. Reimplantation of the ureters can be done in a transtrigonal fashion, or, perhaps preferably, in a cephalotrigonal direction.[57] If necessary, the ureteral hiatus can be relocated more cephalad in combination with high cross-trigonal reimplantations.

The bladder neck reconstruction is begun by outlining a posterior mucosal strip 15 to 18 mm wide by 3 cm in length. This extends from the mid-trigone to the prostatic or posterior urethra. The bladder muscle lateral to this strip is denuded of mucosa. Multiple small incisions in the free edges of these triangles of muscle allows the reconstruction to assume a more cephalad position. The posterior mucosal strip is formed into a tube using interrupted sutures of 4-0 polyglycolic acid. The denuded muscle flaps are overlapped and sutured in place with 3-0 polyglycolic acid sutures to reinforce the neobladder neck. The reconstruction may be performed over an 8F urethral catheter, but this is removed at the end of the procedure.

It is essential to the success of the procedure that the bladder neck be dissected completely free of surrounding structures. This allows suspension of the bladder neck to the anterior fascia. Often, it is advantageous to split the symphyseal bar to enhance visualization.[58] The bar is simply closed at the end of the procedure with heavy sutures of polydioxanone. Patient mobility should be restricted appropriately in the postoperative period to allow healing to occur.

Intraoperative urodynamics is helpful in assessing the adequacy of the reconstruction. Retrospective comparisons of the values of intraoperative urethral pressure profiles demonstrate correlation with eventual continence or incontinence. An intraoperative continence length of 2.5 to 3.5 cm is desirable. Closure pressures of 70 to 100 cm H_2O are required to prevent leakage when the bladder pressure is raised to 50 cm H_2O intraoperatively.[59] Suspension of the bladder neck and proximal urethra in the manner of Marshall and colleagues[59,60] further enhances the urodynamic parameters at the time of surgery. At the end of the procedure, the adequacy of the reconstruction is tested by water manometer. There should be no leakage at 50 cm H_2O. If this degree of resistance is not obtained, the reconstruction should be revised.

Ureteral stenting catheters are left indwelling, as is a suprapubic catheter. No tube is left through the bladder neck, and no instrumentation is performed through the bladder neck for at least 3 weeks. The suprapubic tube prevents stretching or pressure on the bladder neck until it is fully healed. Postoperative bladder spasm can be reduced through the use of benzodiazepines, anticholinergics, nonsteroidal antiinflammatory agents, or epidural analgesia. Intravenous antibiotics are administered for 7 days. Prophylactic antibiotics are then begun and continued indefinitely.

Three weeks postoperatively, a soft 8F catheter is passed through the urethra for calibration. Cultures are taken at this time. The suprapubic tube is clamped before removal to ensure adequate voiding. If voiding does not occur, several measures may be taken. A pediatric cystoscopy may be necessary to identify the passage. A soft, 8F Foley-Dover catheter can be left in place for 24 to 48 hours to help gently dilate the bladder neck. The ability to catheterize through the urethra must be established before removal of the suprapubic tube. If reasonable bladder emptying does not occur, a period of intermittent catheterization is necessary.

After removal of the suprapubic tube, there should be a short dry interval. Postoperative irritation and swelling may result in an extremely small bladder capacity at first. Patients are not familiar with the sensation of bladder filling or the need for a detrusor contraction. Several months of readjustment often are required before a reasonable dry interval can be developed. Hints of initial success are an early dry interval of 10 to 15 minutes and the absence of stress incontinence or continuous urethral dribbling. The patient must learn to use his or her dry interval to develop day, and later nighttime, continence.

Results

The results of functional closure of bladder exstrophy have improved remarkably during the past 3 decades. Standard treatment for exstrophy in this country has evolved from urinary diversion in almost all cases to functional reconstruction in almost all cases. Continence rates after staged reconstruction can be expected to be as high as 75% to 80% with preservation of renal function, as documented by several large series.[42,61–64] Long-term success depends on success at each phase of staged reconstruction. An initial bladder closure can be expected to be successful when performed at a center with a large experience, with osteotomies as needed, and with appropriate pelvic fixation and immobilization.[17] The authors hesitate to advocate short hospital stays and no fixation after osteotomy and exstrophy closure.[65] It has been well documented that the success of the initial bladder closure impacts significantly on the eventual ability to achieve continence.[30,42]

The results of genital reconstruction in boys have improved as well. A review of patients treated up to 1989 at the Johns Hopkins Hospital revealed the major complication of epispadias repair to be urethrocutaneous fistula, which occurred in 38% of patients. All of these were closed successfully at subsequent procedures, with the exception of one, which closed spontaneously.[62] The cosmetic appearance was satisfactory to all 49 parents interviewed by Lepor and associates.[66] In a study of postpubertal patients, most were able to achieve satisfactory intercourse.[67] With the recent introduction of the Cantwell-Ransley epispadias repair, the fistula rate has decreased to 8%, with

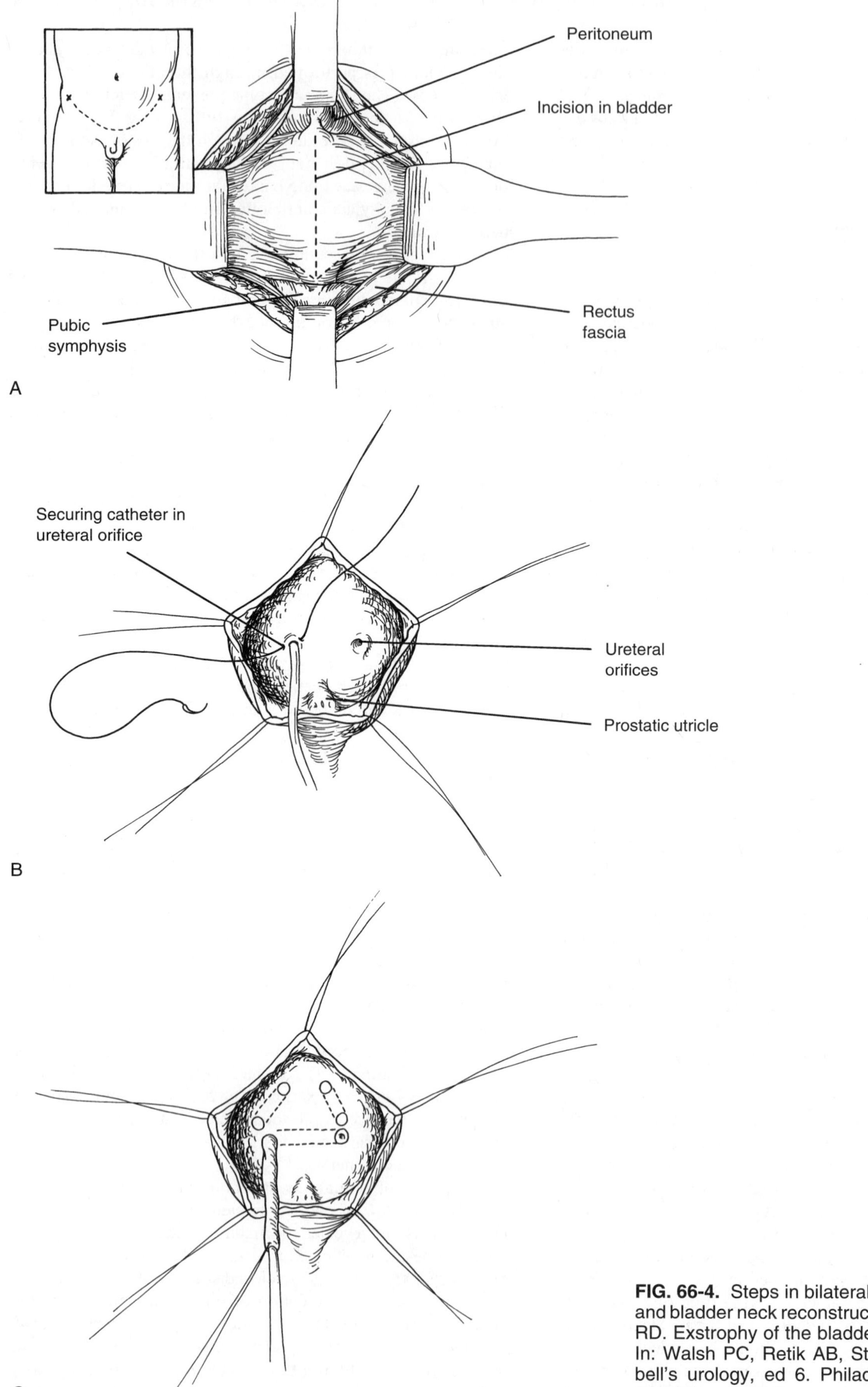

FIG. 66-4. Steps in bilateral ureteral reimplantation and bladder neck reconstruction. (Gearhart JP, Jeffs RD. Exstrophy of the bladder and other anomalies. In: Walsh PC, Retik AB, Stamey JA, et al. Campbell's urology, ed 6. Philadelphia, WB Saunders, 1992) (*continued*)

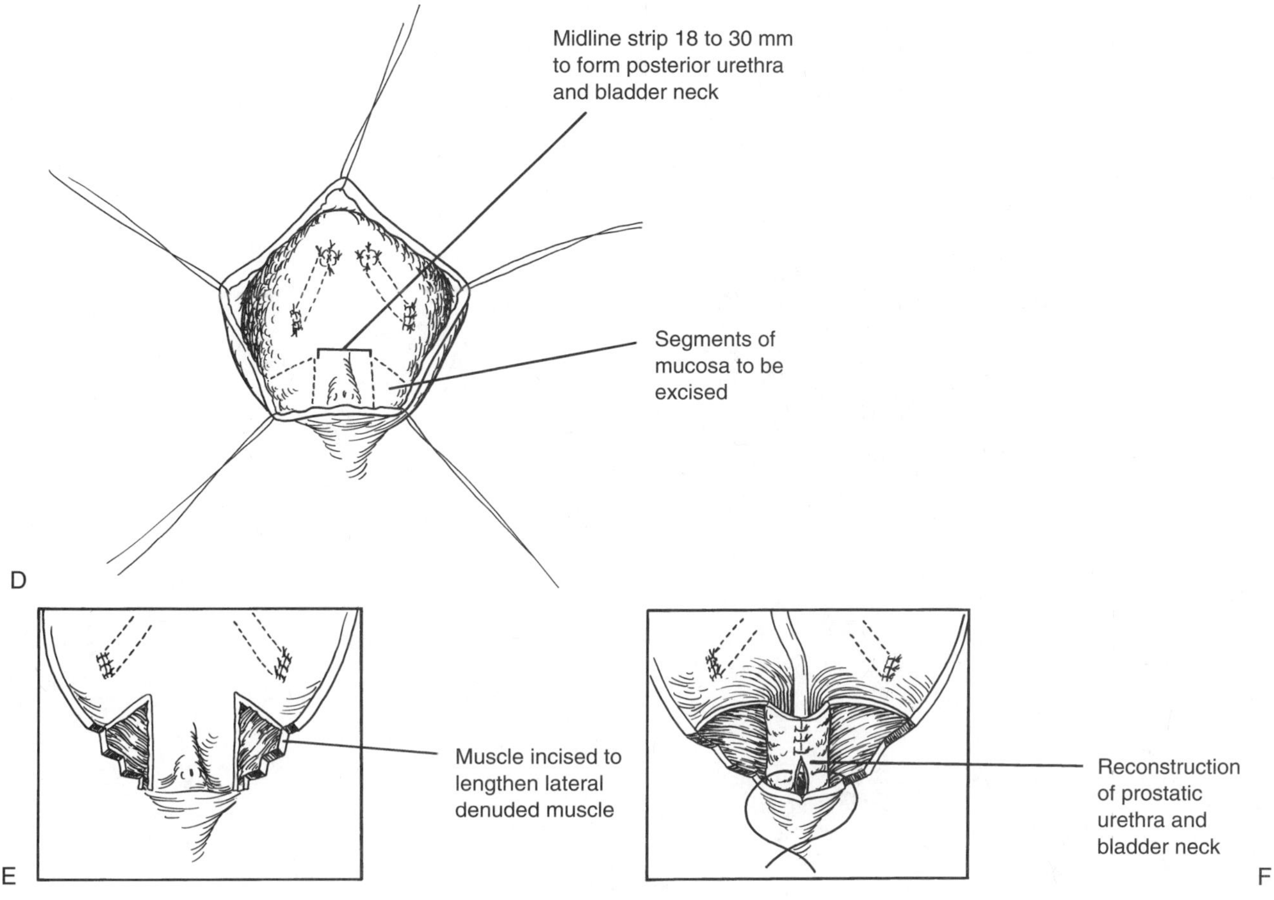

FIG. 66-4. *Continued.*

excellent cosmetic and functional results. The urethra after this repair is straighter and easier to catheterize.[56]

Management of Treatment Failures

Failure of initial bladder closure decreases the likelihood of achieving continence without the use of intermittent catheterization and possibly augmentation. In the past 7 years, 29 boys and 11 girls have been referred to the authors' institution with failure of their exstrophy closure; 38 patients had classic bladder exstrophy, and 2 had cloacal exstrophy. Reclosure was performed for complete bladder dehiscence in 28 cases and for significant bladder prolapse in 10. All reclosure operations were successful.[68] The authors reviewed 47 patients who required reclosure of the bladder, including 28 who underwent a procedure to restore urinary continence. Eighteen patients underwent bladder neck reconstruction, 4 had bladder neck reconstruction along with augmentation, 4 underwent augmentation alone, repeat bladder neck reconstruction was performed in 1, and 1 had reclosure with creation of a continent stoma and augmentation. Nine of 18 patients who underwent primary bladder neck reconstruction are dry on intermittent catheterization, while 8 of the remaining 9 are dry and voiding without catheterization. Four patients who underwent primary bladder neck reconstruction and augmentation and 4 who underwent augmentation after bladder neck reconstruction are dry on intermittent catheteriza-

tion. The patient who underwent reclosure, bladder augmentation, and creation of a continent abdominal stoma is dry on intermittent catheterization. Of 28 patients who underwent salvage procedures, only 1 had upper tract changes. These series demonstrate that despite the formidable nature of the problem, the failed exstrophy closure can be managed with a high expectation for functional reconstruction and urinary continence.[69]

Failure to achieve an adequate bladder capacity for bladder neck reconstruction as assessed by cystogram under anesthesia is an indication to proceed to epispadias repair. As demonstrated, significant increases in bladder capacity can be achieved in this manner.[46] Why bladder capacity should increase, yet hydronephrosis not occur, is not known. Perhaps the bladder gradually pools greater amounts of urine, especially at night, under low pressure. Bladder cycling has not met with success in this population. A promising idea is the use of injectable collagen at the bladder neck before reconstruction to stimulate bladder growth. In five female exstrophy patients who had successful collagen injection 18 months after closure, the average increase in volume before bladder neck reconstruction was 47%.[70]

If, despite these maneuvers, the bladder does not achieve an adequate capacity for bladder neck reconstruction, the main therapeutic alternative is augmentation cystoplasty. Because most of these augmentations produce mucus, the patients must be able to catheterize with a tube of reasonable diameter. This is often difficult through an epispadias repair and bladder neck

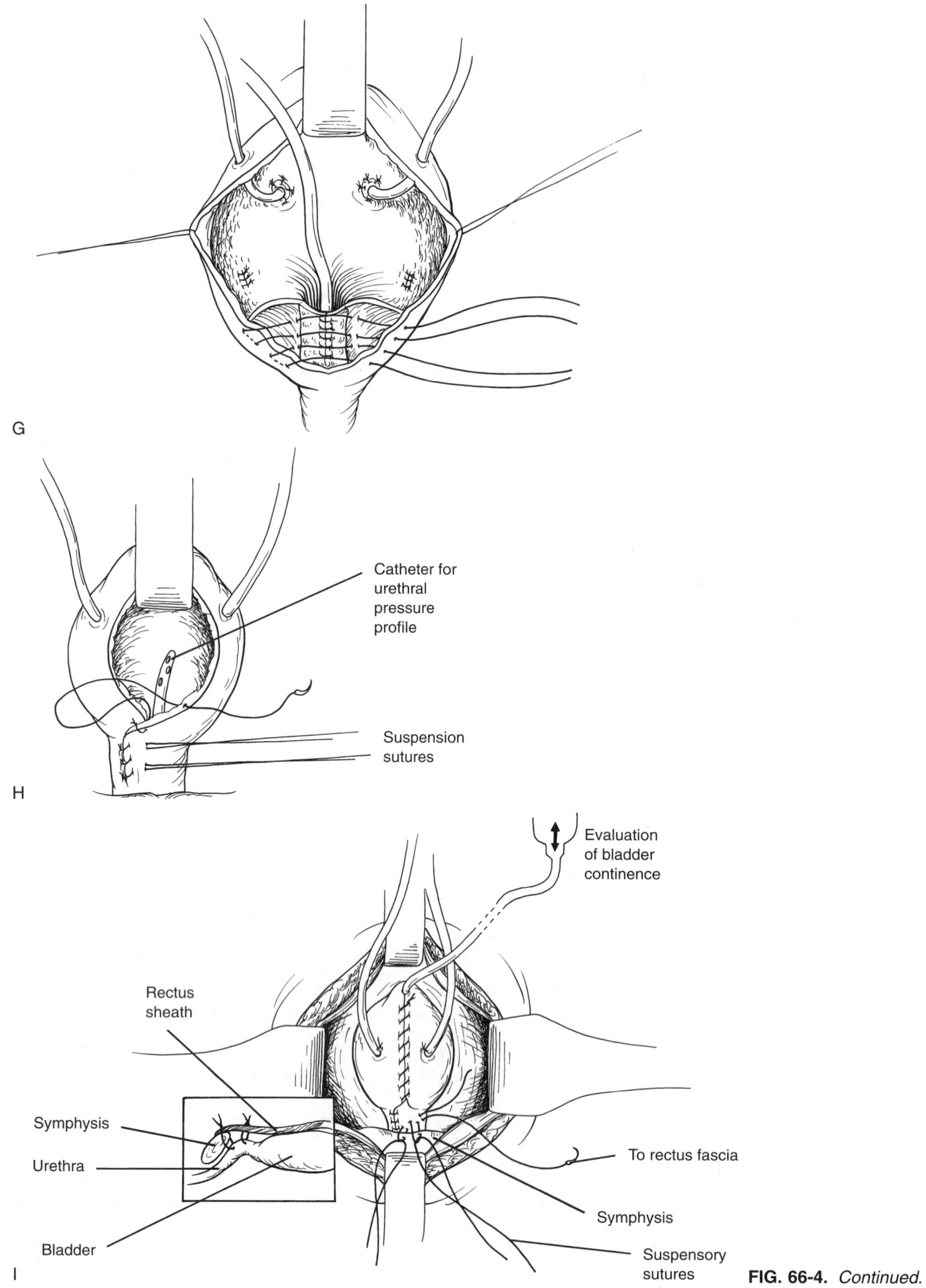

FIG. 66-4. *Continued.*

reconstruction. For this reason, many patients are managed with an abdominal catheterizable stoma with or without ligation of the bladder neck.[71,72]

Urinary continence, defined as a 3-hour dry interval, is usually achieved within 1 year after bladder neck reconstruction. Delayed achievement of urinary continence has been associated with puberty in boys.[73] Magnetic resonance imaging evaluation of prostate size and configuration suggests that there is no anatomic basis for a significant contribution to outlet resistance by the prostate.[74] Patients who do not achieve a 3-hour dry interval within 1 to 2 years after bladder neck reconstruction are unlikely to develop meaningful continence. Options for therapy in these incontinent patients include (1) repeat Young-Dees-Leadbetter bladder neck reconstruction with or without simultaneous bladder augmentation, (2) tubularization of the remaining bladder into a neourethra and bladder augmentation by colocystoplasty,[75] (3) artificial urinary sphincter placement,[76] (4) transection of the bladder neck and augmentation and creation of continent catheterizable abdominal stoma,[72] and (5) as a last resort, urinary diversion.[77]

A patulous bladder neck is best treated by repeating the bladder neck reconstruction.[31] In this series, six of seven patients who underwent repeat bladder neck reconstruction without augmentation are dry for greater than 3 hours and are voiding through the urethra. Despite this, most patients who fail bladder neck reconstruction require bladder augmentation and a continence procedure.[31] The artificial urinary sphincter has been used with some success in these patients, although the revision and erosion rates are significant.[44,76,78] The artificial sphincter may be best used around an Arap-type neourethra[75] or with an omental wrap around the bladder neck. The injection of bovine cross-linked collagen has proved useful in patients after bladder neck reconstruction.[79]

Reconstruction of the phallus and urethra is a formidable task in boys with bladder exstrophy. Despite this, most patients have a functional phallus that is cosmetically acceptable and allows satisfactory intercourse.[67] Formerly, the most common complication of epispadias repair after exstrophy closure in the Johns Hopkins series was urethrocutaneous fistula, occurring in 38% of patients. Using the Cantwell-Ransley technique as discussed previously, the fistula rate has decreased to 8%.[56]

As these boys reach puberty, the three most common problems observed are (1) desire for additional penile length, (2) residual dorsal chordee, and (3) unsightly scars from previous repairs. Lengthening of the mature phallus may require more than simply releasing penile skin. Approaching the base of the phallus through an inverted V incision with the possibility of mobilizing lower abdominal flaps allows access to remaining suspensory tissue.[52] When this tissue, much of which is scar, is taken down, a significant lengthening and chordee release may be effected. If not, other maneuvers, such as a dorsal corporal dermal graft[80] or ventral corporal plication or rotation,[54] must be employed. Further release of the corpora from the inferior ramus of the symphysis pubis is less likely to be effective in this age group.[20] Use of a graft on the dorsum of the corpora generally requires division of the urethra, which then needs to be reconstructed using one of a number of techniques made popular in the repair of hypospadias. Options include free skin or bladder mucosa grafts[50] or buccal mucosa grafts.[81] Pedicle island flaps may be employed in the unlikely circumstance of excess preputial or penile skin.[51] Revision of unsightly scars

may be as simple as excision and plastic closure or may require full-thickness skin grafts. Proximal penile shaft coverage can be facilitated by the use of rhomboid abdominal flaps.[52]

Alternative Techniques of Reconstruction

Unfortunately, not all children with bladder exstrophy are candidates for functional reconstruction, usually because of small bladder plates or hydronephrosis. Many techniques for reconstruction have been attempted over the years, and these previously were considered preferable to functional closure. The most popular of these was the formation of ureterosigmoidostomies. This procedure allowed children continence and, once nonrefluxing ureterocolonic anastomosis was perfected, protection of the upper tracts. There are, however, several potential problems with ureterosigmoidostomy. First, anal continence may be affected by the anterior displacement of the anus and the anterior separation of the puborectal sling. The ability of a child to retain an enema should be assessed before consideration of diversion to the rectosigmoid. The long-term complications of ureterosigmoidostomy have included pyelonephritis, hyperchloremic metabolic acidosis, ureteral obstruction, and late development of colonic malignancy.[82–84] The mechanism of tumor development has not been explained, but in rats, the requirements are urine, feces, ureteral mucosa, and colonic mucosa in contact with each other. Separating the ureters from the colon by a segment of ileum prevented tumors in rats.[85]

Boyce and Vest developed a procedure in which an end sigmoid colostomy was created. A trigonosigmoidostomy was then performed into the isolated rectal segment. This allowed urinary continence through the rectum and collection of feces through a colostomy—considered preferable at the time to urostomy with poor collection devices. A 37-year review of Boyce's patients reveals that most have stable upper tracts with no electrolyte imbalance or malignancy.[86]

Ileal conduit urinary diversion was initially thought to be ideally suited to exstrophy patients. Ten-year to 15-year follow-up studies revealed significant long-term complications, and ileal conduit is no longer considered an acceptable method of urinary diversion in children.[87] An alternative method is the colon conduit, which allows nonrefluxing ureteral anastomoses.[88] The long-term results of colon conduit diversion appear to be better than those of ileal conduit.[89] In addition, secondary anastomosis of the colon conduit to the rectosigmoid can be carried out after the child achieves anal continence.[88]

Another method of undiverting a colon conduit is that of Arap and colleagues.[75] In this technique, the colon conduit is anastomosed to a neourethra consisting of the entire exstrophied bladder formed into a tube. This may be useful in the reconstruction of a failed bladder neck reconstruction or in children with extremely small bladders (less than 3 mL) at birth.

In the Johns Hopkins series, a variety of reconstructive techniques have been used as salvage procedures, including continent urinary diversion using the Mitrofanoff and Benchekroun procedures.[71] All of these procedures should be viewed as salvage procedures for children who have failed or are not candidates for functional closure.

CLOACAL EXSTROPHY

Cloacal exstrophy, also known as vesicointestinal fissure, ileovesical fissure, or splanchnic exstrophy, is the most severe defect that can occur in the formation of the ventral abdominal wall. Fortunately, this entity is extremely rare, occurring in 1 in 200,000 to 400,00 live births. Formerly, the incidence between sexes was thought to be similar; current reports indicate a 2:1 male/female ratio.[17] With newer techniques of prenatal ultrasound, this condition can reliably be diagnosed by the presence of sacral myelomeningocele (usually present in half of patients), ''rocker bottom'' feet, splaying of the pubic rami, and a large cystic mass protruding from the infraumbilical anterior abdominal wall.[90] The mode of inheritance of this condition is unknown because offspring have never been produced from people with this disorder. With reliable prenatal diagnosis, prenatal counseling can be undertaken and perinatal management enhanced.

Anatomy and Embryology

Anatomically, there is exstrophy of the foreshortened hindgut or cecum, which displays its bulging mucosa between the two hemibladders (Fig. 66-5). The orifices of the terminal ileum, the rudimentary tailgut, and a single or paired appendix are apparent on the surface of the everted cecum. The tailgut is blind ending, and the ileum is usually prolapsed. The anatomy of the bony pelvis in cloacal exstrophy was generally described in the past as a widened pubic symphysis with hips that are externally rotated and abducted.[17]

Sponseller and associates[91] have recently described the markedly severe abnormalities of the bony pelvis associated with cloacal exstrophy. Using computed tomographic scans of the pelvis in controls and patients with cloacal exstrophy, the in-

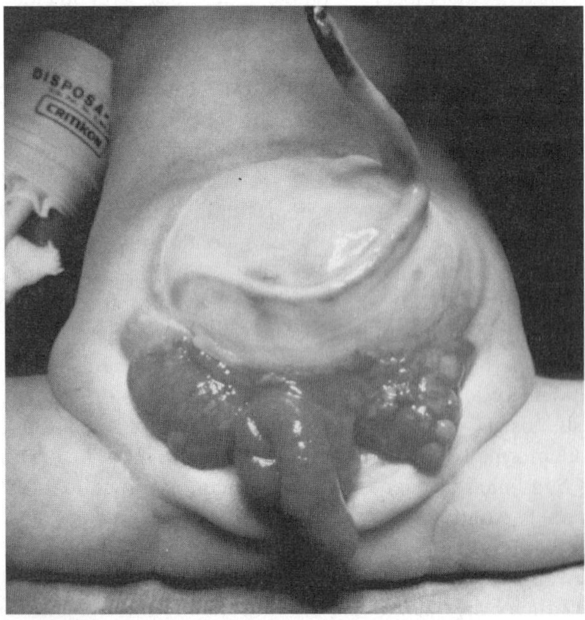

FIG. 66-5. Typical appearance of a newborn with cloacal exstrophy. The large omphalocele and prolapsed terminal ileum may be observed.

terpubic diastasis was found to have a mean of 0.5 cm in controls and 8 cm in cloacal exstrophy patients. The anterior segment length (distance from the triradiate cartilage to the pubis) was 37% shorter in cloacal exstrophy patients than in controls. Also, the angle of the iliac wing was markedly increased at 45 degrees, showing the amount of external rotation. Likewise, the ischiopubic angle was markedly increased in patients with cloacal exstrophy. Overall, patients with cloacal exstrophy have extreme abnormalities of the pelvis as well as asymmetry between the sides, sacroiliac joint malformations, and occasional hip malformations.[91]

The phallus is usually separated into a right and left half with adjacent scrotum or labia. Occasionally, the penis is together in the midline, but the structure is diminutive and the corporal bodies small, so that rearing the child as a girl is appropriate for most of these patients.[92] Husmann and colleagues[92] found that, of eight genotypic boys with cloacal exstrophy, all had phallic inadequacy; and of four who have reached puberty, two are impotent, and three have required intense psychiatric counseling. Thus, sexual conversion should be a part of the treatment plan in all genotypic boys with the cloacal exstrophy syndrome.

Schlegel and Gearhart[93] first defined the neuroanatomy of the pelvis in the child born with cloacal exstrophy syndrome (Fig. 66-6). The autonomic innervation to the bladder halves and corporal bodies arises from a pelvic plexus on the anterior surface of the sacrum. The nerves to the hemibladders travel along the midline on the posteroinferior surface of the pelvis and extend laterally to the hemibladders. The autonomic innervation of the phallic halves arises from the sacral pelvic plexus, travels in the midline, perforates the inferior portion of the pelvic floor, and courses medially to the hemibladder. Duplication of the vena cava is also seen.

Two main theories on the embryology of cloacal exstrophy have been proposed.[17] Patten and Barry proposed that the paired primordia of the genital tubercles are displaced caudally. This permits persistence of the more cephalad cloacal membrane. Thus, if there is incomplete urorectal septal division and disintegration of the unstable cloacal membrane, then both the exstrophied bladder and bowel would be on the ventral abdominal surface. The theory advanced by Marshall and Muecke suggests that the cloacal membrane is overly developed. This overdevelopment prevents migration of the mesenchymal layer between the inner endodermal and outer ectodermal layers. As previously mentioned, the unstable membrane ruptures, and if this occurs before fusion of the genital tubercles and before caudal movement of the urorectal septum, then the ventral abdominal defect arises.

Manzoni and associates[94] have suggested a gridlike schema to describe cloacal exstrophy and to better delineate its variants. In type I classic cloacal exstrophy (Fig. 66-7), the hemibladders may be confluent cranial to the bowel patch, lateral to the bowel (most common), or confluent caudal to the bowel. Type IIA grids show variations of the bladder (covered bladder or hemibladder); type IIB grids show variations of distal exstrophied bowel segments (duplications); and type IIC grids depicts the situation in which both bowel and bladder variations occur. The grid also describes the penis (hemi or united) and the clitoris and vaginal status (duplications). The authors have modified the grid concept to describe the status of the hindgut remnant.[17]

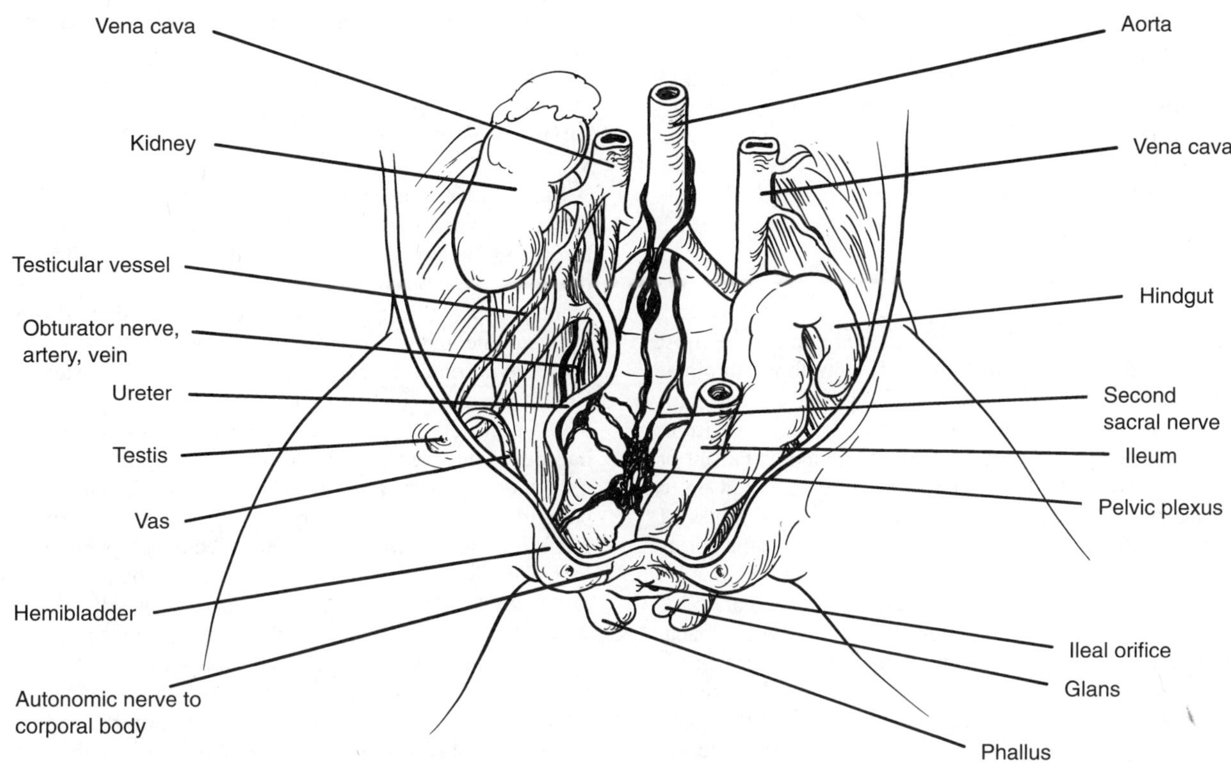

FIG. 66-6. Dissection of the pelvis in a child with cloacal exstrophy. (Gearhart JP, Jeffs RD. Exstrophy of the bladder and other anomalies. In: Walsh PC, Retik AB, Stamey JA, et al. Campbell's urology, ed 6. Philadelphia, WB Saunders, 1992)

Associated Conditions

Although cloacal exstrophy is one of the most severe congenital anomalies compatible with life, these patients have potentially salvageable problems. Certainly, these children face multiple problems, in part owing to the various associated anomalies, including anomalies of the central nervous system, the skeletal system, and the reproductive, gastrointestinal, and upper urinary tracts.

Central Nervous System Anomalies

Of the anomalies associated with cloacal exstrophy, those involving spinal dysraphism associated with myelomeningocele are the most devastating. Besides the neurosurgical management of this anomaly, it has important implications with regard to hydrocephalus, intellect, eventual ambulation, and bladder function in the cloacal exstrophy patient.

The incidence of spina bifida in various series ranges from 29% to 86%, but of course figures include patients with meningoceles and lipomeningoceles.[95] In the series by Howell and associates,[96] the level of the myelomeningocele was 72% lumbar, 14% sacral, and 14% thoracic. In the series by Ben-Chaim and colleagues,[97] the levels were 80% lumbar, 10% sacral, and 10% thoracic. Close consultation with a pediatric neurosurgeon must be established to determine the distinction between meningocele, myelomeningocele, and lipomeningocele and to develop a plan of treatment priorities.

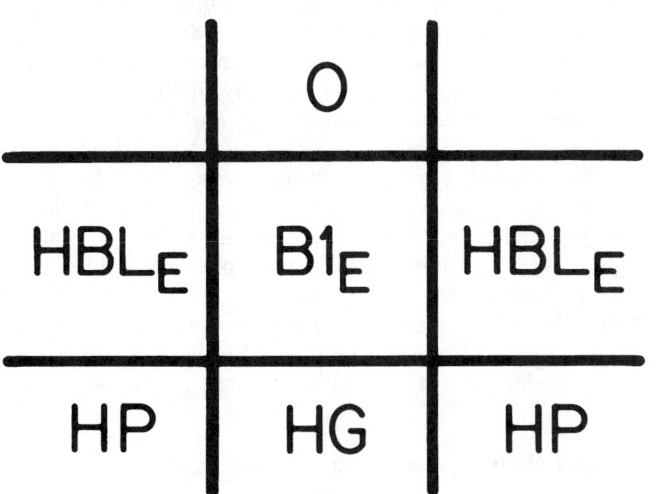

FIG. 66-7. Modified coding grid used to describe classic cloacal exstrophy and variants. O, omphalocele; HBLᴇ, hemibladder; B1ᴇ, everted bowel, HP, hemiphallus; HG, hindgut.

Upper Urinary Tract Anomalies

Because the lower urinary tract is exstrophied, attention is often focused in this area. Several series have demonstrated, however, the common occurrence of upper tract anomalies.[98–100] The most common anomalies are those of pelvic kidney and renal agenesis, occurring in up to one third of patients. Hydronephrosis and hydroureter were one third of patients in Howell's series[96]; while in the series by Ben-Chaim and associates,[97] this defect was found in only 1 of 22 patients. Ectopia of the ureter draining into the vasa in boys and into the uterus, vagina, or fallopian tube in girls has also been reported.[95]

Müllerian and Testis Anomalies

Duplication anomalies of the uterus and vagina are the most commonly found müllerian anomalies. Hurwitz found duplication of the vagina in 43% of patients,[98] while Tank and Lindenauer[99] found this anomaly in 65% of patients. In addition, vaginal agenesis occurs in 25% to 43% of patients.[95] Partial or complete duplication of the uterus has been described in up to 95% of patients.[98] Normal ovarian tissue was found in six of seven female patients in Hurwitz's series.[98] In both the series by Hurwitz and colleagues[98] and Ricketts and colleagues,[100] the testis was undescended and was found in the groin or abdomen in most patients. Because almost all boys with cloacal exstrophy need gender reassignment along with bilateral orchiectomy, the need for orchiopexy is therefore rare. Most müllerian structures, however, should be preserved because these can be used in lower urinary tract reconstructive efforts later in life. Skeletal system anomalies of both the vertebral bodies and lower limb are commonly seen in cloacal exstrophy patients. Vertebral anomalies have been reported in up to 80% of patients.[95] Lower limb abnormalities are seen in from 12% to 65% of patients.[95] These include club foot, congenital hip dislocation, agenesis, and severe deformity of both the foot and leg.[95,98]

Gastrointestinal System Anomalies

Because omphaloceles are so commonly associated with the cloacal exstrophy complex, most surgeons consider them an integral part of the disorder. Most series report an incidence of more than 85% in most cases.[17] Of course, the size of the omphalocele can vary, but immediate closure is required to prevent rupture of the omphalocele with its attendant problems. In the authors' experience, all omphalocele defects were closed primarily, and in no cases were prosthetic materials used. The use of a silicone silo has been reported when the omphalocele is extremely large.[98] Although most attention has been taken to the repair of the omphalocele defect, other serious anomalies of the gastrointestinal tract have been described, including malrotation, bowel duplication, duodenal atresia, and Meckel diverticulum.[98] The short gut syndrome has been variously reported in 25% to 50% of patients in most series.[95] Importantly, this problem has been reported with normal small bowel length, suggesting absorptive dysfunction and emphasizing the absolute need to preserve as much large bowel as possible.

Cardiovascular and Pulmonary Anomalies

Life-threatening anomalies of the cardiovascular and pulmonary systems are extremely rare. Cyanotic heart disease and aortic duplication have been described, as has duplication of the vena cava.[101] A bilobular lung and atretic upper lobe bronchus have been reported.[96]

Surgical Management

Steinbuchel[102] described the first reported surgically reconstructed cloacal exstrophy. The omphalocele was corrected at birth, and the atretic colon was pulled through to the perineum; however, the neonate died at 5 days of age. Formerly, surgical reconstruction of cloacal exstrophy was considered futile, and untreated neonates usually died from prematurity, sepsis, short bowel syndrome, or renal and central nervous system deficits. Remigailo and colleagues[103] reported the most unusual case of a well-adjusted, 18-year-old patient with cloacal exstrophy who had never undergone surgical reconstruction.

In the past, survival was the greatest challenge facing these patients. When the importance of separating the genitourinary tract from the gastrointestinal tract became apparent, survival increased. Rickham[104] reported on the first patient with cloacal exstrophy to survive surgical reconstruction. The omphalocele was repaired, the intestinal strip was separated from the hemibladders, and the blind-ending colon was pulled out through the perineum. The hemibladders were then reapproximated. An ileal conduit was constructed at age 18 months, and a cystectomy was subsequently performed. After early reconstructive efforts, the patient was left with two ostomies: one to collect urine and the other to collect stool. Because survival is no longer the major issue, achieving a good quality of life is now the greatest challenge facing these patients.[100]

Immediate Neonatal Assessment

The authors' approach to the reconstruction of cloacal exstrophy is by staged surgical reconstruction. The infant's condition at birth may be critical, and attempts to reconstruct and repair may be futile or morally or ethically unwise.[17] Often, the severity of cloacal exstrophy is enhanced by the nature and severity of the associated anomalies. The more robust infant will survive, and reparative surgery is initiated at birth. The authors' preference is a one-stage closure when the infant is in excellent condition and has favorable anatomy with minimal associated anomalies.[17] However, many of these infants are premature, are small for gestational age, and have such severe associated anomalies that it is difficult for them to undergo an extensive one-stage procedure in the newborn period.

Surgical management and preoperative assessment should only be undertaken by a multidisciplinary team that includes surgeons who are familiar with the principles of exstrophy treatment, its options, and later reconstructive techniques. Also included in the team should be a neonatologist, a neurosurgeon, and an orthopedic surgeon familiar with the osteotomy techniques needed for a secure pelvic closure.

Surgical Options in the Neonatal Period

Among the important decisions to be made during this period is whether to perform a one-stage or two-stage closure. A one-stage closure is preferred in a select group of patients. During either a one-stage or two-stage procedure, the omphalocele is excised, and the bowel is separated from the bladder halves. The lateral vesicointestinal fissure is closed in continuity, and a short colostomy is created from the end of the distal colon segment. The hemibladders then are reapproximated in the midline to create a single exstrophic bladder. If a one-stage procedure is selected, the entire bladder is closed completely after a bilateral anterior innominate osteotomy has been performed. Also, an anterior osteotomy allows placement of pins for external fixation and is preferred when severe lumbosacral dysraphism is present. With a large omphalocele defect, bladder closure and osteotomy may be delayed until respiratory and gastrointestinal stability are achieved.[17]

Management of the Bowel in Cloacal Exstrophy

The management of the bowel in cloacal exstrophy must be closely integrated with the management of the urinary tract. The traditional approach that cloacal exstrophy is mainly an ileocecal exstrophy separating two hemibladders that is treated with a two-stomal diversion certainly needs rethinking in light of modern reconstructive surgery. The grid coding system for cloacal exstrophy has previously been mentioned and ensures that a precise description of the bowel anomalies is undertaken, that variant patterns are identified, and that appropriate early decisions are made concerning the exstrophied bowel and hindgut.[94]

The principles guiding the management of the bowel in cloacal exstrophy are to conserve all bowel segments, to minimize fluid and electrolyte loss, and to make bowel available both for later urinary tract reconstruction and for vaginal reconstruction in adolescence. Formerly, patients died from fluid and electrolyte loss with a short bowel and terminal ileostomy. The authors have instituted early total parenteral nutrition to help these infants grow so that the short gut syndrome becomes less of a problem as the patients get older. Careful preservation of the hindgut segment is important because this segment can enlarge considerably if it is used initially as a fecal colostomy, and it may help absorption and prevent fluid loss.[105] Also, the hindgut enlarges if used for a fecal colostomy and later can be used as a bladder augmentation or vaginal replacement. In the ideal situation, a long hindgut segment is apportioned to both the bladder and bowel. In this case, the exstrophied segment is left in situ with the bladder, the more distal hindgut is mobilized on its mesentery and anastomosed to the small bowel, and a terminal colostomy is fashioned.

Placement of the colostomy or ileostomy at a favorable location is of prime importance. It should be placed where it can easily be managed with an appliance. In the rare instance in which there is an adequate hindgut and no neurologic deficit, a colostomy can be created with a later posterior sagittal anorectoplasty to bring the colon to the perineum. Ricketts and associates[100] have used this approach in 2 patients with good success, although daily enemas are required. Careful evaluation of neurologic status and magnetic resonance imaging studies of these patients must be accomplished before this approach is chosen. Finally, every effort must be expended to save both of the appendiceal structures for later continent stoma construction if needed.

Management of the Phallic Structures and Vagina

In boys with cloacal exstrophy, the penis is usually represented by two widely separated small phallic structures. Because these structures are rudimentary and wide apart, attempts at reconstruction have been generally unsatisfactory.[92] Therefore, the medial aspects of the bifid phallus are denuded of mucosa and brought together in the midline. This is usually done at the time of bladder closure and osteotomy. If there is a single phallic structure in the midline (20% of patients), the urethral plate is dissected from the corporal bodies and dropped between them to the perineum for a urethral opening. The corpora and glans are then recessed for a more appropriate female appearance, and labial folds are created from the scrotum by a posterior Y-V plasty.

Correction of genital anomalies in girls is usually done at the time of bladder closure and osteotomy. The medial aspect of the hemiclitoris is denuded of mucosa, and the halves are brought together with 5-0 Vicryl for the subcutaneous layer and fine 6-0 Vicryl for the epithelial layer.[17]

Commonly, duplicate vaginas are far apart and on opposite sides of the pelvis. In the unusual case of the vaginas being close together, they should be joined in the midline and used for later reconstruction. The ostia of the vaginas may be difficult to find at the time of the initial closure, and the surgeon should be aware that they can enter the posterior wall of the bladder. It is acceptable to leave the vaginas in situ, but further surgery will be needed to bring one of these to the perineum.

In the genotypic male patient raised as a girl, the vagina is usually created at the time of puberty. In the past, vaginas have been created by anatomic "scraps," such as portions of duplicated bowel, unneeded dilated ureter, or a few centimeters of the distal colonic segment.[98] One of the authors has made two vaginas from a small portion of the distal colonic segment, and both were stenotic and of no use to the child. Therefore, it is probably better to wait until puberty and construct a vagina from intestine or from a free full-thickness skin graft. There is a paucity of literature on the construction of a neovagina in the cloacal exstrophy patient, but as more of these patients reach puberty, experience with this entity will increase, and long-term information will be available.

Reconstruction of the Lower Urinary Tract

Bladder Closure

Whether the bladder is closed at initial operation or as a second procedure, care must be taken when the bowel is separated from the bladder halves to avoid damage to the blood supply of the bowel mesentery and to the autonomic vesical innervation, which becomes exposed at the medial aspect of the hemibladder.[93] The bladder closure is performed much as that of classic bladder exstrophy described earlier.[17] In girls, a double vagina may complicate closure of the urethra. If possible, the vaginas are joined and positioned posteriorly, and the tissue on the anteromedial aspect is tubularized to form a urethra. If this tissue is unavailable, then local tissues are used to form a urethral channel. As mentioned previously, in the genotypic male patient raised as a girl, the urethral plate is raised from the corpora, much as in the initial part of a Cantwell-Ransley repair, and then brought ventral to the corpora as a perineal urethra.

Drainage of the urinary tract is accomplished by ureteral stents and suprapubic catheter all exiting from the abdomen. No urethral stent or catheter is used. After bladder closure, free incontinent drainage of urine through the urethra is expected, but antibiotic suppression and close monitoring are necessary to avoid retention, infection, and reflux nephropathy.

Osteotomy is performed in all of the authors' patients with cloacal exstrophy based on success with this procedure for classic bladder exstrophy.[97] The goal is to achieve tension-free approximation of the widely separated pubic bones and of the anterior abdominal wall. Anterior osteotomy also provides large cancellous surfaces with good healing potential. Furthermore, in cases of extreme pubic diastasis, combined anterior innominate and posterior osteotomy may be done within the periosteum through the same skin incision for better correction. Immobilization is provided by an external fixator and modified Bryant traction or Buck traction for 4 weeks.

The importance of an osteotomy at the time of cloacal exstrophy closure has become more obvious during the past several years. In a series reported by Ben-Chaim and colleagues,[97] nine patients were referred for further treatment after closure elsewhere without osteotomy. Of these cloacal exstrophy patients, six developed dehiscence, one a large ventral hernia, and one a major bladder prolapse. In contrast, of 12 of the authors' patients who underwent osteotomy at the time of cloacal exstrophy closure, there was one dehiscence and one minor prolapse. Therefore, it is clear that osteotomy has a significant role in the closure and success rates of cloacal exstrophy.

Management of Urinary Incontinence

Incontinence of urine is managed by diapering only during the early years. Intermittent catheterization is likely to be needed for emptying after any procedure to enhance outlet resistance. This may be due in part to spinal defects, which can cause a neurologic deficit in bladder function, or to a small bladder capacity, which may require augmentation. In both instances, bladder detrusor activity usually is impaired. Surgery to produce a continent reservoir should be delayed until the child is old enough to participate in self-care.[106] The choice between a catheterizable urethra or an abdominal stoma depends on the adequacy of the urethra and bladder outlet, the intellect and dexterity of the child, and the child's orthopedic status as regards the spine, hip joints, braces, and ambulation.

The time to initiate management of urinary incontinence is determined by the age at which the child can understand and manage the type of bladder emptying required. Social factors, intelligence, school support, and mobility are important considerations for this group.

Occasionally, hindgut is available for bladder enhancement, but ileum has traditionally been used. In an effort to avoid further loss of absorptive surface by preserving both hindgut and ileum, Adams and colleagues[107] have used gastrocystoplasty with good success. Regardless of which bowel segment is chosen, bladder augmentation should be delayed until bowel function is mature and nutrition and acidosis are no longer a problem.

Some patients have a functioning bladder and can void through a reconstructed bladder outlet. Innovative methods may be needed, however, to construct a continent outlet in patients without substantial native urethral tissues.[108] These techniques include use of the vagina to form a urethra, with reimplantation of the vagina into the bladder for continence, or an ileal nipple, as described by Hendren.[109]

Personal Experience With Achieving Continence in the Cloacal Exstrophy Patient

The two senior authors follow 23 patients with cloacal exstrophy, of whom 14 have undergone continence procedures. Four patients underwent Young-Dees bladder neck plasty only; 1 patient had bladder neck suspension; 3 had Young-Dees-Leadbetter plasty and augmentation; 4 had Young-Dees-Lead-

TABLE 66-1. *Staged functional reconstruction of cloacal exstrophy*

IMMEDIATE NEONATAL ASSESSMENT
Evaluate associated anomalies
Decide whether to proceed with reparative surgery

FUNCTIONAL BLADDER CLOSURE (SOON AFTER NEONATAL ASSESSMENT)
ONE-STAGE REPAIR (FEW ASSOCIATED ANOMALIES)
Excision omphalocele
Separation of cecal plate from bladder halves
Joining and closure of bladder halves
Bilateral anterior innominate osteotomy
Gonadectomy in boys with duplicated or absent penis
Terminal ileostomy or colostomy
Genital revision if needed

TWO-STAGE REPAIR—FIRST STAGE (NEWBORN PERIOD)
Excision omphalocele
Separation of cecal plate from bladder halves
Joining of bladder halves
Gonadectomy in boys with duplicated or absent penis
Terminal ileostomy or colostomy

TWO-STAGE REPAIR—SECOND STAGE (AGE 4–6 MONTHS OF AGE)
Closure joined bladder halves
Bilateral anterior innominate osteotomy
Genital revision if needed

ANTIINCONTINENCE OR REFLUX PROCEDURE (4–5 YEARS OF AGE)
BLADDER CAPACITY > 60 ML MINIMUM: (SMALL GROUP OF PATIENTS)
Young-Dees-Leadbetter bladder neck reconstruction
Bilateral Cohen ureteral reimplantations
Marshall-Marchetti bladder neck suspension
BLADDER CAPACITY < 60 ML
Young-Dees-Leadbetter bladder neck reconstruction
Bilateral Cohen ureteral reimplantations
Bowel segment used to augment bladder > or <
Continent diversion with abdominal or perineal stoma

VAGINAL RECONSTRUCTION
Vagina constructed or augmented using colon, ileum, or full-thickness skin graft

(After Gearhart JP. Anomalies of the bladder. In: Kelalis PP, King L, Belman AB, eds. Clinical Pediatric Urology, ed 3. Philadelphia, WB Saunders, 1992)

better plasty, augmentation, and continent abdominal stoma; and 2 had closure of the bladder neck, augmentation, and creation of a continent abdominal stoma. The upper tracts remain normal in 21 patients. Two patients required revision of their continent stomas owing to catheterization difficulties. One patient required injection of collagen into the reconstructed bladder neck, and one patient who had both bladder neck reconstruction and bladder augmentation underwent reoperation with bladder neck closure and ileal Mitrofanoff continent diversion for failure to achieve continence.[110] Overall, 12 patients (86%) experience diurnal continence, while 79% are dry at night. Twelve are on a CIC regimen, and two are voiding spontaneously.[97]

Despite the complexity of this anomaly, a staged approach to lower tract reconstruction can produce urinary continence (Table 66-1). An individualized approach is required to find the most suitable solution for each patient's bladder and bowel anatomy and function, according to their intellectual, neurologic, and orthopedic capabilities. Ricketts and associates[100] have developed a scoring system to analyze both bladder and bowel continence. In the absence of multiple cases, owing to the rarity of this condition, use of this scoring system may allow a collective experience to be analyzed and thus optimization of future management of this complex disorder.

PRUNE BELLY SYNDROME

The prune belly syndrome[111] is known by many other names, including Eagle-Barrett syndrome[112] and, more commonly, the triad syndrome.[113] This syndrome has three distinguishing features: (1) deficient abdominal wall musculature; (2) undescended testes, usually intraabdominal; and (3) urinary tract abnormalities. Strictly speaking, only boys can be affected by all of these findings; a triad of abdominal wall laxity, urinary tract dilation, and genital anomalies, most commonly vaginal atresia or bicornuate uterus, has been described in girls.[114] The incidence of prune belly syndrome is estimated to be between 1 in 29,000[115] and 1 in 40,000 live births.[116]

Prune belly syndrome represents a spectrum of involvement. In the classification popularized by Woodard and Zucker,[117] patients can be divided into three categories. Category I patients have oligohydramnios, pulmonary hypoplasia, possibly urethral obstruction, patent urachus, and often neonatal death. Category III patients have mild or incomplete abdominal wall involvement and a near-normal urinary tract. Most patients fall into category II, with abdominal wall and urinary tract findings characteristic of the syndrome, but with no immediate threat to survival. These are the patients in whom the choice of therapy is often controversial.

Several theories have been advanced to explain the constellation of findings in prune belly syndrome. Theories proposing a disorder of embryogenesis postulate a lateral mesenchymal defect, affecting both the development of the abdominal wall musculature and the smooth muscle of the urinary tract.[113] The association of omphalocele[118] and gastroschisis[119] with prune belly syndrome supports these theories. Another widely held belief is that a transient severe bladder outlet obstruction, perhaps due to prostatic hypoplasia and collapse of the posterior urethra, is the inciting event.[120] This obstruction is thought to cause dilation of the urinary tract, urinary ascites, abdominal wall stretching, and maldevelopment and cryptorchidism owing to obstruction of the inguinal canals by the bladder.[121,122] An animal model of urethral and urachal obstruction in the first-trimester fetal lamb appears to support this theory.[123] Ascites of a nonurinary nature has been associated with the abdominal wall findings of prune belly with no urinary tract abnormalities.[124]

The genetic basis of prune belly syndrome is unclear. Several theories have been proposed, but there is little solid evidence for any of them. Several associations have been reported with prune belly syndrome, and a multifactorial inheritance or a teratogenic mechanism might best explain the range of associations. Prune belly syndrome has been associated with trisomy 13,[125] trisomy 18,[121,126,127] trisomy 21,[128] interstitial deletion of the long arm of chromosome 1,[129] 8q interstitial deletion,[130] 45XO phenotype,[131] Beckwith-Wiedemann syndrome,[132,133] exposure to teratogens,[134] and paucity of interlobular bile ducts.[135] One report has been made of an association between prune belly syndrome and α_1-antitrypsin deficiency.[136] It will take careful study of greater numbers of patients to allow any scientific genetic counseling. Parents should be made aware that prune belly syndrome has occurred in siblings, although the relative risk of this occurrence is unknown.[137]

Anomalies of the Prune Belly Complex

The abdominal wall in the affected patient has a characteristic appearance, especially in the infant[137] (Fig. 66-8). The abdomen is doughy, with bulging flanks. The liver edge is plainly seen, and intestinal peristalsis is often evident. The enlarged upper urinary tract may be palpable, as is the distended bladder. The defect represents a complete or patchy absence of the lower abdominal wall musculature.[113] The umbilicus is displaced upward because the upper abdominal muscles are often relatively spared.[113] Because of the absence of the lower rectus abdominus, these children generally need to assist with their arms when attempting to sit up from a supine position.

The abnormalities of the urinary tract may be divided into those that affect the upper tracts, the bladder, and the urethra. The kidneys are often dysmorphic, with large calyces, long infundibuli, and dilated pelves (Fig. 66-9). Pathologic changes consistent with segmental or total dysplasia are often seen.[113,138] The ureters are tortuous and markedly dilated; usually, this is more pronounced distally. Often, the upper ureters are less dilated and more apt to demonstrate effective peristalsis.[137] A high-resolution color image video analysis system was used to quantify morphometrically the smooth muscle and collagen content of various abnormal ureter types. Collagen content of the lower ureters from prune belly patients demonstrated significantly elevated collagen levels, especially in those demonstrating reflux (62%). It is proposed that this increase in collagen associated with reflux is due either to repetitive stretching stimulating collagen production, or a primary ureteral bud abnormality leading to reflux and increased collagen interdependently.[139] These impressive megaureters are rarely truly obstructed, and the radiographic appearance correlates poorly with renal function. Ureteropelvic junction obstruction, horseshoe kidney, and renal hypoplasia[138] are other upper tract anomalies reported.

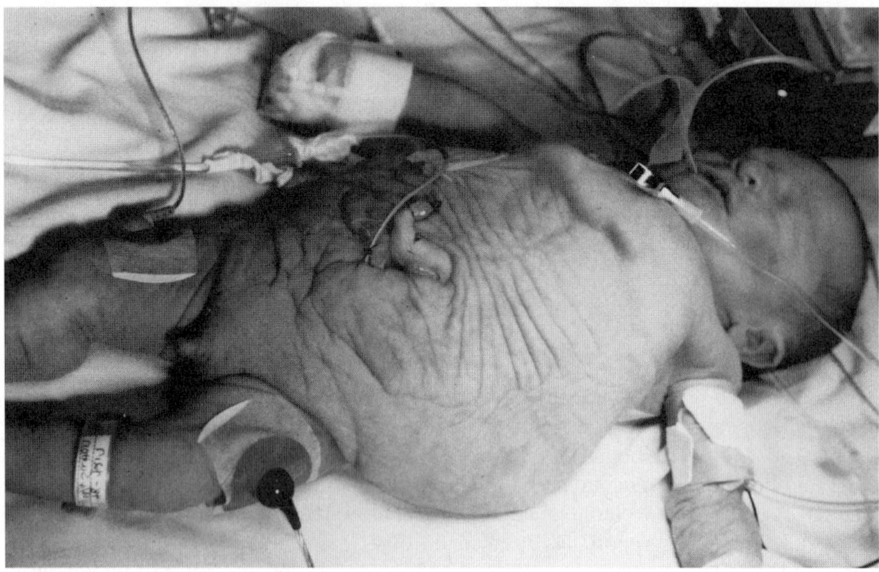

FIG. 66-8. Typical appearance of an infant with prune belly syndrome, characterized by lax abdominal wall and pectus deformity.

The bladder characteristically is large with thickened walls,[113] but trabeculation is generally absent.[137] There is commonly a pseudodiverticulum at the dome, which is conceptually a urachal extension, and occasionally the urachus is patent (Fig. 66-10). In an autopsy study of fetuses with posterior urethral valves and prune belly syndrome, Workman and Kogan found that patients with prune belly bladders can be divided into two groups. The first group of patients have increased muscle mass and connective tissue similar to patients with posterior urethral valves. In these fetuses, bladder outlet obstruction is evident on autopsy examination.[140] The ureteral orifices are laterally placed on a large trigone, and many of these bladders demonstrate vesicoureteral reflux. The second group demonstrated no histological evidence of bladder thickening or outlet obstruction.

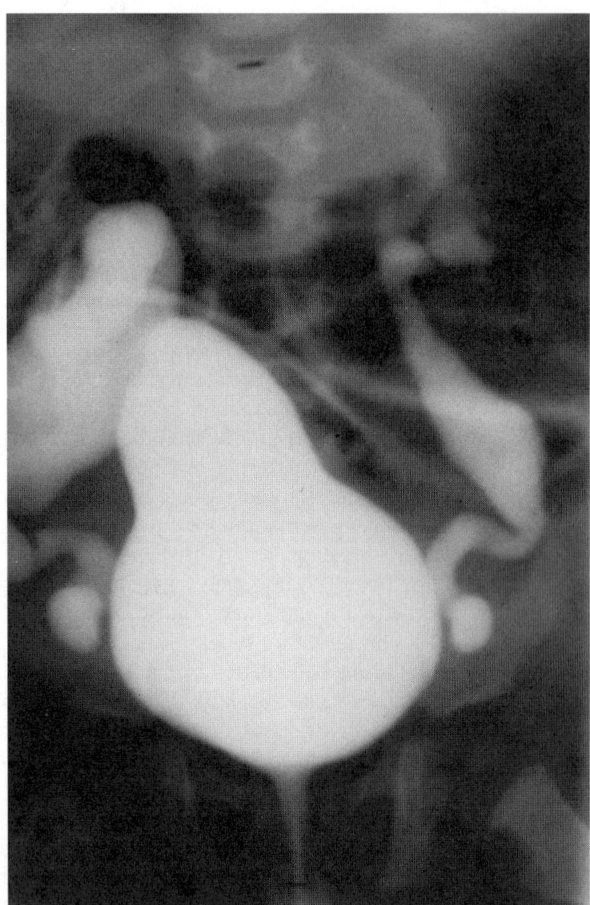

FIG. 66-9. Voiding cystourethrogram demonstrating the bizarre dilated upper urinary tracts typical of the prune belly syndrome.

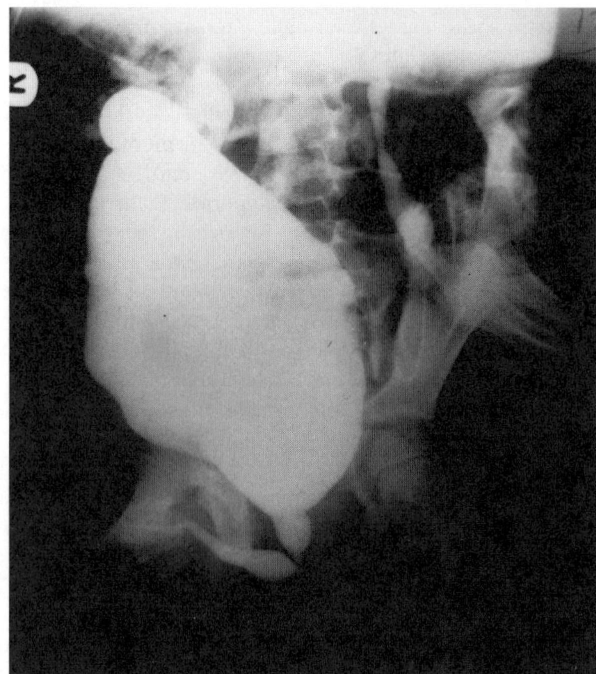

FIG. 66-10. Oblique voiding view of cystogram demonstrating dilated posterior urethra and urachal extension at the dome of the bladder.

The posterior urethra in patients with prune belly syndrome is dilated and may be confused with posterior urethral valves. Valves apparently have been documented in some cases of prune belly syndrome,[141] although they tend to occur in severe cases with oligohydramnios and neonatal death. No valves can be demonstrated in most children with the syndrome.[137] The histology of the dilated posterior urethra is consistent with a deficiency of development of the prostate.[113] The bladder neck is wide, not hypertrophied, as it often is with valves.[141] The verumontanum is usually not apparent radiographically or cystoscopically, but is present on pathologic examination.[141]

The anterior urethra is usually normal, although a narrow, underdeveloped urethra or a megalourethra may be found. Urethral atresia is usually associated with fatal pulmonary hypoplasia but may be compatible with survival in the presence of a patent urachus.[142] Megalourethra comes in two forms: the fusiform deformity involves absence or hypoplasia of all the penile bodies, and the scaphoid megalourethra is due to an isolated defect in the spongiosum. The fusiform megalourethra is generally found in severe cases and is often associated with neonatal death.[143] The scaphoid megalourethra was associated with azotemia or death in more than half of patients reviewed by Appel and colleagues.[144] Megalourethra may be associated with significant urethral obstruction, and improvement of the upper urinary tracts has been seen after megalourethra repair.[143] Hypospadias is rarely associated with the prune belly syndrome but has been reported.[138,145]

One of the defining features of the prune belly syndrome is bilateral cryptorchidism. The testes may be located anywhere along the normal course of descent but are most commonly found in the abdomen. The fertility potential of these testicles is a matter of controversy. The histology of the testes at the time of orchidopexy has been variably described as consistent with Sertoli-cell–only syndrome,[146] or as consistent with age-matched controls.[113] Orvis and colleagues[147] found that spermatogonia are present, but in reduced numbers, in the fetus with the prune belly syndrome. There appears to be a significant risk for testicular malignancy in these cryptorchid testes.[148,149] Massad and associates[150] documented an atypical appearance of the germ cells in early orchidopexy biopsy specimens, suggesting intratubular neoplasia.

Associated Abnormalities

One of the potentially devastating associations with prune belly syndrome is the tendency for respiratory difficulties. Respiratory compromise due either to pulmonary hypoplasia or pneumothorax[138] may be seen in the severely affected neonate. The pulmonary hypoplasia seen is almost certainly related to the occurrence of oligohydramnios[151] rather than to compression by the distended abdomen.[152] In addition, the lack of abdominal muscles to assist in coughing predisposes these children to respiratory infection and postoperative atelectasis.[117] In one study of four patients who developed postanesthesia respiratory distress, three had no prior history of pulmonary compromise.[153]

Gastrointestinal abnormalities are frequently found, especially on autopsy of severe cases. Among these are intestinal malrotation, small bowel atresia, large bowel atresia,[154] megacolon (not due to aganglionosis[154]), and imperforate anus.[138,145]

Imperforate anus occurs most commonly in more severe forms of the complex. Chronic constipation, probably due to lack of abdominal musculature, can be a feature of the syndrome.[153] Fecal impaction has also been noted.[155] Volvulus has been described in eight cases, and a high index of suspicion must be maintained in cases of intestinal obstruction or abdominal pain.[154] Splenic torsion has been reported, presumably due to abdominal wall laxity.[138]

Cardiovascular abnormalities are present in greater than 10% of patients; these include patent ductus arteriosus, atrial septal defect, ventricular septal defect, and bicuspid aortic valve.[138] Orthopedic anomalies occur in most patients, the most common being clubfoot,[145] but also including congenital dislocation of the hip[153] and atresia or agenesis of the lower limb,[145] perhaps due to iliac artery compression by the distended bladder.[156,157] Pectus deformities and scoliosis are also more common in prune belly syndrome than in the general population.[158] Dimpling at the knee is a common finding, even in children who have no other orthopedic deformities.[137]

Presentation and Diagnosis

The prune belly syndrome is frequently diagnosed on prenatal ultrasound examination.[159] The findings are similar to those of posterior urethral valves, with an enlarged bladder, bilateral hydronephrosis, and in some cases, oligohydramnios. One case has been documented in which an apparent transient bladder outlet obstruction was associated with the prune belly phenotype.[160] Other aspects of the syndrome, such as undescended testicles and megalourethra,[161,162] have been detected prenatally.

The diagnosis of prune belly syndrome is usually easily made on the initial examination of the newborn. Physical findings include abdominal wall laxity and bilateral cryptorchidism. The deficient abdominal musculature may allow visualization of the liver edge and intestinal peristalsis. Palpation of the abdomen often reveals the dilated bladder and upper urinary tracts. Examination of the extremities often reveals lateral dimpling of the knees, equinovarus abnormality, and perhaps changes associated with oligohydramnios, including Potter facies.

Initial radiologic evaluation should consist of renal and bladder ultrasound examination. The urinary tract dilation that is evident in most cases is not necessarily obstructive in nature but is always consistent with significant urinary stasis. The voiding cystourethrogram often reveals the entire urinary collecting system owing to bilateral vesicoureteral reflux, but this test may be inadvisable initially, owing to the high risk of urinary tract infection.[137] diuretic renal scintigraphy, which is an invaluable tool for detecting urinary tract obstruction, may be inaccurate owing to pooling in the large pelves and ureters.[163] Intravenous pyelography can give some information regarding function and obstruction but often is inadequate in newborns.

Serial creatinine values should be obtained in the neonate to assess the adequacy of renal function. Often, it becomes apparent that, despite the appearance of the urinary tract, the renal function is within the normal range for age. If creatinine values are rising in a manner consistent with renal compromise, further evaluation and surgical treatment for obstruction may be necessary.

Treatment

Two schools of thought have emerged on the treatment of the urinary tract in prune belly syndrome. Some children do well with no surgical treatment for reflux or gross dilation of the urinary tract.[164] An initial conservative stance is reasonable, keeping in mind that there are indications for aggressive surgical management. The impetus for an aggressive reconstructive approach in these children is the assumption that pooling of urine and reflux lead to progressive renal damage, or the assumption that the appearance of the urinary tract is due to obstruction. Conservative therapy, consisting of prophylactic antibiotics and monitoring of urine cultures and serial renal function studies, is properly undertaken when the urinary tract has a balanced nature.[165] Even a balanced urinary tract can decompensate over time, and serial monitoring is of the utmost importance.

Vesicostomy is occasionally indicated in the management of the child with prune belly syndrome who has recurring infections or a rising creatinine. Vesicostomy addresses the issues of poor bladder emptying and vesicoureteral reflux. If there is obstruction at the vesicoureteral or ureteropelvic junction, a ureterostomy or pyelostomy may be more appropriate. Temporary urinary diversion may be preferable to major reconstruction in the neonate because of the unpredictability of the pulmonary reserve in these infants.[117] Upper urinary tract diversion is rarely necessary because true ureterovesical junction obstruction is rare. When needed, pyelostomy is probably the procedure of choice because it spares the upper ureter, which is needed for later reconstruction of the urinary tract.[137] The lower ureter can also be brought to the skin as an end-cutaneous ureterostomy because this portion of ureter generally is discarded.

Surgery of the dilated ureters can be performed for obstruction at the ureteropelvic or ureterovesical junction, or for reflux with recurrent infection. The stasis of urine in the dilated ureters predisposes to urinary infection, and any surgery to correct reflux or obstruction should address this redundancy.[117] Generally, the lower ureter, which is more dilated and tortuous than the upper, is discarded. The more normal upper ureter is tapered as necessary and then reimplanted into the bladder in a nonrefluxing fashion. Preservation of the vascular adventitia of the ureter is extremely important in this type of reconstruction, especially if correction of ureteropelvic junction obstruction is carried out during the operation.

The function of the urinary bladder in prune belly syndrome can change over time. These bladders may empty poorly, and double voiding, Credé maneuver, or intermittent catheterization should be employed as necessary to reduce postvoid residuals. Urethrotomy is occasionally performed to improve bladder emptying, but it is unclear how often this is actually necessary and effective.[145] Urodynamic evidence of obstruction should be sought before urethrotomy.[117] If urodynamics prove a relative urethral obstruction and decompensation of the bladder on that basis, urethrotomy appears to be of benefit.[165] The function of the urinary bladder can change and potentially decompensate with aging, and it should be followed. Onset of recurrent urinary infections, worsening renal function, urinary incontinence, or frequency should prompt reevaluation of bladder function. The assessment may be as simple as a renal and bladder ultrasound before and after voiding. It seems obvious that the function of the bladder should be improved by removing the large dome

diverticulum often found in these children,[166] but there is no urodynamic evidence that this cystoplasty actually improves emptying ability.[167] Detrusor augmentation using rectus femoris flaps has been recommended to improve bladder emptying, but there are few indications for this extensive procedure when the use of intermittent catheterization appears satisfactory.[155]

The one clear indication for surgical intervention in the child with prune belly syndrome is orchidopexy for the bilaterally undescended testes. It is unknown whether early orchidopexy results in improved spermatogenesis in affected patients, but the ease of orchidopexy decreases after the patient is 1 or 2 years of age.[168] Options for orchidopexy include a conventional transabdominal approach maintaining the integrity of the spermatic vessels. When undertaken early in life, the success rate of this approach is high.[168] The other procedure used frequently in this condition is the Fowler-Stephens long-looped vas orchidopexy, with division of the spermatic vessels. This has been associated with a 20% to 30% atrophy rate in the hands of experienced surgeons.[145] The two-stage Fowler-Stephens approach, involving ligation of the spermatic vessels followed by orchidopexy, may enhance success rates.[169] Microvascular orchidopexy has been performed with reasonable success on boys with prune belly syndrome.[169] These alternatives to conventional transabdominal orchidopexy may be necessary in children who presents for orchidopexy after 1 year of age.

Surgical repair of the abdominal wall defect has been attempted for both cosmetic and functional indications. The psychologic implications of the unusual abdominal appearance in these boys have been stressed.[170,171] Voiding can improve after abdominoplasty, although this does not represent a primary indication for surgery.[167] There are two major alternatives to the reconstruction of the abdominal wall. The first involves vertical plication and overlapping to reduce abdominal girth and to bring the more normally formed lateral muscles toward the midline. This can be done with excision of the midline abdominal wall and preservation of the umbilicus[172] or by overlapping the deficient anterior abdominal fascial layers with or without umbilical preservation.[171,173] The abdominoplasty popularized by Randolph[174] involves a transverse excision of the lower abdominal wall, under the assumption that the upper abdominal musculature is more normally developed and can be brought down to the lower fascia (Fig. 66-11). This can be performed with the adjunct of electromyographic data to optimize the removal of nonmuscular abdominal wall.[168]

Long-Term Results

The long-term outlook for boys with the prune belly syndrome depends in large part on their neonatal course and presentation. Renal function tends to remain normal in children with a balanced or reconstructed urinary tract who start life with reasonable renal function. In severe cases with dysplastic kidneys, there is often early death due to pulmonary or renal failure. Those children who fall somewhere in between often go on to require dialysis or transplantation.[175] The prognosis of renal transplantation is not adversely affected by the diagnosis of prune belly nor by the need for intermittent catheterization.[176] Most patients require preoperative bilateral native nephrectomy.[176] Perhaps the prognosis for renal function will improve

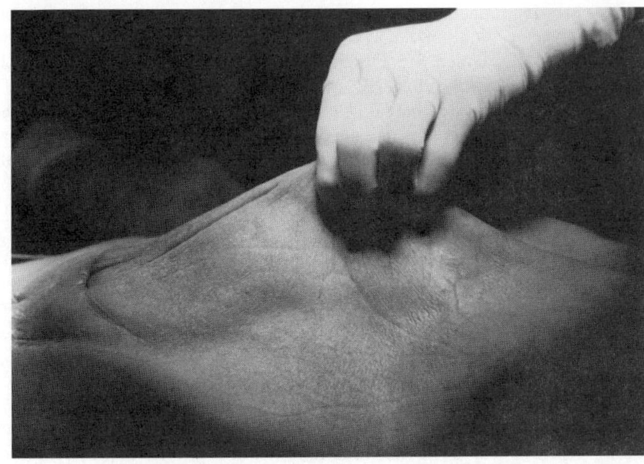
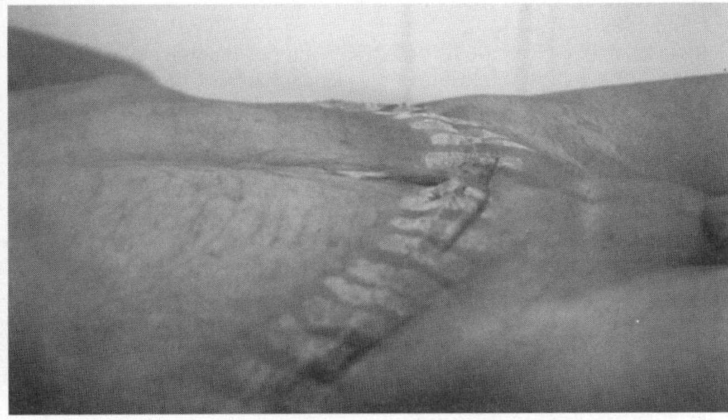

FIG. 66-11. Preoperative (*A*) and postoperative (*B*) views of the abdominal wall in a child undergoing a Randolph-type abdominoplasty.

with a modern understanding of the significance of urinary tract infection and appropriate prophylaxis.[175]

The prognosis for sexual function and fertility is mixed. Boys with prune belly syndrome have several causes of impaired fertility. The first is bilaterally undescended testicles, which, until recently, were not brought to a scrotal position until later in life. Whether the spermatogenic potential of these testicles is normal is a matter for debate. Semen analysis in adults who ejaculate are generally acellular.[177] The question may be answered more definitively as children who have undergone neonatal orchidopexies mature. The other cause of infertility is the hypoplastic nature of the prostate. Most of these men do not ejaculate at all.[177] There has been no documented fertility in men with prune belly syndrome.[145,177] Other aspects of sexual function can be expected to be normal.[177]

REFERENCES

1. Lancaster PAL. Epidemiology of bladder exstrophy and epispadias: a communication from the International Clearinghouse for Birth Defects Monitoring Systems. Teratology 1987;36:221.
2. Jeffs RD, Lepor H. Management of the exstrophy-epispadias complex and urachal anomalies. In: Walsh PC, et al, eds. Campbell's urology. Philadelphia, WB Saunders, 1986:1882.
3. Muecke EC, The role of the cloacal membrane in exstrophy: the first successful experimental study. J Urol 1964;92:659.
4. Muecke EC. Exstrophy, epispadias, and other anomalies of the bladder. In: Walsh PC, et al, eds. Campbell's urology. Philadelphia, WB Saunders, 1986:1856.
5. Ambrose SS, O'Brien DI. Surgical embryology of the exstrophy-epispadias complex. (Review) Surg Clin North Am 1974;54:1379.
6. Thomalla JV, Rudolph RA, Rink RC, et al. Induction of cloacal exstrophy in the chick embryo using the CO2 laser. J Urol 1985;134:991.
7. Mildenberger H, Kluth D, Dziuba M. Embryology of bladder exstrophy. J Pediatr Surg 1988;23:166.
8. Shapiro E, Lepor H, Jeffs RD. The inheritance of the exstrophy-epispadias complex. J Urol 1984;132:308.
9. Ives E, Coffey R, Carter CO. A family study of bladder exstrophy. J Med Genet 1980;17:139.
10. Smith NM, Chambers HM, Furness ME, et al. The OEIS complex (omphalocele-exstrophy-imperforate anus-spinal defects): recurrence in sibs. J Med Genet 1992;29:730.
11. Blickstein I, Katz Z. Possible relationship of bladder exstrophy and epispadias with progestins taken during early pregnancy. Br J Urol 1991;68:105.
12. Gelehrter TD. Lysergic acid diethylamide (LSD) and exstrophy of the bladder. J Pediatr 1970;77:1065.
13. Mirk P, Calisti A, Fileni A. Prenatal sonographic diagnosis of bladder exstrophy. J Ultrasound Med 1986;5:291.
14. Verco PW, Khor BH, Barbary J, et al. Ectopia vesicae in utero. Australas Radiol 1986;30:117.
15. Jaffe R, Schoenfeld A, Ovadia J. Sonographic findings in the prenatal diagnosis of bladder exstrophy. Am J Obstet Gynecol 1990;162:675.
16. Barth RA, Filly RA, Sondheimer FK. Prenatal sonographic findings in bladder exstrophy. J Ultrasound Med 1990;9:359.
17. Gearhart JP, Jeffs RD. Exstrophy of the bladder, epispadias, and other bladder anomalies. In: Walsh PC, et al, eds. Campbell's urology. Philadelphia, WB Saunders, 1986:1772.
18. Gearhart JP, Ben-Chaim JB, Jeffs RD, et al. Criteria for the prenatal diagnosis of bladder exstrophy. 1994 OB2GYN.85:961, 1995.
19. Muecke EC, Currarino G. Congenital widening of the pubic symphysis: associated clinical disorders and roentgen anatomy of affected bony pelves. AJR 1968;103:179.
20. Woodhouse CR, Kellett MJ. Anatomy of the penis and its deformities in exstrophy and epispadias. J Urol 1984;132:1122.
21. Husmann DA, McLorie GA, Churchill BM, et al. Inguinal pathology and its association with classical bladder exstrophy. J Pediatr Surg 1990;25:332.
22. Peppas DS, Connolly JA, Jeffs RD, et al. Prevalence and repair of inguinal hernias in children with classical bladder exstrophy. J Urol 1995;154:1900.
23. Jones HJ. An anomaly of the external genitalia in female patients with exstrophy of the bladder. Am J Obstet Gynecol 1973;117:748.
24. Krisiloff M, Puchner PJ, Tretter W, et al. Pregnancy in women with bladder exstrophy. J Urol 1978;119:478.
25. Shapiro E, Jeffs RD, Gearhart JP, et al. Muscarinic cholinergic receptors in bladder exstrophy: insights into surgical management. J Urol 1985;134:308.
26. Peppas DS, Tchetcen MB, Jeffs RD, et al. A quantitative histological analysis of the bladder in classical bladder exstrophy in various stages of reconstruction utilizing color morphometry. J Urol 1994 (in press).
27. Woodhouse CR, Ransley PG, Williams DI. The patient with exstrophy in adult life. Br J Urol 1983;55:632.
28. Lattimer JK, Hensle TW, MacFarlane MT, et al. The exstrophy support team: a new concept in the care of the exstrophy patient. J Urol 1979;121:472.
29. Ansell JS. Surgical treatment of exstrophy of the bladder with emphasis on neonatal primary closure: personal experience with 28 consecutive cases treated at the University of Washington hospitals from 1962 to 1977: techniques and results. J Urol 1979;121:650.
30. Oesterling JE, Jeffs RD. The importance of a successful initial bladder closure in the surgical management of classical bladder exstrophy:

analysis of 144 patients treated at the Johns Hopkins Hospital between 1975 and 1985. J Urol 1987;137:258.

31. Gearhart JP, Jeffs RD. State-of-the-art reconstructive surgery for bladder exstrophy at the Johns Hopkins Hospital. (Review) Am J Dis Child 1989;143:1475.

32. Sponseller PD, Gearhart JP, Jeffs RD. Anterior innominate osteotomies for failure or late closure of bladder exstrophy. J Urol 1991;146:137.

33. Montagnani CA. Innominate osteotomy in reconstructive surgery for exstrophy of the bladder. J Pediatr Surg 1967;2:583.

34. Gokcora IH, Yazar T. Bilateral transverse iliac osteotomy in the correction of neonatal bladder extrophies. Int Surg 1989;74:123.

35. Aadalen RJ, O'Phelan EH, Chisholm TC, et al. Exstrophy of the bladder: long-term results of bilateral posterior iliac osteotomies and two-stage anatomic repair. Clin Orthop 1980;68:156.

36. McKenna PH, Khoury AE, McLorie GA, et al. Iliac osteotomy: a model to compare the options in bladder and cloacal exstrophy reconstruction. J Urol 1994;151:182.

37. Frey P, Cohen SJ. Anterior pelvic osteotomy: a new operative technique facilitating primary bladder exstrophy closure. Br J Urol 1989;64:641.

38. Duckett JW. Use of paraexstrophy skin pedicle grafts for correction of exstrophy and epispadias repair. Birth Defects 1977;13:175.

39. Gearhart JP, Peppas DS, Jeffs RD. Complications of paraexstrophy skin flaps in the reconstruction of classical bladder exstrophy. J Urol 1993;150:627.

40. Jordan GH, Gilbert DA. Operative procedures for epispadias and exstrophy of the bladder. (Review) Semin Urol 1987;5:243.

41. Ransley PG, Duffy PG, Wollin M. Bladder exstrophy closure and epispadias repair. In: Operative surgery: pediatric surgery. Edinburgh, Butterworth, 1989;620.

42. Husmann DA, McLorie GA, Churchill BM. Closure of the exstrophic bladder: an evaluation of the factors leading to its success and its importance on urinary continence. J Urol 1989;142:522.

43. Lowe FC, Jeffs RD. Wound dehiscence in bladder exstrophy: an examination of the etiologies and factors for initial failure and subsequent success. J Urol 1983;130:312.

44. Hollowell JG, Ransley PG. Surgical management of incontinence in bladder exstrophy. Br J Urol 1991;68:543.

45. Hendren WH. Nonrefluxing colon conduit for temporary or permanent urinary diversion in children. J Pediatr Surg 1975;10:381.

46. Gearhart JP, Jeffs RD. Bladder exstrophy: increase in capacity following epispadias repair. J Urol 1989;142:525.

47. Gearhart JP, Jeffs RD. The use of parenteral testosterone therapy in genital reconstructive surgery. J Urol 1988;138:1077.

48. Kelley JH, Eraklis AJ. A procedure for lengthening the phallus in boys with exstrophy of the bladder. J Pediatr Surg 1971;6:645.

49. Johnston BH. Lengthening of the congenital or acquired short penis. Br J Urol 1974;46:685.

50. Hendren WH. Penile lengthening after previous repair of epispadias. J Urol 1979;121:527.

51. Thomalla JV, Mitchell ME. Ventral preputial island flap technique for the repair of epispadias with or without exstrophy. J Urol 1984;132:985.

52. Kramer SA, Jackson IT. Bilateral rhomboid flaps for reconstruction of the external genitalia in epispadias-exstrophy. Plast Reconstr Surg 1986;77:621.

53. Brzezinski AE, Homsy YL, Laberge I. Orthoplasty in epispadias. J Urol 1986;136:259.

54. Koff SA, Eakins M. The treatment of penile chordee using corporeal rotation. J Urol 1984;131:931.

55. Schillinger JF, Wiley MJ. Bladder exstrophy: penile lengthening procedure. Urology 1984;24:434.

56. Gearhart JP, Leonard MP, Burgers JK, et al. The Cantwell-Ransley technique for repair of epispadias. J Urol 1992;148:851.

57. Canning DA, Gearhart JP, Peppas DS, et al. The cephalotrigonal reimplant in bladder neck reconstruction for patients with exstrophy or epispadias. J Urol 1993;150:156.

58. Peters CA, Hendren WH. Splitting the pubis for exposure in difficult reconstructions for incontinence. J Urol 1989;142:527.

59. Gearhart JP, Williams KA, Jeffs RD. Intraoperative urethral pressure profileometry as an adjunct to bladder neck reconstruction. J Urol 1986;136:1055.

60. Marshall VF, Marchetti AA, Krantz KE. The correction of stress urinary incontinence by simple vesicourethral suspension. Surg Gynecol Obstet 1949;88:509.

61. Jeffs RD, Guice SL, Oesch I. The factors in successful exstrophy closure. J Urol 1982;127:974.

62. Canning DA, Gearhart JP, Oesterling JE, et al. A computerized review of exstrophy patients managed during the past thirteen years (Abstract 219) American Urological Association Meeting, Dallas, May 7, 1989.

63. Mollard P, Basset T, Deseubis M, et al. Results of bladder and urethra reconstruction for exstrophy. (French) Chir Pediatr 1986;27:27.

64. Connor JP, Hensle TW, Lattimer JK, et al. Long-term followup of 207 patients with bladder exstrophy: an evolution in treatment. J Urol 1989;142:793.

65. Allen TD, Husmann DA, Bucholz RW. Exstrophy of the bladder: primary closure after iliac osteotomies without external or internal fixation. J Urol 1992;147:438.

66. Lepor H, Shapiro E, Jeffs RD. Urethral reconstruction in boys with classical bladder exstrophy. J Urol 1984;131:512.

67. Mesrobian HG, Kelalis PP, Kramer SA. Long-term followup of cosmetic appearance and genital function in boys with exstrophy: review of 53 patients. J Urol 1986;136:256.

68. Gearhart JP, Peppas DS, Jeffs RD. The failed exstrophy closure: strategy for management. Br J Urol 1993;71:217.

69. Gearhart JP, Canning DA, Peppas DS, et al. Techniques to create continence in the failed bladder exstrophy closure patient. J Urol 1993;150:441.

70. Caione P, Lais A, de GM, et al. Glutaraldehyde cross-linked bovine collagen in exstrophy/epispadias complex. J Urol 1993;150:631.

71. Leonard MP, Gearhart JP, Jeffs RD. Continent urinary reservoirs in pediatric urological practice. J Urol 1990;144:330.

72. Gearhart JP, Peppas DS, Jeffs RD. Continent catheterizeable stomas in the failed exstrophy reconstruction. Br J Urol 1995;75:87.

73. Kramer SA, Kelalis PP. Assessment of urinary continence in epispadias: review of 70 cases. J Urol 1982;128:290.

74. Gearhart JP, Yang A, Leonard MP, et al. Prostate size and configuration in adults with bladder exstrophy. J Urol 1993;149:308.

75. Arap S, Martins GA, Menezes, J et al. Initial results of the complete reconstruction of bladder exstrophy. Urol Clin North Am 1980;7:477.

76. Decter RM, Roth DR, Fishman IJ, et al. Use of the AS800 device in exstrophy and epispadias. J Urol 1988;140:1202.

77. Gearhart JP, Failed bladder exstrophy repair: evaluation and management. Urol Clin North Am 1991;18:687.

78. Hanna MK. Artificial urinary sphincter for incontinent children. Urology 1981;18:370.

79. Caione P, Capozza N, Lais A, et al. Female genito-urethroplasty and submucosal periurethral collagen injection as adjunctive procedures for continence in the exstrophy-epispadias complex: preliminary results. Br J Urol 1993;71:350.

80. Woodhouse CR. Reconstruction of the epispadiac penis in adolescents. Prog Pediatr Surg 1989;23:165.

81. Burger RA, Muller SC, el DH, et al. The buccal mucosal graft for urethral reconstruction: a preliminary report. J Urol 1992;147:662.

82. Zabbo A, Kay R. Ureterosigmoidostomy and bladder exstrophy: a long-term followup. J Urol 1986;136:396.

83. Stockle M, Becht E, Voges G, et al. Ureterosigmoidostomy: an outdated approach to bladder exstrophy? J Urol 1990;143:770.

84. Strachan JR, Woodhouse CR. Malignancy following ureterosigmoidostomy in patients with exstrophy. Br J Surg 1991;78:1216.

85. Gittes RF. Carcinogenesis in ureterosigmoidostomy. (Review) Urol Clin North Am 1986;13:201.

86. Kroovand RL, Boyce WH. Isolated vesicorectal internal urinary diversion: a 37-year review of the Boyce-Vest procedure. J Urol 1988;140:572.

87. Jeffs RD, Schwartz GR. Ileal conduit urinary diversion in children: computer analysis follow-up from 2 to 16 years. J Urol 1975;114:285.

88. Hendren WH. Exstrophy of the bladder: an alternative method of management. (Review) J Urol 1976;115:195.

89. Gharib M, Engelskirchen R, Bliesener JA, et al. Comparative results of ileal conduit and colonic conduit: analysis of 50 children with bladder exstrophy. (German) Z Kinderchir 1986;41:214.

90. Langer JC, Brennan B, Lappalainen RE, et al. Cloacal exstrophy: prenatal diagnosis before rupture of the cloacal membrane. J Pediatr Surg 1992;27:1352.

91. Sponseller PD, Bisson LS, Gearhart JP, et al. The anatomy of the pelvis in the exstrophy complex. Bone & Joint Surgery 1995;77:177.

92. Husmann DA, McLorie GA, Churchill BM. Phallic reconstruction in cloacal exstrophy. J Urol 1989;142:563.

93. Schlegel PN, Gearhart JP. Neuroanatomy of the pelvis in an infant with cloacal exstrophy: a detailed microdissection with histology. J Urol 1989;141:583.

94. Manzoni GA, Ransley PG, Hurwitz RS. Cloacal exstrophy and cloacal exstrophy variants: a proposed system of classification. J Urol 1987;138:1065.

95. Diamond DA. Management of cloacal exstrophy. Dial Pediatr Urol 1990;13:1.

96. Howell C, Caldamone A, Snyder H, et al. Optimal management of cloacal exstrophy. J Pediatr Surg 1983;18:365.

97. Ben-Chaim J, Peppas DA, Sponseller PD, et al. Applications of osteotomy in the cloacal exstrophy patient. J Urol 1995;154:865.

98. Hurwitz RS, Manzoni GA, Ransley PG, et al. Cloacal exstrophy: a report of 34 cases. J Urol 1987;138:1060.

99. Tank ES, Lindenauer SM. Principles of management of exstrophy of the cloaca. Am J Surg 1970;119:95.

100. Ricketts RR, Woodard JR, Zwiren GT, et al. Modern treatment of cloacal exstrophy. J Pediatr Surg 1991;26:444.

101. Soper RT, Kilger K. Vesicointestinal fissure. J Urol 1964;92:490.

102. Steinbuchel W. Veber nabelschurbruch and blassenbauchspalte mit codken bildung von seiten des dunndormers. Arch Gynaeckol 1900;60:465.

103. Remigailo RV, Woodard JR, Andrews HG, et al. Cloacal exstrophy: 18-year survival of untreated case. J Urol 1976;116:811.

104. Rickham PP. Vesico-intestinal fissure. Arch Dis Child 1960;35:97.

105. Husmann DA, McLorie GA, Churchill BM, et al. Management of the hindgut in cloacal exstrophy: terminal ileostomy versus colostomy. J Pediatr Surg 1988;23:1107.

106. Gearhart JP, Jeffs RD. Reconstruction of the lower urinary tract in cloacal exstrophy. Dial Pediatr Urol 1990;13:4.

107. Adams MC, Mitchell ME, Rink RC. Gastrocystoplasty: an alternative solution to the problem of urological reconstruction in the severely compromised patient. J Urol 1988;140:1152.

108. Gearhart JP, Jeffs RD. Techniques to create urinary continence in the cloacal exstrophy patient. J Urol 1991;146:616.

109. Hendren WH. Ileal nipple for continence in cloacal exstrophy. J Urol 1992;148:372.

110. Longaker MT, Harrison MR, Langer JC, et al. Appendicovesicostomy: a new technique for bladder diversion during reconstruction of cloacal exstrophy. J Pediatr Surg 1989;24:639.

111. Osler W. Congenital absence of the abdominal musculature, with distended and hypertrophied urinary bladder. Bull Johns Hopkins Hosp 1901;12:331.

112. Eagle JF Jr, Barrett GS. Congenital deficiency of abdominal musculature with associated genitourinary abnormalities: a syndrome. Report of 9 cases. Pediatrics 1950;6:721.

113. Nunn IN, Stephens FD. The triad syndrome: a composite anomaly of the abdominal wall, urinary system and testes. J Urol 1961;86:782.

114. Reinberg Y, Shapiro E, Manivel JC, et al. Prune belly syndrome in females: a triad of abdominal musculature deficiency and anomalies of the urinary and genital systems. J Pediatr 1991;118:395.

115. Baird PA, MacDonald EC. An epidemiologic study of congenital malformations of the anterior abdominal wall in more than half a million live births. Am J Hum Genet 1981;33:470.

116. Garlinger P, Ott J. Prune belly syndrome: possible genetic implications. Birth Defects 1974;10:173.

117. Woodard JR, Zucker I. Current management of the dilated urinary tract in prune belly syndrome. Urol Clin North Am 1990;17:407.

118. Walker J, Prokurat AI, Irving IM. Prune belly syndrome associated with exomphalos and anorectal agenesis. J Pediatr Surg 1987;22:215.

119. Short KL, Groff DB, Cook L. The concomitant presence of gastroschisis and prune belly syndrome in a twin. J Pediatr Surg 1985;20:186.

120. Hoagland MH, Hutchins GM. Obstructive lesions of the lower urinary tract in the prune belly syndrome. Arch Pathol Lab Med 1987;111:154.

121. Hoagland MH, Frank KA, Hutchins GM. Prune-belly syndrome with prostatic hypoplasia, bladder wall rupture, and massive ascites in a fetus with trisomy 18. Arch Pathol Lab Med 1988;112:1126.

122. Pagon RA, Smith DW, Shephard TH. Urethral obstruction malformation complex: a cause of abdominal muscle deficiency and the ''prune belly.'' J Pediatr 1979;94:900.

123. Gonzalez R, Reinberg Y, Burke B, et al. Early bladder outlet obstruction in fetal lambs induces renal dysplasia and the prune-belly syndrome. J Pediatr Surg 1990;25:342.

124. Kuruvilla AC, Kesler KR, Williams JW, et al. Congenital cystic adenomatoid malformation of the lung associated with prune belly syndrome. J Pediatr Surg 1987;22:370.

125. McKeown CM, Donnai D. Prune belly in trisomy 13. Prenat Diagn 1986;6:379.

126. Nevin NC, Nevin J, Dunlop JM, et al. Antenatal diagnosis of grossly distended bladder owing to absence of urethra in a fetus with trisomy 18. J Med Genet 1983;20:132.

127. Nivelon CA, Feldman JP, Justrabo E, et al. Trisomy 18 and prune belly syndrome. (French) J Genet Hum 1985;33:469.

128. Amacker EA, Grass FS, Hickey DE, et al. An association of prune belly anomaly with trisomy 21. Am J Med Genet 1986;23:919.

129. Scarbrough PR, Files B, Carroll AJ, et al. Interstitial deletion of chromosome 1 del(1)(q25q32) in an infant with prune belly sequence. Prenat Diagn 1988;8:169.

130. Ramos FJ, McDonald MD, Emanuel BS, et al. Tricho-rhino-phalangeal syndrome type II (Langer-Giedion) with persistent cloaca and prune belly sequence in a girl with 8q interstitial deletion. Am J Med Genet 1992;44:790.

131. Savanelli A, Orfeo L, Stabile M, et al. Prune belly appearance in a Turner subject. J Med Genet 1986;23:92.

132. Watanabe H, Yamanaka T. A possible relationship between Beckwith-Wiedemann syndrome, urinary tract anomaly and prune belly syndrome. Clin Genet 1990;38:410.

133. Knight JA, Palmer WM, Gardner AY, et al. Association of the Beckwith-Wiedemann and prune belly syndromes. Clin Pediatr 1980;19:485.

134. Greene C, Wilson A, Shapiro E. Prune belly syndrome and heart defect in one of monozygotic twins, following exposure to Tigan and Bendectin. Acta Genet Med Gemellol (Roma) 1985;34:101.

135. Aanpreung P, Beckwith B, Galansky SH, et al. Association of paucity of interlobular bile ducts with prune belly syndrome. J Pediatr Gastroenterol Nutr 1993;16:81.

136. Schmittenbecher PP, Endres W. Alpha 1-antitrypsin deficiency and prune-belly syndrome: first report of coincidence. Klin Wochenschr 1990;68:6.

137. Woodard JR. Prune-belly syndrome. In: Walsh PC, et al, eds. Campbell's urology. Philadelphia, WB Saunders, 1986:1851.

138. Manivel JC, Pettinato G, Reinberg Y, et al. Prune belly syndrome: clinicopathologic study of 29 cases. Pediatr Pathol 1989;9:691.

139. Lee BR, Partin AW, Epstein JI, et al. Quantitative histological analysis of collagen subtypes: primary obstructed and refluxing megaureters, ectopia, posterior urethral valves and prune belly syndrome. J Urol 1994;151:336.

140. Workman SJ, Kogan BA. Fetal bladder histology in posterior urethral valves and the prune belly syndrome. J Urol 1990;144:337.

141. Popek EJ, Tyson RW, Miller GJ, et al. Prostate development in prune belly syndrome (PBS) and posterior urethral valves (PUV): etiology of PBS—lower urinary tract obstruction or primary mesenchymal defect? Pediatr Pathol 1991;11:1.

142. Passerini GG, Araguna F, Chiozza L, et al. The P.A.D.U.A. (progressive augmentation by dilating the urethra anterior) procedure for the treatment of severe urethral hypoplasia. J Urol 1988;140:1247.

143. Mortensen PH, Johnson HW, Coleman GU, et al. Megalourethra. J Urol 1985;134:358.

144. Appel RA, Kaplan GW, Brock WA, et al. Megalourethra. J Urol 1986;135:747.

145. Burbige KA, Amodio J, Berdon WE, et al. Prune belly syndrome: 35 years of experience. J Urol 1987;137:86.

146. Uehling DT, Zadina SP, Gilbert E. Testicular histology in triad syndrome. Urology 1984;23:364.

147. Orvis BR, Bottles K, Kogan BA. Testicular histology in fetuses with the prune belly syndrome and posterior urethral valves. J Urol 1988;139:335.

148. Woodhouse CRJ, Ransley PG. Teratoma of the testis in the prune belly syndrome. Br J Urol 1983;55:580.

149. Sayre R, Stephens R, Chonko AM. Prune belly syndrome and retroperitoneal germ cell tumor. Am J Med 1986;81:895.

150. Massad CA, Cohen MB, Kogan BA, et al. Morphology and histochem-

istry of infant testes in the prune belly syndrome. J Urol 1991;146: 1598.

151. Docimo SG, Luetic T, Crone RK, et al. Pulmonary development in the fetal lamb with severe bladder outlet obstruction and oligohydramnios: a morphometric study. J Urol 1989;142:657.

152. Saur L, Harrison MR, Flake AW, et al. Does an expanding fetal abdominal mass produce pulmonary hypoplasia? J Pediatr Surg 1987; 22:508.

153. Geary DF, MacLusky IB, Churchill BM, et al. A broader spectrum of abnormalities in the prune belly syndrome. J Urol 1986;135:324.

154. Wright JJ, Barth RF, Neff JC, et al. Gastrointestinal malformations associated with prune belly syndrome: three cases and a review of the literature. (Review) Pediatr Pathol 1986;5:421.

155. Messing EM, Dibbell DG, Belzer FO. Bilateral rectus femoris pedicle flaps for detrusor augmentation in the prune belly syndrome. J Urol 1985;134:1202.

156. Genest DR, Driscoll SG, Bieber FR. Complexities of limb anomalies: the lower extremity in the ''prune belly'' phenotype. (Review) Teratology 1991;44:365.

157. Perez AA, Graham JM, Hersh JH, et al. Urethral obstruction sequence and lower limb deficiency: evidence for the vascular disruption hypothesis. J Pediatr 1993;123:398.

158. Loder RT, Dayioglu MM. Association of congenital vertebral malformations with bladder and cloacal exstrophy. J Pediatr Orthop 1990; 10:389.

159. Shimizu T, Ihara Y, Yomura W, et al. Antenatal diagnosis of prune belly syndrome. Arch Gynecol Obstet 1992;251:211.

160. Fitzsimons RB, Keohane C, Galvin J. Prune belly syndrome with ultrasound demonstration of reduction of megacystis in utero. Br J Radiol 1985;58:374.

161. Fisk NM, Dhillon HK, Ellis CE, et al. Antenatal diagnosis of megalourethra in a fetus with the prune belly syndrome. J Clin Ultrasound 1990;18:124.

162. Benacerraf BR, Saltzman DH, Mandell J. Sonographic diagnosis of abnormal fetal genitalia. J Ultrasound Med 1989;8:613.

163. Hunter GJ, Gordon I, Sweeney L, et al. 99mTc DTPA scanning with diuretic washout: is it useful in the investigation of obstruction in the presence of gross renal tract dilatation? Br J Urol 1987;59:208.

164. Duckett JW. The prune-belly syndrome. In: Kelalis PP, King LR, Belman AB, eds. Clinical pediatric urology. Philadelphia, WB Saunders, 1976:615.

165. Snyder HM, Harrison NW, Whitfield HN, et al. Urodynamics in the prune belly syndrome. Br J Urol 1976;48:663.

166. Perlmutter AD. Reduction cystoplasty in prune belly syndrome. J Urol 1976;116:356.

167. Kinahan TJ, Churchill BM, McLorie GA, et al. The efficiency of bladder emptying in the prune belly syndrome. J Urol 1992;148:600.

168. Fallat ME, Skoog SJ, Belman AB, et al. The prune belly syndrome: a comprehensive approach to management. J Urol 1989;142:802.

169. Boddy SA, Gordon AC, Thomas DF, et al. Experience with the Fowler Stephens and microvascular procedures in the management of intraabdominal testes. Br J Urol 1991;68:199.

170. Parrott TS, Woodard JR. The Monfort operation for abdominal wall reconstruction in the prune belly syndrome. J Urol 1992;148:688.

171. Ehrlich RM, Lesavoy MA, Fine RN. Total abdominal wall reconstruction in the prune belly syndrome. J Urol 1986;136:282.

172. Monfort G, Guys JM, Bocciardi A, et al. A novel technique for reconstruction of the abdominal wall in the prune belly syndrome. J Urol 1991;146:639.

173. Ehrlich RM, Lesavoy MA. Umbilicus preservation with total abdominal wall reconstruction in prune-belly syndrome. Urology 1993;41: 231.

174. Randolph J, Cavett C, Eng G. Abdominal wall reconstruction in the prune belly syndrome. J Pediatr Surg 1981;16:960.

175. Reinberg Y, Manivel JC, Pettinato G, et al. Development of renal failure in children with the prune belly syndrome. J Urol 1991;145: 1017.

176. Reinberg Y, Manivel JC, Fryd D, et al. The outcome of renal transplantation in children with the prune belly syndrome. J Urol 1989; 142:1541.

177. Woodhouse CR, Snyder H. Testicular and sexual function in adults with prune belly syndrome. J Urol 1985;133:607.

SECTION D

Intestine

Surgery of Infants and Children: Scientific Principles and Practice, edited by
Keith T. Oldham, Paul M. Colombani, and Robert P. Foglia.
Lippincott–Raven Publishers, Philadelphia, © 1997.

CHAPTER 67

Gastrointestinal Bleeding

Michael G. Caty and Richard G. Azizkhan

Gastrointestinal (GI) hemorrhage is an alarming situation for both parent and surgeon. Fortunately, GI bleeding in most children is due to benign causes and is usually self-limited (Table 67-1). Nevertheless, an aggressive diagnostic approach to the child with significant bleeding is warranted. A logical diagnostic approach based on the frequency of age-related causes of bleeding usually results in the establishment of a cause for the bleeding.

INITIAL APPROACH AND RESUSCITATION

The initial steps in the evaluation of the child with GI bleeding are to identify the source as upper or lower, assess the magnitude of the bleeding, and initiate resuscitation of the child.

Upper GI hemorrhage is defined as bleeding that originates proximal to the ligament of Treitz. This is manifested by either hematemesis, melena, or occult blood loss. Lower GI hemorrhage may present with hematochezia, melena, or occult blood loss. Elements of the patient's history that suggest an upper GI source include preexisting liver disease, recent surgical stress, and family history of ulcer disease. A recent diarrheal illness, history of weight loss with abdominal pain, or family history of polyps or colon resections may suggest a lower source of GI bleeding. The initial diagnostic maneuver is to place a nasogastric tube. The absence of blood in the presence of aspirated bile rules out an upper GI source with reasonable certainty. If blood is detected, the nasogastric tube allows lavage of the stomach to assess the rate of bleeding. It also removes blood that would impair endoscopic evaluation.

To direct the diagnostic evaluation and guide the resuscitation, an estimate of the rate of bleeding must be made. An initial impression can be formed from observation of the volume of blood from the nasogastric tube or amount of melenic stool. The most important information comes from the physiologic status of the infant or child. Children tolerate blood loss of less than 10% of blood volume (8 mL/kg) extremely well and may demonstrate only minimal elevation of the pulse rate. Increasing heart rate and the presence of orthostatic hypotension suggest a 10% to 20% loss. The findings of hypotension and poor capillary refill are associated with blood loss in excess of 30% of blood volume. Patients with greater than 10% blood loss should be monitored in an intensive care unit.

The intensity of the resuscitation of the child with GI hemorrhage conforms to the magnitude of the bleeding. A history of the bleeding is obtained and the location and magnitude estimated. A history of medications that affect the coagulation system is elicited. A complete blood count, platelet count, liver function tests, and coagulation studies are obtained. A nasogastric tube is placed. The child with significant GI bleeding should have two large-bore intravenous cannulas inserted, blood type and cross-match obtained, and a urinary catheter placed.

Intravenous resuscitation is accomplished with normal saline or lactated Ringers solution. In addition to a maintenance rate of fluid, boluses of 20 mL/kg are given. A positive response to resuscitation includes improved capillary refill, decreased heart rate, and increased urine output. The decision to transfuse is multifactorial. Patients with inadequate response to crystalloid resuscitation and ongoing bleeding should be transfused. Earlier consideration for transfusion should be made in patients with preexisting heart or lung disease. The hematocrit can be a misleading indicator of early blood loss owing to failure of equilibration. A normal hematocrit in the presence of ongoing bleeding should not prevent blood transfusion. In the presence of ongoing bleeding, several units of packed red blood cells should be immediately available for transfusion.

After the initial approach and resuscitation, the management plan shifts to that of diagnosis and treatment. A discussion of organ-specific sources of GI bleeding is followed by an age-related approach to the diagnostic evaluation of children with upper and lower GI hemorrhage.

SOURCES OF UPPER GASTROINTESTINAL BLEEDING

Anatomic sources of upper GI hemorrhage are discussed in terms of their pathophysiology and treatment. Topics are abbreviated if they are addressed elsewhere in the text.

Esophagitis

Esophagitis is a rare cause of hematemesis. It usually occurs in infancy as a result of gastroesophageal reflux. Although bi-

TABLE 67-1. *Typical causes of gastrointestinal hemorrhage in children*

UPPER GI TRACT

NEWBORN
Gastritis
Swallowed maternal blood

INFANT
Gastritis
Esophagitis
Peptic ulcer disease

PRESCHOOL AGE
Gastritis
Esophagitis
Peptic ulcer disease
Esophageal varices

SCHOOLAGE AND ADOLESCENT
Esophageal varices
Peptic ulcer disease

LOWER GI TRACT

NEWBORN
Necrotizing enterocolitis
Malrotation with midgut volvulus
Anal fissure
Hirschsprung disease with enterocolitis

INFANT
Anal fissure
Allergic proctocolitis
Intussusception
Meckel diverticulum
Lymphonodular hyperplasia
Intestinal duplication

PRESCHOOL AGE
Juvenile polyps
Lymphonodular hyperplasia
Meckel diverticulum
Hemolytic uremic syndrome
Henoch-Schönlein purpura
Infectious colitis

SCHOOLAGE AND ADOLESCENT
Inflammatory bowel disease
Infectious colitis
Juvenile polyps

opsy-proven esophagitis is present in 61% to 83% of patients, clinically apparent bleeding is unusual.[1] Esophagitis usually causes occult blood loss and anemia. Acute bleeding from esophagitis is treated with nasogastric decompression, histamine-2 (H_2) antagonists or oral antacids, and positional therapy. If nonoperative therapy is successful, reflux is documented, and medical management is instituted. If medical management does not control reflux, an antireflux operation is performed. Severity of esophagitis has not been shown to correlate with the need for antireflux surgery.[2]

Esophageal Varices

Variceal hemorrhage is an important cause of upper GI hemorrhage in children and adolescents. Most children with portal hypertension and variceal hemorrhage present before 5 years of age. Portal hypertension in children usually results from either extrahepatic or intrahepatic causes. Among the known causes of extrahepatic portal hypertension are neonatal omphalitis and umbilical vein catheterization. Intrahepatic portal hypertension commonly results from cirrhosis secondary to biliary atresia. Nonoperative management includes endoscopic variceal ligation or injection, placement of a Sengkstaken-Blakemore tube, and use of intravenous vasopressin. Operative management includes shunts, variceal ligation, esophageal division, and esophageal devascularization.

Stress Ulceration and Gastritis

Gastritis may be defined as primary or secondary. Primary gastritis in children is most often due to *Helicobacter pylori* infection. This rarely results in symptomatic gastritis.[3] Its importance lies in its relation to the cause of peptic ulcer disease in children. Secondary gastritis resulting in GI hemorrhage usually occurs secondary to stress ulceration of the stomach. Premature infants and children sustaining trauma, burns, or serious medical illnesses are at risk. The pathophysiology of stress ulceration of the stomach is not fully defined. Important concepts include loss of mucosal barrier function, alterations in gastric microcirculation, back diffusion of hydrogen ions, and duodenogastric bile reflux. Neonates and children present with either "coffee-ground" emesis or hematemesis. Children with significant ongoing bleeding should undergo endoscopy. Initial nonoperative management includes transfusion, correction of any coagulopathy, and the use of antacids, H_2-antagonists, or sucralfate. If correctable causes of stress exist, such as burn wound infection or intraabdominal abscess, they should be treated concurrently. If initial management does not succeed, operative exploration should be performed.

Preoperative endoscopy can identify bleeding sites in the stomach in most patients. The presence or absence of associated duodenal bleeding from either duodenitis or peptic ulcer disease should be established. In the absence of duodenal bleeding, a gastrotomy should be performed and the walls of the stomach inspected. Attempts to do the least ablative surgery should be made. If possible, superficial erosions should be oversewn. Focal ulcers or isolated areas of bleeding can be resected locally or with a standard partial gastrectomy, but this is rarely necessary. Problems arise in patients with life-threatening hemorrhage from all surfaces of the gastric wall. Gastric devascularization has been used successfully to treat this condition.[4] If this fails to stop the bleeding, total gastrectomy remains the only option. It is difficult to identify the appropriate application of vagotomy in these situations, but it can be recommended in children with associated duodenal disease. Having discussed the operative management of the child with stress gastritis, it is important to emphasize the importance of prophylaxis. Stressed children should have aggressive attempts to raise their gastric pH to above 4.5 with either H_2-antagonists or antacids.

Peptic Ulcer Disease

Peptic ulcer disease can afflict children in all age groups. The capacity of the stomach to produce acid is present in the premature and full-term newborn infant.[5] About half of children with acute ulcers present with GI hemorrhage. Fortunately, this bleeding is usually not life-threatening. Endoscopy accurately diagnoses the location of the ulcer. Endoscopic techniques, such as heater probe coagulation or bipolar cautery, may be used to arrest the bleeding focus. If this does not stop the bleeding, an operation is necessary. Standard therapy includes exposure of the ulcer and three-point suture ligation of the ulcer bed. Ligation of the gastroduodenal artery may be beneficial. Vagotomy and a drainage procedure do not appear necessary for acute bleeding ulcers in children. After successful medical or surgical management, children are placed on an H_2-antagonist for 3 to 6 months. The Zollinger-Ellison syndrome should be considered in any child with multiple ulcers or recurrent ulcers. Serum gastrin levels are obtained to rule out this syndrome.

SOURCES OF LOWER GASTROINTESTINAL BLEEDING

Common causes of lower GI hemorrhage are discussed in terms of their pathophysiology and treatment.

Meckel Diverticulum

Lower GI hemorrhage is a common complication of a Meckel diverticulum. Most children affected are younger than 5 years of age.[6] Bleeding results from ulceration of adjacent ileal mucosa by heterotopic gastric mucosa contained in the diverticulum. Bleeding is usually painless. The diagnostic test of choice is a technetium-99m pertechnetate scan (Fig. 67-1). Uptake of the isotope by the heterotopic mucosa allows identification of the bleeding source. The technetium scan is 75% to 85% sensitive for a Meckel diverticulum presenting with hemorrhage. Administration of cimetidine or pentagastrin may increase the diagnostic yield of the scan. Nonbleeding Meckel diverticula can also be diagnosed by visceral angiography.[7] After the child is stabilized, the diverticulum is excised. Care is taken to assess the adjacent ileum for the presence of an ulcer that may need to be resected with the diverticulum. Some diverticula may be amenable to laparoscopic excision.

Intestinal Polyps

Juvenile Polyps

Bleeding from juvenile polyps usually occurs in preschoolage children. These polyps, also known as *hamartomatous* or *retention polyps,* are benign. Bleeding originates from the friable surface of the polyps (Fig. 67-2). The cause of these polyps is unknown. The presence of interstitial eosinophils raises the

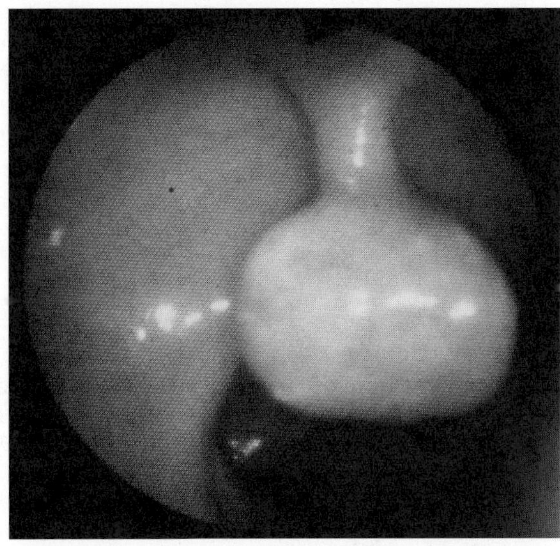

FIG. 67-2. Pedunculated juvenile polyp. (Courtesy of Dr. Thomas Rossi, Children's Hospital of Buffalo)

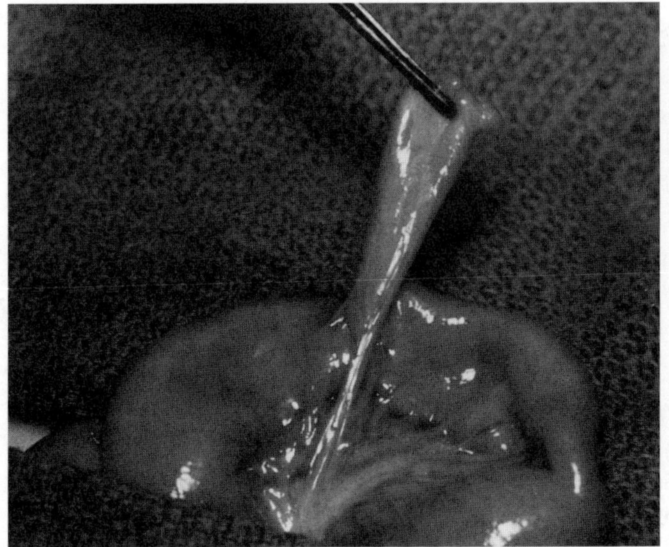

A

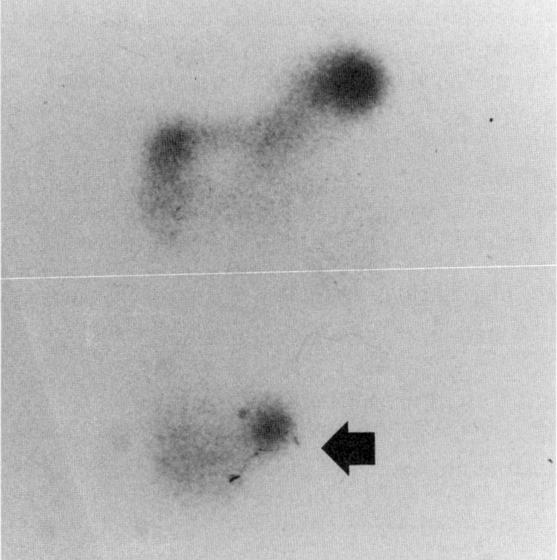

B

FIG. 67-1. (*A*) Meckel diverticulum. (*B*) Technetium scan positive for bleeding Meckel diverticulum (*arrow*).

possibility of an allergic reaction of the colonic mucosa. Past evidence suggested that most of these lesions were confined to the rectosigmoid colon. Recent application of colonoscopy to children has revealed that most juvenile polyps are located proximal to the transverse colon.[8] Colonoscopy has also refuted the assumption that juvenile polyps are usually solitary. Treatment with colonoscopic polypectomy or transanal excision is curative.

Lymphoid Polyps

Lymphoid polyps result from lymphonodular hyperplasia of the colon. They are benign lesions that cause bleeding in infants and preschoolage children. Diagnosis can be made with either sigmoidoscopy or air contrast enema. Endoscopy reveals multiple small friable nodules scattered throughout the colon. Air contrast enema shows raised nodules with a characteristic central umbilication. This entity is thought to be due to an associated systemic illness. These lesions resolve spontaneously without treatment.

Anorectal Lesions

Anal fissures are a common cause of rectal bleeding in infants. Infants present with bright red blood on the outside of the stool or with blood in the diaper. Physical examination reveals a small tear at the anal verge. The fissure is often posterior. Fissures result from a superficial tear of the squamous lining of the anal canal during the passage of a firm stool. Bowel movements cause significant discomfort to the infant. Reluctance to defecate results in worsening constipation and increased pain with bowel movements. Treatment consists of breaking this vicious cycle by softening the stool and using warm Sitz baths. It is unusual for breastfed infants to have anal fissures. Anal fissures may also be a presentation of child abuse. This should be suspected in patients with multiple fissures, perianal condylomata, or other indications of perineal trauma.

Other, less common entities in the anorectum may cause lower GI bleeding. Anorectal varices result from portal hypertension in children and are rarely symptomatic. Treatment includes sclerotherapy, banding, embolization, and portosystemic shunting.

The solitary rectal ulcer syndrome may also cause bleeding in children. Ulceration is thought to be due to either ischemia or degeneration of a rectal polyp. Treatment is conservative and consists of observation and laxative administration.[9]

Heterotopic gastric mucosa in the colon or rectum can also cause bleeding. Lesions are identified by either endoscopy or technetium scan. Treatment consists of local excision.

Intestinal Vascular Malformations

Vascular malformations of the intestine are rare lesions that can involve any part of the alimentary tract. Hemorrhage may be slow and chronic, or massive. Lesions may be associated with the Klippel-Trenaunay or Rendu-Osler-Weber syndrome. Endoscopy can identify vascular malformations in the colon and stomach. Endoscopy may not identify lesions during massive hemorrhage. Radionuclide scanning, selective angiography, or both are useful in this instance. Preoperative localization allows directed resections of prepared bowel. Endoscopic laser ablation has been described as an excellent method of palliation of anorectal lesions.[10]

Miscellaneous Causes of Lower Gastrointestinal Bleeding

Malrotation with midgut volvulus may cause lower GI hemorrhage. This results from mucosal injury secondary to ischemia of the volvulized bowel. This diagnosis must be considered in the newborn with bilious emesis or abdominal distention. An upper GI series identifies the location of the ligament of Treitz and establishes the diagnosis. The child is immediately operated on and the bowel untwisted. Nonviable bowel is resected. The operation concludes with a lysis of Ladd bands and an appendectomy.

The premature infant who has rectal bleeding is evaluated for necrotizing enterocolitis (NEC). Bleeding indicates mucosal ischemia. Findings supportive of the diagnosis of NEC include pneumatosis intestinalis or pneumoperitoneum on abdominal radiograph, abdominal wall erythema, and thrombocytopenia. Initial management includes nasogastric decompression, administration of broad-spectrum antibiotics, and fluid resuscitation. Operation is reserved for patients with pneumoperitoneum or clinical deterioration. Although the stomach is rarely involved in NEC, heme-positive nasogastric aspirates may alert the clinician to the diagnosis in the at-risk newborn.

Intestinal duplications can occur in any part of the intestine along its length from mouth to anus. Among the many complications they cause is bleeding. Because most duplications are located in the ileum, bleeding complications usually result in lower GI hemorrhage. Duplications cause bleeding by one of three mechanisms: (1) the presence of heterotopic gastric mucosa in a duplication can result in local peptic ulceration, (2) necrosis and bleeding of the bowel wall can result from expansion of a duplication, and (3) a duplication can serve as an intussusceptum and cause bleeding from pressure necrosis of the intestine. Duplications containing heterotopic gastric tissue can be diagnosed with a technetium scan. Detection of an abdominal mass in a patient with lower GI hemorrhage should raise the suspicion of a duplication. Surgical excision of the duplication is curative.

Intussusception occurs in infants and young children. Rectal bleeding occurs frequently and is described as ''currant jelly.'' This bleeding is rarely hemodynamically significant; its importance relates to helping recognize the diagnosis of intussusception in the infant with crampy abdominal pain.

Invasive bacteria, such as *Salmonella*, *Shigella*, and *Campylobacter* sp and *Escherichia coli* can cause colitis presenting with hematochezia. A history of vomiting and diarrhea suggests this cause. Stool cultures and the presence of fecal leukocytes confirm it.

Viral infection from cytomegalovirus can cause life-threatening lower GI hemorrhage. Affected children usually have acquired immunodeficiency syndrome. Multiple, deep mucosal ulcerations of the colon and small intestine are the source of the bleeding. Bleeding can be localized by arteriography or colonoscopy. This entity is often fatal.

Allergic proctocolitis is a common cause of hematochezia in young infants. It results from an allergic response to exposure to cow milk, soy milk, or breast milk. Diagnosis is made on clinical grounds after serious illnesses, such as infectious diarrhea and Hirschsprung disease, have been ruled out. The implicated formula is stopped and an alternative formula used. Reinstitution of the previous formula should result in a similar symptom complex. Most cow milk and soy milk allergies resolve by 2 years of age.

Lower GI bleeding may also result from acquired bleeding disorders. The hemolytic uremic syndrome is characterized by fever, hemolytic anemia, and renal dysfunction. Lower GI hemorrhage can result from small vessel occlusion and mucosal ischemia of all segments of the intestine. Henoch-Schönlein purpura causes a diffuse vasculitis that often involves the intestine. Bloody stools result from diffuse mucosal hemorrhage. Intussusception associated with Henoch-Schönlein purpura can also cause GI hemorrhage.

AGE-RELATED APPROACH TO THE DIAGNOSIS OF GASTROINTESTINAL BLEEDING IN CHILDREN

The age at which a child with GI bleeding presents defines the differential diagnosis and guides the diagnostic approach. Age-related approaches to the work-up of GI hemorrhage are discussed. For the sake of simplicity, newborns and infants are considered together, as are preschoolage children, schoolage children, and adolescents. Algorithms outlining these approaches are presented below.

Upper Gastrointestinal Bleeding in Newborns and Infants

Newborns and infants with upper GI hemorrhage present with hematemesis or heme-positive nasogastric aspirates (Fig. 67-3). A hospitalized newborn or infant usually has stress gastritis or ulcer disease as a cause of the bleeding. A nasogastric tube is passed and the stomach lavaged. If the blood clears with irrigation, the nasogastric tube is placed on suction, and the patient is observed. In stressed newborns and infants, intravenous cimetidine or ranitidine is administered, and a blood type and screen is sent for analysis. Failure to clear continued bleeding warrants upper endoscopy for diagnosis. Endoscopy may not be possible in extremely premature infants, but in rare instances, an ultrathin bronchoscope may be used for diagnostic esophagogastroduodenoscopy. If this is unsuccessful, laparotomy serves as the diagnostic procedure. Patients with bleeding that fills the stomach and prevents endoscopic diagnosis and patients that are unstable should also undergo laparotomy. At laparotomy, the stomach and duodenum are inspected. The absence of pathology in the stomach or duodenum warrants examination of the esophagus and gastroesophageal junction for esophagitis or a Mallory-Weiss tear. The full-term infant with hematemesis on the first day of life should be suspected of having swallowed maternal blood. This can be confirmed with the Apt test. This is performed by adding sodium hydroxide to the observed blood. Fetal blood remains pink, while adult blood turns brown.[11] All newborns with bleeding must be considered to have vitamin K deficiency, and 1 mg of vitamin K is administered intramuscularly if indicated.

Upper Gastrointestinal Bleeding in Children and Adolescents

Children and adolescents with upper GI hemorrhage may present with hematemesis or heme-positive nasogastric aspirates. Older children may also demonstrate massive rectal bleeding or melena as a manifestation of upper GI hemorrhage (Fig. 67-4). The history and physical examination contribute important clues to the cause of the bleeding in this age group. The presence of von Willebrand disease and hemophilia should be sought. A history of placement of an umbilical vein catheter,

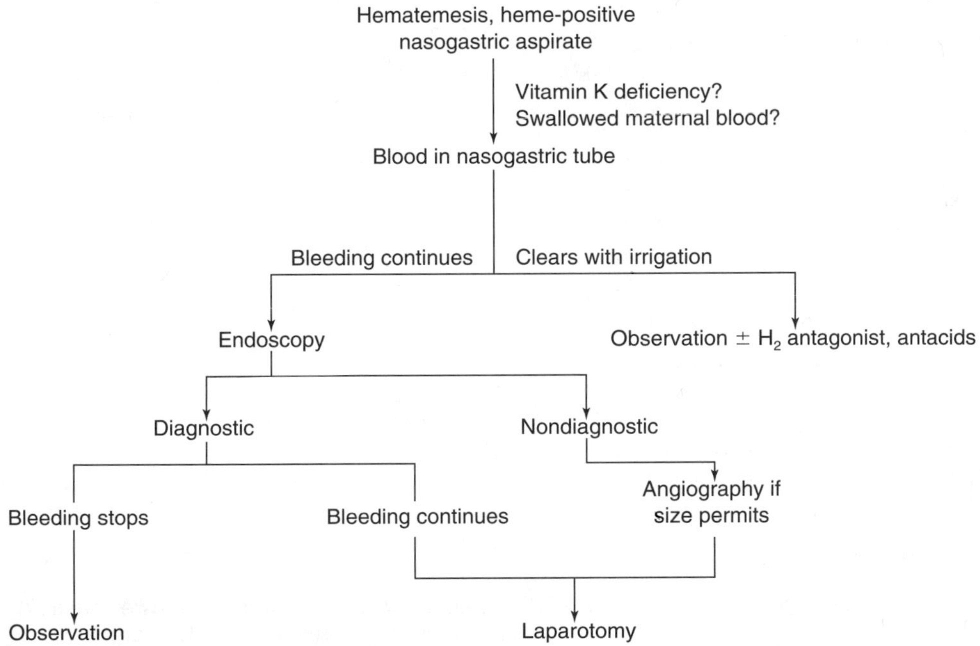

FIG. 67-3. Diagnostic approach to upper gastrointestinal hemorrhage in infants and children.

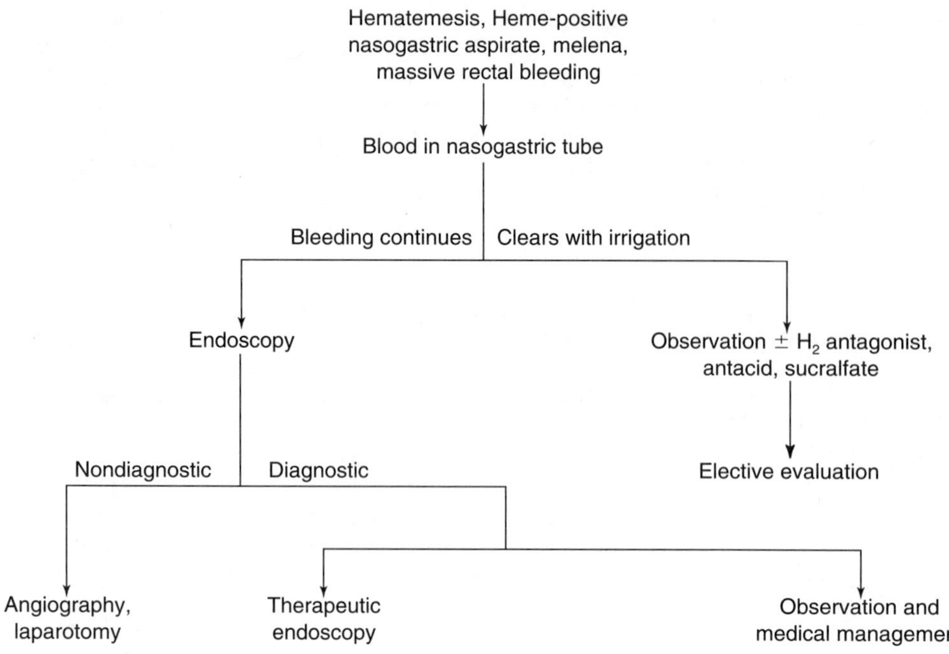

FIG. 67-4. Diagnostic approach to upper gastrointestinal hemorrhage in children and adolescents.

omphalitis, or biliary atresia suggests esophageal varices as a cause. A family history of ulcer disease should be sought. A nasogastric tube is placed, confirming the location of the bleeding and estimating its magnitude. Prompt clearing of the blood merits observation and elective evaluation with endoscopy or an upper GI series. Continued bleeding warrants immediate endoscopy. In these age groups, therapeutic endoscopy should be performed at the initial examination. This should include injection or banding of varices and heater probe or cautery treatment of bleeding ulcers. Laparotomy should be reserved for patients with ongoing bleeding despite therapeutic endoscopy, life-threatening hemorrhage at presentation, or recurrent bleeding.

Lower Gastrointestinal Bleeding in Newborns and Infants

The newborn infant with rectal bleeding should have an upper GI source ruled out by passage of a nasogastric tube. The clinical situation in which the bleeding occurs suggests the diagnosis (Fig. 67-5). The premature infant must be suspected of having NEC. The newborn or infant with bilious emesis must have malrotation ruled out. Intussusception is considered in the older infant with associated crampy abdominal pain. Inspection of the anal area confirms the diagnosis of an anal fissure. Abdominal radiographs help to evaluate for Hirschsprung disease, malrotation, NEC, and intussusception. The infant with significant

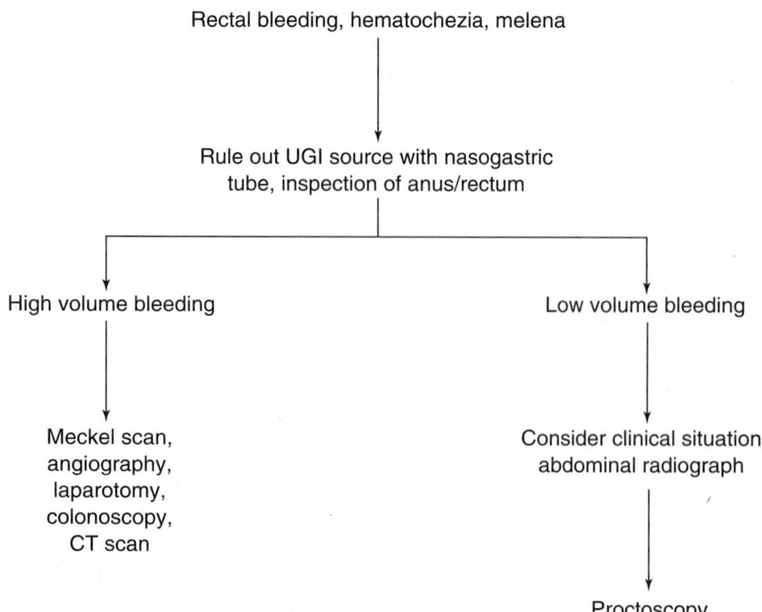

FIG. 67-5. Diagnostic approach to lower gastrointestinal hemorrhage in infants and children.

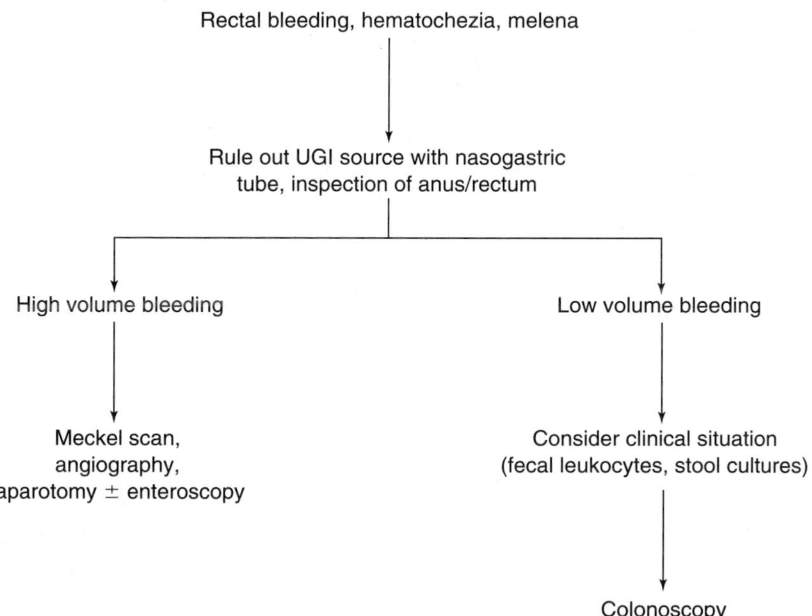

FIG. 67-6. Diagnostic approach to lower gastrointestinal hemorrhage in children and adolescents.

hematochezia should undergo a technetium scan. If this scan is negative, it should be repeated with administration of cimetidine or pentagastrin. If this is again negative, a computed tomographic scan can be performed to evaluate for a duplication. Alternatively, in the presence of significant bleeding, an angiogram can be performed to evaluate for a duplication, vascular malformation, or Meckel diverticulum not detected by nuclear medicine scan. Patients thought to have allergic proctocolitis by history can have this diagnosis confirmed by proctoscopy and biopsy.

Lower Gastrointestinal Bleeding in Children and Adolescents

The evaluation of the child or adolescent with rectal bleeding begins with a thorough history and physical examination (Fig. 67-6). The presence of associated symptoms, such as diarrhea and vomiting, should be ascertained. A family history of inflammatory bowel disease or familial polyposis should be sought. Stool should be inspected for fecal leukocytes and cultures sent when infection is suspected.

Patients with significant bleeding should undergo a technetium scan. If this does not prove diagnostic, colonoscopy should be performed to evaluate for polyps, infectious colitis, and inflammatory bowel disease. If the inflammatory bowel disease is restricted to the small bowel, an upper GI series with small bowel follow-through may be necessary to make the diagnosis. Colonoscopy may not be effective with massive bleeding, and

angiography may be necessary. Angiography can potentially identify bleeding from vascular malformations, Meckel diverticula, and intestinal duplications.

REFERENCES

1. Shub MD, Ulshen MH, Hargrove CB, et al. Esophagitis: a frequent consequence of gastroesophageal reflux in infancy. J Pediatr 1985;12:881.
2. Black DD, Haggitt RC, Orenstein SR, et al. Esophagitis in infants: morphometric histological diagnosis and correlation with measures of gastroesophageal reflux. Gastroenterology 1990;98:1408.
3. Drumm B. Helicobacter pylori in the pediatric patient. Gastroenterol Clin North Am 1993;22:169.
4. Udassin R, Nissan S, Lernau OZ, et al. Gastric devascularization-An emergency treatment for hemorrhagic gastritis in the neonate. J Pediatr Surg 1983;18:579.
5. Brownlee KG, Kelly EJ. When is the fetus first capable of gastric acid, intrinsic factor and gastrin secretion? Biol Neonate 1993;63:153.
6. St-Vil D, Brandt ML, Panic S, et al. Meckel's diverticulum in children: a 20-year review. J Pediatr Surg 1991;25:1289.
7. Routh WD, Lawdahl RB, Lund E, et al. Meckel's diverticula: angiographic diagnosis in patients with non-acute hemorrhage and negative scintigraphy. Pediatr Radiol 1990;20:152.
8. Steffen RM, Wyllie R, Sivak MV, et al. Colonoscopy in the pediatric patient. J Pediatr 1989;115:507.
9. De la Rubia L, Ruiz Villaespesa, Cebrero M, et al. Solitary rectal ulcer syndrome in a child. J Pediatr 1992;122:533.
10. Azizkhan RG. Life-threatening hematochezia from a rectosigmoid vascular malformation in Klippel-Trenaunay syndrome: long term palliation using an argon laser. J Pediatr Surg 1991;26:1125.
11. Apt L, Downey WS. ''Melena'' neonatorum: The swallowed blood syndrome. J Pediatr 1955;46:6.

Surgery of Infants and Children: Scientific Principles and Practice, edited by
Keith T. Oldham, Paul M. Colombani, and Robert P. Foglia.
Lippincott–Raven Publishers, Philadelphia, © 1997.

CHAPTER 68

Stomach and Duodenum

David K. Magnuson and Marshall Z. Schwartz

Congenital anomalies and acquired abnormalities of the stomach and duodenum are common problems in children. The proper management of these abnormalities, many unique to infants and children, requires an understanding of the anatomy and physiology of the proximal gastrointestinal (GI) tract. The stomach is a complex organ with two distinct physiologic functions: a secretory function effected by the cells of the epithelial lining, and a storage, mixing, and propulsive function effected by the three muscular layers of the gastric wall. These functions are regulated by a complex variety of stimulatory and inhibitory feedback mechanisms that employ neurocrine, endocrine, and paracrine components. The duodenum produces a large number of peptides, many with unknown physiologic roles, and contains the structures that convey bile and pancreatic secretions to the intestinal lumen for mixing with the gastric effluent. Although anatomically, histologically, and functionally distinct, the stomach and duodenum are often considered together because of their proximity and their many interrelated physiologic properties and pathophysiologic responses to disease and stress. This chapter reviews the developmental anatomy of the stomach and duodenum, examines the physiology and pathophysiology of gastric secretory and motor activity, and discusses the treatment of both congenital and acquired gastroduodenal abnormalities in children.

ANATOMY AND PHYSIOLOGY

Developmental Gross Anatomy

The primordial digestive tube forms from the lateral and craniocaudad folding of the embryo during gestational weeks 3 and 4. During this process, the germinal endodermal layer forms the interior of the tube and is surrounded by splanchnic mesoderm. Differentiation of endodermal precursors into surface and glandular epithelium, and of mesodermal precursors into smooth muscle and peritoneal attachments, occurs over the next 6 to 8 weeks. Development of the specialized neuroendocrine cell population of the stomach occurs at about the same time.

Grossly, the stomach begins as a dilation of the foregut, which occurs at about 5 weeks' gestation. Both the stomach and duodenum are suspended between the posterior and anterior

body walls by a dorsal and ventral mesentery. During gestational weeks 6 to 10, the stomach undergoes rotation in two planes. A 90-degree rotation occurs around the longitudinal axis in the clockwise direction when viewed from a craniocaudad perspective, and a lessor rotation around the anteroposterior axis occurs in a clockwise fashion when viewed from the front. Differential growth of the ventral wall of the stomach occurs concurrently. These processes result in the following developmental relations: the greater curvature of the stomach migrates inferiorly and to the left of midline; the gastroesophageal junction is placed superior and to the left; the pylorus moves inferiorly and to the right of midline; the dorsal mesogastrium becomes the gastrosplenic ligament and greater omentum and forms the anatomic boundary of the lessor sac; and the ventral mesogastrium becomes the gastrohepatic ligament. Rotation of the vagal trunks results in the left vagus innervating the anterior gastric wall and liver, and in the right vagus innervating the posterior gastric wall, small intestine, and retroperitoneum.

The shape of the stomach and the various epithelial cell types that constitute its mucosal lining create several histologically and functionally distinct zones: the cardia, which surrounds the gastroesophageal junction; the fundus, which projects cephalad from the gastroesophageal junction; the corpus, or body, which represents the largest portion of the gastric reservoir; and the antrum, which describes that portion of the stomach immediately preceding the pylorus (Fig. 68-1). The outer longitudinal and intermediate circular muscle layers (which are concentrated on the greater and lesser curvatures), and the inner oblique layer (concentrated over the anterior and posterior surfaces) compose the three muscular layers of the gastric wall. The gastric wall in the neonate is extremely thin initially but grows rapidly in the postnatal period in response to the propulsive work associated with enteral feeding.

The gastric blood supply is redundant and derived principally from branches of the celiac axis. The left gastric artery supplies the cardia and proximal lesser curvature; the splenic artery gives off short gastric arteries to the fundus, and the left gastroepiploic artery to the proximal greater curvature; the common hepatic artery gives off both the gastroduodenal artery, from which derives the right gastroepiploic artery to the distal greater curvature, and the right gastric artery to the pylorus and distal lesser curvature. Venous return is to the portal vein through the splenic, left gastric (coronary), and superior mesenteric veins.

1133

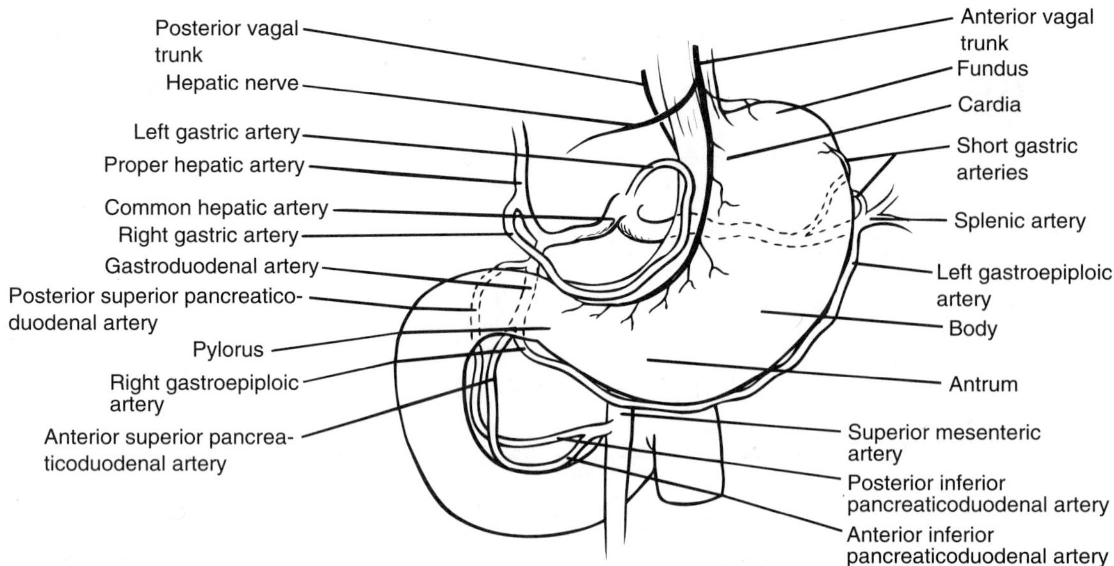

FIG. 68-1. Gross anatomy of the stomach and duodenum.

The duodenum occupies a section of the primitive digestive tube that spans the transition from foregut to midgut. The foregut is proximal to the liver bud and subserved by branches of the celiac trunk, while the midgut is distal to the liver bud and subserved by the superior mesenteric artery. The duodenum also undergoes a rotational process. The proximal duodenum is drawn superiorly and to the right during anteroposterior rotation of the stomach, while the distal duodenum is drawn leftward by the counterclockwise rotation of the midgut as it returns to the abdomen from the umbilical stalk. The net result of these movements is the C-loop configuration of the normal duodenum. Superimposed on these rotational events is a shortening of the dorsal mesoduodenum, which fixes the duodenum in a retroperitoneal location.

During the 6th to 10th weeks of gestation, the proximal duodenum (along with the esophagus and rectum) undergoes a process of rapid epithelial proliferation that obliterates the hollow lumen, converting the duodenum into a solid, cordlike structure. Vacuoles appear in this homogenous epithelial interior after 8 weeks' gestation, and gradual recanalization occurs as these vacuoles coalesce into larger cavities. The distal duodenum is thought not to pass through a solid phase.

The duodenum is divided into four portions corresponding to the curvatures of the C loop. A consistent landmark is the ampulla of Vater, which is located medially in the second portion and represents the confluence of the common bile and pancreatic ducts and their entry into the duodenum. The duodenal blood supply is derived from the celiac axis through superior pancreaticoduodenal branches of the gastroduodenal artery, and the superior mesenteric artery through inferior pancreaticoduodenal branches. Venous drainage is through corresponding branches to the portal vein.

During this same period, the pancreas develops from separate dorsal and ventral anlagen. The ventral anlage arises to the right of midline, and as the intestinal tract undergoes rotation, this structure also rotates posterior to the duodenum and fuses with the dorsal anlage to the left of the duodenal C loop. The two separate ductal systems fuse, forming the main pancreatic duct of Wirsung and a minor accessory duct of Santorini. Abnormalities of pancreatic migration and fusion result in ductal anomalies (pancreas divisum) and parenchymal anomalies (annular pancreas). The frequent coexistence of annular pancreas with congenital duodenal obstruction suggests that the anatomic development of these structures is closely interrelated.

Developmental Neuroanatomy

The stomach is richly innervated by all three components of the autonomic nervous system—sympathetic, parasympathetic, and enteric—although functionally the latter two predominate. Sympathetic fibers in which the postganglionic neurotransmitter is primarily norepinephrine are generally inhibitory to GI function, while parasympathetic pathways mediated by acetylcholine are generally stimulatory. In contrast, the enteric nervous system (ENS) is characterized by a wider variety of neurotransmitters, including dopamine, somatostatin, vasoactive intestinal peptide (VIP), gastrin-releasing peptide (GRP), cholecystokinin (CCK), and a wider variety of effector and regulatory functions. Many of the peptides used by the ENS as neurocrine mediators are also elaborated by enteroendocrine cells as endocrine and paracrine mediators.

The sympathetic and parasympathetic innervation of the stomach is well defined. Sympathetic (predominately adrenergic) innervation emanates from cell bodies within the thoracic spinal cord and extends through presynaptic sympathetic fibers in the greater splanchnic nerve to relay with postsynaptic neurons in the celiac ganglion, whose axonal fibers follow blood vessels into the gastroduodenal wall. This arrangement correlates well with the principal sympathetic function of vasomotor control. Sympathetic innervation of the muscular layers is sparse and is concentrated chiefly in the pyloric sphincter. Parasympathetic presynaptic efferent nerves originate in the brain stem and follow the vagus nerves to the stomach. Interestingly, efferent impulses constitute only about 20% of the total neural traffic in the vagus nerves. The entire gastric wall is richly innervated by terminal vagal fibers branching off the left (anterior) and right (posterior) vagal trunks as they give off their hepatic and celiac divisions, respectively. These presynaptic fibers synapse with intramural ganglia and also integrate at this level with ENS ganglion cells. Parasympathetic innervation mediates predominantly prosecretory and prokinetic functions.

The ENS is a peripheral compartment of the autonomic nervous system that comprises more than 10^8 resident neurons within the walls of the GI tract and their axons. It is distinguished from the sympathetic and parasympathetic systems by its anatomic separation from the central nervous system (CNS). It has long been recognized that the ENS functions more or less independently, but receives modulatory input from the central autonomic system, mostly by way of the vagus (parasympathetic) nerves. When one considers that the efferent fibers of the vagal trunks at the esophageal hiatus number only about 2000, it is clear that most of the ENS neurons receive stimulatory and inhibitory inputs from other ENS neurons.[1] Thus, the inherent myoelectric activity of GI smooth muscle is under both intrinsic (ENS) and extrinsic (CNS) control.

ENS precursors differentiate from neuroblasts located in the vagal area of the neural crest and migrate in the embryonic phase with the vagus nerve to the developing stomach and GI tract. Once incorporated into the gastric wall, these ENS neurons further differentiate, proliferate, and establish connections to each other, to other autonomic pathways, and to developing gastric secretory and muscle cells. Although the migrating precursors transiently express immunoreactivity for catecholamines, once established within the gastric wall, they no longer express catecholamines. ENS plexuses are found within virtually every histologic layer of the stomach, integrating with ganglia found in the mucosa, the intermyenteric plane, and the subserosa.

Developmental Histology of the Gastric and Duodenal Epithelium

The gastric epithelium is an aggregation of diverse cell populations that are distributed in a regionally specialized manner and that account for the various well-regulated secretory functions of the stomach. Seen from the luminal surface, the gastric mucosa is a monotonous sheet of mucus-secreting columnar epithelial cells riddled with tiny openings referred to as *gastric pits*. At the base of these pits are the gastric glands, which are specialized tubular invaginations of the mucosa that contain the effector and regulator cells of gastric secretion (Fig. 68-2). Gastric glands are composed of different cell populations in various regions of the stomach, allowing the stomach to be compartmentalized by histologic and functional characteristics.

Primitive mucosal pits are first seen between gestational weeks 6 and 9. The underlying glands form by the dichotomous branching of an initial invagination beginning during weeks 11 to 13. By weeks 20 to 25, each pit opens into a group of as many as seven glands, which have become greatly elongated and convoluted. Although major differences in cellular composition exist, all gastric glands tend to have a similar morphologic pattern. There is a surface zone that includes the pit and that connects the gastric lumen to the underlying gland. This zone

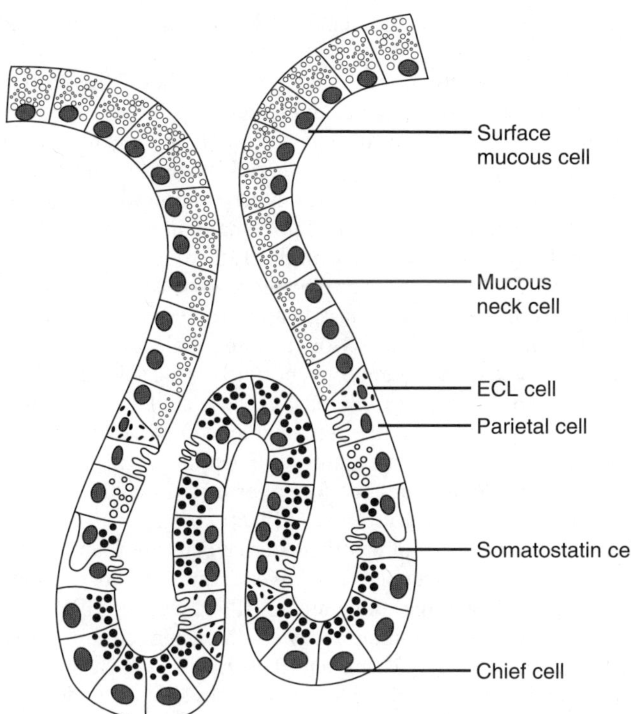

FIG. 68-2. Representative histology of an oxyntic gastric gland from the parietal cell region. ECL, enterochromaffin-like.

leads to a narrow isthmus, followed by a long, tubular neck, and finally the base. The location of a particular gland within the stomach dictates the specific type and density of cells in each of these zones and therefore determines the functional role of the gland.

The cells that occupy the surface zone throughout the entire stomach secrete mucus, which provides a protective barrier between luminal acid and the gastric wall. These surface mucous cells are simple columnar epithelium with projecting microvilli. Immediately subjacent to the villi are mucous granules, which fuse with the apical cell membrane and deliver mucus by exocytosis. An extensive and active Golgi apparatus and rough endoplasmic reticulum are seen in the cytoplasm. These cells continuously recycle every 72 hours. Mucous neck cells are found deeper in the neck of the gland and have a similar morphology and function. They appear to renew every 7 days.

Parietal cells are perhaps the most functionally unique cells found in the gastric epithelium. They produce both hydrochloric acid (HCl) and intrinsic factor (IF) and are under a complicated system of regulatory controls. In the resting state, these cells contain unusual intracellular smooth membranes termed *tubulovesicles*. When stimulated, these structures are replaced by extensive intracellular canaliculi that communicate directly with the glandular lumen at the apical interface and that contain numerous microvilli. These microvilli appear to be the site of greatest concentration of the H^+-K^+-ATPase (proton pump) that drives HCl secretion against a large concentration gradient. Consistent with such an energy-intensive process, these cells contain large mitochondria in a concentration exceeded only by the myocardium. Parietal cells are found throughout the isthmus and neck regions of the glands, predominantly in the gastric fundus and body and less often in the proximal antrum. They can be identified in gastric glands as early as gestational week 10.

Chief cells are found exclusively at the base of the gastric glands. They synthesize, store, and secrete pepsinogen, a zymogen that is hydrolyzed to the active proteolytic enzyme pepsin in the acid environment of the gastric lumen. Pepsinogen is stored in apical zymogen granules in preparation for release by exocytosis. These cells are found principally in the gastric fundus and body, and first appear in the 12th week of gestation.

Enteroendocrine cells are present throughout the stomach and intestine (Fig. 68-3). This classification represents a spectrum of cells that produce a variety of signaling molecules that integrate and regulate the complex events underlying acid secretion, digestion, and motility (Table 68-1). These cells have in common the ability to internalize certain precursor molecules and to produce biologically active amines and peptides by intracellular decarboxylation; they are therefore referred to as *amine precursor uptake and decarboxylation (APUD)* cells.

Many distinct types of enteroendocrine cells are found in the gastric mucosa, producing such diverse amines and peptides as serotonin, histamine, dopamine, VIP, glucagon, GRP, and motilin. The most common and well-characterized are the G cells, which produce gastrin, and the D cells, which produce somatostatin. Because these substances function in endocrine and paracrine regulation, respectively, the cells that produce them tend to have high concentrations of secretory granules at their basolateral (ie, abluminal) membranes. Microvilli on their apical (luminal) membranes contain the chemoreceptors and pH receptors necessary to sense environmental changes and function in feedback inhibition. Another enteroendocrine cell,

the enterochromaffin-like (ECL) cell, produces histamine, perhaps the primary stimulus for acid secretion. Enteroendocrine cells are ubiquitous both within the gastric glands throughout the stomach and also within the duodenal wall. The most common types, the G and D cells, predominate in the gastric antrum.

Enteroendocrine cells are among the first to populate the gastric glands, emerging at 8 to 9 weeks' gestation. The origin of these cells is controversial. Because they share many biochemical and morphologic properties with other APUD cells of neuroendocrine origin, it is presumed that they reach the fetal stomach by migration from the neural crest. A competing theory based on embryo grafting experiments suggests that these cells derive from stem cells located within the base of the gastric gland. Certain cells, referred to as *A cells,* appear to produce glucagon and are only present in fetal and neonatal glands. Such observations, along with the recognition that many GI hormones have trophic effects, have led to the hypothesis that some enteroendocrine cells may participate in the growth and differentiation of the fetal stomach and other regions of the GI tract.

Finally, a large number of undifferentiated cells can be seen interspersed with other cell types in the gastric glands. Their role is postulated to be the regeneration of all cellular components of the epithelium, except the enteroendocrine population, after injury. Enteroendocrine regeneration appears to result from specific precursors.

Based on the cell types previously described, it is possible to segregate the stomach into three histologically and functionally distinct regions characterized by the presence of one of three specific gland types: cardiac, oxyntic, or pyloric. Cardiac glands are devoid of parietal and chief cells and occupy a 1- to 2-cm

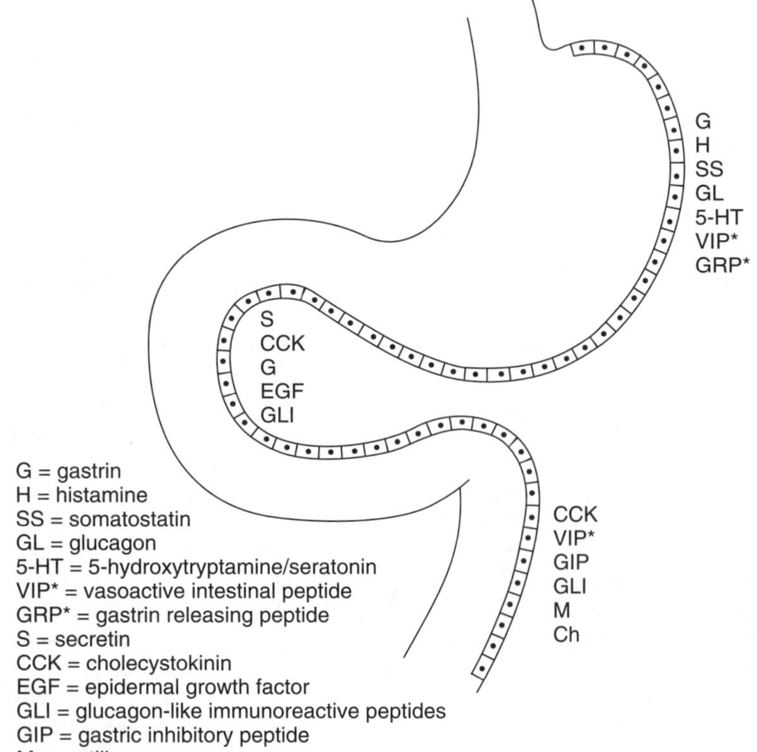

FIG. 68-3. Distribution of selected enteroendocrine and neurocrine (designated by asterisk) cells and their products in the proximal gastrointestinal tract.

TABLE 68-1. *Important intercellular signaling molecules in the stomach and duodenum*

Mediator	Location	Cell type	Primary physiologic effects
GASTRIN FAMILY			
Gastrin	Fetal duodenum; postnatal stomach	G	Stimulates enterochromaffin-like (ECL) cell histamine release and potentiates parietal cell stimulation; trophic effects on mucosal growth
Cholecystokinin	Duodenum	I	Stimulates gallbladder contraction and exocrine pancreatic secretion in response to fatty acids and amino acids
	Stomach	ENS	Possible role in ECL cell inhibition
SECRETIN FAMILY			
Secretin	Duodenum	S	Stimulates bicarbonate production in pancreas, liver, and duodenal mucosa
Vasoactive intestinal peptide	Stomach, duodenum	ENS	Stimulation of G-cell gastrin secretion in response to low-level gastric distention
Gastric inhibitory peptide	Duodenum	K	Inhibits gastric secretory and motor activity; mediates insulin response to enteral sugars
OTHERS			
Somatostatin	Stomach; entire GI tract	D	Inhibits G-cell and parietal cell secretion; inhibits enteroendocrine secretion
Histamine	Stomach	ECL	Final mediator of parietal acid secretion
Gastrin-releasing peptide	Stomach	ENS	Stimulates G-cell gastrin secretion in response to aromatic amino acids
Serotonin (5-HT)	Stomach, duodenum	EC	Poorly defined: may regulate CNS- and duodenal-mediated effects on gastric secretion and motility
Glucagon	Fetal stomach	A	Undefined; possible role in mucosal development
Glucagon-like immuno-reactive peptides (enteroglucagon, oxynto-modulin, glucagonlike peptides)	Duodenum	L	Poorly defined; possible roles in inhibiting gastric secretion and motility, adaptive hyperplasia; mediates insulin response to enteral sugars

ring around the gastroesophageal junction. Oxyntic glands are the most prevalent and occupy the fundus and most of the body. These glands contain all the cell types listed earlier, and are especially rich in parietal and chief cells. Pyloric glands, found in the distal 10% of the stomach, have few parietal and no chief cells, but are well endowed with enteroendocrine cells, especially G and D cells.

The duodenal mucosa is also richly populated with enteroendocrine cells. These cells are stimulated by nutritional substrates delivered from the stomach, and they secrete mediators that regulate a variety of digestive processes. Secretin is produced by duodenal S cells in response to luminal acid, stimulating bicarbonate secretion from the pancreas, liver, and duodenal Brunner glands and mucosal cells. CCK is produced by duodenal I cells in response to certain fatty acids and amino acids and stimulates gallbladder contraction and pancreatic exocrine secretion. Secretin and CCK have also been proposed to have trophic effects on the fetal intestinal tract and pancreas, respectively. Many other enteroendocrine cells are present, and their physiologic significance is under intense investigation. A partial list of these cells and their putative functions is found in Table 68-1.

Physiology of Gastric Motor Function

The coordinated muscular activity of the stomach and duodenum, like that of the rest of the GI tract, is the net result of many complex interactions between mural smooth muscle cells and the ENS. The stomach is divided into two distinct functional zones based on marked differences in motor activity. The proximal stomach, including the fundus and proximal third of the body, exhibits the properties of receptive relaxation and accommodation and serves as a reservoir in which the ingested meal is stored. The ability to distend without a concomitant increase in intraluminal pressure is important during bolus feeding. Additionally, the proximal stomach generates slow, sustained, tonic contractions that elevate mean intragastric pressure above duodenal pressure and provide a constant pressure gradient that controls the passage of liquids through the stomach. These properties are under significant CNS modulation by nonadrenergic, noncholinergic vagal fibers. Therefore, vagotomy significantly impairs these functions and causes rapid emptying of liquids. The remainder of the stomach distal to the first third of the body is functionally and physiologically distinct from the proximal stomach. Motor activity in the distal stomach is characterized by spontaneous myocyte membrane depolarizations that result in phasic, directional contractions. These contractions account for the ability of the distal stomach to mix and grind solid food and to empty mixed food particles into the duodenum in a controlled fashion.

A basic property of smooth muscle cells in the distal stomach and duodenum (but not the proximal stomach) is a spontaneous slow depolarization of their membrane potential from a resting level of -40 to -70 mV toward zero. Since myocytes are physiologically linked through gap junctions, the slow wave depolarizations of one cell are communicated to adjacent and more distant cells through serial connections. This leads to a spreading wave of depolarization in which cells with the most frequent spontaneous membrane depolarizations entrain those with lower frequencies. In the stomach, the cell population with the highest rate of spontaneous depolarization, referred to as the *gastric pacemaker,* is located along the greater curvature at the proximal boundary of the distal zone. Depolarizations spread aborally through the body, antrum, and pylorus without being propagated into the proximal zone. The rhythmic activity of the gastric pacemaker is about 3 to 4 cycles per minute (in the duodenum, which can be considered to be a small intestine pacemaker; slow waves are generated at a rate of about 10 to 12 cycles per minute).

Slow wave depolarizations are electrical events. They are coupled to mechanical contractions only when the depolarizations exceed a threshold potential, at which time a rapid depolarization to 0 mV occurs (termed an *action potential*) and triggers smooth muscle contraction by a rapid increase in intracellular calcium. When an action potential of sufficient magnitude is generated, a series of rapid action potentials follows before repolarization can occur (termed a *spikeburst*); this results in a sustained muscular contraction sufficient to elevate intragastric pressure. The underlying organization of slow wave depolarization dispersion ensures that contractions are organized in a propulsive or peristaltic fashion. The frequency, direction, and magnitude of muscular contraction is under intrinsic and extrinsic neurocrine controls that alter resting membrane potentials, threshold potentials, and action potentials as a means of regulating the translation of slow wave depolarizations into mechanical contractions.

During the fasting state, gastric myoelectric activity follows a repetitive pattern with a period of about 90 to 120 minutes, called the *interdigestive migrating motor* (myoelectric) *complex* (MMC). The MMC can be divided into four phases. Phase I is mechanically silent, without the generation of action potentials or muscular contractions. In phase II, random, low-amplitude contractions occur. Phase III is characterized by regular, intense muscular contractions resulting from the conversion of every slow wave depolarization into an action potential with spikebursts. This phase empties the gastric lumen of all indigestible materials and is responsible for imparting the term *housekeeper* to describe the MMC. A short phase IV is marked by a gradual return to phase I quiescence.

The fed state occurs when the interdigestive MMC is interrupted by the arrival of ingested food in the stomach. The regular pattern of MMC activity is replaced with forceful, nonpropagated contractions in the distal stomach, coupled with coordinated contractions of the pyloric sphincter, that serve to churn and grind food into small particles. Distal gastric motor activity appears to be controlled by multiple factors: vagal cholinergic activity, gastrin, GRP, CCK, neurotensin, and motilin stimulate contractions, while adrenergic and noncholinergic vagal activity, somatostatin, secretin, VIP, and gastric-inhibitory peptide inhibit them.

When the average particle size approximates 1 mm in diameter, chyme is allowed to empty into the duodenum. The particulate composition and osmolality of chyme affects the rate of emptying: carbohydrates empty faster than proteins, which empty faster than fats. Isocaloric amounts of nutrients, however, empty in about equal times. Intraduodenal acid, carbohydrate, and fat stimulate intramural, cholinergic ENS feedback loops that result in pyloric contraction, slowing gastric emptying. This complex set of interactive factors ensures that the rate of gastric emptying is adjusted to provide an isocaloric flow of nutrients into the duodenum over time.

Physiology of Gastric Secretion

Production and secretion of HCl by gastric parietal cells is governed by a complex, highly redundant network of stimulatory and feedback controls that involve neurocrine, endocrine, and paracrine pathways. Establishing a dominant or final common pathway has been difficult because the parietal cell and other regulatory cells have been shown to possess cell-surface receptors for a wide variety of molecular secretagogues. The parietal cell receives input from cholinergic and noncholinergic nerve terminals of the autonomic nervous systems (sympathetic, parasympathetic, and enteric), from hormones delivered through the microvasculature from distant sources (eg, gastrin from antral G cells), and from peptide and amine messengers secreted into the local interstitial environment (eg, histamine from fundic ECL cells). Each of the cells elaborating these regulatory substances are, in turn, subject to regulatory inputs equally complex.

Functions of acid include initiating and facilitating the hydrolysis of peptide bonds during protein digestion by denaturing ingested proteins and exposing specific amino acid sequences to pepsin, an endopeptidase that requires an acidic environment for activation. It is likely, however, that the pH-dependent activation of pepsin evolved in response to this acidic environment, rather than the converse. Because patients with chronic achlorhydria do not often suffer from malabsorption, the importance of acid-peptic digestion may not be critical. Nevertheless, when acid secretion is normal, it plays an integral role in initiating the digestive process.

An additional function of gastric acid is to create a barrier to the entrance of bacteria into the GI tract. Gastric acidity not only protects the upper aerodigestive tract from potentially pathogenic bacteria found in the lower GI tract but also insulates the various populations of indigenous bacteria inhabiting the lower tract from constant challenges by new strains of ingested microorganisms. Chronic neutralization of intragastric acidification results in bacterial overgrowth, which can lead to nosocomial respiratory tract infections, digestive abnormalities, and possibly generation of carcinogenic nitrosamines.

Gastric secretory function evolves early in development. By 10 weeks' gestation, parietal and enteroendocrine cells have begun to differentiate, and by 12 to 13 weeks, gastrin, HCl, pepsin, and IF can all be detected. Mucus and bicarbonate secretion commences later, at about the 16th week of gestation. Further prenatal growth and development is probably under enteroendocrine control. In the newborn, the gastric luminal pH is neutral, owing to swallowed amniotic fluid. Within the first several hours of life, however, acid secretion is sufficient to reduce the pH to 3.5. Further secretion lowers the pH to 1.0 to 3.0 by 48 hours, with little distinction between basal and stimulated outputs. Thereafter, acidity declines until the 3rd week, when HCl secretion begins to increase again. By the age of 3 to 4 years, acid secretion approximates adult levels. Premature infants have a prolonged period of alkalinity, often extending for several days. As expected, the smallest premature infants display the most prolonged delay in acid secretion.

Phases of Gastric Acid Secretion

Acid secretion in response to a meal occurs in four relatively well-defined phases: cephalic, gastric, intestinal, and basal or interdigestive. In the cephalic phase, acid secretion commences when the subject thinks about food. Impulses generated in the CNS are relayed through the parasympathetic system by the vagus nerve to ganglia in the submucosal plexus, and by postganglionic neurons to cellular targets in the antrum and corpus. The fact that this phase is controlled primarily by neurocrine factors is supported by the finding that vagotomy or administration of atropine effectively abolishes this phase. The cephalic phase accounts for 30% to 50% of the acid secretory response to a meal.[2]

The gastric phase of secretion begins when a bolus of food enters the stomach. Intragastric mechanisms that sense distention, elevation in pH, and the chemical composition of the food (particularly amino acids from ingested proteins) stimulate and regulate acid secretion directly at the parietal cell level and indirectly through stimulation of gastrin secretion. These local processes are still under significant control by CNS centers by vagal input.[3] This phase is responsible for 40% to 50% of the secretory response.

The intestinal phase accounts for the remainder of the acid secretory response to a meal. This phase is the least well characterized but is controlled largely by the secretion of hormones and peptides into the circulation by cells at various levels of the GI tract. The duodenum and upper jejunum have been shown to secrete gastrin. Absorbed amino acids have an endocrine effect in stimulating gastric parietal cells. Other, less well-characterized substances, such as enterooxyntin, are secreted by the distal small intestine and may have significant effects on acid secretion.

Between meals, the interdigestive or basal phase of acid secretion appears to be initiated by reacidification of the antrum as buffered food exits the stomach. This decrease in pH results in inhibition of antral G-cell gastrin secretion. Inhibitory peptides from the small intestine, such as secretin, gastric-inhibitory peptide, and enteroglucagon, also effect a negative feedback loop on gastric acid production by gastrin regulation.[4] The interdigestive phase displays a circadian variation that is abolished by vagotomy, implying that basal acid secretion is largely under vagal (CNS) control.

Control of Acid Secretion

Parietal cells in the fundus and corpus display surface membrane receptors for a variety of substances that stimulate or inhibit production and secretion of HCl. Stimulatory substances and their receptors include histamine (H_2 receptor), acetylcholine (M3 receptor), and gastrin (gastrin receptor); inhibitory substances include somatostatin (somatostatin receptor), epidermal growth factor (EGF receptor), prostaglandin E (PGE) series prostaglandins (EP_3 receptor), and possibly adrenergic neurotransmitters (β-adrenergic receptors). Although the heterogeneity of receptors suggests that receptor-mediated acid secretion can be effected through a number of pathways, the observation that competitive inhibition of H_2 receptors can abolish acid output in response to all secretagogues strongly supports a central role for histamine as the final common pathway for most

acid secretion under physiologic conditions. Gastrin alone is a relatively weak activator of isolated parietal cells in culture.[5] The primary function of both acetylcholine and gastrin at the parietal cell membrane is probably to potentiate the effect of histamine, since synergistic responses in acid secretion are seen with combinations of histamine and either gastrin or acetylcholine.[6]

Although the source of gastric histamine was originally presumed to be the mast cell, gastrin has no demonstrable effect on mast cell histamine secretion. It is now widely accepted that the cell responsible for histamine-mediated parietal cell activation is the ECL cell.[7] These enteroendocrine cells are intimately associated with the much larger parietal cells and possess numerous vacuoles containing histamine, which is released by exocytosis. Cell-surface receptors for gastrin and acetylcholine have been purified from ECL membrane preparations, suggesting that the ECL cell directly integrates these inputs and releases histamine in a paracrine fashion (Fig. 68-4). When gastrin receptors are occupied, intracellular calcium concentrations in the ECL cell rise by increased flux across the cell membrane and by release from intracellular stores. Whether acetylcholine and other agonists use calcium or cyclic adenosine monophosphate (cAMP) as their second messengers is undetermined. CCK receptors are also found on human ECL cells, although their function is unclear. β-Adrenergic receptors have been found on rat ECL cells, which respond to epinephrine and are inhibited by propranolol, implying a potential mechanism for stress-induced acid secretion.[8]

The major inhibitory regulator of ECL cell function is somatostatin, which causes receptor-mediated suppression of histamine release in response to the secretagogues mentioned earlier. Somatostatin-secreting D cells also exert a tonic inhibitory effect on acid secretion by directly suppressing parietal cell function. The principal stimulators of D-cell activity are hydrogen ion, resulting in a negative feedback loop, and noncholinergic neurons, releasing VIP in response to low-grade distention. Other stimulators of fundic somatostatin release include gastrin and epinephrine, but their roles have not been clarified. Acetylcholine exerts a negative effect on somatostatin secretion, potentiating cholinergic enhancement of acid secretion by ECL and parietal cell stimulation.

The dominant pathway of parietal cell activation is paracrine stimulation of parietal cells by ECL cell–secreted histamine. The more proximal mechanisms that transduce physiologic stimuli into ECL cell histamine release involve the production of gastrin by antral G cells and the transmission of impulses through gastric effector neurons of the enteric autonomic system directly to the ECL cells. G cells are responsive to two stimulatory neurocrine agents: acetylcholine from cholinergic neurons and GRP from noncholinergic neurons. Vagal cholinergic activity governs gastrin release from both cephalic-phase (CNS) stimulation and high-level gastric distention (ie, after ingesting a meal). GRP appears to mediate gastric-phase activation of G cells by luminal protein fragments, particularly aromatic amino acids.[9] On stimulation by either acetylcholine or GRP, antral G cells secrete gastrin into adjacent capillaries. This neurocrine stimulation accounts for the entire gastrin response to central and local factors.

Gastrin is actually a heterogeneous collection of at least three peptides: big gastrin (34 amino acids), little gastrin (17), and mini-gastrin (14). Big gastrin predominates physiologically be-

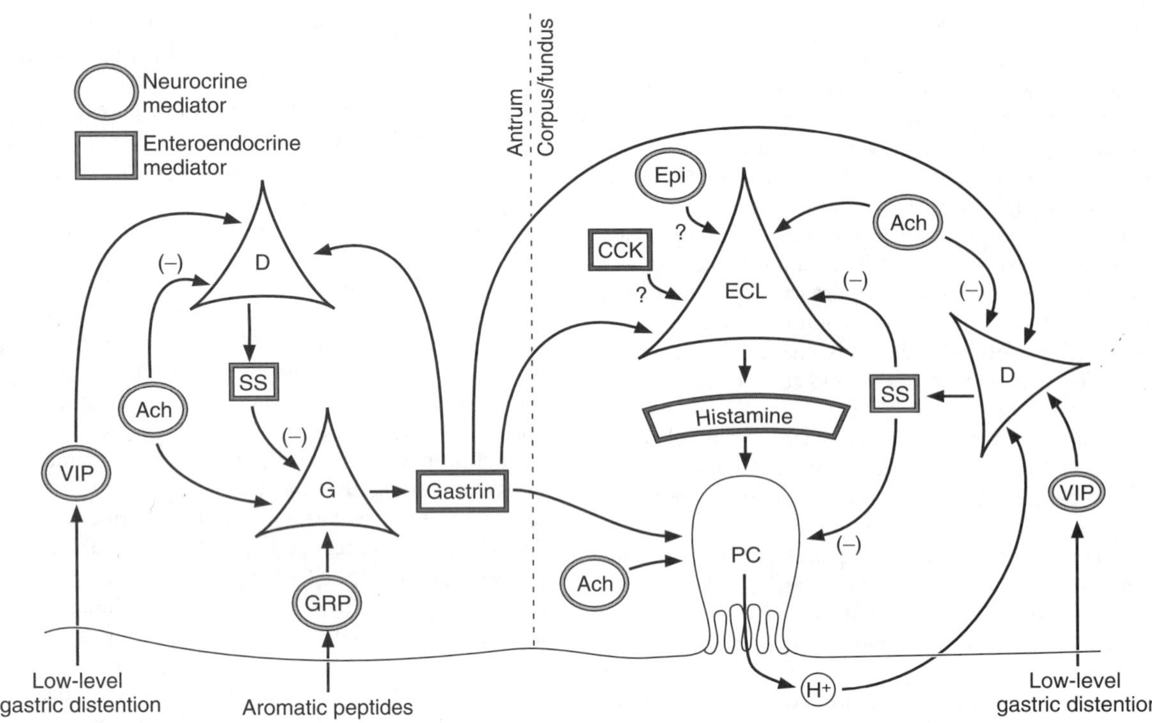

FIG. 68-4. Regulation of gastric acid secretion by neurocrine, endocrine, and paracrine agents. Ach, acetylcholine; CCK, cholecystokinin; ECL, enterochromaffin-like cell; Epi, epinephrine; GRP, gastrin-releasing peptide; PC, parietal cell; VIP, vasoactive intestinal peptide; SS, somatostatin.

cause it has the longest half-life. Actions of gastrin include the direct stimulation of ECL cells and potentiation of the parietal cell response to histamine. Proposed physiologic effects of gastrin are trophic effects on oxyntic gland mucosa, secretion of IF and pepsin, and augmentation of lower esophageal sphincter (LES) pressure, intestinal motility, and pancreatic exocrine secretion.

G cells are under constant, ambient inhibitory influences exerted by somatostatin secreted from adjacent D cells. Histologically, D cells are linked to G cells through cell-membrane processes that abut directly on the G-cell plasma membrane. Somatostatin, released into the interface, binds to receptors on the G cells that down-regulate gastrin secretion. Somatostatin secretion is stimulated by gastrin, resulting in a negative feedback loop. In addition to gastrin, somatostatin secretion is elicited by VIP released from noncholinergic neurons in response to low-level gastric distention (ie, after partial emptying of a meal).[10] This constitutive inhibition by somatostatin must be blocked for maximal stimulation of gastrin secretion to occur. Acetylcholine inhibits somatostatin secretion, potentiating its direct stimulation of gastrin secretion.

Mechanism of Acid Secretion

Activating agents bind with high affinity to parietal membrane receptors that are linked to second messenger systems, resulting in either the generation of cAMP or an increase in the intracellular calcium concentration ($[Ca]_i$). The H_2 receptor appears to be a typical seven-membrane segment, G-protein–coupled receptor that activates adenylate cyclase on the cytoplasmic surface of the plasma membrane, resulting in the hydrolysis of adenosine triphosphate (ATP) and generation of cAMP. Cyclic AMP then triggers the phosphorylation and activation of various cytoplasmic protein kinases.[11] The critical component in this linkage is the stimulatory guanosine triphosphate–binding protein (G_s) that translates external receptor occupation to internal adenylate cyclase activation. Both acetylcholine and gastrin receptors result in increased $[Ca]_i$, presumably owing to phospholipase C–dependent inositol turnover and protein kinase C activation, increased surface membrane Ca^{2+} conductance, or both. Receptors for inhibitory substances (somatostatin, PGE, opioids, EGF) are linked to an inhibitory G protein (G_i) that suppresses adenylate cyclase activity.

When the appropriate stimulatory signals converge on the parietal cell basolateral membrane, a number of distinct morphologic changes occur that coincide with acid secretion from the apical end of the cell. Cytoplasmic tubulovesicles, which have been shown to contain the quiescent proton pump, coalesce into a larger membrane system termed the *secretory canaliculus,* which communicates with the gastric gland lumen at the apical cell surface. At the same time, the K^+-Cl^- channel, which provides exchangeable K^+ ions to the extracellular portion of the proton pump, is also inserted into the membrane of the secretory canaliculus. These changes occur within minutes of activation and persist throughout the entire period of increased acid secretion.

Although the sequence of events after the activation of cAMP is undefined, these events eventually result in the activation of the proton pump—an H^+-K^+-ATPase that effects an electroneutral exchange of H^+ for K^+ at the luminal surface of the secretory canaliculus (Fig. 68-5). This enzyme is a heterodimer

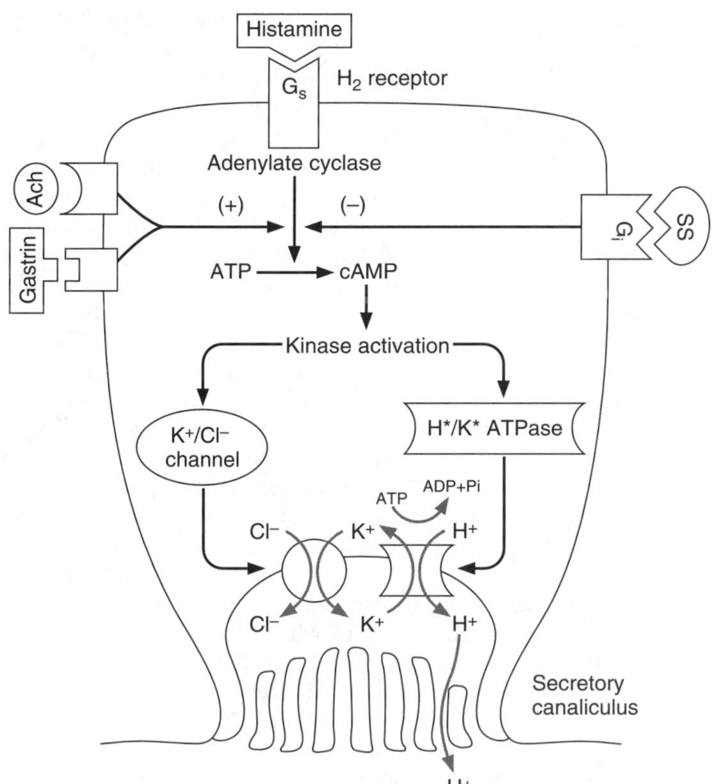

FIG. 68-5. Intracellular mechanism of parietal cell acid secretion. Ach, acetylcholine; SS, somatostatin.

with a 1000–amino acid catalytic subunit and a glycosylated 300–amino acid regulatory subunit, both of which share significant sequence homology with the Na^+-K^+-ATPase. When activated, ATP hydrolysis drives a conformational change in the enzyme that causes vectorial transport of an H^+ ion (or hydronium ion, H_3O^+) through the hydrophilic core of the transmembrane enzyme to the luminal surface, followed by the return of a K^+ ion through the same core to the cytoplasmic surface. Pump activity is dependent on a constant supply of K^+ ions at the luminal surface of the canalicular membrane, making the juxtapositioning of the K^+-Cl^- channel to the proton pump a critical step in acid secretion.[12] Omeprazole, a substituted benzimidizole, is a weak base and becomes protonated and trapped within the low-pH canaliculus. There, it undergoes conversion to a sulfenamide, which reacts with the exposed portions of the catalytic subunit of the H^+-K^+-ATPase pump, forming stable disulfide bonds and preventing the conformational change that allows for ion transport.

Other Gastric Secretory Products

Pepsinogen

Pepsin refers to a family of digestive enzymes synthesized and secreted by the chief and mucous neck cells of the gastric glands. The pepsinogen family can be divided into two groups: A (or I) and C (or II). Pepsinogen A has a molecular weight of about 43 kd and is secreted by the proximal stomach; pepsinogen C is of similar size and is secreted by the entire gastric mucosal surface as well as by the duodenum, prostate, and sem-

inal vesicles. The enzymes are actually synthesized and stored in zymogen granules as prepepsinogens, which undergo intracellular conversion to their zymogen forms, pepsinogens, by cleavage of an N-terminal sequence before secretion through exocytosis. In addition to pepsinogen A and C, two other acid proteinases are secreted by the gastric mucosa: cathepsin D and E. Their physiologic importance is not well defined.

After secretion as an inactive zymogen, an N-terminal sequence is cleaved by acid-mediated hydrolysis, converting pepsinogen to active pepsin. Thereafter, pepsin autocatalyzes its own conversion from pepsinogen. Pepsin is an acid proteinase that has an abundance of aspartate residues at the catalytic site (hence, an aspartic proteinase). At pH below 5, pepsin is progressively more efficient at cleaving internal peptide bonds between aromatic amino acids, thus generating protein fragments with exposed aromatic residues known to stimulate gastrin secretion maximally by GRP-dependent neurocrine stimulation. Pepsinogens can be detected in the fetal stomach by 8 weeks' gestation, but peptic activity is absent until about 16 weeks.

Stimulation of pepsinogen secretion is primarily governed by cholinergic and β-adrenergic inputs. Paracrine and endocrine stimulation also occurs through histamine, CCK, secretin, and VIP. Gastrin does not elicit pepsinogen secretion. Inhibitory regulation is mediated by somatostatin and PGE.

Lipase

Gastric lipase activity is demonstrable at birth. Its optimal pH for activity (5.5) is higher than that of pepsin but is still slightly acidic. Intragastric lipolysis liberates long-chain fatty acids, which stimulate duodenal CCK secretion, and medium-chain fatty acids, which are directly absorbed through the gastric epithelium.

Intrinsic Factor

Intrinsic factor is a 60 kd mucoprotein that is secreted from parietal cells in the fundus and body. Regulatory controls for IF closely parallel those for acid secretion, suggesting a physiologic coupling of IF and acid secretion. In the infant and young child, however, this coupling is dissociated, allowing a constant, basal secretion of IF, which exceeds that of acid.[13]

In the stomach, IF competes with a second ligand, R protein, for binding to vitamin B_{12} cobalamins. Although vitamin B_{12} preferentially binds R protein in the stomach, pancreatic enzymes in the intestine degrade R protein, allowing IF to bind available vitamin B_{12}. The IF–B_{12} complex is then absorbed in the terminal ileum.

Mucus

Mucus is a complex gel consisting of mucin, desquamated epithelial cells, salts, and water. In the stomach, bicarbonate is also secreted and trapped in this gel and is an important protective component of gastric mucus. Mucin, consisting of proteins, glycoproteins, and mucopolysaccharides, is secreted by surface epithelial cells and mucous neck cells in a manner that appears coupled to acid secretion—synthesis and secretion are stimulated by acetylcholine, histamine, and gastrin.[14] The mucus layer is about 180 μm deep and displays a thin layer of hydrophobic phospholipids on its luminal surface.

The physiologic function and importance of mucus is controversial. Previously, the mucus–bicarbonate barrier was considered important in maintaining a pH-neutral environment overlying the surface epithelium by preventing back-diffusion of HCl and pepsin, and by preventing the dissipation of epithelial-secreted bicarbonate. Indeed, a pH gradient of nearly 5 logs exists between the gastric lumen and the epithelial surface. Disruption of the mucus layer by mucolytic agents, however, does not render the underlying epithelium more susceptible to acid-mediated injury, but it does exacerbate epithelial disruption by other injurious agents. It may be reasonable to conclude that the physiologic role of gastric mucus is not in preventing injury, but in protecting of the already injured epithelial surface during the regenerative phase. Other functions of mucus include lubricating the gastric surface to minimize mechanical trauma during mixing, and trapping ingested microbes until they can be processed and phagocytized by immunocompetent cells.

Mucosal Defense Mechanisms

Mucosal defense is a critical ongoing function for an organ whose luminal surface is regularly exposed to a highly acidic environment, a wide range of osmolarities, and activated proteolytic enzymes. The components of mucosal defense, their relative importance, and the precise mechanisms by which they confer protection to the gastric epithelium are, however, poorly understood. Certain mechanisms have been proposed to constitute a hierarchical system of mucosal defense. Those that are best described include: (1) mucus and bicarbonate secretion, (2) epithelial resistance and restitution, (3) mucosal blood flow, and (4) subepithelial activity of immunoinflammatory cells.

Mucus and bicarbonate secretion are the best characterized of mucosal defense components. A thick layer of mucus provides a physiochemical barrier to the diffusion of hydrogen ions from the lumen to the surface epithelial cells. There is speculation that the fine layer of hydrophobic surfactant-like phospholipids at the luminal surface of the mucus layer provides a nonwettable interface that further resists penetration by protons. An additional feature of this barrier is a layer of unstirred bicarbonate interposed between the mucus layer and the underlying cells, which neutralizes hydrogen ions that are successful in penetrating the mucus. The bicarbonate anions originate in the parietal cells deep within the gastric glands and are secreted from their abluminal surfaces into the mucosal capillary network. This network transports them to the surface epithelial cells, which internalize and then resecrete them across their luminal membranes (alkaline tide). This elegant mechanism is attractive as a primary defense mechanism, but recent insights into mucosal injury under circumstances in which the mucus–bicarbonate system is compromised suggest that this system may be of minor importance, or at least redundant.

The surface epithelial cells also contribute to mucosal defense. Monolayers of surface epithelial cells are resistant to exposure of their apical surfaces to a pH of 2, while significant injury occurs when their basolateral membranes are exposed to mildly acidic conditions of pH 5.5. The mechanism underlying this phenomenon is not understood. Senescent cells are removed either by extrusion or through phagocytosis by adjacent epithelial cells. When larger areas of the epithelial surface are injured by acid exposure, they are rapidly replaced by a process referred to as *restitution,* in which the epithelial layer is restored before acid-peptic injury to the basement membrane can occur. This process involves the formation of a mucoid cap—an impenetrable conglomeration of mucus, bicarbonate, desquamated cells, plasma, and fibrin. Under this protective umbrella, new epithelial cells migrate out of the gastric glands along the exposed basement membrane and proliferate. This crucial mechanism limits acid injury to the surface cell layer only.

The importance of mucosal blood flow was mentioned earlier with respect to the delivery of bicarbonate to the surface mucus layer, and of oxygen and other energy substrates to the metabolically active epithelial cells. An additional and perhaps more important function of mucosal blood flow is the rapid removal of noxious substances from the mucosa once they have breached the first lines of defense. This enhanced dispersion of acid and pepsin helps confine the injury to the superficial layers. Alterations in mucosal blood flow are effected by a wide variety of mediators elaborated by immunoinflammatory cells. Mast cells secrete histamine, which causes vasodilation and increased microvascular permeability. Other vasoactive mediators may play a role in regulating perfusion, the most important of these being the prostaglandins. Equally important appear to be ENS neurons using calcitonin gene–related peptide as their primary neurotransmitter, which detect acid and stimulate vasodilation directly.

Impairment of these defense mechanisms appears to play a crucial role in the development of stress-related ulcerations. Although a complete understanding of this process is lacking, several hypotheses are popular. Perhaps the best supported is the role of mucosal hypoperfusion in the setting of hypovolemic shock, in which redistribution of blood flow is effected by mesenteric vasoconstriction. It is attractive to speculate that regional or global reductions in gastric microperfusion may result in deficiencies in the supply of oxygen and other substrates to the metabolically stressed epithelium, leading to accelerated cell death. The delivery of bicarbonate would also be diminished, as would the dispersion and removal of noxious substances. Stress-related alterations in mucus and bicarbonate production, epithelial restitution, and immunoinflammatory cell function are under investigation. Finally, circumstantial evidence for catacholamine-mediated stimulation of acid secretion suggests yet another mechanism of stress-induced mucosal injury.

CONGENITAL ABNORMALITIES OF THE STOMACH AND DUODENUM

Abnormal Gastric Fixation and Gastric Volvulus

Congenital abnormalities of mesenteric fixation of the stomach to the posterior peritoneum predispose to gastric volvulus and can present in two ways. Normally, the stomach is suspended in a peritoneal leaflet that is tethered in four quadrants by the gastrohepatic, gastrophrenic, and gastrosplenic ligaments and the retroperitoneal fixation of the duodenum. The gastrocolic ligament (omentum) may also provide stabilization. Absence or laxity of the gastrohepatic and gastrosplenic ligaments allows the stomach to rotate around its longitudinal axis, producing an *organoaxial volvulus* (Fig. 68-6). Similar abnormalities of the gastrophrenic ligament and duodenal attachments allow rotation around the stomach's transverse axis, referred to as a *mesentericoaxial volvulus.* Organoaxial volvulus is the more common of the two types in infants and children.

A strong association has been found between gastric volvulus and several other anatomic anomalies. These include malrotation, hiatal hernia with a mobile gastroesophageal junction, diaphragmatic hernia or eventration, and asplenia. Because these entities share concurrent abnormalities of the stabilizing peritoneal attachments listed earlier, a causative role is assumed.

Although gastric volvulus can present as either an acute or chronic problem, an acute presentation is usual in children. The classic description of sudden catastrophic epigastric pain, intractable retching without emesis, and failure to advance a nasogastric tube into the stomach may not be reproduced in the actual clinical setting. Children may experience emesis, which can be bilious or nonbilious, and may not have abdominal distention. Any combination of symptoms suggesting a partial or complete high mechanical obstruction may be manifest. Profound physiologic decompensation, hemodynamic instability, or unrelenting metabolic acidosis suggest strangulation, ischemic necrosis, and possibly perforation. Obviously, such a presentation mandates emergent surgical intervention concurrent with ongoing resuscitation. Older children may present with chronic, intermittent volvulus exhibited by postprandial pain, early satiety, and belching.

Radiologic assessment can reveal several characteristic findings. On plain abdominal radiographs, massive gastric dilation usually can be seen, often with a distinct incisura pointing toward the right upper quadrant. The spleen and small intestine may be displaced inferiorly. If a contrast study has been attempted, the contrast column may be confined to the esophagus, with a long, gradual tapering at the bottom. Occasionally, a paraesophageal hiatal hernia is detected (Fig. 68-7).

Operative treatment includes gastric decompression by nasogastric suction or needle aspiration and reduction of the volvulus. Perforations are closed primarily or, depending on their location, around a Malecot tube; more extensive necrosis requires resection. Coexisting anomalies, such as malrotation, should be corrected. Recurrent volvulus is prevented by performing a Stamm-type gastrostomy in the mid-body of the stomach, usually combined with anterior gastropexy. Recurrence is rare.

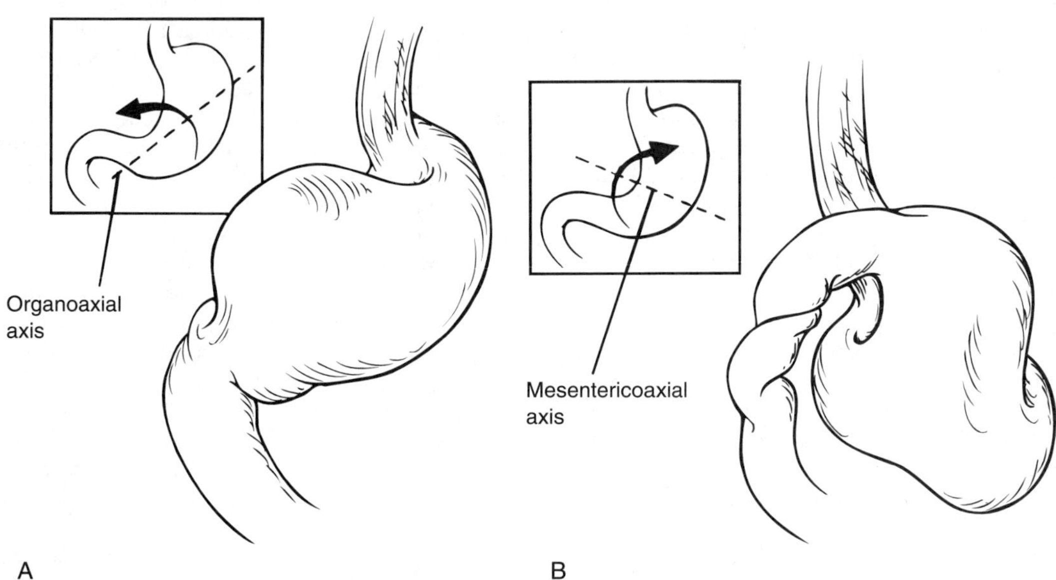

FIG. 68-6. Two variants of gastric volvulus.

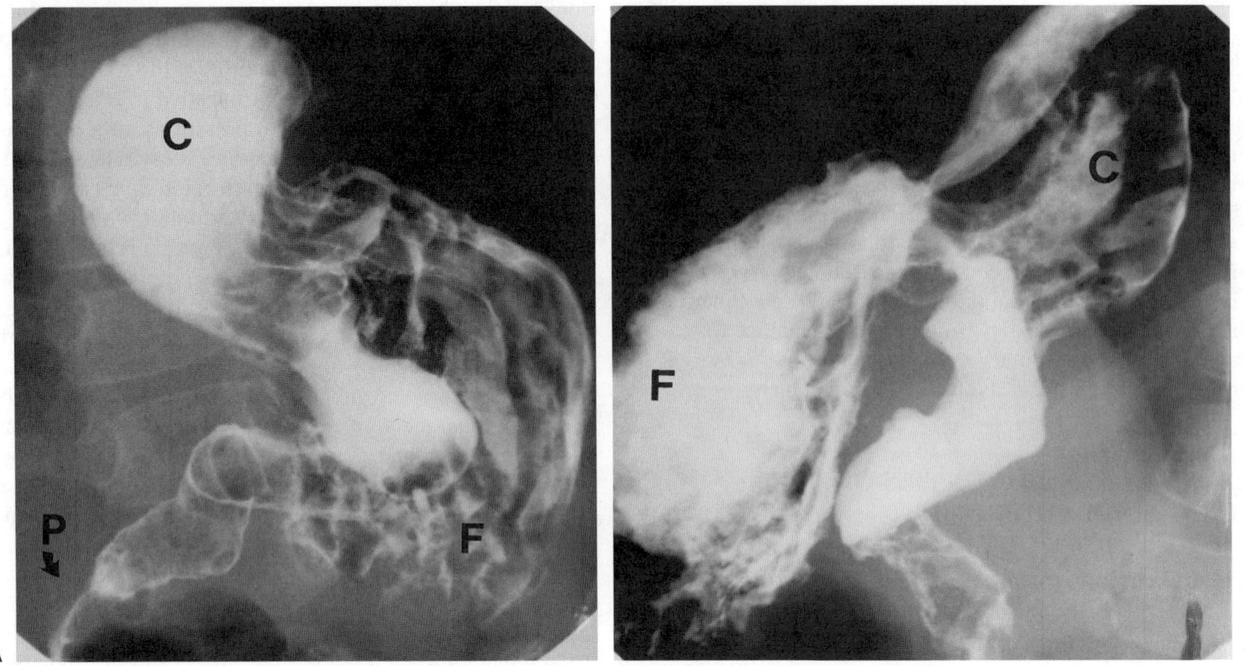

FIG. 68-7. Organoaxial gastric volvulus defined by upper gastrointestinal tract contrast study. (*A*) Antero-posterior projection shows a caudad rotation of the upper corpus and fundus (F), a cephalad rotation of the antrum and lower corpus (C), and a nondisplaced pylorus (P). (*B*) Oblique view reveals that the corpus forms a paraesophageal hernia.

Microgastria

Congenital microgastria is a rare anomaly in which the stomach retains a tubular morphology, fails to develop its normal rotation and fixation, and attains a much smaller volume than normal. Follow-up involving one long-term survivor has documented that the gastric volume remains small indefinitely.[15] Other abnormalities of the abdomen frequently accompany this condition, including megaesophagus, gastroesophageal reflux (GER), intrinsic duodenal obstruction, malrotation, biliary anomalies, situs inversus, asplenia, and skeletal defects.

Microgastria presents with vomiting and failure to thrive in the infant, often associated with persistent diarrhea. Vomiting may be due to duodenal obstruction, GER, or simply a small gastric reservoir. Diarrhea is presumed to be due to rapid gastric transit and a dumping phenomenon. The diagnosis is established by contrast upper GI tract study, which reveals a small stomach with a transverse lie and frequently a large, patulous esophagus (Fig. 68-8). Particular attention should be given to the anatomy of the duodenum and ligament of Treitz.

The initial management of microgastria is usually by continuous drip feeding. This approach has been variably successful in providing both fluids and calories sufficient to meet the infant's needs for growth. In severe cases, parenteral nutritional supplementation is necessary. When continuous feedings can be maintained for several weeks despite reflux, the stomach may undergo significant enlargement, allowing for a gradual transition to bolus and ad lib feeds. Antireflux precautions, including small frequent meals, may be required indefinitely. If this strategy is unsuccessful, surgical correction is indicated. Although case reports of successful management by gastrojejunostomy exist, the favored approach involves construction of a Roux-en-Y jejunal reservoir—the Hunt-Lawrence pouch[16] (Fig. 68-9).

Congenital Antral and Pyloric Obstruction

Congenital partial or complete obstructions of the antrum and pyloric channel are much less common than acquired causes of gastric outlet obstruction in the newborn. They may also be diagnosed in older children after a long period of vague symptoms. Anatomic obstructions that require surgical correction must be distinguished from nonoperative causes, such as neonatal gastroparesis. The obstruction may take the form of a segmental defect (gap), which is sometimes bridged by a fibrous cord, or a membrane (web), which can have one or more apertures through which gastric contents pass. Histologically, such membranes consist of mucosa and submucosa without a muscularis. Prepyloric membranes can become redundant after exposure to antegrade propulsive pressures, creating a "windsock" web that can prolapse through the pyloric channel. This can be the source of considerable confusion and lead to strategic errors in surgical management. Pyloric webs account for two thirds of these obstructions, pyloric atresia accounts for about a quarter, and most of the remainder are antral webs and atresias. Rarely, ectopic pancreatic tissue resides within the submucosa of the pyloric channel, bulging into the lumen and producing a partial obstruction.

The etiology of antral and pyloric atresia is not understood. Unlike jejunoileal atresias, in utero infarction from a vascular accident or volvulus is unlikely, owing to the stomach's multi-

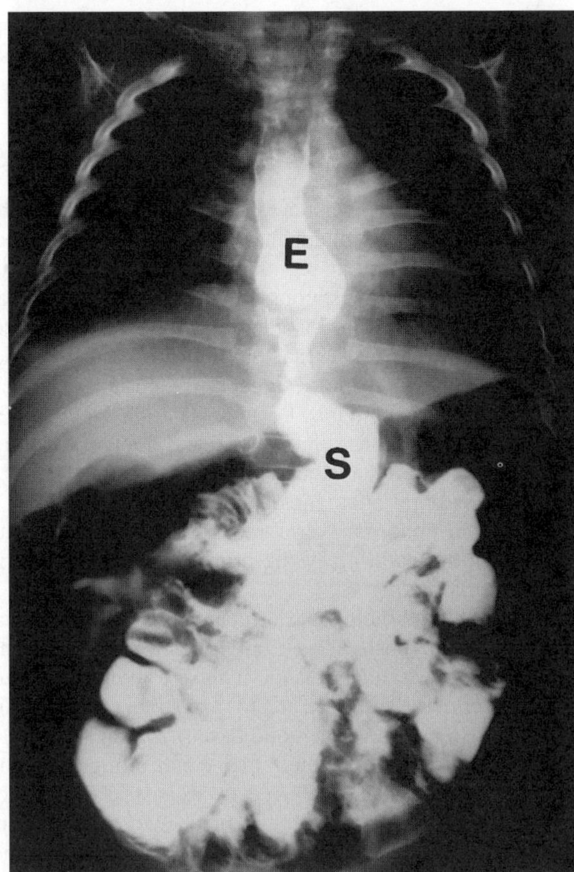

FIG. 68-8. Characteristic upper gastrointestinal tract contrast study findings in congenital microgastria, including a small, tubular stomach (S) and free reflux into a patulous esophagus (E).

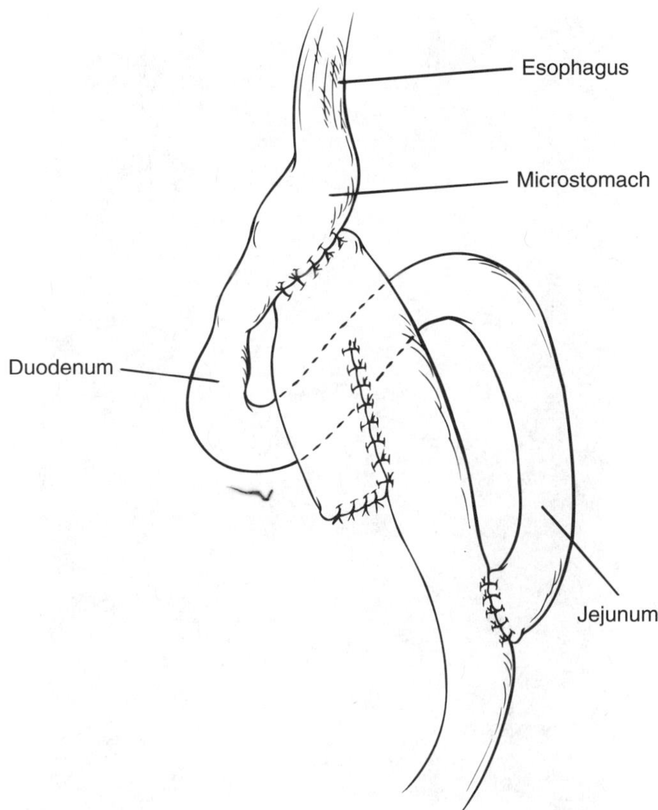

FIG. 68-9. Technique of Roux-en-Y gastrojejunostomy with J-pouch reservoir (Hunt-Lawrence procedure) for microgastria.

ple redundant blood supply and extensive peritoneal fixation. And, because the stomach does not undergo a solid embryonic phase like the duodenum, failure of recanalization cannot account for these anomalies. Instead, some form of foregut segmentation mechanism is proposed but unproved. A genetic cause has been identified for some cases of pyloric atresia that occur in association with epidermolysis bullosa lethalis (Herlitz syndrome), which is inherited in an autosomal recessive manner. A hemidesmosome defect has been identified in the gastric mucosal epithelium in this syndrome, although the causative relation between this observation and the occurrence of pyloric atresia has not been established.

Clinical manifestations depend primarily on the degree of obstruction. Complete membranes or atresias present in the first few days of life as acute gastric outlet obstruction with nonbilious projectile vomiting. There is often a history of maternal polyhydramnios. Gastric distention leading to respiratory compromise can occur, and frank gastric perforation has been reported as early as 12 hours of life. Incomplete gastric outlet obstruction owing to fenestrated membranes or heterotopic pancreatic tissue can present early in the neonatal period or later in childhood, the length of delay depending on the relative degree of obstruction. Epigastric pain, vomiting, and weight loss can all occur in the older child. Adolescents and adults occasionally present with an incomplete prepyloric mechanical ob-

struction, but whether such a web is congenital or acquired from long-standing peptic ulcer disease and mucosal erosion and inflammation is debatable.

Radiologic evaluation characteristically reveals a large gastric air bubble, either without any gas distal to the obstruction (Fig. 68-10), or with a nondistended distal small intestine in cases with a fenestrated membrane. Because neonatal gastric hypotonia can reproduce these radiographic findings, upper GI tract contrast studies are preferable. These studies either show nonfilling of the duodenum or delineate the membrane when viewed laterally (Fig. 68-11). Ectopic pancreatic tissue can cause an eccentric protrusion into the pyloric channel. The typical string sign and bulging muscle of hypertrophic pyloric stenosis (HPS) is absent. In situations in which a contrast study is equivocal, fiberoptic gastroscopy may be helpful.

Preoperative resuscitation and preparation of the infant with antral or pyloric obstruction is similar to that for HPS, but intermittent gastric decompression is necessary in infants with complete gastric outlet obstruction. A chloride-responsive contraction alkalosis is often seen and requires specific measures to restore both intravascular and total extracellular volume as well as to correct chloride and potassium deficits. Prolonged vomiting in the neonate can also lead to profound hypoglycemia, which must be anticipated and corrected.

Surgical management depends on the exact pathology encountered. In general, webs can be excised through a longitudinal incision that bisects them, followed by transverse closure

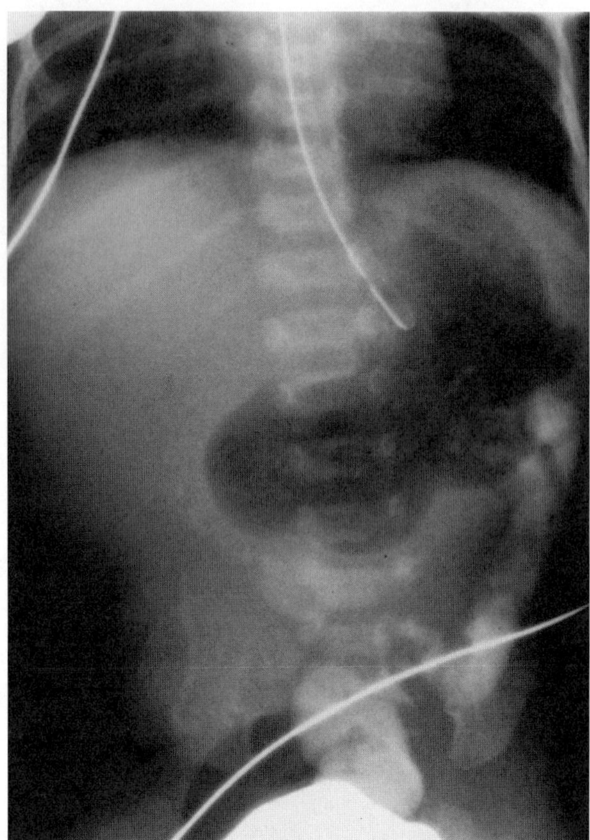

FIG. 68-10. Plain radiograph of isolated gastric distention in pyloric atresia.

to avoid stenosis. Complete atresias with anatomic disconnection can usually be corrected by primary anastomosis, such as gastroduodenostomy. Gastrojejunostomy is poorly tolerated in the neonate and should be avoided. Recognition of windsock deformities and distal atresias by passage of a balloon catheter proximally and distally can be helpful in defining the exact anatomy and in detecting additional distal obstructions. Ectopic pancreatic tissue in the pylorus requires excision of the mass and reconstruction of the pylorus.

Duplications

Duplications of the GI tract are covered in detail elsewhere, so only a brief review is included here. The stomach and duodenum are the least common regions of the GI tract in which duplications occur. For most congenital lesions of the stomach and duodenum included in this category, the term *duplication* may be a misnomer. The actual embryologic cause of these lesions is unknown, but the designation of enterogenous cyst or congenital diverticulum may be more accurate. Nevertheless, it is important to recognize that gastric and duodenal duplications are frequently associated with other GI duplications as well as with vertebral anomalies. Communications with or attachments to an abnormal vertebral column suggest a cause related to aberrant splitting of the primitive notochord during the early embryonic period.

Classically, four pathologic criteria are considered necessary to establish the diagnosis of gastric duplication: (1) contiguity with the stomach; (2) an outer smooth muscle layer; (3) a shared blood supply with the stomach; and (4) a gastric epithelial lining (which may also contain pancreatic tissue). Extragastric cystic structures lined by gastric epithelium and exhibiting a muscular wall, however, are usually referred to as gastric duplications regardless of their proximity to the stomach. Most gastric duplications are cystic, do not communicate with the gastric lumen, and are located along the greater curvature of the stomach. When a luminal communication is present, it may be due to peptic ulceration of the common wall between the two structures. Tubular duplications are less common, frequently communicate with the gastric lumen, and are also most commonly found on the greater curvature (Fig. 68-12). Several case reports of gastric duplications, both adjacent to the stomach and in the retroperitoneum, have described a connection to a normal or abnormal pancreatic lobe. These connections may actually include patent communications with an abnormal pancreatic duc-

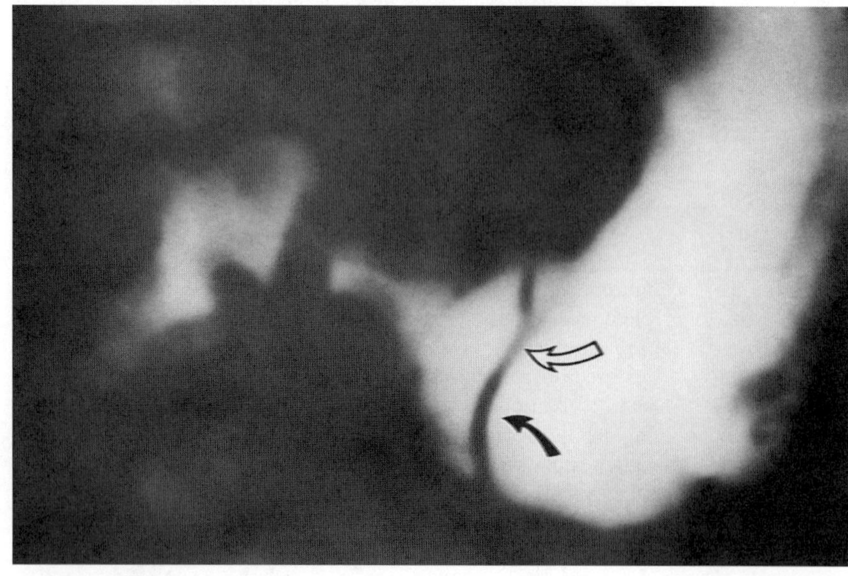

FIG. 68-11. Upper gastrointestinal tract contrast study showing an antral web (*closed arrow*) with a central aperture (*open arrow*).

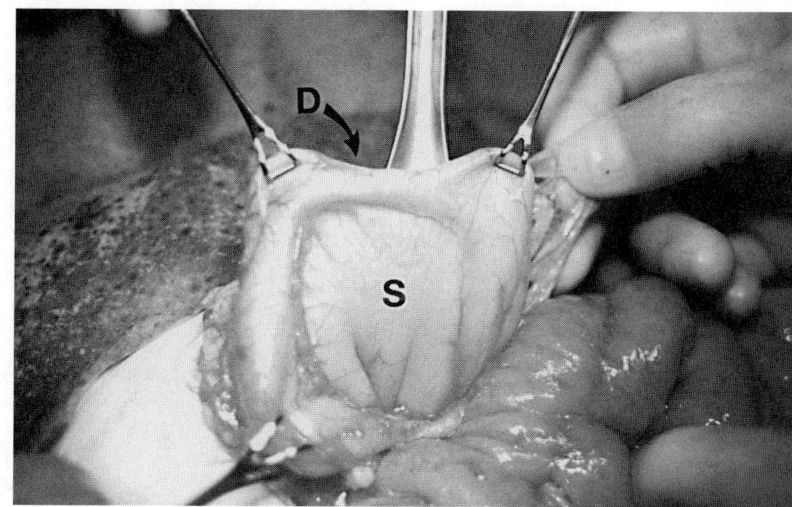

FIG. 68-12. Tubular gastroduodenal duplication (D) adjacent to the greater curvature of the stomach (S).

tal system and have resulted in chronic pancreatitis and pseudocyst formation. Communications with intrathoracic esophageal duplications have also been described. Duodenal duplications most commonly occur in the first or second portion, usually on the posterior surface, and may be lined with gastric mucosa.

Gastroduodenal duplications often present in the neonatal period with symptoms and signs of proximal GI obstruction. Vomiting is common and can be bilious or nonbilious, depending on the location of the extrinsic compression relative to the ampulla of Vater. A palpable mass, failure to thrive, pain, and pancreatitis may also be apparent. Gastroduodenal hemorrhage or perforation secondary to peptic ulceration are the usual emergency indications for surgery; however, hemorrhage secondary to erosion into the transverse colon has been reported. An upper GI tract contrast study may demonstrate an extrinsic compression of the stomach or duodenum, but ultrasound and computed tomography can definitively reveal the mass itself. Technetium-99m scans may identify duplications distant from the stomach if they contain ectopic gastric mucosa but are not specific for duplications per se.

Resection of the entire duplication, either by enucleation or limited gastric resection, is the treatment of choice. With extensive duplications, however, removal of the entire mucosal cyst lining is indicated to avoid potential malignant degeneration. Adenocarcinoma arising from the gastric epithelium has been described in later life.[17] Partial excision of the duplication with stripping of the residual mucosa is acceptable for lesions around the pylorus and duodenum for which en bloc resection of the contiguous gastroduodenal wall would necessitate sacrificing important structures (eg, the common bile duct). Internal drainage into the adjacent duodenum or a Roux-en-Y jejunal limb is reserved for the rare circumstance in which resection or mucosal stripping is not feasible. Partial resection of a contiguous aberrant pancreatic lobe or internal drainage of an associated pseudocyst may also be required. Marsupialization should be avoided.

Congenital Duodenal Obstruction

Congenital duodenal obstruction is a relatively common abnormality in the newborn period and may be complete or partial,

intrinsic or extrinsic. Intrinsic obstructions of a developmental nature are referred to as *atresias* or *stenoses,* depending on whether they are complete or partial. Intrinsic duodenal obstructions are relatively common; a population-based study documented that duodenal atresias and stenoses have an incidence of about 1 in 7000 live births and account for 49% of all small intestinal atresias.[18] Extrinsic obstruction has many causes, including malrotation with Ladd bands, preduodenal portal vein, gastroduodenal duplications, cysts or pseudocysts of the pancreas and biliary tree, and annular pancreas. Annular pancreas is almost invariably associated with an intrinsic cause of duodenal obstruction.

Intrinsic duodenal obstructions and annular pancreas are developmental abnormalities that occur during early development of the GI tract. Duodenal atresia and stenosis are believed to result from a failure of the recanalization process that occurs during the first trimester (Fig. 68-13). Annular pancreas was originally suggested by Lecco[19] to occur when the ventral bud fails to rotate behind the duodenum, leaving pancreatic tissue fully encircling the second portion of the duodenum. This results in a nondistensible ring of pancreatic parenchyma and a functional stenosis (Fig. 68-14). Immunohistochemical studies of the annular tissue have identified pancreatic polypeptide-rich islets, also known to predominate in the ventral anlage, and lend credence to this hypothesis.[20] Annular pancreas frequently coexists with intrinsic duodenal anomalies and anomalies of

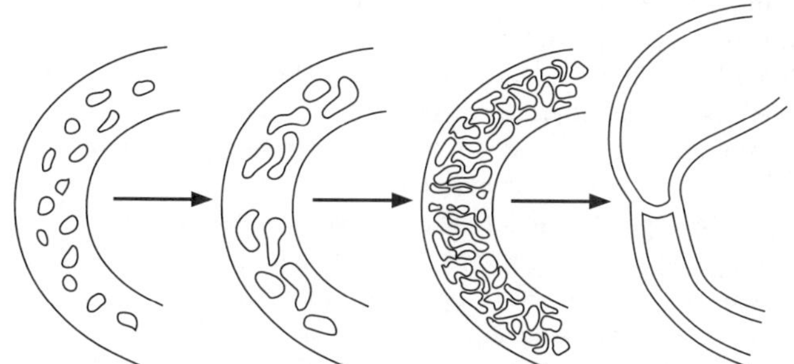

FIG. 68-13. Failure of duodenal recanalization during weeks 8 to 10 of gestation, resulting in a persistent endoluminal membrane.

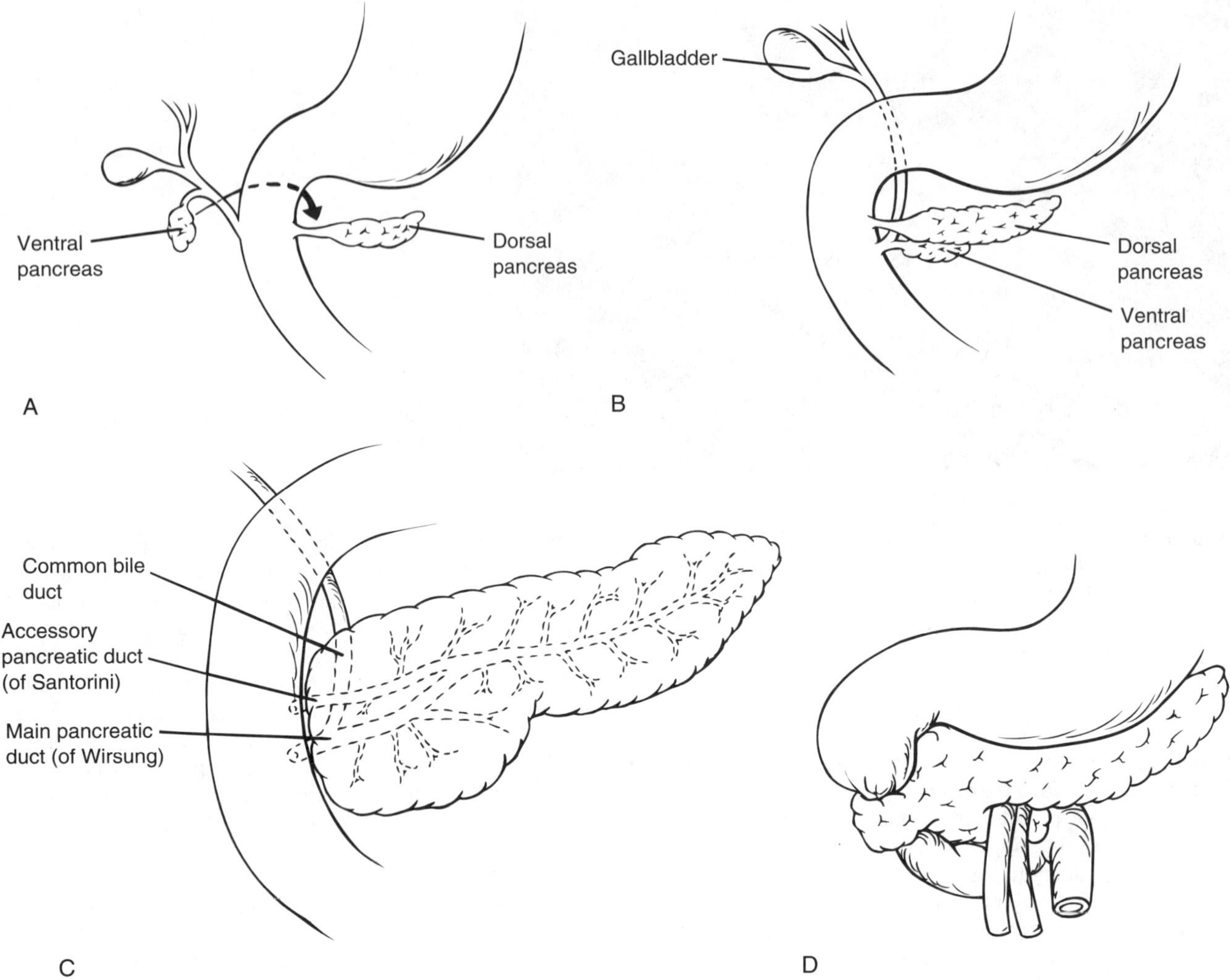

FIG. 68-14. Proposed cause of annular pancreas. (*A* to *C*) Normal process of migration of the ventral pancreas and bile duct behind the duodenum. The ventral pancreatic duct fuses with the dorsal duct, producing the major pancreatic duct (of Wirsung) and the major papilla. (*D*) Persistent annulus of pancreatic parenchyma results from failure of ventral pancreatic migration.

the pancreaticobiliary ductal system, suggesting closely linked mechanisms of pancreatic, duodenal, and biliary development during this stage.

Atresias of the duodenum have three basic morphologic appearances (Fig. 68-15). Type I atresias are characterized by luminal webs or membranes, which include mucosal and submucosal layers. Endoluminal membranes usually span the duodenal lumen at the level where the dilated proximal duodenum changes to a smaller, distal segment. Of particular interest are membranes that take on a windsock morphology, in which the endoluminal membrane extends distally for a variable distance from its origin. An external transition zone then occurs at the leading edge of the windsock; a significant portion of the dilated duodenum may therefore be distal to the point of obstruction. Type II atresias have dilated proximal and diminutive distal segments connected by a fibrous cord. Type III atresias are characterized by a complete discontinuity or gap between the segments. Congenital intrinsic stenoses are caused by luminal membranes identical to Type I atresias, but contain a crescentic

defect or central fenestration of variable size. Large openings can provide a conduit of sufficient size to postpone symptoms until later in life.

The relation between the point of obstruction and the ampulla of Vater is important. Most series document a predominance of postampullary obstructions, approaching 80% in some studies.[21] A European report described a preampullary predominance.[22] Obstructions caused by a membrane are frequently associated with anomalies of the common bile duct. Instead of opening into the medial wall of the duodenum, the common bile duct may terminate with one or more ductules within the membrane itself.

Congenital duodenal obstructions are commonly associated with other serious congenital anomalies, which account for most of the morbidity and mortality in these patients. Various reports put the incidence of associated conditions between 50% and 80%. Structural congenital heart disease and trisomy 21 (Down syndrome) are the most common associated conditions, each occurring in about 30% of cases.[23] Not infrequently, all three

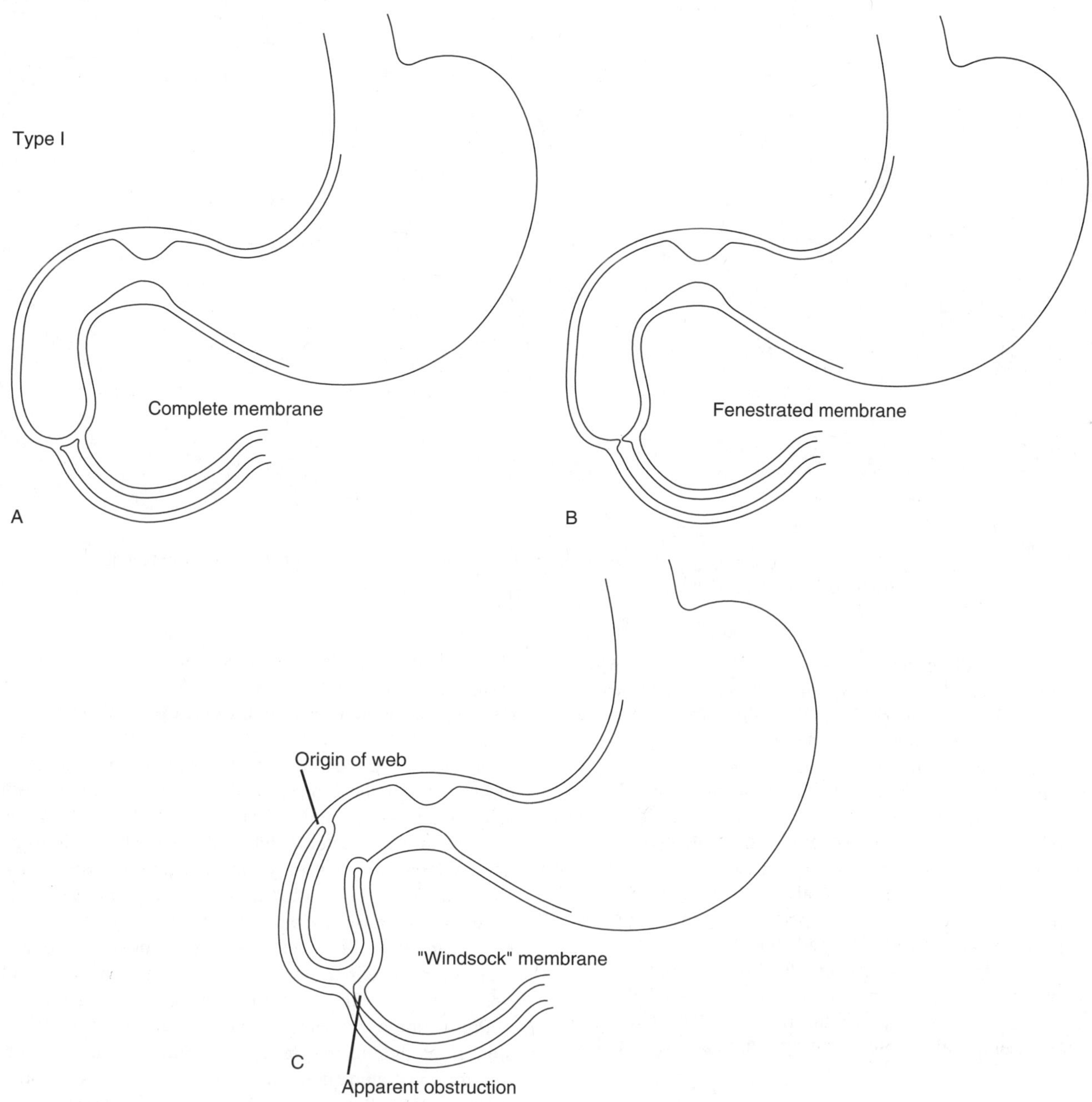

FIG. 68-15. Variants of congenital duodenal obstruction. Type I refers to a luminal membrane, which can be simple, fenestrated, or elongated (windsock). (*Figure continues.*)

conditions coexist in the same patient.[24] In patients with trisomy 21 who underwent prenatal ultrasonography, about 4% were found to have prenatal evidence of duodenal atresia.[25] Other associated anomalies include intestinal malrotation in about 20%, esophageal atresia or imperforate anus in 10% to 20%, corporal asymmetry, and gallbladder agenesis. The outcome for patients with duodenal atresia depends more on the severity and correctability of these associated anomalies than on the surgical management of the obstruction.

The diagnosis of duodenal atresia is often suggested by prenatal ultrasound (Fig. 68-16). A maternal history of polyhydramnios is common in congenital duodenal obstruction, approaching 75% in one series.[26] Prenatal sonographic evaluation of the fetus in these instances can detect two fluid-filled structures consistent with a double-bubble reliably at 22 to 23 weeks' gestation, with the earliest detection having been reported at 18 weeks.[27] About 15% to 20% of patients with duodenal atresia have the diagnosis suggested by prenatal ultrasonography. Reliable data regarding the rate of false-positive examinations for duodenal obstruction in the fetus are unavailable.

The clinical presentation of the infant with congenital duodenal obstruction depends on the presence or absence of a membranous aperture, its size, and the location of the obstruction relative to the ampulla. The classic presentation of a complete postampullary obstruction includes bilious vomiting within 24 hours of birth in an otherwise stable infant with a nondistended

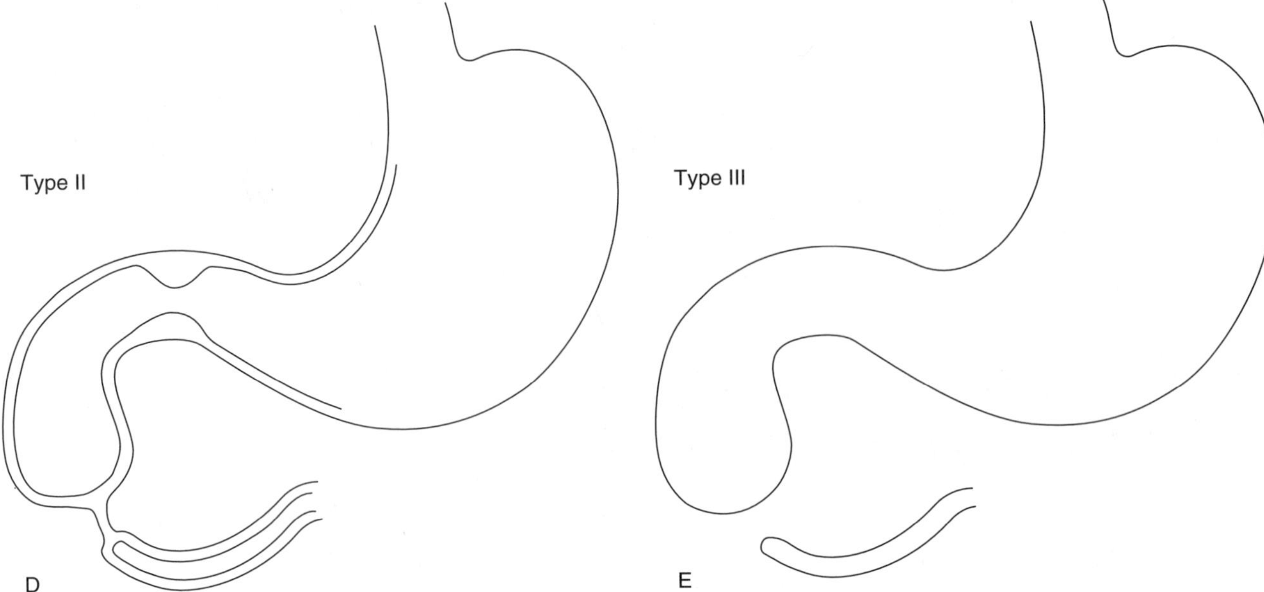

FIG. 68-15. *Continued.* Types II and III describe atresias with complete mural discontinuity with or without a connecting fibrous cord, respectively.

abdomen. Plain radiographs of the abdomen typically show the classic double-bubble sign—two distinct gas collections or air–fluid levels in the upper abdomen resulting from the markedly dilated stomach and proximal duodenal bulb (Fig. 68-17). If the infant's stomach has been decompressed by vomiting or previous nasogastric aspiration, 40 to 60 mL of air may be injected carefully through the nasogastric tube and the double-bubble reproduced. Air makes an excellent contrast agent, obviating an upper GI tract contrast study in routine cases. The distal intestinal tract may be gasless or may reveal a small amount of intraluminal air, owing to a membranous aperture, a microperforation of an otherwise complete web,[28] or a patent, bifid bile duct with ostia on both sides of the obstructing diaphragm.[29]

The importance of differentiating intrinsic duodenal obstruction from intestinal malrotation with a midgut volvulus in the infant who presents with bilious vomiting cannot be overstated. A

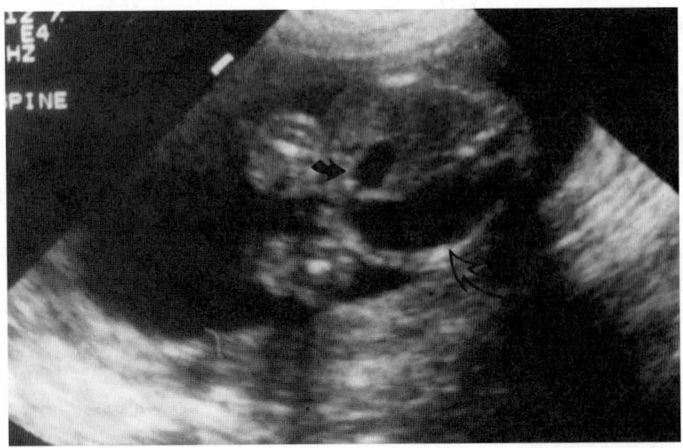

FIG. 68-16. Prenatal ultrasound of a fetus with duodenal atresia showing the dilated duodenum (*closed arrow*) and stomach (*open arrow*).

clue may be derived from the appearance of the duodenum on the plain radiograph. In the classic double-bubble sign, the duodenum appears dilated and round, owing to chronic intrauterine obstruction. When a distended stomach is associated with a near-normal-caliber duodenum, or the obstruction appears to be at the third portion of the duodenum, the diagnosis of malrotation with an incomplete duodenal obstruction secondary to Ladd bands or volvulus must be entertained. Emergent echocardiography and upper GI tract contrast study may be required to establish the correct diagnosis when an infant displays hemodynamic compromise, since therapy obviously differs for congenital heart disease and midgut volvulus. Even when the diagnosis of duodenal atresia is established in the stable patient, cardiac anatomy and function should be evaluated before surgical correction.

Preoperative preparation includes nasogastric decompression, fluid and electrolyte replacement, and a thorough evaluation for associated anomalies. If malrotation is ruled out, surgical correction of duodenal atresia can be temporarily postponed, and more urgent conditions evaluated and treated. Prophylactic perioperative antibiotics, usually ampicillin and gentamicin, are begun preoperatively.

Surgical management of intrinsic duodenal obstruction is commenced through a transverse right upper quadrant incision. The ligament of Treitz is identified to exclude concomitant intestinal malrotation. It may be necessary to mobilize the hepatic flexure of the colon to expose the duodenum. True atresia with mural discontinuity and annular pancreas is easily recognized. More often, mural continuity is maintained, and the presence of an intraluminal membrane is inferred. When a windsock diaphragm is present, however, the transitional region may not coincide with the location of the obstruction.

The most widely accepted surgical management of both true atresia and annular pancreas involves constructing an anastomosis between the dilated proximal duodenum and the diminutive distal duodenum. The long side-to-side duodenoduodenostomy

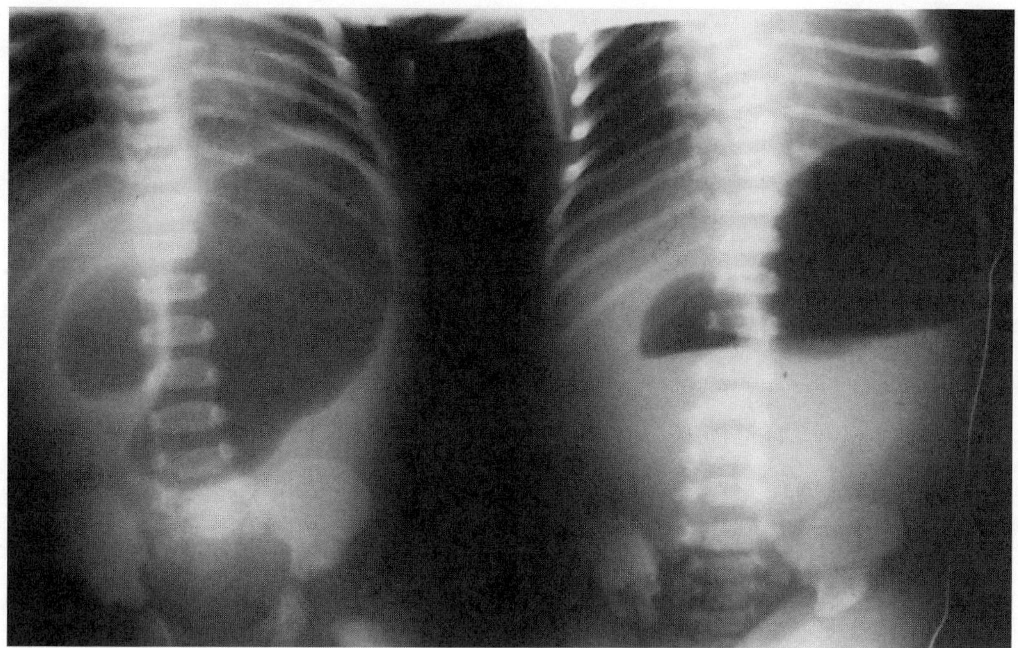

FIG. 68-17. Supine and upright air-contrast radiographs displaying the classic appearance of a double bubble in duodenal atresia.

is an effective procedure but has been associated with a high incidence of anastomotic dysfunction and prolonged obstruction. The duodenojejunostomy, commonly employed in the past, is also associated with greater morbidity and is now reserved for special circumstances, such as the presence of a long gap between proximal and distal duodenal segments or a large ventral pancreatic remnant that prevents apposition of the duodenal segments. Gastrojejunostomy is an unacceptable alternative, given the high incidence of marginal ulceration and bleeding.

The diamond duodenoduodenostomy, as described by Kimura and colleagues,[30] has yielded consistently good results. Limited mobilization of the duodenum distal to the atresia may be necessary to facilitate apposition of the segments. A transverse incision is made in the anterior wall of the distal-most portion of the dilated proximal duodenal pouch, and an incision of similar length is made in a longitudinal orientation on the antimesenteric border of the distal duodenum. The anastomosis is fashioned in such a way as to approximate the ends of one incision to the midpoints of the other incision. The tension resulting from this orientation tends to hold the anastomosis open in a self-stenting manner (Fig. 68-18).

In Kimura's series[30] of patients managed with the diamond-type duodenoduodenostomy, two thirds were followed up with contrast studies and displayed no significant anastomotic dysfunction or residual megaduodenum. In contrast, a contemporary series of standard side-to-side anastomoses reported a 30% incidence of radiographic abnormalities related to anastomotic dysfunction, including megaduodenum with delayed transit.[26] An additional 17% displayed GER, which may have been due, in part, to a relative impairment in gastric emptying. Even with the diamond anastomosis, a persistent megaduodenum with symptomatic partial obstruction and stasis can occur. This complication may be effectively managed by a tapering duodenoplasty.

The surgical management of an intrinsic duodenal web begins

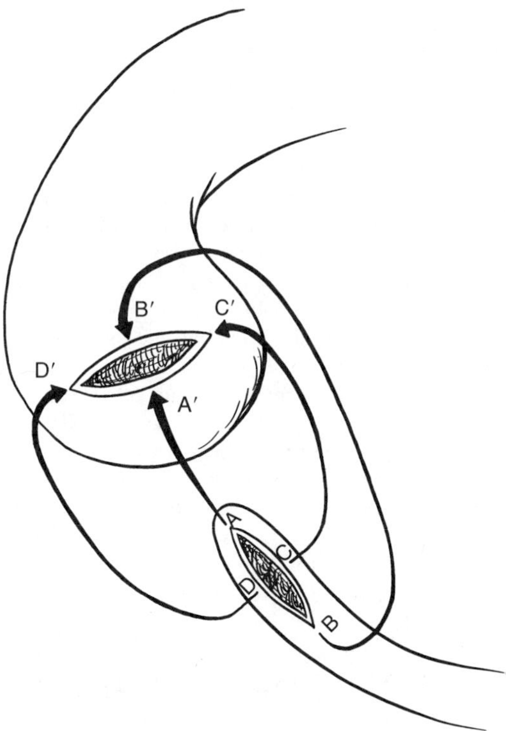

FIG. 68-18. Technique of diamond duodenoduodenostomy as described by Kimura and colleagues. (After Kimura K, Mukohara N, Nashijima E, et al. Diamond-shaped anastomosis for duodenal atresia: an experience with 44 patients over 15 years. J Pediatr Surg 1990;25:977)

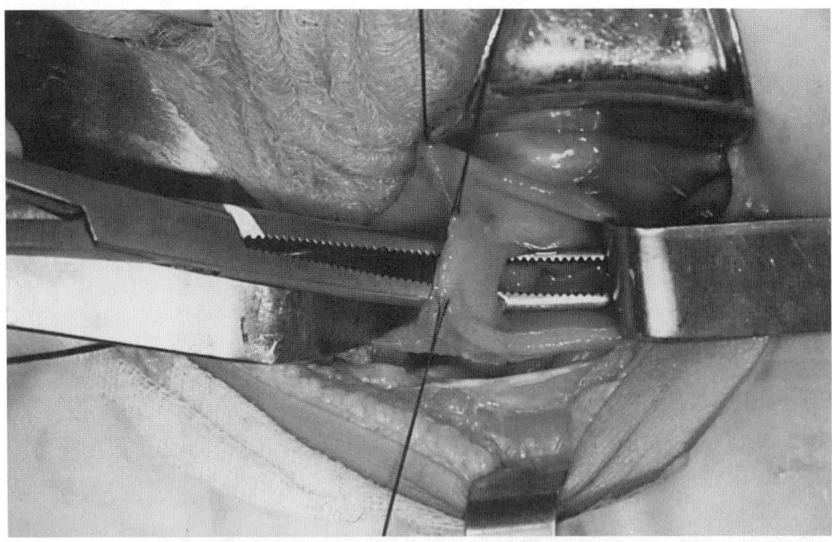

FIG. 68-19. Intraoperative appearance of a fenestrated duodenal web.

with a longitudinal incision centered over the web origin. The site of origin, however, may not be easily identified. Palpation of the duodenal wall may reveal a thickened circumferential ridge. When this is not detected, a catheter can be advanced by the anesthesiologist and guided into the duodenum by the surgeon. When the advancing catheter encounters the web, further advancement produces an indentation on the wall of the duodenum. This may be at or proximal to the actual transition zone. Once the site of attachment has been determined, stay sutures are placed in the antimesenteric wall and the duodenum opened longitudinally for a short distance (less than 1 cm) in both directions (Fig. 68-19).

Because of the high incidence of bile duct anomalies, a thorough search for the ampulla and accessory ductal ostia is important. If these are separate from the membrane, a portion of the web on the antimesenteric aspect of the lumen can be excised. If anomalous bile ducts involve the web itself, the uninvolved portion of the web can be incised from the antimesenteric border to the center. In either case, the longitudinal incision is closed transversely, widening the lumen at that point. An additional option is a diamond anastomosis, bypassing the web to avoid injury to the common bile duct.

A feeding gastrostomy should not be necessary for postoperative management of an uncomplicated duodenal repair. Gastroduodenal function usually returns within 5 to 7 days, at which time enteral feeding can be initiated with small boluses and progressively advanced in volume as tolerated. Results of surgery are generally good. As mentioned earlier, complications related to surgery are directly related to the underlying pathology and choice of operation. Survival rates of 95% are commonly reported in those for whom surgery is deemed appropriate, and virtually all the mortality in these series was due to associated conditions.

ACQUIRED ABNORMALITIES OF THE STOMACH AND DUODENUM

Hypertrophic Pyloric Stenosis

The first accurate clinicopathologic description of HPS in an infant is credited to Hirschsprung in the late nineteenth century, who considered it to be a congenital disease. At that time, surgical management consisted of gastrojejunostomy, which resulted in a mortality rate of 60%. Extramucosal pyloroplasty was unsatisfactory, owing in large part to excessive hemorrhage, which occurred when sutures tore through the edematous muscle that had been closed. In 1911, Ramstedt omitted this unnecessary muscle closure and thus defined the pyloromyotomy procedure that has since been recognized as the definitive standard.

HPS is defined as an acquired condition in which the circumferential muscle of the pyloric sphincter becomes thickened, resulting in elongation and obliteration of the pyloric channel. This produces a high-grade gastric outlet obstruction with compensatory dilation, hypertrophy, and hyperperistalsis of the stomach. The thickening of the smooth muscle results from hypertrophy, not from hyperplasia.

The incidence of HPS ranges between 0.1% and 1% in the general population and appears to be rising. Studies conducted 40 years ago reported rates of 1 in 300 to 1 in 900. More recent population-based studies from the United Kingdom have documented a rise in incidence from 0.1% to 0.2% up to 0.3% to 0.8% during the past several decades. A large population-based study conducted by the Mayo Clinic documented an overall incidence of 0.26% in Olmsted County, Minnesota, from 1950 to 1984, but reported that the rate approached 0.5% by the end of the study period.[31] A longitudinal study employed ultrasonographic evaluation of 1400 randomly selected term neonates.[32] All 9 infants in whom HPS later developed (0.65%) had ultrasonographically normal pyloric dimensions at birth. There is a significant male predominance of about 4 : 1, although the long-held belief that HPS primarily afflicts first-born males has not been confirmed. The incidence in whites exceeds that in blacks by several fold; the incidence in Asian infants is low. The development of HPS appears to involve the variable transmission of an inheritable trait between generations. Transmission from mothers is more common than from fathers: HPS develops in 19% of boys and 7% of girls whose mothers had HPS as infants and in 5% of boys and 2.5% of girls whose fathers were previously affected.[33]

The cause of HPS remains unknown, but several hypotheses have been suggested. One proposal is that dyscoordination between gastric peristaltic activity and pyloric relaxation causes inappropriate pyloric contraction in the face of elevated intragastric pressures. This presumably results in work hypertrophy of the pyloric muscle and initiates a cycle of increasing pyloric obstruction and gastric contractions. Although functional disturbances in gastric emptying in the first weeks of life have not been reported to occur in neonates in whom HPS later develops, a report of in utero gastric dilation in a neonate who later experienced HPS may warrant further investigation.[34]

The pathophysiology of pyloric dysfunction in HPS has not been defined. Observations regarding decreased ganglion cell density in the pyloric region have not been consistently reproduced, nor does such an observation explain the curative role of pyloromyotomy. Attempts to establish a causative link between the hypergastrinemia and hyperacidity seen in these patients and HPS have also been unsuccessful. In fact, gastrin-mediated acid secretion is an expected consequence of any gastric outlet obstruction that produces gastric distention. Elevated levels of certain prostaglandins (eg, PGE_2 and PGF_2-α) have been described in these patients and have been proposed to cause pyloric constriction with the eventual development of HPS. Gastric outlet obstruction due to pylorospasm has been reported in neonates receiving prostaglandin infusions. Pyloric dysfunction in these infants, however, does not lead to muscular hypertrophy.[35]

Perhaps a more promising hypothesis for the pathophysiology of HPS is a primary abnormality of the ENS. Immunohistochemical identification of a variety of neuropeptides, such as GRP, VIP, somatostatin, and substance P, has revealed a marked reduction in these neuropeptides in patients with HPS as compared with normal controls.[36] Another observation has implicated a local decrease in nitric oxide, a ubiquitous mediator of smooth muscle relaxation, as a causative factor in the development of HPS. Nitric oxide synthase, which can be identified in significant concentrations in the pyloric circular and longitudinal muscle layers and the myenteric plexus in normal controls, has been shown to be selectively absent in the circular muscle layer in patients with HPS.[37] Furthermore, ENS axons within the circular muscle layer were morphologically distorted. Another study has reported axonal degeneration in both the myenteric plexus and the intramuscular nerves in patients with HPS.[38] Whatever the primary disorder underlying HPS is, it appears to be transient because recurrence after surgery is rare.

The typical clinical presentation is a term male infant between 3 and 6 weeks of age who has progressive, nonbilious, projectile vomiting. Many infants are initially thought to have a food allergy or GER until the vomiting consistently follows every feeding and is forceful. At the time of presentation, many infants with HPS are significantly dehydrated. Inanition fortunately is no longer a common finding. Serum chemistries reflect a hypochloremic, hypokalemic contraction metabolic alkalosis, which may be associated with paradoxical aciduria when severe. Significant hypoglycemia can also be present and may cause seizures. Unconjugated hyperbilirubinemia is common and correlates with a decrease in hepatic glucuronyltransferase activity. The jaundice is transient and resolves as soon as the gastric outlet obstruction is corrected, making it attractive to speculate that the hepatic defect is secondary to abnormal enteroendocrine feedback between the stomach and the hepatocyte.

The hallmark of the diagnosis is the finding of a small, mobile, ovoid mass referred to as an *olive* (because of its size and shape) in the epigastrium. The process of detecting the olive may difficult. Two or three fingertips are gently placed in the upper abdomen and gently advanced into the deeper tissues below the liver edge. They are then slowly swept inferiorly toward the umbilicus. The olive can be felt to roll under the fingertips during this sweeping motion—no other structure gives this sensation. The art of detecting the olive lies in performing the examination under conditions conducive to deep abdominal palpation in a quiet, cooperative infant. Sometimes considerable time—15 to 20 minutes—may be required to obtain conditions that are conducive for palpation of the hypertrophied pylorus. Prior nasogastric suctioning to empty the stomach followed by removal of the tube allows the surgeon to examine the abdomen while the baby is sucking on a small amount of dextrose water. This often permits a more thorough palpation of the pyloric region. If the pylorus is unequivocally felt, the diagnosis is established, and no further diagnostic maneuvers are necessary.

If the pylorus is not detected and the clinical presentation is sufficiently suggestive to warrant further evaluation, radiologic evaluation can be definitive. Real-time ultrasonography has supplanted barium upper GI tract study as the procedure of choice. Teele and Smith[39] observed the hypertrophied pylorus to have a characteristic appearance on B-mode ultrasound, and subsequently it has been shown that measurement of pyloric dimensions accurately establishes the diagnosis of HPS. Parameters measured include overall diameter, single wall thickness, and pyloric channel length, with the latter two being the most commonly used (Fig. 68-20). Measurements found to have greater than 90% positive predictive value include diameter 17 mm or more, muscular wall thickness 4 mm or greater, and channel length 17 mm or greater. In infants 30 days of age or younger, it has been suggested that diagnostic criteria for wall thickness be reduced to 3 mm.[40] When parameters are equivocal (eg, wall thickness 2 to 3 mm, channel length 12 to 16 mm), especially in younger infants, calculation of the pyloric volume has been reported to have greater diagnostic accuracy than the individual measurements alone.[41] Finally, upper GI tract study can be diagnostic in cases in which ultrasound is equivocal by demonstrating an elongated and narrowed pyloric channel, with the characteristic shoulders of the hypertrophied pylorus bulging into the gastric lumen (Fig. 68-21).

Although an accurate diagnosis based on physical examination should be possible in most cases, and should be attempted in all, it is evident that an increasing reliance on ultrasonography will continue to erode the skills of examiners. A review comparing diagnostic accuracy between two eras in a single pediatric institution found that the sensitivity of physical examination declined by half during a period of increasing reliance on ultrasound.[42] It is likely that ultrasound, a noninvasive, highly accurate, and relatively inexpensive technology, will experience even greater popularity in the future among primary care providers who first evaluate these infants.

Preoperative preparation is critical once the diagnosis is made. HPS is not a surgical emergency, so careful correction of fluid and electrolyte losses should be accomplished before operative intervention. The infant who presents early in the course of the disease with no clinical dehydration, normal serum electrolytes and glucose, and a normal urine output can be operated on at the earliest convenience. Many patients, however, present with dehydration, hypoglycemia, or a contraction alka-

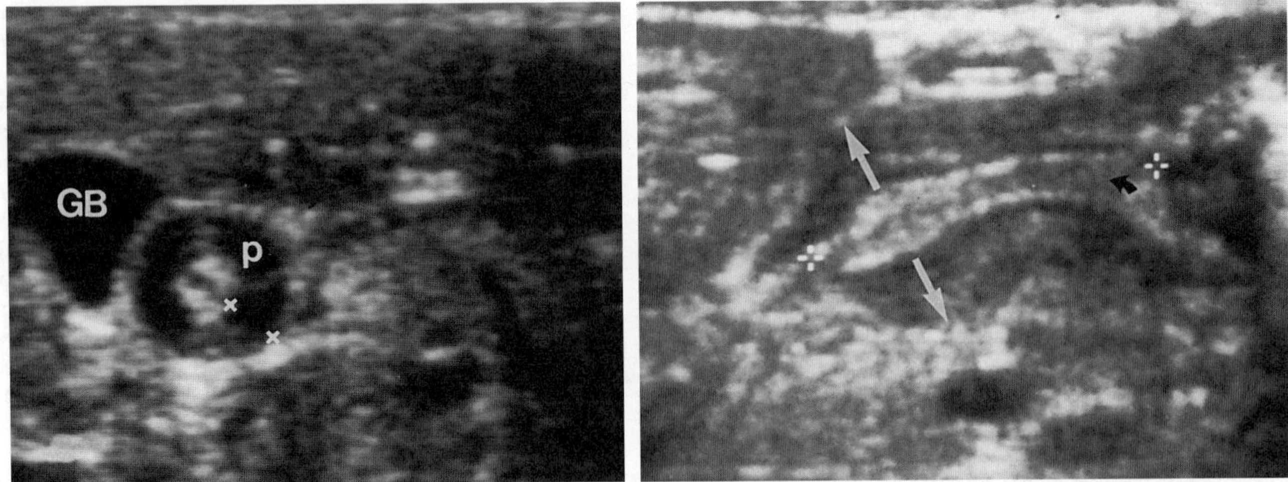

FIG. 68-20. Two-dimensional ultrasonographic findings in hypertrophic pyloric stenosis. (*A*) Transverse view showing cross section of hypertrophied pylorus (P) and adjacent gallbladder (GB). The thickness of the echolucent circumferential muscle layer is measured by the distance between the cursors. (*B*) Longitudinal view showing echolucent muscle walls in profile (*white arrows*). They are separated by two echogenic lines that represent the submucosa and an echolucent core that represents the pyloric channel lumen (*black arrow*). The channel length between the cursors is increased in hypertrophic pyloric stenosis.

losis of sufficient severity to require preoperative resuscitation for 24 to 48 hours. Infants with severe intravascular fluid deficits causing hypoperfusion should first be resuscitated with isotonic lactated Ringer solution in boluses of 10 to 20 mL/kg until hemodynamic stability is documented. Most preexisting deficits can be replaced with 5% dextrose in 0.45% NaCl, which is administered intravenously at 1.5 times the maintenance rate. Because total body potassium and chloride deficits are considerable in these patients, the maintenance fluid is supplemented with KCl at a concentration of 20 to 40 mEq/L. The serum potassium level underestimates the potassium deficit because alkalosis shifts extracellular potassium ions into the intracellular compartment. Once volume status and urine output have normalized, serum chloride and potassium have normalized, and serum bicarbonate is trending below 30 mEq/L, surgery can be conducted safely.

The treatment of HPS is pyloromyotomy. The operation is performed through a transverse right upper quadrant incision over the rectus muscle at or above the liver edge. The rectus muscle is either divided or split longitudinally, and the peritoneal cavity is entered through the posterior rectus sheath. The pylorus may be identified by delivering the greater curvature of the stomach through the wound and using it as a fulcrum to externalize the pylorus. The pylorus usually has a pale white

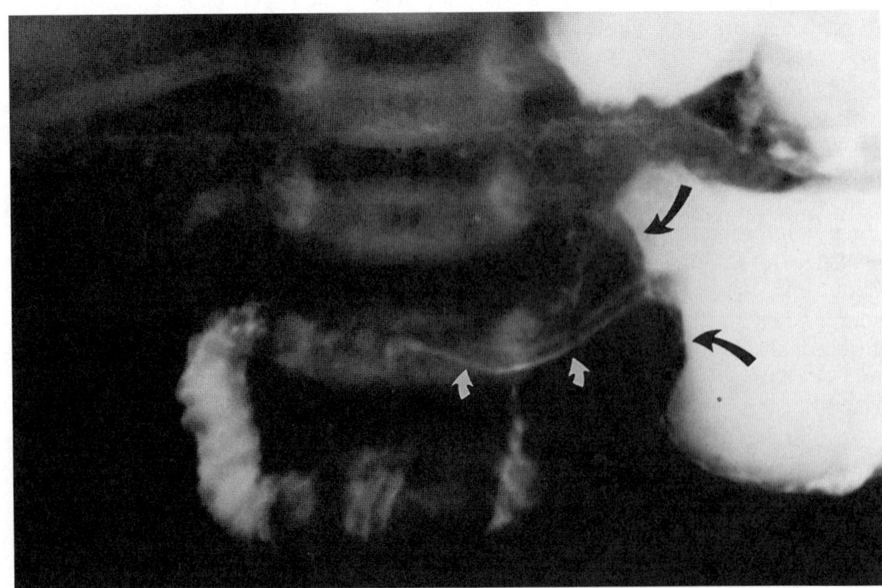

FIG. 68-21. Upper gastrointestinal tract contrast study findings in hypertrophic pyloric stenosis, displaying the "string sign" of a stenotic channel lumen (*white arrows*) and the bulging "shoulders" of the hypertrophic pyloric muscle (*black arrows*).

appearance and a rubbery texture. A superficial incision is made through the serosa on the anterior surface from a point 1 to 2 mm from the duodenal end to the antrum. The duodenal end is usually easily identified by the color change from the pale pylorus to the pink duodenal wall, and is further delimited by the pyloric vein, which is often prominent. Careful definition of the duodenal border is important because the duodenal mucosa prolapses over the shoulder of the distal end of the pylorus. If the initial incision is extended too far distally, the duodenal lumen may be entered as the myotomy is deepened.

The myotomy is commenced where the pylorus is thickest and its fibers most easily split. The myotomy is deepened to the submucosa, extending proximally to the antrum and distally to the pyloric vein. To perform the myotomy, the back of a scalpel handle is a safe instrument; many pediatric surgeons use a pyloric spreader. It is necessary to divide the fibers along the entire length of the pylorus down to the level of the submucosa. Once the submucosa is exposed, the overlying muscle fibers should be gently mobilized off the submucosa to an extent sufficient to allow the submucosa and mucosa to herniate or bulge out (Fig. 68-22). Care must be taken to avoid tearing the underlying mucosa, particularly at the duodenal end. Deliberate attention to the possibility of a mucosal tear is important because the morbidity associated with a recognized injury is minimal, while that associated with delayed recognition is not. When the hypertrophied muscle has been adequately mobilized and the two halves of the pylorus can be moved back and forth in opposite directions producing a rocking motion, the pyloromyotomy is complete, and the pylorus is returned to the abdominal cavity. Venous congestion caused by delivering the pylorus through a relatively small incision under moderate traction can result in venous bleeding from the submucosa and the cut surface of the muscle. This bleeding ceases when the pylorus is returned to the abdomen, and electrocautery is unnecessary. The wound is closed in layers as usual.

If the submucosa or mucosa of the underlying pyloric channel or duodenum is violated, the management of this perforation should be individualized. If the lumen is entered early in the conduct of the pyloromyotomy, the mucosa is closed with fine absorbable sutures; attempts to continue the muscle spreading only enlarge the rent. The muscle is closed over the mucosal repair, and a second myotomy is performed by rotating the pylorus 180 degrees. If the tear occurs at a point when the myotomy is essentially complete, the tear can be closed with fine absorbable sutures and covered with a portion of the gastro-colic omentum, obviating a second myotomy. In this situation, some surgeons prefer to decompress the stomach for several days until GI function fully returns. Others contend that the nasogastric tube represents a risk of reperforation and simply withhold feeding for several days. Water-soluble contrast studies are unnecessary before feeding unless clinically indicated for other reasons.

The postoperative management of an uncomplicated pyloromyotomy is straightforward. A feeding regimen is begun 6 to 8 hours after operation with a small volume of sugar water, advancing volume and osmolarity every 3 hours until the infant is taking formula or milk ad libitum. It is common for occasional emesis to occur after pyloromyotomy; this should not delay the progression of the feeding schedule in most cases. In general, most infants so managed are able to be discharged within 24 to 48 hours of surgery.

Persistent postoperative vomiting beyond 48 hours is uncommon. In this circumstance, the possibilities of an incomplete myotomy or unrecognized perforation should be considered. Contrast studies are of little value in evaluating the completeness of the myotomy because the radiologic and ultrasonographic appearances of the hypertrophied pylorus before and after myotomy are similar. A contrast study should be obtained, however, to exclude a mucosal leak with a peripyloric fluid collection compressing the gastric outlet. In the absence of a leak or complete obstruction, an interval of at least 2 weeks is allowed to pass before the presumptive diagnosis of incomplete myotomy prompts reexploration.

Most children treated for HPS can expect excellent short-term and long-term outcomes. With appropriate resuscitation, expert anesthesia, and a standard surgical approach, mortality has been virtually eliminated. The reported rates of duodenal perforation range from 3% to 30% (depending on whether the procedures were performed by pediatric surgeons), although rates above 10% are unusual. Wound infection and dehiscence,

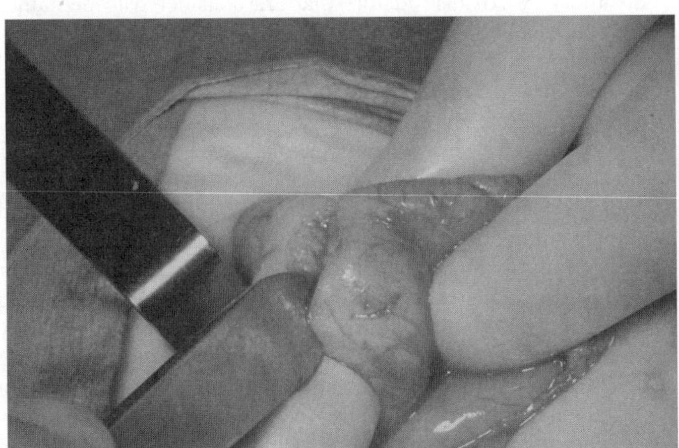
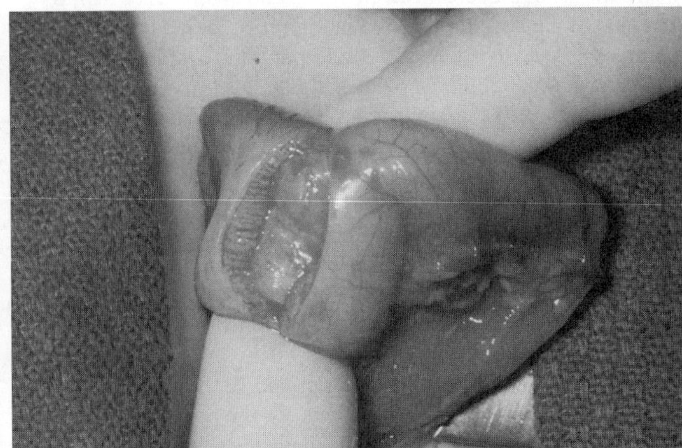

A   B

FIG. 68-22. Operative technique of pyloromyotomy. (*A*) The pyloric muscle is split longitudinally with the blunt end of a scalpel handle. (*B*) Completed myotomy allows the submucosal layer to bulge out to the level of the serosa.

significant problems in previous eras, are relatively uncommon today. A study addressing gastric emptying and abdominal symptoms after pyloromyotomy found no differences between treatment and control groups several decades after surgery.[43]

Acid-Peptic Disease

The most common clinical disorders implicating the stomach and duodenum in human disease involve acid-peptic injury to the mucosa, resulting in inflammation, superficial erosions, and ulcerations. Hence, the physiologic and pharmacologic regulation of acid secretion have become important areas of investigation. Despite significant progress in the understanding of the physiology of acid secretion, the many causes of acid-peptic disease (APD) still lack complete explanation.

Although the incidence of APD in adults is gradually declining, it appears to be increasing in children. This is in part due to the increased use of endoscopy in evaluating children with abdominal symptoms, but there are indications that the prevalence of the disease in children is also increasing. Increased usage of ulcerogenic drugs (eg, nonsteroidal antiinflammatory agents) and an increase in the numbers of children subjected to and surviving physiologically stressful events (eg, trauma, burns, cancer chemotherapy, bone marrow transplantation) may contribute to this increased incidence.

It is commonly accepted that most ulcers follow a progression from mucosal inflammation to superficial erosions to actual ulcers. Superficial erosions are defined as discrete, punctate defects in the mucosa that extend only into the submucosa. An ulcer must extend at least through the submucosa and muscularis mucosa into the muscularis propria. Ulcers are usually accompanied by significant inflammation and edema as well as by thickened ruggal folds that radiate away from the lesion. Both erosions and ulcers can disrupt underlying intramural blood vessels and cause hemorrhage. True ulcers can extend through the entire wall, leading to hemorrhage from major adjacent arteries (eg, the gastroduodenal artery), free perforation, or retroperitoneal penetration (eg, into the head of the pancreas).

The process of peptic ulceration requires an imbalance between the aggressive forces of hydrochloric acid and activated pepsin and the protective mechanisms that serve to defend the gastroduodenal mucosa from chemical and autodigestive injury. Any one of a large number of abnormalities in this homeostatic balance can lead to progressive mucosal injury. Although maximal acid outputs and basal acid outputs are often increased in children with APD, a significant degree of overlap exists between the APD patients and normal controls. Furthermore, the degree of maximal acid output elevation correlates poorly with duration and severity of symptoms (although it correlates somewhat better with prognosis and need for surgical intervention). It is therefore difficult to ascribe a causal relation between hyperacidity and clinical disease. Simple acid hypersecretion is probably the principal cause of APD in only a minority of patients.

Gastroduodenal ulcers in children can be defined as either primary or secondary. Primary ulcers are the result of an intrinsic ulcer diathesis and are not associated either with contributing extrinsic factors or with other acute medical illnesses. They are usually duodenal in location, but concurrent pyloric channel ulcerations can also occur. Primary gastric ulcers in children are rare. These ulcers are chronic and usually present with longstanding complaints of abdominal symptoms. Acute primary ulcers are probably present for a considerable time before causing symptoms.

Although most patients with primary APD do not have any definable underlying condition, a small number of patients have a known cause for acid hypersecretion. The most well characterized of these conditions is the Zollinger-Ellison syndrome (ZES), caused by a secreting gastrinoma. Other conditions associated with primary APD include G-cell hyperplasia, G-cell hyperfunction, and systemic mastocytosis.

Much attention has focused on a possible infectious etiology for primary APD. *Helicobacter pylori* (previously *Campylobacter pylori*), a fastidious spiral-shaped gram-negative rod, has been recovered from antral biopsy specimens in virtually all adults and children with primary gastritis or duodenal ulcers. The organism is occasionally recovered from the duodenum as well, but only from areas of gastric metaplasia. Most or all children with *H pylori*–associated antral gastritis alone do not have symptoms, and their gross endoscopic findings are frequently normal. Those with endoscopic abnormalities display a characteristic antral nodularity but no inflammation. Histopathologic examination of biopsy material in all patients, however, uniformly reveals chronic inflammatory changes with mononuclear cell infiltrates.

The high correlation between *H pylori*–associated chronic gastritis and primary duodenal ulcer suggests a causative link between the two conditions. The virulence factors influencing the ability of *H pylori* to invade and colonize the antral mucosa involve urease production, flagellar-mediated motility, and specific membrane-associated adhesins that allow the microorganism to attach to gastric cells. The pathophysiologic mechanisms that translate antral colonization into duodenal ulceration are unknown but probably involve gastrin hypersecretion by the chronically inflamed antral mucosa. Basal, peak, and 24-hour integrated gastrin levels are increased in patients with *H pylori* gastritis and duodenal ulcer; elevations in basal or stimulated acid outputs, however, have not been consistently observed.[44] Although the causal link has not been firmly established, the prevention of recurrence of primary APD in children appears to require the eradication of *H pylori*–associated antral gastritis.[45]

Secondary APD occurs in association with other unrelated disorders or extrinsic factors that are considered to be pathophysiologically linked to ulcer formation. This association may be through either acid hypersecretion or compromise of mucosal defense mechanisms. These include physiologically stressful events (hence the term *stress ulcer*), such as neonatal hypoxia, sepsis, trauma, head injury (Cushing ulcer), and severe burns (Curling ulcer). Drug-related secondary APD in children most commonly occurs with the use of aspirin and other nonsteroidal antiinflammatory drugs. These compounds decrease mucosal blood flow by inhibiting prostaglandin synthesis; inhibit other defense mechanisms, such as bicarbonate and mucus secretion; and stimulate the elaboration of other cytotoxic inflammatory mediators. Secondary APD is more common in most pediatric series than is primary disease and involves the stomach as often as the duodenum. Additionally, the incidence of complications (ie, hemorrhage and perforation) and death are much higher in secondary APD than in primary APD.[46]

As in adults, the treatment of choice for most children with primary APD is medical management. Strategies to control the adverse effects of gastric acid include acid neutralization (antacids), stimulus inhibition (H_2 blockers such as ranitidine), inhibition of acid production (proton pump blockade such as omeprazole), and mucosal protection (binding resins such as sucralfate). Insights into the mechanism of action of sucralfate suggest that it functions not only by providing a protective physiochemical barrier but also by enhancing mucosal microvascular flow and by the protective binding of basic fibroblast growth factor, a prime regulator of angiogenesis and ulcer healing.[47]

The treatment of secondary APD involves all of these approaches and also includes prostaglandin replacement (eg, misoprostol, a PGE_1 analogue) to restore mucosal perfusion in patients receiving nonsteroidal antiinflammatory drugs. Obviously, the single most important component of stress ulcer management is to remove the precipitating event. This, of course, is not often possible, accounting for the high degree of treatment failure and complications in this group.

Because of the high morbidity associated with stress ulceration, treatment has focused on prevention in high-risk patients. Maintenance of an intragastric pH higher than 4 clearly reduces the incidence of APD-associated hemorrhage. Although this can be accomplished with equal efficacy using antacids or H_2 blockers, H_2 blockade is usually more practical. Evidence also suggests that the incidence of bleeding can be further reduced by administering the H_2 blocker by continuous infusion, reducing the number of episodes of breakthrough hyperacidity. Frequent monitoring of gastric pH to assess the adequacy of acid suppression is important.

Attention has also focused on the beneficial antimicrobial effects of gastric acidity, suggesting that the stomach's acid environment may reduce the incidence of gastric colonization and subsequent nosocomial infections in critically ill ventilated patients. In adults, sucralfate has been shown to prevent stress ulcer–related complications as effectively as H_2 blockade. A concomitant decrease in the incidence of nosocomial pneumonia has not been seen, however.[48] The efficacy of sucralfate compared with H_2 blockers for prophylaxis against nosocomial infections has not been adequately studied in children.

The absolute indications for surgery in children are the same as in adults: perforation, persistent hemorrhage, obstruction, and intractability. A relative indication is recurrence—the risks of surgery and its side effects must be weighed against a life-long dependency on medication. Primary APD in children has an extremely high recurrence rate, exceeding 50% in many series. In the past, such high recurrence rates constituted an indication for definitive surgery in a significant number or patients, approaching 40% in a retrospective series.[49] Today, with a wide variety of effective pharmacologic approaches and an expectation that *H pylori* eradication will lead to a higher cure rate, definitive surgery for primary APD is less commonly performed. Intractability or rapid recurrence off medication should prompt a thorough workup for gastrinoma (see later).

When surgery is performed for APD in children, it is usually performed for hemorrhage or perforation resulting from secondary disease. In the study cited earlier,[46] nearly 50% of children with endoscopically proven secondary APD ultimately required emergent surgical intervention for either hemorrhage or perforation. Historically, hemorrhage and perforation have been relatively equivalent in their frequencies as indications for emergency surgery in children.

The indications for surgical intervention in children with hemorrhage from APD are subjective. Persistent or repeated bleeding in the face of failed medical and endoscopic therapy are noncontroversial indications. Other recommendations include hemorrhage of sufficient magnitude to require transfusion of one half the calculated blood volume in 8 hours, or one total blood volume in 24 hours (some consider one half the blood volume in 24 hours to be an indication). A visible vessel at the ulcer base, identified during endoscopic examination, is associated with a high risk of rebleeding and is commonly considered another indication for surgical therapy. Perforation, marked by pneumoperitoneum and peritonitis, is an absolute indication for surgery. Recommendations in the adult literature regarding nonoperative management of contained perforations in stable patients of advanced age are difficult to translate to children, and experience with such management is anecdotal.

The choice of operation depends on several factors: the indication for surgery, the chronicity of disease, the anticipated need for surgical control of future ulcer diathesis, the stability and preoperative condition of the patient, and the child's age. Most data regarding the efficacy and risks of surgery for APD have been from studies in adults. The application of conclusions and recommendations from these studies to infants, children, and adolescents must be individualized.

For most adolescent and adult patients, the curative options available to the surgeon include truncal vagotomy and drainage (usually by pyloroplasty; VP), truncal vagotomy and antrectomy (VA), or proximal gastric vagotomy (PGV). Mortality, morbidity, and recurrence rates for these procedures performed electively in adults have been well established. All three have minimal mortality rates. Both VP and VA have significant long-term side effects associated with GI denervation and impaired gastric emptying that approach 15% for both procedures. The rate of recurrence for VA (about 2%) is, however, considerably lower than for VP (10% to 15%). Although PGV has a rate of recurrence similar to VP, the virtual absence of side effects, greater acceptance by patients as scored by the Visik grading scale, and availability of effective new drugs to control recurrence makes PGV the procedure of choice whenever possible.[50]

In the rare child with primary APD refractory to medical therapy, or in whom multiple recurrences have occurred after cessation of medications, PGV is the recommended procedure after eliminating ZES as a potential cause. A modification of this procedure, which includes a posterior truncal vagotomy and an anterior PGV (lesser curve seromyotomy), has been reported to be as effective and free of side effects as PGV, while having the additional advantages of preserving the blood supply to the lesser curve and lending itself to laparoscopic techniques.[51] Experience with either of these procedures in children is limited.

More commonly, surgical intervention is necessitated by hemorrhage or perforation occurring in the setting of stress or steroid-related secondary duodenal ulcers. Support can be found both for limited intervention to control the complication and for combining control of the complication with definitive antiulcer surgery. Simple oversewing of the bleeding ulcer followed by pharmacologic suppression of acid secretion is the preferred treatment in infants and young children. Because most older patients who present with uncontrolled hemorrhage do so despite maximal attempts at prophylaxis, antisecretory therapy, and endoscopic control, it is prudent to advocate definitive ulcer surgery in most of these patients. The risk of recurrent bleeding in patients who have failed medical control, and the consequences of repeated life-threatening hemorrhage, argue against limited surgery simply to ligate the involved vessel. VP provides both a simple approach to expose the duodenal ulcer for vessel ligation and relatively effective antisecretory therapy. Although VA is considered to be superior to VP for bleeding duodenal ulcers in stable, healthy adults, there is little enthusiasm for (or experience with) VA in children. In the well-resuscitated stable patient, consideration should be given to ligation of the duodenal ulcer through a pylorus-sparing duodenotomy, followed by anatomic duodenal closure and either formal or modified PGV. This approach has gained favor in adults but is unstudied in children.

For children with perforated duodenal ulcers, most pediatric surgeons support simple closure of the perforation with an omental buttress (Graham patch), relying on aggressive postoperative medical therapy, including continuously infused histamine blockers or omeprazole, to facilitate ulcer healing. Avoidance of a suture line and hiatal dissection in the face of peritonitis are thought to be reasonable tenets. In adults, historical evidence documenting high rates of recurrence and eventual surgery has led to an acceptance of combining PGV with closure of the perforation as a definitive procedure in this setting. The rationale for and results of this approach in children are not defined.

As noted earlier, patients with a particularly aggressive ulcer diathesis should be evaluated for ZES before deciding on the surgical approach. ZES is a condition of severe ulcer diathesis caused by a gastrin-secreting neoplasm. Gastrin levels are markedly and continuously elevated and do not show any evidence of physiologic regulation. Parietal cell hypersecretion and peptic ulceration are severe, and the incidence of multifocal disease, recurrence, and ulcer-related complications is high. Diagnosis relies on the demonstration of elevated gastrin levels, both at baseline and after stimulation with secretin. The primary tumor, or gastrinoma, is usually found in the duodenal wall, the pancreas (as a non-β islet cell tumor), or in the adjacent retroperitoneum. In the familial form of the disease, associated with multiple endocrine neoplasia syndrome type I, there is a high incidence of multicentricity, with multiple tumor nodules dispersed diffusely throughout the pancreas. In the sporadic form, fewer tumors (one to three) are usually observed. Noninvasive imaging has been disappointing in localizing the primary tumor, but computed tomography is recommended to evaluate the liver for metastatic deposits. Angiography and intraoperative ultrasonography may offer improvements in definitive localization. Although total gastrectomy was formerly required to control the effects of hypergastrinemia, management with aggressive H_2 blockade and proton pump inhibitors has largely controlled the severe ulcer diathesis. Surgical management involves extirpation of the gastrinoma, if possible, by tumor enucleation or distal pancreatic resection in the sporadic form. Even though only half of the patients who undergo tumor excision are rendered biochemically free of disease, surgical resection of the primary gastrinoma appears to reduce the incidence of eventual metastasis.[52] In patients with multiple endocrine neoplasia syndrome type I, curative surgery is unlikely given the diffuse nature of the disease. Medical management with antisecretory agents and somatostatin analogues has been successful in achieving long-term survival, in part owing to the indolent nature of the disease. Long-term prognosis in the face of metastatic disease is poor.

Gastric Dysmotility

Rarely, infants younger than 1 year present with persistent nonbilious vomiting and are presumed to have GER. Evaluation for GER by manometric and pH probe studies documents normal LES function. An upper GI tract contrast study reveals a funnel-shaped, atonic antrum with delayed gastric emptying and reflux of contrast. The pylorus is normal. These patients have antral dysmotility, a primary motility disorder of unknown etiology. Usually, the condition is transient and responds to conservative measures, such as altering the feeding regimen. In one series, nearly 40% of patients underwent pyloroplasty with good results.[53] Alternatively, pyloromyotomy can be used and has proved to be effective.

Neonatal Gastric Perforation

The causes of gastric perforation in neonates can be categorized as traumatic, ischemic, or spontaneous. Traumatic perforations are generally caused by pneumatic gastric distention from bag-mask ventilation or positive-pressure ventilation in an infant with a tracheoesophageal fistula, or by puncture of the stomach during gastric intubation. Usually, these appear as short lacerations or discrete puncture wounds.

Ischemic perforations occur in the setting of severe physiologic stress, such as extreme prematurity or birth asphyxia, and sometimes accompany necrotizing enterocolitis involving the distal GI tract. The pathophysiology of these lesions is unknown but is presumed to be associated with locoregional redistribution of blood flow resulting in infarction of a small area of the gastric wall. It is possible that some of these lesions represent perforated stress ulcers. The perforations are often accompanied by a surrounding zone of necrosis and devitalized tissue.

Occasionally, a healthy neonate presents with a spontaneous gastric perforation of unknown cause. Some of these infants are premature or small for gestational age, but otherwise are stable. Therefore, a plausible explanation for the perforation is lacking. One hypothesis suggests that a congenital abnormality of the muscularis causes a focal weakness prone to rupture.[54] The most common location is high on the greater curvature near the gastroesophageal junction.

The most constant diagnostic feature of gastric perforation in the neonate is massive pneumoperitoneum, unless the perforation is posterior and contained within the lesser sac. Exploration requires mobilization to evaluate the gastroesophageal junction and lesser sac to locate perforations that do not occur on the anterior aspect of the stomach. Surgical management is individualized to either simple débridement and closure or closure around a temporary gastrostomy tube. Extensive gastric resections have not been necessary. Perforations of the greater curvature of the stomach at the gastroesophageal junction, which usually resemble ruptures or lacerations, can be difficult to repair because of their location. We prefer to débride the edges and perform a two-layer closure. Outcomes depend on the cause of the perforation and associated disease, such as respiratory failure and complex congenital malformations. Although mortality rates have historically ranged from 25% to 60%,[55,56] current mortality rates should be significantly lower for most types of neonatal gastric perforations.

Foreign Bodies and Bezoars

Foreign bodies within the stomach and duodenum constitute an unusual indication for surgical intervention in the current era. Coins are the most commonly ingested objects and usually lodge in the esophagus. Those that reach the stomach are passed through the GI tract without incident 80% to 90% of the time; most of the remainder are endoscopically retrievable, and a small number (about 1%) require surgical removal.[57] Round objects greater than 2 cm in diameter and linear objects longer than 3 cm in the infant or toddler, or longer than 5 cm in the older child, are unlikely to pass spontaneously. Objects that are sharp at one end are usually passed through with the blunt end in front. Objects that are sharp at both ends are more likely to cause penetration of the bowel wall and have been observed to migrate into the chest, liver, and retroperitoneum. For these reasons, endoscopic removal of gastroduodenal foreign bodies is recommended at the outset for high-risk objects and for those of large size. Others can be managed expectantly with serial abdominal films to follow movement and examination of the stools to detect passage. Objects remaining in the stomach after 4 weeks should be retrieved. If endoscopic removal is unsuccessful, open gastrotomy is indicated.

Disk-shaped batteries used in cameras and other electronic devices represent a special problem. Complications from battery ingestion include pressure necrosis, low-voltage electrical burn, corrosive alkaline injury, and, rarely, mercury toxicity. Although impaction in the esophagus mandates immediate removal, passage into the stomach usually results in spontaneous transit. Some surgeons favor immediate retrieval of all batteries to minimize the risk of mucosal injury. If immediate removal is judged unnecessary, endoscopic or surgical retrieval should be performed if the battery remains in the gastric lumen longer than 48 hours or if abdominal symptoms develop.

Bezoars represent aggregations of multiple foreign bodies ingested over time. The most common type in children is the trichobezoar, which is composed of hair (ingested due to an emotional disorder) and other indigestible fibers from carpets, blankets, toys, and so forth. Less common types include phytobezoars (derived from vegetable matter) and lactobezoars (derived from precipitates of milk and usually occurring in premature infants). Bezoars commonly form a cast of the stomach with a tail that extends a variable distance through the pylorus (Fig. 68-23).

The most common symptoms associated with bezoars relate to gastric outlet obstruction, with abdominal distention, early satiety, pain, and vomiting being common. Less common manifestations include anemia and hypoproteinemia from chronic gastritis, and jaundice, pancreatitis, and steatorrhea from pancreaticobiliary obstruction. Plain radiographs often display a frothy appearance in the gastric lumen. An upper GI tract contrast series and endoscopy are diagnostic.

Treatment depends on the type of bezoar and the associated symptoms. Trichobezoars virtually always require surgical removal. Phytobezoars can often be fragmented endoscopically or partially digested with papain, acetylcysteine, or cellulase.

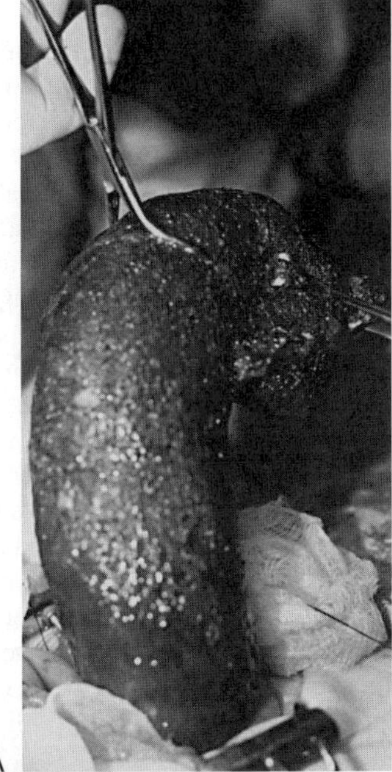

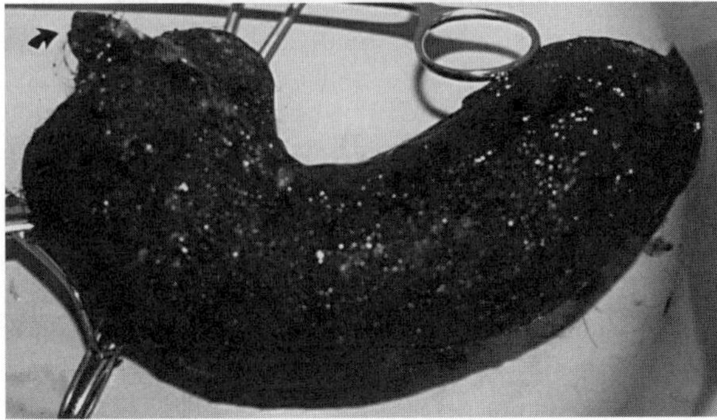

FIG. 68-23. (*A*) Gastric trichobezoar being delivered through a gastrotomy in a 12-year-old child with trisomy 21 and a fenestrated duodenal web. (*B*) The bezoar creates a cast of the gastric lumen and pyloric channel (*arrow*).

Lactobezoars usually respond to nasogastric decompression with intravenous rehydration and parenteral nutrition.[58]

ENTERAL ACCESS FOR NUTRITION

Surgically placed gastrostomy tubes for enteral access have revolutionized the long-term care of many children with neurologic deficits, GI anomalies, complex congenital heart disease, and inanition due to cancer and chemotherapy. The effectiveness of aggressive nutritional intervention in these patients is undisputed, and permanent access to the gastric lumen has simplified the care rendered by nurses, nutritionists, and parents. Gastrostomies, however, are not without considerable complications. Furthermore, although they may be beneficial for feeding, caution must be exercised when they are used for decompression because they may be less reliable than standard nasogastric tubes used for this purpose. For patients who may require permanent gastric decompression, such as the spastic, neurologically impaired child, they offer a distinct advantage over nasogastric placement.

The two open surgical techniques employed for gastrostomy are the Stamm and Janeway procedures. The Stamm gastrostomy is most common and involves placing a mushroom-tipped catheter into the gastric lumen through a double pursestring suture, which inverts the tract (Fig. 68-24). The gastrostomy site is then fixed to the anterior abdominal wall, through which the tube exits, to minimize the risk of leakage. In 2 or 3 weeks, the anterior surface of the stomach fuses with the parietal peritoneum of the abdominal wall, and a secure gastrocutaneous fistula develops through which the feeding tube passes. It is necessary to keep the tube inserted to maintain the tract. Removal of the tube usually results in closure of the fistula within 24 hours. Its reversibility is one of the principal advantages of this procedure.

The Janeway gastrostomy entails creating a gastric tube from the anterior wall or the greater curvature, and bringing the tube through the rectus sheath to be matured as a permanent stoma. Although the stoma is designed to be continent, problems with difficult catheterization and with incontinence plague this procedure in common practice. Furthermore, it is reversible only with a second procedure. Its present use is limited to unusual cases.

The risks and complications associated with gastrostomy tubes are numerous and are usually associated with the medical comorbidity in this patient population. Reported complications include exacerbation of GER with aspiration, tract infections with abdominal wall cellulitis, intraperitoneal leakage, external leakage with cutaneous excoriation, accidental dislodgement and removal of the tube, inadvertent advancement of the tube causing gastric outlet obstruction, internal herniation around the gastrostomy, gastric volvulus, and duodenal perforation. Many of these complications are avoided by immobilization of the tube at the skin level. The reported incidence of significant complications has been between 2% and 10% in most series.

The incidence of GER in these patients merits special attention. The apparent increased incidence of GER after gastrostomy in neurologically impaired children has led many to hypothesize that gastrostomy worsens subclinical GER or produces GER in some previously unaffected patients,[59] apparently by distorting the angle of His and causing incompetence of the LES.[60,61] These observations have led to a recommendation that an antireflux procedure be routinely added to a feeding gastrostomy in these patients.[62] Newer data have supported the selective use of antireflux procedures only in those patients documented to have GER preoperatively.[63] It seems reasonable to evaluate all neurologically impaired children referred for enteral access for GER by upper GI tract study, radionuclide scan, and pH monitoring, and to perform concomitant fundoplication only in those displaying GER before operation. In patients who do not require fundoplication initially, consideration should be given to positioning the gastrostomy on the lesser curvature in an effort to preserve LES function and reduce postgastrostomy GER.[64,65]

In 1980, a percutaneous, endoscopically assisted technique of gastrostomy placement (PEG) was introduced to reduce the need for general anesthesia and to reduce the ileus and discomfort associated with the open procedure.[66] Since its introduction, PEG has become the predominant method of providing enteral access in patients who do not require laparotomy for other reasons. Its safety and efficacy have been well documented.[67] Modifications include the development of a ''push'' technique that obviates transoral passage of the gastrostomy device and may reduce the number of catheter-related infections,[68] as well as nonendoscopic techniques that rely on fluoroscopic guidance.[69] Recognition of GER in many of these patients has generated enthusiasm for percutaneous placement of dual-lumen tubes comprising a gastric decompression port and a transpyloric jejunal feeding port (PEJ). Studies in adults, however, have failed to document a significant difference between PEG and PEJ with respect to reflux episodes and aspiration pneumonia.[70]

Another development in enteral access has been the low-profile tube with a one-way valve—the gastrostomy ''button.'' Several designs are commercially available, and all are relatively effective in preventing tube movement and dislodgement—two problems that lead to many of the complications listed earlier. Acceptance by patients and parents is high because of the practical and cosmetic advantages associated with the lack of an external tube. In the past, a standard gastrostomy was established either by percutaneous or open technique, and the catheter was exchanged for a button about 6 weeks later when the gastrocutaneous fistula was sufficiently secure to tolerate manipulation. This procedure can be done without general anesthesia in most cases. Experience with primary surgical button placement is increasing, and it does not appear to be associated with an increase in the complication rate. A report on a percutaneous technique for primary placement of gastrostomy

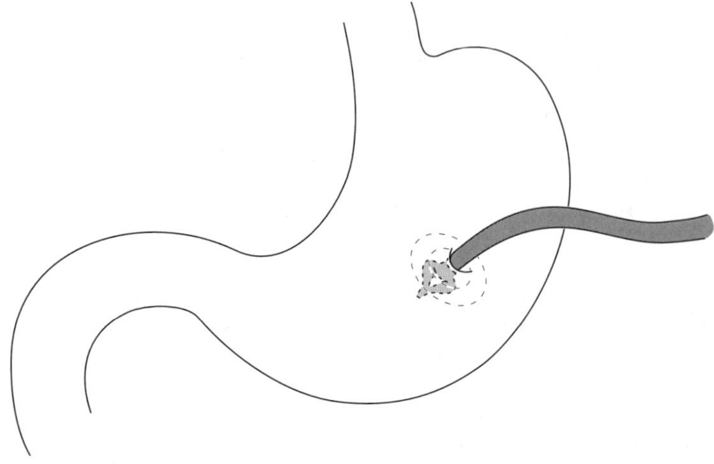

FIG. 68-24. Technique of Stamm gastrostomy.

buttons may indicate the beginning of an era in which permanent enteral access with a convenient appliance is routinely available on an endoscopic basis.[71]

REFERENCES

1. Furness JB, Costa M. Types of nerves in the enteric nervous system. Neuroscience 1980;5:1.
2. Richardson CT, Walsh JH, Cooper KA, et al. Studies on the role of cephalic-vagal stimulation in the acid secretory response to eating in normal subjects. J Clin Invest 1977;60:435.
3. Grotzinger U, Bergegarde S, Olbe L. Effect of atropine and proximal gastric vagotomy on the acid response to fundic distension in man. Gut 1977;18:303.
4. Wolfe MM, Reel GM. Inhibition of gastrin release by gastric inhibitory peptide mediated by somatostatin. Am J Physiol 1986;250:G331.
5. Prinz C, Kajimura M, Scott D, et al. Acid secretion and the H,K ATPase of the stomach. Yale J Biol Med 1992;65:577.
6. Wolfe MM, Soll AH. The physiology of gastric acid secretion. N Engl J Med 1988;319:1707.
7. Hakanson R, Boettcher F, Ekblad E, et al. Histamine in endocrine cells in the stomach. Histochemistry 1986;86:5.
8. Prinz C, Kajimura M, Scott DR, et al. Histamine secretion from rat enterochromaffinlike cells. Gastroenterology 1993;105:449.
9. Schubert ML, Coy DH, Makhlouf GM. Peptone stimulates gastrin secretion from the stomach by activating bombesin/GRP and cholinergic neurons. Am J Physiol 1992;262:G685.
10. Schubert ML, Hightower J. Release of gastric somatostatin during distension is mediated by gastric VIP neurons: a mechanical reflex for inhibition of gastrin. Gastroenterology 1989;96:A455.
11. Gantz I, Schaeffer M, DelValle J, et al. Molecular cloning of a gene encoding the histamine H_2-receptor. Proc Natl Acad Sci 1991;88:429.
12. Sachs G, Chang HH, Rabon E, et al. A nonelectrogenic H^+ pump in plasma membranes of hog stomach. J Biol Chem 1976;251:7690.
13. Agunod M, Yamaguchi N, Lopez R, et al. Correlative study of hydrochloric acid, pepsin, and intrinsic factor secretion in newborns and infants. Am J Digest Dis 1969;14:400.
14. Shimamoto C, Takao Y, Asada S, et al. Regulation of human and rat gastric mucin synthesis: assessment by histochemical and biochemical methods. Gastroenterology 1991;100:A159.
15. Blank E, Chisholm AJ. Congenital microgastria: a case with a 26-year followup. Pediatrics 1973;51:1037.
16. Velasco AL, Holcomb GW III, Templeton JM Jr, et al. Management of congenital microgastria. J Pediatr Surg 1990;25:192.
17. Coit DG, Mies C. Adenocarcinoma arising within a gastric duplication cyst. J Surg Oncol 1992;50:274.
18. Cragan JD, Martin ML, Moore CA, et al. Descriptive epidemiology of small intestinal atresia in Atlanta, Georgia. Teratology 1993;48:441.
19. Lecco TM. Zur Morphologie des Pankreas annulare. Sitzungsb Akad Wissensch Cl 1910;119:391.
20. Suda K. Immunohistochemical and gross dissection studies of annular pancreas. Acta Pathol Jpn 1990;40:505.
21. Fonkelsrud EW, de Lorimier AA, Hays DM. Congenital atresia and stenosis of the duodenum: a review compiled from the members of the Surgical Section of the American Academy of Pediatrics. Pediatrics 1969;43:79.
22. Schier F, Schier C, Waldschmidt J, et al. Duodenal atresia: experiences with 145 patients. Zentralbl Chir 1990;115:135.
23. Grosfeld JL, Rescorla FJ. Duodenal atresia and stenosis: reassessment of treatment and outcome based on antenatal diagnosis, pathologic variance, and long-term follow-up. World J Surg 1993;17:301.
24. Fogel M, Copel JA, Cullen MT, et al. Congenital heart disease and fetal thoracoabdominal anomalies: associations in utero and the importance of cytogenetic analysis. Am J Perinatol 1991;8:411.
25. Nyberg DA, Resta RG, Luthy DA, et al. Prenatal sonographic findings of Down syndrome: review of 94 cases. Obstet Gynecol 1990;76:370.
26. Spigland N, Yazbeck S. Complications associated with surgical treatment of congenital intrinsic duodenal obstruction. J Pediatr Surg 1990;25:1127.
27. Stubbs TM, Horger EO. Sonographic detection of fetal duodenal atresia. (Letter) Obstet Gynecol 1989;73:146.
28. Bickler SW, Harrison MW, Blank E, et al. Microperforation of a duodenal diaphragm as a cause of paradoxical gas in congenital duodenal obstruction. J Pediatr Surg 1992;27:747.
29. Panuel M, Bourliere-Najean B, Delarue A, et al. Duodenal atresia with bifid termination of the common bile duct. Arch Fr Pediatr 1992;49:365.
30. Kimura K, Mukohara N, Nashijima E, et al. Diamond-shaped anastomosis for duodenal atresia: an experience with 44 patients over 15 years. J Pediatr Surg 1990;25:977.
31. Jedd MB, Melton LJ III, Griffin MR, et al. Trends in infantile hypertrophic pyloric stenosis in Olmsted County, Minnesota, 1950–1984. Paediatr Perinat Epidemiol 1988;2:148.
32. Rollins MD, Shields MD, Quinn RJ, et al. Pyloric stenosis: congenital or acquired? Arch Dis Child 1989;64:138.
33. Carter CO, Evans KA. Inheritance of congenital pyloric stenosis. J Med Genet 1969;6:233.
34. Katz S, Basel D, Branski D. Prenatal gastric dilatation and infantile hypertrophic pyloric stenosis. J Pediatr Surg 1988;23:1021.
35. Mercado-Deane MG, Burton EM, Brawley AV, et al. Prostaglandin-induced foveolar hyperplasia simulating pyloric stenosis in an infant with cyanotic heart disease. Pediatr Radiol 1988;24:45.
36. Wattchow DA, Cass DT, Furness JB, et al. Abnormalities of peptide-containing nerve fibers in infantile hypertrophic pyloric stenosis. Gastroenterology 1987;92:443.
37. Vanderwinden JM, Mailleux P, Schiffmann SN, et al. Nitric oxide synthase activity in infantile hypertrophic pyloric stenosis. N Engl J Med 1992;327:511.
38. Dieler R, Schroder JM. Myenteric plexus neuropathy in infantile hypertrophic pyloric stenosis. Acta Neuropathol (Berl) 1989;78:649.
39. Teele RL, Smith EH. Ultrasound in the diagnosis of idiopathic hypertrophic pyloric stenosis. N Engl J Med 1977;296:1149.
40. Lamki N, Athey PA, Round ME, et al. Hypertrophic pyloric stenosis in the neonate: diagnostic criteria revisited. Can Assoc Radiol J 1993;44:21.
41. Westra SJ, de Groot CJ, Smits NJ, et al. Hypertrophic pyloric stenosis: use of the pyloric volume measurement in early US diagnosis. Radiology 1989;172:615.
42. Macdessi J, Oates RK. Clinical diagnosis of pyloric stenosis: a declining art. Br Med J 1993;306:553.
43. Ludtke FE, Bertus M, Voth E, et al. Gastric emptying 16 to 26 years after treatment of infantile hypertrophic pyloric stenosis. J Pediatr Surg 1994;29:523.
44. Levi S, Beardshall K, Haddad G, et al. *Campylobacter pylori* and duodenal ulcers: the gastrin link. Lancet 1989;1:1167.
45. Yeung CK, Fu KH, Yuen KY, et al. *Helicobacter pylori* and associated duodenal ulcer. Arch Dis Child 1990;65:1212.
46. Kumar D, Spitz L. Peptic ulceration in children. Surg Gynecol Obstet 1984;159:63.
47. Folkman J, Szabo S, Stovroff M, et al. Duodenal ulcer: discovery of a new mechanism and development of angiogenic therapy that accelerates healing. Ann Surg 1991;214:414.
48. Maier RV, Mitchell D, Gentilello L. Optimal therapy for stress gastritis. Ann Surg 1994;220:353.
49. Drumm B, Rhoads JM, Tringer DA, et al. Peptic ulcer disease in children: etiology, clinical findings, and clinical course. Pediatrics 1988;82:410.
50. Jordan PH, Thornby J. Twenty years after parietal cell vagotomy or selective vagotomy antrectomy for treatment of duodenal ulcer. Ann Surg 1994;220:283.
51. Taylor TV, Gunn AA, MacLeod DA, et al. Morbidity and mortality after anterior lesser curve seromyotomy with posterior truncal vagotomy for duodenal ulcer. Br J Surg 1985;72:950.
52. Fraker DL, Norton JA, Alexander JR, et al. Surgery in Zollinger-Ellison syndrome alters the natural history of gastrinoma. Ann Surg 1994;220:320.
53. Byrne WJ, Kangarloo H, Ament ME, et al. Antral dysmotility: an unrecognized cause of chronic vomiting during infancy. Ann Surg 1984;193:521.
54. Herbut PA. Congenital defect in the musculature of the stomach with rupture in a newborn. Arb Pathol 1943;36:91.
55. Rosser SB, Clark CH, Elechi EN. Spontaneous neonatal gastric perforation. J Pediatr Surg 1982;17:390.
56. Tan CE, Kiely EM, Agrawal M, et al. Neonatal gastrointestinal perforation. J Pediatr Surg 1989;24:888.

57. Schwartz GF, Polsky HS. Ingested foreign bodies of the gastrointestinal tract. Am Surg 1985;51:173.
58. Yoss BS. Human milk lactobezoars. J Pediatr 1984;105:819.
59. Mollitt DL, Golladay ES, Seibert JJ. Symptomatic gastroesophageal reflux following gastrostomy in neurologically impaired patients. Pediatrics 1985;75:1124.
60. Jolley SG, Tunnell WP, Hoelzer DJ, et al. Lower esophageal pressure changes with tube gastrostomy: a causative factor of gastroesophageal reflux in children? J Pediatr Surg 1986;21:624.
61. Papaila JG, Vane DW, Colville C, et al. The effect of various types of gastrostomy on the lower esophageal sphincter. J Pediatr Surg 1987;22:1198.
62. Jolley SG, Smith EI, Tunell WP. Protective antireflux operation with feeding gastrostomy: experience with children. Ann Surg 1985;201:736.
63. Wheatley MJ, Wesley JR, Tkach DM, et al. Long-term follow-up of brain-damaged children requiring feeding gastrostomy: should an antireflux procedure always be performed? J Pediatr Surg 1991;26:301.
64. Stringel G. Gastrostomy with antireflux properties. J Pediatr Surg 1990;25:1019.
65. Seekri IK, Rescorla FJ, Canal DF, et al. Lesser curvature gastrostomy reduces the incidence of postoperative gastroesophageal reflux. J Pediatr Surg 1991;26:982.
66. Gauderer ML, Ponsky JL, Izant RJ Jr. Gastrostomy without laparotomy: a percutaneous endoscopic technique. J Pediatr Surg 1980;15:872.
67. Marin OE, Glassman MS, Schoen BT, et al. Safety and efficacy of percutaneous endoscopic gastrostomy in children. Am J Gastroenterol 1994;89:357.
68. Crombleholme TM, Jacir NN. Simplified ''push'' technique for percutaneous endoscopic gastrostomy in children. J Pediatr Surg 1993;28:1393.
69. Malden ES, Hicks ME, Picus D, et al. Fluoroscopically guided percutaneous gastrostomy in children. J Vasc Interven Radiol 1992;3:673.
70. Kadakia SC, Sullivan HO, Starnes E. Percutaneous endoscopic gastrostomy or jejunostomy and the incidence of aspiration in 79 patients. Am J Surg 1992;164:114.
71. Treem WR, Etienne NL, Hyams JS. Percutaneous endoscopic placement of the ''button'' gastrostomy tube as the initial procedure in infants and children. J Pediatr Gastroenterol Nutr 1993;17:382.

Surgery of Infants and Children: Scientific Principles and Practice, edited by
Keith T. Oldham, Paul M. Colombani, and Robert P. Foglia.
Lippincott–Raven Publishers, Philadelphia, © 1997.

CHAPTER 69

Small Intestine

William R. Treem

The small intestine is the major digestive and absorptive portion
of the gastrointestinal tract. Any pathologic process that disrupts
the normal function of the small intestine profoundly affects
the normal growth and metabolism of the patient. Pediatric surgeons are involved in the care of patients with chronic conditions of the small intestine that preclude normal enteral nutrition. These include conditions resulting in short bowel
syndrome and protracted diarrhea in infancy; motility disorders
causing pseudoobstruction and bacterial overgrowth; acquired
inflammatory immune-mediated conditions, such as Crohn disease and graft-versus-host disease; and acquired conditions
thought to be triggered by viral or bacterial infections, such
as Henoch-Schönlein purpura and hemolytic uremic syndrome.
Parenteral nutrition has provided a means of supporting these
patients while treating their underlying disease and waiting for
growth, development, and regeneration of the damaged small
intestine. This chapter briefly reviews the ontogeny of small
intestine development, the basic gross and microscopic anatomy, the physiology of nutrient digestion and absorption, and
normal small intestinal motility. The second portion of the chapter highlights some of the disease processes that disrupt normal
function in these areas and lead to the potential need for surgical
intervention to provide parenteral or selective enteral nutrition.

DEVELOPMENTAL ANATOMY

The gut lengthens rapidly between 6 and 12 weeks' gestation.
During this time, the small intestine transiently herniates into
the umbilical cord. On reentry into the abdominal cavity, the
intestine rotates counterclockwise 270 degrees around an axis
formed by the superior mesenteric artery. Further positioning
of the small intestine continues until 20 weeks' gestation, when
the gastrointestinal tract achieves its final anatomic position.
The small intestine continues to lengthen throughout gestation
and measures 200 to 300 cm at birth in a full-term neonate.[1]
Between 26 and 38 weeks' gestation, the overall length of the
gastrointestinal tract doubles. The small intestine does not
achieve its maximum length of 600 to 800 cm until at least 4
years of age. These changes in overall length, the doubling
of the intestinal diameter, and the development of the plicae
circulares, villi, and microvilli, combine to enlarge the absorp-

tive surface area of the small intestine from about 950 cm^2 at
birth to 7500 cm^2 in the adult.[2]

The circular muscles of the small intestine appear at 6 weeks'
gestation, and the longitudinal muscles at 8 weeks' gestation.
Neuroblasts appear at 7 weeks' gestation, and differentiation
into the myenteric and submucosal plexuses occurs at 9 and 13
weeks' gestation, respectively. Peristalsis first occurs shortly
thereafter, but jejunal contractions remain disorganized in the
premature infant before 30 weeks' gestation.[3] When radiographic contrast material is injected into the gastrointestinal
tract of a fetus in utero before 30 weeks' gestation, there is
little movement of the marker out of the stomach.[4] With the
appearance of the migrating motor complexes (MMCs) at 32 to
34 weeks' gestation, duodenal and jejunal contractions become
more coordinated but are still immature. Despite the greater
frequency of MMCs in premature infants, transit time through
the small intestine can be as long as 9 hours, or twice as long
as that in term infants, because of the two-fold shorter propagation rate of the MMCs. By 38 weeks postconception, the MMCs
are fully present, and fasting motor activity is mature.[5] Feedings
increase the number of duodenal contractions in infants as
young as 25 weeks postconception; in very premature infants,
there is often the coexistence of an active fed pattern with an
immature fasting pattern and no MMCs.[6] The administration
of corticosteroids accelerates maturation of neonatal small intestinal motility, whereas ischemia and central nervous system
disease slow maturation.

Villi appear in the duodenum at 8 weeks' gestation and proliferate distally, reaching the terminal ileum by 11 weeks' gestation. The villi acquire their tall, finger-like shape in the proximal
intestine by 14 weeks' gestation but remain shorter in the distal
small intestine, resulting in a four-fold greater absorptive surface area in the jejunum than in the ileum. Microvilli also appear
at 8 weeks' gestation, and by 14 weeks' gestation, enterocytes
are morphologically mature and display a well-organized brush
border. The crypt compartment of the small intestine, which is
the site of enterocyte proliferation, appears in the duodenum by
10 weeks' gestation. The entire process of enterocyte migration
from crypt to villus in the newborn infant is slower than that
in adults and requires at least 6 days for epithelial renewal.

Endocrine cells appear in the gut by 9 weeks' gestation, and
for the next 3 weeks, mature secretory granules containing the

various gut peptide hormones appear in the endocrine cells of the crypts. Several peptide hormones, including enteroglucagon, neurotensin, gastrin, pancreatic polypeptide, and motilin, have been measured in the fetal circulation between 16 and 20 weeks' gestation. The appearance of vasoactive intestinal polypeptide (VIP) in the gut lags behind, appearing in the epithelial cells after 18 weeks' gestation. The concentration of these hormones and neurotransmitters increases throughout gestation and reaches adult levels by term, with the exception of fasting levels of gastrin and VIP, which are significantly higher.[7] The functional significance of many of these hormones during embryologic development remains to be elucidated; however, it has been shown that during the first two postnatal weeks, the basal levels of many of these peptide hormones rise dramatically in response to enteral feedings but remain low in infants who have never been fed.[8] This observation, coupled with studies in newborn animals showing that intestinal growth and functional maturation is delayed by withholding feedings, suggest that elaboration of these hormones is an important stimulus for postnatal development of the small intestine.

ONTOGENY OF DIGESTION AND ABSORPTION

Carbohydrates

Despite the mature appearance of the intestinal epithelium by the end of the second trimester, its brush-border membrane is functionally immature. The disaccharidases lactase and sucrase-isomaltase can be detected by 8 weeks' gestation, but lactase activity remains functionally immature at birth.[9] Peak lactase activity is found during early postnatal life. Within the first few years of life, lactase activity decreases to adult levels (one tenth that at birth). In contrast, sucrase-isomaltase activity rises throughout gestation, so that 70% of adult levels is achieved at 34 weeks, gestation and adult levels are reached at birth. Glucoamylase (maltase) has been detected at 13 weeks' gestation, and the presence of this α-glucosidase together with sucrase-isomaltase allows the premature infant to digest glucose polymers more readily than lactose. Despite the apparent lactase deficiency, term infants tolerate lactose-containing formulas and human milk owing to the process of carbohydrate salvage through fermentation to short-chain fatty acids by colonic bacteria. Infant formulas designed for preterm infants often contain lower lactose and higher glucose polymer concentrations.

The rate of glucose transport is low in the first trimester and increases the number of sodium-coupled transport sites increases first in the jejunum and then in the ileum. The maximal glucose transport rate in the jejunum of infants is 20% to 25% that of adults and increases throughout the first year of life.[10]

Proteins

Most protein hydrolysis occurs in the proximal gut and is dependent on the presence of enterokinase, pancreatic proteases, and brush-border and cytosolic peptidases. Enterokinase initiates the process of protein digestion by the activation of trypsinogen. Enterokinase activity is detected in the duodenum at 24 weeks' gestation and increases during the latter part of gestation to 10% of eventual adult levels, which are finally achieved by about 4 years of age. Despite the relative deficiency of enterokinase, the presence of the pancreatic proteases (trypsin, chymotrypsin, and carboxypeptidase B) permits efficient digestion of protein to peptides. Most of the activities of both the brush-border and cytosolic peptidases are present at 8 weeks' gestation and soon reach levels similar to those found in adults.

Fats

The efficiency of long-chain triglyceride absorption ranges from 70% to 90% in term infants and from 40% to 90% in premature infants. Medium-chain triglycerides are digested and absorbed more efficiently than are long-chain triglycerides because they do not require bile salts for esterification or solubilization in mixed micelles. Medium-chain triglycerides are taken up directly in the portal vein. The multiple factors that contribute to the immaturity of bile acid metabolism and the enterohepatic circulation of bile acids in the newborn are collectively termed *physiologic cholestasis*[11,12] (Fig. 69-1). These factors include decreased rates of bile acid synthesis, a smaller pool size, and the lack of an active transporter of bile salts in the ileum.[13] Although taurine-conjugated bile acids are passively absorbed by the fetal gut, active ileal transport does not begin until after birth. Together, these factors contribute to the relative paucity of bile salts appearing in the infant duodenum; these may not reach the critical micellar concentration necessary for long-chain fat absorption, especially in premature infants. Hormones such as glucocorticoids and thyroxine, growth factors such as epidermal growth factor, and dietary factors including long-chain fatty acids all are thought to regulate and enhance the development of bile acid metabolism and the enterohepatic circulation in the fetus and premature infant.[14]

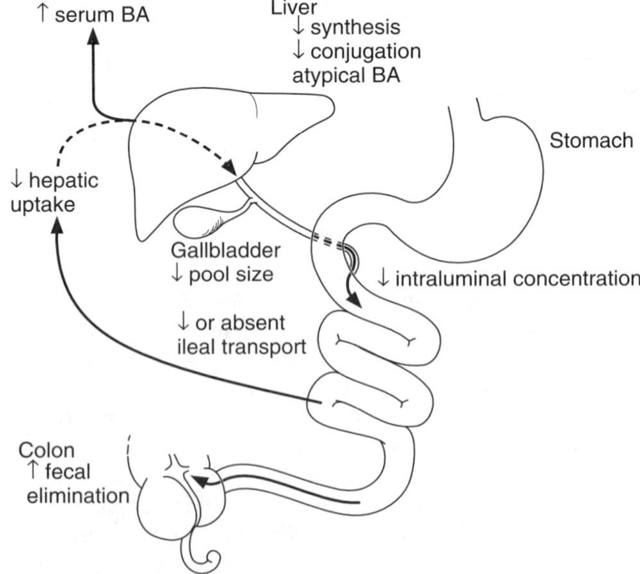

FIG. 69-1. Manifestations of immature bile acid (BA) transport and metabolism in early life. Most facets of the enterohepatic circulation are defective, allowing spillover of bile acids into the systemic circulation (physiologic cholestasis) and loss through fecal elimination.

Trypsin, lipase, and amylase are found in the duodenums of premature infants at 32 weeks' gestation, but their concentrations are lower than those found in term infants.[15] Alternative mechanisms facilitating fat absorption in the infant include both lingual lipase (detected at 26 weeks' gestation) and gastric lipase. In addition, a third compensatory lipase is found in the milk of mothers beyond 26 weeks' gestation and may contribute to the decrease in fat malabsorption noted in breastfed infants.

DEVELOPMENT OF THE IMMUNE FUNCTION OF THE GUT

The components of the intestinal immune system, including lamina propria lymphocytes, organized submucosal collections of lymphocytes known as Peyer patches, and the M cells that overlie Peyer patches and permit uptake of macromolecules and antigenic processing by the gut, are all in place by about 20 weeks' gestation. Antigenic stimulation required for activation of these lymphoid tissues, however, does not develop until several weeks after birth. Several other aspects of the mucosal immune system are immature at the time of birth. Permeability of the infant gut to undigested macromolecules, including cow-milk proteins, is greater than in the adult intestine.[16] A decrease in permeability appears to be enhanced by oral feedings, and the rate of gut closure is more rapid when infants are fed human milk rather than commercially prepared formulas.[17] Small intestinal immunoglobulin-secreting plasma cells and secretory immunoglobulin A (IgA) are both deficient throughout the first 12 days of life. Premature infants younger than 35 weeks' gestation are unable to form antibodies to foreign antigens when fed exogenous proteins.[18] This has led to the preparation of special formulas for premature infants that contain less antigenic forms of milk protein, including hydrolyzed casein and whey.

NORMAL ANATOMY AND PHYSIOLOGY

Gross Anatomy

Although a distinct demarcation between jejunum and ileum is not apparent, structural differences are present that reflect the functional compartmentalization of the small intestine (Table 69-1). The thickness of the small bowel wall, the overall luminal diameter, and the prominence of the circular submucosal folds (plicae circulares) are all greatest in the proximal jejunum and decrease with progression through the ileum. Absorptive surface area, as a consequence, is much greater in the

TABLE 69-1. *Structural differences between the jejunum and the ileum*

Structural element	Jejunum	Ileum
Wall thickness	Increased	Decreased
Luminal diameter	Greater	Less
Plicae circulares	Prominent	Less
Surface area	Increased	Decreased
Peyer patches	Less	Increased
Villi	Taller	Blunt, shorter
Tight junctions	Leaky	Tighter

jejunum than in the ileum. The direct stimulatory effect of nutrients on the growth of the absorptive mucosa is thought to be responsible for the normal proximal to distal absorptive gradient; proximal jejunal villi are taller and have greater absorptive capacity because of abundant exposure to nutrients, most of which are depleted by the time intestinal chyme reaches the distal small intestine. The ileum of animals undergoing jejunectomy experiences marked hyperplasia when exposed to enteral nutrients. Similarly, when a segment of ileum is transplanted proximally and exposed to the jejunal nutrient environment, that segment becomes hyperplastic and takes on the morphologic and functional absorptive characteristics of proximal intestine.[19] Conversely, a jejunal segment transposed to the ileal environment undergoes opposite changes and decreases its mucosal mass.

Four layers make up the wall of the small intestine. From outside inwardly, these consist of the serosa, the muscularis, the submucosa, and the mucosa. The serosa is a simple extension of the peritoneum and mesentery, which envelops this tubular organ. The muscularis is made of smooth muscle cells, which are divided distinctly into two separate layers: an outer, longitudinal layer and an inner, circular layer. The muscular layers are heavily infiltrated with sympathetic and parasympathetic nerves derived primarily from the vagus and mesenteric nerves. The ganglionated nerve plexus, located between the longitudinal and circular layers of the muscle coat, is called the *myenteric* or *Auerbach plexus* and extends without interruption throughout the alimentary tract. The submucosa is a band of dense connective tissue lying just under the mucosa that is richly endowed with numerous arteries, veins, and lymphatic channels to ensure adequate handling of absorbed fluids, nutrients, and electrolytes after a meal. Also located within the submucosa is an extensive network of ganglion cells and nerve fibers constituting the *autonomic submucosal plexus,* or *Meissner plexus,* which communicates with the Auerbach plexus, resulting in complete neuroregulatory control of the small intestine.

The mucosa is the innermost layer of the small intestine and is composed of three distinct layers: the muscularis mucosa, lamina propria, and epithelial cell lining (Fig. 69-2). As noted, the most striking feature of the small intestinal mucosa is the formation of villi, which are about 1.5 mm tall in the jejunum and progressively shorter through the ileum. Surrounding the base of each villus are several pitlike crypts, called the *crypts of Lieberkühn,* which average one third to one fourth the height of the villi.

The muscularis mucosa is a thin sheet of smooth muscle cells, averaging 3 to 10 cells thick, lying immediately adjacent to the submucosa. Continuing luminally from the muscularis mucosa, the lamina propria is next encountered. This is composed of a thin layer of connective tissue that surrounds the crypts and extends into the villus protrusions. Arterioles, capillaries, veins, and lacteals are present within the lamina propria in close proximity to the basal surfaces of the absorptive epithelial cell, the enterocyte. This brings the epithelial absorptive cell in close proximity to the endothelial cell and allows for the rapid transfer of absorbed nutrients, fluids, and electrolytes. Small nerve fibrils are also present in the lamina propria within the core of each villus, along with plasma cells, macrophages, lymphocytes, eosinophils, fibroblasts, and mast cells. Regulation of intestinal transport results from a combination of factors, including cholinergic and adrenergic nerve fibrils, cytokines, his-

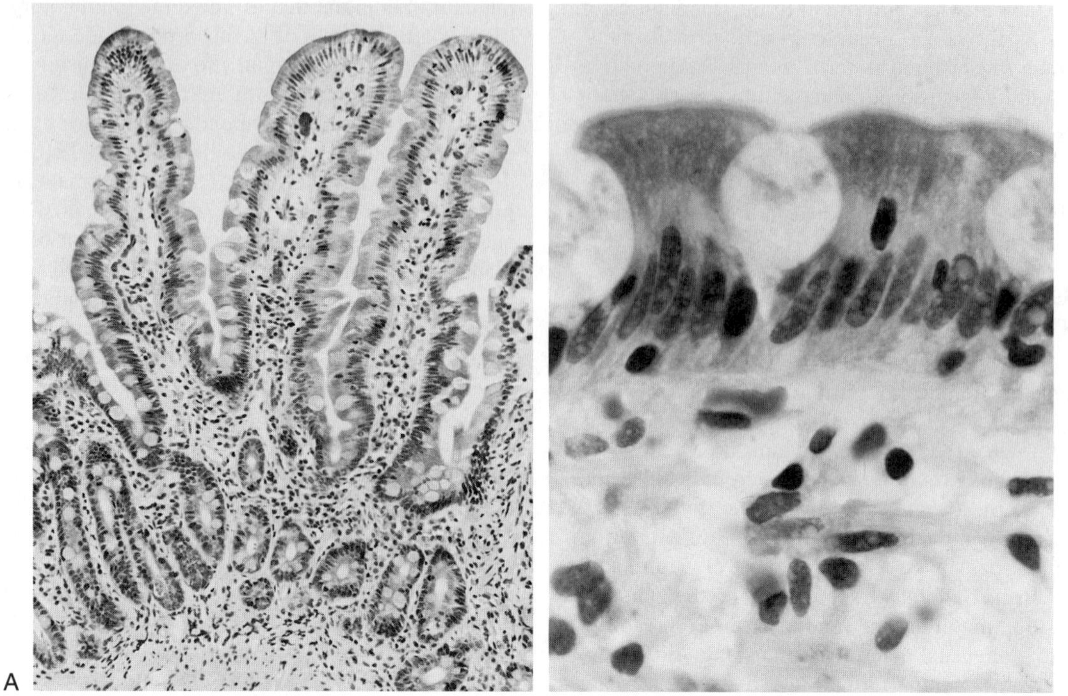

FIG. 69-2. (*A*) Light photomicrograph of the normal mucosa of the human jejunum. The villi are tall, thin, and most prominently developed within the jejunum. In the ileum, the villi are broader and shorter, goblet cells are more prominent, and the lamina propria contains more lymph follicles and lymphoid cells. (Hematoxylin–eosin stain, ×100.) (Courtesy of M. Gottfried, MD) (*B*) High-powered view of brush border showing columnar epithelium with interspersed goblet cells. Deep to the epithelial layer of the mucosa is the lamina propria, a thin layer of connective tissue filled with arterioles, capillaries, veins, lacteals, small nerve fibrils, and numerous additional cellular elements. At the luminal surface of the epithelial cell is the brush border or microvillous membrane, shown here by the lucent band running along the apical enterocytes.

tamine, and prostaglandins released by the cellular elements of the lamina propria, and the secretory products of the enteroendocrine cells of the mucosal epithelium. The lamina propria is also the site of secretory IgA synthesis, an important contributor to the immunologic protection of the host.

Cells that populate the epithelial layer differ depending on whether they overlay the villi, crypts, or the lymphoid aggregates of Peyer patches. The most abundant cells in the crypt epithelium are undifferentiated columnar epithelial cells, with fewer goblet cells, enteroendocrine cells, and Paneth cells. The columnar cells are responsible for cell renewal and can differentiate into all other cellular components. In addition, the columnar cells regulate water and ion secretion. The villus epithelium contains a similar population of cells; however, mature differentiated enterocytes, responsible for absorption, replace the undifferentiated cells of the crypts, and Paneth cells are absent. Structurally distinct M cells that are found in the epithelium overlaying Peyer patches appear to be important in antigen processing and presentation to immunocompetent gut lymphocytes.

The small intestine is in a perpetual state of turnover, with intense mitotic activity in the crypts, uniform migration of all cell types (with the exception of Paneth cells) luminally up the side of the villus, and eventual extrusion at the villus tip. As cells make this journey, they acquire the special structure and intracellular elements needed for their mature function, including the development of specific digestive and absorptive func-

tions. Epithelial cell migration and maturation occur about every 3 to 5 days; the entire mucosal lining is replaced in 1 week.

Cellular Anatomy

Enterocytes are tall columnar epithelial cells that are responsible for absorption. These cells rest tightly on their basal laminae and are attached at the apical pole to adjacent enterocytes by tight junctions. In the jejunum, however, these tight junctions are actually permeable, and back diffusion of fluid and electrolytes into the lumen allows the luminal contents to remain isotonic even as the bulk of nutrients are absorbed. Conversely, in the ileum, the tight junctions are less permeable; there is less back diffusion and an increased concentration of luminal contents. Thus, resection of the ileum has more profound effects on the volume and tonicity of intestinal contents reaching the colon.

The luminal surface of the enterocyte has numerous membrane extensions, termed *microvilli,* which are about 1 mm tall. The microvilli (also known as the *brush border;* Fig. 69-3) are in direct contact with the luminal contents and contain the membrane-bound digestive enzymes, transport proteins, and other elements necessary for nutrient absorption. The brush border can be damaged by multiple small bowel pathogens such

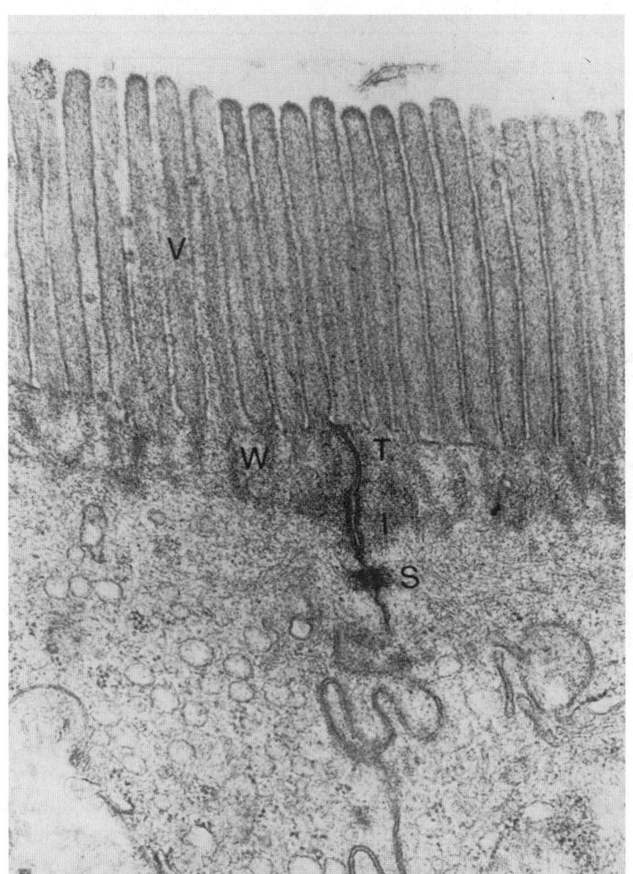

FIG. 69-3. Electron micrograph of adjacent villous absorptive cells. The adjacent cells are tightly adherent through the formation of a junctional complex, containing a tight junction (T), intermediate junction (I), and spot desmosome (S). Thin, supporting central filaments of actin are present within the microvillus (V) and terminate by embedding with filaments in the terminal web (W). (×15,000.) (Antonson D. Anatomy and physiology of the small and large intestine. In: Wyllie R, Hyams J, eds. Pediatric gastrointestinal disease: pathophysiology, diagnosis, and management. Philadelphia, WB Saunders, 1993:477)

as rotavirus or *Giardia sp,* leading to transient reduction in digestive enzyme function. Interposed between and lying on top of the microvilli is a glycoprotein coat called the *glycocalyx* or the "fuzzy coat." Glycoproteins that make up this layer are resistant to removal by enzymatic activity.[20] Fluid and electrolyte trafficking between cells is controlled by the junctional complexes between adjacent cells and the basolateral membrane. This portion of the cell membrane lacks the disaccharidases and peptidases present on the apical membrane but is rich in Na^+,K^+-ATPase, glycosyl transferase, and adenyl cyclase, all of which are involved in the major energy-dependent mechanisms that control fluid and electrolyte transport.

Although the specific functions of the goblet cell are not completely known, it likely serves to provide a protective lubricant barrier to the epithelial surface because of secretion of carbohydrate-rich mucous from mucin-secreting granules. Goblet cell mucus may also act as a hydrating gel between the glycocalyx and the unstirred water layer, and may bind specifi-

cally with bacterial surface antigens to inhibit their attachment to the epithelial cell surface. The most distinctive feature of the enteroendocrine cells, which are scattered sparsely throughout the entire length of the small intestine, is the presence of neurosecretory granules. These are contained within the cytoplasm and are of relatively uniform shape and size. It appears that each of these cells secretes only one or two biologically active amines or peptide hormones, such as secretin, gastrin, VIP, gastric inhibitory polypeptide, neurotensin, cholecystokinin, somatostatin, enteroglucagon, substance P, or pancreatic polypeptide.[21] The major physiologic functions of the peptides are summarized in Table 69-2. Paneth cells are found solely at the base of the crypts and are also secretory cells that appear to have a function in host protection. They are filled with granules that contain lysozyme and have trypsin-like activity, and they can phagocytize bacteria and protozoa.[22]

Small Intestinal Motility

The two functions of small intestinal motor activity are to mix and propel ingested food, promoting effective digestion and absorption of luminal contents, and to sweep the small intestine clear of undigestible food particles, bacteria, and desquamated cells during periods of fasting. Coordinated peristalsis, consisting of contractions and relaxations, is regulated by the intrinsic activity of the smooth muscle together with the modulating actions of the autonomic nervous system and gastrointestinal hormones. The human enteric nervous system (ENS) consists of cell bodies and processes of the neural plexuses within the gut wall. It contains more than 10^8 neurons, which is roughly equivalent to the number of neurons in the spinal cord. The size and complexity of this neural control network account for its being called the "little brain in the gut."[23]

An intestinal peristaltic reflex consists of coordinated contraction above and relaxation below the site of stimulation. Cholinergic and tachykinin motor neurons regulate contraction, and VIP motor neurons are responsible for descending relaxation.[24] Somatostatin-releasing neurons enhance VIP release, and opioid neurons exert a continuous inhibitory effect on VIP neurons.

During fasting, small intestinal motility is organized into a recurrent pattern of sequential periods, which together make up the MMCs. The MMCs have been called the "intestinal housekeeper" because they clear the small intestine of bacteria and undigestible food residue. Absence of MMCs in patients with pseudoobstruction is associated with bacterial overgrowth.[25] MMCs consist of three phases. Phase 1 is a period of quiescence characterized by slow transit and maximal absorption of nutrients. It is followed by phase 2, a period of random, intermittent contractions similar to the normal postprandial pattern, designed for mixing rather than propulsion. Phase 3 is a brief period of high-amplitude contractions occurring at maximal frequency. Phase 3 can start anywhere from the lower esophageal sphincter to the distal jejunum, and propagates at a rate of 5 to 15 cm/min toward the ileum. Phase 3 is also associated with an increase in intestinal secretions, which may aid in clearing the small intestine of bacteria and residue.[26] As one complex reaches the terminal ileum, another starts in the proximal intestine. A complete MMC occurs every 90 to 300 minutes in adults and every 40 to 100 minutes in infants.

Ingestion of a nutrient meal disrupts the cyclic pattern of the

TABLE 69-2. *Human gastrointestinal regulatory peptides: main anatomic source and primary physiologic action*

Regulatory peptide	Main source	Main action
Gastrin	Antrum	Stimulates gastric acid secretion
Cholecystokinin	Upper small intestine and CNS	Gallbladder contraction and pancreatic enzyme secretion
Secretin	Upper small intestine	Pancreatic bicarbonate secretion
Pancreatic glucagon	Pancreas	Stimulates hepatic glucose output
Enteroglucagon	Ileum and colon	Gut mucosal growth, gut motility, and gallbladder contraction
Pancreatic polypeptide	Pancreas	Inhibits pancreatic enzyme secretion and gallbladder contraction
Gastric inhibitory polypeptide	Upper small intestine	Enhances insulin secretion
Motilin	Upper small intestine	Stimulates gastrointestinal motility
Vasoactive intestinal polypeptide	All tissue	Neurotransmitter (secretomotor, vasodilator, and smooth muscle relaxation)
Bombesin	Gut, CNS, and lung	Stimulates gut hormone release
Somatostatin	Gut and CNS	Inhibits hormone release and hormone target tissue
Neurotensin	Ileum and CNS	Inhibits gastric emptying and acid secretion
Substance P	Gut, CNS, and skin	Sensory neurotransmitter (especially pain)
Leu-enkephalin and met-enkephalin	Gut and CNS	Opiate-like (endorphin system)
Peptide HI	Gut and CNS	Unknown
Peptide YY	Gut and CNS	Inhibits gastric acid secretion and gut motility

(Adapted from Aynsley-Green A. Endocrine function of the gut in early life. In: Pediatric gastrointestinal disease: pathophysiology, diagnosis, management. Philadelphia, BC Decker, 1994:238)

MMCs, leading to a prolonged period of irregular activity similar to phase 2 during fasting. The fed pattern, however, has even fewer propagating contractions than phase 2 of the MMC and results in slow transit and more time for intraluminal digestion and absorption of nutrients in the proximal small intestine.[27] The duration of the fed pattern correlates with the time of gastric emptying and is influenced by the characteristics of nutrients ingested. Fat meals are slower to empty the stomach and inhibit the MMC longer than isocaloric amounts of sucrose, which in turn inhibit the MMC longer than protein. Hormonal influences play a role as well. Intravenous infusions of secretin, insulin, glucagon cholecystokinin, or gastrin disrupt the MMC and induce a fed motility pattern, even in the absence of luminal nutrients. Neural control is also important because vagotomy inhibits the fed pattern, suggesting that vagal activity has a role in suppressing the fasting pattern.[28] Local perfusion of anticholinergic compounds disrupts the MMC for a considerable distance proximal and distal to the perfusion site.

The ENS is made up of the myenteric plexus (Auerbach plexus), situated between the longitudinal and circular muscle layers, and the submucosal plexus (Meissner plexus), located in the submucosa. The two plexuses contain networks of neurons, communicate through connecting nerve axons, and generate stereotypic patterns of electrical activity that regulate motility secretion and blood flow. These intrinsic patterns are essential, as illustrated by numerous animal models of extrinsically denervated intestinal segments that retain peristalsis and cycled MMCs. When the small intestine is divided into small segments by multiple transections and reanastomoses, each segment generates its own MMC, which cycles independently from other segments.[29] Stimulation of motilin receptors by erythromycin, which ordinarily induces MMCs in adults, fails to induce similar motility changes in preterm infants who lack a mature ENS necessary for normal intestinal cyclic motor activity.[30]

In the presence of a mature ENS, extrinsic neurogenic, chemical, and hormonal control is important in regulating small bowel motility. The small intestine is supplied by parasympathetic nerves from the vagus and by sympathetic nerves from the thoracolumbar spinal cord. Blocking the parasympathetic input by vagotomy or the administration of atropine reduces the duration of phase 2 of the MMC, and initiating an MMC by injections of motilin into the stomach requires an intact vagus.[31] In contrast, extrinsic sympathetic nerves are important inhibitory efferents to the small intestine and mediate the disappearance of MMCs, as seen in patients who develop a postoperative ileus.[32] Chemical excitatory substances that stimulate small bowel contraction include acetylcholine, tachykinins, and substance P. Likely candidates for postsynaptic inhibitors of contraction include VIP, calcitonin gene-related peptide, nitric oxide, high doses of somatostatin, and β-endorphin. The peptide hormone motilin appears to stimulate MMCs that originate in the stomach, but MMCs that begin below the pylorus do not correlate with plasma motilin variation. Eating a meal produces an increase in the serum concentration of motilin.[33]

Physiology of Water and Electrolyte Absorption

Osmotic differences of as little as 1.6 mOsm/L across the apical enterocyte membrane and of only an additional O.7 mOsm/L across the basolateral membrane are thought to account for the transfer of water from the luminal space to the capillary space in the small intestine.[34] Solute entry into the enterocyte to maintain this small osmotic gradient is achieved primarily by active transport processes. The apical (luminal) membrane of the enterocyte contains numerous active transporters of solutes, including glucose and amino acids, which transfer sodium in an obligatory process. The basolateral membrane contains an active transporter for sodium in the form of the Na^+-K^+-ATPase pump. Together, these processes maintain a small gradient of relative hypotonicity in the lumen, intermediate tonicity in the cell, and mild hypertonicity within the lateral

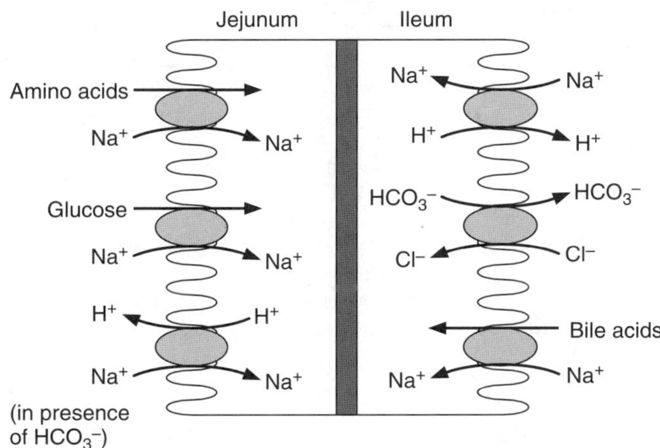

FIG. 69-4. Schematic comparison of the important mechanisms for sodium absorption in the jejunum and the ileum. See text for details.

intracellular space. Increasing hydrostatic pressure in this space helps push water across the freely permeable basal lamina and interstitial space into the capillaries of the lamina propria.

Ion transport across the small intestinal epithelium occurs by passive diffusion down a chemical concentration gradient or because of electrical potential differences, by solvent drag from the passive flow of solutes secondary to water flow, or by active transport carrier-mediated processes that are energy-dependent and move ions against either an electrical or a chemical concentration gradient. In all segments of the small intestine, the final determinant of the driving force for all active ion transport is the Na^+-K^+-ATPase pump located along the basolateral membrane. This pump actively transports sodium out of the cell at the basolateral membrane in exchange for potassium. Absorption of sodium and other ions is regulated by the intestinal epithelium covering the villi, and secretion of chloride is predominantly handled by the crypt cells.

The intestinal epithelium has a number of mechanisms for sodium absorption (Fig. 69-4). In the jejunum, one to three molecules of sodium are cotransported with each glucose molecule. Activation of the sodium-coupled cotransporter by glucose is associated with loosening of the tight junctions between enterocytes and a resultant increase in paracellular transport of small molecules. This may be the major route for assimilation of glucose and other nutrients after a meal.[35] Sodium–hydrogen exchange is also an important mechanism of sodium absorption when bicarbonate is present in the jejunum.[36] This process results in a one-to-one exchange of sodium for hydrogen and can be inhibited by amiloride. Solvent drag likely also plays a significant role in sodium absorption in the jejunum but has a lesser role in the ileum.

In the distal small intestine, sodium absorption occurs primarily through electroneutral sodium chloride absorption, with a dual exchange of sodium for hydrogen and chloride for bicarbonate.[37] Congenital absence of the chloride–bicarbonate exchanger in the ileum and proximal colon results in the rare diarrheal disorder congenital chloridorrhea, in which the patient suffers from a chloride-rich secretory diarrhea.[38] Electrogenic sodium absorption is possible in the ileum, where the less permeable junctions allow maintenance of the electrochemical

gradient, thus favoring sodium transport into the cell by the basolateral Na^+-K^+-ATPase pump. Active bile salt reabsorption also occurs in the terminal ileum, where the bile salt transporter couples sodium to bile salt absorption in a stoichiometric ratio of $1:1$.

Chloride secretion occurs in intestinal crypt cells because of two mechanisms. Chloride is carried into the cell by a cotransporter located in the basolateral membrane, which results in the electroneutral transport of one sodium, one potassium, and two chloride molecules. Chloride carried across the basolateral membrane is then secreted from the cell through chloride-selective channels located in the apical membrane of crypt cells.[39] These chloride-selective channels are generally closed, but they can be opened by activating cyclic AMP, cyclic GMP, or protein kinase C, or by calcium. Cyclic AMP is stimulated by cholera toxin, VIP, and prostaglandins.[40] Cyclic GMP stimulation can result from *Escherichia coli* enterotoxin and calcium. As chloride is secreted across the apical membrane, sodium is lost through the paracellular pathway in response to the outwardly directed electrochemical gradient created by the chloride secretion.

Physiology of Nutrient Digestion and Absorption

Carbohydrates

Starches and oligosaccharides are the major form of carbohydrate in the human diet but must undergo digestion to monosaccharides before they can be absorbed. Table 69-3 summarizes the extraintestinal and brush-border enzymes that participate in carbohydrate digestion to monosaccharides. A small amount of dietary disaccharide and as much as 10% to 20% of starch normally are not absorbed in the small intestine and pass into the colon to be fermented by colonic bacteria to short-chain fatty acids reabsorbed in the colon. This colonic reclamation of carbohydrate prevents loss of energy and the osmotic diarrhea that would result from carbohydrate malabsorption. It is also probably important in limiting diarrhea in patients with lactose intolerance, sucrase-isomaltase deficiency, and short bowel syndrome.

The most important enzyme in the digestion of starch is α-amylase, which acts on the interior α_{1-4} bonds of starch. Salivary amylase makes a minor contribution to overall starch digestion, except perhaps in neonates, because it is inactivated at gastric pH. Human milk, in contrast to cow milk, is rich in α-amylase activity.[41] Pancreatic amylase activity is low in the first months of life, but in older children with normally functioning pancreases, it is present in excess of normal requirements for starch hydrolysis. Therefore, starch digestion is essentially complete when intestinal contents reach the distal duodenum.[42] Exposure of the duodenum to nutrient is the major stimulus for pancreatic amylase secretion. This effect is likely mediated through both the cholinergic nervous system and gut hormones because administration of a cholecystokinin receptor antagonist reduces meal-stimulated pancreatic enzyme secretion by 60%, and atropine causes nearly complete suppression of pancreatic enzyme secretion.[43] Secretin, the major stimulant of pancreatic bicarbonate and fluid secretion, also promotes α-amylase secretion but has less effect on lipase and little effect on pancreatic protease release.

TABLE 69-3. *Extraintestinal and brush-border enzymes of carbohydrate digestion*

Enzyme	Bond cleaved	Substrate	Products
Amylase (human milk, saliva, pancreas)	α_{1-4}-Glucosidase	Starch (amylose, amylopectin)	Maltose, maltotriose, oligosaccharide with terminal 1–6 linkage (α-limit dextrins)
Lactase	β_{1-4}-Galactosidase (β-glucosidase)	Lactose	Glucose, galactose
Sucrase	α_{1-4}-Glucosidase	Sucrose, maltose, maltotriose, α-limit dextrins with terminal α_{1-4} links	Glucose, fructose, maltooligosaccharide with α_{1-6} linkage
Glucomylase	α_{1-4}-Glucosidase	Maltose, maltotriose, maltooligosaccharide (glucose polymers with maximal affinity for chains of 6–10 residues)	Glucose, maltooligosaccharide with terminal α_{1-6} linkage
Isomaltase (α-dextrinase)	α_{1-6}-Glucosidase	Maltose, isomaltose, α-limit dextrins (maltooligosaccharide with terminal α_{1-6} links)	Glucose, maltooligosaccharide
Trehalase	α-and β-glucosidase (tested on renal trehalase)	Trehalose (found principally in mushrooms)	Glucose

(Adapted from Treem WR. Congenital sucrase-isomaltase deficiency. J Pediatr Gastroenterol Nutr in press)

Oligosaccharides, including the hydrolytic products of starch digestion, and the disaccharides lactose and sucrose are hydrolyzed at the luminal surface of the brush border by disaccharidases. These are membrane-bound glycoprotein enzymes that protrude from the microvillus membrane into the small intestinal lumen. Disaccharidase activity is greatest in the enterocytes near the villus tip and in the proximal jejunum. With the exception of lactase, the disaccharidases have the capacity to hydrolyze substrate more rapidly than the resulting monosaccharides are absorbed. Thus, monosaccharide absorption is usually the rate-limiting step in the assimilation of oligosaccharides. The hydrolytic products of starch digestion are digested by the complementary action of sucrase, isomaltase, and glucoamylase; each enzyme is responsible for glucose polymers of different chain lengths.[44] The α_{1-6} bonds of starch hydrolysis products can be cleaved only by isomaltase. Studies in normal volunteers demonstrated that starch and oligosaccharides are completely absorbed before the intestinal contents have reached the distal jejunum.[45]

Fats

Figure 69-5 provides an overview of the major steps of lipid digestion and absorption. Despite the complexity of the process, absorption from the lumen into the enterocyte and then to the lamina propria requires only about 12 minutes, and over 95% of intraluminal fat is normally absorbed. Triglycerides, which make up about 90% of dietary fat intake, are emulsified into tiny particles and stabilized by other dietary components, such as phospholipids and polysaccharides or endogenous bile salts. Bile salts are important in solubilization and in the promotion of pancreatic lipase activity, but 75% of dietary triglyceride can be absorbed without bile salts. Cholesterol and fat-soluble vitamin absorption are affected more severely by bile acid deficiency than is triglyceride absorption.

Multiple lipases have a role in the hydrolysis of the ester bonds of triglycerides and phospholipids, but pancreatic lipase, in conjunction with its cofactor colipase, is responsible for the major proportion of triglyceride hydrolysis. Lingual and gastric lipases initiate hydrolysis in the stomach and can be of great importance in the neonatal period when pancreatic lipase is deficient. Gastric lipase hydrolyzes medium-chain triglycerides five to eight times faster than long-chain triglycerides. In neonates, medium-chain triglycerides disappear more rapidly from the stomach after a meal than do long-chain triglycerides because neonates appear to absorb medium-chain triglycerides directly from the stomach.[46] This factor, in addition to the necessity for bile salts for long-chain triglyceride solubilization, may explain the relative advantage of medium-chain triglyceride–containing formulas for premature neonates. Fat digestion in breastfed infants also benefits from a separate lipase found in human milk.[47] This enzyme is resistant to stomach acid and is activated by bile salts in the duodenum.

In the presence of bile salts and phospholipid in the proximal intestinal lumen, colipase binds pancreatic lipase to the triglyceride emulsion for hydrolysis of fatty acids off the glycerol backbone. Colipase is initially synthesized as procolipase and subsequently activated by trypsin. The functions of colipase are to attach to the ester bond of the triglyceride and to bring lipase close to this bond, facilitating hydrolysis. In patients with steatorrhea secondary to pancreatic insufficiency, fecal fat loss correlates better with colipase secretion than with lipase secretion.[48] As little as 2% of normal lipase secretion can be compatible with normal fat digestion if colipase secretion is adequate. Phospholipase A_2 is a calcium-dependent bile salt–activated lipase secreted by the pancreas. It is the major enzyme in the digestion of intestinal phopholipids, both from the diet and contained in bile.

As a solute passes from the bulk phase within the lumen toward the enterocyte, it first passes through the unstirred water

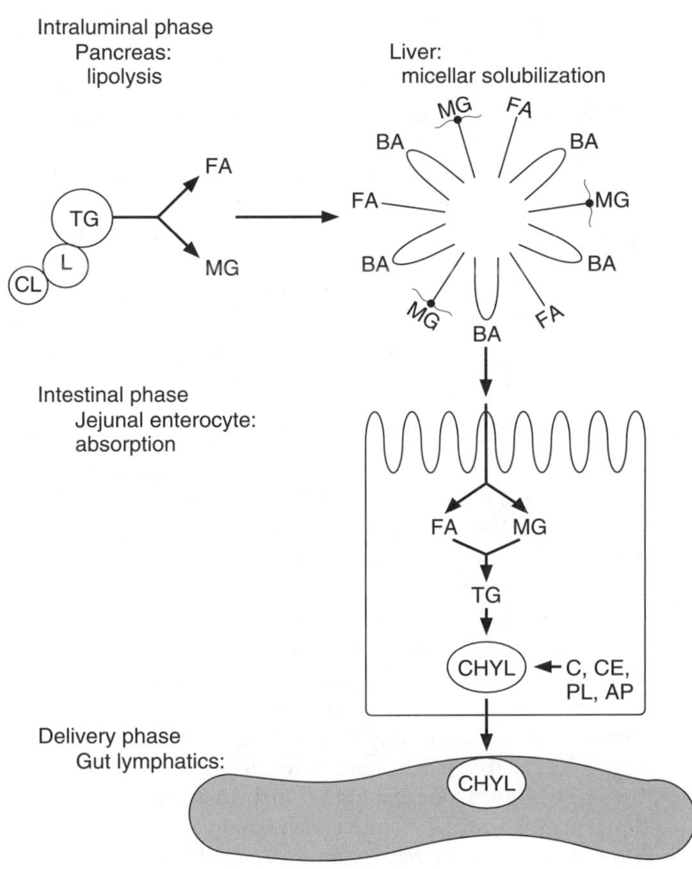

FIG. 69-5. Overview of the major steps of lipid digestion and absorption. (1) Lipase (L) and colipase (CL) bind to the triglyceride (TG) droplet. (2) Intraluminal lipolysis of triglyceride to fatty acids (FA) and monoglycerides (MG). (3) Formation into micelles with bile acids (BA). (4) Absorption of the fatty acids and monoglycerides into the enterocyte. (5) Reesterification into triglycerides and formation of chylomicrons (CHYL) made up of cholesterol (C), cholesterol ester (CE), phospholipid (PL), and apoproteins (AP). (6) Secretion of chylomicrons into intercellular spaces and gut lymphatics in lamina propria.

layer, adjacent to the microvillus membrane. The layer acts as a diffusion barrier and is the rate-limiting step for the absorption of fats in the small intestine.[49] The products of fat digestion are free fatty acids, monoglycerides, phosphatidylcholine (phospholipid), free cholesterol, and free sterols (vitamins), which are solubilized in bile acid micelles. Most absorption of the contents of these mixed micelles occurs in the proximal small intestine at the villus tips and is complete by the mid-jejunum. Dissociation of micelles into an absorbable form is promoted by the acid pH of the microenvironment at the surface of the microvillus membrane.[50] A change in luminal pH can affect the pH of the microenvironment and therefore can affect lipid absorption. Once the products of lipolysis reach the enterocyte membrane, they rapidly diffuse by passive transport into the cell.

A small proportion of the bile acids that previously formed the micelle are absorbed by passive diffusion in the jejunum. The bulk are reabsorbed in a conjugated form by active transport in the terminal ileum. Deconjugation of intraluminal bile acids by small bowel bacterial overgrowth and loss of active transport of bile salts by ileal disease or resection can compromise the enterohepatic circulation of bile acids and adversely affect fat absorption. In addition, jejunal hyperacidity, which occurs in cystic fibrosis and other forms of pancreatic insufficiency, can cause precipitation of bile acids, further compromising fat absorption.

Once inside the enterocyte, the products of lipolysis are bound to fatty acid–binding protein and transported to the smooth endoplasmic reticulum for reassembly into triglycer-

ides, phophatidylcholine, and cholesterol. Chylomicrons, made up of phopholipid and apoprotein surface coats and inner triglyceride, cholesterol esters, and free cholesterol, are synthesized inside the enterocyte and subsequently released across the basolateral membrane. They enter lacteals within the lamina propria and subsequently reach gut lymphatic vessels.

Proteins

Protein digestion begins in the stomach, where gastric acid denatures dietary protein and promotes pepsin digestion of protein into large polypeptides. Pancreatic proteases, secreted into the small intestine, then act to further split large polypeptides into oligopeptides of six or fewer amino acid residues. Pancreatic proteases are initially secreted in an inactive form. Conversion of the inactive pancreatic trypsinogen into trypsin is catalyzed by the brush-border enzyme enterokinase, which is localized to the proximal small intestine. Trypsin then activates the other pancreatic proteases, including chymotrypsin and elastase. Animals with ligation of the pancreatic duct can still absorb nearly 40% of a protein meal, and patients with severe pancreatic insufficiency can still absorb a portion of ingested protein.[51] This ability is due to the presence of three neutral endopeptidases expressed in the mature region of the villus, which can also hydrolyze intact large peptides.[52]

Also present on the brush-border surface of the enterocyte are peptide hydrolases, which split oligopeptides further into component amino acids.[53] Some oligopeptides with three or fewer amino acids enter the cell intact and are cleaved by cytosolic peptide hydrolases. At the luminal surface of the enterocyte are specific carriers for neutral, basic, and acidic amino acids as well as dipeptides and tripeptides. Active transport of amino acids is coupled with sodium transport; the driving electrochemical gradient is maintained by the basolateral Na^+-K^+-ATPase pump. At high intraluminal amino acid concentrations, diffusion becomes quantitatively important as a method of amino acid entry into the enterocyte. Although dietary protein can be identified in the proximal ileal contents, digestion and absorption are nearly completed by the time that the intestinal contents arrive at the terminal ileum. Less than 1 g of protein, oligopeptides, and free amino acids normally pass into the colon each day.

CHRONIC SMALL INTESTINAL DISEASES

This section describes some clinical syndromes and specific disease entities that often are characterized by diffuse involvement of the small intestine and that present with chronic vomiting, diarrhea, failure to thrive, or gastrointestinal bleeding. The pediatric surgeon is frequently involved in the treatment of patients with these problems because of the acute need for surgical intervention, the need for chronic enteral or parenteral nutrition, or consideration of special procedures to relieve strictures of the small intestine, lengthen the intestine, or restore more normal small bowel motility. This discussion concentrates on the recognition of the clinical symptoms and complications that characterize these syndromes and the diagnostic tests available to evaluate them. Treatment of these complicated patients is often a collaborative effort among the pediatric surgeon, pediatric gastroenterologist, and other pediatric subspecialists.

Short Bowel Syndrome

Compromise of the normal anatomic and physiologic mechanisms that facilitate small bowel function is perhaps best illustrated by the complex problems encountered in children with short bowel syndrome. Abnormalities in small bowel motility, digestion, and absorption characterize these patients and contribute to significant morbidity and even mortality in some patients. Two major developments have dramatically altered the prognosis for even the most severely affected infants and children with short bowel syndrome. For more than 20 years, parenteral nutrition has been an indispensable part of the acute and chronic management of short bowel syndrome. More recently, limited success with small intestine transplantation has offered hope to those without sufficient intestinal adaptation to support enteral feedings.[54]

Short bowel syndrome is defined as malabsorption, fluid and electrolyte loss, and malnutrition after massive resection of the small intestine. Wilmore[55] reviewed the case histories of 50 infants younger than 2 months of age and defined short bowel syndrome as less than 75 cm of residual small intestine, or less than 40% of the normal length of the small intestine in a full-term neonate. Resection of more than 75% of the small intestine with preservation of the ileocecal valve invariably produces initial intractable malabsorption and diarrhea. As much as half of the small intestine can be lost, however, without significant long-term problems in sustaining normal nutrition, provided the duodenum, distal ileum, and ileocecal valve are spared.

In contrast, distal ileal resections that include the ileocecal valve can cause severe diarrhea even though only 25% of the small intestine has been resected. This is most likely due to several important functions peculiar to the ileum. First, the ileum is capable of undergoing much more dramatic compensatory hyperplasia in response to jejunal resection than is the jejunum in response to ileal resection. Second, resection of the ileum has more profound effects on the volume and tonicity of intestinal contents reaching the colon because it is only in the ileum that decreased permeability of the intracellular tight junctions allows for increased concentrations of luminal contents. Also, only the ileum and right colon can absorb sodium chloride against a steep concentration gradient. Third, resection of the ileum also causes diarrhea and even steatorrhea if the resection is massive enough, secondary to the malabsorption of bile salts. And finally, loss of the ileocecal valve is one of the major permissive factors in the development of bacterial overgrowth in the small intestine.

In addition to the amount of intestine resected, whether it is predominantly jejunum or ileum, and whether the resection includes the ileocecal valve, other important variables determining the outcome include whether the colon is intact, whether some enteral nutrition can be provided to stimulate intestinal adaptation, and whether there is residual intestinal disease or surgical complications that further compromise nutrient absorption. Patients who have undergone partial or total colectomy in addition to extensive resection of the small intestine are more prone to experience severe dehydration, hypokalemia, hypomagnesemia, and hyponatremia—the *end-jejunostomy syndrome*.[56] The large potential reserve capacity of the intact healthy adult colon has been demonstrated by the absorption of 6 L of water and 800 mEq of sodium, slowly perfused into the cecum of normal healthy adult volunteers.[57] The colon also salvages malabsorbed carbohydrate by bacterial fermentation to short-chain fatty acids, which are absorbed and used as fuel by colonic epithelial cells or exported to the liver for energy-yielding metabolic processes.

Nutrients in the lumen of the small intestine are essential for the maintenance of mucosal mass. Not only starvation but also the provision of adequate protein and calories exclusively by total parenteral nutrition results in mucosal atrophy in humans and experimental animals. Numerous studies in animals have demonstrated that even in the presence of resection of the small intestine (the most potent trigger of small intestinal mucosal hyperplasia), no adaptation occurs unless luminal nutrients are provided. These findings suggest that after intestinal resection, parenteral nutrition should be supplemented with enteral nutrients as soon as possible to stimulate small intestine adaptation. Preliminary work suggests that glutamine supplementation of parenteral nutrition solutions may result in relative preservation of small bowel mucosal mass and function in patients with short bowel syndrome.[58] Growth hormone has been implicated in the response to resection of the small intestine because hypophysectomized animals do not undergo mucosal hyperplasia after enterectomy despite the provision of sufficient enteral calories.[59] Studies using growth hormone supplementation to promote intestinal adaptation are also underway in patients with short bowel syndrome.[60]

TABLE 69-4. *Causes of short bowel syndrome in infants*

Cause	Wilmore, 1972[55]	Bohane et al, 1979[61]	Cooper et al, 1984[62]	Dorney et al, 1985[63]	Grosfeld et al, 1986[64]	Caniano et al, 1989[65]	Goulet et al, 1991[66]
Volvulus	30	2	6	6	5	1	22
Atresia	14	6	3	3	13	5	36
Gastrochisis	5	3	2	1	5	5	10
Necrotizing enterocolitis	0	4	5	2	24	2	11
Other*	1	0	0	1	7	1	8
TOTAL	50	15	16	13	54	14	87

* Meconium peritonitis, extensive intestinal angioma, complicated intussusception, congenital short bowel syndrome.

(Treem WR. Short bowel syndrome. In: Wyllie R, Hyans J, eds. Pediatric gastrointestinal disease: pathophysiology, diagnosis, management. Philadelphia, WB Saunders, 1993:574)

Table 69-4 summarizes the causes of short bowel syndrome in infants.[55,61–66] The most common causes include necrotizing enterocolitis, volvulus, jejunoileal atresia, and gastroschisis. Short bowel syndrome has been reported in 7% to 38% of infants who survive surgical therapy for necrotizing enterocolitis.[54] Midgut volvulus and diffuse small bowel Crohn disease predominate in older children. Less frequent causes of short bowel syndrome include trauma to the gastrointestinal tract and total colonic aganglionosis with proximal extension into the small intestine.

Specific clinical consequences of massive resection of the small intestine include the following:

- Nutrient malabsorption
  Steatorrhea
  Fat-soluble vitamins
  Starch, disaccharides
  Iron, folate, vitamin B_{12}, zinc
- Electrolyte loss
- Hypocalcemia, hypomagnesemia
- Bile acid malabsorption
- Bacterial overgrowth
- Gastric acid hypersecretion
- D-Lactic acidosis
- Hyperoxaluria (renal stones)
- Cholelithiasis
- Total parenteral nutrition–induced hepatotoxicity
- Central venous catheter–related infections

Deficiencies of divalent cations, especially magnesium, are common and lead to symptoms of tetany, osteopenia, osteomalacia, and spontaneous fractures. Luminal absorption of both calcium and magnesium can be compromised by fat malabsorption. Zinc deficiency can also develop in the setting of fat malabsorption and is more prone to occur when the terminal ileum has been resected. Malabsorption of fat-soluble vitamins (vitamins A, D, E, and K) increases with steatorrhea, and iron and folate deficiency occur when proximal small intestine has been lost. Vitamin B_{12} malabsorption is almost invariably present when more than 100 cm of terminal ileum has been resected.

Bacterial overgrowth exacerbates malabsorption of almost all nutrients secondary to its detrimental effects on bile acid reabsorption, vitamin B_{12} absorption, small intestine motility, and the normal turnover and regeneration of the small bowel mucosa and mucosal enzymes. Factors that promote bacterial overgrowth in patients with short bowel syndrome include absence of the ileocecal valve; presence of a partial small intestine obstruction from a tight anastomosis, an ischemic stricture, or an adhesion; presence of a dilated hypotonic intestinal segment with disordered motility; presence of an enteroenteral fistula secondary to an underlying inflammatory disease, such as Crohn disease, or a surgical complication; and relative achlorhydria secondary to the prolonged use of H_2-receptor antagonists to prevent gastric acid hypersecretion. Treatment of bacterial overgrowth consists of periodic use of oral antibiotics, such as trimethaprim-sulfamethoxazole, metronidazole, ciprofloxacin, vancomycin, or gentamicin.

In both adults and children, gastric acid hypersecretion occurs after massive resection of the small intestine. Its magnitude appears to be proportional to the length of intestine resected; gastric acid hypersecretion is more prevalent in patients with less than one third of the small intestine remaining.[67] Treatment with an H_2-receptor antagonist for 6 to 12 months after resection is advisable. Patients with small bowel bacterial overgrowth can develop D-lactic acidosis, a syndrome of encephalopathy and metabolic acidosis brought on by liberalization of the diet to include more lactose and bacterial fermentation of the lactose to D-lactic acid. Effective treatment consists of correction of the acidosis, cessation of enteral carbohydrates, and reduction of the intestinal flora with antibiotics, such as oral vancomycin, neomycin, or metronidazole.

In four recent reviews of short bowel syndrome in infancy and childhood, 20 of 174 patients developed cholelithiasis, and 16 of 20 required cholecystectomy for acute cholecystitis, biliary colic, or both.[63–66] In addition to the increased risk of cholelithiasis in children treated with chronic total parenteral nutrition, ileal resection appears to be another important predisposing factor for this complication.[68] Because of the high incidence of gallstones in children with significant ileal resections, some centers perform cholecystectomy routinely during the initial small intestine resection or at the time of reestablishment of intestinal continuity. Early institution of enteral nutrition to stimulate the elaboration of gut hormones, gallbladder motility, and bile flow, and the use of choleretic agents, such as ursodeoxycholic acid, may prevent bile stasis and the formation of biliary sludge and stones.

Protracted Diarrhea in Infancy

Another group of patients with severe chronic malabsorption and a functional short bowel syndrome are infants with protracted diarrhea from a variety of causes. Protracted diarrhea is defined as greater than 20 mL/kg/d of stool output that begins any time after birth, persists for more than 2 weeks, and requires change not only in the composition but also in the mode of delivery of nutrition. The most frequent causes of protracted diarrhea produce both an osmotic and secretory diarrhea due to severe mucosal injury. These include congenital disorders of enterocyte proliferation and differentiation, disorders of immune regulation, severe intraluminal infections, congenital mucosal ion transport defects, tumors producing intestinal secretagogues, and bacterial overgrowth secondary to functional or mechanical obstruction (Table 69-5).

Diarrhea usually begins in the first few weeks of life and is often initially accompanied by vomiting, poor feeding, and failure to thrive. Dietary manipulation with multiple formula changes and the institution of oral rehydration solutions of half-strength formulas is usually the first intervention and contributes to the spiral of malnutrition that further compromises gut regeneration. In some of these infants, a trial of a hydrolyzed casein formula containing glucose polymers as the carbohydrate source may initially ameliorate the diarrhea, but this improvement is often short-lived. Over time, the persistence of the diarrhea with concomitant fluid and electrolyte problems and protein calorie malnutrition dictates that central venous access be established for parenteral alimentation.

TABLE 69-5. *Differential diagnosis of protracted diarrhea in infancy and childhood*

IMPAIRED INTRALUMINAL DIGESTION

Cystic fibrosis
Biliary atresia (other cholestatic syndromes)
Short bowel syndrome
Crohn disease (with marked small bowel resection)
Bacterial overgrowth
Congenital enterokinase deficiency

IMPAIRED MICROVILLOUS MEMBRANE FUNCTION

FLAT VILLOUS LESION
Celiac disease
Eosinophilic gastroenteritis
Rotavirus (other viral infections)
Giardia sp, *Cryptosporidium* sp, other parasites*
IgA deficiency, severe combined immunodeficiency, common
   variable hypogammaglobulinemia
Graft-versus-host disease
Microvillous inclusion disease

NORMAL VILLI
Congenital chloridorrhea
Primary bile acid malabsorption
Congenital sucrase-isomaltase deficiency
Congenital glucose-galactose malabsorption
Congenital lactase deficiency

IMPAIRED CHYLOMICRON FORMATION AND DELIVERY

Abetalipoproteinemia
Congenital lymphangiectasia

EXTRAINTESTINAL CAUSES (NORMAL VILLI)

Neural crest tumors
Laxative abuse (Munchausen by proxy, anorexia nervosa)
Iatrogenic (sorbitol, fructose in medication)

   * Occurs mainly in immunocompromised hosts.

It is rare that viral gastroenteritis (rotavirus, adenovirus) or enteric bacterial infections cause protracted diarrhea in infancy, unless they are superimposed on previous mucosal injury caused by malnutrition, cow milk or soy protein allergy, or bacterial overgrowth. In patients with congenital or acquired immunodeficiency states, chronic diarrhea can be associated with opportunistic pathogens, including *Cryptosporidium* sp, *Giardia* sp, *Isospora belli, Microsporida* sp, cytomegalovirus, and *mycobacterium avium–intracellulare.* Bacterial overgrowth, particularly with strains of *E coli* that adhere to the enterocyte brush border, can damage the microvillus membrane and cause patchy villus atrophy and depression of brush-border enzymes.[69,70]

A primary immunodeficiency state or acquired immunodeficiency syndrome should be suspected in infants with chronic diarrhea who have persistent shedding of pathogens that usually cause a self-limited diarrhea. These include *Salmonella* sp, *Giardia* sp, adenovirus, and rotavirus. Other potential clues to an underlying immunodeficiency disease include chronic thrush and diarrhea with *Candida albicans;* recurrent otitis media, sinusitis, and bronchopulmonary infections; the presence of opportunistic pathogens in the stool; chronic skin rashes; and recurrent hematologic abnormalities, including hemolytic or aplastic anemia, neutropenia, or thrombocytopenia. In T-cell or combined cellular and humoral immunodeficiency diseases, chronic diarrhea is often a presenting or prominent syndrome. Even in patients with isolated B-cell deficiencies, including isolated IgA deficiency, flat, villus lesions have been described.[71] Unlike patients with gluten-sensitive enteropathy (celiac disease) or cow milk protein allergy, the flat, villus lesion seen in patients with immunodeficiency syndromes usually does not respond to removal of any food protein from the diet.

A number of reports have described a subgroup of infants with intractable diarrhea who have diffuse inflammatory flat, villus lesions of the small intestine and features of autoimmune disease, including circulating enterocyte autoantibodies and concurrent extraintestinal disease.[72–74] Extraintestinal disease can take the form of membranous glomerulonephritis, interstitial nephritis, thyroiditis, hemolytic anemia, autoimmune thrombocytopenia, diabetes mellitus type 1, and polyarteritis nodosa. Circulating antibodies against renal epithelial cells, anti–smooth muscle antibodies, antinuclear antibodies, and antithyroid microsomal antibodies have also been detected in selected cases. Treatment with a variety of immunosuppressive agents, including azathioprine, methylprednisolone, and cyclosporine, has been effective in some cases.[75] In many cases, however, the response is short-lived, and relapses are common once the medication has been discontinued.

Congenital microvillus atrophy is a rare disorder associated with a flat, villus lesion causing intractable diarrhea beginning in the first week of life.[76] The major distinction between this entity and the flat, villus lesions associated with the infectious and immunologic causes mentioned earlier is the lack of inflammatory or regenerative activity noted in the small intestine. Biopsy of the small intestines in these patients show total villus atrophy, normal crypts, but no evidence of mitotic activity in the crypt compartment. The lamina propria shows little increase in cellularity. Electron microscopy reveals shortened and irregular microvilli and dense lysosomal inclusions or cystic structures in the apical portion of the enterocyte. In contrast to the villus cells, the ultrastructure of the crypt cells is normal. The restriction of the abnormality to the absorptive villus tip cells suggests a failure of normal maturation and differentiation of crypt cells. No effective therapy is available.

In the presence of normal small intestinal villus architecture, potential causes of protracted diarrhea include congenital transport defects, secretory tumors, and laxative-induced diarrhea as a manifestation of Munchausen syndrome by proxy.[77] Congenital chloridorrhea is a rare autosomal recessive disorder resulting from a selective defect in the Cl^-, HCO_3^- exchange transport system of the ileum and colon.[78] Abdominal distention and severe secretory diarrhea with a high chloride content are present from birth. Electrolyte disturbances in untreated patients include hyponatremia, hypochloremia, and alkalosis. Protracted diarrhea can also be an important clinical manifestation of neural crest tumors in young children, including ganglioneuromas and neuroblastomas.[79,80] These tumors have been found to contain cells capable of secreting catecholamines, glucagon, gastrin, secretin, and VIP. VIP has been implicated as the main cause of the secretory diarrhea, and often VIP levels are elevated in the blood. Laxative abuse in infants and young children can be a clinical manifestation of child abuse or Munchausen syndrome, as noted. The clinical picture of surreptitious laxative ingestion includes abdominal pain, vomiting, muscle weakness, lassitude, hypokalemia, and nonspecific inflammation, melanosis, or both on rectal biopsy. Protracted diarrhea can also be the result of unsuspected osmotic agents used as vehicles for the suspension of common medications. Sorbitol is such an agent.

Any infant who presents with diarrhea in the first week of life and or any child who is admitted with severe diarrhea of greater than 2 weeks' duration associated with weight loss should be given nothing by mouth and started on intravenous nutrition. It is a mistake to delay nutritional repletion while the diagnostic evaluation is taking place because malnutrition is a potential complicating factor in the perpetuation of severe protracted diarrhea. If the diarrhea ceases within 24 to 48 hours after the child is given nothing by mouth, secretory diarrhea is not present, and an evaluation for a secretory tumor by assaying serum VIP levels or urinary vanillymandelic acid is not called for. Trials of formulas that do not contain cow milk or soy protein are warranted if there are no signs of intestinal obstruction or enterocolitis. Avoidance of lactose or sucrose-containing formulas excludes the rare genetic abnormalities of congenital lactase deficiency and sucrase-isomaltase deficiency. The persistence of the diarrhea with the use of a formula that contains glucose polymers as its sole carbohydrate helps to identify patients who have acquired monosaccharide malabsorption. This usually is secondary to a severe diffuse small intestinal injury from viral gastroenteritis or other causes.

The diagnostic evaluation suggested by the differential diagnosis should include an assessment for infectious causes, immunodeficiencies, and secretory diarrhea. Small intestine and often colonic biopsies are extremely useful in the evaluation and treatment of infants and children with protracted diarrhea. Aside from the routine histologic assessment afforded by such biopsies, special stains can be performed that illuminate infectious organisms, such as cytomegalovirus, *Cryptosporidium* sp, and *Giardia* sp. Electron microscopy is invaluable in the identification of congenital microvillus atrophy, enteroadherent bacterial overgrowth, and certain viral pathogens. Measurement of intestinal disaccharidase activity can be helpful in determining the diagnosis of congenital or acquired problems of carbohydrate absorption and direct the choice of the proper carbohydrate composition of the formula.

Chronic Intestinal Pseudoobstruction

Chronic intestinal pseudoobstruction is characterized by signs of intestinal blockage in the absence of an anatomic obstruction. The most common signs and symptoms are abdominal distention, failure to thrive, abdominal pain, vomiting, and constipation or diarrhea. The following discussion is limited to syndromes that affect the small intestine in childhood. Causes of chronic pseudoobstruction in children are summarized in Table 69-6. These include primary congenital forms and acquired causes related to an underlying chronic disease.

The occurrence of pseudoobstruction in infants with fetal alcohol syndrome and in those who were exposed to narcotics in utero suggests that substances that potentially alter neuronal migration or maturation might affect the development of the myenteric plexus and cause severe small intestine motility problems. Some premature infants with bronchopulmonary dysplasia or with a past history of necrotizing enterocolitis appear to develop severe gastrointestinal motility disturbances, presumably related to ischemia and chronic hypoxemia that causes myenteric plexus injury. In a few cases, chronic intestinal pseudoobstruction results from a familial inherited disease.[81]

Histologic diagnosis can be made only by full-thickness intestinal biopsy; abnormalities may be noted in the muscle, nerve, or rarely, both.[82] In the muscular forms, the muscularis appears thin, and there can be extensive fibrosis within the muscle tissue, especially in the external longitudinal muscle layer. Key features of the neuropathic form of intestinal pseudoobstruction include fewer and smaller neurons in the myenteric plexus or so-called intestinal neuronal dysplasia,[83] characterized histologically by hyperplasia of the parasympathetic neurons and fibers of the myenteric plexus.

Most affected children develop symptoms in the first year of life. Of children presenting with symptoms at birth, about

---

TABLE 69-6. *Causes of chronic intestinal pseudoobstruction in children*

PRIMARY

Familial, sporadic, visceral neuropathies
Aganglionosis affecting the small bowel
Familial, sporadic, visceral myopathies
Neuronal intestinal dysplasia with trisomy 21, neurofibromatosis, multiple endocrine neoplasia type IIb
Megalocystis–microcolon intestinal hypoperistalsis syndrome

ACQUIRED OR ASSOCIATED WITH SYSTEMIC CAUSES

Fetal alcohol syndrome
Infants of cocaine- or narcotic-abusing mothers
Drugs—anticholinergics, opiates, calcium-channel blockers, phenothiazines, tricyclic antidepressants, vincristine
CNS or spinal cord injury
Muscular dystrophies (Duchenne, myotonic)
Scleroderma, other connective tissue disorders
Familial dysautonomia
Diabetes, hypothyroidism
Chagas disease (*Trypanosoma cruzi* infection)

40% have malrotation. Abdominal distention and vomiting are the most common features. Constipation, abdominal pain, and poor weight gain are also present in many patients. Urinary tract smooth muscle is affected in about one fifth of all intestinal pseudoobstruction patients, including those who present at birth with the aptly named megacystis–microcolon intestinal hypoperistalsis syndrome.[84] The radiographic signs are usually those of intestinal obstruction (dilated small intestine loops and air–fluid levels) and the presence of a microcolon because of obstruction at birth.

Antroduodenal manometry is the confirmatory test for the diagnosis of small intestinal pseudoobstruction syndrome. Once true mechanical obstruction has been excluded and the diagnosis of intestinal pseudoobstruction has been made, antroduodenal manometry can help differentiate between neuropathic and myopathic pseudoobstruction, offer prognostic information, and suggest potential responses to pharmacologic intervention.[85] The presence of identifiable MMCs during fasting is associated with the ability to tolerate some form of enteral nutrition in more than 80% of children with intestinal pseudoobstruction despite the presence of abnormal nonpropagating bursts of contractions and complaints of bloating, pain, vomiting, and constipation. In contrast, when MMCs are absent, over 80% of patients require partial or total parenteral nutrition. Children with total enteric aganglionosis have contractions of normal amplitude that are never organized in MMC or fed patterns but that appear only as a monotonous pattern of random events. Other studies of gastrointestinal motility can be informative when evaluating the child with suspected pseudoobstruction. Gastric scintiscans can reveal a delay in the emptying of a liquid or solid meal. Esophageal motility abnormalities, including low-amplitude contractions or high-amplitude aperistaltic contractions, can be demonstrated in about half of patients. Colonic manometry may show few or no colonic contractions in a patient with smooth muscle myopathy and no postprandial gastrocolonic response in a patient with the neuropathic form of pseudoobstruction.[86] Anorectal manometry, however, is normal in chronic intestinal pseudoobstruction; the absence of the rectoanal inhibitory reflex occurs only in those with Hirschsprung disease.

Other Diffuse Diseases of the Small Intestine

Hemolytic–Uremic Syndrome

Strictly speaking, the definition of hemolytic–uremic syndrome includes the triad of microangiopathic hemolytic anemia, thrombocytopenia, and acute renal failure. In many patients in the United States, however, it is most often associated with an enteric infection with the verotoxin-producing bacteria *E coli* 0157:H7, and typically presents with a prodrome of bloody diarrhea before the onset of obvious hemolysis, thrombocytopenia, or oliguria and renal failure.[87,88] The association with *E coli* 0157:H7 is much less striking in other parts of the world. For example, in Argentina, only 2% of children with hemolytic–uremic syndrome are infected with *E coli,* but 55% have evidence of an antecedent infection with *Shigella* sp.[89] Epidemic outbreaks of hemolytic–uremic syndrome have been associated with the ingestion of raw and poorly cooked ground beef and unpasteurized milk.

The pathogenesis of both the intestinal wall and renal injury appears to be caused by endothelial cell damage, intravascular platelet activation, and subsequent ischemic intestinal and renal disease. Endothelial damage may occur by a variety of proposed mechanisms, including direct bacterial cytotoxin-induced cytolysis, systemic endotoxin release, cell membrane lipid peroxidization, or immune complex–mediated injury. In addition to bloody diarrhea, crampy abdominal pain and vomiting may be part of the prodrome. At times, peritoneal signs are prominent, leading to consideration of an exploratory laparotomy. Usually, as the gastrointestinal symptoms subside, the other features of pallor, severe anemia, petechiae, easy bruising, thrombocytopenia, oliguria, edema, hypertension, electrolyte disturbances, and renal failure become evident.

Stool cultures for routine pathogens are usually negative. Many laboratories can culture for *E coli* 0157:H7 if it is specifically requested. A careful examination of the blood smear may reveal early changes of microangiopathic hemolytic anemia and a disproportionately low platelet count in the setting of inflammatory enterocolitis. A flat plate of the abdomen often shows ''thumbprinting,'' indicative of edema and mucosal hemorrhage in the intestinal wall. The endoscopic appearance of the colon is nonspecific, and the mucosa usually appears hyperemic, edematous, and friable.[90] Perforations of the small intestine and colon are recognized complications of the ischemic bowel disease (although the latter can be caused by the insertion of a peritoneal dialysis catheter). Intussusception has also been reported, and intestinal strictures and fistulas are late complications.

Henoch-Schönlein Purpura

Henoch-Schönlein purpura is a vasculitis that primarily affects the postcapillary venules of the intestine, skin, kidneys, and joints. It commonly presents with a prodrome of abdominal pain, a purpuric rash, and then later manifestations of nephritis, arthritis, and edema. Occult gastrointestinal blood loss is common, but only about 3% of children have gross lower intestinal bleeding. Henoch-Schönlein purpura generally affects children younger than 7 years of age, and most cases occur in clusters in the winter and early spring.[91] Almost all pediatric cases are preceded by a viral or bacterial illness, including cases associated with hepatitis A and B and parvovirus.[92]

The central pathogenic mechanism appears to be the deposition of IgA immune complexes on postcapillary venules throughout the body, triggered by some unknown antigen.[93] The alternate complement pathway is activated, resulting in the depletion of plasma C_3 and the deposition of C_3 in immune complexes. The rash has a predilection for the lower extremities and buttocks and is described as *palpable purpura*. Abdominal pain and blood in the stool may appear as early as 1 week before the rash, leading to erroneous diagnoses of infectious colitis, intussusception, or inflammatory bowel disease. Joint pain and overt pauciarticular arthritis occur in more than half of affected patients, with the knees and ankles most commonly involved. Renal involvement with overt hematuria and proteinuria occurs in about 40% of patients. Less common manifestations include central nervous system vasculitis, leading to encephalopathic changes and even seizures[94]; pancreatitis; orchitis; cholecystitis; and pulmonary hemorrhage. Intussusception occurs in a small number of children, with the edematous intestine acting as a lead point; rarely, the intestine perforates or becomes strictured secondary to the transmural ischemic changes in the wall. Both upper and lower gastrointestinal endoscopy reveal purpuric lesions of the stomach, small intestine, and colon that are similar to those seen in the skin. Punctate hemorrhages may also be seen. Biopsy of the skin or intestine shows vasculitis with selective IgA and C_3 deposition on the wall of small veins, a finding that differentiates Henoch-Schönlein purpura from other vasculitides.

Acute Graft-Versus-Host Disease of the Intestine

Graft-versus-host disease is seen in human bone marrow transplant recipients and presents with profuse diarrhea, crampy abdominal pain, nausea, anorexia, vomiting, and intestinal bleeding.[95] Patients may have abdominal distention and peritoneal signs secondary to the transmural inflammation and edema of the small intestine. Often, the gastrointestinal manifestations are accompanied by jaundice, evidence of hepatitis, and a diffuse erythematous skin rash. The findings of large amounts of cellular debris in the stool, occult blood, and fecal leukocytes are all consistent with graft-versus-host disease, but intestinal infection, especially with cytomegalovirus, adenovirus, and other viruses, and the residual effects of conditioning chemotherapy must be ruled out. Enteric protein loss is striking and is reflected in profound depression of serum albumin and other protein levels.

Widespread radiographic changes are often present in the small intestine, including bowel wall edema, thickened folds, and even pneumatosis cystoides intestinalis. Occasionally, mucosal ulcers are seen in the colon. The endoscopic appearance of graft-versus-host disease ranges from normal to patchy erythema to extensive mucosal sloughing with denudation of the villose absorptive surface. These changes are most prominent in the ileum, cecum, and ascending colon, but the stomach and proximal small intestine can also be involved. The most characteristic histologic finding in the gut is individual cell necrosis in intestinal crypts, which is called *apoptosis*.[96] There is little or no inflammatory response around the degenerating cell, in contrast to the occasional apoptotic bodies seen in infectious colitis, inflammatory bowel disease, and chemoradiation injury, in which widespread inflammatory cell infiltrates are seen.

Complications of acute intestinal graft-versus-host disease include massive loss of fluid and electrolytes; profound malabsorption; severe retching, vomiting, and abdominal pain; severe ileus or megacolon; and sepsis. Gastrointestinal bleeding can also become a major problem, particularly in the presence of thrombocytopenia. Patients who suffer these complications invariably require large amounts of total parenteral nutrition. The loss of large amounts of protein through the gut and the increased metabolic demands of the patient make it difficult to maintain a positive nitrogen balance. Because of the diffuse loss of villus tip cells and the absorptive epithelium of the small intestine in severe cases, the diarrhea is both osmotic and secretory. Even when the patient is taking nothing by mouth, massive losses of water and electrolytes can continue, necessitating assiduous monitoring of the fluid and electrolyte status and vigorous replacement therapy.

REFERENCES

1. Siebert JR. Small-intestinal length in infants and children. Am J Dis Child 1980;134:593.
2. Klish WJ, Putnam TC. The short gut. Am J Dis Child 1981;35:1056.
3. Morriss FH Jr, Moore M, Weisbrodt NW, et al. Ontogenic development of gastrointestinal motility. IV. Duodenal contractions in preterm infants. Pediatrics 1986;78:1106.
4. McLain CR. Amniography studies of the gastrointestinal motility in human fetus. Am J Obstet Gynecol 1963;86:1079.
5. Bisset WM. Intestinal motor activity in the preterm infant. In: Milla PJ, Welburn P, eds. Disorders of gastrointestinal motility in childhood. Chichester, John Wiley & Sons, 1988:29.
6. Berseth CL. Neonatal small intestinal motility: motor responses to feeding in term and preterm infants. J Pediatr 1990;117:777.
7. Bryant MG, Buchan AM, Gregor M, et al. Development of intestinal regulatory peptides in the human fetus. Gastroenterology 1982;83:47.
8. Lucas A, Bloom SR, Aynsley-Green A. Metabolic and endocrine consequences of depriving preterm infants of enteral nutrition. Acta Paediatr Scand 1983;72:245.
9. Antonowicz I, Lebenthal E. Developmental pattern of small intestinal enterokinase and disaccharidase activities in the human fetus. Gastroenterology 1977;72:1299.
10. Younoszai MK. Jejunal absorption of hexose in infants and adults. J Pediatr 1986;85:446.
11. Watkins JB, Szczepanik P, Gould JB, et al. Bile salt metabolism in the human premature infant. Gastroenterology 1975;69:706.
12. Heubi JE, Balistreri WF, Suchy FJ. Bile salt metabolism in the first year of life. J Lab Clin Med 1982;100:127.
13. Lester R, Smallwood RA, Little JM, et al. Fetal bile salt metabolism: the intestinal absorption of bile salts. J Clin Invest 1977;59:1009.
14. Henning SJ. Postnatal development: coordination of feeding, digestion, and metabolism. Am J Physiol 1981;241:G199.
15. Zoppi G, Andreotti G, Pajno-Ferrara F, et al. Exocrine pancreas function in premature and full-term infants. Pediatr Res 1972;6:880.
16. Udall JN, Walker WA. The physiologic and pathologic basis for the transport of macromolecules across the intestinal tract. Pediatr Gastroenterol Nutr 1982;1:295.
17. Weaver LT, Laker MF, Nelson R, et al. Milk feeding and change in intestinal permeability and morphology in the newborn. Pediatr Gastroenterol Nutr 1987;6:351.
18. Rieger CHL, Rothberg RM. Development of the capacity to produce specific antibody to an ingested food antigen in the premature infant. J Pediatr 1975;87:515.
19. Mienge H, Robinson JWL. Functional and structural characteristics of the rat intestinal mucosa following ileojejunal transposition. Acta Hepatogastroenterol 1986;25:150.
20. Madara JL. Functional morphology of epithelium of the small intestine. In: Field M, ed. Handbook of physiology, vol 4, sec 6: the gastrointestinal system. New York, Oxford University Press, 1991::83.
21. Solcia E, Capella C, Buffa R, et al. The diffuse endocrine-paracrine system of the gut in health and disease: ultrastructural features. Scand J Gastroenterol 1981;16(Suppl 70):25.
22. Bohe M, Borgstrom C, Ohlsson K. Trypsin-like immunoreactivity in human Paneth cells. Digestion 1984;30:271.
23. Wood JD. Intrinsic neural control of intestinal motility. Annu Rev Physiol 1981;43:33.
24. Grider JR. Identification of neurotransmitters regulating intestinal peristaltic reflex in humans. Gastroenterology 1989;97:1414.
25. Vantrappen G, Janssens J, Ghoos Y. The interdigestive motor complex of normal subjects and patients with bacterial over-growth of the small intestine. J Clin Invest 1977;59:1158.
26. Vantrappen GR, Peeters TL, Janssens J. The secretory component of the interdigestive migrating motor complex in man. Scand J Gastroenterol 1979;14:663.
27. Sarna SK, Soergel KH, Harig JM, et al. Spatial and temporal patterns of human jejunal contractions. Am J Physiol 1989;257:G423.
28. Thompson DG, Ritchie HD, Wingate DL. Patterns of small intestinal motility in duodenal ulcer patients before and after vagotomy. Gut 1982;23:517.
29. Sarna SK, Otterson MF. Small intestinal physiology and pathophysiology. Gastroenterol Clin North Am 1989;18:375.
30. Tomomasa T, Miyazki M, Igarashi T, et al. The effect of erythromycin

on the gastroduodenal motility in human premature infants. J Gastrointest Motil 1991;3:205.

31. Hall KE, Greenberg GR, El-Sharkawy TY, et al. Relationship between porcine motilin-induced migrating motor complex-like activity, vagal integrity, and endogenous motilin release in dogs. Gastroenterology 1984;87:78.

32. Bueno L, Fioramonti J, Ruckebusch Y. Postoperative intestinal motility in dogs and sheep. Dig Dis Sci 1978;23:682.

33. Boivin M, Raymond MC, RiBerdy M, et al. Plasma motilin variation during the interdigestive end digestive states in man. J Gastrointest Motil 1990;2:240.

34. Sullivan SK, Field M. Ion transport across mammalial small intestine. In: Field M, ed. Handbook of physiology, vol 4, sec 6: the gastrointestinal system. New York, Oxford University Press, 1991:287.

35. Madara JL. Loosening tight junctions: lessons from the intestine. J Clin Invest 1989;83:1089.

36. Turnberg L, Fordtran J, Carter N, et al. Mechanism of bicarbonate absorption and its relationship to sodium transport in human jejunum. J Clin Invest 1970;49:548.

37. Turnberg L, Bieberdorf F, Morawski S, et al. Interrelationships of chloride bicarbonate, sodium, and hydrogen transport in the human ileum. J Clin Invest 1970;49:555.

38. Holmberg C, Perheentupa J, Launiala K, et al. Congenital chloride diarrhea: clinical analysis of 21 Finnish patients. Arch Dis Child 1977; 52:255.

39. Field M. Intestinal ion transport mechanisms. In: Diarrheal diseases. New York, Elsevier, 1991:3.

40. Dobbins JW, Laurenson JP, Forrest JN. Adenosine and adenosine analogues stimulate adenosine cyclic 3',5'-monophosphate–dependent chloride secretion in the mammalial ileum. J Clin Invest 1984;74:929.

41. Jones JB, Mehta NR, Hamosh M. Alpha-amylase in preterm human milk. J Pediatr Gastroenterol Nutr 1982;1:43.

42. Fogel MR, Gray GM. Starch hydrolysis in man: an intraluminal process not requiring membrane digestion. J Appl Physiol 1973;35:263.

43. Adler G, Beglinder C. Hormones as regulators of pancreatic secretion in man. Eur J Clin Invest 1990;20:S27.

44. Gray GM, Lally GB, Conklin KA. Action of intestinal sucrase-isomaltase and its free monomers on a α-limit dextrin. J Biol Chem 1979; 254:6038.

45. Dahlqvist A, Borgstrom B. Digestion and absorption of disaccharides in man. Biochem J 1961;81:411.

46. Hamosh M, Bitman J, Liao TH, et al. Gastric lipolysis and fat absorption in preterm infants: effect of medium-chain triglyceride- or long-chain triglyceride-containing formulas. Pediatrics 1989;83:86.

47. Bernback S, Blackberg L, Hernell O. The complete digestion of human milk triacylglycerol in vitro requires gastric lipase, pancreatic colipase-dependent lipase and bile salt–stimulated lipase. J Clin Invest 1990; 85:1221.

48. Gaskin KJ, Durie PR, Lee L, et al. Colipase and lipase secretion in childhood-onset pancreatic insufficiency: delineation of patients with steatorrhea secondary to relative colipase deficiency. Gastroenterology 1984;86:1.

49. Proulx P, Aubry H, Brglez I, et al. Studies on the uptake of fatty acids by brush border membranes of the rabbit intestine. Can J Biochem Cell Biol 1984;63:249.

50. Shiau Y-F, Levine GM. pH dependence of micellar diffusion and dissociation. Am J Physiol 1980;239:G177.

51. Curtis KJ, Graines HD, Kim YS. Protein digestion and absorption in rats with pancreatic duct occlusion. Gastroenterology 1978;74:1271.

52. Guan D, Yoshioka M, Erickson RH, et al. Protein digestion in human and rat small intestine: role of new neutral endopeptidases. Am J Physiol 1988;255:G212.

53. Tobey N, Heizer W, Yeh R, et al. Human intestinal brush border peptidases. Gastroenterology 1985;88:913.

54. Vanderhoof JA, Antonsen DL, Kaufman SS, et al. Combined liver/intestinal versus isolated intestinal transplantation in children. Gastroenterology 1995;108:A221.

55. Wilmore DW. Factors correlating with a successful outcome following extensive intestinal resection in newborn infants. J Pediatr 1972;80:88.

56. Allard JP, Jeejeebhoy KN. Nutritional support and therapy in the short bowel syndrome. Gastroenterol Clin 1989;18:589.

57. Debongnie JC, Phillips SF. Capacity of the human colon to absorb fluid. Gastroenterology 1978;74:468.

58. Hwang TL, O'Dwyer ST, Smith RJ, et al. Preservation of small bowel mucosa using glutamine enriched parenteral nutrition. Surg Forum 1986;37:56.

59. Taylor B, Murphy GM, Dowling RH. Effect of food intake and the pituitary on intestinal structure and function after resection. (Abstract) Gut 1975;16:397.

60. Burne TA, Morrissey TB, Ziegler TR, et al. Growth hormone, glutamine, and fiber-enhanced adaptation of remnant bowel following massive intestinal resection. Surgical Forum 1992;43:151.

61. Bohane TD, Haka-Ikse K, Biggar WD, et al. A clinical study of young infants after small intestinal resection. J Pediatr 1979;94:552.

62. Cooper A, Floyd TF, Ross AJ, et al. Morbidity and mortality of short-bowel syndrome acquired in infancy: an update. J Pediatr Surg 1984; 19:711.

63. Dorney SFA, Ament ME, Berquist WE, et al. Improved survival in very short small bowel of infancy with use of long-term parenteral nutrition. J Pediatr 1985;107:521.

64. Grosfeld JL, Rescorla FJ, West JW. Short bowel syndrome in infancy and childhood. Am J Surg 1986;151:41.

65. Caniano DA, Starr J, Ginn-Pease ME. Extensive short-bowel syndrome in neonates: outcome in the 1980's. Surgery 1989;105:119.

66. Goulet OJ, Revillon Y, Jan D, et al. Neonatal short bowel syndrome. J Pediatr 1991;119:18.

67. Hyman PE, Everett SL, Haranda T. Gastric acid hypersecretion in short bowel syndrome in infants: association with extent of resection and enteral feeding. J Pediatr Gastroenterol Nutr 1986;5:191.

68. Roslyn JJ, Berquist WE, Pitt HA, et al. Increased risk of gallstones in children receiving total parenteral nutrition. Pediatrics 1983;71:784.

69. Sherman P, Drum B, Karmali M, et al. Adherence of bacteria to the intestine in sporadic cases of enteropathogenic *Escherichia coli*–associated diarrhea in infants and young children: a prospective study. Gastroenterology 1989;96:86.

70. Hill SM, Phillips AD, Walker-Smith JA. Enteropathogenic *Escherichia coli* and life-threatening chronic diarrhea. Gut 1991;32:154.

71. Anderson KE, Finlayson NDC, Deschner EE. Intractable mal-absorption with flat jejunal mucosa and selective IgA deficiency. Gastroenterology 1974;67:709.

72. Walker-Smith JA, Unsworth DJ, Hutchins P, et al. Autoantibodies against gut epithelium in child with small intestinal enteropathy. Lancet 1982;1:566.

73. Colletti RB, Guillot AP, Rosen S, et al. Autoimmune enteropathy and nephropathy with circulating autoantibodies. J Pediatr 1991;118:853.

74. Hill SM, Milla PJ, Bottazzo GF, et al. Autoimmune enteropathy and colitis: is there a generalized autoimmune gut disorder? Gut 1991;32: 36.

75. Seidman EG, Lacaille F, Russo P, et al. Successful treatment of autoimmune enteropathy with cyclosporine. J Pediatr 1990;117:929.

76. Cutz E, Rhoads JM, Drumm B, et al. Microvillus inclusion disease: an inherited defect of brush border assembly and differentiation. N Engl J Med 1989;320:646.

77. Ackerman NB, Strobel CT. Polle syndrome: chronic diarrhea in Munchausen's child. Gastroenterology 1981;81:1140.

78. Bieberdorf FA, Gorden P, Fordtran JS. Pathogenesis of congenital alkalosis with diarrhea. J Clin Invest 1985;51:1958.

79. Kaplan SJ, Holbrook CT, McDaniel HG, et al. Vasoactive intestinal peptide secreting tumors in childhood. Am J Dis Child 1980;134:21.

80. Mitchell CH, Sinatra FR, Crast FW, et al. Intractable watery diarrhea, ganglioneuroblastoma and vasoactive intestinal peptide. J Pediatr 1976; 89:593.

81. Mayer EA, Schuffler MD, Rotter JI, et al. Familial visceral neuropathy with autosomal dominant transmission. Gastroenterology 1986;91: 1528.

82. Schuffler MD. Chronic intestinal pseudo-obstruction: progress and problems. J Pediatr Gastroenterol Nutr 1990;10:157.

83. Schofield ED, Yunis EJ. Intestinal neuronal dysplasia. J Pediatr Gastroenterol Nutr 1991;12:182.

84. Vargas JH, Sachs P, Ament ME. Chronic intestinal pseudo-obstruction syndrome in pediatrics: results of a national survey of members of the North American Society of Pediatric Gastroenterology and Nutrition. J Pediatr Gastroenterol Nutr 1988;7:323.

85. Hyman PE, McDiarmid SV, Napolitano JA, et al. Antroduodenal motility in children with chronic intestinal pseudo-obstruction. J Pediatr 1988;112:889.

86. Snape WJ Jr, Sullivan MA, Cohen S. Abnormal gastrocolic response in patients with intestinal pseudo-obstruction. Arch Intern Med 1980; 140:386.

87. Martin DL, MacDonald KL, White KE. The epidemiology and clinical

aspects of the hemolytic-uremic syndrome in Minnesota. N Engl J Med 1991;323:1161.

88. Neill MA, Agosti J, Rosen H. Hemorrhagic colitis with *Escherichia coli* 0157:H7 preceding adult hemolytic uremic syndrome. Arch Intern Med 1985;145:2215.

89. Lopez EL, Diaz M, Grinstein S, et al. Hemolytic uremic syndrome and diarrhea in Argentine children: the role of Shiga-like toxins. J Infect Dis 1989;160:469.

90. Berman W Jr. The hemolytic uremic syndrome: initial clinical presentation mimicking ulcerative colitis. J Pediatr 1972;81:275.

91. Allen DM, Diamond LK, Howell DA. Anaphylactoid purpura in children (Schönlein-Henoch syndrome). Am J Dis Child 1960;99:833.

92. LeFrere J, Courouce A, Soulier J, et al. Henoch-Schönlein purpura and human parvovirus infection. Pediatrics 1986;78:183.

93. Stevenson JA, Leong LA, Cohen AH, et al. Henoch-Schönlein purpura: simultaneous demonstration of IgA deposits in involved skin, intestine, and kidney. Arch Pathol Lab Med 1982;106:192.

94. Belman A, Leicher C, Moshe S, et al. Neurologic manifestations of Schönlein-Henoch purpura: report of three cases and review of the literature. Pediatrics 1985;75:687.

95. McDonald GB, Shulman HM, Sullivan KM, et al. Intestinal and hepatic complications of human bone marrow transplantation. I. Gastroenterology 1986;90:460.

96. Roy J, Snover D, Weisdorf S, et al. Simultaneous upper and lower endoscopic biopsy in the diagnosis of intestinal graft-versus-host disease. Transplantation 1991;51:642.

Surgery of Infants and Children: Scientific Principles and Practice, edited by Keith T. Oldham, Paul M. Colombani, and Robert P. Foglia. Lippincott–Raven Publishers, Philadelphia, © 1997.

CHAPTER 70

Introduction to Neonatal Intestinal Obstruction

Keith T. Oldham

A variety of congenital anatomic defects, inherited metabolic disorders, and acquired physiologic abnormalities are associated with intestinal obstruction in the first month of life. These are discussed in detail in the chapters that follow. The cardinal clinical manifestation of neonatal intestinal obstruction is bilious vomiting, often in conjunction with abdominal distention. These signs in the newborn must be considered to be the result of mechanical obstruction until proved otherwise. Table 70-1 provides an overview of the possible diagnoses, with some important generalizations regarding the history, physical examination, and relevant diagnostic studies. These are discussed in detail later.

Considerable variability exists in the clinical presentations of these disorders. Distal obstructions are almost invariably characterized by abdominal distention, but proximal obstructions are not. Partial obstructions may produce minimal or no physical findings. The anatomic relation of the obstruction to the ampulla of Vater determines whether bile is present in the

TABLE 70.1 *Neonatal intestinal obstruction*

Diagnosis	History	Physical examination	Relevant studies
Intestinal atresia or stenosis	Bilious vomiting	Abdominal distention Acholic meconium	Plain radiograph Barium enema
Congenital duodenal obstruction	Bilious vomiting	Gastric distention Trisomy 21	Plain radiograph Upper GI study
Imperforate anus	Failure to pass meconium Bilious vomiting (late)	Abdominal distention Nonpatent anus	Evaluate for VATER syndrome and cardiac anomalies
Necrotizing enterocolitis	High-risk, premature infant Bilious vomiting	Abdominal distention Guaiac-positive stool	Plain radiograph Contrast studies contraindicated
Meconium ileus	Bilious vomiting Cystic fibrosis	Abdominal distention Acholic meconium	Plain radiograph Barium enema
Malrotation	Full-term, healthy infant Bilious vomiting	No abdominal distention	Plain radiograph Upper GI study Barium enema
Hirschsprung disease	Bilious vomiting Delayed passage of meconium Family history	Abdominal distention Trisomy 21	Barium enema Suction rectal biopsy
Uncommon causes of neonatal obstruction (intussusception, Meckel diverticulum duplications)	Variable	Incarcerated hernia Mass	Variable
Medical conditions associated with bilious vomiting and ileus	Variable	Variable	Sepsis, hypothyroidism, meconium plug syndrome, others

(Oldham KT. The pediatric abdomen: intestinal disorders. In: Greenfield LJ, Mulholland MW, Oldham KT, et al. Surgery: scientific principles and practice. Philadelphia, JB Lippincott, 1993:1839)

stool or in the gastric contents. Generally, clinical clues provide enough information for a preliminary diagnosis and thus direct the diagnostic approach for an individual infant. Because malrotation with midgut volvulus is part of this differential diagnosis, the imaging evaluation must be considered an emergency and must be pursued until malrotation is eliminated as a possibility.

Fortunately, establishment of a diagnosis is ordinarily straightforward by use of a combination of readily available imaging studies, such as plain abdominal radiographs, barium enema, and upper gastrointestinal contrast studies. More complex diagnostic strategies provide little additional information and generally have a limited role. In the absence of specific clinical clues, the imaging sequence for suspected neonatal intestinal obstruction should begin with plain radiographs, followed by a barium enema and an upper gastrointestinal study. The information obtained with each study determines the next requirement. For example, a plain film with pneumatosis intestinalis may be diagnostic of neonatal necrotizing enterocolitis and therefore sufficient. Both Hirschsprung disease and malrotation have classic abnormalities on barium enema that are essentially diagnostic. With many forms of small bowel obstruction, however, the barium enema simply demonstrates a nonspecific microcolon, which is actually an unused but normal colon. Therefore, an upper gastrointestinal study may provide additional information. An upper gastrointestinal series is most helpful in evaluating suspected malrotation or possibly proximal and incomplete obstructions.

Although the classic surgical causes of neonatal bilious vomiting are considered in detail in subsequent chapters, other medical problems and a variety of less common anatomic obstructions also present with a similar clinical picture. These are briefly considered in Table 70-1. Of the less common obstructive lesions noted, only incarcerated hernia is typical in the neonatal age group. This is considered elsewhere in detail and is excluded here because it does not generally present a diagnostic dilemma. Simple inspection ordinarily yields this diagnosis. Infants with a wide variety of medical illnesses may also develop an ileus with bilious vomiting. Underlying diseases may be common, such as sepsis; some are rare, such as congenital hypothyroidism. These topics are not within the scope of this review but do represent important considerations for the clinician once mechanical obstruction is ruled out. The meconium plug syndrome is a benign but important problem relevant to these neonates and is discussed later as well.

Surgery of Infants and Children: Scientific Principles and Practice, edited by Keith T. Oldham, Paul M. Colombani, and Robert P. Foglia. Lippincott–Raven Publishers, Philadelphia, © 1997.

CHAPTER 71

Meconium Syndromes and Cystic Fibrosis

Samuel M. Mahaffey

The meconium syndromes of infancy are a complex group of gastrointestinal diseases with considerable overlap in clinical presentation and management. For purposes of this discussion, the meconium syndromes are separated into distinct entities based on their unique clinical features. *Meconium ileus* is a form of intraluminal obstruction resulting from thick, inspissated, abnormal meconium; meconium ileus is virtually always associated with cystic fibrosis (CF). *Meconium plug syndrome* also presents as neonatal intestinal obstruction; decreased intestinal motility resulting in an inspissated plug of meconium is thought to be the underlying cause of this disease. The obstruction is usually colonic and typically occurs in preterm infants. *Meconium peritonitis* is a form of chemical peritonitis that results from prenatal perforation of the intestine. Meconium ileus, or any of the other causes of neonatal intestinal obstruction, can result in perforation and meconium peritonitis. *Meconium ileus equivalent* is a form of mechanical intestinal obstruction seen in older children and adolescents with CF, and is again the result of obturator obstruction by thick, inspissated stool.

MECONIUM ILEUS

The first description of an association between pathologic changes in the pancreas and newborn intestinal obstruction by inspissated meconium was made by Landsteiner in 1905.[1] CF was described as a clinical entity characterized by pancreatic insufficiency and chronic pulmonary disease by Fanconi in 1936.[2] Meconium ileus was recognized as an early manifestation of CF 2 years later.[3]

Meconium ileus is the earliest clinical manifestation of CF, occurring in 10% to 20% of CF patients. CF is the most common fatal, genetic illness among whites. CF is an autosomal recessive disease and thus is expressed only in homozygotes; the incidence in whites is about 1 in 2500 live births. The estimated frequency of heterozygotes in the white population is 5% to 6%. The disease is rare in African Americans and is almost never seen in native Africans or Asians.

CF is a systemic illness, affecting exocrine glands throughout the body. Tenacious mucous and chronic pulmonary infection are major features of the disease. Damage to the pancreas begins prenatally, with progressive ductal obstruction, acinar hypertro-

phy, and eventually fibrosis of the exocrine pancreatic tissue. Eighty-five to 90% of infants with CF have advanced pancreatic lesions and manifestations of exocrine pancreatic insufficiency. The sweat glands, salivary glands, liver, nasal mucous membranes, and reproductive organs are also affected.

Pathophysiology

The Cystic Fibrosis Gene and the CFTR

Localization of the *CF* gene and identification of the most common mutation were achieved in 1989.[4,5] The gene is located on the long arm of chromosome 7 (Fig. 71-1). The most common mutation, delta F508, results in a three–base-pair deletion from the gene. This leads to an in-frame deletion of a single phenylalanine residue from the transcription product. The delta F508 mutation is present in more than 70% of CF patients of northern European descent. More than 200 additional mutations have been identified since the original report in 1989. The frequency of these CF alleles varies among populations.

The transcription product of the *CF* gene is referred to as the cystic fibrosis transmembrane regulator (CFTR). Expression of the CFTR in cultured cells (Chinese hamster ovary and Sf-9 insect cell lines) results in the appearance of a cyclic adenosine monophosphate (cAMP) activated chloride channel that is not usually expressed by the cells.[6] In HeLa cells and NIH 3T3 fibroblasts, expression of the CFTR induces cAMP-dependent chloride currents, although a single-channel basis for the currents has not been established. Cultured human CF tracheal epithelial cells have no baseline chloride secretion, and the secretory response to cAMP is only 10% of normal. The inability of CF cells to secrete chloride in response to cAMP has been linked to a reduced apical membrane chloride conductance. Early patch-clamp studies strongly suggested that the molecular basis of this reduced conductance was an anion channel that shows outward rectification (ie, has less resistance to outward than inward current flow); more recent studies argue against a role for this channel in cAMP-mediated chloride secretion.[6]

Dysregulation of epithelial electrolyte transport has been observed in many organs from CF patients. O'Laughlin and colleagues[7] reported abnormal chloride secretion and sodium ab-

1183

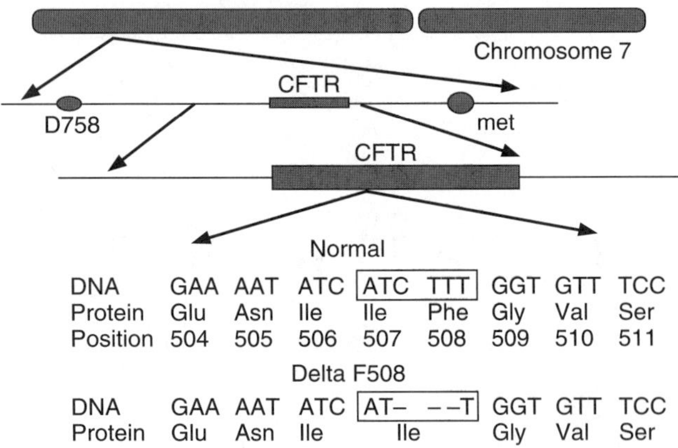

FIG. 71-1. The cystic fibrosis gene and the most common mutation, delta F508. CFTR, cystic fibrosis transmembrane regulator.

sorption in response to a range of secretagogues in in vitro studies of jejunal epithelium from CF patients compared with controls. Many investigators[8] favor the hypothesis that multiple chloride channels exist in the enterocyte: a cAMP-stimulated Cl^- transporter in the apical membrane, and a Ca^{2+}-stimulated Cl^- channel in the basolateral membrane. In contrast, in airway epithelium, the cAMP- and Ca^{2+}-stimulated Cl^- channels are localized on the brush-border membrane. The clinical implications of this primary defect in stimulation of Cl^- secretion by cAMP and Ca^{2+} are not well understood. The decreased Cl^- secretion may, however, lead to relative dehydration of the mucus and deposition of the viscid mucus on epithelial surfaces, leading to malabsorption and luminal obstruction. Analysis of goblet cell mucin reveals that CF mucin has an increased sedimentation coefficient, a higher content of carbohydrates with a longer chain length, and increased proportions of fucose and galactose.[9] The three-dimensional conformation of CF mucins also leads to increased antigenicity.[10] Deposition of immune complexes, complement activation, and recruitment of activated polymorphonuclear leukocytes are believed to be one possible mechanism of ongoing tissue injury in CF patients.

Based on the predicted amino acid sequence of the CFTR, it is estimated to have a nonglycosylated size of 168 kd. Hydrophobicity studies suggest that the CFTR is an integral membrane protein with two arms, each with six transmembrane α-helical segments. The arms are connected to a cytoplasmic body, which differs from other known ion channels by the presence of two nucleotide-binding domains and a highly charged region with multiple potential phosphorylation sites (the regulatory, or R, domain; Fig. 71-2). Most mutations occur in the cytoplasmic body, within the nucleotide-binding folds or the R domain. The mutations presumably disrupt the conformational symmetry of the molecule and prevent phosphorylation of the R domain; without phosphorylation, the chloride channel remains closed.

Manifestations of Cystic Fibrosis

The identification of the genetic abnormality in CF and the resultant dysfunction of the CFTR provide a unifying basic physiologic defect that could explain the multitude of clinical manifestations of the disease. The widespread organ dysfunction in CF and the variability of disease expression among patients, however, suggest that the clinical signs and symptoms of CF result not only from abnormal chloride transport but also from a number of secondary morphologic and biochemical abnormalities.

Diagnosis and Screening

The diagnosis of CF is usually suspected on clinical grounds and is confirmed by quantitative measurement of chloride (or sodium) in sweat collected after stimulation by pilocarpine iontophoresis.[11] It has generally been believed that an adequate volume of sweat cannot be collected in young infants; however, in a large study of infants 1 to 11 weeks old, an inadequate volume of sweat was obtained in only 0.8%.[12] Direct molecular confirmation of the diagnosis is also possible in most patients by analysis of blood samples for delta F508 and the more common alleles. This analysis is limited by the large number of CF alleles and the variable frequency within a given population.

It is also possible to screen newborn infants for CF. The substance screened is immunoreactive trypsinogen (IRT), which can be measured from the same blood sample used for phenylketonuria and hypothyroidism screening, which are mandated in all states. The cause of IRT elevation observed in CF patients in unclear. Unfortunately, many normal infants also

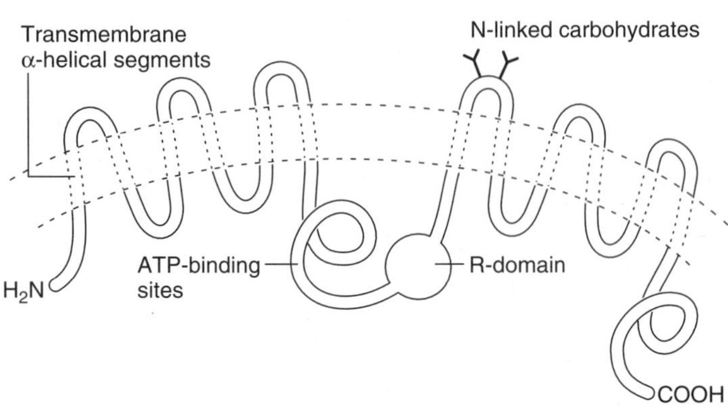

FIG. 71-2. Structure of the cystic fibrosis transmembrane regulator.

have elevated IRT levels. There is controversy about the utility of the screening test, considering the effects on families of infants with a false-positive diagnosis of CF,[13] although the specificity is greatly improved when DNA analysis is added to the screening test.

Also under considerable discussion is DNA analysis for screening of the population to detect the heterozygote (carrier state). A useful screening program to identify the more than 10 million heterozygotes in North America alone would require the resolution of a number of problems, including funding, availability of genetic counselors, potential for abuse of the results by employers and insurers, and the effect of false-negative results. For the time being, screening should be limited to couples who request it, usually relatives of patients with CF.

Pulmonary Manifestations

Pulmonary disease is universally present in patients with CF; more than 95% of patients succumb to complications directly related to pulmonary involvement. Although there is variability in the phenotypic expression of the pulmonary disease, there is no clear genotype–phenotype relation, and the severity of pulmonary disease appears multifactorial. The main clinical feature—thick, tenacious tracheobronchial secretions leading to recurrent infections (particularly with *Pseudomonas aeruginosa*)—has been recognized for years and has been thought to be the most important factor in the progression of pulmonary disease. The mainstays of treatment have been the use of antibiotics for suppression and for the treatment of established infections, and chest physical therapy and postural drainage to promote clearing of the tracheobronchial secretions.[14] Several new therapies directed at the abnormal secretions are under investigation. The sodium pump blocker amiloride has been shown to lessen the electrical abnormalities of CF epithelial tissues.[15] Administered as an aerosol, amiloride has been shown to decrease sputum viscosity and increase cough clearance of mucus and noncoughing mucociliary transport.[16]

Attention has turned to the inflammatory nature of the pulmonary disease. It appears that the balance of protease and antiprotease activity may be skewed in CF airway fluid by an excess of neutrophil-derived elastase.[17] In addition to the nonspecific destruction of airway elastin fibers and stimulation of mucus secretion, neutrophil elastase digests the C3bi opsonin on the surface of *P aeruginosa* bacteria and the receptor for the C3b component of complement on the surface of neutrophils, effectively disabling complement-mediated phagocytosis of *P aeruginosa*. Elastase also cleaves the Fc portion from anti–*P aeruginosa* antibodies, rendering them ineffective. The resulting persistence of *P aeruginosa* in the airway leads to the release of bacterial toxins, recruitment of additional neutrophils, and the creation of a vicious cycle of infection and inflammation.

Several strategies have been devised to attempt to minimize progression of the pulmonary disease by inhibiting the inflammatory response. Deoxyribonuclease aerosols have been used to decrease sputum viscosity and may improve pulmonary function.[18] The effect of deoxyribonuclease is largely on neutrophil degradation products, which are not present in the absence of inflammation. Other protease inhibitors, such as secretory leukocyte protease inhibitor[19] and α_1-antitrypsin, may also play a role. Systemic antiinflammatory drugs, including prednisone

and ibuprofen, are being investigated. Intravenous immunoglobulin G has been used with success in some patients with acute pulmonary exacerbations, perhaps by enhanced phagocytosis of *P aeruginosa*.[20]

The most exciting potential treatment for CF is gene therapy. In vitro, CF cells have been successfully transfected with a "normal" gene at the CF locus using retroviral vectors, resulting in normal chloride-channel activity.[21] Investigators have transfected a functional human α_1-antitrypsin gene into airway epithelial cells of the cotton rat using the adenovirus vector,[22] and have accomplished a similar functional gene transfection with CFTR. A cellular cure awaits the identification of an appropriate vector and demonstration of safety and efficacy in humans.

Gastrointestinal Complications of Cystic Fibrosis

Genetic and Biochemical Basis of Meconium Ileus

The chemical composition of the abnormally viscid meconium in infants with meconium ileus was observed to be different from unaffected infants as early as the 1950s.[23] The meconium contains less carbohydrate and more protein (the concentration of albumin is about 5 to 10 times higher) in infants with meconium ileus than in unaffected infants.[24] Significant increases in γ-glutamyltranspeptidase and 5′-nucleotidase activities have also been reported.[25] These enzymes are produced by the liver and secreted into the fetal bile at about twice the normal concentration. It is suggested that the components present in the duodenum (γ-glutamyltranspeptidase, 5′-nucleotidase, and albumin from the amniotic fluid) are abnormally concentrated in the duodenum and jejunum. Other enzymes secreted into the ileum, such as aminopeptidase M and alkaline phosphatase, are present in the meconium at normal concentrations, suggesting that they are secreted into an already abnormally concentrated meconium. There is not a good correlation between meconium ileus and the severity of pancreatic disease, suggesting that meconium ileus is primarily the result of abnormal intestinal secretion rather than deficiency of pancreatic enzymes.

The phenotypic expression of CF is likely the result of numerous complex genetic and environmental interactions. The identification of the *CF* gene, however, has made it possible to genotype individual patients and to attempt to characterize genotype–phenotype relations in CF. Pancreatic status appears to be genetically determined; patients with the most common mutation, delta F508, almost universally have pancreatic insufficiency.[26] Other specific alleles associated with pancreatic sufficiency have been identified. Patients with these alternative alleles remain pancreatic sufficient, are diagnosed later, have lower sweat chloride values, and have milder respiratory disease than patients with alleles associated with pancreatic insufficiency.

The missense mutation G551D (glycine to aspartic acid missense mutation at codon 551) is the third most common CF mutation, with a worldwide frequency of 3.1% of *CF* genes. Retrospective cohort studies of compound heterozygotes (G551D and delta F508), compared with matched delta F508 homozygotes, showed a lower incidence of meconium ileus in heterozygotes and a trend toward later diagnosis of pancreatic insufficiency.[27] The groups were comparable in all other aspects, and clinical outcome (after survival of meconium ileus) was indistinguishable.

A correlation between the occurrence of meconium ileus and specific CF alleles is also suggested by family studies. Recurrence rates as high as 47% have been reported in subsequent children when the first child of a given couple had meconium ileus, even though the expected occurrence would be only 10% to 20%.[28,29]

Distal Intestinal Obstruction Syndrome

Mechanical intestinal obstruction may develop in the ileocecal region of older children, adolescents, and adults with CF. The most severe form, meconium ileus equivalent, is defined as a postneonatal condition of partial or complete intestinal obstruction due to abnormally viscid feculent material. This was first described in 1941.[30] The reported incidence is up to 40% in patients followed in long-term CF clinics. The patient often presents with an irregular mass in the right lower quadrant, the accumulation of abnormal fecal material. Nausea, vomiting, constipation, and abdominal pain often follow and are due to obstruction. Abdominal radiographs reveal dilated intestinal loops with air–fluid levels. A bubbly, granular appearance may be seen, particularly on the right side of the abdomen.

Meconium ileus equivalent is thought to result from exocrine pancreatic insufficiency, decreased intestinal transit time, and abnormal intestinal mucus. Cessation of pancreatic enzyme supplementation, particularly in older adolescents and young adults, is a precipitating factor in many cases, along with respiratory exacerbations, dehydration, or dietary changes. Contrast studies with diatrizoate are diagnostic and therapeutic (Fig. 71-3). Although intussusception (the inspissated feces acts as a lead point) or volvulus may complicate meconium ileus equivalent, this is not usually the case, and operation is rarely required.

Appendicitis is also a complication associated with distal intestinal obstruction. On occasion, the lumen of the appendix becomes filled with thick intestinal mucus. This is often not associated with inflammation, but it may produce chronic, intermittent, right lower quadrant pain and tenderness. The symptoms usually resolve after appendectomy.[31] In other cases, obstruction of the appendiceal orifice results in acute inflammatory appendicitis, which often progresses to perforation and abscess formation. The presence of a right lower quadrant mass thus often presents the clinician with a diagnostic dilemma.

Liver Disease

Cystic fibrosis patients with intestinal obstruction also appear to be at greater risk for the development of liver disease.[32] Liver disease occurs in up to 20% of CF patients, and hepatocellular failure or portal hypertension is the cause of death in about 5%. The underlying pathology is not clear, although mucus plugging within proliferated bile ducts is commonly observed. Cirrhosis is invariably present when mucus plugs are found in a patient with a history of meconium ileus or meconium ileus equivalent.

Because there is no successful medical treatment for liver disease associated with CF, some patients with end-stage he-

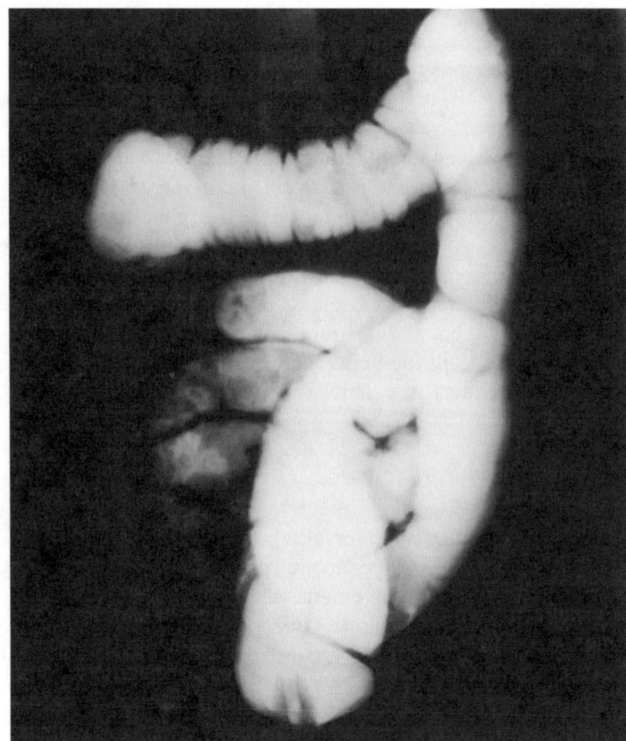

FIG. 71-3. Contrast enema in an adolescent with meconium ileus equivalent showing inspissated fecal plugs in the transverse colon.

patic failure have come to transplantation. The results are comparable to those for other groups undergoing liver transplantation, and pulmonary function actually improves in some cases.[33]

Clinical Features of Meconium Ileus

Meconium ileus is conveniently divided into two categories: uncomplicated and complicated. Simple obturator obstruction of the distal ileum is referred to as uncomplicated meconium ileus. The bowel proximal to the inspissated pellets of meconium in the ileum fills with thick meconium that is plastic or putty-like in consistency. The colon is a small and unused microcolon.

Complicated cases of meconium ileus include volvulus, perforation, atresia, and giant cystic meconium peritonitis. The heavy, meconium-filled bowel proximal to the obstruction may become twisted, resulting in volvulus. Subsequent perforation and egress of meconium into the peritoneal cavity may result in a chemical peritonitis or formation of a giant pseudocyst. Ischemia of the base of the volvulus may result in bowel atresia.

Presentation

Meconium ileus is often diagnosed antenatally by maternal ultrasound, particularly in complicated cases in which there is a mass effect or peritoneal calcification. Maternal polyhydramnios may be seen in cases of high intestinal obstruction. More typically, the presentation is that of a term neonate who develops abdominal distention and bilious vomiting and fails to pass meconium. Signs and symptoms of intestinal obstruction can take 24 to 48 hours to develop; during that time, the infant may tolerate several feedings. Although these infants may be of relatively low birthweight, they are rarely premature. Associated anomalies are uncommon.

Other findings are usually seen in complicated cases. Neonates with perforation or pseudocysts may exhibit abdominal distention or bilious emesis shortly after delivery. An abdominal mass may be present owing to volvulus or pseudocyst. Meconium may be passed through the fallopian tubes and uterus and appear in the vagina in girls; meconium or calcifications may appear in the scrotum of boys as the result of passage through the processus vaginalis.

Abdominal radiographs reveal features of intestinal obstruction, with multiple distended loops of intestine (Fig. 71-4). Often, there is a coarse, granular appearance of the radiograph owing to air bubbles within the meconium; this is referred to as a *soap-bubble* or *ground-glass* appearance. There may be a paucity of intraluminal air or air–fluid levels because the bowel loops are filled with liquid; however, this finding is not unique to meconium ileus. Radiologic signs of a complication include intraperitoneal calcification (meconium peritonitis), a dense mass with flecks of calcium (pseudocyst), ascites, or free intraperitoneal air. Specific radiographic findings are absent in up to one third of neonates with complicated meconium ileus.

In suspected cases of meconium ileus, contrast studies usually confirm the diagnosis. Contrast enema (barium is preferred for the initial examination) reveals a microcolon of normal length but markedly decreased caliber. Reflux into the terminal ileum identifies the site of obstruction and outlines the inspissated pellets of meconium (Fig. 71-5). The barium enema usually differentiates cases of intestinal atresia or midgut volvulus from cases of uncomplicated meconium ileus.

Differential Diagnosis

The differential diagnosis of meconium ileus includes most other causes of neonatal intestinal obstruction. Colonic and ileal atresias, congenital aganglionosis (particularly total colonic aganglionosis), congenital hypothyroidism, and meconium plug syndrome all can have a similar presentation. Complicated meconium ileus with perforation and peritonitis can be difficult to differentiate preoperatively from other causes of perforation.

Management

The initial management of neonates with intestinal obstruction includes intravenous fluid resuscitation, nasogastric decompression, and the administration of antibiotics. Radio-

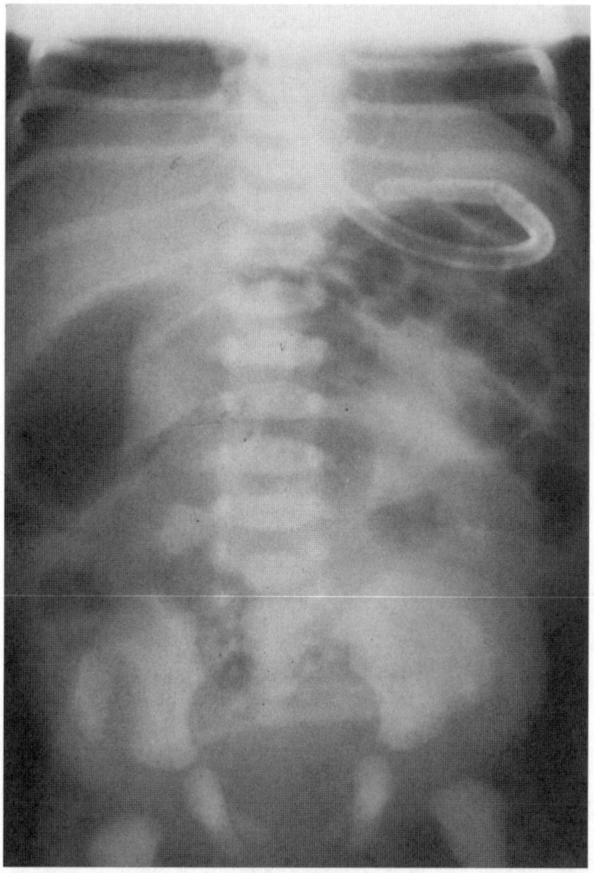

FIG. 71-4. Abdominal radiograph showing the soap-bubble or ground-glass appearance characteristic of meconium ileus.

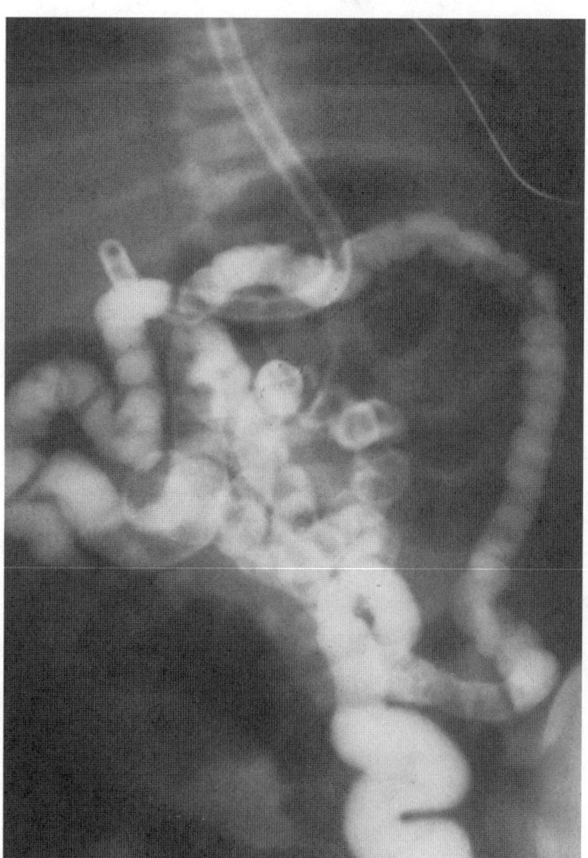

FIG. 71-5. Contrast enema revealing the microcolon and inspissated pellets of meconium in the terminal ileum.

graphic investigation is undertaken after the patient is appropriately stabilized.

Simple Meconium Ileus

In 1969, Noblett[34] introduced the meglumine diatrizoate 0.1% polysorbate 80 (Gastrografin) enema for management of neonates with uncomplicated meconium ileus. Uncomplicated patients are defined as those with no clinical or radiographic evidence of volvulus, necrotic bowel, atresia, perforation, or peritonitis. The hyperosmolar solution (1900 mOsm/L) apparently draws fluid into the bowel lumen from the plasma, helping to liquefy the inspissated meconium and creating an osmotic diarrhea that aids in passage. The neonate must be adequately fluid-resuscitated before and during administration of the enema to avoid hypovolemia due to redistribution of fluid. This technique is successful in relieving the obstruction in most patients, although several enemas may be required.

Potential complications of the technique include perforation, necrotizing enterocolitis, and shock. Perforations can result from overdistention during administration, from the osmotic process, or from mucosal injury by the agent. A review of the literature reveals a success rate of about 55% and an 11% incidence of perforation.[35] Other enema preparations have been used, including Tween 80, N-acetylcysteine, diatrizoate sodium, iothalamate meglumine, and saline; however, these preparations are also associated with complications. It is common to use dilute Gastrografin to decrease the osmolarity and the risk of complications, while achieving the desired effects. It may be necessary to administer sequential enemas to resolve the clinical obstruction.

Complicated Meconium Ileus

Operative management is necessary in patients with complicated meconium ileus and in patients with uncomplicated meconium ileus who fail enema treatment. The goal of operative management in simple meconium ileus is evacuation of the inspissated meconium from the lumen. A number of operative strategies to achieve this end have been advocated over the years (Fig. 71-6), beginning with enterotomy and saline irrigation as described by Hiatt and Wilson in 1948.[36] Various modifications of the irrigation technique have since been described, using N-acetylcysteine,[37–39] Gastrografin,[40] saline, pancreatic enzymes, and hydrogen peroxide. Pancreatic enzymes were shown not to be effective. The use of hydrogen peroxide may result in gas emboli, and its use has been abandoned. In 1953, Gross[41] reported successful relief of the obstruction by resection of the dilated bowel and creation of a Mikulicz enterostomy. In 1957, Bishop and Koop[42] described resection and construction of a proximal end-to-side anastomosis with a distal end ileostomy to allow postoperative irrigation of the ileum. The principal advantage of these two early procedures was that the stoma could subsequently be closed by an extraperitoneal operation.

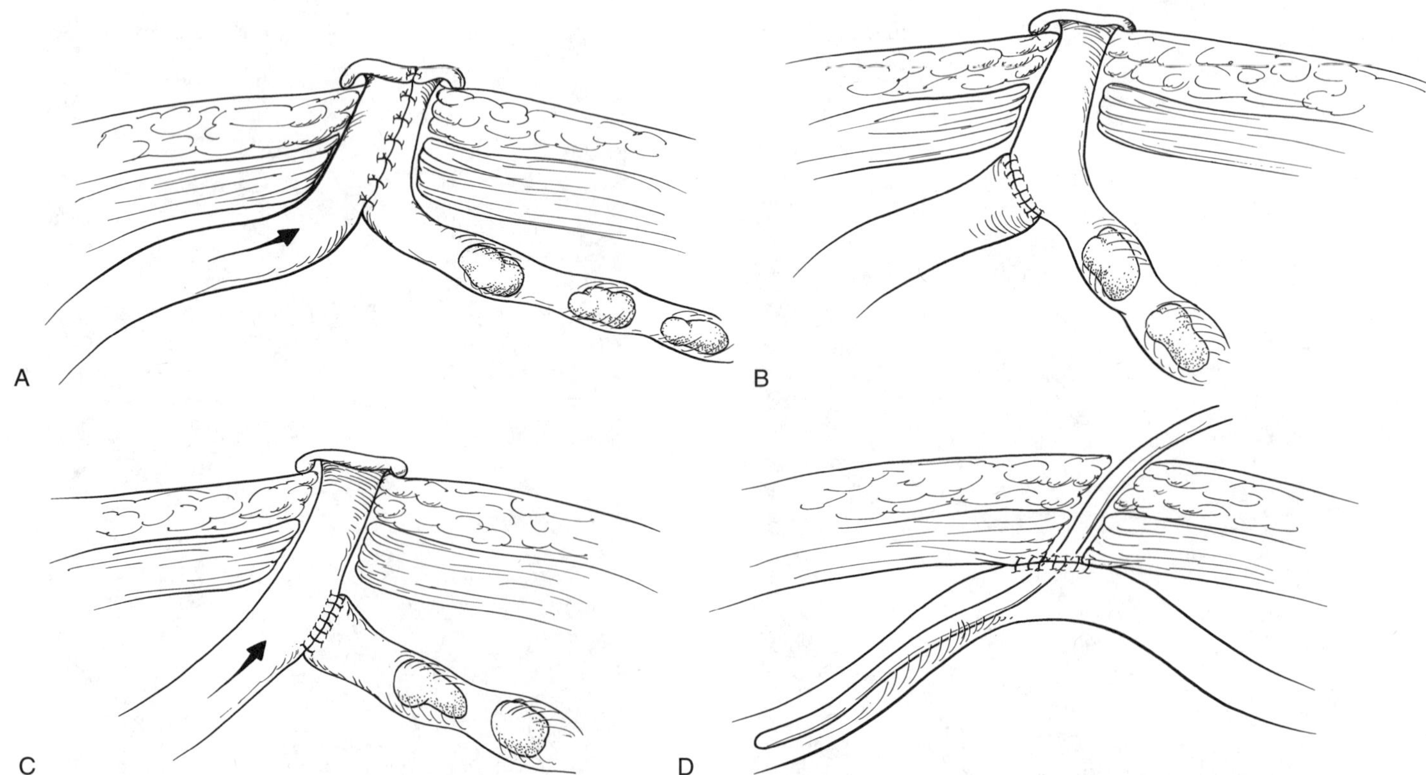

FIG. 71-6. Operative approaches used in the management of meconium ileus. (*A*) Resection and Mikulicz enterostomy. (*B*) Bishop-Koop procedure. (*C*) Santulli-Blanc procedure. (*D*) Enterostomy and irrigation. For infants with uncomplicated meconium ileus who require operation, most investigators advocate enterotomy with irrigation.

In 1961, Santulli and Blanc[43] described resection and side-to-end anastomosis with a proximal "chimney" enterostomy. In 1962, Swenson[44] recommended resection, irrigation, and end-to-end anastomosis; this technique was not widely accepted owing to frequent anastomotic leaks. Placement of a tube enterostomy for postoperative irrigation has been advocated by O'Neill and colleagues[45] and by Harberg and associates.[46]

Contemporary authors generally recommend enterotomy with irrigation as the treatment of choice for meconium ileus that requires operative intervention uncomplicated by volvulus, atresia, or intestinal necrosis. A soft rubber catheter is introduced through a pursestring suture on the antimesenteric border of the bowel, and the bowel is gently irrigated with saline, dilute Gastrografin solution, or dilute (less than 4%) acetylcysteine solution. Excessive manipulation of the bowel can result in serosal tears and is to be avoided. The pellets of inspissated meconium can be removed through the enterotomy or the appendix,[47] or they can be flushed into the colon. The enterotomy is closed at the conclusion of the procedure. Resection is rarely required, and an intraperitoneal anastomosis (with the potential for leaks) or exteriorization (requiring a second operative procedure) is avoided.

Meconium ileus complicated by volvulus, intestinal necrosis, atresia, or giant pseudocyst requires immediate operative intervention. In cases of atresia or volvulus, resection of massively dilated segments, distal irrigation, and exteriorization or primary anastomosis constitute the preferred procedure. In cases of perforation or cystic peritonitis, débridement, resection, and exteriorization constitute the preferred procedure. Enterostomy closure can usually be accomplished 4 to 6 weeks after the initial operation.

Postoperative care includes antibiotics and nasogastric decompression until there is return of intestinal function. Parenteral nutritional support should be instituted; if there is a prolonged period of intestinal dysfunction, the central route should be used to insure adequate caloric support. Adequate pulmonary support is essential to a satisfactory outcome.

Outcome

Operative survival rates have improved dramatically during the past four decades, from 40% to 50% in the 1960s to 90% or higher in contemporary series.[48,49] This improvement in survival is largely attributable to improved supportive care, including high-quality pediatric anesthesia, improved techniques of ventilatory support and management of the pulmonary complications of CF, timely diagnosis and management, and parenteral nutrition.

Overall, the population of patients with CF has changed dramatically during this time period. A review of the registry maintained by the Cystic Fibrosis Foundation[50] revealed a significant shift in the age distribution of CF patients between 1969 (8% adults) and 1990 (33% adults). Median survival age also increased from 14 years to 28 years during that period. With improved care, CF patients are living much longer than in the past, but they still have significant complications related to their disease, including chronic pulmonary infections, endocrine pancreatic insufficiency, and liver disease.

MECONIUM PLUG SYNDROME

Meconium plug syndrome was first described in 1956 by Clatworthy and colleagues.[51] The affected infants were described as "plugged-up babies." Included within this description of meconium plug syndrome are a number of clinical entities that, owing to abnormal composition of meconium or altered intestinal motility, result in inability to clear the meconium mass and distal intestinal obstruction. The terms *functional inertia of prematurity, small left colon syndrome,* and *left-sided microcolon* are also used to describe the meconium plug syndrome.

Pathophysiology

Several factors are regularly associated with colonic hypomotility. Hypermagnesemia, which may result from treatment of maternal eclampsia with magnesium, decreases acetylcholine release, resulting in myoneural depression. Although this association has been reported clinically,[52] it has not been proved in experimental animals.[53] Hypoglycemia in infants of diabetic mothers induces glucagon secretion, which may result in hypomotility.[54]

Clinical Features

Affected infants are often preterm and present with signs and symptoms of distal intestinal obstruction. Abdominal distention is a prominent feature. Little or no meconium is passed. Rectal examination is appropriate and can be both diagnostic and therapeutic. Plain radiographs often reveal multiple, dilated loops of intestine. Water-soluble contrast enema is the diagnostic study of choice. The meconium plug may appear as an intraluminal filling defect (Fig. 71-7), or the contrast may fill a small left colon with an abrupt obstruction in the left colon or splenic flexure. The enema usually stimulates passage of the meconium plug, although additional contrast or saline enemas may be required to evacuate the meconium completely.

A suction rectal biopsy should be performed to rule out Hirschsprung disease. Although the presentation is different from the ileal obstruction seen in CF patients with meconium ileus, the typical presentation of meconium plug syndrome is sometimes seen in patients with CF. Accordingly, it is appropriate to perform a sweat chloride test in these patients. In the absence of associated disease, patients with meconium plug syndrome can be expected to do well; most have no long-term problems.

MECONIUM PERITONITIS

Meconium peritonitis is an aseptic chemical or foreign-body peritonitis that results from prenatal perforation of the intestine.

Pathophysiology

The prenatal intestinal perforation is usually caused by distal intestinal obstruction, which may be due to meconium ileus,

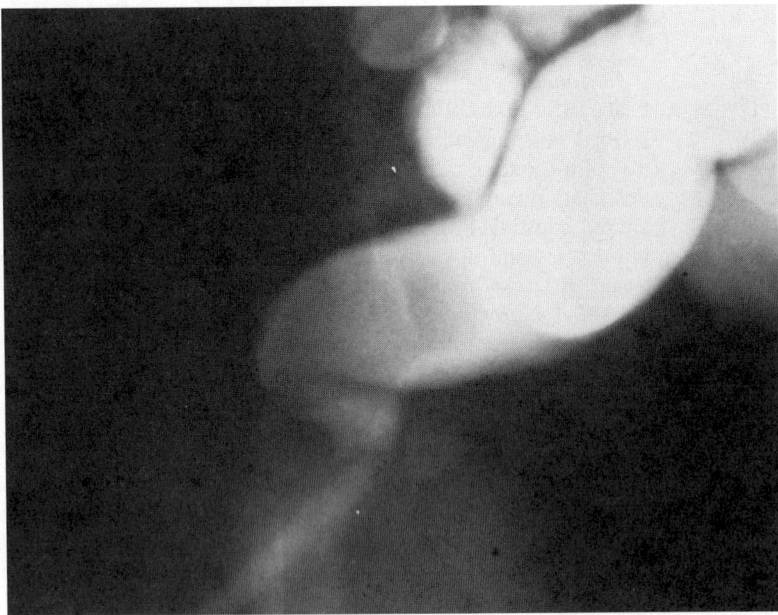

FIG. 71-7. Contrast enema examination showing a meconium plug within the rectum.

intestinal atresia or stenosis, volvulus, internal hernia, peritoneal bands, or intussusception. Volvulus of the meconium-filled segment of bowel proximal to the obstruction in infants with meconium ileus is one cause of complicated meconium ileus; ischemic necrosis of the base of the volvulus may lead to perforation, or the area may heal, resulting in a stricture or atresia. Extravasation and liquefaction of the meconium may result in a pseudocyst (giant cystic meconium peritonitis).[55]

Three pathologic types of meconium peritonitis have been described.[56] Fibroadhesive peritonitis results from the intense chemical reaction induced by the meconium, resulting in dense fibrous adhesions. The site of perforation may be sealed off by the adhesions and calcification (Fig. 71-8). Cystic meconium peritonitis results when the sealing process is not effective, and meconium continues to spill into the peritoneal cavity. A pseudocyst forms, consisting of loops of intestine (which may be partially necrotic) surrounding the liquefied meconium. In generalized meconium peritonitis, the meconium is distributed throughout the peritoneal cavity. The inflammatory reaction is less severe, and the adhesions between loops are more fibrinous. This type of meconium peritonitis apparently results from perforation just before birth.

Clinical Features

Most patients present with intestinal obstruction. Intraperitoneal calcification in patients who have no other symptoms does not require operative intervention. The operative procedure is individualized based on the findings at operation and the cause. Nonviable bowel should be resected. Massively distended bowel should also be resected, although a conservative approach is recommended to avoid malabsorption due to short gut. Many patients require temporary exteriorization of the bowel. Return of adequate motility and absorptive capacity is often delayed, and central venous hyperalimentation is usually required for nutritional support.

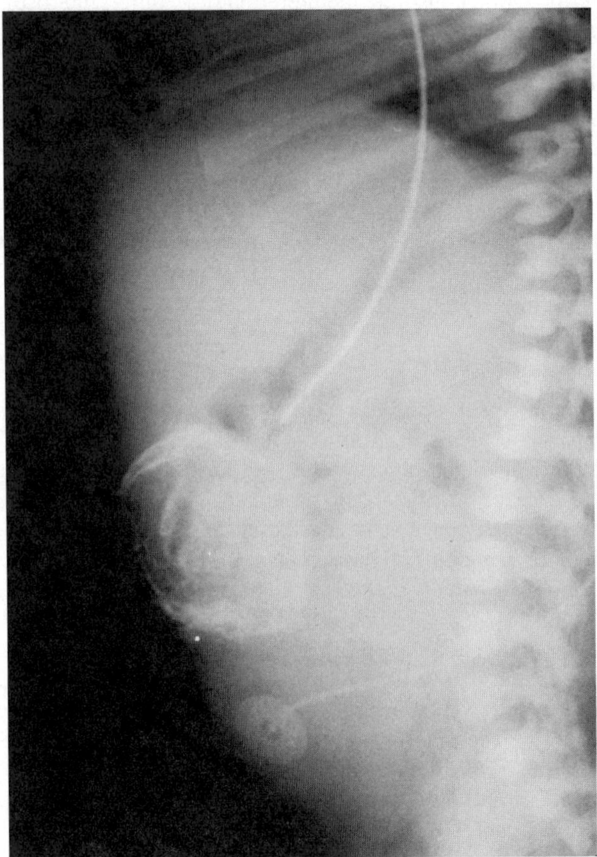

FIG. 71-8. Intraperitoneal calcifications seen with meconium peritonitis.

REFERENCES

1. Landsteiner K. Darmverschluss durch eingedictes Meconium Pankreatitis. Zentralbl Allg Pathol 1905;16:903.
2. Fanconi G, Uehlinger E, Knauer C. Das Coeliakiesyndrome bei Angeborener Zystischer Pancreasfibromatose und Bronchiektasien. Wien Med Wochenschr 1936;86:753.
3. Andersen DH. Cystic fibrosis of the pancreas and its relation to celiac disease: a clinical and pathologic study. Am J Dis Child 1938;56:344.
4. Riordan J, Rommens JM, Kerem BS, et al. Identification of the cystic fibrosis gene: cloning and characterization of complimentary DNA. Science 1989;245:1066.
5. Rommens JM, Iannuzze MC, Kerem BS, et al. Identification of the cystic fibrosis gene: chromosome walking and jumping. Science 1989;245:1059.
6. Widdicombe JH, Wine JJ. The basic defect in cystic fibrosis. Trends Biochem Sci 1991;16:474.
7. O'Loughlin EV, Hunt DM, Gaskin KJ, et al. Abnormal epithelial transport in cystic fibrosis jejunum. Am J Physiol 1991;260:G758.
8. Eggermont E, DeBoeck K. Small-intestinal abnormalities in cystic fibrosis patients. Eur J Pediatr 1991;150:824.
9. Wesley A, Forstner JF, Qureshi R, et al. Human intestinal mucin in cystic fibrosis. Pediatr Res 1983;17:65.
10. Mantle M, Stewart G. Intestinal mucins from normal subjects and patients with cystic fibrosis. Biochem J 1989;259:243.
11. Gibson L, Cooke R. A test for concentration of electrolytes in sweat in cystic fibrosis of the pancreas utilizing pilocarpine by iontophoresis. Pediatrics 1959;23:545.
12. Hammond K, Abman S, Sokol R, et al. Efficacy of statewide neonatal screening for cystic fibrosis by assay of trypsinogen concentrations. N Engl J Med 1991;325:769.
13. Holtzman N. What drives neonatal screening programs? (Editorial) N Engl J Med 1991;325:802.
14. Reisman J, Rivington-Law B, Corey M, et al. Role of conventional physiotherapy in cystic fibrosis. J Pediatr 1988;113:632.
15. Knowles M, Stutts M, Yankaskas J, et al. Abnormal respiratory epithelial ion transport in cystic fibrosis. Clin Chest Med 1986;7:285.
16. Knowles M, Church N, Waltner W, et al. A pilot study of aerosolized amiloride for the treatment of lung disease in cystic fibrosis. N Engl J Med 1990;322:1189.
17. Berger M. Inflammation in the lung in cystic fibrosis. Clin Rev Allergy 1991;9:119.
18. Shak S, Capon D, Hellmiss R, et al. Recombinant human DNase reduces the viscosity of cystic fibrosis sputum. Proc Natl Acad Sci USA 1990;87:9188.
19. Vogelmeier C, Buhl R, Hoyt R, et al. Aerosolization of recombinant SLPI to augment antineutrophil elastase protection of pulmonary epithelium. J Appl Physiol 1990;69:1843.
20. Van Wye J, Collins MS, Baylor M, et al. Pseudomonas hyperimmune globulin passive immunotherapy for pulmonary exacerbations in cystic fibrosis. Pediatr Pulmonol 1990;9:7.
21. Drumm M, Pope H, Cliff W, et al. Correction of the cystic fibrosis defect in vitro by retrovirus-mediated gene transfer. Cell 1990;62:1227.
22. Rosenfeld M, Siegfried W, Yoshimura K, et al. Adenovirus-mediated transfer of a recombinant α_1-antitrypsin gene to the lung epithelium in vivo. Science 1991;25:431.
23. Buchanan DJ, Rapoport S. Chemical comparison of normal meconium and meconium from a patient with meconium ileus. Pediatrics 1952;9:304.
24. Green MN, Clarke JT, Shwachman H. Studies in cystic fibrosis of the pancreas: protein patterns in meconium ileus. Pediatrics 1958;21:635.
25. Brock D. A comparative study of microvillar enzyme activities in the prenatal diagnosis of cystic fibrosis. Prenat Diagn 1985;5:129.
26. Campbell PW III, Phillips JA III. The cystic fibrosis gene and relationships to clinical status. Semin Respir Infect 1992;7:150.
27. Hamosh A, King TM, Rosenstein BJ, et al. Cystic fibrosis patients bearing both the common missense mutation Gly–Asp at codon 551 and the delta F508 mutation are clinically indistinguishable from delta F508 homozygotes, except for the decreased risk of meconium ileus. Am J Hum Genet 1992;51:245.
28. Mornet E, Simon-Bouy B, Serre JL, et al. Genetic differences between cystic fibrosis with and without meconium ileus. Arch Surg 1988;124:837.
29. Kerem E, Corey M, Kerem B, et al. Clinical and genetic comparisons of patients with cystic fibrosis, with or without meconium ileus. J Pediatr 1989;114:767.
30. Rasor GB, Stevenson WL. Meconium ileus equivalent. Rocky Mount Med J 1941;38:218.
31. Coughlin JP, Gauderer MW, Stern RC, et al. The spectrum of appendiceal disease in cystic fibrosis. J Pediatr Surg 1990;25:835.
32. Maurage C, Lenaerts C, Weber A, et al. Meconium ileus and its equivalent as a risk factor for the development of cirrhosis: an autopsy study in cystic fibrosis. J Pediatr Gastroenterol Nutr 1989;9:17.
33. Mieles L, Orenstein D, Toussant R, et al. Outcome after liver transplantation for cystic fibrosis. Pediatr Pulmonol Suppl 1991;6:130.
34. Noblett HR. Treatment of uncomplicated meconium ileus by Gastrografin enema: a preliminary report. J Pediatr Surg 1969;4:190.
35. Rescorla FJ, Grosfeld JL. Contemporary management of meconium ileus. World J Surg 1993;17:318.
36. Hiatt RB, Wilson PE. Celiac syndrome: therapy of meconium ileus. Report of 8 cases with review of the literature. Surg Gynecol Obstet 1948;87:317.
37. Meeker IA, Jr, Kincannon WN. Acetylcysteine used to liquefy inspissated meconium causing intestinal obstruction in the newborn. Surgery 1964;56:419.
38. Kalayoglu M, Sieber WK, Rodman JB, et al. Meconium ileus: a critical review of treatment and eventual prognosis. J Pediatr Surg 1971;6:290.
39. Venugopal S, Shandling B. Meconium ileus: laparotomy without resection, anastomosis, or enterostomy. J Pediatr Surg 1979;14:715.
40. Caniano DA, Beaver BL. Meconium ileus: a fifteen year experience with forty-two neonates. Surgery 1987;102:699.
41. Gross RE. Intestinal obstruction in the newborn resulting from meconium ileus. In: The surgery of infancy and childhood. Philadelphia, WB Saunders, 1953:175.
42. Bishop HC, Koop CE. Management of meconium ileus: resection, Roux-en-Y anastomosis and ileostomy irrigation with pancreatic enzymes. Ann Surg 1957;145:410.
43. Santulli TV, Blanc WA. Congenital atresia of the intestine: pathogenesis and treatment. Ann Surg 1961;154:939.
44. Swenson O. Pediatric surgery, ed 2. East Norwalk, CT, Appleton & Lange, 1962.
45. O'Neill JA, Grosfeld JL, Boles ET, et al. Surgical treatment of meconium ileus. Am J Surg 1970;119:99.
46. Harberg FJ, Senekjian EK, Pokorny WJ. Treatment of uncomplicated meconium ileus via T-tube ileostomy. J Pediatr Surg 1981;16:61.
47. Fitzgerald R, Conlon K. Use of the appendix stump in the treatment of meconium ileus. J Pediatr Surg 1989;4:899.
48. Rescorla FJ, Grosfeld JL, West KW, et al. Changing patterns of treatment and survival in neonates with meconium ileus. Arch Surg 1989;124:837.
49. Del Pin CA, Czyrko C, Ziegler MM, et al. Management and survival of meconium ileus: a 30-year review. Ann Surg 1992;215:179.
50. FitzSimmons SC. The changing epidemiology of cystic fibrosis. J Pediatr 1993;122:1.
51. Clatworthy HW, Howard WHR, Lloyd J. The meconium plug syndrome. Surgery 1956;39:131.
52. Sokal MM, Koenigsberger MR, Rose JS, et al. Neonatal hypermagnesemia and the meconium-plug syndrome. N Engl J Med 1972;286:223.
53. Cooney DR, Rosevear W, Grosfeld JL. Maternal and postnatal hypermagnesemia and the meconium plug syndrome. J Pediatr Surg 1976;11:167.
54. Stewart DR, Nixon GW, Johnson DG, et al. Neonatal small left colon syndrome. Ann Surg 1977;186:741.
55. Moore, TC. Giant cystic meconium peritonitis. Ann Surg 1963;157:566.
56. Lorimer WS, Ellis DH. Meconium peritonitis. Surgery 1966;60:470

Surgery of Infants and Children: Scientific Principles and Practice, edited by Keith T. Oldham, Paul M. Colombani, and Robert P. Foglia. Lippincott–Raven Publishers, Philadelphia, © 1997.

CHAPTER 72

Jejunoileal Atresia

Kurt Newman

The history of the management of neonatal intestinal atresia is a valuable paradigm illustrating the development and success of pediatric surgery as a specialty. In the early 1900s, bowel obstruction in the newborn period meant certain death. Initial progress came with advances and refinements of surgical technique. Novel experimental investigation in the 1950s elucidated the cause and pathophysiology of these malformations. Subsequent advances in supportive care, such as parenteral nutrition, respiratory management, and anesthesia, have made excellent outcomes routine for most infants. For some children, however, difficult problems related to small bowel adaptation and multiorgan system failure remain, constituting a challenge for continuing research and improvement in management. Although small intestinal atresia and stenosis are major causes of bowel obstruction in infancy, they are rare occurrences. Published incidence estimates range from 1 in 300 to 400 births to 1 in 20,000 births. One review using appropriate epidemiologic methodology estimates the incidence at less than 2 in 10,000 births.[1] Regardless of the specific incidence, the event is reasonably uncommon, even at major children's surgical centers. It is, however, an important and classic neonatal surgical emergency that must be recognized and treated efficiently to realize the excellent outcomes that are expected. Up to 20% of infants with one small bowel atresia are found to have one or more additional areas of atresia. Cases have been reported with a familial incidence, and there appears to be a higher incidence in twins, but no clear genetic association has been identified. The male/female ratio is equal in most studies. With the exception of intrauterine intestinal ischemic events, children with jejunoileal atresia do not generally have associated extraintestinal anomalies.

EMBRYOLOGY AND ANATOMY

The embryonic intestine is identified by the third gestational week and is divided into the foregut, midgut, and hindgut. The transverse septum demarcates the caudal extent of the foregut; the hindgut is within the formative tailfold; and the midgut is between the two. The midgut can be considered a simple tubular structure that undergoes elongation, herniation into and reduction from the celoem, rotation, and ultimately fixation to the posterior body wall. The formative gut also undergoes a period of rapid epithelial proliferation between the fifth and eighth gestational weeks. The intestinal lumen may be transiently occluded during this process, and incomplete recanalization is one possible explanation for the development of intestinal webs or diaphragms. Ninety percent or more of infants with congenital jejunoileal obstructions have complete atresia, and the remainder have stenoses or perforated intraluminal diaphragms. The single most common location is in the distal ileum, but any site is possible, and the overall distribution is roughly equal between the jejunem and ileum. Infants with a perforated intraluminal diaphragm may have a small eccentric opening, perhaps only millimeters in diameter. Nevertheless, the diagnosis often is not apparent in the neonatal period because symptoms of incomplete obstruction may be minimal or absent for months or even years. The discrepancy between orifice size and symptoms is often remarkable. This is in substantial contrast to the neonate with a complete obstruction from atresia, in whom the diagnosis becomes inescapable within hours of birth.

PATHOPHYSIOLOGY

Multiple causes of intestinal atresia have been proposed, ranging from a developmental failure of recanalization to intussusception in utero. Several theories are summarized schematically in Figure 72-1.[2] Although these are all possible causes, there is no substantial consensus. The pioneering work of Louw and Barnard implicated an ischemic event as the cause of most atresias. These investigators ligated the intestinal mesenteric blood supply of dog fetuses. After birth, the puppies exhibited the most common anatomic and histologic findings of small bowel atresia. In particular, a V-shaped mesenteric defect was associated with discontinuity between proximal and distal intestinal segments. Other experimental models using the lamb, rabbit, and chick embryo have been developed in which intestinal atresia is produced by ischemia of the fetal intestine. The pathologic and functional results in these animal models are similar to those seen in human infants. These models are widely used for developmental studies of intestinal motility, absorption, and adaptation. Tovar and colleagues[4] produced the entire anatomic spectrum of human intestinal atresia in an avian model by inter-

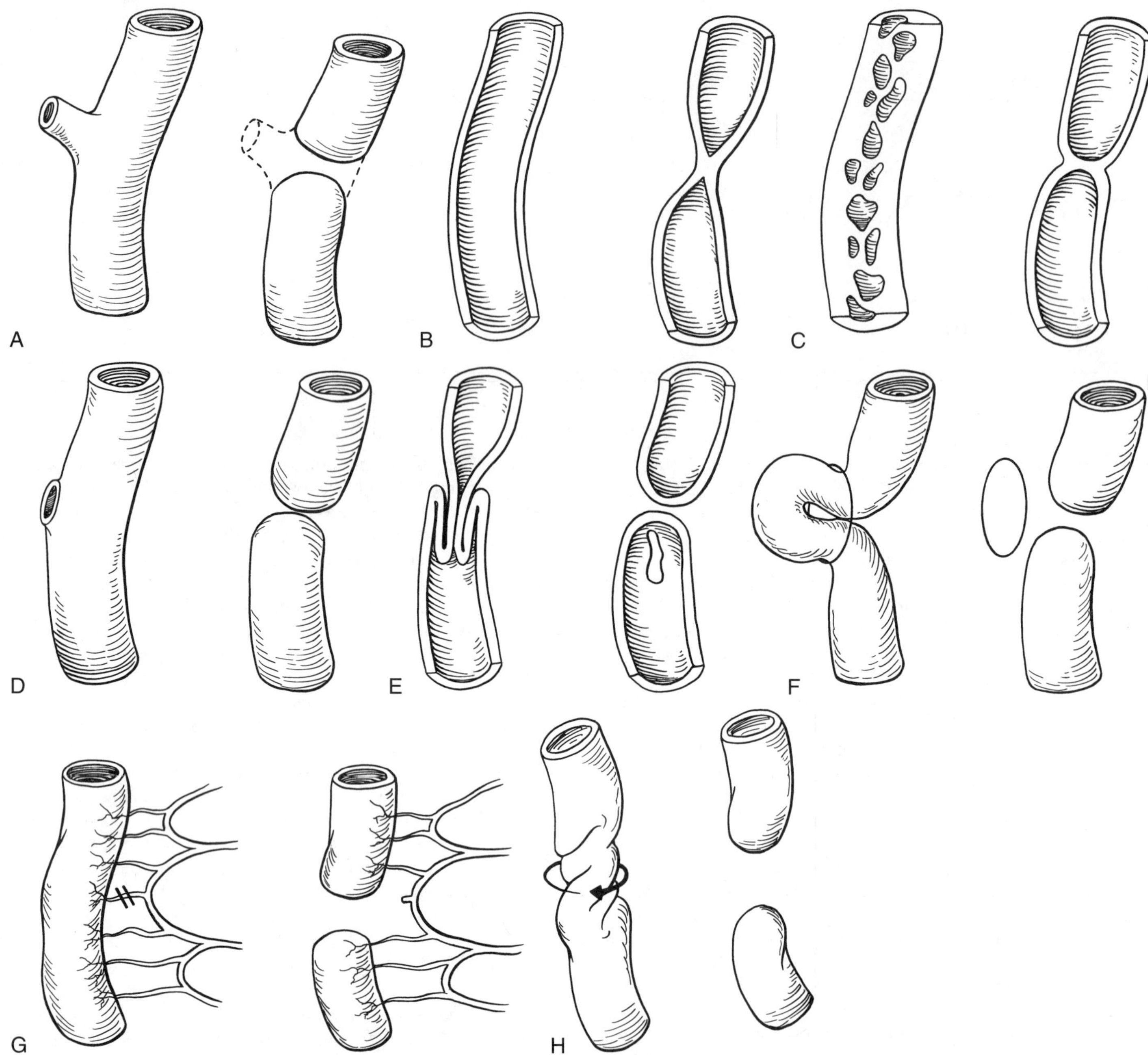

FIG. 72-1. Abnormal organogenesis results in intestinal atresia or stenosis. Several possibilities are depicted in this illustration. (*A*) Excessive resorption of Meckel diverticulum. (*B*) Attenuation, whereby cell proliferation fails to keep up with elongation (stenosis). (*C*) Failure of complete recanalization (stenosis). (*D*) Intestinal perforation in utero. (*E*) Intussusception in utero. (*F*) Entrapment of the intestine in the umbilical ring. (*G*) Thrombosis of vascular supply, with local necrosis and closure of distal and proximal ends. (*H*) Segmental volvulus. (After Skandalakis JE, Gray SW, Ricketts R, et al. Embryology for surgeons: the embryological basis for the treatment of congenital anomalies. Baltimore, Williams & Wilkins, 1994:204)

rupting the vascular supply of the embryonic chick intestine. Touloukian[5] was able to demonstrate adaptive villous hypertrophy as well as other antenatal muscosal compensatory responses after experimental jejunoileal atresia was induced in the lamb. Trahair and associates[6] used a fetal sheep model to demonstrate that fetal amniotic fluid ingestion provides the developing gastrointestinal tract with an important stimulus for growth. The implication of this work and other studies is that trophic growth factors, possibly peptide hormones, play an important role in the ontogeny of the fetal intestine.

Doolin and colleagues[7] found that intestinal motility disturbances result from intestinal atresia in a lamb model. Their findings are from consistent with the clinical observation that the proximal dilated intestinal segment in small bowel atresia is unable to contract efficiently. Evidence from these models suggests that motility may become normal when the mechanical obstruction is relieved. These studies are crucial to future advances in clinical management of these infants.

The clinical correlation of intrauterine events, such as gastroschisis, volvulus, and internal hernias, with bowel atresia suggests that intestinal ischemia is the major cause of jejunoileal atresia.[8] Up to 23% of infants with gastroschisis have associated bowel atresia. An association between immunodeficiency disorders and small bowel atresia has been reported.[9] Therefore, in infants with multiple atresias, a search for immunodeficiency is warranted. Irradiated blood products should be used in these infants until immunodeficiency is ruled out.

Most work has focused on the functional abnormalities of the small intestine in infants with jejunoileal atresia. Serrano and Zetterstrom[10] found altered disaccharidase activity in both the proximal dilated intestinal segment and the distal bowel in patients with congenital intestinal obstruction. Glucose and vitamin A absorption were also impaired. These findings point to deficient intestinal transport as one source of the failure-to-thrive syndrome commonly seen in these patients. Tepas and colleagues[11] demonstrated that altered motor activity in the obstructed bowel may also be a cause of poor intestinal function. Hamdy and associates[12] correlated the poor peristaltic capability of the bowel with histochemical evidence of diminished acetylcholinesterase activity in human specimens. Further work is required to elucidate specific pathophysiologic mechanisms that will permit targeted correction of the corresponding abnormalities.

CLASSIFICATION

Grosfeld[13] developed an anatomic classification system that stratified jejunoileal atresia into four major groups. These are summarized below and in Figures 72-2 and 72-3.

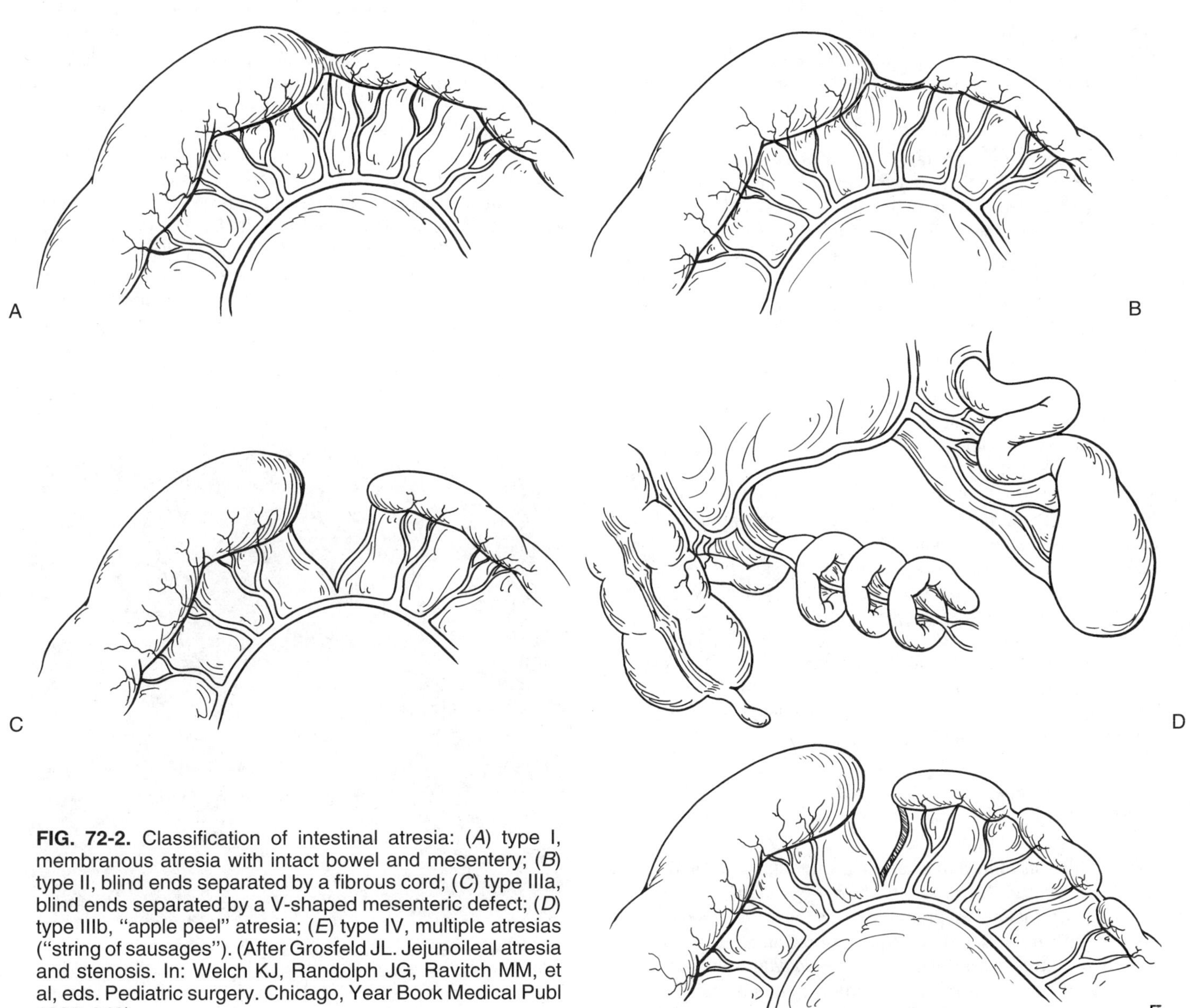

FIG. 72-2. Classification of intestinal atresia: (*A*) type I, membranous atresia with intact bowel and mesentery; (*B*) type II, blind ends separated by a fibrous cord; (*C*) type IIIa, blind ends separated by a V-shaped mesenteric defect; (*D*) type IIIb, "apple peel" atresia; (*E*) type IV, multiple atresias ("string of sausages"). (After Grosfeld JL. Jejunoileal atresia and stenosis. In: Welch KJ, Randolph JG, Ravitch MM, et al, eds. Pediatric surgery. Chicago, Year Book Medical Publ 1986:843)

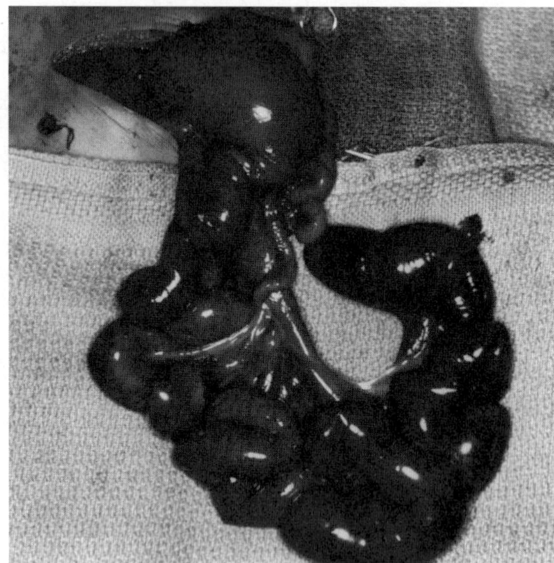

FIG. 72-3. Operative photograph displaying characteristics of type IIIb atresia. Surgical correction presents problems owing to the technical considerations of poor blood supply.

Type I: Membranous atresia with intact mesentery
Type II: Blind ends of the bowel with intact mesentery
Type IIIa: Blind ends with defect in the mesentery
Type IIIb: ''Apple peel'' atresia in which the superior mesenteric blood supply is compromised and the bowel is supplied distally by the ileocecal artery. The bowel corkscrews around the vessel, giving it the classic appearance of an apple peel (see Fig. 72-3).
Type IV: Multiple atresias

The different forms of intestinal atresia suggest several possible patterns of abnormal organogenesis. Type I membranous atresia may result from incomplete recanalization of the embryonic gut. The resulting stenosis or web may be either complete or partially obstructing. Types II and IIIa atresia appear to be caused by intrauterine ischemia resulting from events such as gastroschisis, volvulus, internal hernia, or intussusception. These two groups account for most atresias in most series—generally more than half of any single series. Types IIIb and IV atresia are more complex and unusual. These appear to be related to major or multiple interruptions of proximal mesenteric blood flow during gestation. As noted earlier, more than one jejunoileal atresia is present in up to 20% of infants afflicted. This obviously mandates a complete intraoperative assessment of distal intestinal patency.

DIAGNOSIS

The diagnosis of intestinal atresia is often suspected and confirmed prenatally. Suspicion of a bowel obstruction arises because of maternal polyhydramnios. This results from proximal obstruction with failure of absorption of the amniotic fluid and subsequent excessive accumulation of fluid. Ultrasound examination confirms the presence of polyhydramnios and reveals dilated loops of intestine (Fig. 72-4). During gestation the cause

of the obstruction is difficult to establish with certainty; it can range from meconium ileus to intestinal atresia. Therefore, a prenatal evaluation for conditions such as cystic fibrosis may be warranted. Prenatal counseling and planning are helpful in providing support for the family and in making appropriate decisions regarding obstetric and neonatal care.

Abdominal distention and bilious vomiting are the cardinal signs of jejunoileal obstruction in newborn infants. Usually, infants with these obstructions fail to pass meconium, although this is not an absolute finding. If the atresia developed late in gestation, it is possible to have enough meconium in the colon to pass a small meconium stool. Vomiting occurs promptly after feeding in these neonates. Upper abdominal distention and tympany are generally apparent. As with any cause of complete intestinal obstruction in neonates, the degree of abdominal distention is directly related to the anatomic site of obstruction. Proximal obstructions produce gastric, duodenal, and upper intestinal distention so that the degree of abdominal distention may be limited; more distal obstructions produce a picture of more jejunal or ileal obstruction, hence more dramatic abdominal distention. Rectal examination is necessary in all of these infants, regardless of gestational age. Congenital jejunoileal obstruction generally produces white mucoid material on rectal examination. Although this finding is not specific for atresia, it correlates well with the finding of congenital bowel obstruction between the ampulla of Vater and the anus. Jaundice is occasionally present, although the genesis of this is unknown.

The clinical presentation of jejunal atresia is usually straightforward because of the presence of complete bowel obstruction. The symptoms occur promptly. As noted earlier, with incomplete obstructions from a web, symptoms are usually more subtle, and presentation may not occur until several months or even years of age. Ileal atresia may be more difficult to diagnose in newborns because of the need to differentiate it from other conditions such as meconium ileus or Hirschsprung's disease. Symptoms may be more delayed in onset as well.

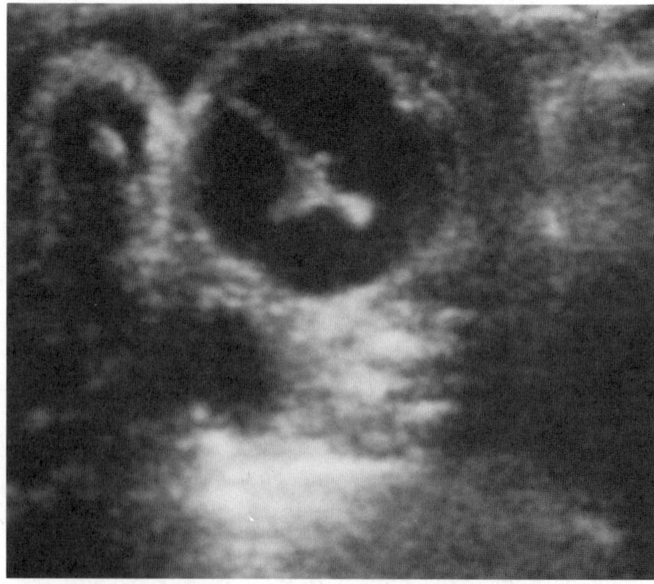

FIG. 72-4. Prenatal ultrasound showing several dilated loops of fetal intestine. This infant proved to have jejunal atresia, although meconium ileus and other causes of neonatal obstruction create similar images.

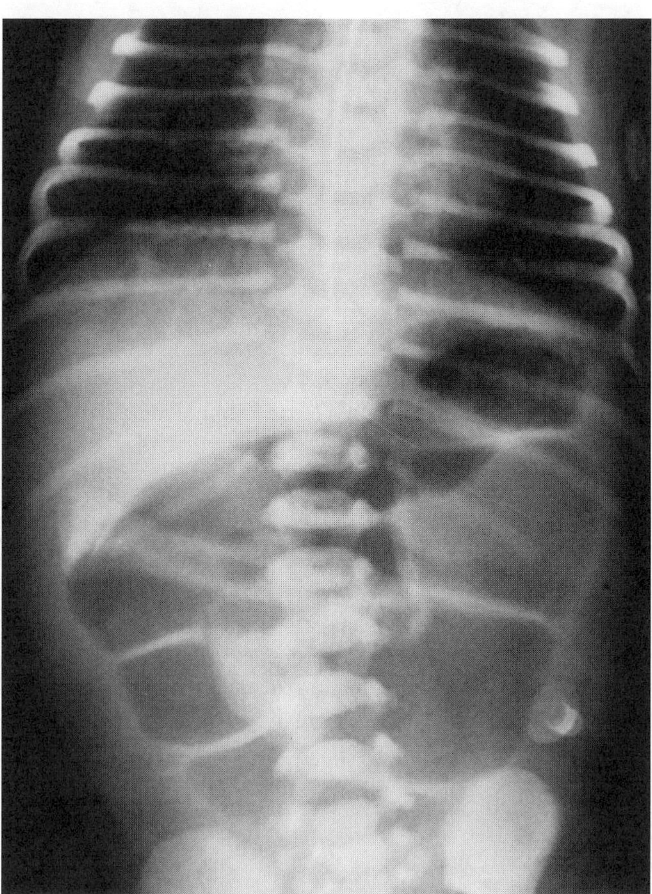

FIG. 72-5. Abdominal radiograph showing dilated bowel loops indicative of obstruction. There is an absence of distal air. The level of the obstruction is difficult to determine from a plain film. This child has jejunoileal atresia.

Plain abdominal radiographs are the initial diagnostic study for neonates with suspected intestinal obstruction. The typical findings of distended air-filled bowel loops and an absence of distal air are shown in Figure 72-5. A contrast enema is employed to confirm the diagnosis of small bowel obstruction and atresia and to exclude meconium ileus, a condition that often responds to nonoperative management. The contrast enema usually shows a microcolon (Fig. 72-6), particularly with distal atresia. If the small bowel atresia is proximal, a microcolon may not be evident because of the accumulation of sufficient intestinal contents in the colon to distend the bowel to a normal diameter. In these infants, the colon is intrinsically normal but is diminutive because of disuse. Upper GI contrast studies are generally unnecessary and probably unwise in view of the impending need for operative intervention. Incomplete obstruction from a partial web or diaphragm may be difficult to diagnose without a more sophisticated approach, such as enteroclysis, but this is typically a problem in infants beyond the neonatal period and children, as noted earlier.

TREATMENT

Preoperative resuscitation of the neonate should be expeditious. Intravenous hydration is essential. Maintenance of appro-priate body temperature is crucial to successful management. Placement of a nasogastric tube permits evacuation of air and intestinal contents. Broad-spectrum antibiotics are routinely given. A careful physical examination should be performed to exclude other anomalies. If the diagnosis of jejunoileal atresia is clear, it is important to correct systemic or associated problems related to issues such as prematurity or congenital heart disease. Once the resuscitation and diagnostic evaluation are complete, surgical exploration should be prompt, particularly if malrotation and volvulus have not been excluded. These perioperative issues are discussed in detail elsewhere in this text.

Generally, the abdomen is explored through an upper abdominal transverse incision. The entire intestine is thoroughly inspected, with particular reference to the possibilities of ischemia and multiple atresias. Determination of whether multiple atresias exist may require passing a rubber catheter or instilling saline into the lumen of the distal bowel to make certain there are no additional anatomic obstructions. Failure to identify an additional area of atresia can lead to the catastrophic complications that result from performing an anastomosis proximal to an unrecognized obstruction. Although once considered a routine component of care, gastrostomy is now rarely performed at initial surgery.

The surgical goal of intestinal reconstruction in these infants is to reestablish intestinal continuity while preserving bowel length and normal anatomy as much as possible. In practice,

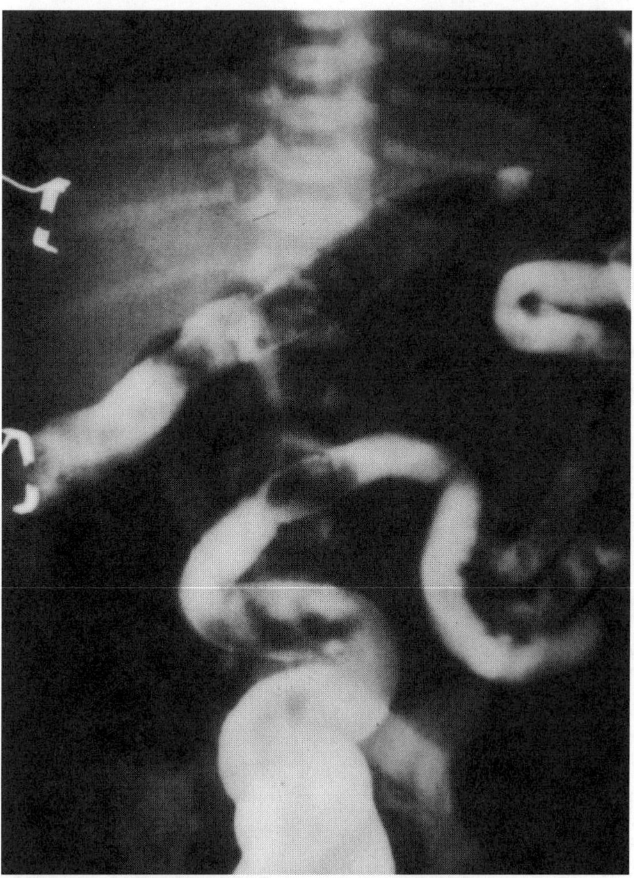

FIG. 72-6. Contrast enema showing a small colon with dilated proximal air-filled loops in an infant with ileal atresia.

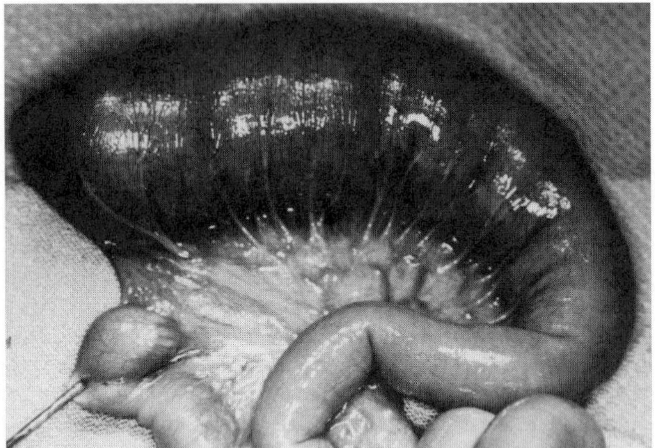

FIG. 72-7. Characteristic appearance of dilated proximal jejunum and the diminutive bowel distal to the atresia. Limited resection of the thickened, dilated proximal segment permits a satisfactory anastomosis and restoration of intestinal continuity.

this requires a delicate balance between preservation of bowel length and resection of abnormal intestine.[14] The proximal bowel is usually dilated (Fig. 72-7). The proximal segment may also be ischemic and dysfunctional, so when bowel length permits, it is best to perform a limited resection of this region.

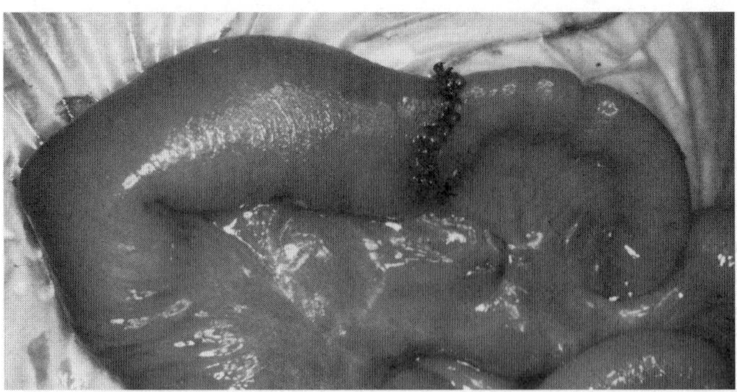

FIG. 72-9. Operative photograph of a completed anastomosis for jejunoileal atresia with a large lumenal mismatch. This anastomosis may be at high risk for functional obstruction because of potential dysmotility of the proximal dilated segment.

Resecting the extremely dilated bowel also facilitates an end-to-end anastomosis, especially when a substantial size mismatch is present. One helpful technique is to bevel the distal bowel so that the orifices are more equal in size and then to proceed with an end-oblique anastomosis (Figs. 72-8 and 72-9). Single-layer anastomoses are simple and efficacious, but some surgeons prefer double-layer anastomoses. Bowel diversion may be necessary if the viability of the bowel is questionable, but this is not

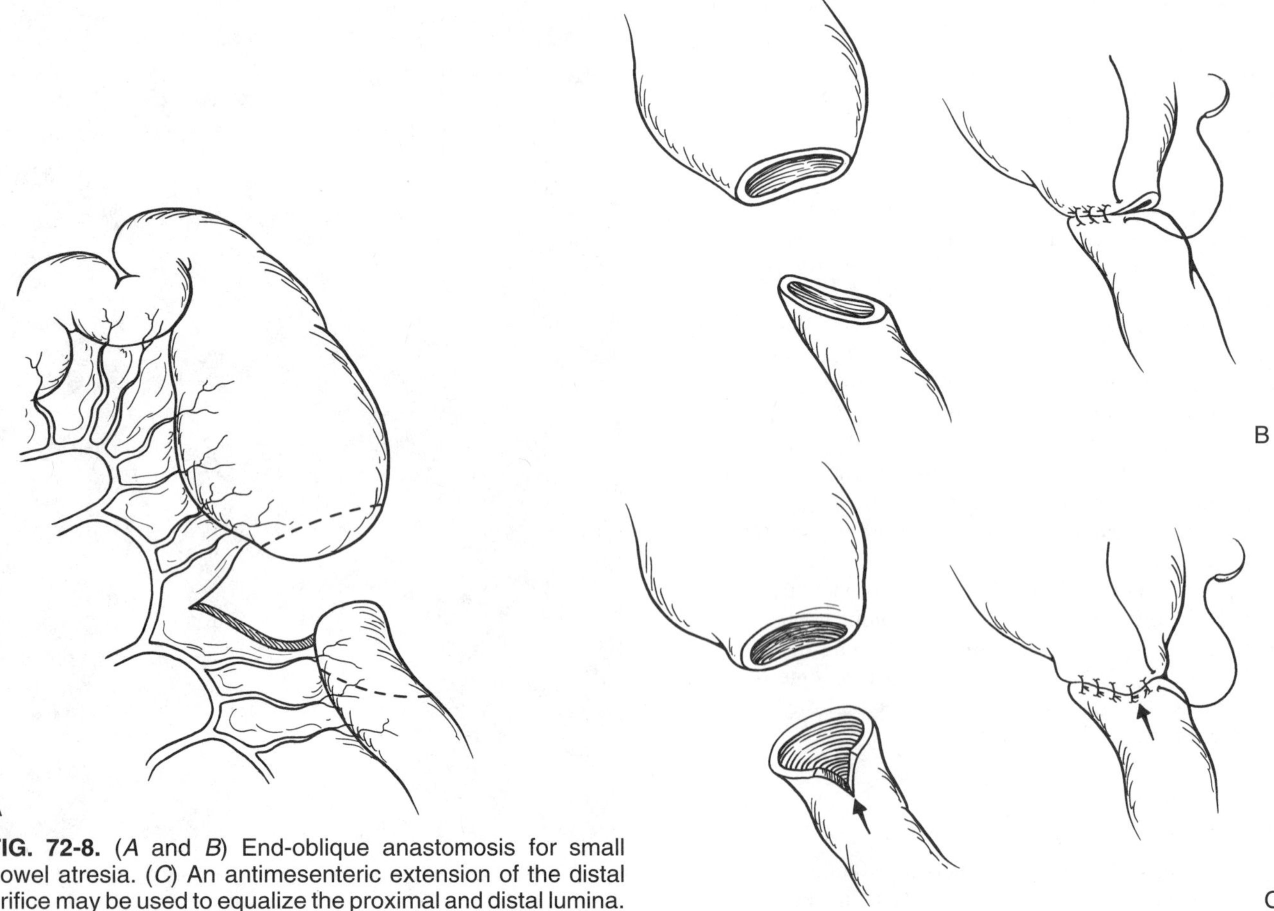

FIG. 72-8. (*A* and *B*) End-oblique anastomosis for small bowel atresia. (*C*) An antimesenteric extension of the distal orifice may be used to equalize the proximal and distal lumina.

done in most cases to avoid unnecessary loss of bowel and secondary operations. Although previously employed broadly and with enthusiasm, exteriorization techniques are rarely required in modern practice.

With a proximal jejunal atresia, it may not be reasonable to resect the dilated segment because of its proximity to the duodenum and pancreas, so alternative strategies are required to preserve bowel length.[15,16] This issue may also arise with complex and multiple atresias elsewhere. Some have advocated tapering this segment by resecting the antimesenteric portion of intestine and constructing a proximal intestinal segment of relatively normal caliber. This tapered end is then sewn to the distal bowel (Fig. 72-10). Others have imbricated the antimesenteric aspect of the dilated bowel, thereby avoiding resection. The role for these proximal tapering enteroplasties is limited, and the potential complications are substantial. These judgments, however, are subjective and controversial. It is prudent, therefore, at initial operation to emphasize the principles of reestablishing intestinal continuity as simply as possible without sacrificing essential gut length.

When jejunoileal atresia occurs in the presence of gastroschi-sis, it may be difficult to identify the specific site of the atresia owing to thickening of the bowel and inflammation. In these cases, it is best to reduce the bowel back into the abdominal cavity and close the abdominal wall defect because it is the lesion of least physiologic significance. Definitive surgery for the atresia delayed for 6 weeks after the abdominal wall closure, at which time the acute inflammation has usually subsided and resection and anastomosis are technically feasible.

Difficult decisions may be required when the bowel length is marginal. The intestine should be carefully measured in this circumstance. The concept of an absolute minimum length of bowel required for survival is still evolving. In the 1970s, 30 to 40 cm of small bowel was thought to be the threshold for survival.[17] Preservation of the ileocecal valve, avoidance of concomitant colon resection, and the potential for bowel growth in premature infants all reduce the minimum length of bowel necessary to sustain life. Ten centimeters of small bowel, including an ileocecal valve, is potentially adequate for survival, but each treatment decision must be individualized.[18] In any event, every attempt should be made to preserve bowel length in these situations. When multiple atresias are present, this may

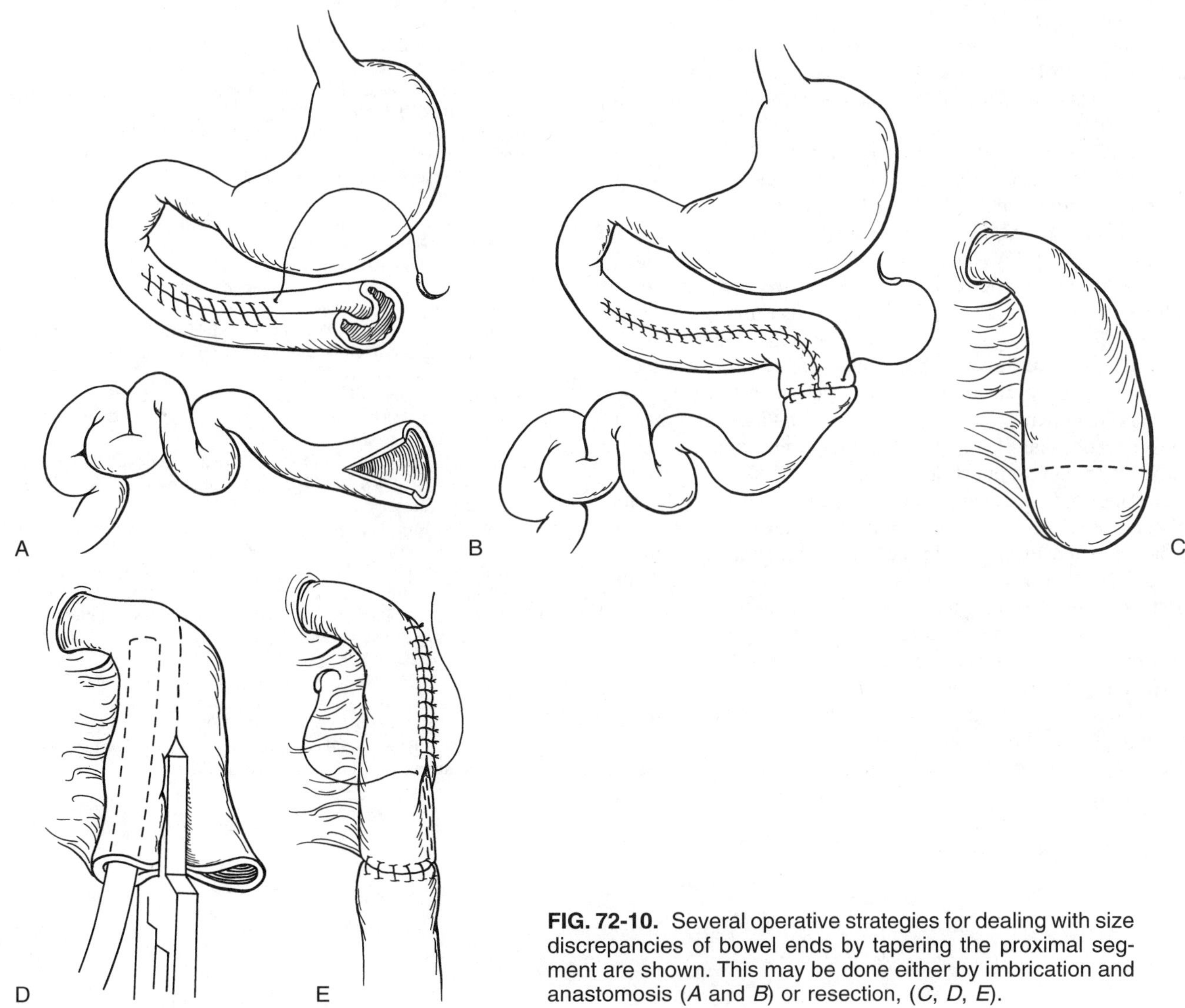

FIG. 72-10. Several operative strategies for dealing with size discrepancies of bowel ends by tapering the proximal segment are shown. This may be done either by imbrication and anastomosis (*A* and *B*) or resection, (*C, D, E*).

require many anastomoses, although rarely are segments less than 4 cm in length salvageable. Children with less than 10 cm of intestine should be evaluated early for potential small bowel transplantation. Postoperative care is directed toward maintaining nutrition parenterally until bowel function appears and adaptation to an enteral diet is accomplished. These issues are discussed in detail elsewhere in this text (see Chapter 69).

The spectrum of potential outcomes is broad. Some infants with uncomplicated anastomoses and adequate bowel length begin passing stools within a few days and can be advanced to a normal breast milk or formula diet within a few weeks. At the other extreme are infants with short gut or difficult anastomoses who require months of parenteral nutritional support and a prolonged adjustment to enteral feedings. The refinement of intravenous and elemental enteral formulas has greatly enhanced the outlook for these children, particularly because much of their care can now be accomplished in the home environment.

OUTCOME

In most neonates with jejunoileal atresia, the prognosis is excellent, with a reported survival rate of 100% in a recent series of infants with isolated atresia.[19] The incidence of technical anastomotic problems, such as leak or stricture formation, is as high as 10% to 15% in some published reports, but the current experience is more nearly 5%, which is probably not different than for other enterostomies. Although once common, wound infections are now relatively rare, probably because of improved nutrition and antibiotics. Vitamin deficiencies, necrotizing enterocolitis, renal calculi, and adhesive small bowel obstruction are potential complications.[20] Children generally require lifetime follow-up because of these possible complications. With the exception of short gut–related problems, morbidity and mortality are largely limited to that imposed by concurrent illness, such as prematurity, congenital heart disease, abdominal wall defects, and associated problems. As noted earlier, prolonged dysfunction of a proximal gut is relatively common and may persist for several months. In this regard, parenteral nutrition is life-saving. Parenteral nutrition, however, carries its own complications, which are discussed elsewhere. Sepsis-induced and parenteral infusion–induced cholestatic jaundice are the most frequent of these. Cholestatic jaundice is to be expected in any infant on total parenteral nutrition for more than 2 to 4 weeks, but it is usually reversed with the establishment of enteral feedings.

The failure of some children to progress promptly to an enteral diet can be a difficult clinical problem. It may relate to dysfunction of the intestine at the site of anastomosis or in the proximal segment. In this instance, upper GI contrast studies are indicated, and reoperation may be required. Functional obstruction may be present owing to the retention of bowel, which was normal in appearance at the original operation, but because of ischemia, intrinsic dysmotility, or absorptive problems, proves inadequate. This is probably more common with the more complex or multiple atresias. In most cases, bowel adaptation can be accomplished over a period of months with monitoring and dietary management. In selected cases, secondary reconstructive procedures, including the tapering enteroplasties, or even small bowel transplantation may be considered.

REFERENCES

1. Cragan J, Martin M, Moore C, et al. Descriptive epidemiology of small intestinal atresia. Teratology 1993;48:441.
2. Skandalakis JE, Gray SW, Ricketts R, Richardson DR. The small intestines. In: Embryology for surgeons: the embryological basis for the treatment of congenital anomalies. Baltimore, Williams & Wilkins, 1994: 184–241.
3. Louw JH, Barnard CN. Congenital intestinal atresia: observations on its origin. Lancet 1955;2:1065.
4. Tovar JA, Sunol M, Lopez-Detorre B, et al. Mucosal morphology and experimental intestinal atresia: studies in the chick embryo. J Pediatr Surg 1991;26:184.
5. Touloukian RJ. Antenatal intestinal adaptation with experimental jejunoileal atresia. J Pediatr Surg 1978;13:468.
6. Trahair JS, Rodgers HS, Cool JC, et al. Altered intestinal development after jejunal ligation in fetal sheep. Virchows Arch A 1993;423:45.
7. Doolin J, Ormsbee HS, Hill JL. Motility abnormality in intestinal atresia. J Pediatr Surg 1987;22:320.
8. Gornall P. Management of intestinal atresia complicating gastroschisis. J Pediatr Surg 1989;24:522.
9. Walker MW, Lovell MA, Kelly TE, et al. Multiple areas of intestinal atresia associated with immunodeficiency and post-transfusion graft vs host disease. J Pediatr 1993;123:93.
10. Serrano J, Zetterstrom R. Disaccharidase activities and intestinal absorption in infants with congenital intestinal obstruction. J Pediatr Gastroenterol Nutr 1987;6:238.
11. Tepas J, Wyllie RG, Shermeta DW, et al. Comparison of histochemical studies of intestinal atresia in human newborn and fetal lamb. J Pediatr Surg 1979;14:376.
12. Hamdy MH, Man DWK, Bain D, et al. Histochemical changes in intestinal atresia and its implications to surgical management: a preliminary report. J Pediatr Surg 1986;21:17.
13. Grosfeld JL. Jejunoileal atresia and stenosis. In: Welch KJ, Randolph JG, Ravitch MM, et al, eds. Pediatric surgery. Chicago, Year Book, 1986:838.
14. Nixon HH, Tawes R. Etiology and treatment of small intestinal atresia: analysis of a series of 127 jejunal ileal atresias in comparison with 62 duodenal atresias. Surgery 1971;69:41.
15. Howard ER, Othersen HB. Proximal jejunoplasty in the treatment of jejunal atresia. J Pediatr Surg 1973;8:685.
16. Weber TR, Vane DW, Grosfeld JL. Tapering enteroplasty in infants with bowel atresia and shortgut. Arch Surg 1982;117:684.
17. Wilmore DW. Factors correlating with successful outcome following extensive intestinal resection in newborn infants. J Pediatr 1972;80:88.
18. Kurkchubasche AJ, Rowe MI, Smith SD. Adaptation in short bowel syndrome: reassessing old limits. J Pediatr Surg 1993;28:1069.
19. Rescorla JF, Grosfeld JL. Intestinal atresia and stenosis: analysis of survival in 120 cases. Surgery 1985;98:668.
20. Lafferty K, Brereton RJ, Wright BM. Necrotizing enterocolitis in small bowel atresia. Z Kinderchir 1983;38:224.

Surgery of Infants and Children: Scientific Principles and Practice, edited by
Keith T. Oldham, Paul M. Colombani, and Robert P. Foglia.
Lippincott–Raven Publishers, Philadelphia, © 1997.

CHAPTER 73

Necrotizing Enterocolitis

Ann M. Kosloske

Necrotizing enterocolitis (NEC) of the neonate emerged in the
1970s as the most common surgical emergency and the most
common gastrointestinal emergency in the neonatal intensive
care unit (NICU).[1–3] It is a syndrome with a predilection for
premature or low-birthweight infants, who comprise 90% of
cases.[3] NEC is characterized by the clinical findings of ileus
and gastrointestinal bleeding, by the radiographic finding of
pneumatosis intestinalis, and by the pathologic finding of crepitant necrosis of the gut. One third to one half of all infants with
documented NEC require operation for gangrenous or perforated bowel. The overall incidence in the United States is 1 to
3 cases per 1000 live births, representing 1% to 7.7% of all
admissions to NICUs.[4] The average annual mortality rate for
1979 through 1985 was 13.1 deaths per 100,000 live births;
reported case fatality rates ranged from 20% to 40%.[3,4]

Although NEC occurs worldwide in developed countries, its
distribution is uneven among these countries. For example,
NEC is a problem in the United States, Canada, the United
Kingdom, and Australia, but it is rarely encountered in Switzer-
land, the Scandinavian countries, and especially Japan, where
a survey of NICUs showed an incidence that was 4 to 28 times
lower than that reported for the United States.[5] In general, countries that enjoy low premature birth rates see few cases of NEC.
In countries in which NICU technology is not available, NEC
is not a problem among neonates. Older infants and children
in these countries, however, may fall victim to *necrotic enteritis*,
a syndrome also characterized by ileus, gastrointestinal bleeding, and crepitant necrosis of the gut. This syndrome, which
may be analogous to NEC, is caused by toxins of certain types
of *Clostridium perfringens*.[6]

ANATOMY AND PATHOLOGY

Necrotizing enterocolitis can affect any segment of the gastrointestinal tract but most often strikes the ileocecal area. A
detailed study of 84 pathologic specimens from operation or
autopsy of infants with NEC showed involvement of both small
and large intestine (usually terminal ileum and proximal colon)
in 44%, small intestinal disease alone in 30%, and colonic involvement alone in 26%.[7] In about half the patients, a continuous segment of intestine was affected; the others had discontin-

uous involvement, with skip areas or subcircumferential
disease. In 14 patients (17%), the entire small and large bowel,
from the ligament of Treitz to the transverse colon, was necrotic[7] (*pannecrosis, NEC totalis*), a lesion which is incompatible with survival (Fig. 73-1).

The ileocolic predilection of NEC is evidence of an ischemic
cause. Because the arteries supplying the ileocecal area are the
most peripheral branches of the superior mesenteric artery, the
intestine in their watershed is most vulnerable to ischemic or
hypoxic injury.

The predominant histologic lesion, coagulation necrosis, is
further support for the role of ischemia in the pathogenesis.
Surgical specimens generally contain areas of full-thickness intestinal necrosis and partial-thickness necrosis. Adjacent areas
may show both acute and chronic inflammation (Fig. 73-2). If
present, reparative tissue changes, such as epithelial regeneration, granulation tissue formation, and fibrosis, suggest ongoing
tissue injury of at least several days' duration. In about half of
specimens, characteristic gas bubbles of pneumatosis intestinalis are found.[7] Table 73-1 lists the prevalence of histologic
findings in acute NEC.

About one in four infants who survive acute NEC develop
late intestinal strictures from injured areas that did not perforate
but rather healed with circumferential scarring[2,8] (Fig. 73-3).

PATHOPHYSIOLOGY

The pathogenesis of NEC is not clearly understood. A multifactorial etiology is usually cited, invoking an interaction of
three essential components outlined by Santulli and colleagues[1]:
(1) ischemic injury of the intestine; (2) bacterial colonization
of the gut; and (3) the presence of substrate, usually formula
feedings, within the gut lumen. These elements may be documented or inferred in most infants who develop NEC. Unifying
theories of pathogenesis fail, however, because the three elements may also be documented or inferred for virtually all infants in an NICU, most of whom never develop NEC.[6] Case-
control studies have failed to identify predisposing factors of
significance, except prematurity.[9]

Ischemic events in the neonatal intestine may occur by various mechanisms. Selective circulatory ischemia (the diving re-

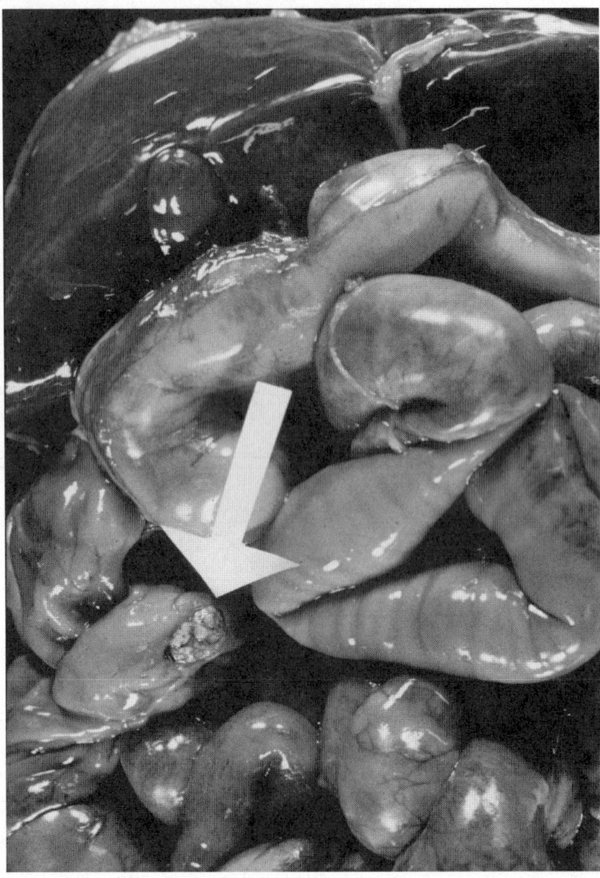

FIG. 73-1. Autopsy specimen of pannecrosis of necrotizing enterocolitis. Extensive intestinal gangrene includes perforation (*arrow*) of the ileum. (Courtesy of Professor H. Becker, Institute of Pathology, Graz, Austria)

TABLE 73-1. *Histologic findings in 84 infants with acute NEC*

Finding	Prevalence (%)
Coagulation necrosis	89
Inflammation	89
Both acute and chronic	60
Acute alone	18
Chronic alone	11
Eosinophils	14
Ulceration	76
Hemorrhage	74
Peritonitis	68
Reparative changes	68
Epithelial regeneration	54
Granulation tissue/fibrosis	28
Villous atrophy	19
Bacterial overgrowth	66
Pneumatosis intestinalis	48
Edema (usually submucosal)	43
Crypt abscesses	12
Pseudomembranes	9.5
Fungal overgrowth	3.5

(Ballance WA, Dahms BB, Shenker N, et al. Pathology of neonatal necrotizing enterocolitis. J Pediatr 1990;117:S6)

flex) diverting blood flow away from the gut during perinatal stress is the most widely held theory.[8,10] Thrombotic or embolic bowel injury may be associated with catheters placed in the infant aorta for monitoring.[11] Low-flow states may result from diverse events, including congenital heart disease, hyperviscosity, cold stress, and certain pharmacologic agents, such as indomethacin or methylxanthenes.

Reperfusion of ischemic tissue triggers a chain of biochemical events leading to necrosis; a key step is the release of free radicals of oxygen, whose toxic chemical reactivity is caused

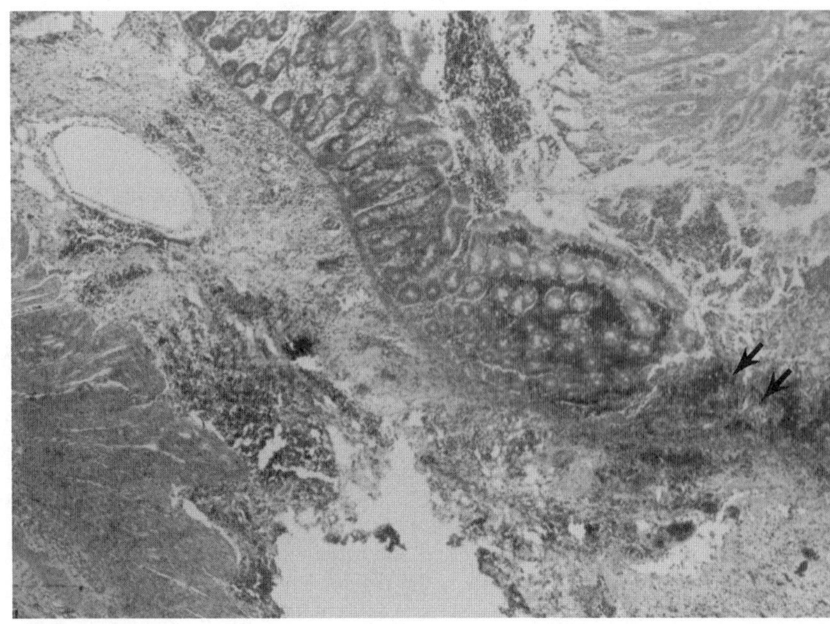

FIG. 73-2. Acute necrotizing enterocolitis with extensive ischemic change of intestinal wall and focus of frank gangrene (*arrows*). (Hematoxylin & eosin; original magnification × 100)

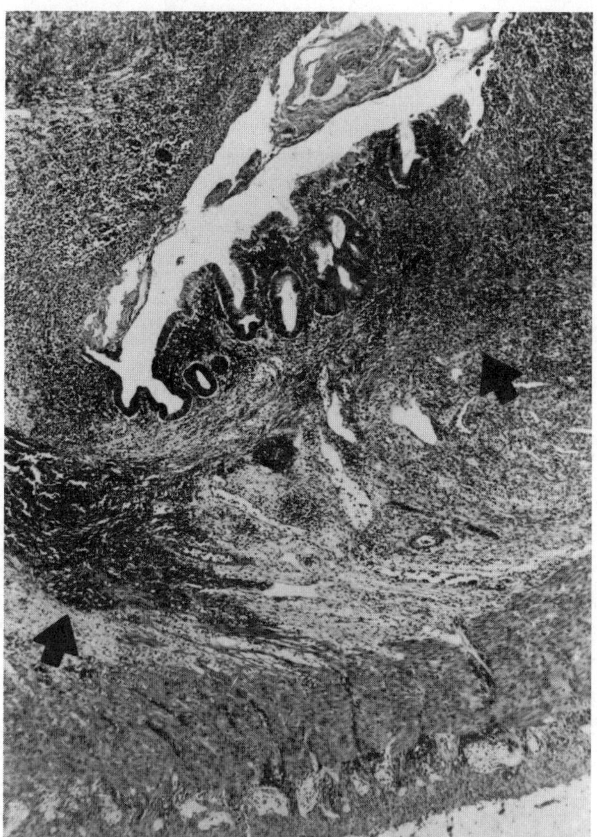

FIG. 73-3. Intestinal stricture in necrotizing enterocolitis. Mucosa at top is destroyed. Submucosa shows acute inflammation (*arrows*). The lumen is obliterated. (Hematoxylin & eosin; original magnification × 50)

by a single unpaired electron in the outer shell.[8] Cytotoxic free radicals include superoxide (O_2^-) and hydroxyl (HO^-), plus hydrogen peroxide (H_2O_2) derived from the superoxide. The two sources of these cytotoxic free radicals in the reperfused tissue are polymorphonuclear neutrophils and the enzyme xanthine oxidase. Strategies for prevention of necrosis induced by ischemia–reperfusion injury include pharmacologic agents, such as free radical anion scavengers (superoxide dismutase[12,13]), inhibitors of xanthine oxidase, (allopurinol[12,14]), and agents that deliver dissolved oxygen directly to the tissues (perfluorocarbons[15]).

Lawrence and associates[16] linked the impaired immunologic defense mechanisms of the premature gut with luminal bacterial toxins. In the NICU environment, which is characterized by frequent antibiotic usage and sterile nursing practices, gut colonization is delayed, with limited numbers and species of bacteria.[16] Intestinal B and T lymphocytes are decreased in numbers as well.[17] The terminal ileum of the premature infant at birth is permeable to the passage of intact macromolecules. Translocation of whole bacteria may occur with little impediment. Closure of the mucosal barrier coincides with the synthesis of adequate levels of secretory immunoglobulin A, which takes 2 to 3 weeks. During this early vulnerable period, toxins from certain bacterial strains, including antibiotic-resistent strains, may damage the enterocyte, thus initiating NEC. Although bacterial colonization in the NICU is delayed and the variety limited, the

bacteria most often associated with NEC (*Klebsiella* sp, *E coli*, and *Clostridia* sp) are members of the normal flora of the neonatal gut, rather than pathogenic strains.[18,19]

Breast milk contains many beneficial factors (macrophages, secretory immunoglobulin A, lactoferrin, and others) that confer passive immunity to the neonatal intestine. In the British multicenter study of Lucas and Cole,[20] NEC was rare among infants born at more than 30 weeks' gestation who were fed breast milk. It was 20 times more common in those fed formula only and had an intermediate incidence in those who received both formula and breast milk.

Spontaneous endotoxemia may occur with enteral feeding of premature infants.[21] Endotoxin, tumor necrosis factor, platelet activating factor, and other inflammatory mediators may be the agents or the by-products of intestinal injury in NEC.[22–24]

Animal models of NEC are generally unsatisfactory, although many have been tried. Tiny rat or mouse pups, weighing less than 10 g, are fragile and unpredictable; germ-free models are cumbersome and may cease to work.[25] Results are more reproducible in mature animals, but the intestinal necrosis achieved in these experiments may not be analogous to NEC. About a dozen such animal models devised in the past 15 to 20 years[16,22,26,27] suffer from conceptual or methodologic flaws; none is recognized as a standard for experimentation. Perfection of an animal model may thus be less fruitful for prevention of NEC than clinical trials of promising interventions.

The epidemiology, pathogenesis, and prevention of NEC have been reviewed.[6,28,29] It appears to be a complex, multifactorial disease process that we do not understand fully. Table 73-2 summarizes six proposed factors in the pathogenesis of NEC and lists 27 selected clinical or experimental studies, most within the past decade, providing data that support (or sometimes challenge) one or more of these factors.

CLINICAL DIAGNOSIS

The clinical signs of NEC are those of intestinal ischemia, including abdominal distention, lethargy, feeding intolerance, bilious vomiting, and rectal bleeding. The early manifestations of NEC may be indistinguishable from those of neonatal septicemia.[3] Plain abdominal radiographs show the pathognomonic finding of pneumatosis intestinalis, that is, air within the bowel wall (Fig. 73-4). The intramural air is produced by gas-forming bacteria from fermentation of formula feedings. Pneumoperitoneum in an infant with NEC signifies intestinal perforation and is an indication for immediate operation. The radiographic finding of portal venous gas is usually associated with extensive gangrene (Fig. 73-5) and a high mortality rate.[30] The initial radiographic findings of NEC predict its outcome (Table 73-3).

A clinical staging system for NEC devised by Bell and colleagues[31] stratified the severity of the illness (Table 73-4), allowing the comparison of series from different centers. Studies of NEC generally adhere to a strict case definition, requiring radiologic confirmation of NEC (pneumatosis intestinalis, gas in the portal venous system, or free air in the abdomen) or a pathologic specimen from operation or autopsy showing intestinal necrosis.

TABLE 73-2. *Selected studies regarding pathogenesis of necrotizing enterocolitis*

Investigators*	Proposed factor	Clinical or experimental	Control group	Description
Lloyd, 1969[10]	Ischemia	Clinical	No	Classic study linking the diving reflex (selective circulatory ischemia) to neonatal GI perforation
Czyrko et al, 1991[56]		Clinical	Yes	Maternal use of cocaine, a potent vasoconstrictor, was associated with NEC
Malcolm et al, 1991[57]		Clinical	Yes	Absent or reversed end-diastolic flow velocity in the umbilical artery was associated with NEC
Parks et al, 1982[12]	Reperfusion	Experimental	Yes	Superoxide dismutase or allopurinol protected cat intestinal mucosa from ischemia
Vohra et al, 1989[13]		Experimental	Yes	Superoxide dismutase protected rabbit ileal mucosa from ischemia
Megison et al, 1990[14]		Experimental	Yes	Allopurinol protected rat intestinal mucosa from ischemia
Oldham et al, 1987[15]		Experimental	Yes	Intraluminal perfluorocarbons protected rat intestine from ischemia
Kosloske et al, 1978[58]	Bacteria	Clinical	No	Fulminant NEC associated with *Clostridia* sp; other cases associated with *Enterobacteriaceae* family
Kosloske et al, 1985[59]		Clinical	Yes	Fulminant NEC associated with *Clostridium perfringens*
Blakey et al, 1985[19]		Clinical	No	No obvious culprit strains cause sporadic NEC; *C perfingens* associated with the most severe cases
Musemeche et al, 1986[27]		Experimental	Yes	In germ-free rat model, bacteria most important factor (versus ischemia, formula) in pathogenesis of bowel necrosis
Hoy et al, 1990[60]		Clinical	No	Quantitative overgrowth of *Enterobacteriaceae* family was antecedent to NEC
Lawrence et al, 1982[16]	Bacterial toxins	Experimental	Yes	Toxin-forming bacteria initiated necrotic enteritis in germ-free rat pups
Lawrence & Bates, 1983[25]		Experimental	No	Toxin-forming bacteria ceased to initiate NEC-like illness in germ-free rat pups
Scheifele et al, 1985[21]		Clinical	Yes	Spontaneous endotoxinemia with feeding of premature infants
Scheifele et al, 1987[61]		Clinical	Yes	Delta toxin of coagulase-negative *Staphylococcus* sp associated with NEC
Sun & Hseuh, 1988[22]	Cytokines	Experimental	Yes	Bowel necrosis in rats from interaction of tumor necrosis factor (TNF) and platelet-activating factor (PAF)
Harris et al, 1994[24]		Clinical	Yes	Infants with bacterial sepsis and NEC had elevated plasma interleukin-6 levels but no elevation of plasma TNF
Caplan & Hseuh, 1990[23]		Clinical	Yes	Infants with NEC had elevated plasma levels of PAF and TNF-α
Barlow et al, 1974[26]	Feedings	Experimental	Yes	Classic study showing protective effect of breast milk in rat pups
Lucas & Cole, 1990[20]		Clinical	Yes	Breast milk protected British infants from NEC (passive immunity)
Book et al, 1975[62]		Clinical	Yes	Hyperosmolar formula feedings associated with NEC
LaGamma et al, 1985[63]		Clinical	Yes	Delayed oral feeding of low-birthweight (LBW) neonates does not prevent NEC
McKeown et al, 1992[64]		Clinical	Yes	Delayed oral feeding of very LBW neonates may prevent NEC
Eibl et al, 1988[65]	Immunologic immaturity	Clinical	Yes	Oral immunoglobulins A and G prevented NEC in LBW infants
Fast & Rosegger, 1994[66]		Clinical	Yes	Oral immunoglobulins A and G did not prevent NEC; oral gentamicin plus lyophilized *Enterobacter* sp more effective
Halac et al, 1990[67]		Clinical	Yes	Corticosteroid administration prevented NEC in LBW infants

* Each study is listed under a single pathogenic factor, although multiple factors could be considered (eg, breast milk provides both feedings and passive immunity).

LBW = low birthweight.

TABLE 73-3. *Radiographic abnormalities and clinical outcomes in 147 infants with necrotizing enterocolitis**

Radiographic abnormality	No. of infants (%)	No. with gangrene (%)	No. with pannecrosis (%)	No. of deaths (%)
Pneumatosis intestinalis				
Mild	51 (35)	23 (45)	4 (8)	9 (18)
Moderate	57 (39)	32 (56)	7 (12)	12 (21)
Severe	32 (22)	29 (91)	18 (56)	20 (63)
Pneumoperitoneum	45 (31)	45 (100)	15 (33)	15 (65)
Portal venous gas	23 (16)	23 (100)	14 (61)	15 (65)
Pneumatosis (severe) and portal venous gas	14 (10)	14 (100)	11 (79)	12 (86)

* The total number of infants is greater than 147 because some infants had two or three radiographic abnormalities. The grading system for pneumatosis intestinalis was: *mild*, a focal area in one quadrant of the abdomen; *moderate*, focal areas in two or three quadrants; or *severe*, focal areas in four quadrants or diffuse pneumatosis. Pannecrosis is necrosis involving 75% or more of total length of jejunum, ileum, and colon.

(Kosloske AM, Musemeche CA, Ball WS Jr, et al. Necrotizing enterocolitis: value of radiographic findings to predict outcome. AJR 1988;151:771)

MEDICAL MANAGEMENT

When the diagnosis of NEC is suspected, medical supportive treatment is begun immediately. The principles of medical management are cardiovascular support, control of sepsis, and close observation for gangrene or perforation. A protocol of medical management is outlined in Table 73-5. Surprisingly large volumes of intravenous fluid may be required to restore organ perfusion in NEC. Infants with ischemic bowel sequester fluid in the injured intestinal wall, in the dilated intestinal lumen, and in the peritoneal cavity. Fluid boluses may be required to

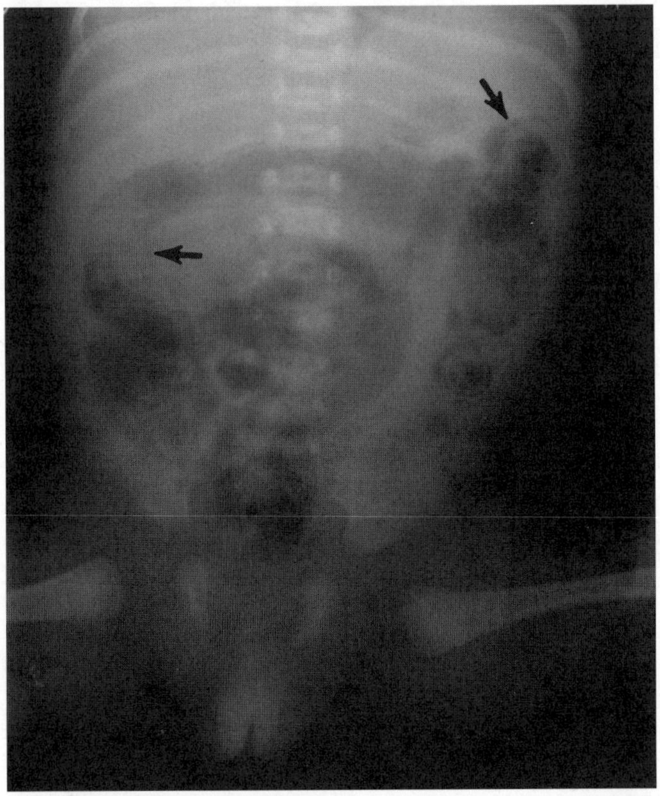

FIG. 73-4. Abdominal radiograph (supine view) showing pneumatosis intestinalis of entire colon (*arrows*). Intramural air appears as bubbles, streaks, or rings.

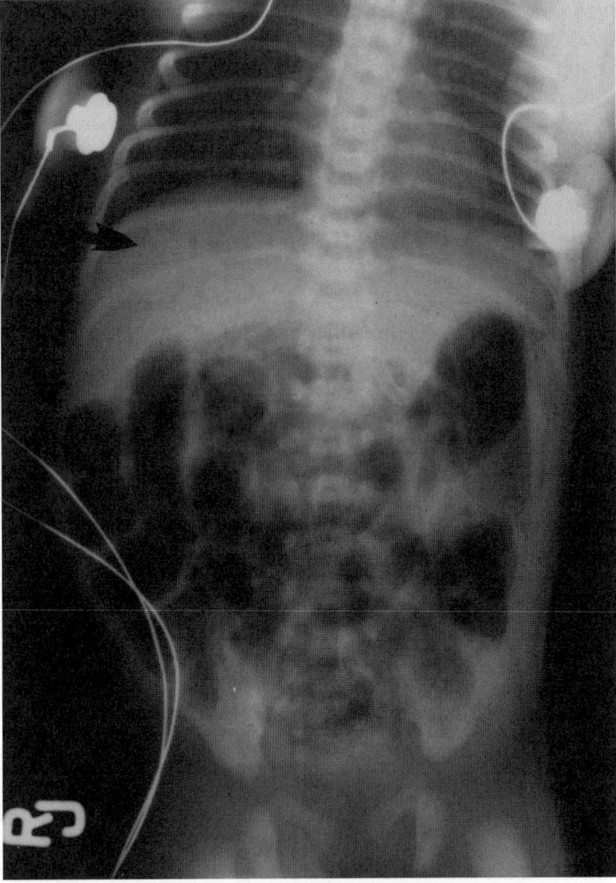

FIG. 73-5. Abdominal radiograph (lateral decubitus view) showing portal venous gas (*arrow*) and widespread pneumatosis intestinalis.

TABLE 73-4. *Clinical staging system for acute necrotizing enterocolitis*

Stage	Clinical findings	Radiographic findings	Treatment	Survival (%)*
I: Suspected NEC†	Mild abdominal distention, poor feeding, vomiting	Mild ileus	Medical, including work-up for sepsis	100
II: Definite NEC	The above, plus marked abdominal distention, GI bleeding	Significant ileus, pneumatosis intestinalis, portal vein gas (9% of cases)	Medical (see text and Table 73-5)	96
III: Advanced NEC	The above, plus deterioration of vital signs, septic shock	The above, plus pneumoperitoneum (60% of cases)	Surgical (see text)	50

* Survival rates are from Bell MJ, Ternberg JL, Feigin RD, et al. Neonatal necrotizing enterocolitis: therapeutic decisions based upon clinical staging. Ann Surg 1978;187:1)

† Most authors omit stage I patients from clinical series of NEC. Infants with NEC may progress to a more severe stage despite appropriate treatment. Infants whose disease progressed from stage II to stage III were considered to have stage III disease.

reverse hypotension, and two or even three times maintenance volume may be needed to maintain vital signs and urinary output. Low-dose dopamine (2 to 5 μg/kg/min) is sometimes useful to augment renal perfusion. Volume resuscitation for restoration of perfusion limits the ischemic damage (although reperfusion may trigger the release of oxygen free radicals). Systemic antibiotics are essential for control of sepsis. The sepsis syndrome may induce complications such as coagulopathy, respiratory arrest, or renal failure, requiring specific treatment. Serial examinations of the infant with serial abdominal radiographs, including supine and left lateral decubitus views, are essential to assess improvement (or deterioration) of the infant.

One half to two thirds of infants with NEC recover with medical management alone. Those who require operation are the sickest infants with advanced NEC.

INDICATIONS FOR OPERATION

The indications for operation in NEC are intestinal perforation or intestinal gangrene. The advent of pneumoperitoneum

TABLE 73-5. *Medical management of necrotizing enterocolitis*

Cultures: blood culture is essential; cerebrospinal fluid, urine, and other sites are cultured as indicated

Gastric suction for decompression of bowel, prevention of aspiration, and control of ileus

Intravenous fluids: 150–250 mL/kg/d of fluid for restoration of tissue perfusion and urinary output

Antibiotics: a penicillin (penicillin or ampicillin), an aminoglycoside (gentamicin), and usually clindamycin or metronidazole for control of sepsis from gut pathogens

Blood and blood products as needed for correction of anemia, coagulopathy

Radiographs of abdomen: supine and left lateral decubitus views every 6–8 h until infant is stable, then less frequently

Reexamination every 6–8 h until infant is stable, then less frequently

Paracentesis performed if the infant worsens or fails to improve after 4–6 h of intensive medical therapy

Operation indicated for evidence of intestinal gangrene or perforation

in an infant with NEC is an unequivocal sign of intestinal perforation, whereas signs of intestinal gangrene before perforation are less exact, and some are controversial. NEC strikes small, ill, premature infants, who rarely exhibit classic evidence of gangrene, such as fever, abdominal tenderness, or leukocytosis, and who cannot complain of pain. Thus, the diagnosis of gangrene may be delayed until perforation and peritonitis have occurred, and the septic process is far advanced. The radiographic finding of pneumatosis intestinalis is not an indication for operation because at least half of infants with this finding recover with medical therapy. Moreover, most pediatric surgeons are reluctant to operate without clear indications of intestinal gangrene because negative exploratory laparotomy is not an acceptable diagnostic procedure for critically ill premature infants. Ideally, operation should be carried out after the advent of intestinal gangrene but before perforation. One study in 1980 documented a mortality rate of 30% for infants with intestinal gangrene operated on before perforation and 64% for those operated on after perforation.[32]

A variety of clinical and radiographic criteria have been proposed as indications for operation for NEC. In a study of 147 infants from the University of New Mexico, 12 proposed criteria were evaluated by standard epidemiologic methods, calculating sensitivity, specificity, positive predictive value, and negative predictive value.[33] The results are summarized in Table 73-6. Pneumoperitoneum was a reliable criterion for intestinal gangrene after perforation. No false-negative results were noted, although pneumoperitoneum may occur from a pulmonary air leak in a ventilated infant. A positive paracentesis (described later) and the radiographic finding of portal venous gas were the most specific and useful criteria for diagnosis of intestinal gangrene before perforation. Grosfeld and associates[34] emphasized the value of portal venous gas as an indication for early operation in NEC. Less common, but highly specific findings associated with intestinal gangrene were a fixed, dilated loop on serial abdominal radiographs (Fig. 73-6), an abdominal mass, and erythema of the abdominal wall. Several other criteria proposed as indications for operation for NEC were less predictive of gangrene because of false-positive results (present in infants without gangrene) or false-negative results (absent in infants who proved to have gangrene). These criteria were as

TABLE 73-6. *Indications for operation in acute necrotizing enterocolitis*

Indication	No. with finding/no. of infants surveyed	Sensitivity (%)*	Specificity (%)†	Positive predictive value (%)‡	Negative predictive value (%)§
Pneumoperitoneum	45/147	48	100	100	52
Positive paracentesis#	26/50	87	100	98	60
Portal venous gas	23/147	24	100	100	43
Severe pneumatosis intestinalis	32/147	31	94	91	43
Dilated loop on serial radiographs	3/61	12.5	100	100	46
Fixed abdominal mass	3/61	12.5	89	100	46
Erythema of abdominal wall	2/61	8	100	100	45
Clinical deterioration¶	7/61	39	89	78	59
Platelet count $<100,000/mm^3$	8/61	38	83	73	54
Persistent abdominal tenderness	7/61	29	72	58	43
Severe GI hemorrhage	3/61	12.5	83	50	42
Plain films: gasless abdomen with ascites	1/61	0	94	0	41

* Number of true positives divided by number of infants with gangrene.
† Number of true negatives divided by number of infants without gangrene.
‡ Number of true positives divided by number of positives.
§ Number of true negatives divided by number of negatives.
# Brown fluid or bacteria on Gram stain.
¶ Clinical deterioration defined as two or more of the following: hypotension, oliguria, lethargy, increasing apnea, or persistent metabolic acidosis.

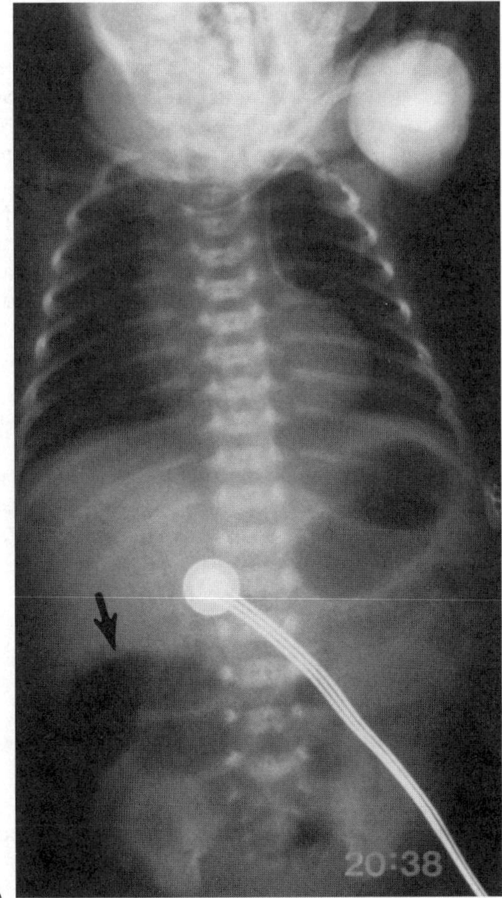

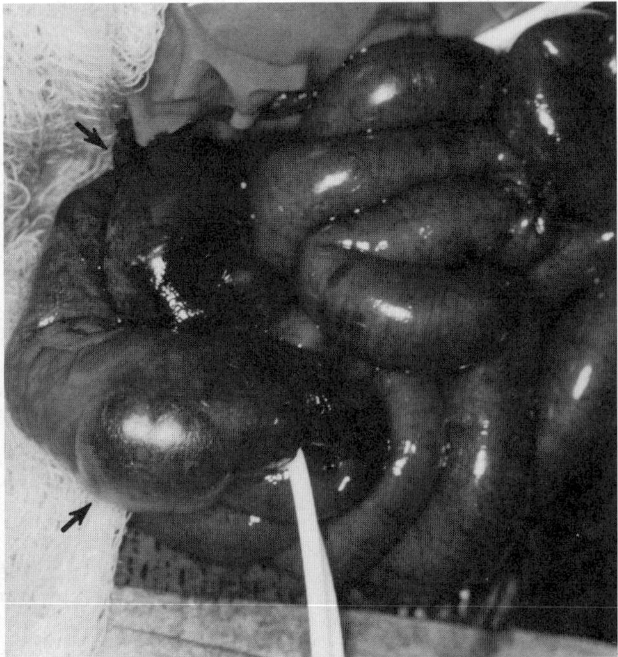

FIG. 73-6. (*A*) Plain radiograph of an infant with necrotizing enterocolitis. Note the prominent loop of intestine in the right mid-abdomen (*arrow*). Persistence of this loop on radiographs taken 4 hours and 8 hours later provided evidence of intestinal gangrene, requiring operation. (*B*) Operative findings. Note the corresponding loop of infarcted, but not yet perforated, intestine (*arrows*).

follows: (1) clinical deterioration, (2) a platelet count of less than 100,000 mm^3, (3) abdominal tenderness, (4) severe gastrointestinal hemorrhage, and (5) a radiologic finding of a gasless abdomen with ascites.

PARACENTESIS

Paracentesis may be performed on infants in whom the diagnosis of intestinal gangrene is suspected. The procedure is unnecessary in infants with suspected NEC (stage I, Bell system[31]), those with definite NEC (stage II) who are improving on medical therapy, or those with pneumoperitoneum, who already have an indication for operation. Paracentesis is optimally done a few hours after the onset of symptoms because the evolution of intestinal gangrene may take several hours. Serial paracenteses may be done in infants who fail to improve on medical therapy.

The technique of paracentesis must be gentle, yet precise. The following procedure should be performed under the direction of the attending pediatric surgeon:

1. Abdomen is palpated for identification of any masses or enlarged viscera.
2. An antiseptic skin preparation is done.
3. A small needle (22 or 25 gauge) is inserted into the flank at a 45-degree angle, advanced slowly, and aspirated gently.
4. The specimen is adequate when 0.5 mL or more of peritoneal fluid flows freely into the syringe. Any volume less than 0.5 mL is a "dry tap," which cannot be interpreted.
5. Color and appearance of the fluid are noted.
6. The fluid is transported (in capped syringe) immediately to the laboratory for Gram stain and cultures for aerobic and anaerobic bacteria.
7. *Positive paracentesis* is indicated by brown fluid or bacteria on Gram stain of the unspun fluid.

The finding of bacteria on Gram stain of an unspun body fluid is roughly quantitated at 10^5/mL or more organisms.[35] Ricketts and Jerles,[36] using a technique similar to that described here, reported 94% sensitivity and 100% specificity rates for paracentesis findings in infants with intestinal gangrene from NEC.

OPERATIVE PROCEDURE

The principles of operation for NEC are as follows: (1) excision of the gangrenous bowel, (2) exteriorization of the marginally viable ends, and (3) preservation of as much intestinal length as possible.

Exploration

The bowel is gently delivered from a transverse supraumbilical incision, generously made to permit good exposure. Retraction on the liver is avoided to reduce the risk of subcapsular hematoma, a rare but devastating complication that can occur during operation for NEC. The bowel is examined from stomach to rectum, although the retroperitoneal duodenum is not routinely mobilized. The ileocecal area is usually the site of the most severe ischemia, often with frank gangrene or perforation.

Injured segments are typically pale gray from ischemic necrosis or purple from hemorrhagic necrosis. Bubbles of intramural air may be seen beneath the serosa. Skip areas of viable intestine between ischemic segments are common.

Resection

Segments that are obviously gangrenous should be resected. Dusky bowel may be preserved because it may have the potential for healing, especially if protected by a proximal enterostomy. Perforations generally should be exteriorized rather than closed. Gangrenous foci that have not yet perforated, usually located on the antimesenteric border of the bowel, may be inverted into the lumen by enteroplasty. Massive intestinal resection, leaving less than 30 cm of viable intestine, should not be done. Surgical options in such cases of extensive NEC are discussed later.

Enterostomy

After resection of the necrotic intestine, the peritoneal cavity is washed with warm saline to remove residual fluid and debris. The bowel ends are then exteriorized as an enterostomy. Figures 73-7 and 73-8 depict two techniques of enterostomy for NEC. The author's preferred method of exteriorization is by the Mikulicz enterostomy, brought (whenever possible) through a separate incision near the laparotomy incision (see Fig. 73-7). The two ends of bowel can be brought out separately through the laparotomy incision (see Fig. 73-8). In a comparative study of 100 infants who underwent enterostomy formation and subsequent closure, there was no difference in the rate of wound or stomal complications between the two methods depicted in Figures 73-7 and 73-8.[37]

Both methods exteriorize the bowel ends in close proximity, which is advantageous because subsequent closure can be performed without a formal laparotomy. Barium enema is necessary before enterostomy closure to rule out distal stricture formation. In the study cited earlier,[37] stricture of the distal bowel occurred more often after separate stomas were formed than after the Mikulicz enterostomy (36% versus 18%), a finding attributed to earlier reestablishment of intestinal continuity in the Mikulicz group. Although there was no statistical difference in complication rates after closure of the two different types of enterostomy, the Mikulicz closure (Fig. 73-9) is a simpler operation than closure of separate stomas.[37] In general, precise technique and meticulous enterostomy care are more important than the method of enterostomy chosen.

OTHER OPERATIONS FOR ACUTE NECROTIZING ENTEROCOLITIS

Resection and Primary Anastomosis

A few pediatric surgeons advocate resection and primary anastomosis for selected infants with NEC, including some with intestinal perforation and peritonitis.[38,39] Although controversial, this is not recommended because of an increased risk of anastomotic leak, a potentially fatal complication. A decision

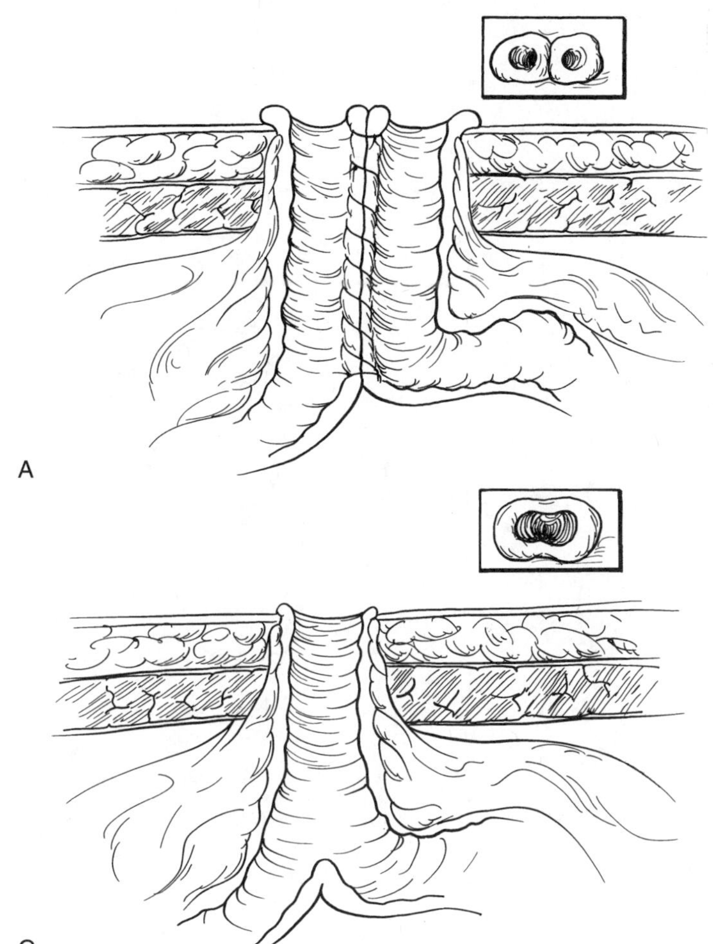

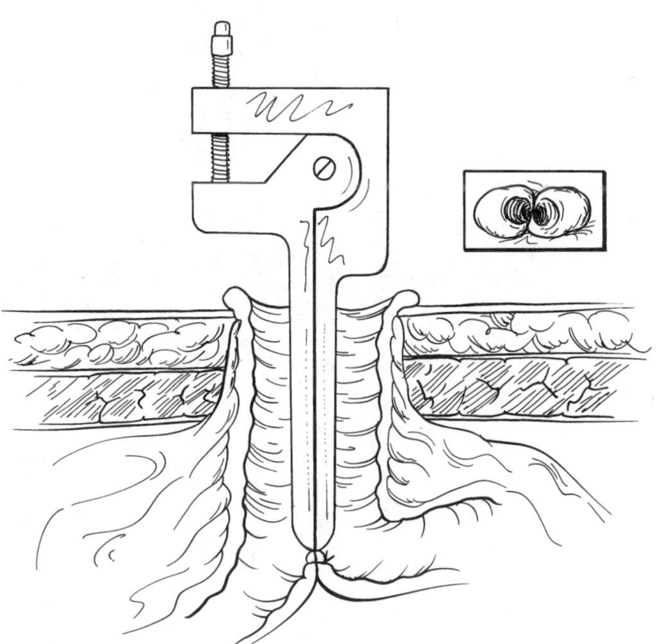

FIG. 73-7. Mikulicz enterostomy. (*A*) Double-barreled enterostomy, with limbs sutured together on antimesenteric border. (Stoma is allowed to mature spontaneously by this technique.) (*B*) Spur-crushing clamp is applied after stoma has matured. Alternatively, the septum may be divided by direct application of a stapling device. (*C*) Intestinal continuity is restored.

for primary anastomosis may also lead to an unnecessarily extensive resection, to ensure that the bowel ends are unequivocally viable. An analysis of 173 infants with advanced (surgical) NEC operated on at Children's Hospital of Philadelphia found no advantage for primary anastomosis in selected patients.[40] The authors observed that a decision for primary anastomosis may actually jeopardize the survival of an infant who should be expected to live. Although the subject is still debated, consensus favors resection and enterostomy as the safer and preferred procedure for acute NEC.[2,8,34]

Peritoneal Drainage

The technique of peritoneal drainage was introduced by Ein and associates[41] at the Hospital for Sick Children in Toronto for very premature and unstable infants who appeared too sick for transport and general anesthesia. The procedure is performed in the NICU under local anesthesia. A small incision is made in the right lower quadrant or above the umbilicus for evacuation of free gas, peritoneal exudate, pus, and feces, and a small drain inserted. Others have used peritoneal drainage as an adjunctive procedure for resuscitation before laparotomy,[42] or as primary therapy in very ill premature infants with bowel perforation,[39] some of whom, remarkably, survived. The author is not an advocate of peritoneal drainage as primary therapy because it violates the surgical principle of excision of necrotic intestine, which is a source of continuing sepsis. Even tiny premature infants can be optimally resuscitated for expeditious laparotomy. Peritoneal drainage may have an adjunctive role during resuscitation, for decompression of a tense abdomen which compromises ventilation.

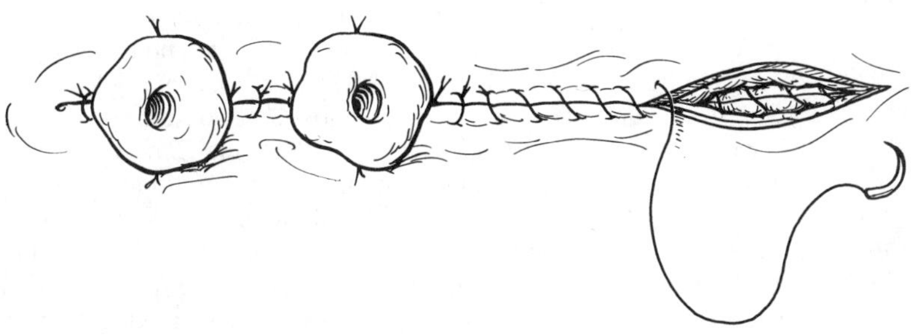

FIG. 73-8. Double enterostomy (Ricketts technique). Proximal and distal stomas are brought through the incision and secured with interrupted sutures, leaving a narrow bridge of fascia and skin between them. Stomas are matured as shown.

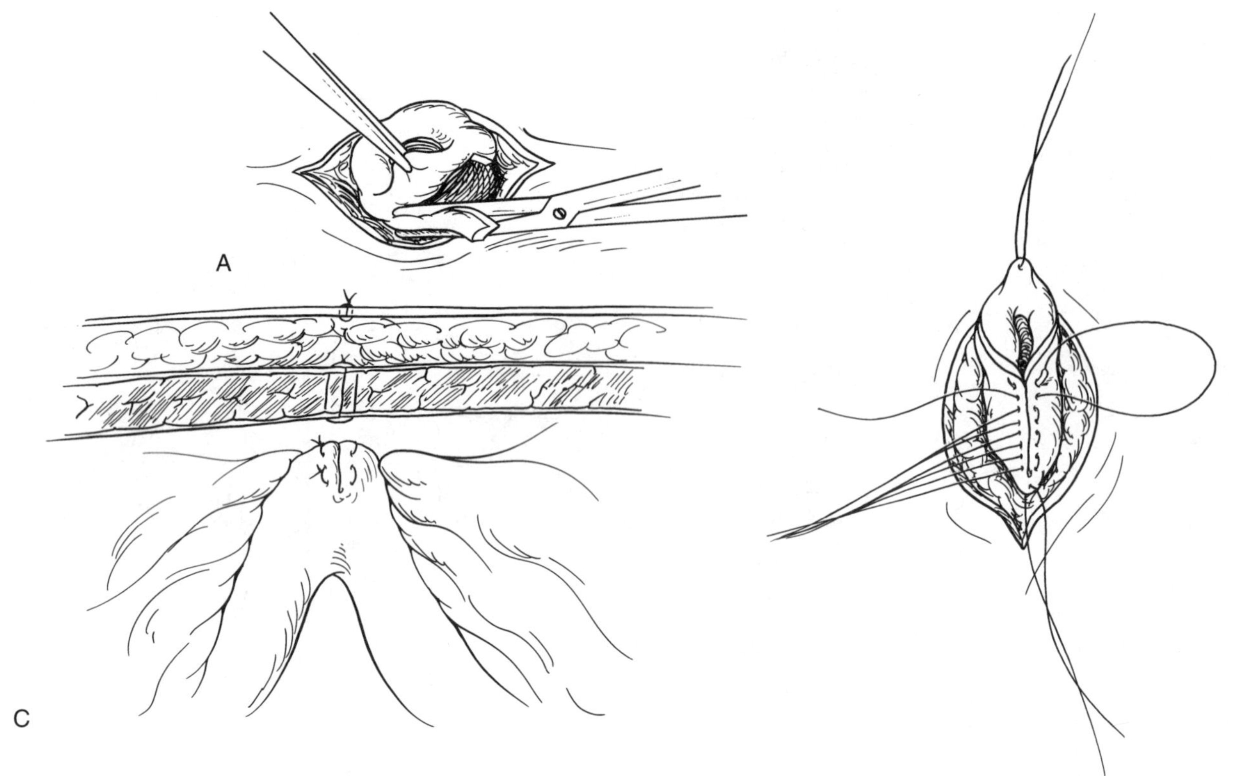

FIG. 73-9. Closure of Mikulicz enterostomy. (*A*) Stoma is mobilized and margins trimmed. (*B*) Single-layer closure. (*C*) Closure completed.

Proximal Jejunostomy and Second-Look Procedure

Massive ischemic injury of the small and large intestine (*pannecrosis* or *NEC totalis*) is found in 18% to 38% of operations for NEC.[34] In these cases, ischemic changes begin a few centimeters beyond the ligament of Treitz, with dusky or purplish areas of infarction or hemorrhagic necrosis, greenish-black spots of frank gangrene, and occasional transparent serosal windows. Surprisingly, skip areas of viable intestine may be interspersed between areas of damage. Rarely, even the stomach, duodenum, or rectum is necrotic. In these patients, the mortality rate approaches 100%, and operative resection has little to offer.

The best option for this worst-case scenario may be a proximal enterostomy, followed by a second-look operation 48 to 72 hours later. If sufficient viable bowel (about 30 cm) remains at second look, the demarcated gangrenous segments can be resected. This approach seems preferable to massive resection, which leaves debilitating short gut syndrome if the patient survives; or an open-and-close laparotomy, followed by inevitable death. Long-term total parenteral nutrition and intestinal transplantation are related subjects discussed elsewhere in this text. Salvage from extensive NEC might be further improved by earlier intervention based on the radiographic abnormalities of severe pneumatosis intestinalis or portal venous gas, which are highly correlated with extensive NEC.[30,34]

POSTOPERATIVE MANAGEMENT

The goals of postoperative management are as follows: (1) control of sepsis, (2) nutritional support, (3) prevention of enterostomy-induced electrolyte deficits, and (4) surveillance for stricture. After operation for acute NEC, the infant receives maximal supportive care in the NICU. Intravenous antibiotics for coverage of aerobic and anaerobic bacteria are continued for at least 7 to 10 days. Gastric suction is maintained until ileus has resolved and the enterostomy begins to function. Total parenteral nutrition is given, usually through a central vein. After sepsis and ileus have subsided, usually in the second week after operation, oral feedings may be cautiously resumed. There is no advantage to a mandatory 2- or 3-week period of withholding enteral feedings; this may predispose to mucosal atrophy and bacterial translocation. An elemental formula is preferred because most infants have malabsorption after NEC. Excessive sodium and bicarbonate losses from the enterostomy may be anticipated, often leading to depletion of total body sodium, metabolic acidosis, or failure to thrive. An abnormally low urinary sodium concentration is diagnostic of sodium depletion; serum sodium may remain deceptively normal. These electrolyte problems are preventable by oral administration of supplements of sodium chloride, sodium citrate, or sodium bicarbonate, or by early closure of the enterostomy. A review of 100 infants who underwent enterostomy and closure found no difference in complication rates between early (infant younger

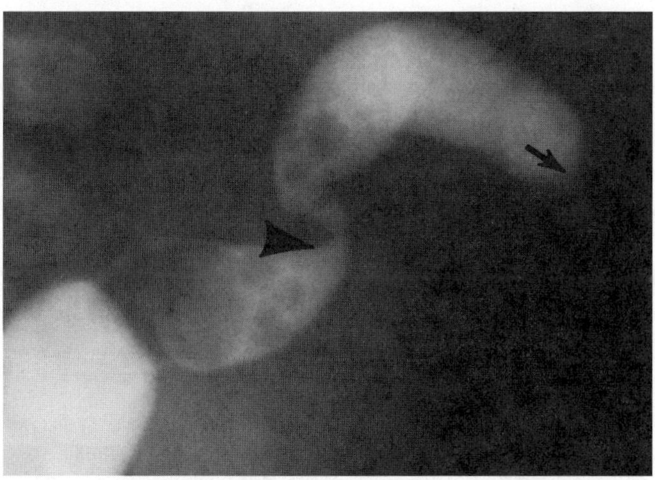

FIG. 73-10. This barium enema illustrates a stricture of the sigmoid colon (*arrow at left*) in an infant with a history of necrotizing enterocolitis. In addition, in this infant, the descending colon could not be filled because of a second stricture, which completely occluded the descending colon (*arrow at right*).

than 3 months or weighing less than 2.5 kg) versus late closure.[37] Thus, early closure of enterostomies is recommended as long as good pediatric anesthesia and special care facilities for premature infants are available.

RECURRENT AND POSTOPERATIVE NECROTIZING ENTEROCOLITIS

A report from the Institute for Child Health (Great Ormond Street, London) noted a recurrent episode of NEC in 16 of 196 neonates (6%) at a mean interval of 37 days from onset of the first episode.[43] Type and timing of enteral feedings had no effect on recurrence rate in this report. Most infants (11 of 16) were successfully managed medically.

Postoperative NEC may occur after surgical correction of congenital anomalies, most commonly gastroschisis[44,45] or meningomyelocele. The mortality rates were high in series from Kansas[45] and Arkansas[46]: 67% and 46%, respectively,

INTESTINAL STRICTURE

One or more strictures develop in 15% to 25% of survivors of acute NEC.[7] The pathogenesis is cicatricial healing of a seg-

ment of intestine injured by ischemia (see Fig. 73-3). The usual location is the colon, most commonly the sigmoid colon, allowing identification of the stricture by contrast enema. Infants recovering from acute NEC should be followed closely for early signs of intestinal obstruction. Surveillance by contrast enema 4 to 6 weeks after acute NEC may also be appropriate because infants with post-NEC stricture occasionally present with sudden onset of life-threatening sepsis or perforation.

Strictures located distal to an enterostomy are asymptomatic; usually, they are discovered on contrast enema before enterostomy closure (Fig. 73-10). Strictures composed of heavy scar tissue must be resected (Fig. 73-11), but smaller focal strictures may not require resection. Dilation of focal strictures under fluoroscopy using the balloon catheter technique has been successful.[47] This technique is recommended only for strictures located distal to an enterostomy that are asymptomatic. It should not be used for symptomatic strictures after medical treatment of NEC; these infants with clinical evidence of intestinal obstruction should be treated with urgent operation.

NECROTIZING ENTEROCOLITIS IN TERM INFANTS

Although NEC usually strikes premature infants, term infants account for about 10% of cases. Predisposing conditions associated with shock and reduced gut perfusion are usually identified, such as birth asphyxia, exchange transfusion, congenital heart disease, maternal cocaine use, and others. Onset of symptoms is earlier in term infants than in premature neonates.

Development of NEC among term infants with gastroschisis or myelomeningocele may be attributed to defective neurocirculatory reflexes or aberrant peristalsis.[44,45] A fulminant form of NEC associated with gut colonization by *Clostridium perfringens* is more common among term infants than premature neonates.[48,49]

OUTCOME

The operative survival rate in large series of NEC has improved during the past two decades. The series of Santulli and colleagues[1] (1955 to 1974) included the earliest, far-advanced cases; only 22% of the infants survived. In the Indiana study by Grosfeld and associates,[34] an improved operative survival rate (from 51% in 1972 through 1982, to 75% in 1983 through 1990) was attributed to early operation and resection of necrotic

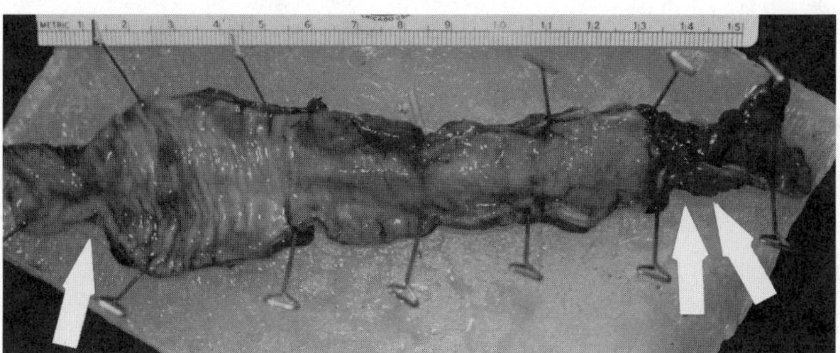

FIG. 73-11. Surgical specimen from same patient as in Figure 73-10, showing strictures of sigmoid colon (*single arrow*) and descending colon (*double arrow*).

bowel as well as technologic advances in neonatal care, such as surfactant therapy and jet ventilators. Ricketts and Jerles'[36] series from Atlanta (1980 to 1987) correlated hospital survival with birthweight: survival was 54% for the group weighing 1000 g or less and 74% for infants weighing 1001 to 1500 g. The highest operative survival rate, 85%, was reported in 1988 from Scotland by Freeman and associates.[50]

Although recovery of normal gastrointestinal function may be anticipated after NEC, serious neurologic problems often remain. A follow-up study from Stanford University tested a group of 40 survivors of NEC at 1 to 3 years of age.[51] Half of these patients were completely normal children; 35% had mild sequelae, such as an abnormal electroencephalogram; and 15% had moderate to severe neurologic impairment, usually spasticity. These neurologic sequelae occurred at the same rate in a matched group of premature infants without NEC and thus were attributed to prematurity and perinatal stress rather than to the specific impact of NEC. Others have confirmed a generally encouraging follow-up for infants surviving NEC, although the surgical survivors have an increased risk of late sepsis from gram-negative bacilli[52] and an increased risk of growth retardation and neurodevelopmental impairment.[53]

PREVENTION

Prevention of NEC awaits a better understanding of its pathogenesis. Because animal models do not duplicate the human syndrome, the greatest hope for prevention may lie with clinical trials of promising interventions. These interventions might accomplish the following: (1) prevent ischemia, (2) diminish colonization with pathogenic bacteria, (3) limit formula-induced bowel injury, (4) enhance immunologic defense mechanisms, and (5) hasten maturity of the mucosal barrier. In the design of a clinical trial, a concurrent control or placebo group is mandatory for documentation of efficacy; historical controls are flawed because NEC occurs both sporadically and in epidemics. Measures tried thus far include oral administration of an immunoglobulin,[54] successful but yet to be repeated; and administration of corticosteroids to mature the mucosal barrier, successful despite potential complications.[55] Prevention of the primary risk factor, prematurity, would require substantial societal and behavioral changes (eg, universal prenatal care, cessation of maternal cigarette smoking and drug abuse). Control of NEC would be better achieved by such public health measures rather than by scientific or technologic advances.

REFERENCES

1. Santulli TV, Schullinger JN, Heird WC, et al. Acute necrotizing enterocolitis in infancy: a review of 64 cases. Pediatrics 1975;55:376.
2. Kosloske AM. Necrotizing enterocolitis in the neonate: collective review. Surg Gynecol Obstet 1979;148:259.
3. Kliegman RM, Fanaroff AA. Necrotizing enterocolitis. N Engl J Med 1984;310:1093.
4. Holman RC, Stehr-Green JK, Zelasky MT. Necrotizing enterocolitis mortality in the United States. Am J Publ Health 1989;79:987.
5. Shimura K. Necrotizing enterocolitis? A Japanese survey. NICU 1990;3:5.
6. Kosloske AM. A unifying hypothesis for pathogenesis and prevention of necrotizing enterocolitis. J Pediatr 1990;117:S68.
7. Ballance WA, Dahms BB, Shenker N, et al. Pathology of neonatal necrotizing enterocolitis. J Pediatr 1990;117:S6.
8. Amoury RA. Necrotizing enterocolitis. In: Ashcraft KW, Holder TM, eds. Pediatric Surgery, ed 2. Philadelphia, WB Saunders, 1993:341.
9. Stoll BJ, Kanto WP, Glass RI, et al. Epidemiology of necrotizing enterocolitis: a case control study. J Pediatr 1980;96:447.
10. Lloyd JR. The etiology of gastrointestinal perforations in the newborn. J Pediatr Surg 1969;4:77.
11. Tyson JE, deSa DJ, Moore S. Thromboatheromatous complications of umbilical arterial catheterization in the newborn period. Arch Dis Child 1976;51:744.
12. Parks DA, Bulkley GB, Granger DN, et al. Ischemic injury in the cat small intestine: role of superoxide radicals. Gastroenterology 1982;82:9.
13. Vohra K, Rosenfeld W, Singh I, et al. Ischemic injury to newborn rabbit ileum: protective role of human superoxide dismutase. J Pediatr Surg 1989;24:893.
14. Megison SM, Horton JW, Chao H, et al. Prolonged survival and decreased mucosal injury after low-dose enteral allopurinol prophylaxis in mesenteric ischemia. J Pediatr Surg 1990;25:917.
15. Oldham KT, Guice KS, Gore D, et al. Treatment of intestinal ischemia with oxygenated intraluminal perfluorocarbons. Am J Surg 1987;153:271.
16. Lawrence G, Bates J, Gaul A. Pathogenesis of neonatal necrotizing enterocolitis. Lancet 1982;1:137.
17. Udall JN Jr. Gastrointestinal host defense and necrotizing enterocolitis: an update. J Pediatr 1990;117:S33.
18. Kosloske AM, Ulrich JA. A bacteriologic basis for the clinical presentations of necrotizing enterocolitis. J Pediatr Surg 1980;15:558.
19. Blakey JL, Lubitz L, Campbell NT, et al. Enteric colonization in sporadic neonatal necrotizing enterocolitis. J Pediatr Gastroenterol Nutr 1985;4:591.
20. Lucas A, Cole TJ. Breast milk and neonatal necrotizing enterocolitis. Lancet 1990;336:1519.
21. Scheifele DW, Olsen E, Fussell S, et al. Spontaneous endotoxinemia in premature infants: correlations with oral feeding and bowel dysfunction. Pediatr Gastroenterol Nutr 1985;4:67.
22. Sun X, Hsueh W. Bowel necrosis induced by tumor necrosis factor in rats is mediated by platelet-activating factor. J Clin Invest 1988;81:1328.
23. Caplan MS, Hsueh W. Necrotizing enterocolitis: role of platelet activating factor, endotoxin, and tumor necrosis factor. J Pediatr 1990;117:S47.
24. Harris MC, Costarino AT, Sullivan JS, et al. Cytokine elevations in critically ill infants with sepsis and necrotizing enterocolitis. J Pediatr 1994;124:105.
25. Lawrence GW, Bates J. Pathogenesis of neonatal necrotizing enterocolitis. Lancet 1983;1:540.
26. Barlow B, Santulli TV, Heird WC, et al. An experimental study of acute necrotizing enterocolitis: the importance of breast milk. J Pediatr Surg 1974;9:587.
27. Musemeche CA, Kosloske AM, Bartow SA, et al. Comparative effects of ischemia, bacteria, and substrate on the pathogenesis of intestinal necrosis. J Pediatr Surg 1986;21:536.
28. Kosloske AM. Epidemiology of necrotizing enterocolitis. Acta Paediatr 1994;(Suppl 396):2.
29. Kosloske AM. Prevention of necrotizing enterocolitis. Semin Pediatr Inf Dis (submitted).
30. Kosloske AM, Musemeche CA, Ball WS Jr, et al. Necrotizing enterocolitis: value of radiographic findings to predict outcome. AJR 1988;151:771.
31. Bell MJ, Ternberg JL, Feigin RD, et al. Neonatal necrotizing enterocolitis: therapeutic decisions based upon clinical staging. Ann Surg 1978;187:1.
32. Kosloske AM, Papile LA, Burstein J. Indications for operation in acute necrotizing enterocolitis of the neonate. Surgery 1980;87:502.
33. Kosloske AM. Indications for operation in necrotizing enterocolitis revisited. J Pediatr Surg 1994;29:663.
34. Grosfeld JL, Cheu H, Schlatter M, et al. Changing trends in necrotizing enterocolitis: experience with 302 cases in two decades. Ann Surg 1991;214:300.
35. Barry AL, Smith PB, Turck M. Laboratory diagnosis of urinary tract infections. Cumitech 2, American Society of Microbiology, Washington D.C., April 1975.

36. Ricketts RR, Jerles ML. Neonatal necrotizing enterocolitis: experience with 100 consecutive surgical patients. World J Surg 1990;14:600.

37. Musemeche CA, Kosloske AM, Ricketts RR. Enterostomy in necrotizing enterocolitis: an analysis of techniques and timing of closure. J Pediatr Surg 1987;22:479.

38. Stringer MD, Spitz L. Surgical management of neonatal necrotizing enterocolitis. Arch Dis Child 1993;69:269.

39. Robertson JRF, Axmy AF, Young DG. Surgery for necrotizing enterocolitis. Br J Surg 1987;74:387.

40. Cooper A, Ross AJ III, O'Neill JA Jr, et al. Resection with primary anastomosis for necrotizing enterocolitis: a contrasting view. J Pediatr Surg 1988;23:557.

41. Ein SH, Marshall DG, Girvan D. Peritoneal drainage under local anesthesia for perforations from necrotizing enterocolitis. J Pediatr Surg 1977;12:963.

42. Cheu HW, Sukarochana K, Lloyd DA. Peritoneal drainage for necrotizing enterocolitis. J Pediatr Surg 1988;23:557.

43. Stringer MD, Brereton RJ, Drake DP, et al. Recurrent necrotizing enterocolitis. J Pediatr Surg 1993;28:979.

44. Oldham KT, Coran AG, Drongowski RA, Baker PJ, Wesley JR, Polley TZ Jr. The development of necrotizing enterocolitis following repair of gastroschisis: A surprisingly high incidence. J Pediatr Surg 1988;23:945.

45. Amoury RA, Goodwin CD, McGill CW, Smith TH, Ashcraft KW, Holder TM. Necrotizing enterocolitis following operation in the neonatal period. J Pediatr Surg 1980;15:1.

46. Mollitt DL, Golladay ES. Postoperative neonatal necrotizing enterocolitis. J Pediatr Surg 1982;17:757.

47. Ball WS Jr, Kosloske AM, Jewell PF, Seigel RS. Balloon catheter dilation of focal intestinal strictures following necrotizing enterocolitis. J Pediatr Surg 1985;20:637.

48. Kosloske AM, Ulrich JA, Hoffman H. Fulminant necrotising enterocolitis associated with Clostridia. Lancet 1978;2:1014.

49. Kosloske AM, Ball WS Jr, Umland E, Skipper B. Clostridial necrotizing enterocolitis. J Pediatr Surg 1985;20:155.

50. Freeman RB, Lloyd DJ, Miller SS, Duffty P. Surgical treatment of necrotizing enterocolitis: A population-based study in the Grampian region, Scotland. J Pediatr Surg 1988;23:942.

51. Stevenson DK, Kerner JA, Malachowski N, Sunshine P. Late morbidity among survivors of necrotizing enterocolitis. Pediatrics 1980;66:925.

52. Walsh MC, Simpser EF, Kliegman RM. Late onset of sepsis in infants with bowel resection in the neonatal period. J Pediatr 1988;112:468.

53. Walsh MC, Kliegman RM. Severity of necrotizing enterocolitis: Influence on outcome at 2 years of age. Pediatrics 1989;84:808.

54. Eibl MM, Wolf HM, Furnkranz H, Rosenkranz A. Prevention of necrotizing enterocolitis in low-birth-weight infants by IgA-IgG feeding. N Engl J Med 1988;319:1.

55. Halac E, Halac J, Begue EF, et al. Prenatal and postnatal corticosteroid therapy to prevent neonatal necrotizing enterocolitis: A controlled trial. J Pediatr 1990;117:132.

56. Czyrko C, Del Pin C, O'Neill JA Jr, et al. Maternal cocaine abuse and necrotizing enterocolitis: outcome and survival. J Pediatr Surg 1991;26:414.

57. Malcolm G, Ellwood D, Devonald K, et al. Absent or reversed end diastolic flow velocity in the umbilical artery and necrotizing enterocolitis. Arch Dis Child 1991;66:805.

58. Kosloske AM, Ulrich JA, Hoffman H. Fulminant necrotising enterocolitis associated with Clostridia. Lancet 1978;2:1014.

59. Kosloske AM, Ball WS Jr, Umland E, et al. Clostridial necrotizing enterocolitis. J Pediatr Surg 1985;20:155.

60. Hoy C, Millar MR, MacKay P, et al. Quantitative changes in faecal microflora preceding necrotizing enterocolitis in premature neonates. Arch Dis Child 1990;65:1057.

61. Scheifele DW, Bjornson GL, Dyer RA, et al. Delta-like toxin produced by coagulase-negative staphyloccocci is associated with neonatal necrotizing enterocolitis. Infect Immunol 1987;55:2268.

62. Book LS, Herbst JJ, Atherton SO, et al. Necrotizing enterocolitis in low-birth-weight infants fed an elemental formula. J Pediatr 1975;87:602.

63. LaGamma EF, Ostertag SG, Birenbaum H. Failure of delayed oral feedings to prevent necrotizing enterocolitis: results of study in very low birth weight neonates. Am J Dis Child 1985;139:385.

64. McKeown RE, Marsh TD, Amarnath U, et al. Role of delayed feeding and of feeding increments in necrotizing enterocolitis. J Pediatr 1992;121:764.

65. Eibl MM, Wolf HM, Furnkranz H, et al. Prevention of necrotizing enterocolitis in low-birth-weight infants by IgA-IgG feeding. N Engl J Med 1988;319:1.

66. Fast C, Rosegger H. Necrotizing enterocolitis prophylaxis: oral antibiotics and lyophilized enterobacteria vs oral immunoglobulins. Acta Paediatr 1994;83(Suppl 396):86.

67. Halac E, Halac J, Begue EF, et al. Prenatal and postnatal corticosteroid therapy to prevent neonatal necrotizing enterocolitis: a controlled trial. J Pediatr 1990;117:132.

Surgery of Infants and Children: Scientific Principles and Practice, edited by
Keith T. Oldham, Paul M. Colombani, and Robert P. Foglia.
Lippincott–Raven Publishers, Philadelphia, © 1997.

CHAPTER 74

Appendix and Meckel Diverticulum

Robert S. Sawin

APPENDIX

ANATOMY

Embryology

The appendix develops from the cecum, which first appears
during the fifth gestational week as a ventral enlargement of
the midgut. The appendix is first visible at 8 weeks' gestation,
apparently the result of disproportionately slow growth of the
terminal cecum compared with the rest of the hindgut. Although
the appendix continues to grow, its diameter is only 20% to
25% of the diameter of the cecum at birth. Absence of this
expected asymmetric growth may explain the few documented
patients with congenital absence of the appendix. The asymmetric growth of the appendix and cecum also causes the appendix
to shift from the apex of the cecum to a more medial position
near the ileocecal valve. The variability of this shift results in
multiple possible positions of the appendix (Fig. 74-1).

Gross Anatomy

In addition to the variable location of the tip of the appendix,
its relation to surrounding structures is quite variable. For instance, the appendix may lie across the psoas muscle or over
the pelvic brim, resting on the pelvic fascia, which overlies
the obturator internus muscle. These positions account for the
physical findings of pain on extension of the hip (psoas sign)
or pain with flexion and internal rotation of the thigh (obturator
sign). Additional variations in appendiceal position result from
the abnormalities of midgut rotation; because the attachment
of the appendix to the base of the cecum is a constant, anomalies
such as malrotation can lead to a left-sided appendix. The size
and shape of the appendix also vary. It may be funnel shaped
or cylindrical with a uniform caliber. The length can range from
0.3 to 33 cm. The appendices of males tend to be slightly longer
than those of females.

The arterial supply to the appendix is derived from the ileocolic artery, a branch of the superior mesenteric artery. One of
four terminal branches of the ileocolic artery, the appendiceal

artery passes posterior to the terminal ileum and gives off multiple short, straight branches to the appendix. The retroileal
course of the appendiceal artery may predispose it to kinking,
with resultant ischemia and inflammation of the appendix. The
venous drainage of the appendix is through the superior mesenteric vein to the portal vein, which accounts for the occasional
findings of pylephlebitis or liver abscess after appendicitis.

Like the rest of the midgut, the appendix is innervated by
branches of the splanchnic nerves, which arise from the lower
thoracic ganglia. Typically, the T-10 ganglia is the one through
which painful stimuli from the appendix are conducted to the
dorsal nerve root, along the spinothalamic tract to the brain.
The umbilical region of the abdominal wall develops from the
same embryonic region, or dermatome, as the appendix; this
explains in part why appendiceal pain initially localizes to the
periumbilical region. This innervation is common to the kidney,
upper ureter, and testicle, accounting for some of the organs that
must be considered in the differential diagnosis of periumbilical
pain.

Histology

Like the rest of the intestinal tract, the appendix has four
layers. In both the mucosa and submucosa, germinal follicles
and lymphoid pulp are prominent in infants and children. The
muscularis and serosal layers are not different than in adults.
The lymphoid tissue gradually atrophies with age. It is speculated that this lymphoid tissue predisposes children to appendicitis by luminal obstruction during periods of inflammation.

APPENDICITIS

Epidemiology

The risk of developing appendicitis is estimated to be 6% to
20% for a person in the United States. Residents of Third World
countries have a substantially lower risk of developing appendicitis than those in developed nations. Hypothesized risk factors
for appendicitis include a diet high in sugar and low in fiber
content, and good hygiene with a resultant decreased exposure

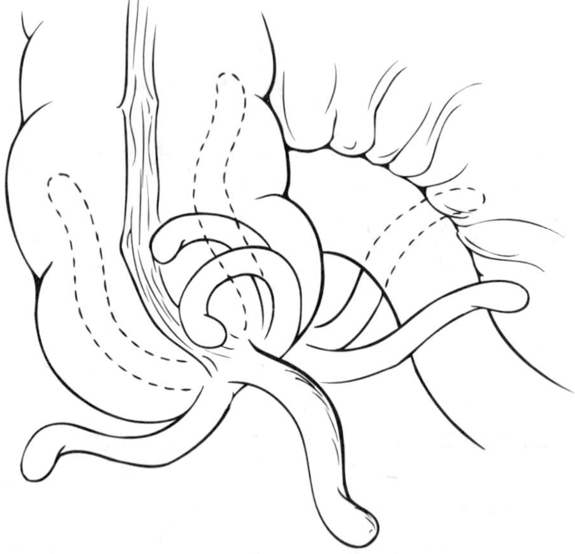

FIG. 74-1. Possible positions of the appendix.

to enteric pathogens at an early age. The epidemiologic literature, however, contains contradictory data. The risk of developing appendicitis is lowest in infancy, perhaps because of the relatively wide base of the appendix at that stage of development. About 1% of all children younger than 15 years of age develop appendicitis, with a peak incidence between 10 and 12 years of age.

The risk of developing appendicitis that progresses to perforation is higher in children than in adults. In most published series of appendicitis from children's hospitals, the incidence of perforation is 20% to 50%. This may be a consequence of the difficulty in making the diagnosis of acute appendicitis in the toddler or preschool-age child who cannot communicate as effectively as the older child. An additional factor is the unfortunate tendency of parents and physicians to attribute all childhood fevers and gastrointestinal symptoms to influenza or other viral illnesses. Some evidence also suggests that easy access to health care providers may reduce the risk of perforation; managed-care patients with private insurance have lower perforation rates than Medicaid and uninsured patients.[1]

Pathophysiology

The pathologic sequence ending in appendicitis is thought to be analogous to that seen with cholecystitis. Although the causes of appendicitis and cholecystitis may be multiple, they often have in common obstruction of the proximal lumen. Wangensteen[2] established the pathophysiologic role of obstruction in appendicitis in an experiment in which the symptoms of appendicitis were replicated by ligating the base of an exteriorized appendix. Fecaliths are the most frequent example of obstructing appendiceal lesions and are present in about 30% to 50% of appendicitis patients. Other obstructing lesions include lymphoid hyperplasia, foreign bodies (Fig. 74-2), parasitic infections, or conditions that cause increased colonic pressure and decreased motility, such as Hirschsprung disease or meconium ileus. Despite the obstruction, the mucosa continues to secrete

mucous, resulting in intraluminal pressure increases that lead to venous congestion and edema. The intramural pressure increases until ischemia and tissue acidosis of the appendiceal wall result. Finally, mucosal ulceration is followed by bacterial invasion, leading to invasive infection of the appendix.

Although this orderly pathologic sequence is consistent with the progressive history and symptoms of appendicitis, the role of obstruction in the pathogenesis of appendicitis is somewhat equivocal. The presence of a fecalith in 30% of incidentally examined appendices at laparotomy suggests that obstruction does not necessarily result in appendicitis. Likewise, the absence of fecaliths in 50% to 70% of appendicitis patients supports the etiologic role of factors other than obstruction.

Microbiology

The possible role of viral infections in appendicitis has been implicated by the frequent prodrome of symptoms with which children with appendicitis initially present. In addition, appendicitis has been described after infection with *Varicella* sp. Cultures of mesenteric lymph nodes and resected appendices may grow adenovirus in children with appendicitis. The viral illness may result in lymphoid hyperplasia or lymphadenopathy, which can obstruct the lumen. Additionally, the viral illness may result in dehydration, leading to a higher likelihood of inspissated stool or mucus, which causes fecalith formation and obstruction. It is also possible that the viral infection is merely coincidental and does not contribute to the development of appendicitis.

Enteric bacteria are the most common organisms associated with appendicitis. In patients with perforation, *Escherichia coli*, *Enterococcus* sp, *Bacteroides* sp, and *Pseudomonas* sp are most frequently isolated. Whether these are the main pathogens in nonperforated appendicitis is not known. Parasitic infections with *Enterobius* or *Ascaris* have also been reported in association with appendicitis. These organisms may cause a local inflammation or may contribute to luminal obstruction, leading to bacterial invasion and suppurative appendicitis.

Pathology

In the early stages of acute appendicitis, the appendix appears thickened and feels turgid, with increased serosal vascularity. The distal portion of the organ is often distended, especially when an obstructing lesion such as a fecalith is present. Histologically, the mucosa is ulcerated and infiltrated with inflammatory cells in early appendicitis. As the bacterial invasion progresses, the inflammatory infiltrate progresses from the mucosa through the muscularis. Cloudy peritoneal fluid filled with polymorphonuclear cells but lacking bacteria may be seen as the inflammation progresses. Necrosis of all the layers or gangrenous appendicitis may occur with or without perforation. If perforation has occurred, cloudy, foul-smelling peritoneal fluid is found. Usually, polymicrobial flora can be cultured from this fluid. Microscopically, dense sheets of polymorphonuclear leukocytes and erythrocytes are seen in the lumen, the muscularis, and the mesoappendix. The site of perforation can be difficult for the pathologist to identify, especially if the appendix has been surrounded by the omentum.

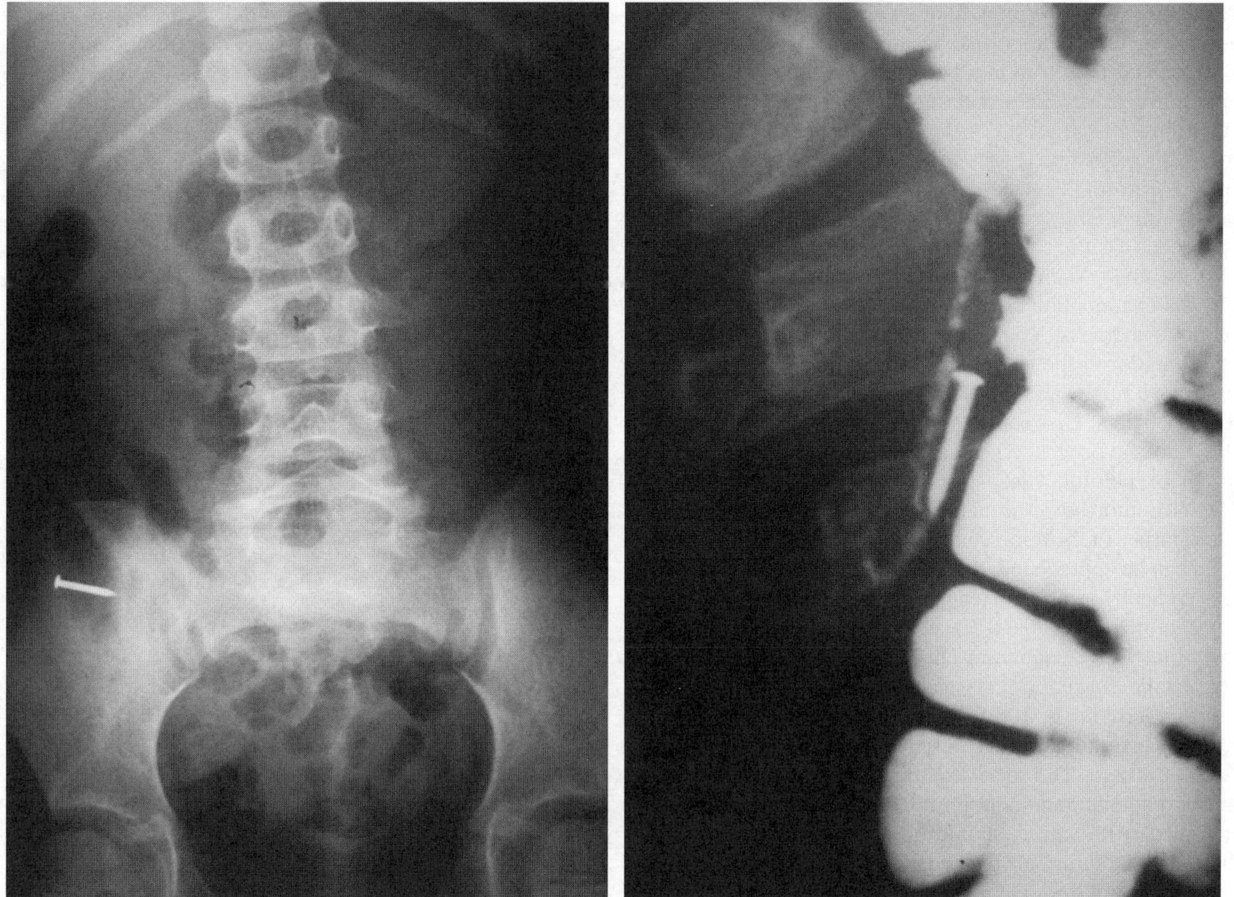

FIG. 74-2. Foreign body in the appendix. This patient had chronic abdominal pain. The barium enema revealed the foreign body in the appendix. Once the appendix was removed, the abdominal pain completely resolved.

Clinical Features

Acute Appendicitis

The child with appendicitis may present with many different symptoms, making appendicitis the most commonly misdiagnosed surgical lesion in the United States. The most frequent symptoms are listed in Table 74-1. The constellation of right lower quadrant abdominal pain, fever, anorexia, and nausea is classically present in children with appendicitis. Unfortunately, fewer than half of children with acute appendicitis present with this complete spectrum of symptoms. The orderly sequence of pathophysiologic events described earlier usually causes a characteristic progression of symptoms. This sequence typically begins with vague abdominal pain, apparently originating in the periumbilical region. This vague localization of pain is termed *referred pain.* The entire midgut shares the same T-10 dermatome with the umbilicus, so that afferent pain stimuli are interpreted erroneously by the brain as originating in the umbilicus. Thus, many painful lesions in the intestinal tract cause a similar periumbilical pain. As the appendix becomes inflamed and the serosa becomes involved, it begins to cause local inflammation of the adjacent peritoneum. With this peritoneal irritation, the pain is usually more localized to the right lower quadrant. As inflammation and distention of the appendix progress, the pain worsens. If the appendix is not removed at this time, the swelling and ischemia progress, culminating in perforation. Thus, physical examination is especially important.

Examining the child with abdominal pain requires a calm, nonthreatening demeanor and careful observation. The child's appearance can be revealing; the appendicitis patient lies quietly, often with the knees drawn up, and resists movement in any way. Shaking the bed or stretcher and having the patient cough may elicit wincing or complaint. Asking the child to get off the bed and walk can be informative. The child with early appendicitis may move reasonably comfortably but complains of pain when asked to walk on the heels or jump to touch the examiner's hand held high.

TABLE 74-1. *Symptoms of appendicitis*

Symptom	Frequency (%)
Anorexia	95
Nausea and vomiting	85
Fever	60–80
Right lower quadrant pain	70
Diarrhea	10–30

Examination should begin with other areas of the body. Auscultation of the lungs is important because pneumonia can present as abdominal pain. Asking the patient to cough may elicit abdominal discomfort. Pain with internal rotation of the thigh (obturator sign) or extension of the hip with the child in a left lateral decubitus position (psoas sign) indicates peritoneal irritation, often the result of retrocecal appendicitis. Before examining the abdomen, the examiner's hands should be warmed. Many surgeons ask the child to point with one finger to the spot that hurts the most. With the knees bent to relax the abdominal muscles, the examination should begin far away from the area of maximal tenderness. Younger children may be more willing to allow palpation if the examiner places the patient's hand or the stethoscope on the abdomen and palpates through these less threatening objects. Distracting the child with questions about family, school, favorite activities, and so forth during the examination can be helpful. Close inspection of the child's facial expressions is more discriminating than asking whether each maneuver hurts. If relaxation can be accomplished, rectus muscle spasm can be appreciated. Sudden withdrawal of the palpating hand to check for rebound tenderness is startling for children and therefore not as reliable a physical sign as in adults. Palpation of the left lower quadrant eliciting right lower quadrant pain, termed the *Rovsing sign,* is a fairly specific sign for appendicitis with referred pain. If diffuse tenderness and guarding are present, free perforation is likely, especially in children younger than 6 years of age. The rectal examination is considered unpleasant by patients and some physicians and is consequently often avoided. Although it should be deferred until last, it is nonetheless an integral part of the examination, particularly in patients who do not have clear anterior abdominal wall tenderness, such as those with retrocecal appendicitis. The child should be gently advised that the rectal examination feels strange but may not hurt. The left lateral decubitus position with the knees drawn to the chest works well. Once the discomfort of the examining finger is tolerated by the patient, the examination should begin away from the right pelvis, leaving it for last. Induration or focal tenderness in the right or midline pelvis are suggestive of appendicitis. If perforation has already occurred, a mass may be palpable on rectal examination, allowing the option of transrectal drainage. A complete 360-degree digital examination should be performed. Patients with appendicitis often have greater tenderness anteriorly than posteriorly. If the examiner's finger elicits as much tenderness posteriorly in the sacrococcygeal region as anteriorly, this may simply indicate the patient's discomfort with the examiner's finger and not peritoneal irritation.

Perforated Appendicitis

Appendicitis with perforation is more common in children than in adults. The large diameter relative to the cecum and the thin wall of the appendix in children may predispose children to more rapid progression of the disease. A more likely explanation of the higher perforation rates is the delay in presentation and the delay in diagnosis. Parents often assume that gastrointestinal symptoms are related to influenza or to digestion and thus are slow to call the physician. Physicians frequently compound the problem with similar rationalization. Indeed, several studies have indicated that most delays in diagnosing appendicitis can be attributed to the health care provider.[3]

This paradigm of the pathophysiologic sequence of appendicitis is a convenient way to assist in the diagnosis. It is reliable only if an accurate history is obtained and if the patient is examined sequentially. Because the goal is to diagnose acute appendicitis before perforation, the key period is the first 24 hours since the risk of perforation within 24 hours of the onset of symptoms is less than 30%. Conversely, if symptoms have been present for more than 48 hours, the probability of perforation exceeds 70%. This time frame is less useful in children younger than 5 years of age because their disease tends to be more virulent, and an accurate history is more difficult to obtain.

The symptoms of perforated appendicitis include severe generalized abdominal pain, temperature often higher than 38°C, worsening anorexia with nausea and vomiting, dehydration, and diarrhea (which can be misleading by suggesting the diagnosis of gastroenteritis). The child may progress through these symptoms and localize the perforation by "walling off" the infection between the surrounding viscera and the omentum. This is particularly true of retrocecal and retroileal appendices. Younger children, with their sparse omentum, are less capable of this localization and are more likely to have generalized peritonitis. The other physical findings with perforated appendicitis are usually similar to those found in nonperforated appendicitis. The absence of bowel sounds or the presence of high-pitched, tinkling bowel sounds may suggest a small bowel obstruction, particularly in children with retroileal appendicitis and in those younger than 6 years of age (Fig. 74-3).

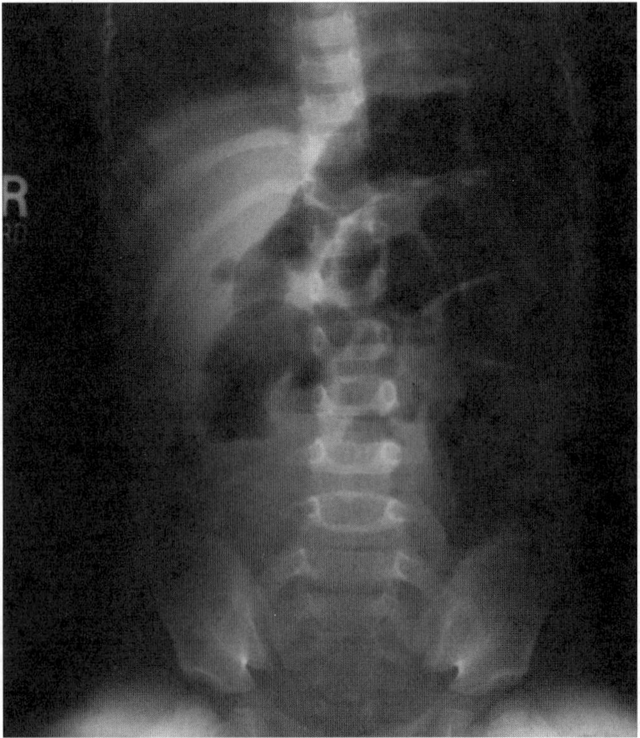

FIG. 74-3. Small bowel obstruction. This 4-year-old child developed a small bowel obstruction from perforated appendicitis. Note the air–fluid levels and appendicolithiasis.

Appendiceal Mass

Appendicitis with a palpable mass is usually a consequence of perforation. The mass may be an abscess or a phlegmon, lacking frank pus and composed of omentum and matted loops of bowel. The treatment of patients who have abdominal masses in addition to appendicitis is controversial. Emergency surgery is seldom indicated because most patients benefit from fluid resuscitation and initiation of broad-spectrum intravenous antibiotics. The standard approach includes limited laparotomy with drainage of the abscess, if present, and appendectomy. Opponents of this approach argue that the acute inflammation of the cecum and surrounding bowel can result in long, difficult operations with more blood loss, increased risk of bowel injury, and inability to perform a complete appendectomy safely.

Alternative approaches depend on whether the mass is an abscess or phlegmon, a distinction that may be resolved with ultrasound or computed tomography (CT). Figure 74-4 shows an algorithm for the delayed laparotomy approach recommended by some pediatric surgeons. If the mass is determined to be a phlegmon, intravenous antibiotics and volume resuscitation without immediate laparotomy are safe and effective treatment, provided the patient shows clinical improvement with lower temperature spikes, decreasing leukocytosis, and decreasing abdominal tenderness. The elective interval appendectomy can be performed 4 to 8 weeks later. If clinical improvement does not occur after 12 to 24 hours of this nonoperative management, laparotomy is indicated. If an abscess is identified, drainage by percutaneous, transvaginal, or transrectal routes is an effective treatment after resuscitation and intravenous antibiotics. Again, as long as clinical improvement occurs, antibiotic therapy is continued until the patient is afebrile, the white blood cell (WBC) count is normal, and the abdominal tenderness is resolved. This postdrainage therapy can be completed on an outpatient basis, reducing the length of hospital stay. Interval appendectomy 4 to 6 weeks later is usually remarkably uncomplicated, with limited inflammatory adhesions and a postoperative hospital stay of 1 day. Whether this delayed operative therapy is superior to immediate appendectomy remains to be proved. It is unlikely that the clinical results will be substantially different, but a comparison of the costs of the two approaches is warranted in the contemporary health care enviroment.

Recurrent Appendicitis

Whether recurrent or chronic appendicitis exists is debated. If the paradigm of progressive pathophysiologic changes discussed earlier in this chapter is accepted, it is difficult to reconcile the possibility of appendicitis resolving without some therapeutic intervention. Nonetheless, about one quarter of patients with surgically proven acute appendicitis report a history of prior episodes of abdominal pain that are similar to the ones that prompted the appendectomy. Histopathology of resected appendices may show both chronic and acute inflammatory infiltrates as well as fibrosis, implicating prior episodes of acute appendicitis. In addition, up to 60% of patients who are successfully treated in a nonoperative fashion for perforated appendici-

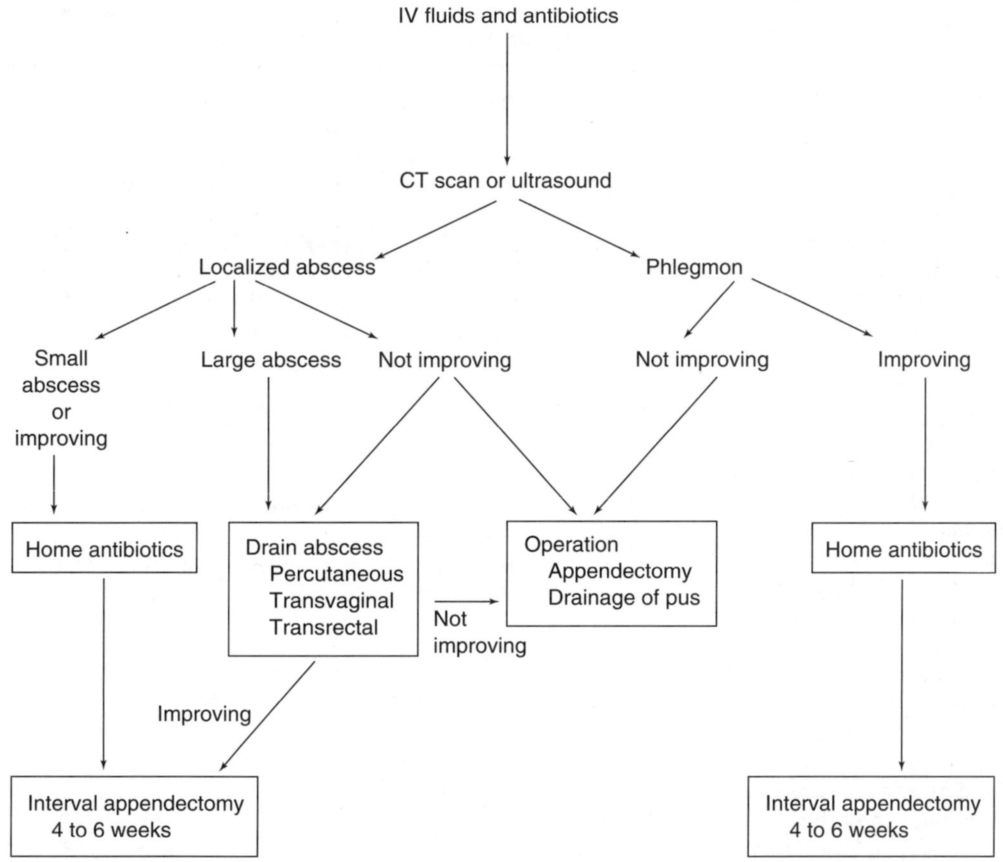

FIG. 74-4. Algorithm for nonoperative management of perforated appendicitis in children with a prolonged history, palpable mass, and no signs of systemic sepsis.

tis have abdominal symptoms suggestive of recurrent appendicitis before the interval appendectomy. The histopathology of the interval appendectomy specimens may show acute inflammation as well as the expected chronic inflammation in these patients.

A more uncommon entity is chronic appendicitis. Children with chronic abdominal pain are difficult to evaluate because many have no apparent physiologic cause for their pain. A small number of these children undergo extensive diagnostic testing, including abdominal ultrasound and gastrointestinal contrast studies. Some of these patients have thickening of the appendix seen on ultrasound or no filling of the appendix seen on barium enema. These findings in the setting of chronic abdominal pain warrant an appendectomy and frequently result in resolution of the symptoms. The diagnosis of chronic appendicitis is inferred, regardless of the absence of histopathologic confirmation. This absence of histologic verification prompts many physicians to attribute the symptomatic improvement to a placebo effect. Like postcholecystectomy syndrome and irritable bowel syndrome, chronic appendicitis can be difficult to define and diagnose, but there are patients whose disease appears to fit the diagnosis.

Special Considerations

Infants

Appendicitis in neonates is uncommon and has a higher mortality rate than in infants and older children. The diagnosis has been recognized at postmortem examination. If identified in the neonatal period, appendicitis should be treated with emergent resection. Because Hirschsprung disease can be the underlying cause, rectal biopsies for frozen-section diagnosis should be done. Colostomy at ganglion cell transition is the only safe option in patients with documented Hirschsprung disease and appendicitis.

Appendicitis also is unusual in infants, who usually present with perforated appendicitis and often manifest complications such as intestinal obstruction and systemic sepsis. It is rare and fortuitous to make the diagnosis of acute appendicitis before perforation in this age group. This is a serious illness in infants, with mortality rates as high as 10%.

Postpubertal Girls

An accurate diagnosis of the source of abdominal pain in postpubertal girls is often difficult to make. In addition to appendicitis, ovarian pathology, such as ruptured ovarian cyst, torsion, and pain with ovulation, or *mittelschmerz,* can be common causes of severe lower abdominal pain. In most series, the rate of appendicitis resulting in perforation is no higher in this group of patients, but the rate of ''negative appendectomies,'' that is, removal of appendices lacking histologic evidence of inflammation, is reported to be as high as 40%. The liberal use of ultrasound examinations may result in lower negative appendectomy rates because ultrasound can be valuable to assess both the ovaries and the appendix. Diagnostic laparoscopy has been touted as an effective way to define the cause of lower abdominal pain in this age group. There is some debate, however, about whether this avoids unnecessary appendectomies,

because many surgeons reason that the appendix should be removed during the laparoscopic procedure regardless of its gross appearance.

Diagnostic Studies

Laboratory Tests

Although many different laboratory tests have been used to help discriminate appendicitis from other causes of abdominal pain, none is consistently definitive.[4] The most reliable blood test is the WBC count and differential; less than 5% of children with appendicitis have both normal WBC counts and differentials without a predominance of polymorphonuclear cells, or so-called left shift. Unfortunately, nonsurgical illnesses, such as gastroenteritis and ruptured ovarian cysts, can also be associated with elevated WBC counts and abnormal differentials. Appendicitis resulting in perforation is almost always associated with leukocytosis or a marked left shift. A normal WBC count in the setting of localized right lower quadrant tenderness or diffuse peritonitis should not dissuade the surgeon from operating for appendicitis. Plasma serotonin levels have been reported to be highly accurate in discriminating early appendicitis from other causes of abdominal pain, but this has not been confirmed on a large scale and probably is not practical in most clinical settings. Other serum tests, including C-reactive protein and erythrocyte sedimentation rate, have been touted as helpful in diagnosing appendicitis. These tests are infrequently needed, have not been evaluated in large clinical trials, and merely add to the expense.

Urinalysis should be routinely performed in children with symptoms suggestive of appendicitis. Elevated urine-specific gravity and ketonuria are common findings in appendicitis but are not diagnostic. The presence of leukocyte esterase, mild to moderate pyuria, or hematuria should raise the question of genitourinary tract pathology, but does not preclude the diagnosis of appendicitis because the inflammation of the appendix can cause irritation of the ureter or bladder. Severe pyuria with more than 25 WBCs per high-power field is much more likely to be associated with pyelonephritis. Ultrasound may help in assessing the kidneys for inflammation and edema suggestive of pyelonephritis and obstruction. In the absence of such evidence or convincing flank tenderness, pyuria should not prevent the surgeon from performing an appendectomy.

Radiologic Examinations

Radiographic studies are frequently unnecessary in evaluating children with abdominal pain and should be reserved for children whose symptoms are atypical or confusing. The features seen on plain abdominal radiographs with acute appendicitis include the following:

- Abnormal gas pattern
- Free peritoneal fluid
- Scoliosis
- Psoas shadow obliteration
- Thickened flank stripe
- Appendicolith (calcified in about 10% of patients)
- Abscess: air–fluid level

Of these, the finding of an appendicolith is the most compelling. If an appendicolith is identified in a child with localized abdominal pain, surgical exploration is indicated because almost all these patients have acute appendicitis. The other features listed are occasionally helpful when evaluating patients with prolonged illness who may have retrocecal or walled-off appendicitis.

Ultrasonography

Advances in ultrasound technology have resulted in its frequent application in the evaluation of patients with abdominal pain. The ultrasound image can detect the thickness of all layers of the bowel wall, luminal caliber, and whether the appendix is compressible. An edematous, distended (more than 6 mm in diameter), or noncompressible appendix accurately predicts the presence of acute appendicitis, especially when its location corresponds to the point of maximal tenderness (Fig. 74-5). The failure to identify these features of acute appendicitis, combined with findings more suggestive of other diagnoses, such as ovarian cysts or tumors, free pelvic fluid, thickened, edematous fallopian tubes, or thickened loops of small intestine, may prevent an unnecessary emergency laparotomy. Multiple studies report sensitivities and specificities of 80% to 95% for the ultrasound diagnosis of acute appendicitis. These studies vary significantly in the type of equipment used, the experience of the ultrasonographers, and the population of patients examined. Several factors predispose to false-negative results, including an obese habitus, recent perforation without the development of an abscess or phlegmon, and gaseous distention of the intestine. In addition, the reliability of the ultrasound study is operator dependent. Thus, a surgeon must weigh the accuracy of the ultrasonographers in his or her own institution. A positive ultrasound examination is infrequently a false-positive result. In contrast, nonvisualization of the appendix is not nearly as accurate in predicting the absence of appendicitis. The inability to identify the appendix over its entire length must be considered a nondiagnostic study and should not dissuade the surgeon from making the diagnosis of appendicitis in the operating room.

Computed Tomography

The use of CT scans to make the diagnosis of acute appendicitis in children should be discouraged because it is expensive and time-consuming. It may be useful, however, in atypical patients with undiagnosed intraabdominal symptoms or in whom satisfactory ultrasound studies are not possible. The latter group may include children who are obese, are immunologically suppressed, are neurologically impaired, or have a protracted illness and lack localizing physical findings. CT scans may also be helpful in patients with perforated appendicitis to distinguish phlegmon from abscess and to plan percutaneous or transrectal drainage of an abscess (Fig. 74-6).

The normal appendix is ordinarily difficult to see with CT imaging. Appendicitis occasionally results in a target-shaped appendix, which is a fairly specific finding. The inflammation associated with acute appendicitis causes edema and streaking of the surrounding fat. These findings are nonspecific and can be seen with other inflammatory lesions of the cecal region, such as neutropenic enterocolitis, inflammatory bowel disease such as Crohn disease, or bacterial enteritis. In small children, who lack the same amount of intraabdominal fat as adults and older children, CT has limited utility unless a discrete abscess is seen.

Barium Enema

Even though several studies have supported the value of barium contrast enema in the diagnosis of appendicitis, this study

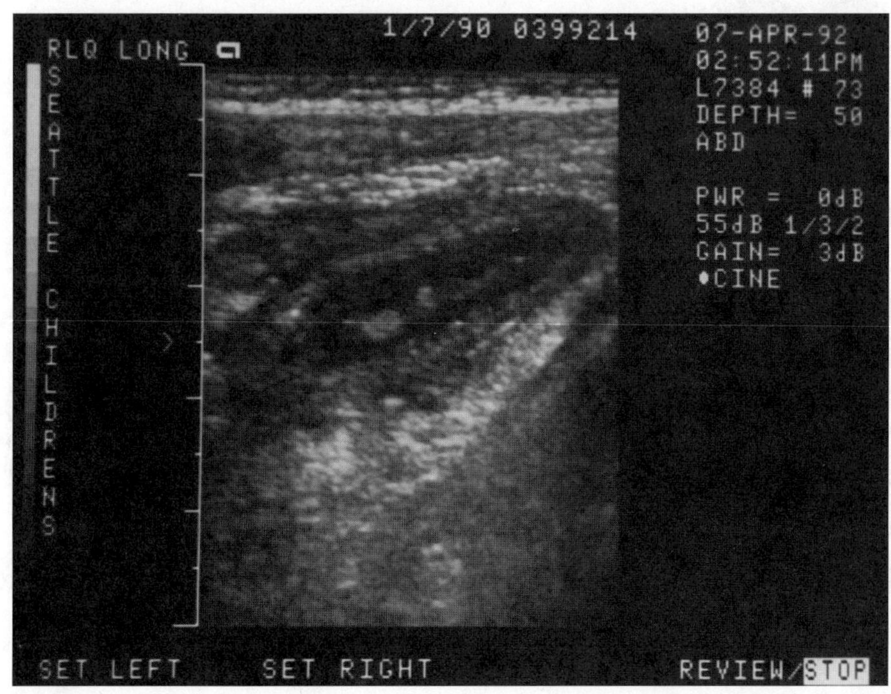

FIG. 74-5. Ultrasound diagnosis of appendicitis. Note the distention (8 mm in diameter) with the hypoechoic area surrounding the appendix, which suggests edema. This appendix was also noncompressible and tender. Histology showed acute appendicitis without perforation.

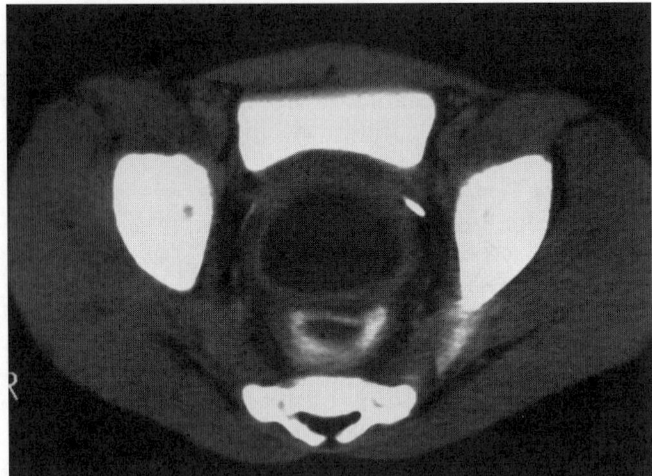

FIG. 74-6. CT scan diagnosis of perforated appendicitis. This intraabdominal abscess developed after several days of abdominal pain, fever, and anorexia. The abscess was drained percutaneously; an interval appendectomy was performed 6 weeks later.

should be used only in the atypical patient with a protracted acute illness or a history of chronic abdominal pain. Barium enema may be useful for these patients if other imaging are nondiagnostic. The barium enema findings that suggest appendiceal pathology are nonfilling or incomplete filling of the appendix and extrinsic compression or distortion of the cecum (Fig. 74-7). The incomplete filling of the appendix is consistent

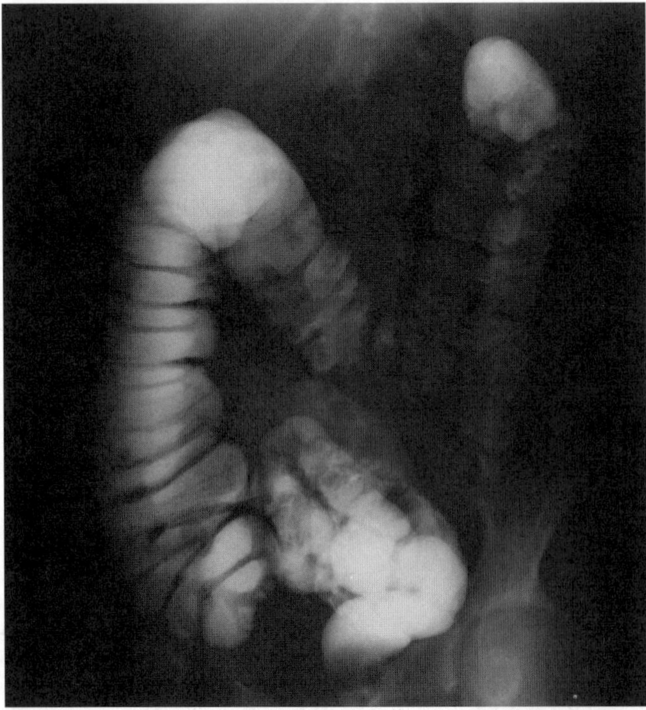

FIG. 74-7. Barium enema findings in appendicitis. Pericecal inflammation and absence of filling of the appendix are diagnostic of appendicitis.

with the hypothesis that luminal obstruction is an important factor in the cause of appendicitis. Unfortunately, up to 20% of normal patients have nonfilling of the appendix. In addition, focal appendicitis of the distal tip may allow nearly complete filling that appears deceptively normal. Like many other imaging studies, the use of barium enema for diagnosing appendicitis is operator dependent. When done with some regularity by experienced pediatric radiologists, barium enema can accurately detect appendicitis. A major benefit of a barium enema is the identification of other causes of right lower quadrant pain and tenderness, such as inflammation of the terminal ileum due to Crohn disease or to infection with *Salmonella*, *Shigella*, or *Yersinia*.

Laparoscopy

The use of the laparoscope is gaining popularity in the treatment of children with abdominal pain consistent with possible appendicitis. The rationale for its use is that identification of some other cause of pathology or a normal appendix would obviate the need for a negative appendectomy with its incumbent risks. Specific patient populations have a high incidence of negative laparotomy, such as the postpubertal girls discussed earlier. Laparoscopy has been especially advocated in that group of patients. Unfortunately, laparoscopy still requires general anesthesia, with its incumbent risks. Furthermore, some advocates of laparoscopy recommend that the appendix be removed through the laparoscope even if the appendix appears grossly normal, eliminating the stated advantage of reducing the negative appendectomy rate. On the other hand, if the cause of the pain is adnexal pathology, the laparoscope allows superior visualization of the pelvic organs compared with the typical appendectomy incision. For this reason, laparoscopy may be most useful when the surgeon is suspicious of other causes of lower abdominal pain. Whether laparoscopic appendectomy is a technically better option in all patients is discussed later.

Surgical Treatment: Appendectomy

The only appropriate treatment for acute appendicitis is appendectomy. Nevertheless, patients occasionally are treated successfully for appendicitis when given antibiotics to treat presumed urinary tract infections or otitis media. These patients usually develop recurrent symptoms and require later appendectomy. The operation is best performed as soon as possible, provided the patient is satisfactorily prepared with fluid resuscitation and perioperative antibiotics. Some researchers have suggested that when a patient presents in the middle of the night, appendectomy for acute appendicitis can be deferred until regular working hours. If one accepts the paradigm presented earlier that appendicitis is a progressive pathologic process and that the incidence of perforation increases with the duration of illness, delaying the appendectomy increases the risk of perforation. If the patient has clearly progressed to perforation already, deferring the operation to complete resuscitation is prudent. Delay beyond this is not. The antibiotics of choice depend on whether perforation has occurred. For perioperative wound prophylaxis in patients with acute appendicitis without perforation, a broad-spectrum intravenous single agent such as a cephalosporin is adequate. For patients with suspected perforation, broad-spectrum coverage directed against gram-negative and anaerobic organisms is necessary. The combination of ampicillin, gentamicin, and clindamycin (or metronidazole) is the standard therapy against which all other antibiotic regimens are compared. Newer single agents have been used in several studies with apparently equal efficacy, although large studies in children with perforated appendicitis have not been reported.

Once antibiotic administration and electrolyte and volume resuscitation are completed, laparotomy should be performed. Unless significant doubt about the diagnosis persists, the incision of choice is transverse, in the right lower quadrant, paralleling the skin line, and placed directly over the point of maximal tenderness or the palpable mass. The incision should be lateral to the rectus muscle but can be extended in a medial direction if greater exposure is needed during the operation. The external oblique is widely incised in the direction of its fibers, exposing the internal oblique, which is split in the direction of its fibers. The transversus abdominis and peritoneum can then be incised and cultures taken of any fluid found. For situations in which the diagnosis is less certain, a lower midline incision is made. Once the peritoneum is opened, the operation is performed in the same fashion.

The cecum is identified first, usually by delivering the most lateral segment of bowel into the wound. If enlarged and inflamed, the appendix may easily be palpable. Otherwise, the appendix can be found consistently by following the taeniae coli to their confluence. If the appendix is retrocecal, encased in inflammatory adhesions, or immobile because of dense retroperitoneal attachments of the cecum, careful blunt dissection usually permits delivery into the wound. Occasionally, the incision needs to be extended to permit safe mobilization of the cecum or appendix. The appendix is mobilized by dividing the mesoappendix; the base of the appendix is ligated, and the organ is amputated at its base. Simple ligation of the base of the appendix is adequate in most cases, but many surgeons also imbricate the appendiceal stump with use of a pursestring suture or Z stitch. The imbrication of too much tissue can lead to a mucocele or can later result in a lead point for an intussusception. Mucoceles can be prevented by cauterizing the residual mucosa at the base of the appendix. After removal of the appendix, the wound is irrigated, and the muscle layers are closed.

Failure to find an obviously inflamed appendix should prompt an exploration for other possible causes of abdominal tenderness. The differential diagnosis is extensive; in children, gastroenteritis, mesenteric adenitis, gynecologic pathology such as hemorrhagic ovarian cysts or torsion, and regional enteritis, both infectious and idiopathic, are the most common sources of this error in diagnosis. Meckel diverticulum should be considered. Consequently, examination of the distal small bowel, mesentery, fallopian tubes, and ovaries is necessary. This can usually be accomplished through the same incision. If purulent or bloody fluid is seen in the peritoneal cavity, extension of the original incision or even a new midline incision is mandated to make a firm diagnosis. Some surgeons have proposed using a laparoscope through the partially closed original incision because this permits excellent visibility of all quadrants of the abdomen. Even if the appendix appears grossly normal, it should be removed because the microscopy may reveal appendicitis. In addition, these patients will have right lower quadrant scars, and physicians in the future will assume that they no

longer have their appendices. An exception should be made for patients with inflammatory bowel disease involving the cecum in the region of the base of the appendix. In these cases, the risk of stump leak and subsequent fecal fistula from the cecum precludes a safe appendectomy.

For patients with suspected perforated appendicitis, broad-spectrum antibiotic therapy and nasogastric decompression are started before laparotomy. The operative technique for perforated appendicitis is essentially the same. Efforts to minimize the incision because of cosmetic concerns are ill-advised because the inflammation and peritonitis make visibility more challenging. Peritoneal pus must be drained as completely as possible. Although it is common practice to culture the pus, the information gained is seldom used to alter the treatment. The organisms cultured and their sensitivities to antibiotics may only partially reflect the bacteriology of the intraabdominal infection, which is almost always polymicrobial. The antibiotic therapy should be kept broad enough to cover the most common gram-negative and anaerobic organisms regardless of the culture results, and it should not be discontinued until the fever, leukocytosis, and abdominal examination have all normalized.

Mobilization of the cecum and appendix can be much more difficult in patients with perforation, occasionally resulting in injury to the neighboring bowel. If the dissection and exposure of the appendix proves unsafe, placement of drains in the abscess cavities and closure of the abdomen is an option, albeit infrequently employed. This must be followed by an interval appendectomy to avoid recurrent appendicitis.

Whether the surgeon should irrigate the pelvic and abdominal peritoneal cavities of patients with appendicitis is controversial. Some studies have suggested that irrigation interferes with normal macrophage function, yet a widely used protocol for pediatric perforated appendicitis includes irrigation with large amounts of saline and yields one of the lowest complication rates in the literature.[5] Although many surgeons include antibiotics in the irrigation, there is no proven advantage. There is also debate about the use of peritoneal drains for these patients.[6–8] Critics argue that no drain can effectively drain the peritoneal cavity, while proponents point to a low rate of residual intraabdominal abscesses when drains are used. No randomized, controlled studies have been performed in the modern antibiotic era comparing the use of drains to no drains in perforated appendicitis. The major complication rates for the two approaches are similar. Wound closure in the face of gangrenous or perforated appendicitis is associated with an infection rate as high as 20%. If drains are not used, some surgeons recommend delayed primary closure, which can be facilitated by leaving widely spaced, nonabsorbable sutures in the skin at the completion of the operation. These sutures can be tied 72 to 96 hours later with a reasonable cosmetic result and a lower risk of wound infection. Other studies have reported wound infection rates of less than 5% with primary closure, even in perforated appendicitis patients.

Laparoscopic appendectomy is gaining popularity, but no real advantage can be documented in children. Some studies have shown slight reductions in the length of hospital stay after laparoscopic appendectomy, but morbidity data show little difference between open and laparoscopic appendectomy. Furthermore, the costs of laparoscopy exceed the cost of laparotomy in most studies. The excellent visibility of laparoscopy may be advantageous in larger or obese children, in whom a large incision would be necessary, or in children with an less certain diagnosis, such as postpubertal females.

During laparoscopy, the mesoappendix can be divided with stainless steel clips or an automatic stapler that fires two parallel sets of staples and cuts between them. The appendix is amputated by use of the stapler or by dividing the base of the appendix between three ligatures of absorbable sutures, which are applied by snaring the appendix. Residual appendiceal mucosa can be carefully cauterized if necessary to prevent mucocele formation. The resected appendix is withdrawn through a port site in a sterile bag. Irrigation of the pelvis and stump region is followed by suture closure of the port incisions. Perforation was initially reported to be a contraindication for pediatric laparoscopic appendectomy. As experience with laparoscopic surgery increases, more surgeons are attempting appendectomy even in the setting of perforation.

Complications

The most common complications and their cumulative incidence in four studies are reported in Table 74-2. Wound infection is the most common complication, with a 1% to 5% (cumulative, 1.4%) incidence in gangrenous or perforated appendicitis. Small bowel obstruction occurs in about 1% to 2% of patients with perforation, but can complicate the recovery of nonperforated patients as well, including those who undergo a negative appendectomy.[9] Operative adhesiolysis is usually necessary. Abscess is seen much more commonly in children with perforated appendicitis. The abscess can be drained percutaneously with ultrasound or CT guidance, or it can be drained through the rectum or vagina. Infertility in women has been attributed to a history of perforated appendicitis in several studies. In a recent longitudinal study of women who had prepubertal perforated appendicitis, however, there was no difference in fertility rates compared with the general population.[10]

Advances in perioperative care and antibiotics have lowered the mortality rate for appendicitis to less than 1%. Intraabdominal sepsis and multisystem organ failure have occurred in children, usually in those younger than 5 years old or who had long illnesses before surgical intervention.

Tumors

Carcinoid tumors are rare in children but may be identified in appendiceal specimens. Most appendices that contain carcinoid tumors are inflamed, often resulting in perforation, presumably because of the high-grade luminal obstruction. The histology of these tumors shows nests of small, uniform cells invading the submucosa and muscularis, often extending to the serosa. These tumors are typically small and, if so, behave in a benign fashion, even with lymph nodes involvement. Consequently, appendectomy alone without adjuvant therapy is generally sufficient treatment in children. Other, more rare tumors include lymphoma, lymphosarcoma, and adenocarcinoid tumor, a much more aggressive malignancy.

Incidental Appendectomy

The wisdom of incidental appendectomy during other abdominal operations has long been debated. Some advocates of incidental appendectomy maintain that the appendix should be removed whenever the exposure allows because it has no function and can cause future morbidity. In addition, microscopy of incidental appendectomy specimens shows inflammation and fibrosis in up to 20%. On the other hand, incidental appendectomy can increase the operative morbidity rate, particularly for wound infections in otherwise clean operations. Available data do not allow definitive resolution of the controversy. Recently described reconstructive procedures involving the appendix have also challenged the wisdom of routine incidental appendectomy. The appendix is well suited as a conduit for urinary drainage (Mitrofanoff procedure)[11] and for biliary drainage. Thus, it should be preserved whenever possible in children with congenital biliary problems, neural tube defects, or genitourinary anomalies who may require reconstructive surgery in the future.

MECKEL DIVERTICULUM

Meckel diverticulum is one of a constellation of congenital anomalies of the midgut that should more accurately be termed *omphalomesenteric duct–related anomalies.* The embryologic midgut is the open ventral portion of the archenteron, which lies between the foregut and the hindgut. During week 3 of gestation, the midgut is opened into the yolk sac, which does not grow as rapidly as the rest of the embryo. Subsequently, by week 5, the connection with the yolk sac becomes narrowed and is termed the *yolk stalk, vitelline duct,* or *omphalomesenteric duct.* Normally, this yolk stalk disappears by the gestational week 9, just before the midgut returns to the abdomen. Persistence of some portion of this omphalomesenteric duct results in a number of congenital anomalies, of which Meckel (or omphaloileal) diverticulum is the most common.

Figure 74-8 shows the variety of omphalomesenteric duct remnants and their associated complications. Some are attached to the small intestine, and most are attached to the umbilicus. The point of attachment to the bowel varies, with about 75% situated within 100 cm of the ileocecal valve. All attachments are located on the antimesenteric side of the bowel. Histologically, the omphalomesenteric diverticulum is a true diverticulum, consisting of all four intestinal layers. The mucosa often contains ectopic gastric and pancreatic mucosa, especially in patients with symptoms. Over 95% of the resected specimens from patients who develop hemorrhagic complications contain gastric mucosa alone or both pancreatic and gastric mucosa. Thirty to 65% of the Meckel diverticula resected from patients without symptoms contain ectopic mucosa. The blood supply

TABLE 74-2. *Complications of perforated appendicitis**

Complication	Incidence (%)
Wound infection	1.4
Bowel obstruction	1.4
Intraabdominal abscess	1.8
Enterocutaneous fistula	0.2

* Based on data from 761 patients.

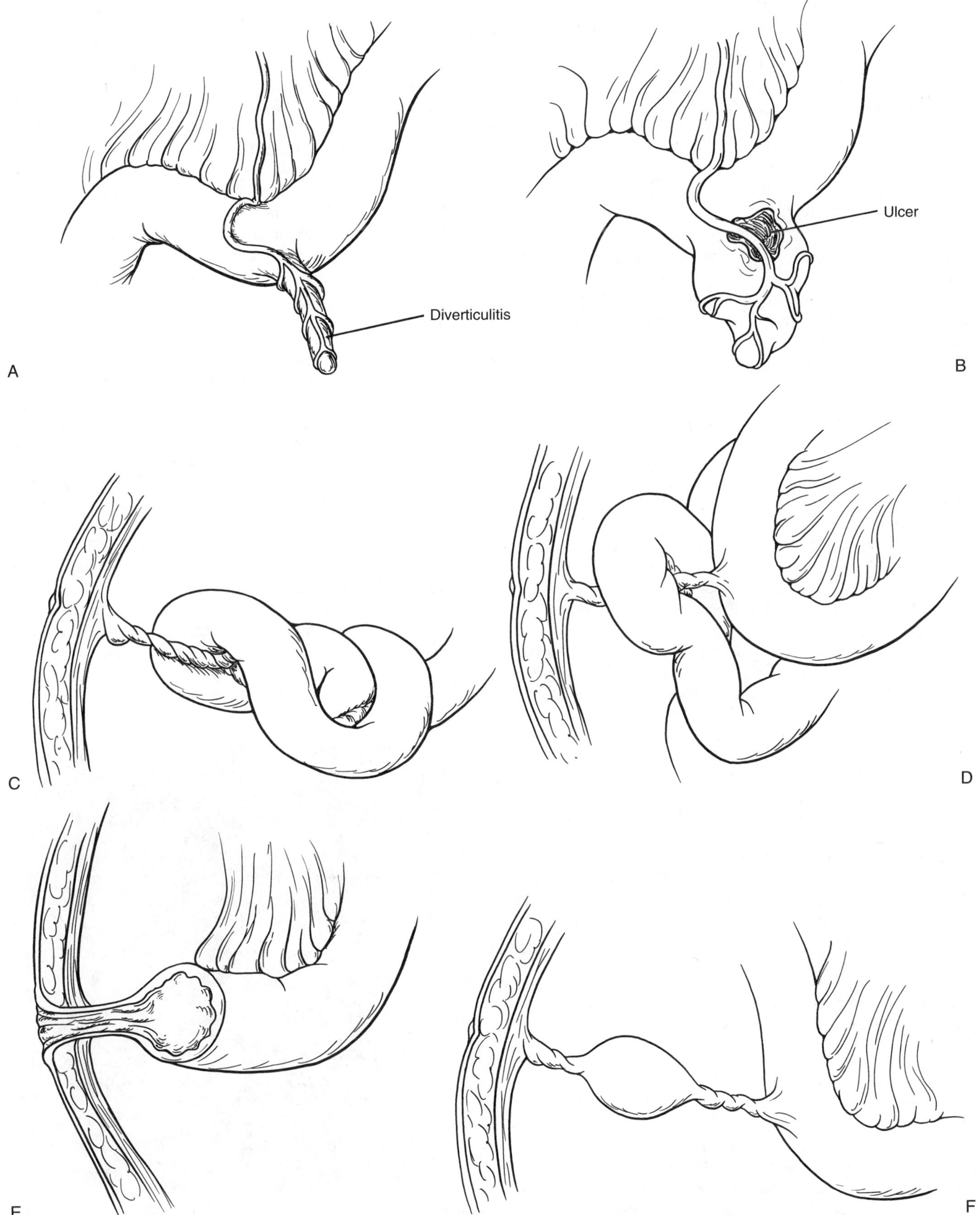

FIG. 74-8. Omphalomesenteric duct remnants. (*A*) Meckel diverticulum with diverticulitis. (*B*) Meckel diverticulum with ulceration and hemorrhage. (*C* and *D*) Bowel obstruction from volvulus around attachment to the abdominal wall. (*E*) Patent omphalomesenteric duct. (*F*) Omphalomesenteric sinus and cyst.

to the omphalomesenteric duct remnant is a vestige of the primitive vitelline artery, which usually arises directly from the mesentery and which can be prominent, especially in patients with bleeding related to ectopic gastric mucosa.

CLINICAL FEATURES

Meckel Diverticulum

Meckel diverticulum is found in about 2% of the population, often incidentally during laparotomy or at autopsy. Estimates of the probability of Meckel diverticulum causing symptoms in a lifetime vary from 4% to 35%, depending on the age of the population studied. Over 60% of patients who develop symptoms from this anomaly are younger than 2 years of age. The most common symptoms of this lesion are bleeding, intestinal obstruction, inflammation, and umbilical drainage. The incidence of each of these problems varies with the age of the patient.[12,13]

Bowel Obstruction

In infants, bowel obstruction is the most likely symptom of a Meckel diverticulum. This can be due either to intussusception with the diverticulum as the lead point or to herniation of the bowel through a patent omphalomesenteric fistula. Obstruction can also occur with volvulus around a fibrous remnant of the omphalomesenteric duct that is attached to the Meckel diverticulum or an internal hernia beneath the vestigial vitelline artery or fibrous remnant. If intussusception has occurred, the diagnosis can be made by barium or air-contrast enema. Enema reduction of the intussusception is seldom successful. If the obstruction is due to prolapse of the intestine through the patent omphalomesenteric fistula, a characteristic ''ram's horn'' appearance may be seen. If obstruction occurs because of volvulus around a fibrous vitelline duct remnant that is not patent, or because of an internal hernia beneath the vitelline artery, the diagnosis can be extremely difficult to make. The onset of pain is usually sudden and severe. In older children, the pain may be out of proportion to the physical findings, a characteristic of intestinal ischemia. Inspection of the umbilicus and barium enema are of little help. Because the volvulus usually involves the distal small bowel, and the obstruction is most often a closed loop, there may be little emesis until late in the course. The sequelae of intestinal ischemia, such as acidosis, peritonitis, and shock, may occur first. In infants and toddlers, this can be a lethal lesion.

Bleeding

Hemorrhage is the most common complication of Meckel diverticulum, occurring in about half of patients with symptoms. Patients who develop bleeding are typically older, with a mean age of about 2 years. The bleeding is rectal, is usually painless, is often massive, and frequently requires transfusion. Hemorrhage from a Meckel diverticulum is the most common cause of serious gastrointestinal bleeding in children. In the era before nuclear scintigraphy, children with massive, painless bleeding or children with unexplained chronic rectal bleeding were assumed to have Meckel diverticula and were taken to the operating room for diverticulectomy after resuscitation. The diagnosis was often correct, but other less common lesions were identified, including juvenile retention polyps, hemangiomas, Peutz-Jeghers polyps, peptic ulcer disease, blood dyscrasias, and inflammatory bowel disease.

The bleeding associated with a Meckel diverticulum originates from ulceration of the ileal mucosa. This ulceration is presumably peptic in origin because the ectopic gastric mucosa contains parietal cells that secrete hydrochloric acid. The ileal mucosa is ill equipped to buffer the resulting low pH and thus is prone to ulceration. The site of ulceration is most often at the junction of the normal ileal mucosa and the ectopic gastric mucosa. A similar situation arises in patients with ectopic gastric mucosa in enteric duplication cysts. The remnant vitelline artery may be prominent in patients who have bleeding from Meckel diverticula.

The technetium-99m pertechnetate isotope scan permits the visualization of the ectopic gastric mucosa. The isotope is taken up by the mucus-secreting cells of the ectopic gastric mucosa as well as by those in the stomach. The remaining isotope is seen in the urinary bladder. Images are exposed every minute for 1 hour (Fig. 74-9). Failure to identify any ectopic gastric mucosa on scintigraphy is associated with only a 5% to 10% error rate. If rectal bleeding persists, a repeat scintigraphy scan is indicated. To enhance the sensitivity of the repeat scan, catheterization of the bladder and intravenous administration of pentagastrin and cimetidine are recommended by some investigators. If the scan is still negative, other studies, such as an isotope-labeled red blood cell scan or angiography, can be con-

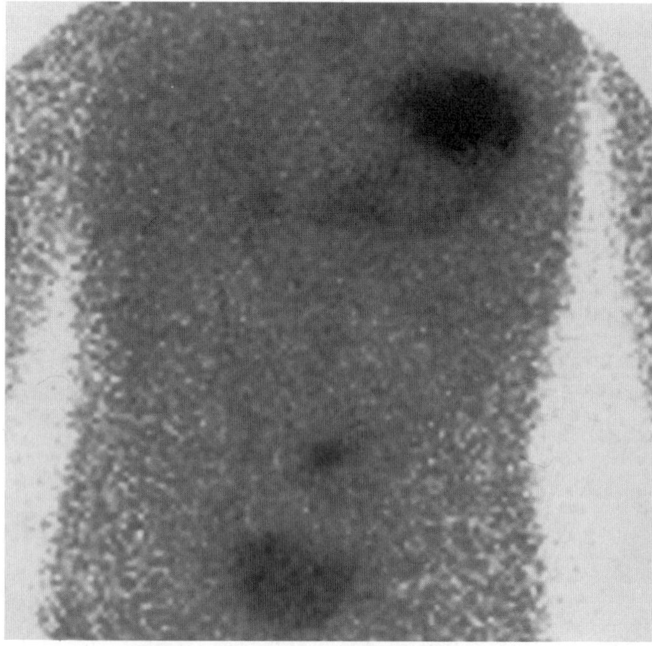

FIG. 74-9. Technetium-99m pertechnetate scintigraphy of a Meckel diverticulum. Radionuclide signal is seen in the stomach, the bladder, and the Meckel diverticulum. Sensitivity of the scintigraphy can be enhanced by bladder catheterization and intravenous administration of pentagastrin or cimetidine.

sidered, but these are rarely needed in children. When no other source of gastrointestinal bleeding is identified, colonoscopy and gastroduodenoscopy, laparotomy or laparoscopy should be considered.

Inflammation

Less commonly, Meckel diverticula become inflamed and result in diverticulitis, which can present in a fashion similar to appendicitis. Like the appendix, the Meckel diverticulum can become inflamed when the lumen is obstructed, resulting in increased pressure with decreased mucosal perfusion, tissue acidosis, and bacterial invasion of the wall. This can lead to progressive inflammation with tissue gangrene and perforation. The role of ectopic mucosa in this process is suggested by its high incidence in resected inflamed diverticula. It is possible that the gastric or pancreatic mucosa contributes to the luminal obstruction; or the gastric mucosa can lead to ileal mucosal ulceration first, which facilitates the bacterial invasion.

The symptoms of Meckel diverticulitis are much like those of appendicitis. With both developing from the same dermatome, the symptoms begin with poorly localized periumbilical pain. Because the omphalomesenteric remnants are variable in their location and may be unattached to the umbilicus, the progressive inflammation of the Meckel diverticulum can cause peritoneal irritation anywhere in the lower abdomen. Right lower quadrant and lower midline are the most common locations for the pain owing to the distal ileal location of most Meckel diverticula. As a result, patients with Meckel diverticulitis are usually assumed to have appendicitis when taken to the operating room. A perforated Meckel diverticulum is potentially more serious than a perforated appendix since the former is more difficult to wall off because of its more mobile position. This may explain why perforated diverticulitis is more likely to result in diffuse peritonitis and pneumoperitoneum detectable on abdominal radiographs. For this reason, it is imperative to search carefully for other causes of peritonitis when a noninflamed appendix is discovered at the time of appendectomy.

Umbilical Drainage

Anomalies of the omphalomesenteric duct can result in umbilical drainage as well. The quantity and character of the drainage may indicate the origin of the lesion. Clear or yellowish drainage signifies a probable urachal anomaly, while an omphalomesenteric duct remnant manifests as feculent drainage. The most common umbilical lesion is probably an umbilical granuloma. This lesion may secrete a mucoid material that can be misleading by suggesting an intraabdominal communication. If the drainage persists despite cauterization of the presumed granuloma with silver nitrate, or if the drainage is copious, imaging studies are indicated. Ultrasound examination may demonstrate a urachal communication or an omphalomesenteric duct. In selected cases, catheterization of the lesion and injection with water-soluble contrast allows radiographic assessment. If the contrast study demonstrates communication with the bladder or gastrointestinal tract, resection is necessary because the omphalomesenteric duct remnants that connect the ileum to the umbilicus can become the focal point of obstruction if not removed.

TREATMENT

Surgical resection of omphalomesenteric duct remnants should be preceded by prompt volume resuscitation for all patients with symptoms, including blood transfusion for those who have hemorrhaged significantly. With the exception of those patients with intestinal obstruction and possible intestinal ischemia, laparotomy can be delayed until after the hematocrit is restored to near-normal levels. Patients with obstructive symptoms should be resuscitated as rapidly as possible, so that relief of the obstruction can be expedited to obviate the need for ischemic bowel resection.

The incision chosen varies with the symptoms and the age of the patient. Infants with feculent umbilical drainage or a ram's horn appearance indicating prolapse of the omphalomesenteric duct remnant can be explored through a relatively small infraumbilical incision. Children with Meckel diverticulitis are most often operated on using a transverse appendectomy incision, which may require medial extension to perform a resection of the involved ileum. A similar right lower quadrant incision works well for resection of a bleeding Meckel diverticulum with ectopic mucosa. Patients with suspected intestinal obstruction should be explored through a generous laparotomy incision to optimize exposure for intestinal decompression and resection of the necrotic sections of bowel in as rapid a fashion as possible.

When possible, omphalomesenteric duct anomalies can be resected without requiring removal of the ileum to which it is attached. Some surgeons use linear staplers applied to the base of the anomaly, allowing complete amputation of the lesion without narrowing the lumen of the ileum. A V-shaped incision at the base of the remnant results in a defect of the antimesenteric wall of the ileum, which can usually be closed in a transverse orientation to avoid stenosis. This can be difficult when a large focus of ectopic mucosa or a resultant ulceration is present near the base of the diverticulum or when the lesion has a wide base. In these instances, resection of the involved portion of ileum is required with an end-to-end anastomosis. Obstructing lesions, such as an omphalomesenteric band, must be destroyed, and the involved bowel may be salvaged. Unfortunately, the difficulty of making the correct diagnosis promptly may result in irreversibly ischemic intestine, which must be resected. In the absence of severe peritoneal soiling or hemodynamic instability, continuity of the small bowel can be safely restored. Meckel diverticulitis, even in the face of perforation, can usually be managed by resection and primary anastomosis as well. The use of laparoscopy for resection of Meckel diverticula, although technically reasonable, provides little advantage over open laparotomy, as discussed in the section on appendectomy.

Controversy exists about what should be done when a Meckel diverticulum is encountered during a laparotomy for unrelated symptoms. The debate focuses on the probability of an omphaloileal diverticulum becoming symptomatic in the future, in contrast to the complications associated with resection.[14,15] Some generalizations can be helpful in making this intraoperative judgment. Lesions with palpable ectopic mucosa, a prominent vitelline artery or fibrous vitelline artery remnant, evidence of inflammation, or a narrow base may all be more likely to cause bleeding, obstruction, or diverticulitis, respectively, and should therefore be resected when discovered. It is also prudent to resect diverticula discovered in patients who present with abdominal pain. Any lesions with attachments to the umbilicus should be detached to prevent distal ileal volvulus. Because omphalomesenteric anomalies can become symptomatic at any age, the age of the patient is not the primary factor in the decision to resect the asymptomatic lesion. If the lesion is not resected, it is imperative to alert the patient's family and primary care physician about the presence of the lesion and its possible symptoms. It is, of course, important to consider this question in the context of the primary operative procedure.

REFERENCES

1. Braveman P, Schaaf VM, Egerter S, et al. Insurance-related differences in the risk of ruptured appendicitis. N Engl J Med 1194;331:444.
2. Wangensteen OH, Dennis C. Experimental proof of the obstructive origin of appendicitis in man. Ann Surg 1939;110:629.
3. Brender JD, Marcuse EK, Koepsell TD, et al. Childhood appendicitis: factors associated with perforation. Pediatrics 1985;76:301.
4. Hoffmann J, Rasmussen OO. Aids in the diagnosis of acute appendicitis. Br J Surg 1989;76:774.
5. Lund DP, Murphy EP. Management of perforated appendicitis in children: a decade of aggressive treatment. J Pediatr Surg 1994;29:1130.
6. Curran TJ, Muenchow SK. The treatment of complicated appendicitis in children using peritoneal drainage: results from a public hospital. J Pediatr Surg 1993;28:204.
7. Neilson IR, Laberge JM, Nguyen LT, et al. Appendicitis in children: current therapeutic recommendations. J Pediatr Surg 1990;25:1113.
8. Karp MP, Caldarola VA, Cooney DR, et al. The avoidable excesses in the management of perforated appendicitis in children. J Pediatr Surg 1986;21:506.
9. Lau WY, Fan ST, Yiu TF, et al. Negative findings at appendectomy. Am J Surg 1984;148:375.
10. Puri P, McGuinness EP, Guiney EJ. Fertility following perforated appendicitis in girls. J Pediatr Surg 1989;24:547.
11. Sumfest JM, Burns MW, Mitchell ME. The Mitrofanoff principle in urinary reconstruction. J Urol 1993;150:1875.
12. St-Vil D, Brandt ML, Panic S, et al. Meckel's diverticulum in children: a 20 year review. J Pediatr Surg 1991;26:1289.
13. Vane DW, West K, Grosfeld JL. Vitelline duct anomalies: experience with 217 childhood cases. Arch Surg 1987;122:542.
14. Soltero JH, Bill AH. The natural history of Meckel's diverticulum and its relation to incidental removal. Am J Surg 1976;32:168.
15. Ludtke FE, Mende V, Kohler H, et al. Incidence and frequency of complications and management of Meckel's diverticulum. Surg Gynecol Obstet 1989;169:537.

Surgery of Infants and Children: Scientific Principles and Practice, edited by Keith T. Oldham, Paul M. Colombani, and Robert P. Foglia. Lippincott–Raven Publishers, Philadelphia, © 1997.

CHAPTER 75

Malrotation

Brad W. Warner

Abnormalities of rotation and fixation of the intestine are of paramount importance since they can be life-threatening and because most anomalies become clinically evident during infancy and childhood. Interruption of any stage of intrauterine intestinal development may result in anatomic defects that set the stage for later obstruction or volvulus. An understanding of the embryology of the intestine is therefore essential in the recognition and appropriate surgical management of these conditions.

The true incidence of rotation or fixation anomalies of the midgut leading to clinical disease is difficult to determine and has been reported to occur with a frequency of 1 in 6000 live births.[1] Complete nonrotation, whereby the entire small bowel is located on the right side of the abdomen and the colon on the left, has been reported in 0.5% of autopsies[2] and as an asymptomatic and incidental finding in 0.2% of barium studies of the gastrointestinal (GI) tract at any age.[3] The validity of this statement with regard to patients who are asymptomatic must be questioned, however, since radiographic contrast studies seldom are performed on patients who do not have symptoms.

EMBRYOLOGY

The growth of the developing midgut is faster than the growth of the body early in gestation. Because of this discrepancy, the midgut normally herniates out of the peritoneal cavity at about the fourth week of development in the human fetus. At at about the 10th week of gestation, the intestine returns to the abdominal cavity. Rotation and fixation of the intestine subsequently occurs, culminating in the final position of the small intestine and colon in the term infant. Interruption or reversal of any of these coordinated movements allows for embryologic explanations for subsequent clinical problems. These intestinal movements are classified into three stages.

Stage 1: Herniation

The midgut begins to buckle ventrally and herniate into the coelom of the body stalk during the fourth week of embryonic life (Fig. 75-1A). The superior mesenteric artery (SMA) is the axis of the herniation and divides the midgut into cranial (prearterial, duodenojejunal) and caudal (postarterial, cecocolic) segments. The rate of growth of the duodenojejunal (prearterial) segment of midgut is greater than the cecocolic (postarterial) segment during this first stage.

Duodenojejunal Limb

As the midgut herniates and continues to grow outside of the body, the duodenojejunal segment is pushed inferiorly by the developing liver and left umbilical vein and undergoes a 90-degree counterclockwise rotation to result in the prearterial limb (for point of reference, the duodenojejunal junction) lying to the right of the SMA (see Fig. 75-1B). With further intestinal development and just before the second stage, the duodenojejunal limb undergoes an additional 90-degree rotation such that the duodenojejunal junction lies directly posterior to the SMA (total of 180-degree rotation thus far; see Fig. 75-1C).

Cecocolic Limb

Rotation of the cecocolic limb of midgut during the first stage directly parallels rotation of the duodenojejunal limb. The ileocecal junction begins inferior to the SMA (Fig. 75-2A), and as the duodenojejunal limb undergoes its first 90-degree rotation to the right of the SMA, the ileocecal junction moves 90 degrees to the left of the SMA in a counterclockwise direction (see Fig. 75-2B). Just before returning to the abdomen (10th week), the ileocecal junction rotates an addition 90 degrees so that it lies directly ventral to the SMA (total of 180-degree rotation thus far; see Fig. 75-2C).

Stage 2: Return to the Abdomen

Duodenojejunal Limb

The developing intestine begins to return to the abdominal cavity during the 10th week (40-mm length) and is completed by the 11th week. The duodenojejunal limb is the first to return to the abdomen and in this process completes an additional 90-degree rotation around the SMA. The final result is a 270-degree

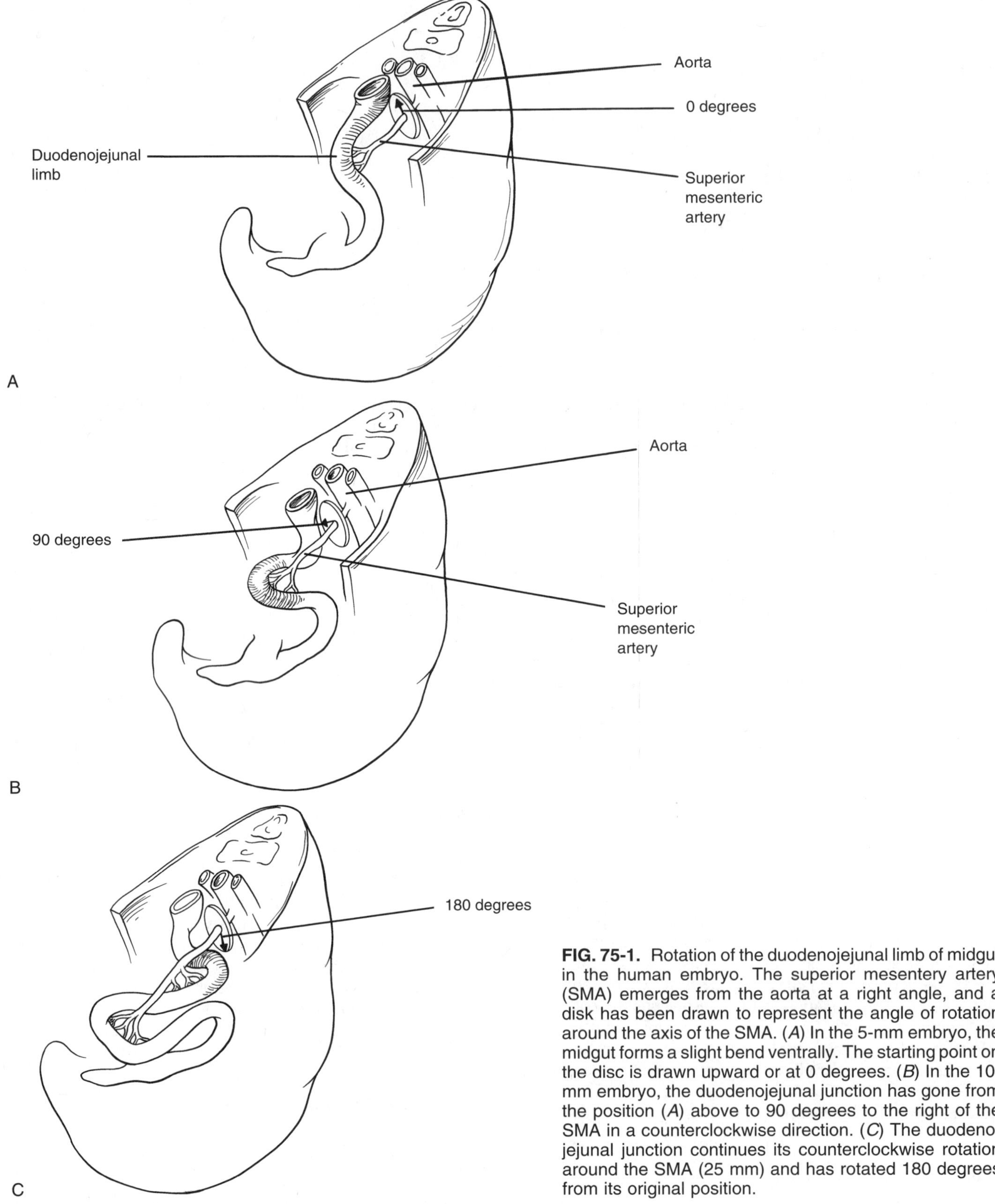

FIG. 75-1. Rotation of the duodenojejunal limb of midgut in the human embryo. The superior mesentery artery (SMA) emerges from the aorta at a right angle, and a disk has been drawn to represent the angle of rotation around the axis of the SMA. (*A*) In the 5-mm embryo, the midgut forms a slight bend ventrally. The starting point on the disc is drawn upward or at 0 degrees. (*B*) In the 10-mm embryo, the duodenojejunal junction has gone from the position (*A*) above to 90 degrees to the right of the SMA in a counterclockwise direction. (*C*) The duodenojejunal junction continues its counterclockwise rotation around the SMA (25 mm) and has rotated 180 degrees from its original position.

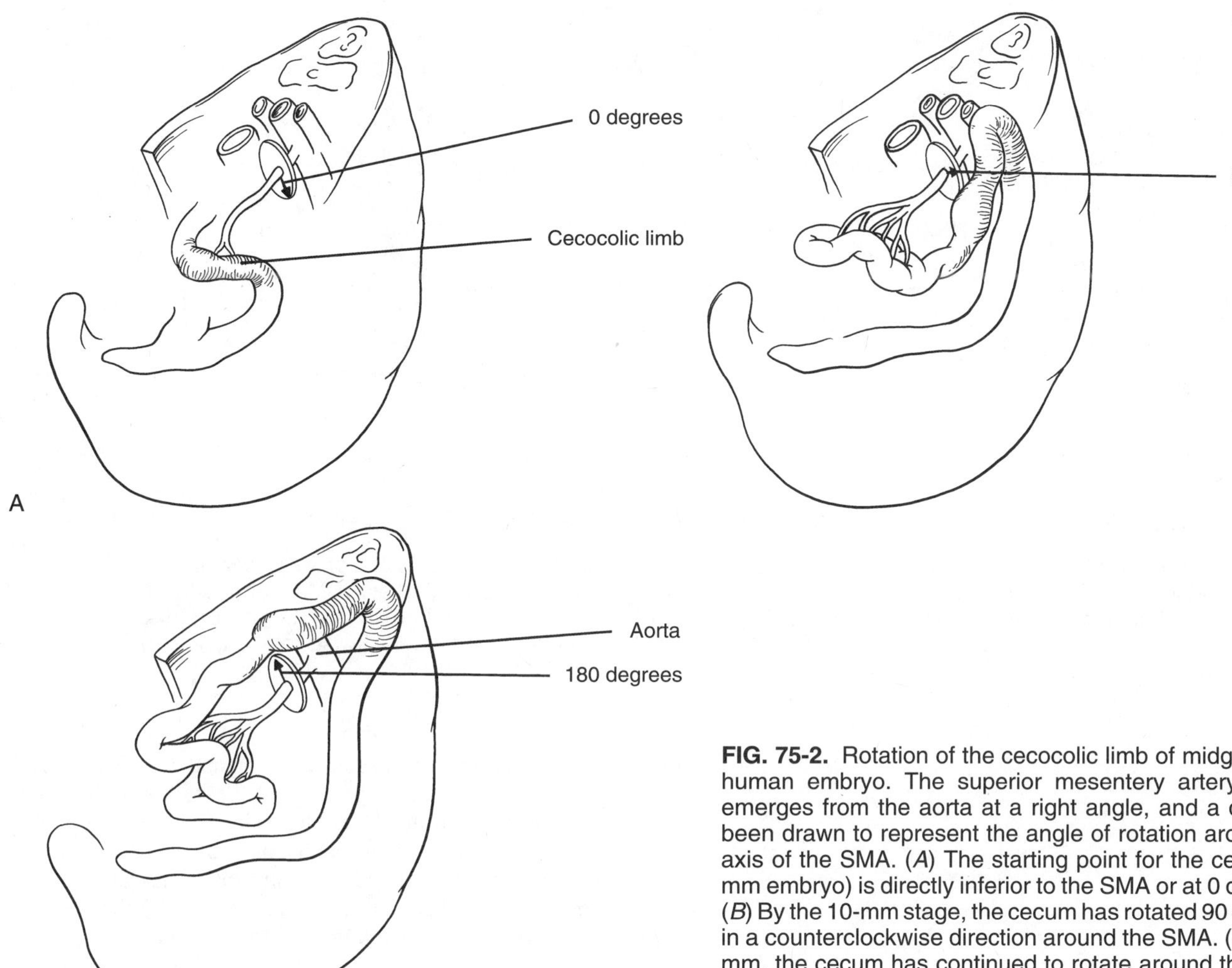

FIG. 75-2. Rotation of the cecocolic limb of midgut in the human embryo. The superior mesentery artery (SMA) emerges from the aorta at a right angle, and a disk has been drawn to represent the angle of rotation around the axis of the SMA. (*A*) The starting point for the cecum (5-mm embryo) is directly inferior to the SMA or at 0 degrees. (*B*) By the 10-mm stage, the cecum has rotated 90 degrees in a counterclockwise direction around the SMA. (*C*) At 40 mm, the cecum has continued to rotate around the SMA; it is at 180 degrees from its starting point and is directly ventral to the SMA.

counterclockwise rotation around the SMA with the duodeno-jejunal junction fixed to the posterior body wall to the left of the SMA at the ligament of Treitz (Fig. 75-3*A*).

Cecocolic Limb

As the cecocolic limb returns to the abdomen, it undergoes an addition 90-degree rotation such that it lies to the right of the SMA. It has thus undergone a total 270-degree counter-clockwise rotation around the SMA (see Fig. 75-3*B*).

Stage 3: Fixation

From the 12th gestational week until after birth, the colon becomes fixed and the mesentery of the ascending and descending portions becomes adherent to the posterior abdominal wall. This process of fixation is not possible unless normal rotation of the midgut has occurred. Peritoneal bands form to anchor the ascending and descending colon respectively in the right and left paracolic gutters. If the cecum and ascending colon do not fully rotate to the right side of the peritoneal cavity, perito-

neal (Ladd) bands secure the ascending colon to the right para-colic gutter, even if the colon is in the middle of the peritoneal cavity. In this event, these pass anterior to the duodenum and may be obstructive.

CLASSIFICATION OF MALROTATION

The spectrum of anatomic abnormalities encountered in patients with malrotation are conveniently classified by separate consideration of the rotations of the duodenojejunal and the cecocolic limbs of the midgut. Abnormalities of fixation generally involve the cecocolic limb only.

Nonrotation

Clinically, complete nonrotation of the midgut is the most frequently encountered anomaly and occurs when neither the duodenojejunal limb nor the cecocolic limb undergo rotation (Fig. 75-4). Normally, the duodenum rotates posterior to the SMA so that the ligament of Treitz is to the left of the midline and at the level of the gastric antrum. If this rotation does not

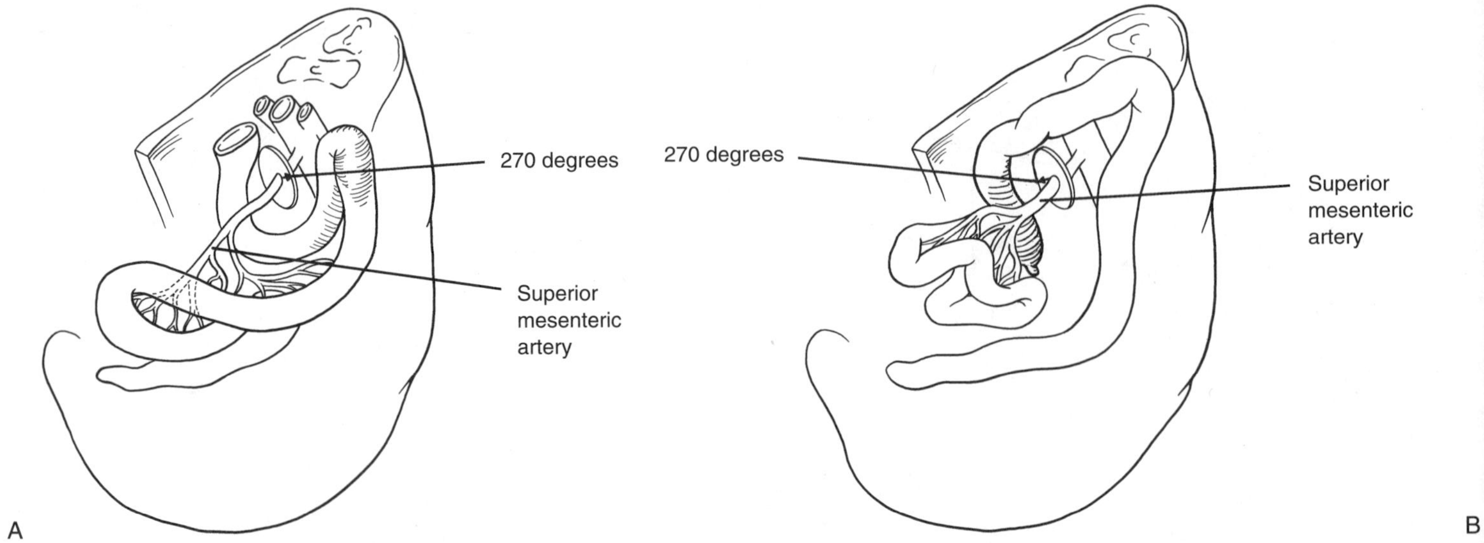

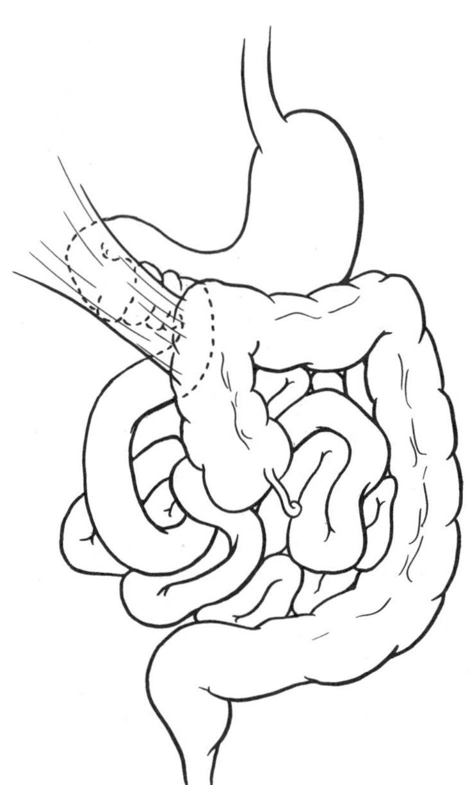

FIG. 75-3. Completed rotation of the midgut in the human embryo. (*A*) Final position of the duodenojejunal junction. Its starting point was directly ventral to the superior mesentery artery (SMA), and, after a 270-degree counterclockwise rotation, lies to the left of the SMA. (*B*) Final position of the cecum. Its starting point was directly dorsal to the SMA, and, after a 270-degree counterclockwise rotation, lies to the right of the SMA.

FIG. 75-4. Complete nonrotation of the midgut. Neither the duodenojejunal junction nor the cecum has rotated around the SMA. All of the small bowel lies to the right of the SMA, and all of the colon lies to the left. The anomaly is the most frequent type of malrotation, and the risk for midgut volvulus is ever present.

occur, the duodenum is truncated, anterior, and often has a corkscrew configuration, all to the right of the midline. This may cause intrinsic partial duodenal obstruction. There may be no fixation of the bowel, and this predisposes the patient to midgut volvulus. The duodenum and colon are fused typically with a common mesentery around the SMA, and this is the pedicle that the midgut twists around. In the normal circumstance, there is a broad-based attachment of the intestinal mesentery, from the ligament of Treitz in the left upper quadrant to the cecum in the right lower quadrant. It is difficult for the mesentery and intestine to undergo axial rotation with normal fixation. In contrast, if the proximal jejunum and distal ileum are both tethered in the mid-abdomen, there is a relatively narrow point of fixation, and the affected intestine can undergo volvulus. This midgut volvulus can completely obstruct the blood supply to the bowel involved.

Rotational Abnormalities of the Duodenojejunal Limb

Nonrotation of the duodenojejunal limb followed by normal rotation and fixation of the cecocolic limb results in duodenal obstruction caused by mesenteric bands from the colon (Fig. 75-5). In this anomaly, the risk for midgut volvulus is low since there is a relatively broad mesenteric base between the duodenojejunal junction and the cecum.

Reverse rotation of the duodenojejunal limb results in the duodenum lying anterior to the SMA rather than in its usual posterior position. If the cecocolic limb also undergoes reverse rotation, the mid-transverse colon lies posterior to the SMA (Fig. 75-6) and creates the potential for colon obstruction. If, on the other hand, the cecocolic limb rotates normally, a right mesenteric pouch (or paraduodenal hernia) is produced (Fig. 75-7). The hernia sac is produced by the mesentery of the right colon as it rotates from the left upper quadrant to the right lower quadrant, passing anterior to the SMA and covering over the duodenojejunal limb of intestine.

Incomplete rotation of the duodenojejunal limb results in the duodenojejunal junction (ligament of Treitz) lying inferior to its usual position in the left upper quadrant. The risk of midgut volvulus may be present if the cecocolic limb is abnormally rotated. The distinction between complete nonrotation of the duodenojejunal limb and incomplete rotation is arbitrary, but the former should be assumed if the ligament of Treitz is anywhere on the right side of midline.

Rotational Abnormalities of the Cecocolic Limb

Even with normal rotation of the duodenojejunal limb, nonrotation of the cecocolic limb has the same potential for midgut volvulus as complete nonrotation (Fig. 75-8). The same type of narrow mesenteric base between the ligament of Treitz and cecum is present, with the SMA running between these two structures.

Incomplete rotation of the cecocolic limb may lead to problems with subsequent fixation of the colon. Incomplete fixation of the hepatic flexure may result in partial obstruction of the duodenum caused by peritoneal bands extending from the colon to the abdominal wall of the right upper quadrant. Incomplete fixation of the cecum may allow for a cecal volvulus to occur.

ASSOCIATED ANOMALIES

Nonrotation or incomplete rotation of the midgut is an important component of congenital diaphragmatic hernia and the ab-

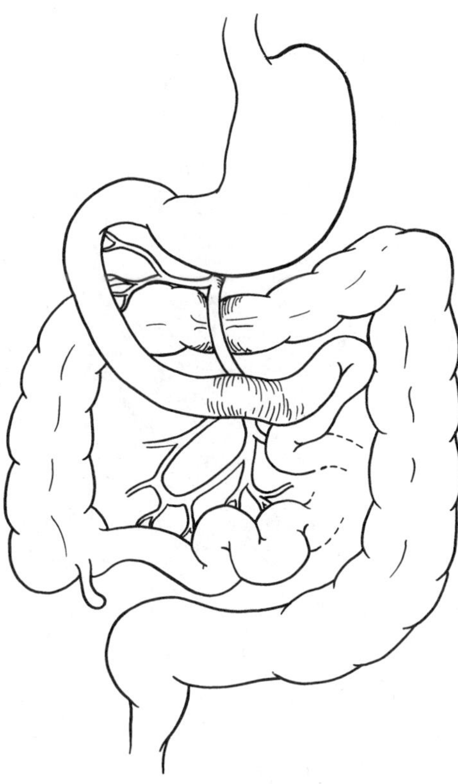

FIG. 75-6. Reverse rotation of the duodenojejunal junction passing ventral rather than dorsal to the superior mesentery artery [SMA]) followed by reverse rotation of the colon (the cecum rotating dorsal rather than ventral to the SMA). This may present clinically as obstruction of the transverse colon.

dominal wall defects: omphalocele and gastroschisis. Other associated conditions are reported to occur in 30% to 62% of patients with malrotation[4–6] and most often are related to the gastrointestinal tract. As many as 50% of patients with duodenal atresia and one third of those with jejunoileal atresia have associated malrotation.[7] One mechanism for this association with jejunal–ileal atresias may be an in utero volvulus with interruption of the mesenteric blood supply and creation of an atresia. Other anomalies include Meckel diverticulum, duodenal web or stenosis, Hirschsprung disease, imperforate anus, esophageal atresia with tracheoesophageal fistula, congenital short gut, biliary atresia, the prune-belly syndrome, cardiac anomalies, situs inversus, and mesenteric cysts. Additional gastrointestinal anomalies such as pyloric stenosis[8] and abnormalities of the gallbladder and extrahepatic biliary system[9] have been described. Familial occurrence of malrotation has been reported,[10] and the association with craniofacial and limb abnormalities[11] has raised the suggestion of a common genetic link.[12]

CLINICAL MANIFESTATIONS

Malrotation can manifest in several ways:

- midgut volvulus
- Duodenal obstruction (partial or intermittent)
- Bilious emesis

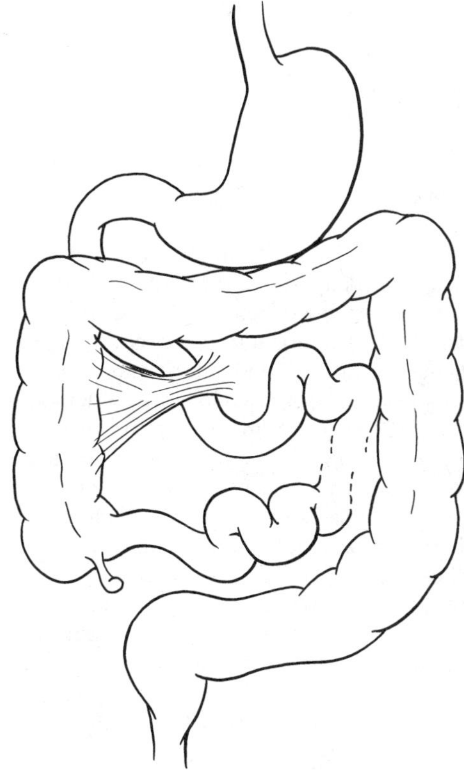

FIG. 75-5. Nonrotation of the duodenojejunal junction with normal rotation of the cecum. This may present clinically as duodenal obstruction from abnormal mesenteric (Ladd) bands from the colon across the anterior duodenum.

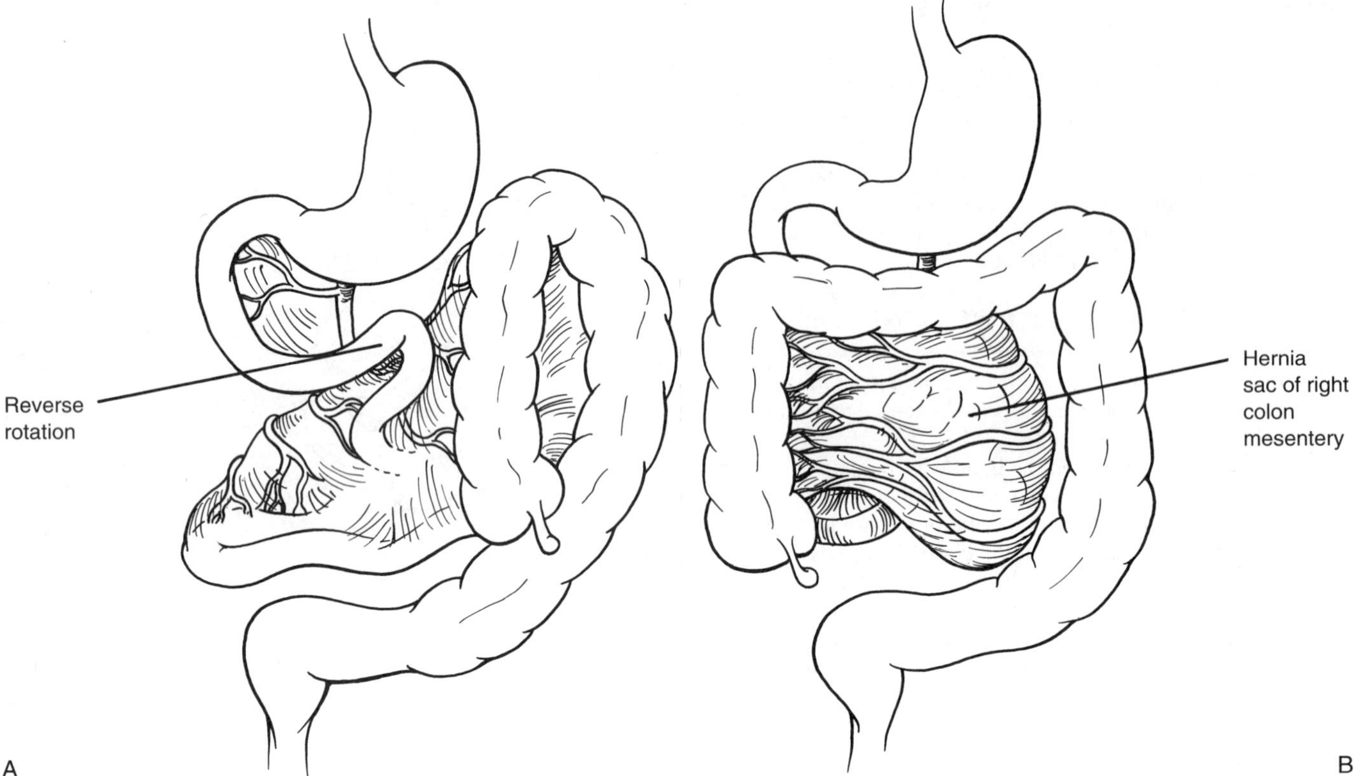

FIG. 75-7. (*A*) Reverse rotation of the duodenojejunal junction (passing ventral rather than dorsal to the superior mesenteric artery [SMA]) followed by normal rotation of the colon. (*B*) A paraduodenal hernia sac is created by the mesentery of the colon as the cecum passes over the small intestine to lie in the right lower quadrant.

- Abdominal pain
- Weight loss or failure to thrive
- Early satiety
- Intermittent diarrhea or blood per rectum
- Asymptomatic

The main symptoms may be grouped together as those related to (1) volvulus, (2) duodenal obstruction, (3) intermittent or chronic abdominal pain, or (4) as an incidental finding in an otherwise asymptomatic patient. Whereas most patients present before 1 year of age[4–6,13,14] (Fig. 75-9), malrotation may be clinically silent until adulthood. Bilious emesis should be assumed to be malrotation until proven otherwise in a child younger than 1 year of age.

Volvulus

Midgut volvulus is a true surgical emergency since delay in operative correction is associated with a high risk of intestinal necrosis and subsequent short bowel or death (Fig. 75-10). The sudden appearance of bilious emesis in a newborn is the classic presentation. Bilious emesis may result from duodenal obstruction caused by the volvulus itself, kinking of the duodenum, or aberrant peritoneal bands (Ladd bands). Whereas bilious emesis frequently results from other causes such as ileus, sepsis, or increased intracranial pressure from hemorrhage, the clinician must expeditiously exclude malrotation as the cause. Observing

the child with bilious emesis while awaiting clinical signs of intestinal strangulation to develop is unacceptable. Once clinical signs of intestinal compromise appear, the ability to salvage the patient or any significant length of small bowel diminishes substantially.

In addition to bilious emesis, the child may have gastric or abdominal distention, dehydration, and irritability. As the intestine begins to strangulate, the patient can become lethargic and develop septic shock. Additional findings may include abdominal wall erythema, peritonitis, and the development of acidosis, thrombocytopenia, and either leukocytosis or leukopenia. Also, hematemesis, melena, or both may result from mucosal ischemia.

Midgut volvulus may be incomplete or intermittent. Typically, patients are older and complain of chronic abdominal pain, intermittent episodes of emesis (which may be nonbilious), early satiety, weight loss, failure to thrive, or malabsorption and diarrhea.[15,16] With partial volvulus, the resultant mesenteric venous and lymphatic obstruction may impair nutrient absorption and produce protein loss into the gut lumen as well as mucosal ischemia and melena as a result of arterial insufficiency.

Duodenal Obstruction

Obstruction of the duodenum may occur as a result of incomplete rotation or nonrotation of the duodenojejunal limb around the SMA. The resultant duodenal position allows for a kinked

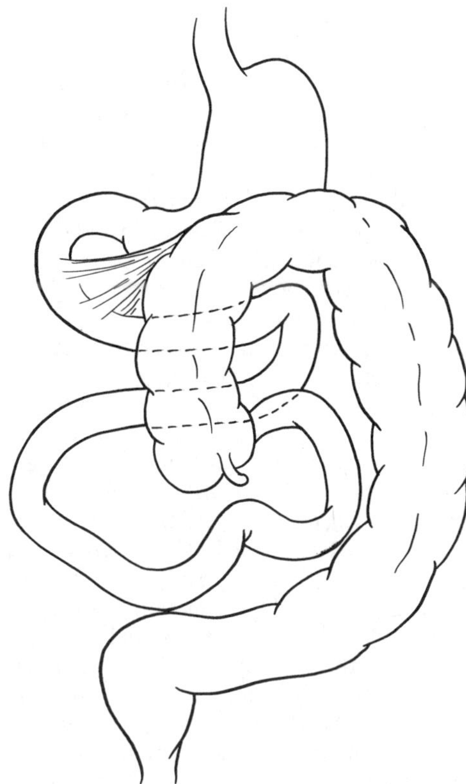

FIG. 75-8. Normal rotation of the duodenojejunal junction with nonrotation of the cecum.These patients are at risk for midgut volvulus.

and tortuous duodenum vulnerable to intermittent obstruction. Additionally, obstruction can result from the congenital bands (Ladd bands) extending from the ascending colon to the posterior parietal peritoneum in the right upper quadrant coursing anterior to the duodenum. These bands may cause extrinsic compression and obstruction of the duodenum. Bilious emesis, abdominal pain or both may be the hallmark of this problem. Occasionally, the emesis may be nonbilious.

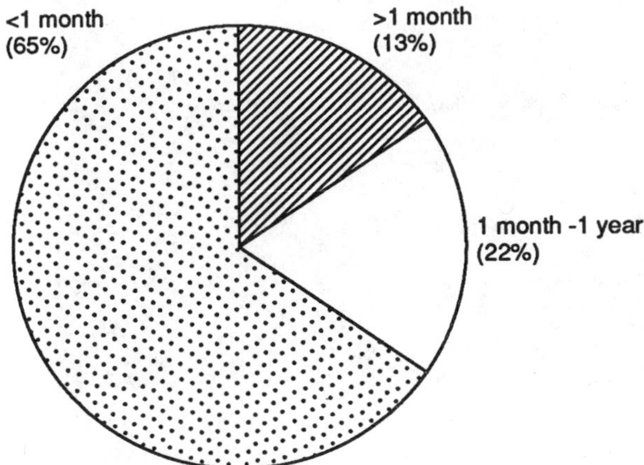

FIG. 75-9. Age distribution of time of clinical presentation of malrotation. Data are compiled from several series, including 527 patients.[8–10,17,18]

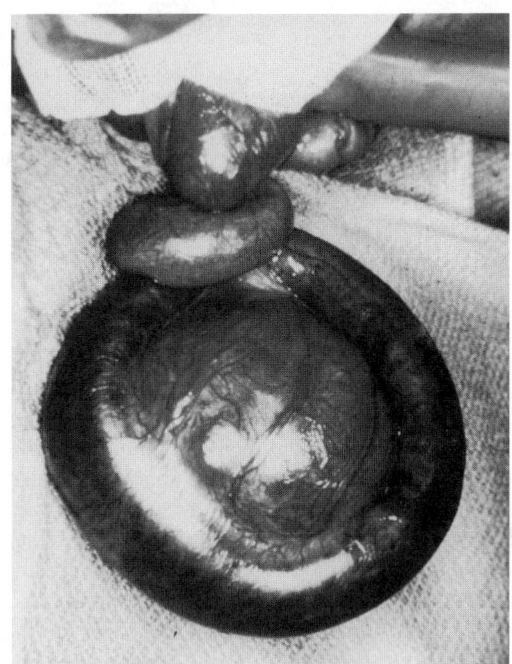

FIG. 75-10. Classic presentation of midgut volvulus.

Intermittent or Chronic Abdominal Pain

The causes of abdominal pain in patients with malrotation are multiple and often coexist. Distention of the bowel produces crampy abdominal pain with vomiting and may occur as a consequence of intermittent volvulus or obstruction from other causes. Partial or intermittent occlusion of the mesenteric venous and lymphatic systems causes edema of the bowel wall, mesentery, and mesenteric lymph nodes. All are potential causes of pain. Chronic arterial insufficiency caused by a partial volvulus may result in diarrhea, chronic pain, worsening pain after meals (intestinal angina), or melena as a result of mucosal ischemia.

Asymptomatic Patient

Malrotation may be discovered as an incidental finding during operation for unrelated reasons or after radiographic contrast administration into the upper or lower GI tract. Midgut volvulus may arise from either complete nonrotation of the both the duodenojejunal and cecocolic limbs or with normal rotation of the duodenojejunal limb and nonrotation of the cecocolic limb. The main anatomic abnormality for both situations is the presence of a narrow mesenteric pedicle that allows for volvulus to occur.

Although midgut volvulus most commonly occurs during infancy and early childhood, it may occur at any age, even into late adulthood. It is impossible to determine which patients with the above two types of malrotation will remain asymptomatic for the duration of their lifetime and which will develop midgut volvulus. Since the consequences of midgut volvulus (need for immediate surgical intervention, short gut syndrome, or death) are potentially so devastating, all patients who are identified to have rotation anomalies known to progress to midgut volvulus should undergo operative correction.

DIAGNOSIS

The preoperative evaluation of malrotation–midgut volvulus is radiologic and includes plain abdominal radiographs and contrast evaluation of either the upper or lower gastrointestinal tract, or occasionally both.

Plain Abdominal Radiography

Any newborn with bilious emesis should undergo urgent imaging evaluation consisting initially of anteroposterior flat and lateral decubitus abdominal radiographs. The plain radiographic findings of malrotation–midgut volvulus are of several general patterns. The first is gastric outlet obstruction. A dilated gastric air bubble is observed and there may be a paucity of distal gas. Duodenal obstruction also may be evident, and the typical ''double-bubble'' sign may be present. These two radiographic patterns are infrequently seen. Normal abdominal radiographs in an infant with bilious emesis do not exclude the diagnosis of malrotation and therefore definitive emergent evaluation is required. Patients with midgut volvulus can have a totally non-specific or normal bowel gas pattern on abdominal plain radiographs. There may be radiographic evidence of a complete small bowel obstruction with multiple dilated loops of bowel with air : fluid levels. This may be associated with intestinal compromise. In patients with plain radiographs demonstrating of bowel obstruction, no further radiographic evaluation is needed. Operative exploration should proceed expeditiously.

Upper Gastrointestinal Series

The upper GI contrast series remains the standard examination when the diagnosis of malrotation is suspected. Barium is considered the contrast agent of choice although water-soluble agents may be used. Little useful information is gained by instilling contrast into a nasogastric tube on the ward and following its progress by serial plain radiographs of the abdomen. The study should be done in the radiology department by a trained radiologist using fluoroscopy. In cases of volvulus, the site of obstruction is typically in the second or third portion of the duodenum and has the appearance of a ''bird's beak'' (Fig. 75-11*A*). If the duodenum is partially obstructed, a spiral or corkscrew configuration may be present (see Fig. 75-11*B*).

In patients with malrotation but without volvulus, the upper GI series is important to document the position of the duodenojejunal junction (ligament of Treitz). The normal position of the duodenojejunal junction is to the left of the spine at the level of the gastric antrum fixed tightly to the posterior body wall. In patients with malrotation, the duodenojejunal junction does not normally rotate around the SMA and is therefore found on the right side of the spine, inferior to the duodenal bulb, and more anterior than expected. Dilated, fluid-filled loops of bowel not evident on plain radiographs may displace the duodenojejunal junction inferiorly and thus mimic malrotation. If this is of concern, further evaluation using a contrast enema to determine the location of the cecum may be indicated. Other findings include all loops of the proximal jejunum on the right side of the abdomen (Fig. 75-12).

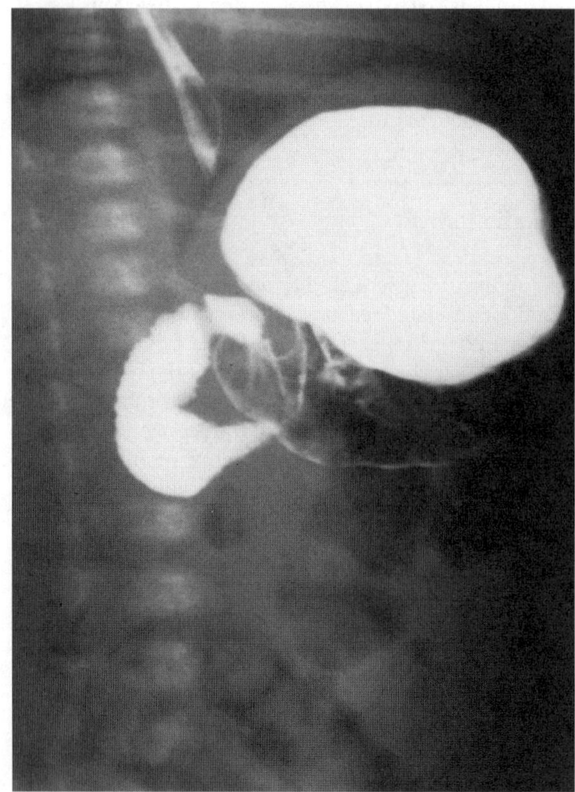

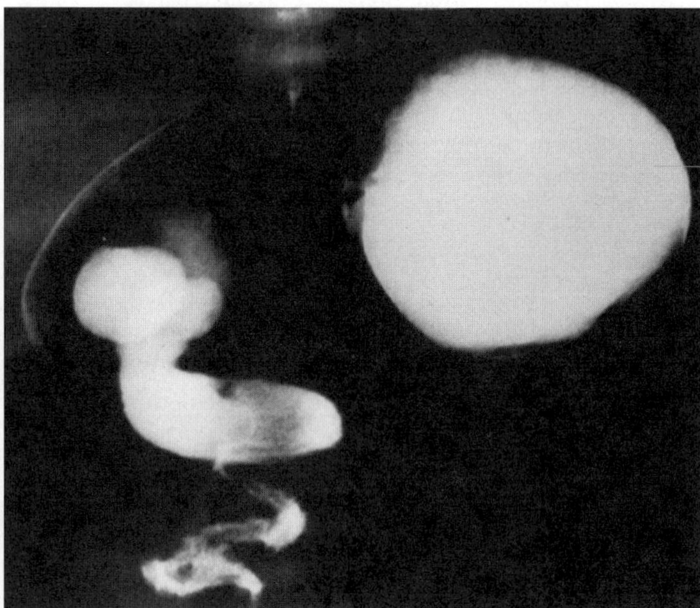

FIG. 75-11. Upper gastrointestinal contrast study in a neonate presenting with bilious emesis and found to have midgut volvulus at laparotomy. Complete obstruction of the duodenum may be observed, with a typical bird's beak configuration at the point of obstruction. (*B*) Corkscrew appearance of the duodenum can be seen in malrotation.

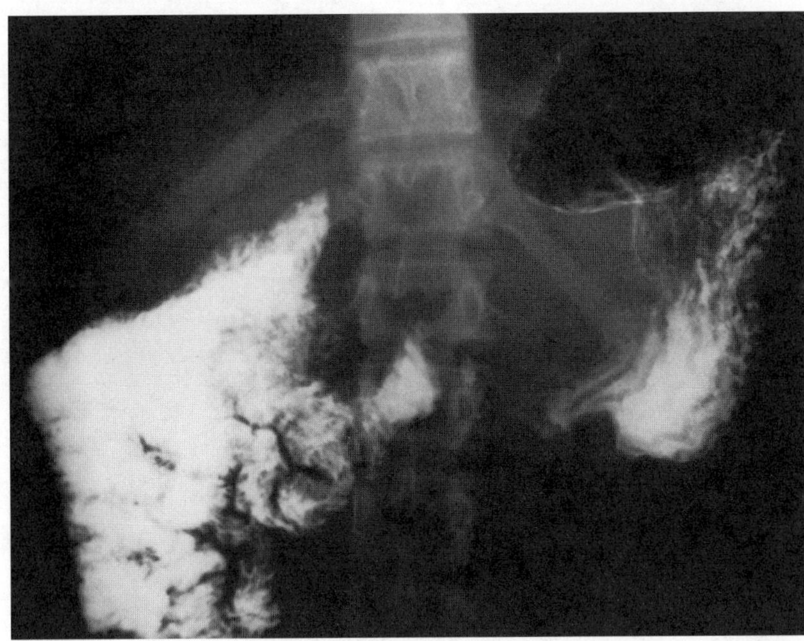

FIG. 75-12. Upper gastrointestinal contrast study of a patient with nonrotation. All of the small bowel is on the right side of the abdomen.

Barium Enema

Although the barium enema has been considered the procedure of choice for the diagnosis of malrotation, its limitations make the upper GI series preferable. The first limitation is that a high and mobile cecum (that suggests malrotation) is found in about 15% of normal infants without malrotation. The spot-film identification of the cecum may be difficult in infants because of the redundancy of the colon. Finally, and more important, duodenal obstruction caused by malrotation may occur in the presence of a normally positioned cecum.

With these limitations in mind, the findings of malrotation by contrast enema include the entire colon within the left abdomen (as seen in complete nonrotation), and an abnormally short ascending colon with the cecum positioned above the right iliac wing.

Ultrasound

Ultrasonography has emerged as an important noninvasive method to evaluate the infant with emesis to exclude the diagnosis of pyloric stenosis. Additional information regarding the orientation of the superior mesenteric vessels also can be obtained by ultrasound and may be useful in suggesting the diagnosis of malrotation. Normally, the superior mesenteric vein (SMV) lies to the right of the SMA. If the SMV lies either anterior or to the left of the SMA, malrotation may be present.

Unfortunately, ultrasonography has not proven to be completely accurate in the diagnosis of malrotation. In one study of nine patients with surgically proven malrotation, abnormal mesenteric vessels were identified in only six.[17] In another study of 249 patients who underwent ultrasonography to exclude pyloric stenosis, abnormal vessel orientation was detected in 9.[18] In 5 patients, the SMV was on the left side of the SMA and all had malrotation. In the other 4 patients, the SMV was ventral to the SMA and 1 had malrotation. Since malrotation may be present in patients with normal mesenteric vessel orientation and abnormal vessel orientation may not be associated with malrotation, ultrasonography must be considered to be suboptimal as a screening tool or definitive test for the diagnosis of malrotation. Its role may be confined to suggesting the need for further evaluation in a vomiting child referred for ultrasonography in whom pyloric stenosis has been ruled out.

MANAGEMENT

In an acutely ill child with midgut volvulus or obstruction, urgent operative correction is indicated and intravenous fluid resuscitation, placing a nasogastric tube and Foley catheter, typing and crossmatching blood, and giving broad-spectrum antibiotics must be done concurrently and expeditiously. Time is critical in terms of intestinal salvage.

In the patient in whom malrotation has been radiographically established but who is asymptomatic, the urgency for operative correction is somewhat lessened. Since it is unpredictable as to when and if a patient with malrotation will develop midgut volvulus, the operation need not be performed emergently. Early operation in neonates seems to be justified. Older children with intermittent symptoms over a prolonged period of time are at lower risk for developing a volvulus within a few days after diagnosis. An operation can be reasonably done electively in this situation.

Operative Technique

The operative technique for the management of midgut volvulus and malrotation involves six principles. The incision generally is made transversely in the right upper quadrant and key elements of the intra-abdominal procedure are diagrammatically illustrated in Figure 75-13.

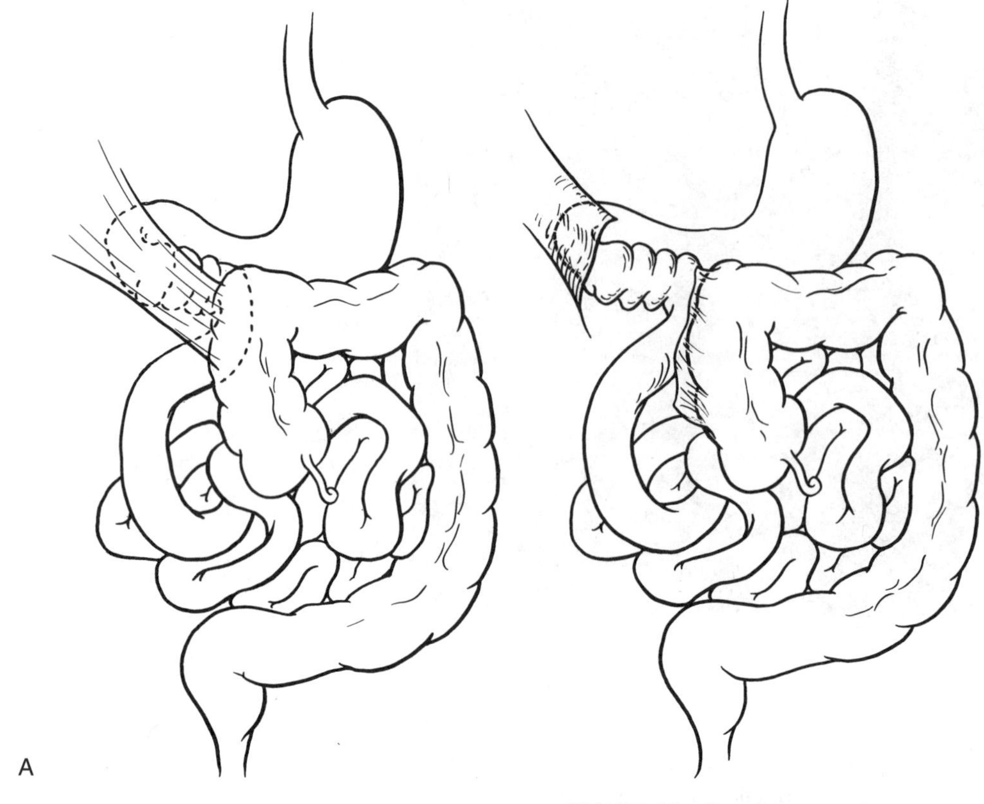

A

B

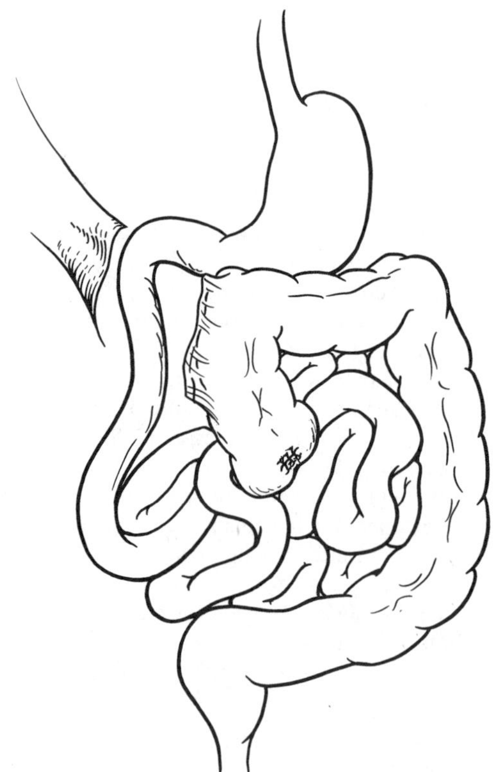

C

FIG. 75-13. Operative repair of malrotation of the intestine. The approach is through a right upper quadrant transverse incision. The entire intestine is eviscerated, and if volvulus is encountered, it is untwisted in a counterclockwise direction. (*A*) This maneuver demonstrates Ladd bands extending from the right colon across the duodenum and attaching to the posterior parietal peritoneum in the right upper quadrant. This component of the duodenal obstruction is relieved by division of the bands along the anterolateral aspect of the duodenum (generous Kocher maneuver). (*B*) A second component of duodenal obstruction is treated by unkinking the duodenum. The colon is separated from the medial aspect of the duodenum and a broad-based mesentery centered about the superior mesenteric artery is created. All adhesions between leaves of the mesentery are divided. The superior mesenteric vessels lie at the base of these bands and must be preserved during the dissection. An incidental appendectomy is then performed, and the small bowel is returned to the right of the abdomen with the colon resting on the left (*C*).

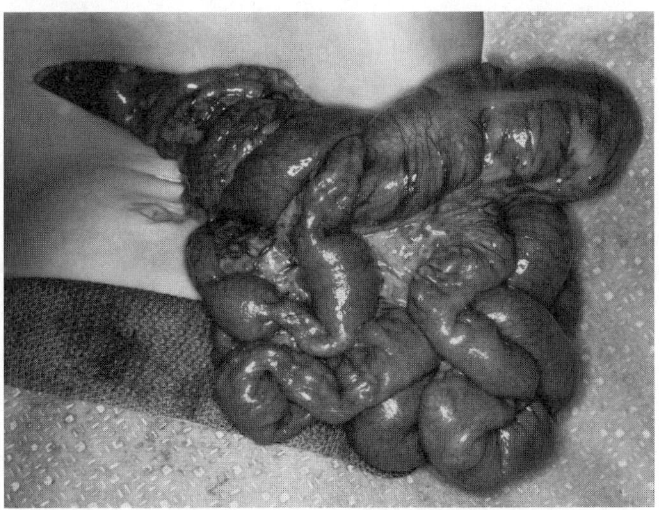

FIG. 75-14. Intraoperative view of midgut volvulus. The proximal jejunum and colon are rotated around the axis of the superior mesenteric vessels in a clockwise direction.

Evisceration

On entering the peritoneal cavity, the entire bowel should be immediately eviscerated to identify the presence or absence of volvulus (Fig. 75-14), to consider obstruction from other causes, to note the position of the cecum, and to enable safe performance of the subsequent steps of the procedure. Cloudy or turbid peritoneal fluid may be encountered and may be chyle as a result of the lymphatic obstruction induced by the volvulus. Alternatively, it may reflect bacterial contamination and purulence from ischemic or necrotic bowel. Peritoneal fluid cultures should be obtained.

Reduction Detorsion of the Volvulus

If no volvulus is encountered, the subsequent steps for correction of the malrotation are undertaken (see later). In most cases, the volvulus twists in a clockwise direction (as viewed from the surgeon's perspective looking down onto the abdomen). The direction of detorsion is therefore counterclockwise. It is helpful to remember the phrase ''turning back the hands of time'' when looking down on the twisted bowel. After detorsion, the intestine may be congested, edematous, and some areas may appear necrotic. Placement of warm sponges and observation for a period of time may improve the appearance of the intestine where the vascular integrity has been compromised. If areas of the bowel are obviously necrotic, resection with creation of one or more stomas is performed. Since as much intestine should be preserved as possible, marginal or questionable segments of bowel should be left in place and a second-look procedure performed within 24 to 36 hours.

Division of Ladd Bands

If Ladd bands are present, they can cause extramural compression of the duodenum and recurrent obstruction. The bands must be lysed completely and on both lateral and medial aspects of the duodenum. To lyse the lateral bands, a generous Kocher maneuver is performed and all bands should be divided to the level of the portal triad superiorly and to the duodenojejunal junction inferiorly. The medial bands then are lysed between the duodenum and the ascending colon.

Widening of Mesenteric Base

The base of the mesentery in patients with malrotation is formed by the SMA running through the space between the duodenum and ascending colon. This mesenteric base is narrow and forms a pedicle on which the midgut can twist. In dividing the bands on the medial aspect of the duodenum, the separation between the duodenum and ascending colon is increased. With further sharp and blunt dissection to separate these structures, the base is maximally broadened such that the tendency to volvulus is lessened. Adhesions generally are present between the leaves of the mesentery, and these should be divided. Although it has been suggested that the cecum and duodenum should be surgically secured into an anatomically normal position,[19] long-term evaluation does not demonstrate any benefit for this.[20]

Relief of Duodenal Obstruction

The duodenum may have a corkscrew configuration from adhesions. This should be fully corrected for the entire length of the duodenum. The entire duodenum from the pylorus to the proximal jejunum should be visualized, with no areas of obstruction observed. If there is significant concern, a Foley or Fogarty embolectomy catheter may be passed through the mouth and advanced beyond the pylorus into the distal duodenum. The balloon is then blown up and the catheter withdrawn into the stomach. Alternatively, the Foley catheter can be introduced via a gastrotomy. This also eliminates the unusual but important possibility of an intrinsic duodenal obstruction. In a child with failure to thrive or known feeding problems, or if a significant amount of intestine must be resected, consideration should be given to placing a gastrostomy tube. It is not necessary in most cases.

Incidental Appendectomy

The cecum ultimately lies on the left side of the abdomen after the Ladd procedure. The potential for diagnostic confusion is great if appendicitis develops at a later date. Incidental appendectomy should therefore be performed. Inversion appendectomy may be performed so that there is no entry into the intestinal tract. The intestine should be replaced into the abdominal cavity with the small bowel lying on the right side while the colon is positioned on the left. Because of the manipulation of the intestine, a paralytic ileus is to be expected and a nasogastric tube generally is required for 1 to 2 days postoperatively.

RESULTS

The mortality rate for the operative correction of malrotation is ranges from 3% to 9%[14,21,22] and is increased in patients with volvulus, intestinal necrosis, prematurity, and the presence of other abnormalities.[21,22] Survival has improved because of the advent of refined pediatric surgical intensive care and parenteral and enteral nutritional support. Further, early diagnosis, heightened awareness of the significance of the presence of a volvulus or rotational anomaly, and urgency in management are the most important factors contributing to favorable outcome.

COMPLICATIONS

Recurrent volvulus is relatively infrequent but should be of prime concern in patients who present with obstructive symptoms at any time postoperatively. Factors contributing to recurrent volvulus include inadequate adhesion formation within the peritoneal cavity to maintain fixation of the small intestine to the right side of the abdomen and the colon on the left, or a mesenteric base that has not been widened sufficiently. The incidence rate of recurrent volvulus has been reported to be between 0% to 10%.[4,20]

GI motility disturbances are common after operative correction of malrotation. Abnormalities characteristic of neuropathic pseudoobstruction raise the possibility of defective intrinsic enteric innervation.[23,24] Other postoperative complications include adhesive bowel obstruction (not caused by volvulus), prolonged ileus, or bleeding related to the operative dissection. Further, the intestine may undergo reperfusion injury after reduction of a significant volvulus. Cytokines, bacteria, and other toxins may be released into the systemic circulation. This may contribute to hemodynamic instability during the intraoperative or early postoperative period.

Finally, midgut volvulus accounts for roughly 18% of cases of short gut syndrome in the pediatric population.[25] Urgent recognition and management of the initial event is the most important factor in preventing this complication.

REFERENCES

1. Byrne WJ. Disorders of the intestines and pancreas. In: Taeusch WH, Ballard RA, Avery ME, eds. Disease of the newborn. Philadelphia, WB Saunders, 1991:685.
2. Skandalakis JE, Gray SW, Ricketts R, et al. The small intestines. In: Skandalakis JE, Gray SW, eds. Embryology for surgeons, ed 2. Baltimore, Williams & Wilkins, 1994:184.
3. Kantor JL. Anomalies of the colon: their roentgen diagnosis and clinical significance. Resumé of 10 years' study. Radiology 1934;23:651.
4. Stewart DR, Colodny AL, Daggett WC. Malrotation of the bowel in infants and children: a 15 year review. Surgery 1976;79:716.
5. Ford EG, Senac MO Jr, Srikanth MS, et al. Malrotation of the intestine in children. Ann Surg 1992;215:172.
6. Filston HC, Kirks DR. Malrotation: the ubiquitous anomaly. J Pediatr Surg 1981;16:614.
7. Smith IE. Malrotation of the intestine. In: Welch KJ, Randolph JG, Ravich MR, et al, eds. Pediatric surgery, ed 4. Chicago, Year Book Medical Publishers, 1986:882.
8. Croitoru D, Neilson I, Guttman FM. Pyloric stenosis associated with malrotation. J Pediatr Surg 1991;26:1276.
9. Campbell KA, Sitzmann JV, Cameron JL. Biliary tract anomalies associated with intestinal malrotation in the adult. Surgery 1993;113:312.
10. Smith SL. Familial midgut volvulus. Surgery 1972;72:420.
11. Barone CM, Marion R, Shanske A, et al. Craniofacial, limb, and abdominal anomalies in a distinct syndrome: relation to the spectrum of Pfeiffer syndrome type 3. Am J Med Genet 1993;45:745.
12. Stalker HJ, Chitayat D. Familial intestinal malrotation with midgut volvulus and facial anomalies: a disorder involving a gene controlling the normal gut rotation? Am J Med Genet 1992;44:46.
13. Kiesewetter WB, Smith JW. Malrotation of the midgut in infancy and childhood. Arch Surg 1958;77:483.
14. Andrassy RJ, Mahour GH. Malrotation of the midgut in infants and children. Arch Surg 1981;116:158.
15. Spigland N, Brandt ML, Yazbeck S. Malrotation presenting beyond the neonatal period. J Pediatr Surg 1990;25:1139.
16. Powell DM, Othersen HB, Smith CD. Malrotation of the intestines in children: the effect of age on presentation and therapy. J Pediatr Surg 1989;24:777.
17. Zerin JM, DiPietro MA. Superior mesenteric vascular anatomy at US in patients with surgically proved malrotation of the midgut. Radiology 1992;183:693.
18. Weinberger E, Winters WD, Liddell RM, et al. Sonographic diagnosis of intestinal malrotation in infants: importance of the relative positions of the superior mesenteric vein and artery. Am J Radiol 192;159:825.
19. Brennom WS, Bill AH. Prophylactic fixation of the intestine for midgut nonrotation. Surg Gynecol Obstet 1974;138:181.
20. Stauffer UG, Herrmann P. Comparison of late results in patients with corrected intestinal malrotation with and without fixation of the mesentery. J Pediatr Surg 1980;15:9.
21. Rescorla FJ, Shedd FJ, Grosfeld JL, et al. Anomalies of intestinal rotation in childhood: analysis of 447 cases. Surgery 1990;108:710.
22. Messineo A, MacMillan JH, Palder SB, et al. Clinical factors affecting mortality in children with malrotation of the intestine. J Pediatr Surg 1992;27:1343.
23. Coombs RC, Buick RG, Gornall PG, et al. Intestinal malrotation: the role of small intestinal dysmotility in the cause of persistent symptoms. J Pediatr Surg 1991;26:553.
24. Devane SP, Smith VV, Bisset WM, et al. Persistent gastrointestinal symptoms after correction of malrotation. Arch Dis Child 1992;67:218.
25. Warner BW, Ziegler MM. Management of the short bowel syndrome in the pediatric population. Pediatr Clin North Am 1993;40:1335.

Surgery of Infants and Children: Scientific Principles and Practice, edited by Keith T. Oldham, Paul M. Colombani, and Robert P. Foglia. Lippincott–Raven Publishers, Philadelphia, © 1997.

CHAPTER 76

Intussusception

Daniel P. Doody

Intussusception, the invagination of the intestine into an adjoining intestinal lumen, is among the most common causes of acute abdominal pain in children younger than 5 years of age. It is a disease primarily of infants and toddlers, although intussusception can occur in utero, in neonates, and in adults. Eighty to 90% of cases of intussusception occur in children between 3 months and 3 years of age.

PATHOGENESIS

The pathogenesis of intussusception has been ascribed to an inhomogeneity of longitudinal forces along the intestinal wall. In the resting state, normal propulsive forces meet a certain resistance at any point. This stable equilibrium can be disrupted when a portion of the intestine does not appropriately promulgate peristaltic waves. Small perturbations provided by contraction of the circular muscle perpendicular to the axis of longitudinal tension result in a kink in the abnormal portion of the intestine, creating a rotary force (torque). Distortion may continue, in-folding the area of inhomogeneity and eventually capturing the circumference of the small intestine. This invaginated intestine then acts as the apex of the intussusceptum.[1]

Intramural, intraluminal, or extramural processes may produce points of disequilibrium. Along with anatomic abnormalities, flaccid areas that follow a paralytic ileus also can create unstable segments as adjoining areas create discordant contractions with the return of bowel activity. Such a model offers an explanation as to the cause of postoperative intussusceptions, which rarely are found to have a surgical lead point but can complicate any procedures that produce an ileus, including thoracotomies and cardiac procedures.

PATHOLOGY

On sectioning, the tumor is composed of the internal layer, the returning middle layer, and the outer ensheathing layer (Fig. 76-1). The entering and returning layers, including the adjacent mesentery, are referred to as the *intussusceptum* and include any surgical lead point. The receiving or ensheathing layer is referred to as the *intussuscipiens*. With normal peristalsis, the

length of the intussusception increases, and the cycle of venous congestion, lymphatic obstruction, and eventual arterial compromise is initiated. The vascular supply at the apex of the intussusceptum is the most compromised, and the mucosa of the apex experiences secondary sloughing, resulting in the passage of "red currant jelly" stools.

ETIOLOGY

The most common cause of intussusception is indeterminate and termed *idiopathic*. In the occasional infant who requires surgical reduction, an enlarged Peyer patch often is identified, which may act as an unstable site for the mechanistic forces.

In 2% to 12% of all pediatric cases, the intussusception has an anatomically identifiable lead point. Children with intussusception secondary to surgical lead points usually require operative treatment because the intussusceptum is rarely reduced by pressure reduction. The frequency of lead points as the cause of intussusception increases with age. This is particularly true in children older than 4 years of age, in whom the prevalence of lead points complicating intussusception has been reported as high as 57%.[2] In adults, the incidence of lead points associated with intussusception is as high as 97%.[3] Meckel diverticulum is the most common anatomic lead point identified in children. Other anatomic lead points include polyps of the ileum and colon, benign hamartomas associated with Peutz-Jeghers syndrome, submucosal hematomas associated with Henoch-Schönlein purpura, lymphoma, lymphosarcoma, enteric cysts ectopic pancreatic and gastric rests, inverted appendiceal stumps, and anastomotic suture lines. In adults, about half of surgical lead points are malignant, and there is a higher incidence of colocolic intussusceptions.

Intussusception is a feature of the gastrointestinal problems associated with cystic fibrosis and Henoch-Schönlein purpura. Together, these medical processes account for 3% to 5% of cases of intussusception.[4]

CLINICAL PRESENTATION

Although intussusception can occur at any age, it is convenient from the clinical perspective to divide these patients into

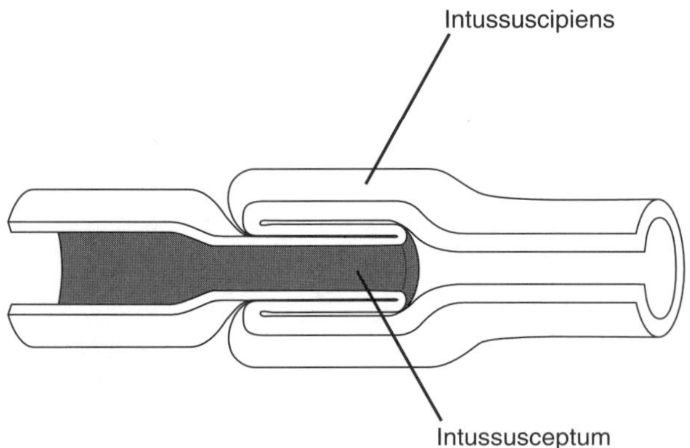

FIG. 76-1. Diagrammatic representation of intussusception.

those occurring in children younger than 3 years of age and those occurring in older children and adults. In children younger than 5 years of age, intussusception accounts for up to 25% of abdominal surgical emergencies, exceeding the incidence of appendicitis. Therefore, the practitioner should always consider intussusception in the evaluation of young children and infants who present with acute abdominal pain.

The typical clinical history is that of a 6 to 2-month-old male infant who suddenly cries out, often drawing his knees up with the abdominal discomfort. Frequently, the child has emesis and often immediately evacuates. The child may appear diaphoretic during the crisis. The abdominal discomfort appears to last briefly, after which the infant is quiet and may appear well. The incident is repetitive, typically occurring in 15- to 30-minute intervals. As time passes, the child may become increasingly ill with abdominal distention, vomiting, and the eventual appearance of red currant jelly stools. With time, shock intervenes, and cardiovascular collapse occurs.

At presentation, the infant often is exhausted and resting quietly. Occasionally and without stimulation, the child may arch and cry out. As the examination begins, the child appears irritable or diaphoretic. Tachycardia or hypotension can be found, even early in the illness, depending on the degree of bowel compromise. Pertinent physical findings are generally confined to the abdomen. A mass may be palpated in the right upper quadrant to mid-abdomen, but this finding may be difficult to appreciate because of the child's irritability. A careful examination of the right lower quadrant shows that the cecum is not palpated in the right iliac fossa (sign of Dance).

Rarely, a cervix-like mass may be seen protruding through the anus. For prolapse of the intussusception to occur, the mesentery is lax, and the progression of the intussusceptum to the rectosigmoid is rapid. The distinction between intussusception and rectal prolapse, an uncommon finding in infants, can often be made by careful examination of the anal crypts at the dentate line. This anatomic landmark is everted in rectal prolapse but is not seen with intussusception. An applicator that passes into the space between the apparent prolapse and the anus is also diagnostic of a prolapsed intussusceptum.

Although hematochezia is not always seen with intussusception, 60% to 90% of children with intussusception have gross or occult blood on rectal examination.[5] Twenty to 50% of infants have passed mucoid, bloody stools (red currant jelly stools), and the remaining infants have occult blood on testing.

The differential diagnosis at presentation includes intestinal colic, gastroenteritis, appendicitis, incarcerated hernia, and more unusual forms of intestinal obstruction, such as internal hernia and volvulus. Radiographic evaluation for the possibility of intussusception begins without establishing intravenous access only if the child is hemodynamically stable.

RADIOGRAPHIC DIAGNOSTIC EVALUATION

Early in the course of the illness, supine and upright abdominal films show a normal or nonspecific bowel gas pattern. As the disease progresses, a more obvious pattern of small bowel obstruction with absence of gas in the colon is noted. The most predictive finding of the disease is the presence of a right upper quadrant soft tissue density, found in 25% to 60% of cases (Fig. 76-2). Other radiographic findings include reduced amount of gas in the jejunum, lateralization of the ileum into the right iliac fossa, indiscernible cecal shadow, and reduced amount of feces in the colon.[6] Even using these radiographic indicators, 50% to 66% of children who undergo a diagnostic enema for suspected intussusception do not have the disease.[7]

Supine cross-table lateral (horizontal-beam) radiographs provide two additional findings that can be helpful in establishing the diagnosis of intussusception.[8] A homogeneous water-density anterior abdominal mass may displace upper abdominal gas inferiorly, or the mass may demonstrate craniocaudal separation into distinct upper and lower bowel gas patterns. One of these

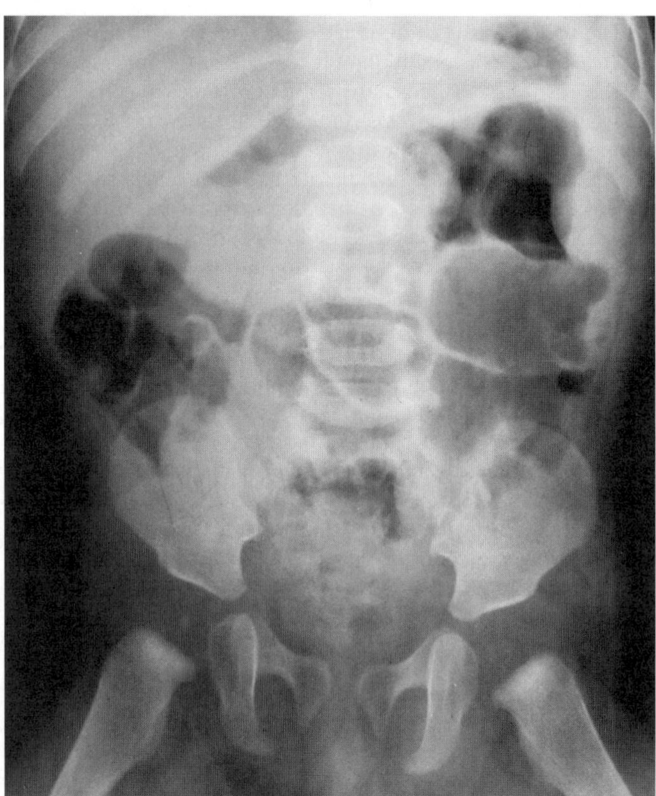

FIG. 76-2. Supine abdominal radiograph showing soft tissue density in right upper quadrant to mid-abdomen. Absence of normal cecal gas shadow can be seen in the right lower quadrant.

two radiographic findings was identified in 75% of intussusceptions in a small series. Others have noted that the intussusceptum may be seen only in this projection and recommend this view as an additional indicator to decide if a diagnostic enema is indicated.[9]

TREATMENT

Often with a clinically suggestive story and nonspecific findings on plain abdominal radiographs, contrast enemas are performed for diagnosis and therapy. Only in children who have clinical peritonitis or radiographic evidence of perforation is an attempt at pressure reduction absolutely contraindicated.

Hydrostatic Reduction

Hydrostatic reduction was proposed by Hirschsprung in 1876 for the treatment of intussusception. The use of contrast enemas allows direct visualization of the reduction under fluoroscopic control and is reported to be successful in 50% to 90% of cases.

A noninflatable rectal tube is inserted in the rectum, and the buttocks are taped to prevent loss of distending pressure. Contrast enters the rectosigmoid by gravity under fluoroscopic guidance. In the usual case, the contrast column meets a concave filling defect in the transverse colon that can be reduced in a retrograde fashion to the cecum.

A radiographic ''rule of threes'' applies to hydrostatic reduction in intussusception to minimize the risk of perforation. The barium contrast column should be no greater than 3 ft above the table (100 cm); each attempt should persist until reduction of the intussusceptum fails to progress for a period of 3 to 5 minutes; and a maximum of three attempts should be made. The purpose of the rule of threes is to prevent the reduction of necrotic bowel while optimizing the care of the infant. Experimentally, hydrostatic columns less than 3.5 ft are unable to reduce gangrenous bowel.[10] At this height, a 60% wt/vol barium suspension generates an intraluminal pressure of 120 mmHg. Dilute water-soluble solutions require a greater height to generate the same intracolonic pressures. A 20% wt/vol meglumine sodium diatrizoate solution (Gastrografin) or 17.2% iothalamate meglumine solution (Cysto-Conray II) achieves an intraluminal pressure of 120 mmHg at a height of 150 cm (5 ft).[11] Because most intussusceptions are reduced within the first two attempts, successful hydrostatic reduction after three attempts is unlikely.[12] The attempted reduction should cease if a progressive reduction of the intussusceptum does not occur after 3 to 5 minutes of constant pressure because the intussusception is unlikely to reduce.

A radiographic finding often associated with irreducible intussusceptions is the dissection sign, which occurs when barium intercalates between the intussusceptum and the intussuscipiens[13] (Fig. 76-3). Although successful reductions of intussusceptions demonstrating this radiographic finding have been reported,[14,15] this feature, coupled with a clinical history greater than 48 hours or radiographic evidence of a complete bowel obstruction, is often associated with intestinal gangrene. Surgery, rather than repeated attempts at hydrostatic reduction, is indicated.

As the intussusceptum is reduced through the ileocecal valve,

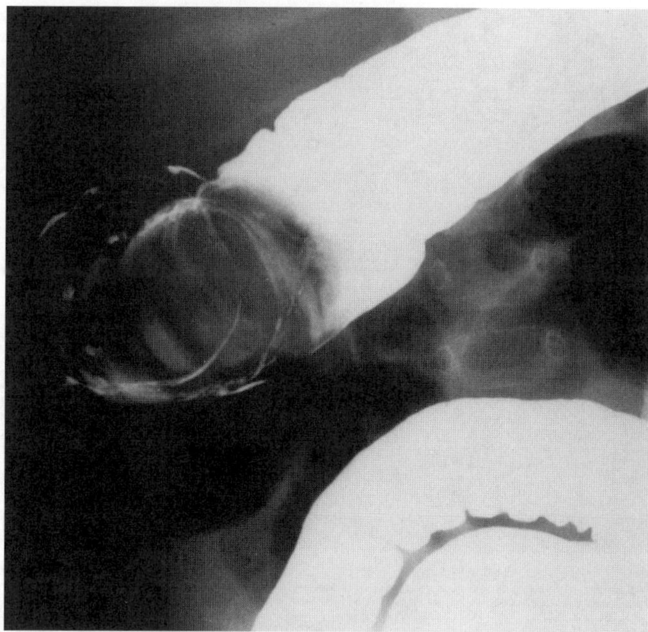

FIG. 76-3. Partial reduction of intussusception demonstrating dissection sign. At surgery, the intussusceptum included a gangrenous Meckel diverticulum as a surgical lead point.

contrast should reflux freely into the small intestine, a radiographic finding considered essential to document a successful reduction. Subtle radiographic features that may indicate an incomplete reduction are complete evacuation of barium without residual contrast in the small intestine and the persistence of small bowel meteorism.

On occasion, inability to reflux into the terminal ileum is ascribed to competency or edema of the ileocecal valve. Some authors propose that observation rather than laparotomy may be appropriate if contrast does not pass into the terminal ileum but the infant becomes asymptomatic. These authors argue that 7% to 20% of intussusceptions are found at laparotomy to be reduced. By reevaluating the stable child after a short period of observation, the morbidity of surgery may be avoided.[16–18]

Ultrasound-Guided Reduction

Ultrasound-guided hydrostatic reduction of intussusception can be performed.[19] Diagnosis of intussusception is established by the ultrasonographic demonstration of target sign on transverse views (Fig. 76-4A) and pseudokidney sign on longitudinal views (see Fig. 76-4B) of the intussusceptum. An enema consisting of saline and water-soluble contrast material (9:1 ratio) is used to reduce the intussusception, and the contrast confirms reflux into the terminal ileum on supine abdominal radiograph. The success rate is comparable to that for pneumatic reduction and may be higher than that for barium enema reduction. Radiographic exposure is lower with ultrasound-guided reduction, and with experienced ultrasonographers, this method may be preferable to fluoroscopically guided reduction. The technique may be limited in those infants with small bowel obstruction because the multiple air–fluid interfaces can interfere with accurate assessment of the reduction.

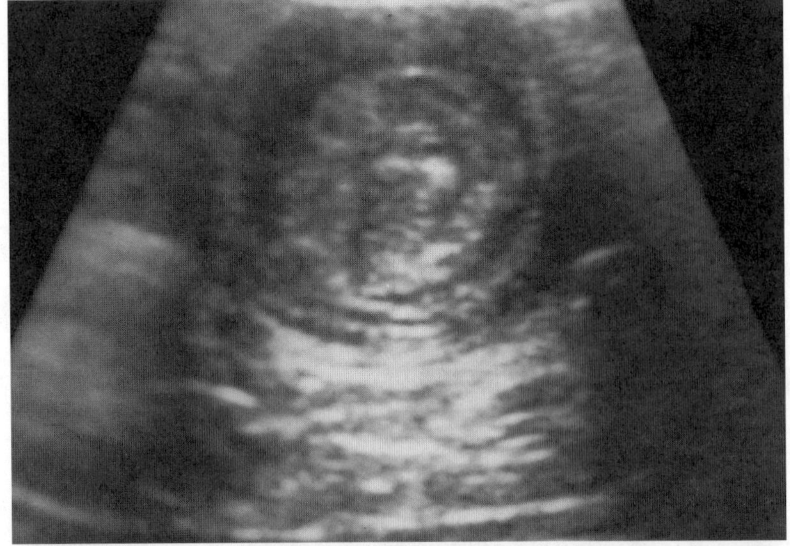

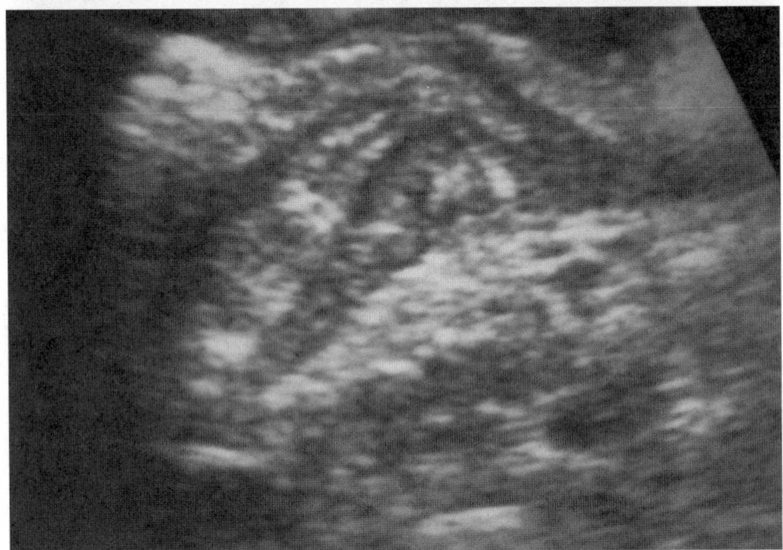

FIG. 76-4. (*A*) Transverse view on ultrasound showing the concentric rings of the intussusceptum within the intussuscipiens (target sign). (*B*) Pseudokidney seen on longitudinal views of the intussusception.

Pneumatic Reduction

Pneumatic reduction of intussusception has been used extensively in China and is receiving increasing acceptance in North America and Western Europe. The contraindications for hydrostatic reduction are equally applicable in evaluating children for pneumatic reduction. If a noninflatable balloon is used for pneumatic reduction, the buttocks are taped firmly to maintain a stable intracolonic pressure to reduce the intussusception (Fig. 76-5). At an initial pressure of 80 mmHg, air is delivered into the colon under fluoroscopic guidance. This pressure can be raised to a maximum of 120 mmHg, equivalent to a 1-M column of barium suspension or a 1.5-M column of a 20% wt/vol meglumine sodium diatrizoate solution. Reflux of air into the terminal ileum signifies complete reduction of the intussusception. Higher rates of reduction are reported with air insufflation (87%) than with hydrostatic reduction (55% to 70%). As the intraluminal pressure is accurately monitored, a more effective mean intracolonic pressure is maintained and may explain the greater success rate with this method.

Technically, the use of air as a contrast medium can be challenging if a small bowel obstruction is present. An additional problem with air reduction is the phenomenon referred to as *pseudoreduction,* whereby air enters the small bowel before complete reduction of the intussusceptum.

Operative Reduction

In children who have clinical evidence of peritonitis or radiographic evidence of perforation, and in those in whom pressure reduction is unsuccessful, surgery is indicated after initiating fluid resuscitation and starting broad-spectrum antibiotic therapy. A right transverse infraumbilical incision is made and carried down through the muscular layers, exposing the right lower quadrant. If necessary, the incision can be extended across the midline to perform a complete evaluation of the abdomen. The intussusception is reduced within the abdomen if possible. As the reduction becomes more difficult, the right colon to the hepatic flexure can be brought into the wound. Warm saline

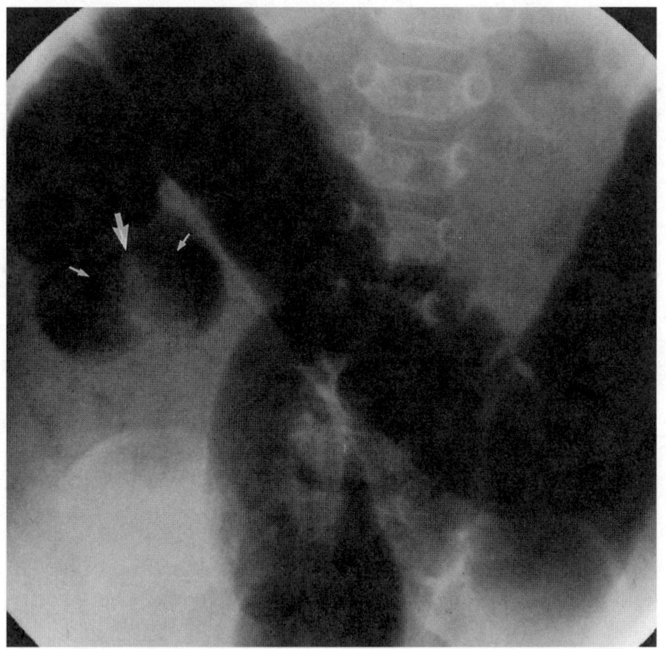

FIG. 76-5. Pneumatic reduction of intussusception to the level of the cecum. Successful reduction was accomplished.

pads are placed around the intussusception, and compression is maintained for 1 to 2 minutes, reducing the tissue edema and facilitating the reduction. The intussusceptum is expressed from the intussuscipiens by placing gentle pressure at the apex of the lesion (Fig. 76-6). The intussusceptum never should be pulled from the intussuscipiens. Traction may disrupt the compromised bowel and force the surgeon to perform resection with anastomosis.

After the intestine is reduced, the bowel is inspected for viability and for surgical lead points. If vascular compromise is a concern 10 to 15 minutes of observation in the operating theater is appropriate before performing a resection. In infants and young children, a large Peyer patch or the ileocecal valve can mimic an intramural or intraluminal mass. Careful palpation of the intestine and awareness of these common findings should prevent unnecessary enterotomies. An incidental appendectomy completes the procedure.

Successful manual reduction can be expected in about 90% of pediatric patients, even if surgical lead points are present. These lead points, if identified, should be removed, and a primary enteroenterostomy should be performed. True irreducibility of the intussusception suggests that gangrenous intestine is present. Even in those instances, a primary resection and anastomosis is appropriate unless the child is so seriously ill that resection and exteriorization are clinically indicated to expedite closure and lessen the anesthetic risk.

Ileocecopexy, suturing the last several centimeters of the terminal ileum to the ascending colon to prevent recurrent intussusception, has not been shown to be beneficial and is no longer recommended. There has been no proven advantage to the additional operative manipulation, and intussusception can occur after ileocecopexy.

Complications

Perforation With Pressure Reduction

In a large international survey,[20] the cumulative incidence of perforation complicating hydrostatic reduction was 0.18%. It remains controversial whether pneumatic reduction is safer than hydrostatic reduction. The incidence of perforation has been higher with pneumatic reduction and varies between 1% and 2.8%. With increasing experience in pneumatic reduction, the incidence of perforation is decreasing.

A more intense inflammatory reaction occurs with the peritonitis complicating a perforation with barium than that seen with water-soluble contrast or air contrast enemas. The mixture of barium and feces can lead to a prolonged septic course. Infants younger than 6 months of age and children with symptoms for longer than 36 hours or with evidence of bowel obstruction are at greater risk for having gangrenous bowel complicating their

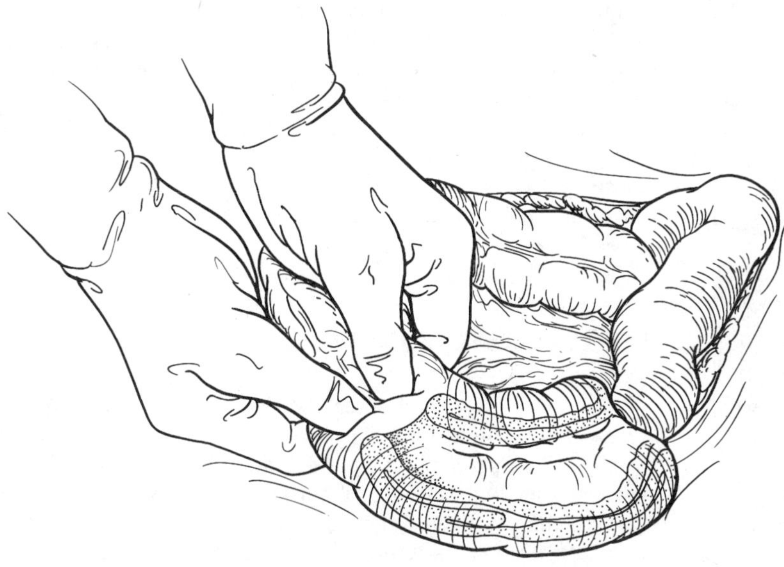

FIG. 76-6. Manual reduction of ileocolic intussusception.

intussusception. They are consequently at greater risk for perforation. If pressure reduction is attempted in these patients, a water-soluble solution or air contrast enema is the more appropriate medium.

Recurrent Intussusception

The rate of recurrent intussusception after successful hydrostatic reduction of intussusception varies between 5% and 11%. Recurrence after surgical reduction is lower but is reported to occur in 1% to 4% of cases. Thirty to 64% of recurrences occur within 72 hours of reduction, although recurrence may occur up to 36 months after successful reduction. Lead points are identified in fewer than 10% of the recurrent cases,[21–23] and hydrostatic or pneumatic reduction is appropriate as the initial treatment (Fig. 76-7).

Celiotomy is indicated for recurrent intussusception only when there is a reasonable expectation of finding a surgical lead point. Children whose presentations place them at greater risk of having an anatomic lead point include those who experience more than one recurrence without prior operation, children older than 3 years of age with recurrences after successful hydrostatic reduction, and children with known intestinal polyposis.[24]

Mortality Rate

Although advances in treatment and increased awareness of the disease have led to a decreased death rate, misdiagnosis, inadequate fluid resuscitation, unrelenting sepsis, and delayed

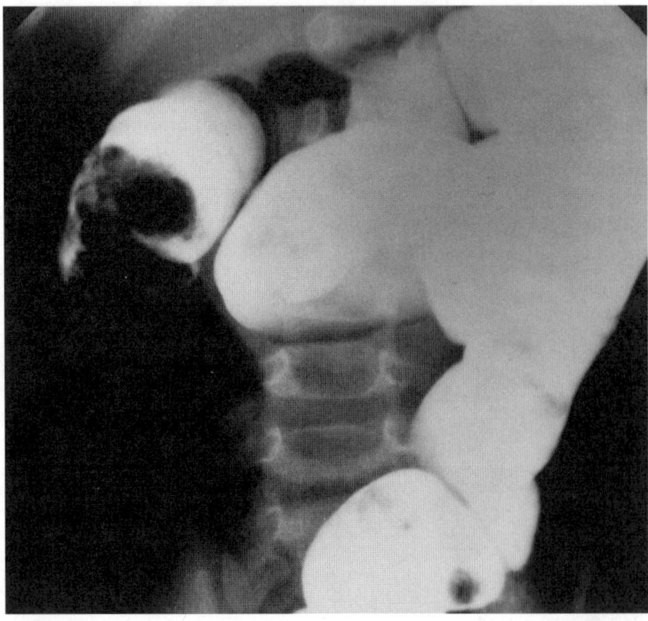

FIG. 76-7. Recurrent intussusception in 22-month-old patient occurring 14 months after uneventful reduction with barium enema. Despite dissection sign of barium around intussusceptum, successful hydrostatic reduction of recurrence was accomplished without surgery.

presentation continue to account for an intussusception-related case-fatality rate of about 1%.[25]

MEDICAL PROCESSES ASSOCIATED WITH INTUSSUSCEPTION

Cystic Fibrosis

Intussusception is among the many intestinal complications associated with cystic fibrosis and occurs in 1% of patients with mucoviscidosis.[26] These children are older than children with idiopathic intussusception, with an average age of 9.75 years (range, 4 to 16 years). The cause of the intussusception is often ascribed to the thick, putty-like material that adheres to the intestinal mucosa. Many times, children with cystic fibrosis who have an intussusception have a chronic and indolent course, and distinguishing among distal intestinal obstruction syndrome (meconium ileus equivalent), an occult appendiceal abscess, and intussusception in a child with cystic fibrosis can be difficult.

Although hydrostatic reduction of intussusception in these patients is possible, operative reduction is required in most cases. Successful manual reduction at laparotomy usually is accomplished, and only rarely is surgical resection required.

Henoch-Schönlein Purpura

Sixty-five percent of patients with Henoch-Schönlein purpura have gastrointestinal symptoms related to the underlying systemic vasculitis.[27] Ninety-five percent of these children have cutaneous manifestations of the disease before the surgical process becomes evident.[28] Abdominal pain and gastrointestinal bleeding are common manifestations of intestinal vasculitis and may mask an intussusception, intestinal necrosis, or perforation. The severity of abdominal pain and the degree of leukocytosis are insignificantly different between patients who have abdominal manifestations of the intestinal vasculitis and those who have surgical complications of the disease.

Intussusception is the most common surgical complication of the disease and occurs in 3% of children with anaphylactoid purpura. In most, if not all, cases, a submucosal hematoma acts as a lead point. Sequential barium enema and upper gastrointestinal series may establish the diagnosis of intussusception, although barium enema reduction is infrequently successful because the lesion typically is enteroenteric and not ileocolic. Surgical reduction of the intussusception is required in most cases.

POSTOPERATIVE INTUSSUSCEPTION

In series from large children's hospitals, postoperative intussusception accounts for 1.5% to 6% of all cases of intussusception.[29,30] The incidence of postoperative intussusception after laparotomy is 0.08% to 0.5%, but this process may complicate cardiac, thoracic, and orthopedic procedures.[31]

After the apparent return of intestinal peristalsis, postoperative intussusception is marked by the gradual appearance of an early bowel obstruction. Abdominal pain is a less prominent symptom, and the most common presenting signs are increasingly bilious nasogastric output and abdominal distention. Unlike adhesive bowel disease, which usually occurs more than 2 weeks after the procedure, obstruction from this form of intussusception occurs early in the postoperative course, on average 8 to 11 days after surgery. The diagnosis of postoperative intussusception infrequently is established by contrast enema, and a contrast meal with small bowel films may identify the obstruction. The intussusception most frequently is located in the small intestine.

The cause of postoperative intussusception is thought to be altered peristalsis due to prolonged or excessive manipulation of the bowel, bruising of the intestine, anesthetic agents, or other neurogenic factors. The higher incidence of postoperative intussusception seen in children who have known dysmotility suggests that abnormal propulsion of the intestine may be an important factor. Lead points from anastomotic suture lines are rarely found.

NONISCHEMIC (CHRONIC) INTUSSUSCEPTION

About 15% of cases of intussusception in children may be described as subacute (symptoms of 4 to 14 days) or chronic (symptoms greater than 14 days).[32,33] Patients with nonischemic intussusception present with recurrent mild to moderate abdominal discomfort and other nonspecific gastrointestinal complaints, including vomiting, diarrhea, rectal bleeding, and failure to thrive. Ischemic compromise of the intussusceptum is found rarely. Abdominal masses are appreciated infrequently in this group.

This nonspecific presentation and frequently normal abdominal examination lead to the common but erroneous diagnosis of gastroenteritis. The presence of a pink mucoid semiloose bowel movement may lead the examiner to suspect the diagnosis of chronic intussusception. Nonischemic intussusception should be included in the differential diagnosis of prolonged cases of vomiting and diarrhea, particularly if stools are positive for occult blood. Awareness of this entity will lead to correct diagnosis, and appropriate therapy can be initiated.

NEONATAL INTUSSUSCEPTION

Neonatal intussusception, with symptoms occurring in the first 30 days of life, is rare.[34] Sixty to 75% of newborn infants who are found to have intussusception are found to have surgical lead points (Fig. 76-8). Once the diagnosis of neonatal intussusception is confirmed, surgery is the preferred treatment option. There is a high incidence of surgical lead points, a low rate of successful enema reduction in small infants,[35,36] and a greater risk of bowel perforation in infants younger than 6 months of age undergoing pressure reduction.[37] Repeated attempts at hydrostatic or pneumatic reduction are not indicated once the diagnosis is established.

INTUSSUSCEPTION IN ADULTS

Intussusception in adults is an unusual problem that may comprise 5% to 15% of all cases of intussusceptions in large

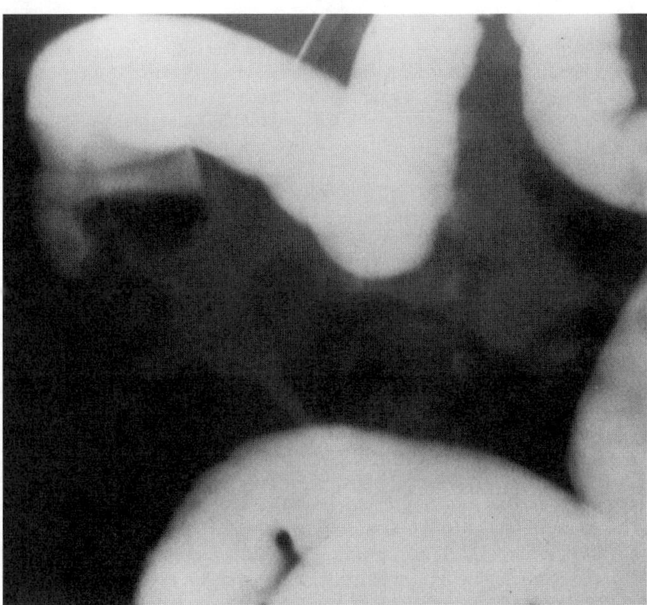

FIG. 76-8. A 6-week-old patient who presented with failure to thrive, feces positive for occult blood, and intermittent symptoms of intestinal obstruction since the first week of life was found to have a nonreducible intussusception with persistent cecal filling defect on contrast enema. At exploration, the infant was found to have a cecal leiomyosarcoma as an intussusception lead point, which was resected.

general hospitals.[3,38] More than 90% of intussusceptions in adults have lead points, and almost half of these lead points are malignant neoplasms. Because of the high associated incidence of surgical lead points, intussusceptions in adults are generally not reducible by air contrast or hydrostatic enemas.

In adults, more than half of colocolic intussusceptions are associated with malignant neoplasms, and primary resection without manual reduction is recommended. Enteroenteric intussusceptions may be associated with postoperative intussusception, congenital anomalies, benign and malignant neoplasms, and enteric tubes passed for feeding. Manual reduction followed by more localized resection is appropriate because the incidence of carcinoma complicating intussusception of the small intestine is low.

In tropical countries, adults account for 40% to 50% of the reported cases of intussusception. Unlike in the United States and Great Britain, most intussusceptions in adults in tropical countries are idiopathic and not related to surgical lead points. This discrepancy has been ascribed to parasitic infestations, amebic ulcers, and diet, but the true cause of tropical intussusception is unknown.

REFERENCES

1. Reymond RD. The mechanism of intussusception: a theoretical analysis of the phenomenon. Br J Radiol 1972;45:1.
2. Ong NT, Beasley SW. The leadpoint in intussusception. J Pediatr Surg 1990;25:640.
3. Pang L-C. Intussusception revisited: clinicopathologic analysis of 261 cases, with emphasis on pathogenesis. South Med J 1989;82:215.
4. West KW, Stephens B, Vane DW, et al. Intussusception: current management in infants and children. Surgery 1987;102:704.

5. Losek JD, Fiete RL. Intussusception and the diagnostic value of testing stool for occult blood. Am J Emerg Med 1991;9:1.
6. Meradji M, Hussain SM, Robben SGF, et al. Plain film diagnosis in intussusception. Br J Radiol 1994;67:147.
7. Eklöf O, Thönell S. Conventional abdominal radiography as a means to rule out ileo-caecal intussusception. Acta Radiol [Diagn] (Stockh) 1984;25:265.
8. Johnson JF, Woisard KK. Ileocolic intussusception: new sign on the supine cross-table lateral radiograph. Radiology 1989;170:483.
9. White SJ, Blane CE. Intussusception: additional observations on the plain radiograph. AJR 1982;139:511.
10. Ravitch MM, McCune RM Jr. Reduction of intussusception by hydrostatic pressure: an experimental study. Bull Johns Hopkins Hosp 1948; 82:550.
11. Kuta AJ, Benator RM. Intussusception: hydrostatic pressure equivalents for barium and meglumine sodium diatrizoate. Radiology 1990; 175:125.
12. Mortensson W, Eklöf O, Laurin S. Hydrostatic reduction of childhood intussusception: the role of adjuvant glucagon medication. Acta Radiol [Diagn] (Stockh) 1984;25:261.
13. Fishman MC, Borden S, Cooper A. The dissection sign of nonreducible ileocolic intussusception. AJR 1984;143:5.
14. Stephenson CA, Seibert JJ, Strain JD, et al. Intussusception: clinical and radiographic factors influencing reducibility. Pediatr Radiol 1989; 20:57.
15. Barr LL, Stansberry SD, Swischuk LE. Significance of age, duration, obstruction and the dissection sign in intussusception. Pediatr Radiol 1990;20:454.
16. Pierro A, Donnell SC, Paraskevopoulou C, et al. Indications for laparotomy after hydrostatic reduction for intussusception. J Pediatr Surg 1993;28:1154.
17. Ein SH, Palder SB, Alton DJ, et al. Intussusception: toward less surgery? J Pediatr Surg 1994;29:433.
18. Connolly B, Alton DJ, Ein SH, et al. Partially reduced intussusception: when are repeated delayed reduction attempts appropriate? Pediatr Radiol 1995;25:104.
19. Riebel TW, Nasir R, Weber K. US-guided hydrostatic reduction of intussusception in children. Radiology 1993;188:513.
20. Katz ME, Kolm P. Intussusception reduction 1991: an international survey of pediatric radiologists. Pediatr Radiol 1992;22:318.
21. Ein SH. Recurrent intussusception in children. J Pediatr Surg 1975;10: 751.
22. Eklöf O, Reiter S. Recurrent intussusception: analysis of a series treated with hydrostatic reduction. Acta Radiol [Diagn] (Stockh) 1978;19:250.
23. Liu KW, MacCarthy J, Guiney EJ, et al. Intussusception: current trends in management. Arch Dis Child 1986;61:75.
24. Beasley SW, Auldist AW, Stokes KB. Recurrent intussusception: barium or surgery? Aust N Z J Surg 1987;57:11.
25. Stringer MD, Pledger G, Drake DP. Childhood deaths from intussusception in England and Wales, 1984-9. Br Med J 1992;304:737.
26. Holsclaw DS, Rocmans C, Shwachman H. Intussusception in patients with cystic fibrosis. Pediatrics 1971;48:51.
27. Cull DL, Rosario V, Lally KP, et al. Surgical implications of Henoch-Schönlein purpura. J Pediatr Surg 1990;25:741.
28. Martinez-Frontanilla LA, Haase GM, Ernster JA, et al. Surgical complications in Henoch-Schönlein purpura. J Pediatr Surg 1984;19:434.
29. Ein SH, Ferguson JM. Intussusception: the forgotten postoperative obstruction. Arch Dis Child 1982;57:788.
30. Holcomb GW III, Ross AJ III, O'Neill JA Jr. Postoperative intussusception: increasing frequency or increasing awareness? South Med J 1991; 84:1334.
31. West KW, Stephens B, Rescorla FJ, et al. Postoperative intussusception: experience with 36 cases in children. Surgery 1988;104:781.
32. Janik JS. Nonischemic intussusception. J Pediatr Surg 1977;12:567.
33. Shekhawat NS, Prabhakar G, Sinha DD, et al. Nonischemic intussusception in childhood. J Pediatr Surg 1992;27:1433.
34. Patriquin HB, Afshani E, Effman E, et al. Neonatal intussusception: report of 12 cases. Radiology 1977;125:463.
35. Jennings C, Kelleher J. Intussusception: influence of age on reducibility. Pediatr Radiol 1984;14:292.
36. Bettenay F, Beasley SW, de Campo JF, et al. Intussusception: clinical prediction of outcome of barium reduction. Aust N Z J Surg 1988;58: 899.
37. Ein SH, Mercer S, Humphry A, et al. Colon perforation during attempted barium enema reduction of intussusception. J Pediatr Surg 1981;16:313.
38. Agha FP. Intussusception in adults. AJR 1986;146:527.

Surgery of Infants and Children: Scientific Principles and Practice, edited by Keith T. Oldham, Paul M. Colombani, and Robert P. Foglia. Lippincott–Raven Publishers, Philadelphia, © 1997.

CHAPTER 77

Tumors of the Small Bowel

Nicholas A. Shorter

Tumors of the small bowel are uncommon at any age. Those that do occur in children are almost all non-Hodgkin lymphomas (NHL). The small intestine contains a mucosal epithelial layer, smooth muscle, connective tissue, and gut-associated lymphoid tissue, all of which, potentially, can give rise to tumors. Why neoplastic transformation of the rapidly dividing mucosal cells is so infrequent, even in adults, is unknown. Primary smooth muscle tumors are also rare in all age groups. This chapter focuses on the small bowel lymphomas of childhood.

CLASSIFICATION

Whereas most cases of NHL in adults are nodal, almost all cases in children are extranodal in origin and are diffuse. The childhood tumors can be divided histologically into three groups[1]:

- Lymphoblastic lymphoma (indistinguishable from acute lymphoblastic leukemia)
- Undifferentiated or small, noncleaved cell lymphoma (indistinguishable from or similar to Burkitt lymphoma)
- Large cell lymphoma

Most lymphoblastic tumors are of T-cell origin, whereas undifferentiated tumors are almost all B-cell–derived, the difference between Burkitt and non-Burkitt being the degree of cellular pleomorphism. Large cell lymphomas can be from either lineage, with an occasional tumor from the histiocytic one. Most tumors arising in the small bowel are of the undifferentiated type, and in the United States 90% of undifferentiated childhood lymphomas present in the abdomen.[2] No doubt it will eventually be possible to divide further each phenotypic group on the basis of precise molecular and genetic differences.

EPIDEMIOLOGY

In the United States, lymphoma is the third most common childhood neoplasm and accounts for about 10% of childhood cancers.[3] NHL is rare in children younger than 5 years of age and the incidence increases with age throughout life.[2] For unknown reasons, the incidence in white children is twice that in blacks, and boys are affected three times as frequently as girls.[2] Thirty to 40% of the cases of childhood NHL originate in the abdomen.[3] In about half of these, the primary site is in the intestinal tract, most commonly in the small bowel and usually the ileum, although a precise figure is difficult to obtain because in extensive abdominal disease it is often impossible to know where the tumor originated.

Etiologic factors are not yet well understood. NHL is more common in other parts of the world, and the incidence of the different subtypes varies in different countries. The association between endemic Burkitt lymphoma and the Epstein-Barr virus is well known, but the specific role of this virus, if any, in the pathogenesis of this disease remains unclear. A role for other viruses is unproven. Immunodeficiency syndromes, including human immunodeficiency virus (HIV) infection, are associated with an increased incidence of NHL. Inherited genetic abnormalities may play a role, as evidenced by the recent identification in Burkitt lymphoma of mutation of the *p53* gene, a tumor suppressor protein.[4] The role of ionizing radiation alone is probably a small one. There is an increased risk for the development of NHL in patients who have been previously treated with combined modality therapy for Hodgkin disease or with chemotherapy for other solid tumors.[2,5]

CELL BIOLOGY

Almost all the childhood lymphomas of the small bowel are of B-cell origin. Most are of the undifferentiated or small, noncleaved cell phenotype, with some being large cell. These tumors bear B-cell markers as well as surface immunoglobulins, almost exclusively IgM. In the majority of Burkitt lymphoma cases, the cells show a specific chromosomal translocation of a portion of the long arm of chromosome 8 to chromosome 14.[1,2] As a result of this molecular rearrangement, the *c-myc* oncogene from chromosome 8 comes to lie next to immunoglobulin heavy chain constant region sequences, resulting in abnormal activation. In a small proportion of cases, the translocation is from chromosome 2 or 22 to chromosome 8, which activates *c-myc* by putting it next to light chain constant region sequences.[2] These translocations probably occur during the normal phase of immunoglobulin gene rearrangement. The subsequent inappropriate production of the c-myc protein presumably maintains the cell in a proliferating state rather than allowing it to enter a resting one. Why these translocations occur is unknown, and it is unclear whether they represent the primary step in the development of the malignancy or only a secondary one. A deficiency in DNA repair has been postulated to be a predisposing factor.[2] The typical chromosome 8 break points are different in different regions of the world.[2]

Mutations in the *p53* tumor suppressor protein have been identified in about a third of Burkitt lymphomas, and the presence of mutation is independent of the geographic origin of the tumor, the 8;14 chromosomal break point locations, and the association of Epstein-Barr virus.[4] The exact role of the Epstein-Barr virus in the development of Burkitt lymphoma is unknown.[6] In 95% of African tumors, the cells carry the genome of this virus, but in North America only 15% of the tumors are positive. When it is present, it is unclear whether it plays an active essential role in neoplastic transformation or merely predisposes to it by producing immortalized clones.

CLINICAL PRESENTATION, DIAGNOSIS, AND STAGING

Small bowel tumors typically present with abdominal pain, bowel obstruction, gastrointestinal bleeding, or perforation. There may be a palpable mass, most commonly in the right lower quadrant, and in extensive cases ascites may occur. The intramural tumor can often act as the lead point of an intussusception. In most cases, symptoms have been present for only a short time, and constitutional symptoms such as fever and weight loss are uncommon.[3]

More than half of the patients with abdominal tumors come to urgent exploration as a result of their presentation with an acute abdomen. The differential diagnosis usually does not include lymphoma, and the operative findings usually are unexpected.[7] In another group, usually those with a palpable mass but without acute symptomatology, the diagnosis is made at the time of a planned laparotomy and biopsy. If ascites is present, paracentesis may yield the diagnosis, and in some patients with abdominal primaries but extensive spread, bone marrow sampling or superficial lymph node biopsy may be diagnostic. The role of laparoscopy likely will increase in the evaluation of a number of these patients. Diagnosis requires obtaining adequate tissue and proper handling of the specimens to ensure that all the necessary immunotyping and cytogenic studies can be done in addition to routine histologic examination. Some patients present only with chronic, often vague, abdominal pain. In the absence of a palpable mass or obstruction, diagnosis of a small bowel lesion can be difficult. A filling defect may be visible on a small bowel barium study, or a small mass may be identified on a CT scan using oral contrast. However, when only nonspecific symptoms are present, even if studies are obtained, the diagnosis may prove elusive until other symptoms appear as a result of further progression of the disease.

It is recognized that all cases of childhood NHL are systemic from the onset and require chemotherapy. Thus, staging plays a different role than it does in Hodgkin disease. The goal is to evaluate overall tumor burden, which is the single most important prognostic factor.[2] A number of staging systems exist, most of which reflect tumor volume. The most widely used are the National Cancer Institute system for Burkitt lymphoma and the St. Jude staging system for NHL (Tables 77-1 and 77-2).[1,2]

Most patients with small bowel tumors will have had a laparotomy, either for diagnosis alone or to treat an acute abdominal process. In addition to obtaining adequate material for diagnosis, a full exploration should be performed at that time to evaluate the extent of intraabdominal disease. For staging purposes, patients with disease localized to the bowel and its mesentery must be distinguished from those with extensive intraabdominal spread. Disease should be looked for in the liver, spleen, kidneys, peritoneal surfaces, ovaries, and retroperitoneum.[8] In most cases involvement can be determined grossly, with sampling of suspect nodes or lesions. A splenectomy is not performed, even if the spleen is involved, and routine liver biopsies are not indicated unless they are requested as part of an ongoing protocol.

Further routine studies include chest radiographs, bone scans, bone marrow sampling, and lumbar puncture. Other studies are obtained on an individual basis. Bone marrow involvement at presentation is seen in about 20% of patients with small, noncleaved cell lymphomas, and may be occult in another 20%.[2] Central nervous system (CNS) involvement at presentation is

TABLE 77-1. *National Cancer Institute staging system for Burkitt lymphoma*

Stage A:	Single extraabdominal site
Stage B:	Multiple extraabdominal sites
Stage C:	Intraabdominal tumor
Stage D:	Intraabdominal tumor with involvement of extraabdominal sites
Stage AR:	Completely resected intraabdominal tumor

TABLE 77-2. *St. Jude staging system for non-Hodgkin lymphoma*

Stage I:	A single tumor (extranodal) or single anatomic area (nodal), with the exclusion of mediastinum or abdomen
Stage II:	A single tumor (extranodal) with regional node involvement
	Two or more nodal areas on the same side of the diaphragm
	Two single (extranodal) tumors with or without regional node involvement on the same side of the diaphragm
	A primary gastrointestinal tract tumor with or without involvement of associated mesenteric nodes only
Stage III:	Two single tumors (extranodal) on opposite sides of the diaphragm
	Two or more nodal areas above and below the diaphragm
	All the primary intrathoracic tumors (mediastinal, pleural, thymic)
	All extensive primary intraabdominal disease
	All paraspinal or epidural tumors, regardless of other tumor sites
Stage IV:	Any of the above with initial central nervous system or bone marrow involvement

uncommon, but spread frequently occurs in the absence of prophylactic therapy.[2]

TREATMENT

Most small bowel tumors are discovered at the time of laparotomy. If the disease is restricted to the bowel, it should be resected (only short resections are necessary because extensive bowel involvement is not seen in the absence of widespread intraabdominal disease), with grossly negative margins and with resection of the associated mesentery.[7,8] Resection in this setting correlates with a favorable prognosis (which may reflect the small volume of disease rather than a therapeutic effect of the resection itself), is associated with minimal complications, and has the additional benefits of eliminating the risk of tumor lysis syndrome and the chance of bowel perforation or gastrointestinal hemorrhage in that segment after the initiation of chemotherapy.[7] With more extensive disease, attempts at tumor resection are not justified because even extensive debulking does not improve survival. Such procedures can lead to complications such as acute renal failure and hemorrhage and can result in a delay in the initiation of chemotherapy.[7,8] Biopsy only is indicated. In this setting, however, a segmental bowel resection may still be necessary to treat the presenting acute abdominal process.

In the setting of an emergent abdominal exploration, intraoperative decision making should be straightforward. Frozen sections may be able to confirm the diagnosis of lymphoma (although not the subtype), but, when negative, cannot be relied on. With extensive disease, the diagnosis is usually self-evident from the gross appearance. In disease limited to the bowel, the diagnosis may be suspected by the experienced eye, but sometimes is not confirmed until the permanent sections are examined. In the latter group, the need for resection usually is obvious from the need to treat the acute abdominal process. On occasion, it may not be possible intraoperatively to distinguish between a nonobstructing inflammatory intestinal mass and a lymphoma. In that situation, resection is justified on clinical suspicion alone. The importance of proper handling of lymphoma specimens cannot be overemphasized. It is mandatory in cases of diagnostic uncertainty to alert the pathologist to the possibility of lymphoma. Inadequate processing of the material results in the loss of critical diagnostic information, which has important therapeutic significance.

Chemotherapy is the mainstay of modern treatment of childhood NHL. Radiation has little if any role and often appears to increase toxicity.[2] Because these tumors grow rapidly, treatment should begin quickly. Any significant delay can worsen prognosis because of the increase in the patient's overall tumor burden. Patients with extensive intraabdominal spread may have significant biochemical abnormalities (elevated uric acid levels, hyperphosphatemia, hyperkalemia) that should be corrected rapidly before the initiation of therapy.[1–3] These children are at risk during therapy for the tumor lysis syndrome, with development of urate nephropathy and renal failure, and sometimes requiring dialysis. Adequate hydration, the maintenance of high urine flow, and allopurinol administration are vital to prevent this.[1–3]

A number of chemotherapy protocols are effective in treating the small, noncleaved cell lymphomas.[2] Patients with limited abdominal disease (ie, completely resected intestinal tumors) require less intensive treatment than those with more extensive disease. CNS prophylactic intrathecal chemotherapy is mandatory except in some patients with completely resected abdominal disease. Short courses of very intensive therapy appear as effective as more prolonged treatment. Abdominal large cell lymphomas are usually treated with the same protocols used for the small, noncleaved cell lymphomas.[2] Refinements are continually being made in all protocols in an attempt to decrease the morbidity of treatment. Local abdominal recurrence is rare as the sole site of disease, so second-look procedures are rarely indicated.[8]

RESULTS

Survival has improved dramatically since the 1970s.[2] A survival rate greater than 90% is now expected in children with totally resected small bowel lymphomas. For more extensive disease, cure rates range between 60% and 90% in those patients without bone marrow or CNS involvement. Although initial bone marrow and CNS involvement have correlated with a worse prognosis, refinements in treatment are now leading to improved survival even in these groups. Recurrence is usually associated with a poor prognosis, although some salvage therapies involving autologous bone marrow transplants appear to show better results.

OTHER TUMORS

Although rare, numerous benign tumors have been reported in the small bowel, including neurofibromas, hemangiomas, juvenile polyps (rare sporadic lesions or in the setting of a juvenile polyposis syndrome), adenomatous polyps (in familial polyposis or Gardner syndrome), hamartomas (especially in Peutz-Jeghers syndrome), inflammatory pseudotumor, and intestinal fibromatosis (nearly exclusively in newborns).[9] When symptomatic, these commonly present with obstruction, sometimes because of intussusception, or bleeding. Appropriate therapy is resection.

Carcinoid tumors are found rarely in the small intestine.[10] These tumors contain argentaffin cells derived from endocrine cells of the bowel. They are most common in the appendix, but, when extraappendiceal, most occur in the ileum, although they have been reported at all levels of the bowel. Most are benign, but malignancy can occur. The carcinoid syndrome is very rare. In tumors restricted to the bowel, resection is curative. Even with metastases, prolonged survival is common because of the indolent nature of these tumors.[11]

Small intestinal smooth muscle tumors, leiomyomas and leiomyosarcomas, are very rare in children.[12] Intestinal obstruction is the most common presentation, and there is often a palpable mass. Bowel perforation is not uncommon. Gastrointestinal leiomyosarcomas are slightly more common in girls, and about one third present in the first month of life. Often the differentiation between the benign and the malignant forms is difficult, based on the mitotic rate, tumor size, and extent of necrosis. For benign lesions, resection alone is adequate. In the malignant form, a favorable outcome is associated with low grade and complete surgical excision.[12] These tumors tend to be locally invasive, and local recurrence is most frequent. Chemotherapy and radiation therapy do not seem to improve survival. There appear to be differences between the behavior of leiomyosarcomas in children and adults, but because of their rarity in children, these have not yet been well characterized. Age may have prognostic implications, with younger patients, especially infants, tending to do better.[13] An unexplained association has been noted between smooth muscle tumors and immune deficiency states, including HIV infection.[14] A translocation has been identified in a childhood leiomyosarcoma that is similar to that seen in adults, suggesting a pathogenic role for this genetic rearrangement.[14]

Adenocarcinoma of the small bowel has been reported in association with the Peutz-Jeghers syndrome.[15] Patients with familial polyposis, Gardner syndrome, and small bowel Crohn disease are also at risk for progression to small bowel malignancy.[11] Metastatic lesions from other tumors can be seen in the small intestine, either as a result of hematogenous spread or direct peritoneal implantation.

REFERENCES

1. Magrath IT. Malignant non-Hodgkin's lymphomas in children. Hematol Oncol Clin North Am 1987;1:577.
2. Magrath I. Malignant non-Hodgkin's lymphomas in children. In: Pizzo PA, Poplack DG, eds. Principles and practice of pediatric oncology. Philadelphia, JB Lippincott, 1993:537.
3. Link MP. Non-Hodgkin's lymphoma in children. Pediatr Clin North Am 1985;32:699.
4. Bhatia KG, Gutierrez MI, Huppi K, et al. The pattern of p53 mutations in Burkitt's lymphoma differs from that of solid tumors. Cancer Res 1992;52:4273.
5. Zarrabi MH, Rosner F. Second neoplasms in Hodgkin's disease: current controversies. Hematol Oncol Clin North Am 1989;3:303.
6. Facer CA, Playfair JHL. Malaria, Epstein-Barr virus, and the genesis of lymphomas. Adv Cancer Res 1989;53:33.
7. LaQuaglia MP, Stolar CJH, Krailo M, et al. The role of surgery in abdominal non-Hodgkin's lymphoma: experience from the Children's Cancer Study Group. J Pediatr Surg 1992;27:230.
8. Shamberger RC, Weinstein HJ. The role of surgery in abdominal Burkitt's lymphoma. J Pediatr Surg 1992;27:236.
9. Dahms BB. The gastrointestinal tract. In: Stocker JT, Dehner LP, eds. Pediatric pathology. Philadelphia, JB Lippincott, 1992:653.
10. Grundy R, Pritchard J. Carcinomas and other rare tumors. In: Voute PA, Barrett A, Lemerle J, eds. Cancer in children. Berlin, Springer-Verlag, 1992:339.
11. Leichtner AM. Intestinal neoplasms. In: Walker WA, Durie PR, Hamilton JR, et al, eds. Pediatric gastrointestinal disease. Philadelphia, BC Decker, 1991:771.
12. Angel CA, Gant LL, Parham DM, et al. Leiomyosarcomas in children: clinical and pathologic characteristics. Pediatr Surg Int 1992;7:116.
13. Goh DW, Raafat F, Gornall P, et al. Intestinal leiomyoma in neonates. Pediatr Surg Int 1990;5:208.
14. Miser JS, Pritchard DJ, Triche TJ, et al. The other soft tissue sarcomas of childhood. In: Pizzo PA, Poplack DG, eds. Principles and practice of pediatric oncology. Philadelphia, JB Lippincott, 1993:823.
15. Cordts AE, Chabot JR. Jejunal carcinoma in a child. J Pediatr Surg 1983;18:180.

Surgery of Infants and Children: Scientific Principles and Practice, edited by Keith T. Oldham, Paul M. Colombani, and Robert P. Foglia. Lippincott–Raven Publishers, Philadelphia, © 1997.

CHAPTER 78

Crohn Disease

Jacob C. Langer

In 1932, Crohn and Ginzburg[1] described a series of patients presenting with transmural inflammation of the terminal ileum, characterized pathologically by the presence of granulomas, and thought to be different from the more prevalent cause of granulomatous ileitis at the time, tuberculosis. Although the authors originally called the disease "terminal ileitis," the name was subsequently changed to "regional ileitis" to avoid the impression of a universally dismal outcome. It was not until almost 30 years later that Lockhart-Mummery and Morson[2] described the colonic form of Crohn disease (termed "granulomatous" colitis) and differentiated it from ulcerative colitis.

Since it was first described, Crohn disease has presented a considerable challenge to physicians and surgeons, as well as to the people afflicted with it. It is a chronic, incurable disease, which in its mildest form may cause inconvenience to the sufferer, but in its severest forms causes ongoing pain, disability, or death. In children, the disease may be particularly devastating, and may interfere with normal growth, social and educational development, and family relationships. This chapter outlines the features and management of Crohn disease, and highlights some of the special issues this disease poses in childhood.

EPIDEMIOLOGY

Crohn disease occurs in all parts of the world, and in all races, but is particularly common in Ashkenazi Jews and is more common in whites than in nonwhites. It occurs with equal frequency in males and females. The peak age of onset is in the late teens and early twenties, although approximately 5% of patients are children younger than 5 years of age. The incidence in the general population is approximately 5.3 per 100,000, with an incidence of 16.0 per 100,000 in the 15- to 19-year-old age range, and 2.5 per 100,000 in children younger than 15 years of age. The prevalence of Crohn disease in children younger than 16 years of age is quoted as 9.5 per 100,000. Although the incidence of Crohn disease increased dramatically between 1950 and 1980, subsequent reports have suggested a decline. It is uncertain whether these observations reflect changes in true incidence or changes in recognition of the disease.

Patients with Crohn disease often report a positive family history, although there is often overlap between Crohn disease and ulcerative colitis in the same families. Siblings of patients with Crohn disease are 17 to 35 times more likely to contract the disease, and children of parents with Crohn disease are subject to a 35- to 70-fold increase in risk.[3]

ETIOLOGY

The etiology of Crohn disease is unknown. However, a number of theories have been proposed, each supported by a body of evidence in both clinical and experimental models. The three most prevalent theories include a transmissable infectious agent, an immunologic mechanism, and genetic predisposition. In all likelihood, Crohn disease is caused by a number of factors, and all three proposed mechanisms may play a role.

Infectious Agent

The similarities in the appearance of Crohn disease with tuberculosis suggested a similar etiology. Support for this theory includes the development of a Crohn-like illness in goats after feeding of a mycobacterium isolated from Crohn patients,[4] and the observation that granulomas form in the foot pads of mice injected with bowel affected by Crohn disease. However, multiple culture and serologic studies have failed to identify a reproducible single agent that is responsible. It is possible, however, that some patients with Crohn disease may have an abnormal response to normal intestinal flora, as suggested by studies documenting inflammation in response to bacterial cell wall components,[5] and immunolocalization of bacterial antigen in tissues of Crohn patients.[6]

Immune Mechanism

The lack of an identifiable infectious agent has focused investigators on the possibility of abnormal immune function. One possibility could be an imbalance between the two normal functions of the intestinal immune system: ability to react to pathogens, and ability *not* to react to normal gut constituents (oral tolerance). Abnormally high activity in the former arm or low activity in the latter arm would result in excessive inflammation, with the intestine representing an ''innocent bystander.'' This theory is supported by findings demonstrating imbalances between helper and suppressor T-cell expression and cytokine production in patients with Crohn disease.[7] Investigators have induced chronic intestinal inflammation in mice by creating specific defects in cytokine and T-cell receptors, further supporting an immunologic basis for Crohn disease.[7]

Genetic Predisposition

Crohn disease occurs with an increased incidence within families, as described earlier. There are also several hereditary conditions, such as glycogen storage disease type Ib and HLA B27, which predispose to the development of inflammatory bowel disease. Several subclinical markers have been identified in members of families of patients with Crohn disease, including complement pathway dysfunction at the level of C3,[8] differences in anaerobic fecal flora,[9] and increased mucosal permeability.[10] These markers suggest either a genetic abnormality predisposing to the disease or an early phase of the disease process that may or may not progress to clinically evident disease. Mapping of genes that predispose to the development of Crohn disease has become a major research thrust.

PATHOLOGY

Pathologically, Crohn disease is characterized by transmural inflammation with edema, lymphocyte and plasma cell infiltration, and noncaseating granulomas in approximately 50% of cases. Cytokines such as tumor necrosis factor and a variety of interleukins have been shown to play an important part in both initiating and perpetuating the inflammation. The clinical course typically follows a waxing and waning pattern, although the factors that incite exacerbations are poorly understood. As the disease progresses, fibrosis becomes evident, particularly in the submucosal region. Crohn disease may involve any part of the intestinal tract from mouth to anus, although most cases involve the distal small bowel and the colon. Skip lesions are characteristic. The distribution of involvement in children is similar to that in adults (Fig. 78-1).

There are many differences between Crohn disease and ulcerative colitis, including age of onset, distribution, pathologic features, and long-term risk of cancer. These differences are summarized in Table 78-1. There is also a third disease group, comprising approximately 10% of patients with colitis, which has features somewhere between those of Crohn disease and ulcerative colitis, and which is termed ''indeterminate colitis.'' Over long-term follow-up, small bowel disease characteristic of Crohn disease goes on to develop in a large proportion of these patients. Because of this trend, children with a pathologic diagnosis of indeterminate colitis should probably be treated as having Crohn disease.

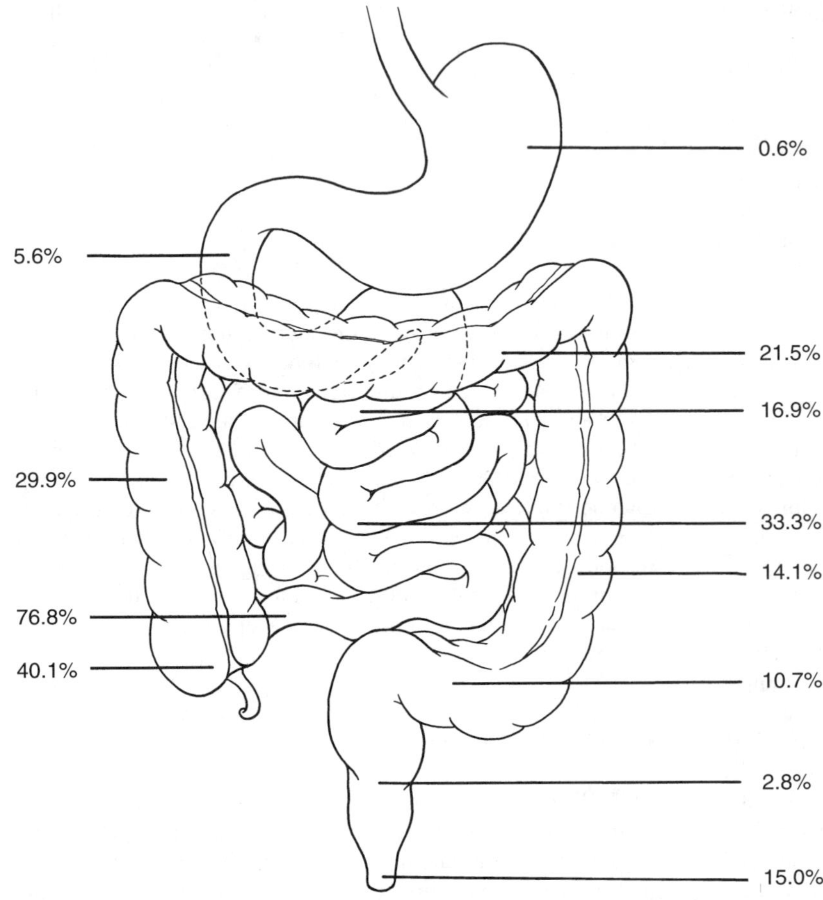

FIG. 78-1. Distribution of bowel involvement in children with Crohn disease. (Adapted from Castile RG, Telander RL, Cooney DR, et al. Crohn's disease in children: assessment of the progression of disease, growth, and prognosis. J Pediatr Surg 1980;15:462.)

TABLE 78-1. *Differences between Crohn disease and ulcerative colitis*

Characteristic	Crohn disease	Ulcerative colitis
Age at onset	Teens and twenties	Bimodal distribution with peaks in twenties and fifties
Distribution	Entire GI tract	Colon only
	Skip lesions	Continuous involvement proximally from rectum
Pathology	Full thickness	Mucosa only
	Granulomas (50%)	No granulomas
Radiology	Entire GI tract	Colon only
	Skip lesions	Continuous involvement proximally from rectum
	Fistulas, abscesses, fibrotic strictures	Mucosal disease only
Presentation		
Bleeding	Uncommon	Common
Obstruction	Common	Uncommon
Fistula	Common	Uncommon
Weight loss	Common	Uncommon
Perianal disease	Common	Uncommon
Cancer risk	Controversial	1%/y starting 10 y from diagnosis (estimated)

CLINICAL PRESENTATION

Crohn disease in childhood may present in many different ways, depending on the area of the gastrointestinal tract involved, the chronicity of the inflammation, and the age of the patient. Most commonly, a child presents during the teenage years with chronic abdominal pain, diarrhea, and weight loss. These complaints are usually caused by inflammation of the terminal ileum, with or without involvement of the ascending colon. Intermittent nausea and vomiting, as well as a significant decrease in energy level, may also occur. Children who have a significant amount of diarrhea may gradually become more isolated, avoiding social situations in which they must frequently excuse themselves to go to the bathroom. In addition,

TABLE 78-2. *Extraintestinal manifestations of Crohn disease in children*

Skin
  Erythema nodosum
  Pyoderma gangrenosum
Joints
  Transient, migratory arthritis
  Ankylosing spondylitis
  Clubbing
Ocular
  Iritis
  Anterior uveitis
  Episcleritis
  Orbital pseudotumor
Stomatitis
Hepatic
  Pericholangitis
  Sclerosing cholangitis
  Fatty liver
  Chronic hepatitis
  Cholelithiasis
Renal
  Calculi (oxalate, urate, and phosphate)
  Hydronephrosis
  Amyloidosis

many children with Crohn disease present because of delay in the onset of puberty, or with secondary amenorrhea.

The most frequent presenting feature in children with Crohn colitis is bloody diarrhea, although abdominal pain, tenesmus, incontinence, and weight loss may also occur. Perianal Crohn disease may be the initial presentation in an individual child, or may accompany the typical symptoms of ileocecal or colonic disease. Perianal Crohn disease should be suspected in any child with recurrent, multiple, or atypical perianal abscesses or fistulas, or in any child with abdominal pain, weight loss, or chronic diarrhea in association with perianal sepsis.

Important physical findings that suggest the presence of Crohn disease include a mass in the right lower quadrant, pallor, evidence of malnutrition such as decreased muscle mass and decreased skin fold thickness, a Tanner stage that is lower than expected for the child's age, and evidence of perianal sepsis such as fissures, skin tags, fistulas, or perianal erythema.

Although it is less common, children may present with a complication of Crohn disease. These may include toxic megacolon, bowel obstruction, intestinal perforation, or fistula formation to skin, bladder, vagina, or bowel. In addition, some children initially present with an extraintestinal manifestation of Crohn disease such as arthritis, erythema nodosum, or a red eye (Table 78-2). Most of the extraintestinal manifestations of Crohn disease occur concomitantly with intestinal symptoms, but occasionally they may exist in an otherwise asymptomatic child.

The severity of Crohn disease varies significantly among patients. In general, it is thought that patients in whom Crohn disease develops early in life have a more virulent form, and are more likely to experience complications and require surgical intervention. Many patients experience a decrease in the severity of their disease as they get older (''burnt out'' Crohn disease). Despite these phenomena, exacerbations can occur at any time in any patient, and the course of Crohn disease is characteristically unpredictable.

DIAGNOSIS

The average time from the onset of symptoms to the diagnosis of Crohn disease in children is approximately 1 year. The diag-

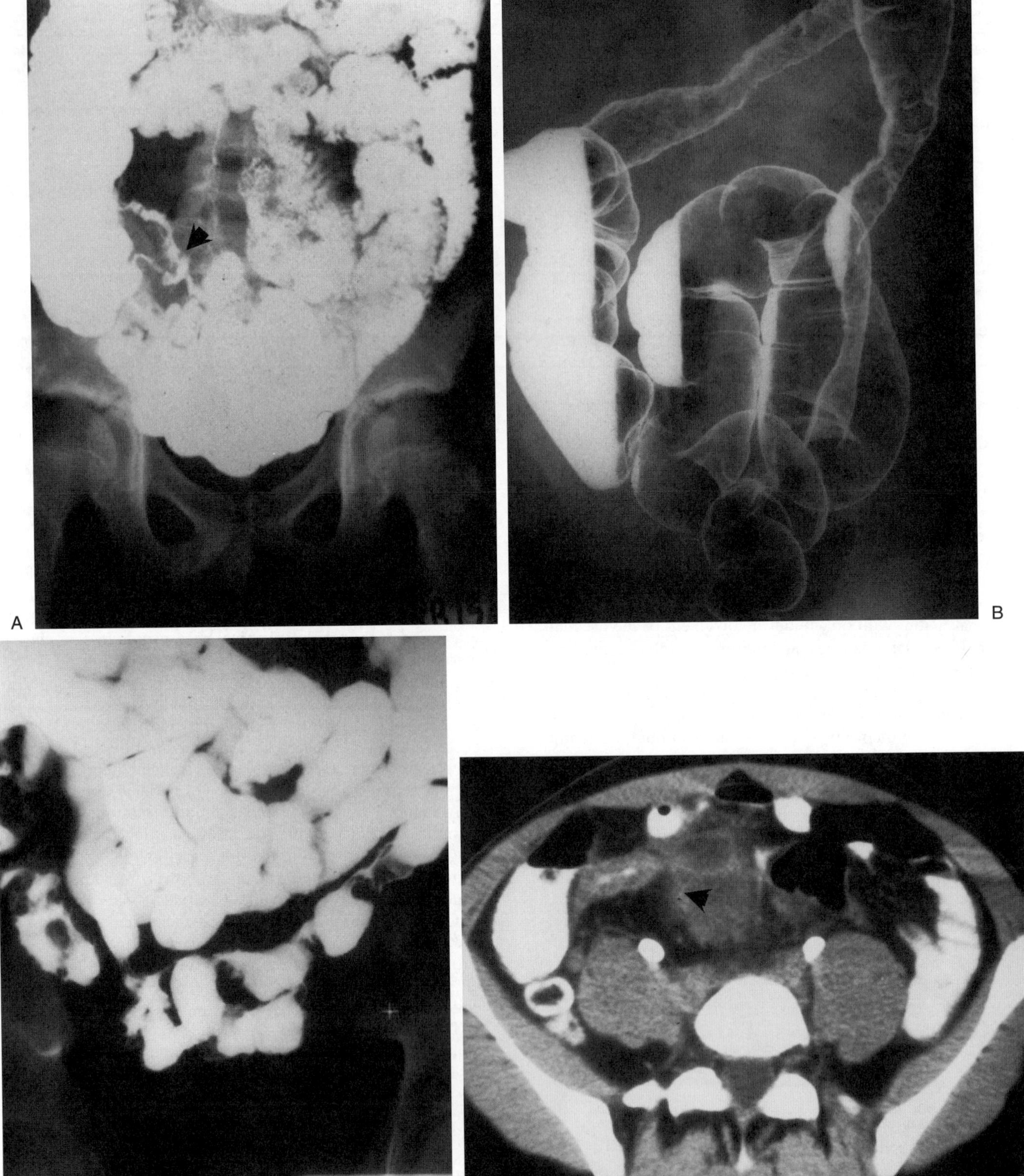

FIG. 78-2. Radiologic appearance of Crohn disease. (*A*) Terminal ileal involvement with typical "lead pipe" appearance and small sinus tract (arrow). (*B*) Colonic involvement with several skip areas. (*C*) Multiple small bowel strictures. (*D*) Abdominal CT scan demonstrating thickening of the terminal ileum with mesenteric inflammation and a localized abscess (arrow).

nosis is often delayed because the symptoms tend to be nonspecific, and the index of suspicion on the part of most primary care physicians may be low. The differential diagnosis includes ulcerative colitis, viral or bacterial gastroenteritis, parasitic infections such as giardiasis and amoebiasis, granulomatous diseases such as tuberculosis or aspergillosis, peptic ulcer disease, celiac disease, and cystic fibrosis. Many children with chronic abdominal complaints are labeled as having a "nervous stomach," chronic abdominal pain syndrome, or irritable bowel syndrome. For patients with a more acute presentation, the differential diagnosis may include appendicitis, cholecystitis, pancreatitis, or intestinal obstruction. The definitive diagnosis of Crohn disease is based on a combination of clinical, laboratory, radiologic, and pathologic criteria.

Laboratory evaluation usually shows anemia, which may be microcytic and microchromic due to chronic blood loss, or may be normocytic and normochromic. In the face of acute inflammation, the leukocyte count and the sedimentation rate may be elevated. Biochemical evidence of malnutrition may include decreased serum albumin, total iron binding capacity, and ferritin.

Radiologic examination is an important part of the diagnostic evaluation (Fig. 78-2), although in some cases it may be falsely negative. Barium examinations of the small bowel or colon may show mucosal disease or strictures, which demonstrate typical skip lesions. The terminal ileum is often narrowed into a "lead pipe" appearance, with dilated proximal loops of bowel. Fissures through the bowel wall are commonly seen, and occasionally a fistula or sinus tract is identified. Computed tomography (CT) may reveal thickening of the bowel wall and the mesentery, and local abscess formation.

Endoscopy also plays an important role in the diagnosis of Crohn disease. Colonoscopy is often used to obtain mucosal biopsy samples, which may be beneficial in differentiating ulcerative colitis from Crohn disease. In cases of ileal Crohn disease, colonoscopy is useful to rule out significant colonic involvement. Upper endoscopy may be important to rule out other conditions such as peptic ulcer disease, and to identify the 20% to 30% of children with small bowel or colonic Crohn disease who have concurrent asymptomatic gastroduodenal involvement.[11]

Once the diagnosis has been made, the severity of Crohn disease can be estimated using the Pediatric Crohn's Disease Severity Index[12] (Fig. 78-3). This index is useful for directing

---

HISTORY (Recall, 1 wk)

Abdominal pain

None	_______ (0)
Mild—brief, does not interfere with activities	_______ (5)
Moderate to severe—daily, longer lasting, affects activites, nocturnal	_______ (10)

Stools (per day)

0–1 liquid stools, no blood	_______ (0)
Up to 2 semiformed with small blood, or 2–5 liquid	_______ (5)
Gross bleeding, or ≥6 liquid, or nocturnal diarrhea	_______ (10)

PATIENT FUNCTIONING, GENERAL WELL-BEING (Recall, 1 wk)

No limitation of activities, well	_______ (0)
Occasional difficulty in maintaining age-appropriate activities, below par	_______ (5)
Frequent limitation of activity, very poor	_______ (10)

LABORATORY

HCT (%)

<10 y:	>33	_______ (0)	11–14 y M:	>35	_______ (0)
	28–32	_______ (2.5)		30–34	_______ (2.5)
	<28	_______ (5)		<30	_______ (5)
11–19 y F:	≥34	_______ (0)	15–19 y M:	≥37	_______ (0)
	29–33	_______ (2.5)		32–36	_______ (2.5)
	<29	_______ (5)		<32	_______ (5)

ESR (mm/h)

	<20	_______ (0)
	20–50	_______ (2.5)
	>50	_______ (5)

Albumin (g/dL)

	≥3.5	_______ (0)
	3.1–3.4	_______ (5)
	≤3	_______ (10)

EXAMINATION

Weight

Weight gain or voluntary weight stable/loss	_______ (0)
Involuntary weight stable, weight loss 1%–9%	_______ (5)
Weight loss ≥10%	_______ (10)

Height

At diagnosis

<1 channel decrease	_______ (0)
1–2 channel decrease	_______ (5)
>2 channel decrease	_______ (10)

or

Follow-up

Height velocity ≥–1 SD	_______ (0)
Height velocity <–1 SD, >–2 SD	_______ (5)
Height velocity ≤–2 SD	_______ (10)

Abdomen

No tenderness, no mass	_______ (0)
Tenderness or mass without tenderness	_______ (5)
Tenderness, involuntary guarding, definite mass	_______ (10)

Perirectal disease

None, asymptomatic tags	_______ (0)
1–2 indolent fistulas, scant drainage, no tenderness	_______ (5)
Active fistula, drainage, tenderness, or abscess	_______ (10)

Extraintestinal Manifestations

(Fever ≥38.5 for 3 days over past week, definite arthritis, uveitis, *E. nodosum*, *P. gangrenosum*)

0	_______ (0)
1	_______ (5)
≥2	_______ (10)

TOTAL SCORE _______________________

FIG. 78-3. Pediatric Crohn disease activity index. HCT, hematocrit; ESR, erythrocyte sedimentation rate (Hyams JS, Ferry GD, Mandel FS, et al. Development and validation of a pediatric Crohn's disease activity index. J Pediatr Gastroenterol Nutr 1991;12:439.)

therapeutic maneuvers, for following response to therapy, and for comparing results of therapy from one center to another.

NONOPERATIVE MANAGEMENT

Once the diagnosis is established, most children with Crohn disease are treated nonoperatively. This kind of therapy can be divided into two types: pharmacologic[13,14] and nutritional.[15] Initially, the goal of therapy is to bring about a remission of the disease, and subsequent therapy is designed to prevent recurrence. A summary of nonoperative strategies appears in Table 78-3.

Figure 78-4 shows a typical algorithm for pharmacologic therapy.

Glucocorticoids

The most commonly used family of drugs in the initial management of Crohn disease is the glucocorticoids. These powerful agents decrease the inflammation of Crohn disease, and are effective in bringing about partial or total remission in virtually all patients. Glucocorticoids can be used intravenously, orally, or topically as an enema. Systemic steroids are associated with significant adverse effects, including cushingoid features, glucose intolerance, osteoporosis, avascular necrosis of the femoral head, cataracts, acne, and psychological derangements (particularly severe mood swings). In children, steroids cause delay in bone maturation, growth retardation, and late onset of puberty. Significant steroid-related complications such as these are usually considered an indication for surgical management. Although steroids are effective in ameliorating a flare of the disease, their role in maintaining remission is less clear. The optimal duration of treatment with high-dose steroids in most cases should be no more than several weeks to months. In some

TABLE 78-3. *Nonoperative strategies in the management of Crohn disease*

PHARMACOLOGIC
Corticosteroids
Aspirin-like compounds
    Sulfasalazine
    5-Aminosalicylic acid (5-ASA)
Immunosuppressives
    Azathioprine and 6-mercaptopurine
    Cyclosporine
Antibiotics (ie, metronidazole)
Specific cytokine blockers (investigational)
Oxygen free radical inhibitors (investigational)

NUTRITIONAL
Elemental feeding
Parenteral nutrition

cases, lower-dose, alternate-day administration of prednisone results in maintenance of remission with minimal risk of adverse effects.

Newer generations of steroids have been developed that are largely inactivated after a first pass through the liver, and therefore may result in fewer side effects. The effectiveness of these agents, such as budesonide, is under study.

Salicylates

The first aspirin-like compound to be widely used in treating inflammatory bowel disease was sulfasalazine, a drug that consists of a 5-aminosalicylic acid (5-ASA) moiety bound to sulfapyridine. The two components are separated by colonic bacteria, and the 5-ASA then acts locally to decrease inflammation. For this reason, sulfasalazine is particularly effective for treating both granulomatous and ulcerative colitis. Unfortunately, this

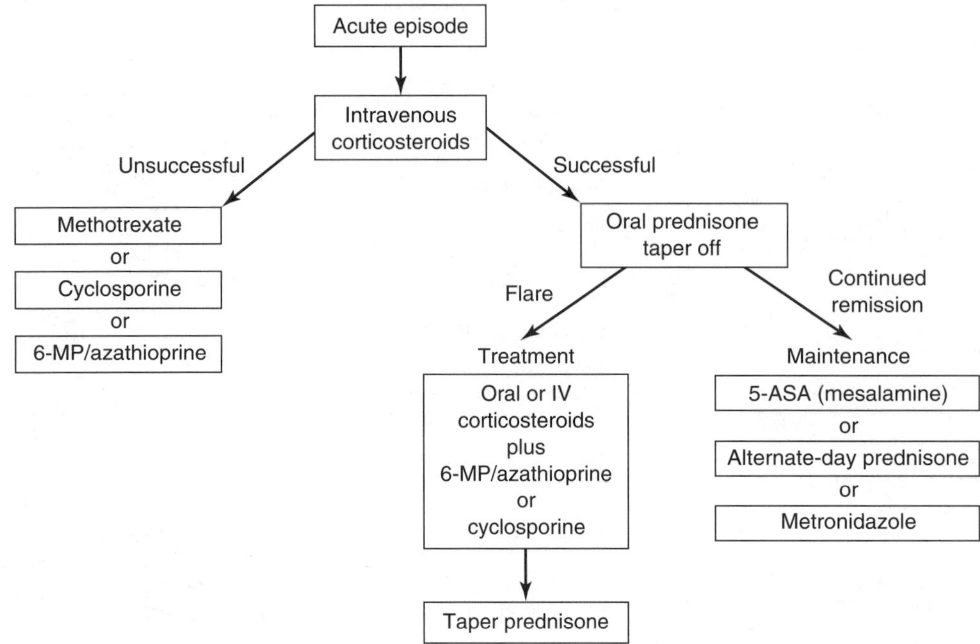

FIG. 78-4. Algorithm for the pharmacologic management of a child with Crohn disease. 5-ASA, 5-aminosalicylic acid; 6MP, 6-mercaptopurine.

drug has been associated with numerous side effects, including bone marrow suppression, skin rashes, nausea, vomiting, and diarrhea, which are largely caused by the sulfapyridine component. For this reason, a new family of drugs was developed that consists of 5-ASA in a variety of delivery systems. Most of them release the active 5-ASA in the terminal ileum or colon based on changes in pH and the action of colonic bacteria. These compounds are used orally or topically in enema form, and have few adverse effects. Evidence is accumulating that 5-ASA may be effective in preventing recurrence in patients with both ileal and colonic Crohn disease.[16]

Immunosuppressive Agents

Immunosuppressive agents[14] such as azathioprine and 6-mercaptopurine are effective in treating active Crohn disease, especially in the presence of persistent fistulas, and have permitted prolonged nonoperative management with low or no doses of steroids in approximately 75% of patients. Despite a relatively low incidence of lymphoreticular malignancy in adult series, use in children has been limited by concerns about long-term adverse effects. Similarly, both cyclosporine and methotrexate have been shown to be more effective than placebo in improving symptoms and decreasing steroid requirements in adults with chronic active Crohn disease,[17,18] but thus far neither of these agents has been used to any extent in children.

Antibiotics

Metronidazole, a nitroimidazole antibiotic, has been used for many years to treat perianal Crohn disease, and its effectiveness in this capacity has been demonstrated in randomized trials.[19] Metronidazole has also been shown to be effective in preventing recurrence after ileocecal resection.[20] Unfortunately, only about 25% of patients who respond to this drug can stop the medication without experiencing a relapse of symptoms. Other antibiotics, such as trimethoprim–sulfamethoxazole, tobramycin, and ciprofloxacin have been reported to be effective in small, uncontrolled trials.

Inflammatory Mediator Blockade

More recent understanding of the role of cytokines in the inflammation of Crohn disease has led to the development of a new generation of agents, most of which are still at the investigational stages.[21] These receptor agonists, monoclonal antibodies, and other agents are designed to block or inhibit the action of specifically targeted cytokines, such as tumor necrosis factor and interleukin-1. Clinical experience with monoclonal antibody to tumor necrosis factor has provided exciting evidence that this line of therapy may improve outcome for many patients.[22] In addition, the important role of free radicals in inducing intestinal damage has prompted development of free radical blockers as possible therapeutic agents. The efficacy of these drugs and their role in children await the results of clinical trials.

Nutritional Therapy

Nutritional therapy is effective for several reasons. First, many of these children are malnourished at the time of diagnosis, and provision of appropriate nutrients makes them feel better and recover more quickly. Second, there is some evidence that bowel rest has a therapeutic effect by decreasing the degree of intestinal inflammation. This is particularly true in maintaining remission after initial treatment with steroids. Nutritional therapy with concomitant bowel rest can be accomplished using either parenteral or enteral routes. Parenteral nutrition, although effective, is associated with risks from metabolic derangements, trace element deficiencies, central line complications, and a much higher cost. For enteral nutrition, most physicians use elemental feeding through a nasogastric or gastrostomy tube. There is, however, no convincing evidence that elemental feeds are preferable to the use of standard enteral formulas.[23]

Because the advantages of bowel rest usually disappear once a normal diet is resumed, this technique is not practical for long-term management. For this reason, nutritional therapy is usually used as a preoperative modality in a child who is on high-dose steroids or who is significantly malnourished. In this capacity, nutritional therapy is effective, safe, and well tolerated.[24]

SURGICAL MANAGEMENT

Indications for surgical management of Crohn disease include the following:

- Failure of medical management
  Complications of steroid or other drug therapy (including growth failure)
  Persistent symptoms despite maximal medical therapy
- Complications
  Perforation
  Fistula formation
  Excessive or uncontrolled bleeding
  Fibrous stricture with intestinal obstruction
  Ongoing sepsis
  Toxic megacolon

Early surgical intervention may rarely be necessary for complications such as free perforation, toxic megacolon, or massive bleeding. In general, however, surgery is indicated for patients with Crohn disease only after nonoperative management has failed. This is particularly true in children, who are at higher risk for recurrence and further loss of bowel length. Although the specific details of preoperative management and indications for surgery depend on the location and nature of the disease, in all cases the goal is to achieve normal nutritional status and to minimize the steroid dose before surgical intervention. This is usually accomplished using bowel rest, nutritional support, and alternate medical therapies during the preoperative period. In addition, it is important carefully to document the extent of disease prospectively using a combination of barium studies and endoscopy.

Ileocecal disease usually responds to high-dose steroids, and remission can often be maintained using 5-ASA or alternate-day, low-dose prednisone. However, this approach may fail because of fixed fibrotic changes, local perforation and abscess

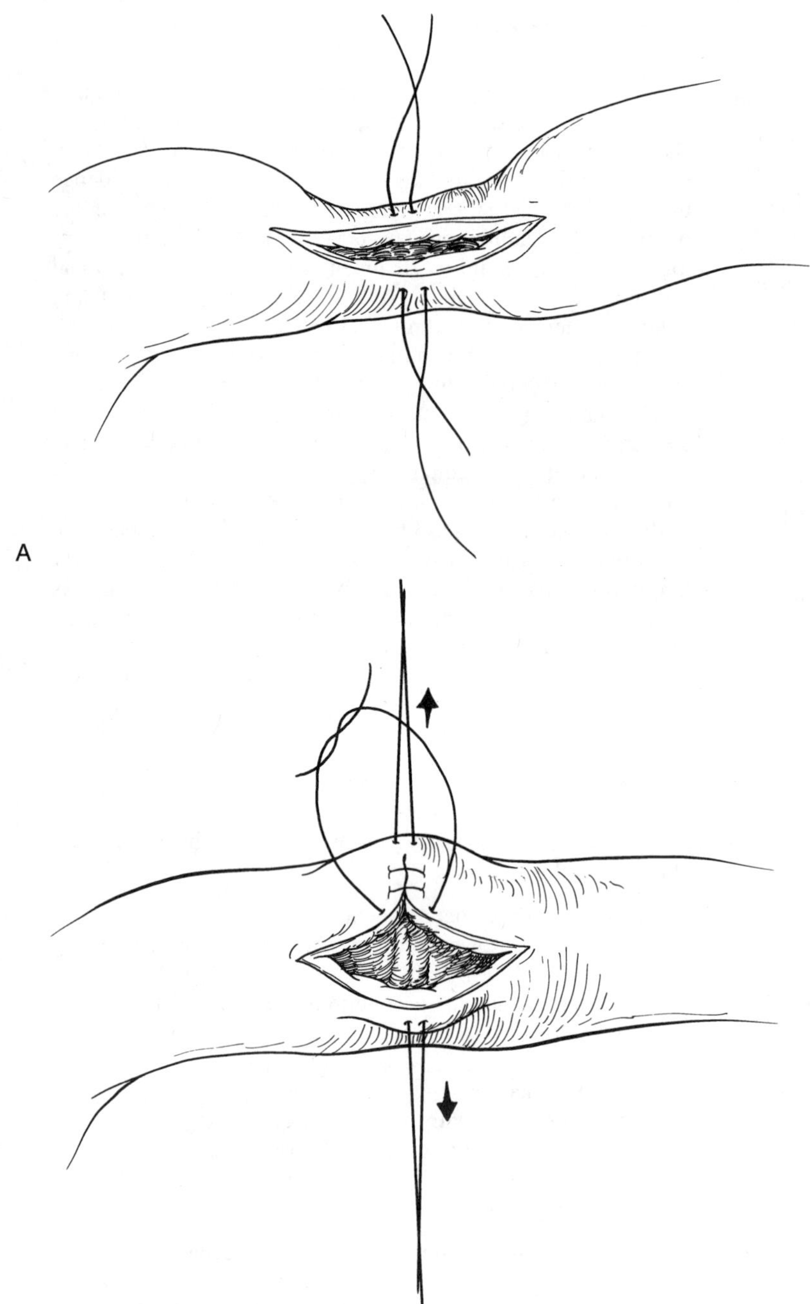

FIG. 78-5. Strictureplasty for multiple strictures in small bowel Crohn disease. The bowel is incised longitudinally across the stricture (*A*), and then closed transversely (*B*). Strictureplasty should be performed on all strictures that cannot permit passage of a 10-mL Foley balloon.

formation, or fistulization to colon, bladder, proximal small bowel, or skin. In addition, some children experience recurrent symptoms once the steroids are tapered, and the disease is controlled only on unacceptably high doses of prednisone. The decision to recommend surgery in these children may be difficult, and should be made collaboratively between the family, the gastroenterologist, and the surgeon. The decision must be based on the balance of surgical risks (including infection, anastomotic leak, adhesions, and recurrent disease) and the risk of long-term high-dose steroids.

Once a decision has been made, the extent of disease must be confirmed, and other studies may be done as necessary. Examples may include a CT scan to assess the possibility of local abscess formation, and renal ultrasound to look for hydronephrosis due to ureteral compression. The surgical goal is removal of the grossly involved bowel. There is no role for frozen section mapping of the resection margins, as was done in the past, because this does not result in a lower recurrence or complication rate.[25] The anastomosis can be hand sewn or stapled. A number of factors may increase the risk of anastomotic leak, including poor nutrition, intraabdominal sepsis, and chronic high-dose steroid administration.[26] For patients in whom anastomotic healing is thought to be compromised, a temporary Brooke ileostomy or a proximal defunctioning stoma should be done.

A small group of patients present with *multiple areas of*

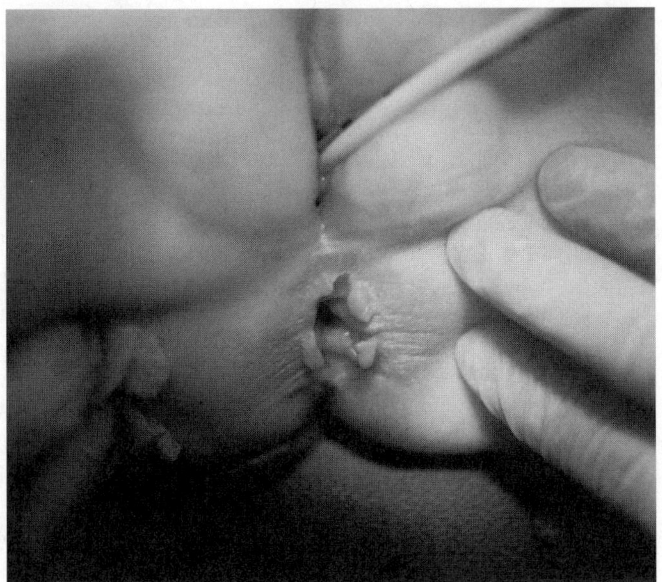

FIG. 78-6. Severe perianal Crohn disease in a 12-year-old child, with multiple fistulas and abscesses. This child ultimately required a proctocolectomy for relief of her symptoms.

symptomatic small bowel disease, with or without ileocecal involvement. Indications for surgery are similar to those enumerated previously, but multiple resections would result in excessive loss of bowel length. In these patients, strictureplasty has been advocated (Fig. 78-5). Results of this procedure in both adults and children have been encouraging, with no evidence of a higher rate of leak, infection, or recurrence.[27]

Crohn colitis often presents a somewhat more complicated picture. Isolated colonic disease can usually be differentiated from ulcerative colitis by the presence of skip lesions or evidence of transmural involvement. Often, both endoscopy and a barium enema are necessary, because endoscopy provides mucosal detail and biopsy tissue, and the barium study permits assessment of distensibility (ie, fibrosis) and fistula formation. In cases where only a small segment of colon is involved, local resection with primary anastomosis can be done. However, most patients have multiple areas of involvement, and at least a subtotal colectomy is necessary. The options for these children are a Brooke ileostomy, an ileorectal anastomosis, or a total proctocolectomy. Sphincter-saving pouch procedures and continent ileostomies are associated with a prohibitive complication rate, and are contraindicated in the presence of Crohn disease. Although functional results in children are extremely good after subtotal colectomy with ileorectal anastomosis, at least 50% of these children ultimately require a permanent ileostomy because of recurrent rectal disease.[28]

Perianal disease also presents a difficult problem in many children (Fig. 78-6). Anal fistulas are often deep and complex, and surgical approaches may lead to permanent sphincter damage. The use of metronidazole and immunosuppressive agents may permit healing of these fistulas without the need for surgery. True perirectal abscesses require surgical drainage, but as conservative an approach as possible should be taken. The use of a defunctioning ileostomy for perianal disease is controversial, and it is likely that the same efficacy can be achieved through the use of elemental feeding or total parenteral nutrition with bowel rest. In extremely severe cases of perianal Crohn disease in which there has been extensive destruction of the anal sphincter, a proctectomy with permanent ileostomy or colostomy may be necessary.

Enteroenteric, enterocutaneous, enterovesical, and rectovaginal fistulas can often be treated medically using bowel rest, steroids, metronidazole, and immunosuppressive agents, al-

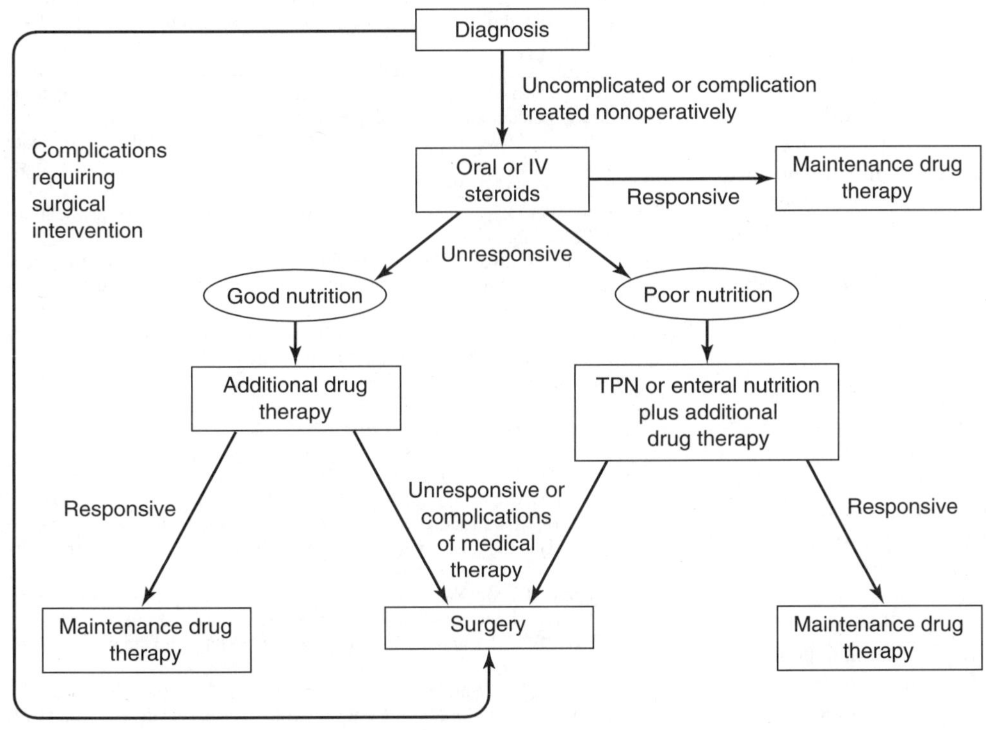

FIG. 78-7. Algorithm for the overall management of a child with Crohn disease. TPN, total parenteral nutrition.

though at least 50% of these recur after therapy is discontinued. In cases in which medical management fails and the fistula is symptomatic, excision of the fistula with local resection of the involved bowel should be done.[29] *Gastroduodenal Crohn disease* can usually be successfully managed using acid-reducing agents such as H_2 blockers or omeprazole. In rare cases in which strictures or severe symptoms persist, most surgeons have recommended gastric bypass, with or without vagotomy.

Figure 78-7 is an algorithm for the overall management of the child with Crohn disease.

COMPLICATIONS AND POSTOPERATIVE MANAGEMENT

As with any abdominal procedure, patients with Crohn disease may have wound infection, adhesions, stoma dysfunction, and ventral hernias. However, the most disturbing complications after surgery for Crohn disease include anastomotic leak and recurrent disease. As previously mentioned, the major risk factor for the development of an anastomotic leak is administration of steroids. Leaks can be diagnosed clinically by the presence of fever, local pain and tenderness, ileus, increasing free intraperitoneal air, and fluid on CT scan. It is rarely necessary to do contrast studies soon after an anastomosis to document a leak, and in fact such a study could potentially make matters worse. Some small leaks, which are not accompanied by systemic sepsis and are well localized, can be managed with bowel rest and antibiotics. In most cases, however, laparotomy and ileostomy are necessary. Primary revision of the anastomosis should never be attempted.

Crohn disease usually recurs in the region of the anastomosis, and may occur weeks to many years after surgery. Early recurrence is highest in patients with active inflammation at the resection margins and in patients with multiple anastomoses.[25] The risk of late recurrence is high, especially in children, and approaches 90% to 100% in series with long-term follow-up.[30] A number of randomized trials in adults have demonstrated that chronic postoperative administration of 5-ASA, metronidazole, or azathioprine results in decreased recurrence rates in patients with both Crohn colitis and ileitis.[31] Overall, patients can be given the ''rule of thirds'' with respect to outcome from surgery: roughly one third will have a relatively prompt recurrence, one third will go 5 to 10 years before their next recurrence, and one third will go more than 10 years or indefinitely without recurrent disease.

PSYCHOSOCIAL CONSIDERATIONS

Crohn disease presents some unique psychosocial issues in childhood, compared to the same disease process in adults. As with any chronic illness in childhood, the disease affects not only the child, but the entire family. It is crucial for the attending physician and surgeon to be aware of this, and to involve the family in discussions and the decision-making process.

Most children with Crohn disease are adolescents, and are going through a normal process of developing independence from their parents and struggling with their self-image.[32] Crohn disease may interfere with this process by imposing dependency on parents; creating self-image problems due to cushingoid features, delay in onset of puberty, and stomas; and socially isolat-

ing the child because of frequent hospitalizations, chronic pain, and diarrhea. Withdrawal from steroid medication, which often occurs during the postoperative period, commonly causes depression, which must be expected and explained to the child and family so that the feelings are not misinterpreted. It is imperative for the health care team to be aware of and sensitive to these issues, because the mental health of the child has a strong impact on physical recuperation.

Finally, quality of life is an important factor in the decision to perform surgery and in the assessment of postoperative results. An index has been described for measuring quality of life in patients with Crohn disease, which can be useful for surgeons in clinical practice.[33] For many children with Crohn disease, the decision to have an operation may revolve more around a quality-of-life issue than a medical one, and the surgeon must be patient and respectful while the child and family struggle to make these difficult choices.

REFERENCES

1. Crohn BB, Ginzburg L, Oppenheimer GD. Regional ileitis: a pathologic and clinical entity. JAMA 1932;99:1323.
2. Lockhart-Mummery HE, Morson BC. Crohn's disease (regional enteritis) of the large intestine and its distinction from ulcerative colitis. Gut 1960;1:87.
3. Fielding JF. The relative risk of inflammatory bowel disease among parents and siblings of Crohn's disease patients. J Clin Gastroenterol 1986;8:655.
4. Chiodini RJ, Van Kruiningen HJ, Thayer WR, et al. Possible role of mycobacteria in inflammatory bowel disease. I. An unclassified mycobacterium species isolated from patients with Crohn's disease. Dig Dis Sci 1984;29:1073.
5. Sartor RB, Cromartie WJ, Powell DW, et al. Granulomatous enterocolitis induced in rats by purified bacterial cell wall fragments. Gastroenterology 1985;89:587.
6. Liu Y, van Kruiningen HJ, West AB, et al. Immunocytochemical evidence of *Listeria*, *Escherichia coli*, and *Streptococcus* antigens in Crohn's disease. Gastroenterology 1995;108:1396.
7. Strober W, Ehrhardt RO. Chronic intestinal inflammation: an unexpected outcome in cytokine or T cell receptor mutant mice. Cell 1993;75:203.
8. Elmgreen J, Both H, Binder V. Familial occurrence of complement dysfunction in Crohn's disease: correlation with intestinal symptoms and hypercatabolism of complement. Gut 1985;26:151.
9. van der Merwe JP, Schroder AM, Wensinck F, et al. The obligate anaerobic faecal flora of patients with Crohn's disease and their first-degree relatives. Scand J Gastroenterol 1988;23:1125.
10. Hollander D. The intestinal permeability barrier. Scand J Gastroenterol 1992;27:721.
11. Lenaerts C, Roy CC, Vaillancourt M, et al. High incidence of upper gastrointestinal tract involvement in children with Crohn's disease. Pediatrics 1989;83:777.
12. Hyams JS, Ferry GD, Mandel FS, et al. Development and validation of a pediatric Crohn's disease activity index. J Pediatr Gastroenterol Nutr 1991;12:439.
13. Linn FV, Peppercorn MA. Drug therapy for inflammatory bowel disease (Part I). Am J Surg 1992;164:85.
14. Linn FV, Peppercorn MA. Drug therapy for inflammatory bowel disease (Part II). Am J Surg 1992;164:178.
15. Stokes MA. Crohn's disease and nutrition. Br J Surg 1992;79:391.
16. Prantera C, Pallone F, Brunetti G, et al. Oral 5-aminosalicylic acid (Asacol) in the maintenance treatment of Crohn's disease. Gastroenterology 1992;103:363.
17. Feagan BG, McDonald JWD, Rochon J, et al. Low-dose cyclosporine for the treatment of Crohn's disease. N Engl J Med 1994;330:1846.
18. Feagan BG, Rochon J, Fedorak RN, et al. Methotrexate for the treatment of Crohn's disease. N Engl J Med 1995;332:292.
19. Sutherland L, Singleton J, Sessions J, et al. Double blind, placebo controlled trial of metronidazole in Crohn's disease. Gut 1991;32:1071.

20. Rutgeerts P, Hiele M, Geboes K, et al. Controlled trial of metronidazole treatment for prevention of Crohn's recurrence after ileal resection. Gastroenterol 1995;108:1617.

21. Hanauer SB. Evolving medical therapies for inflammatory bowel disease. Progress in Inflammatory Bowel Disease 1994;15:1.

22. van Dullemen HM, van Deventer SJH, Hommes DW, et al. Treatment of Crohn's disease with anti-tumor necrosis factor chimeric monoclonal antibody (cA2). Gastroenterology 1995;109:129.

23. Griffiths AM, Ohlsson A, Sherman PM, et al. Meta-analysis of enteral nutrition as a primary treatment of active Crohn's disease. Gastroenterology 1995;108:1056.

24. Blair GK, Yaman M, Wesson DE. Preoperative home elemental enteral nutrition in complicated Crohn's disease. J Pediatr Surg 1986;21:769.

25. Heimann TM, Greenstein AJ, Lewis B, et al. Prediction of early symptomatic recurrence after intestinal resection in Crohn's disease. Ann Surg 1993;218:294.

26. Post P, Betzler M, von Ditfurth B, et al. Risks of intestinal anastomoses in Crohn's disease. Ann Surg 1991;213:37.

27. Oliva L, Wyllie R, Alexander F, et al. The results of strictureplasty in pediatric patients with multifocal Crohn's disease. J Pediatr Gastroenterol Nutr 1994;18:306.

28. Goligher JC. The outcome of excisional operations for primary and recurrent Crohn's disease of the large intestine. Surg Gynecol Obstet 1979;148:1.

29. Pettit SH, Irving MH. The operative management of fistulous Crohn's disease. Surg Gynecol Obstet 1988;167:223.

30. Trnka YM, Glotzer DJ, Kasdon EJ, et al. The long-term outcome of restorative operation in Crohn's disease. Ann Surg 1982;196:345.

31. Sachar DB. Maintenance therapy in ulcerative colitis and Crohn's disease. J Clin Gastroenterol 1995;20:117.

32. Sherkin-Langer F. If this is a test, have I passed yet? Toronto, MacMillan, 1994.

33. Irvine EJ, Feagan B, Rochon J, et al. Quality of life: a valid and reliable measure of therapeutic efficacy in the treatment of inflammatory bowel disease. Canadian Crohn's Relapse Prevention Trial Study Group. Gastroenterology 1994;106:287.

Surgery of Infants and Children: Scientific Principles and Practice, edited by Keith T. Oldham, Paul M. Colombani, and Robert P. Foglia. Lippincott–Raven Publishers, Philadelphia, © 1997.

CHAPTER 79

Intestinal Duplications

Kurt Heiss

Enteric duplications and omental and mesenteric cysts are rare developmental errors. Although complications from these can be significant when left untreated, these lesions are benign and are treated surgically with a goal to preserve function while relieving symptoms. They have been grouped together in one chapter for simplicity. This chapter reviews the incidence, anatomic location, theories of disordered embryology likely to give rise to these lesions, various modes of clinical presentation, and general principles of diagnosis and treatment of duplications in all areas of the gastrointestinal (GI) tract except the esophagus, which is dealt with in Chapter 60.

DUPLICATIONS

Duplications are rare congenital cystic abnormalities of the GI tract that can occur anywhere from the mouth to the anus. Although they can present at any age, greater than 80% of cases present before 2 years of age. The medical literature has recorded many anecdotal reports, but there are few large patient series (Table 79-1). Enteric duplications are named for the associated gastrointestinal structures rather than for the type of mucosa lining the cyst. There are frequently multiple mucosal types found in the same lesion. In addition, the formation of duplications most likely occurs before differentiation of mucosal epithelium into characteristic adult types. Because the frequency of multiple duplications is between 10% and 20%, the diagnosis of one duplication mandates the search for a second lesion elsewhere in the GI tract.

Duplications are classically located in the bowel mesentery, sharing a common muscular wall and blood supply with the associated bowel (Fig. 79-1). The symptoms at presentation are usually acute intestinal obstruction or respiratory possibly distress in the neonate. Older infants and children tend to experience indolent and vague abdominal pain over prolonged periods or intermittent GI bleeding. The large size often attained by these lesions can result in a significant mass effect, resulting in obstruction, torsion, and volvulus of the attached bowel. Finally, ectopic gastric mucosa is found in approximately one third of these lesions, predisposing the cyst mucosa to ulceration. This results in fistulization into the attached bowel with bleeding or free perforation into the peritoneum.

Patients who are symptomatic from an enteric duplication rarely are correctly diagnosed preoperatively. Nausea, vomiting, pain, abdominal distention, and constipation are common symptoms at presentation. Appendicitis, peptic ulcer disease, intussusception, or malrotation are frequent misdiagnoses. Routine abdominal films are often not helpful, except in cases in which a mass effect causes displacement of adjacent air-filled structures, prompting more focused studies. Subsequent contrast studies may demonstrate the impression of a lesion on normal bowel (Fig. 79-2). Communication between the duplication and the lumen of the adjacent bowel is rare, but diagnostic when present (Fig. 79-3).

Ultrasound has proved to be an excellent diagnostic and screening modality for enteric duplications, distinguishing cystic–abdominal masses from solid structures. The classic ultrasound triple-layer effect suggests the diagnosis (Fig. 79-4). Computed tomography (CT) and magnetic resonance imaging scans also demonstrate intraabdominal duplications, but rarely provide additional information that justifies the increased cost or causes a change in therapy. Because of the high incidence of ectopic gastric mucosa in enteric duplications, technetium studies are frequently helpful in diagnosing and locating duplications in the thorax, small bowel, and hindgut.

Duplications that remain undiagnosed into adulthood have been reported to present as malignancies. However, duplications in the pediatric population are benign lesions. Therefore, the surgical therapy should be sufficient to eliminate the patient's symptoms, prevent recurrence, and preserve function. Mortality due to bleeding or sepsis from perforation is related to delay in diagnosis and definitive treatment. The lesions are usually amenable to surgical repair without significant patient compromise. In the 1990s, mortality from this lesion should be rare with proper treatment and diagnosis.

Theories of Embryologic Origin

There are many theories regarding the disordered embryology producing enteric duplications.[8,12] None adequately explains the origin of all locations of duplications, suggesting that more than one theory is correct.

The *split notochord theory* postulates a neural tube traction

TABLE 79-1. *A summary of several reports of enteric duplications*

Investigators	Total number of patients	Location								
		Cervical	Mediastinal	Thoraco-abdominal	Gastric	Duodenal	Jejunal and Ileal	Colonic	Rectal	Other
Gross[1]	68	1	13	3	2	4	32	9	4	
Sieber[2]	25		5		4	2	16	5		
Houston & Lynn[3]	8		1	1			6			
Basu et al.[4]	28		7		1	3	16	4	2	
Mellish & Koop[5]	38	1	6	2	1		18	6	4	
Grosfeld et al.[6]	20		4	2	1		9	4		
Favara et al.[7]	37	3	4		3	4	20	4		
Wrenn	25		3	2	1	2	12	3	4	
Holcomb et al.[9]	96	1	20	3	8	2	47	20		
Ildstad et al.[10]	20		6		1		13			
Bower et al.[11]	78		16		7	5	34	10	2	2
Hudson[12]	90		10		6	8	59	3	3	1
Total	530	6 (1%)	95 (18%)	13 (2%)	35 (7%)	30 (6%)	282 (53%)	68 (13%)	19 (4%)	3 (0.5%)

mechanism as an explanation for the 15% of enteric duplications associated with vertebral defects. Before the formation of the mesoderm in the embryo, the ectoderm and endoderm are in direct contact. An embryologic error may allow a segment of GI endoderm to herniate through the notochord. The roof of the developing gut becomes an entrapped diverticulum as the notochord and endoderm begin to separate during the fourth week of development. As it migrates, the notochord is split by the persistent neurenteric canal, resulting in a vertebral anomaly (Fig. 79-5). The resulting tubular structure may extend through the diaphragm, connecting abdominal viscera to the thoracic or cervical spine. If the connection is lost, an isolated mediastinal duplication, or an intramesenteric abdominal diverticulum may result, and the vertebral anomaly may resolve. Persistent attachment to the notochord may prevent closing of the vertebral bodies, resulting in a spectrum of neurenteric pathology, including occult anterior spina bifida, intraspinal enteric cyst, dorsal enteric sinus, neuroenteric cyst, diastematomyelia, or a complete dorsal enteric fistula.

A second theory suggests that there is a failure of the normal regression of *embryonic diverticula*. Diverticula are common in the developing human GI tract. Their finding at numerous sites around the circumference of the gut wall provides an explanation for small cystic duplications noted in the intestinal wall, and for enteric cysts located in the presacral space. However, this does not explain the propensity for the location of enteric cysts within the leaves of the bowel mesentery, nor the finding of multiple types of mucosa lining the wall of these duplications.

The theory of *median septum formation* suggests that the walls of adjacent fetal bowel may be flattened by extrinsic compression with subsequent adherence and fusion, resulting in doubling of the lumen. Although this would explain the occurrence of adjacent or side-by-side tubular duplications, there is no embryologic evidence for this theory. More likely is the

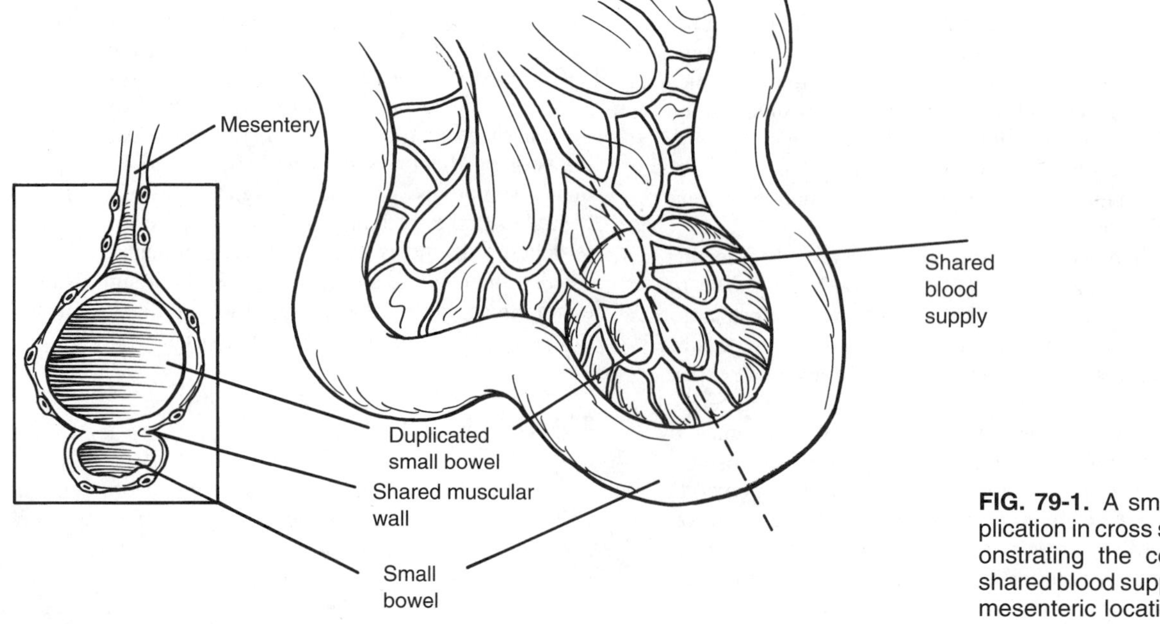

FIG. 79-1. A small bowel duplication in cross section, demonstrating the common wall, shared blood supply, and intramesenteric location.

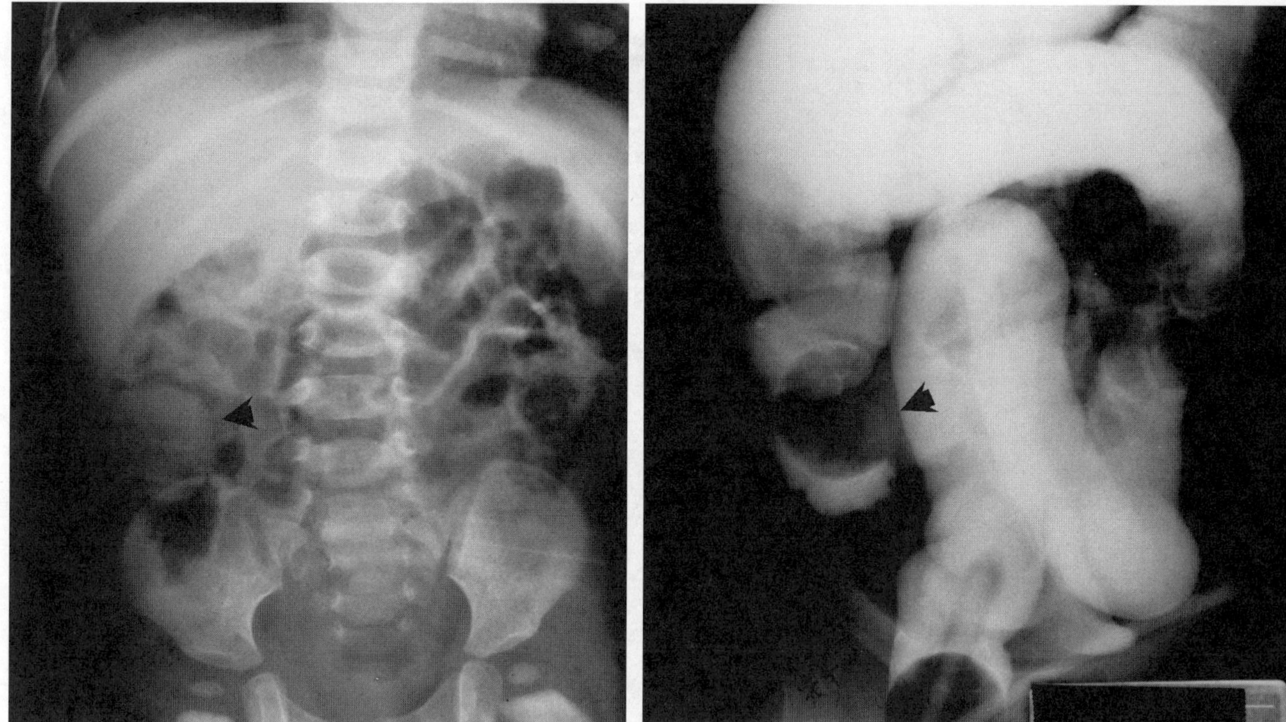

FIG. 79-2. (*A*) A circular mass (arrow) in the cecum suggests the presence of a lesion. (*B*) Subsequent contrast enema demonstrates an intramural duplication cyst (arrow) in this 14-month-old with intermittent obstructive symptoms.

theory of *partial twinning*, which suggests that the axial structures in hindgut duplications are "twinned" because of a split in the primitive streak, resulting in two notochords, separated at their caudal ends, which later fuse during cranial elongation of the embryo. This would result in the duplication of structures derived from the hindgut, including distal ileum, colon, and most of the bladder and urethra. It is speculated that twinning early in the hindgut's caudal growth may result in duplication of other pelvic organs, including genital structures, whereas later twinning may result only in a colorectal duplication.

Finally, the intestinal tract, especially the foregut, has been thought to undergo intense epithelial proliferation between 5 and 8 weeks of gestation. This proliferative period may completely occlude the lumen of the bowel with epithelium for a time. Subsequently, vacuoles form that coalesce to form the definitive lumen and allow recanalization. It has been postulated that there are *errors of epithelial recanalization* that allow formation of cysts located intramurally. This would explain the presence of small submucosal duplications.

Gastric Duplications

Enteric cysts associated with the stomach are the least common form of abdominal duplication, making up less than 5% to 7% in most descriptive series (Fig. 79-6). Although one third present in the newborn period, these lesions tend to present at a mean age of about 3 years, with the incidence in boys being greater than in girls. The most common presenting complaint is vomiting from gastric outlet obstruction. A palpable epigas-

tric mass is present in greater than 60% of patients. Gastric duplications have been associated with congenital pulmonary sequestrations in some reports. This has caused investigators to question whether these are bronchogenic cysts that communicate with the stomach, rather than enteric cysts adjacent to the stomach. Gastric duplications are frequently misdiagnosed, often being confused with pyloric stenosis, or other, more common GI lesions.

Gastric duplications are variable in size, ranging from small, asymptomatic, olive-sized lesions to very large cystic masses that displace adjacent structures (Fig. 79-7). The lesions are usually located on the greater curve or posterior wall of the stomach, but can be located at the pylorus and imitate pyloric stenosis. Pyloric duplications are very rare, and simulate pyloric stenosis by compressing the lumen of the pylorus, causing projectile vomiting with the accompanying electrolyte disturbances and malnutrition. Rarely, gastric duplications are completely separate from the stomach and are located in the retroperitoneum.

Gastric duplications are cystic in nature and do not routinely communicate with the lumen of the stomach. However, penetrating ulceration of the cyst wall and erosion into the stomach, pancreas, or colon, or through the abdominal wall has been reported. Gastric duplications commonly present in an infant with abdominal distention and vomiting as the chief complaint, and should be considered in the differential diagnosis whenever a mass effect displaces the stomach in the pediatric population. Weight loss is frequently present as a result of volume depletion and malnutrition from protracted vomiting. They are often large cysts that are palpable. Pain is secondary to distention of the

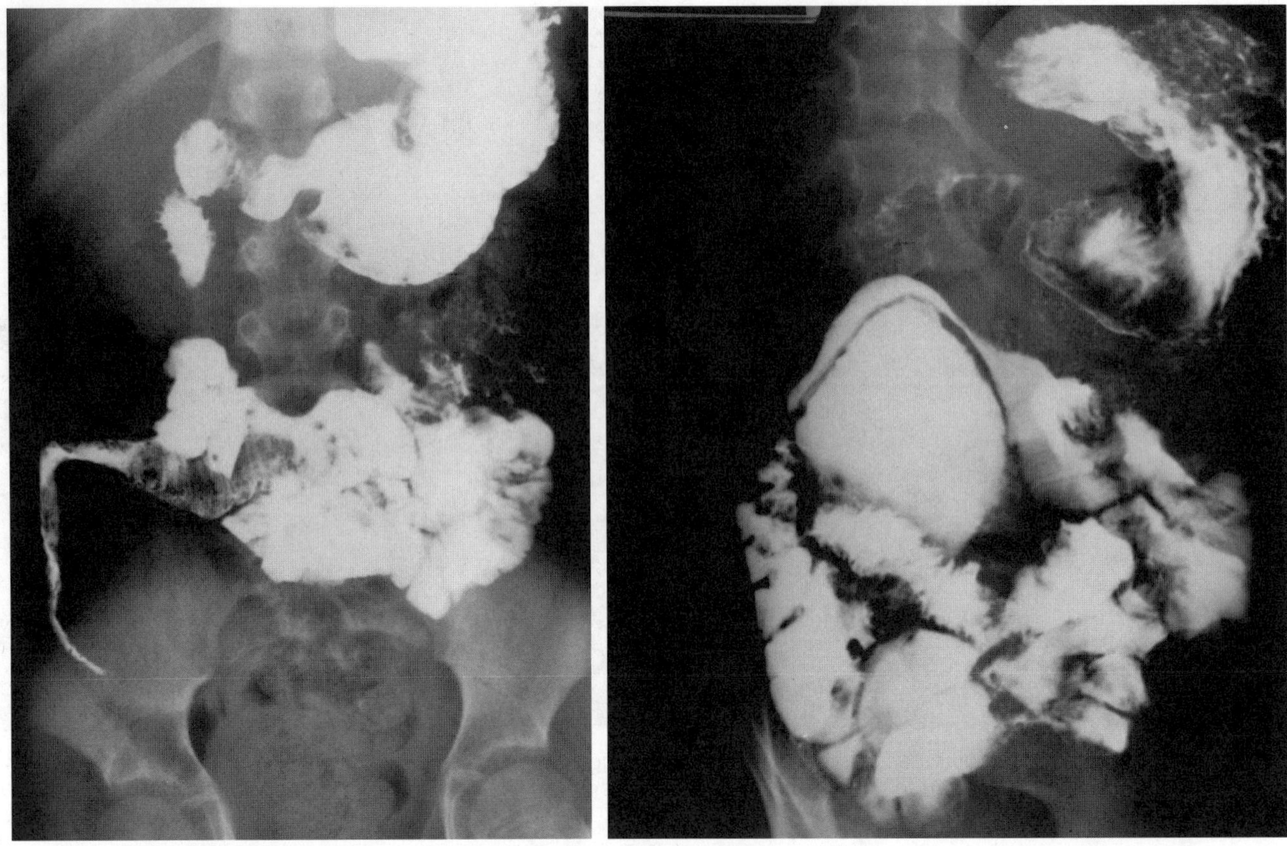

FIG. 79-3. A rare example of a communicating cystic duplication is found in this 10-year-old who presented with bleeding and a mass effect on abdominal flat plate. Upper gastrointestinal contrast study shows an extrinsic mass impression on the bowel (*A*), whereas a later film (*B*) demonstrates filling of the duplication cavity.

cyst or peptic ulceration. Complications associated with undiagnosed gastric duplications occur frequently, with bleeding and perforation being most common. On occasion, these lesions have eroded through the diaphragm, presenting with chest symptoms, including hemoptysis and respiratory distress from lung compression and parenchymal erosion.

Complete resection of the cyst and its common wall with the stomach is usually possible and is the procedure of choice. Internal marsupialization has been reported, but the presence of ulcerated gastric mucosa predisposes the patient to complications. Pyloric duplication cysts are rare and have been treated successfully by submucosal excision of the cyst. Small gastric lesions can be excised and the defect closed primarily. In situations in which removing the entire cyst would result in gastrectomy and put the child at a nutritional risk, subtotal resection should be considered. This requires removal of the free cyst wall, with mucosal stripping from the shared wall between the duplication and the stomach. At this point, efforts should be made to remove all of the cyst lining, regardless of whether the entire cyst wall is removed.

Duodenal Duplications

Duodenal duplications are also rare and comprise less than approximately 6% of enteric cysts of the alimentary tract (see Fig. 79-6). Although the mean age of diagnosis in children is approximately 3 years, they are occasionally not diagnosed until adulthood. Gastric mucosa is occasionally present, but these duplications are usually lined with duodenal mucosa. Duodenal duplications are difficult to diagnose, with the correct diagnosis occurring less than 5% of the time. The patients usually present with symptoms of intermittent upper GI obstruction. Frequently, the time course of the illness is prolonged, because the symptoms are vague and difficult to localize. Anemia from ulceration, bleeding, and fistulization is common. Most of the duodenal duplications are cystic, and approximately 25% of them communicate with the bowel lumen. Vertebral abnormalities and respiratory complaints from transdiaphragmatic erosion are rare. When obtained, barium studies usually demonstrate complete obstruction or narrowing of the duodenal lumen, a widened C-loop, or an intraluminal filling defect of the duodenum. Occasionally, patients with duodenal duplications present with jaundice due to extrinsic compression of the common bile duct. A diiosopropylacetanilide iminodiacetic acid (DISIDA) scan shows good concentration of the tracer in the liver. Failure to fill the cyst suggests that the lesion is not a choledochal cyst.

Most duodenal duplications are located posteromedial to the second or third portion of the duodenum. Complete excision with the attached segment of duodenum is the desired outcome, but this is rarely possible because of the proximity to the ampulla of Vater and the potential of damage to the biliary and pancreatic ducts. Intraoperative cholangiography is important to assess the relation of the mass to the ductal system. If the cyst mucosa is not gastric, internal marsupialization is an acceptable solution. Cystenterostomy, using a Roux loop for drainage, has also been described by some as an acceptable option. In the presence of gastric mucosa, excision of the free duplication wall and stripping of the abnormal mucosal lining from the remaining common wall is the preferred surgical management.

Small Intestinal Duplications

The small intestine is the most common location for enteric duplications, accounting for about 50% of all lesions in large series. Of these, two thirds are ileal in location and one third are jejunal. The lesions are located within the mesentery, sharing a common blood supply and a common muscular wall with the adjacent bowel (see Fig. 79-1). Noncommunicating cystic lesions are most common. One third of small bowel duplications are tubular, and communication with the adjacent bowel is rare. When present, this communication may lie anywhere along the common wall. If the communication is located distally, the lesion may drain into the small bowel and remain asymptomatic. If the communication is proximal, the distal end of the duplication dilates, causing obstruction, perforation, or volvulus (Fig. 79-8).

Small bowel duplications are mobile and often difficult to palpate, with only 25% being noted preoperatively on physical examination. Peptic ulceration with hemorrhage occurs frequently in patients with jejunal duplications because of the high incidence of gastric mucosa in these lesions. Complications from peptic ulceration, such as perforation and melena, are more common in this subgroup of enteric cysts than those in any other portion of the GI tract. In contrast, patients with ileal duplications less frequently experience GI bleeding. Compression from the dilated duplication of the adjacent ileum can result in constipation or obstruction. Newborns with associated atresia are reported to make up 15% of patients presenting with ileal duplications, raising a question as to the embryologic origin of such lesions. The presentation of small bowel duplications tends to occur either as an acute event in the perinatal period, or with a confusing clinical picture after a long period with indolent symptoms. Ileal duplications are often misdiagnosed as appendicitis, Hirschsprung disease, or intussusception, whereas jejunal duplications are confused with Meckel diverticulum, peptic ulcer disease, malrotation, or atresia when the presentation occurs in the newborn period.

Complete excision and primary anastomosis of the cystic lesions is the treatment of choice. Long tubular duplications present a treatment challenge. Simple resection of the duplication and adjacent bowel could result in absorptive deficiencies (Fig. 79-9). Some clinicians have advocated internal drainage by creating a window in the common wall at the distal end of long tubular duplications to avoid the need for massive resection. Patients with gastric mucosa in the small bowel duplication are unable to be treated in this fashion. Stripping of the gastric mucosa through counterincisions along the length of the duplication or marsupialization of the distal end of the duplication to the stomach for drainage has been performed successfully to treat this difficult problem. Long-term follow-up of both these treatment strategies has demonstrated good results (Wrenn EL Jr, personal communication, August, 1994).[13,14]

Colonic Duplications

Enteric duplications of the hindgut are cystic or tubular structures with normal colonic epithelium. In patients with colonic or presacral duplications who remain undiagnosed into adulthood, malignant changes resulting in adenocarcinoma can occur. Constipation, obstruction, and volvulus are the common presenting symptoms because ectopic gastric mucosa is much less common in colorectal duplications. The incidence of neoplastic change in hindgut duplications is much higher than in any other location.[15]

A review of the available cases suggests that there are three types of enteric cysts associated with the hindgut.[16,17] These include midline duplications, bilateral duplications of the colon and rectum, and cystic remnants of the tailgut.

Midline duplications are cystic in nature, lie posterior to the rectum, share a common wall, and have the characteristics of the cystic duplications discussed thus far. Tubular duplications are distinctly uncommon in this location. Midline duplications share a common wall with the normal bowel and may require a large resection for definitive therapy. If attached to the rectum, consideration should be given to protection with a diverting colostomy. Tail-gut remnants should be completely excised, when found, because of the known potential for occasional malignant degeneration in these enterogenous cysts. As is true with sacrococcygeal teratomas, resection of the lesion with the coccyx has been recommended.

Because of their location, cystic duplications are often included with the second type of hindgut duplication, the *tail-gut*

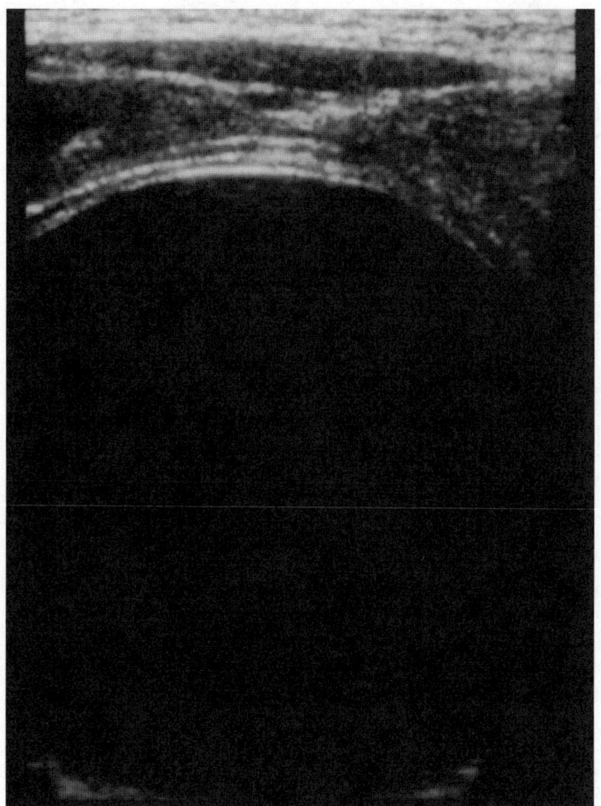

FIG. 79-4. Ultrasound study of a patient with gastric duplication demonstrating the classic findings of triple layering.

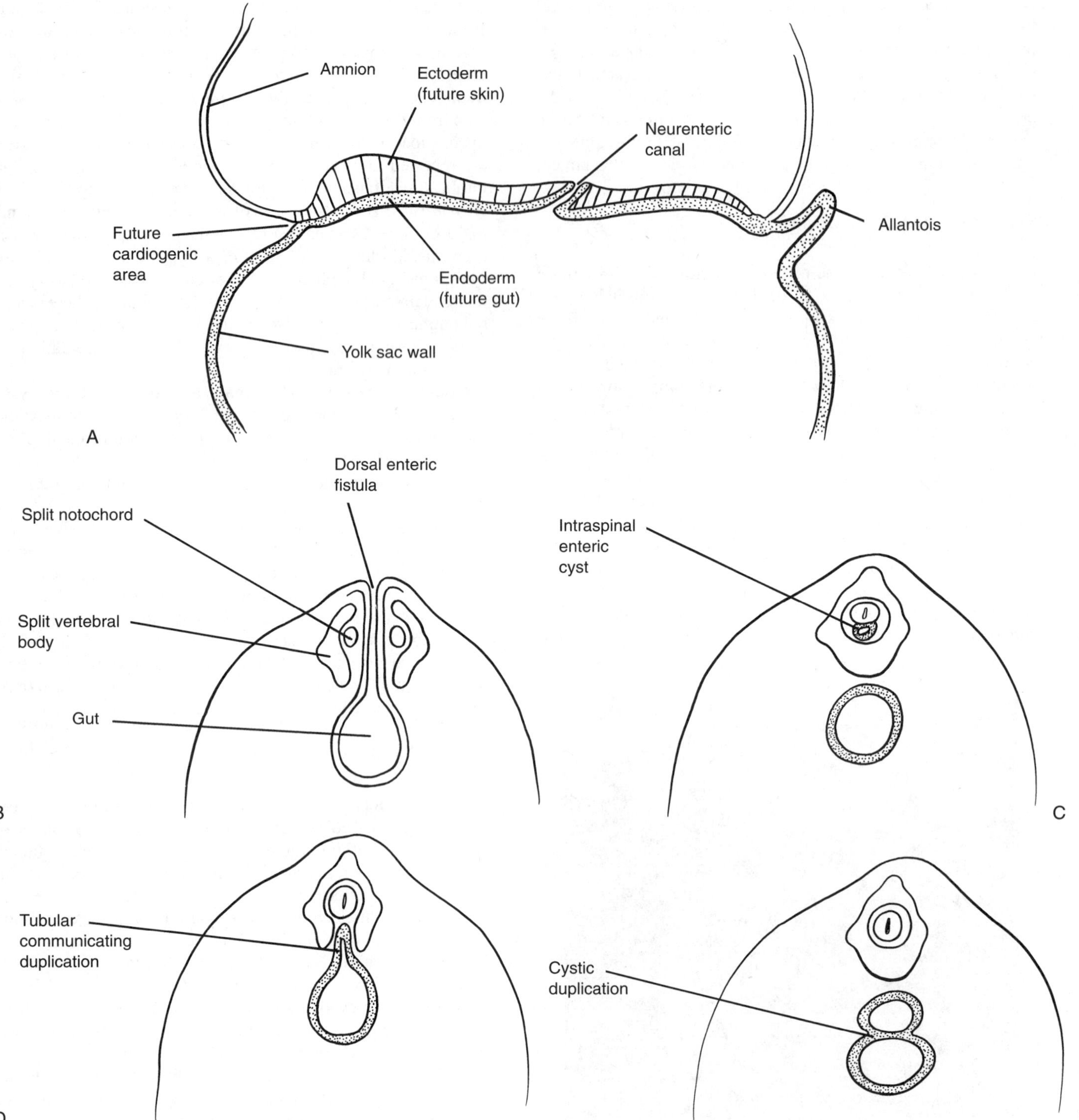

FIG. 79-5. Diagrammatic representation of the split notochord theory of duplication development. (*A*) A sagittal view of the developing embryo illustrating the neurenteric canal. During spinal organogenesis, gastrointestinal endoderm is entrapped, forming a traction diverticulum as the separation begins. A persistent neurenteric canal results in dorsal enteric fistula (*B*), enteric cysts (*C*), tubular communicating duplication (*D*), cystic duplication (*E*), spina bifida, and other vertebral anomalies.

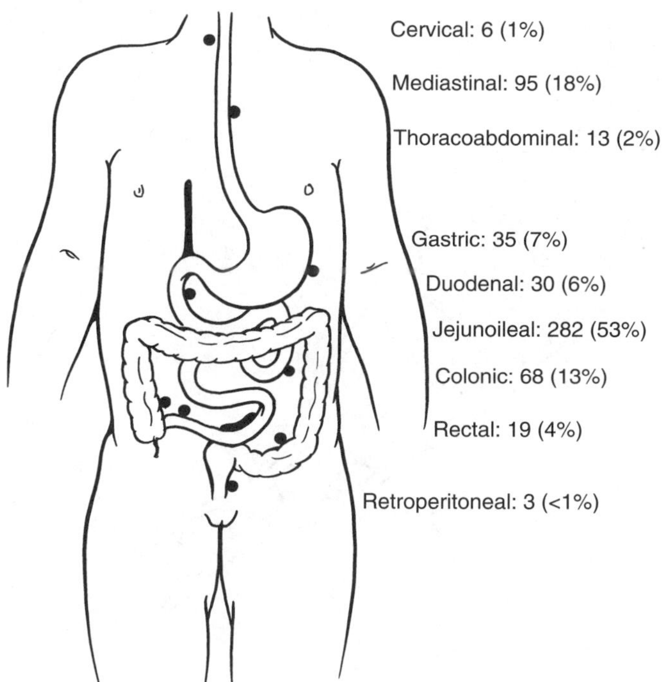

FIG. 79-6. An anatomic representation of the incidence and location of enteric duplications taken from the studies listed in Table 79-1.

cyst. This cystic structure is located between the anus and the coccyx, and contains enteric epithelium. In contrast to the midline variety, it has no common wall and is excised easily without sacrificing the rectum wall. It is considered to be a remnant of the opening between the ectoderm and endoderm at the poste-

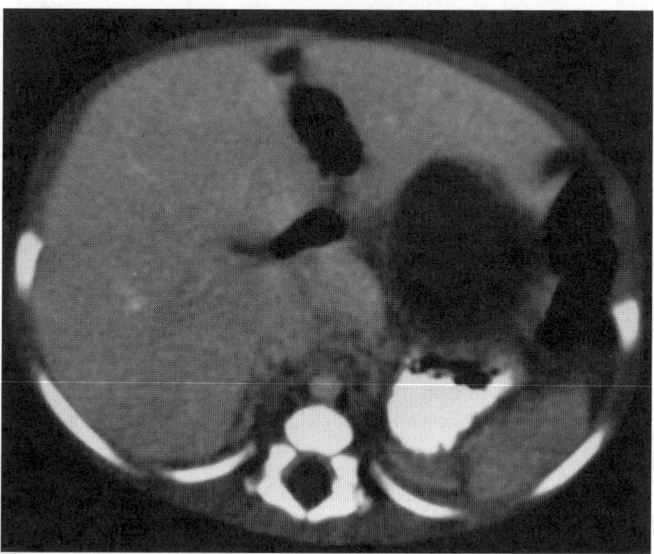

FIG. 79-7. A 1-month-old presented with vomiting and an upper gastrointestinal bleed. A CT scan demonstrates displacement of abdominal viscera by a gastric duplication (no contrast) that does not communicate with the stomach (filled with contrast). (Courtesy of Dr. Francis Blankenburg, Department of Radiology, Packard Children's Hospital at Stanford University, Palo Alto, CA)

rior end of the neural tube. Most midline defects have been attributed to this persistent developmental structure. Presacral tumors with enteric epithelium should probably be considered remnants of this tail-gut abnormality. Obstruction is the most common presenting sign in infants of midline duplications and tail-gut cysts.[18]

The third type of hindgut duplication results from *partial twinning* and is a "side-by-side" rather than an "over-and-under" doubling. The duplication is located next to the normal bowel, rather than within the leaves of the mesentery. This duplication involves the hindgut and structures derived from the hindgut. These patients often have other paired midline structures, such as bladder and uteri. The caudal spinal cord has been found to have anomalies as well, which range from complete duplication of an otherwise normal cord to an anterior myelomeningocele. Duplicated external genitalia and renal abnormalities may be found when extensive hindgut duplication occurs. The pelvis in these infants is wider than normal, and may give rise to an abdominal wall hernia with separated rectus muscles. This is thought to be caused by the presence of extra organs rather than defective development. Finally, the pelvis may be divided by a peritoneal septum arising from the posterior pelvic wall to divide the caudal peritoneal cavity into halves, extending anteriorly up the abdominal wall to the umbilical artery.

Some fully developed cases have demonstrated complete duplication of all caudal intestinal structures, beginning at the Meckel diverticulum, and include two bladders and two vaginas that communicate with two unicornate uteri and open into separate vulvas. In boys, a bifid penis and scrotum have been reported. Two bladders, each with one ureter, empty through two urethras into separate orifices. Sometimes the lumbar vertebrae and the sacrum are doubled or bifid. The uterus and vagina are not derived from the hindgut, but are commonly doubled in severe cases. This failure of fusion of the müllerian-derived structures is considered secondary to the doubling of the urogenital sinus, to which their distal ends attach. There are no reports of a duplicated umbilical vein or arteries, as would be expected with a complete duplication of the allantois. However, cases of three colons have been reported.

Most of these complex hindgut duplications are found in girls (70%). Duplications involving the complete hindgut or colorectum are found in 70%, whereas 10% to 30% have more complex caudal twinning with double bladders, urethras, vaginas, and uteri, and abnormal genitals. The duplicated external genitalia are considered to have normal function, and are often left in place in female patients. Reports exist of women with this hindgut abnormality successfully giving vaginal birth to infants from both vaginas. Boys with the duplicated penes are usually treated surgically to attempt a more normal perineal appearance. The absence of reflux or obstruction allows urologic procedures to be done electively in these patients with completely duplicated caudal twinning. However, obstructive symptoms may require early urologic intervention. Patients who present with doubled genitals usually have no difficulty emptying their duplicated hindgut bowel. In addition, the blood supply to these duplicated colons is separate. However, patients with normal external anatomy and a duplicated hindgut often present with obstruction, with the normal colon being compressed by the blind end of the abnormal obstructed colon. These colons are often densely adherent and share the same blood supply, requiring a drainage procedure to preserve the normal bowel.

The presenting complaints in patients with severe abnormali-

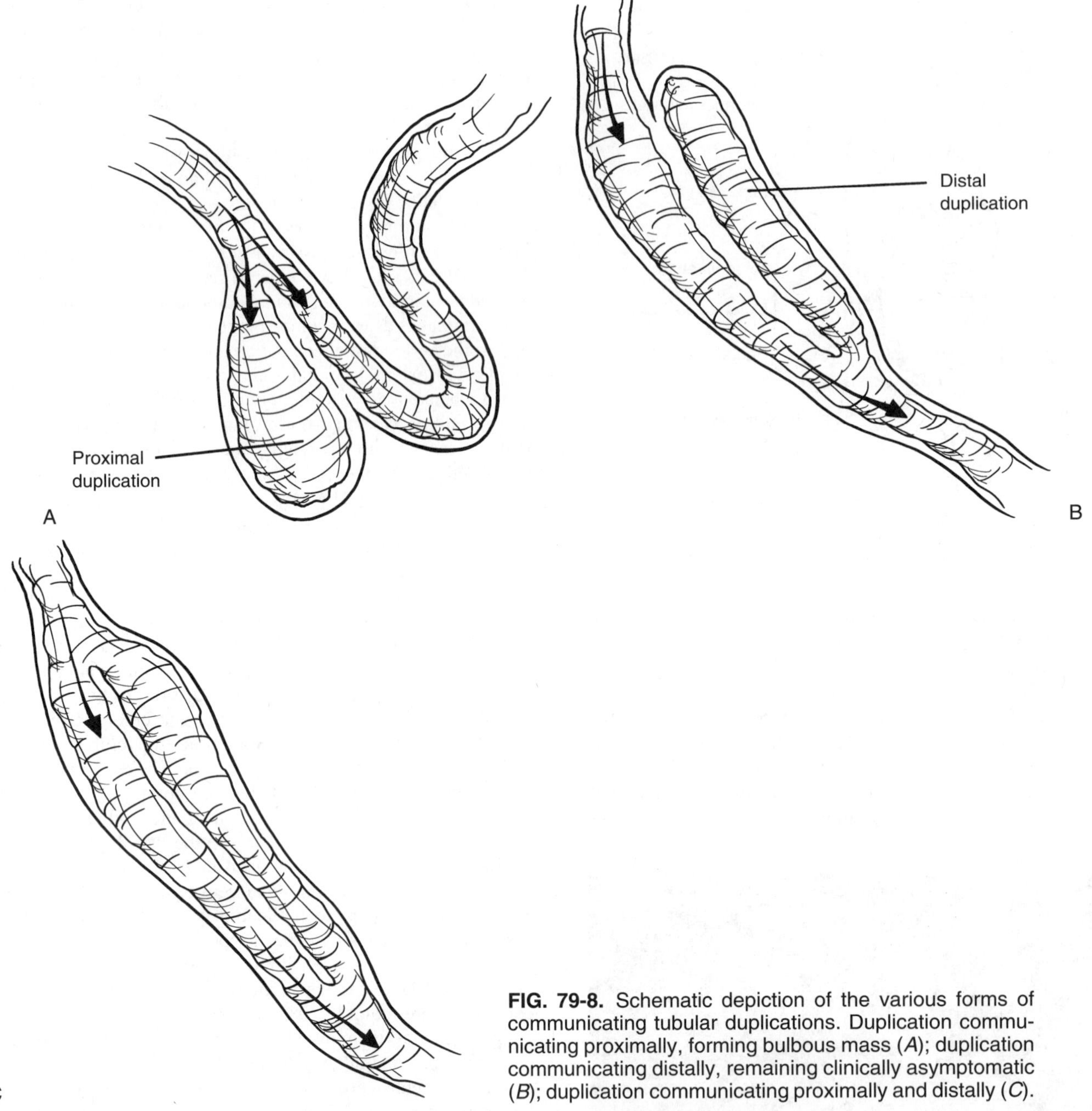

FIG. 79-8. Schematic depiction of the various forms of communicating tubular duplications. Duplication communicating proximally, forming bulbous mass (*A*); duplication communicating distally, remaining clinically asymptomatic (*B*); duplication communicating proximally and distally (*C*).

ties of the hindgut include obstruction of adjacent bowel by the dilated duplication, or complications from the obstruction. Information contributing to the diagnosis can be obtained from barium studies when there are two obvious anal orifices (Fig. 79-10). When only one anus exists, the situation is difficult to diagnose before surgery. *Side-by-side* duplications require an innovative surgical approach directed toward establishing a functional organ, rather than just removing the abnormal segment. Long-segment, blind-ending colonic duplications have been treated by forming a distal communication with the normal colon after repairing the fistula to the genitourinary system system, if present. Excision of an area of the septum between the lumina of the normal bowel and the duplication at their distalmost area of attachment has been successful in creating a communication for the fecal stream to pass through. This functionally results in two long colonic segments, adjacent to each other, sharing a common wall, exiting through a common anus.

MESENTERIC, OMENTAL, AND RETROPERITONEAL CYSTS

Definition and Embryology

Cysts of the retroperitoneum, mesentery, or omentum are uncommon, having an incidence of about 1/100,000 hospital admissions in most series. They may be unilocular or multilocular in nature. The contents of the cysts vary from serum-like to overtly

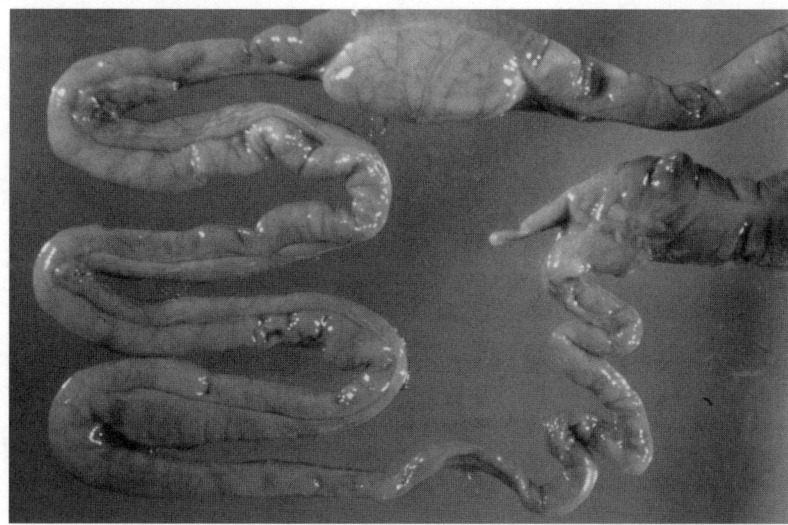

FIG. 79-9. An autopsy specimen showing a tubular small bowel duplication involving a portion of the ileum and much of the jejunum. (Courtesy of Dr. Carlos Abramowsky, Department of Pathology, Egleston Children's Hospital at Emory University, Atlanta, GA)

chylous with a high triglyceride content and high concentrations of lymphocytes. Occasionally, they are bloody because of hemorrhage into the cyst. They are usually thin walled and smooth, with occasional excrescences, forming loculi. The cyst wall is made up of fibrous connective tissue lined by endothelial cells. Dilated lymphatics are often associated with the cyst, and there may be calcification in the wall. Most omental cysts and colonic mesenteric cysts have serous contents, whereas mesenteric cysts located in the small bowel and retroperitoneum are equally divided between serous and chylous.[19–21]

There are many theories as to their origin. Most consider these cysts to be ectopic lymphatic tissue that has disordered production and flow of lymph because of lack of communication with the central lymphatic system. They are associated with embryonic retroperitoneal lymph sacs, making them abdominal equivalents of cystic hygromas of the neck. However, attempts to create lymphatic obstruction in animal models have failed to produce cystic lesions, suggesting a nonlymphatic origin for some cysts.

Mesenteric cysts have been described in all age groups, but about 40% have been in children, suggesting a developmental problem as the etiology.[19] These are rare lesions, as evidenced by an accumulation of 15 to 20 patients from major pediatric centers over a 20- to 25-year period. Mesenteric cysts, of which most are small bowel in location, appear to be more common than omental cysts by a factor of 3 to 1. They are considered to be dynamic but slow growing, which could explain their relative lack of symptoms until presentation in older age groups.

Clinical Presentation and Diagnosis

In studies of both adults and children, these lesions are difficult to diagnose because they are often large and soft in consistency. The correct diagnosis is made preoperatively in less than 25%. More recent studies indicate improved preoperative diagnosis using ultrasound and CT.[20,21] Such cysts can be quite mobile, making a definite abdominal mass difficult to palpate in most cases. The complaint at presentation is commonly abdominal pain due to hemorrhage, obstruction, or volvulus. In addition, acute distention from hemorrhage or bowel infarction, or chronic distention with a gradually enlarging abdomen can also occur. Intestinal obstruction from mesenteric cysts may occur from volvulus, or acute enlargement from hemorrhage into the cyst, or from compression of the adjacent bowel. The jejunum is the most common location of the mesenteric abnormality.

Diagnostic studies are primarily radiologic. Occasionally, a flat plate of the abdomen is useful, demonstrating a mass effect that is gasless and homogeneous, with the appearance of ascites, displacing the abdominal viscera. Ultrasound is usually helpful, demonstrating a unilocular or multilocular fluid-filled structure. A wall can usually be identified, but occasionally, ascites can be difficult to distinguish from a mesenteric cyst. CT scans demonstrate displacement of the bowel by a fluid-filled mass, but rarely add any diagnostic information above that provided by ultrasound. Omental cysts tend to be anteriorly located, displacing the stomach in a posterior or cephalad direction (Fig.

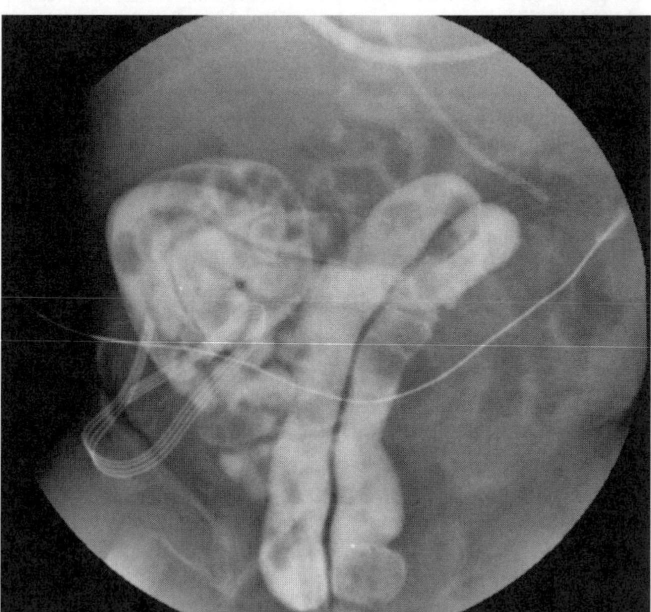

FIG. 79-10. A contrast enema of an infant presenting with doubled anal orifices at birth in addition to other abdominal wall abnormalities.

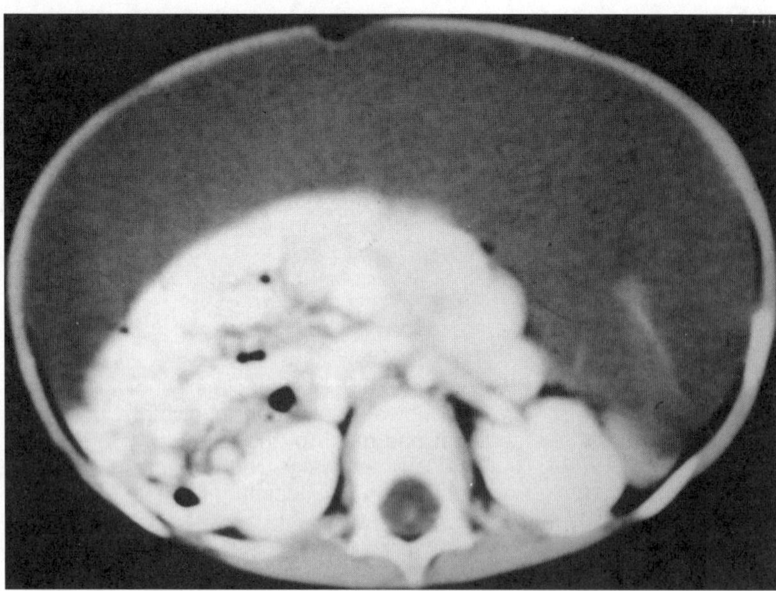

FIG. 79-11. CT scan of a large omental cyst in a 3-year-old boy with abdominal distention.

79-11). Mesenteric cysts may compress the bowel or cause it to appear stretched over an extraluminal mass. There may be difficulty distinguishing a mesenteric cyst from a mass or cyst of ovarian, pancreatic, or enteric origin.

Complete excision of the cyst is the treatment of choice. This is usually possible in cases of mesenteric cysts and always with omental cysts. Occasionally, mesenteric cysts are intimately associated with the blood supply of the bowel, making a bowel resection with primary anastomosis necessary to remove the cyst. This appears to be necessary in about half the cases. Patients in whom the cyst involves the entire mesentery of the bowel or diffusely involves the retroperitoneum may require marsupialization of the cyst, with the breakdown of multiloculated walls and the temporary placement of drains to avoid early recurrence of the cystic process (Fig. 79-12). Recurrence is more common is cases in which complete resection is not possible.

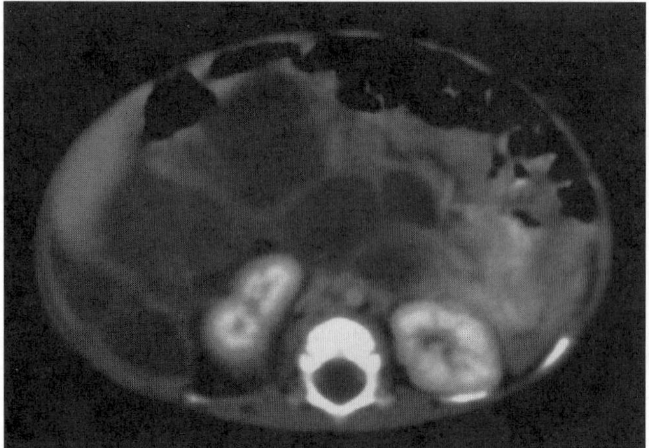

FIG. 79-12. CT scan of a large infant with abdominal distention and a diffuse mesenteric cyst involving the enteric retroperitoneum. The cysts were marsupialized and drained with closed suction drains without recurrence. (Courtesy of Dr. Barry Shandling, Hospital for Sick Children, Toronto, Ontario, Canada)

REFERENCES

1. Gross RE. The surgery of infancy and childhood. Philadelphia, WB Saunders, 1953:221.
2. Sieber WK. Alimentary tract duplication. Arch Surg 1956;73:383.
3. Houston HE, Lynn HB. Duplication of the small intestine in children. Mayo Clin Proc 1966;41:246.
4. Basu R, Forshall I, Rickham PP. Duplication of the alimentary tract. Br J Surg 1960;47:477.
5. Mellish RWP, Koop CE. Clinical manifestations of duplication of the bowel. Pediatrics 1961;27:397.
6. Grosfeld JL, O'Neill JA, Clatworthy HW. Enteric duplications in infancy and childhood: an 18-year review. Ann Surg 1970;172:83.
7. Favara BE, Franciosi RA, Akers DR, et al. Enteric duplications, thirty-seven cases: a vascular theory of pathogenesis. Am J Dis Child 1971;122:501.
8. Wrenn EL Jr. Alimentary tract duplications. In: Ashcraft KW, Holder TM, eds. Pediatric surgery. 2nd ed. Philadelphia, WB Saunders, 1993:421.
9. Holcomb GW, Gheissari A, O'Neill JA, et al. Surgical management of alimentary tract duplications. Ann Surg 1989;209:167.
10. Ildstad ST, Tollerud DJ, Weiss RG, et al. Duplications of the alimentary tract. Ann Surg 1988;208:184.
11. Bower RJ, Sieber WK, Kiesewetter WB. Alimentary tract duplications in children. Ann Surg 1978;188:669.
12. Hudson HW. Giant diverticula or reduplications of the intestinal tract. N Engl J Med 1935;213:1123.
13. Wrenn EL Jr. Tubular duplication of the small intestine. Surgery 1962;52:494.
14. Jewett TC, Walker AB, Cooney DR. A long-term follow-up on a duplication of the entire small intestine treated by gastroduplication. J Pediatr Surg 1983;18:185.
15. Orr MM, Edwards AJ. Neoplastic change in duplication of the alimentary tract. Br J Surg 1975;62:264.
16. Ravitch MM. Hind gut duplication: doubling of colon and genital urinary tracts. Ann Surg 1953;137:588.
17. Beach PD, Brascho DJ, Hein WR, et al. Duplication of the primitive hindgut of the human being. Surgery 1961;49:779.
18. Perry CL, Merritt JW. Presacral enterogenous cyst. Ann Surg 1949;129:881.
19. Kurtz RJ, Heimann TM, Beck AR, et al. Mesenteric and retroperitoneal cysts. Ann Surg 1986;203:109.
20. Chung MA, Brandt ML, St-Vil D, Yazbeck S. Mesenteric cysts in children. J Pediatr Surg 1991;26:1306.
21. Hebra A, Brown MF, McGeehin KM, et al. Mesenteric, omental, and retroperitoneal cysts in children: a clinical study of 22 cases. South Med J 1993;86:173.

Colon

Surgery of Infants and Children: Scientific Principles and Practice, edited by
Keith T. Oldham, Paul M. Colombani, and Robert P. Foglia.
Lippincott–Raven Publishers, Philadelphia, © 1997.

CHAPTER 80

Hirschsprung Disease

Prem Puri

Hirschsprung disease (HD) is characterized by absence of ganglion cells in the distal bowel and extending proximally for varying distances. The aganglionosis is confined to the rectosigmoid colon in 75% of patients; sigmoid, splenic flexure, or transverse colon in 17% of patients, and total colon along with a short segment of terminal ileum in 8% of patients.[1,2] Total intestinal aganglionosis with absence of ganglion cells from the duodenum to the rectum is the rarest form of HD.[3,4] The incidence of HD is estimated to be approximately 1 in 5000 live births.[5] Spouge and Baird[6] studied the incidence of HD in 689,118 consecutive live births in British Columbia and reported an incidence rate for this disease to be 1 in 4,417 live births. The disease is more common in boys with a male to female ratio of 4:1.[7–9] The male preponderance of HD tends to decrease with increasing length of the aganglionic segment. For long segment disease, the sex ratio is 1.5 to 2:1.[5–7]

ETIOLOGY

Neural Crest Cell Migration

It is generally accepted that the enteric ganglion cells are derived from the vagal neural crest cells.[10–12] In the human fetus, neural crest–derived neuroblasts first appear in the developing esophagus at 5 weeks, and then migrate down to the anal canal in a craniocaudal direction during the 5th to 12th week of gestation.[11–12] The neural crest cells first form the myenteric plexuses just outside the circular muscle layer. The mesenchymally derived longitudinal muscle layer then forms, sandwiching the myenteric plexus after it has been formed in the 12th week of gestation. In addition, after the craniocaudal migration has ended, the submucous plexus is formed by the neuroblasts, which migrate from the myenteric plexus across the circular muscle layer and into the submucosa and mucosa. This progresses in craniocaudal direction during the 12th to 16th week of gestation. The absence of ganglion cells in HD has been attributed to failure of migration of neural crest cells.[12] The earlier the arrest of migration, the longer the aganglionic segment.

Studies have suggested that enteric neurons follow a dual gradient of development from each end of the gut to the middle;

vagal neural crest cells provide the main source of enteric neurons, and sacral neural crest cells innervate the distal bowel.[13–15] A dual origin of enteric neurons has been negated by the more recent studies on chick embryo as well as human embryos. Allan and Newgreen[16] isolated bowel segments from embryos at various stages of development, and grew these segments in the chorioallantoic membrane and found that enteric neurons appeared in a craniocaudal sequence demonstrating a vagal source. Meijers and associates[17] transected the bowel *in ovo* at an early stage, before the passage of neural crest cells had occurred, preventing craniocaudal migration of vagal neural crest cells. They found that the hindgut remained aganglionic showing that there was no colonization by sacral neural crest cells. Fujimoto and coworkers[18] studied neural crest cell migration in the developing gut in the human embryo using antineurofilament protein triplet antibody and found that enteric ganglia originated from a single vagal neural crest source. They found that the neural crest–derived cells first appear in the esophagus at 4 weeks and then migrate down along the gut in a craniocaudal direction.

Microenvironmental Alterations

Another hypothesis put forward regarding etiology is that the aganglionosis may result from failure of differentiation because of microenvironmental changes.[19,20] Extracellular matrix proteins have been recognized as important microenvironmental mediators of the neuronal processing pathway in the early embryonal stage and as an important matrix for cell adhesion and movement.[21–23] Fujimoto and coworkers[18] studied the distribution of extracellular matrix proteins and cell–matrix interactions in the migration pathway of neural crest cells in the gut in the early human embryo using a panel of anti-extracellular matrix protein antibodies such as fibronectin, laminin, collagen type IV, and hyaluronic acid. It was observed that enteric neurogenesis is dependent on extracellular matrices; fibronectin, and hyaluronic acid providing a migration pathway for neural crest–derived cells in the developing gut, and laminin and collagen type IV promoting outgrowth and maturation of neurites from settled neural crest–derived cells. Alteration of extracellular matrices in early embryonal stage may either cause the arrest of migration of neural crest–derived cells to their final destination, thus producing HD or result in the abnormal development of enteric ganglia, thereby producing HD-related disorders (e.g., neuronal intestinal dysplasia). Studies of bowel in HD have demonstrated abnormal distribution of extracellular matrix components, laminin and collagen type IV, thus supporting the hypothesis that abnormal microenvironment may have a role in the pathogenesis of HD.[24,25] Shimotake and colleagues[26] reported impaired proliferative activity of mesenchymal cells affecting the migrating pathway for neural crest cells in the developing gut.

MHC Class II Antigen and Intercellular Adhesion Molecule-1 Abnormalities

Recently, Kuroda and associates[27] and Hirobe and coworkers[28] demonstrated marked elevation of major histocompatibility complex (MHC) class II antigens throughout the intestinal wall in aganglionic colon with abnormal localization in the mucosa and lamina propria. The ectopic expression of MHC class II antigen was not seen in any portion of bowel of patients who did not have HD. These authors suggested that ectopic expression of class II antigens may indicate that an underlying immunologic mechanism may be responsible for causing HD. We reported strong expression of intercellular adhesion molecule-1 (ICAM-1) and MHC class II antigen on hypertrophic nerve trunks both in the submucous and myenteric plexuses of aganglionic colon and small ganglia in myenteric and submucous plexuses in the transition zone without histologic evidence of inflammation[29] (Figs. 80-1 and 80-2). However, no staining of ganglia or nerve fibers could be found in the submucous and myenteric plexuses of the colon from controls or the normal ganglionic colon from HD patients. The hypertrohic nerve trunks and abnormal transitional segment ganglia may act as antigen-presenting cells. The antigen-presenting cell function of the hypertrophic nerve trunks and abnormal transitional segment ganglia may be mediated, in part, through ICAM-1 and MHC class II antigen expression.

Genetic Factors

Genetic factors have been implicated in the etiology of HD. HD is known to occur in families. The reported incidence of familial cases varied from 3.6% to 7.8% in different series.[1,2,5] A familial incidence of 15% to 21% has been reported in total colonic aganglionosis[1,30] and 50% in the rare total intestinal aganglionosis.[31]

Schiller and colleagues[32] reported 22 infants belonging to four families from Gaza, who had either documented or clinically suspected HD. Of these infants, 13 underwent laparotomy and multiple intestinal biopsies, 10 had total intestinal aganglionosis, 1 had total colonic aganglionosis, 1 had near total colonic aganglionosis and only 1 had rectosigmoid HD. Engum and associates[33] reported 20 cases of HD in 12 kindreds. The level of aganglionosis was rectal or rectosigmoid in eight cases, left colon in two, transverse or right colon in two and total colonic ganglionosis with variable small bowel involvement in eight.

Although genetic factors are definitely involved, there is no clear pattern of inheritance and most investigators have found a sex-modified multifactorial mode of inheritance. Badner and coworkers[9] performed complex segregation analysis in 487 patients with HD and their families in an attempt to study inheritance patterns. The families were classified according to the extent of aganglionosis. For patients with aganglionosis beyond the sigmoid colon, the mode of inheritance was compatible with a dominant gene with incomplete penetrance, whereas for cases with aganglionosis extending no farther than the sigmoid colon, the inheritance pattern was equally likely to be a result of either multiple factors or a recessive gene with a very low penetrance. Stannard and coworkers[34] described two families with HD where pattern of transmission was consistent with single gene inheritance. In one family, four of the five brothers were affected, two of whom were monozygotic twins. The cluster of affected brothers in this family was consistent with X-linked recessive inheritance. In the second family, members of successive generations were affected by long-segment HD that appeared to have been transmitted in a pattern consistent with autosomal dominant inheritance.

The relation with Down syndrome also tends to suggest a genetic component in the etiology of HD. Down syndrome is the most common chromosomal abnormality associated with aganglionosis and has been reported to occur in 4.5% to 16% of all cases of HD.[35–38] Other chromosomal abnormalities that have been described in association with HD include interstitial delection of distal 13q,[39,40] partial deletion of 2p22 and reciprocal translocation (3:7)(p21:q22),[41] and Trisomy 18 mosaic.[42] A number of unusual hereditary syndromes have been reported in patients with HD. These include Waardenburg syndrome,[43,44] Von Recklinghausen syndrome,[45] type D brachydactyly,[34] and Smith–Lemli–Opitz syndrome.[37]

Recurrence risk to siblings is dependent on the sex of the person affected and the extent of aganglionosis. Badner and associates[9] calculated the risk of HD transmission to relatives and found that the recurrence risk to siblings increases as the aganglionosis becomes more extensive. The brothers of patients with rectosigmoid HD have a higher risk (4%) than sisters (1%). Much higher risks are observed in cases of long-segment HD. The brothers and sons of affected females have a 24% and 29% risk of being affected, respectively.

Segregation analyses have demonstrated that HD is a genetic disorder with autosomal dominant, autosomal recessive, and polygenic forms, whereas some cases are thought to be of environmental origin.[9] An autosomal dominant gene causing this disease was mapped to human chromosome 10q11.2,[46,47] and further localized in an interval of 250-kilobases by physical characterization of three interstitial deletions.[48] This region contains the RET protooncogene whose mutations were recently reported in HD patients.[49,50] Over 70 new RET mutations have been reported in HD since 1994 when RET mutations were first reported in this disease. However, the existence of some autosomal dominant HD families with no linkage to RET suggests that additional susceptibility genes for HD may exist.

In a large inbred kindred with a high incidence of HD, a missense mutation was demonstrated in the endothelin-B receptor (EDNRB) gene,[51] which was mapped to chromosome 13.[52] There also have been reports describing that some HD patients are associated with de novo interstitial deletions of chromosome 13.[39,53,54] Moreover, it has been shown that the interaction of

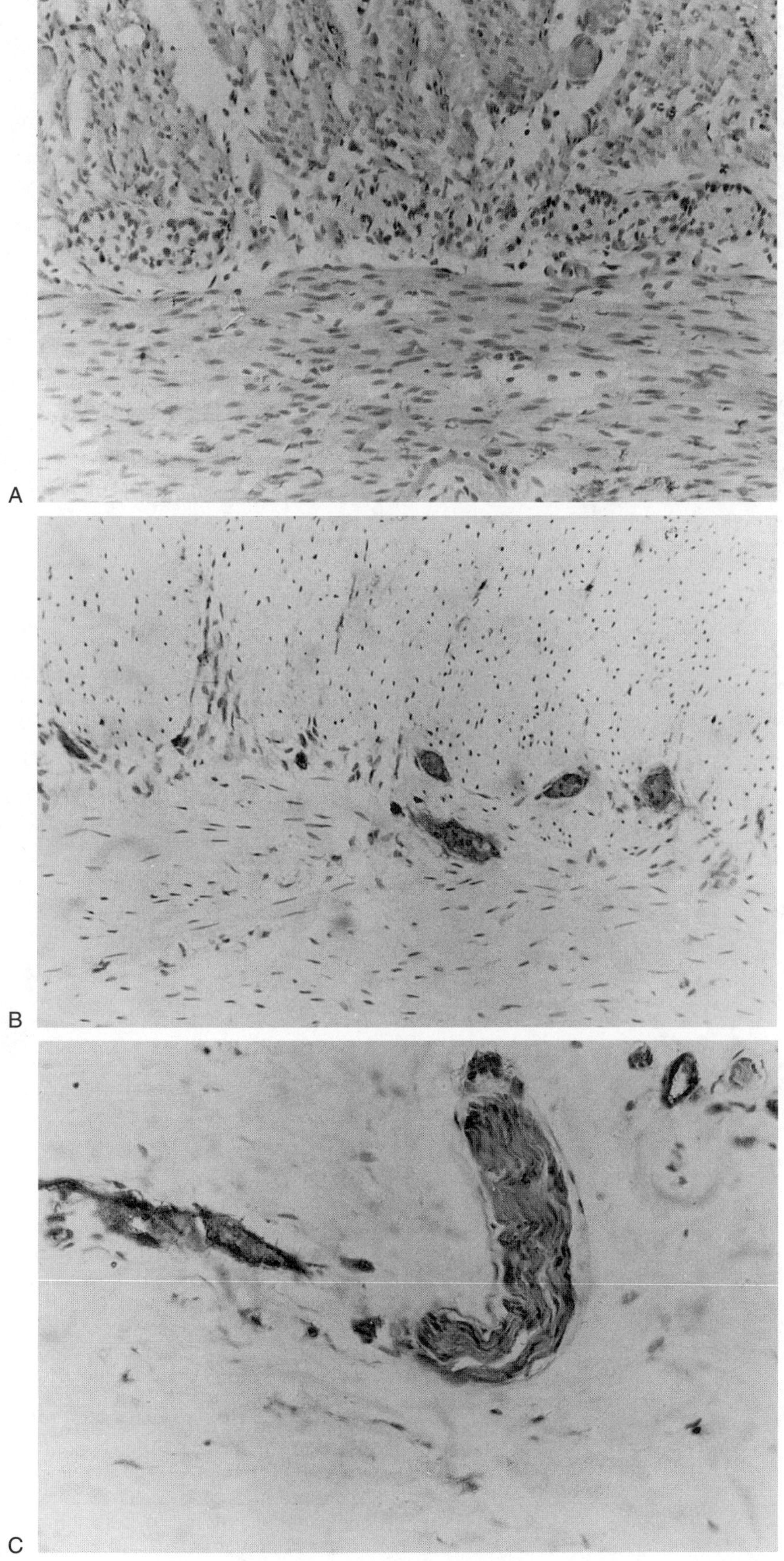

FIG. 80-1 (*A*) ICAM-1 staining of ganglionic colonic segment of a Hirschsprung disease patient. No ICAM-1 staining is seen around or within myenteric ganglia. (×160.) (*B*) ICAM-1 staining of transitional zone. ICAM-1 strongly stained abnormal small ganglion cell and nerve trunks. (×160.) (*C*) ICAM-1 staining of aganglionic segment. Strong ICAM-1 staining around and within the submucosal hypertrophic nerve trunks. (×250.)

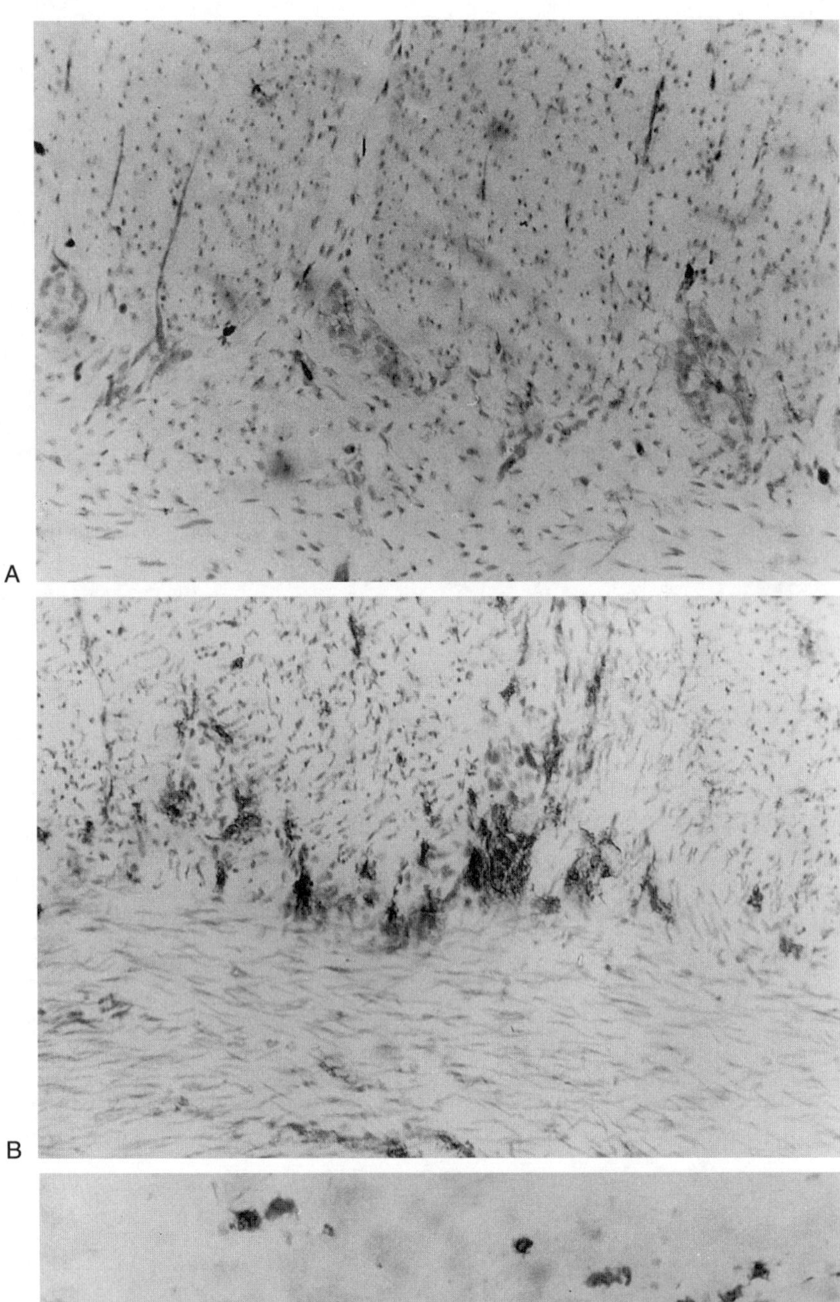

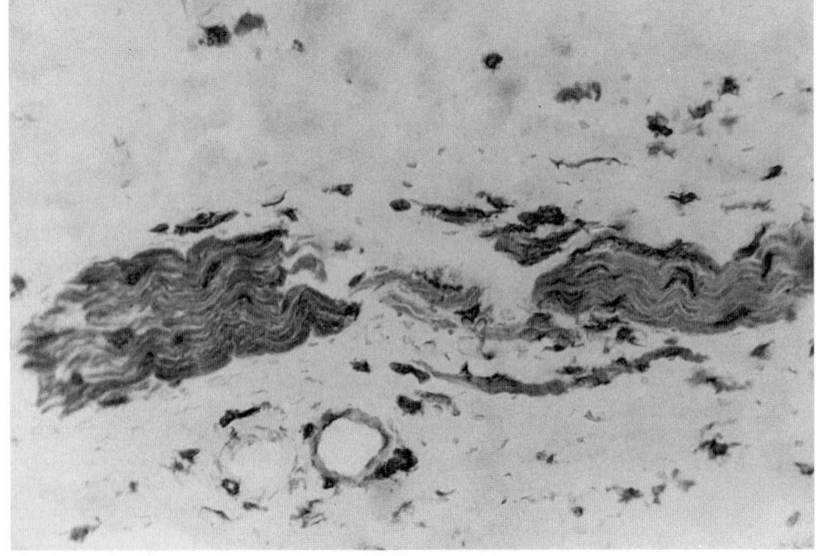

FIG. 80-2. (*A*) MHC class II staining of ganglionic colonic segment in a patient with Hirschsprung disease. A few MHC class II–positive cells seen in the muscle. No MHC class II antigen staining was seen around or within the myenteric ganglia. (×160.) (*B*) MHC class II staining of transitional zone. Strong MHC class II staining of abnormal small ganglia and around nerve trunks. (×160.) (*C*) MHC class II staining in aganglionic segment. Strong MHC class II staining around and within the hypertrophic nerve trunks in the submucosa. (×250.)

endothelin-3 (END-3; ligand corresponding to EDNRB) with EDNRB is essential for development of enteric neurons, using animal models in which EDN-3 or EDNRB was disrupted.[55,56] Disruption of either of these genes impairs normal colonization of myenteric ganglion cells and leads to aganglionosis of the intestine that is analogous to human HD. For two murine mutants, lethal spotted and piebald lethal, which have been described as models for HD and exhibit autosomal recessive phenotype, the gene loci for their mutations have been also confirmed to encode EDN-3[55] and EDNRB,[56] respectively. To date, 13 EDNRB gene alterations, including our two novel mutations, have been identified in sporadic and familial HD.[56a,56b] EDNRB mutations are usually associated with short-segment HD.

PATHOPHYSIOLOGY

The pathophysiology of HD is not fully understood. There is no clear explanation for the occurrence of spastic or tonically contracted aganglionic segment of bowel (Fig. 80-3). The most important histologic finding in aganglionic colon is the absence of ganglion cells, which normally coordinate muscular activity by balancing the motor effects of the preganglionic cholinergic fibers and the inhibitory influence of the postganglionic, adrenergic fibers (Fig. 80-4).

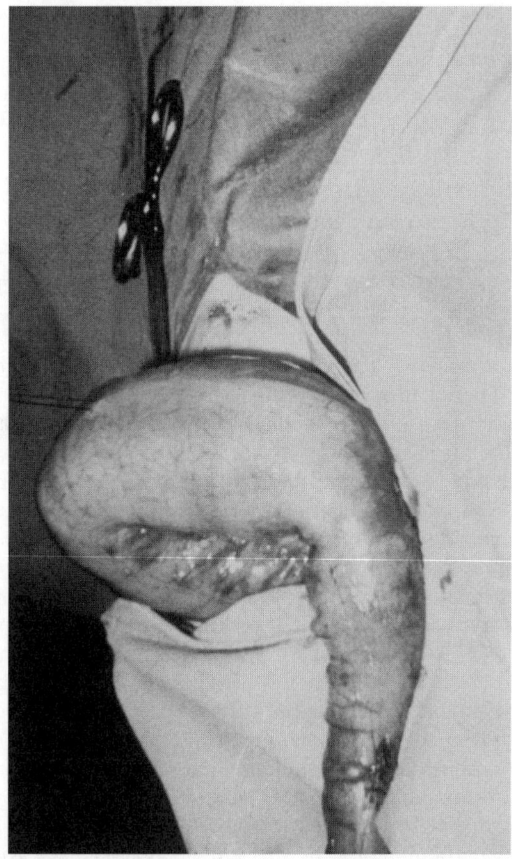

FIG. 80-3. Typical gross pathology in Hirschsprung disease with transitional zone at rectosigmoid level.

Adrenergic Innervation Abnormalities

Ehrenpreis,[57] using fluorescent microscopy, demonstrated a lack of adrenergic nerve fibers in the aganglionic segment of HD and suggested that a state of denervation hypersensitivity (based on Canon's law), induced permanent contraction of smooth muscle in the aganglionic segment. Other investigators, however, have shown that the adrenergic innervation of the aganglionic bowel is increased relative to that of normal bowel.[58,59] The tissue concentration of norepinephrine, the neurotransmitter of adrenergic nerves, is two to three times higher in the aganglionic bowel than in the normal colon;[60,61] and also there is a corresponding increase in tyrosine hydroxylase, an enzyme that regulates norepinephrine biosynthesis.[62] It is proposed that adrenergic hyperactivity of the aganglionic segment contributes to the increased muscle tone and abnormal peristaltic activity observed in HD. Because adrenergic nerves normally act to relax the bowel, it is unlikely that adrenergic hyperactivity is responsible for increased tone in the aganglionic colon.

Cholinergic Hyperinnervation

Cholinergic nerve hyperplasia has been proposed as the cause of spasticity of the aganglionic segment.[63,64] In the absence of ganglion cells, there is an overabundance of acetylcholine, which in turn stimulates an excessive production of the enzyme acetylcholinestrase (AChE). In the aganglionic segment, therefore, an excessive accumulation of the enzyme AChE occurs, resulting from a continuous acetylcholine release from the axons of the extramural parasympathetic ganglion. Pharmacologic investigations of the colon in HD have demonstrated higher acetylcholine release in the aganglionic segment at rest and after stimulation compared with the proximal ganglionic bowel.[65,66] In HD the increased acetylcholine release, the enhanced sensitivity of smooth muscle cells to acetylcholine, and the lack of α_2 adrenoreceptor-mediated noradrenergic modulation of acetylcholine release from cholinergic interneurons might be responsible for the spasm of aganglionic segment. Histochemical staining techniques demonstrate marked increase in AChE activity in the aganglionic segment compared with the ganglionic colon.[67,68]

Abnormal Peptidergic Innervation

Strong evidence has emerged that the enteric nervous system is not only composed of adrenergic and cholinergic nerves but also importantly nonadrenergic, noncholinergic (NANC) autonomic nerves, which contain different peptides; and these peptides act as neurotransmitters, neuromodulators, or both. These nerves have been termed peptidergic nerves.[69,70] Several authors have reported that the contracted state of the aganglionic segments may be a result of abnormal peptidergic patterns of innervation. They noted a decrease of vasoactive intestinal polypeptide–containing fibers in the aganglionic bowel.[71–74] Other investigators have reported absence or reduction of nerve fibers containing substance P[15,73–76] (Fig. 80-5), met-enkephalin[74–78] and gastrin-releasing peptide,[75,76] and peptide histidine isoleucine[78] in aganglionic segments in Hirschsprung disease. The

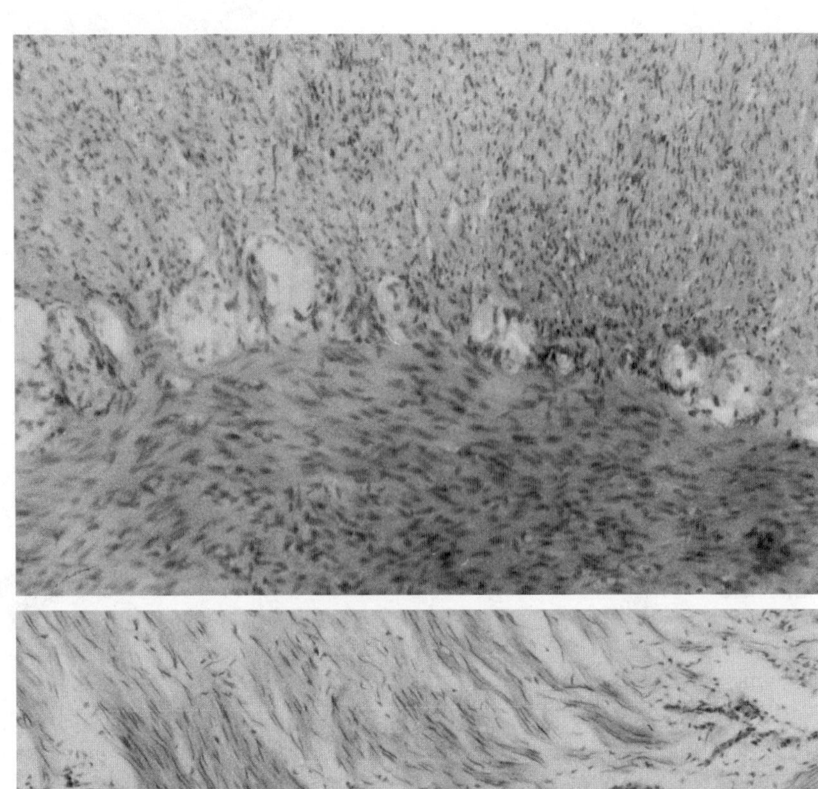

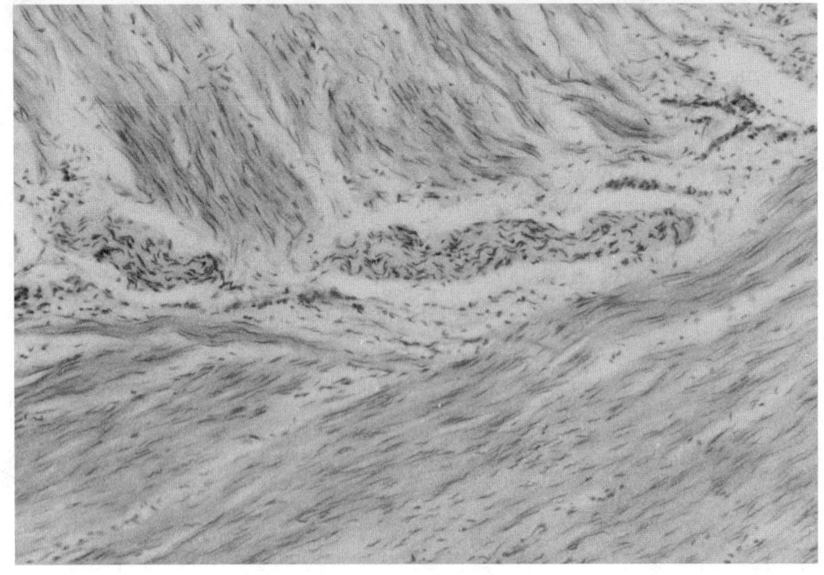

FIG. 80-4. (*A*) Normal myenteric plexus, containing ganglion cells. (*B*) Hypertrophied nerve trunks in an aganglionic colonic biopsy from a patient with Hirschsprung disease.

density of nerve fibers containing galanin or calcitonin gene-related peptide is not overtly changed in the aganglionic bowel compared with aganglionic bowel, whereas fibers containing neuropeptide Y are increased in number in the aganglionic segment.[79–81] Romanska and colleagues[82] reported that the distribution and density of peptide-containing nerves in the aganglionic segment vary greatly from one patient to another. Moreover, abnormal peptidergic innervation is present in the proximal limit of colonic resection in a significant number of patients with HD. The peptidergic nerves play an important role in the neural regulation of gut function, but the precise functional significance of defects in peptidergic innervation in HD has yet to be defined.

Abnormalities of Nerve Supporting Cells

The enteric nervous system is composed of two distinct neural components, extrinsic and intrinsic; and its supporting cells possess some unique characteristics of both central nervous system astrocytes and peripheral nervous system Schwann cells.[33] The intrinsic innervation has two major divisions: the myenteric plexus, which is concerned primarily with motor activity; and the submucous plexus, which receives sensory input from the lumen of the intestine and controls secretomotor function. The supporting nerve cells of the intrinsic enteric nervous system are often referred to as enteric glia.[84,85] These glia have been reported to express various markers for both astrocytes and Schwann cells, such as (1) glial fibrillary acidic protein, a specific marker for astrocytes within the central nervous system;[86,87] (2) S-100, a marker for astrocytes and Schwann cells;[88,89] and (3) D_7, a marker of Schwann cells[90,91] and oligodendrocytes.[92] The nerve-supporting cells permit cell bodies and processes of neurons to be arranged and maintained in a proper spacial arrangement and are essential in the maintenance of basic physiologic functions of neurons.[93]

Abnormalities of nerve-supporting cells have been reported in the aganglionic colon by many investigators.[94–97] We have used antibodies against neuron-specific enolase (NSE), neurofilament, S-100 protein, and D_7 in our laboratory in an attempt to

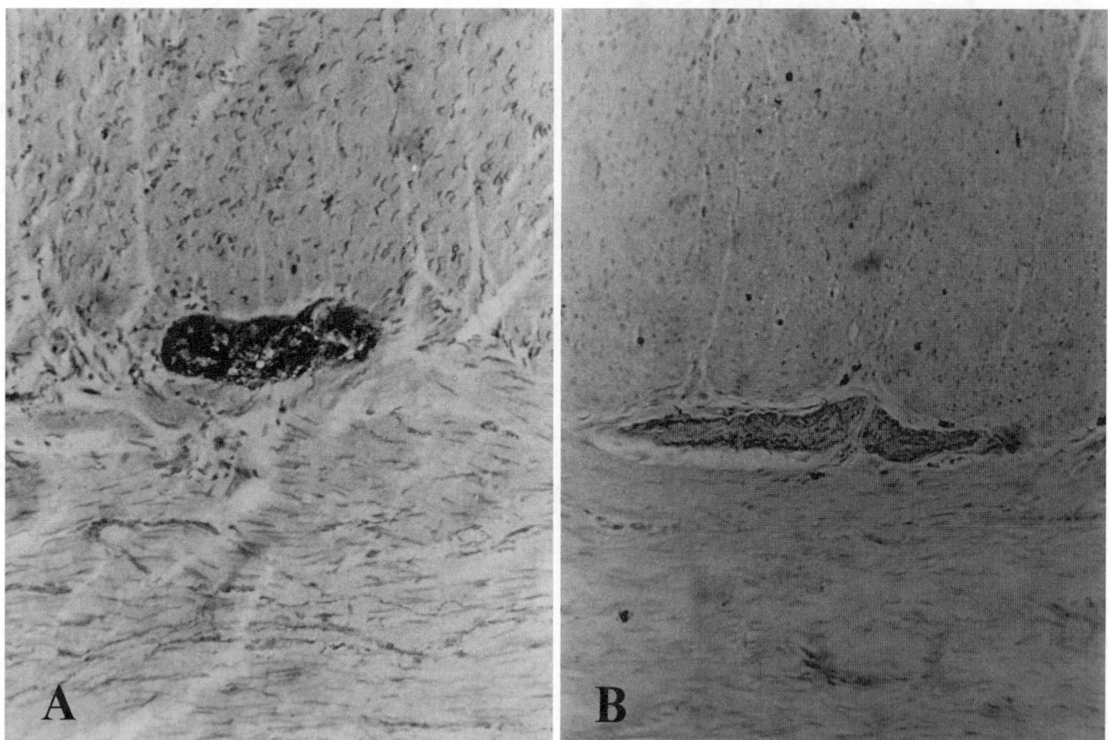

FIG. 80-5. Immunocytochemical staining with substance P. (*A*) Numerous immunoreactive fibers in the muscle and myenteric ganglia in normal colon; (*B*) marked reduction of substance P positive fibers in the muscle of aganglionic colon with hypertrophic nerve trunks in HD.

characterize morphologic changes in neuronal cells in HD.[98–101] Immunhistochemical scanning of the entire resected specimen of colon from patients with HD following Swenson's operation demonstrated the absence of a unique Schwann cell antigen in the circular muscle of aganglionic colon identified by D_7 monoclonal antibody produced in our laboratory. Comparative studies with other antineuronal cell antibodies showed that while neurofilament, NSE, and S-100 protein–positive fibers in the circular muscle were present in abundance in the ganglionic colon and reduced in number in aganglionic bowel, D_7 monoclonal antibody alone identified a neuronal cell antigen (Schwann cell antigen) in the circular muscle that is present in abundance in the ganglionic segment but is completely absent in the aganglionic colon. Ultrastructural serial examination of the entire resected specimen of colon from these patients demonstrated grossly swollen monoaxonal or oligoaxonal Schwann cell units with loss of cellular contents in the circular muscle of aganglionic colon.[101] The decreased intensity of NSE and neurofilament protein-immunoreactive fibers corresponded with the ultrastructural finding of markedly reduced numbers and morphologically abnormal axons in the circular muscle of aganglionic colon. The combination of abnormal immunoreactivity with Schwann cell markers, D_7 monoclonal antibody, S-100 protein, and glial fibrillary acidic protein; and the presence of pathologic Schwann cells in the circular muscle of aganglionic colon on electronmicroscopy suggest that degenerative changes in Schwann cells and axons within the circular muscle coat of aganglionic segment may be a factor in the pathogenesis of HD. A central question arising from these observations is whether absence of axonal sprouting can or cannot lead to the

morphologic and immunologic alterations in Schwann cells seen in the circular muscle of aganglionic colon. If the central role of the Schwann cell is to provide a supporting structure for axons, then the absence or diminution of such axons could significantly alter the environment within the Schwann cell and thereby lead to abnormal morphologic changes.

Mucosal Neuroendocrine Cell Abnormalities

It has become evident that the gastrointestinal tract and its glandular derivatives contain a variety of neuroendocrine (NE) cell types that are dispersed along the mucosa. Each NE cell type synthesizes, stores, and secretes a specific neuropeptide, biogenic amine, or both that act as a chemical messenger in orchestrating the various secretory, motor, and absorptive functions of the gut. The NE cells modulate gut function by endocrine, paracrine, or neurocrine routes. By the use of immunocytochemistry and serial tissue sectioning, we have shown that the number of endocrine cells in the aganglionic colon in patients with HD is significantly increased compared with the numbers in the normal ganglionic segment.[102] The oligoganglionic or transitional segment of bowel showed an intermediate number of NE cells. These results were seen both with the generic endocrine cell markers, chromogranin A and synaptophysin that stain all or virtually all endocrine cells, and with the specific markers, 5-hydroxytryptamine peptide YY and somatostatin that identify distinct subpopulations of endocrine cells. In contrast with the absence of ganglion cells and many peptidergic nerve fibers in HD, the peptide- and amine-containing mucosal endocrine cells are increased in the aganglionic compared with the ganglionic colon of HD. This suggests that endocrine cells are not intimately associated with these nerve fibers and probably have an independent derivation. Although the precise physiologic function of the individual NE cells is unclear, as a group they are believed to influence secretion, absorption, and motility.

Abnormalities of Nitric Oxide–Producing Neurons

In 1990, Bult and colleagues[103] provided evidence that nitric oxide (NO) is released on stimulation of enteric NANC nerves. Since then, substantial evidence has emerged indicating that NO acts as a NANC neurotransmitter in the gut and mediates relaxation of the smooth muscle of the gastrointestinal tract.[104–106] Several investigators have reported lack or deficiency of NO synthase–containing nerves in the smooth muscle of aganglionic colon in HD patients[107–111] (Fig. 80-6). The lack of NO-producing nerve fibers in the aganglionic colon probably contributes to the inability of the smooth muscle to relax, therby causing lack of peristalsis in HD.

Hypertrophic Nerves in Hirschsprung Disease

Hirschsprung disease is characterized histologically by the absence of ganglion cells in the myenteric and submucous plexuses and the presence of hypertrophied nerve trunks in the space normally occupied by the ganglion cells. There is no explanation for the occurrence of hypertrophied nerve trunks in the myenteric and submucous plexuses.

Many investigators have attempted to determine the nature and origin of the hypertrophic nerve trunks found in the aganglionic segment of colon in patients with HD.[112–115] It has been suggested that hypertrophic nerve trunks originate from intrinsic nerves and that the abnormality of nerve hypertrophy in aganglionic segments results from an increased number of nerve fibers instead of an increase in their size.[114] In contrast, whole-mount studies have suggested that the hypertrophic nerve trunks are blind-ending, bulbous terminations of extrinsic nerves.

Nerve growth factor (NGF) and its receptor (nerve growth factor receptor [NGFR] are neurotrophic proteins that play an essential role in the normal development and survival of neurons in the peripheral and central nervous system.[116] During development, NGF is necessary for outgrowth of axons and establishment of synapses, and NGFR is the transmembrane protein that binds NGF and brings it into the cell.[117] Cholinergic nerve hyperplasia is a consistent finding in the aganglionic segment of the bowel. Studies have shown that the effect of NGF on the development and integrity of neurons is predominantly confined to the cholinergic system, and that the effects of NGF are transmitted via receptors localized within the cholinergic neurons.[118–120]

We have investigated the pattern of NGFR immunoreactivity in the normal and aganglionic colon.[121] The most striking finding in this study was the strong expression of NGFR immunoreactivity on the perineurium of hypertrophic nerve trunks in the submucous and myenteric plexuses (Fig. 80-7). Although NGFR immunoreactivity was present in the nerve fibers of the hypertrophic trunks, the perineurium was the region in which

NGFR expression constituted most reactivity in the form of a thick ring surrounding the hypertrophic nerve trunk. These results showed that the pattern of NGFR perineural staining of hypertrophic nerve trunks in the aganglionic segment was identical to that seen in the serosal (mesenteric) nerves of the bowel.[121] The strong NGFR perineural staining of serosal (mesenteric) nerves in the normal bowel was confined only to extrinsic nerves and was not present in the nerves of the muscle or submucous layer. This suggests that the hypertrophic, nerve trunks originate from extrinsic enteric nerves.

Enterocolitis

Enterocolitis remains the most serious complication of HD, resulting in high morbidity and mortality. The reported incidence ranges from 20% to 58%.[122–125] Relapses of enterocolitis can occur despite a defunctioning colostomy and after a definitive pull-through operation.[124,126–129] It has been reported that patients with enterocolitis-complicating HD have persistent inflammatory changes in the excluded large bowel after diversion of the fecal stream by colostomy.[130,131] The pathogenesis of enterocolitis remains poorly understood. Many theories have been advanced; these include mechanical dilatation and fecal stasis,[132] alterations of mucin components,[124,131,133] increased prostaglandin E1 activity,[134] *Clostridium difficile* infection,[135,136] and (more recently) rotavirus infection.[137]

Mucosal Immune Defense Mechanisms in Enterocolitis

Imamura and coworkers[138] reported significant changes in the mucosal immune response throughout the resected colon in patients with persistent enterocolitis-complicating HD. Immunoglobulin A (IgA), IgM, and J chain–containing plasma cells were significantly increased in the lamina propria along the entire length of resected bowel in enterocolitis patients, compared with nonenterocolitis patients and controls. Luminal secretory component staining of the aganglionic segment of colon from enterocolitis cases was markedly reduced. Lamina propria CD68-positive monocyte and macrophages and CD45RO-positive lymphocytes were increased in all enterocolitis patients compared with nonenterocolitis patients.

Although there was a general increase in all inflammatory cell types investigated, there was a disproportionate increase in natural killer (NK) cells infiltrating the ganglionic segment of bowel in enterocolitis compared with nonenterocolitis patients. NK cell levels in aganglionic segment of colon in both enterocolitis and nonenterocolitis patients were similar to those in controls. Previous studies have suggested that enterocolitis occurs only in the dilated ganglionic bowel of patients with HD.[139–141] Although this study demonstrated inflammatory changes throughout the resected segment in enterocolitis patients, increased NK cell infiltration was confined to the ganglionic segment of bowel in these patients.

The major biologic functions of NK cells are those of antitumour and antiviral responses, as well as their potential regulation of antibody production.[142–144] If we are to attach particular significance to the differential pattern of NK cell infiltration in enterocolitis patients, then their function as effector cells of antiviral immunity is their most likely role in this condition.

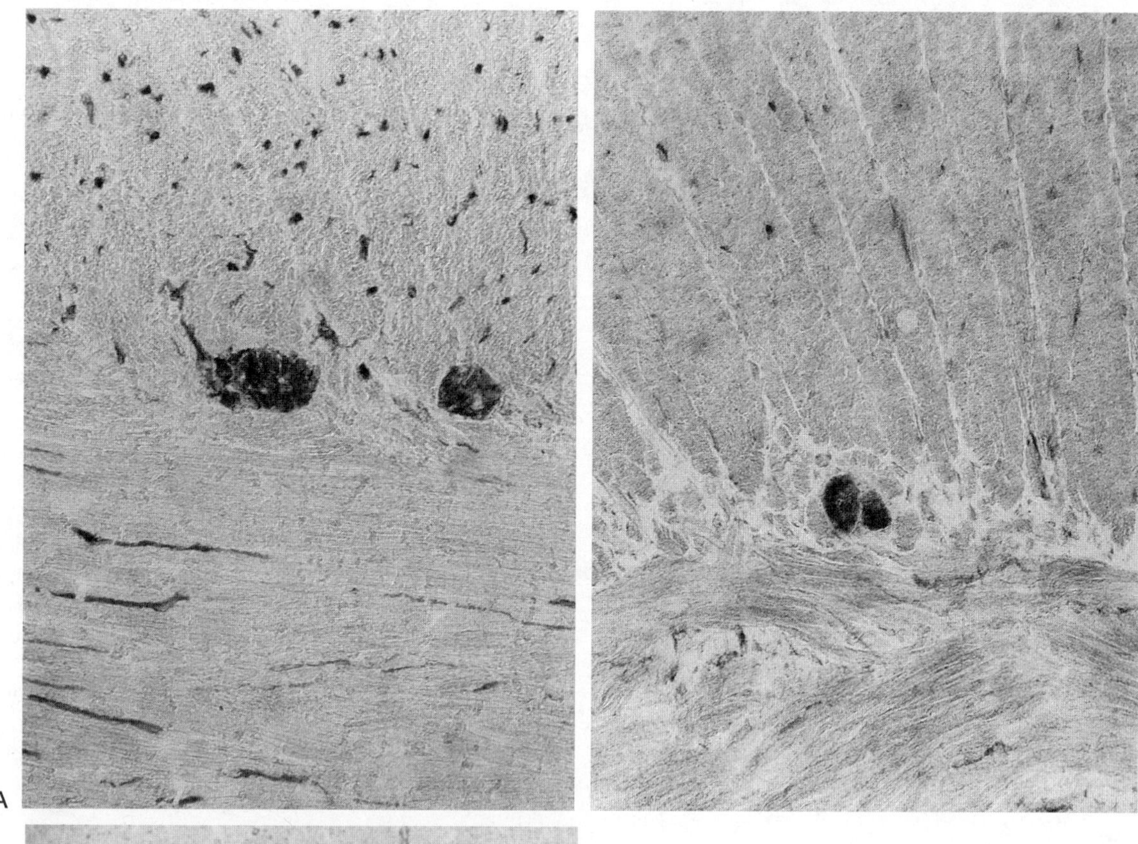

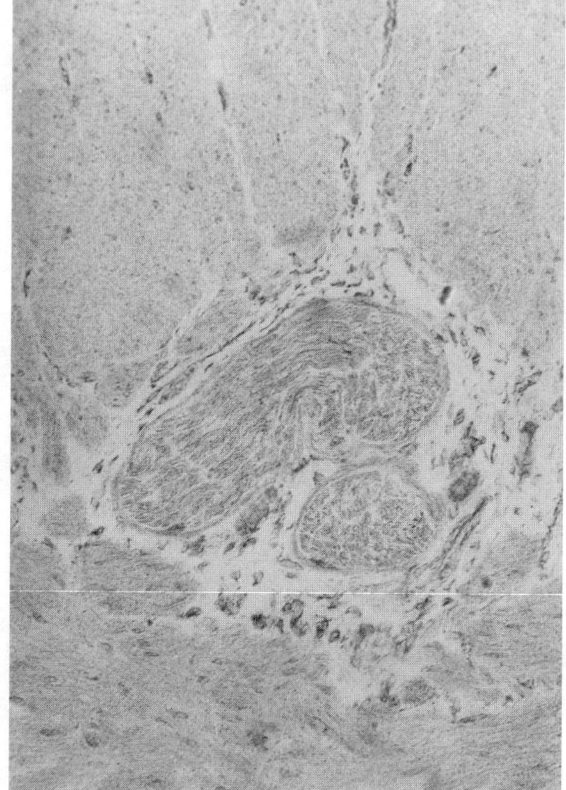

FIG. 80-6. (*A*) Ganglionic segment of bowel from HD patients. There are many nerve fibers in circular and longitudinal muscle layers. Myenteric ganglia stain strongly (NADPH-diaphorase colocalizes with neuronal nitric oxide synthase). (×160.) (*B*) Transitional segment of bowel. Markedly reduced nerve fibers are seen in circular and longitudinal muscle layers. Small myenteric ganglion cells stain strongly (NADPH-diaphorase histochemistry). (×160.) (*C*) Aganglionic segment of bowel. There is total lack of nerve fibers in circular and longitudinal muscle layers. Hypertrophic nerve trunks stain weakly (NADPH-diaphorase histochemistry). (×160.)

Several peptides described as neurotransmitters have been shown to modulate the immune response in the gastrointestinal tract.[145] Because of the known abnormalities in peptidergic nerves in HD, it is possible that the regional abnormality of NK cell infiltration may be related to regional abnormalities in neuropeptides.

This concept has provided further support for a possible infectious etiology of the enterocolitis. Increased NK cell responses confined to the ganglionic bowel, the site which has been considered by many investigators to be the primary focus of enterocolitis,[140,142] are consistent with a possible local viral infection. The reduction of luminal secretory IgA in the aganglionic bowel may be a further predisposing factor to a microbial pathogenesis. However, this reduction of secretory IgA is confined to the aganglionic portion only, and does not represent a primary deficiency in secretory IgA transport across epithelial cells. It is probable that the luminal IgA deficiency is more a reflection of damage to the mucosal surfaces or of changes in mucin composition, leading to diminished IgA adherence to the mucosal surface. The diversity of altered local immune responses seen may be reflective of a multifactorial microbial etiology in enterocolitis associated with HD.

Kobayashi and colleagues[146] demonstrated a strong expression of ICAM-1 in the endothelial lining of the submucosal vessels in both aganglionic and ganglionic segments in patients with enterocolitis-complicating HD. They emphasize the importance of endothelial cell activation in the pathogenesis of enterocolitis. Fujimoto and Miyano[147] have demonstrated strong expression of blood group–associated antigen Le^b throughout the entire length of the crypts of aganglionic bowel. This Le^b antigen is absent under normal circumstances in the distal rectum and colon and is only present in fetal colon. They report that the colonic mucosa of aganglionic bowel represents a persistence of the fetal stage of development and speculate that the abnormalities of the mucosal endothelium may be a factor in the pathogenesis of enterocolitis.

The etiology of HD-associated enterocolitis remains a complex issue. Ongoing immunohistochemical studies along with in situ hybridization using specific probes provide further insights into our understanding of the pathophysiologic basis of enterocolitis-complicating HD.

CLINICAL FEATURES

Eighty to ninety percent of all cases HD produce clinical symptoms and these are typically diagnosed during the neonatal period.[148,149] Delayed passage of meconium is the cardinal symptom in neonates with HD. Over 90% of patients fail to pass meconium in the first 24 hours of life.[150,151] The usual presentation of HD in the neonatal period is with constipation, abdominal distension (Fig. 80-8), and vomiting during the first few days of life. In many cases, a rectal examination or rectal irrigation causes passage of meconium and relief of acute intes-

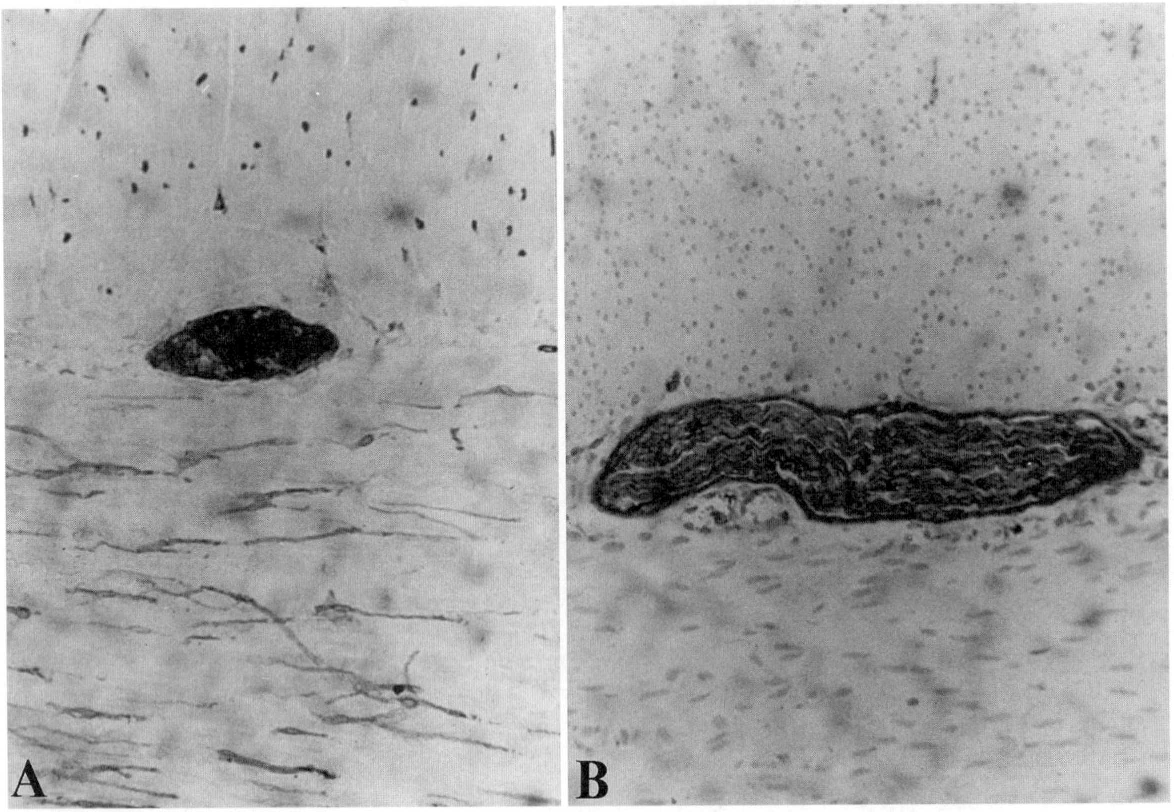

FIG. 80-7. Immunoperoxidase staining for nerve growth factor receptor: (*A*) myenteric ganglia and nerve fibers in smooth muscle in normal colon are stained, (*B*) hypertrophic nerve trunk in aganglionic segment of Hirschsprung disease showing intense perineurial and axonal staining. There are no NGFR-positive fibers in the muscle.

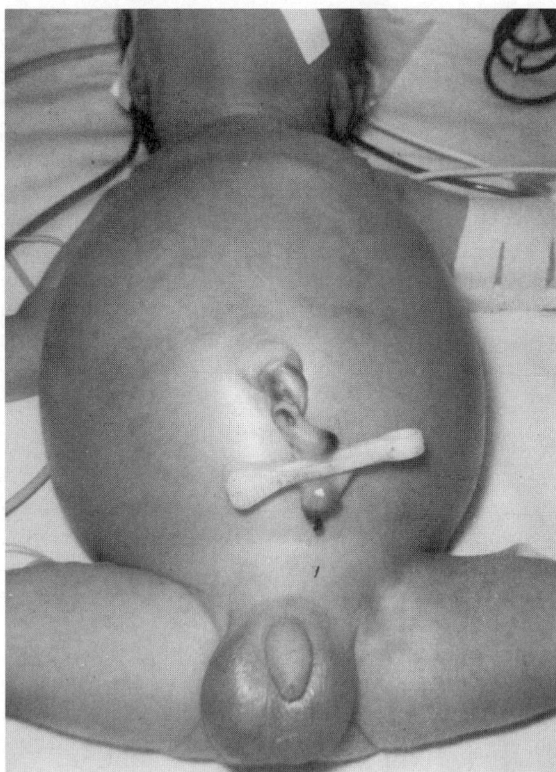

FIG. 80-8. Two-day-old infant with marked abdominal distension and failure to pass meconium. Suction rectal biopsy confirmed Hirschsprung disease.

tinal obstruction. These babies may have normal bowel movements for a few days or weeks and then present again with signs and symptoms of intestinal obstruction. Some babies may have normal health for several months or years in response to changes in feeds, laxatives, suppositories, or enemas; and develop a chronic form of congenital aganglionosis manifested by chronic constipation with or without abdominal distension.

About a third of the babies with HD present with diarrhea.[152] Diarrhea in HD is always a symptom of enterocolitis, which remains the most common cause of death in this disease. Enterocolitis may resolve with adequate therapy or it may develop into a life-threatening condition, the toxic megacolon, characterized by the sudden onset of marked abdominal distention, bile-stained vomiting, fever and signs of dehydration, and shock.[153] Rectal examination or introduction of a rectal tube or a thermometer results in the explosive expulsion of gas and foul-smelling stools.

DIAGNOSIS

The diagnosis of HD is usually based on clinical history; radiologic studies; anorectal manometry; and, in particular, histologic examination of the rectal wall biopsy specimens.

Radiologic Diagnosis

Plain abdominal films in a neonate with HD will show dilated loops of bowel with fluid levels. Occasionally, one may be able to see a small amount of air in the undistended rectum and a dilated colon above it. This should raise the suspicion of HD. We have found the prone lateral view with buttocks elevated and use of the horizontal beam invaluable in demonstrating gas in the undilated rectum in HD. The main advantage of this view is the lack of discomfort to the baby who can be kept in this position for 10 minutes or longer to allow gas to ascend from the colon into the rectum.

In patients with enterocolitis-complicating HD, plain abdominal radiographs may show thickening of bowel wall with mucosal irregularity or a grossly dilated colon loop indicating toxic megacolon. Pneumoperitoneum may be found in those with perforation. Spontaneous perforation of the intestinal tract has been reported in 3% of patients with HD.[8] A strong correlation was noted between the length of aganglionic bowel and spontaneous perforation; half of the perforations occurred in those patients with long-segment HD.

A barium enema performed by an experienced radiologist using careful technique should achieve a high degree of reliability in diagnosing HD in the newborn. It is important that the infant should not have rectal washouts or even digital examinations prior to the barium enema because such interference may distort the transitional zone appearance and give a false-negative diagnosis. A soft rubber catheter is inserted into the lower rectum and held in position with firm strapping across the buttocks. A balloon catheter should not be used because of the risk of perforation and the possibility of distorting a transitional zone by distension. The barium should be injected slowly in small amounts under fluoroscopic control with the baby in the lateral position. A typical case of HD demonstrates the flow of barium from the undilated rectum through a cone-shaped transitional zone into the dilated colon (Fig. 80-9). Some cases may show an abrupt transition between the dilated proximal colon and the distal aganglionic segment, leaving the diagnosis in little doubt.

In some cases, the findings on a barium enema are uncertain and a delayed film at 24 hours may confirm the diagnosis by demonstrating the retained barium and often accentuating the appearance of the transitional zone (Fig. 80-10).

In the presence of enterocolitis-complicating HD, a barium enema may demonstrate spasm, mucosal edema, and ulceration (Fig. 80-11). The characteristic finding of the transitional zone of HD is not present because of impairment of muscular function by inflammation.

Anorectal Manometry

In the normally innervated bowel, distention of the rectum produces relaxation of the internal sphincter.[154] In 1964, Callaghan and Nixon[155] reported the absence of internal sphincter response to rectal distention in HD. The absence of internal sphincter relaxation is the basis for the manometric differentiation of HD from other causes of constipation.[156–159]

Investigators use different materials (air or water) for recording anorectal motor activity and rectal sensation. There are no significant differences in anorectal manometry between the results of rectal balloon inflation with water or air.[160]

In normal persons, when the rectal balloon is distended with air, the rectum immediately responds with a transient rise in

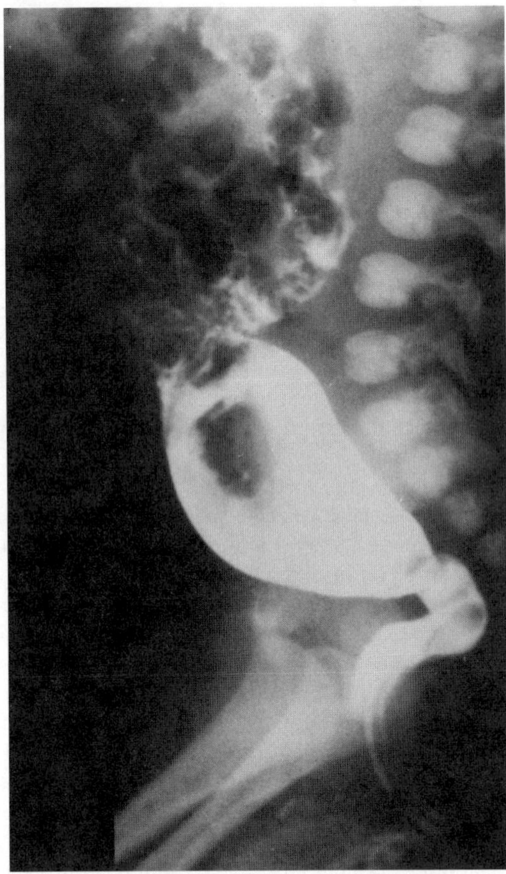

FIG. 80-9. Hirschsprung disease. Barium enema in this patient reveals transitional zone in the sigmoid colon.

to be accurate in the newborn infant for the diagnosis of HD.[166–169] Tamate and colleagues[168] reported manometry findings in 60 normal neonates and 17 neonates with gastrointestinal obstructive symptoms. They showed that all 60 healthy neonates had a normal rectosphincteric reflex regardless of postnatal age and birth weight. Among the 17 patients, 5 were diagnosed as having HD based on absence of the rectosphincteric reflex. There were no false-negative or false-positive results among these cases. They suggested that the failure to detect the rectosphincteric reflex in premature and term neonates is probably a result of technical difficulties and not of immaturity of ganglion cells. We have found anorectal manometry to be an excellent screening method for the exclusion of HD.

Rectal Biopsy

The diagnosis of HD is confirmed on examination of rectal biopsy specimens. Prior to the use of suction rectal biopsies, a full-thickness rectal biopsy specimen that included both muscle coats and submucosa provided enough tissue to make a relatively easy diagnosis.

Although the introduction of the suction rectal biopsy technique makes the procedure less traumatic for the patient, it has made the diagnosis more difficult for the pathologist. Many histopathologists are reluctant to make a positive diagnosis of HD on the basis of suction rectal biopsies using conventional

pressure lasting 15 to 20 seconds; and at the same time the internal sphincter rhythmic activity is depressed or abolished and its pressure falls by 15 to 20 cm, the duration of relaxation coinciding with the rectal wave. In patients with HD, the rectum often shows spontaneous waves of varying amplitude and frequency in the resting phase. The internal sphincter rhythmic activity is more pronounced. On rectal distention with an increment of air, there is complete absence of internal sphincter relaxation.

Although in older children anorectal manometry has proved to be a reliable method for diagnosing HD, considerable controversy exists as to the diagnostic accuracy of manometry in neonates. Holschneider[161] has reported that the development of the normal rectosphincteric reflex is completed on 12th day of life and therefore absence of the reflex could be diagnostic only after that. Ito and associates[162] reported that the normal reflex does not occur in the premature or infants who are younger than 39 weeks in maturational age (gestational plus postnatal age) and who weigh less than 2.7 kg. The absent or atypical rectosphincteric reflex is thought to be related to immaturity of ganglion cells, as demonstrated by Smith[163] and Bughaighes and Emery.[164] Little is known of the state of anatomic maturity at which the neurons become effective. In an experimental study, Puri and coworkers[165] showed that function can precede anatomic maturity of the ganglion cells.

Other investigators have demonstrated anorectal manometry

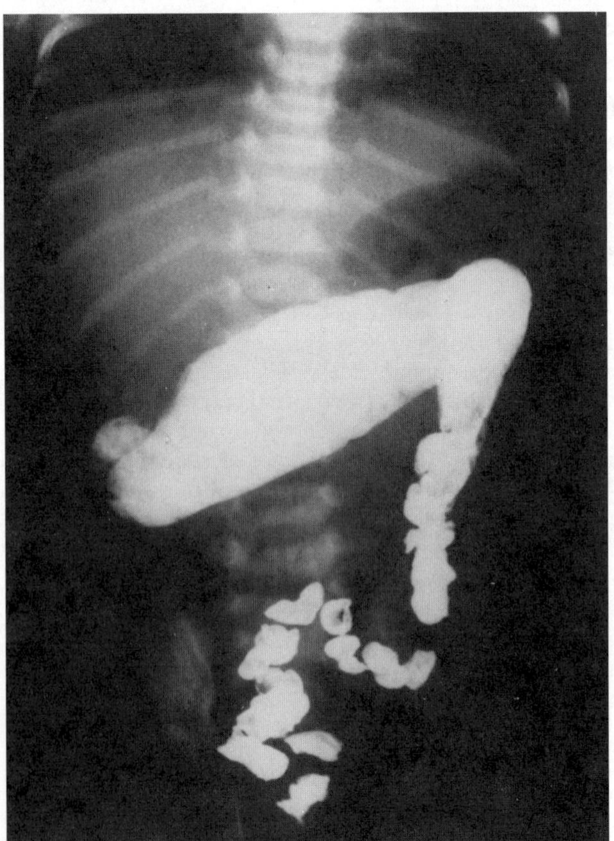

FIG. 80-10. Delayed 24-hour film in lateral position showing barium retention with accentuated transition at the splenic flexure level in a 10-day-old baby with HD.

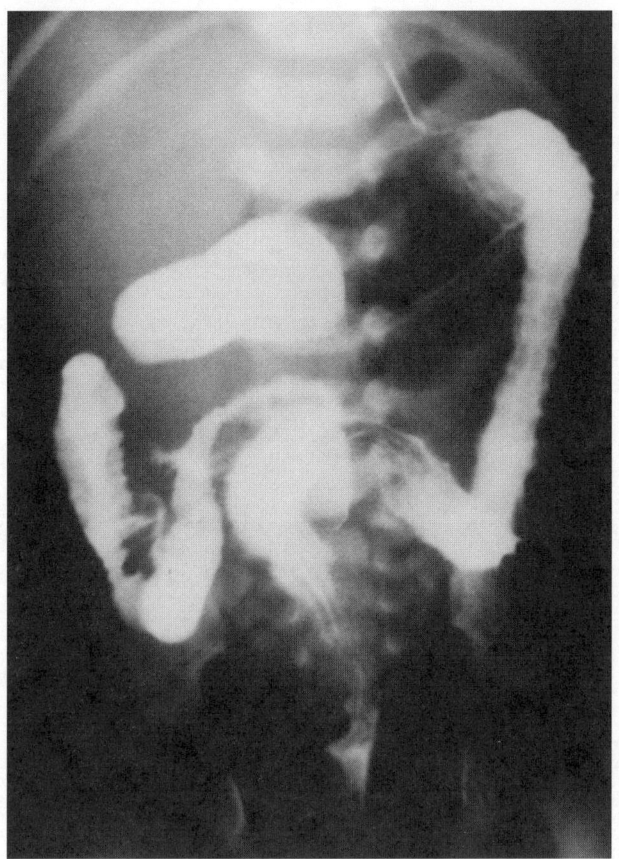

FIG. 80-11. Enterocolitis-complicating HD in rectosigmoid colon on barium enema. Fine mucosal ulceration and mucosal edema give a cobblestone appearance.

hematoxylin and eosin stains. This is a result of both doubt as to the amount of submucosa that must be scanned before absence of ganglion cells can be confirmed and relative difficulty of accurate identification of smaller and sparse submucosal ganglion cells by comparison with the more compact and familiar ganglion cells of the intermuscular plexus.

The development of histochemical and immunohistochemical staining techniques using suction rectal biopsies for the diagnosis of HD represents a considerable advance in the investigation of this disease, particularly in the newborn. Meier-Ruge and associates[67] described a histochemical staining technique of Karnovsky and Roots for the detection of AChE in rectal suction biopsies. Lake and coworkers[68] reported an improved method of staining using Hankers modification of Karnovsky and Roots' method, which stains cholinergic fibers almost black, making them easily noticeable. In normal persons, barely detectable AChE activity is observed within the lamina propria and muscularis mucosa, and submucosal ganglion cells stain strongly for AChE. In HD, there is marked increase in AChE activity in lamina propria and muscularis, which is evident as coarse, discrete cholinergic nerve fibers stained brown to black (Fig. 80-12). By using a supplemental oxidation step, we have modified the AChE histochemistry technique of Karnovsky and Roots to produce staining of cholinergic nerve fibers in 10 minutes instead of 2 hours as required with the conventional technique.[170,171] The rapid AChE technique is simple and reliable

method for the diagnosis of HD and for intraoperative evaluation of the extent of the aganglionic segment.

At our hospital, we usually take three biopsy specimens at 2, 3, and 5 cm above the dentate line. One specimen is stained by conventional hematoxylin and eosin staining to ascertain the presence or absence of ganglion cells; one specimen is stained histochemically for the detection of AChE; and the third specimen is processed for immunocytochemistry using general neuronal markers such as PGP9.5, NGFR, neural cell adhesion molecule, and neurofilament protein (Fig. 80-13). Most investigators have found the histochemical staining technique for the detection of AChE in rectal suction biopsies to be a reliable and simple method for diagnosing HD.[68,170–175] Occasionally, false-negative results have been reported in newborns and in patients with total colonic aganglionosis.[176]

MANAGEMENT

Once the diagnosis of HD has been confirmed by rectal biopsy examination, the infant should be prepared for laparotomy. Biopsies for frozen sections are taken to determine the level of transition, and the colostomy is placed just proximal to the transition zone.

If newborns have enterocolitis-complicating HD, they require correction of dehydration and electrolyte imbalance by infusion of appropriate fluids. Thomas and associates[135] have demonstrated a relationship to the *Clostridium difficile* and its toxin in about 30% of patients with enterocolitis in HD and have suggested treating these patients with vancomycin during acute episodes. It is essential to decompress the bowel as early as possible in these babies. Deflation of the intestine may be conducted initially by rectal irrigations, and when the baby is clinically stable, a colostomy can be performed.

Traditionally, a definitive pull-through operation for HD has been performed when the infant is 6 to 12 months old. This approach evolved during the 1950s when major operations on neonates were considered unsafe and neonatal HD was associated with a high mortality.[177–179] Advances in neonatal anesthesia, monitoring, and surgical care together with parenteral nutrition and effective antibiotics have allowed primary prolonged reparative procedures to be undertaken safely in the neonate. In recent years, most cases of HD are diagnosed in the neonatal period. Many centers are performing one-stage pull-through operations in the newborn with minimal morbidity and encouraging results.[149,180–183] The advantages of operating in the newborn are that the colonic dilatation can be quickly controlled by washouts and the caliber of the pull-through bowel is near normal, allowing for an accurate anastomosis that minimizes leakage and cuff infection.[149]

A number of different operations have been described for the treatment of HD. The three most commonly used operations are the rectosigmoidectomy developed by Swenson and Bill,[183] the retrorectal transanal approach developed by Duhamel,[184] and the endorectal procedure developed by Soave.[185] The basic principle in all these procedures is to bring the ganglionic bowel down to the anus. Long-term results of any of these operations are very satisfactory if they are performed correctly.[150,151,181,186,187]

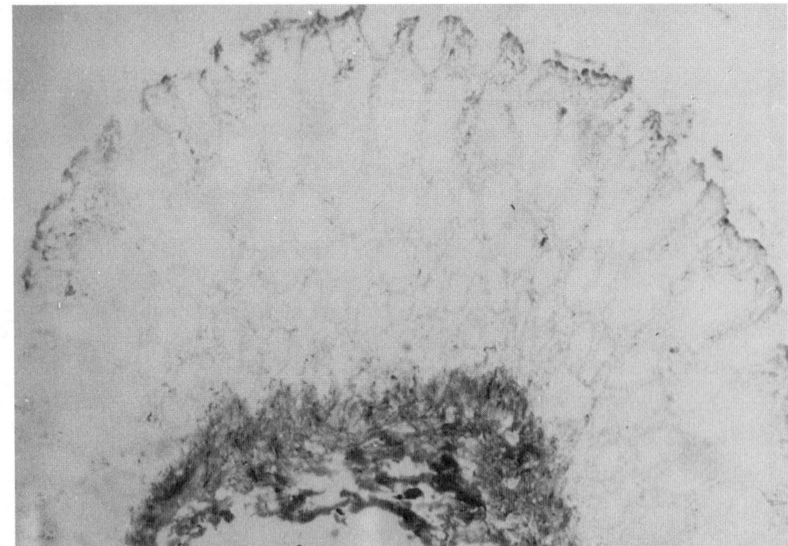

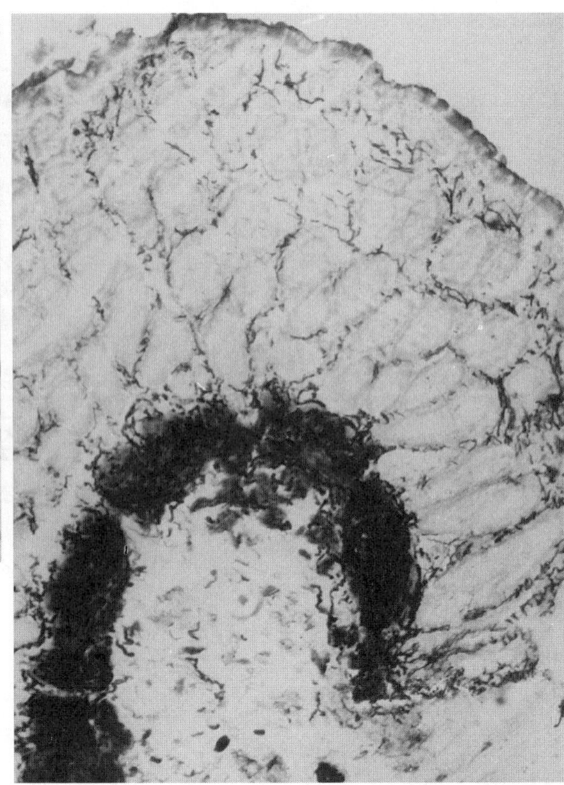

FIG. 80-12. Acetylcholinesterase staining of suction rectal biopsy. (*A*) Normal rectum showing minimal acetylcholinesterase staining in mucosa, lamina propria, and muscularis mucosae. Darkly stained ganglion cells in the submucosa may be seen. (×160.) (*B*) Hirschsprung disease characterized by marked staining of cholinesterase-positive nerves in the lamina propria and muscularis mucosae. (×40.)

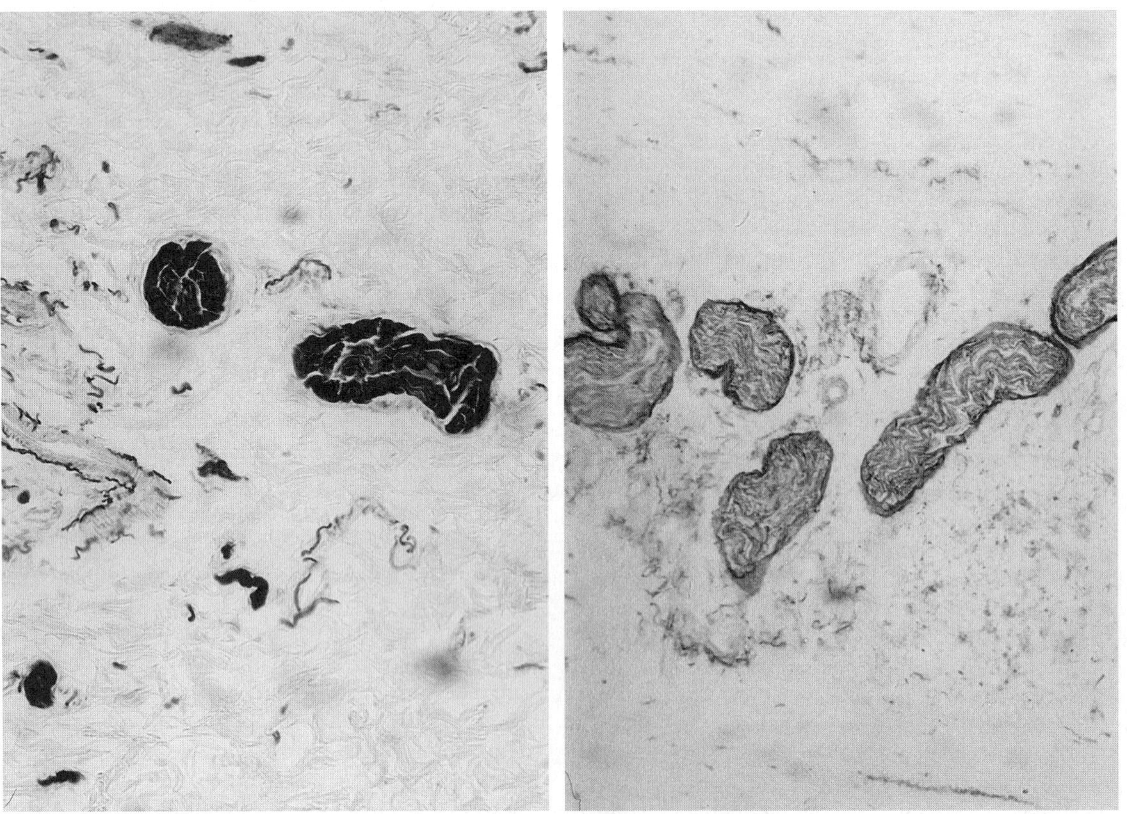

FIG. 80-13. Suction rectal biopsy from a Hirschsprung disease patient showing hypertrophic nerve trunks. (*A*) Stained for neural cell adhesion molecule. (*B*) Stained for NGFR.

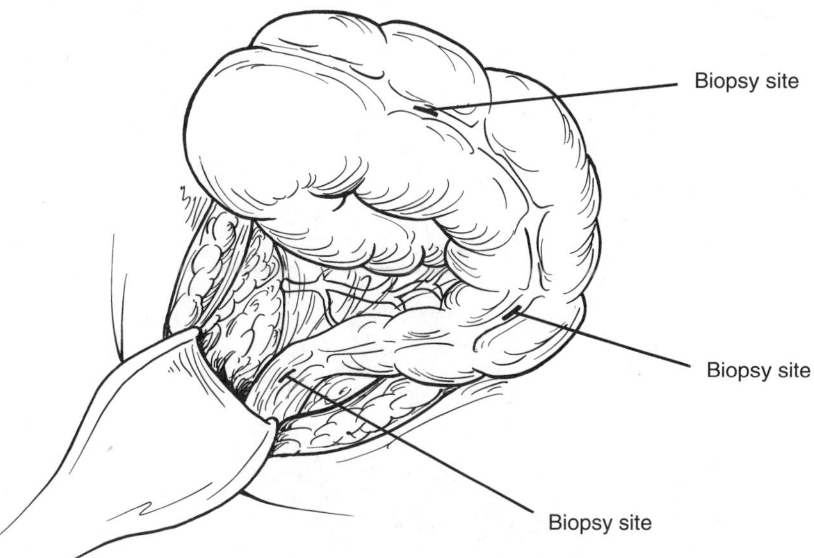

FIG. 80-14. Typical biopsy sites to establish the level of transition between ganglionic and aganglionic bowel.

Colostomy

Many surgeons prefer right transverse colostomy. Others advocate performing a colostomy just above the transition to the ganglionic bowel. Ileostomy is indicated in patients who have total colonic aganglionosis. The abdomen is opened via a left paramedian incision. The biopsy site is selected by observing the apparent transitional zone. In a normal case of rectosigmoid aganglionosis, three seromuscular biopsies are taken along the antimesenteric surface without entering the lumen (Fig. 80-14). One biopsy is taken from the narrowed segment of bowel, a second biopsy is taken from the transition zone, and a third biopsy is obtained from the dilated portion above the transition zone. Biopsies are assessed intraoperatively by frozen section to determine the level of ganglionic bowel.

A right transverse colostomy is very convenient in usual cases. We perform a loop colostomy over a skin bridge. A V-shaped incision is made in the right upper quadrant (Fig. 80-15*A*). The V-skin flap is reflected upward. The external oblique is split, and the internal oblique and transverse abdominis muscles are divided with diathermy. The peritoneum is opened. An opening is made in the mesocolon of the selected segment of the transverse colon (Fig. 80-15*B*). The skin flap is pulled through the opening in the mesocolon and sutured to the opposite skin margin (Fig. 80-15*C*). A few interrupted sutures of 4–0 or 5—0 silk are placed between the peritoneum, muscle layers of abdominal wall, and seromuscular layer of colon. The colon is opened longitudinally along the antimesenteric border using diathermy (Fig. 80-15*D*). The bowel is sutured to the skin using interrupted 4–0 silk sutures (Fig. 80-15*E*).

Primary Pull-Through Operation

Many surgeons have reported good results with a primary neonatal pull-through operation for HD. Some surgeons have recently reported good results using laparoscopic technique for pull-through operations. The author, like many others, prefers Swenson's pull-through operation in the neonatal period be-

cause of its simplicity and lack of complications. We have not used a divertionary colostomy for usual cases.

Once the diagnosis of HD is confirmed, the neonate is started on total parenteral nutrition 2 to 3 days prior to the operation. Rectal irrigations are conducted twice a day for 3 days before surgery. Intravenous gentamicin and metronidazole are started on the morning of the operation.

Operative Technique

The patient is positioned on the operating table to provide simultaneous exposure of the perineum and abdomen. The pelvis is allowed to drop back over the lower end of the table and legs are strapped over sandbags. A Foley catheter is inserted into the bladder.

The abdomen is opened via a left paramedian incision. We, like some other surgeons prefer a Pfannenstiel incision (Fig. 80-16*A* and *B*). When performing a Swenson's pull-through operation in the neonate. A Denis–Browne retractor is applied, and the urinary bladder is lifted forward out of the abdomen by stay sutures. Extramucosal biopsies are taken at intervals along the antimesenteric border and assessed by frozen section to determine the level of ganglionated bowel as outlined earlier. Sigmoid colon is mobilized by dividing sigmoid vessels and retaining the marginal vessels. It may be necessary to mobilize the splenic flexure to obtain adequate colonic length. The proximal level of resection above the ganglionated previously determined by frozen section is selected and the bowel is divided between intestinal clamps or staples (Fig. 80-16*C*).

The peritoneum is divided around its lateral and anterior reflection from the rectum, exposing the muscle coat of the rectum. At this point, the bowel is divided at the rectosigmoid junction and removed. Dissection extends around the rectum, keeping very close to the bowel wall (Fig. 80-16*D*). It is essential to maintain the dissection close to the muscular wall to prevent damage to the pelvic splanchnic innervation. All vessels are electrocoagulated under direct vision. Sufficient tension-free length is obtained by dividing the inferior mesenteric pedi-

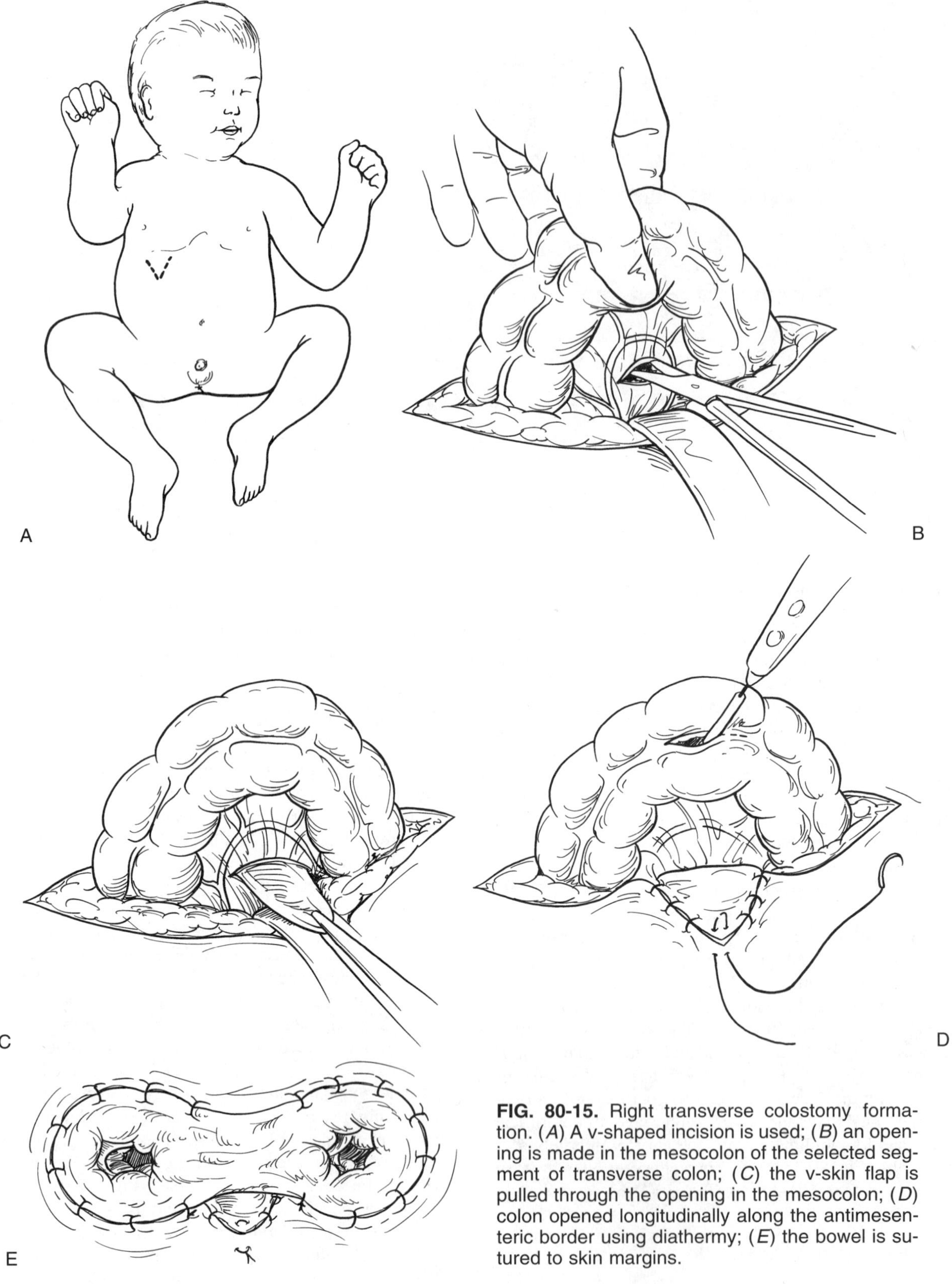

FIG. 80-15. Right transverse colostomy formation. (*A*) A v-shaped incision is used; (*B*) an opening is made in the mesocolon of the selected segment of transverse colon; (*C*) the v-skin flap is pulled through the opening in the mesocolon; (*D*) colon opened longitudinally along the antimesenteric border using diathermy; (*E*) the bowel is sutured to skin margins.

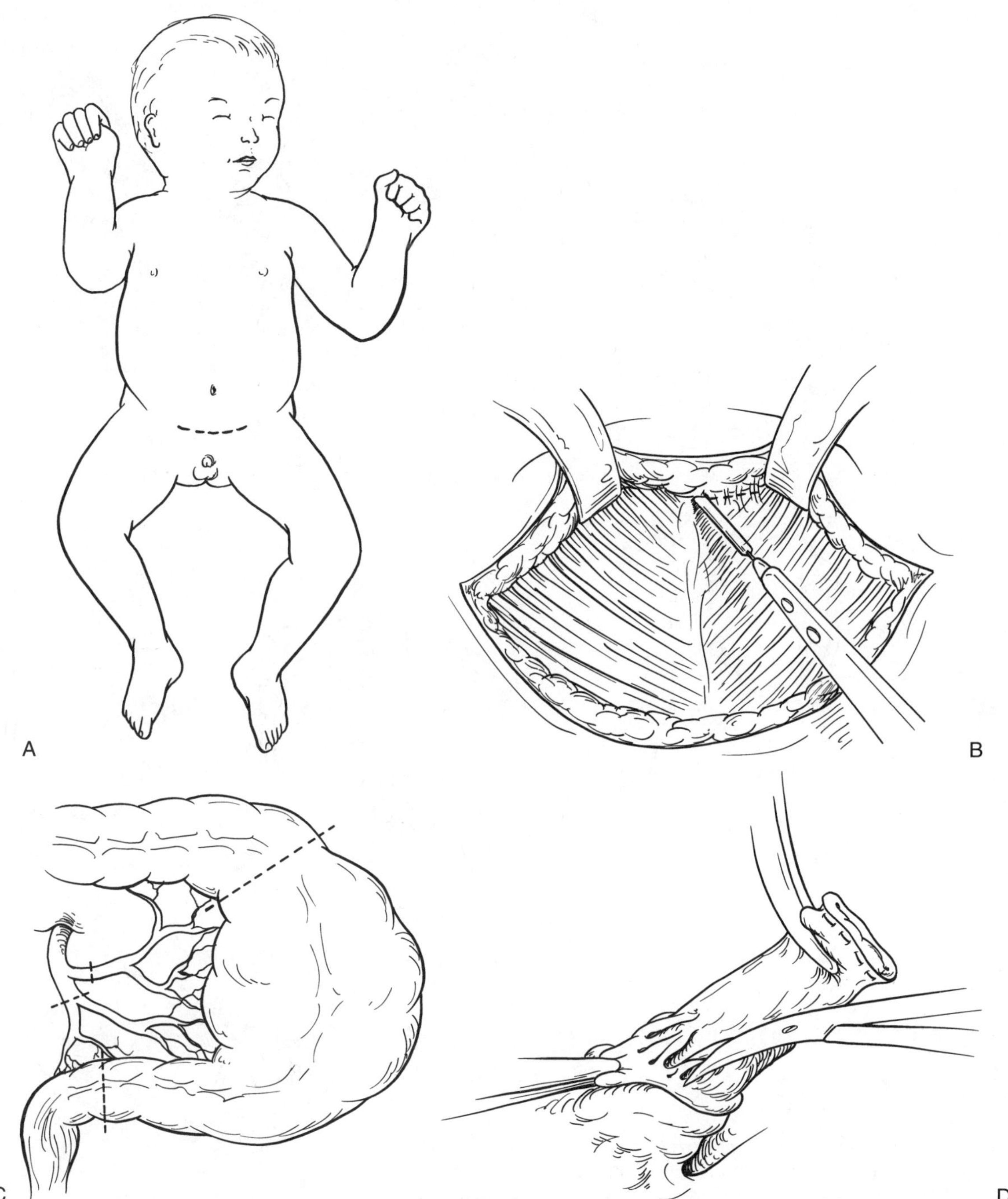

FIG. 80-16. Swenson's pull-through operation. (*A*) Pfannensteil incision; (*C*) proximal and distal level of resection of colon to provide more room for dissection in the pelvis; (*D*) it is essential to maintain dissection close to rectal wall in order to prevent damage to splanchnic nerves (*continued*).

cle, carefully preserving the marginal vessels. Dissection is carried down to the level of external sphincter posteriorly and laterally but does not extend as deeply anteriorly, leaving around 1.5 cm of intact rectal wall abutting against the vagina or urethra. The extent of dissection can be confirmed by putting a second glove over that on one hand and by manual palpation with a finger in the anus.

The mobilized rectum is intussuscepted through the anus by passing a curved clamp or a Babcock forceps through the anal canal, and an assistant places the closed rectal stump within the jaws of the clamp (Fig. 80-16E). The mucosal surface is cleaned with betadine. When the dissection has been completed, it should be possible to evert the anal canal completely when traction is applied on the rectum. An incision is made anteriorly through the rectal wall about 1 to 2 cm from the dentate line, extending halfway through the rectal circumference. A clamp

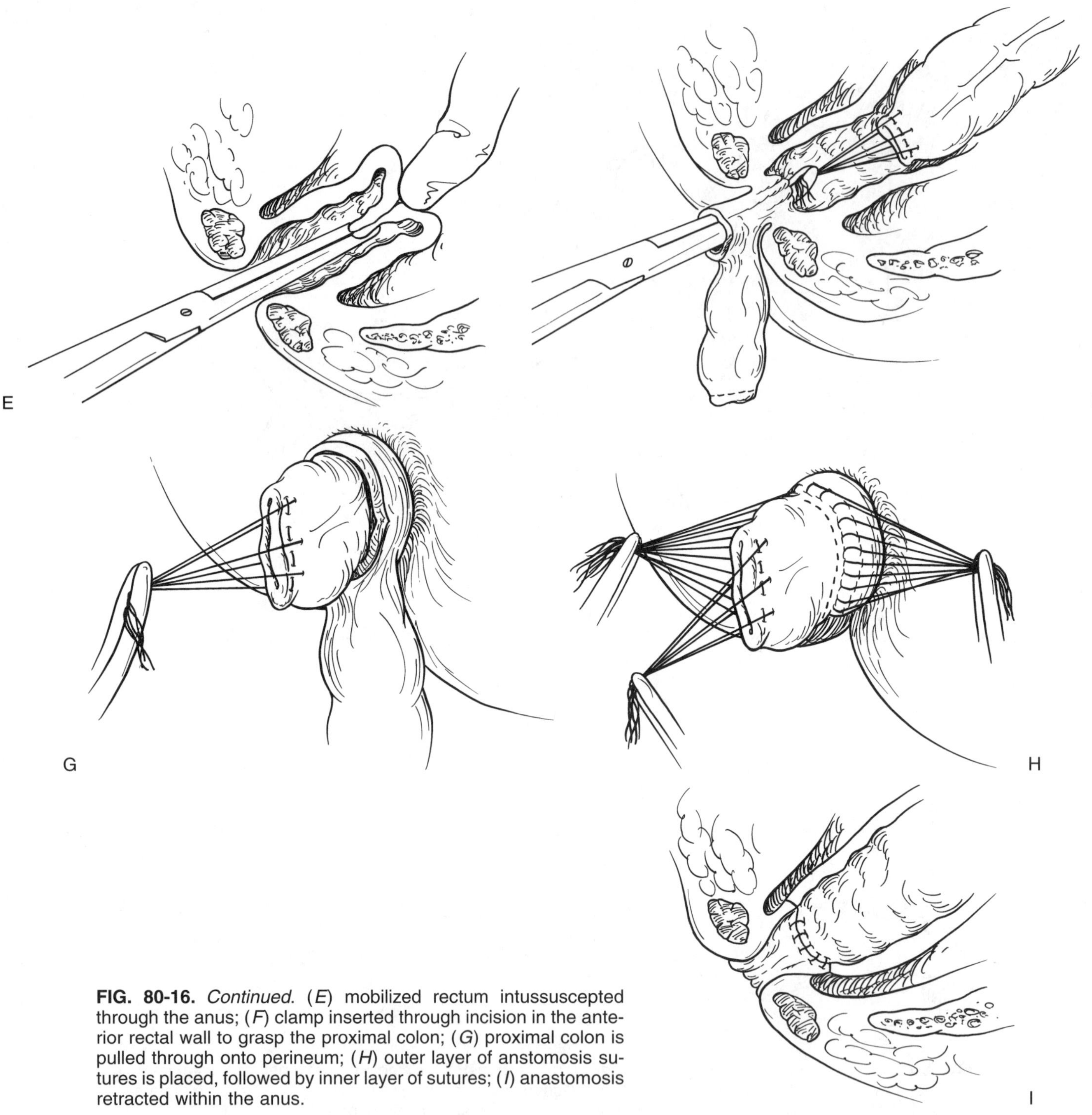

FIG. 80-16. *Continued.* (*E*) mobilized rectum intussuscepted through the anus; (*F*) clamp inserted through incision in the anterior rectal wall to grasp the proximal colon; (*G*) proximal colon is pulled through onto perineum; (*H*) outer layer of anstomosis sutures is placed, followed by inner layer of sutures; (*I*) anastomosis retracted within the anus.

is inserted through this incision to grasp multiple sutures placed through the cut end of the proximal colon (Fig. 80-16*F* and *G*). An outer layer of interrupted 4-0 Vicryl sutures are placed through the cut muscular edge of the rectum and the muscular wall of the pull-through colon (Fig. 80-16*H*). When the outer layer has been completed, the proximal bowel is opened and an inner layer of interrupted 4-0 Vicryl sutures is placed. When anastomosis is completed, the sutures are cut, allowing the anastomosis to retract within the anus (Fig. 80-16*I*).

Postoperatively, we keep the infant on total parenteral nutrition for 7 days and then gradually start oral feeds. The urethral catheter is removed after 3 days. Antibiotics are discontinued after 5 days. Rectal examination is performed 2 weeks later during an outpatient visit.

The procedures initially described by Duhamel and Soanes are comparable in terms of technical difficulty and outcome. Generally the choice of procedure is determined by the surgeon's training and personal preferences. Recently, a laparoscopically assisted pull-through technique was described in neonates as a single-staged procedrue. It is premature to judge this procedure at present.

OUTCOME

The attainment of normal postoperative defecation is dependent on intensity of bowel training, social background, and respective intelligence of the patients. Mental handicap, including Down syndrome, is invariably associated with long-term incontinence. Those patients with preoperative enterocolitis would also seem to have a marginally higher long-term risk of incontinence. The length of disease segment does not usually influence outcome.

There is no doubt that many patients do have disturbance of bowel function after surgery for HD, and this may persist for many years before disappearing. Some of these patients may never have a completely normal bowel habit.

INTESTINAL NEURONAL DYSPLASIA ASSOCIATED WITH HIRSCHSPRUNG DISEASE

The advances in the management of HD afford most patients a satisfactory outcome after definitive corrective surgery. However, some patients continue to have persistent bowel dysfunction despite adequate resection of the aganglionic bowel segment. The postoperative bowel dysfunction may include enterocolitis, constipation, and incontinence. Postoperative enterocolitis occurs in 6% to 20% of patients, and its incidence is unrelated to the timing or type of definitive surgery. Constipation and soiling have been reported to occur in 11% to 35% of patients after pull-through operations. It is not known why these postoperative persistent bowel problems occur. Some investigators have suggested an association between increased risk of complications and a particular type of pull-through operation. Others have not observed any correlation between postoperative bowel symptoms and the type of definitive procedure. Similarly, the length of the aganglionic segment does not appear to influence the clinical outcome. Persistent bowel problems after pull-through operations have led to an increasing realization that within the pulled-through segment, the presence of normal ganglion cells is not sufficient as an indicator of satisfactory outcome.

In 1977, Puri and associates[189] reported the first case (in the English literature) of intestinal neuronal dysplasia (IND) immediately proximal to a segment of aganglionic colon. Since then, there have been several reports of the combined occurrence of these disorders. Some investigators have reported that 25% to 35% of patients with aganglionosis have associated IND.[190,191] Others have rarely encountered IND in association with HD.[192]

IND has been classified into two distinct morphologic and clinical subtypes. Type A, seen in less than 5% of all cases, is congenital aplasia or hypoplasia of the sympathetic innervation and presents acutely with enterocolitis in the neonatal period. Type B, seen in 95% of cases, is characterized by a malformation of the parasympathetic submucous nerve plexus. IND associated with HD is usually type B. Attempts to define the diagnostic features of IND have identified the following as suggestive of IND: hyperganglionosis; giant ganglia (containing more than seven ganglion cell; ectopic ganglion cells in the lamina propria; and increased AChE activity in the mucosa, muscularis mucosa, and surrounding submucosal vessels.[190–194] Kobayashi and associates[195] reported IND in the proximal margin of the resected segment in 10 of the 31 patients with HD. All 10 patients with IND had persistent bowel symptoms such as enterocolitis, soiling, or constipation after definitive operations for HD. Their study emphasizes the importance of histochemical examination on the resected segment to predict postoperative bowel function in patients with IND.

REFERENCES

1. Kleinhaus S, Boley SJ, Sheran M, et al. Hirschsprung's disease: a survey of the members of the surgical section of the American Academy of Pediatrics. J Pediatr Surg 1979;14:588.
2. Ikeda K, Goto S. Diagnosis and treatment of Hirschsprung's disease in Japan: an analysis of 1628 patients. Ann Surg 1984;199:400.
3. Ziegler MM, Ross AJ III, Bishop HC. Total intestinal aganglionosis: a new technique for prolonged survival. J Pediatr Surg 1987;22:82.
4. Senyuz OF, Danismend N, Erdogan E, et al. Total intestinal aganglionosis with involvement of the stomach. Pediatr Surg Int 1988;3:74.
5. Passarge E. The genetics of Hirschsprung's disease. N Engl J Med 1967;276:138.
6. Spouge D, Baird PA. Hirschsprung's disease in large birth cohort. Teratology 1985;32:171.
7. Russell MB, Russell CA, Niebuhr. An epidemiological study of Hirschsprung's disease and additional anomalies. Acta Paediatr 1994; 83:68.
8. Sherman JO, Snyder ME, Weitzman JJ, et al. A 40 year multinational retrospective study of 880 Swenson's procedures. J Pediatr Surg 1989; 24:833.
9. Badner JA, Seiber WK, Garver KL, et al. A genetic study of Hirschsprung's disease. Am J Hum Genet 1990;46:568.
10. Yntema CL, Hammond WS. The origin of intrinsic ganglia of trunk viscera from vagal neural crest in the chick embryo. J Comp Neurol 1954;101:515.
11. Huther W. Die Hirschsprungsche Krankhiet als Folge einer Entwicklungsstorung der intramuralen Ganglien. Beitr Pathol Anat 1954; 114:161.
12. Okamoto E, Ueda T. Embryogenesis of intramural ganglia of the gut and its relation to Hirschsprung's disease. J Pediatr Surg 1967;2:437.
13. LeDouarin NF. Migration and differentiation of neural crest cells. Curr Top Dev Biol 1980;16:31.
14. Gershon MD, Epstein MC, Hegstrand L. Colonization of the chick gut by progenitors of enteric serotonergic neurons. Dev Biol 1980; 77:41.
15. Tam PKH. An immunohistochemical study with neuronspecific enolase and substance P of human enteric innervation: the normal development pattern and abnormal deviations in Hirschsprung's disease and pyloric stenosis. J Pediatr Surg 1986;21:227.
16. Allan IJ, Newgreen DF. The origin and differentiation of enteric neurons of the intestine of the fowl embryo. Am J Anat 1980;157:137.
17. Meijers JHC, Tibboel D, Van der Kamp AWM, et al. A model for aganglionosis in the chicken embryo. J Pediatr Surg 1989;24:557.
18. Fujimoto T, Hata J, Yokoyama S, et al. A study of the extracellular matrix protein as the migration pathway of neural crest cells in the gut: analysis in human embryos with special reference to the pathogenesis of Hirschsprung's disease. J Pediatr Surg 1989;24:550.
19. Kamagata S, Donahoe PK. The effect of fibronectin on cholinergic differentiation of the fetal colon. J Pediatr Surg 1985;20:307.
20. Ueno S. The role of extracellular matrices during the development of intramural ganglion cells in the gut. J Jpn Soc Pediatr Surg 1987;23: 491.
21. Bernfield M, Banerje S, Koda J, et al. Remodelling of basement membrane as a mechanism of morphogenetic tissue interaction. In: Trelstadt RL, ed. The role of extracellular matrix in development. New York, Alan RL Liss, 1984:545.
22. Greenberg JH, Seppa S, Seppa H, et al. Role of collagen and fibronec-

tin in neural crest cell adhesion and migration. Dev Biol 1981;87:259.

23. Brauer PR, Markwald RR. Attachment of neural crest cells to endogenous extracellular matrices. Anat Rec 1987;219:275.

24. Parikh DH, Tam PKH, Velzen DV, et al. Abnormalities in the distribution of lamina and collagen Type IV in Hirschsprung's disease. Gastroenterology 1992;102:1236.

25. Parikh DH, Tam PKH, Lloyd DA, et al. Quantitative and qualitative analysis of the extracellular matrix protein laminin, in Hirschsprung's disease. J Pediatr Surg 1992;27:991.

26. Shimotake T, Iwai N, Yanghara E, et al. Impaired proliferative activity of mesenchymal cells affects the migratory pathway for neural crest cells in the developing gut of mutant murine embryos. J Pediatr Surg 1995;30:445.

27. Kuroda T, Doody DP, Donahoe PK. Aberrant colonic expression of MHC class II antigens in Hirschsprung's disease. Aust NZ J Surg 1991;61:373.

28. Hirobe S, Doody DP, Ryan DP, et al. Ectopic class II major histocompatibility antigens in Hirschsprung's disease and neuronal intestinal dysplasia. J Peditar Surg 1992;27:357.

29. Kobayashi H, Hirakawa H, Puri P. Overexpression of intercellular adhesion molecule-1 (ICAM-1) and MHC class II antigen on hypertrophic nerve trunks suggests an immunopathologic response in Hirschsprung's disease. J Pediatr Surg 1995;30:1680.

30. Boix-Ochoa J, Casasa JM, Marhuenda C, et al. Total colonic aganglionosis: surgical treatment and long term follow-up. Pediatr Surg Int 1991;6:198.

31. Caniano DA, Ormsbee HS III, Polito W. Total intestinal aganglionosis. J Pediatr Surg 1985;20:456.

32. Schiller M, Levy P, Shawa RA, et al. Familial Hirschsprung's disease: a report of 22 affected siblings in four families. J Pediatr Surg 1990;25:322.

33. Engum SA, Petrites M, Rescorla FJ, et al. Familial Hirschsprung's disease: 20 cases in 12 kindreds. J Pediatr Surg 1993;28:1286.

34. Stannard VA, Fowler C, Robinson L, et al. Familial Hirschsprung's disease: report of autosomal dominant and probable recessive x-linked kindreds. J Pediatr Surg 1991;26:591.

35. Goldberg E. An epidemiological study of Hirschsprung's disease. Int J Epidemiol 1991;13:479.

36. Lister J, Tam PKH. Hirschsprung's disease. In: Lister J, Irving IM, eds. Neonatal surgery. London, Butterworths, 1990:523.

37. Polly TZ, Coran AG. Hirschsprung's disease in the newborn. Pediatr Surg Int 1986;1:80.

38. Caniano DA, Teitelbaum DH, Qualman SJ. Management of Hirschsprung's disease in children with Trisomy 21. Am J Surg 1990;159:402.

39. Lamont MA, Fitchett M, Dennis NR. Interstitial deletion of distal 13q1 associated with Hirschsprung's disease. J Med Genet 1989;26:100.

40. Kiss P, Osztovics M. Association of 13q deletion and Hirschsprung's disease. J Med Genet 1989;26:763.

41. Webb GC, Keith CG, Campbell NT. Concurrent de novo interstitial deletion of band 2p 22 and reciprocal translocation (3:7) (p21:q22). J Med Genet 1988;25:125.

42. Passage E. Genetics of Hirschsprung's disease. Clin Gastroenterol 1973;2:507.

43. Omenn GS, McKusick VA. The association of Waardenburg syndrome and Hirschsprung's megacolon. Am J Med Genet 1979;3:217.

44. Badner JA, Chakravarti A. Waardensburg syndrome and Hirschsprung's disease: evidence for pleiotropic effects of a single dominant gene. Am J Med Genet 1990;35:100.

45. Clausen N, Andersson P, Tommerup N. Familial occurrence of neuroblastoma, Von Recklinghausen's neurofibromatosis, Hirschsprung's aganglionosis and jaw-winking syndrome. Acta Paediatr Scand 1989;78:736.

46. Lyonnet S, Bolino A, Pelet A, et al. A gene for Hirschsprung's disease maps to the proximal long arm of chromosome 10. Nat Genet 1993;4:346.

47. Angrist M, Kauffman E, Slauenghaupt SA, et al. A gene for Hirschsprung's disease (megacolon) in the pericentromeric region of human chromosome 10. Nat Genet 1993;4:351.

48. Yin L, Ceccherini I, Pasini B, et al. Close linkage with the RET proto-oncogene and boundaries of deletion mutations in autosomal dominant Hirschsprung's disease. Hum Mol Genet 1993;2:1803.

49. Romeo G, Ronchetto P, Yin L, et al. Point mutations affecting the tyrosine kinase domain of the RET proto-oncogene in Hirschsprung's disease. Nature 1994;367:377.

50. Edery P, Lyonnet S, Mulligan LM, et al. Mutations of the RET proto-oncogene in Hirschsprung's disease. Nature 1994;367:378.

51. Puffenberger EG, Hosoda K, Washington SS, et al. A missense mutation of the endothelin-B receptor gene in multigenic Hirschsprung's disease. Cell 1994;79:1257.

52. Arai H, Nakao K, Takaya, et al. The human endothelin-B receptor gene: structural organization and chromosomal assignment. J Biol Chem 1993;268:3463.

53. Kiss P, Osztovics M. Association of 13q deletion and Hirschsprung's disease. J Med Genet 1989;26:793.

54. Bottani A, Xie Y, Binkert F, et al. A case of Hirschsprung's disease with a chromosome 13 microdeletion, del (13) (q32.3q33.2): potential mapping of one disease locus. Hum Genet 1991;87:748.

55. Baynash A, Hosoda K, Giaid A, et al. Interaction of Endothelin-3 with Endothelin-B receptor is essential for development of epidermal melanocytes and enteric neurons. Cell 1994;79:1277.

56. Hosoda K, Hammer RE, Richardson JA, et al. Targeted and natural (piebald lethal) mutations of endothelin-B receptor gene produce megacolon associated with spotted coat colour in mice. Cell 1994;79:267.

56a.Kusafuka T, Wang Y, Puri P. Novel mutations of the endothelin-β receptor gene in isolated patients with Hirschsprung's disease. Hum Mol Genet 1996;5:347.

56b.Kusafuka T, Wang Y, Puri P. Mutational analysis of the RET, the endothelin-β receptor, and endothelin-3 genes in sporadic patients with Hirschsprung's disease. J Pediatr Surg (in press).

57. Ehrenpreis T. Some newer aspects of Hirschsprung's disease and allied disorders. J Pediatr Surg 1966;1:329.

58. Bennett A, Garrett JR, Howard ER. Adrenergic myenteric nerves in Hirschsprung's disease. Br Med J 1968;1:487.

59. Gannon BJ, Noblett HR, Burnstock G. Adrenergic innervation of bowel in Hirschsprung's disease. Br Med J 1969;3:338.

60. Touloukian RJ, Aghajanian G, Roth RH. Adrenergic hyperactivity of the aganglionic colon. J Pediatr Surg 1983;8:191.

61. Baumgarten HG, Holstein AG, Stelzner F. Nervous elements in the human colon of Hirschsprung's disease. Virchows Arch 1973;358:113.

62. Touloukian RJ, Morgenroth VH, Roth RH. Sympathetic neurotransmitter metabolism in Hirschsprung's disease. J Pediatr Surg 1975;10:593.

63. Kamijo K, Hiatt RB, Koelle B. Congenital megacolon: a comparison of the spastic and hypertrophic segments with respect to cholinestrase activities and sensitivities to acetylcholine, DFP and barium ion. Gastroenterology 1953;24:173.

64. Meier-Ruge W. Das Megacolon: Seine Diagnose and Pathophysiologie. Virchows Arch 1968;344:67.

65. Frigo GM, Del Tacca M, Lecchini S, et al. Some observations on the intrinsic nervous mechanism in Hirschsprung's disease. Gut 1973;14:35.

66. Vizi ES, Zseli J, Kontor E, et al. Characteristics of cholinergic neuroeffector transmission of ganglionic and aganglionic colon in Hirschsprung's disease. Gut 1990;31:1046.

67. Meier-Ruge W, Lutterbeck PM, Herzog B et al. Acetylcholinesterase activity in suction rectal biopsies of the rectum in the diagnosis of Hirschsprung's disease. J Pediatr Surg 1972;7:11.

68. Lake BD, Puri P, Nixon HH, et al. Hirschsprung's disease: an appraisal of histochemically demonstrated acetylcholine estrase in suction rectal biopsy specimens as an aid to diagnosis. Arch Pathol Lab Med 1978;102:244.

69. Bloom SR, Polak JM. Peptidergic versus purinergic. Lancet 1978;1:93.

70. Polak JM, Path MRC, Bloom SR. Neuropeptides of the gut: a newly discovered major control system. World J Surg 1979;3:393.

71. Bishop AE, Polak JM, Lake BD, et al. Abnormality of the colonic regulatory peptides in Hirschsprung's disease. Histopathology 1981;5:679.

72. Tsuto T, Okamura H, Fukui K, et al. An immunohistochemical investigation of vasoactive intestinal polypeptide in the colon of patients with Hirschsprung's disease. Neurosci Lett 1982;34:57.

73. Taguchi T, Tanaka K, Ikeda K, et al. Peptidergic innervation irregularities in Hirschsprung's disease. Virchows Arch 1983;401:223.

74. Larsson LT, Malinfors F, Sundler F. Peptidergic innervation in Hirschsprung's disease. Z Kinderchir 1983;38:301.

75. Larsson LT, Malmfors G, Sundler F. Defects in peptidergic innervation in Hirschsprung's disease: immunocytochemical observation in 14 cases. Pediatr Surg Int 1988;3:147.

76. Tsuto T, Okamura H, Fukui K. Immunohistochemical investigations of gut hormones in the colon of patients with Hirschsprung's disease. Z Kinderchir 1983;38:301.

77. Tam PK, Boyd GP. New insights into peptidergic abnormalities in Hirschsprung's disease by wholemount immunocytochemistry. J Pediatr Surg 1991;26:595.

78. Wattchow DA, Furness JB, Costa M, et al. The distribution and coexistence of peptides in nerve fibres of large bowel affected by Hirschsprung's disease. Pediatr Surg Int 1991;6:322.

79. Larsson LT, Malmfors G, Sundler F. Neuropeptide Y, calcitonin gene-related peptide, and galanin in Hirschsprung's disease: an immunocytochemical study. J Pediatr Surg 1988;23:342.

80. Hamada Y, Bishop AE, Federici G. Increased neuropeptide Y-immunoreactive innervation of aganglionic bowel in Hirschsprung's disease. Virchows Arch A 1987;411:369.

81. Kawana T, Nada O, Hirose R, et al. Distribution of neuropeptide Y-like immunoreactivity in the normo-ganglionic and aganglionic segments of human colon. Acta Neuropathol 1990;80:469.

82. Romanska HM, Bishop AE, Brereton RJ, et al. Immunocytochemistry for neuronal markers shows deficiencies in conventional histology in the treatment of Hirschsprung's disease. J Pediatr Surg 1993;28:1059.

83. Kato H, Yamamoto T, Yamamoto H, et al. Immunocytochemical characterization of supporting cells in the enteric nervous system in Hirschsprung's disease. J Pediatr Surg 1990;25:514.

84. Gabella G. Glial cells in the myenteric plexus. Z Naturforsch 1971;266:244.

85. Gabella G. Ultrastructure of the nerve plexuses of the mammalian intestine: the enteric glial cells. Neuroscience 1981;6:425.

86. Jessen KR, Mirsky R. Glial cells in the enteric nervous system contain glial fibrillary acidic protein. Nature 1980;286:736.

87. Eng LF. The glial fibrillary acidic (GFA) protein. In: Bradshaw R, Schneider D eds. Proteins of the nervous system. New York, Raven, 1980:85.

88. Ferri GL, Probert L, Cocchia D, et al. Evidence for the presence of S-100 protein in the glial component of the human enteric nervous system. Nature 1982;297:409.

89. Muller CM. Astrocytes in cat visual cortex studied by GFAP and S-100 immunocytochemistry during postnatal development. J Comp Neurol 1992;317:309.

90. Fujimoto T, Reen DJ, Puri P. Immunohistochemical characterization of abnormal innervation of colon in Hirschsprung's disease using D$_7$ monoclonal antibody. J Pediatr Surg 1987;22:246.

91. Fujimoto T, Puri P, Reen DJ. A study of specificity of the anti-glial fibrillary acidic protein like monoclonal antibody D$_7$ Biochem Soc Trans 1987;15:279.

92. Kempstead J. Imperial Cancer Research Fund, personal communication, November 1991.

93. Sugimura K, Haimoto H, Nagura H, et al. Immunohistochemical differential distribution of S-100α and S-100β in the peripheral nervous system of the rat. Muscle Nerve 1989;12:919.

94. Taguchi T, Tanaka K, Ikeda K. Immunohistochemical study of neuron specific enolase and S-100 protein in the Hirschsprung's disease. Virchows Arch 1985;405:399.

95. Kawana T, Nada O, Ikeda K. An immunohistochemical study of glial fibrillary acidic (GFA) protein and S-100 protein in the colon affected by Hirschsprung's disease. Acta Neuropathol 1988;76:159.

96. Kawana T, Nado O, Ikeda K, et al. Distribution and localization of glial fibrillary acidic protein in colons affected by Hirschsprung's disease. J Pediatr Surg 1989;24:448.

97. Kato H, Yamamoto T, Yamamoto H, et al. Immunocytochemical characterization of supporting cells in the enteric nervous system in Hirschsprung's disease. J Pediatr Surg 1990;25:514.

98. Scallon C, Puri P, Reen DJ. Identification of rectal ganglion cells using monoclonal antibodies. J Pediatr Surg 1985;20:37.

99. Fujimoto T, Reen DJ, Puri P. Immunohistochemical characterization of abnormal innervation of colon in Hirschsprung's disease using D$_7$ monoclonal antibody. J Pediatr Surg 1987;22:246.

100. Fujimoto T, Reen DJ, Puri P. A study of the specificity of the anti-

101. Puri P, Fujimoto T, Sheppard B. Ultrastructural demonstration of abnormal multiaxonal Schwann-cell units in Hirschsprung's disease. Pediatr Surg Int 1989;4:326.

102. Soeda J, O'Brian DS, Puri P. Mucosal neuroendocrine cell abnormalities in the colon of patients with Hirschsprung's disease. J Pediatr Surg 1992;27:823.

103. Bult H, Boeckxstaens GE, Pelckmans PA, et al. Nitric oxide as an inhibitory non-adrenergic non-cholinergic neurotransmitter. Nature 1990;345:346.

104. Boeckxstaens GE, Pelckmans PA, Bult H, et al. Non-adrenergic non-cholinergic relaxation mediated by nitric oxide in the canine ileocolonic junction. Eur J Pharmacol 1990;190:239.

105. Stark ME, Bauer AJ, Sarr MG, et al. Nitric oxide mediates inhibitory nerve input in human and canine jejunum. Gastroenterology 1993;104:398.

106. Burleigh DE. N^g-nitro-L-arginine reduces nonadrenergic, noncholinergic relaxations of human gut. Gastroenterology 1992;102:679.

107. Vanderwinden JM, De Laet MH, Schiffman SN, et al. Nitric oxide synthase distribution in the enteric nervous system of Hirschsprung's disease. Gastroenterology 1993;105:969.

108. Kobayashi H, O'Brian DS, Puri P. Lack of expression of NADPH-diaphorase and neural cell adhesion molecule (NCAM) in colonic muscle of patients with Hirschsprung's disease. J Pediatr Surg 1994;29:301.

109. Bealer JF, Natuzzi ES, Buscher C, et al. Nitric oxide synthase is deficient in the aganglionic colon of patients with Hirschsprung's disease. Pediatrics 1994;93:647.

110. O'Kelly TJ, Davies JR, Tam PKH, et al. Abnormalities of nitric-oxide-producing neurons in Hirschsprung's disease: morphology and implications. J Pediatr Surg 1994;29:294.

111. Larsson LT, Shen Z, Ekblad E, et al. Lack of neuronal nitric oxide synthase in nerve fibers of aganglionic intestine: a clue to Hirschsprung's disease. J Pediatr Gastroenterol Nut 1995;20:49.

112. Okamoto E, Satani M, Kuwata K. Histologic and embryologic studies on the innervation of the pelvic viscera in patients with Hirschsprung's disease. Surg Gynecol Obstet 1982;144:823.

113. Mackenzie JM, Dixon MF. An immunohistochemical study of the enteric neural plexi in Hirschsprung's disease. Histopathology 1987;11:1055.

114. Deguchi E, Iwai N, Goto Y, et al. An immunohistochemical study of neurofilament and microtubule-associated tau protein in the enteric innervation in Hirschsprung's disease. J Pediatr Surg 1993;28:886.

115. Tam PKH, Boyd GP. Origin, course and endings of abnormal enteric nerve fibres in Hirschsprung's disease defined by whole mount immunohistochemistry. J Pediatr Surg 1990;25:457.

116. Barde YA. Trophic factors and neuronal survival. Neuron 1989;2:1525.

117. Thoenen H, Barde YA. Physiology of nerve growth factor. Phys Rev 1980;609:1284.

118. Hefti F, Hartikka J, Salvatierra A, et al. Localization of nerve growth factor receptors in cholinergic neruons of the human basal forebrain. Neurosci Lett 1986;69:37.

119. Kordower JH, Bartus RT, Bothwell M, et al. Nerve growth factor receptor immunoreactivity in the nonhuman primate (Cebus apella): distribution, morphology, and colocalization with cholinergic enzymes. J Comp Neurol 1988;277:465.

120. Koliatsos VE, Clatterbuck RE, Nauta HW, et al. Human nerve growth factor prevents degeneration of basal forebrain cholinergic neurons in primates. Ann Neurol 1991;30:831.

121. Kobayashi H, O'Briain DS, Puri P. Nerve growth factor receptor immunostaining suggests an extrinsic origin for hypertorphic nerve in Hirschsprung's disease. Gut 1994;35:1605.

122. Nixon HH. Hirschsprung's disease in newborn. In: Holschneider AM, ed. Hirschsprung's disease. Stuttgart, Hippokrates Verlag, 1982:103.

123. Bill AH, Chapman ND. The enterocolitis of Hirschsprung's disease: history and treatment. Am J Surg 1962;103:70.

124. Fujimoto T, Puri P. Persistence of enterocolitis following diversion of faecal stream in Hirschsprung's disease: a study of mucosal defense mechanism. Pediatr Surg Int 1988;3:141.

125. Surana R, Quinn FMJ, Puri P. Evaluation of risk factors in the development of enterocolitis complicating Hirschsprung's disease. Pediatr Surg Int 1994;9:234.

126. Sherman JO, Snyder ME, Weitzman JJ, et al. A 40 year multinational retrospective study of 880 Swenson procedures. J Pediatr Surg 1989; 24:833.

127. Nixon HH. Hirschsprung's disease: progress in management and diagnostics. World J Surg 1985;9:189.

128. Shanbhogue LKR, Bianchi A. Experience with primary Swenson resection and pull-through for neonatal Hirschsprung's disease. Pediatr Surg Int 1990;5:446.

129. Carneiro PMR, Brereton RJ, Drake DP, et al. Enterocolitis in Hirschsprung's disease. Pediatr Surg Int 1992;7:356.

130. Lifschitz CH, Bloss R. Persistence of colitis in Hirschsprung's disease. J Pediatr Gastroenterol Nutr 1985;4:291.

131. Teitelbaum DH, Caniano DA, Qualman SJ. The pathophysiology of Hirschsprung's associated enterocolitis: importance of histologic correlates. J Pediatr Surg 1989;24:1271.

132. Bill AH, Chapman ND. The enterocolitis of Hirschsprung's disease: its natural history and treatment. Am J Surg 1962;103:70.

133. Akkary S, Sahwy E, Kandil W, et al. A histochemical study of the mucosubstances of the colon in cases of Hirschsprung's disease with and without enterocolitis. J Pediatr Surg 1981;16:664.

134. Lloyd-Still JD, Demers LM. Hirschsprung's enterocolitis, prostaglandins and response to cholestyramine. J Pediatr Surg 1978;13:417.

135. Thomas DFM, Fernie DS, Bayston R, et al. Enterocolitis in Hirschsprung's disease: a controlled study of the etiologic role of Clostridium difficile. J Pediatr Surg 1986;21:22.

136. Hardy SP, Bayston R, Spitz L. Prolonged carriage of Clostridium difficile in Hirschsprung's disease. Arch Dis Child 1993;69:221.

137. Wilson-Storey D, Scobie WG, McGenity KG. Microbial studies of enterocolitis of Hirschsprung's disease. Arch Dis Child 1990;65:1338.

138. Imamura A, Puri P, O'Brian DS, et al. Mucosal immune defense mechanisms in enterocolitis complicating Hirschsprung's disease. Gut 1992;33:801.

139. Kleinhaus S, Boley SJ, Sheran M, et al. Hirschsprung's disease: a survey of the members of the surgical section of the American Academy of Pediatrics. J Pediatr Surg 1979;14:588.

140. Swenson O, Sherman JO, Fisher JH, et al. The treatment and postoperative complications of congenital megacolon: a 25 year follow-up. Ann Surg 1975;192:266.

141. Sieber WK. Hirschsprung's disease. In: Welch KJ, Randolph JG, Ravitch MM, et al. eds. Pediatric surgery, Chicago, Year Book Medical, 1986:995.

142. Roberston MJ, Ritz J. Biology and clinical relevance of human natural killer cells. Blood 1990;76:2421.

143. Meuer SC, Dienes HP. Lymphocytes mediated cell lysis. Virchows Arch B 1989;57:1.

144. Priebe T, Ruiz L, Nelson JA. Role of natural killer cells in the modulation of primary antibody production by purine nucleosides and their analogs. Cell Immunol 1990;130:513.

145. O'Doriso MS. Neuropeptides and gastrointestinal immunity. Am J Med 1986;81:74.

146. Kobayashi H, Hirakawa H, O'Brian DS, et al. Intercellular adhesion molecule-1 (ICAM-1) in the pathogenesis of enterocolitis complicating Hirschsprung's disease. Pediatr Surg Int 1994;9:237.

147. Fujimoto T, Miyano T. Abnormal expression of blood group-associated antigen (BGA) in colon of Hirschsprung's disease. Pediatr Surg Int 1994;9:242.

148. Helbig D. Hirschsprung's disease in infancy and childhood. In: Holschneider AM, ed. Hirschsprung's disease. Stuttgart, Hippocrates Verlag, 1982:93.

149. Cass DT. Neonatal one-stage repair of Hirschsprung's disease. Pediatr Surg Int 1990;5:341.

150. Swenson O, Sherman JO, Fisher JH. Diagnosis of congenital megacolon: an analysis of 501 patients. J Pediatr Surg 1973;8:587.

151. Nixon HH. Hirschsprung's disease: progress in management and diagnosis. World J Surg 1985;9:189.

152. Nixon HH. Hirschsprung's disease in the newborn. In: Holschnedier AM, ed. Hirschsprung's disease. Stuttgart, Hippocrates Verlag, 1982:103.

153. Menardi G. Toxic megacolon. In: Holschneider AM, ed. Hirschsprung's disease. Stuttgart, Hippocrates Verlag, 1982:125.

154. Gowers WR. The automatic action of the sphincter ani. Proc R Soc Med 1877;26:77.

155. Callaghan RP, Nixon HH. Megarectum: physiological observations. Arch Dis Child 1964;39:153.

156. Lawson JON, Nixon HH. Anal pressures in the diagnosis of Hirschsprung's disease. J Pediatr Surg 1967;2:544.

157. Schnaufer L, Talbert JL, Haller JA. Differential sphincteric studies in the diagnosis of anorectal disorders of childhood. J Pediatr Surg 1967;2:538.

158. Aaronson IA, Nixon HH. A clinical evaluation of anorectal pressure studies in the diagnosis of Hirschsprung's disease. Gut 1972;13:138.

159. Loening-Baucke VA. Anorectal manometry: experience with strain gauge pressure transducers for the diagnosis of Hirschsprung's disease. J Pediatr Surg 1983;18:595.

160. Sun WM, Read NW, Prior A, et al. Sensory and motor responses to rectal distension vary according to rate and pattern of balloon inflation. Gastroenterology 1990;99:1008.

161. Holschneider AM, Kellner E, Streibl P, et al. The development of anorectal continence and its significance in the diagnosis of Hirschsprung's disease. J Pediatr Surg 1976;11:151.

162. Ito Y, Donahoe PK, Hendren WH. Maturation of the rectoanal response in premature and perinatal infants. J Pediatr Surg 1977;12:477.

163. Smith B. Pre and postnatal development of ganglion cells of the rectum and its surgical implications. J Pediatr Surg 1968;3:386.

164. Bughaighis AG, Emery JL. Functional obstruction of the intestine due to neurological immaturity. Prog Pediatr Surg 1971;3:37.

165. Puri P, Blake N, Carroll R, et al. Relationship between functional and histologic appearances of developing ganglion cells in the guinea pig rectum. J Pediatr Surg 1980;15:42.

166. Boston VE, Scott JES. Anorectal manometry as a diagnostic method in the neonatal period. J Pediatr Surg 1976;11:9.

167. Loening-Baucke V, Pringle KC, Ekiro GG. Anorectal manometry for the exclusion of Hirschsprung's disease in neonates. J Pediatr Gastroenterol Nutr 1985;4:596.

168. Tamate S, Shiokawa C, Yamada C, et al. Manometric diagnosis of Hirschsprung's disease in the neonatal period. J Pediatr Surg 1984; 19:285.

169. Verder H, Peterson W, Mauritzen K. Anal tonometry in the neonatal period for the diagnosis of Hirschsprung's disease. Acta Paediatr Scand 1991;80:45.

170. Kobayashi H, O'Brian DS, Hirakawa H, et al. A rapid technique of acetylcholinesterase staining. Arch Pathol Lab Med 1994;118:1127.

171. Kobayashi H, Wang Y, Hirakawa H, et al. Intraoperative evaluation of extent of aganglionosis by a rapid acetylcholinesterase histochemical technique. J Ped Surg 1995;30:248.

172. Kurer MH, Lawson JON, Pambakion H. Suction biopsy in Hirschsprung's disease. Arch Dis Child 1986;6:83.

173. Ikawa H, Kim SH, Hendren HW. Acetylcholinesterase and manometry in the diagnosis of the constipated child. Arch Surg 1986;121:435.

174. Lake BD, Malone MT, Risdon RA. Acetylcholinesterase in the diagnosis of Hirschsprung's disease, including a comment on intestinal neural dysplasia. Pediatr Pathol 1989;9:351.

175. Schofield DE, Devine W, Yunis EJ. Acetylcholinesterase stained suction rectal biopsies in the diagnosis of Hirschsprung's disease. J Pediatr Gastroenterol Nutr 1990;11:221.

176. Athon AC, Filipe MI, Drake DP. Problems and advantages of acetylcholinesterase histochemistry of rectal suction biopsies in the diagnosis of Hirschsprung's disease. J Pediatr Surg 1990;25:520.

177. Klein RR, Scarborough RA. Hirschsprung's disease in the newborn. Am J Surg 1954;88:6.

178. Sieber WK, Girdany BR. Management of symptomatic aganglionic megacolon in early infancy. Arch Surg 1957;75:388.

179. Grosfeld JL, Balantine TVN, Csicsko JF. A critical evaluation of the Duhamel operation for Hirschsprung's disease. Arch Surg 1978;113:454.

180. So HB, Schwartz DL, Becker JM, et al. Endorectal "pull-through" without preliminary colostomy in neonates with Hirschsprung's disease. J Pediatr Surg 1980;15:470.

181. Carcassonne M, Guys JM, Morrison-Lacombe G, et al. Management of Hirschsprung's disease: curative surgery before three months of age. J Pediatr Surg 1989;24:1032.

182. Shanbhogue LKR, Bianchi A. Experience with primary Swenson resection and pull-through for neonatal Hirschsprung's disease. Pediatr Surg Int 1990;5:446.

183. Swenson O, Bill AH. Resection of rectum and rectosigmoid with

preservation of sphincter for benign spastic lesions producing megacolon. Surgery 1948;24:212.

184. Duhamel B. A new operation for the treatment of Hirschsprung's disease. Arch Dis Child 1960;35:38.

185. Soave F. Hirschsprung's disease: a new surgical technique. Arch Dis Child 1964;39:16.

186. Puri P, Nixon HH. Long term results of Swenson's operation for Hirschsprung's disease. Prog Pediatr Surg 1977;10:87.

187. Heij HA, de Vries X, Bremer I, et al. Long term anorectal function after Duhamel operation for Hirschsprung's disease. J Pediatr Surg 1995;30:430.

188. Cilley RE, Statter MB, Hirschi RB, et al. Definitive treatment of Hirschsprung's disease in the newborn with one stage procedure. Surgery 1994;115:551.

189. Puri P, Lake BD, Nixon HH, et al. Neuronal colonic dysplasia: an unusual association of Hirschsprung's disease. J Pediatr Surg 1977; 12:681.

190. Scharli AF. Neuronal intestinal dysplasia. Pediatr Surg Int 1992;7:2.

191. Fadda B, Pistor G, Meier Ruge W, et al. Symptoms, diagnosis and therapy of neuronal intestinal dysplasia masked by Hirschsprung's disease. Pediatr Surg Int 1987;2:76.

192. Smith W. Isolated intestinal neuronal dysplasia: a descriptive histological pattern or a distinct clinicopathological entity? In: Hadziselimovic F, Herzog B eds. Inflammatory bowel disease and morbus Hirschsprung's disease. Dordrecht, The Netherlands, Kluwer Academic, 1992:203.

193. Munakata K, Morita K, Okabe I, et al. Clinical and histological studies of neuronal intestinal dysplasia. J Pediatr Surg 1985;20:231.

194. Borchard F, Meier-Ruge W, Wiebecke B, et al. Innervationsstorungen des dicksarmes-klassifikation und diagnostik. Pathologe 1991;12:171.

195. Kobayashi H, Hirakawa H, Surana R, et al. Intestinal neuronal dysplasia is a possible cause of persistent bowel symptoms after pull-through operation for Hirschsprung's disease. J Pediatr Surg 1995;30:253.

Surgery of Infants and Children: Scientific Principles and Practice, edited by
Keith T. Oldham, Paul M. Colombani, and Robert P. Foglia.
Lippincott–Raven Publishers, Philadelphia, © 1997.

CHAPTER 81

Ulcerative Colitis

David L. Dudgeon

Ulcerative colitis is a relatively rare disease in childhood. The overall incidence varies, dependent on geographic location, but is 3.5 to 8.0 per 10^5 in the general population with approximately 15% of these patients diagnosed prior to 16 years of age.[1] An early occurrence can, however, be a sign of a more ominous clinical course. Children with a history of ulcerative colitis for 10 years have a 3% incidence of colon cancer and this increases by 20% for every subsequent decade.[2] Ulcerative colitis is a surgically curable disease if a total colectomy with proctectomy is utilized. However, most parents are reluctant to subject young children to a permanent ileostomy and it has an even more devastating effect when suggested as therapy to a body conscious teenager. Fortunately, anal-sparing curative surgical therapy is now available.

HISTORICAL PERSPECTIVE

Diarrheal disease has always been a significant health problem, as described in the early writings of Hippocrates (circa 400 BC).[3] Some of these early patients could have had ulcerative colitis, but diarrhea associated with ulcerative colitis was first reported by Bailey, a British pathologist (1761 to 1823).[4] He reported autopsy descriptions of intestinal pathology suggesting that ulcerative colitis was killing patients in the late 18th century.[5] There still was no differentiation between the more common infectious diarrhea and the nonspecific ulcerative colitis variety, however, until the 19th century. Crohn,[5] in an historical note on ulcerative colitis in 1962, noted that the autopsy description of 200 cases of diarrhea and dysentery in the Union Army during the Civil War were probably ulcerative colitis. This term was first applied to these patients.[5] Sixteen years later in 1875, Wilks and Moxon published their classic anatomic description of ulcerative colitis and differentiated it from dysentery.[5] In 1907, Lockhart Mummery[6] first reported an increased incidence of carcinoma of the colon in 7 of 36 ulcerative colitis patients. Kirsner[7] first recommended the routine chronic surveillance of ulcerative colitis patients with the electrically illuminated proctosigmoidoscope.

Medical therapy in this era consisted mostly of dietary restrictions and homeopathic medications. The original surgical therapy for ulcerative colitis, according to Goligher and associates[8]

was a sigmoid colostomy first described by Pennel in 1850. Subsequently, in 1902, an irrigation appendicostomy was described, followed by the use of an ileostomy as a complete diversion in 1913. The latter was used in conjunction with partial resection of the diseased colon with colonic irrigations used via the appendicostomy or the ileostomy. Total colectomy, with or without a proctectomy, and an ileostomy were not considered as definitive therapy until 1940. The resultant high output ileostomy was associated with a significant peristomal complication rate until Brooke[9] described surgical maturation of the stoma in 1952. This technique permitted effective appliance application and reduced many of the associated peristomal skin complications.

The modern era of surgical therapy for ulcerative colitis was ushered in by the unique anus-saving technique described by Ravitch and Sabiston[10] in 1947. However, it resulted in an unacceptable acute and chronic postoperative complication rate and was largely ignored in favor of the subsequently developed Kock continent ileostomy. This development permitted both stoma fecal continence and, in great measure, freedom from the associated problems of a stoma appliance.[11] This, too, had a potentially high acute and chronic complication rate and still resulted in the necessity of an abdominal stoma.

This undesirable situation led to a reevaluation of the rectal mucosectomy procedure and the intestinal pull-through procedure. A modification of the Soave technique commonly used for the correction of Hirschsprung disease was used for the treatment of ulcerative colitis by Martin and LeCoultre.[12] They emphasized that extensive preoperative preparation and precise intraoperative technique were required for its utilization as an operation for ulcerative colitis. This resulted in an acceptable complication rate and good functional results. However, the operation, using an ileal pull-through procedure with anal anastomosis and a temporary backup ileostomy, still resulted in significant postoperative morbidity. There was an undesirable high stool frequency rate and nighttime incontinence after closure of the ileostomy.[13] These complications prompted the further addition of several types of surgically constructed ileal reservoirs or pouches that could be used in conjunction with the pull-through procedure.[14–18] All of the pouch techniques offered potentially less frequent stooling and faster postoperative recovery, and facilitated an earlier return to a more normal pattern of daily living. They also resulted in an increased incidence of reservoir inflammation dubbed "pouchitis." This common complication produces bleeding and pain, and requires chronic antibiotic therapy in 26% to 40% of the patients.[17–20] The incidence of stool frequency and nighttime soilage 1 year after an ileoanal pull-through procedure without a pouch in most patients is essentially the same as an ileoanal pull-through technique with an added reservoir pouch. This has prompted some pediatric surgeons to avoid the use of the added pouch in younger pediatric patients who seem to have less morbidity in the early postoperative period. This modification would reduce most potential acute or chronic pouchitis complications.

ETIOLOGY

Ulcerative colitis, a diffuse inflammatory disease of the colonic and rectal mucosa, does not have a clear etiology. It is a disease that occurs with equal sex distribution but is four times more frequent in Caucasians than in other races. It also occurs four times more frequently in the Jewish versus non-Jewish population.[22] However, there is a comparatively lower incidence in Jews in Israel but a higher incidence in Jewish people who have emigrated from North America or Europe. There is a lower ulcerative colitis incidence in other Mediterranean regions, as well as in Africa and Asia. The incidence is increased in the United States and Europe, especially in Scandinavia and England.[23–25] This suggests a strong genetic risk of ulcerative colitis but with a potential environmental or socioeconomic factor precipitating the increased incidence in certain geographic areas. Although the incidence of ulcerative colitis exceeded that of Crohn disease in the first half of the 20th century, they are now about equal.

The etiology of inflammatory bowel disease (IBD) has been related to other environmental factors, but no conclusive evidence has been reported to implicate diet, as has been previously suggested. Cigarette smoking and the incidence of IBD have been widely studied. Harries and colleagues[26] first linked a lower incidence of ulcerative colitis with smoking in a 1982 survey. Crohn disease risk is doubled but the incidence of ulcerative colitis is reduced 50% in smokers. At least one adult case has been reported in which a sustained remission of ulcerative colitis has been related to chewing nicotine gum. However, the risk of ulcerative colitis is greater among exsmokers than in individuals who have never smoked.[27] This could be of importance in the future because there is a continued increase in the incidence of teenage smoking.

As noted, a genetic predisposing factor for ulcerative colitis could help explain both the geographic distribution as well as race and culture predilection. Approximately 15% of ulcerative colitis patients have one or more family members who have a form of IBD. Ulcerative colitis patients who have complicating idiopathic ankylosing spondylitis and uveitis have an increased incidence of the major antigen type HLA-W27.[28] Several other potential candidate genes have also been suggested with an association of HLA-DR2 confirmed in American ulcerative colitis patients. In a comparable population, Crohn disease was associated with a HLA-DR1/DQw5 phenotype.[30] Antineutrophilic cytoplasmic antibodies have been detected in healthy family members of ulcerative colitis patients. This also suggests a genetic susceptibility for ulcerative colitis.[31]

Recently, an abnormal plasma polyunsaturated fatty acid pattern with an increase in n3 and decrease in n6 fatty acid levels were noted during periods of either active or inactive IBD, and in both ulcerative colitis and Crohn disease.[33] These abnormal levels could also be a result of a primary genetic defect.

A specific infectious origin was originally suspected in all IBD. However, despite extensive investigations, the search for a single agent or a combination of etiologic, viral, or bacterial agents has been inconclusive.[32] Although the development of Crohn disease may be related to *Mycobacterium paratuberculosis*, and in some cases the disease appears to respond to antituberculous drugs,[34] conclusive etiologic evidence is still lacking.[35,36] Likewise, no specific relation between an infectious etiology and ulcerative colitis has been demonstrated.

Mucin abnormalities have been suggested as a predisposing factor in ulcerative colitis either related to a secondary infection or to other toxic agent invasion. However, a deficiency in mucin class IV, which was determined in ulcerative colitis patients, has also been measured in patients without IBD.[37]

The histologic appearance, the associated clinical conditions, and the changes in measurable immune system function suggest that an immunocellular response could be producing the mucosal changes of IBD.[38] Any or all of several potential pathogenic factors such as genetic, dietary, environmental, or even microbiologic influence could be critical factors in inciting this immune response. The specific effector cell type (i.e., plasma cells, T cells, macrophages, neutrophils), or the role of their secreted products (i.e., antibodies, eicosanoids, cytokines, and oxygen radicals) has not been delineated. Therefore, the most important factors in producing the mucosal response in ulcerative colitis are not known.[33]

Most attention has been focused on mucosal T cells, with more recent efforts directed toward the process of identification of antigens by T-cell receptors. Specifically, the varying utilization of the α- and β-chain regions of the T-cell receptor that occurs in response to the specific molecular structure of the presenting antigen and the associated HLA surface molecules is being defined. This is the so-called trimolecular complex.[33] The over- or underutilization of variable (β) regions of the T-cell receptor has been identified in other recognized autoimmune diseases such as rheumatoid arthritis and autoimmune thyroiditis. It is hypothesized, therefore, that restricted or predominant antigens could trigger specific T cells with a selected response in IBD.[33] Evidence of abnormal utilization of the T-cell receptor has been identified in ulcerative colitis with a decreased expression of the V β 2 genes in lamina propria T cells and expression of V δ 3 genes in intraepithelial lymphocytes.[39,40]

The soluble mediators released by cells during the IBD inflammatory response are also being studied extensively. Fiocchi and coworkers[41] have reviewed and described the current level of understanding of the complex intestinal mucosal cytokine network that exists in IBD. In Crohn disease but not in ulcerative colitis, circulating plasma levels of interleukin-6 (IL-6) are elevated.[42] Also the Crohn disease activity index correlates closely with elevated serum levels of soluble IL-2 receptor.[43] Tumor necrosis factor (alpha) (TNF-α) occurs in increased amounts in both the stool and peripheral blood of pediatric IBD patients.[44,45] There is a demonstrated imbalance of IL-1, a proinflammatory cytokine, and its receptor antagonist (Il-lra), an antiinflammatory protein, in IBD mucosa.[46] It is hypothesized that correction of this imbalance could have therapeutic implications.[33] It is also possible that these mediators could be utilized diagnostically to differentiate ulcerative colitis from Crohn disease.

Nonimmune cells may also play an important role in the pathogenesis of the intestinal IBD response. These include epithelial, muscle, and endothelial cells, as well as intestinal fibroblasts, all of which influence the immune response. These cells can function during antigen presentation, during immune regulation, or as secretors of soluble mediators. Gut epithelial cells display and functionally present class II (HLA-DR) antigen.[47] An abnormality of this function could be an etiologic factor in IBD.[48] Epithelial cells can also produce a potent proinflammatory lipid mediator platelet-activating factor that is produced in excessive amounts in ulcerative colitis.[49] Intestinal fibroblasts, particularly those from strictured areas of Crohn disease, produce large amounts of collagen that could be important in the intestinal response of IBD.[50] Intestinal muscularis mucosa cells and mucosal fibroblasts proliferate in response to immune derived cytokines.[33] These cytokines are obtained from cultured lamina propria and include separately, or in combination, IL-1, IL-6, and TNF-α.[51] It appears, therefore, that the intestinal immune response is not limited to activated immune cells, but that an interaction of immune cells, cytokines, epithelial cells, muscle cells, endothelium, fibroblasts, and the secretions of these cells are involved in the IBD inflammatory response. This interaction, when completely defined, probably holds the key to selective and, therefore, effective therapeutic ablations of the IBD intestinal response.

HISTOLOGIC CHARACTERISTICS

Ulcerative colitis and Crohn disease are clinical entities with a significantly different clinical prognosis that can be difficult to differentiate using either anatomic or histologic criteria. Ulcerative colitis involves the rectum (95%) with frequent proximal contiguous extension without skip areas.[52] When pancolitis is present in ulcerative colitis, the most severely involved areas are the rectum and sigmoid. Crohn disease, on the other hand, usually occurs only in the small intestine, but can affect only the colon and be confused with ulcerative colitis. In 10% of ulcerative colitis patients, there is also mild distal ileal inflammation with edema, the so-called "backwash ileitis."[52] The inflammatory response of ulcerative colitis is limited to the colonic mucosa and submucosa. Grossly, there appear to be healing superficial ulcers over a very vascular and friable mucosa. More advanced disease will have mucosal fissures with some patients having islands of mucosa resulting in a "cobblestone" or polypoid appearance. Ulcerative colitis produces mucosal ulcers with submucosal undermining that results in this characteristic appearance of the colon. These gross mucosal changes can revert to a more normal nonpolypoid appearance during periods of remission.[53]

As previously noted, the typical ulcerative colitis patient has a mucosal–submucosal process, not a transmural granulomatous disease as in Crohn colitis. Ulcerative colitis, however, can appear histologically to involve more than the mucosa. Unfortunately, the nonspecific ulcerative colitis microscopic picture also cannot be fully differentiated from the microscopic appearance of some colonic infectious and inflammatory conditions such as shigellosis, amebiasis, and gonorrheal colitis.[53]

The earliest ulcerative colitis microscopic change is an infiltration of round cells and polymorphonuclearocytes into the crypts of Lieberkuhn at the base of the mucosa with resultant abscesses. The overlying epithelial cells stain poorly and have vacuolization by light microscopy. Transmission electron microscopy demonstrates that the mitochondria are swollen, the interstitial spaces are widened, and the endoplasmic reticulum is broadened. The crypt abscesses coalesce and mucosal ulcers are formed with undermining of the adjacent areas producing the gross appearance of "pseudopolyps" and cobblestoning, as previously described. The ulcerated areas contain collections of collagen and granulation tissue that descend to, but rarely through, the muscularis layer. Full thickness intestinal wall inflammation occurs only in fulminant ulcerative colitis (15%), and in toxic megacolon (3%).[28]

CLINICAL PRESENTATION

Although ulcerative colitis is a disease that is usually diagnosed in young adults, approximately 4% occurs in patients under 10 years of age.[52] It is usually an insidious disease, presenting with persistent diarrhea, rectal bleeding or both, with associated pus or mucus (Table 81-1). It is easier to comprehend the significant rectal bleeding that can occur when the gross and microscopic picture of ulcerative colitis is considered. The mucosal edema and ulcerations along with the exuberant granulation tissue preclude normal colonic absorption, and the resultant diarrhea irritates and produces disruption of the friable mucosal surface. Cramping lower abdominal pain or tenesmus can be a presenting complaint but this tends to occur with a more chronic disease course. Other chronic symptoms include anorexia, weight loss, and growth retardation. Growth retardation is probably related both to the intestinal inflammation with resulting poor nutrition and to the effects of the steroid therapy that is commonly utilized. Decreased growth velocity is the

TABLE 81-1. *Clinical presentation of ulcerative colitis*

Diarrhea
  Mucous
  Exudate
  Bleeding
Pain
  Lower abdominal cramping
  Tenesmus
  Arthralgia
  Arthritis
Anorexia
  Weight loss
  Growth retardation
Anemia
Uveitis
Skin lesions
  Oral ulcerations
  Pyoderma gangrenosum
  Erythema nodosum
Liver disease
  Abnormal liver function tests
Nephrolithiasis
Osteoporosis
Mental depression

most important aspect of the developmental problem and approximately 14% of the patients have decreased height percentiles at the time of diagnosis of ulcerative colitis.[54] These short stature patients have demonstrated normal growth hormone levels. Pediatric ulcerative colitis patients have delayed sexual maturation with lower measured urinary gonadotropin levels.[55]

The patients may have other nonintestinal symptoms that include arthralgia and arthritis, skin lesions,[57] liver disease,[58] anemia, osteoporosis, nephrolithiasis, uveitis, and oral ulcerations. Arthralgia may be a presenting symptom of ulcerative colitis and commonly affects the wrists, knees, and ankles. The skin lesions include both pyoderma gangrenosum and erythema nodosum. The liver disease is manifested by abnormal liver function tests and can be a result of either fatty infiltration or sclerosing cholangitis. It has been suggested that the nephrolithiasis is related to chronic fluid loss and poor oral intake.[28] Chronic and severe ulcerative colitis tends to produce emotional changes with feelings of inferiority and depression in the pediatric patient. Although emotional stress has never been established as an etiologic factor in ulcerative colitis, exacerbations of the disease can occur in association with episodes of severe emotional stress.

DIAGNOSIS

The diagnosis and extent of ulcerative colitis involvement in a child with the preceding symptoms are usually dependent on radiologic or endoscopic examination of the rectum and lower colon. Sigmoidoscopy with mucosal biopsies will suggest the presence of ulcerative colitis. The endoscopic and histologic characteristics of ulcerative colitis are not specific; therefore, stool specimens must be obtained to rule out a specific infectious pathogen. These include *Salmonella, Shigella,* and *Campylobacter cultures,* and analysis for Clostridium difficile toxin, and *Entamoeba histolytica.* Unless the child presents with severe disease (i.e., toxic megacolon), further evidence for the presence and the extent of the disease is determined by air contrast barium enema, flexible colonoscopy, or both. The presence of toxic megacolon is a contraindication for the use of contrast enemas or high endoscopic evaluation because colonic perforation is a potential complication.

MANAGEMENT

Nonoperative

Ulcerative colitis is treated based on an arbitrary classification of mild, moderate, or severe disease (Table 81-2). Mild disease is diagnosed in children with less than six stools per day; and without fever, hypoalbuminemia, or anemia. If children have more than six stools daily, have a fever of greater than 38°C, are hypoalbuminemia or anemic, they are diagnosed as having moderate disease. Severe disease is diagnosed when the child is having eight or more stools per day (with marked abdominal pain, cramping, abdominal tenderness, high fever, anemia) and has leukocytosis. Toxic megacolon is included in the severe disease classification.[59]

Mild or moderate disease is treated with oral agents such as sulfasalazine, olesalazine, mesalamine and other forms of 5′

TABLE 81-2. *Clinical classification of ulcerative colitis*

MILD (<6 STOOLS DAILY)
No fever
Normal hemoglobin
Normal serum proteins

MODERATE (>6 STOOLS DAILY)
Fever >38°C
Anemic, hypoalbuminemic, or both

SEVERE (?TOXIC MEGACOLON) (≥8 STOOLS DAILY)
Severe abdominal tenderness
High fever
Anemia
Leukocytosis

ASA, the active component of sulfasalazine. Topical steroids and nonsteroidal enemas are also used.[60] Systemic intravenous cortiosteroids have been used for over 40 years for moderate to severe disease. Short-term immune suppression is now being added in association with systemic steroids in unresponsive patients.[61] Although other oral and intravenous antibiotics, metronidazole and tobramycin, respectively, have been advocated for use during acute attacks of ulcerative colitis, their efficacy has not been proved.[62] It is estimated that less than 10% of children who develop acute symptoms of ulcerative colitis will recover without further relapses. Complete bowel rest is indicated in the treatment of acute ulcerative colitis symptoms. Because a poor nutritional state is frequently present at the time of diagnosis, total parenteral nutrition (TPN) is an important therapeutic modality to be used in association with other therapy. This is particularly true in children who require operative therapy. However, the use of TPN in severe ulcerative colitis does not produce as high a success rate in achieving an acute remission as noted in Crohn disease.[63,64]

As previously stated, 15% of the children can present with acute fulminating ulcerative colitis. These children have profuse bloody diarrhea, abdominal cramps, fever, and usually sepsis. Approximately 3% to 5% will present with, or acutely develop, signs and symptoms of toxic megacolon. This is fulminating ulcerative colitis in association with abdominal distention and the roentgenographic appearance of pancolonic dilatation. These findings signify an emergent situation because a subsequent acute colonic perforation is common. Rapid preoperative resuscitation with crystalloids and colloids, including broad-spectrum antibiotics and an emergency total colectomy, is required in toxic megacolon.

Surgical

Surgery is indicated in ulcerative colitis for failure of medical management, hemorrhage, perforation or impending perforation, toxic megacolon, or severe toxicity (Table 81-3). Acute ulcerative colitis should respond to medical management within the first 12 days of therapy. An unacceptable complication rate results with further continued medical therapy. The definition of failure of chronic medical management includes persistent symptoms of diarrhea, hematochezia, abdominal pain, anemia, and hypoproteinemia. Growth failure and delayed sexual matu-

TABLE 81-3. *Indications for surgical management of ulcerative colitis*

ACUTE
Hemorrhage
Intestinal perforation or impending perforation (i.e., toxic megacolon)

CHRONIC
Failed medical management (i.e., socially or physically dysfunctional)
Growth failure
Delayed sexual maturation
Histologic dysplasia

ration as well as other side effects of long-term steroid therapy and chronic poor nutrition must also be considered as indications for surgical therapy.[55] Long-term active disease can result in colonic mucosal aneuploidy leading to histologic dysplasia and possible neoplastic transformation.[65] As previously noted, children have a 20% colon cancer risk per decade after 10 years of active ulcerative colitis disease.[2] Approximately 25% to 30% of all diagnosed ulcerative colitis children will require a surgical resection within 10 years.[66] Because ulcerative colitis is limited to the colon, however, as opposed to Crohn disease, surgical colectomy is curative.

Preoperative

In children, surgical therapy consists of a total colectomy, usually in association with an added procedure to produce stool continence. Preoperative preparation for elective or urgent surgical procedures is extremely important in these frequently debilitated and malnourished patients who have been receiving long-term steroid or immunosuppressive therapy. Unless the patient has toxic megacolon, which requires emergent surgical management, adequate preoperative therapy includes both restoration of metabolic balance and possible nutritional repair. This may require 2 to 6 weeks of TPN. This also permits attempt at reduction of immunosuppressive medications or corticosteroids. Blood transfusions should be judiciously utilized during this period. The child should receive a preoperative mechanical bowel preparation if possible. The use of a balanced hyperostotic oral solution such as Golytely at a dose of 25 mL/kg given 24 hours prior to the planned procedure is recommended. This can be given by mouth if tolerated, but frequently it must be administered by a nasogastric tube. In small children, care must be exercised that intravascular volume depletion with dehydration does not result during this treatment. Broad-spectrum intravenous antibiotics, in a dosage based on patient weight and including coverage for anaerobic organisms, are started at least 1 hour prior to the surgical procedure. A preoperative dose of hydrocortisone, 2 mg/kg, is also given at this time. Corticosteroids must also be given intraoperatively and then tapered during the postoperative recovery period usually returning to preoperative dosages within 5 to 7 days.

SURGICAL PROCEDURES

The choice of surgical procedure to be used in conjunction with a total colectomy is dependent on the child's preoperative condition and the desires of the patient or family (Table 81-4). In rare pediatric patients, either the child or the parents will elect to have placement of a permanent noncontinent Brooke ileostomy. A standard continent Kock ileostomy, using a pouch reservoir with a nipple for intermittent cannulation, is one surgical option.[67] However, the acute and chronic mechanical complication rate, a high incidence of chronic pouchitis, and the need for a visible stoma with required maintenance make this a less desirable choice for most children and their families. Although abdominal colectomy with ileorectostomy has been utilized in adults, potential complications of rectal recurrence and malignant potential make it an inappropriate choice for pediatric patients.

An alternative procedure that offers improved stool continence without a permanent abdominal wall stoma is a modification of the pull-through technique first used by Ravitch and Sabiston[10] and refined by Martin and Le Coultre.[12] This is an abdominal colectomy along with a rectal mucosectomy and an ileoanal anastomosis. This procedure can be performed in stages with an initial colectomy and temporary ileostomy. After a reasonable period for postoperative recovery, cessation of the ulcerative colitis chemotherapy, and full nutritional restoration, a second-stage rectal mucosectomy and ileoanal anastomosis is performed utilizing a backup ileostomy. Again, after a recovery period to allow complete healing of the ileoanal anastomosis, the backup ileostomy is closed as a third procedure. Although the acute postoperative morbidity is acceptable, there is a high chronic morbidity associated with this procedure that is related to the ensuing postoperative diarrhea. For the first weeks or months, 15 to 20 stools daily are not uncommon. Nighttime incontinence is universally encountered and results in sleep deprivation for the first few postoperative weeks to months. This usually results in a severe perianal rash and a drastically altered lifestyle for the child and family. It leads to emotional upheaval and frequently depression in older teenage patients.

This morbidity has led to the use of an ileal pouch reservoir in association with the ileoanal anastomosis. This modification reduces the stooling frequency to four or six times daily within 1 month following ileostomy closure. Although it decreases the frequency of nighttime incontinence, it does not eliminate the problem in the initial postoperative period.[19] Several types of surgically constructed pouches have been utilized, but the most popular versions are the J-pouch[67] and the S-pouch.[17] These are different techniques in which the terminal ileum is folded on itself and the contiguous loops are joined after opening up the adjacent common wall or walls. This results in a large volume

TABLE 81-4. *Surgical options for ulcerative colitis patients*

Pancolectomy with
  Brooke ileostomy
  Kock (continent) ileostomy
Abdominal colectomy with ileorectostomy (not appropriate for pediatric patients)
Abdominal colectomy with rectal mucosectomy
  With ileoanal anastomosis (no reservoir)
  With ileal pouch-anal anastomosis
    J-pouch (two ileal loops)
    S-pouch (three ileal loops plus spout)
    Lateral reservoir (two ileal loops plus spout)
    W-pouch (four ileal loops plus spout)

terminal ileal reservoir that reduces the degree of urgency and stooling frequency. Initially, this was done as a three-stage procedure, but with appropriate precautions, the two-stage procedure has a comparable complication rate. The a-stage procedure consists of total abdominal colectomy, rectal mucosectomy, and construction of the ileal pouch and ileoanal anastomosis, with a backup ileostomy placed as the first step. The second step is the takedown of the ileostomy. However, the two-stage procedure is not advocated for patients who require urgent surgical management of ulcerative colitis complications or for cases where malignancy or the possibility of Crohn disease cannot be ruled out. If the patient has a low hemoglobin value, a low serum albumin, and is on therapeutic steroid doses, the two-stage procedure is also more hazardous.[68] There is no definitive evidence for, or against, the use of an ileoanal pull-through technique with a reservoir procedure for indeterminate colitis (i.e., gross and histologic features of both ulcerative colitis and Crohn disease) in pediatric patients. In adult patients, with a relatively short clinical follow-up, there is no difference in the complication rate for this procedure between indeterminate colitis and ulcerative colitis.[69] However, the pouch–anal pull-through technique is contraindicated in established Crohn disease.[70]

Acute complications of the pouch reservoir technique include leakage, infection, and stenosis. Adult females have been reported to develop a 6.5% incidence of ileal pouch vaginal fistula; however, this has not been noted in the pediatric female population.[71] If the reservoir, regardless of the type (i.e., number of contiguous loops), is not contained within the pelvis, poor stool evacuation can also be a complication. This has resulted in the need for intermittent transrectal catheter drainage or surgical revision of the reservoir.[72,73] The major chronic reservoir complication is *pouchitis*, which requires antibiotic therapy in many patients,[74] and in some instances requires the placement of a temporary or permanent ileostomy. The use of the reservoir is primarily intended to overcome the early morbidity of the ileoanal anastomosis because the stooling frequency with or without a pouch diminishes in both procedures after 1 to 2 years. Be-

cause pouchitis is a significant complication in children, with the unknown potential of long-term complications, some surgeons utilize only the ileoanal anastomosis. They have attempted to overcome some of the early postoperative morbidity encountered with this procedure by instituting balloon dilatation of the terminal ileum after the ileoanal anastomosis and prior to the closure of the protecting ileostomy. They feel this increases the reservoir capacity of the neorectum.[75] This procedure has resulted in marginal improvements in stooling frequency and nighttime incontinence. A small percentage (<5%) of ileoanal pull-through patients with or without a reservoir become dissatisfied and elect to have a permanent ileostomy constructed. However, most pull-through patients are satisfied with the procedure and have accommodated themselves to their stooling habits by maximizing dietary, medicinal, and lifestyle changes.

Emergency Procedure

Emergent colectomies for toxic megacolon or severe colitis demand prompt preoperative repair of intravascular volume deficits, correction of anemia and hypoalbuminemia, use of intravenous broad-spectrum antibiotic coverage and intravenous steroid replacement, and placement of a urinary Foley catheter. The total abdominal colectomy is done with distal closure of the retained sigmoid colon as a Hartmann pouch with an ileostomy.

Postoperative medical treatment of the involved rectum usually allows a second procedure, a rectal mucosectomy and ileoanal pull-through, as an anus-sparing procedure.

Elective Procedures

Total Proctocolectomy and Permanent Ileostomy

The preoperative preparation for elective colectomy includes the previously mentioned oral bowel cleansing (Golytely), total

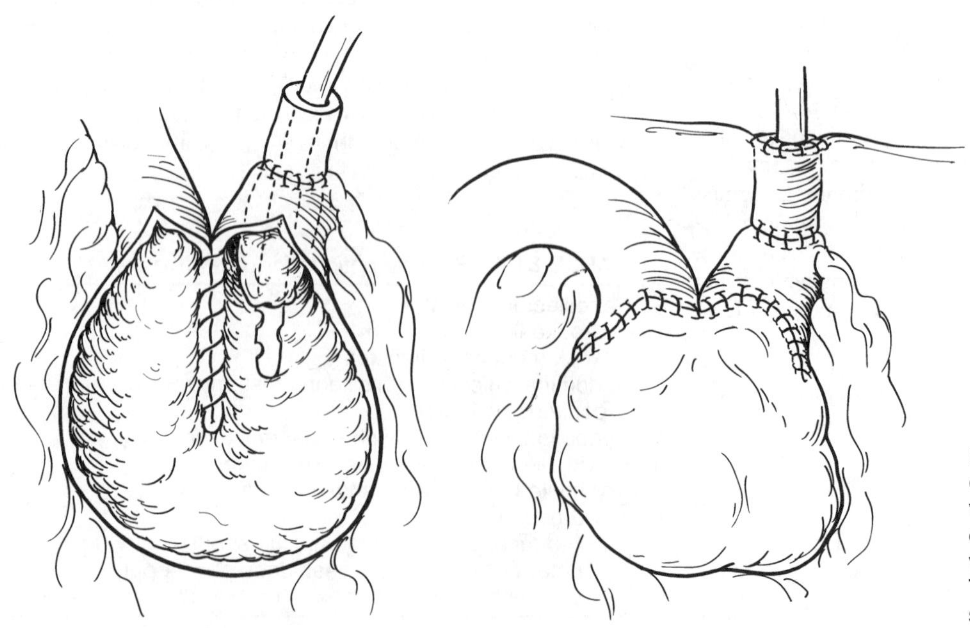

A,B

FIG. 81-1. The Kock pouch is a distal ileal double-loop reservoir with the distal outlet loop intussuscepted and sutured to form a nipple valve for intermittent cannulation. The spout is sutured flush to the skin.

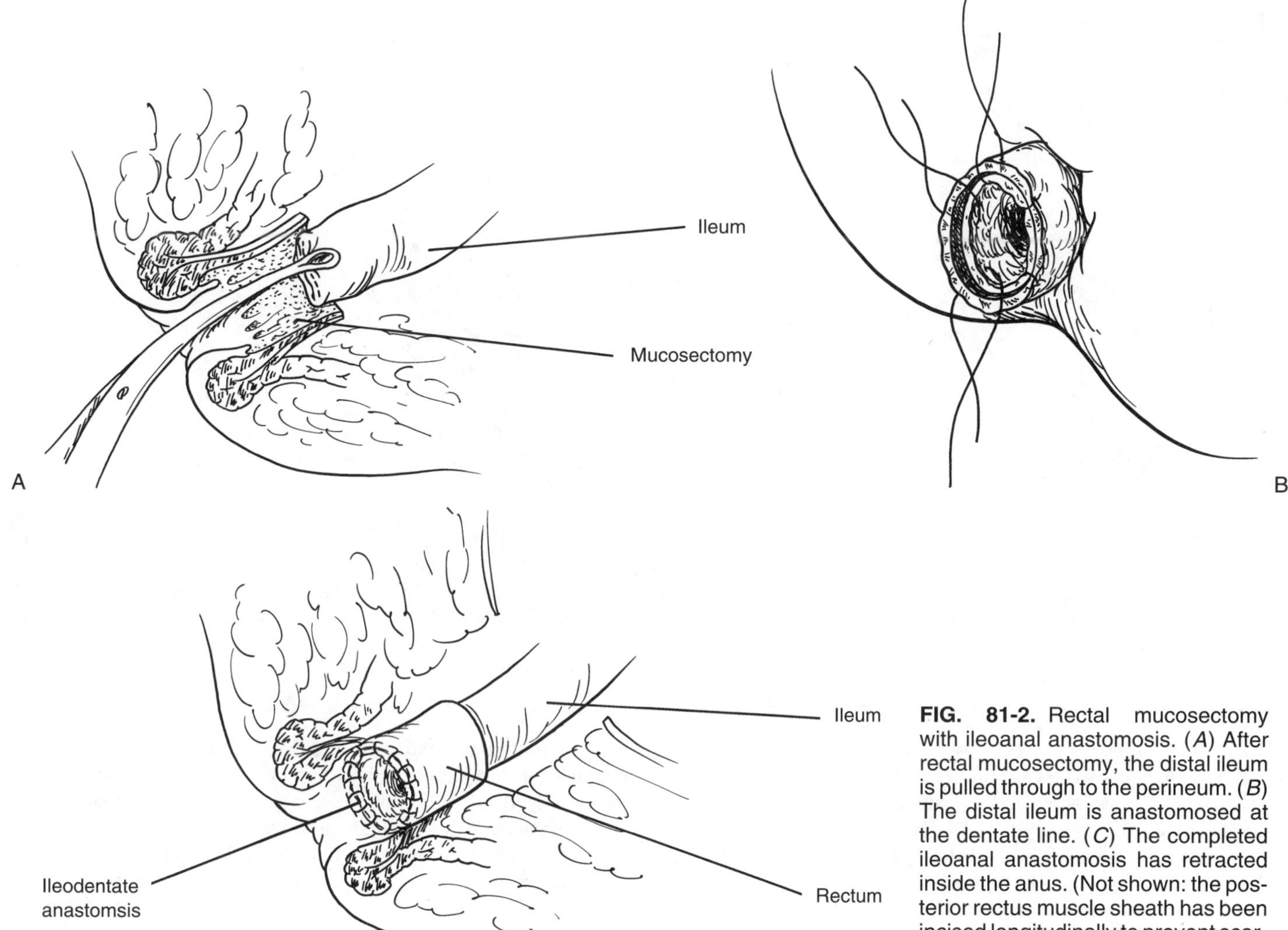

FIG. 81-2. Rectal mucosectomy with ileoanal anastomosis. (*A*) After rectal mucosectomy, the distal ileum is pulled through to the perineum. (*B*) The distal ileum is anastomosed at the dentate line. (*C*) The completed ileoanal anastomosis has retracted inside the anus. (Not shown: the posterior rectus muscle sheath has been incised longitudinally to prevent scarring and constriction.)

parenteral nutrition, and the metabolic resuscitation emphasized for emergent procedures. After induction of general anesthesia and adequate intravenous access has been achieved, a midline abdominal laparotomy incision is made. Not only does this afford good exposure but also the incision is far enough separated from the premarked ileostomy site to facilitate good appliance placement. The colon is mobilized in standard fashion and divided at the level of the mid-sigmoid colon with a stapling instrument. The colonic mesenteric vessels are isolated, ligated with absorbable suture, and divided. The pelvic dissection is begun by opening the peritoneal reflection at the rectum. Careful cautery dissection of this area and division of all vessels near the bowel wall minimize division of the sacral parasympathetic nerves. Sexual or bladder dysfunction are minimized with proper attention to these details. The dissection should proceed extramurally distally to within 4 or 5 cm of the dentate line. The rectum is thoroughly irrigated with either a dilute iodine skin preparation solution or a nonabsorbable antibiotic solution. An anal encircling incision is made approximately 1 cm distal to the dentate line and dissection is conducted proximally to the previous dissection, again staying extramural and on the bowel wall maintaining careful cautery hemostasis. After re-

moval of the colon and rectum, the pelvis is again irrigated copiously and the muscle approximated with absorbable sutures. The skin is closed loosely with nonabsorbable sutures. The area is drained with one or two small-caliber silastic suction catheters that exit through the lower abdominal wall.

The permanent ileostomy is constructed by removing skin, subcutaneous tissue, and the underlying muscle–fascial disk in the previously marked right lower quadrant site. The distal ileum is cleared of mesenteric vessels for approximately 3 to 5 cm. This end is brought through the prepared site and sutured to the surrounding fascia with absorbable sutures. Although some surgeons prefer not to mature the stoma, a carefully performed Brooke ileostomy with interrupted seromuscular, full-thickness, and dermal placement sutures give the best appliance fit early in the postoperative period. A temporary stoma appliance is applied immediately.

Continent Ileostomy

To form a continent ileostomy, approximately 45 to 50 cm of distal ileum is required depending on the size of the patient

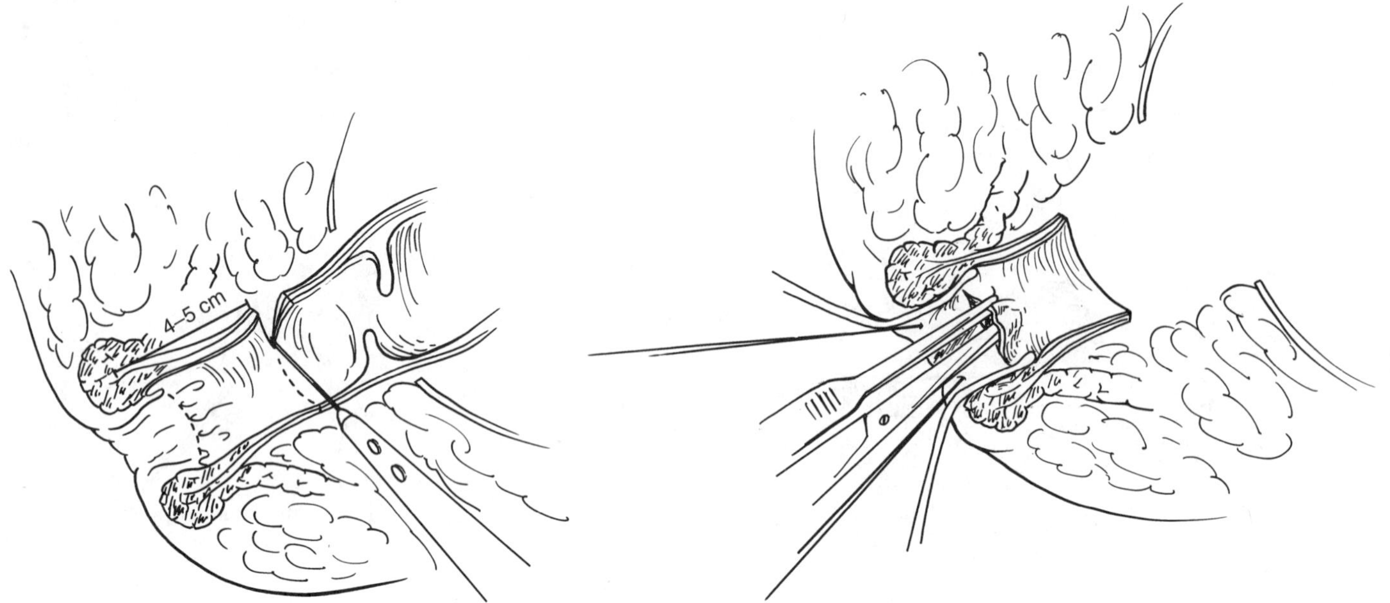

FIG. 81-3. Division of rectum prior to distal mucosectomy.
(*A*) Active or inactive rectal disease can make division of the rectum prior to mucosectomy an easier procedure. (*B*) If division of the rectum is necessary, the distal to proximal mucosectomy is started from the perineum.

(Fig. 81-1). The proximal 30 to 35 cm is used to create a double-loop pouch to serve as the reservoir. The distal end of the outflow loop is intussuscepted and sutured in place to produce a nipple valve. The remaining protruding distal ileum is sutured to the muscle–fascia with the distal ''spout'' sutured flush to the skin. The high complication rate of this technique has relegated its use primarily to patients who have already had a proctocolectomy with Brooke ileostomy and now desire a continent stoma.

Abdominal Colectomy, Rectal Mucosectomy, and Ileoanostomy

The patient is anesthetized and placed in lithotomy position, and both the abdomen and perineum are prepared as a single sterile field. A standard abdominal colectomy with a stapled division at the lower sigmoid colon is conducted. The ileum is mobilized to the origin of the superior mesenteric artery. The mobilized ileum should reach the anal–perineal area without tension. The rectum is mobilized distally, opening the peritoneum as previously described, and dissecting extramurally along the bowel wall (Fig. 81-2). This dissection proceeds distally to a point approximately 4 to 5 cm above the anus. Two different techniques to complete the rectal mucosectomy are used. The rectum is irrigated copiously and either it is divided at this level or a submucosal dissection is begun (Soave technique). In the latter technique, the bowel wall is infiltrated with a 1:100,000 dilution of epinephrine in saline. An incision is made carefully in the rectal muscle and a submucosal dissection is conducted distally and circumferentially. Frequently, if the patient has had severe rectal disease either quiescent or active at this time, this is an impractical approach. In this case, the

rectum is divided proximally, and the submucosal dissection is begun from the perineum near the dentate line and extended proximally (Fig. 81-3). This requires digital rectal dilatation and the placement of traction sutures and self-retaining retractors. The traction sutures are placed distal to the dentate line, and with moderate tension the dentate line is visualized and the incision is made circumferentially with a cautery device. Previous injection with the dilute epinephrine–saline solution will aid in a less bloody proximal submucosal dissection. It is essential that all mucosa is removed to prevent a chronic pelvic infection with a draining fistula. The pelvis is again thoroughly irrigated and a careful check for hemostasis is made. The ileum is brought down through the muscular sleeve and sutured to the dentate line by full-thickness ileum to seromuscular wall absorbable sutures. Careful and meticulous approximation with multiple interrupted sutures is required. The muscular sleeve is divided longitudinally in the midline posteriorly to avoid stenosis. The proximal abdominal edge of the sleeve is loosely sutured to the contiguous ileal wall to roughly reconfigure the sphincter muscle.

A temporary backup, completely diverting ileostomy is constructed by dividing the ileum at least 15 to 20 cm proximal to the anastomosis with a stapling instrument. The proximal end is brought out through through a preoperatively marked site in the right lower abdomen in a standard fashion. Although the ileostomy should be completely diverting, the closed distal ileal stump (Hartmann pouch) can be loosely sutured alongside the exiting ileal wall to facilitate recovery for an ileal reapproximation in 3 to 4 months. The pelvis is drained with two small silastic suction drains placed bilaterally in or near the muscular sleeve and exiting the abdominal wall. They can be withdrawn on the fourth or fifth postoperative day. The intravenous antibiotics are discontinued after the pelvic drains have been removed. After the intravenous antibiotics are stopped, oral antibiotics (i.e., metranidazole) are used for a total of 3 weeks after the operation. Three weeks after the procedure, the anal anastomosis is examined while the patient is anesthetized. No rectal medications or manipulation are permitted prior to this examination. Daily home rectal dilatations using a smooth uterine dilator (size depending on the patient) are begun subsequently. Weekly or biweekly office visits for physician evaluation are required. As noted, the temporary ileostomy is closed approximately 3 to 4 months after the ileoanal anastomosis and only if there is no significant anastomotic stricture. Prophylactic application of stoma skin preparation to the perianal area for

at least 1 week prior to ileostomy closure seems to improve the perianal rash that complicates the initial use of this new anal connection. In this procedure, without a reservoir, judicious use of antidiarrheal medications may be required in the early postoperative period. However, their use requires caution to avoid inducing stasis enteritis.

Abdominal Colectomy and Ileoanal Anastomosis With Ileal Reservoir

The initial diarrhea, stooling, urgency, and excessive night-time incontinence encountered with the ileoanal pull-through

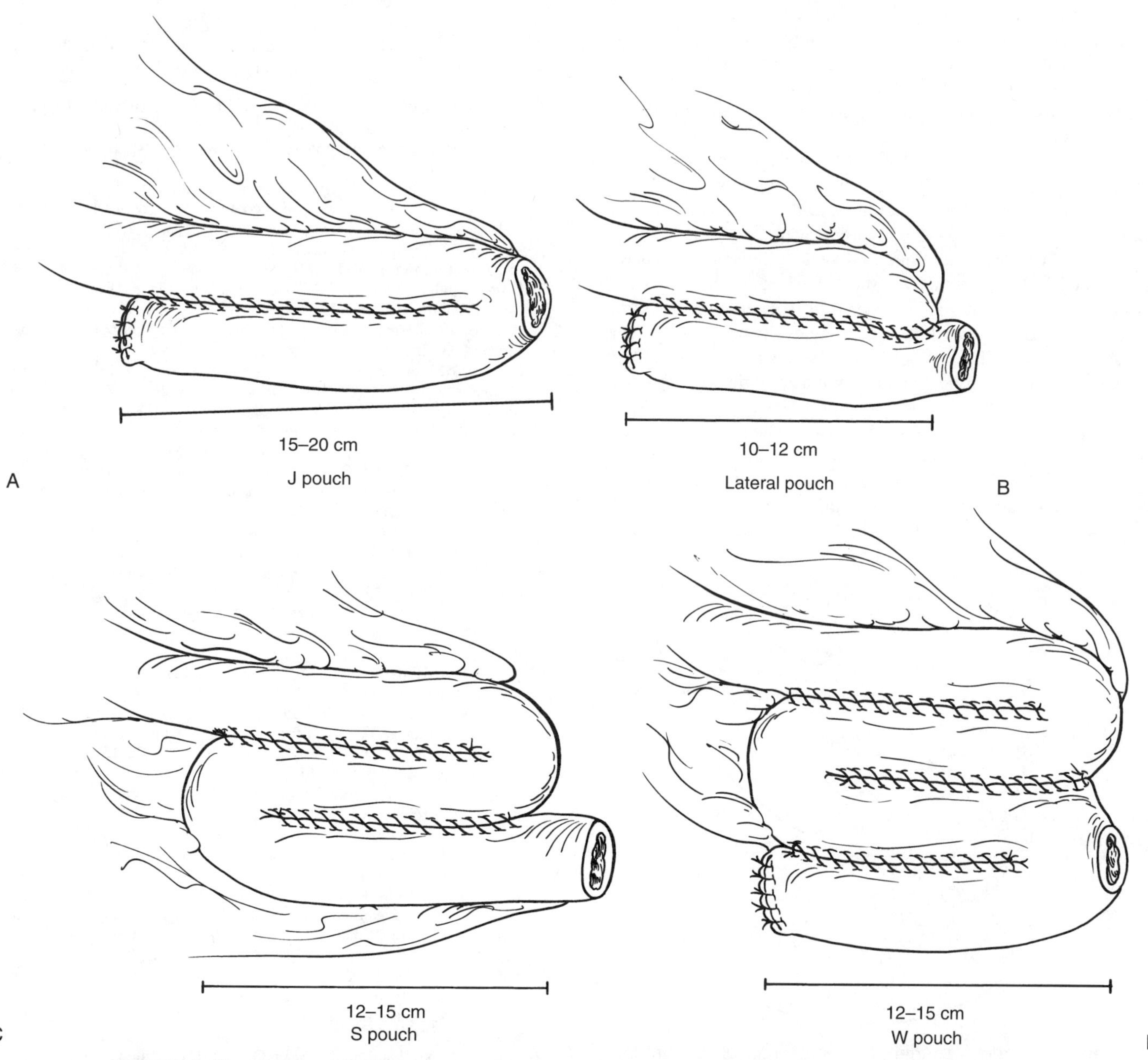

FIG. 81-4. Four types of ileal reservoirs. The J-pouch is the most commonly used pouch in pediatric patients. The lateral reservoir, S-pouch, and W-pouch can also be used.

procedure has encouraged the addition of an ileal reservoir. There are four major types of pouches, two that utilize two loops (the J-pouch and lateral reservoir), one that includes three loops (S-pouch), and one that requires four loops (W-pouch); (Fig. 81-4). The lateral, S- and W-pouches all require a spout that is anastomosed to the anus. This contributes to potential complications such as poor vascularity, stenosis, and (if too long) poor emptying. The S- and W-pouches require 35 to 60 cm of distal ileum for construction. This potentially can add to malabsorption problems. The multiple loop pouches also are more difficult to construct and have a higher postoperative leakage and infection rate than the straight pull-through or J-pouch. Vascularity is also more likely to be compromised. The J-pouch is the most popular reservoir used in ulcerative colitis surgery for pediatric patients, but some surgeons prefer the lateral reservoir.[76]

The J-pouch is formed by doubling the distal ileum back on itself and anastomosing the two communicating loops together over a 15-cm distance (Fig. 81-5). A stapling instrument is used to construct the pouch through the opening at the distal end of the two loops. The loop is pulled into the pelvis, and this distal opening is anastomosed to the anus. The majority of the length of the pouch suction should be in the pelvis. The peritoneal reflection is sutured loosely to the suction pouch wall with absorbable sutures. The area is drained with two silastic suction catheters exiting the lower abdominal wall, as in the straight ileoanal pull-through technique. A diverting ileostomy is placed proximally just as previously described. The anastomosis is examined under anesthesia 3 weeks following its construction. Again dilatations are performed at home by the patient or parent on a daily basis. The ileostomy is closed 3 to 4 months later when the area is well healed and no anastomotic strictures are present. The antibiotic coverage, both intravenous and by mouth, is handled as previously described. The use of the pouch does not affect the length of the initial hospitalization. Patients who have ileoanal anastomosis with or without an associated reservoir have an average postoperative stay of 7 or 8 days. The pouch technique has the primary advantage of returning the patient to his or her daily routine activities in about 6 weeks after ileostomy closure; whereas, the patients who have an anastomosis without a pouch usually require at least 3 months or longer to resume daily functions after the ileostomy closure. Prolonged stool urgency and excessive nighttime stooling frequency in a patient with an ileoanal pouch should make the physician suspicious of pouchitis, possibly as a result of an underlying stricture. Antidiarrheal medications should be used with extreme caution and only after endoscopy and mucosal biopsy of the pouch have been used to rule out pouchitis.

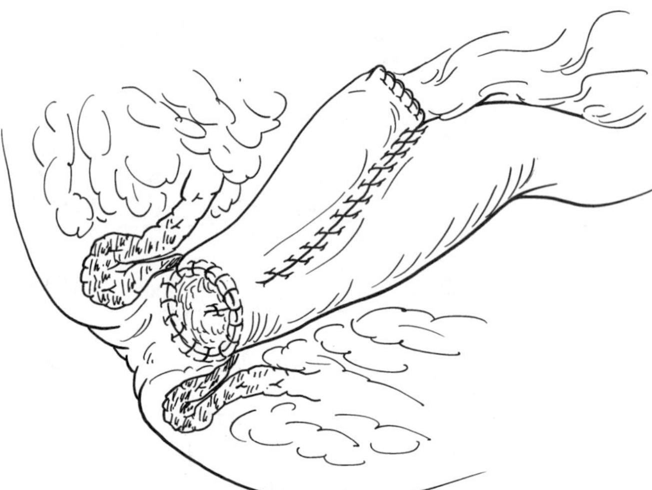

FIG. 81-5. J-pouch ileoanal anastomosis for ulcerative colitis. The two-loop ileal J-pouch anastomosed near the dentate line is the preferred reservoir procedure in pediatric patients.

REFERENCES

1. Farmer RG, Easley KA, Rankin G. Clinical patterns, natural history, and progression of ulcerative colitis: a long term followup of 1116 patients. Dig Dis Sci 1993;38:1137.
2. Devroede GJ, Taylor WF, Saurer WG, et al. Cancer risk and life expectance of children with ulcerative colitis. N Engl J Med 1971;285:17.
3. Adams F. The genuine works of Hippocrates. Baltimore, Williams & Wilkins, 1939.
4. Morson BC, Current concepts of colitis: the 1970 Lettsomian lectures. Trans Med Soc Lond 1970;86:159.
5. Crohn, BB. An historical note on ulcerative colitis. (Letter) Gastroenterology 1962;42:366.
6. Lockhart Mummery JP. The causes of colitis: with special reference to its surgical treatment, with an account of 36 cases. Lancet 1907;1:1638.
7. Kirsner JB. The historical basis of the idiopathic inflammatory bowel diseases. Inflamm Bowel Dis 1995;1:2.
8. Goligher JC, De Dombal FT, Watts JM, Watkinson G. Ulcerative colitis. Baltimore, Williams & Wilkins, 1968.
9. Brooke BN. Management of ileostomy including its complications. Lancet 1952;2:102.
10. Ravitch MM, Sabiston DL Jr. Anal ileostomy with preservation of the sphincter: a proposed operation in patients requiring total colectomy for benign lesions. Surg Gynecol Obstet 1947;84:1095.
11. Koch NG. Historical perspective, in Dozois RR, ed. Alternatives to conventional ileostomy. Chicago, Year Book Medical, 1985:133.
12. Martin LW, LeCoultre C. Technical considerations in performing total colectomy and Soave endorectal anastomosis for ulcerative colitis. J Pediatr Surg 1978;13:762.
13. Becker JM. Anal sphincter function after colectomy, mucosal proctectomy and endorectal ileoanal pullthrough. Arch Surg 1984;119:526.
14. Parks AG, Nicholls RJ. Proctolectomy without ileostomy for ulcerative colitis. Br Med J 1978;2:85.
15. Utsunomiya J, Iwama T, Imajo M, et al. Total colectomy, mucosal proctectomy, and ileoanal anastomosis. Dis Colon Rectum 1980;23:459.
16. Wong WD, Rothernerger DA, Goldberg DM. Ileoanal pouch procedures. Curr Probl Surg 1985;22:1.
17. Nicholls RJ, Pezim ME. Restorative proctocolectomy with ileal reservoir for ulcerative colitis and familial adenomatous polyposis: a comparison of three reservoir designs. Br J Surg 1985;72:470.
18. Fonkalsrud EW, Stelzner M, McDonald N. Experience with the endorectal ileal pullthrough with lateral reservoir for ulcerative colitis and polyposis. Arch Surg 1988;123:1053.
19. McIntyre PB, Pemberton JH, Wolff BG, et al. Comparing functional results one year and 10 years after ileal pouch-anal anastomosis for chronic ulcerative colitis. Dis Colon Rectum 1994;37:434.
20. Lobo AJ, Sagar PM, Rothwell J, et al. Carriage of adhesive Escherichia coli after restorative proctocolectomy and pouch anal anastomosis: relation with functional outcome and inflammation. Gut 1993;34:1379.
21. Salesmons JMJI, Nagengast FM, Lubbers EJC, et al. Postoperative and long-term results of ileal pouch-anal anastomosis for ulcerative colitis and familial polyposis coli. Dig Dis Sci 1992;37:1882.
22. Burakoff R. Update on the epidemiology of IBD. Prog Inflamm Bowel Disc 1994;15:1.
23. Kidebro S, Nordgaard K, Aronsen O, et al. The incidence of ulcerative colitis in Northern Norway from 1983–1986. Scand J Gastroenterol 1990;25:890.

24. Stowe SP, Redmond SR, Stormont M, et al. An epidemiological study of inflammatory bowel disease in Rochester, New York, hospital incidence. Gastroenterology 1990;98:104.

25. Yoshida Y, Murata Y. Inflammatory bowel disease in Japan: studies of epidemiology and etiopathogenesis. Med Clin North Am 1990;74:67.

26. Harries AD, Baird A, Rhodes J. Nonsmoking: a feature of ulcerative colitis. Br Med J 1982;284:706.

27. Jick H, Walker AM. Cigarette smoking and ulcerative colitis. N Engl J Med 1983;308:261.

28. Fonkalsrud EW. Pediatric surgery. In: Ashcraft K, Holder T, eds. Inflammatory bowel disease. Philadelphia, WB Saunders, 1993:440.

29. Rotter JI. Immunogenetic susceptibilities in inflammatory bowel disease. Can J Gastroenterol 1990;4:261.

30. Rotter JI, Wang S-J, Yang H, et al. Genetic heterogeneity between ulcerative colitis (UC) and Crohn's disease (CD) identified by molecular HLA class II association. Gastroenterology 1992;102:A688.

31. Shanahan F, Duerr RH, Rotter JI, et al. Neutrophil autoantibodies in ulcerative colitis: familial aggregation and genetic heterogeneity. Gastroenterology 1992;103:456.

32. Esteve-Comas M, Minez MC, Fernandez-Banares F, et al. Abnormal plasma polyunsaturated fatty acid pattern in non-active inflammatory bowel disease. Gut 1993;34:1370.

33. Fiocchi C, Strong SA, West GA, et al. IBD: progress in pathogenesis. Can J Gastroenterol 1993;7:110.

34. Kohn A, Prantera C, Mangiarotti R, et al. Antimycobacterial therapy and Crohn's disease: a randomized placebo controlled trial. Gastroenterology 1992;102:A647.

35. Sanderson JD, Moss MT, Tizard MLV, et al. Mycobacterium paratuberculosis DNA in Crohn's disease tissue. Gut 1992;33:890.

36. Rosenberg WMC, Bell JI, Jewell DP, et al. Mycobacterium paratuberculosis DNA cannot be detected in Crohn's disease tissues. Gastroenterology 1991;100:A611.

37. Tysk C, Riedelsen H, Lindberg EE, et al. Colonic glycoproteins in monozygotic twins with inflammatory bowel disease. Gastroenterology 1991;100:419.

38. Fiocchi C. Immunology of inflammatory bowel disease. Curr Opin Gastroenterol 1991;7:654.

39. Duchmann R, Strober W, Fiocchi C, et al. TCR V(beta)2 gene expression is selective in control but not in IBD lamina propria lymphocytes. Gastroenterology 1992;102:A617.

40. Landau SB, Balk SB, Yang L, et al. T-cell receptor (TCR) delta variable region utilization is altered in ulcerative colitis. Gastroenterology 1992;102:A650.

41. Fiocchi C. Cytokines. In: MacDermott RP, Stinson W, eds. Inflammatory bowel disease. New York, Elsevier, 1992:137.

42. Mahida YR, Kurlak L, Gallagher A, et al. High circulating levels of interleukin 6 in active Crohn's disease but not ulcerative colitis. Gut 1991;32:1531.

43. Mueller C, Knoflach P, Zielinski CC, et al. T-cell activation in Crohn's disease: increased levels of soluble interleukin-2 receptor in serum and supernatants of stimulated peripheral blood mononuclear cells. Gastroenterology 1990;98:639.

44. Murch SH, Lamkin VA, Savage MO, et al. Serum concentrations of tumour necrosis factor in a childhood chronic inflammatory bowel disease. Gut 1991;32:913.

45. Braegger CP, Nicholls S, Murch SH, et al. Tumour necrosis factor alpha in stool as a marker of intestinal inflammation. Lancet 1992;339:89.

46. Cominelli F, Fiocchi C, Eisenberg SP, et al. Imbalance of IL-1 and IL-1 receptor antagonist in the intestinal mucosa of Crohn's disease and ulcerative colitis patients. Gastroenterology 1992;100:3.

47. Mayer L, Eisenhardt D, Salomon P, et al. Expression of class II molecules on intestinal epithelial cells in humans: differences between normal and inflammatory bowel disease. Gastroenterology 1991;100:3.

48. Mayer L, Eisenhardt D. Lack of induction of suppressor T cells by intestinal epithelial cells from patients with inflammatory bowel disease. J Clin Invest 1990;86:1255.

49. Ferraris L, Klein J, Fiocchi C, et al. Both epithelial and lamina propria nonnuclear cells contribute to the enhanced platelet activating factor generation in inflammatory bowel disease. Gastroenterology 1992;102:1920.

50. Stallmach A, Schuppan D, Riese HH, et al. Increased collagen type III synthesis by fibroblasts isolated from strictures of patients with Crohn's disease. Gastroenterology 1992;102:1920.

51. Strong SA, West GA, Klein JS, et al. Inflammatory cytokines stimulate proliferation of intestinal mucosa mesenchymal cells. Gastroenterology 1992;102:A701.

52. Sloan WP, Bargen JA, Gage RP. Life histories of patients with chronic ulcerative colitis: a review of 2,000 cases. Gastroenterology 1950;16:25.

53. Becker JM, Moody FG. Ulcerative colitis. In: Sabiston DC Jr, ed. Textbook of surgery. Philadelphia, WB Saunders, 1986:1011.

54. Markowitz J, Daum F. Growth impairment in pediatric inflammatory bowel disease. Am J Gastroenterol 1994;89:319.

55. McCaffery TD, Khosrow N, Lawrence AM, et al. Severe growth retardation in children with inflammatory bowel disease. Pediatrics 1970;45:386.

56. Korelitz BI, Gribetz D, Danziger I. The prognosis of ulcerative colitis with onset in childhood. I. The presteroid era. Ann Intern Med 1962;57:582.

57. Edwards FC, Truelove SC. The course and prognosis of ulcerative colitis. III. Complications. Gut 1964;5:1.

58. Lagercrantz R, Winberg J, Zetterstrom R. Extracolonic manifestations in chronic ulcerative colitis. Acta Paediatr Scand 1958;47:675.

59. Kirschner BS. In: Rudolph AM, ed. Chronic inflammatory bowel disease: ulcerative colitis and Crohn's disease. Norwalk, Appelton & Lang, 1987:933.

60. Mantzaris GJ, Hatzis A, Petraki K, et al. Intermittent therapy with high-dose 5-aminosalicylic acid enemas maintains remission in ulcerative proctitis and proctosigmoiditis. Dis Colon Rectum 1994;37:58.

61. Lichtiger S, Present DH, Kornbluth A, et al. Cyclosporine in severe ulcerative colitis refractory to steroid therapy. N Engl J Med 1994;330:1841.

62. Mantzaris GJ, Hatzis A, Kontogiannis P, et al. Intravenous Tobramycin and Metronidazole as an adjunct to corticosteroids in acute, severe, ulcerative colitis. Am J Gastroenterol 1994;89:43.

63. Elson CO, Layden TJ, Nemchausky BA, et al. An evaluation of total parenteral nutrition in the management of inflammatory bowel disease. Dig Dis Sci 1980;25:42.

64. Dickinson RJ, Ashton MG, Axon ATR, et al. Controlled trial of intravenous hyperalimentation and total bowel rest as an adjunct to routine therapy of acute colitis. Gastroenterology 1980;79:1199.

65. Befrits R, Hammarberg C, Rubio C, et al. DNA aneuploidy and histologic dysplasia in long-standing ulcerative colitis. Dis Colon Rectum 1994;37:313.

66. Sedgwick DM, Barton JR, Hamer-Hodges DW, et al. Population-based study of surgery in juvenile onset ulcerative colitis. Br J Surg 1991;78:176.

67. Ein SH. A ten-year experience with the pediatric Kock pouch. J Pediatr Surg 1987;22:764.

68. Nicholls RJ, Holt SDG, Lubowski DZ. Restorative proctocolectomy with ileal reservoir: comparison of two-stage vs. three-stage procedures and analysis of factors that might affect outcome. Dis Colon Rectum 1989;32:323.

69. Pezim ME, Pemberton JG, Beart RW Jr, et al. Outcome of ''indeterminant'' colitis following ileal pouch-anal anastomosis. Dis Colon Rectum 1989;32:653.

70. Deutsch AA, McLeod RS, Cullen J, et al. Results of the pelvic-pouch procedure in patients with Crohn's disease. Dis Colon Rectum 1991;34:475.

71. Wexner SD, Rothenberger DA, Jensen L, et al. Ileal pouch vaginal fistulas: incidence, etiology, and management. Dis Colon Rectum 1989;32:460.

72. Galandiuk D, Scott NA, Dozois RR, et al. Ileal pouch-anal anastomosis: reoperation for pouch-related complications. Ann Surg 1990;212:446.

73. Stone MM, Lewin K, Fonkalsrud, EW. Late obstruction of the lateral ileal reservoir after colectomy and endorectal ileal pullthrough procedures. Surg Gynecol Obstet 1986;162:411.

74. Fonkalsrud EW. Update on clinical experience with different surgical techniques of the endorectal pull-through operation for colitis and polyposis. Surg Gynecol Obstet 1987;165:309.

75. Telander RL, Perrault J. Colectomy with rectal mucosectomy and ileoanal anastomosis in young patients: its use for ulcerative colitis and familial polyposis. Arch Surg 1981;116:623.

76. Fonkalsrud EW, In: Cameron JL, ed. Current surgical therapy. St. Louis, Mosby-Yearbook, 1992:150.

Surgery of Infants and Children: Scientific Principles and Practice, edited by
Keith T. Oldham, Paul M. Colombani, and Robert P. Foglia.
Lippincott–Raven Publishers, Philadelphia, © 1997.

CHAPTER 82

Colon

Aviva L. Katz

The colon is divided into the cecum, vermiform appendix (see Chap. 74), and the ascending, transverse, descending, and sigmoid colon. The cecum lies below the level of the ileocolic valve, which consists of two horizontal folds of mucous membrane that project around the orifice of the ileum. The cecum is completely peritonealized. The ascending colon lies in the right iliac region and extends upward from the cecum to the inferior surface of the right hepatic lobe, where it turns, forming the right colic flexure and becoming continuous with the transverse colon. In contrast to the cecum and transverse colon, peritoneum covers only the anterior and lateral aspects of the ascending colon. This is sufficient to secure the ascending colon to the posterior abdominal wall. The transverse colon extends across the abdomen, from the right to the left colic flexures, suspended by the transverse mesocolon. The posterior border of the greater omentum is also attached to the transverse colon. The descending colon lies in the left iliac region and extends from the left colic flexure, suspended from the diaphragm by the phrenicolic ligament, to the pelvic brim, where it is continuous with the sigmoid colon. As with the ascending colon, the descending colon is bound to the posterior abdominal wall by peritoneum. The sigmoid colon is continuous with the descending colon and joins the rectum anterior to the third sacral vertebrae.

Significant features of the external anatomy of the large intestine include the concentration of the longitudinal muscle coat into three bands—the *teniae coli.* These teniae create sacculations, called *haustra,* which are separated by semilunar folds, allowing the differentiation of large from small intestine radiologically after infancy. Additionally, the colon has fatty appendages, called *appendices epiploicae,* attached to the muscular wall. The colonic mucosa is characterized by crypts of Lieberkuhn, which are lined with absorptive, goblet, and endocrine cells. The colon has two basic functions: (1) the absorption of water and electrolytes and (2) the storage and elimination of feces. Its absorptive function is significant; the colon absorbs over 80% of the water left after passage through the small intestine.

The arterial supply to the colon is derived from the superior and inferior mesenteric arteries. The superior mesenteric artery provides the blood supply to the colon from the ileocecal area to the distal third of the transverse colon. The cecum is supplied by the anterior and posterior cecal arteries, the ascending colon by the ileocolic and right colic branches, and the transverse colon by the middle colic artery. The distal transverse colon, descending colon, and sigmoid colon are all supplied by the superior and inferior left colic branches of the inferior mesenteric artery. There is communication among arterial branches through the marginal arteries, which extend from the ileocolic junction to the distal sigmoid colon (Fig. 82-1).

POLYPS AND POLYPOSIS SYNDROMES

Juvenile Polyps and Polyposis Syndromes

Juvenile, or retention, polyps are the most common polypoid lesion of the colon in children, accounting for almost 90% of colorectal polyps in this population. They are the most common cause of rectal bleeding in children older than 1 year of age. These lesions are usually large, erythematous, and glistening, and they contain large fluid- or mucus-filled cystic spaces. The epithelial surface is often ulcerated and friable, and these patients characteristically present with mild asymptomatic hematochezia, although profuse rectal bleeding can occur. The origin of these polyps is unknown, although an inflammatory or hamartomatous cause is most often suspected.

Knowledge of the natural history of these polyps continues to evolve. Although early reports indicated that juvenile polyps were usually solitary, in recent studies, the incidence of multiple polyps on colonoscopic examination has significantly increased. More than half of patients have more than one lesion. Additionally, an increased number of polyps are seen proximal to the transverse colon. This change in the distribution and number of polyps throughout the colon is thought to be due to the extensive use of colonoscopy (Fig. 82-2) and its sensitivity in the evaluation of hematochezia, rather than a true change in the nature of the disease.

In addition to the changes in the distribution of juvenile polyps, reports also document adenomatous changes in some juvenile polyps (Fig. 82-3). The presence of adenomatous areas raises concern for the risk of developing colorectal carcinoma. Because of this finding of adenomatous changes, especially in the setting of multiple juvenile polyps, colonoscopic removal

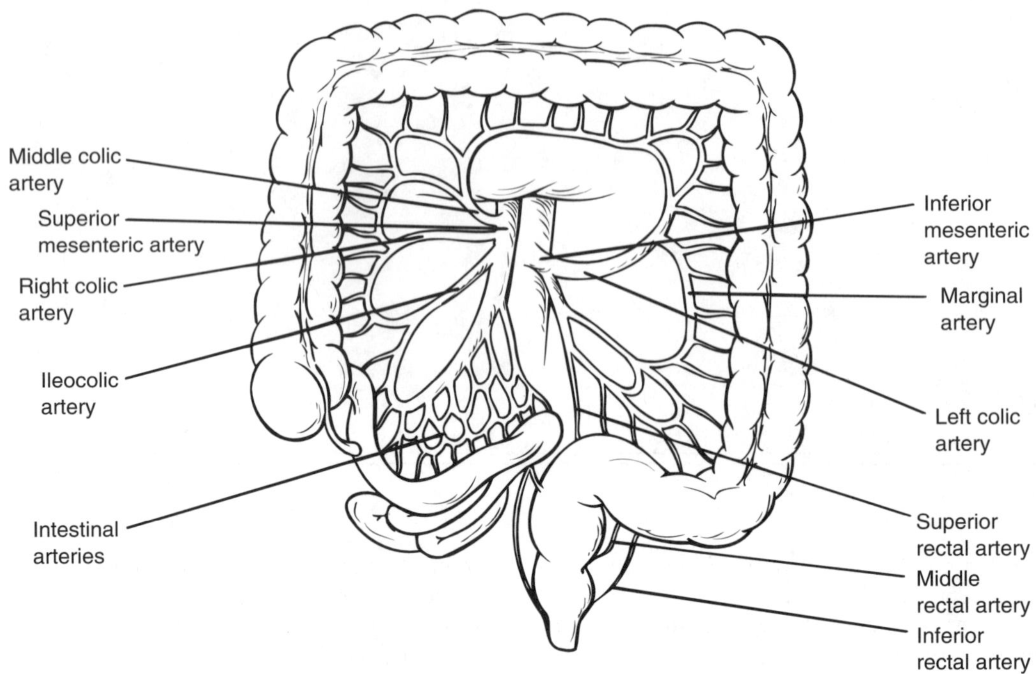

FIG. 82-1. The anatomy and blood supply of the colon.

of all juvenile polyps may be warranted, but available data do not justify prophylactic colectomy solely for the risk of colorectal carcinoma.

The rare familial syndromes involving juvenile polyps include juvenile polyposis, infantile juvenile polyposis, and generalized or diffuse gastrointestinal polyposis. The most common of these is juvenile polyposis, associated with multiple polyps throughout the colon and a positive family history in up to half of patients, suggesting autosomal dominant transmission. Infantile juvenile polyposis occurs in children younger than 2 years of age and can present with severe rectal bleeding, diarrhea with associated protein loss, malnutrition and failure to thrive, rectal prolapse, and intussusception, rarely leading to death. In generalized or diffuse polyposis, there are multiple polyps throughout the gastrointestinal tract and an associated family history in about 25% of patients, suggesting an autosomal recessive inheritance. Because of the risk of adenomatous change with the occurrence of multiple polyps, it is prudent to treat juvenile polyposis with scheduled surveillance colonoscopy and removal of all polyps.

Peutz-Jeghers Syndrome

Peutz-Jeghers syndrome, mucocutaneous pigmentation with intestinal polyposis, is a familial disease with autosomal dominant inheritance associated with high penetrance and variable expression. The abnormal pigmentation most commonly involves the lips and oral mucosa but can also be seen on the hands, feet, digits, perineum, and around the eyes. Multiple hamartomatous polyps are found in most cases, most frequently in the small intestine, particularly in the jejunum. Polyps have also been noted in the colon, stomach, and duodenum. About one third of patients are diagnosed during childhood, the most common presenting complaint being intermittent abdominal pain thought to be due to transient but recurrent intussusception.

Gastrointestinal cancer has been reported in these patients, particularly in those with gastric or duodenal polyps, and some polyps have been noted to contain areas of adenoma or carcinoma. It appears that although the risk of cancer is less than in other inherited polyposis syndromes, it is still significant. Removal of gastric or duodenal polyps is recommended because of the higher risk of malignant transformation. Pathologic evaluation of excised polyps appears to support a hamartoma–adenoma–carcinoma sequence. The true risk of cancer has been difficult to determine in this population and probably requires

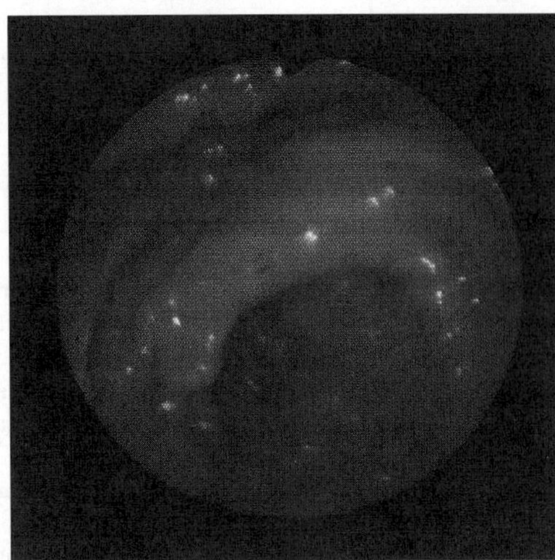

FIG. 82-2. Multiple adenomatous polyps are apparent in this photograph obtained during colonoscopy in a patient with familial adenomatous polyposis. (See Color Figure 82-2.)

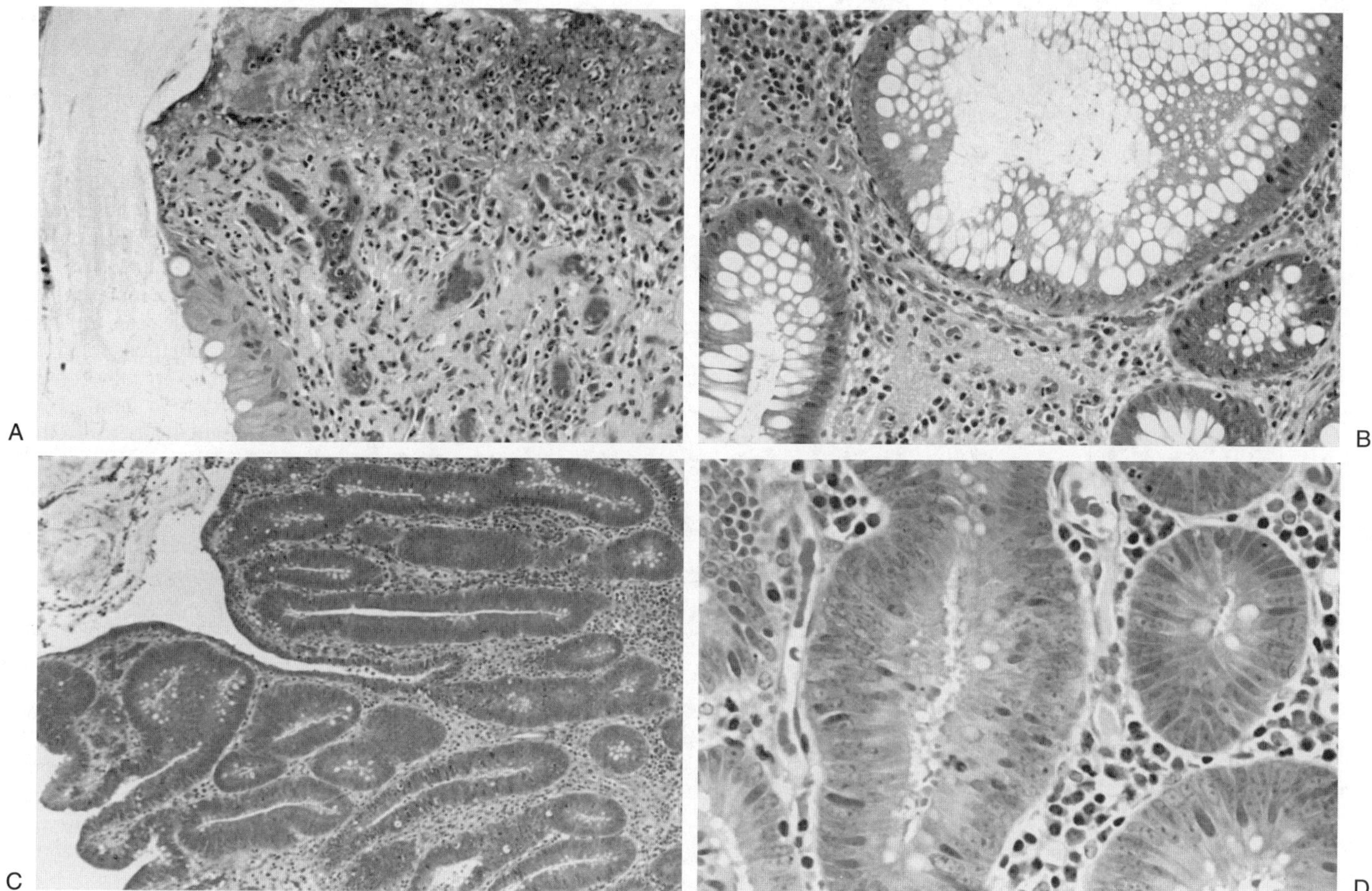

FIG. 82-3. (*A*) Photomicrograph of a juvenile polyp with an ulcerated epithelial surface. (*B*) Normal glandular morphology with a large mucus-filled central cystic space is apparent, as is a juvenile polyp. (*C*) In contrast, a photomicrograph of an adenomatous polyp illustrates the characteristic frondlike glandular structure and, at higher magnification (*D*), exuberant epithelial proliferation. (See Color Figure 82-3.)

long-term prospective evaluation of a large registry of Peutz-Jeghers patients. A review of reported malignant tumors suggest that the most frequent site of gastrointestinal cancer is the colon, followed by the duodenum, jejunum, and stomach. It has been estimated that between 3% and 20% of patients develop a gastrointestinal malignancy. Uterine, breast, and more frequently, ovarian sex cord tumors are also reported in female Peutz-Jeghers patients. Compared with the general population, Peutz-Jeghers patients have a relative risk of death from gastrointestinal malignancy of 13 and a relative risk of death from any malignancy of 9.[1,2]

Familial Adenomatous Polyposis

Familial adenomatous polyposis (FAP) is an inherited autosomal dominant polyposis syndrome with high penetrance. It occurs in 1 in 10,000 live births. In addition to the familial cases, about 40% of patients represent new mutations. Gardner syndrome, which can include the extraintestinal features of mesenteric fibromatosis, desmoid tumors, epidermoid cysts, osteomas, and dental abnormalities, appears to be a clinical and genetic variant of FAP.

Colonic polyps appear most frequently in the second decade of life, with cancer developing at an average age of 40 years in the natural history of unresected disease (Fig. 82-4). The polyps are adenomatous and are associated with the near certain development of malignant colorectal carcinoma. Hyperplastic gastric polyps with no malignant potential are found in half of patients, and adenomatous duodenal polyps with a significant associated risk of periampullary carcinoma is found in 90% of patients. Despite the clear risk of malignant transformation, there is no consensus on screening guidelines. Colonoscopy beginning at 10 to 12 years of age and continuing yearly until 35 years of age in all first-degree relatives of the index patient appears prudent because the age at which the polyps first appear varies. The probability of finding polyps at 10 years of age is 15%, but this increases to 98% by 30 years of age. In addition to colonoscopy, screening should include yearly surveillance with a side-viewing endoscope for gastric and duodenal polyps once colonic polyps have appeared. Epidemiologic surveys have shown a 750-fold to 7500-fold increased incidence of hepatoblastoma in infants and children with FAP, although there are no clear screening guidelines for children from families at risk.[3]

A predictive test that would accurately determine the risk

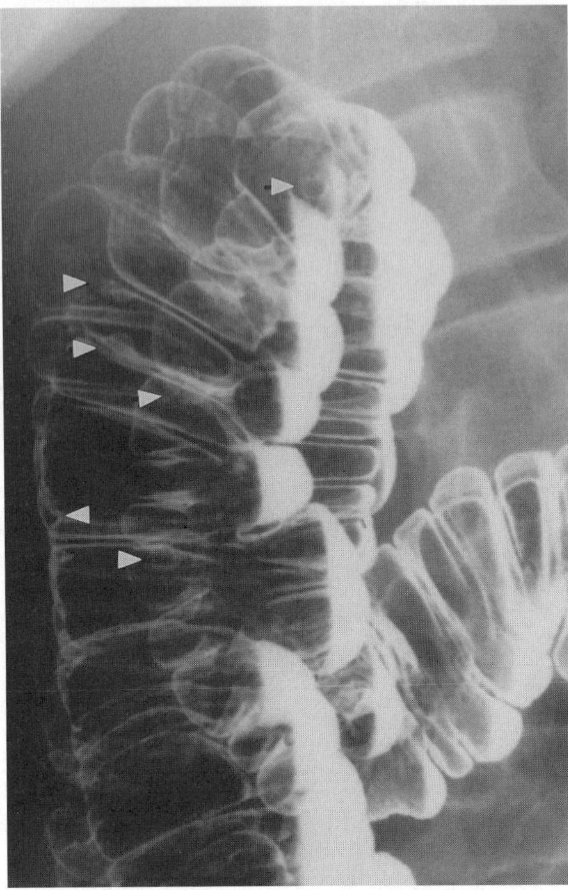

FIG. 82-4. Radiograph after an air-contrast barium enema demonstrates multiple adenomatous polyps (*arrows*) in a patient with familial adenomatous polyposis.

of developing FAP would eliminate the need for surveillance endoscopy in those not affected, decreasing discomfort, anxiety, and expense. It might also allow for earlier resection in the affected population. Because the age of onset of polyps is variable, to exclude the presence of FAP safely, surveillance colonoscopy must continue to 35 years of age. In contrast, congenital hypertrophy of the retinal pigment epithelium appears to be present at birth in patients with phenotypic FAP, even those without other extraintestinal findings. The ophthalmologic examination is a direct, noninvasive, and inexpensive screening test. Although the sensitivity and specificity of these fundic lesions are high as a predictive phenotypic marker, and thus may allow earlier detection of FAP, negative eye signs in young, unaffected first-degree relatives cannot safely preclude surveillance screening.[4,5]

Once the adenomatous polyposis coli (*APC*) gene—the gene responsible for FAP—was mapped to the long arm of chromosome 5, attempts were made at linkage analysis to provide presymptomatic diagnosis. Despite the availability of flanking markers, it may be a minority of families that benefit from polymorphic probe DNA analysis. The difficulties encountered include the inherent inaccuracy of the probe due to its recombination fraction, the death of families members before tissue analysis, and the occurrence of new mutations.[6,7] Additionally, linkage analysis, when available, can give only an estimation of risk, not an absolute diagnosis, and can therefore safely reduce, but not eliminate, surveillance screening.

Identification of the *APC* gene might allow direct genetic testing when this gene is found to be mutated in the germline in patients with symptoms, and therefore might allow a more exact calculation of cancer risk in family members. Most mutations of the *APC* gene result in truncations of the gene product due to frameshifts, nonsense mutations, and splice-site changes. An in vivo synthesized protein assay that can pick up truncated APC protein, combined with an allele-specific expression assay that can identify mutations as an imbalance in the representation of alleles at the RNA transcription level, can scan the entire *APC* transcript for mutations and identify mutations in 87% of tested kindred with FAP.[8,9] Linked DNA markers may continue to have a place in presymptomatic diagnosis in families with mutations that are difficult to type. Additionally, because there is a wide range of phenotypic presentations associated with inheritance of mutant *APC* alleles, appropriate treatment and counseling will remain difficult.

Although germline mutations in *APC* result in FAP, somatic mutations can result in colorectal tumors in the general population. Of the tumor-suppressor genes, *APC* mutations appear earliest in the pathway of progression of colorectal tumorigenesis. The APC gene product normally binds to β-catenin and can modulate the interaction between cadherins and catenins, affecting the pathway through which intercellular interactions control cell growth and differentiation. Mutant, truncated APC proteins have a reduced or absent affinity for β-catenin, and this deficiency can contribute to the development of the phenotype. Formation of polyps can result from a loss of intercellular contact inhibition dependent on interaction between *APC* and β-catenin.[10,11]

Colectomy with endorectal proctectomy and ileal pullthrough is the most favored option for the surgical therapy of FAP in childhood. Removal of the entire rectal mucosa to the dentate line does not interfere with anorectal sphincter function nor the ability to differentiate gas from liquid or solid stool.[12] Ileorectal anastomosis leaves the patient at risk for future carcinoma and requires long-term surveillance, and the conversion from ileorectal to ileoanal anastomosis can be complicated by the higher rate of development of desmoid tumors in this population. At long-term follow-up of patients who underwent ileorectal anastomosis for FAP, a significant number developed cancer in the rectal segment. Chronologic age, not the number of years of follow-up, appears to be the significant risk factor, with a 10% probability of rectal cancer by 50 years of age, a 30% risk by 60 years of age, and a mean age of onset of 48 years. Unfortunately, few of these patients had symptoms before detection, and most were compliant with every 6-month screening. Because the ileorectal anastomosis provides a functional result similar to that of an ileoanal anastomosis with pouch reconstruction, it appears that ileorectal anastomosis does not adequately fulfill the requirements for surgical therapy of FAP—that it be safe, that it allow the preservation of function, and that it eliminate the risk of cancer.[13,14]

Sulindac, a long-acting nonsteroidal antiinflammatory agent, has been noted to cause regression of polyps in FAP. Sulforeduction by anaerobic bacteria results in an increased colonic intraluminal concentration of the active sulfide form, which can inhibit the signaling cascade that controls growth and cell proliferation. Randomized, placebo-controlled trials in patients with FAP either before any surgery or after ileorectal anastomosis demonstrated rapid regression in the number and size of colorectal polyps with the oral administration of sulindac. Unfortunately, complete resolution of polyposis was not always reached, and the polyps reappeared shortly after discontinuing treatment. Additionally, the correlation between regression of polyps and a decrease in malignant transformation is unknown.[15,16]

Turcot Syndrome

Turcot syndrome is a rare, autosomal recessive disorder that represents the association between FAP and central nervous system tumors. Management of the colonic polyposis is as outlined earlier for FAP.

Lymphoid Polyposis

Nodular lymphoid hyperplasia can give rise to polyps in the colon or rectum. These submucosal nodules are often multiple and small with a central umbilication and represent simple aggregates of lymphoid follicles. Although generally a benign, self-limited entity, lymphoid polyps can be a cause of rectal bleeding or a lead point for intussusception, requiring excision.

COLON CARCINOMA

Colorectal carcinoma is the most common carcinoma of childhood, although only about 1% of all colorectal malignancies are found in patients less than 30 years of age. Although adenocarcinoma can complicate FAP or ulcerative colitis, most cases in childhood arise in previously healthy children without known underlying pathology. The signs and symptoms of colon carcinoma—abdominal pain, vomiting, constipation, weight loss, and melena or hematochezia—are similar in children and adults. The rarity of carcinoma in childhood, however, leads to the expectation of alternative diagnoses and often delays the diagnosis of cancer.

The most important prognostic factor in patients with colorectal cancer is the depth of invasion of the primary tumor. The first practical staging system to incorporate this observation was the Dukes classification. It was originally designed for the classification of rectal tumors but has been expanded with modification to allow the classification of colon carcinoma.

MODIFIED DUKES CLASSIFICATION

Stage A—extension of the lesion from the mucosa through the muscularis propria without serosal involvement
Stage B—extension of the lesion from the mucosa through the serosa into the perirectal or pericolonic fat
Stage C$_1$—extension of the lesion from the mucosa through the serosa to involve extracolonic tissues and lymph nodes
Stage C$_2$—extension of the lesion from the mucosa through the serosa to involve extracolonic tissues and lymph nodes as high as the point of ligature of the major vessels at the aorta
Stage D—evidence of distant organ (hematogenous) involvement

Several significant differences can be found in the nature of the colon carcinomas found in children and adults. Although

TABLE 82-1 *Five-year survival rate of patients with colorectal carcinoma*

Stage	Patients <40 years old		Patients >40 years old	
	With tumors (%)	Survival rate (%)	With tumors (%)	Survival rate (%)
A and B	46	96	68	78
C and metastatic disease	54	23	32	21
Overall		51		75

mucinous adenocarcinoma is seen in only about 5% of adults, this more poorly differentiated aggressive carcinoma accounts for about 50% of cases in children. There is also a shift from the pattern of left-sided lesions seen in adults to a more even distribution of tumors throughout the colon in children. Because of these differences, and the frequent delay in diagnosis, children and adolescents tend to present with more advanced disease than adults. Most patients have modified Dukes stage C or D disease at presentation, with involvement of regional lymph nodes and distant metastases preventing curative resection. Incomplete tumor removal is associated with an extremely poor prognosis and few long-term survivors. Young adults and children have a significantly lower overall 5-year survival rate than do older patients, owing to the increased incidence of advanced disease at presentation[17,18] (Table 82-1).

The goal of surgery for colon carcinoma is to maximize the chance for cure through en bloc removal of tumor and lymph node basins with adequate margins. The most significant factors affecting prognosis reflect the stage of disease at the time of presentation and are not under the control of the surgeon. Factors of possible prognostic significance that are under the surgeons' control include the extent of margins of resection, extent of lymphatic resection, timing and level of vascular ligation, intraluminal use of cytotoxic solution, anastomotic technique, and prevention of colonic perforation during resection. The results of adjuvant therapy, to prevent dissemination of disease at the time of surgery and to control distant disease, have been disappointing. No adjuvant therapy is recommended for Dukes stage A lesions, therapy in defined clinical trials is recommended for Dukes stage B lesions, and either treatment with levamisole plus 5-fluorouracil or entry into clinical trial is indicated for Dukes stage C lesions.

COLITIS

Pseudomembranous Colitis

Pseudomembranous colitis is almost invariably caused by toxin-producing *Clostridium difficile* infection after antibiotic usage. Toxigenic *Clostridium perfringens* type C and *Shigella dysenteriae* type 1 may also be responsible for the development of pseudomembranous colitis. Nearly all antimicrobial agents have been implicated in the disorder, including antifungal, antiviral, and antimicrobial agents to which *C difficile* is susceptible, including vancomycin and metronidazole. Pseudomembra-

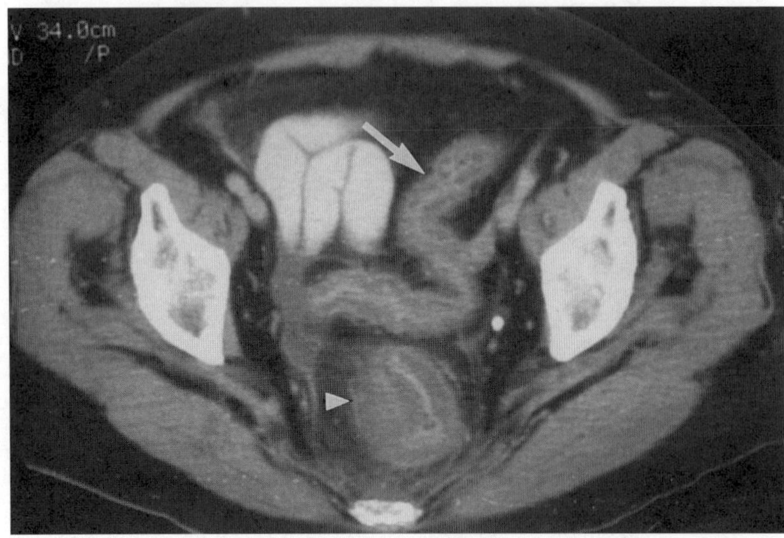

FIG. 82-5. Pseudomembranous colitis. CT scan shows thickening of the bowel wall in the sigmoid colon (*arrow*) and rectum (*arrowhead*). Mucosal edema and "thumbprinting" are apparent.

nous colitis has also been reported in infants whose only exposure to antibiotics was through breast milk. The risk of development appears unrelated to the dose or duration of antibiotic treatment. The protection against *C difficile* proliferation provided by normal intestinal flora can be disrupted by antibiotic usage, increasing susceptibility to pseudomembranous colitis.

The pathogenicity of *C difficile* is due to its production of toxins. Toxin A is an enterotoxin that binds to receptors on the mucosal epithelial surface, resulting in severe inflammation and fluid secretion. Toxin B is a cytotoxin that induces alterations in cell shape and causes diffuse enterocyte cell damage. Although the production of toxin is necessary for the development of colitis, the titer of toxin found in a patient's stool does not necessarily correlate with the severity of disease. Extraintestinal circulation of toxin after mucosal and submucosal invasion may be responsible for the shock state and sudden death that infrequently accompany severe disease.

Pseudomembranous colitis most frequently presents with mild to moderate, watery, nonbloody diarrhea beginning 7 to 10 days after the initiation of antibiotics, although the spectrum of disease can vary widely. Some patients present with fulminant disease and an acute abdomen with signs of toxic megacolon or perforation, even in the absence of preceding diarrhea. In unrecognized and untreated catastrophic disease, mortality rates are as high as 20%. The diagnosis should also be considered in any child with a severe, protracted course of debilitating diarrhea, especially after antibiotic treatment. The diagnosis can be established by visualizing classic yellowish white, placque-like pseudomembranes on endoscopy. More frequently, the diagnosis is made noninvasively in the appropriately suspicious clinical setting. Plain films of the abdomen may reveal "thumbprinting," reflecting a markedly edematous colonic wall. Computed tomography of the abdomen may demonstrate colonic wall thickening and inflammation (Fig. 82-5). The most sensitive method to establish a diagnosis of pseudomembranous colitis is by *C difficile* toxin detection. The most accurate method of toxin detection remains the cytotoxin tissue culture assay. The latex agglutination test is less reliable, although it can be used as a rapid screening test.

Patients who have mild pseudomembranous colitis, typically with fever, mild abdominal pain, and diarrhea, may respond to discontinuation of the implicated antibiotic. In more severe disease, treatment should include oral vancomycin, 40 mg/kg/d in three divided doses, or metronidazole, 20 to 30 mg/kg/d in three divided doses, continued for 7 to 10 days. The addition of this specific therapy allows for continued treatment with the inducing antibiotic if necessary. Enteral administration of these therapeutic antibiotics, by rectal or stomal irrigation if the oral route is unavailable, is much more effective than intravenous administration in reaching effective intraluminal concentrations. When parenteral therapy must be given, as in the case of severe ileus, intravenous metronidazole achieves therapeutic fecal concentrations; intravenous vancomycin is less effective and does not reach adequate intraluminal concentrations. Relapse after treatment occurs in 10% to 20% of patients and is most often due to sporulation of *C difficile*. These spores are resistant to treatment, and either longer courses of treatment or pulsed doses of antibiotics may be effective.

Children who have undergone definitive therapy for Hirschsprung disease appear to have an increased incidence of pseudomembranous colitis. The increased frequency of asymptomatic colonization with *C difficile* in infants younger than 1 year of age has interfered with the study of this population. Of children who have undergone definitive surgical treatment for Hirschsprung disease, significantly prolonged carriage of *C difficile* and an increased rate of toxin production are seen only in those with recurrent enterocolitis and diarrhea. The cause of this increased sensitivity to pseudomembranous colitis is unclear. Suspected mechanisms include intestinal stasis; a change in the character of the intestinal epithelial mucins, allowing adherence of *C difficile*; incompletely resolved chronic intestinal injury; and immunologic defects, with increased lymphocyte accumulation in the lamina propria and decreased immunoglobulin A transfer across the epithelium.[19,20] Because the clinical picture of pseudomembranous colitis can be indistinguishable from that of Hirschsprung enterocolitis, with fever, abdominal pain, and diarrhea, empiric therapy should be started while awaiting results of stool evaluation in patients who are seriously ill.

Diversion Colitis

Diversion colitis is an inflammatory process in a bypassed colorectal segment after surgical diversion of the fecal stream. The colonic inflammation must be distinguished from changes related to the underlying disease state requiring formation of the stoma. The development of colitis may be due to a difference in the microflora in the bypassed segment, with a decrease noted in both the total number of bacteria and in the number of strict anaerobes. Alternatively, mucosal injury and inflammation may be secondary to a deficiency of short-chain fatty acids, specifically butyric acid, leading to nutritional deprivation of the colonocytes. When studied in children with long-term stomas for the management of Hirschsprung disease or motility disorders, which are well-defined diseases with no inflammatory component, no correlation was noted between the severity of the colitis and the duration of diversion or age at time of diversion. Almost all children studied had microscopic evidence of diversion colitis, even in the absence of clinical signs or symptoms. Findings included mucosal inflammation, nodular hyperplasia of the lymphoglandular complexes and germinal centers, an expanded submucosa with chronic inflammatory cells in the lamina propria, and cryptitis and crypt abscesses. This may be a particularly difficult condition in patients who require long-term total parenteral nutrition because the chronically inflamed, bypassed intestine can be a source of bacterial translocation and recurrent sepsis, occasionally prompting resection rather than bypass.[21,22] Generally, this problem resolves spontaneously when intestinal continuity is restored.

ENTERIC INFECTIONS

Viral gastroenteritis is the second most common illness in the United States, where it accounts for 300 to 400 annual childhood deaths. Worldwide, viral gastroenteritis is responsible for more than 4 million childhood deaths per year. Rotavirus is responsible for more cases of diarrheal disease in infants and children than is any other single cause. Norwalk virus and enteric adenoviruses are other relatively common viral pathogens that cause acute gastroenteritis. Rotavirus is responsible for the winter peak in childhood gastroenteritis, while the enteric adenoviruses are responsible for the summer peak. Both tend to affect children younger than 2 years of age, are accompanied by significant diarrhea, and not uncommonly result in dehydration. Treatment is supportive; oral rehydration solutions are extremely useful and are often life-saving in cases of dehydration.

Whereas viral agents invade villus enterocytes along the entire span of the small intestine, infecting bacterial agents often act in the colon. Several bacterial virulence mechanisms act specifically on the colon, causing cytotoxin injury, direct epithelial cell invasion, and enteroadhesive activity. *Salmonella* sp is the most common cause of bacterial diarrhea in children in the United States, and the incidence of this disease appears to be increasing. Because of the invasiveness of this organism, infection can result in colitis and bacteremia, especially in patients with lymphoproliferative diseases and sickle cell anemia. Antibiotic treatment, with ampicillin or trimethoprim-sulfamethoxazole, is recommended in patients at high risk for the development of disseminated disease, those who appear septic, neonates, and those with complicated cases of gastroenteritis. *Shigella* sp is the second most common pathogen identified in cases of bacterial diarrhea in children, and is an especially common cause of outbreaks of diarrhea in daycare settings. Although *Shigella* sp most frequently causes a mild, self-limited diarrhea, antibiotics are sometimes appropriate for patients who are severely ill to shorten the course of disease and to decrease the period of shedding of the organism. Nonpathogenic strains of *Escherichia coli* are among the most common bacteria in the normal flora of the human intestine, but pathogenic strains are an important cause of diarrheal disease. Enterohemorrhagic *E coli* can occur in sporadic cases and in food-borne outbreaks. These bacteria produce a range of symptoms from watery diarrhea to hemorrhagic colitis. Verotoxic serotype 0157:H7 is implicated in the development of the hemolytic–uremic syndrome, characterized by microangiopathic hemolytic anemia, uremia, and thrombocytopenia (see Chap. 69). It is the most common cause of acute renal failure in children. Antibiotic treatment does not hasten resolution of this disease, but aggressive, supportive measures are required because hemolytic–uremic syndrome is associated with high morbidity and mortality rates. Significant medical complications include encephalopathy, pancreatitis, cardiomyopathy, hypertension, and seizures. Most patients can be treated successfully nonoperatively, but surgery may be required to support dialysis or for treatment of the acute abdomen with colonic injury leading to acidosis, peritonitis, or obvious perforation or obstruction. Resection for late stenosis after resolution of the acute illness has also been reported.[23]

Gastrointestinal manifestations of acquired immunodeficiency syndrome are often like colitis, with abdominal pain and bloody diarrhea. Cytomegalovirus is the most common associated colonic pathogen and can cause necrotizing lesions that can lead to hemorrhage or perforation. Treatment with ganciclovir is often effective, although relapses are common.[24]

CHRONIC IDIOPATHIC INTESTINAL PSEUDOOBSTRUCTION

Chronic idiopathic intestinal pseudoobstruction (CIIOP) is a clinical syndrome defined by the presence of signs and symptoms characteristic of intestinal obstruction in the absence of anatomic obstruction. Patients most frequently present with abdominal pain and distention, failure to thrive, and vomiting and constipation. Most cases are congenital, are of either myopathic or neuropathic origin (rarely both), and arise sporadically, with no obvious family history. Histologic findings can include muscle fibrosis, vacuolar degeneration and disorganization of myofilaments, maturational arrest of myenteric plexuses, neuronal intestinal dysplasia, and a completely normal intestinal wall. In addition to these idiopathic cases, pseudoobstruction can be seen in association with Down syndrome, neurofibromatosis, multiple endocrine neoplasia type 2B, Russell-Silver syndrome, Duchenne muscular dystrophy, acute viral gastroenteritis, and extreme prematurity.

The clinical presentation is one of abdominal distention and vomiting (Fig. 82-6). More than half of affected infants develop symptoms within a few days of birth. Of these, about 40% have associated malrotation. Some less severely affected infants present with vomiting and failure to thrive within the first few months of life, so that more than three quarters of affected infants present during the first year of life. Although laparotomy for biopsy alone is not indicated, many of these children

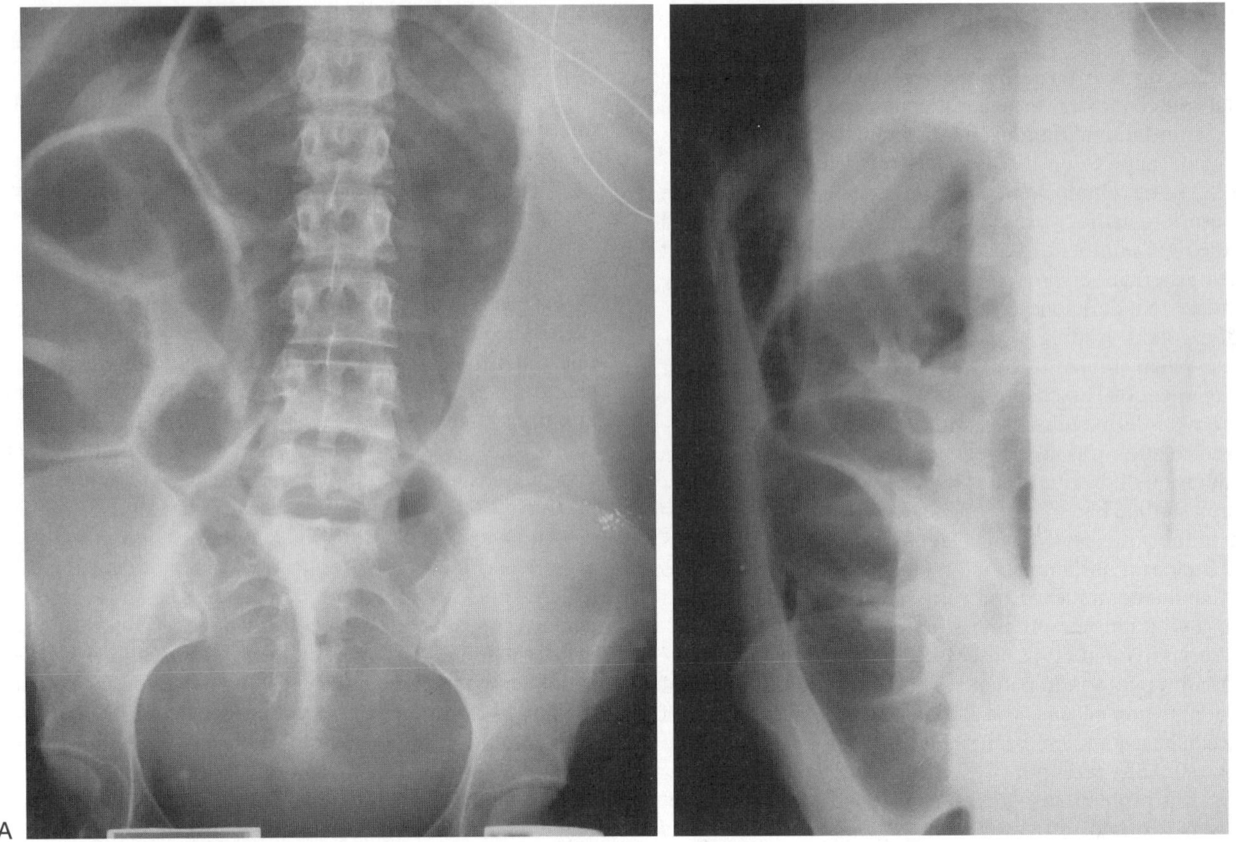

FIG. 82-6. Supine (*A*) and decubitus (*B*) abdominal radiographs of a child with chronic idiopathic intestinal pseudoobstruction demonstrate marked bowel distension.

undergo surgery for treatment of malrotation or evaluation of intestinal obstruction. At this time, a biopsy of full-thickness bowel wall should be obtained. The tissues should be processed for conventional histology, appropriate histochemistry, electron microscopy, and silver stains to evaluate for myopathic or neuropathic processes.

Although CIIOP is a clinical diagnosis, manometric studies can be useful in documenting abnormalities in amplitude or coordination of contractions. Esophageal, antroduodenal, colonic, and anorectal manometry can help determine the site and type of pseudoobstruction and assist in evaluating the response to therapy. Prokinetic drugs are helpful in a minority of children with CIIOP. A trial of cisapride is indicated in most patients, although it brings significant relief only to a select few without dilated intestine. Erythromycin is not effective for generalized motility disorders or those with colonic involvement but can bring relief in neuropathic gastroparesis. Nutritional support is vital because the clinical course is often characterized by remissions and exacerbations, and malnutrition can cause exacerbations. Most children tolerate all or some of their nutrition enterally, which causes significantly less morbidity than parenteral nutrition. Surgery should play a small role in the long-term treatment of CIIOP. Although gastrostomy tube placement can be useful in allowing a convenient access for long-term tube feeding or venting, other procedures, such as fundoplication, pyloroplasty, or gastrojejunostomy, have proved less useful. Colectomy has been helpful in the few children with isolated colonic pseudoobstruction. Prolonged postoperative ileus is to

be expected in these patients, and the development of adhesions makes evaluation of future episodes of acute pseudoobstruction increasingly difficult.

A relatively well-defined subset of CIIOP patients includes neonates with megacystis–microcolon intestinal hypoperistalsis syndrome. This rare cause of functional neonatal intestinal obstruction has associated hypoperistalsis, malrotation, dilated proximal ileum, narrow distal ileum and colon, and bladder distention. The cause of this syndrome is unknown, but possible mechanisms include visceral myopathy, imbalance in gut peptides, defective autonomic inhibitory neuroeffector activity, and destruction of hollow, viscus smooth muscle and neural network by an in utero intramural inflammatory process with resultant fibrosis. This disorder appears to be autosomal recessive and is usually lethal; most deaths occur by 6 months of age. Prenatal ultrasound diagnosis allows counseling in subsequent pregnancies in affected families.[25,26]

ANATOMIC CONGENITAL ANOMALIES

Colonic Atresia

Of the gastrointestinal tract atresias, only gastric atresia is more uncommon than colonic atresia. Acquired obstruction of the colon, usually secondary to necrotizing enterocolitis, is significantly more common than congenital atresia. Isolated colonic atresia may be associated with ophthalmologic defects,

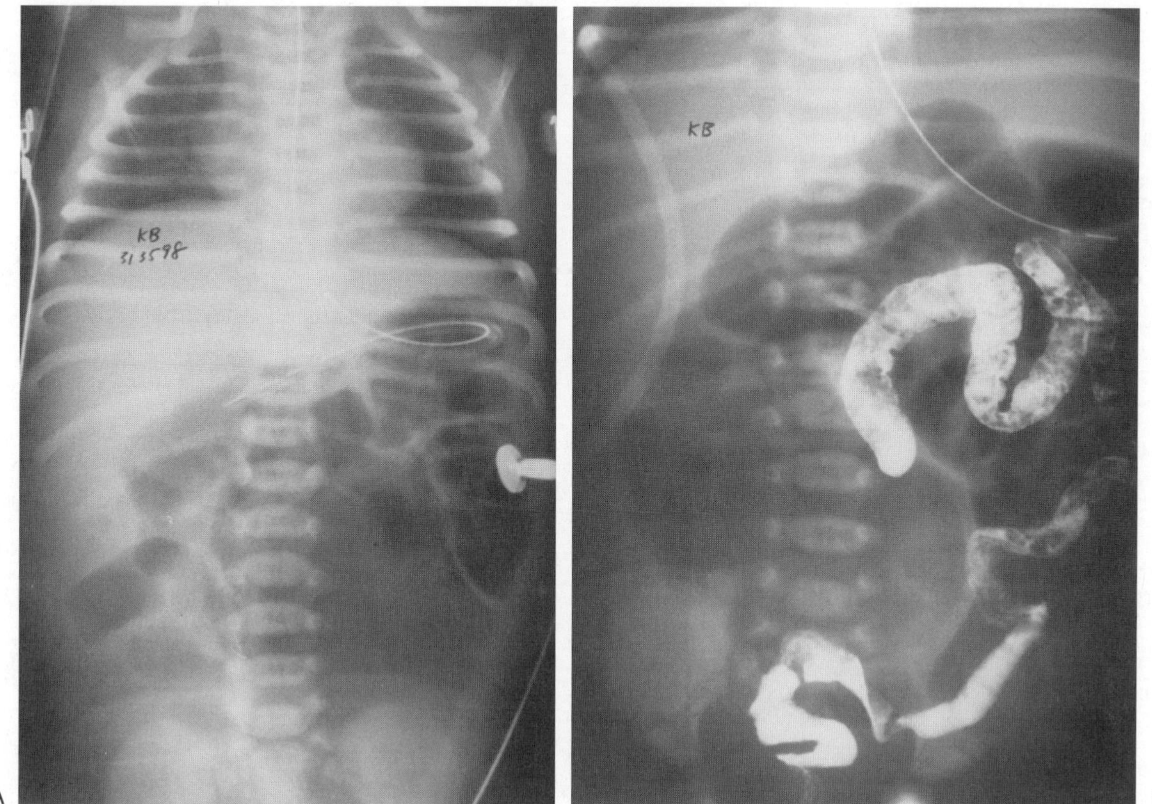

FIG. 82-7. (*A*) Plain abdominal radiograph of an infant with colonic atresia. (*B*) Radiograph after barium enema in the same patient. Note the contrast-filled distal microcolon and the cutoff in the mid-transverse colon.

skeletal anomalies, jejunal atresia, aganglionosis, and abdominal wall defects. Colonic atresia presents as a low intestinal obstruction in the neonate, with abdominal distention, bilious emesis, and absent passage of meconium. It must be differentiated from other causes of ileal or colonic obstruction. Barium enema is vital to the evaluation of these neonates, revealing a distal microcolon with incomplete colonic filling. Importantly, in neonates with clinically apparent proximal small bowel atresia, barium enema reveals the colonic atresia, if present, and allows concurrent repair, preventing a potential postoperative disaster (Fig. 82-7).

Optimal management techniques are determined by the location of the atretic segment and other medical problems. Generally, atresia of the colon is managed by limited segmental resection of the dilated proximal segment and with primary end-oblique anastomosis to the distal mesocolon. Occasionally, exteriorization as a colostomy with mucous fistula is necessary to prepare for future colocolostomy if there are confounding medical or technical problems. Resection is required because of the size discrepancy and concerns about abnormalities in vascularity and innervation adjacent to the atretic segment. Obviously, management of the more complicated forms of colonic atresia must be individualized.

Rotational Anomalies

Abnormalities of intestinal rotation represent a diffuse spectrum of incomplete or nonrotation of either (or both) the duode-nojejunal or cecocolic intestinal limb. Although the duodenojejunal limb completes its rotation before the cecocolic limb, multiple combinations of failure of rotation are possible. Malrotation is associated with several other anomalies, including congenital diaphragmatic hernia, omphalocele, gastroschisis, and intestinal atresia. Most patients with symptoms attributable to malrotation present with duodenal obstruction or small bowel volvulus. Rarely do patients present with colonic symptomatology. In reverse rotation, the duodenum and jejunum lie anterior to the superior mesenteric vessels, which may then obstruct the posteriorly placed transverse colon. This can result in chronic colonic obstruction, which usually responds to reflection of the colon and reversal of the rotation. Cecal volvulus, with associated obstruction and distention, can result from the inadequate fixation of the cecum, terminal ileum, and proximal ascending colon. Treatment includes reduction of the volvulus, followed generally by resection and possibly by fixation.

REFERENCES

1. Hizawa K, Iida M, Matsumoto T, et al. Peutz-Jeghers polyposis. Dis Colon Rectum 1993;36:953.
2. Spigelman AD, Murday V, Phillips RKS. Cancer and the Peutz-Jeghers syndrome. 1989;30:1588.
3. Hughes LJ, Michels VV. Risk of hepatoblastoma in familial adenomatous polyposis. Am J Med Genet 1992;43:1023.
4. Berk T, Cohen Z, McLeod RS, et al. Congenital hypertrophy of the retinal pigment epithelium as a marker for familial adenomatous polyposis. Dis Col Rectum 1988;31:253.

5. Morton DG, Gibson J, MacDonald F, et al. Role of congenital hypertrophy of the retinal pigment epithelium in the predictive diagnosis of familial adenomatous polyposis. Br J Surg 1992;79:689.

6. MacDonald F, Morton DG, Rindle PM, et al. Predictive diagnosis of familial adenomatous polyposis with lined DNA markers: population based study. BMJ 1992;304:869.

7. Dunlop MG, Wyllie AH, Steel CM, et al. Linked DNA markers for presymptomatic diagnosis of familial adenomatous polyposis. Lancet 1991;337:313.

8. Powell SM, Petersen GM, Krush AJ, et al. Molecular diagnosis of familial adenomatous polyposis. N Engl J Med 1993;329:1983.

9. Liu ET. From the molecule to public health. N Engl J Med 1993;329:2028.

10. Rubenfeld B, Souza V, Albert I. Association of the APC gene product with B-catenin. Science 1993;262:1731.

11. Su L-K, Vogelstein B, Kinzler KW. Association of the APC tumor suppressor protein with catenins. Science 1993;262:1734.

12. Fonkalsrud EW, Loar N. Long-term results after colectomy and endorectal-ileal pullthrough procedure in children. Ann Surg 1993;215:57.

13. Ambroze WL Jr, Dozois RR, Pemberton JH. Familial adenomatous polyposis: results following ileal pouch-anal anastomosis and ileorectostomy. Dis Colon Rectum 1992;35:12.

14. Nugent KP, Phillips RKS. Rectal cancer risk in older patients with familial adenomatous polyposis and an ileorectal anastomosis: a cause for concern. Br J Surg 1992;79:1204.

15. Labayle D, Fischer D, Vielh P, et al. Sulindac causes regression of rectal polyps in familial adenomatous polyposis. Gastroenterology 1991;101:635.

16. Giardiello FM, Hamilton SR, Krush AJ. Treatment of colonic and rectal adenomas with sulindac in familial adenomatous polyposis. N Engl J Med 1993;328:1313.

17. Marble K, Banerjee S, Greenwald L. Colorectal carcinoma in young patients. J Surg Oncol 1992;51:179.

18. LaQuaglia MP, Heller G, Filippa DA, et al. Prognostic factors and outcome in patients 21 years and under with colorectal carcinoma. J Pediatr Surg 1992;27:1085.

19. Bagwell CE, Langham MR Jr, Mahaffey SM, et al. Pseudomembranous colitis following resection for Hirschsprung's disease. J Pediatr Surg 1992;27:1261.

20. Hardy SP, Bayston R, Spitz L. Prolonged carriage of clostridium difficile in Hirschsprung's disease. Arch Dis Child 1993;69:221.

21. Ordein JJ, DiLorezzo C, Flores A, et al. Diversion colitis in children with severe gastrointestinal motility disorder. Am J Gastroenterol 1992;87:88.

22. Hague S, Eisen RN, West B. The morphologic features of diversion colitis: studies of a pediatric population with no other disease of the intestinal mucosa. Hum Pathol 1993;24:211.

23. Brandt ML, O'Regan S, Rousseau E, et al. Surgical complications of the hemolytic-uremic syndrome. J Pediatr Surg 1990;25:1109.

24. Dolgin SS, Larsen JG, Shah KD, et al. CMV enteritis causing hemorrhage and obstruction in an infant with AIDS. J Pediatr Surg 1990;25:696.

25. Anneren G, Meurling S, Olsen L. Megacystis-microcolon intestinal hypoperistalsis syndrome (MMIHS), an autosomal recessive disorder: clinical reports and review of the literature. Am J Med Genet 1991;41:251.

26. Srikanth MS, Ford EG, Isaacs H Jr, et al. Megacystis-microcolon intestinal hypoperistalsis syndrome: late sequelae and possible pathogenesis. J Pediatr Surg 1993;28:957.

Surgery of Infants and Children: Scientific Principles and Practice, edited by
Keith T. Oldham, Paul M. Colombani, and Robert P. Foglia.
Lippincott–Raven Publishers, Philadelphia, © 1997.

CHAPTER 83

Rectum and Anus

Charles N. Paidas and Alberto Peña

For more than 100 years, surgeons around the world have been grappling with the morphologic consequences of events involving the caudal end of the embryo which occur between the fourth and eighth weeks of gestation. The anomalies are known as anorectal malformations (ARMs). As the embryologic and genetic sequencing of events continue to unfold, the questions of how and why these caudal defects occur are to be answered. For the time being, the pediatric surgeon is consulted for antenatal counseling, postnatal and perioperative opinions, and definitive operative correction of ARMs. Ultimately, the pediatric surgeon must manage the sequelae of these defects including constipation, fecal and possibly urinary incontinence, and sexual inadequacies, regardless of how impeccable the initial operative correction. What we have learned thus far is that there is an intimate relation among muscle, bone, and nerves at the caudal end of the embryo demanding a clinical management algorithm that considers this embryologic trio.

For centuries, an anal orifice was blindly created by making an incision in the perineum of children with imperforate anus. Many of these children did well, probably because these were defects with an anus located very close to the skin of the perineum (low defects). In contrast, most children with higher defects did not survive. In Paris in 1835, Amussat[1] actually performed the first surgical anoplasty by suturing the wall of the rectum to the skin edges without a colostomy. This procedure became the standard for what we now call a low imperforate anus. Until 1953, a key recommendation for the repairs of high imperforate anus was to stay close to the sacrum to avoid damage to the urinary tract during the dissection. Cadaveric dissections by Stephens[2] led him to use a combined sacral and abdominoperineal approach whereby he pulled the rectum down as close to the genitourinary tract as possible in an effort to preserve the puborectalis sling. In contrast to pre-1953, preservation of the puborectalis sling became the theme for many subsequent operative approaches to ARMs.[3–5] As more was learned about ARMs, not only the existence of the puborectalis sling but also the role (if any) such a muscle might play in bowel continence were both questioned.

A posterior sagittal approach to ARMs was introduced in 1982.[6,7] Through a wide posterior sagittal incision and with electrical stimulation of muscle, the surgeon can more correctly identify a spectrum of anorectal anomalies and tailor the reconstruction of the perineum. The posterior sagittal anorectoplasty (PSARP) approach to ARMs hopefully facilitates correlations of the anatomy of these malformations to the clinical results obtained for each type of male and female defect.

EMBRYOLOGY

In the past 10 years, the science of embryology has evolved from the mere study of isolated events in development to a two-stage process that links the formation of the body plan with the organs and tissues that belong in the respective regions of this body plan. We now know there are a set of genes that "pattern" the embryo such that organs and tissues appear where they are spatially meant to be, and an additional set of genes that are responsible for the actual formation of these organs and tissues.[8] As a result of a process called gastrulation (see later), this body plan is set up by the end of the third week of gestation. There is substantial literature identifying the genes responsible for the patterning of the cranial region of the embryo and the tissues these genes specify.[9] However, there is a paucity of data describing patterning of the caudal region of the embryo.[10–14]

Anomalies of the anorectum have been previously explained on the basis of an arrest of the caudal descent of the urorectal septum toward the cloacal membrane during the fourth week and ending by the eighth week of gestation.[15] The urorectal septum is composed of mesoderm. The growth, migration, and differentiation of this mesoderm constitute a critical pathway for normal descent of the urorectal septum as well as other mesodermally derived tissues in its vicinity. For example, formation of the muscular and skeletal systems also derive from mesoderm. Furthermore, it is quite likely that embryonic induction of a specific developmental pathway in one group of cells (i.e., movement of the urorectal septum) may induce adjacent tissue (i.e., sacral somites) to transform into muscle, bone, and skin. Substances that might alter this induction of organs or disrupt cell–cell interaction following specification by a genetic code include proteins of the extracellular matrix (laminin, fibronectin, and collagen types I and IV)[16,17] and growth factors. Activation of a sequential family of genes or intracellular biochemical changes may further affect the induction of these tissues. Thus, in addition to the spectrum of anorectal anomalies

TABLE 83-1. *Timetable of embryologic events leading to formation of the anorectum*

Week	Event
3	Gastrulation and formation of caudal eminence
4	Mesoderm forms somites; neural crest migration; formation of lumbosacral spinal nerves
4–6	Cloaca forms; somites differentiate
5	Sclerotome cells migrate around neural tube
6	Tourneux and Rathke mesoderm form and migrate; septation of cloaca into a urogenital sinus and anorectal canal; caudal end of embryo develops from the caudal eminence
7	Sacrum and caudal spinal cord completely formed
7–8	Striated muscle of perineum (levator ani, external sphincter) formed
8	Fusion of anal membrane (ectoderm) and the superior two-thirds (mesoderm) of anorectal canal give rise to dentate line and canalization of anus

that result from dysmorphogenesis of the mesodermally derived urorectal septum, important consideration must be given to the induction of the caudal regional triad of muscle, bone, and nerve in weeks three through eight of gestation (Table 83-1).

In general, ARMs are not related to either the preimplantation or fetal period but instead to the embryonic period of gestation (2 to 8 weeks). During the third week of embryogenesis, the process of gastrulation transforms the bilaminar germ disk into a trilaminar disk by ingress of epiblasts into the hypoblasts in an area called the primitive streak. Three definitive layers of the newly formed trilaminar germ disk are called ectoderm, endoderm, and mesoderm. The trilaminar germ disk forms the basis for the body plan, both cranially and caudally.[18,19] Gastrulation then is synonymous with formation of mesoderm and thus, the body plan. The implication of dysmorphogenesis this early in gestation is that patterning of the embryo is altered. Also, if something abnormal occurs this early in gestation, we should look regionally for other anomalies. There are, however, some malformations that almost never have associated defects (see Anatomy, Classification, and Description of Defects). This has clinical relevance because we know that with ARMs there is a 40% to 50% overall incidence of associated malformations.[20,21]

At either end of the embryo, the ectoderm and endoderm fuse, excluding the mesoderm in these areas, and give rise to a cranial buccopharyngeal and caudal cloacal membrane. The buccopharyngeal membrane breaks down in the fourth week to form the mouth. It is thought that the cloacal membrane fuses and canalizes in humans by the eighth week to give rise to the anus and distal urethra. However, formation of the cloacal membrane and an anal opening from the dorsal segment of the cloacal membrane has been identified as early as 10 days postcoitus in mice. Absence of any of the dorsal part of the developing cloaca and its membrane (as opposed to the urorectal septum) seems to give rise to a spectrum of fistulas or communications of the hindgut with the urogenital tract.[22] These findings lend credence to the notion that the events leading to formation of ARM can be ascribed to a much earlier time in gestation (i.e., gastrulation) and not solely the result of the movement of

the urorectal septum. Although these early embryologic errors were observed in a mutant mouse strain (Sd mouse), it is quite possible that this early sequence of dysmorphogenesis can also occur in humans.[23] Further examination of the Sd mouse reveals that it has an abnormal notocord resulting in reduced number of caudal vertebrae and abnormal cloaca and caudal gastrointestinal and genitourinary pathology.[24] These data suggest that there are very early links in the genetic code of the caudal body plan and the set of genes that subsequently form organs.

During the third week of embryogenesis as gastrulation proceeds, the primitive streak regresses caudally. In the caudal region of the embryo, the streak disappears giving rise to a mass of mesoderm cells called the caudal eminence. The caudal eminence gives rise to two very intimately related areas including the caudal somites of the body and the caudal end the neural tube. Mesoderm inferior to the second sacral level fuses with the more cranial neural tube. The caudal region of the body plan is dependent on the formation, differentiation, and migration of the caudal eminence and its derivatives. This process is complete by 6 weeks of development.

In the latter part of the third week of embryogenesis, the mesoderm cells on either side of the regressing primitive streak give rise to paraxial, intermediate, and lateral plate mesoderm. Paraxial mesoderm yields axial skeleton, voluntary muscle, and skin dermis. The intermediate mesoderm produces the urinary system and elements of the genital anatomy. The ventral layer of the lateral plate mesoderm gives rise to visceral mesoderm, and the dorsal layer of the lateral plate gives rise to parietal mesoderm, parts of the limbs, and most of the dermis.

Paraxial mesoderm gives rise to somitomeres, all during the third and fourth weeks, starting in the cranial end and terminating caudally. In humans, somitomeres form somites numbering 39 pairs in a cranial–cauded direction. Somites give rise to axial skeleton, vertebral columns, skull bones, voluntary muscles (i.e., levator muscle complex, external sphincter), and dermis (perineal skin).[25] They also give rise to the segmental pattern within the body wall that eventually gives rise to other structures such as blood vessels and nerves. The five pairs of sacral somites form the sacrum and associated musculature of the pelvis (levator ani group and external sphincter). The three pairs of coccygeal somites form the coccyx and probably contribute to induction of paraxial mesoderm in the perineum.

Somites subdivide into three types of mesoderm: myotomes, dermatomes, and mesenchymal sclerotomes. Sclerotomes (ventral portion of the somite) develop first and differentiate into vertebrae at all levels of the developing embryo. The adhesion molecule, N-cadherin, has been reported to be important for dissolution of the somite and formation of the sclerotome.[26] The remainder of the somite that remains forms the dermatomyotome (dorsal half of the somite). The dermatomes contribute to fat and connective tissue. The myotomes differentiate into muscle cells. Along the ventral surface of the body, these myotomes are called hypomeres. These hypomeres migrate into lateral plate mesoderm along with their respective dermatome and spinal nerves.[27] The muscles of the perineal region differentiate from hypomeres of the sacral and coccygeal regions of the embryo. As expected, dermatomes and spinal nerves also migrate along with the hypomeres giving rise to the levator ani musculature, external anal sphincter, and voluntary muscles of the external genitalia and their corresponding nerves.[28] Thus, in the caudal region of the developing embryo, like in the cranial region of the body plan, organization and migration of these mesodermally derived somites give rise to the triad of muscle, bone, and nerve.

Regionalization of the postgastrulation mesoderm in the area of the sacrum and coccyx is probably regulated by pattern formation. In the case of the anorectum, pattern formation facilitates localization of the urinary tract anterior to the rectum as well as a series of migrations that culminate in separate genital, urinary, and gastrointestinal tracts. In addition, the correct position of muscle with respect to the bones of the perineum is also probably dependent on pattern formation. This process is thought to be controlled in part by a class of genes called homeobox genes[29–33] and other families of homeotic genes all of which are genes that regulate the expression of other genes by producing transcriptional factors. The pharyngeal arches in the cranial region of the embryo are a prototype of patterning regulated by a homeobox genes.[34] The homeobox or *Hox* gene expression may specify a code for postgastrulation mesoderm differentiation such as the paraxial mesoderm and simultaneously all three germ layers surrounding this area.[35,36]

During the fourth week, the neural plate folds into the neural tube by a process called neurulation. Special subpopulations of cells that arise from the lateral regions of the developing neural tube are called neural crest cells. These specialized detached cells give rise to a variety of components of the peripheral nervous system that ultimately innervate the developing gut (including the hindgut). In fact, peripheral sensory neurons and parasympathetic and sympathetic peripheral motor neurons are all neural crest derivatives. An important neurologic milestone related to ARMs, during the fourth week of embryogenesis, is the formation of the spinal nerves from sacral levels 2, 3, and 4, which contributes to the peripheral parasympathetic nervous system. In contrast to the failure of migration and thus absence of ganglion cells observed in Hirschsprung disease, abnormal matrix, cell-to-cell communication, or an abnormal induction pathway of neural crest development may be the basis for rectosigmoid propioceptive and motility problems associated with ARMs. In the absence of any gross anatomic abnormality, the clinical manifestations of such a molecular embryologic phenomenon may include postoperative complaints of constipation and incontinence.

The caudal end of the neural plate (flanked by somites) gives rise to the lower end of the spinal cord. Secondary neurulation takes place once the neural plate has closed (primary neurulation) over a period of 7 weeks and is defined as the formation of the spinal cord at the caudal limit or tail bud of the embryo.[37] The tail bud contributes to the sacral and coccyx levels of the spinal cord. The caudal eminence also induces both spinal cord and other paraxial mesoderm cells so that ultimately this area forms the nervous system of the caudal part of the body. Defects in the caudal eminence give rise to sacral agenesis and the fatal dysmorphogenic caudal regression syndrome of Duhamel[38] (Fig. 83-1). Muscle, bone, and nerve pathology is associated with this lethal condition that may be the result of abnormal gastrulation in a very specific area of the primitive streak. It is possible that defects in the derivatives of the mesodermally derived caudal eminence are caused by macromolecules of the extracellular martix.[16] In addition, cell surface glycoproteins and cell adhesion molecules (N-CAM) participate in the transformation of the caudal eminence.[39] These disturbances may

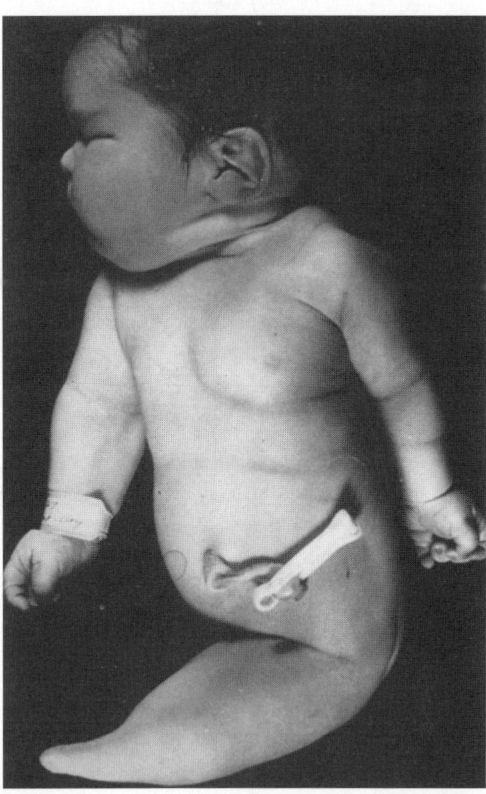

FIG. 83-1. Sirenomelia, the most severe form of the Duhamel caudal regression or dysplasia syndrome, is characterized by a constellation of congenital anomalies that includes muscle, bone, and nerve derived from the caudal eminence.

have a multifactorial etiology and include both genetic and environmental causes.

It is widely held but never has been proved that between weeks four and six the primitive gut tube at the level of the cloacal membrane gets canalized and partitioned into an anterior urogenital sinus and a posterior anorectum by the cranial caudal growth of a mesodermally derived partition called the urorectal septum (see Fig. 83-2). Ultimately, the urorectal septum fuses with the cloacal membrane and the fusion site is called the perineal body.

Overgrowth of the cloacal membrane prevents the lateral mesoderm from forming the anterior abdominal wall and the cloaca ruptures. If the cloacal membrane ruptures after complete descent of the urorectal septum, exstrophy of the bladder occurs, whereas rupture before descent of the septum yields cloacal exstrophy.

The urorectal septum is a composite of two mesoderm structures: the midline Tourneux fold and two lateral Rathke folds (see Fig. 83-2). In contrast to the superior two thirds of the anal canal, the inferior third is derived from ectoderm called the anal pit or proctodeum (Fig. 83-3). The anal membrane resorbs by the eighth week, and this area when fused with the descending mesoderm of the hindgut is called the pectinate or dentate line. Some authors feel that proof of this process of septation or caudal migration of a septum is lacking and the partitioning of the cloaca is the result of normal dorsal–ventral cloacal development.[22,40]

The failure of Rathke folds to develop results in arrest of

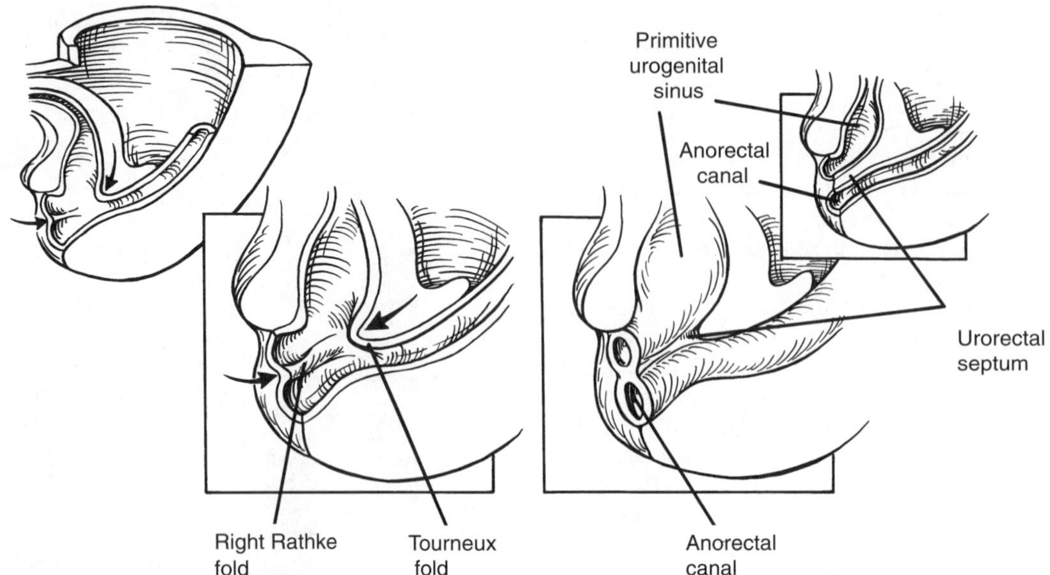

FIG. 83-2. Septation of the cloacal membrane by the urorectal septum. Craniocaudal and lateral mesoderm of the urorectal septum partition the cloaca into an anterior urogenital sinus and posterior anorectum.

the inferior part of the urorectal septum and thus rectourethral (prostatic) fistulas in the male and a common channel (cloaca) for the urethra, vagina, and rectum in the female (Fig. 83-4).

In females, the distal end of the urogenital sinus forms the vestibule and distal third of the vagina. The proximal vagina and uterus are formed following fusion of the paramesonephric ducts (müllerian ducts) and union of these structures with the proximal urogenital sinus. It is thought that formation of the uterus, vagina, and fallopian tubes requires the absence of anti-müllerian hormone or müllerian-inhibiting substance.[41]

The arrest of Rathke folds usually takes place just below the paramesonephric ducts, but a slightly more caudal failure of Rathke folds could result in a high rectovaginal fistula in the female (see Fig. 83-4).

The failure of both Tourneux and Rathke folds results in rectobladder neck fistulas in both sexes (Fig. 83-5). We suspect that this is not true because we have not seen a rectovesical fistula in a female with normal genitalia. Instead, failure of both folds is more likely to be a cloacal anomaly in the female. In the female, failure of formation of both folds can also result in duplicated vaginas and uteruses that empty into one bladder. This concept is consistent with what we find in the spectrum of cloacal anomalies.

Malalignment of Tourneux and Rathke folds may result in formation of a rectourethral (bulbar) fistula in males and a low vaginal or vestibular fistula in females (Fig. 83-6).

Imperforate anus without fistula results from the anal pit not forming. Mesodermally derived Tourneux and Rathke folds are

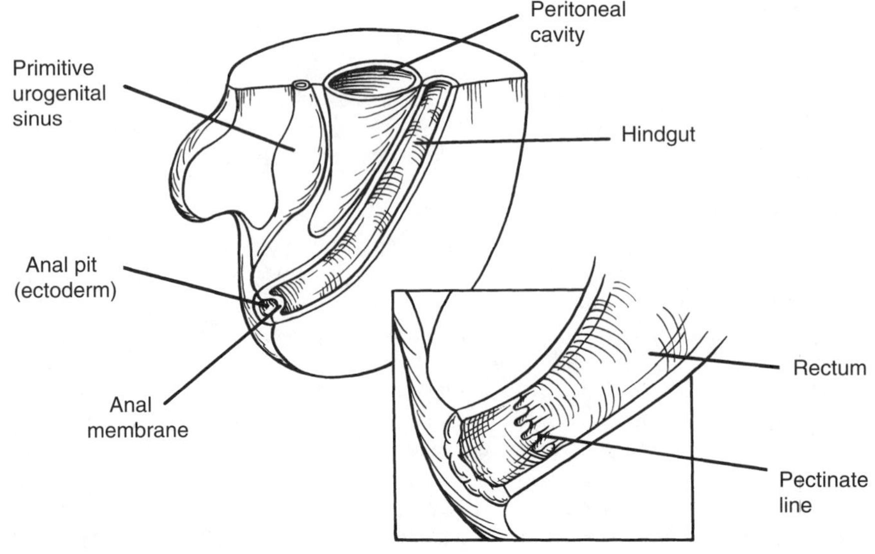

FIG. 83-3. Formation of the anal canal. The lower third of the anorectum is derived from ectoderm. As the anal membrane is resorbed, the ectoderm fuses with the more proximal mesoderm at an area called the pectinate or dentate line.

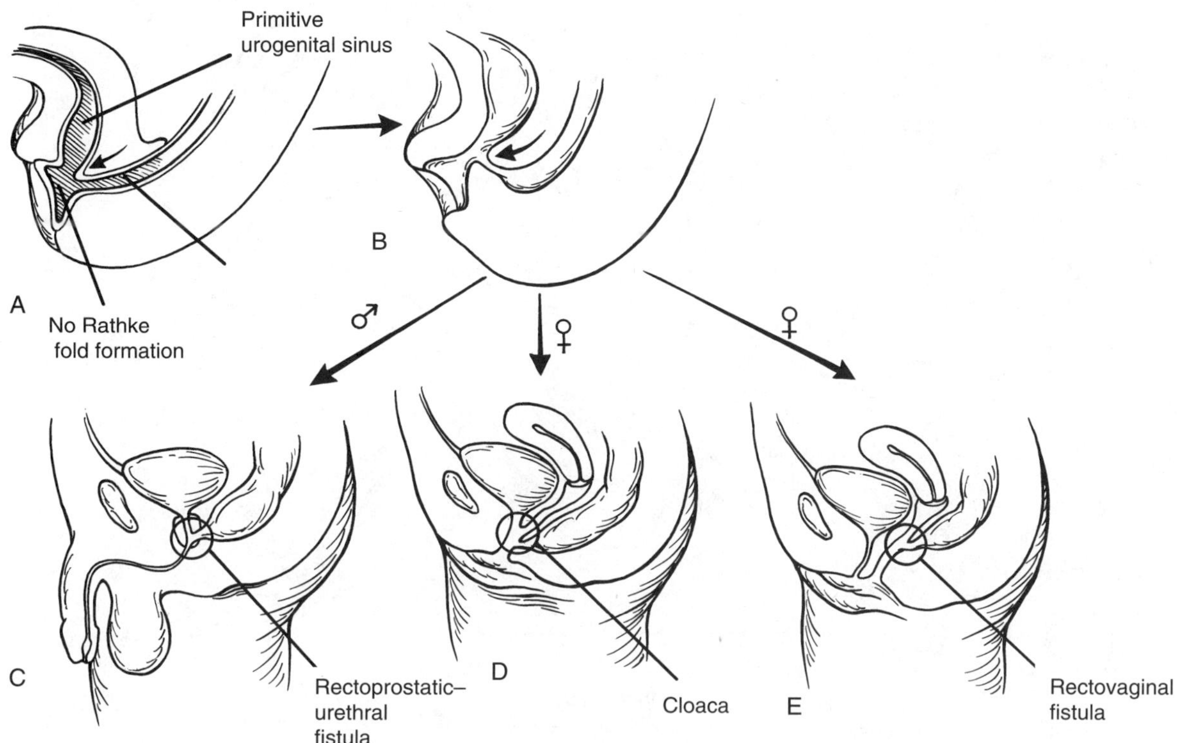

FIG. 83-4. Fate of the embryo following failure of Rathke fold development. Arrest of this mesoderm probably results in a rectoprostatic fistula in the male and a common cloaca or the rare high rectovaginal fistula in the female.

aligned but the ectodermally derived anal pit has not fused with the mesoderm. Thus, the result is an imperforate anus but no fistula to the skin (Fig. 83-7).

Formation of the anal pit but failure of the anal membrane to resorb or resorb incompletely results in rectal atresia or anal stenosis, respectively. This fusion defect consists of cloacal ectoderm and descending rectal mesoderm (Fig. 83-8).

Fusion of the genital folds gives rise to a covered anus. This does not happen in females because in the absence of testosterone there is no fusion of the genital folds, but instead they

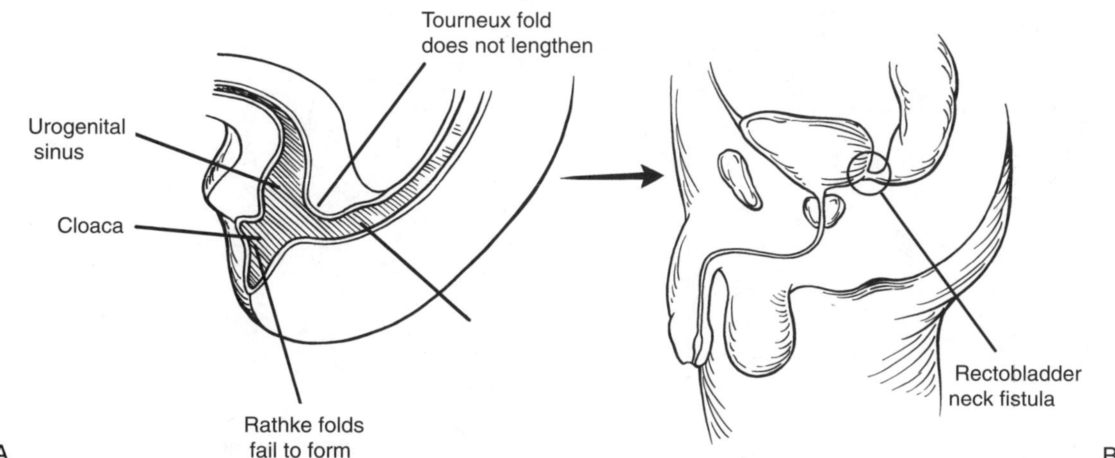

FIG. 83-5. Failure of both Tourneux and Rathke folds. In all likelihood this probably results in a rectovesical (bladder neck) fistula in the male and a common cloaca in the female. We have never seen a rectovesical fistula in a female.

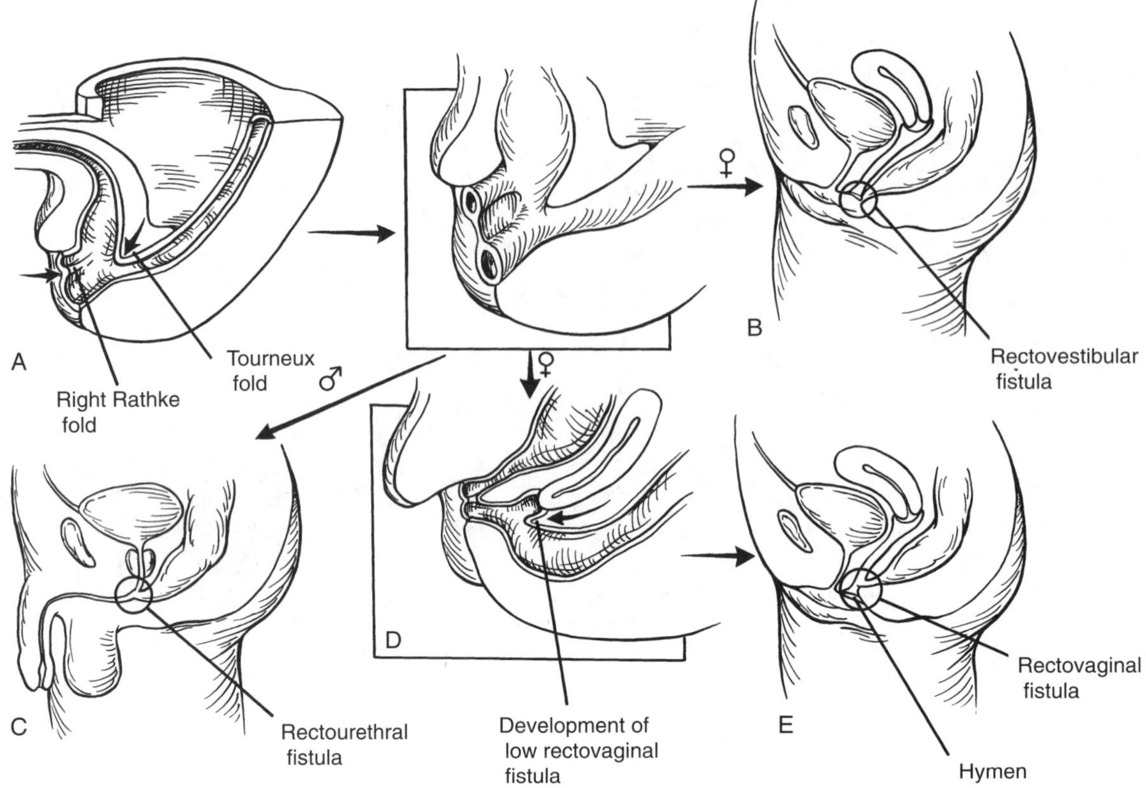

FIG. 83-6. Malalignment of Tourneux and Rathke folds. In males (*C*), a rectobulbar urethral fistula occurs; by contrast, in the female, a low vaginal or rectovestibular fistula occurs. We suspect that most low vaginal fistulas are more appropriately classified as either a vestibular fistula (*B*) or a cloaca because a true rectovaginal fistula is so rare.

remain separate to form the labia. Defects in the mesoderm at the level of the perineal body where fusion of the ectoderm and endoderm is taking place result in a misplaced anal opening, called a perineal fistula (Fig. 83-9).

In the next few years, it should not be surprising to find genetic literature linking the formation of the body plan (gastrulation) with postgastrulation organ formation in the caudal region of the embryo. Ultimately, these data should give rise to the regionalized phenomenon of caudal patterning of muscle, bone, and nerve. The Sd mouse is an excellent model for com-

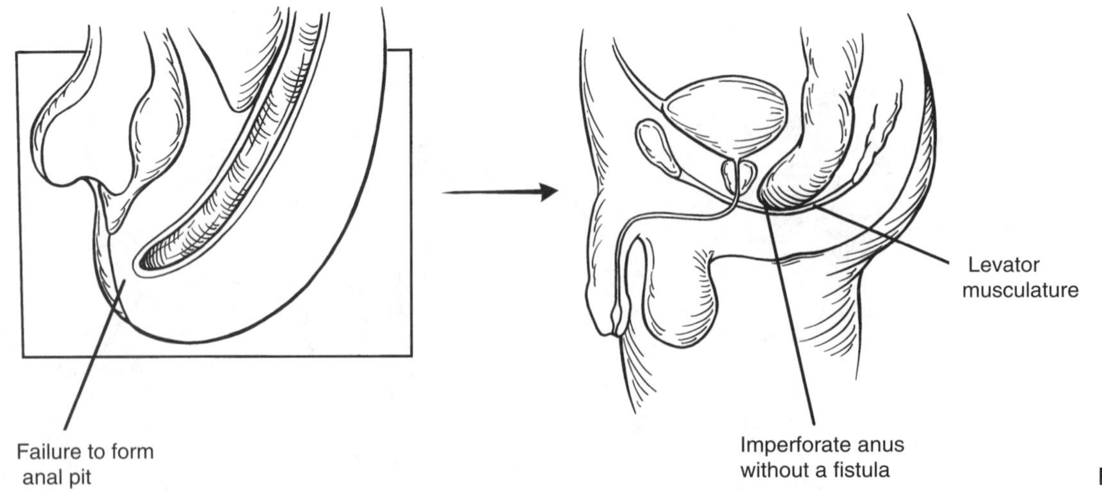

FIG. 83-7. Dysmorphogenesis causing imperforate anus without a fistula. Arrest of formation of the anal pit causes imperforate anus without a fistula.

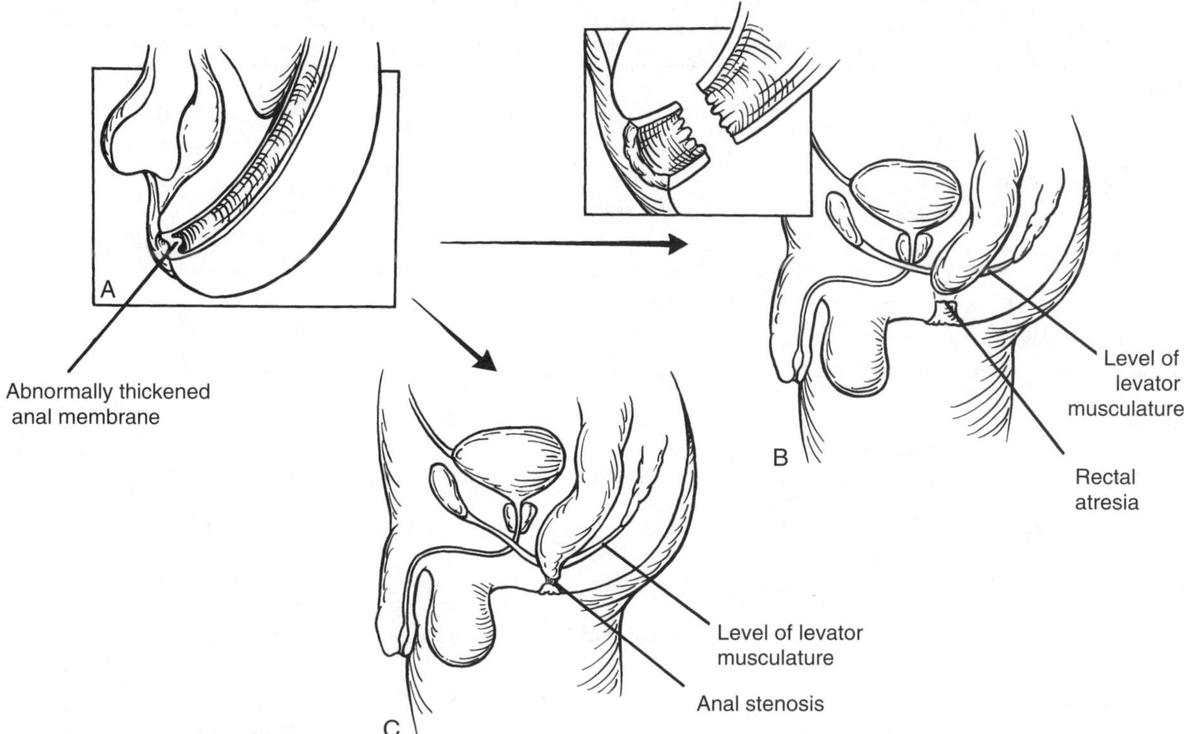

FIG. 83-8. Cause of rectal atresia or anal stenosis is illustrated. Failure of the anal membrane to resorb and fuse with the descending mesoderm results in rectal atresia. Incomplete resorption gives rise to varying degrees of anal stenosis.

plex ARMs and may be used in the future to probe the two-stage process involving the origin, fate, and interaction of meso-derm (the body plan) and regional organ formation.

GENETICS

As early as 1950, records were compiled about congenital anomalies, their incidence, and their overall contribution to ma-

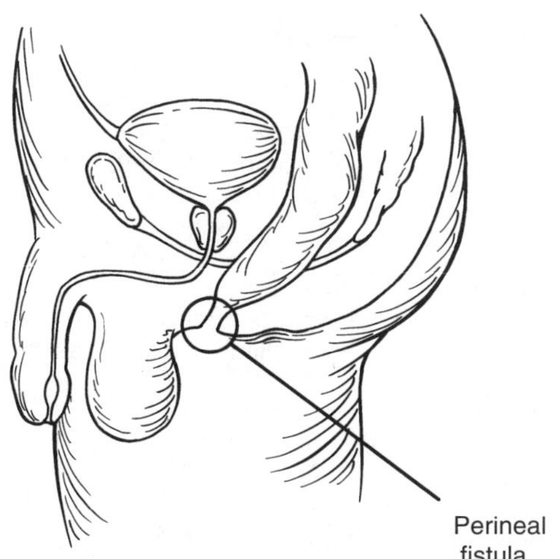

FIG. 83-9. The perineal fistula. Deficient or abnormally situated mesoderm at the level of the perineal body in both sexes results in an anal opening anterior to the striated muscle of the external sphincter.

ternal and fetal morbidity and mortality. Over 90% of congenital anomalies occur in the first 8 weeks of gestation and more than half of these occur in the first 4 weeks or just after gastrulation.[42] As for ARMs, the overall incidence approaches 1 in 5000 live births[43] and the risk for future pregnancies in a mother of a patient with ARM is 1 in 100 or 1%.[44] Relative to all types of caudal regression anomalies, ARMs are much more common if one separates out the incidence of persistent cloaca (1:40,000 to 50,000) and cloacal exstrophy (1:200,000).[45] Yet, we suspect that the real incidence of persistent cloaca is much higher based on the fact that so many alleged rectovaginal fistulas are cloacas. In general, males slightly outnumber females by about three to one and there seems to be no ethnic predilection.

The genetic basis of ARMs is multifactorial, meaning there is no one single cause,[46] ARMs can be caused by a sporadic or an inherited event. Sporadic events are isolated and probably induced by some as yet unknown genetic or environmental cause. It is unclear if a sporadic case is inherited. If, however, another sibling or descendent has an ARM, then one can infer that the malformation is inherited either as an isolated event or as part of a syndrome. The patterns of ARM inheritance include the mendelian disorders (autosomal dominant, recessive, etc.), chromosomal abnormalities (i.e., cat eye syndrome), or environmental teratogens (i.e., maternal diabetes). Some syndromes that include ARMs can be inherited as a result of multiple gene mutations, hence, the term *hetrogeneous causation*. The actual incidence of sporadic versus inherited ARMs is unknown despite literature quotes supporting a higher incidence of isolated ARMs.[47] Based on the fact that there is a reported range of associated anomalies between 22% and 72%, it is very possible

TABLE 83-2. *Anorectal malformations (ARMs) in association with extraanal anomalies*

Syndrome	Prominent features	Causation*
ARM ALONE		
Isolated imperforate anus	None	Heterogeneous, AR, XLR, and AD
ARM AND NEUROLOGIC ANOMALIES		
Anosacral defect	Anterior sacral meningocele, teratoma, or cyst	Heterogeneous, AD (176450), XLD (312800)
FG	Macrocephaly, broad forehead, frontal hair upswept, hypotonia, mental retardation	XL (305450)
ARM AND SKELETAL ANOMALIES		
Baller–Gerold	Craniosynostosis, radial defect, short stature	AR (218600)
IVIC	Radial defects, strabismus, thrombocytopenia, deafness	AD (147750)
Jarcho–Levin	Rib and vertebral defects, respiratory failure in infancy	AR (277300)
Presacral teratoma	Sacral dysgenesis	AD (176450)
Saldino–Noonan	Short ribs, short limbs, postaxial polydactyly, visceral abnormalities, lethality	AR (263530)
Say	Preaxial polydactyly, malformed vertebral bodies and ribs (may be the same as PIV syndrome)	Sporadic
Thanatophoric dysplasia	Micromelia, platyspondyly, early death	Sporadic (187600)
Townes–Brocks	Deafness, triphalangeal thumbs, overfolded helices, flat feet	AD (107480)
ARM AND CHROMOSOMAL ANOMALIES		
Cat eye	Ocular coloboma; ear, cardiac, and renal anomalies; variable mental retardation	Heterogeneous; have an extra small metacentric chromosome, possibly rearranged chromosome 2
Tetrasomy 12p	Coarse face, sparse anterior scalp hair, hypertelorism, epicanthus, hypotonia, hypomelanotic spots, severe mental retardation	Chromosomal anomaly
ARM AND CARDIOVASCULAR ANOMALIES		
Fuhrmann	Polydactyly, heart defect	Uncertain
ARM AND UROGENITAL ANOMALIES		
Hypertelorism-hypospadias	Hypertelorism, hypospadias (may be the same as Opitz G syndrome)	XLR (313600)
Opitz BBB	Same as Opitz G	
Opitz G	Hypertelorism, hypospadias, swallowing defects	AD (145410)
ARM AND MULTIPLE ANOMALIES		
Ankyloblepharon filiforme	Fused eyelids and normal globe endocardial cushion defects, fused digits, cleft lip and palate, esophageal atresia	AD (106250)
Adnatum		Chromosomal anomaly
ASP association	Anal anomalies, sacral defect, presacral mass (teratoma, cyst, or meningomyelocele)	AD (176450)
Axial mesodermal defect	Sacral dysgenesis; dysfunction of lower limbs, bladder, and bowel; aphalangy, spinal, and rib abnormalities	AR
Caudal regression	Dysgenesis of lower spine; variable dysfunction of bladder, bowel, and lower limbs	Heterogeneous, maternal diabetes mellitus in some cases AD (182940)
Christian skeletal dysplasia	Metopic ridge, cervical fusion, dysplastic spine, abducens palsy, mental retardation	XLR (309620)
Cryptophthalmos	Palate, ear, renal, laryngeal, genital, digital, and eye malformations	AR (219000)
Diabetes, maternal	Fetal overgrowth; increased incidence of neural tube defects, cardiac anomalies, caudal dysgenesis, and renal defects	Exposure of abnormal glucose metabolism during pregnancy
Johanson–Blizzard	Hypoplastic alae nasi, exocrine pancreatic insufficiency, deafness, hypothyroidism	AR (243800)

TABLE 83-2. *Continued.*

Syndrome	Prominent features	Causation*
Kaufman–McKusick	Congenital heart defects, polydactyly, hydrometrocolpos	AR (236700)
Lowe	Sensorineural deafness, nephritis	AD
Meckel	Encephalocele, polydactyly, cystic kidneys	AR (249000)
OEIS	Omphalocele, exstrophy of the bladder, imperforate anus, spinal defects	Uncertain, may have vascular causation
Pallister–Hall	Hypothalamic hamartoblastoma, hypopituitarism, postaxial polydactyly	Sporadic (146510)
Pallister: ulnar-mammary	Ulnar ray defects, delayed puberty, oligodactyly or polydactyly, hypoplasia of apocrine glands and breasts, genital anomalies	AD (181450)
PIV	Polydactyly, imperforate anus, vertebral anomalies	Sporadic (174100)
Potter variant	Renal, lung, thymic, parathyroid, dysplasia	AR (?), chromosomal anomaly
Rieger	Ocular anterior chamber anomalies, hypodontia	AD (180500)
Sirenomelia	Single, lower limb, renal agenesis, genital agenesis	Sporadic, based on vascul steal
VACTERL	Vertebral, anal, cardiac, tracheo-esophageal, renal, and radial limb defects	Sporadic (19235)

* Number in parentheses represents the Online Mendelian Inheritance in Man classification[51] on-line data base.

AD, autosomal dominant; AR, autosomal recessive; ASP, anal anomalies, sacral defect, presacral mass; PIV, polydactyly, imperforate anus, vertebral anomalies; VACTERL, vertebral, anal, cardiac tracheo-esophageal, renal, and radial limb defects; XL, X linked; XLR, X linked recessive; XLD, X linked dominant.[114,144]

that sporadic cases are in fact part of a syndrome.[21] Granted we have multiple examples of hindgut dysmorphogenesis that can account for these associations, it is compelling to consider a syndromic etiology as advances in molecular genetics occur. There is some evidence, albeit scant, that isolated low anal malformations (perineal fistula, covered anus) may be inherited, whereas isolated high ARM lesions are likely to be sporadic embryologic events with little to no risk of familial recurrence.[48,49] Similar to the sporadic ARMs, the familial-related ARMs carry a 50% incidence of associated malformations.[50]

Both from a reproductive counseling perspective and for postnatal care, the potential for inheriting an ARM must be considered. Because it is nearly impossible to make an antenatal diagnosis of the more common ARMs, detailed family pedigree may provide a clue to potential hereditary mechanisms. Risks of recurrence within a family can then be based on the pattern of inheritance. For example, if an autosomal dominant condition is identified, it carries a 50% incidence of recurrence, whereas a recessive condition occurs in 25% of offspring. Family genetic counseling about ARMs should also include the potential for association with other system anomalies and chromosomal defects. A prenatal karyotyping should be performed in all cases in which there is a family history of ARMs.

Postnatal physical examination should alert physicians to the possibility that the baby has a syndrome. Table 83-2 is a helpful guide for the extraanal anomalies associated with ARMs. The mendelian inheritance in man (MIM) number is an on-line computerized data base[51] that can be accessed for a more complete update of each diagnosis. The vertebral, anal, tracheoesophageal, renal, and radial limb anomalies (VATER)[52,53] or vertebral, anal, cardiac, tracheoesophageal, renal, and nonradial limb anomalies (VACTERL)[54,55], associations should not be the sole extraanal associations ruled out when evaluating a patient with an ARM. This is especially important from an embryologic perspective when we consider that the mesoderm involved in the VATER and VACTERL associations as well as all compo-

nents of the other anomalies listed in Table 83-2 are present by the fifth week of gestation. Likewise, if a baby has skeletal, visceral, or neurologic anomalies, one should look for the constellation of bowel, bladder, or bone anomalies.[56]

ANATOMY, CLASSIFICATION, AND DESCRIPTION OF DEFECTS

In general, the frequency of ARMs is slightly higher in males compared with females and this also includes the potential for associated anomalies. A rectourethral (bulbar and prostatic urethra) fistula is the most frequent defect in newborn males followed by a perineal fistula. Higher defects, such as the rectobladder neck fistula, occur in less than 10% of male series.[57,58]

In females, by far the most frequent defect is an imperforate anus with a rectovestibular fistula followed in frequency again by the perineal fistula. Most cases of rectovaginal fistulas are probably misdiagnosed rectovestibular fistulas or cloacas because in Pena's series of more than 800 cases, rectovaginal fistulas were virtually nonexistent. The common cloaca comprises about 10% of the defects in females and ranks third in frequency.[57,58]

Imperforate anus without a fistula occurs in less than 5% of cases in both sexes and has a high association with Down Syndrome.[57,58]

Although there is a long history of proposed classifications for ARMs, the 1984 Wingspread classification[59] of high, intermediate, and low defects has been used extensively.[60,61] With respect to therapy and prognosis, however, the classification falls short of implications and utility. A therapy-oriented classification is shown in Table 83-3. This proposed categorization combines diagnosis and treatment, and therefore should facilitate more homogeneous communication about specific malformations among pediatric surgeons.

TABLE 83-3. *Proposed classification of defects*

MALE

NO COLOSTOMY
Rectoperineal (cutaneous) fistula

COLOSTOMY
Rectourethral fistula (bulbar, prostatic)
Rectobladder neck
Imperforate anus without fistula
Rectal atresia and stenosis

FEMALE

NO COLOSTOMY
Rectoperineal (cutaneous) defects

COLOSTOMY
Vestibular fistula
Rectovaginal fistula (extremely unusual)
Persistent cloaca
Imperforate anus without fistula
Rectal atresia and stenosis

Male Defects

Perineal Fistula

Perineal fistula is a low defect (Fig. 83-10). The lowest part of the rectum opens on the perineum anterior to the center of the external sphincter. The more proximal rectum remains within the muscles of the sphincter. A subepithelial rectoperineal fistula can be found along the midline raphe from the base of the scrotum or penis (Fig. 83-11*A*). Occasionally a skin tag is encountered (bucket handle deformity, (Fig. 83-11*B*) below which meconium may be seen coming from the fistulous tract. Male and female patients with a perineal fistula have a well-developed midline groove and anal dimple, normal sacrum, ample sphincter musculature, normal rounded contour of their buttocks, and minimal urinary and neurologically associated anomalies.

Rectourethral Fistula

The rectourethral fistula defect (Fig. 83-12) is characterized by the rectum communicating with the posterior part of the urethra at its lower (bulbar, Fig. 83-12*A*) or upper segment (prostatic, Fig. 83-12*B*). In general, the patients with a bulbar fistula have a substantial sphincter mechanism, normal sacrum, prominent midline groove, and well-defined anal dimple. In contrast, those males with a rectoprostatic urethral fistula have a more flat contour buttock, poor sphincter mechanism, abnormal sacrum, and poorly defined anal dimple. Most males fit these observations but there are exceptions such that a rectoprostatic fistula can be associated with a normal sacrum, defined anal dimple, and good muscle.

Above the rectourethral fistula, the rectum and urethra share a common wall. As expected, the common wall is longer in cases of a bulbar fistula in contrast with a prostatic fistula. The rectum in both types of rectourethral fistulas is usually surrounded by the funnel-shaped voluntary striated muscle mechanism innervated by the sacral plexus (sacral levels 2, 3, and 4).

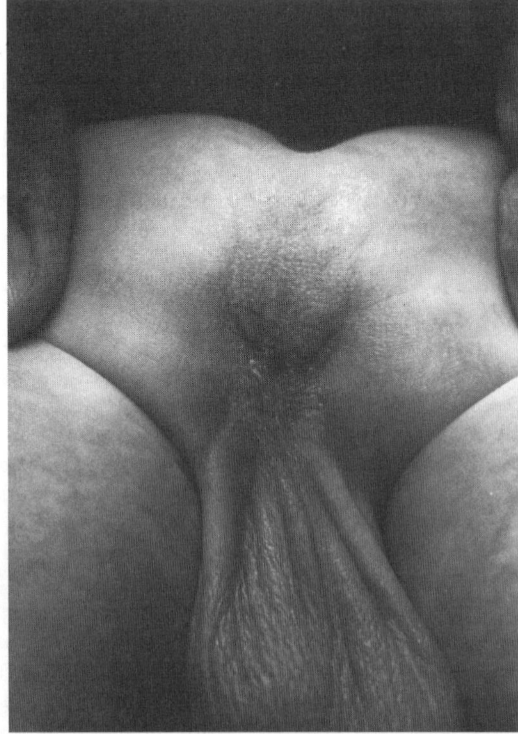
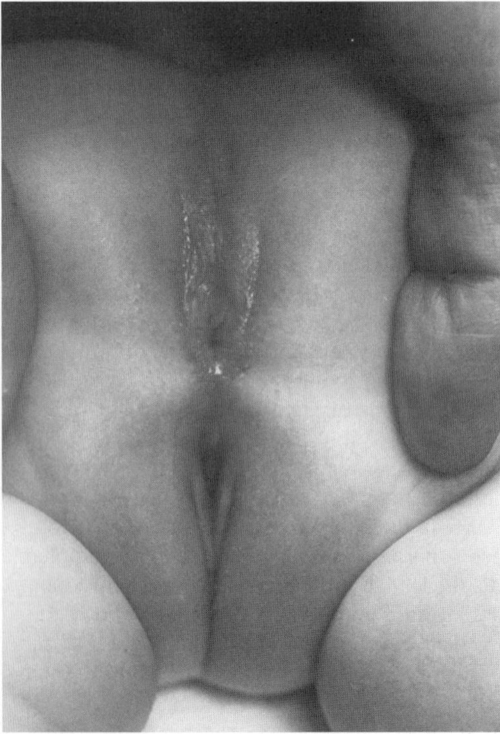

FIG. 83-10. Perineal fistula in (*A*) male and (*B*) female. Electrical stimulation of perineal skin shows that the anal opening is anterior to the external sphincter muscle.

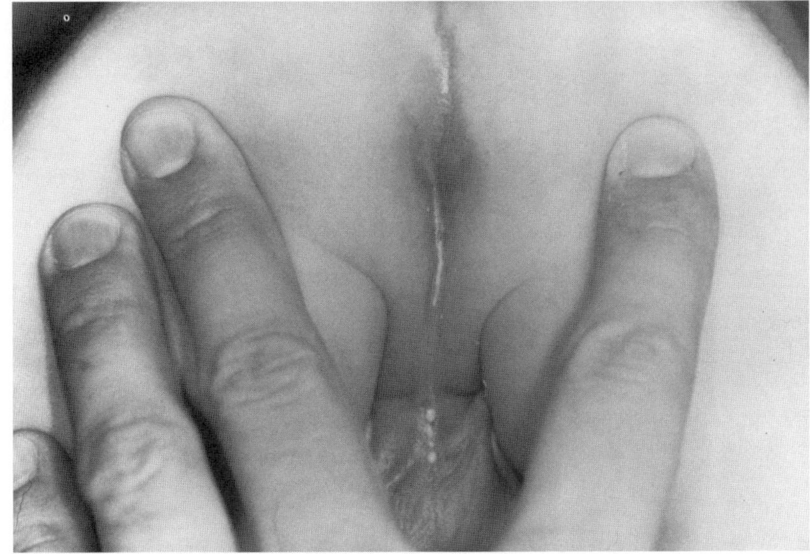

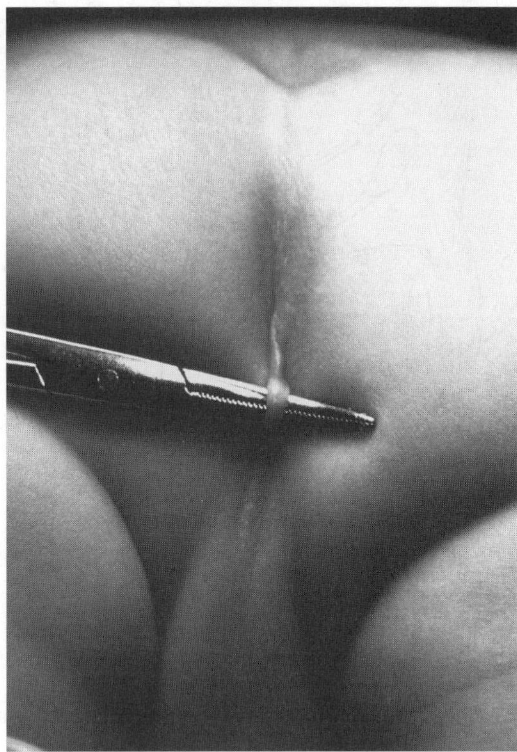

FIG. 83-11. (*A*) Subepithelial rectoperineal fistula. (*B*) Bucket handle deformity.

Rectobladder Neck Fistula

In the case of rectobladder neck fistula defect (Fig. 83-13), the rectum opens at the bladder neck in a T configuration. In contrast with a rectourethral fistula common wall, patients with a bladder neck fistula do not share a common wall. In these defects, the rectum is located above the funnel-shaped levator musculature. Ectopic ureters usually open into the bladder close to the site of the fistula. The perineum is usually flat, there is a paucity of perineal muscle, and the sacrum is dystrophic and frequently absent. This ARM has a high frequency of associated anomalies.

Imperforate Anus Without Fistula

In the imperforate anus without fistula defect, (Fig. 83-14), the rectum ends approximately 2 cm from the perineal skin.

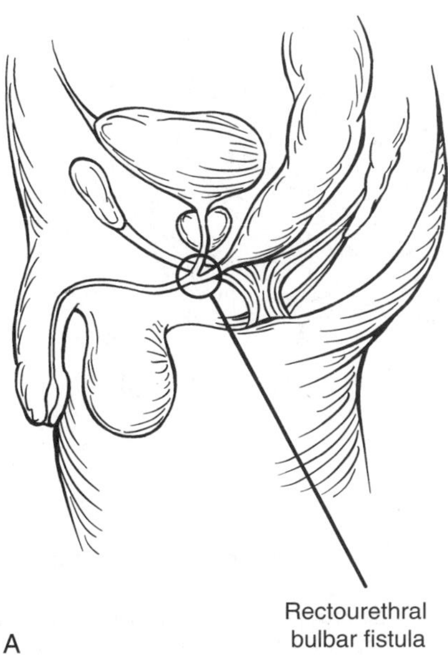

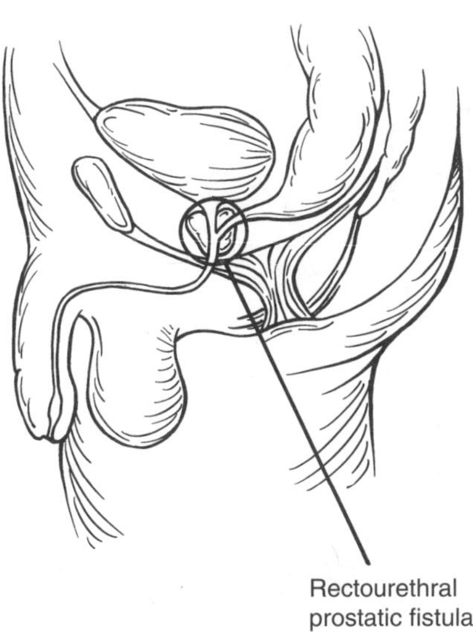

FIG. 83-12. (*A*) Rectourethral bulbar fistula. (*B*) Rectourethral prostatic fistula.

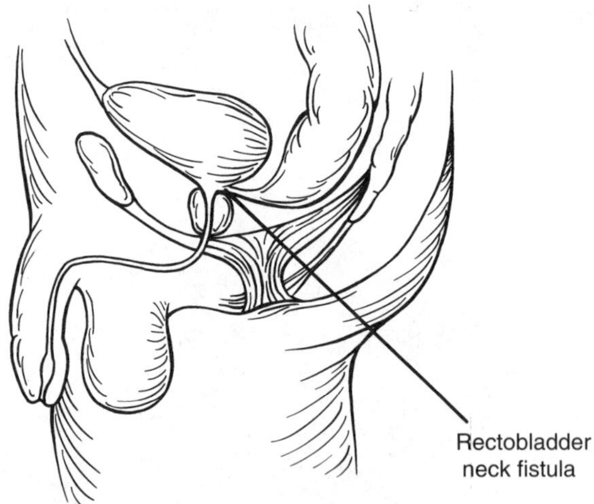

FIG. 83-13. Rectobladder neck fistula.

The sphincter mechanism, muscles, and sacrum are all usually present, and thus bowel function is predictably good. Even though there is no direct communication between the urethra and anus, however, there is a very thin common wall between these structures.

Rectal Atresia and Stenosis

In the cases of rectal atresia (Fig. 83-15) and stenosis, the rectum ends blindly (atresia) or partially communicates with the distal anal canal (stenosis). Typically these patients have a normal-looking anus that ends blindly 1 to 2 cm above the perineal skin. The atresia or stenosis occurs at the embryologic junction of the anal canal with the rectum. These two structures are separated by a thin membrane or fibrous band. Following repair, continence and sensation are usually excellent. Voluntary muscles, sacrum, and perineum are nearly normal.

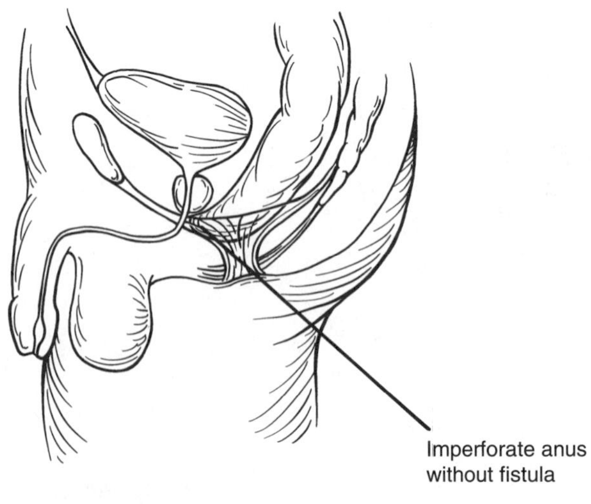

FIG. 83-14. Imperforate anus without fistula.

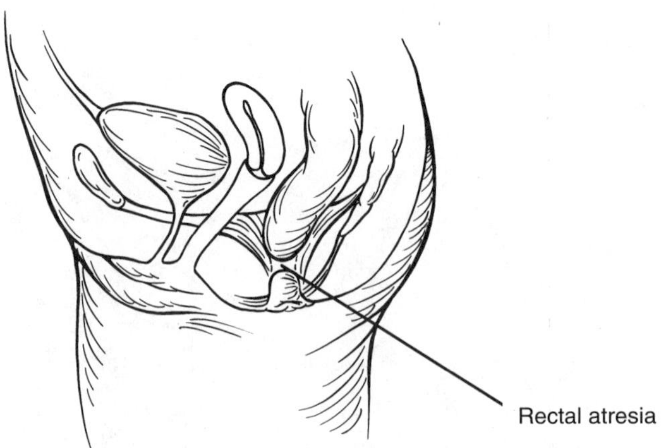

FIG. 83-15. Rectal atresia.

Female Defects

Rectoperineal Fistula

The rectoperineal fistula malformation is the equivalent to the low-lying male cutaneous fistula because it is also surrounded by skin. The anus opens onto the perineal body anterior to the external sphincter, yet, the opening is posterior to the vestibule of the vagina. These patients have an excellent anal dimple and buttock contour. The sacrum in this defect is normal as is the presence of the levator musculature. Rectum and vagina are also well separated and thus there is no shared common wall.

Rectovestibular Fistula

The rectovestibular fistula ARM is characterized by the rectum opening immediately behind the hymen within the vestibule of the vagina (Fig. 83-16). This defect is frequently erro-

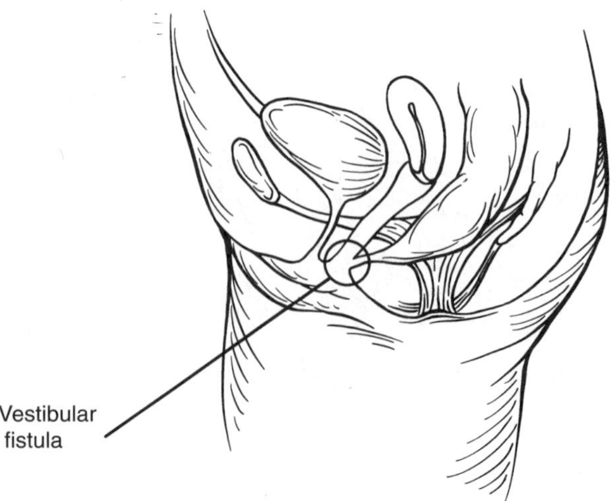

FIG. 83-16. Rectovestibular fistula in parasagittal plane and photo of introitus. The fistula is anterior to the hymenal ring, yet within the introitus. We do not consider this a low defect and as such bring up a colostomy prior to definitive repair.

neously diagnosed as a rectovaginal fistula. Just above the fistula the rectum and vagina are separated by a thin common wall. Yet, these patients usually have excellent musculature, normal sacrum, and anal dimple.

Imperforate Anus Without Fistula and Rectal Atresia and Stenosis

The imperforate anus without fistula and rectal atresia and stenosis malformations have similar anatomic, diagnostic, therapeutic, and prognostic implications in males and females (see Figs. 83-14 and 83-15). Imperforate anus without a fistula has a slightly higher incidence in females compared with males.

Persistent Cloaca

The persistent cloaca (Fig. 83-17) defect is characterized by fusion of the rectum, vagina, and urethra into a single common channel.[62] The length of the common channel varies between 1 and 10 cm. A short common channel is usually defined as shorter than 3 cm, whereas common channels longer than 3 cm are considered long-channel malformations. Figure 83-17B shows a child with cloaca with a common channel of approximately 3 cm. Figure 83-17A is the perineum in a female baby with imperforate anus, small genitalia, and single perineal orifice. In contrast, Figure 83-17C shows a case in which the common channel is much longer. In this situation, separation and mobilization of the three structures, creating two walls out of

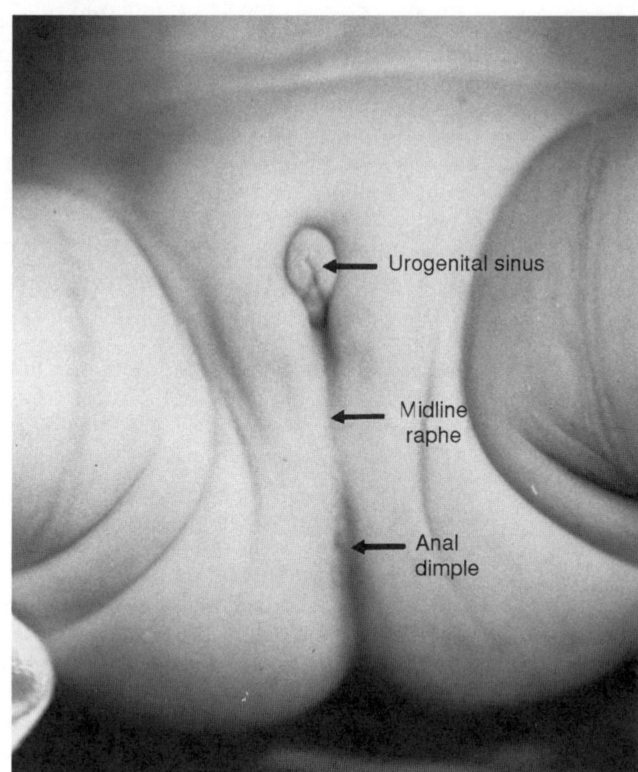

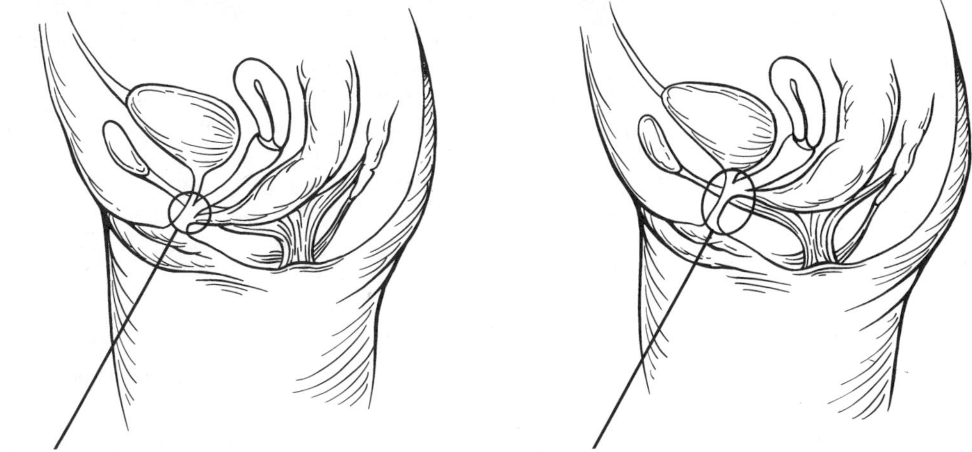

FIG. 83-17. (*A*) Persistent cloaca, external topography. (*B*) Common channel cloaca shorter than 3 cm. (*C*) Common channel cloaca longer than 3 cm.

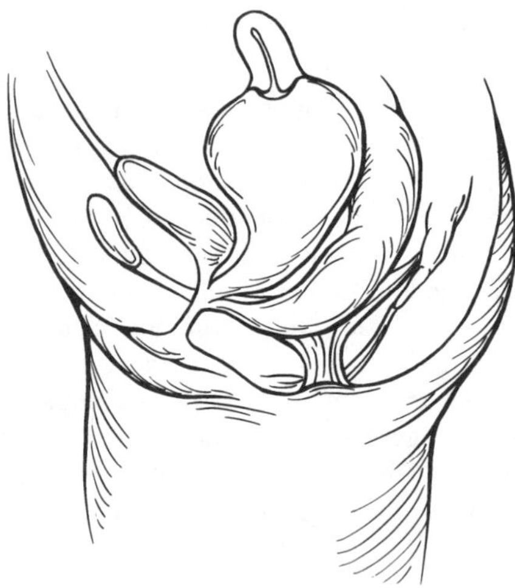

FIG. 83-18. Hydrocolpos in a cloaca.

each common wall between the urethra and vagina as well as the vagina and rectum, is difficult and most likely requires some form of vaginal replacement and probable laparotomy. Urinary function may be compromised in these long-channel defects. The perineum is usually well developed, and musculature, sacrum, and innervation are adequate in cases of short common channels. Frequently, the vagina in cases of persistent cloaca is distended and full of secretions (hydrocolpos) (Fig. 83-18). In some series, the incidence of a hydrocolpos approaches 40%.[61,62] The hydrocolpos may compress the trigone of the bladder and interfere with drainage of the ureters. In addition, the vagina and uterus frequently suffer from different degrees of septation or even complete separation of two hemivaginas or two hemiuteruses. Patients with persistent cloaca have a high incidence of associated anomalies.

ANATOMY AND PHYSIOLOGY

For the pediatric surgeon, pertinent aspects of the anatomy and physiology of the anorectum should include knowledge of the normal process of defecation and continence and how these processes can be affected by the spectrum of ARMs. With respect to both defecation and continence, we must focus on the sphincteric mechanism, anorectal sensation, propioception, and finally rectosigmoid motility. These areas comprise the functional elements of normal defecation and fecal continence. It is incumbent on the surgeon to realize how defecation and fecal continence can exist, given a spectrum of ARMs, a spectrum of anatomy, physiology.

Anatomy of Normal Children

Sphincter Mechanism

In normal children, the muscle groups of the sphincter mechanism include the voluntary striated muscles of the external sphincter and the levator musculature, and the involuntary, smooth muscle, internal sphincter (Fig. 83-19).

The striated external sphincter follows a circular path around the anus and is organized into three parts: subcutaneous, superficial, and deep[64] (Fig. 83-19). It is believed that the external sphincter is in a tonic state of contraction at rest. Because it can both relax and augment its baseline state of contraction at rest, it is possible that the striated muscle composition of the external sphincter is not homogeneous. This concept of differing cell types of striated muscle within the external sphincter, however, has not as yet been elucidated. The external sphincter is innervated by the pudendal nerve as well the autonomic nervous system. The pudendal nerve is derived from the sacral plexus roots S2 to S4. This nerve is both motor to the external sphincter and sensory to the skin around the anus. Autonomic innervation of the external sphincter is via the nervi erigentes, derived from segments S2 to S4 of the spinal cord. This parasympathetic pelvic splanchnic nerve provides afferent information about the degree or magnitude of rectal fullness. Sympathetic innervation of the external sphincter probably exists, but as yet no studies have identified its specific role.

The levator ani muscle is a series of striated muscle groups composed of ischiococcygeus, ileococcygeus, pubococcygeus, and puborectalis (Fig. 83-20). The levator ani muscle extends from the pubic bone, the lowest portion of the sacrum, and the middle of the pelvis downward and medial to join with the external sphincter.[64] This muscle group is usually depicted as a funnel-shaped sling. In contrast with the innervation of the external sphincter, the motor innervation of the levature musculature is from only S3 and S4. It is also innvervated by the autonomic system (both sympathetic and parasympathetic).

The internal sphincter has been described as a continuation of the circular smooth muscle inner layer of the muscularis propia of the bowel wall (see Figs. 83-19 and 83-20). The internal sphincter is under sympathetic (resting tone) and parasympathetic (relaxation) control.[64]

Pain, touch, temperature, and pressure are felt through sensory afferents located in the anal mucosa, including a zone slightly more than 1 cm above the dentate line.[65] The rectum is devoid of these sensory afferents except for pacinian corpuscles that are pressure receptors located in the rectum between internal and external sphincters and in the presacral space as well as the submucosa of the anal canal.[66]

These anal mucosa sensory afferents traverse the spinal cord and then to the cortex, all with the feelings of fullness and ultimately a desire to defecate. Each sensory nerve ending is responsible for one kind of stimulus. Proprioceptive stretch receptors exists within the muscle spindles of the voluntary striated muscle mechanism. These receptors carry afferent impulses stimulated in response to rectal distention. These sensory afferents are derived from the neural crest in contrast with the mesodermal origin of the caudal eminence muscle, bone, and nerve.[65,67]

Anatomy of Children With Anorectal Malformations

Children with ARMs challenge the traditional concept of the gross anatomy of the sphincter mechanism. After many years

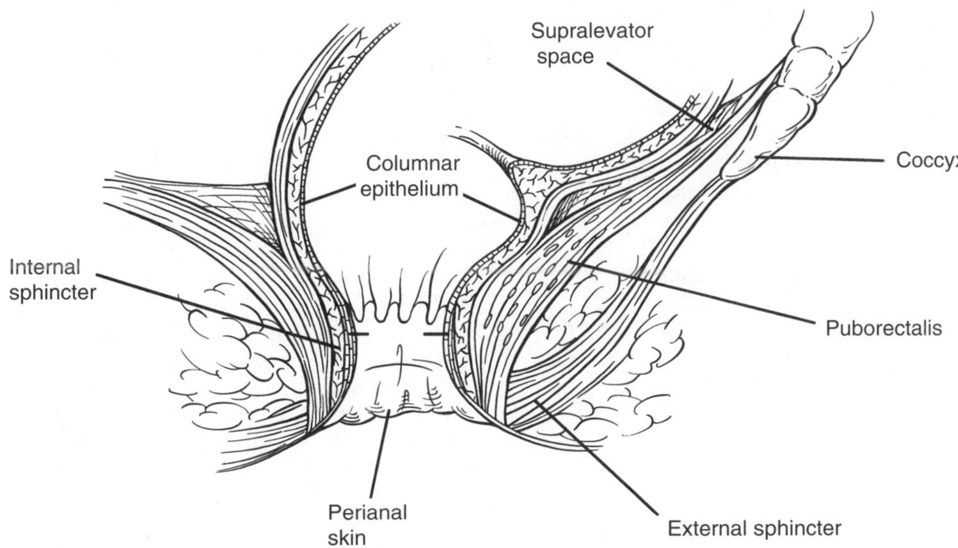

FIG. 83-19. Normal parasagittal anatomy of the perineal musculature. Voluntary striated muscle includes the external sphincter (parasagittal fibers) and levator musculature. The internal sphincter is composed of involuntary smooth muscle. (See also Figure 83-20.)

using the posterior sagittal approach to repair ARMs, it is our concept that the external sphincter runs in a paramedian instead of a circular direction. In addition, the muscular boundaries of the external sphincter are fused; and, thus, we are unable to distinguish the components of the external sphincter.

During a posterior sagittal dissection, the junction of levator musculature with external sphincter is defined by a vertical group of striated muscle fibers called the muscle complex[68] (Fig. 83-21). Electrical stimulation of the upper end of the levator group pulls the rectum forward. Stimulation of the muscle complex (vertical fibers) elevates the anus and the paramedian fibers of the external sphincter close the anus.

Furthermore, in children with ARMs there are varying degrees of striated muscle development from almost normal-looking striated muscle to virtually no muscle seen at operation. In very high defects, the rectum may rest at the upper part of the funnel-shaped voluntary striated muscle; and, in lower defects, the rectum may traverse the base of the muscular funnel.

Once again, the internal sphincter is said to be a continuation of the outer circular smooth muscle of the bowel wall. In children with ARMs, however, we have never seen what is referred to as the limits or for that matter the actual internal sphincter. Instead, if surgeons biopsy a segment of the wall of the rectum during an operative dissection for ARM, they obtain histologic reference to smooth muscle. When subjected to electrical stimulation and drugs, this type of biopsy seems to respond as though it was, in fact, bowel sphincter type of smooth muscle but there has been no clear evidence for a definable internal sphincter in patients with ARMs.[69]

Physiology of Normal Children

Continence in the normal child requires intact sphincter function, anal canal sensation and propioception, and coordinated colonic as well as rectosigmoid motility. Unfortunately, much of the mechanism that underlies all these events is unclear. Moreover, the movement of stool from the rectosigmoid down

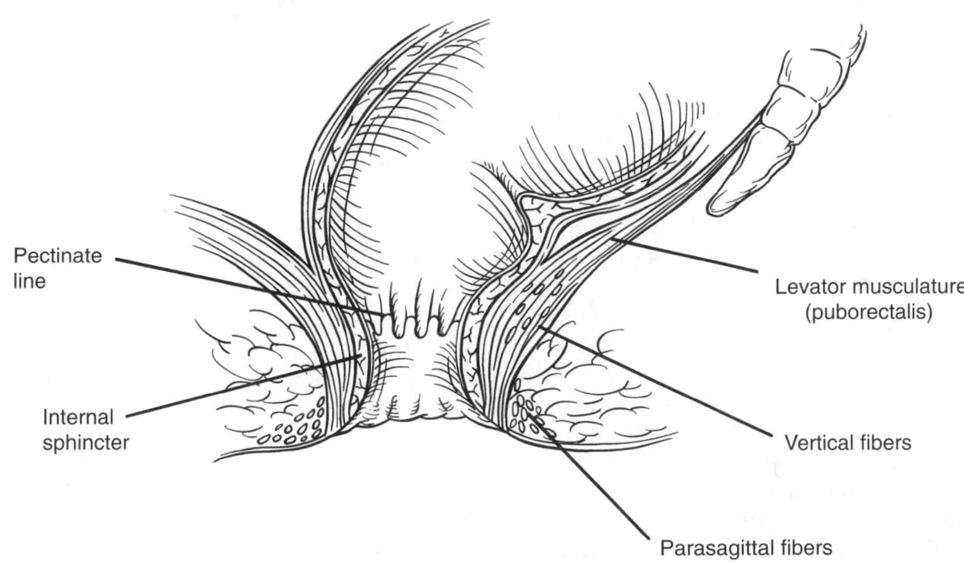

FIG. 83-20. Normal anatomy of the perineum. The voluntary striated mechanism is composed of the external sphincter, vertical fibers (muscle complex), and the levator muscle. This muscle represents a funnel-shaped continuum that is not truly separable into distinct parts.

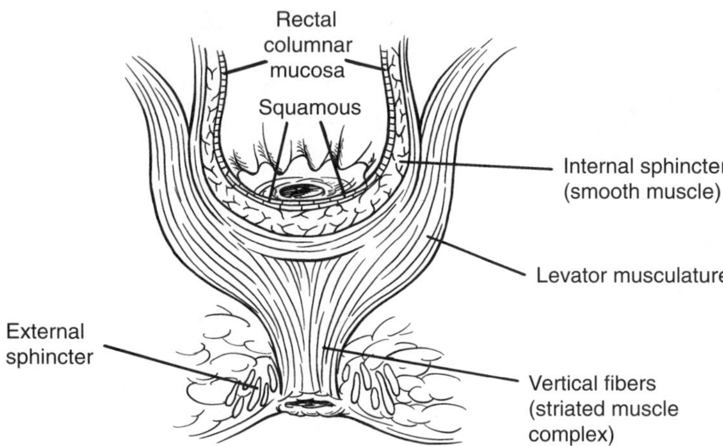

FIG. 83-21. The muscle complex. The muscle complex consists of vertical striated muscle fibers connecting the external sphincter with the levator muscle. In patients with imperforate anus, there are varying degrees of loss of the funnel-shaped striated muscle.

to the anus, namely, the process of defecation, is even less well defined. As such, it is difficult to provide answers to pathologic conditions when normal physiology has not been elucidated.

Sphincter Function

The two normally present types of sphincters include the voluntary external sphincter and the involuntary internal sphincter. Rectal manometric studies assume that the internal sphincter provides the majority of resting pressure in the rectum by virtue of its near maximal contraction in the basal state.[70] In response to rectal distention, during manometry, there is a fall in the pressure of the lower rectum and the anal canal that is called the *relaxation reflex*.[71] It is assumed that relaxation of the internal sphincter provokes this fall in the intraluminal pressure. Relaxation is followed by a brief increase in pressure that is interpreted as a contraction of the external sphincter. This rectoanal inhibitory reflex (RAIR) is a manometric finding and may not be entirely extrapolated to defecation. In view of the fact that both these structures (internal and external sphincters) are superimposed anatomically (see Figs 83-19 and 83-20), we do not understand how these conclusions were reached. In other words, how can we say that it is the internal or the external sphincter relaxing when they are both superimposed?

Nitric oxide has emerged as the neurotransmitter that mediates the RAIR. It has been assumed that the nonadrenergic, noncholinergic parasympathetic nerves in the wall of the internal sphincter produce relaxation of the sphincter in response to rectal distention. The inhibitory nerve cell bodies lie in the rectal myenteric ganglia and their processes pass to the sphincter.[72] The RAIR does not require connection to the spinal cord but instead is transmitted via the ganglion cells in the internal sphincter's intermuscular plexus of Auerbach. This reflex is classically absent in patients with Hirschsprung disease and variably present in patients with a high imperforate anus who have undergone operative correction.[73]

In adults, anal endosonography provides definition of the voluntary striated external sphincter and involuntary smooth muscle internal sphincter.[74] It is also possible to determine the status of the pudendal nerve by using electroneurography.[75] These techniques may have future benefit for postoperative evaluation of incontinence following repair of ARMs.

Sensation and Proprioception

It is thought that in normal children innervation of the anus and anal skin is not present at birth, but is acquired as the child learns to defecate and, therefore, toilet train.[76] These receptors are not necessary for keeping the external sphincter contracted because normal newborns have an external sphincter reflex.[77] The presence or absence of these receptors and the status of the voluntary muscle in newborns has not been elucidated. Furthermore, it is difficult to assume that innervation of the anus and anal skin is not present early in life as evidenced by the facial grimaces that these children use when wanting to defecate. Moreover, there are many additional unanswered questions about the role of and presence of sensory nerve endings in the newborn as well as the contribution, if any, of the anal mucosa to continence and defecation.

Colonic and Rectosigmoid Motility

It is well-known that it takes between 3 and 6 hours for the gastric content to transit the small bowel. The intestinal content reaches the cecum in a liquid state. It then takes about 20 to 24 hours for that fecal material to reach the rectum and become formed (solid). The rectosigmoid acts as a reservoir and keeps the fecal material for variable periods of time. The anal canal (below the pectinate line), however, is usually empty because of the action of the surrounding sphincteric mechanism. Occasionally, however, there are peristaltic waves that push the fecal material toward the anus. The voluntary sphincter can be voluntarily relaxed, allowing sampling to occur. The rectal content moves distally and touches the exquisitely sensitive tissue of the anal canal, providing the individual with valuable information related to the nature of the rectal content (gas, solid, liquid). Depending on the surrounding social circumstances, the individual may let the rectal content escape or may contract the sphincteric mechanism pushing stool or gas back into the rectum. The distention of the rectum produces a vague sensation of fullness or even a colicky pain (proprioception) but does not provide specific information concerning the physical characteristic of the content.

We know very little about the mechanism that triggers the peristalsis of the rectosigmoid to defecate but certainly we know that the degree of rectal fullness has a definite role. Thus, when the time comes, the rectosigmoid generates waves of peristalsis aiming to empty the lumen. Individuals can restrain this temporarily by using the voluntary sphincter. With a voluntary decision to allow the stool to come out, the sphincter is relaxed and the individual waits for the next peristaltic wave. Normal defecation allows a massive emptying of the rectosigmoid followed by another resting period of about 24 hours, during which the rectosigmoid acts again as a reservoir.

The importance of rectosigmoid motility has been highly underestimated in the past for a variety of reasons, not the least of which are a suitable animal model and proper equipment for the study of children. Tonic, phasic, and high-amplitude propagated contractions (HAPCs, those greater than 80 mmHg); and rectal motor complexes (RCMCs) are the hallmarks of normal colonic motility in children but they are not necessarily representative of rectosigmoid motility. These responses are intrinsic to the bowel wall and are derived from brain–gut connections.[78] With age in normal children, the number of HAPCs falls and this parallels the decrease in daily bowel movements.[79] The RMC is the only colonic activity that occurs distal to the rectosigmoid.[80] Colonic motility as defined by both the HAPCs and the RMCs should be stimulated after eating. This colonic response to food is diagnostic of normal colonic motility and forms the basis for future studies of abnormal colonic motility in children with pseudo-obstruction.[81] None of these colonic motility studies evaluate the propogation of a wave through to the anal canal. Most of these studies stop at the rectosigmoid, which is the area where most HAPCs stop. Furthermore, the role of the more distal RMCs is unknown.

Physiology of Children with Anorectal Malformations

Sphincter Function

Some studies suggest that for children with high imperforate anus, nerve cell numbers in the medial ventral horn of the spinal cord, corresponding to the external anal sphincter and muscle complex, are reduced.[82]

In contrast with the spectrum of voluntary striated muscle abnormalities in children with ARMs, the status of the smooth muscle does not seem to affect prognosis. Some authors suggest the internal sphincter is crucial for bowel control. Although postoperative manometry in some patients with ARMs shows that there is occasional preservation of the RAIR, there is no evidence that absolutely links the presence or absence of the internal anal sphincter to normal bowel control.

Sensation and Propioception

Children born with ARMs have a spectrum of sensation and propioception. Agenesis of these nerve endings, such as occurs in high imperforate anus, may mean that for whatever spectrum of voluntary striated musculature is present there may also be a defect in sensation and propioception. In children with ARMs, a feeling of fullness (propioception) may be accompanied by a spectrum of exquisite or rudimentary sensation to no sensation at all. Thus, when dealing with a high imperforate anus, it is imperative to appreciate all the musculature and its symmetry in an effort to relocate the neoanus between the fibers of the voluntary striated mechanism.[66] Only in this optimally relocated anatomic scenario can distention and propioception help the child have fecal continence. In these children, sensation is a consequence of distention of the neoanus. They cannot rely on an intact voluntary striated muscle mechanism because by definition there is a paucity of this muscle mass and its innervation. Therefore, many of these children cannot hold stool or have a normal bowel movement when liquids are present in their neoanus. Solid feces will distend the rectum but liquid stools do not; thus, liquid stools must be avoided at all costs.

Colonic and Rectosigmoid Motility

Children with ARMs have a spectrum of rectosigmoid motility disorders. Children with ARMs subjected to surgical techniques that preserve rectosigmoid suffer from constipation. Constipation, one of the most important functional sequelae of ARMs, is probably the result of hypomotility of the rectosigmoid. The hypomotility is self-perpetuating and self-aggravating to the point that if left untreated, megasigmoid develops.[83] In extreme cases, children may develop fecal impaction and encopresis or overflow pseudo-incontinence. Analysis of results after PSARP shows that constipation is worse in the lower defects (see Results). Knowing this and the fact that hypomotility can begin a vicious cycle leading to megasigmoid, it is incumbent on the pediatric surgeon to avoid the cycle of hypomotility, constipation, and megasigmoid. In fact, aggressive patient follow-up using dietary, mechanical, and pharmacologic treatment prevents this cycle. Usually, suppositories, enemas, or colonic irrigations suffice. Constipation from functional, postoperative, and neurologic etiologies has been treated with the prokinetic agent cisapride.[84,85] It stimulates the smooth muscle of the entire gastrointestinal tract by releasing acetylcholine, shortening transit time, and causing improved sensitivity to distention. What cannot be overemphasized is the concept that constipation, especially for the lower ARM defects is expected, and, thus, all precautions should be taken to avoid aggravating this problem.

In contrast with the problem of constipation secondary to hypomotility, children with ARMs who for whatever reason have lost their rectosigmoid suffer from the exact opposite (i.e., tendency for diarrhea). These children have no reservoir capacity, are highly sensitive to fruits and vegetables, and worst of all suffer from incontinence. They have a spectrum of hypermotility dysfunction with the most severe complaints in children with no colon.

Unfortunately, there is a paucity of data in the literature concerning the normal mechanism of rectosigmoid motility and even less information in patients with ARMs. The clinical findings in children treated for constipation and incontinence, however, are compelling for the importance of rectosigmoid motility.

ASSOCIATED ANOMALIES

Because arrest of migration of mesoderm within the caudal eminence and abnormal resorption of the cloacal membrane are likely embryologic causes of ARMs, it follows that other mesodermally derived tissues should be affected. These tissues include derivatives of the paraxial and lateral plate mesoderm that consist of the genitourinary, skeletal, muscular, and gastrointestinal systems. The incidence of associated malformations depends on the type of anorectal defect but a specific type of associated malformation does not seem to correlate with a specific ARM.

Genitourinary System

The most common associated malformations are derivatives of the genitourinary system, with an incidence in the range of 20% to 54%.[86–88] They include the following:

- Absent, dysplastic, or horseshoe kidneys
- Vesicoureteral reflux
- Hydronephrosis
- Hypospadias
- Bifid scrotum

The triad of penile agenesis, complete absence of the median raphe, and imperforate anus is incompatible with life.[89]

In general, the higher the ARM the greater the likelihood of an associated genitourinary anomaly. For example, patients with a persistent cloaca or a rectobladder neck fistula have a 90% chance of associated genitourinary anomaly. Rectourethral or rectovestibular fistulas have an associated incidence of 30% but a child with a perineal fistula has less than a 10% chance of an associated genitourinary anomaly.[88] This information is important for the neonatal management of these children. Therefore, it should be mandatory for all newborns with an ARM to undergo an abdominopelvic ultrasound. If hydronephrosis is found, a voiding cystourethrogram (VCUG) should be done before the colostomy is created.[90] In so doing, appropriate additional decompression of bladder, vagina, or both may be performed when indicated along with the colostomy under a single episode of anesthesia. Patients with a rectobladder neck fistula (flat bottom) and patients with cloacas represent potential urologic emergencies and should undergo colostomy without a prior urologic diagnosis. Deteriorating renal function from hydronephrosis, urosepsis, or uncorrectable metabolic acidosis is the most frequent cause of morbidity and mortality in patients with ARMs. Associated genitourinary reflux should be treated with suppressive antibiotics.

Patients with symptomatic voiding pathology (vesicoureteral reflux) usually have a high imperforate anus (rectourinary fistulas) and bony sacral and spinal cord anomalies (44%). Yet, these may exist in the absence of sacral agenesis. On the other hand, patients without voiding symptoms tended to have a low imperforate anus and minimal or no bone anomalies (8%).[91]

Skeletal System

In general, the higher the ARM the more likely there is an associated skeletal anomaly. Such anomalies include the following:

- Partial or complete lumbosacral agenesis
- Hemivertebrae
- Agenesis of thoracic vertebrae
- Scoliosis
- Hemisacrum or scimitar sacrum
- Asymmetric sacrum
- Posterior protruding sacrum
- Agenesis of the coccyx

Up to 45% of patients with ARMs have sacral abnormalities.[92] There appears to be an excellent correlation between the degree of skeletal sacral anomaly and the functional prognosis of the newborn with an ARM. Absence of one of the five sacral vertebrae does not seem to correlate with function or outcome.[93] Two or more absent vertebrae, however, have been shown to represent a poor prognostic sign of bowel function.[94] Many times it is difficult to actually count the number of sacral vertebrae. Thus, the sacral ratio technique seems to be a useful method to help the surgeon predict functional prognosis. In addition, sometimes children have five sacral vertebrae, yet, the sacrum may be very short and looks obviously abnormal. As a result, a more accurate way to evaluate the sacrum was perfected. After placing the newborn either in an anteroposterior or a lateral position, three lines are drawn (Fig. 83-22). Line A extends across the uppermost portion of the iliac crest; line B unites the inferior–posterior iliac spines; line C runs parallel to lines A and B and passes through the lowest sacral point visible on the radiograph. Normal children have an average sacral ratio (BC:AB) of 0.7:0.8, in contrast with children with severe ARMs whose ratio may be as low as zero.[58] Low ratios correlate with poor functional prognosis (i.e., incontinence). The sacral ratio seems to be a predictor of functional outcome when comparing types of ARMs.

Absence of any portion of the spine from the mid-thoracic level or higher is probably not compatible with intrauterine life. The absence of the coccyx is invariably asymptomatic, but absence of any lumbosacral vertebrae may have associated anomalies such as the limbs and genitourinary system in addition to ARMs.[95] The Currarino triad is an example of a specific anomaly of the sacrum instead of agenesis that is found in association with two other anomalies.[96] The triad consists of a scimitar sacrum, anal stenosis, and presacral mass (i.e., lipoma, lipomeningocele) (Fig. 83-23). All children with anal stenosis as well as an ARM should have a lumbosacral spine x-ray to rule out this triad. If indeed a scimitar sacrum is found, then an ultrasound of the pelvis or a magnetic resonance (MR) scan of the spine should be obtained to exclude a presacral mass.

Factors that may influence the normal development of the vertebral column include insulin-dependent maternal diabetes, trauma to the fetus, and prolonged fever during pregnancy.[97] Overall causes of sacral anomalies like the etiology of ARMs are multifactorial and include both environmental and hereditary factors. Interestingly, characteristics of patients with isolated lumbosacral deformities are similar to those with ARMs. These similarities include flattening of the buttocks, shortening of the intergluteal cleft, loss of perineal muscle mass, and motor deficits of the levator (S2 to S5) and gluteal muscles (L5 to S1). Sensation is derived from dorsal root ganglia and peripheral sensory nerves, both of which are derived from neural crest tissue. In contrast with isolated ARMs, where we find abnormalities not only in motor ability but also in neural crest–derived perineal sensation; sensation in children with lumbosacral agenesis is relatively unaffected.[98] When compared with abnormalities of the sacrum alone or sacrum and limb deformities,

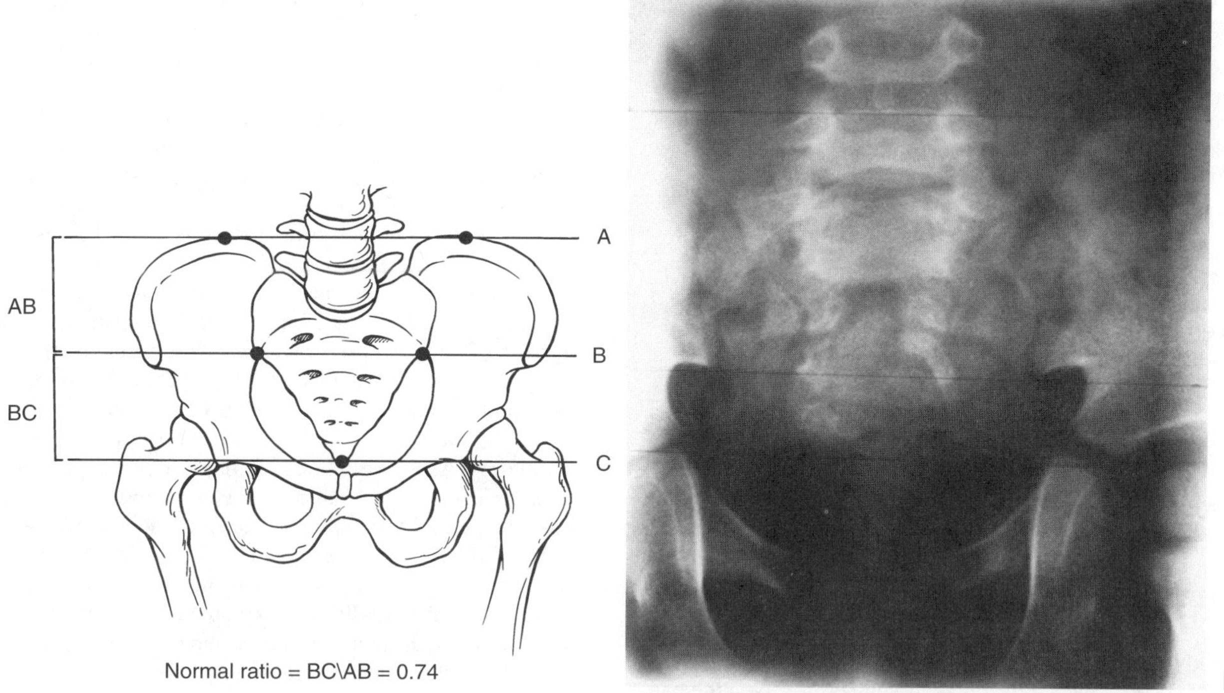

FIG. 83-22. (*A*) Sacral ratio. Three lines are drawn in either the anteroposterior or lateral position. Line A extends across the uppermost portion of the iliac crest. Line B unites the inferior–posterior iliac spines, line C is parallel to lines A and B, and passes through the lowest sacral point visible on radiograph. (*B*) Actual radiograph showing an abnormal ratio of 0.31.

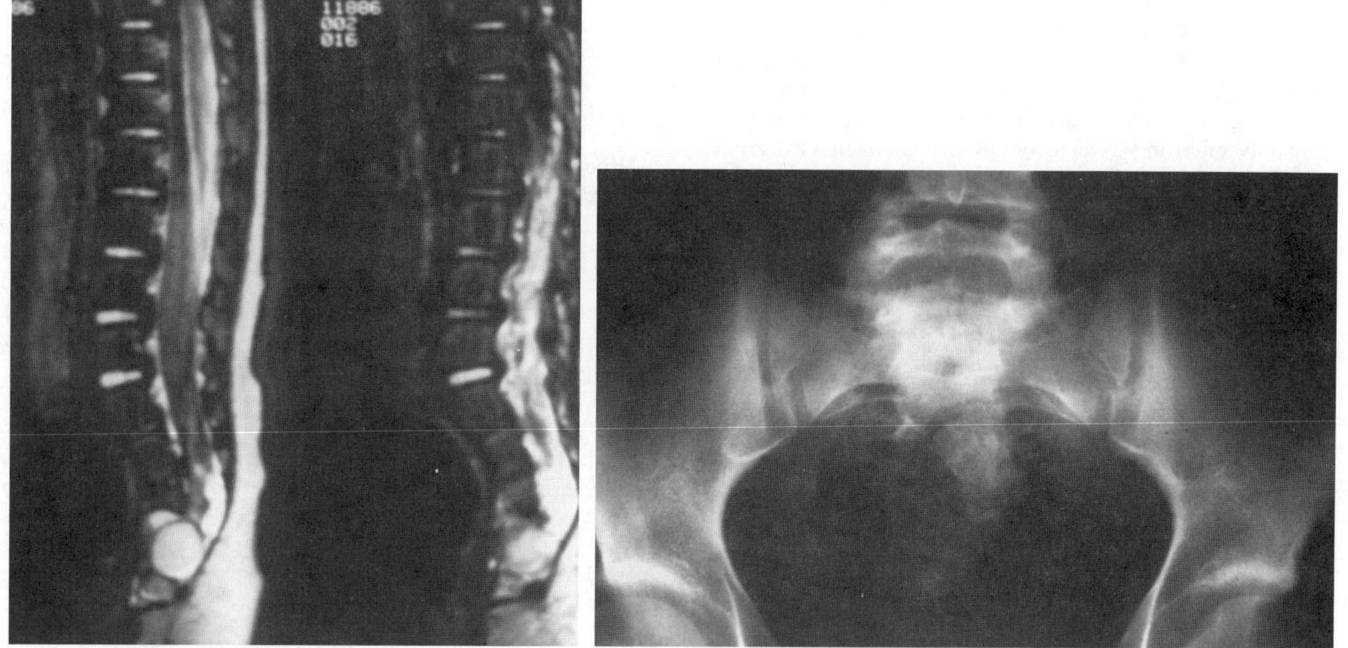

FIG. 83-23. The Currarino triad. These children have anal stenosis, presacral masses, and scimitar sacrum. (*A*) MR scan shows the presacral mass, which in this case is a lipomeningocele. (*B*) The plain radiograph is a scimitar sacrum.

TABLE 83-4. *Indications for screening for tethered cord with ARMs*

MANDATORY
Myelodysplasia
Abnormal sacral ratio (AP < 0.4 or LAT <0.6)
Complex defect
Cloacal exstrophy

RECOMMENDED
Rectobladder neck fistula
Persistent cloaca (common channel >3 cm)
Presacral mass
Hemivertebrae
Genitourinary anomaly
Poor result despite good prognosis

AP, anteroposterior; LAT, lateral.

sacral agenesis associated with any visceral anomalies (such as ARMs) constitutes the worst functional prognosis.[99]

Nervous System

A study performed on 94 patients with all forms of ARMs showed a 38% incidence of spinal anomalies.[100] Given the paucity of data in the literature, however, the frequency of spinal anomalies with ARMs is at best an approximation, and, in addition, it is difficult to speculate who should not undergo screening for spinal anomalies. As such, all patients with ARMs should have their lumbosacral spine evaluated with plain radiographs. Screening with a magnetic resonance scan should be *mandatory* for some children and *recommended* for others (Table 83-4). There are no data to support the notion that spinal dysraphism (i.e., tethered cord), except in severe cases, is directly linked to the functional outcome in patients with ARMs. It appears, however, that the higher the ARM the more likely it is for the child to have associated neurologic and skeletal problems. Therefore, it is mandatory for all patients with ARMs to undergo a pelvic ultrasound to rule out the possibility of spinal dysraphism.[101] Magnetic resonance imaging (MRI) may also be used, including in the neonate, as the sole study to evaluate potential associated anomalies.[102] Radiologists claim that they can make the diagnosis of a tethered cord with ultrasound in patients before 3 months of age; older patients require MRI. The MR scan is difficult in babies because it requires remote anesthesia services for heavy sedation and sometimes intubation to keep the baby immobile. In addition, the baby is relatively inaccessible for the duration of the scan, which makes monitoring cumbersome. We recommend going directly to an MR scan for the evaluation of the postoperative patient with constipation, incontinence, or bladder dysfunction that cannot be explained by the nature, type, and height of the original ARM.[103]

Various associated spinal anomalies have been reported:

- Tethered cord
- Dural sac stenosis
- Narrow spinal canal
- Diastematomyelia
- Myelomeningocele, meningocele
- Intraspinal teratoma
- Neurogenic bladder

Prevention of rostral migration of the spinal cord during development because of an abnormal point of fixation secondary to bony deformities results in a shortened cauda equina and low-lying conus medullaris. During an axial growth spurt, the spine grows faster than the cord; and this may provoke stretching, traction, and eventual infarction of the cord above the point of fixation. Normally the conus is at the level of L3 at birth, ascends to the upper border of L2 by age 5, and remains there through adulthood. Detecting the conus below L3 suggests tethering. Although metrizamide computed tomographic (CT) scans have been used in the past, the MR scan for definitive diagnosis and ultrasound for screening (in patients less than 3 months of age) are used today.[104] Knowledge of the presence of a tethered cord instead of operation for correction should be the standard of care. On the other hand, there is clear benefit from untethering a spinal cord in patients with progressive symptoms. As the vertebral columns lengthens with age, symptoms are usually radicular pain, myelopathies, and foot deformities. Postoperative constipation or fecal incontinence as isolated symptoms have not been shown to be associated with a tethered cord. If a pelvic ultrasound, performed before 3 months of age, detects any abnormalities of the spinal canal or the vertebrae, then an MR scan should be performed to rule out any possibility of an associated neural abnormality.

Gastrointestinal and Cardiovascular Systems

Gastrointestinal anomalies are probably fourth in the frequency of potential anomalies associated with ARMs, followed by intracardiac defects. All of the following associated anomalies can occur separately or as VATER and VACTERL associations:

- Esophageal atresia
- Duodenal atresia
- Ventricular or atrioseptal defects
- Tetrology of Fallot
- Hirschsprung disease

Keep in mind that none of these associated gastrointestinal and cardiac anomalies have contributed to the overall prognosis of the ARM. These associations, however, have made it mandatory for an echocardiogram to be performed and an orogastric tube to be inserted. If bilious drainage is discovered in the newborn period, a contrast study should be performed. Likewise, if the orogastric tube does not pass, there should be a high index of suspicion for esophageal atresia.

Concerning the possible association of Hirschsprung disease and ARMs, one can submit a piece of the pulled-through bowel at the time of definitive repair or perform a suction rectal biopsy of the distal limb of the colostomy at any time.[105] The authors, however, have never seen a child with concurrent ARMs and enterocolitis from Hirschsprung disease, yet, there are many children with ARMs and constipation who probably have been misdiagnosed with associated Hirschsprung disease.

PRENATAL DIAGNOSIS

In general, gastrointestinal anomalies occur as isolated in utero events in 65% to 70% of cases, and multiple organ systems are involved in the remaining 30% to 35%.[106] In cases of lower gastrointestinal tract anomalies such as ARMs, the incidence of associated anomalies approaches 50%.[20,21] In contrast with the most gastrointestinal anomalies, few, if any ARM cases are diagnosed prenatally. Although this is a shortcoming, ARMs should not be included in a list of congenital anomalies that cause major long-term disability or death.[107] Antenatal diagnosis of ARMs is at best included in a list of possible diagnoses. This problem is operator dependent, limited technically, and finally nonspecific unless dramatic in presentation (i.e., sirenomelia). Nonspecific prenatal ultrasound findings include the following[108]:

- Dilatated, U-shaped colon in the lower abdomen or pelvis
- Highly distended vagina
- Calcified intraluminal meconium or enterolithiasis
- Normal or diminished amniotic fluid volume (associated bilateral renal disorders)
- Absence of a circular rim of hypoechogenicity in perineum with a central linear echo running sagittally
- Septated, cystic pelvic mass, oligohydramnios, and impaired fetal growth in girls in the case of cloaca

Prenatal anal ultrasonography has identified the normal anal canal by the presence of a circular rim of hypoechogenic tissue in the perineum together with a central linear echogenic stripe. The absence of these findings is suggestive but not as yet pathognomonic for ARMs.[109] Caudal regression syndromes[110] ranging from lumbosacral agenesis to the mermaid-like caudal features in association with ARM, genitourinary, central nervous system, and cardiorespiratory anomalies are easier to identify in contrast with isolated ARMs.

Dilated colon is gestational age dependent (usually not seen prior to 24 to 26 weeks) and nonspecific because it can also be associated with meconium plug syndrome, Hirschsprung disease, small left colon syndrome, or atresia.[111] Dilated colon in the lower abdomen or pelvis has a long list of differential diagnoses including ovarian cyst, hydrometrocolpos, obstructive uropathy, megacystis–microcolon intestinal hypoperistalsis syndrome, urachal cyst, and ARMs including a cloacal malformation. In general, effort should be made to identify kidneys, liver, spleen, and bladder before considering a sonolucent pelvic mass to be an ARM.

Polyhydramnios implies either a misdiagnosis or an additional anomaly such as esophageal atresia. In fact, 1 out of 15 healthy pregnancies with polyhydramnios is associated with proximal instead of distal gastrointestinal tract obstruction.[112] Polyhydramnios then should not imply a hindgut anomaly.

Microvillar disaccharidase activity is diminished, presumably because like most intestinal atresias there is an obstruction to the passage of colonic contents.[113–115] These intestinal enzymes may be present in amniotic fluid in response to desquamation of intestinal cells in utero. Fetal intestinal disaccharidases (α- and β-glucosidase, β-galactosidase) within amniotic fluid are detectable during the 10th week of gestation, peaking by the 17th week, and finally are found at very low levels by the 22nd week.[116] Reasons for this evolution are unclear, but may be related to the formation and recanalization of the intestinal tract and its patency both in the cranial and caudal axes. As amniotic fluid volume increases during the third trimester, the enzymes may be diluted or the disaccharidases may be

cleared by fetal swallowing. In general, institutions using the intestinal enzyme activity as an aid to the diagnosis of bowel obstruction restrict their sampling to a gestational age of 14 to 21 weeks.[117]

The diagnosis of a cloacal malformation has been established by identifying a septated cystic mass in the pelvis, no evidence of bladder, oligohydramnios, and hydronephrosis by ultrasound.[118]

NEONATAL DIAGNOSIS AND MANAGEMENT OF ARMs

Male Algorithm

As for clinical evaluation, the patient with an ARM should not present as an intestinal obstruction; instead, the diagnosis should be made during clinical examination of the newborn[119] (Fig. 83-24).

The needs to perform a diverting colostomy and to manage any life-threatening–associated anomalies (such as cardiac and urinary tract) are the two most important issues in the newborn period, regardless of sex. Inspection of the male perineum should allow a diagnosis and thus direct the need for a diverting colostomy in 80% to 90% of cases. Questionable cases rely on the presence of meconium in the urine, and invertogram or perineal ultrasound at 24 hours of life. A perineal ultrasound performed after 24 hours may also provide similar diagnostic information, but this is highly operator dependent and thus not always available. The invertogram can pinpoint the bowel as close as 5 mm from the skin provided the radiograph is performed after 18 hours of life. It usually takes 16 to 24 hours for the newborn intestine to pass meconium through a fistula communicating with the skin or the urethra. Thus, decisions about performing a diverting colostomy should not be made before 24 hours of life. In the interim, a gauze can be placed on the tip of the penis looking for filtered meconium and an ultrasound of the abdomen must be performed to rule out kidney pathology and hydronephrosis. An echocardiogram should also be performed.

Low defects include subepithelial midline passage of meconium through fistula or prominent skin tag (bucket handle deformity) (see Fig. 83-11). These ARMs are usually treated with a perineal anoplasty either via a posterior sagittal approach or an anterior approach using a cutback V-Y anoplasty.

Higher defects on inspection are characterized by a very flat bottom, meconium in the urine, or air in the bladder. All high defects require a diverting descending colostomy in the newborn period and definitive repair usually by 3 months of age provided there has been consistent weight gain and associated malformations have been managed. Prior to creation of the colostomy in the newborn period, the need for urinary diversion should be ruled out, because if indicated, this procedure can be performed simultaneously.

In questionable cases, instead of a traditional invertogram, a cross-table lateral with the baby in the prone position and the pelvis elevated can be used to determine the distance between perineal skin and the blind rectal pouch.[120] If the rectum is located less than 1 cm from the perineal skin, this is considered a low-lying ARM. In such cases, in retrospect, most likely a perineal fistula was missed during the examination of the peri-

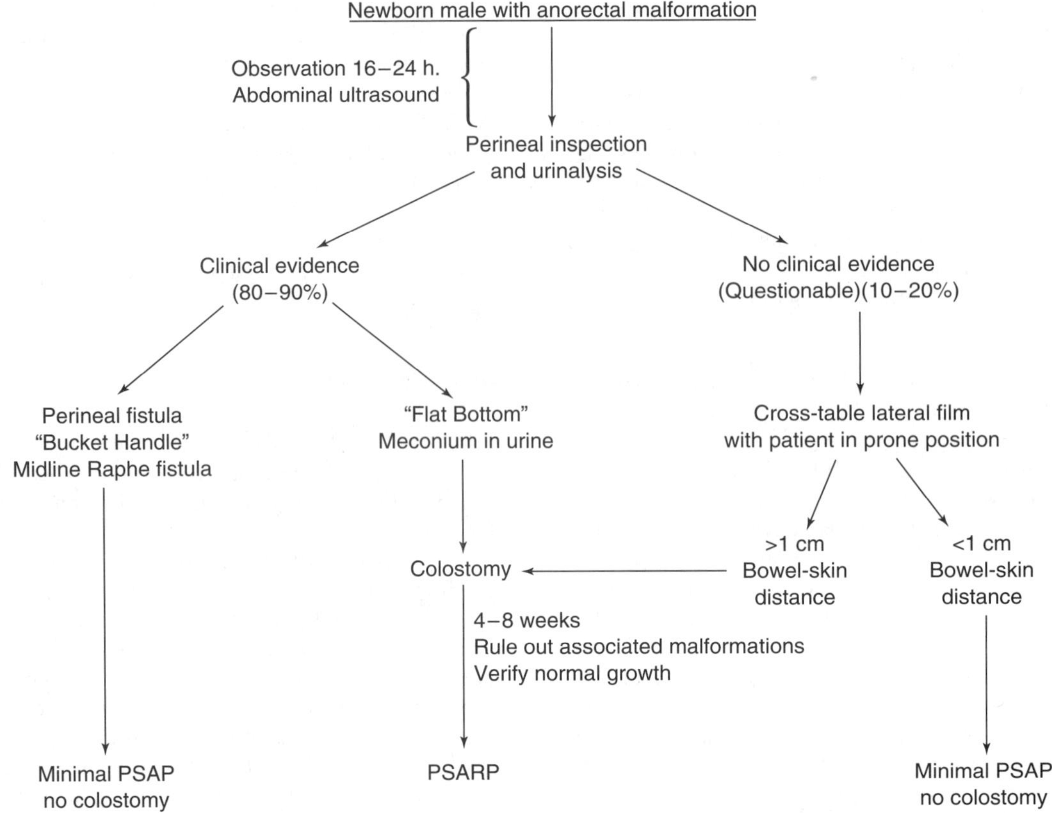

FIG. 83-24. Algorithm for the neonatal management of anorectal malformations in a male.

neum. All lesions higher than 1 cm are high ARMs and require a diverting colostomy.

Invertogram CT is not necessary to establish the diagnosis.[121] Other modalities include ultrasonograms, CTs, and invertograms, which may be used for the evaluation of a low-lying lesion. Lesions less than 1 cm from the skin may be treated by perineal anoplasty.[122]

Female Algorithm

Simple perineal inspection provides the diagnosis in virtually 90% of ARMs in females (Fig. 83-25). For example, cutaneous and vestibular fistulas are readily identified during a perineal exam. One must immobilize the baby's legs and use good lighting. A rectovestibular fistula orifice can usually be identified just outside the hymen, whereas a rectovaginal fistula is identified by meconium coming from inside the vagina through the hymen. A perineal (cutaneous) fistula has the same prognostic and therapeutic significance as in males. A vestibular or vaginal fistula tends to be competent and to remain patent with serial dilatations. In these cases, a colostomy can, and in our opinion should, be performed prior to discharge. Passage of stool through this fistula for prolonged periods of time can induce varying degrees of megacolon and potential constipation. A single perineal orifice means the baby has a persistent cloaca. In most of these cases, there is an associated urologic emergency that requires prompt evaluation. Thus, these babies will most likely receive a colostomy, a vaginostomy or vesicostomy, or

any other urinary diversion. A midline, lower abdominal mass in these newborns is pathognomonic for a hydrocolpos, which must be diagnosed and managed with decompression during the opening of the colostomy.

If a female does not pass meconium in the first 16 to 24 hours of life, then again an invertogram or cross-table lateral radiograph is indicated. In addition, an abdominal ultrasound to evaluate the kidneys and ureters is also required.

Perineal Fistula

Special consideration is given to this variant of ARM because it is frequently discovered in the pediatrician's office for the workup of constipation.[123,124] Usually, the sphincteric mechanism is present and functioning. The anal orifice, however, is well forward of the muscles and a posterior shelf and pocket or cul-de-sac is palpable during rectal examination. The clinical picture is remarkably consistent. Chronic constipation persists despite all medical management using formula changes, laxatives, and stimulants. The referral to pediatric surgeons is usually to rule out Hirschsprung disease, and in most of these patients, there is no aganglionic bowel. These patients need a thorough physical examination that includes the rectum. In fact, the diagnosis can be suspected merely by inspection. The anus should normally be positioned at the midpoint of a line drawn between the base of the vagina or scrotum and the tip of the coccyx. The perineal fistula is anterior to this midpoint position. Not all these patients require repositioning operatively. Those

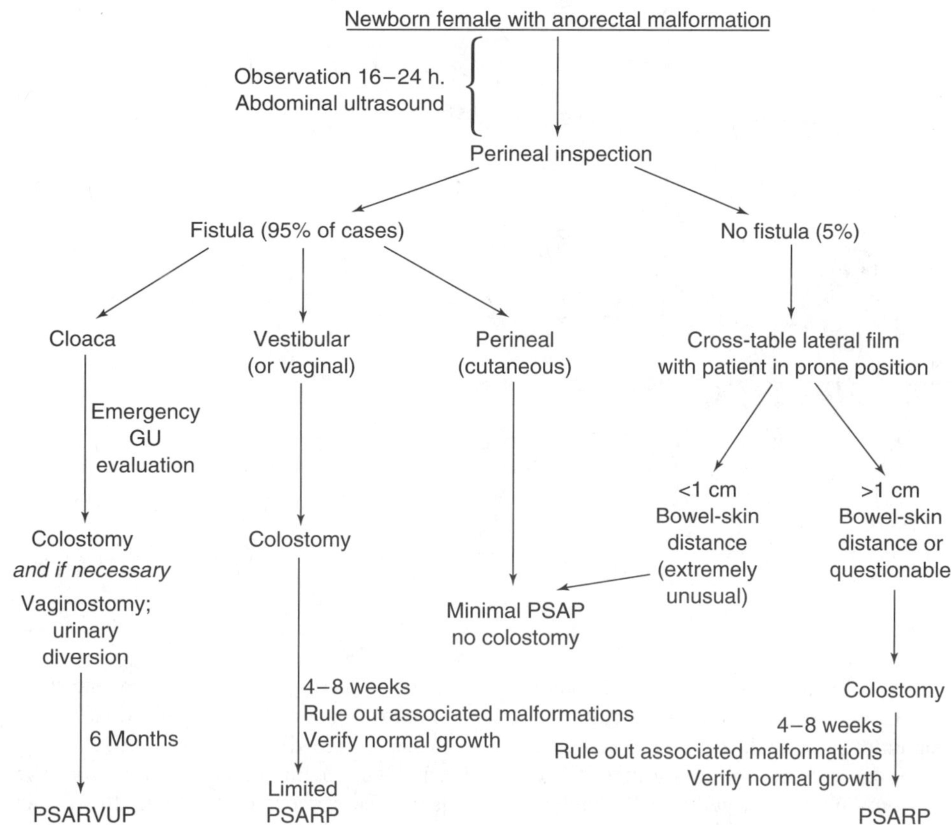

FIG. 83-25. Algorithm for the neonatal management of anorectal malformations in a female.

who fail medical treatment with stool softening and have recurrent urinary tract infections probably should undergo anoplasty. A minimal posterior sagittal approach facilitates exposure of the external sphincter and its junction with the muscle complex. Restoration of the perineal body and positioning of the anus within these structures is all that is required. A colostomy is not indicated. In newborns, no bowel preparation is required. However, in older patients a very strict bowel preparation is mandatory, along with 5 to 7 days of nothing-by-mouth status that usually means peripheral alimentation.

Anoplasty

The indication for some form of anoplasty includes cases of male and female perineal fistulas (Fig. 83-26). Regardless of the type of operation performed, the goal is to restore the anus to its normal anatomic position within the external sphincter. Because postnatal bacteria flora usually takes 3 days to be present in the baby's stool, no bowel preparation is necessary if the anoplasty is performed during this time period. Prophylactic antibiotics are given, and in males a Foley catheter in the bladder is mandatory. The most frequent complication is urethral injury because even in the low defects the rectum and urethra are intimately attached. The operations include the minimal posterior sagittal anoplasty (Fig. 83-27), a cutback procedure, or a Y-V transplant anoplasty.

The minimal posterior sagittal anoplasty not only uses the nerve stimulator but also takes advantage of the direct visualiza-

tion of the external sphincter from anterior to posterior. Multiple 6–0 traction sutures are placed around the perineal orifice, and then a dissection is performed circumferentially around the rectum. The sphincters should not be mobilized. It is the bowel that is to be dissected. Just enough bowel is mobilized to allow placement of the neoanus within the confines of the sphincter. In females, there is little to no morbidity with this procedure. Maintaining a plane immediately beyond the anus and not traveling beyond these limits facilitates protection of the bulbar urethra. Prior to the neoanoplasty, the perineal body should be restored using interrupted absorbable suture material. Two weeks after the minimal PSARP, a schedule of dilatations is begun (Table 83-5).

The cutback procedure involves an incision usually using a scissor at the posterior border of the perineal fistula and extended to the posterior border of the external sphincter. The neoanoplasty is matured with absorbable sutures using anus and skin. In the supine position, the Y-V anoplasty starts with nerve stimulation to identify the external sphincter. Skin is then incised in a Y shape around the perineal orifice and the anal skin is sutured around the new orifice in a V-shaped configuration. After these procedures, anal dilatations are begun 2 weeks after repair (see Table 83-5).

Colostomy

A descending colostomy is the procedure of choice for ARMs.[125] In general, a completely diverting descending colos-

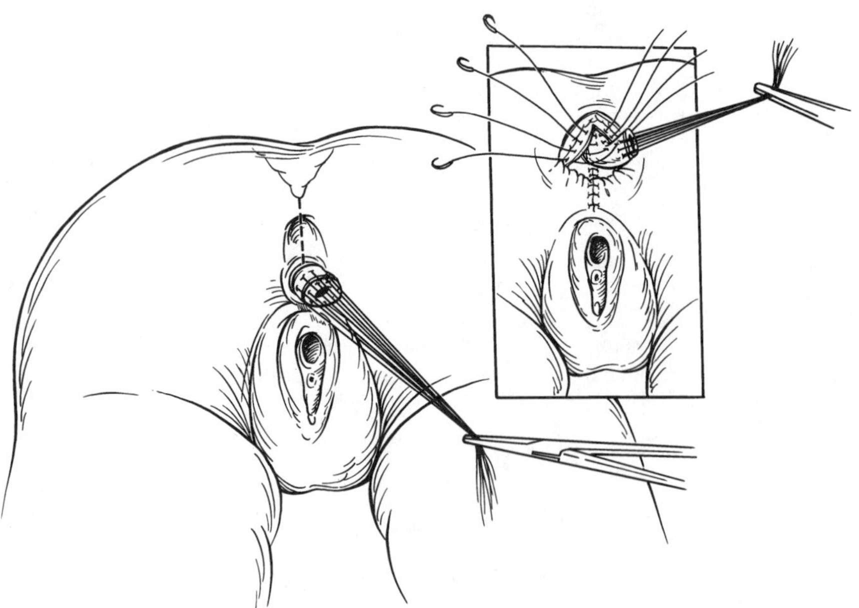

FIG. 83-26. The minimal posterior sagittal anoplasty.

tomy or a descending loop colostomy can be created in a newborn with a high ARM. Complete diversion is difficult, if not impossible, with a loop colostomy, and, thus, the potential for continued communication between rectum and urinary tract is high. Also, a loop colostomy in contrast with a completely diverting colostomy predisposes the child to urinary tract infections. The propensity for continued overflow into the distal bowel and consequent abnormal bowel distention can compromise the definitive repair as well as bowel motility. Postoperative constipation can be associated with megarectum, secondary to fecal impaction, created by this overflow into the distal bowel. If a loop colostomy is created too loosely, there is the potential for prolapse of the proximal stoma. The most common error is opening the colostomy too distally, leaving one with an incomplete length of bowel for the definitive repair, and thus forcing the surgeon to gain length by performing a laparotomy.

The descending colon double-barrel colostomy is our procedure of choice. Both types of stomas should be created through an oblique left lower quadrant incision using two layers of long-term absorbable sutures, one incorporating the posterior sheath and the second layer using the anterior sheath. Either stoma should be created so that the distal stoma is narrow to avoid prolapse. The distal stoma (mucous fistula) should be irrigated with warm saline in the operating room so that the distal bowel is cleared of meconium. Again, this maneuver facilitates cleaning the bowel; however, if a loop is created, one must be vigilant about checking for overflow and distention of the distal bowel. A right transverse colostomy is preferable prior to a redo operation.[126]

Preoperative Colostography

A preoperative colostogram is usually performed 3 to 4 weeks following creation of the stoma. It is commonly performed on an outpatient basis because the baby has likely been discharged from the hospital. The purpose of the colostogram is to define the anatomy of the distal bowel and establish the site of fistulous connection with the urinary tract. Thus, the procedure is called a distal colostogram. The single most important limitation to an adequate study is the fact that the distal rectum is surrounded by the sphincteric mechanism, which even in patients with ARMs exerts enough tone to collapse the rectum. For adequate filling of the distal bowel, enough hydrostatic pressure must be exerted to overcome the resting muscle tone and ultimately fill the distal bowel and fistula site. Therefore, we recommend injection of contrast material into the distal bowel using a Foley catheter with 2- to 3-mL inflation of the balloon. The lumen of the mucous fistula is occluded by pulling on the catheter and hand injecting a radiopaque water soluble contrast using fluoroscopy. The anal dimple with a piece of lead. In the anteroposterior position, the first piece of information to be obtained is the measurement of available length of distal bowel. Next, in the lateral projection, the fistula site is determined again by injection of contrast. The contrast material that passes into the urethra usually goes into the bladder. To complete the study, contrast should distend the bladder and the patient should be seen voiding.[127] A voiding cystourethrogram

TABLE 83-5. *Anal dilatations recommended with sizes and schedule*

Age	Dilator size (mm)
1–3 months	12
4–8 months	13
9–12 months	14
1–3 years	15
4–14 years	16
14 and older	17

Schedule
Once a day for 1 month
Every third day for 1 month
Twice a week for 1 month
Once a week for 1 month
Once a week for 3 months

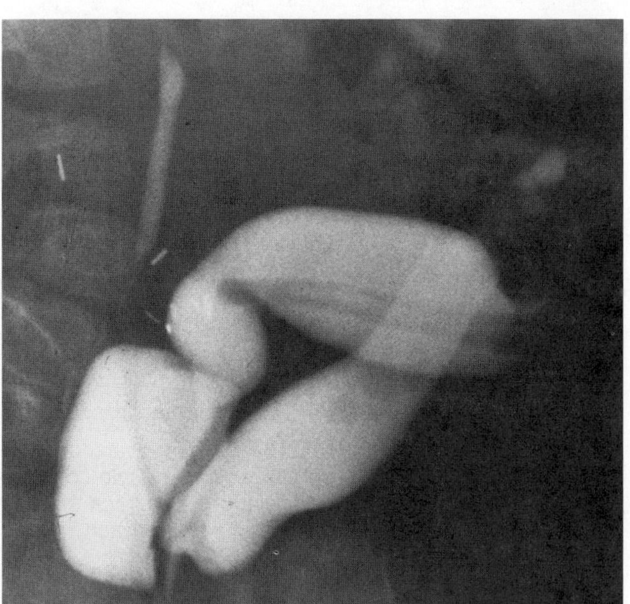

FIG. 83-27. Distal colostogram of cloaca showing connection between bladder, vagina, and bowel. The length of the common channel is determined during cystoscopy.

(VCUG) is not necessary because the distal colostogram, if done as outlined, provides all the essential information. The bladder, urethra sacrum, and anal dimple should be visualized in all projections. Failure of a colostogram is frequently the result of lack of back pressure while injecting the contrast or muscle action around the distal rectum.

In patients with a common cloaca, contrast should be injected through the common channel on the perineum, the distal colostomy, and the vesicostomy and vaginostomy when present (Fig. 83-27). A VCUG in children with cloacas is very difficult to obtain, except in those with a cystostomy or vesicostomy.

DEFINITIVE REPAIR

General Concepts

The indications for definitive repair of an imperforate anus include all patients with nonlife-threatening–associated anomalies and nonlife-threatening chromosomal defects. Myelomeningocele, high cloaca, and absent sacrum are not contraindications to definitive repair. Absence of the colon, however, is a contraindication to PSARP.

Although a variety of abdominoperineal approaches have been advocated for the repair of ARMs, the authors recommend the posterior sagittal approach for all defects. In cases of a rectobladder neck fistula and a persistent cloaca with a common channel longer than 3 cm, a laparotomy may also be required.

Patient Positioning

The prone position with the pelvis elevated is the optimal position for the posterior sagittal approach to ARMs. A Foley catheter is inserted into the bladder prior to positioning the patient. It is not uncommon for the catheter to follow the fistula tract into the rectum and end up in the field during the operation. It should be redirected once the rectum has been opened.

Electrical Stimulation

Although the patient is paralyzed, electrical stimulation of the perineum can be conducted through a series of reflex arcs directly via muscle. Stimulation facilitates maintaining a symmetry of muscle during the dissection. When stimulating on the skin, 100 to 200 mA may be required, whereas current of 20 to 40 mA is all that should be required directly on muscle.

Incision

A midline incision facilitates keeping the sphincter mechanism symmetrically about the midline. Direct regional periodic electrical stimulation of the sphincteric mechanism ensures equal distribution of the voluntary striated muscle. There have been no published reports of nerves and vessels crossing the midline in this part of the body. Thus, staying in the midline raphe that seems to divide whatever spectrum of muscle is present is a prudent maneuver. Exposure using using a sharp, self-retaining retractor should only be performed in a superficial plane.

Anatomy

From the posterior sagittal approach, the anatomy of a normal child is different compared with the potential paucity of muscle in children with ARMs (see Figs. 83-19 to 83-22). One should be able to identify an external sphincter (parasagittal fibers), vertical fibers of the striated muscle complex, and the levator. Smooth muscle, but no discrete internal sphincter, has been identified.

Posterior Sagittal Anorectoplasty

Operative Approach for Males

Rectourethral Fistula (Bulbar and Prostatic)

The incision for the rectourethral fistula procedure usually extends from just above the coccyx through to and including the center of the anal dimple and perineal body (see Fig. 83-12). The *parasagittal fibers* of the external sphincter are meticulously divided in their parallel course to the midline. This dissection is facilitated by electrical stimulation of these fibers, which usually run anteriorly and posteriorly to the anal dimple. Remember that ARMs are a spectrum of defects, thus, a spectrum of this voluntary striated muscle density will be encountered.

Medial to the parasaggital fibers and running perpendicular to them is the *muscle complex* composed of voluntary striated fibers. This muscle is really the distal (caudal) continuum of the levator muscle (Fig. 83-28).

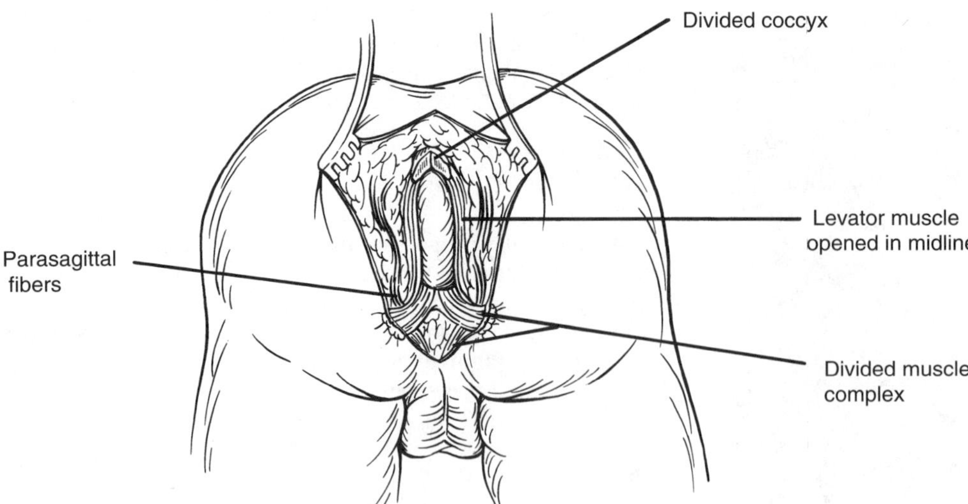

FIG. 83-28. Exposure of parasagittal fibers, muscle complex, and levator muscle via the posterior sagittal approach.

Deep to the parasagittal fibers is ischiorectal fat. If the surgeon does not stay in the midline, a small hernia of this fat can protrude into the operative field. The midline raphe in this area is very thin, and, thus, the potential for this fat to herniate is common. As the dissection continues deep to the ischiorectal fat, the midline *levator musculature* comes into the field (Fig. 83-29). The levator fibers run parallel to the skin incision.

Electrical stimulation of all three groups of muscle produces distinctive contraction of the anal dimple. For example, stimulation of the levator muscle contracts the anus in a forward motion. Stimulation of the muscle complex moves the anal dimple up toward the pelvis. The parasagittal fibers circumferentially contract the anus. Suture markers can be placed at the junction of the muscle complex and parasagittal fibers because these points form the posterior and anterior limits of the neo anus.

At this point in the procedure, the surgeon needs to have a sense of how extensive a dissection must be performed to find the rectum. Distal colostography provides the most valuable information to delineate the anatomic position of the bowel to ultimately approach the fistula. Thus, for example, the location of the rectum in a rectourethral bulbar fistula should be evident distally in the operative field after the levator muscle has been divided, whereas in cases of a prostatic fistula the bowel is located much higher in the field. Based on distal colostography,

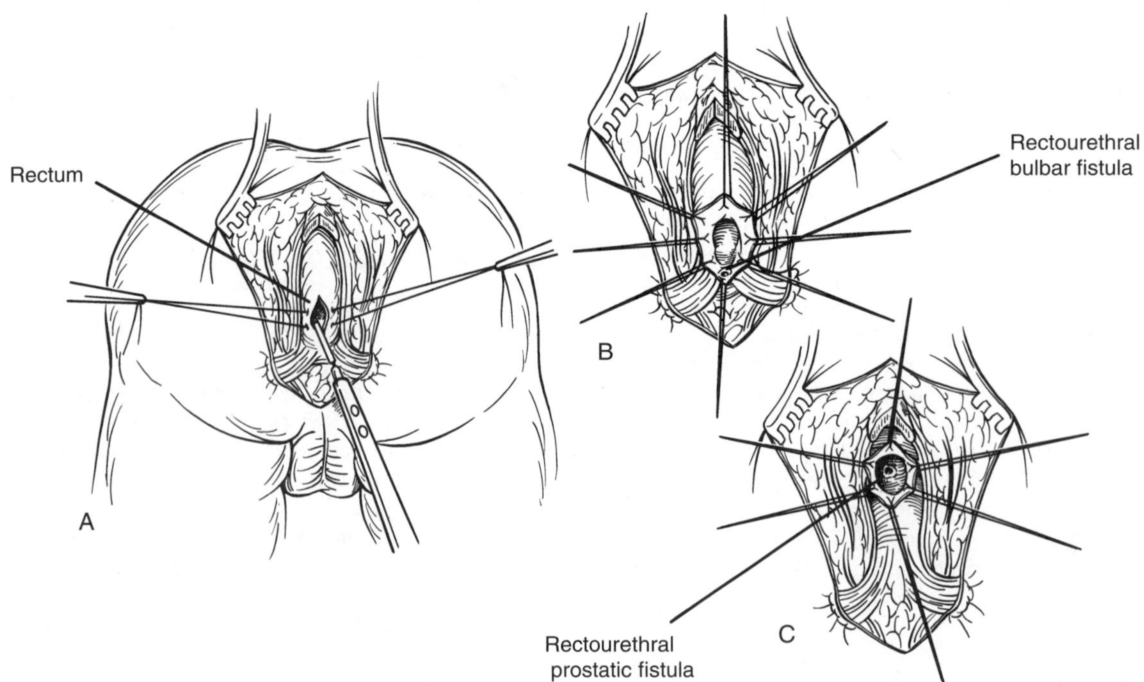

FIG. 83-29. Locating the fistula via the posterior sagittal anorectoplasty approach. Stay sutures on either side of the rectum facilitate opening the rectum. (*A*) In cases of bulbar fistula (*B*) and prostatic urethral fistula (*C*), the stay sutures provide access to the fistula opening.

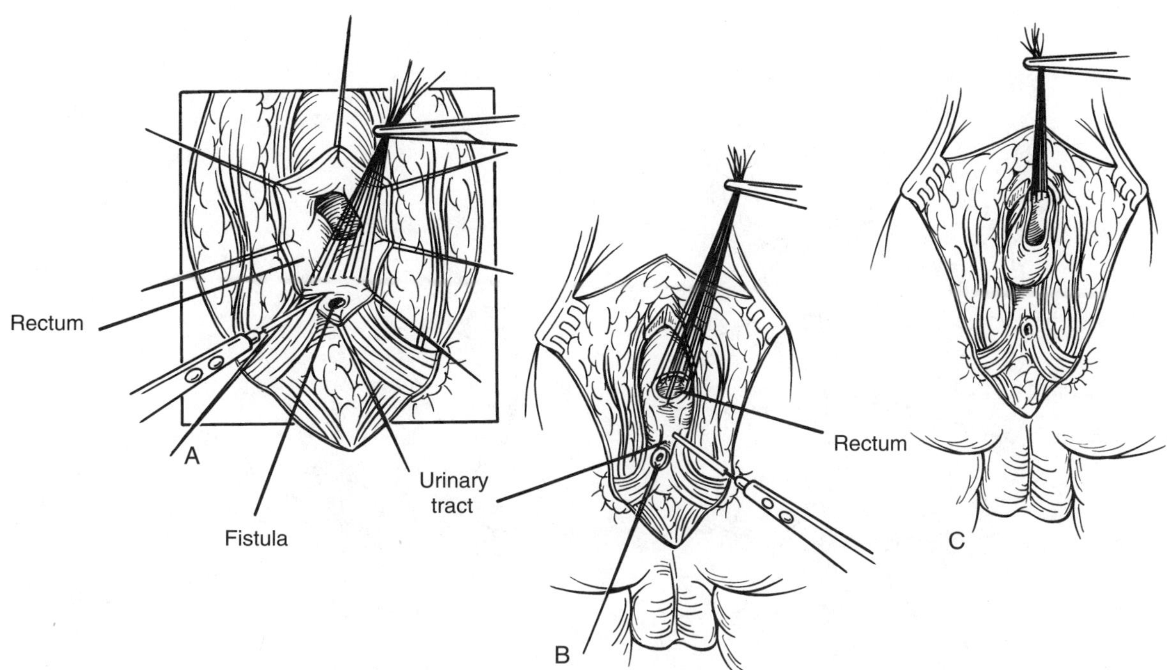

FIG. 83-30. Separation of rectum and urethral fistula via the posterior sagittal anorectoplasty approach. Traction sutures are used to begin a submucosal dissection (*A*) that ultimately separates the rectum (*B*) from the urinary tract (*C*).

one can readily appreciate that the rectum in a bladder neck fistula cannot be seen or reached from a posterior sagittal approach; and therefore it must be found and mobilized through an abdominal incision. Once the rectum is identified, a series of posterior stay sutures facilitate opening the rectum in the midline. The rectal incision is extended until the fistula site, usually anterior in location, is found (see Fig. 83-29).

Above the fistula there is no plane of dissection between the urethra and rectum. Therefore, a submucosal dissection must be performed separating these two structures. Silk stay sutures will facilitate this dissection. Uniform traction can be exerted on these stay sutures while dissecting between rectum and urethra for a distance of 6 to 8 mm above the fistula (Fig. 83-30). A plane is encountered that independently separates the urethra and rectum. The urethral fistula is sutured with interrupted absorbable sutures. At this point in the procedure, circumferential dissection of the rectum is performed to mobilize and gain enough length to reach the perineum. Nerves, fascia, and blood vessels outside the circular outer wall layer of the rectum must be divided to gain adequate length. The consequences of this denervation are unclear. Recall that the rectum has an excellent intramural blood supply, and, therefore, the rectal wall must remain intact to avoid devascularization of the rectum. If the rectum is entered at multiple sites, however, the potential for ischemia and fibrosis is increased. A tension-free neoanoplasty must be assured after an adequate mobilization. The size of the rectum (frequently ectatic), the available space, and the limits of the external sphincter dictate the need for a posterior tapering of the rectum. In general, this tapering is not necessary, but, if the rectum cannot be tailored to rest within the limits of the sphincteric mechanism, then tapering should be performed.

After the rectum is dissected and placed in its new position, the fistula is closed, and all bleeding is cauterized, the recon-

struction can proceed. The perineal body is first created by reapproximating the tissue anterior to and including the anterior limits of the external sphincter. Electrical stimulation should facilitate localizing this anterior limit. Next, the levator musculature behind the rectum is reapproximated from the cut edge of the coccyx to the posterior limit of the muscle complex. The rectal wall is not included in these bites. The posterior limit of the muscle complex is sutured together with the posterior wall of the rectum (Fig. 83-31). This maneuver usually prevents prolapse of the rectum. The ischiorectal fat and subcutaneous tissue are sutured with careful attention to avoid any dead space. Skin is closed using a subcuticular stitch or interrupted absorbable sutures. Ultimately, the anoplasty is performed using 16 absorbable 5–0 sutures in a circumference that incorporates skin and full-thickness bowel within the boundaries set forth by stimulation of the muscle complex and external sphincter (Fig. 83-32).

Rectobladder Neck Fistula

In the case of a rectobladder neck fistula, a laparotomy along with a posterior sagittal approach is required (see Fig. 83-13). Therefore, we recommend a total body preparation extending from the nipples, including both the anterior and posterior body walls through to and including both lower extremities. The operation begins by posteriorly dividing the sphincter mechanism in the midline as detailed above. A red rubber catheter is useful as a marker and should be positioned in front of the levator muscles and in the presacral space, simulating the desired position of the rectum (Fig. 83-33). The surgeon can then elect to reconstruct the perineal musculature, the levator muscle, and muscle complex, and to close the wound as in the case of the

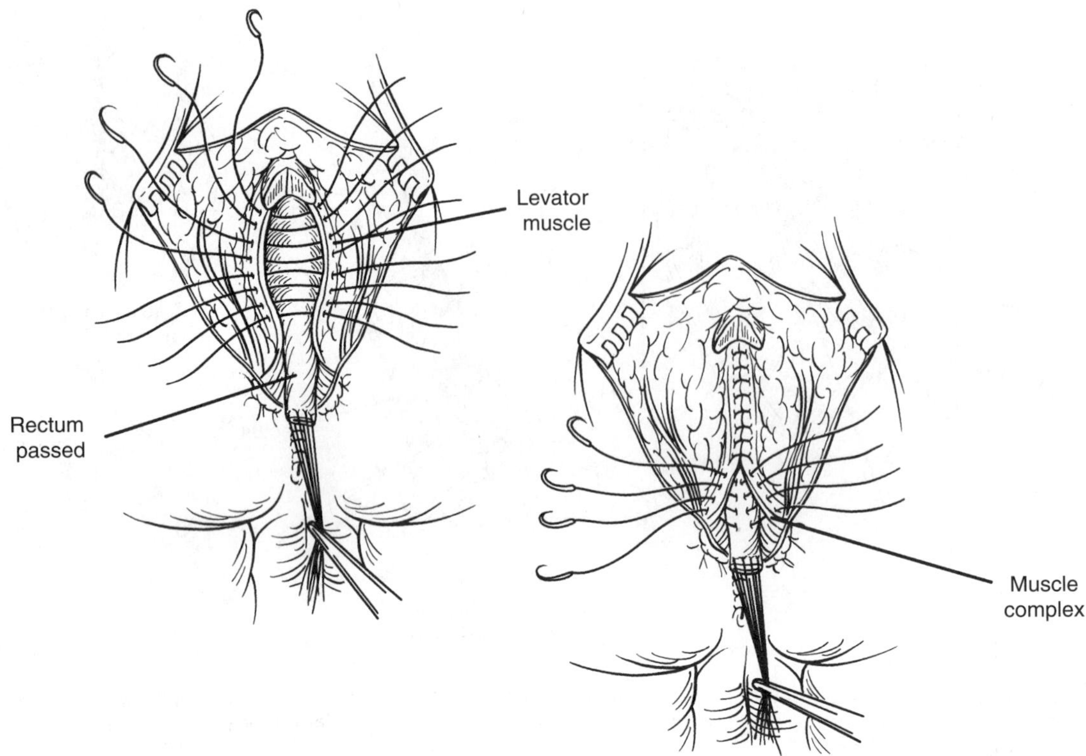

FIG. 83-31. Suturing the voluntary striated muscle mechanism. (*A*) The levator muscle is reapproximated from the coccyx to the posterior limit of the muscle complex. (*B*) The posterior limit of the muscle complex is sutured to the posterior rectal wall.

rectourethral fistula around the rubber catheter. The patient can then be turned and the abdomen is opened; the sigmoid colon is identified and the dissection proceeds to the bladder neck. In general, the junction of the bladder neck and the sigmoid colon is at most 2 cm below the peritoneal reflection. There is usually no requirement for an endorectal dissection. It is important to stay as close to the rectal wall as possible because any lateral dissection runs the risk of damage to the vas deferens

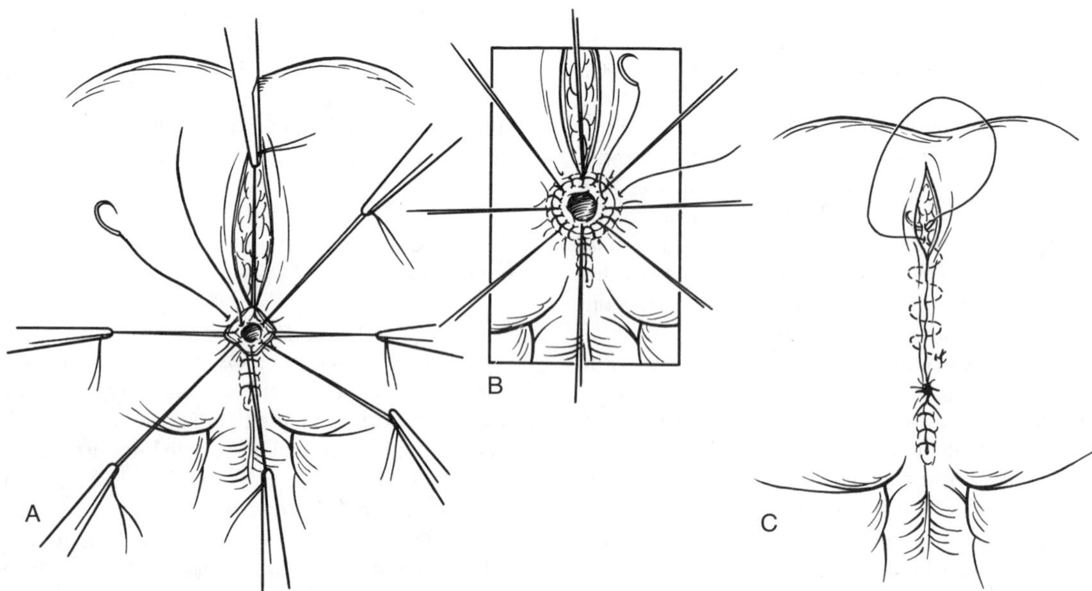

FIG. 83-32. Anoplasty. The anoplasty incorporates full-thickness bowel to skin and is located within the boundaries of the muscle complex and external sphincter fibers.

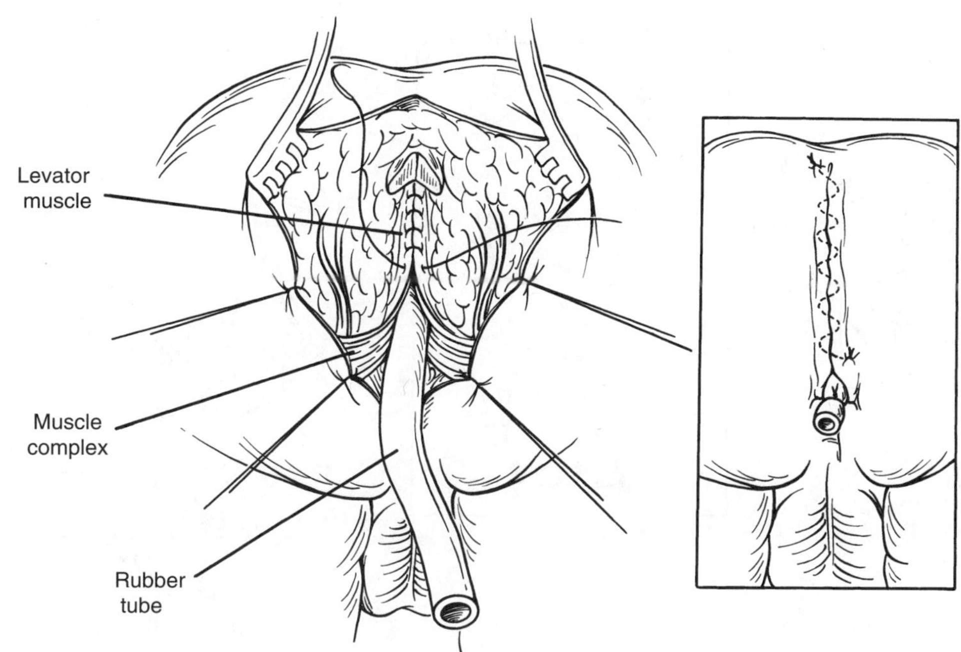

FIG. 83-33. Posterior sagittal anorectoplasty approach for recto-bladder neck fistula. A catheter can be positioned in front of the levator musculature into the presacral space. The musculature can then be reconstructed, the wound closed, and the child turned for the abdominal portion of the procedure.

and ureters. The rectosigmoid usually narrows as it approaches the bladder and ultimately inserts in a T fashion into the trigone. The rectum is divided and the bladder is closed with 2–3 absorbable sutures. Next, the red rubber catheter is found in the retroperitoneum and is anchored to the bowel (Fig. 83-34). If there is significant disparity in the size of the bowel such that it appears that the bowel cannot be pulled onto the perineum, then a posterior tapering of the rectum can be performed. In addition, if the mobilization of the rectum is limited by the vasculature, the necessary length can be obtained by dividing the peripheral branches of the inferior mesenteric vessels. The major blood supply to the rectum is via its intramural blood supply. Once the bowel is pulled through the presacral space to the perineum, an anoplasty can be performed as previously described.

Imperforate Anus Without Fistula

In the case of imperforate anus without fistula, the rectum is usually located at the level of a bulbar urethral fistula (see Fig. 83-14). Here the rectum is intimately associated with the posterior urethra, and meticulous dissection to separate the two

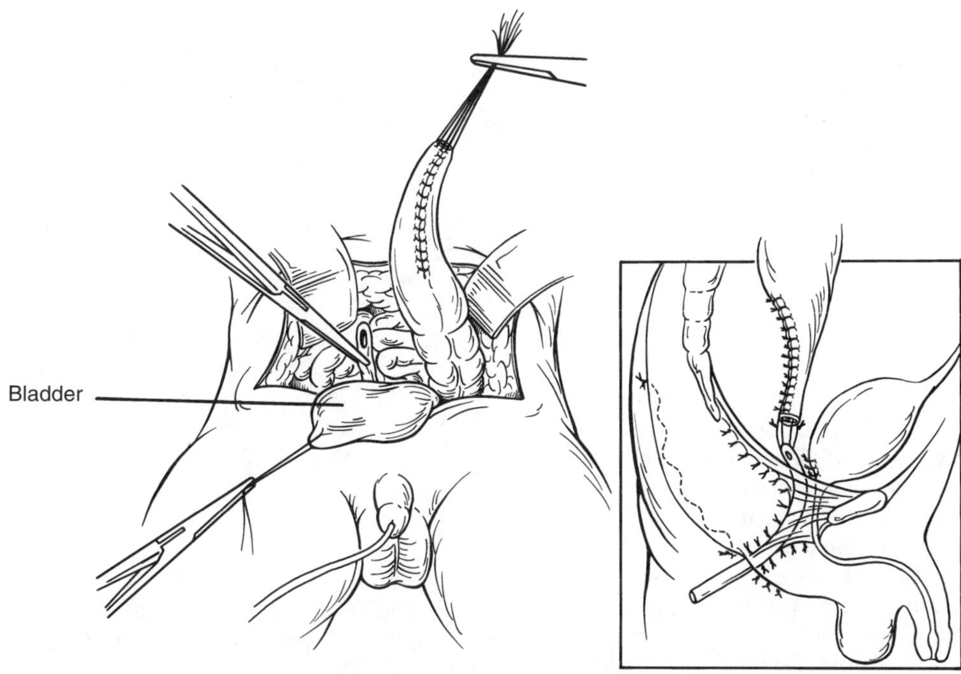

FIG. 83-34. Posterior sagittal anorectoplasty completion bladder neck repair. The rectosigmoid usually enters the bladder at the level of the trigone. After dividing the rectum and closing the bladder, the rectum can be anchored to the catheter and pulled through the presacral space.

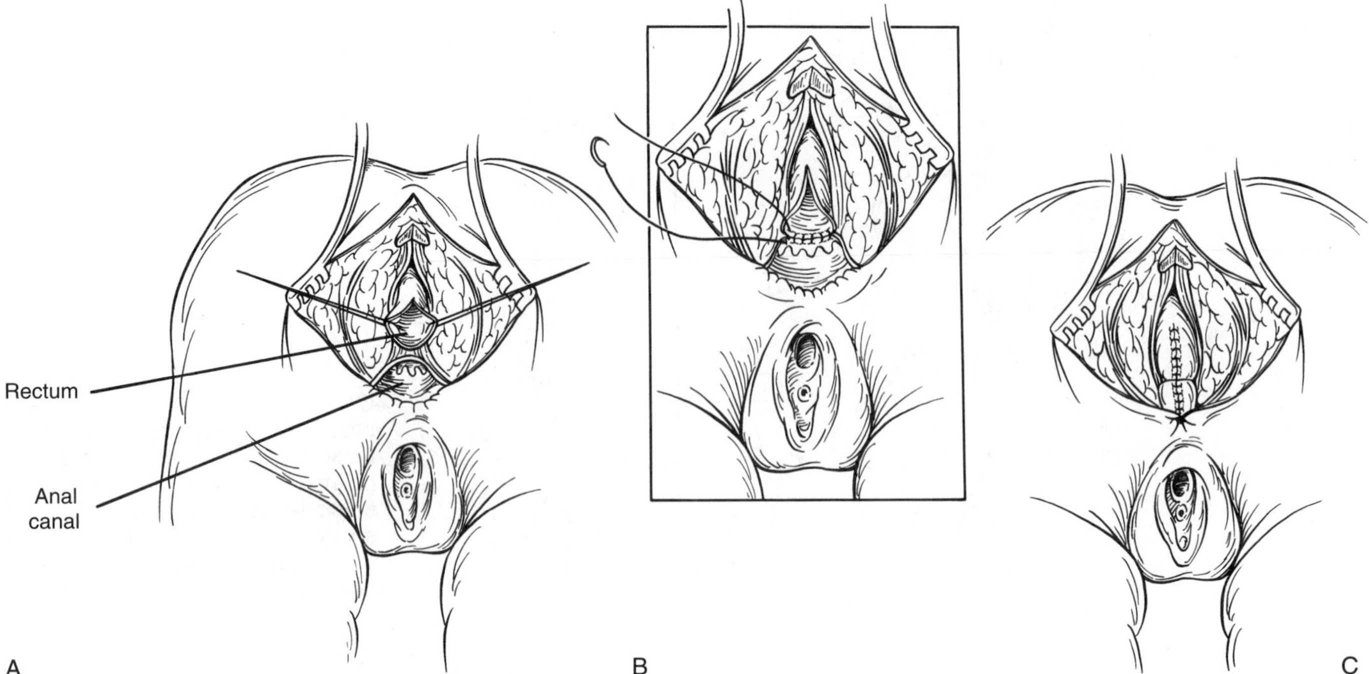

FIG. 83-35. Posterior sagittal anorectoplasty repair of rectal atresia. The distal end of the bowel is sutured end-to-end to the blind-ending rectum (*A, B*), and then the rectum is closed (*C*).

must be performed. The remainder of the operative procedure follows the techniques described for rectourethral fistula defects.

Rectal Atresia and Stenosis

We recommend a posterior sagittal approach for the rectal atresia and stenosis defect (see Fig. 83-15). The distal end of the anal canal must be sutured end-to-end to the blind-ending rectum (Fig. 83-35). In general, the two structures are usually separated by at most a distance of 1 cm. Minimal mobilization is required because usually the upper rectum lies very close to the anal canal. A strict protocol of bowel dilatation must be followed to avoid a stricture because one must remember that after the operation, the anastomosis is going to be constantly compressed by an almost normal sphincteric mechanism.

Operative Approach for Females

Rectovestibular Fistula

There is an obvious disagreement in the pediatric surgical literature concerning the appropriate management of the recto-vestibular fistula[129–132] (see Fig. 83-16). In part, this is because of a fundamental underestimation of the complexity of the defect. There is no question that this ARM can be repaired without a colostomy but the functional prognosis should be excellent. Yet in the absence of a protective colostomy, the repair of the vestibular fistula carries a significant morbidity characterized by wound dehiscence and infection that can jeopardize the final

functional prognosis. Therefore, a protective colostomy is advised and a limited PSARP is performed at 1 month of age provided the baby is otherwise healthy.

A limited posterior sagittal anoplasty incision begins anterior to the coccyx and is continued to and around the fistula in the vestibule anterior to the hymen (Fig. 83-36). Multiple 6–0 sutures are placed around the fistula site to exert a uniform traction, and this parachute technique is used to facilitate dissection of the rectum. The posterior wall of the rectum is identified

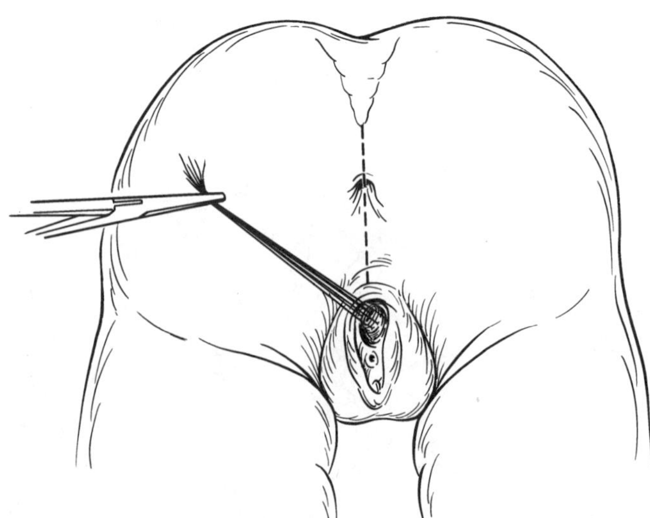

FIG. 83-36. Posterior sagittal anorectoplasty repair of recto-vestibular fistula. This procedure should begin with control of the fistula using traction sutures.

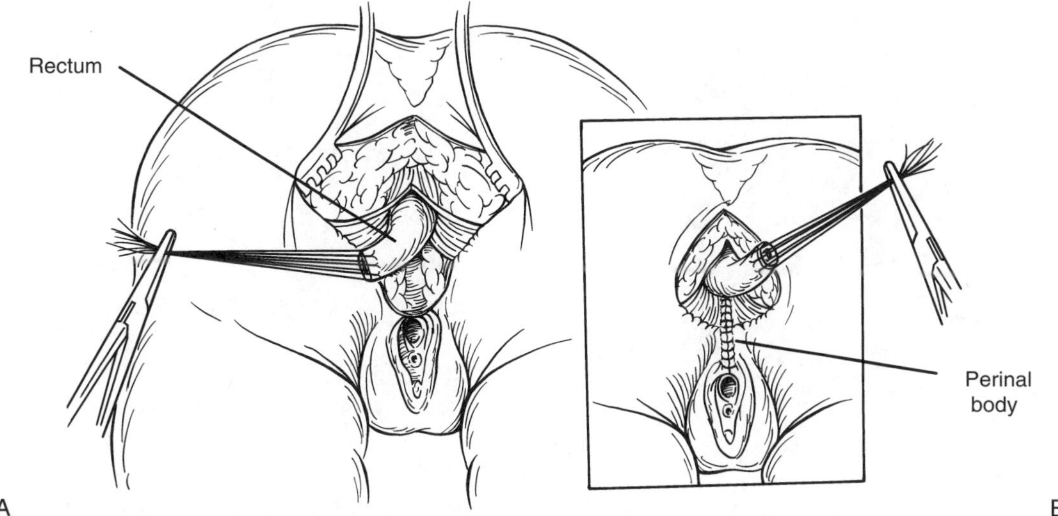

FIG. 83-37. Separation of rectum from vagina. (*A*) The rectum is separated from the vagina until two common walls exist. (*B*) The perineal body is reconstructed.

and the dissection proceeds laterally. Inferior hemorrhoidal vessels are cauterized as the dissection proceeds laterally. Separation of the rectum and vagina is facilitated by pulling on the stay sutures surrounding the fistula (Fig. 83-37). Anteriorly, there is an extensive common wall between the rectum and vagina but two walls must be created until complete separation into a definable rectal and vaginal wall plane develops. Tension resulting from too small a dissection predisposes to dehiscence.

Using electrical stimulation, the limits of the neoanus are identified and marked with sutures (see Operative Approach for Males, Rectourethral Fistula). Restore a perineal body is restored with one or two layers of tissue separating the rectum and vagina and including the anterior limits of the muscle complex (see Fig. 83-38). The muscle complex is reconstructed incorporating the posterior edge of bowel in the midline (Fig. 83-38). The levator muscle usually is not exposed. An anoplasty

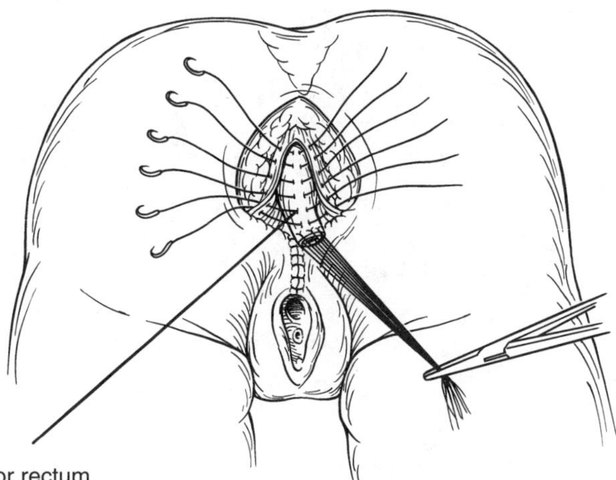

FIG. 83-38. Reconstruction of the voluntary striated muscle. In these cases, the levator is usually not exposed, instead the muscle complex must be reapproximated and anchored to the rectum.

and skin closure are performed as previously described (see Operative Approach for Males, Rectourethral Fistula).

In cases of the rare vaginal fistula, the dissection is similar except here the levator is divided because the rectum must be mobilized to reach the perineum.

Persistent Cloaca

The repair of persistent cloaca, is the most technically challenging of all types of ARMs (see Fig. 83-17). The common channel represents the confluence of urinary tract, vagina, and rectum. The operative procedure begins with a long mid-sagittal incision extending from the middle of the sacrum through the perineum and into the common single opening. A mid-sagittal incision is performed; and parasagittal fibers of the external sphincter, then the muscle complex, and finally the levator muscle are divided as mentioned above. The rectal wall should be opened in the midline distally and held open with stay sutures. The rectum must be separated from the vagina (Fig. 83-39), and then the vagina must be separated from the urinary tract (Fig. 83-40). Ultimately, all structures should reach the perineum. The rectum and vagina have a common wall as described in cases of vestibular fistula. A more complex relation is the attachment of the vagina and urethra, in fact, the separation of these structures is the most difficult part of the operation. The vagina and urinary tract have a more extensive common wall such that the vagina surrounds the posterior urethra about 270 degrees, ultimately creating two cul-de-sacs on either side of the urethra (see Fig. 83-40). The neourethra should be reconstructed using two layers of interrupted sutures (Fig. 83-41*A*). Then the vagina must be mobilized and placed behind the urethra such that there are no facing suture lines (Fig. 83-41*B*). The vagina can be rotated 90 degrees to avoid this. Likewise, any damaged urethral wall should be repaired and again suture lines should not be in opposition. A perineal body should be created after the urethra and vagina have been reconstructed and the rectum should be situated within the limits of the sphincter and muscle complex as previously described.

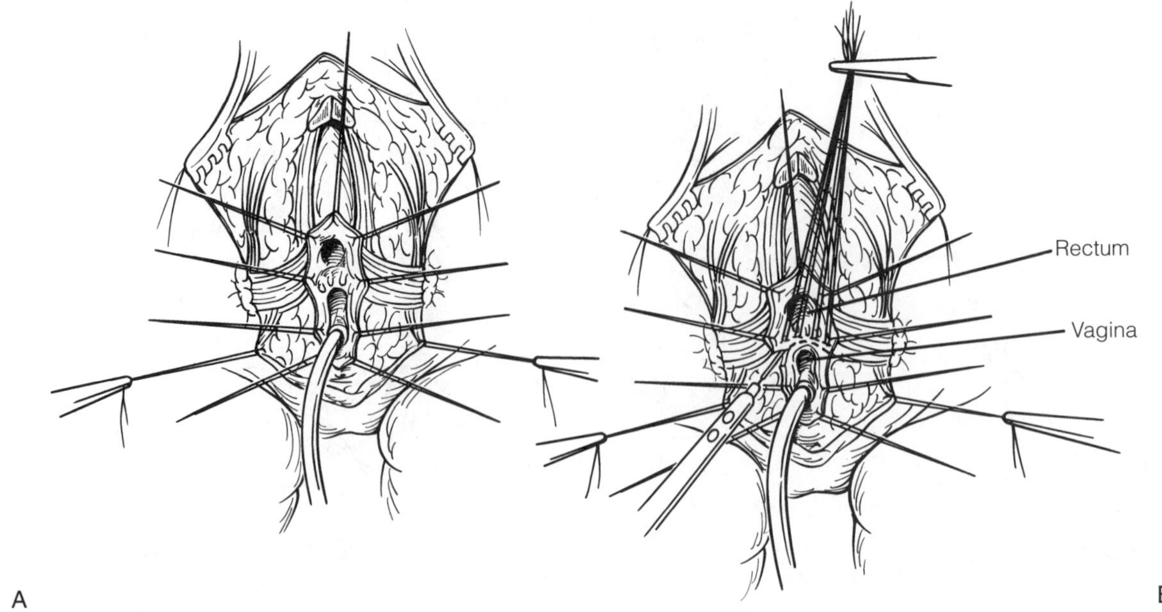

FIG. 83-39. Separation of rectum from vagina in cloaca. (*A*) Opening the cloaca. (*B*) Separation of rectum from vagina.

On the basis of the senior author's experience, a common channel less than 3 cm and normal-sized vagina means the vagina can be repaired via the posterior sagittal approach without any special maneuvers. However, a common channel longer than 3 cm with an associated small or absent vagina presents significant difficulties for adequate vaginal length. Vaginal replacement or augmentation are useful procedures for lengthening the vagina.

For cases involving vaginal atresia or a small vagina, a piece of small intestine or colon can be used to obain enough length for the vagina to be situated behind the urethra and reach the perineum.[132–134] A laparotomy is performed and a piece of bowel is chosen with a fairly long mesentery so that its vascular arcades can be manipulated through the pelvis posterior to the neourethra. The fate of the upper end of the replacement de-

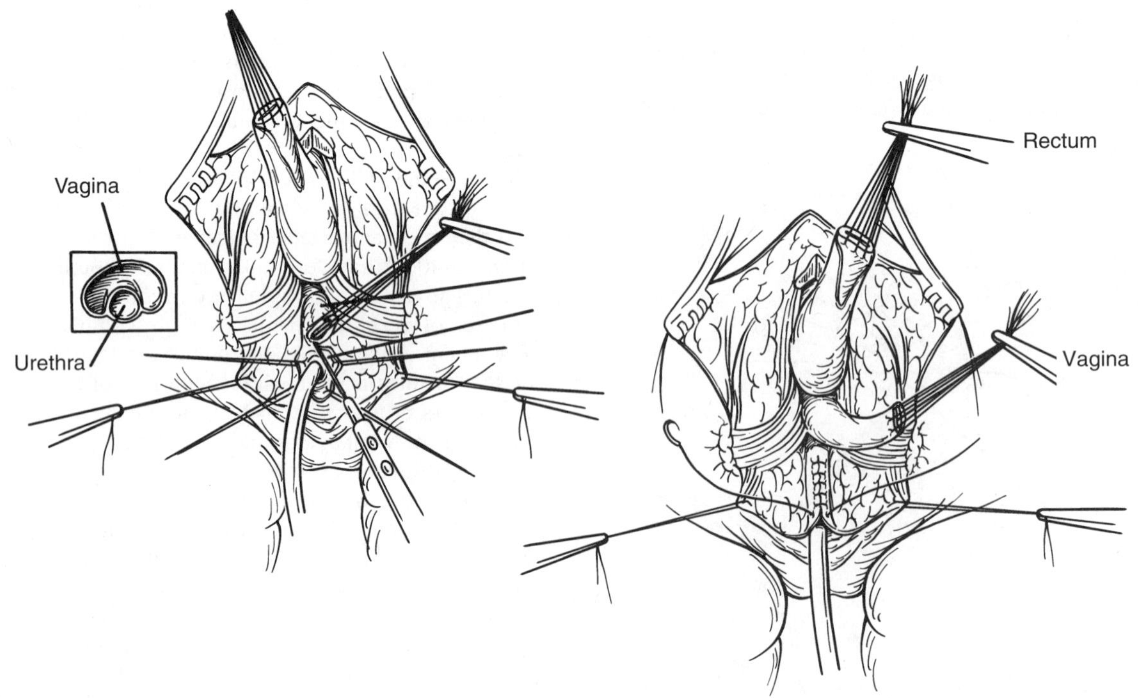

FIG. 83-40. Separation of vagina from urethra and urethral reconstruction. (*A*) Separation of vagina from urethra. Note how the vagina surrounds the posterior half of the urethra. (*B*) Urethral reconstruction.

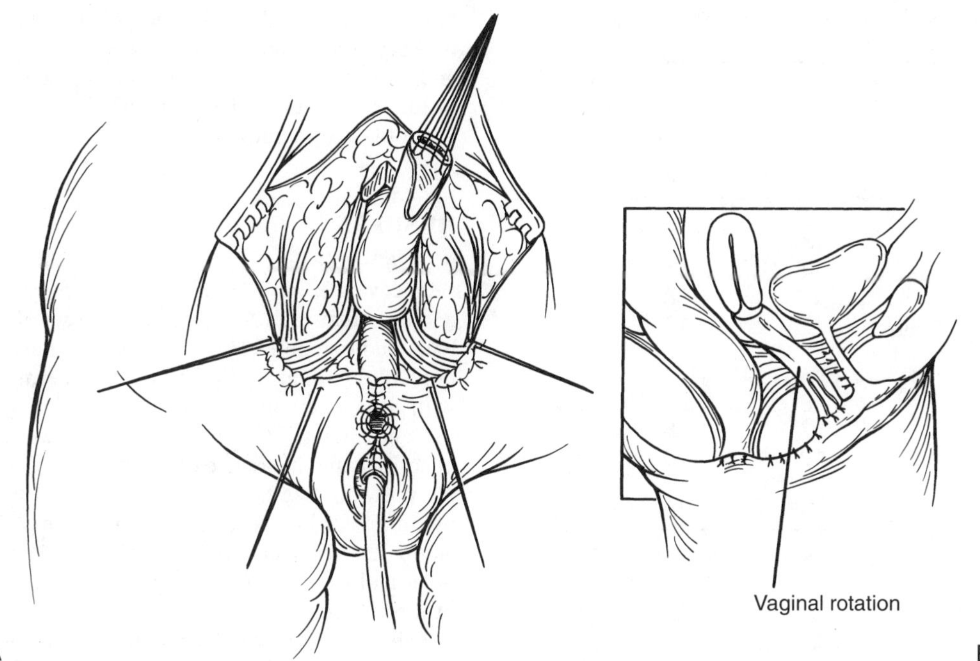

FIG. 83-41. Neourethra and vagina reconstructed. (*A*) Reconstruction of both urethra and vagina and the limits of the neoanus identified. (*B*) To avoid suture lines facing each other, the vagina is rotated 90 degrees before reconstruction.

pends on the anatomy. It either is sewn shut as a blind pouch in cases of vaginal atresia, or is sewn to the atretic portion of the vagina. The main disadvantage in using bowel to replace the vagina is excess mucus secretions. Skin flaps for any type of vaginal reconstruction should be avoided because of the high incidence of fibrosis, retraction, and scar formation.

In cases of two large hemivaginas, bilateral hydrocolpos, and two hemiuteruses, the potential for ischemic injury during the attempt to mobilize the vaginas is high. If the horizontal length of the vaginas is longer than the vertical length, the blood supply of one hemivagina is sacrificed and the hemiuterus on the same side is excised. Next the common septum separating both hemivaginas is excised and the vaginas are tubularized into a single vagina that is switched onto the perineum.

A vaginal dome flap can be created in those instances where the vagina is very large. This flap off the dome of the vagina can be tubularized to reach the perineum.

POSTOPERATIVE MANAGEMENT

In general, postoperative ARM children have little pain except for those who undergo laparotomy. Patient-controlled anesthesia instead of epidural pain control is advisable. In cases of rectourethral or bladder neck fistula, the Foley catheter remains for 4 to 5 days. After a cloacal repair, the Foley catheter remains for 10 to 14 days. Suprapubic drainage is indicated in cases of cloacas with a common channel longer than 3 cm. Perioperative intravenous antibiotics are given for 2 to 3 days and a topical antibiotic ointment can be used for the wound. Sitz baths are usually started by postoperative day 3 to 4.

Timing the Colostomy Closure

In general, 2 to 3 weeks after repair anal dilatations are started. The operating surgeon should perform the first one, then twice daily dilatations should be performed by the family or health care worker. Each week the dilator can be advanced by 1 mm in caliber until the desired size is reached. Once the desired size is achieved, the stoma can be closed. Dilatations, however, must be continued twice daily until the dilator can be passed easily. Then dilatations proceed once daily for a month followed by every third day for the next month, twice a week for a month, once a week for one month, and finally once a month for 3 months. A systematic program of postoperative anal dilatation to avoid anal strictures cannot be overemphasized.

After closure of the colostomy, children may suffer from a diaper rash secondary to multiple daily bowel movements. A typical paste used for the diaper rash consists of vitamin A and D ointment, aloe, neomycin, Desitin, and Mylanta. Nystatin is added if the rash is the result of yeast. We encourage the use of a constipating diet to add bulk to the stool. The surgeon, however, must be cognizant of the fact that these children were born with no anus and some element of rectal atresia; thus, the major postoperative physiologic problem is a hypomotility disorder of the pulled-through bowel. In the unfortunate situation in which the rectum and colon were resected, hypermotility and intractable diarrhea may be the chief post operative complaint.

Bowel Training Program

We encourage families of children about 2 years of age with a good prognosis type of ARM to begin a bowel training program

TABLE 83-6. *Voluntary bowel movement and type of defect*

Defect	Cases (No.)	Voluntary bowel movement No.	%
Rectal atresia or stenosis	5	5	100
Perineal fistula	14	14	100
Vestibular fistula	44	41	93.2
Bulbar fistula	47	38	80.9
Imperforate anus without fistula	17	13	76.5
Vaginal fistula	4	3	75
Cloaca	38	27	71.1
Prostatic fistula	57	38	66.7
Bladder neck fistula	19	3	15.8
Total	245	182	74.3

(Pena A. Anorectal malformations. Semin Pediatr Surg 1995;4:35).

(BTP) of using the potty after each meal. If the family is unsuccessful in toilet training by the time the child is ready to attend school, then we recommend delaying the start of school and continuing with the BTP or beginning a bowel management program (BMP) for the temporary period of 1 year. We do not recommend that children with repaired ARM be allowed to suffer in diapers at school while their peers are toilet trained.

Bowel Management Program

The BMP is designed to keep artificially clean all those children who suffer temporary or permanent fecal incontinence. Therefore, the BMP is usually indicated in children with high defects and poor anatomy. Obviously, children with ARMs have a spectrum of defects and thus we should expect a spectrum of results regardless of how impeccable an operation. The basic principle of this program involves cleaning the colon once a day and keeping the colon quiescent (i.e., no motility or little motility) for 24 hours. This is conducted using enemas (Fleet) and colonic irrigations (via Foley catheter using Fleet enema or saline), as well as dietary manipulation and medications (i.e., Lomotil or Imodium).

RESULTS

The single most important concept in analyzing series of results is that each ARM has its own set of postoperative problems and outcome. Thus, the authors must stress that expectations of continence in a child with a perineal fistula compared with a bladder neck fistula must be different. In general, results can and should focus on voluntary bowel movements, degree of soiling, and incidence of constipation. Some authors feel that the posterior sagittal approach has not changed the prognosis of children with anorectal malformations.[128,135–137] The senior author has critically reviewed his ARM patients ages 3 and older and who are at least 6 months postoperative from closure of their stoma.[58]

Table 83-6 shows the number of patients who achieved a voluntary bowel movement in each type of defect. Overall, 245 children were interviewed and the incidence of a voluntary bowel movement was 74.3%. Children with a perineal fistula and rectal atresia or stenosis had the best results followed by repair of the vestibular fistula. To emphasize the importance of the mesodermal derivation of hindgut bone, muscle, and nerve it is interesting that the three patients with a vestibular fistula who did not have a voluntary bowel movement also had abnormal sacra. Children who had a bulbar fistula and an ARM without a fistula had similar rates of voluntary bowel movements. The poorest prognosis for a voluntary bowel movement is seen in children with a bladder neck fistula. In these children, there was only a 15% incidence of voluntary bowel movements.[58]

Children who soil are represented in Table 83-7, again related to type of defect. Of the cohort interviewed, 57% had some degree of soiling. Grade 1 soiling (19%) is defined as a nondisturbing event and is considered normal by parents. Anything more than a grade 1 is a problem both for the child and parents (38%). Soiling was not a problem for children with rectal atresia

TABLE 83-7. *Soiling and type of defect*

Defect	Cases	Soiling Grade 1*	Grade >1*	Total	%
Rectal atresia or stenosis	5	0	0	0	0
Perineal fistula	14	0	0	0	0
Vestibular fistula	43	9 (20.9)	4 (9.3)	13	30.2
Imperforate anus with no fistula	18	1 (5.5)	6 (33.3)	7	38.9
Bulbar fistula	48	14 (29.1)	17 (35.4)	31	64.6
Cloaca	38	9 (23.6)	17 (44.7)	26	68.4
Prostatic fistula	58	11 (18.9)	32 (55.1)	43	74.1
Bladder neck fistula	23	1 (4.3)	18 (78.2)	19	82.6
Vaginal fistula	4	2 (50.0)	2 (50.0)	4	100.0
Total	251	47 (18.7)	96 (38.2)	143	57.0

* Percentage in parentheses.
(Pena A. Anorectal malformations. Semin Pediatr Surg 1995;4:35).

TABLE 83-8. *Totally continent patients and type of defect*

Defect	Cases	Totally continent*	
		No.	%
Perineal fistula	14	14	100
Atresia or stenosis	5	5	100
Vestibular fistula	44	29	65.9
Imperforate anus with no fistula	17	9	52.9
Bulbar fistula	47	16	34
Cloaca	38	12	31.6
Prostatic fistula	57	15	26.3
Vaginal fistula	4	0	0
Bladder neck fistula	19	0	0
Total	245	100	40.8

* Voluntary bowel movement and no soiling.
(Pena A. Anorectal malformations. Semin Pediatr Surg 1995;4:35).

or perineal fistula. Instead, children with high ARMs such as bulbar and prostatic, bladder neck, cloaca, and vaginal fistulas had the highest incidence.

Children who are totally free of soiling and have a voluntary bowel movement are shown in Table 83-8. These children are called totally continent. Overall, 41% of the children surveyed were totally continent. This included all children with perineal fistulas and rectal atresia or stenosis and none of the children with bladder neck or vaginal fistulas. Of those with vestibular fistulas, 66% were totally continent, but only 26% of males with prostatic fistulas fit in this category.

In contrast, constipation was found most frequently in children with a vestibular and bulbar fistula and least in patients with higher defects (Table 83-9). Grade 1 constipation can be managed with diet alone, and 15% of the cohort had this degree of constipation. A more severe form of constipation was experienced by 27%, and overall some degree of constipation was experienced by 43%.

The preceding results would indicate that children with a perineal fistula, rectal atresia, or stenosis (the low ARM) should be totally continent yet have a high incidence of constipation.

In contrast, the bladder neck, cloaca, or vaginal fistulas (the high defects) have the lowest incidence of constipation and highest frequency of incontinence.

Urinary incontinence seems to be most frequent in children with poor sacrums and a persistent cloaca.[58] In general, excluding the persistent cloaca, if a child has a normal sacrum and an isolated ARM, we should expect normal urinary function.

For patients with a persistent cloaca, the groups separate out based on the length of the common channel (Table 83-10). A short common channel (<3 cm) and good sacrum mean a better prognosis than a long common channel and an associated abnormal sacrum.[58]

COMPLICATIONS

Table 83-11 lists the complications following PSARP. They can be divided into early and late problems and should not be confused with functional sequelae of the original ARM but instead are operator dependent. Early complications include infection and dehiscence secondary to ischemia from damage of the intramural blood supply of the bowel. A neurogenic bladder can be the result of not staying in the midline during the dissection. In cases of long-channel cloacas (>3 cm), a neurogenic bladder may be an unavoidable sequela of the anomaly. Other early complications include transient femoral nerve palsy from defective cushioning of the child's groin. Additional complications include intraoperative injury to the urethra and vas deferens and complete necrosis of a mobilized vagina in the case of a cloaca.

Late complications include vaginal and neoanus anastomotic strictures, narrow introitus (cloaca), urethrovaginal fistula (cloaca), persistent rectourethral fistula, and prolapse of the pulled-through bowel. A posterior urethral diverticulum found post-operatively on a VCUG may represent retained rectum. This complication has never been seen following a PSARP. It may cause urinary dribbling despite a normally reconstructed anus and takedown of the fistula. This late complication has been seen after the abdominoperineal type of pull-through procedure.

TABLE 83-9. *Constipation and type of defect*

Defect	Cases	Constipation			
		Grade 1*	Grade >1*	Total	%
Vestibular fistula	44	15 (34.1)	12 (27.3)	27	61.4
Bulbar fistula	45	5 (11.1)	20 (44.4)	25	55.5
Imperforate anus with no fistula	18	3 (16.7)	6 (33.3)	9	50.0
Prostatic fistula	58	9 (15.5)	15 (25.9)	24	41.4
Atresia or stenosis	5	1 (20.0)	1 (20.0)	2	40.0
Perineal fistula	14	3 (21.5)	1 (7.1)	4	28.6
Cloaca	36	1 (2.7)	9 (25.0)	10	27.7
Vaginal fistula	4	0	1 (25.0)	1	25.0
Bladder neck fistula	22	1 (4.6)	3 (13.6)	4	18.2
Total	246	38 (15.4)	68 (27.6)	106	43.1

* Percentage in parentheses.
(Pena A. Anorectal malformations. Semin Pediatr Surg 1995;4:35).

TABLE 83-10. *Clinical results in cloacas and importance of length of common channel and sacral ratio**

Common channel length	Sacral ratios		No. voluntary bowel movement (% cases)	Soiling (% cases)	Constipation (% cases)	Urinary incontinence (% cases)
	Anterior-posterior	Lateral				
<3 cm	0.558	0.657	23.8	71	19	19
>3 cm	0.556†	0.551††	37.5	69	40	69

* This series consisted of 39 cases.
† Difference not significant.
††$P=0.2$.
(Pena A. Anorectal malformations. Semin Pediatr Surg 1995;4:35).

EVALUATION, MANAGEMENT, AND RECOMMENDATIONS FOR POSTOPERATIVE FUNCTIONAL DISORDERS

Problems Following Posterior Sagittal Anorectoplasty

After an ARM is repaired, the goal is fecal continence of the patient. Most normal children toilet train between the ages of $2\frac{1}{2}$ to 3 years of age. Prior to this age in children with ARMs, there are some signs that indicate the possibility for toilet training. Good prognostic signs include 1 to 3 bowel movements per day and no soiling in between, evidence for sensation when passing stool (such as pushing or making faces), good quality sacrum, well-formed and contoured buttocks, and urinary control. Early postoperative signs of poor prognosis include constant soiling of stool, absence of any sensation during defecation, dribbling or urinary incontinence, flat bottom, and poor quality sacrum (more than two sacral vertebrae missing).

The most common postoperative sequelae seen in children with imperforate anus following PSARP include constipation, soiling, and absence of voluntary bowel movements.

Constipation

Constipation occurs a few days or even weeks after the colostomy is closed. These children are not close to toilet-training age, so this problem is not associated with continence. Constipa-

TABLE 83-11. *Complications*

EARLY
Infection
Dehiscence
Neurogenic bladder
Transient femoral nerve palsy
Intraoperative injury to urethra, vas deferens
Complete necrosis of the mobilized vagina

LATE
Anastomotic stricture
  Neoanus
  Vagina
Narrow introitus
Urethrovaginal fistula
Persistent rectourethral fistula
Prolapse of bowel
Retained rectum

tion should be diagnosed and treated very early in the postoperative care of a child with ARMs. After PSARP, constipation should be expected, especially with the lower defects (see Results), and therefore prevented. Most doctors or parents make the diagnosis of constipation if a child does not have a bowel movement in 4 to 48 hours. On the other hand, constipated children frequently have multiple small loose tiny bowel movements during the day, which confuses the parents and physicians. In reality, these children never empty their rectosigmoid colon and may be suffering from fecal impaction. Postoperative constipation is thought to be caused by a hypomotility disorder of the ectatic rectum. Iatrogenic causes of postoperative constipation following PSARP include loop and transverse colostomies that allow passage of stool into the distal segment of bowel as well as delays in definitive PSARP repair (i.e., operation 1 year after creation of the colostomy). If untreated, hypomotility results in incomplete emptying of the rectosigmoid colon, constipation, and impaction.

Denervation of the rectal pouch, provoked by its dissection and mobilization, and tapering of the rectum have been invoked as causes of constipation. This proved not to be the case in our series, however.[58,83] Instead, we have seen post-PSARP constipation associated with lower defects (by definition minimal dissection and no tapering). By contrast, patients with higher defects (by definition more dissection) suffer from less constipation.

Post-PSARP constipation is treated with laxatives. We have found that each child suffers from a different degree of constipation and therefore the amount and type of laxative regimen must be individualized. In general, we first start with dietary awareness (benefits of fresh fruit and vegetables) and proceed from natural fiber-based laxatives (pear and prune juices, bran) to active medication such as stimulants (lactulose, mineral oil) and cathartics (senna). If by the end of the day the child has not had a bowel movement, enemas are introduced as a last resort. The amount of laxative must be increased daily until we find the appropriate dose for the child, but in the meantime the rectum must be emptied everyday by the use of an enema. Once we can provoke a bowel movement using the laxatives, then the child does not need enemas any longer.

The literature is replete with the use of behavior modification and biofeedback techniques to help keep the colon clean, but these have not been used in cases of constipation after repair of ARM.[138,139] The authors have no personal experience with the use of these techniques for ARMs. Biofeedback is dependent on rectal sensation, but because the child must be able to make a response, age is crucial. Anal manometry is helpful for biofeedback techniques.[140] Children who are in the process of toilet training, having two to three bowel movements per day and soiling in between, may also benefit from behavior modification techniques.

Soiling

Soiling is either associated with voluntary or involuntary bowel movements. Soiling associated with a voluntary bowel movement should be viewed as a symptom of constipation. Children with a defect that has a good prognosis may soil between bowel movements. This sign must alert the clinician about the presence of chronic impaction. Thus, this type of soiling is usually treated and eliminated with laxative therapy. Generally, these children will respond successfully. Children with involuntary bowel movements and soiling should be considered totally incontinent. In children with a poor prognosis, soiling indicates incontinence and is expected. Because of their original poor prognosis, we recommend a trial of BMP. If this is not successful, we offer the child a permanent diversion or a continent appendicostomy.

No Voluntary Bowel Movements

In children with a poor prognosis, having no voluntary bowel movements, despite a good PSARP repair, this is expected and signifies incontinence. These children can be helped with the BMP (see Postoperative Management). In children with a good prognosis, lack of voluntary bowel movements may represent overflow pseudo-incontinence secondary to constipation or real incontinence resulting from poor operative technique. Treating these children with laxatives will elucidate the differential problem.

Problem of Fecal Incontinence After ARM Repair

The pediatric surgeon is frequently called in consultation for a child suffering from fecal incontinence after an operation for ARMs performed at another institution. The initial evaluation should consist of a detailed history (including a review of the actual x-rays and pathology), knowledge of the type of operation performed (endorectal, rectosigmoid resection), and physical examination. Accuracy of classification of the original defect facilitates a more realistic appraisal of the prognosis. A physical examination should verify that the rectum is in proper position to describe the contour of the buttocks. Radiographs of the lumbosacral spine should be evaluated for abnormalities and the sacral ratio should be calculated (see Associated Anomalies). A contrast enema identifies a megasigmoid colon and shows exactly how much colon is remaining after the pull-through procedure. The postevacuation film gives an idea of the type of motility that the patient has. An MRI study determines the position of the anus in relation to the voluntary striated mechanism and identifies a tethered cord.[141,142] Voiding cystourethrography and kidney ultrasound examination should be performed even if there are no associated complaints or urinary incontinence. This is done because sometimes children have asymptomatic urethral and bladder problems as a consequence of an ARM repair. Finally, a rectal exam should be performed.

A decision-making algorithm for postoperative fecal incontinence is shown in Figure 83-42. After the children have been evaluated as described, they fall into four major categories.

Incontinence With Bad Prognosis (Not Operable)

The first group consists of patients who have a bad prognosis and thus they would not benefit from any type of reoperation. In this group are children with a poor sacrum (more than two sacral vertebrae missing), flat bottom, paucity of muscle, high defects, absence of perineal sensation, poor bowel movement pattern, and possibly associated urinary incontinence. A further reason for not reoperating on a child with postoperative incontinence is the problem of a short colon (i.e., children missing the rectosigmoid colon for whatever reason, which is verified with a contrast study. Children with short colons have an inability to form solid stool and, thus regardless of the status of their voluntary muscle mechanism, never gain bowel control. This bad prognosis, not operable group of children can be helped by a BMP. This program involves teaching the parents to clean the child's colon once daily through the use of enemas or colonic irrigations. The goal is to keep the colon quiescent between enemas.

If the child is incontinent and also suffers from constipation, he or she probably requires only large-volume enemas to remain completely clean for 24 hours. If, however, the child is incontinent and suffers from episodes of diarrhea (resulting from a lost rectosigmoid colon, as occurs in children who undergo an endorectal pull-through procedure), we recommend both a constipating diet and medication to slow the colon. Again, the goal is to keep the colon clean between enemas.

The BMP is successful in 95% of these cases. If the BMP is successful but children are dissatisfied with the enemas given in the BMP, they may be candidates for a continent appendicostomy as they get older.[143] In contrast, if the BMP is unsuccessful, as in the case of nonmanageable diarrhea, which occurs in approximately 5% of cases, a permanent colostomy should be recommended.

Candidates for Reoperation

The second group of patients with postoperative fecal incontinence includes children who are candidates for reoperation. These are children with a well-formed sacrum, good-looking perienum, good muscles, and sensation, with a mislocated rectum after repair of a rectourethral fistula in males or a rectovestibular fistula in females. Relocating the neoanus within the limits of the voluntary striated mechanism allows many of these children to become toilet trained. If, however, there is no postoperative improvement, a BMP should be instituted.

Megasigmoid

The third category of patients with postoperative fecal incontinence is characterized by those children with severe constipation and fecal impaction resulting in a megasigmoid colon. This

Algorithm for fecal incontinence post repair ARM

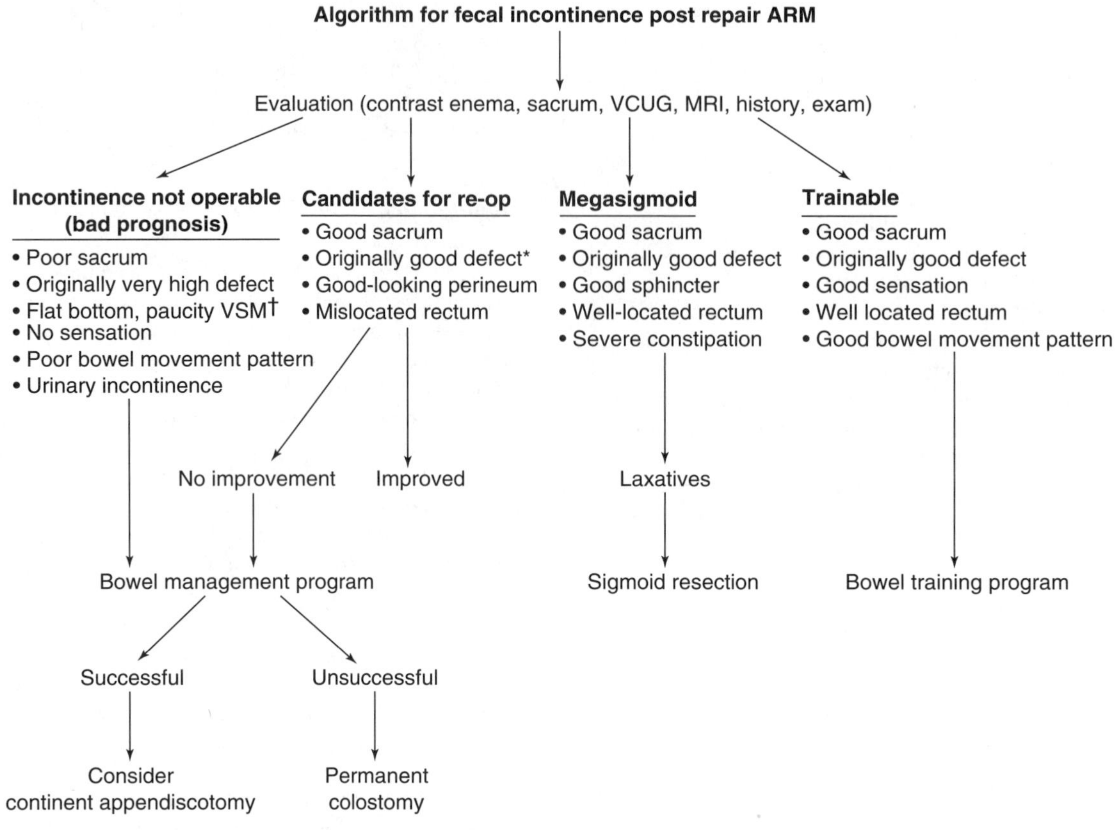

FIG. 83-42. Algorithm for fecal incontinence postrepair of anorectal malformations.

is a very specific group of children who are characterized by a properly located rectum and good sphincters and sacrum but troubled by severe constipation and subsequent incontinence. The surgeon is consulted for fecal incontinence in spite of the fact that the child should be continent.

Because these patients originally had a good prognosis, there is a strong suspicion that the child is not really incontinent but instead is continent while suffering from overflow pseudo-incontinence. How do we know that a child such as this is indeed continent? Perhaps the child is constipated and suffers from fecal incontinence. These children should first be managed using laxatives. Enemas should be avoided because they will obscure your ability to determine if the patient is continent. If these children are continent, laxative therapy should work and be titrated to avoid impaction. If the child becomes continent, the child and family then have two options. The child may continue laxative therapy for life (provided this keeps the child continent) or undergo a sigmoid resection and thus eliminate or diminish the need for laxatives altogether.[83] The resection of the sigmoid (with preservation of the rectum because the child had a good operation and one does not want to eliminate the patient's reservoir) cures or alleviates a great deal of the constipation and makes the child continent. If diarrhea is a problem after sigmoid resection, then we recommend small-volume enemas to keep the colon clean and a constipating diet to decrease colonic motility.

If the child remains fecally incontinent despite resolving the constipation, he or she suffers from real incontinence. In this situation, we take advantage of the fact that the child is consti-

pated (has hypomotility of the rectum), and discontinue all laxatives and use large-volume enemas. Under these circumstances, by keeping the rectosigmoid clean using daily enemas, the child should stay clean because he or she is constipated.

Trainable

The final category includes those children who are deemed trainable. These are children who were born with a good prognosis type of defect and underwent a good, uncomplicated operation. All indications are that they will have bowel control, but they are slightly delayed in becoming toilet trained and therefore a BTP is indicated.

REFERENCES

1. Amussat JZ. Gustiure d'une operation d'anus artificial practique avec succes par un nouveau procede. Gaz Med Paris 1835;3:735.
2. Stephens FD. Imperforate anus: a new surgical approach. Med J Aust 1953;1:202.
3. Kiesewetter WB. Imperforate anus II: the rationale and technique of sacroabdominoperineal operation. J Pediatr Surg 1967;2:106.
4. Louw JH, Cywes S, Cremin BJ. The management of anorectal agenesis. S Afr J Surg 1971;9:21.
5. Rehbein F. Imperforate anus: experiences with abdomino-perineal and abdomino-sacro-perineal pull-through procedures, J Pediatr Surg 1967;2:99.
6. Pena A, DeVries P. Posterior sagittal anorectoplasty: important technical considerations and new applications. J Pediatr Surg 1982;17:796.
7. DeVries PA, Pena A. Posterior sagittal anorectoplasty. J Pediatr Surg 1982;5:638.
8. Carlson B. Human embryology. St. Louis, Mosby, 1994.

9. Larsen WJ. Human embryology. London, Churchill Livingstone, 1993:369.
10. Duhamel B. Embryology of exomphalos and allied malformations. Arch Dis Child 1963;38:142.
11. Hartwig N, Steffelaar JW, et al. Abdominal wall defect associated with persistent cloaca: the embryologic clues in autopsy. Am J Clin Pathol 1991;96:640.
12. Shenefelt RE. Morphogenesis of malformations in hamsters caused by retinoic acid: relation to dose and stage at treatment. Teratology 1972;5:103.
13. Chen Y, Huang L, Russo AF. Retinoic acid is enriched in Hensen's node and is developmentally regulated in the early chicken embryo. PNAS 1992;89:10056.
14. Cohen AR. The mermaid malformation: cloacal exstrophy and occult spinal dysraphism. Neurosurgery 1991;28:834.
15. Fitzgerald MJT, Fitzgerald M. Human embryology, Bailliere Tindall, Philadelphia, Saunders, 1994.
16. Griffith CM, Sanders E. Effects of extracellular martix components on the differentiation of chick embryo tail bud mesenchyme in culture. Differentiation 1991;47:61.
17. Spemann H. Embryonic development and induction. Reprinted by Hafner, New York, 1938.
18. Rosa F, Roberts AB, Danielpour D, et al. Mesoderm induction in amphibians: the role of TGF-BZ like factors. Science 1988;239:783.
19. Faust C, Magnuson T. Genetic control of gastrulation in the mouse. Curr Opin Genet Dev 1993;3:491.
20. Santulli TV, Schullinger JN, Kiesewetter WB, et al. Imperforate anus: a survey from the members of the surgical section of the American Academy of Pediatrics. J Pediatr Surg 1971;6:484.
21. Hasse W. Associated malformations with anal and rectal atresia. Prog Pediatr Surg 1976;9:99.
22. Kluth D, Hillen M, Lambrecht W. The principles of normal and abnormal hindgut development. J Pediatr Surg 1995;30:1143.
23. Kluth D, Lambrecht W, Reich P, et al. SD-mice: an animal model for complex anorectal malformations. Eur J Pediatr Surg 1991;1:183.
24. Sd, Danforth's short tail, semidominant. In: Lyon MF, Searle AG, eds. Genetic variants and strains of the laboratory mouse, ed 2. New York, Oxford University Press, 1989:324.
25. Christ B, Wilting J. From somites to vertebral column. Ann Anat 1992;174:23.
26. Duband JL, Durfour S, et al. Adhesion molecules during somitogenesis in the avian embryo J Cell Biol 1987;104:1361.
27. Hamilton WJ, Boyd JD, Mossman HW. Human embryology, ed 3. Baltimore, Williams & Wilkins, 1962:414.
28. Patten BM. Human embryology, ed 3. New York, MacGraw-Hill, 1968:248.
29. Scott MP. Vertebrate homeobox gene nomenclature. Cell 1992;71:551.
30. Gamer L, Wright C. Murine Cdx-4 bears striking similarities to the Drosophila caudal gene in its homeodomain sequence and early expression pattern. Mech Dev 1993;43:71.
31. Krumlauf R. Hox genes in vertebrate development. Cell 1994;78:191.
32. Zhou X, Sasaki H, Lowe L, et al. Nodal is a novel TGF-B-like gene expressed in the mouse node during gastrulation. Nature 1993;361:543.
33. Takada S, Stark K, et al. Wnt-3a regulates somite and tailbud formation in the mouse embryo. Genes Dev 1994;8:174.
34. Hunt P, Gulisano M, Cook M, et al. A distinct Hox code for the branchial region of the vertebrate head. Nature 1991;353:861.
35. Joly J, Maury M, et al. Expression of a zebrafish caudal homeobox gene correlates with the establishment of posterior cell lineages at gastrulation. Differentiation 1992;50:75.
36. Joly JS, Joly C et al. The ventral and posterior expression of the zebrafish homeobox gene evel is perturbed in dorsalized and mutant embryos. Development 1993;119:1261.
37. O'Rahilly R, Muller F. Neurulation in the human embryo: neural tube defects. Ciba Symp 1994;181:70.
38. Duhamel B. From the mermaid to anal imperforation: the syndrome of caudal regression. Arch Dis Child 1961;36:152.
39. Griffith CM, Wiley MJ, Sanders E. The vertebrate tail bud: three germ layers from one tissue. Anat Embryo 1992;185:101.
40. Van der Putte SCJ. Normal and abnormal development of the anorectum. J Pediatr Surg 1986;21:434.
41. Larsen WJ, ed. Development of the urogenital system. In: Human embryology. New York, Churchill Livingstone, 1993:235.
42. Stevenson SS, Worcester J, Rice RG. 677 congenitally malformed infants and associated gestational characteristics. I. General considerations. Pediatrics 1950;6:37.
43. Stephens FD, Smith ED. Anorectal malformations in children. Chicago, Year Book Medical Publishers, 1971.
44. Anderson RC, Read SC. The likelihood of recurrence of congenital malformations. Lancet 1954;74:175.
45. Jones KL. Smith's recognizable patterns of human malformations, Philadelphia, WB Saunders, ed 4. 1988.
46. Fraser FC. J Chron Dis 1959;10:97.
47. Stevenson RE. In: Stevenson RE, Hall JG, Goodman RM, eds. Rectum and anus in human malformations and related anomalies, vol 2. New York, Oxford University Press, 1993:chap. 20.
48. Reid IS, Turner G. Familial anal abnormality. J Pediatr 1976;88:992.
49. Cozzi F, Wilkinson AW. Familial incidence of congenital anorectal anomalies. Surgery 1968;64:669.
50. Murken JD, Albert A. Genetic counseling in cases of anal and rectal atresia. Prog Pediatr Surg 1976;9:115.
51. Online Mendelian Inheritance in Man, OMIM (TM). Center for Medical Genetics, Johns Hopkins University (Baltimore, MD) and National Center for Biotechnology Information, National Library of Medicine (Bethesda, MDF), 1996. World Wide Web URL: http//www3.ncbi.n1m.nih.gov/omim/
52. Quan S. The VATER association: a spectrum of associated defects. J Pediatr 1973;82:104.
53. Temtamy M. Extending the scope of the Vater association. J Pediatr 1974;85:345.
54. Kaufman RL. Birth defects and oral contraceptives. Lancet 1973;1:1396.
55. Nora A, Nora L. Arch Environ Health 1975;30:17.
56. Blumel J, Evans EB. Partial and complete agenesis or malformation of the sacrum with associated anomalies. J Bone Joint Surg 1959;41:497.
57. Pena A. Results in the management of 322 cases of anorectal malformations. Pediatr Surg Int 1988;3:105.
58. Pena A. Anorectal malformations. Semin Pediatr Surg 1995;4:35.
59. Stephens FD, Smith ED. Classification, identification and assessment of surgical treatment of anorectal anomalies. Pediatr Surg Int 1986;1:200.
60. Raffensperger JG, ed. Anorectal anomalies. In: Swenson's pediatric surgery, ed 5 Norwalk, CT, Appleton & Lange, 1990:583.
61. Templeton JM, O'Neill JA. Anorectal malformations. In: Welch KJ, Randolph JG, Ravitch MM, et al. eds. Pediatric surgery. Chicago, Yearbook Medical Publishers, 1986:1022.
62. Pena A. The surgical management of persistent cloaca: results in 54 patients treated with a posterior sagittal approach. J Pediatr Surg 1989;24:590.
63. Gardner E, Gray DJ, O'Reilly R. Anatomy, ed 3. Philadelphia, WB Saunders, 1966:506.
64. Devroede G, Lamarche J. Functional importance of extrinsic parasympathetic innervation to the distal colon and rectum in man. Gastroenterology 1974;66:273.
65. Duthie HL, Gairns FW. Sensory nerve-endings and sensation in the anal region of man. Br J Surg 1960;47:585.
66. Li L, Li Z, Hou H-S, et al. Sensory nerve endings in the puborectalis and anal region: normal findings and changes in anorectal anomalies. J Pediatr Surg 1990;25:658.
67. Boemers TM, et al. Urodynamic evaluation of children with the caudal regression syndrome. J Urol 1994;151:1038.
68. Pena, A. Figure of muscle complex. In: Atlas of surgical management of anorectal malformations. New York, Springer-Verlag, 1989:2.
69. Pena A, Hedlund H. Does the distal rectal muscle in anorectal malformations have the functional properties of a sphincter? J Pediatr Surg 1990;25:985.
70. Orr WC, Schuster MM. Clinical applications of anorectal manometry. In: Barkin J, O'Phelan CA, eds. Advanced therapeutic endoscopy. New York, Raven Press, 1990:147.
71. Schuster MM, Hendrix TR, Mendelhoff AI. The internal anal sphincter response: manometric studies on its normal physiology, neural pathways, and alteration in bowel disorder. J Clin Invest 1963;42:196.
72. O'Kelly TJ, Davies JR et al. Distribution of nitric oxide synthase containing neurons in the rectal myenteric plexus and anal canal. Dis Colon Rectum 1994;37:350.
73. Meunier P, Louis D, Jaubert de Beaujeu M. Physiologic investigations of primary constipation in children: comparison with the barium enema study. Gastroenterology 1984;87:1351.

74. Alexander AA, et al. High-resolution endoluminal sonography of the anal sphincter complex. J Ultrasound Med 1994;13:281.

75. Jost W, Schimrigk K. Dis Colon Rectum 1994;37:697.

76. Zheng L, Hong-shen L, et al. Sensory nerve endings in the puborectalis and anal region of the fetus and newborn. Dis Colon Rectum 1992; 35:552.

77. Ming Y, Zheng L. Electromyography of external anal sphincters in the child. Chin J Pediatr Surg 1988;9:31.

78. Altschuler SM. Neurology of the gut. In: Wylie R, Hyams JS, eds. Pediatric gastrointestinal disease pathophysiology: diagnosis management. Philadelphia, WB Saunders, 1993:74.

79. Weaver LT. Bowel habits from birth to old age. J Pediatr Gastroenterol Nutr 1988;7:637.

80. Orkin BA, Hanson RB, Kelly KA. The rectal motor complex. J Gastrointest Motil 1989;1:5.

81. DiLorenzo C. Colonic manometry in pediatric gastrointestinal motility disorders. Hyman P, ed. New York, Academic Professional Information Services, 1994:215.

82. Li L, et al. J Pediatr Surg 1993;28:880.

83. Pena A, El Behery M. Megasigmoid: a source of pseudoincontinence in children with repaired anorectal malformations. J Pediatr Surg 1993;18:199.

84. Staiano A, et al. Dig Dis Sci 1991;36:733.

85. Staiano A, DelGuidice E. Pediatrics 1994;94:169.

86. Belman BA, King LR. Urinary tract abnormalities associated with imperforate anus. J Urol 1972;108:823.

87. Parrott TS. Urologic implications of anorectal malformations. Urol Clin North Am 1985;12:13.

88. Rich MA, Brock WA, Pena A. Spectrum of genitourinary malformations in patients with imperforate anus. Pediatr Surg Int 1988;3:110.

89. Gilbert J, Clark R, Koyle M. Penile agenesis: a fatal variation of an uncommon lesion. J Urol 1990;143:338.

90. Sheldon C. Occult neurovesical dysfunction in children with imperforate anus and its variants. J Pediatr Surg 1991;26:49.

91. J Urol 1994;151:1041.

92. Greenfield, Fera. Urodynamic evaluation of the patient with an imperforate anus: a prospective study. J Urol 1991;146:539.

93. Pena A. Posterior sagittal anorectoplasty: results in the management of 332 cases of anorectal malformations. Pediatr Surg Int 1988;3:94.

94. Pena A. Imperforate anus and cloacal malformations. In: Ped Surgery, Ashcraft & Holder, Philadelphia, WB Saunders, 1993:372.

95. Freedman B. Congenital absence of the sacrum and coccyx: report of a case and review of the literature. J Surg 1950;37:299.

96. Currarino G, Coln D, Votteler T. Triad of anorectal, sacral and presacral anomalies. Am J Roentgenol 1981;137:395.

97. Sarnat HB, Case ME, Graviss R. Sacral agenesis. Neurology 1976; 26:1124.

98. Pang D, Hoffman HJ. Sacral agenesis with progressive neurologic deficit. Neurosurgery 1980;7:118.

99. Banta JV, et al. Sacral agenesis. J Bone Joint Surg 1969; 51A:693.

100. Denton J. Clin Orthop 1982;162:91.

101. Karrer FM, Flannery AM, Nelson MD, et al. Anorectal malformations: evaluation of associated spinal dysraphic syndromes, J Pediatr Surg 1988;23:45.

102. Davidoff AM, et al. Occult spinal dysraphism in patients with anal agenesis. J Pediatr Surg 1991;26:1001.

103. Sachs T, et al. Use of MRI in evaluation of anorectal anomalies. J Pediatr Surg 1990;25:817.

104. Carson JA, Barnes PD, et al. Imperforate anus: the neurologic implication of sacral abnormalities. J Pediatr Surg 1984;19:838.

105. Watanatittan S, et al. Association of Hirschsprung's disease and anorectal malformations. J Pediatr Surg 1991;26:192.

106. Barss VA, Benacerraf BR, Frigoletto FD. Antenatal sonographic diagnosis of fetal gastrointestinal malformations. Pediatrics 1985;76:445.

107. Morrison I. Perinatal mortality: basic considerations. Semin Perinatol 1985;9:144.

108. Nyberg, DA, Mahony BS, Pretorius DH. Diagnostic ultrasound of fetal anomalies: text and atlas. Chicago, Year Book Publications, 1990: Chap 10.

109. Guzman E, Ranzini A, Day-Salvatore D. The prenatal ultrasonographic visualization of imperforate anus in monoamniotic twins. J Ultrasound Med 1995;14:547.

110. Loewy, JA, Richards DG, Toi A. In-utero diagnosis of the caudal regression syndrome: report of three cases. J Clin Ultrasound 1987; 15:469.

111. Harris RD, Nybeerg DA, Mack, LA, et al. Anorectal atresia: prenatal sonographic diagnosis. Am J Roentgenol 1987;149:395.

112. Duenholter JH, et al. Prenatal diagnosis of gastrointestinal tract obstruction. Obstet Gynecol 1976;47:618.

113. Rudd N, Klimek ML. Familial caudal dysgenesis: evidence for a major dominant gene. Clin Genet 1990;38:170.

114. Pinsky L. The syundromology of anorectal malformation (atresia, stenosis, ectopia). Am J Med Genet 1978;1:461.

115. Benzie RJ, Doran TA. The fetoscope: a new clinical tool for prenatal genetic diagnosis. Am J Obstet Gynecol 1975;121:460.

116. Potier M, Dallaire L, Melancon SB. Biol Neonate 1975;27:141.

117. Romero R, Pili G, Jeanty P, et al. Prenatal diagnoses of congenital anomalies, Norwalk, CT, Appleton & Lange, 1988:233.

118. Landle IM, Hamilton EF. The antenatal sonographic visualization of cloacal dysgenesis. J Ultrasound Med 1986;5:275.

119. Carty H, Brereton RJ. The distended neonate. Clin Radiol 1983;34: 367.

120. Narasimharao KL, Prasad GR, Katariya S. Prone cross table lateral view: an alternative to the invertogram in imperforate anus. Am J Roentgenol 1983;140:227.

121. Leighton DM, de Campo M. CT invertograms. Pediatr Radiol 1989; 19:176.

122. Donaldson J, Black CT, et al. Ultrasound of the distal pouch in infants with imperforate anus. J Pediatr Surg 1989;24:465.

123. Leape LL, Ramenofsky ML. J Pediatr Surg 1978;13:627.

124. Hendren H. J Pediatr Surg 1978;13:505.

125. Pena A. Atlas of surgical management of anorectal malformations. New York, Springer-Verlag, 1990:19.

126. Wilkins S, Pena A. The role of colostomy in the management of anorectal malformations. Pediatr Surg Int 1988;3:105.

127. Gross GW, Wolfson, PJ, Pena A. Augmented-pressure colostogram in imperforate anus with fistula. Pediatr Radiol 1991;21:56.

128. Bliss DP, Tapper D, Anderson JM, et al. Does posterior sagittal anorectoplasty in patients with high imperforate anus provide superior fecal continence? J Pediatr Surg 1996;31:26.

129. Zivkovic SM, Kristie ZD, Vukanic DV. Vestibular fistula: the operative dilemma-cutback, fistula transplantation or posterior sagittal anorectoplasty? Pediatr Surg Int 1991;6:111.

130. Moore TC. Advantages of performing the sagittal anoplasty operation for imperforate anus at birth. J Pediatr Surg 1990;25:276.

131. Goon HK. Repair of anorectal anomalies in the neonatal period. Pediatr Surg Int 1990;5:246.

132. Pena A. The surgical management of persistent cloaca: results in 54 patients treated with a posterior sagittal approach. J Pediatr Surg 1989; 24:590.

133. Hendren WH. Further experience in reconstructive surgery for cloacal anomalies. J Pediatr Surg 1982;17:695.

134. Hendren WH. Repair of cloacal anomalies. Curr Tech J Pediatr Surg 1986;21:1159.

135. Langemeijer RATM, Molenaar JC. Continence after posterior sagittal anorectoplasty. J Pediatr Surg 1991;26:587.

136. Brain AJL, Kiely EM. Posterior sagittal anorectoplasty for reoperation in children with anorectal malformations. Br J Surg 1989;76:57.

137. Smith D. The bath water needs changing but don't throw out the baby: an overview of anorectal malformations. J Pediatr Surg 1987;22:335.

138. Loening-Baucke V. Functional constipation. Semin Pediatr Surg 1995;4:26.

139. Berquist WE. Biofeedback therapy for anorectal disorders. Semin Pediatr Surg 1995;4:48.

140. Orr W, Schuster MM. Clinical applications of anorectal manometry: advanced therapeutic endoscopy. New York, Raven Press, 1990:147.

141. Taccone A, et al. New concepts in preoperative imaging of anorectal malformations. Pediatr Radiol 1992;22:196.

142. Sato Y, et al. Congenital anorectal anomalies: MR imaging. Radiology 1988;168:157.

143. Malone PS, Ransley PG, Kiely EM. Preliminary report: the antegrade continence enema. Lancet 1990;336:1217.

144. Stevenson R. Rectum and anus in human malformations and related anomalies, vol 2. New York, Oxford University Press, 1993:Chap 20.

Liver, Biliary Tract, and Pancreas

Surgery of Infants and Children: Scientific Principles and Practice, edited by
Keith T. Oldham, Paul M. Colombani, and Robert P. Foglia.
Lippincott–Raven Publishers, Philadelphia, © 1997.

CHAPTER 84

Liver Physiology and Pathophysiology

Jean Pappas Molleston, Theodoros Ziambaras, and David H. Perlmutter

The liver is the largest organ in the body. Composed of a complex array of cell types, it participates in many essential bodily functions. A number of disease processes affect it; in many the liver is the primary tissue involved and in others it is one of several tissues involved by a systemic disorder. This chapter reviews some of the principles of anatomy, physiology, and pathophysiology of the liver, giving particular attention to those issues unique to the pediatric patient.

ANATOMY

The function of the liver depends on a dual blood supply. Approximately one third of this supply is derived from the hepatic artery, and the remainder comes from the portal vein. Through the portal vein, the liver receives the venous outflow of the intestine, rich in hormones and substrates for energy metabolism. In addition, the liver is potentially capable of translocating toxins and microbes from the intestinal lumen. Although the liver accounts for 2% of the body weight, it receives approximately 25% of the cardiac output through this dual blood supply. Venous blood leaves the liver through the hepatic veins and is directed into the vena cava.

The liver parenchyma is organized into anatomic-functional units, referred to as *lobules* (Fig. 84-1). Each lobule contains a branch of the hepatic vein, called the *central vein*, cords of hepatocytes, each one-cell layer thick and radiating toward peripherally located *portal tracts*. Each portal tract contains a branch of the hepatic artery, portal vein, and bile duct and is surrounded by a *limiting plate* of connective tissue. A single cord of hepatocytes is lined on both sides by a sinusoid. This hepatic lobular architecture allows blood flow from the hepatic artery and portal vein to percolate through the sinusoids toward the central vein, and ultimately into the vena cava. The lobular architecture is also specially designed for relatively efficient delivery of molecules from the blood to hepatocytes: in each hepatocyte, a large proportion of the surface area faces the sinusoidal blood, which is separated from the hepatocyte's sinusoidal surface by only a densely fenestrated endothelium, a relatively incomplete basement membrane, and the space of Disse.

Opposite to the sinusoidal surface of each hepatocyte, a canalicular surface is arranged in microvilli and separated from

the sinusoidal domain by tight junctions. Adjacent hepatocytes, connected by tight junctions, come together to form bile canaliculi at this pole. Bile acids, cholesterol, phospholipids, and products of liver cell metabolism, such as xenobiotics, are excreted as bile into these biliary canaliculi. The biliary canaliculi direct bile into the right and left hepatic bile ducts, which are drained by the common bile duct, eventually reaching the upper small intestine. The cystic duct, which provides drainage from the gallbladder, joins the common bile duct just outside the liver capsule.

PHYSIOLOGY

Of the numerous, diverse, and critical functions of the liver, energy metabolism is one of the most important. In terms of carbohydrate, the liver is the portal of entry for fructose and galactose metabolism. The liver is an important site of glycolysis, breaking down glucose to form energy, as well as gluconeogenesis, producing glucose from lactate and amino acids. Energy is shuttled between muscle and liver in the form of alanine or pyruvate, depending on the energy needs of the body. The liver also serves as a storehouse for glycogen; in starvation, the liver releases glycogen reserves as needed.

The liver is also an important site for protein metabolism. Amino acids derived from dietary protein or from tissue protein turnover are converted to glucose by gluconeogenesis, to keto acids by a number of biochemical pathways, and to ammonia and urea by the urea cycle pathway. In some cases, such as the Krebs–tricarboxylic acid pathway, protein metabolic activity in the liver is essential for energy generation.

De novo synthesis of proteins, such as albumin and clotting factors, is another hallmark of liver function. The hepatic production of albumin each day supplies the circulation with colloid oncotic pressure as well as carrying capacity for fatty acids and other substances. The liver is responsible for synthesizing many of the proteins involved in coagulation, fibrinolysis, and complement activation as well as proteins such as antithrombin III, protein C inhibitor, and C1 inhibitor that regulate these pathways. Because the vitamin K–dependent coagulation factors II, VII, IX, and X have the most rapid turnover, their plasma levels are most acutely affected by liver failure. The prothrombin time, which depends on these clotting factors, and albumin levels are therefore used in clinical practice to assess liver synthetic function.

The liver is a critical determinant of lipid metabolism. Its functions include synthesis of cholesterol, phospholipids, and lipoproteins, especially in the fed state. During starvation, the liver is involved in uptake and oxidation or metabolic conversion of free fatty acids essential for ketone body and free energy generation. The liver plays a major role in catabolism of lipoproteins and transport and excretion of cholesterol and phospholipids into the bile.

The liver is also responsible for biotransformation of drugs. This is especially important for drugs that are poorly soluble in water and therefore inefficiently excreted in urine or by respiration. Hepatic drug metabolism usually involves two phases. Phase I renders most drugs more polar by means of enzymes in the microsomes, particularly cytochrome P450 enzymes. These enzymes are induced by drugs and their function in any single individual may be affected by inherited polymorphic variation. Some of the products of phase I biotransformation are more toxic than the untransformed drug. Thus, phase II biotransformation reactions are important. These reactions involve enzymes that generally conjugate drugs with moieties that render them hydrophilic, thus facilitating their excretion in bile or urine, for example, glutathione-S-transferases, glucuronyl transferases, epoxide hydrolase, sulfotransferase, and N-acetyl transferase. Although concentrations of many phase I and phase II enzymes are lower in neonates, concentrations reach adult levels in infancy and hepatic clearance of drugs is more rapid in children. Specific enzymes are also affected by development. Because glucuronidation develops slowly in the neonate, bilirubin is not conjugated efficiently.

Another critical function of the liver is excretion of bile, which elimates many endogenous and exogenous compounds, such as bilirubin, cholesterol, and drugs, and promotes the digestion and absorption of dietary fat and fat-soluble vitamins in the intestine. Bile is a complex secretory product consisting of bile acids, cholesterol, lecithin, bilirubin, protein, electrolytes, water, and metabolites. Bile acid secretion is the principle driving force of overall bile secretion. Bile acids are synthesized in hepatocytes by conversion from cholesterol. The primary bile acids are conjugated with glycine or taurine before excretion. Since glycine conjugation develops slowly, bile acids are preferentially conjugated to taurine during the newborn period. Once excreted from the liver, bile is concentrated as much as 18-fold, depending on active transport mechanisms in the gallbladder. Bile is also modified in the biliary system as a result of the secretion of chloride and other anions by biliary epithelial cells. The cystic fibrosis transmembrane conductance regulator is one of the molecules involved in bile modification

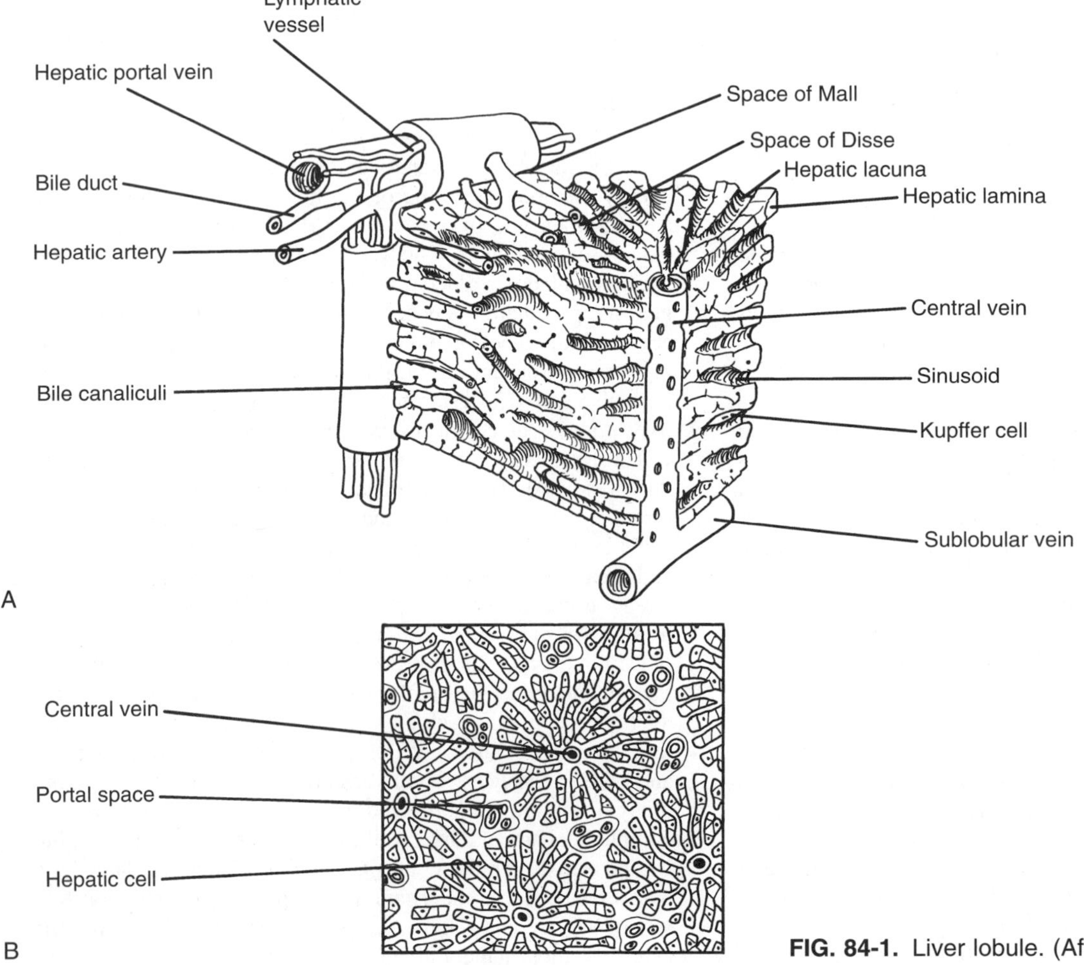

FIG. 84-1. Liver lobule. (After Anatomical Charts, Co.)

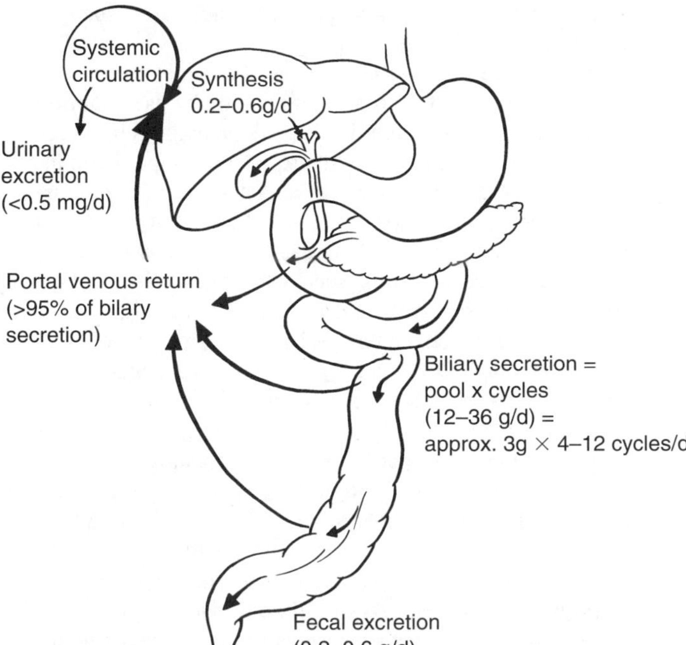

FIG. 84-2. Enterohepatic circulation of bile acids. (Carey MC. The enterohepatic circulation. In: Arias IM, Popper H, Schacter D, et al, ed. The Liver: Biology and Pathobiology. New York, Raven Press, 1982:430)

within the biliary system. After a meal, cholecystokinin stimulates the release of bile from the gallbladder into the intestine. Bile acids are conserved by a system referred to as the *enterohepatic circulation* (Fig. 84-2). In this system, a specific transporter in the ileum delivers bile acids to the portal circulation, and the bile acids are ultimately subjected to re-uptake by the hepatocyte sinusoidal bile acid transport system. This mechanism allows 94% of the bile acid pool to be reabsorbed and reduces the energy required for de novo bile acid synthesis.

Although not strictly a part of the immune system, the liver is an important participant in the immune response in that it contains the largest collection of fixed macrophages in the body, the Kupffer cells. Kupffer cells reside in the hepatic sinusoids and are in direct contact with hepatocytes because of the fenestration of the sinusoidal endothelium. Kupffer cells are thought to be responsible for phagocytosis of particles and microbes that penetrate the portal venous blood, pinocytosis of endotoxins, antigen processing, secretion of bioactive molecules such as cytokines and reactive oxygen intermediates, and clearance and catabolism of senescent cells, lipids, and many other protein degradation products.

PATHOPHYSIOLOGY

Cholestasis

Cholestasis is defined as a decrease in bile flow. It is manifest clinically by accumulation in blood and extrahepatic tissues of substances normally excreted in bile: accumulation of bilirubin results in jaundice; accumulation of cholesterol is associated

with hypercholesterolemia and xanthomatosis; and accumulation of bile acids is associated with pruritus.

Although secretion of other organic and inorganic anions contributes to a small extent, bile acid secretion is the major physiologic determinant of bile flow.[1] The rate-limiting step in bile acid secretion is transport across the hepatocyte canalicular membrane. It is not yet known whether one or more adenosine triphosphate–dependent transporters are involved in this step, but the recently described rat liver canalicular bile acid transporter–ectoATPase–cell cam 105 is one of these.[2] Subsequent transport through the intrahepatic and extrahepatic bile ducts allows for delivery of sufficient bile acids to the upper small intestine to facilitate the micellar solubilization of fat and fat-soluble vitamins from the diet. Bile acids are also subject to re-uptake in the ileum by a specific carrier-mediated transport system and are delivered back to the liver by enterohepatic circulation. The hepatocyte sinusoidal membrane has a distinct bile acid transporter for uptake of recycled bile acids.[3] Hepatocytes also have a pathway for de novo synthesis of bile acids in which cholesterol is the precursor.

Biliary tract obstruction, most notably extrahepatic biliary obstruction, is a major cause of cholestasis in infants. Cholestasis is also a prominent feature in many disorders of the liver parenchymal cells. This is especially true for liver injury in the neonate or infant. Congenital infections, acquired infections, metabolic disorders, parenteral nutrition, drugs, hypoperfusion, infiltrative disorders, and idiopathic cholestatic syndromes such as arteriohepatic dysplasia all cause cholestasis in this age group.

There is a growing body of evidence that cholestasis itself exacerbates liver parenchymal injury. This probably involves the accumulation of abnormal, hepatotoxic bile acid intermediates and accounts for the improvement in serum transaminases in several liver diseases with ursodeoxycholic acid treatment.

Liver Failure

Most studies of liver failure have involved primarily adult patients. The definition of fulminant liver failure in these studies is onset of hepatic encephalopathy within 8 weeks of the onset of liver disease in an individual with no history of preexisting liver disease. Because the incidence of encephalopathy is lower in infants and children, and the rate of development may be lower, the term *fulminant liver failure* or *acute liver failure* is used for a child without preexisting liver disease who develops severe derangement of the vital functions of the liver within several months.

There are many causes of acute liver failure in infants and children, but the underlying etiology is usually not discovered. In most of the cases in which an etiology is identified, viral infections are responsible. The etiology of acute liver failure depends on age. In neonates, common considerations include herpes virus, metabolic disorders such as galactosemia, tyrosinemia, and neonatal hemochromatosis, and ischemic hepatitis associated with perinatal asphyxia or congenital heart disease. In infants, hepatitis B virus, virus, and drug-induced or toxic liver injury, including that associated with valproate, acetaminophen, isoniazid, or mushroom poisoning, are more likely. In children, occasional cases of malignant or infiltrative disorders, including leukemia, lymphoproliferative diseases, and erythrophagocytic conditions, cause acute liver failure. Reye syndrome only rarely has been identified in recent years. In teenagers, one must consider autoimmune hepatitis, Wilson disease, and acute fatty liver of pregnancy in the differential diagnosis of acute liver failure.

The pathogenesis of liver failure is still poorly understood and depends on the underlying etiology. The offending agent or the host reponse to that agent usually causes severe hepatocyte necrosis. Occasionally, severe functional impairment of the hepatocyte occurs without overt necrosis. In these cases, derangement in specific subcellular organelles and fatty infiltration usually occur, as in acute fatty liver of pregnancy or tetracycline poisoning. High levels of growth factors that mediate liver regeneration, such as hepatocyte growth factor and transforming growth factor α, are usually present during acute liver failure, but liver regeneration may not be possible because of the release of factors that inhibit hepatocyte replication or the loss of the connective tissue matrix and collapse of the liver's infrastructural integrity.[4] Derangements in specific systems may also potentiate liver injury, including perturbation in prostaglandin or nitric oxide metabolism, inappropriate release of tumor necrosis factor, and exhaustion of liver-derived actin scavengers such as group-specific component protein, permitting polymerization of actin and platelet aggregation in the peripheral circulation.[5]

Histopathologic examination of the liver usually shows necrosis of hepatocytes, collapse of the liver's reticulin framework, and infiltration of micro- and macrovesicular fat. The severity of the histologic abnormalities does not correlate with the severity of the clinical course or outcome of individual cases, and liver biopsy is therefore sometimes not informative or misleading.[6] In fact, because risk of liver biopsy in these patients is usually significant, it may not be undertaken in many cases.

Acute liver failure usually begins with a flulike illness, but the child does not get better over the usual interval of several days to a week. The child becomes lethargic, can become somnolent, and may have bleeding complications or jaundice, or both. Biochemical abnormalities including elevated transaminases, hyperbilirubinemia, elevated blood ammonia, prolonged prothrombin time, and low platelet counts are usually more severe than anticipated.

The most devastating complication is hepatic encephalopathy. It is often manifested in infants, initially, as irritability and sleep disturbance. In stage II encephalopathy, the child becomes more drowsy and lethargic with gross motor impairment including ataxia, dysarthria, and apraxia. Asterixis, a flapping tremor present during voluntary movement but not at rest, is almost always present by this stage. It may be difficult to elicit in small children because it is best seen when the patient voluntarily stretches his or her arms and hyperflexes the wrists. Stage III encephalopathy is characterized by deepening somnolence, stridor, extreme agitation, and rage. In stage IV hepatic encephalopathy, the patient loses responsiveness to all stimuli, and coma progresses to the point of decerebrate posturing and loss of brain stem responses. Nonspecific electroencephalographic changes may occur, but neuropathologic abnormalities are not seen. Improvement in patients undergoing liver transplantation for acute liver failure indicates that hepatic encephalopathy is reversible. The pathophysiologic basis of hepatic encephalopathy is still poorly understood (Fig. 84-3). There is evidence for accumulation of neurotoxic or neurodepressant substances including ammonia, mercaptans, fatty acids, phenols, neurotransmitters (serotonin, catecholamines, glutamate, aspartate), and endogenous ligands for the γ-aminobutyric acid (GABA) receptor.[7] Although ammonia is almost certainly involved, it is clearly not the only responsible neuroactive substance. Moreover, blood ammonia levels do not correlate with the development or degree of hepatic encephalopathy. Activation of GABA receptors, which results in depression of neuronal activity and benzodiazepine receptor ligands, is an alternative mechanism that has been intensely studied.[8]

Another devastating complication of acute liver failure is cerebral edema. This condition is characterized by deep coma with abnormal reacting pupils, muscular rigidity, decerebrate posturing, and loss of brain stem reflexes. Seizures may occur. Intracranial pressure exceeds 30 mm Hg. Ventricular size is reduced and gyrae appear flattened on computed tomographic scan or magnetic resonance imaging. Altered integrity of cere-

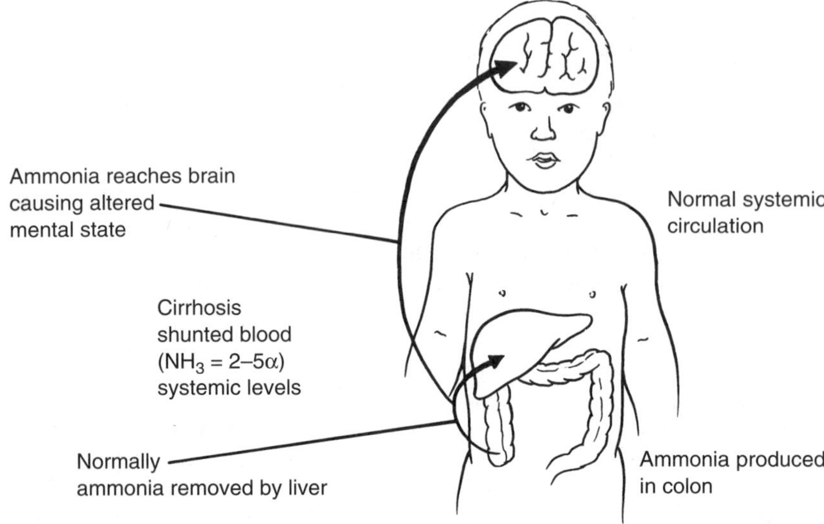

FIG. 84-3. Hepatic encephalopathy. (Iber F. The undergraduate teaching project in gastroenterology and liver disease. American Gastroenterology Association, Bethesda, MD.)

bral microcirculation allows excessive solute and water to pass into the brain. Homeostatic mechanisms, such as sodium efflux pumping, may be impaired. Finally, iatrogenic factors such as fluid overload and cerebral hypotension may contribute to cerebral edema.

The bleeding diathesis of acute liver failure is a result of disturbances in hemostasis and fibrinolysis. It is associated with depressed synthesis of coagulation factors and fibrinolytic proteins, alteration in clearance and catabolism of these factors, hypersplenism, disturbances in platelet function, and intravascular consumptive coagulopathy. Children may bleed profusely from needle puncture sites, from the upper gastrointestinal (GI) tract (gastritis, ulcers, nasogastric tube trauma), and occasionally develop intracranial hemorrhage.

Biochemical abnormalities include hypoglycemia, hyponatremia, and hypokalemia. Hypoglycemia results from failed glucose synthesis and release, hyperinsulinemia, increased glucose utilization, and secondary bacterial infections. Hyponatremia is a result of deranged renal water excretion. Hypokalemia is usually a sign of secondary hyperaldosteronism. Early in the course of acute liver failure, central hyperventilation leads to respiratory alkalosis. Potassium depletion is later associated with metabolic alkalosis. In severe cases, metabolic acidosis reflects metabolic failure with release of acetate, free fatty acids, and organic acids.

Renal dysfunction is also common in acute liver failure. This may be as mild as azotemia and oliguria from decreased intravascular volume or as severe as functional renal failure, the so-called hepatorenal syndrome. This syndrome is characterized by sodium retention, reduced urine output, and normal urinary sediment. Acute tubular necrosis, characterized by oliguria, abnormal urinary sediment, excessive urinary sodium losses, and poor urinary creatinine clearance, may also occur. In acute tubular necrosis, renal dysfunction is usually reversible.

Other complications of acute liver failure include peripheral vasodilatation, defective ventilation, poor oxygenation due to intrapulmonary shunting, and occasionally pulmonary edema or infections. Bone marrow failure has occurred with acute liver failure, especially that caused by non-A, non-B, non-C hepatitis virus. Secondary bacterial and fungal infections complicate the course of acute liver failure in 50% of children. Skin-derived organisms, staphylococci, and streptococci, are most often implicated. Neutropenia, depressed neutrophil function, and defective opsonization have been considered as contributing pathogenetic mechanisms.

Chronic Liver Failure and Cirrhosis

Cirrhosis is the end-stage of many chronic pediatric liver diseases. It is characterized by fibrosis and conversion of normal liver architecture into abnormal nodules. Progression of the cirrhotic process results in gross distortion of liver architecture and compression of hepatic vascular structures.

The pathogenesis of cirrhosis is thought to involve a dynamic interaction between the primary injury to liver cells (necrosis) and the liver's response, which involves elaboration of fibrous tissue (fibrosis) and regeneration (nodule formation). When necrosis dominates, the patient develops signs of liver failure almost identical to those described earlier for acute liver failure. When fibrosis and nodule formation dominate, the patient de-

velops portal hypertension, as described later. Most children with progressive cirrhosis have variable degrees of both liver failure and portal hypertension.

The clinical manifestations of chronic liver failure or cirrhosis in children include poor growth, muscle weakness, fatigability, jaundice, edema, ascites, steatorrhea, GI bleeding, digital clubbing, and splenomegaly. The extrahepatic manifestations of cirrhosis include esophageal and gastric varices, hemorrhoids, and a troublesome form of gastritis known as hemorrhagic portal hypertensive gastropathy. Diarrhea, malnutrition, and fat-soluble vitamin deficiencies result from fat malabsorption. Malnutrition also results from poor caloric intake, caused by anorexia and malaise. Most commonly, vitamin K deficiency worsens the intrinsic tendency for bleeding in these patients, vitamin D deficiency leads to loss of bone density, and vitamin E deficiency causes a spinocerebellar degenerative process with pigmentary retinopathy. Patients with cirrhosis have a higher incidence of gallstones and cholecystitis. Cirrhosis is occasionally associated with intrapulmonary shunting, which results in hypoxemia, cyanosis, and digital clubbing. Rarely, patients with cirrhosis develop pulmonary hypertension. Patients with cirrhosis are also susceptible to hepatic encephalopathy. Cirrhosis, in this setting, is usually chronic, more likely to involve episodic confusion and disorientation rather than coma, and probably has a somewhat more complex pathogenesis than acute liver failure. Cirrhosis is almost always associated with a state of high cardiac output. Dermatologic signs include spider angiomata and palmar erythema. Signs of feminization are not uncommon in teenage boys with cirrhosis, including gynecomastia and delayed pubertal development. Ascites, edema, and hypokalemia may be present. Children with cirrhosis have anemia resulting from GI bleeding, hypersplenism, dilution of red blood cell volume from sodium and water retention, and iron and folic acid deficiency associated with malabsorption. Coagulation disturbances are also common and have complex, multifactorial origins. Deficits in immune function make these patients more susceptible to pneumonia, bacteremia, and spontaneous bacterial peritonitis.

Although the pathophysiology of cirrhosis is still poorly understood, several interesting observations have recently been made. First, cirrhosis is associated with marked changes in constituents of the extracellular matrix.[9] Deposition of collagen, especially types III, IV, V, and VI, and laminin increase significantly in the perisinusoidial and periductular spaces. The increase in perisinusoidal deposition, so-called capillarization of sinusoids, is especially damaging. The matrix becomes a barrier to exchange of constituents between blood and hepatocytes. The altered sinusoids form portal-to-central vein conduits, in effect shunting blood from entire hepatic lobules and causing further ischemic damage to liver cells. Thus, a vicious pathogenic cycle is established in which liver cell necrosis leads to formation of connective tissue bands, further liver cell necrosis, stimulation of regeneration, formation of regenerative nodules, compression of blood vessels by hepatic nodules, and persistent ischemic damage to liver cells. Second, several specific mediators of liver fibrogenesis have been identified. In particular, transforming growth factor β mediates marked increases in hepatocyte collagen synthesis.[10] Third, several specific mediators of liver regeneration have been identified. The most interesting of these is hepatocyte growth factor (HGF), which mediates a marked increase in hepatocyte proliferation. HGF is a plasminogen-like molecule that interacts with a tyrosine kinase growth factor receptor, a product of the *met* protooncogene, and mediates proliferation of many epithelial cells.[11] HGF is not present in normal serum but can be detected in serum and ascites of cirrhotic patients in concentrations that reflect the degree of liver cell damage. Further understanding of the biochemical characteristics determining the interaction between HGF and the *met* protooncogene product and their relationship to the highly coordinated and synchronized hepatic regenerative response should be forthcoming.

Portal Hypertension

Portal hypertension is characterized by elevated portal blood pressure above 5 to 10 mm Hg and results from a dynamic interaction between increased portal blood flow and increased portal resistance (Fig. 84-4). The signs and symptoms of portal hypertension represent manifestations of decompression of the supraphysiologic portal pressure through portosystemic collaterals, including esophageal, gastric, and rectal varices, and through splenic congestion and hypersplenism.

Increased vascular resistance is usually caused by intrahepatic diseases. Hepatocyte swelling, hepatocyte and sinusoidal cell hyperplasia, portal tract inflammation, and deposition of collagen and fibrous tissue all lead to impingement on the intrahepatic portal vein lumen in a wide variety of diseases. Increased portal vascular resistance, however, commonly accompanies extrahepatic diseases also, including Budd-Chiari syndrome and other causes of hepatic vein obstruction, portal vein thrombosis, and cavernous transformation of the portal vein. Hepatic venoocclusive disease, hepatoportal sclerosis, and schistosomiasis cause portal hypertension directly rather than through intrahepatic or extrahepatic disease.

Increased portal blood flow is largely caused by increased cardiac output. This, in turn, results from increased cardiac preload (venous return) and diminished cardiac afterload (arteriolar vasodilatation). In each case, multiple factors are involved. Increased venous return, however, largely reflects expanded total body blood volume. Diminished arteriolar tone is characteristic of portal hypertension but the mechanism is poorly understood, but recent data suggest that derangement in nitric oxide metabolism may be involved. Increased portal blood flow is also seen in arteriovenous fistulae or splenomegaly alone.

The most common clinical manifestations of portal hypertension are hematemesis or melena resulting from ruptured esophageal varices. Most of these children have splenomegaly, but the splenic size does not correlate well with portal pressure. Many episodes of intestinal hemorrhage are associated with upper respiratory tract infections, fever, or aspirin ingestion.

These children also tend to develop ascites (Fig. 84-5). The gradual accumulation of ascites represents a disturbance in distribution of intravascular volume. According to the Starling proposal, increased portal venous pressure and diminished plasma oncotic pressure facilitate the development of ascites. There are three hypotheses for the induction of ascites.[12] In the underfilling hypothesis, increased hepatic sinusoidal pressure is the initiating factor. This results in increased portal venous pressure, increased splanchnic volume, decreased systemic vascular resistance, and decreased "effective" intravascular volume. Renin-aldosterone and vasopressin release increase, and avid renal sodium and water retention occurs. Increased portal venous pressure also causes an increased accumulation of lymph in the ascites fluid. The overflow hypothesis implicates increased renal sodium and water retention as the inciting factors, causing increased sinusoidal pressure as an upstream event, but it is not clear how sodium and water retention is initiated or maintained. The peripheral arterial vasodilatation hypothesis

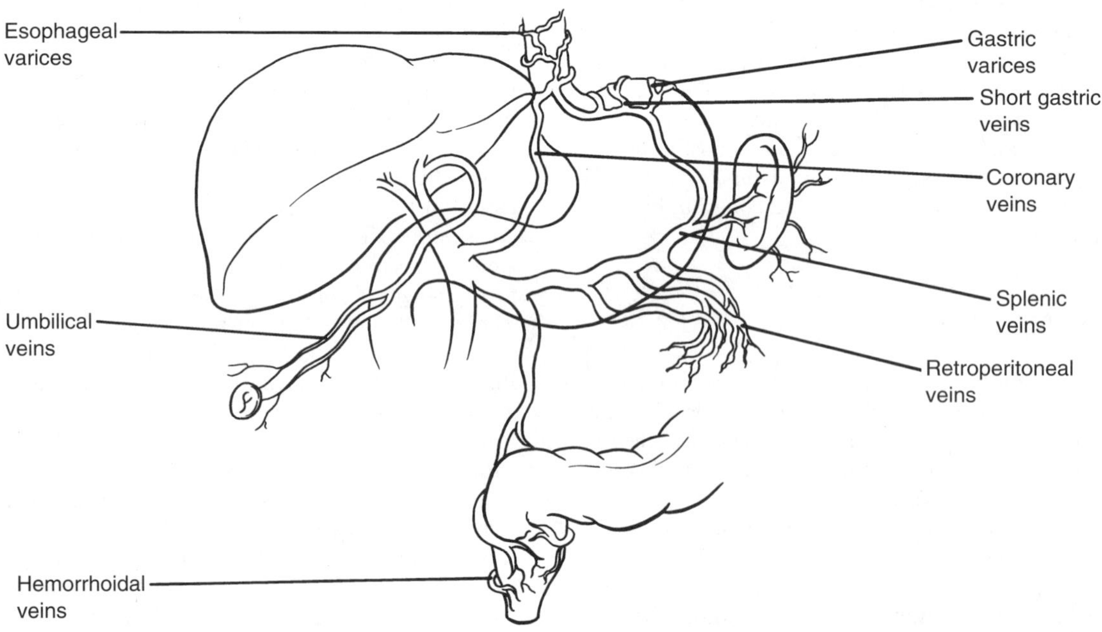

FIG. 84-4. Portal collateral circulation. (Iber F. The undergraduate teaching project in gastroenterology and liver disease. American Gastroenterology Association, Bethesda, MD.)

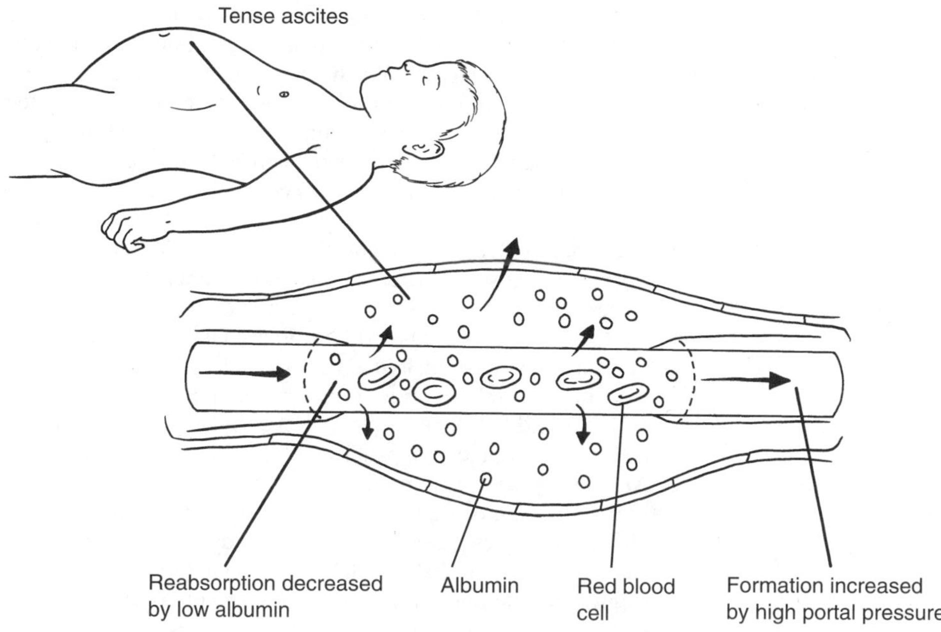

FIG. 84-5. Pathophysiology of ascites. (Iber F. The undergraduate teaching project in gastroenterology and liver disease. American Gastroenterology Association, Bethesda, MD.)

states that vasodilatation leads to sufficient sodium and water retention and increased plasma volume to form ascites but not to refill the expanded vascular compartment. Thus, there is inappropriate lack of suppression of the renin-aldosterone and vasopressin systems.

The clinical manifestations of ascites in children may differ from those in adults. Children are less likely to have accompanying peripheral edema. Shifting dullness may be difficult to elicit in chubby children. The first sign of ascites may be inappropriate weight gain. Later the abdomen is distended with fluid. The flanks are bulging. Distension of the scrotum and abdominal wall veins may be present. In late stages, pleural effusion and peripheral edema arise. The child may be irritable, complain of abdominal pain, and suffer from dyspnea.

Children with portal hypertension and ascites are susceptible to spontaneous bacterial peritonitis (SBP). SBP is defined as a bacterial infection of the peritoneal fluid in the absence of gut perforation or any other secondary source of bacterial contamination. Discussions of its pathogenesis have invoked defects in reticuloendothelial and neutrophil function, low serum and ascitic fluid levels of complement, and opsonic activity. None of these abnormalities is profound, however, and, even together, they cannot account completely for the pathogenesis.[12] SBP is usually caused by a single organism of gut origin. Gram-negative enteric bacteria such as *Escherichia coli, Klebsiella,* and *Enterococcus* sp account for 60% to 80% of adult cases. *Streptococcus pneumoniae, Haemophilus influenzae,* and *Neisseria meningitidis* may cause relatively higher percentages of cases in young children.

SBP should be considered when a child with ascites presents with fever, abdominal pain, and leukocytosis. Infants have poor feeding, lethargy, and abdominal distension. Vomiting, diarrhea, hypotension, and worsening of hepatic encephalopathy may occur. Abdominal tenderness, even rebound tenderness, may be present on physical examination. Several recent studies have shown that SBP occurs in asymptomatic adults. This has not yet been clearly documented in children, but the observation should raise the index of suspicion for this diagnosis in susceptible children. Abdominal paracentesis provides the definitive diagnosis of SBP. It should be done approximately 2 cm below the umbilicus, in the left lower quadrant, slightly anterior to the midaxillary line, but lateral to the rectus muscle. The fluid should be immediately inoculated into blood culture bottles. Neutrophil counts greater than 250 cells/mL^3 are the best predictors of positive cultures.[13] The ascitic fluid protein is usually greater than 1 g/dL, and the glucose level is less than 50 mg/dL in SBP.

NEONATAL HEPATITIS SYNDROME

Neonatal hepatitis syndrome describes hepatocellular dysfunction and bile duct obstruction in infants under 8 weeks of age. The syndrome is broadly defined because many types of insults (infectious, ischemic, obstructive, metabolic, toxic) to the liver, at this age, have similar clinical and histopathologic effects. Clinically, these infants present to the pediatric gastroenterologist or surgeon with jaundice, elevated conjugated bilirubin levels, and often, elevated transaminases.[14] Almost all infants have evidence of cholestasis. The spectrum of histologic abnormalities includes invasion of the periportal region by mononuclear cells, lobular disarray, ballooning degeneration of hepatocytes, and transformation into multinucleated giant cells, with mild to moderate degrees of bile duct proliferation. Because extrahepatic biliary atresia is one of the most common causes of this syndrome, and because the palliative effects of the hepatic portoenterostomy procedure are believed to be better the earlier in life it is done, timely diagnosis of the etiology for the neonatal hepatitis syndrome is essential. Other surgically correctable causes of the neonatal hepatitis syndrome include choledochal cyst, the treatment of which should not be delayed.

In general, multiple diagnostic modalities are used to evaluate infants with this syndrome.

History and physical examination
Laboratory tests
  Basic
    Complete blood count
    Electrolytes
    Glucose
    BUN
    Creatinine
    Liver
    Enzymes
    Bilirubin panel
    Albumin
    PT and PTT
    Vitamin D and E levels
  Diagnostic
    α_1-Antitrypsin phenotype
    T_4 and TSH
    Urine succinyl acetone/organic acids
    Sweat chloride
    GPUT
    Reactive plasma reagent
    Viral serology
    Urinalysis
    Serum and urine bile acids
Radiology
  Liver ultrasound
  HIDA scan
Histology
  Liver biopsy
Operative cholangiogram

Serum transaminases suggest whether hepatocellular inflammation is present, and conjugated bilirubin levels determine whether cholestasis exists. Serum albumin levels and prothrombin time are used to assess liver synthetic function. Malabsorption of fat-soluble vitamins is most easily detected by examining the serum level of vitamin E. Among the fat-soluble vitamins, vitamin E is most susceptible to malabsorption in cholestatic conditions. A series of more specific diagnostic studies is done almost always, to exclude treatable medical causes of neonatal hepatitis. For instance, an *αl-AT* phenotype (*αl-AT* Pi type) is ordered immediately, because variant PiZZ *αl-AT* deficiency, the most common genetic cause of neonatal hepatitis, accounts for as many as 10% of the affected infants, and its diagnosis obviates any more invasive diagnostic evaluation.

A liver ultrasound is used to detect choledochal cyst. At one time, identification of the gallbladder by ultrasound was thought to exclude the diagnosis of biliary atresia. However, it is now known that the gallbladder is detected in 10% or more of infants with biliary atresia.[15] Failure to detect the gallbladder by ultrasound is often a result of technical considerations and therefore is not helpful. Other observations, such as the size of the bile ducts or the presence or absence of bile duct dilatation, usually are not helpful.

Hepatobiliary scintigraphy, using technetium-labeled iminodiacetate derivatives, is useful in examining the infant for biliary tract obstruction. The sensitivity of the test is 100% in most studies, although a few infants reported to have biliary atresia had excretion into the small intestine during an earlier scintigraphic study.[16] Presumably, biliary atresia was an evolving postnatal process in these infants. The study has low speci-

ficity, however, because excretion of isotope into the intestine is absent in more than half of patients with intrahepatic (nonobstructive) cholestasis.[17] Treatment with phenobarbital is reported to improve the specificity, with a decrease in conjugated bilirubin and improved excretion of isotope into the intestine after treatment in several infants.[18] However, this use of phenobarbital has not been subjected to controlled studies.

Percutaneous liver biopsy is frequently used in the diagnostic evaluation of the jaundiced baby. Bile duct proliferation is considered the most characteristic histologic abnormality of extrahepatic biliary tract obstruction, and is often accompanied by intraductal bile plugs and portal fibrosis. Giant cell transformation and hepatic parenchymal necrosis are said to be more common in neonatal hepatitis. Other histologic findings, such as periodic acid Schiff–positive, diastase-resistant globules in α_1-antitrypsin deficiency, paucity of intrahepatic bile ducts in Alagille syndrome, ground-glass hepatocytes in hepatitis B virus infection, or steatosis without inflammation in metabolic disorders, suggest specific diagnoses. However, biopsy results can be misleading. Biliary atresia may occur in the absence of significant bile duct proliferation in as many as 20% of biopsies.[19] Conversely, in up to 30% of patients with neonatal hepatitis bile duct proliferation is seen in the liver biopsy specimen.[20] Giant cell transformation is found in liver biopsy specimens of approximately 10% to 30% of infants with biliary atresia and 65% to 70% of infants with other causes of neonatal hepatitis syndrome.[21] This overlap reduces the predictive value of liver biopsy in discriminating biliary atresia from other causes of neonatal hepatitis, but a direct, systematic, prospective study is needed to definitively demonstrate this impression.

When the diagnostic evaluation suggests or cannot exclude the possibility of extrahepatic biliary atresia, the infant is sent to the operating room for intraoperative cholangiogram and treated by hepatic portoenterostomy, if any portion of the extrahepatic biliary system is not visualized. Even in this case, however, there may be some uncertainty. It has been difficult to visualize the extrahepatic biliary tree directly or by cholangiogram in several infants with intrahepatic bile duct paucity syndromes.[22] Moreover, it may be possible to visualize the biliary system early in the newborn period in an infant in whom extrahepatic biliary atresia later clearly was identified.

Table 84-1 lists the major specific diagnoses that cause the neonatal hepatitis syndrome. As many as 50% of this affected population ultimately are diagnosed with idiopathic giant cell hepatitis. In most cases, this resolves spontaneously over the first year of life, but in an estimated 10% to 20% of cases there is progressive liver dysfunction.[23] Unfortunately, this population has not been subjected to careful and systematic prospective characterization.

Systemic infections may also be responsible for the neonatal hepatitis syndrome. Bacterial sepsis, especially associated with urinary tract infection and gram-negative organisms, causes conjugated hyperbilirubinemia. There is evidence that endotoxin directly inhibits the biliary excretion of conjugated bilirubin.[24] Endotoxin may also affect other phases of bilirubin metabolism. Moreover, hemolysis and hepatic ischemia also contribute to hepatic dysfunction. In some cases, when the affected infant does not appear ill and may have relatively few other signs of systemic bacterial infection, the diagnosis requires a high index of suspicion.

In some studies cytomegalovirus (CMV) infections are a rela-

TABLE 84-1. *Major causes of neonatal hepatitis syndrome*

Surgically correctable obstructive lesions
    Extrahepatic biliary atresia
    Choledochal cyst
    Spontaneous perforation of the bile duct
Idiopathic neonatal giant cell hepatitis
Infection
    Bacterial sepsis, especially urinary tract infection
    Syphilis
    Viral hepatitis A, B, or C
    Cytomegalovirus hepatitis
    Other causes
Metabolic
    α_1-Antitrypsin deficiency
    Galactosemia
    Tyrosinemia
    Fructosemia
    Mitochondrial defects
    Peroxisomal defects
Cystic fibrosis
Hypothyroidism
Syndromic or nonsyndromic paucity of the intrahepatic bile
    ducts
Bile acid synthetic defects
Toxins

tively common cause of the neonatal hepatitis syndrome.[25] When the CMV infection is congenital, other signs may include petechiae and neurologic abnormalities, in addition to jaundice and hepatosplenomegaly. When the CMV infection is postnatal or when congenital CMV develops over a delayed interval, a few other signs of the infection may exist. Hepatosplenomegaly, hypertransaminasemia, and direct hyperbilirubinemia may last for weeks. Liver biopsy shows giant cell transformation and may also show extramedullary hematopoiesis, bile duct proliferation, and fibrosis. In some cases, CMV is thought to cause destruction of biliary epithelium and obliteration of biliary ductules. Neonatal hepatitis associated with CMV does not usually lead to chronic liver disease, but a few cases with prolonged fibrosis or cirrhosis, and rare cases of hepatic necrosis, have been reported. A positive urine culture for CMV suggests, but does not prove, the diagnosis. CMV can be cultured from the urine of otherwise asymptomatic neonates. Seroconversion is also helpful. Although gancyclovir has been used to treat immunocompromised individuals with CMV hepatitis, it has not yet been used in CMV-associated neonatal hepatitis.

Infants may be infected with hepatitis B transplacentally, during delivery, or postnatally. Infection can be prevented if the mother is known to be hepatitis B surface antigen–positive and the infant is given hepatitis B immunoglobulin (HBIG) and immunization. Most infected infants are asymptomatic chronic carriers, although some may develop chronic hepatitis. Acute hepatitis or even fulminant hepatitis failure rarely occurs in the first 5 months of life.[26] At this time, treatment involves supportive measures. Interferon is being studied as a potential treatment for children with chronic active hepatitis B.

Congenital syphilitic hepatitis may present in the first days to weeks of life. Jaundice, hepatosplenomegaly, rash, fever, snuffles, and osteochondritis may be observed.[27] Direct hyperbilirubinemia (with bilirubin ranging from 8 to 30) and transaminases 7 to 150 times normal are present. Histology of the liver

is characterized by inflammation with giant cells. There is very little evidence that the hepatitis is progressive. Penicillin is the treatment of choice. Several authors have reported a transient worsening of hepatic function during treatment.

A variety of other viruses have been associated with the neonatal hepatitis syndrome.[28] Infants with congenital rubella have a characteristic rash, hepatosplenomegaly, and hematologic abnormalities. Herpes simplex virus can also present as neonatal cholestasis. Many infants with neonatal herpes hepatitis have skin or central nervous system manifestations of the infection. Case reports mention echovirus, coxsackie virus, and adenovirus.

A number of metabolic liver diseases cause neonatal hepatitis syndrome, the most common being *α1-AT* deficiency.[29] The clinical manifestations and liver histologic characteristics of *α1-AT* deficiency–associated liver disease are similar to those of other causes of neonatal hepatitis. Low serum concentration of *α1-AT* is consistent with the diagnosis, but levels may be spuriously elevated during an acute-phase response. The presence in liver biopsy specimens of periodic acid Schiff–positive, diastase-resistant globules in the endoplasmic reticulum of liver cells substantiates the diagnosis. If the diagnosis is correct, these globules should stain positively with antibody to *α1-AT* by immunohistochemical analysis. Nevertheless, definitive diagnosis is established by determining serum *α1-AT* phenotype in isoelectric focusing. Although more than 70 phenotypes for *α1-AT* are defined, liver disease is clearly associated with only the homozygous *PiZZ* phenotype. *α1-AT* deficiency may also first reach clinical attention because of portal hypertension during adolescence, chronic hepatitis and cryptogenic cirrhosis, or hepatocellular carcinoma in adulthood. Finally, emphysema may develop late in the third to fourth decades in individuals with this deficiency.

The most important treatment for *α1-AT* deficiency is avoiding cigarette smoking. Cigarette smoking markedly accelerates the destructive lung disease associated with *α1-AT* deficiency, reduces the quality of life, and shortens longevity. Liver disease associated with *α1-AT* deficiency has been treated by orthotopic liver transplantation (OLT). In fact, it is the most common genetic diagnosis for which individuals undergo OLT. Survival rates are approximately 80% at 1 year and 70% at 5 years. Nevertheless, even individuals with *α1-AT* deficiency and moderate to severe liver dysfunction may have relatively low rates of disease progression. Therefore, a selective group of these patients may not require OLT as urgently as do patients with other forms of liver disease. Adults with *α1-AT* deficiency and emphysema have undergone replacement therapy with purified plasma *α1-AT* by the intravenous route or by intratracheal aerosol administration. Serum concentrations of *α1-AT* and concentrations of *α1-AT* and neutrophil elastase inhibitory capacity in bronchoalveolar lavage fluid improved with this therapy. No significant side effects were seen during these trials. Protein replacement therapy is not being considered for individuals with liver disease, because deficient serum levels of *α1-AT* have not been shown to be mechanistically related to liver injury.

Perlmutter reviews the considerable information available on the pathophysiology of liver disease in this deficiency.[29] First, a single amino acid substitution (*glu* to *lys 342*), encoded by a single nucleotide substitution, is found in *Z α1-AT*. Second, an abnormal protein accumulates in the endoplasmic reticulum (ER). Only 15% of the newly synthesized *α1-AT* molecules are able to transverse the secretory pathway to reach the extracellular medium and ultimately the body fluids. Third, the substitution of *lys* for *glu 342* is sufficient to produce this cellular defect. This molecular abnormality presumably results in a change in the conformation or folding of the nascent *α1-AT* polypeptide after translocation into the lumen of the ER. Two studies have raised the possibility that the substitution of *lys* for *glu 342* reduces the stability of *α1-AT* in the monomeric form and increases the likelihood that *α1-AT* polymers are generated by a proposed loop-sheet insertion mechanism.[30,31] Fourth, studies in transgenic animals provide convincing evidence that liver injury is a direct consequence of intracellular retention of the presumably hepatotoxic *α1-AT* molecule. Transgenic mice carrying the mutant (Z) allele of the human *α1-AT* gene develop periodic acid Schiff–positive, diastase-resistant intrahepatic globules and exhibit neonatal hepatitis and growth failure, a syndrome similar to that characterizing liver injury in deficient humans. Because these animals have normal levels of *α1-AT* and, presumably, other antielastases, as directed by the endogenous murine genes, the liver injury cannot be attributed to proteolytic attack.

Any theory for the pathogenesis of liver injury in *α1-AT* deficiency must also consider that only a subpopulation of these individuals develops significant liver injury. This was shown by Sveger, who prospectively screened 200,000 newborn infants in Sweden.[32] One hundred twenty-seven *PiZZ* infants were identified and observed, prospectively. By 12 years of age, more than 75% of these children had normal serum transaminase and no evidence of liver injury.[33]

The observations of Sveger and the demonstration of an uninduced heatshock and stress response in *PiZZ* individuals with liver disease, but not in *PiZZ* individuals without liver disease, have led us to predict that a subset of the *PiZZ* population is more susceptible to liver injury by virtue of a second or several additional inherited traits or environmental factors, which exaggerate the intracellular accumulation of the mutant Z *α1-AT* protein or the cellular pathophysiologic consequences of mutant *α1-AT* accumulation. In a recent study skin fibroblasts from deficient individuals with and without liver disease were transduced with the mutant Z *α1-AT* gene.[34] The results show a lag in endoplasmic reticulum degradation of mutant *α1-AT* protein, resulting in greater net intracellular retention of the abnormally folded hepatotoxic *α1-AT* Z molecule in patients predisposed to liver disease. An understanding of this second defect may allow prenatal prediction of susceptibility to liver disease within the deficient population.

Galactosemia, an autosomal recessive inborn error of carbohydrate metabolism, resulting from a deficiency of galactose-1-phosphate uridyl transferase, occurs in approximately 1 in 20,000 live births.[35] Accumulation of galactose-1-phosphate results in toxic effects in a number of organ systems. In the severe toxicity syndrome, the infant feeds poorly, fails to thrive, is delayed in development, and often, presents with vomiting. Symptoms may develop in the first week of life if the infant is drinking lactose-containing formula or breast feeding. On physical examination, jaundice, hepatomegaly, and cataracts may be evident. Laboratory evaluation is remarkable for hypoglycemia and hyperbilirubinemia, which in early stages is predominantly unconjugated, because of hemolysis, and later is conjugated. A renal Fanconi syndrome is sometimes present. These infants may be first identified during an episode of *E. coli* sepsis.[36] It is not known, however, whether galactosemia predisposes infants to gram-negative sepsis by a disease-specific mechanism.

The major long-term sequelae of galactosemia are cataracts, mental retardation, and cirrhosis. The extent of liver damage depends on age and duration of galactose exposure. Fibrosis and cirrhosis eventually develop in untreated cases. However, severe liver damage can resolve completely on dietary elimination therapy.

The diagnosis of galactosemia is often suggested by the presence of reducing substance in the urine in the absence of glucosuria, the former is measured by the Clinitest tablet, the latter by commercially available glucose oxidase assays. However, detection of galactosuria by these determinations is insensitive and nonspecific. Poor lactose intake or intermittent excretion of excess galactose can be responsible for false-negative results. False-positive results are observed in severe liver disease or after certain medications are administered. Therefore, specific diagnosis relies on determination of red blood cell galactose-1-phosphate uridyl transferase activity.

Treatment of transferase-deficiency galactosemia involves complete elimination of galactose from the diet. All milk and milk products are forbidden. Pregestimil (Mead Johnson, Evansville, IN), Alimentum (Ross Laboratories, Columbus, OH), and Nutramigen (Ross Laboratories, Columbus, OH) are effective substitutes for infants, although some may contain small amounts of lactose from milk preparation. Soy formulas also seem to be adequate substitutes. The galactose-containing oligosaccharides raffinose and stachyose are found in soy formulas, but are not hydrolyzed by intestinal mucosal enzymes. Recent studies have clarified at least a few of the molecular defects in galactosemia. A variety of missense mutations have been found in the transferase gene, resulting in a marked decrease in enzyme activity.[37]

Hereditary fructose intolerance is caused by severe deficiency of fructose-1-phosphate aldolase B to less than 5% of its normal activity.[38] It results in acute episodes of abdominal pain, vomiting, and hypoglycemia shortly after fructose ingestion or with failure to thrive, hepatomegaly, and severe liver dysfunction in the chronic syndrome. The chronic syndrome usually develops when parents have unconsciously removed fructose from the diet, and the patient, at preschool age, develops a strong distaste for sweet food. If neither of these occurs, prolonged ingestion of fructose beginning at the weaning period, when fruits and vegetables are introduced into the diet, leads to poor feeding, vomiting, jaundice, hepatomegaly, renal tubular insufficiency, and eventually hepatic failure. The hypoglycemia is caused by inhibition of glycogenolysis and gluconeogenesis mediated by fructose-1-phosphate. Other metabolic abnormalities include metabolic acidosis with high levels of lactic acid and hyperuricemia. Occasionally, hereditary fructose intolerance is diagnosed in adulthood. Affected individuals develop specific aversions to food containing fructose and sucrose and have a very low incidence of caries, which are known to be promoted by sucrose.

Definitive diagnosis should be determined by enzyme assay on liver tissue. The intravenous fructose tolerance test is discouraged by many investigators who have observed severe toxic effects during the study. Liver biopsy shows diffuse steatosis, necrosis of a few scattered hepatocytes, fibrosis, and sometimes cirrhosis.

The disorder involves an autosomal recessive defect in aldolase B, an enzyme expressed in liver, intestine, and kidney. The gene has been characterized, and a missense mutation within a region critical for substrate binding has been identified in four patients. Genetic heterogeneity exists, however, indicating that other mutations genetic abnormalities will be discovered.[39,40]

When this diagnosis is entertained, sucrose, fructose, and sorbitol should be eliminated immediately from the diet and from medications. Chronic ingestion of even small amounts of these saccharides can be damaging. The salutary effect of the elimination diet is observed within days.

Hereditary fructose-1,6-diphosphatase deficiency is a related abnormality of fructose metabolism in which affected newborns or older infants present with life-threatening episodes of hyperventilation caused by lactic acidosis, apnea, hypoglycemia, and ketosis triggered by fasting or febrile illnesses.[41] These infants may have mild hepatomegaly and hepatic steatosis; however, unlike infants with hereditary fructose intolerance, they do not usually have elevated serum transaminases or other evidence of hepatic dysfunction, and do not have hepatocyte necrosis or fibrosis in liver biopsy specimens.

Hereditary tyrosinemia type I is characterized by progressive liver failure, renal tubular dysfunction, and hypophosphatemic rickets. It is an autosomal recessive defect, most prevalent in French Canadian descendants of Quebec.[42] In the acute form of the disease, the infant may have poor growth, vomiting, diarrhea, a cabbage-like odor, and possibly bleeding complications. If untreated, the disorder results in liver failure within 6 to 8 months. In the chronic form, hepatic dysfunction is evident, but the clinical picture is dominated by renal tubular dysfunction, hypertension, and hypophosphatemic rickets. Patients with this form of the disease may also develop neurologic crises that resemble acute intermittent porphyria. These crises presumably result from competitive inhibition of δ-aminolevulinic acid dehydratase by succinylacetone, a metabolite of tyrosine degradation that accumulates in hereditary tyrosinemia. Patients with this disorder have increased susceptibility to hepatocellular carcinoma, even within the first 5 to 10 years of life. These individuals also have a predilection for hypertrophic obstructive cardiomyopathy.

Laboratory evaluation is remarkable for prolonged prothrombin time, elevated plasma tyrosine, and methionine levels in excess of those associated with chronic liver disease. The plasma α-fetoprotein levels may also be markedly elevated. Liver biopsy is notable for hepatocellular inflammation and necrosis, fatty infiltration, pseudoacinar formation, and marked nodular regeneration. The diagnosis is established by elevated urine succinylacetone and absence of or decreased fumarylacetoacetate hydrolase in liver tissue or skin fibroblasts.

This disorder is associated with a deficiency in fumarylacetoacetate hydrolase, which catalyzes the last reaction in the pathway for degradation of tyrosine (Fig. 84-6). A series of studies examining messenger RNA and protein levels in liver and skin fibroblasts from a number of individuals with the disorder show evidence for genetic heterogeneity.[43]

Dietary restriction of tyrosine and phenylalanine has been used until recently as therapy for this disorder. Liver transplantation has been successful, but needs to be considered before the development of hepatoma. Hematin can be used to treat the neurologic crises.[44] The rationale for this intervention is the capacity of hematin to inhibit aminolevulinic acid synthetase and the production of δ-aminolevulinic acid while the patient

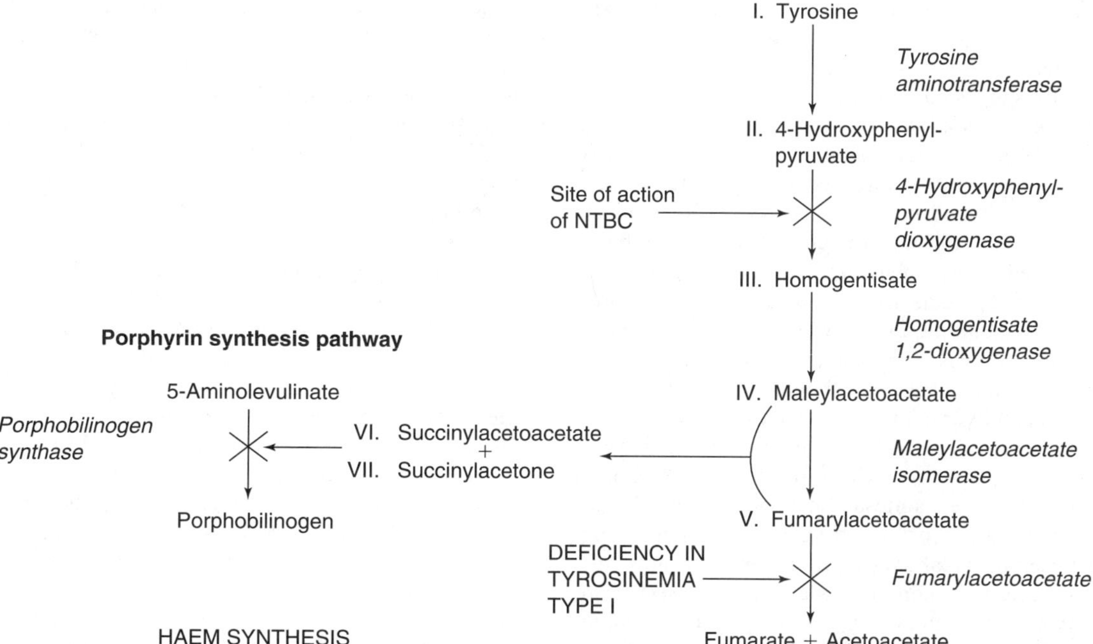

FIG. 84-6. Tyrosine degradation pathway. (Lindstedt S, Holme E, Lock EA, et al. Treatment of hereditary tyrosinaemia type I by inhibition of 4-hydroxyphenylpyruvate deoxygenase. Lancet 1992;340:813)

awaits liver transplantation. Recently, NTBC [2-(2-nitro-4-trifluoro-methylbenzoyl)-1,3-cyclohexanedione], a drug that inhibits tyrosine deoxygenase early in the tyrosine degradation pathway, has been associated with a marked reduction in succinylacetone accumulation and results in amelioration of hepatic and renal injury.[45] The major drawback of this treatment, hypertyrosinemia, with theoretical corneal deposition can apparently be avoided by adhering to a diet with restricted tyrosine and phenylalanine. NTBC also had a remarkable beneficial effect on liver and kidney damage in a recently described animal model of tyrosinemia, characterized by deletion of the *FAH* gene.[46] Long-term effects of NTBC on disease progression or development of hepatoma are unknown.

Abnormalities in peroxisomes or peroxisomal enzymes cause a recently recognized group of genetic disorders. The most well-described of these disorders, Zellweger cerebrohepatorenal syndrome, consists of facial dysmorphism, hypotonia, seizures, failure to thrive, and liver disease.[47] Babies with this syndrome usually survive only a few months. Liver disease may be suspected only with enlargement of the liver. However, some infants already have elevated serum transaminases, coagulopathy, and hypoalbuminemia in the neonatal period. Liver involvement progresses to liver failure in most of the infants who survive beyond the neonatal period. The diagnosis is suggested by elevation of very-long-chain fatty acids in the blood. Liver biopsy shows fibrosis, even frank cirrhosis. Electron microscopy usually shows absence of peroxisomes. A gene for peroxisomal assembly factor-1 that confers peroxisome assembly on a peroxisome-deficient cell line has recently been characterized.[48]

A number of other diagnoses can mimic Zellweger syndrome. In infantile Refsum disease, neurologic dysfunction is less severe, but hepatomegaly and hepatic dysfunction are common. Patients with rhizomelic chondrodysplasia punctate also have liver disease. Like patients with Zellweger syndrome, these patients have elevated serum levels of very-long-chain fatty acids, diminished serum levels of red blood cell plasmalogens, and a liver biopsy specimen that usually shows absence of peroxisomes. Patients with Refsum disease can be distinguished by elevation of phytanic acid levels. Rhizomelic chondrodysplasia punctate is usually suggested by dysmorphic and skeletal features on initial presentation.

Neonatal and X-linked adrenoleukodystrophy may also mimic Zellweger syndrome. Several recent studies have contributed to the elucidation of the pathogenesis of these two disorders. Recently, the peroxisomal bifunctional enzyme has been shown to be deficient in neonatal adrenoleukodystrophy.[49]

A number of other disorders are associated with the neonatal hepatitis syndrome, including cystic fibrosis.[50] Because early diagnosis of cystic fibrosis by sweat test can result in more effective management, a sweat test should be routine in the evaluation of neonatal liver injury. Nevertheless, the characteristic focal biliary cirrhosis–portal hypertension of cystic fibrosis is generally first clinically manifest later in childhood or adolescence and is only rarely the manifestation by which cystic fibrosis is diagnosed in the neonatal period. Of note is a strong association between neonatal liver injury and meconium ileus.

The neonatal hepatitis syndrome has also been observed in hypothyroidism and hypopituitarism.[51] Septooptic dysplasia, in which abnormalities in development of the central facial structure, blindness, and hypopituitarism are manifest as hypoglycemia and hypoadrenalism, is the most common form of hypopituitarism associated with liver injury. Early recognition and treatment of these conditions is essential in preventing mental retardation and severe growth disturbance from hypothyroidism and vascular collapse from adrenal insufficiency in hypopituitarism.

Alagille syndrome, or arteriohepatic dysplasia, is a disorder in which neonatal jaundice is associated with a characteristic facies, vertebral malformations, retarded physical, mental, and sexual development, and peripheral pulmonic stenosis.[52] The characteristic facies consists of a prominent forehead, hypertelorism, and a small pointed chin. Vertebral arch abnormalities and ophthalmologic anomalies such as posterior embryotoxon have been reported. Patients may develop hypogonadism later in life. There is marked cholestasis with pruritus, hypercholesterolemia, and fat-soluble vitamin deficiencies. These children may develop pigmentary retinopathy and spinocerebellar degeneration from severe vitamin E deficiency. Inheritance is autosomal dominant. A deletion on chromosome 20 has been implicated.[53,54] Liver histology demonstrates absence or paucity of bile ducts in most portal areas. Bile stasis and giant cell transformation can be observed. This syndrome is characterized by a chronic, stable cholestasis without progression of the liver injury. Treatment involves symptomatic measures to reduce pruritus and fat-soluble vitamins, especially vitamin E, to prevent fat-soluble vitamin deficiency.

In contrast, Byler syndrome is an inherited cholestatic disease with progressive liver injury,[55] sometimes called progressive familial intrahepatic cholestasis. This disorder may present clinically with jaundice, pruritus, and symptoms of fat-soluble vitamin deficiency. There is an unexplained predilection for reactive airway disease. Laboratory abnormalities include elevated transaminases, elevated serum bile acids, prolonged prothrombin time, reduced serum albumin, and an unexplained reduction in γ-glutamyl transpeptidase and cholesterol. The disorder is inherited as an autosomal recessive trait. It often progresses to liver failure and predisposes to hepatocellular carcinoma. Some patients have benefited from a biliary diversion procedure.[56]

In recent years, bile acid synthetic defects have been reported as causes of the neonatal hepatitis syndrome[57,58] and, perhaps, neonatal hemochromatosis. δ-3-Oxosteroid-5-β-reductase deficiency, an inborn error of bile acid metabolism, results in neonatal cholestasis and severe hepatic dysfunction. This diagnosis is made by assessing the urinary bile acid profile. Three patients have improved during treatment with ursodeoxycholic acid.

Hypoperfusion, or ischemia, is another relatively common cause of liver dysfunction in the neonate. It is usually precipitated by acute illness with dehydration or in congenital heart disease associated with left ventricular failure and decreased cardiac output.[59] The liver is usually enlarged, transaminases elevated, and prothrombin time prolonged out of proportion to the other derangements of liver function. Liver histology may show necrosis with distension of sinusoids. With congestive heart failure be centrilobular congestion and hemorrhage may occur. The liver injury usually resolves when the acute illness or heart failure are treated, but on some occasions, the liver reticulin structure collapses, and progressive liver failure ensues.

Total parenteral nutrition (TPN) is associated with liver injury in the neonate, especially low-birth-weight premature infants. Mild elevation of transaminases and conjugated bilirubin levels may be observed within 2 weeks of initiating TPN.[60]

There are no specific findings on liver histologic examination. Mild nonspecific inflammatory infiltration, bile plugs, and later, portal fibrosis become evident. Carbohydrate, amino acid, and fat constituents of TPN solutions have all been implicated in the liver injury, though this is inconclusive. An interesting series of studies suggests that very high plasma phytosterol levels developing during infusion of lipid emulsions contribute to cholestasis.[61] One of the difficulties in establishing cause-and-effect relationships between components of TPN and liver injury is the exposure of affected infants to other potentially hepatotoxic conditions including hypoperfusion, sepsis, drugs, and metabolic insults.

Metabolic Liver Disease in Older Children

Several genetic or metabolic liver diseases come to clinical attention after the neonatal period, in later infancy, childhood, or adolescence (Table 84-2). For instance, Gaucher disease presents in later childhood or even in adult years. It is associated with deficiency of glucocerebrosidase, a lysosomal enzyme that catalyzes the degradation of glycolipids. The highly insoluble glucocerebrosides accumulate in lysosomes, leading to bone disease, hepatosplenomegaly, and neurologic symptoms.[62]

Patients with the most common form, type I or adult-type Gaucher disease, may be recognized at any age by pathologic fractures, bone pain, thrombocytopenia, easy bruising, and leukopenia. Hepatosplenomegaly and mild hepatic dysfunction occur frequently. In the type II acute neuronopathic form of Gaucher disease, patients develop opisthotonic posturing, seizures, strabismus, marked delay in development, and poor feeding in the first year of life. Many of these infants suffer from respiratory difficulties, particularly stridor. The liver and spleen are also enlarged. Type III juvenile Gaucher disease is associated with mild neurologic symptoms that emerge at 3 to 10 years of age.

The diagnosis is suggested by foam cells in peripheral smear or bone marrow aspirate, flaring of the distal femur on long bone films, and elevation of acid phosphatase and angiotensin-converting enzyme levels. However, definitive diagnosis requires the demonstration of absent or markedly decreased leukocyte glucocerebrosidase. Liver biopsy specimens are characterized predominantly by fibrosis, with foam cells in centrilobular regions.

Gaucher disease is an autosomal recessive defect most prevalent among the Ashkenazi Jewish population. At least 30 genetic abnormalities in the glucocrebrosidase gene have been described.[62] The acute neuronopathic form of the disease is associated with the most severe defects. An animal model of Gaucher disease, from targeted disruption of the mouse glucocerebrosidase gene, has been described and should provide more information about pathogenesis and treatment options.[63]

One of the major advances in treatment of inborn errors of metabolism is the development of targeted enzyme replacement for Gaucher disease. This therapy depends on a purified enzyme

TABLE 84-2. *Clinical presentations of metabolic liver disease*

Disorder	Typical presentation	Diagnostic test	Treatment
Galactosemia	Neonatal jaundice and sepsis	Red blood cell tranferase level	Galactose/lactose-free diet
Fructose aldolase deficiency	Vomiting, hypoglycemia, liver failure	Enzyme level in liver	Fructose/sucrose-free diet
Glycogen storage disease			
I	Hypoglycemia, hepatomegaly		Frequent feeds or cornstarch
III	Hypoglycemia, hepatomegaly		Frequent feeds*
IV	Cirrhosis, central nervous system dysfunction	Enzyme level in liver	None*
VI	Hepatomegaly		None
Tyrosinemia	Liver failure in infancy, Fanconi syndrome, rickets	Urine succinyl acetone	Low tyrosine–low phenylalanine diet* NTBC
Niemann-Pick disease	Jaundice, hepatomegaly, neurologic deterioration	Leukocyte enzyme levels	None
Gaucher disease	Hepatomegaly, neurologic dysfunction	Leukocyte enzyme levels	Enzyme infusion*
Wolman disease	Hepatomegaly, failure to thrive, adrenal calcifications	Leukocyte enzyme levels	None
Cholesterol ester storage disease	Portal hypertension	Leukocyte enzyme levels	Lipid-reducing drugs*
Zellweger disease	Hypotonia, seizures, hepatitis, hepatomegaly	VLCFA, ultrastructure	? Bile acid therapy
Wilson disease	Jaundice, hemolysis, psychomotor abnormalities	Liver copper	Penicillamine Liver transplant
α_1-Antitrypsin deficiency	Neonatal jaundice, portal hypertension	Serum pi type	Avoidance of cigarette smoke Liver transplant

* Liver transplant has been done.
VLCFA, very long chain fatty acid; NTBC, 2-(2-nitro-4-trifluoromethylbenzoyl)-1, 3-cyclohexanedione)

modified so that the carbohydrate moieties are terminated with mannose (Ceredase, Genzyme Corp, Cambridge, MA), allowing for targeting to macrophages via the mannose receptor. More than 30 patients have had improvements in anemia, thrombocytopenia, and the size of the spleen and liver.[62] A few patients showed signs of skeletal improvement over longer intervals of treatment.

Glycogen storage disease (GSD) results from deficiencies in specific enzymes of the glycogenolytic system and is associated with accumulation of glycogen in tissues, especially liver, skeletal muscle, and, in one case, cardiac muscle. More than 10 forms have been reported, each with distinct clinical features.[64] Types I, III, IV, and VI predominantly affect the liver.

Type I GSD, or glucose-6-phosphatase deficiency, has at least two clinical entities, type Ia and Ib. Glucose-6-phosphatase is composed of at least five polypeptides.[65] A catalytic subunit spans the membrane of the endoplasmic reticulum. A regulatory calcium-binding protein and three translocases allow glucose-6-phosphate, phosphate, and glucose to cross the endoplasmic reticulum membrane. In type Ia GSD, glucose-6-phosphatase activity in liver tissue is minimal or totally absent. In type Ib GSD, normal phosphatase activity is present in fully disrupted liver microsome preparations, but not in intact microsomal vesicles. A defect in one of the translocases has been proposed.

In classic type Ia GSD, infants are short but chubby with doll-like faces, poorly developed, flabby musculature, abdominal distension, and hepatomegaly. They are most commonly recognized because of hypoglycemia and metabolic acidosis caused by high circulating levels of lactic acid. Laboratory evaluation may also indicate the presence of elevated triglyceride and uric acid levels. Liver enzymes are usually not elevated, and liver biopsy specimens are remarkable only for evidence of increased glycogen. These patients may develop adenomas and carcinomas of the liver. They also develop progressive renal dysfunction. Determination of glycogen content and glucose-6-phosphatase activity in liver provides a definitive diagnosis.

The prognosis for patients with type Ia GSD has improved dramatically since the introduction of nocturnal nasogastric glucose infusion[66] and oral cornstarch therapy.[67] The latter regimen is based on slow degradation by amylase, which allows maintenance of normal blood glucose levels for up to 6 hours.

In type Ib GSD, patients have the additional burden of recurrent infections resulting from neutropenia. Recurrent pneumonia, oral mucositis, perianal abscesses, and inflammatory lesions of the bowel may dominate the clinical picture. The introduction of recombinant human granulocyte colony–stimulating factor has greatly improved the lives of several patients.

In type III GSD, the glycogen debranching enzyme is deficient. During infancy these patients often are difficult to clinically distinguish from patients with type I GSD. However, they usually do not develop acidosis, hyperuricemia, or hypertriglyceridemia. The liver may be inflamed, as reflected by increased serum transaminases, mild hepatocellular necrosis, and portal fibrosis seen in liver histologic examination. Occasionally, these patients develop cirrhosis and portal hypertension. In other patients with type III GSD, the hepatomegaly tends to recede, and progressive muscle weakness and wasting develop as the patients reach adulthood. Enzyme activity measurements in muscle, liver, skin fibroblasts, and sometimes erythrocytes may establish definitive diagnosis.

Type IV GSD is characterized by deficiency in the glycogen branching enzyme, progressive liver dysfunction, hypotonia,

growth failure, and delayed development. Liver failure is common in the first 3 to 5 years of life. Diagnosis can be made by enzyme assays in leukocytes and skin fibroblasts, as well as in liver and muscle biopsies. Type VI GSD has been diagnosed in asymptomatic children with hepatomegaly, and is thought to represent a genetically heterogeneous deficiency in liver phosphorylase or phosphorylase b kinase.

Wilson disease is an autosomal recessive disorder associated with accumulation of copper in many tissues, specifically damaging to the liver and the brain.[68] Symptoms in childhood are almost always referable to the liver. These symptoms are usually not apparent until after the age of 8 years, but they have been reported in children as young as 5 years of age. Vomiting, malaise, and jaundice are common. Hepatic dysfunction is often much more severe than one would expect for acute viral hepatitis or even autoimmune hepatitis. A considerable number initially present in acute liver failure. Other clinical manifestations include acute hemolytic crisis, arthritis, and renal stones. Neurologic symptoms do not become manifest until later stages of the disease, unless acute liver failure with hepatic encephalopathy exists at the time of initial diagnosis. These symptoms are rarely observed before the age of 12. Dysarthria, poor coordination of voluntary movements, development of involuntary movements, and sometimes disorders of posture and tone are characteristic of the early period.

Kayser-Fleischer rings, a yellow-brown copper deposition on the Descemet membrane at the limbus of the cornea, are seen in 70% of children and almost all adults, even in the absence of neurologic symptoms. At early stages, a slit-lamp examination is required, but later the rings can be seen with an ophthalmoscope or by the naked eye. Absence of these rings does not exclude the diagnosis of Wilson disease. Kayser-Fleischer rings are occasionally seen in other liver diseases.

Laboratory findings are sometimes misleading. Serum ceruloplasmin and serum copper are usually low, and urinary copper is markedly increased, but each of these values can be normal in individual patients. Definitive diagnosis of Wilson disease requires determination of liver copper concentration. Liver copper can be elevated in other forms of chronic liver disease but rarely reaches levels over 300 $\mu g/g$ liver, as occurs in most patients with Wilson disease. Liver histology is relatively nonspecific, with steatosis, hepatocellular necrosis, fibrosis, and sometimes cirrhosis. Ultrastructural abnormalities of mitochondria, microsomes, and lysosomes may be observed.

The disorder is autosomal recessive and has been linked to a gene on chromosome 13, near the esterase D locus.[69] The defective gene is thought to be necessary for transport of copper to intracellular sites required for incorporation into copper-binding proteins. For instance, copper is not efficiently incorporated into ceruloplasmin to allow for secretion into the blood and is not efficiently incorporated into other copper-binding proteins that allow excretion into bile. The defect results in a partial reduction in biliary excretion of copper and, hence, the relatively long time before copper accumulation in the liver is significant. Eventually, copper overflows into other tissues such as cornea, brain, kidney, bones, joints, and cardiac muscle. The Long-Evans Cinnamon rat seems to be an excellent animal model for Wilson disease.[70]

Clinical effects of Wilson disease can be completely reversed by medical treatment, specifically penicillamine, if instituted early. In some patients already affected by liver failure, penicillamine may be ineffective, and liver transplantation may be necessary. Elemental zinc and trientine can be used in patients with hypersensitivity to penicillamine.

AUTOIMMUNE HEPATITIS

Autoimmune hepatitis is characterized by chronic hepatitis, with or without cirrhosis, in association with circulating autoantibodies. It is predominantly observed in adolescents, more prevalent in girls, and associated with anorexia, malaise, weight loss, jaundice, and amenorrhea.[71] On physical examination, it is not uncommon to observe spider angiomata, cutaneous striae, acne, hirsutism, and a rounded face characteristic of cushingism, even before corticosteroid therapy is initiated. The liver may be palpable, but the spleen is almost always enlarged. Laboratory evaluation is characterized by hypergammaglobulinemia, low platelet counts with hypersplenism, elevated transaminases, reduced serum albumin, and prolonged prothrombin time. Serologic tests identify specific subtypes of the syndrome. The classic autoimmune hepatitis is the ANA-positive ''lupoid'' hepatitis. A more recently recognized form is anti–liver-kidney-microsomal (LKM) antibody–mediated chronic active hepatitis. This form of autoimmune hepatitis usually presents in children between ages 2 and 18 years and has a high rate of progression to cirrhosis early in its course.[72,73] Other, less common autoantibodies (e.g., antisoluble liver antigen, antimitochondrial antibody) have been identified in autoimmune hepatitis. Liver biopsy shows periportal inflammation with piecemeal necrosis, fibrosis, and sometimes cirrhosis. Infiltration of plasma cells in the periportal region is frequently a striking finding. Autoimmune hepatitis is also associated with autoimmune disease in other organs, such as thyroiditis and atrophic gastritis or pernicious anemia. Treatment usually involves prednisone and azathioprine.

Autoimmune liver disease in children also takes the form of primary sclerosing cholangitis.[74] Adults typically present with cholestasis, pruritus, and abdominal pain, but children with sclerosing cholangitis may lack prominent cholestasis (and even elevation of alkaline phosphatase levels) and present with mild transaminase elevation. Hypergammaglobulinemia, autoantibodies, and even immunodeficiency may be present. Liver biopsy reveals concentric fibrosis around the bile ductules as well as inflammatory infiltrates. Diffuse bile duct abnormalities (stenosis and dilatation) on endoscopic retrograde cholangiopancreatography are diagnostic. Ursodeoxycholic acid has been used in medical therapy, and the ductal lesions in sclerosing cholangitis are sometimes amenable to surgical or endoscopic intervention. A strong association exists between sclerosing cholangitis and ulcerative colitis. Careful monitoring is necessary because of the high rate (10%) of development of cholangiocarcinoma in this disease.

DRUG-INDUCED AND TOXIC LIVER DISEASE

Drug-induced liver disease is much less common in children than in adults, and toxins associated with liver injury in children are different from those that affect adults. This is mostly because less drug is administered to children, but it may also be related to developmental aspects of drug metabolism.

Drug-induced liver disease is classified into five categories.[75]

The first, hepatitis, predominantly affects hepatocyte necrosis. The patient is often asymptomatic, but has elevated liver enzymes. However, the patient may also have nonspecific symptoms such as fatigue, anorexia, nausea, and vomiting. Second, cholestatic disease is manifested by jaundice, pruritus, and elevated alkaline phosphatase. Oral contraceptives often produce this picture. Third is mixed hepatitis-cholestatic syndrome. This is the pattern of most drug-induced liver disease. An example is the liver disease seen after erythromycin administration. Fourth is hypersensitivity syndrome, with fever and signs of inflammation in other organs such as exanthem, enanthem, lymphadenopathy, renal dysfunction, myocardial dysfunction, eosinophilia, and atypical lymphocytosis. The fifth category, chronic active hepatitis syndrome, or drug reactions that take a subacute or chronic course, with fatigue, anorexia, rash, arthralgia, elevated immunoglobulin G levels, and even positive antinuclear antibody. α-Methyldopa, nitrofurantoin, and oxyphenisatin are drugs that have this effect.

One of the best known causes of drug-induced liver disease is acetaminophen toxicity. Children who ingest single large doses of acetaminophen develop nausea, vomiting, jaundice, and coagulopathy. A disproportionately prolonged prothrombin time is characteristic. Progressive hepatic dysfunction may result in encephalopathy and liver failure. Early recognition is essential, because treatment with N-acetylcysteine is most effective if given within 10 hours of ingestion. The mechanism of hepatic injury is formation of a toxic metabolite after phase II gluronidation and sulfation reactions are saturated. This corresponds to the histologic changes in the zone 3 pericentral region of the liver lobule, because hepatocytes in this region are particularly enriched in phase I cytochrome P450–mediated reactions.

Phenobarbital and phenytoin also cause a characteristic type of liver injury. Each produces severe hepatic dysfunction, jaundice, and coagulopathy associated with a systemic hypersensitivity syndrome. Hepatosplenomegaly, arthralgia, lymphadenopathy, erythema multiform, eosinophilia, and atypical lymphocytosis are found. The mechanism of the hepatotoxicity probably involves formation of toxic arene oxide intermediates, especially in individuals with defective function of the arene oxide detoxifying enzyme, epoxide hydrolase.[76]

Valproic acid hepatotoxicity has been extensively studied. There are two syndromes: one involves asymptomatic elevation of transaminase levels and responds well to decreases in dosage; the second syndrome involves progressive liver failure, with a clinical picture that resembles Reye syndrome. The latter is not related to the dose of valproic acid and may progress after the drug is discontinued. It is more common in infants, especially those with other conditions such as mental retardation and developmental delay. Initially, this syndrome resembles hepatitis, with malaise, anorexia, nausea, and vomiting. Later, jaundice, coagulopathy, hypoglycemia, hyperammonemia, and deterioration of seizure control occur. Liver histology is characterized by zonal hepatocellular necrosis, microvesicular steatosis, and mitochondrial abnormalities. The mechanism of hepatotoxicity is related to a toxic intermediate as well as genetic susceptibility. The toxic metabolite, 4-envalproic acid, is structurally related to hypoglycin A, a hepatotoxin that causes Jamaican vomiting sickness, a Reye-like syndrome in Jamaicans who eat the unripe akee fruit. The genetic susceptibility is probably related to defective mitochondrial β-oxidation.

Oral contraceptives also produce liver injury. This may take the form of prolonged cholestasis, focal nodular hyperplasia or adenoma, poliosis hepatitis with focal dilatation of sinusoids, or hepatic or portal vein thrombosis from the coagulation disorder associated with contraceptive steroids.

Halothane hepatitis may be asymptomatic, with mild elevation of liver enzymes, or it may produce severe hepatic necrosis and liver failure. The incidence of severe halothane hepatitis in children is thought be 1 in 80,000 to 200,000. The mechanism of liver injury is still not completely understood, although several toxic intermediates and autoantibodies have been identified, and evidence for genetic susceptibility has been generated.[77]

Isoniazid is associated with mild elevation of serum transaminases and, rarely, with liver failure in children. In many cases it is dose-related and responds to lowering the amount administered. Slow acetylation of a toxic intermediate has been implicated as the mechanism of liver injury.

Several other antibiotics cause liver injury. Erythromycin and sulfa drugs produce a mixed hepatitis-cholestatic process with anorexia, nausea, jaundice, right upper quadrant abdominal pain, pruritus, and enlargement of liver and spleen. The cholestasis may be prolonged for weeks or months. Because eosinophils are present within portal infiltrates on histologic examination of liver and eosinophilia may be present, an allergic mechanism has been discussed. Ceftriaxone has been associated with biliary sludge formation, probably because it is excreted in bile and forms insoluble complexes with calcium. Patients receiving high doses of this cephalosporin who have bile stasis are at increased risk for this adverse effect.

Antineoplastic drugs also cause liver injury. Most cases include asymptomatic elevation of serum transaminases associated with drugs such as cyclophosphamide, cytosine arabinoside, cisplatin, and 6-mercaptopurine. L-asparaginase can cause severe hepatic necrosis with steatosis. Combination chemotherapy with thioguanine, methotrexate, and cyclophosphamide, or a combination of radiation and chemotherapy, are associated with venoocclusive disease, which presents acutely with an enlarged, tender liver, ascites, and jaundice. There is usually centrilobular subendothelial edema, congestion, and collagen deposition in liver biopsy specimens. The clinical picture resembles the venoocclusive disease originally seen in Jamaicans exposed to pyrolizidine alkaloids in medicinal bush teas containing Senecio.

Hydralazine produces a syndrome resembling chronic active hepatitis. Antinuclear antibodies and anti-liver microsomal antibodies, such as antibody to cytochrome P4501A2, have been identified in several patients with this drug-induced hepatitis.[78]

MEDICAL MANAGEMENT

Gastrointestinal Bleeding

Several conditions predispose children with liver disease to gastrointestinal bleeding. First, portal hypertension leads to esophageal, gastric, duodenal varices, and hemorrhoids. Second, liver disease leads to disturbed hemostasis. Third, chronic gastritis and peptic ulcer disease are frequently associated with chronic liver disease. Finally, increased intraabdominal pressure secondary to hepatosplenomegaly and ascites may exacerbate gastroesophageal reflux and esophagitis, causing occult bleeding from esophagitis or contributing to GI bleeding from esophageal varices.

Variceal bleeding (usually esophageal) is the major cause of GI bleeding in children with portal hypertension, and is the initial manifestation of portal hypertension in many children. In up to one third of patients with esophageal varices, GI bleeding episodes are not related to the varices, but rather are caused by gastritis or peptic ulcer disease.

The major complications of GI bleeding are vascular collapse from decreased intravascular volume, precipitation of acute renal tubular insufficiency–hepatorenal syndrome, and, by leading to hyperammonemia, precipitation of hepatic encephalopathy. Immediate treatment is mandatory. Stabilizing the hemodynamic status with administration of intravenous fluids is the first step. Passage of a nasogastric tube allows monitoring of the severity of GI bleeding and empties the intestinal tract of blood that could precipitate encephalopathy. Fresh frozen plasma may be used. Parenteral administration of vitamin K may correct the coagulation disturbance at least in part. It should be given slowly to avoid anaphylaxis. Empiric administration of ranitidine is indicated because it is the primary treatment of gastritis or ulcer disease, and may reduce the effect of acid reflux on bleeding from esophageal varices.

Because acute GI bleeding, including bleeding from esophageal varices, is often self-limiting in children, endoscopy may not be necessary. If bleeding persists or blood transfusions are required, an upper endoscopy is used for diagnosis and, sometimes, therapy. Endoscopic sclerotherapy may be useful acutely in controlling bleeding from esophageal varices, but it is not effective for varices lower in the GI tract.

For persistent variceal bleeding, intravenous administration of vasopressin and emergency endoscopic sclerotherapy are considered. Vasopressin decreases portal pressure by increasing splanchnic vascular tone. Studies in adults show that somatostatin is also capable of decreasing splanchnic blood flow and has a similar effectiveness in controlling variceal bleeding.[79]

The Sengstaken-Blakemore tube, used to tamponade uncontrollable esophageal varices, is associated with significant complications and a high incidence of rebleeding after the tube is removed. In view of the more benign course of variceal bleeding in children compared to adults, this approach is rarely necessary. A number of emergency surgical approaches for interruption of blood flow though the esophagus are, likewise, rarely indicated. Portosystemic shunting and orthotopic liver transplantation are more definitive and effective measures for preventing further bleeding episodes, and should be considered in the long-term management of these patients.

Cholestasis

Children with cholestatic liver disease are often characterized by poor growth, complications of fat-soluble vitamin malabsorption, and pruritus. Therefore, considerable attention is given to caloric intake and vitamin supplementation. In infancy, this may mean supplementing formula with polycose and medium-chain triglycerides. The latter are directly absorbed into the portal vein, and do not require micellar solubilization by bile acids. In some cases additional calories, provided by nocturnal intragastric infusions of formula, may be necessary. In older children with pruritus and chronic inflammation from their liver disease, appetite is often impaired. In these patients, the diet may need to be liberalized to improve its taste and stimulate appetite. If this involves a greater proportion of long-chain triglyceride in the diet, the child will need to be monitored for loss of trace elements, as a result of increased fat malabsorption.

Most children with cholestasis require treatment with fat-soluble vitamins. Vitamin K supplementation is necessary to prevent excessive bleeding. This usually takes the form of vitamin K_1 in a dose of 2 to 5 mg/d. Vitamin E deficiency is common in cholestatic liver disease, because it is the fat-soluble vitamin that depends most on micellar solubilization by bile acids for intestinal absorption. Vitamin E deficiency is associated with spinocerebellar degeneration, ophthalmoplegia, and pigmentary retinopathy, and it can be extremely debilitating if allowed to progress.[80] If vitamin E deficiency is detected by low serum levels of vitamin E, or by low vitamin E–to–lipid ratios in children with hyperlipidemia, vitamin E supplementation is provided at a dose of 25 IU/kg/d. Some children may require a liquid preparation of the water-soluble ester of vitamin E, d-α-tocopherol polyethylene glycol-1000 succinate (TGPS; Liquid E), at a dose of 15 to 25 IU/kg/d.[81] Vitamin D absorption is also deranged in chronic cholestasis. Supplementation is started at 2500 to 5000 IU/d of vitamin D_3, and may need to be increased on the basis of serum 25-hydroxyvitamin D levels. Vitamin A deficiency is much less common, but children with cholestasis are usually given 5000 to 10,000 IU/d of vitamin A supplement.

Pruritus is the most troubling complication of cholestatic liver disease. Incessant itching can lead to secondary bacterial infection and scarring. General measures to alleviate pruritus include cool baths, skin moisturizers, antihistamines, and sedatives. In some cases pruritus is improved by treatment with bile acid–binding resins, cholestyramine and colestipol. These resins bind bile acids in the intestine and increase fecal bile acid excretion. Presumably, this reduces the systemic accumulation of bile acids. Doses of 0.25 to 0.50 g/kg/d are recommended. Unfortunately, it is difficult to get infants and children to take these resins, even mixed in applesauce or juice. Phenobarbital is thought to decrease cholestasis and pruritus by increasing bile acid–independent bile flow. Its sedative effects make phenobarbital less desirable. In several studies, rifampin has ameliorated pruritus by an unknown mechanism. A dose of 10 mg/kg/d has been recommended. Ursodeoxycholic acid ameliorates pruritus and decreases cholestasis and hepatocellular damage in children with cholestatic liver disease. It is particularly useful in intrahepatic cholestatic syndromes and the liver disease of cystic fibrosis,[82] but it has also been used in cholestatic syndromes caused by parenteral nutrition.[83] When fixed obstruction to bile flow exists, however, it may worsen pruritus and liver dysfunction, and is therefore contraindicated in children with extrahepatic biliary atresia and poor drainage following portoenterostomy. Ursodeoxycholic acid exerts its effects mainly by fecal excretion of toxic bile acids. The currently recommended daily dose is 10 to 20 mg/kg/d divided into two to three doses. Diarrhea is occasionally reported as a side effect in children. Experience in treating children with pruritus and cholestasis with naloxone, partial biliary diversion, phototherapy, or plasmapheresis is relatively limited, although there are reports of use in adults.

ASCITES

It is much more difficult to restrict sodium and water intake for ascites in children than in adults. Sodium restriction exacerbates the tendency for anorexia, and fluid restriction interferes with efforts to increase caloric intake. Diuretics are, therefore, initiated earlier in children than in adults. Potassium-sparing aldosterone antagonists, such as spironolactone, are the first line of therapy. The starting dose of spironolactone is 1 mg/kg/d, increased by increments of 1 mg/kg/d, up to a total 6 mg/kg/d. Monitoring of serum electrolytes, urea, and creatinine during diuretic therapy is important. Thiazide diuretics, such as hydrochlorothiazide, at doses of 2 to 3 mg/kg/d, may need to be added to the regimen. Occasionally loop diuretics, such as furosemide, are necessary. The starting dose is 1 to 2 mg/kg/d, which can be increased by 1 mg/kg/d to a total of 6 mg/kg/d. When ascites is severe enough to produce respiratory compromise or is refractory to diuretic therapy, large-volume paracentesis in conjunction with albumin infusion can be used. Up to 100 mL/kg of ascitic fluid can be removed at an individual session. Albumin is infused at a rate of 6 to 8 g/L of ascitic fluid removed.

HEPATIC ENCEPHALOPATHY

The first priority in treating hepatic encephalopathy is to identify and manage the precipitating event. Conditions such as GI bleeding, dehydration, and infection require prompt attention, because one of these may be precipitating hepatic encephalopathy. Since onset of hepatic encephalopathy may be subtle and progress may be slow, close neurologic monitoring of the patient is important. Specific treatment is primarily directed toward decreasing ammonia production. Protein restriction may be required, but should be balanced against the need for optimal nutrition. Lactulose is often effective in treating children. Its mechanism of action is unknown, but believed to involve a decrease in colonic ammonia absorption. Doses of lactulose for children range from 0.3 to 0.4 mL/kg, three times a day. The dose should be sufficient to acidify the stool (pH less than 6.0) without causing severe diarrhea. Lactulose can be combined with cleansing enemas and neomycin. Neomycin suppresses ammonia-forming bacteria in the gut without affecting the ability of the colonic flora to metabolize lactulose. Sedating drugs should be avoided, because they may also precipitate encephalopathy.

INFECTIONS

Although it is still uncertain, patients with chronic liver disease probably have an increased incidence of infections, especially spontaneous bacterial peritonitis and cholangitis.

Children with biliary system obstruction, such as choledochal cyst, or dilatation, such as in congenital hepatic fibrosis, are more susceptible to cholangitis. However, cholangitis is most frequently observed in children who have undergone hepatic portoenterostomy for biliary atresia. Clinical manifestations include fever, jaundice, right upper quadrant pain, and shock. Laboratory findings include leukocytosis, hyperbilirubinemia, elevation of serum transaminases, and alkaline phosphatase. Blood cultures are positive in 50% of cases. Gram-negative enteric bacteria such as *E. coli, Klebsiella* sp, and *Enterococcus* account for most cases. Anaerobes may also be involved. Empiric treatment with intravenous antibiotics should be initiated at the same time as the hemodynamic state is stabilized and general supportive measures are instituted. An antibiotic regimen including ampicillin, cefotaxime, and an aminoglycoside should be considered to cover a broad spectrum of gram-negative aerobic organisms as well as *Enterococcus*. Further modification of the antibiotic regimen based on culture and sensitivity results is important.

SBP is a common complication of ascites in chronic liver disease. Because enteric gram-negative organisms are the most common cause of SBP, a third-generation cephalosporin-like cefotaxime is the preferred treatment. Cefotaxmine also covers for *Streptococcus pneumoniae*, an organism that occasionally causes SBP in children. The first episode is usually treated for 10 to 14 days, but subsequent episodes may indicate the need for longer treatment periods.

REFERENCES

1. Erlinger S. Secretion of bile. In: Schiff L, Schiff E, eds. Diseases of the liver, ed 6. Philadelphia, JB Lippincott, 1987:77.
2. Sippel CJ, Suchy FJ, Ananthanarayanan M, Perlmutter DH. The rat liver ecto-ATPase is also a canalicular bile acid transport protein. J Biol Chem 1993;268:2083.
3. Hagenbuch B, Stieger B, Foguet M, et al. Functional expression cloning and characterization of the hepatocyte Na + bile acid cotransport system. Proc Natl Acad Sci USA 1991;88:10629.
4. Gove CD, Huges RD. Liver regeneration in relationship to acute liver failure. Gut 1991;32:S92.
5. Jones EA, Schafer DF. Fulminant hepatic failure. In: Zakim D, Boyer TD, eds. Hepatology Philadelphia, WB Saunders, 1990:460.
6. Hanau C, Munoz SJ, Rubin R. Histopathological heterogeneity in fulminant hepatic failure. Hepatology 1995;21:345.
7. Gammal SH, Jones EA. Hepatic encephalopathy. Med Clin North Am 1989;73:793.
8. Basile AS, Jones EA, Skolnick P. The pathogenesis and treatment of hepatic encephalopathy: evidence for the involvement of benzodiazepine receptor ligands. Pharmacol Rev 1991;43:27.
9. Martin GR, Timpl R. Laminin and other base membrane components. Annu Rev Cell Biol 1987;3:57.
10. Fausto N, Mead JE. Regulation of liver growth: protooncogenes and transforming growth factors. Lab Invest 1989;60:4.
11. Tashiro K, Hagiya M, Nishizawa T. Deduced primary structure of rat hepatocyte growth factor and expression of the mRNA in rat tissue. Proc Natl Acad Sci USA 1990;87:3200.
12. Schrier RW. Pathogenesis of sodium and water retention in high-output and low-output cardiac failure, nephrotic syndrome, cirrhosis, and pregnancy, parts I–II. N Engl J Med 1988;319:1065,1127.
13. Runyon BA. Spontaneous bacterial peritonitis: an explosion of information. Hepatology 1988;8:171.
14. Watkins JB, Katz AJ, Grand RJ. Neonatal hepatitis: a diagnostic approach. Adv Pediatr 1977;24:399.
15. Ikeda S, Sera Y, Akagi M. Serial ultrasound examination to differentiate biliary atresia from neonatal hepatitis: special reference to changes in size of the gall bladder. Eur J Pediatr 1989;148:396.
16. Tolia V, Dubois RS, Kagalwalla A, et al. Comparison of radionuclear scintigraphy and liver biopsy in the evaluation of neonatal cholestasis. J Ped Gastroenterol Nutr 1986;5:30.
17. Williamson SL, Seibert JJ, Butler HL, et al. Apparent gut excretion of Tc-99m-DISIDA in a case of extrahepatic biliary atresia. Pediatr Radiol 1986;16:245.
18. Majd M, Reba RC, Altman RP. Effect of phenobarbital on ^{99m}TC-IDA scintigraphy in the evaluation of neonatal jaundice. Semin Nuc Med 1991;9:1994.
19. Hays DM, Wooley MM, Simpler WH, et al. Diagnosis of biliary atresia: relative accuracy of percutaneous liver biopsy, open liver biopsy, operative cholangiography. J Pediatr 1967;71:598.
20. Brough AJ, Bernstein J. Conjugated hyperbilirubinemia in early infancy: a reassessment of liver biopsy. Human Pathol 1974;5:507.
21. Brough AJ, Bernstein J. Liver biopsy in the diagnosis of infantile obstructive jaundice. Pediatrics 1969;43:519.
22. Markowitz J, Daum F, Kahn EI, et al. Arteriohepatic dysplasia: I. Pitfalls in diagnosis and management. Hepatology 1983;3:74.
23. Chang M-H, Hsu MC, Lee CY, et al. Neonatal hepatitis: a follow-up study. J Pediatr Gastroenterol Nutr 1987;6:203.
24. Utili R, Abernathy CO, Zimmerman HJ. Cholestatic effects of Escherichia coli endotoxin on the isolated perfused rat liver. Gastroenterology 1976;70:248.
25. Chang MH, Huang MH, Huang ES, et al. Polymerase chain reaction to detect human cytomegalovirus in livers of infants with neonatal hepatitis. Gastroenterology 1992;103:1022.
26. Dupuy JM, Frommel D, Alagille D. Severe viral hepatitis type B in infancy. Lancet 1975;1:191.
27. Long WA, Ulshen MH, Lawson EE. Clinical manifestations of congenital syphilis hepatitis: implications for pathogenesis. J Pediatr Gastroenterol Nutr 1984;3:551.
28. Watkins JB, Sunaryo FP, Berezin SH. Hepatic manifestations of congenital and perinatal disease. Clin Perinatol 1981;8:467.
29. Perlmutter DH. Alpha-1-antitrypsin deficiency. In: Suchy FJ, ed. Liver disease in children. New York, BC Decker, 1994:686.
30. Lomas DA, Evans DL, Finch JJ, et al. The mechanism of Z α1-antitrypsin accumulation in the liver. Nature 1992;357:605.
31. Mast AE, Enghild JJ, Salvesen G. Conformation of the reactive site loop of α1-proteinase inhibitor probed by limited proteolysis. Biochemistry 1992;31:2720.
32. Sveger T. Liver disease in alpha-1-antitrypsin deficiency detected by screening 200,000 infants. N Engl J Med 1976;294:1216.
33. Sveger T. The natural history of liver disease in alpha-1-antitrypsin deficient children. Acta Paediatr Scand 1988;77:847.
34. Wu Y, Whitman I, Molmenti E, et al. A lag in intracellular degradation of mutant α1-antitrypsin correlates with liver disease phenotype in homozygous PiZZ α1-antitrypsin deficiency. Proc Natl Acad Sci USA 1995;91:9014.
35. Segal S. Disorders of galactose metabolism. In: Stanbury JB, Wyngaarden JB, Frederickson DS, eds. The metabolic basis of inherited disease, ed 6. New York, McGraw-Hill, 1989:453.
36. Levy HL, Sepe SJ, Shih VE, et al. Sepsis due to Escherichia coli in neonates with galactosemia. N Engl J Med 1977;297:823.
37. Reichardt JK, Levy HL, Woo SL. Molecular characterizations of two galactosemic mutations and one polymorphorism: implications for structure-function analysis of human galactose-1-phosphate uridyl transferase. Biochemistry 1992;311:5430.
38. Gitzelmann R, Steinmann B, Van den Berghe G. Disorders of fructose metabolism. In: Stanbury JB, Wyngaarden JB, Frederickson DS, eds. The metabolic basis of inherited disease, ed 6. New York, McGraw-Hill, 1989;399.
39. Cross NCP, Tolan DR, Cox TM. Catalytic deficiency of human aldolase B in hereditary fructose intolerance caused by a common missense mutation. Cell 1988;53:881.
40. Cross NCP, de Franchis RD, Sebastio G, et al. Molecular analysis of aldolase B genes in hereditary fructose intolerance. Lancet 1990;335:306.
41. Baker L, Winegrad AI. Fasting hypoglycaemia and metabolic acidosis associated with deficiency of hepatic fructose-1,6-diphosphatase activity. Lancet 1970;2:13.
42. Goldsmith LA, Laberge C. Tyrosinemia and related disorders. In: Scriver CR, Beaudet AL, Sly WS, et al, eds. The metabolic basis of inherited disease, ed 6. New York, McGraw-Hill, 1989;556.
43. Phaneuf D, Lambert M, Laframboise R, et al. Type I hereditary tyrosinemia: evidence for molecular heterogeneity and identification of a causal mutation in a French Canadian patient. J Clin Invest 1991;90:1185.
44. Rank JM, Pascual-Leone A, Payne W, et al. Hematin therapy for the neurologic crisis of tyrosinemia. J Pediatr 1991;118:136.
45. Lindstedt S, Holme E, Lock EA, et al. Treatment of hereditary tyrosinemia type I by inhibition of 4-hydroxyphenylpyruvate dioxygenase. Lancet. 1992;340:813.
46. Grompe M, Al-Dhalimy M, Finegold M, et al. Loss of fumaryl acetoacetate hydrolase is responsible for the neonatal hepatic dysfunction phenotype of lethal albino mice. Genes Devel 1993;7:2298.
47. Lazarow PB, Moser HW. Disorders of peroxisome biogenesis. In:

Scriver CR, Beaudet AL, Sly WS, et al, eds. The metabolic basis of inherited disease, ed 6. New York, McGraw-Hill, 1989;1479.

48. Tsukamoto T, Miura S, Fujiki V. Restoration by a 35k membrane protein of peroxisome assembly in a peroxisome-deficient mammalian cell mutant. Nature 1991;350:77.

49. Watkins PA, Chen WW, Harris CJ, et al. Peroxisomal bifunctional enzyme deficiency. J Clin Invest 1989;83:771.

50. Gaskin K, Ch B. The liver and biliary tract in cystic fibrosis. In: Suchy FJ, ed. Liver disease in children. New York, BC Decker, 1994:705.

51. Herman SP, Baggenstoss AH, Cloutier MD. Liver dysfunction and histologic abnormalities in neonatal hypopituitarism. J Pediatr 1975; 87:892.

52. Riely CA. Familial intrahepatic cholestatic syndromes. Semin Liver Dis 1987;7:119.

53. Schnittger S, Hofers C, Heidemann P, et al. Molecular and cytogenetic analysis of an interstitial 20p deletion associated with syndromic intrahepatic ductular hypoplasia (Alagille syndrome). Hum Genet 1989;83: 239.

54. Zhang F, Deleuze JF, Aurias A, et al. Interstitial deletion of the short arm of chromosome 20 in arteriohepatic dysplasia (Alagille syndrome). J Pediatr 1990;116:73.

55. Clayton RJ, Iber FL, Ruebner BH, et al. Byler disease. Am J Dis Child 1969;117:112.

56. Whitington PF, Freese DK, Alonso EM, et al. Progressive familial intrahepatic cholestasis (Byler's disease). In: Lentze M, Reichen J, eds. Paediatric cholestasis. Lancaster, PA Kluwer Academic Publishers, 1992:165.

57. Clayton PT, Leonard JV, Lawson AM, et al. Familial giant cell hepatitis associated with synthesis of $3\beta,7\alpha$-dihydroxy- and $3\beta,7\alpha,12\alpha$-trihydroxy-5-cholenoic acids. J Clin Invest 1987;79:1031.

58. Setchell KDR, Suchy FJ, Welsh MB, et al. Δ^4-3-Oxosteroid 5β-reductase deficiency described in identical twins with neonatal hepatitis: a new inborn error in bile acid synthesis. J Clin Invest 1988;82: 2148.

59. Kaymakcalan H, Dowdourekas D, Szanto PB, et al. Congestive heart failure as a cause of fulminant hepatic failure. Am J Med 1978;65:384.

60. Quigley EMM, Marsh MN, Shaffer JL, et al. Hepatobiliary complications of total parenteral nutrition. Gastroenterology 1993;104:286.

61. Clayton PT, Bowron A, Mills KA, et al. Phytosterolemia in children with parenteral nutrition-associated cholestatic liver disease. Gastroenterology 1993;105:1806.

62. Beutler E. Gaucher's disease as a paradigm of current issues regarding single gene mutations of humans. Proc Natl Acad Sci USA 1993;90: 5384.

63. Tybulewicz VL, Tremblay ML, LaMarca ME, et al. Animal model of Gaucher's disease from targeted disruption of the mouse glucocerebrosidase gene. Nature 1992;357:407.

64. Segal S. Disorders of galactose metabolism. In: Scriver CR, Beaudet AL, Sly WS, et al, eds. The metabolic basis of inherited disorders. New York, McGraw-Hill, 1989:453.

65. Burchell A. Molecular pathology of glucose-6-phosphatase. FASEB J 1990;4:2978.

66. Green HL, Slonim AE, O'Neil JA Jr, et al. Continuous nocturnal intragastric feeding for management of type I glycogen-storage disease. N Engl J Med 1976;294:423.

67. Chen Y-T, Cornblath M, Sidbury JB. Cornstarch therapy in type I glycogen storage disease. N Engl J Med 1984;310:171.

68. Danks DM. Disorders of copper transport. In: Scriver CR, Beaudet AL, Sly WS, et al, eds. The metabolic basis of inherited disorders. New York, McGraw-Hill, 1989:1411.

69. Frydman M, Bonne-Tamir B, Farrer LA, et al. Assignment of the gene for Wilson's disease to chromosome 13: linkage to the esterase D locus. Proc Natl Acad Sci USA 1985;82:1819.

70. Li Y, Togashi Y, Sato, et al. Spontaneous hepatic accumulation in Long-Evans Cinnamon rats with hereditary hepatitis: a model of Wilson's disease. J Clin Invest 1991;87:1858.

71. Bearn AG, Kunkel HG, Slater RJ. The problem of chronic liver disease in young women. Am J Med 1956;21:3.

72. Homberg JC, Abuaf N, Bernard O, et al. Chronic active hepatitis associated with anti-liver/kidney microsome antibody type 1: a second type of "autoimmune" hepatitis. Hepatology 1987;7:1333.

73. Manns M, Gerken G, Kyriatsoulis A, et al. Characterization of a new subgroup of autoimmune chronic active hepatitis by autoantibodies against a soluble liver antigen. Lancet 1987;i:292.

74. Sisto A, Feldman P, Garel L, et al. Primary sclerosing cholangitis in children: study of five cases and review of the literature. Pediatrics 1987;80:918.

75. Roberts EA. Drug-induced liver disease in children. In: Suchy FJ, ed. Liver disease in children. New York, BC Decker, 1994:523.

76. Spielberg SP, Gordon GB, Blake DA, et al. Predisposition to phenytoin hepatotoxicity assessed in vitro. N Engl J Med 1981;305:722.

77. Farrell G, Prendergast D, Murray M. Halothane hepatitis: detection of a constitutional susceptibility factor. N Engl J Med 1985;313:1310.

78. Bourdi M, Larrey D, Nataf J, et al. Anti-liver endoplasmic reticulum autoantibodies are directed against human P-450 1A2. J Clin Invest 1990;85:1967.

79. Burroughs AK, McCormick PA, Hughes MD, et al. Randomized, double-blinded, placebo-controlled trial of somatostatin for variceal bleeding: emergency control and prevention of early variceal rebleeding. Gastroenterology 1990;99:1388.

80. Rosenblum JL, Keating JP, Prensky AL, et al. A progressive neurologic syndrome in children with chronic liver disease. N Engl J Med 1981; 304:503.

81. Sokol RJ, Heubi JE, Butler-Simon NA, et al. Treatment of vitamin E deficiency during chronic childhood cholestasis with oral D-alpha-tocopheryl polyethylene glycol-1000 succinate (TPGS). Gastroenterology 1987;93:975.

82. Colombo C, Setchell KDR, Podda M, et al. Effect of ursodeoxycholic acid therapy on liver disease associated with cystic fibrosis. J Pediatr 1990;117:482.

83. Lindor KD, Burnes J. Ursodeoxycholic acid for the treatment of home parenteral nutrition-associated cholestasis. Gastroenterology 1991;101: 250.

Surgery of Infants and Children: Scientific Principles and Practice, edited by Keith T. Oldham, Paul M. Colombani, and Robert P. Foglia. Lippincott–Raven Publishers, Philadelphia, © 1997.

CHAPTER 85

Surgical Liver Disease

C. K. Breuer and J. P. Vacanti

HISTORICAL PERSPECTIVE

The evolution of surgical techniques for hepatic resection closely parallels the development of our understanding of the anatomy of the liver. Early in the evolution of hepatic surgery, sections of the liver were removed without regard to intrahepatic planes, for it was believed that the falciform ligament was the only anatomic division.[1] In 1888, Langenbuch[2] successfully excised a section of the left lobe of the liver and thus performed the first reported elective hepatic resection. In 1898, Cantlie[3] demonstrated that the main lobar fissure extended from the bed of the gallbladder to the inferior vena cava. This work was further extended by others[4,5] who showed that the right lobe of the liver was divided into anterior and posterior segments and the left lobe was divided into medial and lateral segments. This understanding of hepatic anatomy led the early hepatobiliary surgeons to develop the concept of surgical planes of the liver enabling safe hepatic resections.[1] This concept enabled Keen[6] to perform the first successful left lobectomy in 1899 and Wendell[7] to perform the first right lobectomy in 1911. The success of these early hepatobiliary surgeons was based on performing anatomic resections along intersegmental planes. More recently, in the 1950s Couinaud[8] demonstrated that the two lobes of the liver are hemilivers consisting of eight segments (Fig. 85-1). These segments form the smallest anatomic units of the liver. Hepatic segmentation is based on the distribution of the portal pedicles and the position of the hepatic veins.[9] In the right and left lobes, there are two sectors, each divided into two segments. In the right lobe, the anteromedial sector is divided into segment V anteriorly and segment VIII posteriorly. The posterolateral sector is divided into segment VI anteriorly and segment VII posteriorly. In the left lobe, the anterior sector is divided into segment IV and segment III by the umbilical fissure. The posterior sector is composed of only segment II. Segment I's vascularization is independent of portal division and the hepatic veins. Each hepatic segment can theoretically be resected.[10] The replacement of morphologic descriptions of the liver anatomy by descriptions based on a segmental anatomic division allowed for resection of hepatic lesions without excision of an excessive amount of normal liver parenchyma because the boundaries of the resection were based on the segmen-

tal blood supply.[9] This concept ushered in the modern era of hepatic surgery and provides the basis for all modern hepatic resections.

SEGMENTAL ANATOMIC DIVISIONS

The anatomic divisions are the basis of the nomenclature for hepatic resection. Resection of a portion of the liver along intersegmental planes is called a segmentectomy. Unisegmentectomy refers to the excision of one segment and a plurisegmentectomy refers to the excision of two or more segments. There are two major classifications used to describe the four major resections: that of Couinaud[8] and the more commonly applied nomenclature of Goldsmith and Woodburne.[11]

Hepectomies and Lobectomies

The definitions of the classic hepatectomies and lobectomies can be clarified by use of the segmental classification. The terms right and left lobectomies are often used to describe what is in fact a right or left hepatectomy. According to the segmental classification, a right hepatectomy excises segments V through VIII and a left hepatectomy segments II through IV. These hepatectomies can be extended to include resection of segment I. A right trisegmentectomy is a right hepatectomy extended to segment IV and involves resection of a total of five segments. Classic resection of the left lobe, which includes segments II and III, is commonly referred to as a left lateral lobectomy.

We recommend abandoning the imprecise and often confusing traditional nomenclature and instead simply listing the segments to describe an hepatic resection. For instance, an extended medial bisegmentectomy would be more easily understood if referred to as plurisegmentectomy IV/V/VI/VIII, whereas an extended left trisegmentectomy should be referred to as plurisegmentectomy II/III/IV/V/VII/VIII.[9]

Theoretically each of the eight segments can be removed separately, but in practice only certain segmentectomies are commonly performed.[10] Unisegmentectomy of segment I is not performed because removal of this segment requires excision of segments II and III to gain appropriate access.[9] Segment II

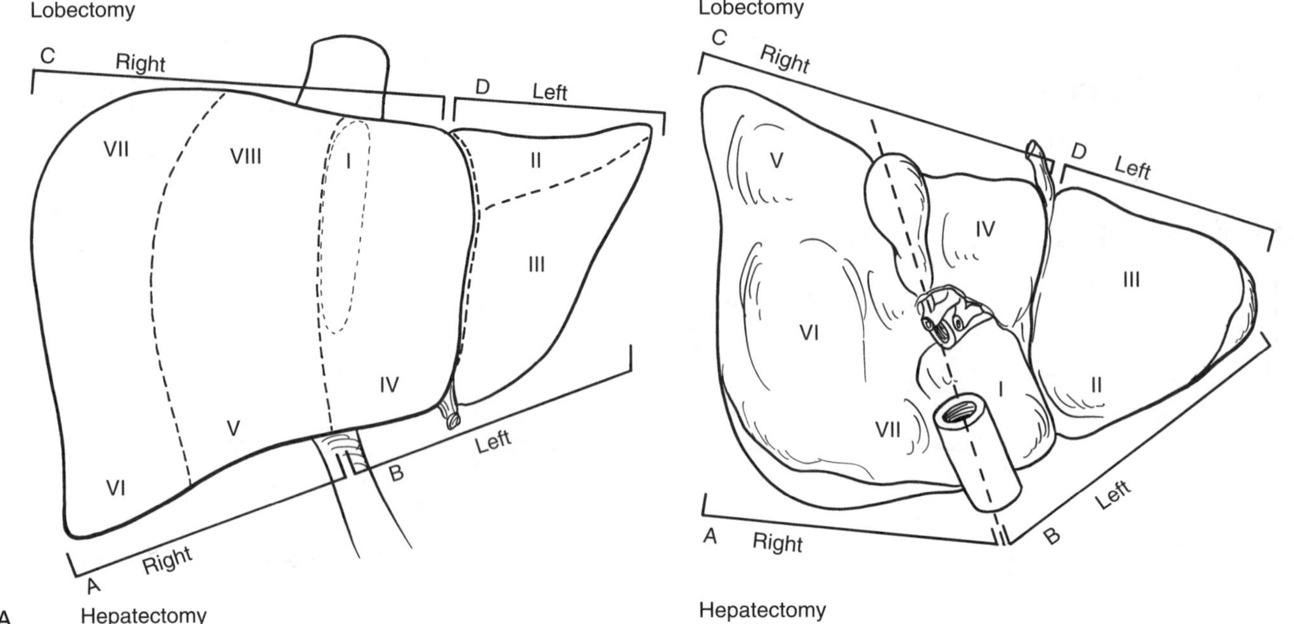

FIG. 85-1. Couinaud's segmental divisions. Anterosuperior (*A*) and posterior (*B*) views of the liver.

or III is usually not removed independently since they can be easily removed together as a left lateral lobectomy.[1] Unisegmentectomy of segment IV usually refers to excision of the anterior part of that segment.[9] Unisegmentectomy of V is feasible, but not usually performed. Bisegmentectomy of IV and V is used for patients with carcinoma of the gallbladder extending into the liver or for Klatskin tumor.[10] Segments IV, V, and VI may be removed as a unit.[1] Resection of segment VI or VII alone is rarely performed, but is possible. Plurisegmentectomy of VI and VII may be called right lateral sectorectomy.[9] Segment VIII is difficult to resect because it is connected with the intrahepatic vena cava and segment I.[1]

Segmental resection of a major portion of the liver incorporates several basic steps. These include an incision to allow for adequate exposure, mobilization of the liver to provide appropriate access, control of the inflow vessels to permit transection of the hepatic parenchyma without excessive blood loss, ligation of intrahepatic vessels and ducts to control hemorrhage, and hemostasis of the raw surface of the liver.[1] An abdominal incision is appropriate in many instances, providing one can achieve adequate exposure. In the case of a large tumor mass, a thoracoabdominal incision can be helpful. To adequately mobilize the liver and permit delivery into the operative field, the ligamentous attachments must be divided. The ligamentum teres is transected and the falciform ligament is divided down to the inferior vena cava. Next, the triangular ligament is divided. Finally, the right and left coronary ligaments are transected, exposing the suprahepatic vena cava (Fig. 85-2).

Plurisegmentectomies

There are two basic techniques for plurisegmentectomies. The first incorporates individual ligation of the structures in the hepatoduodenal ligament supplying the lobe to be resected and ligation of the hepatic vein draining the lobe before transecting the parenchyma.[9] The advantage of the technique is that it reduces intraoperative bleeding and demonstrates demarcation of the devascularized portion of the segments to be excised, thus reducing the excision of excessive amounts of normal tissue.[1] The disadvantage of this technique lies in the potential for injury to the inferior vena cava during dissection of the hepatic veins.[10]

The second technique begins after temporary inflow occlusion has been achieved.[1] This is accomplished using either an atraumatic clamp or an occluding loop that incorporates all structures within the hepatoduodenal ligament.[10] Once proximal control is attained, transection of the parenchyma in the appropriate intersegmental plane can be performed. Occlusion of vascular inflow can be continued for up to 60 min without permanently impairing liver function.[9] Next, the portal elements are sequentially ligated and divided as they traverse the plane of dissection. Last, once isolated, the hepatic vein draining the dissected segments is ligated and divided, or occluded with clamps and oversewn[1] (Fig. 85-3). The advantage of this technique is that it reduces operative time and removes an amount of liver tissue specifically related to tumor size and location.[10] This technique also helps assure preservation of vessels supplying the remaining segments of the liver. The disadvantage of this approach is that intraoperative bleeding may be greater than with the other technique.[9]

TRANSECTION OF THE PARENCHYMA

A variety of technical innovations have reduced the extent of bleeding associated with transection of the parenchyma.[10] These include improving compression of parenchyma to effect tamponade during dissection, improving methods of dissection to skeletonize intraparenchymal vessels, and improving control of bleeding from the raw surface.[1]

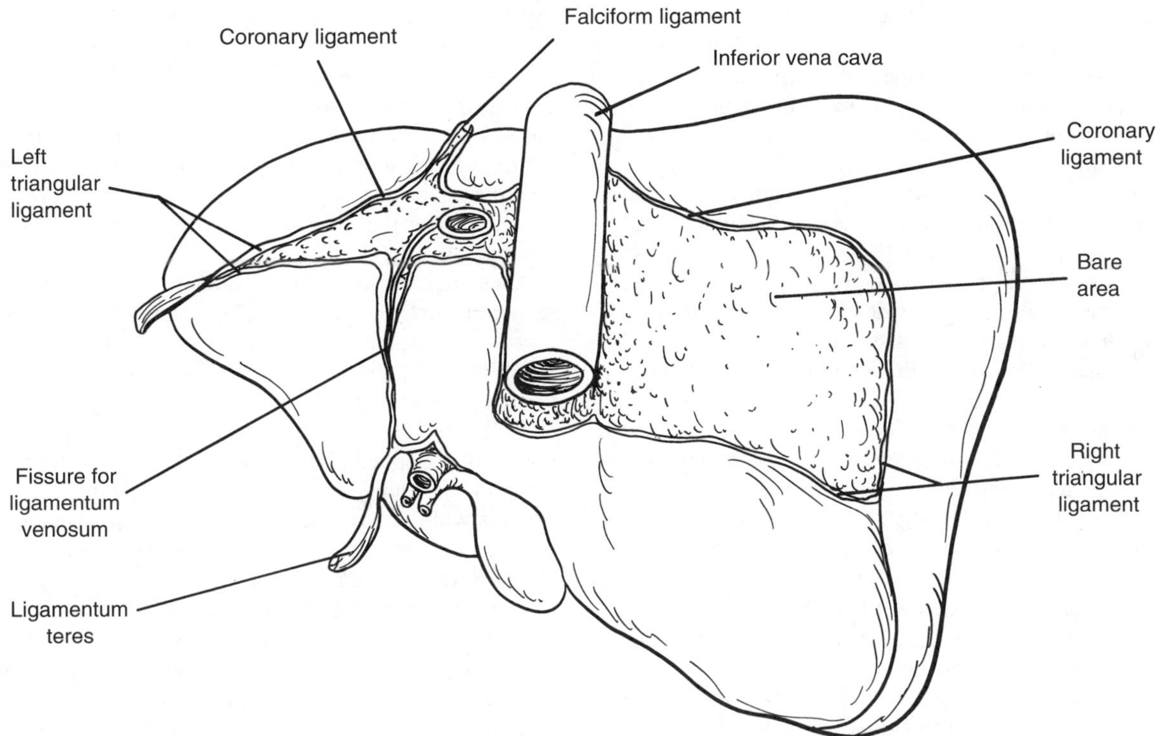

FIG. 85-2. Ligamentous and diaphragmatic attachments of the liver (seen from posteroinferior view).

Several devices have been developed to provide improved parenchymal compression, thereby decreasing intraoperative hemorrhage. In 1971, Storm and Longmire[12] reported the design of a clamp that provided uniform pressure on hepatic tissue and significantly reduced the time required to perform a hepatic lobectomy. In 1973, Lin[13] reported the design of a special hepatic clamp that made hepatic transection almost bloodless without preliminary inflow or outflow occlusion. Several other occlusion devices have been developed and described in the literature.[14,15] All provide temporary inflow and outflow occlusion by compression, thereby diminishing intraoperative bleeding. The most recent modification provides permanent parenchymal compression by a series of interlocking through-and-through sutures placed by means of a mechanical device.[16] In

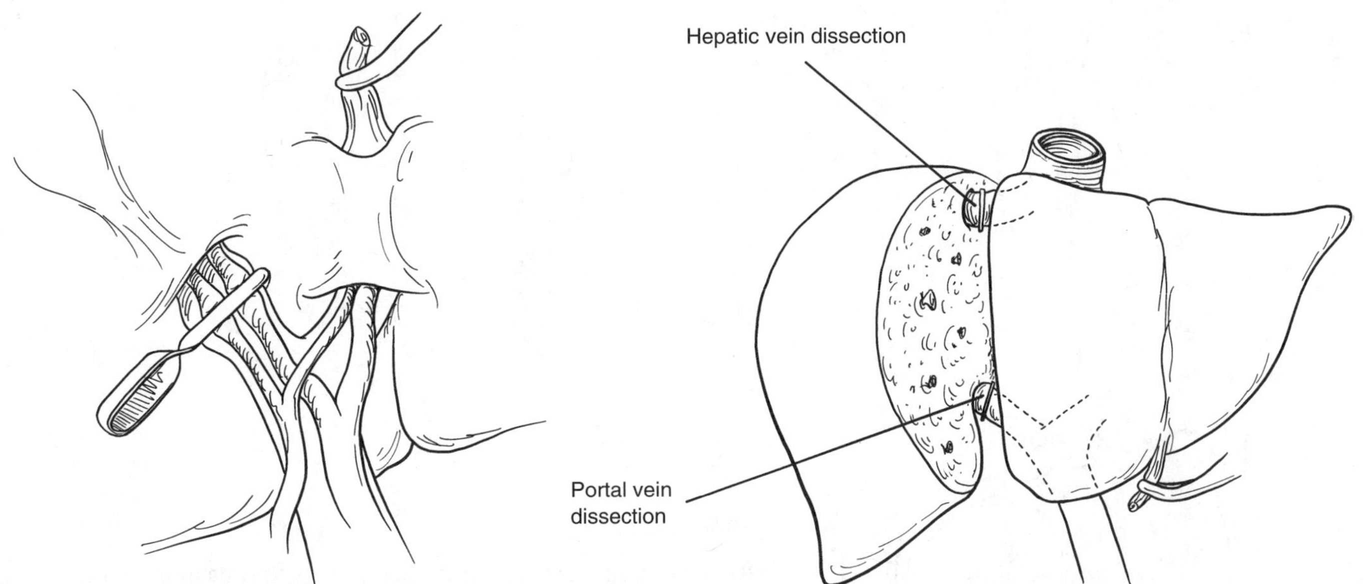

FIG. 85-3. Surgical resection of the right lobe of the liver. (*A*) Vascular inflow occlusion. (*B*) Parenchymal dissection and secondary controlled ligation of portal and hepatic vein branches.

many instances of resection in children, mattress sutures using atraumatic needles in the line of transection allow for minimal blood loss and do not compromise the viability of the liver (Fig. 85-4). We have modified this technique and have used spinal needles as an introducer to create mattress sutures.

A variety of approaches have been introduced as a substitute for finger fracture of the parenchyma. These include Almersjo and Hafstrom's[17] suction knife to facilitate parenchymal transection, Hodgson and DelGuercio's[18] ultrasonic dissector to disrupt liver parenchyma and isolate traversing vessels and ducts, and more recently, a specially designed water jet to fragment and wash away parenchymal tissue, leaving ducts and vessels to be ligated.[19] We believe that finger fracture parenchymal dissection is still the safest, most reliable technique.

Control of oozing from the raw surface of the transected liver can usually be achieved by applying direct pressure to the bleeding surface. When this does not succeed, other methods of hemostasis must be used. The use of local hemostatic agents such as cellulose or collagen can be effective. The use of glues and adhesive sprays has resulted in excessive inflammation. More recently, either laser or microwave application[20] that combines dissection and hemostasis has been utilized. The hemostatic property is related to formation of a thin coagulum on the surface.[20] It is uncertain whether laser or microwave application offers any advantage over other techniques.[21] Again, we recommend the use of mattress sutures for this purpose. Mattress sutures provide permanent compression and decrease the total raw surface area by incorporating and approximating Glissen's

capsule. We have found this to be a safe and effective technique in the pediatric population.

In addition to the use of surgical techniques already discussed, the use of real-time operative ultrasonography has reduced operative bleeding.[22] Although originally introduced to define the extent and multiplicity of tumors, it can be used to map the major intrahepatic vascular anatomy. This serves as a guide, defines the line of transection, and thereby decreases intraoperative blood loss.

A lesion is considered resectable if the amount of liver tissue remaining after resection is sufficient to provide adequate support for the patient. Therefore, any condition requiring hepatic resection that could result in insufficient hepatic parenchyma to provide essential hepatic function should not be considered amenable to surgical intervention unless resection can be coupled with transplantation. Because the liver has tremendous reserve and the ability to regenerate, up to an 80% hepatectomy in patients without baseline hepatic dysfunction is conceivable.[23] Patients with cirrhosis have much less reserve and an impaired ability to regenerate hepatic tissue. Thus, they can tolerate less resection. Patients with Child's class A cirrhosis can usually tolerate about a 50% hepatectomy, whereas those with Child's class B can tolerate only a 25% hepatectomy. Patients with Child's class C cirrhosis cannot tolerate any degree of hepatic resection and therefore have unresectable tumors by definition unless postresection transplantation is a consideration.[23] Owing to the intolerance of hepatectomy, reported cures for malignant tumors are rare in cirrhotic patients.[1] Similarly, even in an other-

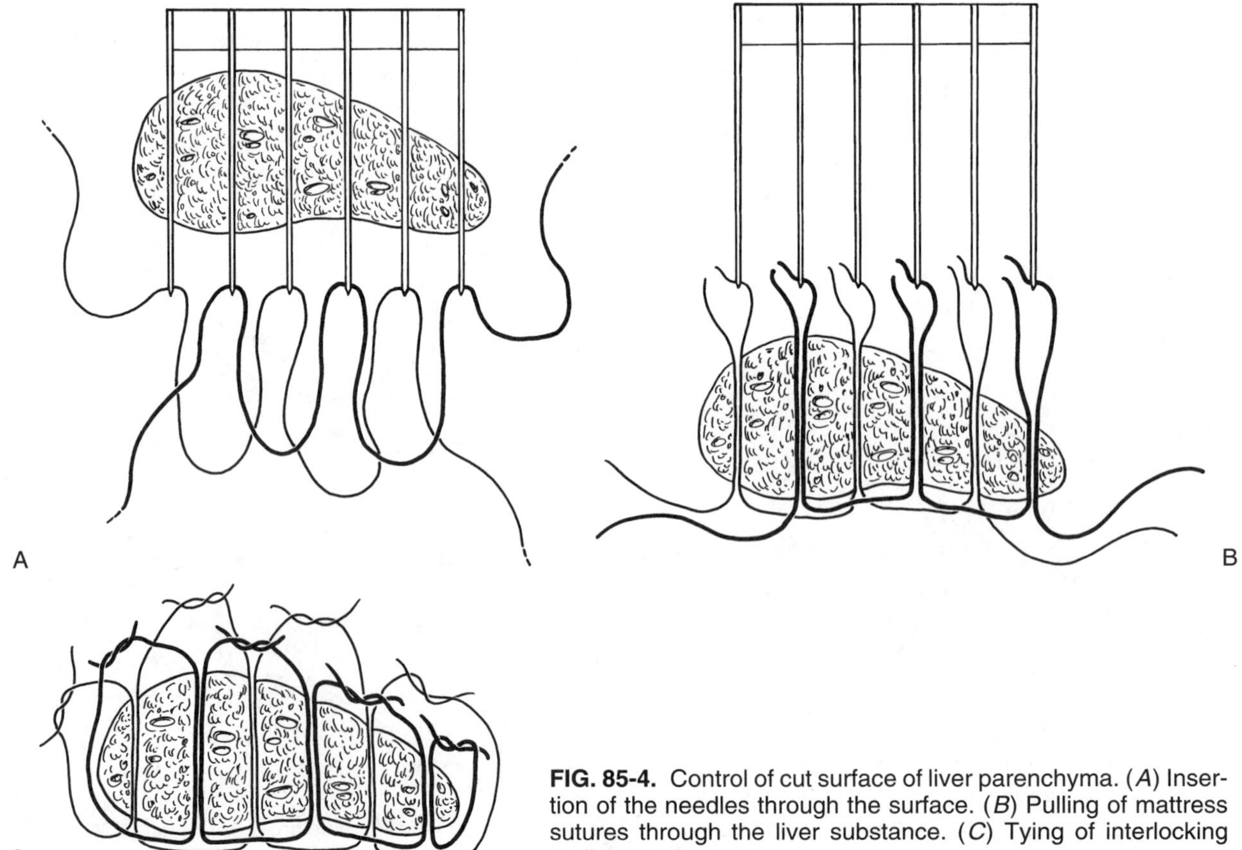

FIG. 85-4. Control of cut surface of liver parenchyma. (*A*) Insertion of the needles through the surface. (*B*) Pulling of mattress sutures through the liver substance. (*C*) Tying of interlocking mattress sutures.

wise healthy liver a tumor may be unresectable if it involves multiple segments of the liver so that the amount of tissue resected would surpass the hepatic reserve and thereby prevent safe excision. Preoperative chemotherapy and radiation therapy can shrink and, in some cases, downstage tumors so that some unresectable tumors may become resectable.

PREOPERATIVE INVESTIGATION

Preoperative investigation is aimed at determining the nature of the hepatic lesion and its potential for resection, as well as assessing baseline liver function.[10] The order in which these processes are undertaken depends on the individual patient and the nature of the lesion.

Ultrasonography is a useful, noninvasive, investigational tool that provides information regarding the size and extent of liver tumors.[24,25] It is limited by being operator-dependent, and its utility varies among ultrasonographers. Computed tomography (CT) complements the information obtained by ultrasonography. In certain situations CT may obviate the need for other invasive studies; for example, the need for angiography can be obviated when a peripherally placed lesion is demonstrated.[24] Determination of the relationship between a lesion and the adjacent vascular structures can be improved with the use of intravenous contrast media. Assessment of vascular invasion is not always possible with these techniques. At this institution, preoperative hepatic angiography is thought to be an invaluable adjunct to careful dissection, because it provides a vascular road map to facilitate surgical resection. Late-phase portal venography is important in that it can be used to assess for the presence of tumor invasion into the vasculature. It can also alert the surgeon to the presence of tumor thrombus.[26] Inferior venacavography is reserved for voluminous tumors involving the right hemiliver and the midline.[24] Magnetic resonance imaging (MRI) and MRI angiography have taken on a more important role in the preoperative evaluation of liver masses, since they provide excellent visualization of the tumor and its vasculature.[24–26] Additionally, they are noninvasive. Very recently, magnetic resonance cholagiography has been reported[27] as a method to delineate intra- and extrahepatic biliary anatomy.

The diagnostic workup should consist of standard hematologic and biochemical determinations. Tumor markers, liver function studies, coagulation studies, and clotting factors should be assessed. Liver enzymes and the α-fetoprotein determination usually are within normal limits with benign tumors but are elevated in approximately half of children with malignancies.[28]

The roentgenographic workup of a suspected hepatic mass should begin with a flat-plate abdominal film to look for calcifications within the lesion. An ultrasound[29] can then be obtained to differentiate a solid mass from a cystic mass. If the tumor is not a simple cyst by ultrasound, a contrast-enhanced CT[24] should be performed. CT can be used to assess the extent and location of the tumor.[30] Whereas standard CT scanning is limited to the axial plane, MRI can provide images in multiple planes. In the coronal plane, MRI can provide useful information regarding hepatic segmental involvement and vascular displacement by the tumor mass.[24,25] Additionally, MRI offers the advantage of being able to distinguish malignant tumors from hemangiomas, because hemangiomas have a prolonged T2 value.[28]

Other imaging techniques that have specific applications for hepatic tumors include the technetium-99m sulfur colloid liver–spleen scan, which is useful in differentiating benign solid tumors from malignant ones. Most benign lesions take up technetium, whereas malignant solid tumors usually do not.[31]

Patients with malignant hepatic tumors should be screened for extrahepatic metastases by chest roentgenography, abdominal and thoracic CT, and a bone scan. Cholangiography may be necessary when patients are jaundiced.

OPERATIVE CONSIDERATIONS

At the time of operation, there should be good understanding and cooperation between the anesthetist and the surgeon. Patients require invasive monitoring and adequate vascular access because of the possibility of intraoperative hemorrhage. Venous return to the heart may be impaired during vascular clamping, and the anesthetist should be prepared to act accordingly. Central venous pressure and arterial lines are used routinely. Core temperature is measured, and blood and other infusion fluids are warmed before transfusion.

There are some special considerations that must be made in caring for patients after a hepatic resection because of the hepatic dysfunction that frequently occurs in the immediate postoperative period. Specifically, these complications include hypoglycemia, hypoalbuminemia, and coagulopathy. The treatment for each of these problems consists of careful monitoring and replacement therapy as needed. Patients should be kept on a constant glucose infusion in the initial postoperative period, and the dextrose concentration of replacement fluids should be adjusted according to frequently measured glucose values. Albumin should be administered in the first few postoperative days to maintain a normal physiologic oncotic pressure and thus avoid excessive third spacing of fluid. Postoperatively, liver resection patients may be placed on a fresh frozen plasma drip in addition to using fresh frozen plasma to replace surgical drainage and prevent a coagulopathy. These complications are usually temporary and are most severe during the first postoperative day. However, in patients with preexisting liver disease, such as those with cirrhosis, those who underwent extensive resections, or those who had excessively long ischemic times, the period of liver dysfunction can be prolonged or, at worst, permanently extended. These unfortunate patients can be temporized with plasma exchange or plasmapheresis, but may ultimately go on to require liver transplantation.

Operative Techniques

As understanding of liver anatomy has improved, effective operative techniques have been developed, so that hepatic resection is now associated with an acceptably low morbidity and mortality rate.[1] This has led to broader indications for resection. Basically, these can be divided into hepatic resections for malignant and nonmalignant causes of surgical liver disease. In general, when attempting a curative operation for a malignant hepatic lesion, the entire lesion, including all portions of any segment in which the tumor is involved, must be excised. Additionally, the remaining margins must be left free of disease if a purely surgical cure is hoped for. Benign tumors, however, can be locally excised, unless segmental resection provides a safer, more controlled, operation without excessive loss of hepatic parenchyma.

INCIDENCE AND ETIOLOGY

Primary liver neoplasms are the third leading cause of malignant abdominal masses after Wilms tumors and neuroblastomas in the pediatric age group.[32] However, the overall incidence of hepatic lesions in a pediatric population is very low, since these lesions are uncommon.[33] A wide variety of benign and malignant tumors of the liver occur. The most common hepatic mass in childhood is the hepatoblastoma.[28] Hepatocellular carcinoma, benign vascular tumors, mesenchymal hamartomas, sarcomas, adenomas, focal nodular hyperplasia, cysts, metastatic lesions, and abscesses constitute the remainder of hepatic masses. The Baggenstoss classification system[34] is the nomenclature used to describe hepatic masses.

Malignant hepatic tumors occur more frequently than benign hepatic tumors in the pediatric population.[32] Most benign liver tumors occur during the first 6 months of life, whereas most malignant liver tumors occur later in infancy or in childhood.[28] Notable exceptions to this rule are hepatic adenomas and possibly hemangiomas, which occur more frequently in the older pediatric population and whose incidence has increased over the past two decades, possibly owing to the use of oral contraceptives.[35]

Ninety-five percent of all hepatic malignancies in the pediatric population are either hepatoblastomas or hepatocellular carcinomas.[28] Even though there is no etiologic association between the two, hepatoblastoma and hepatocellular carcinoma are often combined in clinical trials and reports because both are rare tumors whose surgical management is similar.[25] Other rare malignant hepatic tumors in the pediatric population include hepatic mesenchymoma and rhabdomyosarcoma. Hepatoblastoma and hepatocellular carcinoma are discussed in detail in Chapter 36.

The hepatocarcinoma occurs more frequently in boys than in girls.[36] It appears in children younger than 3 years of age with another peak incidence in children from 12 to 13 years of age.[32] The period of acute onset of symptoms is usually brief. Patients usually present with the development of an abdominal mass or distension. Abdominal pain, anorexia, and weight loss are also frequent presenting symptoms. About 15% to 20% of patients have jaundice or fever at the time of presentation.[28] Approximately 5% of patients present after tumor rupture.[28] Most patients have mild anemia, and more than 10% present with a coagulopathy.[28] The patients frequently have abnormally elevated liver function tests as well as hyperbilirubinemia. The serum α-fetoprotein concentration is elevated in approximately half of children presenting with hepatocellular carcinomas.[28] This tumor is more likely to be found in previously cirrhotic livers.[32] In childhood, almost all types of cirrhosis have an increased incidence of hepatocellular carcinomas. Infants who develop cirrhosis secondary to heredity tyrosinemia, biliary atresia, neonatal hepatitis, glucose-6-phosphatase deficiency, α_1-antitrypsin deficiency, and parenteral nutrition associated liver failure all have an increased risk of developing hepatocellular carcinoma.[37] The hepatocellular carcinoma tends to be multicentric and invasive. Microscopically, the cells are more polygonal, bizarre, and irregular, with a high rate of mitotic figures.

Hepatocellular carcinoma has been associated with hepatitis B virus infection in the pediatric population.[38,39] Hepatitis B surface antigen can be demonstrated in some children with this tumor.[39] Additionally, cases of perinatal transmission of hepatitis B and subsequent development of hepatocellular carcinoma in less than a decade point out the considerably shorter interval before tumor development in children than in adults, in whom it may require 20 years to develop.[40]

Additionally the long-term use of androgenic steroids[41,42] or the consumption of large amounts of alcohol are also associated with the development of hepatocellular carcinoma.[43]

Histologically these tumors are bile-stained. Distinguishing features include large tumor cells, broad trabeculae, tumor giant cells, and nucleolar prominence. One histologic subtype is recognized: the fibrolamellar hepatocellular carcinoma.[28] This subtype is characterized by deeply staining, eosinophilic hepatocytes covered by an abundant fibrous stroma, which separates the cells into nodules. This subgroup may be more amenable to resection and, therefore, have a better prognosis.[28]

The hepatocellular carcinoma tends to be multicentric and invasive. At the time of diagnosis metastatic spread is common.[34] The usual sites of metastasis include regional lymph nodes, lung, and occasionally bone.

The Children's Cancer Study Group classification and treatment protocol[43] is the basis for the staging and treatment of hepatocellular carcinoma (Table 85-1). Potential cure of hepato-

TABLE 85-1. *Children's Cancer Study Group hepatoma III study classification and treatment for hepatoblastoma and hepatocellular carcinoma*

Classification	Treatment
Group I: complete excision of tumor	Vincristine, doxorubicin, cyclophosphamide, 5-fluorouracil
Group II: gross tumor excision with localized microscopic residual tumor	Hepatic irradiation
	Vincristine, doxorubicin, cyclophosphamide, 5-fluorouracil; addition of bleomycin and cisplatin in selected patients
Group III: gross tumor residual or unresectable tumor	Hepatic irradiation in selected patients
	Vincristine, doxorubicin, cyclophosphamide, 5-fluorouracil, bleomycin, cisplatin
Group IV: metastatic tumor	Resection, if possible
	Hepatic irradiation (optional)
	Vincristine, doxorubicin, cyclophosphamide, 5-fluorouracil, bleomycin, cisplatin

(Ablin et al.[42])

cellular carcinoma is primarily dependent on complete surgical excision of the tumor.[33] Although hypothermia and hypotensive anesthesia have been recommended for liver resection, they have not been proved to control hemorrhage.[44] Multimodal chemotherapy has done little to improve the dismal 12% survival rate; however, it has been helpful in shrinking and downstaging tumors preoperatively, thereby improving the chance of successful resection.[42]

A variety of much rarer tumors than hepatoblastomas or hepatocellular carcinomas make up the remaining hepatic malignancies. Malignant mesenchymoma is one such tumor.[41] It usually occurs between the ages of 5 and 10.[45] The chief complaint is usually an abdominal mass; however, abdominal pain or fever may also be seen.[46]

Radiographic workup should begin with an ultrasound of the mass to determine whether it is solid or cystic. Mesenchymoma can present in either way. If a solid mass is visualized on ultrasound, a radionuclide scan should be obtained. Mesenchymoma presents as a cold nodule.[33] Contrast-enhanced CT can be used to outline the margins and extent of the tumor. Angiography may reveal a variable pattern, from hypervascularity to hypovascularity and is useful in planning the surgical resection.[33]

Grossly malignant mesenchymomas present as a mucoid, multicystic mass with areas of hemorrhage. The tumor is usually well demarcated without evidence of gross tumor invasion into the surrounding normal parenchyma; however, microscopic invasion can be present. Histologically, spindle cells are present. The malignant cells may vary from small cells with oval nuclei to multinucleated anaplastic cells.[41]

The treatment for malignant mesenchymomas is primarily surgical and consists of complete excision, adjuvent chemotherapy, and irradiation of the tumor bed.[33] Hepatic irradiation following resection must be done with caution because of the deleterious effects of radiation on liver regeneration.[41]

Sarcomas other than malignant mesenchymal tumors are even rarer in children. Patients usually present with jaundice secondary to biliary tract obstruction by the tumor mass.[47] Microscopically, the tumor is identical with rhabdomyosarcoma elsewhere and appears to originate from the bile duct wall. Despite the apparent success of complete excision, irradiation, and adjuvent chemotherapy, the prognosis is poor, with an average survival less than 6 months after surgery. Some long-term survivors have been reported in the literature.[33]

Angiosarcoma is another rare hepatic neoplasm. Angiosarcomas are thought to be related to exposure to hepatoxins, such as arsenic and thorium dioxide.[46] This lesion is considered to be a malignant form of the common benign vascular tumor, infantile hemangioendothelioma.[33] Many cases of hepatic angiosarcoma arose in children previously irradiated for suspected hemangioendothelioma.[48] The prognosis for this tumor is poor, with most children dying within 2 years of their diagnosis.[49]

Hemangiomas constitute more than half of benign tumors of the liver.[33] The principal hepatic vascular tumors are infantile hemangioendothelioma and cavernous hemangiomas. Cavernous hemagioma is the most common benign hepatic lesion. Cavernous hemangiomas usually present in older children and are usually not associated with hemangiomas elsewhere in the body.[33] Infantile hemangioendothelioma usually presents before 6 months of age.[49] Approximately 40% of patients with this lesion also have cutaneous hemangiomas.[50] Both lesions usually present as either single or multiple asymptomatic masses of varying size. Histologically, hemangiomas are composed of dilated vascular spaces with a flattened, inconspicuous endothelium. Hemangioendotheliomas are derived from endothelial cells, forming vascular channels, but retain a focal or diffuse hypercellular pattern.[33]

Hemangioendotheliomas are derived from endothelial cells, forming vascular channels, with a hypercellular pattern.[51]

Hemangioendotheliomas are not encapsulated. Histologically they present as either lesions with a prominent endothelium closely related to a portal tract, pushing the normal liver parenchyma away instead of infiltrating it, or as lesions that are larger, more tortuous vascular channels with endothelial cells branching into and invading adjacent liver tissue.[52]

Most hepatic hemangiomas remain asymptomatic and therefore are never recognized during life. The vast majority of hepatic hemangiomas run a benign course without the occurrence of major complications, such as intraperitoneal hemorrhage, heart failure or thrombocytopenia. Most infantile hemangiomas spontaneously decrease in size by 12 months of age with regression progressing steadily thereafter.[49] Thus, for asymptomatic hepatic vascular lesions, observation with serial liver–spleen scans, ultrasound, or CT scans is usually all that is recommended.[32]

The diagnosis of a cavernous hemangioma is usually radiographic. Diagnosis is suspected when an infant presents with a hepatic mass and an associated coagulopathy. Diagnosis is confirmed radiographically by the characteristic findings on ultrasonography, liver–spleen scan, or CT scan.[33] Angiography and surgical exploration are rarely needed, except in those rare instances when malignancy can not be ruled out on the basis of radiologic findings alone. The appearance of the liver scan in hemangioendotheliomas is sufficiently characteristic that an accurate diagnosis can almost always be made.[53–56]

MAJOR COMPLICATIONS

In a small subset of patients, major life-threatening complications can occur. This usually happens only in patients with larger forms of hepatic hemangiomas. Major complications include chronic and subacute heart failure secondary to arteriovenous shunting through the vasculature of the tumor, thrombocytopenia, and anemia due to platelet and red blood cell sequestering within the tumor capillaries, or respiratory distress caused by the mass effect of the enlarged liver on the thoracic cavity.[42] Major complications require treatment. Some hemangiomas are surrounded by areas of normal hepatic parenchyma and, therefore, are readily resectable, most tumors large enough to cause a major complication are usually not resectable. If a liver hemangioma is associated with cardiac failure, an arteriogram should be obtained to accurately identify the hepatic artery and the location of the arteriovenous shunt. Additionally, a cardiac catheterization or echocardiogram should be obtained to rule out congenital heart disease.[32] With heart failure, a period of observation along with digitalization and diuretic therapy may stabilize the patient until the time when the tumor will spontaneously regress. Similarly, steroid therapy has been reported to help control the thrombocytopenia and even to promote tumor shrinkage, but the long-term use of steroids in this patient population is fraught with complications, including deleterious effects on patient growth and development.[56] Interferon has recently proved to be effective therapy in treating some hemangiomas.[57] When patients fail medical therapy, surgical intervention may be indicated. Ligation of the hepatic artery can be performed without excessive loss of hepatic function because of the dual blood supply to the liver, and this has been reported to shrink the tumor and control the complications of the hemangioma.[58] More recently, embolic vessel occlusion has become the mainstay of therapy. Embolization of hemangiomas employing a variety of agents has been successful in reducing the size of the tumor, controlling secondary effects.[48,59] The goal of either surgical or medical therapy is to provide enough time for the natural regression of the tumor to occur.[60]

Benign, solid liver tumors are less common than malignant lesions.[61] The distinction between a benign versus a malignant lesion can be difficult. A biopsy is the gold standard technique for differentiating between a benign or a malignant lesion. However, depending on the lesion, the diagnosis can often be made without the use of exploration and biopsy by combining information obtained from the history, physical examination, radiographic findings, and laboratory data.

Benign liver tumors have been associated with systemic disease or with therapy for chronic disease states.[28] For example, hepatic adenomas are associated with the use of oral contraceptives and anabolic steroids.[62] However, this association is most commonly seen in an adult population, possibly owing to the duration of exposure necessary to induce the formation of the adenoma. Patients with von Gierke disease, glycogen storage disease type I, have a predilection for developing liver adenomas.[63] Most children with this metabolic disorder develop one or more adenomas in their lifetimes. In some instances, these tumors have regressed following the cessation of androgen therapy, but this is not routine.[64] Therapeutic measures for the amelioration of the basic disease, such as portacaval shunts and continuous night feeding regimens, have no effect on preventing the formation of adenomas. However, hepatic transplantation does eliminate predilection to adenomas by altering the metabolic derangement in this disease.

Grossly, the hepatic adenoma appears as a well-circumscribed, firm, homogeneous, yellow-brown mass. Adenomas are usually large, solid, solitary masses that occur in the right lobe of the liver. They are encapsulated with a thin capsule. Histologically, they are composed of hepatocytes that appear normal but show no lobular differentiation, instead having a diffuse or acinar arrangement. The absence of mitotic figures or bizarre nuclei differentiates them from hepatocellular carcinoma.

These lesions present clinically as asymptomatic hepatic masses or after intraperitoneal hemorrhage secondary to rupture. In stable patients, diagnosis can be determined radiographically by demonstrating a well-circumscribed lesion on CT or ultrasound with a deficit on liver–spleen scan. Angiographic findings are nonspecific and vary from hypervascular to avascular lesions.

Because of the risk of rupture and occurrence in the same patient population at risk for hepatocellular carcinoma, resection of hepatic adenomas is the treatment of choice.[28] The prognosis after resection is excellent. Enucleation of the adenoma is the preferred therapy; however, partial hepatic resection may be necessary for complete removal in some cases.[33] Recurrence after resection is rare.

Focal nodular hyperplasia is more common in teenage girls who have taken oral contraceptives.[65] The etiology is unknown.

Most children affected with focal nodular hyperplasia present in the first 10 years of life, but most tumors present in adults.[66,67] Females known to have this diagnosis should not use oral contraceptives. Focal nodular hyperplasia produces a nonencapsulated but well-circumscribed, nodular mass in an otherwise normal liver.[32] The mass is usually small and solitary. It is seen most frequently on the inferior surface of the right lobe. There is no evidence of invasion or metastasis. These tumors present microscopically as nodules of hepatocytes that are separated by bands of connective tissue and nests of ducts. Focal nodular hyperplasia of the liver may be histologically similar to normal liver or to a well-differentiated adenoma. Hyperplasia is associated with hemihypertrophy, Wilms tumor, and adrenocortical neoplasm.[28] It usually presents as an asymptomatic mass. This condition has no malignant potential and no propensity for complications such as hemorrhage.[33] If the patient is asymptomatic, focal nodular hyperplasia may be observed.

Radiographic diagnosis of focal nodular hyperplasia depends on a characteristic angiographic pattern of hypervascularity and a liver–spleen scan showing partial uptake of radionucleotide. Ultrasound reveals a solid mass. Use of CT does not differentiate these lesions from adenomas.[37] Definitive diagnosis often requires biopsy.

The diagnosis and treatment are subject to controversy. If diagnosis could be accurately made without operation, no therapy would be indicated. If open biopsy is necessary for diagnosis, a small biopsy should be performed first, although it may be inconclusive and resection of the lesion might be necessary for definitive diagnosis. Radical surgical excision of this lesion should not be necessary.

Another group of benign hepatic tumors of unknown etiology and without association with a systemic disease consists of mesenchymal hamartomas.[28] These lesions consist of epithelial lined fluid-filled cysts of varying sizes, joined by solid, connective-tissue stroma. All tissue types are histologically mature in appearance. Grossly these lesions are cystic and smooth. Mesenchymal hamartomas do not show evidence for invasion of adjacent organs. They usually originate in the anterior aspect of the right hepatic lobe and may be very large. These tumors frequently become massive before the patient becomes symptomatic. The tumors are usually recognized in early infancy because of the mass effect on the function of other abdominal or thoracic structures.[28] Complications, including congestive heart failure, have been reported but are rare. Temporary decompression of the dominant cyst by catheter drainage may be indicated in acutely symptomatic infants.

Diagnosis is radiographic. Ultrasonography can reveal a mixed cystic and solid mass. Hamartomas of the liver have a characteristic appearance by CT.[68] Nuclear scans or CT scans with contrast demonstrate a decreased blood supply, an important point in differentiation of these lesions from malignant tumors or hemangiomas.[55] Angiography is rarely necessary for diagnosis but is useful as an aid to surgery by demonstrating any vascular anomalies and distortion caused by the tumor mass.

Treatment depends on the complications arising from tumor. Tumors may be drained internally or externally. When the cysts extend to the level of the vena cava or into both the major lobes, drainage is the most expeditious form of initial management. Definitive treatment of these lesions consists of frozen section to rule out the possibility of malignancy, followed by surgical excision. Usually these tumors can be enucleated or simply removed by transecting the pedicle. Formal segmentectomies may be necessary to ensure safe removal with minimal excision of normal parenchyma.[9] Recurrence following resection is rare.[33]

Teratomas of the liver are very rare in children.[69] Teratomas may be either benign or malignant and can be differentiated histologically from hepatoblastomas because hepatoblastomas do not contain neuroectoderm or neural crest derivatives.[33] The recommended treatment is complete excision. Prognosis depends on the nature of the tumor and the ability of the surgeon to completely resect it.[33]

Solitary hepatic cysts either are caused by echinococcal infection or are congenital malformations. Congenital malformations may be solitary or multiple (polycystic disease). Approximately half of patients with polycystic hepatic disease have associated polycystic kidney disease.[70] Solitary hepatic cysts are not associated with renal malformations.[71] Microscopically, the cysts may be lined with simple cuboidal, columnar, or squamous epithelial cells. The cysts may be caused by the failure of fusion of intralobar and interlobular ducts.[71] Most patients with congenital hepatic cysts are completely asymptomatic. A large solitary cyst usually presents as asymptomatic hepatomegaly. Ultrasonography demonstrates a solitary cyst with no septa.[55] These lesions are not malignant, nor are they associated with complications, so surgical excision is not indicated. Biopsy is indicated only if the diagnosis is in question. In endemic areas of echinococcal disease, a Casoni intradermal test to exclude hydatid disease of the liver is indicated before any hepatic surgery.[33] Hydatid cysts occur in children from areas endemic for *Echinoccocus*, such as the southwestern United States. Albendazole has proved useful in eliminating the organism.[72] The efficacy of this therapy is potentiated when combined with ultrasound-guided aspiration of the cysts.

Surgical excision is reserved for cysts that are easily accessible and can be removed with minimal morbidity. If the cyst is deeply embedded in the hepatic parenchyma and adheres to major biliary and vascular structures, excision can become hazardous and may be contraindicated. Similarly, extensive resection of normal parenchyma for complete excision of the cyst is also contraindicated. If excision is not possible and the cyst contents are clear, the cyst may be marsupialized and drained into the peritoneal cavity. If the cyst contains bile, suggesting a cyst–biliary tract communication, a Roux-en-Y drainage of the cyst is indicated.[32]

Before the advent of antibiotics, liver abscesses were most often secondary to a perforated appendix.[32] A liver abscess in the neonatal period is usually secondary to umbilical vein catheterization.[74] Other predisposing factors include chronic granulomatous disease, sickle cell anemia, HIV, and intestinal parasites. Liver abscesses may develop secondary to any infectious process.[32]

Abscesses usually present in the right lobe of the liver. Most often liver abscesses are solitary cavities filled with purulent material. Occasionally multiple abscesses can occur. The most common organisms found in liver abscesses have been *Staphylococcus aureus, Streptococcus pyogenes*, and *Escherichia coli*. Other less common pathogens include *Klebsiella* pneumonia and *Corynebacterium* acnes.[32,74]

Presenting signs of an hepatic abscess usually include fever, hepatomegaly, and right upper quadrant pain. Associated symptoms include jaundice, abdominal distention, and anorexia. Radiographic techniques such as CT scan or ultrasound may delineate these masses and are useful in making the diagnosis. In addition, a single abscess may be drained with percutaneous aspiration and catheter placement with either ultrasound or CT guidance. When surgical intervention is required, a transverse upper abdominal incision is made over the mass. Any suspicious soft areas of the liver are aspirated with a syringe and a needle.[32] If pus is found, the area is walled off with moist pads, and the abscess is unroofed by dividing the overlying liver tissue with electrocautery. Necrotic tissue within the cavity is excised, and the area around the abscess is debrided. When there are multiple abscesses, as in chronic granulomatous disease, as many abscesses as possible are unroofed and drained, but the primary treatment is medical, consisting of long-term specific antibiotic therapy based on culture results of the purulent material.

The morbidity and mortality associated with liver abscesses are significant. Morbidity including hematobilia, recurrent abscesses, and biliary obstruction occurs with significant frequency. In patients with chronic granulomatous disease, the mortality rate is approximately 25%. In patients without granulomatous disease, the mortality rate is nearly 45%.[74,75]

The ability to diagnose and treat liver disease is directly related to the underlying understanding of the scientific basis of the diseases being fought. As knowledge in the fields of oncology, immunology, angiogenesis, and infectious diseases continues to grow so will the ability to treat presently incurable diseases.

REFERENCES

1. Schwartz SI. Hepatic resection. Ann Surg 1990;211:1.
2. Langenbuch C. Ein fall von resection eines linksseitigen schurlappens der leber. Berl Klin Wochenscher 1888;25:37.
3. Cantlie J. On a new arrangement of the right and left lobes of the liver. J Anat Physiol 1898;32:4.
4. Hjortsjo CH. The topography of the intrahepatic duct system. Acta Anat 1951;11:599.
5. Healey JE, Schroy PC. Anatomy of the biliary ducts within the human liver. Arch Surg 1953;66:599.
6. Keen WW. Report of a case of resection of the liver for the removal of a neoplasm with a table of seventy-six cases of resection of the liver for hepatic tumor. Ann Surg 1899;267.
7. Wendel W. Beitrage zur chirurgie der leber. Klin Chir Berl 1911;95:887.
8. Couinaud C. Etudes anatomiques et chirugicales. Paris, Masson, 1957.
9. Bismuth H, Castaing D, Garden O. Segmental surgery of the liver. Surg Annu 1988;20:291.
10. Bismuth H, Garden O. Regular and extended right and left hepatectomy for cancer. In: Nyhus L, Baker R, eds. Mastery of surgery, vol 2. Boston, Little, Brown, 1992:864.
11. Goldsmith NA, Woodburne RT. The surgical anatomy pertaining to liver resection. Surg Gynecol Obstet 1957;105:310.
12. Storm FK, Longmire WP. A simplified clamp for hepatic resection. Surg Gynecol Obstet 1971;133:103.
13. Lin TY. Results in 107 hepatic lobectomies with preliminary report on the use of a clamp to reduce blood loss. Ann Surg 1973;177:413.
14. Goldwasser B, Bowers BA, Carson CC, et al. A new clamp for hepatic resection. Surg Gynecol Obstet 1987;164:379.
15. Lee KS, Kim BR. The banding method as a simplified technique for resection of the liver. Surg Gynecol Obstet 1988;167:77.
16. Nagao T, Kawano N, Morioka Y. The surgeon at work: a new instrument for hepatic resection. Surg Gynecol Obstet 1988;166:269.
17. Almersjo O, Hafstrom L. The suction knife. A new device for dividing liver parenchyma. Acta Chir Scand 1974;140:581.
18. Hodgson WJB, DelGuercio RM. Surgical technique. Preliminary experience in liver surgery using the ultrasonic scalpel. Surgery 1984;95:230.

19. Persson BG, Jeppsson B, Tranberg KG, et al. Transection of the liver with a water jet. Surg Gynecol Obstet 1989;168:267.

20. Fidler JP, Hoefer RW, Polanyi TG, et al. Laser surgery in exsanguinating liver surgery. Ann Surg 1975;181:74.

21. Transberg KG, Rigotti P, Brackett KA, et al. Liver resection, a comparison using Nd:YAG laser, ultrasonic aspiration, or blunt dissection. Am J Surg 1985;151:368.

22. Makuuchi M, Hasegawa H, Yamazaki S, et al. The use of operative ultrasound as an aid to liver resection in patients with hepatocellular carcinoma. World J Surg 1987;11:615.

23. Bismuth H, Houssin D, Ornowski J, et al. Liver resections in cirrhotic patients: a western experience. World J Surg 1986;10:311.

24. Miller JH, Greenspan BS: Integrated imaging of hepatic tumors in childhood. II. Benign lesions (congenital, reparative, and inflammatory). Radiology 1985;154:91.

25. Miller JH, Greenspan BS: Integrated imaging of hepatic tumors in childhood. I. Malignant lesions (primary and metastatic). Radiology 1985;154:83.

26. Boechat MI, Kangarloo H, Gilsanz V: Hepatic masses in children. Semin Roentgenol 1988;23:185.

27. Barrows P, Lund D. Magnetic resonance cholangiography private communication.

28. Hays DM: Lesions of the liver. In: Ashcraft KW, Holder TM, eds. Pediatric Surgery. Philadelphia, WB Saunders, 1993.

29. Kaude JV, Felman AH, Hawkins IF: Ultrasonography in primary hepatic tumors in early childhood. Pediatr Radiol 1980;9:77.

30. Chandra RS, Kapur SP, Kelleher J, et al. Benign hepatocellular tumors in the young: a clinicopathologic spectrum. Arch Pathol Lab Med 1984;108:168.

31. Bernardino ME, Lewis E: Imaging hepatic neoplasms. Cancer 1982;50:2666.

32. Baum ES, Raffenssperger JG: Liver tumors. In: Raffensperger JG, ed. Swenson's pediatric surgery. Norwalk, Appleton & Lange, 1990.

33. Randolph JG, Guzzetta PC. Tumors of the liver. In: Welch KJ, Randolph JG, Ravitch MM, ONeill JA, Rowe MI, eds. Pediatric Surgery. Chicago, Year Book Medical, 1986:302.

34. Baggenstoss AH: Pathology of tumors of liver in infancy and childhood. In: Pack GT, Islami AH, eds. Tumors of the liver. New York, Springer-Verlag, 1970.

35. Klatskin G: Hepatic tumors: possible relationship to oral contraceptives. Gastroenterol 1977;73:385.

36. Ishak KG, Glunz PR: Hepatoblastoma and hepatocarcinoma in infancy and childhood: report of 47 cases. Cancer 1967;20:396.

37. Mahour GH, Wogu GU, Siegel, et al: Improved survival in infants and children with primary malignant liver tumors. Am J Surg 1983;146:236.

38. Blumberg BS, London WT: Primary hepatocellular carcinoma and hepatitis B virus. Curr Probl Cancer 1982;6:1.

39. Kew MC, Hodkinson J, Paterson AC, et al. Hepatitis-B virus infection in black children with hepatocellular carcinoma. J Med Virol 1982;9:201.

40. Harvey VJ, Woodfield DG, Probert JC: Maternal transmission of hepatocellular carcinoma. Cancer 1984;54:1360.

41. Weinberg AG, Finegold MJ: Primary hepatic tumors of childhood. Hum Pathol 1983;14:512.

42. Fremond B, Jouan H, Sameh AH, et al: Hepatic tumors secondary to androgenotherapy: report of two pediatric cases. Chir Pediatr 1987;28:97.

43. Ablin AR, Campbell JR, Gooding C, et al. Children's Cancer Study Group, Hepatoma III Study, unpublished data.

44. Hays DM: Anesthesia for pediatric cancer surgery. In: Pizzo PA, Poplack DG, eds. Principles and practice of pediatric oncology. Philadelphia, JB Lippincott, 1989, 209.

45. Dehner LP: Hepatic tumors in the pediatric age group: a distinctive clinicopathologic spectrum. In: Rosenberg HS, Bolande RP, eds. Perspectives in pediatric pathology, vol 4. Chicago, Year Book Medical, 1978.

46. Roat JW, Wald A, Mendelow H, et al. Hepatic angiosarcoma associated with short-term arsenic ingestion. Am J Med 1982;73:933.

47. Stocker JT, Ishak KG: Undifferentiated (embryonal) sarcoma of the liver: report of 31 cases. Cancer 1978;42:336.

48. Trastek VF, van Heerden JA, Sheedy PF, et al. Cavernous hemangiomas of the liver: resect or observe. Am J Surg 1983;145:49.

49. Falk H, Herbert JT, Edmonds L, et al. Review of four cases of childhood hepatic angiosarcoma: elevated environmental arsenic exposure in one case. Cancer 1981;47:382.

50. Dachman AH, Lichtenstein JE, Friedman AC, et al. Infantile hemangioendothelioma of the liver: a radiologic-pathologic-clinical correlation. Am J Roentgenol 1983;140:1091.

51. Abramson SJ, Lack EE, Teele RI. Benign vascular tumors of the liver in infants: sonographic appearance. Am J Roentgenol 1982;138:629.

52. Ishak KG, Rabin I. Benign tumors of the liver. Med Clin North Am 1975;59:995.

53. Brant WE, Floyd JL, Jackson DE et al: The radiological evaluation of hepatic cavernous hemangioma. JAMA 1987;257:2471.

54. Larcher VF, Howard ER, Mowat AP. Hepatic haemangiomata: diagnosis and management. Arch Dis Child 1981;56:7.

55. Larcos G. A typical appearance of an hepatic hemangioma with technetium-99m RBC scintigraphy. J Nucl Med 1989;11:1885.

56. Shannon K, Buchanan GR, Votteler TP. Multiple hepatic hemangiomas: failure of corticosteroid therapy and successful hepatic artery ligation. Am J Dis Child 1982;136:275.

57. Folkman J. Use of interferon in hemangiomas, private communication.

58. deLorimier AA, Simpson EB, Baum RS, et al. Hepatic artery ligation for hepatic hemangiomatosis. N Engl J Med 1967;277:333.

59. Enjolras O, Riche MC, Merland JJ, et al. Management of alarming hemangiomas in infancy: a review of 25 cases. Pediatrics 1990;85:491.

60. Stanley P, Geer GD, Miller JH, et al. Infantile hepatic hemangiomas: clinical features, radiographic investigations, and treatment of 20 patients. Cancer 1989;64:936.

61. Vandza T, Valayer J. Benign tumors of the liver in children: analysis of 20 cases. J Pediatr Surg 1986;21:419.

62. Shapiro P, Ikeda R, Ruebner B, et al. Multiple hepatic tumors and peliosis hepatis in Fanconi's anemia treated with androgens. Am J Dis Child 1977;131:1104.

63. Ehern H, Mahour GH, Isaacs H. Benign liver tumors in infancy and childhood: report of 48 cases. Am J Surg 1983;145:325.

64. Smithson WA, Telander RL, Carney JA. Mesenchymoma of the liver in childhood: five-year survival after combined-modality treatment. J Pediatr Surg 1982;17:70.

65. Christopherson WM, Mays ET. Liver tumors and contraceptive steroids: experience with the first one hundred registry patients. J Natl Cancer Inst 1977;58:167.

66. Knowles DM, Wolff M. Focal nodular hyperplasia of the liver: a clinicopathologic study and review of the literature. Hum Pathol 1976;7:533.

67. Dehner LP, Parker ME, Franciosi RA, et al. Focal nodular hyperplasia and adenoma of the liver: a pediatric experience. Am J Pediatr Hematol Oncol 1979;1:85.

68. Stanley P, Hall TR, Woolley MW, et al. Mesenchymal hamartomas of the liver in childhood: sonographic and CT findings. Am J Roentgenol 1986;147:1035.

69. Todani T, Tabuchi K, Watanabe Y, et al. True hepatic teratoma with high alpha fetoprotein in serum. J Pediatr Surg 1977;12:591.

70. Leese T, Farges O, Bismuth H. Liver cell adenomas: a 12-year surgical experience from a specialist hepato-biliary unit. Ann Surg 1988;208:558.

71. Rogers JV, Mack LA, Freeny PC, et al. Hepatic focal nodular hyperplasia: angiography, CT, sonography and scintigraphy. Am J Roentgenol 1981;137:983.

72. Morris D, Dyke S, Mariner S. Albendazole- objective response in human hydatid cysts. JAMA 1985;253:2053.

73. Tariq A, Rudolph N, Levin F. Solitary hepatic abscess in a newborn infant: a sequel of umbilical vein catheterization and infusion of hypertonic glucose solution. Clin Pediatr 1977;16:577.

74. Lazarchick J, deSouza N, Nichols D, Washington J: Pyogenic liver abscess. Mayo Clin Proc 1973;48:349.

75. Chusid M: Pyogenic hepatic abscess in infancy and childhood. Pediatrics 1978;62:554.

Surgery of Infants and Children: Scientific Principles and Practice, edited by Keith T. Oldham, Paul M. Colombani, and Robert P. Foglia. Lippincott–Raven Publishers, Philadelphia, © 1997.

CHAPTER 86

Biliary Atresia

Frederick M. Karrer and John R. Lilly

Biliary atresia is a disease that results in progressive sclerosing fibrous obliteration of the extrahepatic ducts. It is the most common cause of surgical jaundice in infants, occurring in between 1 in 10,000 and 1 in 20,000 live births. There is a slight female preponderance, but no racial predilection.[1]

Without surgical relief, cholestasis leads to hepatic cirrhosis and death before the age of 2 years.[2] In 1959, Kasai and Suzuki developed the *hepatic portoenterostomy* to establish bile drainage by resecting the obliterated biliary ducts at the liver hilum, where microscopic patency may persist for several months after birth.[3] The importance of early operation has been repeatedly demonstrated. Even with relief of biliary obstruction, many children progress to cirrhosis and develop complications of decompensated liver disease. Largely through the pioneering efforts of Tom Starzl, liver transplantation has become an accepted therapy.[4] As a result of advances in immunosuppression and surgical technique, liver transplantation now offers hope for those who progress despite Kasai's operation. Children with biliary atresia have the promise of long-term survival with a combination of surgical therapies: hepatic portoenterostomy and liver transplantation.

EMBRYOLOGY AND ETIOLOGY

Despite numerous theories and investigations of biliary atresia pathogenesis, the precise etiology remains unknown. Proposed causes include failure of recanalization, a defect in embryogenesis, vascular insufficiency, genetic factors, environmental teratogenesis, and perinatal viral infection. The fetal extrahepatic biliary system develops from the hepatic diverticulum of the embryonic foregut. As the cranial component expands to form the liver cords, the future ductal system becomes a solid cord of cells resulting from epithelial proliferation (similar to the duodenum). Reestablishment of the lumina of the ducts starts caudal, in the sixth week, and progresses cranially. Recanalization of the duct frequently results in two or three lumina, which eventually coalesce.[5] Yllpö, in 1913, postulated a failure of recanalization of the solid epithelial cords as the cause of biliary atresia, but this view is no longer widely accepted.[6]

Approximately 10% to 20% of patients with biliary atresia have an associated complex of anomalies termed *polysplenia syndrome*. In addition to polysplenia, the syndrome may include one or more of the following: absent inferior vena cava, bilobed symmetric liver, preduodenal portal vein, abdominal heterotaxia, malrotation, bilobed lungs, and cardiac defects[7] (Fig. 86-1). The association suggests an early teratogenic event during embryonic development. At approximately the same time as the biliary tree is forming and differentiating, a number of other important events in organogenesis are occurring. The polysplenia association indirectly supports biliary atresia as a result of a defect in biliary tree embryogenesis; however, most infants with biliary atresia have no associated anomalies.

Historically, evidence for vascular insufficiency as a cause of intestinal atresia stimulated efforts to make a similar connection with biliary atresia. A number of investigators attempted to reproduce biliary atresia in animals by making the bile ducts ischemic.[8–10] In some experiments, the extrahepatic ductal system became fibrosed and obstructed, but the intrahepatic ducts typically dilated, a finding inconsistent with biliary atresia. Despite numerous studies using different methods to injure the ducts in rabbits, dogs, and sheep, none has provided a workable model of biliary atresia.

A genetic cause is not supported by large case series, in which no familial case pattern has been seen.[11,12] Although case reports of two siblings with biliary atresia exist, they are rare. There are numerous examples of twins, both identical and fraternal, discordant for biliary atresia. To date, both twins developing biliary atresia has been reported only once.[13] Any influence of genetic factors in this condition is most likely indirect, possibly increasing the susceptibility to infectious or toxic agents.

Lacking evidence for genetic transmission, environmental teratogenesis remains suspect. This suspicion is amplified by two well-documented studies showing time-space clustering of biliary atresia.[11,14] Strickland's finding of cases clustered in the fall in rural northern Texas suggests agricultural activity as a possible environmental source of the increased incidence of biliary atresia.[14] An epidemiologic study by Carmi and coworkers identified two major exposures that exerted independent effects on the risk for biliary atresia: farming or pesticide exposure and maternal infectious illness during the last trimester.[15] Probably the most popular theory is a perinatal viral infection

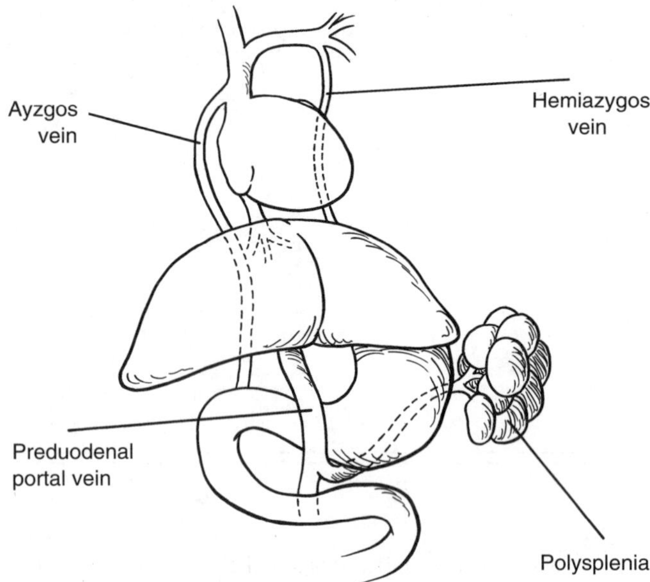

FIG. 86-1. Some of the associated anomalies seen in polysplenia syndrome: symmetric liver, preduodenal portal vein, absent inferior vena cava (with persistence of azygous venous drainage), polysplenia. Situs inversus, cardiac defects, and bilobed lungs are not illustrated.

causing progressive postinflammatory obstruction of the extrahepatic biliary tree.[16] A variety of viruses have been suggested, including hepatitis B, rubella, cytomegalovirus, Epstein-Barr virus, reovirus type 3, and rotovirus. To date, none has been proven to cause biliary atresia in humans.

Schrieber and coworkers postulated that biliary atresia may result from some insult (viral or toxic) that causes the biliary epithelium to become "upregulated" and express new antigens on the biliary cell surface.[17] These antigens are then recognized by the circulating T cells, which initiate a cell-mediated immune reaction. The ensuing fibrosclerotic injury to the bile ducts eventually results in biliary atresia. Whether any of the current theories of biliary atresia pathogenesis are correct remains to be proven. Biliary atresia may not have a single etiologic entity. In our opinion, there are two distinct groups: those with associated anomalies (probably caused by an early embryologic insult), and those that occur in isolation. The latter group may have several inciting events, resulting in a final common pathway of biliary epithelial destruction.

PATHOLOGY

Bile Ducts

In spite of the classic terminology, extrahepatic biliary atresia does not represent congenital agenesis of the bile ducts, but is characterized by progressive inflammatory destruction of all or part of the extrahepatic biliary tree. This gradual sclerotic process is probably not completed until around birth. The old classification into correctable and noncorrectable types, based on the presence of dilated proximal bile ducts, is no longer accurate since both types are correctable. The Japanese Society of Pediatric Surgeons' classification describes three main types:

Type 1—atresia of the common bile duct, which may be associated with a cyst in the porta hepatis
Type 2—atresia of the common hepatic duct
Type 3—atresia of the right and left hepatic ducts

Based on this classification scheme, nearly 90% of patients fall into type 3.[18] It is more clinically relevant to classify biliary atresia into three patterns, according to the operative and cholangiographic findings (Fig. 86-2). In the most common variant, the extrahepatic ducts are replaced by fibrous cords, and the gallbladder is similarly fibrotic, with a minute lumen containing a few drops of "white bile." The next most common group (20%) is characterized by residual patency of the gallbladder, cystic duct, and a common bile duct with proximal hepatic duct obliteration. Infants with the least common variant (10%) have proximal hilar cysts and distal obliteration of the ducts formerly considered correctable type.

Microscopic examination of the obstructed extrahepatic bile ducts shows complete fibrous obliteration resulting from cicatricial granulation tissue with chronic inflammation (Fig. 86-3). At the liver hilus, the remnants of the biliary tree have abundant inflammatory cell infiltrates, fibrosis, and various ductlike structures. Some of these ductal structures represent the residual lumina of the true bile duct, of which the epithelial lining may be damaged or absent. Others are either collecting ducts or residual biliary glands. Kasai and coworkers[19] showed that the intrahepatic ducts communicate with the porta hepatitis through these minute channels, at least during the first months of life. Surgical correction of the disease is based on this precept.

Liver Parenchyma

The liver of infants with biliary atresia is enlarged and firm with dark green discoloration. Later, nodular changes of cirrhosis develop. Microscopically, the hepatic histology is typical of any bile duct obstruction in this age group, with bile pigment in hepatocytes and canaliculi, widening of the portal tracts, and proliferation of bile ductules. If the obstruction is unrelieved, portal and periportal fibrosis progress and begin to bridge between portal tracts, leading to cirrhosis. In contrast to neonatal hepatitis, in biliary atresia the liver architecture is preserved, at least in the early stage. The classic features of neonatal hepatitis are hepatocellular necrosis, giant cell transformation, and mononuclear cell infiltrate in the hepatic parenchyma. Unfortunately, all of these findings may be present in biliary atresia as well, especially in the late stages. Diagnoses based on liver biopsy findings therefore have an estimated 5% to 10% error rate.[20]

DIAGNOSIS

Jaundice in the newborn that persists beyond 2 weeks should no longer be considered physiologic and warrants prompt investigation. There are numerous causes for jaundice in infancy[21] (Table 86-1). The diagnostic evaluation to exclude *every* possibility could take weeks and should not be done. The most important distinction is between mechanical or obstructive causes and jaundice due to hepatocellular dysfunction (infectious, hematologic, metabolic, genetic). Rapid investigation is essential, al-

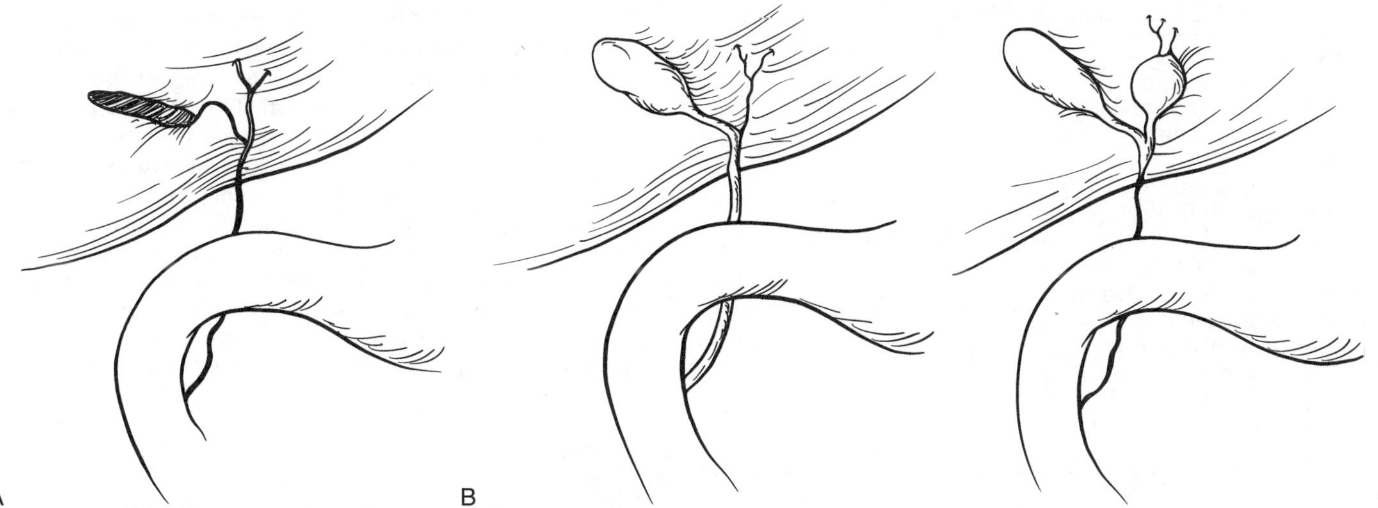

FIG. 86-2. Variants of biliary atresia. (*A*) Totally fibrotic extrahepatic ducts, with a minuscule gallbladder; (*B*) patency of the gallbladder, cystic duct, and distal common bile duct, with proximally fibrotic hepatic ducts; (*C*) patency of the gallbladder and proximal hepatic ducts, forming a cystic dilation, with distal obstruction.

lowing infants with biliary atresia to undergo operation before 8 weeks of age. The cardinal signs of biliary atresia are jaundice, dark urine, pale stools, and hepatomegaly. Jaundice is sometimes present at birth, but in most infants it appears a few weeks later. The stool color is often misleading. According to the Japanese Biliary Atresia Registry, approximately 40% of neonates passed normal meconium at birth, and yellowish feces were observed in about 60%.[22] Infants with biliary atresia are often full-term infants and remain robust for 1 or 2 months, despite development of jaundice. In contrast, infants with hepatocellular causes of jaundice are more often small for gestational age, are commonly jaundiced at birth, and appear sickly. In practice, however, no historic factors or physical findings can accurately identify cases of biliary atresia.

Biochemical Tests

In biliary atresia, the total serum bilirubin is usually 6 to 12 mg/dL at the time of diagnosis, and 50% to 80% is conjugated; however, any jaundiced infant with a conjugated bilirubin fraction greater than 20% requires further investigation. Serum transaminases are elevated, typically two to three times normal levels. The alkaline phosphatase is also elevated, and γ-glutamyl transpeptidase can be markedly high. At an early stage, markers of hepatic synthetic function, such as albumin, are normal. A mild coagulopathy may be present, but should resolve with parenteral administration of vitamin K.

Biochemical tests are most useful for excluding nonobstructive causes of jaundice (Table 86-2). These include serologic

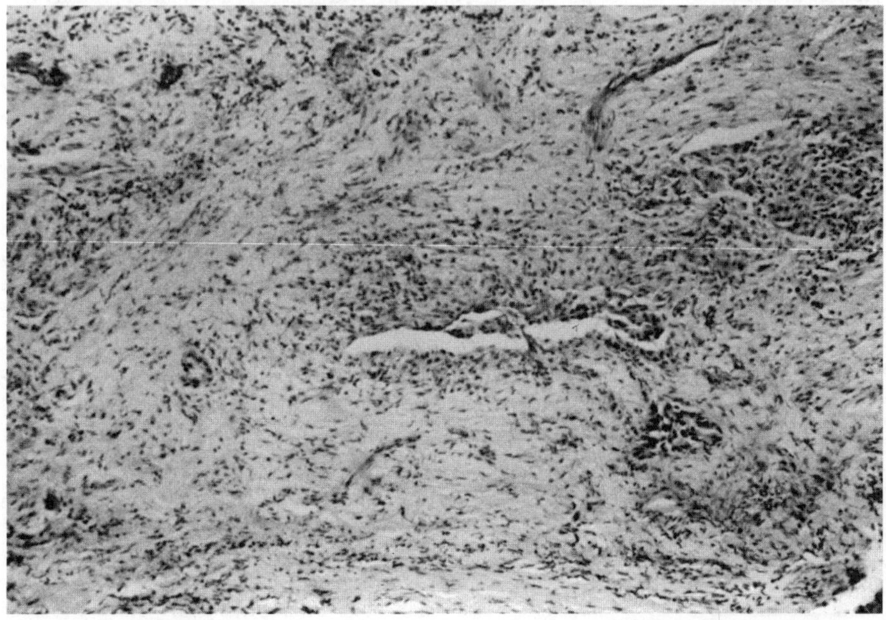

FIG. 86-3. Photomicrograph of the extrahepatic duct of an 8-week-old infant with biliary atresia. Note the concentric fibrosis of the ductal remnant and the degree of inflammatory infiltrate. Some small biliary structures persist in the periphery of the destroyed main duct.

TABLE 86-1. *Causes of jaundice in infancy*

Physiologic
Breast milk feedings
ABO or Rh incompatability
Hemolytic disease (eg, spherocytosis)
Infectious
    Bacterial sepsis
    Protozoan infections (eg, toxoplasmosis)
    Viral infections (eg, cytomegalovirus, hepatitis B, rubella,
       herpes virus, echovirus, varicella, coxsackievirus)
Genetic–Metabolic disease
    Alpha-1-antitrypsin deficiency
    Galactosemia or fructosemia
    Tyrosinemia
    Cystic fibrosis
    Niemann-Pick disease
    Gaucher disease

tests for hepatitis A, B, and C, and TORCH titers (*to*xoplasmosis, *r*ubella, *c*ytomegalovirus, and *h*erpesvirus), to exclude other infectious etiologies. α_1-Antitrypsin deficiency can mimic biliary atresia at exploration and must be excluded by determining the α_1-antitrypsin level. A standard complete blood count with examination of the peripheral smear largely excludes hematologic disorders causing jaundice due to hemolysis (usually associated with an unconjugated hyperbilirubinemia). Serum lipoprotein-X (Lp-X) levels are also advocated for diagnosing biliary atresia. Lp-X greater than 300 mg% strongly suggest biliary atresia, but this threshold is also exceeded in 20% to 40% of patients with neonatal cholestasis.[23] Because of its lack of specificity and universal availability, this test has not been widely adopted, at least in Western countries.

Ultrasonography

Ultrasonography is a simple, noninvasive procedure that should be used in almost all patients with cholestatic jaundice as a first step in the work-up. Using high-resolution and real-time imaging, the radiologist can determine the gallbladder size and contractility, the presence of associated anomalies, and also extra- or intrahepatic biliary dilation. The liver of infants with biliary atresia usually demonstrates increased hepatic parenchymal echoes, and the gallbladder is either absent or small, shrunken, and noncontractile. Demonstration of a decrease in the

TABLE 86-2. *Essentials in evaluation of the jaundiced infants*

Blood tests
    Complete blood count
    Liver panel
    Coagulation times (PT, PTT)
    Hepatitis A, B, C serologies
    TORCH titers
    Alpha-1-antitrypsin level
Ultrasonography
Hepatobiliary scintigraphy–"IDA" scan
Liver biopsy
Cholangiography

gallbladder size following feeding may not be as helpful as thought, because the gallbladder remains continuous with the duodenum through patent cystic duct and common bile duct in 20% of patients, even with proximal atresia.[24] Demonstration of associated anomalies such as polysplenia, preduodenal portal vein, absence of the inferior vena cava, or abdominal situs inversus indicates biliary atresia with polysplenia syndrome, findings never reported in patients with hepatocellular jaundice. Cystic structures or dilation of the biliary tree, seen with choledochal cyst or biliary obstruction from choledocholithiasis or inspissated bile syndrome, are readily identified by ultrasonography. There is no ductal dilatation in biliary atresia; either the extrahepatic tree is not visualized or appears to be of normal caliber.

Nuclear Imaging

Radionuclide hepatobiliary imaging with ^{99m}technetium-labeled derivatives of iminodiacetic acid is commonly used to separate obstructive from parenchymal jaundice. In the normal patient, the labeled compound is rapidly taken up by the liver and excreted through the biliary tree into the gut. In the patient with biliary atresia, the hepatocyte clearance of the isotope is relatively well maintained, and excretion into the bowel is absent, even on delayed images. Visualization of isotope in the bowel excludes biliary atresia. In hepatocellular jaundice, the isotope uptake is delayed by parenchymal disease, and excretion into the gut may or may not be seen. In fact, radioisotope excretion into the bowel was absent in 67% of children with hepatitis syndromes reported by Manolaki and coworkers.[25] Thus, mere absence of gut excretion is not diagnostic of biliary atresia. Phenobarbital, because it increases bilirubin conjugation and excretion, has been used to increase the value of iminodiacetic acid imaging. If administered for a few days before the study (5 to 10 mg/kg/d), it reduces the number of false-positives.[26]

Cholangiography

Exploratory laparotomy with operative cholangiography and open liver biopsy is still the sine qua non diagnostic maneuver. Exploration is performed through a limited right subcostal incision. A generous wedge biopsy of the liver is obtained. In many patients, the gallbladder is contracted and fibrotic. Sometimes there is no gallbladder lumen at all, making cholangiography impossible, or a tiny lumen containing only a few drops of "white bile." If the findings at exploration are consistent with biliary atresia, full surgical exploration is undertaken. If the gallbladder is patent, a cholangiogram is obtained by injecting dilute contrast material under just enough pressure to demonstrate continuity of the biliary tree between the liver and the duodenum. The patent extrahepatic ducts in neonatal hepatitis and biliary hypoplasia are often minute, and inattention to details of the cholangiogram has led to false diagnoses of biliary atresia and unnecessary excision of the extrahepatic ducts. If the gallbladder contains bile, but the common hepatic duct cannot be demonstrated, it is probably wise to close the abdomen, leaving the catheter in the gallbladder for subsequent cholangiography, because biliary hypoplasia is probably medically based.

Cholangiography has been attempted using endoscopic or

percutaneous-laparoscopic techniques. The development of small side-viewing endoscopes (PJE endoscope, Olympus, Keymed, UK) for pediatric patients permits endoscopic retrograde cholangiopancreatography even in young infants. This technique requires general anesthesia and an experienced endoscopist, but it has been used successfully to differentiate biliary atresia from neonatal hepatitis without the need for surgical exploration.[27,28] Percutaneous cholangiography has been used in a few centers, and may receive broader application with the advent of newer laparoscopic techniques.[29,30]

SURGICAL MANAGEMENT

The only therapies that offer hope of cure for biliary atresia are surgical. Following Holmes' observation in 1916[31] that at least 16% of cases were suitable for operation with a bile duct-to-bowel anastomosis, sporadic reports have appeared of success in establishing bile flow in children with the correctable type of biliary atresia.[32] For most patients in whom the bile ducts were occluded at the liver, nothing could be done. A variety of operations for noncorrectable biliary atresia were devised, including partial hepatic resection and drainage of the cut surface,[33] impalement with intrahepatic tubes,[34] and lymphathic drainage procedures.[35] None of the procedures provided long-term success. The dismal results and difficulty in differentiating biliary atresia from neonatal hepatitis led to the recommendation that surgical procedures be postponed until the child is 4 months old.[36] This practice undoubtedly delayed adoption of operations to relieve biliary obstruction earlier, as advocated by Kasai.

Kasai's Portoenterostomy

In 1959, Kasai and Suzuki reported a new operation, hepatic portoenterostomy, which could be applied to infants with non-correctable biliary atresia.[3] The Kasai operation amputates the biliary remnant at the porta hepatis with the plan to find still patent, microscopic ducts communicating with the intrahepatic biliary system and draining bile into a coapted intestinal conduit. After the cholangiogram and liver biopsy are completed and the diagnosis of biliary atresia is confirmed, the incision is widened into a bilateral subcostal laparotomy. The operation begins with mobilization of the gallbladder from the liver and dissection along the cystic duct to the common bile duct. The superficial peritoneum over the hepatoduodenal ligament is opened to expose the hepatic arteries and bile duct remnants. The fibrotic extrahepatic duct is carefully dissected and divided distally. Using the ductal remnants for traction, the dissection proceeds proximally to the hilus of the liver. Magnifying loupes and perfect lighting are essential for this delicate dissection. The fibrous ductal structures tend to widen and enter the liver between the bifurcation of the portal vein. The cone-shaped, fibrous mass is separated from the right and left portal veins, where several small bridging veins must be meticulously divided. Stay sutures are placed laterally and posteriorly at the margins of the duct, as it enters the liver. The fibrous cone is amputated at the level of the posterior surface of the portal vein, flush with the liver substance (Fig. 86-4). The excised cone is sent for frozen section to determine the presence of microscopic bile ducts. If no ductules are identified, traction is applied to the posterior stay suture, and this specific area is reexcised. The procedure is completed by anastomosis of intestine to the porta hepatis, using the previously placed guy sutures. Care must be taken not to place sutures through the transected posterior end of the fibrous cone, in which the minute bile ducts are often present. We prefer a single-layer end-on anastomosis, using a running absorbable suture.

Originally, Kasai and coworkers drained the porta into the gut with a traditional Roux-en-Y jejunal limb. A number of variations are now available for reestablishing GI continuity.[18] These options all stem from attempts to reduce the frequency

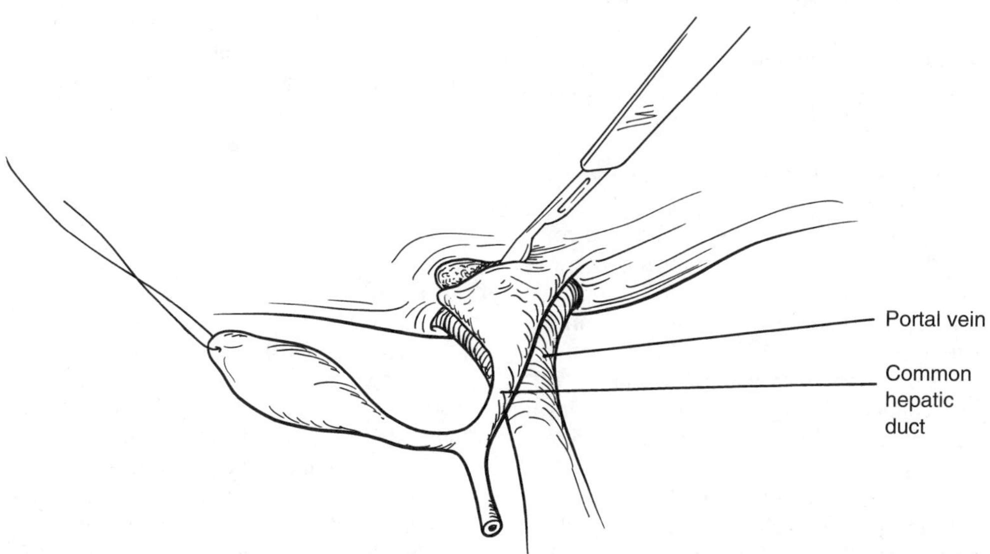

FIG. 86-4. Operative technique of hepatic portoenterostomy. Using the gallbladder for traction, the biliary remnants are dissected proximally. The remnants fan out into a fibrous cone between the bifurcation of the portal vein and posterior to it. The fibrous cone is transected flush with the liver surface.

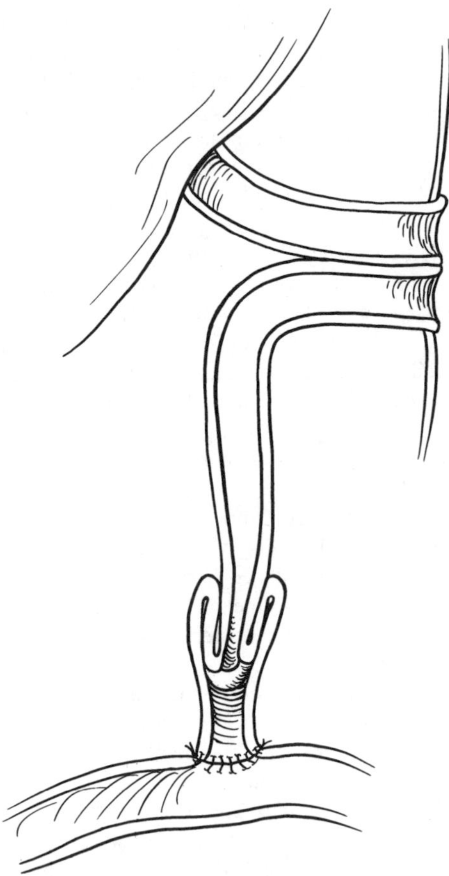

FIG. 86-5. Bilioenteric conduit, as constructed by the authors. The proximal end of the defunctionalized jejunum is anastomosed end-on to the porta hepatis. It is exteriorized as a double-barrel stoma, and an intussusception valve is created in the distal limb.

and severity of postoperative cholangitis. Some surgeons temporarily exteriorize the conduit, and others include an antireflux valve mechanism in the intestinal conduit. Our preference is to use both techniques[37] (Fig. 86-5). Exteriorization permits early assessment of bile flow and quality, for intervention and prognostication. Incorporating an intussusception valve may reduce the incidence of cholangitis in the early critical period after hepatic portoenterostomy. The biliary stoma is closed soon (3 to 6 weeks) after stable bile flow has been established. To complete the operation, a drain is placed into the subhepatic space, and the wound is closed in layers.

Occasionally, a bile cyst is encountered at the liver hilum. In the past, an anastomosis was made directly to the cyst, but long-term bile drainage was only infrequently maintained. Because the cyst has no epithelial lining, anastomotic shutdown occurs.[38] The cyst must be resected and a standard portoenterostomy carried out.

In about 20% of patients, patency of the gallbladder, cystic duct, and common bile duct permits performance of a portocholecystostomy.[39] In these cases, the gallbladder must be carefully mobilized to preserve its blood supply. It is opened longitudinally, and directly anastomosed to the transected porta. Initially, the hypoplastic cystic and common bile duct are sometimes incapable of accepting the full volume of bile drainage. Tempo-

rary tube decompression (leaving the cholangiocatheter in place) permits healing of the anastomosis without leakage until gradual dilation of the distal ducts occurs. If portocholecystostomy is successful, patients rarely experience postoperative cholangitis.[40]

Postoperative Management

Intravenous fluids and nasogastric decompression are continued until bowel peristaltic activity returns. Preoperative broad-spectrum antibiotics are continued for 5 days after operation. Some surgeons then administer oral antibiotics for cholangitis prophylaxis. There is no evidence, however, that prophylactic antibiotics prevent cholangitis, and they may select out resistant strains that are more difficult to eradicate.[41] Oral feedings are usually begun early, to stimulate bile flow. A formula that contains fats in the form of medium-chain triglycerides (e.g., Pregestamil) is preferred, since fat absorption is impaired early in the absence of good biliary excretion. Fat-soluble vitamin (D, E, and K) supplements are also necessary until good bile drainage is well established. If a cutaneous enterostomy is used, bile drainage must be replaced with intravenous fluids until it can be periodically refed into the distal stoma throughout the day.

Liver Transplantation

Improvements in immunosuppression and the technique of liver transplantation have added another option to the treatment of children with biliary atresia. Biliary atresia is the single most common indication for liver replacement in the pediatric age group (see Chapter 43). Some have advocated primary liver transplantation as the initial surgical management of biliary atresia, fearing that Kasai's operation may interfere with the success of the transplant procedure. The concern has been shown to be unfounded,[42] and the consensus among pediatric surgeons worldwide is that Kasai's procedure should be performed initially, unless the presentation is late and success unlikely.[43] Liver transplantation is reserved for those children who are diagnosed late, fail to drain bile after portoenterostomy, or progress to decompensated liver disease and portal hypertension despite partial relief of biliary obstruction.

COMPLICATIONS

Cholangitis

Cholangitis is the most frequent and serious complication after hepatic portoenterostomy, occurring in 40% to 100% of infants.[18,37,39] The two prerequisites for cholangitis, bacteria, and bile stasis are inherent to the disease. Cholangitis presents with fever, leukocytosis, and decreased bile output manifested by rising serum bilirubin levels, acholic stools, or decreased quantity and quality of bile from the cutaneous enterostomy. Early postoperative cholangitis can result in complete cessation of bile flow, and repeated attacks can cause progressive deterioration of hepatic function. Early intervention is therefore essential. Prompt treatment with intravenous broad-spectrum antibiotics (e.g., imipenum-cilastatin) is usually effective. Symptoms usually abate within 24 to 48 hours, but the bilirubin may take several days to return to baseline.

During the early post-Kasai course, refractory cholangitis and threatened bile shutdown are treated with choleretics. We use corticosteroids in a high but rapidly tapering dose (i.e., methylprednisolone 10 mg/kg/d tapered over 4 days). Corticosteriods have a dual action of choleresis, augmenting the bile acid–independent fraction of bile flow, and antiinflammatory effects, which reduce periductular edema bile stasis.[44] Other choleretics such as phenobarbital, glucagon, cholestyramine, dehydrocholic acid, and ursodeoxycholic acid (UDCA) have also been used. We prefer UDCA for long-term use, in an oral dose of 10 to 20 mg/kg/d. UDCA, a bile acid initially used for medical dissolution of cholesterol gallstones, is a potent choleretic. It modifies the composition of the endogenous bile-acid pool, increases bile flow by stimulating bicarbonate excretion, and has an inherent hepatocytoprotective effect. Nittono and coworkers reported beneficial effects of UCDA in biliary atresia patients, and in our experience, it has resulted in reduced incidence of cholangitis and bile shutdown.[45]

Susceptibility to cholangitis wanes over the first year after operation and is unusual beyond the second year. Infants with recalcitrant cholangitis were sometimes treated by reoperation to score the liver hilus, which was generally unsuccessful. The only bona fide indication for reoperation is an infant with good initial bile flow who suddenly experiences bile shutdown unresponsive to steroid therapy. Other causes, such as obstruction of the conduit, should also be entertained at reoperation.

Portal Hypertension

Portal hypertension is a serious complication that occurs even in jaundice-free survivors with biliary atresia. Whether the ongoing fibrosis of the liver is a result of the progression of the initial inflammatory sclerosing of the intrahepatic ducts or the persistent cholestasis is unknown. Some degree of hepatic fibrosis is present in all patients at the time of initial diagnosis, and measurements of portal pressures at portoenterostomy have documented portal hypertension in most. The clinical manifestations of portal hypertension include esophageal variceal hemorrhage, hypersplenism, and ascites. Esophageal varices are identified in 40% to 80% of children by age 5 years; leading to variceal bleeding in 10% to 25%.[46] Management is by endoscopic sclerotherapy or variceal band ligation. Both techniques have been used successfully to control and eliminate esophageal varices.[47,48] The tendency to bleed from esophageal varices seems to diminish with age, particularly in the jaundice-free group.[49] For this reason, continued nonoperative treatment of variceal bleeding is justified as long as hepatic function is preserved. In the setting of jaundice, poor coagulation, and hypoalbuminemia, variceal hemorrhage should initiate referral for liver transplantation.

Many children develop splenomegaly even with sustained bile drainage after Kasai's operation. In most, hypersplenism does not develop. In some, however, hypersplenism progresses to life-threatening leukopenia and thrombocytopenia. In these exceptional cases, partial splenic embolization, with small particles (gel foam) embolized angiographically into the peripheral splenic arteries, has been curative in most patients (10 of 13 in our hands).[50] Complications such as fever and atelectasis are common and take 1 to 2 weeks to resolve.

Ascites is the least common manifestation of portal hypertension. It forms from the serosal surfaces of the GI tract and the liver surface. The problem of increased portal pressure is magnified by reduced plasma oncotic pressure if hypoalbuminemia is present. Conservative management consists of dietary sodium and water restriction, spironolactone, and furosemide (Lasix). Ascites formation is usually accompanied by significant hepatic deterioration, and referral for liver replacement is indicated.

Malnutrition and Fat-Soluble Vitamin Deficiency

Intraluminal bile salts are necessary for micelle formation, permitting normal absorption of fats. Because of the absence of bile flow before and reduced bile flow after operation in children with biliary atresia, inadequate absorption of fat and fat-soluble vitamins (A, D, E, and K) should be anticipated. Rickets (vitamin D deficiency), ataxic neuropathy (vitamin E deficiency), keratopathy (vitamin A deficiency), and coagulopathy (vitamin K) have all been reported in children with biliary atresia. Appropriate supplementation can correct or minimize these sequelae. Metabolism abnormalities of protein, water-soluble vitamins, calcium, iron, zinc, and copper have also been documented in children with chronic liver disease.[51] Until normal bile drainage is achieved, formulas containing fats provided as medium-chain triglycerides are preferred (e.g., Pregestamil). Medium-chain triglycerides are absorbed directly through the intestinal mucosa without the need for emulsification, micelle formation, and hydrolysis.

OUTCOME

Kasai's operation has positively influenced the prognosis for infants with biliary atresia. Without intervention, patients with biliary atresia have an average life expectancy of approximately 12 months.[52] Portoenterostomy offers long-term survival in cases previously thought to be uncorrectable, and results of treatment are gradually improving. Both Ohi and Lilly have shown an improvement in the operative results for biliary atresia over the years. For example, Ohi and coworkers reported a dramatic improvement in the number of children who drained bile from 61% to 94% between 1953 and 1991, and the 10-year survival has increased from 10% to 71%.[18] Lilly demonstrated a tripling of the 5-year survival rate from 19.4% between 1973 and 1978 to 62.4% between 1978 and 1983.[53]

The major determinants of long-term survival are the patient's age at operation, and establishment of postoperative bile flow. In every large series of patients treated with Kasai's portoenterostomy, the patient's age at operation has been an important factor in the long-term success. Most authors have found that infants operated on in the first 2 months of life have the best prognosis. For instance, in the largest series reported from Sendai, Japan, 10-year survival rate were 72% for those operated on before 60 days of age; 41% for those between 61 and 70 days, 24% for those 71 to 90 days, and only 15% for those operated on after 90 days.[18] In the largest Western registry, parallel results have been reported; of infants operated on under 30 days of age 62.5% survived, between 31 and 60 days 43.6% survived, between 61 to 90 days 39.5% survived, and only 28% of infants operated on after 90 days of age survived.[39]

The most significant predictive factors in the prognosis of infants with biliary atresia are establishment of bile flow and resolution of jaundice. Various series have reported bile excretion in 50% to 85% of infants, and earlier operation improved the chances for establishing bile flow.[18,54–56] Several investigators have demonstrated that bile flow exceeding a critical amount of daily bilirubin excretion correlates with prognosis. Stewart used a value of 6 mg bilirubin a day, Houwen used the value of 8.8 mg/d and Ohi used 10 mg/d, but each showed a clear separation between groups above and below these benchmark levels.[56–58] Excretion of bilirubin above a certain watershed level equates with the clinical clearing of jaundice, which occurs in from 25% to 76% of cases. If an infant becomes jaundice-free, the prognosis is markedly improved. Ohi showed that for infants in whom jaundice cleared at any point in their postoperative course, the 10-year survival was 82%, whereas if the infant never become jaundice-free, the 10-year survival was only 10%.

The 10-year survival rate of all infants treated by hepatic portoenterostomy ranges from 30% to 55%.[39,54,59] Unfortunately, survival does not necessarily equate with cure. Many children develop complications related to hepatic cirrhosis and portal hypertension. Laurent reported that of 40 children 10 years or more after successful hepatic portoenterostomy, only 11 were free of portal hypertension and had completely normal liver function.[59] Toyosaka found 9 out of 20 biliary atresia patients more than 10 years old had normal liver function.[60] This means that more than half of the long-term survivors after Kasai's procedure are jaundiced or require treatment for complications of portal hypertension. Despite these deficiencies, the jaundice-free long-term survivors achieve normal growth and have normal motor and mental development. Several have survived into the fourth decade of life, and two have become pregnant and delivered normal children. As a consequence of improvements in operative technique and postoperative management, early results have improved, equating with more and more extended survivors. Combined with advances in liver transplantation, Kasai's operation offers patients with biliary atresia an 80% to 90% chance of long-term survival.

ACKNOWLEDGEMENT

Supported in part by a grant (RR-69) from the General Clinical Research Centers Program at the Division of Research Resources, National Institutes of Health, and the Pediatric Liver Center, University of Colorado/The Children's Hospital, Denver, Colorado.

REFERENCES

1. Shim W, Kasai M, Spence M. Racial influence on the incidence of biliary atresia. Prog Pediatr Surg 1974;6:53.
2. Hays DM, Snyder WH. Life-span in untreated biliary atresia. Surgery 1963;64:373.
3. Kasai M, Suzuki S. A new operation for noncorrectable biliary atresia: hepatic portoenterostomy. Shujutsu 1959;13:733.
4. Starzl TE, Iwatsuki S, Van Thiel DH. Evolution of liver transplantation. Hepatology 1982;2:614.
5. Skandalakis JE, Gray SW, Ricketts R, et al. The extrahepatic biliary ducts and the gallbladder. In: Skandalakis JE, Gray SW, eds. Embryology for surgeons, ed 2. Baltimore, Williams & Wilkins, 1994:296.
6. Yllpö A. Zwei fälle von kongenitalem gallengangsverschluss: fettund bilirubin-stoffwechselversuche bei einen derselben. K Kinder 1913;9:319.
7. Karrer FM, Hall RJ, Lilly JR. Biliary atresia and the polysplenia syndrome. J Pediatr Surg 1991;26:524.
8. Picket LK, Briggs HC. Biliary obstruction secondary to hepatic vascular ligation in fetal sheep. J Pediatr Surg 1969;4:95.
9. Okamoto E, Okasora T, Toyosaka A. An experimental study on the etiology of congenital biliary atresia. In: Kasai M, Shiraki, eds. Cholestasis in infancy. Baltimore, University Park Press, 1980:217.
10. McSherry CK, Morrissey KP, Swarm RL, et al. Chenodeoxycholic acid–induced liver injury in pregnant and neonatal baboons. Ann Surg 1976;184:490.
11. Silverira TR, Salzano FM, Howard ER, et al. The relative importance of familial, reproductive and environmental factors in biliary atresia: etiological implications and effect on patient survival. Braz J Med Biol Res 1992;25:673.
12. Danks D, Bodian M. A genetic study of neonatal obstructive jaundice. Arch Dis Child 1963;38:378.
13. Smith BM, Laberge JM, Schreiber R, et al. Familial biliary atresia in three siblings including twins. J Pediatr Surg 1991;26:1331.
14. Strickland A, Shannon K. Studies in the etiology of extrahepatic biliary atresia: time space clustering. J Pediatr 1982;100:749.
15. Carmi R, Magee CA, Neill CA, et al. Extrahepatic biliary atresia and associated anomalies: etiology heterogeneity suggested by distinctive patterns of associations. Am J Med Genet 1993;45:683.
16. Landing BH. Consideration of the pathogenesis of neonatal hepatitis, biliary atresia and choledochal cyst: the concept of infantile obstructive cholangiopathy. Progr Pediatr Surg 1974;6:113.
17. Schrieber RA, Kleinman RE. Genetics, immunology, and biliary atresia: an opening or a diversion? J Pediatr Gastroenterol Nutr 1993;16:111.
18. Ohi R, Ibrahim M. Biliary atresia. *Semin Pediatr Surg* 1992;1:115.
19. Kasai M, Ohi R, Chiba T. 1980 Intrahepatic bile ducts in biliary atresia. In: Kasai M, Shiraki K, eds. Cholestasis in infancy. Baltimore, University Park Press, 1980:181.
20. Tolia V, Dubois RS, Kagalwalla A, et al. Comparison of radionuclear scintigraphy and liver biopsy in the evaluation of neonatal cholestasis. J Pediatr Gastroenterol Nutr 1986;5:30.
21. Balistreri WF, Schubert WK. Liver disease in infancy and childhood. In: Schiff L, Schiff ER, eds. Disease of the liver, ed 7. Philadelphia, JB Lippincott, 1993:1099–1203.
22. Chiba T, Ohi R, Kamiyama T, et al. Japanese biliary atresia registry. In: Ohi R, ed. Biliary atresia. Toyko, Icom Associates, 1991:79.
23. Tazawa Y, Konno T. Semiquantitative assay of serum lipoprotein-X in differential diagnosis of neonatal hepatitis and congenital biliary atresia. Tohoku J Exp Med 1980;130:209.
24. Weinberger E, Blumhagen JD, Odell JM. Gallbladder contraction in biliary atresia. Am J Roentgenol 1987;149:401.
25. Manolaki AG, Larcher VF, Mowat AP, et al. The prelaparotomy diagnosis of extrahepatic biliary atresia. Arch Dis Child 1983;58:591.
26. Majd M. Radionuclide studies in the evaluation of neonatal jaundice. In: Daum F, ed. Extrahepatic biliary atresia. New York, Marcel Dekker, 1983:22.
27. Heyman MB, Shapiro HA, Thaler MM. Endoscopic retrograde cholangiography in the diagnosis of biliary malformations in infants. Gastroint Endo 1988;34:449.
28. Takahashi H, Kuriyama Y, Maie M, et al. ERCP in jaundiced infants. In: Ohi ed. Biliary atresia. Tokyo, Professional Postgraduate Services, 1987:110.
29. Franken E, Smith W, Smith J, et al. Percutaneous cholangiography in infants. Am J Roentgenol 1978;130:1057.
30. Yamamoto H, Yoshida M, Ikeda S, et al. Laparoscopic cholecystcholangiography in a patient with biliary atresia. Surg Lapa Endo 1994;4:370.
31. Holmes JB. Congenital obliertion of the bile ducts: diagnosis and suggestions for treatment. Am J Dis Child 1916;11:405.
32. Ladd WE. Congenital atresia and stenosis of the bile ducts. JAMA 1928;91:1082.
33. Longmire WP, Sanford MC. Intrahepatic cholangiojejunostomy with partial hepatectomy for biliary obstruction. Surgery 1948;24:264.
34. Sterling JA. Artificial bile ducts in the management of congenital biliary atresia. J Int Coll Surg 1961;36:293.
35. Williams LF, Dooling JA. Thoracic duct–esophagus anatomosis for relief of congenital biliary atresia. Surg Forum 1963;14:189.

36. Thaler MM, Gellis SS. Studies in neonatal hepatitis and biliary atresia. Am J Dis Child 1968;116:257.

37. Lilly JR, Karrer FM, Hall RJ, et al. The surgery of biliary atresia. Ann Surg 1989;210:290.

38. Lilly JR, Hall RJ, Vasquez J, et al. The surgery of correctable biliary atresia. J Pediatr Surg 1987;22:522.

39. Karrer FM, Lilly JR, Stewart BA, et al. Biliary atresia registry, 1976 to 1989. J Pediatr Surg 190;25:1076.

40. Lilly JR, Stellin G. Catheter decompression of hepatic portocholecystostomy. J Pediatr Surg 1982;17:904.

41. Hitch DC, Lilly JR. Identification, quantification and significance of bacterial growth within the biliary tract after Kasai's operation. J Pediatr Surg 1978;13:563.

42. Wood RP, Langnas AN, Stratta RJ, et al. Optimal therapy for patients with biliary atresia: portoenterostomy (''Kasai'' procedures) versus primary transplantation. J Pediatr Surg 1990;25:153.

43. Vacanti JP, Shamberger RC, Eraklis A, et al. The therapy of biliary atresia combining the Kasai portoenterostomy with liver transplantation: a single center experience. J Pediatr Surg 1990;25:149.

44. Karrer FM, Lilly JR. Corticosteroid therapy in biliary atresia. J Pediatr Surg 1985;20:593.

45. Nittono H, Tokita A, Hayashi M, et al. Ursodeoxycholic acid in biliary atresia. Lancet 1988;1:528.

46. Ohi R, Mochizuki I, Komatsu K, et al. Portal hypertension after successful hepatic portoenterostomy in biliary atresia. J Pediatr Surg 1986;21:271.

47. Lilly JR. Endoscopic sclerosis of esophageal varices in children. Surg Gynecol Obstet 1981;152:513.

48. Karrer FM. Portal hypertension. Semin Pediatr Surg 1992;1:34.

49. Odievre H. Long-term results of surgical treatment of biliary atresia. World J Surg 1978;2:589.

50. Brandt CT, Kumpe D, Rothbarth LJ, et al. Splenic embolization in children: long-term efficacy. J Pediatr Surg 1989;24:642.

51. Greene HL. Nutritional aspects in the management of biliary atresia. In: Daum F, ed. Extrahepatic biliary atresia. New York, Marcel Dekker, 1983:133.

52. Adelman S. Prognosis of uncorrected biliary atresia: an update. J Pediatr Surg 1978;13:389.

53. Lilly JR. Biliary atresia: the jaundiced infant. In: Welch KJ, Randolph JG, Ravitch MM, et al, ed. Pediatric surgery. Chicago, Year Book Medical Publishers, 1986:1047.

54. Howard ER. Biliary atresia. In: Blaumgart LH, ed. Surgery of the liver and biliary tract. Edinburgh, Churchill Livingstone. 1994:835.

55. Evans JS. Abnormalities of the bile ducts. In: Wyllie R, Hyams JS, ed. Pediatric gastrointestinal disease. Philadelphia, WB Saunders, 1993:901.

56. Stewart BA, Hall RJ, Karrer FM, et al. Long-term survival after Kasai's operation for biliary atresia. Pediatr Surg Int 1990;5:87.

57. Houwen R, Zwierstra R, Soverijner R, et al. Prognosis of extrahepatic biliary atresia. Arch Dis Child 1989;64:214.

58. Ohi R, Hanamatsu M, Mochizuki I. Progress in the treatment of biliary atresia. World J Surg 1985;9:285.

59. Laurent J, Gauthier F, Bernard O, et al. Long-term outcome after surgery for biliary atresia: study of 40 patients surviving for more than 10 years. Gastroenterology 1990;99:1793.

60. Toyosaka A, Okamoto E, Okasora T, et al. Outcome of 21 patients with biliary atresia living more than 10 years. J Pediatr Surg 1993;28:1498.

Surgery of Infants and Children: Scientific Principles and Practice, edited by
Keith T. Oldham, Paul M. Colombani, and Robert P. Foglia.
Lippincott–Raven Publishers, Philadelphia, © 1997.

CHAPTER 87

Disorders of the Gallbladder and Biliary Tract

Alan W. Flake

This chapter describes a heterogeneous group of diseases that
involve various components of the biliary tract. The spectrum
of biliary tract disorders in children includes abnormalities of
ductal anatomy, physiologic aberrations in bile composition or
flow, primary or secondary inflammatory disease, and neoplastic transformation.

DEVELOPMENT OF THE BILIARY SYSTEM

An understanding of the developmental sequence of events
resulting in formation and maturation of the hepatobiliary system is fundamental to an understanding of most childhood biliary tract diseases. Extensive morphologic and biochemical information about many of these disease processes is available.
A more fundamental understanding of their causes, however,
awaits definition of the regulatory and inductive influences
present at their inception.

Embryology of the Bile Ducts

The liver develops from an endodermal bud in the ventral
floor of the foregut at about 22 days' gestation. The cells of
the cranial portion give rise to mature hepatocytes, intrahepatic
bile ducts, proximal extrahepatic ducts, and gall bladder. The
distal extrahepatic bile ducts are derived from cells in the caudal
portion. Early in development, there appears to be only one
type of endodermal cell in the cranial portion of the liver diverticulum, which serves as a common precursor for both hepatocytes and intrahepatic bile ducts. Immature hepatocytes, or *hep-
atoblasts,* are derived from these early cells and retain the
potential to differentiate into either hepatocytes or intrahepatic
ducts. Evidence suggests that small numbers of these cells may
persist and serve as a facultative stem cell compartment in postnatal life. These cells can be stimulated to proliferate and differentiate under certain pathologic conditions (Fig. 87-1). Neoplastic transformation of these cells is thought to result in
hepatoblastoma.

At about 2 months' gestation, primitive intrahepatic bile
ducts can be distinguished from early hepatocytes by their tendency to form small cysts in close proximity to portal venous

branches. Contiguous bile ducts are formed by the fusion of
biliary cysts, which begins in sequence at the liver hilum and
extends peripherally into the segmental distribution of the developing liver. This occurs after the appearance of the portal
veins and hepatic arteries, to complete the portal triad. At the
hilum, connection is made to the extrahepatic bile ducts. Formation of the major vessels of the biliary tree is completed by 10
to 12 weeks' gestation, but interlobular bile ducts probably do
not completely extend to all regions of the liver until late in
the third trimester.

The development of the distal common bile duct and pancreaticobiliary junction is of particular relevance to pediatric
surgeons. During the fifth week of gestation, the dorsal and
ventral pancreatic buds appear. The dorsal bud forms the body
of the pancreas and empties through what will become the accessory pancreatic duct (Santorini duct) into the duodenum. The
ventral bud arises from the distal common bile duct, rotates
dorsally to join the body of the pancreas as the uncinate process,
and empties through the main pancreatic duct (Wirsung duct)
into the common bile duct. During normal development, the
junction of the main pancreatic duct and common bile duct
migrates distally through the duodenal wall to merge within the
sphincter of Oddi at the ampulla (Fig. 87-2). Variations on this
process account for a variety of anatomically based biliary disorders of childhood.

Physiologic Maturation of the Biliary System

The hepatocyte performs a wide variety of essential physiologic tasks. These include production of plasma proteins, gluconeogenesis and glycogenolysis, biotransformation of toxins and
chemicals, bile acid metabolism and cholesterol regulation, and
bilirubin excretion. During gestation, many of these functions
are performed for the fetus through placental transport and maternal hepatic function. Although plasma protein synthetic capacity is present even in the primitive hepatoblast, many of the
excretory functions of the fetal liver mature only after birth.
The physiologic immaturity of the premature or term newborn
liver undoubtedly plays a role in the pathophysiology of a variety of neonatal diseases characterized by abnormal bile compo-

1405

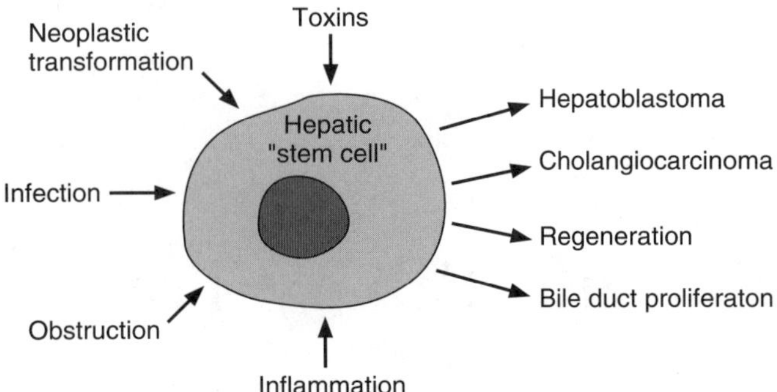

FIG. 87-1. The hepatoblast, or hepatic stem cell, can differentiate into either mature hepatocytes or bile duct epithelium. A variety of environmental and genetic influences result in proliferation or differentiation, which ultimately can be beneficial or detrimental to the patient.

sition or flow. Differences between immature and mature hepatic function are summarized in Table 87-1 and discussed next.

Maturation of Bile Acid Metabolism and the Enterohepatic Circulation

Bile acids are amphipathic sterols formed in the liver by stereospecific additions and modifications of cholesterol. Bile acid metabolism is a critical determinant of cholesterol regulation. Interaction of bile acids, phospholipids, and cholesterol leads to mixed micelle formation, allowing biliary excretion of these lipids and other compounds, such as toxic xenobiotics, and facilitating intestinal absorption of dietary fat. Finally, bile acids are a major driving force for the cellular formation of bile.

The enterohepatic circulation maintains the bile acid pool by recycling of 90% of excreted bile acid. This occurs through a sodium–bile acid cotransport system, present on the ileal brush border, that absorbs bile acid against a concentration gradient. The bile acids then return to the liver through the portal circulation, where they are actively secreted by a second sodium–bile acid cotransporter across the hepatocyte canalicular basolateral membrane. Bacteria present in the jejunum and ileum metabolize a portion of the primary bile acids (taurodeoxycholic, taurochenodeoxycholic, glycochenodeoxycholic, and cholic acids) to secondary bile acids (deoxycholic acid, ursodeoxycholic acid, and lithocholic acid), which are passively absorbed in the colon and reenter the hepatic circulation. Lithocholate (the product of 7α-dehydroxylation of chenodeoxycholic acid) can be hepatotoxic and may contribute to the liver damage associated with various types of cholestasis.

Immaturity of bile acid synthesis, excretion, and enterohepatic circulation has been demonstrated in all fetal animal models studied and in limited human studies. Bile acids are first detected in human fetuses at about 14 weeks' gestation. Increased activity of the synthetic enzymes involved increases bile acid pool size late in gestation, but pool size remains smaller in children than in adults until about 7 weeks of age. Maturation of hepatic and ileal bile acid transport mechanisms does not begin until around the time of birth and is not complete until weaning in animals. Similarly, despite decreased bile acid pool

size and diminished intestinal absorption, serum bile acids remain elevated in human infants younger than 6 months of age, implying ineffective hepatic clearance. In addition, there are qualitative differences in bile acid composition in fetuses and newborns as compared with adults. Fetal bile contains an increased chenodeoxycholic/cholic acid ratio, a predominance of taurine conjugates, and the presence of unusual bile acids with specific hydroxylations seen in adults with cholestasis.

Thus, the preterm or term infant has several predispositions to cholestasis. The diminished bile acid pool and decreased intraluminal concentrations of bile acids result in decreased bile flow. Ineffective hepatic bile acid clearance results in elevated serum bile acid levels and accumulation of bile acids within the hepatocyte. The abnormal bile acid composition may favor the formation of toxic secondary bile acids in circumstances of clinical cholestasis, contributing to hepatic damage. Finally, low bile acid concentrations result in lithogenic bile, which favors the development of sludge or cholelithiasis.

Maturation of Bile Pigment Excretion

Most bilirubin is the end product of heme degradation derived from erythrocytes normally removed from the circulation and destroyed in the reticuloendothelial system. Erythrocyte half-life is shorter in the fetus and neonate, and therefore production of unconjugated bilirubin is greater per kilogram of body weight than in the adult. Most pigment is transferred unaltered across the placenta to the maternal circulation. Bilirubin UDP-glucuronyltransferase activity, which conjugates bilirubin, first detected at about 20 weeks' gestation, remains low until after birth. The enzyme appears to be induced by substrate, and activity rapidly increases after birth after a rise in plasma unconjugated bilirubin levels, regardless of gestational age.

The serum bilirubin concentration normally peaks at levels between 5 and 6 mg/dL on the third to fifth day of life in full-term human newborn infants and gradually declines to adult levels in the first several weeks of life. The reabsorption of unconjugated bilirubin from the intestine may also contribute to the increased bilirubin load after birth. Conjugated bilirubin gradually accumulates in meconium during fetal life. Bacterial flora responsible for the conversion of conjugated bilirubin to urobilin are absent or reduced in the gut of the newborn infant, which allows the enzyme β-glucuronidase to deconjugate the accumulated bilirubin. This process results in the absorption of a significant load of unconjugated bilirubin from the newborn intestine and accounts for the increased jaundice seen in circumstances of delayed passage of meconium, that is, in infants with intestinal obstruction.

DISORDERS OF THE EXTRAHEPATIC BILE DUCTS

Choledochal Cysts

The term *choledochal cyst* has been applied to a heterogeneous group of relatively uncommon cystic disorders of the biliary tract. Choledochal cysts have been categorized according to their anatomic and cholangiographic appearance into five types (Fig. 87-3). Type I (cystic or fusiform dilation of the common

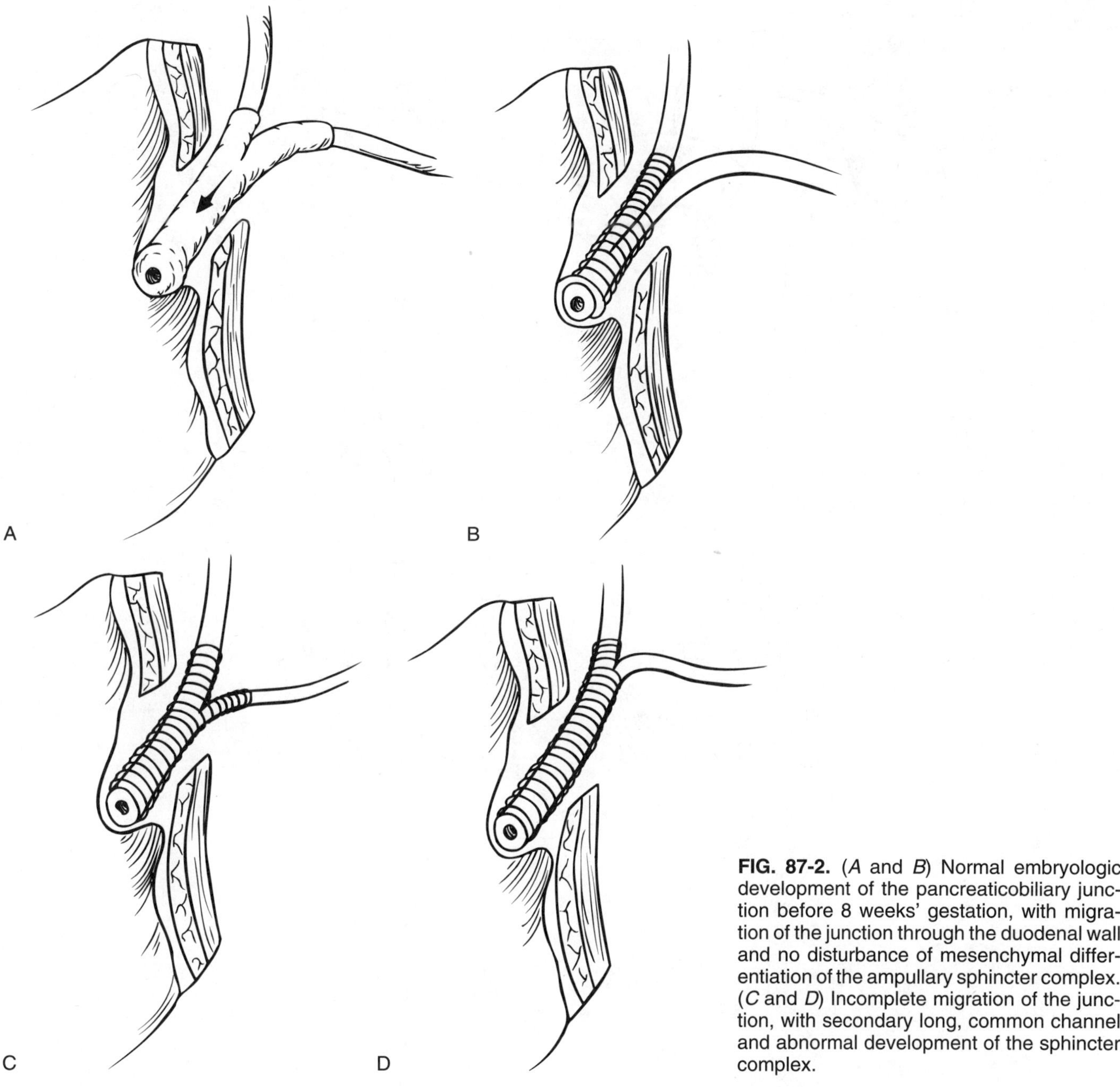

FIG. 87-2. (*A* and *B*) Normal embryologic development of the pancreaticobiliary junction before 8 weeks' gestation, with migration of the junction through the duodenal wall and no disturbance of mesenchymal differentiation of the ampullary sphincter complex. (*C* and *D*) Incomplete migration of the junction, with secondary long, common channel and abnormal development of the sphincter complex.

TABLE 87-1. *Predisposition to cholestasis in preterm and term neonates*

Immature physiology	Result
↓ Bile acid synthesis	↓ Bile acid pool
↓ Canalicula carrier–mediated transport	↑ Hepatocellular (bile acid)
↓ Bile acid secretion	↓ Bile (bile acid)
	↓ Bile flow
Abnormal bile acid profile	↑ Hepatocellular toxicity
↓ Serum bile acid uptake	↑ Serum (bile acid)
↓ UDP-glucuronyltransferase	↑ Hyperbilirubinemia
↑ Bilirubin production	

bile duct) is by far the most common. Type II (diverticulum of the common bile duct) and type III (choledochocele) are relatively rare. Types IV and V (Caroli disease) involve the common bile duct, with either fusiform or saccular dilation of the intrahepatic bile ducts, respectively.

Most cases have been reported from Japan, suggesting a higher incidence in Asia than in the West. A female preponderance of about 4:1 exists, and a number of familial cases have been reported, although no genetic basis has been established.

Pathogenesis

About 20 speculative mechanisms have been proposed as causes for choledochal cysts, most of which are unsubstantiated.

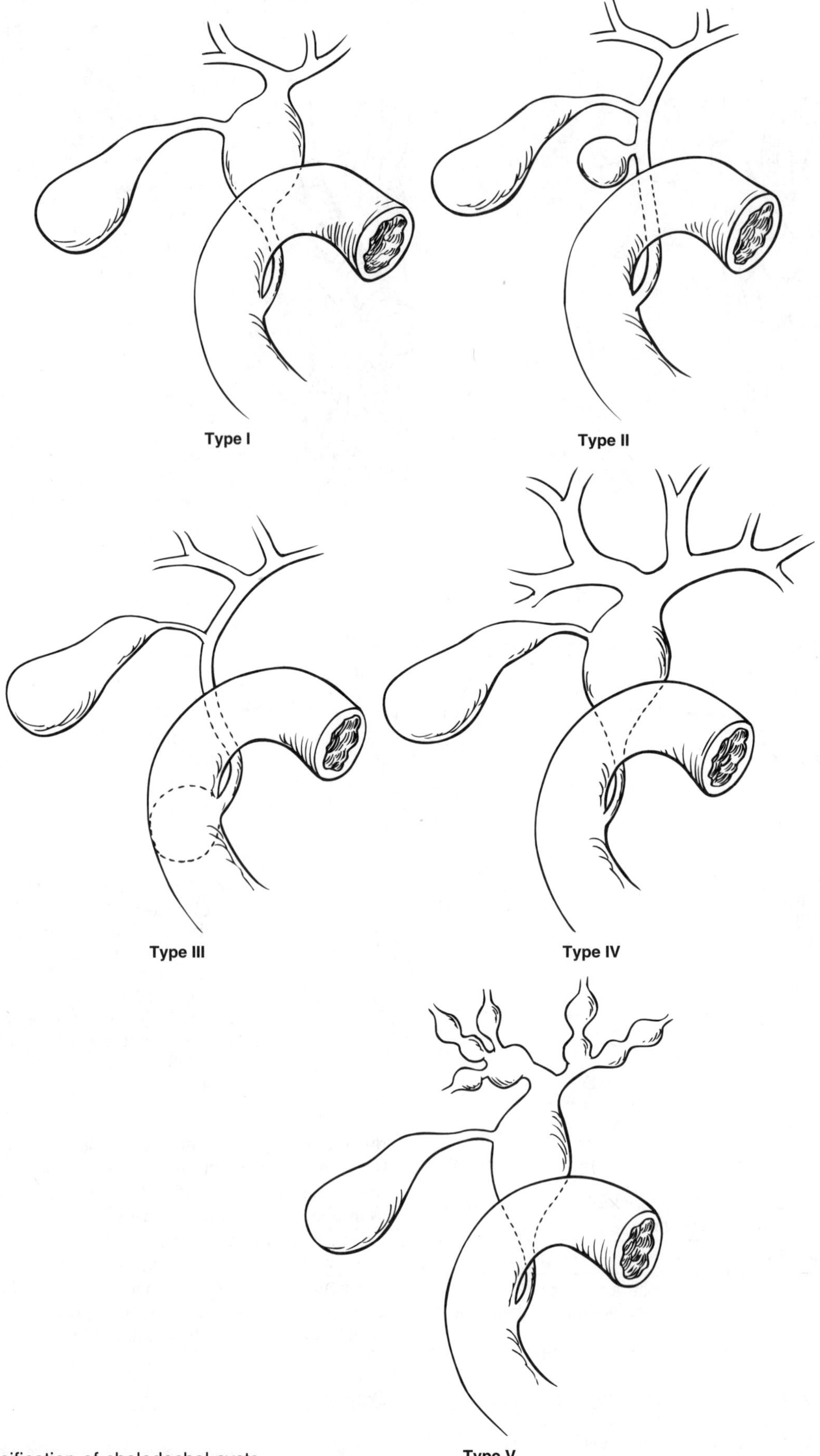

FIG. 87-3. Classification of choledochal cysts.

All of the proposed mechanisms are based on distal obstruction, on a congenital or acquired weakness of the duct wall, or on a combination of the two. In reality, as one might expect from the clinical and anatomic heterogeneity of the disease, there are probably several etiologic factors responsible for choledochal cysts. The following discussion focuses on mechanisms supported by clinical or experimental observation.

The theory of pancreaticobiliary reflux secondary to an anomalous pancreaticobiliary junction has been advanced by a number of investigators. According to this theory, incomplete migration of the choledochopancreatic junction into the duodenal wall results in a proximal insertion of the pancreatic duct into the common duct, that is, a long common channel (see Fig. 87-2). This results in free reflux of pancreatic secretions into the biliary ducts, resulting in activation of proteolytic enzymes, weakening of the duct wall, and cystic dilation. This may be potentiated by varying degrees of functional distal obstruction caused by an associated anomalous or spastic sphincter of Oddi complex. Supporting observations include the following:

- High incidence (80% to 100% in some series) of anomalous pancreaticobiliary junction associated with choledochal cysts
- Common presence of activated pancreatic enzymes (beyond the neonatal period) in choledochal cyst fluid
- Manometric high-pressure zone at the sphincter of Oddi in many patients with choledochal cyst and a long common channel
- Documentation of acquired ductal dilation later in life associated with the aforementioned observations
- Ductal inflammation histologically similar to choledochal cyst in animal studies of surgically created long common channels

Unfortunately, not all patients with choledochal cysts have an anomalous pancreaticobiliary junction, and many patients with anomalous pancreaticobiliary junctions never have symptoms, negating an absolute cause-and-effect relation. In addition, choledochal cysts have been prenatally diagnosed as early as 15 weeks' gestation, a time when acinar development of the pancreas is rudimentary, arguing against a significant role for pancreaticobiliary reflux in these cases. Similarly, activated pancreatic enzymes are rarely documented in bile in newborns and infants with choledochal cysts. Finally, documented stenosis or atresia of the distal common bile duct, with or without associated pancreatic ductal abnormalities, has been described in many cases of choledochal cyst, particularly those presenting early in life. Neonatal cases of choledochal cyst are frequently indistinguishable from ''correctable'' biliary atresia, leading to confusion in classification and unifying theories of pathogenesis. At this point, it is probably most reasonable to consider choledochal cyst to be a spectrum of diseases that can arise from primary developmental obstructive causes or be acquired during life from the sequelae of inflammatory and obstructive influences related to anomalous pancreaticobiliary development.

Clinical Presentation

Choledochal cyst can present at any age, but more than half of patients present within the first decade of life. Although

TABLE 87-2. *Age-related clinical presentation of choledochal cysts*

YOUNGER THAN 1 YEAR
Unrelenting jaundice
Otherwise asymptomatic
Mass: palpable or found during workup for jaundice
Occasional prenatal disease

OLDER THAN 1 YEAR
Pain, jaundice, palpable mass; <30% have the classic triad
Usually intermittant jaundice with or without pain, often overlooked for years
Cholangitis or pancreatitis

presentation is variable, patients generally fit into one of two groups based on age of presentation (Table 87-2). Presentation as a neonate or infant is characterized by asymptomatic, unrelenting jaundice; in the absence of a palpable mass, patients are indistinguishable from infants with jaundice from other causes. The classification of these disorders as choledochal cysts versus correctable biliary atresia is controversial but is probably best determined based on the presence or absence of inflammatory changes in the intrahepatic ducts. In contrast, children older than 1 year of age generally present with one or more components of the classic triad: pain, jaundice, or a palpable mass. The entire triad is present in less than one third of patients, and the typical patient has a history of intermittent jaundice or pain that may have been overlooked for months or years. The intermittent nature of the symptoms is related to recurring episodes of cholangitis or pancreatitis related to variable degrees of outflow obstruction and pancreaticobiliary reflux. As a result, any child with a diagnosis of pancreatitis should be evaluated for choledochal cyst. Undiagnosed choledochal cysts can lead to cholelithiasis, cirrhosis, portal hypertension, cyst rupture, hepatic abscess, or biliary carcinoma. The incidence of associated carcinoma (most commonly cholangiocarcinoma) is between 2.5% and 15% and rises with increasing age.

Pathology

The gross pathology of choledochal cyst is a spectrum of varying degrees of cystic dilation of the common bile duct or the intrahepatic ducts with or without evidence of distal ductal obstruction. The intrahepatic dilation can be fusiform and in continuity with the common bile duct dilation, or there can be defined cysts of the intrahepatic ducts. The former usually resolves with operative drainage, whereas the latter persists. Strictures of the bile duct are common, particularly of the common bile duct just proximal to the long common channel. There is frequently associated sludge, cholelithiasis, or choledocholithiasis.

Histologic analysis of choledochal cysts reveals dense fibrous connective tissue in the wall, with intense inflammation and ulceration of the mucosa and submucosal layers. Intramural glandular structures with mucin-secreting cells and immunoreactive gastrin- and somatostatin-containing cells, similar to intestinal mucosa, are frequently seen, suggesting epithelial metaplasia secondary to repeated destruction and regrowth of the lining of the unexcised cyst. These changes increase with advancing age and are seen in close association with adenocarcinomas, when they are present, suggesting neoplastic transformation. With advanced disease, the mucosal lining is sometimes partially or completely absent. An interesting variant of choledochal cyst has been described as *long common channel syndrome* or *forme fruste choledochal cyst*. These patients have minimal ductal dilation but identical symptoms and histologic changes of the duct wall, and respond well to surgical treatment.

Diagnosis

Choledochal cyst has been diagnosed in a number of patients by prenatal ultrasound. After birth, diagnosis depends on clinical suspicion. The best initial radiologic examination in the postnatal patient is also ultrasound, which is usually definitive. Hepatobiliary scintigraphy may be useful in some patients, particularly in newborns and infants, in whom cholangiography may not be possible and for whom the differential diagnosis includes biliary atresia. The imaging study that provides maximal preoperative information is endoscopic retrograde cholangiopancreatography (ERCP). ERCP provides detailed information on the extent of cystic dilation, the presence of intrahepatic cysts, anomalous or obstructive distal ductal anatomy, and the presence or absence of stones or sludge. In capable hands, ERCP can be performed even in small infants with high success rates and should be obtained if the expertise is available. Other imaging modalities, such as computed tomography and magnetic resonance imaging, are useful in selected patients but generally are unnecessary.

Treatment

Treatment of all types of choledochal cysts, with the exception of diffuse intrahepatic cysts, is surgical. Although cyst enterostomy or partial cyst excision were widely practiced in the past, the contemporary mandate is complete surgical excision of the cyst wall with biliary reconstruction. With modern surgical techniques, complete cyst excision is almost always possible, with acceptable morbidity and no mortality. In older children and adults with long-standing inflammation of the cyst wall, a plane can be developed between the inner and outer linings of the cyst wall, and the outer lining can be left behind on the associated hilar structures. In most cases, the entire cyst wall can be excised, and a safe plane can be established between the outer cyst wall and the portal vein and hepatic artery. This dissection is facilitated by taking the gallbladder down first and developing the plane at the hilum. The duct should be divided proximally and the distal dissection performed under direct vision to facilitate recognition of a high insertion of the pancreatic duct. The common duct is oversewn just above the pancreatic duct to ensure that no residual stump of cyst wall remains. Biliary reconstruction can be performed by Roux-en-Y hepaticojejunostomy or by interposing a segment of jejunum on its mesentery between the hepatic duct and the duodenum. In either case, an intussusception of the drainage conduit can be surgically constructed to prevent reflux of intestinal content into the hilum. Important technical considerations include performing the biliary enteric anastomosis above the proximal extent of the cyst in a mucosa-to-mucosa, end-to-side fashion, using fine absorbable suture. In cases in which the hepatic duct is minimally dilated, a wide anastomosis can be ensured by incising the hepatic ducts laterally. No stents or drains are routinely necessary. In selected cases of ampullary stenosis or stricture, with or without obstructing stones or sludge, a transduodenal sphincteroplasty may also be necessary to prevent pancreatitis.

Caroli disease and choledochocele require special consideration. If the cysts in Caroli disease are confined to one liver lobe, then hepatic lobectomy is curative. Otherwise, treatment is palliative, and liver transplantation may be required. In addition, there may be associated congenital hepatic fibrosis or hepatobiliary fibropolycystic disease, which can further complicate management. Choledochocele is treated by transduodenal unroofing of the choledochocele, with sphincteroplasty of the pancreatic and common bile ducts. Successful endoscopic drainage of choledochoceles has been reported, but the endoscopic approach requires further experience and follow-up.

Results

Earlier series using cystenterostomy were complicated by high rates of anastomotic stricture, recurrent cholangitis and pancreatitis, bleeding, portal hypertension, and malignancy. Recent series employing cyst excision report minimal morbidity and mortality and few late complications. Anastomotic stricture is the most common late complication. Development of carcinoma in residual intrahepatic ducts has been reported after cyst excision and remains a concern that requires long-term follow-up, particularly in patients with type IV disease.

Spontaneous Perforation of the Bile Ducts

Although rare, spontaneous perforation of the common bile duct is second only to biliary atresia as a cause of surgically correctable jaundice in neonates. The perforation always occurs anteriorly on the common bile duct at the junction of the common bile duct and cystic duct, but the pathogenesis remains speculative. Although the consistent location suggests a developmental weakness in the duct wall at that position, normal common bile ducts from neonatal autopsies blow out at this position with increased intraluminal pressure, suggesting that obstruction may play a role. Distal common duct obstruction by stones or sludge has been described in one fourth of reported cases, and it is conceivable that obstructing stones passed or floated out of the perforation site in others. Age at presentation ranges from 1 week to 4 years and 5 months of age, but most patients present between 2 and 6 weeks of age. Clinical presentation is variable, but the diagnosis should be suspected in the presence of jaundice and ascites. The disease can follow a chronic, subacute, or acute course, with varying degrees of peritonitis, fever, intestinal obstruction, sepsis, and cardiorespiratory collapse. Diagnosis may be suspected at ultrasound if subhepatic fluid collections are identified, or abdominal paracentesis may reveal bile-stained fluid, but the best diagnostic study is hepatobiliary scintigraphy, which documents extravasation of bile into the peritoneal cavity.

Treatment is surgical. Findings at the time of exploration are usually of sterile bilious ascites or a loculated bile pseudocyst with a 1- to 3-mm perforation of the common bile duct at the junction, with the cystic duct and varying degrees of ductal and serosal inflammation. Cholangiography may reveal distal common duct obstruction, and sludge or small stones are frequently found either in the bile duct or floating outside the duct. Regardless of the presence or absence of distal obstruction, simple external drainage of the periductal area is all that is required for successful treatment. A cholecystostomy tube should be left in cases of distal obstruction or marked ductal inflammation. If the duct is relatively normal, it is reasonable to close the perforation transversely with fine absorbable sutures. Results of this approach have been excellent, with uniform resolution of distal ductal obstruction. Healing of the duct and the status of distal obstruction can be followed by cholangiography through the cholecystostomy tube, and the tube can be removed when healing is complete and the duct is open. More extensive surgical procedures, such as choledochoduodenostomy, have resulted in higher morbidity rates and occasional mortality.

Bile Duct Tumors

Most bile duct tumors occur after childhood, but they must be included in the differential diagnosis of any child with obstructive jaundice. Presentation is variable, with symptoms of either biliary cholic or painless jaundice. Cholangiocarcinoma occurs in children primarily in association with choledochal cysts. The incidence begins to increase sharply in the third and fourth decade of life, but cases have been reported in patients as young as 12 years of age. The most common primary malignant tumor of the extrahepatic bile ducts in children is rhabdomyosarcoma. The average age of presentation is 4.5 years, 40% have local or distant metastasis at the time of diagnosis, and the average survival time is 6 months. Because complete resection is often technically difficult, treatment should include adjuvant chemotherapy and radiotherapy.

Benign obstructive tumors of the biliary tract are also extremely rare. The histologic type is usually determined after extensive resection for presumed malignancy. Neoplasms include localized hemangioendotheliomas, heterotopic gastric mucosa, benign inflammatory tumors, and biliary granular cell tumors. Resection is curative.

Primary Disorders of the Gallbladder

Gallbladder Hydrops and Acalculous Cholecystitis

Gallbladder hydrops and acute cholecystitis are probably related disorders that occur in the setting of serious systemic disease. Hydrops is classically described as acute, massive dilation of the gallbladder without wall thickening or biliary infection. The most common cause of hydrops is the mucocutaneous lymph node syndrome, also known as Kawasaki disease. About 3% to 5% of patients with mucocutaneous lymph node syndrome develop gallbladder hydrops. The syndrome is recognized by the association of prolonged fever, lymphadenopathy, conjunctivitis and polyarteritis, red mouth and cracked lips, red and swollen palms that peel, and polymorphous rash. Hydrops usually presents as the development of a right upper quadrant mass and pain within the first 2 weeks of the disease but can precede other diagnostic manifestations of the syndrome. The

course is usually benign, indicating an initial conservative management approach, but it can progress to gangrene and perforation, necessitating cholecystectomy or cholecystostomy. Findings in resected specimens suggest vasculitis as the inciting cause. Hydrops has also been described in scarlet fever, Mediterranean fever, and a variety of other systemic diseases.

Acalculous cholecystitis is generally reported as a more fulminant disease that usually occurs during the course of other severe diseases, such as septicemia, bacterial endocarditis, mycoplasma sepsis, typhoid fever, and salmonellosis. Occasionally, it has been described postoperatively, particularly after spinal fusions. On ultrasound, the gallbladder wall is markedly thickened, and the gallbladder contains debris. There can be pericholecystic fluid collections, suggesting perforation. The clinical course is more aggressive than hydrops, with frequent evolution to gangrene and perforation. Bile may be culture-positive. Treatment is surgical if there is progressive gall bladder distention or if clinical deterioration occurs. Cholecystectomy is the preferred procedure.

Miscellaneous Gallbladder Disorders

Anatomic disorders of the gallbladder range from agenesis to duplication. Surgically significant but extremely rare disorders of the gallbladder include septate gallbladder, heterotopic gastric mucosa of the gallbladder, polyposis of the gallbladder associated with metachromatic leukodystrophy, and porcelain gallbladder. These problems usually present as chronic abdominal pain and are treated by cholecystectomy.

DISORDERS OF BILE COMPOSITION OR FLOW

Cholestasis and Cholelithiasis

Cholelithiasis is no longer a rare diagnosis in childhood, and in the estimation of many investigators, the incidence is increasing. In contrast to common perception, a significant portion of gallstones in children are idiopathic—that is, they are not associated with underlying disease. The remainder, however, are associated with predisposing conditions that result in cholelithiasis, either indirectly through chronic illness, fasting, and secondary cholestasis, or directly through alterations of bile composition. Predisposing factors that may at least in part account for the observed increase in cholelithiasis include the following:

- Common use of total parenteral nutrition in fasting premature infants
- Increase in incidence of necrotizing enterocolitis requiring ileal resection
- More frequent use of lithogenic medications
- Improved medical treatment and longer survival of patients with hemolytic disease
- Increase in adolescent pregnancy

Pathogenesis

The pathogenesis of cholelithiasis in children is multifactorial and differs according to age at presentation (Fig. 87-4). In in-

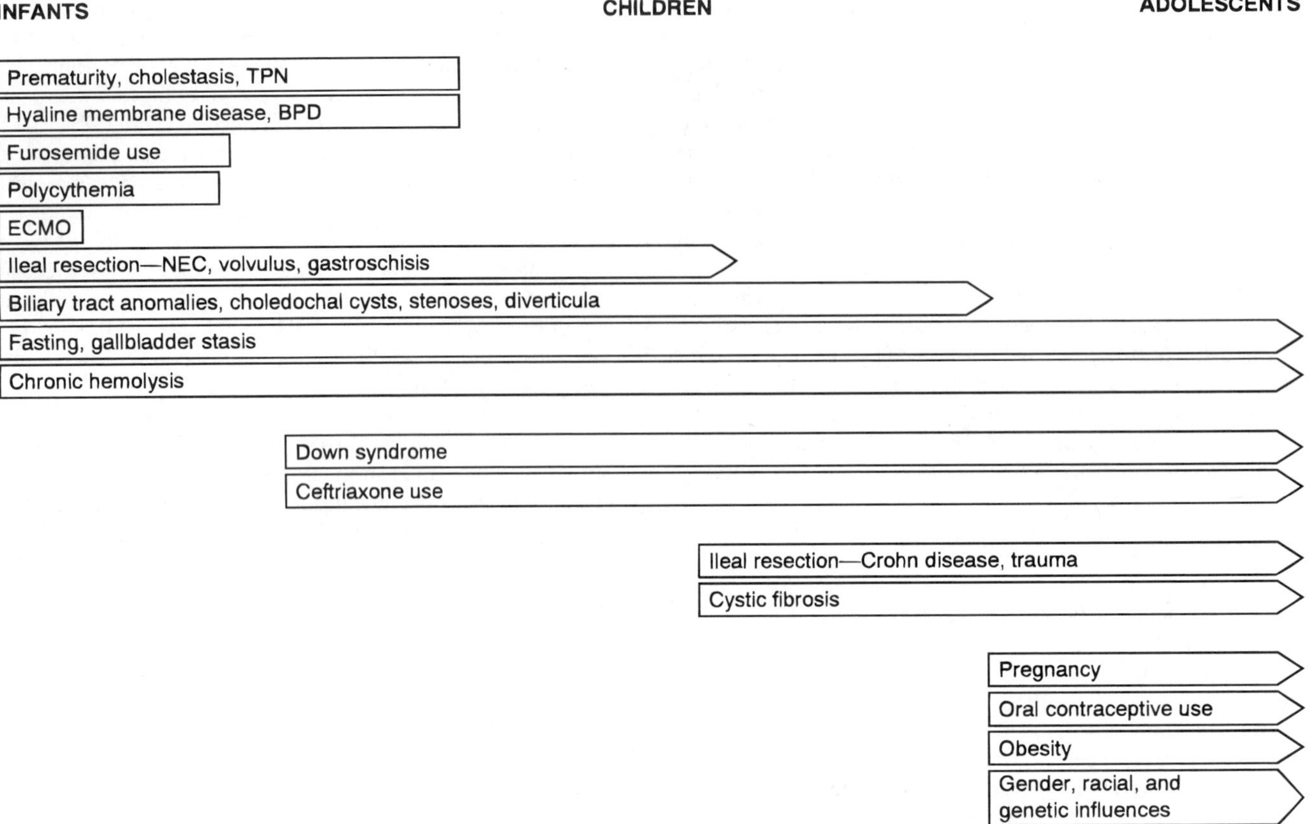

FIG. 87-4. Predisposition to cholelithiasis at different stages of maturation. TPN, total parenteral nutrition; BPD, bronchopulmonary dysplasia; NEC, necrotizing enterocolitis.

fants, the normal immaturity of hepatic excretory function and the enterohepatic circulation lower the threshold for stone formation when combined with other lithogenic influences. These include total parenteral alimentation and fasting, dehydration, furosemide treatment, ileal resection related to nectrotizing enterocolitis or volvulus, biliary tract anomalies, and polycythemia. In this age group, cholestasis can manifest as liver functional abnormality, as biliary sludge, or as true cholelithiasis and is directly related to duration of fasting. The ultrasonographic evolution of sludge to sludge balls to stones has been well documented and is presumably related to absence of gallbladder contraction. In the prepubertal child, stones are more likely to be idiopathic or related to chronic hemolysis, cystic fibrosis, ileal resection or disease, or ceftriaxone therapy. In this age group, stone composition is usually predominantly calcium bilirubinate or calcium carbonate, and the sex incidence is equal. After puberty, as in the adult population, stones are more likely to be predominantly cholesterol, and an increased female/male incidence ratio is seen. Racial and genetic influences, obesity, oral contraceptives, and pregnancy are also more frequent predisposing factors in this age group.

The composition of gallstones is variable and offers a clue to their pathogenesis. Primary types of gallstones include predominantly cholesterol, pigment, or calcium carbonate stones. Cholesterol stones result from cholesterol saturation of bile, followed by a process of nucleation and stone growth. Cholesterol is virtually insoluble in bile and is made soluble by one of two mechanisms. The first is formation of bile acid–lecithin–cholesterol mixed micelles. Although once thought to be the primary mechanism, probably only about 30% of total bile cholesterol is transported in micelles. Most cholesterol is transported in vesicular form. These vesicles are composed of phospholipid bilayers similar to cell membranes and can transport more cholesterol than micelles. The saturation and precipitation of bile cholesterol is believed to depend primarily on the stability of these structures. *Nucleation* refers to the process of crystallization and macroscopic agglomeration of cholesterol. Bile from people without gallstones frequently contains cholesterol crystals, and the factors that promote nucleation are poorly understood. The process of nucleation is much more rapid in bile from patients with cholesterol stones than from patients without stones, but with a similar degree of cholesterol saturation. Pronucleation factors that may be important in gallstone patients include specific heat-labile glycoproteins, calcium, gallbladder stasis, and altered gallbladder absorption. Bile generally does not become saturated with cholesterol until after puberty, when most stones that are predominantly cholesterol are seen.

Pigment stones presumably are due to abnormal solubilization of unconjugated bilirubin with precipitation of calcium bilirubinate and insoluble salts. β-Glucuronidase is required to hydrolyze bilirubin glucuronide to free bilirubin and glucuronic acid. Free bilirubin can then combine with calcium to form a calcium–bilirubinate matrix, which is the primary component of most pigment stones. β-Glucuronidase is released by bacteria, and an endogenous form of it has been identified in human bile. Thus, pigment stone formation may be favored by circumstances of biliary tract infection, conjugated bilirubin excess, and stasis.

Clinical Presentation

Clinical presentation also depends on age. Stones are frequently asymptomatic in all age groups and detected on evaluation for other problems. Diagnosis in infancy requires clinical suspicion because the presentation is nonspecific and sometimes subtle. Hyperbilirubinemia is common in infancy, but persistence of direct hyperbilirubinemia should lead to an evaluation of the biliary tract, including evaluation for cholelithiasis. Jaundice and fever in infants with any of the predisposing factors mentioned earlier should prompt evaluation for stones. In older children, the presenting complaint is almost always abdominal pain. Younger children may not be able to localize abdominal pain; older children have more typical right upper quadrant or subscapular pain. Diagnosis is often delayed because of a lack of suspicion in children and an absence of predisposing conditions. Evaluation of children with recurrent unexplained abdominal pain should include an evaluation for biliary disease. Obviously, abdominal pain in patients with chronic hemolysis or other predisposing factors should prompt immediate biliary evaluation. Presentation in the postpubertal population is similar to that in adults. Pain is usually dull and subcostal in location, sometimes with radiation to the subscapular region. Fatty food intolerance with associated nausea and vomiting may be present. Biliary pancreatitis or cholangitis are relatively infrequent presentations in children but are more common in patients with sickle cell anemia.

Diagnosis

Most gallstones in children are radiolucent, and ultrasonography is the diagnostic modality of choice. In fact, the prenatal diagnosis of biliary sludge and stones by ultrasound has been reported as early as 26 weeks' gestation. Ultrasound diagnosis of stones requires the presence of movable, echogenic structures within the gallbladder, with associated shadowing. Sludge is a fluid substance consisting of calcium bilirubinate, which on ultrasound examination can be seen layering out in the dependent portion of the gallbladder. This results in low-amplitude echoes without acoustic shadowing, although the ultrasonic differential diagnosis of sludge from multiple small stones may be difficult. Ultrasound findings of an impacted stone at the ampulla, associated gall bladder wall thickening, or localized pericholecystic fluid support the clinical diagnosis of acute cholecystitis. Common bile duct dilation suggests choledocholithiasis, although ultrasound is insensitive for the presence of choledocholithiasis. Confirmatory ERCP or operative or transhepatic cholangiography may be required. Biliary scintigraphy can be helpful in confirming cystic duct or common duct obstruction, but false-positive diagnoses are common in fasting patients without biliary disease.

Treatment

Symptomatic or complicated cholelithiasis is treated with cholecystectomy. Laparoscopic cholecystectomy has become the standard of practice in adults for acute or chronic cholecystitis. The increasing experience with this procedure in children suggests that it is equally applicable in both populations. In experienced hands, the laparoscopic approach has been well documented to reduce the discomfort, length of hospitalization, cost, and morbidity associated with cholecystectomy. Indications for open cholecystectomy include multiple previous abdominal procedures, pregnancy, and the inability to adequately visualize the anatomy at laparoscopy. Cholangiography should always be performed in the presence of a dilated cystic or common duct, multiple small stones, or jaundice. Choledocholithiasis can be treated by common duct exploration or endoscopic sphincterotomy. Chemical stone dissolution, mechanical disruption, shock-wave lithotripsy, or combinations of these are occasionally successful in selected patients; however, given the success of laparoscopic cholecystectomy, these procedures are rarely indicated in children.

Treatment of patients who do not have symptoms is controversial and depends on age and associated disease. The prenatal diagnosis of biliary sludge or stones appears to be benign. In most patients, the ultrasound findings resolved after birth; in no reported case did the stones become clinically symptomatic. Simple observation is recommended to allow a better understanding of the natural history of this relatively unknown entity. Several researchers have reported spontaneous resolution of asymptomatic gallstones diagnosed in infants from 2 weeks to 6 months after their initial discovery. For this reason, cholecystectomy should be reserved for patients with persistence of gallstones for more than 12 months or for patients with radiopaque gallstones that are unlikely to resolve. In contrast, patients with cholelithiasis secondary to chronic hemolytic disease who initially do not have symptoms frequently develop symptoms and present with complications. Because of the significant risk of emergency surgery and sepsis in this group, most authors advocate elective cholecystectomy. Patients with cystic fibrosis rarely have biliary complications and should be treated nonoperatively until symptoms develop. Older children without symptoms differ from adults without symptoms in that they have many more years for complications to develop. It is therefore reasonable to offer cholecystectomy to any child who has persistent or enlarged stones after 6 to 12 months of observation. The laparoscopic approach is particularly applicable to patients with relatively normal gallbladders and no symptoms.

BIBLIOGRAPHY

Bishop WP, Kao SCS. Prolonged postprandial abdominal pain following Kawasaki syndrome with acute gallbladder hydrops: association with impaired gallbladder emptying. J Pediatr Gastroenterol Nutr 1991;13:307.

Bucavalis JC. Bile acid metabolism during development. In: Polin RA, Fox WW, eds. Fetal and neonatal physiology. Philadelphia, WB Saunders, 1992:1137.

Debray D, Pariente D, Gauthier F, et al. Cholelithiasis in infancy: a study of 40 cases. 1993;122:385.

Haller JO. Sonography of the biliary tract in infants and children. AJR 1991;157:1051.

Joyce AD, Howard ER. Hepatobiliary tumours of childhood: investigation and management. Prog Pediatr Surg 1989;22:69.

Komi N, Tamura T, Miyoshi Y, et al. Histochemical and immunohistochemical studies on development of biliary carcinoma in forty-seven patients with choledochal cyst: special reference to intestinal metaplasia in the biliary duct. Jpn J Surg 1985;15:273.

Komi N, Takehara H, Kunitomo K, et al. Does the type of anomalous arrangement of pancreaticobiliary ducts influence the surgery and prognosis of choledochal cyst? J Pediatr Surg 1992;27:728.

Megison SM, Votteler TP. Management of common bile duct obstruction associated with spontaneous perforation of the biliary tree. Surgery 1992;111:237.

Okada A, Nakamura T, Higaki J, et al. Congenital dilatation of the bile duct in 100 instances and its relationship with anomalous junction. Surg Gynecol Obstet 1990;171:291.

Quigley EMM, Marsh MN, Shaffer JL, et al. Hepatobiliary complications of total parenteral nutrition. Gastroenterology 1993;104:286.

Reif S, Sloven DG, Lebenthal EL. Gallstones in children. Am J Dis Child 1991;145:105.

Rosenthal P. Bilirubin metabolism in the fetus and neonate. In: Polin RA, Fox WW, eds. Fetal and neonatal physiology. Philadelphia, WB Saunders, 1992:1154.

Schweizer P, Schweizer M. Pancreaticobiliary long common channel syndrome and congenital anomalous dilatation of the choledochal duct: study of 46 patients. Eur J Pediatr Surg 1993;3:15.

Shirai Z, Toriya H, Maeshiro K, et al. The usefulness of endoscopic retrograde cholangiopancreatography in infants and small children. Am J Gastroenterol 1993;88:536.

Watkins JB. Neonatal cholestasis: developmental aspects and current concepts. Semin Liver Dis 1993;13:276.

Surgery of Infants and Children: Scientific Principles and Practice, edited by Keith T. Oldham, Paul M. Colombani, and Robert P. Foglia. Lippincott–Raven Publishers, Philadelphia, © 1997.

CHAPTER 88

Pancreas

Craig Lillehei

The pancreas is a central metabolic organ with key roles in both exocrine and endocrine function. Its proximity to the biliary and gastrointestinal (GI) tracts has important consequences when disease arises.

EMBRYOLOGY

The dorsal pancreatic primordium is first recognized during the fourth week of gestation as an outpouching from the dorsal duodenum. Shortly thereafter, the ventral pancreatic primordium arises from the base of the hepatic diverticulum (Fig. 88-1). With duodenal rotation, there is fusion of these two primordia and their ductal elements by the seventh week of gestation. The ventral primordium gives rise to the head and uncinate process, whereas the dorsal primordium develops into the body and tail. The main pancreatic duct of Wirsung is formed by fusion of the ventral duct with the distal dorsal duct. It drains into the duodenum with the common bile duct at the ampulla of Vater. The proximal dorsal duct may persist as the accessory duct of Santorini, draining through an independent entry into the more proximal duodenum. Secretory acini develop from the epithelial cords during the third month of gestation. The islets of Langerhans are recognized as independent derivatives of these acini by the end of the third month.[1]

ANATOMY

The pancreas is a retroperitoneal organ of the upper abdomen that extends from its head, closely applied within the duodenal concavity, to the tail at the splenic hilum.

The splenic artery supplies the body and tail of the gland and lies along its superior border. The pancreatic head is supplied by parallel branches from the gastroduodenal artery and the superior pancreaticoduodenal arteries, which lie in front and behind the gland. These vessels join with the inferior pancreaticoduodenal vessels arising from the superior mesenteric artery. The pancreaticoduodenal arteries thereby support both the pancreatic head and duodenum. Pancreatic veins drain directly into the splenic vein, which passes behind the body of the gland to join the superior mesenteric vein forming the portal vein.[2]

The uncinate process is an extension of the head that protrudes behind the superior mesenteric vessels. The pancreatic ductal system is variable, depending on the embryologic fusion of the dorsal and ventral ducts. This is discussed below.

Operative assessment of the pancreas can be obtained in several ways. Surgical exposure of the pancreatic head is facilitated by a Kocher maneuver of the duodenum. The ventral surface of the body and tail is accessed by an opening into the lesser sac.

PHYSIOLOGY

Exocrine

The pancreas is the primary source of digestive enzymes. More than 20 different enzymes are synthesized in the rough endoplasmic reticulum and stored within zymogen granules of the secretory acini. The pancreas actually secretes more protein than any other gland in the body except the lactating mammary gland.[3]

The proteolytic enzymes such as trypsin, chymotrypsin, and carboxypeptidase are secreted as inactive proenzymes. On entering the duodenum, they are converted to active enzymes when enterokinase, an intestinal brush-border enzyme, splits off a peptide component. These active proteolytic enzymes may in turn activate more proenzymes. Pancreatic lipase and amylase, in contrast, are secreted in their active forms.

The secretory acinar cells are under complex neural and hormonal regulation. The pancreas is responsive to stimulation of the vagus nerve. This cephalic phase of digestion is mediated by acetylcholine. Cholecystokinin, formerly known as pancreozymin, is a polypeptide hormone that mediates the intestinal phase and causes discharge of the zymogen granules from acinar cells. It is released from the duodenal mucosa in response to luminal amino acids and fatty acids. Feedback regulation is provided by pancreatic proteases within the duodenum.

The ducts that drain the acini are lined by centroacinar and ductular cells. These cells secrete water and bicarbonate. Secretin is a polypeptide hormone released by the duodenal mucosa in response to acid within the lumen. It stimulates fluid and bicarbonate secretion, which raises intestinal pH and thereby facilitates pancreatic enzyme activity.[4]

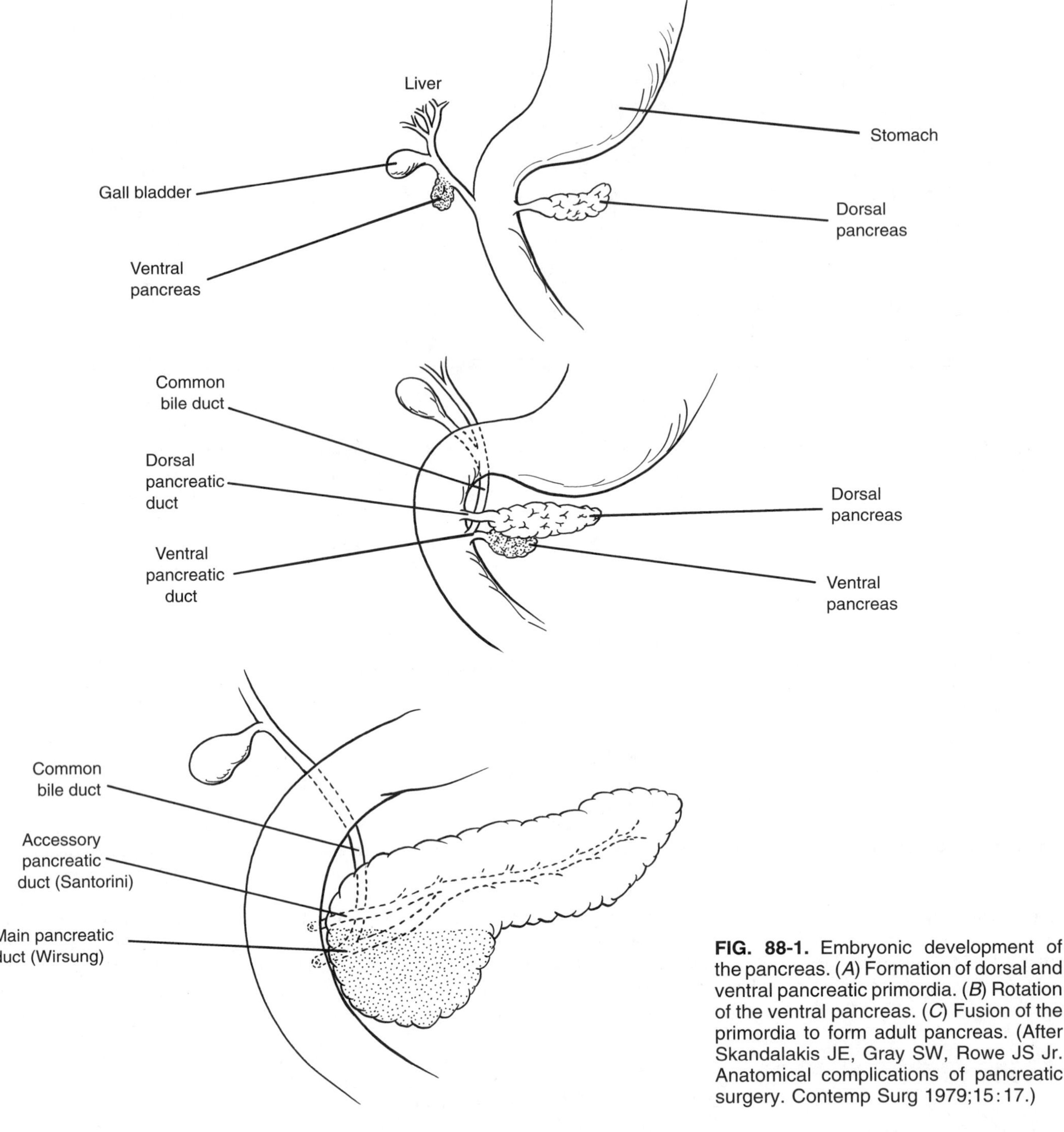

FIG. 88-1. Embryonic development of the pancreas. (*A*) Formation of dorsal and ventral pancreatic primordia. (*B*) Rotation of the ventral pancreas. (*C*) Fusion of the primordia to form adult pancreas. (After Skandalakis JE, Gray SW, Rowe JS Jr. Anatomical complications of pancreatic surgery. Contemp Surg 1979;15:17.)

Evidence of maldigestion is seen only after dramatic (more than 90%) reduction of pancreatic exocrine function. Whereas neonates are born with nearly normal capacity for protein digestion, secretion of amylase and lipase do not reach adult levels until after the first year of life.[5]

Endocrine

The pancreas has an essential role in the hormonal regulation of metabolism and glucose homeostasis. These endocrine func-tions are provided by the islets of Langerhans. Approximately 1% to 2% of the pancreatic mass is comprised by the 1 to 2 million islets. Although present throughout the gland, the islets are more plentiful in the pancreatic tail.[6] The islets are vascular and richly innervated with both sympathetic and parasympathetic fibers. Four distinct cell types are recognized within islets. The α cells are responsible for glucagon production, β cells for insulin, δ cells for somatostatin, and PP cells for pancreatic polypeptide. The β cells form the central core of the islets. The islets appear to respond to both systemic and local (paracrine) influences. Insulin secretion is stimulated by glucagon, whereas glucagon secretion is suppressed by insulin. Somatostatin inhibits both insulin and glucagon secretion.

Insulin is synthesized as a proinsulin molecule. It is converted to active insulin after cleavage of a 33 amino acid portion, termed C peptide. With exocytosis from the cytoplasmic granules, both insulin and C peptide are released into the circulation. Since C peptide is poorly metabolized by the liver, it is a useful indicator of endogenous insulin secretion.

Serum glucose concentration is the primary stimulus for insulin secretion. However, it is also affected by hormonal, neuronal, and biochemical influences. Insulin promotes glucose storage (as glycogen or fat) and protein synthesis by its actions on muscle, liver, and adipose tissue.

Glucagon also responds to glucose concentration by causing increased glycogenolysis and gluconeogenesis.[6]

CONGENITAL ANOMALIES

Annular pancreas arises from interference with free rotation of the ventral pancreatic anlage. The differential diagnosis of antenatal duodenal obstruction should include an annular pancreas. It may be associated with Down syndrome, malrotation, or intrinsic duodenal obstruction.[7] Presentation in infancy usually is secondary to duodenal obstruction, whereas adults are more likely to present with pain or peptic ulceration.[8] Presentation may occur in the first several days of life with a complete duodenal obstruction and a ''double bubble'' sign indicating no passage of material beyond the duodenum. In other cases, obstruction may not develop for several days or weeks. Alternatively, some patients may remain asymptomatic. Surgical treatment of symptomatic patients is achieved with a side–side duodenoduodenostomy or duodenojejunostomy. No attempt is made to divide the pancreatic tissue as this does not reverse underlying abnormalities intrinsic to the duodenum and it also leads to injury of the pancreatic duct.

Ectopic or *heterotopic pancreas* is seen in 1% to 2% of autopsy series.[9] Most cases involve the upper GI tract, which is consistent with the pancreatic origin from the foregut. However, ectopic pancreas may occur anywhere along the GI tract or, rarely, in extraintestinal locations.[10] Most lesions are asymptomatic, but local inflammation with pain, bleeding, or ulceration are the most common symptoms and are seen in Meckel's diverticulum and intestinal duplication.

Pancreatic agenesis, *hypoplasia*, or *dysplasia* may account for malabsorption if less than 5% of functional pancreas remains. Distinction between these lesions may be made by ultrasound or computed tomographic (CT) examination of the pancreas since, in contrast to agenesis, the pancreatic size is normal in the hypoplasia or dysplasia syndromes.[11] Examples of such latter inherited exocrine deficiencies include the Schwachman-Diamond and Johanson-Blizzard syndromes.

Cystic fibrosis is the most frequent lethal genetic disease in North America (see Chapter 71). It is inherited as an autosomal recessive trait and occurs in approximately 1 in 2500 live births, suggesting a carrier frequency rate of almost 5%. It primarily affects secreting epithelial cells. Although its clinical presentation may be variable, pancreatic insufficiency with malabsorption and steatorrhea is encountered in most patients. Exogenous pancreatic exocrine replacement corrects this problem. Flareups of pancreatitis can be seen in these patients. Treatment consists of adjusting the amount of pancreatic enzyme that is given.

Pancreas divisum is a ductal anomaly of the pancreas. In 5% to 10% of patients, the dorsal and ventral pancreatic ducts fail to fuse, resulting in separate and distinct ductal drainage.[12] The dorsal pancreatic duct drains through the proximal accessory papilla, whereas the ventral duct drains with the common bile duct at the ampulla of Vater. Although patients with this anatomic arrangement may be entirely asymptomatic, coexistent stenosis or dysfunction at the minor papilla may produce pancreatic disease typically presenting as recurrent acute pancreatitis.[13] Other ductal anomalies include a common channel of pancreaticobiliary secretion in which the pancreatic duct enters the common bile duct 5 to 15 mm proximal to the ampulla. This arrangement can predispose to pancreatitis or choledochal cysts.[14] Appropriate treatment may consist of sphincteroplasty. In the case of a concomitant choledochal cyst, treatment includes excision of the choledochal cyst with duct–enteric drainage. With closure of the distal common bile duct, pancreatic drainage flows directly into the duodenum.

CLINICAL PRESENTATION

Pancreatitis

Pancreatitis is an important but uncommon cause of abdominal pain in children.[15] Although there are a variety of classifications, the simple distinction between acute and chronic pancreatitis is useful. Many different etiologies have been identified including traumatic, structural, metabolic, infectious, and idiopathic causes. In adults, gallstones or alcohol abuse are responsible for most cases. However, in children, trauma is the leading cause, all too often the result of child abuse.

Acute pancreatitis can be defined by a combination of clinical symptoms (abdominal pain, tenderness, ileus, guarding) and biochemical abnormalities (elevation of amylase and lipase); diagnostic imaging studies can show if pancreatic inflammation is present. The typical clinical presentation of acute pancreatitis is abdominal pain, characteristically epigastric and constant, radiating to the midback. However, the historical specifics may not be evident in young children. Fever, nausea, and vomiting often accompany the discomfort.

The physical examination is remarkable for abdominal distension and tenderness, which may mimic visceral perforation. Rarely, a mass is palpable. In severe episodes, signs of hypovolemic shock may be seen. Measurements of serum and urinary amylase and lipase remain the most useful biochemical tests to confirm the diagnosis. Although less sensitive than amylase, elevations of serum lipase are most specific and remain elevated longer.[16] Secondary laboratory abnormalities may include hemoconcentration, leukocytosis, hypocalcemia, coagulopathy, hyperglycemia, and elevated liver function tests.

Imaging of the pancreas is integral to the delineation of the cause of the abnormality. Ultrasound examination is noninvasive and widely available. If overlying bowel gas does not interfere, it allows visualization of parenchymal edema and ductal dilatation. Pancreatic pseudocysts or associated biliary disease, such as gallstones or a choledochal cyst, may be identified. Computerized tomography scanning is useful to further define the degree of parenchymal destruction or abscess formation (Fig. 88-2). Although endoscopic retrograde cholangiopancreatography may itself pose a risk for pancreatitis in the acute setting, this study offers the best visualization of ductal anomalies.

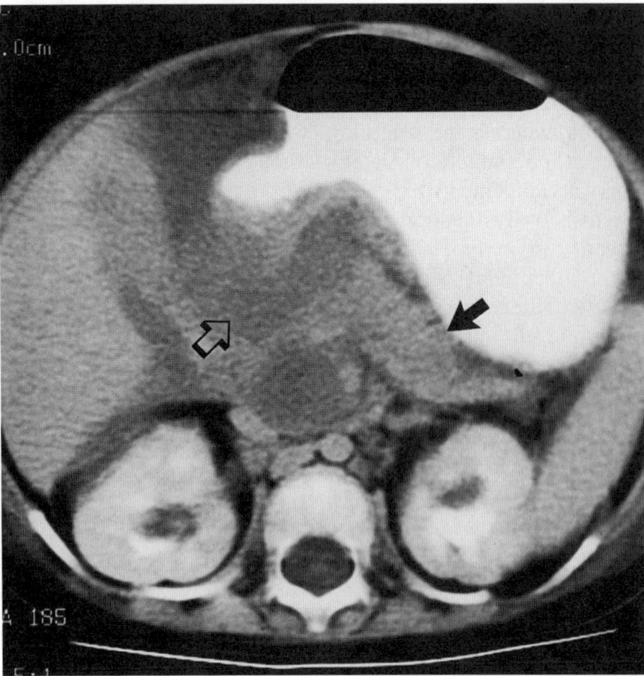

FIG. 88-2. Abdominal CT scan with contrast in a child with severe acute pancreatitis demonstrating thickened distal pancreas (*solid arrow*) and necrotic lucent head of pancreas (*open arrow*).

The exact pathophysiologic mechanism of pancreatitis remains unclear.[17] The injury seems to be caused by disordered release and activation of various enzymes including trypsin, chymotrypsin, elastase, phospholipase, and carboxypeptidase. These enzymes cause autodestruction of the pancreas. The molecular mechanisms for the activation of each of these enzymes is not well defined. However, several routes seem to reach similar endpoints (Table 88-1). The injury may range from edema to hemorrhage or frank necrosis. Proteolytic and other digestive enzymes appear to be activated within the parenchyma producing a local, and occasional systemic, inflammatory response. Trypsin plays a central role in initiating the inflammatory process. Small amounts of this enzyme may activate the elastases, phospholipases, and products of the kallikrein system responsible for the cellular damage. Mechanisms that ordinarily protect the gland from autodigestion are the production of inactive pro-

TABLE 88-1. *Causes of acute pancreatitis*

Anatomic
   Trauma
   Ductal obstruction
   Reflux
Metabolic
   Drugs
   Cystic fibrosis
   Hyperlipidemia
   Diabetes
Systemic
   Sepsis
   Shock
Idiopathic

enzymes, storage of digestive enzymes within zymogen granules, and the presence of protease inhibitors.

The role of ductal obstruction and bile reflux continues to be controversial. Several metabolic causes for acute pancreatitis have been outlined. Hyperlipidemia is much more strongly associated with pancreatitis in adults than in children. In cystic fibrosis, the lack of adequate secretory fluid flow through the pancreatic ducts may predispose to protein precipitation, ductal injury, and the clinical picture of pancreatitis. Many drugs have been associated with pancreatitis. In most cases, a relation with a drug is noted but a specific mechanism is not defined. Drugs known to cause pancreatic inflammation include valproic acid, furosemide, L-asparaginase, 6-mercaptopurine, sulfonamides, and estrogens. Possible relations have been shown with steroids, nonsteroidal antiinflammatory drugs, and azathioprine. In most cases, discontinuing the medication resolves the pancreatitis.

The management of acute pancreatitis primarily is supportive medical therapy, including intravenous hydration and bowel rest. Although no controlled clinical trials in children have demonstrated the efficacy of gastric decompression, most patients are managed with taking nothing orally, and nasogastric drainage often is used to lessen pancreatic stimulation. Careful monitoring of electrolytes, glucose, calcium, and hemoglobin levels is essential. Parenteral nutrition may be required in severe or prolonged bouts of inflammation. Further supportive care may be necessitated, depending on the degree of pancreatic and extrapancreatic organ involvement. Specific treatments aimed to lessen the process of pancreatic autodigestion have not proven effective.

Early recognition of a specific cause is important. Acute interventions may be required for such problems as ductal disruption, an impacted stone, or a potentiating medication. Alternatively, specific anatomic or pathologic conditions may be identified that require future surgical correction to prevent recurrent injury. Surgical intervention usually is reserved for the complications of pancreatitis, namely, hemorrhage, necrosis, pseudocyst, or ductal fistula.

The management of pancreatic pseudocysts remains controversial. Clearly, some pseudocysts resolve spontaneously. Therefore, unless associated problems develop, a trial of observation with sequential cyst measurement is warranted. However, these lesions must be distinguished from other cystic disease of the pancreas. In the absence of a history of pancreatitis or abdominal trauma, a less common pancreatic cystic disease must be suspected, such as unilocular cyst, enteric duplications (Fig. 88-3), retention cyst, or cystic neoplasm. Local resection or biopsy of the cyst wall may be indicated. Internal surgical drainage into the stomach, duodenum (cyst gastrostomy or cyst duodenostomy) or, alternatively, into the small intestine using a Roux-en-Y limb is effective treatment for chronic pseudocysts. However, the role of endoscopic, radiologic, and laparoscopic techniques continues to evolve and adds to the available armamentarium.

Chronic pancreatitis consists of recurrent episodes of acute persistent abdominal pain, pancreatic insufficiency, and destruction of pancreatic tissue. The causes of chronic pancreatitis are not well defined but seem to be related to obstructive causes and those that lead to calcification in the pancreas. Chronic pancreatitis is infrequent in children, and an underlying cause should be sought. Localized anatomic disease may require re-

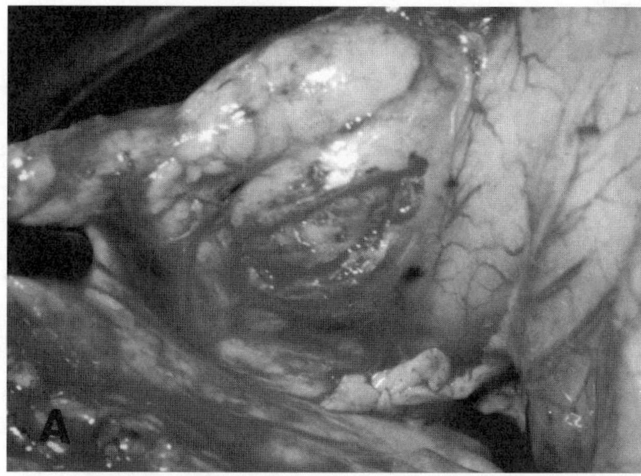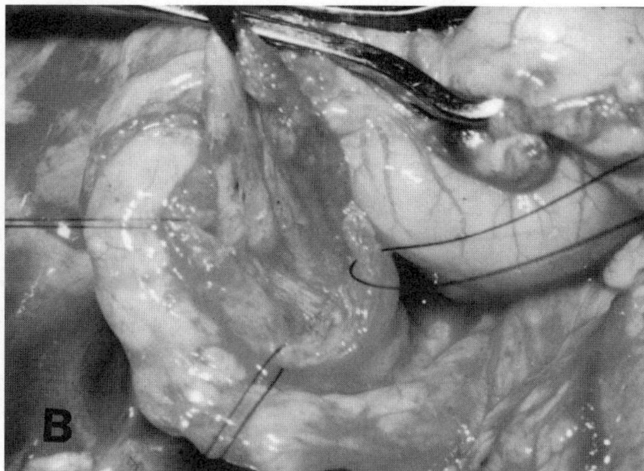

FIG. 88-3. Enteric duplication cyst within pancreatic head. (*A*) Incision into pancreas to expose cyst. (*B*) Removal of mucosal lining.

section or drainage procedures such as sphincteroplasty or lateral pancreaticojejunostomy.

Hypoglycemia

Early identification and treatment of hypoglycemia in infants and young children is essential to avoid permanent neurologic impairment. Symptoms may range from minor behavioral alterations or muscle twitching to frank seizures. Alternatively, children may be entirely asymptomatic except during acute illness.

Prompt diagnostic and treatment efforts need to overlap to minimize injury. A complete evaluation must include extrapancreatic causes for decreased glucose production.[18] Hormone deficiencies (eg, cortisol, growth hormone) or enzymatic defects (eg, glucose-6-phosphate dehydrogenase deficiency, galactosemia) should be excluded. The pancreatic causes of hypoglycemia include nesidioblastosis, islet cell adenomas, and glycogen storage disease. A diagnosis of nesidioblastosis with hyperinsulinemia can be confirmed by demonstration of high plasma insulin and C peptide relative to blood glucose. Provocative testing may be required, and several measurements are recommended to confirm the diagnosis. Simultaneous plasma measurements of free fatty acids and ketones are low because of the inhibition of lipolysis and ketogenesis by insulin. Transient neonatal hypoglycemia should be anticipated in infants who are premature, small for gestational age, born of diabetic mothers, and in those with omphaloceles or with associated Beckwith-Wiedemann syndrome.

Initial medical management is appropriate for infants with hyperinsulinemia since the likelihood of adenoma is low. Intravenous glucose infusions are used to maintain normoglycemia. Raw cornstarch or continuous gastric feedings may provide sufficient enteric glucose support. A trial of diazoxide therapy is useful to inhibit glucose-stimulated insulin secretion, mobilize glucagon, and stimulate catecholamine release. Somatostatin also inhibits insulin release, and analogues such as octreotide have been used for prolonged treatment.[19] Nonetheless, if normoglycemia cannot be maintained, surgical intervention is warranted.

Debate continues as to the pathologic characterization of neo-

natal hyperinsulinemic states. The distinctions between nesidioblastosis, hyperplasia, adenomatosis, or dysplasia may be more apparent than real.[20] Islet cell adenomas can be identified preoperatively by ultrasound, CT scanning, or a vascular blush on angiography. These tumors often are small, difficult to visualize, and islet cell adenomas often are multicentric. Intraoperative ultrasound may be useful to localize nonpalpable adenomas.

If no ectopic or discrete pancreatic tumor is identified, subtotal pancreatectomy is warranted. A 95% pancreatectomy including removal of the uncinate process with preservation of the spleen is recommended, leaving only a narrow rim of pancreatic tissue along the duodenum.[21,22] Care must be taken to avoid injury to the common bile duct. Lesser resections have been associated with a high rate of recurrent hypoglycemia. Although the neonatal pancreas seems to have a capacity for regeneration,[23] there is developing concern regarding late risks of pancreatic insufficiency.

In patients with a glycogen storage disease, sufficient glucose reserve cannot be stored. The patient—particularly an infant—becomes hypoglycemia unless fed frequently or given a parenteral glucose-containing solution. Placing a gastrotomy tube permits nocturnal feeding to avoid the sequelae of hypoglycemia.

Pancreatic Tumors

Pancreatic tumors are rare in children. However, children's tumors display a wide variety of histologic characteristics, and the overall prognosis is actually more favorable than in adults. Patients typically present with a mass, pain, or jaundice, although functional tumors may be revealed by their hormonal effects. Ultrasonography, CT scanning, magnetic resonance imaging, and angiography are useful to characterize these lesions. Distinction from benign and more common pathologic entities such as pancreatic pseudocysts usually can be made. The exocrine pancreas rarely gives rise to benign tumors such as dermoid cysts, adenomas, or cystadenomas.[27] Therefore, most pancreatic tumors are malignant.

Needle biopsy can be used for pathologic identification but carries the risk of sampling error. Complete surgical excision, when possible, provides an accurate diagnosis and offers the best chance for long-term survival. Surgical options, even in infants, include total pancreatectomy or pancreaticoduodenectomy if indicated.

Pathologic distinction is made between tumors of the exocrine and endocrine pancreas (Table 88-2). In adults, ductal cell adenocarcinoma is responsible for more than 90% of the malignancies. Although still the most common histologic type in children, it represents less than 50% of reported cases and the prognosis is poor with this histologic finding.[28]

Other tumors have a more favorable prognosis. Pancreatoblastoma or infantile carcinoma of the pancreas is seen in children ranging from 3 weeks to 8 years of age, with a mean age at diagnosis of 4.3 years. A male preponderance is reported. Wide local excision is associated with long-term survival. The role of radiation or chemotherapy is less certain.

The endocrine tumors represent a fascinating array and larger proportion of pancreatic malignancies in children than adults. They share the cytochemical features of other neuroendocrine cells with amino precursor uptake and decarboxylation, and often are referred to as APUDomas. Complete surgical excision remains the best mode of therapy, but multicentricity is common. Since these tumors can be small and nonpalpable, intraoperative ultrasound may be useful. These tumors are generally slow growing, less aggressive, and carry a good prognosis.

The most frequent functional pancreatic tumor is the β-cell tumor or insulinoma. Unlike the other endocrine cell types, these lesions usually are benign. Hypoglycemic episodes should alert the clinician. These lesions can be treated by enucleation.

The Zollinger-Ellison syndrome has been described in children with refractory peptic ulceration and diarrhea. This results in excessive gastrin release from a gastroma. Contemporary treatment consists of the use of H_2 blockers for symptomatic treatment; surgical excision is used only selectively in children. The watery diarrhea, hypokalemia, and achlorhydria syndrome associated with excessive production of vasoactive intestinal peptide is in association with a ganglioneuroma or neuroblastoma than a pancreatic vipoma. Other functional elements of the islets may produce excessive glucagon or somatostatin.[29]

Identification of an endocrine tumor within the pancreas should alert the clinical to a possible multiple endocrine neoplasia type 1 syndrome. This complex involves tumors or hyperplasia of at least two endocrine organs including pituitary, parathyroid, or pancreas. It is inherited as an autosomal dominant feature with high penetrance. Both the patient and first-order relatives should be screened for disease.

TABLE 88-2. *Pediatric pancreatic neoplasms*

Exocrine
Ductal cell carcinoma
Nonductal carcinoma
  Acinar cell carcinoma
  Pancreatoblastoma
  Solid cyst tumor
Endocrine
  Nonfunctioning islet cell tumors
  Functioning islet cell tumors (insulinoma, glucagonoma, gastrinoma, vipoma, somatostatinoma)
Sarcoma

Diabetes Mellitus

Diabetes mellitus presenting in childhood (type I, juvenile onset) is an autoimmune disorder with destruction of functional pancreatic islets.[24] The insulin deficiency results in increased glucose production by the liver, decreased use of glucose, and breakdown of endogenous fat and protein. Hyperglycemia and glycosuria produce the classic triad of polydipsia, polyuria, and polyphagia. Less commonly, children may present with frank ketoacidosis or insidious lethargy and weakness. Although the acute effects of hyperglycemia and ketoacidosis usually can be controlled with parenteral insulin, the long-term complications of the associated microangiopathy are potentially devastating. Neuropathy, nephropathy, and retinopathy typically progress despite satisfactory glucose regulation.

Pancreatic transplantation offers the possibility of restoring precise glucose homeostasis and averting this microangiopathy. However, these benefits must be balanced against the risks of chronic immunosuppression. The initial experience with pancreatic organ transplantation has been poor secondary to allograft rejection and destructive complications produced by the exocrine secretions. However, with improved immunosuppression and the development of more reliable exocrine drainage through the bladder, successful transplantation can be accomplished. The best results are achieved with simultaneous kidney–pancreas transplantation.[25] Islet cell transplantation offers the prospect of restoring pancreatic endocrine function without the risks associated with exocrine secretions. Furthermore, the procedure itself is a more limited surgical procedure. Unfortunately, monitoring of rejection is problematic, and long-term success limited.[26] Whether diabetes mellitus will be managed in the future by more precise insulin infusions, pancreatic organ or islet transplantation, or gene therapy is controversial.

REFERENCES

1. Skandalakis LJ, Rowe JS, Gray SW, et al. Surgical embryology and anatomy of the pancreas. Surg Clin North Am 1993;73:661.
2. Warwick R, Williams PL, eds. Gray's anatomy, ed 35. Philadelphia, WB Saunders, 1973:1299.
3. Henrix TR. The secretory function of the alimentary canal. In: Mountcastle VB, ed. Medical physiology, ed 13. St Louis: CV Mosby, 1974: 1189.
4. Werlin SL. The exocrine pancreas. In: Walker WA, Duric PR, Hamilton JE, et al, eds. Pediatric gastrointestinal disease. Philadelphia, BC Decker, 1990:335.
5. Hadorn HB, Munch G. The exocrine pancreas: development physiology and disease. In: Anderson CM, Burke V, Gracey M, eds. Pediatric gastroenterology, ed 2. London: Blackwell Scientific Publications, 1987.
6. Ganong WF. Endocrine functions of the pancreas and the regulation of carbohydrate metabolism. In: Review of medical physiology. Norwalk, CT, Appleton & Lange, 1995:306.
7. Kiernan PD, ReMine SG, Kiernan PC, et al. Annular pancreas. Arch Surg 1980;115:46.
8. Merrill JR, Raffensperger JG. Pediatric annular pancreas: twenty years' experience. J Pediatr Surg 1976;11:921.
9. Strobel CT, Smith LE, Fonkalsrud EW, et al. Ectopic pancreatic tissue in the gastric antrum. J Pediatr 1978;92:586.
10. Dolan RV, ReMine WH, Dockerty MB. The fate of heterotopic pancreatic tissue: a study of 212 cases. Arch Surg 1974;109:762.
11. Winter WE, Maclaren NK, Riley WJ, et al. Congenital pancreatic hypoplasia: a syndrome of exocrine and endocrine pancreatic insufficiency. J Pediatr 1986;109:465.

12. Delhaye M, Engleholm L, Crener M. Pancreas divisum: congenital anatomical variant or anomaly? Gastroenterology 1985;89:951.
13. Warshaw AL, Simeone JF, Schapiro RH, et al. Evaluation and treatment of the dominant dorsal duct syndrome (pancreas divisum redefined). Am Surg 1983;93:634.
14. Okada A, Oguchi Y, Kamata S, et al. Common channel syndrome: diagnosis with ERCP and surgical management. Surgery 1983;93:634.
15. Weizman Z, Durie PR. Acute pancreatitis in childhood. J Pediatr 1988;113:24.
16. Steinberg WM, Goldstein SS, Davis NP, et al. Diagnostic assays in acute pancreatitis: a study of sensitivity and specificity. Ann Intern Med 1985;102:576.
17. Marshall JB. Acute pancreatitis. Arch Intern Med 1993;153:1185.
18. Villee D, Najjar S. Hypoglycemia. In: Avery ME, First LR, eds. Pediatric medicine, ed 2. Baltimore, Williams & Wilkins, 1993:1008.
19. Glaser B, Hirsh HJ, Landau H. Persistent hyperinsulinemic hypoglycemia of infancy: long-term octreotide treatment without pancreatectomy. J Pediatr 1993;123:644.
20. Davies MR. Nesidioblastosis: still an enigma. Surg Annu 1992;2:231.
21. Spitz L, Bhargava RK, Grant DB, et al. Surgical treatment of hyperinsulinaemic hypoglycemia in infancy and childhood. Arch Dis Child 1992;67:201.
22. Filler RM, Weinberg MJ, Cutz E, et al. Current status of pancreatectomy for persistent idiopathic neonatal hypoglycemia due to islet cell dysplasia. Prog Pediatr Surg 1991;26:60.
23. Schonau E, Deeg KH, Huemmer HP, et al. Pancreatic growth and function following surgical treatment of nesidioblastosis in infancy. Eur J Pediatr 1991;150:550.
24. Eisenbarth GS. Type I diabetes mellitus: a chronic autoimmune disease. N Engl J Med 1986;314:1360.
25. Sutherland DE, Moudry-Munns K, Gruessmer A. Pancreas transplant results in United Network for Organ Sharing (UNOS). In: Terasaki PI, Cecka JM, eds. Clinical transplants 1993. Los Angeles, UCLA Tissue Typing Laboratory, 1993:47.
26. Broushard BH, Rogers DG. Pancreatic and islet replacement therapy for insulin-dependent diabetes mellitus. Clin Pediatr 1993;32:258.
27. Kissane JM. Tumors of the exocrine pancreas in childhood. In: Humphrey GB, Grindey GB, Dehner LP, et al, eds. Pancreatic tumors in children. The Hague, Martinus Nijhoff, 1982:99.
28. Jaksic T, Yaman M, Thorner P, et al. A 20 year review of pediatric pancreatic tumors. J Pediatr Surg 1992;27:1315.
29. Norton JA. Neuroendocrine tumors of the pancreas and duodenum. Curr Probl Surg 1994;31:79.

SECTION G

Spleen

Surgery of Infants and Children: Scientific Principles and Practice, edited by
Keith T. Oldham, Paul M. Colombani, and Robert P. Foglia.
Lippincott–Raven Publishers, Philadelphia, © 1997.

CHAPTER 89

Spleen

Daniel L. Mollitt and Maryanne L. Dokler

EMBRYOLOGY AND ANATOMY

Normal

The spleen is unique in that it represents the only human organ
of neither midline nor bilateral origin.[1] It arises at about 5
weeks' gestation (8 mm) as a mesenchymal condensation within
the dorsal mesogastrium. With continued development and normal gastric rotation, the spleen is carried into the left upper
quadrant, where it comes to lie dorsal and superior to the stomach, with the diaphragm above and the left adrenal and kidney
posterior. It assumes a wedge or triangular shape, with a convex
parietal surface adjacent to the diaphragm and a concave visceral surface abutting the stomach, colon, and kidney (Fig. 89-
1). The leaves of the dorsal mesentery enveloping the spleen
become its peritoneum, with an inner capsule of connective
tissue containing elastic fibers covered by serous mesothelium.
An extensive network of trabeculae develops from the capsule,
dividing the splenic substance into numerous communicating
compartments. At the splenic hilum, the leaves of the dorsal
mesentery coalesce into the gastrosplenic and splenorenal ligaments, providing primary fixation as well as encompassing the
splenic pedicle. Several lesser attachments develop between the
spleen and the diaphragm, colon, and pancreas.

At birth, the spleen normally weighs 10 to 12 g and measures
about 5 cm at its greatest dimension. Growth parallels body
weight, usually reaching a maximum of 140 to 150 g at puberty
and then gradually declining.

Splenic circulation accounts for 5% of cardiac output but can
vary considerably in normal and pathologic conditions. The
splenic artery, the main arterial blood supply, arises from the
celiac trunk. Additional arterial blood is obtained from several
small branches of the left gastroepiploic artery, the short gastric
arteries (Fig. 89-2). At the hilum, the splenic artery divides
into trabecular arteries that enter the parenchyma within the
trabecula of the spleen. These leave the trabecula to enter the
splenic substance as central arteries, so called because of their
central location in a sheath of white pulp. Within the white
pulp, numerous branches are given off radially. The central
artery then terminates in the penicillate arterioles and capillaries
within the red pulp. Many of the capillaries are characterized

by a terminal sheath of phagocytic cells (the sheathed capillary;
Fig. 89-3). All communicate with the venous system, either
directly through the splenic sinus (closed circulation) or indirectly, ending in the splenic substance (open circulation).[2]

Formal venous drainage begins with the splenic sinuses
within the red pulp. These are relatively large, irregular, endothelium-lined structures interspersed with the splenic cords.
They empty directly into venules and veins coursing with the
trabecular arteries. At the hilum, these join to form a single
splenic vein, which runs parallel to the splenic artery. Near the
tail of the pancreas, it is joined by the inferior mesenteric vein.
It then joins the superior mesenteric vein to form the portal
vein (see Fig. 89-2).

The splenic parenchyma is divided into red and white pulp.
Red pulp forms 75% of the spleen's substance. It is composed
of cords of loose reticular tissue rich in capillaries and reticuloendothelial cells interspersed among the venous sinuses. The
remaining substance, white pulp, is composed of aggregations
of lymphoid tissue within the reticular substance. White pulp
is localized around the central artery and arterioles. There are
distinct areas of T-cell and B-cell predominance. The B-cell
areas are arranged as follicles (malpighian bodies) composed
of a germinal center surrounded by a ring of small lymphocytes
(mantel zone). This, in turn, is surrounded by a ring of larger
cells, both lymphoid and phagocytic (marginal zone), which
lies between the white and red pulp. In contrast, the T-cell areas
are more irregular. Immediately surrounding the central artery,
the T cells are dense, forming a sheath that becomes attenuated
peripherally (see Fig. 89-3). The unique arrangement of both
the spleen's microvascular and parenchymal architecture is vital
to its normal physiologic function.[3]

Abnormal

Asplenia and Polysplenia

Asplenia and polysplenia are both unusual defects that arise
from a failure of normal asymmetric organogenesis and, accordingly, share several common features. In general, they represent
symmetric development of normally asymmetric organs and
isomerism of paired organs.[1]

Congenital asplenia (Ivemark syndrome) occurs as a conse-

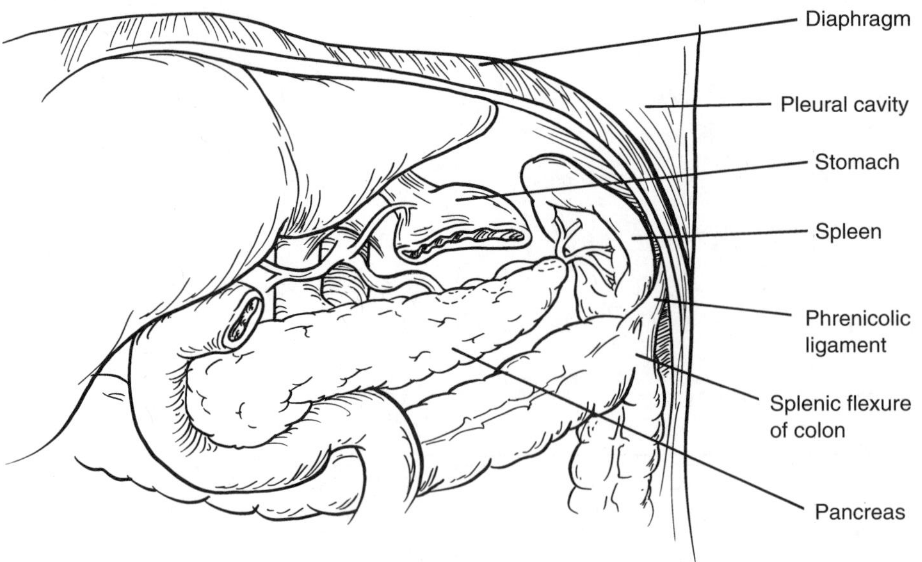

FIG. 89-1. Normal anatomic relations of the spleen in situ.

quence of bilateral right-sidedness. It is associated with bilateral trilobed lungs and a centrally located (bilateral) liver. The stomach is located in the right abdomen, and in slightly more than half of cases, incomplete intestinal rotation is present (Fig. 89-4). The most serious accompanying abnormalities involve the heart, with complex cardiac anomalies generally resulting in cyanosis and early death. Splenic absence is most easily suggested by examination of a peripheral blood smear. Morphologic abnormalities, such as Howell-Jolly bodies, siderocytes, and pocked erythrocytes, are increased.

Congenital polysplenia occurs as a consequence of bilateral left-sidedness. Multiple spleens are located along the greater curvature of the stomach. Situs inversus is present in one third to one half of cases. The lungs generally are both bilobed, and the liver may be bilateral. Cardiac defects are present in up to 75% of cases but are, as a rule, much less severe than encountered in asplenia. Associated lesions of surgical importance include a preduodenal portal vein and biliary atresia. Splenic function in this condition is normal.

Accessory Spleen

Accessory spleen refers to the presence of small (1 to 10 cm) nodules of functioning splenic tissue in addition to an anatomi-

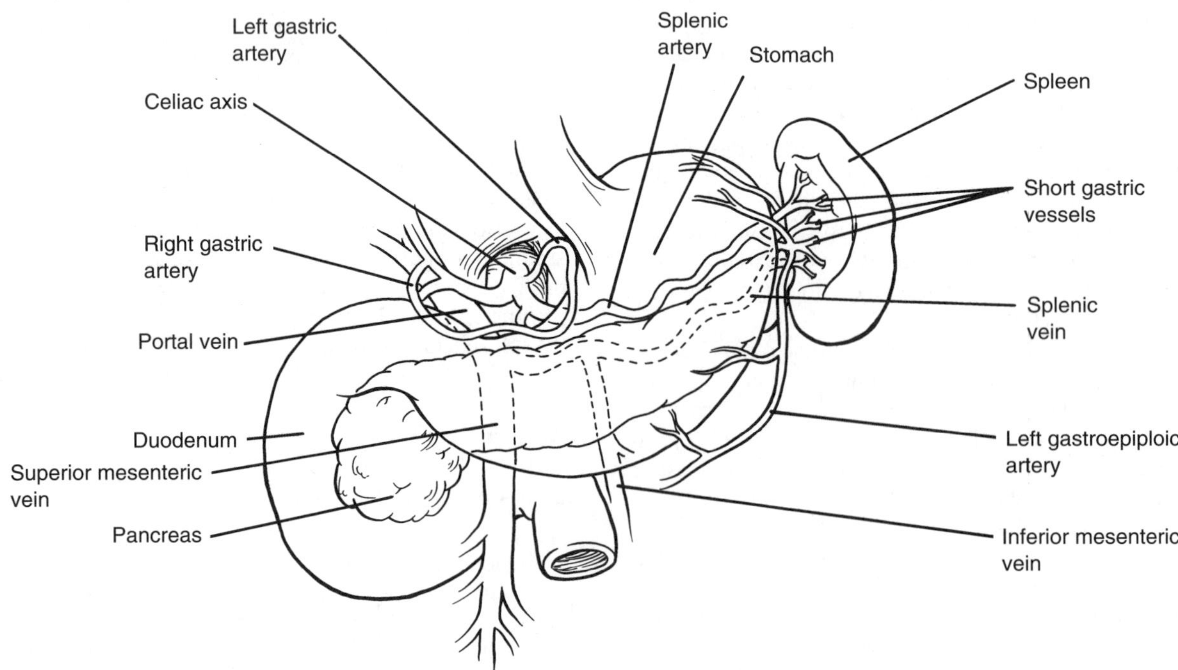

FIG. 89-2. Normal blood supply to the spleen.

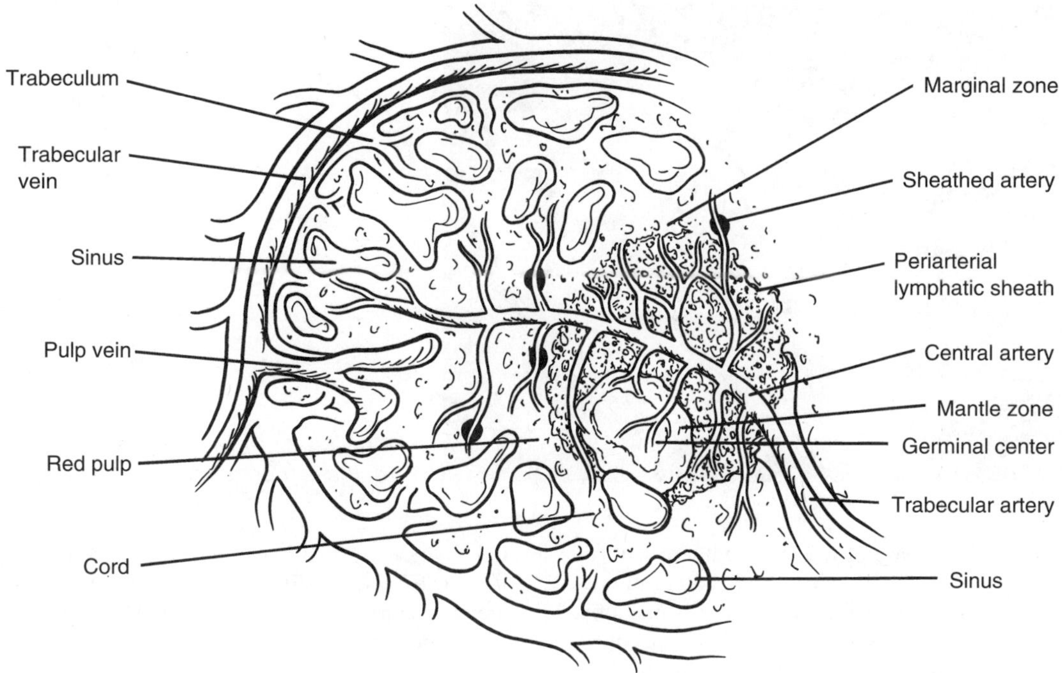

FIG. 89-3. Microscopic anatomy of the spleen.

cally normal spleen. It is, by far, the most common anomaly of the spleen and one of the most common anomalies of the body overall. It is reported to occur in 10% to 30% of the general population. Although a single accessory spleen is present in most cases, multiple accessory spleens have been reported. It is thought to arise as a consequence of failure of fusion of the splenic primordium in the dorsal mesogastrium. Seventy-five percent of accessory spleens are located near the splenic hilum; other locations include the greater or lesser omentum, mesentery, and retroperitoneum. They have clinical significance only in conditions that also affect the normal spleen. Because they share function with their main counterparts, if overlooked dur-

ing splenectomy, accessory spleens can cause recurrent pathology.[1]

Splenogonadal Fusion

Splenogonadal fusion is a rare developmental anomaly that results in the presence of splenic tissue in the left scrotum or adnexa. This aberrant tissue may be connected to the normal spleen by a band of fibrous tissue with or without additional splenic tissue along its course. It most likely is due to adherence of the splenic primordia to the mesonephric ridge. Most patients

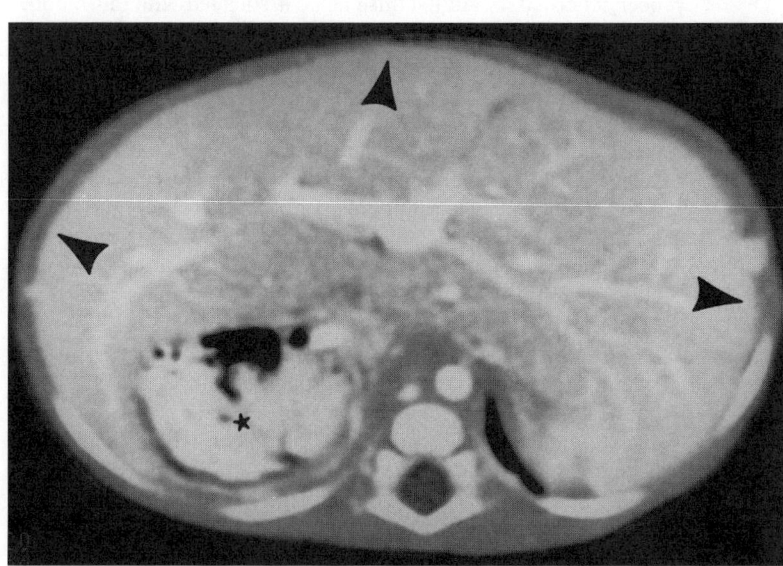

FIG. 89-4. Upper abdominal CT scan of a child with congenital asplenia showing a central bilateral liver (*arrowheads*), a right-sided stomach (*asterisk*), and the absence of a spleen.

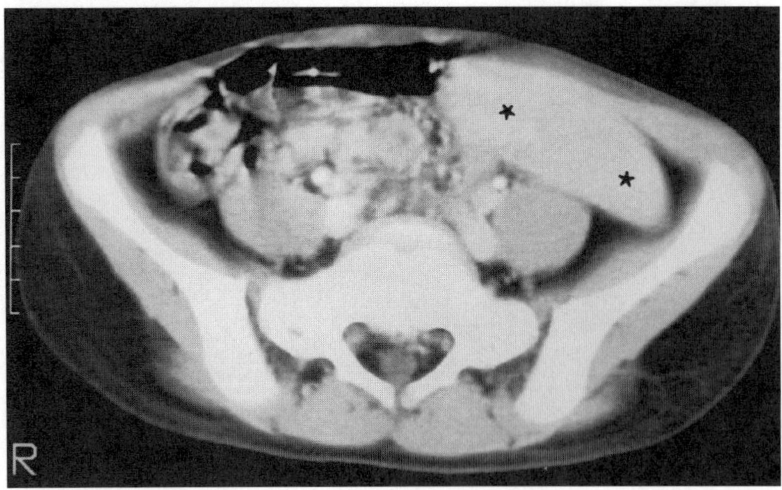

FIG. 89-5. Pelvic location of wandering spleen (*asterisks*) demonstrated on CT.

are male, which may reflect ease of discovery rather than true incidence. It can be associated with micrognathia and limb defects, particularly in cases with a fibrous splenic connection. Left cryptorchidism can occur in association with or as a consequence of splenogonadal fusion. Most cases present as a left scrotal mass with symptoms indistinguishable from an inguinal hernia. Removal of the splenic tissue can be complicated by an actual fusion with testicular tissue beneath the tunica.[1]

Splenic Ectopia (Wandering Spleen)

Splenic ectopia, or wandering spleen, refers to a condition in which the spleen is extremely mobile and located anywhere in the peritoneal cavity other than the left upper quadrant (Fig. 89-5). Although the cause is controversial, this abnormality most likely results from failure of the dorsal mesogastrium to form properly the major supporting ligaments of the spleen. Mobility is enhanced by an associated elongation of the splenic pedicle. Clinical significance is related to the risk of splenic torsion, which can result in infarction, an acute surgical condition. This, in fact, represents the most common presentation in children. Other presentations include chronic abdominal pain and a painless abdominal mass. The characteristic finding on physical examination is a mobile, notched, elliptical abdominal mass. Diagnosis is most easily confirmed by ultrasound of the mass, which demonstrates the characteristic morphologic findings of spleen in the absence of any identifiable spleen in its normal anatomic location. Other diagnostic modalities include radionuclide imaging, computed tomography (CT), and magnetic resonance imaging. Therapy is based, in large part, on the indications for and findings at operation. In the presence of torsion with splenic infarction, splenectomy is required. If the spleen is normal other than its location, splenopexy is performed with use of polyglactin mesh. This is secured to the diaphragm and retroperitoneum, placing the spleen in about its normal anatomic position.[1]

PHYSIOLOGY AND FUNCTION

Normal

The spleen, by virtue of its location, blood supply, and structure, is ideally suited for its function. Although much remains unknown about its physiologic role, it is abundantly clear that it is far from an easily expendable organ. Its primary activities are most conveniently divided into those related to hematologic and immunologic functions.

Hematologic Function

Erythroid precursors are present within the spleen as early as 6 to 8 weeks' gestation. These increase until mid-gestation, contributing to fetal erythropoiesis. Subsequently, the bone marrow gradually assumes predominance, with few hematopoietic cells remaining within the spleen at term. The potential for splenic hematopoiesis remains throughout life, however, with splenic blood formation in a variety of severe hematologic disorders.

Although the spleen serves as a major red cell reservoir in a variety of mammalian species, there is little evidence for such a role in humans. In contrast, however, the human spleen does serve as a reservoir for platelets, with up to 30% of all platelets sequestered within the splenic substance at any time. This proportion is increased in hypersplenic states. Splenectomy may result in a transient thrombocytosis due to the loss of this reservoir, and postoperative platelet counts greater than 10^6 have been recorded. In adults, this can be associated with thrombotic complications involving primarily the mesenteric circulation. This, in turn, has led to the routine use of platelet antagonists, such as aspirin and dipyridamole, in severe cases. Postsplenectomy thrombotic complications have rarely been noted in children, however, and these medications are seldom employed.

The spleen is a major repository of lymphoid cells. Twenty-five percent of the T-lymphocyte pool resides within the spleen normally, along with 10% to 15% of the B-cell population. These populations are transient, constantly exchanging with circulating cells. The spleen also contains a large number of marginated neutrophils.

Aside from storage, the major hematologic function of the spleen is its role in the normal nurture and support of the circulating cellular elements, particularly erythrocytes.[4] Reticulocytes are selectively retained by the spleen where maturation occurs. This is characterized by remodeling of the cell membrane, shrinkage of cell volume, and loss of reticulum. The spleen removes numerous intraerythrocytic inclusions, such as Howell-Jolly bodies, Heinz bodies, and hemosiderin granules.

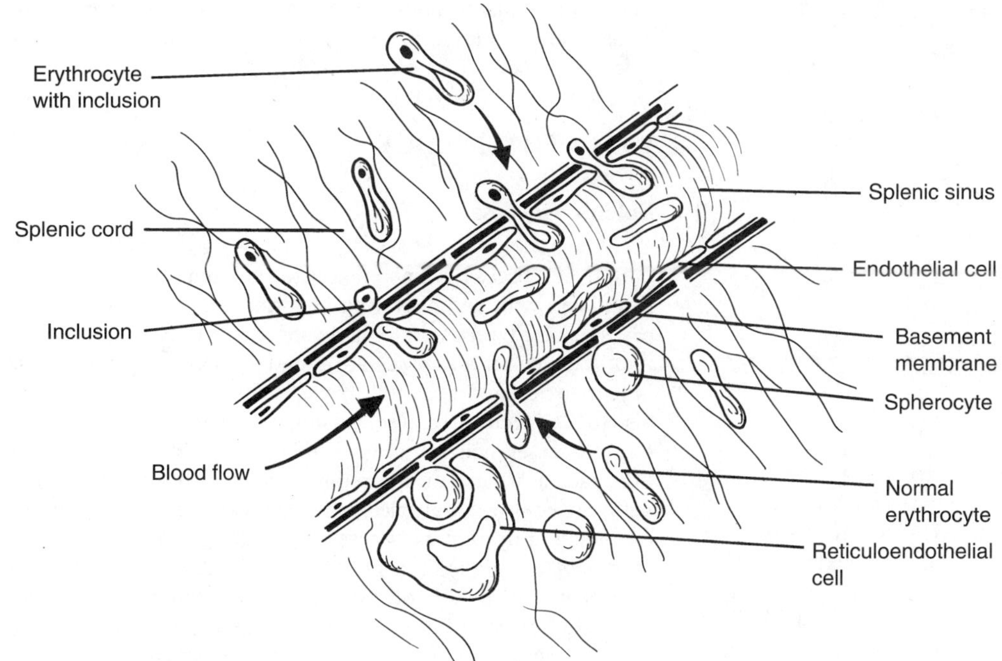

FIG. 89-6. Representation of the microcirculation and function of the spleen. Normal erythrocytes are deformed and pass through interendothelial pores, entering the splenic sinus. Senescent red cells are unable to deform sufficiently to gain access to the sinus. These cells are therefore trapped in the splenic cords until phagocytozed by resident reticuloendothelial cells. Erythrocytes containing noncompressible inclusions pass through the endothelial pores, but the inclusions are pinched off with a portion of cell wall, effectively removing them from the cell (pitting).

This unique splenic function, termed *pitting,* is a consequence of the splenic ultrastructure. Erythrocytes traversing the splenic cords must reenter the circulation by passing through the minute interendothelial cell apertures of the splenic sinus.[5] This is facilitated by the intrinsic deformability of the red cell. Cells containing nondeformable inclusions are impeded in their passage, and the cell membrane is slowly stretched until a small portion containing the inclusion is pinched off at the sinus aperture. So efficient is this function that the presence of inclusions in circulating erythrocytes provides a morphologic indication of diminished splenic function (Fig. 89-6).

Culling refers to the ability of the spleen selectively to remove abnormal erythrocytes from the circulation. This is based on the absence of normal deformability in cells such as spherocytes and poikilocytes. This reduced cell membrane flexibility prohibits passage into the splenic sinus, trapping these cells in the cords, where they are eventually phagocytized by the numerous reticuloendothelial cells. Aged erythrocytes are removed by similar mechanisms. As a normal red cell matures, there is a gradual decrease in adenosine triphosphate content and enzyme activity. This results in a diminished ability to maintain cell membrane deformability, ultimately precluding splenic passage (see Fig. 89-6).

The splenic removal of old red cells also occurs through an immunologic mechanism. Immunoglobulin G (IgG) antibody accumulates on the surfaces of these senescent cells. The specific antigenic site is unclear, but it may be a membrane protein exposed in the normal aging process. Subsequent slow passage through the splenic substance exposes the sensitized cells to the numerous monocytes and macrophages of the splenic reticuloendothelial system, facilitating their phagocytosis.

Immunologic Function

The spleen represents one of the largest collections of both reticuloendothelial cells and lymphoid tissue in the human body. This cellular structure, combined with the vascular anatomy and high-volume blood flow, equips the spleen for a major role in the normal immune defenses.[6,7] Arterial inflow facilitates immunologic filtration. Numerous arterial branches arise at an acute angle off the central artery, effectively filtering the plasma and any suspended particles from the circulation. These arterial branches terminate in white pulp areas rich in both lymphoid and reticuloendothelial cells, enabling antigen processing and phagocytosis. The now concentrated cellular elements that remain flow within the central artery and are directed into the red pulp. Here, the flow slows, allowing cells coated with antibody or opsonins to be presented effectively to the numerous monocytes and macrophages for phagocytosis. Splenic efficiency in this immunologic filtration, on a weight-for-weight basis, far exceeds that of the liver. It is particularly important in the handling of larger particles and those with a low ratio of antibody or opsonin to antigen.

The spleen serves as a major source of IgM antibody, and plasma levels are significantly decreased after splenectomy. The spleen also produces properiden, a protein that activates the alternate complement pathway, as well as tuftsin, a tetrapeptide resulting from cleavage of the Fc fragment of IgG. Tuftsin stimulates both chemotaxis and phagocytosis.

Abnormal

Functional abnormalities of the spleen, regardless of the specific cause, can be classified as either hyposplenism or hypersplenism. Strictly speaking, these terms are devoid of any anatomic or diagnostic significance, describing only a physiologic state. Hyposplenism indicates primarily decreased splenic phagocytosis and immune function. Peripheral blood smears may reflect diminished splenic activity by the finding of increased erythrocyte inclusions. Phase microscopy also demonstrates an increase in pocked red cells. These erythrocytes are

TABLE 89-1. *Conditions associated with hyposplenism*

Inflammatory bowel disease
Lupus erythematosus
Rheumatoid arthritis
Glomerulonephritis
Nephrotic syndrome
Sickle cell disease
Thalassemia
Radiation
Prematurity
Senility
Amyloidosis
Sarcoidosis

characterized by small membrane defects that are rare in normal people. Those affected generally demonstrate an increased susceptibility to infection. Spleen size may be normal or small.

Acquired splenic hypofunction has been described in a variety of conditions (Table 89-1), most of which affect primarily adults. The most common cause of hypofunction in the child is sickle cell disease. In this condition, there is a gradual loss of splenic function for several years, culminating in functional asplenia.

Developmental hyposplenia is present in the normal neonate. Pocked red cells are increased in the newborn circulation, as are intraerythrocytic inclusions and reticulocytes. The marginal zone of the white pulp is deficient at birth. This is the area where splenic macrophages normally process antigens and present them to the lymphocyte. This area appears to be particularly important in the handling of thymus-independent polysaccharide antigens. This may explain the susceptibility of neonates to infection by encapsulated organisms. These deficiencies are proportionately increased in the premature infant.

Hypersplenism refers primarily to the splenic functions of sequestration and cellular destruction.[8] It is characterized by a decrease in one or more of the formed circulating blood elements, in conjunction with a corresponding increase in marrow precursors of that same element or elements. It may or may not be accompanied by splenomegaly. Hypersplenism is rarely primary. Secondary hypersplenism results from any process that increases blood sequestration within the spleen. Most commonly, this is the result of venous outflow obstruction or congestion (Table 89-2). The resulting anemia is secondary to both increased red cell pooling and a diminished survival time.

TABLE 89-2. *Conditions associated with hypersplenism*

Portal hypertension
Splenic vein thrombosis
Congestive heart failure
Leukemia
Lymphoma
Felty syndrome
Lupus erythematosus
Sarcoidosis
Amyloidosis
Gaucher disease
Niemann-Pick disease

Leukopenia and thrombocytopenia result primarily from increased sequestration. In certain instances, patients with hypersplenism benefit from elective splenectomy.

PATHOPHYSIOLOGY

Splenic Abscess

Splenic abscess is uncommon in children and generally is associated with an underlying abnormality.[9] In the past, most cases reported were solitary large abscesses. Recently, however, multiple smaller abscesses are reported more frequently. This is perhaps related not only to better diagnostic capability but also to the spectrum of predisposing pathology in children. Solitary abscesses generally occur after splenic structural disruption, such as trauma or infarction associated with hemoglobinopathy. In contrast, multiple small abscesses are most commonly encountered in immunosuppressed children, particularly those with hematologic malignancy. Concomitant bacterial infection is present in about 30% of children who develop splenic abscess.

Most affected children present with fever and other signs of systemic sepsis, but localizing symptoms depend on the type of abscess present. Solitary lesions are commonly associated with left upper quadrant pain. Left-sided pleuritic chest pain may also be present. In contrast, the complaints associated with multiple abscesses are more generalized and nonspecific. The most frequent physical finding is splenomegaly, but this is present in only half of cases. Diagnosis is most easily confirmed radiographically. Ultrasonography documents a solitary splenic abscess but may not be sensitive enough in cases of multiple smaller lesions. CT or magnetic resonance imaging is more specific.

Causative organisms include *Staphylococcus*, *Streptococcus*, and *Salmonella* species. *Salmonella* sp infection is most frequently associated with an underlying hemoglobinopathy. *Candida* sp infection is an increasing cause of multiple splenic abscesses, particularly in children with leukemia.

Therapy for multiple abscesses is preferably intravenous antimicrobial agents. This is particularly true of *Candida* sp infection, which can represent a manifestation of systemic candidiasis. Splenectomy is reserved for refractory cases. Identification of the causative organism may, however, require splenic biopsy or aspiration because peripheral blood cultures are positive in only 30% to 40% of cases. A solitary splenic abscess may respond to simple drainage, either operative or percutaneous. If the lesion is not amenable to this therapeutic option, formal splenectomy is required.

Infiltrative or Storage Disease

Infiltrative or storage diseases compose a group of inherited disorders characterized by the accumulation of nonmetabolized substrates within the lysosomes of various tissue cells.[10] They result from the deficiency of specific acid hydrolases used in normal intracellular digestion. The individual diseases are classified according to the substance that accumulates abnormally. Splenomegaly or hypersplenism is a prominent component of several specific disorders.

Gaucher disease is a deficiency of the glucocerebrosidase

enzyme, and it results in the accumulation of glucosylceramide in macrophages, primarily in the reticuloendothelial system. Type I Gaucher disease, the chronic nonneuropathic or so-called adult form, not only is the most common variant of this disorder but also represents the most common lysosomal storage disease. Although typically diagnosed in adulthood, it can become symptomatic at any age. The usual presentation is painless splenomegaly with hypersplenism. Hepatomegaly is frequent, and bone involvement may also be present. There are no central nervous system manifestations, and life expectancy can be normal.

The spleen may obtain massive proportions, with weights of 10 kg reported in this disorder. Histologically, there is diffuse infiltration of both sinuses and cords with Gaucher cells, glucosylceramide-laden histiocytes. Fibrosis may be prominent. Hypersplenism is secondary to congestion and may be aggravated by bone marrow involvement. Splenectomy may be indicated to control complications of hypersplenism in Gaucher disease. Traditionally total splenectomy has been done, however, recent reports suggest that partial splenectomy is a reasonable alternative, particularly in children. Regrowth of the splenic remnant occurs, but control of hypersplenism may be adequately maintained.

Splenomegaly may be a prominent feature of type I Niemann-Pick disease, a deficiency of sphingomyelinase. This results in the accumulation of sphingomyelin in macrophages of the spleen, lymph nodes, and bone marrow. The liver, lung, and gastrointestinal tract are also frequently involved. The primary organ of pathology is the brain, with severe progressive neurologic involvement. Death generally occurs in early childhood. Splenomegaly is striking with diffuse infiltration of the red pulp by lipid-laden "foam cells." Because of the lack of any effective therapy for the underlying disorder, as well as its rapid progression and fatal outcome, splenectomy plays no role in the management of this disorder.

A variety of the mucopolysaccharidoses are associated with splenomegaly, secondary to the accumulation of glycosaminoglycans within the red-pulp macrophages. Physiologic dysfunction is determined primarily by the degree of central nervous system or cardiac involvement. Hypersplenism is seldom of any clinical consequence, and there is little role for surgical therapy in the management of the splenomegaly.

Hematologic Diseases

Hemolytic Anemias

Hemolytic anemias result in hyperplastic splenomegaly as the result of an increased rate of removal of abnormal red cells from the circulation.[11] Accelerated sequestration and phagocytosis in the red pulp can occur because of intrinsic red cell defects in spherocytosis, elliptocytosis, and several other rare abnormalities. These are generally the result of specific erythrocyte membrane protein deficiencies that lead to membrane fragility or rigidity, both of which result in splenic culling and shortened erythrocyte survival.

Hereditary spherocytosis is the most common of the hereditary hemolytic anemias. Patients present with varying degrees of anemia, jaundice, and splenomegaly. Pigment gallstones develop frequently and can occur in childhood. Hereditary spherocytosis can be difficult to distinguish from a variety of other diagnoses associated with spherocytes, including immune hemolytic disease, glucose-6-phosphate dehydrogenase (G6PD) deficiency, and sickle cell disease. The autohemolysis test is the most discriminating study. Transfusions are required mainly during crises, which are often associated with a febrile illness. Splenectomy is curative, except in autosomal recessive disease, although red cell survival usually does not completely return to normal. Recurrence of anemia and jaundice should prompt a search for growing splenic tissue in retained accessory spleens.

The clinical course of hereditary elliptocytosis is similar to hereditary spherocytosis. Diagnosis relies on the clinical presentation, family history, and red cell morphology. Although the common mild anemia requires no treatment, splenectomy is beneficial in the transfusion-dependent anemia of homozygous hereditary elliptocytosis.

Hereditary hemolytic anemias can also result from abnormalities of red cell enzymes. Pyruvate kinase deficiency is the most common abnormality involving anaerobic glycolysis. G6PD deficiency affects the normal function of the oxidative pathway of glycolysis and, overall, is the most common metabolic disorder of red blood cells. Both disorders have highly variable degrees of expression. Significant, chronic anemia in pyruvate kinase deficiency benefits from splenectomy to avoid recurrent aplastic crises. The anemia associated with G6PD deficiency is often controlled by avoiding drugs known to precipitate hemolysis. Although occasional transfusion may be needed during episodes of aplastic crises, splenectomy is rarely indicated.

Sickle Cell Anemia

Abnormal red cells associated with hemoglobinopathies also result in anemia because of increased destruction in the spleen. Sickle cell anemia is the most common hereditary hematologic abnormality in the United States, occurring in about 1 in 625 births.[12] Polymerization of HbS in red cells resulting in sickling is promoted by hypoxia, acidosis, cold, dehydration, increased concentrations of HbS, and other factors. Identification of abnormal hemoglobins by hemoglobin electrophoresis is diagnostic. Increased phagocytosis of sickle erythrocytes results initially in splenomegaly, commonly noted by 6 months of age. With recurrent vasoocclusive crises, however, splenic function is gradually lost, and evidence of hyposplenism develops. Even young children with sickle cell disease have an increased susceptibility to overwhelming sepsis. Sudden trapping of blood in the spleen causes a rapid increase in splenic size and an acute splenic sequestration crisis.[13] The volume of blood sequestered within the spleen can be substantial, and shock and death may result. Recurrent episodes are common until adequate splenic fibrosis occurs to limit its expansion, usually by the age of 5 or 6 years; thereafter, splenic sequestration crises are uncommon. Splenectomy prevents recurrences of these crises but must be balanced with the risks of postsplenectomy sepsis in young patients.

Thalassemia

The thalassemias consist of several abnormalities of hemoglobin synthesis and are considered to be the most common genetic disorder worldwide.[14] Thalassemia patients require regular transfusions, and splenomegaly can develop with the sequestration of transfused erythrocytes in the spleen. With progressive enlargement of the spleen, red cell survival decreases and may be accompanied by leukocyte and platelet trapping. The progressive anemia increases the transfusion requirement and accelerates the complications of iron overload. An increasing transfusion requirement, exceeding 200 to 250 mL packed red cells/kg/y, has been recommended as an indication for splenectomy.

Thrombocytopenia

The primary hematologic abnormality of the spleen that presents as thrombocytopenia is idiopathic thrombocytopenic purpura.[15] It results from accelerated destruction of platelets due to an unknown immunologic process. Acute idiopathic thrombocytopenic purpura occurs most commonly in children 2 to 6 years of age, frequently after a viral infection. Spontaneous resolution is common in the acute form, but patients with chronic idiopathic thrombocytopenic purpura have recurrent symptoms of bleeding associated with thrombocytopenia. Clinical bleeding correlates with the platelet count. Most severe hemorrhage occurs with platelet counts less than $10^4/\mu L$. Although rare, intracranial bleeding can be a devastating complication. Evaluation of thrombocytopenia includes ruling out potential drug-related or infectious causes. Bone marrow aspiration is usually needed to exclude bone marrow abnormalities causing thrombocytopenia.

Therapy for chronic idiopathic thrombocytopenic purpura includes a trial of prednisone, 1–2 mg/kg/d for 2 to 4 weeks, followed by gradual tapering. Intravenous immunoglobulin (IVIG) has also been used with some success. Splenectomy is thought to be beneficial by removing the site where antibody-sensitized platelets are destroyed as well as the site of antibody production, if possible. The decision to proceed with splenectomy is individualized, but indications include (1) lack of spontaneous remission after 6 months with moderate bleeding, (2) failure to respond to prednisone or contraindications to steroid use, and (3) problems with compliance. Splenectomy is contraindicated (1) early during the initial episode of bleeding because spontaneous remission is common, especially in children; (2) in children less than 2 years old because of the risk of sepsis; and (3) in pregnant women. A careful search for accessory spleens is necessary at the time of surgery to prevent recurrent idiopathic thrombocytopenic purpura after splenectomy.

Congenital idiopathic thrombocytopenic purpura occurs in neonates from the placental transfer of platelet antibodies. Most infants require no therapy, although platelet transfusions are done if needed to prevent intracranial hemorrhage. The efficacy of steroids or exchange transfusion is controversial.

Histiocytosis

Langerhans cell histiocytosis, or histiocytosis X, refers to a group of disorders characterized by the proliferation or infiltration of histologically specific histiocytes (Langerhans cells) in one or more organs.[16] Clinical heterogeneity is reflected by the various syndromes that encompass this abnormality in children.

These include eosinophilic granuloma, Hand-Schüller-Christian disease, and Letterer-Siwe disease. Eosinophilic granuloma and Hand-Schüller-Christian disease are primarily localized. Letterer-Siwe disease represents disseminated Langerhans cell histiocytosis with characteristic involvement of the skin, visceral organs, and lymphatic and hematopoietic systems. Splenomegaly is common and results from histiocytic infiltration of the red pulp cords and sinuses. Congestive hypersplenism can result with secondary pancytopenia. This may be aggravated by the histiocytic marrow infiltration. Therapy in disseminated disease is primarily systemic, with use of vinblastine or etoposide with or without corticosteroids. Rarely, splenectomy is useful in severe transfusion-dependent pancytopenia.

Malignant histiocytosis is a rare variant of lymphoma, differentiated from Langerhans cell histiocytosis by the marked cytologic atypia of the cells. It is a systemic malignancy involving the entire reticuloendothelial system and is usually seen in older children and adults, who present with symptoms of generalized illness. Splenomegaly is prominent and occasionally is the first sign in a patient who has no other symptoms. The pattern of splenic involvement is similar to that seen in Langerhans cell histiocytosis. Hypersplenism is common, with phagocytosis of the humoral elements by the neoplastic cells. Treatment is multiagent chemotherapy, with median survivals of about 40 months.

Myeloproliferative Disorders

Splenomegaly is a frequent component of myeloproliferative disorders that occur in childhood.[17] All arise as a consequence of the abnormal clonal proliferation of hematopoietic stem cells. Although the cells are multipotential, a single cell lineage generally predominates, enabling differentiation into several distinct syndromes. Each is unique in its clinical and pathologic features.

Chronic myelogenous leukemia is the most common myeloproliferative disorder in children and accounts for about 5% of the childhood leukemias. Ninety percent of cases are associated with the Philadelphia chromosome, a 9:22 translocation. The involved stem cell has a primary commitment to the granulocyte line. The abnormality is characterized by myeloid hyperplasia of the marrow, extramedullary hematopoiesis, mild anemia, and granulocytosis. White blood cell counts are usually in excess of $10^5/\mu L$, with differentials demonstrating all the myeloid elements. Splenomegaly is marked with myeloid metaplasia of the red pulp and obliteration of the white pulp. Maturing hematopoietic precursor cells are prominent. Spontaneous splenic infarction may occur. Splenic irradiation was used in the past as part of routine therapy; it is now considered only for transient palliation of symptomatic massive splenomegaly in children refractory to chemotherapy. Splenectomy may also benefit children with symptomatic splenomegaly and hypersplenism. Additionally, it may be useful in reducing the leukemic burden in children undergoing ablative therapy before bone marrow transplantation. Overall prognosis is poor, despite aggressive chemotherapy. Bone marrow transplantation appears to offer the best chance of disease-free survival.

Polycythemia vera is rare in children. It arises from clonal expansion of erythroid progenitors exquisitely sensitive to erythropoietin. This results in a significant increase in the red cell mass, with the attendant complications of hyperviscosity.

Splenomegaly is present in 70% of cases secondary to congestion, with occasional foci of myeloid metaplasia. Therapy is aimed at reducing hyperviscosity by phlebotomy.

Essential thrombocythemia is characterized by persistent thrombocytosis with no apparent cause. Although predominantly a disease of adults, 10% to 15% of cases occur in children. There is proliferation of megakaryocytes, with peripheral platelet counts commonly exceeding $10^6/\mu L$ and bizarre platelet morphology. Clinically, it manifests with thrombotic complications. The spleen is enlarged in half of cases, with extramedullary hematopoiesis. The myeloid metaplasia involves primarily the splenic sinuses. Spontaneous thrombosis of the spleen with infarction can result in splenic atrophy, which, in turn, aggravates the condition because of the loss of this important site of platelet sequestration. For similar reasons, splenectomy is contraindicated. This condition is generally well tolerated in children, but therapy with hydroxyurea may be required in patients with symptoms.

Solid Neoplasms

Angiosarcomas are exceedingly rare but represent the most frequent primary malignant solid tumor of the spleen.[17,18] These patients most often present with painless splenomegaly. About one third present with spontaneous splenic rupture. These lesions are frequently multicentric, with involvement of the liver. They are highly malignant and evidence both local invasion and metastatic spread.

Metastatic neoplasms to the spleen occur late in disease progression and represent hematogenous spread. They occur primarily in adults. In children, the spleen is more frequently involved by direct extension from contiguous malignant neoplasms, such as neuroblastoma and Wilms tumor.

Hamartoma

Splenic hamartomas can be primarily lymphoid, chordal, or mixed.[17,18] Prominent lymphoid features can make differentiation from lymphoma and Hodgkin disease difficult. Hamartomas, however, contain no Reed-Sternberg cells and compress normal splenic parenchyma rather than invade it. Large lesions are generally multifocal and confluent. They most frequently present as hypersplenism. Splenectomy is curative.

Lymphoma and Leukemia

The lymphomas and acute leukemias account for about half of the malignant diseases in children younger than 15 years of age.[19] In contrast to the nonhematologic neoplasms, the spleen is frequently involved in these disorders[20] (see Chap. 37).

Non-Hodgkin lymphomas are a diverse group of lymphoreticular neoplasms classified on the basis of their presumed cell of origin. In children, these tumors are among the most rapidly growing, frequently presenting with a short duration of symptoms but impressive clinical manifestations. The usual presentation is painless lymphadenopathy. Non-Hodgkin lymphomas can, however, arise in any lymphoid tissue site. Splenic involvement varies with the lymphoma cell type but is characteristically multifocal, affecting primarily the white pulp. Splenomegaly generally accompanies involvement. Small cell lymphoma presents with a miliary nodular pattern of involvement, while the red pulp is essentially intact. In contrast, the large cell lymphomas tend to form large single or multiple tumor masses secondarily involving the red pulp as the white pulp nodules coalesce. Splenectomy plays little role in the management of these neoplasms, except perhaps in the diagnosis of the rare case of primary splenic involvement or in the removal of localized tumor before chemotherapy. Staging is nonoperative, and therapy is primarily multiagent chemotherapy and radiotherapy.

Hodgkin disease is a subset of the malignant lymphomas distinguished by the presence of characteristic large multinucleated cells (Reed-Sternberg cells). The origin of these cells is unclear. Hodgkin disease rarely involves the spleen primarily, but secondary splenic involvement occurs in 30% of cases. Early lesions appear in the periarteriolar lymphoid sheath of the white pulp or the marginal zone between the red and white pulps. With progression, either a miliary nodular pattern or a confluent multinodular tumor mass may predominant. Splenomegaly corresponds to the extent of tumor involvement. Classically, splenectomy is a routine part of the operative staging of Hodgkin disease. This approach has, however, become increasingly controversial, not only with regard to indications for staging but also with respect to the type of splenectomy performed. Generally, the need for this is now determined by specific collaborative investigative protocols. When staging laparotomy is undertaken, total splenectomy is performed in the absence of obvious splenic disease.

Acute lymphoblastic leukemia is the most common malignancy of children in Western countries. It arises from the clonal expansion of malignant lymphopoietic stem cells, with the progressive infiltration of marrow with malignant lymphoblasts. Production of normal hemopoietic cells is suppressed. Splenomegaly is a part of the clinical findings in up to 90% of cases. Tumor cells accumulate in both the white and red pulp, with invasion of the intima of trabecular vessels occasionally noted. Splenic enlargement is noted in half of children with acute myelogenous leukemia. This disorder is characterized by the progressive infiltration of normal marrow with nonmaturing myeloblasts. It represents 20% of the acute leukemias of childhood. Splenic involvement is characterized by the accumulation of cells, primarily in the splenic sinusoids. Splenectomy plays no role in the treatment of either acute myelogenous leukemia or acute lymphoblastic leukemia.

Vascular Abnormalities

Splenic artery aneurysm is exceedingly rare in children.[21] Those cases that have been reported were diagnosed in adolescence. Unusual as they are, they may well represent the most common visceral aneurysm in children. Although of atherosclerotic origin in adults, pediatric cases have most frequently been associated with portal hypertension. Other causes include emboli secondary to bacterial endocarditis and congenital absence or deficiency of the arterial internal elastic membrane. Ehlers-Danlos type III patients are an important consideration with regard to the latter. There is a known association between pregnancy and splenic artery aneurysm, with a risk of rupture as high as 50%; therefore, adolescent girls are at risk. Clinical presentations vary from vague abdominal pain to hemorrhagic shock from rupture. Diagnosis is dependent on angiography or laparotomy. Splenectomy is usually performed.

Splenic vein occlusion is seen most frequently in conjunction with hepatic or portal vein obstruction.[22] When isolated, it is usually the result of pancreatitis. This usually presents as upper gastrointestinal bleeding secondary to esophageal and gastric varices. Splenomegaly is present. Splenectomy is the treatment of choice.

Miscellaneous Lesions

Cystic lesions of the spleen are uncommon and most frequently due to endemic parasitic infections (*Echinococcus* sp).[18] Nonparasitic cysts classically have been categorized on the basis of histology as primary (true cysts with epithelial lining present) or secondary (pseudocysts with no lining present). The cause of primary cysts remains controversial. They are considered congenital in most reports, secondary to embryonic rests of epithelial or mesothelial cells. Several studies suggest, however, that these lesions may be a consequence of trauma, with proliferation of mesothelial inclusions from the disrupted fibrous capsule. The most common true cyst is the epidermoid cyst, lined by stratified squamous epithelium. Dermoid cysts are characterized by squamous epithelium containing skin appendages and are extremely rare. Primary cysts may be single or multiple, unilocular or multilocular. The cyst fluid is clear or cloudy and contains cholesterol crystals. Secondary cysts, or pseudocysts, are the most common nonparasitic cysts of the spleen. They are the result of intrasplenic hemorrhage, with subsequent degeneration and the formation of a fibrotic capsule. They are unilocular and contain brown turbid fluid. Symptomatology is, for the most part, related to size. A painless abdominal mass is the most frequent presentation (Fig. 89-7). Pain, when present, may be localized to the left upper quadrant or be described as a vague, heavy sensation. Complications of both rupture and infection have been reported. Diagnostic adjuncts

include ultrasonography and CT. Small pseudocysts may be unroofed and drained intraabdominally. Large cysts require splenectomy, either total or partial. Drainage of primary cysts can result in recurrence; therefore, splenectomy is recommended. Resection with partial splenectomy is preferable in children, if technically feasible.

A lymphangioma of the spleen is differentiated from a primary splenic cyst only by its endothelial lining. Preoperative and intraoperative findings may be otherwise indistinguishable in larger discrete lesions. Lymphangiomatosis can replace the splenic parenchyma with diffuse involvement. These lesions may be isolated to the spleen alone or part of multivisceral involvement. Complications of hemorrhage, consumptive coagulopathy, hypersplenism, and portal hypertension have been reported with larger lesions. Treatment is similar to that noted for primary splenic cysts.

Hemangioma is the most common benign neoplasm of the spleen. Most of these lesions are small and of little clinical significance; however, large lesions have been noted in children. Most are associated with other visceral lesions. Platelet trapping (Kasabach-Merritt syndrome) occurs in half of cases. CT aids in diagnosis and localization. Splenectomy is generally required.

OPERATIVE TECHNIQUES

The techniques used in the removal of the spleen vary with indication, spleen size, and local expertise. Although the impetus in pediatrics has been on splenic salvage, splenectomy continues to be the procedure of choice for a variety of abnormalities. Laparoscopic techniques and other technical advances have resulted in reports of successful endoscopic splenectomy, adding another option to the operative management of this organ.

Open splenectomy is performed with the child supine. Elevation of the left flank can facilitate exposure in cases of significant splenomegaly. A nasogastric tube is placed to maintain gastric decompression. In nontrauma cases, a left upper quadrant transverse incision is employed. This is carried across the left rectus to the midline. If cholecystectomy is anticipated, the incision can be extended. In cases of trauma, a vertical midline incision is used. On entering the peritoneal cavity, the omentum and small bowel are packed inferiorly. Any adhesions between the anterior abdominal wall or omentum and the spleen are transected. Hemostasis must be meticulous, particularly in cases of portal hypertension. The gastrocolic ligament is opened in an avascular plane, entering the lesser sac. With gentle upward traction on the stomach, the splenic artery is localized along the superior border of the pancreas. The peritoneum overlying the artery is carefully cleared and the artery circumferentially freed. Care must be taken to avoid injury to the splenic vein, which lies immediately below the artery. Once isolated, the artery is ligated in continuity with nonabsorbable suture. After ligation of the splenic artery, the opening in the gastrocolic ligament is extended superiorly through the gastrosplenic ligament. This ligament is transected between clamps, securing the short gastric arteries. The spleen is then gently grasped and retracted medially and inferiorly. Any adhesions between it and the diaphragm are sharply lysed. The splenorenal ligament is exposed and the avascular overlying peritoneum transected, elevating the spleen from its bed. The splenocolic ligament at the

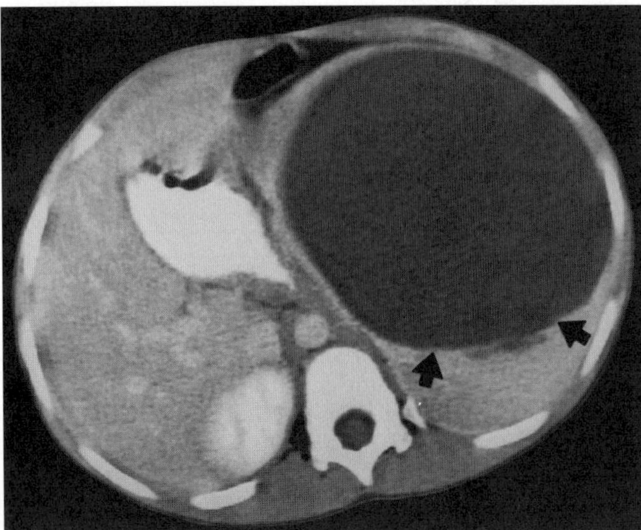

FIG. 89-7. Abdominal CT scan of a primary cyst of the spleen (*arrows*).

inferior pole is divided between clamps and secured for hemostasis. The spleen can now be withdrawn from the abdomen. It is retracted medially; the tail of the pancreas is identified and, if necessary, carefully freed from the splenic pedicle. The splenic vessels are individually separated, clamped, and transected. Each is doubly ligated with a nonabsorbable suture. Any remaining tissue is transected and the spleen removed. The splenic pedicle, ligaments, and bed are carefully examined for hemostasis, which must be ensured.

In circumstances in which it is inadvisable or impossible to ligate the splenic artery in continuity within the lesser sac, the splenorenal ligament and the diaphragm are first incised, the spleen delivered, and the vessels are identified within the pedicle and secured.

After splenectomy, particularly for blood dyscrasia, a careful search for accessory spleens is performed. This includes exploration of the region of the splenic hilum and tail of the pancreas, splenic ligaments, omentum, and small and large bowel mesenteries. If any splenic tissue is encountered, it is removed completely.

Concern for postsplenectomy sepsis has altered the traditional operative approach to the spleen in several conditions. Partial (subtotal) splenectomy is now an accepted technique in a variety of abnormalities and trauma.[23] The spleen is first mobilized by division of all its attachments, except the pedicle, and withdrawn from the abdomen. The main splenic artery and vein are identified and cleared up to their entry into the splenic substance. At this point, they generally divide into three or four branches, which are individually isolated. Each branch of the artery and vein is secured and transected, beginning at either pole. As each pair is ligated, the corresponding portion of spleen turns dark, demarcating the devascularized area. The process is repeated until a sufficient portion of spleen has been excluded. Usually, a single pole is preserved on the final vascular pair within the pedicle. The splenic parenchyma is transected at the line of vascular demarcation, and the raw surface of the viable spleen is compressed with large chromic mattress sutures. Stapling is an option as well. An omental patch or hemostatic agent may be further applied to the raw surface as necessary. The spleen is then returned to its bed and fixed to the diaphragm with several individual absorbable sutures or a polyglactin mesh to avoid torsion of the remaining portion of the spleen.

Further refinement in the surgery of the spleen has been the development of minimally invasive pediatric surgery. The introduction of the laparoscopic tissue morcellator has facilitated removal of solid organs previously not amenable to a laparoscopic approach, while preserving an adequate specimen for histology. Several pediatric centers are routinely performing laparoscopic splenectomy in children.[24] Preparation is the same as for any laparoscopic procedure and includes a nasogastric tube and Foley catheter. The initial trocar is placed through an infraumbilical incision and capnoperitoneum induced. A particularly large spleen mandates that these initial maneuvers be performed under direct vision to avoid injury. After the telescope is introduced, a visual inspection of the intraabdominal contents is conducted. Three to four additional working ports are inserted under direct endoscopic control in the right middle and upper abdomen. The child is then placed in the reverse Trendelenburg position and rolled slightly to the right. The gastrosplenic ligament is visualized and transected between endoscopic clamps or vascular staples. The splenocolic and splenorenal ligaments

are similarly visualized and transected. Visualization may be facilitated by further rolling of the patient. The splenic hilum is exposed laterally by endoscopic manipulation of the spleen. After careful identification of the tail of the pancreas, the splenic pedicle is transected and secured by endoscopic stapler. A reinforced nylon pouch is passed into the abdomen and the spleen manipulated into the bag. The pouch is partially withdrawn through the large port, and the tissue morselator is placed in the bag to cut the specimen sufficiently to permit removal. The splenic bed is carefully reexamined for hemostasis before removal of the ports. The nasogastric tube and Foley catheter are removed in the operating room.

POSTSPLENECTOMY SEPSIS

Morris and Bullock[25] first suggested a possible association between removal of the spleen and infection in 1919. Despite this report, the indications for splenectomy continued to increase, with little note of any significant consequences. Attention was refocused on the risks of splenectomy in 1952 by King and Shumaker,[26] when they reported sepsis in five infants who had undergone splenectomy for hereditary spherocytosis. Subsequent reviews have confirmed the validity of these initial observations and have forever altered the view of the spleen as an expendable organ.[27]

Overwhelming postsplenectomy infection (OPSI) is characterized by septicemia with frequent meningitic involvement. Although generally occurring within 2 years of surgery, it can arise anytime after splenectomy and has been reported from 13 days to 25 years postoperatively. The infection tends to be fulminant, with a mortality rate approaching 50%. Death can occur within 12 to 24 hours of the onset of symptoms and is associated with adrenal hemorrhage (Waterhouse-Friderichsen syndrome). Prodromal signs can be minimal, with the child presenting in cardiovascular collapse. High fever is a characteristic early finding.

The overall incidence is about 4.25% but varies with age and underlying disease. The greatest risk occurs during infancy, gradually decreasing to adulthood, from whence it persists at a low, but constant, level throughout life. The incidence of OPSI in children younger than 4 years of age is twice that in older children. Mortality is similarly increased. The disease process for which splenectomy is performed is also a major factor affecting the risk of OPSI. This may, in part, reflect the underlying immunodeficiency of the disease state. Splenectomy performed for trauma or incidental operative injury carries the lowest incidence of OPSI (1.5% to 2%), but the accompanying mortality rate is still 50 times that of the general population. The risk is greatest after splenectomy for thalassemia and reticuloendothelial disorders, such as histiocytosis (10% to 11%). Splenectomy for the various anemias, idiopathic thrombocytopenia, and portal hypertension is associated with risks between the two extremes (2% to 8%).

Streptococcus pneumoniae (pneumococcus) is responsible for about half of the reported cases of OPSI. Other organisms frequently implicated are *Neisseria meningitidis*, *Escherichia coli*, and *Haemophilus influenzae*. All but *E coli* are characterized by a polysaccharide capsule. These organisms are also characterized by rapid doubling time, which may explain the fulminant nature of OPSI. Blood bacterial contents as high as $10^5/\mu L$ have been noted.

The bacteriology of OPSI highlights the immunologic importance of the spleen, particularly in children. Phagocytosis of encapsulated organisms is enhanced greatly by antibody opsonization. These antibodies are initially acquired passively from the mother, affording protection for the first several months of life. Levels diminish, however, before full active antibody development by the child. During this period of relative antibody deficiency, the spleen plays a critical role in the defense against these encapsulated pathogens. The efficiency of splenic phagocytosis in the face of a low antibody/antigen ratio far exceeds that of other reticuloendothelial organs, making the spleen the primary site of removal of these organisms from the bloodstream. In the absence of the spleen, rapid bacterial proliferation occurs, overwhelming the less efficient macrophages of the remaining reticuloendothelial system. Other contributing factors include impaired antibody production in response to blood-borne antigens after splenectomy as well as decreased levels of tuftsin and properiden.

Treatment is primarily prevention through the avoidance of splenectomy, particularly in children under 4 years of age, as well as the liberal use of partial splenectomy and techniques of splenic salvage. In circumstances in which splenectomy is necessary, polyvalent pneumococcal vaccine is administered 2 weeks before operation. The formulation provides capsular polysaccharide antigens from the 23 most prevalent pneumococcal types, representing about 85% of all clinical pneumococcal isolates. Children younger than 2 years of age do not reliably respond to vaccination, and the response in immunocompromised and immunosuppressed children is variable. With response, however, adequate antibody levels persist for 3 to 5 years. Routine revaccination is controversial, particularly in light of data that show an increased incidence of adverse reactions. Haemophilus influenzae vaccine is also administered to those children not previously immunized.

Prophylactic penicillin is routinely employed after splenectomy to protect against pneumococcal strains not included in the vaccine as well as other susceptible organisms. An oral preparation is administered twice daily, preferably for life. Families are instructed of the potential significance of febrile illness in the splenectomized child and the importance of prompt medical attention.

REFERENCES

1. Skandalakis LJ, Gray SW, Ricketts R, et al. The spleen. In: Skandalakis LJ, Gray SW, eds. Embryology for surgeons: the embryological basis for the treatment of congenital anomalies, ed 2. Baltimore, Wilkins & Wilkins, 1994:334.

2. Chen L-T. Microcirculation of the spleen. Science 1978;201:157.
3. Van Krieken JHJM, te Velde J. Normal histology of the human spleen. Am J Surg Pathol 1988;12:777.
4. Crosby WH. Normal functions of the spleen relative to red blood cells: a review. Blood 1959;14:399.
5. Burke JS, Simon GT. Electron microscopy of the spleen. Am J Pathol 1970;58:127.
6. Bohnsack JF, Brown EJ. The role of the spleen in resistance to infection. Annu Rev Med 1986;37:49.
7. Lockwood CM. Immunological functions of the spleen. Clin Haematol 1983;12:449.
8. Bowdler AJ. Splenomegaly and hypersplenism. Clin Haematol 1983; 12:467.
9. Keidl CM, Chusid MJ. Splenic abscesses in childhood. Pediatr Infect Dis J 1989;8:368.
10. Rubin E, Farber JL. Developmental and genetic diseases. In: Rubin E, Farber JL, eds. Pathology, ed 2. Philadelphia, JB Lippincott, 1994:200.
11. Kelton JG, Brain MC, Hayward CPM. Destruction of red cells by the vasculature and reticuloendothelial system. In: Nathan DG, Oski FA, eds. Hematology of infancy and childhood, ed 4. Philadelphia, WB Saunders, 1993:511.
12. Platt OS, Dover GJ. Sickle cell disease. In: Nathan DG, Oski FA, eds. Hematology of infancy and childhood, ed 4. Philadelphia, WB Saunders, 1993:732.
13. Powell RW, Levine GL, Yang Y, et al. Acute splenic sequestration crisis in sickle cell disease: early detection and treatment. J Pediatr Surg 1992;27:215.
14. McDonagh KT, Nienhuis AW. The thalassemias. In: Nathan DG, Oski FA, eds. Hematology of infancy and childhood, ed 4. Philadelphia, WB Saunders, 1993:783.
15. Davis PW, Williams DA, Shamberger RC. Immune thrombocytopenia: surgical therapy and predictors of response. J Pediatr Surg 1991;26:407.
16. Griffith RC, Janney CG. Hematopoietic system: bone marrow and blood, spleen, and lymph nodes. In: Kissane JM, ed. Anderson's pathology, ed 9. St Louis, CV Mosby, 1990:1373.
17. Burke JS. Surgical pathology of the spleen: an approach to the differential diagnosis of splenic lymphomas and leukemias. II. Diseases of the red pulp. Am J Surg Pathol 1981;5:681.
18. Garvin DF, King FM. Cysts and nonlymphomatous tumors of the spleen. Pathol Ann 1981;16:61.
19. Miller DR. Hematologic malignancies: leukemia and lymphoma. In: Miller DR, Baehner, Miller LP, eds. Blood diseases of infancy and childhood, ed 6. St Louis, CV Mosby, 1990:604.
20. Burke JS. Surgical pathology of the spleen: an approach to the differential diagnosis of splenic lymphomas and leukemias. I. Diseases of the white pulp. Am J Surg Pathol 1981;5:551.
21. Dean RH. Uncommon arteriopathies of childhood. In: Dean RH, O'Neill JA Jr, eds. Vascular disorders of childhood. Philadelphia, Lea & Febiger, 1983:97.
22. Lankisch PG. The spleen in inflammatory pancreatic disease. Gastroenterology 1990;98:509.
23. Guzzetta PC, Ruley EJ, Merrick HFW, et al. Elective subtotal splenectomy: indications and results in 33 patients. Ann Surg 1990;211:34.
24. Lobe TE, Presbury GJ, Smith BM, et al. Laparoscopic splenectomy. Pediatr Ann 1993;22:671.
25. Morris DH, Bullock FD. The importance of the spleen in resistance to infection. Ann Surg 1919;70:513.
26. King H, Schumacker HB Jr. Splenic studies. I. Susceptibility to infection after splenectomy performed in infancy. Ann Surg 1952;136:239.
27. Singer DB. Postsplenectomy sepsis. Perspect Pediatr Pathol 1973;1:285.

SECTION **H**

Adrenal Gland

Surgery of Infants and Children: Scientific Principles and Practice, edited by Keith T. Oldham, Paul M. Colombani, and Robert P. Foglia. Lippincott–Raven Publishers, Philadelphia, © 1997.

CHAPTER 90

Adrenal Gland

Dennis P. Lund

ANATOMY

The adrenal glands are bilateral structures situated high in the retroperitoneum just above and medial to the upper poles of the kidneys. They are triangular and mustard colored and weigh about 5 g each in adults. There are two major divisions of the adrenal gland: the outer portion is the *adrenal cortex,* and the inner portion is the *medulla.* The cortex is the site of sex hormone, mineralocorticoid, and glucocorticoid hormone synthesis. It is divided into three separate zones: the outermost portion is the zona glomerulosa, the middle zone is the zona fasciculata, and the innermost section is the zona reticularis. Each zone and the medulla have separate synthetic functions, which are detailed later.

The arterial supply of the adrenal glands consists primarily of three sets of small arteries. The superior adrenal arteries are branches of the inferior phrenic arteries that arise from either the aorta or the celiac trunk. The middle adrenal arteries arise from the aorta near the origin of the superior mesenteric artery. The right middle adrenal artery runs posterior to the inferior vena cava. Each renal artery gives rise to an inferior adrenal artery. Venous drainage from the glands is largely through a single dominant adrenal vein. On the left, the adrenal vein drains into the left renal vein; on the right, the adrenal vein is short and often of generous caliber. The right adrenal vein drains directly into the inferior vena cava posterior to the right lobe of the liver. The unique anatomic features of the right adrenal vein pose the risk of significant hemorrhage during adrenalectomy by the unwary surgeon (Fig. 90-1*A*).

Adrenal Cortex

The *zona glomerulosa,* the outermost zone of the cortex, consists of small polyhedral cells arranged in rounded groups or curved columns. The cells have deeply staining nuclei and scanty basophilic cytoplasm containing a few lipid droplets. The cytoplasm has abundant endoplasmic reticulum without granules, characteristic of cells that synthesize steroids. It is a

fairly thin layer, and is primarily responsible for synthesis of aldosterone and related mineralocorticoids.

The wider *zona fasciculata,* internal to the zona glomerulosa, contains large polyhedral cells with basophilic cytoplasm. These cells are arranged in characteristic columns two cells wide, containing venous channels coursing parallel to and within the columns. The cells contain large numbers of lipid droplets with fat, phospholipid, and cholesterol. The cytoplasm contains abundant smooth endoplasmic reticulum. These cells are largely devoted to glucocorticoid and sex hormone production.

The innermost cortical zone, the *zona reticularis,* consists of a sheet of branching and intermingling columns of rounded cells. The cytoplasm contains much smooth endoplasmic reticulum, lysosomes, and pigment bodies, which may be the result of cellular degeneration. The cells of the zona reticularis provide a repository for cholesterol, and because this is the precursor for steroidogenesis, this is an important functional zone in both cortisol and sex hormone synthesis. There is probably some overlap between the functions of the cells in the reticularis and fasciculata zones (see Fig. 90-1*B*).

Adrenal Medulla

The adrenal medulla is composed of ectoderm-derived chromaffin cells, or pheochromocytes. The medulla is surrounded by the cortex, and cortical venous blood bathes the medulla before leaving the gland. These cells are located in groups and columns with wide venous spaces between them. Nerve cell bodies and axons are abundant throughout the medulla. The pheochromocytes and nerves cells provide functional capability to the adrenal medulla and also account for the two principal childhood medullary neoplasms, pheochromocytoma and neuroblastoma. Chromaffin cells synthesize norepinephrine and epinephrine. These products are secreted into the venous sinuses under sympathetic nervous control. The cells are large and polarized with intimate anatomic relations to the venous sinuses. The nuclei tend to be situated in the basal aspects of the cells, while the secretory apparatus occupies an apical position adjacent to the venous sinuses. The cytoplasm is basophilic and

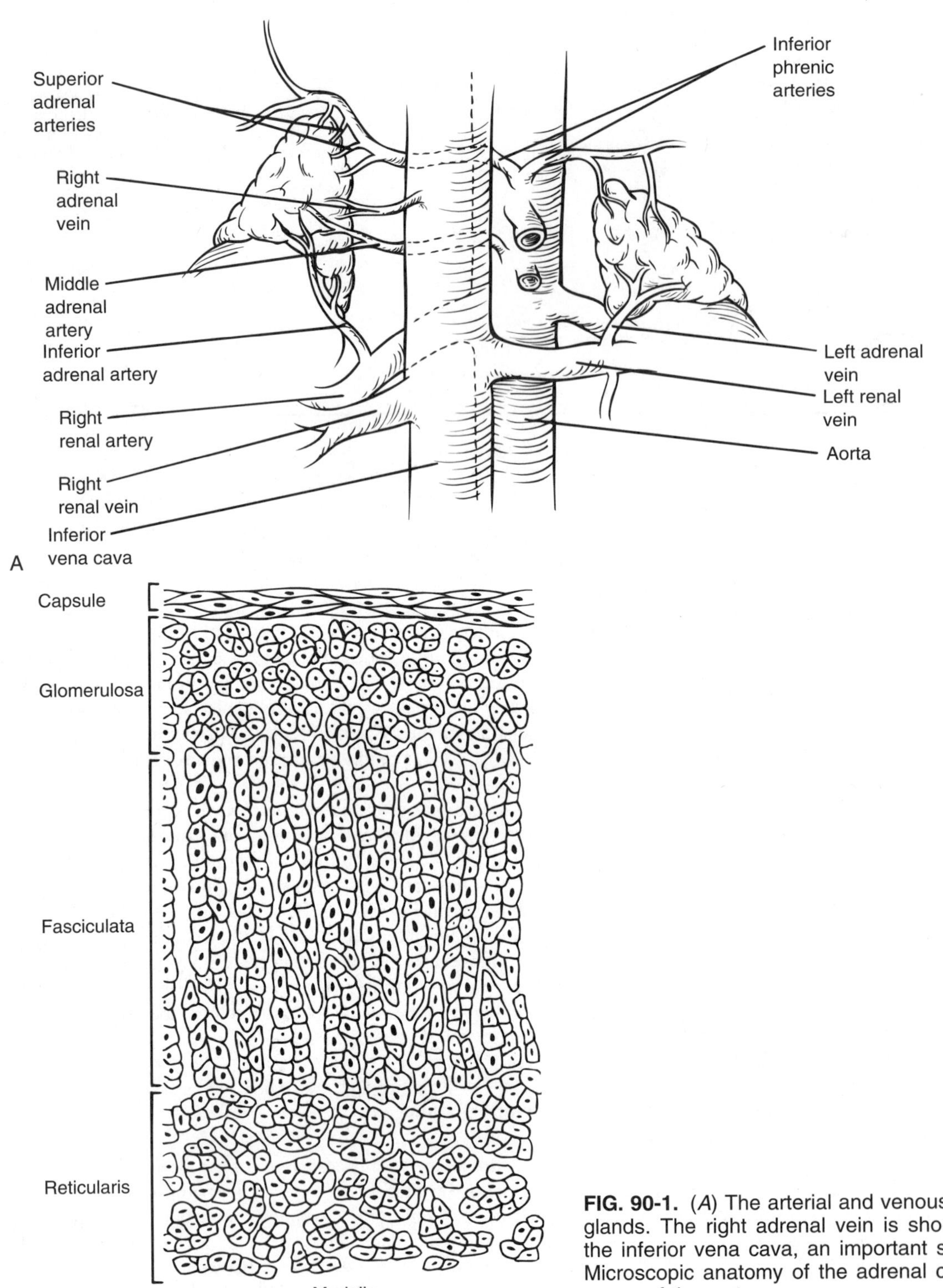

FIG. 90-1. (*A*) The arterial and venous anatomy of both adrenal glands. The right adrenal vein is short and drains directly into the inferior vena cava, an important surgical consideration. (*B*) Microscopic anatomy of the adrenal cortex, including the three zones of the cortex.

contains granular endoplasmic reticulum, mitochondria, and Golgi complexes, all signs of metabolically active cells. Secretory vesicles are plentiful. Abundant innervation to the medulla is through myelinated preganglionic sympathetic fibers, which control epinephrine and norepinephrine secretion in response to various stimuli. Sympathetic synaptic control is through the basal cell membrane.

EMBRYOLOGY AND FETAL ADRENAL FUNCTION

The adrenal gland is one of the earliest identifiable endocrine organs in the human embryo. It plays a unique physiologic role in fetal organogenesis. The adrenal cortex arises from mesodermal elements of the adrenogenital ridge, whereas the medulla arises from neuroectoderm. The primordium of the cortex becomes visible by the 4th gestational week. Undifferentiated cells from the coelomic epithelium, in the space between the mesentery and the head of the mesonephros, elongate, divide, and invade the mesenchyme beneath the epithelial surface. The cells coalesce to form the primordium of the fetal adrenal cortex and are a discrete mass by 34 days' gestation (10 mm). A secondary proliferation of coelomic epithelial cells forms a cap over the primitive cortical cells, becoming the zona glomerulosa of the definitive cortex. At about the same time, primitive cells from the sympathetic primordia, the ganglia of the 6th to the 12th thoracic segments, invade the gland, eventually forming the adrenal medulla. Differentiation into mature chromaffin cells begins at about the beginning of the 3rd gestational month.[1]

At 6 weeks' gestation, the fetal zone of the adrenal cortex appears and eventually occupies most of the fetal adrenal gland. The cells of the fetal zone have limited 3β-hydroxysteroid dehydrogenase, an enzyme essential for biosynthesis of active steroid hormones. This may be because large quantities of estrogens reach the fetus through the placenta and inhibit its expression. Fetal zone cells can, however, sulfurylate and hydroxylate steroids in the 16α position; thus, the products of the fetal adrenal gland are by and large 16α-hydroxylated-D-5-steroids, such as 16α-hydroxydehydroepiandrosterone and its sulfate, which are inactive. Limited production of active steroids leads to high levels of adrenocorticotropic hormone (ACTH) in the fetus, which probably explains the hyperplastic nature of the fetal adrenal gland.[2]

The fetal zone of the adrenal cortex normally disappears in humans within a few weeks or months after birth, and is replaced by adult cortical structure. Cortisol, aldosterone, androstenedione, and other steroid hormones are produced there. Once placental estrogens disappear after birth, plasma glucocorticoids levels rise, ACTH levels fall, and regression of the fetal zone occurs. Rapid regression of this zone may contribute to fetal adrenal hemorrhage, which is not infrequent.

The fetal liver can hydroxylate steroids in the 16α position, so that maternal estrogens reaching the fetus are rapidly converted to estriol, and thus made inactive. The placenta contains enzymes necessary to convert androgens produced by the mother and the fetus to estrogens, but it lacks 16α-hydroxylase and 17,20-desmolase activity; thus, it cannot synthesize estrogens de novo. The fetal adrenal cannot synthesize cortisol de novo, but it can convert placental progesterone to cortisol. This synthetic interplay between the fetal adrenal gland and the placenta has led to the concept of the *fetoplacental unit*. The fetal adrenal and the placenta together regulate fetal homeostasis (Fig. 90-2).

Because the fetus participates normally in estrogen production, maternal blood testing for estrogens, particularly estriol, is useful in assessing the health of the pregnancy. Both fetal adrenal and hepatic insufficiency can lead to abrupt falls in maternal estriol levels, which in turn can signal that the pregnancy is in jeopardy.

Both maternal and fetal glucocorticoids play a role in the differentiation of a number of fetal tissues, including the lung, gut, and retina. Blood flowing from the adrenal cortex to the medulla induces *N*-methyltransferase activity, so that fetal epi-

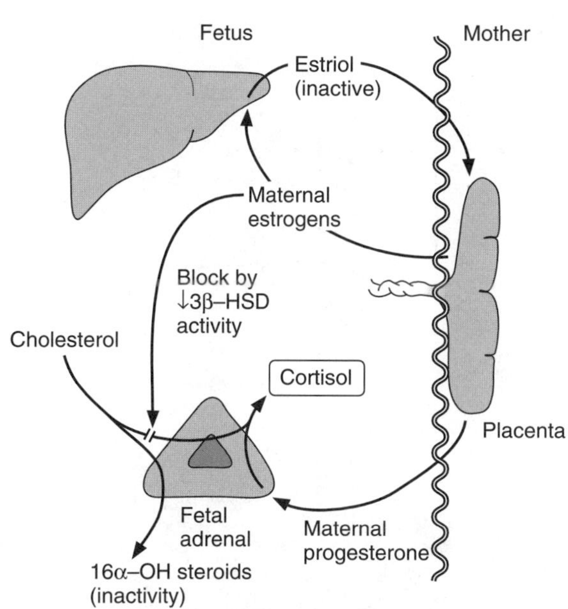

FIG. 90-2. The fetoplacental unit. Maternal estrogens block de novo cortisol synthesis by the fetal adrenal gland and are converted to estriol by the fetal liver. The fetus synthesizes cortisol by metabolism of maternal progesterone. 3β-HSD, 3β-hydroxysteroid dehydrogenase.

nephrine levels rise late in the pregnancy and soon after birth as a result of the enhanced conversion of norepinephrine.

PHYSIOLOGY

Hypothalamic–Pituitary–Adrenal Axis

The principal role of the adrenal glands is the regulation of homeostasis. For this purpose, three types of hormones are synthesized: glucocorticoids, mineralocorticoids, and sex hormones. In general, control of adrenal hormone synthesis and release is through a complex series of feedback mechanisms referred to as the *hypothalamic–pituitary–adrenal* (HPA) *axis*. ACTH stimulates production of all three types of adrenal hormones by binding to a cell-surface receptor, which is internalized; it then activates adenylate cyclase, leading to increased intracellular cyclic AMP (cAMP). cAMP activates phosphoprotein kinases, which stimulate conversion of cholesterol to pregnenolone, the rate-limiting step in steroidogenesis (see later). ACTH is a cleavage product of a larger prohormone that originates from the anterior pituitary gland. The secretion of this molecule is under the control of the hypothalamus, specifically the paraventricular nucleus, by another hormone known as *corticotropin-releasing hormone* (CRH; Fig. 90-3).

CRH is synthesized in the hypothalamus and transported through the pituitary portal system to the adenohypophysis, where it stimulates release of ACTH. Release of CRH is under neural control. The normally diurnal variation of CRH release accounts for the cyclical variation in ACTH and therefore cortisol levels. Typically, these peptides are at peak concentrations in the blood shortly before or at the time of awakening, with a gradual decline during the ensuing 24-hour period. The diurnal

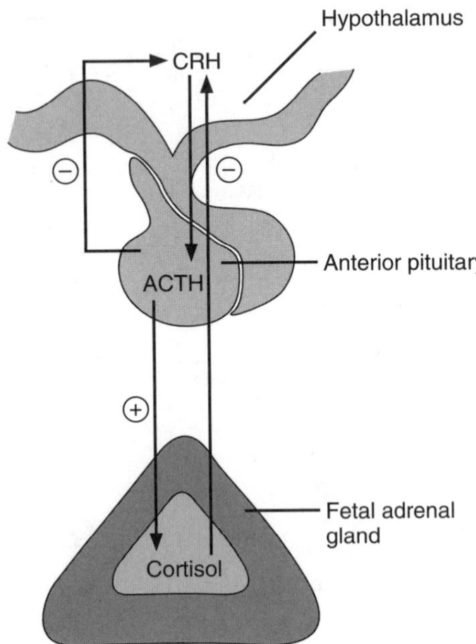

FIG. 90-3. The hypothalamic–pituitary–adrenal axis. Both the adrenal gland and the pituitary have mechanisms of feedback inhibition of corticotropin-releasing hormone (CRH) release from the hypothalamus. ACTH, adrenocorticotropic hormone.

pattern of CRH release can be altered by changing sleep patterns for several days, by manipulating light and dark cycles, and by blindness. In addition, psychologic and physical stress lead to enhanced ACTH release.[3]

Release of CRH is inhibited by cortisol through a negative-feedback loop. There is also evidence for negative feedback by ACTH on CRH release, although this appears physiologically subordinate to cortisol-feedback inhibition. ACTH has a rapid onset of action and a short half-life (measured in minutes), whereas steroid hormones have a longer half-life and slower onset of action. This accounts for the relatively slow physiologic response to cortisol release. The complex interactions of these regulatory loops results in fine homeostatic control of plasma cortisol levels.

Glucocorticoid Synthesis

The biosynthesis of steroid hormones begins with cholesterol as the substrate (Fig. 90-4). The initial event, removal of the side chain from position C-20, is a rate-limiting step and is under the control of ACTH, so that all of steroidogenesis is stimulated by ACTH. Additional intermediate enzymatic steps are also under ACTH control, so that overall synthesis of both glucocorticoids and androgens is regulated by ACTH. Aldosterone synthesis, primarily in the zona glomerulosa, is regulated to a much lesser degree by ACTH.

Cortisol in plasma is bound by two plasma proteins—albumin, with high capacity and low affinity, and cortisol-binding protein with high affinity and low capacity. About 90% of plasma cortisol is bound to cortisol-binding protein, 6% is bound to albumin, and the remainder is free in equilibrium with the bound fraction. Only free cortisol can cross membranes

and exert physiologic control of cellular behavior. Metabolized glucocorticoids are excreted in the urine primarily as 17-hydroxycorticosteroids. A small fraction of free cortisol is also excreted in the urine. Some glucocorticoids undergo side-chain cleavage in the liver, resulting in 17-ketosteroids, which are excreted in the urine as well.

Sex Hormone Synthesis

Adrenal androgens (eg, dehydroepiandrosterone and Δ_4-androstenedione), are biologically weak androgens that can be converted into more active forms, such as testosterone and dihydrotestosterone, in peripheral tissues. Adrenal androgens are secreted in synchrony with cortisol in a cyclical manner. The liver metabolizes androgens, and these compounds are excreted in the urine as 17-ketosteroids. Adrenal androgens are synthesized principally in the zona reticularis, the inner layer of the adrenal cortex; this zone is identifiable by 4 to 5 years of age and becomes biosynthetically active by 6 to 8 years of age. A pituitary regulatory factor, cortical androgen–stimulating hormone has been identified.[4] This hormone appears to stimulate androgen, but not cortisol secretion, from the adrenal gland. Other hormones, such as prolactin, may also play a role in the regulation of adrenal androgen production. In addition, prolactin receptors have been identified in the adrenal gland.[5] This may explain why increased levels of dihydroepiandrosterone are seen in hyperprolactinemic conditions. Finally, blood flow characteristics in the zones of the adrenal may influence the steroid production in different areas. For example, in the zona reticularis, levels of Δ_4-3-ketosteroids may suppress 3β-hydroxysteroid dehydrogenase and thereby shift the synthesis toward production of dehydroepiandrosterone and its sulfate.

In summary, the secretion of adrenal androgens is controlled by ACTH, hormones such as cortical androgen–stimulating hormone and prolactin, and probably intraadrenal mechanisms. Pituitary gonadotropins do not normally affect adrenal production of androgens. Some androgen-producing adrenal carcinomas, however, may be influenced by human chorionic gonadotropin.[6]

The human adrenal gland produces minimal amounts of estrogens. Estrogens may be formed from adrenal androgens by peripheral conversion. Both muscle and adipose tissue can synthesize estrone from Δ_4-androstenedione.

Mineralocorticoid Synthesis

The zona glomerulosa is the principal site of aldosterone synthesis. Although synthetic intermediates, such as deoxycorticosterone, corticosterone, and 18-hydroxycorticosterone, are produced in the other cortical zones and their production is regulated by ACTH, overall production and release of aldosterone is only weakly regulated by ACTH. The major control mechanism for mineralocorticoid release is the renin–angiotensin system (see later).

Aldosterone circulates in plasma bound to corticosteroid-binding globulin (22%), to albumin (41%), and in free form (37%). A small fraction of aldosterone is excreted unchanged in the urine. The major site for metabolism of aldosterone is in the liver, where the A ring is reduced to form tetrahydroaldosterone and is subsequently conjugated with glucuronic acid. Therefore, patients with impaired hepatocellular function are predictably

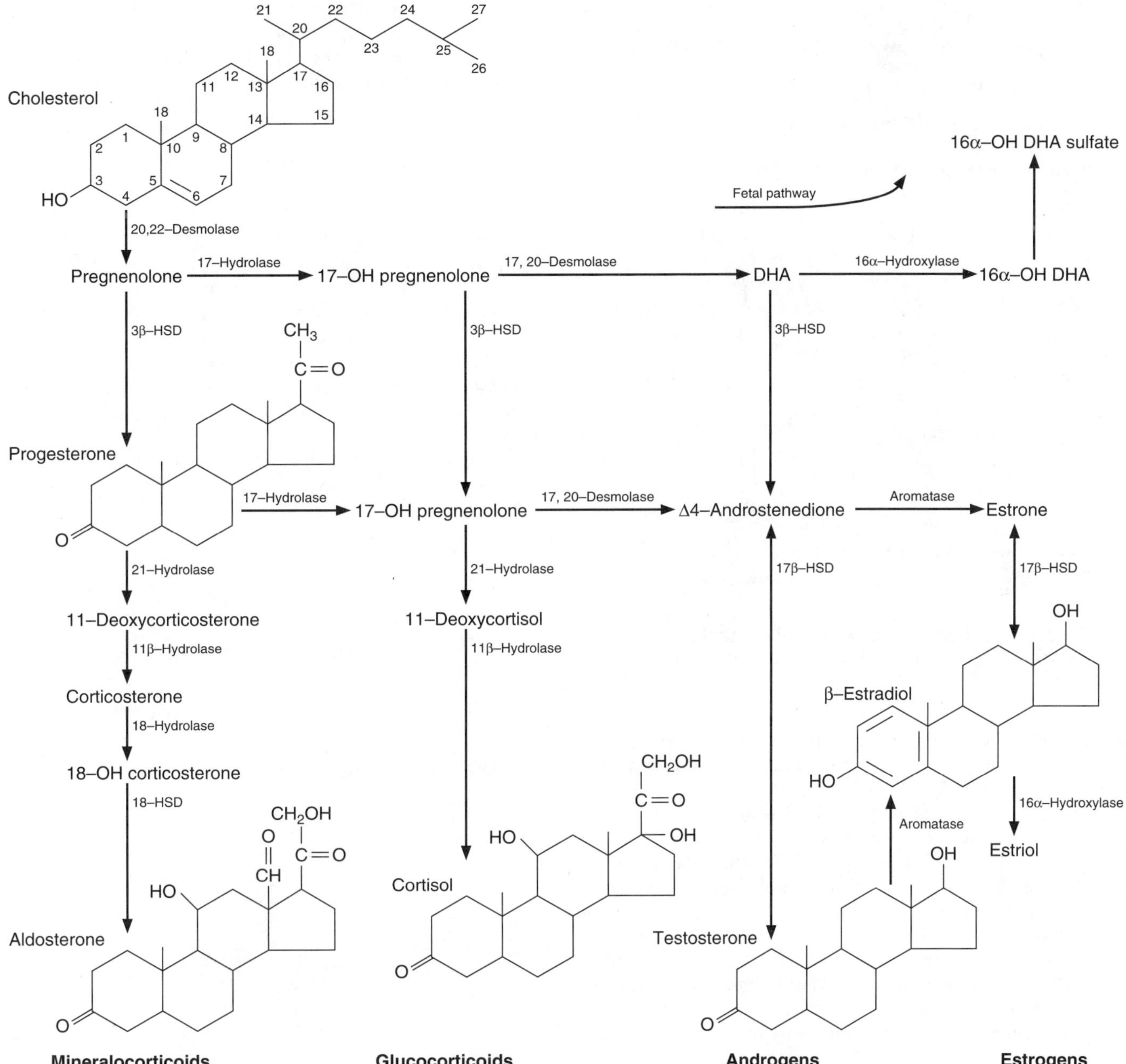

FIG. 90-4. Intermediary metabolism of adrenal steroids. 3β-Hydroxysteroid dehydrogenase (3β-HSD) activity is inhibited in the fetus by maternal estrogens. Thus, the fetal pathway leads to the synthesis of 16α-hydroxy dehydroepiandrosterone (16α-OH DHA) and its sulfate.

subject to clinical problems derived from inadequate metabolic processing, leading to mineralocorticoid excess. An alternative metabolic pathway is present in the liver and the kidney, where the C-18 position can be conjugated with glucuronic acid to form aldosterone glucuronide to aid in excretion.

Renin–Angiotensin System

Primary physiologic control of mineralocorticoid synthesis and secretion resides in the renin–angiotensin system.[7] Changes in blood pressure and serum sodium concentration lead to release of renin from the macula densa of the juxtaglomerular apparatus in the kidney. In particular, diminished perfusion and hyponatremia are powerful stimuli for renin excretion. Specific prostaglandins and the sympathetic nervous system also regulate renin release, but to a lesser degree. Renin is an enzyme that catalyzes conversion of angiotensinogen to angiotensin I. Angiotensinogen is a relatively large peptide synthesized in the liver, and angiotensin I is a decapeptide. Angiotensin I is in turn processed to angiotensin II by a converting enzyme found principally in the lung. Conversion of angiotensin I to angioten-

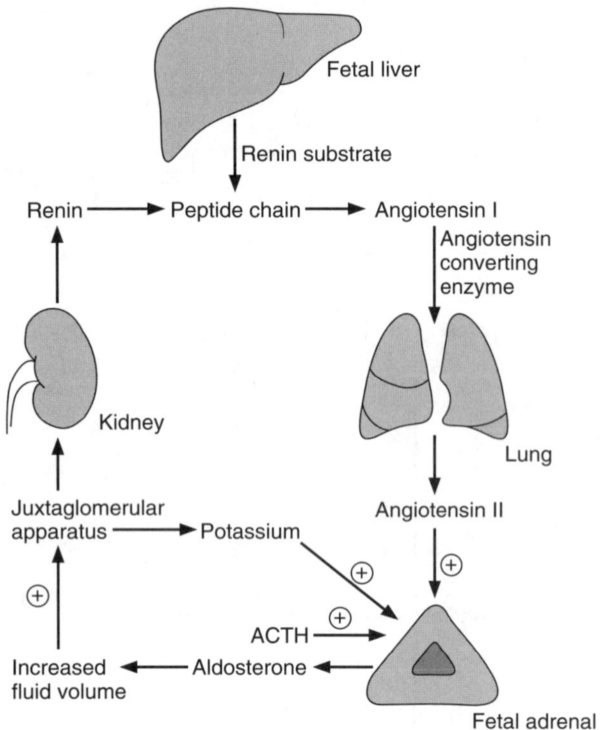

FIG. 90-5. Schematic representation of the renin–angiotensin system. ACTH, adrenocorticotropic hormone.

sin II is 90% complete in a single pass of blood through the lung. This conversion is by an enzyme known as *angiotensin-converting enzyme* (Fig. 90-5).

Angiotensin II acts directly on the adrenocortical cells of the zona glomerulosa by way of a specific cellular receptor to stimulate synthesis of aldosterone. Angiotensin II also acts directly on arterial vessels to increase peripheral vascular resistance and therefore blood pressure.

Calcium has a permissive effect on aldosterone synthesis through a mechanism involving desmolase and the conversion of corticosterone to aldosterone. Hyperkalemia also increases aldosterone synthesis, both by direct effect on the cells of the zona glomerulosa and by renin release by the juxtaglomerular cells.

Other factors are known to effect aldosterone secretion as well, although their specific physiologic functions are not fully understood. A 28–amino acid peptide called *atrial natriuretic peptide* has been isolated.[8] This peptide, from human atria, inhibits aldosterone synthesis by zona glomerulosa adrenocortical cells in vitro, and increased plasma atrial natriuretic peptide levels have been observed in clinical situations such as primary aldosteronism. The anterior pituitary also produces a factor known as *aldosterone stimulating factor*, a glycoprotein found in human urine.[9] This factor causes enhanced aldosterone synthesis in zona glomerulosa cells in vitro.

In general, a decrease in blood pressure or in sodium concentration in the renal tubule leads to increased renin secretion and subsequently increased aldosterone secretion. Conversely, sodium loading, intravascular volume excess, and assumption of the supine position result in diminished renin and angiotensin production with decreased aldosterone production. Hyperka-

lemia increases aldosterone production, thereby promoting potassium excretion in the urine. Likewise, hypokalemia decreases the output of aldosterone and thus provides for potassium conservation in the renal tubule.

Adrenal Medullary Function

Chromaffin cells of the adrenal medulla contain catecholamines localized in cytoplasmic granules. The active catecholamines in humans are dopamine, epinephrine, and norepinephrine. Control of secretion of these compounds resides in the preganglionic sympathetic nerve endings, which secrete acetylcholine. Acetylcholine release is responsible for calcium-dependent exocytosis of these cytoplasmic storage granules and, therefore, for catecholamine release into the circulation. In essence, the adrenal medulla functions as a sympathetic nerve ganglion.

The catecholamine synthetic pathway is outlined in Figure 90-6. The process begins with tyrosine, a nonessential amino

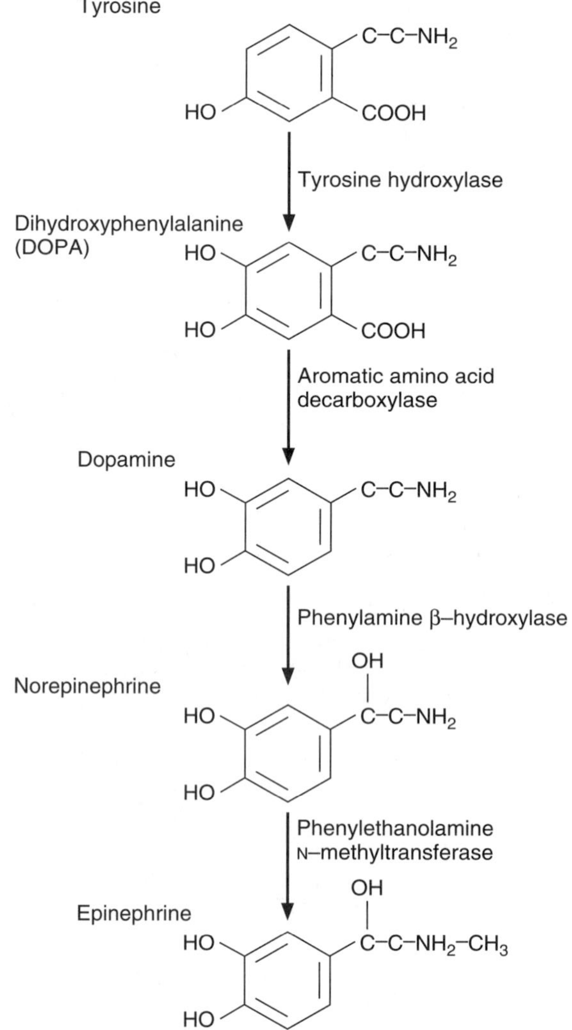

FIG. 90-6. Intermediary metabolism of catecholamines in the adrenal medulla.

acid derived from phenylalanine (which is essential). Tyrosine is converted into dihydroxyphenylalanine (DOPA) by tyrosine hydroxylase. Importantly, tyrosine hydroxylase, the rate-limiting enzyme in the synthetic pathway, is regulated by acetylcholine. DOPA decarboxylase then converts DOPA into dopamine, which is converted to norepinephrine by phenylamine β-hydroxylase. The final step is conversion of norepinephrine to epinephrine by phenylethylamine N-methyltransferase.

A portion of the released norepinephrine and epinephrine is taken up by the chromaffin cells, and some is released into the general circulation. Metabolism of the circulating catecholamines is done by neurons; by enzymatic degradation in other sites, such as liver, gut, and kidney; and by excretion into urine. Catecholamines taken up by neurons are metabolized by monamine oxidase to yield vanillylmandelic acid. Carboxyl-o-methyl transferase acts on the compounds at nonneuronal sites to yield normetanephrine from norepinephrine and metanephrine from epinephrine. A small fraction of the catecholamines are secreted into urine unchanged, and this can be helpful in diagnosing pheochromocytomas.

Catecholamines are released normally into the circulation from the adrenal gland in a ratio of about 80% epinephrine to 20% norepinephrine. About half of plasma catecholamines are loosely bound to protein. The half-life of free epinephrine and norepinephrine is less than 1 minute. Basal levels of epinephrine in plasma range from 20 to 50 pg/mL, but vary considerably depending on the environment and recent stimuli. Predictable, transient rises in plasma levels occur with pain and anxiety. Other stimuli, such as cigarette smoking, upright posture, hypoglycemia, and cold, lead to increases in circulating catecholamine levels.

Two primary feedback inhibitory mechanisms regulate adrenal medullary catecholamine release. First, norepinephrine acts directly on presynaptic, preganglionic α_2-receptors to decrease the release of acetylcholine. Second, high concentrations of norepinephrine inhibit tyrosine hydroxylase activity. Thus, norepinephrine can limit its own production.

PATHOPHYSIOLOGY

Most surgeons concerned with the adrenal gland deal with conditions of hormone overproduction, often as the result of tumors. These are considered later. In addition, the pediatric surgeon must be knowledgeable about conditions of hormone overproduction due to inborn errors of metabolism, such as congenital adrenal hyperplasia. To understand these pathophysiologic states, the surgeon must also understand the normal physiologic functions of the gland and the impact of adrenal hormones on peripheral tissues.

Glucocorticoid Function

Most steroid molecules circulate bound to plasma proteins. The small unbound fraction crosses the plasma membrane of target cells readily because steroids are lipophilic. Specific cytosolic steroid receptors then bind with the hormone, and the steroid–receptor complex is transported to the cell nucleus, where it regulates the synthesis of new messenger RNA and thus the cell protein product. The biologic effects of steroids are often relatively slow, generally taking several hours because of the necessity to synthesize new gene products. Different target cells have different steroid receptors with variable functions and affinities. This accounts for the differential effects of steroids among tissues. For example, cortisol has many effects on basic carbohydrate metabolism, and therefore cortisol receptors are ubiquitous. In contrast, androgens and estrogens have much more limited and specific functions, so that most relevant receptors are concentrated in the tissue of the genital organs, breast, and prostate.

Cortisol has a number of key effects on intermediary metabolism, most of which oppose the effects of insulin. The most pronounced of these may be proteolysis. Glucocorticoids regulate the release of branched-chain and other amino acids from muscle, providing necessary substrate for gluconeogenesis. This effect is present even in the absence of insulin. Cortisol-induced protein breakdown also releases lactate from muscle. Lactate and glycerol released from fat under the influence of epinephrine are also precursors for gluconeogenesis. Cortisol promotes hyperglycemia by two mechanisms: (1) enhanced gluconeogenesis, by generating the necessary substrates and inducing gluconeogenic enzymes in liver; and (2) diminished use of glucose by peripheral tissues when under the influence of cortisol. The latter effect results from decreased insulin binding by insulin-sensitive tissues and also by inhibition of glucose uptake into fat cells.

An additional catabolic effect of cortisol is the enhancement of lipolysis. Serum free fatty acids and triglycerides increase under the influence of cortisol. The characteristic truncal obesity of Cushing syndrome (ie, hypercortisolism) may be explained by the fact that truncal adipocytes may be more influenced by insulin (lipogenesis), whereas extremity adipocytes may be more sensitive to cortisol (lipolysis).

Cortisol also has a number of effects on other tissues relevant to the surgeon. These include its ability to decrease inflammation and immune function and to impair wound healing. Cortisol has both chronotropic and inotropic effects on the myocardium as well as the ability to increase peripheral vascular resistance. These effects, along with the increase in sodium reabsorption in the distal renal tubule, account for the hypertension frequently seen with cortisol excess. In the gastrointestinal tract, glucocorticoids decrease mucosal cell replication and prostaglandin synthesis in the gut and pancreas. These effects may play a role in the development of the peptic ulcers seen with steroid administration and also may explain the more frequent incidence of acute pancreatitis in steroid-treated patients. Cortisol also has an effect on bone, leading to osteopenia as a result of decreased bone formation. This is thought to be due to decreased osteoblast development, which leads to a deficiency of protein in the extracellular matrix.

Every surgeon is aware of the effects of cortisol on inflammation, the immune response, and wound healing. These effects result largely from alterations in both the specific (lymphocyte) and nonspecific (granulocyte) cellular immune response. With regard to the former, cortisol excess appears to act principally by decreasing lymphocyte response to specific antigenic stimulation. This explains the efficacy of glucocorticoids in the prevention of rejection in organ transplantation. This blunted response is responsible, at least in part, for the clinical observation that steroid-treated patients are vulnerable to a variety of opportunistic and conventional infectious organisms. With regard to granulocyte function, leukocytosis occurs in circulating blood as a result of cortisol administration, but both chemotaxis and phagocytosis are impaired. Thus, granulocyte-dependent bacterial killing is less efficient. Wounds have decreased tensile strength in the presence of excess cortisol because both lymphocytes and granulocytes are essential early components of the wound healing process (see Chap. 9). In addition, both epithelialization and scar contraction are impaired. Cortisol also interferes with the production of some soluble mediators of inflammation, although these mechanisms are not fully understood. The net effect of cortisol on the inflammatory process is profound and highly significant for the clinician.

Cushing Syndrome

Elevated levels of glucocorticoids for a prolonged period result in a characteristic combination of clinical features known as *Cushing syndrome.* These features include central obesity, hypertension, muscle weakness and wasting, and thin skin with streaks, called *striae.*[10] Cushing syndrome is rare in children and can be caused by exogenous administration of glucocorticoids or by endogenous overproduction of cortisol or ACTH. Patients with pituitary overproduction of ACTH are said to have *Cushing disease,* a rare entity in children. This is most often the result of an anterior pituitary microadenoma but also can be due to a large, invasive pituitary adenoma. Some of these pituitary adenomas may be the result of excessive hypothalamic stimulation of the pituitary. Whatever the cause of glucocorticoid excess, the syndrome presents in essentially the same form in most patients.

Cortisol hypersecretion can be caused by adrenal tumors, either adenomas or carcinomas. Adrenal carcinomas in children are more likely to produce large quantities of androgens, often in excess of glucocorticoids. Before 6 years of age, excess cortisol production is usually the result of an adrenal tumor. After the early years, the cause is more likely to be excessive pituitary secretion of ACTH, resulting in bilateral adrenal hyperplasia. Rarely, children have excessive ACTH production as a result of an ectopic source, such as a thymoma or pancreatic neoplasm.

The clinical signs and symptoms of Cushing syndrome are as follows:

- Decreased rate of linear growth
- Weight gain
- Hypertension
- Central obesity
- Weakness
- Thin skin with easy bruising
- Striae
- Acne
- Menstrual irregularity
- Osteoporosis
- Glucose intolerance

Muscle wasting is common, especially in the limbs. Frequently, patients have centripetal fat redistribution, and a ''buffalo hump'' is pathognomonic. One of the most important signs of Cushing syndrome in children is impairment of linear growth, which slows or completely ceases. These children continue to gain weight but do not grow longitudinally unless there is also an associated excess production of androgens. Hypertension, glucose intolerance, easy bruising, abdominal striae, and menstrual irregularities can all be present. Patients can also manifest a wide variety of emotional or psychiatric symptoms.

Addison Disease

Insufficient production of steroid hormones from the adrenal glands can lead to a potentially life-threatening entity known as *Addison disease.* The clinical problem can be associated with mineralocorticoid or glucocorticoid insufficiency, or both, depending on the specific cause. The adrenal gland deficiency can be present at birth, secondary to congenital hypoplasia or to pituitary failure. Congenital adrenal hypoplasia can be due to an autosomal recessive disorder in which there is marked lack of development in the fetal zone with a relatively normal adult zone. A second form of congenital adrenal hypoplasia is an X-linked disorder in boys, characterized by abnormal adrenal glands with persistence of the fetal zone architecture. A syndrome of hereditary adrenal resistance to ACTH has also been described. This is probably inherited in an autosomal recessive pattern. This syndrome is not associated with mineralocorticoid deficiency.[11]

Inborn errors of steroid metabolism also can lead to adrenal insufficiency. If these errors occur early in the steroid biosynthetic pathway, they result in insufficient production of all normal steroid hormones. Other metabolic defects can specifically affect production of androgens (Noonan syndrome) or mineralocorticoids (hypoaldosteronism). The most common inborn errors, however, are characterized by defects in glucocorticoid synthesis and are referred to collectively as *congenital adrenal hyperplasia* (see later). Acquired central nervous system lesions involving the hypothalamus or pituitary also can lead to Addison disease through ablation of corticotropin-releasing factor or ACTH secretion.

Finally, there are conditions that can lead to destruction of the adrenal glands. These include hemorrhage, infections, adrenoleukodystrophy, and autoimmune diseases. Formerly, tuberculosis was a leading cause of infectious destruction of the adrenal glands. Today, however, autoimmune disease is a more prevalent cause and can be associated with diseases in other endocrine glands, such as in autoimmune thyroiditis.[12] Overwhelming infection in the newborn or traumatic delivery can lead to acute hemorrhage of the adrenal glands, resulting in acute adrenal insufficiency. Overwhelming postsplenectomy sepsis with pneumococcal organisms, meningococcemia, and other causes of overwhelming sepsis can lead to bilateral adrenal hemorrhages and acute adrenal insufficiency, the Waterhouse-Friderichsen syndrome. Acquired immunodeficiency syndrome can also manifest signs of adrenal insufficiency. In surgical practice, the most common cause of acute adrenal insufficiency is abrupt cessation of long-term exogenous glucocorticoids. Functional adrenal recovery after exogenous steroid therapy may require 6 to 12 months before restoration of normal hypothalamic–pituitary regulation.

Children with Addison disease have a variety of symptoms, including weakness, anorexia, weight loss, fatigue, nausea, vomiting, and diarrhea. If the adrenal insufficiency is due to adrenal insensitivity to ACTH, there is overproduction of ACTH, and this is demonstrable in the serum. Because melanocytes are stimulated to some degree by ACTH, these children have hyperpigmentation. The development of symptoms can be acute or chronic, but if the fatigue and weakness are not diagnosed in a timely fashion, adrenal crisis can ensue. Hypoglycemia associated with adrenal crisis can lead to seizures.

The diagnosis of Addison disease is usually suggested by hyperpigmentation and fatigue. Laboratory tests reveal low serum sodium and chloride levels, while the potassium concentration can be elevated. Fasting glucose levels can be low, and the fasting morning cortisol level is usually low, with an elevated plasma ACTH. An ACTH-stimulation test shows little or no rise in the plasma cortisol levels because the end organ, the adrenal gland, has failed or is unresponsive to stimulation.

Treatment of Addison disease is conceptually simple. Deficient steroid hormones must be replaced. Usually, a glucocorticoid, such as hydrocortisone or, in older children, prednisone, is provided along with a mineralocorticoid, such as fludrocortisone (Florinef). Doses of glucocorticoids need to be increased and often given parenterally during periods of stress or crisis, such as for operations (see later).

Mineralocorticoid Function

Aldosterone, the primary mineralocorticoid in humans, affects sodium, potassium, and hydrogen transport in the distal renal tubule. The major action of aldosterone is to increase distal tubular sodium reabsorption while decreasing the reabsorption of potassium, promoting kaliuresis. Increased sodium reabsorption is also associated with increased hydrogen ion excretion in the urine. As stated earlier, aldosterone secretion is controlled by total body sodium, potassium, and water content around relatively precise physiologic set-points. Increased sodium intake decreases aldosterone output through the renin–angiotensin system. Hyperkalemia can also stimulate aldosterone output and thus lower serum potassium levels by increased urinary potassium loss.

Hyperaldosteronism

Overproduction of aldosterone is termed *hyperaldosteronism*. Causes related to adrenal dysfunction, such as aldosterone-secreting tumors or bilateral adrenal hyperplasia, are termed *primary* hyperaldosteronism. Hyperaldosteronism associated with overproduction of renin (hyperreninemic hyperaldosteronism) is termed *secondary* hyperaldosteronism. Secondary hyperaldosteronism is caused by cirrhosis, renovascular abnormalities such as renal artery stenosis, congestive heart failure, and excess production of renin by a juxtaglomerular cell tumor. A rare condition known as *Bartter syndrome* is associated with hyperplasia of the juxtaglomerular apparatus.[13] Most secondary causes of hyperaldosteronism, with the exception of renovascular disease, are nonsurgical.

Hypertension is characteristic of patients with hyperaldosteronism. This results from increased sodium and water reabsorption. Headaches due to hypertension are frequent, and both systolic and diastolic hypertension are the rule. Other symptoms of hyperaldosteronism include fatigue, weakness, lethargy, poor weight gain, polyuria, polydipsia, and nocturia. Neurologic symptoms, such as paresthesia, tetany, and periodic paralysis,

also can be present. Peripheral edema can be present, but this usually accompanies only secondary forms of hyperaldosteronism.

Hypokalemia is the most frequent laboratory finding associated with hyperaldosteronism. Metabolic alkalosis results from the enhanced loss of hydrogen ions in the urine and is easily demonstrable if sought. In addition to muscle weakness due to hypokalemia, hypoinsulinism and hyperglycemia can also occur because hyperkalemia interferes with pancreatic β-cell insulin release.

Sex Hormone Function

The major adrenal sex hormones are dehydroepiandrosterone, androstenedione, and testosterone. Androstenedione is converted in peripheral tissues to estrogen, and testosterone is the most active masculinizing hormone. Masculinizing effects of androgens include deepening of the voice; deposition of protein in muscle; development of male hair distribution, including facial hair; and coarsening of the skin. Estrogens have the opposite effects and enhance breast tissue development. Fetal exposure to androgens leads to wolffian duct development and elongation of the phallic tubercle as well as fusion of the labioscrotal folds. The urethra migrates to the tip of the phallic tubercle under the influence of androgens. In the normal female fetus, neither the ovary nor the adrenal gland secretes androgens, and the labial folds, phallic tubercle, and urethra remain in the normal female positions. If the female fetus is exposed to androgens, such as in congenital adrenal hyperplasia, the newborn may present with ambiguous or masculinized genitalia. Excess androgen in the male fetus becomes manifest after birth as precocious puberty.

Excessive Sex Steroids

Beyond infancy, patients with excessive androgen or estrogen production by the adrenal gland almost invariably have adrenal carcinoma. Girls with androgen excess develop clitoromegaly and masculinized features and cease menstruating. Boys with excess androgen production develop precocious puberty, but after puberty, this can be a difficult condition to diagnose clinically. The rare adrenal tumor that causes excess production of estrogens in girls produces menstrual irregularities; in boys, it causes breast development and sometimes a more female hair distribution.

Congenital Adrenal Hyperplasia

Congenital adrenal hyperplasia, also known as the *adrenogenital syndrome* in girls, is associated with inherited enzymatic defects in steroid biosynthesis. These defects interfere with the biosynthesis of normal amounts of cortisol and, by loss of negative feedback, lead to enhanced ACTH production. The increased ACTH levels act early in the steroid biosynthetic pathway to yield supranormal levels of androgenic intermediaries. Thus, girls are born with masculinized or ambiguous genitalia, a form of pseudohermaphroditism. The degree of masculinization of the external genitalia is related to the timing and amount of androgen production in the fetus. The spectrum of anomalies ranges from mild clitoromegaly, with a normal-appearing vagina, to a malelike phallus, with a urethra extending to the apex and no perineal vaginal orifice. Usually, the disorder falls between these extremes, with clitoral enlargement, labioscrotal fusion, and a urogenital sinus opening at the base of the clitoris. The internal female organs—uterus, fallopian tubes, ovaries, and upper vagina—are always normal.[14] If mineralocorticoid deficiency is also present, the syndrome may be associated with inability to maintain serum sodium and intravascular volume levels. This is referred to as *salt wasting*. An infant boy has only increased scrotal pigmentation from the ACTH-stimulated melanocytes, and congenital adrenal hyperplasia is usually not diagnosed until adrenal crisis develops 1 to 2 weeks after birth or when he experiences precocious puberty.

At least five enzymatic defects have been described that result in impaired cortisol synthesis, increased ACTH production, and congenital adrenal hyperplasia.[15] About 90% of all cases of congenital adrenal hyperplasia are due to deficiency of 21-hydroxylase, the enzyme that catalyzes the conversion of 17-hydroxyprogesterone to 11-deoxycortisol. It is inherited as an autosomal recessive trait. Certain HLA types are associated with this deficiency, such as A3, BW47, DR7, B14, and DR1 (late-onset form). 11β-Hydroxylase deficiency accounts for 5% of the cases of congenital adrenal hyperplasia, and deficiencies of 3β-hydroxysteroid dehydrogenase, 20,22-desmolase, and 17-hydroxylase account for the remainder of cases (Fig. 90-7).

Congenital adrenal hyperplasia is the most common cause of ambiguous genitalia in newborns. Any newborn with ambiguous genitalia, or any newborn with male external genitalia and bilateral cryptorchid testes, should be screened for this disorder. After a careful history and physical examination, laboratory evaluation should include a buccal smear, karyotype analysis, and serum analysis for specific hormones as outlined later. A detailed diagnostic algorithm for patients with ambiguous genitalia is discussed elsewhere in this text (see Chap. 95). In patients with nonpalpable testes and a buccal smear that is positive

(ie, presence of Barr body), elevated urinary 17-ketosteroids and serum 17-hydroxyprogesterone levels establish the diagnosis of congenital adrenal hyperplasia (21-hydroxylase deficiency.) A simple screen for congenital adrenal hyperplasia is to check baseline and fasting serum steroid levels. An early morning serum 17-hydroxyprogesterone level above 1000 ng/dL almost certainly indicates congenital adrenal hyperplasia. If the diagnosis is in doubt, an ACTH stimulation test can be used. If congenital adrenal hyperplasia is present, precursors of cortisol accumulate out of proportion to cortisol 1 hour after the intravenous administration of ACTH. Prenatal screening with specific molecular probes for congenital adrenal hyperplasia is also possible in families at risk.

Acute treatment for the patient with congenital adrenal hyperplasia is to correct the deficiencies resulting from the salt wasting. This may require intravenous saline administration. Endocrine treatment for congenital adrenal hyperplasia is to provide the patient with adequate exogenous glucocorticoid to suppress the overproduction of ACTH and to provide adequate circulating cortisol levels. Typically, hydrocortisone is used for smaller infants; older children can be given more potent glucocorticoids, such as prednisone or prednisolone. Patients who have the salt-wasting forms of congenital adrenal hyperplasia should also receive mineralocorticoid replacement, usually as fludrocortisone. It is necessary to adjust the hormone levels to suppress ACTH production, control hypertension, and allow for adequate growth. This requires experience and careful surveillance.

Surgical reconstruction for girls with congenital adrenal hyperplasia is done routinely at an early age. For obvious social reasons, it is critical to provide appropriate gender assignment for infants with ambiguous genitalia as soon as possible after birth. Reconstruction consists of clitoral reduction and creation of an adequate vaginal introitus. Most patients have a vagina with a perineal orifice, and a simple cutback procedure may suffice. The patients with a higher vaginal opening and a urogenital sinus, however, require more complex reconstruction to provide an adequate vagina without injuring the urinary sphincter mechanism. Surgical reconstruction for girls with congenital adrenal hyperplasia is discussed in detail in Chapter 95.

The prognosis for children with congenital adrenal hyperplasia is usually good if it is recognized early. Most patients are somewhat short of stature, but this depends on the age at diagnosis and the adequacy of glucocorticoid replacement.[16] In boys, normal puberty and fertility can be expected; however, there is an increased risk of paratesticular tumors in those who do not receive adequate glucocorticoid treatment. These most likely arise from adrenal rests along the course of the spermatic cord. Girls with congenital adrenal hyperplasia can have normal puberty with adequate treatment, although menstrual irregularities are common. They can be expected to be fertile, although the fertility rate is lower than in the normal population and is dependent on the adequacy of hormone replacement and surgical reconstruction.[17]

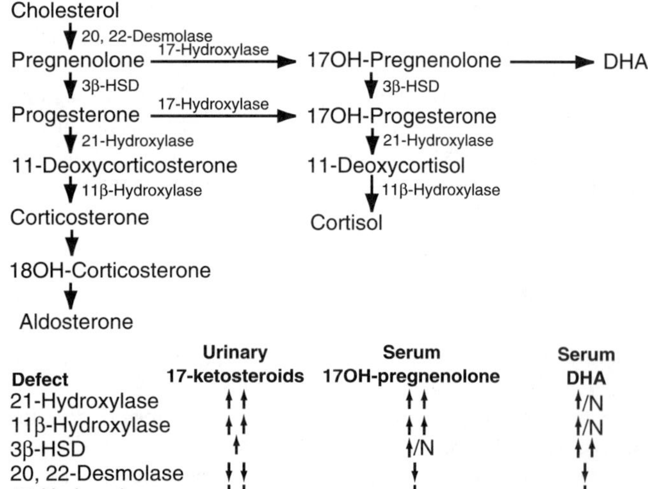

Defect	Urinary 17-ketosteroids	Serum 17OH-pregnenolone	Serum DHA
21-Hydroxylase	↑↑	↑↑	↑/N
11β-Hydroxylase	↑↑	↑↑	↑/N
3β-HSD	↑	↑/N	↑↑
20, 22-Desmolase	↓↓	↓	↓
17-Hydroxylase	↓↓	↓	↓

FIG. 90-7. Metabolic defects in the various forms of congenital adrenal hyperplasia and the resulting urinary and serum metabolites. (After Avery ME, First LR. Adrenal glands. In: Pediatric medicine, ed 2. Baltimore, Williams & Wilkins, 1994:953)

Catecholamine Function

The major active catecholamines are dopamine, epinephrine, and norepinephrine. Unlike steroids, they act through cell-surface receptors. Although receptors for catecholamines exist in many tissues, the initial biochemical characterization of the receptors was done in smooth muscle cells. α-Receptors lead to smooth muscle contraction, while β-receptors lead to relaxation. These two groups of receptors were later subdivided into α_1- and α_2-receptors and β_1- and β_2-receptors. α_1-Receptors lead predominantly to smooth muscle contraction in peripheral vascular beds and in the uterus. α_2-Receptors suppress the release of norepinephrine and acetylcholine from presynaptic terminals and mediate platelet aggregation. β_1-Receptors lead to a variety of effects, including increased inotropy and chronotropy in cardiac muscle, lipolysis in adipocytes, and decreased use of glucose in most cells. The effects of β_2-receptors include smooth muscle relaxation, especially in the conducting airways. β-Agonists include isoproterenol and epinephrine. A variety of specific α- and β-receptor agonists and antagonists are available for clinical use. Epinephrine and norepinephrine both have α-agonist properties, but these effects are both tissue and dose specific.

Other mechanisms can modulate the physiologic effects of catecholamines. Like most ligand-receptor systems, catecholamines down-regulate receptors in the presence of hormone excess; similarly, receptors are up-regulated in the absence of the hormone. This helps explain the phenomenon of tachyphylaxis to high doses of exogenous catecholamines and also hypersensitivity to catecholamines after surgical sympathectomy. Thyroxine also enhances catecholamine effects by increasing intracellular levels of cAMP in receptor cells. Because cAMP is part of the catecholamine signal-transduction process, these target cells have increased sensitivity to catecholamines for a given number of receptors.

Target cells do not require the uptake of the catecholamine ligand to respond. β-Receptor stimulation causes an increase in the intracellular cAMP, which is independent of ligand internalization. α_2-Receptors cause inhibition of cAMP when stimulated. α_1-Receptor stimulation leads to signaling by flux in intracellular calcium levels. All catecholamine effects occur rapidly when compared with the effects of steroid hormones.

Catecholamine Excess

The most common cause of chronic catecholamine excess is overproduction by tumors. In children, neuroblastomas usually secrete catecholamines. In diagnosing or screening for these lesions, it is helpful to check the urine for catecholamine metabolites. Pheochromocytomas are rare tumors that arise from chromaffin tissue. These tumors arise from the adrenal medulla or from extraadrenal chromaffin tissue; in the latter case, they are sometimes referred to as *paragangliomas.* Pheochromocytomas are not functionally under the control of the usual endocrine regulatory mechanisms. They typically produce large quantities of catecholamines.

About 95% of pheochromocytomas occur in adults. In children with pheochromocytomas, there is a preponderance in boys, and the peak incidence is at 9 to 13 years of age. The familial forms of pheochromocytomas, either as a single entity or as part of the multiple endocrine neoplasia (MEN) syndromes, occur more commonly in children. Therefore, any child who presents with a pheochromocytoma should be screened for

TABLE 90-1. *Multiple endocrine neoplasia (MEN) syndromes*

Tumor type	Frequency (%)
MEN I	
Parathyroid tumors	80
Pituitary tumors	75
Pancreatic tumors	65
MEN IIA	
Medullary thyroid carcinoma	97
Pheochromocytoma	30
Hyperparathyroidism	50
MEN IIB	
Medullary thyroid carcinoma	90
Pheochromocytoma	45
Mucosal neuromas	100

MEN types I, IIa, and IIb (Table 90-1; see Chap. 52). Similarly, any patient with MEN should be screened for pheochromocytoma. Malignant pheochromocytomas are rare in children, but there is a higher incidence of bilateral disease.

The symptoms associated with pheochromocytomas include hypertension, headache, intermittent sweating, palpitations, nervousness, weight loss, abdominal or chest pain, and thirst and polyuria. In some cases, these tumors are nonfunctional, but a history of symptoms should be sought if the patient presents with an adrenal mass. The hypertension associated with this disorder can be extreme and episodic, with systolic blood pressure readings in excess of 250 mmHg. On rare occasions, patients present with hypertensive encephalopathy and coma.

DIAGNOSTIC STUDIES

Most patients who come to medical attention for adrenal lesions do so as a consequence of a change in appearance, hypertension, or growth failure, or after discovery as an incidental finding at radiologic or laboratory evaluation. When symptoms arise that suggest an adrenal problem, functional testing is necessary to characterize the problem and to direct further studies to localize the problem. Proper therapy cannot proceed until both the functional and anatomic evaluations are completed. The laboratory evaluations for functional adrenal pathology, as well as the techniques used to localize these problems, are discussed next.

Hypercortisolism (Cushing Syndrome)

Testing for Cushing syndrome entails demonstrating that prolonged, excessive secretion of cortisol is present and that normal feedback regulation is absent.[18] The simplest evaluation is to obtain a fasting serum cortisol level. Serum cortisol levels of 15 to 20 μg/dL are normal. Cushing syndrome can be detected in 80% to 90% of patients by measurement of repeatedly high fasting serum cortisol levels. It is recommended that serum levels be obtained at 8:00 AM and 6:00 PM. Normal diurnal variation of plasma cortisol levels is lost either with hypercortisolism due to a tumor or with Cushing disease. The most sensitive screening method for hypercortisolism is the measurement of urinary free cortisol levels.

After demonstration of cortisol excess, several forms of adrenal suppression testing are commonly used to establish specific causes. These generally use dexamethasone, a synthetic glucocorticoid, to screen for autonomous cortisol production by the adrenal gland. Both high-dose and low-dose dexamethasone suppression tests involve dexamethasone administration followed by measurement of plasma 17-hydroxycorticosteroids, cortisol, and ACTH. The low-dose suppression test consists of administration of a single dose of 1- or 2-mg (child or adult) dexamethasone in the evening. With an intact pituitary–adrenal axis, ACTH, cortisol, and 17-hydroxycorticosteroid levels are suppressed. Normally, the suppression is by 50% or more of baseline levels. In Cushing disease, this stimulus is inadequate to suppress pituitary ACTH production by the adenoma, and therefore serum corticosteroid levels remain unchanged from the baseline. In general, if the fasting cortisol level is only slightly elevated and suppresses to less than 5 μg/dL, it is unlikely that the child has Cushing disease. The high-dose test involves administering oral dexamethasone, 80 mg/kg/d in equal divided doses, every 6 hours for 48 hours. Urine is then collected for 17-hydroxycorticosteroid, 17-ketosteroid, free cortisol, and ACTH levels. If hypercortisolism is due to adrenal hyperplasia, suppression occurs with the high-dose regimen. In patients with autonomous adrenal tumors, however, suppression does not occur with either low- or high-dose dexamethasone.

The metyrapone test is used to differentiate adrenal hyperplasia due to a pituitary adenoma from adrenal tumors or ectopic ACTH production. Metyrapone inhibits adrenal 11-hydroxylase, resulting in decreased cortisol synthesis, increased ACTH secretion, and increased plasma levels of 11-deoxycortisol, the precursor of cortisol. 11-Deoxycortisol and its metabolites are excreted in urine as 17-hydroxycorticosteroids. The test is performed by first obtaining a baseline blood sample and 24-hour urine collection. Metyrapone is then given orally every 4 hours until a total of 300 mg/m^2 is administered. Urine is collected during the 24 hours that the drug is given and again for the 24 hours after administration of the metyrapone; also, blood is sampled 4 hours after the last dose of metyrapone for measurement of cortisol, 11-deoxycortisol, and ACTH. Under normal circumstances, urinary 17-hydroxycorticosteroid levels and blood levels of 11β-deoxycortisol rise about three-fold with metyrapone treatment. If the adrenal glands are hyperplastic under the influence of a pituitary adenoma, they respond with supranormal output of 11-deoxycortisol when the pituitary adenoma increases its output of ACTH in response to declining plasma cortisol levels. If hypercortisolism is due to an adrenal adenoma or ectopic ACTH syndrome, the pituitary output of ACTH is chronically suppressed, and the gland does not respond to inhibition of cortisol synthesis. Thus, 11-deoxycortisol levels do not increase with metyrapone in these cases. An overnight metyrapone test is simpler but not as sensitive.

One final test that is also helpful in defining the cause of Cushing syndrome involves the administration of CRH. In this test, 1 μg/kg of CRH is given intravenously, and serial blood samples are obtained for 3 hours after the drug is given. Normally, there is a moderate increase in ACTH and cortisol levels. With Cushing disease, the increase in ACTH and cortisol in the bloodstream is more marked. There is little overlap between

TABLE 90-2. *Tests used in the diagnosis of Cushing syndrome*

SCREENING
Plasma cortisol—random and diurnal
Urinary 17OH-corticosteroids
Urinary free cortisol
Low-dose dexamethasone suppression test

DETERMINING THE CAUSE
High-dose dexamethasone suppression test
  Suppression with hyperplasia
  No suppression with adrenal tumor
Corticotropin-releasing hormone stimulation
  Accentuated response with pituitary cause
  No response with adrenal or ectopic cause
Metyrapone test
  High response with hyperplasia
  Low or no response with adrenal tumor or ectopic cause
Petrosal sinus sampling
  Lateralizing with pituitary cause
  Nonlateralizing with nonpituitary cause

normal individuals and those with Cushing syndrome in these tests. When high levels of cortisol are due to autonomous adrenal tumors or ectopic ACTH production, there is no response to CRH because the pituitary gland is chronically suppressed. The diagnostic tests for Cushing syndrome are summarized in Table 90-2.

Several syndromes and disease processes are associated with adrenocortical carcinoma. These include the Beckwith-Wiedemann syndrome, MEN I, and other neoplasms such as medulloblastoma and astrocytoma. Hemangiomas, urinary tract malformations and hemihypertrophy have also been linked to this tumor. Although there are rare reports of familial adrenocortical carcinomas as well, most of these patients present with isolated and sporadic tumors.

Hyperaldosteronism

The simplest screening method for hypertensive patients suspected of hyperaldosteronism is measurement of the serum potassium level. Hypokalemia (less than 3.5 mEq/L) is present in more than 90% of cases; frequently there is metabolic alkalosis as well. Any child with hypertension and hypokalemia should be evaluated for hyperaldosteronism, especially if there is excessive urinary loss of potassium with a normal dietary intake. Primary hyperaldosteronism can be diagnosed by measuring high plasma or urine aldosterone levels with simultaneously low plasma renin activity. Plasma renin activity is difficult to interpret in the neonate, however, because a number of other factors can influence its value in this population.

If high aldosterone levels are present, the ability to suppress them should be checked. Generally, this is done in the inpatient hospital setting because of the necessity to control sodium intake and ambulatory status. The patient is given a high sodium diet (150 mEq/d or more) for 3 to 5 days. Plasma aldosterone levels are then measured in the morning before the patient has risen from the supine position. This regimen does not suppress aldosterone levels in the setting of primary aldosteronism but does so normally.

Dexamethasone-suppressible hyperaldosteronism can be detected with a trial of low-dose dexamethasone. These patients have normal cortisol secretion but respond to a salt load just as patients with primary hyperaldosteronism do. Dexamethasone suppresses urinary and plasma aldosterone levels within 48 hours, with a concomitant rise in plasma renin activity. This condition can be due to an adrenal tumor (unilateral) or to hyperplasia (bilateral). Selective adrenal vein sampling may be necessary to differentiate between these two entities and to find the source.

The hypertension of primary hyperaldosteronism responds to surgical intervention only if it is due to a unilateral adrenal tumors. Therefore, differentiating tumor from hyperplasia is of benefit. For unknown reasons, aldosterone-producing tumors are frequently associated with high levels of 18-hydroxycorticosterone (more than 100 μg/dL), an aldosterone precursor, whereas hyperplasia is not. Therefore, if it is not possible to lateralize the source of the hyperaldosteronism to one or the other adrenal gland, but the 18-hydroxycorticosterone plasma level is high, surgical therapy may be worthwhile to cure the hypertension.

Serum renin values are high in conditions of secondary hyperaldosteronism. Bartter syndrome should be considered in children with hypokalemic alkalosis, normal blood pressure, dwarfism, and mental retardation. In addition to high aldosterone levels, these children also can have high blood and urine prostaglandin levels.

Catecholamines

Pheochromocytoma is a tumor that produces excessive amounts of catecholamines. The diagnosis of pheochromocytoma depends on the measurement of elevated blood and urinary catecholamines and their metabolites. A 24-hour urine sample should be collected for norepinephrine, epinephrine, metanephrine, and vanillylmandelic acid analysis. These values vary with age, but most patients with pheochromocytoma have abnormally high urinary output of these compounds. Because some tumors excrete in an episodic fashion, normal plasma levels may be found with blood samples. In urine, this sample-dependent variation is less pronounced because the sample reflects longer time periods, but the studies should be repeated if a pheochromocytoma is suspected and initial screening studies are negative. Tumors arising in an adrenal gland or in the organ of Zuckerkandl are characterized by exceptionally high levels of epinephrine.

The diagnosis of pheochromocytoma is usually not difficult, but localization of the tumor can be. The radiologic tests used to localize these tumors are discussed later. Because pheochromocytoma is more often familial in children, other family members should have urinary catecholamines measured. Also, because pheochromocytoma is associated with MEN II, particularly in children, screening for medullary carcinoma of the thyroid should be done. In the past, this involved provocative testing of plasma calcitonin levels. New molecular probes are now available for definitive kindred analysis (see Chap. 52).

LOCALIZATION STUDIES

The adrenal gland is relatively hidden from view on plain radiographs. Large masses, such as adrenal neuroblastomas or ganglioneuromas with calcifications, can be seen on plain films, but most adrenal masses, particularly those that are functional while small, are not apparent. Occasionally, a patient presents with a mediastinal mass seen on chest radiograph that turns out to be a pheochromocytoma.

Initial screening for a palpable or suspected abdominal mass in infants and children is often with ultrasound. In small children, the adrenal glands are easily seen, and ultrasound can distinguish between solid and cystic masses. Adrenal masses, usually neural tumors, are routinely seen on prenatal ultrasound.[19] Adrenal hemorrhages are also easily demonstrable promptly after birth with ultrasound. Soon after birth, however, the adrenal gland undergoes spontaneous reduction in size. Thus, in most children, computed tomography (CT) and magnetic resonance imaging (MRI) are more helpful than ultrasound in detecting small adrenal lesions.

CT is the radiologic technique most commonly used to define lesions of the adrenal gland. Also, because of the substantial use of abdominal CT for other reasons, incidental lesions of the adrenal gland are frequently found. CT scan can detect lesions of 1 cm diameter with about 80% sensitivity. The sensitivity for lesions of 3 to 4 cm approaches 100% (Figs. 90-8 and 90-9). CT scan can distinguish between solid and cystic lesions but does not provide information about the function of the lesion, nor can it suggest whether the lesion is malignant.

MRI requires more patient cooperation than CT, and frequently small children require general anesthesia so that a high-quality MRI scan can be obtained, although this may be true of CT as well. An important advantage of MRI is derived from T1- and T2-weighted images. Information can be gained about whether a lesion is benign or malignant. In general, carcinomas are brighter, or are said to *enhance*, on T2-weighted images. Another advantage of MRI is that it can better define the tumor's relation to the surrounding tissues, which may assist the surgeon in planning for operation.[20]

Nuclear Medicine Studies

Radiopharmaceuticals that are precursors of hormones can be taken up by adrenal tumors and concentrated. Radioscintigraphy can then be used to localize the tumors. Two such drugs have become useful in the diagnosis and localization of adrenal tumors. An analogue of cholesterol, [131]I-6β-iodomethyl-19-norcholesterol (NP-59), is taken up as cholesterol into the adrenocorticol steroidogenic pathway. This agent can accurately localize the adrenal cortex and functioning adrenocortical tumors. It can differentiate adrenocortical hyperplasia from functioning adenomas or carcinomas. NP-59 can also be used to distinguish unilateral aldosterone-producing tumors from bilateral hyperplasia in cases of primary hyperaldosteronism. NP-59 may be useful in the diagnosis of incidental adrenal masses, where adenomas take up the agent, but carcinomas, either primary or metastatic, do not.

[131]I-methaiodobenzylguanidine (MIBG) is a radionuclide analogue of norepinephrine. MIBG accumulates where norepinephrine is taken up and can be used to detect sympathoadrenal tumors anywhere in the body (Fig. 90-10). It is especially useful for the localization of pheochromocytomas, either primary or metastatic, or in cases of multiple pheochromocytomas. MIBG

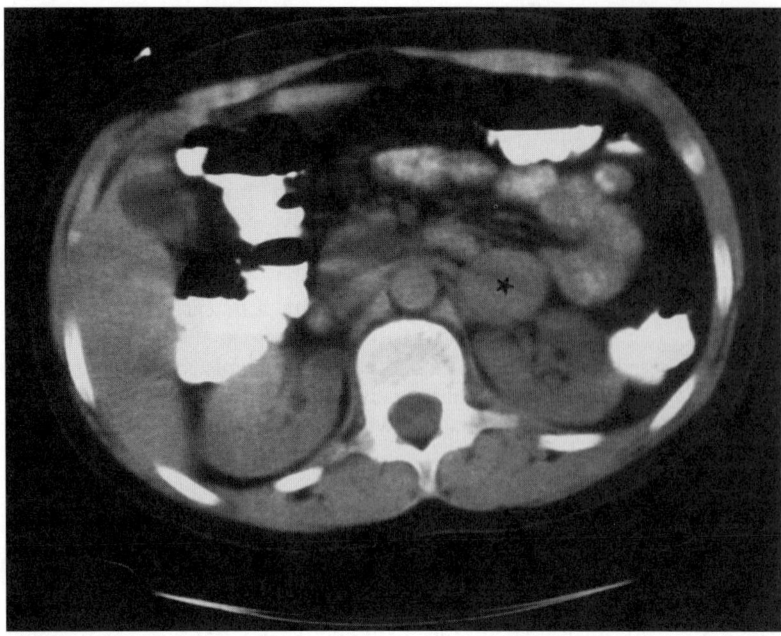

FIG. 90-8. CT image showing a left adrenal mass (*asterisk*) that proved to be a pheochromocytoma.

has also been used in cases of neuroblastoma and is most useful in localizing recurrent or metastatic disease.[21,22]

Invasive Vascular Radiology Techniques

Arteriography, venography, and selective venous sampling have become less necessary as the techniques described earlier have increased in usefulness. Occasionally, however, invasive techniques are needed. Specific sampling of inferior vena cava or selective adrenal vein blood may be helpful to localize the source of primary hyperaldosteronism or an occult pheochromocytoma. It is wise to ensure that a patient with suspected pheochromocytoma has had adequate α-blockade before an in-

vasive vascular radiology procedure because failure to provide α-blockade can result in a hypertensive crisis.

In patients with Cushing disease, MRI of the sella turcica localizes a pituitary adenoma about half of the time. When this fails in occult cases, bilateral simultaneous petrosal sinus ACTH sampling with CRH stimulation is the diagnostic test of choice.

TREATMENT

In most cases, treatment of hyperfunctioning adrenal conditions requires surgical resection of the tumor and the gland. The notable exception to this rule is congenital adrenal hyperplasia. This condition is completely treated with steroid replace-

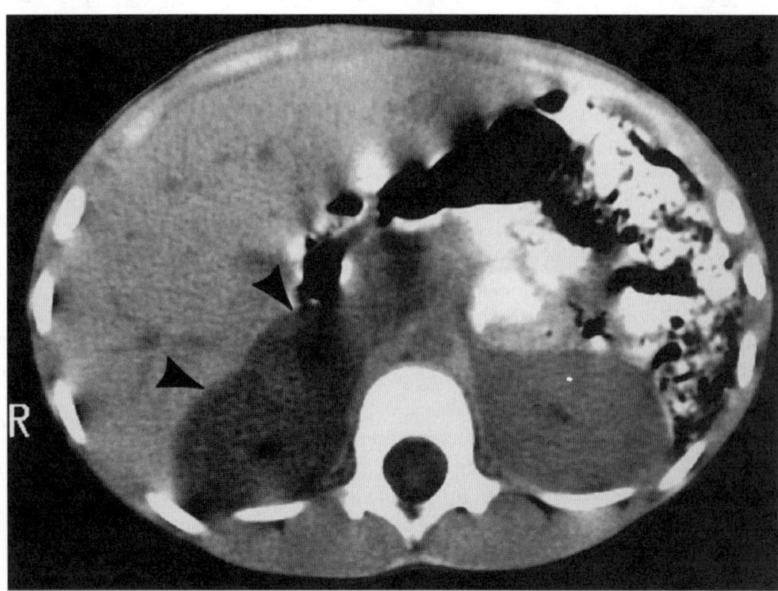

FIG. 90-9. CT image of a right adrenal pheochromocytoma (*arrowheads*) in a patient with familial pheochromocytoma. This lesion extended into the inferior vena cava through the right adrenal vein and was successfully removed by isolating the vena cava after total mobilization of the liver.

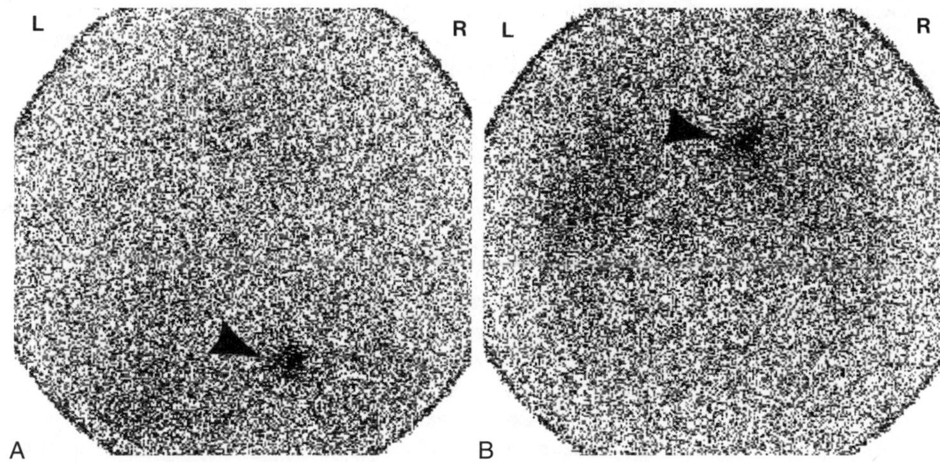

FIG. 90-10. MIBG scan demonstrating a pheochromocytoma in the right adrenal region (*arrowheads*). Both images are posterior views. (*A*) Chest. (*B*) Abdomen.

ment, and the surgical aspects of the disease focus on reconstruction of the genital organs. For some conditions, such as pheochromocytoma, the proper preoperative pharmacologic preparation of the patient is a critical aspect of the overall care of the patient. Furthermore, it is important to recall that conditions of hormone hypersecretion that lead to feedback suppression of the pituitary, such as Cushing disease, cause suppression that does not resolve immediately, and replacement hormones may be necessary for several months postoperatively.

Adrenal Hypercortisolism

Nonoperative Treatment

Long-term medical treatment of children with Cushing disease is not recommended. Cyproheptadine, a serotonin antagonist, has been used with some success in adults, but concerns about efficacy and long-term effects have limited its use in children. Symptoms of cortisol excess from benign functional adrenocorticol lesions can be treated with drugs such as metyrapone and aminoglutethimide, which block adrenal steroidogenesis. They are not useful long-term, however, because of patient noncompliance and drug reactions. Furthermore, adrenal lesions continue to grow while patients take these drugs.

Medical management of congenital adrenal hyperplasia involves glucocorticoid replacement and frequently mineralocorticoid replacement (discussed earlier).

Operative Treatment

In patients with adrenal hypercortisolism of unilateral adrenal origin, the treatment is operative removal of the gland. In adult patients with a large unilateral nonfunctional adrenal tumor (6 cm or more in diameter) or one that is enlarging, adrenalectomy is recommended. No similar recommendation exists for children, although most pediatric surgeons favor removal of any discernible adrenal mass because of the potential for growth over a lifetime.

Preoperative preparation of the patient with unilateral adrenal hypercortisolism is minimal. If there is any question about whether the lesion is functional, it is safest to provide perioperative exogenous glucocorticoid replacement. There is general consensus on this, but specific regimens vary considerably. One such approach is presented later. Patients undergoing operation should receive cortisone acetate, 2.5 to 10 mg/kg/d, or its equivalent parenterally. This is usually given every 6 to 8 hours in divided doses, with the first dose given at the start of the operation. Depending on the operation, this dose is then decreased incrementally by about 50% every 24 to 48 hours until maintenance levels are reached and resumption of oral dosing equivalents is feasible. If hypercortisolism has been present for many months or years, a period of tapering may be necessary over 6 to 12 months.

The surgical approach to the adrenal gland depends on the size of the lesion, the likelihood of malignant disease, the need for bilateral adrenalectomies, and the surgeon's preference. In larger patients, an extraperitoneal approach, either through the bed of the 12th rib or through a flank incision, may limit morbidity. Alternatively, a subcostal incision may be used, but it is necessary to mobilize the liver or the spleen and stomach to approach the glands. It is critical for the surgeon to remember the venous drainage of the glands, especially on the right side, where the broad, short adrenal vein draining directly into the inferior vena cava can create troublesome bleeding if not dissected and controlled adequately. Patients with small glands who require bilateral adrenalectomies are well served by a bilateral posterior approach. Finally, in patients with large lesions or with carcinomas with extensive invasion of surrounding tissues, it may be preferable to use a thoracoabdominal incision.

Children with Cushing disease who require bilateral adrenalectomies require lifelong steroid replacement. These patients have a high incidence of Nelson syndrome, characterized by development of a pituitary adenoma, hyperpigmentation, and markedly high plasma ACTH levels. The tumor of Nelson syndrome may require pituitary irradiation.[23]

Prognosis

Operative removal of benign adrenal tumors causing adrenal hypercortisolism is curative, and patients have excellent long-term prognoses. If the treatment of Cushing disease can be effected before closure of the growth plates, some lost growth can be regained. The earlier the treatment, the less likely is a significant deviation from the predicted height. In patients with adrenocortical carcinoma, the outcome is largely dependent on the resectability of the lesion. There are no effective chemotherapeutic agents against adrenocortical carcinoma.[24] Mitotane, a cytolytic agent, may offer some benefit in decreasing steroid output and therefore in controlling symptoms of cortisol excess, but it has no demonstrated benefit to survival. Its principal role appears to be in the treatment of patients with unresectable disease and symptomatic hypercortisolism.

Hyperaldosteronism

Nonoperative Treatment

Spironolactone is the only pharmaceutical agent of any practical benefit in the treatment of hyperaldosteronism. This drug acts by inhibiting the exchange of potassium for sodium in the distal renal tubule and results in the conservation of potassium and serum pH stability. If tolerated for a long enough period, it can also lead to normalization of the blood pressure. Oral potassium supplementation also helps correct hypokalemia. Spironolactone leads to gynecomastia, however, and large doses may be needed, so it is not well tolerated during the long-term.

Dexamethasone-suppressible hyperaldosteronism can be treated with glucocorticoids, usually with return of the blood pressure to normal levels within 2 weeks of the initiation of therapy. The long-term consequences of exogenous glucocorticoid therapy, however, limit this application.

Operative Treatment

Unilateral adrenalectomy is the treatment of choice in patients with a solitary aldosterone-producing tumors. It is necessary to correct the hypertension and hypokalemia preoperatively. Short-term use of spironolactone can assist in this regard. When the syndrome arises from adrenal hyperplasia, surgical removal of the glands does not correct the hypertension, unless the 18-hydroxycorticosterone level is elevated. Medical therapy with spironolactone is the treatment of choice with bilateral disease, except in selected cases.

Prognosis

After removing a functional tumor, hypoaldosteronism can be present for several weeks. This is due to suppression of the contralateral zona glomerulosa by the tumor. Supplemental sodium chloride should be given during this period either orally or intravenously. Tumor removal should be curative because these tumors are rarely malignant. If bilateral adrenalectomy is undertaken, long-term glucocorticoid and mineralocorticoid administration is necessary.

Pheochromocytoma

Nonoperative Treatment

The treatment of choice for pheochromocytoma is surgical removal of the lesion. As mentioned earlier, these lesions can be extraordinarily active for their size, and accurate preoperative localization of the lesions is essential. These lesions are more often bilateral in children.

Pharmacologic blockade of pheochromocytomas is unsatisfactory in the long run, but this is a critical part of preoperative preparation of the patient. Phenoxybenzamine and prazosin block the α-adrenergic effects of catecholamines. β-Adrenergic blockade with agents such as propranolol and labetalol is used when resting tachycardia is present. This must be delayed until α-blockade is achieved, and then done carefully in patients with hypertensive cardiomyopathy or reactive airway disease to avoid cardiopulmonary decompensation. Generally, providing 2 to 3 weeks of α-adrenergic blockade therapy with phenoxybenzamine, followed by intravenous fluid replacement, is necessary to prepare the patient for operation. The adequacy of the blockade and fluid replacement is apparent when the patient no longer has postural hypotension.[25]

Operative Treatment

Good preparation by the anesthesiologist is essential for successful resection of a pheochromocytoma. In children, preoperative sedation is helpful. An arterial catheter is necessary for real-time blood pressure monitoring because extreme vasoconstriction can occur when the tumor is manipulated, making meaningful blood pressure cuff measurements impossible. Furthermore, the anesthesiologist should have ready access to agents that lower or raise blood pressure as well as to antiarrhythmic drugs. The anesthetic induction should be as smooth as possible.

The operative approach is typically through a transabdominal incision, usually subcostal if the tumor is in the adrenal gland. This makes checking for bilateral adrenal lesions possible, although preoperative MIBG scan usually confirms this diagnosis. The surgical principles involved in removing a pheochromocytoma include minimal direct manipulation of the tumor as it is dissected and early control and ligation of the adrenal vein. Good communication between the surgeon and the anesthesiologist is essential during the operation when it is necessary to manipulate the tumor because this is when arrhythmia and hypertension are most prone to occur. Once the tumor is removed, the blood pressure may fall dramatically, although this is less likely if adequate preoperative hydration has been achieved. Failure to bring the blood pressure down to normal levels after removal of the tumor should prompt a search for other tumors or metastases. The search should include the paravertebral areas, the contralateral adrenal gland, the area of the aortic bifurcation, and the region of the urinary bladder. Occasionally, a tumor also is found along the course of the spermatic cord in the groin or scrotum.

Prognosis

When all functioning pheochromocytomas are removed, the blood pressure returns to normal. Patients with familial pheochromocytomas should be followed carefully for the development of disease in the opposite gland.[26] Although it may seem desirable to preserve part of one gland when there is bilateral disease, experience suggests that there is a high incidence of recurrent disease if this approach is used. In these cases, it is wiser to opt for bilateral total resection and lifelong hormonal replacement therapy.

REFERENCES

1. Skandalakis JE, Gray SW, Scaljon WM, et al. The suprarenal glands. In: Skandalakis JE, Gray SW, eds. Embryology for surgeons, ed 2. Baltimore, Williams & Wilkins, 1994:718.
2. Byrne GC, Perry YS, Winter JSD. Kinetic analysis of adrenal 3β-hydroxysteroid dehydrogenase activity during human development. J Clin Endocrinol Metab 1985;60:934.
3. Chrousos GP. Regulation and dysregulation of the hypothalamic-pituitary-adrenal axis: the corticotropin-releasing hormone perspective. Endocrinol Metab Clin North Am 1992;21:833.
4. Parker LN, Lifrak ET, Odell WD. A 60,000 molecular weight human pituitary glycopeptide stimulates adrenal androgen secretion. Endocrinology 1983;113:2092.
5. Lobo RA, Kletzky OA, Kaptein EM, et al. Prolactin modulation of dehydroepiandrosterone sulfate secretion. Am J Obstet Gynecol 1980;138:632.
6. Wen X, Villee DB, Ellison P, et al. Effects of adrenocorticotrophic hormone, human chorionic gonadotropin, and insulin on steroid production by human adrenocortical carcinoma cells in culture. Cancer Res 1985;45:3974.
7. Newsome HH. Adrenal glands. In: Greenfield LJ, Mulholland MW, Oldham KT, et al, eds. Surgery: scientific principles and practice. Philadelphia, JB Lippincott, 1993:1209.
8. Kangawa K, Matsuo H. Purification and complete amino acid sequence of α-human atrial natriuretic polypeptide (α-hANP). Biochem Biophys Res Commun 1984;118:131.
9. Sen S, Shainoff JR, Bravo EL, et al. Isolation of aldosterone-stimulating factor (ASF) and its effect on rat adrenal glomerulosa cells in vitro. Hypertension 1981;3:4.
10. Jones KL. The Cushing syndromes. Pediatr Clin North Am 1990;37:1313.
11. Kelch RP, Kaplan SL, Biglieri EG, et al. Hereditary adrenocortical unresponsiveness to adrenocorticotropic hormone. J Pediatr 1972;81:726.
12. Neufeld M, MacLaren N, Blizzard R. Autoimmune polyglandular syndromes. Pediatr Ann 1980;9:154.
13. Gill JR Jr, Bartter FC. Evidence for a prostaglandin-independent defect in chloride reabsorption in the loop of Henle as a proximal cause of Bartter's syndrome. Am J Med 1978;65:766.
14. Hendren WH, Crawford JD. Adrenogenital syndrome: the anatomy of the anomaly and its repair: some new concepts. J Pediatr Surg 1969;4:49.
15. Avery ME, First LR. Adrenal glands. In: Pediatric medicine, ed 2. Baltimore, Williams & Wilkins, 1994:953.
16. Kirkland RT, Keenan BS, Holcombe JH, et al. The effect of therapy on mature height in congenital adrenal hyperplasia. J Clin Endocrinol Metab 1978;47:1320.
17. Mulaikal RM, Migeon CJ, Rock JA. Fertility rates in female patients with congenital adrenal hyperplasia due to 21-hydroxylase deficiency. N Engl J Med 1987;316:178.
18. Bickler, SW, McMahon TJ, Campbell JR, et al. Preoperative diagnostic evaluation of children with Cushing's syndrome. J Pediatr Surg 1994;29:671.
19. Ho PTC, Estroff JA, Kozakewich H, et al. Prenatal detection of neuroblastoma: a 10-year experience from Dana Farber Cancer Institute and Children's Hospital. Pediatrics 1993;92:358.
20. Caron KH. Magnetic resonance imaging of the pediatric abdomen. Semin Ultrasound CT MR 1991;12:448.
21. Gelfand MJ. Meta-iodobenzylguanidine in children. Semin Nucl Med 1993;23:231.
22. Paltiel HJ, Gelfand MJ, Elgazzar AH, et al. Neural crest tumors: I-123 MIBG imaging in children. Radiology 1994;190:117.
23. Hopwood NJ, Kenny FM. Incidence of Nelson's syndrome after adrenalectomy for Cushing's disease in children: results of a nationwide survey. Am J Dis Child 1977;131:1353.
24. Neblett WW, Frexes-Steed M, Scott HW. Experience with adrenocortical neoplasms in children. Am Surg 1987;53:117.
25. Pullerits J, Eis S, Balfe JW. Anaesthesia for phaeochromocytoma. Can J Anaesth 1988;35:526.
26. Caty MG, Coran AG, Geagen M, et al. Current diagnosis and treatment of pheochromocytoma in children. Arch Surg 1990;125:978.

Urinary and Genital Systems

Surgery of Infants and Children: Scientific Principles and Practice, edited by Keith T. Oldham, Paul M. Colombani, and Robert P. Foglia. Lippincott–Raven Publishers, Philadelphia, © 1997.

CHAPTER 91

Kidney

Michael A. Keating and Kevin P. McLaughlin

ANATOMY

Familiarity with renal anatomy establishes the basis for understanding and managing many diseases of the kidney, regardless of whether they are surgical, medical, traumatic, or neoplastic.

Gross Anatomy

Location, Size, and Orientation

The kidneys of children share many characteristics with those of adults, although certain differences and clinical implications exist. Positioned slightly above the level of the umbilicus and located on either side of the vertebral column, these paired, bean-shaped organs are well protected in the retroperitoneal space. The right kidney usually is more dependently positioned as a consequence of displacement by the liver. Medially, the organs are buttressed by the paraspinous muscles. Posteriorly, the upper poles are shielded by the lower ribs. However, the softer ribs of children and their underdeveloped abdominal musculature offer the anterolateral surface less effective protection against trauma. Here, an intimate association with several adjacent organs readily explains the high incidence of associated injuries when the kidneys themselves are traumatized[1] (Fig. 91-1).

Each kidney and the adjacent adrenal gland is contained within a thin condensation of connective tissue, Gerota's fascia. This fascial envelope is circumferentially intact, with the exception of an inferior hiatus that allows for exit of the ureter. Although it does not provide mechanical protection, Gerota's fascia is an important anatomic barrier against the extension of primary renal tumors—including Wilms tumor—to adjacent organs. It also effectively contains and controls the hemorrhage of most blunt trauma. Variable amounts of fat also surround the kidneys in either a perinephric (within the fascia) or paranephric (outside of the fascia) position, buttressing them in the retroperitoneum. The paucity of fat in most children makes the organ extremely mobile and much more susceptible to contrecoup, flexion, and deceleration injuries.

The kidneys of the child, especially at an early age, are larger with respect to overall body size than those of an adult. This results in a relative abdominal projection that, again, makes them more susceptible to injury. Nomograms have been developed that estimate normal renal size with respect to age, although concessions should be made with regard to overall size. As a general rule, the length of a normal kidney equals that of the adjacent two and one half vertebral bodies. The absence of growth on serial examination should prompt an investigation into cause. In addition to size, the axis of the pediatric kidney provides a clue to abnormal development. Normally, each upper pole is distinctly medial to the lower pole, and lines drawn along the longitudinal axis of the kidneys typically intersect at the 10th thoracic vertebrae. Vertical or even reversed axes can be caused by upper pole hydronephrosis of duplex collecting systems, tumors of the kidney or adrenal glands, or ectopia from incomplete migration or rotation during embryogenesis (see later).

Parenchyma and Collecting System

Sagittal sectioning allows an appreciation of the kidney's macroanatomy (Fig. 91-2). The integrity of the renal parenchyma is maintained by a thick fibrous capsule that adheres to its entire surface. The capsule is used whenever possible to reinforce the closure of renal wounds since the underlying tissue, like liver, lacks the consistency needed to hold sutures without tearing. Immediately beneath the capsule lies the contiguous outer layer of the kidney, the *cortex*, which contains the glomeruli, proximal and distal tubules, and collecting ducts. Deep to this lies the central renal medulla, composed of straight portions of the tubules, loops of Henle, the vasa recta, and terminal collecting ducts. The *medulla* is divided into discrete pyramid-shaped structures that have their base along the corticomedullary junction and are called, appropriately enough, the renal *pyramids*.

Each pyramid ends at a renal papilla, the macroscopic junction of parenchyma and collecting system (although technically and developmentally the collecting system begins at the level of the more proximal collecting ducts). Extensions of the cortex project between the pyramids into cords known as the columns of Bertin. The mistakenly named medullary rays of Ferrein are actually cortex that extend from the base of the pyramids to the periphery. A renal *lobe* consists of a renal pyramid and its

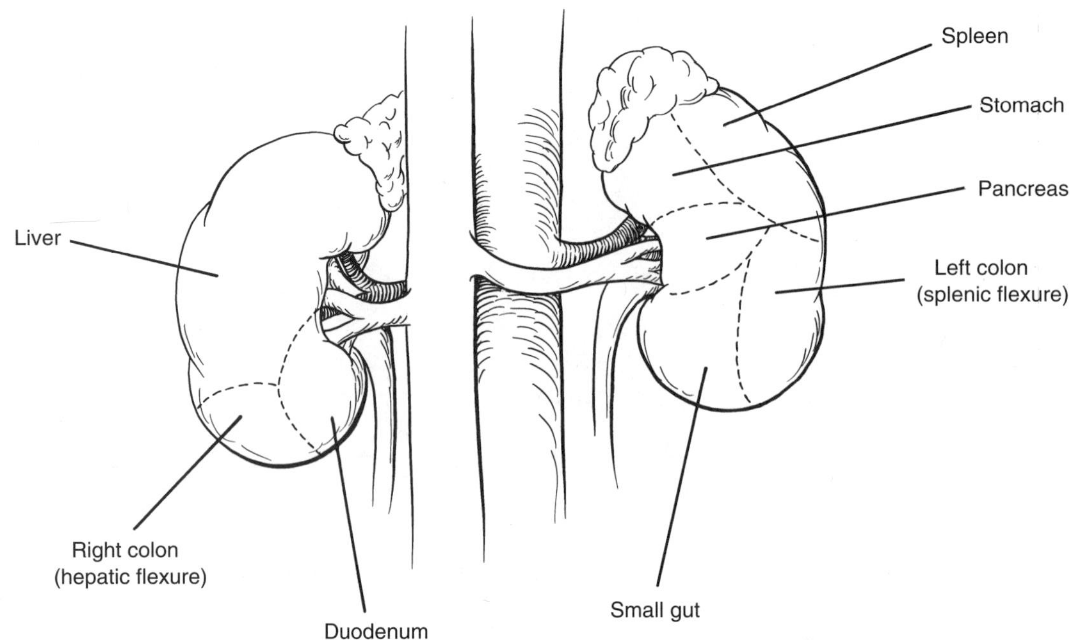

FIG. 91-1. Anterior relations of the kidney.

overlying mantel of cortex. These are unrelated to *lobulations*, which normally occur during fetal development and persist into the first year of life. Lobulations are positioned above the columns of Bertin as opposed to the scars of infection, which occur opposite an affected calyx and its associated pyramid.

The concavity of the medial surface of each kidney is called the *hilum* where the renal vein, artery, and pelvis are positioned in an anterior-to-posterior direction. The fat-filled space surrounding the renal pelvis and overlying kidney is called the renal sinus. The renal pelvis typically branches into two or three major *calyces* as it enters the substance of the kidney. Further

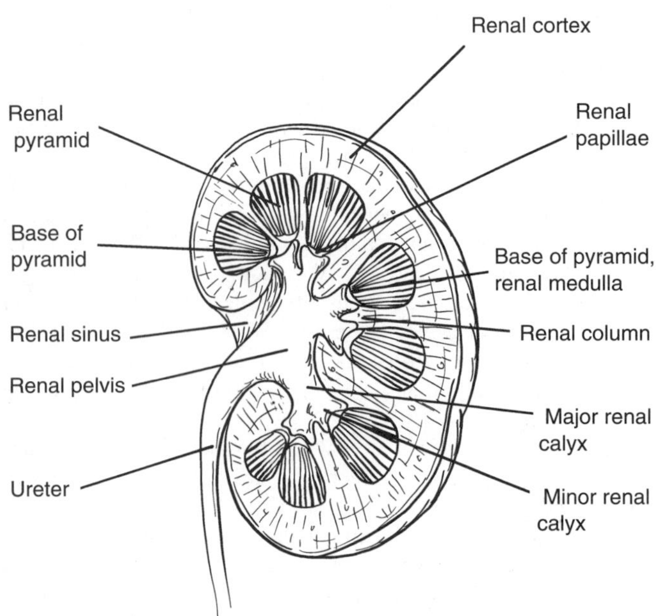

FIG. 91-2. Macroanatomy of kidney on sagittal section.

divisions result in two or three minor calyces. Each renal pyramid (and hence renal lobe) empties into a minor calyx at the papilla, which accounts for convex impressions seen on pyelography (Fig. 91-3).

Vasculature

There can be significant variation in renal vascularity. Normally, the blood supply to each kidney comes from a single main artery that branches off the aorta, just inferolateral to the superior mesenteric artery. Auxiliary arteries from the aorta and adrenal or gonadal arteries frequently supply the superior and inferior poles, especially to the left kidney. These vessels cross the collecting system and are sometimes implicated in obstructions of the ureteropelvic junction. During surgery in infants and newborns, the kidney should be handled gently since its arteries are prone to spasm. In addition, the intima of these vessels is less compliant than its elastic investing layers. This leaves them prone to intimal tears during sudden deceleration (eg, falling from a great height) or flexion.

Within the renal sinus, the main artery gives off a posterior branch that supplies that segment of the kidney exclusive of the poles. Its anterior limb divides into four branches that feed the apical, upper, middle, and lower segments. Despite any variations that might occur with arterial origins and distribution, there is no collateral blood supply between the individual segments. Each segmental artery is an end artery. Brodel's line (Fig. 91-4) defines a plane between the anterior and posterior branches that, in theory, allows a relatively avascular surgical approach to the center of the kidney.

Interlobar arteries, radially oriented from the hilum, branch from the segmental arteries and course toward the cortex along the columns of Bertin. These give off the arcuate arteries at the corticomedullary junction that run parallel to the renal capsule and, in turn, give of the interlobular arteries, which again run

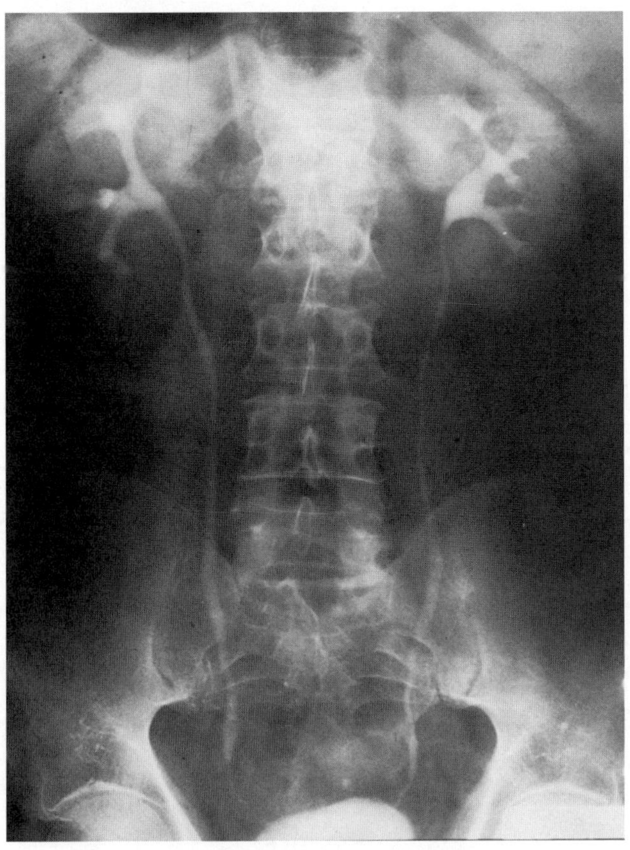

FIG. 91-3. Excretory urogram of normal kidney.

radially toward the capsule. The afferent arterioles branch from the interlobular arteries. Each of these forms a capillary tuft, or *glomerulus*, that supplies an individual nephron. Efferent arterioles carry blood away from the glomeruli with two possible destinations: (1) the rich network of capillaries surrounding the cortical tubules; or (2) the long, straight, descending vasa rectae that provide the main blood supply to the renal medulla. The latter arise predominantly from glomeruli positioned at the corticomedullary junction, and are responsible for the medullary osmolar gradient that permits urinary concentration (see later).

Unlike its arterial supply, the venous drainage of the kidney freely crosses segmental boundaries. After entering the ascending vasa rectae, venous blood drains into the interlobular veins, then retraces the arterial path to the main renal vein. Like its arterial counterpart, the renal vein exhibits a great deal of variation. In most cases, the left renal vein, which is longer, has lumbar, gonadal, and adrenal branches. In contrast, the right renal vein is notoriously short and has no collaterals since the other right-sided veins drain into the vena cava. This difference in drainage gives the left kidney far more resiliency after ligation or thrombosis of its main vein.

Microanatomy and Functional Correlates

At the microscopic level, the kidney becomes a marvel of the interplay between function and structure. The basic unit of function, the *nephron*, is composed of a vascular capillary tuft,

the true glomerulus, and the glomerular or Bowman's capsule. In common usage, however, the term *glomerulus* refers to the combination of capillary tuft and capsule (Fig. 91-5). Each kidney is comprised of about 1 million nephrons whose formation is complete at birth. Parenchymal regeneration through nephron replacement does not occur, and progressive loss can lead to renal insufficiency.

Blood flows to the glomerulus by way of the afferent arteriole and exits through the efferent arteriole. Both vessels enter the glomerulus at the vascular pole or hilum directly opposite the proximal renal tubule at the urinary pole. The glomerulus invaginates the blind-ending renal tubule, and the fenestrated epithelial lining of its capillaries and initiates the ultrafiltration of plasma. Urine ultimately results. Normally, these fenestrations prevent the cellular elements of blood from leaving the intravascular space. The principal driving force regulating glomerular filtration is hydrostatic pressure, a consequence of systemic blood pressure. This is progressively opposed by the hydrostatic pressure in Bowman's space and colloid osmotic pressure of the arteriole until ultrafiltration ceases (Fig. 91-6). A key component to the regulation of hydrostatic pressure is the juxtaglomerular apparatus. This is comprised of specialized cells of the afferent and efferent arterioles responsible for renin production. In addition, components from the mesangium—a centrally located vascular mesentery that supports the capillary network—and adjacent distal tubules play a role in renin and prostaglandin production.

The epithelial component of Bowman's capsule, which surrounds the glomerular tuft and is continuous with the epithelium of the proximal tubule, has both a visceral (lining the capillary tuft) and a parietal (comprising the wall of capsule itself) component. The visceral epithelial cells are called podocytes, which envelope the glomerular capillary tuft and are intimately associated with its endothelial fenestrations. The glomerular basement membrane lies between this endothelial–epithelial border. Once through the slit diaphragms found between adjacent podocytes, the ultrafiltrate enters the urinary or Bowman's space and proceeds into the proximal convoluted tubule. Its composition is identical to that of plasma, with the exception of larger (molecular weight exceeding 68,000) proteins, including globulins and albumin, which normally are unable to traverse the fenestrations. The glomerulus can be injured by immunologic, inherited (presumably biochemical), or coagulation disorders. The response of the glomerulus can include increased capillary permeability, cellular proliferation, immune complex deposition in the basement membrane, and connective tissue replacement. Varying degrees of hematuria, proteinuria, and renal insufficiency result, depending on their severity.

Within the proximal convoluted tubule, the longest portion of the nephron, about 65% of the ultrafiltrate is isotonically reabsorbed. Sodium is actively transported into the peritubular space and chloride and water passively follow. The proximal tubule also is responsible for most (85%) of the urinary acidification and acid–base exchange, as well as the handling of calcium and phosphate under the influence of parathyroid hormone. After passing through the proximal tubule, the ultrafiltrate enters the descending (thin) portion of the loop of Henle accompanied by the adjacent vasa recta. Many loops can extend through the medulla to the tips of the papilla with the collecting ducts. Here a *countercurrent multiplier* acts to increase the osmotic concentration of the medullary interstitium

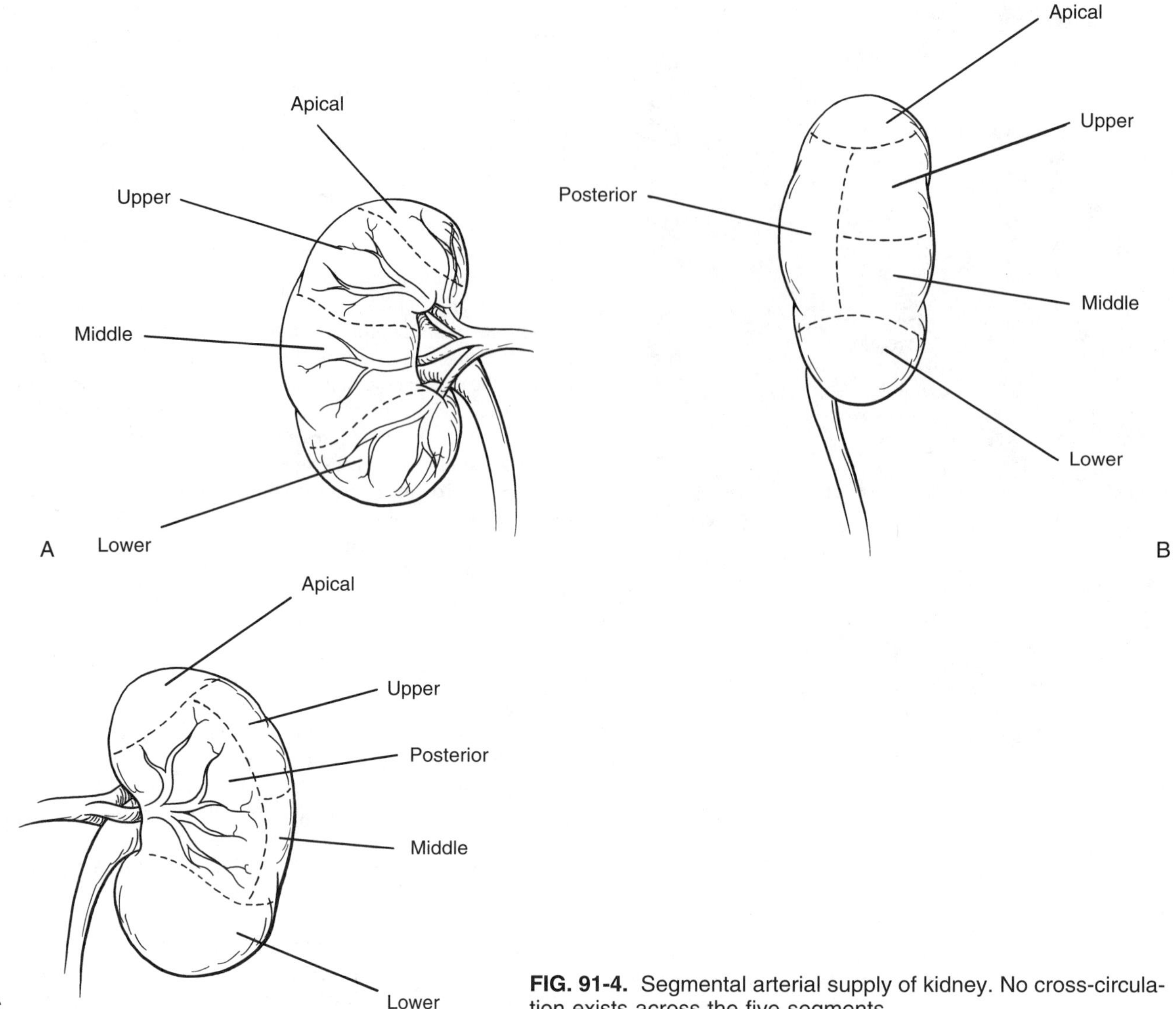

FIG. 91-4. Segmental arterial supply of kidney. No cross-circulation exists across the five segments.

by actively reabsorbing salt. On its upward swing, ultrafiltrate hypotonicity results since the ascending (thick) loop is impermeable to water, yet salts are actively reabsorbed along their elevated osmotic gradients (Fig. 91-7). The distal tubule and collecting ducts ultimately course back through this same hypertonic medullary interstitium, where water reabsorption is mediated largely by antidiuretic hormone. Final sodium handling also occurs here, mediated partly by aldosterone. Damage to this area, especially from the elevated pressures of obstruction, can result in diabetes insipidus and salt wasting.

Henle's loop ascends to the distal convoluted tubule, which courses alongside the glomerulus of origin. The two are functionally linked by the tubule's macula densa, a modified group of cells believed to influence the release of renin by the juxtaglomerular apparatus. Multiple collecting tubules drain into individual collecting ducts that run through the medulla and out to the renal papilla, where other collecting ducts are gathered to give the papilla a porous appearance. The differences in papillary configuration play a role in reflux. Papillae in the midportion of the kidney have a simple cone shape that projects

into the collecting systems and effectively retards the migration of bacteria into the kidney. In contrast, polar papillae are classically flattened or concave and lack a valvular mechanism that negates intrarenal reflux. As a result, the scars of pyelonephritis typically occur in the poles (Fig. 91-8). Renal physiology is discussed in detail in Chapter 6.

EMBRYOLOGY

Congenital anomalies of the urinary tract are common, with a rate as high as 3% cited in asymptomatic infants screened with ultrasound.[2] Understanding the complex interactions required of the renal blastema and its collecting system, the ureteral bud, is a prerequisite to evaluating and managing these children and offers a ready explanation for the frequency of these anomalies.[3]

The mature kidney evolves through three developmental phases. The pronephros, mesonephros, and metanephros are derived from intermediate mesoderm, which coalesces adjacent

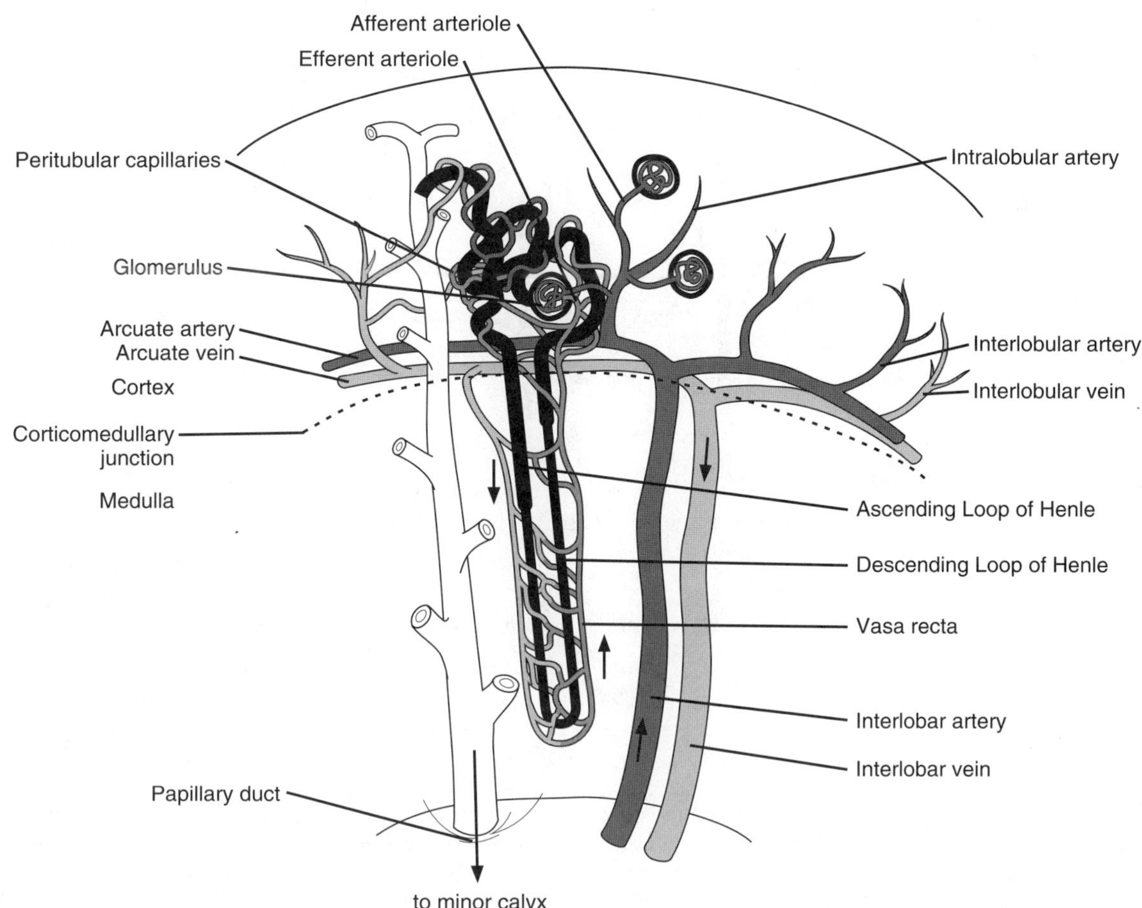

FIG. 91-5. Nephron microanatomy and relation to intrarenal vasculature.

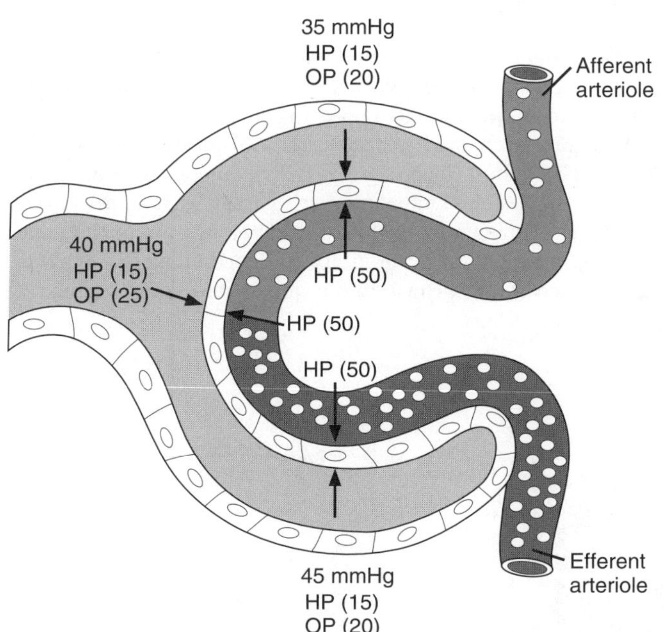

FIG. 91-6. Starling forces. The balance between hydrostatic pressure (HP) in the glomerular capillary and hydrostatic pressure in Bowman capsule in concert with plasma oncotic pressure (OP) dictate net filtration across the glomerulus.

to the second through sixth somites. The superior portion of the primordial anlage or nephrogenic cord is composed of primitive tubules known as the *pronephros*. This appears by the third week of gestation and involutes by week 5.

The medially positioned *mesonephros* is induced from the mesoderm by the descending mesonephric duct, the wolffian duct, which extends caudally to communicate with the anterior cloaca. The union of duct with mesoderm creates about 40 pairs of mesonephric nephrons, which produce urine between the 5th and 10th weeks of development. This probably accounts for expansion of the allantois and rupture of the cloacal membrane. Although the mesonephros gradually involutes, vestigial tubules can be found in both sexes near the reproductive tracts. The mesonephric duct persists as the vas deferens in males. In females, remnants persist as Gartner's duct along the anteromedial vaginal wall. These relations help to explain the insertions of ectopic ureters in the different sexes, which, in females, can bypass the urinary sphincters and cause incontinence.

Formation of the mature kidney depends on the induction of the caudal portion of the nephrogenic cord or *metanephros* by the ureteral bud. The ureteral bud begins to project from the caudal end of the mesonephric (wolffian) duct during the fourth and fifth weeks of gestation. As the bud advances cranially, its end dilates to form an ampulla. The bud's union with the metanephric blastema and its progressive ampullary branching is repeated for 15 generations. The initial 5 generations create the renal pelvis and major calyces. Asymmetry in the branching

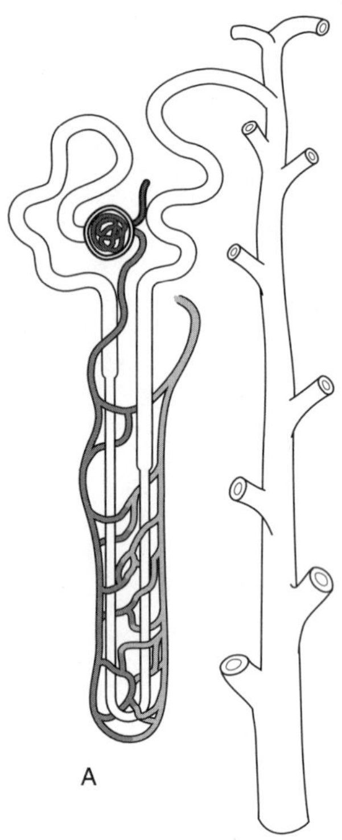

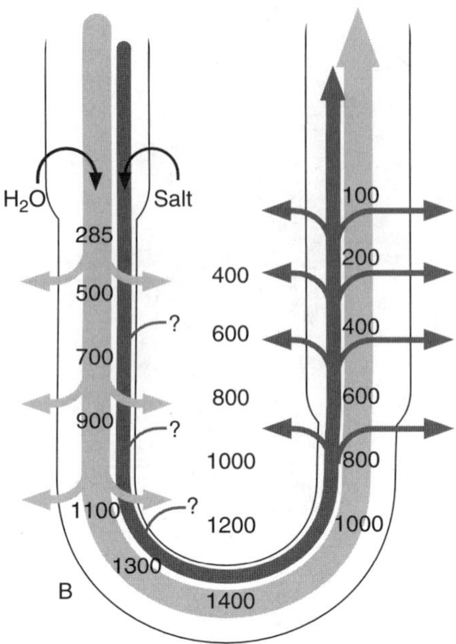

FIG. 91-7. "Countercurrent multiplier" of the loop of Henle. The active transport of salt out of the ascending limb increases medullary osmotic concentration. Water is then reabsorbed by osmotic force if distal tubular and collecting duct permeability, under the influence of antidiuretic hormone, allows.

between the poles and midportion result in the characteristic reniform shape. Minor calyces and medullary collecting ducts are formed between the 6th and 13th generations (7 weeks' gestation). The reciprocal induction of the renal blastema brings about the formation of the nephrogenic structures and supporting tissues. For the remainder of development, one branch of each dividing ampulla differentiates into a nephron, whereas the other continues to bisect and extend to the periphery of the kidney. This progression links a series of successive nephrons by their collecting tubules to a common duct. Additional generations bring about the cortical extension of ampulla–nephrons and the differentiation of discreet masses of blastema to form glomeruli (weeks 15 to 32). After the 32nd week, no further induction of nephrons occurs, although proximal tubule convolution, collecting tubule elongation, and Henle's loop extension into the medulla continue. Each nephron follows a sequential order of maturation in segmentation of glomerulus, proximal tubule, and distal tubule (Figs. 91-9 and 91-10).

Nephrogenesis does not occur if the bud is absent or unable to come into close contact with the metanephrogenic blastema. When the tissues are separated enough to prevent close contact, differentiation does not occur. After being induced by contact, proliferation and morphogenesis of the metanephros continues under the influence of growth factors, extracellular matrix, and proteins. The interactions of fibronectin (which promotes cellular mobility), collagen subtypes, and syndecan (a cell surface proteoglycan that first appears with induction and binds the other two) have received attention. Transferrin, neural cell adhesion molecule, proteoglycans, and laminin (a promoter of cell aggregation) probably also play a role.

Concurrent changes in the position of the fetal kidney also occur. The ureteral bud engages the metanephros in the sacral region, yet the fetal kidney ultimately assumes an upper lumbar position. Explanations for this include elongation of the ureter into the metanephros, migration with lengthening of the parenchyma, and caudal growth of the spine, which causes a relative

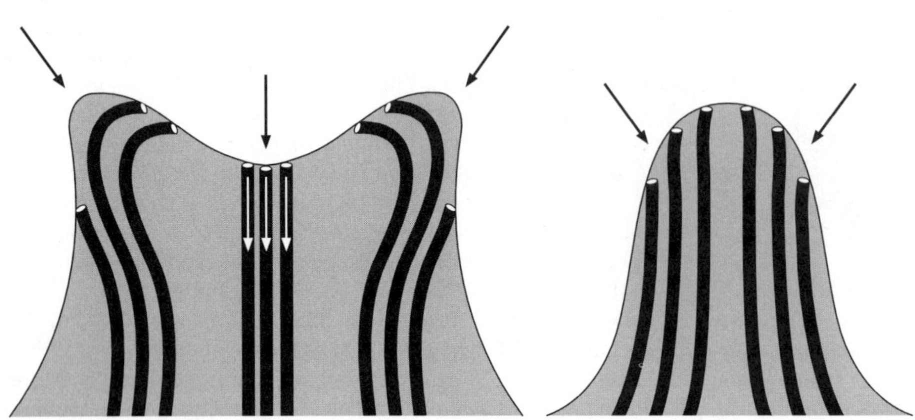

FIG. 91-8. Papillae differ at the poles, whose compound configuration (*left*) more readily allows intrarenal reflux than the simple papillae of the midportion of the kidney.

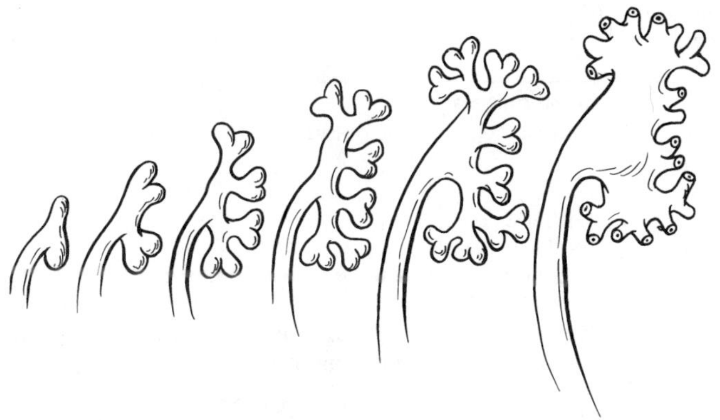

FIG. 91-9. Dichotomous branching of the ureteral bud. Generations 1 through 5 form the pelvis and calyces; 6 through 13, the medullary collecting tubules; and 14 through 15, the cortical collecting tubules.

ascent, especially after the renal moiety becomes fixed to retroperitoneal structures. The last probably is the most important. In addition to ascent, rotation of the kidney also occurs. The pelvis and ureter are initially anteriorly oriented but undergo a medial rotation to face the spine.

Abnormalities in the interplay of the ureteral bud and metanephros are implicated in a number of congenital abnormalities of the kidney (see later). For example, ectopic ureters or severely refluxing ureters positioned off the trigone commonly are associated with renal dysplasia or hypoplasia, findings that are rarely associated with the normal ureter. Calyceal diverticula, some cystic variants, megacalycosis, and renal ectopia also undoubtedly have a embryonic basis where problems with ampullary branching, segmentation of the nephron and renal ascent can occur. Nevertheless, etiologies are difficult to prove.

ANOMALIES OF NUMBER AND POSITION

Renal Agenesis

Unilateral

Unilateral renal agenesis is a fairly common anomaly (1 per 1100 in autopsy series and 1 per 1500 in radiographic reviews) that theoretically results from absence of the mesonephric

(wolffian) duct or ureteral bud, absence of the metanephric blastema, or the failure of a meeting of the two. The 2:1 male predominance seen with renal agenesis probably results from the delicate interplay required of the bud and the wolffian duct. The timing of the error in embryogenesis determines its effects (Table 91-1). As many as half of the patients with one kidney still have a rudimentary ureter on the affected side, an indication that the problem occurred after the ureteral bud has taken off from the wolffian duct, which remains normal. The other half of affected males have an absence of the ureter and ipsilateral hemitrigone of the bladder, as well as absence of the wolffian structures (ejaculatory duct, seminal vesicle, and vas deferens) as indicators of an earlier insult in development. In both instances, the ipsilateral gonad is usually normal.

Similar errors in embryogenesis also affect females for apparently the same reasons. Other than giving off the ureteral bud before they involute, the wolffian ducts play a crucial role in the development of the internal genitalia by guiding the müllerian ducts into position along the urorectal septum. It is easy to implicate abnormalities of this sequence with a unicornuate uterus, where the müllerian duct is never properly positioned, or in uterine didelphys, where the normal fusion and channelization of the two ducts is somehow deterred. Not surprisingly, both anomalies are commonly associated with renal agenesis in female patients. For the same reasons, complete absence or hypoplasia of the vagina also is frequently associated with renal agenesis (*Mayer-Rokitansky-Kuster-Hauser syndrome*).

Unilateral renal agenesis is occasionally discovered during the evaluation of the child with multiple organ system anomalies (eg, syndrome of vertebral defects, imperforate anus, tracheoesophageal fistula, and radial and renal dysplasia [VATER]), serendipitously or in concert with an associated symptomatic genital abnormality such as hydrocolpos. They are more often diagnosed with antenatal ultrasound. After delivery, renal scintigraphy can be used to confirm the diagnosis. Parents also are made aware of the possible genital implications of the finding. Ultrasound can be used to confirm the presence of a cervix and uterus in infants and young girls. Some clinicians also have recommended screening the siblings of affected children, in whom a 10% rate of asymptomatic renal anomalies has been reported.

Until recently, it was believed that children with solitary kidneys experienced no increased nephrologic risk. Compensatory hypertrophy of the single moiety occurs, and life expectancy is assumed to be normal. However, concerns have been raised

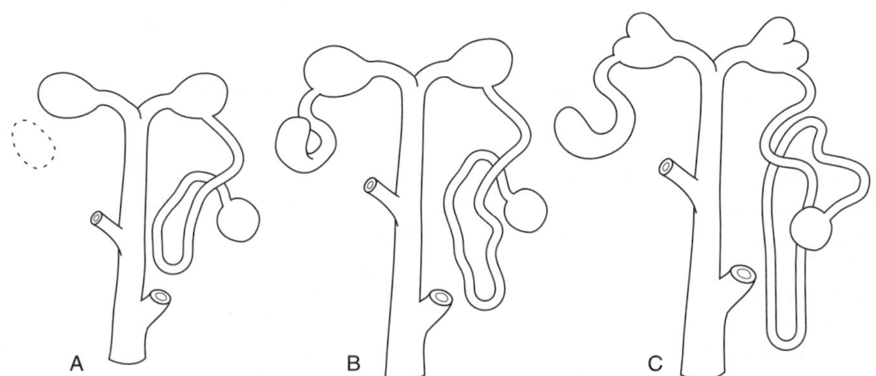

FIG. 91-10. Nephron induction and advancement. Ureteral bud ampulla fuses with metanephric vesicle and then branches. Attached nephron moves peripherally with new branch.

TABLE 91-1. *Common associations with renal agenesis*

	Unilateral	Bilateral
Urologic	Ureteral absence or atresia Asymmetric or hemitrigone Contralateral renal ectopia, malrotation	Ureteral atresia Absent or hypoplastic bladder

Genital	Male
	  Absent vas deferens, seminal vesicle
	Female
	  Unicornuate or didelphic uterus
	  Duplicate or absent vagina
		Male
		  Hypospadia
		  Penile agenesis
		  Undescended testes
		Female
		  Rudimentary, anomalous, or absent uterus, vagina
		  Hypoplastic or absent ovaries

Pulmonary	NA	Pulmonary hypoplasia
Cardiovascular	Septal, valvular defects	Present
Gastrointestinal	Imperforate anus Esophageal stricture, atresia	Imperforate anus
Orthopedic	Vertebral, phalangeal anomalies	Club feet Spina bifida
Other	Syndromes: VATER, Poland, Turner	Characteristic (Potter) facies

VATER, syndrome of vertebral defects, anorectal anomalies, tracheoesophageal fistula, and radial and renal dysplasia.

about the hyperfiltration load assumed by the remaining kidney. Renal function has been adversely affected in animal models, and there have been several reports of proteinuria and focal glomerulosclerosis in patients at risk. Currently, dietary restrictions are not recommended, but this may change with further research.

Bilateral

Bilateral renal agenesis is less common than its unilateral counterpart (1 in 4800 births) and, for obvious reasons, its consequences are more devastating. Male patients are more commonly affected (75%), although the wolffian derivatives usually are normal. Failure of the ureteral bud typically is implicated since an absent or atretic ureter is found in nearly 90% of cases. An increased incidence of imperforate anus and spina bifida suggests a regional disturbance of the cloaca in some children. In the remainder, a 10% incidence of testicular agenesis in the presence of intact wolffian structures implies a dual insult to the renal and gonadal anlages in the dorsal coelom.

Anhydramnios or oligohydramnios during pregnancy usually is the harbinger of bilateral renal agenesis. Antenatal ultrasound confirms absence of the kidneys and nonvisualization of the bladder after a prolonged examination. Although false-positive results have been reported, consideration is given to termination of pregnancy because of the poor prognosis. Intrauterine compression of the fetus results in the classic stigmata of Potter syndrome (clubbed feet, bowed legs, loose skin, and prominent epicanthal fold of the cheek) and severe pulmonary hypoplasia. Stillbirths result in half of the cases, whereas the remainder rapidly die during the first day of life from pulmonary distress. Oliguria and gradual renal failure are predictable for the occasional child who remains alive for a slightly longer period of time. Normal newborns should void during the first 24 hours. Renal agenesis is suggested by more prolonged anuria, especially without a distended bladder. Ultrasound usually is diagnostic, although renal scintigraphy also can be performed for confirmation. The risk of recurrence in subsequent pregnancies

has been estimated at 2% to 5%, underscoring the need for an autopsy of any baby believed to have this diagnosis.

Supernumerary Kidneys

Supernumerary kidneys are extremely rare, with about 75 cases reported in the literature. These accessory organs, which are smaller than normal but have their own blood supply and separate capsule, are usually positioned below an ipsilateral kidney that is normally located. Dual errors in embryogenesis affect both the outpouching of the ureteral bud and simultaneous separation of the metanephros. Hydronephrosis is found in half of the cases, and the associated vascular and ureteral anatomy is widely variable. The latter is equally divided between Y-confluences, with the ureter of the ipsilateral kidney (one orifice) and complete duplications with two separate orifices. Despite these findings, most supernumerary kidneys probably never become symptomatic. Those that do cause urinary tract (UTIs) infections or abdominal pain. Excretory urography or renal scintigraphy usually is diagnostic.

RENAL FUSIONS AND ECTOPIA

Early errors in development can adversely affect the ascent and rotation of the metanephros and result in an impressive array of anomalies in position and configuration.[4] Theories to explain this phenomenon include the following: exaggerated flexion of the fetus causing an anomalous position of the blastema, barriers to ascent by blood vessels; and faulty interplay between the ureteral bud and renal blastema. The latter also could account for the high incidence of vesicoureteral reflux found with these kidneys. Despite their distorted configurations, most of these renal anomalies are never clinically significant. However, they should serve as a caution to clinicians since affected children often have abnormalities of other organs.

Horseshoe Kidney

Horseshoe kidneys are the most common fusion anomaly, with an incidence of 1 in 400 with a 2:1 male prevalence. Fusion of the lower poles are found in more than 90% of cases, a finding that suggests an early error in blastema development before ascent and rotation occur (4 to 6 weeks). An isthmus of functioning renal tissue usually is found anterior to the great vessels just below the inferior mesenteric artery. Renal vasculature is highly variable, and only 30% of horseshoe kidneys have a single renal artery. The remainder are also supplied by other branches from the aorta or the hypogastric, middle sacral, and common iliac arteries.

Most ectopic and fused kidneys, as well as horseshoe kidneys, are malrotated. The ureters are anteriorly directed and draped over the inferior poles and isthmus of the anomaly. Variable degrees of hydronephrosis are the rule, and complete obstruction exists in one third or less of patients. Stasis does present a problem, and calculi ultimately develop in about 20% of patients. When symptoms do occur, vague abdominal pain, a palpable mass, or urinary infection are common presenting signs. A renal scan or intravenous pyelogram (IVP) is diagnostic. Typical radiographic signs include low-lying kidneys, outward deviation of their axes, posterior rather than lateral projection of the calyces, and functioning tissue across the midline (Fig. 91-11).

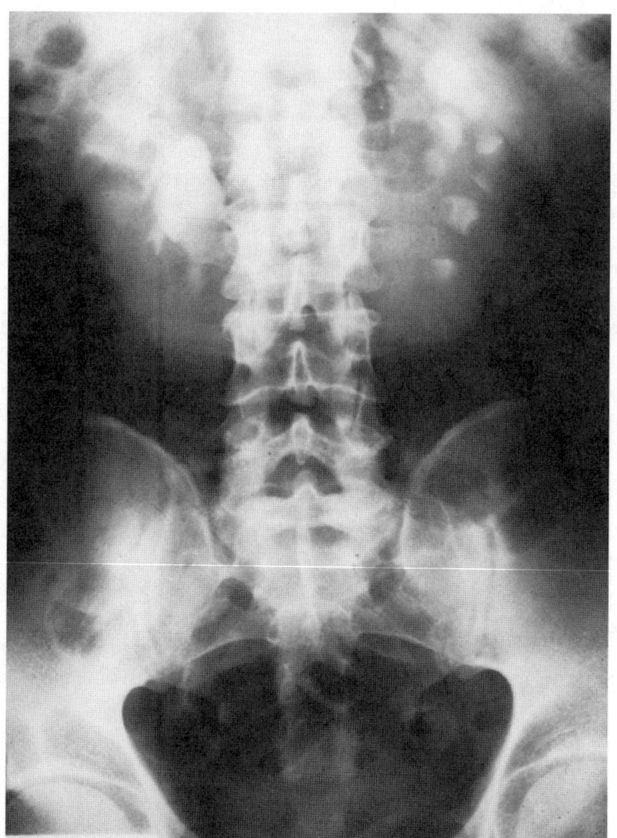

FIG. 91-11. Horseshoe kidney. Excretory urogram shows medial rotation of inferior poles, outward deviation of renal axes, and anteriorly directed renal calyces.

TABLE 91-2. *Common associations with horseshoe kidney*

Musculoskeletal
Spina bifida occulta
Congenital hip dislocation
Webbed neck
Other (polydactyly, club foot)
Central nervous system
Myelomeningocele
Hydrocephalus
Cardiovascular
Ventriculoseptal defects
Gastrointestinal
Imperforate anus
Malrotation
Meckel's diverticulum
Genital
Male patients:
Hypospadias
Female patients:
Bicornuate uterus
Septate vagina
Urologic
UPJ obstruction
Vesicoureteral reflux
Ureteral duplication
Ectopic ureterocele
Renal cystic disease
Chromosomal
Trisomy 18
Turner syndrome

UPJ, ureteral pelvic junction.

Common associations with horseshoe kidneys are summarized in Table 91-2. Long-term survival is unaffected by the presence of a fusion or ectopia. However, these kidneys are more prone to trauma, and it can be difficult to operate on them because of their highly variable vasculature. Depending on the pelvic or renal surgery that is planned, arteriography can provide information about the blood supply to the kidney that may be crucial to success. Voiding cystourethrography also is indicated in any symptomatic child with a horseshoe kidney. Vesicoureteral reflux is seen in one half of these children and presents a risk factor for infection and upper tract damage in an already abnormal kidney.

Crossed Renal Ectopia

Crossed renal ectopia is less common than horseshoe kidney (1 in 1000) and also preferentially affects male patients (2:1). Four categories lend order to what sometimes is bizarre anatomy. In decreasing order of frequency, these include crossed fused (*A*), crossed nonfused (*B*), solitary crossed (*C*), and bilateral crossed (*D*) (Figs. 91-12 and 91-13). Crossed fusions constitute 90% of the variants seen, and the left kidney is the ectopic moiety 75% of the time. In most cases, the orthotopic kidney and ureter are normally positioned. Its lower pole, however, is fused to the upper pole of the crossed ectopic kidney, whose ureter is normally inserted in the bladder on the contralateral side. In less well-defined cases, the ureteral origins remain unchanged but both kidneys meld together on one side in fusions

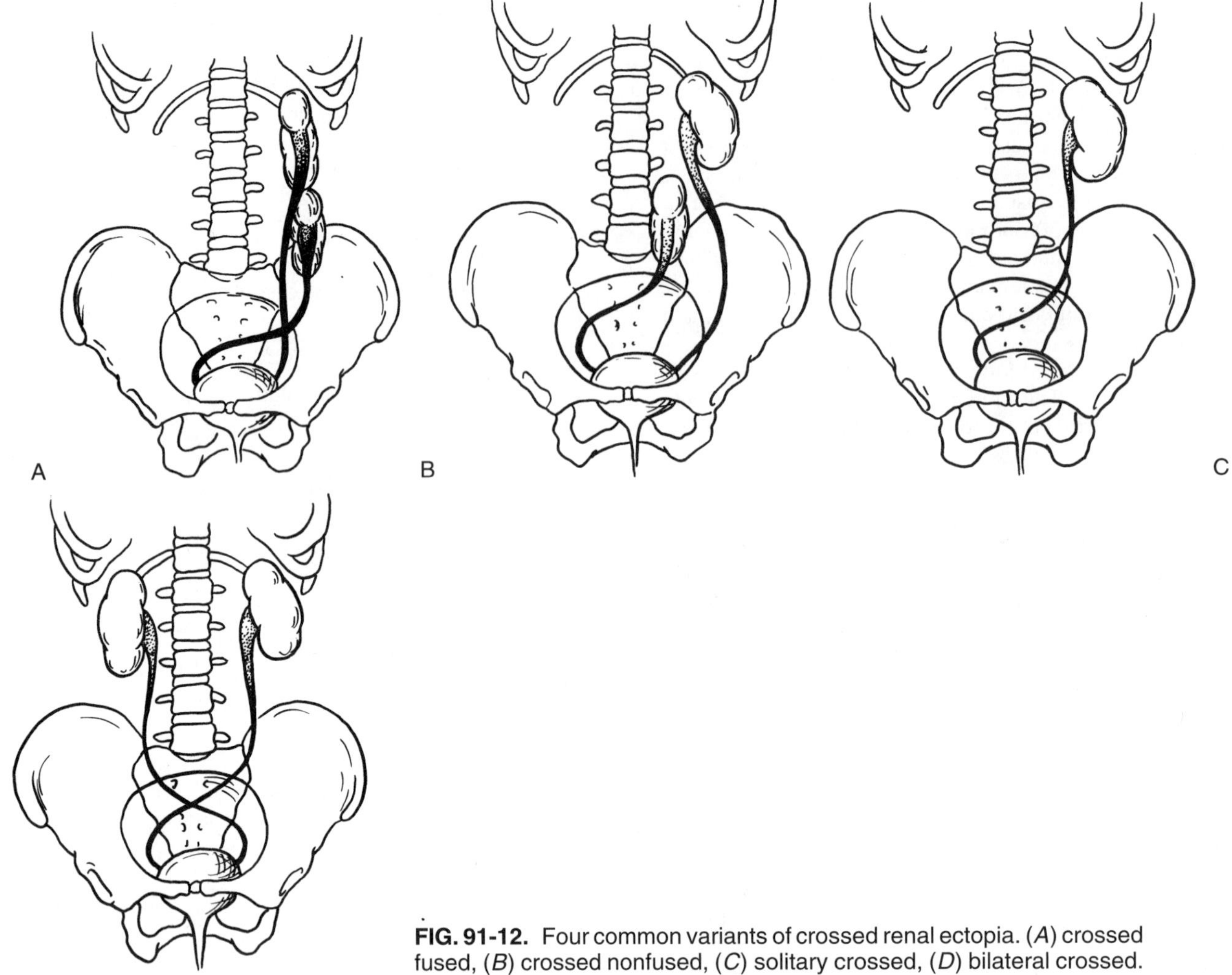

FIG. 91-12. Four common variants of crossed renal ectopia. (*A*) crossed fused, (*B*) crossed nonfused, (*C*) solitary crossed, (*D*) bilateral crossed.

designated as lump, disc, L-shaped, or sigmoid, depending on their shapes.

Other Renal Ectopias

Whenever a kidney occupies an abnormal position, it is classified as ectopic. A compilation of series suggests an overall occurrence of about of 1 in 900. *Pelvic ectopia*, in which the kidney is opposite the sacrum, is the most common type (1 per 3000) (Fig. 91-14). Additional ascent yields *lumbar* (near the sacral promontory) and *abdominal* (above the iliac crest) variants. *Thoracic* ectopia, representing less than 5% of ectopic kidneys, results from either accelerated ascension of the kidney or delayed closure of the foramen of Bochdalek, through which it sometimes projects. Because of its embryologic origin, the adrenal gland is normally positioned, regardless of the position of the kidney.

Ectopic kidneys often are dysmorphic and smaller than normal, yet most are asymptomatic despite their abnormal location. Vascularity typically emanates from anomalous branches of the adjacent great vessels. Like horseshoe variants, ectopic kidneys are malrotated. Presentations include hydronephrosis, obstruction, calculi, infection, vague abdominal pain, and posttraumatic hematuria. When making the diagnosis, a careful examination of the pelvis is made whenever an IVP suggests an ''absent'' kidney. Moieties positioned over the sacrum may be difficult to visualize. Renal scintigraphy, computed tomography (CT), and ultrasonography are other imaging options.

Other anomalies (up to 85%) commonly occur with ectopic kidneys (Table 91-3) for reasons that remain unclear. Since ipsilateral vesicoureteral reflux is a frequent finding (70%), voiding cystourethrography is recommended to complete the work-up of affected children. In addition, the contralateral kidney is abnormal in as many as 50% of patients, causing some investigators to implicate a teratogen in etiology. Finally, the high incidence of müllerian malformations in girls (45%), including duplications of the vagina and a unicornuate or bicornuate uterus, suggests a problem with the ureteral bud early in development.

CYSTIC DISEASES

The categorization of the more common cystic diseases of the kidney can lead to confusion as a consequence of its nomenclature (Table 91-4). The terms *polycystic* and *multicystic* are not synonymous. Instead, polycystic kidney disease (PKD) refers to one of three conditions, two of which are genetically determined and the third acquired. In contrast, the designation of multicystic kidney denotes a histologically distinct entity that is not heritable and generally is devoid of accompanying systemic manifestations.

Polycystic Kidney Disease

Although differing in many ways, the three variants of PKD share the common denominator of cystic development. Theories abound for their appearance, although each remains unproven. Contributions of epithelial proliferation, reversal of the normal secretory–absorptive polarity of tubule cells, and basement membrane abnormalities and nephrotoxins—both exogenous and from endogenous errors of metabolism—all have been implicated by ongoing work.

Although general patterns do exist, the manifestations of PKD comprise a spectrum that can occur across the ages. As a result, its subclassifications (autosomal recessive, autosomal dominant, and acquired) typically are based on modality of acquisition rather than cystic type, their distribution, or the age at presentation.[5]

Autosomal Recessive Disease

Autosomal recessive polycystic kidney disease (ARPKD) is typically diagnosed during childhood, although it can present

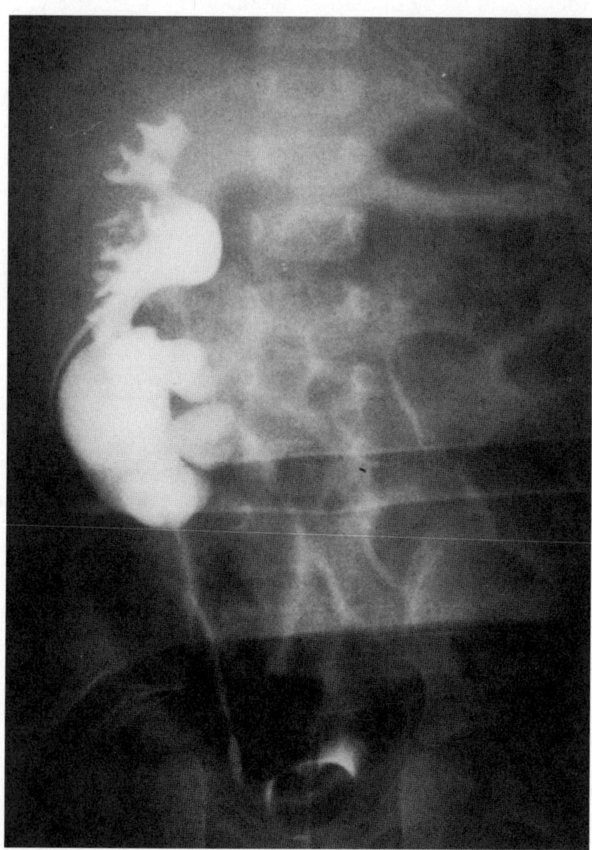

FIG. 91-13. Intravenous pyelogram demonstrates left-to-right crossed ectopia with fusion.

in adolescence. The terms *infantile* or *juvenile* have been discouraged since the dominantly transmitted variant, or the so-called ''adult'' PKD, can occur in children. ARPKD is an uncommon condition whose incidence ranges from 1 in 6000 to 1 in 40,000 in different series. In keeping with its pattern of transmission, 25% of the offspring of carriers are expected to be homozygous and manifest the disease. An alternative diagnosis should be entertained if either parent reports having a ''cystic kidney.'' There is no gender predilection.

Clinical Features

Autosomal recessive polycystic kidney disease is uniformly accompanied by liver abnormalities, ranging from biliary ductal ectasia to periportal fibrosis with portal hypertension and its sequelae. The severity of one organ's involvement usually is inversely related to that of the other. Renal involvement predominates in recessive disease diagnosed during the perinatal period, whereas hepatic dysfunction accounts for detection in later childhood. The clinical presentations follow accordingly.

When the diagnosis is made in utero, fetal kidneys are typically enlarged and diffusely hyperechoic. In some cases, they become large enough to impede labor, making delivery difficult. Some degree of oligohydramnios usually is present and results in pulmonary hypoplasia. Most perinatal mortality is caused by respiratory failure rather than the sequelae of renal involvement. Neonates who survive present with oliguria, abdominal masses, and some degree of pulmonary compromise. Infants who live past the first month of life generally do satisfactorily, although hypertension is almost universal.

Congenital hepatic fibrosis usually is detected later in development. Hepatosplenomegaly, esophageal varices, upper gastrointestinal bleeding, and occasionally ascites all result from periportal fibrosis and portal hypertension. Hepatocyte function is typically unaffected, and jaundice is rare. Renal impairment, concentrating defects, and collecting duct ectasia may be seen.

A third pattern can affect persons at any age and represents a composite of the presentations typical of the newborn and older child. Here, both the liver and kidneys are significantly affected, and the prognosis is uniformly bleak.

Evaluation and Differential Diagnosis

The antenatal diagnosis of ARPKD is suspected when bilateral hyperechoic, enlarged kidneys are seen by ultrasound. Included in the differential diagnosis are multicystic dysplastic kidneys, although they usually show more significant cystic dilatation. There are no known genetic markers for the disease, and its variable presentation can lead to confusion and undue concern. For example, some cases of antenatally diagnosed hyperechoic kidneys demonstrate normal echogenicity and function postnatally. Conversely, fetuses with normal ultrasonic findings early in gestation may demonstrate hyperechoic kidneys typical for ARPKD later in development. In both instances, the presence of oligohydramnios is an ominous prognostic sign.

The kidneys of the neonate with ARPKD are easily palpable, smooth, firm flank masses that often are visible through the anterior abdominal wall. Unlike kidneys affected by massive hydronephrosis, these do not transilluminate because of the

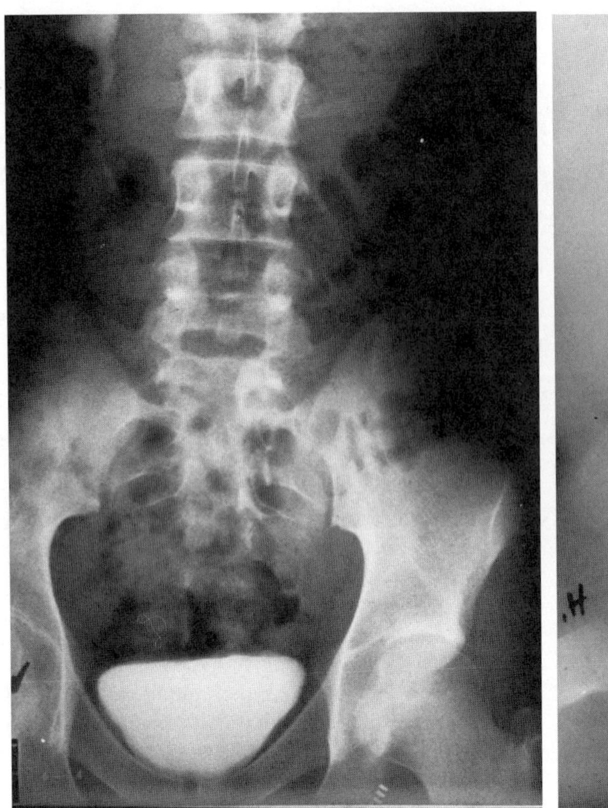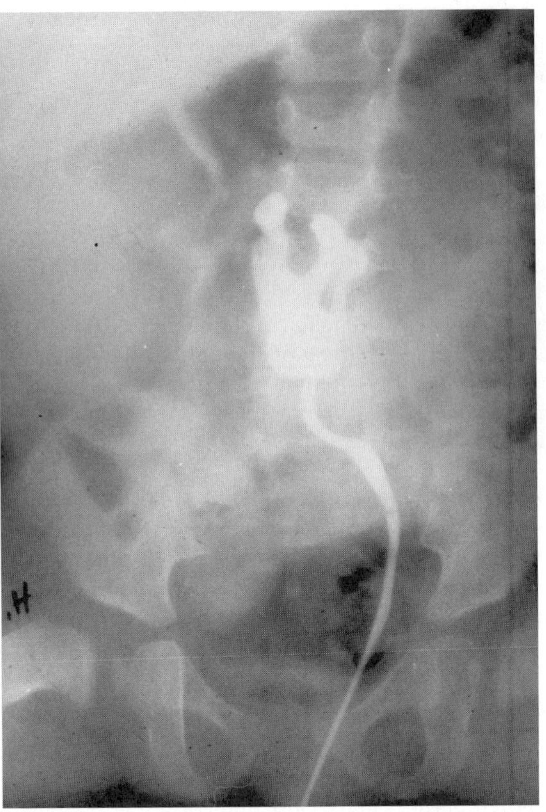

FIG. 91-14. Left pelvic kidney. (*A*) Absence of normally positioned kidney on excretory urography warrants close inspection at the level of the pelvic brim. (*B*) Retrograde study of same patient.

small size of the cysts. They also maintain their reniform shape, despite being as much as 10 times normal size. Newborns affected by oligohydramnios also may exhibit Potter facies, including abnormal ears, beaked nose, and recessed chin.

Ultrasound in affected newborns shows bilateral renal enlargement with dense echogenicity (Fig. 91-15). The cysts are small, but their ubiquity and interface with solid parenchyma give rise to the signature echo-dense pattern of the disease.

Other ultrasonic findings include a particularly echogenic medulla, which is normally echo-free in the neonate, and occasional large, discreet cysts. Additional diagnostic studies offer few other data, although nuclear scintigraphy can help quantify the functional defect.

In older children, the discovery of renal disease usually is made during the evaluation of hepatic dysfunction. Ultrasonog-

TABLE 91-3. *Common associations with ectopic kidney*

Musculoskeletal
   Vertebral, rib anomalies
   Cranial asymmetry
   Absent bones
Urologic
   Vesicoureteral reflux
   UPJ obstruction
   Contralateral agenesis
Genital
   Male patients:
      Undescended testis
      Hypospadia
      Urethral duplication
   Female patients:
      Uterine or vaginal anomalies, atresia, agenesis
Other
   Cardiovascular, gastrointestinal

UPJ, ureteral pelvic junction.

TABLE 91-4. *Cystic disease of the kidney*

GENETIC
Autosomal recessive (infantile) polycystic kidneys
Autosomal dominant (adult) polycystic kidneys
Juvenile nephronophthisis–medullary cystic disease complex
   Juvenile nephronophthisis (autosomal recessive)
   Medullary cystic disease (autosomal dominant)
Congenital nephrosis (autosomal recessive)
Familial hypoplastic glomerulocystic kidney disease (autosomal dominant)
Cysts associated with multiple malformation syndromes

NONGENETIC
Multicystic kidney (multicystic dysplasia)
Multilocular cyst (multilocular cystic adenoma)
Simple cyst
Medullary sponge kidneys (less than 5% inherited)
Sporadic glomerulocystic kidney disease
Acquired renal cystic disease
Calyceal diverticulum (pyelogenic cyst)

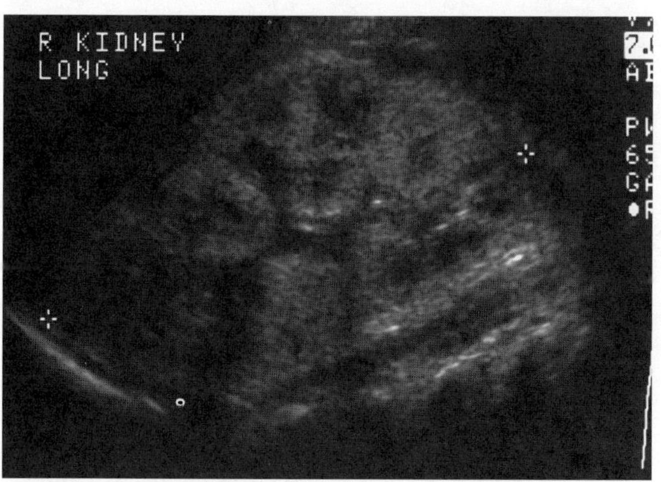

FIG. 91-15. Ultrasonic appearance of autosomal recessive polycystic disease in a newborn shows a large (65 mm) echogenic kidney (normal average, larger than 50 mm).

raphy provides the best screen of the urinary tract. The kidneys generally are large for age, although there may be some shrinkage from their impressive neonatal size. Their sonographic appearance resembles that of the neonate, but often there are several larger discrete cysts. Medullary streaking is characteristic of PKD when an excretory urogram (IVP) is obtained. CT and magnetic resonance imaging may differentiate between the cystic diseases by demonstrating other organ involvement more typical of the dominant variant.

Pathology

The pathologic features of ARPKD mirror its clinical presentation. Regardless of its degree, renal involvement uniformly affects the distal collecting duct of the nephron (Fig 91-16). Cortical involvement is uniformly severe and gives the parenchyma a bubble-like texture if the renal capsule is stripped away. The number and appearance of glomeruli usually are normal, and the architecture of the pyramids and papilla is preserved. Older children have less pronounced cortical changes and a tendency to have larger cysts (2 cm).

The hepatic abnormality affects only the portal area and involves the entire organ. Nonobstructive biliary ductal ectasia (a mimic of Caroli disease) is present in some degree in every child with ARPKD from birth, although the amount of periportal fibrosis increases with age. This progression probably accounts for the predominance of liver-related symptoms in older patients.

Autosomal Dominant Disease

Autosomal dominant polycystic kidney disease (ADPKD) is far more common than its recessive counterpart and occurs in 1 in 1000 live births. It's clinical sequelae are devastating, with an estimated 500,000 active cases accounting for 10% of the chronic hemodialysis patients in the United States. The mechanisms of renal injury probably begin in utero in more severe

cases, and the disease occasionally is diagnosed in younger children. More typically, renal involvement becomes apparent around 40 years of age. A genetic defect has been localized to chromosome 16. Prenatal diagnosis after amniocentesis is possible using molecular probes.

Variable expression occurs among members of the same family. Progeny with the trait have an 80% chance of developing cystic degeneration by their mid-twenties. Offspring with normal findings on renal ultrasound at 35 years of age are no longer considered at risk for the disease. Despite the ominous appearance of cysts, patients with ADPKD have only a 50% chance of developing end-stage renal disease by their 70th birthdays, even if the disease is diagnosed at an early age.

Clinical Features

The diagnosis of ADPKD is made in adults 90% of the time, but the condition is being recognized more frequently in children as awareness increases and imagining techniques improve. There are differences in the pattern of childhood ADPKD compared with that diagnosed in adults, who usually present with hypertension or flank pain. A comparison of ARPKD and ADPKD is shown in Table 91-5.

Although the disease is more commonly discovered during screening of affected families, antenatal diagnosis also is possible. Perinatal ultrasound findings can mimic ARPKD, with bilaterally enlarged, echo-dense kidneys. With the onset of cystic degeneration, concentrating defects of the urine often precede

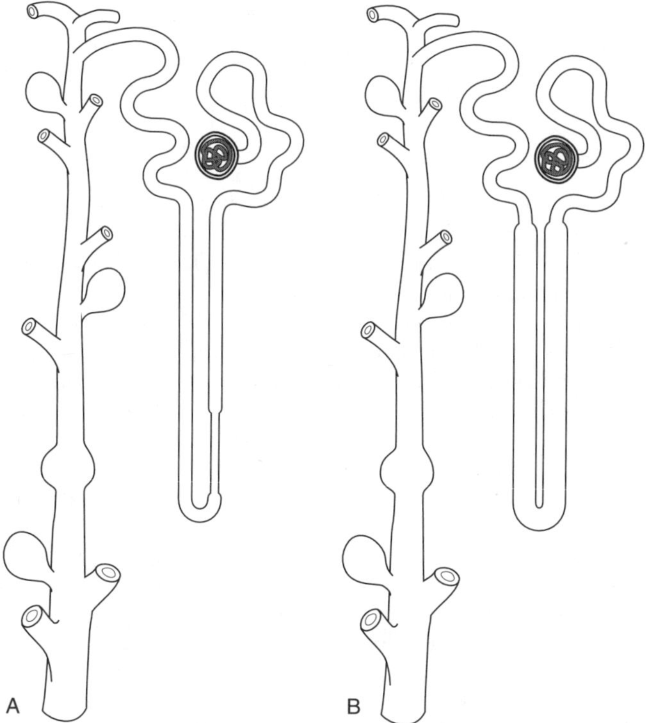

FIG. 91-16. Polycystic kidney disease. (*A*) Recessive type affects global and focal dilatation of the collecting tubules. (*B*) In contrast, the dominant type can involve any portion of the nephron or collecting tubule.

TABLE 91-5. *Comparison of autosomal recessive and dominant polycystic kidney disease*

	ARPKD	ADPKD
Incidence	1 in 6000–40,000	1 in 1000
Inheritance	Autosomal recessive	Autosomal dominant, 100% penetrance, variable expression
Age at diagnosis	0–late adolescence	0–35 y
Imaging	US: Enlarged kidneys with increased echogenicity	US: Multiple large, echolucent cysts
	IVP: Poor function, contrast streaks extend to cortex	IVP: Poor function, distorted collecting system
	CT: Evaluate other organ involvement	CT: Evaluate other organ involvement
Other organs affected	Liver: congenital hepatic fibrosis (with late onset)	Cysts: liver, spleen, thyroid, ovary, endometrium, epididymis, seminal vesicle
		Vascular: circle of Willis aneurysms
Presentation	Younger: renal failure	Renal failure
	Older: liver disease	
Histologic features	Kidney: collecting duct ectasia	Any portion of nephron involved; multiple cysts of varying size
	Liver: periportal fibrosis	

ARPKD, autosomal recessive polycystic kidney disease; ADPKD, autosomal dominant polycystic kidney disease; US, ultrasound; IVP, intravenous pyelogram; CT, computed tomography.

the gradual rises in blood urea nitrogen and creatinine that occur. Rapidly progressive renal failure, hypertension, proteinuria, and hematuria also are common.

Cystic involvement of other organs is common with ADPKD, but cases that become clinically apparent do so at a later age. These can include cysts of the spleen, thyroid, ovary, endometrium, epididymis, and seminal vesicle and diverticula of the colon. Simple cysts of the liver develop in 30% to 50% of patients, although secondary hepatic dysfunction is rare. Berry aneurysms of the circle of Willis present a more serious threat to affected individuals and are found in 10% to 40% of adults. The hypertension that accompanies the condition further increases the risk of intracranial hemorrhage.

Evaluation and Differential Diagnosis

Early ultrasound screening in affected children usually shows normal kidneys, and renal cysts in fetuses or young children are rarely due to ADPKD. With the onset of the disease, both kidneys typically become enlarged. Multiple, variably sized echo-free cysts are seen, and the kidneys lose their reniform shape, unlike the hyperechoic kidneys of the recessive variant (Fig. 91-17). The picture can be confused with multicystic dysplasia (see later), which usually is unilateral, or with other syndromes that feature cysts of the kidneys, including the following:

- Glomerulocystic disease
- Brachymesomelia–renal syndrome
- Orofacial–digital syndrome
- Trisomy 13
- Tuberous sclerosis
- Zellweger syndrome

The family history usually is strongly suggestive.

CT assesses function and other organ involvement. The cysts of the kidneys appear as radiolucent areas, creating a "Swiss cheese" appearance, and puddling of contrast is seen on delayed films. Retrograde studies risk infection and are contraindicated.

Pathology

Since ADPKD can involve any portion of the nephron and can cause cysts of the medulla and cortex that vary widely in size, both kidneys usually are enlarged and distorted, especially

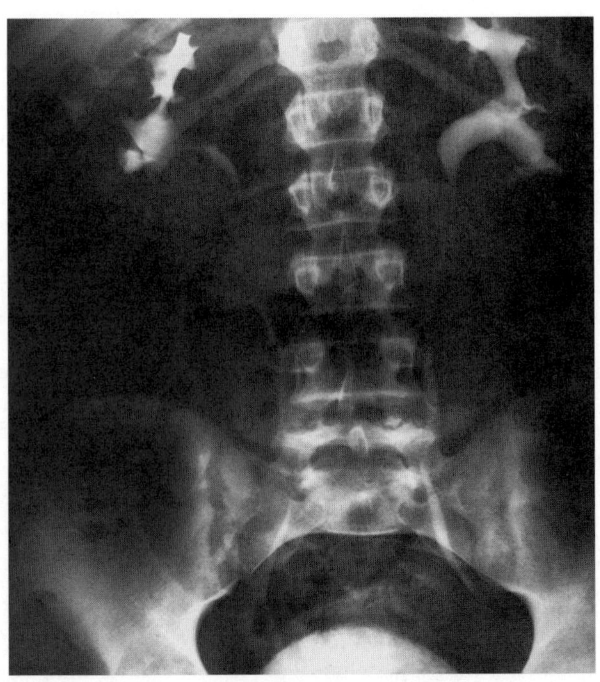

FIG. 91-17. Intravenous pyelogram shows dilated collecting ducts and "brush" appearance of ADPKD. Pooling within ectasia can lead to stone formation.

in adults. When necessary, biopsy can be used to differentiate true glomerulocystic disease from cystic dysplasia.

Acquired Cystic Disease

Patients in end-stage renal failure often develop acquired cystic kidney disease (ACKD). Uremic toxins have been implicated in cyst growth since bilateral involvement is the rule, and cystic regression is noted after successful transplantations. Because of the 3:1 male predominance, a role for a sex-related endogenous growth factor is postulated.

The incidence of ACKD ranges from 35% to 60%. Generally, the cysts are related to the duration of renal failure and length of treatment. Common presentations include fever with infection, flank pain from an intracystic bleed, or hematuria and retroperitoneal hemorrhage, especially in hemodialysis patients on anticoagulants. Cysts develop predominantly in the cortex and reach variable sizes, although most are 0.5 to 1.0 cm in diameter. Some are lined by hyperplastic epithelial cells having irregular nuclei with prominent nucleoli. These may represent the cellular precursors of renal tumors that arise in as many as 25% of patients with ACKD. Tumors usually are multiple, bilateral, and small (less than 2.5 cm in diameter). Because of their size, they receive the designation of benign adenoma. Larger lesions (greater than 3.0 cm) believed to be renal cell carcinomas (RCCs) are rare. Both ultrasound and CT are effective for diagnosis and periodic surveillance.

Multicystic Dysplastic Kidney

Multicystic dysplastic kidneys (MCKs) are the most common cystic disease of the kidney in newborns and infants. With an incidence of 1 in 4300 live births, they represent about 10% of all fetal uropathies. Unlike their polycystic counterparts, MCKs are not genetically transmitted but, instead, seem to result from an early error in embryogenesis. It is plausible that obstruction alone could account for the insult. Some investigators believe that MCKs represent one end of the spectrum of ureteropelvic junction obstruction. Other possibilities include miscommunication between the ureteral bud and renal blastema, an ischemic insult (which might explain the atretic ureter and artery often found with the anomaly), or elements of all three. Similar to ectopic kidneys, there is a 2:1 male predominance. Bilateral dysplasia is extremely rare and incompatible with life.

Clinical Features

Multicystic dysplastic kidney is the most common abdominal mass in newborns, and, until recently, surgical removal has been performed almost uniformly. With ultrasonography, most MCKs are discovered prenatally and the number of children with MCKs has increased in recent years. This has altered the understanding of the anomaly's natural history and its management. The nonoperative management of 260 cases of MCK recently was reported by the Multicystic Kidney Registry.[6] Fifty-four percent of the MCKs became radiographically undetectable when followed for more than 5 years. As cyst fluid is resorbed, the tissue–fluid interface disappears and the kidney progressively decreases in size, which explains why ultrasonic detection is lost. This type of involution is probably responsible for most patients found serendipitously with solitary kidneys before the era of ultrasound.

The risks posed by MCKs that do not involute or by dysplastic renal tissue devoid of its cystic fluid is not fully defined. Urinary infections occur in 2.5%, and hypertension occurs in less than 1% of patients. It is estimated that 8000 nephrectomies of MCKs are necessary to prevent one Wilms tumor. It seems reasonable to follow most MCKs serially (every 3 to 6 months during the first year and once a year thereafter) until involution occurs. Afterward, periodic checks of the blood pressure and urine are appropriate. Nephrectomy is reserved for the uncommon cases that are symptomatic because of size, infection, and hypertension or that enlarge or show cystic changes on ultrasonic follow-up.

Evaluation and Differential Diagnosis

Ultrasound usually is diagnostic, although differentiation from obstructive hydronephrosis can be difficult. In contrast to hydronephrosis, MCKs show multiple cysts of varying sizes that fail to communicate. Typically, there is no identifiable renal parenchyma or centrally located renal pelvis, and there is no uptake of radionuclide on the affected side. When function is seen, the kidney probably is obstructed rather than dysplastic. In poorly developed kidneys, the decision to reconstruct rather than remove sometimes is not made until its parenchyma can be assessed at exploration. Another option with marginal function is to place a nephrostomy tube to allow for recovery. A voiding cystourethrogram also is obtained to complete the evaluation of the urinary tract. Reflux is found in 30% of contralateral solitary kidneys. In addition, hydronephrosis is fairly common and places the patient at risk if obstruction is present.

Pathology

Normal renal parenchyma is replaced by randomly distributed fluid-filled cysts of different sizes lined with normal low cuboidal epithelium. Between the cysts are collections of primitive nephrogenic structures, including immature ducts (pathognomonic for the disease), cartilage, and glomeruli. Both the ureter and artery usually are atretic. Islands of nonproliferative renal blastema have been cited in 2% to 5% of all MCKs.

Other Cystic Conditions

Juvenile Nephronopthisis—Medullary Cystic Disease

Juvenile nephronophthisis (JN) and medullary cystic disease (MCD) initially had been described separately, but generally are designated as a "complex" because of their anatomic and clinical similarities. Whereas about 300 cases have been described, the two differ mainly in age at presentation and mode of transmission. An etiology of the complex remains unclear, but a primary defect of the tubular basement membrane may be at fault. The disease does not recur after transplantation, ruling out the possibility of an inborn error of metabolism.

Clinical Features

The diagnosis of MCD is typically made after the third decade of life and is transmitted in an autosomal dominant pattern. In contrast, JN presents before 20 years of age and is passed in an autosomal recessive fashion. Although less common, JN accounts for 10% to 20% of adolescent renal failure. Consanguineous mating often is recognized in affected families. JN also is more frequently involved in syndromes such as *renal–retinal dysplasia*, where retinitis pigmentosa accompanies the cystic changes of the kidney.

Despite these differences, both conditions share several clinical characteristics. Concentrating defects are predictable and occur in more than 80% of cases. Not surprisingly, polyuria and polydipsia are the usual presenting symptoms. Although less severe than true nephrogenic diabetes insipidus, vasopressin resistance exists and sodium replacement often is necessary. Infection, calculi, and hypertension all are uncommon.

Evaluation

The diagnosis of JN-MDC sometimes is one of exclusion, especially early after the onset of the disease, when renal imaging results usually are normal. An index of suspicion should be raised by the clinical picture and family history. Later in the course of the condition, multiple small medullary cysts can be appreciated by ultrasound. Other studies are of little value in the face of marginal renal function. As with ultrasonography, renal biopsy findings may be normal early on, although most patients eventually develop interstitial nephritis (see later) and atrophic tubular dilatation from the distal convolutions and collecting tubules. Variable alterations in the tubular basement membrane thickness also are found, causing it to be implicated as the primary defect with the condition.

Prognosis

Progression to end-stage renal disease is predictable, and dialysis usually is required within 5 to 10 years after making the diagnosis. In the interim, therapy is supportive. Renal transplantation is an option, provided related donors are well screened to rule out the presence of the same condition in a transplanted kidney.

Medullary Sponge Kidney

Medullary sponge kidneys are affected by *collecting duct ectasia*. As a result, numerous small cysts are found at the papillary tips of the renal pyramids. Unlike JN-MDC, however, medullary sponge kidneys is not an inherited disorder. The disease, whose etiology is unknown, usually is bilateral. Although renal function remains stable throughout life, symptoms are common. Most are discovered after 20 years of age, but childhood disease does occur. Microlithiases form in 60% of patients with sponge kidneys because of stasis, mild acidification defects, and hypercalcuria (30%). Renal colic from their passage is the most common presentation of the condition. Hematuria and urinary infection also can occur.

The cystic dilatations that result usually are too small (1 to 5 mm) to be appreciated by ultrasound, although hyperechogenicity from small calculi may be seen. Instead, excretory urography remains the mainstay of diagnosis. A ''shotgun pellet'' distribution of calcification on the plain film and contrast puddling in dilated tubules is pathognomonic for the disease. Surgery rarely is indicated, and medical management is directed at prevention of calculi and urinary infections.

Simple Cysts

The management of simple cysts in children has changed dramatically because of increased recognition and a better understanding of their natural history. In the past, surgery was the accepted therapy for the entity. It is now understood that true simple cysts can occur in children of any age, including neonates, and that their incidence increases with age. Notably, about 50% of adults aged 50 years have renal cysts.

Most simple cysts are found during the work-up of some other urologic problem (ie, hypospadias, UTI, enuresis). The average age at presentation is 4 years. Other cysts occasionally present as an abdominal mass or with hypertension. Simple cysts usually are single and unilateral. Multiple or bilateral cystic changes suggest a different diagnosis such as PKD.

Ultrasound alone usually is diagnostic. Simple cysts should be smooth walled and filled with anechoic fluid. Exceptions to these criteria should cause concern. The most important differential to exclude is a cystic Wilms tumor variant. Multilocular cysts and calyceal diverticula also can resemble simple cysts. Finally, an upper pole location raises the possibility of a duplicated system associated with a ureterocele or ectopic ureter. Excretory urography can help rule out collecting system anomalies. CT, needle aspiration, and even open exploration sometimes are necessary to confirm a diagnosis if the criteria of simple cyst is not met. When the diagnosis is made in a child, periodic surveillance is all that is necessary to rule out significant change, although long-term compliance with follow-up sometimes is a problem, as with any asymptomatic condition.

Calyceal Diverticulum

A calyceal diverticulum is a cystic cavity peripherally located and connected to an otherwise normal minor calyx. Most are in the upper pole but they can occur anywhere in the kidney. Multiple diverticula are uncommon. An embryologic etiology has been postulated where late generations of the dividing ureteral bud fail to degenerate. Many also are associated with reflux in children. An acquired form of the anomaly is described, which may result from inflammation, obstruction, or trauma. Calyceal diverticula are unusual with an incidence rate of about 0.03%. Most usually are discovered incidentally. They are prone to leave affected patients more susceptible to urinary infections, calculi, and hematuria as a consequence of stasis. Progressive enlargement with pain, abscess formation, and mimics of tumor can result.

Most calyceal diverticula can be diagnosed with excretory urography unless they fail to communicate with the adjacent calyx. Treatment is rarely necessary. Percutaneous management is the treatment of choice for the occasional symptomatic diverticulum, although partial nephrectomy or open nephrotomy provide other options in management.

HYPOPLASIA

Small kidneys having a reduced number of nephrons are termed *hypoplastic*. Anatomically, the reduction can be global or segmental (the so-called Ask-Upmark kidney). Inadequate ureteral bud branching and an aberrant interaction with the renal blastema are the presumed etiology. The differential diagnosis includes renal dysplasia and pyelonephritis. Histologic evidence of chronic pyelonephritis or appreciation of primitive ducts and glomeruli or cartilage as signs of dysplasia help to make the differentiation, although the clinical management is unaffected by designation.

The unilateral hypoplastic kidney usually is asymptomatic and incidentally discovered. Bilateral maldevelopment is rare, although an occasional neonate is affected by *oligomeganephronia*, a variant characterized by small kidneys with a reduced number of giant nephrons. Renal failure results if there are insufficient nephrons to maintain metabolic homeostasis. Hypertension is uncommon with hypoplasia and, in the unilateral setting, more often is indicative of reflux nephropathy.

TUMORS

Renal Cell Carcinoma

Most primary renal tumors in childhood are Wilms tumors and these are discussed in detail in Chapter 33. RCC accounts for less than 10% of childhood renal tumors. The median age at presentation (11 years) is older than that of Wilms tumor, although RCC occasionally occurs during the first few years of life. During the second decade, the incidence of RCC gradually exceeds that of Wilms tumor. Most cases are sporadic, but a familial variant caused by a translocation of chromosomes 3 and 8 has been described. Children with von Hippel-Lindau syndrome and tuberous sclerosis are at increased risk.

The presentation in children is similar to that in adults, with the exception of the absence of paraneoplastic syndromes often seen with RCC in older age groups. Abdominal or flank pain with gross hematuria typically occur. Fever, weight loss, and failure to thrive also are common. Ultrasonography demonstrates a solid renal mass and provides the best assessment of renal vein and caval involvement. CT provides better anatomic resolution of the extent of the tumor. The metastatic work-up evaluates for pulmonary and skeletal disease and includes a chest CT and bone scan.

Prognosis is related to the stage of disease and age at presentation. Localized tumors (stage I) and children younger than 11 years of age have the most favorable outcome. Like adult disease, grade and histopathologic characteristics are less reliable indicators of outcome. Surgery is the mainstay of therapy in children, and 50% are estimated to be cured by radical nephrectomy. Chemotherapy or hormonal manipulation have been ineffective, whereas the benefits of immunotherapy remain unproven. Radiation is used to provide palliation, particularly for bony metastases.

Other Renal Tumors

Other primary malignant tumors of the kidney in children are even less common than RCC. Rhabdomyosarcoma and leiomyosarcoma have been described, and neuroblastoma may involve the kidney primarily. Transitional cell carcinomas of the collecting system are rare in children, although benign fibroepithelial polyps are common. Hematuria and urinary obstruction result. Other benign tumors also arise from fibrous, lymphatic, and vascular elements of the kidney. One example is hemangiopericytoma. A rare renin-secreting tumor that occasionally causes juvenile hypertension.

Secondary renal involvement also occurs, especially with the lymphoproliferative disorders. Lymphoblastic leukemia and non-Hodgkin lymphoma are common tumors. Bilateral or diffuse multinodular infiltration of the kidneys strongly suggests this diagnosis. Recognition is important since treatment in these cases is nonsurgical.

VASCULAR CONDITIONS

Renal Vein Thrombosis

Renal vein thrombosis (RVT) in newborns and children results from low-flow vascular states.[7] Common causes include the following:

- Maternal diabetes
- Severe dehydration (burns, after viral illness)
- Nephrotic syndrome
- Trauma
- Hypercoagulable states (carcinoma)
- Perinephric inflammation

Babies of diabetic mothers are particularly prone because of extracellular dehydration. This results from the osmotic diuresis of glucosuria that compounds the relative oliguria normally seen early after birth. Severe dehydration after burns or viral illness also can cause RVT by inducing hypovolemia and hypoperfusion of the kidney. Children with nephrotic syndrome, particularly that caused by membranous glomerulonephritis, also are at risk but for different reasons. The loss of proteins in the urine, including antithrombin III, which is a potent anticoagulant, sets up a hypercoagulable state in the renal vein.

The prognosis for the kidney depends on the acuteness of the thrombosis and the response of its secondary venous outflow. On occlusion of its main renal vein, the left kidney is more resilient than the right since the adrenal, ureteral, gonadal, and lumbar veins vent the elevated renal vein pressure. On the contralateral side, these same veins drain into the vena cava, leaving the right kidney a relatively isolated organ. When the onset is acute, hemorrhagic infarction results from venous congestion and obstruction. Fortunately, RVT is usually unilateral and renal failure is rare, although some degree of uremia and acidosis is seen in most patients.

The classic presentation of RVT in the newborn is gross hematuria with a palpable mass. RVT accounts for 20% of neonatal hematuria. Red blood cells (RBCs), platelets, and fibrin are destroyed in the evolving clot, and thrombocytopenia, anemia, and increased fibrin split products are commonly seen.

Other findings at any age can include proteinuria, varicocele, pedal edema if the vena cava is involved, and pulmonary embolism. Ultrasonography is the diagnostic test of choice, and in the acute setting shows an enlarged kidney without hydronephrosis and distorted internal architecture. Doppler study and renal scintigraphy document significantly decreased blood flow. Excretory urography should be avoided since further dehydration can result from contrast load, and venography is rarely necessary to confirm the diagnosis.

Treatment is directed at correcting metabolic imbalances, azotemia, and dehydration. Prompt diagnosis and correction of these abnormalities is the key to limiting the progression of thrombosis and avoiding bilateral involvement. The prognosis in most cases of RVT is excellent, although the function of many of the kidneys is impaired, especially when thrombosis affects the right renal vein. The literature is scattered with reports of surgery for RVT. However, the place of surgery, for what is typically small vessel disease, is difficult to defend in the acute setting. Medical management and supportive treatment assume priority. When renovascular hypertension persists, a nephrectomy may become necessary. The use of anticoagulants such as heparin or thrombolytic therapy with agents such as streptokinase or urokinase remains controversial.

Renal Artery Thrombosis

Renal artery thrombosis (RAT) affects two distinct populations of children. The first and more common are neonates with umbilical artery catheters. Mechanical factors such as catheter tip location above the renal arteries and prolonged or traumatic placement are associated with an increased incidence of thrombosis, as is the use of hyperosmolar (ie, radiographic contrast) or sclerosing agents. Systemic conditions such as low perfusion states and sepsis also increase the tendency to thrombosis. Secondary embolization through a patent ductus arteriosus is another common etiology in newborns.

RAT is suspected in any neonate with hematuria and a recent umbilical artery catheterization or who has a heart murmur. Small cortical infarcts may not result in other symptoms, but larger ones can cause proteinuria, decreased renal function, leukocytosis, and fever. Hypertension can initiate congestive heart failure if the condition goes unrecognized. Ultrasonography may show a decrease in size of the affected kidneys, whereas high-resolution color Doppler study is gradually replacing umbilical artery angiography and radionuclide perfusion studies as the diagnostic study of choice.

Since hypertension and congestive failure are poorly tolerated by the neonate, supportive medical treatment must be aggressive and initiated promptly. This includes immediate removal of the offending catheter. Fortunately, most thromboses affect only one kidney and the outcome usually is good. Renal recovery is related to the extent of arterial compromise and the degree of intrarenal collateral circulation. Dialysis may be required if renal failure is present in the rare case of bilateral thromboses. Surgery or thrombolytic agents have been of equivocal value and are avoided for unilateral conditions. Nephrectomy is a last resort when medical management fails.

The second group affected by RAT are older children with preexisting conditions such as heart disease (particularly after cardiac catheterization) or fibromuscular dysplasia of the renal arteries. In addition, the pediatric kidney is particularly susceptible to vascular trauma with sudden deceleration because of its relative mobility. The resultant shear forces can raise intimal flaps that lead to thrombosis. Since hematuria may be absent, a high index of suspicion is important. Treatment is surgical, although renal viability depends on early recognition of the condition.

Arteriovenous Malformations

Renal arteriovenous (AV) malformations can be either congenital or acquired, with the latter accounting for about 75% of the cases. Trauma accounts for most and usually results in a solitary communication between a vein and artery. In contrast, congenital anomalies are tortuous vascular collections having multiple communications within the vascular supply. Symptoms depend on location and size. Most patients have an abdominal bruit, and large fistulas can cause cardiac failure or hypertension from progressive renal ischemia.

Management depends on clinical significance. Most AV malformations are asymptomatic and never come to attention. Others may be responsible for minute amounts of microscopic hematuria or sporadic bouts of gross hematuria. Vascular instability or posttraumatic massive blood loss warrant more immediate attention. If time allows, contrast angiography is the diagnostic test of choice. Embolization usually is effective, although partial or total nephrectomy sometimes is necessary.

HEMATURIA

Hematuria is a common problem, with 3% to 5% of children expected to have at least one episode in their lifetime.[8,9] Although hematuria can be the harbinger of a serious nephrologic or urologic problem, most work-ups yield negative results.

Etiology

There are over 100 causes of hematuria, most of which are medical in origin (Table 91-6). Two major designations based

TABLE 91-6. *Common causes of hematuria in childhood*

Mimics
  Porphyrins
  Beets, blackberries, red food dye
  Pyridium
Hematologic
  Coagulopathies
  Renal vein and artery thrombosis
  Sickle cell disease
Glomerular diseases
  Hemolytic-uremic syndrome
  IgA nephropathy
  Poststreptococcal glomerulonephritis
  Postinfectious nephritis
Stones and hypercalcuria
Anatomic abnormalities and tumors
Trauma
Exercise

on the morphologic features of RBCs can be assigned without reviewing the individual entities. *Glomerular hematuria* distorts cellular morphologic features and tends to be nephrologic in origin, whereas intact RBCs typically accompany *nonglomerular* etiologies. These are largely urologic and related to the collecting system and tubules. Common causes are listed in Table 91-6.

Glomerular Hematuria

Glomerular injury can result from immunologic, inherited, or coagulation disorders. Immunologic injury is the most common and results from the localization of circulating antibody–antigen immune complexes or interaction of antibody with in situ antigen. The process is called *glomerulonephritis* to typify the resulting inflammation of the glomerular capillaries. The pathologic manifestations range from transient proliferation of the glomerular endothelial and mesangial cells caused by immune complex and matrix accumulation, to full-blown fibrin deposition in Bowman's space (crescents) and glomerular sclerosis.

IgA Nephropathy (Berger Disease)

Berger disease is perhaps the most common nephrologic cause of pediatric hematuria. The disease usually presents with recurrent painless hematuria after exercise, respiratory virus, or fever. The bleeding typically resolves and has a favorable prognosis. Biopsy confirmation yields IgA deposits within the glomerular mesangium. Crescentic glomerular changes, later age at presentation, proteinuria, and hypertension are less favorable signs.

Poststreptococcal Glomerulonephritis

Poststreptococcal glomerulonephritis is extremely common and occurs 7 to 30 days after bouts of impetigo or acute pharyngitis caused by group A β-hemolytic *streptococci*. Tea-colored urine containing red cell casts and heavy proteinuria is found. Malaise, hypertension, and edema from hypoalbuminemia also may be present. Antistreptolysin O titers often are nonspecifically elevated, whereas a depressed complement (C3) is more indicative of an active or recent infection. A complete recovery is expected in more than 95% of case with supportive treatment alone.

Hemolytic-Uremic Syndrome

The hemolytic-uremic syndrome is composed of the triad of renal failure, hemolytic anemia, and thrombocytopenia; is believed to be autoimmune in origin; and usually follows a prodrome of intestinal flu-like illness in young children. This is the single most common cause of hematuria among young children. Dialysis may be required to treat the resultant renal failure, although many patients fully recover.

Nonglomerular Hematuria

Tubulointerstitial Disorders

Patients with tubulointerstitial disorders, including the infantile PKD and MCDs discussed earlier, occasionally present with hematuria. Congenital abnormalities of tubular uptake or excretion, including renal tubular acidosis (type 1), cystinuria, and oxalosis, also can be implicated. Acquired tubular disorders have numerous causes that include nephrotoxic agents (aminoglycosides, penicillin derivatives, cimetidine, lithium, and cyclosporine), radiation nephritis, infections, or immune rejection in transplanted kidneys. Nonsteroidal antiinflammatory agents are a particular problem in this regard and cause hematuria in one third of patients who abuse this medication. The term *interstitial nephritis* refers to inflammation between the glomeruli in the areas surrounding the tubules. The pathogenesis remains poorly understood, although hypersensitivity and an immune response may initiate the inflammatory changes seen. In addition to hematuria, proteinuria and urinary concentration defects result.

Hypercalcuria

Hypercalcuria is an increasingly detected cause of microscopic hematuria. The site of bleeding remains undefined. Patients affected with the disorder may be prone to urolithiasis in later life, which is included in the differential diagnosis.

Vascular Causes

Vascular causes include sickle cell disease, RVT, RAT, and AV malformations (see earlier). Patients with bleeding disorders and coagulopathies also are prone to bleed into the urinary tract.

Urinary Tract Infection

Urinary tract infection is the most common urologic cause of hematuria (see later).

Other Common Causes

Other causes of nonglomerular hematuria include tumors, trauma, vesicoureteral reflux nephropathy, and upper urinary tract obstruction with hydronephrosis. Lower tract anomalies include urethral valves, polyps, stricture, prolapse, and meatal stenosis. Another cause is *urethrorrhagia*, a nonspecific inflammation of the bulbar urethra that causes prepubertal boys to spot in their underwear. Culture results are negative, and the condition is uniformly self-limited.

Evaluation

Gross hematuria often suggests a urologic cause and demands further evaluation, although ''pseudohematuria'' from urinary pigments and other causes of bloody diapers should be ruled out. Some RBCs are expected in normal urine as the body rids

TABLE 91-7. *Evaluation of hematuria*

INITIAL SCREENING TESTS
Urinalysis
CBC
BUN/Cr/electrolytes

SECONDARY TESTS
ASO
C3
Urine C & S

OTHER TESTS
ANA
Sickle cell Prep

DIAGNOSTIC STUDIES
Urinary Ultrasound (with rare exception)
Voiding cystourethrogram (only with UTIs)
Cystoscopy (only with persistent bleeding that cannot be explained)

CBC, complete blood cell counts; BUN, blood urea nitrogen; Cr, creatinine; ASO, antistreptolysin O; C & S, culture and sensitivity; ANA, antinuclear antibody; Prep, preparation; UTIs, urinary tract infections.

itself of more than 2 million corpuscles each day. Orthotolidine dipsticks are especially sensitive to the presence of hemoglobin and myoglobin and detect this obligate loss. Positive dipstick results require quantification. More than five RBCs per high-power field in two or three samples warrants further evaluation. Tea-colored urine or microscopic hematuria usually implicate a nephrologic cause. Concomitant proteinuria or cellular casts are more worrisome findings that suggest renal disease. Urinary tumors, the most common cause of hematuria in adults, are uncommon in children. As a result, the diagnostic approach differs markedly in children, where cystoscopy is rarely indicated (Fig. 91-18 and Table 91-7).

A thorough history and physical examination are performed in every child and may aid in the diagnosis. Otherwise, the microscopic and dip-stick analysis of the urine is the cornerstone of the evaluation. Additional laboratory and radiographic testing is directed at differentiating the few serious entities from the remainder, which have no long-term sequelae. Although some variability exists, a urine culture, blood urea nitrogen, creatinine, streptozyme (antistreptozyme O titer), serum complement, and serum protein studies are usually obtained. A spot calcium–creatinine ratio also is used to rule out hypercalcuria, with a ratio of greater than .20 deserving further quantification with a 24-hour urine collection. Other tests that might be obtained, depending on the clinical impression, include a 24-hour clearance of creatinine and protein and complete blood count to evaluate anemia. Nephrologic consultation is helpful in tailoring further evaluation.

Ultrasonography is the best screen of the urinary tract at the least cost and with no invasiveness. The bladder, in addition to the kidneys, should be evaluated. This study result is normal in most instances of uncomplicated hematuria. When the screening result is abnormal, other studies (eg, CT, voiding cystourethrography, renal scintigraphy) become necessary. Pathologic diagnosis can be instrumental to directing therapy of some disease processes, and renal biopsies are used to evaluate persistent hematuria, associated significant proteinuria, or decreasing renal function that occur in the absence of a known cause.

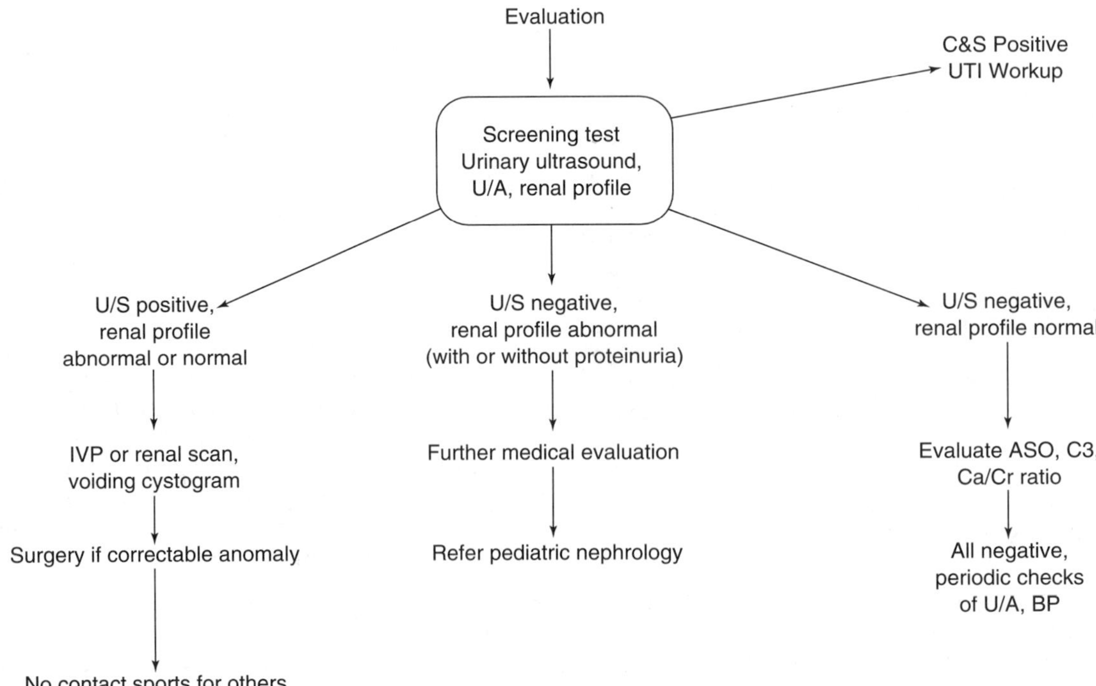

FIG. 91-18. Algorithm for evaluation of hematuria in children. U/A, urinalysis; U/S, ultrasound; IVP, intravenous pyelogram; C&S, culture and sensitivity; UTI, urinary tract infection; ASO, antistreptolysin O; C3, third component of complement; Ca/Cr, calcium/creatinine.

PROTEINURIA

Small amounts (up to 150 mg/24 hours) of protein may be found in the urine of healthy children. Dipsticks are sensitive for albumin but may miss lower weight proteins, including Bence Jones protein and γ-globulins. As a consequence, persistent proteinuria should be quantified with a timed urine collection.

Etiology

Nonpathologic proteinuria usually is serendipitously found incidentally. The most common cause is postural, generally considered a benign condition. The diagnosis is established by finding normal protein excretion in a supine urine collection but increased protein excretion while upright. Other benign causes include fever in excess of 38.3°C and exercise. *Pathologic proteinuria* can be caused by either tubular or glomerular diseases. Glomerulonephritis is the most common and usually is nonselective in its protein loss. The loss of larger proteins such as albumin and IgG typically results in edema. In contrast, tubular causes tend to be more specific, since the proximal tubules reabsorb the bulk of lower weight proteins (ie, light chain immunoglobulins, lysozymes) that are normally filtered by the glomerulus.

Nephrotic Syndrome (Nephrosis)

The most serious form of proteinuria manifests as the nephrotic syndrome, characterized by the appearance of edema, proteinuria, hypoproteinemia, and hyperlipidemia.[10] Most cases are idiopathic and are accompanied by minimal changes in the glomeruli. The remaining cases are attributed to some form of glomerulonephritis. The loss of albumin can cause a decrease in plasma oncotic pressure, which allows fluids to transudate to the interstitial space. The reduced intravascular volume stimulates the renin–angiostensin–aldosterone system, which enhances sodium and water reabsorption, further amplifying water movement to the interstitium. Edema appears when serum albumin levels fall below 2.5 g/dL and protein losses generally exceed 2 g/24 hours. Lipid elevations result from increased liver synthesis in the face of hypoproteinemia and diminished levels of lipoprotein lipase, which normally clears lipid from the plasma.

The diagnosis of nephrotic syndrome is made on the basis of the 24-hour urine collection and evaluation of serum albumin, cholesterol, and triglyceride levels. Most idiopathic disease responds to steroids. Renal biopsy is indicated in patients who do not respond and older children, who more commonly have glomerulonephritis. In addition to steroids and sodium restriction, diuretics, intravenous albumin, antihypertensive agents, and cyclophosphamide occasionally are necessary for fulminant cases or those that continue to cause serious relapses. Fortunately, most children respond to steroids and have no residual renal dysfunction, although recurrent episodes are common until the second decade of life.

URINARY TRACT INFECTION

Clinical Presentation

Most patients with a UTI have symptoms that suggest a specific diagnosis. In contrast, symptoms of newborns are typically nonspecific. Failure to thrive and lethargy are worrisome findings, whereas high fevers are uncommon. Infants and younger children arrive with the more classic signs of fever, malodorous urine, dysuria, urinary frequency, lethargy, and gastrointestinal symptoms including nausea and vomiting. Pyelonephritis usually causes vague abdominal discomfort rather than localized flank pain. Even without infection, children with vesicoureteral reflux, the most common cause of UTIs, may describe abdominal or flank discomfort. When reflux has gone undetected and renal scarring has occurred from significant infection, children can arrive at any age with renal insufficiency, hypertension, and impaired somatic growth.

A urinalysis should be included in the evaluation of any patient who presents with fever or malaise. Unfortunately, urinary infections often are overlooked, and their ill-defined presentations are mistakenly attributed to otitis media, viral gastroenteritis, respiratory infections, or fever of undetermined origin. Until a proper diagnosis is made, severe renal damage continues, especially if reflux is present. If fever is present, the likelihood of having vesicoureteral reflux or some other anatomic abnormality (and presumably, pyelonephritis) is greatly increased. Lower tract infections alone (eg, cystitis) rarely cause serious systemic complaints or symptoms.

Verification

When a UTI is suspected from the clinical history, a culture becomes essential to making the diagnosis. Microscopic study alone might not provide a valid assessment of the urine, although the combined used of dipsticks increases sensitivity. The method of urinary collection also is extremely important. In toilet-trained children, a midstream-voided urine specimen is adequate. The first portion of urine, which contains the bulk of bacterial contaminant of the periurethral region, is omitted. Any growth greater than 100,000 colonies per high-powered field per milliliter of urine (CFU/mL) is significant for a midstream specimen. Catheterization also is an excellent way of obtaining a urine sample with minimal contamination. Bacterial counts greater than 1000 CFU/mL from a catheterized specimen are considered to be significant. Finally, suprapubic aspiration is equally efficient but can be challenging in children older than 1 year of age. Many become anxious and void during the maneuver, making collection difficult. In addition, needle trauma can cause microscopic hematuria, which can cloud the diagnostic picture. When the bladder is not extremely full, ultrasonic guidance is helpful. Any growth from a suprapubic aspiration warrants further evaluation. An adhesive bag urine specimen, although commonly performed, is the least reliable method of collection. It carries a high risk of contamination and probably should be considered suboptimal in the symptomatic patient. About 10% of samples yield growths of greater than 50,000 CFU/mL. Most have no correlation whatsoever with actual urinary infection. Pure

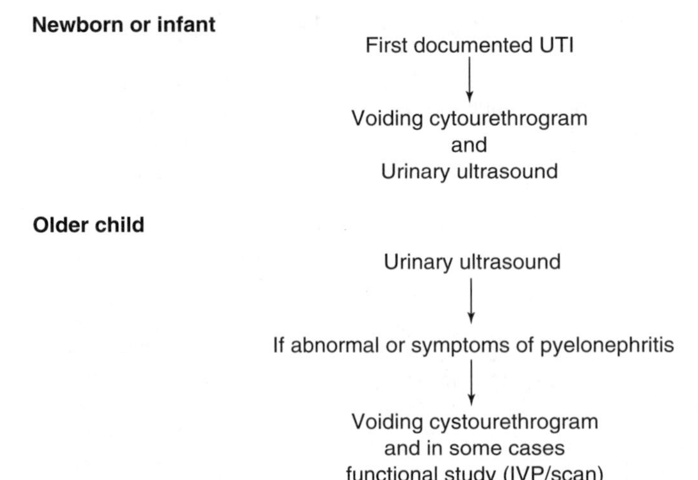

FIG. 91-19. Algorithm for evaluation of urinary tract infection in children.

growths of more than 100,000 CFU/mL have more validity but still can be false-positive because of contamination.

Evaluation

Any study suggests that most (80% to 95%) children who have one UTI are highly likely to have another. As a consequence, it seems reasonable to rule out an anatomic abnormality as early as possible in children who are susceptible to infections. When no anatomic anomaly is present, the tendency to infections usually is related to retentive urinary behavior and improper toilet hygiene. However, the diagnostic yield is significant. For example, vesicoureteral reflux is found in 29% to 50% of children with UTI. About 30% of these patients already have some evidence of renal parenchymal scarring. Unfortunately, there are no reliable clinical features of their infections that distinguish children with reflux or other anatomic abnormalities from those without. Even in the absence of fever, renal scarring can occur after only a single UTI. This type of data amplify the need for a thorough evaluation of any child believed to have a urinary infection.

The evaluation of a child thought to have reflux is tailored to the individual according to the age, gender, and clinical history.[11,12] Any child younger than 5 years of age with a valid, clearly documented UTI should be evaluated for reflux. Children with a UTI and fever, regardless of age, also should be evaluated. In addition, boys of any age with a UTI should be assessed radiographically for the presence of reflux, unless they are sexually active or have a history of urologic disease. An algorithm for evaluation is shown in Figure 91-19. Although this can be tailored somewhat for age and symptom complex, the combination of a voiding cystourethrogram and ultrasonography provides the best screen. In most cases, invasive studies such as a voiding cystourethrogram should be postponed until the urine culture result is negative. Functional studies (IVP,

renal scintigraphy) also occasionally become necessary, depending on the ultrasonic findings.

Treatment

Treatment is directed at the offending organism based on culture and sensitivity results. Infections should be treated for 7 to 10 days regardless of severity, especially since the distinction between upper and lower tract infections sometimes is difficult to make. Studies show that the incidence and severity of renal scarring can be decreased by prompt identification and treatment of pyelonephritis. Radiographic evaluation usually is deferred until the acute phases of the infection have waned. Treatment of the individual entities that might be associated with UTIs is discussed elsewhere in this text.

REFERENCES

1. Guerriero WG. Etiology, classification and management of renal trauma. Surg Clin North Am 1989;68:1071.
2. Arger PH, Coleman BG, Mintz MC, et al. Routine fetal genitourinary tract screening. Radiology 1986;156:485.
3. Larsen WJ. Development of the urogenital system. In: Larsen WH, ed. Human embryology. New York, Churchill Livingstone, 1993:235.
4. Cook WA, Stephens FD. Fused kidneys: morphologic study and theory of embryogenesis. Birth Defects 1977;13:327.
5. Anderson GA, Degroot D, Lawson RK. Polycystic renal disease. Urology 1993;42:358.
6. Wacksman J, Phipps L. Report of the multicystic kidney registry: preliminary findings. J Urol 1993;150:1870.
7. Keating MA, Althausen AF. The clinical spectrum of renal vein thrombosis. J Urol 1985;133:938.
8. Schroeder PL, Francisco LL. Evaluating hematuria in children. Postgrad Med 1990;88:171.
9. Bergstein J. Nephrology. In: Berman RE, ed. Nelson's textbook of pediatrics, ed 15. Philadelphia, WB Saunders, 1996:1480.
10. Rapola J. Congenital nephrotic syndrome. Pediatr Nephrol 1987;1:441.
11. Lebowitz RL. The detection and characterization of vesicoureteral reflux in the child. J Urol 1992;148:1640.
12. Sheldon CA, Gonzalez R. Differentiation of upper and lower urinary tract infections: how and when? Med Clin North Am 1984;68:321.

Surgery of Infants and Children: Scientific Principles and Practice, edited by
Keith T. Oldham, Paul M. Colombani, and Robert P. Foglia.
Lippincott–Raven Publishers, Philadelphia, © 1997.

CHAPTER 92

Collecting System

Jacob Ben-Chaim, John P. Gearhart, and Craig A. Peters

92.1   Upper Urinary Tract

Jacob Ben-Chaim, John P. Gearhart

EMBRYOLOGIC DEVELOPMENT OF THE UPPER URINARY TRACT

The ureter begins development in the end of the fourth week of embryonic life. The ureteric bud originates from the mesonephric (wolffian) duct at the point where the mesonephric duct bends sharply ventrally (Fig. 92-1). If two buds arise close to the normal point of ureteral origin from the mesonephric duct, a complete ureteral duplication results (Fig. 92-2).

As the differentiation of the kidney take place, the ureteral bud grows rapidly and penetrates the metanephric blastema to produce the entire collecting system: ureter, renal pelvis, major and minor calyces, papillary ducts, and collecting ducts. The segment of mesonephric duct from the site of origin of the ureter to the primitive cloaca is known as the *common excretory duct*. By the eighth week of development, the common excretory duct is absorbed into the portion of the cloaca that will become the urogenital sinus, so the ureter and mesonephric duct are separated. The ureteral orifice migrates cephalad and laterally, while the mesonephric duct moves distally and medially. The mesonephric duct enters the posterior urethra at the verumontanum and becomes the epididymis, vas deferens, seminal vesical, and ejaculatory duct. The ureteral bud and the mesonephric duct achieve their final positions by the 12th week of development.[1]

At 4 weeks of development, the ureter is patent in its entire length, but in the 6th week of development, the ureteral lumen obliterates, with gradual reopening of the ureteral lumen caudally and cranially from the middle of the ureter (Fig. 92-3). The lumina at the ureteropelvic junction (UPJ) and ureterovesical junction (UVJ) are the last to become patent again, which may explain why these are common sites for congenital strictures.[2] Muscle begins to appear in the ureter by the end of the 12th week; by 14 weeks, there is transitional epithelium; and at 18 weeks, the ureter shows the normal intrinsic narrowing at the UPJ, pelvic brim, and UVJ.[3]

ANATOMY AND PHYSIOLOGY OF THE URETER

The ureteral musculature is divided into an inner longitudinal layer and an outer layer of spiral smooth muscle fibers (the intravesical ureter has only the longitudinal muscle fibers). These longitudinal fibers of the ureter are in continuity with muscle fibers of the superficial trigone. The entire urinary tract is covered by transitional cell epithelium. Beneath this epithelium is a layer of connective tissue, the lamina propria, which, together with the epithelium, forms the mucosa. The ureter receives blood supply from multiple branches along its course in the retroperitoneum (Fig. 92-4). After reaching the ureter, the arterial branches course longitudinally within the periureteral adventitia in an extensive anastomosing plexus. This structure allows long segments of ureter to be safely mobilized from the surrounding tissues, provided the adventitia is not stripped. The venous and lymphatic drainage of the ureter generally parallel the arterial supply. The ureters are closely adherent to the psoas posteriorly and the colon anteriorly. Thus, both ureters may be endangered during surgical procedures of these organs. Inflammatory or malignant processes of these structures may also affect the ipsilateral ureter and cause hematuria, fistula, or obstruction. The ureter can be divided to three segments: the *upper ureter* extends from the renal pelvis to the upper border of the sacrum; the *middle ureter* then extends to the lower border of the sacrum, which roughly corresponds with the iliac vessels; and the *lower ureter* extends from the sacrum to the bladder. The ureter receives preganglionic sympathetic input from the T-10 to L-2 spinal segments. Postganglionic fibers arise from several ganglia in the aorticorenal, superior, and inferior hypogastric plexuses. Parasympathetic input is received from S-2 to

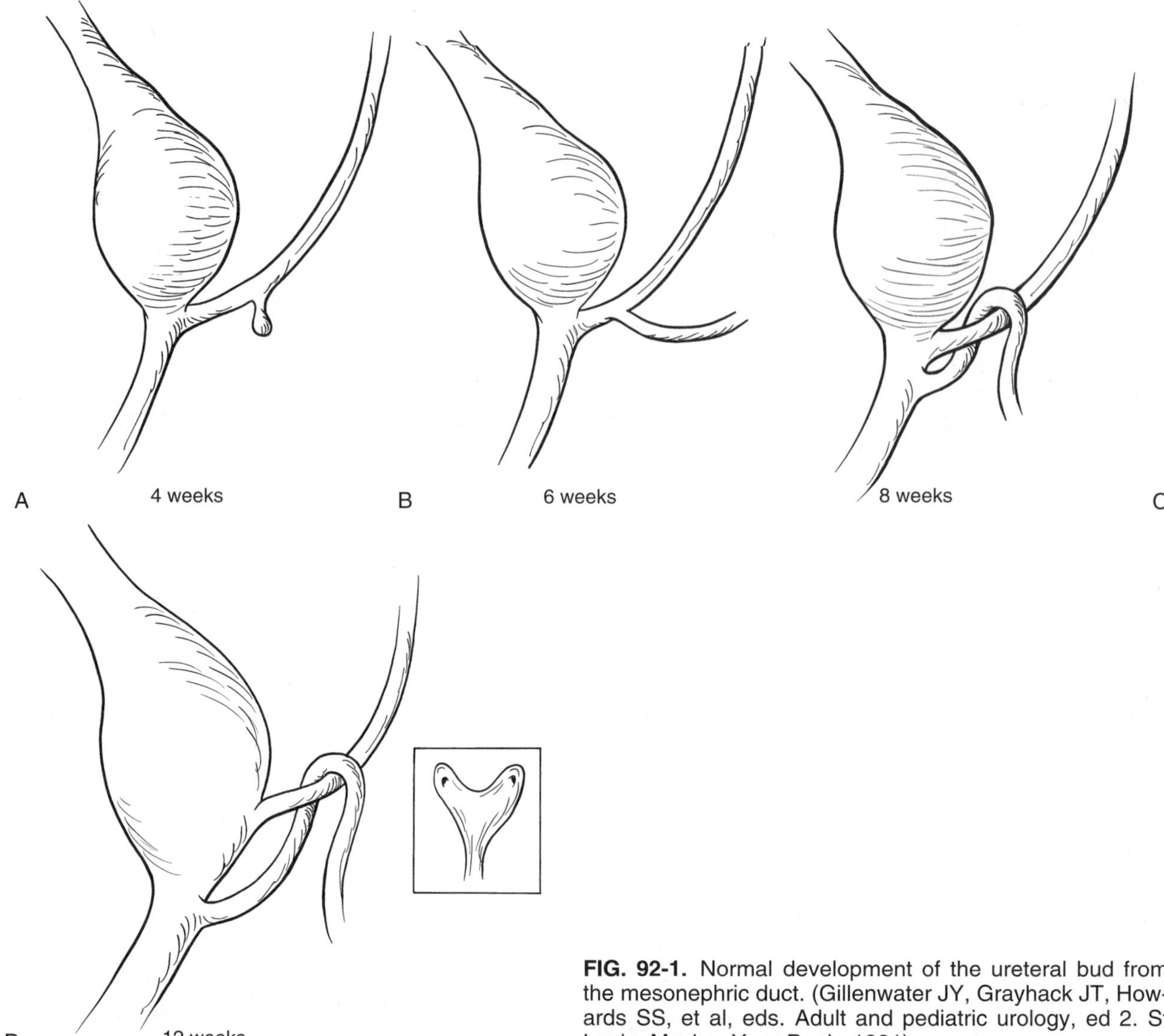

FIG. 92-1. Normal development of the ureteral bud from the mesonephric duct. (Gillenwater JY, Grayhack JT, Howards SS, et al, eds. Adult and pediatric urology, ed 2. St Louis, Mosby–Year Book, 1991)

S-4 spinal segments. Pain fibers are stimulated by nociceptors sensitive to distention of the ureter and to direct mucosal irritation. The resulting visceral pain is felt directly and is referred to somatic distributions that correspond to the spinal segments providing the sympathetic distribution to the ureter. Pain may therefore extend from the ipsilateral flank through the lower lateral quadrant of the abdomen to the groin and hemiscrotum or major labia.[4,5]

The ureter is a muscular conduit that contracts in response to stretch to transport the bolus of urine into the bladder. Normally, ureteral peristalsis originates with electrical activity at the pacemaker. The pacemaker fibers are different in that their transmembrane resting potential does not remain constant but rather undergoes a slow spontaneous depolarization and action potential[6] (Fig. 92-5). The action potential propagates distally along the smooth muscle fibers of the ureter and gives rise to the mechanical event of peristalsis. The pacemaker of ureteral peristalsis is located in the border of the minor calyces and major calyx, but other areas of the ureter may act as latent pacemakers.[7,8] Ureteral peristalsis persists after denervation or transplan-

tation; thus, the ureteral peristalsis can occur without innervation. The nervous system plays a modulating role in ureteral peristalsis by affecting both peristaltic frequency and bolus volume.[9] α-Adrenergic (excitatory) and β-adrenergic (inhibitory) receptors and muscarinic cholinergic receptors have been demonstrated in the ureter.[10–12]

Efficient propulsion of the urinary bolus is dependent on the ability of the ureter to coapt its walls completely (Fig. 92-6). The resting ureteral pressure is 0 to 5 cm H_2O; during ureteral contraction, the pressure ranges from 20 to 80 cm H_2O and occurs two to six times per minute. With increasing urine flow, initially the ureter responds by increasing peristaltic frequency. When the maximum frequency is reached, further increase in urine transport occurs by means of increased bolus volume. If the flow rate continues to increase, several boluses coalesce, the ureteral walls do not coapt and dilate, and a continuous column of fluid is transported rather than a series of boluses, as occurs in perfusion studies (eg, Whitaker test).[13,14] Normally, ureteral contraction pressure exceeds intravesical pressure so that the bolus of fluid passes across the UVJ into the bladder.

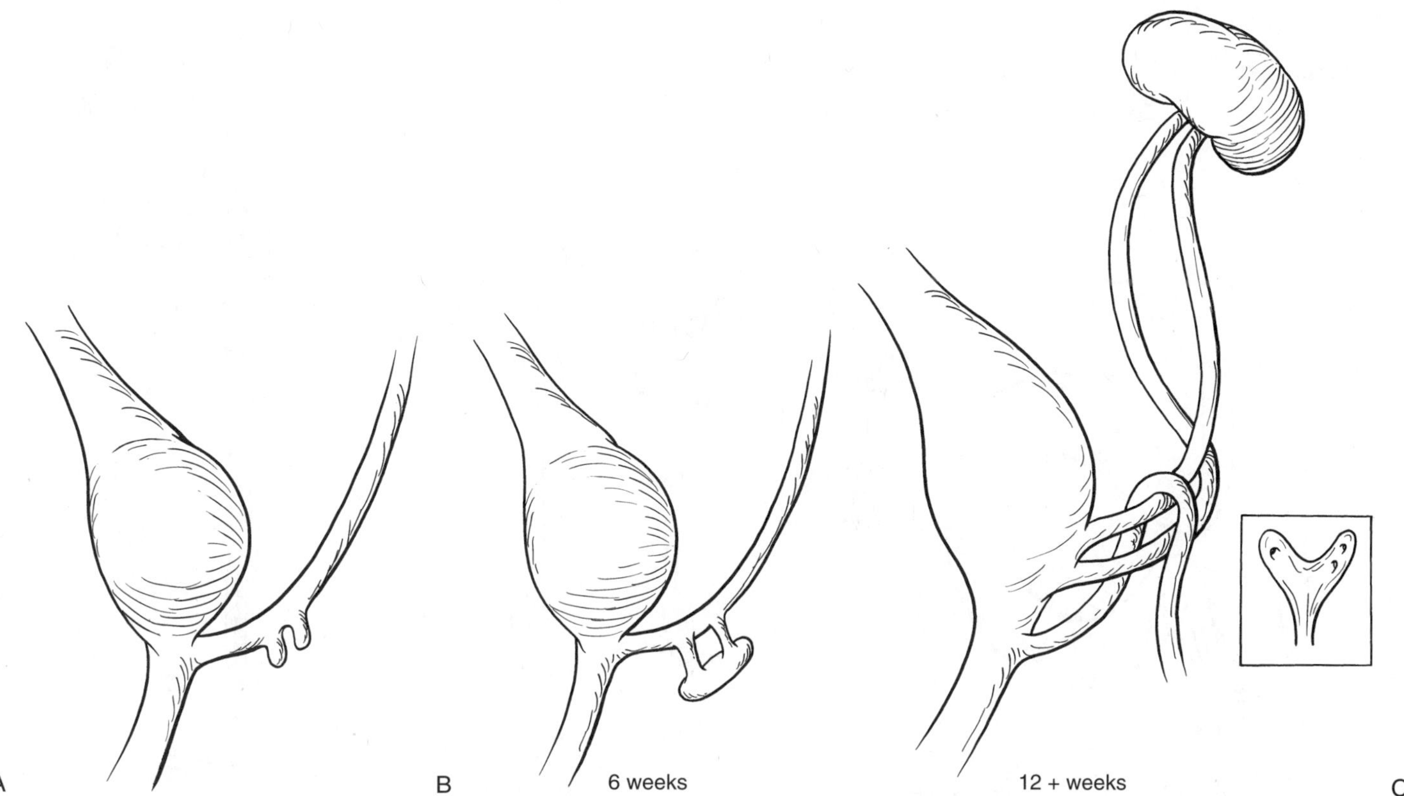

FIG. 92-2. Two ureteral buds at the normal site on the mesonephric duct, leading to complete duplication of the ureter without pathologic sequelae. (Gillenwater JY, Grayhack JT, Howards SS, et al, eds. Adult and pediatric urology, ed 2. St Louis, Mosby–Year Book, 1991)

OBSTRUCTIVE UROPATHY

Pathophysiology

Obstructive uropathy is a common urologic problem. Complete ureteral obstruction eventually destroys kidney function. Chronic partial bilateral ureteral obstruction results in impairment of all measured renal function except urinary dilution, especially in children. Impairment of urinary concentrating ability is one of the first signs of renal damage due to hydronephrosis. Impairment of urinary acidification, including bicarbonate absorption, titratable acidity, and ammonia excretion, was also found secondary to hydronephrosis. The glomerulus and the proximal tubule are the last to show damage from obstructive uropathy on histologic examination. Significant chronic hydronephrosis impairs renal blood flow and glomerular filtration rate (GFR) and usually is detected by elevation of serum creatinine concentration levels.[15,16]

After acute unilateral ureteral obstruction, there is a triphasic relation between renal blood flow and ureteral pressure (Fig. 92-7). The ureteral pressure declines gradually to a level slightly higher than the normal ureteral pressure and then remains stable. The proposed mechanism is glomerular vasoconstriction.

Chronic ureteral obstruction causes an increase in ureteral length and diameter that is manifested clinically by ureteral dilation and tortuousity. The effect of obstruction on ureteral function is dependent on the degree and duration of the obstruction, on the rate of urine flow, on the presence of infection, and on the age of the patient. The neonatal ureter may undergo a greater degree of deformation and dilation in response to obstruction than does the adult ureter.[17]

When there is high resistance to ureteral flow due either to obstruction or an elevation in intravesical pressure, the pressure in the bolus must increase, the contraction can longer occlude some of the ureteral lumen, and some degree of urine backflow occurs.[18] When the resistance to flow is significant enough, the intraureteral pressure increases, the contraction waves become smaller, the ureter dilates, and urine transport becomes dependent on the hydrostatic forces generated by the kidney.[19] The ureteral length and diameter increase as the obstruction persists. The ureteral pressure is relatively low secondary to reabsorption of urine into the venous and lymphatic systems and to a decrease in ureteral wall tension.[20] Obstruction that lasts longer than 2 weeks usually results in irreversible damage to ureter and kidney function.[21]

Prenatal Diagnosis

Maternal–fetal ultrasonography done as part of a routine gestational examination may reveal prenatal congenital obstructive uropathy. The overall incidence of genitourinary defects diagnosed on routine ultrasound screening is between 0.2% and 0.9%. The fetal kidneys can be detected after about 15 weeks' gestation, but the images are not clear until about 20 weeks' gestation. The calyces and collecting system are rarely seen in detail in the absence of some fullness. The fetal bladder may

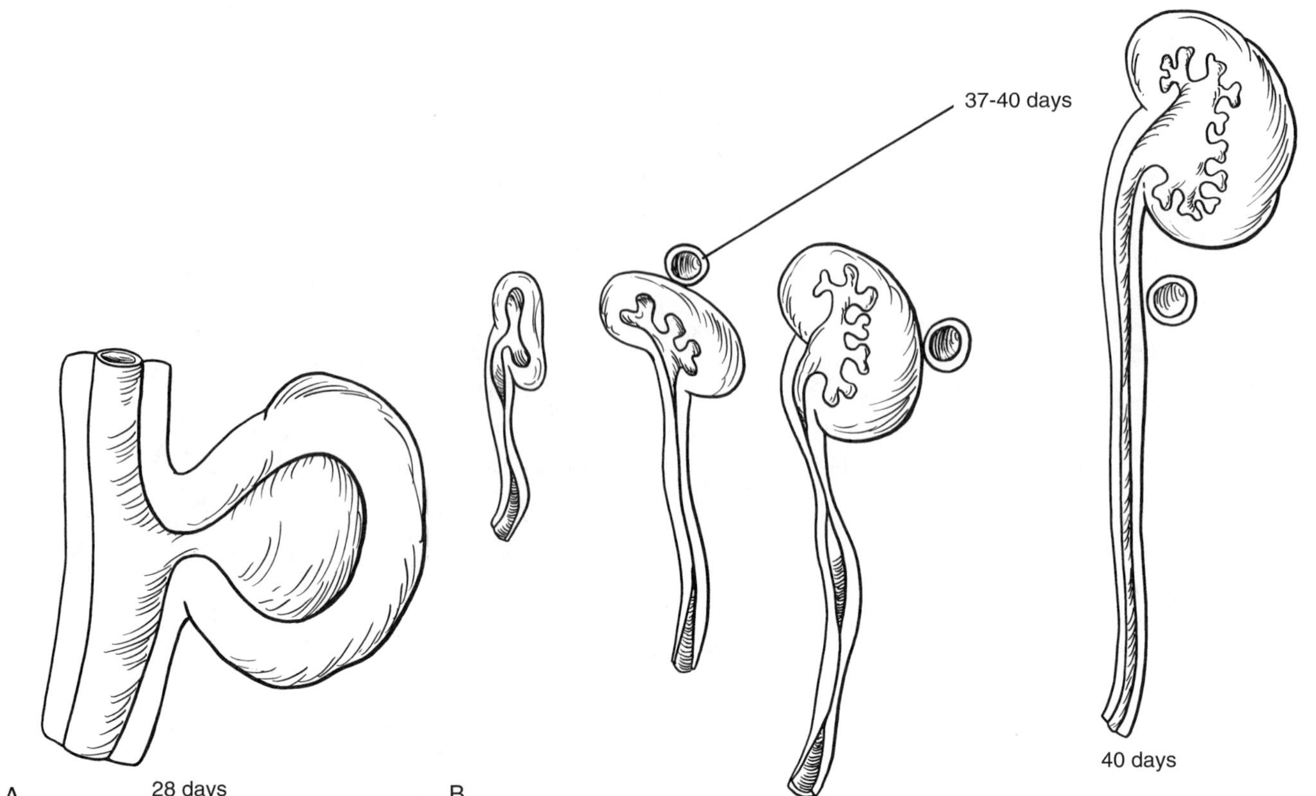

FIG. 92-3. Early development of the ureter. At 28 days' gestation, the ureteral bud appears from the mesonephric duct. Between 37 and 40 days, the lumen of the ureter is first progressively lost, beginning at its mid-portion, then becomes apparent again, beginning at its mid-portion; after 40 days, it is apparent throughout its length. UA, umbilical artery. (Walsh PC, Retik AB, Stamey TA, et al, eds. Campbell's urology, ed 6. Philadelphia, WB Saunders, 1992)

also be detected about the same time as the kidney and can be seen to empty and fill over time. Bladder volume is 4 to 5 mL, and typically the fetus voids hourly. If the bladder is not seen over time, an abnormality should be suspected.[22] Since the amniotic fluid volume after 16 weeks' gestation reflects mainly contribution from fetal urine, evaluation of the amniotic fluid is part of the routine evaluation of the fetal genitourinary system. Severe oligohydramniosis usually reflected the absence of any single area of fluid measuring at least 2 cm on ultrasound[23] (Fig. 92-8). During the prenatal ultrasonography, the degree of hydronephrosis may be assessed subjectively (mild, moderate, severe) or, preferably, by accurate measurements of anteroposterior diameter of the pelvis, and correlated with the age of gestation.[24] It should also be determined whether the hydronephrosis is unilateral or bilateral, symmetric or asymmetric. The quality of renal parenchyma should be estimated (based on cystic changes or hyperechogenicity). The presence or absence of ureteral dilation must be noted. Bladder size, wall thickness, emptying, and the absence or presence of posterior urethral dilation should also be noted. The volume of amniotic fluid and extrarenal fluid collections, the overall growth and development, and the gender of the fetus should also be determined. The most common cause of significant hydronephrosis in utero is UPJ obstruction; this should be suspected in a fetus of more than 20 weeks' gestation with a renal pelvic diameter of more than 10 mm. If caliectasis is present, hydronephrosis should be

considered with a smaller pelvic diameter (Fig. 92-9). In the most severe cases, varying degrees of cystic dysplasia can be seen.

Ureteral dilation in association with pelvic dilation is the next most frequent abnormality seen with hydronephrosis. In the presence of a normal bladder, this finding most often represents either vesicoureteral reflux or UVJ obstruction (Fig. 92-10). The distinction between these conditions prenatally is difficult. If the bladder is dilated, however, the differential diagnosis includes either bladder outlet obstruction (posterior urethral valves) or massive reflux with megacystis–megaureter syndrome.[25,26]

Duplication anomalies should be suspected in the presence of an asymmetric nondilated portion of the kidney. Usually, the ultrasound findings are nonspecific, and the accurate diagnosis is determined postnatally after the prenatal finding of hydronephrosis.[27] A multicystic dysplastic kidney is characterized by multiple cysts of various sizes and shapes without evidence of communication with the collecting system (in contrast to hydronephrosis). Unlike UPJ obstruction, in which the renal pelvis is usually significantly more dilated than the calices, in multicystic kidney, there is not a large, dominant cyst (Fig. 92-11); rather, there is spectrum that ranges from the large multicystic dysplastic kidney to the smaller hypodysplastic kidney, which is more difficult to distinguish antenatally. Available data suggest that prenatal renal ultrasound is sensitive in detecting

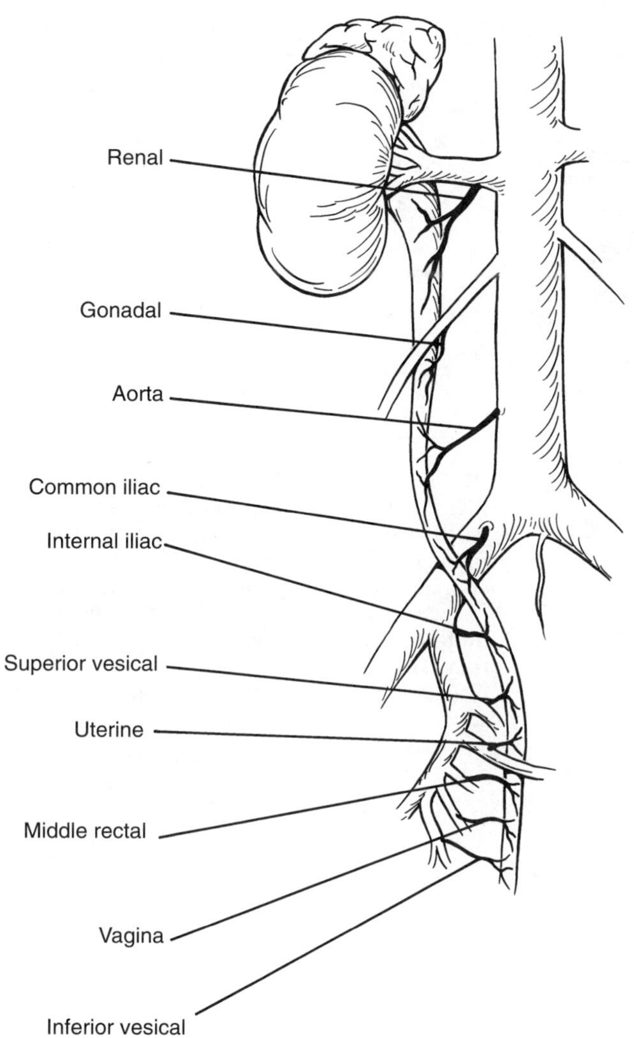

FIG. 92-4. The arterial blood supply of the ureter. (Walsh PC, Retik AB, Stamey TA, et al, eds. Campbell's urology, ed 6. Philadelphia, WB Saunders, 1992)

abnormalities but fails to provide a specific diagnosis in 15% to 70% of cases.[28]

Prenatal Intervention

When a severe bilateral obstructive uropathy is diagnosed prenatally, there are several options for intervention:

- Elective abortion before fetal viability
- Early delivery if the gestational age of the fetus ensures viability; the lecithin/sphingomyelin ratio determines whether steroid supplementation before delivery is needed to enhanced fetal lung maturation
- Percutaneous or open shunting if the gestational stage is before the period of viability
- Needle aspiration of a large cystic mass or severe urinary ascites for therapeutic decompression to prevent dystocia, or for diagnosis
- Needle aspiration of a dilated bladder or hydronephrotic kidney for assessment of fetal renal function

The indications for prenatal intervention are controversial because it is not yet known whether after relief of the obstruction, the amniotic fluid returns to allow lung development or whether the renal impairment is reversible. Furthermore, prenatal intervention carries significant risks to both the mother and fetus. The reported complications include chorioamnionitis, premature delivery, and fetal bowel herniation. Additional risk factors are associated with open hysterotomy, so that percutaneous shunting usually is preferred.[29,30]

Postnatal Diagnosis and Management

A child in whom hydronephrosis was diagnosed on prenatal ultrasound should be started on a course of low-dose prophylactic antibiotics following birth. If bladder outlet obstruction is suspected on prenatal ultrasound, postnatal evaluation with ultrasound examination and voiding cystourethrogram is performed within the first 24 hours. If posterior urethral valves are confirmed, then bladder drainage with urethral catheter and early surgical therapy are performed. Usually, the ultrasound examination should be done after 4 to 5 days of life because neonatal oliguria can mask mild to moderate obstructive lesions. If the neonatal ultrasound did not find the hydronephrosis that was diagnosed prenatally, renal ultrasound should be repeated after 1 month.[31] If hydronephrosis is confirmed on the postnatal ultrasound, voiding cystourethrogram is performed. In the newborn, the ability to concentrate urine and the GFR are relatively

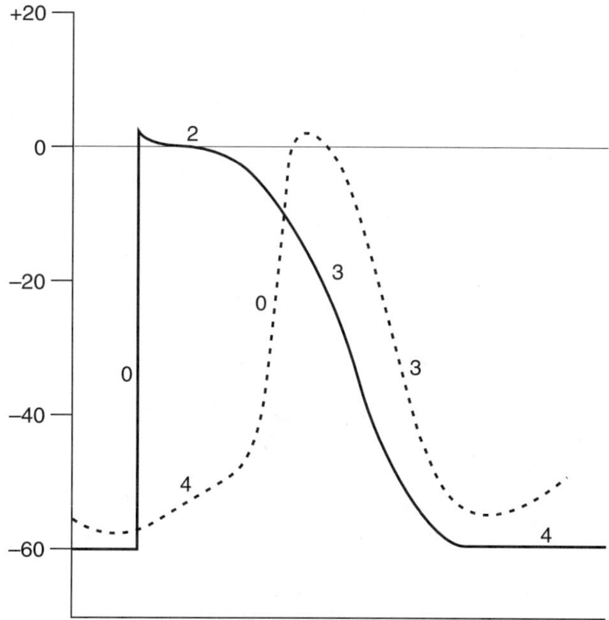

FIG. 92-5. Schematic representation of pacemaker (*dashed line*) and nonpacemaker (*solid line*) action potentials in the ureter: (0) upstroke or depolarization phase, (2) plateau phase, (3) repolarization phase, and (4) resting potential of nonpacemaker cell and spontaneous depolarization phase of pacemaker cell. Spontaneous decrease in transmembrane potential of pacemaker cell accounts for its spontaneous activity. (Walsh PC, Retik AB, Stamey TA, et al, eds. Campbell's urology, ed 6. Philadelphia, WB Saunders, 1992)

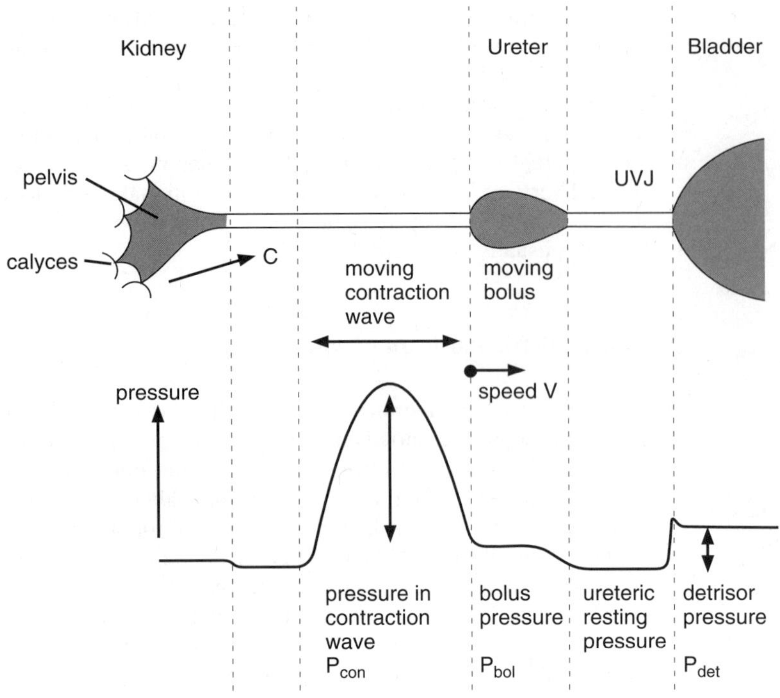

FIG. 92-6. Schematic representation of a single bolus in the ureter moving away from the renal pelvis and toward the bladder. Corresponding distribution of pressure within the urinary tract is shown in the lower tracing. UVJ, ureterovesical joint. (Walsh PC, Retik AB, Stamey TA, et al, eds. Campbell's urology, ed 6. Philadelphia, WB Saunders, 1992)

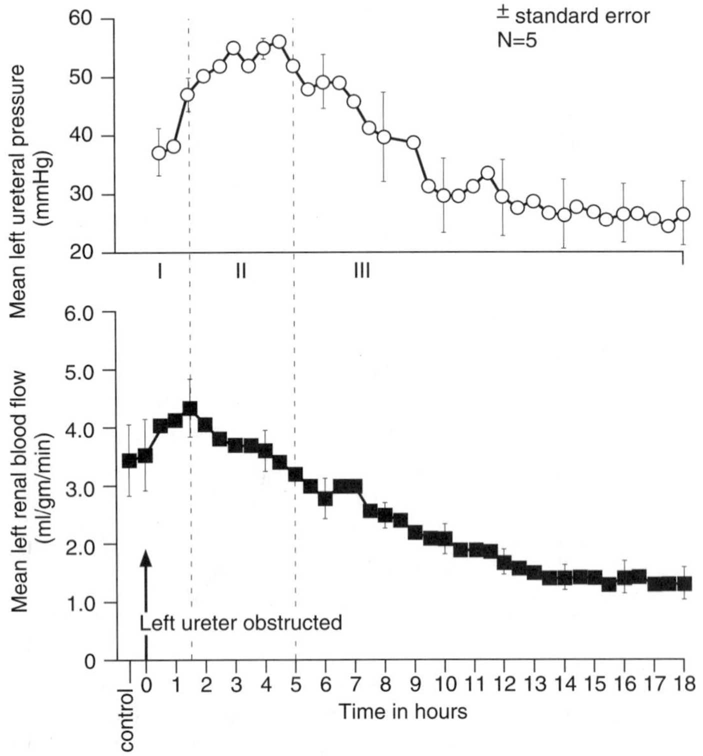

FIG. 92-7. Triphasic relation between ipsilateral renal blood flow and left ureteral pressure during 18 hours of left ureteral occlusion. The three phases are designated by roman numerals and are divided by vertical dashed lines. In phase I, the left renal blood flow and ureteral pressure increase together. In phase II, the left renal blood flow begins to decline, while the ureteral pressure continues to rise. Phase III shows the left renal blood flow and ureteral pressure declining together. (Walsh PC, Retik AB, Stamey TA, et al, eds. Campbell's urology, ed 6. Philadelphia, WB Saunders, 1992)

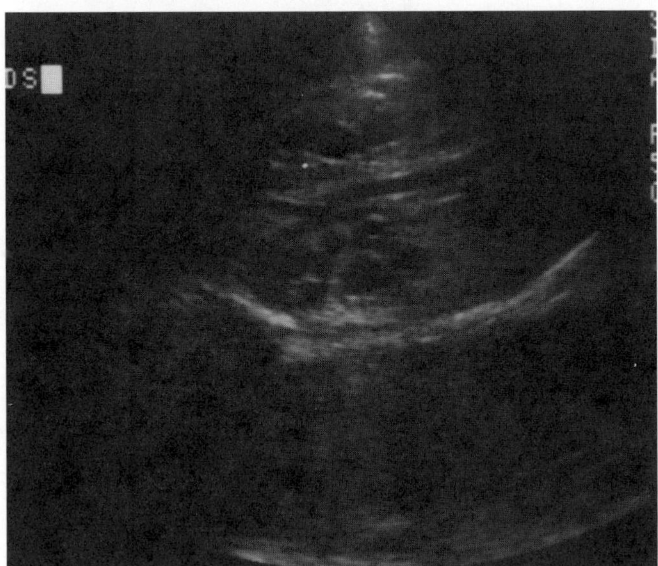

FIG. 92-8. Severe oligohydramnios and bilateral hydrone-phrosis on prenatal ultrasound, secondary to posterior ure-thral valves.

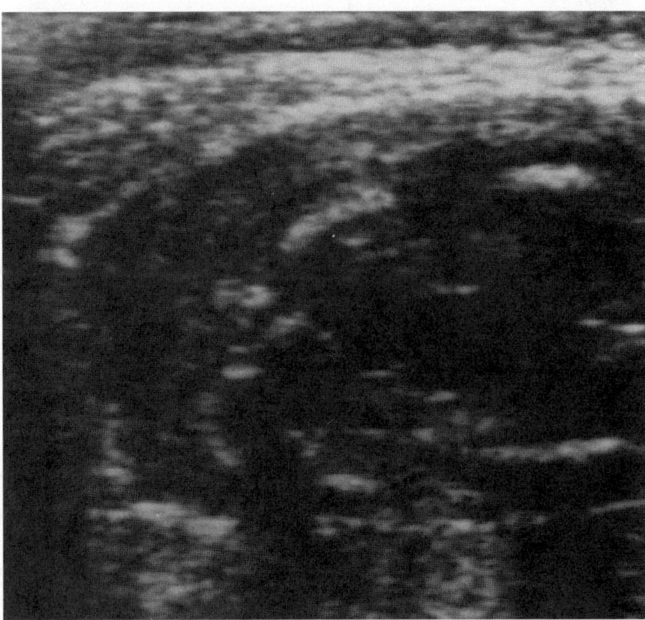

FIG. 92-10. Ureterovesicle junction obstruction due to ectopic ureterocele on prenatal ultrasound at 24 weeks gestation.

low; therefore, the diuretic renal scan and intravenous urography usually are performed at 4 to 6 weeks (Fig. 92-12).

Ultrasonography

Ultrasound usually is done without sedation. The newborn is examined in the supine position, and the kidneys are studied. The neonatal kidney ranges from 3.3 to 5 cm in length, 2 to 3 cm in width, and 1.5 to 2.5 cm in diameter[32] (Fig. 92-13). Attention is then focused on the bladder; supine longitudinal scans of the pelvis are performed to determine bladder volume,

wall thickness, and extravesical or intravesical masses and to follow the course of dilated ureters and posterior urethra, if present. Although ultrasound is the least invasive method of evaluating and following infants with hydronephrosis, other studies, such as voiding cystourethrogram (VCUG), renal scan and, intravenous pyelogram (IVP) are also necessary to establish the accurate diagnosis.

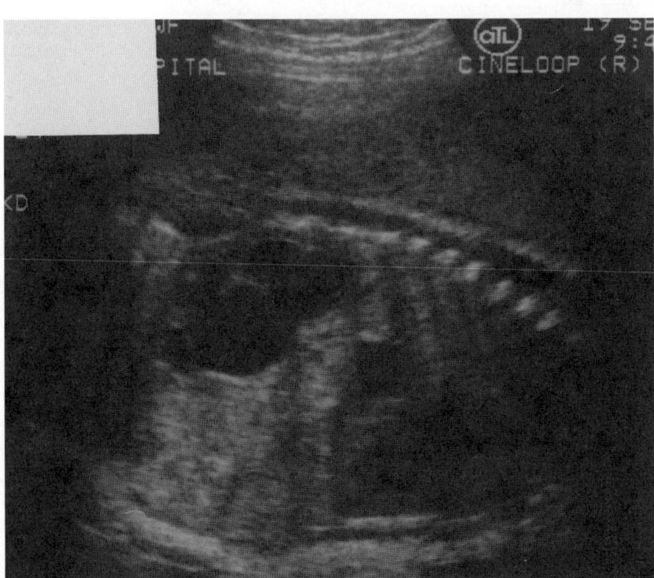

FIG. 92-9. Left hydronephrosis due to ureteropelvic junction obstruction at 35 weeks' gestation on prenatal ultrasound.

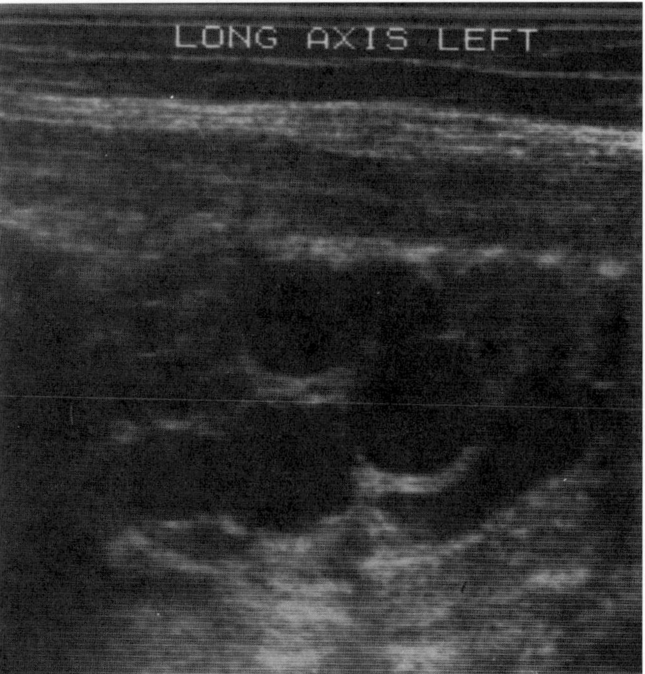

FIG. 92-11. Multicystic dysplastic kidney on prenatal ultra-sound. Multiple cysts are apparent, without evidence of communication with the collecting system.

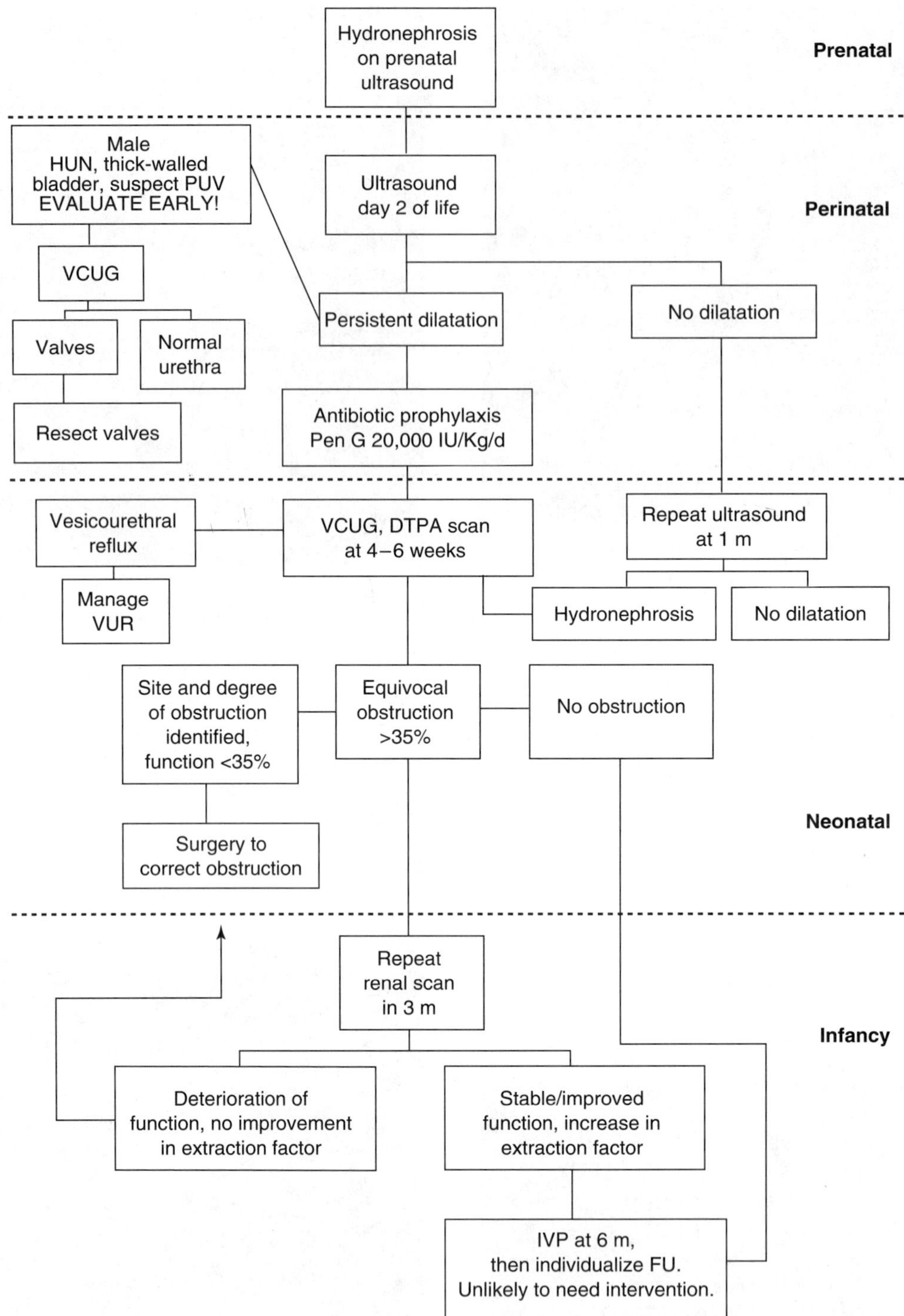

FIG. 92-12. Algorithm for neonatal evaluation of unilateral or mild bilateral hydronephrosis. HUN, hydroureteronephrosis; VCUG, voiding cystourethrogram; VUR, vesicoureteral reflux; PUV, posterior urethral valves; FU, follow-up; interven, intervention. (After Blyth B, Snyder HM, Duckett JW. Antenatal diagnosis and subsequent management of hydronephrosis. J Urol 1993;149:693)

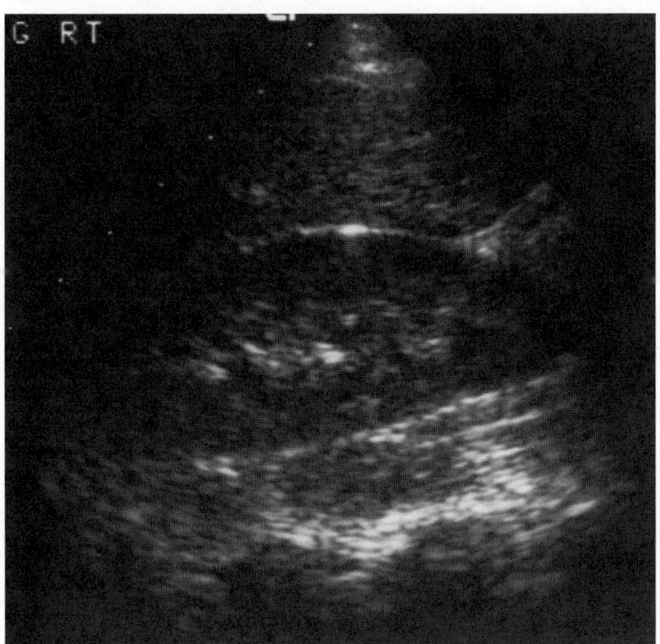

FIG. 92-13. Normal kidney on ultrasound.

Voiding Cystourethrography

A VCUG is performed in newborns through a 5F feeding tube that is inserted into the bladder. Usually, a 15% solution of opaque medium is gradually instilled into the bladder from a drip chamber about 60 to 80 cm above the pubic symphysis until bladder capacity is reached. Capacity is reached when the child become uncomfortable and restless, or when bladder and infusion pressure become equal, and flow ceases or reverses. Normally, the bladder capacity of newborns is 30 to 50 mL. Radiographs are taken with the patient in the supine position and using the right and left lateral oblique projections. Once the catheter is removed, the child starts to void, and films of the urethra filled with contrast material are made (Fig. 92-14). VCUG provides valuable information about the lower urinary tract and usually demonstrates the presence of vesicoureteral reflux, bladder diverticula, bladder capacity, residual volume, trabeculations of the bladder wall, ureterocele, and the site and nature of bladder outlet obstruction.

Intravenous Pyelography

An IVP provides good anatomic and functional information on the upper urinary tract. It has traditionally been used to evaluate hydronephrosis, but it has significant limitations in neonates because gaseous intestinal distention limits the detail of the radiologic images, which are even further impaired in children with poorly functioning or extremely dilated kidneys (Fig. 92-15). Moreover, at birth, renal function is too immature for satisfactory visualization of the collecting system, so an IVP should be done 2 weeks beyond term. In general, 2 to 3 mL/ kg of contrast material is administered, and scout films, 1-minute films, and 10-minute films are obtained. Delayed films may be necessary to visualize a dilated renal pelvis or ureter. Reflux

into a nonfunctioning kidney may cause spurious function, which may be easily prevented by performing the IVP with a catheter draining the bladder. Advances in nuclear imaging have reduced the application of IVP in infants and children.

Nuclear Imaging Studies

Radionuclide studies of the kidneys may be used to assess renal perfusion, glomerular function of each kidney, structural anomalies, and the presence or absence of obstruction.

Technetium-99m diethylenetriaminepentaacetic acid (^{99m}Tc-DTPA) is the primary agent used for determining glomerular function and for diuresis renography. ^{99m}Tc-DTPA is excreted almost exclusively (95%) by glomerular filtration, without significant tubular excretion or retention in the renal parenchyma. Thus, its rate of clearance from the blood is an accurate measure of GFR.

The child is placed supine and restrained for this study, and should be well hydrated because relative dehydration prolongs parenchymal transit time and delays urinary excretion. Bladder catheterization during the study is mandatory to keep intravesical pressure low. ^{99m}Tc-DTPA is injected intravenously as a bolus, and images of the kidneys are obtained each minute. Normally, the parenchyma is well visualized during the first minute; by 2 to 3 minutes, activity is seen in the collecting system; and by 6 to 9 minutes, the bladder is visualized. Calculation of the differential renal function of each kidney is performed 60 to 180 seconds after the injection of ^{99m}Tc-DTPA; this represents parenchymal transit. On computer images, re-

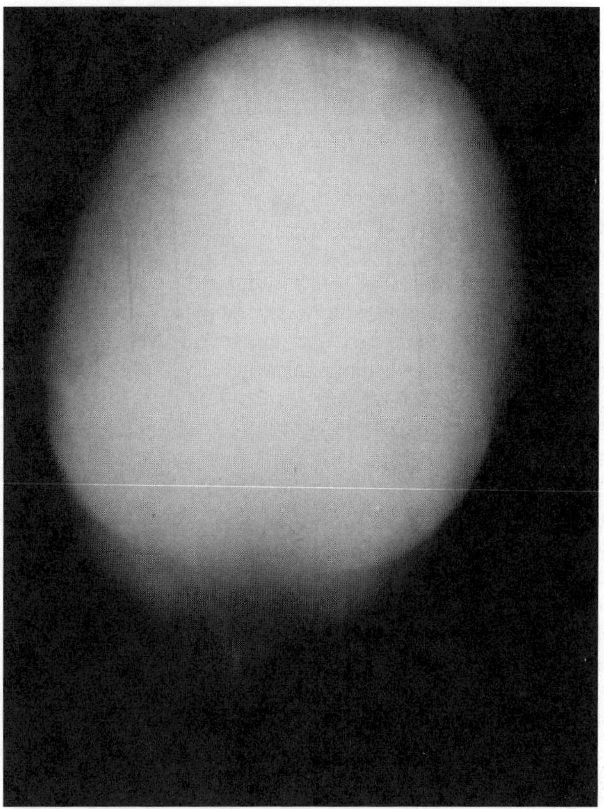

FIG. 92-14. Normal voiding cystourethrogram.

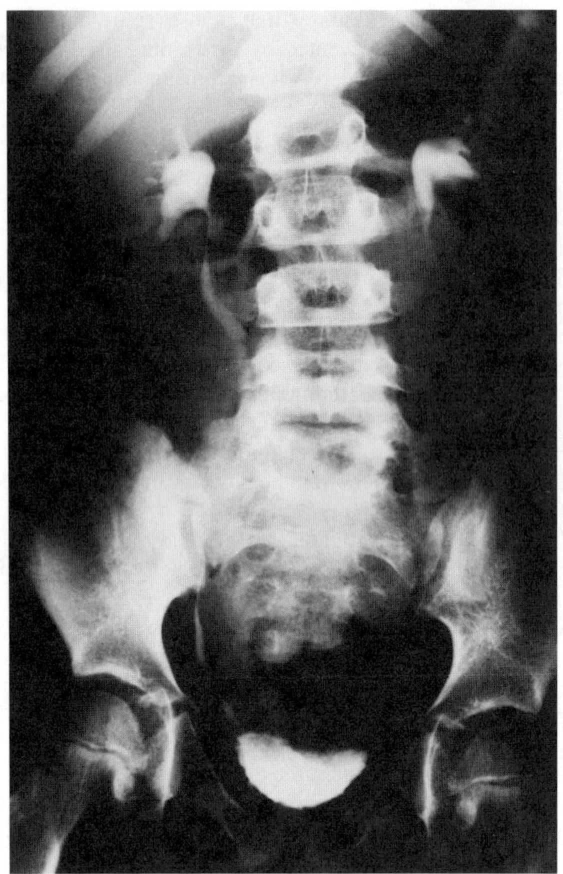

FIG. 92-15. Normal intravenous pyelogram in infant.

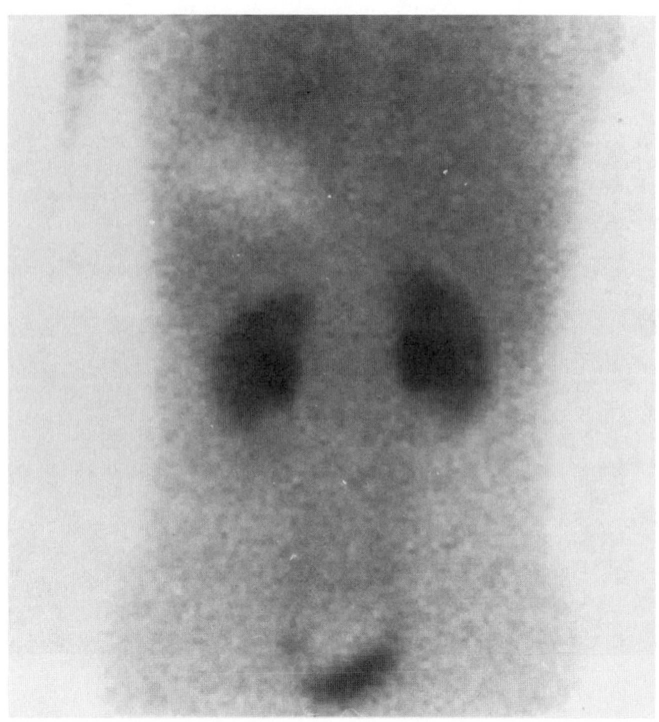

FIG. 92-16. Normal DTPA renal scan.

gions of interest can be selected from each kidney, and background activity is subtracted. The differential activity within each kidney is used to compute differential renal function (Fig. 92-16). In case of duplex a system, in which there is upper pole obstruction, the regions of interest of the affected kidney may be broken down to determine relative function of the upper and lower segments.

A diuretic ^{99m}Tc-DTPA renal scan may be done to determine whether significant obstruction is present. For this test, 1 mg/kg of furosemide is administered intravenously when the hydronephrotic system shows maximal accumulation of radionuclide, but no later than 30 to 60 minutes after ^{99m}Tc-DTPA injection. If the ureter contains a large amount of radionuclide, UVJ obstruction should be suspected before furosemide is given. After administration of furosemide, the activity over each kidney is measured, and the half-time clearance is determined. (*Half-time* represents the number of minutes required for half of the radiopharmaceutical to drain from the collecting system after administration.) A nonobstructed system should have a half-time of less than 10 to 15 minutes; a half-time of greater than 20 minutes suggests obstruction. If the half-time is 15 to 20 minutes, the results are indeterminate, and other studies may be necessary (Fig. 92-17). If the collecting system does not fill completely within 1 hour after injection of ^{99m}Tc-DTPA, or if the kidney has less than 20% of total renal function, the diuretic washout curve may be prolonged, even if the system is not obstructed.[33] In normal newborns, the drainage and the half-time typically

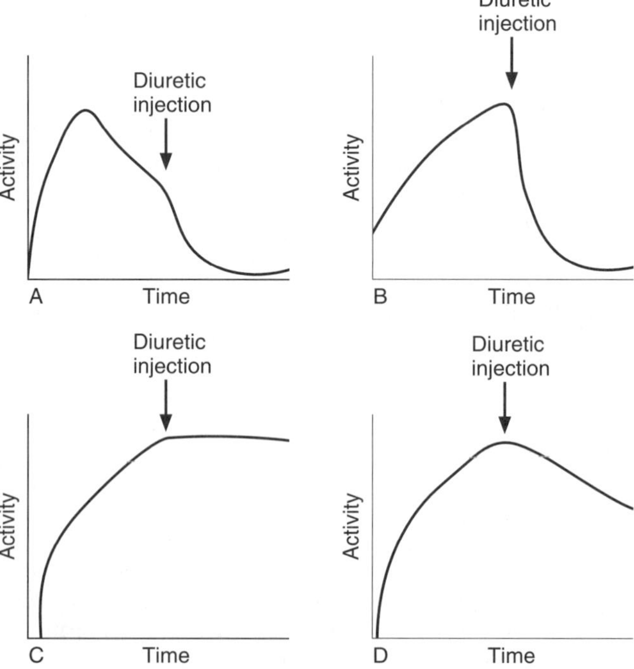

FIG. 92-17. Patterns of response to furosemide in diuretic DTPA renal scan. (*A*) Normal response. (*B*) Dilated nonobstructed system. (*C*) Dilated obstructed collecting system. (*D*) Equivocal response. (Kelalis PP, King LR, Belman AB, eds. Clinical pediatric urology, ed 3. Philadelphia, WB Saunders, 1992)

are delayed compared with drainage in older children, primarily because the GFR is low. Therefore, this study usually should be performed after the child is 4 to 6 weeks of age, when a reasonable GFR is reached.

Another agent that can be used for renal scan is technetium-99m dimercaptosuccinic acid (^{99m}Tc-DMSA), which is tightly bound to the renal tubular cells, with only a small amount is excreted in the urine. ^{99m}Tc-DMSA allows excellent visualization of the renal parenchyma without interference from pelvocalyceal activity and therefore is recommended for detection of cortical lesions, such as acute pyelonephritis, chronic pyelonephritic cortical scars, infarcts, and tumors. Relative renal function can be determined because the ^{99m}Tc-DMSA uptake by each kidney is an accurate measure of relative functioning tubular mass that is well correlated with relative GFR.

Whitaker Test

The Whitaker test, which is a perfusion pressure study, is another way to evaluate the hydronephrotic kidney and usually is performed when other diagnostic tests, such as ultrasound, IVP, and diuresis renography, either do not agree or are inconclusive in establishing the diagnosis. In this test, sterile fluid is infused into the kidney at a constant rate, and the differential increase in the kidney pressure, compared with the pressure in the bladder, is measured (Fig. 92-18). This test is much more invasive than the diagnostic studies mentioned previously because it requires insertion of a needle or small nephrostomy tube into the kidney, with the patient under general anesthesia.

The study is initiated by infusing saline via nephrostomy 5 mL/min for 5 to 10 minutes and checking the renal pressure with manometer or pressure transducer every 5 minutes. If the pressure remains within the physiologic range, the inflow is increased to 10 mL/min for another 5 to 10 minutes. The study also includes performing antegrade pyeloureterography by infusion of contrast medium under fluoroscopy. A measured renal pressure of less than 15 cm H_2O indicates absence of obstruction, pressure greater than 22 cm H_2O is indicative of significant obstruction, and pressure between 15 and 22 cm H_2O is considered indeterminate.[34]

URETEROPELVIC JUNCTION OBSTRUCTION

Hydronephrosis secondary to congenital UPJ obstruction is one of the more common anomalies seen in childhood. Most cases are diagnosed on prenatal ultrasonography. Hydronephrosis accounts for 80% of the dilations of the collecting system in fetuses. The incidence of UPJ obstruction is about 1 in 1000. The male/female ratio exceeds 2:1, and in neonates, more than two thirds occur on the left side. Bilateral UPJ obstruction is present in 10% to 15% of cases, and contralateral anomalies, such as multicystic dysplastic kidney and renal agenesis, are relatively common.[35] UVJ obstruction, a duplicated system, horseshoe kidney, or ectopic kidney may also occur. The causes of UPJ obstruction are classified as intrinsic, extrinsic, and secondary. Intrinsic lesions within the ureteropelvic wall may cause obstruction. Interruption in the development of the circular vasculature and an excessive amount of collagen fibers between muscle cells in the UPJ have been demonstrated.[36] Less common causes of intrinsic UPJ obstruction include congenital valvular mucosal folds, persistent fetal convolutions, and upper ureteral polyps. Extrinsic UPJ obstruction is most commonly caused by aberrant, accessory, or early branching vessels to the lower pole of the kidney that pass anteriorly to the UPJ or upper ureter. Because freeing the involved vessel does not always relieve the obstruction, it is not clear whether the vessel exacer-

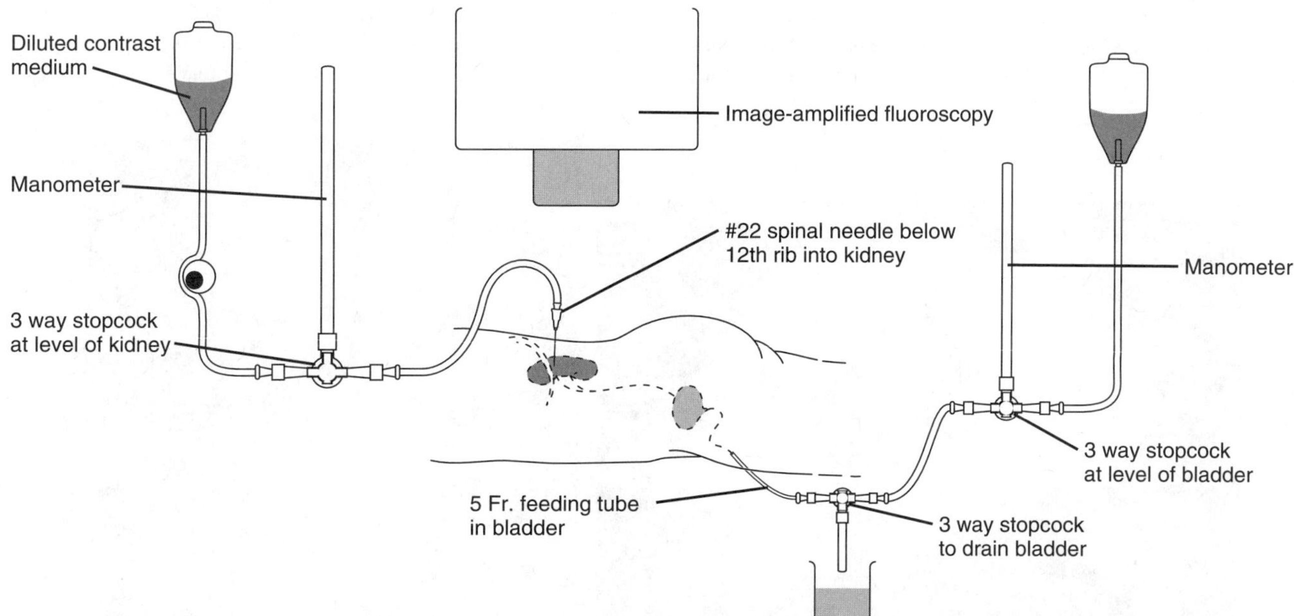

FIG. 92-18. Schematic diagram of antegrade pyelography with pressure–perfusion study (Whitaker test). (Walsh PC, Retik AB, Stamey TA, et al, eds. Campbell's urology, ed 6. Philadelphia, WB Saunders, 1992)

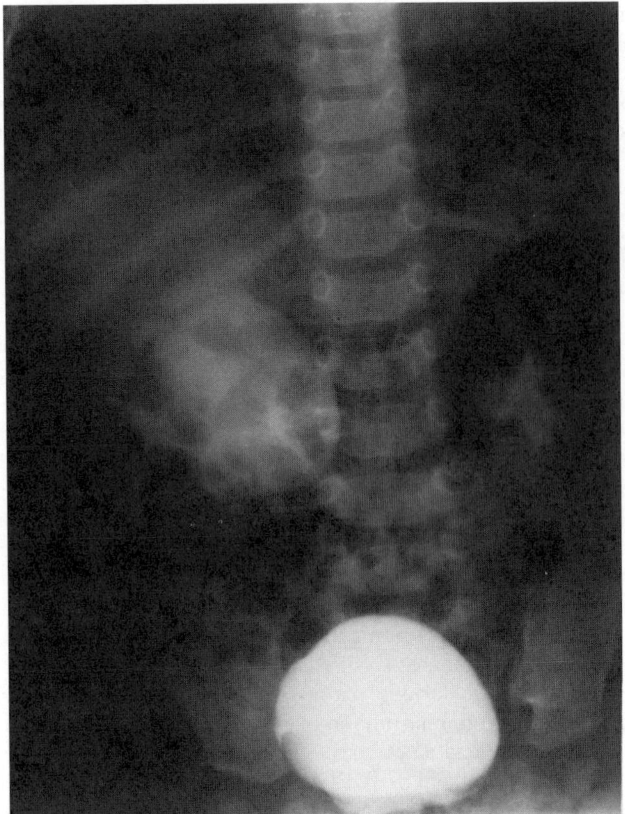

FIG. 92-19. Intravenous pyelogram of an infant with right ureteropelvic junction obstruction.

bates a preexisting intrinsic lesion or causes the intrinsic lesion. Differentiation between intrinsic and extrinsic lesions may be suspected on IVP, but the diagnosis usually is established in the exploration before repair (Figs. 92-19 and 92-20). UPJ obstruction may also be due to severe vesicoureteral reflux and kinking of the UPJ, which coexist in 10% of cases.[37] Most cases of UPJ obstruction present in early infancy as an asymptomatic flank or abdominal mass. Occasionally, schoolage and teenage children experience urinary tract symptoms, and UPJ obstruction is diagnosed.[38]

Whenever the diagnosis of prenatal hydronephrosis is suspected on prenatal ultrasound examination, it must be confirmed by a postnatal examination. Most cases of hydronephrosis detected prenatally resolve either before the end of pregnancy or by 1 year of age.[24] Once the diagnosis of hydronephrosis is confirmed by ultrasonography, evaluation should be completed by VCUG, diuretic ^{99m}Tc-DTPA renal scan, and IVP, as discussed previously. If UPJ obstruction secondary to massive reflux is diagnosed, the secondary obstruction in most cases resolves with correction of the reflux alone. If UPJ obstruction and mild reflux coexist, surgery to repair both anomalies must not be performed at the same time because simultaneous mobilization of the upper and distal ureter risks the ureteral blood supply. Therefore, pyeloplasty and ureteral reimplantation should be separated by an interval of 3 to 6 months when done sequentially. The most common differential diagnoses of hydronephrosis are physiologic hydronephrosis, UPJ obstruction, multicystic kidney, congenital obstructed and nonobstructed megaureter, ectopic ureter, ureterocele, vesicoureteral reflux, prune belly syndrome, posterior urethral valves, and megacalycosis.

Controversy exists whether to perform pyeloplasty soon after birth to prevent further obstructive damage to the developing renal function of the newborn, or to follow the newborn closely and perform the surgical repair when the patient shows deterioration in renal function. Several reports advocate early postnatal reconstruction of UPJ obstruction, showing significant increases in the differential function on ^{99m}Tc-DTPA scan of the involved kidney.[39,40] On the other hand, there is evidence that with prophylactic antibiotics and close follow-up, kidneys with differential function greater than 35% to 40% (normal is 50%) have shown spontaneous improvement. Only 23% of these patients required a pyeloplasty owing to deteriorating differential renal function, urinary tract infection (UTI), or pain. When the renal pelvis diameter of the newborn was less than 12 mm, none of the children required surgical intervention.[41] Cartwright

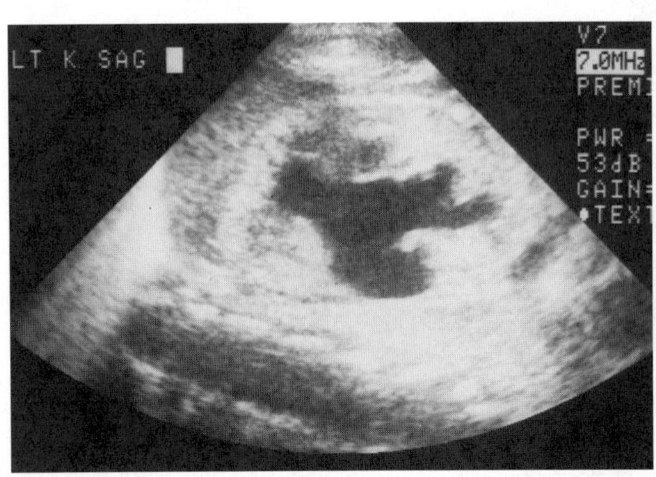

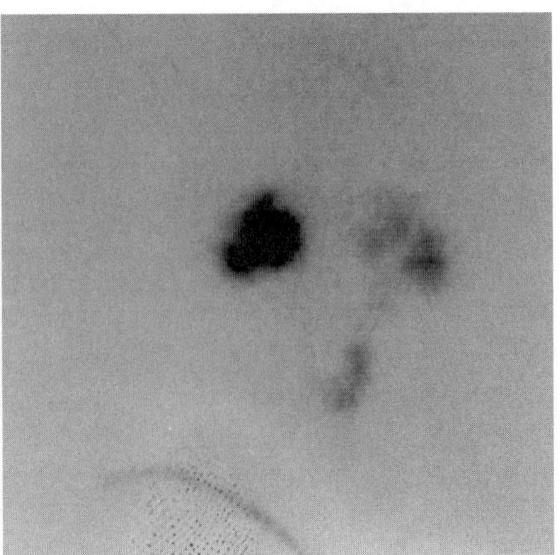

A   B

FIG. 92-20. (*A*) Ultrasound of left hydronephrotic kidney due to ureteropelvic junction obstruction. (*B*) Tc-DTPA renal scan of left ureteropelvic junction obstruction.

and colleagues[42] followed 35 infants with apparent UPJ obstruction. When the initial differential function was greater than 35%, only 6 patients required pyeloplasty, owing to decreasing function in 4 patients, recurrent UTIs in 1 patient, and renal colic symptoms in 1 patient. Koff and Campbell[43] found that many newborn kidneys with severe hydronephrosis were not obstructed despite profound initial decreases in renal function. Therefore, they suggest that diuretic renograms are inaccurate in neonates. The washout curve is influenced by hydration, renal function, volume contractility, compliance of the renal pelvis, and timing of administration of the diuretic. The authors' approach is to perform early pyeloplasty in patients in whom significant obstruction is clearly demonstrated on diuretic ^{99m}Tc-DTPA scan and to follow the other patients.

Open pyeloplasty is the conventional way to repair UPJ obstruction. The most common method of UPJ repair is the dismembered (Anderson-Hynes) pyeloplasty. The pelvis should be exposed by dissecting bluntly in a plane just superficial to its adventitia with the intrinsic blood supply. The dissection of the upper ureter should be minimal, just enough to permit resection of the narrow segment and spatulation. If a large redundant pelvis is present, the pelvis is resected to 1 cm from the edge of the renal parenchyma. If left unresected, a large floppy pelvis may kink at the ureteropelvic anastomosis when filling occurs. The ureteropelvic anastomosis is performed over a catheter with interrupted sutures, allowing for more precise alignment.

When the length of the obstructing segment is more than 1.5 to 2 cm, a nondismembered pyeloplasty using a flap of renal pelvic tissue to enlarge the UPJ can be done. Other repairs, such as the spiral flap and Scardino-Prince vertical flap, can be used to bridge a long, narrow ureteral segment below the UPJ. Ureterocalycostomy usually is reserved for cases in which dependent renal drainage cannot be established by the conventional techniques (eg, fused kidney, previous surgery). In this procedure, amputation of the lower pole cortex should be performed to free the ureter from entrapment by contracting fibrosis of the renal cortex. The most dependent calyx is partially mobilized to allow tension-free mucosa-to-mucosa anastomosis.

Controversy exists regarding whether a nephrostomy and ureteral stent should be used to secure the anastomosis after UPJ repair. Several series have demonstrated that pyeloplasty in the neonate may be safely performed without proximal drainage; nevertheless, nephrostomy is recommended with a solitary kidney, with a bilateral pyeloplasty, and when the ureter is unusually small or thin walled.[44,45] The authors believe that nephrostomy and retroperitoneal drainage are essential. Delayed opening of the anastomosis protected by nephrostomy is common and was reported in up to 45% of infants younger than 1 year of age.[46] If delayed opening occurs, the drainage tubing can be elevated 30 cm to increase the intrapelvic pressure and encourage the anastomosis to open. On follow-up, IVP is performed 3 months postoperatively, and a diuretic renal scan is done after 6 months. The failure rate after pyeloplasty is 8% to 10%, and failure may be secondary to devascularization of the ureter, creation of too tight an anastomosis, or extravasation from an undrained anastomotic leak with subsequent fibrosis.

Another option for treatment of UPJ obstruction is endopyelotomy. Endopyelotomy is an endourologic version of the Davis intubated ureterotomy and is based on the findings that the incised and stented ureteral segment would reepithelialize around a stent with complete mucosal regeneration after 6 days, with muscularis regeneration by 6 to 8 weeks. Thus, incision and stenting of the stenosed UPJ allow the area to heal with a larger lumen (Figs. 92-21 and 92-22). Endopyelotomy has the advantages of no damage to the ureteral blood supply, lower morbidity, and lower cost. The reported success rates in adults are only 80% to 85%, however, and the experience with children is limited, with most reported cases performed on adolescents. Contraindications to endopyelotomy are bleeding diathesis, a long stenotic segment, and a very small child in whom the procedure may not be possible owing to a small-caliber ureter.

Endopyelotomy failures are usually apparent immediately after removal of the stent. The success of an open pyeloplasty in such cases does not appear to be compromised by the primary endopyelotomy.[47] Endopyelotomy has several drawbacks: the reported success rate is lower by 10% to 20% than that for open pyeloplasty, significant bleeding can occur during any

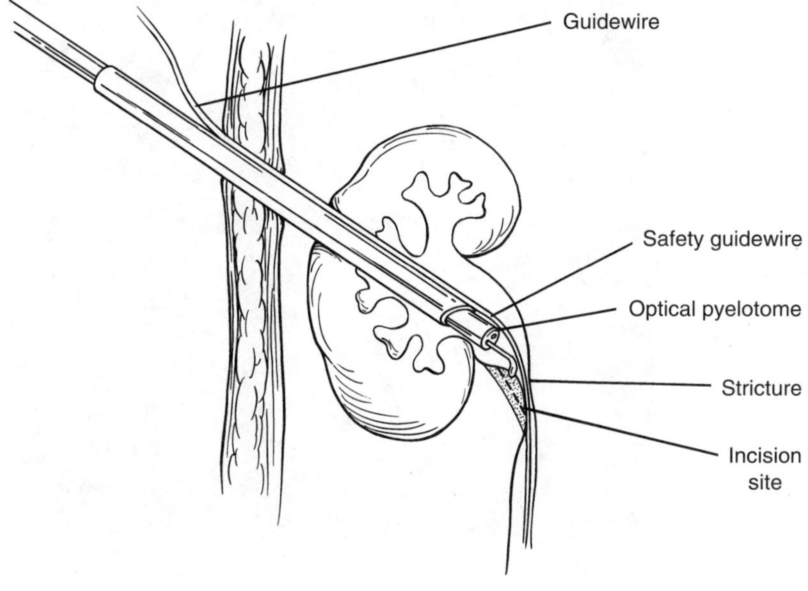

FIG. 92-21. Endopyelotomy approach and technique through a middle or upper posterior calyx, which provides more direct access to ureteropelvic junction obstruction. (Gillenwater JY, Grayhack JT, Howards SS, et al, eds. Adult and pediatric urology, ed 2. St Louis, Mosby–Year Book, 1991)

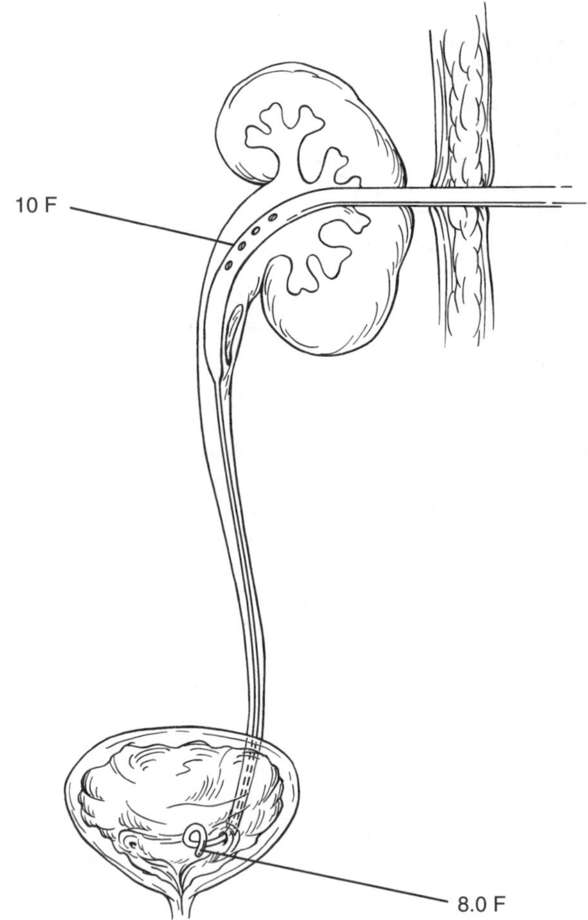

FIG. 92-22. Placement of endopyelotomy stent with proximal segment side holes positioned above ureteropelvic junction within renal pelvis, and distal tapered pigtail within the bladder. (Gillenwater JY, Grayhack JT, Howards SS, et al, eds. Adult and pediatric urology, ed 2. St Louis, Mosby–Year Book, 1991)

percutaneous procedure, there is a potential risk for injury to the aberrant vessel if it was not identified, and a stent is required for 6 to 8 weeks, which many patients find uncomfortable and which can cause persistent UTI.

Laparoscopically dismembered pyeloplasty was successfully performed in an adult patient.[48] This procedure appears to have the advantages of the high success rate of open dismembered pyeloplasty and the decreased morbidity associated with eliminating the need for a large skin incision, as in endopyelotomy. However, experience with this procedure is minimal, it has never been used in small children, it is technically difficult and requires substantial expertise, the operative time is lengthy, and its long-term efficacy is not known yet. The authors perform open dismembered pyeloplasty in all children; endopyelotomy and laparoscopic pyeloplasty may be considered in adolescents.

MEGAURETER

Megaureter simply means big ureter, and the term can be applied to any significant dilation of the ureter. In all dilated ureters, there is lack of effective peristalsis caused by inability of the walls of the dilated ureter to coapt. Lack of peristalsis, however, does not result in renal damage or in failure of the kidney to grow. Therefore, the presence of ureteral dilation even with calyectasis is not absolutely indicative of UVJ obstruction. Megaureter should be considered initially as a radiographic finding (Fig. 92-23) that may be caused by reflux, persistent UVJ obstruction, or transient UVJ obstruction during fetal development that resolved spontaneously. In this scheme, megaureter may be due to obstruction or reflux, or it may be idiopathic. Each of these major categories may then be subdivided into primary and secondary groups. The cause of primary obstructive megaureter is obstruction at or just above the UVJ. In secondary obstructive megaureter, the ureteral dilation is due to infravesical obstruction from valves, prolapsing ureterocele, ureteral stricture, and the like. Primary refluxing megaureter is more likely to be bilateral and is due to short ureteral tunnel or congenital paraureteral diverticulum, and free reflux is demonstrated on VCUG. In secondary refluxing megaureter, reflux is present with another anomaly, such as neuropathic bladder or infravesical obstruction. In primary nonobstructive, nonrefluxing megaureter, the upper tract drainage is good by all functional parameters. The diagnosis of megaureter in this category is one of exclusion. Usually in children, such systems tend to improve in radiographic appearance with growth, although some dilation usually persists. In secondary nonrefluxing, nonobstructive megaureter, the dilation is due to urinary infection, residual dilation from surgery, diabetes insipidus, or other rare causes of high rate of urine production. Rarely, reflux and UVJ obstruction coexist, and this can be diagnosed on delayed film after a cystogram shows poor drainage of one or both upper tracts.[49] Proven obstruction generally requires early surgical correction, whereas reflux is usually treated initially by surveillance. In quantitative histologic studies, the percentage of collagen in refluxing megaureter was significantly higher and the percentage of muscle lower than in controls or obstructing megaureters. In addition, in obstructive megaureter, the percentage of muscle was similar to that in controls, but the percentage

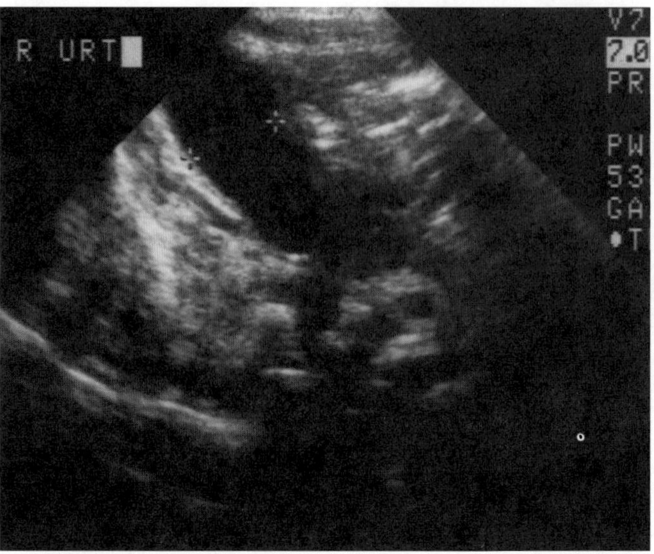

FIG. 92-23. Right megaureter on ultrasonography.

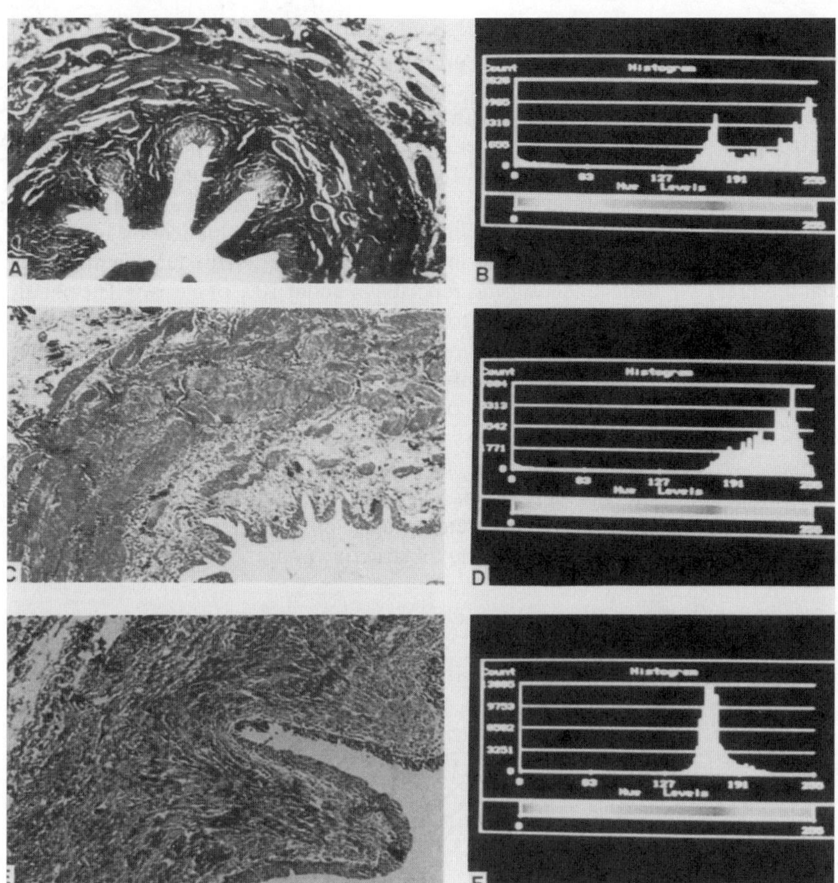

FIG. 92-24. (*A*) Normal ureter. Reduced from original magnification × 10. (*B*) Color image analysis generated histogram of hue component with visible light spectrum as ordinate axis. Band widths within color spectrum correspond to collagen (blue) and smooth muscle (red) components of ureteral muscularis layers. Two distinct populations (collagen and smooth muscle) were quantitated. (*C*) Primary obstructed megaureter. Collagen was localized surrounding smooth muscle bundles of all layers. (*E*) Primary refluxing megaureter. Amount of fibrotic tissue was significantly increased in these patients. (Lee BR, Partin AW, Epstein JI, et al. A quantitative histological analysis of the dilated ureter of childhood. J Urol 1992;148:1482)

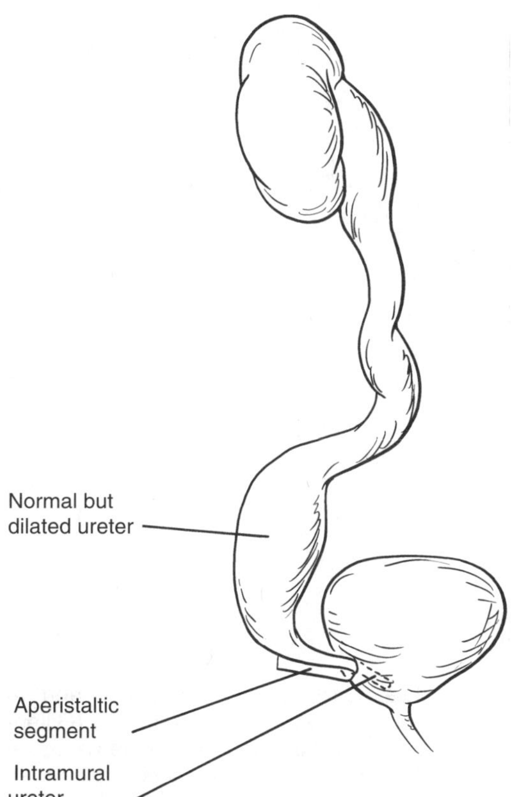

FIG. 92-25. Distal adynamic segment as found in primary obstructive megaureter. (Gillenwater JY, Grayhack JT, Howards SS, et al, eds. Adult and pediatric urology, ed 2. St Louis, Mosby–Year Book, 1991)

of collagen was only slightly higher than in controls (Fig. 92-24). These results suggest that megaureter involves smooth muscle synthesis of excess collagen that is more prominent in the refluxing megaureter. Therefore, the refluxing megaureter that has poor musculature and excessive collagen is likely to have a poorer surgical result than the obstructive megaureter.[50]

Nonobstructive, nonrefluxing megaureter can result from UVJ obstruction that resolved during development or from a primary abnormality of the ureteral musculature. The megaureters in prune belly syndrome are secondary to abnormal ureteral muscular development. The ureter is usually dilated beginning at a point just above the bladder. The dilation may involve the entire ureter or may be segmental, with the lowermost ureter often the widest in appearance. In prune belly syndrome, there is an increase in collagen/smooth muscle ratio, which is especially dramatic in patients who also have vesicoureteral reflux.[51]

Obstructed megaureter usually is caused by a narrowed juxtavesical ureteral segment (Fig. 92-25). The juxtavesical ureter may be normal in caliber and yet be the site of functional ob-

struction. In this case, the undilated segment does not conduct the peristaltic wave, usually owing to deficiency in the muscle fibers and fibrotic rigidity of the ureteral wall.[52] Most patients present with hydroureteronephrosis noted on prenatal ultrasonography. In older children, the presentation is usually with UTI, hematuria, or flank mass. Often, the dilated ureter is found at the time of appendectomy or other abdominal surgery. Bilateral megaureter is found in 25% of these patients. Megaureter is more common in boys and in the left ureter. Contralateral renal agenesis was reported in about 10% of cases.[53] The condition is not known to be hereditary, but families with more than one member with megaureter have been described. Megaureter without reflux or infravesical obstruction is observed on VCUG, but differentiating obstructed from nonobstructed megaureters is more difficult. As was previously described, the exact diagnosis requires a diuretic renal scan; when the results are equivocal, more invasive studies should be considered, such as cystoscopy with retrograde ureterography or Whitaker test with antegrade ureterography. A nonobstructive nonrefluxing megaureter gen-

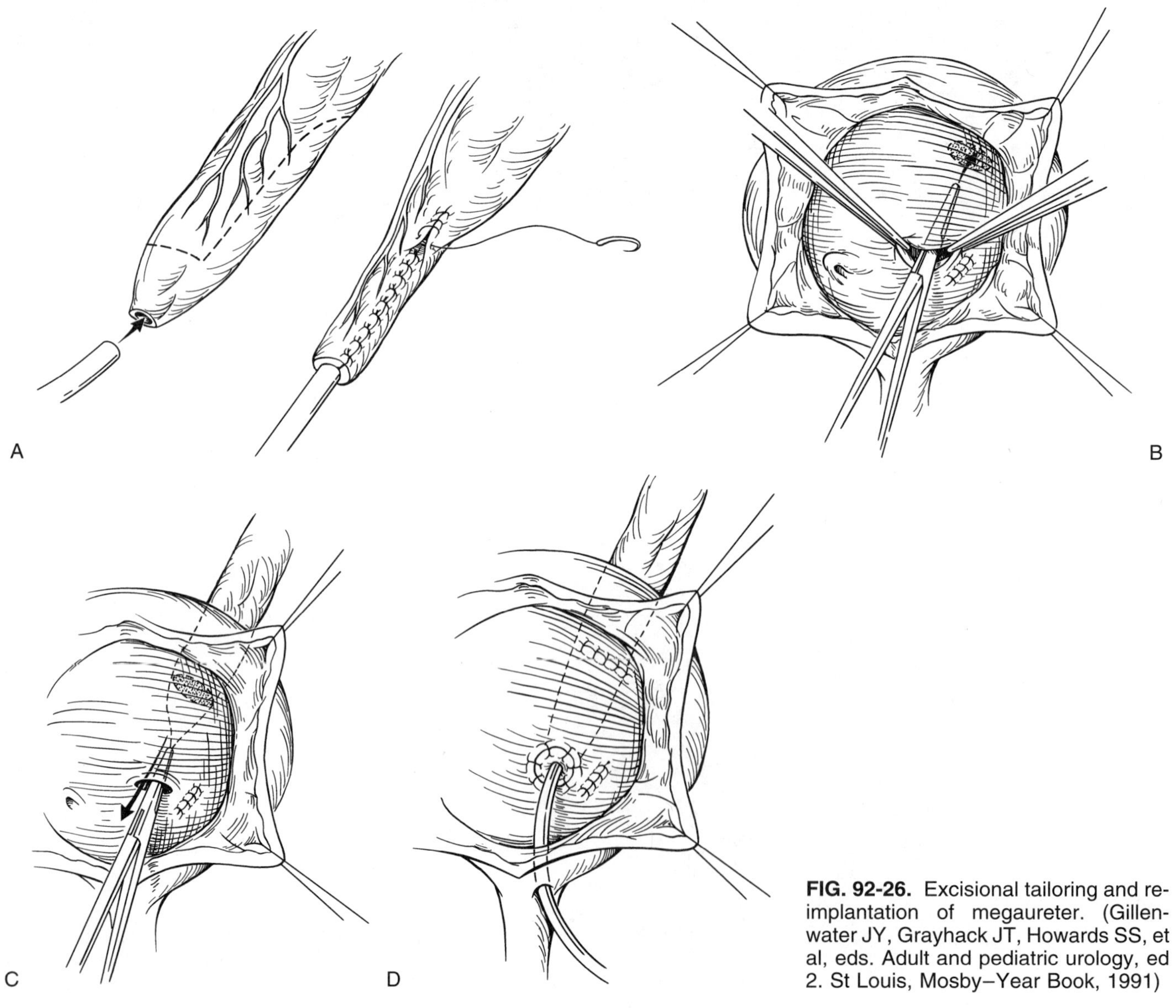

FIG. 92-26. Excisional tailoring and reimplantation of megaureter. (Gillenwater JY, Grayhack JT, Howards SS, et al, eds. Adult and pediatric urology, ed 2. St Louis, Mosby–Year Book, 1991)

erally becomes less dilated as the child grows, and follow-up is essential. Surgery is indicated in cases of deterioration of the upper tract or if recurrent or persistent UTI can be localized to the hydronephrotic system. In a study of 22 asymptomatic children with primary megaureter and good renal function (more than 40% on ^{99m}Tc-DTPA renal scan), regardless of their washout curve, patients were followed conservatively for between 4 months and 8 years. Only one infant showed a slight deterioration in renal function that necessitated surgical repair; all the other patients showed partial or complete regression of the ureteral dilation, with stable good renal function. This study suggests that a diuretic ^{99m}Tc-DTPA scan has a high false-positive rate and that split renal function studies may spare many symptomless infants with primary megaureter from unnecessary surgery.[54]

If refluxing or obstructive megaureter is diagnosed, surgery should be performed in early infancy to improve renal drainage and prevent renal damage from recurrent UTIs.[55] Secondary obstructive megaureter is initially treated by correcting the primary problem. If the bladder is noncompliant secondary to in-

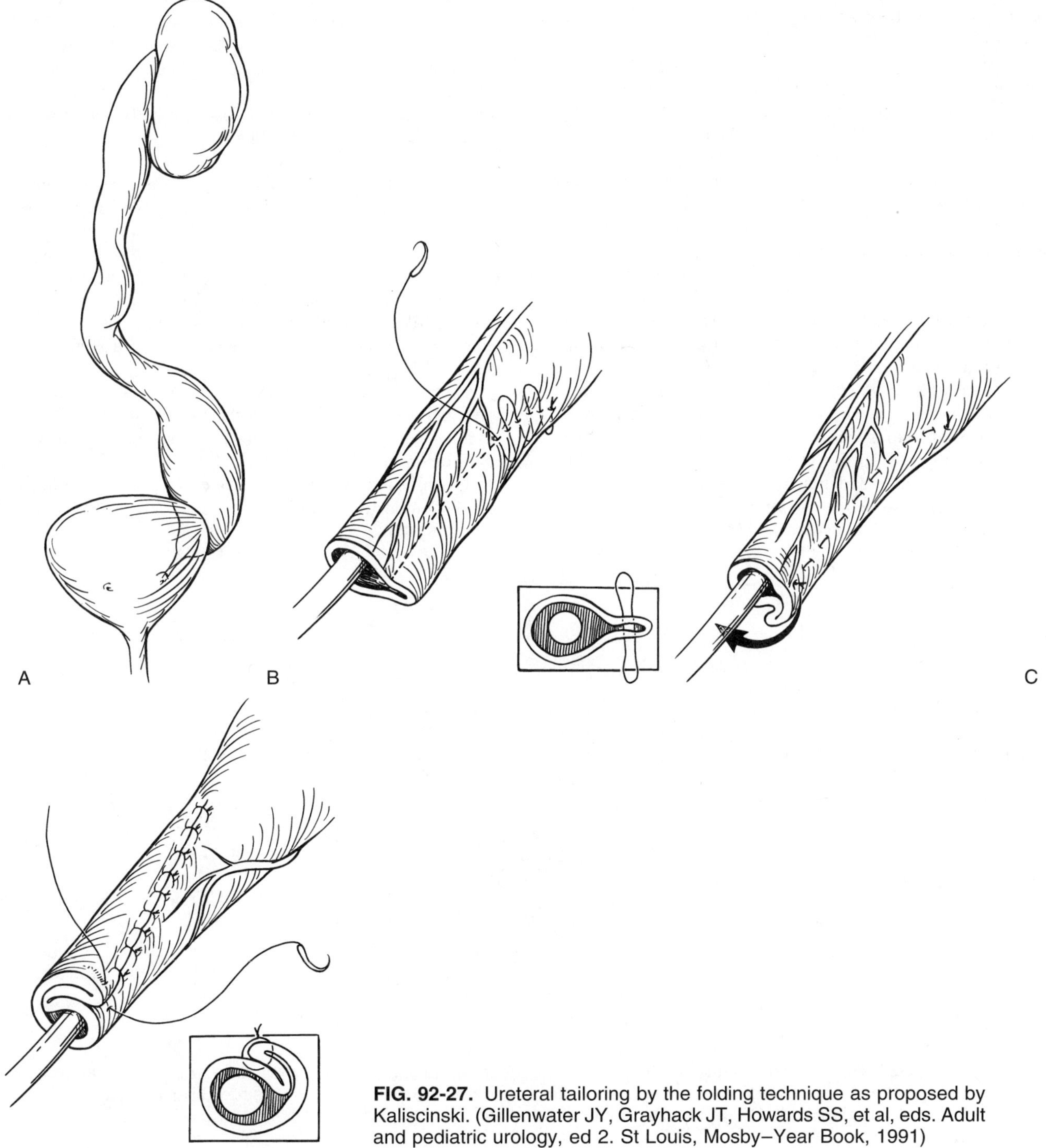

FIG. 92-27. Ureteral tailoring by the folding technique as proposed by Kaliscinski. (Gillenwater JY, Grayhack JT, Howards SS, et al, eds. Adult and pediatric urology, ed 2. St Louis, Mosby–Year Book, 1991)

fravesical obstruction or neurogenic causes, augmentation cystoplasty should be done before reimplantation. In some cases, the reduced bladder pressure results in improvement of ureteral drainage and dilation.

Tailoring and reimplantation of the lowest portion of the megaureter is usually the preferred procedure. The rationale for tailoring of the ureter relates to the inability of the ureteral walls to coapt and propel a bolus of urine. By lowering the radius of the ureter with tailoring, the intraluminal pressure increases, and more efficient propulsion of the urine through the system is achieved. Excisional tailoring has been considered the standard form of therapy for the past 15 years. The obstructive segment of the ureter is resected, and the ureter is shortened. A portion of the lateral wall in the remaining distal 5 cm is excised. This excision is opposite to the vessels that course medially and longitudinally along the ureteral surface, and the ureter is narrowed and tailored to about 12F caliber. The distal part of the ureter is closed by interrupted sutures that allow shortening of the ureter at the time of reimplantation.[56,57] (Fig. 92-26). Alternatively, the ureter can be brought through the original hiatus and reimplanted in a cross-trigonal fashion. Another method is to reduce ureteral caliber by tailoring and folding the ureter, excluding the excess ureteral lumen laterally with running horizontal mattress 5-0 absorbable suture. This lateral portion is then folded over the narrower medial portion of the ureter and secured with interrupted 5-0 absorbable sutures[58] (Fig. 92-27). The advantages of this technique are better preservation of ureteral blood supply and ensured ureteral closure so that the stents can be removed earlier than with excisional tailoring. The excess ureteral bulk can be a problem, however, especially in ureters with poor peristalsis. The success rate of both techniques is about 90%. Complications are primarily either reflux or postoperative obstruction. Obstruction can be due to ureteral angulation, constriction at the hiatus, and ureteral ischemia with atrophy and fibrosis. Although postoperative complications can occur, reoperative procedures are highly successful.[59]

ECTOPIC URETER

An ectopic ureter is one that opens at the bladder neck or more caudally rather than at its normal location on the corner of the trigone. Embryologically, an ectopic ureter forms when the ureteral bud has an abnormally high origin from the mesonephric duct, with delayed or no separation from the duct (Fig. 92-28). Stephens[60] described how an abnormal ureteral bud site may result in obstruction or reflux and abnormal development or dysgenesis of the renal segment by the displaced ureteral bud. The association of segmental renal dysplasia in kidneys with complete duplication of the ureters that arise from cranially or caudally ectopic ureteral buds supports the view that the position at which the ureteral bud contacts the metanephric blastema determines the quality of the resultant kidney (Fig. 92-29). The estimated incidence is 1 in 1900. In girls, more than 80% of ectopic ureters are associated with a duplicated collecting system; whereas in boys, most ectopic ureters drain single systems.[61] Ectopic ureter appears three times more often in girls than in boys, and about 10% are bilateral.[62]

In boys, ectopic ureters terminate in the posterior urethra in 47%, prostatic utricle in 10%, vas deferens and ejaculatory duct in 5% each, seminal vesicle in 33%, and rarely in the epididymis. Therefore, all ectopic ureters in boys terminate above the level of the external urethral sphincter without associated urinary incontinence. Ectopic ureters in boys may remain undiagnosed until symptoms of ureteral obstruction or infection appear. Urgency and frequency may occur as a response to the trickle of urine into the posterior urethra.[62]

When the ectopic ureter ends in the male genital tract, symptoms and signs may include prostatitis, seminal vesiculitis, epididymitis, and pelvic pain. These symptoms usually do not occur until the onset of sexual activity. Prepubertal boys with UTI or epididymitis require evaluation for ectopic ureter by ultrasound, which demonstrates dilation secondary to obstruction of the ectopic system.

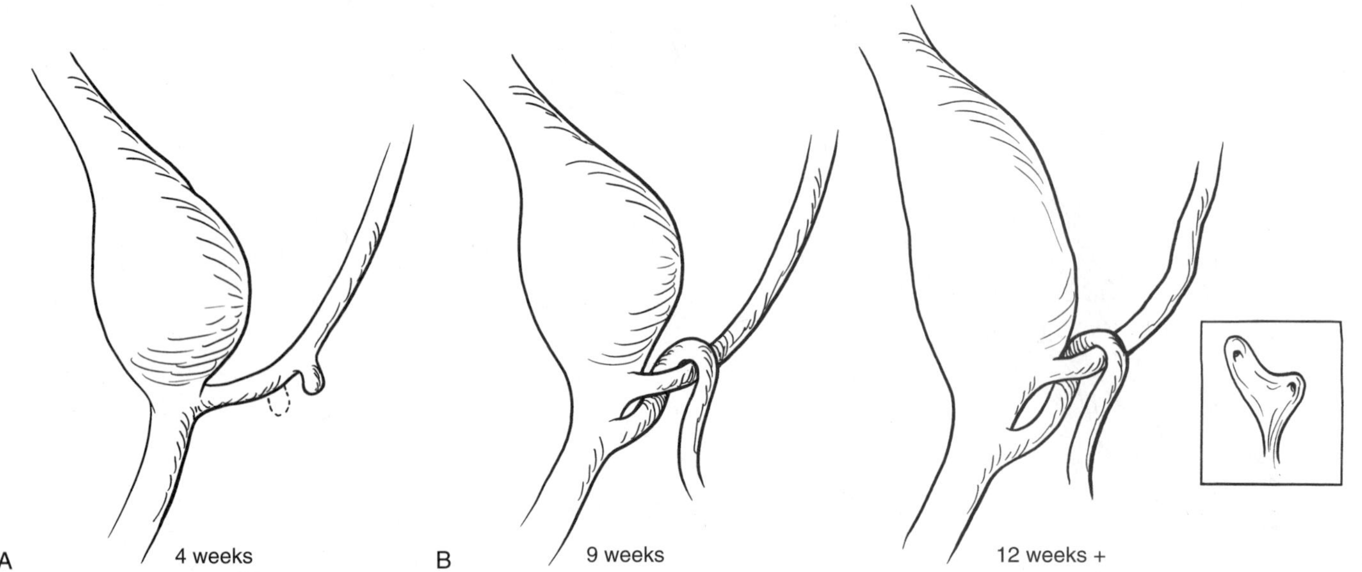

FIG. 92-28. High origin of the ureteral bud from the mesonephric duct leading to mild degree of ureteral ectopia toward the bladder neck, but still on the trigone. Endoscopic view in inset. (Gillenwater JY, Grayhack JT, Howards SS, et al, eds. Adult and pediatric urology, ed 2. St Louis, Mosby–Year Book, 1991)

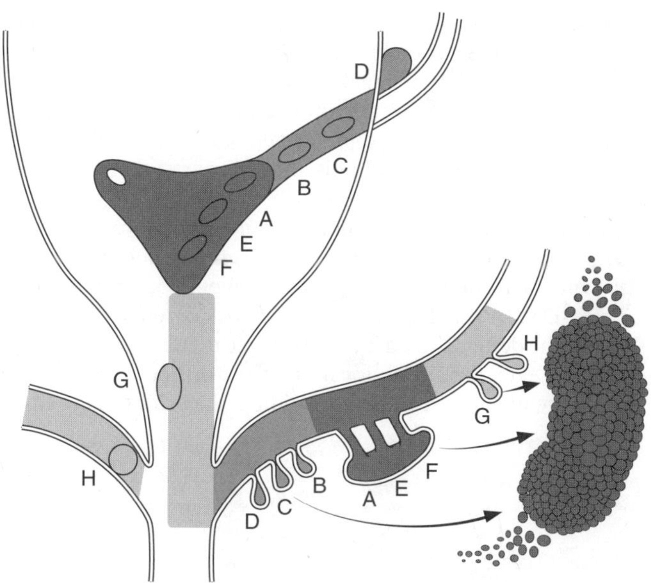

FIG. 92-29. Relation of orifice zones in the bladder and urethra to points of origin from the wolffian duct, and relation of bud positions of wolffian duct to nephrogenic blastema. (Walsh PC, Retik AB, Stamey TA, et al, eds. Campbell's urology, ed 6. Philadelphia, WB Saunders, 1992)

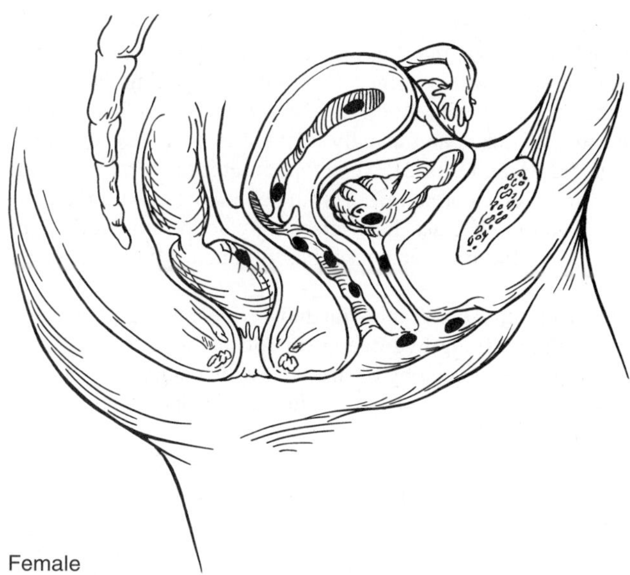

FIG. 92-31. Sites of ectopic ureterocele in female patients. (Gillenwater JY, Grayhack JT, Howards SS, et al, eds. Adult and pediatric urology, ed 2. St Louis, Mosby–Year Book, 1991)

In girls, ectopic ureters commonly exit below the sphincteric control, which accounts for the history of constant wetting from despite normal voiding of urine from ureters terminating in the bladder. The Gartner duct is the remnant of the female mesonephric duct that runs from the broad ligament of the uterus along the lateral wall of the vagina, ending at the vestibule, with secondary rupture of the duct into the urovaginal canal along their common wall. Accordingly, about one third of ectopic ureters in girls open at the level of the bladder neck or slightly more distally in the upper urethra (Fig. 92-30). In less than one third of cases, the ectopic ureter opens in the area of the vaginal vestibule immediately around the urethral orifice, where the end of the Gartner duct may present as a Gartner

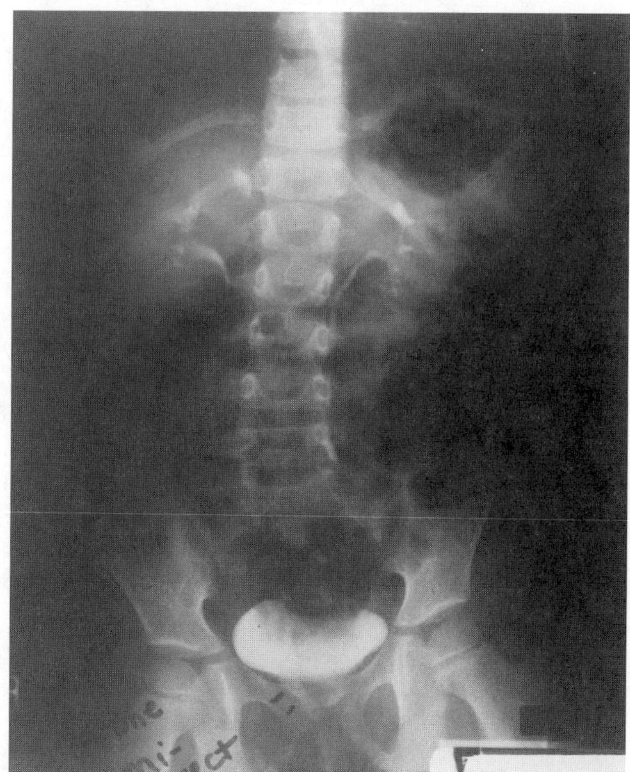

FIG. 92-30. Intravenous pyelogram of a female patient with continuous dribbling of urine. The right ectopic ureter that is opened to the distal urethra is associated with a functioning upper pole.

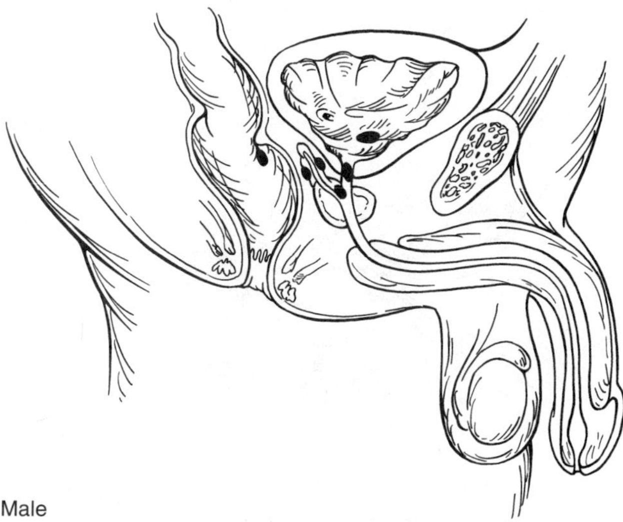

FIG. 92-32. Ectopic ureter sites in boys.

duct cyst.[63] In about 25% of ectopic ureters in girls, the orifice opens into the vagina. Less than 5% of ectopic ureters end at a higher site on the Gartner duct, with an opening at the level of the cervix or even uterus. Ureteral ectopy into the rectum is rare in both sexes and usually is noted incidentally at autopsy (Figs. 92-31 and 92-32). An ectopic ureter that drains into the proximal urethra often refluxes (in about 75%) and drains only during voiding because it traverses a greater portion of the musculature of the bladder neck, thus producing both reflux and obstruction.

Prenatal ultrasonographic diagnosis of ectopic ureters can be done by identifying hydronephrosis of the upper pole of a duplex system produced by obstruction with a completely normal bladder. In girls, a history of continuous urinary dribbling along with normal voiding and an apparent orifice in the urethrovaginal septum suggest ectopic ureter. In most cases, the diagnosis is confirmed by IVP or renal scan that demonstrates a poorly visualized or nonvisualized hydronephrotic upper pole of a duplex system. When an ectopic ureter drains a nonvisualized, diminutive, dysplastic renal unit, the typical radiologic features may not be demonstrated.

The ultrasonographic findings of an ectopic ureter include the dilated pelvis and upper pole ureter behind a normal bladder. The functional status of the upper pole should be assessed with a ^{99m}Tc-DMSA renal scan. On voiding cystourethrography, reflux may be demonstrated into the ectopic ureter during voiding, providing evidence of the location of the orifice. If reflux into the ectopic ureter is seen before voiding, the orifice is proximal

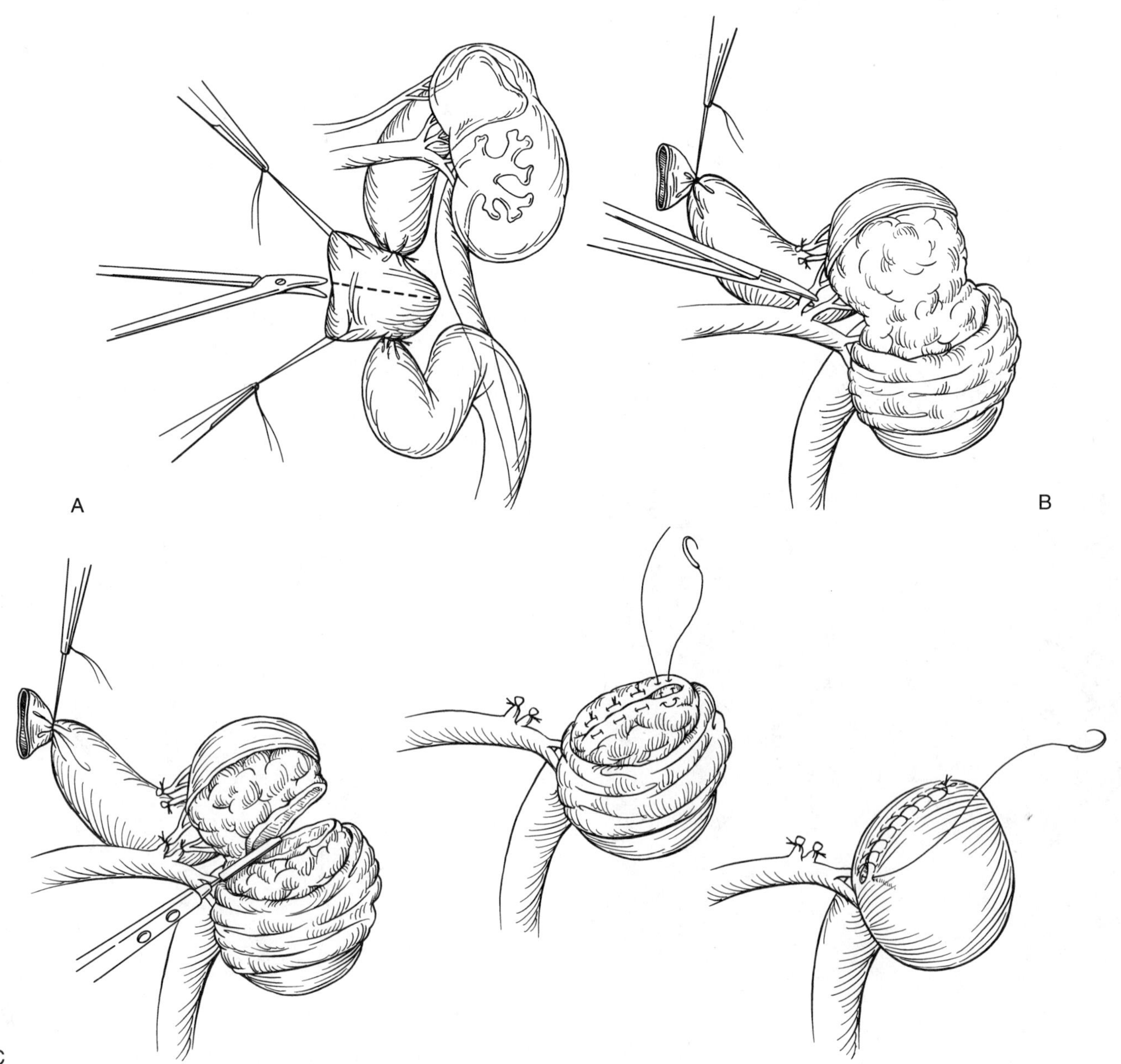

FIG. 92-33. Technique of upper pole nephrectomy. (Walsh PC, Retik AB, Stamey TA, et al, eds. Campbell's urology, ed 6. Philadelphia, WB Saunders, 1992)

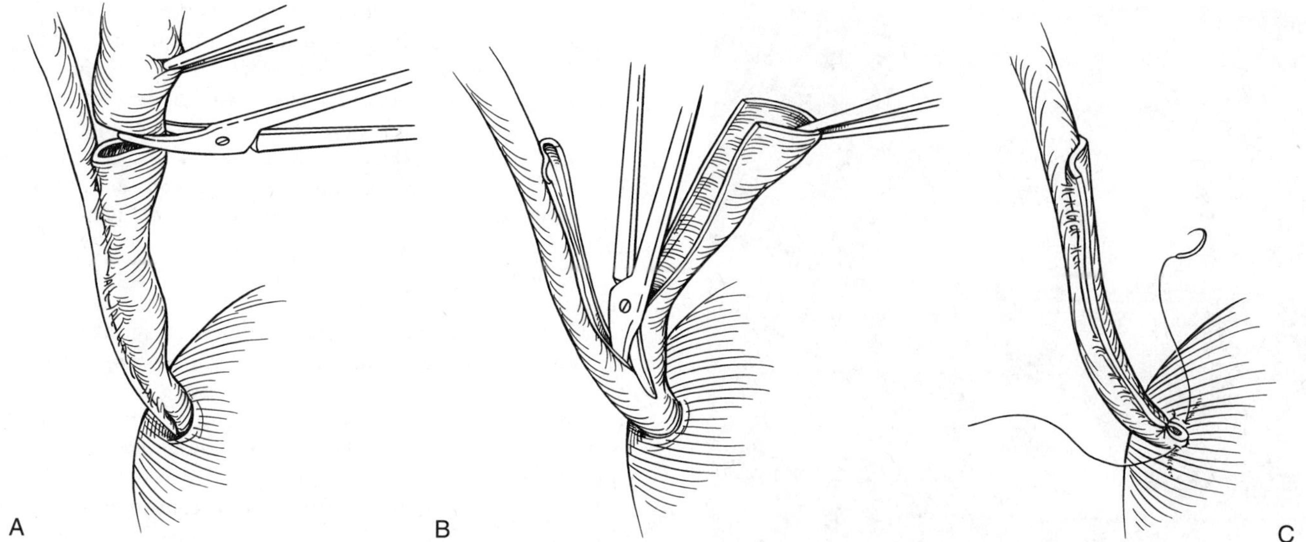

FIG. 92-34. Surgical management of refluxing ureteral stump. (*A*) The ectopic ureter is excised at the point where it is difficult to separate. (*B*) The outer wall of the ectopic ureter is excised to the bladder level. (*C*) A transfixing suture obliterates its lumen, with care being taken not to injure the orthotopic ureter. (Walsh PC, Retik AB, Stamey TA, et al, eds. Campbell's urology, ed 6. Philadelphia, WB Saunders, 1992)

to the bladder neck, while reflux only with voiding suggests an orifice in the urethra. Vesicoureteral reflux into the lower pole ureter is evident in at least half of cases. A large ectopic ureter may press against the bladder, with pseudoureterocele appearance on cystography. Rarely, a computed tomographic scan may demonstrate the small, poorly functioning upper pole segment.[64,65] Ectopic ureteral orifice may be most difficult to identify on cystourethroscopy and vaginoscopy, and injection of indigo carmine usually is not helpful because of the poor function of the ectopic system.

Upper pole nephrectomy with total ureterectomy through a standard flank incision is the usual treatment of an ectopic ureter associated with a poorly functioning upper pole[66] (Figs. 92-33 and 92-34). In rare cases, when the upper pole is not markedly hydronephrotic and has significant function, the upper pole ureter can be anastomosed to the lower pole pelvis or to the proximal lower pole ureter.[67] Common sheath ureteral reimplantation may be performed in instances when reflux to the lower pole ureter is significant and when the ectopic ureter is not severely dilated and drains a renal unit worth saving.

In boys, when the ureter enters the genital tract, even if reflux is not present, total ureterectomy, excision of the common duct, and ligation of the vas are necessary to prevent subsequent epididymitis and pyoureter. Surgical access to the distal ectopic ureter as it enters the genital tract may be facilitated by a transtrigonal approach. When the ectopic ureter opens just distal to the bladder neck, is refluxing, and is associated with a functioning kidney, antireflux surgery is indicated.

URETEROCELE

Ureterocele is a cystic dilation of the terminal intravesical ureter. Simple ureterocele means that the ureterocele is located at the usual location of the ureteral orifice in the trigone (Fig.

92-35). An ectopic ureterocele is located distal to the trigone and may project into the urethra or often means any ureterocele associated with a duplex system. The incidence of ureteroceles was reported to be 1 in 4000 autopsies in children,[68] and it is much more common in whites than in blacks. Ureteroceles are five times more common in girls than in boys, and about 10% are bilateral. About 80% of ureteroceles are associated with the upper pole ureter of a duplex kidney.[69] Ectopic ureterocele is also associated with an increased incidence of duplication on the contralateral side. The ureterocele may vary in size from a tiny cystic dilation of the submucosal ureter to that of a large balloon that fills the bladder (Fig. 92-36). Histologically, the wall of the ureterocele contains varying degrees of attenuated smooth muscle bundles and connective tissue. The ureterocele is covered by vesical mucosa and lined with ureteral mucosa.

Several theories about the embryonic development of ureterocele exist. In Chwalle's theory,[70] a membrane covering the ureteral orifice persists for a prolonged period, leading to the formation of ureterocele. Another theory is that a ureterocele forms when an ectopic ureter is affected by the stimulus to expansion that transforms the bladder into a globular cap, creating an expanded, thin-walled distal ureter.[71] Also, a localized embryonic arrest has been hypothesized as the cause of ureterocele.[72]

Simple ureteroceles are more commonly detected in adults. They usually are associated with single collecting system and rarely with an upper pole ureter of a complete duplication. Most simple ureteroceles have obstructing pinpoint orifices, but the degree of obstruction is probably not significant in most adults.

The Stephens classification[73,74] of ectopic ureterocele is anatomic and commonly used. Stenotic ectopic ureterocele is characterized by a small stenotic orifice and occurs in about 40% of cases. Sphincteric ectopic ureterocele terminates within the internal sphincter and is found in about 40% of all cases. The

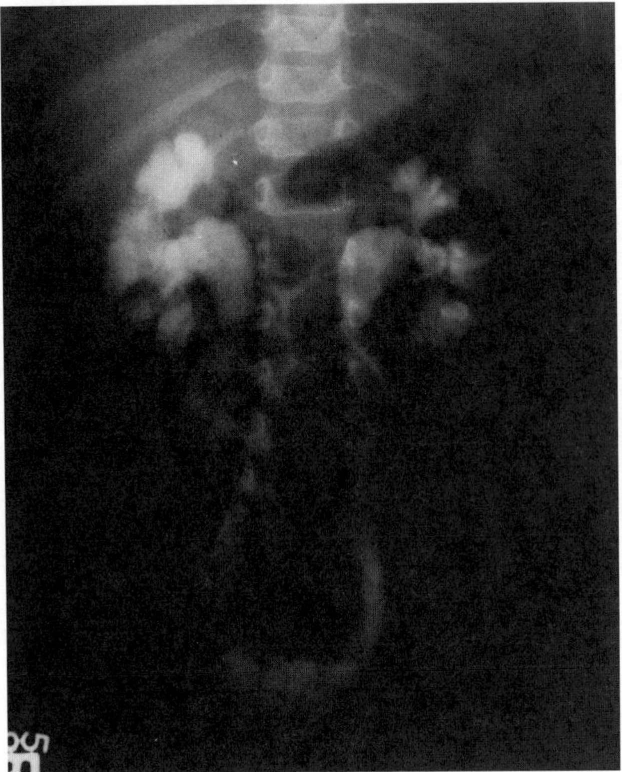

FIG. 92-35. Intravenous pyelogram of a male patient showing bilateral hydronephrosis due to bilateral single system (simple) ureterocele, and the cobra head deformity.

ureteral orifice may be normal or large and may open either in the posterior urethra in boys or distal to the external sphincter in girls. In sphincterostenotic ectopic ureterocele, found in about 5% of cases, the stenotic orifice is located in the urethral floor. Other rare types of ectopic ureterocele include: cecoureterocele, in which the lumen extends distal to the orifice as a long tongue (or cecum); blind ectopic ureterocele, which has no orifice, so that the ureter is completely obstructed; and nonobstructed ureterocele, which has a large orifice in the bladder (Fig. 92-37). Churchill and colleagues[75] proposed a functional classification of ectopic ureterocele.

Ureterocele can be diagnosed on prenatal ultrasonography, and antibiotic prophylaxis should be started soon after birth. Clinically, most children present during the first few months of life with symptoms of UTI or failure to thrive. The stasis and infection predispose the patient to stone formation in the ureterocele and upper collecting system. Rarely, large ureteroceles prolapse through the bladder neck, causing urinary retention owing to bladder outlet obstruction. Some degree of urinary incontinence may occur in girls with large intraurethral ectopic ureteroceles that have rendered the external sphincter lax and inefficient.

Ureterocele can be diagnosed by ultrasonography, but it depends on the degree of bladder filling and the pressure within the ureterocele. If the bladder is overdistended, the ureterocele may collapse, and only dilated ureter may be seen entering the bladder. If the bladder is empty, the dilated ureterocele may fill the entire bladder, giving the impression of a partially full bladder without ureterocele. IVP may demonstrate the characteristic "cobra head" deformity, an area of increased density with a halo or less shadow around it (see Fig. 92-35). Larger uretero-

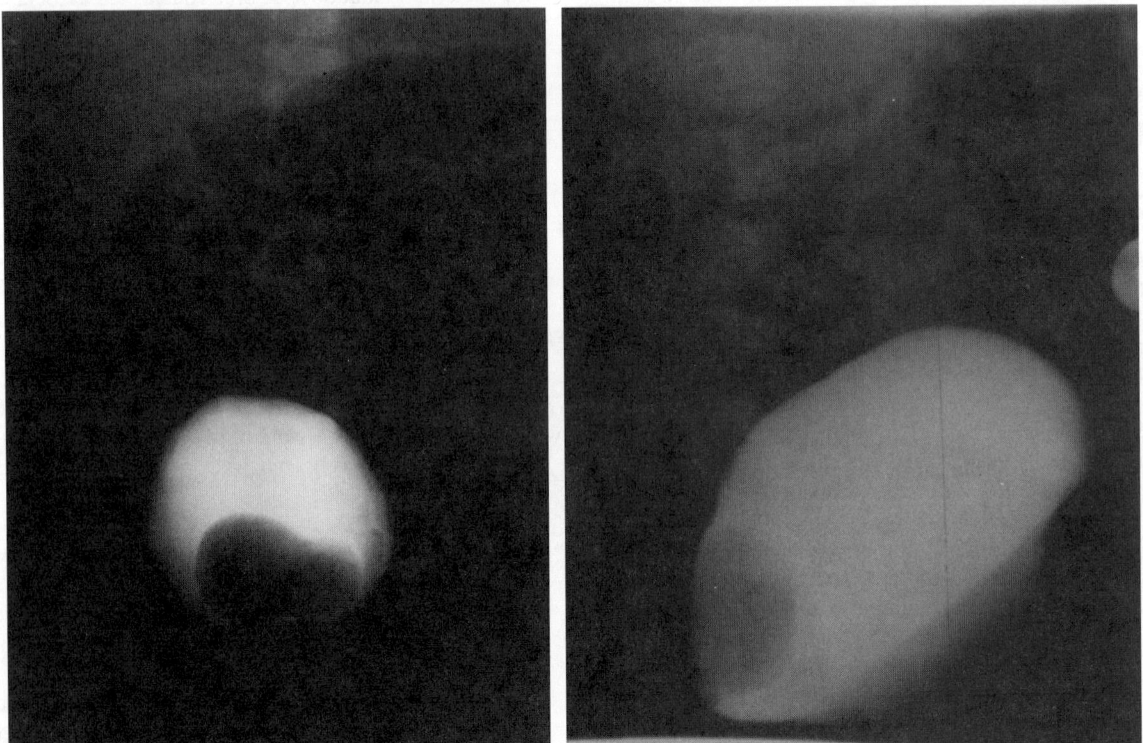

A   B

FIG. 92-36. Voiding cystourethrogram of a female patient with ectopic ureterocele. (*A*) Anteroposterior view. (*B*) Lateral view.

celes may not fill early with contrast material, resulting in a sizable filling defect in the bladder, prostatic urethra in boys, and the entire urethra in the girls. These findings are associated with varying degrees of hydroureteronephrosis. In simple ureterocele, the upper tract changes are less severe than in ectopic ureterocele. In ectopic ureterocele, the upper pole segment is commonly dysplastic and has poor or no function (Fig. 92-38). The ectopic ureterocele may affect the ipsilateral and contralat-

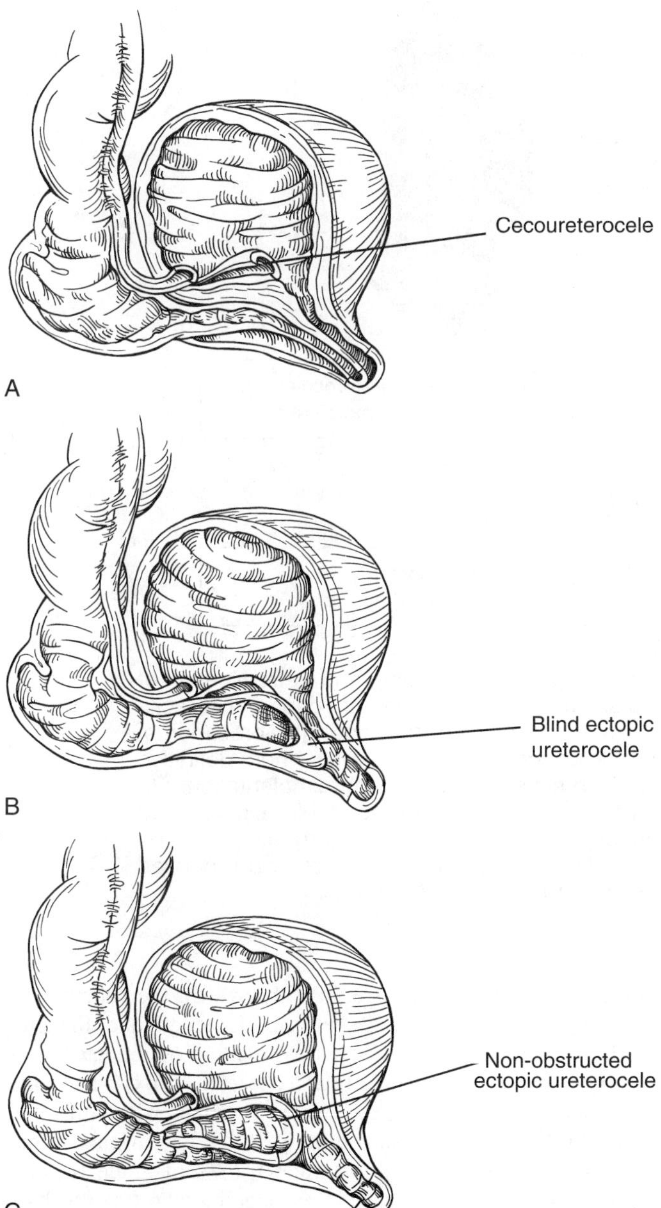

FIG. 92-37. (*A*) Cecoureterocele. The lumen extends distal to the orifice as a long tongue beneath the urethral submucosa. The orifice communicates with the lumen of the bladder and is large and incompetent. (*B*) Blind ectopic ureterocele. There is atrophy of the ureter distal to the ureterocele, which ends blindly. (*C*) Nonobstructed ectopic ureterocele. There is terminal expansion of the ureter, which has a large orifice in the bladder. (Walsh PC, Retik AB, Stamey TA, et al, eds. Campbell's urology, ed 6. Philadelphia, WB Saunders, 1992)

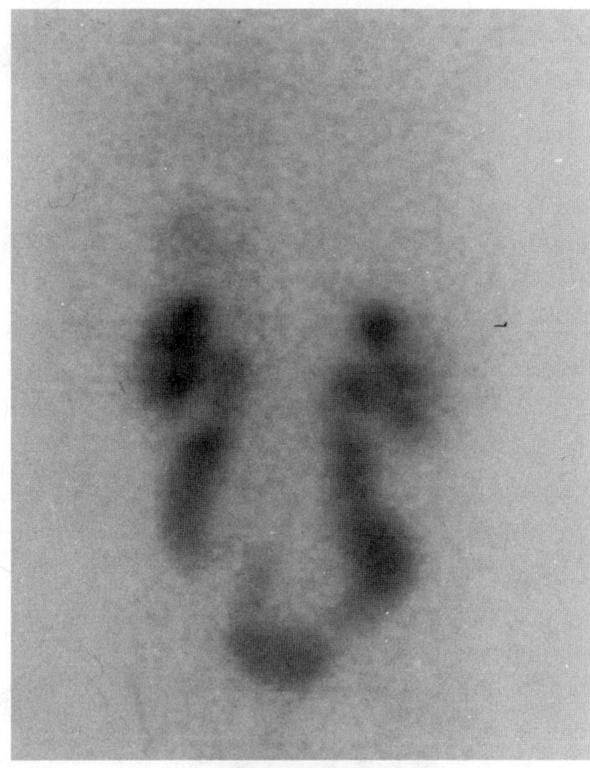

FIG. 92-38. ^{99m}Tc-DTPA renal scan showing poorly functioning left upper pole, secondary to ectopic ureterocele.

eral ureters and renal units. Large ectopic ureteroceles may obstruct the ipsilateral lower pole ureter, and if large and tense enough, they may even obstruct the contralateral side or induce vesicoureteral reflux.[76] Rarely, vesicoureteral reflux is seen with a simple ureterocele. A ^{99m}Tc-DMSA renal scan should be done to assess the function of the involved renal units. At cystoscopy, the ureterocele usually expands rhythmically with each peristaltic wave of urine that fills it, and then shrinks as a thin jet of urine drains through the small orifice.

Because ureteroceles have a broad spectrum of presentations, each case should be treated individually. The primary goal of treatment of ectopic ureterocele is to preserve the renal parenchyma, including the lower pole of the affected kidney, by correcting obstruction and preventing reflux. Simple transurethral incision of a ureterocele with a Bugbee electrode, leaving the intravesical hood of the ureter intact, may be therapeutic and usually does not result in reflux. Transurethral resection of simple ureterocele invariably results in reflux and risk of UTI. In most cases, excision of the simple ureterocele with reimplantation of the involved ureter is the surgical procedure of choice. In ectopic ureterocele with poor kidney function, nephrectomy with partial ureterectomy (as described previously) is indicated. Figure 92-39 outlines the management of ectopic ureterocele and the treatment algorithm based on Churchill and colleagues'[75] classification and grading.

VESICOURETERAL REFLUX

Vesicoureteral reflux allows bladder urine to pass retrograde into the ureter, renal pelvis and calyces. Factors important in

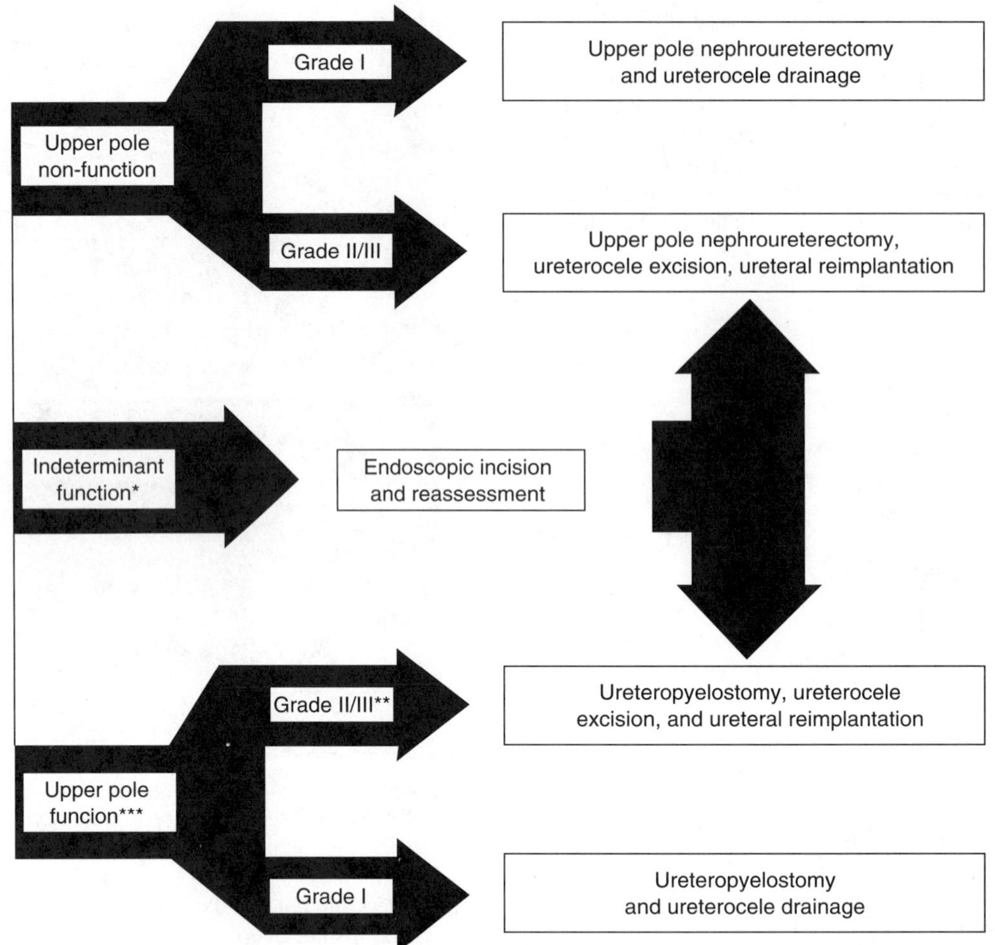

FIG. 92-39. Functional classification of ectopic ureterocele by anatomic grading and determination of upper pole function by DMSA nuclear renography allows selection of a management course that facilitates maximization of renal parenchymal preservation and minimization of multiple operative procedures. *Also considered for unstable infants or infants with multiple congenital anomalies for whom definitive reconstruction is best delayed. Generally obligates patient to subsequent ureteral reimplantation. **In high-risk newborns, the upper pole procedure may be performed only, with ureterocele excision and reimplantation at an older age. ***In the absence of severe ureterectasis, common sheath reimplantation may be considered. (Churchill BM, Sheldon CA, McLorie GA. The ectopic ureterocele: a proposed practical classification based on renal unit jeopardy. J Pediatr Surg 1992;27:497)

the normal absence of reflux in humans are the length of the intravesical ureter relative to its diameter and the intrinsic longitudinal muscular coat of the submucosal ureter that inserts onto the superficial trigone (Fig. 92-40). These factors are reflected in the appearance of the ureteral orifice, which normally resembles a cone, but sometimes resembles a stadium, horseshoe, or golf hole, with increasing tendency toward laterality that results in primary reflux (Fig. 92-41). In addition, the normally low pressure in the resting bladder (8 to 10 mmHg) is sufficient to compress the roof of the intravesical ureter against the underlying detrusor to prevent reflux. A significant increase in bladder pressure, however, due to bladder outlet obstruction or neurogenic low-compliance bladder, or inflammation of the overlying bladder mucosa may result in secondary reflux.[77]

The incidence of vesicoureteral reflux in healthy children is less than 1%.[77] Twenty to 50% of children with urinary tract infection have reflux.[78] In these children, the incidence of reflux correlates inversely with age.[79] With growth, the submucosal ureter elongates and the ratio between the length and diameter of the submucosal tunnel increases, making incompetence of the valve mechanism less likely as a cause of reflux.[60] Thus, the vesicoureteral reflux may disappear spontaneously with time, depending on its extent and severity.[80,81] When urinary infections were prevented, 87% of grade I, 63% of grade II, 53% of grade III, and 33% of grade IV vesicoureteral reflux resolved spontaneously over about 3 years.[82] Reflux is more commonly diagnosed in boys during infancy and in girls during early childhood. Vesicoureteral reflux is more common (30%) in siblings of children with known reflux.[83] Therefore, sibling screening with VCUG or sonography is recommended. The pattern of genetic transmission remains undetermined. Most investigators favor the polygenic mode of inheritance. Also, reflux was found to occur 10 times as frequently in white American girls with infection as in black American girls with infection.[84]

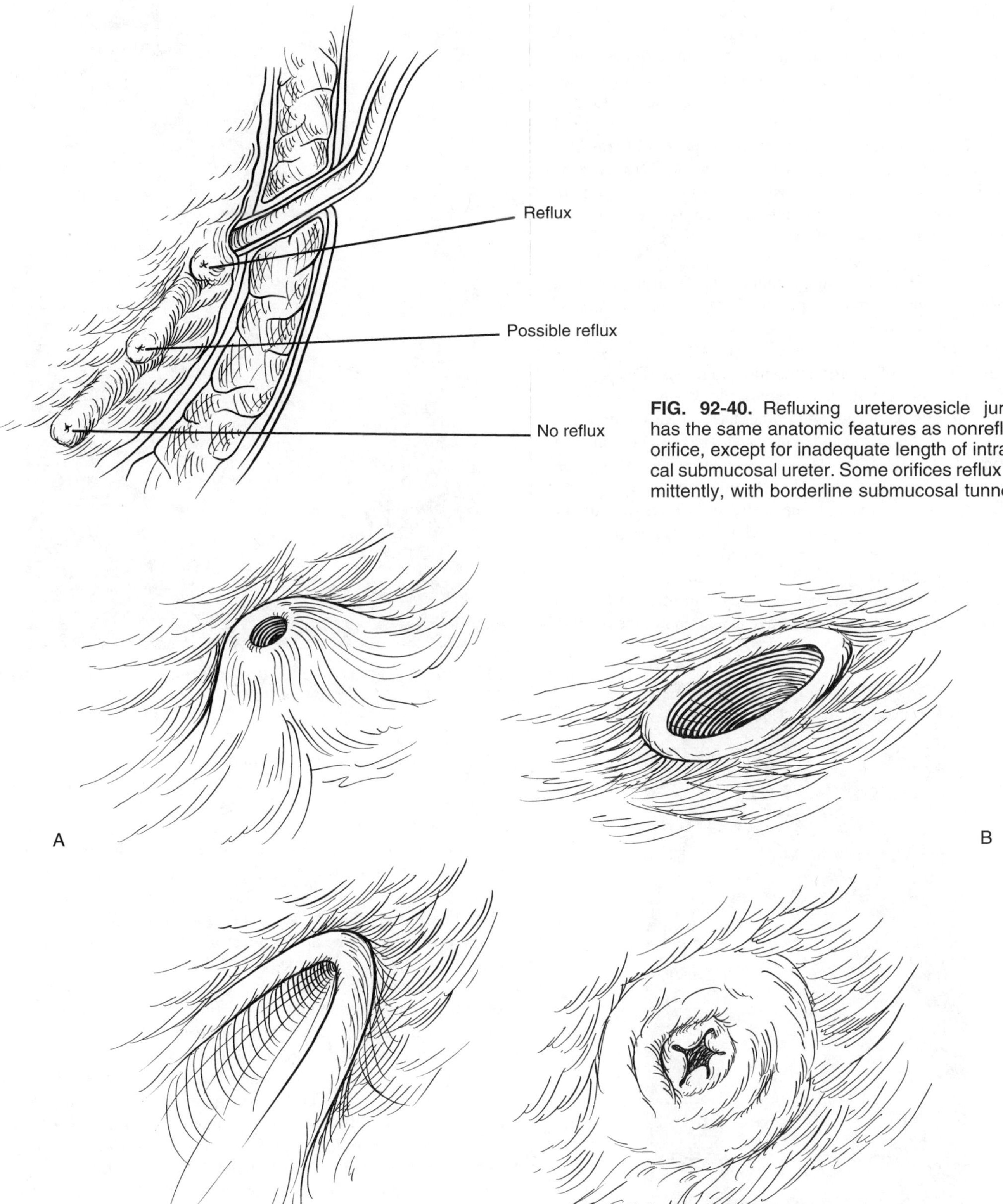

FIG. 92-40. Refluxing ureterovesicle junction has the same anatomic features as nonrefluxing orifice, except for inadequate length of intravesical submucosal ureter. Some orifices reflux intermittently, with borderline submucosal tunnels.

FIG. 92-41. Lyon classification of orifice morphology in primary reflux. (*A*) Normal or volcano-shaped orifice. (*B*) Stadium orifice, which is usually slightly more lateral than the normal orifice and sometimes associated with reflux. (*C*) Horseshoe orifice. (*D*) Golf-hole orifice, which is most lateral in position and lacks any vestige of an intravesical ureter. (Walsh PC, Retik AB, Stamey TA, et al, eds. Campbell's urology, ed 6. Philadelphia, WB Saunders, 1992)

An increased incidence of vesicoureteral reflux occurs in patients with complete duplication of the ureters. Although reflux can affect either ureter, it is much more common in the ureter draining the lower pole because of the more lateral orifice of that ureter and its tendency to have a short submucosal tunnel. Vesical diverticulum is also associated with reflux. The ureteral hiatus represents a potential weak spot in the posterolateral wall of the bladder and is the most common site of diverticula. A diverticulum near or at the hiatus predisposes the patient to reflux. In the presence of such diverticula, spontaneous cessation of reflux is unlikely, and early surgical correction of both lesions is generally indicated.

Reflux may be found during postnatal investigation of hydronephrosis that was diagnosed prenatally or, more commonly, after investigation following an event of UTI. In children, all first UTIs require radiologic evaluation at least with ultrasonography and VCUG to look for anatomic anomalies (Fig. 92-42). Reflux can be suspected on ultrasonography when the ureter appears more dilated during and immediately after voiding. On IVP, reflux can be suspected when a dilated lower ureter, a ureter visible for its entire length, vascular markings on the ureter, hydronephrosis, calyceal distortion, and renal scaring are seen. ^{99m}Tc-DMSA scan is the best way to asses the quality of the kidneys by documenting renal scarring and function. VCUG, however, is the most sensitive and accurate study to detect or exclude reflux (Fig. 92-43). An infection-free interval of 2 to 4 weeks is recommended before the cystogram is performed because the inflammation of the intravesical ureter or the overly-

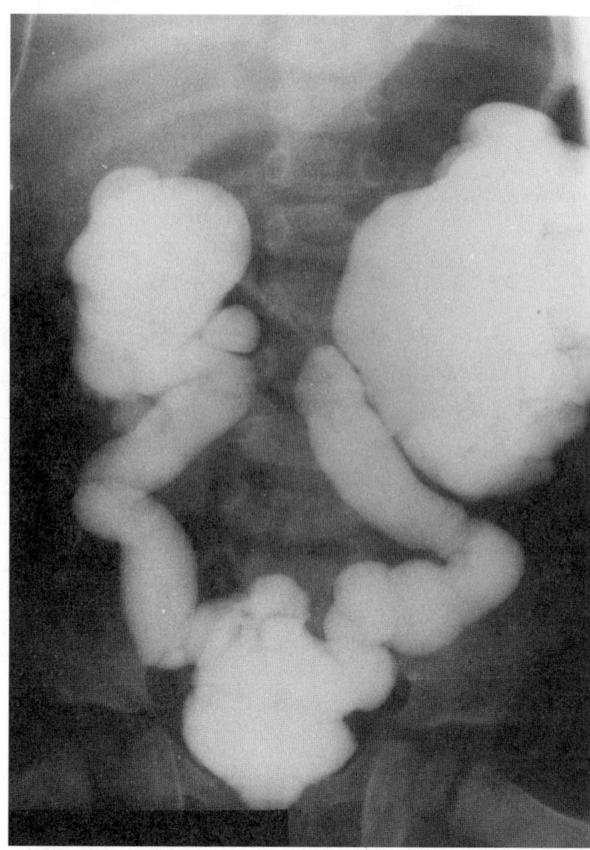

FIG. 92-43. Voiding cystourethrogram showing bilateral grade V reflux to the lower pole.

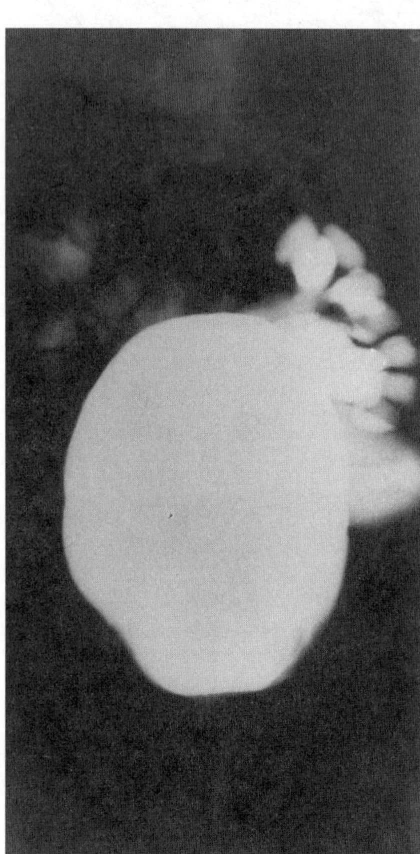

FIG. 92-42. Voiding cystourethrogram of a megalocystis refluxing megaureter in a newborn.

ing mucosa may reduce the compliance of the roof of the ureter and result in transient mild reflux. Radionuclide cystography confers 1% to 2% of the radiation exposure of standard radiographic VCUG. After the diagnosis of reflux is established by VCUG, a nuclear cystogram may be done as follow-up and to verify that reflux is absent after an antireflux procedure.

Several classifications of reflux exist, but the international classification system has come into general use. This system is based primarily on the appearance of the calyces on cystogram (Fig. 92-44) because the degree of dilation of the ureter does not always parallel the degree of dilation of the pyelocalyceal system. Complications that may result from vesicoureteral reflux include acute pyelonephritis, chronic pyelonephritis with renal scaring, hypertension, and chronic renal failure.[85–89]

As was previously mentioned, reflux disappears spontaneously in many children (except grade V reflux or refluxing megaureter), but reflux that persists in adolescence or adulthood is unlikely to resolve spontaneously. Sterile reflux is unlikely to cause renal damage, while persistent reflux of infected urine does cause renal damage in children. In addition, long-term prophylactic antibacterial therapy is usually safe and well tolerated by children. Therefore, continuous prophylactic antibacterial therapy and follow-up is the treatment of choice for low-grade reflux in infants and young children. The indications for surgical therapy include: breakthrough UTIs; high-grade reflux (grade IV or V); persistence of reflux by late childhood or adolescence, especially in girls; and drug allergy or poor compliance of the patient to medical therapy and follow-up.

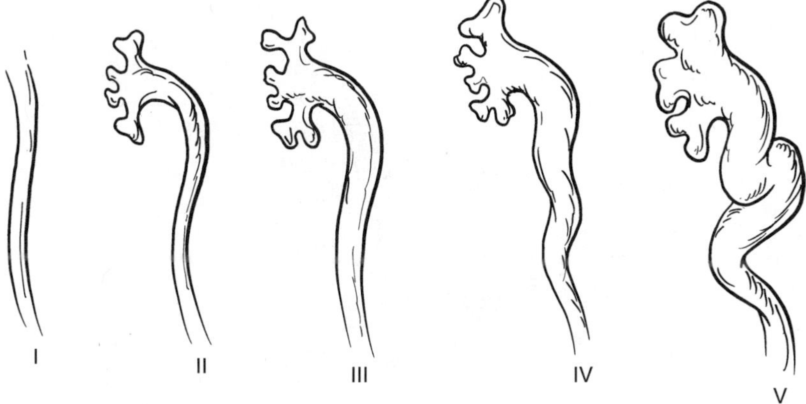

FIG. 92-44. International Reflux Study Classification of grades of vesicoureteral reflux. Grade I, into the ureter only; grade II, into the ureter, renal pelvis, and calices; grade III, mild or moderate dilation of the ureter and renal pelvis with no or minimal forniceal blunting; grade IV, moderate dilation and tortuosity of ureter and pelvis with blunting of the fornices but maintenance of the papillary impressions; grade V, gross dilation and tortuosity of the ureter and pelvis with absence of the papillary impressions. (Walsh PC, Retik AB, Stamey TA, et al, eds. Campbell's urology, ed 6. Philadelphia, WB Saunders, 1992)

Medical Management

Medical management must include an antimicrobial drug that is effective against most gram-negative bacteria, has high urine concentrations, is available, and is well tolerated in liquid forms with minimal cost to the patient. The most common in use are sulfa-trimethoprim, nitrofurantoin, and cephalexin, which are given in one half of the therapeutic dose. The lower prophylactic dose usually causes fewer side effects. The prophylactic medication should be given at bedtime, when the child retains urine the longest and is more likely to develop infection. The antibacterial therapy should be continued until the reflux has resolved. Boys with reflux can be equally well managed with observation alone.[90] Thus, in boys, frequent monitoring of urine without antimicrobial therapy is a viable alternative. All children should be followed every 3 months for history of UTI, and physical examination should include parameters of physical growth and blood pressure. Laboratory studies should include urinalysis and culture every 3 months, white blood cell count every 6 months, and serum creatinine clearance yearly. IVP or ^{99m}Tc-DMSA renal scan to look for renal scarring should be done every 24 months, but sooner if recurrent infections intervene. Contrast VCUG or nuclear cystogram should be done at about 12-month intervals.

Surgical Treatment

Paquin[91] found that the ureter in most normal children has a submucosal tunnel length/ureteral diameter ratio of 5:1. Thus, the goal of antireflux ureteral reimplantation is to reimplant the ureter in a longer submucosal tunnel and to fixate the end of the ureter to the bladder musculature, so that the 5:1 ratio is restored. There are many techniques for surgical repair of reflux; three techniques are commonly used. The Politano-Leadbetter technique[92–94] involves reimplantation of the ureter through a new bladder hiatus (Fig. 92-45). The success of the Politano-Leadbetter procedure is about 95%, comparable with other procedures. The Lich-Gregoire technique[95] (Fig. 92-46) was once popular, with success rates as high as 97%.[96] Associated bladder diverticula and bladders of small capacity may make this repair difficult to use. In addition, megaureter requiring tapering and refluxing duplex ureters with associated pathology, such as ureterocele and ectopia, can not be managed with

this technique. The Cohen,[97] or cross-trigonal, technique has supplanted the other techniques for most pediatric urologists (Fig. 92-47). The advantage of this procedure is that it does not involve creation of new hiatus, and thus an adequate tunnel length can be created to prevent reflux with little chance of obstruction. It also works particularly well in patients with small-capacity bladders. The potential disadvantage is that these ureters can be difficult to catheterize by cystoscopy and are inaccessible to the rigid ureteroscope. The success rate with this procedure is above 97%.

Endoscopic Treatment

The basic principle of endoscopic injection is to provide solid support and backing for the UVJ. With the bladder mostly emptied, the needle is advanced under endoscopic control, and some material is injected beneath the mucosa, 4 to 5 mm distal to the 6-o'clock position of the affected ureteral orifice. As the injection proceeds, the distal ureter flattens, and the orifice closes, assuming an inverted crescentic appearance at the conclusion of the procedure.

The adequacy of the implant is judged by assessing ureteral support (maintenance of the inverted crescentic appearance of the orifice and persistence of the implant under the bladder mucosa) as the intravesical pressure is raised by fluid instillation and application of suprapubic pressure by the operator. Alternatively, intraoperative cystogram can be performed, and if reflux persists, additional paste is injected, usually just medial to the site of the first injection. The patient usually is discharged from the hospital the same day on a suppressive antibiotic regimen. Repeated endoscopic injections are performed if the reflux persists. Surgical reimplantation can be performed in patients with persistent reflux after several endoscopic procedures have failed. Polytetrafluoroethylene (Teflon) was introduced in the early 1970s for successful treatment of incontinence, and Matouschek[98] was first to describe endoscopic correction of vesicoureteral reflux using this material in 1981. Since then, many studies have shown success rates that exceeded 85%, and the technique of subureteric injection for cure of reflux has been widely accepted.[99,100] Polytef is a 50% suspension of Teflon particles in glycerol. This preparation has not been proved safe and is not approved by the US Food and Drug Administration. Several alternative substances were investigated. Ideally, this

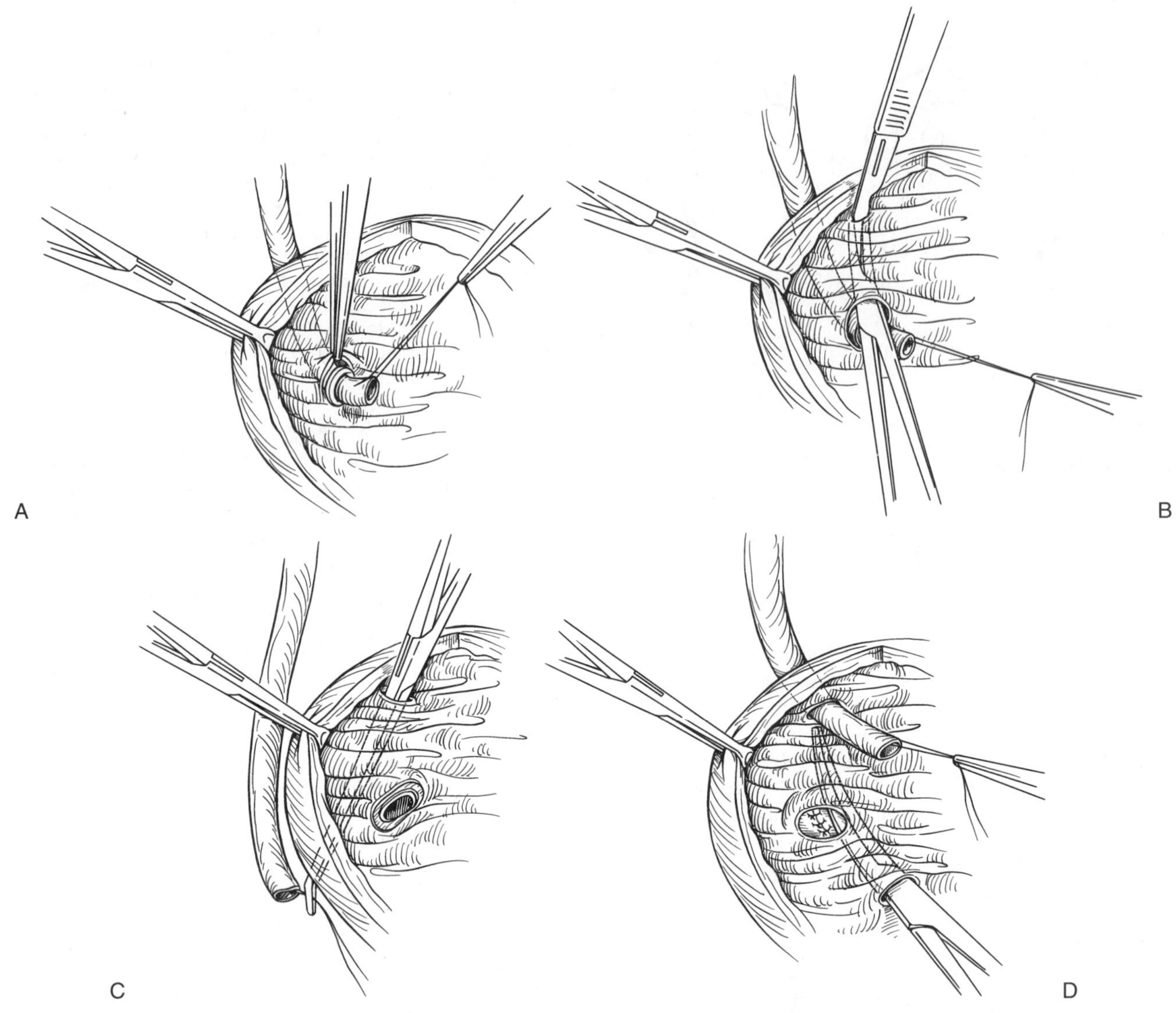

FIG. 92-45. Politano-Leadbetter technique of ureteroneocystostomy. (Walsh PC, Retik AB, Stamey TA, et al, eds. Campbell's urology, ed 6. Philadelphia, WB Saunders, 1992) *(continued)*

substance should be inert, is not reabsorbed, does not migrate, causes minimal or no local tissue reaction, and does not exclude surgical correction of reflux that might be needed in the future. Glutaraldehyde cross-linked bovine dermal collagen meets these criteria and can be injected through a 25-gauge needle with standard endoscopic equipment. All patients should undergo skin testing for collagen sensitivity before initiation of therapy. In the event of a positive reaction, patients are excluded from this procedure. Under this condition, collagen was approved by the Food and Drug Administration for use for endoscopic treatment of vesicoureteral reflux. The results are 65% cure rate at 1-year postoperatively with minimal morbidity.[101] Polyvinyl alcohol foam (Ivalon) was used in the rabbit model and caused giant cell response with fibrotic reaction. This study, however, did not examine the efficacy of this treatment to correct reflux.[102] Other studies have shown that autologous chondrocytes or muscle cells harvested from the auricular surface or the bladder of a minipigs can be successfully used for endoscopic correction of reflux in these animals.[103] The authors have been success-

fully using collagen for endoscopic treatment of grade I to III reflux for the following indications: (1) stable or worsening reflux followed for more than 1 year, (2) breakthrough UTI, (3) patient noncompliance with medical therapy, (4) progressive renal scarring, and (5) failed ureteral reimplantation.[104]

UROLITHIASIS

Urolithiasis is rare in children in industrialized countries, and only 2% to 3% of patients with urolithiasis are children. Urolithiasis in children is often associated with specific metabolic disorders or anatomic abnormalities that often lead to infection or stasis with subsequent stone formation. For crystals to form in urine, the urine must be supersaturated for the precipitating crystal phase. Because the urine is a complex solution, other factors play an important role. Ionic strength and pH influence the availability of ions in urine and affect saturation. Modifiers of crystal formation present in urine can inhibit or promote

(*Text continued on page 1511*)

E F

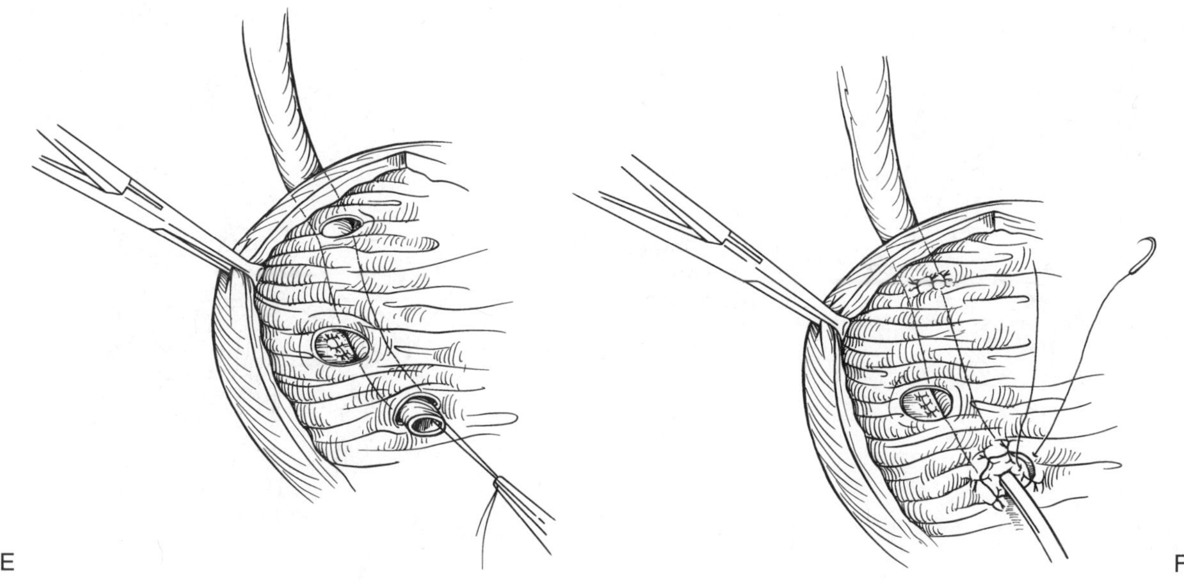

FIG. 92-45. *Continued.*

A B C D

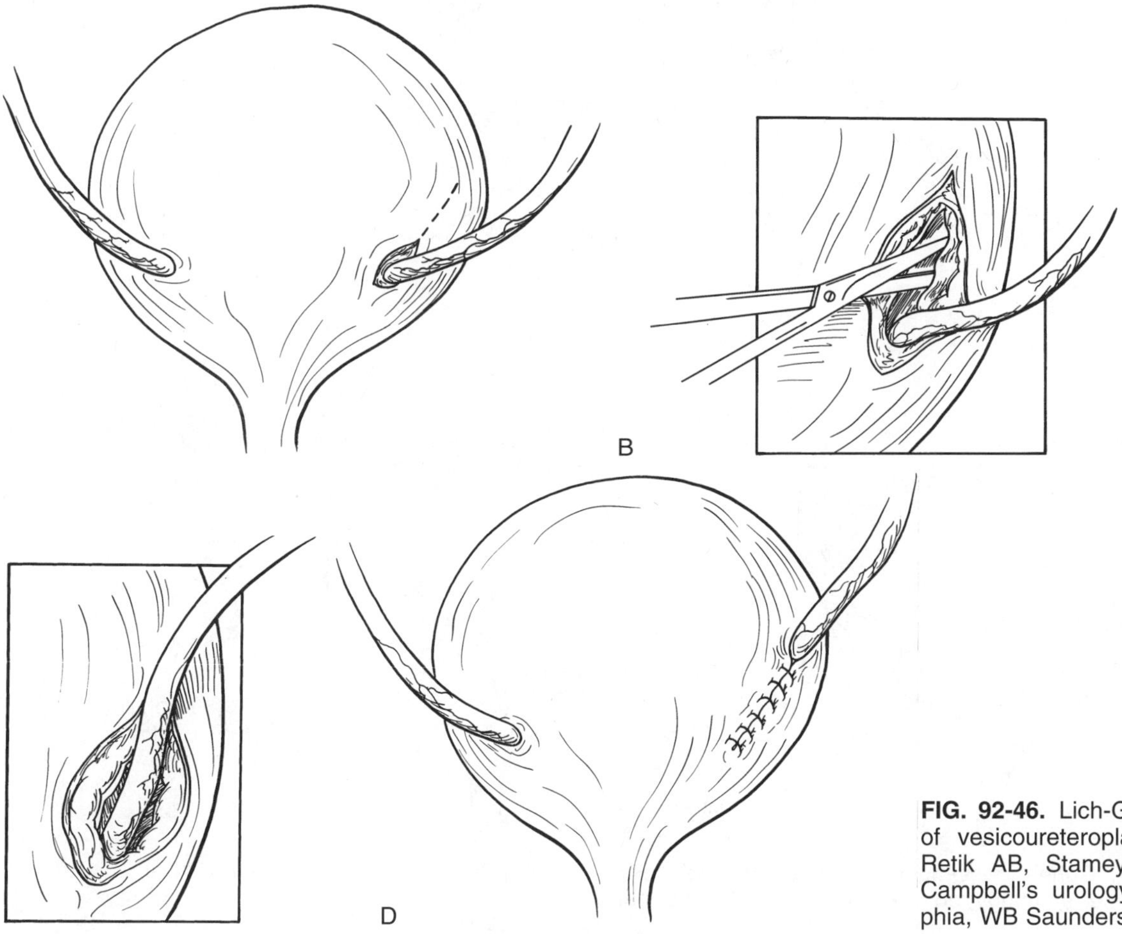

FIG. 92-46. Lich-Gregoire technique of vesicoureteroplasty. (Walsh PC, Retik AB, Stamey TA, et al, eds. Campbell's urology, ed 6. Philadelphia, WB Saunders, 1992)

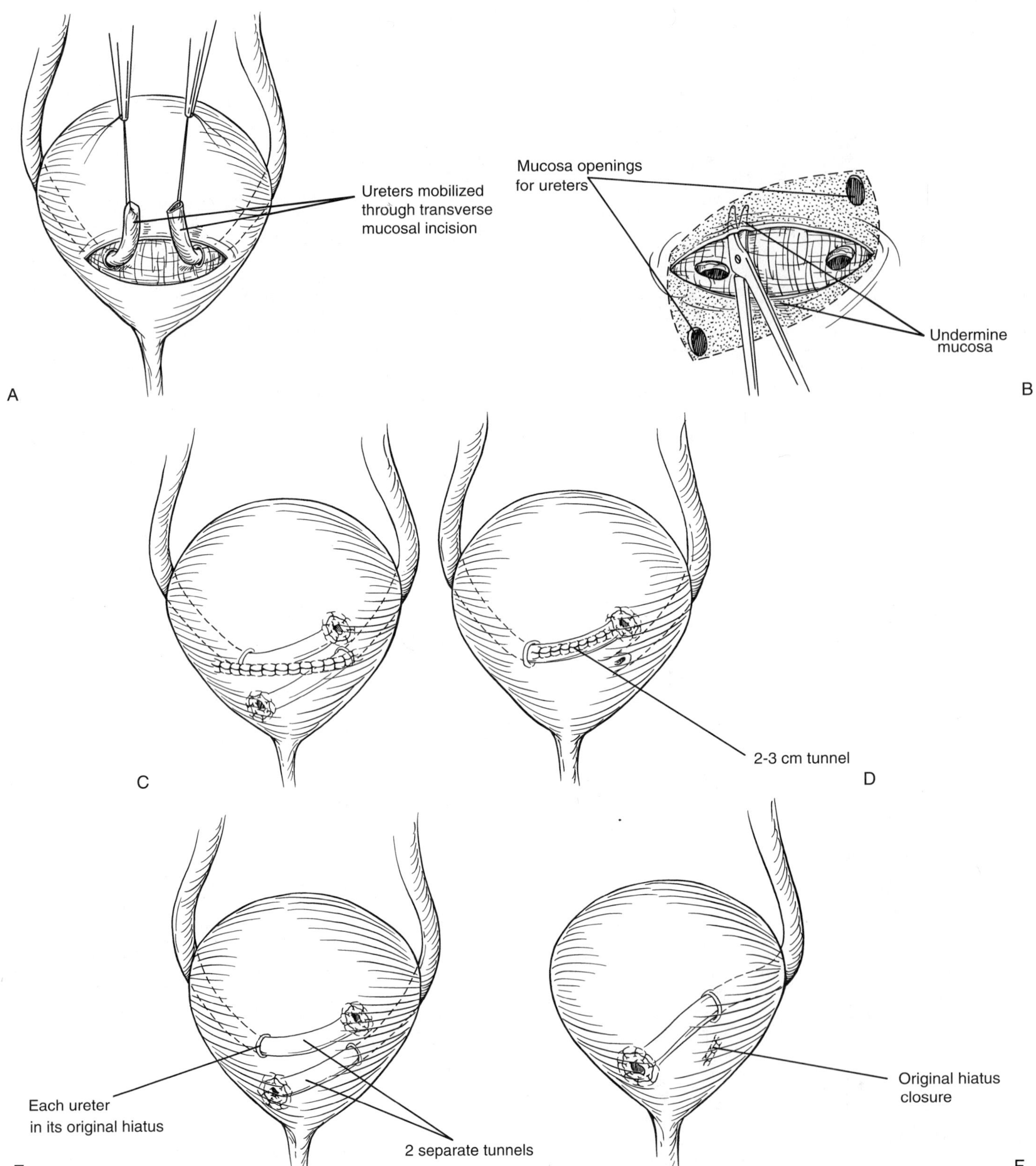

FIG. 92-47. Cohen cross-trigonal reimplantation technique. (Walsh PC, Retik AB, Stamey TA, et al, eds. Campbell's urology, ed 6. Philadelphia, WB Saunders, 1992)

the formation of some common crystals. Inhibitors of calcium phosphate or oxalate crystal formation include magnesium, citrate, zinc, pyrophosphate, and large-molecular-weight substances such as nephrocalcin, glycosaminoglycans, and RNA fragments. Classic renal colic occurs in a minority of children. Gross or microscopic hematuria is the most frequent clinical manifestation, followed by flank or back pain, nausea and vomiting, or irritative bladder symptoms. The more common urolithiasis disorders in children are discussed in this section.

Evaluation of children with urolithiasis should include a family history. Urolithiasis is present in families with cystinuria and primary hyperoxaluria, which are autosomal recessive disorders. Likewise renal tubular acidosis (RTA) or idiopathic calcium oxalate urolithiasis, which are autosomal dominant disorders, have positive family histories. Knowing the age of onset is also helpful. Stone formation beginning in the young child suggests an enzymatic defect, such as primary hyperoxaluria. Cystinuria, idiopathic calcium oxalate urolithiasis, and primary hyperparathyroidism more often begin near puberty or in the middle teenage years. Stone formation secondary to infection and obstruction related to congenital malformations of the urinary tract often present before the age of 5 years. Immobilization secondary to injury in children with active, growing bones may cause mild to moderate hypercalcemia with associated hypercalciuria, leading to stone formation within the urinary tract. Low fluid intake may amplify a tendency to stone formation in patients with underlying idiopathic calcium oxalate urolithiasis. Stone disease is considered surgically active if there is evidence of obstruction, pain, or associated infection. Metabolic activity is considered to be present when there is evidence of new stone formation, stone growth, or passage of documented gravel within the past year. The change in stone formation can be established by reviewing previous radiographs.

Initial laboratory evaluation should include a first morning urinalysis, urine culture, antibiotic sensitivity test, and measurement of serum calcium, phosphorus, sodium, potassium, chloride, bicarbonate, uric acid, and creatinine levels. The anatomy of the urinary tract should be defined by a kidney–ureter–bladder radiograph with tomograms and an excretory urogram. Ultrasonography can help detect obstruction and nonopaque stones. If a stone is available, it should be analyzed. A 24-hour urine collection should be completed when the patient has no symptoms and is on a normal diet with normal fluid intake. Initial studies of the urine should include a measurement of volume, pH, calcium, oxalate, uric acid, citrate, cystine, phosphate, and creatinine.

Enzymatic Disorders

Primary hyperoxaluria is a malignant cause of stone formation within the urinary tract. Sixty-three percent of patients show signs and symptoms of stone disease, and 53% die after 8 years, usually from renal failure with generalized oxalosis. Two specific enzymatic disorders have been described, both are inherited in a autosomal recessive pattern. Type 1 is the most common and is due to a deficiency of alanine-glyoxylate aminotransferase in the membranes of liver cells. Oxalic and glycolic acids are increased in the urine of patients with this defect. Type 2, L-glyceric aciduria, is due to a deficiency of D-glyceric dehydrogenase, which can be demonstrated in leuko-

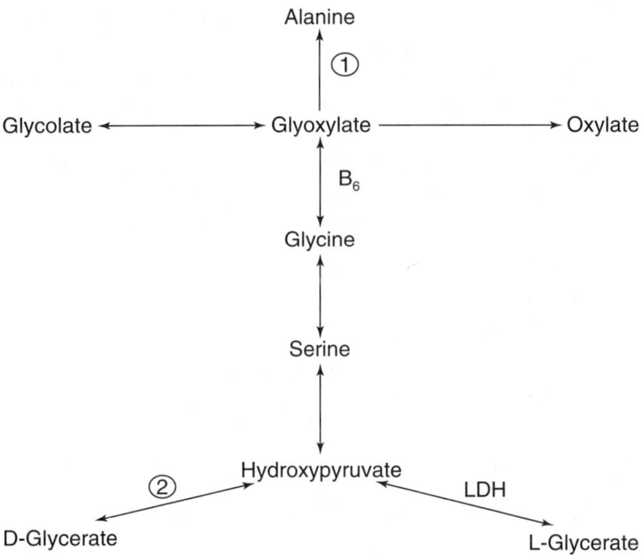

FIG. 92-48. Pathways of oxalate metabolism in humans. The enzyme defect responsible for type 1 primary hyperoxaluria is at 1, and that for type 2 is at 2. Pyridoxine (vitamin B₆) is a cofactor for the conversion of glyoxylate to glycine. (Gillenwater JY, Grayhack JT, Howards SS, et al, eds. Adult and pediatric urology, ed 2. St Louis, Mosby–Year Book, 1991)

cytes. Levels of oxalic and L-glyceric acid are elevated in the urine of patients with this defect (Fig. 92-48). Both defects cause increased endogenous production of oxalate with hyperoxaluria, urolithiasis, nephrocalcinosis, and renal injury. Extrarenal deposition of calcium oxalate (oxalosis) occurs when renal insufficiency is present, with the associated elevation of plasma oxalate. Treatment can prevent progression in many of the patients. In a subset of about 30% of patients with type 1 primary hyperoxaluria, 1.5 to 3 mg/kg/d of pyridoxine may reduce the urinary excretion of oxalate. Magnesium oxide, 6.5 mg/kg/d, has been reported to prevent stone formation and progression of renal disease in these patients. Magnesium forms a soluble complex with oxalate in urine, reducing the free oxalate ion activity and decreasing the level of saturation of calcium oxalate. Orthophosphate, a liquid preparation of sodium potassium phosphate, in combination with pyridoxine is effective for treatment in children with primary hyperoxaluria. When these patients develop renal failure, dialysis is ineffective in preventing the continuing accumulation of calcium oxalate as oxalosis throughout the body (oxalosis). Before significant oxalosis occurs, renal transplantation can be effective in restoring normal kidney function and allowing control of the disease.[105]

Xanthinuria is a rare autosomal recessive disorder caused by the deficiency of the enzyme xanthine oxidase involved in the final steps of purine metabolism and in the production of uric acid (Fig. 92-49). Secondary to this deficiency, there is an increase in the urinary excretion of xanthine and hypoxanthine, with a marked decrease in urinary excretion of uric acid. Serum uric acid levels are less than 1 mg/dL. In about one third of patients, xanthinuria results in formation of radiolucent urinary calculi that resemble uric acid stones. Because xanthine has two pK levels (7.7 and 10.6), pH manipulation in urine has only minor effect on its solubility.

Preventive treatment includes reduction of dietary purines

and high fluid intake.[106] Deficiency of adenine phosphoribosyl-transferase results in disposal of adenine as 8-hydroxyadenine and 2,8-dihydroxyadenine. The second compound is relatively insoluble in the urine, and crystalluria, urinary stones, and renal insufficiency may occur. This is also an autosomal recessive disorder, usually recognized in children with symptoms and signs of urinary stones. These stones resemble uric acid and xanthine stones on radiographs. Treatment includes dietary re-

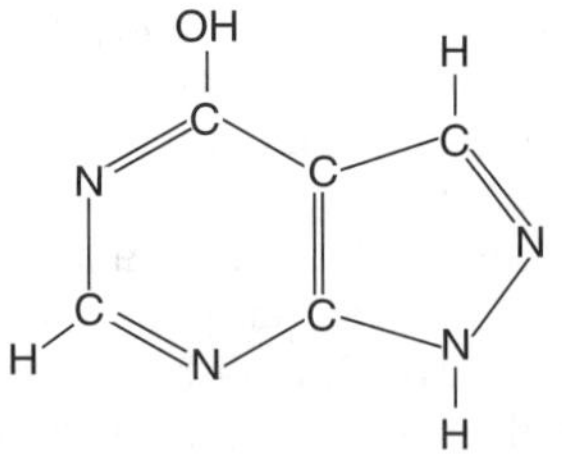

FIG. 92-50. Structure of allopurinol, an analogue of hypoxanthine and xanthine. (Gillenwater JY, Grayhack JT, Howards SS, et al, eds. Adult and pediatric urology, ed 2. St Louis, Mosby–Year Book, 1991)

duction of purine, increased fluid intake, and administration of allopurinol (Fig. 92-50), which blocks the alternative pathway for the oxidation of adenine and thus prevents the production of 2,8-dihydroxyadenine.[107]

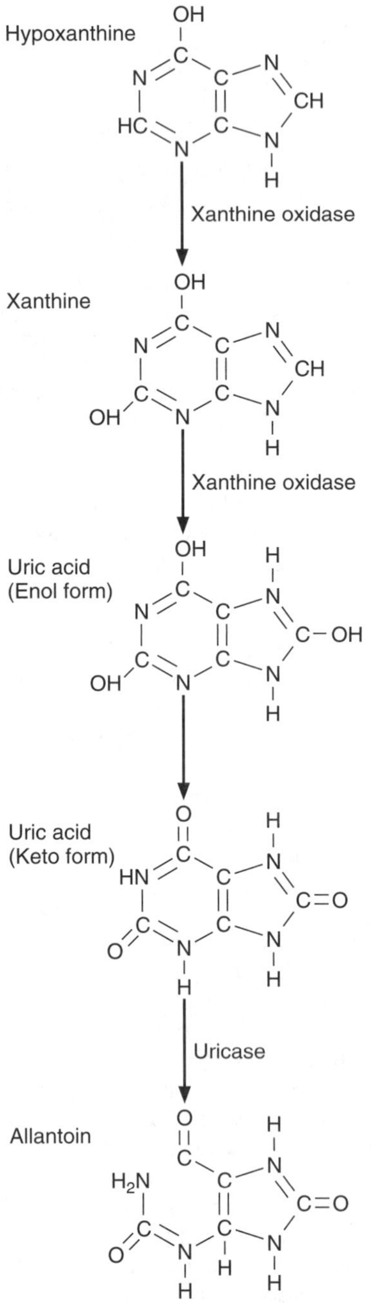

Renal Tubular Syndromes: Cystine Stones

Cystinuria is an autosomal recessive disorder of amino acid transport involving cystine, ornithine, lysine, and arginine. The membrane transport of these amino acids is defective in both the kidney and the intestine. In the homozygote state, the urinary excretion of all four amino acids is significantly increased. Cystine stone formation is the only complication of cystinuria, and the diagnosis is made by demonstrating one of three observations: (1) presence of hexagonal cystine crystals in the urine, usually in the acidic first morning urine, (2) presence of cystine stones on analysis by infrared spectroscopy, or (3) presence of cystinuria (more than 5.7 mg/kg/24 h) with a quantitative analysis of the urine. The goal of treatment is to reduce the level of saturation of cystine in the urine by dilution, diet, increased pH to more than 7.2, and limiting cystine excretion. Patients who excrete less than 800 mg/d of cystine can be controlled by alkalinizing the urine and hydration, maintaining a urine volume of 40 to 50 mL/kg/24 h. Because protein (especially methionine) and sodium can increase cystine excretion, intake of these should be reduced. Alkalinization of urine with potassium citrate to a pH of more than 7.2 significantly increases the solubility of cystine in urine but is associated with a risk of precipitation of calcium phosphate. D-penicillamine and α-mercaptopropionylglycine (Thiola) can reduce the urinary excretion of cystine. Both resemble cysteine in their chemical structures, and they combine with it to form a mixed disulfide that is much more soluble than cystine in the urine. These drugs are associated with serious side effects, such as bone marrow suppression, nephrotic syndrome, epidermolysis bullosa, systemic lupus, and Goodpasture syndrome. In patients whose cystine excretion is greater than 14 mg/kg/24 h, conservative management with fluid, diet, and alkalinization is not enough to prevent stone formation, and one of these drugs is necessary. For prevention of new cystine stone formation, treatment should aim for an excretion rate between 8 and 11 mg/kg/24 h. This can be accomplished with a dosage of 14 mg/kg/24 h with either drug. For dissolution of existing cystine stones, it is desirable to reduce cystine excretion to less than 5 mg/kg/24 h, and a dose as high as 30 mg/kg/24 h may be needed.[108,109]

FIG. 92-49. Metabolic pathway for conversion of hypoxanthine to xanthine and uric acid. Most ureotelic mammals, except humans, have hepatic uricase that converts uric acid into more soluble allantoin. (Gillenwater JY, Grayhack JT, Howards SS, et al, eds. Adult and pediatric urology, ed 2. St Louis, Mosby–Year Book, 1991)

RTA is classified into three types based on the disturbance of acid–base balance within the kidney. Type 1 RTA involves the transport of acid in the distal tubule. Two specific defects have been defined. In the first, the distal tubular cell can secrete hydrogen ion into the lumen, but at that point, it leaks back into the cell, decreasing hydrogen ion excretion and increasing sodium and potassium loss. In the second, the distal tubular cell is unable to secrete hydrogen ion into the tubular lumen. These patients cannot excrete an acidic urine (pH less than 5.4), even in the presence of systemic acidosis. Clinically, in patients with this disorder, muscle weakness, osteomalacia, growth retardation, calcium phosphate urolithiasis, and nephrocalcinosis may develop. Type 2 RTA is associated with a defect in bicarbonate reclamation in the proximal renal tubule and with urolithiasis or nephrocalcinosis in the proximal renal tubule. Patients with type 3 RTA have both proximal and distal tubular defects, and because of the distal tubular component, stones and nephrocalcinosis develop. An example of this is the patient who has been given carbonic anhydrase inhibitor, usually for treatment of glaucoma. Carbonic anhydrase is involved in bicarbonate reclamation in the proximal tubule and hydrogen ion generation in the distal tubule. Its inhibition creates both a proximal and distal defect with associated intracellular metabolic acidosis, hypocitric aciduria, and recurrent calcium phosphate stones in the urinary tract.

Type 1 RTA can be inherited in an autosomal dominant manner; more often, it is an acquired defect. The diagnosis of type 1 RTA is made by demonstrating that the kidney cannot acidify urine below pH 5.4 in the presence of systemic acidosis and in the absence of abnormalities of ammonia and bicarbonate metabolism and transport. If the fasting pH is greater than 5.4, an ammonium chloride load is given as 100 mg/kg/24 h. If the urinary pH remains above 5.4, with a plasma bicarbonate concentration below 20 mEq/L without a bicarbonate leak, the diagnosis of type 1 RTA is confirmed, and the test is discontinued. If the bicarbonate concentration in the plasma is 20 mEq/L or more, a second dose of ammonium chloride is given, and the test is repeated 4 hours later.[110] Treatment of patients with type 1 RTA involves correction of the metabolic acidosis with base and replacement of potassium and sodium loss. Treatment with a sodium potassium citrate solution that provides 2 mEq of base, 1 mEq of sodium, and 1 mEq of potassium per milliliter usually is effective.

Hypercalcemic States

Hypercalcemia of any cause can lead to urolithiasis. Hyperparathyroidism is rare in childhood and almost never occurs before puberty. When hyperparathyroidism does occur, it is often complicated by the formation of urinary stones. Immobilization is more common in childhood, and it can lead to hypercalcemia and hypercalciuria; usually, it is associated with multiple fractures. In this setting, calcium is mobilized from the bone, with resultant hypercalcemia, low levels of parathyroid hormone, and massive hypercalciuria that may result in calcium urolithiasis. This complication can be prevented by high fluid intake, mobilization as rapidly as possible, and the use of orthophosphate. Other, rare causes of hypercalcemia include hypercortisolism, hyperthyroidism, sarcoidosis, hypervitaminosis D, milk alkali syndrome, and malignant neoplasms. It is important to correct these underlying conditions to prevent urolithiasis formation.[111]

Uric Acid Stones

In children, uric acid lithiasis is rare, occurring most commonly in the setting of uric acid overproduction. The pK of uric acid is 5.75; at pH below this level, there is an increased concentration of insoluble uric acid. As pH approaches 7, uric acid exists as a urate salt, which is much more soluble. Children with myeloproliferative disorders, presenting acutely or in relapse, may be associated with gross overproduction of uric acid, with uric acid gravel and stones being formed. In addition, during the early treatment phase, when there is excessive cell breakdown and increased purine metabolism, patients are at risk for uric acid stone formation. Several enzymatic disorders result in an overproduction of uric acid, with uric acid lithiasis, uric acid nephropathy, and gout. Uric acid stones are typically radiolucent, producing a filling defect during the excretory urogram. These stones may be visible, particularly on tomogram, when their size is about 1 cm. Treatment involves the following:

- Dilution by increasing fluid intake to maintain a urine flow between 30 and 40 mL/kg/24 h
- Alkalinization of the urine to pH 6.5 by using a potassium salt of citrate or bicarbonate
- Reduction of uric acid production by the use of the xanthine oxidase inhibitor allopurinol

Enteric Urolithiasis

Intestinal malabsorption from any cause can create a group of abnormalities within the urinary tract that favor the formation of urinary calculi. These include decreased urine volume, increased solute concentration, and decreased urinary excretion of electrolytes with a resulting decrease in ionic strength in the urine. With magnesium malabsorption, the urinary excretion of magnesium decreases, and more of the oxalate present in urine is in the free ionic form. Malabsorption of protein, phosphate, and sulfate decreases the concentration of phosphate and sulfate in urine. Both are important complexors of calcium. Bicarbonate loss causes a mild intracellular metabolic acidosis. This results in a marked reduction in the urinary excretion of citrate. Enteric hyperoxaluria often occurs in patients with intestinal malabsorption when a significant portion of the colon is intact. The fatty acid malabsorption causes saponification with calcium, reducing the concentration of calcium within the intestinal contents. Calcium normally complexes with oxalate to reduce oxalate absorption. If calcium is not available, the oxalate is present as oxalic acid, which is absorbed more easily and this is excreted via the urinary tract.

The second factor that may play a role is the malabsorption of bile acids, which also increase the colon's permeability to oxalate.

Treatment involves increasing the fluid intake to maximum tolerance. The oxalate in the diet should be reduced to the absolute minimum, and dietary calcium should be increased to about 20 mg/kg/24 h. If steatorrhea is present with fatty acid malabsorption, dietary fat should be reduced to about 700 mg/kg/24 h. If bile acid malabsorption is a principal factor in the patient's diarrhea, cholestyramine can reduce the diarrhea and malabsorption. In addition, magnesium replacement and potassium citrate can correct the electrolyte and acid–base disturbances.[112] If uric acid stone formation is a component of the patient's problem, allopurinol can be considered in addition to increasing urinary pH.

Idiopathic Calcium Oxalate Urolithiasis

Idiopathic calcium oxalate urolithiasis is a diagnosis of exclusion, made after other primary metabolic causes of stone formation have been eliminated. It is the most common metabolic cause of urolithiasis in children, often becoming symptomatic after the onset of puberty. Patients usually demonstrate recurrent stone formation. This syndrome occurs commonly in families in an autosomal dominant pattern of inheritance. A classification of this syndrome was proposed by Pak and colleagues.[113] Absorptive hypercalciuria is present when the fasting urine calcium excretion is normal (less than 0.11 mg calcium per 1 mg creatinine) and when hypercalciuria appears with the calcium load. Renal hypercalciuria is present when the urine calcium level is elevated in the fasting state (more than 0.14 mg calcium per 1 mg creatinine). Other abnormalities described in these patients include hyperoxaluria, hyperuricosuria, hypocitruria, and inhibitor deficiencies. Treatment of patients with idiopathic calcium oxalate urolithiasis begins with emphasis on the importance of fluid intake and diet adjustment. The initial agent used to treat hypercalciuria is a thiazide diuretic, such as hydrochlorothiazide, 0.7 mg/kg/24 h in two divided doses. This drug can achieve a 50% reduction of the urinary excretion of calcium. Hypokalemia may develop and should be corrected by potassium citrate. The response to thiazide therapy should be carefully monitored by 24-hour urine collection for calcium, sodium, and citrate, and by kidney–ureter–bladder radiographs with tomograms to assess for new stone formation. If the response is inadequate, the thiazide dose should be doubled. Orthophosphates have been successfully used in patients with idiopathic calcium oxalate urolithiasis who have hypercalciuria, but usually this treatment is reserved for patients who fail to respond to thiazide therapy.[114]

Secondary Urolithiasis

Infection with an organism that produces urease can result in magnesium ammonium phosphate, or struvite, stone formation. The urea-splitting bacteria convert urea into ammonium, raising the pH to greater than 7.2. This allows for precipitation of the constituents and increases the ammonium concentration. These stones are moderately opaque, laminated, and usually large. Often, they branch, forming staghorn calculi. The organisms isolated in this setting are most often *Proteus* sp, although *Klebsiella*, *Pseudomonas*, *Providencia*, *Mycoplasma*, and *Staphylococcus* sp can also produce urease and create this situation. Treatment includes complete surgical removal of all stone material or foreign bodies, correction of the anatomy, and prevention of UTI.[115] Acetohydroxamic acid, 10 to 15 mg/kg/24 h, a urease inhibitor, may be of value in the immediate postoperative period after struvite stone removal to help in the dissolution of small retained fragments that could serve as nidi for recurrent stone formation. This drug is not commonly used, however, owing to severe side effects that include headaches, gastrointestinal disturbances, and neurologic symptoms.[116]

Urinary diversions are commonly associated with infection and stone formation. In the past, when ureterosigmoidostomy was common, metabolic changes caused by bicarbonate loss from the gut created a hyperchloremic hypokalemic metabolic acidosis associated with hypercalciuria and hypocitruria. Ileal conduit and continent urinary diversions are less likely to create these metabolic problems, but ureteral reflux from the conduit to the kidneys and the stasis in a continent pouch may play a role in both infection and stone formation in these cases.[117]

Bladder Stone Disease

Bladder stones in patients in industrialized countries are almost always related to anatomic and functional abnormalities of the bladder that are associated with stasis of urine, such as bladder diverticula, chronic bladder outlet obstruction, and neurogenic bladder. In addition, bowel-augmented bladder and continent pouches are more prone to stone formation due to mucus production and chronic infections. Thus, meticulous bladder emptying and daily irrigation to remove the mucus may prevent stone formation. Etiologic factors important in stone formation include diet, infection, infestation, dehydration, and feeding patterns in young infants. For example, in Thailand, a diet low in milk and early rice supplementation, which is high in oxalate percussors and oxalate and depleted of phosphate, is the major etiologic factor in calcium oxalate crystalluria and stone formation.[118] In these patients, phosphate supplementation corrects the crystalluria and appears to prevent stone formation.[119]

Management of Urolithiasis

The indications for stone removal in children are similar to those in adults and include a symptomatic stone, an obstructing stone, or a stone that is a source of infection. Until recently, almost all stones necessitated an open surgical procedure for removal. In the past 15 years, with the development of percutaneous nephrolithotripsy (PCNL), ureteroscopy, and extracorporeal shock wave lithotripsy (ESWL), the incidence of open surgery has been reduced significantly.

Extracorporeal Shock Wave Lithotripsy

Shock waves are generated and focused by one of four systems: (1) spark-gap generated, ellipsoid focused; (2) piezoelectric generated, spherical dish focused; (3) electromagnetic generated, acoustic lens focused; and (4) explosive-pellet generated, ellipsoid focused. Generally, the spark-gap generated, ellipsoid focused systems are the most powerful. Localization of the stone or placing the stone in the focal point (F2) is effected by fluoroscopy, ultrasonography, or plain radiographs. The procedure is usually done under general anesthesia. It is effective for stones less than 2 cm in the urinary tract and more effective for nephrolithiasis than for ureterolithiasis. In choosing ESWL as a therapeutic tool, its efficacy and risks should be considered. ESWL generates small parenchymal scars in the kidney. In adults, these scars are of no long-term significance. It has been experimentally demonstrated in animals, however, that substantial scars develop in the very young and that these scars are permanent.[120] In children who underwent ESWL, the growth of the kidney appeared normal, and there was no permanent drop in renal function at 3-year follow-up.[121] In general, stones break up well in children, perhaps because the shock wave is less attenuated by body mass than in adults. Moreover, in children, the ureter is more distensible and flexible, so even large fragments usually pass readily, but unresponsive fragments require invasive maneuvers for removal. Cystine stones larger than 1 cm are relatively unresponsive to ESWL; therefore, they should be treated primarily with PCNL. ESWL should be avoided if obstructive uropathy is present because the broken pieces cannot pass spontaneously. Placement of a stent often enables the patient to pass fragments that might otherwise collect in the ureter, forming an obstructive column (stein strasse). Also, ESWL may play a role in patients with residual disease after surgery or PCNL.[122]

Percutaneous Nephrolithotripsy

Percutaneous nephrolithotripsy may be indicated for kidney stones that are larger than 2 cm, staghorn stones, cystine stones, upper ureteral stones that failed ESWL, or as a part of percutaneous endourologic procedure for calyceal diverticula or UPJ obstruction. With the child under general anesthesia, access to the kidney is achieved by insertion of a percutaneous nephrostomy tube, usually under fluoroscopic control. The tract is then dilated to a size sufficient to introduce working instruments (up to 24F). The stone is broken under fluoroscopy and direct vision with direct lithotripsy using ultrasonic, electrohydraulic, or pulse dye laser energy. The smaller the patient, the narrower

is the margin of error[123]; inadvertent fluid absorption generating fluid overload may be the greatest risk. Disability and morbidity after the procedure are minimal, and most patients remain in the hospital for 2 to 4 days.[124]

Ureteroscopy

Transurethral endoscopic access to the ureter usually is indicated for lower ureteral stones that do not pass spontaneously. The limitation of this procedure in children has always been the small size of the child's ureter relative to the available instruments, and the necessity of dilating the ureter, which can result in reflux. Ureteroscopes as small as 6.3F are now available that are suitable for pediatric applications, allowing the lower third of the pediatric ureter to be entered and examined without ureteral dilation. With the child under general anesthesia, the ureteral stone is approached, and the breakdown of the stone is usually achieved with the ultrasonic probe. In selected cases, ureteroscopy can be useful in removing stones that might otherwise require a surgical procedure.[125,126]

Open Surgery

The rate of open surgery for stones in children is higher than in adults because of the limitations of ESWL, PCNL, and ureteroscopy in children. Surgery is rare (about 4%) in children with urolithiasis, however, because urolithiasis in children may be associated with congenital anomalies that should be corrected simultaneously. Generally, lithotomy surgery involves a muscle-splitting abdominal wall incision and opening of the urinary tract through a relatively avascular plane where the stones reside on radiograph. The stones are removed, and the urinary tract is drained with a stent or nephrostomy tube. The urinary tract is closed with fine absorbable sutures (such as chromic catgut 5-0), with retroperitoneal drainage.

92.2   Bladder

Craig A. Peters

Normal bladder function is essential to the physical and psychosocial development of all children. Abnormalities of bladder function can have profound effects on the well-being of a child, ranging from simple family tension as a result of persistent enuresis, to permanent loss of renal function due to hypertonic bladder dysfunction. The work of the bladder rests on two basic functions: storage and emptying. Storage of urine for a socially acceptable period of time requires the bladder to accommodate by enlarging its capacity without increasing its pressure. Bladder compliance is the critical parameter involved in normal storage. Normal emptying of the bladder permits continence of urine between emptying and efficient evacuation of the stored urine in a timely fashion, under voluntary control. This action

requires the coordination of the detrusor muscle of the bladder with the bladder neck or internal sphincter and the skeletal or voluntary sphincter. The contraction must be sustained for a sufficiently long period to permit complete emptying. Discoordination of the activities of the detrusor and sphincter produce significant derangements in bladder function and can produce permanent damage.

A basic understanding of the activity of the bladder is essential to permit clinical assessment and management of various bladder disorders. Bladder dysfunction has become an active area of investigation as the clinical, social, and economic significance of bladder diseases has become evident. Clinical understanding of childhood bladder dysfunction has developed rapidly in the past 15 to 20 years, but the scientific knowledge that should be the basis of clinical understanding is only now emerging.

One reason for the lack of basic scientific knowledge of the pediatric bladder is the influence of development on bladder function and dysfunction, creating a highly dynamic system with multiple interacting factors. Abnormalities of the bladder that occur during development may change the patterns of bladder function and development in mutually interdependent ways. Understanding this relation is critical to the continued investigation of pediatric bladder disease.

This chapter briefly reviews normal bladder anatomy and function, patterns of bladder development, and the manifestations of bladder diseases. The assessment and management of the major categories of bladder dysfunction are presented. Areas of developing knowledge that will influence therapy are also reviewed.

NORMAL BLADDER ANATOMY AND FUNCTION

Although the basic structure and function of the bladder may appear simple, the bladder is an organ dependent on complex interactions of autonomic and voluntary neural regulation as well as smooth and skeletal muscle groups to store and expel a hypertonic solution without significant absorption or inadvertent leakage. Clinically significant bladder disorders are the result of various failures in these processes. The functional anatomy of the urinary bladder has been the subject of vigorous investigation in adults, principally aimed at understanding bladder outlet obstruction in men, incontinence in women, and neurologic bladder disease in spinal cord injury patients. Many of the principles of bladder function in adults are applicable to children, yet this assumption should not be too broadly applied.

Anatomy

The bladder in the young child is an intraabdominal organ that becomes progressively intrapelvic with age. It is extraperitoneal, which permits most surgical exposures to be performed without peritoneal entry. The ureters enter posterolaterally from the deep posterior pelvis and are associated with the obliterated umbilical arteries, the vas deferens in boys, and the uterine ligaments and fallopian tubes in girls. The base of the bladder rests on the pelvic floor, or the urogenital diaphragm, an important structure in the maintenance of continence. The suspension of the bladder neck from the pelvic floor and symphysis pubis is particularly important for continence in girls.

The bladder is usually divided into two anatomic parts, the body or detrusor and the base, including the trigone and bladder neck. As noted earlier, these are of distinct embryologic origin, with functional and neurophysiologic differences. The detrusor is composed of an inner epithelial layer with three cell layers, including a basal cell layer and a relatively impermeable luminal epithelial layer. Beneath the uroepithelium is the lamina propria, consisting of connective tissue elements, which may have significant functional importance as the mediators of bladder compliance.[127] The implications of these preliminary observations is that if the lamina propria is altered by disease processes, changes in bladder compliance may be expected. The

muscular layers of the bladder are not as distinctly organized into longitudinal and circumferential layers as in the intestine. Rather, they are more of an interdigitating meshwork of smooth muscle bundles and connective tissue elements, including fibroblasts, collagen fibers, and elastin, along with several other extracellular matrix components.

Uroepithelium

The biologic properties of the uroepithelium are only recently coming to be recognized. Previously considered impermeable, there is evidence to indicate selective permeability with ion transport that may be influenced by mechanical factors. A layer of glycosaminoglycans probably acts as a protective coat, and disruptions in this layer are thought to be related to several inflammatory conditions, including interstitial cystitis.[128] They are likely to play a role in resistance to infection as well. As noted earlier, the uroepithelium appears to be important in the developmental regulation of bladder formation,[129] and it may continue to play a regulatory role in the function of the detrusor muscle. This relation may be a two-way communication network.

Muscular Components

The muscular layer of the trigone merges inferiorly into the proximal urethra, and taken together, this muscular complex functions as a sphincter. Although there is no anatomically distinct sphincter, its functional existence is supported by urethral pressure studies, by video urodynamic observations, and by the fact that continence may be maintained with its sole presence, or lost with injury. Its function as a sphincter is augmented by soft tissue coaptation and elasticity, loss of which impairs continence. These smooth muscle fibers may be seen to interdigitate with skeletal muscle of the external sphincter.[130,131] The skeletal muscle sphincter is more anatomically distinct and acts to maintain continence with activity and to permit voluntary termination of urination. Discoordination of the activity of the sphincters with that of the detrusor may lead to significant bladder dysfunction (see later).

Innervation and Neural Control of Bladder Function

The bladder is richly innervated by sacral parasympathetic fibers from S-2 to S-4, thoracolumbar sympathetic fibers, and sacral somatic fibers traveling through the pudendal nerves.[132] Bladder function is regulated through the interactions of both autonomic and voluntary neural systems, with both spinal and brain-stem reflex arcs as well as cerebral control over their activity. A variety of neural effectors are active in normal bladder function, and many neurotransmitters have been shown to influence bladder function. The basic bladder functions and their neural control include filling and storage, which requires relaxation of the detrusor and concomitant sphincter contraction, and emptying, which depends on a sustained bladder contraction with coordinated sphincteric relaxation.

Filling and storage of the bladder must be at low pressure. Two primary factors contribute to these properties of the bladder. The smooth muscle of the bladder must relax against a passive stretch induced by increasing bladder volume.[133] Smooth muscle relaxation has been shown to be an active process, mediated at a molecular level by dephosphorylation of myosin light chains as well as by changes in a Ca^{2+}-dependent force maintenance system referred to as a *latch state*.[134,135] Centrally, relaxation is mediated through storage reflexes that increase the inhibitory impulses to the bladder as intravesical pressure rises. These impulses are mostly sympathetic, mediated by the β-adrenergic receptor system. This occurs with increased sphincter activity and is thought to be controlled at the level of the lateral pontine reticular formation. This relation underscores the conceptual notion that bladder function is often determined by balances between excitatory and inhibitory influences. Although bladder function is biphasic (storage and emptying), switching between these phases appears to be the result of alterations in thresholds of activity that are influenced by a dynamic balance of excitatory and inhibitory influences.

The extracellular matrix is also important in bladder storage characteristics, possibly more than the muscular components, and is described by the viscoelastic properties of the connective tissue matrix.[136,137] The importance of this element of bladder compliance is particularly relevant in the child with a non-compliant bladder from prior obstruction because developmental alterations in matrix remodeling have been shown to occur with fetal obstruction.[138] The folding and unfolding of connective tissue bundles, and the properties of individual fibers, such as elastin, contribute to the overall properties of the bladder as it fills with urine.

Bladder emptying requires initiation and maintenance of a detrusor contraction, coordinated with relaxation of the sphincters under voluntary control. The infant demonstrates involuntary or reflex voiding. This is largely without inhibitory influences from the cortex, which develop with toilet training. Central coordination is through the pontine micturition center, which acts as a switch, triggered by a level of afferent or sensory impulses from the bladder as it fills. Activation of the sacral parasympathetics inhibits the somatic pathways to the urethral sphincter and permits relaxation. Sympathetic activity, which permits bladder filling, is inhibited, and parasympathetic activation of the bladder occurs. Cortical inhibition of these reflexes can prevent onset of micturition.

The mediators of bladder neural control have been widely studied. The principal neuropharmacologic mechanisms include the cholinergic and adrenergic systems, and recently described purinergic and peptidergic mechanisms are likely to play an important role in function and dysfunction. Cholinergic receptors in the bladder body are largely muscarinic (M2) and act to stimulate muscle contraction. They are balanced by adrenergic β_2-receptor mechanisms. Purinergic receptors responsive to ATP or adenosine contribute to the contractile response and may serve to initiate a contraction, which is then sustained by cholinergic activity. Adrenergic activity in the bladder neck and urethra is mostly α-receptor mediated and stimulatory. Selective agonists and antagonists have permitted demonstration of site-specific receptor subtype distribution and therefore more specific pharmacologic control over function. Peptidergic neurotransmission has been documented in the bladder, including activity of vasoactive intestinal peptide, neuropeptide Y, substance P, somatostatin, calcitonin gene–related peptide, cholecystokinin, and enkephalin immunoreactive fibers. The functional roles of these neurotransmitters remain unclear, yet are clearly complex and likely to act at several levels of neural control, from smooth muscle contraction to modulation of the effects of other neurotransmitters.

The effect of bladder pathology on neural regulation of function is critical to recognize, particularly in the developing child. Abnormal function, as in obstruction, alters development, which then further affects function. Although there is little α-adrenergic activity in the normal bladder body, increases in α sensitivity have been shown to follow obstruction. Changes in the level of existing receptors occur with both prenatal[139] and postnatal obstruction[140–144] and with abnormal innervation.[145] The functional changes induced by obstruction also affect central neural activity and patterns of innervation.[146–148] This may have long-lasting effects, even after the inducing abnormality has been corrected. The concept of neural plasticity in the regulation of bladder function, particularly in the developing bladder, is critical.

Normal bladder function may be seen as a dynamic balance between the two basic phases of bladder activity: storage and emptying. Neural, muscular, and matrix components contribute to that balance. Abnormalities in those components are the basis for many bladder disorders. Improved understanding of the normal and abnormal integration of those factors and their clinical manifestations will permit more specific therapeutic intervention for children with bladder disorders.

BLADDER DEVELOPMENT

Embryonic Formation and Associations

The bladder forms from the embryonic entoderm and the trigone from the mesoderm.[149] The bladder epithelial surface derives from the entodermal layer and may have a significant role in the induction and maturation of the mesodermal layer as it becomes the detrusor muscle and connective tissues of the bladder wall.[129] As the ventral plate of the embryo infolds, the combined bladder and gut structures take on the form of a tube and become the cloaca as a common channel. At this stage, there is no opening at what will become the perineum, but the allantois is patent and runs parallel to the umbilical vessels. Separation of the ventral bladder and dorsal gut structures occurs between 5 and 8 weeks' gestation, concurrent with separation of the ureter and mesonephric duct and with ingrowth of the urorectal septum. The trigone (triangular area bounded by the ureteral orifices and bladder neck) is initially mesodermal but is ultimately surfaced by entodermal epithelium. The cloacal membrane remains closed at this time but is hypothesized to rupture early in the production of cloacal exstrophy. When fully separate from the hind gut, the bladder begins to receive urine from the metanephric kidneys (8 weeks' gestation). The ureteral structures and associated mesonephric structures are still developing. It is likely that epithelial and mesenchymal interactions similar to the induction of the bladder mesoderm continue to influence maturation of these structures, although little specific evidence is available to prove this.

Development of Musculature

An important element in the bladder that develops in the late embryonic and early fetal period is the bladder musculature.

Muscle cells are first seen at about 7 weeks' gestation, and recognizable bundles are present by 12 weeks' gestation.[150–154] Either bladder myocytes migrate from surrounding mesenchyme, or the undifferentiated mesodermal cells surrounding the bladder epithelium are induced to differentiate in a muscular pattern. It is likely that bladder filling and emptying play a role in modulating this process; bladders that have never functioned (eg, exstrophy of the bladder) have a variety of developmental differences from normal bladders. The onset of this interaction may not occur until closure of the urachus, which occurs at about 16 weeks' gestation. Innervation of the bladder is likely to begin at this point because receptors for various neurotransmitters have been shown in the early fetal bladder.[154–157] Muscularization of the bladder continues with further growth and presumed integration of muscles and nerves. Little is known about the mediators of bladder innervation in the fetus. The functional characteristics of bladder smooth muscle cells in the fetus have been investigated, with focus on the ontogeny of calcium regulation of contractility[158,159] as well as the presumed role of nitric oxide.[157] Sphincter function can be demonstrated at 8 weeks' gestation and is followed by development of the ureterovesical junction. Studies have examined the development of the external urethral sphincter in boys.[160]

The extracellular matrix of the fetal bladder has been examined in a variety of systems. Relative developmental increases of collagen type I have been reported in the bovine fetus[161] and are associated with developmental increases in bladder compliance.[162] These observations differ from those of Swaiman and Bradley[163] and Kim and colleagues[164] in humans, in which the developmental balance between type I and III collagen decreases, which is the reverse of that seen in the fetal calf. The author's laboratory has not been able to identify such alterations in fetal sheep using gene expression analysis.[138] These investigations are useful in the focus on the important functional role of the extracellular matrix in bladder development and function. Other components of the matrix are likely be equally important, particularly elastin.

Fetal Bladder Function

Bladder function is ongoing in the fetus, and it is likely that structural and functional development is dependent on bladder activity. Defunctionalized bladders in fetal sheep have altered patterns of contractile protein isoforms and altered concentrations of muscarinic cholinergic receptors.[139] Connective tissue elements are influenced by this activity, in that defunctionalized bladders show reduced procollagen type III gene expression.[165] Although many of the mechanisms of interaction are unclear, it has been shown that fetal bladder function is a critical aspect of development.

The patterns of bladder function have been described in humans and in more detail in fetal sheep. Ultrasonographic images of the human fetal bladder show continued filling and emptying cycles in later gestation, with contractions every 10 to 15 minutes.[166,167] Bladder emptying appears to be complete in most. In sheep, urodynamic investigations have demonstrated similar cyclic filling and emptying, but the contraction patterns are distinct from those seen postnatally. A phasic pattern of contraction, which may be most consistent with incomplete innervation, can be seen in the near-term sheep.[168] The response to

pharmacologic agents has also been described, including agents commonly used in obstetric practice. Magnesium sulfate, for example, suppresses almost all bladder contractions in the fetus, and postnatal voiding may be impaired until this effect has cleared.

Ultrasonographic Appearances

Maternal–fetal ultrasound can detect many bladder abnormalities, both directly and indirectly. Identification of the bladder on maternal–fetal ultrasound should be possible by 16 to 18 weeks' gestation in the normal fetus. The inability to demonstrate the bladder despite two or more attempts is abnormal and should prompt consideration of severe renal dysfunction, bladder exstrophy,[169,170] or a severe abnormality of the bladder neck or ureteral positioning. Protrusion of tissue at the level of the lower umbilicus without a visible bladder lumen should raise the possibility of bladder or cloacal exstrophy, and this may be associated with a low-set umbilical cord. When visible, the bladder should be filled with echo-transmitting fluid without debris or internal echogenic structures. A ureterocele may be demonstrated prenatally when present (usually associated with upper pole hydronephrosis). Massive dilation of the fetal bladder may be seen with bladder outlet obstruction as from valves, with massive vesicoureteral reflux,[171] and with the prune belly syndrome. Bladder wall thickness, the condition of the renal parenchyma, and the status of the amniotic fluid are useful in distinguishing between these. The bladder affected by posterior urethral valves (PUVs) may not be massively dilated, but may have a thickened wall and be only moderately full. The kidneys and ureters may be dilated, and the renal parenchyma may be echogenic, indicating some degree of dysplasia.[172–174] Male gender should be identified in such cases, and oligohydramnios may be present. The distinction between obstructive and nonobstructive conditions of the bladder is not always reliable in the fetus.

MANIFESTATIONS OF BLADDER DISEASE

The principal manifestations of bladder disorders include incontinence of urine, infection, hydronephrosis, hematuria and dysuria, or an alteration in voiding pattern. Each may be present in a spectrum of severity, with specific characteristics indicative of the underlying condition. Recognition of these signs and symptoms is not always immediate, and in certain situations, they should be specifically sought.

Incontinence

Inadvertent urinary emptying, or incontinence, may be one of the most troubling symptoms to afflict a child after the age of toilet training. Causes range from behavioral patterns to major structural anomalies of the urinary tract or nervous system. The patterns of incontinence serve as the most useful initial tool to define the cause. *Nighttime incontinence,* or nocturnal enuresis, is most often a maturational, self-limiting entity, but it should prompt a thorough history and physical examination to rule out subtle manifestations of more serious disease. *Daytime wetting* is primary if it has always been present, or secondary if it develops after normal training. *Constant dampness* in a girl suggests an ectopic ureter to the distal urethra, introitus, or vagina.[175] *Total incontinence*, wetness without a dry interval, suggests a significant structural defect of the bladder neck (epispadias, bilateral ureteral ectopia) or a neurologic defect. Lesser degrees of these conditions may be manifest by *episodic incontinence*, as with stress or movement. *Urgency incontinence*, in which the child senses the need but cannot inhibit voiding, may be behavioral or neurologic; associated signs and symptoms should be sought. *Overflow incontinence* may be suspected in someone with small to moderate amounts of leakage, usually without urgency to void; a full bladder is identified with examination or catheterization. A structural, neurologic, or behavioral basis may be present and require careful further evaluation.

Infection

Urinary tract infection (UTI) is one of the most common health problems in children[176] and can be a manifestation of bladder dysfunction. Inadequate bladder emptying, with or without obstruction, is the most frequent underlying cause. The association with upper tract infection of the kidney, or pyelonephritis,[177] is largely dependent on the presence or absence of reflux, upper tract drainage, and the nature of the infecting organism. Diagnosis of infection is a critical guide to further evaluation and should be based on a properly collected specimen. In the sick child in whom antibiotics are to be started empirically, a definitive culture must be obtained at the outset, using catheterization or a suprapubic aspirate. Clean voided specimens in trained children with minimal symptoms are acceptable. A bag-collected specimen is of value in a negative culture or if there is unusual pure growth of high colony count. Even so, the false-positive rate is about 50%, and no major therapeutic decision should be based on such a specimen.

The most appropriate evaluation of a child with UTI remains controversial. The clinical distinction between cystitis and upper tract infection remains challenging and unreliable. Infants with a culture-proven infection should undergo ultrasonographic imaging and cystography. Older children may be equally served by ultrasonography alone if normal, although the transition age is not defined. The nature of the infection should guide evaluation. Most major structural and functional abnormalities present with febrile infections, but this is not universal.

Hydronephrosis

Bladder dysfunction may be associated with hydronephrosis as a causative agent or a concomitant factor. Bladder outlet obstruction due to either structural or functional reasons may produce upper tract dilation. Usually, this is bilateral and symmetric (Fig. 92-51), but it may be unilateral. PUVs may cause unilateral high-grade dilation with renal parenchymal disruption (vesicoureteral reflux and renal dysplasia association),[178] in which one renal unit acts as the pressure release of the high-pressure bladder. Very often, obstructed bladders will be thick-walled and hypertrophic. As a result, there may be an element of obstruction at the ureterovesical junction contributing in part

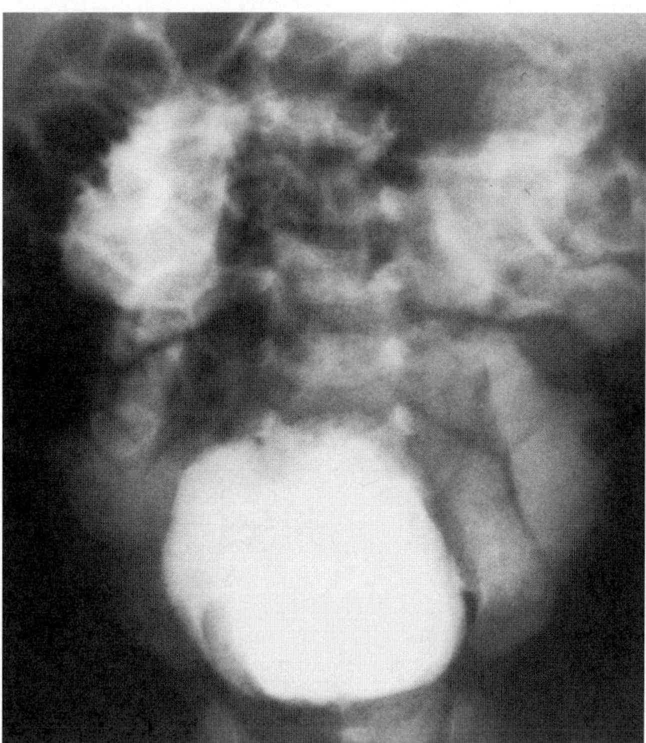

FIG. 92-51. Massive bilateral hydronephrosis due to posterior urethral valves and vesicoureteral reflux in a newborn with prenatally detected valvular bladder obstruction. (Mandell J, Peters CA. Current concepts in the perinatal diagnosis and management of hydronephrosis. Urol Clin North Am 1990; 17:247)

or whole to the upper tract dilation.[179] This factor may be difficult to assess but can be demonstrated by reducing bladder pressures with temporary diversion.

The effect of bladder pressure on upper tract dilation is due to the imbalance between ureteral peristaltic pressure moving urine into the bladder and the pressure within the bladder cavity. Forty centimeters of water pressure is the generally accepted maximal level of pressure generated by the ureter to move urine. Vesical pressures exceeding this cause cessation of flow into the bladder; bladder pressures exceeding this, as during a bladder contraction, can result in increased pressure transmitted to the kidneys. The effect of prolonged elevated pressures on the upper urinary tracts and renal parenchyma has been demonstrated clinically and may produce progressive renal functional deterioration and renal failure. The maximal pressures reached by the bladder with contraction are not the most important factor, however. The total work over time done against the kidney by bladder pressure is most critical and should be assessed to guide management. The product of pressure over the "safe" level of 35 to 40 cm H_2O, and the time during which this occurs, is the work done against the kidney. Normal voiding pressures exceed 35 cm H_2O yet occur only 6 to 8 times per day for 1 to 2 minutes; bladder pressures in the normal range then fall to 5 cm H_2O for the rest of the time. If bladder pressures approach 35 cm H_2O quickly as the bladder refills and stay at that level for most of the bladder filling cycle, the total work against the kidney over a 24-hour period is far greater than normal (Fig.

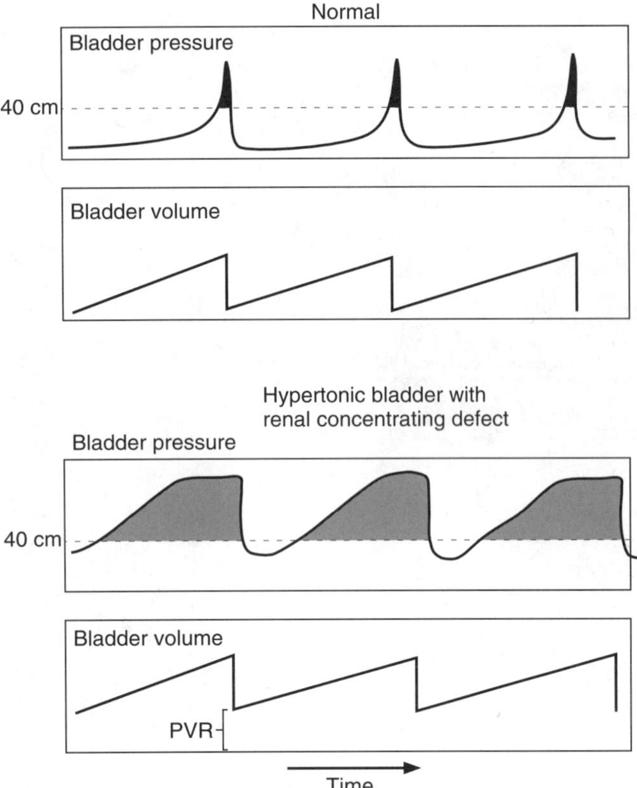

FIG. 92-52. Two schematic representations of bladder pressure and volume curves over several filling and emptying cycles. In the normal bladder, intravesical pressures exceed 40 cm H$_2$O only at the end of filling, near capacity. The work done against the kidneys is small. In contrast, the hypertonic bladder demonstrates an increase in pressure, with small increases in volume due to poor compliance. The pressures reach 40 cm H$_2$O, much sooner than normally. In conjunction with a renal concentrating defect, which is common in boys with posterior urethral valves, high intravesical pressures occur even more quickly owing to rapid bladder filling. If bladder emptying is not complete, as is often the case, the abnormal postvoid residual (PVR) pushes the bladder pressure volume curve further to the right (higher pressures). These factors contribute to a longer period during which intravesical pressures exceed 40 cm H$_2$O and can produce renal damage. Careful evaluation of bladder filling dynamics permits assessment of the safe period of the bladder cycle and serves to guide therapy. (After Peters CA. Congenital bladder obstruction. Curr Probl Urol 1994;8:333)

92-52). This concept of a safe period of bladder filling is critical to determining appropriate bladder management. Hydronephrosis associated with bladder dysfunction should be sought in patients in whom high-pressure bladder patterns may be seen, including those with neuropathic bladders or previously obstructed bladders (so-called valve bladders).[180] When present, hydronephrosis must be dealt with aggressively and monitored diligently by addressing the bladder dysfunction.

Hematuria

Blood in the urine is a dramatic symptom and must be dealt with thoroughly. In children, however, it does not have the same sinister implications as in adults. The pattern of hematuria often provides sufficient clues to permit a diagnosis and guide further evaluation. Total gross hematuria, bloody urine from beginning of voiding to the end, may be associated with flank pain and dysuria or may be painless. Flank pain focuses attention on the ureters and kidneys; dysuria points toward the bladder and urethra; and painless hematuria requires a full evaluation. Ultrasonographic examination of the entire urinary tract is a useful first step and identifies upper tract lesions and most bladder neck lesions, such as tumors or polyps. Viral cystitis in children often is associated with severe voiding pain and urgency and may cause such marked edema of the bladder wall that it mimics a neoplastic process. Occasionally, biopsy is needed to rule this out. Cystoscopy in children is seldom revealing and may serve more to reassure anxious parents. Often, a watchful waiting period is useful because there are few lesions that must be immediately identified that can be missed by a careful physical examination (including rectal examination) and ultrasonography. The nature of the bleeding may serve to guide this decision. Terminal hematuria, occurring at the end of voiding, is indicative of a process at the bladder base or more commonly at the urethra. In peripubertal boys, this is often due to a process termed *benign urethrorrhagia*,[181] a self-limiting condition of unknown cause that does not have long-term sequelae. Cystoscopy is not needed in most cases, and the urethrorrhagia usually resolves within 6 to 8 weeks. Meatal bleeding is most often due to urethral meatal stenosis. This is readily confirmed on examination and by observation of the voiding stream, which typically deviates upward and is thin and jetlike.

Dysuria

Painful urination is a common symptom in children and may be relatively mild or extreme. On occasion, this also is described as suprapubic pain after voiding. Severe abrupt pain during voiding, termed *strangury,* may indicate episodic obstruction as from a stone, particularly if urine flow stops. Dysuria is most often the result of UTI but may also be due to simple perineal irritation, obstruction, or abnormal voiding dynamics. The extreme manifestation of the latter is bladder sphincter discoordination (dyssynergy), which may produce pain in the neurologically intact child. This may be structural or behavioral. In boys with dysuria, it is prudent to rule out a bladder neck obstructive process, such as a tumor, with a rectal examination or ultrasound or both. This is an unusual but sometimes missed diagnosis. Unusual causes of dysuria in children that should be considered include interstitial cystitis, eosinophilic cystitis, and granulomatous disease of the bladder.[182]

Altered Voiding Pattern (Frequency, Decreased Flow, Retention)

Changes in voiding pattern can indicate a variety of problems, most of which can be identified with a careful history and examination. Frequency of urination is most likely due to infection, but it can represent bladder instability due to a neurologic or obstructive process. In kindergarten-age boys, however, this is most often a behavioral, self-limited process termed *poikilouria*.[183] Diminished flow can be the result of outlet resistance, such as a urethral stricture or valves; it also can be due to impaired contractility of the bladder. Urinary retention can result from a semiacute obstructive process, such as tumor of the bladder base or prostate, or from bladder decompensation in a chronic setting of partial obstruction or massive reflux. Unusually, this is due to viral infection (herpes) and rarely is idiopathic or behavioral.

ASSESSMENT OF BLADDER FUNCTION

History

The history of the child's signs and symptoms must be carefully elicited and may serve to focus attention on the appropriate diagnostic possibilities. This serves to guide further evaluation. Important elements of the history were noted earlier in association with the specific signs and symptoms. Other features to consider include pregnancy and birth history of the child, developmental history, and medication exposure. In children with identified diseases or conditions, the surgical history is essential and may be complex; their response to therapy and prior imaging and urodynamic studies are also an essential part of the history.

Imaging

Pediatric urologic imaging is highly specialized and critically important in evaluation and management planning.[184] Ultrasonography has become a mainstay of imaging due to its high resolution and absence of radiation (Fig. 92-53). With careful interpretation, an excellent picture of the anatomy of the entire urinary tract may be obtained, including the urethra in selected cases. Functional inferences may be made, particularly with regard to the bladder if attention is paid to the state of bladder filling, efficiency of emptying, and bladder wall thickness. Ul-

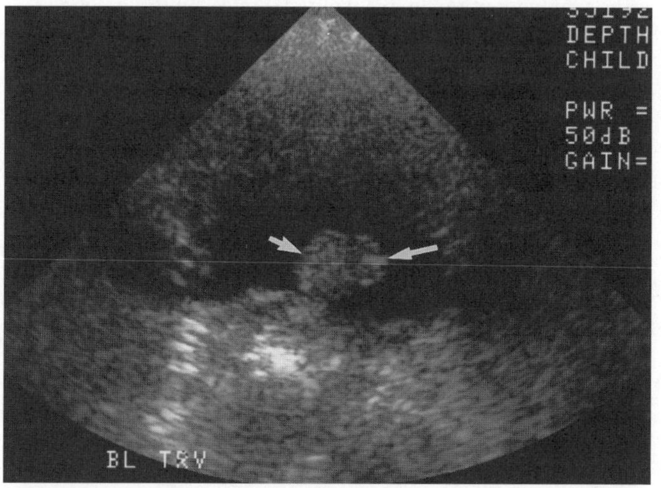

FIG. 92-53. Bladder ultrasound of a bladder neck polyp (*arrows*) in a 4-year-old boy with intermittent bladder neck obstruction, pain, and hematuria. The polyp was fibromuscular and was removed endoscopically by suprapubic access. It could not be removed through the urethra.

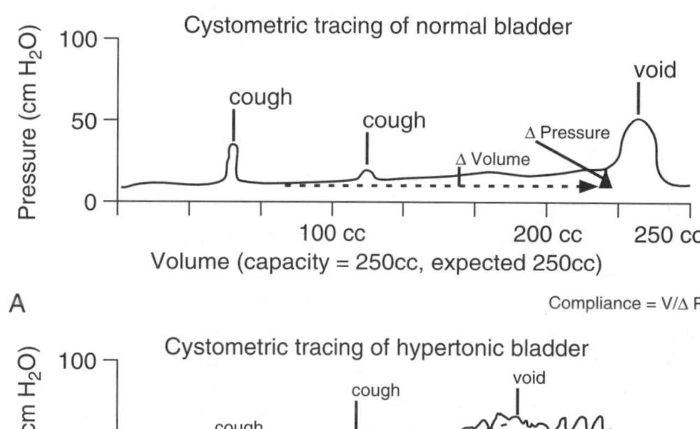

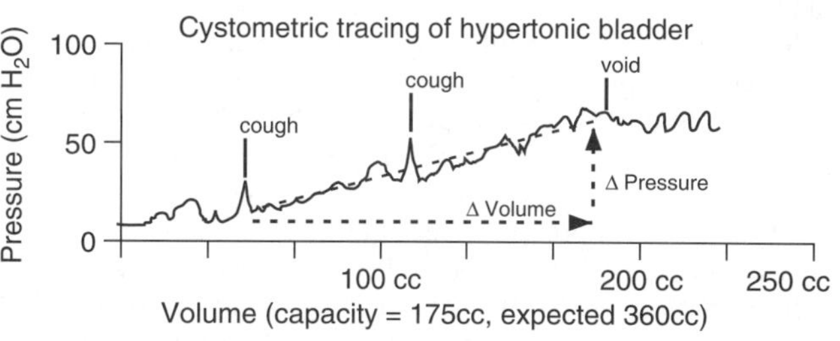

FIG. 92-54. Schematic representation of normal and hypertonic cystometric studies. In the normal bladder, pressure rises little during filling (accommodation), and the compliance (DV/DP) is high. In contrast, the hypertonic bladder often has a reduced capacity, and there are greater rises in pressure with filling; DV/DP is lower than normal.

trasound is particularly useful in long-term follow-up studies. It is important to compare films with prior studies done both immediately before and well before the current study.

Cystography is an important means of bladder evaluation and provides information regarding configuration, emptying, and presence of reflux. The urethra should be well visualized in an adequate study.[185] If voiding cannot be induced, the study should not be considered adequate and should be repeated, if clinically indicated. Radiographic cystography (voiding cystourethrography or micturating cystourethrogram) is usually the best first study to define anatomy; radionuclide cystography is a useful follow-up or screening tool owing to its lower radiation exposure.

Computed tomography and magnetic resonance imaging are important means of defining structural relations of the bladder within the pelvis, particularly in the setting of tumor or trauma.

Urodynamic Evaluation

Functional bladder evaluation is most accurately based on urodynamic studies, which provide objective information regarding the parameters of bladder activity that are the basis for the consequences of bladder dysfunction.[186,187] These include the ability of the bladder to store adequate amounts of urine at low pressures and to empty urine efficiently at appropriate pressures, and the ability of the sphincter mechanisms to retain urine for socially acceptable periods and to relax adequately during voiding. Cystometry is a record of bladder pressure with filling and normally demonstrates low pressures within the bladder as volume increases (Fig. 92-54). As capacity is approached, pressures increase slightly until a voiding contraction is initiated. Pressures then rise rapidly, and if accompanied by sphincter relaxation, voiding occurs. Bladder contractions during filling that cannot be suppressed by the patient are termed *uninhibited contractions* and can be a manifestation of either neurogenic or structural abnormalities. A poorly complaint bladder demonstrates early increases in pressure with filling, and this becomes important when pressures approach the clinically important threshold of 35 to 40 cm H_2O (see Fig. 92-54). Absence of a voiding contraction may be seen with neuropathic bladder dysfunction or postobstructive dysfunction. Abdominal straining can result from trying to empty a noncontracting bladder.

The activity of the bladder sphincter mechanism may be examined using pressure measurements within the urethra, estimating both the level of the pressure and the length over which that pressure is exerted (*functional urethral length;* Fig. 92-55). There is not universal agreement about the interpretation or utility of urethral pressure measurements. An alternative measure of sphincter function is the leak point pressure with either filling or stress such as increased abdominal pressure (Valsalva).[188] These assessments may provide a clinically useful measure of outlet resistance to aid in determination of the basis for urinary incontinence and possible methods of treatment. They must be integrated with an assessment of bladder function and bladder sphincter coordination. Electromyography of the urethral sphincter may permit identification and characterization of neurologic bladder dysfunction and bladder sphincter incoordination (*dyssynergy;* Figs. 92-56 and 92-57).

One of the most important elements of urodynamic evaluations is consistency of application and interpretation. This permits comparisons between patients with similar conditions, and between studies in the same patient, to assess response to therapy or to identify changes in patterns. Most neurologic bladder disorders in children are dynamic, and reliable follow-up is critical to maximize therapeutic outcomes.

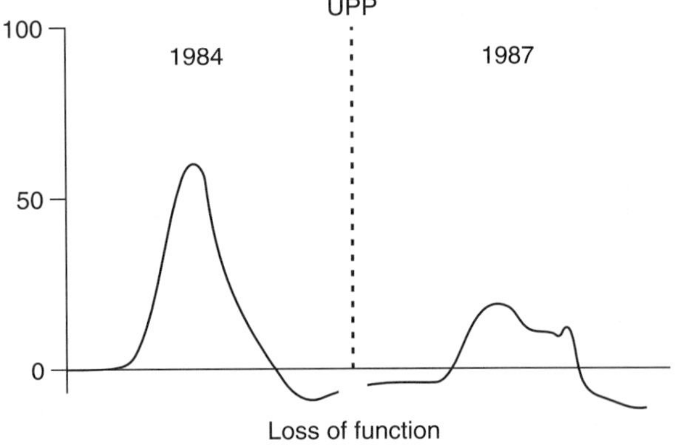

FIG. 92-55. Urethral pressure profiles measured by drawing a urodynamic catheter slowly across the bladder neck and sphincter. The horizontal axis is distance from the bladder neck. The pressure curve (vertical axis in cm H_2O) reflects urethral pressure; the distance along the urethra with elevated pressures is termed the *functional urethral length.* In this child, the urethral pressure profile (UPP) demonstrates decrease in urethral resistance from 1984 to 1987, owing to loss of sphincteric function in the setting of a spinal cord dysraphism. This was associated with increased urinary leakage and was managed with a urethral sling. (Bauer SB, Peters CA, Mandell J, et al. The use of the rectus fascia to manage urinary incontinence. J Urol 1989;142:516)

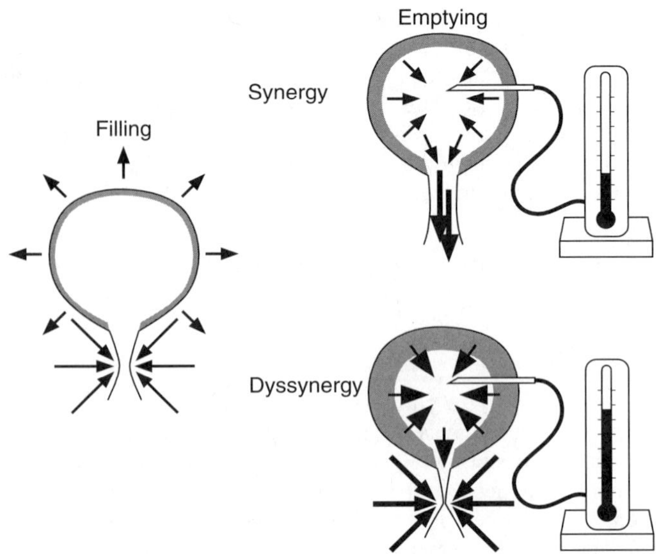

FIG. 92-56. Schematic diagram of normal bladder with outlet relaxation during voiding, contrasted to the dyssynergic bladder in which outlet resistance increases with detrusor contraction. This produces elevated intravesical pressures, which may cause renal damage, as well as bladder hypertrophy and noncompliance.

NEUROGENIC BLADDER DISEASE (TABLE 92-1)

Spinal Dysraphism: Meningomyelocele

Presentation

The child born with meningomyelocele is readily apparent and must be assessed expeditiously. The appearance of a membrane-covered sac along the back is unmistakable (Fig. 92-58). This sac contains neural elements and usually becomes infected if not surgically closed in the first few days of life. Nontreatment is less of an option in the United States but is practiced in certain situations elsewhere. The impact of prenatal screening for α-fetoprotein[189–193] and the use of prophylactic maternal folic acid[194,195] are becoming apparent, and some centers are seeing fewer newborns with this condition. Studies of aborted fetuses with myelomeningocele have shown early changes of bladder wall fibrosis. Whether these changes are due to abnormal innervation affecting bladder development or are the result of abnormal function altering development is unclear. These findings are strong indicators of the profound effect of these lesions on normal bladder development and function.[196]

Neurosurgical closure of the spinal cord defect is usually performed in the first 2 days of life. A basic urologic assessment before closure is optimal, including renal and bladder ultrasound and neurologic examination of the perineum to assess innervation of the sphincter muscles.[182] The presence of hydronephrosis in the newborn indicates abnormal bladder dynamics, usually due to bladder–sphincter dyssynergy. These infants require the most meticulous follow-up to minimize upper tract damage and to preserve bladder compliance. In infants with normal upper urinary tracts, an assessment of bladder emptying is important to determine whether intermittent catheterization

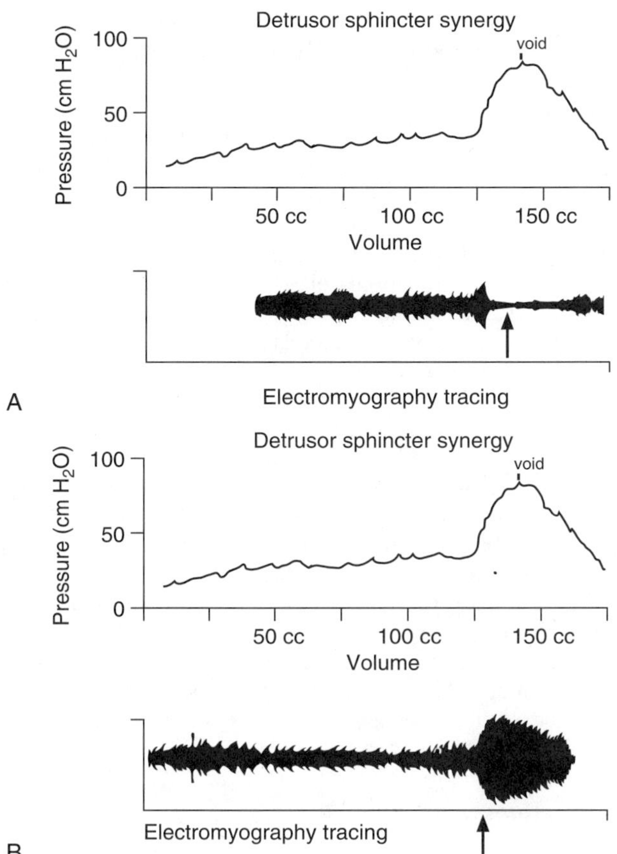

FIG. 92-57. Schematic representation of bladder sphincter electromyographic activity during bladder filling and voiding. (*A*) In the normal bladder, electromyogram activity increases slowly, then slightly moves near capacity, and finally silences during voiding. This indicates coordinated sphincter relaxation during detrusor contraction. (*B*) In contrast, in the abnormal, dyssynergic bladder–sphincter unit, electromyogram activity increases during a detrusor contraction. This corresponds to increased sphincter contraction and elevated voiding pressures (see Figure 92-60).

TABLE 92-1. *Neuropathic bladder disorders*

CONGENITAL

APPARENT
Meningomyelocele
Sacral agenesis

OCCULT
Diastematomyelia
Intradural lipoma
Lipomeningocele
Tight filum terminale
Dermod cyst or sinus
Anterior sacral meningocele

ACQUIRED

Trauma
Ischemic cord injury

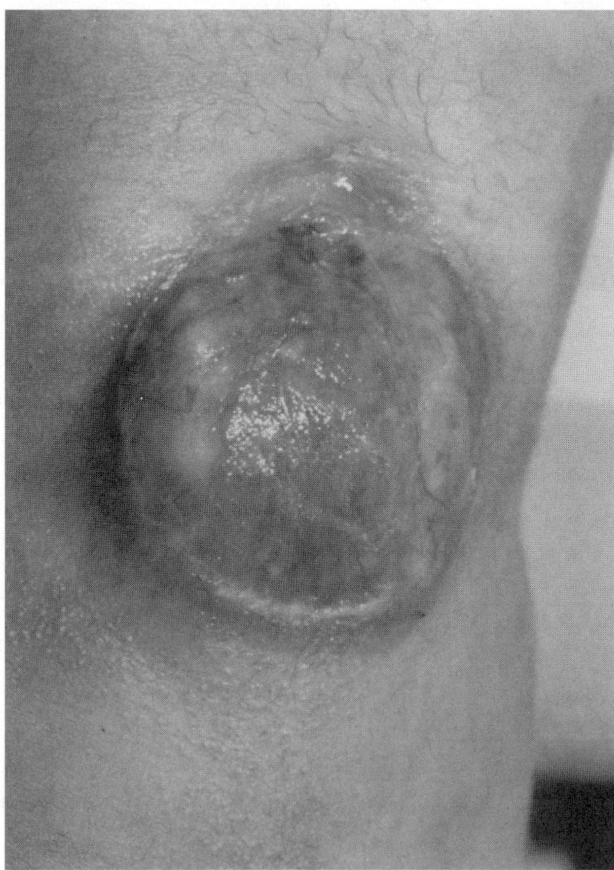

FIG. 92-58. Infant with myelomeningocele before surgical closure. The membrane covers the neural elements. If no neural elements prolapse into the sac, it is termed a *meningocele.*

is needed. Postvoid residual volume measurements by catheter or ultrasound are appropriate.

After neurosurgical closure, some infants experience a period of spinal shock, with bladder flaccidity and poor emptying. Catheterization or Credé emptying for this limited period is appropriate. Urodynamic assessment in this period is seldom useful. After the child has stabilized from the closure, baseline urodynamic assessment should be performed; this may be done when the infant is between 2 and 6 months of life. The principal aim is to identify infants at risk for developing upper urinary tract damage from high bladder pressures. Detrusor–sphincter dyssynergy is the usual cause of this, and when demonstrated on urodynamics, anticholinergic medication to reduce bladder contractile tone (Fig. 92-59) and intermittent catheterization to permit emptying are recommended. This prophylactic treatment avoids upper tract deterioration and may well maintain bladder compliance.[197] Fewer of these children require augmentation cystoplasty than their nontreated counterparts (Fig. 92-60).

Medical Management

The two aims of management of children with myelodysplasia are preservation of renal function and social continence.[187] The first requires normal storage function of the blad-

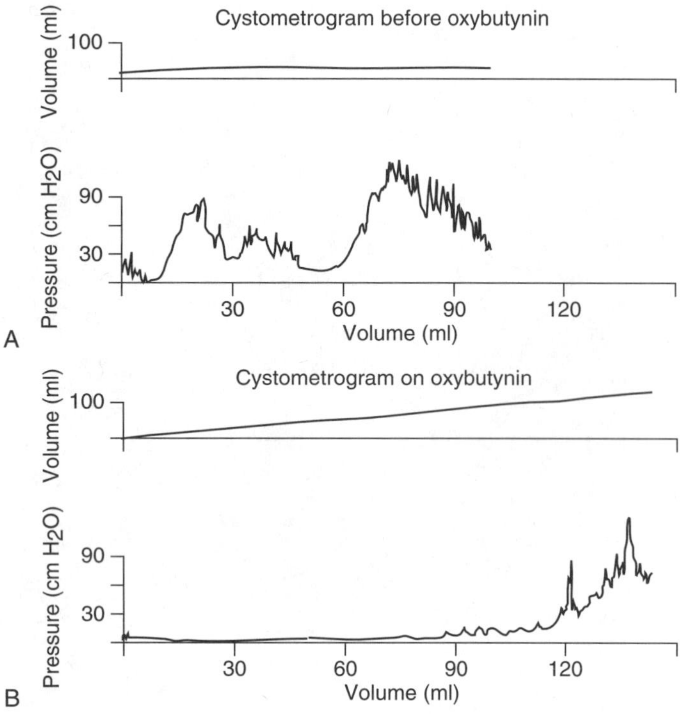

FIG. 92-59. (*A*) Cystometrogram demonstrating a hypertonic bladder with high pressures and small capacity. (*B*) After treatment with oral oxybutynin (Ditropan), the cystomyogram shows a low-pressure filling curve and increased total capacity.

der by maintaining low pressures during bladder filling. With neural abnormalities, the bladder may become noncompliant through two mechanisms. The first is denervation supersensitivity, whereby reduction in nerve input into the bladder muscle leads to an increase in the density of neurotransmitter receptors.[198] The functional consequences of this are bladder instability and hypercontractility. The resting tone of the bladder may be higher than normal. Reduced inhibitory innervation that mediates relaxation also may be active in this context.[199] The second mechanism is from functional bladder outlet obstruction in the setting of detrusor–sphincter dyssynergy. Every time the detrusor contracts, the sphincter contracts with it (see Fig. 92-56). Voiding pressures are elevated, and the bladder behaves as if obstructed. Smooth muscle hypertrophy begins, and increased connective tissue deposition occurs.[200–203] Ewalt and colleagues[127] have shown a redistribution in the subtypes of collagen in the myelodysplastic bladder, with increasing amounts of type III collagen interlacing the smooth muscle bundles in the detrusor. Alterations in elastin concentration and distribution are also seen, reducing the compliance of the bladder wall. The negative effects on the upper urinary tract have been described. Some groups have advocated sphincterotomy by dilation to eliminate this obstructive effect until the child is old enough to be definitively treated.[204] Intermittent catheterization can be taught to parents and may be a more acceptable and lasting solution in these children, without the risk of sphincteric injury.[205]

Surgical Management

Surgical management becomes necessary when one or both of these aims cannot be achieved with medical therapy and

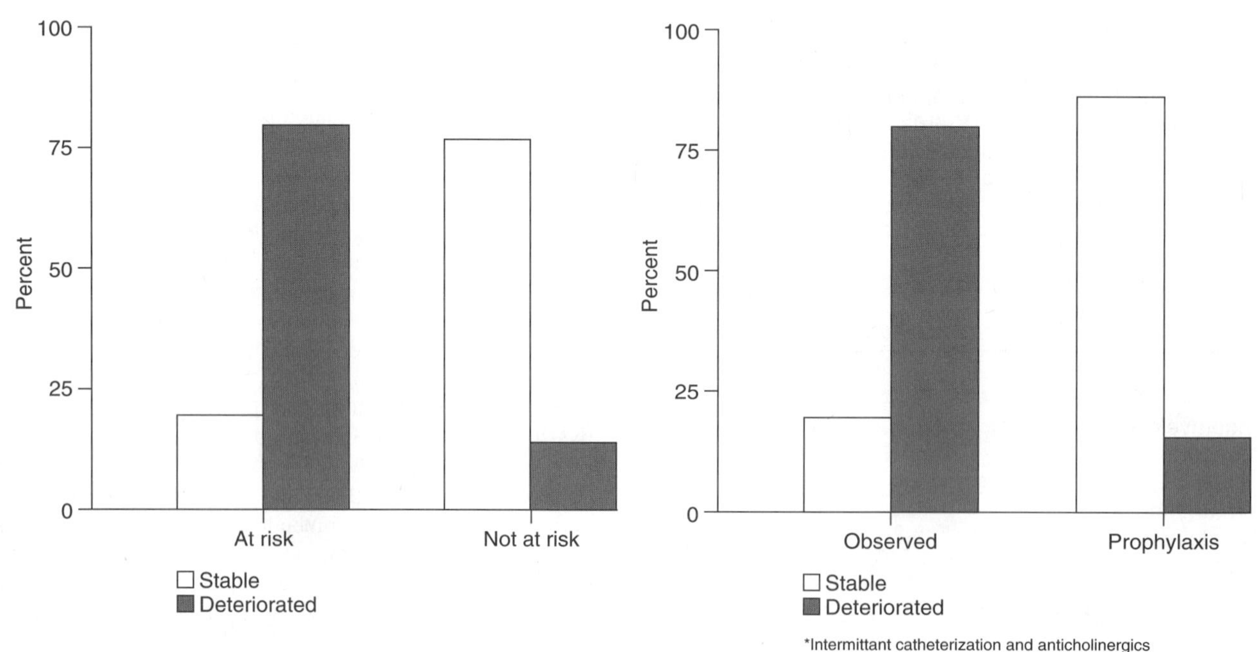

FIG. 92-60. Incidence of urinary tract deterioration (increasing hydronephrosis, reflux, increased postvoid residual urine) in children with myelodysplasia and neuropathic bladder dysfunction. (*A*) In children at risk (ie, with bladder sphincter dyssynergy), a high incidence of deterioration was seen during the first years of life, in contrast to a low incidence in those without risk factors. (*B*) When at-risk children were treated prophylactically with intermittent catheterization and anticholinergic agents to lower bladder pressures, the incidence of deterioration was reduced to a level equal to those children not at risk.

catheterization alone. Bladder hypertonia contributes to incontinence by raising bladder pressures above the resistance level of the sphincter. Even a neurologically abnormal sphincter can maintain continence, depending on the level of the neurologic effect. A totally flaccid sphincter is unlikely to permit continence in any situation, whereas a denervated sphincter may have a level of reflex tone that maintains dryness when bladder pressures are low. Bladder emptying before that resistance pressure is reached ensures continence. Surgical reduction of bladder hypertonia and provision of continence may require bladder augmentation, bladder neck surgery, or both for continence.

Bladder augmentation is a well-established procedure with well-described outcomes.[206–213] It continues to be associated with complications, and the decision to proceed with augmentation cystoplasty must be carefully considered.[214–219] The fundamental principles are to increase the capacity and decrease the pressure of the abnormal bladder by addition of a patch of gastrointestinal tissue onto the bladder. This can be an isolated segment of ileum, sigmoid, right colon, or stomach (Fig. 92-61). Tubular segments must be reconfigured to eliminate the tubular shape, which produces peristaltic contractions and high pressures.[220] Detubularization usually involves cutting the bowel segment along the antimesenteric line and sewing the patch onto the bladder. Gastric segments do not require reconfiguration (Fig. 92-62).

The complications of augmentation cystoplasty include

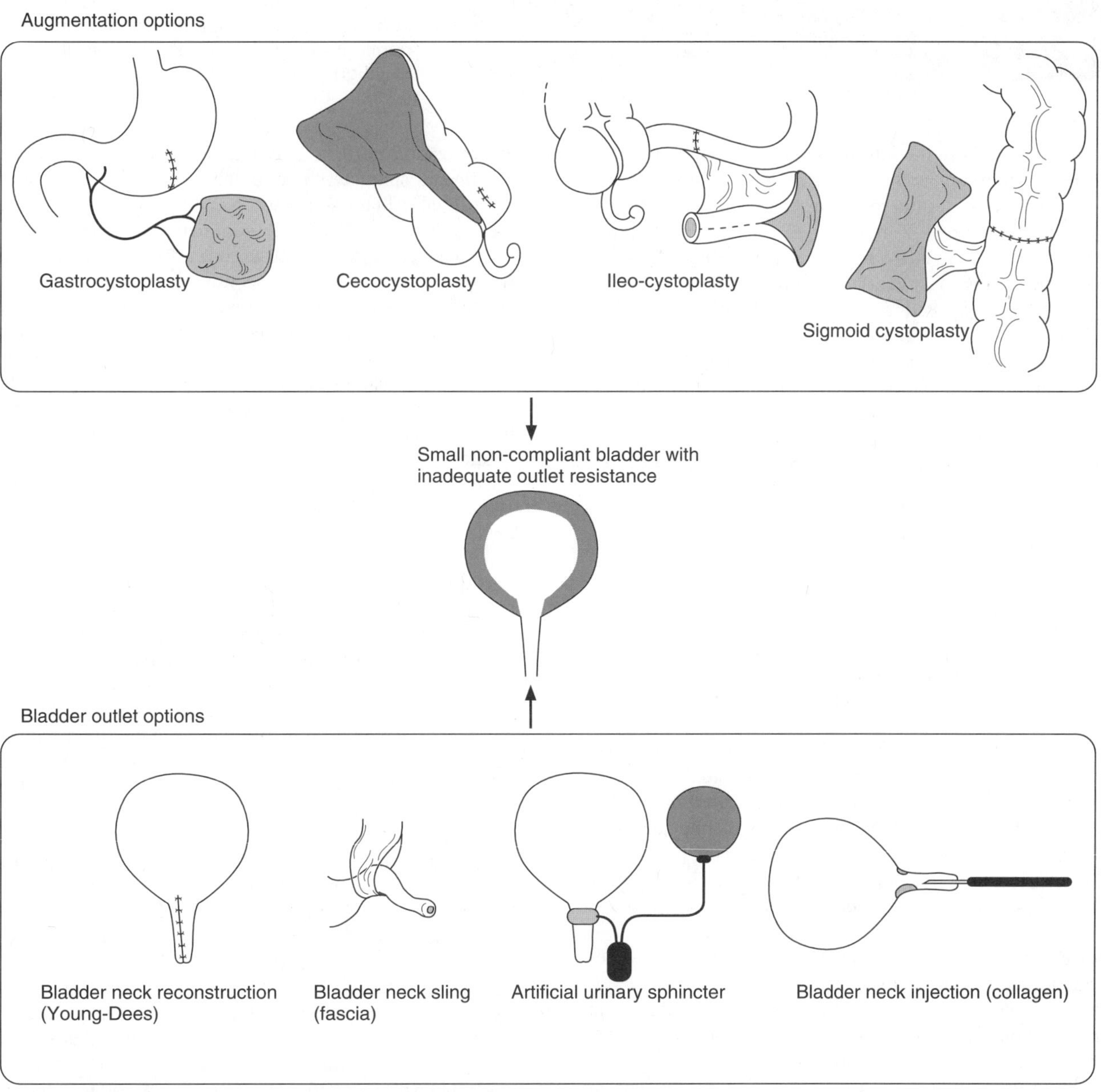

FIG. 92-61. Options for bladder augmentation in the setting of a small-capacity, high-pressure bladder. Any of these enteric segments can be combined with one of the options for increasing bladder outlet resistance, as needed.

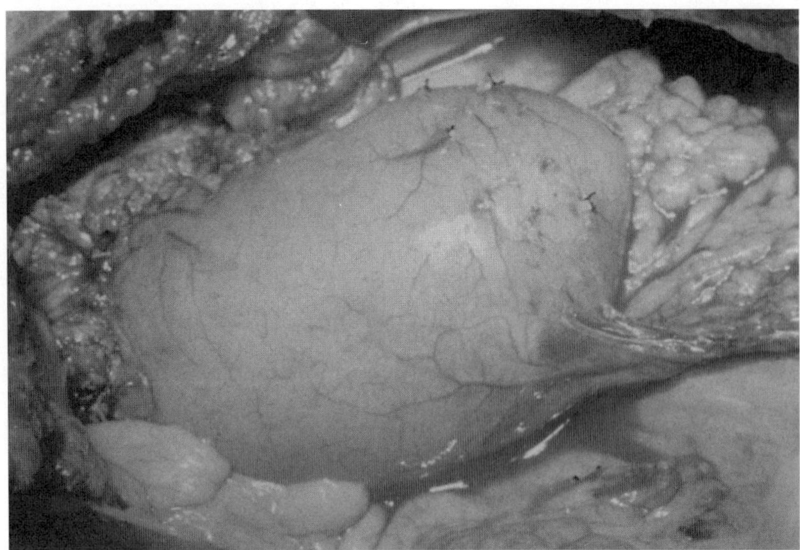

FIG. 92-62. Operative photograph of gastrocystoplasty in a boy with a small-capacity bladder due to epispadias. The gastric patch assumes a spheric shape without reconfiguration. A spheric configuration produces the lowest pressures for the highest volumes.

mucus production from the intestinal segment, which may impair catheter emptying and act as a nidus for stone formation.[215,219] The most serious problem has been perforation of the augmented segment, often in association with infection.[214,221] The specific cause remains unclear, but relative ischemia in the setting of infection and trauma from catheterization have been suggested as possible reasons. The classic clinical presentation of a child with a prior augmentation and a new episode of fever, abdominal pain, and shoulder pain (indicating diaphragmatic irritation from extravasated infected urine in the peritoneum) should be regarded as a bladder perforation until proved otherwise. Early diagnosis, antibiotics, and operative treatment are recommended. This is a potentially lethal condition.

Bladder calculi are an occasional problem with augmentation cystoplasty, likely due to the combination of bacteria and foreign material (mucus, or pubic hair from catheterization) in the urine. Urethral cystolitholapaxy is effective unless this manipulation might injure a reconstructed or artificial sphincter mechanism (artificial urinary sphincter or bladder neck sling). Percutaneous endoscopic stone fragmentation and removal may be performed, but occasionally, the most efficient means of stone removal is through an open cystotomy.

The attainment of social continence is frequently a substantial challenge in the myelodysplastic child. Continence is the result of a balance between intravesical pressure and urethral or bladder neck resistance. When bladder pressures cannot be maintained at a sufficiently low level during most of the bladder filling cycle, incontinence occurs. Inadequate resistance at the bladder neck, even with low bladder pressures, leads to inadequate continence. Stress incontinence, that occurring only with exertion or stress, may be particularly troublesome when wheelchair-bound patients must transfer.

After a thorough evaluation has been performed and the relative contribution of bladder compliance and bladder neck resistance have been identified, it is often necessary to both reduce bladder pressures with an augmentation cystoplasty and increase bladder neck resistance. There are several means of accomplishing the latter. It is unlikely that a child with myelodysplasia can void volitionally, and in all cases, intermittent catheterization must be anticipated and taught. Some children with flaccid sphincters may be able to empty completely with an artificial urinary sphincter, but most need catheterization.

The options available for continence include bladder neck sling, bladder neck reconstruction, artificial urinary sphincter (AUS), collagen or Teflon injection, or diversion to a continent catheterizable stoma on the lower abdomen (see Fig. 92-61). Bladder neck slings, fashioned from a strip of lower rectus fascia and passed around the posterior bladder neck in girls or boys, are a useful option[222–224] (Fig. 92-63). They directly increase urethral resistance and provide stabilization and intra-abdominal fixation of the bladder neck. Bladder neck slings are most useful when intermittent catheterization is planned. Success rates are good, approaching 85% to 90%. Difficulty catheterizing the bladder neck is an occasional problem. Bladder neck reconstruction using the Young-Dees concept is one of the least effective means of providing continence in the myelodysplastic population. The method relies on creating a muscular wrap of the bladder base, which lengthens the functional urethra. Often the tissues, as well as the supporting pelvic floor structures, are poorly developed and ineffective for continence in this arrangement. Modifications of the traditional technique have been able to produce better results, however.[225] The AUS continues to have a role in continence in children, but must be used with caution. When few other options are available, or when the patient may be able to empty completely due to a flaccid bladder neck, the AUS may be appropriate.[226–229] The success rate is about 75%, with a 20% reoperation rate in the latest models of the device. The device includes an inflatable cuff placed around the bladder neck or urethra, attached to a pressure regulating balloon reservoir. The cuff is actuated by a pump device in the scrotum or labia. Infection and erosion of the urethral tissues may occur.

Injection of foreign material to create more urethral resistance has been performed for more than 15 years. One of the original materials, Teflon paste, can be effective in patients with only a slight imbalance in bladder and urethral resistance as well as in patients with stress incontinence. A new collagen paste product has been released for a similar use[230–232] (Fig. 92-64). The collagen does not have the risks that have been tied to Teflon and is easily injectable. It may not remain in place as long as

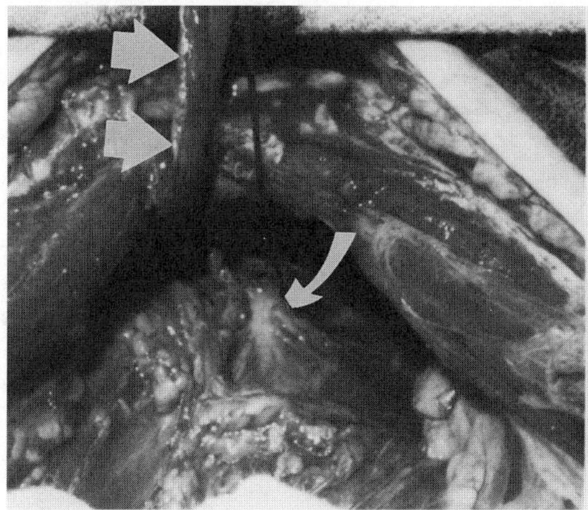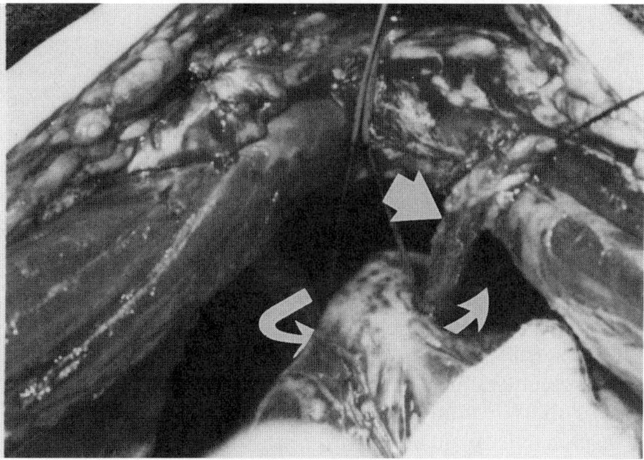

FIG. 92-63. Operative photograph of bladder neck dissection for placement of a fascial sling. The sling (*wide arrow*) is passed through the inferior rectus sheath, and a vessel loop is passed around the bladder neck (*curved arrow*). The sling is then passed around the bladder neck and wrapped around the anterior rectus fascia. The sling should not be tied too tightly, but enough to maintain the bladder base and neck in an intraabdominal position. (Bauer SB, Peters CA, Mandell J, et al. The use of the rectus fascia to manage urinary incontinence. J Urol 1989;142:516)

Teflon but can be easily touched up. The long-term results of this material remain to be defined. It may be useful in patients in whom other methods have not worked completely.

One option that has been gaining acceptance is creation of a continent catheterizable stoma (CCS). This is done in association with bladder neck closure or, preferably, with a bladder neck sling. The purpose of the CCS is to prevent leakage, but it allows catheterization as a back-up and pressure release. In most cases, the CCS has been placed as a back-up catheterization port, yet it is regularly used due to ease and comfort. The stoma can be constructed from appendix, ureter, or a tapered segment of small bowel. The Mitrofanoff principle is used, whereby the tube is implanted into the bladder in a tunneled fashion, as with antireflux surgery, to prevent leakage of urine from the bladder but to permit easy catheterization.[233–235] The stoma can be placed in the umbilicus, where it is concealed, or in the lower abdomen, just above the underwear line. Care must be taken to ensure that the child has the manual dexterity and body habitus to permit such a maneuver.

Occult Spinal Dysraphism

A small subset of patients with spinal dysraphisms do not present with the external manifestations of myelodysplasia, yet may demonstrate some of the same neurologic features.[236,237] The causes of these conditions include tethered spinal cord, diastematomyelia, sacral agenesis, and lipomeningocele. These conditions may cause an insidious deterioration of bladder function, which becomes irreversible by the time of diagnosis. Early diagnosis has generally permitted more recovery of lost function. A high index of suspicion is necessary to detect these patients, whose only manifestations may be minor changes in urinary patterns, minimal neurologic findings of the lower extremities, and subtle physical findings. A lower spinal hairy nevus, vascular malformation, and asymmetric gluteal cleft are all signs of a possible underlying neural defect. The classic finding of a flat buttock should be a clue to sacral agenesis, particularly in the infant of a diabetic mother. Appropriate spinal cord imaging and urodynamic and urologic evaluation usually reveal the specific nature of the condition and permit therapeutic planning. Bladder management is similar to that for myelodysplasia and depends on the neurologic status of the bladder and sphincter as well as on the condition of the upper urinary tracts.

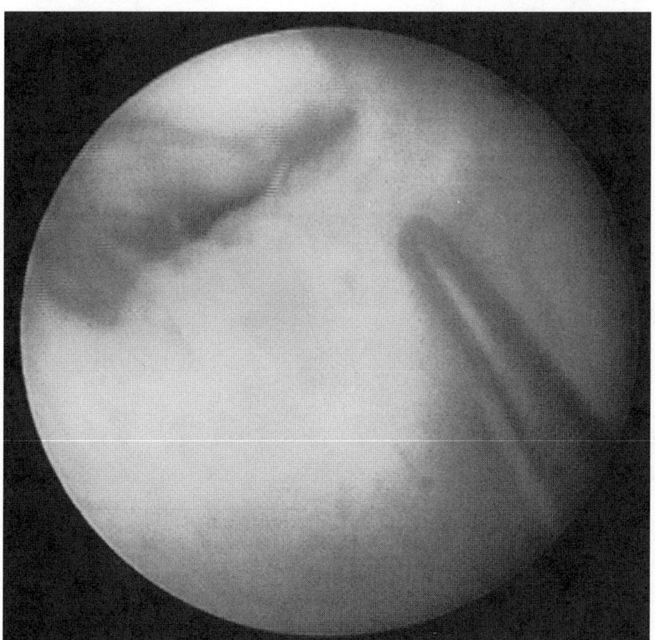

FIG. 92-64. Endoscopic photograph of intraurethral injection of collagen paste (Contigen) in a boy with bladder exstrophy in an attempt to increase outlet resistance to permit bladder growth before definitive bladder neck reconstruction. The injections are made just submucosally.

Associations With Anorectal Malformations

An association between neurogenic bladder dysfunction and anorectal abnormalities has been established and must be recognized to permit adequate urologic management in these patients.[212,238–240] The incidence of spinal cord abnormalities in children with anorectal anomalies is greater than normal, and routine evaluation of the lower spine using ultrasound (younger than 6 weeks of age) or magnetic resonance imaging is recommended. About 40% of children with imperforate anus have evidence of neuropathic bladder dysfunction; most of these patients are children with high imperforate anus. The basis for the bladder abnormality is usually a spinal anomaly, such as tethered cord of diastematomyelia.[238] If anorectal surgery is anticipated, urodynamic evaluation is also prudent before surgery. This serves to identify any underlying abnormality and provides a baseline for comparison in the event of any neural injury during surgery. Although these children do not typically present with urologic symptoms early in life, the identification of a neurologic anomaly permits selective monitoring and early intervention. This may have a benefit in reducing the 55% incidence of neuropathic bladder dysfunction in the adolescent years.[212]

CONGENITAL BLADDER OBSTRUCTION: POSTERIOR URETHRAL VALVES

Posterior urethral valves represent the most pure form of congenital bladder obstruction. Although originally well described in 1919,[241,242] valves continue to challenge the clinician and scientist. Valves are located just below the bladder neck at the level of the verumontanum and are likely the remnants of the migration of the mesonephric ducts to the trigone (Fig. 92-65). The severity of obstruction is highly variable, and the consequences are similarly variable.[243] In the most severe form, congenital bladder obstruction produces renal dysplasia, oligohydramnios, and pulmonary hypoplasia, leading to neonatal

death from respiratory failure.[244] Lesser degrees of obstruction may cause severe renal impairment leading to chronic renal failure and necessitating renal replacement.[245–248] The bladder dysfunction that is produced by PUV and persists long after removal of the obstruction[180] may even impair function of a renal transplant. The relatively recent recognition of chronic bladder dysfunction due to PUV (valve bladder)[80,249,250] has permitted improved management of these children, in whom a steady progression to renal failure was witnessed with frustration despite multiple surgical interventions. Management of PUV begins in utero and can extend well into young adulthood. The patterns of bladder, renal, and pulmonary dysfunction are well described, yet their mechanisms remain undefined; this is the principal challenge to the clinical scientist interested in PUV.[251]

In Utero Posterior Urethral Valves

The prenatal diagnosis of PUV may be made as early as 15 weeks' gestation,[252] although usually this is identified after 18 weeks' gestation. The initial presentation may provide an indication of prognosis. Boys with oligohydramnios, bilateral echogenic kidneys, and a large, thick-walled, dilated bladder have a poor prognosis.[244] Those boys in whom oligohydramnios did not develop and who did not have markedly dysplastic kidneys may survive without significant renal impairment. The uniformly poor prognosis of fetuses with severe obstruction and evidence of evolving renal dysplasia and pulmonary hypoplasia has prompted in utero interventions to relieve the obstruction.[253] This issue is discussed elsewhere. The role of in utero shunting procedures in boys with presumed PUV remains incompletely defined. The principal hindrance to developing effective treatment protocols is the inability to predict neonatal outcomes accurately given current imaging and assessment.[172] As an understanding of the processes and mechanisms of congenital obstructive uropathy develops, markers of the progression of this process will permit more specific assessment of the potential for positive outcomes with intervention. Anecdotal experience

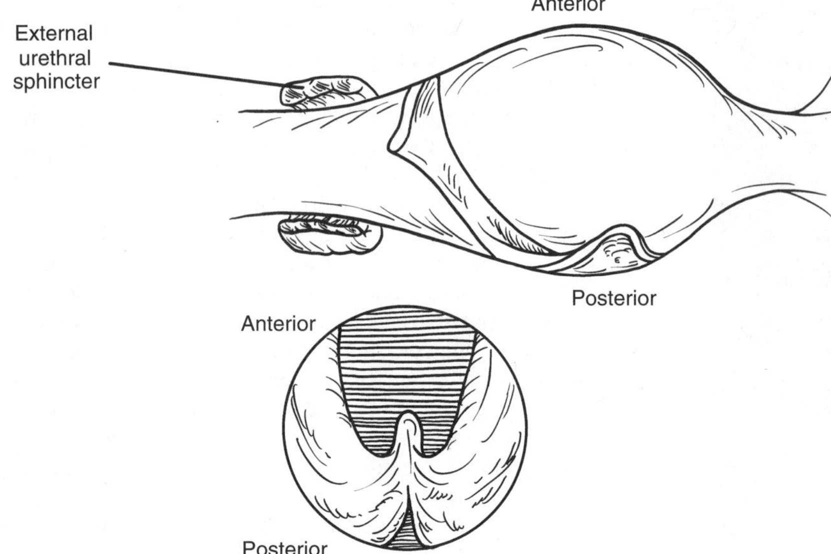

FIG. 92-65. Anatomy of posterior urethral valves. The valves emanate from the distal veru montanum at the apex of the prostate and sweep anteriorly and laterally, forming a dorsal web of tissue. The dorsal web may not be readily visible on an endoscopic view (*inset*), which shows the lower leaflet folds. (Retik AB. Management of posterior urethral valves. In: Glenn JF, ed. Urologic surgery. Philadelphia, JB Lippincott, 1991:812)

indicates that it is possible to salvage an otherwise doomed fetus with an appropriate in utero intervention.[254] The broad application of these technologies, however, is not justified at present. Prenatal diagnosis serves an important role in providing information to the prospective parents and physicians about the possible outcomes and the need for *postnatal* evaluation and intervention.[255]

The fetus with presumed valves should be monitored periodically to follow amniotic fluid status, the condition of the kidneys, and bladder dynamics. Abrupt changes in these parameters may prompt reconsideration of postnatal therapy. It is almost never necessary to suggest a late-gestation intervention. Late-onset oligohydramnios has not been associated with significant pulmonary complications because basic pulmonary development has already occurred.[256] Early delivery in these cases to reduce exposure of the fetal kidney to obstruction has not been demonstrated to have a positive effect. It must be balanced against the risks of pulmonary insufficiency due to prematurity.

Neonatal Management

A child with a prior presumptive diagnosis of valves should be delivered at an institution where the complications of pulmonary insufficiency, sepsis, and renal failure can be handled, and where a thorough evaluation can be obtained. Initial management, particularly if the child is sick, should be catheter drainage of the bladder with a feeding tube. Ultrasound imaging of the upper tracts and bladder at that time may provide a baseline. Cystography to confirm the presence of the valves and to assess the presence of reflux should be performed (Fig. 92-66). The child should be placed on prophylactic antibiotics and monitored for azotemia and acidosis.

The pattern of serum creatinine change in the newborn with

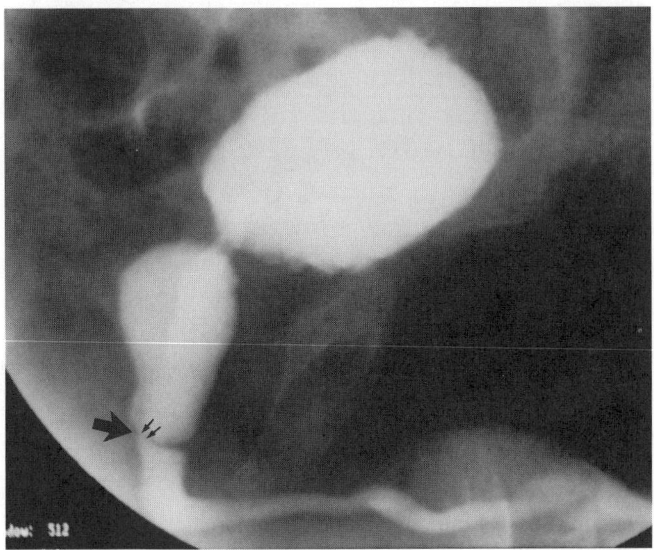

FIG. 92-66. Voiding cystourethrogram of an infant boy with severe posterior urethral valves. The dilated posterior urethra is a characteristic radiographic finding associated with valves. The narrow postobstruction urethral lumen originates inferiorly (*arrows*), consistent with the valvular opening on the inferior aspect of the urethra (see Figure 92-65).

PUV may provide some information about the level of renal function and adequacy of renal drainage. At birth, the creatinine is that of the mother, usually about 0.8 to 1 mg/dL. If it begins to rise in the first days of life, serious renal impairment may be anticipated. This should be addressed aggressively and all efforts to maximize drainage of the upper tracts undertaken. Functional obstruction of the distal ureters can occur as a consequence of bladder hypertrophy due to PUV. In this case, the bladder may remain empty due to catheter drainage or vesicostomy drainage, yet the kidneys remain markedly hydronephrotic. Supravesical diversion may be one option to manage these children[257,258]; another is total reconstruction,[259] which can be a formidable undertaking. A stable serum creatinine or a fall in the initial level suggests more adequate renal drainage. These children are best served by endoscopic valve ablation and close follow-up (Fig. 92-67). In the very premature infant, temporary cutaneous vesicostomy remains a useful option.

The response of the child to valve ablation is critical and must be closely attended. If upper tract dilation persists, and there is any evidence of impaired renal function, such as elevated creatinine level or acidosis, improving upper tract drainage may be necessary by way of upper tract diversion (ureterostomy) or total reconstruction. One third of boys with severe valves who present in the first year of life progress to renal failure[260] (Fig. 92-68). It seems prudent to maximize their potential renal function by providing for the best means of urinary drainage during the first year of life.

Most infants with PUV show rapid improvement in upper tract dilation and evidence of normal renal function. The presence of vesicoureteral reflux is common, yet in nearly half of patients, it resolves spontaneously after valve ablation. A subset of boys have evidence of severe unilateral reflux and a nonfunctioning kidney, the vesicoureteral reflux, renal dysplasia (VURD) association.[178] Unilateral nephrectomy is often indicated to avoid risk of infection. Further monitoring of boys with a rapid response to valve ablation aims to identify any signs of bladder dysfunction before they cause irreversible consequences.

Bladder Dysfunction and Posterior Urethral Valves

The association between PUV and bladder dysfunction has been recognized for the past 15 years.[250] Before that time, the clinical pattern of voiding dysfunction with hydronephrosis in a boy with previously ablated valves was thought to be due to bladder neck hypertrophy and persistent outlet obstruction.[249] Bladder neck surgery was performed, often exacerbating the incontinence. Persistent reflux was treated with repeated ureteral reimplantation, usually without success. The continued high-pressure bladder dynamics caused steady deterioration in renal function. It became apparent that the primary cause of this pattern was a persistently hypertonic bladder, the result of congenital obstruction. Attention was paid to reducing bladder pressures, principally with anticholinergic medication, augmentation cystoplasty, and rigorous voiding regimens to improve emptying.

Three patterns of bladder dysfunction have been identified in association with PUV and may be seen long after valve ablation[180] (Fig. 92-69). These include bladder hypertonia, the most potentially damaging; bladder instability; and a pattern of myogenic failure or contractile failure. Hypertonia may manifest as

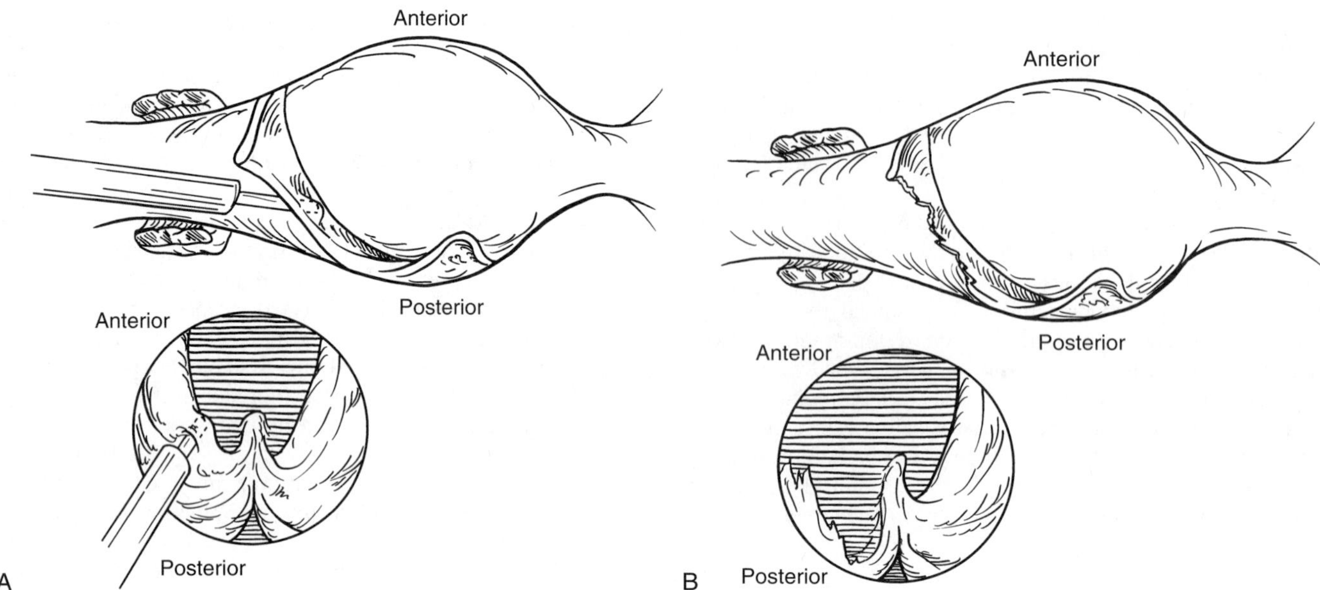

FIG. 92-67. Endoscopic technique for valve ablation. (*A*) A small (3F) ureteral catheter with a metal stylet attached to the electrocautery unit is placed. (*B*) The stylet ablates the valve leaflets, disrupting the sail-like continuity of the valve. (Retik AB. Management of posterior urethral valves. In: Glenn JF, ed. Urologic surgery. Philadelphia, JB Lippincott, 1991:812)

incontinence and hydronephrosis and is usually associated with a small-capacity bladder, often with trabeculation (Fig. 92-70). Instability may produce urge incontinence due to uninhibited bladder contractions and may occur with some hypertonia. Myogenic or contractile failure may represent a decompensated bladder with insufficient contractile coordination to produce a sustained bladder contraction. This leads to high postvoid residuals, infection, overflow incontinence, and occasionally hydronephrosis.

Boys with previously ablated valves and voiding dysfunction should be evaluated carefully to identify the pattern of bladder dysfunction present and to determine appropriate therapy. Mixed patterns may be present. Incontinence in these boys almost never is due to a sphincter abnormality. The fact that incontinence reflects bladder dysfunction, which may injure renal function, is apparent in the report by Parkhouse and colleagues.[261] In their long-term review, 45% of boys with inconti-

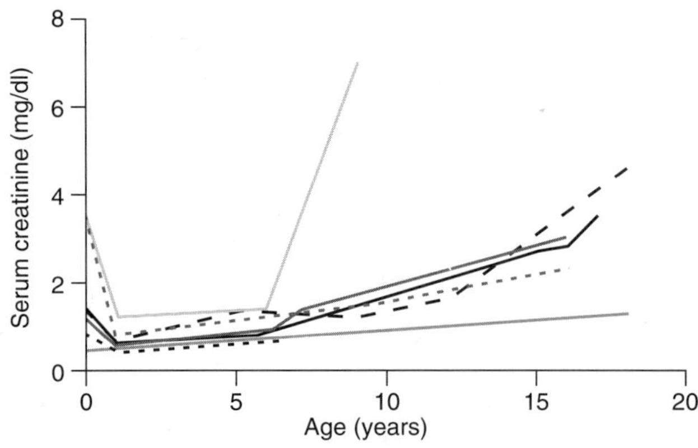

FIG. 92-68. Serum creatinine values in a group of boys with posterior urethral valves diagnosed before 1 year of age, all of whom underwent valve ablation and urinary tract reconstruction. Many had low serum creatinine levels at the end of the first year of life, yet progressed to chronic renal failure. A low nadir creatinine in the first year of life is not a guarantee that the patient is not at risk for renal failure.

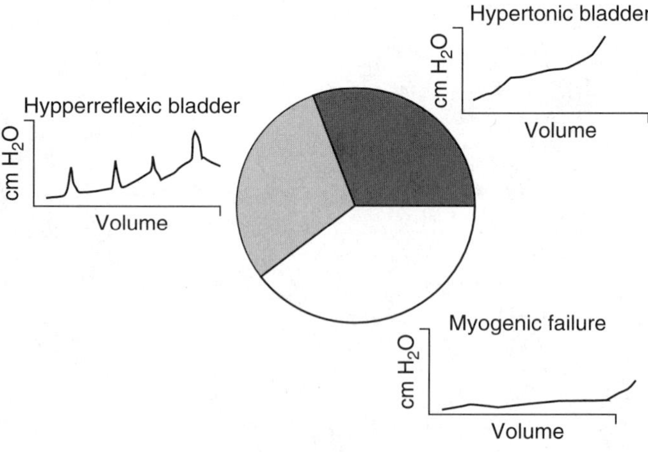

FIG. 92-69. Patterns of bladder dysfunction in a group of boys with previously corrected posterior urethral valves and later onset of voiding dysfunction. Representative cystometric curves correspond to the urodynamic pattern. Boys with bladder hypertonia and noncompliant, small-capacity bladders are at most risk for renal injury. (Peters CA, Bolkier M, Bauer SB, et al. The urodynamic consequences of posterior urethral valves. J Urol 1990;144:122)

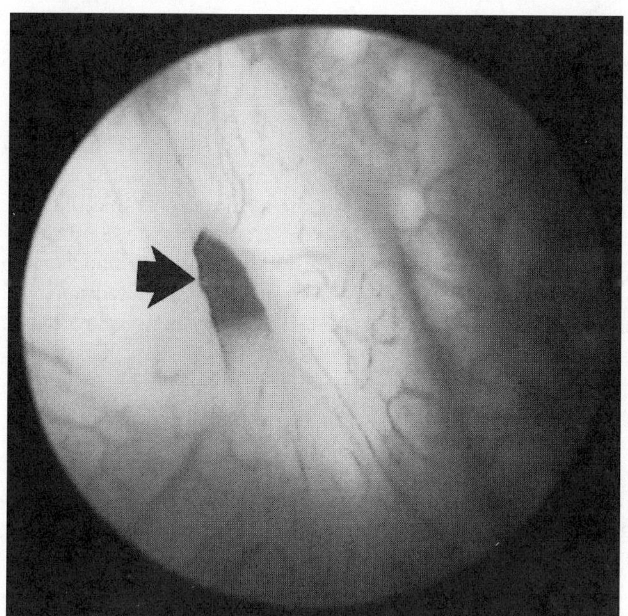

FIG. 92-70. Endoscopic photograph of bladder wall trabeculation in a boy with posterior urethral valves. The mouth of a small diverticulum is indicated by the arrow.

nence also had renal failure, in contrast to only 4% of boys without incontinence.

Older Boys With Valves

The clinical presentation of boys with milder forms of PUV who are not diagnosed until later in life is highly variable. Their presentation is usually a reflection of some element of bladder dysfunction due to chronic obstruction. This may be infection with inadequate emptying, new onset of incontinence due to bladder instability or overflow from a decompensated bladder, or occasionally, azotemia due to high pressure bladder dysfunction. Valve ablation is the most appropriate first intervention, followed by a period of observation to assess the status of the bladder and kidneys with stabilization. The pattern of bladder dysfunction before valve ablation is not always that seen after valve ablation. The need for upper tract reconstruction depends on the presence of reflux and the adequacy of upper tract drainage. It is highly unusual to need temporary diversion, except in boys with sepsis or such severe renal impairment that renal salvage is not appropriate.

Mechanisms of Bladder Dysfunction

More complete understanding of the basis of bladder dysfunction due to PUV is essential to permit more specific therapy of this entity. This would reduce the incidence of surgical reconstruction of the previously obstructed bladder and may reduce the incidence of renal failure in these patients. It may also permit more accurate prediction of the occurrence of bladder dysfunction in any particular child, which might lead to improved outcomes with earlier treatment. The processes active in the devel-

opment of the dysfunctional bladder due to PUV are likely to be similar to other processes in organ systems beyond the bladder. Cardiac hypertrophy and fibrosis due to outflow resistance is an obvious example. Hypertrophy and fibrosis are common pathologic pathways.

Congenital bladder obstruction has been studied to a limited degree in the laboratory.[251] Initial experiments focused on pulmonary effects of PUV and the in utero reversibility of this condition. Harrison's group[253] suggested the possibility of prevention of pulmonary hypoplasia with in utero shunting of an obstructed bladder. A model of obstruction earlier in gestation with greater renal injury was created, and pulmonary morphometry was used as an endpoint to confirm this initial impression.[262] Early oligohydramnios due to bladder obstruction could be reversed to permit more normal lung development,[263,264] but this was dependent in large measure on the response of the kidneys to obstruction and decompression. When the renal effects of early bladder obstruction were not reversed with bladder decompression, pulmonary hypoplasia was present despite effective decompression. This was usually associated with histologic evidence of renal dysplasia.

The bladder consequences of in utero obstruction demonstrated a marked increase in growth and alterations in the developmental regulation of several functional proteins.[139] Bladder growth was due to increases in bladder smooth muscle cells and was both hyperplastic (more cells) and hypertrophic (larger cells; Fig. 92-71). A large increase in connective tissue elements was also demonstrated, which may be a significant factor producing reduced compliance. Functionally, the bladders had less compliance as measured by stress relaxation (Fig. 92-72). Developmental regulation of contractile proteins was affected by obstruction, as were the concentrations of neurotransmitter receptors. Similar findings were reported in a model of moderate partial bladder obstruction, with increased growth and altered developmental regulation.[265]

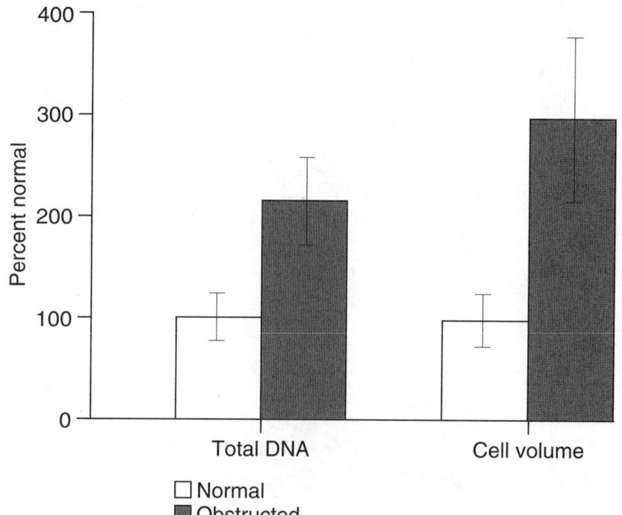

FIG. 92-71. Effect of fetal bladder obstruction in fetal sheep on bladder DNA and bladder smooth muscle cell size. These data indicate that both hyperplasia and cellular hypertrophy occur with prenatal bladder obstruction. (Adapted from Peters CA, Vasavada S, Dator D, et al. The effect of obstruction on the developing bladder. J Urol 1992;148:491)

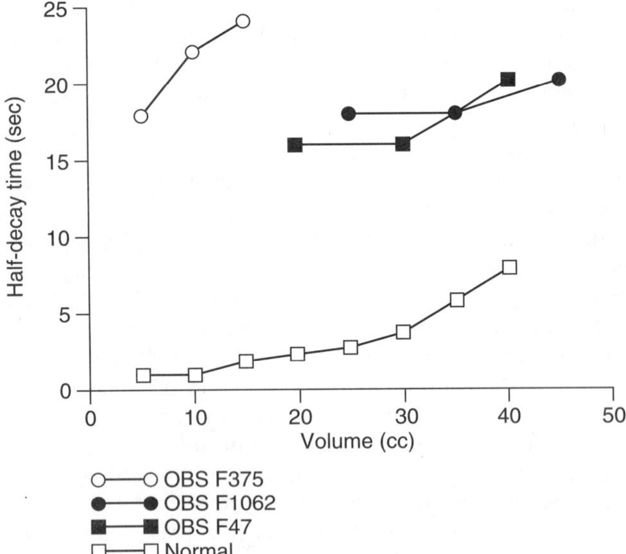

FIG. 92-72. Marked increase in half-decay times in fetal sheep bladders subjected to in utero obstruction. The prolonged stress relaxation time is indicative of impaired passive compliance, largely due to the nonmuscular elements of the bladder wall. This corresponds to the poor compliance often seen in patients with posterior urethral valves. (After Peters CA, Vasavada S, Dator D, et al. The effect of obstruction on the developing bladder. J Urol 1992;148:491)

A model of severe partial obstruction confirms these initial observations and has further examined the metabolism of bladder collagen. Gene expression of the principal bladder interstitial collagens (types I and III) was not changed with obstruction despite an increase in bladder collagen.[138] Activity of the key collagen degradation proteins, the matrix metalloproteinases (MMPs), was shown to be reduced, and activity of the inhibitors of the MMPs (tissue inhibitors of metalloproteinases [TIMPs]) was increased. The increased amounts of collagen may be the result of a shift in the balance of collagen synthesis and breakdown (Fig. 92-73). This balance may potentially be modulated exogenously and suggests possible mechanisms for favorably intervening in the development of bladder dysfunction in the setting of PUV.

Much remains to be learned regarding the evolution of bladder dysfunction due to PUV, from the level of the organism to the bladder muscle cell. It is likely that some of the key principles will be applicable to other systems as well.

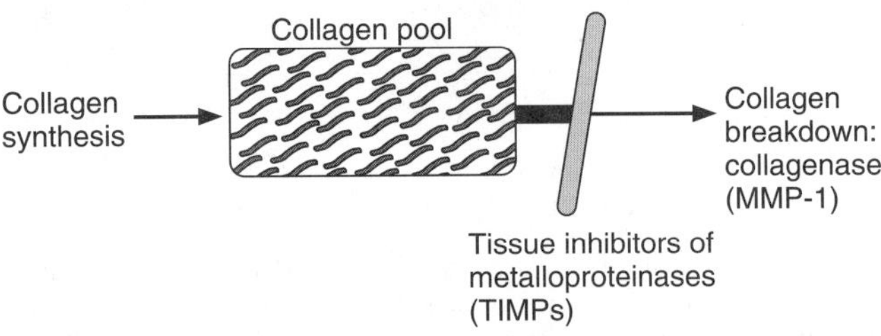

FIG. 92-73. Possible relation among collagen synthesis, degradation, and the regulation of degradation in determining the collagen pool in tissue such as the bladder.

Surgical Management of the Valve Bladder

The basic principles of management of the valve bladder are those involved in the care of the neuropathic bladder. The aim is to achieve low-pressure storage of urine for a socially acceptable period and to permit complete emptying. The surgical options are essentially the same as those for neuropathic bladder, including augmentation cystoplasty. It is unusual to require surgical intervention for sphincteric function. Patients must be able to perform catheterization, and often this is instituted during a trial of pharmacologic therapy with anticholinergic agents in an effort to reduce bladder pressures. Occasionally, patients can learn to empty their bladders with abdominal pressure voiding, even with augmentation cystoplasty. The timing and commitment to surgical bladder augmentation is dependent on the pattern of bladder dynamics, the level of renal function, the commitment of the patient and family, and the response to pharmacologic therapy.

Renal Transplantation in Boys With Posterior Urethral Valves

The boy with prior valves and chronic renal failure presents a special challenge to the transplantation team. These boys require thorough urologic evaluation of bladder function before transplantation.[266–268] Of principal concern is the identification of bladder hypertonia, which may negatively impact on renal graft survival. Cystography is useful to confirm complete valve ablation, and urodynamics should be performed to assess bladder dynamics. It is unusual for a child with chronic renal failure secondary to PUV to have normal bladder function.

Depending on previous surgical interventions, urinary tract reconstruction or undiversion may be necessary before transplantation. If augmentation cystoplasty is found to be necessary, it is best performed before transplantation. Gastrocystoplasty has been widely used in transplant recipients, with added benefits of acid secretion, reduced infections, stones, and mucus.[269] It has been associated, however, with a significant incidence of gastric acid–induced dysuria and hematuria.[269,270] These symptoms occasionally are profound. Attempts to control gastric acid secretion by way of histamine-receptor blockers (ranitidine) or H^+-ion pump inhibitors (omeprazole) have been moderately successful.[271] Often, this condition is self-limiting. Particular attention must be paid to boys with gastrocystoplasty who became anuric with progression of renal failure or from native nephrectomies. They have a high risk of bladder erosion from gastric acid.[272] Appropriate attention to bladder dynamics after transplantation improves the likelihood of graft survival. Episodes of graft failure or dysfunction should prompt a consideration of bladder dysfunction as a possible cause.

NEOPLASMS OF THE BLADDER

Rhabdomyosarcoma

The general management of pediatric rhabdomyosarcoma is presented elsewhere, but several specific issues relating to bladder and prostatic rhabdomyosarcoma (BPR) are relevant to a discussion of pediatric bladder diseases. In particular, the diagnosis of BPR is often made in the context of evaluation of children for voiding dysfunction. The management strategies should be carefully integrated with the outlook for bladder function or, when necessary, surgical replacement of bladder function.

Diagnosis

A high index of suspicion is essential to diagnose BPR in a timely fashion. Initial symptoms may be subtle and considered to be due to infection, behavior, or nonspecific complaints of dysuria or frequency. BPR may be readily detected in most cases with a rectal examination, in which the normal prostate may be barely felt as a smooth, soft midline bump. Ultrasound of the bladder base is also an effective examination in cases of low suspicion. The more apparent clinical presentations of urinary retention and UTI usually are recognized for their true nature. Voiding cystourethrogram and upper urinary tract ultrasound are usually sufficient to provide the diagnosis. Careful cystoscopic and bimanual examination to determine tumor extent and mobility is performed at the time of transurethral or perineal biopsy for tissue diagnosis; biopsies should be performed with a cold-cup biopsy forceps to avoid cautery artifact. Modern imaging usually provides a precise definition of tumor extent. These observations are important in follow-up evaluations.

Integrating Bladder Functional Outlook With Therapy

Controversy exists about the appropriate therapy for BPR in children, but it remains important to anticipate bladder functional needs. This comes into play as early as the time of urinary diversion, if needed, because many options should be kept open to permit future normal bladder function or appropriate replacement of bladder function with continent reservoirs. A temporary period of diversion is often needed, and transverse colon conduits are highly effective and permit later integration into a continent reservoir if the bladder is unusable. The conduit would also be useful if bladder augmentation were appropriate after radiotherapy and complete disease clearance. Extensive radiotherapy may affect sphincter function with fibrosis. Bladder-sparing strategies are appealing, but the functional capacity of a bladder after intensive radiotherapy may not always be normal. Reported results have varied in terms of long-term bladder salvage rates, the most optimistic being about 50%.[273–275]

Urethral-sparing strategies in boys have been fraught with the need for secondary urethrectomy after margins are found to be positive with permanent sections. "Skip lesions" are frequently noted in prostatic rhabdomyosarcomas. This limits the potential for use of the urethra in functional reconstruction.

Reconstructive Options

Continent reconstruction in children after cure of BPR is a formidable challenge. These children may have significant radiation fibrosis of the pelvis, precluding orthotopic reconstruction. Sphincter function may be inadequate, and the therapeutic options in such children are limited. As noted earlier, use of the native urethra must be undertaken cautiously. Continent diversion to a neobladder of gastrointestinal segments is often the most effective means of providing continence without risk to the upper urinary tracts. Construction of reservoirs from the initial diverting segment added to an ileocecal segment with the appendix as a catheterizable conduit is a particularly useful option. The appendix may be kept in situ in the cecum and tunneled into an adjacent tinea. This creates a flap–valve mechanism, much like antireflux surgery, and then provides for continence. The appendix may be brought to the umbilicus, where catheterization is technically easy, and the stoma is concealed. In the absence of appendix, the ureter or tapered ileum may be implanted into the reservoir. A careful evaluation of the effects of radiation must be performed on any segments of bowel considered for integration into a continent reservoir. Concomitant evaluation of rectal function must be performed to avoid limiting options for rectal continence in the setting of radiation proctitis.

In a review of 33 patients with a variety of pelvic rhabdomyosarcomas, 31 patients are alive and well with a combination of urinary diversions and reconstructions.[276] Six of 16 patients with cystectomy have continent diversion, and the others continue with urinary conduit diversion. These continent diversions have relatively few complications and an excellent success rate. In 10 patients undergoing bladder-sparing therapy involving radiation or chemotherapy alone, prostatectomy, or partial cystectomy, 5 required some form of urinary reconstruction or diversion for continence or hydronephrosis. One underwent secondary radical cystectomy, and 1 patient died. Although bladder-sparing therapy may be a worthy and achievable goal in some patients, the need should be anticipated for more extensive urinary reconstruction to ensure continence and upper urinary tract preservation.

Transitional Cell Carcinoma

The most common bladder neoplasm in adults is extremely rare in children and exhibits a distinct biology. The typical behavior of childhood transitional cell carcinoma (TCC) is to be noninvasive and nonrecurring, the two hallmarks of adult TCC.[277] Diagnosis is often by chance because hematuria in the child is not usually evaluated with cystoscopy.[278] No other diagnostic modality is effective in detecting the small papillary lesions typical of pediatric TCC.[279] Ultrasonography may occasionally detect a small lesion of the bladder wall.[280] The low grade lesion is difficult to detect cytologically. Local endoscopic resection is the treatment of choice, with adequate biopsy material to determine the level of invasion. Subsequent follow-up is not recommended unless the tumor is of high grade or demonstrates anything but a superficial pattern.[281] Invasive TCC may be best treated with radical resection as in adults; the role of adjuvant chemotherapy has not been defined in children, given the rarity of the condition.

Adenocarcinoma

Adenocarcinoma of the bladder is rare in adults and children but has an increased incidence in patients with bladder exstrophy.[282–84] The cause is presumed to be due to chronic irritation of the exposed bladder. A possible link has been made to the occurrence of gastrointestinal rests of glandular epithelium, or to a metaplastic response of bladder. Two cases of carcinoma have been reported in patients with closed exstrophy (not closed as newborns), and these were of squamous histology. Chronic monitoring has been recommended by some but is not widely practiced in patients with closed bladder exstrophy.

Neurofibromatosis

Involvement of the bladder lower urinary tract can occur with neurofibromatosis. These children usually have other stigmata of neurofibromatosis or a family history of von Recklinghausen syndrome. Urologic presentation may be that of any mass effect in the bladder, including dysuria, frequency, urinary retention, or infection.[285] Upper tract obstruction may occur. Involvement of the external genitalia may occur. The extent of involvement should be delineated with imaging studies, and a biopsy is recommended to rule out malignancy. Malignant degeneration occurs in 5% to 30% of cases.[286] Management depends on the clinical presentation and extent of involvement. Curative resection is not usually possible. Urinary diversion may be necessary with extreme involvement.

Pheochromocytoma

The bladder is the most common extraadrenal site of involvement of pheochromocytoma in children, who are found to have extraadrenal tumors in more than 30% of cases.[287,288] Usually benign, these tumors may present with the classic findings of pheochromocytoma, including hypertension, dizziness, headache, palpitations, faintness, and pallor. These symptoms may be present with typical urinary symptoms of hematuria, dysuria, and frequency, and they may be exacerbated with urination. Appropriate diagnostic evaluation to assess the functional characteristics of the tumor, as well as searching for other sites, is needed. Vesical pheochromocytomas require the same level of preoperative preparation as adrenal pheochromocytomas, including volume repletion, adrenergic blockade, and intensive anesthesia monitoring. Specific management details discussed in Chapter 90. Local resection is appropriate.

Hamartoma (Nephrogenic Adenoma)

Hamartomas are benign tumors that are usually associated with a source of chronic irritation and may present with irritative symptoms, hematuria, and a history of recurrent UTI. They have a papillary appearance and do not demonstrate evidence of invasiveness.[289] Local resection is curative. Histologically, they have an appearance that resembles a developing kidney (hence the name).

MISCELLANEOUS BLADDER CONDITIONS

Bladder and Urethral Polyps

Polyps of the bladder usually occur at the bladder neck and in the proximal prostatic urethra.[290–293] They may create a ball–valve effect at the bladder neck and cause intermittency of the urinary stream or severe dysuria and strangury. They may also produce gross hematuria. In some children, the symptoms are not as severe and may be attributed to behavioral causes. Ultrasonographic evaluation may detect the polyp (see Fig. 92-53), but voiding cystourethrogram is usually definitive. Cystoscopic diagnosis confirms the diagnosis and usually permits removal. Some large polyps require open bladder removal. This may also be performed using a percutaneous approach with a large (24F to 28F) working sheath.

Urachal Anomalies

Urachal abnormalities are uncommon and may be suspected in the infant with umbilical drainage or inflammation.[294] Uriniferous drainage is typical and diagnostic. A mass may be felt infraumbilically, or the child may present with urinary infection or apparent omphalitis. Ultrasonography can identify a mass or cystic structure behind the midline of the rectus muscles.[295] Voiding cystourethrogram may demonstrate contrast into a urachal sinus. Treatment is surgical removal to avoid infection, which is often staphylococcal. A small infraumbilical incision is usually adequate to identify the urachus at the dome of the bladder and to trace it to the umbilicus. It should be removed in its entirety, with a small cuff of bladder. The peritoneum should not be violated.

Vascular Malformations

Bladder vascular malformations may be isolated or associated with an identified condition of multiple arteriovenous malformations.[296–298] Intravesical varices present with significant gross hematuria and clot. Cystoscopy is diagnostic and is appropriate in the setting of gross hematuria that is not consistent with viral cystitis. The latter is usually abrupt in onset, associated with intense dysuria and frequency, and self-limiting. A diffuse edematous reaction of the bladder wall may be seen ultrasonographically. Varicosities of the bladder, however, are small and discrete. Superficial ulcerations may be noted. Electrocautery and laser fulguration have been successful.[299] More extensive bladder arteriovenous malformations may be seen in conditions such as Klippel-Trenaunay-Weber and Sturge-Weber syndromes.[300] Recurrent gross hematuria may be difficult to control in some patients. Treatment options include local resection, embolization, and sclerotherapy.

Bladder Diverticula

Congenital diverticula of the bladder are uncommon. Identification of a bladder diverticulum should prompt an evaluation for bladder outflow obstruction due to PUV or neurogenic voiding dysfunction. In the setting of a smooth-wall bladder, however, outflow obstruction is usually not found. The basis for the diverticulum is presumed to be a weakness in the bladder wall musculature. Diverticula have been described in children with connective tissue defects, including Ehlers-Danlos syndrome[301] and Menkes kinky-hair syndrome,[302] both characterized by defects in collagen structure. It is possible that abnormal development of the lamina propria permits eventration of the pliable uroepithelium through the muscle fibers. Surgical repair of these diverticula is controversial because it does not deal with the underlying defect and recurrence is reported to be frequent. The author observed two children with Menkes syndrome who went into urinary retention due to the diverticula and were effectively managed with simple diverticulectomies. Intermittent catheterization may not always be effective owing to poor emptying and the risk of subsequent UTIs.

CONTINENT URINARY DIVERSION AND BLADDER RECONSTRUCTION

Indications

Continent urinary diversion involves the creation of a system of urinary storage and emptying other than native bladder, or with a bladder emptying mechanism other than urethra. Its application is appropriate whenever storage of emptying functions cannot be effectively restored with bladder or urethra. This is most often the case in patients with neurogenic bladder dysfunction in whom bladder capacity is markedly limited, sphincter function is inadequate, or both. Other situations involve bladder absence or total unreconstructability as in prior radical excision for tumor, or a small fibrotic bladder as with some bladder exstrophy patients. Causes of urethral unreconstructability include prior surgery and scarring, neurogenic fibrosis, and a severely abnormal body habitus that prevents perineal catheterization. A catheterizable abdominal stoma is often the most appropriate means of attaining continence with adequate emptying.

Continent diversion depends on intermittent catheterization, which must be ensured before reconstruction. It is often more

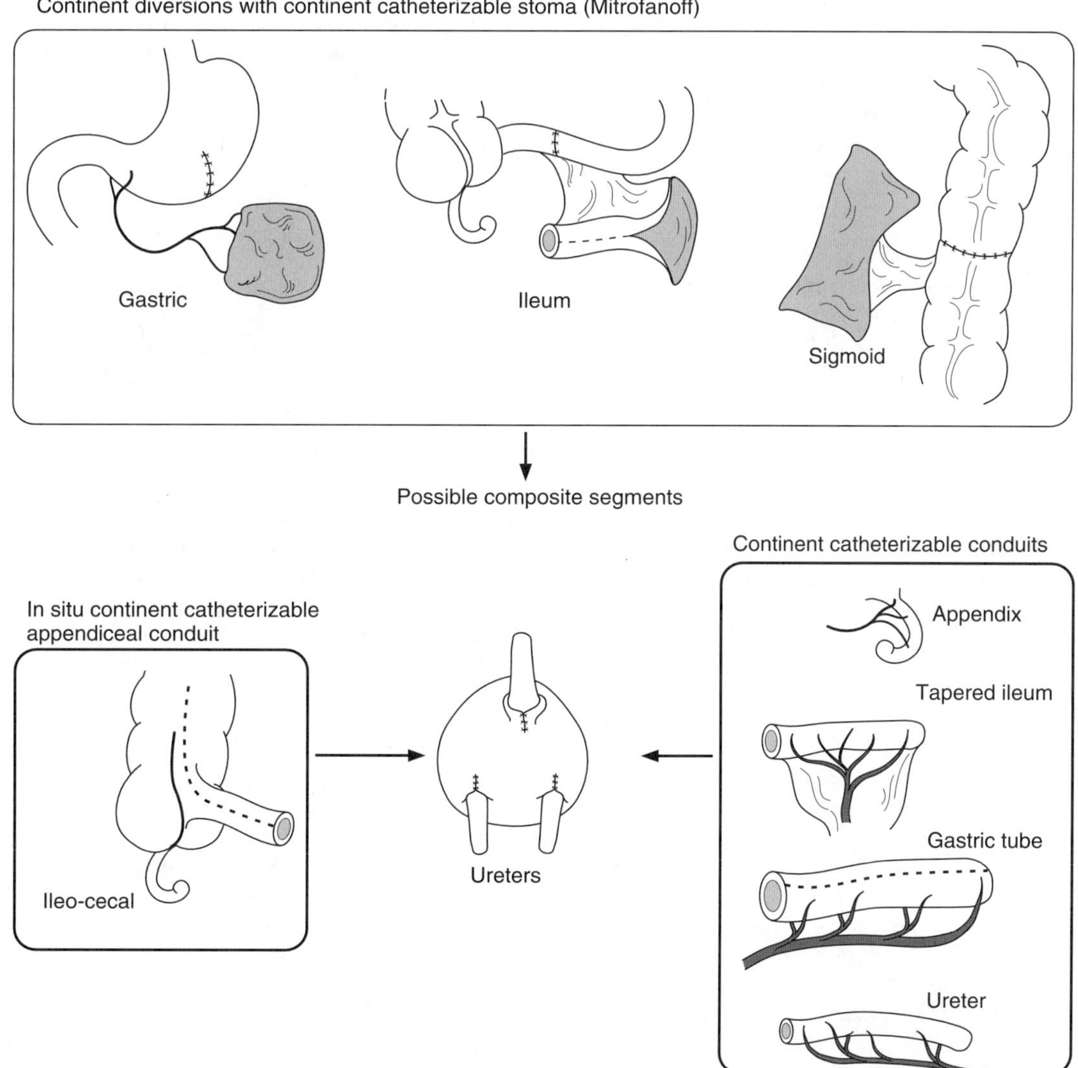

FIG. 92-74. Various options involved in continent diversion using the Mitrofanoff principle. The reservoir can be constructed of a single reconfigured enteric segment or a combination of more than one segment. The ureters are usually tunneled into the wall of the reservoir in an antireflux manner. The reservoir is made continent through the catheterizable conduit, using appendix, ureter, or a constructed tube from the bowel.

acceptable to patients to catheterize an abdominal rather than a perineal urethral stoma.

Techniques

Reservoir

The urinary reservoir for a continent diversion may include native bladder in whole or part[303] (Fig. 92-74). Augmentation of bladder capacity to decrease pressure is usually needed. This can involve segments of ileum, cecum, sigmoid, or stomach. When the bladder is unusable or absent, a reservoir may be constructed by one of a variety of mechanisms, depending on the condition, mobility of bowel segments, and the surgeon's preference. Reconfigured ileocecal reservoirs have been widely used with good results. Complete detubularization and reconfiguration is essential.[220]

Alternative techniques for creation of an adequate-capacity, low-pressure reservoir have been explored, including ureterocystoplasty[304–307] and the use of demucosalized segments of the gastrointestinal tract.[308,309] The principal aim of these techniques is to avoid the application of enteric mucosa in a urinary reservoir.

Continence Mechanisms

A variety of mechanisms to achieve continence are available, based on either a flap–valve technique, tissue pressure, or external compression.[310] The flap–valve technique involves a tubular structure implanted into the wall of the bladder or colonic segment and is generally referred to as the *Mitrofanoff technique.*[311] This approach has an excellent success rate and is efficient to create. Avoidance of too long a catheterizable segment avoids problems with postoperative inability to catheterize. Creation of a V flap of skin into the spatulated end of the tube helps to prevent stomal stenosis. Tissue pressure methods include tapering an ileal segment and reinforcing the ileocecal valve mechanism. The ileum would then be brought out to the skin for catheterization. External pressure techniques include use of an artificial urinary sphincter or Marlex mesh cuff around an intestinal segment.

The flap–valve technique provides continence most effectively but does not permit pop-off if catheterization is not rigorously attended.

Complications

The complications of continent urinary diversions are largely preventable with appropriate attention to detail in the initial creation of the diversion and with postoperative follow-up. Adequate mobilization and detubularization of the intestinal segments prevent ischemic problems and maintain adequately low reservoir pressures. The continence mechanism must be short and easily catheterizable. This should be ensured in the operating room. Postoperatively, the most common problems revolve around inadequate emptying of the reservoir, which can cause infection, perforation,[312] mucus plugging,[312] electrolyte abnormalities,[216,217,313–316] and stones.[215,219] Regular irrigation with

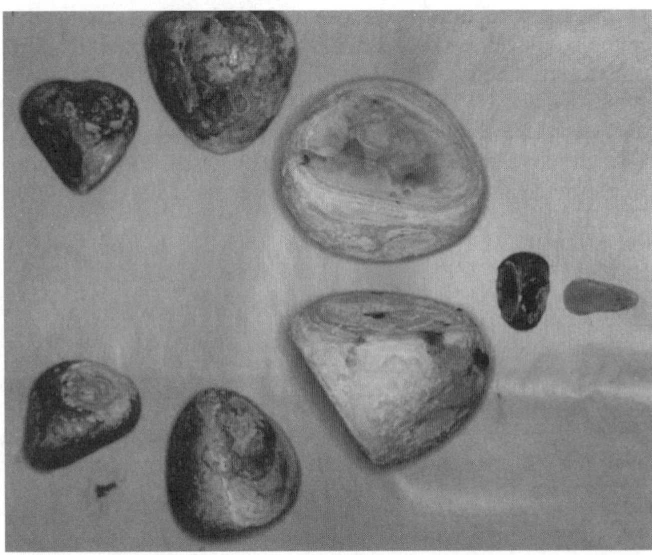

FIG. 92-75. Stones removed from a continent diversion. They weighed 500 g and were asymptomatic. The patient was noncompliant with catheterization and irrigation.

saline solution and a strict emptying regiment are important. Periodic monitoring of the pouch to identify stones early avoids the need for a major procedure to remove any that may form. Percutaneous techniques are useful with small calculi, but larger stones may be most efficiently removed with open surgery (Fig. 92-75). Tumors have not been reported in continent urinary diversions in children, but the possibility has been raised, and investigation and monitoring are ongoing.[317]

Urothelial Culture and Expansion

The principal limitation in reconstructive urologic surgery is the shortage of usable uroepithelium-lined structures. Enteric segments have permitted complete reconstruction of the urinary tract in a wide variety of patients, with generally good success. These procedures are nonetheless complex and still plagued by late complications. These complications are largely the result of the biologic properties of the enteric segment, which was not destined to serve as a urinary reservoir. Attempts to surface enteric segments with uroepithelium have been reported, with anecdotal success. A more appealing alternative appearing on the horizon has been the use of cultured uroepithelial cells constructed into usable replacements for bladder, urethra, or ureter. Tissue engineering may permit more efficient reconstructions without the risk of the late complications of stones, infection, and metabolic aberrations.[318–320]

After harvesting a small number of uroepithelial cells, culturing in vitro and many-fold expansion of the cells provides a new source of uroepithelium for reconstruction. These cells are then attached and supported on a scaffold to permit introduction into the body in a functional configuration, such as a bladder augmentation. The scaffold is biodegradable and serves to support the cells as they become engrafted into the new host. Composite reconstructions that include uroepithelium and smooth muscle may also be possible, although integrated function remains speculative. These strategies may permit complete bladder reconstruction in patients with inadequate or abnormal native bladder tissue, from a small source of cells. Such reconstructions would be preferable to those involving enteric segments. These studies have also permitted investigation of the unique biology of the uroepithelial cell and may ultimately lead to a better understanding of the pathologic processes that affect the bladder.

REFERENCES

1. Snyder HM III. Anomalies of the ureter. In: Gillenwater JY, Grayhack JT, Howards SS, et al, eds. Adult and pediatric urology, ed 2. St Louis, Mosby–Year Book, 1991:1832.
2. Ruano-Gil D, Coca-Payeras A, Tejedo-Mateu A. Obstruction and normal recanalization of the ureter in the human embryo: its relation to congenital ureteric obstruction. Eur Urol 1975;1:293.
3. Matsuno T, Tokunaka S, Koyanagi T. Muscular development in the urinary tract. J Urol 1984;132:148.
4. Williams PL, Warwick R, Dyson M, et al. Gray's anatomy, ed 37. New York, Churchill Livingstone, 1989.
5. Kabalin JN. Surgical anatomy of the genitourinary tract. In: Walsh PC, Retik AB, Stamey TA, et al, eds. Campbell's urology, ed 6. Philadelphia, WB Saunders, 1992:35.
6. Weiss RM. Ureteral function. Urology 1978;12:114.
7. Gosling JA, Dixon JS. Morphologic evidence that the renal calyx and pelvis control ureteric activity in rabbit. Am J Anat 1971;130:393.
8. Morita T, Ishizuka G, Tsuchida S. Initiation and propagation of stimulus from the renal pelvic pacemaker in pig kidney. Invest Urol 1981;19:157.
9. Morita T, Wada I, Saeki H, et al. Ureteral urine transport: changes in bolus volume of flow resulting from autonomic drugs. J Urol 1987;137:132.
10. Rose JG, Gillenwater JY. The effect of adrenergic and cholinergic agents and their blockers upon ureteral activity. Invest Urol 1974;11:439.
11. Wheeler MA, Housman A, Cho YH, et al. Age dependence of adenylate cyclase activity in guinea pig ureter homogenate. J Pharmacol Exp Ther 1986;239:99.
12. Latifpour J, Morita T, O'Hollaren B, et al. Characterization of autonomic receptors in neonatal urinary tract smooth muscle. Develop Pharmacol Ther 1989;13:1.
13. Ross JA, Edmond P, Kirkland IS. Behavior of the human ureter in health and disease. Edinburgh, Churchill Livingstone, 1972.
14. Griffiths DJ, Notschaele C. The mechanics of urine transport in the upper urinary tract. I. The dynamics of the isolated bolus. Neurourol Urodynam 1983;2:155.
15. McCrory WW, Shibuya M, Leumann E, et al. Studies of renal function in children with chronic hydronephrosis. Pediatr Clin North Am 1971;18:445.
16. Winberg J. Renal function in water-losing syndrome due to lower urinary tract obstruction before and after treatment. Acta Pediatr 1959;48:149.
17. Akimoto M, Biancani P, Weiss RM. Comparative pressure-length-diameter relationships of neonatal and adult rabbit ureters. Invest Urol 1977;14:297.
18. Gillenwater JY. The pathophysiology of urinary tract obstruction. In: Walsh PC, Retik AB, Stamey TA, et al, eds. Campbell's urology, ed 6. Philadelphia, WB Saunders, 1992:499.
19. Rose JG, Gillenwater JY. Pathophysiology of ureteral obstruction. Am J Physiol 1873;225:830.
20. Rose JG, Gillenwater JY. Effects of obstruction upon ureteral function. Urology 1978;12:139.
21. Biancani P, Hausman M, Weiss RM. Effect of obstruction on ureteral circumferential force-length relations. Am J Physiol 1982;243:F204.
22. Hobbins JC, Romero R, Grannum P, et al. Antenatal diagnosis of renal anomalies with ultrasound. I. Obstructive uropathy. Am J Obstet Gynecol 1984;148:868.
23. Manning FA, Hill LM, Platt LD. Qualitative amniotic fluid volume determination by ultrasound: antepartum detection of intrauterine growth retardation. Am J Obstet Gynecol 1981;139:354.
24. Mandell J, Blyth B, Peters CA, et al. The natural history of structural genitourinary defects detected in utero. Radiology 1991;178:193.
25. Mandell J, Peters CA, Retik AB. Current concepts in the perinatal diagnosis and management of hydronephrosis. Urol Clin North Am 1990;17:249.
26. Benacerraf BR, Saltzman DH, Mandell J. Sonographic diagnosis of abnormal fetal genitalia. J Ultrasound Med 1989;8:613.
27. Winters WD, Lebowitz RL. Importance of prenatal detection of hydronephrosis of the upper pole. AJR 1990;155:125.
28. Clarke NW, Gough DCS, Cohen SJ. Neonatal urological ultrasound: diagnostic inaccuracies and pitfalls. Arch Dis Child 1989;64:578.
29. Elder JS, Duckett JW, Snyder HM. Intervention for fetal obstructive uropathy: has it been effective? Lancet, 1987;2:1007.
30. Glick PL, Harrison MR, Golbus MS, et al. Management of the fetus with congenital hydronephrosis. II. Prognostic criteria and selection of treatment. J Pediatr Surg 1985;20:376.
31. Dejter SW Jr, Gibbons MD. The fate of infant kidneys with fetal hydronephrosis but initially normal postnatal sonography. J Urol 1989;142:661.
32. McInnis AN, Felman AH, Kaude JV, et al. Renal ultrasound in the neonatal period. Pediatr Radiol 1982;12:15.
33. Kass EJ, Majd M. Evaluation and management of upper urinary tract obstruction in infancy and childhood. Urol Clin North Am 1985;12:133.
34. Elder JS, Duckett JW. Perinatal urology. In: Gillenwater JY, Grayhack JT, Howards SS, et al, eds. Adult and pediatric urology. St Louis, Mosby–Year Book, ed 2, 1991:1711.
35. Johnston JH, Evans JP, Glassberg KI, et al. Pelvic hydronephrosis in children: a review of 219 personal cases. J Urol 1977;117:97.
36. Koff SA, Hayden LJ, Cirulli C. Pathophysiology of ureteropelvic junction obstruction: experimental and clinical observations. J Urol 1986;136:336.
37. Lebowitz RL, Blickman JG. The coexistence of ureteropelvic junction obstruction and reflux. AJR 1983;140:231.
38. Snyder HM III, Lebowitz RL, Colodny AH, et al. Ureteropelvic junction obstruction in children. Urol Clin North Am 1980;7:273.
39. King LR, Coughlin PWF, Bloch EC, et al. The case for immediate pyeloplasty in the neonate with ureteropelvic junction obstruction. J Urol 1984;132:725.
40. Mandell J, Kinard HW, Mittelstaedt CA, et al. Prenatal diagnosis of unilateral hydronephrosis with early postnatal reconstruction. J Urol 1984;132:303.
41. Ransley PG, Dhillon HK, Gordon I, et al. The postnatal management of hydronephrosis diagnosed by prenatal ultrasound. J Urol 1990;144:584.
42. Cartwright PC, Duckett JW, Keating MA, et al. Managing apparent ureteropelvic junction obstruction in the newborn. J Urol 1992;148:1224.
43. Koff SA, Campbell K. Nonoperative management of unilateral neonatal hydronephrosis. J Urol 1992;148:525.
44. Bejjani B, Belman AB. Ureteropelvic junction obstruction in newborn and infants. J Urol 1982;128:770.
45. Roth DR, Gonzales ET Jr. Management of ureteropelvic junction obstruction in infants. J Urol 1983;129:108.
46. Snyder HM III, Lebowitz RL, Colodny AG, et al. Ureteropelvic junction obstruction in children. Urol Clin North Am 1980;7:273.
47. Rich MA, Smith A. Pediatric endourology. In: Gillenwater JY, Grayhack JT, Howards SS, et al, eds. Adult and pediatric urology. St Louis, Mosby–Year Book, ed 2, 1991:2349.
48. Kavoussi LR, Peters CA. Laparoscopic pyeloplasty. J Urol 1993;150:1894.
49. King LR. Megaloureter: definition, diagnosis and management. (Editorial) J Urol 1980;123:222.
50. Lee BR, Partin AW, Epstein JI, et al. J Urol 1992;148:1482.
51. Gearhart JP, Lee B, Partin AW, et al. A quantitative evaluation of the dilated ureter of childhood. II. Prune belly, ectopia and posterior urethral valves. J Urol (in press).
52. McLaughlin AP III, Pfister RC, Leadbetter WF, et al. The pathophysiology of primary megaloureter. J Urol 1973;109:805.
53. Williams DI, Hulme-Moir I. Primary obstructive megaureter. Br J Urol 1970;42:140.
54. Cozzi F, Madonna L, Maggi E, et al. Management of primary megaureter in infancy. J Pediatr Surg 1993;28:1031.
55. Peters CA, Mandell J, Lebowitz RL, et al. Congenital obstructed meg-

aureters in early infancy: diagnosis and treatment. J Urol 1989;142:641.

56. Johnston JH. Reconstructive surgery of megaureter in childhood. Br J Urol 1967;39:17.

57. Hendren WH. Operative repair of megaureter in children. J Urol 1969;101:491.

58. Kalicinski ZH, Kansy J, Kotarbinska B, et al. Surgery of megaureters: modification of Hendren's operation. J Pediatr Surg 1977;12:183.

59. Gearhart JP, Leonard MP. Reoperative ureteral reimplantation: strategies for management. J Pediatr Surg 1991;26:58.

60. Stephens FD. Correlation of ureteric orifice position with renal morphology. Trans Am Assoc Genitourin Surg 1976:53.

61. Schulman CC. The single ectopic ureter. Eur Urol 1976;2:64.

62. Ellerker AG. The extravesical ectopic ureter. Br J Surg 1958;45:44.

63. Mogg RA. The single ectopic ureter. Br J Urol 1974;46:3.

64. Wyle JB, Lebowitz RL. Refluxing urethral ectopic ureters: recognition by cyclic voiding cystourethrogram. AJR 1984;142:1263.

65. Diard F, Chateil JF, Bondonny JM, et al. "Pseudo-ureterocele": buckling of an ectopic megaureter imprinting the urinary bladder. J Radiol 1987;68:177.

66. Smith FL, Ritchie EL, Maizels M, et al. Surgery for duplex kidneys with ectopic ureters: ipsilateral ureteroureterostomy versus polar nephrectomy J Urol 1989;142:532.

67. Gearhart JP, Jeffs RD. The use of topical vasodilators as an adjunct in infant renal surgery. J Urol 1985;134:298.

68. Campbell M. Ureterocele: a study of 94 instances in 80 infants and children. Surg Gynecol Obstet 1951;93:705.

69. Brock WA, Kaplan WG. Ectopic ureteroceles in children. J Urol 1978;119:800.

70. Chwalle R. The process of formation of cystic dilatations of the vesicle end of the ureter and of diverticula at the ureteral ostium. Urol Cutan Rev 1927;31:499.

71. Stephens FD. Caecoureterocele and concepts on the embryology and aetiology of ureteroceles. Aust N Z J Surg 1971;40:239.

72. Tokunaka S, Gotoh T, Koyanagi T, et al. Morphological study of the ureterocele: a possible clue to its embryogenesis as evidenced by a locally arrested myogenesis. J Urol 1981;126:726.

73. Stephens FD. Ureterocele in infants and children. Aust N Z J Surg 1958;27:288.

74. Stephens FD. Congenital malformations of the urinary tract. New York, 1983.

75. Churchill BM, Sheldon CA, McLorie GA. The ectopic ureterocele: a proposed practical classification based on renal unit jeopardy. J Pediatr Surg 1992;27:497.

76. Koyanagi T, Hisajima S, Goto T, et al. Everting ureterocele: radiographic and endoscopic observation and surgical management. J Urol 1980;123:538.

77. Lyon RP, Marshall S, Tanagho EA. The ureteric orifice: its configuration and competency. J Urol 1969;102:504.

78. Ransley PG. Vesicoureteral reflux: continuing surgical dilemma. Urology 1978;3:246.

79. Walker RD, Duckett JW, Bartone F, et al. Screening school children for urologic disease. Pediatrics 1977;60:239.

80. Edwards D, Norman ICS, Prescod N, et al. Disappearance of vesicoureteric reflux during long term prophylaxis of urinary tract infection in children. Br Med J 1977;2:285.

81. Roberts JA. Studies of vesicoureteral reflux: a review of work in a primate model. South Med J 1978;71:28.

82. Berllinger MF, Duckett JW. Vesicoureteral reflux: a comparison of non-surgical and surgical management. Contrib Nephrol 1984;39:81.

83. Noe HN. Screening for familial reflux: an update. Semin Urol 1986;4:86.

84. Askari A, Belman AB. Vesicoureteral reflux in black girls. J Pediatr Nephrol Urol 1981;1:11.

85. Ginsburg CM, McCracken GH Jr. Urinary tract infections in young infants. Pediatrics 1982;69:409.

86. Filly R, Friedland GW, Govan DE, et al. Development and progression of clubbing and scarring in children with recurrent urinary tract infections. Pediatr Radiol 1974;113:145.

87. Jacobson SH, Eklof O, Eriksson CG, et al. Development of hypertension and uremia after pyelonephritis in childhood: 27 year follow-up. Br Med J 1989;299:703.

88. Smellie JM, Normand ICS. Reflux nephropathy in childhood. In: Hodson J, Kincaid-Smith P, eds. Reflux nephropathy. New York, Masson, 1979:14.

89. Walker RD, Richard GA, Dobson D, et al. Maximum urinary concentration: early means of identifying patients with reflux who may require surgery. Urology 1973;1:343.

90. Decter RM, Roth DR, Gonzales ET. Vesicoureteral reflux in boys. J Urol 1988;140:1989.

91. Paquin AJ. Ureterovesical anastomosis: the description and evaluation of a technique. J Urol 1959;82:573.

92. Politano VA, Leadbetter WF. An operative technique for the correction of vesicoureteral reflux. J Urol 1958;79:932.

93. Ben-Chaim J, Shenfeld O, Leibovitch I, et al. Ureteral obstruction after puberty: a case seven years after ureteral reimplantation by the Politano-Leadbetter technique. (submitted)

94. Tocci PE, Politano VA, Lynne CM, et al. Unusual complications of transvesical ureteral reimplantation. J Urol 1976;115:731.

95. Lich R, Howerton LW, Goode LS, et al. The ureterovesical junction of the newborn. J Urol 1964;92:436.

96. Marberger M, Altwein JE, Straub E, et al. The Lich-Gregoir antireflux plasty: experiences with 371 children. J Urol 1978;120:216.

97. Cohen SJ. Ureterozystoneostomie, eine neue Antirefluxtechnik. Akt Urol 1975;6:1.

98. Matouschek E. Die behandlung des vesikorenalen Refluxes durch transurethrale Einspritzung von Teflonpaste. Urologe 1981;20:263.

99. Kaplan WE, Dalton DP, Firlit CF. The endoscopic correction of reflux by polytetrafluoroethylene injection. J Urol 1987;138:953.

100. O'Donnell B, Puri P. Technical refinements in endoscopic correction of vesicoureteral reflux. J Urol 1988;140:1101.

101. Leonard MP, Canning DA, Peters CA, et al. Endoscopic injection of glutaraldehyde cross-linked bovine dermal collagen for correction of vesicoureteral reflux. J Urol 1991;145:115.

102. Merguerian PA, McLorie GA, Khoury A, et al. Submucosal injection of polyvinyl alcohol foam (Ivalon) in rabbit bladder. J Urol 1990;144:531.

103. Atala A, Kim W, Paige KT, et al. Endoscopic treatment of reflux with autologous chondrocytes. Presented at the American Academy of Pediatrics meeting, Washington, D.C., October 1993.

104. Gearhart JP. Endoscopic management of vesicoureteric reflux. Probl Urol 1990;4:639.

105. Wandzilak TR, Williams HE. Hyperoxaluric syndromes. Endocrinol Metab Clin North Am 1990;19:851.

106. Seegmiller JE. Xanthine stone formation. Am J Med 1968;45:780.

107. Witten FR, Morgan JW, Foster JG, et al. 2,8-Dihydroxyadenine urolithiasis: review of the literature and report of a case in the United States. J Urol 1983;130:938.

108. Crawhall JC. Cystinuria: an experience in management over 18 years. Miner Electrolyte Metab 1987;13:286.

109. Singer A, Das S. Cystinuria: a review of the pathophysiology and management. J Urol 1989;142:669.

110. Batlle DC, Sehy JT, Roseman MK, et al. Clinical and pathophysiologic spectrum of acquired distal renal tubular acidosis. Kidney Int 1981;20:389.

111. Stewart AF, Adler M, Byers CM, et al. Calcium homeostasis in immobilization: an example of resorptive hypercalciuria. N Engl J Med 1982;306:1136.

112. Smith LH, Fromm H, Hofmann AF. Acquired hyperoxaluria, nephrolithiasis and intestinal disease: description of a syndrome. N Engl J Med 1972;286:1371.

113. Pak CYC, Kaplan R, Bone H, et al. A simple test for the diagnosis of absorptive, resorptive and renal hypercalciurias. N Engl J Med 1975;292:497.

114. Yendt ER, Cohanim M. Prevention of calcium stones with thiazides. Kidney Int 1978;13:397.

115. Griffith DP, Osborne CA. Infection (urease) stones. Miner Electrolyte Metab 1987;13:278.

116. Williams JJ, Rodman JS, Peterson CM. A randomized double-blind study of acetohydroxamic acid in struvite nephrolithiasis. N Engl J Med 1988;311:760.

117. Muldoon LD, Resnick MI. Secondary urolithiasis. Endocrinol Metab Clin North Am 1990;19:909.

118. Dhanamitta S, Valyasevi A, Susilavorn B. Research report on bladder stone disease, Thailand. In: van Reem R, ed. Idiopathic urinary bladder stone disease. Washington DC, Department of Health, Education and Welfare, Publication DHEW No 77-1063, 1977:151.

119. Srivastava RN, Hussainy AA, Goel RG, et al. Bladder stone disease in children in Afganistan. Br J Urol 1986;58:374.

120. Evan AP, Willis LR, Connors B, et al. SWL induces more severe renal structural and functional changes in juvenile V adult mini-pig kidney. J Endocrinol 1990;4:S58.

121. Adams M, Newman D, Lingeman J, et al. Extracorporeal shock wave lithotripsy in the pediatric age population: short and long term results. J Urol 1989;140:271A.

122. Losty P, Surana R, O'Donnel B. Limitations of extracorporeal shock wave lithotripsy for urinary tract calculi in young children. J Pediatr Surg 1993;28:1037.

123. Hulbert J, Reddy P, Gonzales R. Percutaneous nephrostolithotomy: an alternative approach to the management of pediatric calculus disease. Pediatrics 1985;76:610.

124. Segura JW, Patterson DE, LeRoy AJ, et al. Percutaneous removal of kidney stones: review of 1000 cases. J Urol 1985;134:1077.

125. Thomas R, Ortenberg J, Cerniglia F. Ureteroscopy and ureterolithotripsy in pediatric patients. J Endocrinol 1990;4:S109.

126. Smith LH, Segura JW. Urolithiasis in clinical pediatric urology, ed 3. Philadelphia, WB Saunders, 1992:1327.

127. Ewalt DH, Howard PS, Blyth B, et al. Is lamina propria matrix responsible for normal bladder compliance? J Urol 1992;148:544.

128. Parsons CL, Boychuck D, Jones S, et al. Bladder surface glycosaminoglycans: an epithelial permeability barrier. J Urol 1990;143:139.

129. Baskin LS, Young P, Hayward S, et al. Role of mesenchymal–epithelial interactions in normal bladder development. J Urol 1995;153:264A.

130. Oerlich TM. The urethral sphincter muscle in the male. Am J Anat 1980;158:229.

131. Oerlich TM. The striated urogenital sphincter muscle in the female. Anat Rec 1983;205:223.

132. Steers WD. Physiology of the urinary bladder. In: Walsh PC, Retik AB, Stamey TA, et al, eds. Campbell's urology. Philadelphia, WB Saunders, 1992:142.

133. Brading A. Physiology of bladder smooth muscle. In: Torrens M, Morrison JFB, eds. The physiology of the lower urinary tract. Berlin, Springer-Verlag, 1987:161.

134. Kamm KE, Stull JT. The function of myosin and myosin light chain kinase phosphorylation in smooth muscle. Annu Rev Pharmacol Toxicol 1985;25:593.

135. Kamm KE, Stull JT. Regulation of smooth muscle contractile elements by second messengers. Annu Rev Physiol 1989;51:299.

136. Kondo A, Susset JG. Viscoelastic properties of bladder. II. Comparative studies in normal and pathologic dogs. Invest Urol 1974;11:459.

137. Susset JG, Regnier CH. Viscoelastic properties of bladder strips: standardization of a technique. Invest Urol 1981;18:445.

138. Peters CA, Poppas DP, Freeman MR, et al. Abnormal collagen deposition in fetal bladder obstruction: a role for matrix metalloproteinases and their inhibitors. J Urol 1995;153:264A.

139. Peters CA, Vasavada S, Dator D, et al. The effect of obstruction on the developing bladder. J Urol 1992;148:491.

140. Kitada S, Wein AJ, Kato K, et al. Effect of acute complete obstruction on the rabbit urinary bladder. J Urol 1989;141:166.

141. Levin RM, High J, Wein AJ. The effect of short-term obstruction on urinary bladder function in the rabbit. J Urol 1984;132:789.

142. Kato K, Wein AJ, Kitada S, et al. The functional effect of mild outlet obstruction on the rabbit urinary bladder. J Urol 1988;140:880.

143. Kato K, Wein AJ, Radzinski C, et al. Short term functional effects of bladder outlet obstruction in the cat. J Urol 1990;143:1020.

144. Malkowicz SB, Wein AJ, Elbadawi A, et al. Acute biochemical and functional alterations in the partially obstructed rabbit urinary bladder. J Urol 1986;136:1324.

145. Lepor H, Gup D, Shapiro E, et al. Muscarinic cholinergic receptors in normal and neurogenic human bladder. J Urol 1989;142:869.

146. Steers WD, deGroat WC. Effect of bladder outlet obstruction on micturition reflex pathways in the rat. J Urol 1988;140:864.

147. Steers WD, Ciambotti J, Erdman S, et al. Morphological plasticity in efferent pathways to the urinary bladder of the rat following urethral obstruction. J Neurosci 1990;10:1943.

148. Steers WD, Ciambotti J, Etzel B, et al. Alterations in afferent pathways from the urinary bladder of the rat in response to partial urethral obstruction. J Comp Neurol 1991;310:401.

149. Gyllensten L. Contributions to embryology of the urinary bladder; development of definitive relations between the openings of the Wolffian ducts and ureters. Acta Anat 1949;7:305.

150. Newman J, Antonakopoulos GN. The fine structure of the human fetal urinary bladder: development and maturation. A light, transmission and scanning electron microscopic study. J Anat 1989;166:135.

151. Ayres PH, Shinohara Y, Frith CH. Morphological observations on the epithelium of the developing urinary bladder of the mouse and rat. J Urol 1985;133:506.

152. Cano M, Johansson SL, Wilson RB, et al. Preparation methods for light microscopic and ultrastructural studies of fetal rat bladder. Scan Electron Microsc 1986;4:1357.

153. Matsuno T, Tokunaka S, Koyanagi T. Muscular development in the urinary tract. J Urol 1984;132:148.

154. Hoyes AD, Ramus NI, Martin BGH. Ultrastructural aspects of the development of the innervation of the vesical musculature in the early human fetus. Invest Urol 1973;10:307.

155. Mitolo CD, Schonauer S, Grasso G, et al. Ontogenesis of autonomic receptors in detrusor muscle and bladder sphincter of human fetus. Urology 1983;21:599.

156. Levin RM, Malkowicz SB, Jacobowitz D, et al. The ontogeny of the autonomic innervation and contractile response of the rabbit urinary bladder. J Pharmacol Exp Ther 1981;219:250.

157. Lee JG, Coplen D, Macarek E, et al. Comparative studies on the ontogeny and autonomic responses of the fetal calf bladder at different stages of development: involvement of nitric oxide on field stimulated relaxation. J Urol 1994;151:1096.

158. Zderic SA, Gong C, Snyder HM, et al. Maturational influences on intracellular calcium sequestration in the rabbit: a new assay based on thapsigargin. J Urol 1995;153:263A.

159. Zderic SA, Hypolite J, Duckett JW, et al. Developmental aspects of bladder contractile function: sensitivity to extracellular calcium. Pharmacology 1991;43:61.

160. Bourdelat D, Barbet JP, Butler-Browne GS. Fetal development of the urethral sphincter. Eur J Pediatr Surg 1992;2:35.

161. Baskin LS, Constantinescu S, Duckett JW, et al. Type III collagen decreases in normal fetal bovine bladder development. J Urol 1994;152:688.

162. Baskin L, Meaney D, Landsman A, et al. Bovine bladder compliance increases with normal fetal development. J Urol 1994;152:692.

163. Swaiman KF, Bradley WE. Quantitation of collagen in the wall of the human urinary bladder. J Appl Physiol 1967;22:122.

164. Kim KM, Kogan BA, Massad CA, et al. Collagen and elastin in the normal fetal bladder. J Urol 1991;146:524.

165. Peters CA, Carr MC, Freeman MR, et al. Collagen gene expression in the fetal bladder is altered by in utero bladder functional status. In: American Academy of Pediatrics, Urology Section. San Francisco, 1992.

166. Campbell S, Wladimiroff JW, Dewhurst CJ. Antenatal measurement of fetal urine production. J Obstet Gynecol Br Commonw 1973;80:680.

167. Wladimiroff JW, Campbell S. Fetal urine-production rates in normal and complicated pregnancy. Lancet 1974;1:151.

168. Kogan BA, Iwamoto HS. Lower urinary tract function in the sheep fetus: studies of autonomic control and pharmacologic responses of the fetal bladder. J Urol 1989;141:1019.

169. Barth RA, Filly RA, Sondheimer FK. Prenatal sonographic findings in bladder exstrophy. J Ultrasound Med 1990;9:359.

170. Jaffe R, Schoenfeld A, Ovadia J. Sonographic findings in the prenatal diagnosis of bladder exstrophy. Am J Obstet Gynecol 1990;162:675.

171. Mandell J, Lebowitz RL, Peters CA, et al. Prenatal diagnosis of the megacystis-megaureter association. J Urol 1992;148:1487.

172. Manning FA. Fetal surgery for obstructive uropathy: rational considerations. Am J Kidney Dis 1987;10:259.

173. Stiller RJ. Early ultrasonic appearance of fetal bladder outlet obstruction. Am J Obstet Gynecol 1989;160:584.

174. Seeds JW, Mandell J. Congenital obstructive uropathies: pre- and postnatal treatment. Urol Clin North Am 1986;13:155.

175. Retik AB, Peters CA. Ectopic ureter and ureterocele. In: Walsh PC, Retik AB, Stamey TA, et al, eds. Campbell's urology. Philadelphia, WB Saunders, 1992:1743.

176. Spencer JR, Schaeffer AJ. Pediatric urinary tract infections. Urol Clin North Am 1986;13:661.

177. Roberts JA. Etiology and pathophysiology of pyelonephritis. Am J Kidney Dis 1991;17:1.

178. Hoover DL, Duckett JW Jr. Posterior urethral valves, unilateral reflux, and renal dysplasia: a syndrome. J Urol 1982;128:994.

179. Glassberg KL, Schnieider M, Haller JO, et al. Observations on persistently dilated ureter after posterior urethral valve ablation. Urology 1982;20:20.

180. Peters CA, Bolkier M, Bauer SB, et al. The urodynamic consequences of posterior urethral valves. J Urol 1990;144:122.

181. Kaplan GW, Brock WA. Idiopathic urethrorrhagia in boys. J Urol 1982;128:1001.

182. Bauer SB, Kogan SJ. Vesical manifestations of chronic granulomatous disease in children: its relation to eosinophilic cystitis. Urology 1991;37:463.

183. Koff SA, Byard MA. The daytime urinary frequency syndrome of childhood. J Urol 1988;140:1280.

184. Zawin JK, Lebowitz RL. Neurogenic dysfunction of the bladder in infants and children: recent advances and the role of radiology. Radiology 1992;182:297.

185. Mandell J, Lebowitz RL, Hallett M, et al. Urethral narrowing in region of external sphincter: Radiologic-urodynamic correlations in boys with myelodysplasia. AJR 1980;134:731.

186. Blaivas JG, Labib KL, Bauer SB, et al. Changing concepts in the urodynamic evaluation of children. J Urol 1977;117:778.

187. Bauer SB. Neuropathology of the lower urinary tract. In: Kelalis PP, King LR, Belman AB eds. Clinical pediatric urology. Philadelphia, WB Saunders, 1992:399.

188. Wan J, McGuire EJ, Bloom DA, et al. Stress leak point pressure: a diagnostic tool for incontinent children. J Urol 1993;150:700.

189. Rose NC, Mennuti MT. Maternal serum screening for neural tube defects and fetal chromosome abnormalities. (Review) West J Med 1993;159:312.

190. Loft AG, Hogdall E, Larsen SO, et al. A comparison of amniotic fluid alpha-fetoprotein and acetylcholinesterase in the prenatal diagnosis of open neural tube defects and anterior abdominal wall defects. Prenat Diagn 1993;13:93.

191. Wald NJ, Kennard A. Prenatal biochemical screening for Down's syndrome and neural tube defects. (Review) Curr Opin Obstet Gynecol 1992;4:302.

192. Drugan A, Dvorin E, Obrien JE, et al. Alpha-fetoprotein. (Review) Curr Opin Obstet Gynecol 1991;39:230.

193. Cuckle HS. Screening for neural tube defects. (Review) Ciba Found Symp 1994;181:253.

194. Wald NJ. Folic acid and neural tube defects: the current evidence and implications for prevention. Ciba Found Symp 1994;181:192.

195. Rieder MJ. Prevention of neural tube defects with periconceptional folic acid. Clin Perinatol 1994;21:483.

196. Shapiro E, Becich MJ, Perlman E, et al. Bladder wall abnormalities in myelodysplastic bladders: a computer assisted morphometric analysis. J Urol 1991;145:1024.

197. Kasabian NG, Bauer SB, Dyro FM, et al. The prophylactic value of clean intermittent catheterization and anticholinergic medication in newborns and infants with myelodysplasia at risk of developing urinary tract deterioration. Am J Dis Child 1992;146:840.

198. Mattiasson A, Andersson KE, Sjogren C, et al. Supersensitivity to carbachol in the parasympathetically decentralized feline urinary bladder. J Urol 1984;131:562.

199. Keating MA. The noncompliant bladder: principle in pathogenesis and pathophysiology. Probl Urol 1994;8:348.

200. Dixon JS, Gilpin CJ, Gilpin SA, et al. Sequential morphological changes in the pig detrusor in response to chronic partial urethral obstruction. Br J Urol 1989;64:385.

201. Gosling JA, Gilpin SA, Dixon JS, et al. Decrease in the autonomic innervation of human detrusor muscle in outflow obstruction. J Urol 1986;136:501.

202. Speakman MJ, Brading AF, Gilpin CJ, et al. Bladder outflow obstruction: a cause of denervation supersensitivity. J Urol 1987;138:1461.

203. Uvelius B, Mattiasson A. Detrusor collagen content in the denervated rat urinary bladder. J Urol 1986;136:1110.

204. Bloom DA, Knechtel JM, McGuire EJ. Urethral dilation improves bladder compliance in children with myelomeningocele and high leak point pressures. J Urol 1990;144:430.

205. Joseph DB, BAuer SB, Colodny AH, et al. Clean, intermittent catheterization of infants with neurogenic bladder. Pediatrics 1989;84:78.

206. Atala A, Bauer SB, Hendren WH, et al. The effect of gastric augmentation on bladder function. J Urol 1993;149:1099.

207. Cher ML, Allen TD. Continence in the myelodysplastic patient following enterocystoplasty. J Urol 1993;149:1103.

208. deBadiola FI, Castro DD, Hart AC, et al. Influence of preoperative bladder capacity and compliance on the outcome of artificial sphincter implantation in patients with neurogenic sphincter incompetence. J Urol 1992;148:1493.

209. deCastro R, Pavanello P, Tani G, et al. Further experience with the use of gastrointestinal segments in bladder reconstruction in the complex of exstrophy-epispadias]. Pediatr Med Chir 1993;15:145.

210. Goldwasser B, Webster GD. Augmentation and substitution enterocystoplasty. J Urol 1986;135:215.

211. Khoury JM, Webster GD. Evaluation of augmentation cystoplasty for severe neuropathic bladder using the hostility score. Dev Med Child Neurol 1992;34:441.

212. Ralph DJ, Woodhouse CR, Ransley PG. The management of the neuropathic bladder in adolescents with imperforate anus. J Urol 1992;148:366.

213. Stephenson TP. Techniques and complications of substitution and augmentation cystoplasties. Scand J Urol Nephrol Suppl 1992;142:123.

214. Bauer SB, Hendren WH, Kozakewich H, et al. Perforation of the augmented bladder. J Urol 1992;148:699.

215. Blyth B, Ewalt DH, Duckett JW, et al. Lithogenic properties of enterocystoplasty. J Urol 1992;148:575.

216. Gold BD, Bhoopalam PS, Reifen RM, et al. Gastrointestinal complications of gastrocystoplasty. Arch Dis Child 1992;67:1272.

217. Gosalbez RJ, Woodard JR, Broecker BH, et al. Metabolic complications of the use of stomach for urinary reconstruction. J Urol 1993;150:710.

218. Khoury JM, Timmons SL, Corbel L, et al. Complications of enterocystoplasty. Urology 1992;40:9.

219. Palmer LS, Franco I, Kogan SJ, et al. Urolithiasis in children following augmentation cystoplasty. J Urol 1993;150:726.

220. Hinman FJ. Selection of intestinal segments for bladder substitution: physical and physiological characteristics. J Urol 1988;139:519.

221. Mevorach RA, Hulbert WC, Merguerian PA, et al. Perforation and intravesical erosion of a ventriculoperitoneal shunt in a child with an augmentation cystoplasty. J Urol 1992;147:433.

222. Bauer SB, Peters CA, Mandell J, et al. Fascial slings in the management of incontinence. J Urol 1989;142:516.

223. Herschorn S, Radomski SB. Fascial slings and bladder neck tapering in the treatment of male neurogenic incontinence. J Urol 1992;147:1073.

224. Gormley EA, Bloom DA, McGuire EJ, et al. Pubovaginal slings for the management of urinary incontinence in female adolescents. J Urol 1994;152:822.

225. Jones JA, Mitchell ME, Rink RC. Improved results using a modification of the Young-Dees-Leadbetter bladder neck repair. Br J Urol 1993;71:555.

226. Mitchell ME, Rink RC. Experience with the artificial urinary sphincter in children and young adults. J Pediatr Surg 1983;18:700.

227. Bosco PJ, Bauer SB, Colodny AH, et al. The long-term results of artificial sphincters in children. J Urol 1991;146:396.

228. Aprikian A, Berardinucci G, Pike J, et al. Experience with the AS-800 artificial urinary sphincter in myelodysplastic children. Can J Surg 1992;35:396.

229. Gonzales R, Sheldon CA. Artificial sphincters in children with neurogenic bladders: long-term results. J Urol 1982;128:1270.

230. Shortliffe LM, Freiha FS, Kessler R, et al. Treatment of urinary incontinence by the periurethral implantation of glutaraldehyde cross-linked collagen. J Urol 1989;141:538.

231. Caione P, Lais A, de Gennaro M, et al. Glutaraldehyde cross-linked bovine collagen in exstrophy/epispadias complex. J Urol 1993;150:631.

232. Wan J, McGuire EJ, Bloom DA, et al. The treatment of urinary incontinence in children using glutaraldehyde cross-linked collagen. J Urol 1992;148:127.

233. Duckett JW, Snyder HM. Continent urinary diversion: variations on the Mitrofanoff principle. J Urol 1986;136:58.

234. Mitrofanoff P. Cystostomie continente trans-appendiculaire dans le traitement des vessies neurologiques. Chir Pediatr 1986;21:297.

235. Duckett JW, Lotfi AH. Appendicovesicostomy (and variations) in bladder reconstruction. J Urol 1993;149(3):567.

236. Ritchey ML, Sinha A, DiPietro MA, et al. Significance of spina bifida occulta in children with diurnal enuresis. J Urol 1994;152:815.

237. Keating MA, Rinak RC, Bauer SB, et al. Neurourological implications of the changing approach in management of occult spinal lesions. J Urol 1988;140:1299.

238. Kakizaki H, Nonomura K, Asano Y, et al. Preexisting neurogenic voiding dysfunction in children with imperforate anus: problems in management. J Urol 1994;151:1041.

239. Parrott TS. Urologic implications of anorectal malformations. (Review) Urol Clin North Am 1985;12:13.

240. Sheldon C, Cormier M, Crone K, et al. Occult neurovesical dysfunction in children with imperforate anus and its variants. J Pediatr Surg 1991;26:49.

241. Young HH, Frontz WA, Baldwin JC. Congenital obstruction of the posterior urethra. J Urol 1919;3:289.

242. Campbell MF. Obstruction of the posterior urethral valve in infancy and childhood: a study of eighteen cases. JAMA 1931;96:592.

243. Hendren WH. Posterior urethral valves in boys: a broad clinical spectrum. J Urol 1971;106:298.

244. Nakayama DK, Harrison MR, and de Lorimier AA. Prognosis of posterior urethral valves presenting at birth. J Pediatr Surg 1986;21:43.

245. Egami K, Smith ED. A study of the sequelae of posterior urethral valves. J Urol 1982;127:84.

246. Henneberry MD, Stephens FD. Renal hypoplasia and dysplasia in infants with posterior urethral valves. J Urol 1980;123:912.

247. Hutton KA, Thomas DF, Arthur RJ, et al. Prenatally detected posterior urethral valves: is gestational age at detection a predictor of outcome? J Urol 1994;152:698.

248. Johnston JH, Kulatilake AE. The sequelae of posterior urethral valves. Br J Urol 1971;43:743.

249. McGuire EJ, Weiss RM. Secondary bladder neck obstruction in patients with urethral valves: treatment with phenoxybenzamine. Urology 1975;5:756.

250. Mitchell ME. Persistent ureteral dilatation following valve resection. Dialog Pediatr Urol 1982;5:8.

251. Peters CA. Congenital bladder obstruction: research approaches. Adv Exp Med 1995;385:117.

252. Bellinger MF, Comstock CH, Grosso D, et al. Fetal posterior urethral valves and renal dysplasia at 15 weeks gestational age. J Urol 1983;129:1238.

253. Harrison MR, Nakayama DK, Noall R, et al. Correction of congenital hydronephrosis in utero. II. Decompression reverses the effects of obstruction on the fetal lung and urinary tract. J Pediatr Surg 1982;17:965.

254. Mandell J, Greene MF, Peters CA, et al. Aspiration of bilateral perinephric urinomas and vesicoamniotic shunt placement in fetal bladder outlet obstruction. J Ultrasound Med 1992;11:679.

255. Mandell J, Peters CA. Current concepts in the perinatal diagnosis and management of hydronephrosis. Urol Clin North Am 1990;17:247.

256. Mandell J, Estroff J, Benacerraf BR, et al. Late onset severe oligohydramnios associated with genitourinary abnormalities. J Urol 1992;148:515.

257. Churchill BM, Krueger RP, Fleisher MH, et al. Complications of posterior urethral valve surgery and their prevention. Urol Clin North Am 1983;10:519.

258. Krueger RP, Hardy BE, Churchill BM. Growth in boys with posterior urethral valves. Urol Clin North Am 1980;7:265.

259. Hendren WH. A new approach to infants with severe obstructive uropathy: early complete reconstruction. J Pediatr Surg 1970;5:184.

260. Hendren WH, Peters CA, Ginsburg HB, et al. Severe urethral valves: experience with 77 primary cases. J Urol 1989;141:170A.

261. Parkhouse HF, Barratt TM, Dillon MJ, et al. Long-term outcome of boys with posterior urethral valves. Br J Urol 1988;62:59.

262. Docimo SG, Luetic T, Crone RK, et al. Pulmonary development in the fetal lamb with severe bladder outlet obstruction and oligohydramnios: a morphometric study. J Urol 1989;142:657.

263. Peters CA, Reid LM, Docimo S, et al. The role of the kidney in lung growth and maturation in the setting of obstructive uropathy and oligohydramnios. J Urol 1991;146:597.

264. Peters CA, Docimo SG, Luetic T, et al. Effect of in utero vesicostomy on pulmonary hypoplasia in the fetal lamb with bladder outlet obstruction and oligohydramnios: a morphometric analysis. J Urol 1991;146:1178.

265. Karim OMA, Cendron M, Mostwin JL, et al. Developmental alterations in the fetal lamb bladder subjected to partial urethral obstruction in utero. J Urol 1993;150:1060.

266. Stephenson TP. Lower urinary reconstruction in patients with severely impaired renal function. Scand J Urol Nephrol Suppl 1992;142:127.

267. Burns MW, Watkins SL, Mitchell ME, et al. Treatment of bladder dysfunction in children with end-stage renal disease. J Pediatr Surg 1992;27:170.

268. Sheldon CA, Gonzalez R, Burns MW, et al. Renal transplantation into dysfunctional bladder: role of adjunctive bladder reconstruction. J Urol 1994;152:972.

269. Dykes EH, Ransley PG. Gastrocystoplasty in children. Br J Urol 1992;69:91.

270. Nguyen DH, Bain MA, Salmonson KL, et al. The syndrome of dysuria and hematuria in pediatric urinary reconstruction with stomach. J Urol 1993;150:707.

271. Kinahan TJ, Khoury AE, McLorie, GA, et al. Omeprazole in postgastrocystoplasty metabolic alkalosis and aciduria. J Urol 1992;147:435.

272. Reinberg Y, Manivel JC, Froemming C, et al. Perforation of the gastric segment of an augmented bladder secondary to peptic ulcer disease. J Urol 1992;148:369.

273. Raney BJ, Heyn R, Hays DM, et al. Sequelae of treatment in 109 patients followed for 5 to 15 years after diagnosis of sarcoma of the bladder and prostate: a report from the Intergroup Rhabdomyosarcoma Study Committee. Cancer 1993;71:2387.

274. Kamii Y, Taguchi N, Tsunematsu Y. Primary chemotherapy for children with rhabdomyosarcoma of the "special pelvic" sites: is preservation of the bladder possible? J Pediatr Surg 1994;29:461.

275. Loughlin KR, Retik AB, Weinstein HJ, et al. Genitourinary rhabdomyosarcoma in children. Cancer 1989;63:1600.

276. Duel BP, Hendren WH, Bauer SB, et al. Reconstructive options in genitourinary rhabdomyosarcoma. In: American Academy of Pediatrics Section on Urology, Dallas, 1994.

277. Madgar I, Goldwasser B, Nativ O, et al. Long-term followup of patients less than 30 years old with transitional cell carcinoma of bladder. J Urol 1988;139:933.

278. Quillin SP, McAlister WH. Transitional cell carcinoma of the bladder in children: radiologic appearance and differential diagnosis. (Review) Urol Radiol 1991;13:107.

279. Lalmand B, Avni EF, Simon J, et al. Transitional cell papillary carcinoma of the bladder in a child. Pediatr Radiol 1987;17:77.

280. Wilson SD, Allen AE, Variend S. Transitional cell papillary bladder neoplasm in a girl: an unusual presentation. J Pediatr Surg 1992;27:113.

281. Keetch DW, Manley CB, Catalona WJ. Transitional cell carcinoma of bladder in children and adolescents. (Review) Urology 1993;42:447.

282. Silber SJ. Carcinoma in the bladder left behind. J Urol 1973;110:675.

283. Mortensen PB, Jensen KE, Nielsen K. Adenocarcinoma development in the trigone 34 years after trigonocolonic urinary diversion for exstrophy of the bladder. J Urol 1990;144:980.

284. Kandzari SJ, Majid A, Ortega AM, et al. Exstrophy of the urinary bladder complicated by adenocarcinoma. Urology 1974;3:496.

285. Borden TA, Shrader DA. Neurofibromatosis of bladder in a child: unusual cause of enuresis. Urology 1980;15:155.

286. Clark SS, Marlett MM, Prudencio RF, et al. Neurofibromatosis of the bladder in children: case report and literature review. J Urol 1977;118:654.

287. Albores-Saaverdra J, Maldonado ME, Ibarra J, et al. Pheochromocytoma of the urinary bladder. Cancer 1969;23:1110.

288. Heyman J, Cheung Y, Ghali V, et al. Bladder pheochromocytoma: evaluation with magnetic resonance imaging. J Urol 1989;141:1424.

289. Nold SR, Terry WJ, Cerniglia FR Jr, et al. Nephrogenic adenoma of the bladder in children. J Urol 1989;142:1545.

290. Cendron J, Melin Y, Baviera DE, et al. Polyp of the posterior urethra: apropos of 6 cases. (French) Chir Pediatr 1985;26:356.

291. De Castro R, Campobasso P, Belloli G, et al. Solitary polyp of posterior urethra in children: report on seventeen cases. Eur J Pediatr Surg 1993;3:92.

292. Kearney LP, Lebowitz RL, Retik AB. Obstructive polyps of the posterior urethra in boys: embryology and management. J Urol 1979;122:802.

293. Raviv G, Leibovitch I, Hanani J, et al. Hematuria and voiding disorders in children caused by congenital urethral polyps: principles of diagnosis and management. Eur Urol 1993;23:382.

294. Blichert-Toft M, Nielson OV. Congenital patent urachus and acquired variants. Acta Chir Scand 1971;137:807.

295. Avni EF, Matos C, Diard F, et al. Midline omphalovesical anomalies in children: contribution of ultrasound imaging. Urol Radiol 1988;2:189.

296. Hamsher JB, Farrar T, Moore TD. Congenital vascular tumors and malformations involving urinary tract: diagnosis and surgical management. J Urol 1958;80:299.

297. Hendry WF, Vinnicombe J. Haemangioma of bladder in children and young adults. Br J Urol 1971;43:209.

298. Leonard MP, Nickel CJ, Morales A. Cavernous hemangiomas of the bladder in the pediatric age group. J Urol 1988;140:1503.

299. Smith JA Jr. Laser treatment of bladder hemangioma. J Urol 1990;143:282.

300. Klein TW, Kaplan GW. Klippel-Trenaunay syndrome associated with urinary tract hemangiomas. J Urol 1975;114:596.

301. Levard G, Aigrain Y, Ferkadji L, et al. Urinary bladder diverticula and the Ehlers-Danlos syndrome in children. J Pediatr Surg 1989;24:1184.

302. Daly WJ, Rabinovitch HH. Urologic abnormalities in Menkes' syndrome. J Urol 1981;126:262.

303. Peters CA. Bladder reconstruction in children. Curr Opin Pediatr 1994;6:183.

304. Bellinger MF. Ureterocystoplasty: a unique method for vesical augmentation in children. J Urol 1993;149:811.

305. Churchill BM, Aliabadi H, Landau EH, et al. Ureteral bladder augmentation. J Urol 1993;150:716.

306. Landau EH, Jayanthi VR, Khoury AE, et al. Bladder augmentation: ureterocystoplasty versus ileocystoplasty. J Urol 1994;152:716.

307. Wolf JSJ, Turzan CW. Augmentation ureterocystoplasty. J Urol 1993;149:1095.

308. Kropp BP, Rippy M, Bradylak SF, et al. Small intestinal submucosa: urodynamic and histopathologic evaluation in long-term canine bladder augmentation. J Urol 1995;153:375A.

309. Nguyen DH, Carr MC, Bagli DJ, et al. Demucosalized gastrocystoplasty with autoaugmentation: a clinical experience. J Urol 1995;153:279A.

310. Hinman FJ. Functional classification of conduits for continent diversion. J Urol 1990;144:27.

311. Watson HS, Bauer SB, Peters CA, et al. Comparative urodynamics of appendiceal and ureteral Mitrofanoff conduits in children. J Urol 1995;154:878.

312. George VK, Gee JM, Wortley MI, et al. The effect of ranitidine on urine mucus concentration in patients with enterocystoplasty. Br J Urol 1992;70:30.

313. Champetier D, Haouas T, Hamza T, et al. Cholelithiasis and ileoceco-cystoplasty (study of 39 patients). Prog Urol 1992;2:391.

314. McDougall WS. Metabolic complications of urinary intestinal diversion. J Urol 1992;147:1199.

315. Steiner MS, Morton RA, Marshall FF. Vitamin B12 deficiency in patients with ileocolic neobladders. J Urol 1993;149:255.

316. Bogaert GA, Mevorach RA, Kim J, et al. Physiology of gastrocystoplasty: once a stomach, always a stomach. J Urol 1995;153:1977.

317. Buson H, Diaz DC, Manivel JC, et al. The development of tumors in experimental gastroenterocystoplasty. J Urol 1993;150:730.

318. Cilento BG, Freeman MR, Schneck, FX, et al. Phenotypic and cytogenetic characterization of human bladder urothelia expanded in vitro. J Urol 1994;152:665.

319. Atala A, Freeman MR, Vacanti JP, et al. Implantation in vivo and retrieval of artificial structures consisting of rabbit and human urothelium and human bladder muscle. J Urol 1993;150:608.

320. Hutton KA, Trejdosiewicz LK, Thomas DF, et al. Urothelial tissue culture for bladder reconstruction: an experimental study. J Urol 1993;150:721.

Surgery of Infants and Children: Scientific Principles and Practice, edited by
Keith T. Oldham, Paul M. Colombani, and Robert P. Foglia.
Lippincott–Raven Publishers, Philadelphia, © 1997.

CHAPTER 93

Male Genital Tract

Thomas A. Rozanski and David A. Bloom

Sexual differentiation, a sequential process, begins at fertilization with the determination of chromosomal sex. The karyotype established, XX or XY, depends on the X or Y chromosome contributed by the fertilizing sperm. Chromosomal sex directs gonadal sex; gonads are initially bipotential and indistinguishable, and local factors created by the chromosomal prescription influence differentiation into a testis or ovary. The testis-determining *SRY* gene on the short arm of chromosome Y facilitates differentiation of the gonad to a testis. Gonadal sex ultimately directs phenotypic sex, the appearance of anatomic characteristics. Each step in this sequential process of differentiation depends on the preceding step.

Normal fetal testis function includes production of testosterone by Leydig cells and müllerian inhibiting substance by Sertoli cells. Both substances are crucial for normal male phenotypic development. Müllerian inhibiting substance causes local regression of the paramesonephric ducts (müllerian system), and testosterone stimulates ipsilateral mesonephric (wolffian) duct development. The male genital tract is formed largely between 6 and 13 weeks of gestation. During the latter two thirds of gestation, the testicles descend and the external genitalia undergo differential growth.

Although internal ductal development is testosterone-mediated, virilization of the male external genitalia is governed by dihydrotestosterone (DHT). The enzyme 5-α reductase, which converts testosterone to DHT, and competent androgen receptors are necessary for development of normal external genitalia. Under the influence of DHT, the genital tubercle becomes a penis, the urethral folds fuse, and the genital swellings form into a scrotum.

PHALLUS

Embryology

The genital tubercle forms ventral to the cloaca by the fourth week of gestation, and is identical in both sexes until age 9 weeks. The male genital tubercle enlarges, elongates, and assumes a cylindrical shape. A circumferential groove delineates the glans. Elongation pulls the urethral folds forward, creating the lateral walls of the urethral groove. The folds migrate toward the midline and fuse by 12 weeks forming the penile urethra, the ventral surface of the phallus, and median raphe (Fig. 93-1). Mesenchyme coalesces around the deepening groove to form the corpus spongiosum. The urethral groove (entoderm) does not extend to the tip of the phallus; rather, the distal urethra is formed during the fourth month of gestation, when ectoderm from the glans tip invaginates to form the external meatus, which then joins the lumen of the penile urethra. When urethral formation is almost complete, preputial development begins as an epithelial fold growing over the glans. The surrounding pleat of skin is completed at birth.

Anatomy

The normal male term infant penis measures 3.5 cm in stretched length and 1.1 cm in diameter. Stretched penile length correlates with erect length. Measurement, made from the pubic symphysis to the tip of the glans, should be at least 2.5 cm. Care should be taken to depress the suprapubic fat pad completely to get an accurate measurement. Penile size often increases during the first 6 months after delivery, because of the physiologic surge of testosterone in the male infant at 2 to 3 months of age. From this time until puberty, however, only modest phallic growth occurs (Fig. 93-2). The urethra and external meatus of a premature or infant male should accommodate a 5F feeding tube. An 8F tube should pass without difficulty by age 1 year.

The prepuce protects the delicate urethral meatus from minor trauma. The inner epithelial surface fuses to the glans penis in infancy, obscuring the glans and meatus. This normal anatomic condition should not be confused with phimosis. True phimosis is a pathologic condition seen later in life, when a fibrotic preputial ring develops. During the first 3 to 5 years of life, the natural process of intermittent erections and progressive accumulation of desquamated residue (smegma) separate the inner epithelial surface of the prepuce from the glans. By age 3 years, 90% of foreskins are retractable. However, many boys have persistent isolated areas of adhesion, particularly around the coronal margin. By age 5 years, after the natural process of separation, the prepuce has no major function.

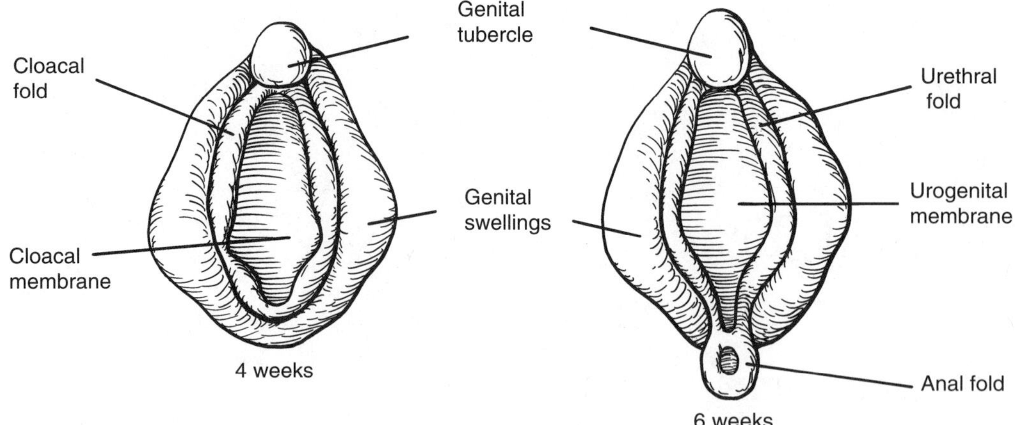

FIG. 93-1. Early stages of embryologic development; the genital swellings.

CIRCUMCISION

Circumcision, the most common surgical procedure in the United States, is usually performed for social reasons. Ritual circumcision is controversial. In 1989 the American Academy of Pediatrics altered its position, concluding that newborn circumcision may have potential benefits.[1] These include prevention of penile carcinoma, phimosis, balanoposthitis, and most important, neonatal urinary tract infection (UTI). An uncircumcised male neonate is 20 times more likely to have a UTI than a circumcised infant, because of colonization of the prepuce by urinary pathogens.[2] The higher incidence of UTI occurs only during the first year of life, and beyond that time, circumcision has not been shown to decrease infections. Circumcision should be discussed with the family of any male infant with a UTI or vesicoureteral reflux, although suppressive antibiotics for the first year of life are an option. Disadvantages of ritual circumcision include meatitis and meatal stenosis, since the protective covering of the prepuce is lost. In addition, a boy may develop chordee or phimosis, and the procedure is not without discomfort.

Circumcision is usually performed in one of two ways. Infants less than 3 months of age undergo a clamp or bell circumcision. A freehand technique by dorsal slit or sleeve method is preferred for older children. Routine circumcision should be avoided in children with hypospadias, chordee, or a prominent dorsal hood prepuce, so that the foreskin can be used for a later reconstructive procedure. Neonatal circumcision should also be deferred in boys with a small penis or a buried or webbed penis. Whenever a circumcision is performed, the surgeon must carefully examine the underlying glans and meatus for occult hypospadias with normal foreskin. If circumcision is not performed, families should be instructed in care of normal foreskin. The American Academy of Pediatrics brochure is a good instructional guide.[3] Forcible retraction of the prepuce is painful, harmful, and unnecessary. Tearing the prepuce places the child at risk for cicatrix formation and phimosis, and is therefore inadvisable.

Neonatal Circumcision

Infant circumcision is not without complications and should be performed by someone experienced in the technique who

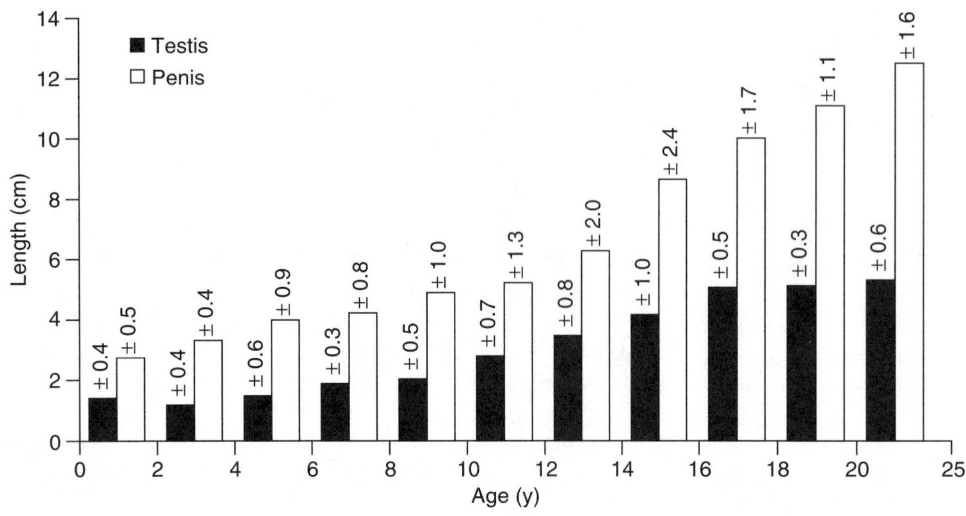

FIG. 93-2. Male genital dimensions. (After Bloom DA, Wan J, Key D. Disorders of the male external genitalia and inguinal canal. In: Kelalis PP, King LR, Belman AB, eds. Clinical pediatric urology, ed 3. Philadelphia, WB Saunders, 1992:1015)

will evaluate the child postoperatively to gauge the results. The child is placed in a papoose board restraint. We believe local anesthesia can be safely administered, with 1 mL or less of 0.25% lidocaine instilled as a dorsal nerve block or circumferential subcutaneous block. The anesthetic must not be injected intravascularly or into the corporal body. A small dorsal slit is usually required to expose the glans, and all adhesions are detached by blunt dissection. The clamp or bell is applied visually; experience helps in judging the proper amount of skin to excise. A suture with surgeon's knot is secured over the bell device, or, with the clamp technique, the clamp is left in place for 10 minutes for hemostasis before redundant skin is excised. Electrocautery should never be used when a metal clamp technique is employed. To guard against meatal stenosis, petroleum or antibiotic ointment should be placed on the meatus at each diaper change for at least 6 months after operation.

Freehand Circumcision

Circumcision after 3 months of age is best performed under general anesthesia with a freehand technique. Adhesions between glans and prepuce are carefully reduced using a clamp dipped in iodine solution, and the location of the meatus should be assessed. The sleeve method begins with a circumferential incision of the prepuce 6 to 8 mm proximal to the coronal sulcus, carried to the relatively avascular subcutaneous plane. The prepuce is then reduced and a parallel incision is made in the distal penile skin overlying the prepuce, at the level of the coronal sulcus. The sleeve of tissue is removed. Compression is applied to the exposed shaft for several minutes, and larger vessels are ligated or fulgurated. Particular attention should be directed to the skin edges, where small vessels may retract. The proximal and distal skin edges are aligned and reapproximated with an interrupted, small (6–0 or 7–0) absorbable suture. Compressive dressing is rarely needed (and usually falls off before the child reaches the recovery room). If ventral skin is deficient or bleeding is difficult to control at the frenulum, this area can be reapproximated with sutures vertically, to control bleeding and create additional ventral skin. Parents should be instructed to apply ointment to the meatus for 6 months following the operation, to prevent meatal stenosis.

Complications

Careful neonatal circumcisions have a low rate of complications (less than .5%).[4] Fortunately, the complications are usually minor and heal with conservative management. Excessive skin resection can lead to tension and skin separation, which usually heals well by secondary intention. Postoperative bleeding often responds to manual pressure or suture ligation and rarely requires exploration. Postoperative dressings are not required, which obviates the chance of urinary retention from a constrictive dressing.

Complications that require intervention include urethrocutaneous fistula, concealed penis, dense adhesions between glans and shaft, and meatal stenosis. A fistula is often associated with unrecognized deficient spongiosum. Concealed penis occurs following overzealous skin excision, or when a scarred preputial ring forms distal to the glans. Dense adhesions may cause pain

with erection, and should be divided. Meatal stenosis may ensue because of irritation of the unprotected meatus; liberal use of ointment postoperatively prevents this complication.

Prepuce Abnormalities

True phimosis refers to a circumferential preputial ring that prevents foreskin retraction. This differs from the physiologic inability to retract the foreskin in male infants. Preputial tears or cracks from natural erection, forcible retraction, or infection can lead to cicatrix formation and narrowing of the preputial aperture (Fig. 93-3). Circumcision or dorsal slit effectively corrects the abnormality.

Phimosis is the leading cause of preputial inflammation, or posthitis. Balanitis is inflammation or infection of the glans penis. The terms posthitis and balanitis are often used interchangeably, and often coexist when posthitis progresses to involve the glans. The inflammation is usually self-limited and responds to topical or oral antibiotics. Recurrent episodes are managed with circumcision following resolution of acute inflammation. Infection that spreads to the penile shaft and abdominal wall should be managed with parenteral antibiotics. Uncontrolled cellulitis may progress proximally, along tissue planes, to form a necrotizing fasciitis that requires operative intervention.

STRUCTURAL ABNORMALITIES

Aphallia

Absence of the penis is rare, with fewer than 100 reported cases. These are otherwise normal XY males. The scrotum is usually fully formed with descended testes, although these boys are likely to have concurrent genitourinary as well as nonurinary anomalies. A small skin tag is often present anterior to the anus, and the urethra usually opens onto the perineum near the anus. The urethra may drain into the rectum, and the more proximal the urethral meatus, the higher the incidence of associated anomalies and neonatal mortality. Gender reassignment should be considered, since penile reconstructive surgery is often unsatisfactory. Orchiectomy and feminizing genitoplasty can be performed in the neonatal period, and vaginoplasty at a later age.

Diphallia

A duplicated phallus is a rare anomaly that results from incomplete fusion or branching of the genital tubercle shortly after the fifth week of gestation. The two varieties of duplication are bifid penis and true duplication. Bifid penis implies separation of the corpora so that each unit has a single corporal body and hemiglans penis. A single hypospadiac meatus may lie at the base of the two penile shafts. This entity is often associated with the exstrophy-epispadias complex. True diphallia may be glans duplication or total penile duplication. Independent voiding and erectile function occur in the individual shafts, with complete duplication. Treatment is individualized to create an acceptable functional and cosmetic result.

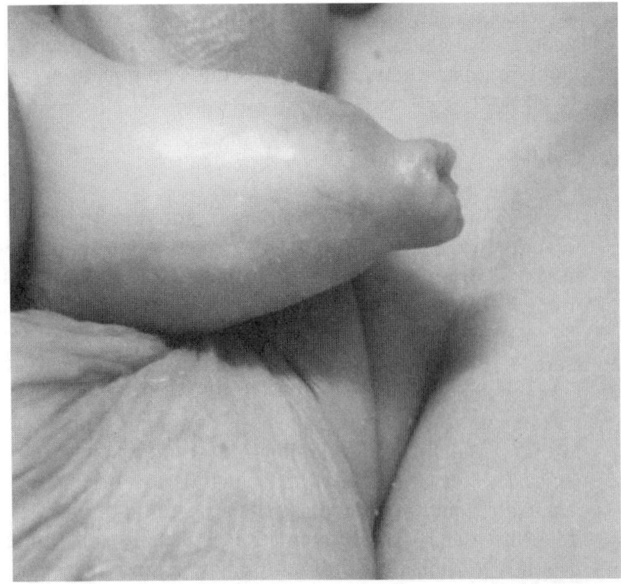

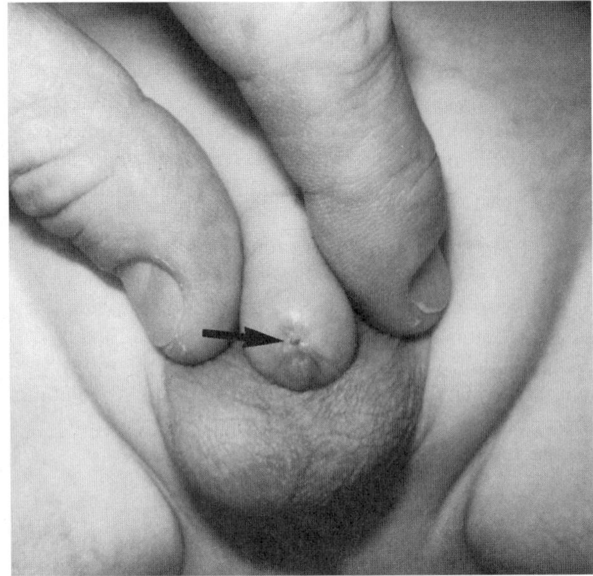

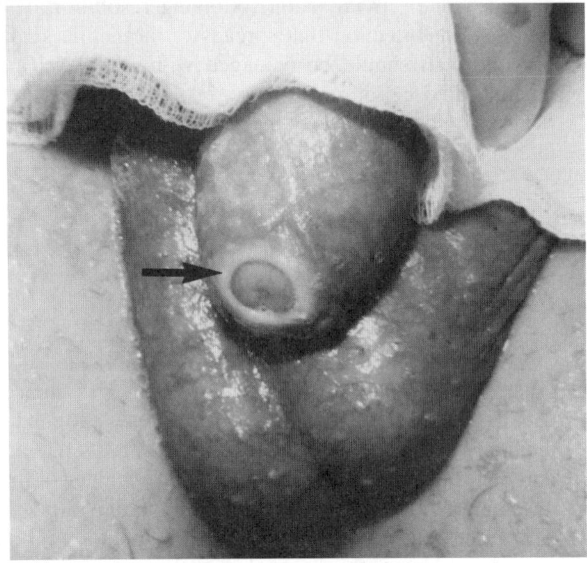

FIG. 93-3. Phimosis in boys. (*A*) Normal, nonretractile prepuce of infancy. (*B*) True phimosis with tiny preputial aperture (*arrow*) in a 3-year-old boy. (*C*) True phimosis in a 16-year-old male with scarred phimotic ring (*arrow*) from previous recurrent posthitis. (Bloom DA, Wan J, Key D. Disorders of the male external genitalia and inguinal canal. In: Kelalis PP, King LR, Belman AB, eds. Clinical Pediatric Urology, ed 3. Philadelphia, WB Saunders, 1992:1015)

Microphallus

A penis smaller than two standard deviations below mean normal length is a microphallus.[5] Normal neonatal mean stretched penile length is 3.5 cm, and an infant male penis should measure at least 2.5 cm. This definition excludes hypospadias and ambiguous genitalia. During the second and third trimester, fetal androgens stimulate penile growth. Any condition that interferes with fetal testicular testosterone production after organogenesis is complete (first trimester) can cause micropenis. Hypogonadism also produces an underdeveloped scrotum and small, undescended testes.

An abnormality in the hypothalamus–pituitary–testis axis can result in testicular failure. *Primary* testicular failure (end-organ disease) can be assessed by measuring serum testosterone before and after human chorionic gonadotropin (hCG) is administered. The normal response is a four-fold increase in testosterone within 24 hours of the final dose of hCG. *Secondary* gonadal failure (hypogonadotropic hypogonadism) with microphallus occurs with conditions such as anencephaly, pituitary agenesis, and Kallman, Noonan, and Prader-Willi syndromes. Microphallus is described as idiopathic when no deficit is found in the endocrine axis. Because differential diagnosis includes the intersex disorders, an appropriate evaluation should include karyotype and endocrine status.

The growth potential of the penis must be assessed by evaluating for a response to androgen administration. Testosterone may be given as a topical or parenteral preparation. Since the absorption of testosterone creams is variable, a 3-month trial of monthly intramuscular testosterone enanthate, 25 to 50 mg, is more appropriate. Such a short course of androgens does not result in premature closure of the epiphyseal growth plates. Gender reassignment is considered when there is no response in penile growth. Management of boys who do respond is controversial, since many show no dramatic response to the androgen surge at puberty. Many men with microphallus are sexually active and well adjusted, however, showing that penile function is satisfactory despite the small size.[6]

Webbed Penis

The webbed penis is a phallus of normal length that appears short because scrotal skin extends onto the ventral shaft. The ventral portion of the shaft is buried in the scrotum or tethered to the scrotal cleft by a frenulum (Fig. 93-4). The congenitally webbed penis usually has a normal urethra, and the scrotum is otherwise normal. Since cavernosal and spongiosal tissue are normal, the penis is straight when erect. Although the condition is asymptomatic, the cosmetic appearance usually warrants surgical repair. This condition can also occur following an overaggressive circumcision, when excess ventral skin is excised. Surgical correction is performed with a Heinecke-Mikulicz–type procedure, using a transverse incision and vertical closure.

Buried and Concealed Penis

The terms *buried penis* and *concealed penis* are often used interchangeably; however, they describe different conditions.[7] A buried penis is normally developed and appears small because of an overlying generous suprapubic fat pad, which hides the normal penile shaft. Occasionally a large hydrocele obscures the shaft, resulting in a buried penis. Manual depression of the fat pad, an important maneuver when measuring penile length, reveals the normal penis. For many of these boys, the genital lengthening and pubic hair growth of adolescence solve the cosmetic dilemma. For some boys and parents, however, the potential embarrassment and emotional trauma of an obscured penis mandate repair. Successful surgical correction can produce enormous improvement in a boy's self-esteem. Circumcision unmasks the glans, and liposuction or excision of the suprapubic fat address the underlying etiology. Occasionally, additional surgical maneuvers are required, including release of dysgenetic Scarpa's fascia extending below the fat pad, where it continues as the dartos layer of the penis, and anchoring su-

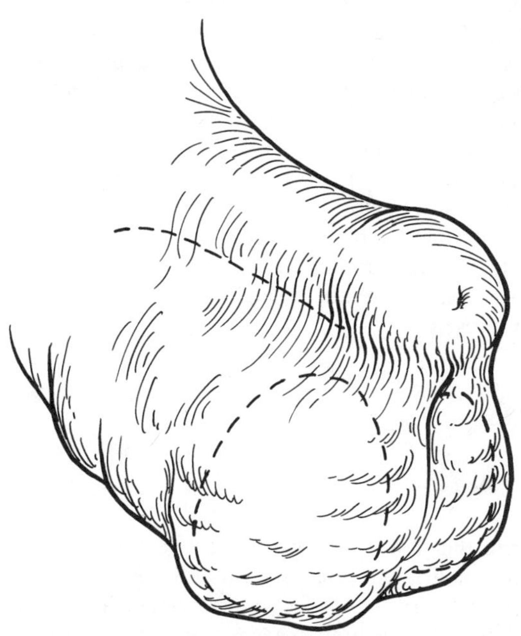

FIG. 93-4. Webbed penis.

prapubic skin to the fascia overlying the pubis and anterior abdominal wall.

Concealed (trapped) penis occurs after circumcision. A cicatrix forms at the anastomotic line, and the penis retracts proximal to the scar. Surgical revision is often challenging, since a limited amount of shaft skin remains. Dorsal slit or removal of the cicatrical ring is required.

FUNCTIONAL DEVIATION

Penile Torsion

Penile torsion is a rotational defect of the penile shaft that is usually of greater cosmetic than functional significance. The defect occurs in 1% to 2% of males, and is more common in patients with hypospadias. The median raphe spirals obliquely around the shaft, producing a rotation that is usually less than 90 degrees. Mild forms are repaired by penile degloving and skin reorientation. On rare occasions, the rotational defect is 90 to 180 degrees. Severe defects are repaired by mobilizing penile skin to the base of the penis and incising any chordee; they may require resection of Buck's fascia. Torsion also occurs iatrogenically following circumcision or hypospadias repair. Most cases are minimally rotated, not associated with chordee, and rarely a functional problem.

Penile Bending (Chordee)

The term *chordee* refers to a ventral bend of the shaft on erection. Chordee occurs normally in embryonic penile development; the ventral bend may persist in premature male infants, but it usually corrects spontaneously within several months. Chordee is usually associated with hypospadias, in which deficient ventral penile development includes skin, spongiosum, Buck's fascia, and urethra. Hypospadias should not be corrected without fixing the chordee.

Chordee may also occur in spite of a normal urethra, although a preputial dorsal hood and thin ventral skin often coexist. Such chordee result from skin tethering, a urethral bowstring defect, or corporal disproportion. Vaginal penetration is difficult with an erect penile bend of greater than 45 degrees. Release of skin and dysgenetic bands may not completely straighten the penis. In such cases, dorsal plication or elliptical wedge excision of the corporal body at the point of maximum bend may be required (Fig. 93-5). Should urethral tethering exist, mobilization of the urethra within the spongiosum corrects the bend. Occasionally the urethra must be divided and repaired. Intraoperative erections induced by saline injection of the corpora must be performed to gauge the defect and repair.

Lateral Curvature

Lateral curvature of the shaft probably has an etiology distinct from chordee; it most likely results from overgrowth or hypoplasia of one corporal body. The lesion is congenital, but it is not recognized until later in life, when erections occur, because the penis appears entirely normal in the flaccid state. Significant lateral bending is repaired with degloving of penile

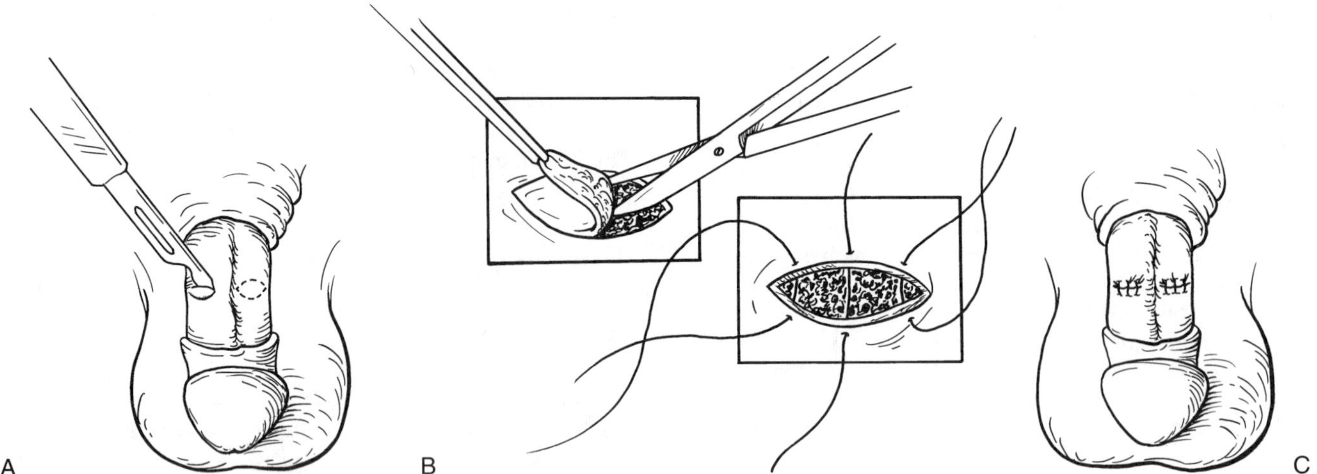

FIG. 93-5. Penile straightening by elliptical wedge excision of the corporal body.

skin and plication or elliptical resection of the corporal body at the point of maximum bend. In spite of perfect correction, as assessed by intraoperative erection testing, the bending may recur, requiring secondary repair. These patients should be monitored for at least several years before successful correction is assumed. Depending on where the corporal defect is located, the urethra or dorsal neurovascular bundle may require mobilization.

MEATAL STENOSIS

Stenosis of the urethral meatus usually occurs years after neonatal circumcision. The delicate meatus is susceptible to inflammation from local trauma such as from a wet diaper. Meatitis progresses to cicatrix formation, with narrowing of the orifice. Deflected urinary stream and prolonged voiding times are typically noted by parents after a child is toilet trained. A fine, forceful stream may emanate from a pinpoint meatus. Irritative voiding symptoms, such as dysuria and urgency, rarely occur without a concomitant UTI. Isolated meatal stenosis without infection does not require radiographic assessment of the urinary tract or cystoscopy. When stenosis is suspected, the meatus can be calibrated with small catheters or sounds. If stenosis is not severe, parents can be taught to perform daily obturation with a feeding tube or the tip of an ophthalmic ointment tube. Significant stenosis should be surgically corrected by a ventral incision, followed by a 3-month program of daily calibration of the urethra with a catheter, to ensure adequate opening.

Balanitis xerotica obliterans is an idiopathic condition that can produce meatal stenosis. A characteristic white patch on the prepuce and glans may extend to the urethral meatus, and occasionally progresses into the fossa navicularis. The meatus appears white, indurated, edematous, and stenotic. The histologic appearance of this chronic inflammatory condition is similar to that of lichen sclerosis et atrophicus, found elsewhere on skin. The lesion is best treated with meatotomy. Topical steroids applied to the meatus in the postoperative period reduce the otherwise high recurrence rate. Severe, diffuse lesions may require excision of the tissue and urethroplasty.

PRIAPISM

Priapism is involuntary, prolonged erection of the corpora cavernosa, with flaccid glans penis and spongiosum. Extended or recurrent episodes lead to corporal fibrosis and impotence. Sickle cell patients account for most pediatric priapism; about 5% of these patients experience priapism. The erection occurs as part of a diffuse sickle crisis or as an isolated event. Sickle crisis is managed by transfusion to dilute the hemoglobin S, oxygenation, hydration, alkalinization, and pain control. When conservative management fails to relieve an associated priapism, a shunt is required to drain the engorged corpora cavernosa. Aspiration with irrigation of the corporal bodies is unsuccessful in sickle cell patients. Shunts connecting the corpora cavernosa to the spongiosum are effective, but may result in impotence.

Leukemia is another cause of childhood priapism. Although chronic granulocytic leukemia accounts for only a small percentage of pediatric leukemias, half of all leukemic priapism occurs in these patients. Leukemic cells probably sludge within the corporal bodies, but other possible factors include leukemic infiltration of the sacral nerves or central nervous system as well as abdominal and pelvic venous obstruction. Treatment is directed at lowering the white blood cell count. Shunts may be necessary for refractory cases. Other etiologies for priapism in the child include blunt perineal trauma, spinal cord injury, medications, and retroperitoneal fibrosarcomas. As with sickle cell disease and leukemia, treatment is aimed at the underlying disease process.

TESTIS

Embryology

During the first 3 to 5 weeks of gestation, gonadal ridges constitute indifferent gonads. Primordial germ cell migration from the entodermal yolk sac lining to the genital ridge is complete by week 6, resulting in a bipotential gonad. The *SRY* gene facilitates gonadal differentiation into a testis such that Sertoli cells develop in weeks 6 and 7, and shortly thereafter produce Müllerian inhibiting substance, which causes ipsilateral müllerian duct regression. By the ninth week, Leydig cells produce testosterone, which stimulates wolffian duct development. The testis and caput epididymis arise from the genital ridge, whereas the epididymal body and vas deferens originate from mesonephric tubules. Canalization of the rete testis and mesonephric tubules begins about week 12 of gestation, and is complete by puberty. Testicular descent is a third-trimester event; prenatal ultrasounds typically show no descent prior to 28 weeks. Many theories have been proposed to explain testis descent, including gubernacular traction, differential somatic growth, intraabdominal pressure, epididymal maturation, and hormone milieu. In all likelihood, a combination of events and influences under androgen regulation leads to normal testis descent.

Anatomy

The average length of the infant testis is 1.4 to 1.6 cm. The testis grows minimally in the prepubertal years; significant growth is not noted until onset of puberty (see Fig. 93-2). In boys with monorchidism, a solitary testis may undergo compensatory hypertrophy, and any solitary infant testis longer than 2 cm suggests contralateral testicular absence.[8]

Appendages of the testis and epididymis are vestigial embryologic remnants (Fig. 93-6). An appendix testis, present on approximately 90% of testes, is a remnant of the müllerian ducts. The müllerian system completely regresses in males except for its cranial remnant, which persists as the appendix testis, and the extreme lower end remnant, which forms the prostatic utricle. The appendix testis is located on the cranial surface of the testis, and occasionally at the testis–epididymal junction. The remaining appendages are vestigial remnants of the mesonephric tubules. An appendix epididymis is located on the globus major of the epididymis in 34% of males. The paradidymis is a remnant structure found at the junction of the epididymis and vas deferens. These remnants serve no known function, except to confound the differential diagnosis of an acute scrotum.

Physiology

The infant testis is hormonally active and is not as quiescent as was once believed. Normal activity in the first 6 months of postnatal life seems to be crucial for the testis to develop normal adult function. A postnatal surge of gonadotropins at 60 to 90 days results in proliferation of Leydig cells by 3 months.[9] Leydig cells respond with a testosterone surge that triggers germ cell development. The first step in postnatal germ cell development is the transformation of gonocytes to adult dark (Ad) spermatogonia, which is completed by 6 months. These spermatogonia may represent the pool of stem cells that replenish germ cells throughout life. The second stage of development occurs around 3 years of age, when the Ad spermatogonia transform to primary spermatocytes. Alterations in this normal cascade of events may result in a dysfunctional adult testis.[9] Later in childhood, spermatogonia populate the base of the seminiferous tubules, and spermatogenesis begins at puberty.

ABNORMAL SIZE

Microorchidism (Hypoplasia)

The testis changes little in size from birth until the onset of puberty. Spermatic tubules comprise 90% of testicular volume, and this volume increases enormously when spermatogenesis ensues at puberty. Small testes result from congenital disorders or secondary to various insults. Klinefelter syndrome (47,XXY) is an example of primary hypogonadism. Testes may be small even in the prepubertal years, and the pubertal growth surge does not occur. Secondary hypogonadism occurs with any pituitary or hypothalamic deficiency that results in lack of gonadotropin stimulation of the testes (Kallman syndrome). These testes may be normal at birth, but remain small after puberty. Insults to the testis (mumps orchitis, epididymitis, trauma, hernia repair with vascular embarrassment, torsion, chemotherapy, radiation therapy, sickle cell crisis) severely damage parenchyma, resulting in growth retardation or atrophy. Failure of normal growth occurs with a varicocele and uncorrected cryp-

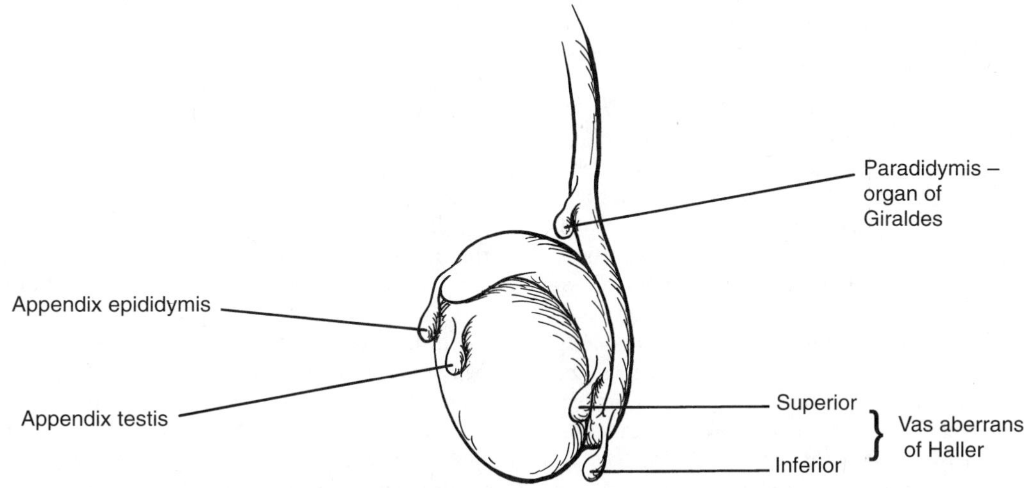

FIG. 93-6. Testis and epididymal appendages.

torchid testis. Varicocele-induced growth retardation is probably the most reversible insult; many testes undergo significant growth after successful varicocele repair.

Macroorchidism

Testicular enlargement is sometimes the result of atrophy or absence of the contralateral testis, when the monorchid testis undergoes compensatory hypertrophy. A tense hydrocele can be mistaken for gonadal enlargement; however, transillumination or ultrasonography settles the issue. Primary testis tumors or metastatic neoplasms to the testes enlarge the gonad. Ultrasound examination is helpful to rule out neoplasm. When tumor is considered, the serum tumor markers α-fetoprotein and βhCG are obtained, and surgical exploration should be inguinal, with early vascular control.

Adrenal hyperplasia may produce unilateral or bilateral macroorchidism, with nodularity from islands of benign hyperplastic adrenal tissue within the testes. Juvenile hypothyroidism or an intracranial mass lesion stimulate precocious puberty, with resultant bilateral macroorchidism. Mental retardation and the fragile-X syndrome are also sometimes associated with enlarged testes. Some cases of bilateral macroorchidism are described as idiopathic, provided that gonadotropin and thyroid hormone evaluation, as well as the scrotal ultrasound, are normal.

ABNORMAL NUMBER

Testicular Absence

Intrauterine or perinatal vascular accidents, with loss of a formed fetal testis, probably account for most absent testes. True agenesis is rare, and implies total developmental failure of the embryonic gonadal ridge. Laparoscopy has demonstrated that müllerian structures or remnants are rare in monorchid and anorchid boys, indicating the presence of a fetal testis before 14 to 15 weeks' gestation, at which time Sertoli cells have elaborated enough müllerian inhibiting substance to promote müllerian regression. The laparoscopic or open surgical finding of blind-ending spermatic vessels suggests testis loss. The frequent histologic finding of hemosiderin, calcium, and hyalinization in testicular remnant nubbins supports the supposition of vascular accident.

Anorchia, or vanished testes syndrome, implies absent testicular tissue in an otherwise normal XY male. Endocrine evaluation in patients with bilateral nonpalpable testes may help ascertain whether testes are present. βHCG stimulation normally causes a more than four-fold increase in serum testosterone, whereas anorchid patients have no testosterone response. Basal levels of gonadotropins are usually elevated three standard deviations above mean values in prepubertal anorchid boys.[10] Negative βhCG stimulation and elevated follicle-stimulating hormone strongly suggest anorchism, although false-negative values have been reported in boys found to have testes present at exploration. Laparoscopic exploration is an excellent alternative to multiple endocrinologic assays. Blind-ending vessels confirm the diagnosis of anorchia. Visualization of spermatic cord structures entering the internal ring mandates inguinal ex-

ploration, which is performed under the same anesthetic. Since malignancy can occur in abdominal testes, a negative inguinal exploration alone is insufficient to confirm testicular absence. Testicular prosthesis placement at an early age is recommended for anorchid boys, to avoid a flat hypoplastic scrotum throughout childhood.

Monorchid testes undergo compensatory hypertrophy, although the increase in volume is too variable to diagnose monorchidism on the basis of ipsilateral testis measurement alone. Hormone assays are not useful for diagnosing monorchidism. For unknown reasons, solitary fetal testis loss is more likely on the left side. When laparoscopic evaluation confirms unilateral testis absence, prophylactic orchiopexy of the contralateral solitary testis is indicated. No study has shown that monorchidism portends a higher risk of testis torsion, however, loss of the solitary testis for any reason is catastrophic. Monorchid boys and their parents should be counseled about the risks of contact sports and the need for scrotal protection, the requirement for immediate medical evaluation for acute scrotal pain or swelling, and the importance of testicular self-examination. With one normal testis in the scrotum, placement of a prosthesis is discretionary.

Polyorchidism

The presence of more than two testes in a male is rare. Polyorchidism usually describes a single supernumerary testis, which is located in the scrotum in half of cases, and undescended in the remainder. A division of the genital ridge early in embryonic development is the presumed etiology for the condition. The ipsilateral testes usually share a common epididymis and vas deferens, and may have separate vascular pedicles that join proximally. Few of these gonads are completely duplicated. Testis parenchyma are structurally normal or abnormal, and both malignancy and torsion have been reported in the supernumerary testis. These gonads are usually discovered as a painless inguinal or scrotal mass; surgical exploration confirms the diagnosis. The extra testis can be removed unless orchiectomy jeopardizes the vascular or ductal system of the ipsilateral mate.

ABNORMAL LOCATION

Cryptorchidism

Cryptorchidism means hidden or obscure testis, and is generally synonymous with undescended testis. The incidence at birth is about 4%, with bilateral involvement in 15% of these cases. Testes may descend within several months of birth, and the incidence drops to about 1% by 1 year of age, where it remains throughout childhood and beyond puberty. Two important reasons for moving the testis to a scrotal location are the psychologic disadvantage of an empty scrotum and the accessibility of the testis for self-examination later in life. In addition, orchiopexy may improve fertility potential. Testes require the cooler thermal environment of the scrotum for normal spermatogenesis. Infertility is increased in men with a history of cryptorchidism. Bilateral undescended testes portend a worse fertility potential than unilateral cryptorchids.

Surgical intervention is recommended before 18 to 24 months

of age. Theoretically, early orchiopexy preserves fertility; however, substantive data are lacking. Most undescended testes are smaller than their contralateral descended mate, and this volume loss is evident within the first year of life. Biopsy of undescended testes reveals the number of spermatogonia per tubule to be higher in boys under the age of 1 year, compared with older cryptorchids.[13] Similarly, the seminiferous tubule diameter is larger in biopsies from boys less than a year old with undescended testes.[14] These findings suggest that damage to the germinal epithelium is acquired, progressive, and irreversible because of higher local temperatures. Early intervention is therefore recommended, with the hope of improving fertility.

Subnormal fertility may be multifactorial in cryptorchid males, and not a result of thermal injury alone. Defective germ cell maturation, noted within the first year of life, may be a result of an abnormal hypothalamic–pituitary–testis endocrine axis. Many cryptorchid boys do not have the normal postnatal surge of gonadotropins at 2 to 3 months of age, which should stimulate Leydig cells to respond with a surge in testosterone. This cascade of events may be important to prime normal germ cell maturation. In addition, one fifth to one third of undescended testes have a defect in epididymal–testis fusion or epididymal suspension. Abnormal sperm transport may result in infertility, despite normal spermatogenesis. Therefore, orchiopexy alone may not improve paternity rates, because of the multiple potential factors for infertility in these patients.

Cryptorchid testes have a greater risk of malignancy than normal descended testes. The chance of a cryptorchid patient developing a testicular tumor is almost 10 times that of the general male population. Six percent to 10% of all testicular cancers originate in a cryptorchid testis. When tumors develop in a cryptorchid patient, 20% occur in the contralateral descended testis.[15] Orchiopexy does not alter the malignant potential of a cryptorchid testis; however, scrotal position allows self-examination and early detection of a tumor.

A cryptorchid testis may be substantially intraabdominal (at least 1 cm above the internal ring), high annular (at the internal ring), canalicular (in the superficial inguinal pouch), distantly ectopic (perineal, femoral, or penopubic), or high scrotal. Some of these locations suggest migration arrest during the normal course of testis descent, whereas ectopic testes are found outside the usual anatomic path of descent. Whether the superficial inguinal pouch, which is the most common location for an undescended testis, is ectopic or the result of migration arrest is a matter of debate.

The basic principles of standard orchiopexy are gonad identification, mobilization, cord dissection, isolation of a patent processus vaginalis, and relocation of the testis to the scrotum. An important innovation in orchiopexy is the method of scrotal fixation. Since sutures placed through the tunica albuginea of the testis may damage parenchyma, one can place the testis in a subdartos pouch, using absorbable sutures to fix the tunica vaginalis to the dartos.[11,12]

The nonpalpable testis is a special circumstance of cryptorchidism in which a gonad is impalpable in spite of a deliberate set of diagnostic maneuvers. It is usually not difficult to examine an awake child who is relaxed and cooperative. In a warm room, examination begins over the area of the internal inguinal ring, gently walking the fingers down the inguinal canal toward the scrotum. If a testis is not identified, reexamination in a cross-leg sitting or squatting position, using lubricating jelly to decrease the tactile friction, may reveal an elusive gonad. Nonpalpable testes account for 10% to 20% of undescended testes. Ultimate assessment of nonpalpable testes reveals absence in 45%, an intraabdominal location in 30%, and a lower testis missed to palpation in 25% of cases.

Radiographic evaluation for an undescended testis is unreliable. Generally, thorough physical examination by an experienced surgeon is more valuable and reliable than ultrasound, computed tomographic scan, or magnetic resonance imaging. These techniques may discern a gonad in older children, but rarely does radiographic assessment influence management or prognosis enough to justify the expense. Venography is more successful, although it requires anesthesia or sedation. We believe that laparoscopy is the best first step in localizing a nonpalpable testis or proving it absent; accuracy exceeds 95%.[16] Laparoscopic findings define the next operative step, which may take further advantage of the laparoscopic access. The three likely findings at laparoscopy are blind-ending spermatic vessels above the internal ring, an intraabdominal testis, and normal cord structures entering the internal inguinal ring. When blind-ending or atretic vessels are identified above the inguinal ring, no further evaluation or surgery is indicated. If a high intraabdominal testis is found, therapeutic options include traditional Fowler-Stephens orchiopexy, first-stage vasal-pedicle orchiopexy with laparoscopic ligation of the gonadal vessels, laparoscopic orchiopexy, and orchiectomy. If vessels enter the inguinal ring, then regardless of findings at subsequent inguinal exploration, one is assured that further retroperitoneal or abdominal exploration is unnecessary.

Long-term follow-up is imperative for cryptorchid boys. Parents must be aware of the issues of infertility and tumorigenesis. When they reach puberty, boys should be taught monthly testicular self-examination. Fertility issues can be discussed at an adult follow-up visit. Cryptorchidism has far-reaching ramifications, and surgeons must ensure the education and long-term follow-up of these patients.

Retractile Testis

The retractile testis is a normally descended gonad that retracts so readily and vigorously that the condition is confused with cryptorchidism. The ipsilateral scrotum is normally developed, and may invert during retraction at the gubernacular attachment. Retractile testes have normal volumes, may be bilateral, and once manipulated to the dependent portion of the scrotum, tend to remain without tension. The cremasteric reflex is weak or absent for several months after birth; therefore eliciting a history of a normal scrotal examination in infancy. Subsequent evaluation suggests retractile testis. Because the cremasteric reflex is dampened during general anesthesia, a testis in an abnormal position under anesthesia is likely to be cryptorchid. No treatment is necessary for the retractile testis; parents should be reassured and the child examined annually. Failure to recognize the retractile testis may explain why the number of orchiopexies performed exceeds the expected incidence of cryptorchidism.[17]

Testis Ascent

The retractile testis has been implicated in the phenomenon of testis ascent; however, inaccurate normal examinations recorded during infancy and retractile testes probably do not account for all cases of ascent. An additional explanation is that spermatic cord elongation may not keep up with somatic growth, resulting in relative ascent. We think that, in some instances, ascent is the result of unrecognized minimally undescended testes in a low-lying, superficial inguinal pouch, which extends into the scrotal inlet. With somatic growth, relatively less of the pouch lies within the scrotum, and the testis appears to ascend.

ACUTE SCROTUM

Testis Torsion (Intravaginal)

Testis torsion, the most frequent cause of an acute scrotum in children, is often, mismanaged. Detorsion within 6 hours affords a good chance of salvage, 12 hours or more of ischemia before reduction of torsion is usually associated with loss of the gonad. Classic torsion of the testis usually occurs in adolescents and young adult males, but it can occur in younger children. Some boys have an anatomic predisposition to torsion. High insertion of the tunica vaginalis on the cord structures allows for a horizontal testis position and mobility similar to a bell clapper within a bell (Fig. 93-7). This allows the distal cord to twist within the tunica vaginalis, hence the designation *intravaginal torsion.*

Patients usually have a sudden onset of severe pain, often associated with abdominal discomfort, nausea, and vomiting. In some instances, however, a gradual onset of testicular and abdominal pain is the primary complaint. The evaluation of any male with abdominal pain should include a thorough scrotal examination. Half of symptomatic boys describe similar tran-

sient, prior episodes of scrotal pain, consistent with intermittent torsion-detorsion. Physical examination reveals a tender testis, scrotal erythema, new hydrocele, and loss of the cremasteric reflex. Anatomic landmarks are often not distinguishable because of edema and inflammation. If the history and examination are consistent with testis torsion, prompt surgical exploration and reduction is the next step, without need for further tests and delay. Loss of the testis ensues without spontaneous or surgical reduction. Treatment is surgical detorsion and fixation orchiopexy.

An important part of the surgical procedure is fixation of the contralateral uninvolved testis. For many patients, the window of opportunity for salvaging the symptomatic gonad has passed, and contralateral orchiopexy protects the surviving testis. In addition, the bell-clapper deformity is often bilateral, and the contralateral testis is at higher risk for torsion later. Orchiopexy is not a guarantee against future torsion, but it does decrease the odds. The child and parents must be made aware that subsequent scrotal pain or swelling can still result from torsion and must be evaluated promptly. Our bias is to remove a testis only when it is necrotic and nonviable. Theoretic concerns that a damaged testis remaining in the scrotum may be detrimental to its mate have not been substantiated. If there is restoration of blood flow or the chance of viable parenchyma, we proceed with orchiopexy. The involved testis can be reduced and observed while contralateral fixation is performed.

Manual reduction of a torsed testis can be attempted with or without narcotic analgesia. Successful detorsion alleviates acute symptoms and may obviate emergent exploration; however, it is not a definitive treatment. Testes usually torse in an inward or medial direction, with an anteromedial rotation of the spermatic cord. Manual detorsion should proceed with two or three lateral or outward (viewing the scrotum from the feet) rotations. Dopp-

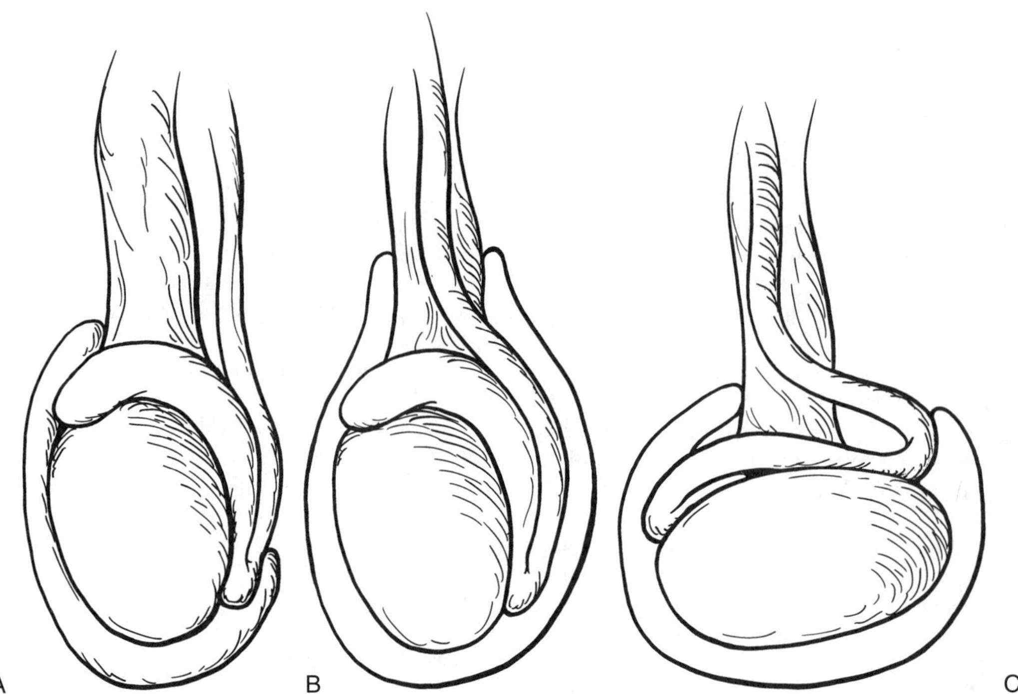

FIG. 93-7. Testis position within tunica vaginalis. (*A*) Normal anatomy. (*B*) Bell-clapper deformity. (*C*) Bell-clapper deformity with horizontal testis lie.

ler pulse evaluation may suggest successful detorsion if distal pulses return; however, the physician usually notes release and elongation of the cord followed by a marked diminution in symptoms. Successful manual reduction should be followed by elective orchiopexy. A pitfall to manual detorsion is partial reduction of a 720-degree or greater twist. Partial detorsion may relieve symptoms and improve the examination, but not relieve the ischemia.

Color Doppler and nuclear scrotal scans are of little benefit when torsion is suspected. These modalities are costly in dollars and time. They are a poor substitute for a well-performed history, clinical evaluation, and judgment. These examinations are often obtained in patients for whom torsion is a low priority, only to confirm the diagnosis of nontorsion.

Neonatal Torsion

Extravaginal torsion is a variant in which torsion occurs proximally in the inguinal portion of the spermatic cord, or just below the canal, above the insertion of the tunica vaginalis. The entire tunica vaginalis and contents torse. This occurs in utero, during delivery, or in the postnatal period (within the first 30 days of life). The pathogenesis is unknown; however, weak attachments between the tunica vaginalis and scrotal wall may predispose the young to this process. Extravaginal torsion occurs much less frequently than intravaginal torsion, and unlike the latter, is usually asymptomatic in the neonate. Bilateral in utero torsion is the likely etiology for the vanished testes syndrome. Salvage of the extravaginally torsed testis is rare; most gonads are necrotic at exploration. Primary reasons for intervention are to confirm diagnosis, for orchiectomy, and for contralateral testis fixation. Although unilateral extravaginal torsion is not associated with a higher incidence of contralateral intravaginal torsion, loss of a single remaining testis would be devastating, and prophylactic orchiopexy should be considered. Exploration in the neonate should be by inguinal incision, since torsion may occur within the canal, and concomitant inguinal hernia may exist.

Torsed Appendages

The appendix testis is a müllerian duct remnant, whereas epididymal appendages are vestigial remnants of the wolffian duct system. The etiology for appendiceal torsion is not known; however, the process mimics testis torsion. The onset of pain is usually gradual over a day or 2, but it may be acute and severe. A reactive hydrocele often confounds the examination, and extrascrotal symptoms such as nausea and emesis are infrequent. Physical examination reveals the classic blue dot sign, in which the infarcted appendage can be visualized through thin scrotal skin or palpated as the point of isolated tenderness at the upper pole of the testis. Certainty of diagnosis precludes exploration, and the symptoms resolve with scrotal support, antiinflammatory agents, and bed rest over several days to a week. If the diagnosis is in doubt, spermatic cord torsion must be ruled out with surgical exploration.

Acute Scrotum Without Torsion

Acute scrotal pain sometimes occurs in the child for reasons other than torsion. Infection of the epididymis is uncommon in the prepubertal male. Inflammation of the epididymis results from UTI, trauma, chemical irritation, autoimmune phenomenon, vasculitis, or granulomatous disease. Pyuria suggests epididymitis; however, since torsion is the most frequent cause of acute scrotal pain and swelling, the diagnosis of epididymitis should be made with great caution. Epididymitis often occurs secondary to a UTI, and these children need to be evaluated for underlying urinary tract anomalies such as ectopic ureter, ectopic vas deferens, and bladder outlet abnormalities. Foley catheter drainage, intermittent catheterization, and other forms of urinary tract instrumentation predispose a child to infection, and therefore epididymitis. Despite the many diagnostic modalities available, torsion must be considered, and surgical exploration is often required to confirm the diagnosis of epididymitis. Orchitis is rare in the pediatric population. Mumps orchitis is strictly a postpubertal disease.

An acutely symptomatic hydrocele develops for a variety of reasons, including trauma, torsion, infection, tumor, or presentation of a previously asymptomatic indirect inguinal hernia, or it may be idiopathic. The underlying condition must be considered, and surgical exploration may be required to secure a diagnosis. If the testis cannot be adequately palpated and the diagnosis of tumor is entertained, the approach to the scrotum should be inguinal. Malignant lesions in the scrotum do not usually present with acute pain or swelling; however, hemorrhage and necrosis in a testis tumor cause symptoms, and tumor-bearing testes are susceptible to torsion. Idiopathic fat necrosis is a condition sometimes seen in obese prepubertal boys after strenuous physical activity. The prepubertal scrotum contains fat, and indurated masses of adipose tissue may be found around the testis at exploration. The etiology of fat necrosis is unknown.

The sudden onset of unilateral or bilateral scrotal edema may result from acute idiopathic scrotal edema. Erythema and mild tenderness can accompany the edema. Patients are typically under 10 years of age. Urinalysis and blood studies are unremarkable. Symptoms and edema resolve spontaneously. The cause of the edema is not known; proposed etiologies include unrecognized insect bite, perianal infection, allergic reaction, contact dermatitis, and angioneurotic edema. Acute idiopathic penile edema is a similar condition in which edema is confined to the penile shaft.

Henoch-Schonlein purpura is a systemic vasculitis that usually presents with nonthrombocytopenic purpura, abdominal pain, arthralgias, and bloody diarrhea. Involvement of the genitourinary system includes vasculitic changes of the renal parenchyma (nephritis, hematuria) and the spermatic cord and scrotum. As many as a third of boys develop acute pain and swelling of the scrotum. Most children are under age 7 years, and the duration of illness averages 4 to 6 weeks. The initial dermatologic manifestation is urticaria, with subsequent macular and maculopapular lesions. The characteristic rash is usually present well before the onset of scrotal symptoms. Nuclear scan or Doppler studies may confirm normal or increased testicular perfusion and obviate exploration, but concomitant testis torsion has been reported in these children. Treatment for Henoch-Schonlein purpura is supportive, although corticosteroids may be indicated in renal disease.

Incarcerated hernia, traumatic hematocele, varicocele, and splenogonadal fusion also cause scrotal pain or swelling. A patent processus vaginalis may test a surgeon's diagnostic skill when intraabdominal processes such as ruptured appendicitis, meconium peritonitis, and intraperitoneal bleeding gain access to the scrotal cavity. The tip of a ventriculoperitoneal shunt can migrate through a patent processus, causing scrotal discomfort or palpable mass.

TESTICULAR TUMORS

Prepubertal testicular tumors represent a small, but controversial aspect of testicular lesions.[18] The tumors account for only 1% of all pediatric solid tumors and are the seventh most common pediatric malignancy. Germ cell tumors comprise 95% of adult testicular tumors, but only 75% of prepubertal testicular tumors.

Since these tumors are rare and the published series are few, it is sometimes difficult to define natural history and optimal treatment regimens. The Prepubertal Testis Tumor Registry was established in 1980 to address these issues.[19] A painless mass is the most common manifestation of a prepubertal testicular tumor. These lesions are sometimes misdiagnosed as a hydrocele, which delays treatment. Yolk sac tumor is the most common prepubertal testicular tumor, although it is a rare isolated lesion in adults. In contrast, seminoma is the most common adult testicular tumor, but is extremely rare in the prepubertal population. For these reasons, application of adult testicular tumor classification schemes to the pediatric population is unsatisfactory. The Section of Urology of the American Academy of Pediatrics devised a classification for unilateral testicular tumors composed of eight categories:

Germ cell tumors—yolk sac, teratoma, teratocarcinoma, seminoma
Gonadal stromal tumors—Leydig cell, Sertoli cell, mixed
Gonadoblastoma
Tumors of supporting structures—fibroma, leiomyoma, hemangioma
Leukemia and lymphoma
Tumorlike lesions—epidermoid cyst, hyperplastic nodules due to congenital adrenal hyperplasia
Secondary tumors
Paratesticular tumors

The serum tumor marker α-fetoprotein (AFP) is produced by yolk sac cells and is useful in managing prepubertal testicular tumors. AFP is elevated in 90% of yolk sac tumors, and has a half-life of 5 days. Postoperative elevation beyond the half-life calculations suggests residual tumor. AFP is normally elevated in neonates, and the physiologic elevation may persist for up to 12 to 15 weeks. βHCG is not elevated in prepubertal testicular tumors. In addition to tumor markers, metastatic evaluation should include chest radiologic examination and computed tomography scan or ultrasound of the abdomen. The retroperitoneum and lungs are the most common sites of metastases.

The examination of any child with a scrotal tumor must include assessment of the stage of sexual development and the presence or absence of gynecomastia. If the testis cannot be palpated, ultrasound examination may characterize the underlying gonad. Tumor markers should be obtained, and an inguinal approach used, with early control of the spermatic vessels.

Yolk Sac Tumor

Yolk sac tumors account for 70% of all prepubertal testicular tumors. Mean age at diagnosis is 3 years. This germ cell tumor is *not* of yolk sac origin; the name originated from the histologic similarity to the endodermal sinus of rat yolk sac. Other names have been used, such as endodermal sinus tumor, infantile embryonal carcinoma, and orchidoblastoma. Yolk sac tumor should *not* be confused with the embryonal cell carcinoma of postpubertal males, although the tumors are histologically similar, their clinical behavior is different. The histologic sine qua non of yolk sac tumor is the Schiller-Duval body, a glomerular-like cluster of cells that contain AFP.

Preorchiectomy levels of AFP do not correlate with tumor volume and are not prognostic. If levels do not fall as projected by the 5-day half-life following orchiectomy, however, residual metastatic disease is likely. Metastases have been described despite normal AFP. Staging for yolk sac tumor is similar to the adult staging system. Stage 1 tumors are limited to the testis, stage 2 implies regional lymphatic disease (retroperitoneum), and stage 3 is supradiaphragmatic spread. Yolk sac tumors metastasize through both the vascular and lymphatic systems, though they seen to have a predilection for hematogenous spread; more patients with metastatic disease have pulmonary lesions than retroperitoneal metastases. Treatment begins with orchiectomy. Few centers have extensive experience with yolk sac tumor, and routine retroperitoneal lymph node dissection is controversial. Since AFP is an excellent tumor marker and chemotherapy is effective, close observation of stage 1 tumors after orchiectomy with frequent AFP determinations, chest radiologic studies, and computed tomographic scan or ultrasounds is reasonable. Metastatic disease is best managed with a team approach, using chemotherapy, retroperitoneal lymph node dissection, and radiation. Mortality rates for yolk sac tumor are 10% to 30%.

Teratoma

Teratoma is the second most frequent prepubertal testicular tumor, and is one of the few tumors of the neonatal period. The mean age at presentation is 18 to 20 months. Unlike adult teratoma, this lesion is benign, with no reported metastases in the prepubertal population. Tumor tissue represents the different germinal layers—entoderm, mesoderm, and ectoderm—with variable distribution for individual patients. Multiple cystic areas are characteristic enough that the diagnosis can often be suggested preoperatively with ultrasound. Orchiectomy is curative in young children. Peripubertal and postpubertal boys should probably be treated and followed as adults. Histologic diagnosis rests on the recognition of fetal or adult tissue from all three germ cell layers.

Gonadal Stromal Tumors

Sometimes referred to as interstitial tumors, gonadal stromal tumors are the most common non–germ cell tumor in boys. These tumors arise from the stromal component of the testis. The vast majority are of Leydig and Sertoli cell origin; however, the stroma, on rare occasions, gives rise to ovarian stromal tumors.

Leydig cell tumors usually occur in 5 to 10 year olds, with the latter part of a bimodal distribution occurring in the third to sixth decades. Leydig cell tumors are hormonally active and usually present with precocious puberty, gynecomastia, or both. Feminization is more common in postpubertal tumors. Functional prepubertal tumor cells secrete testosterone, which causes virilization. Differential diagnosis for virilization in the prepubescent male also includes congenital adrenal hyperplasia, adrenal carcinoma, and idiopathic precocious puberty. Improperly treated congenital adrenal hyperplasia produces hypertrophied Leydig cell nodules in the testis, which are treated medically rather than by orchiectomy. Despite the many mitotic figures, Leydig cell tumors are usually benign, and orchiectomy is sufficient treatment. Malignancy, defined by the presence of metastases, occurs in fewer than 10% of patients.

Sertoli cell tumors are rare lesions best treated by orchiectomy. Occasionally patients present with feminization and gynecomastia. The vast majority of Sertoli cell tumors are benign. Malignancy is defined by the presence of metastases, a feature seen more commonly in adult patients.

Gonadoblastoma

Gonadoblastoma, a rare tumor that usually occurs in the postpubertal male, is a mixture of germ cell and stromal cell elements, and is usually associated with the dysgenetic testes of intersex patients. Nearly all patients with a gonadoblastoma have an underlying gonadal abnormality. As a general rule, streak or dysgenetic gonads should be removed before a tumor develops. Gonadoblastoma occurs bilaterally in a third of patients. The tumors are usually benign; however, malignant degeneration resembling a dysgerminoma, and similar to a seminoma, can occur.

Leukemic Infiltrate

The testis is a potential sanctuary for leukemic cells. A blood–testis barrier may protect tumor cells from chemotherapeutic agents. Acute lymphocytic leukemia is the most common type of leukemia to infiltrate the testis, occurring in up to 25% of patients. The usual presentation is a painless testicular swelling, however, the testis may be entirely normal to palpation, despite leukemic infiltration. Testicular biopsies were once routine because occult testicular leukemia occurs in 10% to 20% of boys who are otherwise in remission following treatment for acute lymphocytic leukemia. In the past several years, pediatric oncologists have abandoned routine testis biopsies for two reasons. New multidrug chemotherapy regimens including methotrexate are more effective in preventing testicular relapse, and survival has been shown to be similar whether a boy is treated for occult testicular disease or gross recurrence elsewhere. Currently, testis biopsies are performed for acute lymphocytic leukemia only when a scrotal examination suggests a mass or tumor in the testis.

Tumorlike Lesions

Epidermoid cysts are rare, benign lesions that are monolayer (ectoderm) expressions of teratomas. Dermoid cysts are composed of two germ cell layers, usually ectoderm and mesoderm. Tumor excision is usually adequate treatment. Tunica albuginea cysts are small, asymptomatic lesions that are benign and can be locally excised. They probably represent retention cysts or capsule formation following resolution of a traumatic hemorrhage. Ectopic adrenal rests are usually paratesticular or in the spermatic cord, but occasionally they occupy a testicular position. The lesions are harmless, though when exposed to high levels of adrenocorticotropic hormone, the rests enlarge and become hormonally active.

Paratesticular Rhabdomyosarcoma

Paratesticular rhabdomyosarcoma, although extratesticular, is usually included in the classification. Up to 10% of intrascrotal tumors in prepubescent boys are rhabdomyosarcomas, and these are the most common spermatic cord tumors in children and adults. Paratesticular rhabdomyosarcomas represents 7% of all rhabdomyosarcomas. A tumor marker does not exist for rhabdomyosarcomas. Similar to Wilms tumor, two histologic types are described, favorable and unfavorable. Fortunately, the vast majority of paratesticular lesions are of the embryonal (favorable) subtype. Alveolar patterns portend an unfavorable prognosis. The cord and testis should be excised with a high inguinal orchiectomy. If the scrotum has been violated by incision, biopsy, or previous scrotal surgery, hemiscrotectomy should be performed. Staging evaluation should include imaging of the retroperitoneum and chest. The Intergroup Rhabdomyosarcoma Study III evaluated the role of routine retroperitoneal lymph node dissection in 121 boys with localized paratesticular tumors. The value of retroperitoneal lymph node dissection in overall survival was not established, and significant surgical complications were reported. The Intergroup Rhabdomyosarcoma Study IV recommendation for a child with localized, completely resected tumor whose retroperitoneal imaging studies are normal is observation with close monitoring for nodal relapse.[20] Multimodal treatment using chemotherapy, radiation, and surgery has resulted in a 90% overall survival rate for paratesticular rhabdomyosarcoma.

SCROTUM

Genital swellings form as ridges of tissues lateral to the cloacal folds. During the fourth month of gestation, the ipsilateral genital swelling and cloacal fold migrate caudally, fuse, and form a hemiscrotum. The two hemiscrota unite at the midline, caudal to the fused urethral folds. An internal septum separates each intrascrotal compartment.

The scrotal wall consists of skin and the dartos tunic of smooth muscle and fascia. The dartos tunic is continuous with the superficial fascia of the anterior abdominal wall. Dartos smooth muscle contracts and relaxes in response to various stimuli and comprises a precise thermoregulatory mechanism for the testes. The scrotal wall in a child contains fat as a continuation of the fatty layer of superficial fascia in the abdomen, but an equivalent component of adipose tissue is not present in the adult male scrotum. A median raphe extends anteriorly from the anus along the posterior and anterior surface of the scrotum to the base of the penis, and then continues along the ventral penile surface.

Abnormalities of the scrotum result from a defect in the normal posterior and caudal migration of the genital swellings (labioscrotal folds). Since the scrotum develops simultaneously with fusion of the urethral groove, scrotal anomalies tend to be associated with hypospadias, chordee, and urogenital sinus anomalies. Intersex disorders and exstrophy are also associated with abnormal scrotal development. Hormonal and mechanical influences probably contribute to the maldeveloped scrotum. There are three major types of scrotal abnormality: bifid scrotum, penoscrotal transposition, and ectopic scrotum.

Bifid scrotum occurs if the genital swellings fail to fuse at the scrotal septum, allowing the two hemiscrotal compartments to separate. This is commonly seen with intersex and severe hypospadias with chordee, and probably represents a less severe form of penoscrotal transposition. Isolated bifid scrotum, in the absence of other genital anomalies, is rare.

Transposition of the penis and scrotum, or scrotal engulfment, occurs in conjuction with proximal hypospadias and chordee. The transposition can be partial or complete. The less severe, incomplete lesions including the doughnut scrotum and shawl scrotum, are likely to have a normal urethra. Embryologically, abnormal development of the genital tubercle is associated with delayed fusion of the urethral folds, which retards the caudal migration and fusion of the genital swellings. Surgical correction is usually performed in two stages, since simultaneous scrotal recession may compromise the vascularity of preputial flaps used for hypospadias repair. The transposition is corrected with rotational flaps, dropping the scrotum below the penis. Proximal hypospadias can be repaired using a transverse preputial island flap procedure or a free graft of skin, bladder epithelium, or oral mucosa.

Scrotal ectopia is a rare anomaly in which one hemiscrotum is located in an aberrant position, such as the inguinal region, perineum, or medial thigh. Proximal ectopic locations are variants of unilateral penoscrotal transposition, and result from a failure of migration. Perineal ectopia probably results from abnormal migration of the ipsilateral genital swelling. The ectopic scrotum often occurs in conjunction with cryptorchidism, inguinal hernia, and exstrophy. The ipsilateral testis can be normal or dysplastic, and is usually located within or in close proximity to the ectopic hemiscrotum. The gubernaculum is present before migration of the genital swellings, and directs the descent of the testis to the abnormal locus. Treatment involves scrotoplasty and orchiopexy. Evaluation of the kidneys is warranted in these children because of the high incidence of ipsilateral upper urinary tract anomalies, such as agenesis, dysplasia, and ectopic ureter.

Hypoplasia of the scrotum occurs with testicular maldescent and anorchism. Local diffusion of testosterone from the gonad stimulates ipsilateral hemiscrotal development. Without a descended testis, the scrotum is deficient, flat, poorly developed, and lacks the normal deep rugal folds. Orchiopexy may be technically difficult; however, the scrotum usually expands to accommodate the testis. Prostheses should be placed in anorchid boys; placement early in childhood to allow scrotal distention and easier access for an adult prosthesis after puberty. Application of testosterone cream to the scrotum perioperatively may be beneficial.

EPIDIDYMIS–VAS DEFERENS–SEMINAL VESICLES

The mesonephric (wolffian) ducts extend from the mesonephros to the cloaca, and give rise to the internal male genital ducts. The cranial portion of the ducts serve an excretory function early in fetal development, and eventually regress. The distal segment may persist as a vestigial appendix epididymis. The portion of the mesonephric duct adjacent to the testis contacts the rete testis, forming efferent ducts of the testis. The epididymis is formed by elongation and convolution of the ducts distal to the testis efferent ducts. The midportion of the mesonephric duct becomes the vas deferens, and the caudal aspect gives rise to the seminal vesicles.

The epididymis is a single tubule, approximately 6 m long, with many convolutions, in which sperm are stored and mature before transport to the vas deferens. Sperm undergo biochemical and molecular changes as they pass through the epididymis. The vas deferens has a thick muscular layer, and the greatest wall-to-lumen ratio of any tubular structure in the body. Muscular contractions propel sperm through the vasal lumen. The seminal vesicle is not a storage organ for sperm, as was once believed, but secretes fluid crucial to sperm survival and function. The seminal vesicle duct joins the vas deferens to form the ejaculatory duct, which traverses the prostate and empties into the urethra on either side of the utricle.

Abnormalities of the epididymis are usually found in association with undescended testes. Approximately one third of cryptorchid testes have maldeveloped testis-epididymal fusion or abnormal epididymal suspension. Fusion abnormalities include loss of continuity between the testis and epididymis, and absent or atretic epididymal segments. Suspension defects are a widened epididymal mesentery and long epididymal tail or long, looped vas deferens (Fig. 93-8). Such abnormalities contribute to the infertility noted in cryptorchid men, and make the epididymis and vas deferens susceptible to iatrogenic injury during scrotal or inguinal surgery.

Epididymal cysts (spermatoceles) are uncommon in prepubescent boys, and are usually acquired lesions. The cysts occur primarily in the globus major and are readily diagnosed by physical examination and transillumination or by ultrasound. The incidence of epididymal cysts is increased in the male children of mothers treated with diethylstilbestrol during pregnancy. Epididymal tumors are rare in children; the most common is the benign adenomatoid tumor.

Congenital unilateral absence or atresia of the vas deferens occurs in .5% to 1% of the general male population, with a strong left-sided predominance. Bilateral absence or atresia accounts for 1% to 10% of azoospermic men. Males with cystic fibrosis are infertile and often have bilateral vasal agenesis. Most abnormalities of the vas deferens are associated with epididymal abnormalities. The vas deferens and ureteral bud are mesonephric duct derivatives in close embryologic proximity, which explains the high incidence of ipsilateral renal agenesis with absence of the vas deferens. An ectopic vas deferens may enter the ureter or bladder, often causing recurrent UTIs and epididymitis.

Seminal vesicle abnormalities in children are rare. Incomplete ductal differentiation results in seminal vesicle cysts. The seminal vesicle, a wolffian derivative, is in close approximation to the ureteral bud, at the caudal end of the mesonephric duct. As with abnormalities of the vas deferens, absence or a lesions of the seminal vesicle results in a high incidence of ipsilateral renal agenesis and dysplasia.

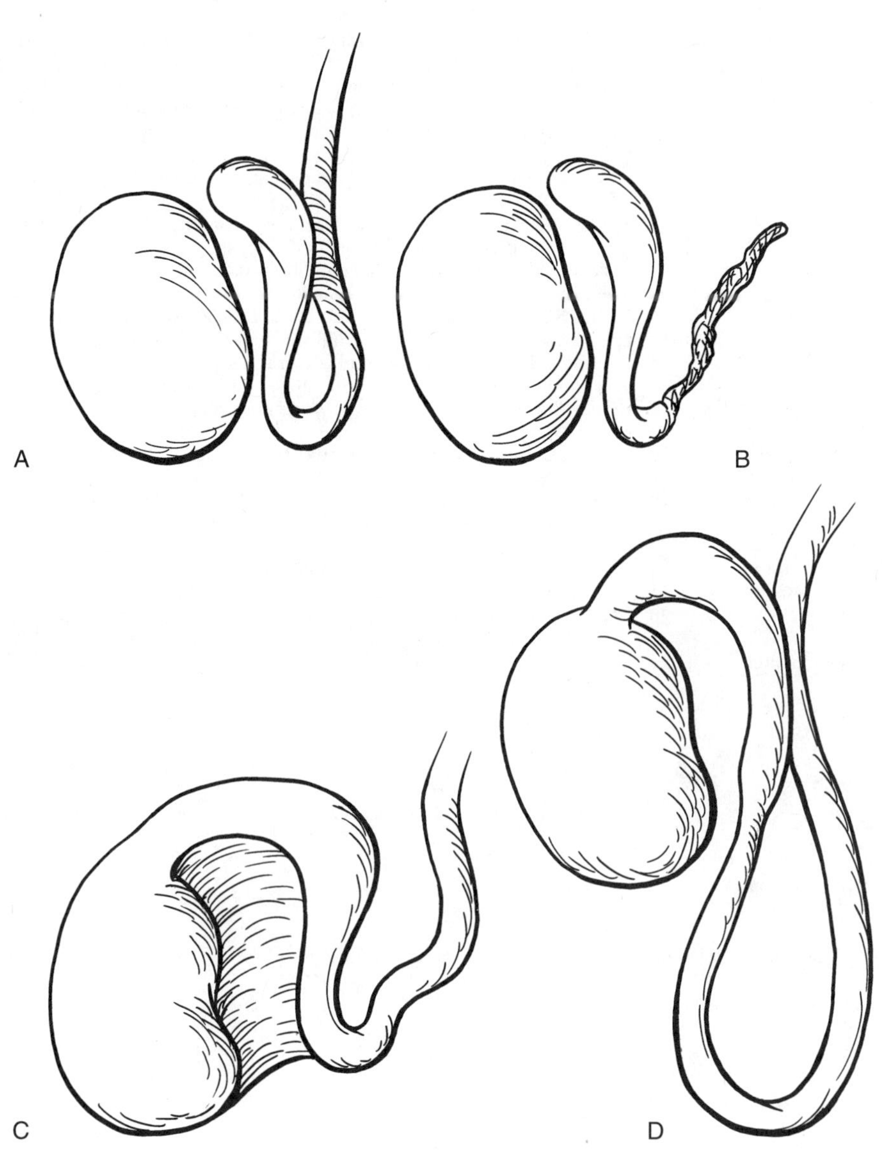

FIG. 93-8. Abnormalities of the epididymis. Fusion abnormalities: loss of continuity (*A*) and atretic segment (*B*) Suspension defects: wide mesentery (*C*) and long looped vas deferens (*D*).

VARICOCELE

A varicocele is an abnormal dilation of the spermatic veins within the scrotum, and although it is not specifically an abnormality of the male genital tract, it warrants discussion here because of its presentation and effects on the reproductive system. A varicocele occurs in 15% of the adult male population, but is uncommon before puberty. Older children may present with heaviness or scrotal discomfort, an ill-defined scrotal mass, or growth retardation of the ipsilateral testis. Left-sided lesions predominate, probably because the left gonadal vein is 8 to 10 cm longer than the right, inserts at a right angle into the left renal vein, and has a higher incidence of incompetent valves. Physical examination is notable for the classic bag of worms appearance and consistency of the lesion. Varicocele is graded with the patient in the standing position:

Grade I—palpable varicosities with Valsalva maneuver
Grade II—visible varicosities with Valsalva maneuver
Grade III—visible varicosities without Valsalva maneuver

The dilated veins should reduce when the patient is placed in the supine position. Varicocele is the most readily identifiable cause of subnormal fertility in the male, and is often associated with oligoasthenospermia and a small ipsilateral testis. Surgical repair of the varicosities can result in significant improvement in semen quality.

A proposed mechanism for the subfertility is that the venous dilation causes increased intratesticular pressures and blood flow, leading to an increase in testicular temperatures and resultant detrimental effect on spermatogenesis. Adolescents with a large varicocele may have a significant decrease in ipsilateral testicular volume. One third of boys with grade II lesions and more than half of those with grade III varicoceles have measurable testis hypoplasia. Because of the potential for altered spermatogenesis, testis growth retardation is an indication for varicocelectomy in the adolescent.[21] One arbitrary standard for intervention is a 4-mm difference in length, or 20% volume loss, in the ipsilateral gonad compared to the contralateral mate. Significant testicular growth often occurs after successful repair. Interruption of the spermatic veins can be accomplished with open surgery in the high scrotum, inguinal canal, or retroperitoneum, the laparoscope or with venographic techniques. In addition to testicular growth retardation, symptomatic varicoceles and grade III lesions are indications for intervention.

REFERENCES

1. American Academy of Pediatrics Task Force on Circumcision. Report of the Task Force on Circumcision. Pediatrics 1989;84:388.
2. Wiswell TE, Smith FR, Bass JW. Decreased incidence of urinary tract infections in circumcised male infants. Pediatrics 1985;75:901.
3. Newborns: care of the uncircumcised penis. Elk Grove Village, IL, American Academy of Pediatrics Division of Publications, 1990.
4. Wiswell TE, Geschke DW. Risks from circumcision during the first month of life compared with those for uncircumcised boys. Pediatrics 1989;83:1011.
5. Aaronson IA. Micropenis: medical and surgical implications. J Urol 1994;152:4.
6. Reilly JM, Woodhouse CRJ. Small penis and the male sexual role. J Urol 1989;142:569.
7. Dwoskin JY. Management of the ''concealed'' penis. Dialog Pediatr Urol 1993;16:1.
8. Koff SA. Does compensatory testicular enlargement predict monorchism? J Urol 1991;146:632.
9. Huff DS, Hadziselimovic F, Snyder HM, et al. Early postnatal testicular maldevelopment in cryptorchidism. J Urol 1991;146:624.
10. Jarow JP, Berkovitz GD, Migeon CJ, et al. Elevation of serum gonadotropins establish the diagnosis of anorchism in prepubertal boys with bilateral cryptorchidism. J Urol 1986;136:277.
11. Bellinger MF, Abromowitz H, Brantley S, et al. Orchiopexy: an experimental study of the effect of surgical technique on testicular histology. J Urol 1989;142:553.
12. Bloom DA, Key DW. Orchiopexy. In: Fowler JE Jr, ed. Urologic surgery, ed 1. Boston, Little, Brown, 1992:556.
13. Canavese F, Lalla R, Linari A, et al. Surgical treatment of cryptorchidism. Eur J Pediatr 1993;152(Suppl 2):S43.
14. Kogan SJ, Tennenbaum S, Gill B, et al. Efficacy of orchiopexy by patient age one year for cryptorchidism. J Urol 1990;144:508.
15. Johnson DE, Woodhead DM, Pohl DR, et al. Cryptorchidism and testicular tumorigenesis. Surgery 1968;63:919.
16. Bloom DA, Semm K. Advances in genitourinary laparoscopy. Adv Urol 1991;4:167.
17. Cooper BJ, Little TM. Orchiopexy: theory and practice. Br Med J 1985;291:706.
18. Wan J, Bloom DA. Testicular tumors in children. In: Crawford ED, Das S, eds. Current genitourinary cancer surgery, ed 1. Philadelphia: Lea & Febiger, 1990:429.
19. Kaplan GW. Testicular tumors in children. AUA Update Series 1983;2:lesson 12.
20. Wiener ES, Lawrence W, Hays D, et al. Retroperitoneal node biopsy in paratesticular rhabdomyosarcoma. J Pediatr Surg 1994;29:171.
21. Kass DA. The management of the asymptomatic varicocele in adolescence. Prob Urol 1990;4:690.

Surgery of Infants and Children: Scientific Principles and Practice, edited by Keith T. Oldham, Paul M. Colombani, and Robert P. Foglia. Lippincott–Raven Publishers, Philadelphia, © 1997.

CHAPTER 94

Female Genital Tract

E. Stanton Adkins

The pediatric general surgeon is often confronted with problems in the female child that in an adult fall in the purview of the obstetrician or gynecologist. The problems range from disorders in the development of the female genital system to infections, tumors, and sexual abuse. The pediatric surgeon must be adept in the diagnosis and treatment of these various problems. Endoscopic techniques such as urethroscopy, vaginoscopy, and laparoscopy, as well as improvements in radiologic imaging, have advanced the ability to evaluate and treat children with disorders of the genital system.

EMBRYOLOGY

Embryology of the female genital tract may be considered based on the origin of the genital structures. The ovary arises from genital ridge mesenchyme and is populated by germ cells.[1] The fallopian tubes, uterus, and upper vagina descend from the müllerian ducts. The lower vagina and external genitalia are derived from the urogenital sinus and ridge. Some minor structures are attributable to the wolffian ducts.[2]

DEVELOPMENT OF THE OVARY

The ovary consists of germ cells and the supporting stroma. Until the embryo has reached an age of 7 weeks, the ovary is morphologically indistinguishable from a testis and is rightly termed a gonad. Germ cells may be seen in a 24-day embryo in the caudal portion of the yolk sac near the allantoic stalk. During the fifth week of gestation, these germ cells migrate dorsally along the wall of the yolk sac and the gut until by the end of the week they reach the genital ridge. The migrating cells increase in number from between 30 and 50 to approximately 10,000 by the process of mitosis during this time.

The genital ridge gives rise to the supporting stroma of the ovary. It is composed of mesenchyme from the ventral medial aspects of the mesonephros and the coelomic epithelium overlying the mesenchyme. The best evidence indicates that the genital ridge releases factors which attract germ cells to the gonad. Agar blocks impregnated with a mesodermal homogenate attract migrating germ cells when the native genital ridge has

been destroyed. Germ cells leave transplanted gonads to migrate to the genital ridge of appropriately aged recipient embryos.

Germ cells are likewise necessary for the differentiation of gonadal stroma into an ovary or testis. Arrest of the migration of germ cells leads to failure of development of the ovary.

As the embryo grows, epithelial cords of cells, the sex cords, grow into the mesenchyme. By the eighth week, some differentiation has occurred. In males, the sex cords develop into seminiferous tubules and the rete testis; in females, the sex cords regress. Testis determining factor appears to be a necessary element for growth and differentiation of the sex cords. In its absence, the sex cords in the medullary portion of the gonad regress over several months. They are absent at full-term gestation.

Once germ cells reach the ovary, they are termed oogonia. They increase in number by the process of mitosis, numbering 6 to 7 million by the 20th week of gestation. Starting at approximately the 15th week, oogonia enter into prophase of the first meiosis. This process starts deep within the ovary and then proceeds to more superficial portions. Once the cells enter into prophase, they are termed oocytes. The process is essentially complete by the 4th postnatal month.

Concurrent with the formation of oocytes, primary follicles develop. The oocytes become enclosed or encased with granulosa cells and mesenchymal theca cells. Follicles deep within the ovary become atretic, whereas superficial follicles (those formed most recently) are preserved to form the ovarian cortex. The follicles remain dormant for many years, with oocytes arrested in their first prophase of meiosis until puberty. With each estrous cycle, several of the primary follicles mature and complete the first meiosis with ovulation. The second meiosis does not occur until after ovulation when a sperm encounters the ovum.

MÜLLERIAN DUCT

The Müllerian ducts, also known as the paramesonephric ducts, appear in embryos of both sexes late in the sixth week. Each duct originates as a groove lateral to the developing gonad and kidney, which tubularizes as the edges of the groove come together. In its more caudal aspect, the müllerian duct arises

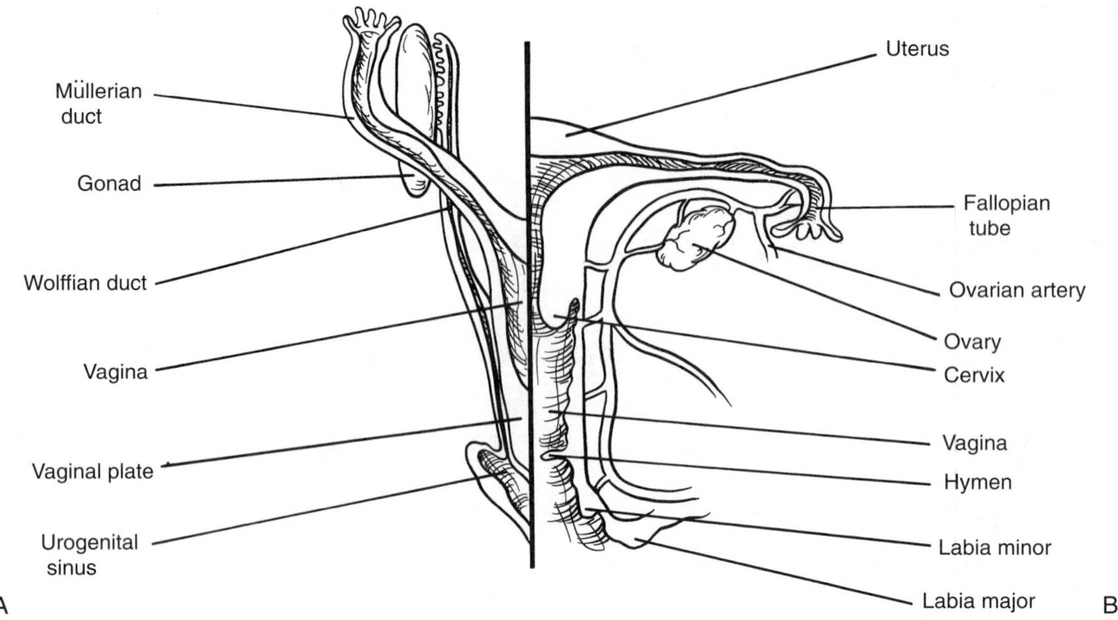

FIG. 94-1. (*A*) Female genitalia at 3 months gestation, immediately before atrophy of the wolffian duct and before completion of müllerian duct fusion. (*B*) Adult anatomy.

from a nest of cells medial to the basement membrane of the wolffian duct and the overlying epithelium. The origin of the müllerian duct depends on the presence of the wolffian duct.

The paired müllerian ducts lie lateral to the wolffian ducts scranially and at the more caudal extent are medial to the wolffian ducts (Fig. 94-1). Soon after their development, the caudal portion of the müllerian ducts fuse to form a single canal. The lumen of these fused ducts is initially V-shaped. As the fusion proceeds cranially, the müllerian duct system develops first a Y and then a T shape.

As the embryo grows, the point of fusion with the urogenital sinus elongates. This portion has no lumen and gives rise to the vagina. The vagina itself develops when this vaginal plate recanalizes at approximately the sixth month. It appears that the proximal two thirds of the vaginal plate is of müllerian duct origin and the lower one third is of urogenital sinus origin. The hymen might seem to be a logical point of division, but it is lined on both its lower and upper surfaces with urogenital sinus epithelium.

The uterus, cervix, and fallopian tubes arise from the persistently patent portions of the müllerian ducts. The uterine tubes originate from the unfused lateral extensions of the müllerian ducts. The uterine body and cervix develop from the fused portion of the müllerian ducts. A small constriction indicates the division between the uterus and the cervix. The cervix is larger in the fetus relative to the uterus than it is in the adult and may measure as much as two times the length of the body of the uterus. The epithelium of the uterus and cervix, which is columnar, becomes increasingly higher in the few weeks before birth. The columnar epithelium of the cervix is later replaced by squamous vaginal-type epithelium after birth.

The uterine muscle develops from the mesenchyme surrounding the uterus and vagina at the 11th week. These cells differentiate into true smooth muscle to form two longitudinal

and one circular muscle layers. Myometrial development is complete by the seventh month.

UROGENITAL SINUS

The urogenital sinus gives rise to the external genitalia and the lower third of the vagina. External genitalia arise from the cloacal membrane starting at the fourth gestational week. On the anterior margins of this membrane are two genital swellings; posteriorly are paired anal swellings. The cloacal membrane diminishes in size to become a groove between urogenital folds at the sixth week. At this stage, the perineal body forms, separating the anus from the urethral groove. The fusion anterior to the groove becomes the phallus. During the eighth week, labioscrotal swellings lateral to the phallus move caudally to form the labia minora. The clitoris develops from the phallus and extends posteriorly into two corpora cavernosa of erectile tissue.

WOLFFIAN DUCT

The wolffian ducts originate as the duct system for the primitive kidney, the pronephros. These are associated with the mesonephros, the first functional kidney, sometime after the fifth week of life. Each duct connects with the urogenital sinus. It persists as a defined structure for only a short time in the female. By the ninth week, the mesonephros ceases any excretory function, and its duct begins to regress. By the middle of the fourth month, the opening into the urogenital sinus closes. Regression is not complete, however, so some structures of wolffian origin persist into adulthood. These structures include the pedunculated hydatid of Morgagni, the appendix vesiculosa, the epoöphoron and, for a short time, the paroöphoron.

One structure, Gartner's canal, persists in the wall of the

cervix and upper vagina in approximately 20% of adults. It represents the caudal portion of the wolffian duct. In situations where the ureter fails to make a normal connection with the bladder, Gartner's canal may become an ectopic opening for the ureter.

HOMEOBOX GENES

The homeobox gene complex is a phylogenetically well conserved set of instructions for the longitudinal development of higher animals. There is spatial cephalocaudal organization of the expression of these genes. Evidence from the mouse indicates that these genes play a role in the mesenchymal development of the genitourinary system.[3] In female mice, homeobox 4.8 (*HOX 4.8*) is expressed in the urinary bladder and distal uterus. *HOX 4.7* is expressed in the entire uterine wall, whereas *HOX 4.6* and *4.5* are found in the oviduct and to a small extent in the ovary. Certain malformations may be due to abnormal expression of a homeobox sequence. Cloacal disorders may arise when *HOX 4.8* is affected. Nonetheless, the exact role of these genes in the developing genitourinary system remains to be determined.

ANATOMY, GROWTH, AND DEVELOPMENT

The ovary migrates from its position at the genital ridge to a position at the pelvic brim during the first 12 weeks of gestation. It remains an abdominal structure until birth. Thereafter, it descends into the ovarian fossa and rotates laterally to a vertical position on the posterior surface of the broad ligament. The ovary is attached by the uteroovarian ligament to the uterus. The round ligament extends from the upper uterine cervix through the inguinal ring and terminates diffusely in the labia majora. The uteroovarian ligament and the round ligament of the uterus represent female derivatives of the gubernaculum. Unlike the male gubernaculum, the female gubernaculum does not shorten during ovarian migration.

The uterus is a three-layered muscular organ. The normal position is anteflexed relative to the cervix and anteverted relative to the vagina, so that it rests on the dome of the bladder. Retroversion and retroflexion as well as extreme anteversion and anteflexion, are variants that may often be seen. The adnexa consists of the fallopian tubes, ovaries, and broad ligaments, which are lateral on either side. The fallopian or uterine tubes lie anterior to the uteroovarian ligament and posterior to the round ligament of the uterus. They are enveloped in the broad ligament. The broad ligament extends from the uterus to the pelvic side wall. The lateral-most portion is termed the infundibulopelvic ligament, or suspensory ligament of the ovary.

The vagina lies just posterior to the bladder and urethra. It extends from the vestibule to the uterine cervix. Its three layers of muscle are lined with squamous epithelium. The course of the vagina parallels that of the pelvic brim and is essentially horizontal. The uterine cervix penetrates the anterior wall of the vagina near its apex. The surface of the vagina forms a collapsed H-shape tube that when distended possesses a series of horizontal folds, or rugae.

Sizes and shapes of the pelvic viscera are age dependent (Table 94-1).

The external genitalia include the labia majora, which extend anteriorly from the mons pubis posteriorly to the labial commissure at the perineal body. The labia majora are covered with skin. The labia minora lie medial to the labia majora and are covered with squamous mucosa. At their anterior extent, the labia minora join to form the prepuce of the clitoris. The labia minora form the lateral margins of the vestibule. Within the vestibule is found the urethra in the anterior midline. Slightly posterior to this is the vaginal orifice, which is covered by a membrane, the hymen. Through the aperture in the hymen, the vagina may be visualized.

In the infant, the labia majora, labia minora, and clitoris are relatively larger and more prominent than they are later in life. The hymen is a membranous fold that may protrude between the labia minora. In the average full-term infant, the vaginal orifice has a 5-cm circumference and is more deeply positioned than in later life. The vaginal mucosa, which at birth may be up to 20 cell layers in depth, rapidly thins to one or two cell layers and is redder than in the adult. With the onset of puberty, the labia majora and mons pubis become covered with hair. The labia minora remain hairless. The vestibule may become slightly more shallow, and the vaginal mucosa once again proliferates. The vagina is moistened with cervical mucus, since the vagina has no glands of its own. With puberty, the vagina becomes colonized by *Lactobacillus acidophilus*, which metabolizes glycogen into lactic acid and lowers the pH of the vagina.

At birth, when the female child leaves the maternal environment, estrogen levels which had been high, begin to fall. The levels stay low until shortly before puberty. Growth of the genitalia is largely hormonally dependent and therefore does not parallel the linear growth of the child.

The ovary doubles in size in the first 6 weeks of life. Thereafter it grows very slowly until just before puberty, when the growth rate increases (see Table 94-1). The newborn ovary often has follicles present and may have some follicular cysts. In most situations, the cysts resolve by the time girls are several months old.

The uterus, which at birth has a length of approximately 3.5 cm and volume of 3.5 cc, two thirds of which is the cervix, decreases in size following estrogen withdrawal. Length may decrease by one third and volume by 50%. Uterine volume stays relatively constant for the first 6 years of life and then gradually increases until the onset of puberty when there is a rapid increase in size.

The fallopian tubes do not decrease in size as the corpus of the uterus does. At birth they measure approximately 3 cm in length and gradually increase in length to a full adult length of 7.5 cm. The vagina gradually lengthens as the child grows, reaching a final adult length of approximately 9.0 cm on the posterior wall and 7.5 cm on the anterior wall.

Vascular Supply

Ovarian arteries arise from the aorta bilaterally. The ovarian veins arise from the vena cava on the right and the renal vein on the left. The vessels cross the iliac vessels at the iliac bifurcation and travel with the ureters initially. They then enter the broad ligament and course to the ovaries. The remaining blood

TABLE 94-1. *Ultrasound measurement of genital organ volume and size by age*

	Ovary	Fallopian tube	Uterus	Vagina
VOLUME (cc)				
Birth	0.3		3.5	
2 y	0.7		2.0	
6 y	1.2		1.8	
12 y	3.8		16.2	
Adult	6.5		50.0	
SIZE (cm)				
Birth				
Length	1.5–3.0	3.0	2.5–5.0	2.5–3.5
Width	0.4–0.8	0.5	2.0	1.5
Thickness	0.4–0.8		1.3	
6 y				
Length			3.3	
Width			1.5	
Thickness			0.7	
12 y				
Length			5.4	
Width			4.5	
Thickness			1.7	
Adult				
Length	2.5–3.5	10.0	7.5	7.5 anterior
Width	2.0		5.0	9.0 posterior
Thickness	1.0		2.5	

(After Orsini LF, Salardi S, Pilu G, et al. Pelvic organs in premenarcheal girls: real-time ultrasonography. Radiology 1984;153:113; and Crelin ES. Functional anatomy of the newborn. New Haven, Yale University, 1973:67).

supply of the deep organs comes from the hypogastric arteries, with the largest branch being the uterine artery that proceeds toward the uterine cervix and then branches to send one marginal artery along the lateral aspect of the uterus and one along the vagina. Spiral arteries extend from this vessel anteriorly and posteriorly. There is a separate vaginal branch of the hypogastric artery. The external pudendal artery (a branch of the external iliac), the internal pudendal artery (a branch of the hypogastric), and the hemorrhoidal vessels supply the vulva and lower third of the vagina. There is an extensive collateral blood supply in this vicinity, so much so that a pregnancy may be supported following ligation of both hypogastric arteries. With the exception of the ovarian veins, the genital venous drainage parallels that of the arterial supply.

Lymphatic Vessels

Lymphatic drainage of the genitalia has been well described. The perineum, vulva, and lower anterior abdomen drain toward the ipsilateral subinguinal and inguinal nodes, first entering the superficial nodes then draining more deeply through the fossa ovalis to the deep inguinal nodes. From there, drainage proceeds up the iliac chain. The internal drainage proceeds to the ipsilateral hypogastric, common iliac, and occasionally aortic or periaortic nodes. Only occasionally do the pelvic viscera drain to the inguinal nodes.

PUBERTY

Puberty is the transition from childhood to adulthood during which a child develops into a physically mature and reproduc-

tively capable adult. Maturation of the primary sexual characteristics, genitals and gonads, is heralded by the appearance of axillary and pubic hair and the development of breast buds. The hormonal control of puberty begins with the release of an increased amount of gonadotropin-releasing hormone (Gn-RH) from the hypothalamus, which stimulates the pituitary to produce luteinizing hormone (LH) and follicle-stimulating hormone (FSH). These, in turn, stimulate the ovary. Estrogen and progesterone synthesis and secretion increase markedly with the onset of puberty. It is these steroids that lead to the development of the secondary sexual characteristics.

The regulation of the hypothalamic pituitary ovarian axis is an intricate process with positive and negative feedback loops. Gn-RH synthesis secretion and feedback control are regulated by steroid levels as well as several neurotransmitters, including epinephrine, norepinephrine, dopamine, endorphins, and neuroactive amino acids. Gn-RH is released in discrete bursts, which are as great at birth as they are during puberty and adulthood. Downregulation of Gn-RH secretion occurs during the first year of life and remains diminished throughout childhood. Consequently LH and FSH are present, but in significantly reduced quantities during childhood. The signals which stimulate the increased secretion of Gn-RH are not known. There may be a loss of prepubertal inhibitory controls or the secretion of new stimulators.

PRECOCIOUS PUBERTY

Precocious puberty is defined as the development of secondary sexual characteristics before the age of 8 years or the onset of menarche before the age of 10 years. Precocious puberty may be either central, which is Gn-RH–dependent; peripheral, which is Gn-RH–independent; or incomplete, which involves the expression of some primary or secondary sex characteristics but not others.

Central precocious puberty may be idiopathic but is generally due to central nervous system dysfunction. The dysfunction may originate from congenital defects, tumors, other space-occupying lesions, hydrocephalus, inflammation, trauma, or radiation. Central precocious puberty is always isosexual. It is diagnosed by performing a Gn-RH challenge and seeing marked increases in both serum FSH and LH. It may be treated surgically by removing the inciting cause or medically using a Gn-RH analogue to suppress pituitary release of LH and FSH.

Peripheral, Gn-RH–independent precocious puberty is due to the presence of inappropriate levels of circulating sex steroids. These steroids may be either exogenous or endogenous. Exogenous steroids include oral contraceptives, anabolic steroids, and rarely estrogen-like environmental chemicals. The endogenous causes include ovarian tumors or cysts as well as some feminizing adrenal tumors. There may be an association with McCune-Albright syndrome. Peripheral precocious puberty may be isosexual or heterosexual, depending on which steroids are present in greatest concentration. Serum LH and FSH levels are normal or low for age. Once exogenous sources of steroids have been ruled out, workup involves search for a tumor. The tumor may arise from the ovary or adrenal gland. Imaging with CT scan or MRI can locate and define the lesion. Surgical resection of the tumor is usually curative. Adjuvant chemotherapy and radiation may be necessary for malignancies.

Incomplete sexual precocity may involve premature thelarche, premature pubarche, or premature menarche. Premature thelarche, or early breast development, is a common problem in infants and young children. It presents with subareolar nonprogressive breast development that may be unilateral or bilateral. There are no areolar changes associated with this self-limited process. If the breast development is progressive or does not show signs of regression after 1 to 2 years, an endocrine evaluation is indicated. Premature pubarche involves the early development of pubic hair and is a sign of androgen excess. Pubarche does not normally occur before the age of 8 years, though some blacks may have a normal physiologic pubarche several months earlier. If the age of onset is sufficiently early or signs of virilization should appear, endocrinologic evaluation is indicated. Androgen-producing tumors or adrenal hyperplasia may be responsible.

Premature menarche or vaginal bleeding is a normal event in some newborns with the withdrawal of maternal estrogen stimulation. Estrogen-producing cysts may lead to bleeding when they rupture, and estrogen levels fall. Otherwise isolated menarche is rare. Vaginal bleeding from nonendocrine causes such as vulvovaginitis, trauma, abuse, or malignancy is more common and must be excluded. A thorough history and physical examination can detect most of these causes.

OVARIAN DISORDERS

Ovarian disorders typically present with pain or a mass. Pain is often due to rupture of a cyst and requires no therapy. Occasionally pain is a symptom of torsion of the ovary and requires emergent surgery. Ovarian masses may be found on physical examination of the abdomen or pelvis, or incidently during ultrasound or CT examination. Rapid assessment and intervention may prevent ovarian loss and preserve fertility.

Ovarian Cysts

Functional ovarian cysts occur when a follicle or corpus luteum fails to regress. In the prenatal period, ovarian cysts are often discovered during maternal ultrasound. Following these cysts with serial ultrasound shows resolution of the cyst as newborn hormone levels fall (Fig. 94-2). In pubertal females cysts

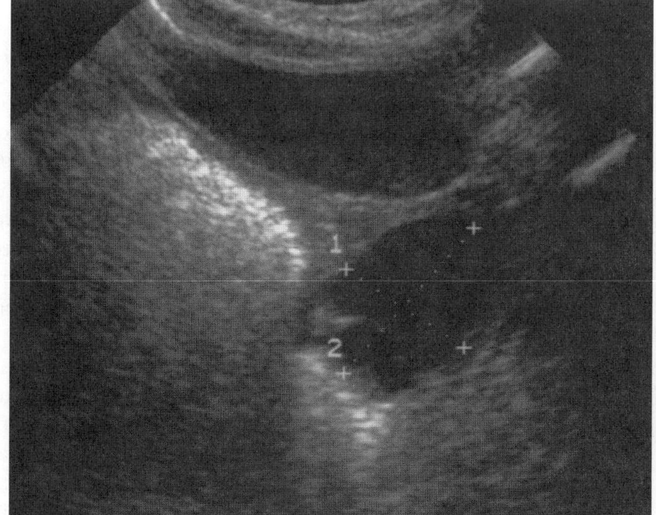
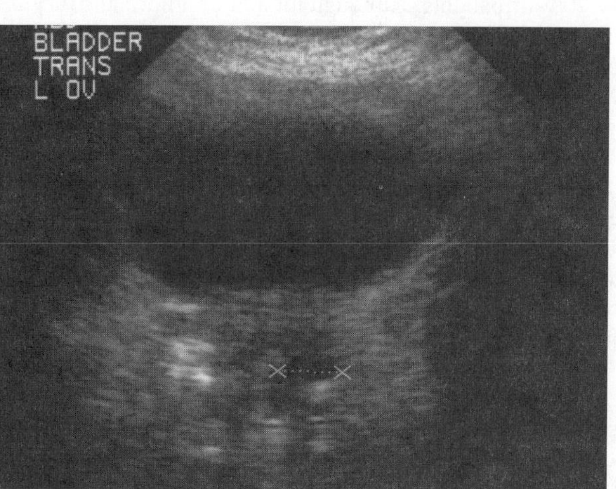

FIG. 94-2. Ultrasound images of an infant with a benign cyst of the ovary as a newborn (*A*), and at the age of 4 months (*B*). The cyst largely resolved over the 4 months between the ultrasound sessions. Prenatal ultrasound regularly reveals these benign cysts, which result from estrogen influences. It is important to recognize the benign, self-limited nature of the finding.

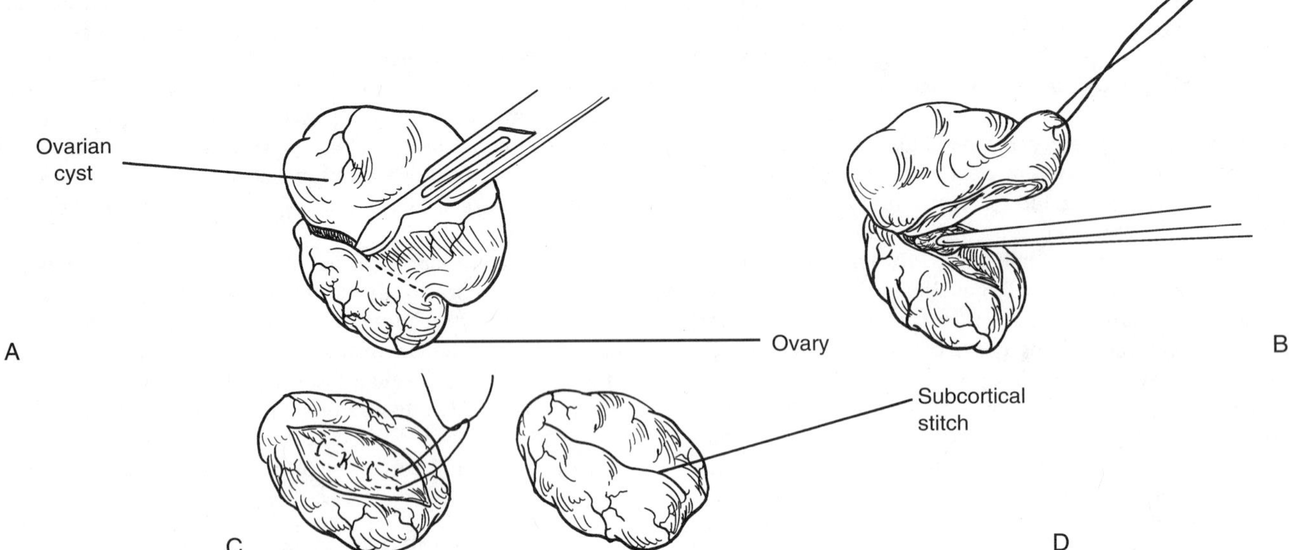

FIG. 94-3. Ovarian cyst removal. (*A*) An incision is made near the base of the cyst. (*B*) A plane is developed to bluntly dissect the cyst from the ovary. (*C*) Deep tissues are approximated with an absorbable monofilament suture. (*D*) The ovarian surface is closed with subcortical stitch.

3 to 8 cm in diameter may be seen. Observation of cysts less than 6 cm in diameter over two menstrual cycles often shows regression. If enlargement occurs or the cyst persists beyond 3 months, surgical resection is indicated. The incidence of infertility following ovarian cystectomy is high. Reconstruction of the ovary with atraumatic technique to minimize adhesion formation may lessen the incidence of infertility thereafter (Fig. 94-3).

Ovarian Torsion

Ovarian torsion is one of the few gynecologic emergencies a pediatric surgeon may encounter. Prompt diagnosis and treatment is likely to result in salvage of a viable ovary in approximately 70% of patients. Although torsion of a normal ovary is possible, the vast majority of torsed ovaries are enlarged with one or more cysts or a tumor.

Ovarian torsion presents with acute onset of intense lower abdominal pain. There is sometimes a history of similar pain that resolved spontaneously. Anorexia or nausea often accompany the pain. Focal tenderness and a mass may be appreciated on pelvic exam. Plain films sometimes reveal the calcifications of a teratoma and nonspecific ileus. When further information is required, ultrasound with color flow Doppler (Fig. 94-4) can demonstrate the mass and occasionally demonstrate loss of perfusion. Unfortunately, the presence of flow within the mass does not prove the converse, that the adnexa is not torsed.

At operation via a Pfannenstiel or midline incision, the involved ovary is detorsed. If perfusion is questionable, fluorescein can demonstrate reperfusion in a viable ovary. When tumor is present, salpingo-oophorectomy is indicated. Cysts should be resected, the ovary repaired, and oophoropexy performed. The contralateral ovary must be inspected. Since contralateral torsion with consequent castration has been described, many surgeons recommend fixation of the opposite ovary.

OVARIAN TUMORS

Ovarian tumors in childhood may originate in any of the three components that make up the ovary. Ninety percent of these are of germ cell origin of which two thirds are benign teratomas. Approximately 4% are of stromal origin derived from the sex cords, those being granulosa-theca cell tumors and androblastomas. Only 3% are of epithelial origin. This contrasts with the adult experience in which 90% of all ovarian tumors are epithelial in nature.[4]

Germ Cell Tumor

Tumors develop from germ cell precursors. The tumors may be located at any point in the migration of germ cells from the yolk sac to the ovary and occasionally beyond the normal migration path. Germ cell tumors of the ovary account for 3% of all childhood malignant disease. The incidence is approximately 4.2 new malignant germ cell tumors per million children below the age of 15. Malignant germ cell tumors are more common among young females than young males in contrast with the higher male incidence in older adolescents and adults.

Recent advances in molecular biology have revealed structural chromosome changes in the majority of germ cell tumors. These involve abnormalities primarily of chromosomes 1 or 12 but may also involve chromosomes 5, 7, 9, 17, 21, and 22. The isochromosome 12p [I{12p}] is one of the most common anomalies and has been found in all histologic subtypes. Karyotype studies of tumor cell lines indicate that the anomalies occur before the first meiotic division. Concurrent or posttreatment hematologic malignances are sometimes seen with the same chromosomal defects.

The majority of these tumors arise spontaneously; however, there are well-described instances of familial germ cell tumors. Within a given family the tumors may not necessarily be of the

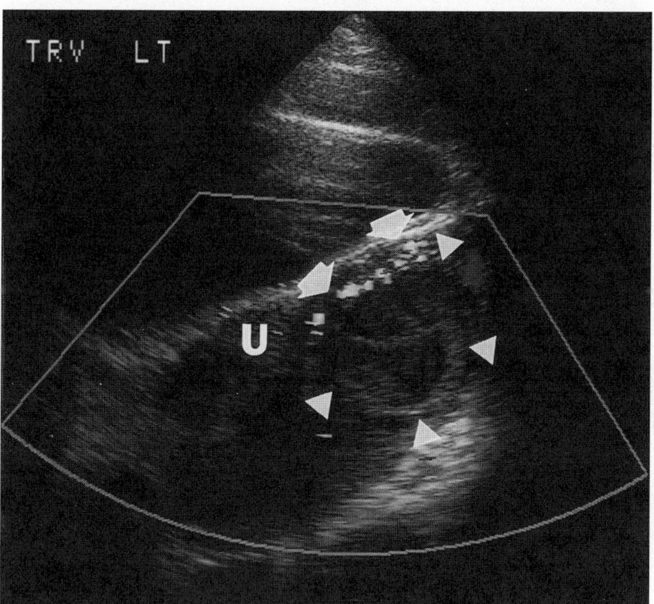

FIG. 94-4. Color Doppler image of a painful lower quadrant mass in a 5-year-old girl shows the characteristic features of ovarian torsion: ovarian enlargement with cysts (*arrowheads*) and increased peripheral blood flow with lack of flow through the parenchyma (*arrows*). (See Color Figure 94-4.)

same histologic type. The Li-Fraumeni cancer family syndrome has been associated with germ cell tumors in addition to bone and soft tissue sarcomas. Other conditions such as 46XY gonadal dysgenesis and mosaic Turner syndrome are highly associated with the development of gonadoblastomas.

The germ cell tumors are histologically classified based on the developmental stage they most closely resemble. The ontogeny of the germ cell tumors is described in Table 94-2 and these are discussed as well in Chapter 38.

Germinoma

Germinoma is the current terminology designating the most primitive of the germ cell tumors. It includes tumors which

TABLE 94-2. *Ontogeny of germ cell tumors*

	Tumor	Marker
Primordial germ cell	Germinoma	PLAP
Embryonic differentiation	Embryonal carcinoma	HCG, AFP
Extraembryonic differentiation	Endodermal sinus tumor	AFP, LDH-1 HCG
	Choriocarcinoma	
Complete differentiation	Teratoma	—
Dysgenetic gonad	Gonadoblastoma	—

PLAP, placental alkaline phosphatase; AFP, α-fetoprotein; HCG, β-human chorionic gonadotropin; LDH-1, lactate dehydrogenase isomer 1.
(Ablin A, Isaacs H. Germ cell tumors. In: Pizzo PA, Poplack DG, eds. Principles and practice of pediatric oncology, ed 2. Philadelphia, JB Lippincott, 1993:867).

were previously termed seminomas when they developed in the testis, dysgerminomas when they developed in the ovary, and germinomas at extragonadal sites. Germinomas are present in 10 percent of all ovarian tumors in children. They are rarely found in pure form, more often in combination with other germ cell tumors. Histologically, the germinomas consist of large round cells with vesicular nuclei and a clear to eosinophilic cytoplasm. The cells resemble primordial germ cells. Placental alkaline phosphatase is present in most germinomas. Markers for α-fetoprotein and β-human chorionic gonadotropin (β-HCG) are negative in pure germinomas.

Embryonal Carcinoma

Embryonal carcinoma is histologically poorly differentiated with anaplastic elements and extensive necrosis. Areas may resemble endodermal sinus tumor; however, the cells are larger with more abundant cytoplasm and large nucleoli. The tumors are uniformly negative for α-fetoprotein, but may be focally positive for placental alkaline phosphatase and β-HCG. Chemotherapy occasionally causes these tumors to mature.

Endodermal Sinus Tumor (Yolk Sac Tumor)

The endodermal sinus tumor is the most common malignant germ cell tumor of childhood. In infants it is most frequently involved with sacrococcygeal teratomas. The ovarian location is seen more frequently in later childhood and adolescence. Gross appearance is that of a pale tan-yellow slimy tumor with foci of necrosis. The tumors are friable. The pathology may be papillary, reticular, solid, or polyvesicular. α-Fetoprotein is typically elevated in the sera of patients with this lesion.

Choriocarcinoma

Choriocarcinoma histologically resembles placental tissue with two components, cytotrophoblasts and syncytiotrophoblasts. The cytotrophoblasts are large, round cells with clear cytoplasm and vesicular nuclei, and the syncytiotrophoblasts represent syncytia with abundant cytoplasm. There are frequent foci of hemorrhage and necrosis. β-HCG is produced by these tumors.

Gonadoblastoma

Gonadoblastoma is a tumor that arises in dysgenetic gonads in association with the Y-chromosome karyotype. The patients are phenotypic females with either a 46XY or mosaic 46XY/45XO karyotype. One third of these patients will develop gonadoblastomas. Pure gonadoblastomas do not metastasize; however, one third of the tumors are associated with germinomas, which do metastasize. Microscopically, the tumors consist of large germ cells surrounded by smaller Sertoli cells containing hyaline bodies and calcium. No markers are known for this tumor.

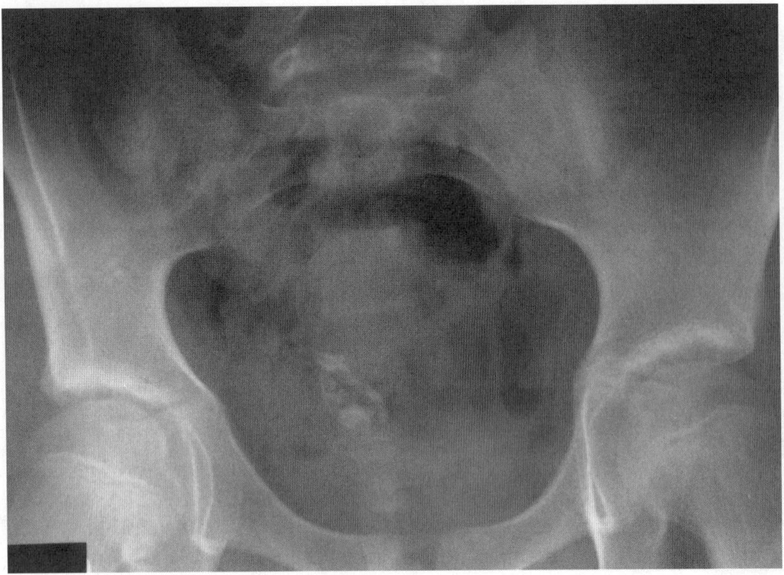

FIG. 94-5. Plain pelvic radiograph of an 11-year-old girl showing the classic calcification of a benign teratoma of the right ovary.

Teratoma

The teratoma is the most common germ cell tumor of childhood and is benign in more than 90 percent of cases. The most common sites are the sacrococcygeal area and the ovary. Classically, the tumor is composed of endoderm-, mesoderm-, and ectoderm-derived tissues foreign to the organ or anatomic site from which they originate. Teratomas may be grouped into three subtypes—mature, immature, and teratomas with malignant components. Mature teratomas show fully developed tissues such as brain, skin with hair, teeth, and the aerodigestive tract. Calcification is common (Fig. 94-5). Immature teratomas differ in that they possess neuroglial or neuroepithelial elements which are not fully differentiated. The incidence of malignancy is associated with degree of immaturity of the tumor.

The malignancies most commonly found within teratomas are germinomas or other germ cell tumors. Occasionally somatic cell malignancies may be found. Prognosis and therapy are based on the tissue type of the malignancy. A mature teratoma does not manufacture α-fetoprotein or HCG. These may be found in tumors with malignant germ cell elements, however.

SURGICAL CONSIDERATIONS

Simple ovarian cysts without any solid intracystic component are benign and may be treated by drainage without oophorectomy. Solid and complex masses are potentially malignant. Tumors are staged according to Children's Center Group/Pediatric Oncology Group (CCG/POG) guidelines (Table 94-3). Small masses may be treated with excisional biopsy and frozen section. Large tumors should be managed according to intergroup surgical guidelines (Table 94-4). Occasionally, a benign-appearing teratoma is found to have immature or malignant elements within it after completion of the operation. In such a case, reexploration for staging is required.

Surgery is curative for mature teratomas and may be curative in immature teratomas. However, among adults, survival in immature teratomas depends on histologic grade. Five-year survival decreases from approximately 80% with grade I to 30% with grade III tumors. Among immature teratomas α-fetoprot-

ein may be a poor prognostic marker. Children with this marker in particular may benefit from chemotherapy. Ongoing clinical trials seek to clarify the prognosis in children.

RADIATION THERAPY

Germinomas are quite sensitive to radiation and may be treated with therapeutic radiation with quite good results. The response of other germ cell tumors to radiation as an adjunct to chemotherapy is unclear.

CHEMOTHERAPY

The chemotherapy of germ cell tumors is a product of clinical experience over the last 25 years. Treatment has evolved from single-agent treatment with less than 50% response rates to the current standard of bleomycin, etoposide or vinblastine, and a platinum agent. With this regimen, survival is typically between 60% and 100% at 5 years. Current therapeutic trials are seeking

TABLE 94-3. *Staging of ovarian germ cell tumors*

Stage	Extent of disease
I	Limited to ovary or ovaries Negative peritoneal washings Tumor markers fall to normal May include gliomatosis peritonei
II	Microscopic residual tumor or Lymph nodes positive (<2 cm) Negative peritoneal washings
III	Gross residual tumor on biopsy Lymph node involvement (>2 cm) Contiguous visceral involvement Positive peritoneal washings
IV	Distant metastases

(Ablin A, Isaacs H. Germ cell tumors. In: Pizzo PA, Poplack DG, eds. Principles and practice of pediatric oncology, ed 2. Philadelphia, JB Lippincott, 1993:867).

TABLE 94-4. *Surgical guidelines for ovarian germ cell tumors*

GENERAL

Evaluate extent of disease
  Palpate and visualize all peritoneal surfaces particularly
    Omentum
    Liver
    Subphrenic space
  Collect ascitic fluid or peritoneal fluid for cytology
  Perform complete omentectomy
  Biopsy (sample) bilateral retroperitoneal lymph nodes
    Internal iliac
    Common iliac
    Low paraaortic
    Perirenal
  Mark biopsy sites with titanium clips

STAGE I–II
Unilateral oophorectomy

STAGE III–IV
Unilateral oophorectomy with debulking as feasible
Wedge biopsy contralateral ovary
Biopsy peritoneal seeding

BILATERAL DISEASE
Bilateral oophorectomy

(Haase GM, Wiener ES, Albright AL, et al, eds. Surgical guidelines. Arcadia, CA, Childrens Cancer Group Operations Center, 1994).

to determine whether these response rates may be preserved while reducing toxicity from the chemotherapy.

EPITHELIAL TUMORS

Epithelial tumors are staged according to the American Joint Committee on Cancer (Table 94-5). They include adenocarcinoma, endometrioid tumors, clear cell tumors, and undifferentiated carcinomas. The prognosis in younger women is more favorable than it is in older women. Rodriguez and colleagues[5] found that among women younger than 25 years of age with epithelial ovarian malignancies the majority presented with

TABLE 94-5. *Staging of ovarian epithelial tumors*

Stage	Extent of disease
IA	Limited to one ovary with intact capsule
IB	Limited to both ovaries with intact capsule
IC	Limited to one or both ovaries with either capsule rupture, tumor on ovarian surface, or positive washings
II	Tumor involves one or both ovaries with pelvic extension
III	Tumor involves one or both ovaries with metastatic tumor outside the pelvis or regional lymph nodes
IV	Distant metastases

(American Joint Committee on Cancer. Ovary. In: Beahrs OH, Henson DE, Hutter RVP, Kennedy BJ, eds. Manual for staging of cancer, ed 4. Philadelphia, JB Lippincott, 1992: 167)

early disease: stage I 58.5%, stage II 8.9%, stages III and IV 28.9%. The majority were also low-grade tumors. Survival is, in general, excellent, with 96% of stage I, 90% of stage II, 78% of stage III, and 70% of stage IV tumors surviving 5 years. As with many other malignant diseases, the trend is toward more conservative surgery, as adjuvant therapy has become more effective. The tumor marker CA-125 is found in many epithelial malignancies.

Adjuvant therapy, stage related chemotherapy given in two to four drug combinations, has achieved 40% to 75% complete response in patients with advanced disease. The chemotherapy may be given intravenously as well as intraperitoneally. Most chemotherapeutic regimens contain platinum. Taxol has proved useful for those patients who are resistant to platinum-based chemotherapy.

STROMAL TUMORS

Stromal tumors include the androblastoma, otherwise known as the Sertoli-Leydig cell tumor, and the granulosa–theca cell tumors. These tumors are commonly hormonally active. Granulosa cell tumors are the most common cause of isosexual precocity in childhood. After menarche, they typically present as menstrual irregularity. They may present with signs of peritonitis, ascites, or an abdominal or pelvic mass. Tumors are rarely bilateral. Surgical therapy consists of unilateral salpingo-oophorectomy with appropriate staging (see Table 94-5). For disease that is truly confined to the resected ovary (stage IA), resection should be curative. Response to chemotherapy and radiotherapy has been disappointing in more advanced tumors. Juvenile granulosa cell tumors differ in several ways from adult granulosa tumors. They are primarily prepubertal at presentation. On pathology there are no Call-Exner bodies, nuclei are dark and nongrooved, and luteinization is present. The recurrence pattern is much earlier in the juvenile than the adult variety.

Androblastomas are less common. They most typically exhibit androgenic activity and thus present with hirsutism, severe acne, or deepening voice. Occasionally these tumors exhibit no endocrine activity, or in rare situations they may produce estrogen or progesterone. They are sometimes microscopic at presentation but are most typically 5 to 15 cm in diameter. They are usually cystic with irregular intraluminal papilla on ultrasound. Resection is usually curative for early disease.

PRESENTATION

Ovarian tumors may present in various ways. Age at presentation may give some clue as to the type of tumor. Teratoma may occur at any age, whereas malignant germ cell tumors are rare before the age of 10 and have a median age at presentation of 13 years. This corresponds with the onset of puberty. The stromal tumors are more typically prepubertal at presentation, and epithelial tumors increase in frequency with patient age.

The symptoms associated with tumors include pain, which is usually chronic and not severe. Occasionally ovarian enlargement leads to torsion with acute severe lower abdominal pain. This pain may be accompanied by nausea, vomiting, fever, constipation, and dysuria. Premature menarche or pseudopregnancy may be seen in β-HCG-producing germ cell tumors, though this is more commonly a sign of a granulosa cell tumor. Hirsutism, acne, occasionally clitoromegaly, and secondary amenorrhea most typically accompany an androblastoma.

Evaluation should include thorough history and physical examination, including bimanual examination of the pelvis. In a virginal female, this may be accomplished with one finger in the rectum and one on the abdomen. A nontender pelvic mass is often detectable in this fashion. An abdominal flat radiograph of the abdomen should be taken in the nonpregnant female. The characteristic calcifications associated with ovarian teratomas are often discovered. Abdominal ultrasound is useful for non-calcified masses or clinical dilemmas.

FALLOPIAN TUBE, UTERUS, AND VAGINA

Fusion Defects

The paired müllerian ducts normally fuse in the midline to form a single upper vagina, cervix, and uterus. If this process is arrested, a spectrum of anomalies can result (Fig. 94-6). In the uterus, complete failure of fusion results in uterus didelphys, in which two separate hemiuteri form and lie side by side. Bicornuate uterus involves a single cervix with two uterine horns. A uterine septum may persist in situations where two ducts have fused but the common wall has failed to involute, with the mildest form termed arcuate uterus. A longitudinal vaginal septum often accompanies uterine fusion defects. Typically these defects manifest with infertility and are not discovered in the pediatric age group. However, a significant number of the defects are asymmetric and can be associated with obstruction of one or both systems. Such an obstruction may become evident in the neonatal period or at the time of puberty.

In situations where midline fusion is complete, atresias may result along the longitudinal axis. This may occur as a result of failure of recanalization of the vaginal plate or a primary failure of the müllerian anlage to reach the urogenital sinus. Manifestations include imperforate hymen, transverse vaginal septum, and cervical atresia.

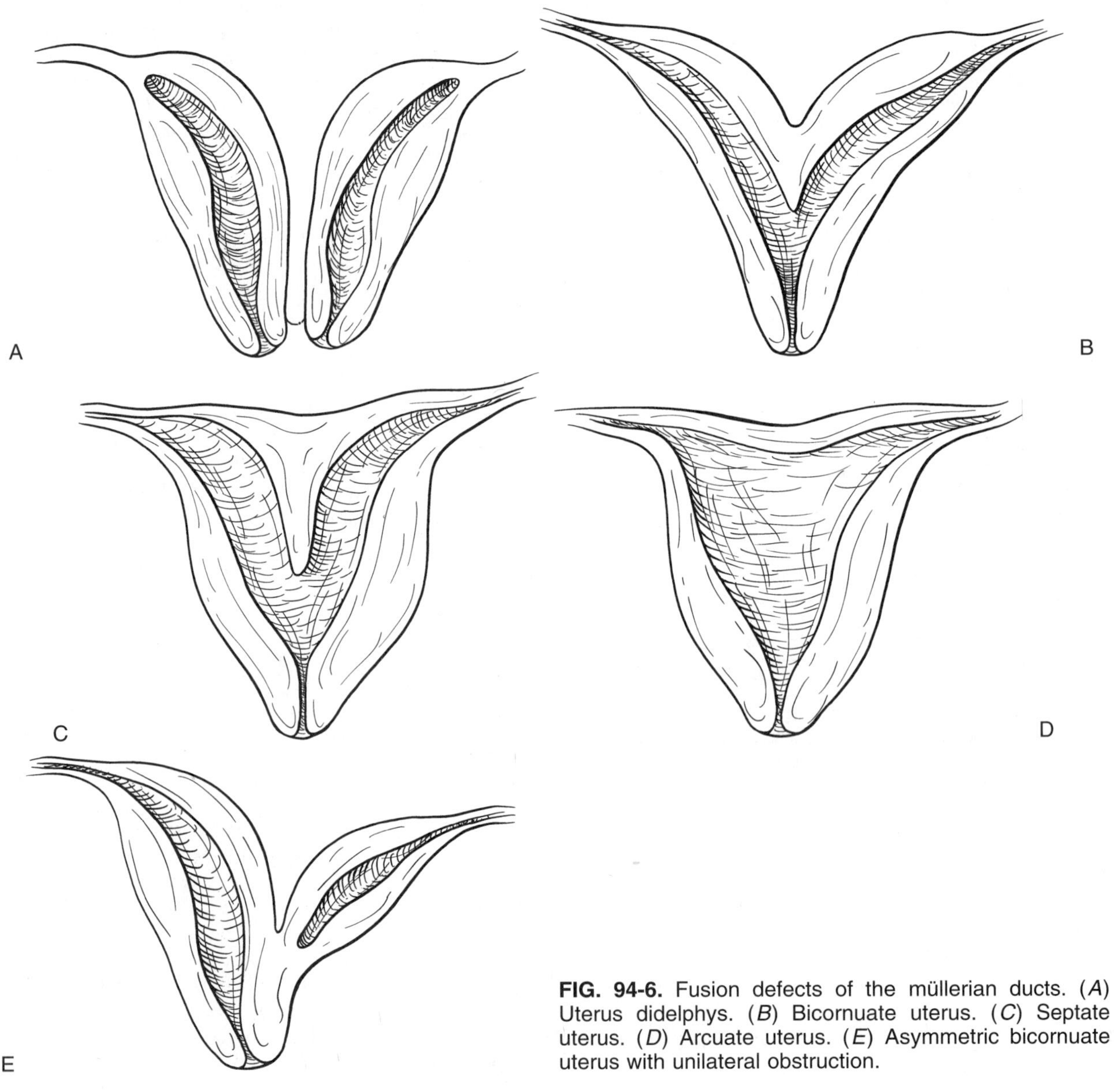

FIG. 94-6. Fusion defects of the müllerian ducts. (*A*) Uterus didelphys. (*B*) Bicornuate uterus. (*C*) Septate uterus. (*D*) Arcuate uterus. (*E*) Asymmetric bicornuate uterus with unilateral obstruction.

Any of the obstructive syndromes may present in the neonatal period when circulating maternal estrogens are still high and withdrawal bleeding leads to distention of the obstructed structure. This distention is occasionally severe, with a large midline mass causing urinary obstruction. This is a surgical emergency and requires urgent drainage to prevent permanent renal damage. More typically the obstructions manifest at the time of puberty with cyclic pain and a pelvic mass. In the case of an imperforate hymen or distal vaginal atresia, a bulging membrane may be seen within the introitus. The membrane appears bluish black from shed menstrual blood. Cruciate incision is definitive therapy for imperforate hymen. For a more proximal atresia, complete excision of the vaginal septum with a sutured anastomosis between the proximal and distal vagina is necessary to prevent an annular cicatrix and consequent dyspareunia.

More proximal atresias of the vagina and particularly of the cervix are more difficult to deal with surgically. An abdominal perineal approach may be necessary. Hysterectomy is the most common treatment for a cervical atresia. If an adequate uterine cavity can be demonstrated with ultrasound or MRI, an operation to create a cervix and preserve the uterus can be performed. Some patients undergoing this procedure have given birth successfully.

In situations where a uterine septum obstructs one half of the uterus, excision of the septum relieves symptoms. When uterine development is asymmetric, only one side of the bifid uterus may be obstructed. Resection of the obstructed uterine horn relieves the patient's symptoms without diminishing reproductive capacity.

Rokitansky-Kuster-Hauser Syndrome

In patients with a congenital absence of the vagina, a constellation of other defects is also present. Typically, the uterus is hypoplastic or atretic and in some patients is associated with shortness of stature, bony anomalies involving the spine, and sometimes deafness. Differentiation on physical examination between this condition and imperforate hymen may be difficult. Only at the time of puberty may the difference become evident with bulging of the hymen due to menstrual blood. Testicular feminization may show similar prepubertal findings. Ultrasound or MRI can establish the correct diagnosis. In the Rokitansky syndrome, the uterus is nonfunctional, but the ovaries are normal. Puberty progresses normally, but menses never commence. The atretic uterus does not possess a hormonally responsive endometrium and so does not become distended and painful.

Treatment involves the creation of a vagina to permit normal sexual intercourse. The use of a series of dilators to both lengthen and widen the posterior depression in the vestibule has been proposed. After many weeks, this depression may be of such a size as to permit satisfactory intercourse. Timing is important. By late adolescence, the patient is often motivated enough to perform 20-min dilations three times each day. Adolescent tissues are elastic and dilate well.

Other patients require surgical creation of a vagina. In the procedure described by McIndoe, a vagina is created from a tubularized skin graft. A transverse incision is made in the posterior vestibule, and a space is developed between the rectum and bladder. Meticulous hemostasis is achieved. Then an intermediate thickness skin graft approximately $^{18}\!/_{1000}$ of an inch in thickness is harvested and sutured to form a tube around a soft Silastic and foam form. The form with the overlying skin graft is then placed into the perineal space and secured with heavy sutures. After approximately 10 days, the form may be removed and the lower end of the tube graft trimmed and sutured to the vestibular skin. A second inflatable mold needs to be reinserted at this time. Once the skin graft is fully adherent, dilation is still needed for several months to prevent a contracture. Graft take is typically quite good. Sexual intercourse may begin after a few months, provided an adequate lubricant is used.

Alternative procedures involve vaginal creation from colon or cecum grafts. They have the advantage of lesser scar contracture and do not require lubricants for intercourse. They have the disadvantage of continuous mucous production, which leads to soiling or odor.

Endometriosis

One possible cause of cyclic abdominal pain and dysmenorrhea in the adolescent female is endometriosis. Ectopic uterine endometrium enlarges and sheds in response to systemic LH and FSH. The endometrial tissue is found within the peritoneal cavity most typically, but may be found elsewhere. Whether this is a developmental problem originating with metaplasia of the coelomic epithelium or is due to expulsion of endometrium from the uterine tubes with subsequent implantation is unresolved. There is evidence to support both beliefs. Endometriosis can be a sign of an obstructed uterine horn. On occasion endometriosis may be diagnosed with ultrasound, but more often laparoscopy or laparotomy is required to secure the diagnosis. Darkly pigmented lesions in the peritoneal surface are classic, though red, purple, blue, or white coloration is sometimes noted. Hormonal treatment with androgens, progesterone, danazol, or Gn-RH agonists is often effective. Surgical treatment with excision or cautery may be necessary when hormonal treatments have failed.

Tumors

Tumors of the uterus and tube are quite rare in childhood and early adolescence. Cervical intraepithelial neoplasia and consequent cervical cancer have been linked to human papillomavirus infections. Thus they are found primarily in sexually active adolescents and adults.

Clear cell carcinomas are exceedingly rare tumors of the vagina and cervix. The majority of these tumors developed as a consequence of in utero exposure to diethylstilbestrol (DES) and certain other synthetic estrogens. Only one third of the patients have no such history. Approximately 1 of 1000 women exposed to DES develop this disease. Sixty percent of the lesions are vaginal, and 40% are cervical. Treatment consists of local excision with adjuvant chemotherapy. Radiation is reserved for more aggressive advanced disease. Five- and ten-year survival for early lesions (stage I or stage II disease) approaches 80% to 90%. Ninety percent of patients present at such an early curable stage. Long-term follow-up is necessary to detect recurrence early.

Rhabdomyosarcoma of the female genital tract is the most

common malignant tumor in this region. It differs from rhabdomyosarcomas of other sites by having generally favorable histology of the botryoidal type with infrequent nodal or metastatic disease. The treatment of these tumors has evolved over the last several years toward less aggressive surgical therapy. Chemotherapy with vincristine, actinomycin D (Dactinomycin), and cyclophosphamide (VAC) may lead to such impressive response that radical surgery is no longer required. Second-look surgery to obtain a complete response is now the standard treatment. When the tumor originates in the uterus, hysterectomy is necessary, but preservation of the distal vagina and ovaries is possible.

VULVA

The vulva, or external genitalia, derive from the urogenital sinus and urogenital ridge. They include the labia majora, labia minora, clitoris, vestibule, and hymen. The abnormalities that we may see with the vulva include ambiguous genitalia, labial fusion or agglutination, trauma, infections, and various dermatologic disorders.

Intersex Anomalies

Gender assignment is one of the first tasks performed at birth. The appearance of the external genitalia determines the gender assignment. There are four situations that present at birth where anatomic gender is not obvious. These include female pseudohermaphroditism, true hermaphrodism, male pseudohermaphrodism, and mixed gonadal dysgenesis. Maternal ultrasound may occasionally detect an anomaly before birth. In such cases, definitive gender assignment should wait until confirmatory studies are performed at birth. Diagnosis and treatment of intersex anomalies is dealt with in Chapter 95.

Labial Fusion

True labial fusion is an uncommon intersex problem that is present from birth. A more common situation is that of labial agglutination, which is not present at birth but which can develop a month to a few years after birth. The development depends on atrophy of the labial epithelium as maternal estrogen stimulation is withdrawn. Clinically significant adhesions are present in a small minority of girls, though a small degree of posterior adhesion was found in 39% of normal prepubertal females.[6] Most instances of labial adhesion are self-limited and therefore require no treatment. Other cases are so severe as to result in urinary discomfort and occasionally urinary tract infection. In these cases, a more aggressive therapeutic approach is indicated.

Topical therapy with either estrogen (Premarin) or estradiol (Estrace) cream for no more than 3 weeks is often adequate to release the fusion. The estrogens stimulate the mucosa to proliferate, and the gentle force of application lyses some of the adhesion with each application. In situations where hormonal therapy alone is not effective, surgical lysis may be necessary. Even after surgical lysis, recurrence is common. The incidence of recurrence may be reduced with perioperative application of hormone cream. In the absence of obstructive urinary problems and infection, multiple attempts at surgical lysis are not indicated.

Trauma

Vulvar trauma may be accidental, sports-related, or the result of voluntary intercourse or sexual assault. Accidental injuries are likely to be confined to the vulva, since the deeper structures are protected. The most common injury is a blunt injury to the labia from a fall. Ecchymoses, abrasions, and hematomas are typical. Occasionally a midline tear may be sustained in an extreme straddle injury. Most of these injuries are self-limited. Even a sizable vulvar hematoma will resolve on its own given time. After the injury, an ice pack may be useful to prevent tissue swelling, which causes the major morbidity in the situation. In situations where the hematoma continues to grow despite conservative therapy, incision of the hematoma with ligation of the bleeding points might be necessary.

Occasionally a vulvar hematoma may be only the outward manifestation of a more serious deep injury such as a pelvic fracture. The clinician should look for any signs of such an injury as part of the evaluation.

Vulvar lacerations are often superficial and do not bleed substantially. When a laceration is deep, surgical repair may be necessary. Although blood loss from vulvar injury may be small, there may be enough bleeding into periurethral tissues to cause urethral spasm and urinary retention. Sitz baths may successfully relax the area to permit voiding. Urethral catheterization is necessary if the child is unable to void.

In situations where sexual abuse has caused injury, the damage is often deep, involving the hymeneal ring and vagina. In the absence of deep injuries, diagnosis of abuse is less certain and relies as much on history as on physical findings.

Inflammations and Infections

The vulva is often the site for local skin infections, which may range from diaper rash in the infant to streptococcal cellulitis and staphylococcal abscesses. Vulvar infections with herpes simplex virus, human papillomavirus, and molluscum contagiosum may be related to sexual abuse.

Neoplasms

Neoplasms of the vulva are rare. Neurofibromatosis occasionally presents in the vulva. More common in this area are hemangiomas or lymphangiomas. Hemangiomas typically resolve without therapy; lymphangiomas require resection. Lipomas may also be present in this area. Premalignant lesions such as vulvar intraepithelial neoplasia may be found. These typically accompany cases of sexual abuse and human papillomavirus infection. Cases have been reported even in toddlers. Squamous cell carcinoma is exceedingly rare in children. Melanomas have occasionally been reported in the vulvar region.

VAGINAL BLEEDING

Vaginal bleeding requires investigation whenever it occurs in the prepubertal child. It may be caused by inflammatory conditions, trauma, or tumors. Determining the cause of bleeding is often a challenge.

Vulvovaginitis

The bleeding associated with vulvovaginitis is a secondary effect of scratching the perineum. The vulva and vagina are easily soiled in childhood, the mucosa is thin and does not offer much protection, and the acidic pH of the mature vagina is absent. Infections, therefore, are common in prepubertal girls. Evaluation will show a foul-smelling discharge with a considerable amount of redness originating near the vagina, sometimes extending into the perineum. Proper hygiene is preventive. Broad spectrum antibiotics are curative. Topical estrogen for no more than a week may speed mucosal healing in extreme cases.

Foreign Bodies

Foreign bodies are often found as the root cause of vaginal infection. Wads of toilet paper, paper clips, pen caps, and other items have been found. Vaginoscopy is necessary to remove foreign bodies. Recurrence may be seen. Foreign bodies may also be associated with child abuse.[7]

Urethral Prolapse

Occasionally on genital examination a mass is associated with bleeding. The most common bleeding mass in the area is a prolapsed urethra. The mass is typically small, edematous, and circular. The urethral orifice is seen to exit through the center of the mass. The mass is always anterior to the vagina. Minimal cases may resolve with topical estrogen therapy. However, many cases require resection of the prolapsed tissue. Foley catheter drainage is necessary for 24 h.

Genital Tumors

Occasionally, bleeding hemangiomas are seen in the perineum. Bleeding from capillary hemangiomas is controllable with pressure. Cavernous hemangiomas sometimes require therapy when they are large and have failed to involute spontaneously. Cryotherapy, excision, or injection are effective. α-interferon has also been used with some success. Vaginal rhabdomyosarcomas present with bleeding and a visible tumor mass protruding into the vagina and occasionally into the vestibule. Treatment consists of chemotherapy followed by surgery, as previously outlined.

Endometrial Bleeding

Occasionally a child presents with vaginal bleeding that cannot be attributed to previously mentioned causes and may be the initial manifestation of precocious puberty. Hormonally in-

duced bleeding is normal in the early neonatal period and after the age of 10 years. All other instances require evaluation. Evaluation includes estrogen levels, Gn-RH stimulation test, pelvic ultrasound or CT scan, and a CT scan of the head. In the adolescent, increasingly irregular bleeding should be investigated. It may signify ectopic pregnancy, trophoblastic disease, or impending loss of pregnancy. Tumors, trauma, or infection are also possible. In rare cases, excessive bleeding may be related to coagulation disorders or liver or renal failure. Among adolescents anovulatory uterine bleeding is frequent in the first several years after menarche. It may take 5 years or more for the menstrual cycle to become regular. The patient's own history is the best clue as to whether an extensive work-up is necessary.

SEXUALLY TRANSMITTED DISEASE

Sexually transmitted diseases are fortunately rare in childhood. When present, they often signify sexual abuse. Sexually transmitted diseases are also increasingly prevalent in adolescence. Goals are to make the diagnosis, determine the mode of acquisition, and treat the illness. The presentation may involve several syndromes, urethritis, vaginitis, cervicitis, genital lesions, pelvic inflammatory disease, and systemic illness.

Epidemiology

In the United States the traditional bacterial sexually transmitted diseases (syphilis and gonorrhea) have become less prevalent in the last decade. This decrease parallels decreases in the rest of the Western world. *Chlamydia* and the viral diseases, however, are increasing. Their prevalence now exceeds that of syphilis and gonorrhea. There is a substantial incidence of perinatal transmission of these diseases.

The human immunodeficiency virus (HIV), or AIDS virus, has grown in just 15 years from a disease which affected primarily gay men and drug addicts to involve a large number of people from all walks of life.[8] HIV seroprevalence among patients in sexually transmitted disease clinics rose from 0.23% to more than 5% from 1979 to 1989. Male predominance has vanished. There has been a greater than 10-fold increase in the disease among teenagers. The rate is now greater in blacks than in whites. These increases are particularly alarming, given the absence of a cure for the disease. Life-prolonging treatments with multiple drugs are available, but they have not altered the ultimate outcome.

All sexually transmitted diseases have the same risk factors: early age at initiation of sex, multiple sexual partners, and inconsistent or lack of use of condoms. Use of oral contraceptives may alter the microenvironment of the cervix and vagina and increase the risk of cervicitis and pelvic inflammatory disease. Ignorance of the way these diseases are spread is a common finding in patients in sexually transmitted disease (STD) clinics. Education can help control their spread, so efforts should be directed at teaching teenagers before they establish high-risk sexual behavior.

Urethritis

Urethritis is a common finding in children and sexually active adolescents. Most cases are due to superficial infection with a common bacterial organism. Occasionally gonorrhea or *Chla-*

mydia are the infectious agents. In cases where gonorrhea is found on culture, single-dose therapy with ceftriaxone is sufficient. To assure treatment of *Chlamydia*, a common co-pathogen, 7 days of tetracycline or erythromycin should be given.

Vaginitis

Isolated vaginitis may be caused by hypersensitivity to laundry soap or bubble bath, or by a local infection of the vagina with bacterial organisms. Abnormal vaginal discharge is the most frequent presentation. Preadolescents are at increased risk for vaginitis because the vaginal epithelium is thin and vaginal pH is neutral. In this age group, the infection is polymicrobial and resolves with improved perineal hygiene, antibiotics, or short-course topical estrogen therapy. Among adolescents, the causative organisms include *Candida, Gardnerella,* and *Trichomonas.* The appearance of candidal vaginitis is a reddened mucosa with curdlike plaques. *Gardnerella* discharge is thin and gray with a "fishy" odor. Vaginal pH is elevated, and mixing the fluid with 10% KOH enhances the fishy odor. Trichomonas is suspected when drainage is frothy and malodorous. The "strawberry cervix" is characteristic of this infection. *Candida* responds to topical antifungal therapy. Both *Gardnerella* and *Trichomonas* may be cured with a 7-day course of metronidazole.

Genital Lesions

Lesions of the vulva and perineum often lead to surgical consultation. Raised and polypoid perineal warts are signs of human papillomavirus infection. A chancre, or condyloma latum, signifies syphilis. Small vesicles that may become confluent connote genital herpes. These are painful or pruritic. The presence of each of these infections in a child is often secondary to abuse. In adolescents, consensual sex is becoming a more frequent source.

Pelvic Inflammatory Disease

The classic triad of low abdominal pain, cervical motion tenderness, and adnexal tenderness are the sine qua non of pelvic inflammatory disease (PID). These signs and symptoms are often accompanied by fever, leukocytosis, and elevated erythrocyte sedimentation rate. There may or may not be a vaginal discharge noted. Culdocentesis may show white blood cells and microorganisms. The infections are typically polymicrobial and may not have the same organisms as are present in vaginal or cervical cultures. Cultures should be obtained but should not limit antibiotic therapy.

Patients most at risk for PID have multiple sexual partners, are younger than 25 years, have a history of previous gonorrheal or candidal cervicitis or PID, cannot afford care, and have delayed coming for medical attention. Many adolescents fall into these categories. The Centers for Disease Control has established hospitalization criteria for PID. The criteria include adolescent age group, uncertainty in diagnosis (rule out appendicitis), suspected pregnancy, concurrent HIV infection, severe illness with nausea and vomiting, inability to tolerate therapy

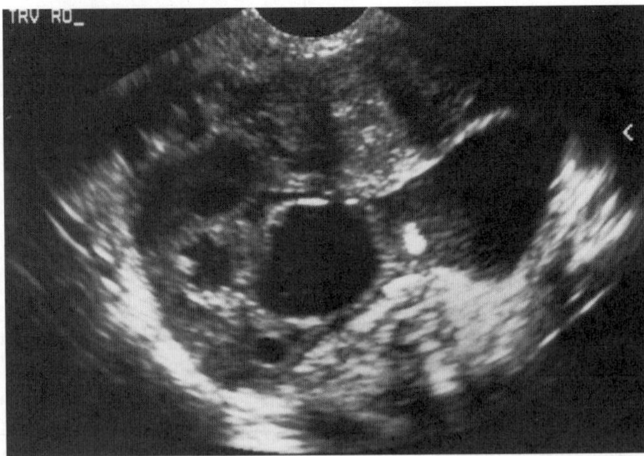

FIG. 94-7. Transvaginal ultrasound scan showing a complex cystic mass surrounding the left ovary in a 14-year-old girl with a tuboovarian abscess.

or failure to respond as an outpatient, and inability to follow up in 72 h.

Treatment of the infection includes intravenous ceftriaxone and oral or parenteral tetracycline. In PID complicated by abscess (Fig. 94-7), percutaneous or surgical drainage leads to quicker resolution of symptoms and shorter overall hospitalization.

Systemic Infection

Syphilis and HIV become systemic infections shortly following acquisition. Syphilis manifests with a local, painless ulcer, a chancre, at the site of infection, but soon the total body rash of secondary syphilis appears. If treatment is delayed, the central nervous system may be affected. Therapy is directed at prevention of this latter stage.

HIV is an RNA virus that, by means of reverse transcriptase, is able to make DNA copies of itself and then propagate using host DNA and RNA replicative reactions. The virus attacks T lymphocytes and vastly compromises the host's ability to fight infection. Coexisting HIV infection necessitates prolonging the course of treatment for other sexually transmitted disease. No effective vaccine has been developed. Contact with blood or bodily secretions may transmit the infection. Various studies estimate the rate of transmission from 1 in 100 to 1 in 1000 exposures. Current control measures include celibacy, barrier contraception with condoms, and experimental virucidal agents. Treatment of the disease involves drug therapy directed against the virus as well as prevention and treatment of opportunistic infections. Most antiviral agents interfere with reverse transcriptase to slow viral propagation. Current multidrug regimens including recently developed protease inhibitors offer the prospect of effective therapy, although they have not yet altered the ultimate outcome. There is evidence that treatment of pregnant HIV carriers and their newborn children reduces the likelihood of infection in those children.

SEXUAL ABUSE

There is a growing recognition of sexual abuse of children. The abused child may be either a male or female, though females outnumber males by two to four times. The National Center on Child Abuse and Neglect estimates that the number of abused children may be more than 200,000 in the United States. The laws regarding sexual abuse and child protection vary considerably from state to state and from year to year. It is the responsibility of physicians who are examining and treating abuse victims to know and understand the laws within their state to best protect the welfare of the abused child.

History

When a sexual assault is suspected, a careful history of what has happened should be obtained. Ideally, the victim should be interviewed in a safe, comfortable environment in terms that he or she might understand. There should be no time pressures on the interview. Care should be taken to avoid putting words in the child's mouth. Open ended, nondirective questioning is preferable. Particularly in young children, the verbal skills necessary to adequately describe the act may be missing. Anatomically correct dolls may be used to help the child be more specific. Because abuse is often not a single isolated assault, the interviewer should ask questions to establish a relationship between the attacker and victim.

Physical Examination

The physical examination begins with observation of the child during the interview. The examination includes a complete skin examination, looking for bite or suction marks, examination of the oral cavity for signs of trauma, and examination of the perineum and pelvis. In many instances, adequate examination may be obtained in a doctor's office or emergency room. In the less frequent cases where penetration of the anus or vagina is suspected or discovered, an examination under general anesthe-

sia is necessary to establish and treat deeper injuries. After an assault, one may see findings ranging from contusions, ecchymoses, and hematomas to superficial and deep lacerations. If the time between abuse and examination is prolonged, the findings are likely to be more subtle. These may involve healing or healed tears of the posterior fourchette, hymen, vagina, and anus. More often than not, a late physical examination shows no signs of physical abuse.

Because there are no well-defined criteria to classify the physical findings, detailed description with drawings is advised. Nonspecific abnormalities suggestive of abuse include redness of the genitalia, increased vascularity in the vestibule and labial mucosa, vaginal discharge, and small mucosal tears. McCann and coworkers,[6] in examining 93 unabused girls, found erythema in 56%, labial adhesions in 40%, and superficial posterior fourchette injuries in 25%. Hymeneal diameter in these patients covered a wide range, with a general trend toward wider opening at later ages (see Table 94-6).

Foreign bodies in the vagina of prepubertal girls may be a marker of sexual abuse. In 12 girls seen by Hermen-Giddens[7] with vaginal foreign bodies, eight were confirmed victims of abuse, and in three more abuse was suspected.

Specific findings strongly suggestive of abuse include deep lacerations of the hymen and vagina, proctoepisiotomy, teeth marks in the perineum, and laboratory confirmation of sexually transmitted disease. The presence of sperm or pregnancy is definitive.

The examination should be considered incomplete if any forensic evidence is overlooked. This includes a collection of specimens that may be used later as evidence (Table 94-7). All specimens should be handled as specified by law and the rules of evidence. This usually requires proper labeling with patient identification, specimen, site from which the specimen was collected, the date and time collected, and the initials of the examiner. Specimens should be placed into containers and sealed appropriately. If local laws require, they should be processed by a police laboratory.

TABLE 94-6. *Colposcopic transhymenal diameter by age and examination method*

Age group	Method	Plane	N	Mean + SD (mm)	Range (mm)
Preschool (2–4$^{11}\!/_{12}$ y)	Separation	Vert	21	5.5 + 2.2	2.5–10.0
		Horiz	21	3.9 + 1.4	1.0–5.5
	Traction	Vert	24	5.5 + 1.7	3.0–8.5
		Horiz	24	5.2 + 1.4	2.0–8.0
	Knee-chest	Vert	29	6.3 + 1.7	3.0–10.0
		Horiz	29	4.6 + 1.3	2.5–7.5
Early school age (5–7$^{11}\!/_{12}$ y)	Separation	Vert	39	5.6 + 2.3	1.0–11.0
		Horiz	39	4.2 + 1.7	1.0–8.0
	Traction	Vert	43	6.1 + 2.1	1.0–10.0
		Horiz	43	5.6 + 1.8	1.0–9.0
	Knee-chest	Vert	41	7.0 + 2.0	3.0–11.5
		Horiz	41	5.6 + 1.5	2.5–8.5
Preadolescent (8 y to Tanner II)	Separation	Vert	19	8.4 + 2.2	5.0–13.5
		Horiz	19	5.7 + 1.6	3.0–8.5
	Traction	Vert	20	8.3 + 2.8	2.0–15.0
		Horiz	20	6.9 + 2.0	2.5–10.5
	Knee-chest	Vert	21	8.7 + 2.6	5.0–15.0
		Horiz	21	7.3 + 1.7	4.0–11.0

(McCann J, Wells R, Voris J. Genital findings in prepubertal girls selected for nonabuse: a descriptive study. Pediatrics 1990;428). Horiz, horizontal; Vert, vertical.

TABLE 94-7. *The forensic evaluation: specimens to be collected*

GENERAL

Outer and underclothing worn during or immediately after the assault
Fingernail scrapings
Dried or moist secretions and foreign material on the body, anus, and genital area (Wood lamp to detect semen)

ORAL CAVITY

Swabs for semen (two) within 6 h of assault
Culture for gonorrhea and other sexually transmitted diseases

GENITAL AREA

Comb pubic hair; collect all loose hair and foreign material
Vaginal swabs (three)
Wet mount slides
Dry mount slides (two)
Culture for gonorrhea and other sexually transmitted diseases

ANUS

Rectal swabs (two)
Dry mount slides (two)
Culture for gonorrhea and other sexually transmitted diseases

BLOOD OR URINE

Blood type
Syphilis serology
HIV serology
Pregnancy test (blood or urine)
Alcohol/toxicology evaluation (blood or urine)
Urinalysis

OTHER

Saliva: use clean gauze or filter paper
Head hair: cut and remove sample
Pubic hair: cut and remove sample

(Muram D. Child sexual abuse. In: Sanfilippo JS, Muram D, Lee PA, et al, eds. Pediatric and adolescent gynecology. Philadelphia, WB Saunders, 1994:376)

Now that HIV is a pathogen found in the community at large, testing of sexual assault victims should include HIV cultures or serology. These should be obtained at the time of the assault as well as 6 months later. In the rare instances where HIV infection occurs, additional therapy should be directed toward this life-threatening illness.

Treatment

The treatment of sexual assault injuries should follow the general principles of wound care. Superficial injuries may be managed with sitz baths; deep injuries require operative repair with absorbable suture. All bite wounds and wounds older than 6 to 12 h should be treated as dirty, in open fashion with irrigation and debridement.

Antibiotics are used as appropriate to treat the wound, but prophylaxis for sexually transmitted disease is not recommended. Should a sexually transmitted disease be found, the treatment consists of coverage for the identified organism as well as the common co-pathogens *Chlamydia* and gonorrhea.

Treatment also involves prevention of further abuse by re-moving the child from the site of abuse. Psychological sequelae of abuse often require psychotherapy. In most areas, therapists are available who have been trained to help the child and the family deal with the trauma of the event as well as with the demands of the examination, medical treatment, and investigative interviews by child protective services and law enforcement agencies.

IMAGING

Some of the major advances in the care of female genital disorders have been possible because of advances in noninvasive imaging. Color flow Doppler and transvaginal ultrasound have made it possible to determine the function and fine structure of uterine and adnexal masses. Spiral computer tomography has enabled examination of the abdomen and pelvis without the need for deep general anesthesia. Magnetic resonance imaging has enabled surgeons to know in advance the structure of a congenital duplication or atresia without laparotomy. The age of the patient and the expected pathology determine which of these modalities is used.

In the neonate, radiologic imaging is needed for three reasons: confirmation of a prenatal finding, investigation of a palpable abdominal mass, and evaluation of a child with ambiguous genitalia. In most situations a simple ultrasound examination will provide the clinician with all the needed information.[9] A prenatally diagnosed cyst must be characterized after birth as simple or complex, and measured. If the cyst is small and without internal echoes, it should be followed with regular examinations to assure its resolution as estrogen levels fall. CT or MRI should not be needed in this instance. A palpable abdominal mass should be studied with ultrasound and treated similarly. Whenever a cyst is excessively large or complex, operative intervention is indicated. A suspected vaginal atresia or uterine anomaly should be studied with ultrasound or MRI to define the anomaly and provide a road map for surgical repair.

Evaluation of the child with ambiguous genitalia is a pediatric emergency. Imaging should discern the presence of ovaries or testes and determine whether the uterus is normal, atretic, or absent. Simple ultrasound can answer all these questions.

The older child requires evaluation for precocious puberty, tumor or mass, abdominal pain, and vaginal discharge. The imaging in precocious puberty involves measuring the size of each ovary and the uterus looking for both a source and the effect of elevated hormonal levels. This may be performed with ultrasound, but CT or MRI scans are more efficient, since they allow better visualization of the adrenal glands as well. A mobile abdominal mass is most likely a teratoma at this age. Plain radiographs or ultrasound are sufficient to establish this diagnosis. Other tumors, such as a pelvic rhabdomyosarcoma, are best visualized with MRI. Local extent, invasion of surrounding structures, and metastases can be seen quite readily. Tissue planes are more easily seen than with CT. Sagittal views show the extent of invasion more clearly.

The evaluation of abdominal pain involves differentiation between ovarian cysts, adnexal torsion, and appendicitis. Adnexal torsion may be suspected because of the acute onset of pain in the lower abdomen. Ultrasound shows an enlarged, lucent, or complex ovary. CT and MRI add little to this information and are rarely indicated. Color flow Doppler may show diminished or absent flow to the involved ovary, with minimal signal within the mass. The symptomatic child with a positive scan should be explored promptly.

Vaginal discharge, if chronic and watery, may signify a wolffian duct anomaly with ectopic ureteral entry into the vagina, often at Gartner's duct. Intravenous urography may be the most efficient evaluation of this phenomenon. Ultrasound often shows renal dysplasia and may show ureteral or vaginal dilatation.

In the adolescent, primary or secondary amenorrhea, pregnancy, sexually transmitted disease, and malignant ovarian tumors are the common problems. Primary amenorrhea may be due to gonadal dysgenesis, testicular feminization syndrome, or Rokitansky-Kuster-Hauser syndrome. In the first instance, small gonads with müllerian structures present or absent are seen; in the second, no ovarian tissue or müllerian structure is present; and in the third, ovaries are normal, but the müllerian structures are atretic. Ultrasound may establish the etiology, but MRI is advisable when Rokitansky syndrome or other atresia is suspected.

Ultrasound of the pelvis is the initial test needed to evaluate the potentially pregnant patient. An intrauterine pregnancy may be seen and dated. For suspected ectopic pregnancy, transvaginal ultrasound with color Doppler is a better modality. Resolution and sensitivity are increased. Unfortunately, most pediatric facilities do not possess transvaginal capabilities because few patients can accommodate the probe.

Pelvic inflammatory disease is a clinical diagnosis, the treatment of which is antimicrobial. Ultrasound shows blurring of the tissue planes, adnexal enlargement, and pelvic fluid (see Fig. 94-7). Follow-up scans performed for failure to improve often show abscesses that require drainage. Percutaneous drainage may be guided by ultrasound or CT.

Ovarian masses in the adolescent should be evaluated first by ultrasound. Simple cysts may be followed with ultrasound. MRI or CT are helpful if malignancy is suspected. They can show the local extent of disease and screen for metastases. MRI is able to distinguish between scar tissue and tumor after resection of a primary tumor.

LAPAROSCOPY

Surgical laparoscopy began in earnest with the report of 250 cases by Raoul Palmer, a French gynecologist, in 1947. Infertility, pelvic pain, endometriosis, and neoplasia may be evaluated and treated in many cases without ''open'' surgery. Tubal pregnancy may be treated with coagulation, segmental excision, linear salpingotomy, tubal aspiration, or salpingectomy. Ovaries may be biopsied; cysts may be aspirated; and torsed ovaries may be untorsed and pexed or excised. The procedure has aided in the differentiation of appendicitis and pelvic inflammatory disease.

Laparoscopy in the prepubertal female typically requires two ports. One port is used for viewing and insufflation, the other for manipulation of the pelvic viscera. For complex procedures, an additional port may be necessary for insertion of instruments. In older adolescents, manipulation may be performed by means of a uterine cannula or mobilizer inserted transvaginally. The use of such a cannula is contraindicated when uterine anomalies prevent safe access via the cervix and when intrauterine pregnancy is suspected.[10]

Progress in the last decade suggests that increasing numbers of procedures will be performed laparoscopically. Telescopes and instruments are shrinking, and techniques are evolving rapidly. Soon, even the smallest patients may be candidates for laparoscopic evaluation and treatment.

REFERENCES

1. Skandalakis JE, Gray SW, Parrott TS, et al. Ovary and testis. In: Skandalakis JE, Gray SW, eds. mbryology for surgeons. ed 2. Baltimore, Williams & Wilkins, 1994:736.
2. Gray SW, Skandalakis JE, Broecker BH. Female reproductive system. In: Skandalakis JE, Gray SW, eds. Embryology for surgeons. ed 2. Baltimore: Williams & Wilkins, 1994:816.
3. Dolle P, Izpisua-Belmonte J-C, Brown JM, et al. *Hox-4* genes and the morphogenesis of mammalian genitalia. Genes and Dev 1991;5:1767.
4. Ablin A, Isaacs H. Germ cell tumors. In: Pizzo PA, Poplack DG, eds. Principles and practice of pediatric oncology. ed 2. Philadelphia, JB Lippincott, 1993:867.
5. Rodriguez M, Nguyen HN, Averette HE, et al. National survey of ovarian carcinoma XII: epithelial ovarian malignancies in women less than or equal to 25 years of age. Cancer 1994;73:1245.
6. McCann J, Wells R, Voris J. Genital findings in prepubertal girls selected for nonabuse: a descriptive study. Pediatrics 1990;86:428.
7. Herman-Giddens ME. Vaginal foreign bodies and child sexual abuse. Arch Pediatr Adolesc Med 1994;148:195.
8. Quinn TC, Groseclose SL, Spence M, et al: Evolution of the human immunodeficiency virus epidemic among patients attending sexually transmitted disease clinics: a decade of experience. Infect Dis 1992; 165:541.
9. Teele RL, Share JC. Ultrasonography of the female pelvis in childhood and adolescence. Radiol Clin North Am 1992;30:743.
10. Gomel V, Taylor PJ, Yuzpe AA, Rioux JE. Laparoscopy and hysteroscopy in gynecologic practice. Chicago, Year Book Medical, 1986.

Surgery of Infants and Children: Scientific Principles and Practice, edited by
Keith T. Oldham, Paul M. Colombani, and Robert P. Foglia.
Lippincott–Raven Publishers, Philadelphia, © 1997.

CHAPTER 95

Intersex States

Curtis A. Sheldon

Nowhere in the craft of surgery does an in-depth understanding of the pertinent basic sciences contribute so greatly to one's approach to diagnosis and therapy as in the surgical management of intersex states. This extremely complex discipline requires prompt and accurate decision-making with regard to one of the most important determinants of a child's future, his or her sex of rearing.

The social impact of giving birth to a child with ambiguous genitalia is overwhelming to the family and must be approached with reassurance and compassion. The parents are immediately faced with the first question asked of any new parent: Is it a boy or a girl? Extensive guidance is necessary from the outset in helping the parents cope with the pressures applied by family and friends.

Once the initial dilemma has been addressed, the parents and physicians must address multiple potential adverse sequelae—life-threatening metabolic complications, the risk of malignancy, the potential impact of inadequate genitalia, the psychological impact of the diagnosis on the child with maturation, and finally, the risk that further children may be born with similar malformations.

DEVELOPMENT OF SEXUAL CHARACTERISTICS

Transcriptional Control Over Morphogenesis

The sex of an individual may be defined by a number of criteria. We speak of *genetic sex* (a male or female chromosomal pattern), *gonadal sex* (whether testes or ovaries are present), and *phenotypic sex*. Of these, the most important is the phenotypic sex, for this alone determines whether an individual can experience adequate sexual intercourse and often determines if healthy, nurturing adult relationships are achievable.

Every individual begins with common, indifferent gonadal and genital primordia. An inherent tendency to feminize dominates unless specific developmental influences are present to direct male morphogenesis. Three specific but closely interrelated developmental sequences are required for normal sexual development, each governed by unique embryologic influences. These are gonadal, genital ductal, and external genitalia development.

While numerous genes located on both the sex chromosomes and autosomes are essential for morphogenesis, the earliest and most critical are those that control the structure and function of the gonad. Much can be inferred, with respect to genetic composition, from systematic analysis of the metaphase chromosomes—the *karyotype*. The normal human cell contains 22 autosomes and 2 sex chromosomes. Females have two X chromosomes, whereas males have an X and a Y chromosome. Each pair of chromosomes may be identified by differential staining banding techniques.

Anomalies of chromosomal composition may profoundly influence sexual development and are best understood with reference to the biology of cell division, which has been reviewed in detail by Simpson and Rebar[1] and by Grumbach and Conte.[2] Generally, cell division results in two progeny cells that receive identical copies of the parental cell chromosomes, a process known as *mitosis*. Each chromosome consists of two chromatids connected at the centromere. The centromere divides into two centrioles, which migrate to opposite poles of the nucleus (*prophase*). The mitotic spindle forms between the centrioles as the nuclear membrane disappears (*metaphase*). The centromere subsequently divides longitudinally, and the sister chromatids migrate to opposite poles (*anaphase*). Subsequently, the mitotic spindle disappears and new nuclear membranes form as the cell completes its cycle of division (*telophase*). During this process, the progeny cells retain their *diploid* state—each cell containing 23 pairs of chromosomes, each member of which is derived from a maternal and a paternal source.

Germ cells undergo a unique form of cell division (*meiosis*) in which the progeny cells contain half the number of chromosomes—a *haplotype* state. This enables the fertilization of an oocyte by a spermatozoon to result in a single diploid cell, the progeny of which culminates in a fully developed organism. The process of meiosis involves two sequential cell divisions, but DNA replication occurs only once. During the first division (meiosis I), DNA replication again results in two sister chromatids attached by a centromere. Each analogous pair of chromosomes becomes aligned during metaphase. During anaphase, the pairs separate, the members migrating to opposite poles, each with its centromere intact. The second division (meiosis II) progresses with the formation of a mitotic spindle, longitudinal division of each centromere, polar migration, and cell division.

The result is four haplotype progeny cells from each parental germ cell. Tremendous potential for genetic variation and gamete diversity is built into this process. Independent assortment and recombination of the 23 pairs of maternal and paternal chromosomes allows for a potential of 2^{23} different gamete chromosomal compositions. Additionally, the close prophase alignment of the replicated chromosomes during meiosis I allows DNA exchange between homologous chromosomes—a process known as *crossing over*, which tremendously amplifies the potential for diversity.

The complex nature of cell division also provides potential for the generation of chromosomal anomalies. Common abnormalities in chromosomal number include aneuploidy and mosaicism. *Aneuploidy* refers to any deviation from the expected number of chromosomes. Proposed mechanisms include meiotic or mitotic nondisjunction and anaphase lag. Nondisjunction during meiosis results in aneuploid gametes. With fertilization, the resultant zygote is aneuploid, with an identical chromosomal constitution in all cells. Nondisjunction during mitosis produces two or more cell lines in the zygote, which is referred to as *mosaicism*. Aneuploid states associated with abnormal sexual development include 47,XXY (Klinefelter syndrome), 45,X (Turner syndrome), and 45,X/46,XY mosaicism associated with gonadal dysgenesis. The existence of two or more cell lines within an individual is termed *chimerism*. Placental admixture of hemopoetic and primordial germ cells between twin fetuses of opposite sex is responsible for the relatively commonly observed hermaphrodite state in cattle, termed the freemartin. Other postulated mechanisms to explain chimerism without true twinning include double fertilization of a binucleate ovum, double fertilization of an ovum and its polar body, and fusion of two morulae or zygotes before implantation.[3] Presumably, 46,XX/46,XY and 46,XX/47,XXY true hermaphroditism may arise from mosaicism or chimerism. Structural chromosomal abnormalities are not uncommon and include *deletions* (loss of any part of a chromosome), *translocations* (the transfer of chromosomal material from one chromosome to another), *isochromosomes* (chromosomes with identical arms, arising from horizontal rather than vertical centromere division), *dicentric chromosomes* (a chromosome with two centromeres), *ring chromosomes*, and *duplications*. 46,XX sex-reversed males and 46,XX true hermaphrodites may represent examples of translocation of Y chromosomal material, whereas 46,XY sex-reversed females may represent examples of deletion of Y chromosomal material. An isochromosome involving the long arm of the X chromosome, 46,X,i(Xq), may be associated with gonadal dysgenesis, while dicentric chromosomes are occasionally seen in

45,X/46,XY mosaicism. On a molecular level, alterations in DNA sequence may result in sufficient genetic alteration to compromise gene product function and produce abnormal sexual development[4] (Table 95-1).

The Y chromosome is central to the control of gonadal determination. In the absence of a Y chromosome, except in conditions involving translocation, the indifferent gonad develops into an ovary. That 47,XXY individuals have testes and 46,X individuals do not demonstrates that the presence of the Y chromosome and not the absence of two X chromosomes determines testicular organogenesis. The additional observation that 46,X,i(Yq) individuals are female in appearance further suggests that the determinants of testicular development are located on the short arm of the Y chromosome.

In 1955, an antigen present on the cell surface of male cells and capable of inducing skin graft rejection in female animals of the same strain was identified and termed H-Y antigen.[5] Later, antibodies to H-Y antigen were identified and have led to serologic assays.[6] Because the H-Y antigen was found to be strongly conserved among vertebrates, was invariably associated with the heterogametic sex, and appeared extremely early in male embryos (eight-cell), this substance was considered to be responsible for testicular organogenesis.[7,8] The demonstration of H-Y antigen in 46,XX males and true hermaphrodites supported this conclusion. Importantly, however, the demonstration that the gene for H-Y antigen is located on the paracentromeric region of the long arm of the Y chromosome, whereas the gene for sex determination is located on the short arm of the Y chromosome, excludes this hypothesis.[9]

Another postulated testis-determining factor was the zinc-finger Y (ZFY) gene, which codes for a zinc-finger containing protein.[10,11] However, the finding of a homologous gene (*ZFX*) on the X chromosome, as well as the demonstration of 46,XX males without *ZFY*, eliminated this factor as a viable candidate for testis determination.[12]

Importantly, a series of 46,XX males negative for *ZFY* but with evidence of Y- to X-chromosomal translocation involving Y chromosomal sequences distal to the *ZFY* locus on the short arm have been reported.[13,14] Within this Y chromosomal sequence, between the *ZFY* gene and the pseudoautosomal region, lies a highly conserved gene that is currently favored as the true testis-determining gene—the *SRY* gene. This concept is supported by the finding of phenotypic females with 46,XY gonadal dysgenesis who have specific *SRY* gene mutations.[15,16] Additionally, transgenic *Sry* (murine *SRY* analogue) insertion into XX female mouse embryos has resulted in male differentiation, implicating *Sry* as the only known Y-linked gene required

TABLE 95-1. *Chromosomal location of genes pertinent to sexual development*

Chromosome	Location	Gene product
1	Short arm (*1p13–p11*)	3β-hydroxysteroid dehydrogenase
6	Short arm (*6p21.3*)	21α-hydroxylase
8	Long arm (*8q21–q22*)	11β-hydroxylase
10	—	17α-hydroxylase, 17,20-lyase
15	—	Side-chain cleavage enzyme
19	Short arm (*19p13.3*)	Antimüllerian hormone
X	Short arm (*Xq12*)	DHT receptor
Y	Short arm (*Yp11.3*)	Testis-determining factor

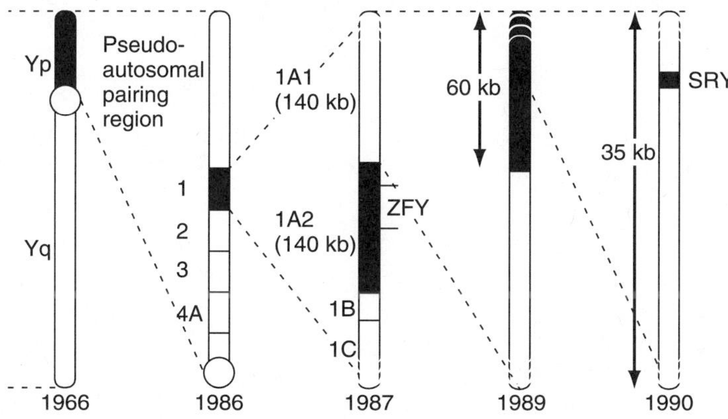

FIG. 95-1. Thirty-one years of hunting the testis-determining factor. The chromosomal region thought to include the elusive factor is shaded. The search was narrowed from 30 to 40 million bases (1959) to less than 250 bases encoding the conserved 80-amino-acid motif of SRY (1990). (McLaren A. What makes a man a man? Nature 1990;346:216.)

to induce male development.[17] Figure 95-1 outlines the chronology of the search for the testis-determining factor.[18] Figure 95-2 provides a conceptual outline of gene locations on a G-banded Y chromosome. Note the presence of a pseudoautosomal region at the distal end of the short arm of the Y chromosome, which is analogous to the distal end of the short arm of the X chromosome. These regions are thought to provide necessary alignment during meiosis. A large portion of the long arm of the Y chromosome is believed not to be engaged in gene transcription, containing highly repetitious DNA sequences.

Strong evidence exists to suggest that other genes are required to effect testicular organogenesis, with both X-chromosomal and autosomal influences implicated. These could be involved in *SRY* regulation or could be downstream targets of *SRY*. Data exist to suggest that some 46,XX males and 46,XX true hermaphrodites may in fact be negative for *SRY*.[19–21] Additionally, individuals with 46,XY gonadal dysgenesis are reported with present and unaltered *SRY* sequences.[22–25] Such determinations are difficult to interpret, however, given the observations that potentially undetected mosaicism with a Y-bearing cell line may explain some cases of 46,XX males[19] and that postzygotic *SRY* mutations in portions of gonadal tissue may result in 46,XY true hermaphroditism.[26] Vilain and colleagues[27] have analyzed the histologic findings in a series of patients with 46,XY gonadal dysgenesis. Individuals with streak gonads composed of exclusively ovarian-like stroma were found to have *SRY* mutations, whereas those with streak gonads containing undifferentiated stroma harboring either tubules or a rete structure had no detectable mutation in the *SRY* gene.

In the absence of a Y chromosome, ovarian differentiation generally occurs. However, the X chromosomes play a critical role in ovarian organogenesis. Individuals with monosomy X (45,X) demonstrate early ovarian development. In the absence of a second X chromosome, oocytes usually do not survive meiosis, and folliculogenesis fails to occur or is defective. The result is dysgenetic (streak) gonads. Because similar events are noted for individuals with deletion of either the short or long arm of the X chromosome, both arms are thought to contain important ovarian maintenance determinants. As reviewed by Simpson and Rebar,[1] individuals with deletions in the *Xp11.2–11.4* and *Xq11.3–21* regions create a high risk for primary amenorrhea. Deletions in the *Xp21* and *Xq25–26* regions also cause significant ovarian dysfunction. In each instance, the more proximal region is where the most critical genes are located.

A unique event occurs involving the X chromosome, the formation of the *Barr body*. In 1949, Barr and Bertram[28] described a chromatin mass located at the periphery of the nucleus and found in female but not in male cells. In the past, this observation was used clinically to help suggest an infant's chromosomal content and aid in the evaluation of intersex states. An analysis of buccal mucosal smears was employed. A female 46,XX karyotype was generally associated with at least a 20% identification rate of Barr bodies within the nuclei (*chromatin-positive*). Barr bodies are also identifiable in 47,XXY males, and multiple Barr bodies may be identified in both males and females with more than 2 X chromosomes. Conversely, a relative absence of Barr bodies implied a 46,XY karyotype, but could also be seen in individuals with 45,X and 45,X/46,XY. Such individuals are referred to as *chromatin-negative*.

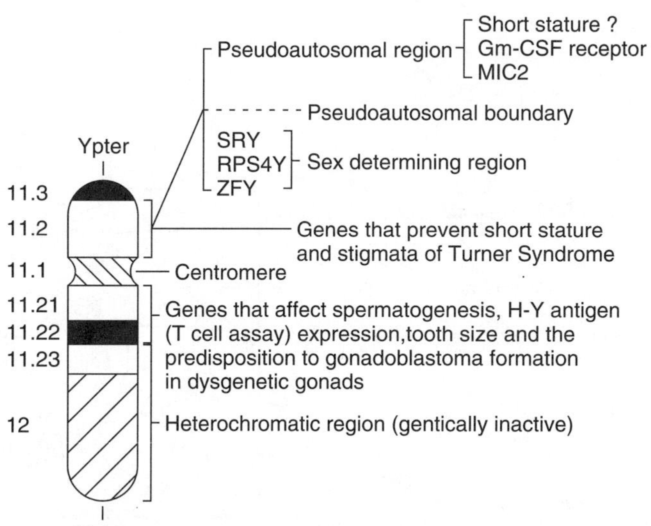

FIG. 95-2. Diagrammatic representation of a G-banded Y chromosome. Y-linked genes are shown. ZFY, zinc finger Y; SRY, sex-determining region Y; GM-CSF, granulocyte-macrophage colony-stimulating factor; M1C2, gene for a cell-surface antigen recognized by monoclonal antibody 12E7; RPS4Y, ribosomal protein S4. (Grumbach MM, Conte FA. Disorder of sex differentiation. In: Wilson JD, Foster DW, eds. Williams textbook of endocrinology. Philadelphia, WB Saunders, 1992:858.)

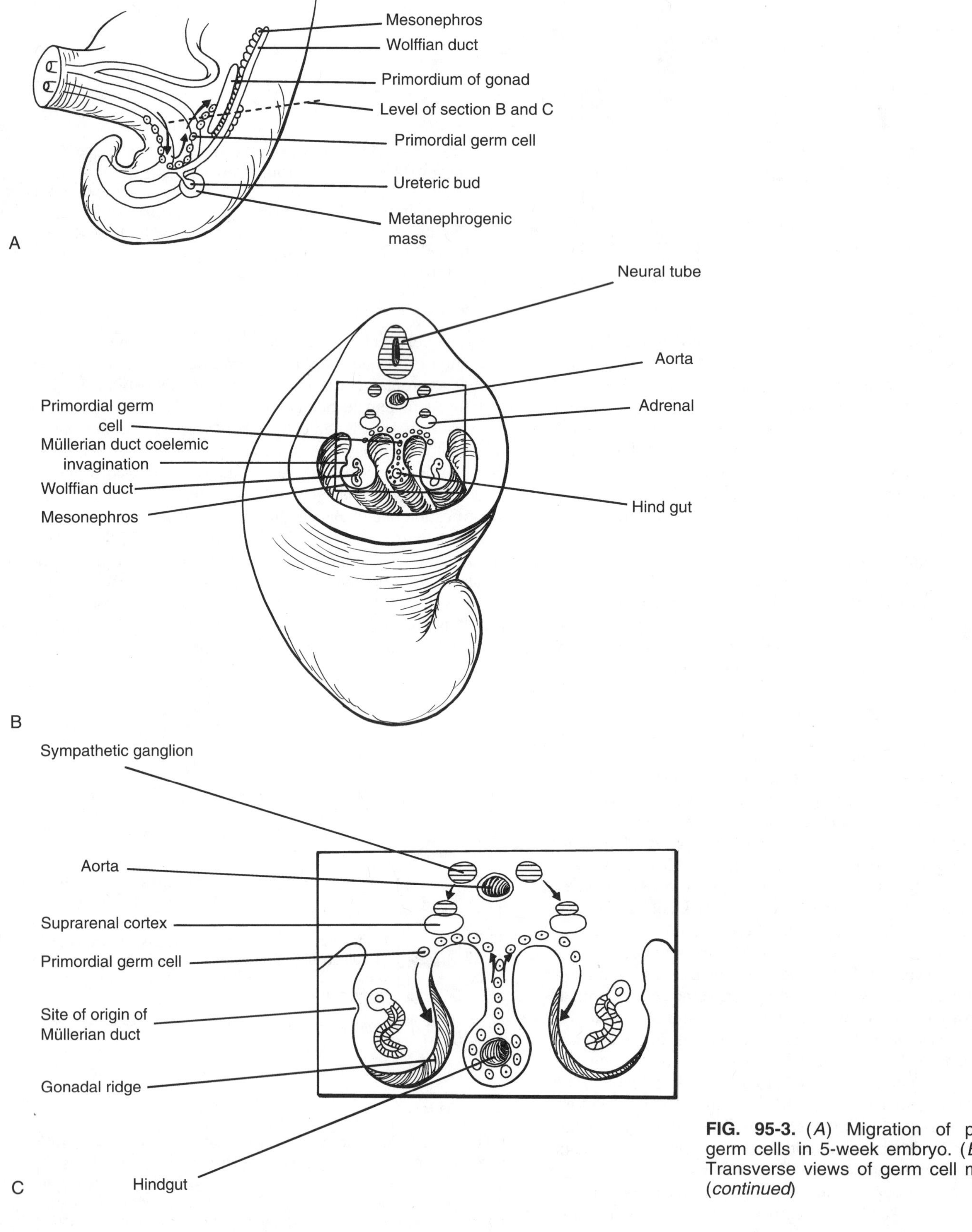

FIG. 95-3. (*A*) Migration of primordial germ cells in 5-week embryo. (*B* and *C*) Transverse views of germ cell migration. (*continued*)

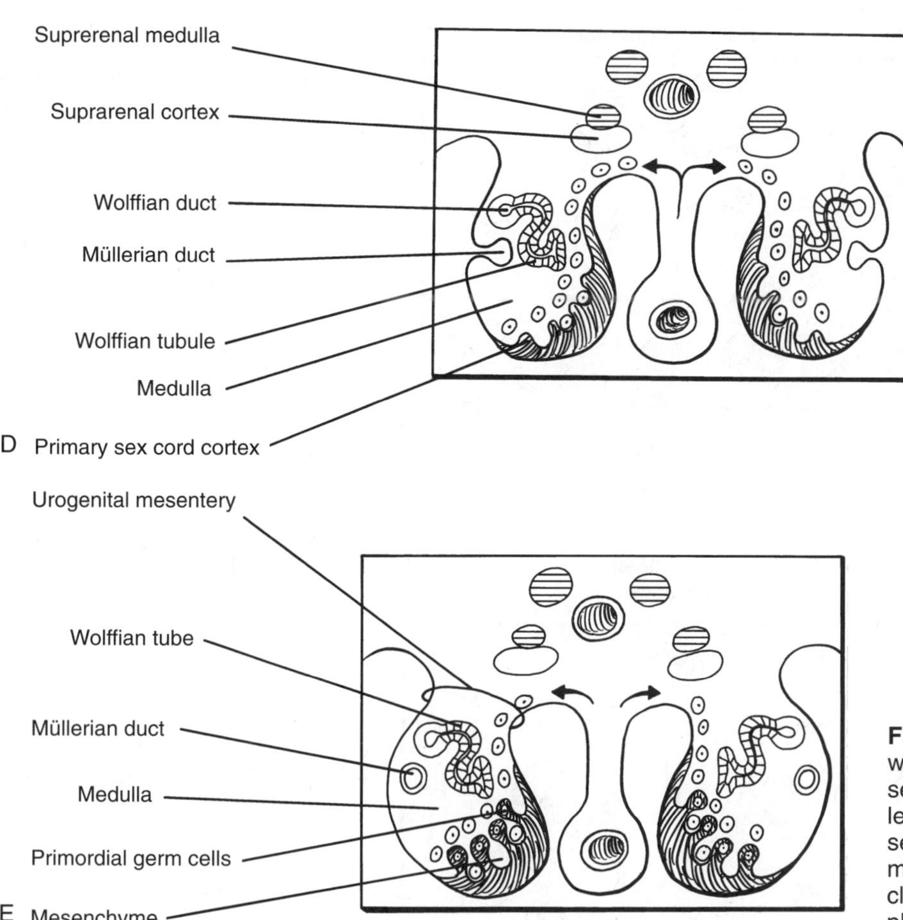

FIG. 95-3. *Continued.* (*D*) Six-week embryo with developing müllerian ducts and primary sex cords. (*E*) Further development of the müllerian and wolffian ducts as well as the primary sex cords. Arrows indicate primordial germ cell migration. (Moore KL. The developing human: clinically oriented embryology, ed 3. Philadelphia, WB Saunders, 1982:271.)

Gonadal Development

Early in embryogenesis, the gonads of both sexes are both *indifferent* and *bipotential*. Germ cells are identifiable in the dorsal endoderm of the yolk sac near the origin of the allantois. During weeks 4 and 5 of gestation, they migrate along the dorsal mesentery of the hindgut to the gonadal ridges. Invasion of the underlying mesoderm during week 6 allows them to become incorporated into the developing primary sex cords. These events are depicted in Figure 95-3. At approximately 40 days of gestation, divergent gonadal differentiation becomes evident (Fig. 95-4). Recent work has provided insight into these processes.[29]

In the human testis, seminiferous cords are differentiated by 7 weeks. Differentiation of the supporting cells is observed during weeks 8 to 11. *Sertoli cells* demonstrate ultrastructural evidence of intense protein biosynthesis as early as 8 weeks. The product of this biosynthesis would appear to be the antimüllerian hormone (AMH) as evidenced by the observation of coincident regression of müllerian ducts and the detection of AMH in the rough endoplasmic reticulum.[30] The multipotent Sertoli cell is thought also to secrete *inhibin* (provides negative feedback for follicle-stimulating hormone [FSH] secretion), *activin* (provides positive feedback for FSH secretion), and *follistatin* (provides inhibition of FSH release), and in addition is believed to nurture the germ cells and is postulated to prevent meiosis, possibly by the production of a meiosis-inhibiting substance.

Similarly, *Leydig cells* acquire ultrastructural features that suggest active steroid synthesis as early as 8 weeks, coincident with the onset of testosterone formation and metabolism in the human fetus.[31,32] Human chorionic gonadotropin (hCG)-luteinizing hormone (LH) cell membrane receptors are detected by week 12 of gestation.[35,36] Peak testosterone levels in the human fetus circulation is reached at approximately 16 weeks.[33,35] It is suggested that hCG secreted by the syncytiotrophoblast stimulates testosterone secretion during the critical period of male sexual development. The dependence of fetal testosterone biosynthesis on placental hCG has, however, been brought into question.[36,37]

As the *primitive germ cells* become incorporated into the primitive seminiferous tubules, they undergo a series of mitotic divisions resulting in multiple *prespermatogonia*, which then enter a long phase of quiescence during childhood. These prespermatogonia enter into active mitosis prior to puberty. Further mitotic division results in the *primary spermatocyte* series, which is still euploid in chromosomal composition. Following the first meiotic division, these primary spermatocytes give rise to a haploid series of *secondary spermatocytes*. The second

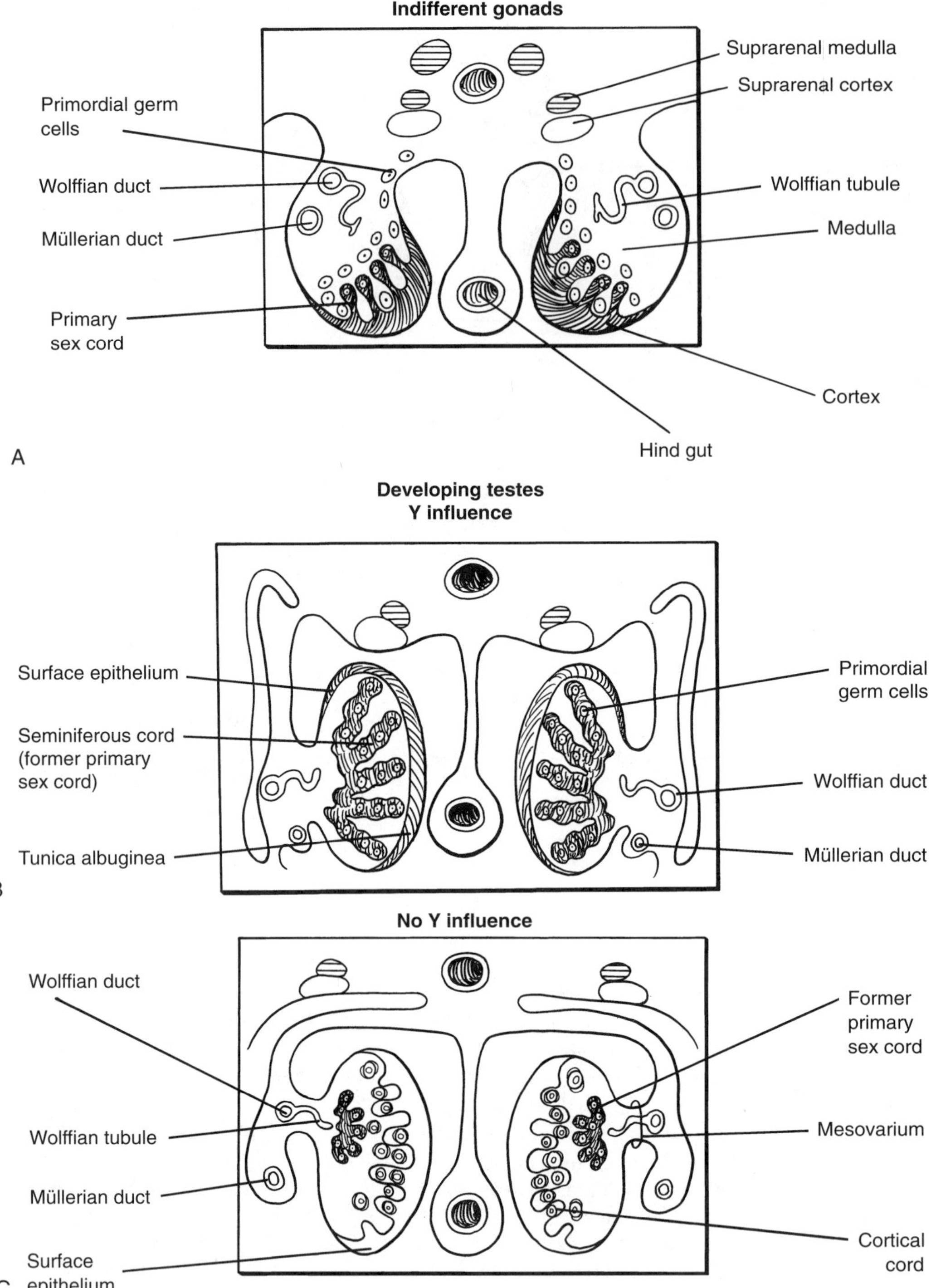

FIG. 95-4. Ovarian and testicular differentiation. (*A*) Indifferent 6-week gonad. (*B*) Primary sex cords develop into seminiferous cords, and the tunica albuginea becomes detectable at 7 weeks. (*C*) Twelve-week ovary. Cortical cords have extended from the epithelium. Primary sex cords are displaced into the mesovarium, forming rudimentary rete ovarii. (*continued*)

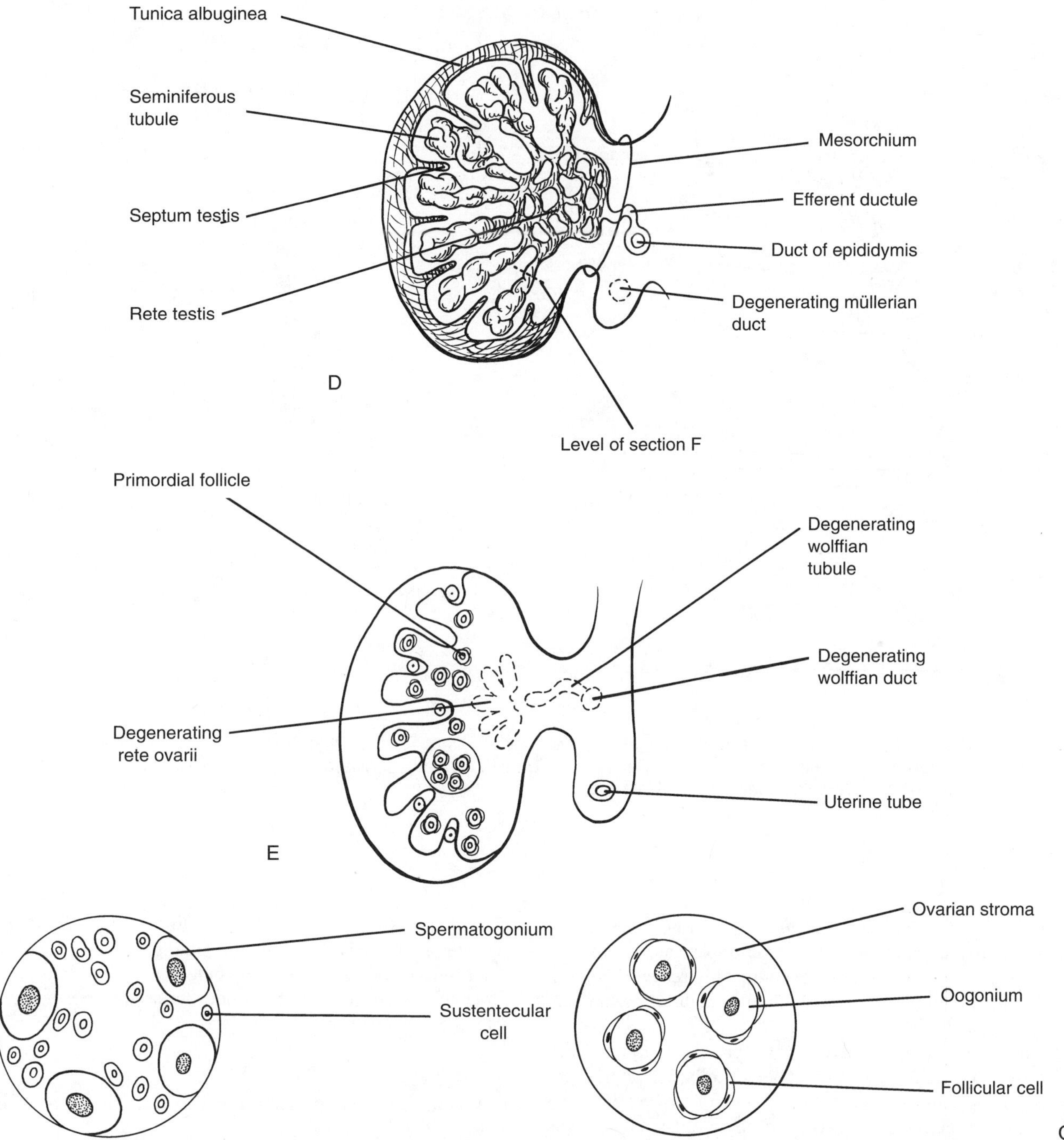

FIG. 95-4. *Continued.* (*D*) Twenty-week testis. The seminiferous tubules and rete testis have developed from seminiferous cords. Wolffian tubules develop into efferent ductules, and the wolffian duct gives rise to the duct of the epididymis. (*F* and *G*) Section of the testis and ovary in the 20-week fetus. (Moore KL. The developing human: clinically oriented embryology, ed 3. Philadelphia, WB Saunders, 1982: 271.)

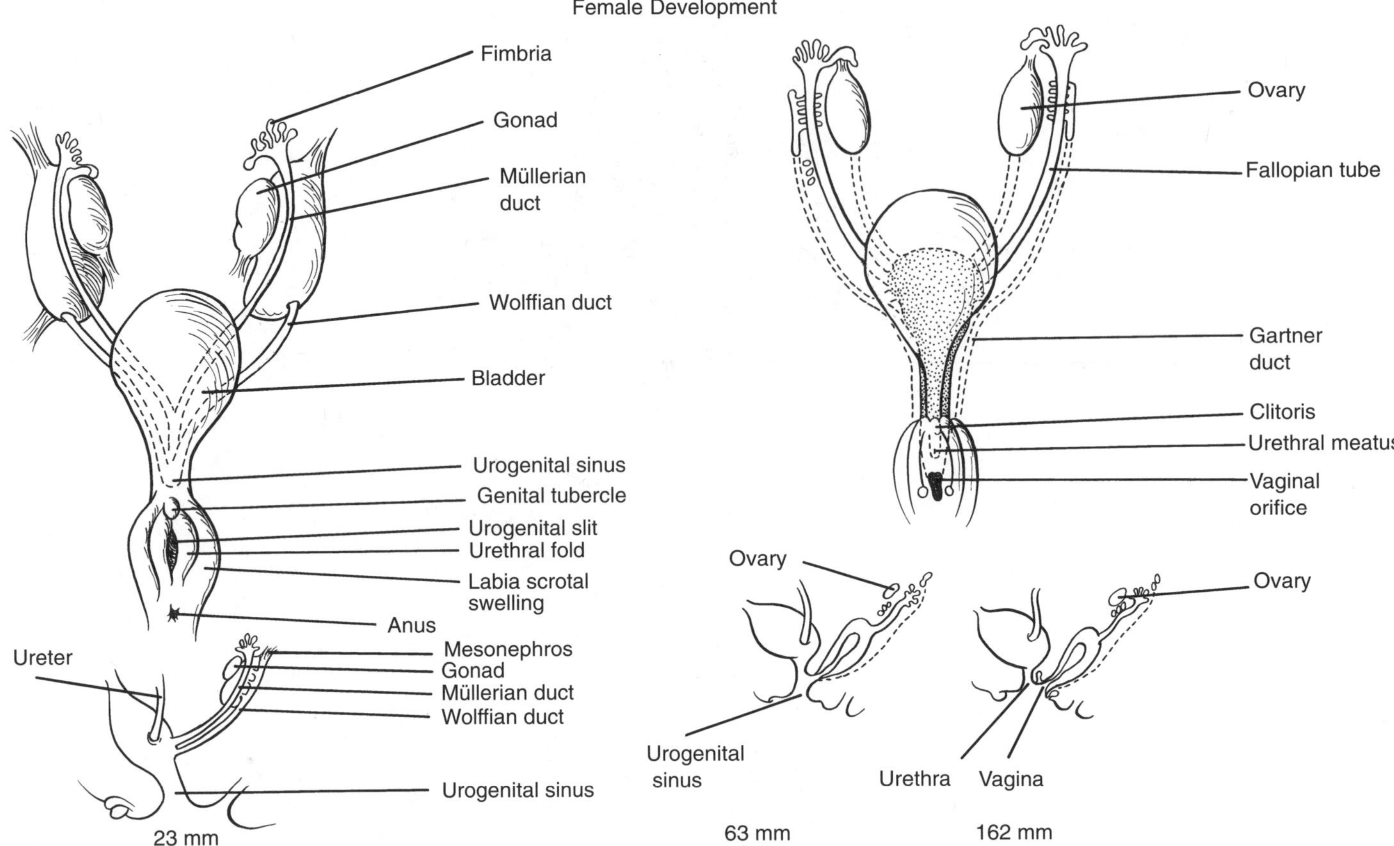

FIG. 95-5. Embryonic differentiation of female genital ducts (see text). (Grumbach MM, Conte FA. Disorder of sex differentiation. In: Wilson JD, Foster DW, eds. Williams textbook of endocrinology. Philadelphia, WB Saunders, 1992:871.) (*continued*)

meiotic division results in *spermatids*, which do not undergo further cell division but rather mature into spermatozoa. In contrast to the female, the adult male continually renews his germ cell population with a spermatogonium-to-mature sperm cycle of approximately 69 to 79 days.

In the female fetus, ovigerous cords are noted during week 7.[29] Oogonia are surrounded by cuboidal cells with long overlapping cytoplasmic processes that are thought to be precursors of granulosa cells. This early cytologic differentiation is matched by the ability of the human fetal ovary to aromatize androgens, documented as early as 8 weeks of gestational age.[38] Like the Sertoli cell, the granulosa cell is found to produce inhibin, activin, and follistatin. In contrast, however, the fetal ovary does not contain hCG receptors nor detectable quantities of AMH.

In contrast to the male fetus, organization of ovigerous cords does not impede the mitotic activity of the germ cells. Germ cells enter meiosis early, at about 11 to 12 weeks of gestation. The primary oocyte is arrested in the diplotene stage of the first meiosis and surrounded by granulosa cells, to give rise to primary follicles by week 20 to 25. There is a progressive decrease in the number of germ cells over time, from approximately 7 million at 5 months' gestation to 2 million at birth

and 300,000 at 7 years of age.[39] Just prior to ovulation, the first polar body is extruded, completing meiosis I. This haploid secondary oocyte immediately enters meiosis II but remains in metaphase and does not extrude the second polar body until the ovum is penetrated by a sperm cell.[2]

Development of the Internal Genital Ductal Systems

The development of the genital ductal systems and urinary tract have several critical anatomic and functional correlates and have recently been reviewed.[40] Figure 95-5 diagrammatically depicts these events. From the intermediate mesoderm arises the nephrogenic cord from which the *mesonephros* (the temporary kidney) and *metanephros* (the permanent kidney) develop. Cranially, the nephrogenic cord gives rise to the mesonephros as mesonephric vesicles develop that are connected by mesonephric tubules to the mesonephric duct. The latter develops initially as a solid rod beneath the surface ectoderm, ultimately opening into the developing cloaca. Within the mesonephros, tufts of capillaries give origin to primitive glomeruli, which begin to produce urine by week 6 of gestation.

Mesonephric differentiation occurs in a cranial-to-caudal di-

Male Development

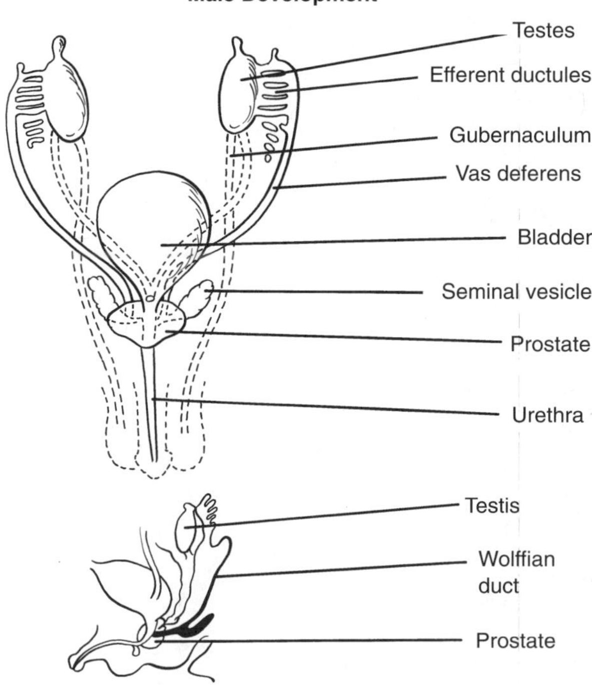

FIG. 95-5. *Continued.*

rection, during which the more cranially located nephrons progressively degenerate. Further caudally, the metanephros originates from the metanephric blastema of the nephrogenic cord and the ureteric bud and its branches. The latter develops as a diverticulum from the caudal mesonephric duct and is thought to induce development of the metanephric tubules. It becomes branched, giving origin to the ureter, renal pelvis, calyces, and collecting tubules. Late in the first trimester, the mesonephros ceases to be functional and excretion is taken over by the metanephros. Only a few caudal-most mesonephric tubules persist in the male to become the efferent ductules of the testis. These ductules drain into the mesonephric (*wolffian*) duct, which gives origin to the epididymis, vas deferens, seminal vesicles, and ejaculatory ducts.

The paramesonephric (*müllerian*) ducts arise as coelomic invaginations in the mesonephros (see Fig. 95-3). This process is believed to be induced by the mesonephric duct and begins cranially at a site that represents the future abdominal ostium of the uterine (*fallopian*) tube. The paramesonephric ducts grow caudally, fuse, and ultimately drain into the urogenital sinus. The unfused portions give rise to the fallopian tubes, while the fused portion develops into the uterus and upper vagina. Because müllerian duct differentiation fails to occur in the absence of a wolffian duct, renal aplasia is often associated with anomalies of the fallopian tubes, uterus, and vagina.

The differentiation of the internal genital ductal system is critically dependent on gonadal influences. Both the mesonephric and paramesonephric ducts are present in the fetus at 7 weeks' gestation in both males and females. In the absence of testicular influence, whether or not an ovary is present, mesonephric ducts regress and paramesonephric ducts mature. These influences, AMH produced by fetal Sertoli cells, and testoster-

one produced by fetal Leydig cells are local and hence principally unilateral in character and occur during the third month of fetal life.

Experimentally, gonadectomy of either male or female fetuses early in gestation results in wolffian regression and müllerian development. Further, unilateral castration of a male fetus results in ipsilateral wolffian regression and müllerian development, while the contralateral genital ducts develop in a normal masculine fashion.[41] Conversely, testicular grafts placed in female fetuses result in müllerian regression and wolffian stimulation. The local implantation of androgens in female fetuses causes unilateral wolffian ductal maturation, whereas müllerian ductal development is unaltered.[41,42]

AMH is a glycoprotein composed of two identical 72-kd subunits, connected by disulfide bonds,[43] that is encoded by a gene on the short arm of chromosome 19.[44] Work by Donahoe and associates[45] has suggested that AMH acts by blocking tyrosine phosphorylation on membrane proteins. AMH is thought to be the mediator responsible for the bovine freemartin, having origin in the Sertoli cell of the male twin and gaining access to the female twin via placental anastomoses.[46,47] The freemartin (the female twin) demonstrates müllerian regression and inhibition of ovarian development with the presence of seminiferous tubule-like cords. A similar finding has been reported in transgenic female mice expressing the human AMH gene, further implicating AMH as the source of these phenotypic changes.[48] As recently reviewed, AMH appears to have multiple potential functions, including not only müllerian duct regression but also germ cell maturation and gonadal morphogenesis, lung maturation, testicular descent, and growth inhibition of certain transformed cells.[49]

Similarly, local androgen production by the fetal testis promotes ipsilateral wolffian duct maturation. This effect appears to require high local testosterone concentration because wolffian differentiation is not induced by systemic androgen administration in early gestation. Because 5α-reductase is not present in wolffian ducts, it is testosterone, not dihydrotestosterone, that binds to the cytosolic androgen receptor to induce these phenotypic changes.[31]

These embryologic phenomena explain many observations made clinically.

1. Female fetuses with congenital virilizing adrenal hyperplasia do not demonstrate müllerian regression or wolffian maturation.
2. 46,XY women with testicular feminization (complete androgen insensitivity) have regression of müllerian ducts, but wolffian ducts remain rudimentary.
3. Genetic males with severe defects in steroid biosynthesis that result in androgen deficiency have rudimentary wolffian derivatives.
4. Genetic males with isolated deficiency of AMH have persistence of müllerian derivatives, but wolffian development proceeds normally.
5. In individuals with asymmetric gonadal development such as 45,X/46,XY mixed gonadal dysgenesis and true hermaphroditism, genital ductal development follows that of the homolateral gonad; the presence of testicular tissue results in ipsilateral müllerian regression and wolffian development.

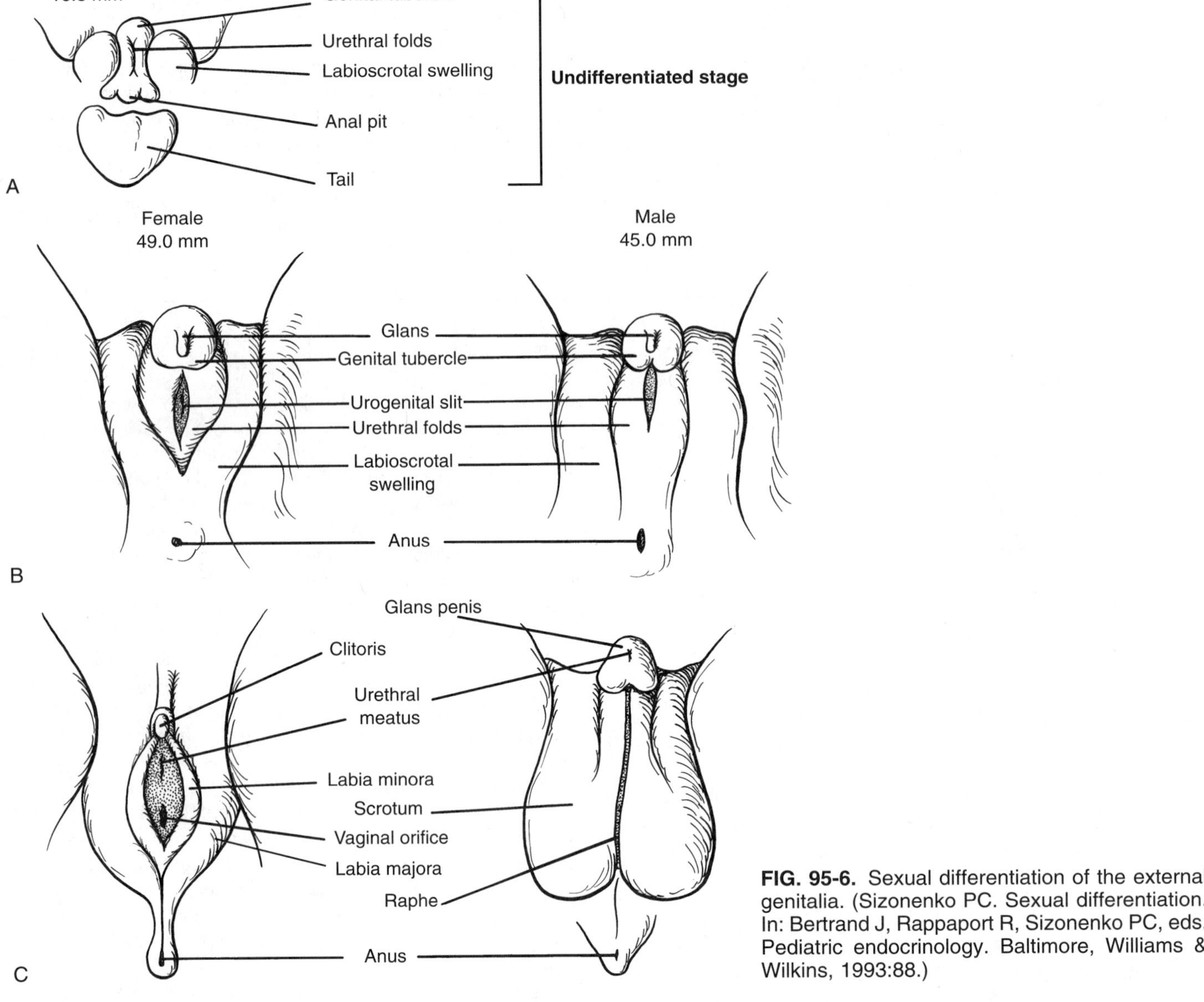

FIG. 95-6. Sexual differentiation of the external genitalia. (Sizonenko PC. Sexual differentiation. In: Bertrand J, Rappaport R, Sizonenko PC, eds. Pediatric endocrinology. Baltimore, Williams & Wilkins, 1993:88.)

Development of the Urogenital Sinus and External Genitalia

At week 8 of gestation, the external genitalia of both males and females are identical and remain uncommitted. Figure 95-6 outlines the differentiation of male and female external genitalia. In males, the *genital tubercle* becomes the penis, while the *urethral folds* fuse to become the floor of the penile urethra and the corpus spongiosum that encloses the penile urethra. In analogous fashion, the *labioscrotal swellings* fuse in the midline to become the scrotum. In the female, the genital tubercle becomes the clitoris and the urethral folds and labioscrotal swellings do not fuse, becoming the labia minora and the labia majora respectively.

Sexual differentiation of the urogenital sinus is illustrated in Figure 95-7. As with the external genitalia, the urogenital sinus is similar in both sexes up to week 8 or 9 of fetal life. The müllerian tubercle protrudes from the posterior wall of the urogenital sinus between the two wolffian duct orifices. This contact of the urogenital sinus with the fused müllerian ducts is critical to normal development of the vagina.[50,51] Although this interpretation is controversial, the lower vagina appears to be of urogenital sinus origin and the upper vagina of müllerian origin. Expansion of the tissue composing the vesicovaginal septum allows for spatial separation of the vagina and urethra. In the male, the urogenital sinus undergoes elongation to form the prostatic and perineal urethra.

In analogous fashion to the differentiation of the internal genital ducts, masculinization of the urogenital sinus and external genitalia requires the presence of a testis. In contrast, however, this effect occurs in response to exposure to *dihydrotestosterone* (DHT) and can be induced by systemic androgen exposure (Fig. 95-8). Testosterone enters the cell by diffusion, whereupon it may bind to a high-affinity androgen receptor

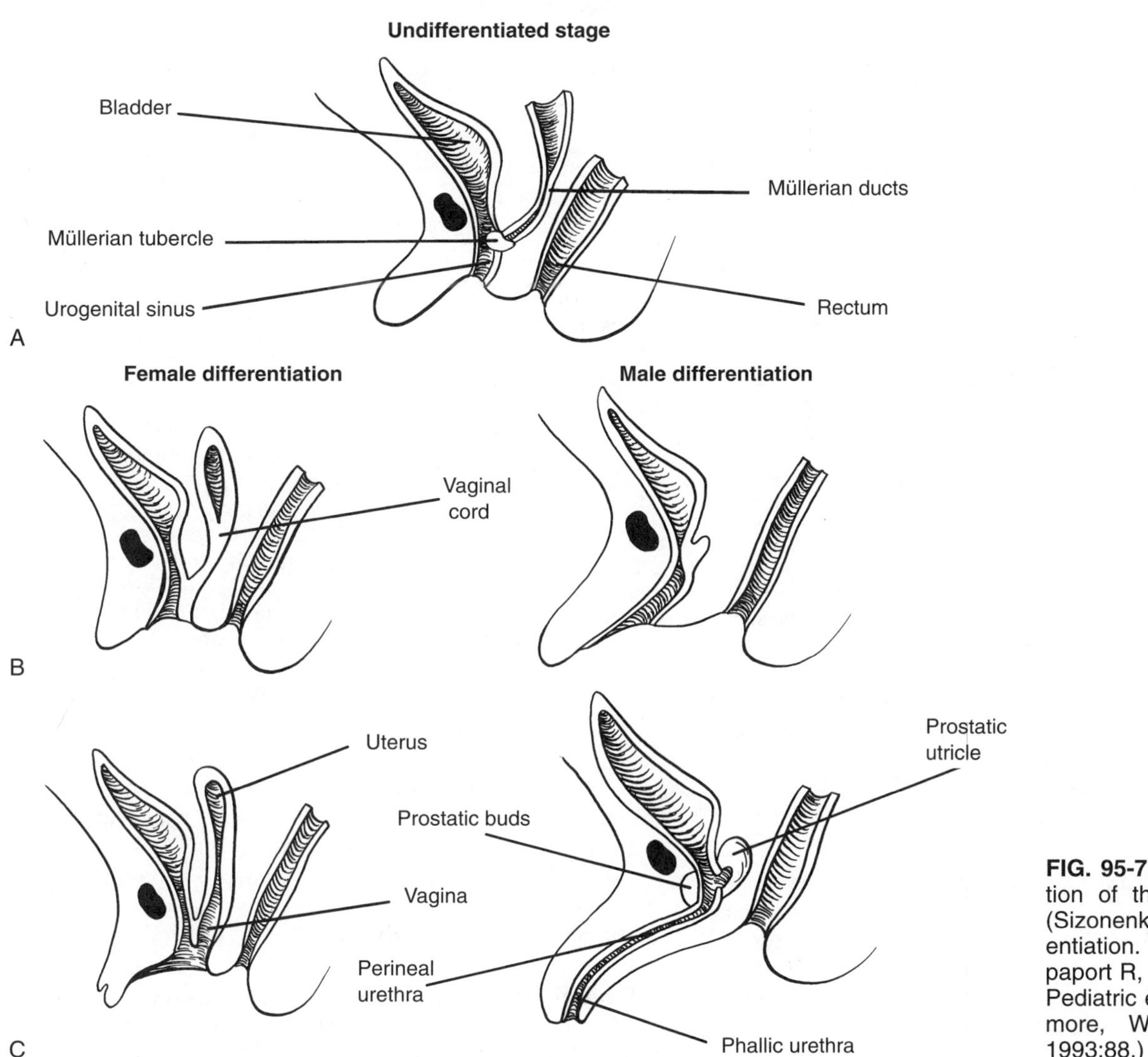

FIG. 95-7. Sexual differentiation of the urogenital sinus. (Sizonenko PC. Sexual differentiation. In: Bertrand J, Rappaport R, Sizonenko PC, eds. Pediatric endocrinology. Baltimore, Williams & Wilkins, 1993:88.)

protein, be aromatized to estradiol, or be converted to DHT by the action of *5α-reductase*. While both testosterone and DHT may bind to the androgen receptor protein, the binding affinity of the receptor for DHT is much greater. As with several members of the steroid receptor superfamily, the DNA binding site is occupied by an inhibitory (eg, heat shock) protein.[52] Binding of the androgen to the receptor leads to dissociation of the inhibitory protein by conformational change, enabling the receptor to bind to specific sites on the DNA, referred to as receptor-dependent transcriptional enhancers. The result is transcription and processing of mRNA, which is then translated, allowing the synthesis of new proteins that mediate the androgenic effects involved with masculinization of the urogenital sinus and external genitalia.

Psychosexual Development

It has been generally assumed that gender identity (the identification of one's self as either male or female) is largely a learned process, and that this gender identity is firmly established by 1.5 and 2.5 years of age.[53] Clearly, the assignment of the sex of rearing is the single most critical event in this process. Reinforcement of this assignment is crucial and requires unambiguous genital anatomy and unambiguous family interactions. One must not, however, overlook the importance of endocrine effects during prenatal development and puberty. Gender-related behavior, including gender role, has been demonstrated to be influenced by prenatal sex hormone exposure.[54,55] Further, pubertal hormonal influences producing phenotypic changes counter to that of the original gender assignment have been reported to induce not only doubts about gender identity but to cause alterations in gender behavior in some individuals.[56] Males with a small penis, followed into adulthood, do not in general experience altered gender identity, altered desire for heterosexual activity, or alterations in other activities generally considered to be predominantly male.[57] This and other studies, however, have demonstrated that life with inadequate or compromised genitalia is often confounded by debilitating emotional disturbances.

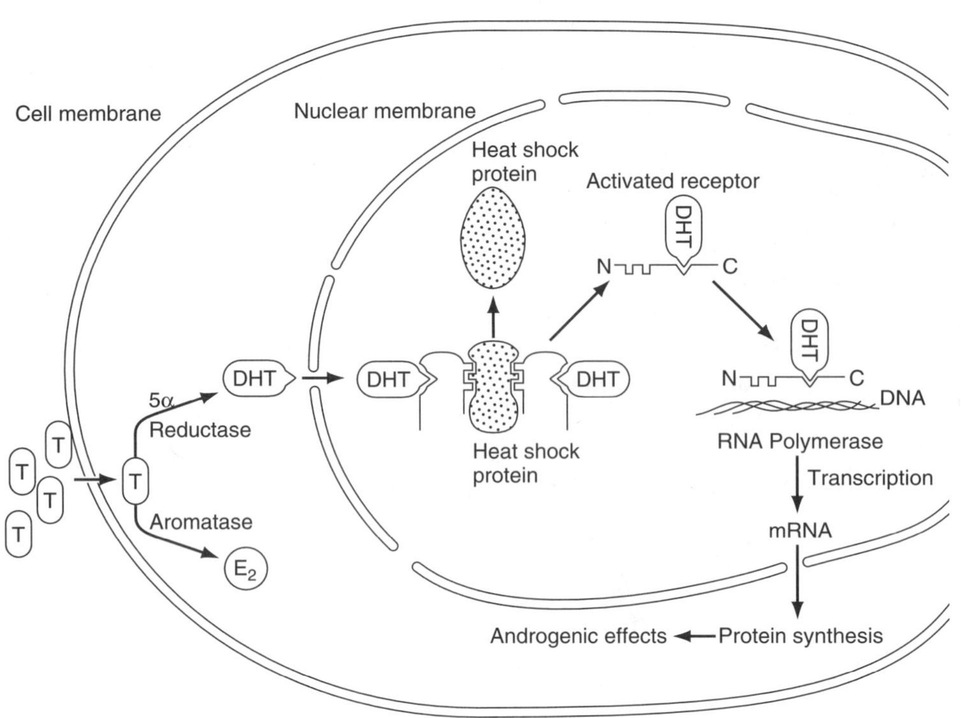

FIG. 95-8. Mechanism of action of androgens on cell function (see text). T, testosterone; DHT, dihydrotestosterone. (Grumbach MM, Conte FA. Disorder of sex differentiation. In: Wilson JD, Foster DW, eds. Williams textbook of endocrinology. Philadelphia, WB Saunders, 1992:875.)

Developmental Temporal Sequence

An understanding of the temporal sequence of the development of the reproductive tract is helpful clinically. As illustrated in Figure 95-9, one may conceptualize this process as a series of interrelated steps. Chromosomal sex is determined at the time of conception. This is followed by an indifferent phase of embryogenesis that lasts approximately 7 weeks. Thereafter, divergent development is progressive with the sequential differentiation of the gonads, followed by the internal genital ducts, followed by the urogenital sinus and external genitalia.

Evidence exists to suggest that during the period of organogenesis, inclusive of the differentiation of the external genitalia, fetal Leydig cell activity is driven by placental hCG rather than by LH from the fetal pituitary.[33,35] The pattern of testosterone secretion during early gestation reflects that of hCG and the fetal testicular hCG binding capacity.[35,58,59] Additionally, the expression of several steroidogenic genes appears to be directly regulated by circulating hCG.[60–63] Fetal pituitary LH appears to take over the modulation of testosterone synthesis after midgestation and, along with placental hCG, appears to play a critical role in the growth of the differentiated penis and scrotum as well as descent of the testes.[58]

These observations, coupled with the facts that after about 12 weeks of gestation the vagina has separated from the urogenital sinus, and the urethral folds and labioscrotal swellings are unable to fuse even with intense androgenic stimulation, explain several important clinical observations: (1) females exposed to androgens after the period of organogenesis develop clitoromegaly, but urethral fold and labioscrotal fusion does not occur; (2) the diagnosis of congenital virilizing adrenal hyperplasia generally does not explain clitoromegaly in the absence of midline fusion; and (3) males with congenital hypopituitarism or selective gonadotropin deficiency often present with microphallus, but the penis and scrotum are generally well differentiated.

Summary of Reproductive Tract Differentiation

Figure 95-10 summarizes the events leading to normal sexual development in both males and females. In the presence of two normal X chromosomes, two normal ovaries develop. In the absence of testosterone and AMH, paramesonephric ducts mature into fallopian tubes, uterus, and upper vagina, whereas mesonephric ductal elements regress. Similarly, in the absence of androgenic stimulation, feminine differentiation of the urogenital sinus and the external genitalia occurs. (1) In the absence of an X chromosome or a critical portion of an X chromosome, important ovarian developmental failure may result. Additionally, 46,XX males with *SRY* translocations and 46,XX males with undetected mosaicism with a Y-bearing cell line are reported and are associated with testicular organogenesis. 46,XX and 46,XX/46,XY true hermaphroditism is similarly associated with development of some testicular tissue. (2) Once present, testicular tissue may produce sufficient testosterone and AMH to result in mesonephric development and paramesonephric regression, which if unilateral, is restricted to the side where testicular tissue is located. (3) Exposure of the fetus to either exogenous (eg, maternal ingestion) or endogenous (eg, congenital virilizing adrenal hyperplasia) androgen may result in various degrees of virilization of the urogenital sinus and the external genitalia.

In the presence of a normal Y and X chromosome, testicular development follows. The production of AMH by Sertoli cells and the production of testosterone by Leydig cells results in paramesonephric regression and mesonephric development, re-

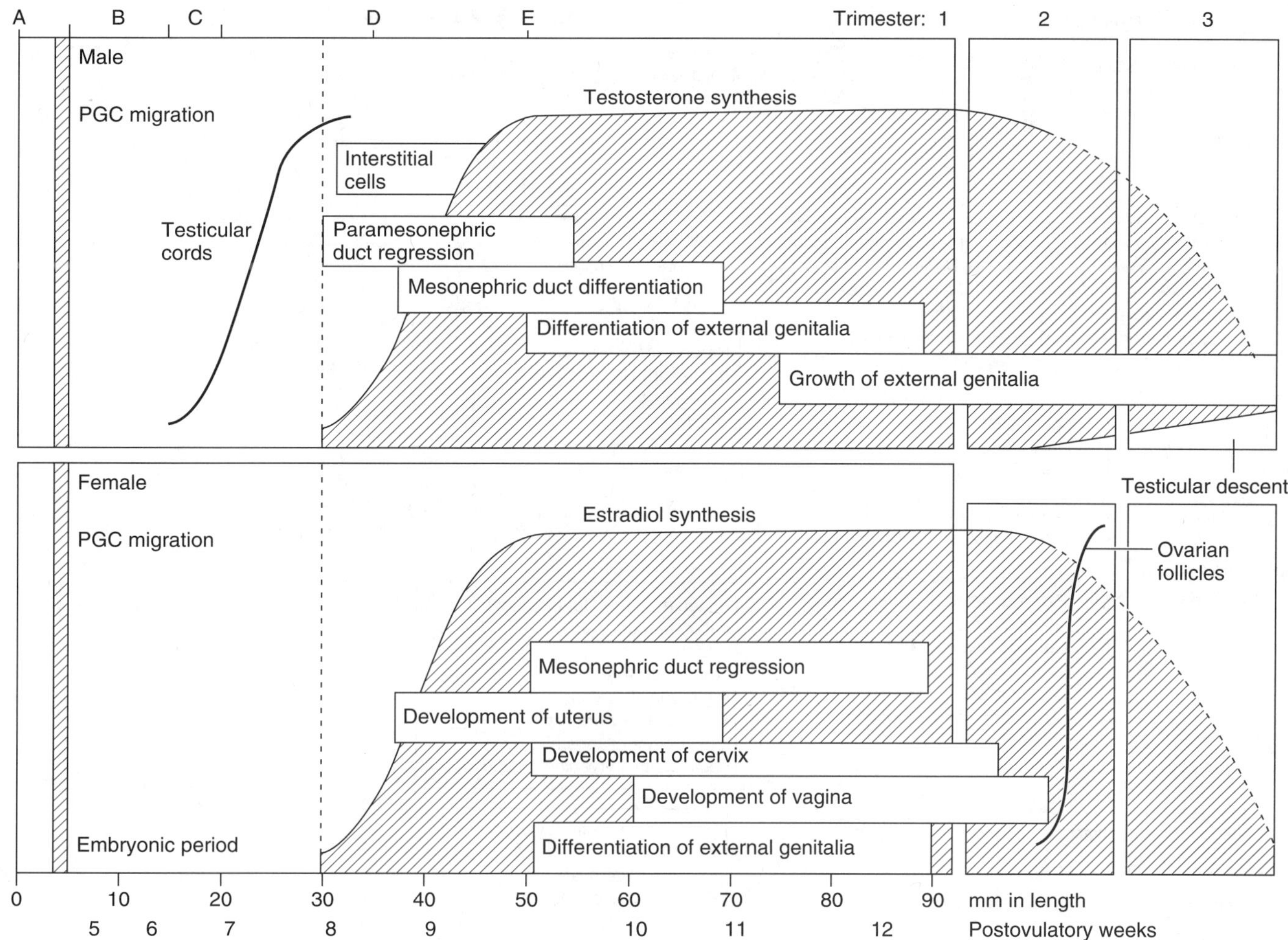

FIG. 95-9. Prenatal development of the reproductive system as a function of embryonic/fetal length and age. (*A*) Chromosomal sex established. (*B*) Indifferent phase. (*C*) Gonadal differentiation. (*D*) Genital ductal differentiation. (*E*) External genitalia differentiation. (See text.) (O'Rahilly R, Muller F. Human embryology and teratology. New York, Wiley-Liss, 1992:207.) PGC, primordial germ cell.

spectively. During the period of organogenesis, Leydig cell steroid synthesis is driven by placental hCg and thereafter by fetal pituitary LH. Testosterone is converted to DHT by 5α-reductase, which, in the presence of the cytosolic androgen receptor protein encoded by a gene on the X chromosome, causes masculinization of the urogenital sinus and external genitalia. (4) In the absence of a Y chromosome (eg, 45,X/46,XY) or (5) a critical portion of the Y chromosome (*SRY*), defective testicular development may occur. (6) AMH deficiency may occur in isolation or as part of more complete testicular failure and results in persistence of paramesonephric structures. (7) Leydig cell steroid synthetic failure may occur as a result of specific enzymatic deficiency or as part of more complete testicular failure and results in incomplete masculinization of the internal genital ducts, urogenital sinus, and external genitalia. (8) Partial androgen receptor deficiency may result in incomplete masculinization, whereas complete deficiency may result in a nearly normal female phenotype. Because AMH production is normal, paramesonephric structures are rudimentary. (9) 5α-reductase

deficiency results in insufficient DHT production, which produces only partial virilization. (10) Congenital hypopituitarism or isolated gonadotropin deficiency may result in inadequate stimulation of Leydig cell function. The result is a small but completely formed penis and scrotum.

Defects in Steroid Biosynthesis

The subject of steroid biosynthesis has been extensively reviewed by Grumbach and Conte.[2] Defects can result in either masculinization of genetic females, female sexual infantilism, undermasculinization of the genetic male, or excessive masculinization of the genetic male. These defects are often overlooked because of the wide variability of phenotypic expression. They must be understood by surgeons because the first level of referral may be to the surgeon for correction of what may appear as a relatively common anomaly such as hypospadias.

The steroid biosynthetic pathways are diagrammed in Figure

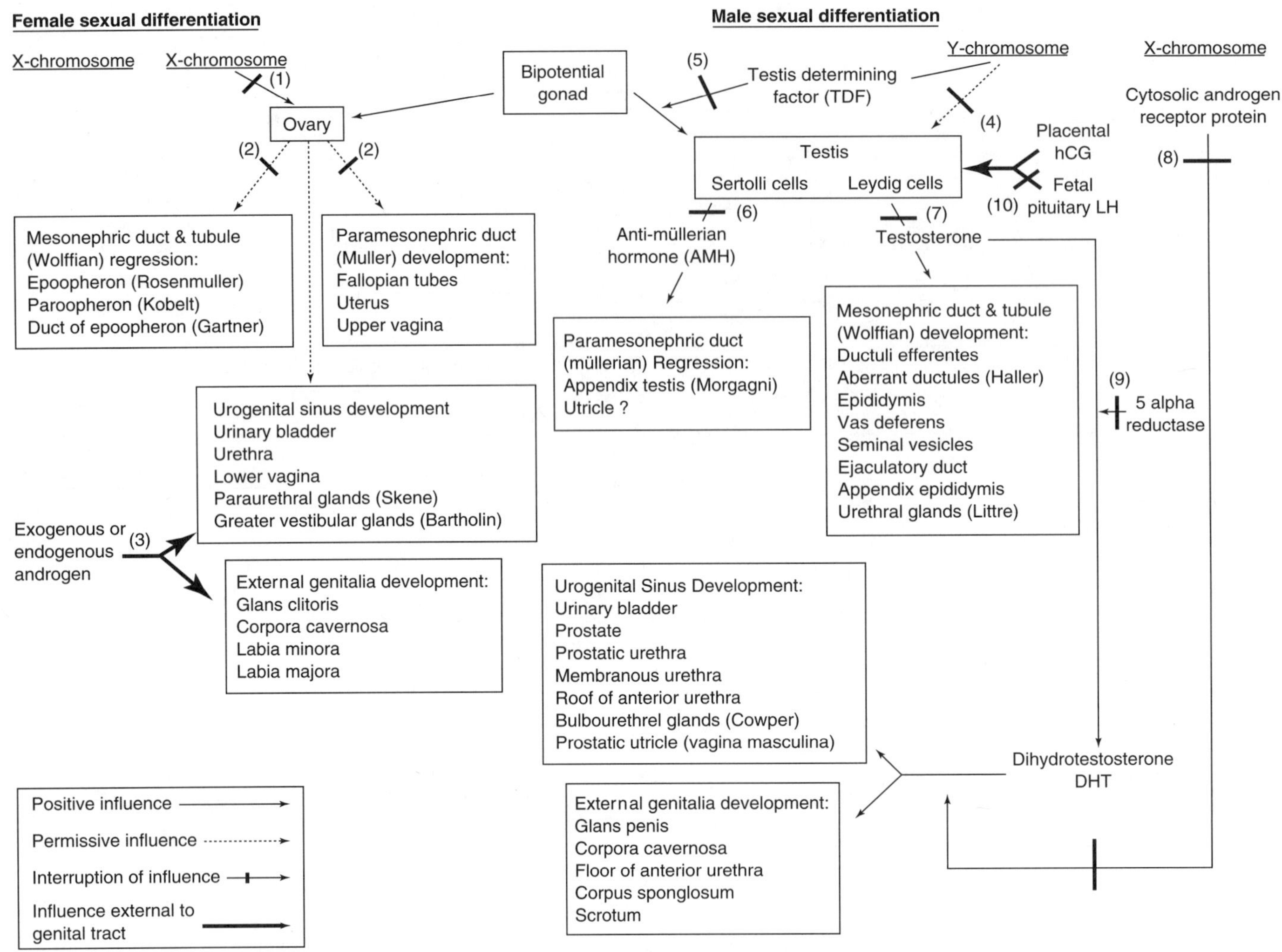

FIG. 95-10. Diagramatic depiction of events involved with normal and abnormal male and female sexual differentiation. Interruptive influences are numerically labeled and referred to in text. Adult derivatives and vestigial remnants of embryonic genital structures are outlined. Commonly encountered eponyms are noted in parentheses.

95-11. Congenital adrenal hyperplasia is responsible for the majority of cases of female pseudohermaphroditism and accounts for approximately half of ambiguous genitalia cases. The most common enzymatic defect is *21-hydroxylase deficiency*. This enzyme is encoded by a gene on *chromosome 6*, occurring between the *HLA-B* and *HLA-DR* foci. Consequently, this deficiency is inherited in an *autosomal recessive* fashion, and its inheritance is intimately associated with that of the major transplant antigens. Analysis of human histocompatability antigens may therefore be helpful in genetic counseling. The incidence of classic 21-hydroxylase deficiency is about 1 in 15,000 to 40,000 newborns.[64]

The defective enzyme in 21-hydroxylase deficiency is a cytochrome P-450 enzyme. Both the phenotypic expression and the biochemical expression of 21-hydroxylase deficiency is remarkably variable. Females may present with very mild degrees of masculinization or be sufficiently masculinized to appear to have hypospadias with bilateral cryptorchidism (Fig. 95-12).

The classic presentation of 21-hydroxylase deficiency is that of hyponatremic dehydration, hyperkalemic acidosis, and ultimately vascular collapse. It is particularly important for the surgeon to be cognizant of this presentation, as it may be confused with other lesions for which surgical consultation may be obtained, such as sepsis and bowel obstruction, including hypertrophic pyloric stenosis. Females characteristically present with ambiguous genitalia, whereas males may develop excessive masculinization.

Nonclassic presentations for 21-hydroxylase deficiency exist. These include late-onset and cryptic varieties. Such individuals may have completely normal genitalia in the newborn period and then demonstrate signs of androgen overproduction in later childhood. Cryptogenic deficiencies may demonstrate biochemical changes in the absence of signs or symptoms.

Figure 95-13A demonstrates the biochemical changes that may be assayed to determine the diagnosis. Blockage of 21-hydroxylase activity impairs the conversion of progesterone and 17-hydroxyprogesterone to deoxycorticosterone and 11-deoxycortisol, respectively. The result is an accumulation of proges-

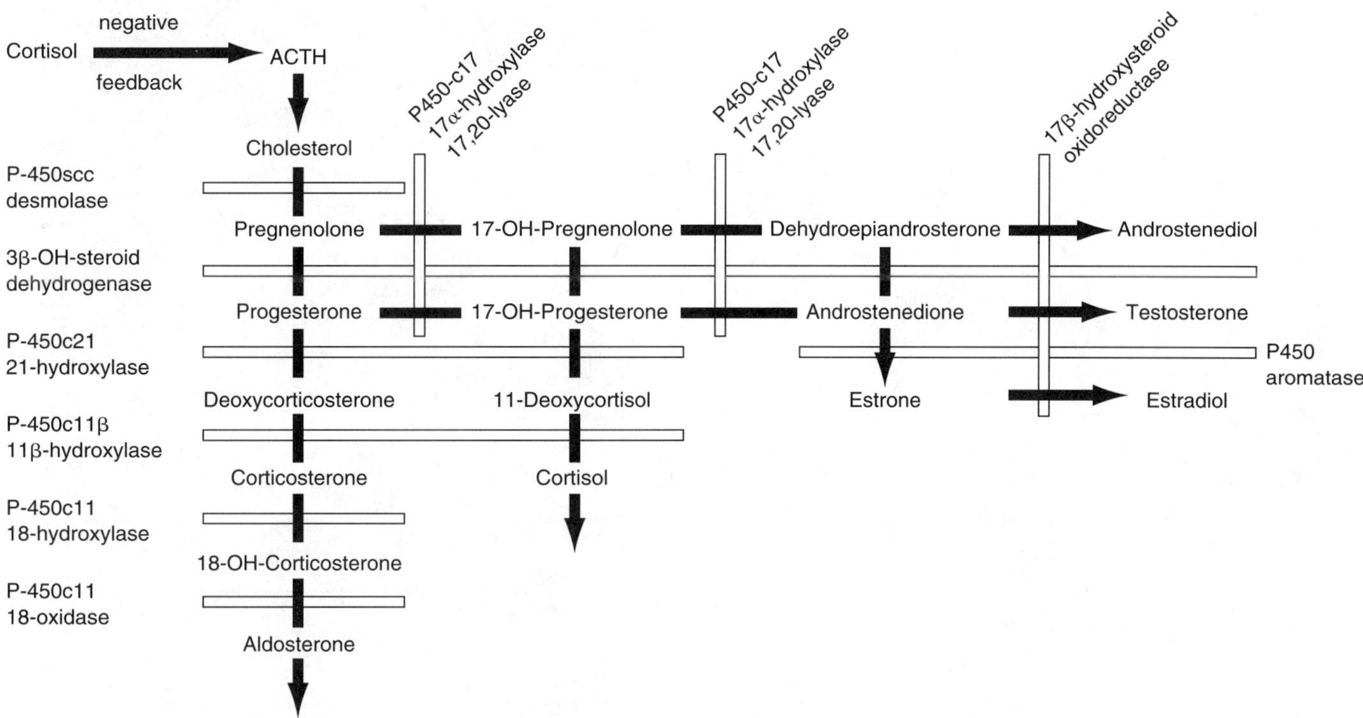

FIG. 95-11. Steroid biosynthetic pathways. Note separate pathways required for the synthesis of mineralocorticoids, glucocorticoids, and the sex steroids.

terone and 17-hydroxyprogesterone. The buildup of these precursors results in lateral metabolism toward the production of androgenic compounds. Traditionally, biochemical assays included the measurement of urinary 17-ketosteroids (urinary metabolites of the excessively produced androgenic compounds) and urinary pregnentriol, a specific metabolite of 17-hydroxyprogesterone. Currently, serum 17-hydroxyprogesterone is the preferred biochemical marker for this disease.

Treatment acutely involves volume resuscitation and steroid loading. Chronically, patients are maintained on cortisone and flucortisol supplementation for glucocorticoid and mineralocorticoid maintenance, respectively. Of greatest concern from a surgical perspective is strict attention to providing stress-level steroid supplementation with surgical procedures, and any acute illness.

Individuals with *11β-hydroxylase* deficiency (see Fig. 95-13B) demonstrate a defect in the conversion of deoxycorticosterone and 11-deoxycortisol to corticosterone and cortisol, respectively. As with 21-hydroxylase deficiency, deficient cortisol production results in increased ACTH stimulation of adrenal biosynthesis. The gene for this enzyme is located on *chromosome 8*, resulting in an *autosomal recessive* inheritance pattern. Like 21-hydroxylase deficiency, classic, mild, late-onset, and cryptic forms are reported.

Again, precursor metabolites accumulate, providing substrate for the overproduction of androgenic steroids, which cause inappropriate masculinization of females and excessive masculinization of males. Elevated serum deoxycorticosterone and 11-deoxycortisol levels may be assayed. Elevated deoxycorticosterone, which has mineralocorticoid activity, results in volume

expansion and low-renin hypertension, which often manifests itself beyond 2 years of age. Pertinent diagnostic findings include elevated serum deoxycorticosterone and 11-deoxycortisol as well as their urinary metabolites, tetrahydrodeoxycorticosterone and tetrahydro-11-deoxycortisol. Additionally, urinary 17-ketosteroids are elevated.

Another enzymatic deficiency resulting in congenital adrenal hyperplasia is *3β-hydroxysteroid dehydrogenase deficiency*. This enzyme is encoded by a gene on *chromosome 1*, and its deficiency is also inherited in an *autosomal recessive* pattern. This deficiency (see Fig. 95-13C) results in impaired conversion of pregnenolone and 17-hydroxypregnenolone to progesterone and 17-hydroxyprogesterone, respectively. Additionally, the conversion of dehydroepiandrosterone to androstenedione and of androstendiol to testosterone is impaired. The result is mild masculinization of the genetic female and feminization of the genetic male. Males may demonstrate poor virilization and the development of gynecomastia at puberty.

As with 21-hydroxylase deficiency, impaired glucocorticoid production results in increased ACTH stimulation of the adrenals and hyperplasia. Impaired mineralocorticoid production results in salt wasting, hyponatremia, and volume contraction. Again, this defect is potentially life-threatening in the newborn period. Non–salt-losing, mild, and late-onset forms of this disease are described. Elevated serum 17-hydroxypregnenolone and dehydroepiandrosterone, as well as their urinary metabolites, dehydroepiandrostendione sulfate and 17-ketosteroids, are characteristic.

Figure 95-14 outlines the characteristic findings with the side-chain cleavage defect. This abnormality, also known as

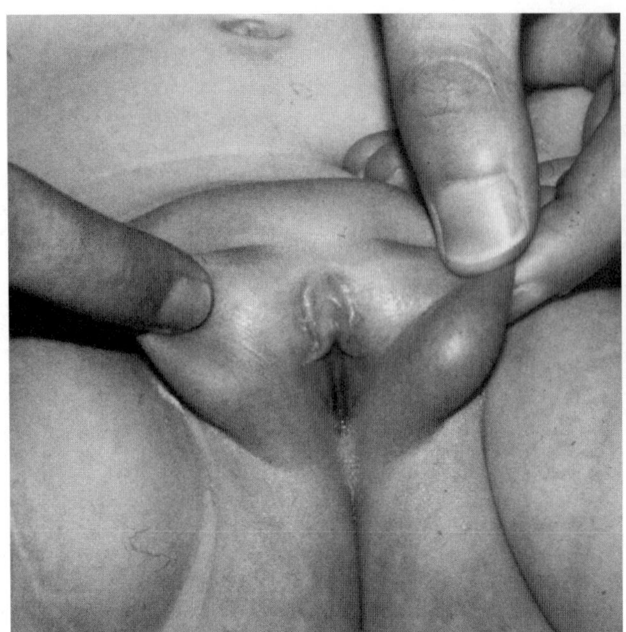

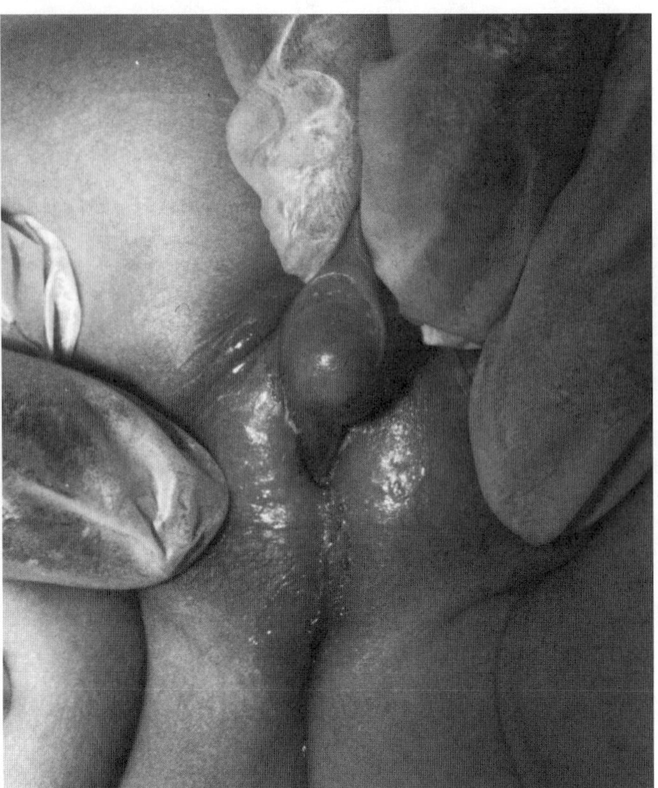

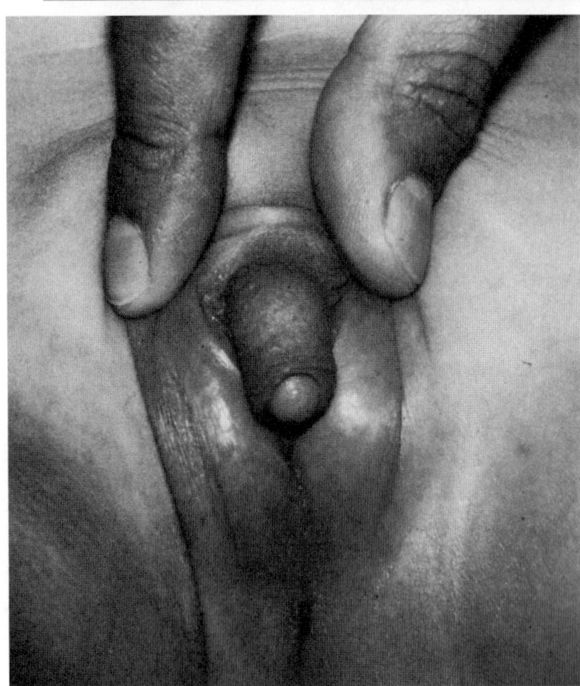

FIG. 95-12. Spectrum of abnormalities encountered with 46,XX congenital adrenal hyperplasia due to 21-hydroxylase deficiency.

lipoid adrenal hyperplasia and 17,20-desmolase deficiency, is due to a defect of the enzymatic complex that results in the conversion of cholesterol to pregnenolone. Recent data have raised questions as to whether an abnormality in the P450$_{SCC}$ side-chain cleavage enzyme is truly responsible for this disease.[65] These patients have severe deficiencies in glucocorticoid and mineralocorticoid activity and diminished levels of multiple steroid compounds. The enzyme is encoded by a gene on chro-

mosome 15, and again autosomal recessive inheritance is noted. Females have normal internal and external genital tracts, whereas males are often severely feminized, with female external genitalia and a blindly ending vaginal pouch. Secondary sexual characteristics of puberty are severely blunted in both sexes.

Another cause of congenital adrenal hyperplasia is *17α-hydroxylase deficiency* (Fig. 95-15). The deficiency of this en-

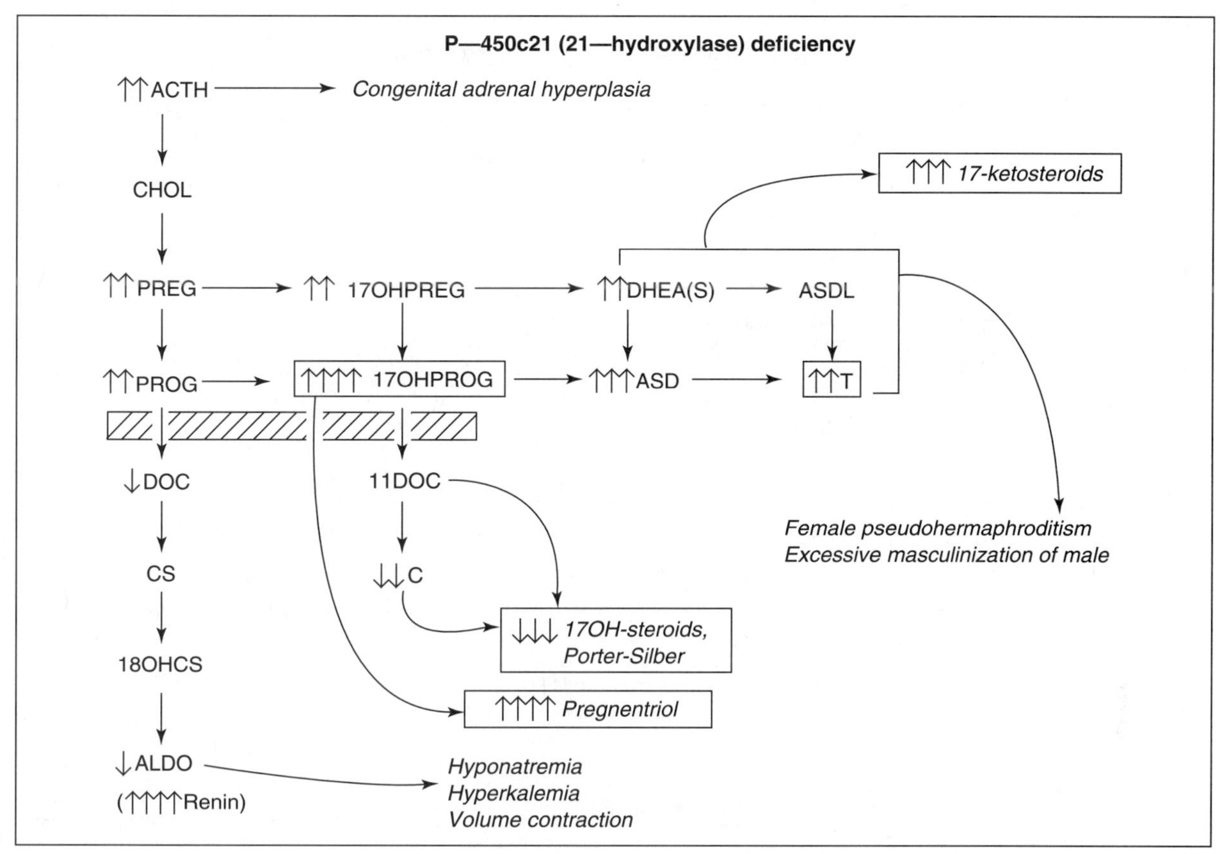

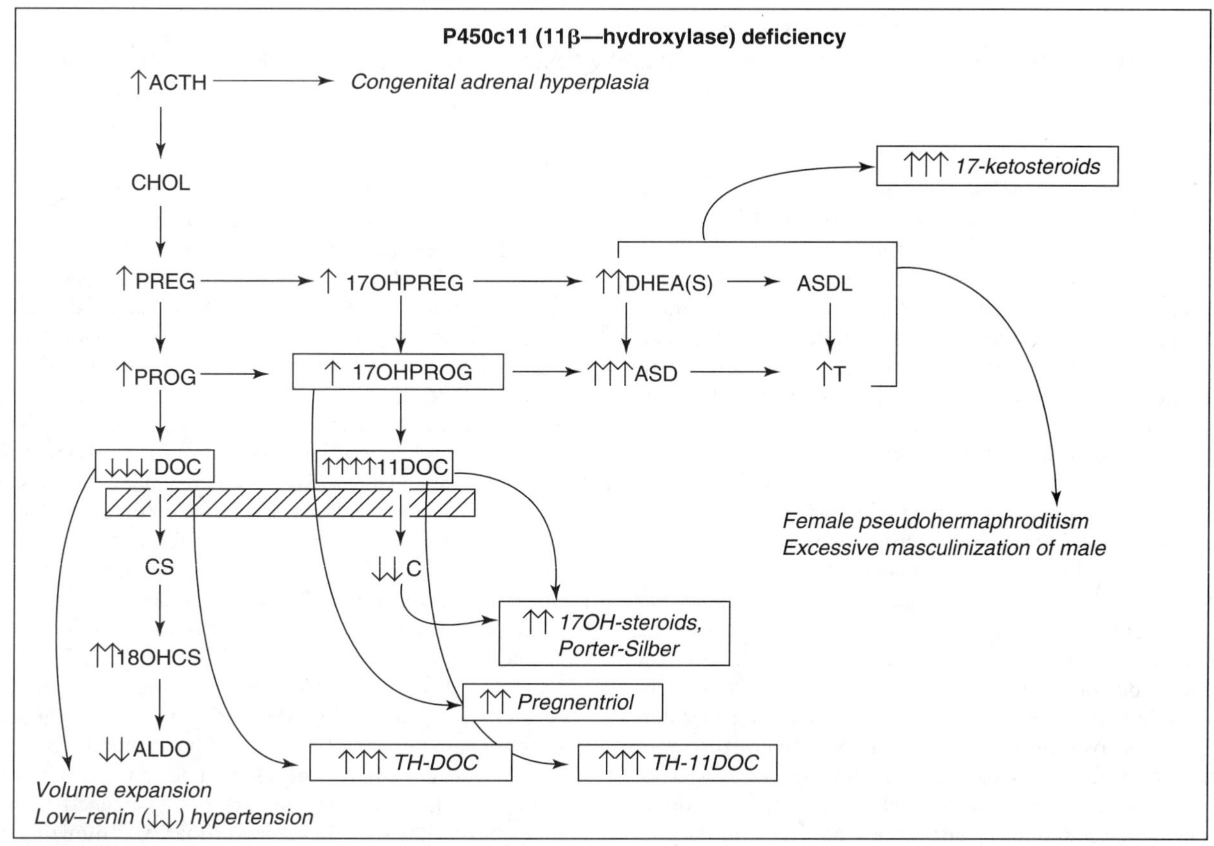

FIG. 95-13. (*A*) Consequences of 21α-hydroxylase deficiency. (*B*) Consequences of 11β-hydroxylase deficiency. (*continued*)

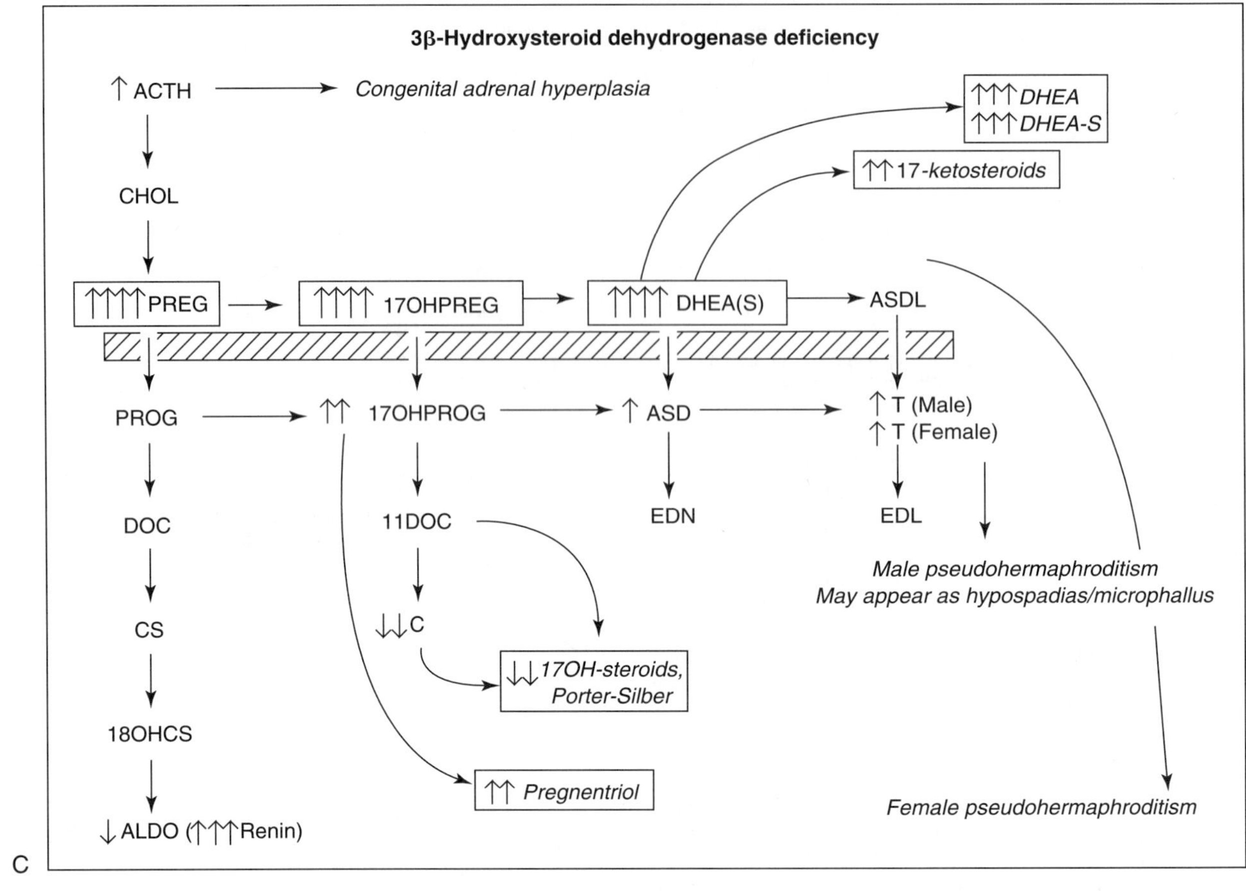

FIG. 95-13. *Continued.* (*C*) Consequences of 3β-hydroxysteroid dehydrogenase deficiency. (See also Fig. 95-11 and text.)

zyme, encoded by a gene on chromosome 10, results in impaired conversion of pregnenolone and progesterone to 17-hydroxy-pregnenolone and 17-hydroxyprogesterone, respectively. Deficient cortisol production results in excessive ACTH stimulation and resultant adrenal hyperplasia. Note, however, that mineralocorticoid production is elevated, and accumulation of mineralocorticoid precursors are identifiable. These individuals experience volume expansion and low-renin hypertension. Females exhibit sexual infantilism, whereas males are often severely feminized, even appearing to have normal female external genitalia.

The conversion of 17-hydroxypregnenolone and 17-hydroxy-progesterone to dehydroepiandrosterone and androstenedione, respectively (*17,20-lyase* activity) is mediated by the same enzyme that provides 17α-hydroxylase activity. Both activities are therefore inherited in an autosomal recessive pattern. Mutations in the *P-450*$_{C17}$ gene may cause either 17,20-lyase deficiency alone or in combination with 17α-hydroxylase deficiency. As demonstrated in Figure 95-16, 17-hydroxyprogesterone and 17-hydroxypregnenolone are elevated, while the serum testosterone level as well as those of dihydroepiandrosterone and androstenedione are depressed. Note that cortisol production is not impaired, and congenital adrenal hyperplasia does not occur. Female sexual infantilism and male pseudohermaphroditism are characteristic.

Figure 95-17 depicts the biochemical changes associated with

17β-hydroxysteroid oxidoreductase deficiency. Here, conversion of dehydroepiandrosterone and androstenedione to androstendiol and testosterone, respectively, is impaired. The result is increased levels of androstenedione and estrone, while levels of testosterone and estradiol are depressed. Clinically, males appear as highly feminized male pseudohermaphrodites.

The biochemical changes associated with *P-450* aromatase deficiency are outlined in Figure 95-18. This defect is associated with marked impairment in estrogen production by the fetoplacental unit and subsequent virilization of the female fetus.

In summary (Table 95-2), five enzymatic deficiencies may result in congenital adrenal hyperplasia, of which two are primarily virilizing, two are primarily feminizing, and one may have mixed effects on phenotypic expression. Three may present with salt wasting and vascular collapse, whereas two tend to cause salt retention and hypertension.

One type of congenital adrenal hyperplasia, side-chain cleavage deficiency, results in markedly enlarged adrenals with lipid density radiographically. Radiographically enlarged adrenals are not characteristic of the other four forms of adrenal hyperplasia, but a cerebriform ultrasound pattern has been described.[66] Three deficiencies are not associated with adrenal hyperplasia. Two of these are primarily feminizing and one primarily virilizing. Figure 95-19 demonstrates the relative frequencies of enzymatic deficiencies associated with congenital adrenal hyperplasia.

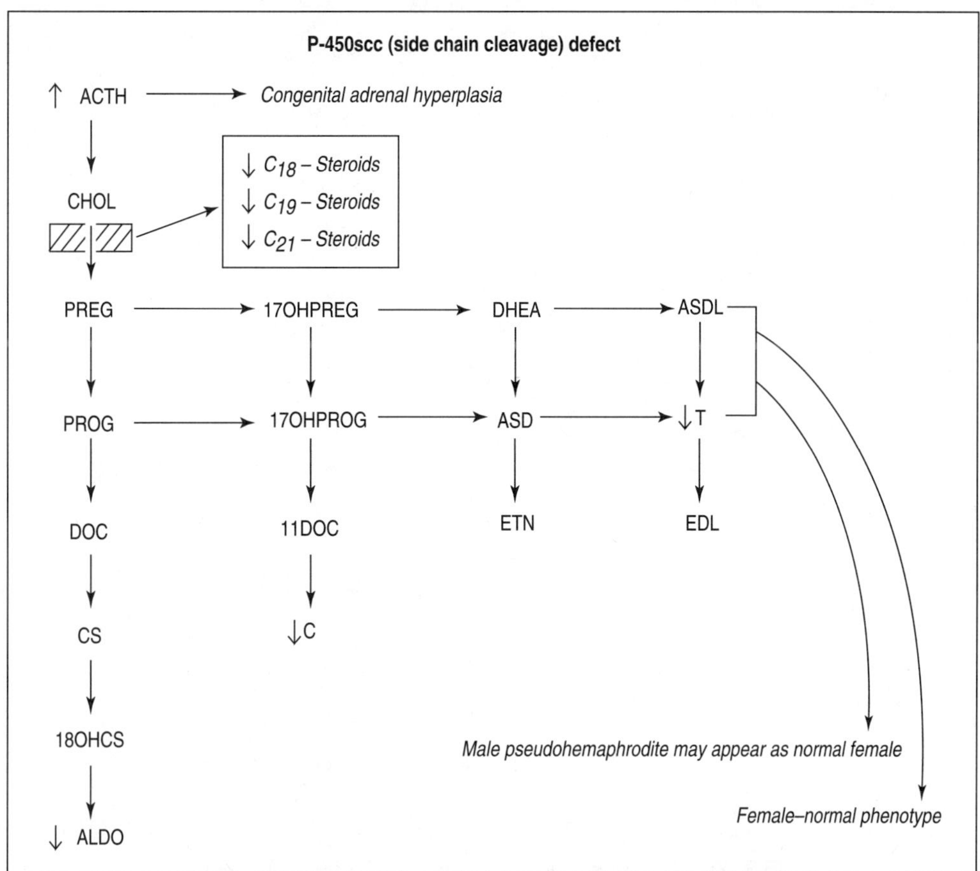

FIG. 95-14. Consequences of cholesterol desmolase (side chain cleavage) deficiency.

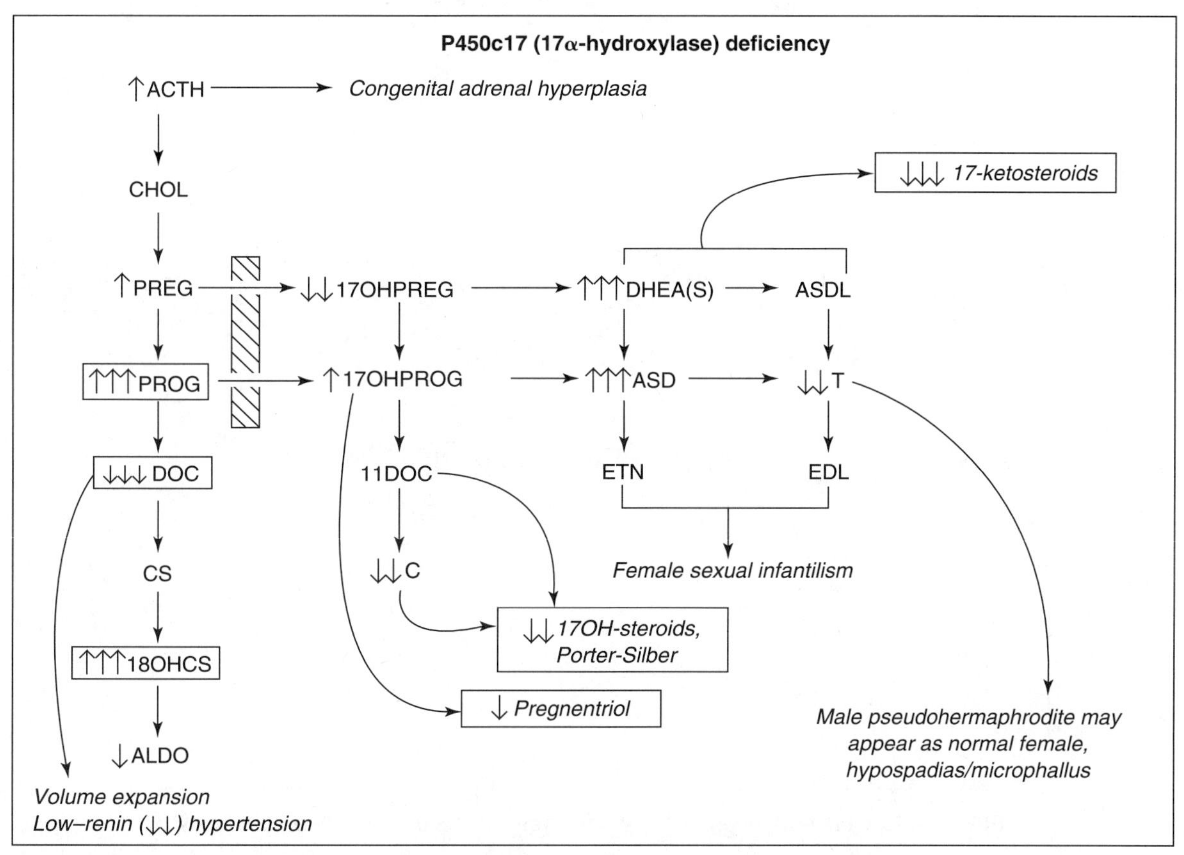

FIG. 95-15. Consequences of 17α-hydroxylase deficiency.

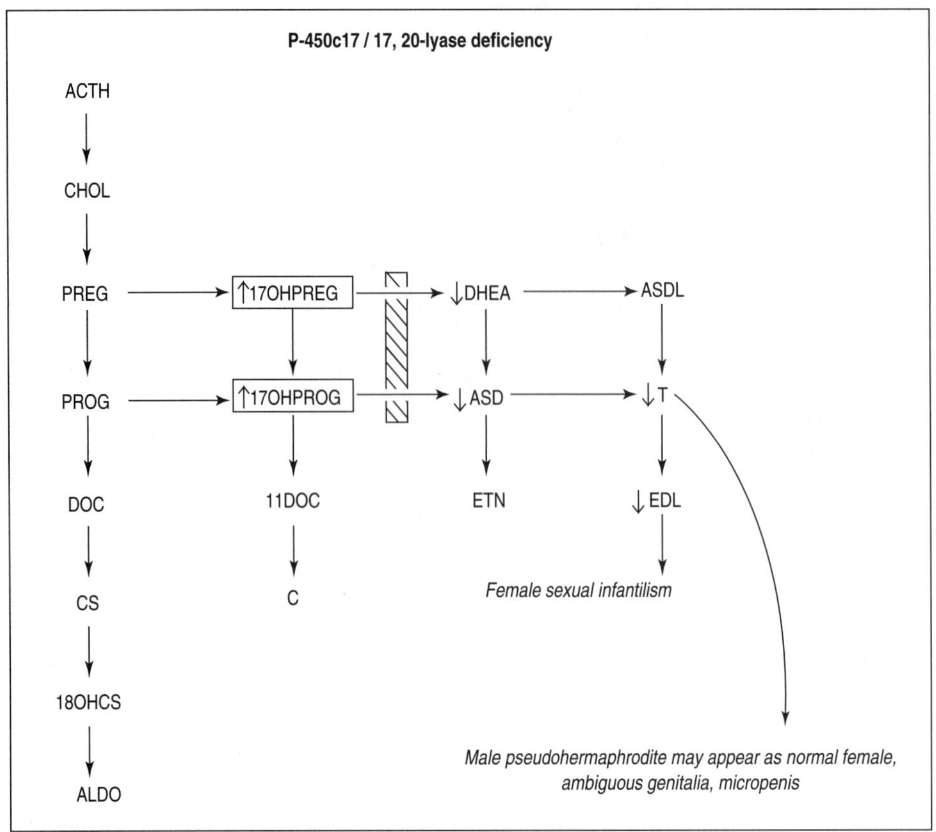

FIG. 95-16. Consequences of 17–20-lyase deficiency.

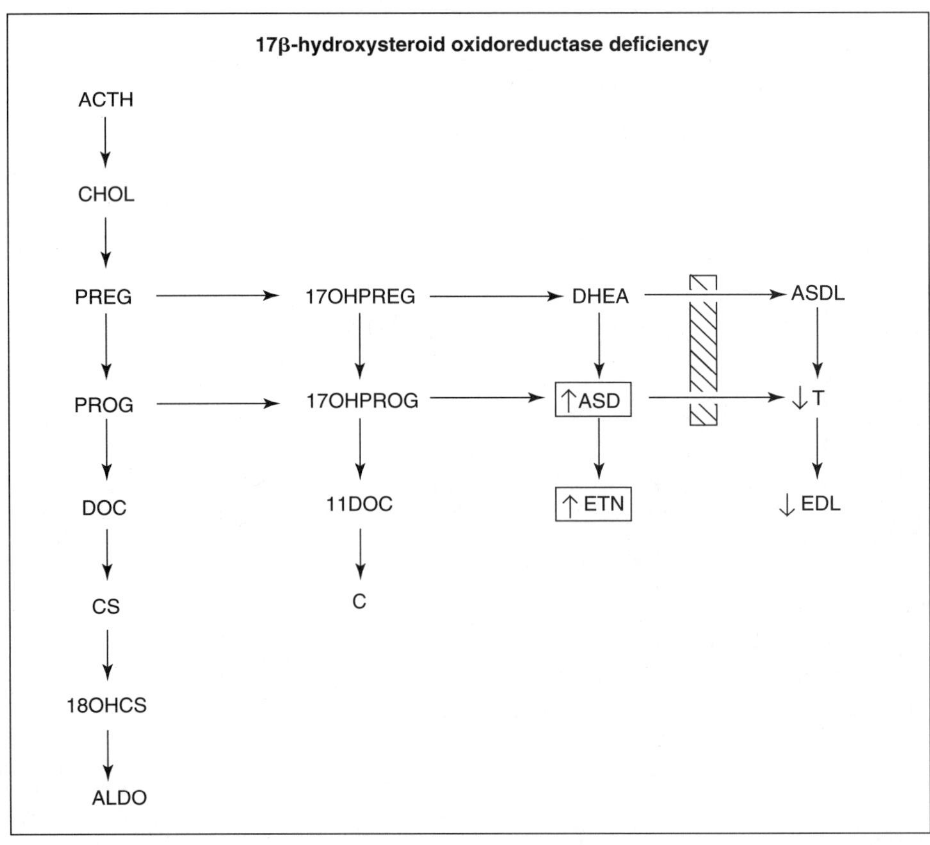

FIG. 95-17. Consequences of 17β-hydroxysteroid oxidoreductase deficiency.

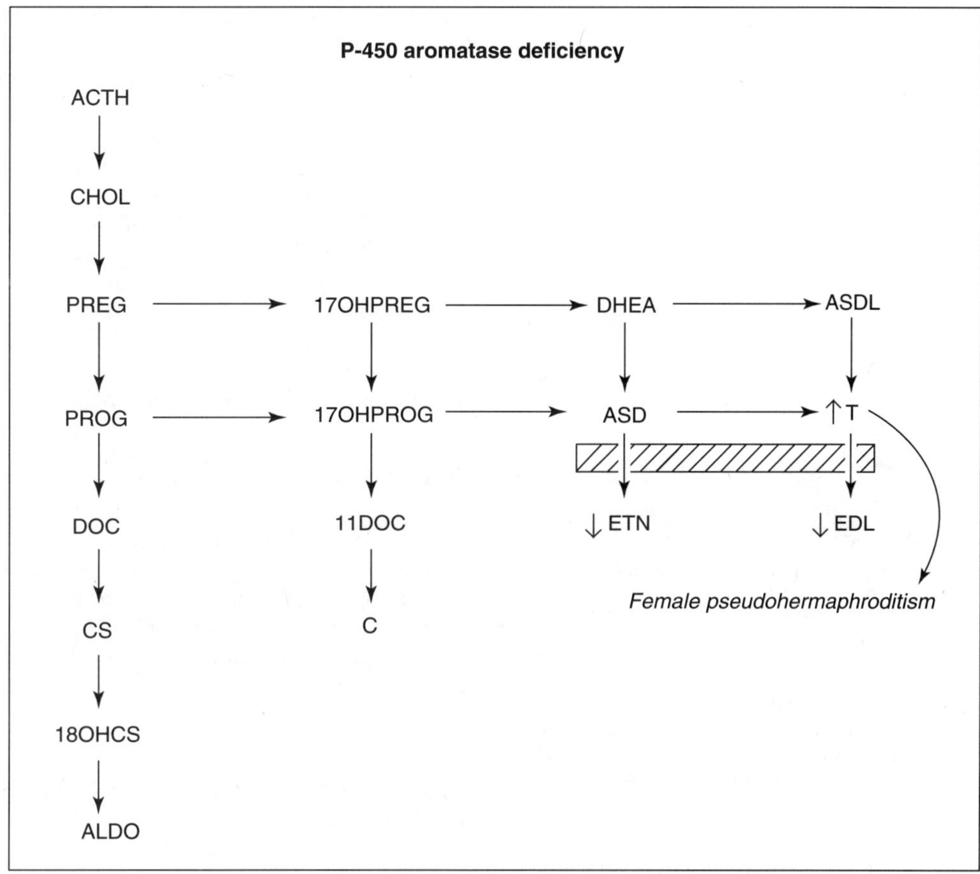

FIG. 95-18. Consequences of P-450 aromatase deficiency.

Five defects in steroid biosynthesis are associated with male pseudohermaphroditism, of which three (3β-hydroxysteroid dehydrogenase deficiency, side-chain cleavage deficiency, and 17α-hydroxylase deficiency) are associated with adrenal hyperplasia, and two (17,20-lyase and 17β-hydroxysteroid oxidoreductase deficiencies) are not.

CLASSIFICATION

An organized approach to classification of intersex anomalies is essential for effective application of diagnostic and therapeutic modalities. Patients may be classified according to the etiology of the anomaly, clinical presentation, or need for surgical

TABLE 95-2. *Defects in steroid biosynthesis*

Category	Phenotypic effect	Enzymatic defect
Congenital adrenal hyperplasia	Virilizing	21α-hydroxylase
	Virilizing	11β-hydroxylase
	Mixed	3β-hydroxysteroid dehydrogenase
	Feminizing	Side-chain cleavage
	Feminizing	17α-hydroxylase
Salt-wasting syndrome	Virilizing	21α-hydroxylase
	Mixed	3β-hydroxysteroid dehydrogenase
	Feminizing	Side-chain cleavage
Salt retention, hypertension	Virilizing	11β-hydroxylase
	Feminizing	17α-hydroxylase
No adrenal hyperplasia	Feminizing	17,20-lyase
	Feminizing	17β-hydroxysteroid oxidoreductase
	Virilizing	Aromatase

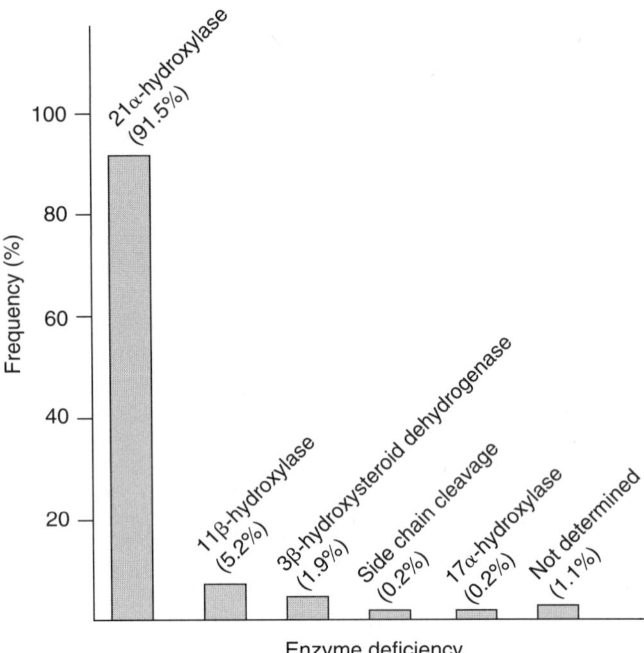

FIG. 95-19. Relative frequencies of enzymatic deficiencies associated with congenital adrenal hyperplasia. (Bois E, Mornet E, Chompret A, et al. L'hyperplasie congénitale des surrénales (21-OH) en France. Arch Fr Pediatr 1985;42:175.)

intervention. Table 95-3 presents a typical, inclusive approach to classification, which incorporates diagnoses in neonates with ambiguous genitalia and also diagnoses in children born with unambiguous genitalia. In the latter instance, individuals often have other somatic abnormalities or may appear quite normal until a problem arises at an older age for which therapy is sought. Not all these diagnoses benefit from surgical intervention.

Indications for Diagnostic Evaluation

The surgeon must maintain a high index of suspicion for disorders of sexual differentiation, because failure to establish a diagnosis may result in a lost opportunity to provide genetic counseling, prevent malignancy, prevent inappropriate virilization at puberty, and prevent medical crisis from steroid metabolic abnormalities. Clearly, all neonates with ambiguous genitalia require complete diagnostic evaluation. Diagnostic evaluation is also indicated in the presence of any salt-wasting syndrome, especially if associated with abnormal genitalia. Any degree of hypospadias associated with any degree of cryptorchidism requires a karyotype, as does bilateral nonpalpable testes. Micropenis with or without hypospadias requires evaluation of karyotype and hormonal profile. A palpable mass in the inguinal canal or the labia majora in phenotypic females must be evaluated to ensure that a testis is not present.

Older children requiring diagnostic evaluation include those presenting with stigmata of Turner syndrome, primary amenorrhea, and sexual infantilism. Unexplained virilization in females and gynecomastia in males (especially if bilateral and associated with testicular atrophy) require diagnostic evaluation as well.

SURGICAL CONSIDERATIONS

Of greatest importance to the surgeon are those instances where surgical intervention is anticipated. Such intervention is critical to patient management not only from a reconstructive perspective but also for diagnostic purposes. This is particularly true from the perspective of sexual assignment for ambiguous genitalia, because the ability to surgically achieve unambiguous and functional genitalia is the fundamental criterion for sex assignment. Table 95-4 outlines the most common reasons for which individuals with intersex states may be seen by surgeons. Surgical involvement may include pediatric surgeons, pediatric urologists, adult urologists, and gynecologists. Consequently, an awareness of these entities is crucial for all such individuals.

AMBIGUOUS GENITALIA

Table 95-5 outlines a diagnostic classification framework for patients with ambiguous genitalia. Similarly, Table 95-6 provides a conceptual framework for the diagnosis of children with anomalous sexual development but with unambiguous genitalia. A great deal of information can be attained simply by addressing the karyotype and the nature of the gonads and internal ductal systems.

Masculinization of the Genetic Female (Female Pseudohermaphroditism)

Female pseudohermaphroditism is characterized by a 46,XX karyotype and by the presence of ovaries and müllerian ductal structures bilaterally. Most cases are due to congenital virilizing adrenal hyperplasia. Occasionally, masculinization of the female fetus may be due to maternal androgen-producing ovarian or adrenal tumors, a luteoma of pregnancy, or arrhenoblastoma. Iatrogenic causes are primarily due to exogenous administration of hormonal agents during pregnancy, such as testosterone, danazol, methylandrostenediol, norethindrone, ethisterone, norethynodrel, methoxyprogesterone, and 6a-methyltestosterone.

Congenital adrenal hyperplasia accounts for approximately half of patients presenting with ambiguous genitalia, and over 90% of cases of congenital adrenal hyperplasia are due to 21α-hydroxylase deficiency (see Fig. 95-19). Genetic females with ambiguous genitalia secondary to either congenital adrenal hyperplasia or exogenous androgenic compounds should be given a female gender assignment and undergo feminine reconstruction, because they have the potential for both normal sexual function and fertility.

Although only surgical therapy is required for exogenous virilization, medical therapy assumes great importance in cases of congenital adrenal hyperplasia. Treatment is directed at correcting cortisol deficiency and suppressing the overproduction of adrenal androgens. Careful monitoring of therapy is essential to avoid the adverse effects of excessive glucocorticoid therapy (diminished growth, short stature, obesity) and insufficient therapy (adrenal crisis with stress, pituitary hyperplasia–Nelson's syndrome, and adrenal carcinoma in both males and females; menstrual pathology, hirsutism, acne, and polycystic ovarian disease in females; and hypertrophied adrenal rests simulating testis tumors in males).

TABLE 95-3. *Classification of anomalous sexual development*

I. Disorders of Gonadal Differentiation
  A. Seminiferous tubular dysgenesis (Klinefelter syndrome)
  B. Syndrome of gonadal dysgenesis and its variants (Turner syndrome)
  C. Complete and incomplete forms of 46,XX and 46XY gonadal dysgenesis
  D. True hermaphroditism
II. Female Pseudohermaphroditism
  A. Congenital virilizing adrenal hyperplasia
  B. *P-450* aromatase (placental deficiency)
  C. Androgens and synthetic progestogens transferred from maternal circulation
  D. Associated with malformations of intestine and urinary tract (non–androgen-induced female pseudohermaphroditism)
  E. Other teratologic factors
III. Male Pseudohermaphroditism
  A. Testicular unresponsiveness to hCG and LH (Leydig cell agenesis or hypoplasia)
  B. Inborn errors of testosterone biosynthesis
    1. Enzyme defects affecting synthesis of both corticosteroids and testosterone (variants of congenital adrenal hyperplasia)
      a. $P\text{-}450_{scc}$ (cholesterol side-chain cleavage) deficiency (20–22 desmolase deficiency, congenital lipoid adrenal hyperplasia)
      b. 3β-Hydroxysteroid dehydrogenase deficiency
      c. $P\text{-}450_{c17}$ 17α-hydroxylase) deficiency
    2. Enzyme defects primarily affecting testosterone biosynthesis by testes
      a. $P\text{-}450_{c17}$ (17,20-lyase) deficiency
      b. 17β-hydroxysteroid oxidoreductase deficiency
  C. Defects in androgen-dependent target tissues
    1. End-organ resistance to androgenic hormones (androgen receptor and postreceptor defects)
      a. Syndrome of complete androgen resistance and its variants (testicular feminization and its variant forms)
      b. Syndrome of partial androgen resistance and its variants (Reifenstein syndrome)
      c. Androgen resistance in infertile men
      d. Androgen resistance in fertile men
    2. Defects in testosterone metabolism by peripheral tissues: 5α-reductase deficiency, pseudovaginal perineoscrotal hypospadias
  D. Dysgenetic male pseudohermaphroditism
    1. X chromatin—negative variants of syndrome of gonadal dysgenesis (e.g., 45,X/46,XY,46,XYp-)
    2. Incomplete forms of XY gonadal dysgenesis
    3. Associated with degenerative renal disease
    4. "Vanishing testes" (embryonic testicular regression syndrome; 46,XY agonadism; 46,XY gonadal agenesis; rudimentary testes; anorchia)
  E. Defects in synthesis, secretion, or response to AMH
    1. Female genital ducts in otherwise normal men—herniae uteri inguinale; persistent müllerian duct syndrome
  F. Maternal ingestion of progestogens
IV. Unclassified Forms of Abnormal Sexual Development
  A. Hypospadias/cryptorchidism
  B. Ambiguous external genitalia in patients with multiple congenital anomalies
    a. Cloacal exstrophy
    b. Fetal trimethadone or hydantoin effects
    c. Fraser syndrome
    d. Reiger syndrome
    e. Ectodermal dysplasia
    f. Robinow syndrome
    g. Smith-Lemili-Opitz syndrome
    h. Aarskog syndrome
    i. De Lange syndrome
    j. Chromosomal anomalies: 9q, 10q, 13q, 18q, 20q
  C. Absence or anomalous development of vagina, uterus, and fallopian tubes (Mayer-Rokitansky-Küster-Hauser syndrome)

(Grumbach MM, Conte FA. Disorder of sex differentiation. In: Wilson DJ, Foster DW, eds. Williams textbook of endocrinology. Philadelphia, WB Saunders, 1992:853; Rappaport R, Forest MG. Disorders of sexual differentiation. In: Bertrand J, Rappaport R, Sizonenko PC, eds. Pediatric endocrinology. Baltimore, Williams & Wilkins, 1993:447.)

Medical management of 21-hydroxylase deficiency has been extensively reviewed.[2,67] Neonatal management consists of volume and sodium resuscitation and administration of glucocorticoid in the form of hydrocortisone sodium succinate. Following resuscitation, maintenance steroid therapy is begun. Often, this takes the form of hydrocortisone, 12 to 20 mg/m^2/d, divided into three oral doses. Patients with salt-wasting forms of congenital adrenal hyperplasia receive mineralocorticoid supplementation in the form of fluorocortisone, 70 to 90 μg/m^2/d orally. Glucocorticoid therapy is monitored by serum 17-hydroxyprogesterone, androstendione, and testosterone levels and by urinary pregnentriol (21α-hydroxylase deficiency). Mineralocorticoid levels are monitored by plasma renin activity.

These pharmacologic concepts are prudent to the surgeon. Elective surgery should not be undertaken unless adequate glucocorticoid suppression has been achieved. Additionally, increased dosages of glucocorticoids are required in the periopera-tive period (Table 95-7). A similar increase in dosage is required for emergent surgical or nonsurgical stress. Note that even in the absence of stress, during periods where oral intake is impossible or unreliable, parenteral therapy is needed. Table 95-8 outlines the dosage equivalents for various glucocorticoid preparations.

Surgical reconstruction in the form of feminizing genitoplasty is undertaken at 6 to 12 months of life. Best results are obtained when clitoroplasty and vaginoplasty are combined as a single-staged reconstruction. Surgical outcome plays a critical role in terms of patient well-being. This fact is emphasized by the observations of Mulaikal and colleagues,[68] who reported a 75% incidence of homosexual, bisexual, or absent sexual activity in women who had an inadequate introitus, as opposed to a 25% incidence in those whose introitus was adequate. Reduction clitoroplasty is preferred over clitorectomy in order to preserve clitoral sensation and is also preferred over clitoral

TABLE 95-4. *Reasons for seeking pediatric surgical specialist involvment*

I. Ambiguous Genitalia
II. Hernia as an Isolated Clinical Finding
    A. Female: Testicular feminization, Leydig cell agenesis
    B. Male: Herniae uteri inguinale
III. Hypospadias, Cryptorchidism
IV. Micropenis
    A. Real
    B. Apparent
        1. True concealed penis
        2. Obesity
V. Need for Orchiectomy
    A. To prevent virilization with female sexual assignment
        1. True hermaphroditism
        2. Male pseudohermaphroditism
    B. To prevent or treat malignancy
        1. Mixed (46,X/XY) gonadal dysgenesis
        2. Testicular feminization
        3. Pure 46,XY gonadal dysgenesis
        4. Dysgenetic male pseudohermaphroditism
        5. True hermaphroditism
VI. Evaluation of Scrotal Mass
    A. Gonadal malignancy
        1. Germ cell
        2. Non–germ cell
    B. Hypertrophied adrenal rests from congenital adrenal hyperplasia
VII. Evaluation of Mass in Inguinal Canal or Labia of Female
VIII. Gynecomastia
IX. Need for Masculine Reconstruction
X. Need for Feminine Reconstruction

recession because it avoids the potential for uncomfortable erection, as is seen when recession techniques are employed.

True Hermaphroditism

True hermaphroditism is a relatively uncommon disorder of sexual development. Its presentation is quite variable, ranging from an unambiguous neonatal female phenotype to what appears to be a male with hypospadias. Although the majority have ambiguous genitalia, most are quite virilized. Common presentations are cryptorchidism with hypospadias and hernia.

Patients with true hermaphroditism have by definition both ovarian and testicular tissue. Approximately 60% of patients have a 46,XX karyotype, followed by 46,XX/46,XY and 46,XY karyotypes, which represent 13% and 12% of individuals, respectively.[69] Proposed mechanisms include mosaicism (mitotic or meiotic errors), chimerism (double fertilization, fusion, etc), and translocation of Y chromosomal material to an autosome or to the X chromosome.

The key to the clinical diagnosis and management of true hermaphroditism is the gonad. Several caveats regarding the gonads of these individuals are critical. As depicted in Figure 95-20*A* the most common gonad in true hermaphroditism is the ovotestis. However, there is important variation with respect to the side of occurrence. On the right, the ovotestis clearly predominates. On the left, the incidence of an ovary actually slightly exceeds that of the ovotestis. The ovary is generally encountered in the pelvis, although it may rarely be encountered in the inguinal canal in the presence of a significant inguinal hernia. Half of ovotestes are intraabdominal, with the remainder

TABLE 95-5. *Classification of commonly encountered ambiguous genitalia*

Category	Gonad	Internal ducts	Karyotype	Diagnosis

Female PsH	O-O	M-M	46,XX	Congenital adrenal hyperplasia
				   21α-hydroxylase deficiency
				   11β-hydroxylase deficiency
				   3β-hydroxysteroid dehydrogenase deficiency
				Transfer of maternal androgens
				   Maternal ingestion
				   Androgen-producing neoplasms

True hermaphroditism	O-T OT-T OT-O OT-OT	M-W M/W-W M/W-M M/W-M/W	46, XX 46,XX/46,XY 46,XY	True hermaphroditism

Male PsH	T-T	W-W	46,XY	Incomplete androgen insensitivity
				5α-reductase deficiency
				Defects in androgen synthesis
				   Side chain cleavage deficiency
				   3β-hydroxysteroid dehydrogenase deficiency
				   17α-hydroxylase deficiency
				   17,20-lyase deficiency
				   17β-hydroxysteroid oxidoreductase deficiency

Primary gonadal disorders	T-S X-X DT-DT	W-M/W X-X M-M	45,X/46,XY 46,XY 46,XY	Mixed gonadal dysgenesis Embryonic testicular regression Dysgenetic male pseudohermaphroditism

PsH, pseudohermaphrodite; O, ovary; T, testis; OT, ovotestis; S, streak; DT, dysgenetic testis; X, absent, M, müllerian; W, wolffian.

TABLE 95-6. *Diagnosis of intersexuality in children despite unambiguous genitalia*

External genitalia	Palpable gonads	Karyotype	Diagnosis	Symptoms, neonate	Symptoms, childhood
Female	Yes (+/−)	46,XY	Testicular feminization	Inguinal hernia	Primary amenorrhea
	Yes (+/−)	46,XY	Leydig cell agenesis	Inguinal hernia	Pubertal failure
	Yes (+/−)	46,XY	17β-hydroxysteroid oxidoreductase deficiency		Virilization, primary amenorrhea, ± gynecomastia
	Yes (+/−)	46,XY	Side chain cleavage	Salt wasting	Pubertal failure
	Yes (+/−)	46,XY	17α-hyroxylase deficiency		HTN, primary amenorrhea ± gynecomastia, sexual infantilism
	Yes (+/−)	46,XY	17,20-lyase		Sexual infantilism
	No	45,X	Turner syndrome	Lymphedema	Short stature, pubertal failure
	No	XX or XY	Pure GD		Pubertal failure
Male	Yes	46,XY	Persistent müllerian duct	Inguinal hernia	Inguinal hernia
	No	46,XX	21α-hydroxylase	Salt wasting, hypospadias	Virilization, hematuria
	No	46,XX	11β-hydroxylase	Hypertension, hypospadias	Virilization, hematuria
	Yes (+/−)	46,XX, etc	True hermaphroditism	Micropenis, hypospadias	Virilization, gynecomastia
	Yes	46,XX	XX male syndrome		Atretic testes infertility

GD, gonadal dysfunction; HTN hypertension.
(Rappaport R, Forest MG. Disorders of sexual differentiation. In: Bertrand J, Rappaport R, Sizonenko PC, eds. Pediatric endocrinology. Baltimore, Williams & Wilkins, 1993:447.)

approximately equally distributed between the inguinal canal and the labioscrotal fold. In contrast, a testis is most commonly encountered in the labioscrotal fold and relatively uncommonly (22%) in an intraabdominal position. These relationships are outlined in Figure 95-20*B*.

As demonstrated in Figure 95-21, there is a relationship between the karyotype and gonadal distribution. In the presence of a Y chromosome, the incidence of a testis, ovotestis, and ovary is 61%, 52%, and 68%, respectively. In contrast, in the absence of a Y chromosome, the relative incidences are 29%, 80%, and 56%. Among individuals with a 46,XX karyotype, the diagnostic gonad present is either an ovotestis (80%) or a testis with a contralateral ovary (20%). Of individuals with a

46,XX/46,XY karyotype, 60% have an ovotestis and 40% a testis with contralateral ovary. Of patients with a 46,XY karyotype, 46% have an ovotestis and 54% a testis with contralateral ovary. Other reported karyotypes are 46,XY/47,XXY (5.6%), 45,X/46,XY (3.5%), and other (6.2%).

As would be expected, the internal ducts are determined by the character of the ipsilateral gonad. Müllerian development is generally observed in the presence of either an ovary or ovotestis, whereas wolffian development is usually encountered in the presence of a testis. The majority of individuals have significant müllerian elements, a fact that has significant therapeutic implications.

From a diagnostic perspective, short of gonadal biopsy, those findings most suggestive of true hermaphroditism are a

TABLE 95-7. *Glucocorticoid therapy guidelines for elective surgery in patients with congenital adrenal hyperplasia*

	Day	Agent	Dosage
Before surgery	−2	Cortisone acetate, hydrocortisone	20 mg/m^2 IM bid or 20 mg/m^2 PO tid
	−1	Cortisone acetate, hydrocortisone	20 mg/m^2 IM bid or 20 mg/m^2 PO tid
During surgery	0	Cortisone acetate, hydrocortisone	40 mg/m^2 IM bid IV as needed
After surgery	+1	Cortisone acetate, hydrocortisone	20 mg/m^2 IM bid or 20 mg/m^2 PO tid
	+2	Hydrocortisone	Maintenance if surgical stress over

(Modified from Morel Y, Bertrand J, Rappaport R. Disorders of hormonosynthesis. In: Bertrand J, Rappaport R, Sizonenko PC, eds. Pediatric endocrinology. Baltimore, Williams & Wilkins, 1993:305.)

TABLE 95-8. *Mean estimated optimal dose of glucocorticoid for growth in patients with congenital adrenal hyperplasia*

Glucocorticoid	Dosage mg/m^2/d	Equivalent dosage
Dexamethasone	0.23	1
Methylprednisolone	2.4	10
Prednisone	3.7	16
Hydrocortisone	18.4	80
Cortisone acetate (IM)	13.9	60
Cortisone acetate (PO)	22.0	96

(Grumbach MM, Conte FA. Disorders of sex differentiation. In: Wilson JD, Foster DW, eds. Williams textbook of endocrinology. Philadelphia, WB Saunders, 1992:853; Mulaikal RM, Migeon CJ, Rick JA. Fertility rates in female patients with congenital adrenal hyperplasia due to 21-hydroxylase deficiency. N Engl J Med 1987;316:178.)

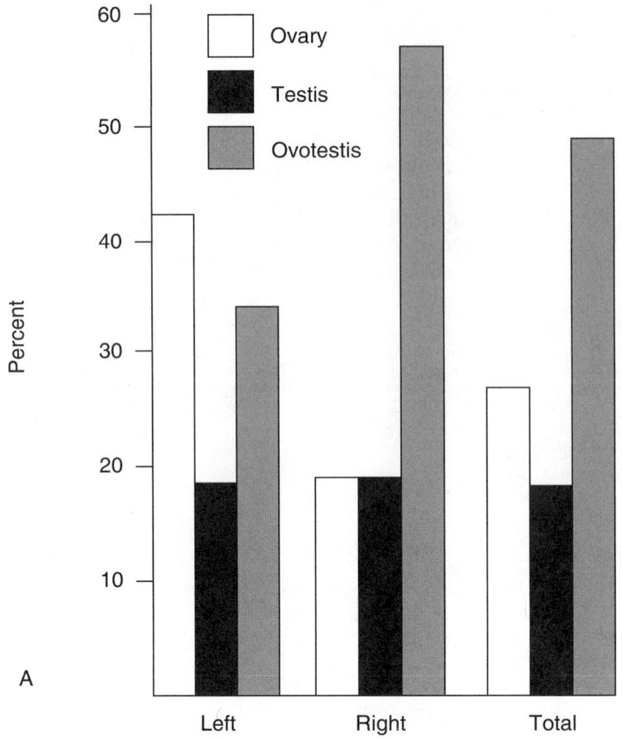

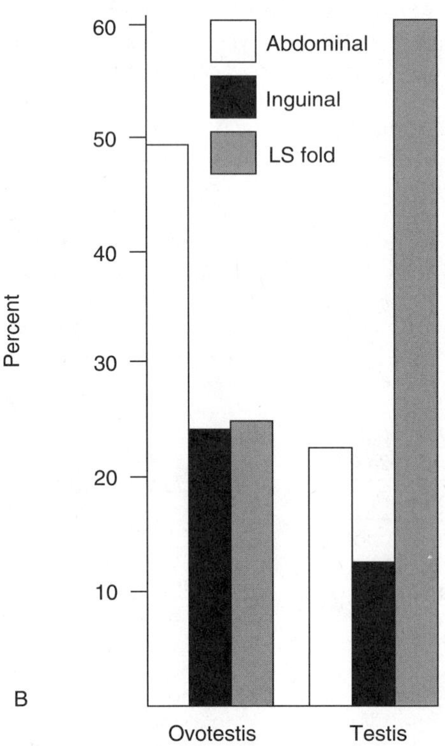

FIG. 95-20. (*A*) Relative incidence of gonads encountered in true hermaphroditism. (*B*) Position of ovotestes and testes in true hermaphroditism.

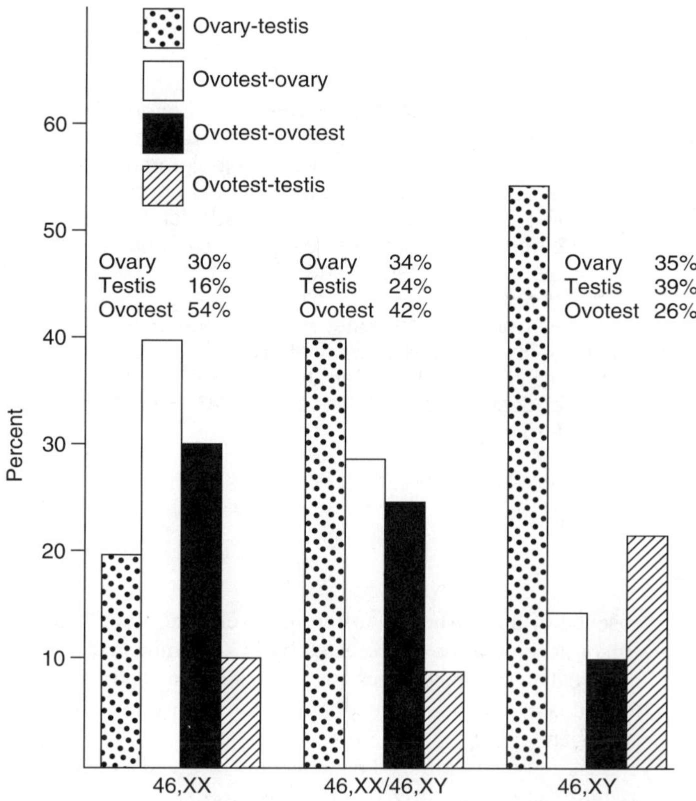

FIG. 95-21. Gonadal distribution as a function of karyotype in true hermaphroditism.

46,XX/46,XY karyotype; the palpation of an elongated, lobulated gonad; and an elevated testosterone level that rises with hCG stimulation in the face of a 46,XX karyotype. Also suspicious is the individual with hypospadias and an undescended testis who is found to have a 46,XX or 46,XX/46,XY karyotype.

Traditionally, the majority of patients have been given a masculine gender assignment, but recent data question the wisdom of this policy. In individuals raised as males, spermatogenesis is characteristically deficient. Additionally, at puberty, gynecomastia is not uncommon, and periodic hematuria (menstruation) may be encountered. In contrast, individuals raised as females may ovulate, become pregnant, and deliver normal offspring. The potential for transmission of the disorder to offspring is thought to be small. Because females may virilize at puberty, it is critical to remove all testicular tissue when this gender assignment is given. Clearly, prompt neonatal diagnosis is important.

Surgical management of such patients is determined by the sex of rearing, which in most cases should be female. Those with a male gender assignment require removal of ovarian tissue and müllerian remnants. Because the testicular component of the ovotestis is generally dysgenetic, the entire gonad is removed. Often testes in this setting are dysgenetic as well, and if documented to be so, should be removed. Testes that can achieve a scrotal position and do not demonstrate dysgenetic features by biopsy may be retained. Otherwise, a program of penile reconstruction, gonadectomy, testicular prosthesis placement, and hormonal replacement therapy appears most warranted. Patients given a female gender assignment must have all testicular tissue removed, including both testes and the testicular component of ovotestes.

Inadequate Masculinization of the Genetic Male (Male Pseudohermaphroditism)

As outlined in Table 95-3, male pseudohermaphroditism may be due to impaired testicular responsiveness to hCG and LH, inborn errors of testosterone biosynthesis, end-organ resistance to androgenic hormones, defects in testosterone metabolism, disorders of testicular development, and defects in the synthesis or secretion of or response to antimüllerian hormone. Many of these, however, do not result in genital ambiguity. Disorders of testicular development are discussed in a separate section. Characteristically, these patients have two testes and, with the exception of isolated antimüllerian hormone deficiency, müllerian elements are absent and wolffian ductal development is evident.

Inborn Errors of Testosterone Biosynthesis

Inborn errors of testosterone biosynthesis have been discussed in detail previously. While cholesterol side-chain cleavage, 3β-hydroxysteroid, 17α-hydroxylase, 17,20-lyase, and 17β-hydroxysteroid oxidoreductase deficiencies all cause incomplete masculinization of the genetic male, 3β-hydroxysteroid dehydrogenase is most likely to result in true genital ambiguity. Some defects such as 17α-hydroxylase, 17,20-lyase, and 17β-hydroxysteroid oxidoreductase deficiencies may result in ambiguous genitalia. However, these lesions usually result in primarily highly feminized individuals.

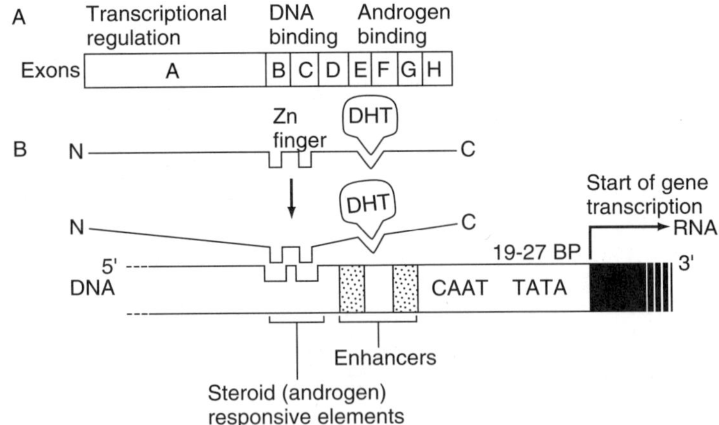

FIG. 95-22. (*A*) Diagrammatic representation of the androgen receptor gene divided into its nine exons. Exon A codes for the NH2-terminal domain and regulates transcription. Exons B and C code for two zinc fingers. Exons D through H code for the androgen-binding domain of the receptor. (*B*) Organization of a steroid-responsive gene. Ligand binding activates the receptor, which then binds to the steroid response elements of the gene, resulting in activation. (Grumbach MM, Conte FA. Disorder of sex differentiation. In: Wilson JD, Foster DW, eds. Williams textbook of endocrinology. Philadelphia, WB Saunders, 1992: 925.)

End-Organ Resistance to Androgenic Hormones

End-organ resistance may be complete (testicular feminization) or incomplete. Patients with complete androgen insensitivity generally present with normal-appearing female external genitalia. They tend to have inguinal hernias or palpable inguinal masses in early childhood or primary amenorrhea in adolescence. Characteristically, normal pubertal female body habitus changes, including breast development, are noted with puberty. Axillary and pubic hair is usually minimally developed or occasionally completely absent. Pelvic examination reveals a short, blind-ending vagina with no cervix. Patients with incomplete androgen insensitivity characteristically have ambiguous genitalia. These individuals have been previously referred to by a number of eponyms, including Reifenstein, Lubs, and Gilbert-Dreyfus.

Significant genetic heterogeneity exists within these patient populations. Androgen insensitivity may be due to defects either in androgen receptor quantity or quality, including affinity and lability. Figure 95-22 depicts the androgen receptor gene and the mechanism of action of its product. The molecular biology of this receptor has been reviewed in detail.[2] Pertinent points include the following: (1) the androgen receptor is encoded by a gene on the X chromosome, only 3% (8 exons) of which is actually translated; (2) the NH_2-terminal domain of the androgen receptor is encoded by exon A and is thought to have a transcriptional regulation function; (3) exons B and C code for 2 zinc fingers that are responsible for binding to DNA, with consequent stimulation of transcription of mRNA and translation of new protein, which then mediates androgenic effects; (4) this binding is made possible by a conformational alteration in the androgen receptor induced by DHT binding. These events are similar to other proteins in the steroid receptor superfamily. Both deletions and point mutations resulting in altered receptor function have been described.

Individuals with incomplete androgen insensitivity present with ambiguity (small hypospadic phallus and occasionally undescended testes) and a 46,XY karyotype. This condition is distinguished from disorders of testosterone biosynthesis by the absence of diminished testosterone levels and absence of precursor accumulation exacerbated by hCG administration. Supportive data include the measurement of diminished DHT binding capacity and a blunted clinical response to exogenous androgen.

Strikingly masculinized patients may be given a male gender assignment, particularly if a response to exogenous androgen can be demonstrated. Otherwise a feminine gender assignment would seem most appropriate. Individuals raised as males may develop gynecomastia at puberty, whereas those raised as females may experience some masculinization. Consequently, females should undergo early orchiectomy and should have estrogen replacement therapy at puberty.

Defects in Testosterone Metabolism

Deficiency of 5α-reductase activity is an unusual form of 46,XY male pseudohermaphroditism. It most typically presents with severe hypospadias involving a small phallus and the presence of a blind vaginal pouch that may open into a urogenital sinus or onto the perineum, hence the descriptive name *pseudovaginal perineoscrotal hypospadias*. Diagnosis is confirmed by the measurement of diminished 5α-reductase activity and is suggested by an elevated testosterone/DHT ratio and diminished basal and hCG-stimulated 5α/5β urinary steroid ratios.

As with incomplete androgen insensitivity, patients may be raised as males if they are heavily masculinized, particularly if the phallus is of adequate dimension and responds to DHT administration. Otherwise, a female gender assignment is most prudent. Because of a strong tendency toward masculinization with puberty, early orchiectomy is mandatory in females.

Disorders in Testicular Development

Syndromes associated with defective ovarian formation or persistence (eg, 45,X Turner syndrome, its karyotypic variants, and 46,XX pure gonadal dysgenesis) are associated with unambiguous female genitalia. In contrast, syndromes associated with defective testis formation or defective testicular persistence may result in ambiguous genitalia. Examples include mixed gonadal dysgenesis, dysgenetic male pseudohermaphroditism, and embryonic testicular regression syndromes. Some primary testicular defects such as Leydig cell agenesis and 46,XY pure gonadal dysgenesis result in a female phenotype, whereas others, such as congenital anorchia, result in an unambiguous male phenotype.

Mixed Gonadal Dysgenesis

Mixed gonadal dysgenesis is characterized by the presence of asymmetric ambiguous external genitalia, a streak gonad on one side with a testis on the other, and a 45,X/46,XY karyotype. Often the testis is dysgenetic, and, as a result, internal ducts may be müllerian on both sides. If the testis is not dysgenetic, ductal development may be müllerian on one side and wolffian on the other.

The tremendous phenotypic variation associated with this syndrome may result in a female presentation with clitoral hypertrophy or a male with hypospadias accompanied by cryptorchidism. In addition to a relatively characteristic karyotype, such clinical clues as the presence of Ullrich-Turner stigmata (facial asymmetry, high palate, low hairline, webbed neck, short metacarpus, multiple nevi) may aid in diagnosis. Testosterone levels tend to be depressed, with elevated LH and FSH levels.

An important clinical correlate of mixed gonadal dysgenesis is the high incidence of gonadoblastoma seen in these individuals, making its diagnosis very important. A confounding observation, however, is that this syndrome may be associated with other mosaic karyotypes and even a 46,XY karyotype. In the latter circumstance, presumably 45,X cell lines occur in low proportion and are consequently undetected.

The preferred sex assignment is female. However, heavily masculinized individuals may be raised as male, provided the testis is scrotal (available for palpation) and not dysgenetic on biopsy. Streak gonads are removed, as are dysgenetic testes, regardless of the sex of rearing. Bilateral orchiectomy is performed in all individuals raised as females.

Dysgenetic Male Pseudohermaphroditism

The category of dysgenetic male pseudohermaphroditism contains individuals with a 46,XY karyotype and bilateral dysgenetic testes associated with Leydig and Sertoli cell functional deficiency. This does not appear to be an etiologically distinct syndrome. An association with Drash syndrome and Frasier syndrome has been described. Gonadoblastoma risk is present, and the preferred sexual assignment is female.

Testicular Regression Syndromes

The category of testicular regression syndrome contains a spectrum of clinical entities with marked phenotypic variability, a 46,XY karyotype, and evidence of testicular formation followed by testicular regression. Congenital anorchia is relatively common. These individuals exhibit a normal male phenotype with absent müllerian derivatives. In contrast, patients with rudimentary testes present with tiny atrophic testes and a micropenis, whereas patients with true agonadism (embryonic testicular regression) present with ambiguous genitalia. In both of the latter diagnoses, müllerian elements may be absent or rudimentary.

46,XX Males

A 46,XX male karyotype may be associated with ambiguous genitalia, a hypospadic male phenotype, or occasionally a normal male phenotype. Careful gonadal examination is imperative to exclude the presence of true hermaphroditism.

HERNIA AS AN ISOLATED CLINICAL PRESENTATION

An inguinal hernia is one of the most common presentations of intersex states associated with normal or near-normal male or female external genitalia. The most common intersex state to present in this fashion is testicular feminization or complete androgen insensitivity. Also encountered are such abnormalities as Leydig cell agenesis, which is associated with a female phenotype, and hernia uteri inguinale, a deficiency of antimüllerian hormone, which presents with a male phenotype.

Both testicular feminization and Leydig cell agenesis are identifiable by encountering either a testis or the absence of müllerian derivatives at herniorrhaphy. In contrast, hernia uteri inguinale is identified by the unexpected encounter of müllerian remnants (i.e., a fallopian tube) at the time of herniorrhaphy in a male.

Testicular feminization occurs with sufficient frequency to warrant exclusion with every female inguinal hernia encountered. Figure 95-23 demonstrates the typical finding at surgery. Every female hernia should be approached with this potential diagnosis in mind. The hernia sac is opened, the most prominent peritoneal fold grasped with forceps, and the fallopian tube delivered for inspection. This is an easy step that adds only seconds to the procedure.

Identification of a fallopian tube excludes the diagnosis of testicular feminization. If this structure is not identified, further examination may reveal a testis (Fig. 95-23). Otherwise, on completion of the herniorrhaphy, the vagina should be examined employing an infant cystoscope. Again, identification of a cervix excludes the diagnosis of testicular feminization. If a blind-ending vagina without a cervix is encountered, a karyotype analysis is indicated.

If unexpectedly encountered, testes are not removed at that setting. Time is required for parental counseling, and the parents are given the option of retaining the testes through puberty with removal later. It is appropriate, however, to electively return to the operating room for orchiectomy during infancy because of the potential risk of losing the patient to follow-up and the subsequent potential for malignant degeneration of the testis.

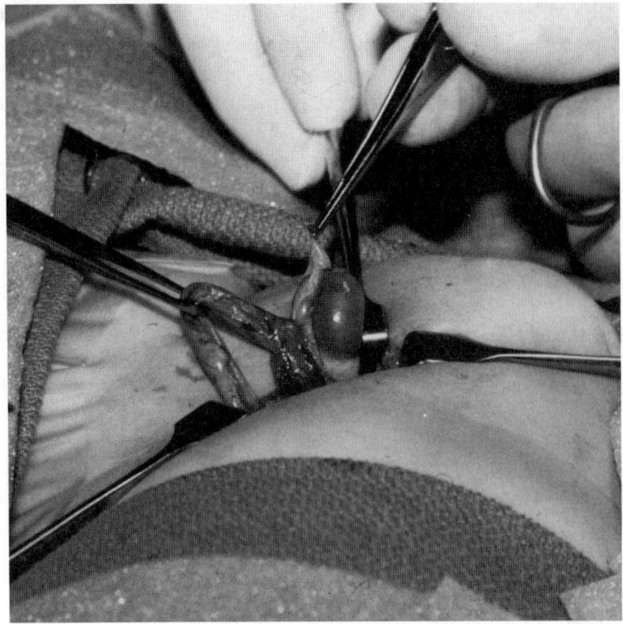

FIG. 95-23. Infant with androgen insensitivity presenting with inguinal hernia. The testis is present in the inguinal incision at the time of hernia repair in this phenotypic female.

HYPOSPADIAS AND CRYPTORCHIDISM

Any degree of hypospadias associated with any degree of bilateral or unilateral gonadal undescent requires evaluation to exclude an intersex state.[70] All such instances require a karyotype analysis. The diagnoses most commonly encountered are mixed gonadal dysgenesis and true hermaphroditism. Cystourethroscopy or ultrasonography (looking for müllerian remnants), diagnostic laparoscopy, or gonadal biopsy may be indicated in selected instances.

MICROPENIS

The terms *micropenis* and *microphallus* have generally been used synonymously. It is important to distinguish between the small penis (true micropenis), which is otherwise normally developed, from that which is associated with a hypospadic meatus and chordee (often referred to as microphallus), which falls under the classification of ambiguous genitalia.

Also confused in the literature are other diagnostic entities associated with the appearance of a small penis. These include the buried penis, the trapped penis, and the webbed penis. These entities are readily distinguished on physical examination by the experienced surgeon. Rarely, extremely masculinized forms of congenital adrenal hyperplasia or other intersex abnormalities may present with a small phallus that is otherwise well developed. Generally, however, careful examination reveals an abnormality in urethral development, even if relatively minor. This differential must not be excluded during the diagnostic evaluation of such an infant.

The true micropenis is primarily an endocrinologic problem and secondarily a surgical problem if an adequate penile growth response is unattainable by hormonal therapy. The differential diagnosis of true micropenis involves abnormalities at several levels of the hypothalamic-pituitary-gonadal axis (Table 95-9). Examples include hypopituitarism (panhypopituitarism, isolated growth hormone deficiency, and isolated gonadotropin deficiency). Additionally, congenital adrenal hypoplasia has been reported as a cause of micropenis. An occasional report has implicated primary testicular failure developing after the first trimester (organogenesis complete) as an etiology.

The evaluation of a newborn with a micropenis begins with a karyotype and a renal and pelvis ultrasound examination. In addition, basal and hCG-stimulated testosterone levels are obtained. Serum is saved for basal and stimulated steroid precursor analysis as well. Depending on the results of these studies, other biochemical assays may be required. In the vast majority of instances, 46,XY infants with micropenis have an attempt made toward a male sexual assignment. Of critical importance is the response to exogenous androgen (testosterone enanthate, hCG, or DHT) administration in terms of penile growth.

It is important to maintain close follow-up of these individuals and monitor their penile growth as compared to normal

TABLE 95-9. *Etiology of micropenis*

ENDOCRINE CAUSES

Isolated growth hormone deficiency (frequently associated with hypoglycemia)
Panhypopitiuitarism
Laron syndrome
Hypogonadotropic hypogonadism
  Isolated with anosmia
  Associated with anosmia (Kallmann or de Morser syndrome)
  Prader-Willi-Labhart syndrome
  Rud syndrome with ichthyosis
  Anencephaly
Hypergonadrotropic hypogonadism
  Klinefelter syndrome
  Other XXXY syndromes
  Anorchidism
  Rudimentary testes syndrome
Male pseudohermaphroditism
  Testosterone biosynthesis defect
  Incomplete androgen insensitivity
  Gonadal dysgenesis syndrome
Fetal exposure to exogenous progestins during pregnancy

NONENDOCRINE CAUSES (POORLY DEFINED ETIOLOGIES)

Noonan syndrome
Smith-Lemli-Opitz syndrome
Cornelia de Lange syndrome
Laurence-Moon-Biedly-Bardet syndrome
Fanconi anemia
Fetal intoxication to hydantoins
Deletion of the long arm of chromosome 18
Williams syndrome

(Sizonenko PC. Disorders of the testes. In: Bertrand J, Rappaport R, Sizonenko PC, eds. Pediatric endocrinology. Baltimore, Williams & Wilkins, 1993:430.)

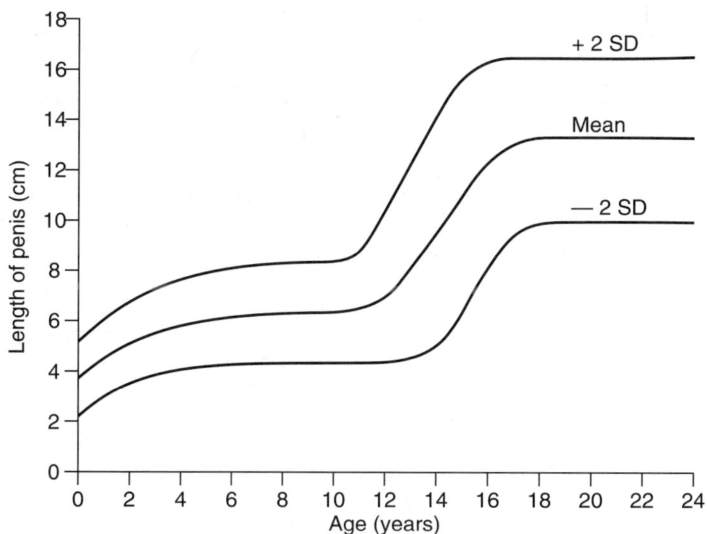

FIG. 95-24. Mean length of phallus ($\pm$ 2 SD) as a function of age. (Schonfeld WD. Primary and secondary sexual characteristices, with biometric study of penis and testes. Am J Dis Child 1943;65:535.)

control populations (Fig. 95-24). Re-dosing may be required to optimize outcome. Males with a small but otherwise normal-appearing penis may tolerate their abnormality quite well. Sexual reassignment in nonresponders must, however, be considered.

NEED FOR ORCHIECTOMY

Orchiectomy may be indicated to prevent malignancy or to prevent unwanted endocrine changes during puberty. It is critically important to remove any testicular tissue in patients raised as females. Failure to do so may result in inappropriate virilization with the onset of puberty. Consequently, patients with male pseudohermaphroditism and mixed gonadal dysgenesis raised as females require bilateral gonadectomy. Similarly, true hermaphrodites raised as females require removal of testes or the testicular component of ovotestes if encountered.

The risk of malignancy in some gonads is also significant. As mentioned previously, patients with mixed gonadal dysgenesis raised as females require bilateral gonadectomy. In instances where a male gender assignment is made, the streak gonad is always removed. If the testis is histologically not dysgenetic and if it has or can be made to have a scrotal position, it can be retained. Otherwise, removal and testicular prostheses along with endocrine maintenance is most satisfactory. If a testis is retained, careful follow-up palpation is mandatory.

Similarly, individuals with testicular feminization and either pure or partial varieties of 46,XY gonadal dysgenesis require bilateral orchiectomy. As with mixed gonadal dysgenesis, the testes and testicular components of ovotestes in true hermaphroditism are often dysgenetic. Patients raised as females have all testicular tissue removed. Individuals raised as males should have all ovotestes and ovaries removed. A testis that is not dysgenetic on biopsy and which has, or can be made to have, a scrotal position can be retained, provided good follow-up is obtained.

EVALUATION OF THE SCROTAL MASS

As with any male, the first consideration for an intersex patient with a scrotal mass is the potential for gonadal neoplasia. A high index of suspicion is warranted. Such neoplasms may be either germ cell or non–germ cell in nature. Evaluation and management are similar to that of other testicular neoplasms. A chest radiograph as well as serum β-hCG and α-fetoprotein (α-FP) are obtained. In the intersex setting, an additional blood sample is stored because some neoplasms may excrete steroid substances, which may be useful in follow-up.

Management consists of an inguinal exploration with early control of the cord vasculature, followed by delivery of the scrotal mass or testicle. If tumor is evident, the cord structures are divided at the level of the internal inguinal ring and the gonad removed. In equivocal cases, the testis may be biopsied, but meticulous attention must be directed at avoidance of tumor spillage.

An important exception to this aggressive surgical approach to the scrotal mass involves the male with congenital virilizing adrenal hyperplasia. Such children, if poorly controlled by steroid maintenance therapy, may develop scrotal masses secondary to hypertrophy of adrenal rests. Often these children present with excessive virilization or pseudoprecocious puberty. *Pseudoprecocious puberty* is generally due to the peripheral excretion of sex steroids independent of true hypothalamic-pituitary control, which induces secondary sexual characteristics that are either isosexual (consistent with genetic sex) or heterosexual (opposing genetic sex). It should be contrasted to *true precocious puberty*, which in general is induced by premature activation of the hypothalamic-pituitary-gonadal axis.

Such hypertrophied adrenal rests are often intratesticular and bilateral. An important differential diagnosis is the Leydig cell tumor, which presents as a scrotal mass (which occasionally is quite subtle) and, because of excessive testosterone excretion, causes isosexual pseudoprecocious puberty. Other entities presenting with excessive virilization of the male child and enlarged testes must be considered in this setting. Table 95-10

TABLE 95-10. *Diagnosis of precocious puberty and pseudoprecocious puberty in boys*

Testes	Possible diagnosis	Pituitary gonadotropins	Testosterone	Additional tools
Both enlarged	True precocious puberty Idiopathic CNS tumors	Low or normal	Moderately elevated	
	Pseudoprecocious puberty Gonadotropin-secreting tumor	Low	Moderately elevated	High α-FP and β-hCG
	Overlap syndrome* Hpothyroidism	Moderately elevated	Moderately elevated	TSH and thyroid hormones
	Congenital adrenal hyperplasia	Low	Moderately elevated	Elevated 17OH progesterone and adrenal androgens; mass on US exam
One enlarged	Benign tumor Leydig cell tumor	Low	Elevated	Mass on US exam
	Malignant tumor Chorioepithelioma	Low	Elevated	High β-hCG; mass on US exam
Both small	Congenital adrenal hyperplasia	Low	Moderately elevated	Elevated 17OH progesterone and adrenal androgens; mass on US exam
	Primary cortisol resistance	Low	Moderately elevated	High cortisol and high ACTH
	Adrenal tumor	Low	Moderately elevated	Elevated adrenal androgens
	Exogenous androgen administration	Low	Usually low	

* Generalized stimulation of tropic hormones secondary to hypothyroidism.
  TSH, thyroid-stimulation hormone; US, ultrasonographic.
Sizonenko PC: Precocious puberty. In: Bertrand J, Rappaport R, Sizonenko PC, eds. Pediatric endocrinology. Baltimore, Williams and Wilkins, 1993:430.

outlines the differential diagnosis of precocious and pseudoprecocious puberty in males. Many of these conditions are associated with enlarged testes. Of additional diagnostic benefit is that the hypertrophied adrenal rests and Leydig cell tumors generally both show discrete intratesticular masses on ultrasonography. An additional important diagnostic point is that Leydig cell tumors are usually unilateral, whereas hypertrophied adrenal rests are generally bilateral.

EVALUATION OF THE MASS IN THE INGUINAL CANAL OR LABIA OF THE FEMALE

An unexplained mass within the inguinal canal or the labia of the female requires urgent surgical evaluation. Masses within the labia are at risk of being either a testis or ovotestis and should be removed. An irreducible mass within the inguinal canal most commonly represents either a lymph node or an incarcerated hernia (usually ovary). However, occasionally testes or ovotestes are encountered.

The diagnostic approach depends on the degree of clinical suspicion. If a lymph node is suspected, ultrasonography can be diagnostic. This study reveals an echolucent center of the inguinal mass and also shows the presence of two ovaries within the pelvis. A lymph node thus confirmed may be treated by antibiotic therapy alone.

If an incarcerated ovary is suspected, prompt surgical exploration and reduction is indicated to reduce the risk of ischemic ovarian injury. The management of a testis or ovotestis, if encountered, is as described.

GYNECOMASTIA

Gynecomastia is commonly encountered in intersex patients raised as males. Examples include true hermaphroditism, some types of male pseudohermaphroditism (eg, defects in testosterone synthesis and incomplete androgen insensitivity), and mixed gonadal dysgenesis.

It is critical to avoid any situations that may raise questions regarding sexual identity and possibly lower self-esteem. Consequently, gynecomastia in such settings warrants surgical intervention. In the setting of mixed gonadal dysgenesis, a retained gonad, and gynecomastia, consideration should be given to the potential presence of a gonadoblastoma, which may induce gynecomastia secondary to estradiol secretion.

NEED FOR MASCULINE RECONSTRUCTION

In the majority of instances, masculine reconstruction can be performed in a single-stage procedure. However, without question, better results are attained in some individuals employing a staged approach. Attention is directed toward urethral reconstruction, correction of chordee (which may be due to cutaneous tethering, true fibrous chordee, or corporal disproportion), and scrotoplasty to correct scrotal tethering or penoscrotal transposition. Such reconstruction is optimally performed prior to 1 year of age.

Urethral reconstruction may be performed employing either vascular pedicle flap or free-graft techniques or a combination. Correction of cutaneous or fibrous chordee is readily attained, whereas chordee due to corporal disproportion can be more

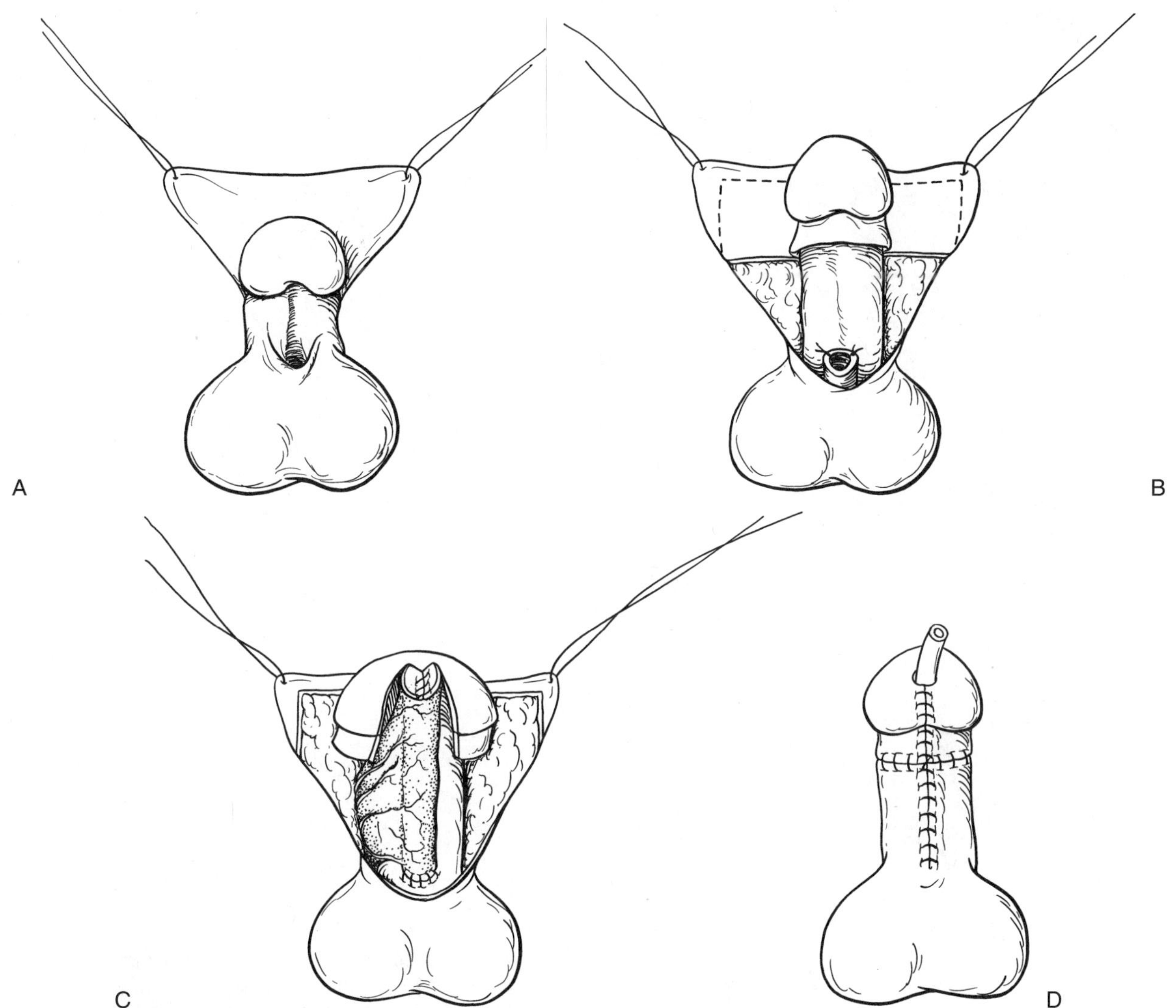

FIG. 95-25. (*A*) Penoscrotal hypospadias associated with chordee. A circumferential incision coursing approximately 5 mm from the coronal sulcus allows the penile shaft skin to be mobilized and the associated fibrous chordee tissue to be excised, resulting in a straight shaft. (*B*) Dissection between the urethra and corpora is generally necessary to optimize chordee release, resulting in further caudal displacement of the urinary meatus. A rectangular flap of inner preputial skin is developed, tubularized (*C*), and mobilized on its vascular pedicle to extend the urethra to the tip of the glans. (*D*) Glans flaps are developed and approximated ventrally to the neourethra, and the cutaneous defect is closed by transposing the remaining dorsal foreskin ventrally.

difficult. Corporal disproportion can be corrected by either dorsal plication (dorsal shortening) or ventral corporoplasty (ventral lengthening) techniques. In the setting of ambiguous genitalia, where penile length is generally compromised, lengthening techniques are often most appropriate.

Figure 95-25 demonstrates a common single-stage procedure used to correct severe hypospadias. This tubularized vascular pedicle preputial flap procedure described by Duckett may be used alone or in conjunction with interposition procedures to achieve a very satisfactory functional and cosmetic result.

Very often in intersex patients, there is insufficient skin to allow both urethral replacement and penile resurfacing. The surgeon must choose between a composite urethral reconstruction (Fig. 95-26) or a staged reconstruction. Composite urethral reconstruction may involve tubularization of a perimeatal-based

flap extending either distally (see Fig. 95-26*A*) or caudally (see Fig. 95-26*B*). Alternatively, a tubularized free graft of bladder mucosa or skin offers an excellent alternative (see Fig. 95-26*C*).

The Durham-Smith staged procedure is a particularly powerful reconstructive alternative in severe cases (Fig. 95-27). Chordee is released as described, and glans flaps are developed (see Fig. 95-27*A*). The dorsal foreskin is incised in the midline and transposed ventrally to cover the penile shaft and, in addition, the exposed glandular surfaces (see Fig. 95-27*B*). After approximately 3 to 6 months, the second stage of the reconstruction begins with an extended U-shaped incision (see Fig. 95-27*C*). The neourethra is created by tubularization of the resultant midline strip of skin (see Fig. 95-27*D*) and the resultant cutaneous defect is closed (see Fig. 95-27*E*). Not uncommonly, insufficient skin at the ventral base of the penis prevents closure with-

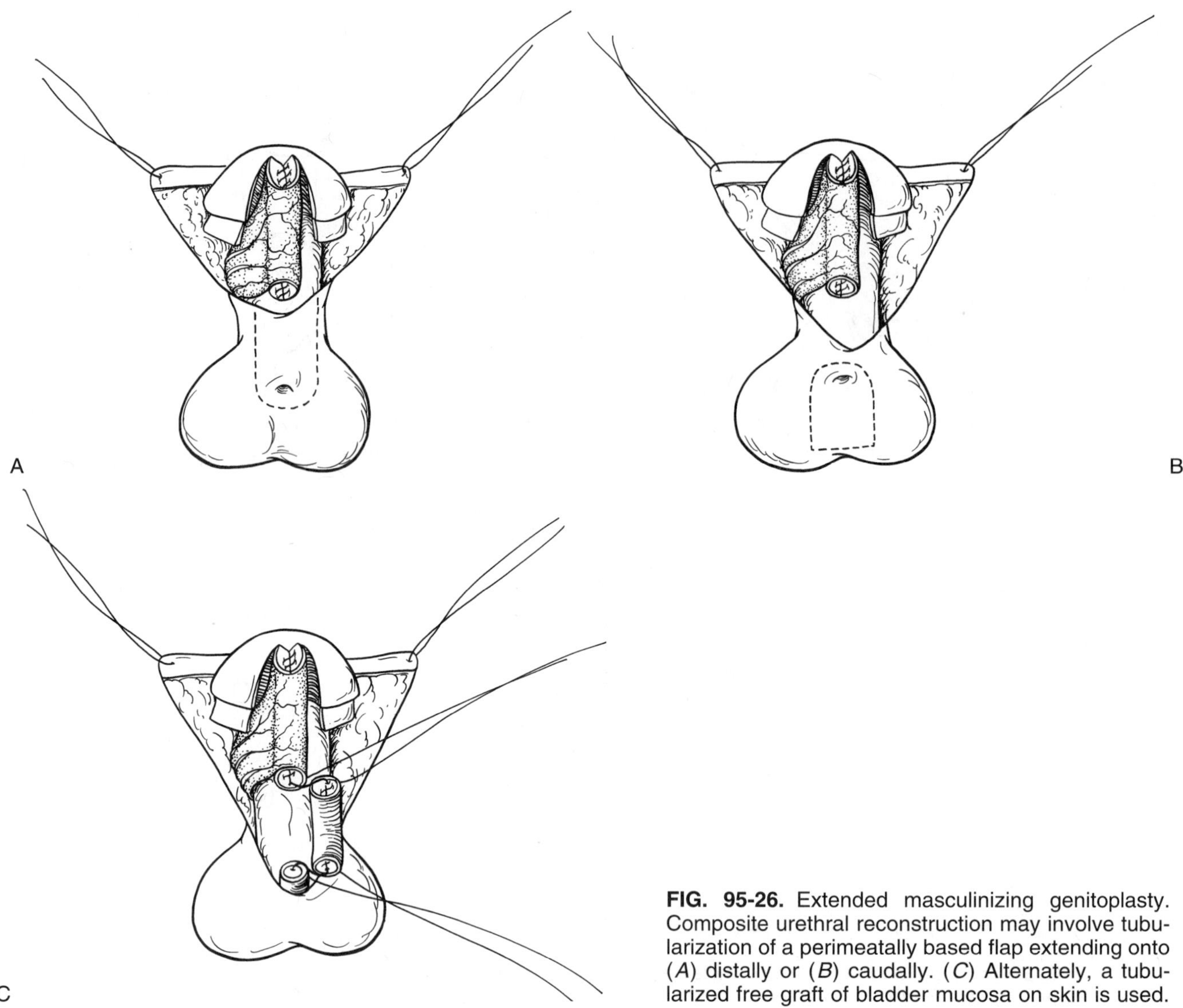

FIG. 95-26. Extended masculinizing genitoplasty. Composite urethral reconstruction may involve tubularization of a perimeatally based flap extending onto (*A*) distally or (*B*) caudally. (*C*) Alternately, a tubularized free graft of bladder mucosa on skin is used.

out tension. This is circumvented by the development of a scrotal interposition flap.

The most difficult cases are those that involve corporal disproportion (Fig. 95-28). After complete cutaneous mobilization and excision of fibrous chordee, a severe ventral curvature persists (see Fig. 95-28*A*). If the curvature is mild or the penile length adequate, a dorsal plication may be considered. Very often, in the intersex patient, this is not a reasonable alternative, and ventral lengthening is required. This begins with the excision of the defective corporal tissue (see Fig. 95-28*B*), which generally gives dramatic straightening and lengthening of the penis (see Fig. 95-28*B*). The resultant defect is resurfaced employing a vascular pedicle flap of tunica vaginalis. Alternatively, a free dermal graft or lyophilized dura has been used.

NEED FOR FEMININE RECONSTRUCTION

Feminizing genitoplasty represents the most common surgical reconstruction for individuals with ambiguous genitalia. Re-

construction of female genitalia with the potential for good function can range from a relatively straightforward to an extremely complex procedure. Such reconstruction should be undertaken by committed, experienced reconstructive surgeons, and long-term follow-up is necessary. Detailed preoperative counseling is critical. Parents must understand the risk of vaginal stenosis, the need for close follow-up, and the need for routine vaginal dilatation until sexual maturity has been reached. Optimal results are achieved employing a single-stage approach, which is ideally completed prior to 1 year of age. Reconstruction consists of clitoroplasty, vaginoplasty, and labioplasty.

The goals of clitoroplasty are threefold. The first is to cosmetically reduce the size of the phallic structure to that expected for a clitoris. Additionally, it is important to preserve sensation and eliminate the potential for problematic future corporal erection. A successful vaginoplasty should achieve a satisfactory cosmetic appearance and a vaginal vault of adequate dimension to allow intercourse on reaching sexual maturity, and should allow the egress of uterine secretions. Vaginal delivery may

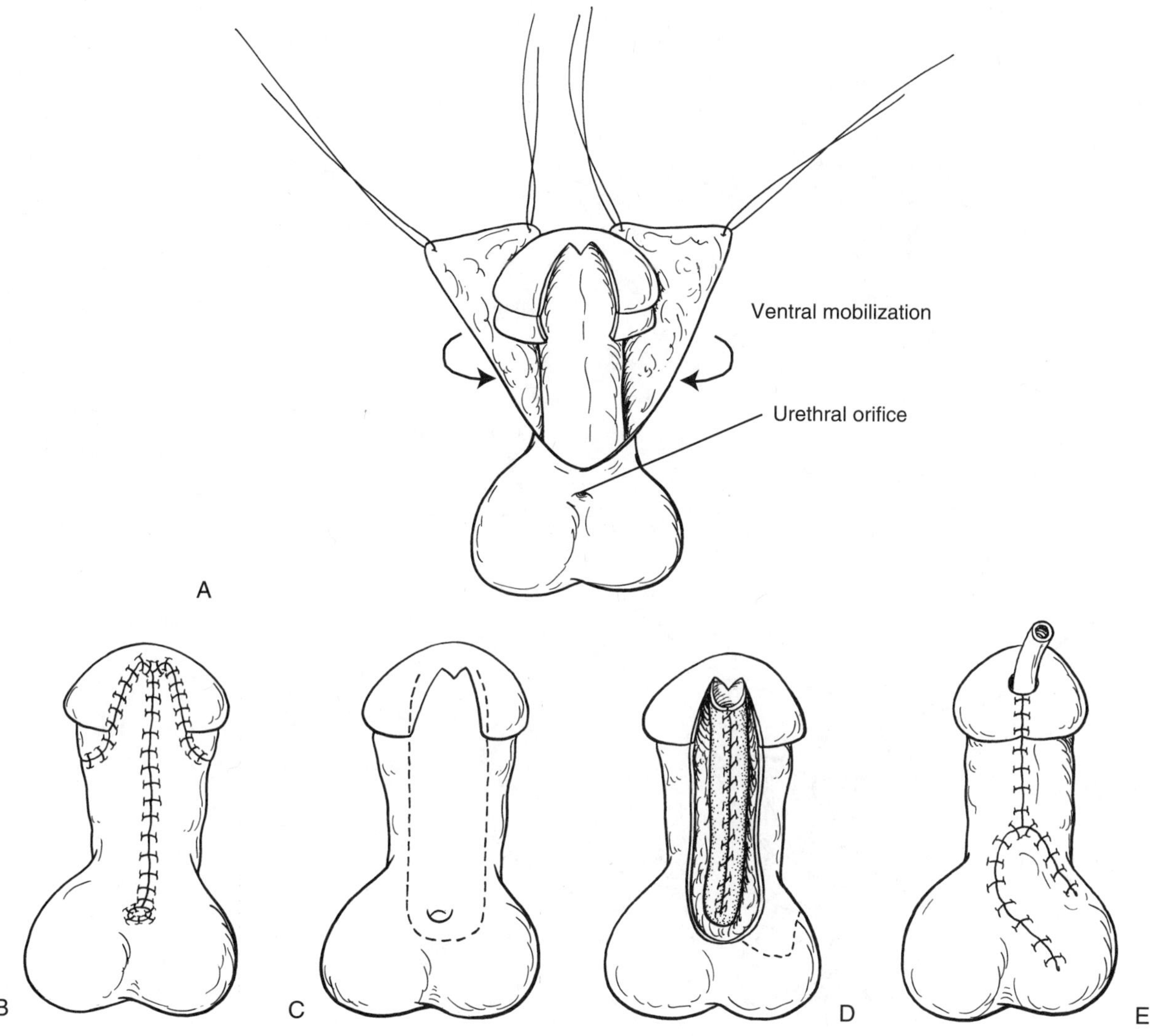

FIG. 95-27. Staged masculinizing genitoplasty (see text).

not be possible without permanent vaginal trauma, however, and cesarean should be considered depending on the extent of surgical reconstruction performed. Vaginal patency and dimension are preserved by routine vaginal dilatation. When the patient reaches sexual maturity, intercourse is often facilitated by a small introitoplasty, which is well tolerated and clearly preferable to the performance of the total vaginoplasty at an older age.

As demonstrated in Figure 95-29, clitoroplasty begins with a circumferential incision 3 to 5 mm proximal to the coronal sulcus, which is interrupted ventrally to allow preservation of the urethral plate and maximization of glandular blood supply (see Fig. 95-29A). The phallic shaft skin is totally mobilized, and the urethral plate and dorsal neurovascular bundles are carefully dissected free from the adjacent corpora cavernosa (see Fig. 95-29B). A strip of tunica albugenia may be left with the neurovascular bundles to prevent injury to these structures. The corpora are dissected throughout their length and ligated and divided at their insertion into the glans and their origins on the inferior pubic ramus and removed. The clitoris is partially

deepithelialized, leaving only a portion of the distal glans comparable with the size of a normal clitoris with epithelium. The clitoroplasty is completed by approximating the oversewn edge of the corpora to the prepubic fascia to secure its final position (see Fig. 95-29C).

The technique of vaginoplasty used depends solely on the individual's internal and external genital anatomy, which is assessed preoperatively by careful endoscopic examination. Of particular importance is the determination of the level of entry of the vagina into the urogenital sinus relative to the striated urinary sphincter. Low anomalies (vaginal confluence distal to sphincter) may be managed by inlay flap techniques, whereas high anomalies (confluence proximal to sphincter) require alternative approaches.

Figure 95-29 A and D demonstrate the most widely applicable technique of feminizing vaginoplasty for low urogenital sinus anomalies, performed in the dorsal lithotomy position. An inverted (D) U or M-shaped incision in the labioscrotal fold outlines a vaginal insertion flap. The underlying urogenital sinus is exposed and incised in the midline, unroofing the urethral meatus

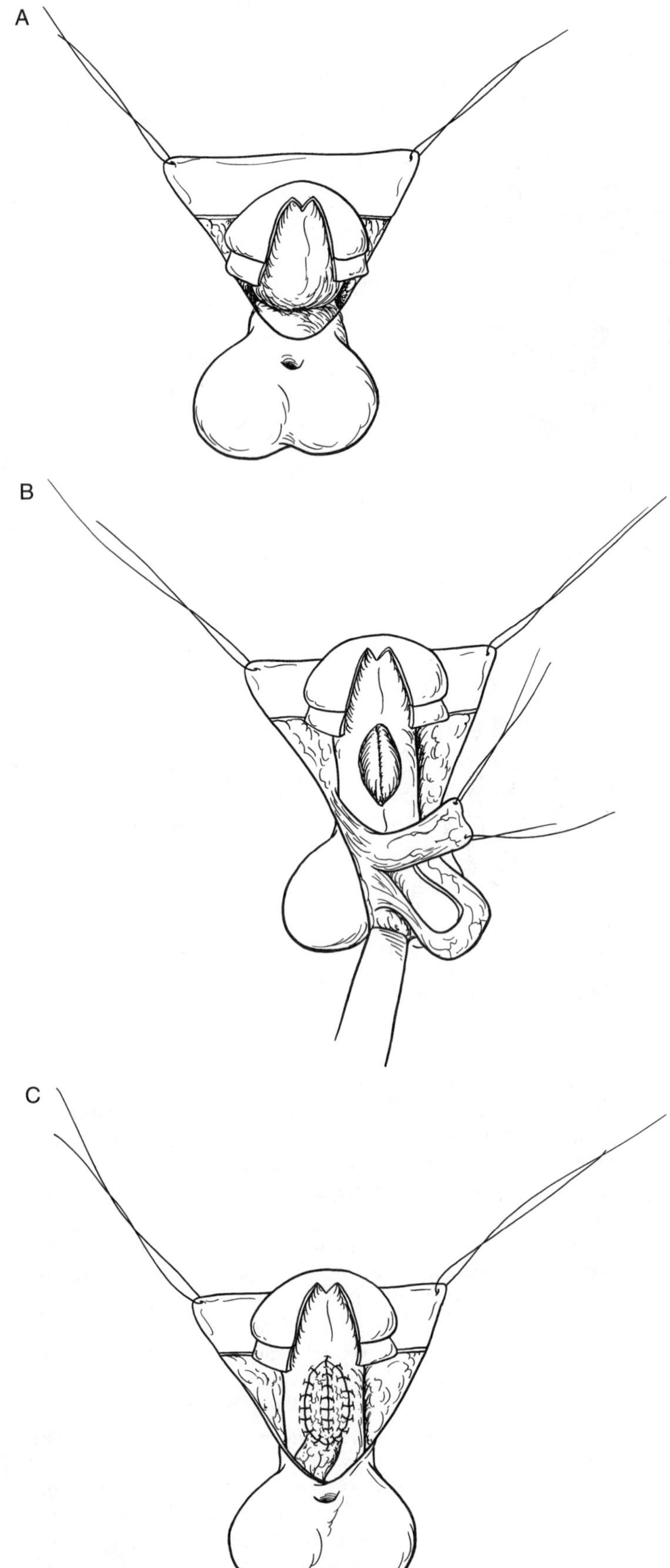

FIG. 95-28. Correction of corporal disporoportion by tunica vaginalis graft. (See text.)

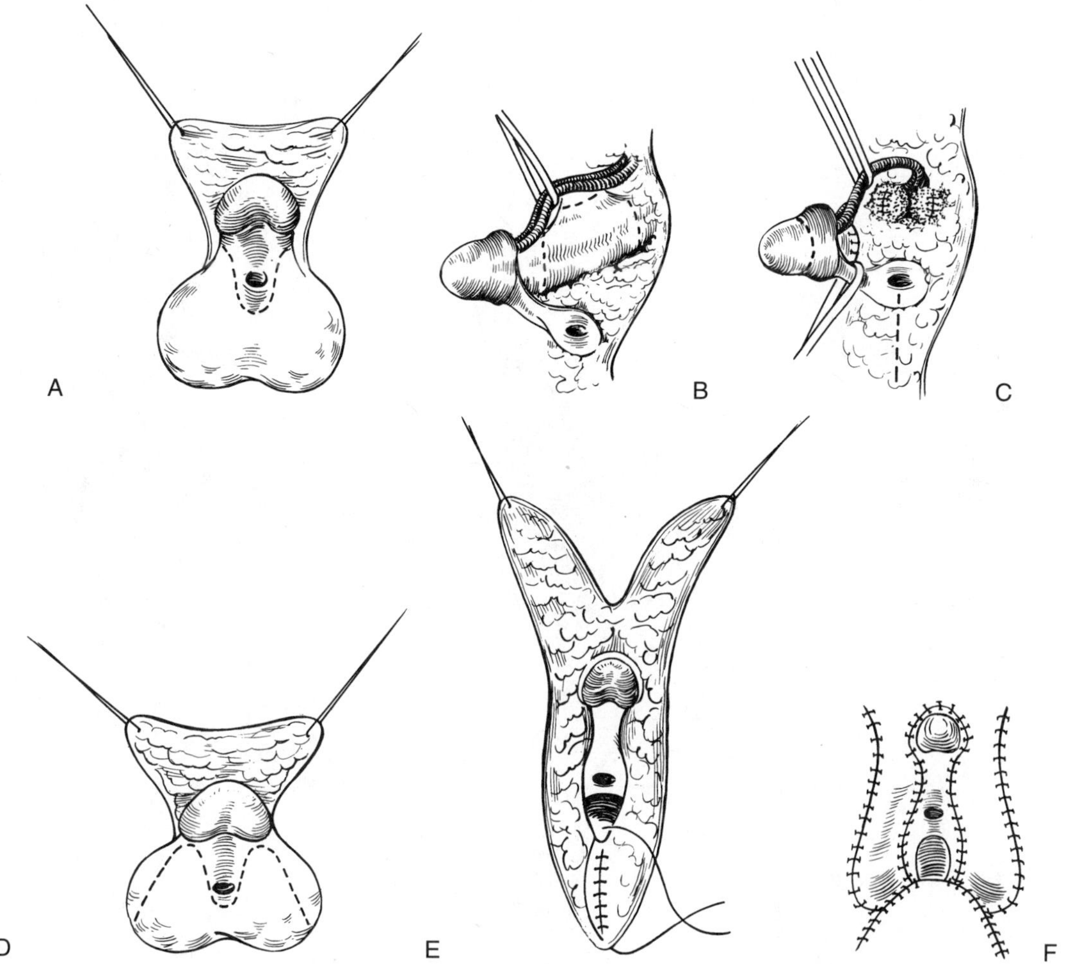

FIG. 95-29. Clitoroplasty and feminizing genitoplasty, low lesion (see text).

and vagina introitus as separate orifices (*E*). The labioscrotal flap is then sutured into place as an insertion flap and the prepuce is incised in the midline. This results in a wide and slightly posteriorly directed orifice[71], and each half of the prepuce is rotated caudally to allow creation of labia (labioplasty) (*F*).

Occasionally, the labioscrotal folds may be sufficiently separated or be associated with a sufficiently posterior urogenital sinus orifice that a U-shaped incision is ineffective. In this setting, an M-shaped incision is created and the two resultant flaps approximated in the midline to create a single posteriorly based insertion flap, as described. The M-shaped incision is extremely versatile and can be used in many cases where the vagina has a high insertion or where the vagina is completely absent.[72]

A considerably more difficult reconstruction is required for the high vaginal insertion. Most surgical variations are based on the work of Hendren.[73] Typically, this involves a vagina that opens into the urogenital sinus at the level of what would otherwise be the utricle in the verumontanum. In this instance, the use of an inlay flap would not only result in an unacceptable cosmetic appearance, but potentially result in urinary inconti-

nence. Many authors have suggested that such cases are best managed by a staged procedure. A single-staged procedure, however, allows greatest reconstructive versatility. Again, this procedure is performed in the dorsal lithotomy position. A Foley catheter is placed in the bladder, and a Fogarty catheter is placed in the vagina to allow palpation. A M-shaped or occasionally a U-shaped incision is created, and the underlying pelvic floor musculature is divided in the anatomic midline, guided by muscle stimulation (see Fig. 95-30*A* and *B*). Clitoroplasty is performed as previously described. The vagina, thus exposed, is divided from its insertion and the urethral defect oversewn (see Fig. 95-30*C*). The vagina is spatulated, the labioscrotal flap is tubularized, and the two structures are sutured together (see Fig. 95-30*D, E,* and *F*). The pelvic floor musculature is reapproximated around the newly reconstructed vagina. An alternate approach, which includes a transvesical approach to vaginal mobilization, may be considered in occasional circumstances.[74]

Some individuals, such as most male pseudohermaphrodites, have no vaginal remnants and no uterine structures requiring drainage. Such patients may be reconstructed employing labio-

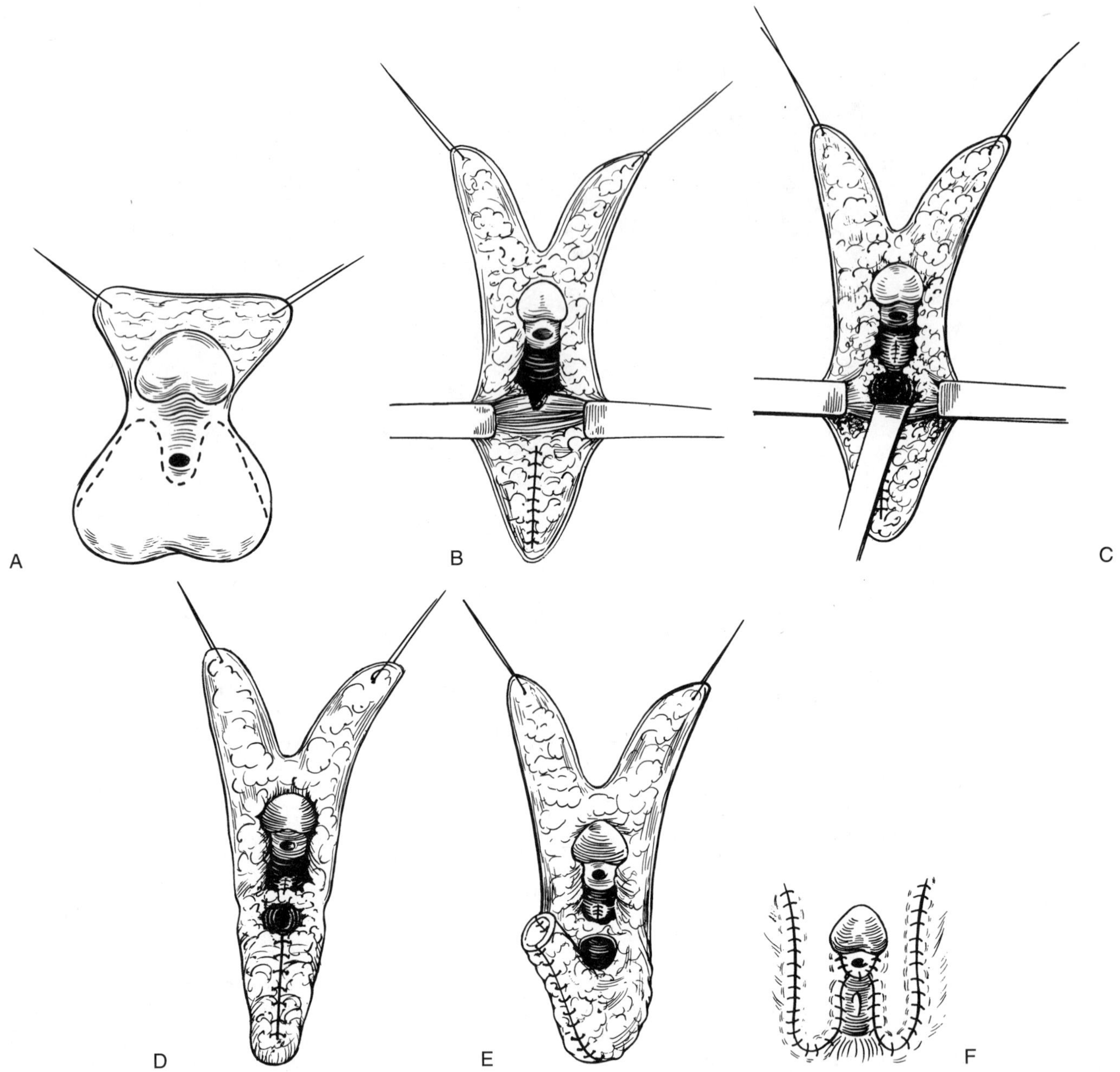

FIG. 95-30. Feminizing genitoplasty, high lesion (see text).

scrotal flaps, or, if insufficient, visceral substitution (colon or occasionally ileum) or skin graft techniques.

Reoperative vaginoplasty is considerably more difficult. Uncomplicated vaginal stenosis is readily managed by perineal inlay flap techniques with high success. Obliteration of the vaginal introitus may be associated with destruction of a large amount of vaginal tissue. In this setting, visceral substitution techniques, myocutaneous flaps, and perineal flaps following tissue-expander procedures are generally successful.

REFERENCES

1. Simpson JL, Rebar RW. Normal and abnormal sexual differentiation and development. In: Becker KL, et al. Principles and practice of endocrinology and metabolism. Philadelphia, JB Lippincott, 1990:710.

2. Grumbach MM, Conte FA. Disorders of sex differentiation. In: Wilson JD, Foster DW, eds. Williams textbook of endocrinology. Philadelphia, WB Saunders, 1992:853.

3. Ford CE. Mosaics and chimaeras. Br Med Bull 1969;25:104.

4. Buyse ML. Birth defects encyclopedia. Cambridge, Blackwell Scientific Publications, 1990.

5. Eichwald EJ, Silmser CR. Untitled communication. Transplant Bull 1955;2:148.

6. Goldberg EH, Boyse EA, Bennett D, et al. Serological demonstration of H-Y (male) antigen on mouse sperm. Nature 1971;232:478.

7. Wachtel SS. H-Y antigen and the biology of sex determination. New York, Grune Stratton, 1983.

8. Ohno S, Nagai Y, Ciccarese S, et al. Testis-organizing H-Y antigen and the primary sex-determining mechanism of mammals. Recent Prog Horm Res 1979;35:449.

9. Simpson E, Chandler P, Goulmy E, et al. Separation of the genetic loci for H-Y antigen and testis determination on the Y chromosome. Nature 1987;326:876.

10. Page DC, Mosher R, Simpson EM, et al. The sex-determining human Y chromosome encodes a finger protein. Cell 1987;52:1091.

11. Lau YFC, Chan K. The putative testis-determining factor and related genes are expressed as discrete-sized transcripts in adult gonadal and somatic tissues. Am J Hum Genet 1990;45:942.

12. Palmer MS, Sinclair AH, Ellis NA, et al. Genetic evidence that ZFY is not the testis-determining factor. Nature 1989;342:937.

13. Sinclair AA, Berta P, Palmer MS, et al. A gene from the human sex-determining region encodes a conserved DNA-binding motif. Nature 1990;346:240.

14. Fukutani K, Kajiwara T, Nagafuchi S, et al. Detection of the testis determining factor in an XX man. J Urol 1993;149:126.

15. Berta P, Ross-Hawkins J, Sinclair AH, et al. Genetic evidence equating SRY and the testis determining factor. Nature 1990;348:448.

16. Jager RJ, Anvret M, Hall K, et al. A human XY female with a frame shift mutation in the candidate testis-determining gene SRY. Nature 1990;348:452.

17. Koopman P, Gubbay J, Vivian N, et al. Male development of chromosomally female mice transgenic for Sry. Nature 1991;351:117.

18. McLaren A. What makes a man a man? Nature 1990;346:216.

19. Fechner PY, Marcantonio SM, Jaswaney V, et al. The role of the sex-determining region Y gene in the etiology of 46,XX maleness. J Clin Endocrinol Metab 1993;76:690.

20. McElreavey K, Rappaport R, Vilain E, et al. A minority of 46,XX true hermaphrodites are positive for the Y-DNA sequence including SRY. Hum Genet 1992;90:121.

21. Toublanc JE, Boucekkine C, Abbas N, et al. Hormonal and molecular genetic findings in 46,XX subjects with sexual ambiguity and testicular differentiation. Eur J Pediatr 1993;152:S70.

22. Berta P, Morin D, Poulat F, et al. Molecular analysis of the sex-determining region from the Y chromosome in two patients with Frasier syndrome. Horm Res 1992;37:103.

23. Pivnick EK, Wachtel S, Woods D, et al. Mutations in the conserved domain of SRY are uncommon in XY gonadal dysgenesis. Hum Genet 1992;90:308.

24. Affara NA, Chalmers IJ, Ferguson-Smith MA. Analysis of the SRY gene in 22 sex-reversed XY females identifies four new point mutations in the conserved DNA binding domain. Hum Molec Genet 1993;2:785.

25. Fechner PY, Marcantonio SM, Ogata T, et al. Report of a kindred with X-linked (or autosomal dominant sex-limited) 46,XY partial gonadal dysgenesis. J Clin Endocrinol Metab 1993;76:1248.

26. Braun A, Kammerer S, Cleve H, et al. True hermaphroditism in a 46,XY individual, caused by a postzygotic somatic point mutation in the male gonadal sex-determining locus (SRY): molecular genetics and histological findings in a sporadic case. Am J Hum Genet 1993;52:578.

27. Vilain E, Jaubert F, Fellous M, et al. Pathology of 46,XY pure gonadal dysgenesis: absence of testis differentiation associated with mutations in the testis-determining factor. Differentiation 1993;52:151.

28. Barr ML, Bertram EG. A morphological distinction between neurona of the male and female, and the behavior of the nucleolar satellite during acceleration of nucleoprotein synthesis. Nature 1949;163:676.

29. Francavilla S, Cordeschi G, Properzi G, et al. Ultrastructure of fetal human gonad before sexual differentiation and during early testicular and ovarian development. J Submicrosc Cytol Pathol 1990;22:389.

30. Tran D, Josso N. Localization of anti-mullerian hormone in the rough endoplasmic reticulum of the developing bovine Sertoli cell, using immunocytochemistry with a monoclonal antibody. Endocrinology 1982;111:1562.

31. Siiteri PK, Wilson JD. Testosterone formation and metabolism during male sexual differentiation in the human embryo. J Clin Endocrinol Metab 1974;38:113.

32. Reyes FI, Boroditsky RS, Winter JSD, et al. Studies on human sexual development. II. Fetal and maternal serum gonadotropins and sex steroid concentration. J Clin Endocrinol Metab 1974;38:612.

33. Kaplan SL, Grumbach MM. Pituitary and placental gonadotropins and sex steroids in the human and sub-human primate fetus. J Clin Endocrinol Metab 1978;37:487.

34. Huhtaniemi IT, Korenbrot CC, Jaffe RB. hCG binding and stimulation of testosterone biosynthesis in the human fetal testis. J Clin Endocrinol Metab 1977;44:963.

35. Molsberry RL, Cau BR, Mendelson CR, et al. Human chorionic gonadotropin binding to human fetal testis. J Clin Endocrinol Metab 1982;55:791.

36. Word RA, George FW, Wilson JD, et al. Testosterone synthesis and adenylate cyclase activity in the early human fetal testis appear to be independent of human chorionic gonadotropin. J Clin Endocrinol Metab 1989;69:204.

37. Huhtaniemi IT, Korenbrot CC, Jaffe RB. Content of chorionic gonadotropin in human fetal tissues. J Clin Endocrinol Metab 1978;46:994.

38. George FW, Wilson JD. Conversion of androgen to estogen by the human fetal ovary. J Clin Endocrinol Metab 1978;47:550.

39. Baker TG. A quantatative and cytological study of germ cells in human ovaries. Proc R Soc Lond Biol 1963;158:417.

40. O'Rahilly R, Muller F. Human embryology and teratology. New York, Wiley-Liss, 1992.

41. Jost A. Embryonic sexual differentiation (morphology, physiology, abnormalities). In: Jones HW Jr, Scott WW eds. Hermaphroditism, genital anomalies and related endocrine disorders. Baltimore, Williams & Wilkins, 1971:16.

42. Jost A. Problems of fetal endocrinology: the gonadal and hypophyseal hormones. Recent Prog Horm Res 1953;8:379.

43. Cate RL, Mattalian RJ, Hession C, et al. Isolation of the human gene in animal cells. Cell 1986;45:685.

44. Cohen-Haguenauer O, Picard JY, Mattei MG, et al. Mapping of the gene for anti mullerian hormone to the short arm of human chromosome 19. Cytogenet Cell Genet 1987;44:2.

45. Donahoe PK, Cate RL, MacLaughlin DT, et al. Mullerian inhibiting substance: gene structure and mechanism of action of a fetal regressor. Recent Prog Horm Res 1987;43:431.

46. Vigier B, Tran D, Legeai L, et al. Origin of anti-müllerian hormone in bovine freemartin fetuses. J Reprod Fertil 1984;70:473.

47. Vigier B, Watrin F, Magre S, et al. Purified bovine AMH induces a characteristic freemartin effect in fetal rat prospective ovaries exposed to it in vitro. Development 1987;100:43.

48. Behringer RR, Cate RL, Froelick GJ. Abnormal sexual development in transgenic mice chronically expressing mullerian inhibitory substance. Nature 1990;345:167.

49. Lee MM, Donahoe PK. Mullerian inhibiting substance: a gonadal hormone with multiple functions. Endocrine Rev 1993;14:152.

50. Forsberg JG. Origin of vaginal epithelium. Obstet Gynecol 1965;25:787.

51. Cunha GR. The dual origin of vaginal epithelium. Am J Anat 1975;143:387.

52. O'Malley B. The steroid receptor superfamily: more excitement predicted in the future. Mol Endocrinol 1990;4:363.

53. Money J, Ehrhardt AA. Man and woman, boy and girl: the differentiation and dimorphism of gender identity from conception to maturity. Baltimore, Johns Hopkins Univ Press, 1972.

54. Ehrhardt AA, Meyer-Bahlburg HFL. Effects of prenatal sex hormones on gender-related behavior. Science 1981;211:1312.

55. Money J, Schwartz M, Lewis VG. Adult heterosexual status and fetal hormonal masculinization and emasculinization: 46,XX congenital virilizing adrenal hyperplasia and 46,XY androgen-insensitivity compared. Psychoneuroendocrinology 1984;9:405.

56. Imperato-McGinley JL, Peterson MD, Gautier T, et al. Androgens and the evolution of male-gender identity among male pseudohermaphrodites with 5α-reductase deficiency. N Engl J Med 1979;300:1233.

57. Reilly JM, Woodhouse CRJ. Small penis and male sexual role. J Urol 1989;142:569.

58. Kaplan SL, Grumbach MM, Aubert ML. The ontogenesis of pituitary hormones and hypothalamic factors in the human fetus: maturation of the central nervous system regulation of anterior pituitary function. Recent Prog Hormone Res 1976;32:161.

59. Mosberry RL, Carr BR, Mendelson CR, et al. Human chorionic gonadotropin binding to fetal testes as a function of gestational age. J Clin Endocrinol Metab 1982;55:791.

60. Voutilainen R. Hormonal development in the fetal gonad. In: Sizonenko PC, Aubert ML, eds. Developmental endocrinology. New York, Raven Press, 1990:27.

61. Reyes FI, Winter JSD, Faiman C. Studies on human sexual development. I. Fetal gonad and adrenal sex steroids. J Clin Endocrinol Metab 1973;37:74.

62. Reyes FI, Boroditsky RS, Winter JSD, et al. Studies on human sexual development. II. Fetal and maternal serum gonadotropin and sex steroid concentrations. J Clin Endocrinol Metab 1974;38:612.

63. Tapanainen J, Kellolumpu-Lehtinen P, Pelliniemi L, et al. Age-related

changes in endogenous steroids of human fetal testis during early and mid-pregnancy. J Clin Endocrinol Metab 1981;52:98.

64. Pang SY, Clark A. Newborn screening, prenatal diagnosis, and prenatal treatment of congenital adrenal hyperplasia due to 21-hydroxylase deficiency. Trend Endocrinol Metab 1990;1:302.

65. Saenger P, Lin D, Gitelman SE, et al. Congenital lipoid adrenal hyperplasia-genes for P450SCC, side chain cleavage enzyme, are normal. J Steroid Biochem Molec Biol 1993;45:87.

66. Avni EE, Rypens F, Smet MH, et al. Sonographic demonstration of congenital adrenal hyperplasia in the neonate: the cerebriform pattern. Pediatr Radiol 1993;23:88.

67. Morel Y, Bertrand J, Rappoport R. Disorders of hormonosynthesis. In: Bertrand J, Rappaport R, Sizonenko PC, eds. Pediatric endocrinology. Baltimore, Williams & Wilkins, 1993:305.

68. Mulaikal RM, Migeon CJ, Rick JA. Fertility rates in female patients with congenital adrenal hyperplasia due to 21-hydroxylase deficiency. N Engl J Med 1987;316:178.

69. Van Niekerk WA, Retief AE. The gonads of human true hermaphrodites. Hum Genet 1981;58:117.

70. Raifer J, Walsh PC. The incidence of intersexuality in patients with hypospadias and cryptorchidism. J Urol 1976;116:769.

71. McC Snyder H, Retik AB, Bauer SB, et al. Feminizing genitoplasty: a synthesis. J Urol 1983;129:1024.

72. Sheldon CA, Gilbert A, Lewis AG. Vaginal reconstruction: critical technical principles. J Urol 1994;152:190.

73. Hendren WH. Surgical management of urogenital sinus abnormalities. J Pediatr Surg 1977;12:339.

74. Passerini-Glazel G. A new one-stage procedure for clitorovaginoplasty in severely masculinized female pseudohermaphrodites. J Urol 1989; 142:565.

Surgery of Infants and Children: Scientific Principles and Practice, edited by Keith T. Oldham, Paul M. Colombani, and Robert P. Foglia. Lippincott–Raven Publishers, Philadelphia, © 1997.

CHAPTER 96

Skin

Bernard A. Cohen

ANATOMY OF THE SKIN

The skin is a complex and dynamic organ composed of many parts and appendages (Fig. 96-1). The outermost stratum corneum provides an effective barrier to irritants, toxins, and organisms. It also protects against excessive loss of fluids and electrolytes. The remainder of the skin manufactures this outer layer. Melanocytes in the basal layer of the epidermis produce melanin, the pigment that is dispersed to the epidermal keratinocytes to protect against ultraviolet light–induced injury. The dermis is composed primarily of fibroblasts and collagen, which form a tough leathery mechanical barrier, and a collagenous matrix, which supports a number of skin appendages. Elastic fibers add resilience. Hair grows from follicles deep in the dermis and is important protection against sunlight and particulate matter. Sebaceous glands arise as an outgrowth of the hair follicle and produce sebum, which lubricates and protects the skin surface. The nails are special organs of manipulation that also protect sensitive digits. Thermoregulation is controlled by sweat produced by eccrine glands as well as by changes in cutaneous blood flow, which are regulated by glomus cells. The skin also contains receptors for heat, pain, touch, and pressure. Sensory input from these structures helps to protect the skin against environmental injury. Beneath the dermis, subcutaneous fat acts as a source of stored energy and as a soft, protective cushion.

EVALUATION OF A RASH

The skin is the largest and most easily accessible organ and often is the most frequent concern of the patient and parents. Consequently, all practitioners must be able to recognize common dermatologic disorders and cutaneous clues to underlying systemic disease.

Information on the duration of the rash, evolution of lesions, presence or absence of pruritus, and topical treatment regimens that have altered primary lesions aid in the diagnosis of skin and related disorders. Details of the child's medical history, including recent and chronic medical conditions and systemic medications, also can provide clues. A family history can help to identify cutaneous infections and infestations, genodermatoses, and disorders with multifactorial inheritance. A review of nurs-

ery records and family photographs can help guide therapeutic decisions by confirming the history of congenital pigmented nevi, hamartomas, and malformations.

A thorough examination of the skin should include a perusal of the scalp, hair, palms, soles, nails, and mucous membranes. Dental, ocular, and bony anomalies may be associated with neurocutaneous disorders and ectodermal dysplasias.

Attention should then turn to the distribution and pattern of the rash. *Distribution* refers to the location of the cutaneous findings; *pattern* defines a specific anatomic or physiologic arrangement. For example, the distribution of skin lesions may include the face, neck, arms, and legs, while the pattern may be sun-exposed sites. Other patterns include intertriginous or flexural surfaces, clothing-covered sites, acrally distributed rashes, pityriasis rosea, and acneform eruptions.[1]

The clinician next should consider the *organization* of the lesions, which defines the relation of primary and secondary lesions to one another in a given location. Are the lesions diffusely scattered or clustered (herpetiform)? Are they linear, annular, serpiginous, or dermatomal?

Finally, the practitioner should examine the morphology of the lesions. Primary lesions, which usually arise de novo, include flat macules (smaller than 1 cm) and patches (larger than 1 cm), elevated papules (less than 1 cm) and plaques (more than 1 cm), fluid-filled vesicles (smaller than 1 cm) and bullae (larger than 1 cm), and deep-seated nodules (less than 1 cm) and tumors (more than 1 cm). Secondary lesions, including pustules, crusts, excoriations, erosions, ulcers, and scars, evolve from primary lesions or develop as a complication of manipulation of primary lesions by the patient.

The most common dermatoses that the pediatric practitioner is likely to encounter fall into the papulosquamous (bumpy, scaly) and vesiculopustular categories. These disorders are reviewed next, with a focus on early diagnosis, treatment, and implications for surgical management. Then, several specific dermatologic disorders for which the surgeon may be consulted are discussed.

PAPULOSQUAMOUS DISORDERS

Although papulosquamous disorders share morphologic features (Table 96-1), they are produced by a number of different

1619

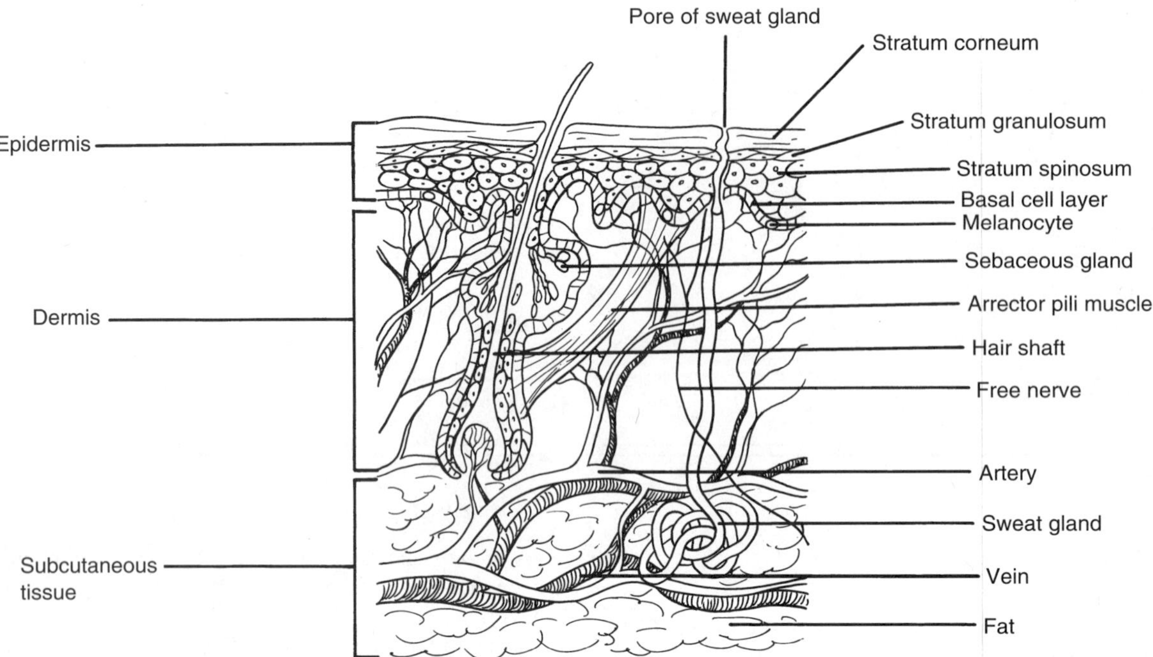

FIG. 96-1. Schematic illustration of the skin. (Holbrook KA, Sybert V. Structure and biochemical properties of the skin of adults, children, and newborn infants. In: Schachner LA, Hansen RC, eds. Pediatric dermatology. New York, Churchill Livingstone, 1988:30)

mechanisms. In psoriasis, a rapid increase in proliferation of basal cells results in a markedly thickened epidermis and stratum corneum. In dermatitic processes, such as contact dermatitis, atopic dermatitis, seborrheic dermatitis, pityriasis rosea, and fungal infections, inflammation results in thickening of the epidermis, dermal and epidermal edema, and occasionally crusts, erosions, and vesiculation. Although these disorders do not usually interfere with the treatment of surgical patients, bacterial colonization of the skin lesions can result in an increased risk of wound infections, and some of these disorders can be exacerbated by surgery.

Psoriasis

Although it is often stated that psoriasis is rare in children, nearly one third of patients develop their first lesions during the first two decades of life, and 2% exhibit lesions before 2 years of age.[2,3] Round, itchy, red plaques with thick, adherent, silvery scales typically develop in a symmetric distribution on the scalp, elbows, knees, lumbosacral area, and genitals. The nails can have pitting, yellowing, onycholysis (separation of the nail from the underlying nail bed, giving an oil droplet appearance), subungual scale, and increased friability. Children

TABLE 96-1. *Papulosquamous eruptions*

Disorder	Skin lesions	Distribution	Diagnostic studies
Irritant dermatitis	Papules, vesicles, scale, crusts	Face, trunk, extremities	
Contact allergic dermatitis	Papules, vesicles, scale, crusts	Face, trunk, extremities	Patch testing
Atopic dermatitis	Papules, scale, crusts, lichenification, pigmentary change	Flexures, face, generalized	None, increased immunoglobulin E
Seborrheic dermatitis	Erythema, papules, scale, pigmentary change	Face, scalp, creases	
Scabies	Papules, scale, vesicles, pustules, burrows	Hands, wrists, axillae, genitals, breasts; infants—scalp, palms, soles	Scabies preparation
Ringworm	Papules, scale, pustules	Face, scalp, trunk, extremities	Potassium hydroxide preparation
Pityriasis rosea	Papules, scaly patches, Christmas tree pattern	Trunk, proximal extremities	Syphilis serology
Psoriasis	Papules, plaques, scale, changes	Scalp, trunk, extremities	Throat culture (in guttate psoriasis)

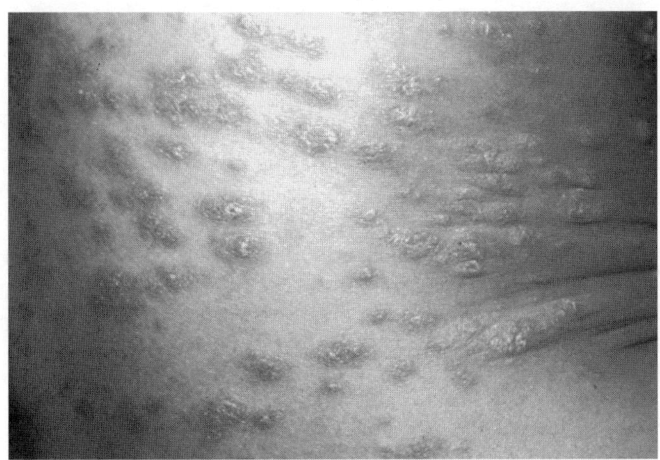

FIG. 96-2. Guttate psoriasis. One- to 2-cm minimally scaly, bright red plaques with central scale erupted on the trunk of this 6-year-old boy after streptococcal pharyngitis. (See Color Figure 96-2.)

tend to present acutely with small guttate disseminated plaques, which may be triggered by streptococcal or viral infections. In infants, psoriasis can masquerade as a recalcitrant diaper dermatitis (Fig. 96-2).

Most patients at some time during the course of their disease demonstrate the Koebner, or isomorphic, phenomenon, in which cutaneous lesions appear at sites of trauma, such as surgical wounds, casts, and external fixation devices. Although the risk of infection is relatively low because of the rapid turnover of epidermal cells at the surface, the disruption of the integument occasionally results in secondary bacterial infections. These can be difficult to distinguish from the primary lesions of psoriasis, in which the presence of small pustules is a common finding. Culture of the suspicious lesions and treatment with antistaphylococcal antibiotics may be necessary.

Medium-potency steroids and emollients are the mainstay of topical therapy. Preparations containing anthralin, tar, and keratolytics, such as salicylic and lactic acid, are useful adjuncts. Psoriatic lesions usually clear in the summer sun, and artificial ultraviolet light therapy can be accomplished during the winter. Sunburns can cause a Koebner reaction and should be avoided.

In most children, psoriasis is mild and remains localized. In others, however, the course is prolonged and severe, with periodic relapses and remissions.

Irritant Contact Dermatitis

Irritant contact dermatitis is the most common dermatitis in childhood. In infants, irritation from urine, stool, and topical medications can produce an acute or chronic dermatitis.[4,5] In acute dermatitic reactions, painful, well-demarcated bright red patches that can quickly become blistered and eroded develop over the thighs, buttocks, genitals, and perineum. Protected areas, such as the skin creases, are usually spared. Chronic diaper rash presents with thickened, scaly red patches frequently associated with increased or decreased pigmentation. When a diaper dermatitis has secondary candidal infection, the eruption

spreads to the skin creases, and discrete papules and pustules appear beyond the confluent areas in the diaper region. When streptococcal or staphylococcal infection complicates diaper dermatitis, blisters, pustules, erosions, and crusts usually expand from the skin folds to involve the entire area and can disseminate to the trunk and extremities.

After abdominal or intestinal surgery, the development of constipation or diarrhea can trigger diaper dermatitis, which may be exacerbated by the administration of antibiotics. Children with chronic diarrhea (eg, short bowel syndrome) and those with fecal and urinary incontinence are particularly prone to persistent diaper dermatitis. Similar lesions can erupt around ostomies and other appliances.

Initial management of diaper dermatitis includes frequent diaper changes and application of occlusive topical barrier preparations (eg, petrolatum, zinc oxide ointment, Corya paste). When the area of involvement is completely surrounded by normal skin, bioocclusive dressings can be applied for several days to permit rapid reepithelialization. Low- or medium-potency topical steroids used intermittently twice a day for 3 to 5 days decrease the erythema and improve symptoms quickly when necessary. When candidal infection is present, an anticandidal agent, such as nystatin, or a broad-spectrum antifungal agent, such as naftifine, cyclopirox, clotrimazole, miconazole, or econazole, should be applied with each diaper change until the lesions clear.

Irritant dermatitis on the cheeks and mouth occurs at some time in almost all children, probably in response to water, juices, food, and saliva. A generalized rash with marked involvement of the skin folds can result from contact with soaps, detergents, fabric softeners, and bleach.[6] Surgical soaps, antiseptic scrubs, and particularly iodophors should be carefully removed from the skin after surgery and should be used only with caution in premature infants and in patients with preexisting skin rashes. The location and type of lesions and a history of exposure to inciting agents aid in diagnosis and avoidance of the irritant.

Tap water or aluminum acetate compresses can be used to relieve acute lesions. Emollients and medium-potency steroid ointments (eg, triamcinolone 0.1%, betamethasone valerate 0.1%) are generally effective in chronic dermatitis, but only low-potency steroids (eg, hydrocortisone 1% to 2.5%) should be used on the face or intertriginous areas. All steroids should be tapered as lesions clear, but emollients can be continued indefinitely.

Allergic Contact Dermatitis

Poison ivy typifies acute contact dermatitis produced by a delayed type IV hypersensitivity reaction (Fig. 96-3). After a period of sensitization lasting 1 week or longer, the eruption can be elicited by exposure to small quantities of the antigen. Acute lesions are recognized by linear vesicular morphology and associated erythema, vesiculation, and intense pruritus. Chronic lesions are indistinguishable from other forms of dermatitis, although a localized asymmetric distribution may suggest the diagnosis.

Tape, latex, rubber, adhesives, topical antibiotics, and other topical agents can trigger an allergic contact dermatitis in the surgical setting.[7] Latex has been implicated in the development of acute immunoglobulin E–mediated urticaria and anaphylac-

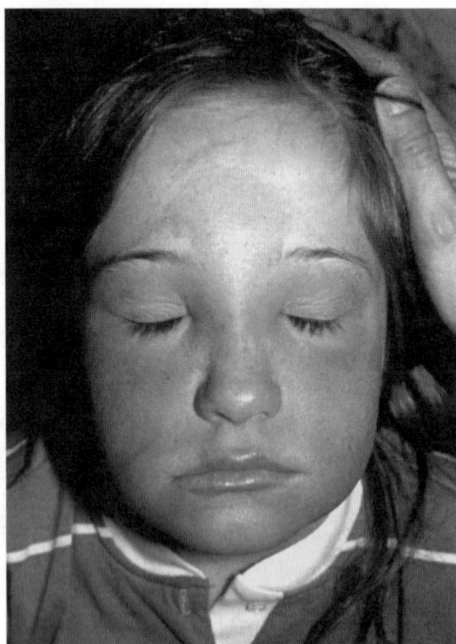

FIG. 96-3. Acute contact dermatitis. An intensely pruritic poison ivy dermatitis developed on the face of this 7-year-old girl after camping. An area of sparing is visible under her bangs on her forehead. (See Color Figure 96-3.)

tic reactions. This is a particularly important concern in patients with spina bifida.[8]

Immediate recognition and discontinuation of the inciting agent are imperative to treat allergic contact dermatitis, regardless of the cause. Topical corticosteroids may be required for several weeks while the reaction subsides. In severe reactions involving large areas of the body surface or strategic areas, such as the hands, face, or genitals, a tapering course of systemic prednisone, 0.5 to 1 mg/kg/d, produces relief of symptoms in 24 to 48 hours. Therapy should be continued for at least 10 days to avoid a rebound of lesions, which frequently occurs when steroids are tapered too quickly. After the acute episode has cleared, patch testing can be performed to help identify a specific agent when the sensitizer is unclear.

Atopic Dermatitis

Although atopic dermatitis often develops during the first year of life, months of observation may be necessary to establish the diagnosis.[9] Scaling, lichenification, excoriations, and hyperpigmentation are often present. With acute flares of disease activity, red papules, vesicles, and crusting may be superimposed. Older children and adolescents present with flexural involvement; in infants, the lesions can disseminate to the face, trunk, and extremities.

A family history of atopic conditions (allergic rhinitis, sinusitis, asthma, eczema, food allergy) is found in 75% of affected infants and children. Although no specific laboratory study confirms the diagnosis, atopic dermatitis should be considered in any child with a family history of atopic conditions and a chronic, recurrent pruritic eruption with the typical distribution.

After adolescence, atopic dermatitis resolves in more than half of patients and improves in most others. Some patients, however, continue to have relapses into adulthood.

In many children, the anxiety associated with surgery and hospitalization can result in increased itching and can trigger eczema. Irritation from bed linens and interference with home skin management routines during hospitalization also can exacerbate the disease. Moreover, the skin of children with atopic dermatitis is often colonized with *Staphylococcus aureus,* which may increase the risk of postoperative infections.

Good skin care requires the aggressive use of lubricants on a routine basis, particularly after bathing, and judicious use of topical steroids. During flare-ups, patients respond quickly to twice-daily applications of medium-potency topical steroid ointments; to oral antihistamines, such as diphenhydramine, 5 mg/kg/d in divided doses every 6 hours, or hydroxyzine, 5 to 10 mg every 6 hours; and to 15-minute cool tap water compresses or tub soaks two or three times a day followed by lubricants. As lesions subside, parents should taper topical steroids and antihistamines. Patients with secondary impetiginization require appropriate oral or parenteral antibiotics. Widespread primary herpes simplex infection (eczema herpeticum; Fig. 96-4) should be considered in any child who fails to respond to treatment or who has a recent history of exposure to the virus. Fever, itching, and skin lesions associated with viral infection may clear quickly with the administration of acyclovir.

Seborrheic Dermatitis

Seborrheic dermatitis is a red, scaly, oily eruption that occurs in areas where sebaceous glands are most highly concentrated (ie, scalp, face, ears, and intertriginous areas).[10] Although the cause is unclear, data suggest a role for the *Pityrosporum* sp yeast, which is found commonly on the involved areas.[11] Histology demonstrates a dermatitis and normal sebaceous glands. Often, the first manifestation is ''cradle cap,'' a thick, scaly rash on the scalp that appears during the first several weeks of life. Red, greasy, scaly patches associated with hypopigmentation can develop on the face, ears, axillae, and diaper area. Occasionally, infantile seborrheic dermatitis becomes generalized, but despite the eruption, patients continue to eat and grow normally. The condition usually improves spontaneously by 6 months of age.

A seborrheic dermatitis-like rash with erosive or hemorrhagic lesions in the skin folds in an infant with poor weight gain, diarrhea, and alopecia should suggest histiocytosis X[12] or a nutritional deficiency (eg, zinc deficiency dermatitis, acrodermatitis enteropathica,[13] essential fatty acid deficiency, biotin deficiency). Nutritional deficiency rashes occur in the setting of inborn errors of metabolism (eg, acrodermatitis enteropathica, biotinodase deficiency), inadequate nutritional intake (eg, total parenteral alimentation without adequate trace element, protein, or essential fatty acid replacement), or malabsorption (eg, cystic fibrosis, short gut syndrome).

Scabies

The diagnosis of scabies should be considered in any child with a chronic itchy rash of unclear cause and when newly

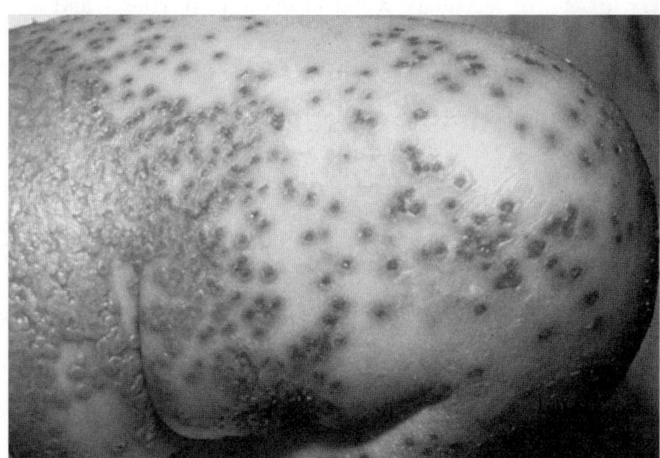

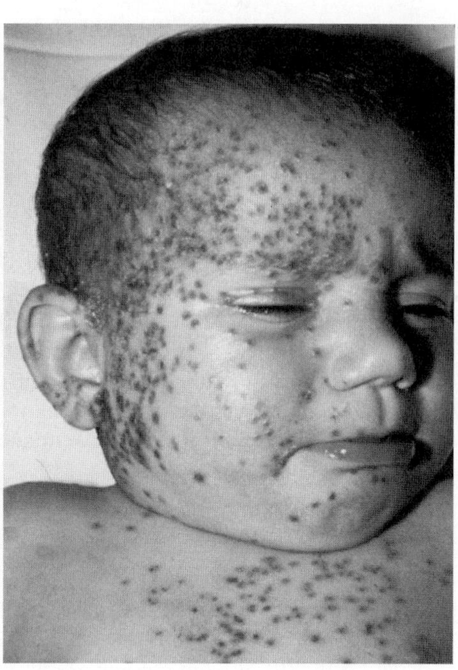

FIG. 96-4. (*A*) Eczema herpeticum spread quickly over the skin of this infant from a primary site on the thigh. (*B*) The uniform, clustered, 3-mm vesicles and erosions are typical of herpes simplex virus infection seen here on the face and chest. (See Color Figure 96-4.)

A

B

diagnosed contact or atopic dermatitis fails to respond to therapy.[14] Transmission requires close physical contact, which occurs frequently in hospitalized surgical patients. Early recognition of the infestation is critical to prevent epidemics among staff and patients.

In older children and adolescents, papules, vesicles, and pustules typically appear on the hands, wrists, and intertriginous areas. Once the patient becomes sensitized to the mite, a generalized acute dermatitis can disturb the primary lesions, making diagnosis difficult. Although burrows are pathognomonic, they are found in only 10% to 25% of cases. Unlike adults, infants frequently have papules, pustules, vesicles, and burrows on the palms, soles, scalp as well as on the trunk. Mites and eggs are readily identified by low-power microscopic examination of material scraped from burrows.

Permethrin 5% cream is the treatment of choice and is approved for use in infants as young as 2 months old. A single overnight application for the child, family members, and all close contacts is safe and effective. γ-Benzene hexachloride is an effective alternative, but it has been associated with significant transcutaneous absorption and central nervous system toxicity and should be used with extreme caution in infants and compromised hosts of all ages.

Ringworm

Dermatophyte (ringworm fungus) infections also produce dermatitis. The rash typically begins as a single papule or multiple papules or pustules on a scaly, red base.[15] Within several days, lesions enlarge to form annular plaques with red papular, scaly borders and flattened, hyperpigmented, or violaceous centers (Fig. 96-5). The eruption is extremely pruritic and can involve the trunk (tinea corporis), the feet (tinea pedis), the face (tinea faciale), the nails (tinea unguium), and the scalp (tinea capitis).

Tinea capitis is extremely common in childhood and can become epidemic in schools and daycare centers.[16] In many children, subtle, minimally scaly patches in the scalp are often dismissed as seborrheic dermatitis. Inflammatory tinea capitis (kerion) with associated edema, pustules, and crusts can be misdiagnosed as impetigo and occasionally heals with scarring alopecia. Patients with kerions may be referred for incision and débridement. Surgical intervention should be avoided because of the increased risk of scarring. The treatment of choice is oral griseofulvin, 10 to 20 mg/kg/d, given as a single or two divided doses with meals. Oral steroids in a tapering dose for 10 to 14 days decrease the inflammatory response and, subsequently, the risk of permanent hair loss.

Chronic tinea pedis (athlete's foot) can occur in children and

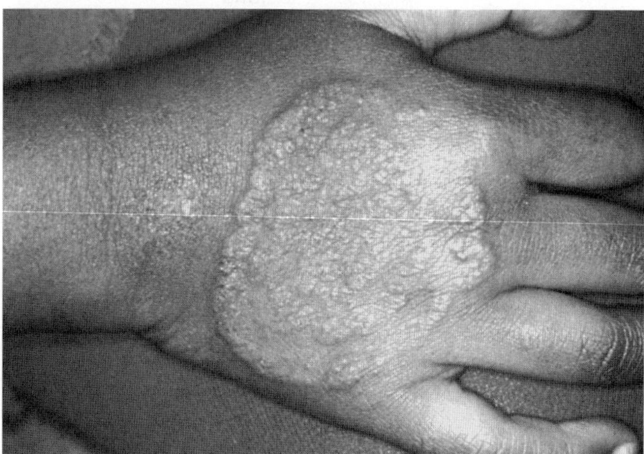

FIG. 96-5. An expanding annular plaque started as a small red papule a week earlier on the back of the hand of a 7-year-old boy. A KOH preparation showed hyphae diagnostic of tinea corporis. (See Color Figure 96-5.)

can be a source of recurrent bacterial cellulitis.[17] Tinea corporis appears acutely and must be diagnosed and treated quickly to avoid an epidemic in an institutional setting.

A potassium hydroxide preparation can be used for microscopic examination of scrapings from the scalp, trunk, extremities, or nails. Fungal cultures should be ordered when the scraping is negative but the clinical pattern is highly suggestive of dermatophyte infection.

Topical antifungal agents (eg, clotrimazole, miconazole, naftifine, econazole) are effective on glabrous skin and should be applied until scale, pustules, and crusts are gone and then for an additional 7 to 10 days. Patients with recalcitrant tinea pedis or widespread tinea corporis usually respond within 2 to 4 weeks to oral griseofulvin and can then switch back to topical agents. Associated bacterial cellulitis should be treated with appropriate antibiotics.

Pityriasis Rosea

Symptomatic papulosquamous disorders must be differentiated from pityriasis rosea, a self-limiting papulosquamous eruption that occurs primarily in children and young adults.[18] Oval, pink, scaly patches appear in a diffuse Christmas tree pattern on the trunk. Lesions occasionally disseminate to the extremities and face. In 40% to 50% of patients, a large (3 to 10 cm) herald patch on the trunk marks the onset of the rash.

Early diagnosis of pityriasis rosea is important to reassure the family and avoid unnecessary treatment. Patients need not be excluded from school, and surgical admission to the hospital can proceed as scheduled.

In the rare case when pityriasis rosea is pruritic, symptoms may respond to emollients, topical steroids, antihistamines, sunlight, or artificial light. Lesions persist for 2 to 3 months and heal spontaneously without scarring. In adolescents, the rash of secondary syphilis can mimic pityriasis, and serology should be checked to exclude this diagnosis.

VESICULOPUSTULAR ERUPTIONS

Vesiculopustular rashes can be benign, self-limiting conditions or rapidly fatal diseases (Table 96-2). Early diagnosis is mandatory, especially in infants. Through careful physical examination and a few bedside techniques, these disorders can be readily differentiated.

Viral Eruptions

Herpes Simplex

Herpes simplex is a common cause of oral lesions in toddlers and older children.[19] Herpetic gingivostomatitis begins with extensive perioral vesicles and pustules and intraoral vesicles and erosions. Lesions can also be scattered on the face and upper trunk; in infants and toddlers, lesions are frequently autoinnoculated onto the hands. Herpetic whitlow, a primary infection involving the distal aspect of one or several fingers, may be mistaken for a deep soft tissue infection because of the intense pain, edema, and fever (Fig. 96-6). Vesicles dry and desquamate, and erosions usually heal without scarring in 7 to 14 days. In immunocompromised children and those with primary skin conditions such as eczema, seborrheic dermatitis, and immunobullous disorders, herpes simplex can disseminate over the entire cutaneous surface and occasionally to the lungs, viscera, and central nervous system. Indolent herpetic ulcers on the skin

TABLE 96-2. *Vesiculopustular eruptions*

Disorder	Skin lesions	Distribution	Diagnostic studies
Herpes simplex	Vesicles, pustules, erosions; mucous membrane lesions	Face, trunk, extremities	Tzanck preparation, viral culture
Varicella	Papules, umbilicated vesicles, crusts; occasional mucous membrane lesions	Face, trunk, extremities	Tzanck preparation, viral culture
Herpes zoster	Dermatomal pattern	Dermatomal	Tzanck preparation
Insect bites	Papules, urticaria, vesicles	Trunk, extremities	Tzanck preparation Gram stain—negative
Miliaria	Papules, vesicles	Occluded areas	Tzanck, potassium hydroxide, Gram stain—negative
Impetigo			
Streptococci	Crusts, scale	Face, trunk, extremities	Gram stain, culture-positive
Staphylococci	Crusts, scale, bullae	Increased on exposed surfaces, but any site	Gram stain, culture-positive
Staphylococcal pustolosis	Papules, pustules	Trunk, diaper area	Gram stain, culture-positive
Staphylococcal scalded skin syndrome	Sunburn-like erythema erosions, crusting	Face, extremities, generalized; mucous membranes spared	Skin biopsy
Toxic epidermal necrolysis	Bullae, erosions, crusts	Generalized; mucous membrane lesions	Skin biopsy
Erythema multiforme	Target lesions, erosions	Extremities, generalized; mucous membrane lesions	Skin biopsy

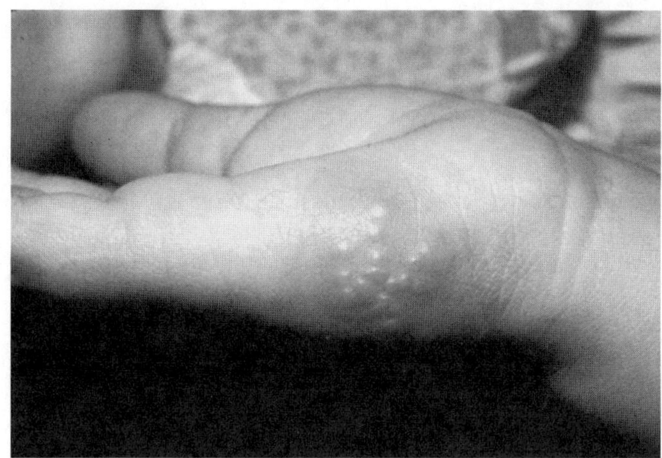

FIG. 96-6. A herpetic whitlow was mistaken for a bacterial cellulitis on the lateral aspect of the hand of this 14-month-old boy, who also had a primary herpes labialis infection. A Tzanck smear from intact vesicles revealed multinucleated giant cells typical of a viral infection. (See Color Figure 96-6.)

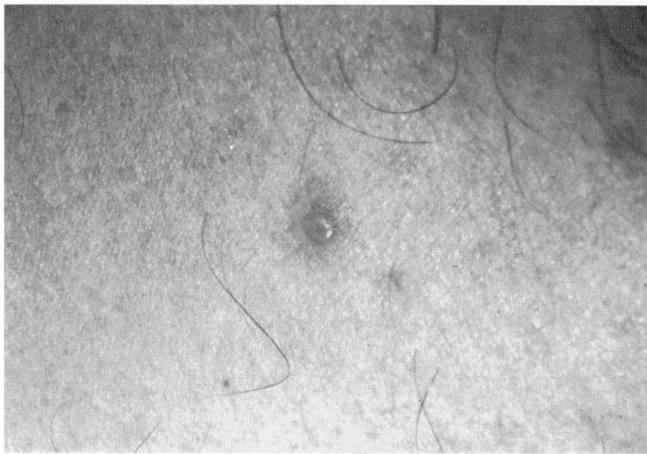

FIG. 96-7. A "dew drop on a rose petal" represents the typical chickenpox vesicle on an inflammatory red base, which is virtually diagnostic for the infection. (See Color Figure 96-7.)

or mucous membranes can persist for weeks and occasionally months in patients with the human immunodeficiency virus. Tzanck smears and viral culture help to exclude herpes simplex virus in this setting.

Herpes simplex virus can also produce devastating disease in the nursery. Primary herpes infection develops in half of infants exposed to herpesvirus at delivery, and half of those children, if untreated, die or develop severe systemic disease. Early treatment of infected infants with acyclovir decreases the risk of morbidity and mortality. Therefore, vesicles, pustules, and eroded areas should be evaluated immediately with a Tzanck smear, which demonstrates multinucleated giant cells in two thirds of patients with fresh herpetic lesions. The physician must obtain confirmatory viral cultures, but these results can require 24 to 48 hours.

In older children and adolescents, patterns of primary and recurrent herpes simplex virus are similar to those seen in adults. Symptomatic treatment with tap water compresses, sitz baths, and analgesics is sufficient. In prepubertal children with genital herpes, the possibility of sexual abuse must be considered.

Varicella

Varicella (chickenpox) is a mild disease in most children. Neonates who contract the infection in utero shortly before delivery or during the first 2 weeks of life, however, are at risk for the development of disseminated disease, which causes neurologic damage or death in 25% to 50% of affected infants.[20] Disseminated disease is also seen in older children receiving immunosuppressive therapy. Early administration of varicella zoster immunoglobulin to immunocompromised children exposed to varicella can be preventative, and antiviral therapy in patients with disseminated lesions can be life-saving. The US Food and Drug Administration recently approved a varicella vaccine; if widely used, it should substantially reduce the risks of this ubiquitous disease.

Fever, sore throat, decreased appetite, and malaise precede the skin lesions by several days. Early cutaneous findings vary from a few scattered, pruritic, red papules to generalized papules that evolve within 24 hours to vesicles on a bright, red base (Fig. 96-7). Central umbilication of vesicles follows quickly, and crusting and desquamation occur within 1 week. New lesions continue to appear for 3 to 4 days. Although the lesions usually heal without scarring, some develop sterile pustules or become secondarily infected and heal with pitted scars. Secondary infection and cellulitis are the most frequent causes of hospitalization (Fig. 96-8). Fasciitis and disseminated intravascular coagulation occur rarely.

Pruritus responds to cool compresses, calamine lotion, and antihistamines. Secondary infection is usually caused by *S aureus* or group A β-hemolytic streptococci and should be treated with systemic antibiotics.

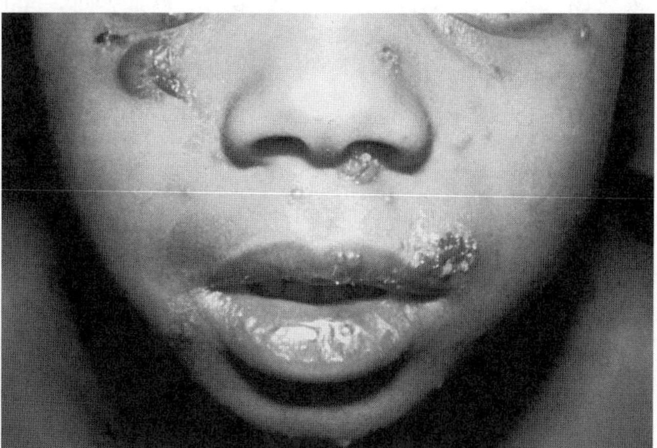

FIG. 96-8. A 7-year-old boy developed large crusts and 1- to 2-cm pustules characteristic of impetiginized chickenpox. (See Color Figure 96-8.)

FIG. 96-9. A unilateral dermatomic vesicular eruption typical of shingles appeared on the trunk of an otherwise healthy girl. (See Color Figure 96-9.)

Herpes Zoster

Reactivation of varicella in a dermatomal pattern (shingles) is a common, self-limiting eruption in children. The risk of dissemination is increased in the immunocompromised child. Although the primary lesions of herpes zoster are indistinguishable from those of chickenpox, the presence of a unilateral rash restricted to one or several contiguous dermatomes is diagnostic (Fig. 96-9). In both varicella and zoster, a positive Tzanck smear can be especially important when the diagnosis is uncertain because viral culture identification requires 7 to 14 days.

Recurrent herpes zoster, like herpes simplex, can be triggered by sunburn, trauma, radiotherapy, surgery, and a number of other nonspecific factors. If surgery is planned in an area that has been subject to herpes simplex or zoster, prophylactic oral acyclovir may be useful to reduce the risk of recurrent skin disease.

Hand, Foot, and Mouth Syndrome

A number of enteroviruses, particularly echovirus and coxsackievirus, can trigger a mild, self-limited papulovesicular eruption involving the hands, feet, mouth, and occasionally the trunk.[21] Lesions start as red papules on the palms and soles and quickly develop into elongated, deep-seated vesicles on a bright red base. Vesicles and small, punched-out erosions on a red base appear on the hard palate, and red papules can develop on the buttocks, back, and abdomen. Symptoms include fever, diarrhea, and vomiting and are usually brief. It is important to recognize this entity, especially in complicated surgical or medical patients, so that skin lesions are not confused with bacterial infections or drug reactions.

Miliaria

Miliaria crystallina may be mistaken for herpes simplex or chickenpox. Obstruction of sweat ducts in the outer layer of the epidermis results in the formation of 2- to 3-mm noninflammatory vesicles that are readily ruptured by the examiner.[22] When the sweat duct obstruction occurs in the middle or deep dermis, an erythematous, papulopustular eruption called *miliaria rubra* is produced. This rash occurs commonly in infants and young children as a result of tight-fitting clothing or use of occlusive topical lubricants, especially during the spring and summer. Loose-fitting clothing and elimination of greasy topical preparations allow for rapid clearing of lesions. Miliaria also frequently erupts in surgical patients when they are immobilized postoperatively. Dependent areas are usually most severely affected, and ventilation and cooling of involved skin is curative.

Impetigo and Staphylococcal Scalded Skin Syndrome

In classic impetigo, honey-colored crusts are found overlying infected abrasions, insect bites, and other primary skin rashes. Bullous impetigo, however, is characterized by slowly enlarging blistered rings surrounding central umbilicated crusts (Fig. 96-10). These lesions, which can reach 10 cm in diameter, are caused by certain strains of staphylococci that elaborate an exotoxin known as *epidermolysin*.[23,24] Epidermolysin produces flaccid bullae by cleaving the skin high in the epidermis.

In infants and young children with low antibody titers against epidermolysin and decreased renal excretion of the exotoxin, widespread bulla formation can occur, resulting in staphylococcal scalded skin syndrome (Fig. 96-11). Blistering is preceded by a generalized, tender, sunburn-like erythema, and patients are febrile and irritable. In localized bullous impetigo, the bacteria are readily obtained directly from skin lesions. In scalded skin syndrome, however, the primary site of infection may not be apparent. In these cases, noncutaneous sources of infection (eg, sinuses, nares, lungs, surgical wound) must be sought.

Although oral penicillin is effective against classic impetigo caused by group A β-hemolytic streptococci, several surveys

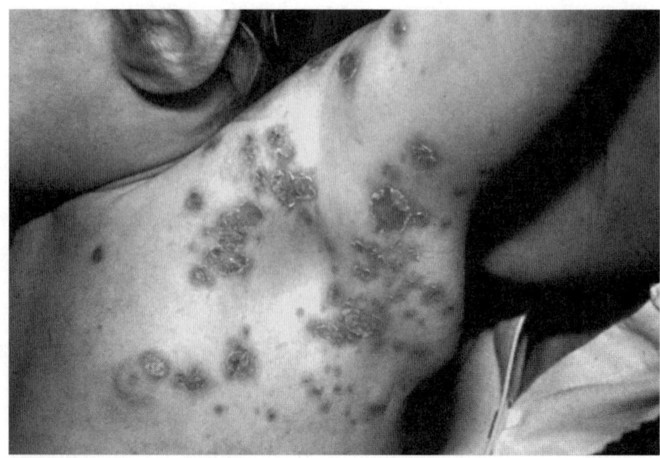

FIG. 96-10. New superficial blisters and crusts continued to spread across the upper chest of a toddler with bullous impetigo. (See Color Figure 96-10.)

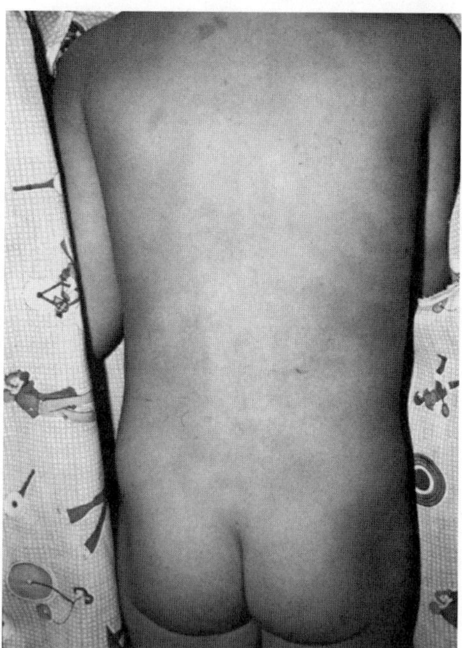

FIG. 96-11. Total-body sunburn-like erythema erupted in a toddler after a day of low-grade fever and upper respiratory symptoms. The Nikolsky sign (epidermal stripping), typical of staphylococcal scalded skin syndrome, can be seen on the upper back. It developed after the boy's father lifted him onto the examining table. (See Color Figure 96-11.)

demonstrate the emergence of *S aureus* as the predominant organism in most cases. Therefore, oral cephalosporins (eg, cephalexin, cephadroxyl), amoxicillin and clavulanic acid, and dicloxacillin are the drugs of choice. Small, localized patches of impetigo can also be treated effectively with topical mupirocin. Most children with staphylococcal scalded skin syndrome respond quickly to oral antibiotics. Seriously ill children should be admitted to the hospital and treated parenterally.

Toxic Epidermal Necrolysis

Although originally described in adults, toxic epidermal necrolysis has been reported in children and adolescents, especially in association with drug hypersensitivity reactions.[25] Children have fever, sore throat, malaise, and generalized erythema, followed by sloughing of large areas of skin. Unlike staphylococcal scalded skin syndrome, the bullae of toxic epidermal necrolysis form by cleavage of the skin at the dermal–epidermal junction, with resultant full-thickness necrosis. Intensive supportive therapy in an intensive care unit or burn unit is required to avoid fluid and electrolyte losses and secondary bacterial infection.[26] Mucous membranes, including the pharynx, conjunctivae, urethra, and perianal and vaginal areas are involved.

Erythema Multiforme

Erythema multiforme can progress to Stevens-Johnson syndrome, with a clinical picture indistinguishable from that of toxic epidermal necrolysis.[27] The lesions generally remain discrete, however, and extensive mucous membrane involvement occurs in fewer than 10% of children (Fig. 96-12).

The hallmark of erythema multiforme is the target or "bull's eye" lesion formed by a central bluish purple macule or vesicle surrounded by alternating pale and violaceous rings. Erythematous papules, annular plaques, and urticarial wheals are usually present. Lesions occur most frequently on the extremities, but the entire skin surface can become involved. Although the lesions heal without scarring, both hypopigmented and hyperpigmented macules can remain, and the eruption can recur with exposure to triggering factors, including certain drugs, toxins, and infectious agents.[28]

Therapy is supportive, but hospitalization may be appropriate, especially when mucosal involvement is severe. The efficacy of systemic corticosteroids in severe erythema multiforme and toxic epidermal necrolysis has never been substantiated in a controlled clinical trial, and steroids may actually prolong hospitalization by producing serious adverse reactions.

Child Abuse

Sharply demarcated blisters or denuded areas of skin consistent with hot water injuries on the distal extremities or diaper area of infants and young children should be considered child abuse until proved otherwise.[29,30] A vague history that is not compatible with the cutaneous findings and that varies with different caretakers or the same caretaker at different times is typical of physical abuse. The presence of bruises, edema, abrasions, and the imprint of the object that caused the injury in

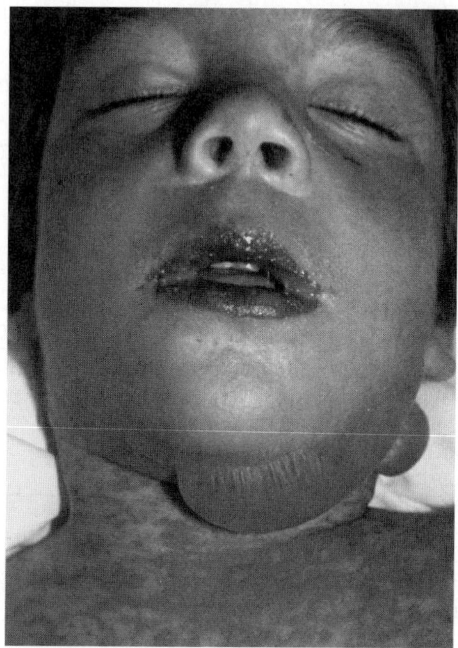

FIG. 96-12. Stevens-Johnson syndrome. A widespread rash associated with severe blistering of the skin and mucous membranes developed in this 6-year-old girl during a course of trimethoprim-sulfamethoxazole for an ear infection. (See Color Figure 96-12.)

an unusual location, such as the middle of the back, buttocks, genitals, upper arms, ears, and feet, should also raise the specter of abuse. Other red flags include a delay in presentation for medical care of injuries, inappropriate parental concern, and a history of repeated visits to the emergency room or physician's office for accidents, fractures, lacerations, or ingestion of foreign objects or poisons.

Whenever physical or sexual abuse is suspected, the child deserves a careful cutaneous and medical examination. Deep soft tissue, intracranial, abdominal, and pelvic injuries must be excluded. Historical data from the emergency room, nursery, and primary care records should be reviewed. All abused children must be reported to the appropriate authorities and released only to caretakers who can ensure their safety.

SUPERFICIAL LUMPS AND BUMPS

Although most superficial tumors in children are innocent and self-limiting, primary cutaneous malignancies and metastatic tumors appear in the skin rarely (Table 96-3). Benign self-limiting tumors, including warts, molluscum contagiosum, and granuloma annulare; epidermal inclusion cysts and adnexal tumors; hamartomatous nevi and pigmented nevi; and cutaneous malignancies are reviewed. Hemangiomas and vascular malformations are discussed in Chapter 32.

Warts

Patients and parents frequently arrive for surgical consultation and demand aggressive therapy for warts. Almost everyone experiences at least a few lesions caused by human papillomavirus (HPV). More than 60 virus types have been identified in a number of clinical settings.[31] Verruca vulgaris, most commonly associated with HPV 2 and 4, is ubiquitous in children and probably spreads directly by skin-to-skin contact and indirectly by contaminated scale. Similarly, plantar warts are caused by HPV 1, flat warts by HPV 3, and condyloma acuminata by HPV 6 and 11 (less commonly by HPV 16, 18, and 42 to 45).

TABLE 96-3. *Histologic diagnosis of 775 superficial lumps excised in children*

Type	Occurrence
Epidermal inclusion cysts	459 (59%)
Congenital malformations (pilomatricoma, lymphangioma, brachial cleft cyst)	56 (7%)
Benign neoplasms (neural tumors, lipoma, adnexal tumors)	56 (7%)
Benign lesions of undetermined origin (xanthomas, xanthogranulomas, fibromatosis, fibromas)	50 (6%)
Self-limiting processes (granuloma annulare, urticaria pigmentosa, insect bite reaction)	47 (6%)
Malignant tumors	11 (1.4%)
Miscellaneous	35 (4%)

(Modified from Knight PJ, Reina CB. Superficial lumps and bumps in children: what, when, and why? Pediatrics 1983; 72:147)

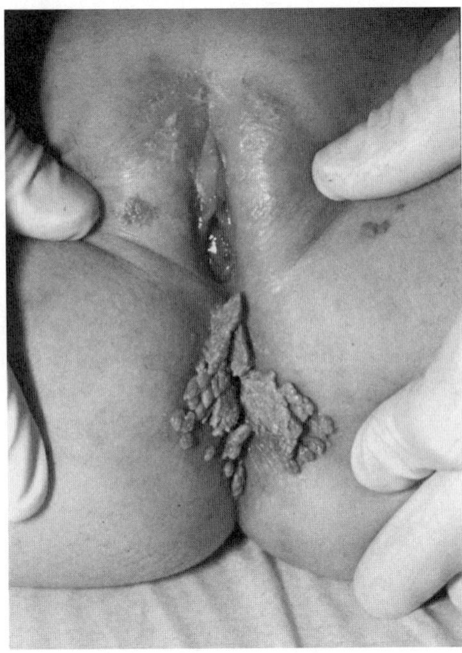

FIG. 96-13. This 1-year-old girl developed extensive anogenital warts at 4 months of age. Her mother had genital warts when the child was delivered. (See Color Figure 96-13.)

The recent epidemic of anogenital warts in children is of special interest to clinicians involved in pediatric care (Fig. 96-13).

Before 1980, fewer than 20 cases of anogenital warts were reported in children, and most were known or suspected to have been acquired from sexual abuse. During the past decade, there has been an explosion in pediatric case reports that has followed the epidemic of condyloma in young sexually active adults.[32] Moreover, several large series of carefully investigated children have demonstrated that most pediatric infections are acquired by an innocent, nonvenereal route. Although the clinician must raise the issue of sexual exposure in any child who presents with anogenital warts, other sources, particularly perinatal contact with maternal condyloma, should be considered. Unfortunately, maternal lesions may be subclinical or regress spontaneously before the diagnosis is made. Indirect contact with maternal or paternal HPV can occur during bathing, diaper changes, and toileting in infants and toddlers.

The risk of recurrence of warts after surgical excision is high, and less aggressive measures, such as the use of topical keratolytics (eg, lactic acid, salicylic acid, retinoic acid) with adhesive tape occlusion or liquid nitrogen freeze, should be attempted first in cooperative children. Fortunately, nearly 85% of warts regress without treatment within 3 years. Recalcitrant warts may respond to intralesional bleomycin, electrocautery, or carbon dioxide laser surgery. All of these modalities are painful and require at least local anesthesia, and they are all associated with a risk of scarring and recurrent lesions. In compromised hosts with large, rapidly growing, or painful lesions, laser or excisional surgery may be necessary for patient comfort or because of recurrent problems with bleeding or secondary bacterial infection. Anal warts in particular require more than one operative session to avoid circumferential operative injury to the anus with stricture formation.

Molluscum Contagiosum

Although the large DNA pox virus that causes the pearly papules of molluscum contagiosum is spread primarily by sexual contact in teenagers and adults, nonvenereal skin-to-skin contact is the usual route of infection in children.[33] These lesions first appear as tiny 1- to 2-mm papules on virtually any skin or mucous membrane site and can grow to 5 to 10 mm, especially in intertriginous areas such as the diaper area or axillae. Scratched molluscum can resolve or develop multiple lesions in lines around the primary papule. Larger lesions develop a characteristic scaly central umbilication through which the core, or molluscum body, which contains the infected keratinocytes, can be expressed.

Immunologic recovery without treatment occurs in most healthy children within 6 months to 3 years. Symptomatic lesions can be curetted painlessly after a 2-hour application of EMLA (eutectic mixture of lidocaine and prilocaine) cream under plastic wrap occlusion.[34] Vesicants, such as cantharidin, can also be used effectively and painlessly. Unfortunately, the risk of new lesions appearing is high, and painful, aggressive procedures should be avoided.

In children with hereditary or acquired immunodeficiency states, widespread and recalcitrant molluscum or HPV may be the earliest manifestation of the underlying disorder.[35] Consequently, otherwise healthy children with disseminated skin lesions that are resistant to treatment deserve screening for decreased cellular and humoral immunologic parameters. Careful history taking may reveal evidence of other chronic or opportunistic infections.

Granuloma Annulare

Parents may seek a surgical consultation for granuloma annulare when this innocent, chronic, self-limiting process is mistaken for a potentially serious tumor. When fully erupted, granuloma annulare presents with annular dermal nodules caused by a characteristic dermal infiltrate of lymphocytes and histiocytes. Typically, lesions begin as one or several papules or nodules that expand over weeks to months to form rings from 1 to 4 cm in diameter. The overlying epidermis is usually intact and the same color as adjacent skin but sometimes is slightly red or hyperpigmented. Most lesions are asymptomatic. Granuloma annulare commonly appears on the extensor surfaces of the lower legs, feet, fingers, and hands, but other areas can be involved.

Granuloma annulare is commonly confused with ringworm. Ringworm, however, produces epidermal changes, such as scale, vesicles, and pustules, and the lesions are itchy or painful. A subcutaneous variant that can involve the extremities as well as the face and scalp can be mistaken for rheumatoid nodules, lymphoma, or other tumors. A small punch biopsy can be performed to demonstrate the typical pathology and reassure the family. Lesions can remit and recur for years, but spontaneous healing is the rule.

Epidermal Inclusion Cysts and Adnexal Tumors

Dermoid cysts and epidermal inclusion cysts are the most common tumors removed from children by surgeons.[36] Dermoid cysts develop as 1- to 4-cm rubbery mobile subcutaneous masses along the lines of embryonic cleavage. They are usually discovered at birth, but subtle lesions may not become apparent for several years. The forehead and scalp are the most common locations, but dermoids also can be found on the chest, lumbosacral area, and scrotum. Dermoid cysts contain mature adnexal structures, including eccrine, apocrine, and sebaceous glands, surrounded by a epidermal sac. Although they have no malignant potential, excision may be indicated because of erosion of the underlying bone and for cosmetic reasons.

Epidermal inclusion cysts are slow-growing dermal or subcutaneous tumors 1 to 3 cm in diameter that arise from the infundibular portion of the hair follicle. Although they commonly appear on the head and neck, they can develop at any site, and unlike dermoid cysts, they do not contain adnexal structures. Although some epidermal inclusion cysts are present at birth, most follow trauma or inflammation. Most of the cysts are solitary; multiple lesions should suggest the diagnosis of Gardner syndrome, in which increasing numbers of cysts are associated with osteomatosis and colonic polyposis with a high risk of malignant transformation. Milia represent miniature superficial epidermal inclusion cysts and are commonly found in newborns as well as after trauma. They typically appear along surgical suture lines and after deep abrasions.

Other tumors arise from follicular and ductal epithelium of adnexa as well as glandular structures. Although some of these tumors have characteristic clinical findings, most are diagnosed at the time of biopsy. In children, adnexal tumors are invariably benign, and only symptomatic lesions are excised.

Nevi

Nevi appear at birth or during the first month of life. They are composed of mature or nearly mature cutaneous elements organized in an abnormal fashion, and they can arise from any structure in the skin. Nevi are usually of only cosmetic importance. Some lesions, however, have malignant potential, while others provide clues to the diagnosis of systemic disorders.

Vascular nevi account for most hamartomatous lesions in newborns and infants. For a discussion of hemangiomas and malformations, see Chapter 32.

Epidermal Nevi

Epidermal nevi, composed of proliferating epidermal keratinocytes, must be distinguished from sebaceous nevi.[37] The epidermal nevus presents at birth as a linear group of warty papules (Fig. 96-14). Epidermal nevi can be small or extend over large portions of the trunk, face, and extremities. Dermatomal distribution patterns are common. Both large and small lesions can be markers for neurologic, bony, ocular, and dental anomalies. Epidermal nevi do not carry a risk of malignant degeneration. The disfiguring warty overgrowth can be associated with heavy bacterial colonization, foul odor, and secondary infection. Small lesions are easily vaporized with carbon dioxide laser therapy or excised and closed primarily. Large nevi respond at least temporarily to the application of topical keratolytics, such as urea, lactic acid, glycolic acid, and salicylic acid. Some of these lesions are amenable to superficial carbon diox-

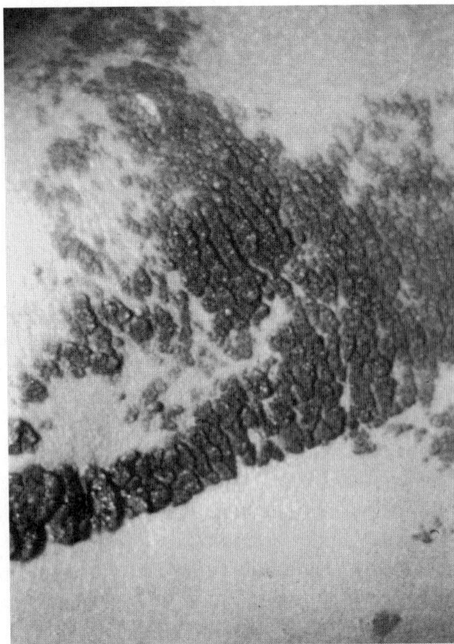

FIG. 96-14. Epidermal nevus. A large, linear, warty plaque was observed on the trunk at birth. (See Color Figure 96-14.)

ide laser therapy or pigmented lesion laser ablation, but surgical excision is not usually feasible.

Sebaceous Nevi

Sebaceous nevi are recognized in the newborn as irregularly shaped but well-demarcated yellow, hairless, cobblestone-like plaques[38] (Fig. 96-15). Most lesions are between 5 mm and 5 cm in diameter and involve the head or neck. Any cutaneous site can be involved, however, and rare lesions extend over large areas of the head, trunk, and extremities. Extensive lesions, especially over the face, neck, and scalp, can be associated with

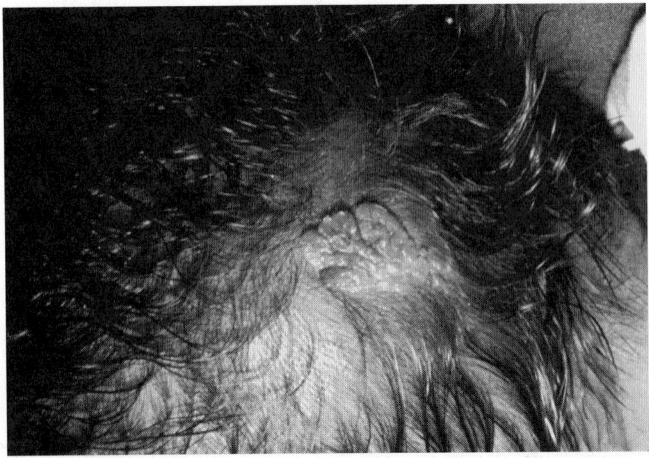

FIG. 96-15. A yellow cobblestone-like plaque is visible on the scalp of this newborn. His neurologic examination was normal. (See Color Figure 96-15.)

multiple neuroectodermal and mesodermal anomalies, similar to epidermal nevus syndrome. Evaluation and management of sebaceous nevi are as for epidermal nevi. Sebaceous nevi, however, have a propensity to develop cutaneous neoplasms that are typically benign and rarely malignant. Most of these hypertrophy under the influence of the pubertal hormonal surge. As a consequence, removal under a local anesthetic is advocated in later childhood or adolescence.

Pigmented Nevi

Acquired pigmented nevi begin to appear during the first few years of life, primarily on sun-exposed areas of skin as 1- to 2-mm brown macules.[39] They are also known as *pigmented moles* or *nevomelanocytic nevi* because they contain nevomelanocytic cells, which are neural crest–derived cells that share with normal melanocytes the ability to produce pigment. In the early flat nevi, nevus cells are located near the dermal–epidermal junction, giving the histologic picture of a junctional nevus. The nevi slowly enlarge and become papular. In these elevated lesions, nevus cells are also found in the deeper dermis, resulting in compound nevi. Over many years, compound nevi become fleshy or pedunculated, particularly on the upper trunk, head, and neck, and many lose pigment. Histologically, the nevus cells are restricted to the dermis, typical of the so-called intradermal nevus.

Most changes in nevi are innocent and do not require biopsy.[40] During puberty, nevi often increase in size and number and darken in color. Most normal nevi, however, do not exceed 0.5 cm in diameter, and they retain their regularity in color, borders, and texture. Sudden enlargement of a nevus with bruising, redness, or tenderness can follow trauma or folliculitis. This usually subsides in several days. The appearance of a well-defined white halo around an otherwise innocent-looking nevus requires close observation. These benign self-destructing nevi demonstrate a lymphocytic dermal infiltrate in the pigmented border but no atypical nevus cells. The nevus disappears during a period of weeks to months, and the skin usually repigments uneventfully.

A number of changes in a pigmented nevus can suggest the development of melanoma and should prompt close observation and possibly biopsy. These changes include the following:

- A change in size or appearance of irregular, scalloped, or poorly defined borders
- A change in the texture of the nevus, such as the development of papules or nodules, scale, ulcerations, or bleeding
- A change in color, with an admixture of black, brown, white, red, and blue
- The presence of burning, itching, or tenderness that results from an inflammatory reaction in a melanoma

Fortunately, melanomas are rare in children and account for less than 2% of all cases.[41] Most prepubertal melanomas arise in large congenital nevi. Other risk factors include inability to tan, light hair and eye color, and severe sunburns, especially in early childhood. Family history of malignant melanoma, particularly if multiple family members have large numbers of big, irregularly shaped nevi, carries a lifetime risk of melanoma that approaches 100% in affected patients. Malignant melanoma in this hereditary setting is referred to as *familial dysplastic nevus syndrome*. During early childhood, affected children develop innocent-looking nevi. The inheritance of this predisposition for the development of malignant melanoma is autosomal dominant, resulting in a 50% risk to children of an affected parent. The presence of large numbers of nevi in sun-exposed as well as protected sites, such as the scalp and lower trunk, may be an early marker in children. These patients require frequent evaluation of nevi beginning in adolescence and immediate biopsy of any unusual or changing nevi to exclude malignant degeneration.

Four types of malignant melanoma have been identified, three of which have a relatively long radial or horizontal growth phase within the epidermis before growing vertically into deeper tissue. Superficial spreading melanomas account for 70% of all melanomas and can arise on sun-exposed as well as covered areas. The most commonly involved sites include the upper back, especially in men, and the lower legs, especially in women. The development of a dark papule or nodule in a broad melanotic plaque that does not usually exceed 2.5 cm may suggest the development of invasive tumor in a slowly expanding, superficial spreading melanoma. Acral lentiginous melanomas develop on the palms and soles and beneath and around the nails. Although they account for less than 10% of all melanomas, acral lentiginous lesions represent a large proportion of melanomas in Asians, Hispanics, and African Americans. Lentigo maligna melanoma begins as an irregularly shaped pigmented patch, lentigo maligna, which can slowly expand peripherally for years before it evolves into a melanoma. These lesions appear on sun-exposed sites of elderly patients and can exceed 4 cm in diameter.

In patients with stage II disease, that is, with regional lymph node involvement, long-term survival is dismal. Most patients diagnosed with malignant melanoma, however, present in clinical stage I, without evidence of lymph node involvement or disseminated disease. In these patients, tumor thickness is the most important factor in determining prognosis.

Originally, the depth of tumor invasion in stage I patients was defined by Clark's five levels[42] (Table 96-4). Breslow tumor thickness, however, measured microscopically from the top of the epidermal granular layer to the deepest extension of the tumor, generally provides the most reliable prognostic data. Many practitioners use a combination of these parameters. Low-risk melanomas with a Breslow thickness of less than 0.76 mm and Clark level II or III can be cured by local excision with a 1-cm margin. Wide margins are unnecessary and do not improve on the 98% 5-year disease-free survival rate. Moderate-risk lesions include melanomas less than 0.76 mm but with

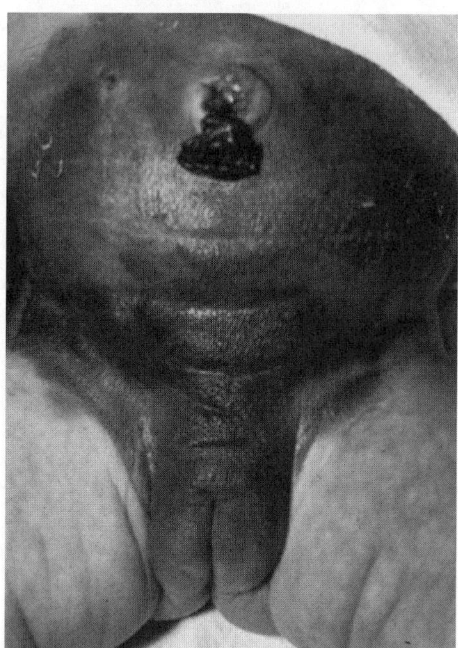

FIG. 96-16. Congenital pigmented nevus. A large pigmented nevocellular nevus covered the lower half of the trunk of this 3-month-old girl at birth. (See Color Figure 96-16.)

characteristics of Clark level IV, melanomas between 0.76 and 1.5 mm thick, and melanomas more than 1.5 mm thick and Clark level III. The 5-year mortality rate for these tumors approaches 25%. Finally, high-risk melanomas more than 1.5 mm thick carry a mortality rate of about 40%. Breslow[43] found that regional lymph node dissection was unnecessary in patients with thin lesions; in intermediate lesions, the results were inconclusive. Long-term survival rates doubled in patients with lesions greater than 1.5 mm who underwent regional lymph node dissection.

Congenital pigmented nevi are noted at birth or within the first few months of life in 1% of infants[44] (Fig. 96-16). At birth, these nevi appear flat and light brown with only vellus hairs. During infancy and early childhood, the nevi often darken, become elevated, and the hair becomes dark and coarse. Occasionally, darkly pigmented nevi lighten during the first few years of life, but in many cases, small dark macules and papules appear within the borders.

Although there is an increased risk of malignant degeneration in small congenital nevi compared with moles that appear later in life, the incidence has not been established, and routine removal of nevi cannot be justified in childhood. Regular reevaluation of nevi should be coordinated with the child's pediatrician. Unusual and irregular changes in borders, pigmentation, or texture may prompt an immediate biopsy. Most congenital nevi can be left alone until the child is old enough to participate in the management decision and cooperate with local anesthesia. Unfortunately, giant lesions carry a significant risk of malignant change even during childhood, and aggressive surgical intervention has not been shown to reduce this risk. Giant nevi that extend over the scalp, neck, or middle back may be associated with leptomeningeal melanocytosis and a high risk of malignant melanoma. In these patients, inaccessible tumors may arise in

TABLE 96-4. *Histologic findings in malignant melanoma*

Clark level	Extent	Breslow thickness (mm)
I	Confined to epidermis	<0.76
II	Extension into papillary dermis	
III	Tumor fills papillary dermis, but does not invade reticular dermis	0.76–1.5
IV	Invasion of reticular dermis	>1.5
V	Invasion of subcutaneous fat	

the central nervous system, and careful radioimaging studies to diagnose meningeal involvement should be performed before extensive cutaneous surgery is planned.

REFERENCES

1. Cohen BA. Atlas of pediatric dermatology. London, Wolfe, 1993.
2. Beylot C, Puisant A, Bioulac P, et al. Particular clinical features of psoriasis in infants and children. Acta Derm Venereol 1979;87(Suppl): 95.
3. Nyfors A, Lemholt K. Psoriasis in children. Br J Dermatol 1975;93: 437.
4. Jordan WE, Blaney TL. Factors influencing diaper dermatitis. In: Maibach HI, Boisits EK, eds. Neonatal skin structure and function. New York, Marcel Dekker, 1982:217.
5. Stein H. Incidence of diaper rash when using cloth and disposable diapers. J Pediatr 1982;101:721.
6. Cronin E. Contact dermatitis. Edinburgh, Churchill Livingstone, 1980.
7. Weston WL. Allergic contact dermatitis in children. Am J Dis Child 1984;138:932.
8. Blanco C, Carillo T, Castillo R, et al. Latex allergy: clinical features and cross-reactivity with fruits. Ann Allergy 1994;73:309.
9. Cohen BA. Atopic dermatitis: breaking the itch-scratch cycle. Contemp Pediatr 1992;9:64.
10. Yates VM, Kern RE, Frier K, et al. Early diagnosis of infantile seborrheic dermatitis and atopic dermatitis: clinical features. Br J Dermatol 1983;10:633.
11. Skinner RB, Noah PW, Taylor RM, et al. Doubleblind treatment of seborrheic dermatitis with 2% ketoconazole cream. J Am Acad Dermatol 1985;12:852.
12. Esterly NB, Maurer HS, Gonzales-Crusi F. Histiocytosis X: a seven year experience at a children's hospital. J Am Acad Dermatol 1985; 13:481.
13. Campo AG Jr, McDonald CJ. Treatment of acrodermatitis enteropathica with zinc sulfate. Arch Dermatol 1976;112:687.
14. Cohen BA. When to think of scabies. In: Contemporary pediatrics: focus on pediatric dermatology and ophthalmology, special edition. Masters of Pediatrics. Montvale, NJ, Medical Economics, 1994:15.
15. Jacobs PH. Fungal infection in children. Pediatr Clin North Am 1978; 25:357.
16. Herbert AA. Tinea capitis: current concepts. Arch Dermatol 1988;124: 1554.
17. McBride A, Cohen BA. Tinea pedis in children. 1992;146:844.
18. Cavanaugh RM. Pityriasis rosea in children. Clin Pediatr 1983;22:200.
19. Corey L, Spear PG. Infection with herpes simplex virus. N Engl J Med 1986;314:686.
20. Baba K, Yabuvehi H, Jakahashiti M, et al. Immunologic and epidemiologic aspects of varicella infection acquired during infancy and early childhood. J Pediatr 1982;100:881.
21. Cherry JD. Viral exanthems. Curr Prob Pediatr 1983;13:1.
22. Holzle E, Kligman AM. The pathogenesis of miliaria rubra: role of the resident microflora. Br J Dermatol 1978;99:117.
23. Elias PM, Fritsch P, Epstein EH Jr. Staphylococcal scalded skin syndrome. (Review) Arch Dermatol 1977;113:207.
24. Ginsburg CM. Staphylococcal toxin syndromes. Pediatr Infect Dis J 1983;23(Suppl):2.
25. Mark RJ, Stower JS, Damon RS. Toxic epidermal necrolysis in a 6-week-old infant. Pediatr Dermatol 1985;2:197.
26. Taylor JA, Grube B, Heimbach DM, et al. Toxic epidermal necrolysis: a comprehensive approach to multidisciplinary management in a burn center. Clin Pediatr 1989;28:404.
27. Nethercott JR, Choi BCK. Erythema multiforme (Stevens-Johnson syndrome): chart review of 123 hospitalized patients. Dermatologica 1985; 171:383.
28. Schofield JK, Tatnall FM, Leigh IM. Recurrent erythema multiforme: clinical features and treatment in a large series of patients. Br J Dermatol 1993;128:542.
29. Helfer RE, Kempe RS, eds. The battered child, ed 4. Chicago, University of Chicago Press, 1987.
30. Krugman RD, ed. Child abuse and neglect. Pediatr Ann 1992;21:471.
31. Androphy EJ. Human papillomavirus: current concepts. Arch Dermatol 1989;135:683.
32. Cohen BA, Honig PG, Androphy EJ. Anogenital warts in children. Arch Dermatol 1990;126:1575.
33. Pierard-Franchimont C, Legrain A, Pierard GE. Growth and regression of molluscum contagiosum. J Am Acad Dermatol 1983;9:669.
34. de Waard-vanderSpek FB, Oranje AP, Lillieborg S, et al. Treatment of molluscum contagiosum using lidocaine/prilocaine cream (EMLA) for anesthesia. J Am Acad Dermatol 1990;23:689.
35. Pandy CR, Artis WM, Jones HE. Atopic dermatitis, impaired cellular immunity, and molluscum contagiosum. Arch Dermatol 1978;114:391.
36. Knight PJ, Reina CB. Superficial lumps and bumps in children: what, when, and why? Pediatrics 1983;72:147.
37. Eichler C, Flowers FP, Ross J. Epidermal nevus syndrome: case report and review of clinical manifestations. Pediatr Dermatol 1989;6:316.
38. Marioka S. The natural history of nevus sebaceous. J Cutan Pathol 1985;12:200.
39. Maize JC, Foster G. Age related changes in melanocytic naevi. Clin Exp Dermatol 1979;4:49.
40. National Institutes of Health Consensus Development Conference. Precursors to malignant melanoma. J Am Acad Dermatol 1984;10:683.
41. Pratt CB, Palmer ME, Thatcher N, et al. Malignant melanoma in children and adolescents. Cancer 1981;47:392.
42. Balch CM, Murad TM, Soong SJ, et al. Tumor thickness as a guide to surgical management of clinical stage I melanoma. Cancer 1979;43: 883.
43. Breslow A. Prognostic factors in the treatment of malignant melanoma. J Cutan Pathol 1979;6:208.
44. Everett MA. Histopathology of congenital pigmented nevi. Am J Dermatopathol 1989;11:11.

Surgery of Infants and Children: Scientific Principles and Practice, edited by Keith T. Oldham, Paul M. Colombani, and Robert P. Foglia. Lippincott–Raven Publishers, Philadelphia, © 1997.

CHAPTER 97

Plastic and Reconstructive Surgery

Craig A. Vander Kolk

Plastic surgery takes its name from the Greek word *plastikos*, which means to mold and shape. Just as we mold and shape plastic, which is also derived from *plastikos*, the plastic surgeon molds and shapes tissue to improve function and appearance. The quest to restore or improve form and function has been a driving force in plastic surgery for decades. Many major advances in the field occurred in war time, to repair the devastating combat injuries. During World War I, in England, Sir Harold Gillies reconstructed complex head and neck wounds using many of the reconstructive principles of his day. He revolutionized the treatment of these deformities by expanding techniques and applying the principle of tissue replacement with similar tissue. This was the beginning of plastic surgery.

In the United States, at Johns Hopkins Hospital, John Staige Davis was the first surgeon to dedicate his career to plastic surgery. He also expanded the new field by correcting war deformities, and his textbook was the first in the United States devoted to plastic surgery. A few of the techniques he refined, such as skin grafting, are recorded in this text, and are still used today.

During the early and middle part of this century, many advances were made. The early discoveries in transplantation occurred in plastic surgery laboratories studying the feasibility of transplanting skin to reconstruct severe burn injuries. Approximately 25 years ago, an explosion of technical knowledge and advances in all fields of medicine occurred. Plastic surgery was changed forever with the development of such new techniques as tissue expansion, muscle flaps, microsurgery, and craniofacial surgery. Many of the techniques used by Gillies and Davis, other than skin grafting and some small local flaps, are no longer used. However, the principles of wound reconstruction reviewed in this chapter, form the basis of contemporary plastic surgery.

WOUND HEALING

Wound healing occurs whenever tissues are damaged. It is easy to observe on the skin surface, following lacerations, abrasions, contusions, and surgical procedures such as incisions and harvesting of skin grafts. However, it also occurs below the skin, in structures that are surgically altered for exposure or treatment, exploration of the abdomen, anastomosis of a major blood vessel or intestine, or resection of a viscus. It occurs following damage related to disease such as stroke, hemorrhage, thrombosis, and myocardial infarction. It is also important to consider the principles of wound healing when treating these medical problems even when no surgical incision is made.

Briefly, wound healing is a carefully orchestrated sequence of events involving cells, cell products, and intercellular signals. Wound healing is divided into three stages. First is the inflammatory phase, followed by the collagen phase, and then the maturation phase. These phases are based on the ability of researchers to examine the cellular and molecular events of each stage. The inflammatory (lag) phase is now called the substrate phase, in which cells are recruited for the healing process. White blood cells form a major portion of this response. This phase typically lasts 4 days in primary healing, or until the wound is closed in secondary and tertiary healing. The proliferative (collagen or fibroblastic) phase, in which the initial fibrin is laid down and subsequently replaced by collagen, usually lasts from day 4 to day 42. It is associated with a gradual increase in the wound's tensile strength. At the end of this period, the wound has reached 90% of its maximum tensile strength. Further increase in wound strength occurs in the remodeling (maturation) phase. This involves intermolecular cross-linking of collagen, which also results in flattening of the wound. This phase is continual, since collagen is constantly broken down and replaced in response to the dynamics of the wound. Maximum improvement in the appearance of the wound usually takes at least 1 year. However, the visible scar is a permanent reminder of the injury or surgery.

When aberrations in wound healing occur, hypertrophic and keloid scars may form. Hypertrophic scars result from excess collagen production. These scars are typically red, raised, and firm. A patient frequently reports annoying pruritus. Treatment consists of massage, elastic pressure, and if the pruritus is severe, steroid injection. Typically, a small amount of Kenalog, 10 mg/mL, accelerates the healing process and decreases the thickening and red appearance of the scar. If treatment is unsuccessful, scar revision may be indicated. Keloids differ from hypertrophic scars in that they are caused by both overproduction of collagen and diminished collagen breakdown. By definition, they grow outside the margin of the original wound; thus they are tumorous growths. They typically occur in dark-skinned individuals. Hypertrophic scars occur more frequently in individuals of Asian heritage. Treatment consists of Kenalog injection and administration of pressure. This is frequently unsuccessful, and intralesional excision with steroid injection may be necessary. Rarely, excision and radiation must be performed.

When scars form against the natural flexion and extension creases of the body (Fig. 97-1), a noticeable contracted scar occurs. Frequently, this scar limits motion and function but can be improved with a Z-plasty or other revision. Z-plasties reorient the scar into favorable lines of relaxation. They actually increase the overall size of the scar, but by allowing it to fall into natural skin creases, both function and appearance are improved (Fig. 97-2).

When the healing process breaks down, wound dehiscence occurs and a complex wound is encountered. This breakdown of the wound is caused by an abnormality in blood supply, infection, metabolic abnormalities, or trauma. In particular, the blood supply can be altered by previous radiation treatment, resulting in fibrosis of the microvasculature. Tension compromises the blood supply resulting in ischemic edges of the wound and subsequent dehiscence. A hematoma makes a wound ischemic, resulting in breakdown and even necrosis of the overlying skin. Infection can delay the healing process and, in severe cases such as necrotizing fasciitis, results in rampant tissue destruction. A metabolic abnormality such as diabetes results in abnormalities not only in the cellular response to injury, but also in the microvasculature, predisposing patients to wound complications. Nutritional abnormalities can delay the cellular response to the healing process. Finally, trauma on either a cellular level or organ level results in a disruption of the wound. When these abnormalities occur or even have a high likelihood of occurrence, reconstructive principles and techniques should be considered.

COMPLEX WOUND EVALUATION

Complex wounds requiring reconstruction result from a myriad of etiologies. Wounds or deformities may occur, during fetal development, resulting in congenital abnormalities involving missing or malformed tissues that require repositioning or replacement. This is illustrated by such deformities as cleft lip, cleft palate, amniotic bands, and gastroschisis. Each of these requires a separate coordinated approach to reconstructing the missing elements and deformity. Traumatic wounds frequently result in extensive tissue destruction from lacerations and abrasions, with loss of a multitude of tissue components, along with fractures and even amputations. Neoplasms not only destroy normal tissue, but their resection results in large defects. These defects are closed primarily or may heal faster, with less morbidity, using the principles of plastic surgery. Finally, wound healing complicated by wound breakdown benefits from plastic surgery.

The evaluation of a wound first requires analysis of the patient's age and health. The healing process cannot be improved specifically at present, but healing problems can be avoided by preventing complicating factors. Nutritional status needs to be maximized for normal healing to occur. The size of the wound is then evaluated. The wound's location is also a significant factor. Both the remaining structures and structures missing from the wound need to be identified.

The location of the wound is one of the most important factors in the evaluation process. Aesthetic concerns are significant in head and neck wounds. The functions of many vital structures in the area need to be preserved. In addition, it is a small area with limited tissue available for reconstruction. The trunk, including the chest and back, contains vital organs. Superficial structures need to be soft and pliable to allow for chest expansion and abdominal movement. Abundant tissue is available in this region, however, wounds can be quite massive. The abdomen and pelvis, including the genital and buttock regions, each has its own particular characteristics that are important for form and function. Significant muscular forces are in these areas. When weakening occurs, hernias can form. The vital structures also need protection from the overlying skin. The buttock region is exposed to shearing and pressure forces that require padding and mobility. Similarly, the extremities, particularly the foot and plantar surface, require soft tissue padding to counteract shearing and weight forces. They need to stay soft and supple for adequate motion. In the extremities, small defects are difficult to reconstruct because of the limited tissues available. The extremities have very little intervening tissue between the skin and the underlying structures. This is more common the more distal on the extremity the injury is.

The size of the wound encountered is often related to its location and the available tissue. Small wounds with exposed underlying structures such as tendons, nerves, or bone may require an extensive reconstructive procedure compared with a small wound on the trunk, which has a large amount of available

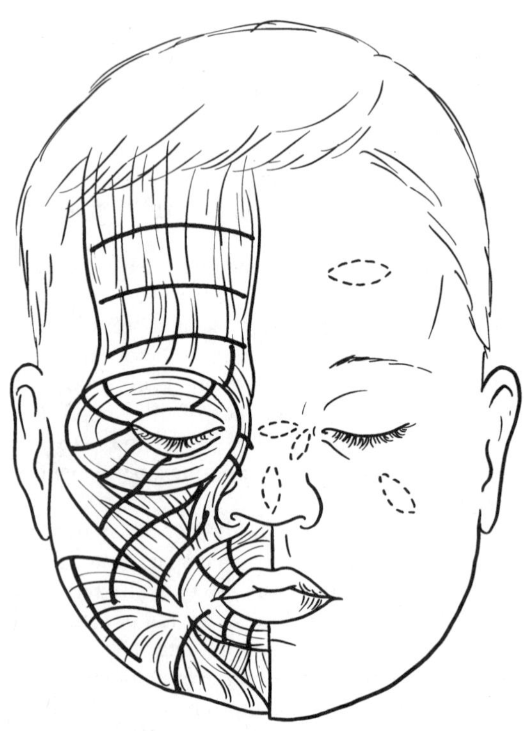

FIG. 97-1. The lines of minimum tension are perpendicular to the underlying facial muscles. On the left, these lines are demonstrated in relation to the muscles, and on the right the direction of elective incisions is shown. When lacerations or incisions are perpendicular to these lines of minimum tension, noticeable scars occur.

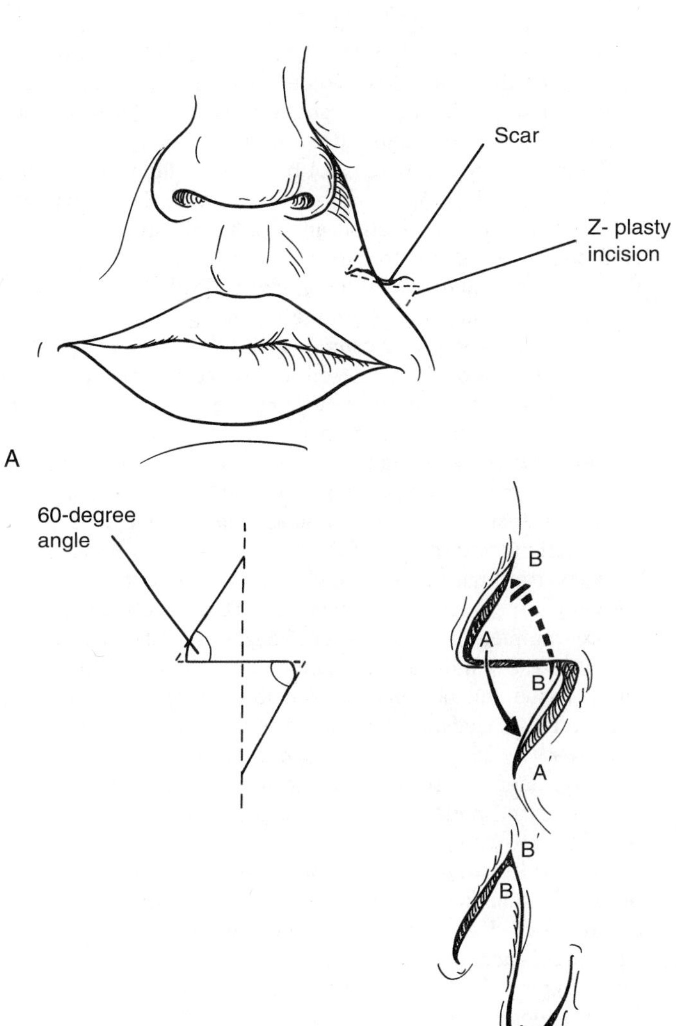

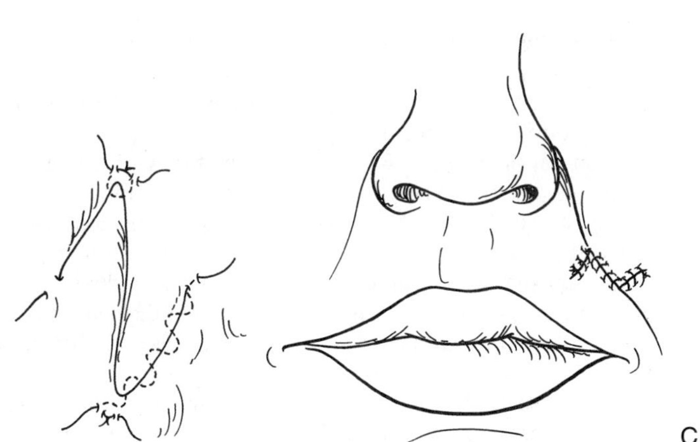

FIG. 97-2. An example of a thick and noticeable scar crossing the nasal labial fold (*A*), which when revised, allows the central portion of the Z to lie within the skinfold, making it less noticeable (*B* and *C*). The Z-plasties are usually at 60-degree angles through the central scar, which ultimately becomes transposed 90 degrees, reorienting the scar along the lines of minimal tension.

tissue. The composition of the wound is related to its size and location. Specific structures that need to be evaluated include the skin, subcutaneous tissue, underlying fascia, and muscle. Vital structures such as tendons, nerves, bone, and other important organs also need to be evaluated. Missing structures should ideally be replaced, and those that remain should be preserved.

The age of the patient affects the overall healing and also the care required for rehabilitation. The best healing occurs at a young age, usually between birth and 1 year. Good healing occurs between the ages of 1 and 4; however, following the age of 4 until adolescence, hypertrophic scars are common. Finally, in adolescence the patient is developing a healing process similar to that of an adult. In general, incisions, abrasions, skin graft donor sites, and specialized tissue such as bone heal faster in children. Rehabilitation of patients needs to be carefully considered and individually structured. This is important since children of different ages have different abilities for cooperation in ambulation, hand movements, and structured therapy during the healing process.

Many miscellaneous factors influence the choice of reconstruction. A child's hobbies or athletic activities may influence

a particular type of reconstruction. A scar may be better tolerated in one place than in another. Many psychological factors also need to be considered when reconstructing individual wounds. In this age of health care reform, the costs of reconstruction and hospitalization need to be carefully considered as well.

RECONSTRUCTIVE PRINCIPLES

For wounds to heal, there must be healthy tissue within the wound as well as any tissue transferred or used in reconstruction must be healthy. Débridement should be done to cleanse the wound of contused, desiccated, or necrotic tissue (Fig. 97-3). Ischemic tissues need to be débrided. In addition, the best treatment for infection is frequently surgical cleansing and débridement. Once a wound is surgically clean, reconstruction can be done primarily or delayed. When reconstruction is delayed, dressing changes should be used. Dressing changes assist in cleansing a wound when surgical debridement is no longer required. Wet-to-dry dressing changes with an antibiotic or antiseptic solution helps clean a contaminated wound. Solutions

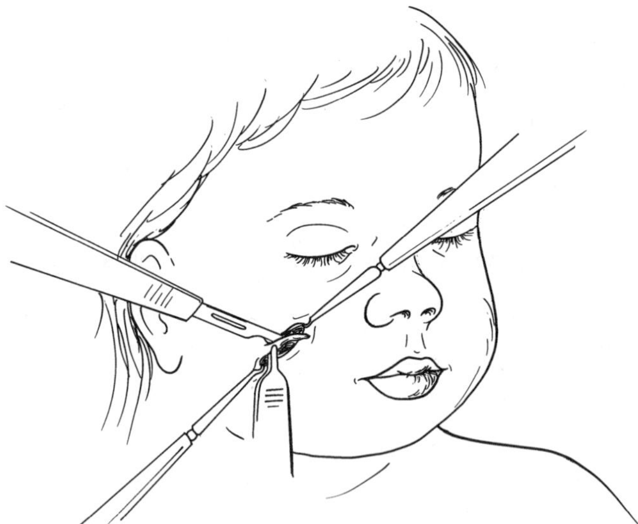

FIG. 97-3. Débridement of a laceration before closure, to promote the best possible healing.

that are available include Betadine, Chlorpactin, Dakin's solution, and Silvadene. These solutions should be used for only a short time, since they damage normal tissues. Once the wound is clean, normal saline wet-to-dry dressings are appropriate for final light débridement of the wound. Once the wound begins to granulate, this tissue needs to be preserved, and a moist environment should be created. This can be accomplished with moist dressings that are not allowed to dry. Occasionally, a nonadherent dressing is appropriate to promote epithelialization. The time between dressing changes varies depending on the wound and the associated pain with the dressing change. Contaminated or infected wounds require dressings every 4 hours, whereas those that are granulating, contracting, and subsequently epithelializing require less frequent dressing changes two or three times daily.

RECONSTRUCTIVE TECHNIQUES

The reconstructive options available for treating a wound either primarily or secondarily involve consideration of the reconstructive ladder. This ladder begins with the easiest, most straightforward closure options and extends to the most complex. Which reconstruction is required depends on the wound and goals. The goal is to maximize function and appearance, keeping in mind the total patient needs. Maximizing form and function usually requires replacing missing tissue with like tissues. When skin is removed, it should therefore be used for the reconstruction, that is, as a skin graft. When skin, muscle, and bone are removed, all three structures frequently need to be reconstructed, either as local or microvascular compound (skin, muscle, and bone) flaps.

Primary closure is the choice for most surgical procedures. Even minimal surgery, such as endoscopic procedures, requires primary closure of the incisions. The small size of the scope allows direct primary approximation of the tissues on withdrawal from the cavity. Primary closure of most incisions is indicated as long as a tension-free closure can be accomplished

with well-vascularized tissue. Dead space, which results in opening of the wound, is avoided with deep primary suture closure or suction drains. The goal is to approximate each level and type of tissue, to allow uneventful healing.

When primary closure cannot be done, or the wound breaks down, secondary closure is the next option. This healing is accomplished by contraction and epithelialization. It is most commonly considered for superficial wounds such as partial-thickness burns and skin graft donor sites. Both of these wounds heal by epithelialization from the wound edges and hair follicles. Secondary wound closure is also used with deep wounds complicated by dehiscence, seroma, or hematoma formation. The goal is to promote healing from the deep portion, of the wound to the superficial portion, through dressing changes, contraction, and epithelialization. Occasionally, secondary healing is used for small wounds in patients who are too sick for an extensive operation or with wounds that do not need a skin graft or flap for closure.

Delayed primary closure is occasionally accomplished after allowing a period of secondary healing with contraction but before complete closure and epithelization. When the wound begins to show signs of granulation and contraction, the granulation tissue can be removed and the wound edges approximated. This speeds up the healing process but may add to the total cost of patient care, with operating room charges. Occasionally, patients are unwilling to undergo a second surgical procedure and prefer dressing changes at home.

Skin grafts can be used to heal almost any wound. They are most useful for large, superficial wounds, because of the loss of skin or subcutaneous tissue. On the other hand, any wound can be grafted as long as the blood supply to the underlying structures is adequate. Bone can be grafted if there is periosteum overlying it. Tendons and nerves can be grafted as long as there is peritendon and perineuron, respectively. Even deep thoracic and abdominal organs can be grafted, if necessary. Skin grafts, in these situations, do not provide much padding or strength, but they do close the wound temporarily or permanently, depending on the health of the patient.

Skin grafts can be thin or thick partial-thickness grafts, full-thickness grafts, or composite grafts in which skin and underlying tissue such as cartilage are transplanted. Thin skin grafts have an excellent potential for successful revascularization. The success rate gradually decreases as thicker grafts of skin, full-thickness skin grafts, and finally, composite grafts are selected. On the other hand, the thicker the graft, the less it contracts and the more durable the reconstruction. In addition, full-thickness skin grafts bring some of the associated adnexal structures (hair follicles, sebaceous glands, and sensory nerve endings) and color, to improve the appearance of the reconstruction (Fig. 97-4).

A successful graft requires a good, well-vascularized recipient site and contact between the graft and the recipient site, allowing for subsequent imbibition and inosculation. Grafts survive through imbibition, that is, local transfer of oxygen through diffusion. Inosculation occurs when blood vessels from the recipient site connect directly to blood vessels in the donor graft, bridging a defect and allowing for early blood flow. After 48 to 72 hours of successful imbibition, inosculation normally occurs. Skin grafting is the mainstay for burn treatment, degloving traumatic injuries, large scalp wounds, and occasionally, large congenital nevi.

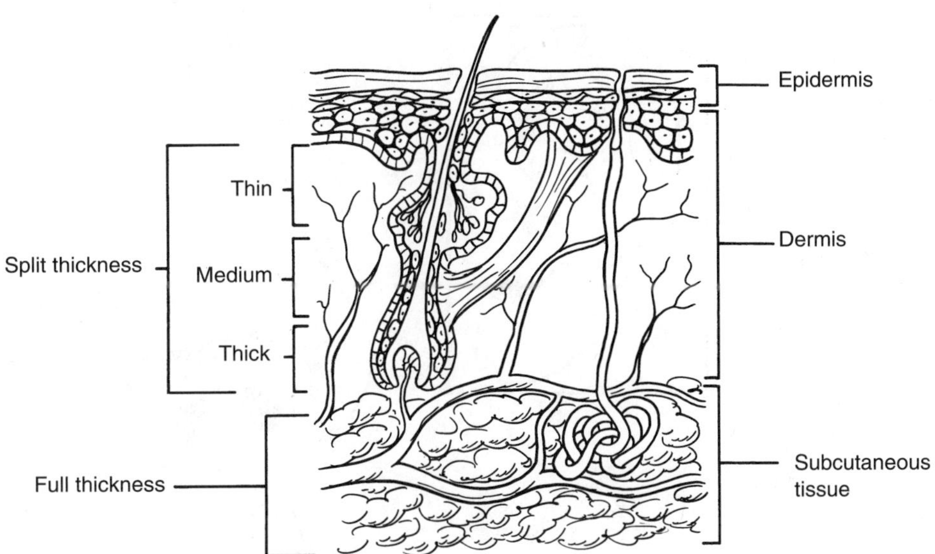

FIG. 97-4. Skin graft thickness, as it relates to the layers of skin and subcutaneous tissue.

Split-thickness skin grafting begins with the preparation of the recipient site. It requires less than 10^5 organisms per gram on quantitative wound cultures. Granulation tissue, which harbors bacteria, should be débrided. In a fresh, surgically created wound, the subcutaneous tissue, with its diminished blood supply, should be removed down to fascia or underlying muscle, to improve the vascularity of the recipient bed. Hemostasis is important in preventing hematoma formation or large clots from elevating the graft itself.

The skin graft is harvested with a dermatome. Choice of donor site is based on the amount of skin required. The buttocks offer a concealed donor site, but it is painful during the postoperative period because the patient is laying and sitting on the site. The upper thigh, below the iliac crest, can be used, since this area is usually covered when the patient wears shorts. For larger amounts of skin, the upper lateral thigh is the best donor site. The amount of tissue required is measured accurately with a template. Mineral oil is placed on the donor site, and traction and countertraction are accomplished with either skin hooks, towel clamps, or an assistant compressing the area. The dermatome is set to a depth of 0.015 inches for most grafts. In babies, the skin is thin and requires a graft to be harvested at 0.08 to 0.010 inches in depth. To prevent contraction and increase durability, a thicker graft is required, of 0.018 to 0.020 inches in depth. The power dermatome is carefully placed over the donor site, and the graft is elevated with smooth, continuous motion. The graft is preserved on a normal saline sponge, and the donor site is covered with a moist gauze. With smaller donor sites, a gauze soaked in lidocaine with epinephrine assists in vasoconstriction and early pain control.

The graft itself is usually meshed. This allows it to follow the contours of the defect and provides for drainage through its interspaces. A mesh ratio of $1:1.5$ is usually the best option, although $1:3$ can be used when donor sites are limited or the burn wound is large. Adherence is usually noted shortly after the graft is positioned on the wound. Tacking sutures are then placed with chromic sutures, and chromic is run around the entire graft. The center of the wound occasionally needs sutures to keep it in position. A tie-over bolster dressing, comprised of xeroform and cotton soaked in mineral oil, is sutured on. This dressing includes sutures at the periphery of the wound, which are tied over the top. Large donor sites are usually treated with nonadherent gauze, and smaller donor sites with an occlusion dressing such as Op-site. Op-site frequently leaks but is associated with less discomfort. Xeroform has no significant drainage but causes more discomfort.

Postoperative care of a skin graft involves protecting of the site for 2 to 5 days. The dressing is taken down, preferably at 5 days, although earlier examination is necessary if an odor is present, drainage occurs, or infection is suspected. Once the bolster dressing is removed, wet-to-dry dressings can be used to debride any crusting. Nonadherent dressings are used later, to promote epithelialization of small areas where the graft did not take or the interspaces of a meshed graft. The donor site usually heals in 7 to 14 days. Xeroform is allowed to dry, and the edges are gradually elevated and trimmed as epithelization occurs beneath the gauze. Epithelialization occurs rapidly in the moist environment under the op-site, and it can be observed for signs of infection or other secondary complications that occur.

Full-thickness skin grafts are used when contraction must be avoided and for small wounds in which color match and adnexal structures are important, most commonly in facial wounds. Limiting contraction is also necessary on the extremities, particularly the hands and feet, to allow for maximum flexibility. In addition, full-thickness skin grafts are appropriate for small skin lesion reconstruction or as part of complex reconstructions, such as an ear reconstruction or the release of finger syndactyly.

The principles of full-thickness grafts are similar to those of split-thickness skin grafts, except that the entire thickness of skin is removed in an area that has excess skin. This is typically in a region of the groin, where a 3-cm by 8-cm graft can be harvested in an older child or a 2-cm by 4-cm graft in infants, with primary closure. Postauricular full-thickness grafts provide the best color match for the face. Contraction of the graft occurs after elevation because of the elasticity of the skin. An accurate template of the wound to be reconstructed is therefore important. In addition, the fat on the undersurface of the graft needs to be removed, because it obstructs the revascularization of the full-thickness skin graft.

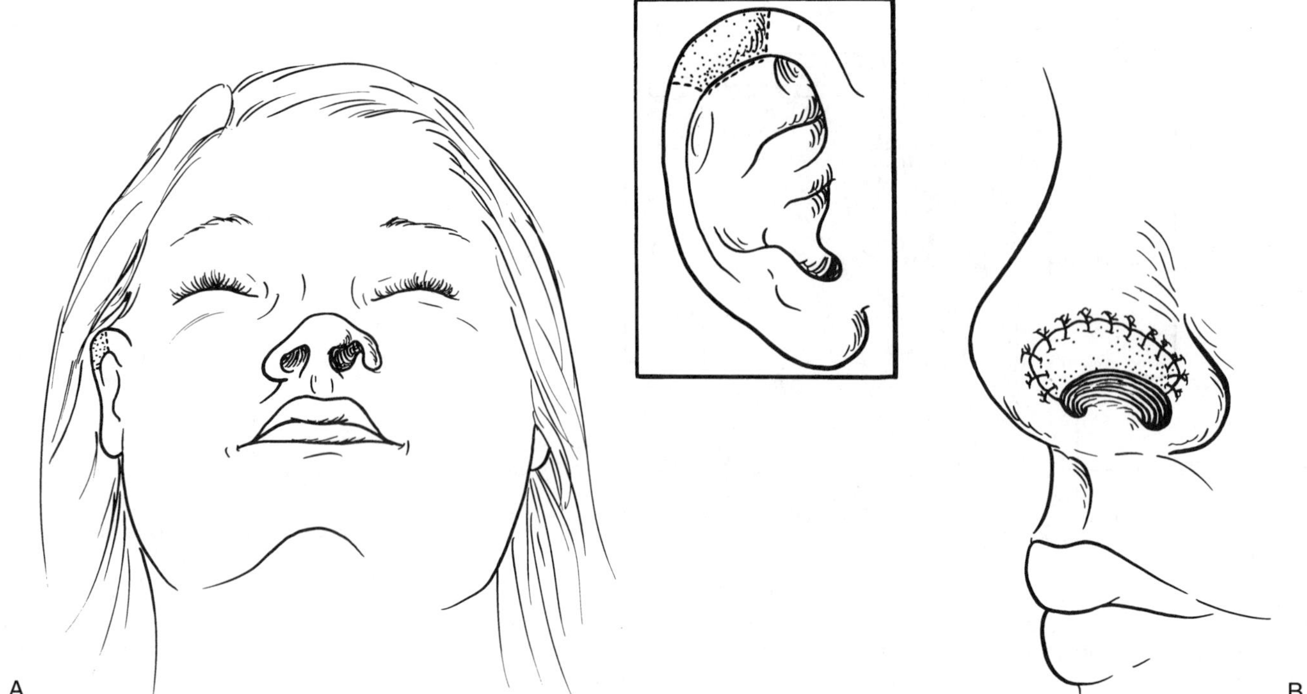

FIG. 97-5. (*A*) A composite graft can be used to reconstruct a traumatic nasal deformity. (*B*) Skin and cartilage are harvested from the helical rim of the ear.

Small, complex composite wounds require small amounts of tissue for reconstruction. A good example is a traumatic wound or defect secondary to tumor resection of nasal skin and cartilage, which needs both the skin and cartilage reconstruction. The helix of the ear can provide this thin skin with associated cartilage (Fig. 97-5). Up to 1 cm of tissue can be transferred to the tip of the nose, with a good chance of revascularization and a successful take.

FLAP RECONSTRUCTION

Flaps are the mainstay of complex tissue reconstruction. Defects requiring reconstruction are larger, deep, and complex. In addition, flaps can provide composite tissues to reconstruct lost muscle, tendon, nerve, and even bone (Fig. 97-6). There are three general types of flaps: skin flaps, fasciocutaneous flaps, and musculocutaneous flaps. Each can be used for local reconstruction or distant reconstruction, using microvascular techniques.

Skin flaps have been used for decades. Originally, large segments of skin and subcutaneous tissue were rolled into a tube and transferred to all parts of the body, through multistage operations. These flaps are now used for small or superficial wounds, most frequently in the head and neck region. Three general categories of skin flaps are based on the underlying blood supply: random flaps, axial flaps, and island flaps. The type of blood supply incorporated in the flap determines the flap's size and ability to be mobilized and positioned for reconstruction.

Random flaps rely on the vascular pattern in the subdermal plexus and, to a lesser extent, the underlying subcutaneous vascularity. The size is usually limited, and the base of the flap usually is slightly greater than 50% of the length of the flap. This size depends on the flap's location; greater length is available in the well-vascularized head and neck region.

Random flaps are designed as advancement flaps or rotation flaps, depending on the location of the defect and the surrounding available skin. Advancement flaps take the available tissue and allow for straightforward movement to fill the defect. When the skin around the base of the flap tethers mobilization, small segments of skin, called burrows triangles, are removed (Fig. 97-7). Rotation flaps and transposition flaps can be rotated to close a defect. Both of these flaps are usually more versatile than advancement flaps. A rectangular (transposition flap, Fig. 97-8) or round (rotation flap, Fig. 97-9) flap of tissue is rotated through a gentle arc, filling the defect. Burrows triangles may also be removed to allow for slight advancement. The flap usually leaves a larger defect, which must be skin grafted if it cannot be primarily closed. There are many variations of rotation flaps, including rhomboid flaps (Fig. 98-10).

Axial flaps and island flaps are based on a dominant blood supply containing a main artery and vein, along with small branches from this central vascular pedicle. In the axial flap, the base is left in place, whereas with the island flap, the base is divided, except for the vascular pedicle. These flaps are viable to a much greater length. Occasionally, a length-width ratio of 4:1 can be accomplished in the head and neck region. This larger flap allows for more versatile reconstruction. Knowledge of the anatomy of the superficial vessels of the skin and subcutaneous tissue is needed to plan these flaps. Usually, the vascular pedicle is identified by palpation and confirmed with Doppler ultrasound. The flap can then be accurately designed. Elevation requires preservation of the underlying structures. As the flap is rotated and positioned, care must be taken not to compromise the vascular pedicle. Donor sites are either closed primarily or skin grafted. Island flaps are more tenuous, since the only tissue holding them in position is the vascular pedicle; on the other hand, they allow for extensive mobilization and reconstruction of more complex defects.

Musculocutaneous flaps have done the most to revolutionize plastic surgery. The underlying anatomy of muscles and their associations with skin was described years ago, but the importance of the communication of vessels between muscle and skin was not appreciated or used until the late 1960s and early 1970s. Once perforating musculocutaneous branches from the deep muscle to the superficial skin were extensively investigated,

complex flaps based on this vascular system could be created. Accurate descriptions of a muscle's anatomy and the position of its blood supply allow mapping of the overlying skin, and this can be elevated and used for reconstruction. The key concept of musculocutaneous flaps is that once the skin distribution of musculocutaneous perforators and the anatomic location of the muscle and its pedicle are known, the arc of rotation around the vascular pedicle can be determined, for precise planning of the reconstructive options (Fig. 97-11). Almost any muscle and its overlying skin can be used for flap reconstruction. Muscles with one dominant vascular pedicle are most easily used, however.

The primary advantage of a musculocutaneous flap is the

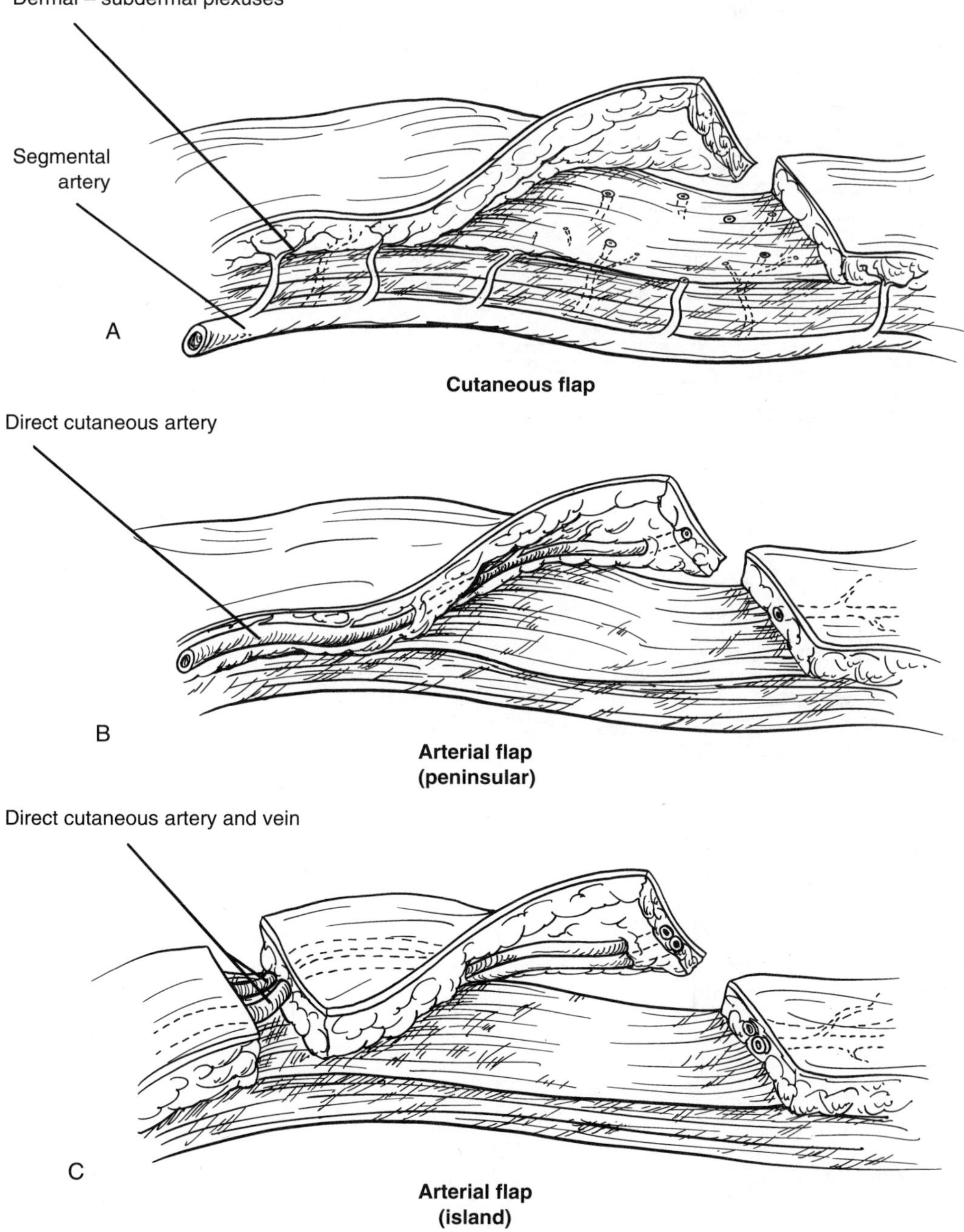

FIG. 97-6. Types of flaps. (See text.) (*continued*)

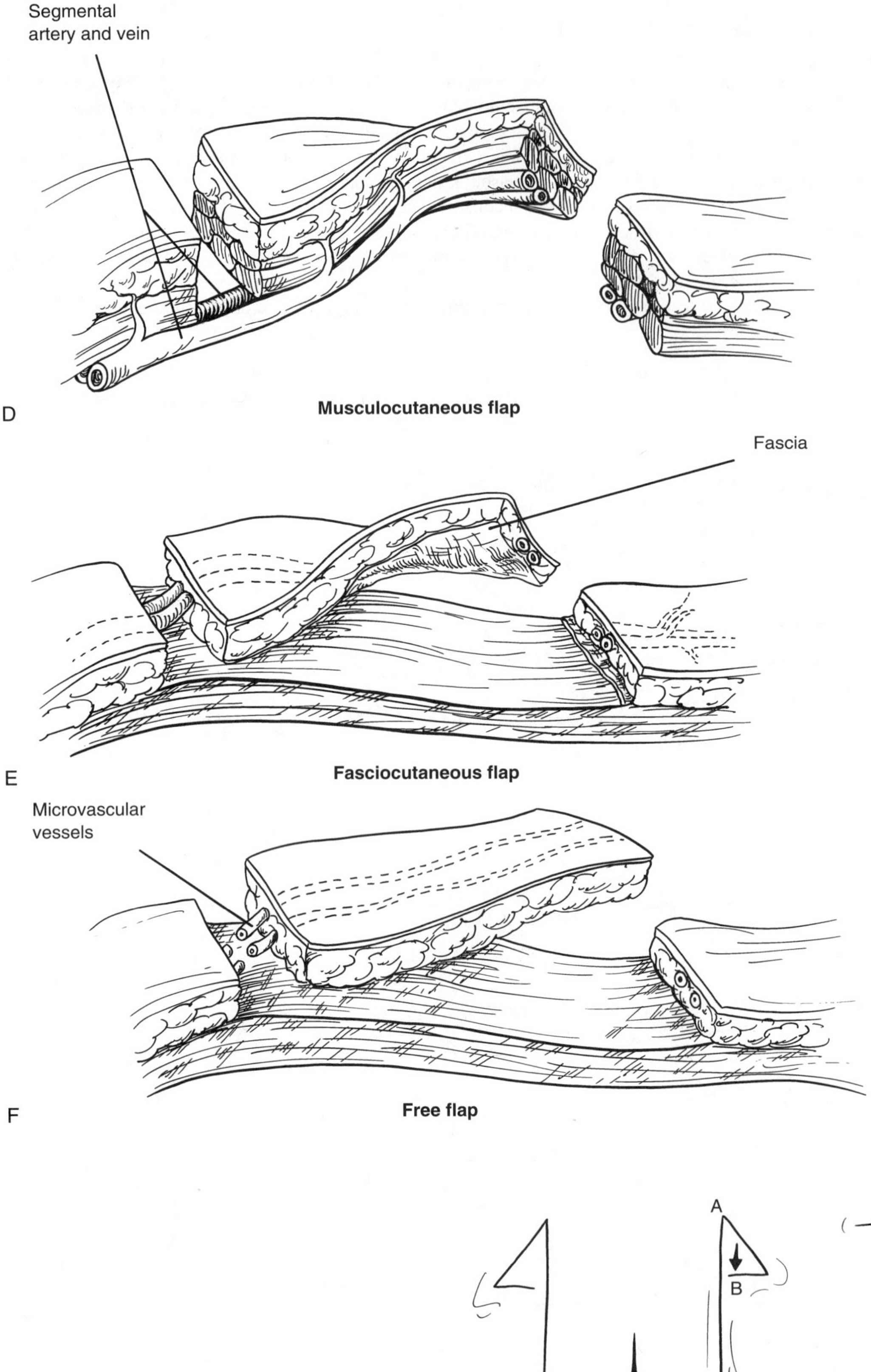

FIG. 97-6. *Continued.*

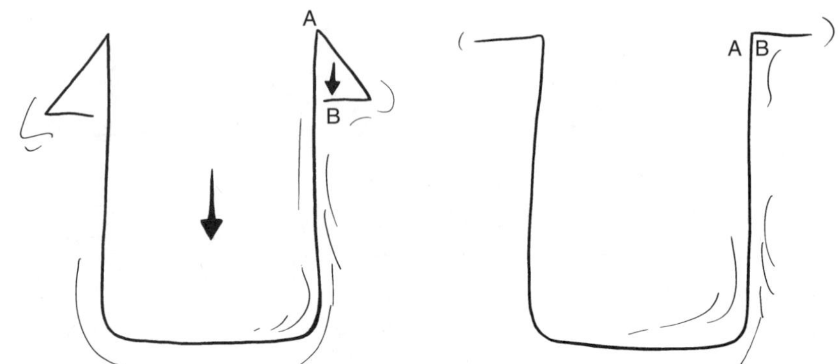

FIG. 97-7. Advancement flap, demonstrating the burrows triangles, excised to allow the flap to be advanced into the defect.

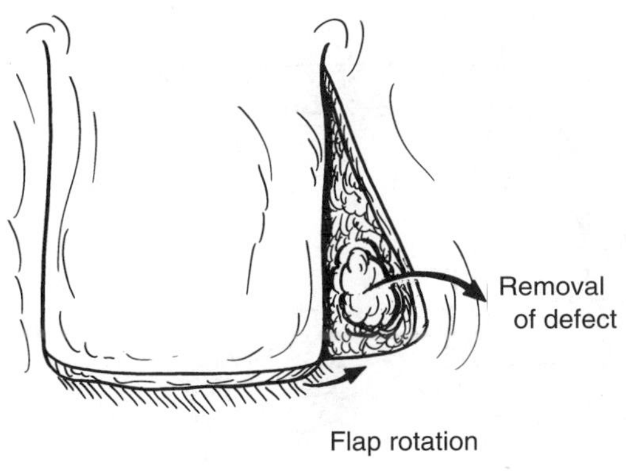

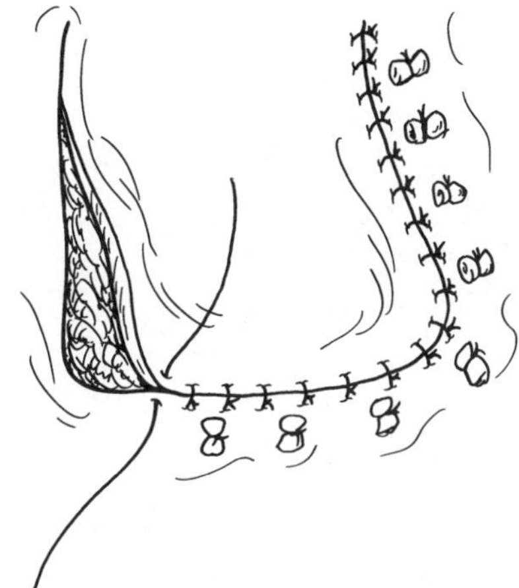

FIG. 97-8. Transposition flap, in which a rectangular flap is rotated to fill a nearby defect.

reliability, the blood supply is relatively easy to identify and dissect compared to random or island flaps. In addition, musculocutaneous flaps are pliable, with adequate tissue to fill large defects. In large defects, they obliterate dead space and bring in a new blood supply. In contaminated or infected wounds, the blood supply brings in additional oxygen, white blood cells, and antibiotics.

The flap itself can be a composite, including nerves for sensation, muscle and tendons for muscular contraction, and bone for support or motion. This results in a wide variety of recon-

structive options. The donor site can usually be closed primarily, since the skin, subcutaneous tissue, and the underlying muscle are removed.

In the head and neck region, reconstructions using pectoralis major muscle or trapezius muscle are good examples of musculocutaneous flaps. These muscles have vascular pedicles high in the neck region. Their origin is along the midline, with insertions into the proximal extremity. Based on their vascular pedicle, these flaps can be rotated easily into the head and neck region for reconstruction. For chest wall reconstruction, the pectoralis major and rectus abdominis muscles are useful. When sternal wound infections occur following median sternotomy, the rectus abdominus muscle obliterates the dead space between the edges of the debrided sternum (Fig. 97-12). In addition, it brings in additional well-vascularized tissue to treat the infection. Complex abdominal closures are accomplished with the rectus femoris muscle and, occasionally, the tensor fascia lata. In the back, the latissimus dorsi bipedicle flap is available for treatment of midline back defects such as a myelomeningocele. In the lower extremity, the gastrocnemius muscle and, soleus muscle are used to cover complex grade III tibial and fibular fractures, in which exposure of the fracture site requires coverage with healthy tissue.

FASCIOCUTANEOUS FLAPS

Fasciocutaneous flaps fill a need midway between the skin flaps and the musculocutaneous flaps. Like musculocutaneous flaps, they have a dominant blood supply from the fascia to the skin. They can therefore be accurately planned and reliably transferred. The blood supply, however, is usually less extensive than that of a musculocutaneous flap because of the smaller size of the vascular pedicle. In this respect they are more like axial skin flaps. With a less robust blood supply than musculocutaneous flaps, fasciocutaneous flaps provide less vascularity to reconstruct ischemic, contaminated or infected wounds. In addition, they are less pliable and do not fill defects as well. Furthermore, the donor site is difficult to close, frequently requiring a skin graft. In elevation and transfer characteristics, fasciocutaneous flaps fall between skin flaps and musculocutaneous flaps.

Muscle flaps are commonly used in the trunk region, because of their overall size and origin in a more proximal position,

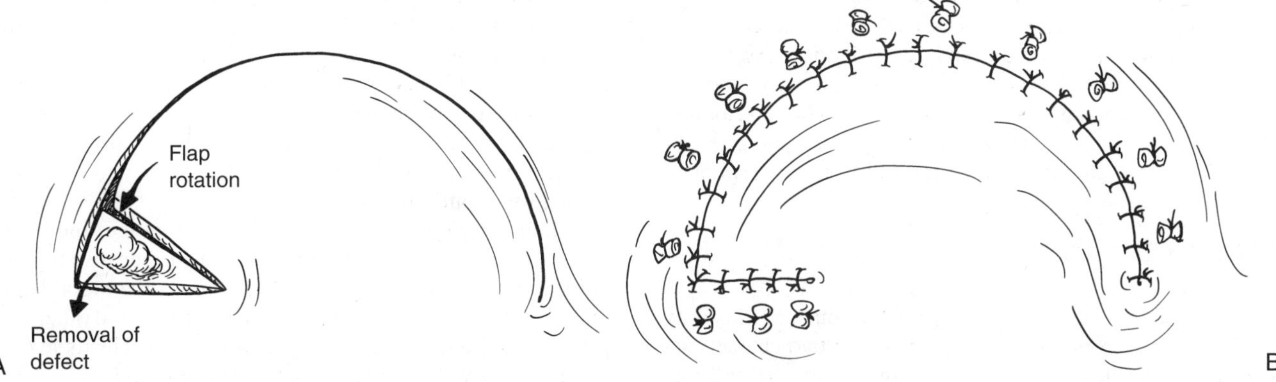

FIG. 97-9. A rotation flap, in which a circular flap is rotated around its axis to fill a defect.

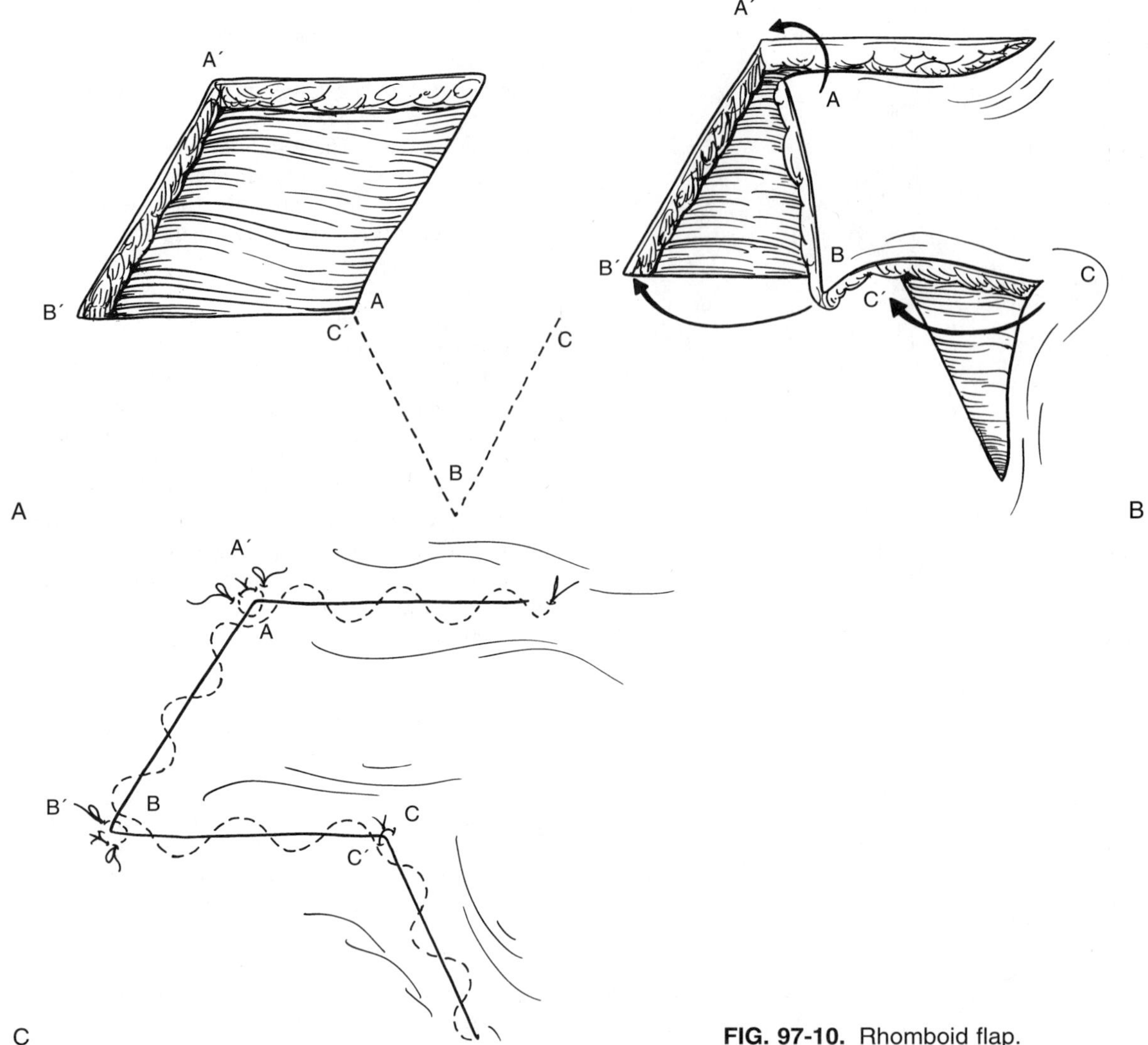

FIG. 97-10. Rhomboid flap.

extending to a more distal insertion. Moving from the trunk to the extremities or head and neck region, muscles become less common. In these regions, fasciocutaneous flaps are more commonly used for reconstruction. Examples of fasciocutaneous flaps include the temporal–parietal–fascial flap, which is used as a thin, well-vascularized flap for head and neck reconstruction. In the upper extremity, the radial forearm flap is a versatile flap used with surrounding bone, tendon, and nerve for reconstructing extremity defects. This is used as well as a microvascular-free tissue transfer. The dorsalis pedis flap is a fasciocutaneous flap along the dorsum of the foot, which corrects distal lower extremity wounds. As with many of the other fasciocutaneous flaps, however, it requires a split-thickness skin graft for the donor site, which carries some morbidity in this region.

TISSUE EXPANSION

Tissue expansion takes advantage of the inherent elasticity and regenerative properties of the skin. These two characteristics make it possible to stretch the skin in a controlled fashion, making more skin available for reconstruction through advancement and rotation flaps. Natural stretching or expansion of the skin occurs during pregnancy or with massive obesity, and new epidermis appears to be created as the dermis is stretched. In extreme cases of obesity, new dermis is manufactured. Mechanical expansion has been performed for centuries in South America, where primitive Indian cultures stretch ear lobes and lips with sequentially larger disks. Surgical expansion is similar. It involves elevating the skin and subcutaneous tissue and inserting a silastic prosthesis. This prosthesis is connected to a remote reservoir through a tube system. After closure of the skin, the prosthesis, which is like a silastic balloon, is sequentially filled with saline to stretch the overlying skin and subcutaneous tissue. After 6 to 12 weeks, enough tissue is usually recruited or stretched to accomplish reconstruction of the defect or surgical wound without a donor site defect.

The advantage of tissue expansion is that it is more reliable than rotated or advanced skin flaps. This is because the capsule of scar tissue around the implant improves the blood supply to the flap. In addition, color match is improved, and other adnexal structures are included in the reconstruction. This is in contrast with ordinary skin grafts, which are usually lighter in color and contain no hair or sebaceous glands. Skin grafting of the donor

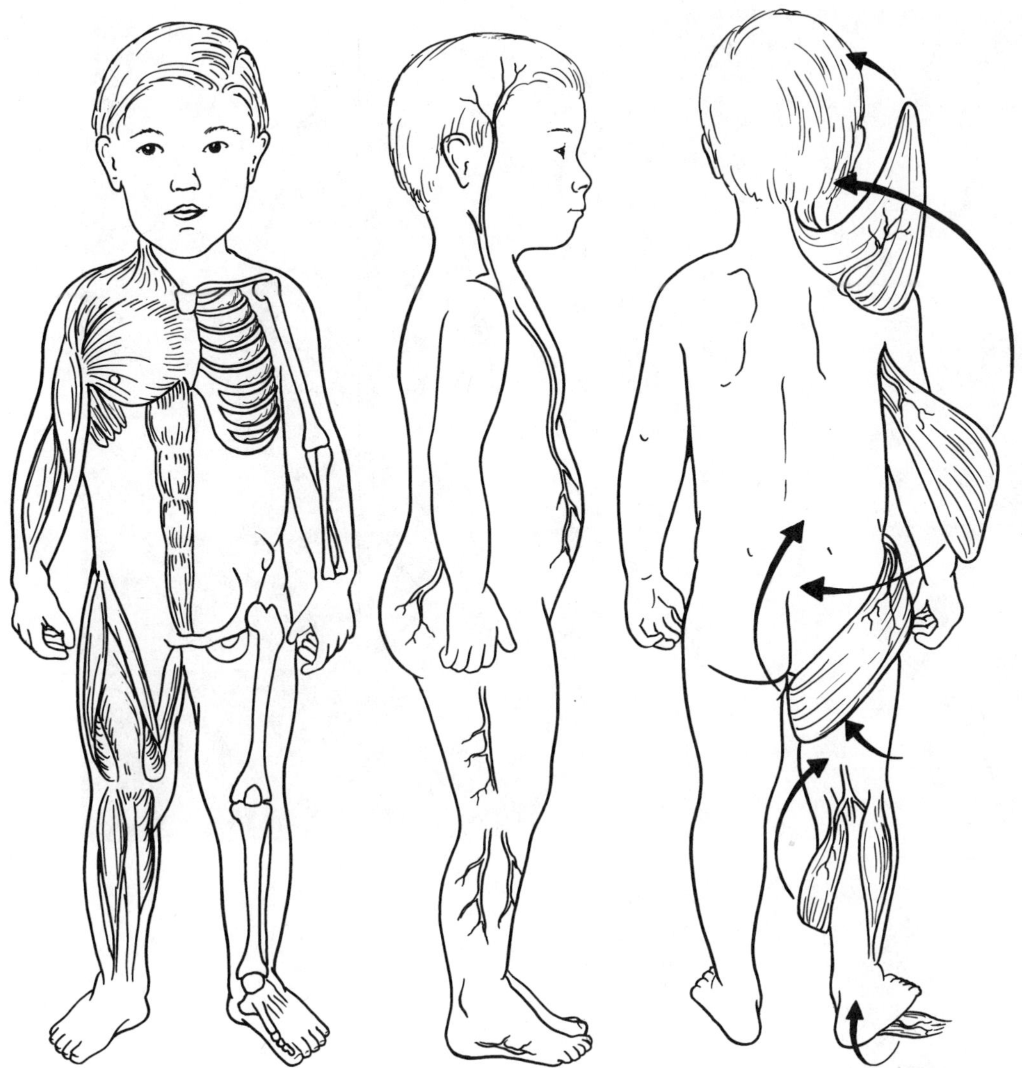

FIG. 97-11. Principles of safe muscle flap transposition are illustrated and the relevant muscular anatomy, blood supply, and some arcs of rotation demonstrated.

site is often required following large rotation flaps but is not needed with tissue expansion, nor are the special surgical techniques or the complex anatomy of musculocutaneous flaps required. The disadvantages of tissue expansion are that it requires two surgical procedures, and multiple office visits are required for serial expansion, although parents or pediatricians can assist in this process. There is also a potential for infection and extrusion of the implant. Finally, the cost of the expanders and two surgical procedures needs to be considered.

Tissue expansion is used in reconstruction of birth defects of the face and trunk, traumatic scalp and facial defects, and congenital defects of the trunk. The decreased vascularity and the thinner tissues of the extremities in relation to the trunk or head and neck region present more difficulty with extrusion.

MICROSURGERY

Microsurgery began with the first replantation of severed digits through the re-anastomosis of 1-mm digital arteries and veins. It was then extended to small vessels that supply islands of skin known as axial skin flaps. Subsequently, microtransfer of musculocutaneous flaps allowed more versatility for reconstruction. They provided a combination of skin and muscle, along with tendon, nerve, and bone. Later, bone based on its own segmental microvascular pedicle, became available for transfer.

Microsurgery is the top of the reconstructive ladder for two reasons. First, it is the most complex. It has a 90% to 95% success rate, but the chance of problems in the reconstruction is greater. It is technically demanding, and requires a microscope and specialized instruments and techniques. It is a long surgical procedure, requiring complex postoperative care, including intensive nursing and extensive rehabilitation.

The second reason microsurgery is at the top of the reconstructive ladder is that it is the most versatile technique and offers results that were impossible 25 years ago. Almost any combination of tissues of any size can be transferred to any area to reconstruct a defect. This affords a precision not possible

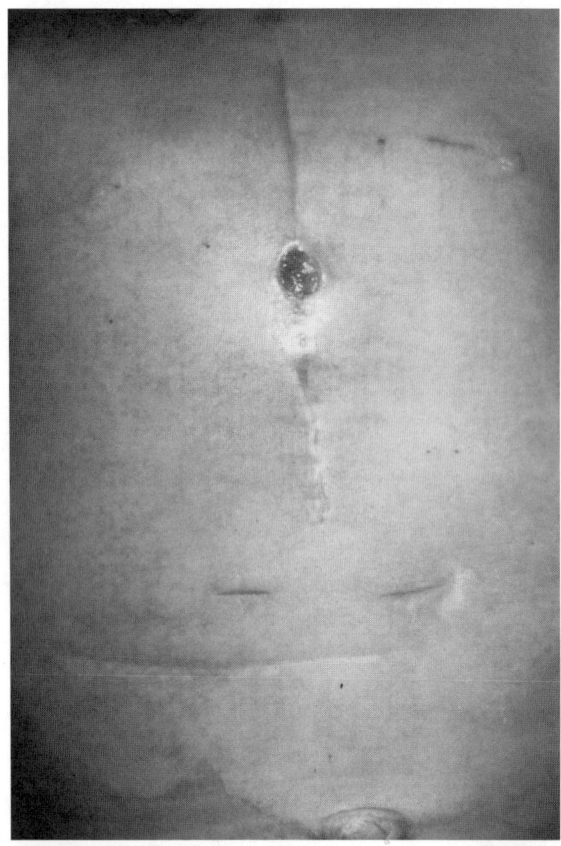

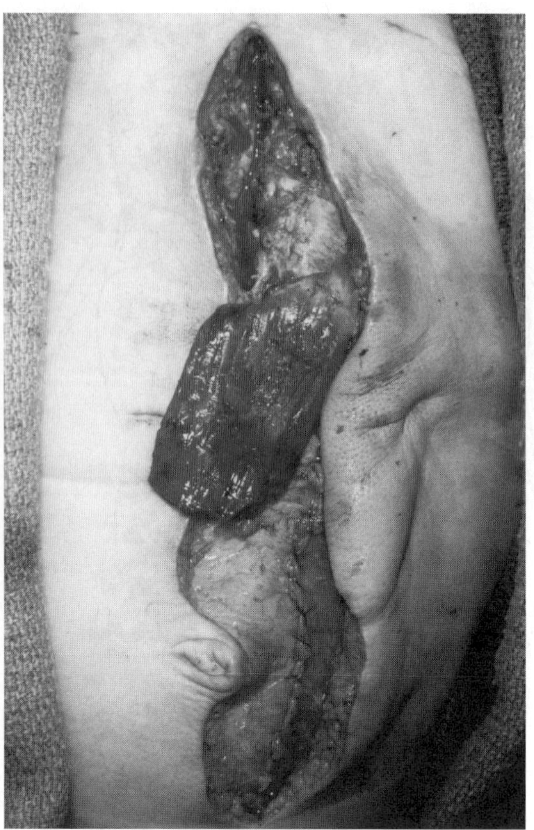

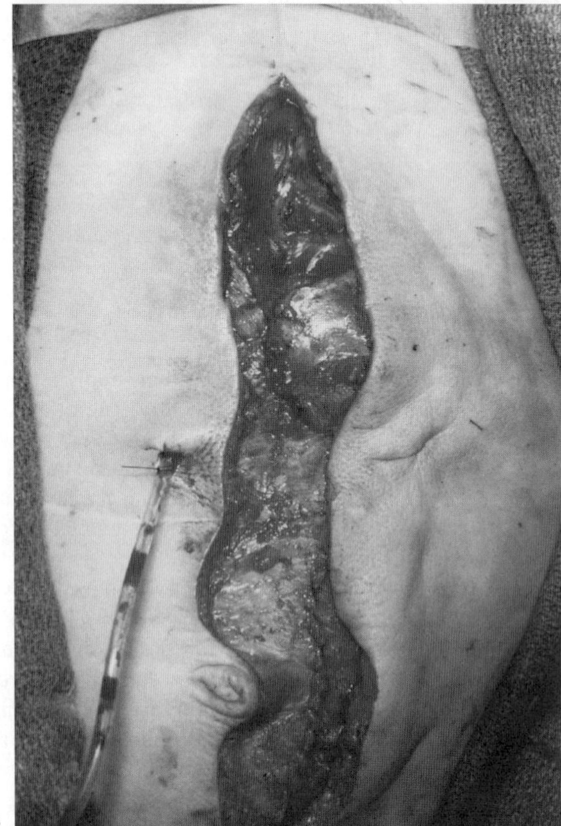

FIG. 97-12. Sternal wound infection demonstrating muscle flap reconstruction. (*A*) At presentation. (*B*) After débridement, with left rectus abdominus muscle elevated. (*C*) Flap rotated into position to obliterate dead space.

with local skin flaps, muscle flaps, fasciocutaneous flaps, or tissue expansion. Hundreds of types of flaps provide a variety of tissue to promote rapid healing of the wound and return form and function. This is often accomplished with minimal cosmetic sacrifice from the donor site.

Although there are many examples of microvascular reconstruction, probably the most common is lower extremity salvage. Complex tibial and fibular fractures frequently injure the thin overlying soft tissue. The upper two thirds of the leg has adequate surrounding posterior soft tissue for coverage of the damaged anterior soft tissue. This is usually accomplished with a soleus or gastrocnemius muscle flap covered with a split-thickness skin graft. Occasionally, a fasciocutaneous flap is also successful. The lower third of the leg has no available soft tissue to cover the anterior wound. Therefore, undamaged, well-vascularized tissue must be transferred to the injured area with microvascular techniques. The two most frequently used sources of tissue are the latissimus dorsi muscle and the rectus abdominus muscle flaps. These two muscles have relatively large vascular pedicles with sufficient length to reach any distal-third defect to be reconstructed. Both muscles have enough bulk to completely fill a complex wound with well-vascularized tissue that augments the local vascularity and assists in fracture healing.

BIBLIOGRAPHY

Davis JS. The story of plastic surgery. Ann Surg 1941;113:641.

Kernahan DA, Thompson HG, Bauer BS. Symposium on pediatric plastic surgery. St. Louis, CV Mosby, 1982.

Kraissl CJ. The selection of appropriate lines for elective surgical incisions. Plast Reconstr Surg 1951;8:1.

McGregor IA, Morgon G. Axial and random pattern flaps. Br J Plast 1973; 26:202.

Mathes SJ, Nahai F. Clinical atlas of muscle and musculocutaneous flaps. St. Louis, CV Mosby, 1979.

Mustarde JC. Plastic surgery in infancy and childhood. Edinburgh, Churchill Livingstone, 1979.

Radavan C. Tissue expansion in soft-tissue reconstruction. Plast Reconstr Surg 1984;74:482.

Rudolph R, Fisher JC, Ninneman JL. Skin grafting. Boston, Little, Brown, 1979.

Sefafin D, Buncke HJ. Microsurgical composite tissue transplantation. St. Louis, CV Mosby, 1979.

Skiles MS, Chaglassian T. Simple geometric flap for closure of skin defects. Surg Gynecol Obstet 1979;149:249.

Tolhurst DE, Haesek B, Zeeman JJ. The development of the fasciocutaneous flap and its clinical application. Plast Reconstr Surg 1983;71:597.

Surgery of Infants and Children: Scientific Principles and Practice, edited by Keith T. Oldham, Paul M. Colombani, and Robert P. Foglia. Lippincott–Raven Publishers, Philadelphia, © 1997.

CHAPTER 98

Central Nervous System

Herbert Edgar Fuchs

The surgeon who works with the developing central nervous system (CNS) must have a thorough knowledge of the embryology of the nervous system to understand and effectively treat the vast array of complex malformations, tumors, and developmental disorders that can occur. This chapter reviews the spectrum of nontraumatic disorders that can affect the developing nervous system.

NORMAL DEVELOPMENT

Human embryonic development is divided into 23 morphologic stages, each of which lasts 2 to 3 days.[1] These stages encompass the period from fertilization to about 60 days' gestation. Table 98-1 depicts the correlation of these stages with gestational age and crown–rump length. These stages have also been correlated with those in animals, particularly rodents and birds. Although there are some important interspecies differences in CNS development, animal model systems have provided great insight into the processes involved in human CNS development and therefore are included in this discussion.[2]

By stage 6, the developing embryo has assumed a two-layer structure with a dorsal epiblast and a ventral hypoblast. The amniotic cavity lies between the epiblast and the trophoblast, and the yolk sac lies below the hypoblast. The primitive streak first appears at the caudal end of the developing embryo, elongates cranially during the next 3 days until stage 7, and then begins to regress toward the caudal end of the embryo. The primitive streak continues cranially with the primitive knot or Hensen's node. In the center of Hensen's node is a small indentation, the primitive pit. Along the length of the primitive streak is the primitive groove, through which cells of the epiblast migrate: first, prospective endodermal cells, and then, prospective mesodermal cells come to lie between the endoderm and the epiblast. The remaining epiblast cells migrate medially to replace the cells that have migrated through the primitive groove. These cells then become the ectoderm (both neuroectoderm and surface ectoderm). This process, by which the two-layered embryo becomes a three-layered embryo, is known as *gastrulation.*

As the primitive streak regresses, the notochord is formed as mesodermal cells are added from Hensen's node. At stage 7, the notochordal cells are arranged around a central lumen, the notochordal canal, which extends dorsally to the amniotic cavity and ventrally to the yolk sac to form the neurenteric canal.

The neural tube forms by a process termed *neurulation,* during embryonic stages 8 to 12, at 18 to 27 days' gestation. During this phase, the most severe, open forms of cranial and spinal dysraphism occur. In the later stages of embryonic development, the caudal neural tube is formed by canalization and regression. During this period, the occult forms of dysraphism can develop.

Neurulation

The notochord induces the overlying ectoderm to form the neural plate, which is contiguous laterally with the superficial ectoderm, by the end of the 3rd week of gestation. During the next several days, the lateral portions of the neural plate begin to elevate and to form the neural folds as the midline portion becomes the neural groove (Fig. 98-1). As this process continues, the neural folds fuse in the midline to form the neural tube, beginning in the cervical region and proceeding both cranially and caudally. The anterior and posterior neuropores close at about 23 and 25 days' gestation, respectively. Immediately after fusion of the neural folds, the superficial ectoderm fuses in the midline and then separates from the neural ectoderm (see Fig. 98-1). Mesenchymal cells then migrate between the skin and the neural tube, ultimately to form the meninges, neural arches, and paraspinal muscles.

Caudal Regression

After neurulation is complete, by day 25, the distal spinal cord begins to form as the caudal end of the neural tube blends into the caudal cell mass, a large mass of undifferentiated cells. The caudal cell mass eventually gives rise to components of the nervous, urogenital, and digestive systems. This accounts for the common joint occurrence of distal vertebral, neural, anorectal, and urogenital anomalies. Within the caudal cell mass, small vacuoles form, coalesce, and eventually connect with the central canal of the spinal cord, in the process known

TABLE 98-1. *Developmental stages in the human embryo*

Stage	Gestational age (d)	Crown–rump length (mm)	Selected features
1	1		Fertilization
2	2–3		2- to 16-cell stage
3	4–5		Blastocyst
4	5–6		Blastocyst attaches to uterine wall
5	7–12	0.1–0.2	Implantation to uterine wall
6	13–15	0.2	Primitive streak
7	15–17	0.4	Notochordal process
8	17–19	1.0–1.5	Neural plate, neurenteric canal
9	19–21	1.5–2.5	1–3 somites, neural folds
10	22–23	2–3.5	4–12 somites, first fusion of neural folds
11	23–26	2.5–4.5	13–20 somites, anterior neuropore closes
12	26–30	3–5	21–29 somites, posterior neuropore closes
13	28–32	4–6	Arm and leg limb buds
14	31–35	5–7	Optic cup, lens invagination
15	35–38	7–9	Cerebral vesicles, hand develops
16	37–42	8–11	Retinal pigment, foot develops
17	42–44	11–14	Finger rays
18	44–48	13–17	Toe rays
19	48–51	16–18	Trunk straightening, limbs extend
20	51–53	18–22	Elbows bent
21	53–54	22–24	Vascular plexus on head is half the distance to normal position
22	54–56	23–28	Hands overlap
23	56–60	27–31	Hands erect, scalp plexus near vertex

(Adapted from Lemire RJ, Siebert JR, Warkany J. Normal development of the central nervous system. In: McLaurin RL, Venes JL, Schut L, et al, eds. Pediatric neurosurgery: surgery of the developing nervous system, ed 2. Philadelphia, WB Saunders, 1989)

as *canalization* (Fig. 98-2). The surrounding cells differentiate toward glial cells, elongating the spinal cord well into the tail fold of the embryo. The most cephalic portion of this distal spinal cord forms the tip of the conus medullaris. The distal spinal cord then begins the process of involution or retrogressive differentiation, leaving a remnant of piaarachnoid, the filum terminale. From this point, the spinal cord and developing vertebral column elongate, with the vertebral column growing faster than the spinal cord. Thus, the conus medullaris appears to ascend from its initial position in the coccyx, to lie at the L2-3 interspace by birth. By 3 months postpartum, the tip of the conus medullaris is nearly at the adult level of the L1-2 interspace.[3]

Formation of the Brain

By embryonic stage 10 (days 22 and 23), the cephalic neural folds distinguish the future brain from the future spinal cord. Two constrictions divide the developing brain into three regions: the prosencephalon (forebrain), mesencephalon (midbrain), and rhombencephalon (hindbrain). By 35 days, the prosencephalon has divided into the telencephalon (future cerebral hemispheres) and the diencephalon, while the rhombencephalon has formed the metencephalon (future pons) and the myelencephalon (future medulla oblongata). Both cerebral hemispheres contain a cavity, the lateral ventricle. Glial and neural precursor cells begin to form around this cavity and migrate radially outward toward the surface of the cerebral hemisphere. The lateral, third, and fourth ventricular cavities are contiguous

with the central canal of the spinal cord at this stage; later development obliterates the site of communication at the obex in the fourth ventricle. The cerebellum forms from a complex series of buckling and folding in the rhombencephalon, initially lying within the fourth ventricle, and eventually coming to lie dorsal to the fourth ventricle.

The choroid plexus first appears in the fourth ventricle at days 43 to 44, in the lateral ventricles at days 45 to 46, and in the third ventricle at days 48 to 49. The caudal roof of the fourth ventricle perforates to form the foramen of Magendie at days 47 to 48; at the same time, the choroid plexus begins to produce cerebrospinal fluid (CSF). This CSF loosens the meshwork of mesenchymal cells surrounding the brain to form the subarachnoid space, beginning at the cisterna magna, and spreading over the cerebral hemispheres and the spinal cord.

Formation of the Skull and Vertebral Column

The skull is formed in two sections: the skull base is formed by endochondral ossification, and the cranial vault is formed as membranous bone. The first chondrification begins during stage 17 (days 40 to 44). The vertebral column originates from the medial portion of the somites in three stages: membrane formation (days 22 to 39), cartilage formation (days 40 to 64), and bone formation, which extends through the fetal portion until well after birth. The notochord appears to direct formation of the vertebral bodies, and the neural tube directs formation of the posterior vertebral elements. Remnants of the notochord remain in the intervertebral disks and in the clivus of the skull.

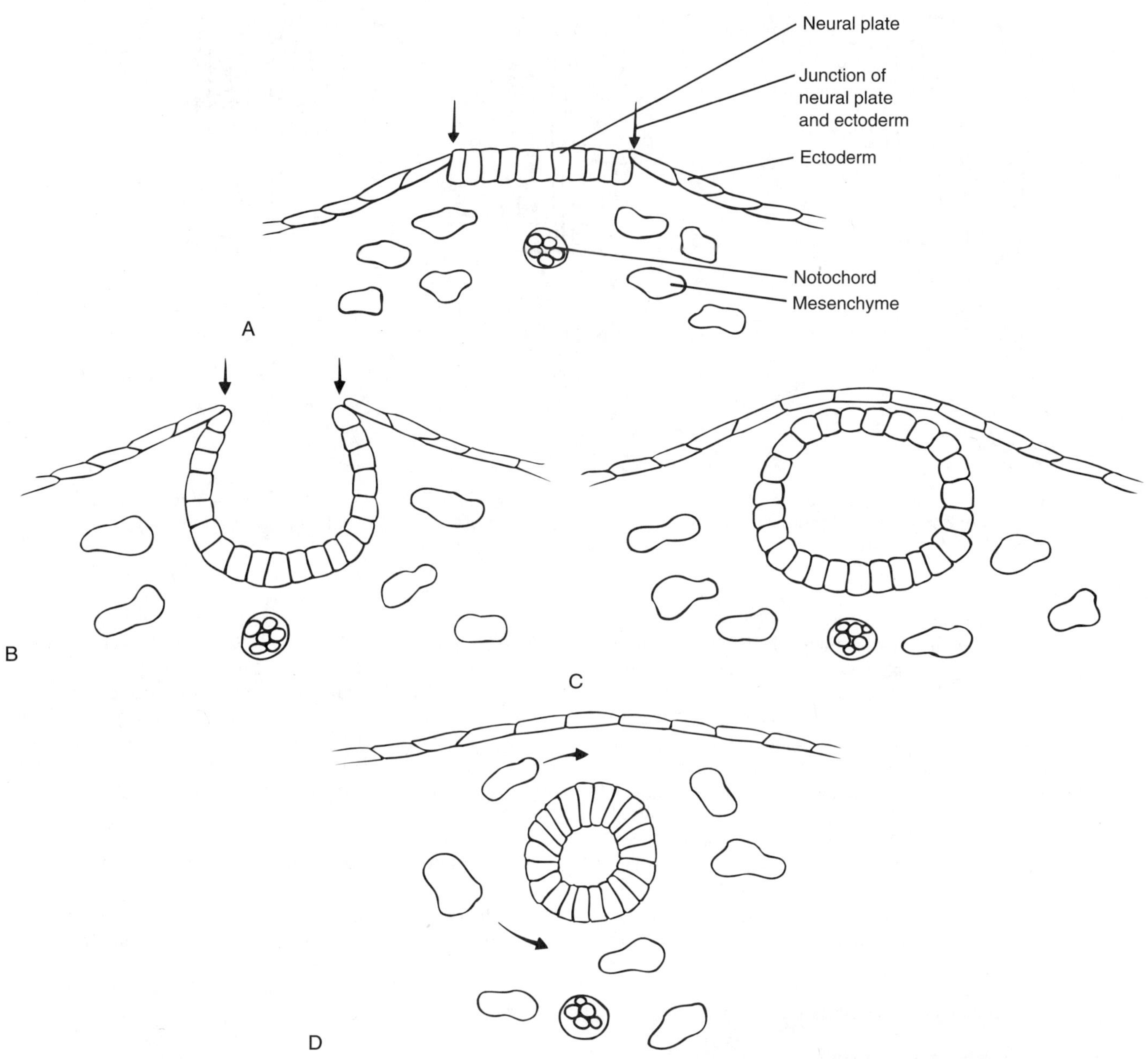

FIG. 98-1. Neurulation. (*A*) Cross section of an embryo, showing the neural plate. (*B*) Formation of the neural folds (*arrows*). (*C*) Formation of the neural tube. (*D*) Separation of the neural tube from the superficial ectoderm by mesenchymal cells.

CONGENITAL MALFORMATIONS

Congenital malformations of the CNS are best understood as derangements of the developmental processes discussed earlier (Table 98-2).

Derangements of Neurulation

Myelomeningocele is the most common derangement of neurulation, occurring in about 1 in 1000 live births. This incidence appears to be decreasing with emphasis on prenatal maternal care, particularly folate supplementation. In this malformation, a focal segment of the spinal cord fails to roll up and form a tube. Because the neural tube does not fuse, the cutaneous ectoderm does not come to cover the neural tube but remains attached, and lateral to, the neural plate, leaving a cutaneous defect (Fig. 98-3). Mesenchymal cells are also prevented from their proper migration, and thus the laminal arches and muscles develop in an abnormal lateral position. The raw, exposed surface of the neural plate represents the interior of the spinal cord. The midline neural groove is also seen. Surrounding this neural placode is a thin layer of skin and arachnoid tissue, below which is the subarachnoid space. The nerve roots lie inferior to the neural placode, with the ventral roots lying medial to the dorsal roots. Because the neural placode is attached to the skin, it is

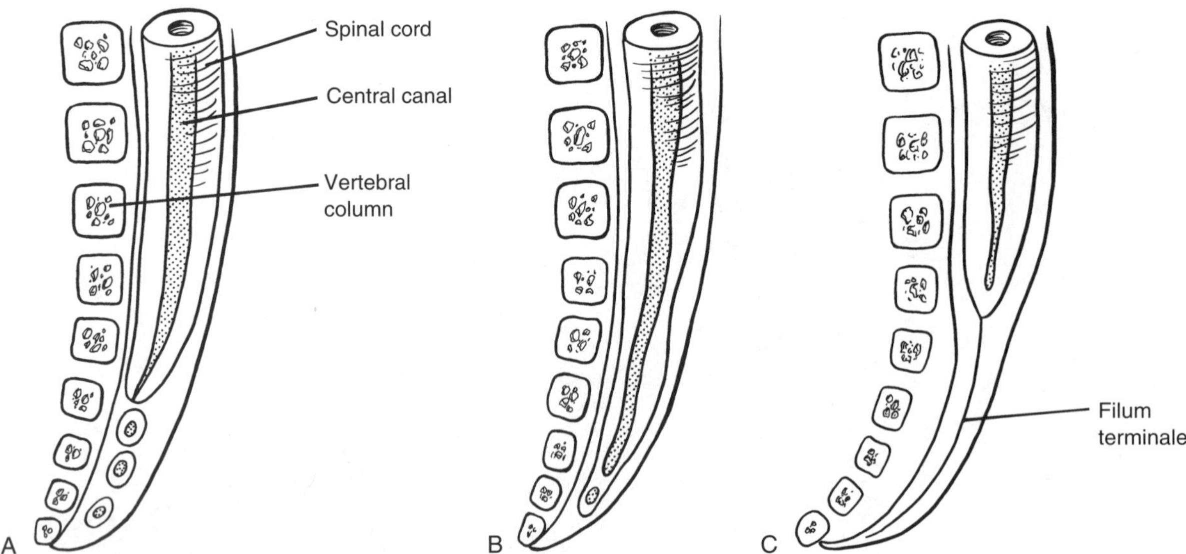

FIG. 98-2. Formation of the caudal spinal cord and filum terminale. (*A*) Vacuolization. (*B*) Vacuoles coalesce; canalization occurs. (*C*) Differential growth and retrogressive differentiation cause the conus medullaris to rise and the filum terminale to lengthen.

tethered and relatively immobile. A number of CNS anomalies have been associated with myelomeningocele, including Chiari II malformation and hydrocephalus, which are discussed later.

Lipomyelomeningocele is believed to form by focal premature dysjunction of neuroectoderm from cutaneous ectoderm, allowing access of mesenchymal cells to the dorsal surface of the unclosed neural tube.[4] The mesenchymal cells then give rise to fat. The anatomy is therefore similar to myelomeningocele, with the exception that the cutaneous ectoderm is able to close over the neural tube. The lipoma may extend from the spinal cord and merge with the subcutaneous fat (Fig. 98-4).

In contrast to lipomyelomeningocele, dermal sinus tract results from incomplete dysjunction of the neural tube and cutaneous ectoderm. As the spinal cord becomes buried beneath the surface and elongates, the localized connection with the skin becomes an elongated tract (Fig. 98-5). The incidence of dermal sinus is highest in the lumbosacral region, the site of posterior neuropore closure, but this derangement also can occur in the cervicooccipital and nasal regions. It can extend to variable depths, ending in the subcutaneous tissues or the dura, or retaining its attachment to the spinal cord or brain stem. Dermoid or epidermoid tumors may be found along the course of the dermal sinus tract.

Derangements of Retrogressive Differentiation

The tight filum terminale or fatty filum terminale syndrome is a condition in which the spinal cord is tethered by an abnormally

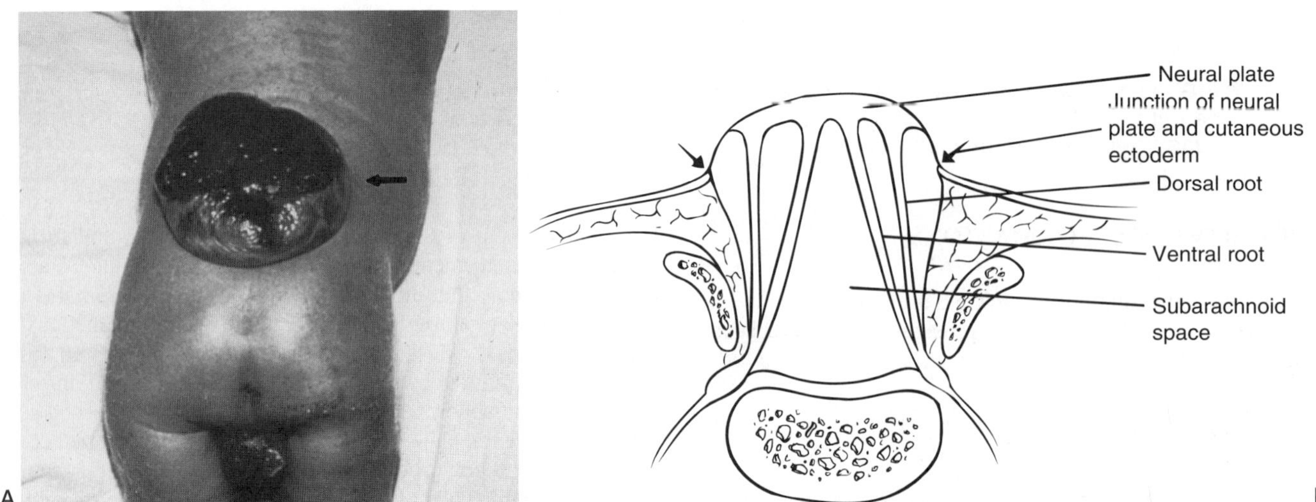

FIG. 98-3. Myelomeningocele. (*A*) Myelomeningocele in a newborn (*arrow*). The anal sphincter is flaccid, and the lower extremity musculature is poorly developed. (*B*) Schematic depiction of a myelomeningocele in cross section.

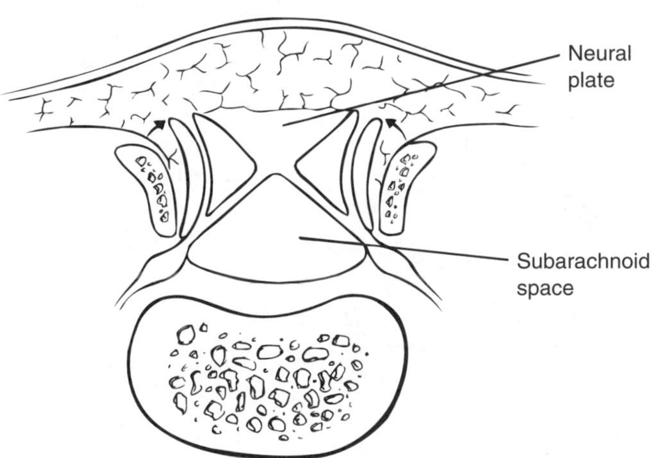

FIG. 98-4. Cross-sectional drawing of a lipomyelomeningocele.

TABLE 98-2. *Congenital malformations of the central nervous system*

DERANGED NEURULATION
Myelomeningocele
Lipomyelomeningocele
Dermal sinus

DERANGED RETROGRESSIVE DIFFERENTIATION
Lipoma of filum terminale or tight filum terminale
Terminal myelocystocele

OTHER MECHANISMS
Diastematomyelia
Neurenteric cyst
Chiari malformations
Dandy-Walker malformation
Meningocele
Arachnoid cyst

short, thickened filum terminale. The terminal myelocystocele is a complex malformation that is believed to be caused by dilation of the central canal in the caudal neural tube, forming a cyst. This cyst distends the arachnoid lining of the distal spinal cord, forming a meningocele. This anomaly is commonly associated with extrophy of the bladder.

Other Embryologic Derangements

Diastematomyelia is a condition in which the spinal cord is split in a sagittal plane into two hemicords that may or may not be symmetric. Diastematomyelia is most common in girls and is usually heralded by a hairy patch overlying the site of the cleft. The cause of this malformation has been a subject of great debate, but studies by Dias and Walker[5] and Pang and colleagues[6] support the concept that these malformations are due to disorders of gastrulation. Pang classified these lesions as type I or II split cord malformation (SCM). Type I SCM is the classic diastematomyelia, with a bony septum lying between two hemicords, each lying in its own dural sac. The type II malformation consists of two hemicords in a single dural sac, with a thin sagittal fibrous septum. These malformations can be caused by splitting of the notocord, either by duplication or by persistence of the neurenteric canal, which effectively causes a localized split of the notocord. The development of mesenchymal elements between the two hemicords then determines the type of SCM formed. A thicker mesenchymal tract gives rise to the bony septum and meninges, whereas a thinner tract may only form a thin fibrous septum (Fig. 98-6).

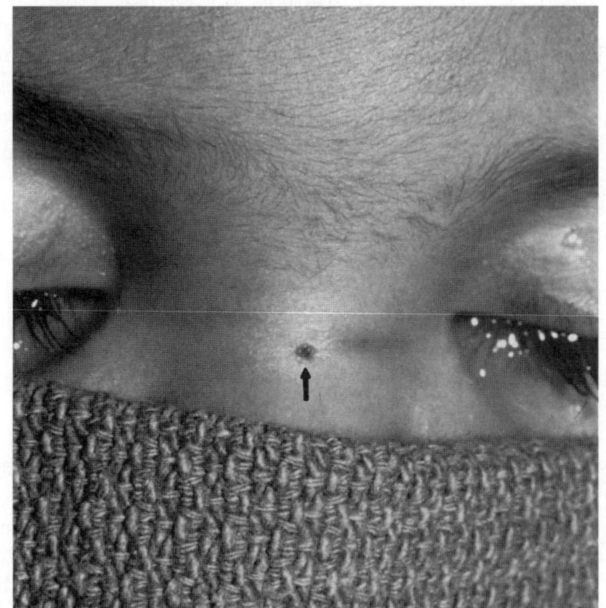

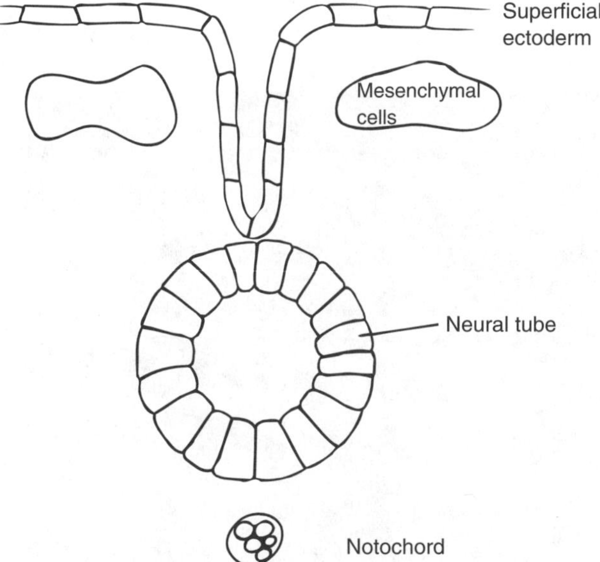

FIG. 98-5. Dermal sinus tract. (*A*) Nasal dermal sinus tract (*arrow*). (*B*) Cross-sectional drawing of a dermal sinus tract.

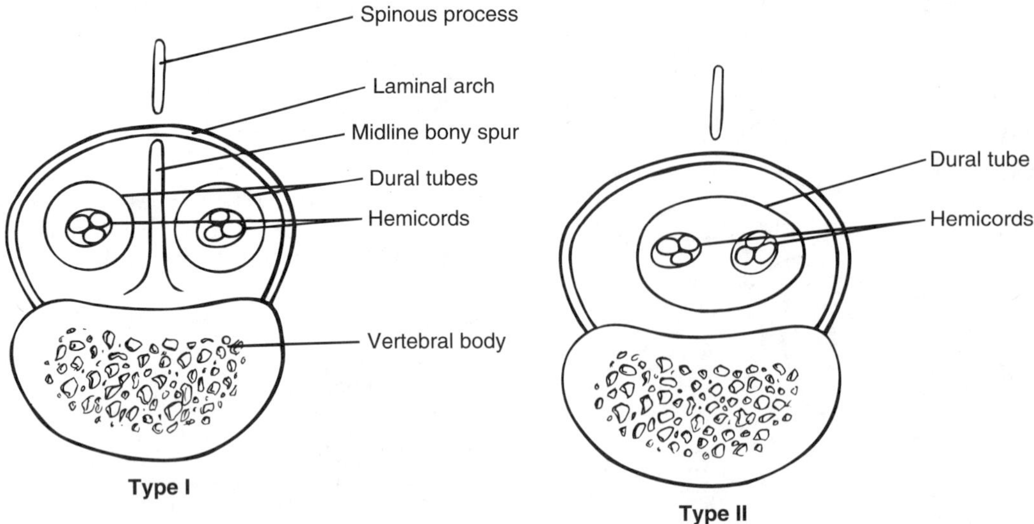

FIG. 98-6. Split cord malformations depicted in cross section.

A neurenteric cyst can also result from persistence of the neurenteric canal and is often associated with SCM. This rare lesion is most often seen as only a partial fistula and is most common in the cervicothoracic region of the spinal cord.

Meningoceles are thought to be due to postneurulation disorders involving cutaneous ectoderm and mesenchyme because the neural tube is normally formed beneath the cutaneous and mesenchymal defect, which contains CSF (Fig. 98-7).

The embryology of encephaloceles has been reviewed by Chapman and associates.[7] Encephaloceles were originally thought to be caused by failure of closure of the anterior neuropore. These lesions, however, contain well-developed neural and mesenchymal structures, which cannot be the result of failure of neural tube closure. Therefore, these lesions are thought to be due to herniation of fully neurulated neural tissue through a mesenchymal defect (Fig. 98-8).

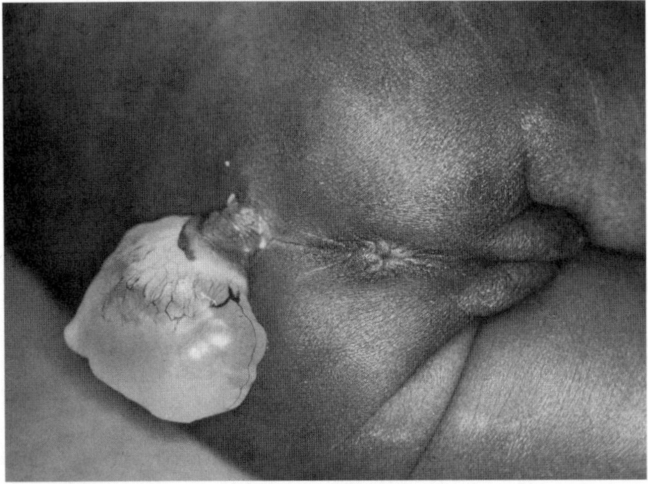

FIG. 98-7. Infant with a sacral meningocele. The sac does not contain any neural elements.

The Chiari II malformation is a complex disorder associated with myelomeningocele. This malformation consists of caudal displacement of the cerebellar vermis and tonsils into the cervical canal; elongation, kinking, and caudal displacement of the lower brain stem into the cervical canal; and upward displacement of the superior cerebellum through a low-lying tentorial incisura, with a small posterior fossa (Fig. 98-9A). McLone and Knepper[8] proposed a unifying theory of pathogenesis of these malformations, in which the open neural placode of the myelomeningocele allows escape of CSF, which interferes with the normal distention of the ventricular system and development of the skull base. Incomplete distention of the fourth ventricle fails to stimulate growth of the skull base, resulting in a smaller posterior fossa that is unable to respond during the later phase of rapid cerebellar growth and development. This results in herniation of neural tissue from the posterior fossa and impairs flow of CSF, resulting in hydrocephalus. The Chiari I malformation, involving caudal displacement of the cerebellar tonsils with a normal posterior fossa, must have its embryologic origin at a later stage than the more severe Chiari II malformation, but the exact mechanisms responsible remain to be elucidated (see Fig. 98-9B).

The Dandy-Walker malformation is a developmental abnormality in which the roof of the fourth ventricle fails to perforate to form the foramen of Magendie. The resultant cystic dilation of the fourth ventricle expands the posterior fossa, elevates the tentorium, and causes hydrocephalus due to obstruction of the aqueduct of Sylvius with concomitant hypoplasia of the cerebellar vermis (Fig. 98-10).

Arachnoid cysts are arachnoid-lined cavities filled with fluid similar in composition to CSF. They can create a disturbance in intracranial dynamics due to shift and displacement of surrounding structures, and can cause intracranial hypertension. Their pathogenesis is unknown. Arachnoid cysts appear to form early in development and may communicate to varying degrees with the surrounding subarachnoid space. The most common locations for arachnoid cysts are the sylvian fissure, suprasellar, and posterior fossa.

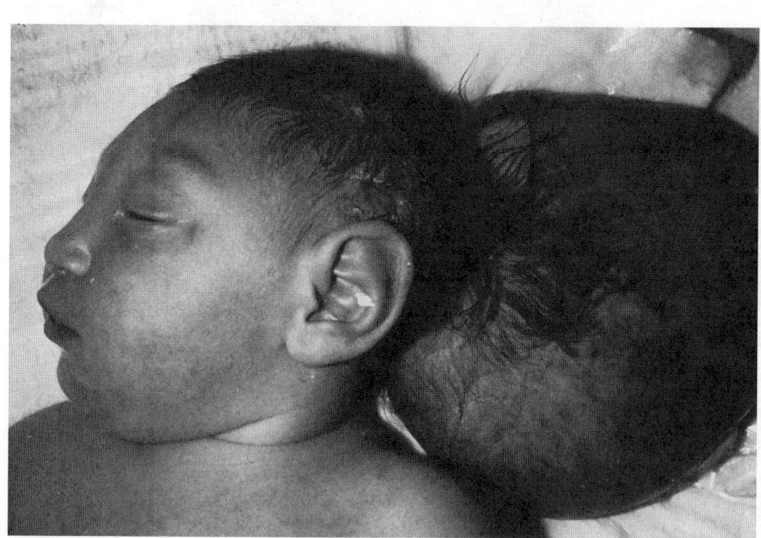

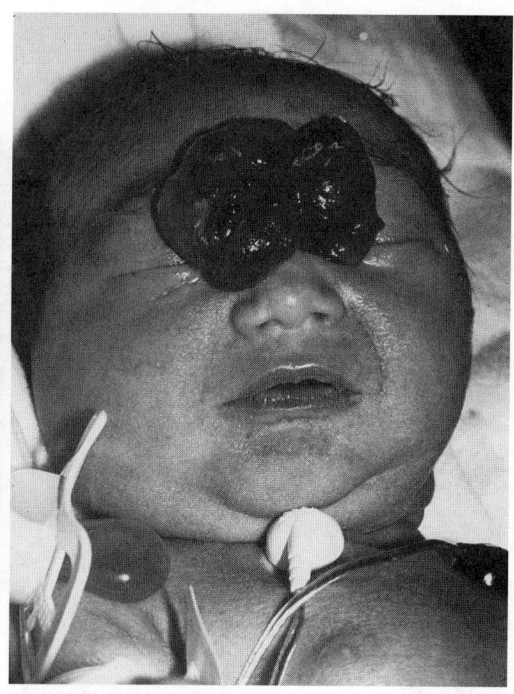

FIG. 98-8. Encephalocele. (*A*) Infant with an occipital encephalocele. (*B*) Infant with a nasal encephalocele.

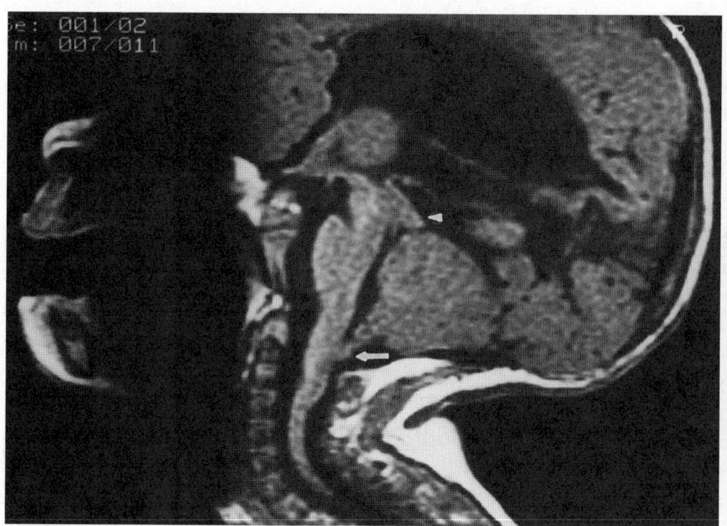

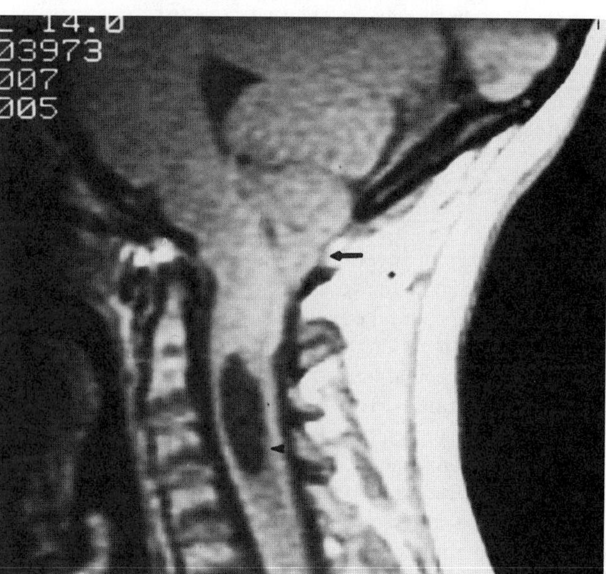

FIG. 98-9. MR images of Chiari malformations. (*A*) Chiari II malformation. The cerebellar vermis is displaced caudad (*arrow*), and the midbrain tectum is beaked (*arrowhead*). (*B*) Chiari I malformation. In contrast to *A,* the brain stem is normal, and only the cerebellar tonsils are descended into the cervical canal (*arrow*). A cervical syrinx (*arrowhead*) is present.

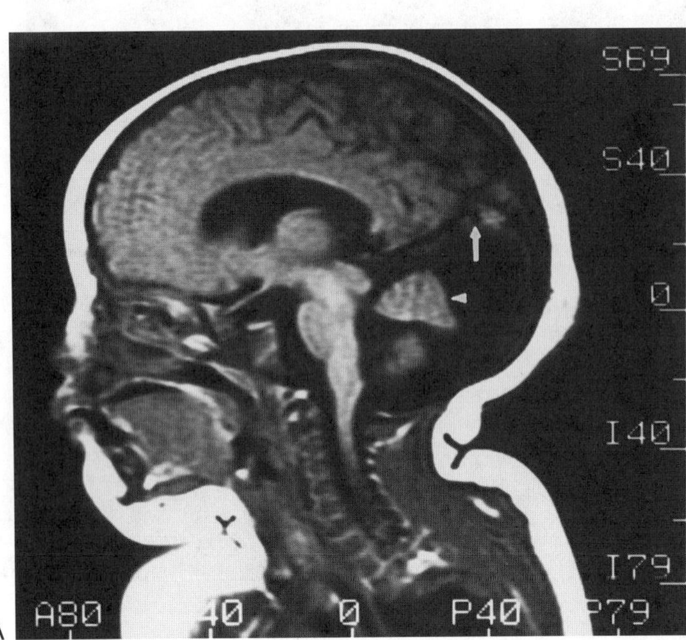
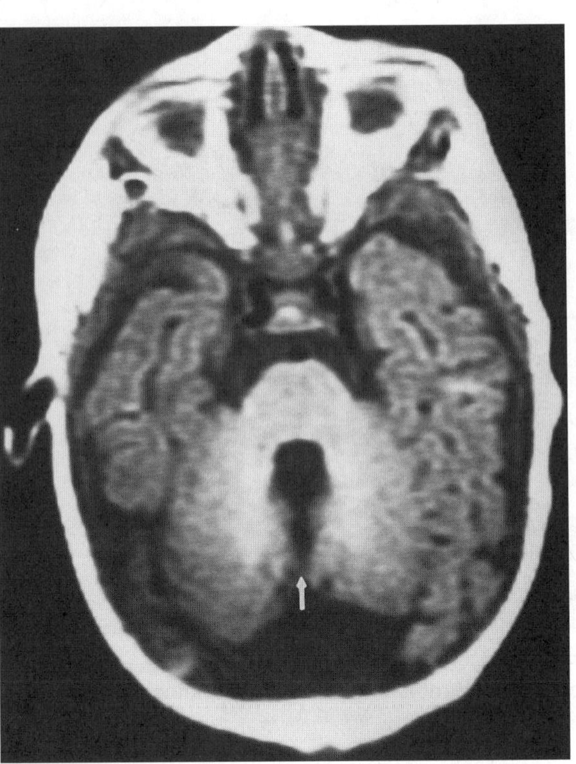

FIG. 98-10. MR images of Dandy-Walker malformation. (*A*) Sagittal image shows an enlarged posterior fossa with a large cyst, elevated tentorium (*arrow*), and absent inferior cerebellar vermis. The superior vermis is indicated by an arrowhead. (*B*) Axial image shows absent inferior vermis and communication with the fourth ventricle (*arrow*).

Diagnosis and Management

Myelomeningocele

The diagnosis of myelomeningocele is obvious at birth. For initial management, the lesion is covered with sterile, saline-soaked dressings, and the patient is kept prone. After a general assessment, the location of the lesion is noted, and a neurologic examination is performed to assess sensorimotor function in the lower extremities. Hip flexion requires function of L-1 to L-3. Hip adduction requires L-2 to L-4 function. Hip abduction, hip extension, and knee extension require L-5 to S-2 function. Plantar flexion requires function of sacral roots. Anal sphincter tone should be assessed because more than 90% of children with myelomeningocele have bowel and bladder dysfunction. Head circumference should be measured and the anterior fontanelle palpated to assess for hydrocephalus. After medical stabilization, and preferably within 24 hours of birth, the child should be taken to the operating room for closure of the myelomeningocele. This procedure involves meticulous anatomic reconstruction of the neural tube, dural sac, and overlying cutaneous tissues, with great care taken not to further injure neural tissue. Postoperatively, the child is monitored for development of hydrocephalus, which is treated with a ventriculoperitoneal shunt, and nursed prone, while the closure heals. During this time period, further orthopedic and urologic work-up can be completed, along with evaluation of brain-stem function to assess the associated Chiari II malformation. The long-term outcomes

for these children have been reported in depth by McLone and coworkers.[9] The survival rate for these children followed for 8 to 12 years was 85%, with 62% having an IQ of 80 or greater. With the development of clean intermittent bladder catheterization, 85% of children with myelomeningocele can achieve social continence of urine. The development of improved leg braces has allowed children with motor levels of at least L-3 function to be community ambulators. McLone's studies have shown that children with myelomeningocele can be functional and that the natural history of this disease is not one of relentless deterioration, as some prior studies had suggested. Any neurologic deterioration seen in children with myelomeningocele should be promptly investigated and treated.

The congenital spinal cord lesions with intact skin are termed *spina bifida occulta* and share a common presentation, owing to tethering of the spinal cord. These lesions also can be associated with an overlying skin lesion such as the dermal sinus, a subcutaneous lipoma, a hemangioma, or a hairy patch. The most common signs and symptoms of tethered cord include changes in gait, weakness, orthopedic deformity, and pain. The most common orthopedic deformities seen include varus and valgus, and cavus changes of the foot. In addition, recurrent hip dislocation and scoliosis may also be seen. Pain and sensory loss are common features of the tethered spinal cord, and both can be asymmetric and nondermatomal. In addition, changes in bowel and bladder function may be missed in young children. Neurologic dysfunction results from traction on the conus medullaris, with stretching and deformation of vessels overlying the tethered cord, resulting in ischemia of the conus.[10] Spinal flexion or growth can result in chronic, repetitive ischemia to the spinal cord. With modern magnetic resonance imaging (MRI) techniques, the diagnosis of spina bifida occulta is straightforward. The treatment of all these lesions is centered around release of the tethered cord, with restoration of more normal anatomic relations of the spinal cord and surrounding structures. With early recognition and treatment, pain, sensory loss, and motor weakness are likely to improve, but if treatment is deferred until bowel or bladder dysfunction occurs, improvement of these functions is unlikely.

Spina Bifida Occulta

Lipomyelomeningocele

The subcutaneous component of the lipomyelomeningocele lies cephalad to, and can distort, the intergluteal crease. The MRI scan confirms the diagnosis and assists in surgical planning (Fig. 98-11). Surgical repair of lipomyelomeningoceles consists of debulking of the lipoma down to the interface with the spinal cord using the CO_2 laser, reformation of the neural tube if possible, and reconstruction of the dura, creating a capacious subarachnoid space to prevent retethering. The remainder of the wound is then closed in layers. In modern series, 40%

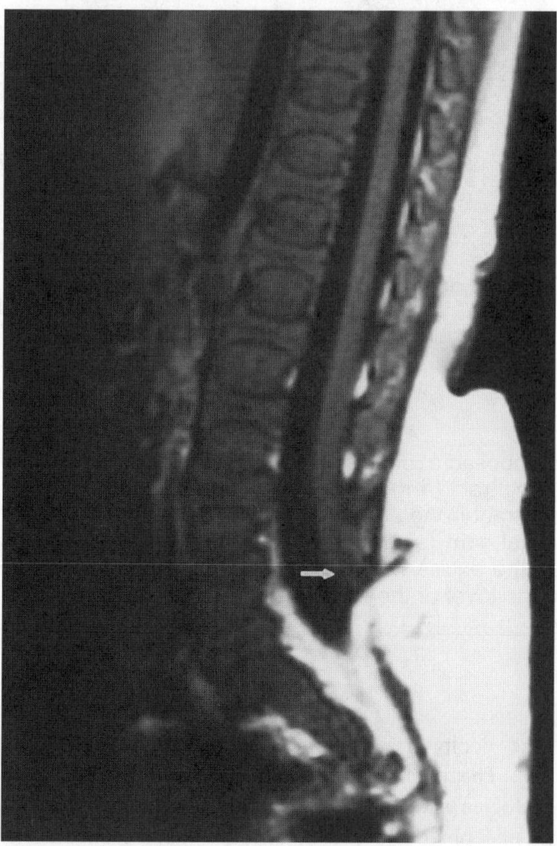

FIG. 98-11. MR image of lipomyelomeningocele. Sagittal image shows tethered cord merging into lipoma (*arrow*), which is contiguous with subcutaneous fat.

of patients with motor deficits and 12% of patients with incontinence recovered normal function after surgery.

Dermal Sinus Tract

A dermal sinus tract can occur in a variety of locations in the CNS. It is usually recognized as a midline cutaneous orifice with hairs in it, with or without an associated hemangioma. It also can present with localized cutaneous infection, meningitis, or brain abscess. The dermal sinus tract can be distinguished from the pilonidal sinus by location because the latter typically lies within the gluteal crease, overlying the tip of the coccyx, and has no connection with the CNS. MRI scan provides the diagnosis and may provide evidence of the extent of the sinus tract (Fig. 98-12). Even without MRI evidence of either intracranial or intraspinal extension, these lesions should be explored because a narrow sinus tract may be missed on imaging studies. Surgery for lumbosacral lesions potentially involves exploration from the site of the cutaneous orifice to the level of the conus. All dermal elements should be removed. Nasal and occipital dermal sinus tracts may require formal craniotomy in addition to excision of the cutaneous portions of the tract to remove the entire tract.

Tethered Cord–Fatty Filum Terminale

The tethered cord–fatty filum terminale syndrome has classically been described as an abnormally low-lying conus medullaris and a thickened, fatty-infiltrated filum terminale. Warder and Oakes[11] described the tethered cord syndrome in patients with the conus in normal position. The clinical presentation, along with the presence of fat in the filum terminale, are the key elements in the diagnosis of tethered cord–fatty filum terminale syndrome. The treatment consists of a limited lumbosacral laminectomy for sectioning of the filum terminale.

Diastematomyelia

As discussed earlier, diastematomyelia is often heralded by a cutaneous hairy patch overlying the cleft spinal cord. MRI confirms the diagnosis and can distinguish the type I and II SCM (Fig. 98-13). Surgery involves complete release of the spinal cord from all tethering lesions, which may include a tight filum terminale, the bony septum, and fibrous bands adherent to the dorsal dura. The dura is then closed to create a capacious subarachnoid space, and the remainder of the wound is closed in layers.

Meningocele

The neural elements are intact, with a CSF-filled sac protruding through a cutaneous defect. Repair is accomplished by localizing the dural defect, amputating the herniating sac, and closing the dura. The remainder of the wound is then closed in layers.

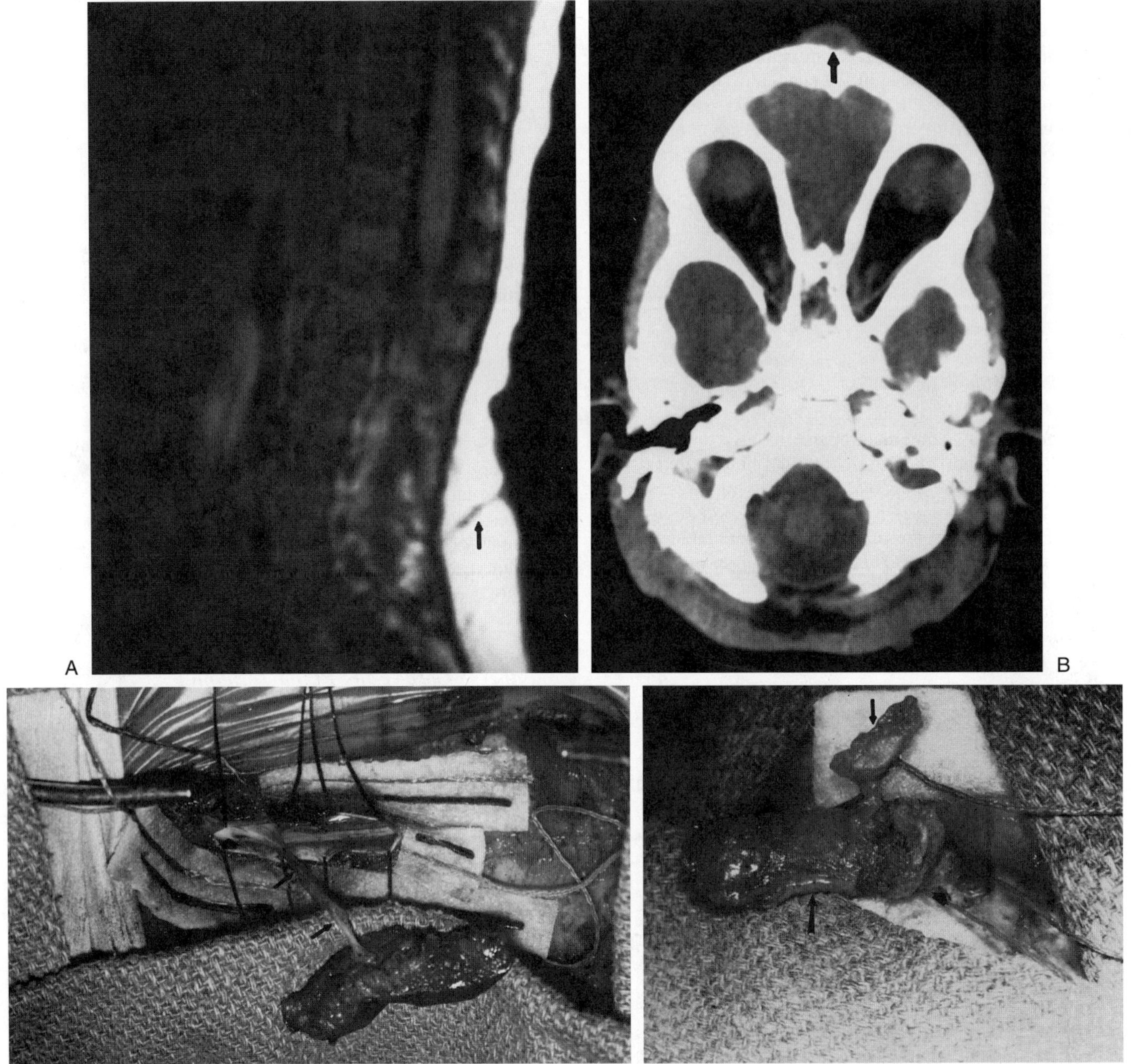

FIG. 98-12. Dermal sinus tracts. (*A*) Sagittal MR image of lumbosacral dermal sinus tract (*arrow*). (*B*) Axial CT scan of nasal dermal sinus shows a dermoid cyst along tract (*arrow*). (*C*) Intraoperative photograph of lumbosacral dermal sinus shown in *A* demonstrates tract (*long arrows*) leading from excised segment of skin into the dural sac and merging with the spinal cord (*short arrow*). (*D*) Intraoperative photograph of nasal dermal sinus shown in *B* demonstrates the excised skin (*arrow at top*), dermoid cyst (*long arrow*), and sinus tract (*short arrow*) extending to the level of the dura.

Encephalocele

The incidence of encephalocele varies according to geographic region, from as high as 1 in 5000 live births in Southeast Asia to as low as 1 in 10,000 live births in North America. The location of the encephalocele also exhibits geographic variability, with frontonasal encephaloceles more common in Southeast Asia and occipital encephaloceles more common in North America. The degree of herniation of neural tissue into the encephalocele sac can be highly variable. MRI classifies the type of encephalocele and determines the presence of neural tissues within the sac (Fig. 98-14). The treatment of encephaloceles is surgical resection, with removal of the lesion at its base, repair of the dura, and bone grafting to cover the calvarial

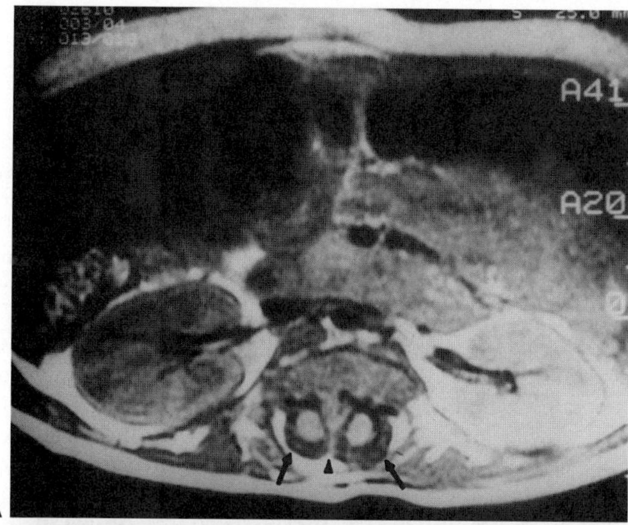

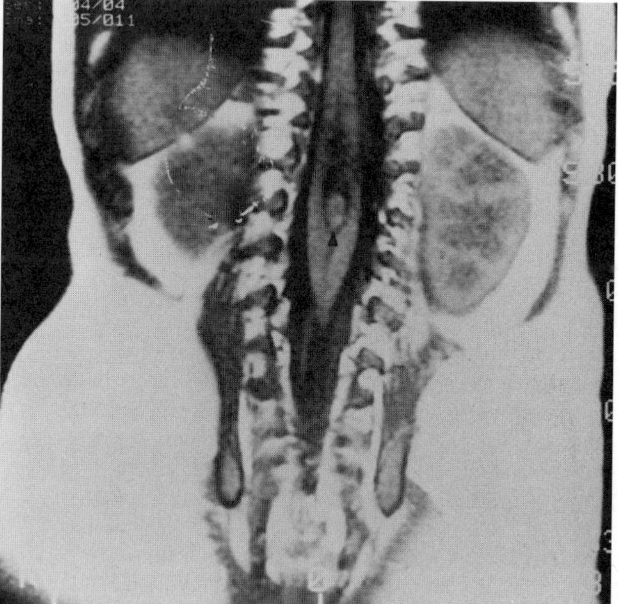

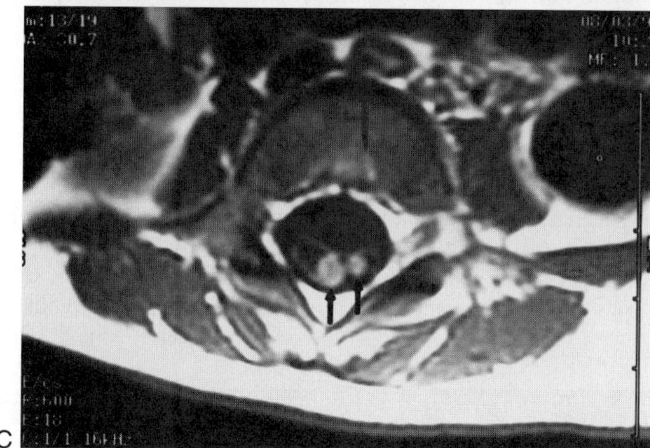

FIG. 98-13. MR images of split cord malformations. (*A* and *B*) Type I split cord malformation shows two hemicords and two dural sacs (*arrows*), separated by a bony septum (*arrowhead*), in axial and coronal sections, respectively. (*C*) Type II split cord malformation reveals two unequal hemicords (*arrows*) contained in a single dural sac.

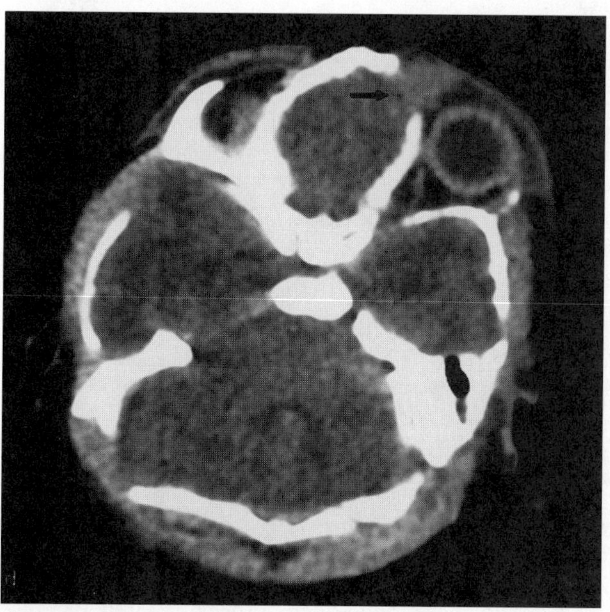

FIG. 98-14. CT scan of a frontal encephalocele shows nasal mass extending into the left orbit (*arrow*).

defect. In some occipital encephaloceles, the sac contains vital neural or vascular structures, and such repair is not possible. The outcome of surgical treatment depends on the location of the encephalocele and the amount of neural tissue remaining within the cranial vault. In general, occipital encephaloceles are more commonly associated with hydrocephalus and have a worse cognitive outcome.

Chiari II Malformation

In children with myelomeningocele, the Chiari II malformation is invariably present. Despite impressive imaging studies, however, the patient may not have symptoms. Typical Chiari II symptoms and signs include occipital pain, nystagmus, upper extremity weakness, lower cranial nerve dysfunction, hypotonia or spasticity, and scoliosis. Hydromyelia (dilation of the central canal of the spinal cord) may also be present. A shunt malfunction must be ruled out before any consideration of cervical decompression. The surgical treatment of Chiari II malformation involves decompression of the brain stem or cervical spinal cord and restoration of normal CSF flow from the fourth ventricle. This is accomplished by a limited suboccipital craniectomy, cervical laminectomies encompassing the extent of the cerebellar herniation, opening and stenting of the foramen of Magendie, and duroplasty. The Chiari II malformation that becomes symptomatic in infancy is the leading cause of death in children with myelomeningocele. Repetitive aspiration and wheezing are particularly worrisome symptoms. Less severe symptoms frequently stabilize by 1 year of age. Older children with Chiari II malformation do more favorably with cervical decompression. Results of Chiari II decompression have been good, with improvement reported in 60% to 80% of patients.[12]

Chiari I Malformation

The Chiari I malformation usually presents in a more delayed fashion than the Chiari II malformation, commonly later in the first decade or even into adulthood. Symptoms of Chiari I malformation include headache (often induced by coughing), upper extremity numbness and loss of pain and temperature sensation, lower extremity spasticity, and eventually lower cranial nerve dysfunction. MRI scan confirms the diagnosis and the extent of any associated hydromyelia. Surgery consists of a suboccipital craniectomy, cervical laminectomy (usually involving C1), stent placement into the fourth ventricle, and duroplasty. This procedure restores normal CSF flow dynamics across the craniocervical junction and usually results in resolution of the hydromyelia (Fig. 98-15). Patients presenting with more mild symptoms do well, with 70% to 80% having improvement. Patients with lower cranial nerve dysfunction do not do as well, with only 35% to 65% having significant improvement from surgery.[12]

Arachnoid Cyst

The presentation of intracranial arachnoid cysts is dependent on the age of the patient. Infants commonly present with increased head circumference, full fontanelle, and signs of increased intracranial pressure. Older children may present with headache, seizures, or focal neurologic deficits. The signs and symptoms also vary with the site of the arachnoid cyst: posterior fossa cysts commonly present with obstructive hydrocephalus; sylvian fissure cysts present with seizures or hemiparesis; and suprasellar cysts present with visual disturbances. Sudden deterioration may be seen, with development of obstructive hydrocephalus, sudden cyst rupture, or bleeding into the cyst, either spontaneous or traumatic. Computed tomography (CT) or MRI can provide the diagnosis; MRI is preferred, owing to multiplanar imaging. Therapy of symptomatic arachnoid cysts is controversial, with some authors recommending simple shunting of the cyst and other recommending cyst fenestration or excision.[13]

HYDROCEPHALUS

Hydrocephalus is a condition in which there is a discrepancy between the rate of formation and absorption of CSF, causing the cerebral ventricles to dilate.[14] CSF is normally formed from the choroid plexus in the lateral third and fourth ventricles. CSF flows through the ventricular system; exits the fourth ventricle

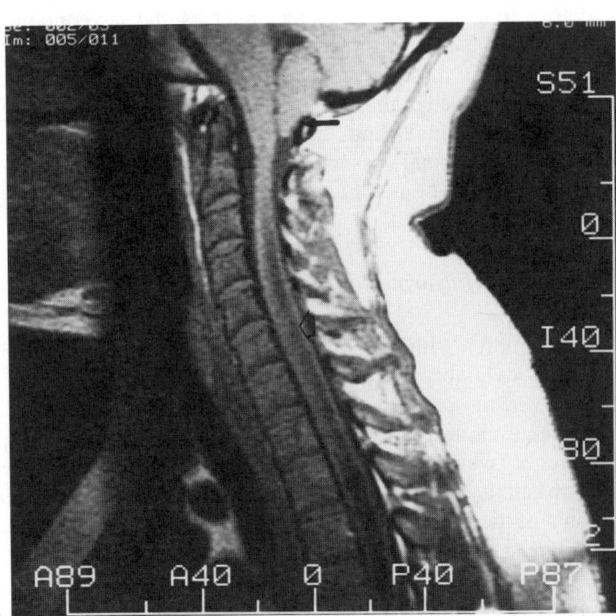
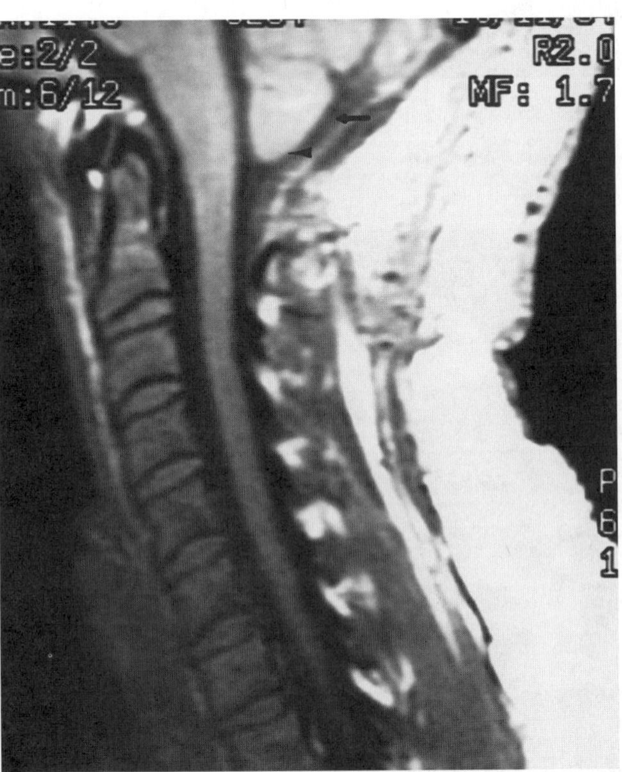

FIG. 98-15. MR images of Chiari I malformation. (*A*) Preoperative image shows tonsillar herniation (*solid arrow*) and large syrinx (*open arrow*). (*B*) Postoperative image shows good decompression of the foramen magnum (*arrow*) and resolution of the syrinx. The tonsil has a more rounded configuration (*arrowhead*).

TABLE 98-3. *Classification of hydrocephalus*

NONCOMMUNICATING

CONGENITAL
Aqueductal obstruction
Atresia of foramen of Monro
Arnold-Chiari malformation
Dandy-Walker malformation
Neoplasms
Benign cysts
Vein of Galen aneurysm

INFLAMMATORY
Infectious ventriculitis
Intraventricular hemorrhage

NEOPLASTIC

COMMUNICATING

CONGENITAL
Dandy-Walker malformation
Arnold-Chiari malformation
Incompetent arachnoid villi
Encephalocele
Benign cysts

INFLAMMATORY
Infectious meningitis
Subarachnoid hemorrhage

NEOPLASTIC

through the foramina of Magendie and Luschka; circulates around the base of the brain, cerebral hemispheres, and spinal cord; and is reabsorbed into the bloodstream through arachnoid villi located primarily along the superior sagittal sinus. Blockade of CSF flow results in noncommunicating hydrocephalus. A defect in the absorptive process leads to communicating hydrocephalus. A summary of conditions that can cause hydrocephalus is listed in Table 98-3. Note that some conditions can cause both noncommunicating and communicating hydrocephalus.

Because the open sutures of the infant skull allow cranial expansion, which helps to dissipate increased intracranial pressure, the clinical presentation of hydrocephalus is dependent on the age of the patient. The young infant with hydrocephalus typically presents with increased head circumference and a full, bulging fontanelle. Normal head growth charts are shown in Figure 98-16. The head circumference should be measured and plotted on the chart with each visit, and deviations from the normal curve should be noted immediately. The fontanelle should be inspected with the patient in the upright position and quiet. Other symptoms of hydrocephalus in the young infant include poor feeding, vomiting, and lethargy. Physical signs also may include cranial sutural diastasis, prominence of scalp veins, and the "sun-setting sign," with a forced downward gaze due to compression of the midbrain tectal plate. Macrocephaly can have a variety of causes in infants, and imaging studies discussed later help distinguish them. Older children with fused sutures cannot dissipate increased intracranial pressure through cranial expansion and often have a more acute presentation of hydrocephalus. Severe headache, vomiting, and lethargy are common. Children with obstructive hydrocephalus secondary to a colloid cyst or tumor may require urgent intervention. Papilledema is commonly seen in patients with more chronic intracranial pressure elevation. The character of the headache is important because headaches from increased intracranial pressure

are characteristically worse at night or early in the morning, often waking the child from sleep, and are associated with vomiting. In these cases, cranial imaging studies should be done to rule out hydrocephalus before embarking on a gastrointestinal work-up. These symptoms may be seen before the development of other neurologic signs.

Evaluation

Radiologic imaging studies are essential in the diagnosis of hydrocephalus. The most commonly used is CT. CT allows rapid screening of the child with macrocephaly, serving to assess ventricular size, brain development, and other intracranial pathology, such as subdural hematomas. In addition, with the administration of contrast agents, intracranial tumors or vascular lesions may be better visualized. Multiple scans can be performed to assess progression of hydrocephalus or treatment efficacy. Ultrasonography is particularly useful in the young infant with an open fontanelle. Because the required equipment is portable, the test can be performed in the intensive care nursery, simplifying the care of the seriously ill infant. In addition, there is no radiation. Ultrasonography is limited in its ability to evaluate structural lesions, particularly in the posterior fossa, and extracerebral fluid collections. MRI has become more widely available during the past several years and provides some advantages over CT. The anatomic detail is superior to that of CT, particularly in the posterior fossa, where CT is limited by bone artifacts. In addition, the ability of MRI to provide imaging in axial, coronal, and sagittal planes allows for a better understanding of structural lesions. The aqueduct may be visualized directly, along with loculations within the ventricular system. Technologic advances have also allowed imaging of CSF flow, particularly through the aqueduct, and of the foramen magnum. Ventriculography and cisternography were used in the past to evaluate patients with suspected obstructive lesions or loculations, but MRI is gradually supplanting these techniques.

Examination of CSF by lumbar or ventricular puncture also provides useful information in the patient with hydrocephalus. An opening pressure is measured and the CSF examined for evidence of hemorrhage or infection before treatment with a shunt. In addition, in the shunted patient, a shunt tap can provide important information on shunt function or infection.

Neuropsychologic testing in the older child and developmental assessment in the younger child also provide useful information in the evaluation of hydrocephalus. Deterioration in performance on these tests can indicate progression of hydrocephalus or shunt malfunction.

Specific Hydrocephalus Syndromes

Congenital

Congenital hydrocephalus is associated with a variety of malformation syndromes discussed earlier. Children born with a myelomeningocele have an 85% incidence of hydrocephalus. Ventricular enlargement may not be present at birth but may develop after closure of the myelomeningocele. With elimination of this CSF reservoir, the ventricles subsequently dilate. This same mechanism is often seen in patients with occipital encephaloceles. Aqueductal stenosis may present in the new-

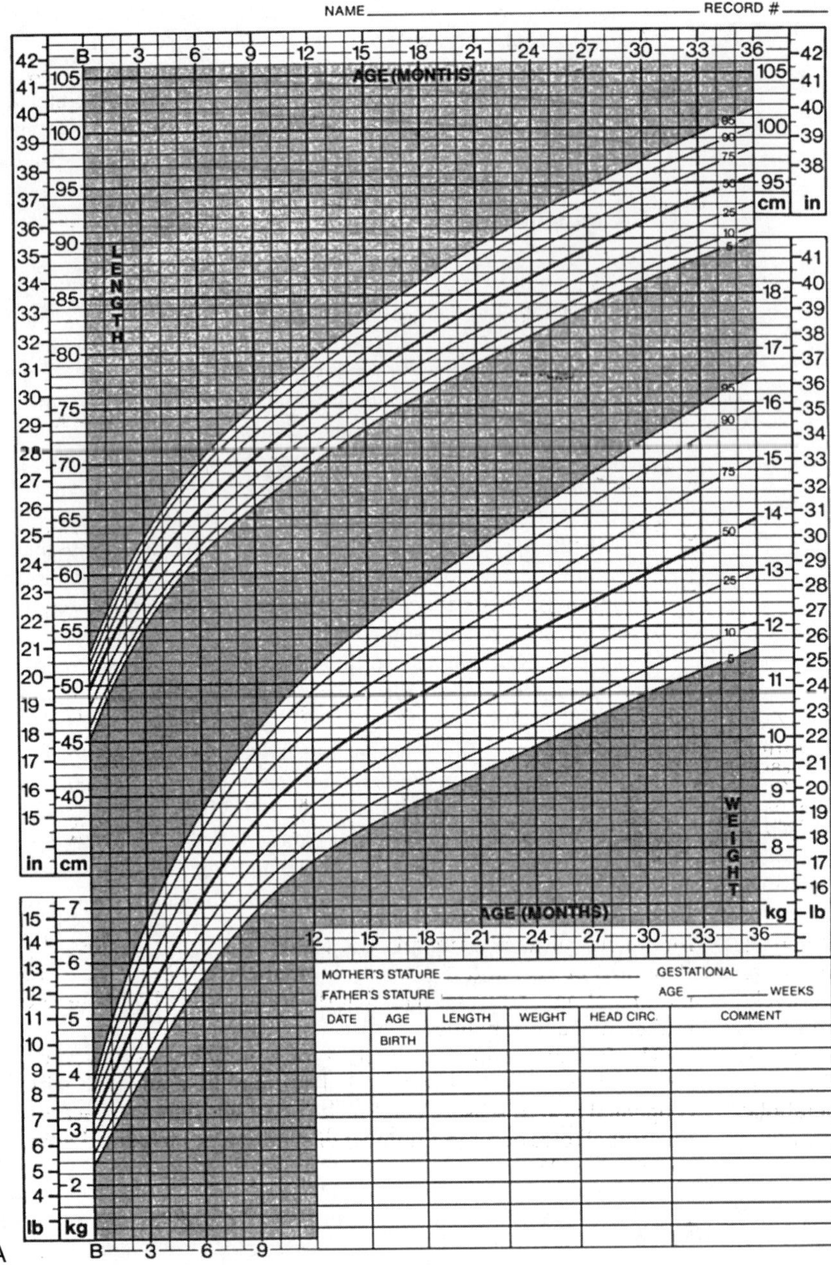

FIG. 98-16. Normal head growth charts for girls (*A*) and boys (*B*). (Courtesy of Ross Laboratories, Columbus, OH) *(continued)*

born or young infant but often presents at later ages as well. Dandy-Walker syndrome may also present at later ages but is most frequently seen early in infancy. Vein of Galen aneurysms may present with hydrocephalus and a cranial bruit. Dilation of ependymal veins and a great potential for hemorrhage account for the high complication rate seen in these patients.

Inflammatory

Posthemorrhagic hydrocephalus is most commonly seen in premature infants. A germinal matrix hemorrhage results in hydrocephalus, owing to obstruction of the ventricular system by clot, aseptic meningitis, and clogging of the arachnoid villi. In full-term infants and older children, hemorrhage can be caused by birth trauma, vascular malformation, tumor, or intracranial injury. Meningitis is also a common cause of hydrocephalus. In young infants, the most common organisms include and *Escherichia coli* and *Staphylococcus aureus.* In 3-month-old to 3-year-old children, the most common organisms include *Haemophilus influenzae, Streptococcus pneumoniae, Neisseria meningitides,* and *S aureus.* After 3 years of age, the most common organisms include *Meissena meningitides, S pneumoniae,* and *Streptococcus* sp. With postmeningitic hydrocephalus, ventricular loculations can be seen, complicating treatment of the resulting hydrocephalus.

Neoplasms

Tumors can cause obstructive hydrocephalus in a variety of locations. Most common is the fourth ventricular tumor. Cranio-

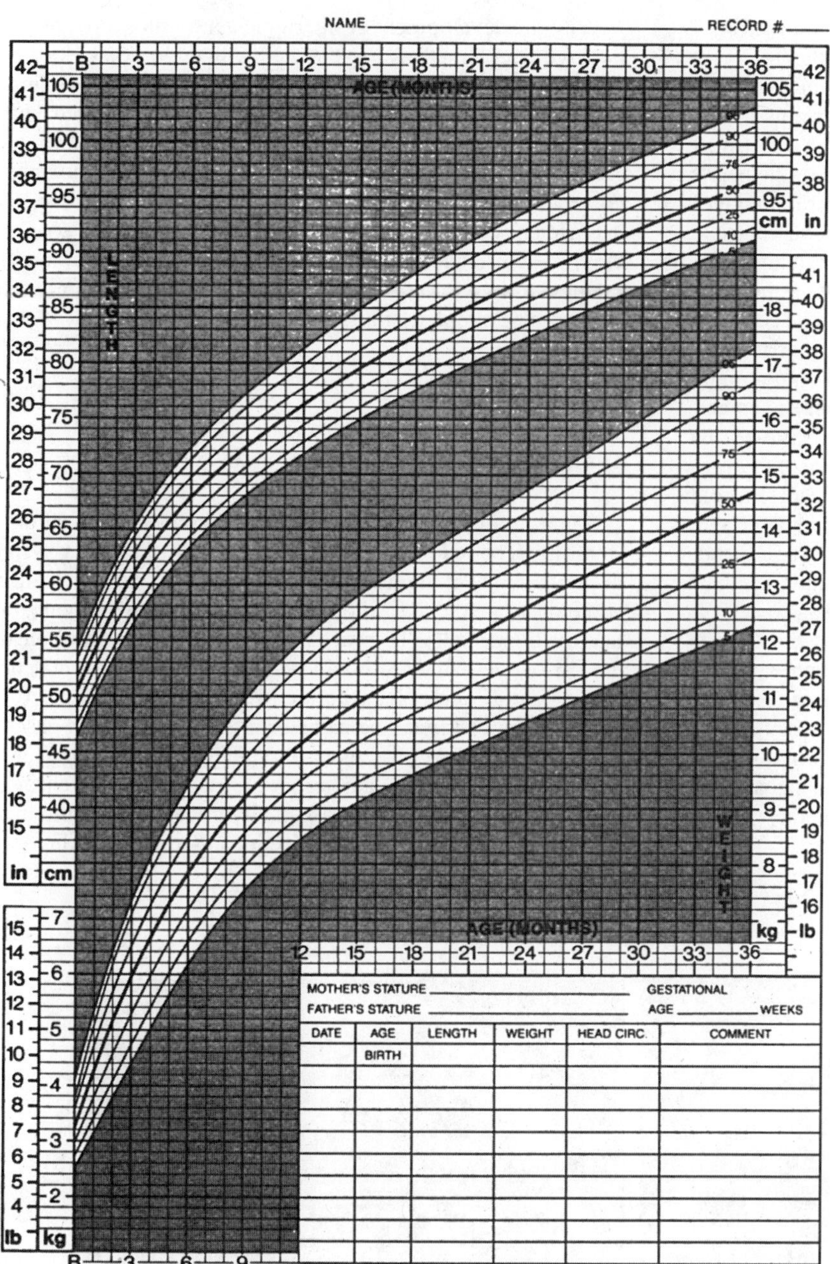

FIG. 98-16. *Continued.*

pharyngiomas can block flow at the level of the third ventricle. Choroid plexus tumors can oversecrete CSF in addition to producing obstruction.

External Hydrocephalus

One condition that must be distinguished from hydrocephalus is external hydrocephalus. This condition is characterized by macrocrania, with the head circumference crossing percentile lines and remaining elevated until 18 to 24 months of age. Development is generally normal, with the exception of poor head control, which can cause a delay in sitting. The fontanelle is normal. The CT scan demonstrates a normal to mildly dilated ventricular system, with pronounced extraaxial fluid spaces.

This external hydrocephalus is believed to be caused by immaturity of the CSF absorption system at the level of the arachnoid villi and resolves in virtually every case.

Treatment

The treatment of hydrocephalus is primarily surgical. Drugs, such as acetazolamide, which reduces CSF production, or mannitol and furosemide, which decrease brain extracellular fluid, may provide temporary relief of increased intracranial pressure from hydrocephalus. In addition, corticosteroids may decrease brain edema associated with some tumors or other lesions and thereby provide temporary relief of increased intracranial pressure. The long-term management of hydrocephalus, however, requires surgical intervention. The development of valve-regulated shunt systems provided the major advance in the treatment of hydrocephalus. A variety of shunt systems are available, each with its own advocates. The key feature of all systems is that the drainage of CSF from the ventricle to a distant site (most commonly the peritoneal cavity or the right atrium of the heart) is controlled by a valve mechanism to prevent overdrainage of CSF. The ventricular catheter is placed into the lateral ventricle from either a frontal or occipital approach. The remainder of the system is tunneled subcutaneously to either the abdomen for a peritoneal shunt or the neck for cannulation of the common facial or other vein to gain access to the right atrium for an atrial shunt. The goals of shunting are to normalize the intracranial pressure and to allow a reexpansion of the brain tissue to constitute a cortical mantle at least 3.5-cm thick to maximize the child's development (Fig. 98-17). Complete collapse of the ventricular system is not desired because this can lead to shunt malfunctions due to obstruction of the ventricular catheter and, with the elimination of the CSF volume buffer, chronic headaches. Patients with posthemorrhagic hydrocephalus are best managed initially with implantation of a subcutaneous reservoir system, which can be tapped intermittently, until the CSF is cleared of blood products that can obstruct the shunt system.

In patients with compartmentalized hydrocephalus, such as the Dandy-Walker syndrome, or with ventricular loculations, multiple ventricular catheters may be required to provide complete CSF drainage. These catheters are usually connected to a single valve system to equalize the pressures in the various compartments and to avoid dangerous brain shifts.

With the development of fiberoptic ventriculoscopy, obstructive hydrocephalus has been treated with endoscopic third ventriculostomy. This procedure involves creating an opening in the floor of the third ventricle into the subarachnoid space, thereby bypassing the obstruction to CSF flow. Reports have generally shown a 70% success rate in treating aqueductal stenosis without the need for a shunt. Failure usually is due to an insufficiency in the development of the subarachnoid spaces in these patients. These techniques also can be used to communicate the various compartments in loculated ventricles, allowing the use of a simpler, single ventricular catheter shunt system.

Complications

Shunting

Shunt malfunction is the most common complication of shunting. This can be due to obstruction of the shunt system, disconnection, or migration. The ventricular catheter can become obstructed due to choroid plexus, brain parenchyma, protein, or tumor cells. To prevent obstruction by choroid plexus, the tip of the catheter should be placed into the frontal horn of the lateral ventricle, anterior to the choroid plexus. Brain parenchyma obstructs the catheter most commonly in cases of suboptimal catheter placement. Protein plugs can occur at either the proximal or distal catheter and are commonly seen in patients shunted for posthemorrhagic hydrocephalus in the initial months after shunting. Disconnections can occur at any point

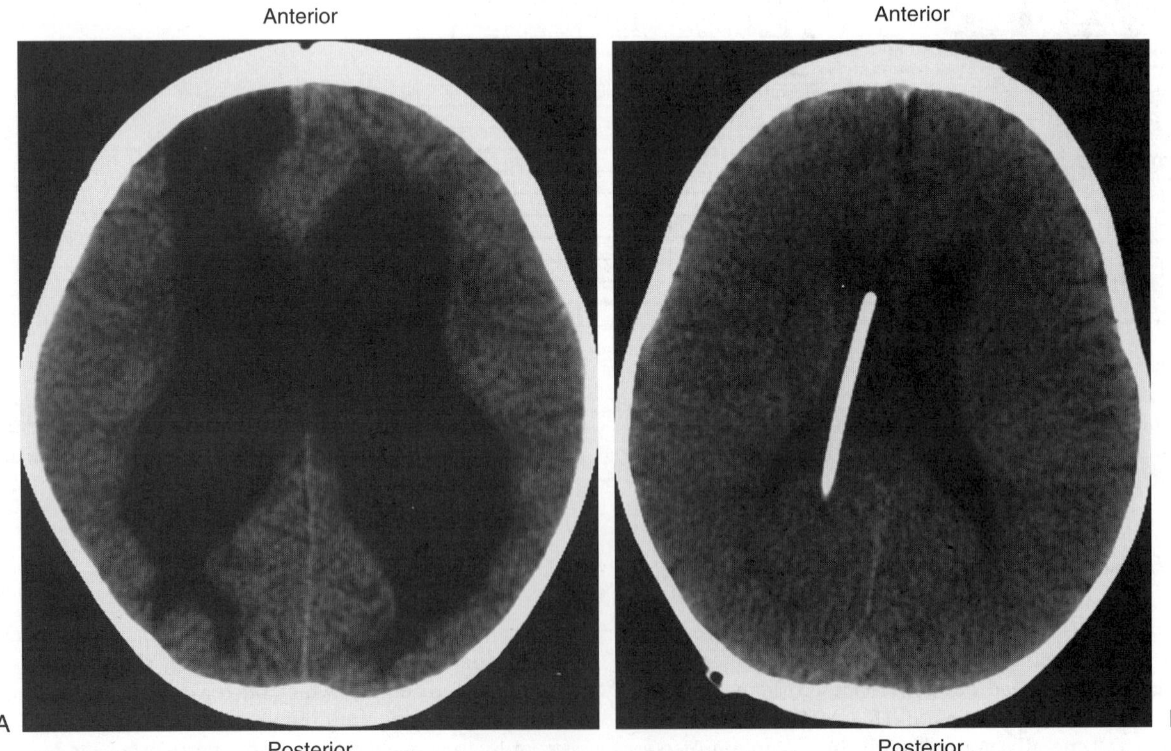

FIG. 98-17. Effects of shunt insertion. (*A*) Preoperative CT scan shows ventricular dilation of hydrocephalus. (*B*) Postoperative scan made 6 months after shunt insertion shows normalization of ventricular size. Shunt catheter is in right lateral ventricle with tip in frontal horn.

in the system but are most common at sites of connection and mobility. Disconnection can be confirmed with radiographic evaluation because the barium impregnated shunt tubing is visualized by plain radiographic studies.

Distal Catheter Malfunctions

Shunt malfunctions associated with the distal catheter depend on the site chosen for distal drainage. The peritoneal catheter is the most common, owing to the ease of access to the peritoneal cavity and the ability to place redundant tubing into the abdomen to allow for future growth of the child. A CSF-filled pseudocyst can form around the distal catheter, resulting in shunt malfunction and abdominal pain. A smaller cyst is more commonly associated with shunt infection, and the larger pseudocyst may be sterile. In addition, small bowel obstruction, abdominal viscus perforation by shunt tubing, and an acute abdomen may be complications of abdominal shunting.

Atrial shunts have their own associated complications. Although the atrial shunt is effective, it is more difficult to revise, and additional tubing cannot be inserted to allow for growth. In addition, pulmonary embolism, septicemia, shunt nephritis, cardiac arrhythmia, and pulmonary hypertension have been reported in patients with atrial shunts.

Shunt infection is the second most common complication of shunting, with a reported incidence of 2.6% to 38%. The most common pathogens in shunt infections are skin flora, especially *S aureus* and *S epidermitis.* Bacterial contamination occurs at the time of surgery or shunt tap, so that meticulous attention to sterile technique and skin preparation are essential to avoid shunt infection. The clinical presentation of these patients is often nonspecific, with low-grade fever, irritability, and shunt malfunction. Patients with atrial shunts can present with septic emboli. In younger patients, gram-negative enteric bacteria are also common, and this problem commonly occurs in an acutely ill patient. The diagnosis of shunt infection is made on shunt tap; lumbar puncture is positive in only half of cases. Shunt infection should be managed with removal of infected hardware, appropriate intravenous antibiotics, and placement of an external ventricular drain as needed. Once the CSF is cleared, a new shunt system can be installed. The morbidity of shunt infection is severe, with a single episode lowering the IQ by 10 to 30 points.

The slit ventricle syndrome is characterized by episodic headaches due to increased intracranial pressure in patients with small or slitlike ventricles. A variety of mechanisms have been proposed to account for this syndrome, including intermittent obstruction of the ventricular catheter, overdrainage of CSF, and decreased ventricular compliance. Medical therapy includes furosemide, acetazolamide, and steroids. Studies of antimigraine medications, including propranolol, dihydroergotamine, and cyproheptadine, have suggested that the slit ventricle syndrome may have at least an element of acquired migraine headache. Surgical options for slit ventricle syndrome include upgrading the resistance of the valve and possibly incorporating a siphon control device to eliminate overdrainage of CSF.

Subdural collections are another complication of overshunting. The thinned brain collapses away from the skull, resulting in disruption of bridging veins and subdural hematoma formation. Most of these patients do not have symptoms. Over time, with growth of the brain, these collections may resolve. In patients with symptoms, incorporation of a subdural catheter into the shunt system (distal to the valve) results in resolution of the subdural collections.

CRANIOSYNOSTOSIS

Craniosynostosis, or premature closure of the cranial sutures, is commonly seen in pediatric neurosurgery. Most cases are sporadic, but up to 10% are familial. Separation of the bones of the calvarium by the cranial sutures allows progressive enlargement of the skull to occur with growth of the brain. Brain weight doubles by 6 months of age and triples by 10 months. Brain growth is virtually complete by 2 years of age, and the cranial sutures are fused by 6 to 8 years of age. When one or more sutures close prematurely, there must be compensatory growth at the remaining open sutures, resulting in recognizable patterns of deformity. When skull growth cannot keep pace with brain growth, increased intracranial pressure results, with the potential for cognitive impairment. Sagittal synostosis results in scaphocephaly; coronal synostosis results in plagiocephaly if unilateral and brachycephaly if bilateral; metopic synostosis results in trigonocephaly; and multiple suture stenosis results in cloverleaf deformity (Kleeblattschädel). Multiple causes may be involved in craniosynostosis. Metabolic conditions affecting bone formation, intrauterine deformation, genetic abnormalities, and syndromic causes, such as Crouzon or Apert syndrome, have all been invoked in cases of craniosynostosis.[15]

Evaluation

The skull deformities that result from closure of the various sutures are recognizable to the trained clinician. The abnormality is usually present at birth, and with time, it may become more severe. Ridges along the fused sutures are obvious to palpation. Skull radiographs confirm the diagnosis of craniosynostosis and may show indentations of the inner table as evidence of increased intracranial pressure. CT scan also demonstrates sutural fusion and allows examination of the underlying brain. Three-dimensional reconstruction of CT images may also facilitate surgical planning. The therapy of craniosynostosis varies with the involved suture.

Scaphocephaly (Sagittal Synostosis)

Isolated sagittal synostosis is by far the most common form of craniosynostosis and is most commonly sporadic. The scaphocephalic appearance is obvious at birth along with compensatory frontal bossing. A bewildering variety of surgical approaches to scaphocephaly have been devised, ranging from suturectomy to complete calvarial reconstructions. In general, the simpler procedures can be effective if performed as early as 2 to 3 months of age because removal of the skull growth constraint allows further brain growth to reshape the calvarium, resulting in excellent cosmetic results. In older children, more complex procedures are often necessary, owing to the more limited remaining brain growth. Figure 98-18 shows a typical child with scaphocephaly before and after surgical correction.

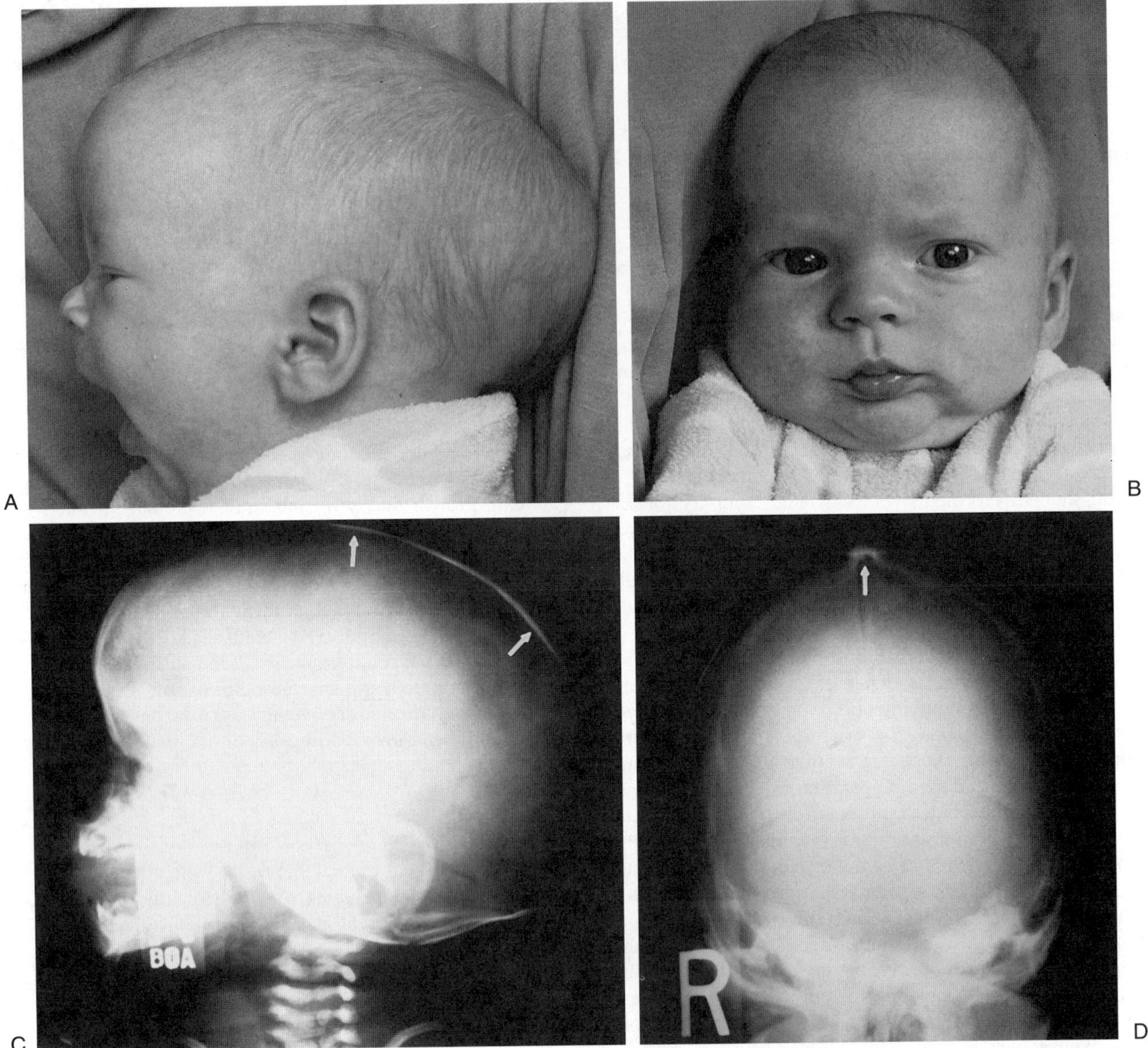

FIG. 98-18. Scaphocephaly. (*A*) Preoperative lateral photograph of a patient with scaphocephaly shows the elongated skull configuration with frontal prominence. (*B*) Preoperative frontal photograph of a patient with scaphocephaly illustrates frontal bossing. (*C*) Preoperative lateral skull radiograph of the same patient shows sclerotic sagittal suture (*arrows*). (*D*) Preoperative anteroposterior skull radiograph shows sclerotic sagittal suture (*arrow*). *(continued)*

Coronal Synostosis

Unilateral Coronal Synostosis

The characteristic deformity of unilateral coronal synostosis is ipsilateral frontal bone and orbital flattening, with ridging of the affected suture (Fig. 98-19*A* and *B*). The contralateral frontal region frequently displays compensatory bossing. Skull radiographs demonstrate the characteristic harlequin orbit deformity on the affected side. Surgery consists of *bilateral* frontal craniotomy and frontal bone reconstruction, with supraorbital bar advancement as well.[16] If only a unilateral procedure is performed, the cosmetic result immediately after surgery may be acceptable, but further growth may be asymmetric, producing an unacceptable result.

Bilateral Coronal Synostosis

Bilateral coronal synostosis is frequently seen as part of a syndrome complex, such as Apert or Crouzon syndrome. There may be significant involvement of the facial bones, and surgical correction may be much more complex than for unilateral coronal synostosis. There is a characteristic brachycephalic appearance, with bitemporal widening, ocular protrusion, and towering

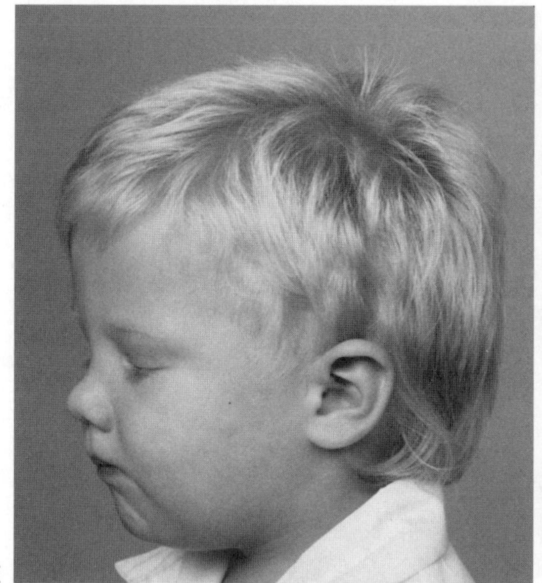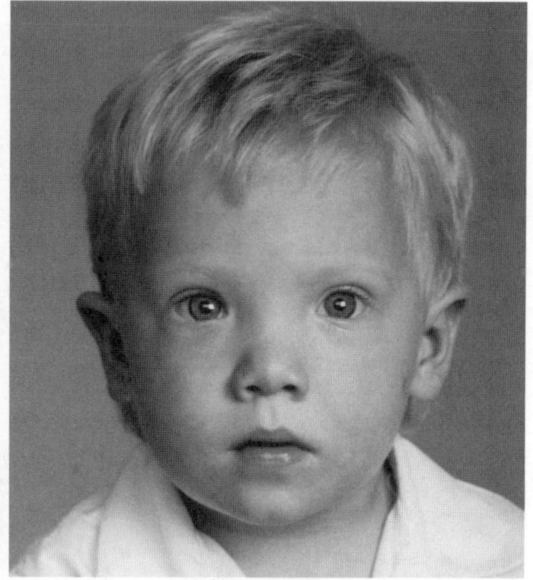

FIG. 98-18. *Continued.* (*E* and *F*) Postoperative photographs of the same patient taken 6 months after extended strip craniectomy for scaphocephaly reveal normalization of head shape, with resolution of frontal bossing.

of the skull (see Fig. 98-19*C* and *D*). The surgical procedure involves bilateral frontal craniotomy and frontal bone reconstruction along with supraorbital bar advancement. Midface retrusion should be treated in a separate facial procedure.

Metopic Synostosis

The characteristic deformity of metopic synostosis is trigonocephaly, with a pointed forehead and a triangular shape to the skull (Fig. 98-20). The surgical procedure involves bilateral frontal craniotomy, with complete reconstruction of the frontal bone and bilateral lateral canthal advances.

Lambdoid Synostosis

The characteristic deformity of lambdoid synostosis is occipital flattening, which is most frequently unilateral. In addition, protrusion of the ipsilateral frontal bone and forward displacement of the ear and petrous bone may be seen. It is important to distinguish true lambdoid synostosis from positional molding, the most common cause of occipital flattening. In patients with positional deformities, a history of lying on one side for prolonged periods and a progressive flattening help make the diagnosis. Even in patients with positional molding, however, there may be an acquired lambdoid synostosis, which can be confirmed with skull radiographs. In young patients with lambdoid synostosis, suturectomy with wide removal of bone relieves the growth constraint on the skull and allows further brain growth to round out the skull.

Multiple Suture Synostoses

When multiple cranial sutures are fused prematurely, increased intracranial pressure must be anticipated, and restora-

tion of the normal cranial vault/brain mass ratio is crucial if blindness and cognitive dysfunction are to be avoided. Treatment consists of total calvarial remodeling and may require multiple operative procedures.

TUMORS

Primary tumors of the CNS are the most common solid neoplasms in children (Table 98-4). Major technologic advances in diagnostic imaging, anesthetic techniques, surgical techniques, radiotherapy, and chemotherapy have brought about improved survival in children with brain tumors, but many problems remain. Often, difficulties in treatment relate more to location within the brain limiting surgical resection, or radiation dosage (due to toxicity to neighboring vital structures), than to intrinsic biologic malignancy of a given tumor. Intracranial tumors can be categorized by their location with respect to the tentorium cerebelli, with supratentorial and infratentorial tumors occurring with nearly equal frequency in children.

Infratentorial Tumors

Cerebellar Astrocytoma

Cerebellar astrocytomas are the most benign brain tumors of childhood in both histology and prognosis.[17] With surgical resection of tumors not invading the brain stem, the 25-year tumor-free survival rate is about 90 percent. Cerebellar astrocytomas are the most common pediatric tumors, accounting for up to 28% of pediatric brain tumors and one third of all posterior fossa tumors. The clinical presentation is typically insidious, with morning headache frequently associated with vomiting. Tumor growth may produce obstructive hydrocephalus, and

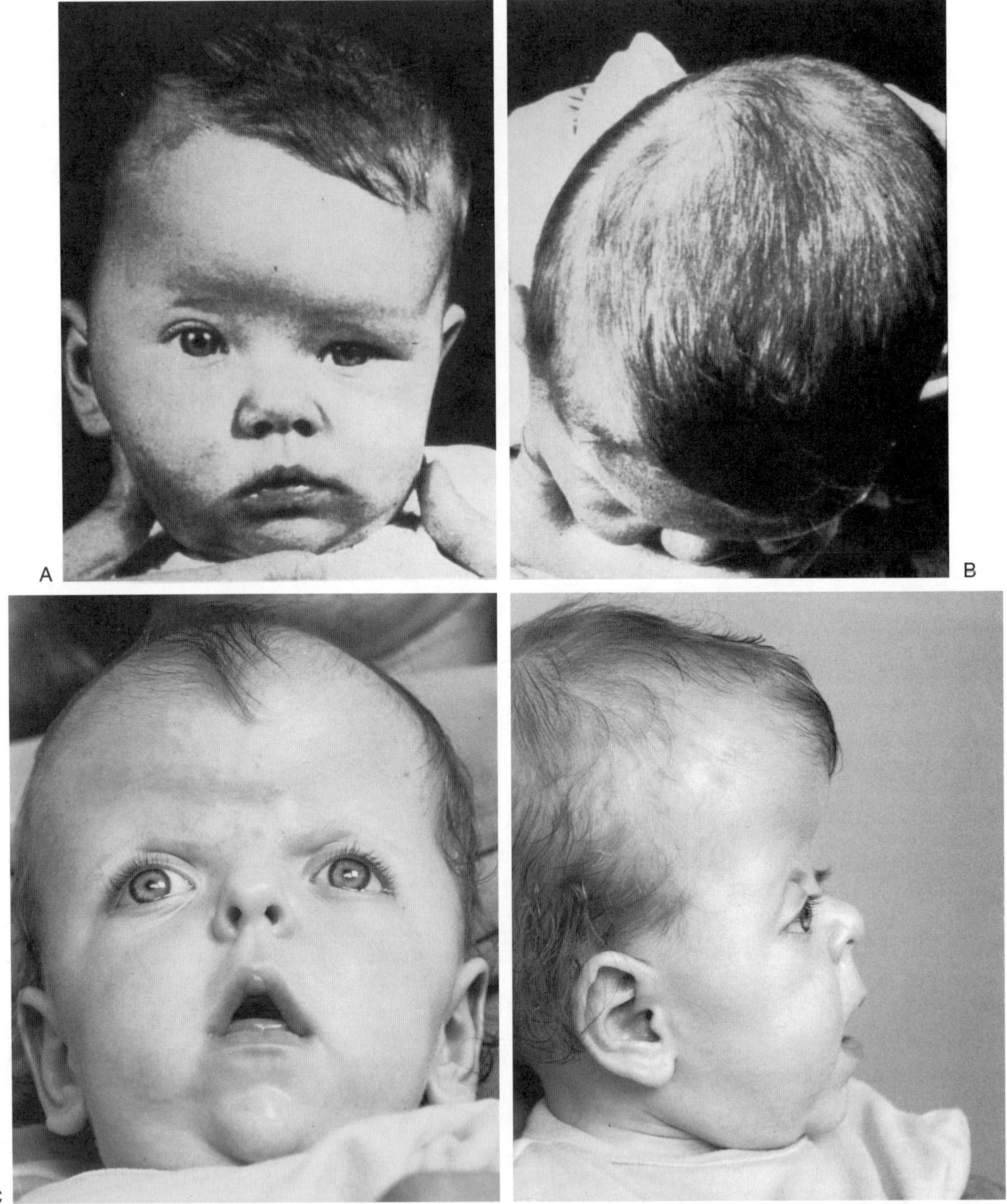

FIG. 98-19. Coronal synostosis. (*A* and *B*). Unilateral. The right side of the forehead is flattened, and the left side is prominent. (*C* and *D*) Bilateral. There is bilateral canthal retrusion and compensatory prominence of upper forehead in this patient, who has Apert syndrome.

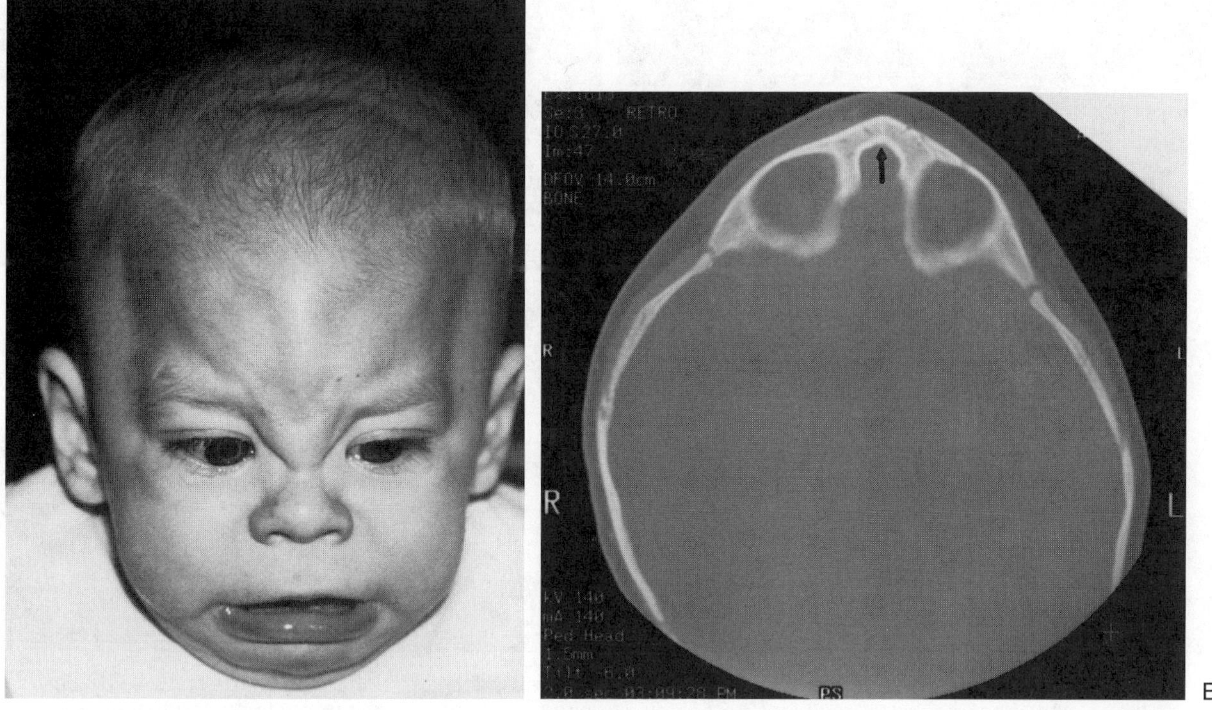

FIG. 98-20. Trigonocephaly. (*A*) The forehead is pointed and towering. (*B*) Axial CT scan reveals fused metopic suture (*arrow*).

TABLE 98-4. *Summary of childhood brain tumors*

Tumor	Incidence*	Treatment	Outcome
POSTERIOR FOSSA			
Medulloblastoma	20%	Surgery, craniospinal irradiation, and chemotherapy for high-risk patients	More than 50% 10-y survival rate with improved chemotherapy
Cerebellar astrocytoma	10%–20%	Surgery alone	95% 25-y survival rate
Brain-stem glioma	10%–20%	Radiotherapy and chemotherapy. No role for surgery in diffuse pontine glioma	Less than 30% 5-y survival rate
Ependymoma	10%	Surgery and radiotherapy	Prognosis depends on extent of surgical resection; much improved if gross total resection can be obtained
SUPRATENTORIAL TUMORS			
Astrocytomas	30%	Surgery, followed by radiotherapy or chemotherapy for more malignant tumors. Observation for benign lesions.	Varies by histology; with benign tumors, prognosis can be excellent
Choroid plexus papilloma	1%–3%	Surgery; radiotherapy and/or chemotherapy reserved for carcinomas	Nearly 100% 5-y survival rate for papilloma; only 50% 5-y survival rate for carcinoma
Hypothalamic or optic pathways glioma	3%	Surgery for biopsy, debulking, followed by radiotherapy or chemotherapy	80%–95% 5-y survival rate
Craniopharyngioma	6%–8%	Surgery and radiotherapy	90% 5-y survival rate
Pineal region tumors	3%–8%	Surgery, radiotherapy, and chemotherapy, depending on histology. Germinoma especially radiosensitive	Varies with histology; most favorable for germinoma with 5-y survival of 70%; malignant histologies much worse

* Incidence is indicated as percentage of total childhood brain tumors.

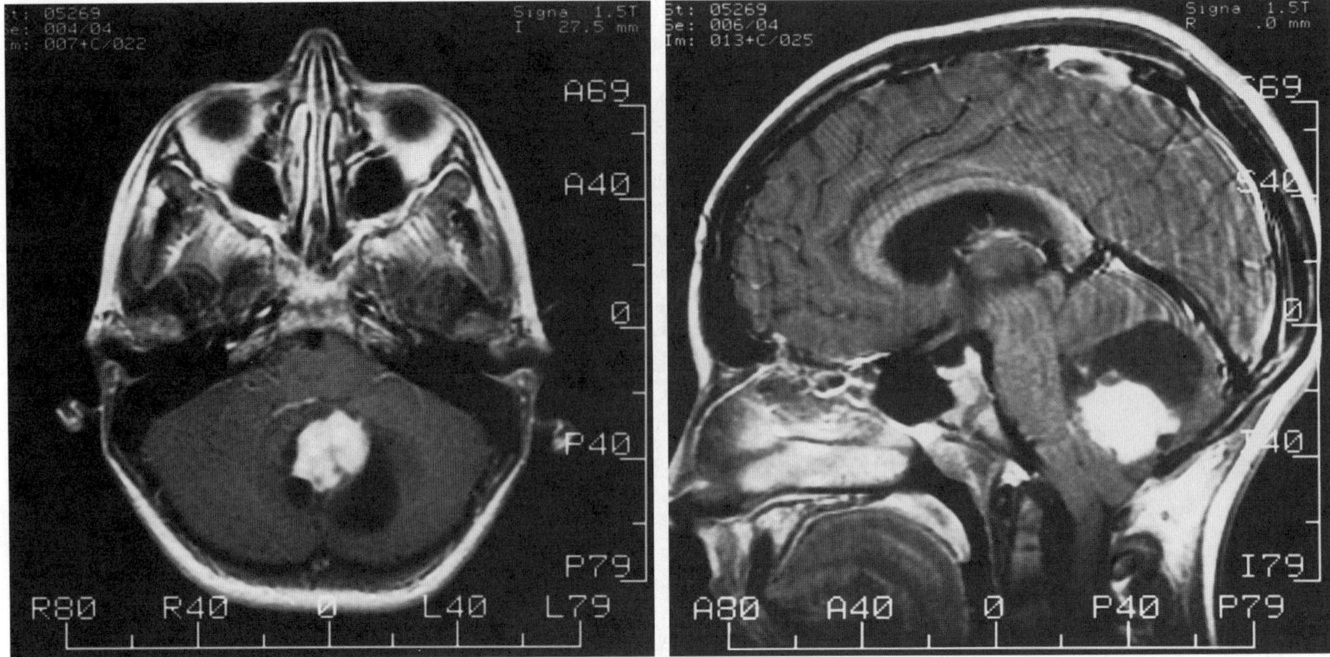

FIG. 98-21. MR images of cerebellar astrocytoma. (*A*) Axial gadolinium-enhanced image shows a cystic lesion with enhancing mural nodule. (*B*) Sagittal image reveals relation of the tumor to the fourth ventricle and brain stem.

papilledema may be seen. Ataxia may be seen at presentation and is a clue to tumor location; tumors in the cerebellar hemisphere typically cause peripheral ataxia, and tumors in the cerebellar vermis cause truncal ataxia. An increase in head circumference may be seen in younger patients. Imaging studies with CT or MRI may provide the diagnosis, most commonly showing a cystic lesion with an enhancing mural nodule (Fig. 98-21). Vermian tumors may be solid. Treatment is surgical, with a goal of gross total tumor removal using a suboccipital craniotomy. Hydrocephalus can be managed perioperatively with an external ventricular drain. If hydrocephalus fails to resolve with tumor removal, a permanent shunt may be required. Perioperative corticosteroids are useful to prevent peritumoral swelling and to minimize postoperative edema. If total tumor resection is achieved, no further therapy is indicated because these tumors recur in only 2.5% of patients. Subtotal resection may also be compatible with long-term survival. If further resection is not feasible, radiotherapy is indicated. Malignant recurrence is extremely rare.

Medulloblastoma

Medulloblastomas are most commonly found in the fourth ventricle, arising within the cerebellar vermis. One characteristic of medulloblastoma is spread in the CSF pathways to the subarachnoid space in the cranial and spinal compartments. This may be present at the time of initial diagnosis or may occur later. Children with medulloblastoma typically present with vomiting, and lethargy from associated hydrocephalus. Because of the midline location of these tumors, ataxia, if present, is of truncal nature. Nystagmus may also be present. The duration of symptoms before diagnosis is typically

6 to 7 weeks, which is much shorter than for cerebellar astrocytomas. This reflects the more rapid growth rate of medulloblastomas. If diffuse subarachnoid spread is present, the child may present with meningeal signs or spinal cord or cauda equina compression. Imaging with either CT or MRI demonstrates a tumor within the fourth ventricle, which enhances brightly with contrast agents. MRI is preferred because the relation to the brain stem can be more precisely defined, and subarachnoid spread of tumor is easily detected (Fig. 98-22). Patients are managed with corticosteroids and perioperative external ventricular drainage. Suboccipital craniotomy is then performed with the goal of total tumor excision. If tumor is invading the brain stem, total excision cannot be achieved, and the tumor is thinned down as close as possible to the level of the brain stem. Postoperatively, the external ventricular drain is removed after progressive elevation of the drainage pressure. Patients who are unable to tolerate decreasing CSF drainage undergo shunt placement. Staging work-up includes postoperative cranial MRI to assess completeness of resection, spinal MRI if not performed preoperatively, CSF cytology, and bone marrow biopsy. Chang and colleagues[18] developed a staging system for patients with medulloblastoma based on tumor size, spread outside the fourth ventricle and throughout the neuraxis, and age. Good-risk patients are those with small tumors located within the fourth ventricle. With gross total resections and age greater than 4 years, these patients have a 60% to 70% 5-year survival rate. Poor-risk patients have disseminated disease, larger tumors with subtotal resections, and are younger than 4 years of age. These patients have only a 36% 5-year survival rate. Postoperative therapy in patients older than 3 years includes radiotherapy to the entire neuraxis and chemotherapy. Children younger than 3 years are treated with chemotherapy alone.

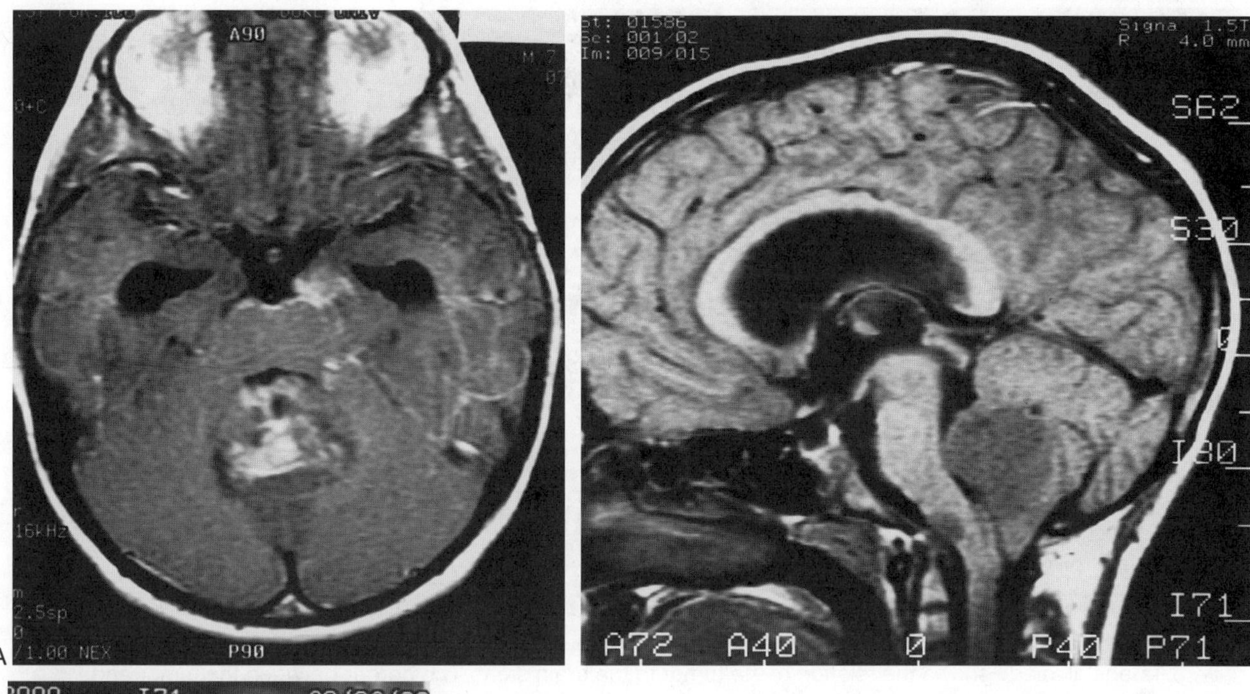

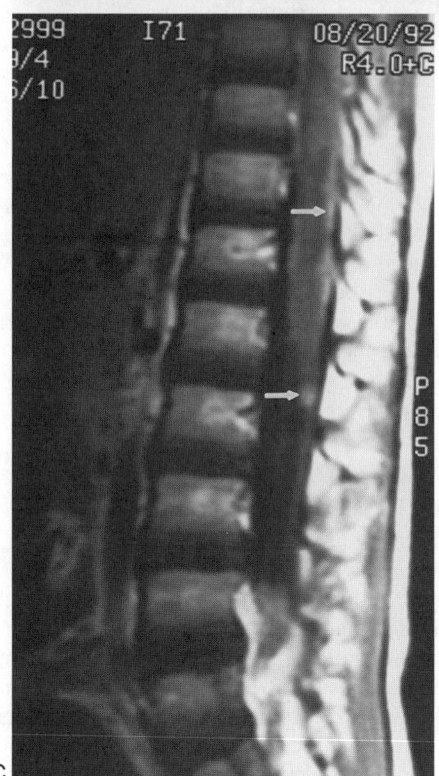

FIG. 98-22. MR images of medulloblastoma. (*A*) Axial image with gadolinium shows the fourth ventricular tumor. (*B*) Sagittal image shows the relation of the tumor to the fourth ventricle and brain stem. (*C*) Spinal image reveals enhancement along the length of the spinal cord, indicating leptomeningeal spread of tumor (*arrows*).

Ependymoma

Ependymomas occur in a variety of locations in children, but the most common location is within the posterior fossa. Presenting symptoms are similar to those described earlier for cerebellar astrocytomas and medulloblastomas, and are most commonly related to associated hydrocephalus due to obstruction of the fourth ventricle. Ependymomas can also extend through the fourth ventricular outlet foramina, into the cerebellopontine angle, and through the foramen magnum. Ependymomas frequently adhere to or invade through the floor of the fourth ventricle. Imaging studies demonstrate a fourth ventricular mass with a less uniform appearance than medulloblastoma. MRI is superior to CT, especially in its ability to provide sagittal imaging to demonstrate the tumor–brain stem interface. Contrast enhancement may be heterogeneous, and cysts may be

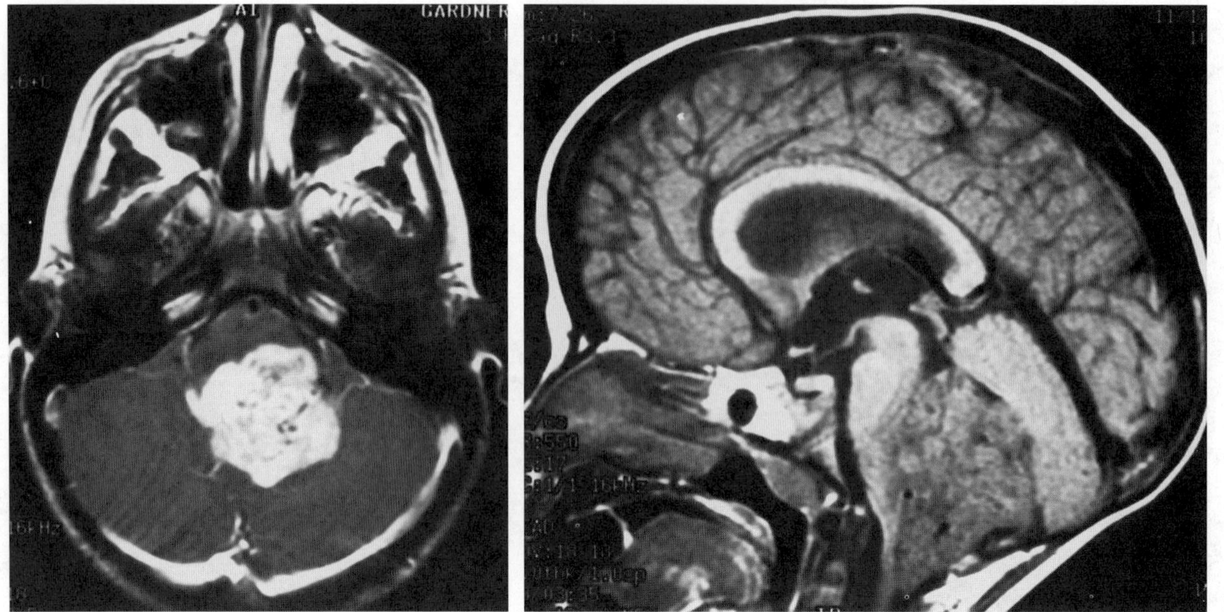

FIG. 98-23. MR images of ependymoma. (*A*) Axial image shows the tumor filling the fourth ventricle. (*B*) Sagittal image shows the relation of the tumor to the brain stem. The border between the tumor and the brain stem is indistinct in this patient. At surgery, the tumor was found to be grossly invasive into the brain stem.

present (Fig. 98-23). Management is as described for medulloblastoma, but great care must be taken not to injure the brain stem because tumor adhesion and invasion of the brain stem are common. If possible, gross total resection should be undertaken. Postoperatively, external ventricular drainage is managed as described earlier. Postoperative cranial and spinal MRI studies are obtained. Radiotherapy to the tumor bed is administered in patients older than 3 years of age. Younger patients are treated with chemotherapy. Extent of resection is the single most important prognostic factor, with patients who have gross total resection faring much better than patients who have subtotal resections.

Brain-Stem Glioma

Intrinsic tumors of the brain stem are common in children, accounting for 10% to 20% of CNS tumors. Modern imaging methods have demonstrated that brain-stem gliomas are a heterogeneous group, with a wide range of clinical features and prognoses.

The classic brain-stem glioma is the diffuse pontine glioma. These tumors typically present with a rapid clinical evolution of symptoms, including gait instability and multiple cranial nerve palsies, most commonly involving cranial nerves VI, VII, IX, and X. CT or MRI demonstrates an expanded pons. MRI characteristically reveals a much more extensive neoplasm because the T2-weighted signal abnormality, which extends far beyond the region of contrast enhancement, has been shown to represent the true extent of tumor (Fig. 98-24). These tumors are invariably highly malignant glioblastoma multiforme, and surgical intervention is not indicated.[19] Treatment is radiotherapy, chemotherapy, or both, but the prognosis remains dismal.

Focal brain-stem tumors are characterized by a clinical presentation that depends on tumor location and a focal lesion seen on MRI. These tumors are typically lower grade than the diffuse tumors and may be amenable to surgical resection.[19] Cystic tumors may be analogous to cerebellar astrocytomas. A subtype of focal tumor is the dorsally exophytic tumor, which extends into the fourth ventricle and can present in the same way as medulloblastoma (described earlier). Surgical resection of the exophytic portion of these low-grade tumors offers a distinct survival advantage for these patients.

Supratentorial Tumors

Tumors of the Cerebral Hemispheres

Tumors of the cerebral hemispheres account for 10% to 20% of childhood brain tumors. Most of these tumors are low grade, particularly pilocytic and fibrillary astrocytomas, oligodendrogliomas, ependymomas, and gangliogliomas. About 20% of supratentorial tumors are malignant, particularly anaplastic astrocytomas and glioblastoma multiforme. The malignant tumors predominate in the first 2 years of life, with a high incidence of teratomas, primitive neuroectodermal tumors, and choroid plexus tumors. Supratentorial tumors may be associated with phakomatoses. Tuberous sclerosis is associated with subependymal giant cell astrocytomas, while neurofibromatosis is associated with optic pathway gliomas, hemispheric astrocytomas and hamartomas, and meningiomas. The initial treatment of all of these tumors is surgical resection, with the intent of achieving gross total resection.

Astrocytoma

The signs and symptoms of supratentorial astrocytic tumors are dependent on tumor location and histologic grade, with more

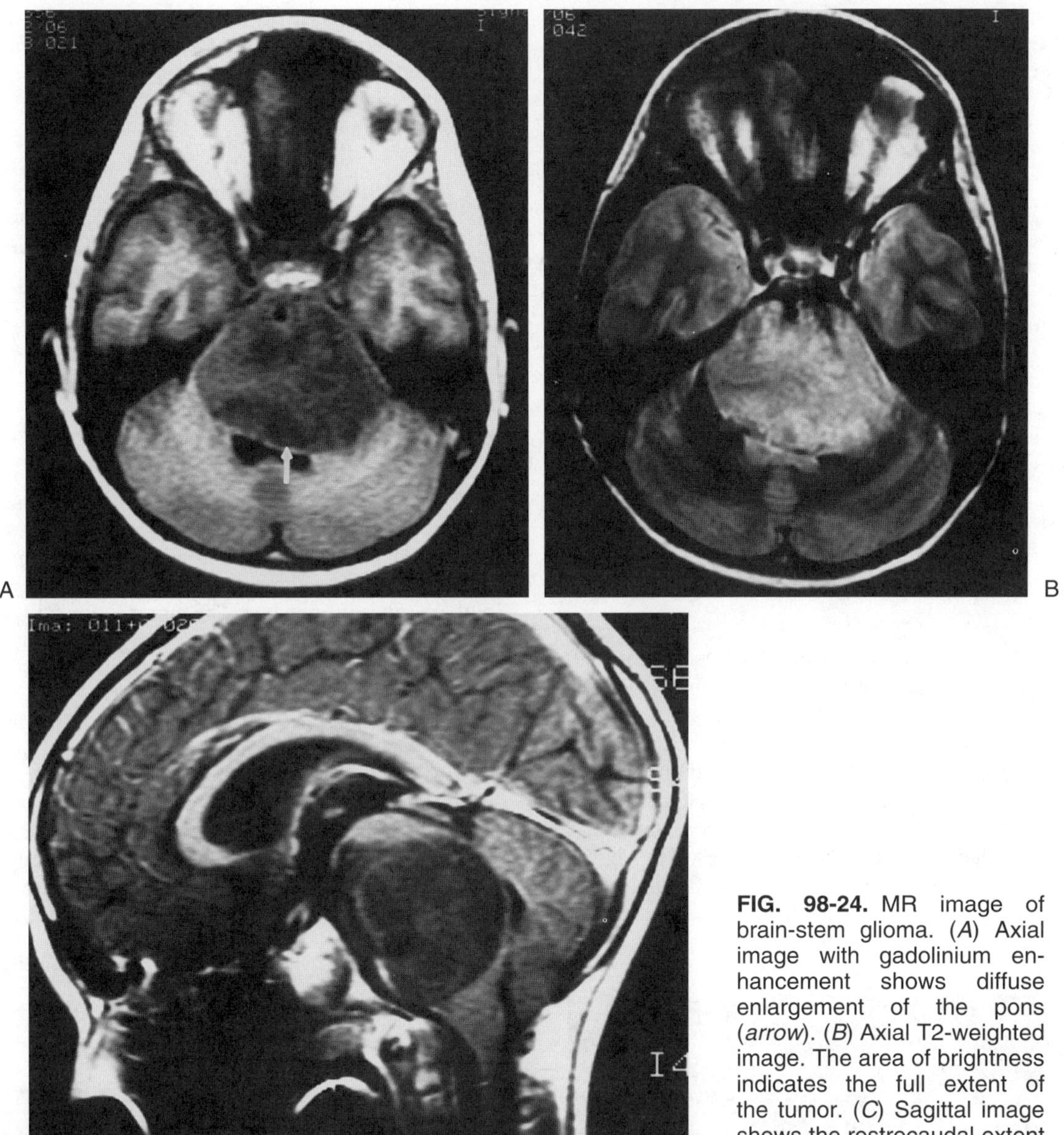

FIG. 98-24. MR image of brain-stem glioma. (*A*) Axial image with gadolinium enhancement shows diffuse enlargement of the pons (*arrow*). (*B*) Axial T2-weighted image. The area of brightness indicates the full extent of the tumor. (*C*) Sagittal image shows the rostrocaudal extent of tumor.

malignant tumors having a shorter symptom duration. Focal signs localize a tumor. Seizures are present in about half of patients. CT or MRI provides the diagnosis. Surgical resection should be performed to the extent possible. Radiotherapy is reserved for high-grade tumors and for low-grade tumor recurrence. Chemotherapy can significantly improve survival rates of children with malignant astrocytomas.

Ependymoma

Supratentorial ependymomas arise within the parenchyma of the cerebral hemisphere, adjacent to the ventricles, in contrast to the fourth ventricular ependymomas, which occur within the fourth ventricle. Macrocysts occur in half of cases. Presentation is similar to the astrocytomas described earlier. The goal of surgery is gross total removal, which provides the best long-term survival, approaching an 85% 5-year survival rate. Postop-

erative radiotherapy is given to the tumor bed, or to the entire neuraxis in the case of anaplastic ependymoma.

Oligodendroglioma

Oligodendrogliomas are rare in children. These tumors are most commonly found in the frontal lobe and present with seizures. Calcification is commonly seen on CT scan. Radical surgical excision is the most effective therapy for these tumors; radiotherapy is of some use in subtotally resected tumors. Chemotherapy may also be of benefit, particularly in anaplastic tumors.

Ganglioglioma

Gangliogliomas are composed of neoplastic ganglion cells and astrocytes. They most commonly occur in the mesial temporal lobe and present with seizures. CT or MRI demonstrates a cystic-appearing lesion. Gross total resection is curative, with long-term disease-free survival rates of 75% to 90%.

Primitive Neuroectodermal Tumors

Primitive neuroectodermal tumor of the cerebral hemisphere is an uncommon tumor that is histologically similar to medulloblastoma, with small, undifferentiated tumor cells. Symptom progression is rapid, with focal signs and signs of increased intracranial pressure. MRI reveals a relatively well-demarcated lesion (Fig. 98-25), which may contain calcifications and cysts. Radical surgical resection should be followed by craniospinal radiation and chemotherapy, as for poor-risk medulloblastoma. Children younger than 3 years are treated with chemotherapy alone. Prognosis is still poor, with 5-year survival rates of about 30% in most series. Studies of hyperfractionated radiotherapy and chemotherapy offer somewhat more encouraging results.

Choroid Plexus Tumors

Choroid plexus tumors occur within the cerebral ventricles, most commonly the lateral ventricles in children, and present with hydrocephalus. The choroid plexus papilloma resembles normal choroid plexus and is typically found in the trigone of the lateral ventricle. The choroid plexus carcinoma is more variegated in appearance. These tumors are vascular, and prevention of intraoperative hemorrhage is of utmost importance in children with relatively small blood volumes. The choroid plexus papilloma is amenable to gross total resection, but the carcinoma is more invasive and difficult to resect. Choroid plexus carcinoma carries a poor prognosis even with postoperative radiotherapy. Gross total resection alone is considered curative for choroid plexus papilloma.

Hypothalamic Glioma

Gliomas that involve the hypothalamus and optic chiasm generally present with symptoms and signs of increased intracranial pressure and hypothalamic dysfunction. These tumors are often large and may be partially cystic. Surgical therapy is often restricted to biopsy or subtotal resection because radical surgery is associated with significant morbidity and mortality. Radiation and chemotherapy are therefore the primary treatments for hypothalamic gliomas.

Craniopharyngioma

Craniopharyngioma is the most common nonglial tumor of childhood. Craniopharyngiomas can occur at any point along the pituitary stalk and commonly grow to compress the optic chiasm anteriorly, the third ventricle superiorly, and the diaphragm sellae inferiorly.[20] The tumor is typically adherent to the tuber cinereum of the hypothalamus, making surgical resection difficult. The tumors are commonly cystic, containing yellow-green fluid loaded with cholesterol crystals. Solid portions may contain calcifications. Presenting symptoms of craniopharyngioma include headache, endocrine dysfunction (most commonly short stature, diabetes insipidus, obesity, and hypothyroidism), visual disturbance, and hydrocephalus. CT and MRI demonstrate the relation of the tumor to the third ventricle and the presence of calcifications (Fig. 98-26). A complete endocrinologic evaluation is imperative before operation, and any necessary hormone supplementation should be initiated. The treat-

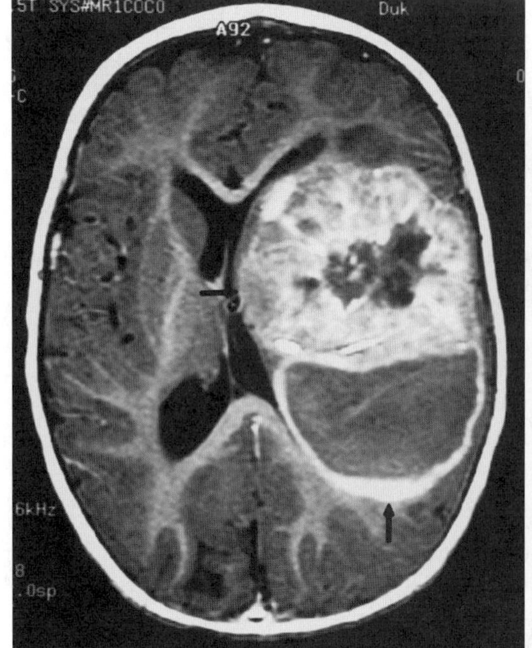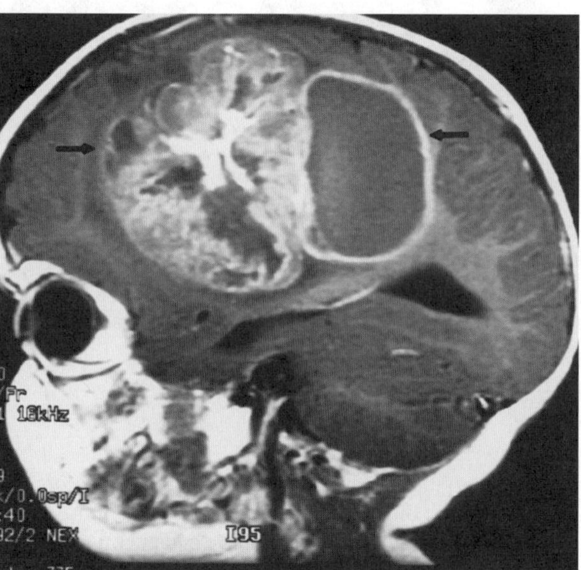

FIG. 98-25. MR image of cerebral primitive neuroectodermal tumor. Axial (*A*) and sagittal (*B*) images with gadolinium enhancement show huge, partially cystic lesion (*arrows*) occupying most of the left cerebral hemisphere, with significant mass effect and shift.

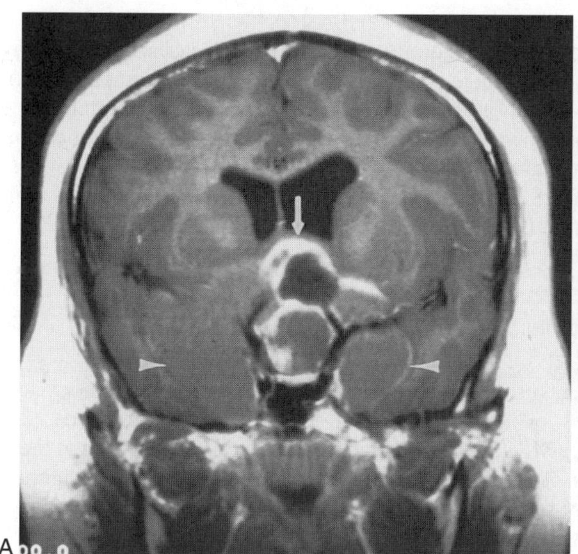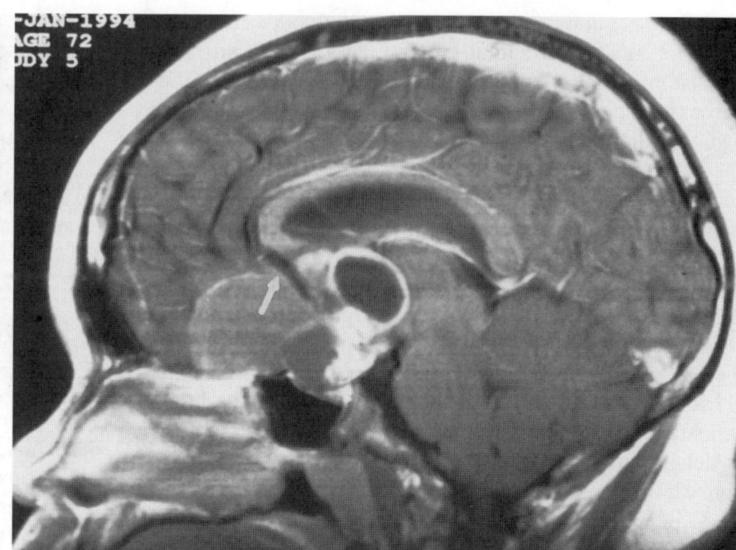

FIG. 98-26. MR image of craniopharyngioma. (*A*) Coronal scan with gadolinium shows a large suprasellar lesion with multiple cystic components invaginating into the third ventricle (*arrow*) and extending into both middle fossae (*arrowheads*). (*B*) Sagittal scan with gadolinium further delineates the tumor and demonstrates the anterior cerebral artery displaced upward by the tumor (*arrow*).

ment of craniopharyngioma has been a matter of great debate: some authors argue for an attempt at gross total resection, with its greater morbidity and mortality; others insist that subtotal resection and radiotherapy provide equivalent results. Postoperatively, endocrine function must be monitored closely because significant endocrine deficits, particularly diabetes insipidus, may be present. Despite the benign histologic appearance of the craniopharyngioma, the clinical behavior is much more aggressive, primarily owing to the involvement of vital centers by the tumor. In addition, radiotherapy of craniopharyngioma carries significant risk of visual and cognitive deterioration, and may not arrest tumor growth. More focal radiotherapy techniques have been applied to these tumors with some success.

Pineal Region Tumors

Pineal region tumors account for 3% to 8% of childhood brain tumors. Germinomas and astrocytomas make up 53% to 78% of these tumors, with the remainder encompassing a wide variety of histologic types. The typical presentation of a pineal region tumor is of hydrocephalus, and shunting is generally required. Germinomas are responsive to radiotherapy, and if a diagnosis of germinoma can be made from CSF cytology, direct surgery of the pineal lesion is not required. Tumor markers in CSF and blood may help to identify germ cell components of the tumor. In general, the treatment of these tumors is surgical, with an attempt at gross total resection for benign tumors identified on frozen section, and subtotal resection for malignant tumors. Postoperative radiotherapy is necessary for germinomas and subtotally resected tumors. Chemotherapy is important in non–germ cell pineal tumors.

Tumors of the Spine

Tumors of the spine can be classified as intramedullary, within the substance of the spinal cord, or extramedullary. Intra-

medullary tumors in children are most commonly ependymomas, with a clear interface between tumor and spinal cord. In contrast, astrocytomas have a much less distinct cleavage plane. These tumors commonly present with a gradual neurologic deterioration, with symptoms based on level of the lesion in the spinal cord. Pain along the spine is common. Weakness of the lower extremities may be subtle. MRI is the diagnostic procedure of choice, owing to its ease of imaging the entire neuraxis and ability to define the relation of the tumor to the spinal cord in great detail. The treatment of these tumors is initially surgical; total resection of ependymomas is possible with modern surgical techniques. Astrocytomas can be more problematic, with some tumors imperceptibly merging into cord tissue and some more malignant astrocytomas with frank cord invasion. In these cases, biopsy alone is performed. Radiotherapy is of uncertain benefit in benign astrocytomas but may slow tumor progression in the more malignant tumors. The long-term outlook for children with these tumors is still uncertain.

Extramedullary spinal tumors in children are a diverse group of tumors that includes meningiomas, nerve sheath tumors, neural crest tumors, and primary bone tumors.

Meningiomas are rare in childhood and are usually intradural or extramedullary, but can be extradural. Histologically, these lesions are usually benign, but they can behave more aggressively in children than in adults. MRI is the diagnostic test of choice. Treatment is surgical resection.

Nerve sheath tumors include schwannomas and neurofibromas. Schwannomas are composed of Schwann cells. Neurofibromas are composed of a mixture of Schwann cells, fibroblasts, and abundant collagen fibers. Pain is the most common presenting complaint, with motor weakness also present in 20% of patients. About 25% of cases are associated with von Recklinghausen disease. These tumors are generally benign but can undergo malignant degeneration, becoming sarcomas. MRI demonstrates these tumors with variable contrast enhancement. Treatment is total resection if possible. Subtotal resection results in recurrence.

Neural crest tumors are common in childhood, accounting for 10% to 20% of all spinal tumors. This group consists of neuroblastomas, ganglioneuromas, and ganglioneuroblastomas. All three types commonly originate from the sympathetic chain or from the adrenal medulla, involving the spinal canal by direct extension.

Neuroblastoma is the most malignant of this group and is most commonly found in younger patients. Neuroblastomas can spread to involve the posterior mediastinum and retroperitoneal space. The spinal canal is involved in 4% to 17% of cases. Metastasis is common to the liver, lymph nodes, and bone. These tumors are frequently seen as paraspinal masses. CT and MRI clearly define the tumor and demonstrate intraspinal extension. MRI offers the benefits of multiplanar imaging and direct visualization of the spinal cord, whereas CT provides better bony detail. The treatment of neuroblastoma with spinal cord compression consists of laminectomy. In these cases, it is preferable to perform a combined procedure with sequential tumor excision. First, the neurosurgeon clears the spinal canal, freeing the thecal sac and nerve roots and decompressing the spinal cord. Then, the pediatric surgeon removes the paraspinal portion of the tumor. In this way, a more complete removal can be obtained than in a staged approach with two separate procedures. The principal treatment of neuroblastoma, however, consists of radiotherapy and chemotherapy.

Ganglioneuroblastomas represent an intermediate tumor type in this group. They rarely involve the spinal canal, unless there is direct extension or metastasis to the vertebra. They are characterized by the presence of mature ganglion cells along with neuroblasts. The behavior of ganglioneuroblastoma is somewhat unpredictable, with some tumors behaving more aggressively. In the presence of spinal cord compression, laminectomy is indicated.

Ganglioneuromas are the most benign of these tumors and are more common in older children. They are slow growing and can be asymptomatic until reaching a large size. If the spinal canal is involved, laminectomy is the treatment of choice.

VASCULAR MALFORMATIONS OF THE BRAIN

Vascular malformations of the brain are common causes of intracerebral hemorrhage in children. The classic arteriovenous malformation (AVM) is the most common, with cavernous angiomas and venous angiomas less commonly associated with hemorrhage. The vein of Galen aneurysm deserves special mention because its presentation varies, depending on the age of the patient.

Arteriovenous Malformation

The classic AVM represents a defect in the formation of the primitive arteriolar capillary network interposed between cerebral arteries and veins. The resulting tangled arteriovenous complex, with its low resistance, invites high blood flow rates and increases the risk of hemorrhage. Most AVMs have a characteristic wedge shape, pointing to the ventricle. The most common presentation of an AVM is intracerebral hemorrhage, which can be catastrophic. Seizures may also be present. CT is the diagnostic modality of choice when acute hemorrhage is suspected. Arteriography delineates the lesion and identifies feeding arteries and draining veins. In some cases, arteriography after a hemorrhage is negative, owing to either compression of the AVM or obliteration of the AVM with the rupture. The ideal treatment of AVM is total surgical removal. Surgical resection may be limited, however, by an eloquent location in the brain. Stereotactic radiosurgery may provide benefit in nonresectable deep lesions.

Cavernous Angioma

The cavernous angioma typically presents with hemorrhage, seizures, or neurologic deficit. Modern imaging methods, particularly MRI, have greatly increased our understanding of these lesions. As imaging techniques have improved, the diagnosis of these lesions before hemorrhage has been possible. These lesions are characterized as a dark blue mass, which is well encapsulated and surrounded by hemorrhage-stained white matter. For lesions that have hemorrhaged, treatment is surgical excision. Lesions that have not hemorrhaged can be excised if easily accessible surgically. Deep lesions that have not hemorrhaged are not approached surgically.

Venous Angioma

The venous angioma is the most common vascular malformation of the brain and the least likely to cause symptoms. It consists of dilated medullary veins separated by normal brain parenchyma. The veins of the angioma drain centripetally into the venous channels around which they are arranged, and they are important for venous drainage of the surrounding brain. The risk of hemorrhage from a venous angioma is uncertain but is clearly less than that associated with a AVM or cavernous angioma. Most venous angiomas can be diagnosed on contrast-enhanced CT. Surgery is not indicated for venous angiomas because the venous drainage they provide is essential for the surrounding normal brain tissue.

Vein of Galen Aneurysm

The presentation of vein of Galen aneurysms depends on patient age. Infants presenting with vein of Galen aneurysms commonly have high-output cardiac failure due to the tremendous arteriovenous shunting. This shunting can also cause cerebral ischemia. The dilated vein of Galen can cause obstructive hydrocephalus, and macrocephaly may be obvious. The treatment of these children is aimed at reduction of the arteriovenous shunt, thereby relieving the cardiac failure. This must be accomplished in a gradual fashion, or the risk of hemorrhage is high. Mickle and Quisling[21] reported on the transtorcular approach to embolization of these lesions. These authors advocate the graded, multisession treatment approach. Older children with vein of Galen malformations commonly present with subarachnoid hemorrhage or hydrocephalus. In these children, direct surgical therapy is possible, but transtorcular embolization has also met with considerable success.

INFECTIONS

The treatment of infections of the CNS has been greatly improved with the development of modern imaging techniques and new antibiotics. The most important aspect in the treatment of these infections is early recognition, with identification of the causative organism and administration of appropriate antibiotics to eradicate the infection.

Intracranial Infections

Brain Abscess

Brain abscess is uncommon in children. The most common causes of brain abscess include contiguous infection, such as sinusitis or mastoiditis; hematogenous spread, such as with congenital heart disease; or direct introduction through a penetrating wound. The formation of a brain abscess proceeds through a well-recognized series of stages. First, the organism produces an inflammatory reaction, termed *cerebritis,* with infiltration of polymorphonuclear leukocytes. Next, the involved tissue becomes necrotic, leading to suppuration in the center of the lesion. The brain attempts to wall off the infection, and fibroblasts deposit a collagen wall around the lesion. Edema is present in the tissue surrounding the capsule. Brain abscess is rare in infants. In older children, congenital heart disease, purulent infection such as sinusitis, or chronic otitis media is often present. A history of penetrating trauma should arouse considerable suspicion of this problem. Patients may present with neurologic signs and symptoms of increased intracranial pressure and focal signs owing to the location of the abscess. CT is the diagnostic study of choice, allowing visualization of the brain, paranasal sinuses, and skull. With contrast administration, a ring-enhancing lesion with considerable edema is commonly seen. Treatment should consist of abscess aspiration (stereotactic techniques may be used for deeper lesions) to obtain adequate material for culture. Drainage of the abscess also helps normalize intracranial pressure and reduce local effects of the abscess. Broad-spectrum antibiotics are started, including coverage for anaerobic bacteria, and can be modified when culture results are available. Antibiotic coverage should continue for 4 to 6 weeks. With early diagnosis and treatment, the morbidity and mortality rates of brain abscess have improved considerably. With increasing numbers of survivors of brain abscess, long-term effects, including seizure disorders, are being seen with increasing frequency.

Subdural Empyema

Subdural empyema is an uncommon infection that occurs primarily in children and adolescents. It is usually secondary to paranasal sinus or middle ear infection but can also result from hematogenous seeding of a subdural hematoma. It is most commonly seen over the cerebral convexities. CT or MRI provides the diagnosis, and lumbar puncture should not be performed. Treatment consists of surgical drainage and antibiotic therapy. If the purulent material is thick, a craniotomy may be necessary to débride purulent material. Complications of subdural empyema include cortical vein thrombosis, brain abscess, and meningitis. Seizures are common in patients with subdural empyema and can persist for years.

Epidural Abscess

Epidural abscess is almost always secondary to another infection of the sinuses, postoperative bone flap, or compound wounds of the head. Local symptoms, such as pain, erythema, and swelling, are common. Treatment consists of surgical drainage (with removal of infected bone), followed by intravenous antibiotics, as described earlier.

Spinal Epidural Abscess

Spinal epidural abscess is rare in children. It occurs most commonly in the thoracic or lower lumbar region. *S aureus* is the most common causative organism, which gains access to the epidural space through hematogenous spread. Back pain is common, and spinal cord compression with lower extremity weakness is often present at the time of clinical presentation. MRI is the diagnostic procedure of choice. Treatment consists of laminectomy with irrigation of the epidural space and culture. A drain is left in place for 24 to 48 hours. Intravenous antibiotics are continued for 4 to 6 weeks. With early diagnosis and treatment before significant neurologic deficit occurs, the prognosis should be good.

REFERENCES

1. O'Rahilly R. Developmental stages in human embryos, including a survey of the Carnegie collection. A. Embryos of the first three weeks (stages 1 to 9). Washington DC, Carnegie Institution of Washington, 1973;631.
2. Lemire RJ, Siebert JR, Warkany J. Normal development of the central nervous system. In: McLaurin RL, Venes JL, Schut L, Epstein F, eds. Pediatric neurosurgery: surgery of the developing nervous system, ed 2. Philadelphia, WB Saunders, 1989.
3. Barson AJ. The vertebral level of termination of the spinal cord during normal and abnormal development. J Anat 1970;106:489.
4. McLone DG, Mutluer S, Naidich TP. Lipomeningoceles of the conus medullaris. In: Imondi AJ, ed. Concepts in pediatric neurosurgery, vol 3. Basel, S Karger, 1982.
5. Dias MS, Walker ML. The embryogenesis of complex dysraphic malformations: a disorder of gastrulation? J Pediatr Neurosurg 1992;18:229.
6. Pang D, Dias MS, Ahab-Barmada M. Split cord malformation. I. A unified theory of embryogenesis for double cord malformations. Neurosurgery 1992;31:451.
7. Chapman PH, Swearingen B, Caviness VS. Subtorcular occipital encephaloceles: anatomical considerations relevant to operative management. J Neurosurg 1989;71:375.
8. McLone DG, Knepper PA. The cause of the Chiari II malformation: a unified theory. Pediatr Neurosurg 1989;15:1.
9. McLone DG, Dias L, Kaplan WE, et al. Concepts in the management of spina bifida. In: Humphreys RP, ed. Concepts in pediatric neurosurgery, vol 5. Basel, S Karger, 1985:97.
10. Yamada S, Zinke DE, Sanders D. Pathophysiology of tethered cord syndrome. J Neurosurg 1981;54:494.
11. Warder DE, Oakes WJ. Tethered cord syndrome: the low-lying and normally positioned conus. Neurosurgery 1994;34:597.
12. Oakes WJ. Chiari malformations, hydromyelia, syringomyelia. In: Wilkins RH, Rengachary SS, eds. Neurosurgery. New York, McGraw-Hill, 1985.
13. Raimondi AJ, Choux M, DiRocco C, eds. Intracranial cyst lesions. New York, Springer Verlag, 1993.

14. Butler AJ, Mclone DG, eds. Hydrocephalus. Neurosurg Clin North Am 1993;4.
15. Hoffman HJ, Kestle JRW. Craniofacial surgery. In: McLaurin RL, Venes JL, Schut L, et al, eds. Pediatric neurosurgery: surgery of the developing nervous system, ed 3. Philadelphia, WB Saunders, 1994.
16. Persing JA, Jane JA, Edgerton MT. Surgical treatment of craniosynostosis. In: Persing, JA, Edgerton MT, Jane JA, eds. Scientific foundations and surgical treatment of craniosynostosis. Baltimore, Williams & Wilkins, 1989.
17. O'Brien MS, Krisht A. Cerebellar astrocytomas. In: McLaurin RL, Venes JL, Schut L, et al, eds. Pediatric neurosurgery: surgery of the developing nervous system, ed 3. Philadelphia, WB Saunders, 1994.
18. Chang C, Housepian E, Herbert C Jr. An operative staging system and a megavoltage radiotherapeutic technique for cerebellar medulloblastomas. Radiology 1969;93:1351.
19. Abbott R, Ragheb J, Epstein FJ. Brainstem tumors: surgical indications. In: McLaurin RL, Venes JL, Schut L, et al, eds. Pediatric neurosurgery: surgery of the developing nervous system, ed 3. Philadelphia, WB Saunders, 1994.
20. Hoffman HJ, Kestle JRW. Craniopharyngiomas. In: In: McLaurin RL, Venes JL, Schut L, et al, eds. Pediatric neurosurgery: surgery of the developing nervous system, ed 3. Philadelphia, WB Saunders, 1994.
21. Mickle JP, Quisling RG. The transtorcular embolization of vein of Galen aneurysms. J Neurosurg 1986;64:731.

Musculoskeletal System

Surgery of Infants and Children: Scientific Principles and Practice, edited by Keith T. Oldham, Paul M. Colombani, and Robert P. Foglia. Lippincott–Raven Publishers, Philadelphia, © 1997.

Chapter 99

Principles of Orthopedics

Paul D. Sponseller

Surgeons caring for children should be familiar with the principles of pediatric orthopedics in order to deal with trauma, recognize skeletal manifestations of systemic diseases, and evaluate congenital or developmental abnormalities. This chapter is intended to help in the initial understanding of the broad range of orthopedic conditions encountered in children and is therefore intended for breadth of coverage. Conditions isolated to one anatomic region are presented first, followed by generalized musculoskeletal conditions. The reference list can serve as a guide for further study of any particular condition.[1-4]

Orthopedic terminology is not always straightforward; the following are a few definitions to assist the reader. The term *physis* refers to the growth plate (Fig. 99-1), and therefore the *epi*physis is the portion of a bone ''on top of'' the physis (i.e., nearer the joint); *meta*physis is the widened portion of the shaft adjacent to and arising from the growth plate, and the *dia*physis is the narrow portion of a tubular bone midway between two physes. The skeleton is largely formed from a cartilaginous precursor, with ossification of the cartilage beginning in the diaphysis. Secondary ossification centers at the ends of each long bone. The small bones of the wrist and foot begin from a single ossification center.

The Greek root *genu* refers to knee, *coxa* to hip, and *pes* to foot. When two bones or two fracture fragments form an angle, they are in *varus* when the apex of the angle points away from the midline (Fig. 99-2) and *valgus* when it points toward the midline. Alternatively, *angulation* may be stated in any of the three standard anatomic planes by the direction of the apex—that is, genu valgus is medial angulation of the lower extremity at the knee. *Dislocation* refers to complete loss of contact of two joint surfaces, and it is specified by the direction of displacement of the most distal part. *Subluxation* is an incomplete dislocation. For example, in a dislocated hip, the femoral head is completely out of the acetabulum; a subluxated hip has been only partially offset. *Abduction* refers to movement away from the midline; *adduction*, toward the midline.

ABNORMALITIES BY REGION

Foot

Isolated idiopathic *adduction* of the forefoot or metatarsals is designated by the terms *metatarsus adductus, metatarsus*

varus, or *C-foot*. In contrast to clubfoot, the hindfoot and ankle are normal. The ankle joint itself has normal dorsiflexion and plantar flexion. The etiology may be increased medially directed pressure in the uterus. Children with metatarsus adductus also may have an increased incidence of other molding deformities, such as developmental dislocation of the hip or torticollis. To measure the degree of adduction, one should draw an imaginary line bisecting the sole of the hindfoot and project it forward to see where it intersects the toes. Normally, the line falls between toes 2 and 3, whereas in severe metatarsus adductus, it is lateral to the fourth toe.[5]

The outcome of untreated metatarsus adductus is spontaneous correction in 85% of children. In 10% of children, mild adduction persists, and in only 5% is it severe.[6] It is, unfortunately, not possible to predict which cases will resolve spontaneously by looking at severity or rigidity. Manipulative correction is equally successful beginning in the first 8 months of life.[5] Therefore, the preferred treatment is observation and stretching for the first 4 to 6 months, with corrective casts or splints if metatarsus adductus persists beyond this time. The casts are changed every 1 to 2 weeks until the adduction is clinically corrected, then followed by holding casts or shoes. Surgery (osteotomy) for very late deformities, in children over 3 years, is only rarely necessary.

Clubfoot, or equinovarus congenita, is a more complex disorder that includes not only metatarsal adduction but also abnormalities of the hind part of the foot: malrotation of the calcaneus under the talus and equinus (plantar flexion) of the ankle. The incidence of clubfoot is 1 per 1000 births, and it is more common in males than in females. Clubfoot may be unilateral or bilateral. Etiology is unknown. Abnormalities have been found in the leg muscles or tarsal bones. Muscle biopsies done for experimental purposes are abnormal, which is consistent with the clinical observation that the leg muscles are underdeveloped even in treated patients.

The clubfoot appears smaller than normal for age, and the combination of deformities results in a 90-degree rotation of the forefoot in all planes so that the leg and foot truly resemble a club (Fig. 99-3). There is a deep crease on the medial border of the foot. The deformity may be correctable to neutral only in the neonatal period, and the range of motion is limited in all directions. Radiographs show an abnormal parallelism of the

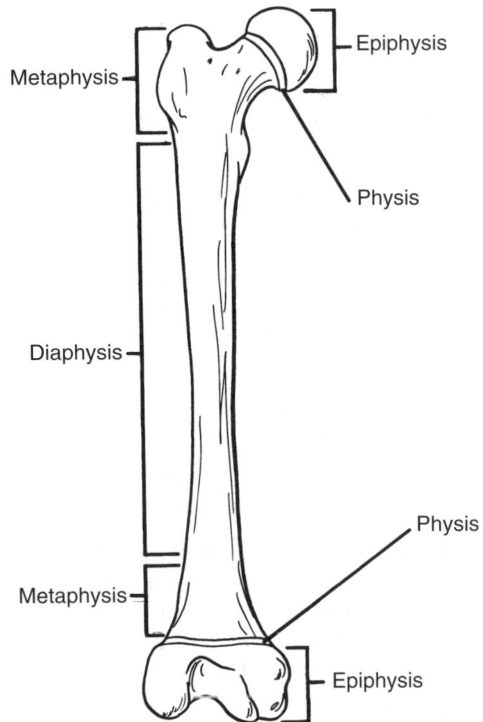

FIG. 99-1. Regions of a long bone. The physis or growth plate is the main reference point. The epiphysis refers to the segment on top of the physis, and so forth.

talus and calcaneus. Neuromuscular disorders (especially lipomeningocele, myelomeningocele, spasticity, or arthrogryposis) may produce similar deformities. Also, diastrophic dwarfism includes a clubfoot-like deformity.

Clubfoot ranges from a mild, postural and easily correctable form to a severe and resistant form. However, a trial of cast correction is indicated in all. This is most successful in the perinatal period when ligamentous laxity is greatest. The casts are changed every few days. Overall, casting is effective in about one third of patients. Surgery is indicated in the others and involves complete correction of all bony malalignments and tendon contractures; it is performed most commonly at ages 6 to 12 months.[7] In older patients or those with recurrent deformity, osteotomy or fusion may be indicated.

Flatfoot (planovalgus) should be divided into flexible and rigid types. The flexible type is a normal variant in children and is usually asymptomatic. Development of an arch occurs spontaneously in the first 8 years of life in most children. The arch of the foot is restored. When the child is on tiptoes or when weight bearing is relieved, varus-valgus motion is normal. As a herald to a more serious condition, *rigid* flat foot may be due to tarsal coalition, vertical talus, neuromuscular imbalance, or arthritis of the foot. These should be considered in the differential diagnosis.

The cause of the usual type of flexible flatfoot is ligamentous laxity. There is no primary muscle abnormality. Occasionally a tight heel cord may contribute to producing flatfoot by pulling the foot into greater valgus. Treatment is not indicated in cases of flexible flatfoot; prospective studies[8] have shown that no orthotic or special shoe can produce a lasting change in pediatric flatfoot. Such devices may be indicated for neuromuscular flat-

feet, but not in asymptomatic children with flexible flatfeet. The heel cord should be stretched if it is tight. Rarely is soft tissue reconstruction or osteotomy indicated.

General principles to stress to parents when they ask about shoes are summarized in an article by Staheli[9]:

- Shoes are primarily for protection.
- Corrective shoes have no effect on flat feet.
- Shoes should be flat, flexible, well aerated, and high topped if needed to keep them from slipping off.

These characteristics should be found in most reasonably priced footwear available in regular shoe stores.

Tarsal coalition involves the bones of the hindfoot, with persistence of a bridge or coalition between two of them. This bridge may be fibrous, cartilaginous, or bony. Tarsal coalition is transmitted as autosomal dominant and is present in approximately 5% of the population.[10] Many persons with tarsal coalition are asymptomatic. The presence of symptoms seems to be related to the degree of valgus, which places more strain on the abnormal coalition. Tarsal coalition usually presents during the second decade as an ankle sprain with persistence of pain longer than expected, or as spontaneous onset of pain in the ankle. The reason for this presentation is probably that the ossification that occurs at this time, near skeletal maturity, makes the coalition stiffer and therefore symptomatic. The hindfoot shows limitation of varus-valgus motion, but it is usually tender to palpation. The foot appears to be in valgus more often than not. Sometimes pain manifests over the peroneal muscles, which overcontract to stabilize the foot.

A plain oblique radiograph of the foot can reliably show the most common type of coalition, the *calcaneonavicular* bar, if it has ossified.[10] It is not evident on the anteroposterior (AP) or lateral view, however. If it is fibrous or cartilaginous, there may not be a bony connection, but an irregularity of the adjacent cortices may be seen. Normal films in the presence of physeal findings of a coalition indicate the need for a coronal computed tomographic (CT) scan of the foot to search for a *talocalcaneal* coalition, the other common type of coalition. Talonavicular and calcaneocuboid coalitions are rare.

With rest or casting, many coalitions develop enough stability to ossify and become painless. If pain persists, however, the coalition can be excised if it is not large and if no arthritic change has occurred.[11] If these conditions are not met, fusion of the hindfoot is the best treatment for the symptomatic foot.

Tibia

Internal tibial torsion is the most common cause of in-toeing between 1 and 3 years of age.[12–14] Tibial torsion is measured by the angle between the foot and thigh, with the ankle and knee bent at 90 degrees. Normally, the foot turns out more with increasing age. Differential diagnosis includes metatarsus adductus, femoral anteversion, or neuromuscular disorders. To differentiate these conditions, the foot itself and the hip should also be examined. Tibial torsion naturally improves with growth, but this often takes years. Because the benign natural history of this condition is now known, braces, such as the Denis-Browne bar, are rarely used any longer.[13] Studies have shown that braces cannot apply significant rotational force to

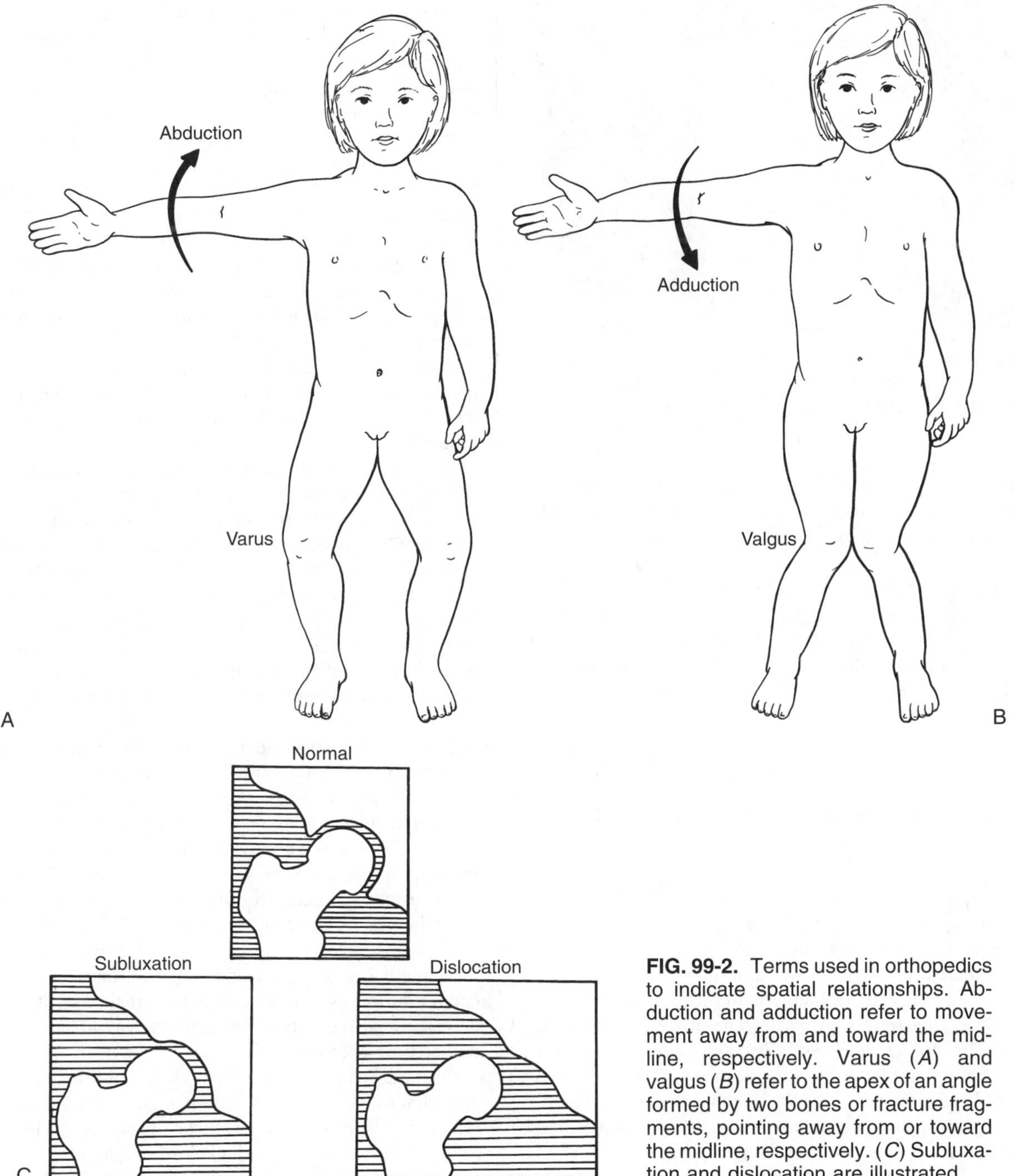

FIG. 99-2. Terms used in orthopedics to indicate spatial relationships. Abduction and adduction refer to movement away from and toward the midline, respectively. Varus (*A*) and valgus (*B*) refer to the apex of an angle formed by two bones or fracture fragments, pointing away from or toward the midline, respectively. (*C*) Subluxation and dislocation are illustrated.

the tibia, since the force is dissipated through the foot, knee, and hip joints. The improvement attributed to the brace in years past is now thought to be due to normal growth patterns. Correction through growth is a gradual process and often frustrates parents. Prior traditional use of braces, reinforced by comments from grandparents and friends, often drive anxious parents to visit the doctor to make sure they are not missing a golden opportunity to prevent deformity. The physician should be confident in allaying the anxiety. The use of a graph may prove convincing. Minor persistent internal torsion has not been shown to be detrimental.

External tibial torsion is less common. These children often appear clumsy for their age. There is little data on the course of this condition, but no treatment is indicated, and some spontaneous improvement can be expected.

Mild *anterior and lateral* bowing of the tibia are common in infancy and should be observed to be sure that they correct spontaneously. Focal, sclerotic defects in the tibia may be seen with marked anterolateral bowing. Such patients may present with or develop a fracture (*congenital pseudoarthrosis*), and patients may be found to have neurofibromatosis. If the severe anterolateral bow is present but the tibia is not fractured, it should be braced for protection. If it is fractured, attempts to gain union by electrical stimulation, rod insertion, vascularized

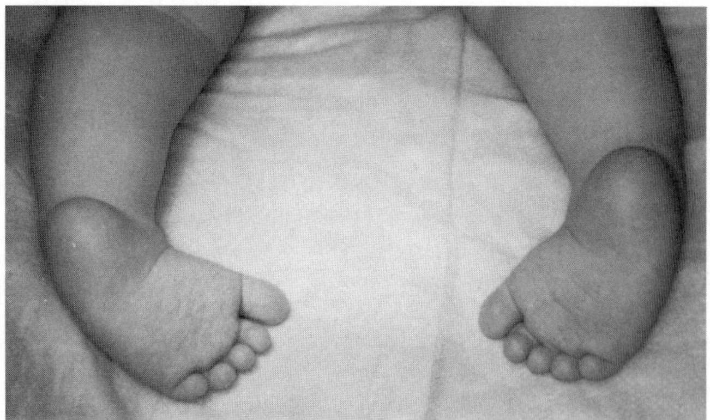

FIG. 99-3. Uncorrected clubfeet in a 7-month-old, seen from the plantar surface. Note the equinus of the ankle and varus, adduction, and malrotation of the rest of the foot.

fibula grafting, or bone grafting have similar success rates of 50% to 75%.[15] An anterolateral bow may also be seen with congenital absence of the fibula, but this does not progress to fracture.

Posterior/medial bowing of the tibia is fortunately more benign; this usually straightens by age 4 and is not associated with fracture. However, there may be 2 to 6 cm of shortening by maturity. Treatment is stretching of the tight dorsiflexor muscles and length equalization as indicated later in childhood.[16]

Knee

Extensor Mechanism Disorders (Patellofemoral Problems)

In children and adolescents a number of conditions involving this region have been described. They are treated by attempting to improve the basic biomechanical forces.

Chondromalacia is a nonspecific term that refers to the appearance of softening and degeneration of the patellar cartilage. *Patellar subluxation* refers to partial lateral *displacement* of the patella. The terms *patellofemoral stress syndrome, patellar malalignment*, and *excessive lateral pressure syndrome* refer to the abnormal *mechanics* causing stress concentration and pain.

The quadriceps-patella mechanism is in valgus, as measured by the Q (quadriceps) angle from anterior superior spine to patella to tibial tubercle. Possible factors contributing to patellar pathology include increased valgus of the knee, increased anteversion of the femur or external torsion of the tibia, a high patella (patella alta), abnormal shape or development of the quadriceps, or flattening of the femoral groove. Underdevelopment of the medial side of the quadriceps restraints contributes to subluxation or dislocation. Females normally have slightly greater valgus of the knee than males. Cartilage degeneration occurs beginning in the deep layers and becoming visible later.

Clinically, patellar problems cause symptoms of aching in the anteromedial region of the knee. This is usually worse with stair-climbing or prolonged sitting, since flexion increases patellofemoral force. Crepitus may be felt, but this may be painless in some patients and is not in itself pathologic. ''Catching'' or ''locking'' may be noted. A feeling of ''giving way'' may be

related, especially with subluxation of the patella. On physical examination, the most reliable way to test patellar tenderness is by direct compression of the patella against the femur. Palpation under the patella is not diagnostic. Effusion is present only if patellar degenerative changes or extreme overuse have occurred. In most cases, there is no effusion. Reproducing patellar subluxation by laterally directed pressure may produce apprehension (the apprehension test). Radiographs are usually nonspecific, but occasionally lateral displacement or tilt of the patella may be seen on the sunrise view.

The natural history of patellofemoral stress disorders is that they are common between the ages of 10 and 20 years but often become less bothersome after these years, and they do not usually progress to arthritis.

Differential diagnosis includes a synovial fold or plica, a medial meniscus tear, tendinitis of the quadriceps or patellar tendon, and osteochondritis dissecans of the patella or distal femur.

Treatment consists of decreasing activities performed with knees flexed, such as stair-climbing and prolonged sitting. Temporary rest from sports and use of nonsteroidal antiinflammatory agents may be necessary. Exercises to strengthen the medial (stabilizing) part of the quadriceps include extension from 0 to 30 degrees, by lifting weights within this range or extending the knee on a pillow to compress it. Hamstrings and rectus femoris muscles should be stretched if they are tight. Arch supports may help if flexible flatfeet are contributing to tibial torsion. Surgical measures are rarely needed, but they include release of a tight lateral patellar retinaculum, medial soft tissue tightening, tibial tubercle transfer, or correction of valgus, anteversion, or patella alta. These all produce satisfactory pain relief in 75% to 90% of cases.

Patellar dislocations may be acute or recurrent. The patella usually dislocates laterally. An acute dislocation is associated with significant swelling and medial knee pain and follows valgus or rotating force. This should be treated for 4 to 6 weeks with the knee extended, using a knee immobilizer, except in cases with bony avulsion. Recurrent *subluxation* is common; the patient has less pain and swelling, and subluxation often occurs during everyday activities. A realignment operation as described earlier is the only effective way to stop frequent and bothersome episodes.

Osgood-Schlatter disease, patellar tendinitis (jumper's knee), and quadriceps tendinitis are all manifestations of excessive, repetitive stresses on the extensor mechanism. They are listed in order of decreasing frequency in children.

Osgood-Schlatter ''disease'' is a traction-induced inflammation of the tibial tubercle, not really a disease. It is a reaction of the bone and growth cartilage of this region to repetitive stress. The tibial tubercle is a distal extension of the proximal tibial epiphysis. It develops an ossification center between ages 9 and 12 but does not completely ossify until ages 15 to 17 years. It is within this age range that repetitive stresses can gradually deform the tubercle, causing enlargement of the tubercle and local inflammation. Tenderness and swelling are localized to the tubercle only and do not extend to the joint. Running, jumping, or kneeling exacerbates symptoms. Treatment involves decreasing activity to a level at which symptoms are minimal, occasionally using a knee immobilizer, crutches, and ice after activity in severe cases. The patient may be vulnerable to recurrence for up to 2 years until the tubercle matures. If he or she is educated about this likelihood, individual regulation of activities can be effective. Complete avulsion of the tubercle is extremely rare and seems more related to sudden stress than to apophysitis.

Patellar tendonitis, inflammation at the *origin* of the patellar tendon (at the inferior pole of the patella), is related to the same type of overuse as Osgood-Schlatter apophysitis. It is most often seen in basketball players, and is therefore known as jumper's knee. Pain present during both rest and activity is more worrisome than pain occuring just after activity. Treatment is the same as for Osgood-Schlatter disease. Warm packs before and cold packs after activity may be of help also. Rarely, pain may occur at the proximal pole of the patella and is termed *quadriceps tendinitis*.

Popliteal cysts in children are localized on the medial side of the popliteal region. They occur most commonly in boys under age 9 years. Unlike popliteal cysts in adults, these cysts in children are usually not associated with any intraarticular pathology,[17] and they usually regress spontaneously with time. The recurrence rate is higher after surgical excision than after observation. The origin of these cysts is a slitlike communication through the joint capsules, between the knee joint and the gastrocnemius-semimembranous bursa on the medial side of the popliteal region.

These cysts often present as tumors but can usually be differentiated clinically by their characteristic location, firm consistency, discrete encapsulation, and slight mobility. Transillumination is helpful, as the whole contents of the mass lights up when the room is darkened, distinguishing it from a blood-filled or a solid tumor. Biopsy should rarely be necessary.

A *discoid meniscus* is an acquired flattening and deformation of the normally semilunar lateral meniscus. In some cases this flattening occurs because of the absence of normal peripheral attachments. Symptoms such as pain, clicking, and locking often develop in the absence of trauma in children from age 2 to adulthood.[18] The meniscus should be trimmed or excised if symptoms become severe.

Bowed leg or genu varum of up to 20 degrees is normal in children until the age of 18 months. Bowing normally does not increase significantly after walking begins.[12] After the age of 24 months, valgus of the knee begins to develop instead.[19] Radiographs are indicated if varus is present after this age or is progressive after 1 year, if it is unilateral, if it appears to be severe, or if it occurs in a high-risk group such as heavy black children who walk early.[12] Radiographic findings of benign genu varum include bowing of the tibia and femur; a normal-appearing growth plate physis, without narrowing or step-off; and a generalized, rather than focal, varus angle.

Treatment of physiologic genu varum is observation until resolution. On physical examination, the measurement should be performed with the child standing and may also be confirmed by measurement of the distance between the femoral condyles. These methods are not as accurate as radiographs, but they are a practical way of following change in patients when the presumptive diagnosis is physiologic genu varum.

Differential diagnosis of physiologic genu varum includes Blount disease, rickets, post-traumatic growth plate disturbance, enchondromatosis, achondroplasia, or other skeletal dysplasias.

Blount disease (tibia vara) is an idiopathic, mechanical overload of the medial tibial growth plate that may be unilateral or bilateral. It presents initially in two different age groups, childhood and adolescence.

If untreated, infantile tibia vara is almost always progressive; along with the varus, it includes flexion and internal rotation and often increased lateral knee laxity. Radiographs demonstrate progressive depression of the medial metaphysis, growth plate, and epiphysis. Eventually the medial metaphysis fuses to the epiphysis in severe cases. A helpful early distinction unique to tibia vara is the focal nature of the change (Fig. 99-4), with sharp angulation of the *proximal* tibial metaphysis, resulting in a metaphyseal-diaphyseal angle of 11 to 16 degrees or more. This is a specific sign, since such localized angulation occurs in fewer than 5% of children with *physiologic* varus but in essentially all cases of Blount disease.[20]

Treatment with a night brace, although not scientifically proven to be effective, is usually used for the mild but definite cases of Blount disease up until about age 3 years. Valgus-rotational osteotomy of the tibia is indicated if the angulation progresses, if growth plate depression occurs, and if the patient is older than 3 years. Recurrence is a risk if treatment begins after 4 years of age, if the epiphysis is fragmented, or if the child is obese. Persistent varus leads to early knee arthritis.

Adolescent tibia vara has onset after 9 years of age. It is to be distinguished from persistent cases of infantile tibia vara. It is most common in obese males. It is believed to be due to decreased growth of the medial tibial physis from excessive medial stresses. Radiographs show medial femoral and tibial bowing. Treatment is osteotomy to realign the limb, or closure of the lateral growth plate to allow catch-up growth medially.

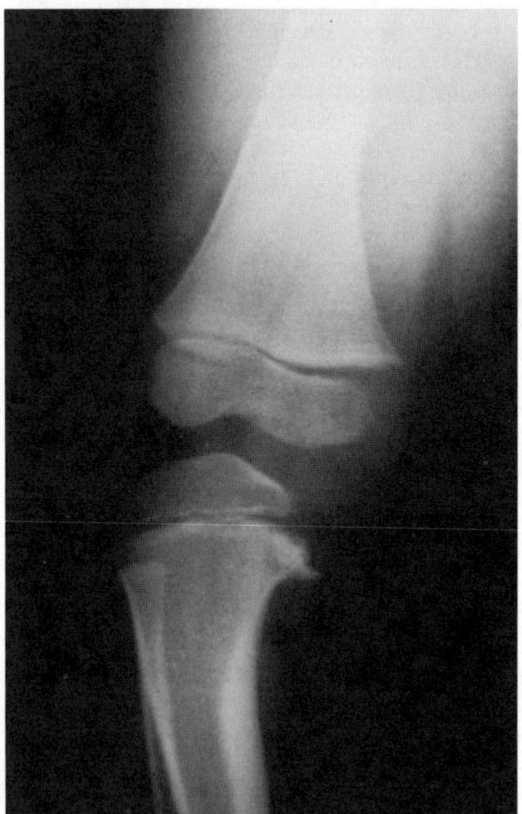

FIG. 99-4. Infantile tibia vara is characterized by focal depression of the medial proximal tibia.

The knee goes through a series of phases of normal alignment. Varus is common before age 2. *Valgus* of the knee is normal after age 2, reaches a mean of 12 degrees at 3 years, and remains at a mean of approximately 7 degrees in boys and 9 degrees in girls after 8 years of age. If valgus remains over 15 degrees at 10 years, early growth plate stapling or later osteotomy of the affected region may be indicated to prevent patellofemoral problems and degenerative changes. Valgus of the proximal tibia often develops after medial tibial metaphyseal fractures, but usually it spontaneously corrects at least partially.

Hip

Developmental Dysplasia of the Hip (DDH)

The hip develops from a common cartilage anlage resulting from reciprocal contact between the femur and acetabulum during growth. Loss of this contact may occur at any point in development as a result of abnormal in utero positioning, neuromuscular abnormalities such as myelodysplasia, arthrogryposis, Larsen syndrome, or intrinsic abnormalities in the connective tissue. The earlier this loss of relationship occurs, the more severe are the femoral and acetabular abnormalities; the earlier it is corrected, the more the remodeling potential and the better the potential outcome.

The etiology of dislocation of the hip in an otherwise normal child is multifactorial. Mechanical factors play a role, and the frequency is greatly increased in breech presentation (a factor in 30% of all DDH), in firstborn children, and in oligohydramnios. Breech position causes the hip to be hyperflexed and the muscle forces to be increased, causing the femur to be directed out over the edge of the acetabulum. The left hip is slightly more commonly involved than the right. These factors are associated with increased force across the hip or positioning or both. Hormonal factors may play a role, because there is generalized ligamentous laxity around the time of birth due to increased circulating estrogens and relaxin. The incidence of DDH is sixfold greater in girls than in boys. Evidence for hereditary control of these and other factors is that over 20% of patients have a positive family history.

There are three degrees of hip dysplasia: subluxable, dislocatable, and dislocated hips, in order of increasing severity. In the first type (subluxable), the femoral head rests in the acetabulum and can be partially dislocated by examination. A dislocatable hip is also located normally when at rest, but it can be fully dislocated. A dislocated hip rests in the dislocated position. The combined incidence of these three types is about 1 in 60 births; incidence of a true dislocation is only 1.5 in 1,000. Because of this variability, a change in terminology from congenital dislocation to developmental dysplasia of the hip has become widely accepted. *Dysplasia* better describes the *spectrum* of severity, from malformation to dislocation of the hip. *Developmental* is meant to acknowledge that some cases are not detectable at birth, and may occur later; the anatomic findings are continually evolving. The pathologic anatomy includes laxity of the capsulae, which progresses to capsular contraction with time if the hip remains out. The acetabulum becomes shallow because of lack of concentric contact with the femoral head. A false acetabulum may form where the femoral head contacts the lateral wall of the ilium above the normal location. The outer rim of the acetabulum becomes rounded during the period when the femoral head is able to slide in and out of the acetabulum. The movement over this ridge is felt as the "clunk" of the Ortolani and Barlow tests. The proximal femur remains anteriorly rotated (anteverted) as the head rests against the lateral iliac wall.

Physical examination remains the most important means of diagnosis. A general rule is that the signs in the newborn period usually consist of instability without significant fixed deformity, whereas in the later months, an untreated dislocation becomes more fixed, and there is less instability and more limitation of certain motions. The Barlow and Ortolani signs should be sought in the newborn (Fig. 99-5). A positive Barlow sign consists of the ability to dislocate the hip; a positive Ortolani sign is the ability to relocate the hip with easy physical manipulation. When performing the tests, the child should be relaxed by keeping him or her warm and on the parent's lap, and using a pacifier. Only one hip should be examined at a time. The pelvis should be held by one hand of the examiner, while the other hand controls the femur with fingers on the greater and lesser trochanters. With adduction and posteriorly directed pressure, the femur can be felt to slide posterosuperiorly over the deformed acetabulum in the abnormal hip. (Barlow sign; see Fig. 99-5*A*) and back in with abduction, causing a dull clunk (Ortolani sign; see Fig. 99-5*B*). Thus these signs, dislocation and relocation, are both aspects of the same condition of hip instability.

Possible errors include examining both hips at once, which impairs proprioception, and mistaking insignificant soft tissue "clicks" for the more important and palpable "clunk." These innocent clicks may be due to movement of fascia over the greater trochanter, clicking of the meniscus or the patella, or the stretch of a normal labrum.

Routine screening of neonates in the past three decades has resulted in a dramatic increase in early diagnosis of DDH, and thus more successful treatment. Approximately 60% of all unstable newborn hips spontaneously become normal within the first 2 to 4 weeks as perinatal laxity resolves. A severely dysplastic hip may have a negative examination because of lack of an acetabular shelf. It is important to stress, however, that not all hips are reducible at birth. This is presumably because of development of dislocation earlier in utero, with evolution of fixed joint contractures. Similarly, it is believed that a few cases of dysplasia may develop after birth. In most large series, it has been shown that not all abnormal hips can be detected by screening, even by skilled examiners.[23] This is because the physical findings are variable and may fall within the range of normal. If the hip remains dislocated, contractures develop, so that by the age of about 6 months most cases cannot be relocated on physical examination in the awake patient. Findings of asymmetry, such as limitation of abduction and of full extension as well as apparent shortening of the thigh, are more sensitive at this time. This last sign, known as the Allis or Galeazzi sign, is noted by comparing the lengths of the two flexed thighs when held together. Asymmetry of skin folds by itself is unreliable and not a highly specific sign, although it is a supportive finding. When the child begins to walk, a positive Trendelenburg sign is noted during gait: when weight is borne on the dislocated side during gait, the pelvis inclines downward, dropping on the other side. Pain is not present, and walking may begin at about the normal age.

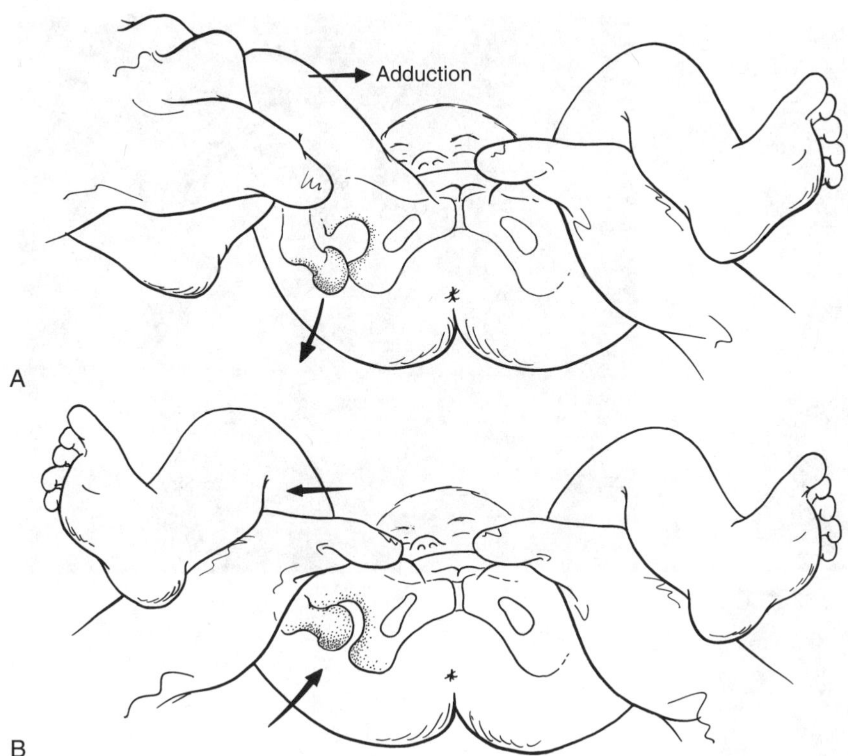

FIG. 99-5. Examination of the hip for DDH. (*A*) Barlow sign, or subluxation with adduction and axial pressure. (*B*) Ortolani sign, or reduction of the hip with abduction.

The surgeon should be especially alert to the possibility of DDH in children with connective tissue disorders, genetic syndromes, or neuromuscular disease.

Except in teratologic conditions, radiographs are not commonly used before 6 months of age because interpretation is more difficult during this time; physical examination remains more reliable. Many centers are using ultrasonography as an objective tool, but interpretation requires much experience and should be done by a pediatric radiologist or orthopedist who is familiar with the technique. Ultrasound is indicated for diagnosis if the neonatal examination is abnormal or questionable, as well as to guide initial treatment[22] (Fig. 99-6*A* and *B*). As the infant grows, plain films may more clearly show cephalad and lateral migration of the femur with a break in the Shenton line (see Fig. 99-6*C*), delayed appearance of the femoral ossific nucleus, a shallow and more vertical acetabulum, and, later, formation of a false acetabulum.

Treatment involves different measures at different ages. The aim of all of these measures is to restore contact between femoral head and acetabulum. Because a high percentage of patients experience spontaneous improvement of lax hip capsules in the early perinatal period, most orthopedists recommend observation of a mild subluxable type of hip, with reexamination at 3 weeks. Dislocated hips are treated at the time of diagnosis. An abduction-flexion device such as a Pavlik harness is most often used. This allows some motion while maintaining the appropriate femoral-acetabular contact. The alignment should be checked by ultrasound or radiography in 1 to 2 weeks.[23] The brace is worn until the clinical and radiologic examinations are normal, a duration approximately equal to one to two times the child's age at diagnosis. If treatment is begun *after* 6 months of age, the child is usually too large and active to tolerate the brace. Then reduction must be preceded by traction to bring the femoral head *down* toward the acetabulum, decreasing the muscle forces that could contribute to avascular necrosis. A manipulative (closed) reduction is thus attempted under general anesthetic.[24] If closed reduction is not successful, open surgical reduction should be carried out. This involves tightening the lax superior capsule and releasing the tight psoas tendon and inferior capsule, allowing the femoral head to be brought down to its appropriate location.

If there is extensive bony deformation, such as a shallow acetabulum or rotated femur, a femoral or pelvic osteotomy as well as open reduction might be indicated. This is more common after the age of 2 years.

Possible complications include persistent dysplasia from failure of normal development, redislocation, and avascular necrosis of the femoral head. The last condition is due to impairment of the epiphyseal vessels by excess pressure or capsular stretch. It is the most serious complication. Its occurrence is more likely if the hip is reduced under excessive tension, or if excessive abduction is used.

The earlier treatment is carried out, the better is the resultant hip development and the safer each of the steps in treatment. Early detection, when possible, can decrease the need for complex orthopedic procedures later on.

Transient (toxic) synovitis of the hip is a diagnosis of exclusion; it is a self-limited condition that is the most common cause of an irritable hip in children. The usual presentation is a painful limp or hip pain of acute or insidious onset, usually occurring unilaterally. The most common ages are 2 to 6 years, but patients from 1 to 15 years have been reported.[25] There is moderate spasm on testing of hip range of motion, particularly internal rotation. Temperature, white blood cell count, C-reactive protein, and erythrocyte sedimentation rate may be normal or slightly elevated. The etiology is unknown; an immune mecha-

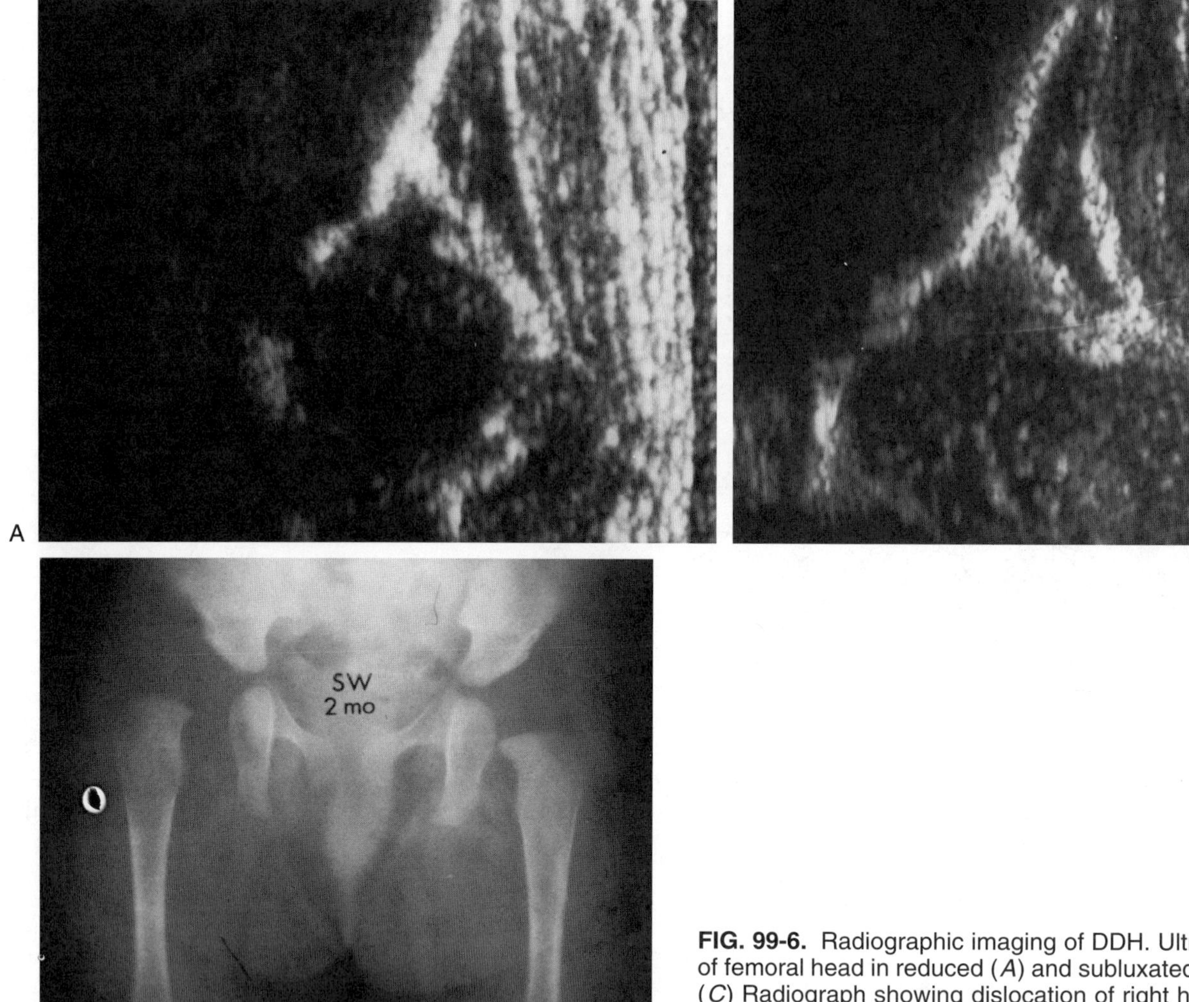

FIG. 99-6. Radiographic imaging of DDH. Ultrasound scans of femoral head in reduced (*A*) and subluxated (*B*) positions. (*C*) Radiograph showing dislocation of right hip is difficult to interpret in first 6 months of life due to lack of ossification of epiphysis.

nism and viral infection have been postulated. Some examples of viral-associated anthropathy have been described. Differential diagnosis should include septic arthritis, osteomyelitis, and Legg-Calvé-Perthes disease, which usually has a subchondral crescent of lucency or further changes in the femoral head on radiograph. Juvenile rheumatoid monarthritis and slipped capital femoral epiphysis should also be considered. Admission to hospital, observation, and early aspiration should be performed if septic arthritis cannot be ruled out. Treatment consists of bed rest with oral analgesics as needed for 2 to 7 days. This can sometimes be done on an outpatient basis with frequent follow-up if septic arthritis is ruled out. Persistence of symptoms beyond 1 week should prompt the physician to perform reevaluation, although persistence of symptoms for as long as 1 month has occasionally been reported.

Legg-Calvé-Perthes disease was first differentiated from tuberculosis within a decade after clinical use of radiography at the turn of the century, but its etiology is still unknown. This disorder consists of ischemia of the proximal femoral epiphysis.[26] The amount of the femoral epiphysis rendered ischemic is variable, and affects the outcome. The ischemia is followed by resorption, then reossification with or without col-

lapse of the femoral head. It most commonly affects children 4 to 8 years old, although exceptions are often seen. Males are affected four times as often as females. Affected patients as a group have slightly shorter stature and delayed bone age compared to peers. Fifteen percent of cases are bilateral, although both sides are not usually affected at the same time.

Clinical presentation is usually a limp, such as abductor lurch, with minimal pain of either short or long duration. The pain is not as acute or severe as that of transient synovitis or septic arthritis. Motions that are especially limited are internal rotation and abduction of the hip. Internal rotation is performed with the patient supine, the hip flexed, measuring the angle to which the leg may be rotated laterally. These movements may be resisted by mild spasm or guarding. At the earliest stage, radiographs may be normal or may reveal slightly smaller size of the affected femoral epiphysis compared to the other side due to its temporary inhibition of growth.[27,28] Later, there may be a narrow crescentic lucency, best seen on the lateral view,[28] which is due to a microfracture of the bone just underneath the joint surface. This reveals the extent of bone involved. In some cases revascularization may occur without collapse of the epiphysis, but in others, revascularization of the femoral head is accompanied by progressive resorption and deformation (Fig. 99-7). Reossification follows, and the femoral head continues to grow. Whether this further growth occurs spherically depends on the patient's age, the amount of collapse, and the method of treatment.

Differential diagnosis should include transient synovitis, septic arthritis, hematogenous osteomyelitis, sickle cell infarct, hemoglobinopathies, steroid-induced necrosis, Gaucher disease, hypothyroidism, and the epiphyseal dysplasias. The last two are often synchronous bilaterally, whereas Legg-Calvé-Perthes is not. Avascular necrosis may also be a serious complication of femoral neck fracture or hip dislocation.

Treatment follows two principles: containment of the femoral head within the acetabulum and maintenance of range of motion. In the early stages of Perthes disease, the avascular portion of the femoral head is less likely to become deformed and more likely to regrow spherically if contained within the mold of the acetabulum by abduction. Children younger than 6 years of age or with involvement of less than one half of the femoral head may be followed without active treatment if a full range of motion is preserved; patients in this age group have a good prognosis.[26] More aggressive treatment is indicated in patients with involvement of more than half of the femoral head or age over 6 years.

Containment may be achieved by a brace or by surgery. The most commonly employed brace is the Scottish Rite brace, which holds the legs abducted and does not extend below the knees. The child may be allowed to play in the brace. The brace should be worn until early reossification of the femoral head takes place. Surgical treatment is used if a brace is not accepted because of the size of the child, an anticipated long duration of wear (up to 18 months in the older child), or lack of acceptance. Either a femoral osteotomy to redirect the involved portion within the acetabulum, or an innominate osteotomy to better redirect the acetabulum may be performed. The two procedures have approximately equal results. Treatment of avascular necrosis that occurs after femoral neck fracture or

dislocation follows similar principles and has a poorer prognosis with increasing age of the child.

Slipped Capital Femoral Epiphysis

Slipped capital femoral epiphysis (SCFE) is a disorder of mechanical overload of the growth plate that occurs near the age of skeletal maturity; it involves a three-dimensional displacement of the epiphysis posteriorly, medially, and inferiorly. In other words, the lower femur is externally rotated from under the head of the femur. The etiology seems to involve mechanical as well as biological factors. SCFE usually occurs without severe sudden force or trauma. Mechanically, there is increased stress because of obesity in most affected children and because of abnormal retroversion (posterior rotation) of the femoral head and neck. The periosteum and growth plate at this age are thin and less able to resist the shearing forces. Possible biologic factors include delayed growth plate maturation and hormonal factors that may be related to the obesity. Increased growth hormone has been associated with decreased physeal shear strength, and hypothyroidism has been found in some cases. SCFE usually occurs during the growth spurt, and before menarche in girls. SCFE is uncommon, with a frequency of 1 to 10 per 100,000. It is more common in males and in blacks. Approximately one quarter to one third of affected children have bilateral involvement,[29] but not usually simultaneously.

Clinical presentation varies with the acuity of the process. Most children with subacute or chronic SCFE present with a limp or pain or both. The discomfort may be in the groin but is very often referred to the thigh or knee. Many patients with thigh or knee complaints are dismissed when no cause is found, only to have the true hip pathology discovered later when the slip worsens. This paradoxical pain distribution is due to referral within the cutaneous distribution of the femoral nerve, which also involves both the hip and knee joints. Other patients have

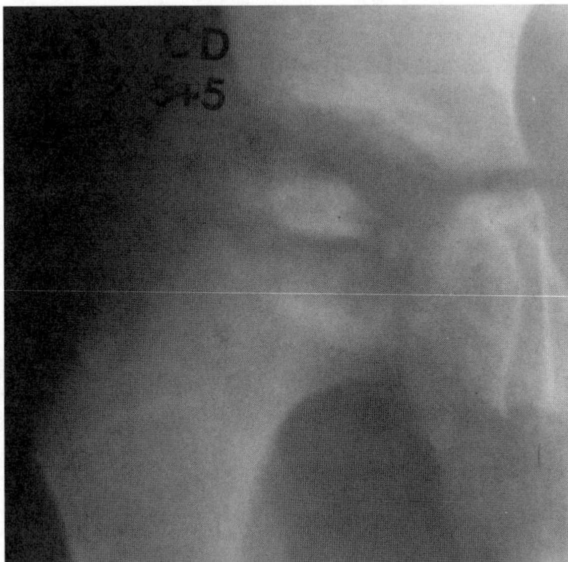
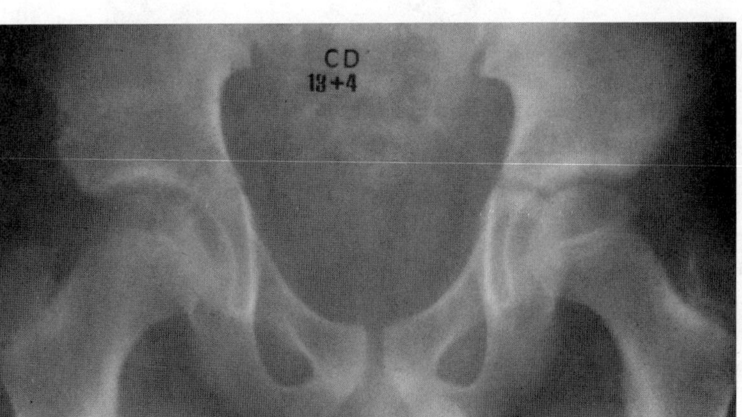

FIG. 99-7. Legg-Calvé-Perthes disease is manifested radiographically by fragmentation and collapse of the femoral head during the initial phase of the disorder (*A*). Later, reossification takes place and can lead to a more spherical femoral head (*B*).

a more acute, sudden presentation, usually following mild to moderate trauma, with severe pain and inability to walk or move the hip. This is more like an acute growth plate fracture. Again, abduction, internal rotation, and flexion are the motions most limited. The involved hip is externally rotated at rest compared to the opposite side. There may be mild limb shortening because of the upward displacement of the metaphysis.

The first radiographic findings are widening and irregularity of the growth plate and osteopenia of the femur (Fig. 99-8). Later, there is displacement of the epiphysis posteriorly, inferiorly, and medially. This is best seen on the frog-leg lateral radiograph of the pelvis. A line on the AP film drawn along through the upper margin of the narrowest portion of the neck should intersect at least 20% of the epiphysis after age 10 years. This is an important point, because with the remodeling that occurs in a chronic slip, there may not be an obvious step-off at the junction of epiphysis and metaphysis or a gap to suggest a fracture. The severity of the slip is graded as mild (less than 33%), moderate (33% to 50%), or severe (more than 50%). Later changes may include avascular necrosis of the epiphysis (seen in 5% to 10%) or chondrolysis, that is, joint space narrowing (seen in 1% to 2%).

Treatment is to prevent further slip, usually by immediately placing the patient at bed rest and arranging prompt orthopedic consultation. The patient should not be allowed to go home once the diagnosis is made. Surgical management is intended to stabilize the upper femur and cause closure of the weakened growth plate. Realignment of the slip and femoral head is not safe in chronic cases, as this may produce avascular necrosis by disrupting the blood supply to the epiphysis. The gold standard of treatment is fixation in situ with a screw. Long-term follow-up shows some remodeling of the slip. The screw should not penetrate into the joint. Open epiphyseal fusion using bone graft avoids the risk of pin penetration and produces more rapid growth plate closure,[29] but it is a longer surgical procedure and requires cast stabilization in acute slips. Osteotomy of the femoral neck to correct the deformity has been occasionally performed, but it carries a risk of avascular necrosis. Later,

osteotomy at the subtrochanteric level, away from the vessels serving the epiphysis, will produce realignment, but it might make later hip replacement, if this should become necessary, more difficult by changing the shape of the proximal femur. The contralateral hip should be monitored for SCFE also and fixed early if symptoms occur. Long-term follow-up shows no early degenerative change unless chondrolysis or avascular necrosis occur; each has an incidence of 1% to 5%. Later arthritis in middle age is still more common than in persons without history of SCFE.

Femoral anteversion is one of several rotational deformities that affect the alignment of the knee and foot with the body. Other causes of in-toeing include internal tibial torsion and foot deformity such as metatarsus adductus. Increased anteversion of the femur is defined as an increase in the angle between (forward rotation of) the plane of the femoral neck and the plane of the posterior femoral condyles. This normally declines with age. The pressure of the anterior hip capsule, as the child stands upright, causes the change. Increased femoral anteversion persists in some neuromuscular conditions because of a lack of these remodeling forces. The type discussed here is idiopathic femoral anteversion.

On physical examination, the patient appears to toe in. The patellae also face medially. Internal rotation of the hip is much greater than external rotation. Anteversion is not usually clinically noticeable or significant unless external rotation at the hip is less than 15 degrees.

On radiographs, the femoral head and neck appear to be in valgus on an AP film. CT scan is best for directly quantitating femoral anteversion in the infrequent situations where this is necessary.

The natural history of femoral anteversion is benign. Anteversion later in life has been found to be unrelated to arthritis of the hip or knee. Anteversion does not impair function or athletic skills. Treatment of increased anteversion consists of observation at least until age 8 and prevention of W-sitting, which may impair remodeling. The child should instead sit in a chair or in the tailor position. Braces employing cables and bars are not effective in derotating the femur; no orthotic method of treatment affects anteversion. In fact, most of these children need no treatment. Femoral osteotomy, proximally or distally, is the only truly effective treatment. It is rarely needed, however, and only in children over 8 who have functional disability due to patellar malalignment, or, rarely, persistent concern with appearance.

Spine

Back problems in children generally fall into two categories: spinal deformity, and back pain. When these conditions exist in the same child, one must first determine the cause of the pain before treating the deformity (Fig. 99-9).

Childhood Back Pain

Back pain in a child is often indicative of a problem that requires further attention and evaluation. Low back pain in the adult age group is very common and often has no demonstrated etiology, but approximately 75% of pediatric cases are found

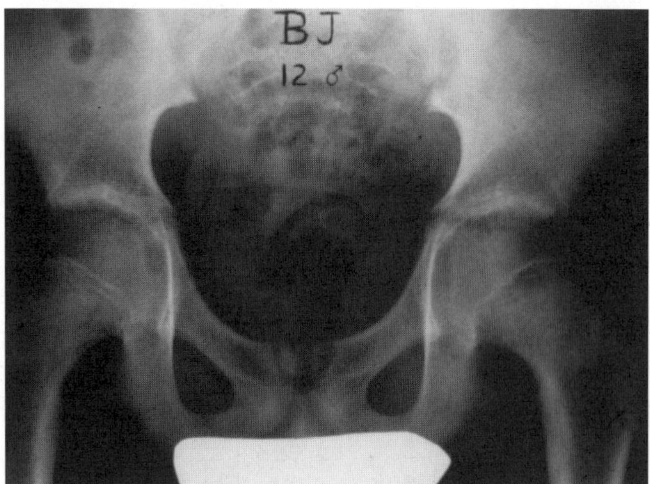

FIG. 99-8. A slipped capital femoral epiphysis is present on the left hip in this radiograph, as manifested by a widening of the growth plate and slight inferior displacement of the epiphysis.

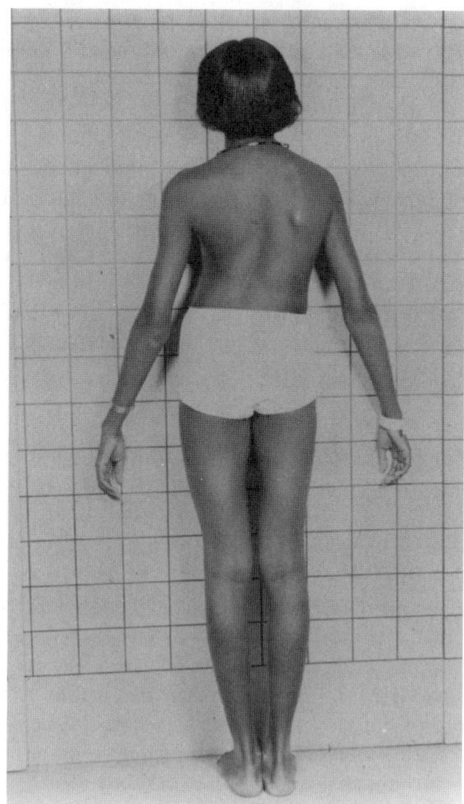

FIG. 99-9. Physical findings in scoliosis include asymmetry of the shoulders, scapulae, and waistline, as well as a midline curve in the spine itself.

to have a definite cause. Factors that increase the index of suspicion for a serious problem include interference with school or play, need for medication, or age under 4. Careful neurologic examination is a must when evaluating children for back pain, as is an assessment of spinal flexibility and deformity. The differential diagnoses listed below are the most commonly encountered conditions.

Musculoligamentous Pain

All components of a child's spine—discs, ligaments, muscles, and joint capsules—are flexible and conform easily to spinal positions encountered daily in the schoolyard or playing field. After about the age of 12, the spine generally loses some of its flexibility, and during the teenage years, further stiffening may take place. Below the age of 10, muscular or ligamentous back pain is rare. This diagnosis should be reserved for the older child, who may be involved in a new physical activity, and who has pain in the lumbar area for which no other specific cause can be determined. This is really a presumptive diagnosis. To merit this diagnosis, the child should have pain localized to the lumbar area, a normal neurologic examination, normal radiographs of the lumbar spine, and, in some instances, a normal bone scan.

Once the diagnosis of musculoligamentous pain has been made, the treatment is rest from any activity that causes pain. Use of ice or heat is efficacious. Once the pain has resolved,

exercises to strengthen the abdominal and lumbar muscles should be used before returning to sports. A lumbosacral corset may be worn in the acute stage and thereafter when participating in sports to protect the lower back and its muscles from extremes of spinal movement. A long-term corset or other brace is rarely needed if this diagnosis is correct. Once low-back pain has resolved, it is important to stress to the child that warming up prior to sports activity is more necessary for him or her than for other children. Exercises may need to be continued indefinitely. Persistence of pain should lead to a search further for unusual causes of back pain.

Spondylolysis and Spondylolisthesis

Spondylolysis, a relatively common cause of childhood back pain, is usually a stress fracture of the pars interarticularis of the vertebra.[30] This thin segment of bone between the facet joints is subjected to high forces, especially with marked lordosis of the lumbar spine or with heavy lifting. The overall incidence in the general population is about 6%. Most of these stress fractures probably occur in early school years, although symptoms appear most frequently when the children are in their early teens. There is a much higher frequency of spondylolysis in children who participate in gymnastics, wrestling, and weight lifting, at times approaching 20% of participants in these sports.

Symptoms most commonly are pain in the lumbar area after or during a sports activity and a concomitant limitation of lumbar spine motion. If the child has a chronic spondylolysis, the pain is often intermittent; if the spondylolysis is acute, the pain is more severe. Radiation of pain along the sciatic nerve distribution into the lateral calf or dorsum of the foot may occasionally be present.

Physical examination may not be remarkable. Usually there is limitation of lateral spine flexion toward the side of the spondylolysis, often associated with limited forward flexion from back pain. Back pain may be produced by straight-leg raising, but radiation of pain into the legs by this maneuver is rare. Neurologic examination is normal.

The diagnosis can usually be made by lumbar spine radiographs (Fig. 99-10). The most common location is at L5, with L4 the next most common. Spondylolysis can sometimes be visualized by the lateral view, but oblique views are usually more definitive. In addition, the oblique views allow one to determine the unilaterality or bilaterality of the defect. If a lytic defect is observed, the age of the lesion should be determined if possible. The spondylolysis is generally old if there are sclerotic edges to the defect. Spondylolysis may occasionally be caused by acute trauma in the adolescent, but more often this represents a preexisting lesion that is simply brought out by the trauma. A technetium-99 bone scan with collimated views is helpful to determine the age of the stress fracture. If the scan is cold and sclerotic edges are present on radiograph, the lesion is old, and it will not be possible to obtain bone union nonoperatively. However, if the scan shows increased uptake at the lytic area and the radiographs show no sclerotic edges, there may be enough reparative activity that the stress fractures might heal if the child is placed in a body jacket brace or cast.

If the scan shows no increased uptake, the treatment of spondylolysis is much like that of a musculoligamentous problem.[30] First, rest from activity is recommended. A lumbosacral corset

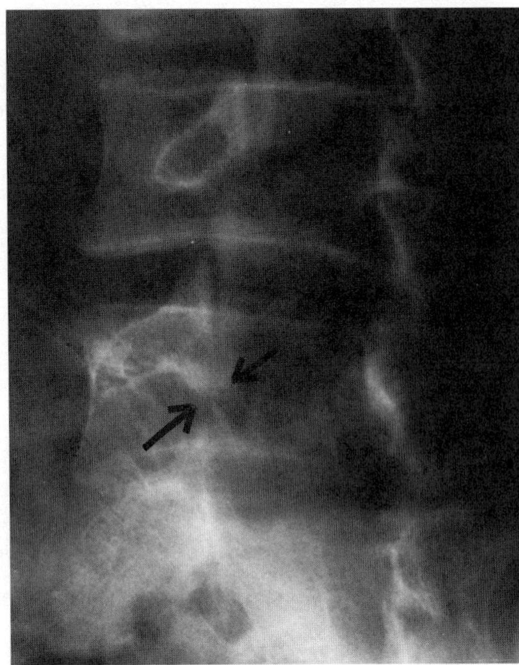

FIG. 99-10. Spondylolysis is shown radiographically as a break in the pars interarticularis of the vertebra (*arrows*) on this oblique radiograph.

is often helpful for a few weeks until pain resolves. Some teenagers with spondylolysis prefer to wear the corset during sports activities as added protection even after acute back pain resolves. Fusion for spondylolysis without significant spondylolisthesis is generally not needed. With the exception of occasional episodes of low-back pain, teenagers can be allowed to participate in sports if they do not repeatedly experience back pain after playing.

Spondylolisthesis follows spondylolysis in some children. This condition is a forward slip of a superior vertebra on the inferior vertebra, most commonly a slip of L5 on the sacrum. Worsening of this slip may occur with growth of the spine, and there is generally little worsening once growth is completed. As the vertebra slips forward, the posterior elements remain behind, attached to the adjacent vertebrae by their ligaments. The combination of excessive motion of the posterior elements and the forward vertebral slip may lead to irritation of L5 or S1 nerve roots. As the slip is usually slow, the nerve root irritation may present only as progressive tightness of the hamstrings, manifested by difficulty in touching the toes or in reaching objects on the floor. If one side of the spine is affected more than the other, scoliosis may also be present.

On physical examination, the main finding is limitation of straight-leg raising because of the hamstring spasm. Radiation of pain into the calf or foot with straight-leg raising may indicate more advanced nerve root irritation. Rarely, the ankle jerk reflex may be diminished.

The diagnosis of spondylolisthesis can be made by plain radiographs and is most easily seen on the lateral view. The amount of slip should be quantified using the terms grade 1 to grade 4 (grade 1, up to 25%; grade 2, up to 50%; and so forth). If the slip is greater than 50%, posterior spinal fusion of the involved level is indicated. If the slip is less than 50%, initial

management is directed to relief of back pain and hamstring spasm, using rest and corset therapy followed by exercises as with spondylolysis. If the pain does not respond to conservative treatment, fusion may be needed. If the pain improves with conservative treatment, follow-up lateral lumbosacral radiographs at 6- to 9-month intervals are recommended until growth is complete or until a worsening slip can be identified. If there is an increase in the percentage of slip, fusion is indicated.

If a child does not have hamstring tightness and is pain free, there is usually no need to restrict activities, provided the child and the parents are aware that periodic low-grade back pain is likely. There is no evidence that increased physical activity causes an increase in vertebral slip.

Intervertebral Disc Herniation (Herniated Nucleus Pulposus)

Herniation of the intervertebral disc is common in the young and middle-aged adult as a cause of back and leg pain. In this adult age group, disc protrusion occurs posteriorly, with the protruded disc compressing the nerve roots or the cauda equina. If similar forces are applied to the spine of a skeletally immature child, the disc does not rupture posteriorly, but the stress leads to a fracture of the growth plate of the vertebral body, causing extrusion of disc material anteriorly or into the vertebral body itself (Schmorl nodes). Most of these children present with back pain without radiation into the lower leg or calf. If nerve root pain also occurs, a small avulsion fracture of the ring apophysis posterolaterally might be present in such a position to cause nerve root compression. The diagnosis of an old disc injury in a child can be confirmed by radiographic findings of a narrowed lumbar disc adjacent to an irregular vertebral end plate.

If no neurologic defect is present, treatment consists of symptomatic care, usually rest, until the pain resolves. If the condition is the result of a vehicular accident, evaluation for development of an ileus should be performed. If there is leg pain as well as back pain, a magnetic resonance imaging (MRI) scan or CT/myelogram should be performed to localize any neural compression, which may be relieved by surgical treatment, with 90% satisfactory results after 5 years.

Discitis

Severe back pain with limitation of back movements is common in the older child, while the younger children may simply present with stiffness, refusing to walk, or limping. Bacterial infection is the most commonly suspected cause. Just as in long bones in children, the vascular anatomy of the growing disc varies from that of the adult, and common bacteremias of childhood can more readily infect the disc than the vertebral body itself. Approximately 50% of these children have positive blood cultures at the time of their acute pain, the most common organism being *Staphylococcus aureus*. Despite this, discitis in its milder forms often appears to resolve without the need for antibiotics.

On physical examination, the most common finding is marked stiffness of the spine on forward bending. Abdominal pain or guarding may occur. Fever is often present. Neurological examination is normal. Early in the course, radiographs of

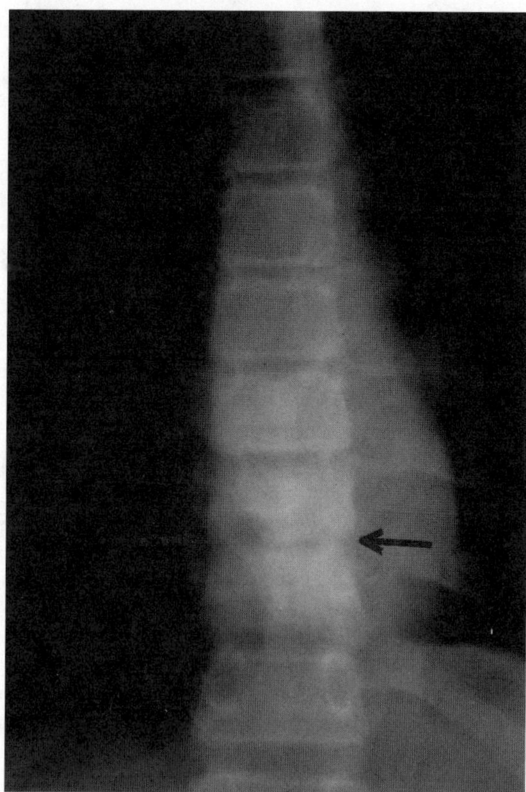

FIG. 99-11. Discitis, in the advanced stages, may be indicated by sclerosis and narrowing of the intervertebral disc as seen here at T10 to 11 (*arrows*).

the spine are normal. Technetium-99 bone scan shows increased uptake at the involved disc early on, before radiographic changes are seen; this scan should be performed whenever discitis is suspected. A few weeks after onset of pain, sclerosis and narrowing of a single disc may be seen on radiograph (Fig. 99-11). The lumbar or thoracic spine may be involved. The sedimentation rate and white blood cell count are often elevated. If the bone scan is positive or the clinical presentation is usual for discitis, needle aspiration or open biopsy of the involved disc is generally not necessary.

Treatment options include antibiotics, bed rest, and body brace or cast, depending on the severity of findings at presentation. If a positive blood culture has been obtained, antibiotics should be given for 3 to 6 weeks. The author's preference is to give antibiotics in children with a positive bone scan, even if no bacteremia has been demonstrated. Bed rest may be helpful as an adjunct if there is severe pain or spasm. If the spasm persists for more than a few days, a trunk brace or cast relieves symptoms by immobilizing the spine and allowing ambulation on a limited basis. The infection is usually cleared with 6 to 8 weeks of treatment. Discitis rarely develops into vertebral osteomyelitis with local bone destruction.

Spinal Cord Tumors

Back pain and limitation of spine movement also may be seen as the presenting problem in spinal cord tumors, even without a neurologic deficit. In spinal cord tumors, the presenting complaint is back pain or scoliosis or both in almost a third of children. The most striking finding on the physical examination is severe limitation of forward flexion of the spine. Pain may be worsened by neck flexion. Neurologic changes may be very subtle and difficult to detect.

In patients with back pain and marked limitation of spinal motion, especially if scoliosis is also present, an MRI is needed if the bone scan and plain radiographs do not elucidate the cause.

The most common tumor to present in this fashion is an ependymoma. Treatment is neurosurgical. If the tumor is benign and can be removed, the pain, scoliosis, and back stiffness generally resolve.

Spinal Deformity

Spinal deformity of minor or significant degree occurs in up to 1 of 20 children. Differentiating those that require treatment is important. Scoliosis, a lateral curvature of the spine, is the most common. The age at development of most spinal curvatures, early adolescence, is a time when parents may not be likely to see the child's back frequently. School screening programs for spinal deformity, mandatory in many states, have served to increase awareness of these conditions. Although school programs are generally targeted toward children in the 6th grade, routine evaluation of the back should also be a feature of each child's annual examination.

Scoliosis

The two forms of scoliosis are postural and structural. *Postural* scoliosis results from factors outside the spine, such as leg length discrepancy. In these cases, if the leg lengths are equalized or if the child sits, the spine becomes straight, indicating that there is no structural abnormality. The more important type of scoliosis is termed *structural*, and it involves not only a lateral spinal curvature, but also a rotation of the vertebrae as well. While numerous conditions are associated with scoliosis, the most common causes include idiopathic (80%), congenital (5%), neuromuscular (10%), and miscellaneous (5%). The miscellaneous group includes connective tissue disorders, genetic diseases, and other less common conditions.

Congenital scoliosis is defined as that due to a primary vertebral malformation, such as a hemivertebra or a wedged vertebra. It is present at birth, although the diagnosis is often not made at that time (Figure 99-12). This may be associated with other birth defects or may be an isolated condition. Because the genitourinary (GU) system arises embryologically from the same region as the spine, about 30% of children with congenital spinal deformity have an associated GU abnormality. The most common anomaly is unilateral renal agenesis, so a sonogram or intravenous pyelogram should be performed on all patients with congenital scoliosis or kyphosis. Active treatment of unilateral kidney absence may not be necessary, but appropriate cautions against contact sports that may lead to kidney injury are important. Tracheoesophageal fistula, imperforate anus, and congenital cardiac defects are often associated with congenital scoliosis. These components make up the VATER syndrome, although not all components are seen in every patient. The spine should

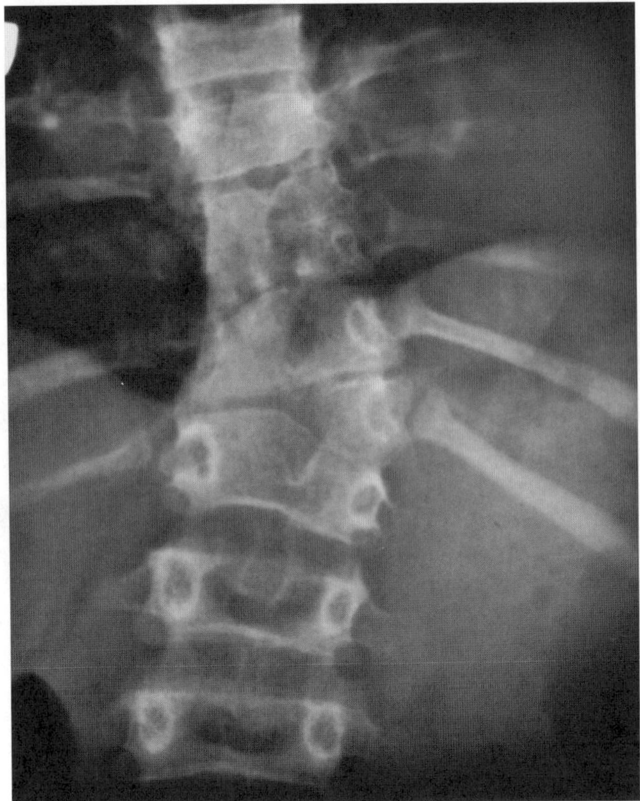

FIG. 99-12. Congenital scoliosis is due to a primary bony malformation, as shown here by this hemivertebra.

be examined radiographically early in all these patients. Management of congenital scoliosis consists of serial radiographic follow-up every 6 to 12 months to determine if the deformity is worsening. If no increase in the curve occurs, further treatment is generally not needed. If worsening of 5 to 10 degrees or more is documented while there is growth remaining, surgical fusion is necessary, no matter what the age of the child. Brace treatment for the congenital scoliosis itself is seldom successful or indicated, because a brace cannot change the shape or growth of a malformed vertebra.

Neuromuscular scoliosis is a deformity that may be associated with almost any neurologic or muscular disease which affects the trunk, such as quadriplegic cerebral palsy, muscular dystrophy, high spina bifida, and poliomyelitis. A spinal curvature secondary to muscular imbalance is classically C-shaped and extends to include the pelvis (Figure 99-13); these features are not commonly seen in idiopathic scoliosis. Scoliosis is more often present and worsens most quickly in patients who are nonwalkers as a result of their neuromuscular disease. With continued worsening of the curve, sitting balance becomes further impaired, and function may be limited by the need to use one arm or hand to assist in sitting. Treatment centers on preservation of the ability to sit and to be transported, and to minimize decline in pulmonary function. Many of these patients have feeding and swallowing problems such as malnutrition and reflux with risk of aspiration. It has been shown that prior treatment of these conditions can decrease risk of complications after major spine corrections. Pediatric general surgical consultation is often required. Methods used for feeding may include oral, tube, or gastrotomy feeds or fundoplication or jejunos-

tomy. Although brace wear is often useful, surgical fusion is frequently indicated to preserve function.

Idiopathic scoliosis is generally found in otherwise healthy children. While idiopathic scoliosis requiring treatment is about eight times more frequent in girls than in boys, the incidence of mild curves is approximately equal between the sexes.[30] In other words, girls seem to have more tendency to worsening of the curves.

A family history of curvature of the spine is found in about two thirds of children with scoliosis, although the exact mode of inheritance has not been determined. The etiology of idiopathic scoliosis remains unknown, but it is currently thought that a combination of neurohormonal and connective tissue factors is important. Scoliosis is also more likely to develop in children who have had thoracotomy or pectus repair or cardiac surgery. It may develop several years after these index procedures, so the surgeon should examine for this and also alert the pediatrician. Marfan syndrome and neurofibromatosis are also associated with an increased risk of scoliosis and should be ruled out. Curves worsen most during the rapid adolescent growth spurt, a time when most curves are diagnosed. Muscles, discs, and bone appear to be normal in the young idiopathic scoliosis patient.

The key to early detection of scoliosis is to carefully assess the entire trunk for asymmetry. The child should be examined with the back clearly exposed. The examination should include evaluation of shoulder height, scapular position and prominence, waistline symmetry, and level of height of the two sides of the pelvis. Asymmetry in any of these areas may indicate a

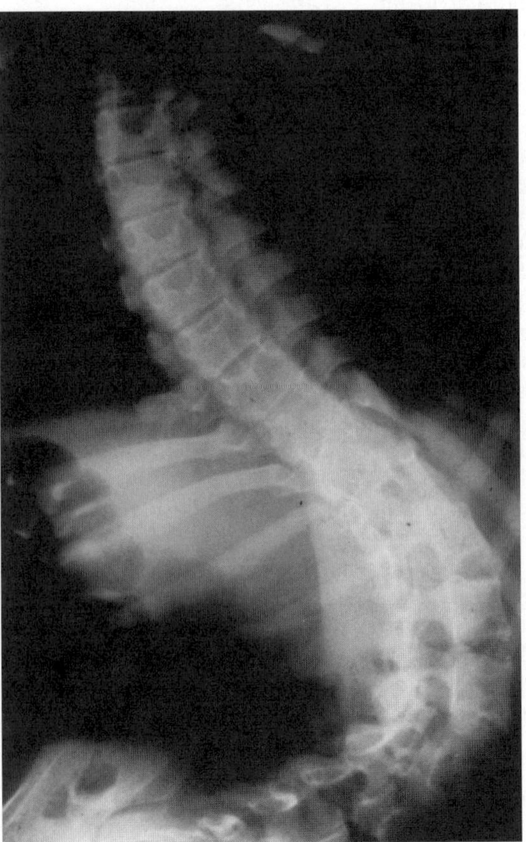

FIG. 99-13. In neuromuscular scoliosis, there is usually a long, sweeping curve with pelvic obliquity.

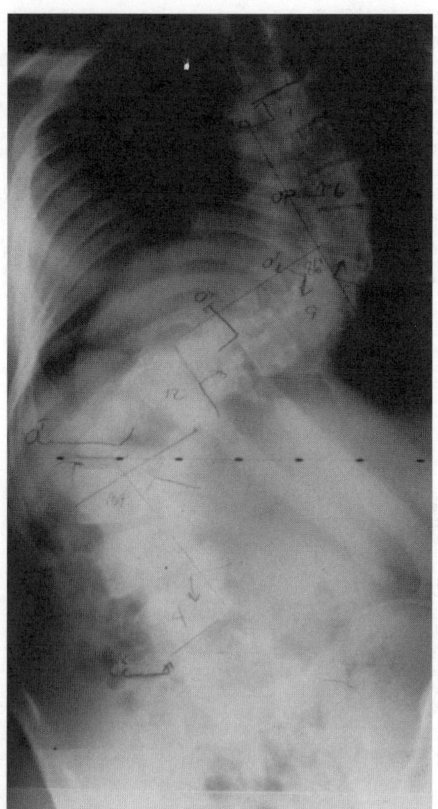

FIG. 99-14. Typical radiographic appearance of a double-major idiopathic scoliosis. Notice that the two curves balance each other, so there is a level pelvis. The curves are 8 to 9 degrees by the Cobb measurement.

scoliosis. However, in about 50% of children with uneven shoulder height, no spinal deformity is present on radiograph. To define further whether or not a structural scoliosis is present, a more sensitive and specific examination is the forward-bend test. The patient should stand with legs straight and together, arms collapsed in front of the body, and slowly bend forward to touch the toes. The examiner, positioned in front and in back of the patient, can see the profile, in sequence, of the thoracic and lumbar regions. It is possible to quantitate the amount of rib prominence by means of an inclinometer placed at the apex of the curve with the child bending forward. If the inclinometer measurement is 5 degrees or less, the scoliosis is rarely significant and radiographs are usually not needed. If the inclinometer reading exceeds 7 degrees, a standing posteroanterior radiograph is indicated for better assessment.

The magnitude of the scoliosis is measured radiographically by the Cobb method. The angle between the end plates of the upper and lower most inclined vertebrae is drawn. This measurement should always be performed on a standing spine radiograph (Figure 99-14). The error of measurement for this method is approximately $\pm$ 5 degrees. No active treatment is needed until the curve reaches 25 degrees. During the adolescent growth spurt, maximum annual curve progression is 10 to 15 degrees or about 1 degree per month.

Completion of growth or skeletal maturity can be assessed most accurately by the bone age on radiographs of the hand and wrist. From the clinical standpoint, girls who have been menstruating for 2 years have essentially completed their spinal growth.

Treatment of scoliosis is based on three fundamental principles.

1. Curves over 25 degrees are likely to increase if the child is still growing.
2. Curves over 40 to 50 degrees are likely to increase even after growth is complete.
3. Some degree of clinically significant pulmonary restriction may begin in association with thoracic curves over about 75 degrees.

Therefore, if a child is skeletally mature and has curvature of under 25 degrees, no further evaluation or treatment of scoliosis is needed. If the scoliosis is 25 degrees or more and the child has growth remaining, brace treatment is generally recommended. It is successful in about 80% of the patients who wear the brace as prescribed. Spinal exercises alone do not stop the curve from worsening. Once brace treatment begins, it is continued until growth is complete. The brace is usually worn 18 to 20 hours daily. There are no limitations of physical activity because of the scoliosis. Success in brace wear is defined as prevention of further increase in the curve progression and not curve correction, as long-term follow-up studies have shown that the final curvature size is virtually the same as before brace treatment began. While the child and parents are often dismayed by the inability to straighten the spine nonoperatively, if curves can be kept below 35 to 40 degrees by the completion of growth, most scolioses do not worsen in adult life and do not cause problems. If the thoracic curve is over 50 degrees or the lumbar curve is over 40 degrees at the completion of growth, increase in the curve usually continues at the rate of about 1 degree annually, and surgery is usually needed.

Surgical treatment is recommended for curves over 40 degrees, particularly if the child is not fully grown. The surgical treatment usually consists of instrumentation (rods) to correct the curved area of the spine, combined with bone graft to promote spinal fusion of the instrumented area (Figure 99-15). This may be done anteriorly or posteriorly or both, according to the judgment of the surgeon. Posterior spine fusion is done through an incision down the middle of the back and can be extended to include the entire spine if needed. Anterior fusion is done through a thoracotomy for thoracic curves and through a retroperitoneal incision for lumbar curves, and may include peripheral detachment of the diaphragm for thoracolumbar curves. Sometimes, if the patient is malnourished or several staged sequential surgeries are planned, central venous hyperalimentation in between stages may be used. Correction of the scoliosis is generally possible to about 50% of the initial curve measurement. Ileus is common for a few days after surgery. Failure of fusion occurs in only about 1% of teenagers. Fusion is complete by 6 to 12 months after surgery, at which time the teenager can return to almost all physical activities, except tackle football, wrestling, and gymnastics. Patients should be encouraged to return to activity, including gym in school, to reduce the psychological potential for disability following this surgery.

If the thoracic scoliosis exceeds 50 to 75 degrees, it is common to have diminished vital capacity and residual lung volumes on pulmonary function testing. Arterial blood gases and forced expiratory volume in 1 second (FEV_1) are normal except in patients

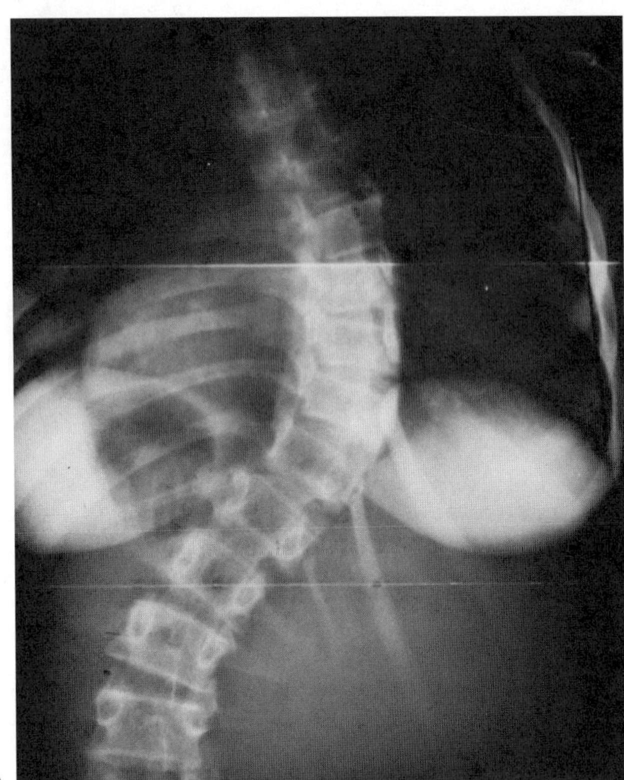
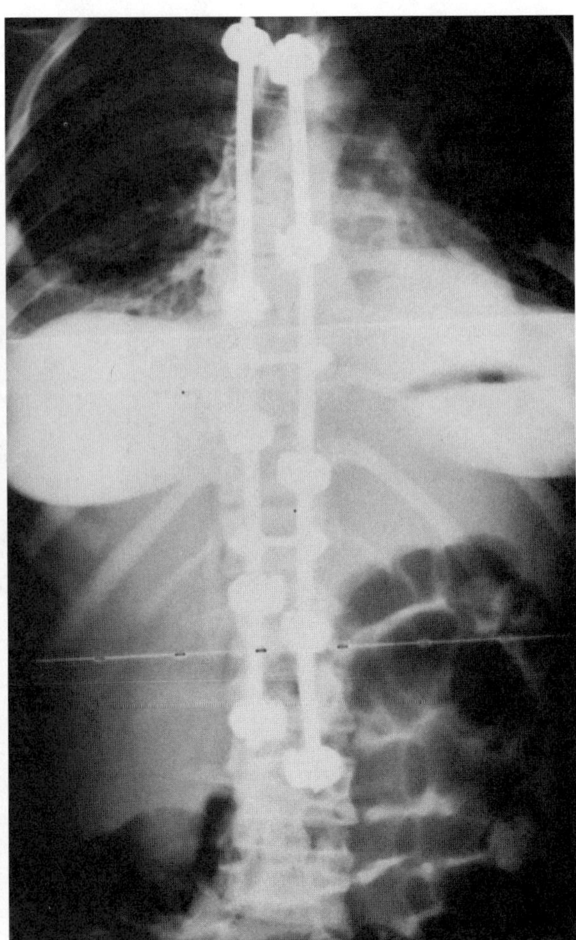

FIG. 99-15. Right thoracic idiopathic scoliosis measuring 57 degrees before correction (*A*). After correction with Cotrel-Dubousset rods (*B*), the curve measures 8 degrees.

with severe curves. Vital capacity is decreased further if there is a thoracic lordosis in association with the scoliosis. Even with the surgical correction of the scoliosis, pulmonary function postoperatively is almost unchanged from preoperatively, because of the persistence of chest wall or rib deformity that has occurred secondary to the scoliosis. It is obviously preferable to prevent scoliosis from progressing to that point.

Pain is rare during adolescence with idiopathic scoliosis. Although in middle age pain may result from degenerative changes, if pain is present during adolescence, further evaluation is indicated. If the neurologic examination is normal, a technetium-99 bone scan is necessary to screen for discitis, stress fracture, osteoid osteoma, or other bone tumors. If there is limited spinal flexion or a neurologic deficit, an MRI is indicated to rule out intraspinal pathology such as a syrinx. All these conditions may cause scoliosis, but the scoliosis usually resolves once the underlying cause is treated appropriately. One should be thoroughly familiar with treatable causes of scoliosis before diagnosing idiopathic scoliosis and instituting brace treatment or recommending spinal fusion.

Kyphosis

Normal spinal sagittal (lateral) contours include lordosis in the cervical and lumbar spinal segments to balance the kyphosis in the thoracic area. The term *kyphosis* is sometimes used to describe abnormal conditions in which there is an increased rounding of the back in the thoracic or thoracolumbar area. The parents usually notice the child's poor posture. The assessment of apparent excessive kyphosis should include a forward bending examination, viewed from the side, to determine if the back is flexible or rigid.

The least serious of cause of kyphosis is *postural roundback*. This most commonly is seen in the preadolescent years. It is seen more often in children who are taller than their peers. This condition is a flexible kyphosis that can be straightened voluntarily by the child and can be well corrected with hyperextension positioning. Kyphosis is one spinal deformity that can be treated by exercises alone. Active hyperextension of the trunk and sit-ups to decrease lumbar lordosis are useful in improving trunk control. Provided no fixed deformity is established, as the teenager's body image improves, so does the rounding of the upper back.

A more fixed and less flexible thoracic or thoracolumbar kyphosis with irregular vertebrae endplates is usually referred to as *Scheuermann disease*. This condition occurs most commonly in teenage boys. Attempts to passively correct Scheuermann kyphosis are unsuccessful, and there is often an associated increased lumbar lordosis. A lateral radiograph of the spine demonstrates irregularity of numerous disc spaces and anterior vertebral body wedging. To establish the diagnosis of Scheuermann kyphosis radiographically, at least 5 degrees of wedging in three adjacent vertebrae should be demonstrated.[30] The Cobb method is employed to quantitate the amount of kyphosis present. The amount of kyphosis present in a normal individual from T3 to T12 is between 20 and 45 degrees. If the kyphosis is present in the thoracolumbar area (T10 to T12), which is normally straight on a lateral radiograph, measurements over 25 degrees are abnormal.

If wedging is present, if there is little correction with thoracic spine hyperextension, and if the thoracic kyphosis is 50 to 65 degrees, bracing is indicated, provided the patient still has remaining growth. A Milwaukee brace, which employs a neck ring in addition to trunk pads, should be used. Unlike scoliosis, where little correction results from bracing, in kyphosis, approximately 10 to 20 degrees improvement in the kyphosis can be anticipated after one year of full-time brace wear. Once this correction is obtained, nighttime brace wear until growth is complete is generally sufficient.[30]

Increased thoracic kyphosis does not cause abnormalities in pulmonary function. The principal problem that may be caused by Scheuermann disease is pain in the thoracic spine. In rare cases, if the kyphosis exceeds 70 degrees by the completion of growth, spinal instrumentation and fusion are performed.

Congenital kyphosis is less common than congenital scoliosis but almost always requires early spinal fusion surgery. If the congenital kyphosis progresses unchecked, spinal cord compression at the apex of the kyphosis may occur. As with congenital scoliosis, evaluation for associated genitourinary abnormalities should be performed.

Cervical Spine

The pediatric cervical spine, owing to its many normal variations on radiographs, is often a confusing area to evaluate. On the lateral cervical spine radiograph, the anterior and superior corner of each vertebral body is normally the last part to ossify, sometimes giving the appearance of a small compression fracture. Full ossification and development of the odontoid process is not complete in the young child and may give the appearance of being maldeveloped. The spine of the child under 10 years is much more flexible than in teenagers or older adults. Up to 3 mm anterior movement of C2 on C3 with flexion (termed pseudosubluxation) is normal in this age group; in adults, none should be present. In fact, when subjected experimentally to stretch, the newborn spine can stretch approximately 2 inches before failing, whereas the spinal cord stretches only one-half inch before it ruptures. Because of this difference in elasticity, infants may sustain spinal cord injury without apparent spinal fracture during birth or during auto accidents. The proper use of car seating supports for these very young children decreases the risk of these devastating injuries. (See Section B: Trauma.)

Children with Down syndrome are a special group. They commonly have instability of the occipitoatlantoaxial region. If this instability persists unrecognized, spinal cord compression with myelopathy may result, leading to leg weakness and impaired walking ability. Lateral cervical flexion/extension radiographs should be performed at age 3 to 4 years in all children with Down syndrome. Approximately 15% of these children show some evidence of atlantoaxial instability, but the majority

do not need fusion surgery; they can be followed periodically by neurologic exam.[31] Gait, strength, reflexes, and clonus should be checked. If the first radiograph showed increased laxity, it should be repeated every 2 years. Atlantoaxial posterior fusion is recommended if a neurologic deficit or excessive instability (greater than 5 to 8 mm translation on flexion-extension) is present.[31]

Instability of the upper cervical spine may also be seen with os odontoideum or from odontoid hypoplasia. Os odontoideum is most likely the result of an early childhood fall that caused a fracture through one of the growth plates of the odontoid process. This unrecognized fracture develops into a fibrous nonunion, which gradually becomes unstable over the ensuing months and years. The diagnosis usually comes to light when evaluating the child with neck pain, or as an incidental finding following head or neck trauma. Neurologic examination may be normal, but if the area is unstable, atlantoaxial fusion is generally indicated to stabilize this region and to protect the spinal cord from sudden, catastrophic and possibly fatal injury. After successful fusion, normal activity can be allowed, although the child has mild limitation of head rotation. Odontoid hypoplasia occurs in normal children periodically, but it is most often associated with genetic disorders, such as Morquio syndrome and spondyloepiphyseal dysplasia congenita. The C1 to C2 segment is often unstable in these conditions, as seen on flexion-extension films. If so, fusion is necessary.

Torticollis is most commonly present at or near the time of birth, being due to a contracture of one sternocleidomastoid muscle. The child's head is tilted toward the side of contracture, with the chin rotated away from the contracted side, because the origin of the contracted muscle is on the mastoid process. The etiology is not well defined, but it may be due to stretch of the involved muscle, or a compartment syndrome developing in utero. The incidence is higher in children with breech presentation and forceps delivery. Commonly, a fusiform firm mass is palpable in the body of the contracted sternocleidomastoid muscle. These children often have plagiocephaly, or asymmetry of facial and skull development. If the neck range of motion can be returned to normal by the age of 1 year, this facial asymmetry disappears. If the torticollis is untreated until later in childhood, the craniofacial bones have less chance of remodeling to become level. This is discussed in Chapter 51.

Cervical spine radiographs should be evaluated to ensure that the head position is not due to congenital spine abnormalities, such as hemivertebrae. If the bony cervical spine is normal, stretching exercises should be instituted shortly after birth. These exercises are designed to stretch the contracted sternocleidomastoid muscle and should be taught to the parents by a knowledgeable physical therapist. While one of the parents should be asked to administer these stretching exercises at home, initial weekly checks by the therapist can help ensure compliance. If, despite stretching exercises, there continues to be a significant contracture by the age of 1 year, surgical treatment to lengthen the sternocleidomastoid is appropriate. This is done at the distal border of the sternocleidomastoid, with proximal lengthening near the mastoid added if needed. Even after surgical release, some stretching and, at times, bracing will continue to be needed as growth continues.

Torticollis due to C1 to C2 rotatory subluxation may present later in childhood following an upper respiratory infection or after trauma. Torticollis following an upper respiratory infection is thought to result from retropharyngeal inflammation and edema that leads to ligamentous laxity allowing subluxation at the atlantoaxial level, causing a rotatory deformity. Similarly, after muscular neck trauma, the child may have a persistent torticollis for several days or weeks, secondary to an unsuspected rotatory subluxation at the atlantoaxial level. CT imaging C1 to C2 is the best means of making this diagnosis. It should be done with the head as close to straight as the patient allows. If torticollis from either of these causes persists, the child is treated with traction, which usually reduces the subluxation, followed by either bracing or atlantoaxial fusion. Fusion is reserved for cases that do not reduce, or that develop recurrent subluxation. The likelihood of need for surgical fusion increases with increasing duration of symptoms, so prompt treatment is recommended. Other causes of torticollis to be ruled out include eye muscle imbalance, spinal cord tumor, or cervical abscess.

Klippel-Feil Syndrome

Failure of normal vertebral development in the cervical spine is known as Klippel-Feil syndrome. In the milder forms, when only two or three vertebrae are fused, diagnosis may not be made until the neck undergoes radiographs for other reasons. However, in children with more levels fused, the neck is very short, and the child appears to have webbing of the base of the neck. Often Klippel-Feil syndrome is associated with Sprengel deformity, a failure of normal descent of the scapulae. Associated GU abnormalities may be present, and a sonogram or IVP is indicated when the diagnosis of Klippel-Feil syndrome is made. There is little specific treatment for this syndrome. Because of the congenital fusion of several segments, excessive strain and thus instability may occur at the levels that move. If this instability is excessive or if neurologic deficits are present, it is necessary to fuse the unstable segment. Surgical fusion may also be needed in adult life for degenerative changes at the mobile segments.

Particularly in the more intensive cases, contact sports, diving, or manual labor are best avoided. Any neck injury in a child with Klippel-Feil syndrome is apt to be serious, because of the limited flexibility of the cervical area.

Upper Extremity

Congenital and developmental abnormalities of the upper extremities of children are less common than those of the lower extremity, perhaps partly because of the lower stresses imposed on the upper extremity in utero and later during standing. They are therefore not covered as extensively in this review. The reader is referred to the texts by Dobyns and colleagues[32] and by Bora[33] and to complete monographs.

Obstetric (Brachial Plexus) Palsy

The brachial plexus is normally composed of nerve root contributions from C5 to T1. Most severe injuries to the area involve lateral flexion of the neck or downward pressure on the shoulder, such as occur during a difficult delivery. Therefore, the upper portions of the plexus (C5 to C7) are most commonly stretched in a manner similar to the pathogenesis of ''burners'' seen in football players. This stretching causes denervation of the shoulder abductors and elbow flexors, resulting in gradual joint contractures if untreated.[34] This is known as Erb-Duchenne palsy. The lower plexus (C7 to T1) can be affected by hyperabduction-traction and has a poorer prognosis; this is the rarest type and is called Klumpke palsy. In these cases, loss of function of the elbow extensors and wrist flexors and finger muscles and possibly Horner syndrome result. The entire plexus may occasionally be involved.

Factors associated with brachial plexus palsy include shoulder dystocia, breech position, high birth weight, and prolonged labor. The incidence is 1 to 3 per 1000 births. Incidence and severity have gradually declined as obstetric care has improved. The site of injury may be at any level from the origin of the nerve roots to the plexus itself, but even root lesions may sometimes resolve spontaneously. On physical examination, the early typical Erb palsy presents with an arm that is internally rotated at the shoulder, extended at the elbow, and flexed at the fingers. Passive range of motion should be full in the early months.

Skeletal injuries such as clavicle fractures and proximal humeral separations should be ruled out radiographically, although they can often be differentiated because they cause guarding on passive motion and by the presence of the Moro response. Testing for the Moro reflex simulates some shoulder and elbow flexion even in the presence of a fracture, but not in the presence of a palsy. Because of the trauma, palsy and skeletal injury may coexist.

Treatment involves maintenance of motion and tendon transfers for those rare, severe cases without spontaneous return of function. However, with current obstetric practice, 92% of palsies completely resolve by 3 months of age, and 95% fully recover eventually.[35] Physical therapy should be used initially to maintain range of motion. For patients with persistent weakness at 3 months of age, electromyography and possibly myelography may help identify those rare cases requiring brachial plexus repair or grafting. Patients presenting later may benefit from osteotomies or contracture release and tendon transfer, to restore external rotation of the shoulder.[34]

Other Deformities

Sprengel deformity, or congenital elevation of the scapula, actually represents embryonic failure of descent, rotation, and development of the scapula. This realignment normally occurs predominantly between the 9 and 12 weeks of gestation.[36] Etiology of the malformation is unknown.

On physical examination, the upper pole of the scapula may be visible at the base of the neck. Abduction is limited because the scapula is rotated inferiorly. The pectoralis major muscle may be underdeveloped. Scapular winging may occur due to serratus anterior palsy. The scapula may be connected to the vertebrae by an abnormal omovertebral bone, named for the two structures it connects. Associated congenital anomalies such as cervical or thoracic vertebral fusions, anal atresia, or cardiac abnormalities may coexist. Treatment is indicated in moderate and severe cases to improve shoulder abduction and appearance. The most effective method involves detaching and lowering the midline origins of the rhomboids and trapezius (Woodward procedure) to correct the scapular malposition.[36]

Congenital pseudoarthrosis of the clavicle is a tapered defect in the continuity of this bone, presumably due to pressure from the more cephalad position of the right subclavian artery. It almost always involves the right clavicle unless the patient has dextrocardia or a cervical rib. Bone grafting and pin fixation before age 6 are usually indicated.

Radial club hand is a longitudinal failure of formation of many tissues on the radial side of the forearm and hand. The severity varies. Approximately 50% are bilateral. Associated abnormalities may include components of the VATER syndrome, hydrocephalus, and clubfoot. The upper arm may also be short and the shoulder girdle underdeveloped. The radial-sided muscles, radial carpal bones, thumb, and radial artery may be absent. The hand is deviated radially up to 90 degrees because it lacks its normal radial support, and the ulna may be bowed. Treatment involves centralization of the wrist on the ulna, tendon transfer, and possibly ulnar straightening and creation of a thumb, as long as reasonable elbow flexion is present.[37] Untreated cases are cosmetically problematic, although functionally less so. Congenital absence of the ulna is only one third as common. In most cases, there is some remnant of the proximal ulna for elbow stability.

Radioulnar synostosis (fusion), often inherited, results in a fixed position of forearm rotation, usually in pronation. At times the synostosis may be only fibrous. Shoulder motion can usually compensate for the lack of rotation, and rotational osteotomy should be done only if clearcut functional deficit can be demonstrated.[38]

Congenital constriction bands (Streeter bands) are most likely due to intrauterine encirclement by amniotic bands or the umbilical cord. They may be located anywhere, and may also be associated with amputation of body parts. The bands can be released with Z-plasties after age 2, or emergently if they are associated with neurocirculatory compromise.

Polydactyly, the presence of an extra digit, varies in spectrum from a hypoplastic soft-tissue-only addition to a fully developed digit with all phalanges and metacarpals. Fifth finger polydactyly is 10 times more common in blacks than whites. A white child with this finding should be examined for other abnormalities, especially of the cardiovascular system. Simple, small, nonskeletal duplications can be excised or tied off. If there is significant skeletal stability, all digits should be reexamined to determine which is the least functional, and this should be excised.

Congenital *trigger thumb* presents as a clenched digit and is not always recognized at birth. It is usually due to excessive tightness of the annular ligament at the metacarpal head. This causes swelling of the tendon, which later becomes firm. Treatment consists of 6 to 8 weeks of stretching if the condition is diagnosed early, and surgical release if it persists or is diagnosed later.

Nursemaid's elbow, or radial head subluxation, refers to elbow pain following longitudinal traction on a pronated, extended elbow in children 2 to 7 years old. A snap may or may not be heard with motion. Radiographs usually show no bony abnormality or displacement. Only one case report, that of Solter and Zaltz,[39] describes actual exploration of this pathology. This report and laboratory studies suggest that the annular ligament of the radial head slips partially over the radial head, the narrowest portion being prominent when pronated. A radial fracture or septic arthritis should be ruled out. Treatment is usually reduction by stabilizing the elbow with one hand, with a finger over the radial head for palpation, followed by gentle firm flexion until a click is felt. The child should begin using the elbow within minutes. Immobilization is usually not necessary in the initial case. It can be done with 2 to 3 weeks in a cast if the episode has recurred. Parent education about the mechanism is most important.

LIMB LENGTHENING, DISTRACTION OSTEOGENESIS, AND DEFORMITY CORRECTION

The challenge of lengthening an obviously short limb has intrigued orthopedic surgeons for generations. The process has gone through an evolution and is now approaching a mature state.

Clinical research has suggested that discrepancies of over 2.5 cm in the lower extremity may cause gait and back problems, and those over 5 cm most often benefit from surgical equalization of the limb lengths. Upper extremities can tolerate much greater discrepancies without causing functional problems. Lengthening a shortened limb poses problems of not only skeletal elongation but also matching distraction of muscles, nerves, and vessels. Initial attempts at limb lengthening involved stimulating the bone by causing inflammation or irritation such as by injection or cautery or causing arteriovenous fistulas. More predictable effects have been achieved, however, by osteotomy and gradual distraction. Initially, this was done by traction in a bed with a frame. However, external fixation techniques have matured, and currently the lengthening process is accomplished by an external distractor. Wagner, in the late 1970s, was the first to popularize leg lengthening. He used a compact, unilateral device that allowed lengthening with less physical encumbrance. He realized that lengthening of approximately 1 mm per day is the maximum tolerated, and that an increase of approximately 10 to 15 percent of the length of the limb can be achieved safely without a high risk of nerve or artery damage. However, the gap where the lengthening occurred often required bone grafting and plating, a second major surgery. It remained for the pioneering Siberian orthopedic surgeon, G. Ilizarov, to recognize that bone would form spontaneously in the gap if conditions were right. This included a stretching or distraction sequence of 0.25 mm 4 times a day. Performance of the procedure in a child often resulted in spontaneous bone formation to resemble a normal bone. This phenomenon is termed distraction osteogenesis. It is now used to lengthen limbs, correct angular deformities, lengthen overall stature, and even stretch soft tissues. This principle of forming new bone has been applied by orthopedic and reconstructive surgeons. The appropriateness of this technique versus standard osteotomies is now being determined.

Different types of devices can now be used to produce the same effect. They can be uniplanar devices (ie, placed only on one side of the limb) or the more cumbersome circular devices, which are more bulky but provide the ability to rotate, distract, and angulate.

Current indications for use of distraction osteogenesis include regeneration of large bone defects following tumor resection, infection, or trauma; major limb length inequality greater than 5 cm; significant soft tissue scarring; and angular deformities that may require adjustment, such as in obese patients. The process of distraction usually takes about 1 month per cm to be obtained. If safe limits of distraction are exceeded, or there is significant local scarring, nerve stretch is a risk.

GENERALIZED ABNORMALITIES

Bone Dysplasias

Osteocartilaginous exostoses (osteochondromas), single or multiple, are sessile or pedunculated excrescenses located on the metaphysis and directed away from the growth plate (Figure 99-16). These outgrowths have their own growth plates. Osteochondromas are thought to arise from defects in the perichondral ring that encircles the growth plate, permitting lateral growth rather than the usual organized distal growth. The condition with multiple exostoses is usually distinct; it is transmitted as autosomal dominant, and affected persons are usually somewhat short.

Any bone with endochondral growth may be affected, but most often the long bones of the extremities are involved. Because of asymmetrical growth plate activity, angulatory growth often ensues, resulting in valgus of knees and ankles and ulnar deviation of forearm and wrist. These should be corrected by partial epiphyseal stapling in young children, or osteotomy in older ones. Leg length inequality is significant in 50% of patients.

The indication for excision of the lesions themselves is pain or compromise due to pressure on tendons, nerves, or spinal cord. Malignant transformation should be suspected if continued growth occurs after skeletal maturity or if new pain occurs. A bone scan may be helpful because absence of uptake indicates

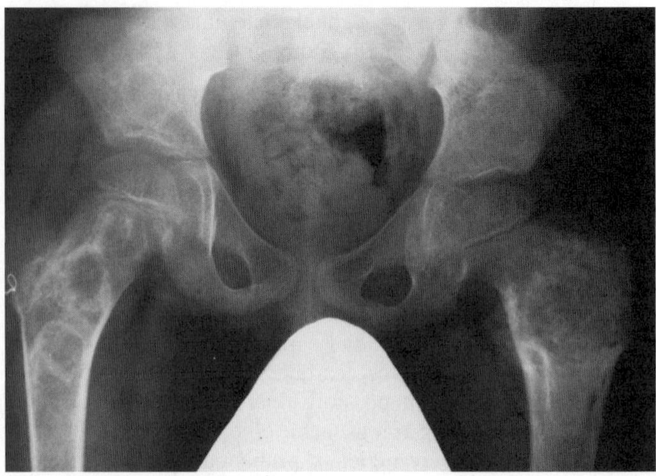

FIG. 99-17. Fibrous dysplasia may affect multiple bones, and may cause cortical thinning and internal alterations as well as bony deformation.

a benign lesion, but increased uptake does not always mean malignant change.[40]

Fibrous dysplasia is a disorder in which bone formation in the medulla and cortex is altered, and the marrow contains much fibrous tissue. Radiographically the bone has a uniform "ground glass" consistency, and the cortex is thin and often deformed (Figure 99-17). One bone (in monostotic form) or several bones (polyostotic form) can be affected. Pathologic fractures occur often but usually heal in a normal period.[41] Proximal femoral (shepherd's crook) bowing is the most difficult to manage.[41] Deformities and fractures of the lower extremities usually require internal fixation, whereas fractures in the upper extremity require only cast treatment.

Irregular "café-au-lait" spots occur in 30% of patients with the polyostotic form. When polyostotic lesions and café-au-lait spots are associated with precocious puberty, the condition is called McCune-Albright syndrome. Other endocrinopathies (thyroid, parathyroid, or adrenal problems) may occur.[41] Malignant transformation to fibrosarcoma or osteosarcoma is rare.

Osteogenesis imperfecta is a spectrum of diseases that are the end result of defects in collagen or proteoglycan synthesis. These result in bones with thin cortices and multiple fractures. Short stature, blue sclerae, middle ear deafness, abnormal dentition, and thin skin may coexist. Inheritance is usually dominant and occasionally recessive, but is frequently due to spontaneous mutation. Microfractures occur to cause the bowing of long bones and scoliosis.[42] Child abuse should be considered in the differential diagnosis, and the absence of pelvic deformity or wormian cranial bones in child abuse may be helpful.

Mobility aids and preventive bracing can be very helpful in preventing fractures.[43] Occasionally, intramedullary rods that elongate with growth are needed. Fortunately, the frequency of fractures diminishes with age.

Tumors

A complete discussion of musculoskeletal tumors is beyond the scope of this section; rather, an attempt is made to describe an appropriate differential diagnosis and evaluation.

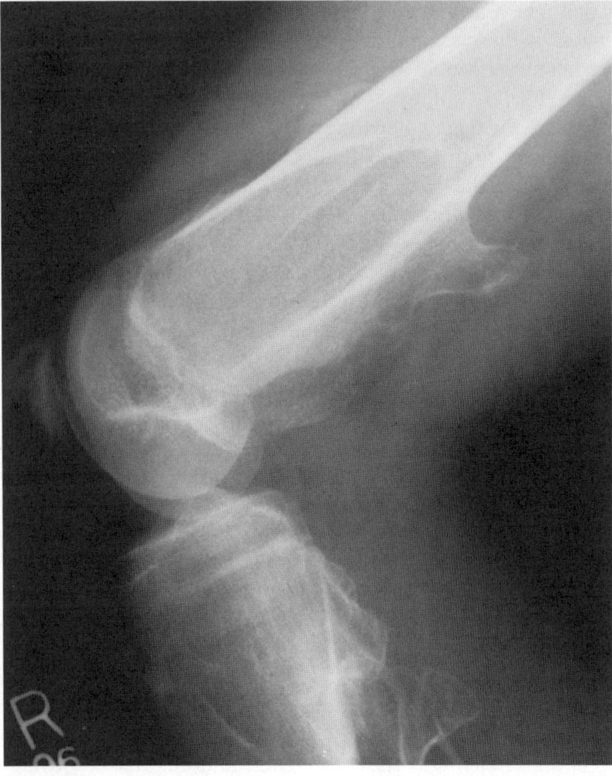

FIG. 99-16. Osteochondromas may be multiple in the inherited form. Note that in this lateral radiograph of the knee, the cortex is continuous with that of the host bone, and they project away from the joint.

Benign or malignant musculoskeletal tumors can be classified according to their tissue of origin.

History and physical examination are rarely definitive. Many tumors become evident following trauma, when a new prominence is noted, or when pathologic fracture occurs through weakened bone. For example, osteoid osteoma, a benign condition, frequently produces pain that is relieved by nonsteroidal antiinflammatory agents. Very early sarcoma may be painless. Unexpected presentations may occur for lesions such as Ewing sarcoma, the histiocytoses, and leukemia, which may each present with fever and malaise.

Some idea of the benign or malignant nature of a tumor can be gained from the following radiographic features. Lesions associated with rapid enlargement and lack of local containment should heighten the suspicion of malignancy. A vague zone of transition between lesion and normal bone is worrisome, as is a soft tissue mass in the presence of a bone tumor. Periosteal lamellation is a response to spread outside the cortex and may occur with benign or malignant tumors. Rapid growth is suggested when periosteal lamellation is extensive and there is no formation of definite new cortex. Thinning of the cortex itself is not pathognomonic of malignancy; this also occurs with fibrous cortical defect and aneurysmal or unicameral cysts. Internal stippling suggests calcification of a cartilage matrix; fluffy opacification usually represents new bone formation, as in osteosarcoma (Figure 99-18). Lesions crossing the epiphyseal plate are usually infections or malignant tumors. Leukemia presents with musculoskeletal complaints 20% of the time; radiographic findings include osteopenia, sclerotic or lytic lesions, lucent metaphyseal bands, or periosteal new bone.[44]

Certain general radiographic studies can be helpful.[45] Radiographic studies must be tailored to the differential diagnosis. CT scans may show internal consistency, soft tissue spread, and extent of the lesion. Technetium bone scans show lesions in the remainder of the skeleton, bony involvement with soft tissue lesions, and bone turnover or activity of questionable lesions. Angiograms may be helpful to determine if the tumor involves a vascular bundle. Laboratory studies generally are not specific; sedimentation rate and complete blood count are abnormal in several of these tumors, and alkaline phosphatase is often elevated in osteogenic sarcoma.

Treatment of musculoskeletal tumors defies simplification. The most important generalization is that any tumor requiring surgery should be cared for by a surgeon who has had experience in this area. Errors related to biopsy placement or specimen adequacy are three to five times more frequent when performed by surgeons in nontumor centers.[46]

Osteogenic sarcoma is the most common primary malignant bone tumor. It usually affects patients during the ages and at the sites of most rapid growth: in teenagers, in the metaphysis of the distal femur, proximal humerus, and proximal tibia. This suggests a focal error in bone remodeling. Treatment involves chemotherapy as well as wide excision with an intact rim of normal tissue, if this can be done without resecting major nerves. The missing skeletal structures are then reconstructed with allograft, autograft, or endoprosthetic implants. Such procedures are called limb salvage. If salvage of a functional limb is not possible, amputation is performed. Recent studies have shown that limb salvage yields results of local recurrence and long-term survival that are as good as with amputation.

Ten-year survival rates have improved from 19% before the era of chemotherapy to over 70%. This gain is the result of improved imaging and surgical technique, adjuvant chemotherapy, and early resection of lung metastases. The prognosis is best for lesions of the proximal humerus and proximal tibia; it is worst for the pelvis and spine.

Ewing sarcoma affects a slightly broader age range (usually ages 4 to 18). It commonly involves the diaphysis of long bones. The tumor is radiosensitive. Traditional treatment has been radiation and chemotherapy. Recently, however, improved survival rates and decreased local complications have been shown with wide surgical excision instead of radiation, when feasible. The long-term survival rate (approximately 60% at 5 years) is not quite as good as for osteosarcoma.

Two common benign bone tumors require brief mention. A *unicameral bone cyst* is a smooth, well-marginated lucency fairly centrally located near the growth plate in the metaphysis of a child 2 to 15 years of age, especially in the humerus or femur (Figure 99-19). The lesion can be observed if it is small and in a non–weight-bearing bone; otherwise it can be curetted or injected with cortico-steroids. The latter two treatments have approximately equal results. The natural history of these defects is spontaneous regression during adolescence.

Fibrous cortical defects are well-marginated lucencies located in, and slightly expanding, the cortex. Usually one radiographic view shows that these lesions are not central in bone (Figure 99-20). They are present in up to one third of all young children at some time and disappear with age. In a weight-bearing bone, the risk of fracture is appreciable if the lesion is

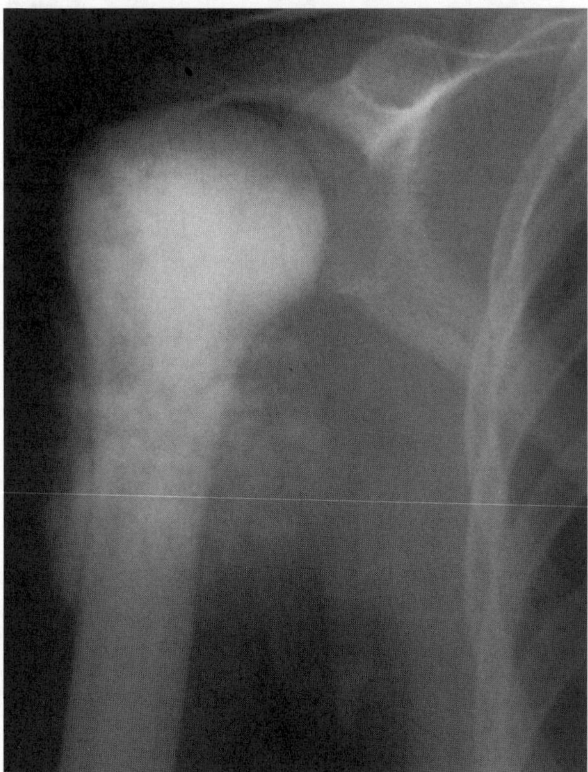

FIG. 99-18. Osteogenic sarcoma is shown here involving the proximal humerus. There is intraosseous and extraosseous spread with no margination, as well as periosteal reaction.

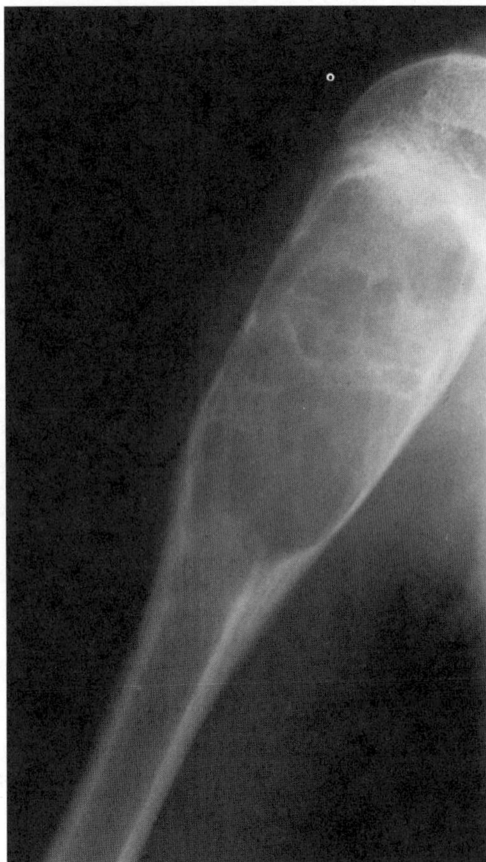

FIG. 99-19. Unicameral bone cyst is a centrally located, lucent lesion, most common in the proximal humerus, as seen here.

greater than approximately 3 cm in length and greater than half the width of the bone. Lesions this large should be protected by limiting activities, if possible, or bone grafted.

Neuromuscular Disorders

Cerebral Palsy

Cerebral palsy is a collective term for a group of nonprogressive conditions affecting the upper central nervous system. This results in two types of musculoskeletal problems: disorders of control for which little can be done, and bone and joint deformities resulting from continued muscle imbalance, which can be managed.[47,48] As a consequence, the athetoid features that predominate in a few children are difficult to modify, except for supportive bracing, but the more common spastic features are more amenable to modification. Assessment of the patient should always include identification of current functional problems and goals. Gait, if possible, may be marked by a crouched position due to knee or hip flexion contractures. The ankle may tend toward plantar flexion or dorsiflexion.

Trial bracing or gait studies may help determine which is the primary problem. Ankle plantar flexion can often be controlled with bracing if the foot can be brought up to a right angle with the tibia. If this is not possible, the tight heel cord should be lengthened; tight hamstring and hip flexors also may be lengthened when indicated. The "scissoring" of the legs while walking or lying may be due to tight adductor muscles.

Hip dislocation occurs with increasing frequency as the severity of involvement increases. This is due to imbalance between the strong adductors and flexors and the underactive extensors and abductors. It is acquired, not congenital, and usually occurs after several years of age. This should be checked every 6 to 12 months in diplegic or quadriplegic patients. The child is at risk for progressive hip subluxation, if abduction is less than 30 degrees with the hip extended. Dislocation and subluxation cause difficulty by interfering with perineal care and balanced sitting, and by causing degenerative joint disease, pain, and increased spasm. Consequently, they should be treated aggressively even in severely involved patients. They can be prevented by early muscle release or later by osteotomy.[47]

Scoliosis is also more frequently encountered with increasing severity of cerebral palsy. It is present in up to 69% of severely involved children, perhaps because of persistent primitive reflexes, an inclined pelvis, or asymmetric muscle tone. Bracing should be tried, but it is less effective than in idiopathic scoliosis. Surgery may be necessary.

The upper extremity may be flexed at the elbow, wrist, and fingers. Whether this should be corrected depends on the patient's intelligence, ability to voluntarily control the hand, and

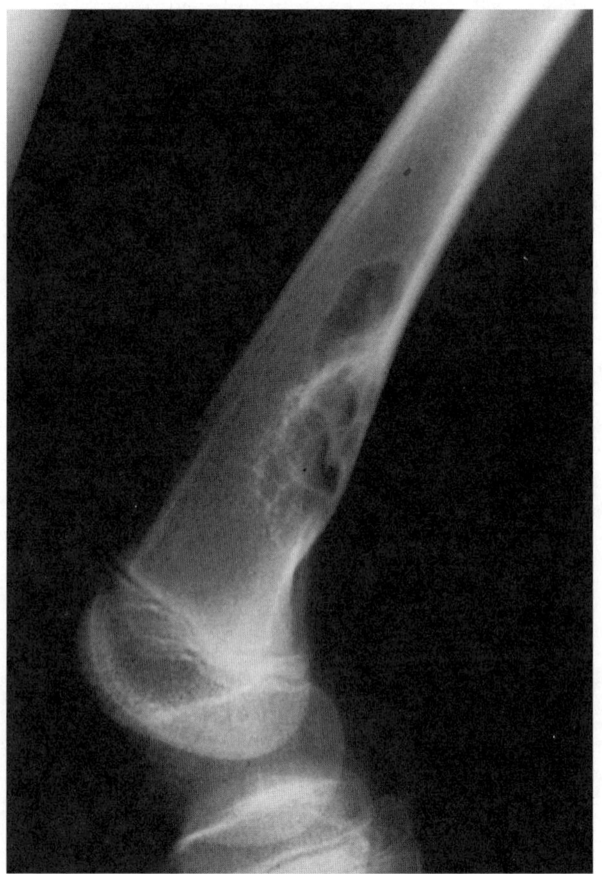

FIG. 99-20. Fibrous cortical defect is more eccentrically located than unicameral bone cyst. As seen here, it is centered in the cortex.

sensation. The thumb may be clenched, and early bracing may be helpful, with surgery performed later if the thumb has potential for use.

The benefits of physical therapy in general are debated. Positioning and hand and heel-cord stretching may produce increased range. However, severity of neurologic involvement is probably more important than therapy in determining walking ability.

Myelodysplasia or spinal dysraphism involves malformation of the embryonic neural tube with paralysis below a certain thoracic or lumbar level of innervation.[49] The functioning muscles usually have more control than in cerebral palsy. The goal of orthopedic management is optimizing mobility and socialization, and this does not always mean walking. The quadriceps are the most important muscles for mobility. Severely involved children with poor intelligence and weak quadriceps are more mobile in wheelchairs. In most cases, joint deformities are treated by releases and bracing. In contrast to cerebral palsy, hip dislocations are not usually painful and should not be reduced unless they are unilateral or the child has good quadriceps. Scoliosis may also occur, especially with higher-level spinal defects. One of the most important roles for the physician is to monitor the child for loss of lower-extremity muscle power as he or she grows. This loss of muscle strength may be due to a tethering of the spinal cord distally as the child grows or to a disturbance of cerebrospinal fluid pressure.

Infections

Hematogenous Osteomyelitis

The incidence and presentation of this condition are changing following the introduction of newer imaging and treatment methods, but there are certain constant principles.[50,51]

Acute hematogenous osteomyelitis by definition includes processes occuring for a week or less at the time of diagnosis.[52] It occurs more frequently in males than in females, presumably because trauma may play a role in increasing susceptibility. The peak ages of occurrence are under 1 year and in the preadolescent years 9 to 11. The incidence declines in adulthood because of the change in vascular supply of bone.[53] The most common sites affected are the femur and tibia, each accounting for one third of the cases, followed by humerus, calcaneus, and pelvis. Any bone may be affected, however. The metaphysis is the most common region involved, and spread may occur from this point to involve any other portion. Rarely, the infection process may begin in the epiphysis.

The pathophysiology is incompletely understood. The metaphyseal vascular channels form loops near the growth plate.[53] Blood flow is slowed, and the capillary basement membrane and reticuloendothelial system is deficient in these regions. Experimental bacteremias have been shown to produce foci of infection only in these regions. Trauma likely has more than a circumstantial role, as experimentally traumatized areas are more susceptible to developing osteomyelitis. Only about one quarter of cases have a demonstrable source, such as cutaneous, aural, or respiratory seeding. Direct traumatic inoculation is a different disease process.

After a focus of infection is initiated, local inflammation is followed by spread up and down the medullary canal. The

growth plate in children has no bridging vessels and acts as a barrier to spread in most cases. The growth cells are on the epiphysial side and are therefore spared. However, in the first year of life, transphyseal vessels do exist that allow spread up to the epiphysis and into the joint.[51] These facts have two implications. First, growth-plate damage is more likely during the first year of life. Second, in children of this age, septic arthritis may follow osteomyelitis in any metaphyseal location, whereas in older children without transphyseal vessels, it occurs only in locations where the joint capsule extends over the growth plate, that is, the shoulder, elbow, and hip. At skeletal maturity with growth-plate closure, this barrier is again eliminated, although hematogenous osteomyelitis is rare after this point. As intramedullary pressure increases, pus dissects through the haversian system to elevate the periosteum and produce a subperiosteal, then soft tissue abscess. The elevated periosteum may be radiographically apparent within 1 to 2 weeks.

Unlike in septic arthritis, the organisms involved vary slightly with age. In all age groups the predominant organism is *S aureus*, although *Streptococcus pneumoniae* and *Haemophilus* must be considered. *Staphylococcus* is associated with a higher recurrence rate than other organisms. *Salmonella* should be considered in patients with sickle cell anemia, although *Staphylococcus* is still more common than *Salmonella* in these patients. Blood cultures in the acute phase are positive approximately 40% to 50% of the time, and direct cultures of pus or bone only 60% to 80% of the time. This may be due to prior antibiotic use, errors in sampling or processing, or auto eradication of the organism.

Clinical diagnosis remains key despite new imaging techniques. The child may appear well or may have systemic involvement ranging from malaise to shock. Often refusal to bear weight is an early symptom. The very earliest sign is fever and local bone tenderness, followed later by fluctuance if a subperiosteal or soft tissue abscess has developed. Spread to adjacent joints should be ruled out by palpation and range-of-motion evaluation. Passive motion of the extremity is usually not significantly resisted unless a soft tissue abscess or joint involvement is present. Increased suspicion should be aroused with neonates, who are more often afebrile, and who may first be noted to have a swollen or motionless limb. Vertebral or pelvic osteomyelitis may present as abdominal pain and can resemble the more common septic arthritis of the hip.

Differential diagnosis primarily includes neoplasm, contusion, undisplaced fracture, and sickle cell crisis. Elevated white blood cell count and sedimentation rate are helpful but not diagnostic. Serum antibody titers may be helpful, but sensitivity is a problem. Radiographs at the earliest stage may show soft tissue swelling. Osteopenia or lysis may appear after 7 to 10 days, followed by new bone formation at the borders of the process. Bone scan has been widely used in the past two decades, but the subtleties of its use have only recently been recognized. The tracer most widely used is ^{99mm}Tc methylene diphosphonate because of its speed, cost, and sensitivity. Immediate scans for flow and blood pool, as well as later skeletal images, should be obtained. The scan may be normal in the very early stages. It should be repeated after 48 hours if clinically indicated.

Cold or photopenic areas are important because they may indicate areas of avascularity, especially when accompanied by adjacent areas of increased uptake. Cellulitis may cause confusion but usually does not show bony localization on delayed images. The overall accuracy of nuclear imaging is approximately 60% to 90%. However, it may be much lower in neonates, according to some reports. Gallium citrate may be sensitive but requires a minimum of 24 hours; indium-labeled white cell studies require similar amounts of time, including preparation of tracer. Because of these limitations, radionuclide scans should not be relied on in all instances, especially when the clinical diagnosis is clear. These studies have their greatest value when localization for aspiration is difficult. The role of MRI has yet to be defined.

Aspiration is indicated in all cases to identify the pathogen and in some cases to decompress localized purulence. It should be performed with a large-diameter needle. The anesthetic may be local, intravenous sedation, or general, as indicated. In sequence, the extraosseous soft tissues, periosteum, and, if necessary, intramedullary canal should be assessed for purulent localization. Fluoroscopy may be useful in deep lesions if radiographic changes are evident. Experiments in animals have shown that aspiration of bone does not by itself cause a bone scan to become positive.

Treatment involves delivery of appropriate antibiotic to all infected tissue. Abscesses with avascularity may therefore require surgical decompression if aspiration cannot accomplish this. Antibiotic therapy can be divided into initial and definitive periods. In the initial phase, broad-spectrum antibiotic agents, including antistaphylococcal agents, are indicated. Vancomycin should be used if resistance is suspected. In neonates, an aminoglycoside should be added. In children younger than 3 years who have osteomyelitis associated with septic arthritis, chloramphenicol or cefuroxime may be used to cover *H influenzae*. In the definitive period, the most effective, least toxic antibiotic for the isolated organism should be given for 4 to 6 weeks. This may be by the oral route if the patient is clinically improved and is compliant, and if adequate serum drug levels can be documented.

Surgery is reserved for those cases in which the child is systemically ill, is worsening under medical treatment, or in whom an abscess has been demonstrated. Abscess or avascular tissue should be removed to allow antibiotic penetration, and the wound is usually closed over a drain. Complications include recurrence, minor growth acceleration, growth plate damage, and fracture through weakened bone.

Subacute osteomyelitis is a more subtle condition. No systemic signs may be evident, and in one series fewer than one fifth of patients had a fever, elevated white blood count, or positive blood count.[51] However, an abnormal radiograph and bone scan were more common than in the acute form. Treatment follows the principles discussed above.

Chronic recurrent multifocal osteomyelitis is a rare syndrome involving low-grade systemic manifestations that are ongoing for several years, with reports of up to 12 areas of lytic-sclerotic juxtaepiphyseal involvement. No organism has been isolated, and treatment is supportive.

Fungal osteomyelitis may be disseminated (sporotrichosis, candidiasis) or direct (eumycetoma). Aggressive debridement is more important in these conditions than in bacterial infections.

Puncture wounds to the foot are significant in that they may be followed by *Pseudomonas* infection. This is because *Pseudomonas* often colonizes the shoe and sock. The wound should be inspected and foreign material removed.[50] The patient should be seen in 3 to 5 days or at least instructed to return if symptoms of infection occur.

Septic arthritis is slightly more common than hematogenous osteomyelitis, and it may potentially have more disastrous long-term consequences if effective treatment is delayed. Most cases occur in infants and younger children, with nearly half of the cases occuring before age 30. A high index of suspicion for septic arthritis should be maintained in sick neonatal patients, for they show few signs.[54] The hip is the most commonly involved joint in the infant, and the knee is the most common site in the older child. The spread may be from the bloodstream or from an adjacent osteomyelitis, especially in the hip and shoulder, where the capsular insertion extends over the growth plate onto the metaphysis. Many theories have been advanced for the pathogenesis of joint destruction, including toxins from both the neutrophils and bacteria.

The spectrum of causative organisms is somewhat broader than that of hematogenous osteomyelitis,[54] which may have some relation to the greater frequency of this condition. Overall, *S aureus* is still the most common causative organism. However, in the age group from 1 month to 5 years, *H influenzae* is more common than *Staphylococcus*. The streptococci, *Escherichia coli, Proteus*, and other organisms should also be considered. The yield of organisms from aspiration is approximately 60% to 80%.

Clinical findings vary with age. In the infant, there may be fever, failure to feed, and tachycardia. Subtle changes in position may serve as clues, as well as unilateral swelling of an extremity or a joint, asymmetry of soft tissue folds, and pain with range of motion. In the older child, the signs are more localized.

Aspiration with a large needle should be performed if there is any reasonable suspicion of septic arthritis, both for diagnosis and in some cases for treatment. In deep joints such as the hip, guidance with ultrasound or fluoroscopy should be used to confirm position of the needle. This assures that joint fluid was actually obtained, and it also helps distinguish joint infection from septic involvement of the bursa underneath the nearby psoas muscle. The white-cell count in fluid obtained in septic arthritis ranges from 25,000 to 250,000/mm^3. Elevated lactate levels may be helpful in cases where white cell counts are borderline.

Differential diagnosis includes toxic synovitis of the hip, in which pain, fever, leukocytosis, and spasm are more moderate and do not escalate on serial observations. However, at times the two are indistinguishable, and aspiration should be performed. Rheumatoid arthritis, cellulitis, traumatic synovitis, and the migratory polyarthralgias of rheumatic fever should be considered. A sympathetic effusion may also occur from adjacent osteomyelitis.

The role of arthrotomy versus aspiration in confirmed cases of septic arthritis is controversial. The key feature is removal of deleterious enzymes and restoration of effective synovial perfusion. Because the decision not to operate requires the ability to monitor and repeatedly aspirate as needed, it is probably preferable to use arthrotomy in joints that are deep and difficult to assess, such as the hip and shoulder; in young patients who are difficult to examine; and when the fluid obtained is viscous.

The surgical procedure should include irrigation, drainage, and closure. This may be done arthroscopically in the knee, shoulder, and ankle. Direct instillation of antibiotics has no benefit. Some investigators believe the femoral metaphysis should be drilled whenever the hip is aspirated to decompress any possible femoral osteomyelitis.

Early effective treatment is very important. Good results decline dramatically if treatment is initiated after 4 days of symptoms. Antibiotics should be continued for 4 to 6 weeks. Contractures should be prevented, and abduction of the hip decreases the likelihood of dislocation. Complications include permanent destruction of cartilage, and in the hip, avascular necrosis with resorption of the femoral head or overgrowth of the femoral head. Complications are more frequent in young infants.

Gonococcal arthritis also occurs in children.[55] It should be distinguished from the more frequent gonococcal migratory polyarthralgia or tenosynovitis. On average, 2 to 3 joints are affected; the most commonly involved are the wrists and knees. Treatment is aspiration and closed irrigation followed by 3 days of intravenous penicillin, and 4 days of ampicillin or amoxicillin. Oral treatment alone with one of these drugs for 7 days is acceptable in reliable patients after a loading dose.

Injuries

A comprehensive discussion of musculoskeletal trauma is beyond the scope of this chapter. The reader is referred to Chapter 35 for further information. Basic principles of injury evaluation and common injuries and emergencies are discussed here.

Children's bones differ from those of adults both biomechanically and physiologically. Mechanically, immature bone is more porous, and the pores serve to limit crack propagation. Instead of complete fractures, children often have involvement of only part of the cortex, such as in a buckle fracture from compression or a greenstick fracture from tension. The most extreme example is plastic deformation of bone without fracture. This should be corrected if it is 20 degrees or more.[56]

Another biomechanical feature of the child's skeleton is that the ligaments are stronger than either bone or growth plate. Injuries that would produce dislocations or sprains in adults, such as elbow dislocation or medial collateral ligament tear of the knee, produce different patterns in children, such as supracondylar humeral fractures or femoral physeal separations, respectively. Thus, the presence of undisplaced fractures and separations should be sought on physical examination and radiographs. In the knee, gentle stress radiographs may show an undisplaced separation that should be immobilized.

Physiologic differences include union rates, remodeling, overgrowth, and growth plate injuries. Nonunion is nearly unheard of in children, occurring only in open fractures with extensive soft tissue loss and periosteal stripping. Bone union times range from 2 weeks in infants to 3 months in adolescents. Remodeling of angulation and displacement is an impressive tendency up until the early teen years (Figure 99-21). This occurs through alterations in physeal growth as well as local periosteal

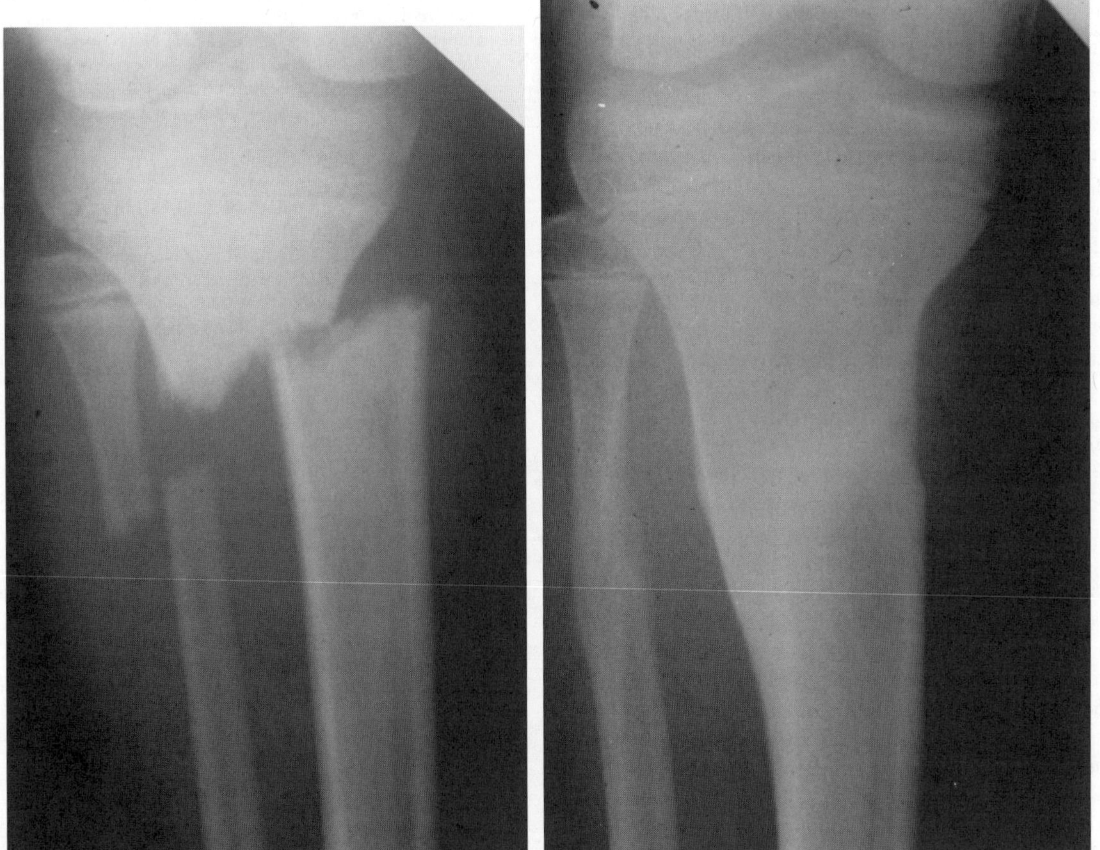

FIG. 99-21. Remodeling of fracture. This proximal tibial metaphyseal fracture (*A*) was held in parallel alignment, but with significant step-off. The periosteum bridging the two fragments filled in the fracture gap (*B*).

resorption on the convex side and deposition on the concave side. This is most effective in the metaphysis, where angulation does not create as much deformity as in the midshaft.

The compensation for any residual deformity is much better if it is in the plane of joint motion. For example, posterior angulation of a distal femur fracture can be compensated for by knee flexion, whereas there is no ability for the knee to compensate for varus angulation at this site. In the upper extremity, overlap of fracture segments is acceptable as long as the angulation is not excessive.

Another physiologic feature of the child's fracture is growth stimulation. This occurs because of hyperemia and continues for approximately 18 months post fracture. It is most significant in the femur, where it averages 1 cm, but it occasionally becomes significant in the tibia. By contrast, growth arrest may occur if the growth plate is crushed or crossed by the fracture.

Hand injuries are common. Fractures of the phalangeal and metacarpal shafts can be splinted if they are minimally angulated and stable, but rotational alignment should be checked by observing the fingernails with the fingers flexed and extended. They should be similarly aligned if there is no malrotation. ''Buddy-taping'' helps minimize malrotation. Growth plate or epiphyseal fractures may be splinted if they are undisplaced but should be referred if they are displaced. Dorsally dislocated interphalangeal joints may be reduced and radiographed to rule out fracture. If stable enough to allow active range of motion, they should be splinted for 3 weeks with an aluminum splint. Immobilization of the metacarpophalangeal joints should be in 50 to 90 degrees of flexion to minimize stiffness, and the interphalangeal joints should be in mild flexion of approximately 20 degrees.

One problem injury is an avulsion of the base of the nail bed, which is often associated with open separation of the nearby phalangeal growth plate; this may then become infected and stop growing. This should be definitively distinguished from a Kirners deformity, which is a bilateral, idiopathic irregularity of the distal phalangeal growth plate.

The scaphoid bone ossifies at age 6. *Scaphoid fractures* may occur in children and develop nonunion if they are not recognized. However, this occurs more rarely in children than in adults. Laceration of the palm and digits may sever a flexor tendon, and active range of motion of each joint should be checked to ensure that this has not occurred.

Muscle contusions occur most frequently in the quadriceps, upper arm, or shoulder. They may be intensely painful. Compartment syndromes are rare in these regions. Treatment consists of limitation of hemorrhage by rest, ice packing, and Ace wrapping. Active range of motion should be instituted in 1 to 3 days, but passive range of motion, such as stretching, should be avoided because it may cause further damage.[57] Strength rehabilitation is instituted after motion is regained. Myositis ossificans, that is, intramuscular calcification and ossification, may follow but usually does not limit function.

Child abuse affects approximately 1% of all children. Most victims are under 3 years of age. In children under age 1, fractures more often than not are nonaccidental. One third of victims are reinjured if the initial diagnosis is missed. Fractures occur in about one third to one half of abused children. The most common areas include long bones, skull, and ribs. Most specific fractures for abuse are those of the metaphysis near the growth plate, posterior ribs, scapula, or sternum. Unfortunately, there are no completely diagnostic signs of abuse on radiograph. It is most helpful to use radiography to look for inconsistency and to guide the investigation into the mechanism. Although long bone fractures may occur from a spontaneous fall out of bed or from a counter, they are rare. It is useful to get an idea of the age of a fracture by radiograph. Periosteal new bone formation occurs 4 to 10 days after a fracture in infants. At 10 to 14 days, there is blurring of the fracture lines and soft, mobile (poorly defined) callus. Hard callus occurs at 14 to 21 days. Differential diagnosis includes osteogenesis imperfecta, Caffey disease, syphilis, scurvy, rickets, leukemia, and congenital insensitivity to pain.[58]

If abuse is suspected, reporting is mandatory, and the reporter is protected by law. The initial search for other fractures should be done by skeletal survey (AP and lateral radiographs of skull and spine, AP radiographs of extremities) with bone scan in selected cases. Admission to hospital is usually the best way to protect the child and further evaluate the family. Careful documentation and willingness to advocate for the child may be the most important things physicians can do to help these children.

REFERENCES

1. Morrissy RT. Pediatric orthopaedics, ed 3. Philadelphia: JB Lippincott, 1996.
2. Rang M. Children's fractures. Philadelphia: JB Lippincott, 1983.
3. Rockwood CA, Wilkins KE, King RE. *Fractures in children.* Philadelphia: JB Lippincott, 1991.
4. Staheli LT. Children's orthopaedics. New York: Raven, 1994.
5. Bleck EE. Metatarsus adductus: classification and relationship to outcomes of treatment. J Pediatr Orthop 1983;3:2.
6. Rushforth GF. The natural history of hooked forefoot. J Bone Joint Surg 1978;60B:8.
7. Simons GW. Complete subtalar release in club feet. J Bone Joint Surg 1985;67A:1044.
8. Wenger DR, Mauldin D, Speck G, Morgan D. Corrective shoes as treatment for flexible flatfoot. J Bone Surg 1989;71(A):800.
9. Staheli LT. Shoes for children: a review. Pediatrics 1991;88:371.
10. Mosier KM, Asher M. Tarsal coalitions and peroneal spastic flat foot. J Bone Joint Surg 1984;66A:976.
11. Scranton PE Jr. Treatment of symptomatic talocalcaneal coalition. J Bone Joint Surg 1982;69A:533.
12. Kling TF, Hensinger RN. Angular and torsional deformities of the lower limbs in children. Clin Orthop 1976;176:136.
13. Staheli LT, Corbett M, Wyss C, et al. Lower extremity rotational problems in children. J Bone Joint Surg 1985;67A:39.
14. Staheli LT. Torsional deformities. Pediatr Clin North Am 1977;24:799.
15. Morrissy RT. Congenital pseudarthrosis of the tibia. J Bone Joint Surg 1981;63B:367.
16. Pappas AM. Congenital posteromedial bowing of the tibia and fibula. J Pediatr Orthop 1984;4:525.
17. Dinham JM. Popliteal cysts in children. J Bone Joint Surg 1975;57B:69.
18. Dickhaut SC, DeLee JC. The discoid lateral meniscus syndrome. J Bone Joint Surg 1982;64A:1068.
19. Salenius P, Vankka E. The development of the tibiofemoral angle in children. J Bone Joint Surg 1975;57A:259.
20. Levine AM, Drennan JC. Physiological bowing and tibia vara. J Bone Joint Surg 1982;64A:1158.
21. Ilfeld W, Westin GW, Making M. Missed or developmental dislocation of the hip. Clin Orthop 1986;203:276.
22. Harcke HT, Kumar SJ. Role of ultrasound in diagnosis and management of congenital dislocation and dysplasia of the hip. Curr Concepts, J Bone Joint Surg 1991;73A:622.
23. Mubarak S. Pitfalls in use of Pavlik harness for treatment of congenital dysplasia, subluxation and dislocation of the hip. J Bone Joint Surg 1981;63A:1239.

24. Zionts LE, MacEwen GD. Treatment of congenital dislocation of the hip in children between the ages of one and three years. J Bone Joint Surg 1986;68A:829.

25. Haueisen DC, Weiner DS, Weiner SD. The characterization of transient synovitis of the hip in children. J Pediatr Orthop 1986;6:11.

26. Catterall AM. Legg-Calvé-Perthes disease. Edinburgh: Churchill Livingstone, 1982.

27. Salter RB. Current concepts review: the present status of surgical treatment for Legg-Perthes disease. J Bone Joint Surg 1984;66A:961.

28. Salter RB, Thompson GH. Legg-Perthes disease. CIBA Clinical Symposia, vol 1986.

29. Weiner DS, Weiner S, Melby A, et al. A thirty-year experience with bone graft epiphyseodesis in the treatment of slipped capital femoral epiphysis. J Pediatr Orthop 1984;4:145.

30. Bradford DS, Lonstein JE. Scoliosis and other spinal deformities. Philadelphia: WB Saunders, 1994.

31. Tredwell SJ, Newman DE, Lockitch G. Instability of the upper cervical spine in Down syndrome. J Pediatr Orthop 1990;10:602.

32. Dobyns JH, Wood V, Bayne LG. Congenital hand deformities. In: Green D, ed. Textbook of hand surgery. New York: Churchill Livingstone, 1982.

33. Bora WF. Pediatric upper extremity. Philadelphia: WB Saunders, 1986.

34. Hoffer MM, Wickenden R, Raper B: Brachial plexus birth palsies. J Bone Joint Surg 1978;60A:691.

35. Tada K, Tsuyuguchi Y, Kawai H. Birth palsy: natural recovery course and combined root avulsion. J Pediatr Orthop 1984;4:279.

36. Carson WF, Lovell WW, Whitesides TE Jr. Congenital elevation of the scapula. J Bone Joint Surg 1981;63A:1199.

37. Bora FW. Radial clubhand deformity. J Bone Joint Surg1981;63A:741.

38. Cleary JE, Omer GE. Congenital radioulnar synostosis. J Bone Joint Surg 1985;67A:539.

39. Salter RB, Zaltz C. Anatomic investigations of the mechanism of injury and pathologic anatomy of ''pulled elbow'' in young children. Clin Orthop 1971;77:134.

40. Lange RH, Lange TA, Rao BK. Correlative radiographic, scintigraphic and histologic evaluation of exostoses. J Bone Joint Surg 1984;66A:1454.

41. Harris WH, Dudley R, Barry RJ. The natural history of fibrous dysplasia. J Bone Joint Surg 1962;44A:207.

42. Albright JA. Management overview of osteogenesis imperfecta. Clin Orthop 1981;159:80.

43. Bleck EE. Nonoperative treatment of osteogenesis imperfecta. Clin Orthop1981;159:111.

44. Lange TA. Ultrasound imaging as a screening study for malignant soft-tissue tumors. J Bone Joint Surg 1986;69A:100.

45. Mankin HJ, Lange TA, Spanier SS. Hazards of biopsy in patients with malignant primary bone and soft tissue tumors. J Bone Joint Surg 1982; 64A:1121.

46. Rogalsky RJ, Black GB, Reed MH. Orthopaedic manifestations of leukemia in children. J Bone Joint Surg 1986;68A:494.

47. Bleck EE. Orthopaedic management in cerebral palsy. Philadelphia, JB Lippincott, 1987.

48. Bleck EE. Locomotor prognosis in cerebral palsy. Develop Med Child Neurol 1975;17:18.

49. Menelaus MB. Orthopaedic management of spina bifida cystica. Edinburgh: Churchill Livingstone, 1980.

50. Green NE. *Pseudomonas* infections of the foot following puncture wounds. Am Acad Orthopaed Surg Instructional Course Lectures 1983: 43.

51. Jackson MA, Nelson JD. Etiology and medical management of acute suppurative bone and joint infections in pediatric patients. J Pediatr Orthop 1982;2:313.

52. Nade S. Acute hematogenous osteomyelitis in infancy and childhood. J Bone Joint Surg 1983;65B:109.

53. Scoles PV, Aronoff SC. Current concepts review: antimicrobial therapy of childhood skeletal infections. J Bone Joint Surg 1984;66A:1487.

54. Green NE. Disseminated gonococcal infections and gonococcal arthritis. Am Acad Orthopaed Surg Instructional Course Lectures 1983:48.

55. Nade S. Acute septic arthritis in infancy and childhood. J Bone Joint Surg 1983;65B:234.

56. Jackson DW, Feagin JA. Quadriceps contusions in young athletes. J Bone Joint Surg1973;55A:95.

57. Sanders WE, Heckman JD. Traumatic plastic deformation of the radius and ulna. Clin Orthop 1984;188:58.

58. Dent JA, Paterson CR. Fractures in early childhood: osteogenesis imperfecta or child abuse? J Pediatr Orthop 1991;11:184.

Surgery of Infants and Children: Scientific Principles and Practice, edited by
Keith T. Oldham, Paul M. Colombani, and Robert P. Foglia.
Lippincott–Raven Publishers, Philadelphia, © 1997.

CHAPTER **100**

Hand

Terry R. Light

The infant's hand is a wondrously adaptable organ that allows the baby to reach out to explore and touch his or her environment. The hand enables the older child to express herself or himself with activities such a finger painting, climbing a jungle gym, or playing the piano. Abnormal hand form or compromised hand function can frustrate normal use. Early anticipation of the long-term consequences of hand malformation, deformity, and injury allows proper parental counseling and timely reconstruction of the child's hand.

ANATOMY AND EMBRYOLOGY

During embryonic growth, the upper limb develops in advance of the lower extremity. Events in the development of the arm and hand precede analogous events in the leg and foot. Within the limb, a proximal–distal gradient enables proximal segments to gain definition before distal portions of the limb. The hand develops from the arm bud, which is evident at day 26 of gestation. The hand paddle appears at day 33. At day 41, the digital rays gain definition as five separate mesenchymal condensations. Separation of the individual fingers begins at day 47 and is complete by day 54 of gestation.

The short tubular bones of the cartilaginous hand model defined during embryonic development begin to ossify during the fetal period.

Postnatal ossification of the carpal bones proceeds in an orderly fashion until skeletal maturity. Although the joints of the hand and wrist actively move during intrauterine development, patterns of functional activity are established during the postnatal period.

CONGENITAL HAND DIFFERENCES

Congenital hand deformities and malformations can be categorized into seven groups of abnormalities based on the nature of the presumed developmental failure[1]:

- Failure of formation of parts
- Failure of differentiation of parts
- Duplication
- Overgrowth
- Undergrowth
- Early amniotic rupture sequence (congenital constriction band syndrome)
- Generalized skeletal abnormalities

Most congenital hand abnormalities represent malformation, reflecting a failure of the normal orderly embryologic definition of the hand. Early amniotic rupture sequence (congenital constriction band syndrome) represents intrauterine disruption and deformation of initially properly formed digits or limbs by the ensnaring fetal membranes.

Congenital hand abnormalities occur in about 1 in every 1500 live births.[2] The two most common hand abnormalities are *syndactyly,* webbing together of fingers, and *polydactyly,* hands consisting of more than the usual five digits. Although the cause of most hand differences cannot be determined, some are the result of syndromes with genetic implications.[3] Multilimb and multisystem abnormalities suggest the possibility of a syndrome. When a syndrome is suspected, referral of families to a geneticist is essential to address questions regarding the likelihood of subsequent offspring being born with similar problems and to evaluate the possibility that the patient's children will have similar involvement. The geneticist also can help parents understand the heterogeneity of the possible phenotypes of a single syndrome.

The motions of the shoulder, elbow, and wrist govern the patient's ability to place the hand in space. Hand reconstruction is undertaken only if the child is able to place his or her hand in space. Surgical treatment aims to achieve a hand with the maximal functional capabilities consistent with the retained elements. *Prehension,* the ability of the hand to securely grasp and release objects, depends on both the mobility and stability of the thumb and fingers.

Aesthetic considerations are vital and should be acknowledged from the outset because the hand is a highly visible, unclothed portion of the body. It is often wise to remove awkward, functionless nubbins that may attract the unwanted attention of classmates. Parental concerns and guilt should be dealt with in an open, sympathetic, and nonjudgmental manner.

Duplication

Duplication of the thumb is the most common form of polydactyly encountered in whites and Asians. In most cases, neither of the two thumb components is normal. Each is hypoplastic. Simple deletion of one digit is rarely satisfactory. Surgical reconstruction requires the merging of soft tissue and occasionally the merging of bone elements of the two thumb components to create an optimal composite digit (Fig. 100-1). The skeleton of the more ulnar digit is usually retained, while the radial digital skeleton is removed. When bifurcation occurs at the level of the metacarpophalangeal or interphalangeal joint, the retained ulnar digit lacks a radial collateral ligament at the level of bifurcation. A collateral ligament can be reconstructed from the remnant of the ligament that formerly secured the deleted radial digit. Intrinsic muscle insertions may need to be removed, and extrinsic flexor and extensor tendons must be repositioned along the reconstructed central digital axis.

Duplication of the little finger (ulnar polydactyly) is an inherited hand abnormality seen frequently in black children. In white children, ulnar polydactyly may be sporadic or associated with syndromes. Small, pedicled, duplicated little fingers can be simply excised or ligated. More substantial little finger duplications require bone and joint reconstruction in addition to soft tissue recontouring.

Syndactyly, the webbing together of adjacent digits, is usually the result of a failure of the normal intrauterine interdigital resorption process. The webbing of the embryologic hand paddle persists, tethering adjacent fingers together. Surgical separation liberates fingers for independent function. Fingers are separated by incisions that create well-vascularized local flaps. Flap tissue is rotated to create a floor for the interdigital web space and to partially cover the adjacent sides of adjacent fingers (Fig. 100-2). Full-thickness skin graft is used to resurface remaining open areas on the sides of the separated digits.

Absence or hypoplasia of the radius can occur as an isolated abnormality or as a part of a syndrome with systemic implications, such as Holt-Oram syndrome or thrombocytopenia–absent radius syndrome. Without the normal radial support of the carpus, the hand deviates radially, assuming an awkward position at a right angle to the longitudinal axis of the forearm. Splinting, casting, or stretching should be instituted at birth to stretch the soft tissues along the radial border of the limb. Between 6 and 12 months of age, the hand and carpus is surgically centralized or repositioned on the end of the distal ulna articular surface. With time, the distal ulna broadens, providing support to the hand and carpus.

Digital Deficiencies

Absence or inadequacy of the thumb substantially limits the ability of the child to hold large objects securely in one hand. If the thumb is hypoplastic but of near-normal length and possesses a mobile carpometacarpal joint, thumb function can be improved by opponensplasty muscle or tendon transfer combined with metacarpophalangeal joint stabilization and first web space release.

When the thumb is absent or when a hypoplastic thumb lacks a carpometacarpal joint, ablation of the thumb and pollicization of the index finger should be considered. Pollicization shortens and rotates the index finger into the thumb position of radial and palmar abduction (Fig. 100-3). The transferred index finger's distal interphalangeal joint takes on the role of the thumb's interphalangeal joint, while the proximal interphalangeal joint assumes the role of the thumb's metacarpophalangeal joint. Removal of the index metacarpal shaft allows the proximally shifted metacarpal head to represent the trapezium, and the former index metacarpophalangeal assumes the role of the thumb's carpometacarpal joint. The tendinous insertions of the first dorsal interosseous and the first palmar interosseous muscles are advanced distally to mimic the function of the abductor pollicis brevis and adductor pollicis muscles, respectively. The extensor indicis proprius and the index extensor digitorum communis

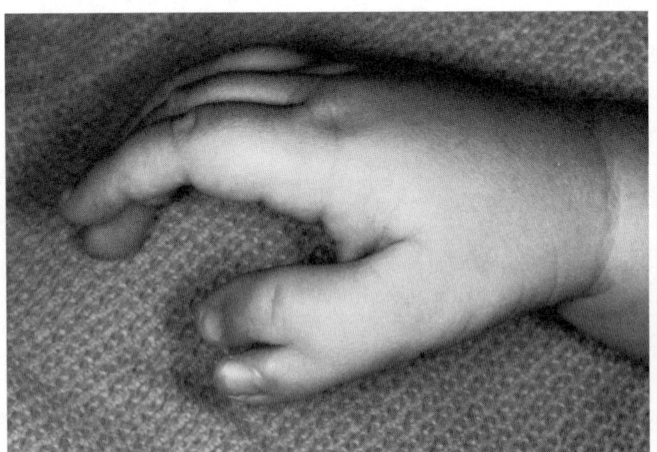

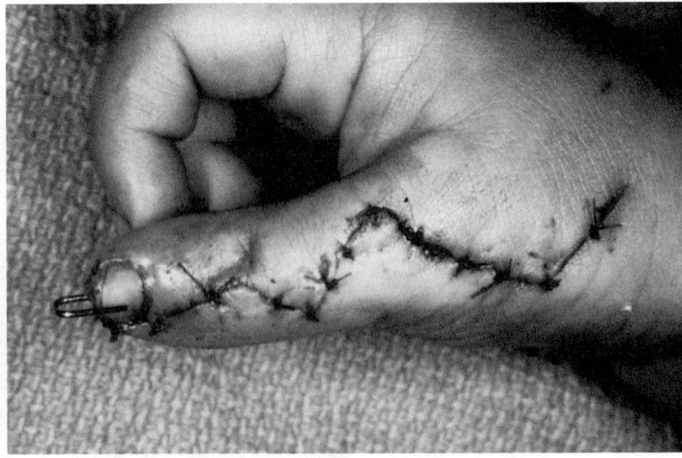

FIG. 100-1. Thumb duplication. (*A*) Wassel type IV duplication consists of two thumb components, each with a proximal and distal phalanx sitting on a common metacarpal. (*B*) Surgical reconstruction removes more radial proximal and distal phalanges, centers more ulnar digit on metacarpal head, and joins soft tissues from both thumb components to improve resultant digit contour. (Light TR, Manske P: Congenital hand malformations and deformities. AAOS Instr Course Lect 1987;37)

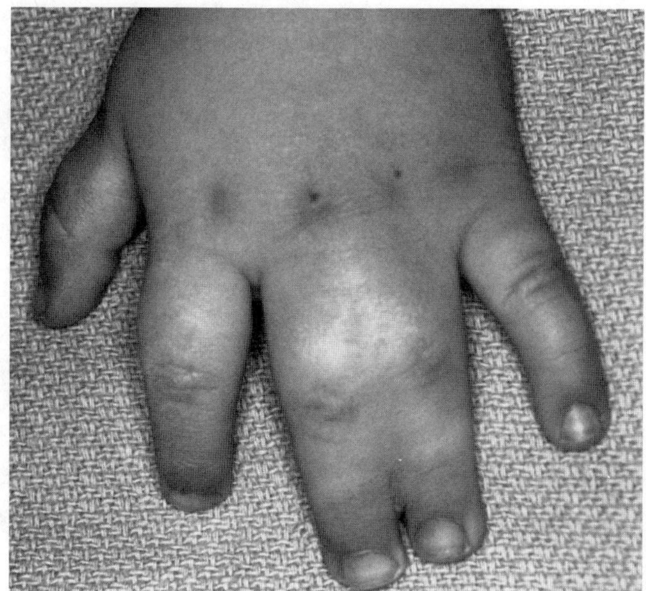
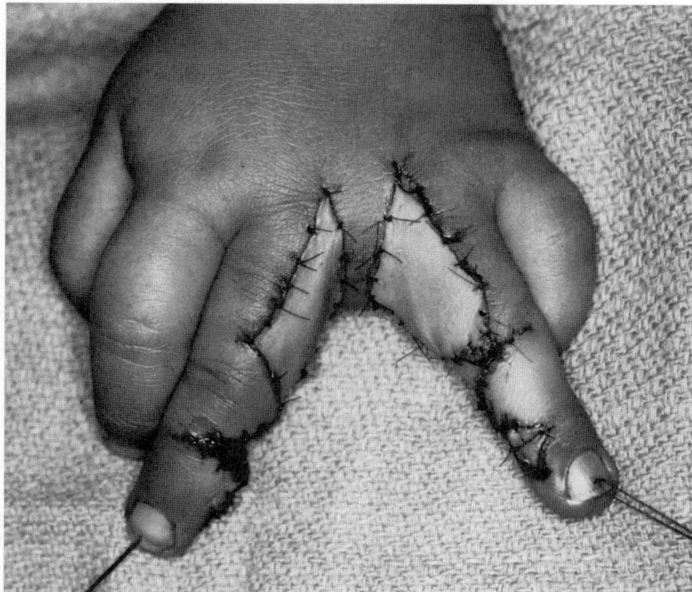

FIG. 100-2. Syndactyly. (*A*) Preoperative dorsal view of incomplete simple syndactyly of middle and ring fingers. (*B*) Syndactyly has been released, with dorsal flap creating a floor to interdigital web space, while full-thickness groin skin grafts surface residual open areas on adjacent sides of separated fingers.

tendons are shortened, and the extrinsic flexor tendons are allowed to shorten gradually.

Short fingers that possess actively mobile proximal phalanges make a useful contribution to hand function. When the digital soft tissue envelope of a short finger is redundant because of phalangeal absence in the presence of a metacarpal, nonvascularized toe phalanx transfer can be employed. Confluent extrinsic flexor and extensor tendon insertions can be separated and reattached to the transferred phalanx to create a mobile digit.

When a hand consists of a mobile thumb but lacks fingers, microvascular transfer of a second toe to a central position provides a growing digit. The thumb is thereafter able to achieve prehension against this stable digit. In cases of intrauterine thumb amputation (early amniotic rupture sequence) at the proximal phalangeal or distal metacarpal level, the carpometacarpal joint, intrinsic musculature, and digital neurovascular structures are normal. In these cases, microvascular toe transfer effectively augments thumb function.

TRAUMA

Fractures and Dislocations

The immature hand is well vascularized and consequently usually heals rapidly. Metacarpal and phalangeal fractures securely heal in a few weeks in the immature hand. Residual angulation usually corrects over ensuing months if rotational malalignment is prevented.[4]

At the metacarpophalangeal joint, the collateral ligament inserts into the epiphysis of the proximal phalanx at a point proximal to the physis. Because this insertion point focuses stress at the physis, proximal phalangeal physeal fractures are common.

Conversely, because the broader insertion of the collateral ligaments of the interphalangeal joints extends distally beyond the physis of the middle phalanx, the middle and distal phalangeal physes are shielded from stress. Consequently, physeal fractures are uncommon in the middle phalanx.

In children, dislocations of the interphalangeal joints are usually treated by closed reduction, while dislocations of the metacarpophalangeal joint are rarely reducible by closed techniques. When the metacarpophalangeal joint of a child is forcibly hyperextended, the volar plate is usually avulsed from its insertion on the proximal phalanx. The resilient, intact periarticular soft tissues tether the proximal phalanx to the metacarpal head, and the volar plate becomes caught between the adjacent displaced articular surfaces (Fig. 100-4). Open surgical extrication of the volar plate from the joint is necessary to achieve congruent reduction of the metacarpophalangeal joint.

Because the carpus is largely cartilaginous during the first decade of life, the carpal bones are relatively resistant to fracture. Fractures in children younger than 10 years of age are uncommon and usually the result of massive trauma. As in adults, fracture of the scaphoid is the most common carpal fracture in children. Treatment of nondisplaced pediatric scaphoid fractures with cast immobilization usually results in solid fracture union.

Pain along the ulnar aspect of the wrist in an adolescent gymnast is often the result of an earlier asymptomatic distal radial physeal injury.[6] Disruption of longitudinal radial growth results in relatively greater growth in the distal ulna. The prominent distal ulna causes pain as it impinges on the ulnar aspect of the carpus. If the area of physeal tether is limited and substantial growth remains, resection of the physeal bar can be attempted. More often, the area of physeal bridge is extensive, or little radial growth remains. In such cases, the distal ulnar physis

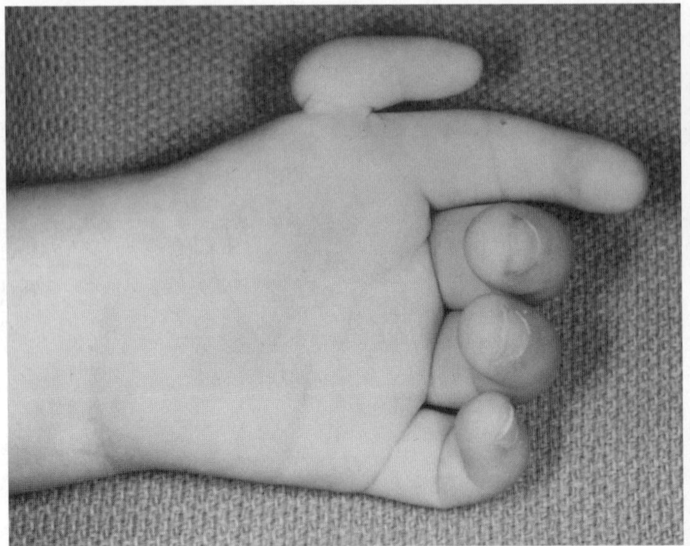

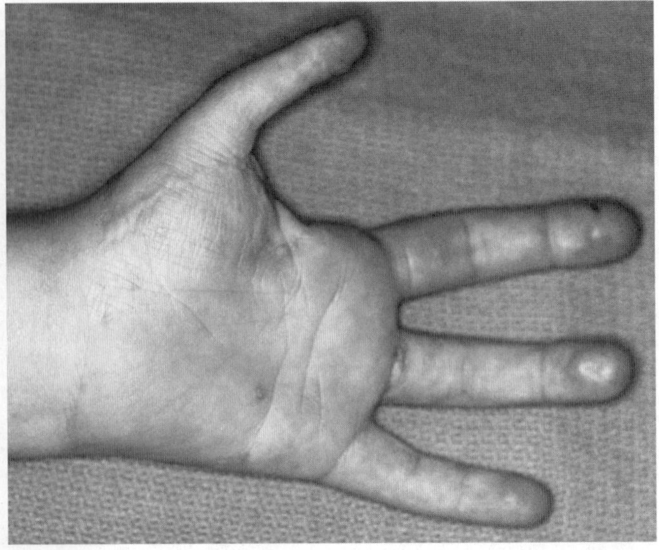

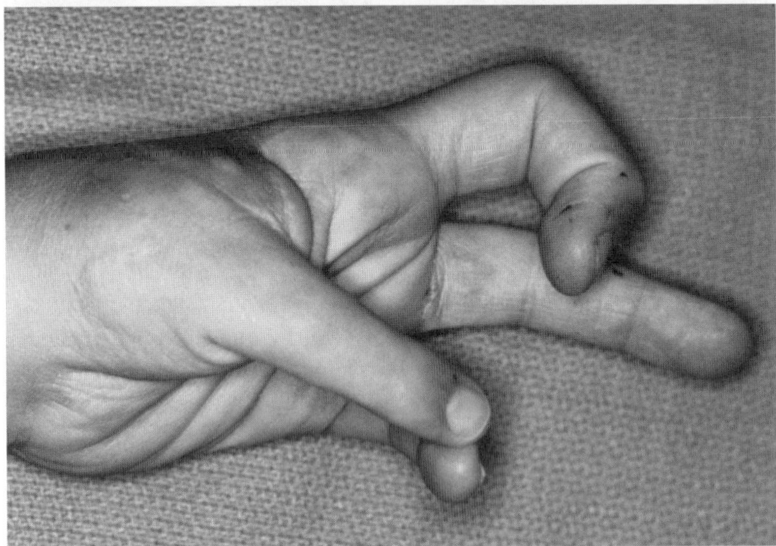

FIG. 100-3. Hypoplastic thumb. (*A*) Hypoplastic thumb contains no bony connection to the hand and no musculotendinous units. Index finger is stiff. (*B* and *C*) Seven years after ablation of hypoplastic thumb and pollicization of index finger, hand function is excellent, with good mobility of pollicized index finger.

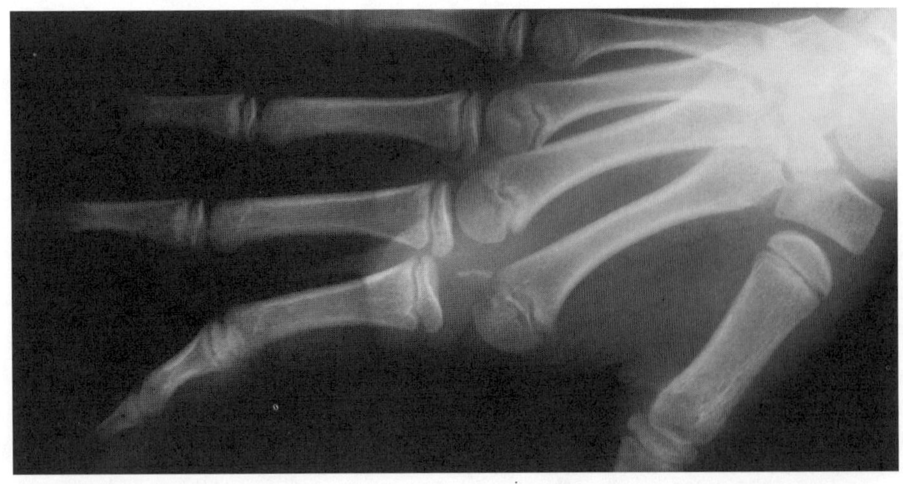

FIG. 100-4. Complex dislocation of index metacarpophalangeal joint associated with dorsal metacarpal head fracture. This injury requires open reduction. (Light TR. Trauma and infections of the hand and wrist in children. In: Manske P, ed. Hand surgery update. Englewood, CO, American Society for Surgery of the Hand, 1994)

should be ablated and the ulna shortened through the diaphysis, retracting the distal ulna to the level of the distal radius.

Fingertip injuries are common in children because young hands are perpetually exploring.[5] Fingertip amputations through the distal phalanx in children can be treated either by reattaching the amputated tissue as a composite tissue graft or by applying serial adhesive bandages over the débrided open wound.

Thermal Injuries

Although frostbite rarely causes total necrosis of digital soft tissues, exposure to cold can cause cellular injury to the physis. Because physeal arrest is not immediately apparent, the injury may appear innocuous. With time, however, nail dysplasia and altered longitudinal growth of the distal and, less commonly, the middle phalanges of the fingers are apparent. Because the child's thumb is usually flexed into the palm with the fingers wrapped around it when it is cold, the physes of the thumb are usually spared from frostbite injury.

Burn injuries in younger children are often the result of direct-contact palmar burns that occur when a child grasps a hot object such as a space heater or an iron. Dorsal scald wounds can also occur in young children injured by pulling a pot of boiling water off a stove. Scald burns usually produce more superficial injuries. Flame burns are somewhat deeper and can occur in children of any age caught in a house fire. Flame burns usually involve the thinner dorsal skin rather than the palmar skin. Treatment of deep burns requires excision and grafting; more superficial burns can be treated with local wound care.

Tendon Injuries

Tendon injuries usually occur as the result of laceration by a sharp instrument, most often a knife or a piece of broken glass. For example, when a child tries to carve a pumpkin, the knife may become stuck, allowing the hand to slip forward toward the pumpkin and exposing the flexor surface of the fingers to the sharp edge of the knife.

Pediatric tendon injuries, particularly flexor tendon injuries, can be difficult to diagnose in a timely fashion. The inability of a small child to move a finger precisely on command and the unlikeliness that a child will complain of the specific aspect of hand function facilitated by a given tendon often obscure the diagnosis of tendon injuries in children. The diagnosis of a flexor tendon injury often is suggested by the posture of the fingers (Fig. 100-5). Disruption of the normal cascade of increasing digital flexion from the index finger to the little finger and disturbance of the tenodesis effect on digital posture as the wrist is passively moved from flexion to extension suggest tendon disruption. When diagnosis is in doubt, surgical exploration should be undertaken.

Although operative repair of flexor tendons in children is similar to adult repairs, the postoperative protocol may need to be modified. In adults, postoperative care usually involves protected early digital motion with a dynamic traction apparatus. In children deemed too young or immature to cooperate with the adult regime, the surgeon may elect to immobilize the finger in a cast with the wrist flexed for 3 or 4 weeks after repair. After the cast is removed, the aid of an experienced hand

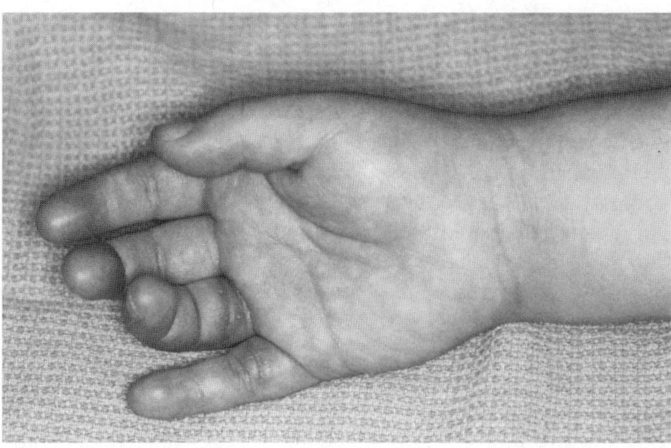

FIG. 100-5. Laceration of ring and little fingers spared ring finger flexor tendons but transected flexor digitorum profundus and flexor digitorum superficialis in the little finger. Alteration in the normal cascade of digital flexion is disrupted. (Light TR. Trauma and infections of the hand and wrist in children. In: Manske P, ed. Hand surgery update. Englewood, CO, American Society for Surgery of the Hand, 1994)

therapist is invaluable in assisting the child to recover maximal active motion.

Nerve Injuries

Nerve injuries can be difficult to identify in young children because of their inability to report numbness. The immersion of the hand in water normally leads to wrinkling of the digital pulp. When the pulp is denervated, the normal wrinkling is absent, and the texture of the denervated skin is dry. As with tendon injuries, early exploration of questionable lacerations is preferable to delayed diagnosis.

Nerve repair is particularly worthwhile in children because children possess an extraordinary ability to reprogram the brain to interpret sensory information properly from repaired nerves.

Replantation

The total severance of a digit or a hand is an unusual pediatric injury. In adults, not all detached parts are reattached. In contrast, in children, attempts are usually undertaken to reattach and revascularize most divided parts, even isolated fingers. Technical difficulties in replantation can be encountered in children because of their relatively smaller-caliber vessels. Additionally, their greater sympathetic tone can result in an increased incidence of intraoperative and postoperative vasospasm. When vascularity is successfully restored, growth in reattached parts averages 80% of the growth of the corresponding contralateral normal part. Because neural recovery is usually good in children, the clinical results of viable pediatric replanted parts are usually good.

Compartment Syndrome

The pediatric hand and forearm are particularly vulnerable to the development of a compartment syndrome. Unrecognized compartment syndromes result in permanent loss of muscle function and secondary deformity due to muscle fibrosis and contracture. Many different mechanisms can lead to elevated pressure within the flexor compartment of the forearm, the extensor compartment of the forearm, or the intrinsic compartments of the hand. When the interstitial pressure within the compartment exceeds the venous pressure, further vascular engorgement ensues. Although arterial pressure may remain high enough to allow detection of a distal pulse, the elevated pressure within the compartment may prevent tissue perfusion and block venous outflow.

Compartment syndromes can occur as the result of a direct crush injury, such as occurs when a child's hand and arm are pulled between the closely spaced rollers of an old wringer washing machine. In children with coagulopathy (eg, hemophilia, leukemia), spontaneous bleeding from the forearm muscles can precipitate a compartment syndrome. The inadvertent infusion of fluid through a misdirected catheter usually results in spontaneously resolving subcutaneous swelling. Infusion beneath the forearm fascia can have grave consequences.

Pain, the usual early indicator of an evolving compartment syndrome, may be misinterpreted or ignored in a young child. Pain with passive stretch of ischemic muscle should be sought. In young children with suspicious findings, the measurement of compartment pressure is helpful in establishing the diagnosis. Because of the permanent effect of ischemia on muscle, early decompression of the involved compartment by open fasciotomy is essential.

CHILD ABUSE

The hand may be injured as the result of child abuse inflicted by a parent or by another caregiver. In young children, the hand may be the focus of abuse. The hand of a child may be injured by mechanisms as diverse as immersion in hot water or by burns inflicted by a lit cigarette. Immersion injury can present as a clear, circumferential, glovelike definition of injured tissue. Cigarette burns produce a series of uniform-diameter circular scars.

The hands of children older than 3 years of age are often incidentally injured when the child tries to protect or shield his or her face from a direct blow or from being struck by a strap or belt buckle.

If child abuse is suspected, the child should be unclothed and thoroughly examined for evidence of other skin or musculoskeletal injuries. Evidence of multiple injuries or fractures of variable age suggest a pattern of repeated abuse. Referral of all suspected instances for social service evaluation is the legal responsibility of the treating physician.

HERPETIC INFECTIONS

Herpetic infections can occur in children younger than 6 years of age. Most often, coexistent oral lesions are noted. Herpetic infections of the finger are characterized initially by a cluster (crop) of clear fluid–filled vesicles. Erythema and swelling are common and can occur in the absence of concomitant bacterial infection, although superinfection has been noted in up to half of cases.[6] Fluid aspirated from a bleb can be cultured for viral growth and examined microscopically (Tzanck smear) to confirm the clinical diagnosis.

Areas of herpetic viral infection should not be incised and drained; rather, a simple protective dry dressing is applied to the involved area. Within 2 weeks, the blisters spontaneously open, and a crust forms on the finger. Skin lesions are usually entirely resolved within 3 to 4 weeks. Broad-spectrum antibiotics may prevent bacterial superinfection.

REFERENCES

1. Swanson AB. A classification for congenital limb malformations. J Hand Surg 1976;1:8.
2. Dobyns JH, Wood VE, Bayne LG. Congenital hand deformities. In: Green DP, ed. Operative hand surgery, vol 1, ed 3. New York, Churchill Livingstone, 1993:251.
3. Light TR, Manske P. Congenital hand malformations and deformities. AAOS Instr Course Lect 1989;37.
4. Beatty E, Light TR, Belsole RJ, et al. Wrist and hand skeleton injuries in children. Hand Clin 1990;6:711.
5. Engber WD, Clancy WG. Traumatic avulsion of the fingernail associated with injury to the phalangeal epiphyseal plate. J Bone Joint Surg 1978; 60A:713.
6. Light TR. Trauma and infections of the hand and wrist in children. In: Manske P, ed. Hand surgery update. Englewood, CO, American Society for Surgery of the Hand, 1994.

Vascular System

Surgery of Infants and Children: Scientific Principles and Practice, edited by
Keith T. Oldham, Paul M. Colombani, and Robert P. Foglia.
Lippincott–Raven Publishers, Philadelphia, © 1997.

CHAPTER 101

Arterial Disease

Philip C. Guzzetta, Jr.

VASCULAR EMBRYOLOGY

The origin of the arterial vascular system has been extensively
studied for more than a century. There is general agreement
that the vessels are mesodermal derivatives that begin as cords
of angioblast cells. These cords orient themselves into tubes
and eventually develop along a capillary net formed by existing
vessels that appear to have preferred paths of development. The
development of paired aortic arches early in gestation reflects
the human evolution from aquatic vertebrates, which use the
aortic arches for blood flow through gills developed from the
branchial clefts adjacent to the paired aortic arches. In humans,
at the end of the first month of gestation, the six pairs of aortic
arches have been formed.

By gestational week 7, there is a single aorta posteriorly.
Many of the paired aortic arches regress, and some persist as
head and neck arterial branches. The left aortic arch IV develops
into the aortic arch, and the left aortic arch VI becomes the
ductus arteriosus. Aortic arch V is not shown and may not even
exist in humans (Fig. 101-1). The location of the aortic arches
during this stage of development is actually within the neck
region, and the descent of the arch into the thorax occurs later
with the development of the heart. Detailed discussion of cardiac development and its relation to various anomalies can be
found in *Embryology for Surgeons* by Skandalakis and Gray.[1]

TECHNIQUES TO DIAGNOSE ARTERIAL
DISEASE IN CHILDREN

Any new technique for imaging the arterial system in children
must be compared with transarterial angiography for safety,
quality of image, need for sedation or general anesthesia, and
cost.

Ultrasound

Real-time ultrasound, particularly when combined with color
Doppler ultrasound, has the attractive features of being a safe,
noninvasive, and inexpensive technique to image vessels. The
images may not be attainable, however, if there is overlying

bone or intestine that contains a great deal of gas, which seriously limits its use for the chest and abdomen. In addition,
simultaneous viewing of vessels within a large area in different
planes, such as the entire abdominal aorta and its branches, is
not possible with ultrasound, which limits its use as a guide for
the correction of problems in these vessels. For evaluation of
a single vessel, such as the renal artery after repair, Doppler
ultrasound has a definite role to ensure patency and flow but
has little place in the initial evaluation of children with suspected arterial disease.

Magnetic Resonance Imaging

The technology of magnetic resonance (MR) imaging is developing rapidly, and many of its limitations for arterial evaluations may soon be overcome. MR imaging can be effective in
assessing venous structures and is the technique of choice in
assessing patency of subclavian veins and the superior vena
cava. The anatomy of vascular anomalies, such as double aortic
arch or aberrant subclavian artery, can be visualized easily by
MR imaging. For small visceral vessels, such as the renal artery,
MR imaging does not allow adequate detail and should not
be depended on solely in making operative decisions. As MR
angiography progresses, it may replace transarterial angiography for diagnosing many diseases. MR imaging has a role in
the assessment of vascular anomalies of the extremities, for
which it shows the relation of the vessels and the soft tissue.
Motion artifact is a serious problem with MR imaging, and
many children require heavy sedation or general anesthesia for
the study.

Computed Tomography

Like ultrasound, computed tomography (CT) does not give
a composite picture of the vascular system but requires piecing
together views of the arterial system. With the standard 1-cm
cuts, important information may be missed, but the cuts can be
narrowed considerably. Unfortunately, narrower cuts mean a
longer scan time and more radiation exposure. The use of intravascular contrast adds the risks of allergic reaction to the contrast or renal dysfunction. As with MR imaging, movement
must be prevented to make CT worthwhile, and sedation or

1717

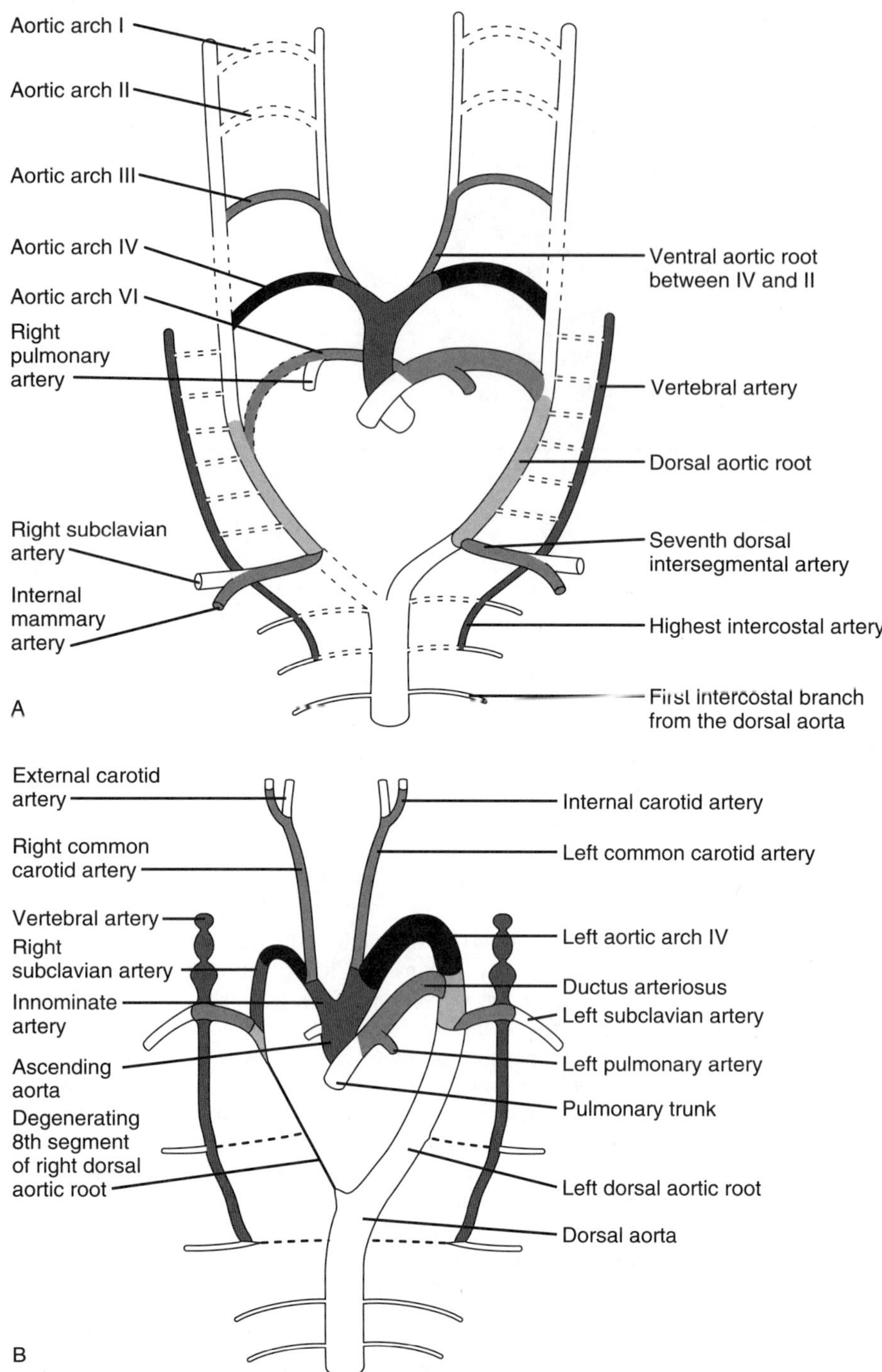

FIG. 101-1. Development of the aortic arch in the human embryo.

anesthesia is usually required in children. With the possible exception of the incidental vascular information obtained during CT assessment of trauma, there is little use for CT in arterial disease in children.

Intravenous Digital Subtraction Angiography

Intravenous digital subtraction angiography was developed to obtain images with the quality of transarterial angiography images without an arterial puncture. Advances in the equipment and expertise of transarterial angiography, however, have greatly reduced the risks of arterial cannulation in children. Therefore, this technique has lost favor with most angiographers because the images are not as clear as transarterial angiography and the contrast load and radiation exposure are high. The need for the patient to remain stationary for a long time is another problem with this approach in children.

Transarterial Angiography

Transarterial angiography remains the gold standard for imaging the arteries of children. The ability to view whole segments of the arterial system at once, magnify the area of interest, and obtain excellent detail of the vascular lumen make this the modality of choice for assessing pediatric arterial disease. Improvements in invasive radiographic treatment of arterial diseases allow the transarterial approach to be therapeutic as well as diagnostic in some cases. Major risks of this approach include damage to the artery used to access the arterial system, potential allergic reactions to the contrast, radiation exposure, and the need for sedation. As the technology improves, MR imaging may be most useful for screening patients for arterial disease, with the transarterial angiography used to confirm the problem in selected patients, especially those who can be treated by invasive radiographic techniques.

ARTERIAL ANEURYSMS

Congenital Aneurysms

Arterial aneurysms have been diagnosed by prenatal ultrasound and have even been implicated in a fetal death. Congenital aneurysms are almost always found in the abdominal aorta, contain all three layers of the involved artery, and show no sign of arteritis. They usually present in children younger than 5 years of age as painless abdominal masses without evidence of distal vascular disease or distal embolus. The form of the aneurysm may be saccular or fusiform. Treatment is resection of the aneurysm and reconstruction with autogenous tissue, if possible. Because many of these aneurysms involve the abdominal aorta, prosthetic graft replacement has been the most common technique, with expected growth of the normal vessel on either side of the graft to accommodate the longitudinal growth of the child.[2]

Acquired Aneurysms

Acquired aneurysms can be separated into those due to an arteritis, syndromes causing medial degeneration, direct arterial infection, trauma (false aneurysms), and arterial dysplasia.

Aneurysms Due to an Arteritis

Arterial aneurysms may develop in children as the result of Kawasaki disease, giant cell arteritis, Takayasu disease, or polyarteritis nodosum. Kawasaki disease (also known as *mucocutaneous lymph node syndrome*) is a disease with a median age of onset of 3 years and is characterized by high fever, cervical adenopathy, conjunctivitis, stomatitis, and generalized erythema, which is frequently most intense on the soles and palms. Coronary artery aneurysms develop in up to 15% of children who are not treated with aspirin or IV γ-globulin. Rarely, aneurysms develop in locations other than the coronary arteries with Kawasaki disease. The coronary artery aneurysms frequently improve with medication, seldom rupture, and may require surgical resection only when they are *giant aneurysms,* defined as greater than 8 mm in diameter. Persistent giant aneurysms tend to cause stenosis or thrombosis of the involved coronary, leading to myocardial ischemia distal to the aneurysm, which requires surgical bypass of the diseased artery.

Giant cell arteritis most commonly involves the aorta, but it may also cause peripheral artery aneurysm formation. Takayasu

arteritis and polyarteritis nodosum most often cause stenosis rather than aneurysm formation, although aneurysms may develop in the aorta or its main branches. Operative correction of an aneurysm due to an arteritis has a high complication rate. Unless the aneurysm is large or threatens to rupture, initial treatment of these patients should be with glucocorticoid therapy rather than surgery.

Aneurysms Due to Syndromes Causing Medial Degeneration

Type IV Ehlers-Danlos syndrome, characterized by an abnormal or absent type III collagen, is associated with medial degeneration of the large arteries with associated aneurysm formation or rupture. The aorta is the most common site of aneurysm formation, but any artery with substantial amounts of collagen is at risk for this problem. Marfan syndrome is an autosomal dominant disease characterized by cystic medial degeneration of the ascending aorta; thin, elongated extremities; chest wall deformities; and dislocation of the lens. The enlarging ascending aorta places the Marfan syndrome patient at significant risk for aneurysmal dissection and rupture or severe aortic valvular insufficiency due to dilation of the aortic root.

Other conditions that deposit abnormal substances into the media of the aorta, such as tuberous sclerosis or cystinosis, may predispose the aorta to aneurysm formation and rupture. Treatment of these children can be complicated by poor tissue integrity at the suture line when a prosthetic graft is placed, leading to false aneurysm formation. Children with some types of Ehlers-Danlos syndrome have abnormal bleeding times, making major surgical procedures hazardous. Nonetheless, the best chance for survival for a patient with one of these syndromes and an aneurysm is resection of the aneurysm and prosthetic graft placement.

Aneurysms Due to Direct Arterial Infection

Most aneurysms that are reported in children are caused by bacterial or fungal infection of a structurally normal arterial wall. An arterial wall, particularly that of the aorta, is generally resistant to bacterial seeding unless there is trauma to the intima or an abnormal flow pattern that potentially weakens the wall. Patients at greatest risk for aneurysm formation due to direct arterial infection are older children with thoracic aortic coarctation and infants with umbilical artery catheters in place.

Children with this type of aneurysm are usually very ill, with signs of bacteremia similar to those seen in patients with acute endocarditis. The most common organism causing this type of aneurysm is *Staphylococcus aureus,* although fungi and other bacteria have also been cultured from infected aneurysms. Histologic examination of the aneurysm reveals inflammation of the arterial wall, with media disruption and aneurysm formation. These aneurysms must be resected because they are at high risk for rupture. Although arterial replacement with autogenous tissue would be ideal, most aortic reconstructions must be done with prosthetic grafts, accepting the potential of graft infection in the future. If the child is large enough to consider extraanatomic bypass of the aorta at the time of aneurysm resection, that should be recommended instead of suturing prosthetic material into a grossly infected area.

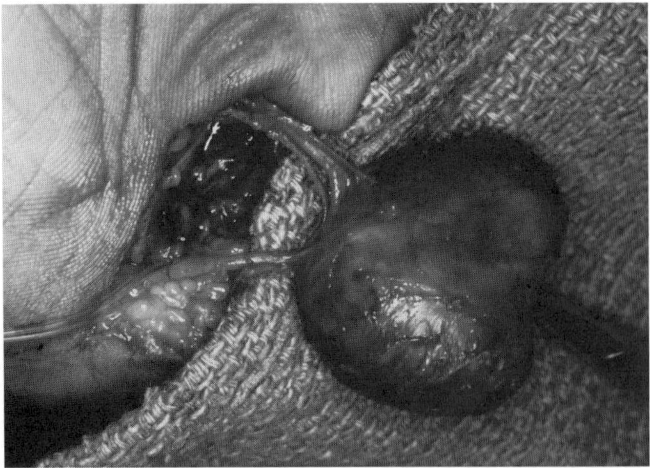

FIG. 101-2. False aneurysm of the superficial palmar artery of the left hand due to a laceration that occurred 6 months earlier.

Aneurysms Due to Trauma (False Aneurysms)

Although they are probably the most common aneurysms in children, the true incidence of aneurysms due to trauma is unknown. These aneurysms are reported infrequently because they are often seen in the distal extremities and are easily cared for by vessel ligation. Most of these aneurysms are caused by penetrating trauma, particularly lacerations of the hands or feet (Fig. 101-2). The trend of nonoperative treatment of ''minimal'' vascular injuries with normal distal pulses[3] will likely increase the appearance of these in the future. Optimal treatment is aneurysm resection with ligation or repair of the artery, depending on the artery involved.

Aneurysms Due to Arterial Dysplasia

In children, aneurysms due to arterial dysplasia are found almost exclusively in the renal arteries, associated with renal artery stenosis and renovascular hypertension. Recognition of the aneurysm is usually made when the patient has an angiogram for hypertension. The aneurysms commonly occur at branch points of the renal artery (Fig. 101-3) and should be distinguished from the poststenotic dilation that is frequently seen in the main renal artery. Treatment of the aneurysm may include resection and suturing of the distal end of the bypass graft to the aneurysm site if the aneurysm is near the main renal artery. No treatment is employed if the aneurysm is small and peripheral. An excellent classification of aneurysms in children was developed by Sarkar and colleagues[4] (Table 101-1).

ARTERIAL OCCLUSIVE DISEASE DUE TO ARTERIOPATHY

Takayasu Arteritis

Takayasu arteritis is an inflammatory condition of unknown cause. It usually involves the aorta and its major branches and can lead to stenosis or occlusion of the involved vessels. The condition is most commonly seen in adolescent girls but can affect boys or girls at almost any age. The sites of involvement usually are the aortic arch vessels or the mid-abdominal aorta and its branches. Diffuse major arterial occlusion can develop, which has led to the name *pulseless disease.* The pulmonary artery is involved in more than half of patients.

The presenting complaints depend on the vessels involved. Hypertension is a common finding in Takayasu arteritis, particularly with abdominal aorta and renal artery involvement. Patients with involvement of the aortic arch may present with signs of cerebral or upper extremity ischemia or evidence of congestive heart failure. It is important to differentiate abdominal aortic Takayasu arteritis from congenital middle aortic syndrome because the appropriate therapy for Takayasu arteritis is steroid administration, whereas treatment of middle aortic syndrome is surgical revascularization. Use of the erythrocyte sedimentation rate or other inflammatory markers should help in diagnosing Takayasu arteritis.

Despite the use of steroids to stabilize the vascular disease in Takayasu arteritis, there is often long-term arterial occlusion as the involved artery heals by fibrosis. Operative therapy in

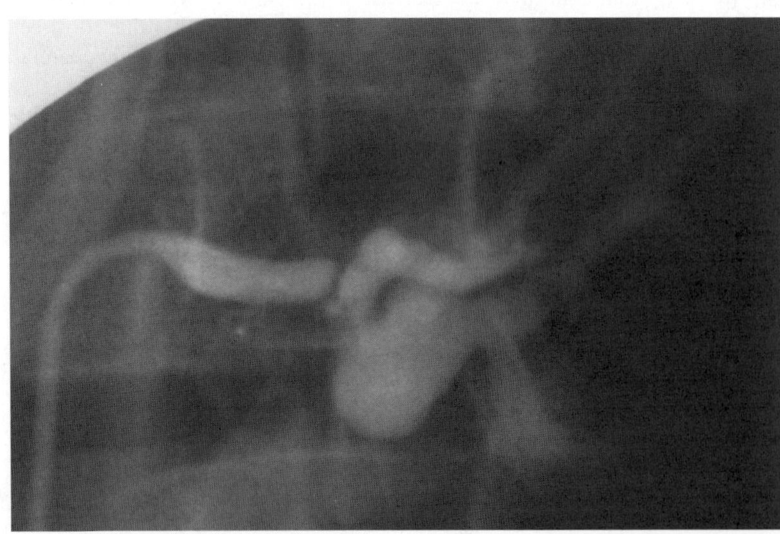

FIG. 101-3. Aneurysm of a branch of the left renal artery associated with high-grade stenosis of the main renal artery.

TABLE 101-1. *Classification of aneurysms in children**

Class	Description	Principal arteries affected	Histologic and morphologic character	Clinical characteristics
I	Arterial infection	Aorta (particularly thoracic), iliac	Acute inflammatory infiltrates present initially, then chronic inflammation and fibrotic changes; saccular aneurysms	Cariovascular anomalies and umbilical artery catheterization predisposing factors; dyspnea, cough, chest pain with progression to ruption and death if untreated
II	Giant cell aortoarteritis	Aorta (peripheral arteries, rare)	Chronic inflammation with giant cells, vessel wall necrosis; saccular aneurysms	Signs and symptoms vary from being absent to shock; untreated aortic lesions progress to rupture
III	Autoimmune vasculitis	Renal, hepatic, and splenic arterial branches	Chronic panmural inflammation and degeneration, late fibrosis; multiple small saccular aneurysms	Usually asymptomatic but may cause hematuria, perirenal hematomas, or death with ruture
IV	Kawasaki disease	Coronary (20%–30%), axillobrachial, iliofemoral, hepatic	Medial degeneration and fibrosis; multiple small saccular aneurysms	Often asymptomatic; myocardial infarction or tamponade (coronary), limb ischemia (extremity), and obstructive jaundice (hepatic) may occur
V	Medial degeneration: Marfan and Ehlers-Danlos syndromes	Aorta	Medial elastic tissue disorganization, mucinous deposits (cystic medial necrosis); solitary saccular or fusiform aneurysms	Aortic rupture or dissection common; arteriography and vascular reconstruction hazardous in type IV Ehlers-Danlos syndrome
VI	Medial degeneration: other forms	Aorta (peripheral arteries, rare)	Medial elastic tissue disorganization, mucinous deposits (cystic medial necrosis); solitary saccular aneurysms	Associated with other cardiac (biscuspid aortic valve) and aortic (coarctation) anomalies; often present with aortic dissection or rupture
VII	Arterial dysplasias	Renal	Medial thinning and fibroplasia; solitary and multiple saccular aneurysms affecting arterial bifurcations most often	Usually asymptomatic, detected during arteriography for renovascular hypertension
VIII	Idiopathic, congenital	Iliofemoral, brachial, aorta	Secondary intimal fibroplasia; saccular, usually solitary, symmetric if multiple	Often asymptomatic but may cause limb ischemia; rupture unreported
IX	Extravascular causes	Aorta, visceral, and extremity arteries	Disruption of usual three layers of artery, fibrosis, and mural thrombus; saccular aneurysms	Protean manifestations; aortic aneurysms often rupture; peripheral lesions often asymptomatic; visceral lesions may cause gastrointestinal bleeding

*Based on a review of 135 reported cases and those in the current report. Excludes aneurysms of the intracranial and coronary arteries.

(Adapted from Sarkar R, Coran AG, Cilley RE, et al. Arterial aneurysms in children: clinicopathologic classification. J Vasc Surg 1991;13:47)

acute Takayasu arteritis should be avoided because of the high failure rate of revascularization; even in "healed" Takayasu arteritis, the success rate is not good.[5]

Giant Cell Arteritis

Giant cell arteritis is an extremely uncommon cause of arterial occlusion in children. It involves the aorta and is treated similarly to Takayasu arteritis, with steroids. The only way to differentiate giant cell from Takayasu arteritis is with histologic evaluation of the vessel, which is seldom necessary.

Other Forms of Arteriopathy

Autoimmune diseases such as polyarteritis nodosum can cause arterial disease in children, but these are rarely of clinical significance. Vasospastic disorders, such as Raynaud syndrome and reflex sympathetic dystrophy, can occur in older children. These disorders are usually responsive to biofeedback or medical therapy and seldom are improved long-term by surgical sympathectomy.[6] Atherosclerosis associated with type II hyperlipoproteinemia can cause severe arterial disease in childhood, but early recognition and treatment of this familial disease should make peripheral vascular disease uncommon before adulthood.

Intracranial arterial occlusive disease in children without a definite cause has been called *moyamoya disease*. The Japanese term moyamoya is derived from the angiographic appearance of the collaterals that form because of extensive stenoses and occlusions of vessels within the circle of Willis. There may be many causes of moyamoya disease because the distribution of lesions and clinical signs vary considerably in different areas of the world. Unfortunately, the diagnosis often is made only after a major stroke has occurred. If the diagnosis is made early enough, however, extracranial-to-intracranial arterial bypass may benefit some children with moyamoya disease.

RENOVASCULAR HYPERTENSION

Hypertension in childhood is defined as three blood pressure measurements, taken in a quiet environment, that are above the 95th percentile for the child's age and gender. Unfortunately, routine blood pressure measurements are not done by all physicians as a part of yearly examinations in children. As a result, most hypertensive children come to the attention of a pediatric nephrologist or pediatric surgeon because of hypertension identified serendipitously when the child is seen in an emergency room for another reason and routine vital signs have been taken. A small percentage of hypertensive children have symptoms; some of these children present with congestive heart failure due to hypertensive cardiomyopathy, chronic irritability, headaches, or even stroke.

With the heightened awareness of the potential for thoracic coarctation in the newborn period, renovascular hypertension is the most common form of surgically correctable hypertension in children older than 1 year of age. A child with hypertension who is younger than 10 years of age has a greater than 50% chance of having a surgically correctable form of hypertension. In teenagers, essential hypertension is the most common form of hypertension; 20% of these patients have surgically correctable elevated blood pressures.[7]

Pathophysiology

The cause of renovascular disease is unknown in most children. Some patients with the middle aortic syndrome have histories consistent with arteritis, but most do not and probably have congenital aortic or renal artery disease. Renovascular hypertension can be associated with neurofibromatosis; it is usually bilateral in those cases. The most common site of stenosis is the renal ostium, particularly when the lesions are bilateral, part of the middle aortic syndrome, or associated with neurofibromatosis. The main renal artery is the next most common site of stenosis; the segmental arteries are the least common location for stenosis.

The histologic evaluation of the stenotic lesions invariably shows fibromuscular dysplasia in the medial or perimedial muscular layers, with intimal hyperplasia of variable degrees. Stanley proposed that the disease within the muscular layer is a developmental one and that intimal hyperplasia is secondary to abnormal flow through the stenotic artery.[8]

Evaluation of the Hypertensive Child

A careful history and physical examination is important in the evaluation of children with hypertension. The history may reveal subtle symptoms of hypertension, such as irritability in the young child or a decreased energy level when cardiomyopathy is present. In the child with abdominal aortic coarctation, there may be a history consistent with leg claudication. On physical examination, the presence of diminished femoral pulses may be due to thoracic or abdominal aortic coarctation. About 15% of children with renovascular hypertension have associated abdominal aortic coarctation and may also have superior mesenteric artery and celiac artery stenosis as a part of the middle aortic syndrome (Fig. 101-4). Abdominal bruits are common in children with middle aortic syndrome but less so in simple renal artery stenosis.

Presence of an abdominal mass in the area of the kidney should alert the examiner to the possibility of a retroperitoneal tumor, such as Wilms tumor, pheochromocytoma, or neuroblastoma. A hydronephrotic kidney may also present with hyperten-

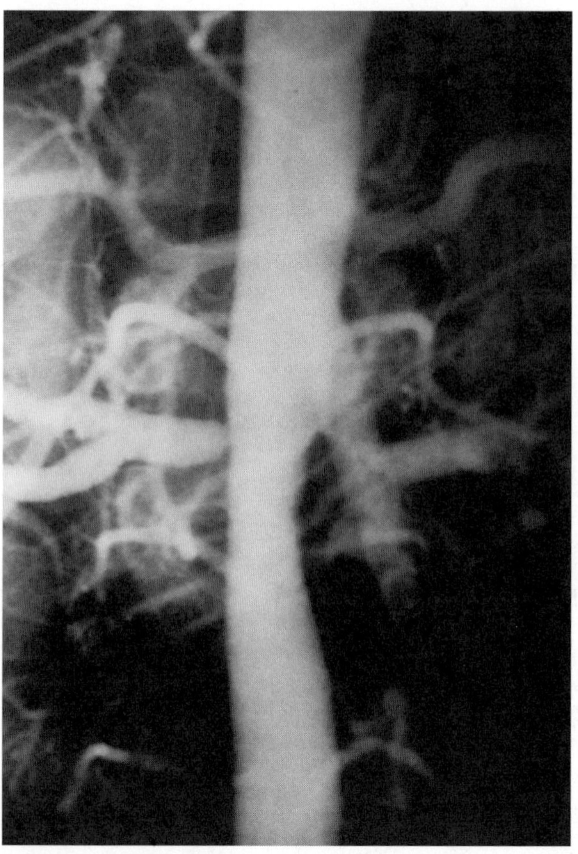

FIG. 101-4. Aortic stenosis and bilateral renal artery stenosis in an 8-year-old girl with middle aortic syndrome.

sion and an abdominal mass. In these patients, abdominal ultrasound followed by CT or MR imaging is appropriate.

Given that the most common medical cause of hypertension in children is renal disease, renal function is evaluated with serum blood urea nitrogen and creatinine and urinalysis. Most children with renovascular hypertension, even when it is bilateral, have normal renal function tests. Peripheral vein renins are elevated from many causes of hypertension and thus are not helpful in differentiating the source. Most children seen are already on antihypertensive medications, which further obfuscates the importance of peripheral vein renins.

Radiographic studies should begin with an ultrasound of the kidneys and abdomen and with Doppler ultrasound assessment of the aorta and renal vessels. The DTPA renal scan is helpful in identifying patients at high risk for renovascular hypertension when it is done without, and then with, pretreatment with the angiotensin-converting enzyme inhibitor captopril. If there is decreased function after the captopril challenge, the likelihood of renovascular stenosis is high. If the scan in patients pretreated with captopril is normal, renovascular disease is not ruled out completely; in fact, it may be present bilaterally.

Selective renal arteriography remains the most accurate method for diagnosing renovascular disease in children. It also may serve as a method of treatment by angioplasty (discussed later). The use of selective renal vein renins in children is seldom necessary, except to decide which side to do first when bilateral disease is to be corrected in separate procedures. In contrast to those in adults, the excellent collateral vessels of children make the renal vein renin ratios less predictive of successful control of the hypertension by correction of the renal artery stenosis. Correction of stenosis cures or improves blood pressure management in over 90% of children who have hypertension and a radiographic renal artery stenosis of greater than 50%, regardless of their renal vein renin levels.

Treatment

Medical Management

All children with hypertension are treated with antihypertensive medications. Patients with renovascular hypertension are at risk for decreased renal function on the side, or sides, with renal artery stenosis when the blood pressure is controlled with angiotensin-converting enzyme inhibitors. Although the renal dysfunction seen after the use of these agents typically is reversible, it is best to avoid them before definitive therapy for renal artery stenosis. The excellent long-term results of renal artery dilation and surgical revascularization in children with renovascular hypertension has made life-long antihypertensive medication, without attempted correction of the stenosis, an unacceptable option.

Percutaneous Transluminal Angioplasty

Dilation of the stenotic renal artery has a definite place in the treatment of renovascular hypertension in children. The lesions that appear to be most amenable to dilation are those within the main renal artery, away from secondary branches. The stenotic lesions that are located at the renal artery ostium

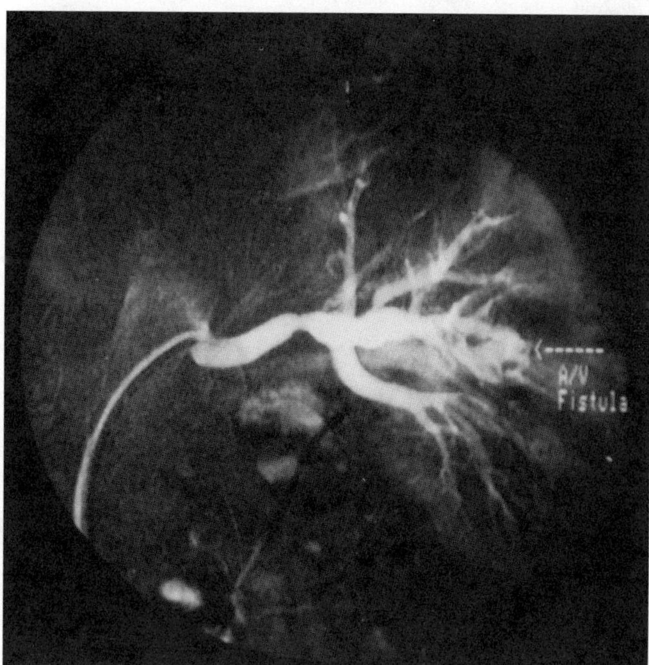

FIG. 101-5. Intraparenchymal renal arteriovenous fistula due to guide-wire injury during attempted percutaneous transluminal angioplasty for renal artery stenosis.

(especially those associated with the middle aortic syndrome) or those adjacent to an aneurysm should not, and often cannot safely, be dilated. These lesions should be surgically repaired. Although complications, such as arterial occlusion, arterial perforation, and renal arteriovenous fistulas, can occur with percutaneous transluminal angioplasty (PTA; Fig. 101-5), success rates of over 80% have been obtained in some children with renovascular hypertension when appropriate lesions have been selected for PTA (Fig. 101-6).

Surgical Revascularization

Any therapy for renal artery stenosis in children must be compared with reported results of greater than 90% cured or improved with surgical revascularization.[8,9] The goal of surgery is correction of the hypertension with preservation of renal function. The high rate of bilateral disease in children (40% in the author's experience) mandates that every effort be made to preserve the kidney with renal artery stenosis.

For unilateral renal artery stenosis, a transverse, transperitoneal incision is used. Approach to the renal artery is direct, with little dissection of the kidney to minimize disruption of the collateral vessels, which maintain some renal perfusion during occlusion of the renal artery for bypass. In patients with the middle aortic syndrome, a left thoracoabdominal incision for aortoaortic bypass grafting done extraperitoneally gives the best exposure to the proximal aorta for anastomosis and is well tolerated.

The technique of renal artery revascularization is best managed in children by renal artery bypass with autogenous tissue. When the lesion is unilateral, use of a hypogastric artery free graft is the first choice for the following reasons: (1) the hypogastric artery is usually a good size match with the renal artery; (2) it is capable of withstanding arterial pressure without the risk of aneurysmal dilation long-term; and (3) it can be harvested through the same incision as the renal artery repair. The second choice for graft material to bypass a stenotic renal artery is a saphenous vein graft. The risk of aneurysmal dilation with use of the saphenous vein graft (Fig. 101-7) may be overcome by wrapping it with a Dacron net, as advocated by O'Neill.[10]

In patients who have middle aortic syndrome in conjunction with left renal artery stenosis, the left renal artery can be reimplanted directly into the prosthetic graft that is used to bypass the aortic narrowing (Fig. 101-8). The prosthetic graft used for the aortic bypass is polytetrafluoroethylene, size 10 mm, and no attempt is made to leave extra length for growth. The author's preference is to stage the revascularization of bilateral renal artery stenosis by repairing the two sides about 6 weeks apart, although some surgeons recommend bypassing both sides at the same procedure.[10] The anastomosis is performed with monofilament, absorbable sutures placed in an interrupted fashion.

Renal reimplantation or autotransplantation techniques with use of "bench" surgical repair of the renal vessels[11] may be applicable for branch renal artery stenosis but otherwise has little use in children with renovascular hypertension.

Two thirds of children with renal artery stenosis have their hypertension cured (normotensive, no medications) when PTA and surgical revascularization are used in combination. Another 25% achieve improved blood pressure control on less medica-

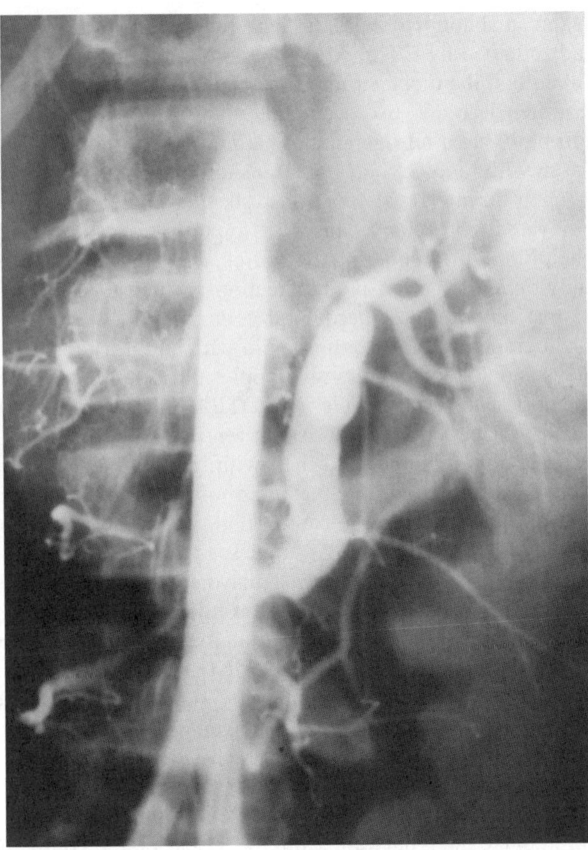

FIG. 101-7. Aortorenal saphenous bypass graft with significant dilation of the graft 1 year after revascularization in an 11-year-old boy.

tion. Less than 10% do not see improvement with this aggressive approach to correct stenosis. Nephrectomy for failed revascularization occurs in 5% to 15% of these patients.[8,9]

ARTERIOVENOUS MALFORMATIONS

Congenital

Congenital arteriovenous malformation (AVM) remains the least satisfactorily treated vascular lesion in childhood. The cause of these lesions is most likely an anomaly of development in which the arterial and venous systems communicate without passing through the capillaries. It is uncertain why some patients present in the newborn period while others not until adolescence with these congenital lesions. The presenting symptoms may be pain or a sensation of excessive warmth in the area of the AVM, hypertrophy of the tissue or limb involved with the AVM, congestive heart failure because of high cardiac output, or hemorrhage into the AVM or externally if the lesion has a component in the skin.

Congenital AVM can occur in any location, but pediatric surgeons are most often asked to see those on the trunk or extremities. Physical examination is helpful in identifying the location of the AVM but commonly results in underestimation of the extent of the lesion. The development of limb hypertrophy

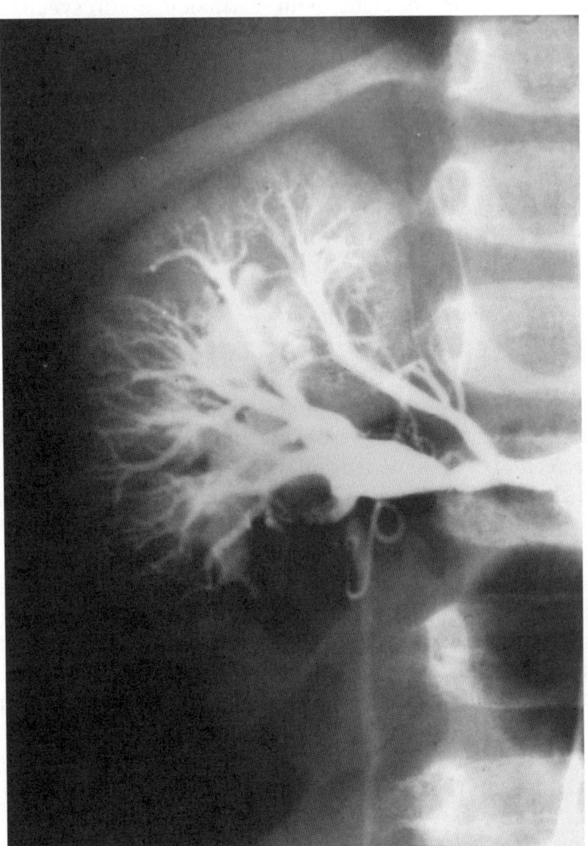

FIG. 101-6. Study made after percutaneous transluminal angioplasty of main renal artery stenosis in a 6-year-old boy. Long-terms results were excellent.

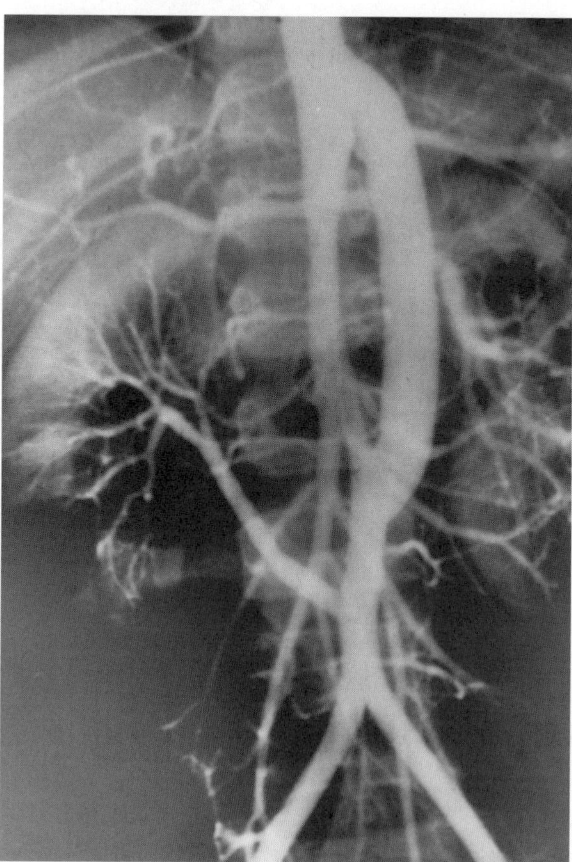

FIG. 101-8. Aortoaortic bypass graft with polytetrafluoroethylene, left renal artery implantation directly into the graft, and right aortorenal bypass with hypogastric artery in a 6-year-old girl with middle aortic syndrome.

the functional result of the treatment should be compared with function before treatment; (3) the flow thorough the fistula may be great enough to cause long-term cardiac problems; and (4) the proposed treatment may effect future treatment options if the AVM recurs.

For the rare situation in which the AVM is well localized and involves nonvital structures, complete surgical excision is the procedure of choice. Some surgeons prefer preoperative AVM embolization to minimize blood loss, but it may make it difficult to determine whether the resection has been complete, and it is not necessary for smaller lesions. In the usual AVM, embolization is useful because the lesion is extensive, and complete surgical excision would require removal of large amounts of normal tissue, such as an amputation. Embolization of the extensive lesions may be the sole form of therapy or may be used in preparation for excision. Embolization is most effective when done into the small arteries of the AVM because embolization of the major arteries may lead to ischemia of distal normal tissues and has no better success rate than embolizing the smaller vessels. When the AVM occurs in an organ that is expendable, such as a pulmonary lobe, resection is the procedure of choice.

Unless wide excision of normal-appearing tissues is performed, recurrence is likely. Even in patients who undergo amputation, recurrence may develop in the tissue that appeared to be entirely normal by previous studies. The high likelihood of recurrence has encouraged a conservative approach to most of

distal to an AVM in a child has never been adequately explained because a great deal of the blood flow to the extremity is diverted through the AVM. Some evidence suggests that limb hypertrophy is due to the elevated pressure and stasis on the venous side of the AVM.

A rough assessment of the amount of flow through the AVM can be obtained if the main artery feeding the malformation can be temporarily occluded by external compression. Patients with over 20% of their cardiac output going through the AVM have tachycardia, and compression of the feeding artery decrease their pulse rates by over 10% and often increases their blood pressures (the Branham sign). Although patients with hemodynamically significant AVM may have a negative Branham sign,[12] a positive sign correlates well with a significant proportion of the cardiac output going through the AVM. A thrill is often palpable over these lesions, and a characteristic bruit can be auscultated.

MR imaging has become an integral part of the evaluation of children with AVM because of its ability to define extent of disease and relation to other structures, particularly muscles. Angiography is still important in refining the MR data and may also be used in some patients for treatment with embolization.

Treatment strategies must be individualized and must be done with the following factors in mind: (1) complete ablation or excision is infrequently possible; (2) if an extremity is involved,

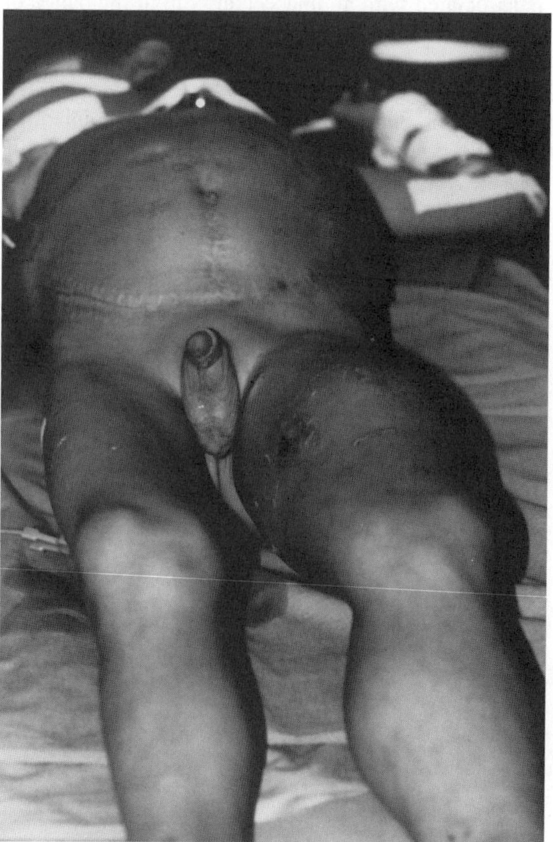

FIG. 101-9. Left leg hypertrophy in an 8-year-old boy with a left femoral artery–femoral vein prosthetic fistula created for hemodialysis.

congenital AVMs, particularly those of the extremity that can be compressed with tight stockings if the cardiac function is not compromised by the AVM. In the future, approaches to control angiogenesis (see Chap. 32) may also be applicable in these children.

Acquired

Acquired AVMs are the result of penetrating trauma or surgical procedure for hemodialysis access. In penetrating trauma of the extremity, there is a trend to avoid exploration of the extremity in the absence of ongoing hemorrhage or pulse deficit.[3] This approach may lead to an increased number of children with acquired AVMs. This type of AVM may be due to injury of the vein and artery adjacent to each other or to an arterial false aneurysm that later decompresses into a vein.

In children with renal failure who are on hemodialysis, it is important to know the type and location of the arteriovenous fistula to prevent too much flow through the fistula, which can lead to cardiac decompensation and limb hypertrophy. The use of autogenous tissue, usually a radial artery–to–cephalic vein fistula, remains the best vascular access for hemodialysis, with the lowest complication rate. If a prosthetic graft must be used because of small vessel size, it is best to stay as distal as possible and to use the upper extremity as the access site. The formation of a femoral–femoral arteriovenous fistula with prosthetic material provides excellent hemodialysis access but in small children is associated with an unacceptably high incidence of cardiac complications and limb hypertrophy[13] (Fig. 101-9).

If the acquired AVM is due to trauma, it should be surgically repaired when identified. If the AVM is created for hemodialysis access, the options for dialysis must be weighed against the risks of the arteriovenous fistula. All children on dialysis are candidates for renal transplantation; when transplant recipients are taken off dialysis, it is important to assess the arteriovenous fistula to determine whether it is causing cardiac or extremity problems.

REFERENCES

1. Skandalakis JE, Gray SW, Symbas P. The thoracic and abdominal aorta. In: Skandalakis JE, Gray SW, eds. Embryology for surgeons, ed 2. Baltimore, Williams & Wilkins, 1994:976.
2. Guzzetta PC. Congenital and acquired aneurysmal disease. Semin Pediatr Surg 1994;3:97.
3. Frykberg ER, Crump JM, Dennis JW, et al. Nonoperative observation of clinically occult arterial injuries: a prospective evaluation. Surgery 1991;109:85.
4. Sarkar R, Coran AG, Cilley RE, et al. Arterial aneurysms in children: clinicopathologic classification. J Vasc Surg 1991;13:47.
5. Beale PG, Meyers KEC, Thomson PD. Management of renal hypertension in children with Takayasu's arteritis using renal autografting or allograft transplantation in selected circumstances and total lymphoid irradiation. J Pediatr Surg 1992;27:836.
6. Athreya BH. Vasospastic disorders in children. Semin Pediatr Surg 1994;3:70.
7. Lawson JD, Boerth R, Foster JH, et al. Diagnosis and management of renovascular hypertension in children. Arch Surg 1977;112:1307.
8. Stanley JC. Pathologic basis of macrovascular renal artery disease. In: Stanley JC, Ernst CB, Fry WJ, eds. Renovascular hypertension. Philadelphia, WB Saunders, 1984:46.
9. Guzzetta PC, Potter BM, Ruley EJ, et al. Renovascular hypertension in children: current concepts in evaluation and treatment. J Pediatr Surg 1989;24:1236.
10. O'Neill JA. Renovascular hypertension. Semin Pediatr Surg 1994;3:114.
11. van Bockel JH, van den Akker PJ, Chang PC, et al. Extracorporeal renal artery reconstruction for renovascular hypertension. J Vasc Surg 1991;13:101.
12. Graff KG, Frederick DS, Singh JB. Branham's sign revisited. N Engl J Med 1977;297:509.
13. Guzzetta PC, Salcedo JR, Bell SB, et al. Limb growth and cardiac complications of fistulas in children. Int J Pediatr Nephrol 1987;8:167.

Surgery of Infants and Children: Scientific Principles and Practice, edited by Keith T. Oldham, Paul M. Colombani, and Robert P. Foglia. Lippincott–Raven Publishers, Philadelphia, © 1997.

CHAPTER 102

Lymphatic and Venous Disorders

Peter Dillon

VENOUS DISORDERS

Venous disorders in children present a broad spectrum of clinical challenges to the pediatric surgeon. Complex congenital lesions encountered in the newborn or early infancy period dominate the pathology. However, acquired processes that are more commonly diagnosed in the older patients may also be found. The proper diagnosis and management of these pathologic disorders serves to minimize the morbidity and long-term consequences of these problems.

Embryology

By the fourth week of gestation, vascular channels have formed from endothelium-lined spaces within the mesenchymal tissue of the embryo. The resulting venous plexus can be divided into two systems—visceral and parietal (Fig. 102-1).

The visceral system is composed of the paired vitelline and umbilical veins. These four veins terminate in the region of the septum transversum and contribute to the sinus venosus. Initially existing as paired veins on either side of the developing gastrointestinal tract, the vitelline veins completely disappear except for the sections surrounded by developing liver parenchyma. The right vitelline vein forms the right branch of the portal vein and its sinusoids. The left vitelline vein contributes to the formation of the main portal vein and its left branch. The left umbilical vein leaves the placental circulation and joins the left vitelline vein in the septum transversum to form the ductus venosus, which is a crucial structure for circulation in utero. The right umbilical vein completely disappears.

The parietal system consists of the paired precardinal and postcardinal veins. These veins are connected by right and left common cardinal veins at the level of the sinus venosus in the region of the developing heart. The precardinal veins drain the cranial half of the developing embryo and eventually form the internal jugular veins. The right precardinal and common cardinal veins also form the superior vena cava, whereas the left precardinal and common cardinal veins atrophy. The left brachiocephalic vein develops from a connection between the two precardinal systems, whereas the subclavian and upper extremity veins develop from the limb buds. Inferiorly, the postcardinal veins drain the caudal half of the embryo, which includes the venous drainage of the lower limb buds, the body wall, and the mesonephric ridges. The right postcardinal vein and its associated plexus contribute in a large part to the development of the inferior vena cava, and there is regression of the left postcardinal system. Lower limb veins develop from limb bud mesenchyme and fuse with the postcardinal structures to establish the right and left iliac systems.

Physiology

The architecture of the vein wall comprises intimal, medial, and adventitial layers composed of endothelium, collagen, elastic tissue, and smooth muscle. Venous tone and capacity are directly influenced by the innervation of the smooth muscle layers by the sympathetic nervous system as well as circulating catecholamine levels. The net result is a system capable of vasoconstriction with a decrease in venous volume and cross-sectional area. Vasodilation appears to be due to the withdrawal of sympathetic stimulation.

One half to two thirds of the body's circulating blood volume can be contained within the venous system, depending on the tone of the vessels. Blood flow through this system is dependent primarily on the driving force of cardiac contractions. However, venous flow is also aided by the negative intrathoracic pressure gradients created during inspiration and the contraction of skeletal muscles resulting in peripheral vein compression and flow augmentation. Valves throughout the venules and larger veins promote unidirectional blood flow toward the heart. In the veins of the lower extremity, the tibial vessels have 10 to 15 valves each, the superficial femoral vein has no more than four, the internal iliac vein has one, and the vena cava has none.[1] These valves in the lower extremity are particularly important, since venous blood flow is also dependent on gravity. During quiet standing, venous pressure at the ankle in an adult can approach 100 mmHg owing to the hydrostatic pressure of the column of blood. Loss of function by these valves leads to inefficient pumping action by the skeletal muscles and contributes to venous hypertension in the extremity. The consequences of persistent venous hypertension in the lower extremity can be quite debilitating. As a result of the increased pressure, Starling forces

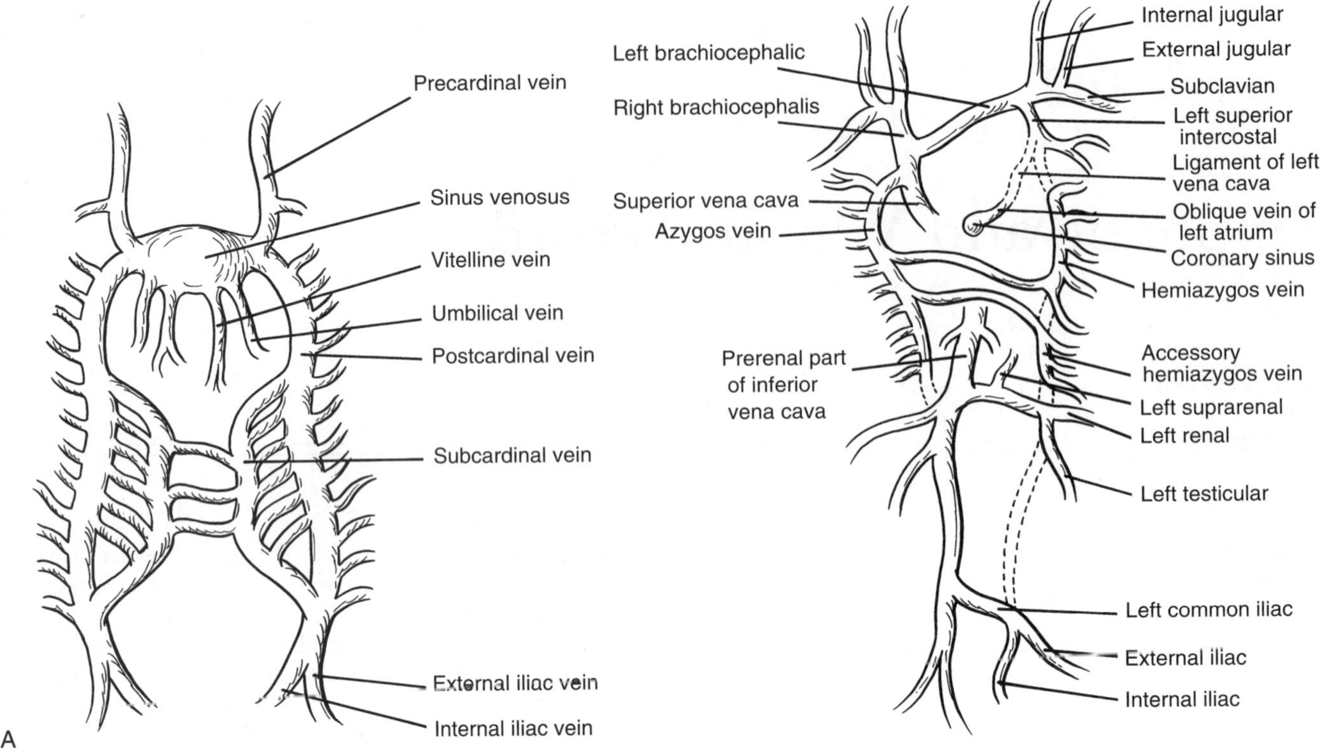

FIG. 102-1. (*A*) Schematic representation of the early fetal venous system involving the visceral and parietal systems. (*B*) Final development of the systemic venous system.

are altered at the capillary level and lead to the formation of chronic edema with protein extravasation, inadequate tissue oxygen transfer, and eventually venous stasis ulcers—a condition found more frequently in adults but which can occur in children.

Venous endothelial cells have a number of important functions affecting the physiology of blood flow through these vessels. It has been shown that an intact endothelial layer is required to mediate vasomotor response to a number of circulating agents.[2] Additionally, the endothelium is capable of producing agents such as endothelium-derived relaxing factor, identified as nitric oxide, which causes vasodilation, and endothelin, which causes local vasoconstriction. Endothelial cells also play a crucial role in regulating thrombosis and blood coagulation by synthesizing and expressing on their surfaces a number of coagulant and antithrombotic agents (Table 102-1). Heparan sulfate is synthesized by the endothelium and binds to antithrombin III to increase its affinity for thrombin as well as to factors VII, IX, and X, resulting in their neutralization. Thrombomodulin, which blocks the protelytic activity of thrombin and activates proteins C and S to inactivate factor Va, is also synthesized and secreted by endothelial cells. In addition, tissue plaminogen activator (TPA) is synthesized and stored in the vein wall. It is responsible for degrading fibrin by activating plasminogen to plasmin. A number of factors that promote coagulation are also synthesized by the endothelium and include von Willebrand factor, factor VIII, and an inhibitor of plasminogen activator. As a result of these biochemical activities, the pathologic processes encountered in a number of vascular disorders may be affected by the endothelial lining of the venous system.

Congenital Venous Disorders

Anomalies can result from abnormal vascular embryogenesis during the course of development. Congenital abnormalities of the central veins are more common and likely to be asymptomatic, whereas those of peripheral veins are usually symptomatic because of associated defects.

Superior Vena Cava Abnormalities

The most common congenital abnormality of the major veins of the thorax is agenesis of the left innominate vein associated with the persistence of the left precardinal vein.[3] A double or duplicated superior vena cava system develops with the right superior vena cava (SVC) draining directly into the right atrium and the left SVC draining into the coronary sinus. If the right precardinal vein undergoes regression rather than the left, a solitary left SVC will develop. This vessel empties directly into the coronary sinus on the posterior wall of the heart and then into the right atrium. These abnormalities are clinically asymptomatic and present no functional impairment to blood flow. However, the anatomic arrangement of superior vena caval blood return to the heart is of significant concern when planning

TABLE 102-1. *Factors regulating important physiologic functions of intact venous endothelium*

VASODILATATION
Arachadonic acid
Adenosine triphosphate
Adenosine diphosphate
Acetylcholine
Bradykinin
Cholecystokinin
Histamine
Norepinephrine
Serotonin
Thrombin
Vasopressin
Vasoactive intestinal polypeptide
Nitric oxide

VASOCONSTRICTION
Endothelin

ANTICOAGULATION
Heparan sulphate
Thrombomodulin
Prostacyclin
Plasminogen
Tissue plasminogen activator

COAGULATION
von Willebrand factor
Plasminogen activator inhibitor
Factor VIII

cardiopulmonary bypass for cardiac surgery, extracorporeal membrane oxygenation for respiratory support, or central venous catheter insertion. These anomalies are usually discovered during the course of a cardiac evaluation by echocardiography or catheterization. Associated cardiac septal abnormalities have been found in one third of the patients.

Inferior Vena Cava Abnormalities

Malformations of the inferior vena cava (IVC) have been reported in 1% to 4% of the population.[4] With the complex pattern of postcardinal development leading to the formation of the IVC, a spectrum of anomalies can be seen. Similar to abnormalities of the SVC, most malformations of the IVC are asymptomatic and discovered during the course of radiographic evaluation or abnominal surgery for other reasons. Such anomalies may include duplication of the inferior vena cava, a left-sided inferior vena cava, or agenesis. When the inferior vena cava fails to develop, the azygous vein becomes the major route of venous blood flow to the heart from the lower extremities. This azygous continuation is associated with the asplenia-polyspenia syndrome and with congenital heart disease.

Congenital obstruction of the IVC has been reported from an internal web in the suprahepatic vena cava or a persistent right atrial eustachian valve.[5] Symptoms of caval and hepatic vein obstruction gradually develop over years. Radiographic evaluation with an inferior vena cavogram or an MRI will confirm the diagnosis. Cavocaval bypass or excision of the web have been successful treatments for this anomaly.

Portal Vein Malformations

Portal vein anomalies are extremely rare and usually discovered while evaluating for other conditions. The spectrum of anomalies includes agenesis, duplication, and malposition. Agenesis of the portal vein results in a direct connection of the mesenteric veins to either a renal vein or the IVC. An appreciation of this anomaly is crucial when planning hepatic surgery or transplantation. Malposition is most typified by the portal vein presenting as a preduodenal vascular structure and is associated with duodenal obstruction and atresia. No vascular intervention is necessary.

Peripheral and Deep Vein Malformations

Abnormalities of the peripheral and deep venous systems include agenesis, duplication, valvular agenesis, varicosities, anomalous position, and compression syndromes. Varicosities of the superficial veins of the lower extremities are the most common vascular abnormalities in adults and are usually due to valvular dysfunction. Such problems have been reported in older children and teenagers. Atresias of the iliac, femoral, or axillary veins are extremely rare. They are seen as part of the Klippel-Trénaunay syndrome. Compression syndromes of the axillary and iliac veins may result in thrombosis. Axillary vein compression is caused by a fibrous or muscular band at the thoracic outlet. Axillary vein thrombosis occurs following strenuous activities (effort thrombosis) or after prolonged extremity immobilization. Abnormalities at the origin of the left iliac vein have been documented and include intraluminal septations or external compression by the crossing right iliac artery. Most cases are isolated to the left iliac system. In general, symptomatic venous obstruction is surgically eliminated if possible. Most patients, however, are best treated with conservative strategies, such as compression garments and extremity elevation.

Thrombotic Venous Disorders

Venous thromboembolic disease in the pediatric population is assuming greater clinical significance as a result of aggressive therapeutic advances in such areas as neonatology, oncology, and gastroenterology and with the attendant use of long-term venous catheters. Previously thought to be rare in children, deep venous thrombosis and its most severe complication, pulmonary embolism, are now recognized with increased frequency. In the past, clinical parameters for the diagnosis and management of these problems had been extrapolated from adult experience. A number of studies now document important differences in venous thromboembolic disease between children and adults, and emphasize the age and developmental status in determining the responses to various therapeutic interventions.

Etiology

The principles of stasis, endothelial damage, and hypercoagulable state (Virchows triad) are applicable to the pathophysiology of pediatric venous disorders. In contrast to adults, all infants and children with thrombosis of either the central or peripheral venous systems have a serious underlying disorder

TABLE 102-2. *Factors associated with venous thrombosis in children and adolescents*

Disorder	%
Indwelling catheter	21
Surgery	13
Trauma	9
Infection	6
Tumor	6
Total parenteral nutrition	6
Hereditary disorder	4
Athletic activity	4
Obesity	2
Paralysis	2

(After David M, Andrew M. Venous thromboembolic complications in children. J Pediatr 1993;123:338)

or predisposing factor (Table 102-2). Risk factors for vascular, thrombosis in the neonatal period include asphyxia, shock, dehydration, polycythemia, sepsis, and maternal diabetes. In infants and children, underlying conditions contributing to venous thrombosis are cancer, congenital heart disease, and venous system interventions such as with catheters, trauma, and surgery.[6] The most common cause of deep-vein thrombosis in children of all ages is the use of long-term indwelling vascular access devices for total parenteral nutrition (TPN) or chemotherapy administration. In contrast, inherited disorders of coagulation as a predisposing cause of venous thrombosis in children are relatively rare.

Infants younger than 1 year are at high risk for thrombotic events, regardless of associated conditions, and premature infants may be at the highest risk of all. Until approximately 6 months of age, the neonate exists in a relatively hypercoagulable state with immature mechanisms of hemostasis and fibrinolysis. Plasma concentrations of a number of coagulation and fibrinolytic factors are dependent on gestational age.[7] Factors I, V, and VIII reach their maximum levels during the last trimester of development. However, the vitamin K–dependent factors II, VII, IX, and X and the factors XI, XII, and III are at 50% of adult levels in a full-term infant at birth. The anticoagulant factors antithrombin III, protein C, and protein S are also at about 50% of adult plasma levels at the time of birth. These imbalances in the control of the coagulation cascade result in a predisposition for thrombosis in the neonate that may be exacerbated by associated factors such as polycythemia, asphyxia, and indwelling catheters. Additionally, the fibrinolytic system of full-term neonates is immature, with only 50% to 70% of adult plasminogen levels typically demonstrable. In contrast, there are normal levels of plasmin inhibitors. The resulting imbalance in the endogenous fibrinolytic system favors thrombosis in the neonate.

Hereditary disorders of the proteins antithrombin III, protein C, protein S, and plasminogen are known to increase the risk of thromboembolic disease.[8] Antithrombin III is a serine protease inhibitor that binds preferentially to thrombin and factor Xa. Protein C is a vitamin K–dependent serine protease that binds to its cofactor protein S to ultimately inactivate factors Va,

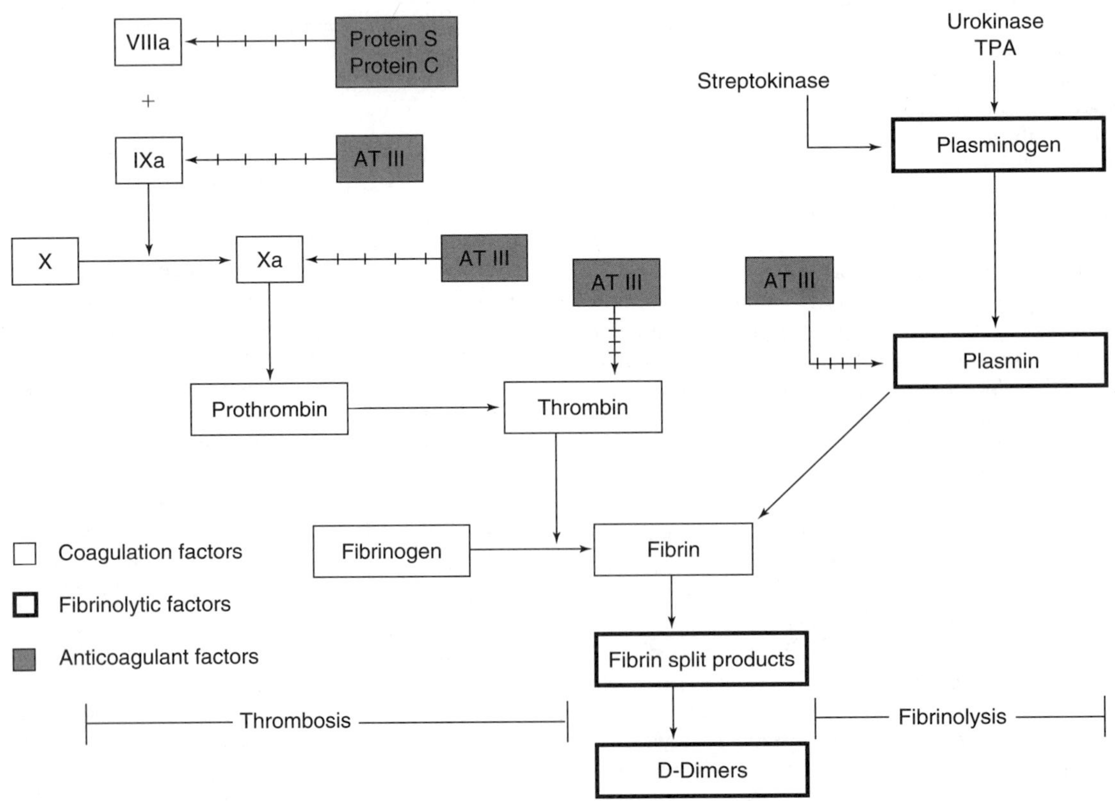

FIG. 102-2. Final common pathways for coagulation and thrombolysis.

VIIIa, and plasminogen activator inhibitor (Fig. 102-2). Plasminogen is normally converted into plasmin to induce clot dissolution. At normal levels of activity, these proteins interrupt the coagulation process and promote thrombolysis. Inherited coagulation deficiencies are responsible for approximately 4% of venous thrombotic events in both adults and children. Patients with an inherited antithrombin III deficiency have a greater risk of thrombosis than those with congenital deficiencies in the other proteins.[9,10] The clinical risk of thrombosis in a patient with hereditary antithrombin III deficiency is 5% in the first decade of life and increases to 65% by 30 years of age.[11]

Acquired deficiencies of these anticoagulation factors are seen in neonatal and pediatric patients.[12] Reduced levels of protein C and protein S have been detected after a number of infections because of the selective consumption of these proteins.[13-15] The most frequent viral infection has been varicella. In a number of patients, severe protein S deficiencies have been attributed to autoantibodies formed during the course of illness. Alterations in hemostasis have also been reported in patients with leukemia receiving chemotherapy.[16] Thrombotic events related to L-asparaginase chemotherapy have been reported in up to 3% of patients and appear to result from an abnormality in the regulation of platelet adherence to the vascular endothelium.[17]

Diagnostic Evaluation

The diagnosis of venous thrombosis in a child is complicated by the size of the patient, associated conditions, and number of anatomic locations potentially involved. No single diagnostic test has proved reliable in documenting the process in children, and so the evaluation has followed parameters established from adult studies.

Contrast venography remains the standard for the diagnosis of venous thrombosis, particularly in the deep veins of the pelvis and lower extremity. In adults, this is accurate in diagnosing thrombus formation in the superficial and deep veins of the calf and thigh.[1] Though its accuracy in children has never been proved, it remains the most widely used test to confirm this diagnosis.[18] Because it is invasive, carries a risk of contrast reaction and phlebitis, and may be difficult to perform in infants and small children, noninvasive diagnostic tests should be used for the initial evaluation.

The primary noninvasive diagnostic study is duplex ultrasonography. Duplex spectral or color Doppler ultrasonography permits pulsed Doppler blood flow velocity measurements with concomitant visualization of the target vessel. The technique allows for the anatomic assessment of vessel morphology and the functional assessment of vascular blood flow. It is highly effective in the detection of major vessel thrombosis in the neonate, including portal vein, renal vein, hepatic vein, and inferior vena cava.[19] In adult studies, it has been found to be 95% sensitive in diagnosing iliofemoral thrombosis.[1] Although it requires experience, it should replace invasive diagnostic tests. Impedance plethysmography is a fairly reliable test in adults for proximal deep vein thrombosis. Its efficacy in children has not been studied, and Doppler ultrasonography has supplanted it as the test of choice for evaluation of possible thrombosis. At the bedside, the use of a Doppler ultrasonogra-

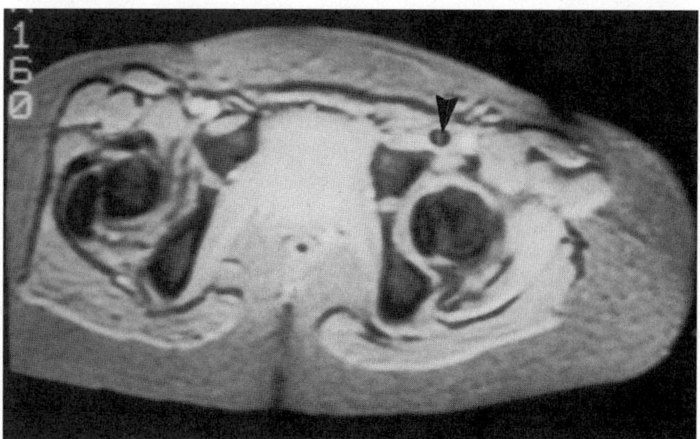

FIG. 102-3. MRI of pelvic region showing femoral vein thrombosis (*arrow*) in an 8-year-old boy.

phy to assess femoral vein flow is helpful. Normally, there should be respiratory variation in femoral venous flow. If this is lost, it is highly suggestive of inferior vena caval or iliofemoral thrombosis.

The ability of MRI to detect blood flow and assess soft tissue structures has led to the emergence of magnetic resonance venography as an important method for noninvasive vascular evaluation in children.[20,21] Using both spin echo and gradient-recalled echo techniques, studies have shown that the veins of the upper extremities, lower extremities, pelvis, abdomen, and thorax can be adequately visualized and examined for thrombosis (Fig. 102-3). In adult studies, magnetic resonance venography has been found to be 97% sensitive, 95% specific, and 96% accurate in diagnosing iliofemoral vein thrombosis when compared to venography. Additionally, MRI for superior vena cava obstruction has been shown to have an accuracy of 100% when compared with venography. In children, this technique is already utilized for inferior vena cava analysis in patients with Wilms tumors. Potential advantages of magnetic resonance venography include visualization of thrombus within the deep veins of the pelvis and thigh when venography is ineffective and routine bilateral extremity examinations for structural comparisons. This technique is especially useful in patients with inadequate venous access or in patients suspected of being unable to tolerate contrast administration because of inadequate renal function or allergic sensitivity.

Therapeutic Interventions

Most protocols for the treatment of venous thrombotic disorders in children have been extrapolated from adult studies without clinical evaluation. Recent coordinated studies have been designed to assess therapeutic interventions for pediatric venous thrombosis.

No matter what venous system is involved by the thrombotic process, the success of any therapeutic intervention must be measured in terms of three clinical goals: The therapy must prevent further extension of the thrombus within the venous system, minimize the risk of thrombus detachment and resultant pulmonary embolism, and permit the gradual dissolution or lysis of the clot with restoration of vessel continuity. For venous thrombotic disorders, pharmacologic therapy has become the primary form of intervention in both adults and children. Therapeutic options include anticoagulant therapy with heparin and warfarin (Coumadin) (1) and (2) thrombolytic therapy with streptokinase, urokinase, or recombinant TPA. There are important differences in the activities and pharmacokinetics of anticoagulant and thrombolytic agents between children and adults.

Heparin has both antithrombotic and anticoagulant activities. In adult studies, it has been shown to prevent the extension of a thrombotic process and lower the risk of a pulmonary embolus while inhibiting the coagulation cascade. In both experimental and clinical studies, children require a higher rate of heparin administration to achieve a therapeutic level because of increased clearance rates. Therefore, anticoagulating heparin therapy should be started with a loading dose of 75 units/kg administered over 10 minutes and then followed by an initial continuous infusion at 22 U/kg/h[18] (Table 102-3). Four to six hours after the loading dose, an activated partial thromboplastin time (APTT) should be obtain to determine the efficacy of heparin therapy. Subsequent changes in heparin administration should be guided by APTT values obtained every 6 to 8 hours while on therapy. Adequate anticoagulation therapy is indicated by an APTT value between 55 and 85 seconds. If a child appears to be unresponsive to heparin administration as determined by APTT values, then heparin levels should be measured directly by protamine titration analysis. Therapeutic heparin levels range between 0.2 and 0.4 U/mL. In children younger than 1 year, initial maintenance heparin administration should be increased to 28 U/kg/h. As in adults, a 5- to 7-day course of therapy is usually sufficient in conjunction with the initiation of oral anticoagulant therapy. When heparin administration is within these guidelines, the risk of hemorrhage ranges from 2% to 7%.[22]

Few studies exist to guide the administration of warfarin in children and infants.[23] To make clinical management more difficult, infants are often on formulas supplemented with vitamin K, and children may be on medications such as antiseizure drugs that influence warfarin pharmacokinetics. It is recommended that warfarin therapy be started with a daily dose at 0.2 mg/kg for 2 days then at 0.1 mg/kg/d, with subsequent doses determined by following the international normalized ratio (INR) computed from the prothrombin times (PT).[18] The INR is calculated as the PT (in seconds) divided by the control PT to the power of the international sensitivity index. This value corrects for the varying sensitivities of reagents in the prothrombin time assay. The overall optimal range for oral anticoagulation as determined by INR values is 2.1 to 3.25 and by PT values is 1.2 to 1.5 times control. Oral anticoagulation therapy can usually be stopped after 3 months.

In children, thrombolytic therapy may be clinically appropriate for a thrombotic disorder unresponsive to heparin, a massive thrombotic process with threatened loss of function, a massive pulmonary embolus, or an occluded central venous catheter. The goal of such therapy is the degradation of fibrin and the subsequent dissolution of the fibrin thrombus. The thrombolytic agents clinically available accomplish this goal by directly or indirectly converting plasminogen to plasmin, since plasmin is the proteolytic enzyme essential for fibrinolysis. Plasminogen exists freely within the plasma or complexed to fibrinogen. It becomes incorporated into a thrombus as the fibrinogen is converted to fibrin. Fibrinolytic agents that act as plasminogen activators can interact with either form of plasminogen. Within a clot, the resulting plasmin will degrade the fibrin structure and dissolve the clot. However, if free plasmin is generated in the circulation, it degrades not only fibrin but also fibrinogen and coagulation factors V and VII, resulting in the generation of a diffuse coagulopathic state.

Streptokinase was one of the earliest agents clinically available for thrombolytic therapy. It is a protein isolated from β-hemolytic streptococci. Streptokinase does not directly convert plasminogen to plasmin. It binds to plasminogen with the subsequent formation of a protein complex capable of activating other plasminogen molecules to plasmin.[24] In children, it has been used to treat superior and inferior vena cava thromboses, arterial thromboses, prosthetic graft occlusions in congenital heart disease, and cardiac valve thromboses.[25–30] A number of therapeutic regimens exist for its administration. A standard loading dose of 2000 U/kg is given, followed by a maintenance dose of 1000 to 4000 U/kg/h for 6 to 12 hours.[18] Recently, low-dose therapy at 50 U/kg/h for as long as several days has been utilized.[31,32] Because of the potential systemic effects, fibrinogen levels, PT, APTT, and fibrin split products should be closely monitored. Antibodies to this protein resulting in allergic and toxic reactions may limit its administration.

The other nonspecific thrombolytic agent is urokinase—a protein synthesized by human renal and vascular endothelial cells. It directly converts plasminogen to plasmin both in the circulation and within the thrombus.[33] Because it is not anti-

TABLE 102-3. *Anticoagulant and thrombolytic therapy in children: recommended agents and doses*[18,42]

	Loading dose	Maintenance dose
ANTICOAGULATION		
Heparin	75 U/kg	22 U/kg/h ($>$1 year)
		28 U/kg/h ($<$1 year)
Coumadin	0.1–0.2 mg/kg	adjusted according to PT/INR
		0.32 mg/kg (infants)
		0.09 mg/kg (teenagers)
THROMBOLYSIS		
Streptokinase	2000 U/kg	1000–4000 U/kg/h
		50 U/kg/h (low dose)
Urokinase		
Catheters	5000 U	200 U/h $\times$ 24 h
Systemic	4400 U/kg	4400 U/kg/h
Tissue plasminogen activator		0.1–0.5 mg/kg/h

genic, its use in pediatric patients is preferred over streptokinase. It is widely used in cases of catheter thrombosis where it is locally instilled into the occluded lumen. Its systemic administration has successfully treated extensive caval thromboses, renal vein thrombosis, and arterial obstructions.[34–40] For occluded catheters, a bolus of 5000 U in 1 or 2 mL should be left into the catheter for 2 hours. If initially unsuccessful, one or two additional volumes can be attempted. The use of continuous low-dose infusions of urokinase at 200 U/h for 24 hours has been reported.[41] For systemic therapy, a loading dose of 4400 U/kg should be given over 20 to 30 minutes followed by a maintenance infusion at 4400 U/kg/h.[18] Infusions for 24 to 48 hours have been well tolerated in children. Coagulation parameters including fibrinogen levels, fibrin split products, APTT, and PT should be followed. To avoid coagulopathy, fibrinogen levels should not be allowed to fall below 100 mg/dL. A number of hemorrhagic complications have been reported with both urokinase and streptokinase administration and include bleeding from intravenous and needle puncture sites, spontaneous retroperitoneal hemorrhages, and intracranial hemorrhage in a newborn.

TPA is a fibrin-specific agent. It binds poorly to circulating plasminogen or fibrinogen but strongly to fibrin. As such, it actively converts plasminogen to plasmin only when bound to fibrin on the surface of a thrombus.[33] Because TPA induces a minimal systemic proteolytic state while inducing thrombolysis within the local environment of the clot, it has theoretic advantages over other thrombolytic or anticoagulant agents in critically ill infants and children. It is being used increasingly in infants and children for venous and arterial occlusive disorders.[42] Current recommendations for its administration suggest a continuous infusion of 0.1 to 0.5 mg/kg/h over 24 to 48 hours.[18,42] Coagulation parameters should be followed every 6 to 8 hours during the infusion. Bleeding complications have been reported with the concomitant administration of heparin.

Surgical thrombectomy in children may be precluded by the vessel size and its flow state, even with microvascular surgical techniques. In adults, venous thrombectomy has been associated with a high rate of rethrombosis even with heparinization or the creation of distal arteriovenous fistulas.

Renal Vein

The renal vein is a common site of thrombosis in the neonate.[43,44] Associated risk factors include asphyxia, shock, dehydration, polycythemia, sepsis, and maternal diabetes. The condition is usually unilateral. Extension of the clot into the IVC with caval occlusion and adrenal hemorrhage can also develop with these patients.[45] The diagnosis should be considered when a palpable flank mass is detected in the neonate. Concomitant signs and symptoms include hypertension, oliguria, anuria, hematuria, hemolytic anemia, or thrombocytopenia.

The diagnosis can be confirmed by a number of radiographic investigations. The intravenous pyelogram (IVP) is abnormal in 80% of cases and characterized by delayed parenchymal opacification and renal enlargement. A venogram of the IVC may visualize thrombus within the cava or renal vein orifice. However, both tests are difficult in the neonate. Doppler ultrasound and MRI are the best methods for diagnostic evaluation of a suspected renal vascular problem. Either of these examina-

tions can exclude other causes of a flank mass, which include multicystic kidney, hydronephrosis, isolated adrenal hemorrhage, and renal or adrenal tumor. The intravenous pyelogram and IVC venogram are used less frequently.

Initial management is directed at treating fluid and electrolyte abnormalities, hypoxia, and sepsis. Therapy for the renal vein thrombosis itself is controversial. Surgical intervention with attempted thrombectomy has been universally unsuccessful. Aggressive medical management with heparin anticoagulation is the current recommendation for treatment of this process. Thrombolytic therapy with systemically administered urokinase or locally instilled tissue plasminogen activator has been reported. Despite such interventions, structural and functional abnormalities in the affected kidney have been reported in up to 90% of the survivors.[46]

Portal Vein

Thrombotic occlusion of the portal vein may develop in a number of different clinical situations with devastating consequences for the lifetime of the child. In the neonatal period, cannulation of the umbilical vein has been associated with portal vein thrombosis in 20% to 61% of cases.[47] Infections of the remaining umbilical stalk with the development of omphalitis have also resulted in neonatal portal vein thrombosis. In older children, thrombosis has occurred in cases of complicated appendicitis and after splenectomy for hematologic disease.[48] Teenagers with massively enlarged spleens are at risk for a thrombotic process following splenectomy for hematologic disease.

Abdominal Doppler ultrasound or MRI of the abdomen outlines vessel anatomy, intravascular obstruction, and confirms the diagnosis.

Most cases of portal vein thrombosis are detected late in the clinical course when cavernous transformation of the vein and hepatofugal portal blood flow develop. Clinical signs and symptoms are consistent with presinusoidal portal hypertension. Treatment is ineffective by this time. Symptoms in the acute setting are often vague and nonspecific, with abdominal pain being the dominant complaint. If diagnosed in the acute setting, portal vein thrombosis should be treated with systemic heparin anticoagulation followed by at least 3 to 6 months of oral anticoagulation. Any child who develops abdominal pain after undergoing a splenectomy should be suspected of developing portal vein thrombosis and should undergo a Doppler ultrasound. Aspirin prophylaxis has been proposed for teenage patients undergoing removal of enlarged spleens.

Deep Vein Thrombosis

Thrombosis of the deep venous system (DVT), including the iliac, femoral, axillary, and subclavian veins, has been thought to be a rare clinical event in children. However, it is now realized that DVT is a serious pediatric clinical problem. In a prospective study involving Canadian children's hospitals, the incidence of DVT was 5.3 per 10,000 hospital admissions, or 0.07 per 10,000 children.[6] Though all ages were reported, infants under 1 year and teenagers were the largest groups affected. Thrombotic events occurred in both upper and lower extremity venous systems, with the lower system predominating by almost a 2:1 ratio. Associated conditions were identified in 96% of the children and included cancer, congenital heart disease, trauma, total parenteral nutrition, and infection. In these clinical settings, central venous access either through a temporary central venous catheter, implanted catheter, or subcutaneous port was the most common cause of vessel thrombosis in one third of all patients and three-quarters of the upper extremity cases.

The aggressive use of central venous catheterization in newborns and premature infants has led to increased problems of vascular thrombosis in this age group.[49] The true incidence of catheter-related thrombosis is not known since asymptomatic infants often are not studied, but incidence reportedly varies from 2% to 22% of catheterized neonates. The risk appears to be greatest in infants less than 28 weeks' gestational age and in those with birth weights under 1000 g.[50]

An additional group of children at risk for the development of DVT involves teenagers disabled following spinal cord injury. The incidence of iliofemoral vein thrombosis in these patients may be as high as 10%, whereas the risk in patients with debilitating closed head injuries or other neurologic disease processes is minimal.[51]

The diagnosis is usually suspected from the clinical examination. Signs and symptoms may include swelling of the involved extremity with associated discoloration, unilateral facial or chest wall edema, diffuse cervical swelling, and pain. Pathologic clinical problems of pulmonary embolism, SVC syndrome, and IVC occlusion may subsequently develop and require treatment. Phlegmasia cerulea dolens, or venous gangrene, is a very rare complication of DVT and represents an extensive thrombotic process within the entire extremity that compromises arterial blood flow.[52] Tissue ischemia and necrosis then develop. Postphlebitic syndrome can develop as a long-term consequence in 25% of children with DVT. Recurrent DVT has been documented in 18.5% of affected children.[18]

Treatment protocols for children with DVT have evolved from adult studies and have included observation alone, intravenous and oral anticoagulation, and thrombolytic therapy. Heparin anticoagulation has been the predominant form of therapy for most children. In cases of catheter-associated thrombosis, particularly when symptoms are minimal, simple removal of the device is sufficient treatment. However, when severe symptoms such as pulmonary embolism, SVC thrombosis with cardiac decompensation, or plegmasia cerulea dolens threaten the patient, serious consideration should be given to thrombolytic therapy or surgical thrombectomy.

Pulmonary Embolism

Pulmonary embolism (PE) is rarely diagnosed in the pediatric population.[53] In autopsy studies, it has been reported to occur in 3% to 4% of children. However, in a recent clinical study PE was found in 3 of 50 children with DVT in the upper extremity venous system and in 11 of 79 children with thrombosis in lower extremity venous veins.[6] Five risk factors identified in children with PE. These include central venous catheterization, immobility, heart disease, surgery, and infection. The diagnosis can usually be made by a ventilation–perfusion scan as in adults. A pulmonary angiogram is infrequently necessary in a child unless thrombolytic therapy is to be used.

Long-term anticoagulation, initially with intravenous heparin followed by oral warfarin, is the standard clinical treatment. Successful thrombolytic therapy with either urokinase or recombinant TPA has been reported, but its overall efficacy in treating this problem in children has not been evaluated. Those children who are not candidates for either long-term anticoagulation of thrombolytic therapy should be considered for cava interruption or placement of an intraluminal filter device if the source of the embolus is identified in the lower extremities.

LYMPHATIC DISORDERS

Most disorders of the lymphatic system encountered in infants and children result from a congenital lymphatic maldevelopment rather than an acquired process such as trauma, malignancy, or infection. These malformations can develop in any region of the body but have a predilection for the sites of the primitive lymph sacs that develop during organogenesis. The clinical manifestations of these anomalies result from obstruction or aplasia of the developing lymph channels.

Embryology

The development of the lymphatic system first becomes evident in the sixth week of gestation with the appearance of primitive lymph sacs associated with the venous system in the embryo. Two theories exist as to the origin of these initial structures. The centripetal theory proposes that the lymphatic spaces start as clefts within the mesenchymal tissue that develop endothelial lined extensions.[54] The centrifugal theory of lymphatic development proposes that capillary buds containing endothelial cells from venous structures form plexuses that eventually coalesce to form lymph sacs.[55] Both theories have supporting embryologic and anatomic models for support. In the human embryo, a total of six lymph sacs develop (Fig. 102-4). Two of the sacs, the jugular and posterior, are paired, and two, the cisterna chyli and the retroperitoneal lymph sac are solitary. The jugular sacs are the first to appear. At 6 weeks of gestation, they develop at the junction of the subclavian and precardinal veins. The posterior sacs develop at the confluence of the iliac veins and the postcardinal venous system. In the retroperitoneal region, the cisterna chyli develops at the level of the third and fourth lumbar vertebrae, while the retroperitoneal sac is found at the base of the small bowel mesentery at the level of the suprarenal glands. By the ninth week of gestation, a chain of small lymph sacs along the dorsal body wall develops into the thoracic duct, eventually linking the cisterna chyli and ilioinguinal lymph sacs to the left jugular lymphatic trunk. Valves develop within this structure by the fifth gestational month.

Peripheral lymphatics develop from lymph sacs by the outgrowth of solid endothelial channels that follow the course of embryonic blood vessels. As these channels lengthen, they become hollow to form lymph vessels. Lymph nodes then develop in areas of connective tissue ingrowth in both vessels and sacs. They subsequently become colonized by the circulating lymphoblasts of the developing immune system.

Physiology

The lymphatic system is designed to control the interstitial fluid volume and its composition. Lymphatic fluid flow is de-

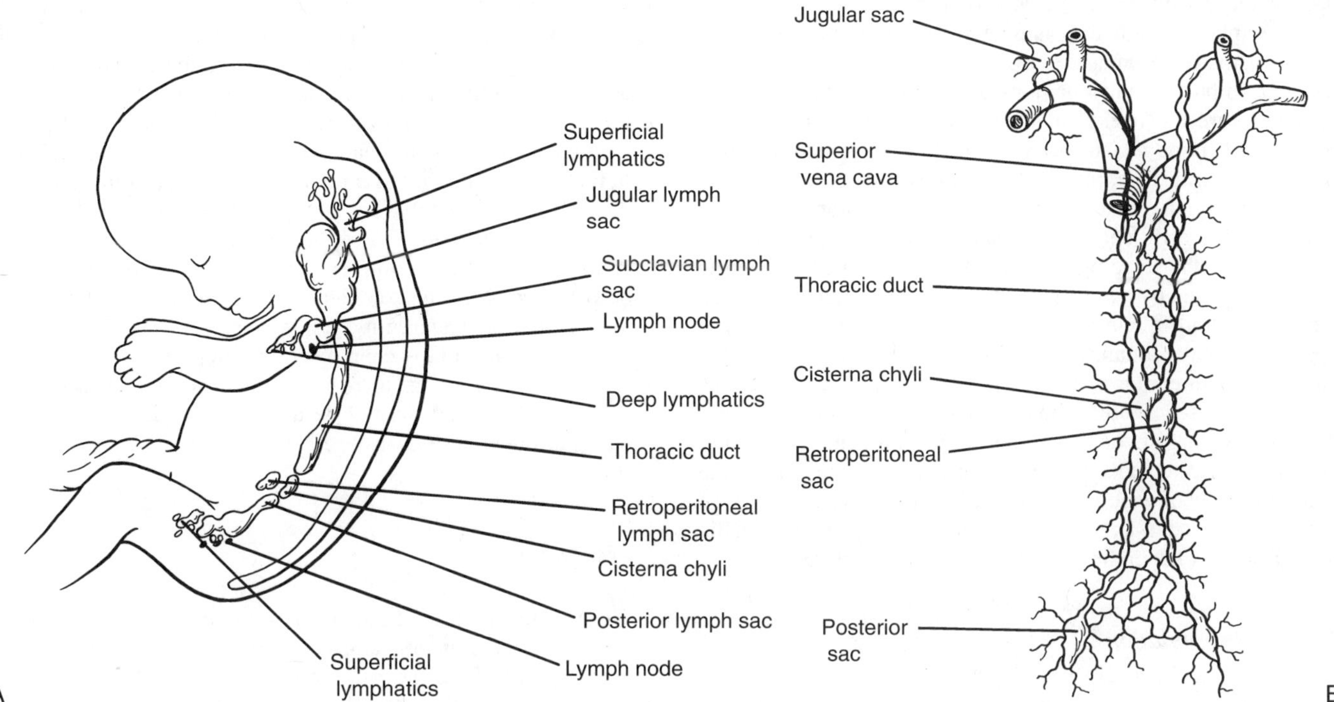

FIG. 102-4. Schematic representation of lymph sac and thoracic duct development in the fetus.

pendent on a number of independent events. Contractions occurring in the walls of the ducts are the principal mechanism driving lymph flow. Valves within the ducts promote unidirectional flow of interstitial fluid toward the central lymphatic system. This process is aided by the contractions of surrounding skeletal muscles and the negative intrathoracic pressure around the thoracic duct during inspiration. The formation of lymphatic fluid is directly dependent on the interstitial fluid volume. This volume is determined by the balance of Starling forces within the accompanying capillary circulation. These forces include the filtration pressure and the osmotic and oncotic pressure gradient across the capillary system.[56]

Lymphatics are permeable to macromolecules, although the protein content of lymph is generally lower than that of plasma. In the intestines, the lymphatics are the main pathways of systemic fat absorption. Fatty acids containing more than 10 to 12 carbon atoms are reesterified into triglyceride structures and are formed into chylomicrons to enter the lymphatics. The lymph in the thoracic duct is milky in appearance because of this fat content. In addition, lymph fluid cell counts are quite high, particularly in the thoracic duct. The lymphatic system is the principal mechanism by which circulating lymphocytes reenter the bloodstream after exiting the circulation at endothelial venules in lymph nodes and organs.

Lymphatic Malformations

The study of lymphatic anomalies is burdened by a confusing and cumbersome array of classification systems and perhaps even inappropriate terminology. Traditionally, lymphatic abnormalities have been divided into four broad categories: lymphangioma simplex, cavernous lymphangioma, lymphangioma circumscriptum, and cystic lymphangioma or cystic hygroma. However, many clinical lesions have histologic elements of two or three categories, and discrete stratification becomes difficult. Since altered lymphatic architecture resulting in functional obstruction to lymph flow is common to all the abnormalities, they should be thought of as a spectrum of developmental anomalies ranging from the microcystic lymphangioma with cystic spaces usually less than several millimeters in size to the macrocystic cystic hygroma.

Furthermore, the use of the term *lymphangioma* to describe these lesions may be incorrect.[57] In classic pathology, the appendix *-oma* implies a collection of cells into a tumor with hyperplastic characteristics and the potential for growth and invasion by cellular proliferation. To date, no biochemical or molecular studies exist that indicate active cellular proliferation or turnover in these lesions. Expansion or enlargement of these lesions represents continued fluid accumulation within the cysts or recruitment of additional abnormal lymphatics in the surrounding tissues. Growth of these lesions generally matches the child's growth. Therefore, a more precise designation of these lesions should be lymphatic malformations or lymphatic anomalies rather than lymphangiomas.[58,59]

Pathology

Defects occurring at different stages in early lymphatic embryogenesis result in the spectrum of anomalies seen clinically. The large cystic malformation, the cystic hygroma, may result from an error in development of the primitive lymph sacs shortly after 6 weeks of gestation. An interruption later in gestation would result in the maldevelopment of the smaller and more peripherally situated lymphatic vessels. The anatomic location of the lesion may determine its structure and morphology.[60] Lymphatic malformations occurring in areas of redundant tissue are able to expand into large cystic structures because of minimal tissue resistance, whereas lymphatic anomalies in tissues with limited expansile capabilities may be constrained to form the microcystic lymphangioma-type lesions.

Despite the different macroscopic appearances of these various lesions, the histology is remarkably similar. Each cystic structure is lined by a layer of flattened endothelium containing lymphatic fluid. Connective tissue is present throughout the cysts and may contain lymphoid aggregates. Fibrosis and chronic inflammation may be noted in the cyst walls. Hemorrhage can be seen within the cysts and is often the reason for the rapid enlargement sometimes noted clinically. Vascular anomalies may coexist within the abnormal lymphatic tissue and are usually of venous origin. These combined anomalies are properly referred to as lymphatic–venous or venous–lymphatic malformations depending on the dominant structure.[59]

Clinical Presentation

The actual incidence of lymphatic malformations in the pediatric population is unknown, but these are relatively unusual lesions. In one study conducted over 15 years, 48 malformations were identified among 768 benign tumors (6.3%).[61] They occur in all races and almost equally in both sexes. The majority of lymphatic malformations are evident early in life with 65% present at birth, 80% evident within the first year of life, and 90% diagnosed by the age of two.[60]

Lymphatic anomalies can assume a number of different clinical presentations, depending on the nature of the malformation. Lesions can vary in size from tiny cutaneous blebs or blisters to large multilocular cysts. In general, surgical consultation is sought because of the discovery of a mass lesion. Associated symptoms such as pain or discomfort are rare unless there has been hemorrhage or infection in the lesion. An increase in the size of the lesion is often due to further obstruction of lymph drainage. Abrupt enlargement can result from hemorrhage into the lesion and has been noted in 8% to 12% of the reported cases. The most common anatomic locations for lymphatic malformations are the head and neck, the extremities, and then the mediastinum and trunk. In the neck, the posterior cervical triangle is the most common location for a cystic hygroma. The malformation is more frequently seen on the left side, possibly due to drainage of lymphatics into the thoracic cavity on the right side. Approximately 10% of cervical lymphatic malformations have extension into the chest.

Diagnostic Evaluation

Lymphatic malformations can be detected by routine prenatal ultrasonography as early as the end of the first trimester of pregnancy[62] (see section on posterior cervical abnormalities). However, since most lesions are detected after birth, radiographic evaluation can involve any one of several imaging studies, depending on the complexity and location of the lesion. This is especially true when attempting to ascertain extension

of the lesion from one body space to another, as from the neck to the mediastinum. For most lesions in any anatomic region, plain radiographs should be obtained as the initial studies to document possible associated anomalies or structural abnormalities. For simple, superficial lesions an ultrasound with concomitant Doppler flow examination will define the extent and nature of the anomaly as well as pinpoint important surrounding structures. It is less valuable for demonstrating extensive lesions in the neck, mediastinum, or retroperitoneum. If the malformation is quite extensive or complex, a CT scan or MRI study should be obtained. MRI is excellent for head and neck, thoracic or mediastinal, and extremity lesions (Fig. 102-5). T2-weighted images are particularly characteristic in defining lymphatic malformations in relation to neurovascular and soft tissue structures.[63] MRI or CT should be used to evaluate abdominal or retroperitoneal lesions as well as solid organ involvement[64] (Fig. 102-6).

Treatment

An understanding of the benefits, limitations, and complications of each therapeutic intervention is crucial to proper clinical management of the spectrum of lymphatic malformations. Surgical resection is the treatment of choice for all lymphatic anomalies. Complete excision of the lesion is performed whenever technically possible. However, only three fourths of the lesions can be totally excised, whereas the others must undergo partial excision.[65] Such partial resection most often is mandated by the involvement of vital structures within the lymphatic malformation. This is most often seen in cystic hygromas of the head and neck region that may involve major cranial nerves and vessels, as well as soft tissue structures such as the hypopharynx, parotid, and trachea. These lesions are not malignancies and should not be subjected to radical extirpative procedures resulting in loss of function or severe deformity. For extensive and complex lesions, staged excisions with each surgical procedure limited to a defined area should be planned.

For small or superficial lesions, primary excision may be easily performed. Often a well-demarcated plane of dissection can be established between the boundary of the malformation and surrounding soft tissue structures that makes its mobilization uncomplicated. Vascular involvement is minimal unless there is a concomitant hemangioma.

The postoperative complication rate can be 30% or higher and usually involves recurrence or operative damage to important neurologic structures.[65] Recurrence rates vary widely, depending on the type of surgical procedure, and range from 10% to 27% for complete resections to 50% to 100% for partially resected lesions. Significant neurologic problems can result from these resection of cervical cystic hygromas; usually involve damage to the facial nerve or its branches. Damage to the ninth, tenth, eleventh, and twelfth cranial nerves has also been reported. Horner syndrome due to sympathetic chain damage and diaphragmatic paralysis from phrenic nerve injury may follow resection of mediastinal and thoracic lesions. Persistent chylothorax has also been noted following thoracic procedures. Mortality following surgery is rare, with the greatest risk in patients with giant head and neck cystic hygromas.

Other surgical interventions have included needle aspiration as well as incision and drainage of the cysts. Both techniques

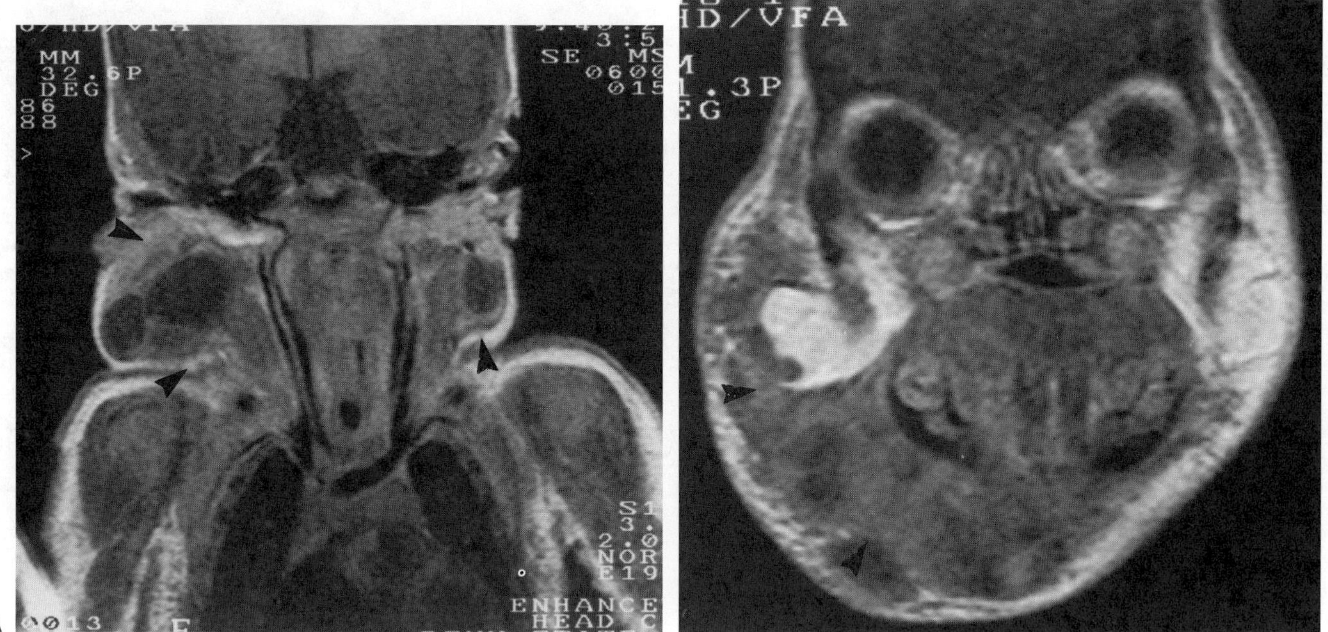

FIG. 102-5. Coronal (*A*) and axial (*B*) MRIs of 2-month-old infant with extensive bilateral cervicofacial lymphatic malformation (*arrows*). Lymphatic involvement extends from the thoracic inlet to the base of the skull.

may be used for emergency decompression of a lesion if respiratory obstruction is imminent or for the management of an acutely infected cyst. However, neither one is acceptable for the long-term therapy of these lesions, since most lesions consisting of large multiloculated structures or small microscopic cysts are inadequately drained and fluid reaccumulates. Extirpative surgery is required to minimize the problems of recurrence.

The direct intracystic injection of various sclerosing agents has had mixed success. Agents that have been tried and found to be ineffective have included boiling water, sodium morrhuate, hypertonic saline, and hypertonic glucose solutions. Two additional compounds may hold promise as possible therapeutic agents but have not been subjected to rigorous clinical trials.

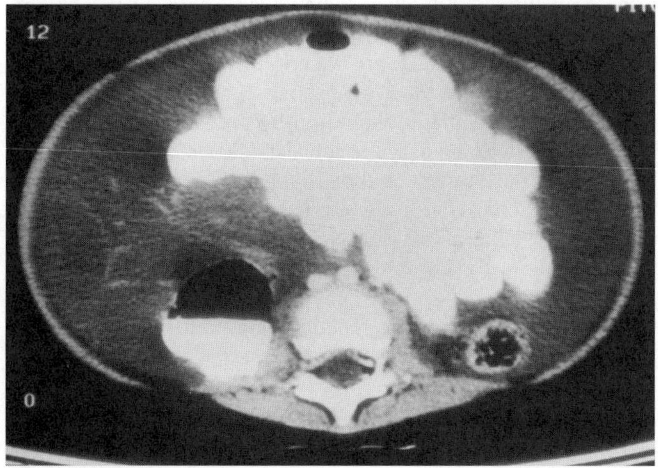

FIG. 102-6. Abdominal CT scan with contrast of an 8-year-old with extensive abdominal lymphatic malformations.

Bleomycin therapy administered in a microsphere-in-oil fat emulsion has been tried in a limited number of patients.[66,67] This type of emulsion is easily transported into the lymphatic system and results in a high concentration of the drug at the site of administration. When injected into a lymphatic malformation, its mechanism of action is thought to be an inflammatory reaction involving the endothelial lining of the cyst. The best response to this form of sclerotherapy has been seen in cystic hygromas. It is administered by injecting 0.3 to 0.6 mg/kg of body weight of the drug into the cavity of the cyst after aspiring as much fluid as possible. Transient swelling develops in the lesion as a result of the inflammatory reaction for up to 2 weeks after the injection. This swelling can result in airway compromise and thus makes this form of therapy contraindicated in lesions with preexisting airway involvement and in giant cervical or mediastinal malformations with this potential. Administration of the drug is also contraindicated in infants under 6 months of age. Possible long-term effects of bleomycin sclerotherapy have not been studied.

A second sclerosing agent with reported beneficial effects in treating lymphatic malformations is OK-432.[68,69] It is a lyophilized mixture obtained by incubating group A *Streptococcus pyogenes* with penicillin G potassium and has been used in a number of studies in Japan. Its mechanism of action involves the initiation of an inflammatory reaction within the cystic spaces of the lymphatic malformation resulting in the destruction of the endothelial cell layer and fibrous of the cyst. It is administered by injecting 0.1 mg of OK-432 in 10 mL of saline solution into the lesion after aspirating as much fluid as possible. In the limited studies to date, all types of lymphatic malformations reportedly have responded to this sclerotherapy. Side effects have included fever for several days and induration at the site of injection. A rigorous clinical evaluation of this therapy has not been done.

Radiation therapy has been tried in the past for these lesions but is currently not considered an acceptable intervention. No study has demonstrated any substantial beneficial effect, and a great deal of concern exists regarding the potential complications of this therapy in infants and children.

Conservative management with expectant observation has been proposed by a number of surgeons.[70] Regression of lymphatic anomalies has been noted in several reports but has involved a very small number of cases. Though the overwhelming majority of surgical opinion is in favor of excision, not all lymphatic malformations require aggressive intervention. A course of observation can be followed if the patient's life is not put at risk by the presence of the lesion, particularly if unresectable.

Laser therapy has been the most effective modality for lymphatic malformations that involve the larynx and airway. The CO_2 laser should be used to minimize damage to surrounding laryngeal structures.

Specific Lymphatic Malformations

Cystic Hygroma

Cystic hygromas are multiloculated lymphatic cysts that can be quite large in size and are one of the most common causes of neck masses in children. They occur with equal frequency in both sexes and have an incidence of 1 in 12,000 births. Hygromas vary tremendously in size and usually present as soft, well-demarcated, asymptomatic masses. About 75% of these malformations develop in the posterior neck area with almost a 2 to 1 predominance of lesions on the left side. This left-sided predominance is believed to result from the embryologic development of the thoracic duct junction with the left subclavian vein. Twenty percent of cystic hygromas occur in the axillary area, with the remained found in the mediastinum, retroperitoneum, and pelvis. Giant cystic hygromas can develop in the cerviofacial area that extend into both sides of the neck and face, involving multiple structures such as the mouth, tongue, parotid, and larynx (Fig. 102-7). In about 15% of cases, the malformation may extend into the mediastinum. In rare instances, if there has been rapid enlargement of the lesion caused by hemorrhage or infection, signs and symptoms of respiratory obstruction can develop such as stridor, dysphagia, apnea, and cyanosis.[58]

Surgical excision is considered the treatment of choice for these lesions. For the large cervicofacial malformations, complete excision often is not possible. Staged procedures and multiple operations are often necessary. For completely asymptomatic lesions with little chance of airway encroachment, a period of observation can be followed to see if spontaneous regression will take place. However, for those lesions with obvious airway involvement or for those giant lesions with the potential for rapid enlargement and airway compromise, early surgical intervention is warranted. This may involve surgery in the neonatal period. Consideration should always be given to the insertion of a tracheostomy and possible gastrostomy to aid in the safe management of the infant or child. Outside the United States, sclerotherapy is becoming increasingly popular in selected cases.

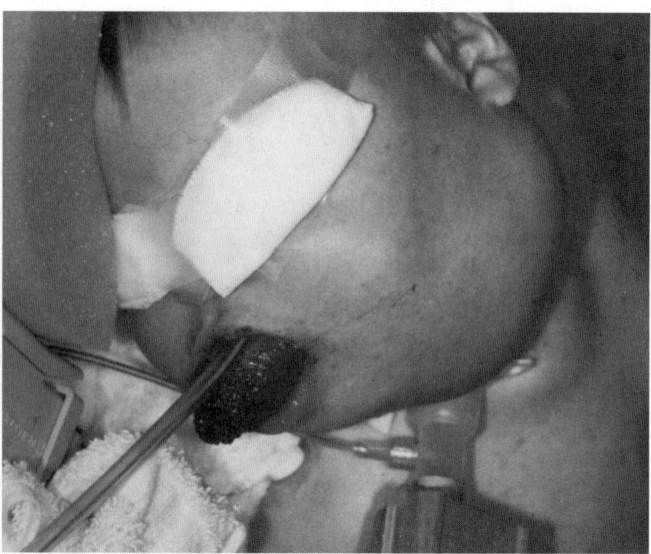

FIG. 102-7. Giant lymphatic malformation of the neck and face requiring a tracheostomy for airway management. The protrusion of the tongue is caused by involvement with the malformation.

Fetal Cystic Hygromas

With the advent of widespread prenatal sonography, it is now recognized that the diagnosis of a cystic hygroma in the fetus represents a different clinical entity than one discovered at birth or thereafter.[62,71] Fetal cystic hygromas diagnosed before 30 weeks' gestational age tend to be located in the posterior cervical region. They are associated with the presence of fetal hydrops and diffuse lymphangiomatosis. Approximately one half of the cases have abnormal genetic karyotypes. Fetuses with abnormal karyotypes most commonly have Turner syndrome, but trisomy 13, trisomy 18, trisomy 21, partial 11q/22q trisomy, and trisomy 22 mosaicism have been reported. In addition, Noonan syndrome, fetal alcohol syndrome, distichiasis-lymphedema, and familial pterygium colli have been associated with fetal cystic hygromas. Spontaneous resolution of these hygromas during the second trimester of pregnancy has been noted with serial ultrasounds also. It has been proposed that many cystic hygromas associated with Turner and Noonan syndromes spontaneously regress and are the etiology of the webbed neck seen in children with these syndromes.

If a cystic hygroma is diagnosed by prenatal testing before 30 weeks' gestational age, the fetus should be carefully examined for hydrops, ascites, and pleural and pericardial effusions, as well as structural cardiac and renal abnormalities. If hydrops is found, the chance for survival is minimal. Amniocentesis should be done for chromosomal analysis. A fetal cystic hygroma discovered late in the pregnancy does not appear to be associated with hydrops or genetic abnormalities and behaves clinically like a lymphatic malformation discovered at birth.

Oral Pharynx

Lymphatic malformations may involve the tongue, floor of the mouth, and associated salivary glands, including the parotid gland, and can be very difficult to manage. The pathology most often involves multilocular microcysts and associated abnormal lymphatic channels infiltrating these structures. Lymphatic malformations are the most common cause of macroglossia and may result in such a degree of enlargement that the tongue constantly protrudes from the mouth. Maxillofacial skeletal hypertrophy and distortion may develop and result in complex problems of malocclusion. The protruding tongue may be repeatedly traumatized, resulting in bleeding and ulceration, and has a high risk of recurrent infections and inflammation. Several surgical resections may be required to shape the tongue to allow it to fit within the confines of the oral cavity.

Lymphatic malformations can be found in both the superficial and deep lobes of the parotid gland. These lesions are often associated with large cystic hygromas of the cervical-facial region. Isolated intracapsular lesions of the parotid may have a vascular hemangioma component that dominates the malformation in the first year of life. A period of observation to see if there is any spontaneous decrease in size is reasonable. The goal of surgical therapy is to excise as much of the cyst as possible without injuring the facial nerve. Excision of the superficial portion of the parotid gland with drainage or sclerosis of the deeper components is currently recommended.

Abdominal Lymphatic Malformations

Based on the ontogeny of the lymphatic system, the abdominal cavity and in particular the retroperitoneum and intestinal mesentery can be sites of lymphatic malformations.[72] These are usually asymptomatic cystic masses encountered during a routine physical examination or during the course of a radiographic or surgical evaluation for an unrelated problem. A small number of these cysts can cause symptoms related to their size or location. Clinical presentations can include abdominal distension, a mass, intestinal and ureteral obstruction resulting from compression, intralesional hemorrhage following trauma, perforation, torsion, volvulus with intestinal infarction, and peritonitis (Fig. 102-8).

Diagnostic evaluation with ultrasonography or CT with oral and intravenous contrast is recommended. Complete excision of the lesion should be attempted if possible and may involve a limited resection of intestine. Extensive mesenteric or retroperitoneal involvement may preclude such an approach. In that case, as much of the malformation is removed as safely as possible. The remaining cysts are opened widely and marsupialized to drain into the abdomen. During the postoperative period, the patient should be followed closely by ultrasonography for the possible recurrence of the malformation or the development of chylous ascites.

Solid Organ Malformations

Abnormalities of the lymphatic system in solid organs tend to involve multiple organ systems.[73] The pathology consists of diffusely dilated lymphatic channels with scattered cystic components. Isolated lesions are rare. These lesions are generally referred to as lymphangiectasia.

Pulmonary lymphangiectasia can be a cause of neonatal respiratory failure and consists of diffuse involvement throughout

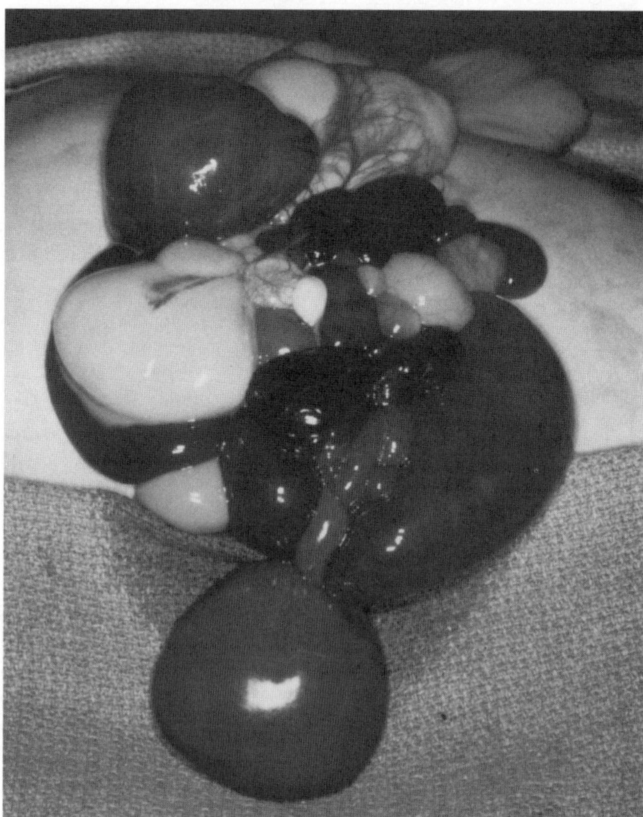

FIG. 102-8. Complex cystic masses of an abdominal lymphatic malformation.

both lungs with the abnormal lymphatic channels.[74] Fluid accumulation within the pleural cavity may occur as a hydrothorax. Three different clinical groups have been proposed to classify pulmonary lymphangiectasia.[75] In the first group, the pulmonary component is part of a larger multiorgan pattern of lymphatic maldevelopment. The second group involves isolated lymphatic maldevelopment solely within the lung, and the third group results from functional pulmonary venous hypertension or obstruction. Chest radiography shows a diffusely hazy parenchymal pattern that has a characteristic CT appearance. Treatment options are limited. Multiple aspirations or tube thoracostomy are usually adequate to control pleural effusions.

Lymphatic malformations of the intestine are rare and consist of abnormal lymphatic structures throughout the bowel and mesentery. The functional consequence of this abnormality is significant impairment of fat absorption. Clinically, symptoms may include diarrhea, steatorrhea, abdominal pain, and vomiting. In addition to severe problems with fat malabsorption, a protein-losing enteropathy may develop because of altered intestinal villus architecture. Severe malnutrition with failure to thrive and growth retardation can result.

An upper gastrointestinal contrast series with complete examination of the small bowel should be performed to evaluate the bowel. Pathologic diagnosis can be made by intestinal biopsies obtained endoscopically or surgically. No surgical therapy exists for this disorder, and treatment is supportive. A low-fat, high-protein diet should be followed and supplemented with medium-chain triglycerides to maximize intravenous fat absorption. Total parenteral nutrition may be required if enteral requirements cannot be met otherwise.

Lymphatic malformations of the spleen and liver are usually seen together and associated with a diffuse pattern of maldevelopment also involving lung, skin, and bone. Solid organ involvement is detected on CT scan, whereas plain radiographs may show diffuse skeletal involvement manifested by multiple, sclerotic destructive lesions. No therapy has been successful, and patients usually die within 5 to 10 years of the diagnosis.

Chylothorax

The appearance of chyle within the thoracic cavity indicates a disruption in the thoracic duct along its course from the aortic hiatus at T10 to T12 to its junction with the left subclavian vein at the thoracic inlet. Within the posterior mediastinum, the duct ascends along the anterior border of the vertebral column and then passes to the left of the spine and esophagus inferior to the aortic arch at fourth thoracic vertebra before continuing its ascent to the base of the neck. Multiple communications exist with mediastinal and chest wall lymphatics and vascular structures to provide a complex pathway for lymph flow, and in 40% of patients a duplication of the thoracic duct has been identified.

A chylothorax can result from a number of different mechanisms. Congenital chylothorax is diagnosed in the newborn period in the absence of birth trauma or other factors and is caused by a malformation within the thoracic duct system.[76] Nontraumatic chylothorax results from a pathologic obstruction of the thoracic duct and associated lymphatics by mediastinal fibrosis from an inflammatory or infectious process, by a mediastinal neoplasm, or by a vascular anomaly such as superior vena cava thrombosis or an aortic aneurysm.[77] Finally, the most common cause of chylothorax is traumatic, from either surgical or nonsurgical injuries.[77,78] A chylothorax can occur after any type of thoracic operation and has been reported after subclavian vascular access procedures. It occurs in almost 1 of 200 pediatric cardiac operations.[78] The lesion can also develop after peritonitis, blunt thoracic injury, and spinal cord injuries.

When evaluating a pleural effusion, the diagnosis of a chylothorax can be made immediately on obtaining the characteristic milky pleural fluid on thoracentesis. If the patient is a newborn or has had no enteral intake for some time, the pleural fluid can appear clear. Laboratory analysis shows that chyle has the following characteristics[79]:

Fat: 0.4 to 0.6 g/dL
Protein content: 2.2 to 5.9 g/dL
Albumin to globulin ratio: 3:1
Lymphocyte count: 400 to 6800/μL
Triglyceride level: >500 mg/dL

Sudan red stain can identify the fat globules and chylomicrons within the fluid to confirm the diagnosis of a chylothorax.

Nonoperative management is successful 75% to 90% of the time.[80] In congenital chylothorax, serial aspirations combined with formula feedings containing medium-chain triglycerides such as Portagen may be effective. For most cases of traumatic chylothorax, tube thoracostomy and total parenteral nutrition

should be employed. To minimize chyle formation and lymph flow within the damaged thoracic duct system, no enteral feedings are given. Such a treatment protocol has been effective in almost 90% of children with traumatic chylothorax. Even the oral administration of water has been found to significantly increase thoracic duct flow.[81] Nonoperative therapy is more likely to fail when there is systemic venous hypertension from superior vena cava thrombosis or increased right-sided cardiac pressures impeding venous return.

Surgical intervention should be considered for patients with persistent pleural drainage unresponsive to conservative management. Most studies indicate that few thoracic duct fistulas will close spontaneously after three weeks of unsuccessful nonoperative management. A thoracotomy on the side of the effusion with ligation of the involved lymphatic channels is the standard approach. Minimally invasive surgery with video-assisted thoracoscopy and clipping of the thoracic duct is an alternative approach. Fibrin glue has also been successfully used to seal the leaking lymphatic area. Visualization of the leaking lymphatics can be improved by the administration of heavy cream to the patient 2 to 4 hours before the operation. Pleuroperitoneal shunts have been successfully used in a small number of infants with refractory nontraumatic chylothoraces.[82] Chemical pleurodesis has been generally ineffective in treating these problems (see Chap. 56).

Chylous Ascites

Most lymph flowing into the cisterna chyli and thoracic duct originates in the liver or intestine. Any disruption in this system can result in the formation of chylous ascites. The etiology of pediatric chylous ascites is idiopathic in 40% of cases, may result from congenital causes, and is rarely due to a malignant condition.[83] It can be due to midgut volvulus, congenital bands with mesenteric constriction, lymphatic malformations, retroperitoneal inflammation, peritonitis, intussusception, and incarcerated hernias.

Chyle accumulation within the peritoneal cavity leads to progressive abdominal distention. The diagnosis is confirmed by paracentesis and examination of the milky fluid (see earlier section on chylothorax). Radiographic evaluation should include plain films, an upper gastrointestinal series with complete small bowel follow-through, and a CT scan with contrast to examine mesenteric and retroperitoneal structures. In rare instances, exploratory laparotomy may be required.

Because chyle formation and lymphatic flow are directly dependent on intestinal fat and fluid absorption, initial therapeutic regimens for treating chylous ascites involve enteral dietary interventions. A fat-restricted, high-protein diet with medium-chain triglycerides can be attempted. However, if ascites continues to form and multiple paracenteses are required, complete enteral rest and total parenteral nutrition should be imposed. Such therapy generally is required for a minimum of 3 to 4 weeks. Surgical exploration should be undertaken if no response is seen after this time. The goal of the surgery is the removal of any structural cause for the ascites and the ligation of the involved lymphatic pathways. As with a chylothorax, the administration of heavy cream several hours before the surgery may improve the visualization of the leak. Temporary success has been noted in controlling the ascites by the insertion of a peritoneovenous shunts. However, because of the high cellular and protein content of the fluid, these shunts tend to obstruct with time.

The consequences of persistent chylous ascites can be devastating and result in severe malnutrition, hypoproteinuremia, and fluid and electrolyte imbalances. A mortality rate of 21% has been reported. Improved nutritional management has improved the outlook for these patients.

Lymphedema

In contrast to the structural abnormalities that result in the malformations discussed earlier, the buildup and persistence of lymph fluid in tissues from lymphatic channel maldevelopment, obstruction, or destruction results in the condition known as lymphedema. Clinically, it most often involves the subcutaneous tissues of the extremities but can affect the perineum and scrotal area as well. It is divided into two types of disorders—primary and secondary. Secondary lymphedema can be caused by any acquired process that blocks or destroys subcutaneous lymphatic channels by such processes as parasitic infestation, infection, trauma, and malignancy. Iatrogenic causes include radiation therapy and extensive axillary, femoral, or pelvic lymph node dissection. This problem is relatively rare in the pediatric population.

Primary lymphedema has been classified as congenital, praecox, or tarda. In pediatric studies, 35% of children have the congenital variety. A rare inherited form of this type of lymphedema is known as Milroy disease.[84] However, the most common type of primary lymphedema is lymphedema praecox, with a peak incidence in the second and third decades of life and a 2:1 female prevalence. The familial form of this disease is known as Meige disease. Pathologic studies have shown that the condition results from a diffuse hypoplastic underdevelopment of channels in the subcutaneous lymphatic network. Aplastic and hyperplastic patterns have also been found.[85] Lymphedema tarda is seen in patients over 30 to 35 years of age.

A number of conditions have been associated with primary lymphedema and include diffuse lymphangiectasias, chylothorax, chylous ascites, congenital heart disease, Fabry disease, and the genetic anomalies of Noonan and Turner syndromes.

With congenital lymphedema, the physical examination characteristically shows swelling on the dorsum of the foot extending up the calf to the knee but no further. It can be bilateral in one third of patients. Occasionally, a hand or forearm may be involved.[86] The edema is soft and nonpitting with no cutaneous abnormalities. With lymphedema praecox and lymphedema tarda, the upper extremities are infrequently involved; and the edema in the lower extremity may extend into the proximal thigh.

Radiographic studies are not helpful in confirming the diagnosis. Lymphangiograms are painful and difficult studies, and radionuclide, vascular contrast studies, and CT scans provide little additional information from the physical examination. The use of MRI with T1- and T2-weighted image comparisons may be beneficial in determining the extent and depth of the abnormality and possible involvement of deep structures within the extremity.

Treatment of primary lymphedema should be as conservative as possible, with surgical intervention reserved for only the severe cases. Early intervention for congenital edema should consist of compression of the involved extremity with either elastic wraps or custom fitted stockings. Because of the rapid growth of the infant, multiple orders of custom stockings can become expensive. Lymphedema praecox and lymphedema tarda both should be treated with custom-fitted elastic stockings. Pneumatic compression at night has also been recommended for these patients with good results, though compliance is always a problem. In all these patients, the risk of cellulitis and skin infections is significant. Skin care requires constant vigilance and the prompt institution of antibiotic therapy.

Surgical options are limited. The primary operation is subcutaneous lymphangiectomy in which full thickness skin flaps are raised and reapplied after the underlying abnormal subcutaneous tissue is excised down to the fascia. Closed suction drains in the subcutaneous space, and compression dressings aid the healing of these skin flaps. The application of split thickness skin grafts following the excision of all abnormal tissue including skin and fascia has also been reported. Microscopic lymphatic grafting, lymphaticovenous anastomosis, and omental grafting have all been tried with little success.

COMBINED VENOUS AND LYMPHATIC MALFORMATIONS: KLIPPEL-TRENAUNAY SYNDROME

The most common combined lymphatic and vascular abnormality was first described in 1900 and is composed of cutaneous capillary (venous) malformations, varicose veins, and limb hypertrophy.[87] Associated abnormalities can include deep-vein abnormalities due to either agenesis or hypoplasia and lymphatic malformations varying from congenital lymphedema of the involved extremity to intrapelvic and intrabdominal cysts associated with the vascular malformations. Intestinal lymphangiomatosis has been found in several cases. A lower limb is involved in 95% of cases, whereas an upper limb is affected 5% of the time. Most cases are unilateral (85%), but in rare cases the whole trunk may be involved.[88] The lesion is usually present at birth, and three fourths of the patients who will develop symptoms will do so before 10 years of age.

In the past, radiographic evaluation included arteriography to rule out coexisting arteriovenous malformations (Parkes-Weber syndrome), venography, and lymphangiography. MRI evaluation of the involved extremity has now superseded these invasive procedures and allows for the examination of the contralateral extremity as well as the pelvis and the abdomen at the same time (Fig. 102-9).

Treatment is largely for symptomatic problems. Multiple episodes of bleeding from ruptured superficial varices, ulcers, or traumatized areas can occur. Compressive dressings and at times the topical application of hemostatic agents such as fibrin glue, topical thrombin, hemostatic collagen, or cellulose may be required. Superficial and deep thrombophlebitis may develop with localized areas of pain and swelling. Low-dose aspirin therapy has proved beneficial for minimizing such episodes. Local infections through breaks in the skin can result in cellulitis or lead to severe sepsis. Aggressive wound care and antibiotic therapy is mandatory for any area of skin breakdown or trauma.

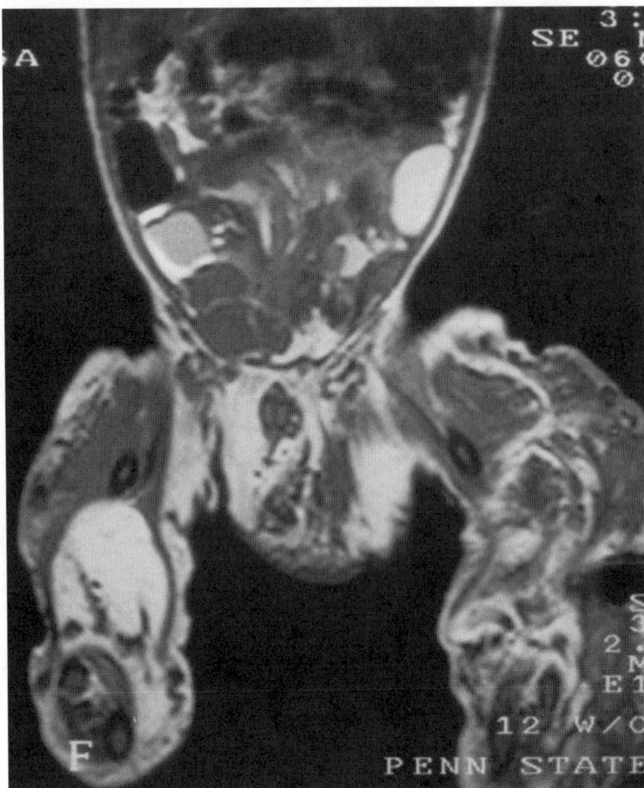

FIG. 102-9. MRI of a 3-month-old male infant with severe Klippel-Trenaunay syndrome involving both lower extremities, the perineum, and the pelvis extending into the lower abdomen. The image displays the grossly disordered mesenchymal development resulting from this process.

Long-term treatment plans involve supportive care and compressive therapy to minimize the problems of lymphedema. Pneumatic compression and elastic stockings have been recommended. Surgical intervention is usually reserved for orthopedic procedures to modify problems of excessive hypertrophy and leg-length discrepancies that may interfere with gait and weight bearing.[89]

REFERENCES

1. Sternbergh III WC, Sobel M. Venous and lymphatic diseases. In: Levine BA, Copeland III EM, Howard RJ, et al, eds. Current practice of surgery, vol 12, sec 9. New York, Churchill Livingstone, 1993.
2. Lindenauer SM. Venous physiology and disorders of the superficial veins. In: Greenfield LJ, Mulholland MW, Oldham KT, et al, eds. Surgery, scientific principles and practice. Philadelphia, JB Lippincott, 1993:1757.
3. Humphrey PW, Spadome DP, Silver D. Vascular disorders of the upper torso. In: Wells Jr SA, ed. Current problems in surgery, vol 30, no. 9. St. Louis, CV Mosby, 1993:819.
4. Sarma KP. Anomalous inferior vena cava—anatomical and clinical. Br J Surg 1966;53:600.
5. Smith BM, Venous disease. In: Welch KJ, Randolph JG, Ravitch MM, et al, eds. Pediatric surgery, ed 4. Chicago, Year Book Medical, 1986:1518.
6. Andrew M, David M, Adams M, et al. Venous thromboembolic complications (VTE) in children: first analysis of the Canadian registry of VTE. Blood 1994;83:1251.
7. Kothari SS, Varma S, Wasir HS. Thrombolytic therapy in infants and children. Am Heart J 1994;127:651.
8. Tabernero MD, Thomas JF, Alberca I, et al. Incidence and clinical characteristics of hereditary disorders associated with venous thrombosis. Am J Hematol 1991;36:249.
9. Finazzi G, Barbui T. Different incidence of venous thrombosis in patients with inherited deficiencies of antithrombin III, protein C and proteins. Thrombos Haemo 1994;71:15.
10. Sequin J, Weatherstone K, Nankervis C. Inherited antithrombin III deficiency in the neonate. Arch Pediatr Adolesc Med 1994;148:389.
11. Hirsch J, Piovella F, Pini M. Congenital antithrombin III deficiency: incidence and clinical features. Am J Med 1989;87(Suppl 3B):34S.
12. Andrew M, Brooker L, Leaker M, et al. Fibrin clot lysis by thrombolytic agents is impaired in newborns due to low plasminogen concentration. Thrombos Haemo 1992;68:325.
13. Francis RB. Acquired purpura fulminans. Sem Thromb Hemost 1990;16:310.
14. Madden RM, Gill JC, Marlar RA. Protein C and S levels in two patients with acquired purpura fulminans. Br J Haematol 1990;75:112.
15. Powars DR, Rogers ZR, Patch MJ, et al. Purpura fulminans in meningococcemia: association with acquired deficiencies of protein C and S. N Engl J Med 1987;317:571.
16. Priest JR, Ramsay NK, Latchaw RE, et al. Thrombolytic and hemorrhagec strokes complicating early therapy for children acute lymphoblastic leukemia. Cancer 1980;46:1548.
17. Shapiro AD, Clarke SL, Christian JM, et al. Thrombosis in children receiving L-asparaginase. Am J Ped Hem Onc 1993;15:400.
18. David M, Andrew M. Venous thromboembolic complications in children. J Ped 1993;123:337.
19. Stringer DA, Krysl J, Manson D, et al. The value of Doppler sonography in the detection of major vessel thrombosis in the neonatal abdomen. Pediatr Radiol 1990;21:30.
20. Carpenter JP, Holland GA, Baum RA, et al. Preliminary experience with magnetic resonance venography: comparison with findings at surgical exploration. J Surg Res 1994;57:373.
21. Spritzer CE. Venography of the extremities and pelvis. In: Finn JP, ed. Magnetic resonance angiography of the body. Magnetic resonance imaging clinics of North Am. Philadelphia, WB Saunders, 1993;239.
22. Andrew M, Marzinotto V, Massicotte P, et al. Heparin therapy in pediatric patients: a prospective cohort study. Pediatr Res 1994;35:78.
23. Evans DI, Rowlands M, Poller L. Survey of oral anticoagulant treatment in children. J Clin Pathol 1992;45:707.
24. Hare WD. Pharmacology of fibrinolysis. Chest 1992;101S–91S.
25. LeBlanc JG, Culham JA, Chan KW, et al. Treatment of grafts and major vessel thrombosis with low-dose streptokinase in children. Ann Thorac Surg 1986;41:630.
26. Kirk CR, Bhrolchain CN, Qureshi SA. Streptokinase for aortic thrombosis. Arch Dis Child 1988;63:1086.
27. Richardson R, Applebaum H, Touran T, et al. Effective thrombolytic therapy of aortic thrombosis in the small premature infant. J Pediatr Surg 1988;23:1198.
28. Wessel DL, Keane JF, Fellows KE, et al. Fibrinolytic therapy for femoral arterial thrombosis after cardiac catheterization in infants and children. Am J Cardiol 1986;58:347.
29. Kirk CR, Qureschi SA. Streptokinase in the management of arterial thrombosis in infancy. Int J Cardiol 1989;25:15.
30. Ino T, Benson LN, Freedom RM, et al. Thrombolytic therapy for femoral artery thrombosis after pediatric cardiac catheterization. Am Heart J 1988;115:633.
31. Lacey SR, Zaritsky AL, Azizhkan RG. Successful treatment of Candida-infected caval thrombosis in critically ill infants by low-dose streptokinase infusion. J Pediatr Surg 1988;23:1204.
32. Pritchard SL, Culham JA, Rogers PC. Low-dose fibrinolytic therapy in infants. J Pediatr 1985;106:594.
33. Holden RW. Plasminogen activators: pharmacology and therapy. Radiol 1990;174:993.
34. Griffin MP, Casta A. Successful urokinase therapy for superior vena cava syndrome in a premature infant. Am J Dis Child 1988;142:1267.
35. Bromberg WD, Firlit CF. Fibrinolytic therapy for renal vein thrombosis in the child. J Urol 1990;143:86.
36. Duncan BW, Adzick NS, Longaker MT, et al. In utero aterial embolism from renal vein thrombosis with successful postnatal thrombolytic therapy. J Pediatr Surg 1991;26:741.
37. Reznik VM, Anderson J, Griswold WR, et al. Successful fibrinolytic

treament of arterial thrombosis and hypertension in a cocaine-exposed neonate. Pediatr 1989;84:735.

38. Belkin M, Belkin B, Bucknam CA, et al. Intra-arterial fibrinolytic therapy. Efficacy of streptokinase vs urokinase. Arch Surg 1986;121:769.

39. Curnow A, Idowu J, Behrens E, et al. Urokinase therapy for silastic catheter-induced intravascular thrombi in infants and children. Arch Surg 1985;120:1237.

40. Suarez CR, Ow EP, Lambert GH, et al. Urokinase therapy for a central venous catheter thrombus. Am J Hematol 1989;31:269.

41. Bagnall HA, Gomperts E, Atkinson JB. Continuous infusion of low-dose urokinase in the treatment of central venous catheter thrombosis in infants and children. Pediatrics 1989;83:963.

42. Dillon PW, Fox PS, Berg CJ, et al. Recombinant tissue plasminogen activator for neonatal and pediatric vascular thrombolytic therapy. J Pediatr Surg 1993;28:1264.

43. Nuss R, Hays T, Manco-Johnson M. Efficacy and safety of heparin anticoagulation for neonatal renal vein thrombosis. Am J Pediatr Hem/Onc 1994;16:127.

44. Ricci MA, Lloyd DA. Renal venous thrombosis in infants and children. Arch Surg 1990;125:1195.

45. Demirci A, Selcuk MB, Yazicioglu I. Bilateral adrenal hemorrhage associated with bilateral renal vein and vena cava thrombosis. Pediatr Radiol 1991;21:130.

46. Mocan H, Beattie TJ, Murphy AV. Renal venous thrombosis in infancy: long-term follow-up. Pediatr Nephrol 1991;5:45.

47. Gault DT. Vascular compromise in newborn infants. Arch Dis Child 1992;67:463.

48. Skarsgard E, Doski J, Jaksic T, et al. Thrombosis of the portal venous system after splenectomy for pediatric hematologic disease. J Pediatr Surg 1993;28:1109.

49. Mehta S, Connors AF, Danish EH, et al. Incidence of thrombosis during central venous catheterization of newborns: a prospective study. J Pediatr Surg 1992;27:18.

50. Alkalay Al, Mazkereth R, Santulli Jr T, et al. Central venous line thrombosis in premature infants: a case management and literature review. Am J Perinatol 1993;10:323.

51. Radecki RT, Gaebler-Spira D. Deep vein thrombosis in the disabled pediatric population. Arch Phys Med Rehabil 1994;75:248.

52. Villavicencio JL, Gonzalez-Cerna JL. Acute vascular problems of children. In: Ravitch MM, Steichen FM, eds. Current problems in surgery, vol 22. Chicago, Year Book Medical, 1985:53.

53. Evans DA, Wilmott RW. Pulmonary embolism in children. In: Wilmott RW, ed. Pediatrics Clinics of North America. Respiratory medicine II, vol 41. Philadelphia, WB Saunders, 1994:569.

54. Huntington GS, McClure CF. The anatomy and development of the jugular lymph sac in the domestic cat. Am J Anat 1910;10:177.

55. Sabin FR. The lymphatic system in human embryos, with a consideration of the morphology of the system as a whole. Am J Anat 1909;9:43.

56. Ganong WF. Dynamics of blood and lymph flow. In: Ganong WF, ed. Review of medical physiology, ed 10; chap 30. Los Altos, CA, Lange, 1981:152.

57. Mulliken JB. Classification of vascular birthmarks. In: Mulliken JB, Young AE, eds. Vascular birthmarks, hemangiomas and malformations, chap 2. Philadelphia, WB Saunders, 1988:24.

58. Fonkalsrud EW. Congenital malformations of the lymphatic system. In: Gans SL, Grosfeld JL, eds. Seminars in pediatric surgery. O'Neill JA, guest ed. Pediatr vascular disorders. Orlando: WB Saunders, 1994; 3:62.

59. Mulliken JB. Vascular malformations of the head and neck. In: Mulliken JB, Young AE, eds. Vascular birthmarks, hemangiomas and malformations, chap 16. Philadelphia, WB Saunders, 1988;301.

60. Bill AH, Sumner DS. A unified concept of lymphangioma and cystic hygroma. Surg Gynecol Obst 1965;120:79.

61. Anderson DH. Tumors of infancy and childhood. Cancer 1951;4:890.

62. Langer JC, Fitzgerald PG, Desa D, et al. Cervical cystic hygroma in the fetus: clinical spectrum and outcome. J Pediatr Surg 1990;25:58.

63. Siegel MJ, Glazer HS, St Amour TE, Rosenthal DD. Lymphangiomas in children: MR imaging. Pediatr Radiol 1989;170:467.

64. Davidson AJ, Hartman DS. Lymphangioma of the retroperitoneum: CT and sonographic characteristics. Radiol 1990;175:507.

65. Hancock BJ, St-Vil D, Luks FI, et al. Complications of lymphangiomas in children. J Pediatr Surg 1992;27:220.

66. Tanigawa N, Shimomatsuya T, Takahashi K, et al. Treatment of cystic hygroma and lymphangioma with the use of bleomycin fat emulsion. Cancer 1987;60:741.

67. Tanaka K, Inomata Y, Utsunomiya H, et al. Sclerosing therapy with bleomycin emulsion for lymphangioma in children. Pediatr Surg Int 1990;5:270.

68. Ogita S, Tsuto T, Tokiwa K. et al. Intracystic injection of OK-432: a new sclerosing therapy for cystic hygroma in children. Br J Surg 1987; 74:690.

69. Ogita S, Toshiaki T, Deguchi E, et al. OK-432 therapy for unresectable lymphangiomas in children. J Ped Surg 1991;26:263.

70. Williams HB. Lymphangioma. In: Marsh JL, ed. Current therapy in plastic and reconstructive surgery, vol 1. St Louis, CV Mosby, 1989: 57.

71. Chervenak FA, Isaacson G, Blakemore KJ, et al. Fetal cystic hygroma. N Engl J Med 1983;309:822.

72. Mollett DL, Ballantine TVN, Grosfeld JL. Mesenteric cysts in infancy and childhood. Surg Gynecol Obstet 1978;147:182.

73. Asch MJ, Cohen AH, Moore TC. Hepatic and splenic lymphangiomatosis with skeletal involvement: report of a case and review of the literature. Surgery 1974;76:334.

74. Gardner TW, Domm AC, Brock CE, Pruitt AW. Congenital pulmonary lymphangiectasis. Clin Pediatr 1983;22:75.

75. Noonan JA, Walters LR, Reeves JT. Congenital pulmonary lymphangiectasis. Am J Dis Child 1970;120:314.

76. Randolph JE, Gross RE. Congenital chylothorax. Arch Surg 1957;74: 405.

77. Servelle M, Nogues C, Soulie J, et al. Spontaneous, postoperative and traumatic chylothorax. J Cardiovasc Surg (Torino) 1980;21:475.

78. Higgins CB, Mulder DG. Chylothorax after surgery for congenital heart disease. J Thorac Cardiovasc Surg 1971;61:411.

79. Stringel G. Hemangiomas and lymphangiomas. In: Ashcraft KW, Holder TM, eds. Pediatric surgery, ed 2. Philadelphia, WB Saunders, 1993;802.

80. Bond SJ, Guzzetta PC, Snyder ML, et al. Management of pediatric postoperative chylothorax. Ann Thorac Surg 1993;56:469.

81. Crandall LA, Barker SJ, Graham DG. A study of the lymph flow from a patient with a throacic duct fistula. Gastro 1943;1:1040.

82. Azizhan RG, Canfield J, Alford BA, et al. Pleuroperitoneal shunts in the management of neonatal chylothorax. J Pediatr Srug 1983;18:842.

83. Sanchez RE, Mahour GH, Brennan LP, et al. Chylous ascites in children. Surgery 1971;69:183.

84. Milroy WF. An undescribed variety of hereditary oedema. NY Med J 1892;56:505.

85. Kinmouth JB. The lymphatics. ed 2. London, Edward Arnold, 1982.

86. Fonkalsrud EW. A syndrome of congenital lymphedema of the upper extremity and associated systemic lymphatic malformations. Surg Gynecol Obstet 1977;145:228.

87. Klippel M, Trenaunay P. Noevus variquex osteohypertrophique. J Practiciens Feb 3, 1900.

88. Young AE. Combined vascular malformations. In: Mulliken JB, Young AE, eds. Vascular birthmarks, hemangiomas and malformations, chap 14. Philadelphia, WB Saunders, 1988:246.

89. McGrory BJ, Amadio PC. Klippel-Trenaunay syndrome: orthopedic considerations. Ortho Review 1993;10:41.

Surgery of Infants and Children: Scientific Principles and Practice, edited by Keith T. Oldham, Paul M. Colombani, and Robert P. Foglia. Lippincott–Raven Publishers, Philadelphia, © 1997.

CHAPTER 103

Vascular Access

John R. Wesley

BACKGROUND AND PATIENT SELECTION

Early pediatric parenteral fluid therapy was marked by technical difficulties that led to the widespread use of subcutaneous clysis or crude intraosseous infusion. Early pediatric intravenous therapy was characterized by difficulty of percutaneous access and a high frequency of intravenous cutdown procedures. Intravenous access was frequently limited by the size of the patient, the crude technology of stainless steel needles and plastic cannulas, and the rudimentary infusion devices available. Since the 1980s, however, there has been a marked improvement in technology for smaller catheters made of less reactive and more reliable materials, with delicate and safe infusion pumps. All of this has contributed to the safety and reliability of vascular access and markedly increased the armamentarium of devices, materials, and techniques available to the surgeon. In the 1990s, the type of vascular access can be tailored to the clinical problem, the size of the patient, and the expected duration of intravenous therapy.

PERIPHERAL VENOUS ACCESS

The goal of all indwelling catheters is to allow patient movement with the lowest possible risk of dislodgement, infiltration, and infection. Indwelling catheters are made of Teflon, Silastic, polyurethane, and other new materials that are less thrombogenic, more flexible, and less likely to promote bacterial adherence and infection than in the past. The four basic approaches to placing an indwelling catheter are over a needle, through a needle, over a guide wire, and direct implantation.

Indications

Peripheral vein cannulation is usually the easiest and safest method of vascular access, and it is the preferred method. If there are no specific indications for central venous access, peripheral venous cannulation should be sufficient. Short-term needs, moderate fluid requirements, multiple uses, and adequate peripheral veins are all consistent with peripheral cannulas. The most accessible sites are the basilic, cephalic, and median cubi-

tal veins in the antecubital fascia, and the interdigital veins of the hand, scalp veins, and the saphenous veins at the ankle. (Fig. 103-1). The external jugular vein is an excellent cannulation site but is sometimes difficult to immobilize effectively.

Advantages and Disadvantages

The principal advantages of peripheral venous access are ease of availability, safety, and a lower incidence of sepsis.

The principal disadvantages and complications of peripheral venous access include infiltration and phlebitis, with or without skin sloughing or necrosis; limited flow rate and therefore limitation of caloric infusion for patients receiving peripheral parenteral nutrition; and discomfort with the need for frequent cannula change. Some authors suggest that peripheral intravenous cannulas in children be replaced after 3 days, but no data support this recommendation. With meticulous insertion, systematically monitored dressing technique, and careful catheter removal at the first sign of infiltration or occlusion, many complications can be avoided.

Technical Considerations

Palpitation or visualization of peripheral veins can be enhanced with tourniquet application, dependent positioning, exercise of the limb, local heat application, and transillumination. The most important considerations are careful matching of the cannula size to the caliber of the vein and insertion of the cannula as illustrated in Figure 103-2.

CENTRAL VENOUS ACCESS

Indications

Central venous catheterization[1] is indicated for (1) rapid infusion of large volumes of fluids or blood products, (2) secure delivery of drugs to the central circulation, (3) administration of parenteral alimentation in high concentration, (4) central venous pressure monitoring, (5) alternative route for parenteral fluid

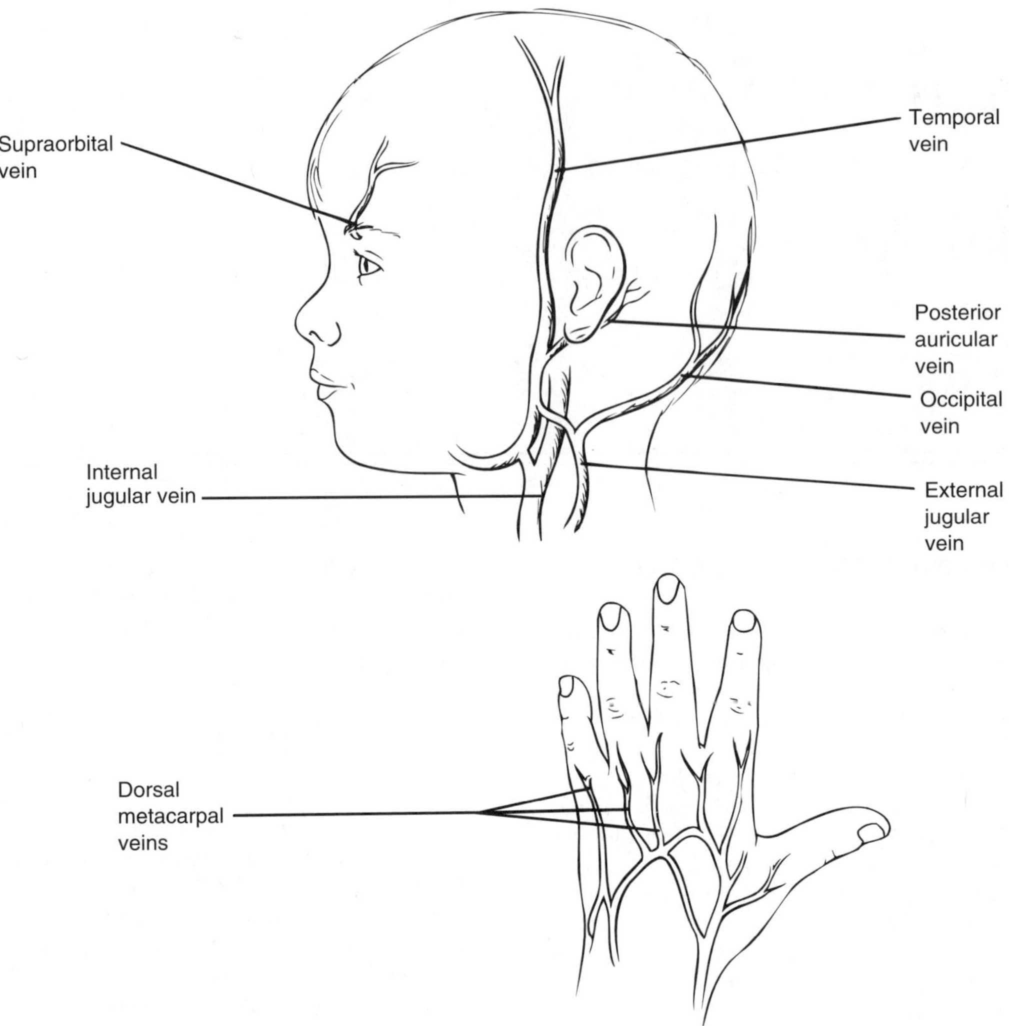

FIG. 103-1. Potential sites for peripheral and central venous access. (*continued*)

or drugs in patients for whom peripheral venous access is no longer possible, and (6) long-term continuous or intermittent access for blood sampling or therapy.

Advantages and Disadvantages

With the advent of subclavian central venous access,[1] central venous catheters were available for use in place of peripheral catheters in older children and adults. They were particularly useful during resuscitation, making possible the infusion of large volumes of blood products and intravenous fluids over short periods of time. Central venous catheters also enabled the administration of hyperosmolar solutions, making total parenteral nutrition (TPN) possible and practical. Once the technical aspects of insertion are mastered, central venous catheters are relatively easy to insert rapidly, with an acceptably low complication rate. Central venous catheter longevity is also much greater than that of peripheral lines, and they are better tolerated by patients, who are left unencumbered by immobilization boards and dressings, thereby retaining use of their hands and feet. Central venous catheters also have the advantage of enabling periodic blood sampling without the necessity of separate peripheral venipunctures. The early 1970s witnessed the evolution of the subclavian technique, so that it is now safe for infants and small children. In 1986, Newman and colleagues[2] demonstrated the efficacy and safety of percutaneous central venous catheters in a prospective study comparing the subclavian or jugular approach with peripheral venous cutdown. They concluded that percutaneous central intravenous catheterization is the method of choice for venous access other than routine short-term situations.

The main disadvantage of central venous catheter placement is that complications are generally more serious than those associated with peripheral venous access. Only physicians well experienced in the techniques of subclavian and internal jugular venipuncture should insert central venous catheters. Except in an emergency, central venous catheters should be inserted only under planned circumstances with sufficient help available and with careful attention to aseptic technique. Possible complications at the time of catheter insertion are discussed in the concluding section.

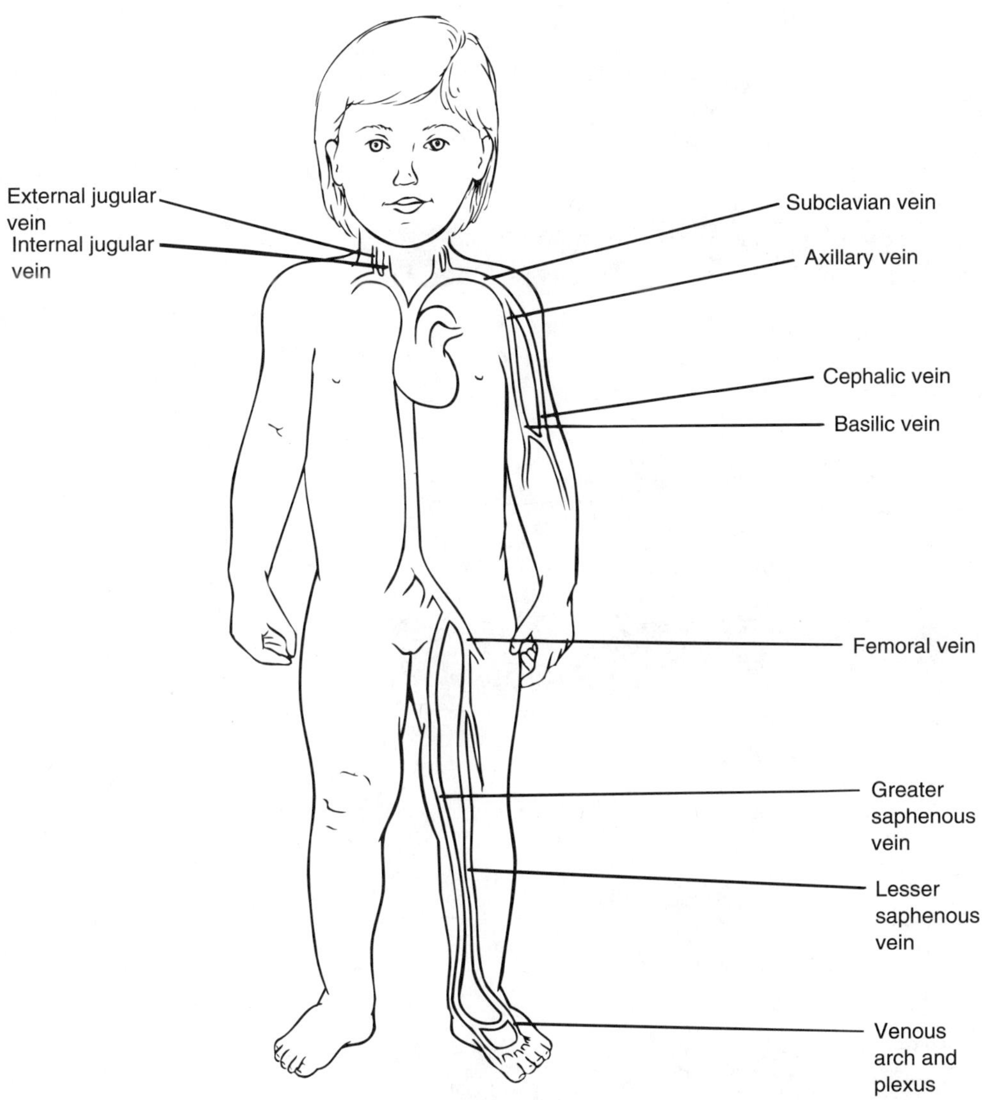

FIG. 103-1. *Continued.*

Technical Considerations

Landmarks for subclavian and internal jugular vein catheter insertion are indicated in Figure 103-3. In children younger than 5 years of age, the subclavian vein is located closer to the superior border of the clavicle, and the needle insertion angle should be adjusted accordingly. Once the needle has been inserted and the angle established, the course should not be changed unless the needle is completely withdrawn for danger of lacerating the vein, artery, or other mediastinal structures, such as the phrenic nerve.

BROVIAC-TYPE SILASTIC CATHETERS: PERMANENT RIGHT ATRIAL CATHETERS

Indications

The first generation of indwelling central venous catheters were made of polyvinyl chloride and were relatively stiff and thrombogenic. They were associated with a number of mechani-

cal and septic complications. In 1973, Broviac and colleagues[3] introduced the Silastic catheter, an indwelling silicone rubber catheter that can remain in place for extended periods. The Silastic catheter is much more flexible and inert and is associated with fewer complications than polyvinyl catheters with respect to mechanical occlusion, venous perforation, and infection. Commercial versions of these catheters have evolved to the widely used permanent right atrial catheter (PRAC).[4] These catheters are manufactured from radioopaque soft silicone rubber, in varying calibers and lengths, and have a small Dacron felt cuff 30 cm from the external end. The cuff allows fibrous ingrowth, which serves to anchor the catheter and to act as a barrier to infection (Table 103-1). Indications for PRAC use in children include any condition requiring long-term venous access for the administration of fluids, antibiotics, antineoplastic drugs, TPN, and blood products, or the need for frequent blood sampling. Appropriate candidates for PRAC placement include in-hospital patients, such as infants recovering from gastroschisis or necrotizing enterocolitis, or outpatients, such as adoles-

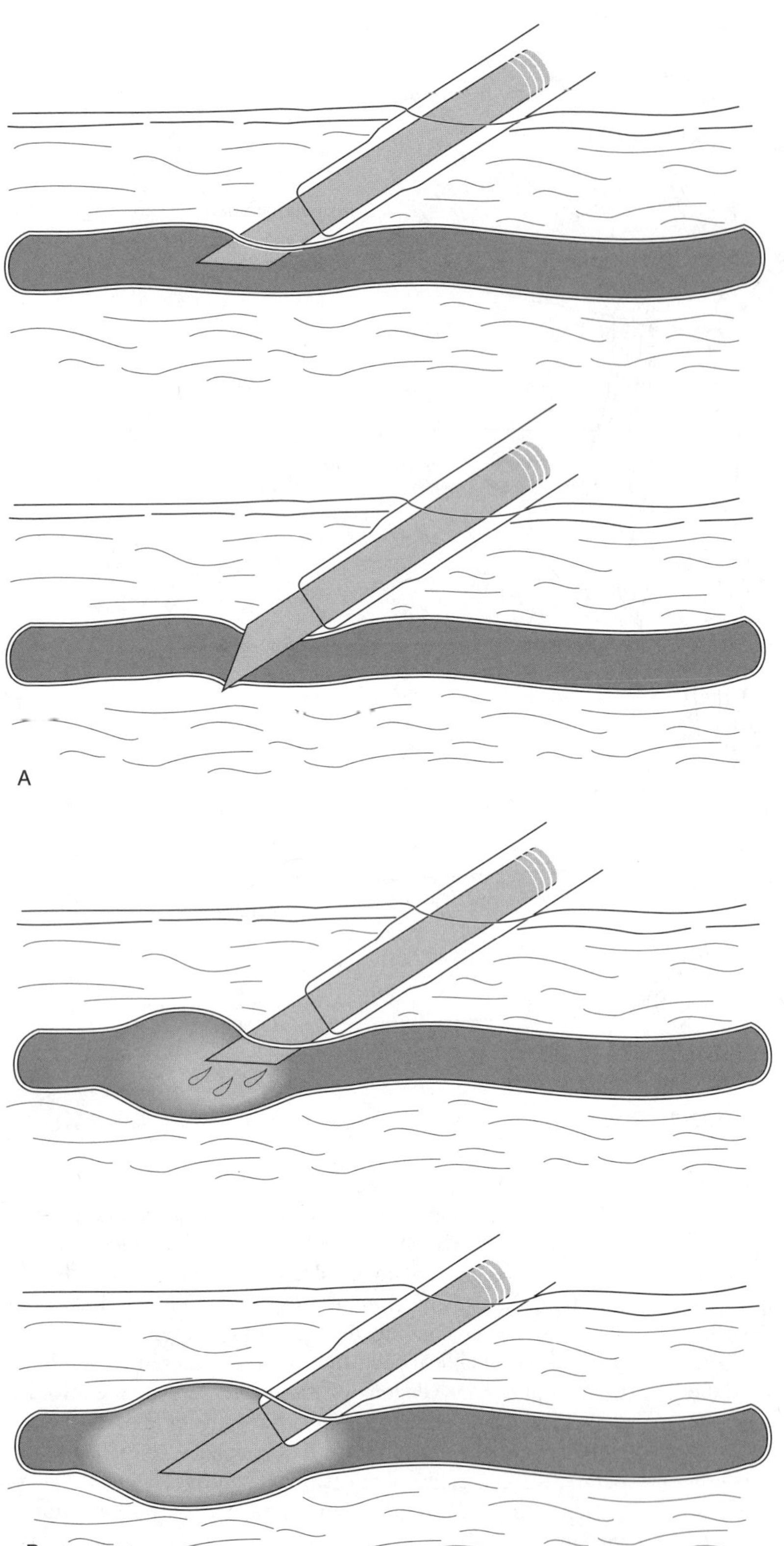

FIG. 103-2. (*A*) When the needle point is inserted up (*top*), the orifice of the needle enters the mid-lumen of the vein. When the needle point is inserted down (*bottom*), the bevel of the needle can puncture the deep wall of the vein before blood return is apparent, and a venipuncture is "blown." (*B*) Gentle injection of sterile saline expands the vein, allowing room for further advancement of the needle. The cannula lip can then enter the lumen of the vessel without the needle perforating the deep wall of the vein.

cents with neoplastic disease requiring chemotherapy or patients with short bowel syndrome on home parenteral nutrition.

Advantages and Disadvantages

Advantages of the external PRAC include freedom of activity when the catheter is heparinized and capped off, no discomfort when hooking up, repair without replacement if a leak develops in the external portion of the catheter, no need for sacrifice of the vein, and decreased septic complications as a result of the tunneled approach, as discussed later.

Disadvantages include the need for anesthesia at the time of insertion, mandatory occlusive aseptic dressing at all times, a high probability of contamination and infection if the dressing and catheter site get wet, the need for periodic catheter irrigation when the catheter is not in use, and disturbance of body image, especially important in adolescents.

Technical Considerations

The catheter is usually placed under general anesthesia, although local anesthesia can be used for infants on ventilators

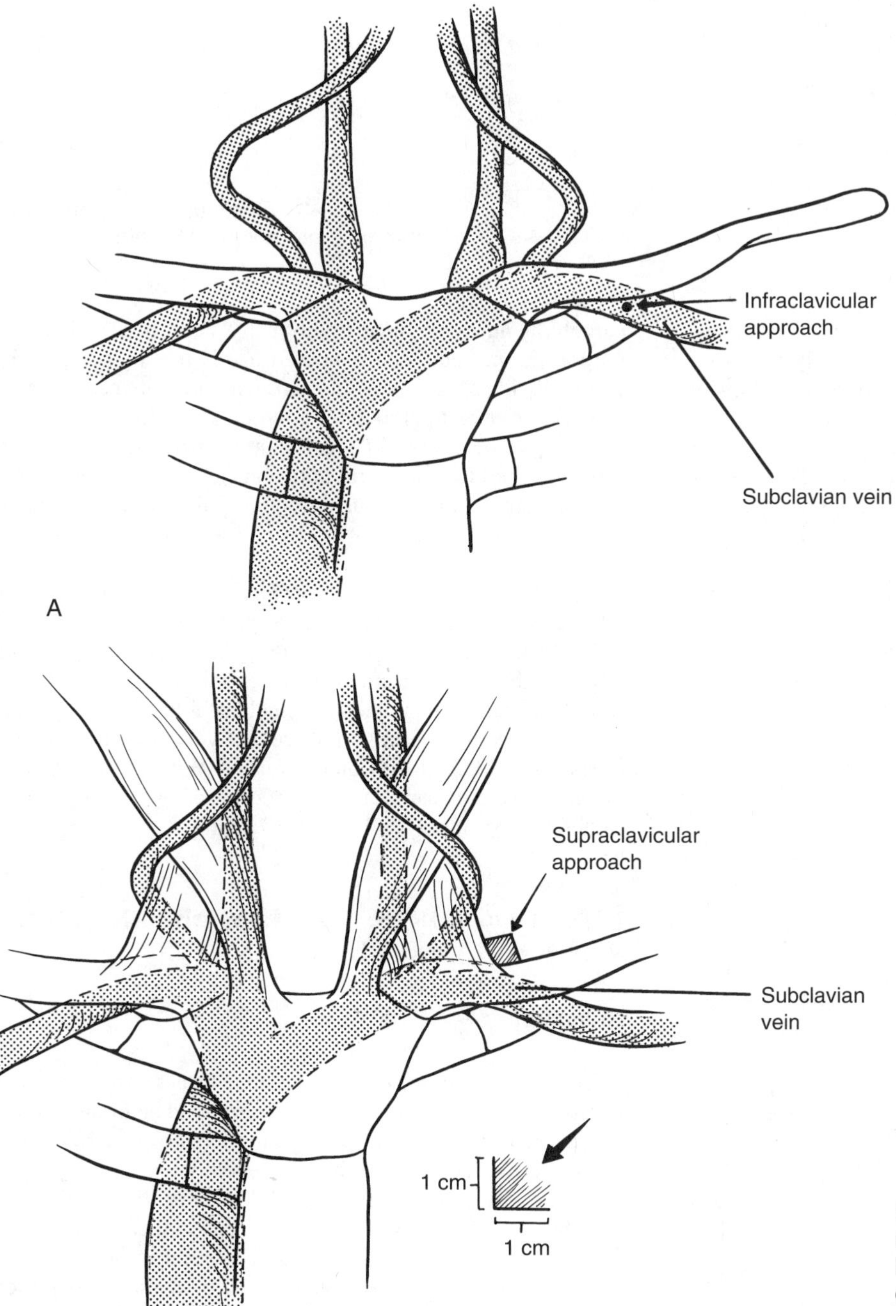

FIG. 103-3. Subclavian and internal jugular vein catheterization. (*A*) Infraclavicular approach, subclavian vein. (*B*) Supraclavicular approach, subclavian vein. *(continued)*

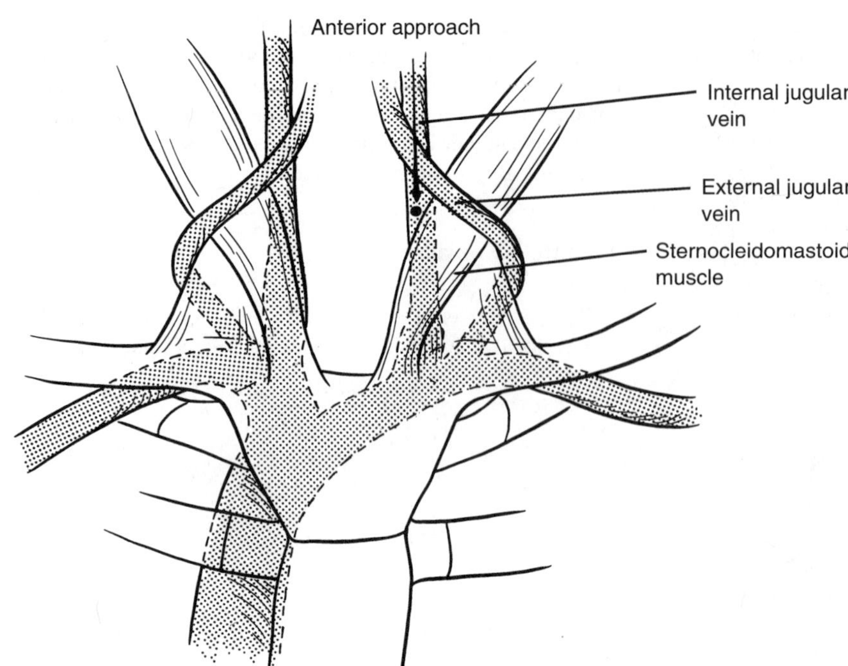

FIG. 103-3. *Continued.* (*C*) Anterior approach, internal jugular vein.

and for older, cooperative patients. (Fig. 103-4). The percutaneous infraclavicular subclavian approach is generally preferred in most age groups and is facilitated by use of a peel-away plastic sheath available in several sizes. The external jugular vein cutdown approach is used in newborns and very young infants, and the internal jugular vein, the facial vain, the saphenous vein, and other veins can be used if other approaches fail. Knowledge of the local venous anatomy and careful dissection can reveal the middle thyroid vein or the common facial vein, which are routes to the internal jugular vein and are preferable to direct ligation. Proximal and distal control should always be obtained when accessing the internal jugular vein by an open approach, and, if possible, the catheter should be placed without ligating the vessel. This allows repeated use of the vessel after catheter removal for malfunction or thrombosis, and it maintains patency of the vein after the catheter is no longer needed and removed. One of the key elements for success identified by several groups is the placement of a portion of the Silastic catheter, usually 4 to 8 cm, in a subcutaneous tunnel, extending from the venotomy site to a more distant site on the anterior chest wall or in the scalp behind the ear.[5]

The PRAC can be used immediately, once proper placement is confirmed by a chest radiograph, which also rules out technical complications such as pneumothorax. Catheters used for parenteral nutrition have traditionally been reserved for that purpose alone, but such restricted use is not always possible, especially in patients in whom no other vascular access is available. Some investigators have found that the infection rate for multiuse catheters is not significantly different from that for catheters used for parenteral nutrition alone.[6] Therefore, central venous catheters can be used for multiple purposes if careful attention is given to sterility and if a well-defined protocol is used.

The Dacron cuff serves as a barrier to infection. Improved catheter longevity and decreased septic complications are well documented in a retrospective study by Holmes and colleagues.[5] These authors demonstrated that central venous catheters inserted through a subcutaneous tunnel last four times longer than catheters inserted directly into a central vein. The latter are four times more likely to become infected. With proper attention given to catheter care and to sterile dressing technique, these catheters have lasted as long as 18 years.

INJECTION PORTS: TOTALLY IMPLANTABLE VENOUS ACCESS DEVICES

Indications

The need to provide reliable vascular access during long-term intermittent parenteral therapy for cancer and other diseases and the desire to further reduce the complications of Broviac-type PRACs provided the stimulus for development of a totally implantable venous access device (TIVAD; Fig. 103-5). Repeated peripheral venipuncture to administer chemotherapeutic agents, antibiotics, and other parenteral medication is uncomfortable for the patient and, over the long-term, damages peripheral veins, posing a high risk of chemical inflammation, infection, and thrombosis. Intermittent extravasation of certain types of

TABLE 103-1. *Comparison of silicon rubber catheters*

Catheter	Unit volume (mL/cm)	Total length (cm)	Total volume (mL)
Hickman	0.02	95	1.90
Broviac	0.008	90	0.70
Pediatric Broviac	0.004	71	0.30
Baby Broviac	0.002	71	0.15

drugs also damages tissue adjacent to the vein or artery, commonly resulting in a prolonged, painful search by the nurse or physician for a suitable vein. Also, delayed or interrupted peripheral venous access leads to wastage of expensive drugs, and regimens involving repeated infusion often cannot be completed in a timely manner. Although centrally placed venous catheters, such as the Broviac-type PRAC, are often used for long-term intermittent infusion therapy, they have obvious drawbacks, many of which were mentioned in the preceding section. Because the catheter receptacle exits through the skin,

infection remains a major problem, and scrupulous attention to sterile technique during periodic dressing change is necessary. In addition, catheter occlusion occurs in up to 25% of patients, despite frequent irrigation with heparinized saline. Finally, the external portion of the catheter restricts daily activities, such as bathing. It is psychologically and aesthetically disturbing to many patients, particularly teenagers. A variety of totally implantable devices, consisting of small-volume subcutaneous injection ports and Silastic catheters, are now available.[7,8]

Indications for TIVADs are similar to those for PRACs, in-

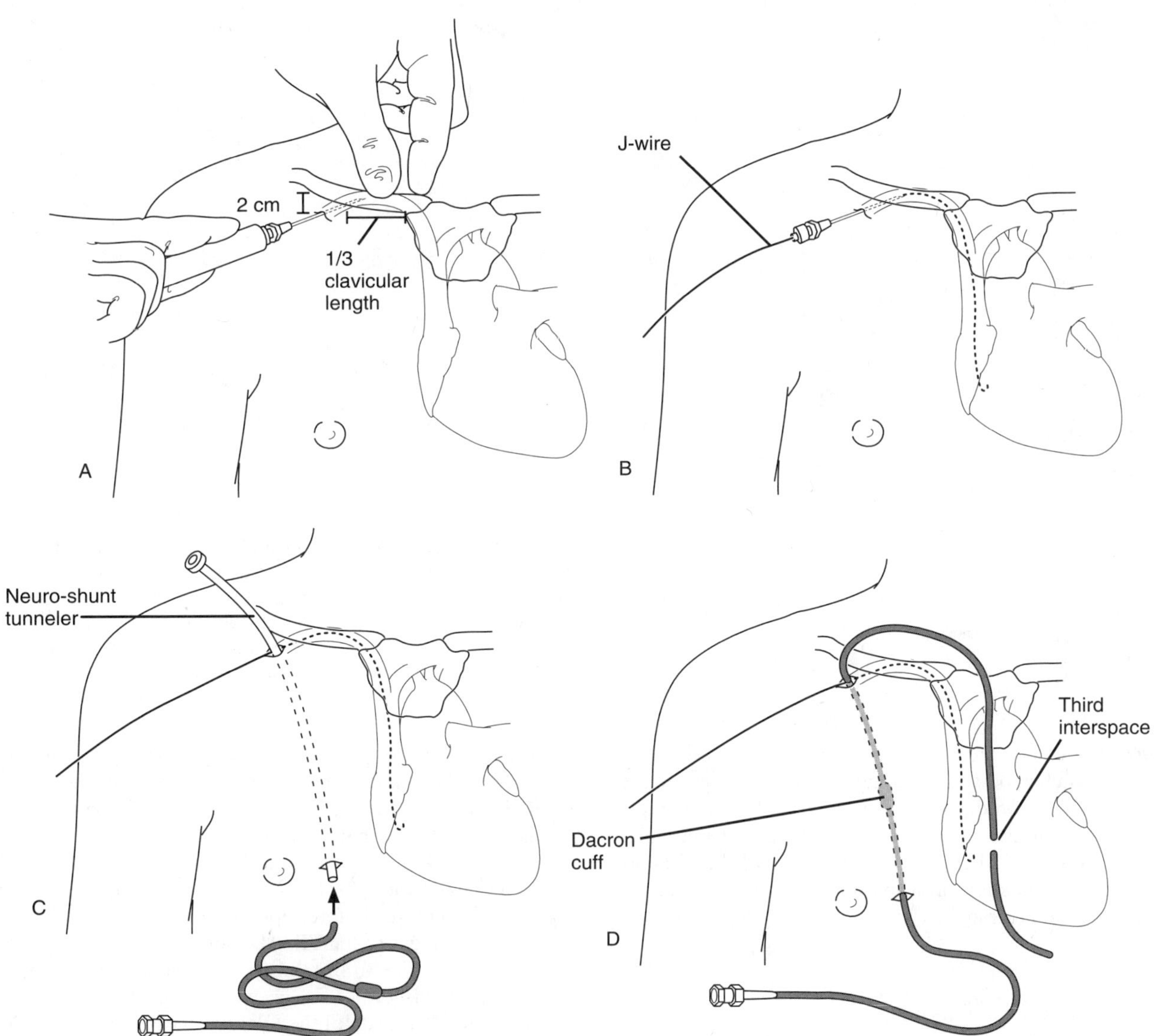

FIG. 103-4. (*A*) Infraclavicular subclavian venous puncture techniques for a patient younger than 5 years old. The subclavian vein tends to be more cephalad beneath the clavicle in children than in older patients. As the needle is advanced, the course should not be changed unless the needle is completely withdrawn because of the possibility that the vein or artery may be lacerated. (*B*) Insertion and advancement of flexible J-wire. Proper position should be confirmed by fluoroscopy or with plain chest radiograph. (*C*) A neurosurgical shunt catheter introducer, a 25-cm tendon passer, or a fine intestinal probe is used to place the catheter in a subcutaneous tunnel. (*D*) The catheter is placed on the anterior chest wall to simulate its intravascular position. Dividing the catheter at the level of the third intercostal space ensures final placement at the junction of the superior vena cava with the right atrium. The Dacron cuff should be positioned at least 3 cm proximal to the exit site. Placement halfway between the vein entry and skin exit sites minimizes the risk of catheter-cuff migration. *(continued)*

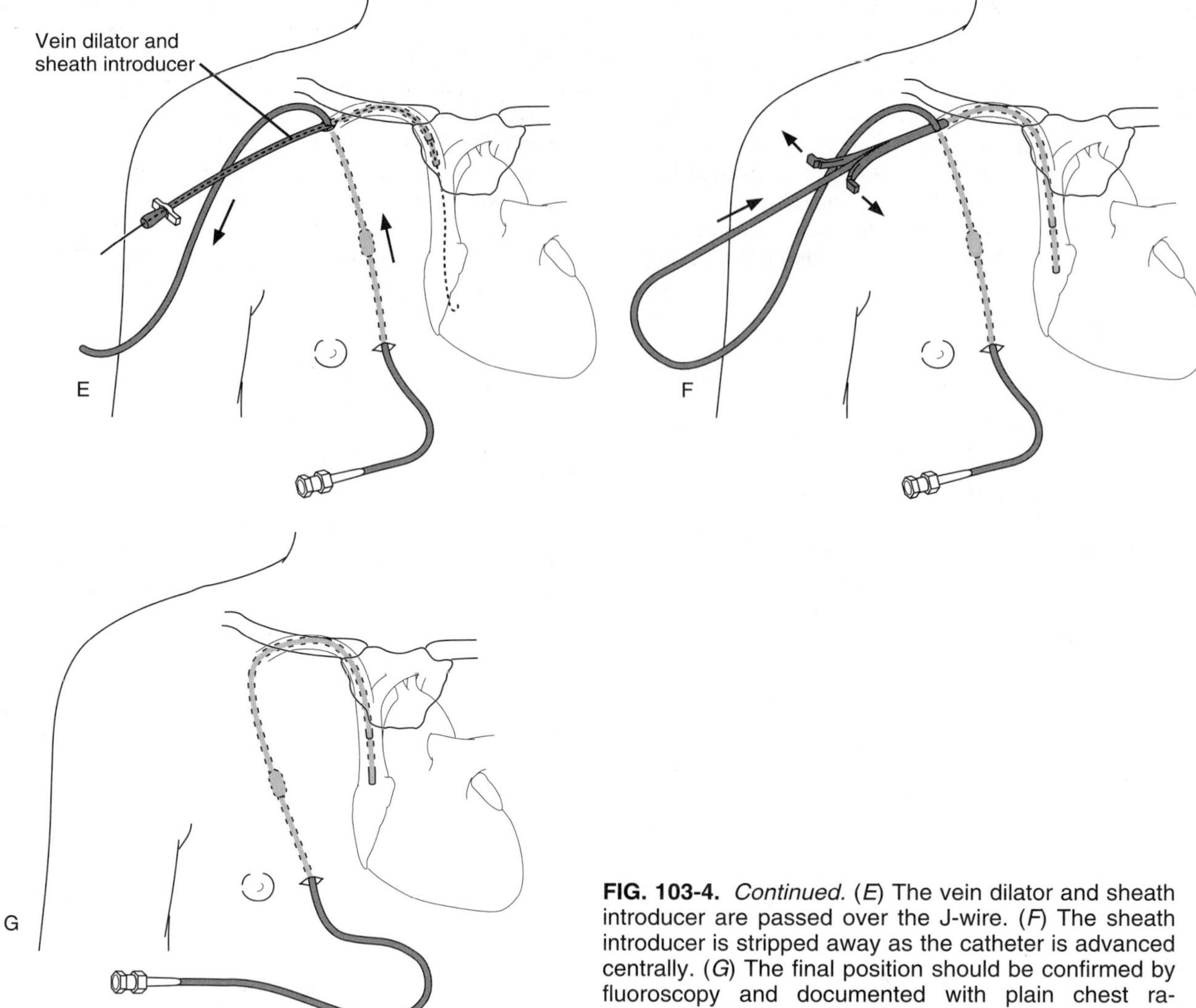

FIG. 103-4. *Continued.* (*E*) The vein dilator and sheath introducer are passed over the J-wire. (*F*) The sheath introducer is stripped away as the catheter is advanced centrally. (*G*) The final position should be confirmed by fluoroscopy and documented with plain chest ratiographs. (Courtesy of the Mayo Foundation)

cluding conditions that require long-term venous access for administration of chemotherapeutic agents, antibiotics, parenteral nutrition, and blood products and the need for intermittent blood sampling. Miniaturization of these devices has extended their use to infants and small children. In-hospital patients destined for intermittent outpatient infusion and outpatients scheduled for interval chemotherapy are particularly appropriate candidates.

Advantages and Disadvantages

Because the TIVAD is implanted under the skin, it spares the peripheral vasculature, decreases the risk of infectious complications, minimizes care and maintenance, facilities ambulatory treatment, and does not interfere with the patient's normal daily activities. The most significant advantage to the patient is that the subcutaneous injection port requires no dressing change and few, if any, heparin flushes between uses. It permits bathing and swimming. It has the added psychologic advantage of being out of sight, except when being used. Clinical experience has demonstrated a marked decrease in catheter sepsis

with TIVADs. A prospective study reported by Ingram and associates[9] documented a significantly lower catheter infection rate in pediatric hematology and oncology patients with subcutaneous ports compared with external venous catheters. The device has also been shown to be effective and safe for home parenteral nutrition; the Silastic diaphragm can receive as many as 2000 punctures before replacement.[10]

Disadvantages of the TIVAD include limitations in the duration of access due to instability of the noncoring Huber needle in the port, discomfort of access through the overlying skin, and limited longevity of the Silastic access septum. In addition, removal usually requires general anesthesia. With the development of the right-angle Huber needle with wings, the access apparatus lends itself to a more secure and stable dressing than with the original straight Huber needle (Fig. 103-6). Consequently, the incidence of dislodgement of the Huber needle apparatus is low, and overnight and long-term access is much safer, leading to applications such as nightly infusion of parenteral nutrition. The Luer-Lok intrinsic to the Broviac-type PRACs is definitely more fail-safe, however, so that PRACs are preferred by some patients and physicians. Access to the Luer-Lok is painless and much less threatening to children than

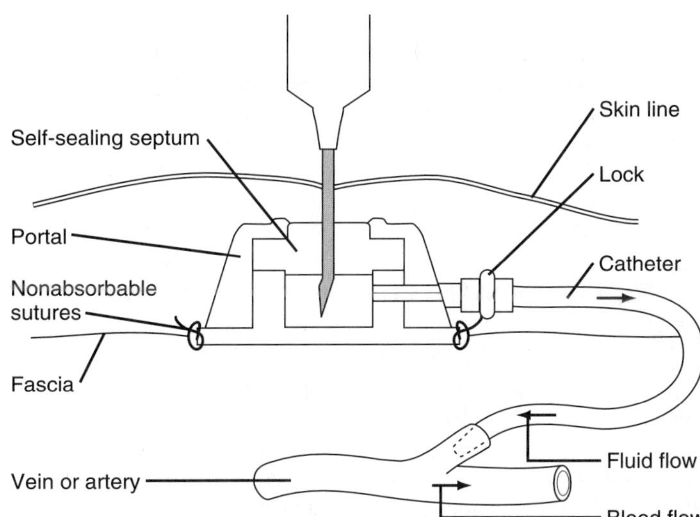

FIG. 103-5. Totally implantable venous access device (TIVAD). Delivery of fluids and drugs using a Huber needle.

the nurse or parent approaching the TIVAD with a Huber needle. These reasons notwithstanding, discomfort of port access to the overlying skin is effectively aborted by application of a topical analgesic, which is especially helpful and appropriate for infants and children. With an upper limit of 2000 system punctures before failure (5 years at one access per day), the limited life-span of the Silastic septum is of theoretic importance only: most TIVADs last until the patient no longer requires the device. For patients who require life-long venous access, the Broviac-type PRAC may be preferred because it is no longer unusual to maintain a single PRAC for 6 to 12 years.

Technical Considerations

After inserting the Silastic catheter into the central vein by either percutaneous or cutdown technique, as described in the preceding section, the catheter is passed through a subcutaneous tunnel into a subcutaneous pocket created on the chest wall or a bony prominence for stability. The location should be selected preoperatively to ensure that it is convenient and comfortable for the patient and family. The port is anchored to the underlying fascia by permanent sutures. After closure, chest radiography documents the correct position of the catheter tip (previously determined by fluoroscopy) and rules out other technical complications, such as pneumothorax or kinks in the subcutaneous catheter. If the port is to be used immediately, the right-angle Huber needle is placed while the patient is in the operating room. Otherwise, 24 hours should elapse before accessing the port to allow the initial stages of healing to proceed undisturbed.

Dressings are not required once the incisions have healed except during the time of infusion. Access should be gained only with a 22-gauge, side-fenestrated, noncoring Huber needle (see Fig. 103-6) to avoid damage to the Silastic self-sealing septum. Use of a conventional needle removes a core from the septum, which is likely to leak.

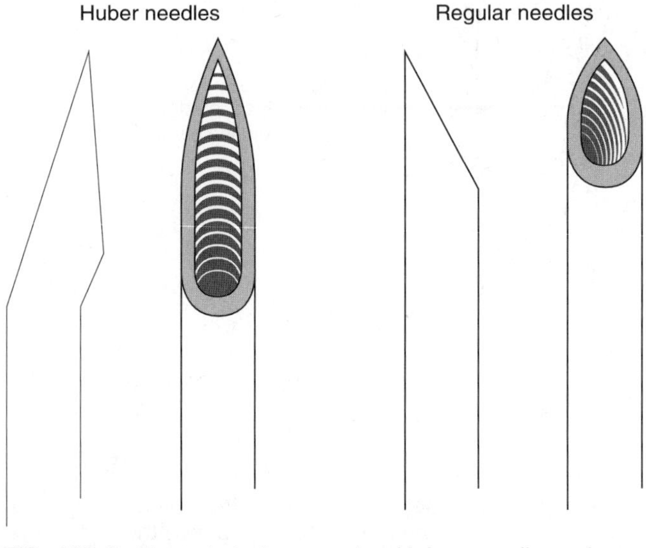

FIG. 103-6. Fenestrated, noncoring Huber needle and conventional needle.

MULTILUMEN CATHETERS

Indications

Multiple-lumen venous access catheters have been developed for both PRAC and TIVAD access systems. The indications are limited to patients who require long-term access for simultaneous administration of two or more parenteral solutions, such as antibiotics, chemotherapeutic agents, fluid for hydration, or parenteral nutrition. Use of a triple-lumen catheter enables concurrent monitoring of the central venous pressure. Double- and triple-lumen PRACs are available commercially, as are double-lumen TIVADs.

Advantages, Disadvantages, and Management

The advantages of double-lumen catheters or double-port systems accrue from the economy of venous access sites and the avoidance of disruption of infusion schedules otherwise necessary if only one access site is available. Disadvantages relate to the potential complications that accompany an increased number of central venous invasive events. These complications are avoided by strict adherence to a detailed protocol, in which each lumen is treated as a separate catheter and in which the access device is reduced to a single-lumen type as soon as the multilumen type is no longer required.

ALTERNATIVE SITES FOR CENTRAL VENOUS ACCESS

Placement of central venous catheter systems most commonly involves access by the percutaneous infraclavicular and supraclavicular approach to the subclavian vein and by the percutaneous or cutdown approach to the external jugular, internal jugular, facial, saphenous, cephalic, and basilic veins. When these sites are infiltrated, thrombosed, infected, or otherwise unavailable, physicians must resort to higher-risk sites, which, by the pressure of necessity, have evolved during the past 10 years. These are reasonably safe alternatives that have documented success records. These include percutaneous femoral venous catheterization,[11] the cutdown approach to the deep inferior epigastric vein in the groin[12] (Fig. 103 7), the cutdown flank approach to the lumbar veins[13] (Fig. 103-8), the thoracotomy approach to the azygos, hemizygous, and intercostal venous systems[14] (Fig. 103-9), and the thoracotomy and direct canalization of the right atrial appendage.[15] In addition, a variety of direct percutaneous approaches are available by the invasive radiologist using ultrasound or other localization techniques. Long-term success of all of the alternative approaches depends on a detailed understanding of regional anatomy, meticulous technique, and well-established protocols for occlusive dressings. With careful adherence to successful principles and protocols, such as tunneling Silastic catheters placed in the groin of infants above the diaper line on the abdominal wall or on the chest wall, mechanical and septic complications can be minimized, and even the most difficult vascular access is made safe.

PERMANENT PERIPHERAL CENTRAL VENOUS CATHETERS

A peripherally placed central venous catheter has been developed with the goal of providing the beneficial features of both peripheral and central lines. The prime benefactor of this effort has been the neonatal patient, particularly the premature or small-for-gestational-age infant who weighs less than 1500 g. The limitations of peripheral access (eg, phlebitis, subcutaneous fluid extravasation, skin slough, restricted use of high-osmolarity solutions, and short-term patency) and the complications of surgically placed PRACs (eg, sepsis, pneumothorax, pericardial effusion, and superior vena cava thrombosis) have been especially difficult in this age group. In 1982, Dolcourt and Bose[16] reported successful use of Silastic percutaneous central venous catheters in 15 neonates, with a mean catheter longevity of

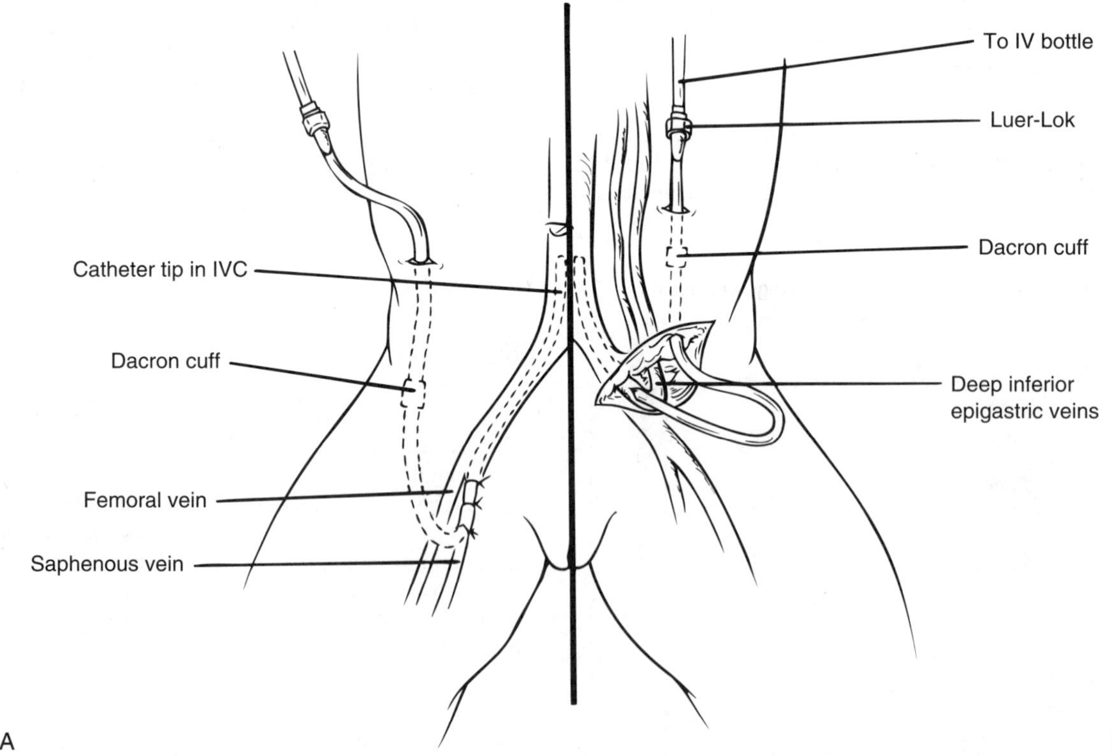

FIG. 103-7. Saphenous vein and deep inferior epigastric vein are accessed to enter the inferior vena cava (IVC). (*A*) Placement of saphenous vein cutdown, with tunneling of catheter to exit site above the diaper line. The exit site is placed over the lower thorax, if possible, because this affords a stable site that simplifies nursing care. (*B*) Deep inferior epigastric vein access. (Courtesy of the Mayo Foundation)

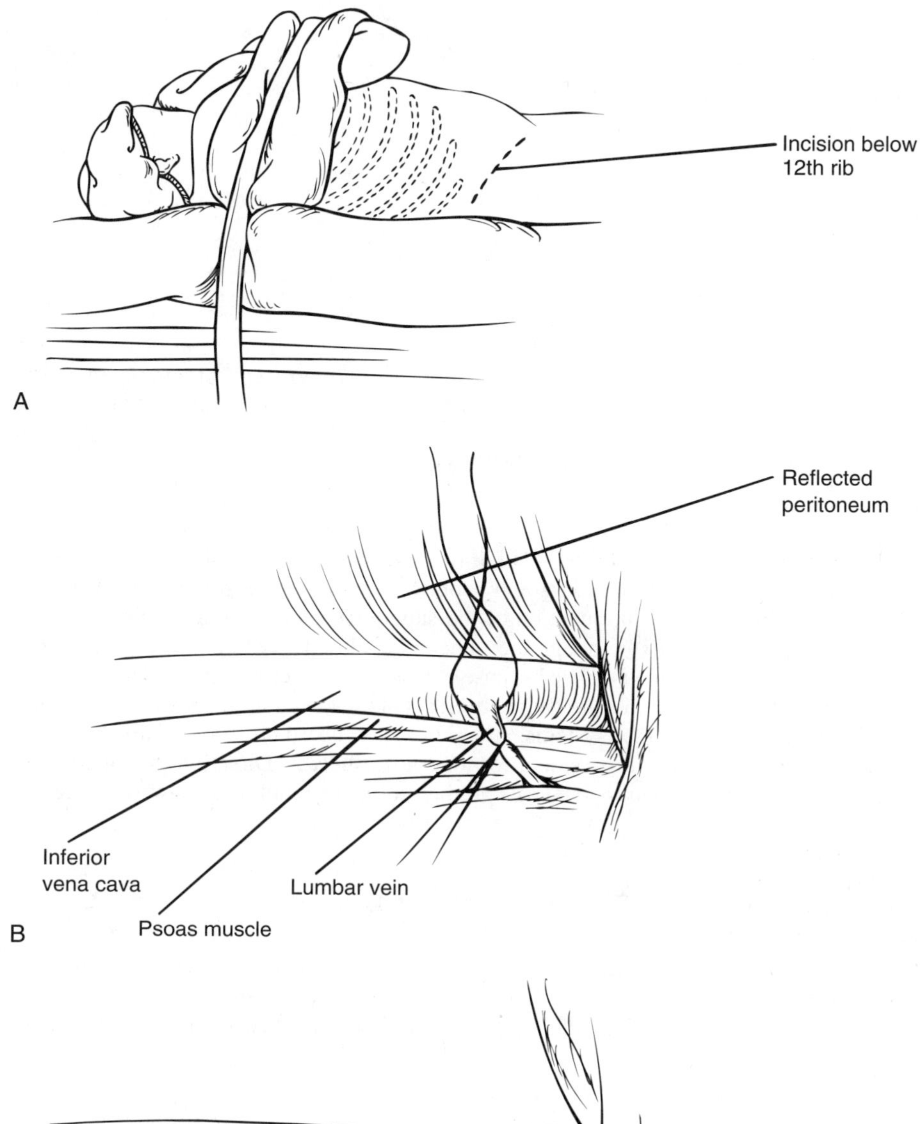

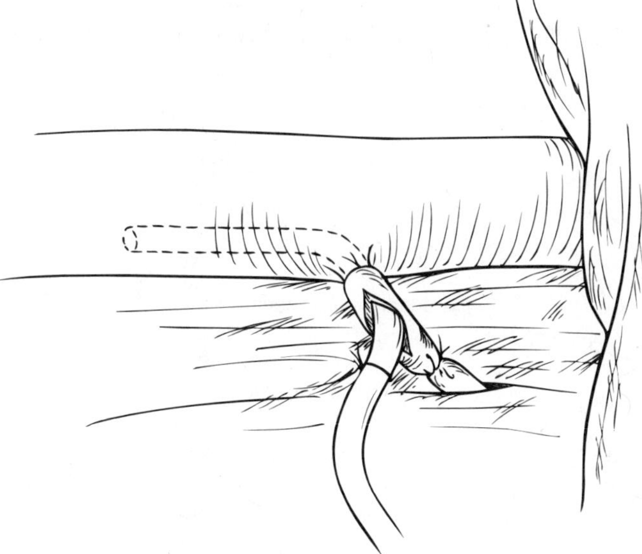

FIG. 103-8. Lumbar vein access to the inferior vena cava (IVC) can be achieved using either an open or percutaneous approach. (*A*) Positioning for flank incision below the 12th rib, with the right side elevated at 20 degrees. (*B*) IVC and lumbar vein are exposed. (*C*) Silastic catheter is placed into IVC through lumbar vein and secured to ileopsoas fascia. *(continued)*

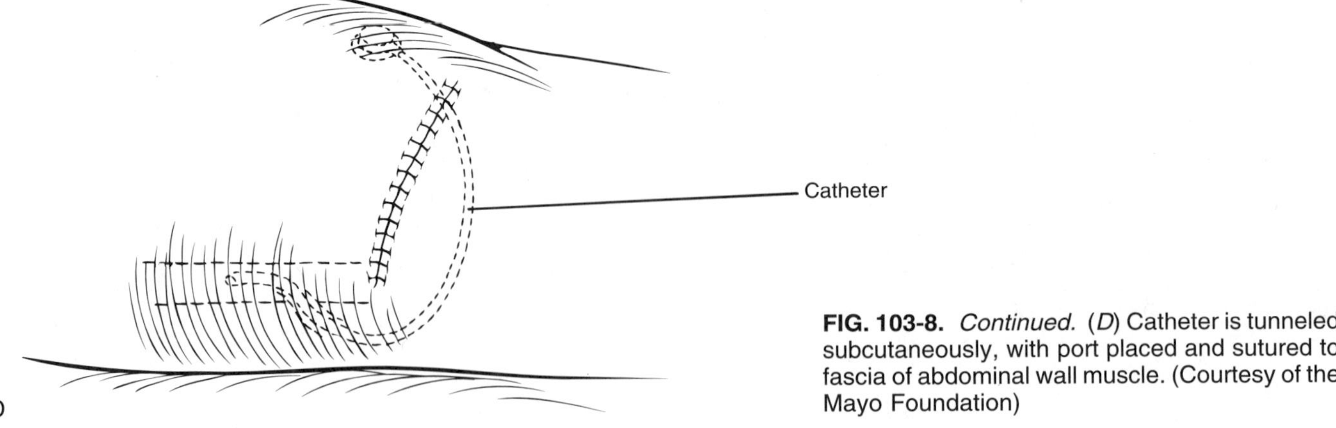

FIG. 103-8. *Continued. (D)* Catheter is tunneled subcutaneously, with port placed and sutured to fascia of abdominal wall muscle. (Courtesy of the Mayo Foundation)

24.8 ± 15.9 days and no catheter sepsis, thrombophlebitis, or caval obstruction. This compares favorably with two studies[17,18] documenting that peripheral intravenous catheters remained functional for a mean of 30.1 and 33 hours, respectively, in neonates of similar weight and gestational age and with reports[19,20] of PRAC catheter sepsis of 31.6% and 25.6% in infants receiving TPN. Other reports have confirmed the effectiveness of permanent peripheral central venous catheters in cohorts of 62 and 45 infants, respectively. The main drawback of this device appears to be a high incidence of mechanical problems, especially with difficulty passing the catheter and occlusion (as high as 28% in one series[21]), related to small caliber, relatively long length, and delicate consistency of the Silastic catheter. Several types of percutaneous catheters are commercially available.

The catheter is placed gently through the introducer needle using a nontoothed, iris thumb-type forceps, and the introducer is carefully withdrawn. An occlusive dressing is placed, and chest radiography confirms the proper position of the catheter at the junction of the superior vena cava and the right atrium. Even though the catheter is radioopaque, the tip can be difficult to visualize because of its small caliber, and it may be necessary to fill the catheter with radioopaque contrast material. As with other systems, attention to a standard protocol for insertion and care is critical for long-term success. Directions supplied with commercial kits are helpful and should be reviewed before attempting catheter placement.

INTRAOSSEOUS ACCESS

The technique of intraosseous infusion has received substantial interest in emergency situations when immediate access to the vascular system is required and when attempts at peripheral

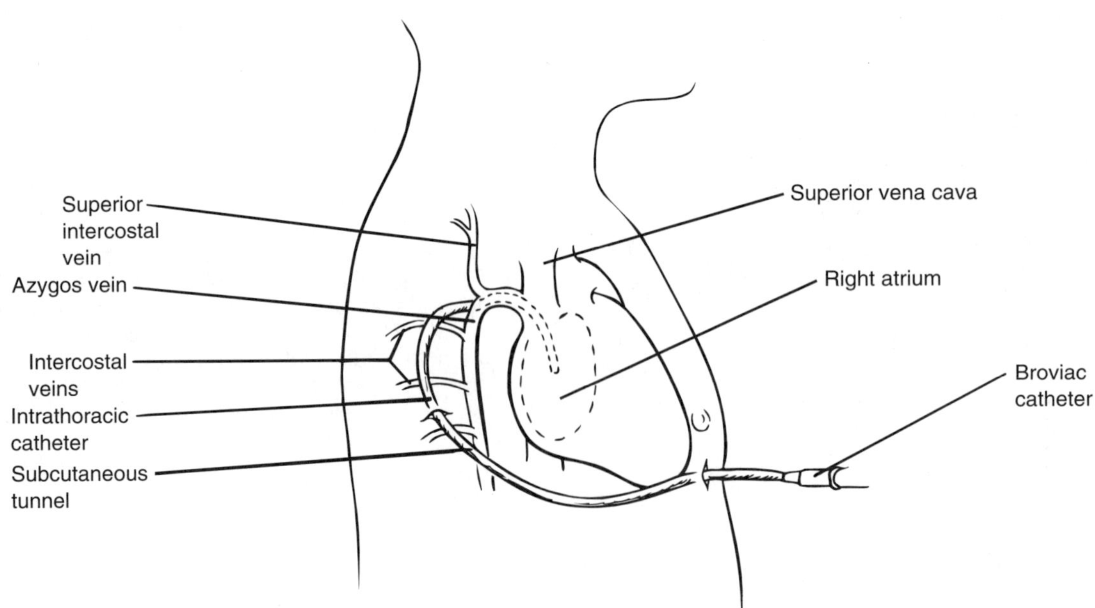

FIG. 103-9. Right thoracotomy approach for azygos vein access to the right atrium. (Courtesy of the Mayo Foundation)

or central venous access have failed or proven too slow. The technique was used extensively in the 1940s and faded into obscurity with improvements in the techniques and quality of intravascular catheter access. Indications include cardiopulmonary arrest, burns, life-threatening status epilepticus, and shock due to trauma, sepsis, or dehydration. In the tibias and femurs of infants and children, the marrow sinusoids drain into the medullary venous channels, and nutrient and emissary veins drain into the systemic venous system. Therefore, substances injected into the bone marrow are absorbed almost immediately into the general circulation.[22] The marrow cavity functions as a rigid vein that does not collapse in the presence of hypovolemia and profound peripheral circulatory shock. Fluids, blood products, and a wide variety of pharmacologic agents have been administered successfully through the marrow cavity. In addition, bone marrow aspirates can be obtained before fluid or blood infusion and can be analyzed for blood chemistry values, PCO_2, pH, hemoglobin level, culture for bacteria, and typing and cross-matching. When used for temporary vascular access in emergency situation, there are few absolute contraindications for intraosseous infusions. These include osteoporosis, osteogenesis imperfecta, and an ipsilateral fractured extremity with the accompanying risk of subcutaneous extravasation. Use of the marrow cavity of long bones for infusion is usually limited to young children because of the physiologic replacement of the red marrow by less vascular yellow marrow at about 5 years of age.

The proximal tibia is the optimal site for insertion of an intra-osseous access needle in children, followed by the distal tibia and the femur. Disposable bone marrow aspiration needles (15 to 18 gauge) with adjustable lengths are preferred. Intraosseous needles have a short shaft with a protective sheath to prevent the tip of the needle from being forced too deep into or through the bone (Fig. 103-10). The needle is directed at an angle of 60 to 90 degrees away from the growth plate to avoid injury to the structure, and is advanced with a boring or screwing motion. Entry into the marrow space is confirmed by noting a lack of resistance after the needle has passed through the cortex. Marrow should aspirate easily into a syringe, and fluid should infuse freely. Although the needle can stand upright without support, it must be secured by taping the phalanges to the skin to prevent dislodgement. The infusion site should be observed for evidence of extravasation. With proper equipment available, virtually all intraosseous catheters can be placed in 3 to 5 minutes.

Although the sternum and the ilium were used as intraosseous infusion sites in the past, they are considered less suitable and can be dangerous. The marrow space in the sternum is inadequate in children under 3 years of age, and insertion into the sternum can be technically difficult as well as dangerous, particularly during chest compressions, when there are substantial risks of mediastinal puncture and injury to the myocardium. Complications of intraosseous infusion are infrequent and generally consist of subcutaneous and subperiosteal infiltration of fluid or leakage from the puncture site. Clotting of marrow in the needle can result in loss of access. Localized cellulitis, with

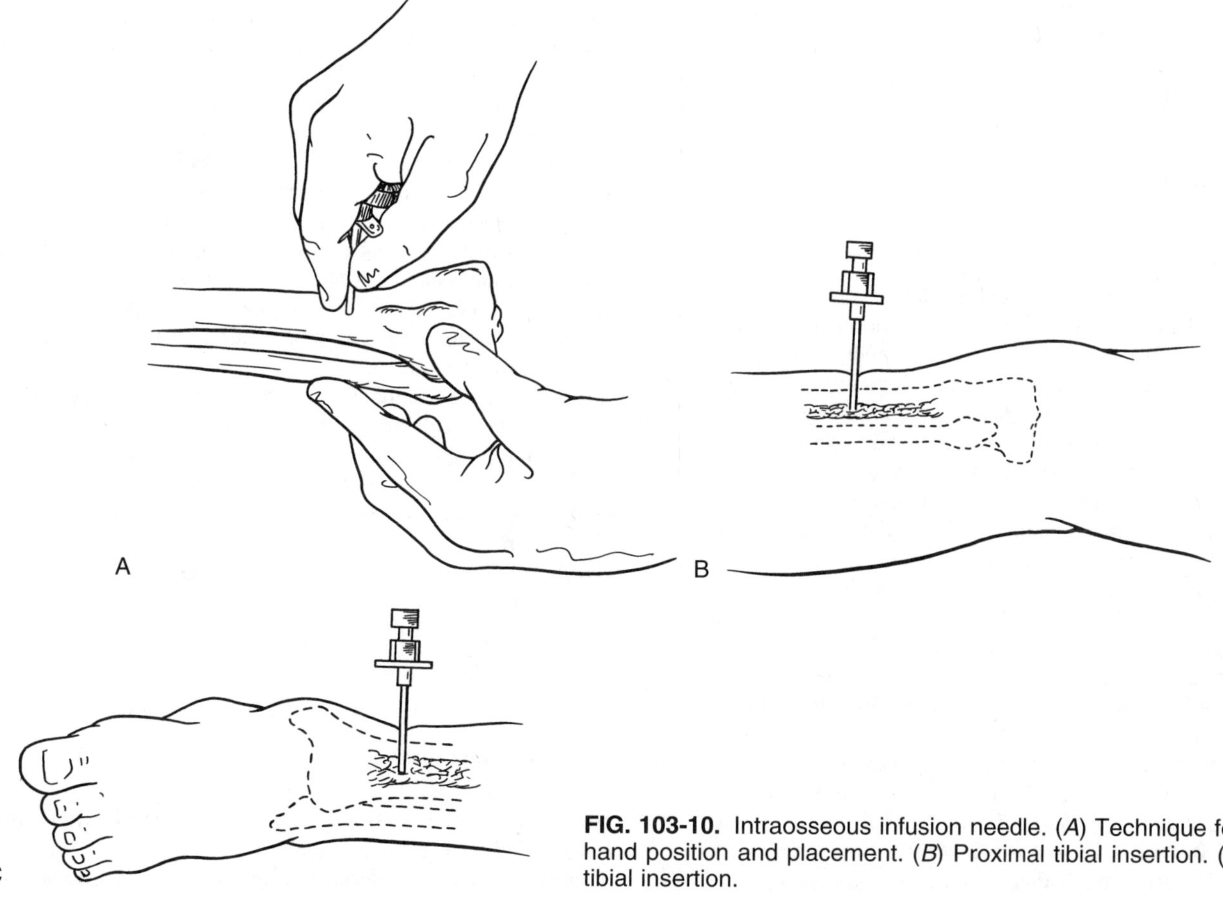

FIG. 103-10. Intraosseous infusion needle. (*A*) Technique for proper hand position and placement. (*B*) Proximal tibial insertion. (*C*) Distal tibial insertion.

the occasional formation of subcutaneous abscesses, has been reported in 0.7% of patients in a collected series.[22] Of greater concern is the risk of osteomyelitis. A 1985 review, however, documented only 27 cases of osteomyelitis in 4270 intraosseous infusions (0.6%).[23] Most reported infections occurred when the catheter remained in place for a prolonged period, or was placed in a patient with bacteremia or who had received hypertonic infusions.

COMPLICATIONS AND THEIR PREVENTION

Many technical, mechanical, and septic complications associated with PRAC and TIVAD use have been reported. These are minimized or prevented when recommended protocols for catheter placement, dressing care, administration of solutions, and monitoring are carefully followed.

Technical Complications

Possible complications at the time of catheter insertion include the following:

- Pneumothorax
- Hemothorax
- Hydromediastinum
- Subclavian artery injury
- Thromboembolism
- Innominate or subclavian vein laceration
- Carotid artery injury
- Catheter embolism
- Thoracic duct laceration
- Cardiac perforation and tamponade
- Brachial plexus injury
- Horner syndrome
- Phrenic nerve paralysis
- Air embolism

Even with experienced personnel and under the best circumstances, complications can occur. Pneumothorax is the most prevalent complication of subclavian venipuncture, occurring in up to 5% of attempted catheterizations. It can be asymptomatic and resolve or require needle aspiration or tube thoracostomy. Instructing patients to hold their breath on deep expiration or temporarily stopping positive-pressure mechanical ventilation in anesthetized patients decreases the incidence of pneumothorax. A chest radiograph should be obtained after every catheterization or unsuccessful attempt. The radiograph alerts the physician to the possible occurrence of complications and confirms the position of the catheter before infusion of medications or parenteral nutrition. Puncture of the subclavian artery, the next most frequent complication, can be minimized by maintaining the angle of entry as close to the horizontal plane as possible. If arterial blood is returned on insertion of the catheter needle, the needle should be withdrawn and direct pressure applied for at least 5 minutes. Puncture of the carotid artery is the most common complication of percutaneous internal jugular vein catheterization. Applying pressure directly to the puncture site is usually sufficient. If this complication is unrecognized,

the resulting hematoma of the neck can lead to tracheal compression and respiratory compromise. Air embolism is a potentially fatal complication of percutaneous catheterization of the subclavian and internal jugular veins. To minimize its occurrence, the patient should be placed in Trendelenburg position during removal of the syringe from the needle trocar and passage of the guide wire and the catheter into the vein. Alternatively, the transition should be made rapidly during deep expiration in the awake patient or with mechanical ventilation temporarily interrupted in an anesthetized patient. Air can also be introduced into the venous system during tubing changes or if the patient is inadvertently disconnected from the intravenous tubing. If the physician suspects that air has been introduced during catheter insertion or during tube-changing maneuvers, the immediate management should consist of clamping the catheter and placing the patient in Trendelenburg position, with the left side down. If the catheter is in place, an attempt should be made to aspirate the air within the right atrium. If the tubing becomes disconnected above the filter, the filter acts as an air lock, preventing the patient from syphoning air into the vascular system.

Mechanical Complications

Mechanical complications of central venous catheters are common and include inadvertent removal, rupture of the catheter, and occlusion. Inadvertent catheter removal is a function of the security of catheter fixation. It is important to maintain an occlusive dressing where the catheter enters the skin and to tape-tether the catheter to the dressing and body site. Rupture of the catheter is almost always confined to the external portion. The site usually is readily identified and repaired with a commercially available kit. Catheter occlusion is most commonly caused by formation of a fibrin sheath either in or at the tip of the catheter, by precipitates of TPN ingredients (eg, calcium, magnesium, or phosphate salts) in the line, or by precipitates of certain types of chemotherapeutic agents. If diagnosed early, formation of a fibrin sheath can be treated successfully by instilling urokinase or streptokinase, according to the protocol outlined in Table 103-2.[24] Precipitates that do not respond to streptokinase or urokinase may be cleared by administration of 0.01 N hydrochloric acid.[25]

Thrombosis of the subclavian, innominate, or internal jugular vein can lead to occlusion of the catheter or to serious vascular complications (eg, superior vena cava syndrome). Suspected thrombosis in patients with catheter malfunction, cardiopulmonary dysfunction, or sepsis can be documented by echocardiography; but routine screening of symptom-free patients is not rewarding.[26] Removal of the catheter with change to a different site and heparinization for 7 to 10 days generally is adequate treatment; clearing of the thrombosed vessel with thrombolytic agents is usually not indicated.

Septic Complications

Septic complications in a patient with a central venous line are suggested by various combinations of temperature increase or decrease, glucose intolerance, oliguria, hypotension, or gen-

TABLE 103-2. *Techniques for treating central venous catheter occlusion with streptokinase, urokinase, or hydrochloric acid*

	Streptokinase	Urokinase	Hydrochloric acid
Diluent	Sodium chloride injection USP	Sterile water injection with preservatives	1 mL 0.1 N HCl plus 10 mL heparin (10 U/mL)
Fluid concentration	125,000 IU/mL	5000 IU/mL	0.01 N
Administration	Fill catheter and clamp for 2 h; aspirate or irrigate and repeat twice, as needed	Instill 1 mL into catheter; wait 5 min and withdraw; if poor results, repeat aspiration attempts every 5 min for 30 min; if no success, cap catheter for 30–60 min and attempt instillation and aspiration again	Draw 0.5 mL into tuberculin syringe and irrigate back and forth for 2 min; clamp and repeat hourly until patency is restored

eral deterioration in clinical condition. Protocol for the work-up of possible catheter sepsis includes an initial investigation of all possible sources of infection (ie, pulmonary, genitourinary tract, gastrointestinal tract, wounds, sputum, urine). If the catheter site demonstrates evidence of infection (eg, purulence), it should be removed. In some patients with localized infection at the catheter–cutaneous junction (and a cuff to help limit proximal spread), local cleansing with hydrogen peroxide followed by antibacterial ointment and administration through the catheter of antibiotics directed to the organism may salvage the catheter. Infections of the tunnel generally require catheter removal. Quantitative blood cultures (for aerobes, anaerobes, and fungi) should be drawn through the catheter and from one peripheral site. After obtaining blood for cultures, appropriate broad-spectrum antibiotics should be administered through the catheter, unless the patient is toxic, in which the case the antibiotics should be started but the catheter removed and the tip cultured. Because of difficulty in obtaining blood cultures from either a peripheral vein or the catheter, many physicians apply the principle that any unexplained signs of infection are catheter related. This leads to overreporting of infections, hinders comparisons, and results in salvageable catheters being removed unnecessarily. If possible, antibiotics should be administered for 24 hours before reinsertion of the catheter. Optimal management after catheter removal due to sepsis requires that blood culture results be normal before another Broviac-type catheter or TIVAD is placed. Colonization of the catheter lumen most commonly results from lapses in techniques in catheter care and use. Faubion and colleagues[6] and Puntis and associates[27] showed that a well-trained vascular access and nutrition support team and a strict protocol for catheter care markedly decreases infection rates. The cost savings and decrease in patient morbidity justify the commitment of institutional resources.

REFERENCES

1. Aubaniac R. L'injection intraveineuse sous-claviculaire: avantages et technique. Presse Med 1952;60:1456. (English translation: The subclavian vein puncture: advantages and technique. Nutrition 1990;6:139.)
2. Newman BM, Jewett TC Jr, Karp MP, et al. Percutaneous central venous catheterization in children: first line choice for venous access. J Pediatr Surg 1986;21:685.
3. Broviac JW, Cole JJ, Scribner BH. A silicone rubber atrial catheter for prolonged parenteral alimentation. Surg Gynecol Obstet 1973;136:602.
4. Hickman RO, Buckner CD, Clift RA, et al. A modified right atrial catheter for access to the venous system in marrow transplant recipients. Surg Gynecol Obstet 1979;148:871.
5. Holmes SJK, Kiely EM, Spitz L. Vascular access. Prog Pediatr Surg 1989;22:133.
6. Faubion WC, Wesley JR, Khalidi N, et al. Total parenteral nutrition catheter sepsis: impact on the team approach. J Parenter Enter Nutr 1986;10:642.
7. Niederhuber JE, Ensminger W, Gyves JW, et al. Totally implanted venous and arterial access system to replace external catheters in cancer treatment. Surgery 1982;92:706.
8. Bothe A Jr, Piccione W, Ambrosino JJ, et al. Implantable central venous access system. Am J Surg 1984;147:565.
9. Ingram J, Weitzman S, Greenberg ML, et al. Complications of indwelling venous access lines in the pediatric hematology patient: a prospective comparison of external venous catheters and subcutaneous ports. Am J Pediatr Hematol Oncol 1991;13:130.
10. Howard L, Claunch C, McDowell R, et al. Five years of experience in patients receiving home nutrition support with the implanted reservoir: a comparison with the external catheter. J Parenter Enter Nutr 1989;13:478.
11. Abdulla F, Dietrich KA, Pramanik AK. Percutaneous femoral venous catheterization in preterm neonates. J Pediatr 1990;117:788.
12. Donahoe PK, Kim SH. The inferior epigastric vein as an alternate site for central venous hyperalimentation. J Pediatr Surg 1980;15:737.
13. Boddie AW Jr. Translumbar catheterization of the inferior vena cava for long term angioaccess. Surg Gynecol Obstet 1989;168:55.
14. Torosian MH, Meranze S, McLean G, et al. Central venous access with occlusive superior central venous thrombosis. Ann Surg 1986;203:30.
15. Hayden L, Stewart GR, Johnson DC, et al. Transthoracic right atrial cannulation for total parenteral nutrition: case report. Anaesth Intens Care 1981;9:53.
16. Dolcourt JL, Bose CL. Percutaneous insertion of Silastic central venous catheters in newborn infants. Pediatrics 1982;70:484.
17. Tabin CR. The Teflon intravenous catheter: incidence of phlebitis and duration of catheter life in the neonatal patient. J Obstet Gynecol Neonatal Nurs 1988;17:35.
18. Johnson RV, Donn SM. Life span of intravenous cannulas in a neonatal intensive care unit. Am J Dis Child 1988;142:968.
19. Sadiq F, Devaskar S, Weber T, et al. Life threatening complications of Broviac catheterization. (Abstract) Pediatr Res 1985;19:361A.
20. Loeff DS, Matlak ME, Black RE, et al. Insertion of a small central venous catheter in neonates and young infants. J Pediatr Surg 1982; 17:944.
21. Durand M, Ramanathan R, Martinelli B, et al. Prospective evaluation of percutaneous central venous Silastic catheters in newborn infants with birth weights of 510 to 3,920 grams. Pediatrics 1986;78:245.
22. Fiser DH. Current concepts: intraosseous infusions. N Engl J Med 1990;322:1579.
23. Rosetti VA, Thompson BM, Miller J, et al. Intraosseous infusion: an alternative route of pediatric intravascular access. Am Emerg Med 1985;14:885.
24. Faubion WC, Bollish SJ, Wesley JR. Central venous catheter occlusion treated by thrombolytic agents. Nutr Supp Serv 1983;3:24.
25. Shulman RJ, Reed T, Pitre D, et al. Use of hydrochloric acid to clear obstructed central venous catheters. J Parenter Enter Nutr 1988;12:509.
26. Ross P Jr, Ehrenkranz R, Kleinman CS, et al. Thrombus associated with central venous catheters in infants and children. J Pediatr Surg 1989;24:253.
27. Puntis JWL, Holden CE, Smallman S, et al. Staff training: a key factor in reducing intravascular catheter sepsis. Arch Dis Child 1991;66:337.

Section N

Conjoined Twins

Surgery of Infants and Children: Scientific Principles and Practice, edited by
Keith T. Oldham, Paul M. Colombani, and Robert P. Foglia.
Lippincott–Raven Publishers, Philadelphia, © 1997.

CHAPTER 104

Conjoined Twins

Robert M. Filler

Konig[1] recorded the first successful separation of conjoined
twins in 1689. These twins were joined at the umbilicus, and
the division was accomplished by necrosing the band of tissue
between the two children with a constricting ligature. Kiesewetter[2] reviewed 24 surgical attempts at separation that appeared
in the literature from 1689 to 1962. More than 200 reports of
successful separations can now be found in the medical literature or lay press.

The inappropriate term *Siamese twins* was coined by P.T.
Barnum, who promoted the exhibition of Chang and Eng
Bunker, conjoined twins born in Siam in 1811. An early medical
description of these most famous conjoined twins, who lived
unseparated until they died at 63 years of age, can be found in
the works of Warren.[3]

INCIDENCE

The exact incidence of conjoined twins is not known, but
estimates have varied from 1 in 25,000 to 50,000 births.[4,5] In
Africa, reports indicate that this anomaly occurs in as many as
1 in 14,000 births, suggesting an increased incidence among
blacks.[6,7] About 70% of conjoined twins reviewed by Rudolph
and colleagues[8] were female. Maternal age and parity do not
appear to influence the occurrence of conjoined twins. Prenatal
diagnosis of conjoined twins has led to increased delivery by
cesarean section and salvage of twins that would not have survived vaginal delivery.[9,10] Polyhydramnios is associated with
this anomaly in about half of cases. In a series from the United
States, 40% of conjoined twins were stillborn, and an additional
35% survived only 1 day.[11]

CLASSIFICATION AND ANATOMY

Conjoined twins may be joined at a variety of anatomic sites,
and complex classifications have been developed to describe all
the possibilities. The nomenclature in use clinically, however, is
derived from the most prominent site of conjunction. The common twin types include thoracopagus, xiphopagus or omphalopagus, pyopagus, ischiopagus, and craniopagus. In some cases,
the distinction between types is blurred because more extensive

unions involve structures ordinarily assigned a different nomenclature, for example, an ischiopagus union with sharing of structures up to and even beyond the level of the diaphragm. The
likely sites of musculoskeletal and visceral sharing or union for
each type are listed in Table 104-1.

Thoracopagus (Fig. 104-1) is the most common type of conjoined twin and, with omphalopagus (or xiphopagus), represents
about 75% of cases reported. The two twins lie face to face
and share a common sternum, diaphragm, and upper abdominal
wall from xiphoid to umbilicus. Nichols and colleagues[12] published an extensive review of the anatomy of thoracopagus
twins. According to data compiled from 42 cases, 75% of these
twins have conjoined hearts. Because of the abnormal ventricular arrangements and associated anomalies of the great arteries
and veins when the hearts are joined, successful surgical division often is not possible. In about half of these cases, the intestinal tract is also joined. Occasionally, the esophagus and stomach are single, but usually the union starts in the distal
duodenum and ends in a pouch at the site of a Meckel diverticulum. Joining of the biliary tree occurs in 25% and should always
be suspected when the duodenum in the region of the ampulla
of Vater is single. A bridge of liver between the twins has been
found in all cases.

Xiphopagus or omphalopagus twins (Fig. 104-2), usually
considered a subgroup of thoracopagus twins, also face each
other and usually have the least complicated union of all conjoined twins. In most instances, they are joined at the anterior
abdominal wall from xiphoid to umbilicus. The peritoneal cavity of one communicates with that of the other, but the upper
intestinal tracts are usually separate. A bridge of liver connects
the children in most cases (Fig. 104-3). In a smaller number of
omphalopagus twins, only the mid-portion of the abdominal
wall and umbilicus are joined. In those with fusion of the abdominal wall below the umbilicus, the terminal ileum from each
child may join and empty into a single shared colon, which
often ends as an imperforate anus. A bridge of bladder may
also be present in the band of tissue joining the two children
(Fig. 104-4). Evaluation of the single umbilical cord in twins
joined at the umbilicus (thoracopagus, xiphopagus, omphalopagus) has revealed the presence of two to seven umbilical vessels.
An omphalocele is often present at the umbilical cord insertion
and may rupture during delivery.

TABLE 104-1. *Possible visceral unions in different types of conjoined twins*

Type	Appearance	Heart & liver	Liver & biliary tract	Upper gastrointestinal tract	Lower gastrointestinal tract	Genitourinary tract	Nervous system
Thoracopagus		Yes	Yes	Yes	—	—	—
Xiphopagus		—	Yes	Yes	Yes	Yes	—
Pygopagus		—	—	—	Yes	Yes	Yes
Ischiopagus		—	Yes	Yes	Yes	Yes	—
Craniopagus		—	—	—	—	—	Yes

Pygopagus twins represent about 20% of cases of conjoined twins. They are joined at the buttocks and perineum and face away from each other. A significant length of one sacrum may be fused; as a result, these twins often share the sacral spinal canal. A single lower rectum and anus is common, and often the lower genital tract and external genitalia are fused.

Ischiopagus twins accounts for 5% of cases. Because these children share organs that can be separated or share structures that are not essential to sustain life, they are amenable to separation in almost all cases. These twins are united at a single bony pelvis (see Fig. 104-4*B*). Four normal lower extremities (ischiopagus tetrapus) may be attached to the ringlike pelvis, but often two of the four lower extremities are fused into one malformed limb (ischiopagus tripus; Fig. 105-5). The intestinal tracts usually join at the terminal ileum, which empties into a single colon (see Fig. 104-4*C*). The rectum and anus may not open onto the perineum, and as in other children with imperforate anus, proximal diversion may be necessary shortly after birth, well before separation is undertaken. Although four kidneys and two bladders usually are present, one ureter from each twin frequently crosses the midline and empties into the bladder of the other (see Fig. 104-4*A*). Female ischiopagus twins commonly have two uteri, four ovaries, and two sets of external genitalia on either side of a single anal opening. Vaginal anomalies and rectovaginal communications, however, are frequent. Male twins may have four gonads, but fusion of the genitourinary

tract distal to the bladder is relatively common, as seen in Figures 104-4*A* and 104-5.

Craniopagus is the least common type of conjoined twin and accounts for 2% of cases. There is always fusion of the skull, and often these children share large dural sinuses and other important vascular structures. A classification into partial or total forms, having a junction at either brow, vertex, or parietal bone, has been devised.[13] In partial forms, the brains are separated by bone or dura, and each brain has separate leptomeninges. In the total form, the brains of each twin are connected, or they are separated only by the arachnoid. Separation of the total type is extremely difficult, and feasibility is often determined by the presence of a superior sagittal sinus for each brain, which provides adequate venous drainage.

Congenital anomalies are fairly frequent in conjoined twins, even in those organs that are not shared. Congenital heart disease, renal and genitourinary abnormalities, intestinal duplication, omphalocele, and imperforate anus have all been reported. In some cases, marked differences in the size and vigor of the two children is noted, and occasionally one is stillborn.

EMBRYOLOGY

Although there is no known collection of conjoined twins embryos, most investigators believe that conjoining represents

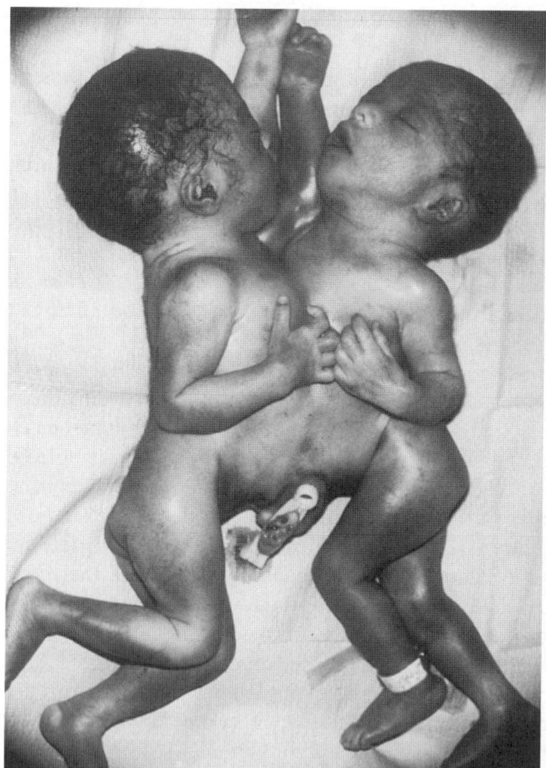

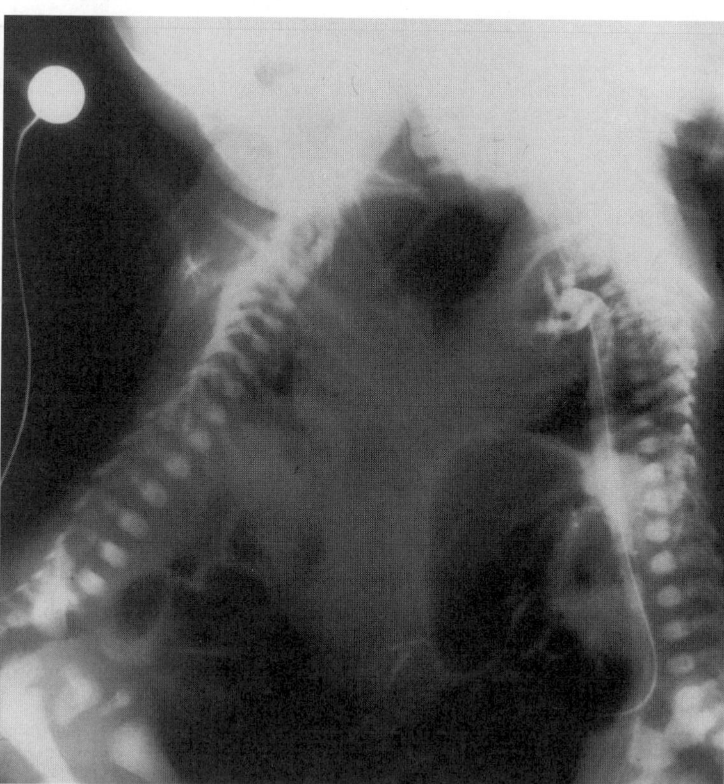

FIG. 104-1. (*A*) Thoracopagus twins who died at 24 hours of age. They shared atria and ventricules and had serious intracardiac anomalies. Because the shared heart has intrinsic abnormalities, twins of this type usually cannot be separated even when one is planning to save only one twin. (*B*) Lateral radiograph taken in newborn nursery shortly after birth. On first look, the hearts may appear separate. The aorta of the twin on the right is filled with radiocontrast media that had been injected through an umbilical artery catheter.

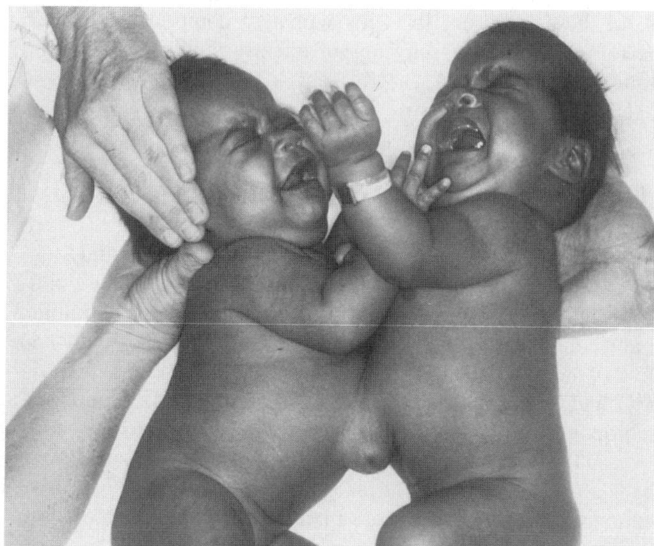

FIG. 104-2. Omphalopagus twins at 2.5 months of age, just before separation. The livers were joined in these children, but other viscera were separate. The separation was uncomplicated.

an aberration of the normal twinning process. Conjoined twins are considered to be monozygotic, monochorionic twins of the same sex with identical chromosome patterns.[14] The teratogenic event is thought to occur at about 20 days' postovulation, although some evidence suggests that the phenomenon may occur a few days earlier.[15,16] At this embryonic stage of twinning, the inner cell mass is splitting into two separate and nearly equal halves, each capable of forming a normal person. According to one theory, in conjoined twinning, complete separation of the inner cell mass within the chorionic vesical does not occur, and nonseparated parts of the otherwise normal twins remain attached throughout the remaining period of development. An alternate theory suggests that the inner cell mass separates, but then reunion occurs, and twins who are attached are formed.

PRENATAL DIAGNOSIS

Suspicion of conjoined twinning is raised in pregnancy complicated by polyhydramnios. With the routine use of ultrasonography in pregnancy, the presence of conjoined twins is usually discovered before delivery and can be made as early as the week 12 of gestation.[17,18] In addition to diagnosing the presence of conjoined twins, ultrasound is useful in describing the extent of joining of the cardiovascular system in thoracoabdominally joined twins. Prenatal echocardiograms correctly diagnosed

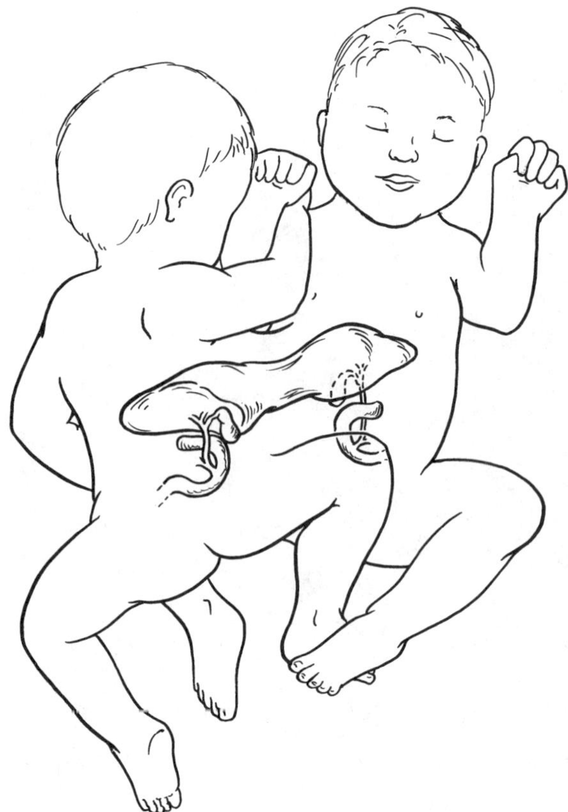

FIG. 104-3. Schematic depiction of the union of the liver and upper abdomen in the twins shown in Figure 104-2. The livers were joined in the midline. Total liver volume was sufficient for both children, and the biliary tracts were separate. This arrangement is the one most often described for this type of conjoined twins.

major cardiac anomalies, although certain important features were missed because of an inability to detect abnormal systemic pulmonary venous connections in four pairs of thoracoabdominally joined twins.[19] In utero echocardiogram is thought to be more thorough than a postpartum study because more views can be obtained, and the examination is not hampered by the presence of an omphalocele. Because mortality and the ability to separate thoracopagus twins are directly related to the union of two hearts and associated cardiac abnormalities, reliable antepartum evaluation may have significant value in deciding whether to recommend termination of pregnancy.

POSTNATAL EVALUATION

Except for life-threatening emergencies, which must be treated by immediate separation of the twins, surgery should be delayed at least until an accurate assessment of shared structures is completed.

A knowledge of the potential visceral and bony unions in a particular set of twins serves as a guide to obtaining the appropriate diagnostic imaging studies (see Table 104-1). Table 104-2 lists the important diagnostic studies, the structures that each study best evaluates, and the type of twin that requires each study. Computed tomography and magnetic resonance imaging

are especially important to understand complicated bony unions and organ sharing.

Comprehensive evaluation of the cardiovascular system is necessary in all thoracopagus twins. If the cardiovascular status has not been assessed prenatally, these studies should begin immediately after birth because of the likelihood of an abnormality that is incompatible with life in one or both children. The most important factor in prognosis is the degree of separation of the two hearts. With one exception,[20] separation has been successful only when all heart chambers were unattached, mainly because of the presence of intrinsic anomalies in the attached hearts.

The presence of separate hearts can be established by finding two separate pulse rates on physical examination and by demonstrating two independent QRS complexes on simultaneous electrocardiograms.[21] In twins with fused hearts, only a single QRS is present. The single QRS usually appears in one twin as a mirror image of that seen in the same standard limb lead of the other. Ordinarily, chest radiographs cannot be used to determine whether the heart is single because in the views that can be obtained, superimposition of shadows makes two separate hearts appear as one. As mentioned, echocardiography has proved to be extremely useful for cardiac evaluation.[19] Angiocardiography can be used to supplement the information obtained from the ultrasound study; Freedom[22] described the angiographic approach to these twins in detail.

Before surgery, an estimate of the degree of admixture of the two circulatory systems can be of practical importance because it allows the surgeon and anesthetist to anticipate an unusual response to drug, anesthetic, or blood administration. In addition, evidence indicating a rapid mixing of circulations suggests the existence of a significant vascular communication, which must be found and properly divided at surgery. By injecting isotope-tagged albumin, methylene blue, or indigo carmine into one twin and monitoring its appearance in the other, the rate of blood exchange can be calculated.[23] The rate of mixing is greatest in thoracopagus twins, especially in those with conjoined hearts. Complete blood exchange may occur every minute in these children. In twins with less complicated unions, the rate of exchange may be sufficiently slow that it has no clinical importance. A careful search for major anomalies at sites other than the sites of fusion should be made in all cases.

TIMING OF SURGICAL SEPARATION

Of the conjoined twins who are born alive, the potential long-term survivors fall into two groups. In the first group are children who thrive despite being joined. No significant physiologic abnormalities related to the union are apparent. Growth and development proceed normally, since cardiovascular, respiratory, and gastrointestinal function is unimpaired. Pygopagus, ischiopagus, and xiphopagus twins usually fall into this category. In these children, there is sufficient time to evaluate organ sharing and to plan the intricate and often complex operative separation. Although there are many pressures to proceed with surgery soon after these studies have been completed, separation probably should be delayed several months, at least in those with complex unions. The infants then are larger, important congenital anomalies not obvious at birth are apparent, and the risks of surgery and anesthesia are lower. In a personal experi-

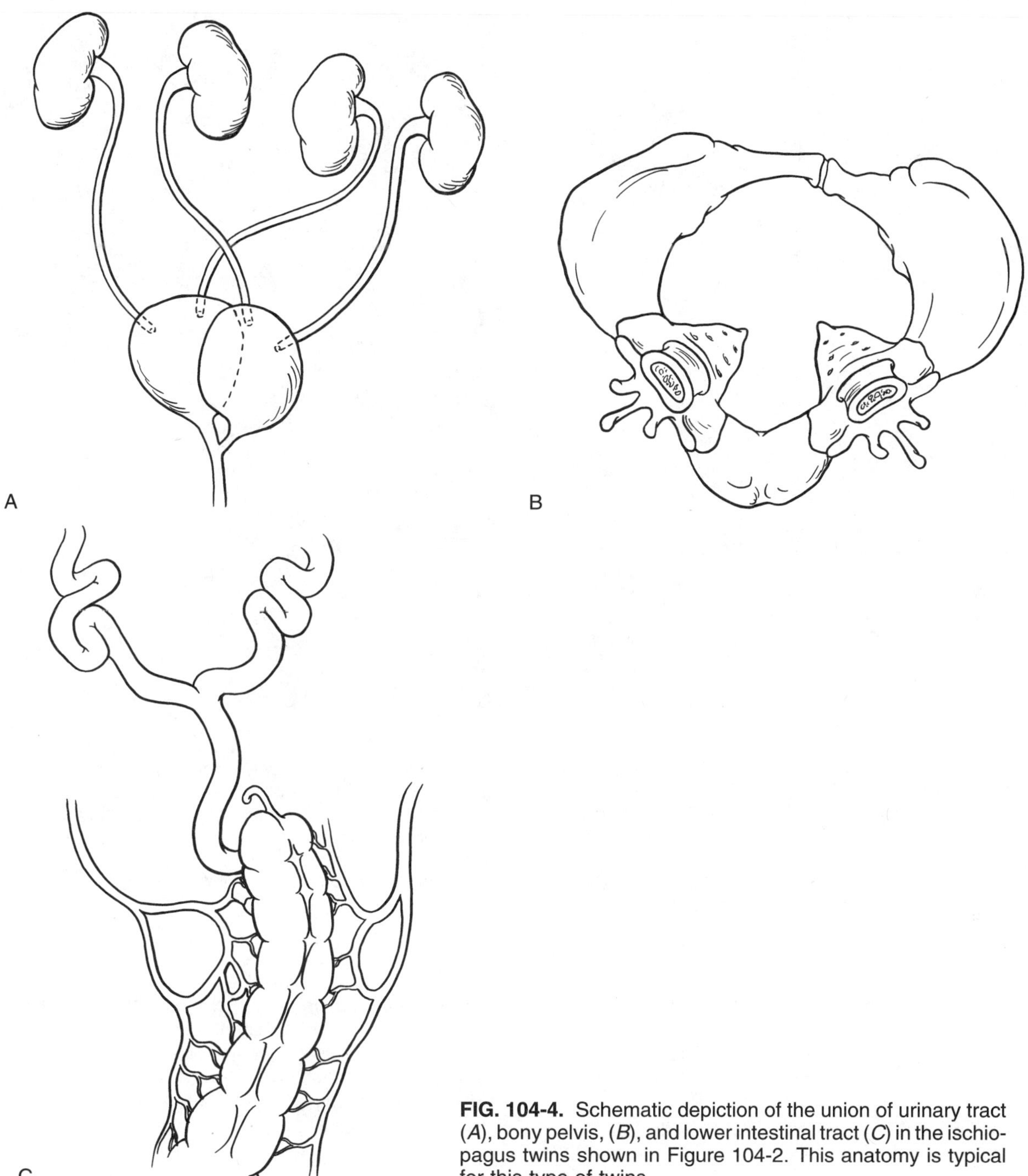

FIG. 104-4. Schematic depiction of the union of urinary tract (*A*), bony pelvis, (*B*), and lower intestinal tract (*C*) in the ischiopagus twins shown in Figure 104-2. This anatomy is typical for this type of twins.

ence with five separations, a delay was clearly beneficial. In one case, separation of omphalopagus twins was postponed for 2.5 months until the infants' combined weight had risen from 2.4 kg at birth to 7.8 kg (see Fig. 104-2). The children had completely recovered from the respiratory distress syndrome that was present during the first week of life. They were vigorous and healthy and tolerated surgery without complications. In another case, separation of ischiopagus twins with complex skeletal, gastrointestinal, and genitourinary sharing was delayed until the infants were 16 months old and weighed 13 kg.[24] During this delay, an intermediate operation was performed to

fashion a skin and muscle flap from a useless fused lower extremity to cover a large abdominal wall defect that was created when the twins were separated. These infants withstood a complicated 9-hour long separation without difficulty and had no serious problems postoperatively. Similarly, in three other separations of abdominoischiopagus twins, definitive separation was delayed for 6 to 10 months. During this waiting period, a colostomy or ileostomy was performed for imperforate anus in all, and a left pyeloplasty was performed in one twin for ureteropelvic obstruction. The abdominal cavity was enlarged by pneumoperitoneum in one pair of twins and by intraperitoneal tissue

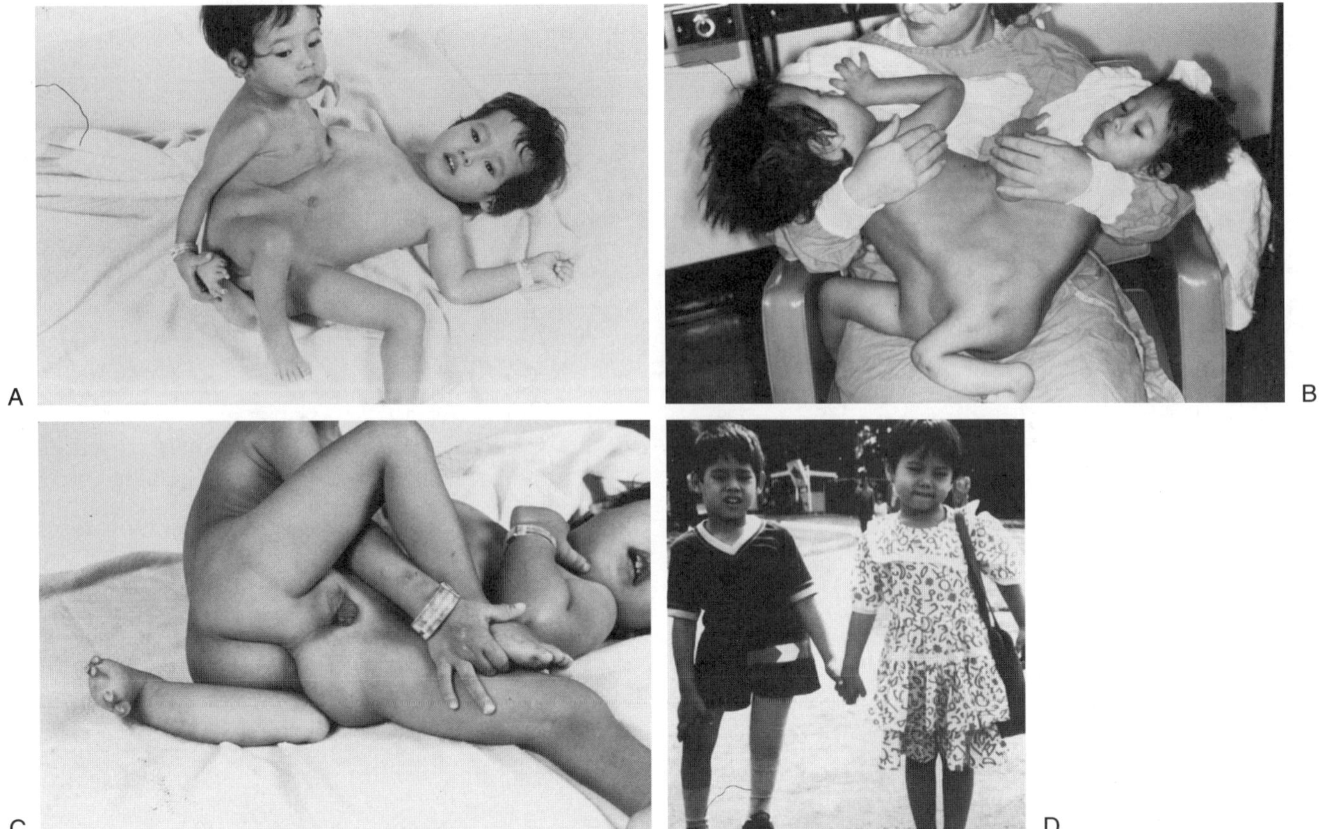

FIG. 104-5. Ischiopagus tripus twins. (*A*) These twins were joined from the upper abdomen to a common pelvis. Their livers were joined, and they shared a terminal ileum and colon. One kidney from each twin drained into the other's bladder. The lower limbs were joined to the fused pelvic ring, which contained elements from each child. (*B*) The abnormal third limb can be seen. The bone from this functionless limb was removed at the time of separation, and the musculocutaneous remnant was used to cover a portion of the defect in one twin's abdominal wall created by the division. (*C*) The single penis was given to one twin, and the other child was raised as a girl. (*D*) Two years later, each child has adjusted to one normal and one artificial lower limb.

expanders in the other two pairs. In addition, tissue expanders were inserted subcutaneously in all before separation to increase the amount of skin, muscle, and fascia available for closure after separation. The use of expanders requires at least two months for maximal expansion.

In the second group are twins whose lives are threatened because of the union or coexistent congenital anomalies. In these children, emergency operation with or without separation may be required before appropriate diagnostic studies can be completed. Urgent operation is indicated in three clinical situations: (1) when the existence of one twin threatens the life of the other[25]; (2) when a potentially correctable life-threatening anomaly is present, such as ruptured omphalocele, severe congenital heart disease, or intestinal obstruction; and (3) when

TABLE 104-2. *Diagnostic studies*

Test	Structures evaluated	Type of union in twins
CT or MR scan	Bony union, kidneys, urinary tract, central nervous system	All types
Radionuclide scan	Liver, spleen biliary tract	Thoracoabdominal
Cystogram, urethrogram	Bladder, urethra	Abdominal pelvic
Barium studies of GI tract	Small bowel, colon	Abdominal pelvic
Angiogram	Heart and major blood vessels	Thoracoabdominal, cranial
Echocardiogram, electrocardiogram with cardiac catheterization*	Heart and great vessels	Thoracoabdominal

*Prenatal test appears to be especially useful.

surgical intervention is necessary for a traumatic injury to the bridge of tissue and underlying viscera joining the twins.

PLANNING THE SURGICAL SEPARATION

The operating team, consisting of duplicate anesthesiologists, surgeons, and nursing personnel, should meet before surgery to clarify and delegate responsibilities. Rehearsal of the operating event by team members is essential. Anesthesia teams should be responsible for setting up methods of continuous but separate physiologic monitoring and for coordinating information obtained.[25] Marking of infants, hospital records, laboratory requisitions, and equipment with colored tape is a practical and useful method to avoid confusion and error. Preoperative calculation of blood and respiratory volumes is useful. Plans should be made to modify existing operating tables because standard tables are not properly designed for the separation of conjoined twins. Modifications to accommodate duplicate teams, operating equipment, and monitoring devices depend on the type of union to be separated.[2,24,26,27]

Serious moral and ethical dilemmas arise in cases in which it is not possible to achieve separation without sacrificing the life or the quality of life of one of the two children. Pepper[28] discusses these issues from the viewpoint of the physician and theologian. Because separation is always of great public interest, preoperative preparation must include the establishment of proper lines of communication with the news media to avoid confusion, frustration, and irritation.

ANESTHETIC MANAGEMENT

Preoperative medication should be minimal. Because of cross-circulation, drugs given to one infant may act on the other.

During surgery, body temperature of the infants must be maintained by controlling room temperature or by the use of heating blankets. Adequate venous routes for fluid and drugs should be ensured in each twin before the induction of anesthesia. Temperature, electrocardiogram, blood pressure, pulse oximeter, and chest sound monitoring are necessary in all cases. Arterial cannulation for direct arterial blood pressure monitoring and blood gas determination is desirable for separation of all complex unions. Anesthesia is best induced after awake endotracheal intubation. Preoxygenation of one infant should be maintained while the other is intubated. Intubation may be difficult in thoracopagus and omphalopagus twins because they face one another and because cervical lordosis is usually present. When possible, placement of one infant above the other should be avoided to prevent hypotension, which can occur when blood drains from the upper to the lower child. To avoid overdoses due to cross-circulation, the less active twin should be anesthetized first. Placement of a nasogastric tube and esophageal stethoscope should follow adequate stabilization of the endotracheal tube. It may be difficult to maintain uniform adequate depth of anesthesia in both twins, particularly if cross-circulation is excessive. In these cases, muscle-paralyzing drugs may be helpful if used cautiously. Fluid and electrolyte balance is controlled precisely by calculation of base deficit from blood gas data. For maintenance fluid requirements during surgery, 5% dextrose in .25% normal saline is administered to each infant at a rate of

4 mL/kg/h, and an additional 10 to 15 mL/kg/h of lactated Ringer solution is given for estimated third-space losses. Colloid and blood are given as necessary. For complex and long procedures, transfusion of 5 to 10 blood volumes may be necessary. The effects of cross-circulation must always be considered during all intravenous infusions until the twins are separated. Several researchers recommend that corticosteroids be given prophylactically because intraoperative shock can be caused by adrenal insufficiency.[29] This thesis has never been well documented, however. The details of anesthetic management in an 18-hour separation of omphaloischiopagus tripus twins clearly shows how the application of these principles can result in a smooth and uneventful operation despite the complexity and duration of the procedure.[30]

SURGICAL CONSIDERATIONS

The surgeon is faced with two major technical problems at surgery. First, separate, shared structures must be separated, leaving each child with a functional residual when possible. Second, the skin, muscle, and bony defect at the site of union must be closed after separation is completed.

Many descriptions of surgical procedures to separate different types of conjoined twins appear in the literature.[2,6,10,20,24,30–40] Although it is beyond the scope of this chapter to review these individual operations in detail, several generalizations seem appropriate. Division of a bridge of liver between two twins can be associated with a moderate degree of blood loss because of the many vessels that traverse this bridge. Bleeding can be minimized by the placement of mattress sutures on either side of the planned line of division before incision. The volume of liver remaining for each twin after separation has been adequate to sustain life in reported cases. On the other hand, for children who share extrahepatic biliary ducts, it may not be possible to leave each child with a satisfactory bile drainage system, and innovations such as portoenterostomy may be necessary.

Separation of a ureter from the bladder of one twin and reimplantation into the other is usually necessary in ischiopagus twins.[24] Implantation can be accomplished by standard techniques, and urinary diversion is not necessary in most cases.

Surgeons planning to separate thoracopagus twins must be prepared to employ cardiopulmonary bypass and hypothermic circulatory arrest, especially when there is evidence that the hearts are joined.

Closure of defects created by separation can be relatively simple when the defect is small, as in the case of omphalopagus twins. When the defect is large, closure can be extremely difficult and can result in complications that seriously threaten the outcome of surgery. In general, wound closure is best achieved by the use of viable tissue. In twins with small defects, this is almost always possible, but even in those with large defects, a flap of skin and muscle is sometimes available for coverage. For example, Koop[35] used a buttock flap to close a peritoneal defect in pygopagus twins, and Mestel and colleagues[24] employed skin and muscle from a useless lower limb for abdominal wall coverage in ischiopagus twins. Others have used local skin flaps from the head and neck to cover the brain in two sets of craniopagus twins.[33] In other cases, however, especially those with a defect in the underlying supporting skeleton, adequate closure has not been possible by these means, and various prosthetic materials have been used successfully. Others have used Teflon mesh,[31] an acrylic prosthesis for skull replacement in craniopagus twins,[37] a combination of polypropylene mesh and Silastic to temporarily cover an abdominal defect, and polyglycolic acid mesh.

In a pair of abdominoischiopagus twins,[41] seven Silastic tissue expanders were inserted into the peritoneal cavity and subcutaneous tissues 8 weeks before separation. The expanders were filled with saline to a total volume of 5 L. This technique provided additional skin and muscle, which greatly aided the closure. Tissue expanders also have been used in the scalp for craniopagus twins.[42] An alternative to intraabdominal tissue expanders to expand the peritoneal cavity has been the creation of pneumoperitoneum beginning 6 to 8 weeks before separation.[24] I resorted to this maneuver when an intraabdominal tissue expander caused intestinal obstruction and bowel perforation and had to be removed prematurely.

RESULTS OF SURGERY

The outlook for omphalopagus and xiphopagus twins is exceptionally good.[13,40] Even 20 years ago in a review of 11 such sets of twins, 19 of the 22 children survived. Of the deaths, one was stillborn and another, its sibling, died 35 hours after separation. Cardiovascular collapse occurred 1 hour after surgery in the third fatality, and adrenal insufficiency was suspected as the cause. When omphalocele is present in this type of twins, the prognosis appears to be somewhat worse. Votteler[43] reviewed the results of separation in seven sets of omphalopagus twins with associated omphalocele treated between 1963 and 1981. The omphalocele had ruptured in four sets. One twin in three of the four sets died. One twin from two of the three sets with intact omphalocele also succumbed.

Except for the successful separation of a set of twins who shared a right atrium,[20] thoracopagus twins sharing hearts have not been long-term survivors. In those with a single pericardium, however, survival of one or both children has been relatively frequent.[11] Infections in and around the heart, cardiac abnormalities, and respiratory failure have been the main causes of death. In most failures, closure of the chest wall has contributed to the poor outcome either because tight closure restricted chest motion or because a defect in the sternum allowed paradoxical respiratory motion.

Survival in craniopagus separations appears to depend on whether the union is total or partial and on how the cerebral vasculature and brain tissue are shared. In a review of 11 sets of craniopagus twins in which one or both twins survived, 5 had a partial union and 6 had a total union.[43] Eight of the 10 children joined by a partial union survived, whereas only 7 of 12 with total union lived. Even though many craniopagus twins survive, as many as half have residual neurologic abnormalities.

The outlook for pygopagus twins has been good, which is not surprising considering that the joined structures usually are not essential for life.[35,44,45] In most cases, both twins have survived.

The separation of ischiopagus twins is usually complex because typically both the intestinal and urinary systems are joined. There is only one pelvic ring and often only three lower extremities. Votteler[43] compiled a list of 12 ischiopagus separations from 1955 to 1981 in which one or both ischiopagus twins survived. Since that report, I have successfully separated three sets of ischiopagus twins, and Ross and colleagues[46] and Grantzow and colleagues[47] have successfully separated two other sets. Successfully separated ischiopagus twins require long-term rehabilitation because of residual orthopedic, gynecologic, urologic, and intestinal disabilities. Despite these problems, separation can result in happy, intelligent, and potentially productive youngsters (see Fig. 104-5).

In a personal experience with one set of omphalopagus and four sets of ischiopagus twins, all children have survived. The omphalopagus twins have no disabilities. Two sets of ischiopagus twins, who are 25 and 10 years old, respectively, each use a prosthesis for an absent lower extremity and each have colostomy. They have adjusted to their disabilities extremely well and are leading productive lives. The third set (ischiopagus tetrapus) are now 9 years old. They each have a colostomy but normal lower extremities. Their urinary tracts are functioning well, and their development is normal, although deformities of the lower chest wall at the site of union are significant but have not affected their lives to date.

REFERENCES

1. Konig G. Sibi invicem adnati feliciter separati. Ephemerid Natur Curios. Dec II, Ann VIII Obs 1689;145.
2. Kiesewetter WB. Surgery on conjoined (Siamese) twins. Surgery 1966; 59:860.
3. Warren JC. An account of the Siamese twin brothers united together from their birth. Am J Med Sci 1829;52:255.
4. Freedman HL, Tafeen CH, Harris H. Conjoined thoracopagus twins. Am J Obstet Gynecol 1962;84:1904.
5. Siegel I. Thoracopagus: vaginal delivery without destructive operation. Illinois Med J 1950;97:40.
6. Bland KG, Hammar B. Xiphopagus twins. Cent Afr J Med 1962;8:371.
7. Bhettay E, Nelson MS, Beighton P. Epidemic of conjoined twins in southern Africa. Lancet 1975;2:741.
8. Rudolph AJ, Michaels JP, Nichols BL. Obstetric management of conjoined twins. The National Foundation—Birth Defects: Orig Art Series 1967;3:28.
9. Gore RM, Filly RA, Parer JT. Sonographic antepartum diagnosis of conjoined twins: its impact on obstetric management. JAMA 1982; 247:3351.
10. Grossman HJ, Sugar O, Greeley PW, et al. Surgical separation in craniopagus. JAMA 1953;153:201.
11. Edmonds LD, Layde PM. Conjoined twins in the United States, 1970–1977. Teratology 1982;24:301.
12. Nichols BL, Blattner RJ, Rudolph AJ. General clinical management of thoracopagus twins. The National Foundation—Birth Defects: Orig Art Series 1967;3:38.
13. O'Connell JEA. Craniopagus twins: surgical anatomy and embryology and their implications. J Neurol Neurosurg Psychiatry 1976;39:1.
14. Zimmermann AA. Embryologic and anatomic considerations of conjoined twins. The National Foundation—Birth Defects: Orig Art Series 1967;3:18.
15. Benirschke K, Temple WW, Bloor C. Conjoined twins: nosology and congenital malformations. Birth Defects 1978;16:179.
16. Streeter GL. Formation of single ovum twins. Bull Johns Hopkins Hosp 1919b;30:235.
17. Schmidt W, Heberling D, Kubli F. Antepartum ultrasonographic diagnosis of conjoined twins in early pregnancy. Am J Obstet Gynecol 1981;139:961.
18. Maggio M, Callan NA, Hamobka KA, et al. The first trimester ultrasonographic diagnosis of conjoined twins. Am J Obstet Gynecol 1985; 152:833.
19. Sanders SP, Chin AJ, Parness IA, et al. Prenatal diagnosis of congenital

heart defects in thoracoabdominally conjoined twins. N Engl J Med 1985;313:370.

20. Synhorst D, Matlak M, Roan Y, et al. Separation of conjoined thoracopagus twins joined at the right atria. Am J Cardiol 1979;43:662.

21. Leachman RD, Latson JR, Kohler CM, et al. Cardiovascular evaluation of conjoined twins. The National Foundation—Birth Defects: Orig Art Series 1967;3:52.

22. Freedom RM. The angiocardiographic approach to thoracopagus conjoined twins. In: Freedom RM, Culham JAG, Moes CAF, eds. Angiocardiography of congenital heart disease. New York: MacMillan, 1984: 655.

23. Spencer RP, Rockoff ML, Nichols BL. Radioisotopic flow studies in conjoined twins. The National Foundation-Birth Defects: Orig Art Series 1967;3:120.

24. Mestel AL, Golinko RJ, Wax SH, et al. Ischiopagus tripus conjoined twins: case report of a successful separation. Surgery 1971;69:75.

25. Graivier L, Jacoby MD. Emergency separation of newborn conjoined (Siamese) twins. Tex Med 1980;76:60.

26. Simpson JS, Pelton DA, Swyer PR. The importance of monitoring during operations of conjoined twins. Can Med Assoc J 1967;96:1463.

27. Savickis J. The separation of conjoined twins: an OR nursing perspective. Can Nurse 1984;80:21.

28. Pepper CK. Ethical and moral considerations in the separation of conjoined twins. The National Foundation—Birth Defects: Orig Art Series 1967;3:128.

29. Aird I. The conjoined twins of Kano. Br Med J 1954;1:841.

30. James RD, McLeod ME, Relton JES, et al. Anesthetic considerations for separation of omphalo-ischopagus tripus twins. Can Anaesth Soc J 1985;33:402.

31. DeVries PA. Separation of the San Francisco twins. The National Foundation—Birth Defects: Orig Art Series 1967;3:75.

32. Eades JW, Thomas CG. Successful separation of ischiopagus tetrapus conjoined twins. Ann Surg 1966;164:1059.

33. Jayes PH. Plastic repair after separation of craniopagus twins. Br Med J 1964;1:1340.

34. Kling S, Johnston RJ, Michalyshyn B, et al. Successful separation of xiphopagus-conjoined twins. J Pediatr Surg 1975;10:267.

35. Koop CE. The successful separation of pyopagus twins. Surgery 1961; 49:271.

36. Spencer R. Surgical separation of siamese twins: case report. Surgery 1956;39:827.

37. Wilson H. Surgery in Siamese twins: a report of three sets of conjoined twins treated surgically. Ann Surg 1957;145:718.

38. Woolley M, Joergenson E. Xiphopagus conjoined twins. Am J Surg 1964;108:277.

39. Zuker RM, Filler RM. Intra-abdominal tissue expansion: an adjunct in the separation of conjoined twins. Presented to The American Pediatric Surgical Association 17th Annual Meeting, Toronto, May 14–17, 1986.

40. O'Neill JA, Holcomb GW, Schnaufer L, et al. Surgical experience with thirteen conjoined twins. Ann Surg 1988;208:299.

41. Gans SL, Morgenstern L, Gettelman E, et al. Separation of conjoined twins in the newborn period. J Pediatr Surg 1968;3:565.

42. Shively RE, Bermant MA, Bucholz RD. Separation of craniopagus twins utilizing tissue expanders. Plast Reconstr Surg 1985;76:765.

43. Votteler TP. Conjoined twins. In: Welch KJ, Randolph JG, Ravitch MM, et al, eds. Pediatric surgery, vol 2. 1986:771.

44. Votteler TP. Necrotizing enterocolitis in a pygopagus conjoined twin. J Pediatr Surg 1982;17:555.

45. Cloutier R, Levassiur L, Copty M, et al. The surgical separation of pygopagus twins. J Pediatr Surg 1979;14:554.

46. Ross AJ, O'Neill JA, Silverman DG, et al. A new technique for evaluating cutaneous vascularity in complicated conjoined twins. J Pediatr Surg 1985;20:743.

47. Grantzow R, Hecker WC, Holschneider AM, et al. Separation of an asymmetric xipho-omphalo-ischopagus tripus. Langenbecks Arch Chir 1985;363:195.

Index

Page numbers followed by t or f indicate tables or figures, respectively; "cf" indicates color figures.